Cecil – Loeb

TEXTBOOK OF MEDICINE

Thirteenth Edition

Edited by

PAUL B. BEESON, M.D.

Nuffield Professor of Clinical Medicine,
University of Oxford

WALSH McDERMOTT, M.D.

Livingston Farrand Professor of Public Health,
Cornell University Medical College

W. B. SAUNDERS COMPANY   PHILADELPHIA – LONDON – TORONTO

W. B. Saunders Company: West Washington Square
Philadelphia, Pa. 19105

12 Dyott Street
London, WC1A   1DB

1835 Yonge Street
Toronto 7, Ontario

Listed here is the latest translated edition of this book, together with the language of the translation and the publisher.

Serbo-Croat (11th Edition) — Medicinska Knjiga, Belgrade, Yugoslavia
Spanish (12th Edition) — Nueva Editorial Interamerican S. A., de C. V., Mexico

Cecil-Loeb Textbook of Medicine   SBN   0-7216-1657-7

Print No.:   9   8   7   6   5   4   3   2

ASSOCIATE EDITORS

GENETIC PRINCIPLES AND HEREDITARY DISEASES

ALEXANDER G. BEARN, M.D.

Professor and Chairman, Department of Medicine,
Cornell University Medical College

ENDOCRINE AND METABOLIC DISEASES

NICHOLAS P. CHRISTY, M.D.

Clinical Professor of Medicine,
Columbia University College of Physicians and Surgeons

HEMATOLOGIC AND HEMATOPOIETIC DISEASES

CARL V. MOORE, M.D.

Busch Professor of Medicine,
Washington University School of Medicine

DISORDERS OF THE NERVOUS SYSTEM AND BEHAVIOR

FRED PLUM, M.D.

Anne Parrish Titzell Professor and Chairman, Department of Neurology,
Cornell University Medical College

DISEASES OF THE DIGESTIVE SYSTEM

MARVIN H. SLEISENGER, M.D.

Professor and Vice Chairman, Department of Medicine,
University of California, San Francisco

PREFACE

In his Preface to the first (1927) edition of this textbook, Dr. Russell Cecil said:

> In internal medicine, as in other branches of human knowledge, the age of specialism has of necessity arrived, and some of our ablest practitioners even devote themselves in great measure to one disease. In order that physicians and students of medicine might have the benefit of an authoritative and up-to-date treatise on every medical subject, it seemed desirable to prepare a textbook of medicine in which each disease, or group of diseases, would be discussed by a writer particularly interested in that subject.

His judgment of the need for multiple authorship in the vast area of general medicine has now come to be universally accepted and is in fact no longer "news." The Cecil—later the Cecil-Loeb—textbook has served as a standard reference work throughout the professional lives of most physicians now in active practice. As we introduce the thirteenth edition, the third under our editorship, we would like to air some of our views about the organization and function of a textbook for the study and practice of medicine.

The pace of clinical investigation is such that the book needs to be largely rebuilt every four years in order to incorporate new concepts, new methods of diagnosis, and new treatments. In preparing a new edition one of our most important responsibilities is selection of contributors, because about one article in three is written by an author not previously associated with the book. In all such matters we consult extensively with the Associate Editors: Drs. Bearn, Christy, Moore, Plum, and Sleisenger. Before a new author is invited, we have together decided on the area to be covered and on the number of text pages that can be allocated to it. We try, by written instructions and by our own editing, to attain a reasonably uniform style of presentation without sacrificing all individuality of expression. Contributors to previous editions are encouraged to rewrite completely if they wish to. The intent is that each article will not only stand by itself but will also serve as an entry-point to a larger body of knowledge. With that object in mind, special attention is given to selection of references.

As we look back on successive editions, we are struck by the continual need to alter the method of presenting specific topics. At various times, for example, the disease sarcoidosis has been looked upon as affecting principally the bones, skin, or lungs, but now it is recognized as a truly multisystemic disease which justifies the hackneyed phrase: "protean manifestations." Contrarily and even more often, the changes must be in the direction of further splintering. Note the present intricate classification of disorders of lipid metabolism, and the need to speak of "glomerular diseases" instead of what was once pigeon-holed as "glomerulonephritis."

Reviewers' comments on past editions have of course been interesting to us. In the main they have been commendatory, but it is obvious that people see different roles for something which bears the title "textbook of medicine." Some have felt that an undergraduate medical student would be better served for his first tour of the field by a sort of primer which would provide concise descriptions of major diseases. Certainly the Cecil-Loeb textbook is not intended to be read cover-to-cover. One can argue, nevertheless, that the undergraduate often wishes to obtain knowledge in depth about a subject, just as does the mature clinician.

One reviewer thought that because weakness is among the most common of symptoms, a textbook should contain an article devoted to that one manifestation. We agree that people often complain of weakness, but we are not convinced that an article about it would contain much useful information. Speaking more generally, we question whether the logic of the clinician often turns on the differential diagnosis of a single manifestation. Instead we think the diagnostic computer is usually turning out possibilities on the basis of concurrence of several manifestations, together with such factors as age, sex, and the sequence of events. If that be the case, many entities are likely to suggest themselves, and the clinician will receive more help from a reference work that provides good discussions of each possibility.

The present edition contains much new material and extensive revisions throughout. One major section, Respiratory Disease, is wholly new, and another, Environmental Factors in Disease, has been reorganized, expanded, and preceded by an introductory article, "Man in his Environment," by H. E. Lewis. This represents an extension of the theme developed by R. J. Dubos in one of the Forewords to the last edition. But the struggles of man in modern society are so varied and the subject so limitless that in a textbook of clinical medicine one can do little more than characterize the major issues and provide guidance to more extended considerations. In this spirit the reader is now introduced to the text proper by a brief essay on medicine in modern society.

We hope that this new work will once again serve the needs of students of all ages. We thank our Associate Editors for their many suggestions as well as for their own important discussions. We are grateful to all contributors for authoritative writing. We must acknowledge special indebtedness to Mrs. Helen W. Miller for her faultless handling of hundreds of manuscripts and proofs; she has been the focal link between contributors, editors, and publishers. As always, we have found it a pleasure to work with the able and devoted people who are the W. B. Saunders Company.

PAUL B. BEESON

WALSH McDERMOTT

CONTRIBUTORS

ALBERT J. AGUAYO, M.D.

General Considerations of the Architecture of the Spinal Cord, Roots, and Spine; Symptoms of Compression of the Nerve Roots and Spinal Cord; Laboratory Aids to Investigation; Arteriovenous Malformations and Other Vascular Lesions of the Spinal Cord; Spinal Epidural Hematoma; Spinal Arachnoiditis; Herpes Zoster; Spinal Cord Tumors

Assistant Professor of Neurology, McGill University, Montreal; Assistant Physician, Department of Medicine, Division of Neurology, Montreal General Hospital, Montreal, Canada.

MARGARET J. ALBRINK, M.D.

Obesity

Professor of Medicine, West Virginia University School of Medicine. Member of Medical and Dental Staff, West Virginia University Hospital, Morgantown, West Virginia.

THOMAS P. ALMY, M.D.

Disorders of Motility

Nathan Smith Professor of Medicine, Dartmouth Medical School; Director of Medicine, the Dartmouth Medical School. Hitchcock Affiliated Hospitals, Hanover, New Hampshire.

HARRY L. ARNOLD, Jr., M.D.

Leprosy

Clinical Professor of Medicine (Dermatology), University of Hawaii School of Medicine. Consultant in Dermatology, Tripler General U.S. Army Hospital, Shriners' Hospital, Maui Memorial Hospital, Wilcox Memorial Hospital, Molokai General Hospital, Leahi Hospital, Honolulu, Hawaii.

GERALD D. AURBACH, M.D.

Parathyroid

Chief, Section on Mineral Metabolism, National Institute of Arthritis and Metabolic Diseases, National Institutes of Health, Bethesda, Maryland.

K. FRANK AUSTEN, M.D.

Connective Tissue Diseases Other Than Rheumatoid Arthritis: Introduction; Periarteritis Nodosa

Professor of Medicine, Harvard Medical School. Physician-in-Chief, Robert B. Brigham Hospital; Physician, Peter Bent Brigham Hospital, Boston, Massachusetts.

ALEXANDER G. BEARN, M.D.

Genetic Principles: Introduction; Analysis of Human Pedigrees; Inborn Errors of Metabolism and Molecular Disease; Polygenic and Multifactorial Inheritance; Pharmacogenetics; Population Genetics; Heredity and Environment; Congenital Malformations; Albinism; Chediak-Higashi Syndrome; Acatalusia; Lipoid Proteinosis; The Mucopolysaccharidoses; The Marfan Syndrome; Pierre Robin Syndrome; Wilson's Disease; Laurence-Moon Syndrome; Dysautonomia

Professor and Chairman, Department of Medicine, Cornell University Medical College. Physician-in-Chief, The New York Hospital, New York, New York.

MARGARET R. BECKLAKE, M.B., B.Ch., M.D.

Chemical and Physical Irritants

Associate Professor in the Departments of Experimental Medicine and Epidemiology and Health, McGill University; Associate of the Medical Research Council of Canada. Associate Physician, Royal Victoria Hospital, Montreal, Canada.

PAUL B. BEESON, M.D.

Granulomatous Diseases of Unproved Etiology: Introduction; Lethal Midline Granuloma; Wegener's Granulomatosis; Some Uncommon Eosinophilic Syndromes; Cranial Arteritis and Polymyalgia Rheumatica; Fibrosing Syndromes; Weber-Christian Disease; Bacterial Endocarditis; Pyelonephritis; Familial Mediterranean Fever; Viral Diseases (Presumptive)

Nuffield Professor of Clinical Medicine, University of Oxford, Oxford, England.

ERNEST BEUTLER, M.D.

Galactosemia

Clinical Professor of Medicine, University of Southern California. Chairman, Division of Medicine; Director, Department of Hematology, City of Hope Medical Center, Duarte, California.

PHILIP K. BONDY, M.D.

Diabetes Mellitus; Hypoglycemic States

C.N.H. Long Professor and Chairman, Department of Internal Medicine, Yale University School of Medicine. Chief of Medicine and Attending, Yale-New Haven Hospital; Consultant, West Haven Veterans Hospital, West Haven, Connecticut.

EUGENE BRAUNWALD, M.D.

Chronic Valvular Heart Disease

Professor and Chairman, Department of Medicine, University of California at San Diego School of Medicine, La Jolla; Chief of Medicine, University Hospital of San Diego County, San Diego, California.

NEAL S. BRICKER, M.D.

Acute Renal Failure

Professor of Medicine, Director of Renal Division, Washington University School of Medicine. Associate Physician, Barnes Hospital, St. Louis, Missouri.

WALLACE BRIGDEN, M.D.

Disease of the Myocardium

Lecturer in the London Hospital Medical College and Institute of Cardiology, University of London. Physician, The Cardiac Department, The London Hospital; Physician to the National Heart Hospital, London, England.

STANLEY A. BRILLER, M.D.

Cardiac Arrhythmias: General Principles

Associate Professor of Medicine, University of Pennsylvania School of Medicine; Associate Professor of Electrical Engineering, Moore School of Electrical Engineering, University of Pennsylvania. Staff Member of the Robinette Foundation for the Study of Cardiovascular Disease, Hospital of the University of Pennsylvania, Philadelphia, Pennsylvania.

ELMER B. BROWN, M.D.

Hypochromic Anemias

Associate Professor of Medicine, Washington University School of Medicine. Director, Division of Hematology, Washington University School of Medicine; Assistant Physician, Barnes Hospital; Director, Hematology Clinic, Washington University Clinics, St. Louis, Missouri.

L. J. BRUCE-CHWATT, M.D.

Malaria

Professor, London School of Hygiene and Tropical Medicine; Director, Ross Institute, London, England.

HOWARD B. BURCHELL, M.D.

Congenital Heart Disease

Professor of Medicine, University of Minnesota Medical School, Minneapolis, Minnesota.

HUGH CHAPLIN, Jr., M.D.

Hemoglobinuria; Transfusion Reactions

Professor of Medicine and Preventive Medicine, Washington University School of Medicine. Associate Physician, Barnes Hospital, St. Louis, Missouri.

F. S. CHEEVER, M.D.

Diphtheria

Professor of Microbiology, University of Pittsburgh School of Medicine; Vice Chancellor, Health Professions, University of Pittsburgh. Active Staff in Medicine, Presbyterian-University Hospital; Senior Staff in Medicine, Magee-Womens Hospital, Pittsburgh, Pennsylvania.

NICHOLAS P. CHRISTY, M.D.

Diseases of the Endocrine System: General Considerations; Anterior Pituitary; Endocrine Syndromes Associated with Neoplasms of Nonendocrine Tissue; Diseases of Metabolism: General Considerations

Clinical Professor of Medicine, Columbia University College of Physicians and Surgeons. Chairman, Department of Medicine, Roosevelt Hospital; Visiting Physician, Francis Delafield Hospital; Associate Attending Physician, Vanderbilt Clinic, New York, New York.

LEIGHTON E. CLUFF, M.D.

Shigellosis; Cholera; Diseases Caused by Malleomyces; Anthrax; Listeriosis; Erysipeloid of Rosenbach

Professor of Medicine, Chairman of the Department of Medicine, Physician-in-Chief, University of Florida College of Medicine, J. Hillis Miller Health Center, Gainesville, Florida.

JAY D. COFFMAN, M.D.

Diseases of the Peripheral Vessels

Professor of Medicine, Boston University School of Medicine. Visiting Physician, University Hospital, Boston, Massachusetts.

C. LOCKARD CONLEY, M.D.

The Hemoglobinopathies and Thalassemias

Professor of Medicine, The Johns Hopkins University School of Medicine. Head, Hematology Division, The Johns Hopkins University and Hospital, Baltimore, Maryland.

REX B. CONN, M.D.

Normal Laboratory Values in Clinical Medicine

Professor of Laboratory Medicine, The Johns Hopkins University School of Medicine. Director of Laboratory Medicine, The Johns Hopkins Hospital, Baltimore, Maryland.

ROBERT B. COUCH, M.D.

Mycoplasmal Pneumonia

Associate Professor of Microbiology and Medicine, Baylor College of Medicine, Houston, Texas. Associate Attending Physician in Medicine, Ben Taub General Hospital; Attending Physician, The Methodist Hospital, Houston, Texas.

ALEXANDER CRAMPTON SMITH, M.A., M.B.

Tetanus

Nuffield Professor of Anaesthetics, Oxford University. Consultant Anaesthetist, United Oxford Hospitals, Oxford, England.

LESLIE J. De GROOT, M.D.

Diseases of the Thyroid

Professor of Medicine, University of Chicago, Chicago, Illinois.

ROGER M. DES PREZ, M.D.

Tuberculosis; Extrapulmonary Tuberculosis

Professor of Medicine, Vanderbilt University Medical School. Chief, Medical Service, Veterans Administration Hospital; Attending Physician, Vanderbilt Hospital, Nashville, Tennessee.

PHILIP R. DODGE, M.D.

Introduction to Infections and Inflammatory Diseases of the Nervous System and Its Covering; Aids to Diagnosis in Intracranial and Intraspinal Inflammatory

Disease; Neurologic Aspects of Meningitis; Spinal Epidural Infections; Diffuse Inflammatory Diseases of the Brain and Spinal Cord; Syphilitic Infections of the Central Nervous System

Professor of Pediatrics and Neurology; Head, Edward Mallinkrodt Department of Pediatrics, Washington University School of Medicine. Medical Director, St. Louis Children's Hospital; Pediatrician-in-Chief, Barnes Hospital, St. Louis, Missouri.

WILBUR G. DOWNS, M.D., M.P.H.

Yellow Fever; Lassa Fever

Professor of Epidemiology, Yale University School of Medicine, New Haven, Connecticut. Associate Director, Rockefeller Foundation.

PIERRE M. DREYFUS, M.D.

Nutritional Disorders of the Nervous System

Professor and Chairman, Department of Neurology, University of California, Davis School of Medicine. Chief, Neurology Service, Sacramento Medical Center, Sacramento, California; Consultant Neurologist, David Grant USAF Hospital, Travis Air Force Base, California.

PETER J. DYCK, M.D.

Diseases of Nerve Roots, Plexuses, and Peripheral Nerves

Associate Professor of Neurology, Mayo Graduate School of Medicine, University of Minnesota. Consultant in Neurology, Mayo Clinic, St. Mary's Hospital, Rochester Methodist Hospital, Rochester, Minnesota.

RICHARD V. EBERT, M.D.

Abnormal Air Spaces; Diffuse Lung Disease

Professor and Chairman, Department of Medicine, University of Minnesota Medical School, Minneapolis, Minnesota.

HAROLD V. ELLINGSON, M.D., Ph.D.

Motion Sickness and Problems of Air Travel

Professor and Chairman, Department of Preventive Medicine, Ohio State University College of Medicine, Columbus, Ohio.

ALVAN R. FEINSTEIN, M.D., M.S.

Neoplasms of the Lung

Professor of Medicine, Yale University School of Medicine. Chief, Clinical Biostatistics and Eastern Research Support Center, West Haven Veterans Administration Hospital, West Haven, Connecticut.

F. ROBERT FEKETY, Jr., M.D.

Staphylococcal Infections

Associate Professor of Internal Medicine; Head, Division of Infectious Diseases, University of Michigan Medical School, Ann Arbor, Michigan.

HARRY A. FELDMAN, M.D.

Meningococcal Disease

Professor and Chairman of Preventive Medicine, State University of New York, Upstate Medical Center. Attending Physician, State University and Silverman Hospitals; Consultant, Syracuse Veterans Administration Hospital and Chenango Memorial Hospital, Norwich, New York.

THOMAS F. FERRIS, M.D.

Toxemia of Pregnancy

Associate Professor of Medicine, Ohio State University School of Medicine. Director, Division of Renal Diseases, Ohio State University Hospital, Columbus, Ohio.

CLEMENT A. FINCH, M.D.

Hemochromatosis

Professor of Medicine, University of Washington School of Medicine. Head, Division of Hematology, University of Washington Hospital, Seattle, Washington.

ALFRED P. FISHMAN, M.S., M.D.

Heart Failure; Shock and Circulatory Collapse

Professor of Medicine, University of Pennsylvania. Director, Cardiovascular-Pulmonary Division; Attending Cardiologist, Hospital of the University of Pennsylvania, Philadelphia, Pennsylvania.

ROBERT A. FISHMAN, M.D.

Intracranial Tumors and States Causing Increased Intracranial Pressure

Professor and Chairman, Department of Neurology, University of California, San Francisco. Attending Neurologist, San Francisco General Hospital; Consulting Neurologist, Veterans Administration Hospital, San Francisco, California.

EDMUND BERNEY FLINK, M.D., Ph.D.

Heavy Metal Poisoning

Professor and Chairman of Medicine, West Virginia University Medical School. Chief of Medical Service, West Virginia University Hospital, Morgantown, West Virginia.

JOHN P. FOX, M.D., Ph.D.

Sandfly Fever; St. Louis Encephalitis; Japanese B Encephalitis; Murray Valley Encephalitis; Russian Spring-Summer Encephalitis and Louping Ill; Omsk Hemorrhagic Fever and Kyasanur Forest Disease

Professor of Epidemiology and Associate Dean, School of Public Health and Community Medicine, University of Washington, Seattle, Washington.

DONALD S. FREDRICKSON, M.D.

Gaucher's Disease and Niemann-Pick Disease

Director of Intramural Research, and Chief, Molecular Disease Branch, National Heart and Lung Institute, Bethesda, Maryland.

NORMAN GESCHWIND, M.D.

Focal Disturbances of Higher Nervous Function

James Jackson Putnam Professor of Neurology, Harvard Medical School. Director, Neurological Unit, Boston City Hospital, Boston, Massachusetts.

GILBERT H. GLASER, M.D., Med. Sc.D.

The Epilepsies

Professor of Neurology, Head of Section of Neurology, Yale University School of Medicine. Attending Physician (Neurology), Yale-New Haven Medical Center, New Haven; Consultant in Neurology, Veterans Administration Hospital, West Haven, Connecticut.

HERMAN A. GODWIN, M.D.

Deficiency of Folic Acid; Miscellaneous and Megaloblastic Anemias

Assistant Professor of Medicine, Harvard Medical School. Assistant Physician, Thorndike Memorial Laboratory; Assisting Physician, Harvard Medical Service, Boston City Hospital, Boston, Massachusetts.

DAVID H. GOLDSTEIN, M.D.

Electric Shock; Carbon Monoxide Poisoning

Professor of Environmental Medicine, New York University Medical Center. Attending Physician, University Hospital, New York University Medical Center; Associate Visiting Physician, Bellevue Hospital, New York, New York.

ROBERT A. GOODWIN, Jr., M.D.

Pulmonary Tuberculosis; Diseases Due to Mycobacteria Other Than M. Tuberculosis and M. Leprae

Associate Professor of Medicine, Vanderbilt University Medical School. Chief, Pulmonary Disease Service, Veterans Administration Hospital; Attending Physician, Vanderbilt Hospital, Nashville, Tennessee.

MELVIN M. GRUMBACH, M.D.

Determination of Sex and Sexual Differentiation; Human Sexual Anomalies; The Testes

Professor of Pediatrics; Chairman, Department of Pediatrics, University of California, San Francisco. Director of Pediatric Services, University of California Hospitals, San Francisco, California.

THORSTEIN GUTHE, M.D., M.P.H.

Treponemal Diseases; Relapsing Fevers; Phagedenic Tropical Ulcer; The Rat-Bite Fevers

Chief Medical Officer, Venereal Diseases and Treponematoses, World Health Organisation, Geneva, Switzerland.

ROBERT J. HAGGERTY, M.D.

Common Accidental Poisoning

Professor and Chairman, Department of Pediatrics, University of Rochester School of Medicine and Dentistry, Pediatrician-in-Chief, Strong Memorial Hospital, Rochester, New York.

WILLIAM J. HARRINGTON, M.D.

Hemorrhagic Disorders

Professor and Chairman, Department of Medicine, University of Miami School of Medicine. Chief of Medical Service, Jackson Memorial Hospital; Consultant in Medicine, Miami Veterans Administration Hospital, Miami, Florida.

EDWARD D. HARRIS, Jr., M.D.

Systemic Sclerosis (Scleroderma)

Assistant Professor of Medicine and Director, Connective Tissue Disease Unit, Dartmouth Medical School, Hanover, New Hampshire.

RICHARD J. HAVEL, M.D.

Disorders of Lipid Metabolism

Professor of Medicine, Associate Director, Cardiovascular Research Institute, University of California, San Francisco. Attending Physician, University of California Hospitals, San Francisco, California.

ROBERT P. HEANEY, M.D.

Diseases of Bone

Professor of Internal Medicine, Creighton University School of Medicine. Head, Section of Endocrinology and Metabolism, Creighton University School of Medicine and Creighton Memorial St. Joseph Hospital, Omaha, Nebraska.

LOUIS H. HEMPELMANN, M.D.

Radiation Injury

Professor of Experimental Radiology, University of Rochester School of Medicine, Rochester, New York.

ALBERT HEYMAN, M.D.

Lymphogranuloma Venereum; Syncope and Hyperventilation

Professor of Neurology, Duke University Medical Center, Durham, North Carolina.

HOWARD H. HIATT, M.D.

Fructosuria and Hereditary Fructose Intolerance; Pentosuria

Herrman L. Blumgart Professor of Medicine, Harvard Medical School. Physician-in-Chief, Beth Israel Hospital, Boston, Massachusetts.

JOHN B. HICKAM, M.D.

Circulatory Disorders

Late Professor and Chairman, Department of Medicine, Indiana University School of Medicine, Indianapolis, Indiana.

EDWARD W. HOOK, M.D.

Bacteroides, Anaerobic Streptococcal, and Fusaspirochetal Disease; Disease Caused by Salmonella

Henry B. Mulholland Professor and Chairman, Department of Medicine, University of Virginia School of Medicine. Physician-in-Chief, University of Virginia, Charlottesville, Virginia.

DOROTHY M. HORSTMANN, M.D.

Mumps; Viral Meningitis

Professor of Epidemiology and Pediatrics, Yale University School of Medicine. Attending Pediatrician, Yale-New Haven Hospital, New Haven, Connecticut.

JOHN BERNARD LLOYD HOWELL, Ph.D.

The Diaphragm; The Chest Wall; Airway Obstruction

Professor of Clinical Science in Medicine, University of Southampton. Honorary Consultant Physician, Southampton General Hospital, Southampton, England.

J. WILLIS HURST, M.D.

Diseases of the Aorta

Professor and Chairman, Department of Medicine, Emory University School of Medicine. Chief of Medicine, Grady Memorial Hospital, Atlanta, Georgia.

HARRIS ISBELL, M.D.

Drug Dependence; Alcohol Problems and Alcoholism; Amphetamine Type of Dependence; Cocaine Dependence; Hallucinogenic Dependence (LSD Type); Dependence on Cannabis (Marihuana, Hashish); Bromides; Poisoning of the Atropine Type

Professor of Medicine and Pharmacology, University of Kentucky College of Medicine. Senior Physician, University of Kentucky Hospital; Consultant, National Institute of Mental Health Addiction Research Center, Lexington, Kentucky.

GEORGE GEE JACKSON, M.D.

The Common Cold; Nonbacterial Pharyngitis, Laryngitis, and Bronchitis; Infections with Rhinovirus; Adenoviral Infections of the Respiratory Tract; Infections with Parainfluenza Viruses; Infections with Respiratory Syncytial Virus

Professor of Medicine, Head, Section of Infectious Diseases, Department of Medicine, Abraham Lincoln School of Medicine, University of Illinois College of Medicine. Attending Physician, University of Illinois Hospital and West Side Veterans Administration Hospital, Chicago, Illinois.

ERNST RICHARD JAFFÉ, M.D.

Methemoglobinemia and Sulfhemoglobinemia

Professor of Medicine, Albert Einstein College of Medicine. Visiting Physician (Medicine), Bronx Municipal Hospital Center and Lincoln Hospital, Bronx, New York.

JAMES H. JANDL, M.D.

Megaloblastic Anemias: Introduction; Pernicious Anemia; Intestinal Malabsorption

George Richards Minot Professor of Medicine, Harvard Medical School. Director, Harvard Medical Unit, Boston City Hospital, Boston, Massachusetts.

ERNEST JAWETZ, M.D., Ph.D.

Trachoma and Inclusion Conjunctivitis

Professor of Microbiology and Medicine, University of California, San Francisco Medical Center, San Francisco, California.

GRAHAM H. JEFFRIES, M.B., Ch.B., D.Phil. (Oxon.)

Diseases of the Liver

Professor and Chairman, Department of Medicine, The Milton S. Hershey Medical Center, Pennsylvania State University College of Medicine. Chief, Medical Service, The Milton S. Hershey Medical Center Hospital, Hershey, Pennsylvania.

KARL M. JOHNSON, M.D.

Arthropod-Borne Viral Fevers, Arthropod-Borne Viral Encephalitides, and Arthropod-Borne Hemorrhagic Fevers: Introduction; Dengue; Hemorrhagic Fever Caused by Dengue Viruses; Hemorrhagic Fever of South America: Argentine and Bolivian Hemorrhagic Fever; Epidemic Hemorrhagic Fever: Hemorrhagic Nephroso-Nephritis

Director, Middle America Research Unit, National Institute of Allergy and Infectious Diseases, National Institutes of Health, U.S. Public Health Service, Balboa Heights, Canal Zone.

RICHARD T. JOHNSON, M.D.

Slow and Latent Viral Infections and Neurologic Diseases

Eisenhower Professor of Neurology and Associate Professor of Microbiology, The Johns Hopkins University School of Medicine. Neurologist, The Johns Hopkins Hospital, Baltimore, Maryland.

ROBERT L. JOHNSON, M.D.

Alterations in Atmospheric Pressure

Deputy Chief, Biomedical Laboratories Division, NASA, Manned Spacecraft Center, Houston, Texas.

FRED S. KANTOR, M.D.

Serum Sickness; Drug Allergy

Associate Professor of Internal Medicine, Yale University School of Medicine. Attending Physician, Yale-New Haven Hospital, New Haven, Connecticut.

ALBERT Z. KAPIKIAN, M.D.

Coxsackie and Echoviruses: General Considerations; Herpangina; Hand, Foot, and Mouth Disease; Acute Lymphonodular Pharyngitis; Epidemic Pleurodynia or Bornholm Disease; Cardiac Manifestations of Coxsackie Virus Infections: "Aseptic Meningitis" Due to Coxsackie and Echoviruses; Exanthemata and "Aseptic Meningitis with Rash" Due to Coxsackie and Echoviruses; Coxsackie and Echoviruses in Diarrheal Diseases of Infants

Head, Epidemiology Section, Laboratory of Infectious Diseases, National Institute of Allergy and Infectious Diseases, National Institutes of Health, Bethesda, Maryland.

NATHAN KASE, M.D.

The Ovaries

Professor and Chairman, Department of Obstetrics and Gynecology, Yale University School of Medicine. Attending, Clinical Laboratories, Yale-New Haven Hospital; Chief of Service, Ob-Gyn, Yale-New Haven Hospital; Staff Consultant, Griffin Hospital, Derby, Connecticut, New Britain General Hospital, New Britain, Connecticut, St. Raphael Hospital, New Haven, Connecticut, Stamford Hospital, Stamford, Connecticut, Norwalk Hospital, Norwalk, Connecticut.

CALVIN F. KAY, M.D.

Cardiac Arrhythmias: Clinical Principles

Professor of Medicine, Chief of Cardiac Section, Cardiopulmonary Division, Department of Medicine; Director of the Heart Station, Hospital of the University of Pennsylvania. Attending Physician, Hospital of the University of Pennsylvania, Philadelphia, Pennsylvania.

DONALD KAYE, M.D.

Gonococcal Disease

Professor and Chairman, Department of Medicine, The Medical College of Pennsylvania, Philadelphia, Pennsylvania.

C. HENRY KEMPE, M.D.

Variola and Vaccinia: Introduction and History; Variola; Vaccinia

Professor of Pediatrics, University of Colorado Medical Center. Consultant, Fitzsimons General Hospital, Children's Hospital, Veterans Administration Hospital, Denver, Colorado.

DAVID NICHOL SHARP KERR, M.S.

Investigation of Renal Function; Chronic Renal Failure

Professor of Medicine, University of Newcastle upon Tyne, England. Consultant Physician, Royal Victoria Infirmary, Newcastle upon Tyne, England.

EDWIN D. KILBOURNE, M.D.

Introduction to the Viral Diseases; Influenza; Measles; Rubella; Exanthemata Associated with Enteroviral Infections; Herpesvirus Infections: General Considerations; Cytomegalovirus Infections

Professor and Chairman, Department of Microbiology, Mount Sinai School of Medicine of the City University of New York, New York, New York.

THOMAS KILLIP, M.D.

Ischemic Heart Disease

Roland Harriman Professor of Medicine, Cornell University Medical College. Attending Physician and Head, Division of Cardiology, The New York Hospital, New York, New York.

PRISCILLA KINCAID-SMITH, M.D., B.Sc.

Treatment of Irreversible Renal Failure by Dialysis and Transplantation

Reader in Medicine, University of Melbourne. Physician in Charge, Medical Renal Unit, Royal Melbourne Hospital, Melbourne, Australia.

JOSEPH B. KIRSNER, M.D., Ph.D.

Acid-Peptic Disease

Louis Block Professor of Medicine, University of Chicago. Attending Professor, Chief of Gastroenterology, Albert Merritt Billings Hospital, Chicago, Illinois.

VERNON KNIGHT, M.D.

Toxoplasmosis; Brucellosis

Professor of Microbiology and Medicine, Baylor College of Medicine, Texas Medical Center. Senior Attending Physician, The Methodist Hospital, Houston, Texas.

M. GLENN KOENIG, M.D.

Food Poisoning

Associate Professor of Medicine, Vanderbilt University School of Medicine. Visiting Staff, Vanderbilt University Hospital; Attending Physician and Consultant in Infectious Diseases, Nashville Veterans Administration Hospital, Nashville, Tennessee.

HILARY KOPROWSKI, M.D.

Rabies

Director, The Wistar Institute of Anatomy and Biology, Philadelphia, Pennsylvania.

O. DHODANAND KOWLESSAR, M.D.

Diseases of the Pancreas

Professor of Medicine, Jefferson Medical College of Thomas Jefferson University. Director, Division of Gastroenterology; Director, Clinical Research Center, Jefferson Medical College and Thomas Jefferson University Hospitals, Philadelphia, Pennsylvania.

RICHARD M. KRAUSE, M.D.

Rheumatic Fever

Professor, Rockefeller University. Senior Physician, Rockefeller University Hospital, New York, New York.

CALVIN M. KUNIN, M.D.

Enteric Bacterial Infections (Including Urinary Tract Infections)

Professor of Medicine, University of Wisconsin School of

Medicine. Chief of Medicine, Veterans Administration Hospital; Associate Chairman, Department of Medicine, University of Wisconsin, Madison, Wisconsin.

HENRY G. KUNKEL, M.D.

Immune Mechanisms in Disease

Professor, Rockefeller University. Senior Physician, Rockefeller University Hospital, New York, New York.

LAWRENCE EDWARD LAMB, M.D.

Gravitational Changes

Professor of Medicine, Baylor College of Medicine, Houston, Texas.

ALEXANDER LEAF, M.D.

Posterior Pituitary

Jackson Professor of Clinical Medicine, Harvard Medical School. Chief of Medical Services, Massachusetts General Hospital, Boston, Massachusetts.

AARON B. LERNER, M.D., Ph.D.

Disorders of Melanin Pigmentation

Professor of Dermatology, Yale University School of Medicine. Chief of Dermatology, Yale-New Haven Medical Center, New Haven, Connecticut.

HAROLD E. LEWIS, B.Sc., M.B., Ch.B.

Introduction to Environmental Factors in Disease

Senior Member of Scientific Staff, National Institute for Medical Research, Hampstead, London. Member of Faculty of Environmental Studies, University College of London, England.

HERBERT L. LEY, Jr., M.D., M.P.H.

Rocky Mountain Spotted Fever; Tick-Borne Rickettsioses of the Eastern Hemisphere; Rickettsialpox; Scrub Typhus; Trench Fever; Q Fever; Bartonellosis

Medical Consultant in Foods and Drugs.

GRANT W. LIDDLE, M.D.

Adrenal Cortex

Professor of Medicine and Chairman of the Department, Vanderbilt University. Physician-in-Chief, Venderbilt University Hospital, Nashville, Tennessee.

HAROLD I. LIEF, M.D.

Medical Aspects of Sexuality

Professor of Psychiatry, University of Pennsylvania School of Medicine. Director, Division of Family Study; Director, Marriage Council of Philadelphia, Philadelphia, Pennsylvania.

PHILIP D. MARSDEN, M.D.

Protozoan and Helminthic Diseases: Introduction; Syndromes Associated with Malaria; Amebiasis; Other Intestinal Protozoa; Helminthic Diseases: General Considerations; The Cestodes; The Hermaphroditic Flukes; Paragonimiasis; Intestinal Flukes; The Nematodes; Tropical Pyomyositis; Eosinophilia in Relation to Helminthic Infections; Arthropods and Leeches as Agents of Disease

Senior Lecturer, London School of Hygiene and Tropical Medicine. Visiting Professor of Public Health, Cornell Medical Center, New York, New York; Assistant Medical Unit, Hospital for Tropical Diseases, London, England.

FRED R. McCRUMB, M.D.

Plague

Professor of International Medicine, University of Maryland School of Medicine, Baltimore, Maryland.

WALSH McDERMOTT, M.D.

Medicine in Modern Society; Chemical Contamination of Water and Air; Introduction to Microbial Diseases; Foot-and-Mouth Disease; Bacterial Diseases: Introduction; Pneumonia; General Considerations; Granuloma Inguinale

Livingston Farrand Professor and Chairman, Department of Public Health, Cornell University Medical College. Attending Physician, The New York Hospital, New York, New York.

WILLIAM V. McDERMOTT, Jr., M.D.

Diseases of the Peritoneum

Cheever Professor of Surgery, Harvard Medical School. Director, Fifth (Harvard) Surgical Unit and Sears Surgical Laboratory, Boston City Hospital, Boston, Massachusetts.

FLETCHER H. McDOWELL, M.D.

Cerebrovascular Diseases

Professor of Neurology, Cornell University Medical College. Attending Neurologist, The New York Hospital; Associate Attending Physician, Memorial Hospital, New York, New York.

PAUL R. McHUGH, M.D.

Dementia; Psychologic Illness in Medical Practice

Associate Professor of Psychiatry and Associate Professor of Neurology, Cornell University Medical College. Attending Psychiatrist, The New York Hospital, Westchester Division, White Plains, New York; Associate Attending Neurologist, The New York Hospital, New York, New York.

GORDON MEIKLEJOHN, M.D., C.M.

Colorado Tick Fever

Professor of Medicine, Chairman, Department of Medicine, University of Colorado Medical Center. Chief of Medical Service, Colorado General Hospital, Denver, Colorado; Affiliated, Denver General Hospital, Veterans Administration Hospital, Denver, Colorado.

SHERMAN A. MINTON, M.D.

Venom Diseases

Professor of Microbiology, Indiana University School of Medicine, Indianapolis, Indiana.

CARL V. MOORE, M.D.

Hematologic and Hematopoietic Diseases: Introduction; The Anemias: Introduction; Normocytic Mormochromic Anemias; Diseases of the White Blood Cells and Reticuloendothelial System: Introduction; The Leukemias; Leukemoid Reactions; Conditions Primarily Affecting the Lymph Nodes; Histiocytosis X; The Concept of Myeloproliferative Disorders; Diseases of the Spleen

Busch Professor of Medicine, Washington University School of Medicine. Physician-in-Chief, Barnes Hospital, St. Louis, Missouri.

STEPHEN I. MORSE, M.D.

Whooping Cough

Professor and Chairman, Department of Microbiology and Immunology State University of New York, Downstate Medical Center, Brooklyn, New York.

HARRY MOST, M.D., D.T.M. and H., D. Med. Sc.

Leishmaniasis

Professor and Chairman, Department of Preventive Medicine, New York University School of Medicine. Attending Physician, University Hospital, New York, New York; Visiting Physician, Bellevue Hospital, New York, New York; Consultant in Tropical Medicine, Veterans Administration, United States Public Health Service, Surgeon General, U.S. Army.

EDWARD S. MURRAY, M.D.

Rickettsial Diseases: Introduction; The Typhus Group

Professor of Microbiology, Harvard School of Public Health, Cambridge, Massachusetts.

JAMES R. NELSON, M.D.

Hearing Loss; Vertigo

Associate Professor and Vice Chairman, Department of Neurosciences. Neurologist-in-Chief, University of California, San Diego, California.

W. E. ORMEROD, M.A., D.Sc., D.M.

African Trypanosomiasis

Reader in Medical Protozoology, London School of Hygiene and Tropical Medicine, London, England.

ELLIOTT F. OSSERMAN, M.D.

Plasma Cell Dyscrasias

American Cancer Society Professor of Pathology (Immunology and Oncology), College of Physicians and Surgeons, Columbia University; Associate Director, Institute of Cancer Research, Columbia University. Visiting Physician, Francis Delafield Hospital, New York, New York.

RUSSEL H. PATTERSON, Jr., M.D.

Injuries of the Head and Spine

Associate Professor of Surgery (Neurosurgery), Cornell University Medical College. Associate Attending Surgeon, The New York Hospital; Consulting Associate Neurosurgeon, Memorial Hospital for Cancer and Allied Diseases, New York, New York.

W. S. PEART, F.R.S., M.D.

Arterial Hypertension

Professor of Medicine, St. Mary's Hospital Medical School, London, England.

ROBERT G. PETERSDORF, M.D.

Bacterial Meningitis Other than that Caused by Meningococci and Mycobacteria

Professor and Chairman, Department of Medicine, University of Washington School of Medicine. Physician-in-Chief, University of Washington Hospital; Consultant Physician, Seattle Veterans Administration Hospital, United States Public Health Service Hospital; Attending Physician, Harborview Medical Center, Seattle, Washington.

MALCOLM L. PETERSON, M.D.

Neoplastic Diseases of the Alimentary Tract

Director, Health Services Research and Development Center, The Johns Hopkins Medical Institutions; Associate Professor of Medicine, The Johns Hopkins School of Medicine; Associate Professor of Medical Care and Hospitals, The Johns Hopkins School of Hygiene and Public Health. Assistant Physician, The Johns Hopkins Hospital, Baltimore, Maryland.

FRED PLUM, M.D.

Introduction to Disorders of the Nervous System and Behavior; Introduction to Consciousness and Its Disturbances; The Pathogenesis of Stupor and Coma; Sleep and Its Disorders; The Management of Acute Depressive Drug Poisoning; Phenothiazine Toxicity; Headache; The Management of Severe Neurologic Disability; Idiopathic Autonomic Insufficiency; Abnormalities in Respiratory Control

Anne Parrish Titzell Professor and Chairman, Department of Neurology, Cornell University Medical College. Neurologist-in-Chief, New York Hospital, New York, New York.

JEROME B. POSNER, M.D.

Delirium and Exogenous Metabolic Brain Disease; Nonmetastatic Effects of Cancer on the Nervous System

Professor of Neurology, Cornell University Medical College. Chief, Neuropsychiatric Service, Memorial Hospital for Cancer and Allied Diseases; Attending Neurologist, The New York Hospital, New York, New York.

JOSEPH M. QUASHNOCK, M.D., Ph.D.

Heat and Cold

Colonel, United States Air Force Medical Corps; Commander, USAF School of Aerospace Medicine, Brooks Air Force Base, Texas.

OSCAR D. RATNOFF, M.D.

Coagulation Defects: Introduction; Heritable Disorders of Blood Coagulation; Acquired Disorders of Blood Coagulation

Professor of Medicine, Case Western Reserve University; Career Investigator of the American Heart Association. Physician, University Hospitals of Cleveland, Cleveland, Ohio.

SEYMOUR REICHLIN, M.D., Ph.D.

The Control of Anterior Pituitary Secretion; The Pineal

Professor of Medicine, Head, Department of Medical and Pediatric Specialties, University of Connecticut School of Medicine.

EDWARD H. REINHARD, M.D.

Polycythemia

Professor of Medicine, Washington University School of Medicine. Associate Physician, Barnes Hospital; Director of the Medical Service, Unit II, Barnes Hospital, St. Louis, Missouri.

DONALD J. REIS, M.D.

Degenerative and Heredofamilial Diseases of the Central Nervous System

Associate Professor of Neurology, Associate Professor of Neurology in Psychiatry, Cornell University Medical College. Associate Attending Neurologist, The New York

Hospital; Associate Attending Neurologist in Psychiatry, The Westchester Division of the New York Hospital, White Plains, New York.

WILLIAM DODD ROBINSON, M.D.

Diseases of Joints

Professor and Chairman, Department of Internal Medicine, The University of Michigan.

HEONIR ROCHA, M.D.

Chagas' Disease

Professor of Internal Medicine, University of Bahia School of Medicine. Hospital Prof. Edgard Santos, Salvador, Bahia, Brazil.

DAVID E. ROGERS, M.D.

Psittacosis

Professor of Medicine, Dean of The Medical Faculty, Vice President (Medicine), The Johns Hopkins University School of Medicine. Medical Director, The Johns Hopkins Hospital, Baltimore, Maryland.

FRED S. ROSEN, M.D.

Immunologic Deficiency States

Assistant Professor of Pediatrics, Harvard Medical School. Chief, Immunology Division, Children's Hospital Medical Center, Boston, Massachusetts.

LEWIS P. ROWLAND, M.D.

Diseases of Muscle and Neuromuscular Junction

Professor and Chairman, Department of Neurology, University of Pennsylvania School of Medicine. Attending Neurologist, Hospital of the University of Pennsylvania; Consultant Neurologist, Children's Hospital of Philadelphia, Graduate Hospital of the University of Pennsylvania, Philadelphia General Hospital, Philadelphia, Pennsylvania.

JAY P. SANFORD, M.D.

Klebsiella and Other Gram-Negative Bacterial Pneumonias; Leptospirosis

Professor of Internal Medicine, University of Texas (Southwestern) Medical School at Dallas. Senior Attending Physician and Chief, Microbiology Laboratory, Parkland Memorial Hospital, Dallas, Texas; Consultant in Internal Medicine, Dallas and Temple Veterans Administration Hospitals, U.S. Army Brooke General Hospital, San Antonio, Texas, Wilford Hall USAF Hospital, San Antonio, Texas.

LABE C. SCHEINBERG, M.D.

The Demyelinating Diseases

Professor of Neurology, Albert Einstein College of Medicine of Yeshiva University. Attending Neurologist, Bronx Municipal Hospital Center and Montefiore Hospital and Medical Center, Bronx, New York; Director of Neurology Services, Hospital of the Albert Einstein College of Medicine, Bronx, New York.

RUDI SCHMID, M.D., Ph.D.

Porphyria

Professor of Medicine, University of California, San Francisco, California.

RICHARD P. SCHMIDT, M.D.

Neurologic Diagnostic Procedures

Dean of the College of Medicine, State University of New York, Upstate Medical Center, Syracuse, New York.

GEORGE E. SCHREINER, M.D.

Obstructive Nephropathy; Toxic Nephropathy; Cysts of the Kidney; Tumors of the Kidney; Miscellaneous Renal Disorders

Professor of Medicine, Georgetown University School of Medicine. Director, Division of Nephrology, Georgetown University School of Medicine, Washington, D.C.

PETER H. SCHUR, M.D.

Systemic Lupus Erythematosus

Assistant Professor of Medicine, Harvard Medical School. Visiting Physician, Robert B. Brigham Hospital; Associate in Medicine, Peter Bent Brigham Hospital, Boston, Massachusetts.

WILLIAM B. SCHWARTZ, M.D.

The Nephropathy of Potassium Depletion; The Nephropathy of Hypercalcemia; Renal Tubular Acidosis; The Nephropathy of Acute Hyperuricemia; Balkan Nephritis; Disorders of Fluid, Electrolyte and Acid-Base Balance

Professor of Medicine, Tufts University School of Medicine. Chief, Renal Service, New England Medical Center Hospitals, Boston, Massachusetts.

NEVIN S. SCRIMSHAW, M.D., Ph.D.

Nutrient Requirements; Assessment of Nutritional Status; Nutrition and Infection; Kwashiorkor, Marasmus, and Intermediate Forms of Protein-Calorie Malnutrition; Undernutrition, Starvation, and Hunger Edema; Nutritional Anemias; Anorexia Nervosa; Deficiencies of Individual Nutrients: Vitamin Diseases

Professor and Head, Department of Nutrition and Food Science, Massachusetts Institute of Technology, Cambridge, Massachusetts.

CHARLES ROBERT SCRIVER, M.D., C.M.

Inborn Errors of Amino Acid Metabolism

Professor of Pediatrics, Associate Professor of Genetics, McGill University. Research Unit Director (Biochemical Genetics), McGill University-Montreal Children's Hospital Research Institute; Physician, Montreal Children's Hospital, Montreal, Canada.

MARGERY W. SHAW, M.D.

Cytogenetics; Numerical Variations in Human Chromosome Complement; Structural Variations; Inherited Chromosome Breakage; Genetic Counseling

Professor of Biology, University of Texas Graduate School of Biomedical Sciences. Medical Geneticist, M.D. Anderson Hospital and Tumor Institute, Houston, Texas.

WILLIAM B. SHERMAN, M.D.

Hay Fever and Allergic Rhinitis; Urticaria; Angioneurotic Edema

Late Associate Clinical Professor of Medicine, College of Physicians and Surgeons, Columbia University. Late Director, Institute of Allergy, Roosevelt Hospital, and Associate Attending, Presbyterian Hospital, New York, New York.

SOL SHERRY, M.D.

Thromboembolic Diseases; Fibrinolysis and Fibrinolytic Disorders

Professor and Chairman, Department of Medicine, Temple University School of Medicine. Physician-in-Chief, Temple University Hospital, Philadelphia, Pennsylvania.

J. B. SIDBURY, Jr., M.D.

Glycogen Storage Diseases

Professor of Pediatrics, Duke University Medical Center, Durham, North Carolina.

LOUIS E. SILTZBACH, M.D.

Sarcoidosis

Clinical Professor of Medicine, The Mount Sinai School of Medicine, New York, New York. Head of Thoracic Diseases Division, The Mount Sinai Hospital; Attending Physician, Pulmonary Division, Montefiore Hospital; Consulting Physician, The Rockefeller University Hospital, New York, New York.

ALBERT SJOERDSMA, M.D., Ph.D.

Sympatho-Adrenal System; The Carcinoid Syndrome

Chief, Experimental Therapeutics Branch, National Heart and Lung Institute. Clinical Center, National Institutes of Health, Bethesda, Maryland.

MARVIN HERBERT SLEISENGER, M.D.

Diseases of the Digestive System: Introduction; Diseases of Malabsorption; Diseases of the Gallbladder and Bile Ducts

Professor and Vice Chairman, Department of Medicine, University of California, San Francisco. Chief, Medical Service, San Francisco Veterans Administration Hospital, San Francisco, California.

LLOYD H. SMITH, Jr., M.D., D.Sc. (hon.)

Diseases of Purine Metabolism; Primary Hyperoxaluria

Professor of Medicine and Chairman of the Department of Medicine, University of California School of Medicine. Physician-in-Chief of the Medical Staff, University of California Hospitals, San Francisco, California.

CHARLES J. STAHL, M.D.

Drowning

Assistant Chief, Military Environmental Pathology Division; Chief, Forensic Pathology Branch; Chief, Marine Biopathology Branch; Registrar, Registry of Forensic Pathology, Armed Forces Institute of Pathology, Washington, D.C.

WILLIAM W. STEAD, M.D.

Diseases of the Pleura

Professor of Medicine, Marquette School of Medicine, Milwaukee, Wisconsin. Director of Chest Services, Marquette School of Medicine; Medical Director, Muirdale Sanatorium, Milwaukee, Wisconsin.

GENE H. STOLLERMAN, M.D.

Streptococcal Diseases: General Considerations; Group A Streptococcal Infection; Clinical Syndromes of Group A Streptococcal Infection; Treatment of Group A Streptococcal Infection and Chemoprophylaxis of Nonsuppurative Complications; Prophylaxis of Streptococcal Infection

Professor and Chairman, Department of Medicine, The University of Tennessee College of Medicine. Physician-in-Chief, City of Memphis Hospitals, Memphis, Tennessee.

JOHN F. SULLIVAN, M.D.

Acute Spinal Intervertebral Disc Disease; Chronic Spinal Intervertebral Disc Disease

Professor of Neurology, Tufts University School of Medicine. Neurologist-in-Chief, New England Medical Center Hospitals, Boston, Massachusetts; Consultant, Neurological Unit, Boston City Hospital; Consultant, St. Elizabeth's Hospital, Brighton, Massachusetts.

AUGUST G. SWANSON, M.D.

Pain

Professor of Medicine for Neurology, University of Washington School of Medicine, Seattle, Washington.

MORTON N. SWARTZ, M.D.

Parameningeal Infections

Associate Professor of Medicine, Harvard Medical School. Visiting Physician and Chief, Infectious Disease Unit, Massachusetts General Hospital, Boston, Massachusetts.

WILLIAM C. THOMAS, Jr., M.D.

Renal Calculi

Professor of Medicine, University of Florida College of Medicine. Chief, Medical Service, Veterans Administration Hospital, Gainesville, Florida.

H. RICHARD TYLER, M.D.

Polymyositis and Dermatositis

Associate Professor of Neurology, Harvard Medical School. Physician, Peter Bent Brigham Hospital, Boston, Massachusetts.

JOHN P. UTZ, M.D.

The Mycoses

Professor of Medicine, Medical College of Virginia. Chief of Infectious Diseases, Medical College of Virginia Hospitals, Richmond, Virginia.

WILLIAM N. VALENTINE, M.D.

The Leukopenic State and Agranulocytosis; Infectious Mononucleosis

Professor and Chairman, Department of Medicine, University of California School of Medicine; Physician-in-Chief, Medicine, University of California Center for Health Sciences, Los Angeles, California.

ROBERT R. WAGNER, M.D.

Herpes Simplex

Professor and Chairman of Microbiology, University of Virginia School of Medicine, Charlottesville, Virginia.

BYRON H. WAKSMAN, M.D.

Encephalomyelitis and Other Neurologic Lesions as Sequelae to Viral Infections and Viral Vaccines

Professor of Microbiology, Yale University School of Medicine, New Haven, Connecticut.

JAMES V. WARREN, M.D.

Pericarditis

Professor of Internal Medicine, Ohio State University College of Medicine. Chairman, Department of Medicine, Ohio State University Hospitals, Columbus, Ohio.

KENNETH S. WARREN, M.D.

Schistosomiasis

Associate Professor of Geographic Medicine, Case Western Reserve University School of Medicine. Assistant Physician, University Hospitals, Cleveland, Ohio.

LOUIS WEINSTEIN, M.D., Ph.D.

Poliomyelitis

Professor of Medicine, Tufts University School of Medicine, Lecturer on Infectious Disease, Harvard Medical School. Chief of the Infectious Service and Senior Physician, New England Medical Center Hospitals; Associate Physician, Medical Service, Massachusetts General Hospital, Boston, Massachusetts.

THOMAS H. WELLER, M.D.

Varicella; Herpes Zoster

Richard Pearson Strong Professor of Tropical Public Health, Director of the Center for the Prevention of Infectious Diseases, and Chairman of the Department, Harvard School of Public Health. Consultant in Tropical Medicine, Peter Bent Brigham Hospital; Consultant, Virus and Parasitic Diseases, Children's Hospital, Boston, Massachusetts.

CLAYTON E. WHEELER, Jr., M.D.

Certain Cutaneous Diseases with Significant Systemic Manifestations: Introduction; Cutaneous Manifestations of Internal Malignancy; Erythemas; Contact Dermatitis; Behçet's Disease; Pemphigus; Acanthosis Nigricans; Mast Cell Disease; Lethal Cutaneous and Gastrointestinal Arteriolar Thrombosis; Angiokeratoma Corporis Diffusum; Incontinentia Pigmenti; Hereditary Anhidrotic Ectodermal Defect; Neurofibrosis of Von Recklinghausen; Ainhum; Warts; Orf; Molluscum Contagiosum; Ehlers-Danlos Syndrome; Pseudoxanthoma Elasticum

Professor of Dermatologic Medicine, University of North Carolina School of Medicine. Chief, Division of Dermatology, North Carolina Memorial Hospital, Chapel Hill, North Carolina.

M. HENRY WILLIAMS, Jr., M.D.

Introduction to Respiratory Disease; Pulmonary Structure and Function; General Considerations; Ventilatory Function; Conducting Airways; Alveolar Structure and Function; Pulmonary Circulation; Disability Evaluation; Hypoxemia

Professor of Medicine, Albert Einstein College of Medicine. Director, Chest Service, Albert Einstein College of Medicine, Bronx Municipal Hospital Center, New York, New York.

EMANUEL WOLINSKY, M.D.

Clostridial Diseases: General Considerations; Clostridial Myonecrosis; Other Clostridial Diseases; Clostridial Gastroenteritis

Professor of Medicine and Associate Professor of Microbiology, Case Western Reserve University. Chief, Infectious Disease Service, Cleveland Metropolitan General Hospital, Cleveland, Ohio.

W. BARRY WOOD, Jr., M.D.

Pneumococcal Pneumonia

Late Boury Professor of Microbiology, The Johns Hopkins University School of Medicine, Baltimore, Maryland.

THEODORE E. WOODWARD, M.D.

Tularemia

Professor and Head, Department of Medicine, University of Maryland School of Medicine. Physician-in-Chief, University of Maryland Hospital, Baltimore, Maryland.

TELFORD H. WORK, M.D.

Semliki Forest-Mayoro Virus Disease; West Nile Fever; Rift Valley Fever; Arthropod-borne Viral Encephalitides: General Considerations; Western Equine Encephalomyelitis; Eastern Equine Encephalomyelitis; Venezuelan Equine Encephalomyelitis; California Encephalitis

Professor of Infectious and Tropical Diseases, University of California at Los Angeles, School of Public Health and School of Medicine, University of California Medical Center, Los Angeles, California.

OLIVER M. WRONG, D.M.

Glomerular Disease

Professor of Medicine, Dundee University. Consultant Physician, Dundee General Hospitals, Dundee, Scotland.

MELVIN D. YAHR, M.D.

Introduction to The Extrapyramidal Disorders; The Parkinsonian Syndrome; Essential Tremor; Senile Tremor; The Choreas; Tics; Athetosis; Dystonia Musculorum Deformans; Spasmodic Torticollis; Hemiballism

Professor of Neurology, Columbia University College of Physicians and Surgeons. Attending Neurologist, New York Neurological Institute and The Columbia-Presbyterian Medical Center, New York, New York.

LAWRENCE E. YOUNG, M.D.

Hemolytic Disorders: General Considerations; Intracorpuscular Abnormalities; Extracorpuscular Hemolytic Agents and Mechanisms

Dewey Professor of Medicine and Chairman, Department of Medicine, University of Rochester School of Medicine and Dentistry Physician-in-Chief, Strong Memorial Hospital, Rochester, New York.

LOUIS ZETZEL, M.D.

Inflammatory Diseases of Intestine

Clinical Professor of Medicine, Harvard Medical School. Visiting Physician and Consultant to Gastroenterology Department, Beth Israel Hospital, Boston, Massachusetts.

CONTENTS

HEMATOLOGIC AND HEMATOPOIETIC DISEASES

DISEASES OF BONE

DISEASES OF JOINTS

NORMAL LABORATORY VALUES OF CLINICAL IMPORTANCE, 1914

MEDICINE IN MODERN SOCIETY

Walsh McDermott

Medicine is not a science but a learned profession deeply rooted in a number of sciences and charged with the obligation to apply them for man's benefit. So complex a process could hardly be reduced to a neat symmetrical design and fitted within the covers of a book. Yet this subject, the beneficial uses of medical science, is not without any design at all—it has a conceptual base on which all medical teaching and all medical books should rest. To consider this base, or certain aspects of it, therefore seems proper at the start of a textbook of medicine. Although the book itself is addressed to medical students and graduate physicians of all ages, this Introduction is presented primarily to those now entering the profession.

One part of the conceptual base is set forth in the opening sentence above that ends ". . . to apply them for man's benefit." Traditionally this applying is made with compassion and in accord with a widely recognized moral and ethical code. Thus the responsibilities of medicine are threefold: to generate scientific knowledge and to teach it to others; to use the knowledge for the health of an individual or a whole community; and to judge the moral and ethical propriety of each medical act that directly affects another human being. These three areas of responsibility command the efforts of individuals from a wide range of scientific disciplines and professions, but the physicians who are involved in the actual applying of the knowledge are of two sorts: those who care for one patient at a time and those who deal with people as groups.

The activities of both sorts of physicians are based on the concept that each disease entity has its own pathogenic chain—the whole series of events that determine its causation and maintenance—and that understanding this chain for a particular disease not only permits clearer recognition of its clinical manifestations, but reveals any weak links that might be exploited for prevention or therapy.

Approach to the body of knowledge organized in this way (both in books and elsewhere) is made from one of two viewpoints. The physician in public health or community medicine is constantly reaching for ways in which pathogenic chains can be broken by some continuing intervention that affects a number of people at once, e.g., to reduce the incidence of goiter by putting iodine in table salt. By contrast, physicians acting within the other system—the clinical system—will search the same knowledge sectors and with educated discrimination will extract those elements appropriate for the solution of a problem in an individual. The viewpoints from which the knowledge is scrutinized are different, but the body of knowledge about each disease is the same in either case. Textbooks about diseases and their pathogenic chains serve both these viewpoints and form important instruments for this process of the beneficial uses of science.

The physician who treats one patient at a time and the physician who deals with a community as a whole both exert compassion, but it is of two quite different sorts. The compassion exercised by the physician who treats individuals takes the form of a cultivated instinct to lend support and comfort to a particular fellow human being. The "group" compassion of the public health or community physician necessarily takes the form of what the writer has previously termed "statistical compassion," meaning an imaginative compassion for people whom one never gets to see as individuals and, indeed, can know only as data on a graph. This compassion—the deep-seated instinct to try to help those whom one never gets to see—is a characteristic form of motivation for political leaders and other social activists, and "statistical" successes bring them major satisfactions. Such is really not the case with most physicians, who usually do not derive as much satisfaction from seeing improvement on a graph as they do from seeing improvement in an individual. Indeed, part of the self-selection in choosing medicine as a career seems to be a self-image of a person whose professional activities are to relate directly with individuals rather than with groups. Thus the system of public health or community medicine—based on physicians *not* seeing patients as individuals—runs contrary to most medical instincts. Yet until we have significant numbers of physicians for whom "statistical compassion" is as rewarding as it is to other types of leaders in our society, we will fail as a society to derive the full measure of the benefits of our medical science.

The scientific basis of medicine had been building up throughout the whole nineteenth century, but the *uses* of that science in the sense of decisively altering or preventing disease were largely accomplished through the nonclinical or "community" physicians who dealt with people as groups. Chlorination of water supplies and the pasteurization of milk are cases in point. It was not until the discovery of insulin 50 years ago, and not really until the advent of the modern antimicrobial era 35 years ago, that the clinical physicians had much in the way of decisive therapies or preventives derived from science. Since that time most of the practical uses of biomedical science and technology have been of a nature fitted to the clinical or personal system, and the other system has been allowed to languish. Indeed, the evolution of the highly complex and extraordinarily effective instrument that is today's medical center has been almost exclusively devoted to the one system—the clinical physician system of one patient at a time.

We could tolerate this so long as what medicine had to offer was technologically simple and physicians were spread out much more evenly than they are now across the whole of society. But the coincidence of massive scientific innovation and wide social change has created a situation in which the application of medical science for man's benefit can no longer be managed by just one of the two systems—we desperately need both.

For there are two critically different populations involved, each of which is the primary responsibility of one of the systems. These two populations are the *constituency* and the *community*. The members of the constituency represent a progressively selected group, in part self-selected, and the selection is based on the presence of a medical problem, frequently one that is quite complex. Each member, in effect, has *voted* to obtain the services of a physician (or center or medical group) and has cast this vote as an individual without reference to others. The constituency is thus a collection of individuals who share in common only the fact that each has perceived a self-problem of illness or disease. It is the group known familiarly as the physician's "practice." The community, by contrast, is made up of people distinguished by the possession in common of some factor not directly related to disease. Usually, but not invariably, this common factor is a domicile located within some geographically defined boundary. In health terms, therefore, the community is a wholly unselected group, and at any one point in time many more of its members are well than are sick. The community and the constituency thus differ strikingly in the prevalence of significant illness and disease. Because of this difference, an institutional form appropriate to meet the needs of one group should be markedly different from the form appropriate for the other.

What the properly sifted members of the constituency need is an institution that can offer a complete array of talents appropriate for the solution of any currently soluble medical problem, no matter how rarely occurring or complicated it might be. What the community needs is recognition of weaknesses in pathogenic chains that may be exploited in the prevention of disease. For nonpreventable disease the community needs straightforward medical care close to home, safeguarded by continuous mechanisms for identifying those who need care in the first place and mechanisms for sifting the few who need complex care from the many who do not. The actual provision of the care is the responsibility of the clinical or personal physician system in either case. Community medicine (or the larger public health system of which it is a part) is thus responsible *not* for the delivery of personal health services to the members of a community, but for ensuring that the community receives proper health serv-

ices of all sorts. And prominent among these are the invention of better mechanisms than we have now for both the continuous community scan of who needs care at any moment and appropriate entry points for the care of those identified. Neither of these two systems is inherently of greater social value than the other, but in the course of developing the personal physician system to its present high point of technologic effectiveness for the individual, we have failed to mount a comparable effort for the nourishment of the other system responsible for the medical welfare of every member of the group. The speedy correction of this imbalance is the critical challenge facing medicine today, and how well we meet it will determine the role of the physician in society. For the imbalance of the two systems affects our efforts for the beneficial uses of science not only at the level of medical care for the community and the constituency, but in those even larger matters that have to do with how the developing individual can be aided in his or her continuous interaction with the environment.

It is not possible to do justice to all these issues in this Introduction or even in this book. Some are considered in the book, notably in the article titled Man In His Environment, by H. E. Lewis. For others, certain key references to the valuable literature that has been developing in recent years are set forth below. There remain a few, however, that are so vital to the conceptual base forming the theme of this article that they deserve special mention.

Moral judgments must be made by the physician engaged in individual patient care, but they are to be made on his own professional acts and those of his colleagues, not on the actions of those who have sought his care. Any moral judgments he might make on his patients' behavior are private matters to be kept within himself; he must not permit them to influence his own professional acts. This has long been the medical tradition, and it is important that it not be forgotten in the tumult of today's world of clashing value systems. The prospect of moral and ethical problems of an essentially new type is also now emerging before us. There is general awareness that advances in medical science are leading to various ethical conflicts that have to be faced by the clinical physician. What is less well recognized, however, is that this situation will become much more widespread and socially serious as advances in biology and medicine, now on the immediate horizon, become more generally applicable through the nonclinical system, whether it be called public health or community medicine. Critical phenomena in human development formerly thought to represent the hand of fate are now found to be, at least in part, environmentally determined, and hence manipulable—such matters as basic intelligence or perhaps the degree of educability. If we develop the power to significantly influence such critical matters—and scientifically we are getting closer to it every day—we may find ourselves faced with seeking to protect the "interests" of an unborn or newborn child to receive a particular intervention against the "rights" of its own parents to be free from outside interference. And this question of how to ensure the best opportunity for the individual without destroying family structure in the process will not be an ethical problem to be faced by medicine once in a while, but one that will involve whole societies. Yet we cannot run away from such questions, for it is the wise application of our science and technology, made with either form of compassion, that allows us to approach one of our major goals — that of ensuring that every child born into the world has the maximal chance to make his run through life's most productive years.

Finally, we must heed a concept of medicine that is ageless. In the life of an individual there ultimately may come a time when all the knowledge so carefully presented by the contributors to this book no longer has usefulness, yet life must go on, at least for a time. Whenever this happens, and it happens every day, it is up to each of us to follow to the fullest measure the charge laid down long ago for "the physician to become himself the treatment."

Crowe, B. L.: The tragedy of the Commons revisited. Science, 166:1103, 1969.

Ethical Aspects of Experimentation with Human Subjects. Daedalus, Spring 1969.

McDermott, W.: Demography, culture, and economics and the evolutionary stages of medicine. In Kilbourne, E. D., and Smillie, W. G. (eds.): Human Ecology and Public Health. 4th ed. New York, The Macmillan Company, 1969.

Morison, R. S.: Where is biology taking us? Science, 155:429, 1967.

The Changing Mores of Biomedical Research: A Colloquium on Ethical Dilemmas from Medical Advances. Forty-eighth Annual Session of the American College of Physicians, San Francisco, April 12, 1967. Ann. Intern. Med., Suppl. 7, Part II, September, 1967.

Tumulty, P. A.: What is a clinician and what does he do? New Eng. J. Med., 283:20, 1970.

Wolfle, D.: Dying with dignity. Science, 168:1403, 1970.

GENETIC PRINCIPLES

INTRODUCTION

Alexander G. Bearn

It is a convenient if misleading abstraction to consider that all diseases of man are due either to the action of environmental agents or to hereditary influences. This simplistic view has been nurtured by innumerable studies that purport to relegate a disease into one or the other category. It is more correct, however, as well as more rewarding, to consider that both environmental and hereditary influences play a role in the etiology of disease. In some conditions genetic influences are clearly decisive, whereas in others the disease appears to be independent of the genetic constitution of the patient. In the majority of diseases, both genetic and environmental factors play a detectably influential role. The science of human genetics is concerned primarily with the recognition of hereditary variations in man. Most of these variations are not harmful; indeed they are beneficial, for they confer on the species the capacity to adapt to an ever-changing environment. But when these variations are associated with clinical disease they come within the realm of the physician. Since medical genetics is an applied science, certain general genetic principles will be discussed before considering in detail the direct application of genetics to clinical medicine.

Following the establishment of the principle of genetic transmission by Gregor Mendel, Johansen, in 1909, introduced the word *gene* to denote a unit of heredity. A structural gene is now defined, operationally, as a functional unit of inheritance situated on a chromosome and responsible for the synthesis of a specific polypeptide. It has been estimated that there are probably no less than 100,000 genes in man. The chemical nature of a gene was unrecognized until 1944, when a soluble extract derived from pneumococci of one genotype was found to effect a stable heritable change when added to a growing culture of pneumococci of another genotype. The prompt definition of the transforming substance in the extract as deoxyribonucleic acid (DNA) launched the present era of molecular biology. The genetic information encoded in the DNA that determines polypeptide structure is transcribed through the synthesis of another macromolecule, ribonucleic acid (RNA). Part of this RNA is termed *messenger RNA* (m RNA), and the linear amino acid sequences in the polypeptide chain are precisely determined by the linear sequences of the coding units (*codons*) in the m RNA. These relationships are often referred to as the central dogma of molecular biology, and can be depicted schematically:

$$DNA \xrightarrow{\text{transcription}} RNA \xrightarrow{\text{translation}} \text{polypeptide.}$$

Deoxyribonucleic Acid. Deoxyribonucleic acid is constructed from three essential components:

the pentose sugar 2-deoxy-D-ribose, phosphoric acid, which confers on DNA its acidic properties, and nitrogenous bases. Two of the bases are purines, adenine (A) and guanine (G), and two are pyrimidines, thymine (T) and cytosine (C). In 1953 Watson and Crick assembled the available physical and chemical data on DNA into the present model for the structure of DNA. Two polynucleotide chains are twisted together to form a double helix. The two chains are held together by hydrogen bonds between the bases which face inward forming the core, and the phosphate-sugar groups form the backbone. The most important feature of the model is the physical-chemical requirement for specific base pairing. Adenine must always pair with thymine (A-T), and guanine with cytosine (G-C). The result of this pairing leads to a precise complementary relationship between the bases on the two chains. Thus, if part of the base sequence of one chain were TTGCC the corresponding portion of the complementary strand would read AACGG.

Replication of DNA. One of the chief attractions of the Watson-Crick model for DNA is a built-in system for self-replication. As the double helix unwinds, each strand acts as a template for the synthesis of a new strand catalyzed by the enzyme DNA polymerase. The replication has been termed *semiconservative* since one of each parental strand is conserved in the next generation when it will pair with its newly synthesized complementary partner.

Ribonucleic Acid. Ribonucleic acid differs from deoxyribonucleic acid in three important ways. (1) The sugar D-ribose replaces the 2-deoxyribose of DNA. (2) The pyrimidine base uracil replaces the thymine of DNA. (3) RNA is a single-stranded polymer in contrast to double-stranded DNA.

Messenger Ribonucleic Acid (m RNA). Messenger RNA is synthesized directly on the DNA template. Adenine pairs with uracil, guanine with cytosine, and single-stranded m RNA is formed. The transcription of one of the strands of DNA to form RNA is catalyzed by the enzyme RNA polymerase (transcriptase). Thus, single-stranded RNA carries into the cytoplasm the genetic information encoded in nuclear DNA in the form of a base sequence complementary to that of DNA. In bacteria, m RNA has a half-life of about two minutes, and it has been calculated that during this time 10 to 20 molecules of protein can be synthesized. In cells of higher organisms the messenger appears to be much more stable, and may remain functional for two to three days and synthesize several thousand molecules.

Ribosomal Structure. More than 80 per cent of the cellular RNA is found in small cytoplasmic particles, closely associated with the endoplasmic reticulum, called ribosomes. These ribosomal particles are the protein synthetic machinery of the cell. Mammalian ribosomes have a diameter of

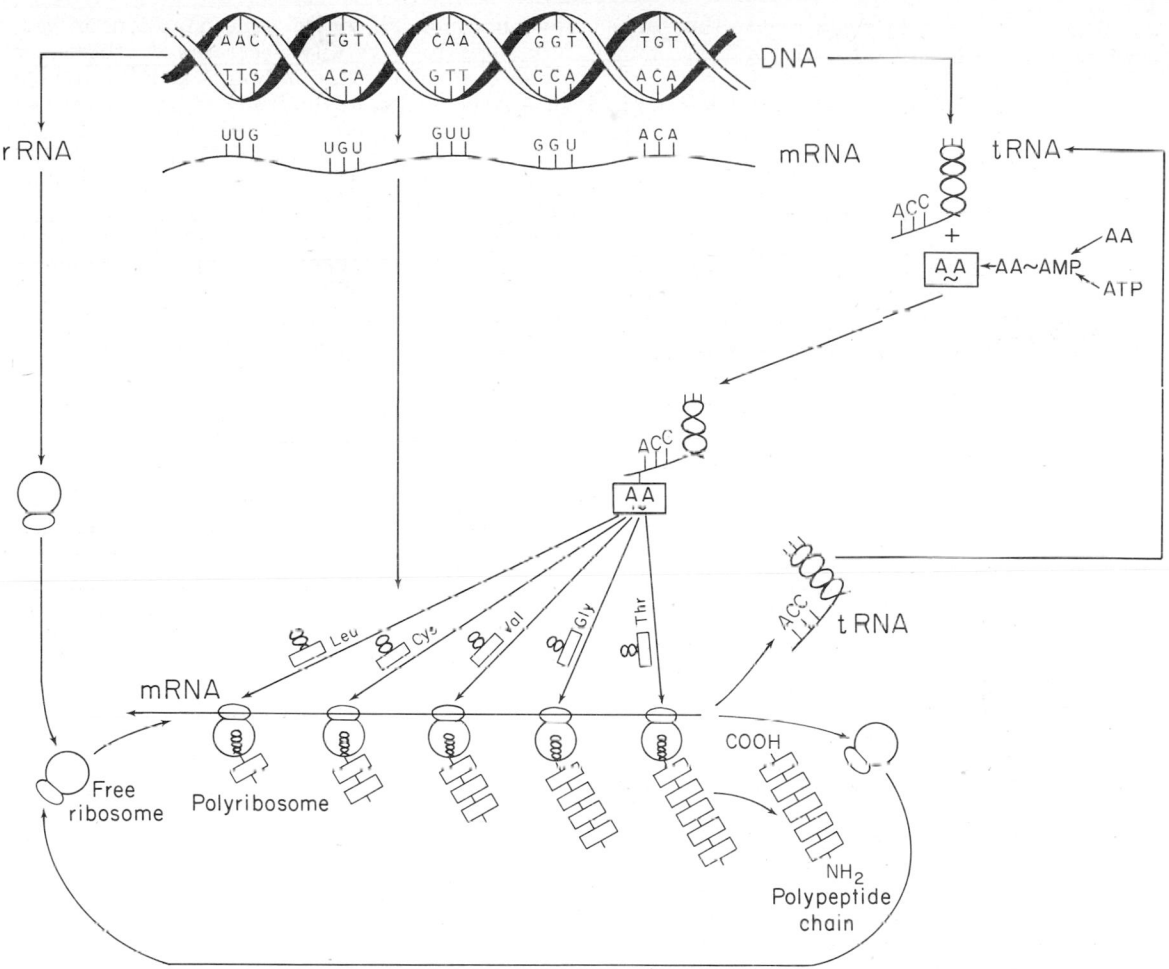

FIGURE 1. A schematic diagram of the genetic control of protein synthesis. A = adenine, T = thymine, G = guanine, C = cytidine, U = uracil. The codons indicated represent code words for the amino acids indicated. The messenger RNA (mRNA) moves across the ribosomes in the direction of the arrow. tRNA = Transfer RNA; rRNA = ribosomal RNA. (Details, see text.)

approximately 200 Å and a sedimentation coefficient of 80S, and dissociate into 60S and 40S subunits in low concentrations of magnesium. Messenger RNA bearing the instructions for protein synthesis attaches itself to the 80S ribosomal particles.

Protein Synthesis, Translation, and Transfer RNA. The first step in protein synthesis requires activation of the amino acids by the enzyme aminoacyl-t-RNA synthetase. This activation is initiated by the reaction of the carboxyl group of an amino acid with the phosphate group of adenylic acid to form amino-acyl-adenylate. Subsequent polymerization of the amino acids into polypeptides requires ribosomes, m RNA, and a number of enzymatic reactions. Mammalian cells contain more than 20 different transfer RNAs, and at least one transfer RNA is specific for each of the 20 amino acids. Each transfer RNA molecule has two recognition sites. One site binds the amino-acyl-t-RNA to the ribosome-m RNA complex, and the second site recognizes the m RNA codon. The fidelity of translation is assured by specific binding of the amino acid with the t-RNA catalyzed

by the specific activating enzyme and by complementary pairing of the anticodon of t-RNA with the codon in the m RNA. Thus, the synthesis of the final polypeptide chain can be summarized in the following steps. As soon as m RNA becomes bound to the ribosomes, translation is initiated. In bacteria the initiation of translation is effected by the codon AUG, which binds a specific t RNA, formylmethionyl-t-RNA, to the ribosome complex. The second codon then recognizes its specific t-RNA, and the second amino acid in sequence is brought into alignment. A peptide bond is formed between the two amino acids, and the ribosome moves along the m RNA so that the third codon, recognizing its t-RNA, brings the third amino acid into position with further elongation of the peptide chain. The information that a polypeptide chain is completed and that its synthesis must be terminated is specified by a special chain-terminating codon.

Codons. Because most proteins normally contain 20 different amino acids and DNA has only four different nucleotide bases, it is evident that more than one base is required to prescribe for a particular amino acid. It is now known that three bases (a codon) are needed to code for each amino acid, and that the code is nonoverlapping. Thus, a gene with 1500 nucleotide pairs would determine the sequence of a polypeptide chain consisting of 500 amino acids. Since the four-letter code is triplet in nature, there would be 64 $(4 \times 4 \times 4)$ possible codons, of which 61 have been shown to code for one of the 20 amino acids. Three codons (chain-terminating codons) represent signals that the polypeptide chain is completed, and two codons (chain-initiating codons) are signals for the initiation of polypeptide synthesis as well as for the insertion of amino acids. The genetic code is said to be *universal* in the sense that all plant and animal species probably use the same genetic code, and *degenerate* because certain amino acids can be specified by more than one triplet.

Certain acridine-induced mutants in bacteriophage insert an extra nucleotide base into the code, and the reading frame becomes altered distal to the point of insertion of the new base leading to a disruption of normal protein synthesis. The correct reading frame of the code can be restored by a deletion of another base distal to the insertion. This model makes the prediction that a double mutant, consisting of an insertion followed by a deletion, will result in a polypeptide chain with an altered amino acid sequence between the two mutations. If the segment of DNA between the two mutations is short, and does not code for amino acids vital for functional specificity, a protein with normal or nearly normal function may be produced.

Structural and Control Genes. The most extensive understanding of genetic regulatory mechanisms stemmed from the investigations of Jacob, Monod, and their collaborators on the β-galactosidase enzyme system in *Escherichia coli*. These studies have led to the formulation of new concepts of regulation in bacteria according to which a hierarchy of *control genes* and *structural genes* has been established. Thus, whereas certain genes (structural genes) are responsible for the actual synthesis of specific protein and enzymes, and contain the DNA code which specifies their amino acid sequences, other genes (control genes) are responsible for the regulation of their production.

A dramatic example of a structural gene mutation in man was most clearly demonstrated when Ingram reported in 1956 that sickle-cell hemoglobin differed from normal hemoglobin in a single amino acid substitution. During the subsequent 15 years a considerable number of structural mutants have been identified in man, and in many instances the precise amino acid substitution disclosed. The question of whether there are mutations in man which affect the synthesis of a protein such that a small amount of the normal structural protein is formed is less easy to document. Although many of the hereditary diseases studied by Garrod are characterized by the synthesis of a decreased quantity of an enzyme of apparently normal structure, rigorous structural studies have not been performed. Moreover, although almost all control gene mutations in bacteria lead to a greatly decreased synthesis, or absence, of a particular protein, it is quite possible for a structural gene mutation to have so altered the code that no protein is synthesized, or that the protein synthesized has become immunologically, enzymatically, and chemically unrecognizable. Thus, although the distribution between control gene mutations and structural mutation can be resolved in micro-organisms by tracing the mutation to a locus within or outside the structural gene, techniques for a similar analysis in man are not yet available. It can be assumed that in man the regulation of gene function is far more complex than in bacteria, and the application of the Jacob-Monod model is undoubtedly a misleading oversimplification. It seems likely that in certain inherited diseases the primary biochemical abnormality resides in a decreased or defective synthesis of messenger RNA, or may be due to ambiguities in the reading of the messenger on the ribosome. The primary abnormality in thalassemia has been ascribed to defective synthesis of m RNA. A disturbance in the regulatory mechanism of the level of translation cannot be excluded (see Hematologic and Hematopoietic Diseases).

ANALYSIS OF HUMAN PEDIGREES
Alexander G. Bearn

Inspection and analysis of human pedigrees form the basis for an understanding of the application of the laws of Mendel to human disease. Analysis of a pedigree begins with the affected individual, who is referred to as the propositus or proband. Using the propositus as the point of departure, a pedigree is constructed, and the pattern of the pedigree is analyzed. It is worth emphasizing, however, that the construction of human pedigrees beyond first and second degree relatives is an occupation more likely to please the physician than illuminate a genetic understanding of the patient's disease. Human memories are notoriously untrustworthy, and when very large pedigrees are recorded and reproduced, the only secure statement that usually can be made is that they are probably incorrect.

Autosomal Inheritance. When there are two alleles A and a, at a locus, three possible genotypes exist, which can be represented AA, Aa, and aa. The genotypes AA and aa are called *homozygotes*; Aa is a *heterozygote*. A gene can be recognized only by the effect it produces; thus in the strictest sense it is incorrect to speak of dominant or recessive genes. If the phenotype Aa cannot be easily distinguished from the phenotype AA, but is clearly different from aa, the effect of gene A is said to be dominant over the effect of gene a. In this circumstance there are only two phenotypes corresponding to the three genotypes AA, Aa, aa. However, the failure to detect a phenotypic difference between the genotypes AA and Aa is usually testimony to the insensitivity of the methods employed.

If the gene product of A and a can both be detected in the heterozygote Aa, the genes are said to exert an effect which is co-dominant. In many ways it would be preferable to discard the terms "dominant" and "recessive" and instead to state whether the genes concerned are expressed in a single or double dose; for the sake of conveneince, however, the terms are often retained.

Autosomal Dominant Traits. Autosomal genes are those genes situated on chromosomes other than the X and Y. Dominant traits are defined as those traits that are fully manifested by the presence of a gene in the heterozygous state. Thus far, approximately 350 well established autosomal dominant traits have been identified in man. Satisfactory examples of dominant traits are those responsible for the formation of certain blood group antigens. In the ABO system, the genes controlling the formation of A and B substances are dominant over O. Thus, it is not ordinarily possible to distinguish serologically AA from AO individuals, or BB from BO individuals. However, heterozygous individuals of type AB can be recognized because the product of genes A and B can be detected. The autosomal dominant trait can be recognized in human pedigrees by its transmission from one generation to the next. Except for mutation, and if illegitimacy can be excluded, every affected individual has at least one affected parent and may have affected offspring (Fig. 2). According to mendelian laws, a heterozygous affected individual married to a normal homozygote will, on the average, transmit the trait to half his offspring, both sexes being equally affected. Considerable variation in the expression of a dominant trait is common; in some instances the expression may be so weak that a generation apparently can be skipped because the carrier of the abnormal gene is clinically normal. Ectrodactyly (lobster claw deformity), chondrodystrophy, neurofibromatosis, and Huntington's chorea are examples of dominant traits of clinical significance. Many dominant traits in man frequently exert only mild effects. When a gene that can be clinically expressed in the heterozygous condition occurs in the homozygous state, the effect is usually more

severe and may be lethal. Examples, although common in species in which experimental matings can be constructed, are exceptional in man since marriage of two affected heterozygotes is rare.

Autosomal Recessive Traits. In an autosomal recessive trait, the father and the mother of the affected individual are usually normal, as are more distant ancestors. On the average, one fourth of the brothers and sisters (sibs) of the affected individual will be affected. If the trait is rare, an increased consanguinity will be observed among the parents of those affected. According to mendelian laws, the offspring of two normal parents, both heterozygous for a recessive trait, will be, on the average, one quarter homozygous for the normal allele, one quarter homozygous for the abnormal allele and thus affected, and one half heterozygous for the abnormal allele, like the parents. Affected individuals usually have phenotypically normal offspring who are necessarily all carriers of the abnormal gene. If an affected individual marries an individual heterozygous for the same gene, one half of the offspring will be affected and one half will be heterozygous carriers (Fig. 3). Approximately 300 well established recessive traits have been identified in man.

Certain aspects of these proportions must be emphasized. Because of the small size of families and because ascertainment of the family is usually through an affected member, the mean observed proportion of affected individuals will be greater than expected. Only when the size of the sibships is large will the expected ratio of one affected to three unaffected be realized in pooled data. Thus, the analysis of the expected ratio in families of various sizes requires a correction factor whose magnitude depends on the number of children in the sibship. The simplest correction is to subtract in each family the index case (propositus) from the total number of affected individuals and then determine the proportion of affected children among the remaining sibs. The disadvantage of the term "recessive" is emphasized by the increasing number of instances in which refined biochemical observations enable the recognition of the trait in the clinically normal heterozygote. Indeed, because of its importance in genetic counseling, the detection of healthy heterozygous carriers of genes that in the homozygous condition cause severe disease is becoming one of the most significants aspects of medical genetics.

Autosomal Dominant

Autosomal Dominant (mutation)

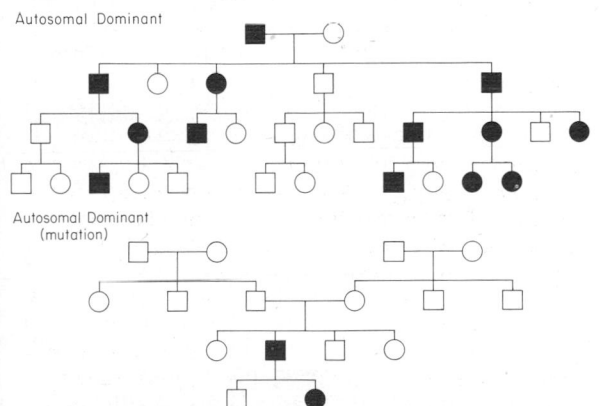

FIGURE 2. Pedigrees of autosomal dominant traits. In the lower pedigree the normal parents of the affected individual suggest the possibility of a new mutation.

Autosomal Recessive

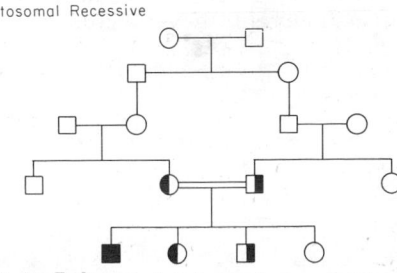

FIGURE 3. Pedigree of autosomal recessive trait. Note: Both parents are heterozygous. One sib is affected, two are carriers, and one is normal. Double line (═══) indicates that parents are related by descent.

X-Linked Inheritance. *Dominant X-Linked Traits.* This mode of inheritance is uncommon. Heterozygous affected females will transmit the trait to both sexes with a frequency of 50 per cent. Affected males will transmit the trait to all their daughters, but to none of their sons (Fig. 4). This rule of X-linked dominant inheritance enables critical distinction from traits inherited in an autosomal dominant fashion, in which an affected male transmits the trait to both sons and daughters. If the trait is uncommon, the incidence in females is approximately twice that in males. The erythrocyte antigen Xg^a, the serum α_2 macroglobulin antigen Xm, and vitamin D-resistant rickets (hypophosphatemic rickets) are inherited as X-linked dominant traits. A total of 70 loci have been identified on the human X chromosome.

Recessive X-Linked Traits. Recessive X-linked traits are relatively common. On the average, half the sons of normal heterozygous females will be normal, and half will be affected. If the trait is rare, parents and relatives will be normal except for male relatives in the female line; for instance, on the average, one half of the maternal uncles will be affected. An affected male married to a normal female will have normal offspring. All their daughters will be carriers and they, in turn, can transmit the trait to the next generation. The rare event of an affected male married to a carrier female will result in equal proportions of affected male and female offspring. The unaffected males will be also genotypically normal; the unaffected females, however, will be heterozygous carriers (Fig. 5). The common red-green color blindness is inherited as an X-linked recessive trait; other, less common traits include hemophilia, pseudohypertrophic muscular dystrophy, congenital agammaglobulinemia (Bruton), and the Aldrich syndrome. In the general population the frequency of affected females will be roughly the square of the frequency of affected males.

Y-Linked Inheritance. If a trait is determined by a gene in the Y chromosome, it will be transmitted through the father to all his sons and none of his daughters. Thus far, the only genes that have been shown to be located in the Y chromosome are those that determine "maleness" and those responsible for the clinically trivial trait of hairy ears. (See also XYY Syndrome, Gonads.)

Sex-Limitation. Autosomal genes that are expressed only in males may mimic sex-linkage but can be formally distinguished if affected individuals reproduce. If the gene is on an autosome,

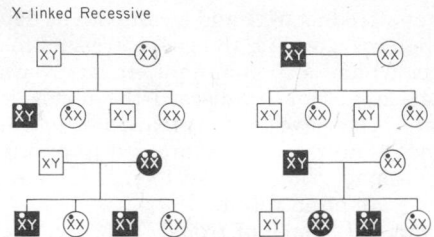

FIGURE 5. Pedigrees of recessive X-linked trait. The X chromosome, being the abnormal gene, is designated by a small circle.

affected males can transmit the trait to their sons; if the gene is on the X chromosome, they cannot.

Modification of Gene Expression. The manifestation of an abnormal gene is influenced not only by its normal allele, but also by alleles at other loci, and no doubt by environment. The terms expressivity and penetrance have been employed to describe the variable manifestation of a gene. These vague words are usually best avoided. Some genetically determined traits such as those determining the blood antigens are present at birth, whereas others such as Huntington's chorea appear only in adult life. A negative correlation between the age of onset of a trait in parents and sibs suggests that the expression of the gene may be influenced by the type of normal allele present. The effect can be seen in certain dominant diseases such as the nail-patella syndrome and in the dominant form of muscular dystrophy. The phenomenon of anticipation—that hereditary diseases tend to have progressively earlier age of onset with successive generations—is a statistical artifact.

Consanguinity. It should be standard procedure in taking a family history to inquire whether there is parental consanguinity. Rare autosomally inherited recessive diseases are found much more frequently among the offspring of cousin marriages than among those whose parents are not related by descent. In all autosomal recessive disorders the affected individual has inherited one abnormal gene from each parent. It is thus evident that an individual will be more likely to inherit the same allele from each parent if the two parents have genes inherited from a common ancestor. First cousins have, on the average, one eighth of their genes derived from a common ancestor. When two first cousins marry, their offspring will have, on the average, one sixteenth of their genes derived from the common ancestor. It is frequently of interest to calculate the expected frequency of first-cousin marriages among parents of a patient with a rare autosomal recessive disorder. Providing that the frequency of the disease in the population can be estimated, and if the frequency of first-cousin marriages in the general population is known, the calculation can be made according to the following formula. If k is the frequency of first-cousin marriages in a rare recessive disease, then as a first approximation $k = \dfrac{c}{16q}$, where c is the frequency of first-cousin marriages in the general population (usually

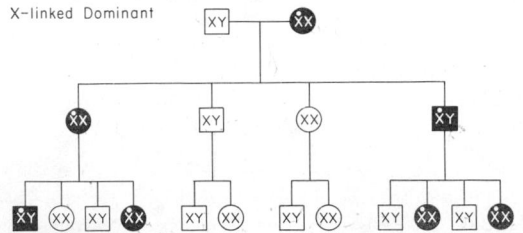

FIGURE 4. Pedigree of dominant X-linked trait. The X chromosome, being the abnormal gene, is designated by a small circle.

about 0.5 per cent) and q is the frequency of the abnormal gene. Let us suppose a recessively inherited disease has a frequency in the population of 1 in 10,000 (q^2); then the frequency of the gene which in double dose causes the disease is 1 in 100 (q). If the frequency of consanguinity in the general population is 0.5 per cent, then k, the frequency of cousin marriages, in the parents is 3 per cent, a sixfold increase over normal. If the disease is much rarer, 1 in 100,000, then 10 per cent of the individuals affected by the disease will have parents who are first cousins. As the frequency of c increases, the expected frequency of parents who are first cousins will also increase. In some geographically isolated populations c may reach 2 per cent. If a recessively inherited disease in such an isolate has a frequency of 1 in 100,000, 40.0 per cent of the parents of the affected individuals will be first cousins. It is important to realize that an increased frequency of consanguinity in the parent is usually not observable if the recessive disease is common. Thus, in cystic fibrosis of the pancreas, which has a frequency of approximately 1 in 2500, no increase in parental consanguinity can be detected. Although the frequency of albinism in the general population is approximately 1 per 20,000, the unexpectedly high consanguinity in the parents (k = 20 per cent) is due to the existence of more than one gene for this condition. No increase in consanguinity would be expected as a correlate of the expression of dominant or X-linked traits.

Association. The occurrence of two traits in the same person more often than would be expected by chance is called association. A consistent positive association between blood group A and carcinoma of the stomach, and between duodenal ulceration and blood group O, has long been recognized. Such an association may be due to many causes, and does not indicate that the genes controlling blood group antigens are on the same chromosome as those associated with the development of duodenal ulceration. If an association is found between two characters in the general population, it is important to determine whether the association persists when the two characters are examined in sibships. If geographic or social stratification is the cause of the association, the correlation will disappear. If, for example, a mixed population of Africans and Europeans is examined, a positive association between cDe Rhesus blood group (common in Negroes) and dark skin color would be found. This association would disappear if individual sibships were examined.

Sometimes two characters are associated because they are due to the action of a single gene. Thus clouding of the cornea and mental retardation are two traits that are associated in Hurler's syndrome. The two traits are not caused by two genes, but are due to a single gene with a so-called pleiotropic effect. When a gene causes a pleiotropic effect the association found in the general population persists when sibships are examined. Pleiotropic effects of genes are common,

and may be of clinical importance. Familial intestinal polyposis is an early consequence of the effect of a gene that later commonly leads to carcinoma of the colon.

Autosomal Linkage. The site of a gene on a chromosome is termed a *locus*. Alternate forms of genes which occupy corresponding sites on homologous chromosomes are called alleles. Applied to human genetics, Mendel's law of independent assortment states that traits controlled by two or more pairs of allelic alternatives will be transmitted to the children of the next generation, either together or separately, by chance alone. The law holds only for genes situated on different chromosomes or at widely separated loci on the same chromosome. However, if two genes occupy closely adjacent sites on the same chromosome, they tend to segregate together and are said to be linked. The occasional segregation of linked genes is due to crossing over at meiosis. The frequency of crossing over gives an estimate of closeness of the linkage. It is important to remember that even if two genes are present on the same chromosomes, they will appear unlinked if they are so far apart that free (50 per cent) recombination between the two loci can take place.

Linkage of two genes, that is, close enough proximity of their loci on the chromosome that crossing over between the two loci is insufficient to lead to independent segregation, does not cause association of the two characters in the general population. In any one sibship the two characters may be associated, in which case the genes are on the same chromosome and are said to be in coupling, or they may be dissociated; that is, they are distributed on each of the two homologous chromosomes, in which case they are described as being in repulsion. A common error is to suppose that the association of two characters in a single sibship implies genetic linkage. If true linkage exists and enough pedigrees are collected, an equal number of sibships will be found in which the two characters are not associated. There are several known instances of autosomal linkage in man including the ABO blood group locus and the locus for the nail-patella syndrome; the Rh blood groups and one form of elliptocytosis; and Lutheran blood group and the Secretor locus (which determines whether soluble ABO substances are present in saliva and other body fluids). The loci determining the β and δ chains of hemoglobin are also very closely linked (see Diseases of Blood). The mathematical procedures devised to detect linkage are complicated, and lie outside the scope of this article.

Linkage has one important practical consequence for clinical medicine. If a mutant causing a serious inherited disease is closely linked to one causing a common trait, healthy carriers of the disease may be detected in unaffected members of the family by the presence or absence of the common trait. It would, of course, be important to know whether the two linked genes in the family under investigation were in the coupling or repulsion phase. Accurate information regarding the phase often can be obtained from studies of the distribution of the two traits in three generations.

INBORN ERRORS OF METABOLISM AND MOLECULAR DISEASE

Alexander G. Bearn

Development of the concept of an inborn error of metabolism by Archibald Garrod in the first decade of this century was one of the most brilliant insights in the history of genetics, for it introduced the hypothesis that the primary action of a gene is to control the synthesis of a specific enzyme. Subsequent work has fully confirmed Garrod's original tenet that an inherited metabolic block is usually ascribable to an inability to carry out a particular reaction because of a deficiency of a

specific enzyme. More recently the term has been extended to include hereditary alterations in proteins that have no enzymatic functions.

The development of precise chemical methods that enable a comparison to be made between normal and genetically altered proteins led to the introduction of the term *molecular disease*, to emphasize that the difference between a normal and an affected individual might reside in the substitution of a single amino acid residue in the primary sequence of a protein molecule. Although the metabolic block may affect protein, carbohydrate, lipid, nucleic acid, porphyrin, or pigment metabolism, the *primary* abnormality invariably lies in the genetic specification of the synthesis of a protein.

Some of the clinical conditions for which a demonstrated abnormality in a specific protein has been observed are listed in Table 1. In most of these a deficiency in a specific enzymatic activity is demonstrable, whereas in others a normal amount of a structurally abnormal protein is synthesized. The classic example of a "molecular

TABLE 1. INBORN ERRORS OF METABOLISM

Condition	Deficiency
Carbohydrate metabolism:	
Hepatorenal glycogenosis	Glucose-6-phosphatase
Hepatic glycogenosis	Liver phosphorylase
Muscle glycogenosis	Muscle phosphorylase
Cardiac glycogenosis	α-glucosidase
Limit dextrinosis	Amylo-1,6-glucosidase
Amylopectinosis	Amylo-$(1,4 \rightarrow 1,6)$ transglucosidase
Pentosuria	L-xylulose reductase
Essential fructosuria	Fructokinase
Fructose intolerance	Fructose 1-phosphate aldolase
Galactosemia	Galactose-1-phosphate uridyl transferase
Juvenile cataracts	Galactokinase
L-glyceric aciduria	D-glyceric dehydrogenase
Amino acid metabolism:	
Familial goitrous cretinism (deiodinase defect)	Deiodinase
Phenylketonuria	Phenylalanine hydroxylase
Albinism	Tyrosinase
Tyrosinemia	p-Hydroxyphenylpyruvic acid oxidase
Tyrosinosis	Tyrosine transaminase
Alcaptonuria	Homogentisic acid oxidase
Maple syrup urine disease	Branched chain keto-acid decarboxylase
Hartnup disease	Tryptophane pyrrolase
Histidinemia	Histidinase
Hyperprolinemia, Type I	Proline oxidase
Type II	Δ'-pyrroline-5-carboxylic acid dehydrogenase
Hydroxyprolinemia	Hydroxyproline oxidase
Citrullinuria	Argininosuccinic acid synthetase
Argininosuccinic aciduria	Argininosuccinase
Hyperammonemia	Ornithine transcarbamylase
Cystathioninuria	Cystathionase
Homocystinuria	Cystathionine synthetase
Isovaleric acidemia	Isovaleric acid CoA dehydrogenase
Hypervalinemia	Valine transaminase
Lipid metabolism:	
Type I hyperlipoproteinemia (primary hyperchylomicronemia)	Lipoprotein lipase
Gaucher's disease	Glucocerebroside-cleaving enzyme
Niemann-Pick disease	Sphingomyelin-cleaving enzyme
Tay-Sachs disease	β-D-N-acetylhexosaminidase
Fabry's disease	Ceramide trihexosidase
Refsum's disease	Phytanic acid hydroxylating enzyme
Generalized gangliosidosis	β galactosidase
Congenital adrenocortical hyperplasia	21-hydroxylase
	11β-hydroxylase
	3β-hydroxysteroid dehydrogenase
Metachromatic leukodystrophy	Arylsulfatase A

TABLE 1. INBORN ERRORS OF METABOLISM (*Continued*)

Condition	Deficiency
Purine or pyrimidine metabolism:	
Xanthinuria	Xanthine oxidase
Lesch-Nyhan syndrome	Hypoxanthine-guanine ribosyl transferase
Hyperoxaluria	2-oxoglutarate gyloxalate carboligase
Orotic aciduria	Orotidylic acid pyrophosphorylase and decarboxylase
Porphyrin and heme pigment metabolism:	
Acute intermittent porphyria	Increase of γ-aminolevulinic acid synthetase
Familial nonhemolytic jaundice (Crigler-Najjar)	Glucuronyl transferase
Erythrocyte protein:	
Congenital methemoglobinemia	Diphosphopyridine nucleotide diaphorase
Favism; drug-induced hemolytic anemia	Glucose 6 phosphate dehydrogenase
Congenital nonspherocytic anemia A	Pyruvate kinase
B	2,3-diphosphoglycerate mutase
Acatalasia	Catalase
Hereditary hemolytic anemia (congenital nonspherocytic hemolytic anemia)	Glutathione peroxidase
	Glutathione reductase
	Glutathione synthetase
	6-phosphogluconate dehydrogenase
	Triose phosphate isomerase
	Hexokinase
	Glucose phosphate isomerase
	Phosphoglycerate kinase
	Adenosine triphosphatase
Sulfur metabolism:	
Neurological disease and cataracts	Sulfite oxidase
Plasma proteins:	
Analphalipoproteinemia (Tangier disease)	α-lipoprotein (high density)
α_1 Antitrypsin deficiency	α_1 Antitrypsin
Abetaliproteinemia (acanthocytosis)	β-lipoprotein (low density)
Agammaglobulinemia	γ-globulin
Afibrinogenemia	Fibrinogen
Wilson's disease (hepatolenticular degeneration)	Ceruloplasmin
Hereditary angioneurotic edema	Inhibitor of C' 1 esterase
Hypophosphatasia	Alkaline phosphatase
Clotting mechanisms:	
Hemophilia A	Antihemophilic globulin
Hemophilia B	Plasma thromboplastin component
Plasma thromboplastin deficiency	Plasma thromboplastin antecedent
Absence of other specific clotting factors	Prothrombin, Hageman factor, Stuart-Prower factor, factor V, von Willebrand's factor

disease" is sickle-cell anemia, in which the only difference between normal and sickle-cell hemoglobin is the substitution of a valine for a glutamic acid in the β chain of hemoglobin.

Although many of the inborn variations in metabolism are unassociated with clinical disease, they represent conspicuous examples of the importance of human biochemical diversity. In some instances they provide a critical genetic background for the expression of an environmentally controlled disorder; in others the physiologic effect of the genetic variation is not apparent.

The concept of *balanced polymorphism* has been defined as the existence of two or more discontinuous forms of a species in such proportion that the rarest of them cannot be maintained at its frequency in the population by recurrent mutation. As a general proposition, if the rarer of the two allelic forms occurs in a frequency that is greater than 1 per cent, the existence of balanced polymorphism should be entertained. It is postulated that the high frequency of the gene for sickle-cell hemoglobin is maintained in certain populations because, under conditions in which falciparum malaria is endemic, the heterozygote is more biologically fit than either homozygote. With the exception of malaria, the forces required to maintain most of the balanced polymorphisms are unknown, and, in recent years, the possibility that many of the inherited biochemical polymorphisms are essentially neutral has been raised.

Genetic Heterogeneity. It is becoming increasingly recognized that an identical or closely deviant phenotype may be due to different mutant genes. Thus, there are at least two forms of recessive albinism which are clinically similar. Proof that these two clinical syndromes are caused by two different genes stems from the observation that two albinos may marry and produce normally pigmented offspring. It is safe to assume that many genetic diseases presently regarded as homo-

TABLE 2. A SELECTION OF COMMON INHERITED BIOCHEMICAL POLYMORPHISMS

Blood groups, e.g., ABO, MNS, Rh
Erythrocyte enzymes
Leukocyte groups
Platelet groups
Glucose 6-PO_4 dehydrogenase
Serum proteins
Haptoglobin
Pseudocholinesterase
α_2 macroglobulin (Xm)
β lipoproteins (Ag, Lp)
Ceruloplasmin
Transferrin
Gamma globulin (Gm and Inv)
β Aminoisobutyric aciduria
Phenylthiocarbamide tasting
Color blindness

geneous entities represent the clinical effects of different mutant (allelic or nonallelic) genes.

Now that it is firmly established that genes control the specificity of particular proteins, genetic heterogeneity can also be detected using techniques to discriminate between closely similar protein molecules. The application of electrophoretic techniques to serum protein and red cell enzymes has disclosed a surprising degree of normal heterogeneity. Any estimate of genetic heterogeneity based on the application of electrophoretic techniques will be too low since it seems probable that only half the mutational events leading to amino acid substitutions result in an altered net charge of the protein.

Screening for Inborn Errors of Metabolism. The primary purpose of any screening program is the detection of individuals in whom it is likely that a specific hereditary disease will develop against which preventive or therapeutic measures are available. Screening for genetic diseases can be performed at three principal phenotypic levels. In many instances the early recognition of clinical disease represents the only phenotypic level at which the inborn error can be presently recognized. Thus, in Huntington's chorea no biochemical abnormality has been found to be characteristic of the disease, and early recognition of signs and symptoms represents the only means to arrive at a diagnosis. Early recognition of polyposis of the colon, however, is important because of the frequency of malignant transformation. The recognition of genital abnormalities at birth in females may aid in early detection of the adrenogenital syndrome. Inborn errors can also be recognized by the presence of an abnormal metabolite in physiologic fluids. The enzymatic deficiency may lead to an accumulation of the substrate for the reaction catalyzed by the normal enzyme and to a deficiency of the product. An increased level of blood galactose in galactosemia and of phenylalanine in phenylketonuria are examples in which the disturbance of the normal metabolic relationships leads to detection of disease.

Since genes control the synthesis of proteins, the most direct way of identifying an inborn error is to utilize a screening program which detects a qualitative change in the structure of the protein, e.g., electrophoretically, or by its altered enzymatic or immunologic activity. Mass screening for inborn errors of metabolism in the general population would be expensive and time-consuming, and a careful estimate of the cost of such a program must be balanced against the potential gains. Long-term social and biologic consequences of screening programs have not been considered in any detail. For the moment it seems wise to limit screening to pilot studies and to focus sharply on those individuals in families and in populations who are particularly at risk and for which effective therapy for the inborn error investigated is available. The recently demonstrated usefulness of amniocentesis to identify certain inborn errors of metabolism before birth can be expected to increase sharply in the years ahead.

POLYGENIC AND MULTIFACTORIAL INHERITANCE
Alexander G. Bearn

Traits determined by the collaborating action of many genes at different loci are called polygenic in contrast to those traits which are determined by a single gene (monogenic). Most of the differences among normal people are determined by the interaction of many genetic and environmental factors (multifactorial inheritance).

Polygenic inheritance, in which many genes contribute a minor effect, is best established for those traits which show continuous variation in the form of a "normal" distribution curve. Height is an example of a polygenic (and multifactorial) trait in which the extremes of the normal distribution are not considered abnormal. The degree of resemblance among relatives can be deduced from the number of genes they share in common. Thus, monozygotic twins have 100 per cent of their genes in common. Dizygotic twins, however, will have 50 per cent of their genes in common as will all sibs. Parents and children also have 50 per cent of their genes in common. Thus it would be expected that if one parent was 6'0" and the other 5'6" all the children, on the average, would be 5'8". Polygenic models have been advanced for inheritance of high blood pressure, diabetes mellitus, and rheumatoid arthritis, as well as a variety of congenital defects.

PHARMACOGENETICS
Alexander G. Bearn

It has long been recognized that certain people react unusually to the administration of drugs. In some instances the altered reaction has an immunologic basis; in others it appears to be idiosyncratic without any obvious cause; and in some the difference appears to be contingent on genetic variations of the host. Pharmacogenetics is concerned with those deviant responses to specific drugs that are genetically determined. The breakdown and disposal of drugs in the body are usually dependent on a series of specific gene-controlled enzymatic reactions. Mutant genes in the population that alter these reactions by mutation can result in serious clinical consequences.

Inherited Diseases Discovered or Precipitated by the Use of Drugs. A number of diseases have been disclosed or precipitated as a direct result of the development of drugs which for their proper metabolic disposal require an intact enzyme system. In the absence of the additional pharmacologic overload, the defective enzyme system does not cause disease.

Glucose-6-Phosphate Dehydrogenase Deficiency. A severe hemolytic anemia may be produced by the ingestion of the broad bean *Vicia fava*. The anemia is due to deficiency of the X-linked enzyme glucose-6-phosphate dehydrogenase in the erythrocytes of susceptible subjects (favism). It is of interest that a deficiency of the enzyme is a necessary but not sufficient cause for the anemia following ingestion of fava beans. Additional genetic factors, presently poorly identified, are also required if the disease is to be manifest. Neonatal jaundice in the Mediterranean basin and Far East may also be associated with glucose-6-phosphate dehydrogenase deficiency.

Persons with glucose-6-phosphate dehydrogenase deficiency are particularly susceptible to hemolytic reactions following administration of the antimalarial drug primaquine and of certain other drugs, including phenacetin. In general, the Mediterranean glucose-6-phosphate dehydrogenase deficiency individuals are sensitive to a wider range of drugs than their Negro counterparts. Interestingly, a severe hemolytic anemia may occur during the course of acute viral hepatitis in individuals with glucose-6-phosphate dehydrogenase deficiency. The trait is present in about 10 per cent of U. S. Negroes and may reach as high as 35 per cent in certain African and Mediterranean populations. Possession of the deficiency trait provides some protection against falciparum malaria and accounts for the persistence of the gene at a very high level in these populations. The relationship of glucose-6-phosphate dehydrogenase deficiency and susceptibility to falciparum malaria affords one of the better examples of a balanced polymorphism.

Isoniazid. The administration of a standard dose of isoniazid to a group of normal subjects disclosed that they could be divided into two subpopulations on the basis of the blood levels of isoniazid attained after a fixed time interval. Those with high levels have been designated "slow inactivators," and those with low levels "rapid inactivators." The basis for the difference lies in the possession by the "rapid inactivator" group of an isoniazid-acetylating enzyme that is absent in the "slow inactivators." Genetic studies indicate that the gene for "slow inactivation" has a low frequency in Eskimos and Japanese populations (10 per cent), but is quite common in Negro and Caucasian populations (60 per cent). The relatively common toxic polyneuropathy associated with isoniazid occurs only in "slow inactivators." The clinical response of patients with tuberculosis to this drug is independent of the patient's genotype. The rate of metabolism of sulfamethazine also depends on the amount of acetylating enzyme.

Suxamethonium (Succinylcholine). Prolonged, occasionally fatal apnea may follow the use of the muscle relaxant suxamethonium in persons who are homozygous for a gene controlling pseudocholinesterase levels. This increased sensitivity, which occurs in about 1 in 3000 patients, can be caused by a number of different allelic genes which influence the activity of pseudocholinesterase.

Hemoglobin Zürich. This abnormal hemoglobin was recognized because two members of a Swiss family developed severe hemolytic reactions following sulfonamide administration.

The cause of the shortened erythrocyte life span in persons with this abnormal hemoglobin is not fully understood.

Anticoagulant Resistance. A family in which some members are extremely resistant to warfarin and other anticoagulants has been reported. Approximately ten times the usual dose of warfarin was needed to increase the prothrombin time to the expected level. This represents an example in which resistance to a drug is genetically determined. The frequency of the trait is unknown.

Glaucoma. The rise in intraocular pressure which follows the instillation of glucocorticoids (Betamethasone alcohol, 0.1 per cent) into the conjunctival sac is under the control of a pair of allelic genes. It seems likely that those genetically susceptible homozygous individuals who respond to the instillation of glucocorticoids with an unusually brisk increase in intraocular pressure are particularly liable to develop glaucoma in later life.

Porphyria. The well known sensitivity of individuals with porphyria to barbiturates, particularly the short-acting barbituate thiopental (thiopentone), is a classic example of a genetically determined altered response to a drug.

POPULATION GENETICS

Alexander G. Bearn

Gene Frequency. Although genes are expressed in individuals, it is often of interest to consider the distribution of mutant genes in the general population. The basis of population genetics is the Hardy-Weinberg law, which was formulated in a context of concern that a dominant trait would eventually displace a normal trait in the population. In particular, it arose in response to the fallacious assertion that if brachydactyly is a dominant trait then, "in the course of time, one would expect in the absence of counteracting factors to get three brachydactylous persons to one normal."

If the frequency of a particular gene A is p, then its alternate allele a is $(1 - p) = q$; the population will consist of individuals of three genotypes: those who are homozygous AA, those who are heterozygous Aa, and those who are homozygous aa. The frequency of these genotypes in a randomly mating population will be in the proportion p^2 (AA), $2pq$ (Aa), and q^2 (aa). One important consequence of this formulation is that whatever the initial frequency of the genes A and a in the population, the proportion of the three genotypes will tend to remain constant during succeeding generations, providing that the three genotypes are equally fertile. If the mating in the population is not random or if there is not equal viability of the three genotypes, the frequency calculations require considerable adjustment and in small populations substantial changes in gene frequency may occur simply as a matter of chance. In any case, the rigorous formulation of population genetic principles shows no necessary relation of dominance or recessiveness to allelic frequency.

A practical consequence of the Hardy-Weinberg law is that if the frequency of a certain rare recessive disease is known, the frequency of the abnormal gene as well as the frequency of heterozygous carriers can be calculated. For a recessively inherited disease aa (q^2) with a frequency of 1 per 10,000, the frequency of the gene a (q) will be the square root of 1/10,000 or 1/100. The frequency of heterozygous carriers will be $2 \times p \times q = 2 \times 99/100 \times 1/100$ or approximately 1/50. Thus, for this trait there will be 200 clinically normal carriers of the abnormal gene in the population for every affected individual. Cystic fibrosis of the pancreas has a frequency (q^2) of approximately 1 in 2500; thus the frequency of heterozygous carriers is approximately 1 in 25 (2pq).

Mutation and Selection. A mutation is a stable heritable change in the genetic material. This change may affect a single locus, or it may consist of chromosome breakage with loss or rearrangement of the fragments. In molecular terms, a point mutation can be regarded as an alteration, addition, or deletion of one of the bases of the DNA molecule. The effect of a mutation in a somatic cell is restricted to the life of an individual, whereas mutation in germ cells can be transmitted to future generations. The natural mutation rate can be greatly increased by x-rays, ultraviolet rays, increased temperature, and various chemical mutagens such as nitrogen mustard, ethylene sulfonate, and 5-bromouracil. Chemical mutagens are thought to achieve their effects by direct structural modification of a purine or pyrimidine base, or by substitution of a base analogue for one of the normal bases.

The germinal mutation rate is usually expressed as the number of mutations per locus per generation. Present estimates of spontaneous mutation rates for a number of traits vary between 0.5×10^{-5} and 10×10^{-5}. One common, often unavoidable, error in estimating mutation rates in man is the failure to recognize that indistinguishable clinical syndromes can be caused by different genes (see Genetic Heterogeneity). Thus, the frequencies deduced by the elegant studies of Haldane on mutation rate for hemophilia must be revised downward because Christmas disease, another bleeding trait on the X-chromosome, had not been discovered when the original calculations were made. Hurler's syndrome (gargoylism) is an example of a disease that, because it can be caused by a gene on the X-chromosome or by one on an autosome, requires an estimate of the mutation rate for each gene. Nonhereditary conditions which mimic mutations are termed phenocopies and also lead to over-estimation of mutation rates.

The frequency of most genes in the population is relatively stable. When a gene is rare and severely disadvantageous, the mutation rate is balanced by the elimination of the disadvantageous gene by natural selection. The frequency of the disadvantageous gene, however, can be stabilized at a high level if the heterozygotes are slightly favored and leave a greater number of progeny than either homozygote (balanced polymorphism). An example of such a balance is the increased resistance of individuals heterozygous for sickle-cell trait to falciparum malaria. Although patients with sickle-cell disease (homozygotes) usually die before they can reproduce, and thus cannot transmit the gene to the next generation, the incidence of the sickle-cell trait may reach 40 per cent in certain West African populations. Theoretically, the high frequency of the sickle-cell gene could be maintained if the heterozygote were 25 per cent more fit than the so-called normal homozygote. It has now been shown unequivocally that death from falciparum malaria is much less frequent in carriers of the sickle-cell trait than in noncarriers, and thus the heterozygote does have an advantage. How much of the advantage is due to differential mortality and how much to differential fertility is uncertain, but this example serves to emphasize that the effect of genes can be assessed only in relation to a particular environment.

Muller introduced the term *genetic load* to describe the total genetic disability of a population. It is composed of the *mutational load*, the load due to recurrent mutations from a normal to a lethal or sublethal gene, and the *segregational load*, which is due to the segregation of harmful genes from favorable heterozygotes. The sickle-cell gene is maintained in the population because of its heterozygous advantage, and thus contributes to the segregational load. It has been estimated that, on the average, every person has three to six genes that, if homozygous instead of heterozygous, would be lethal. The relative contribution of the segregation and mutational load to the total load is unsettled.

HEREDITY AND ENVIRONMENT

Alexander G. Bearn

Disentangling the role of environmental and genetic influences in the causation of disease is a perplexing and precarious problem. In many diseases, the genetic influences are major and environmental influences are trivial, whereas in others the environment plays a major role and the genetic constitution is unimportant. For example, the genetic constitution is solely responsible for the appearance of erythrocyte antigens, the environment being without detectable influence. Many of the inborn errors of metabolism are determined by a single gene that is necessary for their expression. However, the phenotypic expression of recessive disease such as phenylketonuria and galactosemia can be considerably modified by alteration of the diet.

Paradoxically, the greatest difficulty in assessing relative roles of genetic and environmental influences is encountered with the common diseases of man. In disorders such as hypertension and rheumatic fever several genes probably influence the disease, but environmental factors are also relevant. It is worth stressing that a familial concentration of cases will be expected even when the trait is multifactorially inherited. If the frequency of a multifactorially determined trait is n, it can be calculated that the frequency of the trait in first-degree relatives (parents and sibs) will be approximately $\sqrt{n}$. Although in many infections the environmental agent is crucial, the importance of the genotype of the host should not be discounted. It seems likely that, in the past, infectious diseases were powerful selective agents, and the ability to survive epidemic disasters was probably dependent, at least in part, on the individual's genotype.

Comparative studies of identical and non-identical twins, although traditionally regarded as being of great pertinence, have not enabled sharp distinctions between hereditary and environmental influences to be drawn. Even when identical twins are reared apart, they have shared a similar environment before birth, and dogmatic conclusions are treacherous. Nevertheless, with proper regard for their limitations, studies on twins are frequently informative.

More recently, the nature-nurture polemic has been illuminated from fundamental studies on gene regulation. Now good evidence suggests that, at any given time, as much as 80 per cent of the genetic material in the cells of higher organisms is inactive. This inactivation can be reversed by certain environmental influences, and the previously inactive genes can be restored to activity. Particular steroid hormones possess the capacity to influence gene activity, and estrogens have been shown to directly influence the synthesis of m RNA and t RNA. Indeed, the administration of estrogen to a rooster can activate genes in the rooster's liver cells so that it synthesizes egg yolk proteins for which it clearly has no overwhelming need. Additional examples indicate the possibility that the environment may influence the activity of the genetic material. Soon after birth the hepatic levels of the enzyme phenylalanine hydroxylase are equally low in patients with phenylketonuria and in normal people. Normally, the gene for the synthesis of this enzyme becomes fully activated during the early weeks of life, and a healthy child develops. In contrast, children with phenylketonuria appear to be incapable of activating (or derepressing) the structural gene for the synthesis of phenylalanine hydroxylase, with the result that the clinical syndrome of phenylketonuria develops. These observations raise the possibility that some genetically determined diseases may, in the future, be controlled by environmental agents that act directly on the DNA.

CONGENITAL MALFORMATIONS
Alexander G. Bearn

The term congenital malformations is usually applied to important structural defects present at birth that are not caused by a birth injury. The relative importance of congenital malformation has increased as more effective control has been exercised over the environmental agents of disease. In 1900, in the United States, approximately 3.3 per cent of the total infant mortality could be ascribed to congenital malformations, whereas in 1964 congenital malformations accounted for 25 per cent of the total infant mortality. During the first 15 years of life congenital malformations are responsible for approximately 15 per cent of the annual death rate. It has been estimated that 7 per cent of children by the age of one year have a congenital malformation of consequence, yet only 43 per cent of such malformations are detectable at birth. In most malformations no major etiologic factor can be identified, and it must be presumed that their existence depends on complicated interactions of genetic and environmental influences or on particular genetic combinations. The frequency of many congenital malformations is compatible with a polygenic model with a threshold beyond which there is a risk of malformation. Thus, the well known observation that first-degree relatives of an individual with a congenital malformation are more at risk than the general population can be accounted for by the fact that they will have a curve of distribution approximately halfway between the general population and those affected. As an example, in cleft lip and cleft palate, as compared with the population at large, the first-degree relatives (sibs and children) of an affected individual will be 40 times as likely to develop the malformation. The approximate frequency of the major malformations per 1000 births is illustrated in Table 3.

Genetic Factors. With the exception of mongolism (trisomy 21), relatively few congenital

TABLE 3. APPROXIMATE FREQUENCY AND SEX RATIO OF COMMON CONGENITAL MALFORMATIONS

Malformations	Frequency/1000 Births	Sex Ratio, Male:Female
Congenital heart disease	4.0	1.0
Talipes equinovarus	4.0	2.0
Pyloric stenosis	3.0	5.0
Spina bifida	3.0	0.8
Hydrocephalus	3.0	1.0
Down's syndrome (mongolism)	2.0	1.0
Anencephaly	2.0	0.4
Congenital dislocation of the hip	1.0	0.5
Cleft lip ± cleft palate	1.0	1.8

malformations can be ascribed to specific genes or autosomal chromosomal abnormalities. Twin studies and pedigree patterns seldom provide any useful genetic information in the common malformations. Congenital hydrocephalus is occasionally inherited in an X-linked fashion. The offspring of consanguineous marriages show a slight increase in the frequency of congenital malformations. Congenital pyloric stenosis is five times more frequent in males, and hare lip and cleft palate twice as common. Congenital dislocation of the hip and spina bifida are more frequent in females.

Environmental Factors. Contrary to popular belief, there is little direct evidence that environmental factors such as virus diseases, maternal ingestion of drugs, or maternal irradiation make a significant contribution to the *common* malformations, although each of these factors materially increases the frequency of certain *specific* malformations. Recent evidence suggests that approximately 70 per cent of mothers exposed to rubella during the first trimester give birth to children with severe congenital defects such as cataracts, deafness, heart disease, and neonatal thrombocytopenic purpura.

Some evidence indicates that first-born children are more likely to have a congenital defect than later children. This is particularly true of anencephaly, congenital dislocation of the hip, talipes equinovarus, and pyloric stenosis. Striking regional differences in congenital defects have been recognized, and have been well documented for anencephaly and spina bifida. An increased frequency of congenital dislocation of the hip in Lapps and certain American Indians is well recognized. Marked seasonal variation in the incidence of certain malformations has also been reported. It has been estimated that nearly one third of the pregnancies that are complicated by hydramnios result in congenital malformations.

The risk that a congenital malformation will recur with subsequent pregnancies depends on the specific abnormality and its etiology. For the three most common neurologic malformations, anencephaly, hydrocephalus, and spina bifida, the recurrence rate in subsequent children is approximately 4 per cent after the first malformation, but much higher after two malformations.

Drug-induced Embryopathy. Fetal malformations can be regarded as the consequence of developmental unpunctuality, and are liable to follow environmental insults during the first three months of fetal life. There is growing evidence that errors in embryonic development are particularly likely to arise between the sixth and eighth weeks. It is, therefore, clearly prudent to minimize unnecessary medication during the first three months of pregnancy. The importance of drugs as possible etiologic agents in congenital malformations has been emphasized, and perhaps overemphasized, by the thalidomide tragedy. Indeed, it is virtually impossible to specify any drug that will *not* result in an increased frequency of congenital malformations when administered in

a certain dose to a sufficiently large panel of different laboratory animals. To assume that a drug that causes a congenital malformation in one species will necessarily cause one in man is as misguided as to assume that if a drug is harmless in animals, it will be harmless in man. Moreover, it is worth emphasizing that if thalidomide, instead of producing the striking malformation of phocomelia, or so-called "seal extremities" had increased the frequency of a common malformation such as cleft lip or cleft palate, recognition of the causal association might have been long delayed. During the two- to three-year period during which thalidomide (alpha-phthalimidoglutarimide) was freely available, approximately 7000 infants throughout the world were born with thalidomide-induced deformities. Only thalidomide and the antitumor drug Aminopterin (4-aminopteroyl glutamate) have been reported to be definitely teratogenic in humans.

Harris, H.: The Principles of Human Biochemical Genetics. New York, American Elsevier Publishing Company, 1970.
McKusick, V. A.: Human Genetics. 2nd ed. Englewood Cliffs, N.J., Prentice-Hall, Inc., 1969.
Penrose, L. S.: Outline of Human Genetics. 2nd ed. New York, John Wiley & Sons, Inc., 1963.
Porter, I. H.: Heredity and Disease. New York, McGraw-Hill Book Company, 1968.
Steinberg, A. G., and Bearn, A. G. (eds.): Progress in Medical Genetics. Vols. 1-7. New York, Grune and Stratton, 1961–1970.
Stern, C.: Principles of Human Genetics. 3rd ed. San Francisco, W. H. Freeman, 1971.

CYTOGENETICS

Margery W. Shaw

Introduction. The possibility that certain human malformations and inherited defects might be due to chromosomal aberrations has long been adumbrated. However, until 1956 serious technical difficulties in the analysis of human chromosomes prevented this possibility from being systematically investigated. In that year owing to technical improvements, the human chromosomal complement was established by Tjio and Levan to be 46, and this finding initiated a growing interest in the relationship of chromosomal aberrations to disease processes. Of the 46 chromosomes, 44, or 22 pairs, are termed *autosomes*, and are identical in both sexes. The remaining two are the *sex chromosomes*, XX in the female and XY in the male.

Incidence of Cytogenetic Disease. In 1959 Lejeune and others in Paris discovered that patients with Down's syndrome (mongolism) carry an extra autosome in each of their cells. Since that time numerous other examples of chromosomal disease have been discovered, some of which are discussed below. The prevalence of chromosomal aberrations has been estimated through surveys of adult populations, newborns, and spontaneous abortuses. Approximately 7 per 1000 liveborns carry a chromosomal defect. It is also known that

30 per cent of all spontaneous abortions are afflicted with a numerical chromosomal anomaly. Since 15 per cent of detectable pregnancies are aborted, it is calculated that at least 5 per cent of all conceptuses suffer from chromosomal disease, and the majority of these are lethal.

Chromosomal aberrations should be suspected in patients with bizarre congenital abnormalities affecting several systems, mental retardation, or disturbance in growth and development. A familial concentration of cases not conforming to a simple mendelian pattern may occur. In many of these familial clusters one of the parents may have a benign chromosomal structural change which results in a tendency to produce gametes with unbalanced chromosome complements. Sterility, spontaneous abortion, and abnormal offspring may occur. Aberrations of the sex chromosomes often underlie fertility problems and urogenital abnormalities.

Methods of Chromosome Analysis. Several technical innovations have made chromosome analyses so simple to perform that karyotyping has become a common laboratory procedure in the physician's diagnostic armamentarium. Perhaps the single most important advance was the addition of colchicine to cell cultures, which enables the cells to accumulate in metaphase—a stage in the life cycle at which the chromosomes are clearly visible and most easily distinguished from one another. Hypotonic salt solutions are used to swell the cells and spread the chromosomes. Air-dried slide preparations tend to flatten the cells so that the chromosomes have sharp outlines and clear features.

Chromosomal analyses have been performed on cells derived from many somatic tissues and, to a lesser extent, on testicular material. The two most commonly studied tissues are peripheral lymphocytes and cultured skin fibroblasts. Cultured fibroblasts can be examined after many cell generations, and they faithfully retain their original chromosomal complement. Studies utilizing peripheral blood are, however, more convenient and quicker to perform. The lymphocytes derived from a few milliliters of blood can be induced to divide in vitro under the influence of the mitogenic agent phytohemagglutinin. The cells that undergo mitosis are transformed lymphocytes, and superficially resemble plasma cells. Lymphocyte cultures cannot be maintained in vitro for more than a few cell divisions. Although it is frequently sufficient to perform a human karyotype analysis on cultured lymphocytes, examination of the chromosomal complement of dividing fibroblasts or other tissues is important when mosaicism is suspected.

Amniocentesis. Amnion cells are amenable to both cytologic and biochemical analyses, and allow prenatal diagnosis of many chromosomal diseases and inborn errors of metabolism (*vide infra*). A small sample of amniotic fluid can be aspirated through a transabdominal needle and the specimen centrifuged. Some of the desquamated cells thus collected are viable and capable of mitosis in vitro, providing metaphases for karyotype analysis.

Chromosomal Morphology, Identification, and Classification. When the dividing cells are examined during metaphase, the chromosomes appear double with a constricted region at the point of spindle fiber attachment, the *centromere*. Each longitudinal strand of the chromosome is termed a *chromatid* and occurs in duplicate. The position of the centromere is characteristic, and enables the chromosomes to be classified into those in which the centromere is centrally placed, *metacentric chromosomes*, and those in which the centromere is terminal, *acrocentric chromosomes*.

Morphologic identification of only four autosomal pairs is possible by present techniques. Nos. 1, 2, 3, and 16 are unique by the criteria of chromosome length and centromere position. All other chromosomes are grouped according to the brackets shown in Figure 1. Considerable difficulty is encountered with the medium size metacentric chromosomes (6 to 12). The X chromosome cannot be morphologically distinguished from the autosomes in this size group. Satellites, which are small bodies attached by a short stalk to one end of a chromosome, can often be seen on the acrocentric chromosomes 13, 14, 15, 21, and 22. The small Y chromosome in the male can be distinguished from pairs 21 and 22 by its shape and the absence of satellites.

Autoradiographic techniques have aided in the identification of some chromosomes which cannot be distinguished by morphology alone. This method employs the use of the isotope, tritiated thymidine, which is incorporated into the DNA strands at the time of chromosome replication during interphase (period of DNA synthesis). Grains are developed on photographic emulsion which has been layered over the radioactive chromosomes and allowed seven to ten days exposure in the dark. Since DNA synthesis is asynchronous but occurs in an orderly sequential profile in specific chromosome regions, a characteristic labeling pattern emerges. One X chromosome in the female replicates later than any other chromosome and can thus be differentiated from the members of the 6–12 group of autosomes. The early replicating X in the female and the single X in the male cannot be identified, however. Pairs 4–5, 13–14–15, and 17–18 can be distinguished by autoradiography, but pairs 19–20 and 21–22 cannot.

More recent techniques which show promise in advancing our identification of the human karyotype include electron microscopy, computer image processing, and the analysis of meiotic chromosomes. Electron microscope images have been obtained from both sectioned material and whole mounts. Increased magnification provides greater detail of normal structures such as satellites, secondary constrictions, and centromeres. Photographic images of metaphase spreads can be analyzed by a flying-spot scanner connected to a computer. Chromosome counts, measurements, and karyotypes are thus automatically

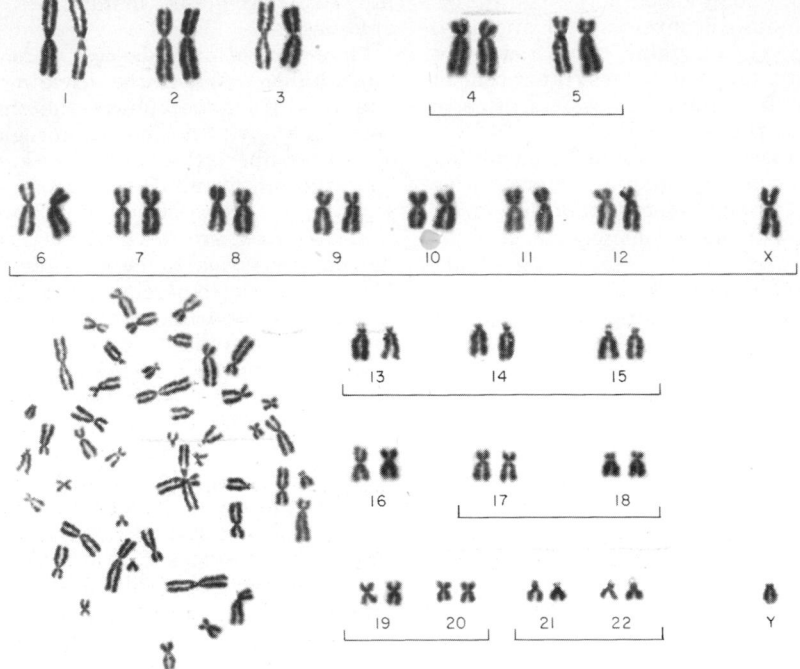

FIGURE 1. Normal male karyotype (enlarged × 2200). The chromosomes are arranged in groups according to size. The approximate length of chromosome number 1 is 7μ. The somatic cell from which the karyotype was constructed is also shown.

processed. Until recently, meiotic chromosome preparations have been disappointing, but newer technical methods have made early prophase of the first division of spermatogenesis from testicular biopsies amenable to study. Cytologic preparations of meiosis in ovarian material in the last trimester of pregnancy and in the first few months of postnatal life also appear promising.

Mitosis. Chromosomal disturbances may occur during meiosis or mitosis. During mitosis or somatic cell division, the distribution of chromosomes to each daughter cell is precise, and each cell receives the normal complement of 46 chromosomes. Although for a brief period the parent cell has 92 chromosomes, the chromosomes with their paired centromeres soon arrange themselves on the spindle and separate, and 46 chromosomes are allocated to each daughter cell.

Meiosis. In order for the diploid content of somatic cells to remain constant, a halving of the number of chromosomes must occur during spermatogenesis and oogenesis. Fertilization of the ovum with a spermatozoon will thus restore the normal somatic diploid number. In the first meiotic division the chromatids are doubled, but the centromere remains single. Thus, when cell division takes place, both cells receive 23 chromosomes, each with duplicated chromatids. In the second meiotic division the centromeres split, and a complete set of 23 chromosomes is deployed to each of the four daughter cells (Fig. 2). Since there is no fixed rule that governs the arrangement of parental chromosomes on the spindle, there is independent assortment of maternal and paternal chromosomes during meiosis. When the chromosomes pair they may exchange homologous

1st meiotic division

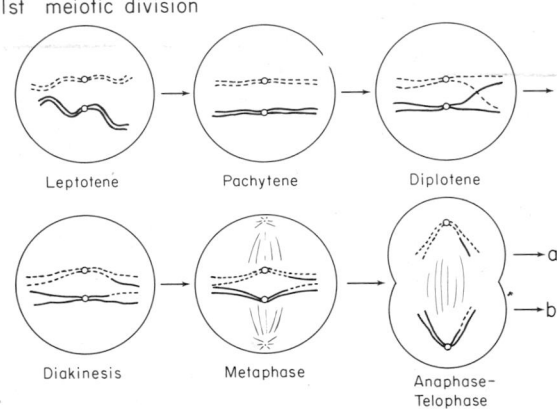

2nd meiotic division

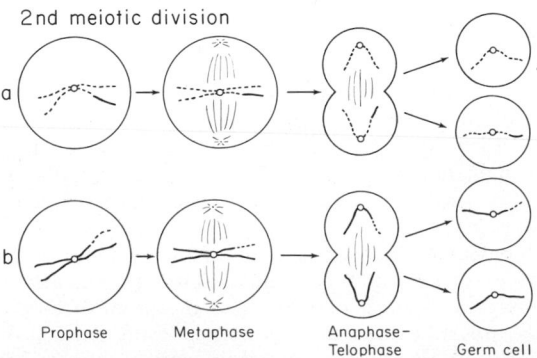

FIGURE 2. Diagrammatic representation of meiosis. Note that four germ cells each with 23 chromosomes have resulted from the meiotic division of a single spermatogonium (or oogonium) with 46 chromosomes.

segments, a process known as *crossing over*. The genetic effect of crossing over is to increase the genotypic diversity of the gametes, already guaranteed by independent assortment. Thus, meiosis and crossing over ensure for the species an almost infinite variety of genetic constitutions.

NUMERICAL VARIATIONS IN THE HUMAN CHROMOSOMAL COMPLEMENT

Margery W. Shaw

Nomenclature. Chromosomal aberrations in man are of two general types: variation in the number of chromosomes and alteration in structure. Cells containing multiples of the normal chromosome number are called *polyploid*, those with irregular numbers *aneuploid*. *Trisomy*, in which a particular chromosome is represented in the somatic cells in triplicate, may cause clinical disease. Complete *monosomy*, in which there is one chromosome less than normal, has been found only in connection with the sex chromosomes.

Etiology. Abnormal segregation of human chromosomes may take place during mitosis or during the first or second meiotic divisions. Abnormal segregation is known as *nondisjunction*. When nondisjunction takes place the chromatids or homologous chromosomes fail to separate, but remain attached at the centromere instead of one going to each of the two daughter cells. Thus when the cell divides, one daughter cell receives both chromosomes, and the other acquires none (Fig. 3). Meiotic nondisjunction produces an ovum containing 24 chromosomes, which is usually viable on fertilization, and one with 22, which is usually inviable except for the XO individual with Tur-

ner's syndrome (see under Human Sex Anomalies in section on Diseases of the Endocrine System). The phenomenon of *anaphase lag*, which results in the loss of a chromosome during mitosis or meiosis, gives rise to two daughter cells, only one of which has an abnormal chromosome number.

If nondisjunction occurs at the first mitotic division of the fertilized ovum, the zygote develops into a mosaic individual, half of whose cells contain 45 chromosomes and half 47. If nondisjunction occurred at the second division or later, and all cell lines were equally viable, a mosaic of 45, 46, and 47 chromosomes would result. If the monosomic cell line of 45 chromosomes were inviable, as is usually the case, a chromosomal mosaic of 46/47 would result. To detect mosaicism it is important to examine the karyotype of the skin as well as that derived from lymphocyte cultures. Mosaicism may be suspected when the clinical manifestations of a disease, known to be caused by chromosomal aberrations, appear relatively mild. Thus the presence of a nearly normal intelligence in a child with mongolism would suggest the presence of a population of cells with a normal chromosomal constitution as well as some with 47 chromosomes. An increased liability to nondisjunction with increasing maternal age appears well established. Moreover, in some families an unusual concentration of chromosomal abnormalities strongly suggests the possibility that genetic factors may predispose to chromosomal aberrations. Consanguinity in one of the parents would strengthen such a supposition.

Mongolism (Down's Syndrome, Trisomy 21). In 1866 Langdon Down described this syndrome, which is characterized by mental retardation, congenital abnormalities, and a pathognomonic facies. Cardinal features include an upward, outward slant of the palpebral fissures, epicanthal folds, flat nose bridge, downward slant of the

FIGURE 3. Diagram of normal and abnormal segregation of chromosomes during cell division.

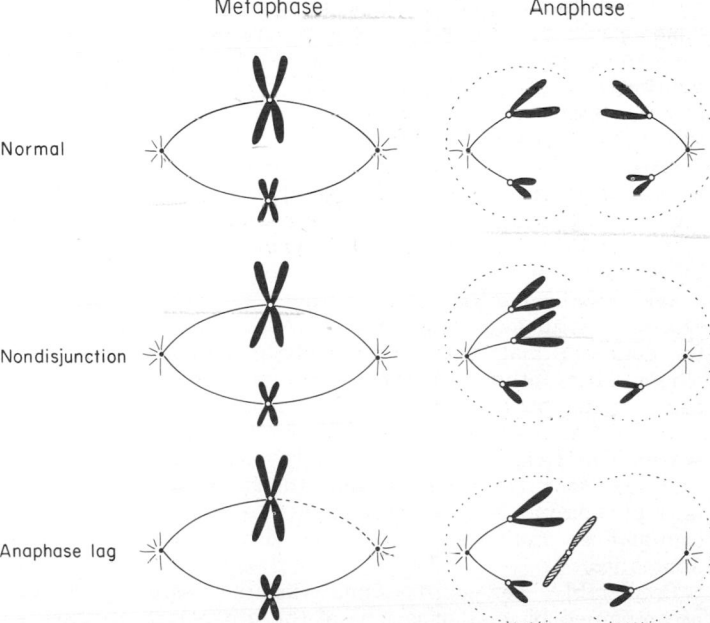

Metaphase   Anaphase

Normal

Nondisjunction

Anaphase lag

mouth, microcephaly, flattened occiput, high arched palate, micrognathia, low set ears, short stature, incurved little fingers, and characteristic dermatoglyphic patterns. Mild skeletal anomalies, particularly a shallow acetabulum, are common, and approximately 25 per cent of mongols have a congenital heart defect, frequently affecting the atrioventricular septum.

There is delayed growth, and mental retardation is almost universal. Approximately 15 per cent of all institutionalized retardates are mongols. There is a familial recurrence in approximately 3 per cent of the cases. Increased maternal age is noteworthy; the average age of mothers at birth of the mongol child is about 33 years compared with 26 years for mothers of normal children. There is a slight excess of males. Some female mongols are fertile, and half their offspring are mongols. Male mongols, however, are sterile. Their testes are small, and spermatogenesis is absent or incomplete.

All but 3 per cent of mongols have 47 chromosomes in each of their body cells—the extra chromosome is No. 21. The remainder result from mosaicism or translocations (vide infra).

Trisomy 13. Clinically this rare syndrome, which has a frequency of approximately 1 per 5000 live births, is characterized by severe central nervous system defects, anophthalmia (rarely, cyclopia), harelip, cleft palate, congenital heart disease, polydactyly, microcephaly, and mental retardation. Arhinencephaly and clubbed feet with prominent elongated heels are common. Over 100 cases have been described; the patients die before six months of age unless they are chromosomal mosaics. There is a strong maternal age effect.

Trisomy 18. This chromosomal abnormality has a frequency of approximately 1 per 3000 live births. The condition is characterized by severe mental retardation, low-set malformed ears, and congenital heart disease. The hands are held in a flexed position with the index and little fingers overlapping the central digits; in the first few months of life this sign in invariably found. The great toes are usually short. Instead of the usual whorls or loops, the fingerprints show several arches, usually more than six. The chin and pelvis are characteristically small. All patients die before one year of age. There is a strong maternal age effect. Confusion with Turner's syndrome must be avoided.

Sex Chromosome Variation. Turner's syndrome (45, XO), Klinefelter's syndrome (47, XXY), and the double Y male (47, XYY) are discussed elsewhere. Many other numerical variants of the X chromosome have been described, including 49 XXXXX females and 49 XXXXY or 49 XXXYY males. The Y chromosome is strongly male-determining; without a Y chromosome the individual is a phenotypic female. Mosaicism is especially common in individuals with sex chromosome anomalies.

Predictably, sex chromosome variations are accompanied by malformations of the urogenital system. Frequently growth disturbances, skeletal malformations, and endocrine defects occur. With increasing numbers of sex chromosomes mental retardation is common. Infertility accompanies the XO and XXY conditions, but XXX and XYY individuals are fertile. The latter produce only children with normal karyotypes.

STRUCTURAL VARIATIONS

Margery W. Shaw

Nomenclature. During meiotic crossing over, homologous chromosomes break and rejoin. Normally, however, the exchange is exact since the breakage point on the two chromatids is the same. Thus, although exchange of genetic material has taken place between the two homologous chromosomes, the total amount of genetic information is unaltered. If, however, the break occurs at different points of the chromosome, one chromosome will have excess genetic material (*duplication*), and the other chromosome will have less (*deletion*). Terminal deletions may be difficult to distinguish from translocations (*vide infra*). If a chromosome is broken in two places and the interstitial segment rotates 180 degrees and rejoins, an *inversion* occurs. When the inverted segment includes the centromere region, it is called a *pericentric inversion*; when it is confined to one arm of the chromosome, it is termed a *paracentric inversion*. All these structural rearrangements are stable and may be inherited.

Etiology. Chromosome breaks may be spontaneous or induced by physical, chemical, or biologic agents. Physical agents include temperature shock, gravity changes, electromagnetic disturbances, and various forms of radiation, e.g., x-rays, gamma rays, and ultraviolet light. Over 200 chemicals are known to alter chromosome structure. These chemicals fall into many classes, but the largest number are nucleic acid analogues and alkylating agents. There is increasing concern that an unidentifiable number of drugs may affect chromosome structure. Antimicrobials and drugs affecting the central nervous system are under particular scrutiny.

There is growing evidence that certain viral infections may cause chromosomal aberrations. Three types of morphologic change have been noted: chromosomal breakage, complete fragmentation and pulverization of the chromosomes, and cell fusion with abnormal spindle formation. Abnormalities can be detected in vitro with measles virus, herpes virus, and certain oncogenic viruses, and have been reported in vivo in certain epidemics of measles, infectious hepatitis, and infectious mononucleosis. The single chromosome breaks, and dicentric chromosomes following viral infection are similar to those that may follow diagnostic or therapeutic irradiation. Several examples of structural chromosome changes, some of which are discussed below, are illustrated in Figure 4.

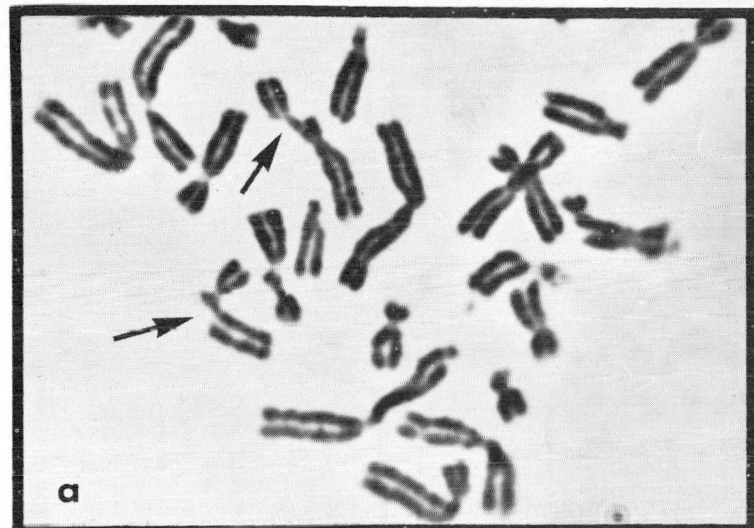

FIGURE 4. Some examples of structural aberrations of human chromosomes. *a,* Chromatid breaks and gaps, typical of cytologic abnormalities seen in Fanconi's anemia and Bloom's syndrome. *b,* Inherited chromosome break in proximal segment of long arm of chromosome No. 2 (note how distal displacement causes chromosome to appear longer than its homologue). *c,* Chromosomes of pairs 4 and 5 in cri du chat syndrome, showing deletion in short arm of chromosome 5. *d,* Philadelphia chromosome compared to normal autosomes in group 21-22. *e,* Ring chromosome.

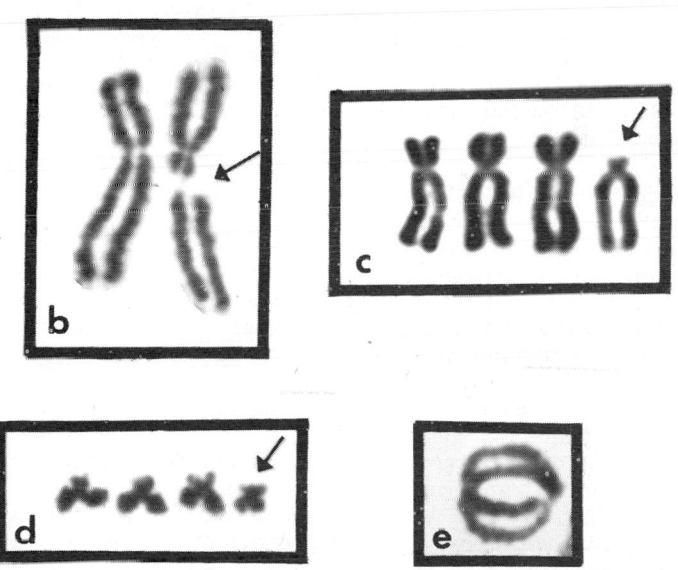

Deletion in the Short Arm of Chromosome 5 (Cri du Chat Syndrome). This syndrome is characterized by hypertelorism, microcephaly, severe mental deficiency, and a characteristic plaintive "catlike" cry. This sign, which disappears after the age of two, has given the syndrome its descriptive name. Approximately 10 per cent of patients suffer from congenital heart disease, and the patients usually die in childhood.

Deletion in the Long Arm of Chromosome 18. Fewer than ten cases of this syndrome have been described. Symmetrical dimples on the shoulders, fusiform fingers, and severe mental deficiency are common.

Deletion in the Long Arm of Chromosome 21 (Philadelphia Chromosome). A partial deletion of the long arm of chromosome 21 has been a constant finding in chronic myelogenous leukemia. The abnormal chromosome is confined to the erythrocytic, thrombocytic, and granulocytic series of hematopoietic cells. During remission the deleted chromosome may disappear from the circulation to reappear during relapse (see Chronic Myelogenous Leukemia).

Rings. A ring configuration results if breaks occur at both ends of one chromosome and the proximal broken ends join. This results in loss of genetic material (deletion) distal to the breaks. Since any chromosome can undergo ring formation, there is no simple phenotype associated with rings. One outstanding characteristic is absence of the thumbs in some patients with a ring chromosome in the 13-14-15 group. Rings are unstable during cell division. They are variable in size and may be lost entirely in some cells.

Translocations. The chromosomal aberration in which a fragment of one chromosome becomes attached to a nonhomologous chromosome is

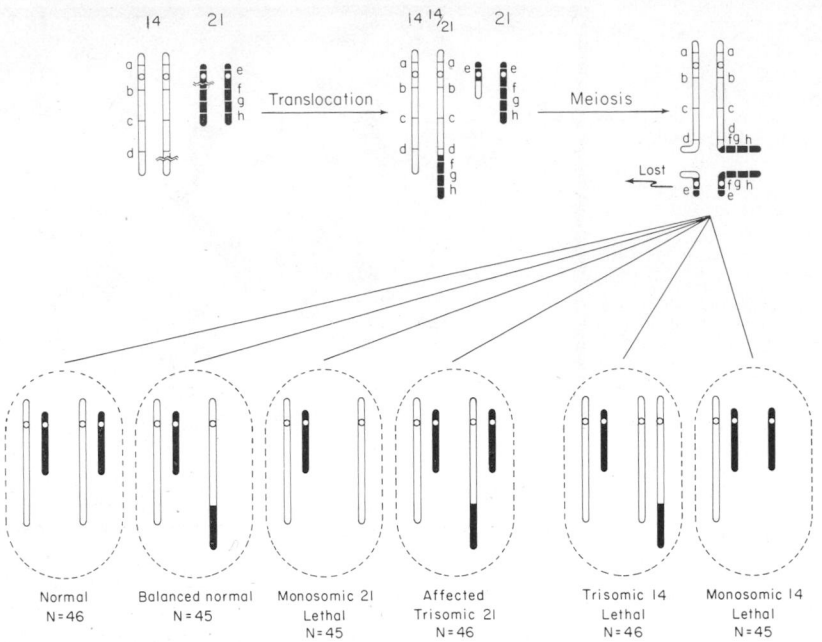

FIGURE 5. Diagram illustrating translocation between chromosomes 14 and 21. Two of the four chromosomes depicted in each zygote are derived from the normal parent. The affected trisomic 21 is a classic mongol even though total chromosomal complement is 46. For details, see text.

termed a translocation. Translocations occur when two chromosomes break and are followed by mistaken reunion of the broken ends.

In order for the homologous segments to pair at meiosis, translocated chromosomes assume cruciform configurations. When the chromosomes separate, six possible gametes are produced. One of these gametes is entirely normal, one has essentially the same amount of genetic information as a normal gamete, but the genetic material is abnormally distributed between the two chromosomes (balanced translocation), and four gametes are unbalanced (Fig. 5). It is apparent that a normal person with a balanced translocation may be phenotypically normal and yet have 45 chromosomes. A person with a balanced translocation may transmit the abnormal chromosomes to his offspring. Only three of the six types of offspring have been observed: normal persons, persons with the balanced translocation who are similar to the parents, and affected persons with 46 chromosomes who are essentially trisomic and have an abnormal phenotype. Individuals who are monosomic and lack the translocation chromosome are not seen; it is presumed that the condition is lethal. It is evident that a concentration of abnormal persons may occur in families in which there is a translocation chromosome. Patients with mongolism who have a chromosomal complement of 46 and possess a translocation chromosome are relatively common. The translocation is usually a 14:21 translocation (2 per cent of mongols), or, more rarely, 21:22 translocation (1 per cent of mongols). In 14:21 translocations the condition is usually transmitted through the mother, whereas the 21:22 translocation is transmitted equally by both sexes.

Minor Structural Variants. In addition to the major rearrangements associated with pathology, a number of minor chromosomal changes are being recognized in normal, healthy, fertile individuals. These include giant satellites on an acrocentric chromosome, deletion of the short arm of an acrocentric chromosome, accentuation of normally occurring secondary constrictions, and variable length of the Y chromosome. Although these variations are believed to be benign, there is some speculation that they occur more frequently in relatives of patients with frank chromosomal abnormalities. Individuals with minor structural variants may be predisposed to nondisjunction, chromosomal breakage, and rearrangements.

INHERITED CHROMOSOME BREAKAGE

Margery W. Shaw

Bloom's Syndrome. This disease is characterized by congenital telangiectatic erythema appearing primarily in the butterfly region of the face, other regions of the head, forearms, and dorsa of the hands. Sun sensitivity is common, and the erythema abates with protection from sunlight. Low birth weight, microcephaly, and stunted growth are universal features of the syndrome. Few patients live beyond the age of 20, and the incidence of leukemia and other malignancies is unusually high.

Bloom's syndrome is caused by homozygosity for an autosomal recessive gene. Consanguinity between parents of affected children, high incidence among Jews, and frequent occurrence of affected sibs attest to the genetic cause of the disease. Multiple chromosome breaks and structural abnormalities are commonly found in skin fibroblasts as well as cultured lymphocytes. In addition to breaks and gaps, dicentric chromosomes, acentric fragments, and chromatid exchanges occur. Parents of affected children may also exhibit a moderate increase in chromosome breakage.

Fanconi's Anemia. Pancytopenia caused by bone marrow hypoplasia is the cardinal sign of this disease. There is a high incidence of congenital anomalies, particularly of the skeletal and urogenital systems. Growth retardation is accompanied by microcephaly, although the intellect is usually normal. Hyperpigmentation of the neck, abdomen, axillae, and groin occurs.

Fanconi's anemia is an autosomal recessive disease. It is usually fatal in childhood or early adulthood from complications of the hematologic defect such as hemorrhage or infection. There is an increased risk of leukemia and other malignancies. The basic genetic defect is unknown, although a disturbance in hexokinase metabolism has been reported.

A tendency to increased chromosome breakage and rearrangement is similar to that in Bloom's syndrome. The chromosomal lesions are found in cultured lymphocytes, direct bone marrow preparations, and skin fibroblasts. Cells cultured from patients with both diseases are particularly susceptible to transformation by the SV40 virus.

Other Hematologic Syndromes. Several other conditions with bone marrow hypoplasia, dysgammaglobulinemia, telangiectasia, and/or congenital anomalies have been suspected of having chromosomal lesions similar to those reported in Bloom's syndrome and Fanconi's anemia. These include ataxia-telangiectasia, Blackfan-Diamond syndrome, multiple myeloma, Wiskott-Aldrich syndrome, and Rothmund-Thomson syndrome. Cytogenetic reports of these conditions are inconsistent, however, and definite conclusions await further evidence.

Familial Specific Chromosomal Breakage. Recently several families have been described in which a specific region of a specific chromosome is particularly susceptible to attenuation and breakage. These patients do not have a pathognomonic phenotype. In fact the condition may occur in healthy, fertile adults.

Four families have been described in which the lesion occurs in the proximal long arm of chromosome No. 2. Other families exhibit a tendency to breakage in the distal long arm of No. 16 or one of the members of the 6-12 group. Pedigree analysis indicates a typical autosomal dominant pattern. The cause of the defect is unknown, but a curious disturbance of replication occurs in the abnormal chromosome. The segment distal to the site of breakage may undergo endoreduplication, whereas the remainder of the chromosomal complement is normal.

GENETIC COUNSELING
Margery W. Shaw

There are two aspects to genetic counseling: the estimate of the genetic risk and the humane presentation of the risk to the patient, taking into consideration all the social and psychologic implications of the probability estimate. Most of those who seek advice from a genetic counseling clinic suffer from predominantly nongenetic disorders. The taking of careful family history is mandatory, and an accurate clinical diagnosis, based on personal examination of the patient, is a prerequisite. The pedigree should include parents, sibs, uncles and aunts, grandparents, and cousins. Specific inquiry concerning the possible existence of consanguinity should be made. An increased consanguinity among the parents of individuals affected with a recessive disease is frequently observed. When a careful family history discloses that a condition is inherited in a clear-cut dominant, recessive, or X-linked fashion, the genetic risk for subsequent offspring, given one affected, can be calculated. Frequently, however, genetic counseling has to rely on approximate "empiric risk figures," which are continually changing as heterogeneous conditions are separated into discrete homogeneous entities. In some recessive diseases it is possible to recognize the healthy carrier of the abnormal gene by appropriate biochemical or tissue culture techniques. Requests for counseling are common in clinical medicine; unfortunately, the information upon which to base a helpful opinion is frequently lacking.

New diagnostic techniques such as karyotype analysis provide some insight into risks for chromosomal disease. Mongolism may be used as an example. With a negative family history, the empiric risk of mongolism is 1/650. If the mother is age 25, the risk is 1/2000, but at age 45 it is increased to 1/50. If the parents have had one mongol child, their risk of recurrence is about 1 to 2 per cent and independent of maternal age. Chromosome studies of the parents will sharpen these predictions. If the mother carries a 14:21 translocation, the odds are about 1 in 3, but if the father is the translocation heterozygote, the odds drop below 1 in 20. If amniocentesis is performed during pregnancy, then a karyotype gives the *exact* diagnosis on the fetus. The physician and parents can then consider a therapeutic abortion. The ultimate aim in genetic counseling is to take the guesswork out of predictions and to be able to provide therapy for individuals with genetic afflictions.

Bartalos, M., and Baramki, T.: Medical Cytogenetics. Baltimore, Williams & Wilkins Company, 1967.
Turpin, R., and Lejeune, J.: Human Afflictions and Chromosomal Aberrations. International Series of Monographs in Pure and Applied Biology, Modern Trends in Physiological Sciences, Vol. 32. Oxford, Pergamon Press, 1969.
Yunis, J. J.: Human Chromosome Methodology. New York, Academic Press, Inc., 1965.

ENVIRONMENTAL FACTORS IN DISEASE

Introduction: Man in His Environment

Harold E. Lewis

In a foreword to the preceding edition of this text, and in other writings, Dubos has reminded us that man is more the product of his environment than of his genetic endowment, and that human populations of diverse mixtures usually acquire the disease pattern of the locale and of the social group. Thus, whereas genes determine fundamental reactions and responses, it is the environment that determines characters and traits. In fact, a large part of the practice of medicine is devoted to treating disorders of body and mind which are expressions of inadequate or inappropriate responses to environmental influences.

The purpose of this introduction is to sketch some of these environmental circumstances, so that the articles that follow may be read in better perspective. For example, the clinical emergency of acute poisoning, whether by heavy metals, gases, contaminated food, or radiation injury, may represent the tip of an iceberg, the submerged portion representing an insidious pollution of our over-all environment. By the same token, we have not always appreciated the effects on our environment brought by attempts to eradicate disease caused by poisonous plants, animals, and insects, which otherwise represents a laudable contribution to the public health. Similarly, research in human physiology has enabled man to overcome problems of gravity, motion sickness, alterations in atmospheric pressure, and problems of heat and cold. These successes have allowed man the widest exploration of our world and of space, but the long-term impact of these travels on man's environment has received insufficient attention.

The practice of medicine teaches us a great deal about the individual as a patient in hospital. We now need to know much more about his environment and background away from the hospital context, as he faces the reality of his daily life. (Edholm). There are two important reasons for knowing about man's habitual activity. The first is to give some idea about man himself, anticipating and, if possible, avoiding the hospital situation. The second is to see what effect man's activities have on his environment.

A wider understanding of man in his environment can only come from interdisciplinary research and imaginative teaching.

page 24

HUMAN ECOLOGY

The word ecology is derived from the Greek "oikos" – a dwelling place. The term refers to study of living things in their environment, their interaction with the physical world, and their relationship with other forms of life. It records the constant adjustment to change, which is in turn the basis of natural selection and the evolutionary process as described classically by Charles Darwin in 1859.

Originally, ecology was the study of plants and trees throughout the world; then it enlarged to include mammals and birds, and their populations. The relationship between food production and population growth was noted by the political economist Malthus (1766–1834), to whom it seemed that food production followed a linear rate of expansion whereas population growth was geometric. In the animal world, there is always a dynamic equilibrium between food production and consumption. When food runs short, the population depending on it must decrease in number; the alternative is migration or starvation. Malthus predicted that the same pressures would apply to human populations.

The concepts of demography, Darwinian evolution, and the genetic theories of Mendel (1822–1884) developed into the science of population genetics; with the use of mathematics, further sophistication was obtained so that adaptation and evolution could be expressed quantitatively in the form of indices.

The organism and the environment are delicately balanced in an ecosystem, which is primarily driven by solar energy. Through photosynthesis, plants are the basic producers; herbivores eat the plants; carnivores eat the herbivores and the plants. The waste from these processes is handled by lower orders such as bacteria and fungi, and simple organic substances and minerals are returned to the environment for recycling. Although all these substances are conserved in the ecosystem, energy is dissipated as heat, and this is constantly replenished by the sun.

Thus, it is apparent that modern ecology is essentially an interdisciplinary subject which probes into the manner of the practical organization of living things in our biosphere. Without this ecologic perspective, many discoveries at the molecular level could be without meaning; and in our search for the understanding of life, it is necessary to realize that both reductionist and interdisciplinary approaches are important.

Man has a special place in the ecosystem because he has learned to cultivate his food sources deliberately and improve the productivity of the land with irrigation and with fertilizers. This behavioral asset has given him dominance in the ecosystem, and has allowed him to adapt easily to ever-changing environmental circumstances. Physiologic adaptation alone would not have given him this unique position. Although man has made a dramatic impact on his own environment, this aspect has hardly been a feature of medical education. The physician and the ecologist are both devoted to the welfare of a species, but there the contact ends. The medical man's traditional primary concern has been for the individual; the applied biologist is more concerned with the population. Their different philosophies may be seen in their attitudes, for example, on the assessment of a pesticide. The medical man is prepared to accept the results of acute or chronic toxicity tests, and will of course be concerned when individuals receive fatal doses by misuse or accident; the ecologist does not consider these physiologic criteria to be adequate, and is more anxious to assess the situation on a population basis and in terms of the other disciplines which make up ecology.

The ecologist has the advantage of seeing the picture as a whole, and the community will increasingly rely on him for early warning signals; his data must therefore be intelligible and precise enough to form the basis of action by the community.

MAN'S ADAPTABILITY

Man has remarkable capacity to adapt to diverse environments, and as long as he continues to adapt there will be little to see at the cellular or molecular level. When changes are detected at these levels, it is as if the last bastions of adaptation have fallen; in retrospect, we would have done better to comprehend the various forces that had been assailing the cell. If, in the examination of an adverse environment, one reads that "no lethal or toxic effect has been shown," this may merely mean that, at present, biologic and statistical techniques are too crude to detect anything except death of the cell. Such a report would have us believe that the effect is not harmful; this use of null hypothesis — which denies that the phenomenon exists unless it can be proved — has a special appeal for those who are responsible for legislation. For example, in spite of the evidence of clinical intuition and obvious loss of amenity in early stages of a noise nuisance, legislation tends to be delayed until there is proved damage to cochlear tissue and subsequent deafness.

How does one translate from the cell to the individual and to society?

This concept is one of level of organization and was studied by Rudolf Virchow (1821-1902), who had already established the cellular basis of disease. Virchow extended these ideas to include the organization of living matter at the level of the organ and at the level of the individual. He recognized that cells in whatever groups — organs, individuals, societies or populations — depend for their survival on their environment, i.e., their organization; moreover, he saw that there was a human analogy and believed it his own civic responsibility to ensure that attention was given to *human* organization at various levels. After being a cellular pathologist and physician, he involved himself in epidemiology and public health, which led him logically to politics and anthropology.

THERMAL ENVIRONMENT

We have briefly mentioned some characteristics of living material at various levels of organization. It is worth summarizing also the nature of man's thermal environment, because it is the starting point of his progress, first for survival and latterly as master. Later, we shall discuss the responsibilities of this privileged position.

In the thermal environment, radiation, conduction, convection, and vaporization are balanced against an individual's own metabolic heat production to achieve constancy of internal body temperature of about 37° C.

Radiation: The human body, irrespective of skin color, radiates heat to the atmosphere if the temperature of surrounding surfaces is lower. The amount of radiation is roughly proportional to the difference in surface temperatures. Out of doors, radiation is received from the sun in three ways: (1) directly, depending on infiltration through the atmosphere and clouds, and elevation of the sun; (2) by reflection from the surface, e.g., snow, water, rocks; and (3) by re-radiation from a heated surface, such as a hot pavement.

Convection: A thin layer of air is constantly in motion upward as it is heated and humidified by the skin, and is replaced by cooler, drier air. The heat transfer of this natural convection depends on the temperature difference between skin and air, and it may be increased by driving the air by a fan. This convecting envelope may properly be considered an example of the human micro-environment. Within its laminar and turbulent layers, particles and micro-organisms are entrained from the skin or the ambient air, or both; it is the driving force which presents polluted air to the respiratory system, and it may also be a link in the spread of infection (Lewis et al., 1969).

Evaporation: Cooling is greater if convected air passes over wet skin surfaces. There is constant transpiration of tissue fluid to the surface, representing a loss of 400 to 500 ml. per day. This is insensible perspiration, quite apart from secretion from sweat glands, which can amount to as much as 11 liters per day in the desert. Cooling is achieved only if the sweat actually evaporates from the surface. There is no benefit if the fluid merely drips away from the skin; this constitutes useless loss of an essential body constituent.

Conduction: Heat passes from the deeper tissues to the surface by conduction. If there is a minimal blood supply, fat, skin, and muscle, in that order, act as relative insulators; but when there is vasomotor activity, these thermal properties are of much less significance compared with heat transfer by blood flow. From the skin surface there is relatively little heat lost to the air, because air has low thermal conductivity. By comparison, the situation is dramatically changed when the individual is immersed in water, the high thermal conductivity of which causes maximal heat flow.

Controlling these physical routes of heat exchange are the physiologic functions of vasomotor activity, sweating and shivering, but the ultimate control is behavioral, viz., the wearing of clothes, the building of shelter, and the use of fire. Man as a naked animal is best suited to the tropical forest where he is protected from solar radiation and extremes of temperature. If he moves to a hotter environment, e.g., the desert, his physiologic functions will have to undergo a process of adjustment so that he can function efficiently. Before he has acclimatized, he will find mental and physical work difficult; he may faint easily, and he will be generally more distressed than the indigenous people. His skin is flushed and dry. Within 10 to 14 days, however, he is more comfortable in the heat. and has an increased capacity for work; his reactions are now the same as those of the resident population.

The initial discomfort is due to a combination of increased peripheral vasodilation and increased pulse rate, providing a disproportionate amount of the cardiac output for cooling the body, which is a preponderant requirement. There is some sweating in the early stages, but it is inadequate. Later, sweating begins at a lower body temperature; it becomes more profuse as the sweat glands have a higher output for longer periods, and evaporative cooling now more effectively allows the transfer of heat to the surface. There is lowering of the body temperature, and a greater proportion of the cardiac output can be used for physical work.

If naked man moves toward the temperate zones, he approaches the limit of adaptation to cold. There is vasoconstriction and shivering, and he will now have to resort to the use of clothing and shelter to be comfortable.

Whereas acclimatization to heat is a well-defined efficient physiologic response, there is no clear evidence for useful acclimatization to cold.

For his migration from the equatorial to the temperate and colder zones of the world, man has had to create a protection, which we may term the built environment. In the tropical regions, this need, though desirable, is not essential for survival. Nonetheless, man requires something better of his environment than mere survival. If he is to

function efficiently and creatively, the built environment emerges as a feature in both the hot and cold parts of the world—but with this difference; its creation has been relatively simple in the former. In cold areas, the built environment is much more elaborate to serve the requirements of vigorous technologic civilizations such as those found as far north as the circumpolar regions of the world.

MANIPULATION OF THE ENVIRONMENT

If we now trace man's progress, we will find certain inevitable consequences which today demand urgent attention.

Man was originally a nomadic hunter; he discovered fire and employed burning to drive game, and possibly to condition the native vegetation to produce more edible plants; he then moved away from the impoverished soil to new land.

Man then learned to domesticate, breed, and cultivate plants and animals; he was assured of a regular food supply and was freed from the necessity of hunting and gathering so that his numbers increased, and he was gradually obliged to change from eating meat provided by his grass-fed animals to eating cereals as well. This situation prevails today as a result of land shortage and overpopulation.

The next development was the discovery of metal ores, and the invention of smelting, which required extra fuel. Forests were accordingly denuded. Early man was a despoiler of the environment, but these losses were on a small scale. However, the invention of steam power in the nineteenth century caused a massive effect on the environment. More and more power was needed; this was now obtained from the store of fossil fuel. In addition to coal mining, there were other extractive processes to provide the raw materials for the newly developed chemical industry. Around these natural resource sites, cities developed.

In the industrialized world, before the eighteenth century, men worked in their cottages; but with the industrial revolution, they were required to work together in factories which contained the expensive machinery.

Settlements had developed in other ways, e.g., transport cities depended on the presence of docks, rivers, warehouses, railroads, and highway intersections, and a concentration of universities, gambling houses, government offices, or resorts produced other types of settlements. These associations of skills, which provide new ideas and tools for the country as a whole, are the essence of industrial cities, the human environment of which is the developing theme of this essay.

With the aggregation of people it becomes practicable to provide transport, social services, and other facilities. Unfortunately, each of these benefits has a less attractive side: the overgrowth of towns and roads occurs at the expense of the countryside. The sewage of the householders and their domestic animals must be disposed of; this requires expensive plants, but in many cities, the effluent is untreated and is simply allowed to flow into rivers and lakes. The presence of nitrates and phosphates alters the ecology of these waters by causing overgrowth of algae, which depletes the water of its oxygen and leads to the death of fish and other river life. A similar disruption is caused by detergent pollution. Another serious problem is the disposal of rust-proof cans, junk automobiles, and inert packaging plastic, which is almost impossible to degrade.

Food must be provided for city people, and in advanced countries this must be achieved by an industrial approach. To produce the quantity that is required at a reasonable price, fertilizers and pesticides are needed. Though not directly toxic, they persist in the soil and are absorbed by animals in whose fat they remain unchanged. In wild life there may be long-term effects on fertility, and in this way man's manipulation of the environment further interferes with the ecologic balance. The massing of animals and mechanized feeding methods raise problems of waste disposal that are much larger than those caused by human population, perhaps five to ten times as great. Los Angeles has a pile of manure 50 feet high, spread over 4 acres, which remains that size in spite of efforts to dispose of it. This would be a valuable commodity in an agricultural area, but in a metropolis it is an embarrassment.

To provide heat, domestic fires are used, but the smoke is responsible for smog, which is especially lethal to people already suffering from chronic respiratory or cardiovascular disorders. In London, the passing of a clean air act considerably improved matters, although power station stacks and domestic fires still produce sulfur dioxide. Chronic bronchitis is particularly prevalent in industrial cities.

The use of the internal combustion engine produces carbon monoxide, lead, and unburnt fuels which produce smog when they react with dust and sunlight, as in Los Angeles and east coast cities.

When man applies himself to industry, the problems are much more serious. By means of central heating, air conditioning, motor exhaust, and decreased ultraviolet radiation, man has changed the properties of the free atmosphere within and above the city. Each house, factory, railway station, wall, and pavement combine to produce a substantial climatic entity—the urban micro-environment (Chandler). Together with the human micro-environment (vide supra), this is the true climate affecting urban man, because we know, from studies of his habitual activities, that most of his time is spent in the built environments of his home and work, and in traveling between the two in closed transport.

BIOSPHERE AND TECHNOSPHERE

It is useful now to consider the relationship between the biosphere and this man-made environment, the technosphere, which also picks up water, fossil fuels, minerals, and biologic products for processing to meet modern technologic needs.

The *biosphere* is a complete, self-contained, permanently balanced system organized to provide all its own needs and to break down, disseminate, and reuse its waste material through natural processes of dissolution and decay. Unfortunately it is a balance that can be upset. The *technosphere* is dependent on the biosphere not only for much of its input but also for its effluents (Nicholson). It was created by historic, social, economic, and scientific developments; it has its own anatomy, its inputs and outputs, and its hazards—accidental or deliberate disturbances to ecologic systems which may result in a chain reaction that man is often powerless to control. This applies particularly to nuclear pollution. The final result is often irrecoverable loss, such as dust bowls and desolation.

Man has a special relationship to the biosphere; at worst he is the greatest and most destructive of predators—but he can seek after solutions, and, by his decisions, determine his own destiny only if there is help from his own institutions: government, industry, agriculture, communities, and education.

We mentioned earlier the curious lack of contact between the ecologist and the conventionally trained physician, and the fact that unfortunately the problems most difficult to evaluate are not the acute ones but the subtle ones accruing from insidious deterioration of the environment. There has been relatively little help from biologists here, because biology instructors themselves have turned away from field work—where the reality of life is to be studied—in favor of the reductionist trend in education, and have concentrated on problems at the cellular or molecular level, as perhaps more convenient to teach in a classroom.

DEMOGRAPHY

Many environmental problems of health are man made, and there is a danger that they may well overtax his capacity to adapt. By far the worst pressure on the environment comes from the growing flood of humans. This demographic "explosion" started in the mid-nineteenth century, and is still accelerating. In both the developing and the industrialized countries there was a rise in the birth rate after World War II; in the developing countries there was, in addition, a fall in the death rate.

After slow growth, over hundreds of thousands of years, the population at the beginning of the nineteenth century reached 1000 million; barely 130 years after that it doubled (2×10^9); and in 1960, after 30 years, it was 3×10^9. By 1975, the population will be 4×10^9, and before the end of the century, unless there is a dramatic change, the population will reach 6×10^9. Extrapolated further, there would by 2500 A.D. be only one square meter of dry land for every human being!

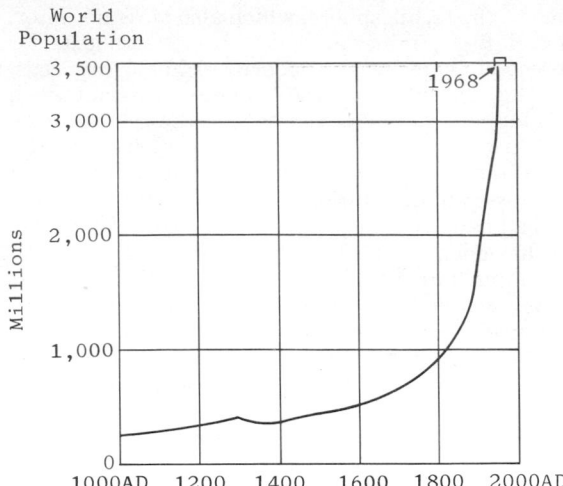

World
Population

The world's population. There was a fairly steady level until about 1400 A.D., and then an increase which has become exponential. In the shape of this curve, there is the most serious threat to mankind today (see text).

This basic process is threatening to change the entire quality of human existence for the worse, and has been likened to a cancer (Huxley). In the developing world, the population is multiplying much faster (from 2 to 4 per cent per year) than the world average. Although the rich nations are becoming richer, the poor nations, in spite of technical aid and assistance, are becoming poorer, largely because their population is increasing so fast. The birth of so many babies is in fact standing in the way of economic development and industrialization, because the nation's capital is taken up with feeding, housing, and educating them.

When animal populations exceed the limits of their environment, the result is disease, strife, starvation, and lack of cover. There is no convincing evidence that man is excused from the same ecologic laws.

Originally, the main argument for reform was Malthusian, from those who saw the problem as one of food shortage. This point of view was immediately countered by certain agricultural economists who calculated that modern agricultural and food technology could provide enough food for many decades to come, and therefore denied the need for family limitation. These calculations did not take into account the problems of national boundaries, food prejudices, and distribution; nevertheless, useless polemic was generated which deflected the urgency away from the equally important problems of shortage of water, educational and health services, raw materials, space for housing and amenities, noise, waste, and pollution (Mayer).

Even with the most successful family planning, in 40 years the population will reach 6 billion by 2000 A.D. It could be more, because the deep instinct of motherhood may insist on more than two children per family. This implies that the

rising expectations of a large part of the world will be frustrated; the people will continue to live in squalor, and may never reach the standards enjoyed by advanced western society. In the United States, $200 per head is devoted to health and welfare today; by 2000 A.D., it is calculated to be $350. In parts of Africa the present budget is 75 cents; in 2000 A.D., it will only be $2 per head.

EDUCATION AND RESEARCH IN HUMAN ECOLOGY

During man's visits to the moon, he obtained a clear insight into the contrast between its inanimate lithosphere and the living biosphere of Earth. He also realized that the biosphere was indeed finite. This has crystallized a public realization that has grown at a remarkable rate over only the last two years: that for all man's achievements in space, the Earth is our home, and it will be a very remote chance indeed that in any numbers we will be able to reach, let alone live on, another planet, if we wear out, eat up, or defile our Earth.

Although conservationists have discussed these problems for a century, the popular writing is recent. Two influential works are Rachel Carson's *Silent Spring* (1962), and Huxley's *Age of Overbreed* (1965), one intriguing aspect of which was the site of its original publication. Public opinion was mobilized probably more by the threat to animals than to humans, viz., DDT found in Antarctic penguins and polar bears, death of fish in the Rhine in 1969, death of birds in the Irish Sea, and death of sheep from nerve gas in Utah.

The environment is now thoroughly discussed by every medium, and there is a danger that the public will become bored by the word "ecology" before they know what it means (Fraser Darling). It has become a noncontroversial issue at the highest political level, and has also inspired student protest in favor of conservation—a welcome form of patriotism. There is a feeling of alarm against man's helplessness against the demands of a new technologic system which he has created but neither understands nor effectively controls. The problem is not of nature threatened by man, but of man and nature, in the same boat, equally threatened by the uncontrolled workings of the technosphere.

Completely new attitudes are needed in order to understand the intricacies of ecologic strategy. The old-fashioned pretechnologic state of thinking is not adequate for the purpose. The problem is not one of confrontation, but of cooperation between those who manage the technosphere and those who guard the biosphere. In describing cost-benefit, economists will have to learn to include human ecologic problems in their balance sheets.

Two examples will serve to emphasize the need for closer understanding among physicians, ecologists, engineers, and agriculturists. During the great anti-malarial activities since World War II, emphasis was placed on vector destruction and chemotherapy. Excessive hopes were founded on the new insecticides with long-lasting effects. Unfortunately, the early hopes for eradication were overoptimistic, and we now cannot assess the real effectiveness of otherwise admirable public health measures because there was little or no attempt to establish baseline data on the local epidemiology of the disease or on human differences with respect to the immunologic reactions induced by the parasites.

Irrigation schemes may have serious ecologic consequences for the public health. In Egypt, schistosomiasis has always been endemic, not made worse by seasonal flooding of the Nile. But in areas of perennial flooding, such as in the Delta, there is total infestation of the population. With the new Aswan Dam, there will be large new areas of perennial flooding, which may greatly increase the spread of this disease.

Before understanding of these factors can be achieved, ecology has to be widely taught. It should be part of a liberal arts education for the chemist, physicist, engineer, lawyer, teacher, forestry and agricultural student, and particularly for those whose careers will take them into public administration. Ecology, in the form of human biology, is now taught at many universities, but only in small aspects; the sanctity of specialized academic departments has tended to discourage interdisciplinary studies, and there are very few universities in the world where interdisciplinary studies have Man at the center, in the Benthamite sense — "the greatest good for the greatest number of people."

One imaginative pioneering exception should be mentioned: the new Green Bay campus of the University of Wisconsin, with its four colleges. It has a broad structure for studying real situations at first hand — problems of urbanization, racial crisis, population explosion, transportation, effects of automation, pollution, and the exhaustion of natural resources. The colleges of Environmental Sciences and of Community Sciences emphasize the problems of the natural resources environment. The other two colleges are also concerned with man: The College of Human Biology centers its attention on human adaptability, i.e., on the way the environment impinges on an individual, and the College of Creative Communication emphasizes the problem of human identity.

Research into problems of man in his environment must be guided by an important principle: although we have stressed the unity of the biosphere, research should be undertaken only in small regions, rather than in a whole country, because common characteristics of regions may be found in many parts of the world, whereas generalization from one country to another is too complex for honest analysis. Thus a pilot project in environmental sciences has selected Dane County, Wisconsin, as an analogue for an American megalopolis, and Iowa County, Wisconsin,

for country and small-town life. Within the International Biological Program, for example (Weiner and Lourie), there is a continuing interdisciplinary study of the small population (circa 300) of Tristan da Cunha, in the South Atlantic. This includes their history, anthropology, nutrition, and medical and dental state. The genealogy of this closed community, accurate for six generations, provides a rare opportunity to use advanced computer methods to predict the genetic properties of the population and the individuals who comprise it. After almost a decade of research, it will now be possible to look more closely also into the interplay between the islanders and their environment — more specifically, the investigation of zoonoses, allergens, and the possible health hazards of their land and marine crops. To this could be added micro-economic studies, in order to obtain a quantitative understanding of the reality of their lives and prosperity. The point is that Tristan is not an "untouched" island; it is an area of human settlement, and the value of such studies is their pertinence to problems in the larger world. Tristan da Cunha may be considered analogous to regions in developing countries which are themselves far too large and complex for micro-studies (Lewis et al., 1970).

Most of our awareness of the need for the new education in ecology has come from the failures seen in our technosphere. It should be clearly stated that the successes are all around us. It is not technology that may be ruining our biosphere, but the mishandling of our technologic capabilities. How to strike the right balance will be the future challenge of human wisdom. Except for the problem of mounting population, there is every reason for optimism and a spirit of affirmation of human capability. As Medawar has observed, one must recognize that all past civilizations or cultures had their ups and downs, and went through a life cycle of degeneration and regeneration. There was never a truly golden age. "We wring our hands over the miscarriages of technology and take for granted the benefactions of antibiotics, DDT and pesticides. We are dismayed by air pollution — the result of improving our standard of living — but not proportionately cheered by the virtual abolition of poliomyelitis. The deterioration of the environment produced by technology is a technological problem for which technology has found, is finding and will continue to find solutions. It is true that we cannot point to a single definitive solution to any one of the problems that confront us — political, economic, social or moral. We are still beginners, and for that reason may hope to improve."

Carson, R. L.: Silent Spring. New York, Houghton Mifflin Company, 1962.
Chandler, T. J.: The Climate of London. London, Hutchinson & Company, 1965.
Dubos, R. J.: Man Adapting. New Haven, Yale University Press, 1965.
Edholm, O. G.: The changing pattern of human activity. Ergonomics, 13 (No. 6), 1970.

Fraser Darling, F.: Wilderness and Plenty. London, B.B.C. Publications, 1970.

Huxley, J.: The age of overbreed. Playboy Magazine, 12:103, 1965.

Lewis, H. E., Edwards, A. E., and Roberts, D. F.: Historical Population Studies. London, Edward Arnold, Ltd. (to be published in 1972).

Lewis, H. E., Foster, A. R., Mullan, B. J., Cox, R. N., and Clark, R. P.: Aerodynamics of the human microenvironment. Lancet, 1:1273, 1969.

Mayer, J.: Towards a non-Malthusian population policy. Columbia (University) Forum, 12:5, 1969.

Medawar, P. B.: On the effecting all things possible. Advance. Sci., 26:70, 1969.

Nicholson, M.: The Environmental Revolution. London, Hodder & Stoughton, Ltd., 1970.

Weiner, J. S., and Lourie, J. A.: Human Biology—A Guide to Field Methods. International Biological Program. Oxford and Edinburgh, Blackwell Scientific Publications, Ltd., 1969.

Heat and Cold

Joseph M. Quashnock

The human body is a heat-producing engine that must maintain its temperature within rather narrow limits through careful regulation of the flow of heat between the body and the environment. The bodily mechanisms concerned include the rate of metabolic heat production, the effectiveness of circulation, skin temperature, and sweating. A crude but useful concept is to consider the body to be made up of a core and a shell. Strictly speaking, no single temperature can be called a core temperature, but it is customary in clinical literature to refer to the rectal measurement of body temperature because the rectum is a readily accessible part of the core or heat-producing part of the body, where temperature varies little from part to part at a given moment. The shell regulates the temperature gradient between the core and the environment and varies both in thickness and in rate of perfusion with blood.

Environmental conditions affecting heat regulation include air temperature, wind, humidity, and radiant temperature. Man's ability to perform in a given environment can be related to an integration of the measurements of these climatic factors into the commonly used Wet Bulb Globe Temperature Index. This index must be used with caution at extremes of temperature and exercise. Furthermore, there is no single universal index.

Acclimatization occurs when man is exposed to high temperatures and can perform hard work with the least physiologic embarrassment. Significant physiologic adjustments take place in about five days: lower pulse and respiratory rate, lower body temperature, dilution and increase in volume of sweat. These changes are complete within two weeks and are maintained by continued periodic exposure.

Acclimatization to cold is less dramatic than to heat, and the subject is controversial. Acclimatized persons are able to elevate metabolic heat production without resorting to shivering. Also, shivering begins at a lower temperature than in the unacclimatized. Shivering is a protective mechanism that results in as much as a four- or fivefold increase in metabolic rate. Acclimatization to cold is slow, taking two months or more, and may very well be a manifestation of the improved state of physical fitness that most people experience when chronically exposed to low temperature environments.

HEAT DISORDERS

Heat-induced illness is the result of disordered physiology that is a byproduct of thermoregulation. Not all disorders are due to accumulation of body heat; some may be caused by indirect physiologic failures such as salt and water imbalance or circulatory collapse. To attempt to classify these as specific syndromes serves no real purpose, for the basic physiologic mechanisms must be given primary attention. However, heat stroke is one disorder that must be treated as a disease entity resulting from collapse of the temperature regulatory mechanism.

Heat Stroke. Heat stroke is an acute and dangerous form of heat disorder. It is characterized by high body temperature of at least 40.6° C., convulsions or coma, and cessation of sweating. These are the result of positive heat storage.

In most cases the onset of symptoms is with sudden delirium or coma. Headache, numbness and tingling, dizziness, restlessness, or mental confusion may be experienced for varying lengths of time before collapse. Cessation of sweating may also be noted as a prodromal symptom. Most patients are in coma, but the central nervous system features may range from disorientation to involuntary limb motions or coarse tremors. The respiratory rate may be at least double normal, and can lead to respiratory alkalosis and tetany. The pulse rate may be as high as 150, and usually there is an elevated blood pressure. Shock commonly follows. The hallmarks of heat stroke are anhidrosis, hyperpyrexia, and coma.

The treatment of heat stroke must include supportive management as well as establishment of negative heat balance. Speed is essential in lowering body temperature to avoid brain damage. A cold water bath or spray is the most effective and rapid method for body cooling. Wet sheets may be wrapped around the body and evaporative cooling accelerated with fans. Rapid cooling of the skin results in peripheral vasoconstriction and stagnation, which must be corrected by vigorous massage of the extremities. Rest and sedation are useful in reducing metabolic heat production.

Untreated heat stroke is fatal. In about one third of the uncomplicated treated cases the patients may die, but there seems to be some correlation between the prognosis and the height of fever, as well as its length. Treatment should be aimed at reducing the temperature to 40° C. within one hour. The temperature will continue to fall after cessation of cooling, but a secondary rise to 40° C. may occur within the first day, and must be corrected with cooling techniques. As much as a week may be necessary for stabilization of the body temperature and return of sweating. When treatment has been delayed for more than four hours or has not been immediately effective, there may be shock or residual damage such as pulmonary edema, cerebral ataxia, hepatic or renal failure, or myocardial damage.

The prevention of heat stroke is approached through identifying the environments in which the disorder has occurred or is expected to occur, adapting human activity to limits of safety within the environment, and taking advantage of the acclimatization capability of man.

Circulatory failure may occur in the presence of successful thermoregulation. The cardiovascular system may have accomplished its important function of transferring heat from the core to the periphery, but the blood is a dual-purpose fluid, since it must also transport metabolites for working tissues. When man works at high temperature, the working muscles place greater demands on the circulation, and less blood is available for cooling the body through heat dissipation at the skin. As perspiration becomes profuse, as much as 3 or 4 liters per hour, dehydration develops and further embarrasses the circulation through reduction in blood volume and increase in blood viscosity.

Heat Syncope. Heat syncope is a disorder ranging in severity from simple lightheadedness to severe fatigue and loss of consciousness. Hypotension with some degree of cerebral anoxia results from peripheral venous pooling. Vasomotor tone is decreased, as evidenced by a fall in both systolic and diastolic pressures, but the diastolic falls less so that the pulse pressure is decreased. The pulse rate is increased slightly. Sweating is visible, and the temperature may be elevated to about 39° C., especially if the episode is induced by exercise. Pallor is marked, and the muscles are flaccid. The patient should be removed from the heat and allowed to rest in a recumbent position. Recovery should occur in a few minutes, but if the patient remains in hot surroundings, more than an hour may be necessary for a return to a sense of well-being. The episode is self-limiting.

Heat Exhaustion. A more serious circulatory disorder is a form of heat exhaustion, which is associated with a depletion of both salt and water. The concentration of body fluids is not altered remarkably, but a decrease in blood volume accounts for the manifestations, which develop insidiously over several days. Early symptoms include headache, fatigue, confusion, and drowsiness. Anorexia, visual disturbances, and vomiting follow and, if persistent, lead to circulatory collapse. However, the patient is usually incapacitated in the early stages of the illness, so that treatment is begun early; hence, the illness is rarely fatal. The picture is one of peripheral vascular collapse with pallor, profuse sweating, decrease in blood pressure, and little, if any, elevation of temperature. Treatment includes removal of the patient to cool surroundings, rest in bed, and replacement of salt and water. Drinking of isotonic saline is useful, but a patient can seldom take more than 20 grams of salt per day orally. At least that amount of salt should be given for several days until the urine chloride content reaches 3 or more grams per liter. Intravenous isotonic saline is necessary when there is coma or severe vomiting.

Heat Cramps. Heat cramps are the result of electrolyte imbalance alone. This disorder occurs in persons working at high temperature and drinking large quantities of water. The basic pathophysiologic change is a dilution of body fluids, which is really a form of *water intoxication*. Body fluid volume is relatively well maintained. Without any prodrome, the voluntary muscles begin fibrillary twitching and then proceed to spasm, which may be very painful. The abdominal wall and extremities are most often involved. The episode usually occurs late in a workday and is accepted by some workers as a nonserious occupational hazard. Since the cramps are corrected promptly by salt replacement, workers rarely seek medical care. Diagnosis is based on a history of an abundant intake of water during sweat-producing work at high temperature followed by characteristic muscle cramps. Temperature is normal and cardiovascular function is unimpaired. Severe cases may require intravenous isotonic saline. Salted foods or fluids are usually adequate. Prevention is dependent upon a sufficient intake of salt, usually about 3 grams extra per day. This requirement can be met for most persons by the liberal use of the salt shaker at mealtimes. Limitation of water intake during work in hot surroundings will prevent cramps, but may result in the more serious consequences of thermoregulatory failure.

HYPOTHERMIA

Hypothermia is an abnormally low body temperature resulting from a negative balance between body heat productivity and heat loss. When the body temperature falls below 35° C., physiologic changes can be expected.

Diminished production of body heat rarely reduces body temperature to seriously low levels. In some debilitating states, narcosis, prolonged unconsciousness, fatigue, and metabolic disorders, the body temperature may fall to 25° to 30° C. However, the hypothermia resulting from accelerated loss of body heat to the environment is considerably more serious, especially when man is immersed in a medium of high heat capacity such as cold water. The inadequately protected man exposed to water at about 0° C. will lose consciousness in about 5 to 15 minutes and will die in 30 to 60 minutes. Most cases of accidental hypothermia result from long exposure to cold air or snow of people who have become unconscious from inebriation, diabetes, epilepsy, or other illness.

The most valuable clinical and research data have been obtained from studies of patients in whom hypothermia was induced as a special technique in cardiovascular surgery and neurosurgery. In such cases, medical support and control are critical.

In hypothermia below 35° C., there is gradual diminution in all physiologic activities. The pulse rate, blood pressure, and metabolic rate fall, and uncontrollable shivering begins. As the body temperature approaches 30° C., disorders of consciousness, such as hallucinations or narcosis, appear. This is the zone of maximal benefit in the surgical patient since the oxygen requirement is reduced to about 40 per cent of normal, allowing safer occlusion of the circulation. The systolic blood pressure is usually lowered to about 90 mm. of mercury. Moderate acidosis appears, owing probably to CO_2 retention.

The most dangerous consequence of hypothermia is ventricular fibrillation. This arrhythmia has commanded most attention and has set the lower limits for the hypothermia used in surgery. It is generally agreed that 28° C. permits occlusion of the circulation for about eight minutes. However, some groups achieve as much as 15 minutes' occlusion with body temperatures of 25° C.

The treatment of hypothermia requires that the negative heat balance of the body be corrected. Rapid rewarming in a water bath of 40° to 45° C. is most desirable. Artificial respiration with oxygen is necessary for the unconscious, apneic patient. The use of 5 per cent CO_2 and 95 per cent oxygen is valuable in stimulating respiration and correcting the metabolic acidosis. Antifibrillating drugs such as quinidine or procaine amide are of doubtful use, whereas electrical defibrillation or cardiac massage is most consistently effective. Ventricular fibrillation must be guarded against for several hours after the body temperature returns to normal.

Clinical reports of accidental hypothermia demonstrate high mortality rates, 80 per cent or more. An important contributory cause is persistent neurologic damage. Brain damage is characterized by disturbances in consciousness or memory,

hypotonia of large postural muscles, and brain stem dysfunction. Little or no residual brain damage is reported at temperatures above 24° to 30° C.

ACCIDENTAL (SPONTANEOUS) HYPOTHERMIA IN THE AGED

In the last decade, British clinicians have drawn attention to the spontaneous development of hypothermia among elderly patients. Usually the subjects have been living alone in underheated homes during the cold weather, unable to obtain assistance. There is evidence that those affected have defective mechanisms for conserving body heat, and the suggestion has also been made that therapy with chlorpromazine accentuates the defect. Patients with body temperatures ranging down to 32° C. usually regain normal temperature within a day or two after being removed to a comfortable environment. However, when body temperature falls to 25° to 32° C., a serious medical problem is presented. Consciousness is impaired, and shivering has ceased. Pulse, respiration, and blood pressure are depressed, and subcutaneous edema may be present. Neurologic signs are sluggish. Commonly, this clinical picture is at first misdiagnosed as cerebrovascular accident. It has been estimated that as many as 2000 deaths may occur annually in Great Britain among elderly patients with accidental hypothermia.

Treatment by rapid rewarming may lead to sudden loss of peripheral vasoconstriction and circulatory failure. It is thought best to reduce body heat loss by the use of thermal insulation and to allow gradual and spontaneous accumulation of metabolic heat. Parenteral fluids in the form of 5 per cent glucose or plasma may be required, but must be administered with caution because of the tendency to pulmonary edema. These patients are liable to respiratory infection and may need antimicrobial therapy.

Adolph, E. F.: Physiology of Man in the Desert. New York, Interscience Publishers, Inc., 1947.

Conference on Hypothermia. Ann. N. Y. Acad. Sci., 80:285, 1959.

Duguid, H., Simpson, R. G., and Stowers, J. M.: Accidental hypothermia. Lancet, 2:1213, 1961.

Hardy, J. D.: Physiology of temperature regulation. Physiol. Rev., 41:521, 1961.

Leithead, C. S., and Lind, A. R.: Heat Stress and Heat Disorders. Philadelphia, F. A. Davis Company, 1964.

MacMillan, A. L., Corbett, J. L., Johnson, R. H., Crampton-Smith, A., Spalding, J. M. K., and Wollner, L.: Temperature regulation in survivors of accidental hypothermia of the elderly. Lancet, 2:165, 1967.

Shibolet, S., Coll, R., Gilat, T., and Sohar, E.: Heatstroke: Its clinical picture and mechanism in 36 cases. Quart. J. Med., 36:525, 1967.

Alterations in Atmospheric Pressure

Robert L. Johnson

GENERAL CONSIDERATIONS

The physiologic and pathologic effects of alterations in atmospheric pressure are governed by the physical behavior of gases. The individual gaseous molecules of the earth's atmosphere have mass and therefore weight due to the effect of gravity. Atmospheric pressure represents the weight of the mass of air extending upward from the earth's surface. At sea level this amounts to 14.7 pounds per square inch, 760 mm. of mercury, or 1 atmosphere. Atmospheric air (dry) contains 20.94 per cent oxygen, 0.03 per cent carbon dioxide, and approximately 79 per cent nitrogen at all altitudes. However, the partial pressures of the individual gases of the atmosphere, in accordance wih Dalton's law, vary directly as the total atmospheric pressure. At sea level, where atmospheric pressure is 760 mm. of mercury, the partial pressures of oxygen, carbon dioxide, and nitrogen are 159 (760 × 0.2094), 2.3 (760 × 0.0003), and 600 (760 × 0.79) mm. of mercury, respectively, in dry air.

Water, being much denser than air, exerts a much greater pressure because of its weight. The weight of a 33-foot column of sea water equals that of a like-sized column of air extending through the entire atmosphere. Since water is incompressible, pressure increases in linear fashion with further descent, each 33 feet adding an additional atmosphere of pressure.

The medical problems created by changes in atmospheric pressure may be grouped into direct and indirect effects. The former result from mechanical forces created when pressure differentials develop across the walls of air-containing spaces within the body or upon its surface. Indirect effects result from alterations in partial pressures of the individual gases of the atmosphere.

DIRECT EFFECTS OF CHANGES IN ATMOSPHERIC PRESSURE

Gases respond to pressure changes in accordance with Boyle's law. Their volume varies inversely and their density, or molecular concentration, directly as the absolute pressure. The fluids and solids of the human body, being incompressible, transmit pressure freely and thus assume the pressure exerted upon the body's surface. Any alteration in the latter is reflected almost instantly by an identical pressure change in body fluids and tissues. Pressure within air-containing spaces of the body can be maintained equal to external pressure only by appropriate adjustments either of the number of molecules of gas within the space or of the volume of the space. No medical difficulties arise as long as air can pass freely between such spaces and the environment. If additional air cannot enter such a space to increase its pressure during descent, fluids and tissues of the surrounding walls, whose pressure is increasing with increasing ambient pressure, tend to move in to reduce its volume and eradicate the pressure differential. The lining of the walls becomes hyperemic and swollen. Serum or blood may move into the relative vacuum. Conversely, during ascent, pressure within the tissues surrounding the space declines with declining environmental pressure. Unless air can be vented from the space, an increasing pressure gradient creates a distending force against the walls.

The natural air-containing spaces of the body are the paranasal sinuses, the middle ear, the airways and lungs, and the gastrointestinal tract. Small pockets of air may also exist beneath fillings or in diseased teeth. In addition, pockets of air against various surfaces of the body may be produced by goggles, tight-fitting hoods, ear plugs, or wrinkles in diving suits. The middle ear is very susceptible to barotrauma during descent. The sinuses are much less frequently affected, but may also incur barotrauma during ascent. Respiratory infection greatly increases the likelihood of injury. Descent in water may damage tissues beneath air-containing structures closely applied to the surface of the body. All these injuries, including barotitis with ruptured tympanic membranes, tend to heal spontaneously.

The most serious mechanical injuries resulting from pressure changes involve the lungs. If the breath is held during diving, the increasing pressure compresses the thoracic cage to the position of maximal expiration. On further descent air within the lungs can no longer be compressed to counter the increasing external pressure. The relatively negative intrapulmonary pressure results eventually in pulmonary congestion, edema, and hemorrhage, a condition known as "thoracic squeeze." Breathing the denser air at depth through equipment with excessive air flow resistance or breathing through a snorkel tube which is too long may also create a relatively negative pressure within the lungs, leading to similar consequences.

After breathing the denser air at depths, air must be released from lungs during ascent to prevent expanding air from building up sufficient pressure to overdistend or rupture lung tissue; if this occurs, pneumothorax, mediastinal emphysema, or air embolism may ensue. Air embolism has been reported during ascents of as little as 9 feet and is said to be exceeded in frequency only by drowning as a cause of accidental death among divers. Lung tissue distal to a poorly communicating diseased bronchial passage may be similarly damaged even if the diver vents his excess air during ascent. The air traveler with such bronchopulmonary disease, or one who happens to be holding his breath, may be similarly injured during a sudden loss of cabin pressure at high altitude.

Knowledge of the character of the dive, including depth, duration, air supply, and patterns of descent and ascent in relation to symptoms, often simplifies the problem of diagnosing lung injury in divers. Frothy, bloody sputum may be produced in either thoracic squeeze or lung rupture. If the victim has been skin-diving or using a snorkel tube, thoracic squeeze is likely. In a scuba diver, however, the first consideration must be lung rupture with potentially fatal aeroembolism. (The term "scuba" is derived from "self-contained underwater breathing apparatus.") The unconscious diver must be presumed to have aeroembolism or decompression sickness. Either aeroembolism or serious decompression sickness requires treatment by recompression at the earliest possible moment. Transport to a recompression chamber should be by the fastest method available. The gain from prompt treatment far outweighs the potential danger of further decompression during air transportation at low altitudes. Meanwhile artificial respiration by the mouth-to-mouth method should be carried out if necessary, and oxygen should be administered. Placing the victim on his left side may be beneficial if aeroembolism is suspected. Thoracic squeeze usually requires no more than supportive measures.

INDIRECT EFFECTS OF CHANGES IN ATMOSPHERIC PRESSURE

Only brief mention can be made here of the effects of increases in the partial pressures of nitrogen, oxygen, and carbon dioxide. At 4 atmospheres absolute pressure (100 feet in water), divers or occupants of hyperbaric chambers may show the narcotizing effect of nitrogen. Judgment, thought processes, and motor ability may become impaired and deteriorate with further increases in atmospheric pressure. Fortunately, the symptoms clear rapidly and completely on return to lower atmospheric pressure.

Hypercapnia normally produces subjective distress and stimulation of respiration, but may cause unconsciousness without warning. Scuba divers who restrict their breathing in an attempt to conserve their air supply expose themselves to this potential hazard. Loss of consciousness in skin divers resulting from "shallow-water blackout" is attributed to a large rise in partial pressure of carbon dioxide associated with an inadequate subjective or respiratory response to hypercapnia.

Convulsive seizures and coma may occur with little warning during exposure to high partial pressures of oxygen. The minimal partial pressure of oxygen capable of producing convulsions appears to be less than 2 atmospheres ($Po_2 = 1520$ mm. Hg). Divers breathing air are at little risk of oxygen convulsions. If they use pure oxygen, however, depths below 25 feet become hazardous.

Hyperbaric oxygenation is achieved by increasing atmospheric pressure within sealed chambers to levels varying from 2 to 4 atmospheres absolute ($Po_2 = 320$ to 640 mm. Hg). Increased oxygenation of tissues occurs chiefly as a result of increased solution of oxygen in plasma. Hyperbaric oxygenation has been reported to be of value during surgical correction of certain congenital cardiovascular disorders and in the treatment of carbon monoxide poisoning and certain anaerobic infections. Precautions must be taken to protect the patient and medical personnel from all of the direct and indirect effects of altered atmospheric pressure.

DECOMPRESSION SICKNESS
(Caisson Disease)

In decompression sickness the manifestations are due to formation of nitrogen bubbles in body tissues and fluids. On exposure to lower atmospheric pressure the partial pressure of nitrogen dissolved in body fluids and tissues exceeds nitrogen partial pressure in the lungs. If this pressure reaches the point where nitrogen evolves from tissues and fluids faster than it can be transported by blood to the alveolar membrane to diffuse into alveolar air, bubbles will form. Bubbles large enough to produce symptoms develop when the partial pressure of nitrogen in tissues rapidly becomes more than twice as great as nitrogen partial pressure in the atmosphere. This situation can arise in a diver whose tissues are saturated with nitrogen at a depth somewhat in excess of 33 feet who surfaces rapidly, or by a flier who rapidly ascends from sea level to higher than 18,000 feet.

In keeping with Henry's law, gases in contact with liquids dissolve in direct proportion to their partial pressures. The processes of nitrogen diffusion and transport necessary for equilibration between tissues and alveolar air require time. Since nitrogen must be transported by blood, equilibration in highly vascular tissues occurs more rapidly than in those that are poorly vascularized. Fatty tissue is not only poorly vascularized but in addition takes up larger volumes of nitrogen since nitrogen is far more soluble in lipids than in water.

The complete elimination of excess nitrogen from the body after exposure to a lower partial pressure of nitrogen in the atmosphere requires about 12 hours. About 75 per cent of the total is eliminated within 2½ hours, mainly from aqueous solution in plasma and interstitial tissue. The slower component arises mainly from tissues high in lipid content such as fat deposits, bone marrow, and spinal cord.

The total amount and the rate at which nitrogen is taken into solution during a dive will depend not only upon the depth but the time spent at depth. The magnitude of this depth-time factor and the rate of ascent determine whether decompression sickness occurs. Beyond certain depth-time values, it is necessary to ascend in stages with time to allow an adequate amount of denitrogenation to occur before ascending further. Stage decompression is based on never exceeding the 2:1 ratio of alveolar to tissue partial pressure of nitrogen. These general principles also apply in altitude decompression sickness, in which tissues are saturated at 1 atmosphere when ascent begins.

Manifestations. The symptoms produced depend primarily upon the site of bubble formation. The size of the bubbles and their rate of growth influence the severity of symptoms. Although bizarre clinical pictures may occur, certain patterns occur frequently, suggesting a predilection to bubble formation in some tissues and organs. The most common and familiar manifestation is "*bends.*" This consists of deep, boring, and usually constant pain in the vicinity of large joints, the knees and shoulders being most frequently involved. Pain may be so severe as to be incapacitating. Most cases of bends occur within the first 30 minutes after decompression, that is, after reaching a critical altitude or after surfacing following a dive in which the depth-time factor was exceeded. Bends in flight disappear completely during descent.

Subjective skin manifestations, usually prickling or burning sensations, termed the "itches" or "creeps," occur rather commonly in fliers. Although objective skin manifestations occur uncommonly, a characteristic pale, cyanotic mottling of the skin sometimes appears, usually over the upper trunk and typically later than bends.

Chokes, believed due to bubbles in the pulmonary vasculature, occurs later than bends, and consists of burning retrosternal distress and cough. Relieved at first by shallow breathing, the symptoms progress in severity until coughing becomes paroxysmal and uncontrollable. Recompression by descent produces partial relief, but symptoms may persist for several days. Often associated with cyanosis and syncope, the syndrome has ominous significance because shock and coma may ensue.

Homonymous scintillating *scotomas* are neurologic manifestations of decompression sickness. Although apparently not observed in divers, they are common manifestations at high altitude. They are transient, and frequently disappear while still at altitude.

One or more of the manifestations already mentioned usually precede more serious stages of decompression sickness, which are characterized by neurologic manifestations and sometimes vasomotor instability that may progress to circulatory collapse with cyanosis, shock, and coma. Almost every possible neurologic sign has been observed, including motor paralysis. In altitude decompression sickness, neurologic findings are usually limited to transient paresis and dysthesias. The lower segments of the spinal cord are most frequently involved in divers, and permanent residuals may occur. In altitude decompression sickness a period of apparent recovery from the earlier manifestations may precede the appearance of circulatory collapse and shock. During this latent period vague symptoms can usually be elicited, and signs of instability of blood pressure and heart rate and at least minor focal neurologic signs can be detected. Hemoconcentration, with hematocrit as high as 60 to 70 per cent, is a characteristic finding that presumably results from widespread vascular injury and loss of plasma into tissues.

Treatment. All the varied manifestations of decompression sickness respond rapidly to early and adequate treatment by recompression. Descent from altitude produces sufficient recompression to abolish the early manifestations, but merely retards the appearance of the more slowly developing serious forms of decompression sickness. In such cases widespread bubble formation has presumably already occurred, and descent is entirely analogous to inadequate recompression therapy during which symptoms subside only temporarily. The clinical picture of decompression sickness in divers and fliers might also be expected to differ because of the greater volumes of nitrogen that must be eliminated in divers on decompression.

Divers can prevent decompression sickness by knowing and following established limits for depth and time at depth. Limitations of air supply unfortunately often prevent ascent in stages after depth-time limits have been exceeded. Adequate denitrogenation by breathing 100 per cent oxygen prior to and during ascent is an effective preventive measure in fliers. Because inadequate cabin pressurization is rarely anticipated, the procedure is often neglected. Divers should avoid the increased hazard of repeating a dive before adequate time at surface to eliminate excess nitrogen from the previous dive. Similarly, fliers who have experienced decompression symptoms during a flight should delay return to even relatively low altitudes because the expansion of bubbles still present in tissues may cause a rapid recurrence of more serious symptoms. The hazard of exposure to altitudes as low as 7000 feet after even safe depth-time dives should be recognized.

OTHER DIVING HAZARDS

Diving, by its nature, either with or without scuba, involves certain respiratory patterns that are potentially hazardous under water. Hyperventilation and breath-holding, for example, may initiate cardioinhibitory and vasodepressor reflexes capable of causing syncope, cardiac arrhythmias, and arrest. Bradycardia, apparently more pronounced than might occur simply from breath-holding and the head-down position, and various cardiac arrhythmias have also been reported during breath-hold diving. Vigorous hyperventilation by skin divers prior to a dive may lead to lowering of arterial P_{CO_2} sufficient to abolish the stimulus to breathe and may allow dangerous levels of hypoxemia to develop. In addition, compression of air within the lungs during descent may maintain adequate alveolar P_{O_2} levels despite a diminishing oxygen supply. Distress from air hunger may not occur because alveolar P_{CO_2} has been reduced by prior hyperventilation. During ascent the expansion of the air remaining within the lungs results in a sharp reduction in P_{O_2}, possibly to levels that result in loss of consciousness before the diver is able to reach the surface, and he may drown unless help is available for prompt rescue and resuscitation. Divers using properly functioning open-circuit scuba are unlikely to experience hypoxia if they restrict their dives to well within the limits of their air supply. The rate of air utilization increases in proportion to the increase in absolute pressure when using open-circuit scuba. Total duration of air supply is, for example, only one third as long at 66 feet as at the surface. Increased utilization from heavy exertion causes a proportionately greater expenditure of air.

The availability of scuba has enabled large numbers of untrained people to enter an unfamiliar and hostile environment previously restricted to trained professional divers. The increasing number of serious diving accidents attests to a general lack of understanding of basic underwater principles. As in any sport, accidents are unavoidable, but most scuba-diving casualties can be prevented. The greatest medical problem is education of those who participate in this sport. Physicians in almost any locality may now be called upon to manage a diving emergency. Excellent publications concerning this subject, such as the United States Navy Diving Manual and others, should be available for this purpose.

HYPOXIA

Hypoxia refers to the reduced partial pressure of oxygen at altitude. It thus represents an indirect effect of altered atmospheric pressure. The clinical manifestations at a given altitude are influenced primarily by duration of exposure, rate of ascent, and individual tolerance. However, the level of physical activity, the degree of health, physical conditioning, altitude acclimatization, and such factors as temperature, wind, and humidity may all modify the response in varying degrees.

The transfer of gases between lung, blood, and tissues depends upon differences in partial pressures. Alveolar air is saturated with water vapor, which exerts a constant pressure of 47 mm. of mercury. Carbon dioxide normally contributes about 40 mm. of mercury pressure to total alveolar pressure. Although total alveolar pressure is in equilibrium with atmospheric pressure, the space available for oxygen and other components of inspired air is approximately 87 mm. of mercury less than existing atmospheric pressure. Mixing of inspired with residual air further reduces alveolar partial pressure of oxygen from that in the atmosphere. The alveolar pressure constantly contributed by water vapor and CO_2 occupies an increasingly large proportion of alveolar pressure as atmospheric pressure declines. At sea level (alveolar $P_{O_2} = 103$ mm. of mercury) hemoglobin is normally 95 to 98 per cent saturated. Not until altitudes of 10,000 feet ($P_B = 523$ mm. of mercury and alveolar $P_{O_2} = 61$ mm. of mercury) does hemoglobin saturation begin to fall below 90 per cent. Thereafter saturation declines rapidly with further increase in altitude and decline in alveolar partial pressure of oxygen.

Manifestations. The first important physiologic effect of hypoxia occurs at about 5000 feet, when night vision begins to be impaired. Ventilatory and cardiovascular adjustments are minimal until about 10,000 feet, above which respiratory rate and depth and heart rate increase progressively to increase alveolar P_{O_2} and cardiac output. Exertional dyspnea may appear, and in some people mental concentration becomes difficult. Vagal cardioinhibitory reflexes may lead to bradycardia and sometimes ectopic cardiac rhythms, and may precipitate syncope. Headache, slight giddiness, and restlessness are common.

Above 15,000 feet some persons experience lassitude and indifference whereas others exhibit increased activity, irritability, euphoria, and other disturbances of affect. The impairment of judgment that begins at these altitudes jeopardizes the safety of fliers and mountain climbers. Cyanosis, loss of peripheral vision, dimming of vision, and variable degrees of muscular incoordination appear at altitudes of around 18,000 feet. Somewhere between this level and 25,000 feet, consciousness can no longer be retained for more than a few minutes. Rapid descent or administration of oxygen is essential to prevent death. If corrective action is taken soon enough, recovery is rapid and complete.

High-flying jet aircraft make it possible for many people of various ages and states of health to be exposed to the potential hazard of sudden hypoxia from rapid decompression. Should cabin pressure be abruptly lost at high altitudes, only a short period of consciousness would be possible with the breathing of ambient air. At altitudes between 30,000 feet and 45,000 feet oxygen transfer across alveolar walls would be reversed, and the duration of consciousness would shorten progressively from about 1 minute to 15 seconds, or the lung-to-brain circulation time of about 9 seconds plus around 6 seconds from oxygen already present in brain tissue. Rapid donning of oxygen masks and descent of the aircraft would shorten the period of severe hypoxia and minimize the possibility of serious injury.

Acute Mountain Sickness

This is a clinical syndrome observed in unacclimatized persons usually within a few hours after rapid exposure to high altitude. Individual tolerance varies widely. Some experience symptoms at altitudes as low as 7000 to 8000 feet, although others tolerate altitudes of 14,000 feet with minimal symptoms. There appears to be no way to predict unusual susceptibility, but rapid ascent, physical exertion, and poor physical condition increase the likelihood. Initial symptoms are usually mild to incapacitating headache, exertional dyspnea, malaise, and weakness. Insomnia, anorexia, nausea, vomiting, diarrhea, and abdominal pain may occur. Mental capacity and judgment may be impaired. Inability to sleep is a common problem. Cyanosis of the lips and nail beds, Cheyne-Stokes breathing and tachycardia are usually present. These manifestations usually subside gradually over a period of several days, but may recur at higher altitudes. In some instances the symptoms are severe and unrelieved except by oxygen or descent to a lower altitude. Gradual ascent with periodic halts of several days to allow acclimatization will prevent or reduce the severity of symptoms. Acetazolamide, given in dosages of 250 mg. every eight hours prior to and during exposure to altitude, has been reported to reduce the frequency and severity of symptoms. The mechanism of its effect is not clear, but increased ventilation and alveolar oxygen tension, decreased carbon dioxide tension and serum bicarbonate, and absence of alkalosis were observed in treated subjects.

High Altitude Pulmonary Edema

Acute pulmonary edema is an uncommon but serious and sometimes fatal complication of rapid exposure to altitudes above 9000 feet. Hypoxia is considered the primary etiologic agent. Many earlier fatal cases were erroneously diagnosed as pneumonia. Young unacclimatized persons and acclimatized residents who have sojourned at lower altitudes for a few days or weeks appear most susceptible. Recurrences are common in those who have experienced an attack. Rapid ascent and heavy physical exertion increase susceptibility.

Autopsy findings have included wet lungs congested with serosanguineous edema fluid. Bronchiolar and alveolar edema with hyaline membranes, resembling those seen in hyaline membrane disease of the newborn, over the internal walls of alveoli, alveolar sacs, and alveolar ducts have been characteristic findings. Dilatation of preterminal arterioles and thrombosis of septal capillaries and of small and medium-sized pulmonary arteries have also been observed. The exact pathogenic mechanism is conjectural. A comparative increase in capillary pressure is thought to be responsible for the alveolar edema. In a few cases pulmonary artery pressure has been elevated and electrocardiograms have suggested acute right ventricular overloading. The hyaline membrane formation, not a characteristic finding in death due to simple hypoxia, has not been explained, but a deficient pulmonary fibrinolysis system has been postulated.

Symptoms usually appear 6 to 36 hours following exposure to altitude and may be preceded by acute mountain sickness. Exertional dyspnea, weakness, malaise, and a persistent, dry, irritating cough are the characteristic initial symptoms. Later, noisy respiration, rales, cyanosis, orthopnea, and hemoptysis develop. Unless continuous oxygen therapy is carried out or the patient descends to a lower altitude, these symptoms progress, and death occurs. Gradual acclimatization and avoidance of undue physical exertion during the early period of exposure to altitude are important preventive measures.

Chronic Mountain Sickness
(Monge's Disease)

Chronic mountain sickness is a clinical syndrome that occurs in residents at high altitudes, usually over 14,000 feet, characterized by loss of tolerance to hypoxia in a previously acclimatized person. The cause is not known, but associated are increased polycythemia, decreased pulmonary ventilation, increased Pco_2, lowered arterial saturation, and impaired sensitivity of the respiratory center as compared with asymptomatic residents at high altitude. Hemoglobin and hematocrit may be increased to as much as 25 grams per 100 ml. and 80 per cent, as compared with 21 grams and 60 per cent in native residents. Hyperplasia and hyperactivity of marrow erythroid cells and pulmonary hypertension are greater than in the healthy residents.

The clinical manifestations are similar to those of erythremia. They include marked cyanosis, dyspnea, cough, palpitations, headache, giddiness, muscular weakness, pain in the extremities, sensory and motor changes, and episodic stupor. The condition can be cured only by returning to a lower altitude or to sea level.

Monge also described a less severe form of chronic mountain sickness in mountain residents that he called *subacute mountain sickness*. Many of the symptoms resemble those of acute mountain sickness, but they persist unless the patient descends to sea level or receives oxygen. The marked cyanosis and alveolar hypoventilation of chronic mountain sickness does not occur, and the laboratory findings are like those in asymptomatic natives.

Arias-Stella, J., and Kruger, H.: Pathology of high altitude pulmonary edema. Arch. Path. (Chicago), 76:147, 1963.

Armstrong, H. G.: Aerospace Medicine. Baltimore, The Williams & Wilkins Company, 1961.

Dewey, A. W., Jr.: Decompression sickness, an emerging recreational hazard. New Eng. J. Med., 267:759; 812, 1962.

Duffner, G. J., and Lanphier, E. H.: Medicine and science in sport diving. *In* Johnson, W. R. (ed.): Science and Medicine of Exercise and Sports. New York, Harper and Brothers, 1960, p. 348.

Ferris, E. B., and Engel, G. L.: The clinical nature of high altitude decompression sickness. *In* Fulton, J. F. (ed.): Decompression Sickness: Caisson Sickness, Diver's and Flier's Bends and Related Syndromes. National Research Council, Committee on Medical Sciences. Philadelphia, W. B. Saunders Company, 1951, p. 4.

Forward, S. A., Landowne, M., Follansbee, J. N., and Hansen,

J. E.: Effect of acetazolamide on acute moutain sickness. New Eng. J. Med., 279:839, 1968.

Lamb, L. E.: Aerospace medicine. *In* Dock. W., and Snapper, I. (eds.): Advances in Internal Medicine, vol. XII. Chicago, Year Book Medical Publishers, Inc., 1964, p. 175.

Lambertsen, C. J. (ed.): Proceedings of the Third Symposium on Underwater Physiology. Baltimore, The Williams & Wilkins Company, 1967.

U. S. Navy Diving Manual. United States Bureau of Ships, Department of the Navy. NAVSHIPS, 538:250, 1959.

Weihe, W. H. (ed.): Physiological Effects of High Altitude. New York, The Macmillan Company, 1964.

Gravitational Changes

Lawrence E. Lamb

Every planet influences the mass of other objects by the property of gravity, which causes mass to have weight. Gravity may be compared to acceleration. The relationship of force, mass, and acceleration may be expressed by the equation

$$force = mass \times acceleration$$

Since weight is a force, the equation may be expressed

$$weight = mass \times gravity$$

Gravitational forces are perpendicular to the planet surface. Since man developed in the gravitational field of earth, the near earth environment is used as a standard gravitational unit or 1 g. The gravitational fields of other planets are expressed in relation to the 1 g field of earth. The moon, with a mass one sixth that of earth, has a one sixth g field.

The gravitational force perpendicular to the surface of the earth may be described as a vector. Its effect upon the body is described in terms of the orientation of the gravitational vector to the three mutually perpendicular axes of the body: vertical, lateral, and anterior-posterior. These effects have been designated by symbols. While a person is standing upright, the gravitational vector is parallel with the vertical axis of the body, and there is associated pooling of blood below the diaphragm. This is designated $+G_z$. The effect of hanging head-down is designated $-G_z$. While a person is lying on his back, the gravitational vector is perpendicular to the anterior chest wall, creating a $+G_x$ effect. While he is lying prone (face down), the gravitational vector is perpendicular to the back and has a $-G_x$ effect. If the subject is lying on his left side, the gravitational vector has a $+G_y$ influence, and if he is lying on the right side, the gravitational vector has a $-G_y$ effect. The same symbols are applied to the orientation of the body in relationship to an acceleration vector; thus, forward acceleration in the seated position, as encountered during driving an automobile, produces a $+G_x$ effect. Acceleration upward in an elevator produces a $+G_z$ effect. Application of g force or acceleration force in these directions is a major consideration in aerospace flight.

Gravity is responsible for the property of body weight, the weight of organs, and the weight of fluid columns. Movement of body mass in the gravitational field requires work or energy expenditure. In this sense work is required to achieve simple standing or perform any body movement. An absence of gravity would result in a decreased work load for body movement. The weight of fluid columns also alters physiology by changing pressure gradients within closed spaces. This is illustrated by the changes in intravascular pressure at different regions of the body associated with simple standing.

Vertical g (G_z). The illustration of simple standing explains many of the physiologic effects of $+G_z$ force. Additional energy must be expended to maintain the upright position, thereby creating a work load. Certain adaptations must be made in the circulatory system. The weight created by upright columns of blood changes intravascular pressure as compared with the pressure found at the level of the aortic valve. In a male of average height the intra-arterial and intravenous pressure at the ankle may be 100 mm. of mercury higher than that noted at heart level. Conversely, intravascular pressure falls above the heart level and may be 25 mm. of mercury less within the vessels of the brain than noted at the level of the aortic valve. The latter effect is due chiefly to the length of the column of blood between the aortic valve and the occiput, which is commonly 30 cm. A column of blood of this height creates a pressure of 25 mm. of mercury. The changes in intravascular pressure may be altered by changing body position. In the seated position the column of blood from heart to ankle is shortened, and the changes in hydrostatic pressure at the ankle are lessened. Similarly, if one leans forward while in the seated position, the height of the column of blood between heart and the brain is decreased, diminishing the changes in pressure between the heart and brain.

There are many circulatory adaptations to the g force encountered in simple standing. Changes in arteriolar tone are affected by peripheral arteriolar constriction, principally in regions below the diaphragm. These changes control the distribution of blood flow or cardiac output in an effort to maintain adequate cerebral blood flow. The mechanisms controlling peripheral arteriolar tone are complex and involve both reflex mechanisms and humoral factors. Failure to increase peripheral arteriolar tone while standing may result in inadequate cerebral blood flow and loss of consciousness. Standing increases the amount of blood pooled below the diaphragm. Commonly, the blood volume in the lower extremities increases 15 per cent. This diminishes the available circulating blood volume. Since the venous reservoir is readily expansile, factors that are associated with increased tone of the venous wall or extravascular pressure in the form of tissue tension or muscle tone tend to control the amount of venous pooling. In the absence of adequate extravascular pressure or diminished venous tone, venous pooling may be excessive, resulting in diminished venous return to the heart, and fainting. Methods of applying external pressure, such as elastic bandages, elastic stockings, or the anti-g pressure garment used in aerospace activities, all serve to limit the expansion of the venous reservoir and venous pooling. By adequate control of this factor, major deficiencies in arteriolar tone can be tolerated.

The increased intravascular pressure in both the arteriolar and the venous circulatory components results in diffusion of water from the intravascular to the extravascular spaces. The normal reabsorption of fluid by the venous circulation due to the osmotic pressure of plasma proteins and the extravascular tissue tension is not effected as readily since the intravascular pressure gradient exceeds their combined influence. This results in a gradual increase in hydration of extravascular spaces and skeletal muscles. Those muscles that have tight fascial sheaths increase their tension and apply external pressure to the venous reservoir, thereby eventually tending to balance the pressure gradients and deter loss of fluid from the intravascular compartment. The loss of fluid to the extravascular spaces results in gradual decrease in plasma volume, which contributes to fainting after prolonged standing. This adverse effect can be counteracted by body movements or muscular contraction that tends to massage the venous reservoir and decrease intravenous pressure.

The circulatory adaptations described above are frequently associated with increased heart rate, fall in systolic pressure, and narrowing of pulse pressure. When these are severe, they may be associated with symptoms of orthostatic intolerance or simple fainting. During aerospace flight or human centrifuge studies, advantage may be taken of body position and other factors that decrease the vertical height of the column of blood. Normally, man cannot tolerate increased acceleration loads above 4 to 5 g. As the g load increases, the pressure created by the column of blood between the aortic valve and the base of the brain is gradually increased. At 2 g's the column of blood exerts the pressure of approximately 50 mm. of mercury. At 4 g's the 30 cm. column of blood exerts the pressure of approximately 100 mm. of mercury. When $+G_z$ loads are sufficiently increased (3 to 4 g's), visual disturbances occur. These are noted prior to fainting because the naturally occurring intraocular pressure causes a lower pressure gradient than noted in the brain. Peripheral vision is lost first,

and finally circulation to the eye may be sufficiently impaired that vision is lost, but the person may still be conscious. A further increase of approximately 1 g usually results in loss of consciousness; this is noted at levels between 4 and 5 $+G_z$. The lunar environment of $1/6$ g has an effect similar to that of being in a bed tilted upright 10 degrees. The 30 cm. column of blood would exert a pressure of only 6 mm. of mercury, and the difference between the pressure at heart level and in the brain would be minimal.

Other minor alterations in circulation are noted during $+G_z$ loads. These include clearing of blood from the apices of the lung and diminished cardiac size. Upon cessation of the g load the cardiac rate may slow abruptly with a cardioinhibitory response. This may result in bradycardia or such disturbances as nodal rhythm with A-V dissociation.

Tolerance to $+G_z$ loads may vary because of such factors as anxiety, fasting, fatigue, and level of physical fitness. Physical stature also influences g tolerance. The short, stocky person with a short neck commonly has a shorter column of blood between the heart and the base of the brain, and usually tolerates increased g loads better than a tall, thin person.

Transverse g (G_x). When an automobile starts from a standing position or an airplane accelerates for take-off, a person seated in it experiences $+G_x$ acceleration. The astronaut lying on his back in the space vehicle during rocket firing experiences forces oriented in the same direction. Under these circumstances the long axis of the major vessels of the circulatory system is perpendicular to the direction of g force application. The absence of any significant vertical height in the fluid columns prevents extensive weight change in long columns of blood. The application of acceleration forces in this direction allows man to tolerate forces of a much greater magnitude. The major load is placed on the respiratory system. Breathing is difficult or impossible while high levels of transverse acceleration are sustained. Normally, for short periods of time man can tolerate $+G_x$ loads of 10 g's. This principle has enabled man to tolerate acceleration forces of sufficient magnitude to achieve orbital velocity for space vehicles and manned space flight. At high g loads there is compression of the posterior region of the lungs and overexpansion of the alveoli in the anterior regions of the lungs. These variations, however, have not been noted to be sufficiently great to create problems within the range of g loads encountered for manned space flight.

In addition to the influence upon the lungs, $+G_x$ forces sustained through a period of time may precipitate supraventricular cardiac arrhythmias. Usually these are in the form of sporadic atrial premature contractions. In some instances short bursts of atrial tachycardia may be observed. The arrhythmias are thought to be secondary to distention of the atria associated with sudden increase in venous return secondary to pressure on the abdomen.

Weightlessness. Energy expenditure during weightlessness secondary to body movement is not entirely absent since much energy is expended in overcoming the muscle viscosity during its contraction. This factor is not dependent on weight. The more rapid the movement, the greater will be the percentage of energy required to overcome muscle viscosity. Decreased energy requirement decreases the work load on the circulatory and musculoskeletal system and, secondarily, may influence the blood volume and hemopoietic activity. These effects are independent of hydrostatic factors related to gravity. In many ways simple bed rest is analogous to the influence of weightlessness since in both circumstances significant increases in intravascular pressure secondary to increased vertical height of any blood column are prevented. In the normally active person simple bed rest and weightlessness appear to induce *"recumbency diuresis."* This has been repeatedly observed in human studies. Recumbency diuresis is caused by a shift of blood volume into the thorax, resulting in distention of the left atrium, which in turn causes reflex inhibition of secretion of antidiuretic hormones, thereby inducing diuresis.

Blood volume is partially maintained by migration of water into the vascular bed from the well hydrated tissues and the high tissue tension. The process continues until a new homeostatic level of hydration is achieved. This usually represents a water loss of 1 to 2 liters and a weight loss of 1 or 2 kg. Larger weight losses have been repeatedly observed during the longer manned space flights even when other factors contributing to dehydration have apparently been controlled. Decreased hydration results in weight loss, decreased tissue tension, decreased plasma volume and, consequently, decreased blood volume. The mean plasma volume loss during simple bed rest is approximately 500 ml., which usually occurs within 24 to 48 hours after the beginning of recumbency. The decreased blood volume and tissue tension or the decreased level of hydration has an immediate effect upon orthostatic tolerance.

Continued bed rest of four weeks' duration or other forms of inactivity are accompanied by a *decreased red cell mass* of approximately 300 ml. The decreased red cell mass and decreased plasma volume result in an average decrease of 800 ml. of blood volume after four weeks of simple bed rest. It is assumed that bone marrow activity is also curtailed.

Urinary calcium excretion increases progressively through the fourth week of bed rest. The values are below those commonly associated with an increased incidence of stone.

Inferences as to what may be expected from longer manned space flights than those achieved today are drawn from laboratory study modes of the influence of bed rest on normal human subjects. In addition to the changes described above, *decrease in heart size, increase in heart rate,* and *decrease in exercise tolerance* are observed. *Foot pain* after absence of weight bearing is real and a matter of practical importance for post-flight activity. It is of equal importance for the patient who has been kept at bed rest for prolonged periods of time.

Human centrifuge studies have demonstrated that four weeks of bed rest, and presumably weightlessness, does not significantly prevent tolerance to de-orbit requirements that expose men to $+G_x$ loads. To prevent fainting in the post-orbital flight period, time-honored procedures may be used; these include advantageous body position (head between the knees, feet above the head) and muscle contraction, the latter to milk blood back to the heart and prevent excessive venous pooling.

The anti-g suit has proved successful in preventing fainting and significant changes in heart rate or blood pressure associated with decreased orthostatic tolerance during tilt-table studies performed after prolonged bed rest. Its action is to prevent venous pooling by external compression of the venous reservoir. Increased physical fitness prior to bed rest helps prevent deconditioning, but for basic physiologic reasons associated with transport of fluid across the capillary membrane it may not prevent recumbency diuresis. Exercises in the recumbent position cannot maintain the level of hydration noted during the ambulatory state unless they are carried out nearly continuously. Various forms of exercise can be used to maintain a high level of cardiac function in the absence of the work load imposed by gravity. Other devices are currently under study as means of preventing the physiologic changes noted with bed rest and encountered in prolonged weightlessness. These include the use of hypoxia to stimulate bone marrow in maintaining erythropoietic action and red cell mass. Hypoxia may also provide some means of controlling the mobilization of calcium. The use of devices to produce negative pressure or suction over the external surface of the lower body is being studied as a means of simulating the circulatory changes encountered with standing on earth. Such a device used with the subject at bed rest when adequate salt and water are administered is capable of rehydrating him to the level of hydration noted during the ambulatory state. The increased hydration by such a device while the subject is still recumbent prevents decreased orthostatic tolerance and fainting when the subject assumes the upright posture or stands in the normal g field. The use of salt-retaining hormones and other devices offers promise in this area. The basic principles in maintaining an optimal state compatible with upright posture and upright activity in the normal g field are to maintain the level of hydration by devices or other means that prevent decrease in level of hydration associated with recumbency, to maintain normal erythropoiesis and bone marrow activity, to maintain cardiac function and skeletal muscle tone, and to prevent significant losses of skeletal calcium or excessive excretion of high calcium loads in the urine.

Lamb, L. E.: Aerospace medicine. *In* Advances in Internal Medicine, Vol. XII. Chicago, Year Book Medical Publishers, Inc., 1964, p. 175.

Lamb, L. E.: Aerospace cardiology. *In* Proceedings of the Second National Conference on Cardiovascular Diseases. Washington, D. C., November 22, 1964.

Lamb, L. E.: Hypoxia — An anti-deconditioning factor for manned space flight. Aerospace Med., 36:97, 1965.

Lamb, L. E., Stevens, P. M., and Johnson, R. L.: Hypokinesia secondary to chair rest from 4 to 10 days. Aerospace Med., 36:755, 1965.

Lamb, L. E., and Stevens, P. M.: The influence of lower body negative pressure on the level of hydration during bed rest. Aerospace Med., 36:1145, 1965.

Miller, P. B., Johnson, R. L., and Lamb, L. E.: The effects of four weeks of absolute bed rest on circulatory functions in man. Aerospace Med., 35:1194, 1964.

Miller, P. B., and Leverett, S. D., Jr.: Tolerance to transverse ($+G_x$) and headward ($+G_z$) acceleration after prolonged bed rest. Aerospace Med., 36:13, 1965.

Torphy, D. E., Leverett, S. D., Jr., and Lamb, L. E.: Cardiac arrhythmias occurring during acceleration. Aerospace Med., 37:52, 1966.

Motion Sickness and Problems of Air Travel

Harold V. Ellingson

MOTION SICKNESS

Manifestations and Occurrence. Motion sickness is a syndrome characterized by pallor, sweating, salivation, and nausea that frequently progresses to vomiting. Prostration may be severe if exposure to precipitating factors is prolonged. It may occur in persons riding in airplanes, ships, automobiles, or trains, or sometimes in children following prolonged or vigorous sessions in playground swings. Among air travelers, the incidence has declined with introduction of newer jet transports that fly at altitudes above the layers of most turbulent air. The disorder still remains a problem among passengers in small aircraft and others flying at low altitudes in stormy or hot weather, when turbulence may be severe.

Etiology. Causative factors are not completely understood. Labyrinthine stimulation resulting from repetitive pitching, rolling, rotating, or up-and-down motion is clearly a most important factor, since persons with nonfunctioning labyrinths are often totally insusceptible to motion sickness, and since incidence and severity are commonly proportional to severity and duration of the motion. Psychic factors also appear to be important. Apprehension undoubtedly predisposes to motion sickness; a few unfortunates feel nauseated on stepping aboard a motionless airplane or a ship at a pier. Some people can tolerate motion without distress until they smell an unpleasant odor such as that of cigar smoke or the vomitus of a fellow passenger. Visceral sensations of motion appear to be contributory, since abdominal restraint reduces incidence of reactions. Visual stimuli apparently may play a part; symptoms sometimes occur in an immobile subject who watches moving pictures depicting motion.

Prevention and Treatment. Prophylaxis may often be achieved by the use of any of a number of drugs, given 30 minutes to an hour before the trip begins. Hyoscine, 1.2 mg., with d-amphetamine, 20 mg., meclizine (Bonine), 25 to 50 mg., cyclizine (Marezine), 50 mg., and dimenhydrinate (Dramamine), 50 mg., are among the most effective agents. For prolonged journeys, the same dose of meclizine or hyoscine-d-amphetamine should be given every 24 hours; doses of cyclizine or dimenhydrinate should be repeated every four to six hours as required. A traveler who senses the onset of an attack may often avert nausea and vomiting by reclining as far as possible, by holding his head firmly against a pillow or head rest, by closing his eyes or fixing his gaze on a point, and by increasing his ventilation with cool air. In treatment, the same drugs mentioned above are useful, though retention may be difficult if vomiting has already occurred. Fortunately, symptoms usually disappear soon after the journey is concluded or motion has ceased. Recovery following prolonged vomiting may be hastened by fluid replacement.

PROBLEMS OF AIR TRAVEL

For the normal person, and for most ambulatory patients under a physician's care, air travel is no more trying than is travel by any other means. However, a physician should be informed of factors encountered in flight that may have an influence on his patient's welfare. Besides accepting as passengers many ambulatory patients under the care of physicians, most airlines are prepared to carry litter patients; special litters can be accommodated by adjustment or removal of several seats. In remote areas, private flying agencies sometimes provide air ambulance service to large medical centers. Before a patient travels or is moved by air, the physician should consider the hazards mentioned below and should, if necessary, discuss the case with a medical official of the carrier. The patient's condition, the altitude and duration of the flight, the cabin pressure altitude, and the availability of oxygen in flight all have a bearing on suitability of air travel by, or movement of, a patient. With proper precautions, all but a few patients can safely be carried by air.

Factors to be Considered. Aside from the possibility of motion sickness, the two most important factors to be considered in air travel by patients are reduction in air pressure and reduction in oxygen content of air at altitude. Cabin pressurization in larger and newer aircraft minimizes these changes, but hazards may be present for a few persons.

In pressurized airplanes, cabin pressure is normally maintained at a fixed excess over that of the outside air. The amount of excess varies with the type of aircraft, but the differential is commonly in the neighborhood of 8 pounds per square inch. This gives a cabin pressure that does not fall below that of sea level until the aircraft reaches 22,000 feet. Above this, internal pressure falls until at 40,000 feet the cabin has an "altitude" of 7000 feet above sea level. In older aircraft, pressure differentials are smaller, and cabin pressures on some flights may be equivalent to as much as 9000 feet. Only a few light aircraft are pressurized; these are often flown at 10,000 to 12,000 feet, or even more over mountainous terrain.

Hazards of Reduced Pressure. A bubble of gas trapped within the body will expand as air pressure is reduced. At an altitude of 5000 feet, trapped gas expands to 125 per cent of its sea level volume, and at 10,000 feet to 150 per cent of its sea level volume. Expansion causes pressure on surrounding tissues; this may jeopardize blood supply, and may cause rupture of containing walls.

Persons with *unreduced hernia* should not fly, since if gas is trapped it may expand and interfere with circulation. A *perforating wound of the eyeball or the skull* may allow entrance of a bubble of air that might expand at altitude. Patients with these injuries should not travel or be moved by air until absorption is complete. Patients with *pneumothorax* should not fly until all air has been absorbed. The same caution applies following *pneumoencephalography.* Expansion of abdominal gas causes some distention, and patients who have had *abdominal surgery* should not fly for two weeks following surgery. A patient with a *colostomy* may expect filling of the bag on ascent. Patients with *acute upper respiratory tract disease* may have discomfort in the sinuses or middle ear because of closure of the ostia of the sinuses or the eustachian tube and consequent failure of pressure adjustment during ascent or descent; use of decongestant nose drops or inhalers before flight may avert difficulty. A similar precaution is useful for the patient with *chronic sinusitis* or *allergic rhinitis.* Patients with *lung cavities, abscesses,* or *bullous emphysema* should not fly because of the danger of rupture.

Hazards of Reduced Oxygen. Oxygen content of alveolar air is reduced at increasing altitudes. Though oxygen saturation of the blood is less markedly reduced, patients whose tissue oxygenation is marginal for any reason (whether from impaired pulmonary function, reduced oxygen-

carrying capacity of the blood, or impaired tissue circulation) should not fly unless prior arrangement has been made with the airline for oxygen to be continuously available in flight. Patients should not fly following *myocardial infarction* until they are symptom-free with moderate exertion, usually at least six weeks after an attack. Patients with *angina pectoris* that is symptomatic on climbing a flight of stairs should have supplemental oxygen available during flight. *Anemia,* when the hemoglobin is less than 50 per cent, should preclude flight unless oxygen is available. A person with *sickle-cell disease* or *sickling trait* is vulnerable to hemolytic crisis and splenic infarction with reduced oxygen tension, and should not fly without oxygen in flight. Patients with *developing gangrene* or *carbon monoxide poisoning* should not be moved without supplemental oxygen in flight. Any *pulmonary disease,* when severe enough to cause cyanosis at ground level, to seriously impair exercise tolerance, or to reduce vital capacity below 50 per cent of normal, is a contraindication to flight unless supplemental oxygen is made available.

Aerial movement is sometimes considered for a patient who has recently suffered from an attack of *poliomyelitis.* In general, such a patient should not be moved by air until his condition has become stabilized. If respiratory paralysis has occurred, the patient who is able to be out of a respirator for 8 to 12 hours a day can usually be moved safely by air. For those requiring a respirator continuously, portable equipment is available that can be carried in aircraft. Such patients should be observed carefully in flight by an experienced attendant, with special attention to the maintenance of normal ventilatory exchange and the avoidance of dehydration, as this tends to make secretions thicker and more difficult to aspirate. If bulbar involvement has caused difficulty in swallowing, a tracheostomy should be performed prior to flight to ensure adequacy of the airway.

Time Zone Changes. Subjective fatigue and delays in adjustment to time zone changes following east-west or west-east travel are matters of common observation. Not only sleeping habits, but more profound cycles of deep body temperature, water and electrolyte excretion, plasma lactic dehydrogenase, and other physiologic measures are involved. The time required for a traveler to "get on schedule" at the destination depends upon many factors, including individual characteristics, the number of time zones passed, the opportunities for rest before and after flight, and, for some, the direction of flight. A traveler to the west is not likely to have trouble in going to sleep at night in the new time zone, but he may have morning insomnia; one traveling several time zones to the east is likely to experience evening insomnia and retarded awakening. If the traveler has a tendency toward insomnia, travel may cause a troublesome accentuation.

Studies have indicated some actual impairment of psychologic performance in the 24 hours immediately following travel through 7 to 12 time zones. Performance has commonly returned to normal following one good night's sleep. Adjustment of sleeping habits and the overcoming of subjective fatigue may take several days; the deeper physiologic cycles require longer periods—from four to eight days for adjustment to a time differential of 7 to 12 zones.

Travelers can minimize problems by giving special attention to rest before and after long flights. If circumstances permit before the trip, the prospective traveler may benefit from modifying his sleep schedules toward those of the destination. Trusted somnifacients for a few nights after arrival may speed the adjustment. Some experienced travelers recommend that "million dollar decisions" be avoided in the first 24 hours after a long flight.

Other Hazards. Prolonged sitting and inactivity may be hazardous for persons with a history of *thrombophlebitis* or other circulatory disorder of the lower extremities. These patients should be advised to move about frequently during long flights. A patient with a *fractured jaw* treated by fixation should not fly because of the danger of aspirating vomitus in case of motion sickness. If he must fly, a quick-release fixation should be devised.

Common Questions. Physicians are often asked questions about flying. *Normal infants* tolerate air travel well, but feeding should be given during descent, to facilitate aeration of the middle ear by swallowing. *Old age* in itself is no contraindication to flight, if significant disease is not present. *Pregnancy* is no contraindication to flight, but if the mother is near term, the airline may require a physician's statement that delivery is not likely to occur during the flight. There is no evidence that the mild oxygen deficit in the atmosphere is harmful to the fetus. *Hypertension* is not adversely affected by air travel, though preflight sedation may be appropriate. Patients with *communicable diseases* should, of course, not travel when hazards of transmission to others exist. *Patients whose conditions make them objectionable to others,* such as those with urinary incontinence or malodorous discharges, should not travel in the crowded cabins of commercial aircraft. *Mild asthma* is not ordinarily adversely affected by flight. Patients subject to severe asthmatic attacks should carry their tested medications, and should ensure in advance the availability of oxygen if needed. In *epileptics,* oxygen deficiency and hyperventilation attending excitement in flight may precipitate seizures. Persons subject to frequent seizures should have proper medication, including sedation, prior to travel by air and if possible should be accompanied by an attendant. *Psychiatric disorders* require individual evaluation; the likelihood of disturbance or agitation under the minimal stress of travel and the safety and comfort of fellow passengers should be considered. Questions regarding other conditions should be referred to the airline's nearest medical official. Indeed, it is advisable to discuss with the airline's medical official any prospective passenger whose condition might be unfavorably influenced by flight.

Beighton, P. H., and Richard, P. R.: Cardiovascular disease in air travelers. Brit. Heart J., 30:367, 1968.

Bergin, K. G.: Transport of invalids by air. Brit. Med. J., 3:539, 1967.

Buley, L. E.: Formula for determining rest periods on long distance air travel. Aerospace Med., 41:680, 1970.

Committee on Medical Criteria: Medical criteria for passenger flying. Arch. Environ. Health (Chicago), 2.124, 1961.

Hauty, G. T., and Adams, T.: Phase shifts of the human circadian system and performance deficit during periods of transition. Aerospace Med., 37:668, 1029, 1966.

Wood, C. D., and Graybiel, A.: Evaluation of sixteen antimotion sickness drugs. Aerospace Med., 39:1341, 1968.

Electric Shock

David H. Goldstein

Electricity may damage the body in three ways: (1) Its effect upon the central nervous system or the heart may briefly stun the victim, produce reversible loss of consciousness or death. (2) The heat may coagulate tissue, with resultant necrosis. Arcing of the current may scorch or even metallize the skin, or there may be flame burns from clothing. (3) Powerful tetanic muscular contractions may lead to injury of bones or soft tissue.

Passage of electric current through the body may produce various effects, depending upon the intensity of the current. The latter in turn depends on the voltage and the resistance of the tissues, chiefly the skin. Skin resistance increases with thickness and is diminished by moisture. Perspiration, by reducing skin resistance to the flow of current through the body, is a factor in the higher fatality rate from electric shock observed during summer months. Electrocution in the bath tub from house current is attributable to the reduction of body skin resistance by water from approximately 3000 ohms to about 500 ohms, together with the ready grounding through the pipes. If the body is well insulated, it may not be damaged even by a high-tension voltage (currents in excess of 1000 volts). Small currents of the order of one milliampere produce a slight tingling sensation. Contraction of the muscles takes place as the current intensity increases. Muscular contractions may be of such severity as to prevent the victim from freeing himself from the circuit. In general, men can free themselves from currents of 9 or less milliamperes, whereas the top "let go" value for women is 6 milliamperes. Failure to let go may result in a reduction in skin resistance through secondary perspiration or blistering, with a consequent rise in current intensity to lethal levels. A current of 0.1 ampere flowing from hands to feet is sufficient to produce ventricular fibrillation.

Not only do the pathways of the current and the duration of the shock influence outcome, but the frequency of alternation plays a role. The 60 cycle frequency of house current in the United States is in a very harmful range. Fatal shocks have been reported with as little as 25 volts A.C. Diathermy, in contrast, produces currents that oscillate at one million cycles a second, involves currents of 20,000 to 40,000 volts at 1 to 2 milliamperes, but does not shock. Direct currents are less harmful than alternating currents. The outcome following contact with high tension currents is often not fatal because the victim is jolted free from the power source.

Electric current diffuses through the body from the point of entrance to the point of exit, usually the feet. The entrance and exit sites may exhibit focal burns because the skin, in offering resistance to the passage of the current, converts electrical energy into heat. Perforations may be seen in clothing or shoes at the points of exit. Should the current enter and leave the body over wide areas of low resistance, as provided by water and good grounding, neither current marks nor burns will be found.

If harmful effects are to be exerted on the heart, it must be in the pathway between the entrance and exit of the current. Once the skin barrier is penetrated, the body offers little resistance to the passage of current, and the waterways, the blood vessels, and intravascular spaces provide an excellent conduction system.

Lightning is a special form of current characterized by a rapid discharge of enormous potential. The currents involved are of the order of thousands of millions of volts and an estimated 20,000 amperes, operating over an average time of 30 microseconds. Although capable of tremendously powerful disruptive force, lightning can be capricious, and is by no means invariably fatal. There are accounts of one person struck by lightning and merely stunned, while a companion who received the discharge from the elbow of the survivor was killed. Victims have had their clothes torn from them and been only stunned or rendered briefly unconscious. On the other hand, a "direct hit" can produce instantaneous death.

Incidence. Approximately 150 persons are killed each year by lightning in the United States, and an equal number die from accidental electrocution in the home. Approximately 700 persons are killed by accidental electrocution at work annually.

Pathology. Aside from those cases with evidence of trauma or burns, the microscopic findings may be limited to a few petechial hemorrhages in the brain and elsewhere. The blood is often dark and uncoagulated. These scanty findings are reported even in those cases of penal electrocution subjected to sustained currents of 1700 volts at 7

amperes. Hughes concluded from this and other laboratory evidence that death in cases of electric shock (without other trauma) is due to ventricular fibrillation and not paralysis of the respiratory center. This conclusion is contested by others, however, who hold the opposite view.

Clinical Manifestations. Electric shock may induce violent muscular spasms and immediate death. In some cases the patient survives the immediate shocking effect of the current but dies later of burns or blunt-force injury. Burns usually are limited to the skin, but with high intensity currents the damage may be deep and extensive, requiring amputation.

Frequently, survivors of electric shock are in an acute state of fear, approaching panic. They are trembling, pale, and sweating. Paralysis of an affected limb may persist up to four hours, and subsequent muscular pain and stiffness may continue for weeks or months as may mild personality changes. There are usually no permanent effects in those recovering from shock. It is rare to find late changes in the electrocardiogram. In severe burns, delayed hemorrhage must be watched for. Cataract formation days or months after the electrical accident has been recorded.

Prognosis. Recent developments in resuscitation, and, more specifically, in external cardiac massage (closed chest) have improved the prognosis in electric shock. No precise case fatality rate or figures on the success of artificial resuscitation can be given. The variations in circumstances of electric shock, the current exposure, the wearing of protective clothing, the proficiency by which resuscitation is administered, and the time between shock and therapy all influence the outcome. In the electric utility industry, the Oesterreich Pole Top Method described by Franco has yielded a 60 per cent successful resuscitation rate when instituted within one minute, based on unpublished data. Recovery falls to 45 per cent when instituted at three minutes and 27 per cent in four minutes.

Treatment. As soon as the victim is freed from the current, artificial respiration and external cardiac massage should be started if spontaneous respiration has ceased. Both artificial respiration and artificial circulation should be maintained simultaneously until satisfactory central nervous system and cardiac function has returned. The mouth-to-mouth method of artificial respiration is employed. Reference should be made to publications of Jude, Kouwenhoven, and their associates, who report successful resuscitation by their method, and outline the steps in treatment to be followed: (1) rapid diagnosis, (2) artificial ventilation, and (3) artificial circulation (external massage), (4) cardiotonic drug therapy, (5) electrocardiogram, (6) defibrillation if necessary, (7) continued cardiovascular and pulmonary support, and (8) postresuscitation therapy.

The treatment of burns will depend on their extent, but for burns confined to the skin a conservative approach is advocated.

In high voltage electrical accidents, it is recommended that efforts to effect alkalinization of the urine be instituted at once. To those who are conscious, sodium bicarbonate can be given by mouth in doses of 4 to 6 grams of bicarbonate in about 300 ml. of water every 15 minutes prior to hospitalization, when intravenous therapy may be instituted. Nephrosis with oliguria or anuria is a common complication, and calls for the usual treatment of renal failure, described elsewhere in this text.

Fischer, H.: Pathologic effects and sequelae of electrical accidents. Electrical burns (secondary accidents, renal manifestations, sequelae) J. Occup. Med., 7:564, 1965.

Franco, S. C.: Electric shock and cardiopulmonary resuscitation. Arch. Environ. Health (Chicago), 19:261, 1969.

Gonzales, T. A., Vance, M., Helpern, M., and Umberger, C. J.: Legal Medicine—Pathology and Toxicology. 2nd ed. New York, Appleton-Century-Crofts, Inc., 1954.

Jude, J. R., Kouwenhoven, W. B., and Knickerbocker, G. G.: Cardiac arrest. J.A.M.A., 178:1063, 1961.

Maclachlan, W.: Electrical shock. Canad. Med. Ass. J., 80:210, 1959.

Proceedings of the International Symposium on Electrical Accidents, Paris, May 2–5, 1962. Geneva, International Occupational Safety and Health Information Center (CIS), ILO, 1964

Ravitch, M. M., Lane, R., Safar, P., Steichen, F. M., and Knowles, P.: Lightning stroke. New Eng. J. Med., 264:36, 1961.

Drowning

Charles J. Stahl

Definition. Drowning is a cause of death that may result from asphyxia by inhalation of fluid into the respiratory tract, or from the complex biochemical and hemodynamic changes that follow the inhalation of fluid during immersion.

Etiology. Accidents account for most drownings, and victims of drowning are often children or other persons who have not learned to swim. Less frequently, drowning may result from suicide or homicide. The circumstances for accidental drowning may include the following: (1) disasters such as floods and tidal waves, as well as shipwrecks and vehicular accidents; (2) hazardous environmental conditions of aquatic sports or occupational activities; and (3) disability while swimming when there is pre-existing illness, intoxication by ethanol or drugs, exhaustion, or overexertion.

Incidence and Prevalence. Each year in the United States, there are over 6000 deaths by drowning and approximately the same number of near-drownings. Drowning is the fourth most common type of accidental death. When underwater accidents are considered alone, drowning is the most common cause of death. It occurs more frequently than deaths from barotrauma, including air embolism and decompression sickness, discussed in the article titled Alterations in Atmospheric Pressure. Several million Americans engage in the sport of underwater swimming, using either self-contained underwater breathing apparatus (scuba) or snorkel. Aquatic accidents may constitute a public health problem in certain geographic areas where underwater swimming is prevalent.

Pathogenesis. Survivors of near-drowning and studies with laboratory animals have provided knowledge of the sequence of events that occur during drowning. The victim of drowning or near-drowning usually experiences panic at the time of complete immersion, and struggles to reach the surface. Small amounts of water may be inhaled or swallowed. It is common to hold the breath and to persist in this until accumulation of carbon dioxide stimulates the respiratory center. At the time it is no longer possible to restrain the urge to breathe, pulmonary carbon dioxide tension is high and pulmonary oxygen tension is low. Gasping, inhalation of water or other liquid, and loss of consciousness are associated with coughing, vomiting, convulsions, and finally death. In about 10 to 15 per cent of cases, however, the initial aspiration of fluid causes laryngospasm and closure of the glottis, resulting in reflex cardiac inhibition, cardiac arrhythmia, or asphyxia. Rescue prior to the terminal inhalation of fluid, as well as appropriate treatment, may interrupt the course of fatal events and bring on spontaneous recovery. Prompt action is required, for death may occur within several minutes after the victim experiences distress during immersion.

The pathophysiologic changes in drowning, based upon studies with laboratory animals, were poorly understood until the work reported by Swann and Spafford in 1951. They demonstrated that the hemodynamic changes during drowning of dogs depend upon the type of fluid medium. When drowning occurs in fresh water, rapid absorption of hypotonic water from the lungs into the circulation results in hypervolemia, hemodilution, and hemolysis. Serum electrolytes, except for potassium produced by hemolysis, are decreased. The alteration in the ratio between sodium and potassium, as well as anoxia, may cause ventricular fibrillation. The mechanism for drowning in sea water, however, is probably different. As the result of the aspiration of sea water, salts pass into the circulation and fluids diffuse into alveoli. Serum electrolytes, particularly chloride and magnesium, increase markedly. Hypovolemia, hemoconcentration, and hypoproteinemia occur. Increased vascular permeability, endothelial damage, and diffusion of plasma into the alveoli are manifested by pulmonary edema and production of frothy white foam in the airway. Studies by Modell and others in 1968 indicate that the amount of fresh water or sea water aspirated by laboratory animals is directly related to the changes in serum electrolytes. At least 20 ml. of water per pound of body weight must be aspirated by dogs to cause persistent changes in electrolytes, as well as ventricular fibrillation.

In persons who survive near-drowning and in human victims of drowning, the pathophysiologic mechanisms seem less well understood and may differ from experimental findings. The majority of human victims of drowning aspirate 10 ml. of fluid or less per pound of body weight. Although biochemical and hemodynamic changes have been stressed previously, clinical evaluations of near-drowning victims suggest that fluid and electrolyte balance is restored rapidly. Significant changes in serum electrolytes and volume of blood have been uncommon. Hemodilution has not been demonstrated, but hemoconcentration may be evident in victims of near-drowning in both fresh water and sea water.

Nonspecific electrocardiographic changes, as well as cardiac arrhythmias, may occur, but ventricular fibrillation is uncommon in human victims. Pulmonary edema, aspiration of foreign material with the water, and hypoxia serve as the basis for the signs and symptoms of the post-immersion syndrome. These cases of near-drowning are frequently complicated by infections of the respiratory tract, leading to pneumonia, lung abscess, or empyema. Instead of profound changes in electrolytes or cardiac arrhythmia, it is more likely that human deaths may be attributed to asphyxia that results in respiratory insufficiency, arterial hypoxemia, and metabolic acidosis.

The pathologic findings are often nonspecific. The white or bloody foam, usually seen in the mouth, nose, and tracheobronchial tree, may not be evident after attempts at resuscitation. Often the skin of the palms and soles is wrinkled and pale. These changes, known as "washerwoman's skin," are consistent with immersion but they are not pathognomonic of drowning. Lacerations or incised wounds of the skin, without evidence of vital reaction, reflect the effects of tides, collision of the body with underwater obstacles, and postmortem injuries inflicted by sharp objects such as motorboat propellors. Mutilation of a body by aquatic animals, particularly the soft tissues about the eyes, nose, and lips, is common. The lungs are heavy and edematous. Foreign material from the aquatic environment may be seen in the tracheobronchial tree. Hemorrhage is frequently observed in the middle ear and mastoid air cells. Microscopic unicellular or colonial algae, containing silica and known as diatoms, offer evidence that death resulted from drowning when demonstrated in organs of the systemic circulation, as well as in the water in which the body was found. After prolonged immersion in water, the changes of decomposition and the effects of aquatic life obscure the usual anatomic findings. Except for pulmonary edema and demonstration of diatoms, the microscopic findings in the lungs are nonspecific. In laboratory animals (rats), differences have been observed in the ultrastructural changes of lungs in fresh-water and sea-water drownings. With sea water, cellular swelling and vacuolation, as well as discontinuity of alveolar lining cells, were noted. After drowning in fresh water, the lungs of rats showed endothelial destruction, mitochondrial swelling, and cellular disruption. Histochemical changes have also been observed in rats. An acute perivasculitis, consisting mainly of neutrophils, is seen in the lungs after drowning in sea water. Similar changes, but to a lesser extent, are seen in fresh-water drowning. The distribution and amount of peroxidase-positive granules in the histologic sections parallel the density of the neutrophilic infiltration around vessels. These findings may serve as the basis for a distinction between drowning in sea water and drowning in fresh water. Numerous chemical and physical tests have been applied to the diagnosis of drowning. These tests include concentrations of chloride or magnesium in whole blood, plasma, or serum; specific gravity of whole blood; and refractive index, electrical conductivity, and osmolarity of blood. The period of reliability and usefulness for these tests is limited to several hours after death. They are usually not reliable after the onset of decomposition. Determination of the specific gravity of plasma from the right and left sides of the heart seems more reliable and subject to less variability than other studies.

Clinical Manifestations. The victim of drowning usually experiences breath-holding and burning suffocation, as well as loss of consciousness and inhalation of fluid. On occasion, the victim appears tranquil, and shows passive behavior. After rescue, the patient is usually unconscious, flaccid, cold, and cyanotic. Respirations are absent, and the pulse is imperceptible. If the patient is conscious, tinnitus and visual abnormalities are often reported. Frothy fluid may be seen in the nose and mouth, and examination of the chest may disclose signs of pulmonary edema. If a significant amount of water has been swallowed, nausea and vomiting may occur, and gastric distention may be evident. Electrocardiographic changes are often nonspecific, and they are related to myocardial anoxia. Cardiac arrhythmias such as atrial fibrillation and ventricular fibrillation, as reported for animals, are uncommon. Studies of gas in the blood may provide evidence of arterial hypoxemia and metabolic acidosis. Changes in serum electrolytes, on the other hand, may not appear significant. With appropriate therapy, there may be uneventful recovery. The postimmersion period, however, may be complicated by pneumonia, hemoglobinuria, or nephrosis of the lower nephron. Occasionally, there may be brain damage from prolonged cerebral anoxia.

Diagnosis. When the patient is a victim of near-drowning, other physical causes for disability should be considered. The diagnosis of near-drowning is usually not difficult after the circumstances are known. Diagnostic studies should include chest films, an electrocardiogram, serial determinations of gas in arterial blood, and appropriate laboratory tests, including determinations of hematocrit, hemoglobin, leukocytes, serum electrolytes, and serum protein. When chest films show diffuse or nodular hazy opacification, the patient is febrile, and leukocytosis is evident during the postimmersion period, respiratory complications, particularly pneumonia, are invariably present. In the differential diagnosis of near-drowning and drowning, other causes of aquatic accidents, especially air embolism and decompression sickness, must be considered. These untoward effects of barotrauma, discussed elsewhere, are usually associated with underwater swimming, diving, or the use of self-contained underwater breathing apparatus (scuba). Recognition of barotrauma and differentiation from near-drowning are extremely important, for recompression, the appropriate method of treatment, may bring dramatic and life-saving results.

When the body of a dead person is found immersed in water, the diagnosis of drowning depends upon exclusion of other possible causes for death. Failure to find an injury or evidence of pre-existing disease, as well as the presence of evidence that the person was alive during the period of immersion, results in the presumption that death was caused by drowning. A careful appraisal of the circumstances of death and of findings from pathologic and toxicologic studies and from postmortem chemical and physical tests is required.

Treatment. Survival depends upon the health of the victim, the duration of immersion, and the amount of water inhaled. Prompt rescue and first aid, including artificial resuscitation, offer the greatest chance for survival. The airway should be clear of any obstructions, and dentures should be removed prior to artificial resuscitation. If a heart beat and carotid pulse are not detectable, closed-chest cardiac massage is required. Artificial resuscitation should be continued until spontaneous breathing occurs or signs of death are evident. In 1963 Krittingen and Naess reported recovery of a child who had drowned in a river. After resuscitation for two hours, heart beat and spontaneous respirations were noted.

After the immediate period, further treatment should be carried out in either an intensive-care unit or a recovery room. If the patient survives the first 24 hours, it is likely that he may recover. Aspiration of the airway or tracheostomy may be necessary. Recurrent vomiting and aspiration of vomitus may be prevented by gastric decompression. Intermittent positive-pressure breathing of 100 per cent oxygen and administration of antifoaming agents may be helpful. As the patient improves, oxygen may be administered by mask or catheter and reduced to 40 per cent in concentration. Based upon serial determinations of gas in arterial blood, arterial hypoxemia and acid-base levels are corrected by effective ventilation, oxygenation, buffers, or bicarbonate. Steroids and antimicrobials are used for pneumonia. It may be necessary to use bronchodilators; digitalization; tranfusions of whole blood, plasma, or packed red cells; hypothermia; or forced diuresis, as indicated.

Fuller, R. H.: The clinical pathology of human near-drowning. Proc. Roy. Soc. Med., 56:33, 1963.

Modell, J. H., and Davis, J. H.: Electrolyte changes in human drowning victims. Anesthesiology, 30:414, 1969.

Modell, J. H., Davis, J. H., Giammona, S. T., Moya, F., and Mann, J. B.: Blood gas and electrolyte changes in human near-drowning victims. J.A.M.A., 203:337, 1968.

Reidbord, H. E., and Spitz, W. U.: Ultrastructural alterations in rat lungs: Changes after intratracheal perfusion with fresh water and sea water. Arch. Path. (Chicago), 81:103, 1966.

Spitz, W. U., Hebel, J. R., and Michaelis, M.: Enzymatic changes in asphyxia, experimental pulmonary edema, and drowning. Amer. J. Clin. Path., 51:102, 1969.

Spitz, W. U., Silverman, B. A., and Michaelis, M.: Histochemical changes in experimental drowning, pulmonary edema and asphyxia. J. Forensic Med., 16:79, 1969.

Timperman, J.: Medico-legal problems in death by drowning. Its diagnosis by the diatom method. J. Forensic Med., 16:45, 1969.

Wiggins, C. E., and Luke, J. L.: The pathology, diagnosis and medical-legal aspects of death by drowning. J. Okla. Med. Ass., 63:3, 1970.

Radiation Injury

L. H. Hempelmann

Definition. Radiation injury is manifested in a number of ways, depending upon the nature of the exposure. Massive radiation exposure causes injury that may be evident within minutes or days, whereas small or repeated exposure induces a response that may not be apparent for years. If the entire body or a large portion thereof is irradiated with a large dose of penetrating radiation, an acute generalized illness called the acute radiation syndrome results. If a small portion of the body is exposed to an excessive dose, a localized injury occurs perhaps with little, if any, systemic reaction. Such localized injuries are usually named after the organ affected, e.g., radiation dermatitis, radiation nephritis, etc. Although acute radiation injuries have distinctive characteristics, the delayed manifestations or late effects of radiation injury (terms preferable to delayed radiation injury) may be indistinguishable from spontaneously occurring diseases, such as leukemia.

Ionizing radiations responsible for radiation injuries are distinct from nonionizing radiations, such as visible and infrared light. They are given off by naturally occurring or artificially produced radioisotopes, by nuclear reactions, or by man-made radiation-producing equipment. Certain radiations, such as x-rays, gamma-rays, and neutrons, emitted from sources outside the body, can penetrate tissues readily and can damage internally placed radiosensitive organs. Other radiations, such as alpha-rays and low energy beta-rays, have a limited range in tissues; they are injurious only if given off by radioactive isotopes deposited within the body.

Definitions for the basic units of radiation and of radioactivity can be found in the textbooks of radiation physics. Roentgens now refer to exposure (not to absorbed dose), and rads indicate the amount of radiation energy absorbed per gram of tissue. When referring to radiation exposures, the amount and type of exposed tissue as well as the dose should be given; for example, total body or abdominal exposure to 500 roentgens. Exposures are usually considered to be single exposures at relatively high dose rates (5 to 50 r per minute). Other types of exposure, e.g., very slow dose rates or fractionated exposures, are less effective and should be so designated. It is interesting that roentgens or rads represent infinitesimal quantities of energy compared with those involved in biologic processes. The energy involved when a cell absorbs one rad of x-rays is less than one four hundred millionth of that expended in the cell's daily metabolism.

Etiology. Known instances of radiation injury in man are usually the result of exposure to radiation from radiation sources. In peacetime, such exposures are almost exclusively medical or industrial and, in the case of late manifestations, may have occurred so long before as to have been forgotten. As knowledge of radiation hazards has been gained, it has become evident that exposure to doses formerly thought to be harmless may have unfortunate late consequences. It is possible that exposure to any amount of radiation produces some biologic effect, but serious acute radiation injury or death occurs only after exposure to relatively large doses.

Large-scale epidemiologic surveys in man indicate a linear relationship between dose and incidence of certain types of late radiation effects, e.g., certain radiation-induced neoplasms. Furthermore, the data give no indication of a threshold dose below which such damage does not occur. Although data in the very low dose range are admittedly meager, to be conservative one must assume that there is no threshold for certain types of somatic damage. Recent studies, however, indicate that radiation-induced damage to the DNA of cultured mammalian cells can be repaired and that mouse ova can recover from point mutations. This allows us to hope that the linear relationship between radiation effects and dose may not hold in the very low dose range or at very low dose rates. The nonthreshold concept does not apply to the acute radiation syndrome or acute localized injury. Such injuries occur only after the threshold dose has been exceeded.

To put the nonthreshold hypothesis into proper perspective, it should be emphasized that this becomes important only when applied to large groups. For example, total body exposure of a large population would cause a finite number of cases of leukemia estimated at one to two cases per year for every million people exposed to one rad each. As far as any individual is concerned, the small increase (approximately 2 to 4 per cent per rad) in his chance of developing spontaneous leukemia (roughly 1 in 20,000 per year) is insignificant compared to everyday hazards.

Incidence. Since radiation injury, as we know it, usually results from exposure to radiation emitted by radiation sources, its incidence depends upon the number of such sources and the care with which they have been used. As information about risks of radiation exposure has been gained, there has been increasing restraint in the use of radiation-producing sources. However, with the widespread use of such sources in medicine and industry, large segments of our population are now exposed to small, controlled amounts of radiation. Furthermore, as a result of nuclear testing, the entire world population has been irradiated by radioactive fall-out, though with doses that are small compared to medical exposures in highly industrialized countries.

Acute radiation injuries in peacetime are surprisingly infrequent. Up to the end of 1969, 97 persons had been irradiated in radiation accidents, and 297 persons had been exposed to excessive radiation due to fall-out from nuclear tests in the Pacific Ocean. Nine persons in the first group were fatally injured, and the others suffered acute injuries of varying degrees of severity. Radiation injury in wartime is another matter. Radiation combined with blast and heat from nuclear explosions could cause the death or serious injury of a large proportion of the world's population.

The incidence of late radiation effects in the general population is difficult to assess, because the relationship between the disease and prior exposure is often obscure. In two epidemiologic studies, however, minimal incidence values are available. In one series of 236 persons exposed to radium, 23 osteogenic sarcomas and 8 carcinomas of the paranasal or mastoid sinuses have occurred; in another series of 268 young adults treated with several hundred roentgens of x-rays for thymic enlargement, 20 thyroid neoplasms (9 malignant) have been discovered. Other forms of radiation-induced malignancy are probably not so frequent. Only 87 cases of leukemia were reported in x-ray workers up to 1959. Although the size of the exposed population is now known, it must number in the hundreds of thousands, indicating a rather low incidence of radiation-induced leukemia.

Pathology. After total body exposure of animals to the usual doses responsible for the acute radiation syndrome, histologic examination reveals a prompt disappearance of mitotic figures. This is followed by the gradual return of mitotic activity, some of the dividing cells showing obvious chromosomal abnormalities. Many of these injured cells, after an interval that tends to vary with the dose and the tissue, die following division or, in some instances, form giant cells before dying. An exception to this so-called reproductive death is the adult lymphocyte, which undergoes prompt intermitotic death and disintegration. Cell damage and death are most extensive in rapidly proliferating tissues, such as blood-forming tissues and intestinal and germinal epithelium, which soon become depleted of almost all radiosensitive cell species. Except after massive radiation exposure, which causes prompt intermitotic death of all cell types, slowly proliferating or nondividing tissues, such as liver and brain, show little or no evidence of acute injury.

Primary radiation damage to blood-forming and intestinal tissues, i.e., depletion of cells and temporary loss of ability of stem cells to repopulate the tissues, inevitably leads to secondary complications. Prominent among these is bacterial invasion with septicemia as a consequence of granulocytopenia, depressed immunologic capabilities, and damage to the intestinal barrier. Infection and toxemia resulting from tissue breakdown lead to a pronounced inflammatory reaction in many tissues, particularly in the oropharynx and intestines, where extensive ulceration may occur. The inflammatory reaction is distinctive in being almost devoid of granulocytes. Another complication is hemorrhage, varying from microscopic extravasation of erythrocytes to gross bleeding at the height of the illness. Late in the syndrome, epilation, particularly of the scalp, may be observed.

In acute localized radiation injury, both intermitotic and reproductive cell death occur, accompanied by a secondary inflammatory response. Upon recovery, endarterial thickening and extensive fibrosis develop gradually. In the case of late radiation effects, such as neoplastic disease, there may be no microscopic features indicative of prior radiation exposure.

Pathogenesis. Although the total radiant energy dissipated in an irradiated cell is small, that involved in the interaction of radiation with individual molecules is sufficient to cause ionization and to break chemical bonds. The resultant chemical alteration of certain biologically important molecules, such as deoxyribonucleic acid (DNA) and chromosomal proteins is probably the basic lesion responsible for the so-called reproductive type of radiation death of cells. It has been calculated that exposure of a mammalian cell to one roentgen of x-rays results in three single-strand breaks and three tenths of a double-strand cut in its DNA molecules. This type of molecular damage may be compatible with life in nondividing cells, but may become evident when the cells recover from the temporary radiation-induced suppression of mitotic activity. The chromosomal aberrations seen in mitotic cells may result in an imbalance of genetic material in daughter cells that is incompatible with continued life and reproduction; such abnormal cells die after one or two mitoses. Rapidly proliferating tissues are radiosensitive in part because their widespread mitotic activity results in rather prompt death of the descendants of many cells with severe chromosomal abnormalities. In contrast to the reproductive

death, the mechanism of intermitotic cell death after massive exposure is poorly understood.

In the *acute radiation syndrome*, cell damage and death in most tissues contribute to clinical manifestations of the illness, but signs and symptoms resulting from intestinal and marrow damage usually predominate. Cell death and interference with the normal mechanisms of cell renewal lead to cell depletion in these tissues. Since some stem cells escape death even after exposure to large doses, recovery of the irradiated patient depends upon whether life can be sustained until the surviving stem cells regain their ability to repopulate these vital tissues with normal cell types. After very large doses, destruction of the nondividing cells of the central nervous system may be so rapidly fatal that death of the patient occurs before symptoms of marrow and intestinal damage seriously complicate the clinical picture.

Chromosomal damage in irradiated cells is believed to be largely repaired by a process involving intranuclear protein synthesis, and this probably explains why repeated or protracted exposure to a given dose of radiation is less damaging than the same dose given in a single exposure. Chromosomal repair is not complete, however, except possibly with very small doses or very low dose rates, and aberrations in slowly dividing tissue can be demonstrated long after exposure. For example, chromosomal abnormalities are reported in long-lived species of lymphocytes in the blood of persons given radiation therapy up to 20 years previously. Residual chromosomal lesions of this type combined with factors that stimulate cell proliferation are suspected of being responsible for malignant change in irradiated tissues. On theoretical grounds it has been suggested that similar lesions might lead to shortening of life. Subtle DNA damage in germ cells compatible with continued life and reproduction can be transmitted to offspring in the form of point or chromosomal mutations.

Clinical Manifestations. The clinical manifestations of the acute radiation syndrome vary with the dose, and reflect damage to the three key organ systems, namely, bone marrow, intestine, and sometimes the central nervous system. With doses in the lethal range or below, the signs and symptoms are primarily those of marrow damage and secondarily of intestinal injury. With higher doses, the illness is more acute, and symptoms of severe intestinal damage overshadow those of marrow depletion. With very high doses, the clinical picture is one of acute central nervous system destruction with resultant disorientation, convulsions, hypotension progressing to shock, and fever. Skin erythema may appear promptly. Death occurs within hours or days before marrow and intestinal damage can significantly influence the manifestations.

Except in the fulminating central nervous system type of injury, the classic *acute radiation syndrome* can be divided into four phases. The first phase develops within minutes or hours after exposure and consists of nausea, vomiting, and, perhaps, diarrhea and weakness. A day or so later, symptoms subside, and the illness enters the second phase, a period of relative well-being. After an interval of one or more weeks, depending upon the severity of the illness, the third or critical phase occurs, primarily as a result of marrow failure and infection. Fever increases in a stepwise fashion, and vomiting and anorexia recur. There may be stomatitis, which can progress to oropharyngeal ulceration. The abdomen may become distended, and there may be severe and sometimes bloody diarrhea. Petechial hemorrhages may be noted in the skin. The patient is obviously toxic, perhaps dehydrated, and shows evidence of marked weight loss. Epilation, particularly of the scalp, may occur during the third week. Death, primarily due to intestinal damage, may occur during the second week before the period in which bleeding and septicemia develop. Following the critical phase, those patients who survive enter the fourth or recovery phase. Recovery almost inevitably begins before the sixth week, and convalescence is slow, residual weakness persisting for months. Temporary sterility may develop during convalescence, and cataracts may occur years later, particularly after neutron exposure.

Hematologic data reflect damage to the radiosensitive blood-forming tissues. The lymphocyte count falls within a matter of hours, reaching a minimal value within four days. After exposure to large doses, lymphocytes may virtually disappear from the blood. An initial granulocytosis lasting a day or so is followed by a fall in granulocytes, in severe cases reaching very low levels early in the second week. With less severe injury, the granulocyte count levels off about the eighth day, and may even show an abortive rise lasting up to 10 to 12 days. The count falls again during the critical phase of the illness, reaching a minimum during the fourth or fifth week in those patients who recover. In such patients, the platelet count begins to fall a few days after exposure, reaching a minimum at 28 to 32 days. The erythrocyte count falls gradually until the twenty-sixth to thirty-eighth day unless there is gross bleeding.

Other laboratory findings, none of which is pathognomonic of radiation injury, may be useful in evaluating severity of the illness. There is an increase in bleeding time during the thrombocytopenic period. Blood cultures during the critical phase may yield enteric bacteria. Analysis of the urine may show creatinuria and increased excretion of beta-aminoisobutyric acid, taurine, and other amino acids and deoxycytidine. Following neutron irradiation, induced radioactivity may be detected in sodium and phosphorus of the plasma and in sulfur of the hair.

The clinical manifestations of *localized irradiation* depend upon the tissues involved. In the skin, erythema develops within days or weeks after acute exposure, and may progress to epidermolysis. Following recovery, there may be atrophy of the skin with underlying fibrosis, telangiectasia, and eventual malignant degeneration. In *radium poisoning*, the first sign of injury may be aplastic anemia. Later, pathologic fractures and/or osteo-

genic sarcomas may develop. Similarly, malignant change can be the ultimate fate of almost any heavily irradiated tissue.

The late manifestations of whole-body exposure include life-shortening, acute or chronic myelocytic (not lymphocytic) leukemia and, possibly, other myeloproliferative disorders. These illnesses do not differ from those that occur spontaneously.

Diagnosis. Acute radiation injury is rarely a diagnostic problem. The history of excessive radiation exposure is usually but not always obvious, particularly in persons occupationally exposed. There have been instances of unsuspected occupational exposures and even unwitting exposure of an entire family. Therefore, the possibility of radiation injury should be entertained in patients with aplastic anemia or pancytopenia of unknown origin, or other illness showing damage to blood-forming tissues.

With late manifestations of radiation injury, the exposure history may be obscure. In the case of malignant conditions, perhaps the only reason for suspecting irradiation is the unusual age at onset, e.g., osteogenic sarcoma in an older person or acute leukemia or thyroid cancer in an adolescent. The presence of internally deposited radioactive materials responsible for some late radiation effects can usually be demonstrated only by sophisticated radiochemical or physical techniques.

Treatment. Treatment of the acute radiation syndrome is symptomatic, directed at preventing and combating infection, controlling bleeding, replacing fluids and electrolytes and, when necessary, correcting anemia. Cronkite, Bond, and their associates, using the following regimen, have succeeded in sustaining life in dogs exposed to supralethal doses of x-rays: (1) administration of broad-spectrum antimicrobials at onset of fever in the critical phase of the illness; as resistance to one antimicrobial developed, usually in three to five days, another was substituted; (2) fresh platelet or blood transfusions to stop bleeding; and (3) fluid and electrolyte replacement. Other symptoms, such as hypotension, shock, and pain, should be treated symptomatically as they occur.

The current ideas about treatment of acute radiation injuries, including use of sterile hospital facilities, can be found in the article by Andrews and his associates. Bone marrow transplantation does not seem justifiable at present, except in those rare circumstances in which the patient's own marrow had been stored prior to exposure or when marrow from an identical twin is available. For patients who recover, a period of convalescence may be required and further occupational exposure should be avoided.

Treatment of localized forms of radiation injury is also symptomatic, for there is no way to undo or modify the injury once it has occurred. When certain bone-seeking, radioactive substances have been taken into the body, however, the possibility of injury can be reduced by administration of chelating agents, which increase their excretion rate.

Prognosis. If a patient is known to have had

total-body exposure to a very high or very low dose of radiation, it is possible to predict with a fair degree of certainty the outcome of his illness. In the case of exposure in the lethal range, it is impossible to differentiate on the basis of dose alone between patients who will survive and those who will die. Limited information about dose response in man and individual variation in response restrict the value of radiation doses in predicting the course of the illness. In accidental exposures, there may be further uncertainty as to the actual dose and/or nonuniform exposure of the body. The prognosis of each patient's illness therefore must be based on clinical grounds.

After a careful analysis of all reported accidental exposures, Bond et al. have classified the acute radiation syndrome into four categories according to the probability of recovery. In the first category, survival virtually impossible, the estimated radiation doses exceeded 500 to 600 rads (total-body exposure). In the second category, survival possible, the estimated dose range was 200 to 450 rads. In the third, survival probable, the range was 100 to 200 rads. Exposures in the fourth category, survival virtually certain, were less than 100 rads. The patients in category I have severe central nervous system damage or predominantly intestinal symptoms. Their blood studies showed severe depression of all formed elements by the second week of the illness. The patients whose survival was considered virtually certain (category IV) had mild symptoms, if any, and no evidence of severe marrow damage. The patients in the survival possible (II) or survival probable (III) categories could not be differentiated early in the illness, although lymphocyte counts below 1000 to 1200 cells per cubic millimeter, severe diarrhea, and skin erythema were ominous signs. Even in the critical phase it was difficult to be certain whether the patient would live. Once the marrow began to recover, usually not later than the fifth week, survival was almost certain. Except for an increased chance of developing late manifestations of exposure, recovery from the illness was virtually complete in all survivors.

The prognosis for localized injuries can be found in radiation therapy textbooks; that for late manifestations is the same as in the spontaneously occurring diseases.

Prevention. Occupational radiation injury is minimized and largely prevented by rigorous enforcement of strict operating regulations. These procedures are designed to avoid accidental overexposure and to limit unavoidable exposure to radiation levels that are not believed to cause detectable bodily damage. The present maximal permissible levels for total-body exposure to x-rays recommended by the National Committee on Ra-

diation Protection is 0.1 roentgen per week with a maximal accumulated dose of 3 roentgens per three months or 5 roentgens per year. The maximal permissible levels of exposure to other radiations and to radioisotopes can be found in the appropriate handbooks published by the National Bureau of Standards, U.S. Department of Commerce. Careful exposure records are kept for each person occupationally exposed, and periodic physical examinations are conducted in accordance with standard industrial practice. Periodic blood counts, formerly regarded as a means of radiation monitoring, have been abandoned except when indicated on medical grounds or after known overexposure.

Because medical roentgenologic procedures are responsible for the major share of the total exposure of our population, it is the duty of every physician to keep patient exposures to the minimum compatible with good medical practice. As mentioned earlier, the risk to any individual is so small that patients should not be denied roentgenographic examinations that could be beneficial. The physician must weigh the risks against the possible benefits in each case. Radiation therapy of benign disease in persons with long life expectancy should be avoided in favor of other forms of treatment. Since the fetus is radiosensitive, particularly during the first eight weeks of gestation, abdominal exposure should be avoided in pregnant women if possible. Some experts recommend that elective abdominal fluoroscopy of women of childbearing age should be done only during the first two weeks after menstruation to avoid irradiation of unsuspected fetuses.

Andrews, G. A.: Criticality accidents in Vinca, Yugoslavia, and Oak Ridge, Tennessee. J.A.M.A., 179:191, 1962.

Andrews, G. A., Balish, E., Edwards, C. L., Knisely, R. M., and Lushbaugh, C. L.: Possibilities for improved treatment of persons exposed in radiation accident. International Atomic Energy Agency, SM 119/56, 1969.

Bacq, Z. M., and Alexander, P.: Fundamentals of Radiobiology. 2nd ed. New York, Pergamon Press, 1961.

Bond, V. P., Fliedner, T., and Archambeau, J. O.: Mammalian Radiation Lethality, a Disturbance in Cellular Kinetics. New York, Academic Press, Inc., 1965.

Hempelmann, L. H., Lisco, H., and Hoffman, J. G.: The acute radiation syndrome—A report of nine cases and a review of the problem. Ann. Intern. Med., 36 (Part II):279, 1952.

Mathé, G., Amiel, J. L., and Schwartzenberg, L.: Treatment of acute total body irradiation injury in man. Ann. N.Y. Acad. Sci, 114:368, 1964.

Sorenson, D. K., Bond, V. P., Cronkite, E. P., and Perman, V.: An effective therapeutic regimen for the hematologic phase of the acute radiation syndrome in dogs. Radiat. Res., 13: 669, 1960.

Report of the United Nations Scientific Committee on the Effects of Atomic Radiation. Supplement No. 14 (A/5814). New York, United Nations, 1964.

The Treatment of Radiation Injury. Publication 1134, National Academy of Sciences, National Research Council, 1964.

Chemical Contamination of Water and Air

Walsh McDermott

Like so many problems in medicine today, the one presented by chemical contamination of our air and water is only partly medical. The effects of contaminants on an individual would be medical; yet the forces that expose the individual to the contaminants would be technologic, economic, or cultural. As modulation of these forces requires social action on a broad scale, the physician's role has to be chiefly one of educator and counsellor for those of his patients who are concerned citizen activists and for the public authorities. But the physician is frequently "a concerned citizen" too. It is imperative, therefore, that while serving as counsellor or educator he be able to distinguish between his advice given as a physician based on scientific and professional evidence relating to *human health*, and his advice given as a concerned citizen—albeit one with a fairly broad background in biology.

The crux of the matter is that with one exception (*vide infra*) the risks to health posed by chemical contamination of our air or water are not tangible disease realities of the sort with which the physician is accustomed to deal. Instead the fact that there are health risks at all is an intellectual judgment based mainly on biologic analogies rather than on evidence established by direct medical observations. To be sure, the physician is well schooled in making judgments among offsetting risks, but he is usually dealing with risks all of which loom for the immediate future of his patient. In weighing chemical threats from the environment, however, he must frequently offset health gains that are clear and immediate against health risks that are far off and theoretical, and indeed might become a problem only for some future generation.

A splendid example of such offsetting threats may be seen in the chemical contamination of our streams and lakes, some of which serve as community water supplies. The availability of this water made it possible to build the United States as an urbanized society, but to do so required the development of a technology whereby the water could be decontaminated of its threats to health. These threats were all actual disease-producing agents. Because they were living organisms they had the property of death and dissolution, and a highly effective technology was based on these biologic properties. For the past 50 years or so, however, on an increasing scale, we have been contaminating the water not only with our microbes but with the direct or indirect products of our chemical industry. Whereas our microbes are bio-degradable, many of these chemicals are not; indeed some are not simplified at all, either by biologic degradation or any other process of decay. Technologic solutions for this part of the

problem are to be expected in the form of substituting more readily degradable pesticides and detergents. The over-all problem, however, cannot be solved purely through technologic means. For the chemical contamination, like that by man's microbes, is part of his aura and is derived from his presence and way of life. To change the aura significantly would require major changes in the way of life; yet it is only the microbial part of his aura that can be clearly incriminated as producers of disease.

The many offsetting factors that must be weighed in a judgment on the health risks of chemical contamination of water are well illustrated by the story of chlorophenothane (DDT). Indeed the DDT situation may be regarded as a fine prototype of the whole problem. As a pesticide this chlorinated hydrocarbon has been marvelously effective in enhancing agricultural productivity; unfortunately it is relatively stable chemically over a wide range of conditions and thus persists for long periods in the environment. Here it produces a number of unsought ecologic effects. These include critically harmful disturbances of the calcium metabolism of predatory birds; interference with various forms of marine life; and persistence in the food chain whereby it can accumulate in the tissues of a number of organisms, including man. All these effects are reason enough for insisting on strict controls on the use of DDT and on an intensive effort to develop less stable but comparably effective substitutes. Moreover, the property of accumulation in human tissue is obviously disquieting from the standpoint of human health. Thus far, however, there is no evidence that this accumulation has led to recognizable disease in humans. The World Health Organization in a 20-year experiment involving more than 200,000 DDT spraymen has received no reports of toxic effect except from accidental swallowing, and even that caused no deaths. No adverse effects were observed in a clinical study of chronic low-grade exposure in which a group of volunteers received daily for 18 months a dosage 200 times the estimated usual exposure from food (Hayes, W. S., et al., 1956).

The physician must offset the theoretic risk that these accumulations might ultimately lead to human disease against the demonstrable health gains from controlling some of the world's major diseases such as malaria (or filariasis) and those caused by arboviruses and rickettsia. And at the present time, there is no wholly satisfactory substitute for DDT in disease control. Faced with this choice between the clear and present danger of vector-borne diseases and the theoretic risk that tissue accumulation of low concentrations of DDT might lead to disease a few decades hence, the physician has no choice but to opt for continued use of DDT under proper control. Yet in making this choice — and the DDT situation can be viewed as the prototype of many more — he must be keenly aware of the critical nature of the factors it was *not* possible to include in the decision.

For to say that low-grade continued exposure to DDT has produced no recognizable disease in man is not to say that it exerts no *physiologic effects*. On the contrary, it is a potent inducer of the microsomal enzyme system of the liver. As this system plays a critical role in the metabolism of drugs and other chemicals introduced to the body from the outside, it serves as a major protective mechanism against chemical threats from the environment, and hence consideration of its workings is appropriate.

The activity of the microsomal enzyme system is minimal at birth and in early life but increases steadily throughout adulthood. It is inducible; and the buildup of enzymatic capability as the individual grows older is thought to be a reflection of increasing experience with chemicals from the environment, acting as inducers. Activity of the system induced by one chemical may also be effective on another. Consequently when more than one drug (or adventitious chemical) are being taken into the body simultaneously, the metabolic disposition of one of the drugs can be significantly altered by the presence and inducing capabilities of the other drug or adventitious chemical. Such "cross-over" effects have obvious implications for multiple drug therapies and conceivably might also attain significance when one of the chemical compounds was an environmental contaminant. The only endogenous materials metabolized via the hepatic microsomal system are the steroid hormones, and their hydroxylation can be considerably enhanced when the system is induced. In theory, therefore, it could be imagined that the presence of DDT with its known potency as an inducer of the hepatic microsomal system could lead to an increased demand for the synthesis of some hormone. There is no evidence that such a DDT phenomenon with steroid hormones actually occurs. But the postulated phenomenon can serve as an imaginary example of how an adventitious chemical in the environment could alter the course of bodily metabolic activities *through an adaptive hepatic system that is known to exist.*

The question arises whether the decades-long stimulation of such an adaptive mechanism in an individual carries with it a risk to the total organism or whether, on balance, such continued stimulation is a good thing. In general, the many bodily systems that work toward homeostasis are regarded as normal processes whose continued operation is not harmful in itself. But some of these systems require the synthesis of protein, and this requires an allocative process involving protein precursors. In effect, therefore, as emphasized by V. R. Potter, there is a "physiologic cost" involved in each of these adaptive enzymatic processes in the sense that one is accomplished at some cost to all possible others. When the "triggering" of the system comes chiefly from the external environment, as in the hepatic microsomal system, the long-continued engagement with a wealth of chemical stimuli conceivably might result in "physiologic costs" that would be harmful to the organism. This could be so; conversely, as our knowledge advances, the notion may prove to have been ridiculously naive. Our current state of knowledge simply does not permit judgment of the question at this time. It is really the fact that we are dealing with so many "unknowns" that serves to temper any tendency to complacency based on the present absence of detectable disease resulting from chemical contamination of water. For any situation in which a variety of chemicals pass through a series of living systems that at some stage may include the human body is bound to be not only complex but a situation that is continuously subject to change. It is this fact — that the door is wide open for trouble rather than that trouble has already occurred — that characterizes our present situation with respect to possible adverse effects on health from chemical contaminants of our water.*

One expressed fear about pesticides in the water also concerns contamination of the air, specifically that the world's newly released oxygen content might be undergoing subtle reduction. Approximately 60 per cent of the world's newly released oxygen each year comes from the activity of oceanic plant life which it was feared might be harmed by the pesticide pollution of the oceans. However, careful studies of Machts and Hughes (1970) have revealed that there has been no change in the world atmosphere's content of oxygen in the 60-year period from 1910 to 1970. Their "negative" data can now serve as a baseline for monitoring this question throughout the future. Fears of reduction in the global oxygen supply from combustion on land can be set completely to rest by examining the quantitative aspects of the question.

With respect to chemical contamination of the air, the challenge to the physician is the same as with water, namely, he must learn to distinguish at any one point in time between what are presently demonstrable health hazards and what are *current stimuli* that conceivably might be generating health effects to be recognized only several decades later. In broad terms two distinct types of widespread† chemical contamination exist: a "London type," composed principally of sulfur compounds from burning coal, and a "Los Angeles" type, composed mainly of petroleum products introduced into the atmosphere principally from automobiles, and consisting chiefly of carbon

---

*A case in point is the revelation that mercury, a substance formerly considered as too valuable to be treated as waste, is now being discarded via the water route in several parts of the United States.

†As distinguished from *localized* forms of air pollution, such as the contamination by asbestos to which building wreckers are exposed and which is associated with pleural endothelioma (Wright, G.: Asbestos and Health in 1969. Amer. Rev. Resp. Dis., 100:467, 1969).

monoxide, carbon dioxide, oxides of nitrogen, lead, and unburned or partially oxidized hydrocarbons. None of these chemicals are present in concentrations sufficiently high in themselves to produce acute toxicity in man. In the Los Angeles type of contamination the visible and palpable "smog" is a result of *sunlight* acting on certain of these discharged chemicals to produce more reactive chemicals, whereas in London it frequently results from *fog* physically trapping the sulfur compounds from the coal. Both types exist in both countries, but in the United States it is the hydrocarbon type that is our basic problem. It is overlaid in certain localities by the sulfur type, for the use of coal varies considerably from region to region. It is highly probable that with both types, one of the important end-results—irritation of certain body and plant cells—is much the same.

In terms of presently demonstrable effects on health the evidence is convincing that the irritation from chemicals in the air is definitely harmful to persons who have sustained damage to their cardiovascular or bronchopulmonary systems, notably that apparently enlarging number of patients with chronic obstructive pulmonary disease (see Respiratory Diseases). A definite correlation between reported excess mortality from cardiopulmonary diseases and levels of common pollutants in the air was observed by Hodgson in New York City. He also found some evidence to indicate that sudden increases in the level of contaminants were associated with excess mortality even when the absolute level of pollution was not unusually high. The physician is on quite solid ground, therefore, in attempting to protect his patients with damaged lungs or bronchi from the aggravating effects of chemically polluted urban air. Sometimes this can be accomplished by emigration, sometimes by window fans with filters. Often, however, particularly among urban poverty groups, it cannot be accomplished at all. For these unfortunates, and indeed for the majority of those with chronic pulmonary disease in all socioeconomic groups, protection, if it is to come, will have to come from the community efforts now in progress in many localities to reduce chemical contamination of the air.

In terms of presently demonstrable effects it must be appreciated that virtually the entire "health case" for reducing the chemical contamination of the air rests on the protection of this population with damaged cardiopulmonary systems. For no convincing case has yet been assembled to the effect that bronchopulmonary disease with its frequent cardiac sequels can be *initiated* by continued exposure to the chemical contamination of urban air. This is not to say there is no medical case at all for continued efforts to minimize contamination of the air for the sake of the far larger population with undamaged bronchopulmonary structures. On the contrary, such a case does exist. The physician must recognize clearly, however, that the case for action to protect the population at large is of quite a different nature from when action is to protect those already damaged. For those damaged the evidence is of a conventional medical sort, i.e., it is based on systematic clinical, laboratory, and epidemiologic observations. For the population at large, however, the case is not derived from actual scientific observations. On the contrary, *as in the case of chemical contamination of the water,* the argument for decontaminating the air can be no more than an intellectual judgment based mainly on biologic analogies.

There is one difference between the problems with air and with water. As mentioned previously, at present there is no recognized disease of unknown pathogenesis that seems to have any relationship to widespread chemical contamination of water. By contrast, in the disease complex of bronchitis and emphysema (chronic obstructive pulmonary disease), there *is* a commonly occurring disease grouping of unknown pathogenesis that starts in early middle age, is clearly aggravated by chemicals in the air, and hence might also be *initiated* by them. But to demonstrate convincingly that such a causative relationship exists is a difficult task that has not yet been accomplished despite careful and intensive studies of laboratory animals and man. The epidemiologic problems involved have to do with the great difficulties in separating for analysis the various factors of conceivable relevance such as cigarette smoking and degree of exposure to particular chemicals in the air.

Above all is the problem of how to study what are in effect "water dripping on stone" effects. The chemicals now contaminating the air, taken singly or collectively, are not present in quantities that produce detectable bronchopulmonary damage in the short run. Thus if the "current stimuli" represented by these chemicals play a significant role in the pathogenesis of such a major disease grouping as chronic bronchopulmonary disease, the effects presumably would take the form of steady but individually minute episodes of damage that ultimately fail to heal completely and emerge to significance only when accumulated over decades. Questions of this type, i.e., 30- to 40-year effects in humans, are far more difficult to answer than questions of the role of environmental contaminants on plant life or other elements of the nonhuman ecology.

To be sure, the physician in his role of public educator and counsellor should support well organized efforts to develop the new methods and new research institutional arrangements necessary for the productive study of these medical questions of this essentially new type. But he should also not fail to stress that because of the very nature of these questions as they apply to *human health*, it seems highly unlikely that answers concerning air pollution as an initiator of disease will be forthcoming in the near future. Whatever action is to be taken, therefore, must be based on the medical information that is available now. From the standpoint of health, therefore, we are left with the following dilemma. On the one hand, most of the actions necessary to abolish air pollution as a potential danger to health are costly and likely to prove quite disruptive to the economy and the whole style of life. To campaign for these actions in the name of health without a convincing scientific case that the evils to be corrected represent a widespread danger to health might be unwise. On the other hand, if, a few decades hence, it were shown convincingly that long-continued chemical contamination of the air *of the present sort* did have the property of initiating chronic bronchopulmonary disease, the proportion of the population of any industrialized country that would by then have been irreversibly affected would be large indeed.

There seems to be no obvious solution for this dilemma so long as the major case for minimizing air pollution is viewed as being primarily a "health matter" and health is considered principally in terms of detectable disease. But there are more subtle aspects to health than definable disease, including even definable mental disease. There is the whole affect involved in one's response to one's environment. The intense love of their city shown by so many Leningraders when it was under seige in World War II is a case in point. These are not the kinds of phenomena that lend themselves readily to comparative weighing in the scale against the major economic factors that might be disrupted in "air reform." Nevertheless, they deserve attention too.

What it comes down to is that, except for those already afflicted with cardiopulmonary disease, the present chemical pollution of urban air is not really a health problem in the orthodox sense; it is a widespread *social* evil that is quite unacceptable on a number of counts, of which the possible health effects are only one (Dubos, 1970). Viewed in this way it becomes the physician's role to characterize continuously what is known or seems highly probable about the health aspects of the matter. Included should be encouragement of attempts to develop more sensitive methods for the essentially permanent monitoring of the possible effects of long-continued chemical stimuli. The physician presents this knowledge not as a determining reason in itself for air control, but as but one portion of a total argument for cleansing this part of our external environment. Once the medical contribution can be regarded as but one contribution to a much larger total effort, the physician can escape from the trap of seeming to be minimizing the significances of a particular form of contamination of the air on the grounds that it is not a *known* danger to health. For the physician to operate in such a cooperative professional-social role is not new; most of the impressive twentieth century accomplishments of medicine in extending life expectancy from birth were made in exactly this way.

Burns, J. J.: Interaction of environmental agents and drugs. Envir. Res., 2:352, 1969.

Conney, A. H., et al.: Effects of pesticides on drugs and steroid metabolism. Clin. Pharmacol. Ther., 8:2, 1967.

Dubos, R.: Reason Awake! Science for Man. New York, Columbia University Press, 1970.

Dubos, R.: So Human an Animal. New York, Charles Scribner's Sons, 1968.

Goodman, L. S., and Gilman, A.: The Pharmacological Basis of Therapeutics. New York, The Macmillan Company, 1965.

Hodgson, T. A., Jr.: Short-term effects of air pollution on mortality in New York City. Envir. Science Tech., 4:589, 1970.

Machta, L., and Hughes, E.: Atmospheric oxygen in 1967 to 1970. Science, 168:1582, 1970.

Royal College of Physicians: Air Pollution and Health. London, Pitman Medical and Scientific Publishing Company, Ltd., 1970.

Diseases Due to Chemical Factors

COMMON ACCIDENTAL POISONING

Robert J. Haggerty

Definition. The term "accidental poisoning" usually is limited to clinical illness that results from the introduction of exogenous chemicals into the body. These chemicals may be medications in excessive dose, other chemicals not intended for human metabolism, or biologic products, both plant and animal. The term, however, generally excludes disease produced by toxic products of the growth of endogenous micro-organisms. An accident is usually defined as (1) an observable tissue or biochemical injury that is (2) unplanned. This definition is not strictly applicable in accidental poisoning, for in many instances the physician is called upon to treat patients who have only ingested a poison but do not yet have any observable symptoms or signs of tissue or biochemical injury. Also, whereas most poisonings are unplanned in children, the same tissue or biochemical damage occurs when a chemical is introduced for homicidal or suicidal intent, and it would seem appropriate to consider these together in this article.

Etiology. Accidental poisoning is best understood as a problem of multiple causes—the interaction of an agent (the poison) with a host (the patient) in a particular environment. The major agents and the number of accidental poisoning deaths caused by each are listed in Table 1, together with the number of suicides and homicides due to poisons. In nonfatal accidental poisoning the agents responsible are quite different from

TABLE 1. MORTALITY: AGENTS RESPONSIBLE FOR ACCIDENTAL POISON DEATHS IN THE UNITED STATES, 1966

	Number of Deaths
Solids and liquids	2283
Medications	
Barbiturates	553
Analgesics and soporifics	437
Alcohol	200
Salicylates	176
Other	402
Household products	
Lead	61
Corrosives (lye, etc.)	39
Petroleum products	40
Solvents	45
Other	330
Gases and vapors	1648
Suicide by all poisons	5588
Homicide by all poisons	47
Total poison deaths	9566

those in fatal cases. The most common agents responsible for nonfatal accidental poisoning are listed in Table 2, together with the number of such accidents in different age groups. Strictly speaking, these are the etiologic agents, but to understand why a particular poisoning occurs requires knowledge of the interaction of the agent, environment, and host; this is discussed under Pathogenesis. It is evident from Table 2 that over two thirds of all accidental poisonings occur in preschool children. Not so evident in this table is the second peak in the late teens and early twenties owing to suicide attempts.

The route of access of the poison (agent) is most often oral for solids and liquids, but may occasionally be by absorption through skin, rectum, or lung or by parenteral injection.

Incidence. Over 3000 accidental poison fatalities occur each year in the United States from solids, liquids, and gases. About one quarter of these occur in children, and 80 per cent of all childhood poisonings are limited to the "age of curiosity," one to four years. In children there are from

300 to 1000 nonfatal poison ingestions for each poison fatality. Some estimates place the total number of nonfatal poisonings as high as 300,000 to 500,000 per year in children in the United States. It is the most common medical, i.e., nonsurgical, emergency seen in childhood. In one study, 12 per cent of all two-year-old children had experienced an accidental poisoning within the previous year. In addition to differences in the agents responsible for fatal as compared with nonfatal poisoning, the agents responsible for accidental poisoning vary considerably in their frequency between children and adults. Salicylates are the most common agent involved in children, whereas barbiturates and carbon monoxide are more common in adults. A multitude of household products (such as cleansers, solvents, and insecticides) are potentially poisonous and are available in the American home. They are more likely to be the cause of childhood than of adult poisonings.

Epidemiology. There are more epidemiologic data available on the role of the agent in causing accidental poisoning than on the host and environmental factors, and very few data on the complex interrelations of these three factors in causing accidental poisoning. Most of the available information is of the retrospective epidemiologic type for accidental poisoning in children. It documents incidence by age (peak childhood age one to four years), sex (males more than females except for the poison suicides of the late teens and early twenties), socioeconomic class (no difference), season (no over-all significant variation, although there are some special variations such as medications that are more frequent in the winter and pesticides in the summer), hour of day (peak in midmorning), geographical area (lye and petroleum distillates more common in the South), and place where poisoning occurred (kitchen, bedroom, bathroom are most common). Unfortunately, this information has not led to effective prevention, for the death *rate* for all age groups from accidental poisoning has remained for the past two decades at about 1 per 100,000 for all age groups. There has been a significant decrease in both the *actual number* of deaths in

TABLE 2. MOST COMMON AGENTS RESPONSIBLE FOR ACCIDENTAL POISONING (NONFATAL) REPORTED TO THE NATIONAL CLEARINGHOUSE FOR POISON INFORMATION CENTERS, 1968

	All Ages	Under 5 Yrs.	5–14 Yrs.	15+ Yrs.	Unknown
Medicines	60,021	38,354	3077	15,695	2895
Aspirin	18,560	15,523	859	1772	406
Other internal	35,522	18,235	1916	13,435	1936
External	5939	4596	302	488	553
Cleaning and polishing agents	13,110	10,349	590	817	1354
Petroleum products	4363	3573	267	224	299
Cosmetics	4924	4286	127	116	395
Pesticides	5739	3965	391	574	809
Turpentine, paints, etc.	4991	3947	267	294	483
Plants	3798	2740	422	114	522
Gases and vapors	630	64	63	257	246
Miscellaneous	6081	3688	850	548	995
Unknown	1521	597	98	686	140
	105,178	71,563	6152	19,325	8138

*Data from National Clearinghouse for Poison Information Centers Bulletin, September-October, 1969.

children under five years of age from accidental poisoning (from 422 in 1958 to 325 in 1968) and in the *rate* (from 2.5 per 100,000 in 1958 to 1.9 in 1968). The reasons are probably multiple, but are likely to be from public and professional education, better therapy, safety enclosures for dispensing medicines, and limitation of the number of tablets in children's aspirin (1 1/4 grains) to 36 per bottle.

Greatly needed are prospective epidemiologic studies with special emphasis upon host and environmental as well as on agent factors. In the few studies so far completed these host and social environmental factors appear to be the important variables, since poisonous agents such as aspirin are available in nearly every home. The very real question is why more children are not poisoned when one considers the ubiquity of potentially poisonous agents.

Some children seem peculiarly susceptible to accidental poisoning. A child with a history of one poisoning episode is nine times as likely to have a second episode in the following year than is a child from a matched control group. Poisoned as compared to nonpoisoned control children appear to have different personalities. They are more impulsive and overactive and are likely to strike back when disciplined, to have disturbed relationships with their parents, and to have other behavior problems. Their social environment is also different, for their parents are more likely to have marital problems, to be suffering acute illness at the time of the ingestion, or to show a more distant and tense family relationship. Whether this knowledge can lead to identification of the high-risk group before poisoning occurs and whether one can change the incidence of poisoning in this high-risk group are not known; prevention has never been documented. Among adults, suicide and homicide by poisoning obviously present a very different epidemiologic picture. Unlike immunization for infectious diseases, no one method of control can be expected to be effective for all types of poisoning.

Prevention. Prevention of accidental poisoning, in spite of these negative statements about its effectiveness, should be attempted by many groups, including physicians. Better labeling of household products and prescriptions is of importance, but it should be remembered that children of the age most often poisoned cannot read. Parents should store such medications in safe places. Physicians treating adults should especially warn grandparents that the digitalis, quinidine, or other potent drugs they are receiving are toxic to small children and are often taken by the child from the grandmother's pocketbook. When prescribing analgesics, especially aspirin, for an acute illness in adults, the physician should warn that these are poisonous to children and should prescribe only the minimal amounts needed for an illness. A mother with an influenzal syndrome may have aspirin prescribed; she may fall asleep, and her two-year-old child may easily ingest a fatal amount of aspirin left on the bedside table. Other acute family crises, social as well as

medical, also seem to be factors in the pathogenesis of childhood poisoning. The physician who cares for such adult crises may be the most likely person to prevent childhood accidental poisonings by seeing that adequate supervision of children is arranged when parents are sick or upset.

The physician caring for children should be even more active in prevention by educating parents to the dangers of poisoning, especially the parents of high-risk children. Perhaps even more important is the treatment of the social and psychologic problems in many of the high-risk families—problems that seem to be underlying causes of many of these poisoning episodes.

Community aspects of poison prevention include public education concerning the hazards of poisons. The Federal Hazardous Substances Labeling Act requires special labeling of hazardous substances and the listing of toxic ingredients on the label. This important step is but one of many that have been taken by the community in an effort to reduce the frequency of accidental poisoning.

Safety enclosures, such as the "Palm 'n Turn bottles" which preschool children have difficulty opening, have been clearly demonstrated in military installations to decrease the incidence of accidental poisoning in this most vulnerable age group. Universal dispensing of medicines in these enclosures could almost eliminate deaths from medicines, which account for about half of all accidental poisoning deaths in children under five years of age.

National Poison Prevention Week during the third week in March serves as a focal point for health education programs. But to have any chance of success such measures should be carried out throughout the year. The rapid development of poison information centers since the first one was formed in Chicago in 1953 to the now more than 500 in the United States is another important community action. The National Clearinghouse for Poison Information Centers of the Public Health Service coordinates activities of the local centers and is a valuable repository of information, both for treatment of poisoned patients and for preventive programs. The Association of Poison Control Centers, a voluntary national group, has produced educational material designed to prevent poisonings, has established standards for operation of poison control centers, including an approved list of antidotes, their indications, and doses, and has promoted scientific study of poisonings. It seems clear that these multiple approaches to prevention of poisoning need to be continued, but there is a need to critically evaluate their effectiveness and to add imaginative new programs aimed at prevention.

Diagnosis. Diagnosis of accidental poisoning is made from (1) the label on the poison container, (2) the characteristic signs and symptoms in the patient, and (3) chemical analyses, in that order of importance. In most cases of acute poisoning, especially in children, there is no problem in determining that ingestion of a poison has occurred. The patient is often observed to ingest the poison or is found with the empty container. Here the problem is only to determine the chemical ingredients of the compound ingested, how much was taken, and what toxicity is to be expected. On the other hand, unlabeled prescriptions or trade-name household products (of which there are estimated to be over 250,000 potentially poisonous ones available in American homes) may present a serious problem in identification of the precise chemical involved. Poison information centers are especially equipped to deal with this aspect of diagnosis, for they keep on file trade names of potentially poisonous products and their ingredients. Most operate 24 hours a day and are listed in the telephone book. Information on management will also be provided by these centers. Of great use to the physician in diagnosis of poisoning, as well as in therapy, is the book by Gleason, Gosselin, and Hodge, which contains a section with over 17,000 trade-name household products, their ingredients, toxicity, symptoms, and treatment.

When the label is missing, identification of the poison may be aided by knowing that certain ingredients are common to household products used for the same specific purpose; e.g., most solvent cleansers contain ketones or hydrocarbons. The new Federal labeling legislation, which requires most hazardous household chemicals to bear a label that plainly lists ingredients, has helped in diagnosis. *The label on the container is the single most useful diagnostic bit of information in accidental poisoning.*

When the patient has not been observed to ingest a poison, the problem of diagnosis may be great. Although some poisons produce pathognomonic signs or symptoms, most do not. Almost any acute disease may be simulated, and the range of symptoms and signs that may result is so vast that one can only advise that any symptoms or signs of unknown cause must be suspected of being due to poisoning until proved otherwise. Lists of such symptoms and signs with the various poisons that can produce them are available in standard texts.

Toxicologic analysis of body fluids or of the ingested substance itself plays a numerically small but important role in the diagnosis of accidental poisoning. Its main usefulness is for certain common medications—e.g., the ferric chloride urine screening test for salicylates and phenothiazines, or barbiturate determinations of blood specimens—and for some heavy metal determinations (lead, thallium, mercury). It is usually impossible for a chemist to analyze a specimen of a completely unknown poison. Even when analysis is possible, the results will not be available for several hours or days; and, except for certain patients with chronic poisoning, treatment must be begun much sooner than that. In those few instances in which analysis is useful, it is usually much easier to analyze the remains in the container from which the poison came than to analyze body fluids in which great dilution of the poison has occurred. Recent developments suggest that chemical analysis may play a more important role in the future. Such techniques as thin-layer and gas chromatography make possible the identification of the minute amounts of poisons present in body fluids. Few laboratories are presently equipped to perform such analyses as routine measures, and it seems likely that development of special regional toxicologic laboratories will be necessary in order to make this resource a reality for the practicing physician.

Once the poison that was ingested has been identified, there remains the problem of determining its potential for harm to the patient. This depends on the amount ingested and the toxicity of the agent. The amount can sometimes be estimated by observers who may have seen the patient ingest the poison and by the amount remaining in the container. The toxicity of a particular poison can be assessed by reference to known data on LD_{50} and minimal lethal dose. A table has been prepared that is most useful in then estimating the degree of risk to the patient (Table 3).

Treatment. A common mistake in the therapy of acute poisoning is to search for a specific antidote, of which there are very few, and to delay general therapy, which may be very effective and is all that is available for the majority of poisonings.

General principles of therapy are (1) elimination of the poison from the body, (2) inactivation of the poison, and (3) supportive measures.

Elimination of the Poison. Induced Emesis. One of the most common poison problems brought to the physician is that of a child who has just ingested a potential poison but is still asymptomatic. The most important part of therapy is removal of the poison from the stomach before significant absorption can occur. It is now clear that gastric lavage, the time-honored method for removal of gastric contents, is much *less* effective than induced vomiting because the stomach normally traps large quantities of material in several pouches, inaccessible to the lavage tube. The most effective way to induce vomiting is to administer a large dose of syrup of ipecac (15 ml. for a child one to four years old) followed by another 10 to 15 ml. if no vomiting occurs within 20 minutes. This dose is considerably larger than recommended in older texts, but it has been found safe and much more rapidly effective than smaller doses. Many physicians now prescribe a 1-ounce

TABLE 3.   TOXICITY RATING

Rating	Probable Lethal Dose	
	mg./kg.	*For 70 kg. man*
6 super toxic	<5	A taste <7 drops
5 extremely toxic	5–50	7 drops to 1 tsp.
4 very toxic	50–500	1 tsp. to 1 oz.
3 moderately toxic	500–5 gm.	1 oz. to 1 pint
2 slightly toxic	5–15 gm.	1 pint to 1 quart
1 practically nontoxic	>15 gm.	>1 quart

(From Gleason, M., Gosselin, R., and Hodge, H.: Clinical Toxicology of Commercial Products. 2nd ed. Baltimore, The Williams & Wilkins Company, 1963.)

bottle of syrup of ipecac for all children at age one in order that parents will have it on hand in case of need. Vomiting is more complete if the patient drinks several ounces of fluid after administration of the syrup of ipecac. Mechanical induction of vomiting by gagging, although having the merit of speed, is so often not effective that it is not the first choice of methods. Parenteral administration of apomorphine (1 mg. for a one- to three-year-old, 6 mg. for an adult) has received renewed interest as a very effective emetic, especially if levallorphan (0.02 mg. per kilogram) is then used as an antidote for the depressant effects once vomiting has occurred. Vomiting should be induced even if several hours have elapsed after ingestion, for many poisons remain for long periods in the stomach when ingested in large quantities. Other methods of inducing vomiting are use of a solution of powdered mustard or soap suds. None of these is very effective.

Cautions Regarding Induced Emesis. The only contraindications to induced emesis in the treatment of accidental poisoning are in patients who have ingested caustics (lyes, acids, etc.), strychnine, and hydrocarbons, and in the comatose patient. Whether one should remove hydrocarbons by careful gastric lavage is still a disputed point. A collaborative study suggests that it may be of slight advantage. At least lavage does not seem to be dangerous, but emesis should not be used to remove hydrocarbons.

Gastric Lavage. Even though less effective than emesis, gastric lavage is indicated for comatose poisoned patients to remove the poison from the stomach with less risk of aspiration into the lungs than with emesis. A large-bore gastric lavage tube should usually be employed, and the stomach should be irrigated with copious amounts of water, dilute solution of sodium bicarbonate, or physiologic saline. Aspiration can be prevented by having the patient lie on his side.

Other Methods of Poison Removal. No data are available on the *effectiveness* of *catharsis* or *colonic irrigations.* Many people induce catharsis by giving 2 to 3 grams of sodium sulfide (for the preschool child), but the risk of serious fluid loss from the treatment does not usually make the risk worthwhile.

Exchange transfusion has proved useful for removal of some poisons when plasma protein binding makes any form of dialysis less effective, i.e., with boric acid and some barbiturates.

Peritoneal dialysis and *hemodialysis* are effective means of removing many poisons. For preschool children, and even for many adults, peritoneal dialysis is preferred because proper equipment and an experienced team for hemodialysis are rarely available. Use of commercially prepared solutions that contain properly balanced electrolytes and albumin, together with simple multiple-holed polyethylene tubing for insertion into the peritoneal cavity, provides a relatively convenient and simple technique. In certain adult patients in whom renal failure from the poisoning is the major problem, e.g., ethylene

glycol poisoning, or for whom prolonged dialysis is needed, hemodialysis has proved very useful.

The kidney is the most effective organ for removal of many poisons. If renal function was normal prior to the poisoning, this route of excretion should be facilitated by adequate fluids, usually intravenously, and in some situations by the use of *osmotic diuretics,* such as mannitol. In salicylate poisoning renal excretion is enhanced as much as twentyfold by making the pH of the urine alkaline with sodium bicarbonate. For patients who are seriously ill several of these routes of elimination of the poison should be used simultaneously, i.e., gastric lavage, enhancement of urinary excretion, and peritoneal dialysis.

Inactivation of the Poison. A time-honored agent designed to inactivate many poisons has been the "universal antidote" made of two parts charcoal, one part tannic acid, and one part magnesium oxide. Most people now believe that this mixture, as usually prepared, is of little value, but there has recently been a renewed interest in, and new data to support, the use of specially prepared activated charcoal to absorb poisons in the intestinal tract. Five to 6 teaspoonfuls of such charcoal mixed in a glass of water should be swallowed or administered by gastric tube and then, after adsorption has occurred, within 30 minutes, removed from the stomach. Neutralization of ingested acids or alkalies is probably of little value since the tissue necrosis that results from such poisons occurs almost immediately upon contact. The use of demulcents, such as olive oil or milk, makes the patient who has ingested an irritant poison more comfortable but probably does little else and should be avoided if the poison is fat-soluble.

Supportive Measures. More lives are likely to be saved by careful, early, symptomatic treatment of complications such as peripheral vascular collapse, respiratory obstruction, urinary retention, fluid imbalance, and central nervous system excitement or depression than by frantic and usually unsuccessful search for specific antidotes. All these complications are treated by the standard methods that are used when they are due to other causes.

Poisonings for Which Specific Antidotes Exist. *Cyanide poisoning* produces death within minutes. Specific antidotes are available, but unless poisoning occurs in a laboratory there is rarely time to administer them. The antidotes are sodium nitrite injected intravenously (6 to 8 ml. per square meter of body surface of a 3 per cent solution at a rate of 2.5 to 5 ml. per minute), which produces methemoglobinemia, followed by sodium thiosulfate intravenously (50 ml. of a 25 per cent solution). Amyl nitrite inhalation may be of value immediately while the sodium nitrite is being prepared.

Heavy metal poisoning can often be successfully treated by various chelating agents—BAL, EDTA, or penicillamine. (See article on Toxic Nephropathy.)

Iron salts produce acute gastroenteritis, shock, liver necrosis, and, frequently, death. As few as 10 tablets of the usual size (0.3 gram) may be fatal. The specific antidote, desferrioxamine, is probably useful both orally to absorb iron in the stomach and prevent systemic absorption (8 to 12 grams in 40 to 60 ml. of distilled water) and intravenously to bind absorbed iron (2.0 grams in 5 per cent of levulose solution intravenously); 140 mg. of desferrioxamine can bind about 1 gram of ferrous sulfate — 200 mg. of iron, dose 90 mg. per kilogram. Fluid replacement, including blood plasma, should be used for shock.

Morphine and other opium derivatives can be successfully antagonized by levallorphan, 0.02 mg. per kilogram subcutaneously. (See article on Drug Dependence.)

Phosphate ester insecticides such as parathion are powerful anticholinesterases. In addition to peripheral parasympathetic stimulation they produce voluntary muscle paralysis, the most serious being to the muscles of respiration. Atropine in very large doses of 1 mg. subcutaneously for a child, 2 to 3 mg. for an adult, every 15 to 60 minutes until symptoms subside will antagonize these peripheral parasympathomimetic toxic effects. 2-Pyridine aldoxime methiodide (PAM), a cholinesterase regenerator, is dramatically effective in relieving skeletal muscle paralysis (1 gram intravenously over a five- to ten-minute period and repeated as a slow intravenous drip as needed for respiratory paralysis). Airway obstruction must be treated by aspiration, positioning, and occasionally by tracheostomy.

Treatment of Specific Common Poisons. A few words should be said about general management of the most common poisoning, but reference to standard texts is necessary for details of treatment of these as well as for the many poisonings that cannot be discussed here.

Amphetamine poisoning is common from an overdose of reducing pills or pep pills. After removal from the stomach, chlorpromazine should be administered in full dose to counteract mania and delirium. Barbiturates should not be used because the late-stage depression that occurs with amphetamines may be compounded.

Atropine poisoning may be produced by overdose or accidental ingestion of the drug or by accidental ingestion of one of several plants, such as the jimson weed. Symptoms include those of parasympathetic blocking, intense erythema, fever, and delirium. Peripheral parasympathetic blockade can be treated with pilocarpine, but this will not counteract the more serious central nervous system symptoms, which must be treated symptomatically with sedatives such as chloral hydrate or paraldehyde.

DDT and other chlorinated hydrocarbon insecticides are relatively uncommon causes of acute poisoning, for fatal doses in man are in the range of 250 mg. per kilogram, and this amount is difficult to ingest. Central nervous system stimulation and convulsions are the most serious symptoms. Treatment is entirely symptomatic.

Hydrocarbon ingestion, especially of gasoline and kerosene, produces a severe pneumonia due mainly to direct aspiration into the lung rather than to blood-stream transport to the lungs. Most of the aspiration probably occurs during the initial swallow, but some may also occur during subsequent vomiting. *Emesis is therefore contraindicated.* If large amounts have been ingested, careful lavage is useful. The head should be lower than the chest to prevent aspiration, and the procedure should be performed with a small Levin tube passed through the nose. This is most effective if done before vomiting and consequent aspiration can occur. Varying degrees of central nervous system depression occur but this rarely needs therapy. Probably the only effective therapy for the patient with severe pneumonia is oxygen. Although adrenocortical steroids and prophylactic antimicrobials have been used, there is little evidence that they are the crucial element in successful therapy of this poisoning.

Carbon tetrachloride produces prompt central nervous system depression and abdominal pain. Early death is due to depression of vasomotor and respiratory centers and convulsions. If the patient survives this period he may develop renal and hepatic necrosis. The management at this stage is the same as for other causes of failure of these organs.

Methyl alcohol can cause severe metabolic acidosis and blindness with a fatal dose from as little as 2 ounces. Treatment includes emesis, ethyl alcohol to inhibit the metabolic oxidation of methanol (whiskey, 30 ml. every three to four hours for adults), and sodium bicarbonate intravenously for the metabolic acidosis.

Lye and other caustics produce severe, deep burns of the esophagus that may perforate or may later cause esophageal stenosis. Initial pain, airway obstruction, and shock are treated symptomatically. Early esophagoscopy, to determine whether burns have occurred, is followed by cortisone if burns are found. After several days for healing to progress, careful dilatation of the esophagus can be begun. Management should be a team effort with the esophagoscopist.

Salicylate poisoning is by far the single most common cause of poisoning in children. Emesis should always be carried out if the patient is awake, even though several hours have elapsed after ingestion. Salicylates produce an initial respiratory alkalosis that is transient in children but less so in adults, followed by severe metabolic acidosis, dehydration, and loss of body potassium. The degree of seriousness of the poisoning can be estimated by reference to a nomogram prepared by Done and reproduced in the accompanying figure. With severe poisoning several routes of elimination may have to be used, i.e., by increasing urinary excretion and by peritoneal dialysis. Initial hydration should be vigorous to initiate brisk diuresis, and the fluids should include sodium bicarbonate, 14 to 20 ml. of 7.5 per cent solution per 500 ml. of fluid. Once diuresis has begun, potassium salts, approximately

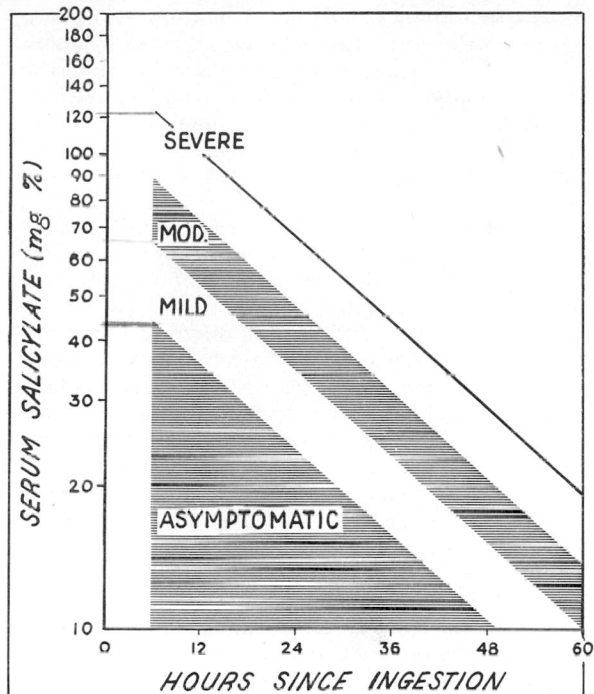

Nomogram relating serum salicylate concentration and expected severity of intoxication at varying intervals following the ingestion of a single dose of salicylate. (From Done, A. K.: Salicylate intoxication: Significance of measurements of salicylate in blood in cases of acute ingestion. Pediatrics, 26:800, 1960, with permission.)

35 mEq. per liter of fluid, should be added to the solution. Monitoring of serum pH and electrolytes and adjustment of fluid and electrolyte administration appropriately are important for optimal therapy. Milder degrees of poisoning can usually be treated with alkali and intravenous fluids alone. Other symptoms, such as respiratory depression or convulsions, are treated symptomatically.

Cirksena, W. J., Bastian, R. C., Malloy, J. P., and Barry, K. G.: Use of mannitol in exogenous and endogenous intoxications, New Eng. J. Med., 270:161, 1964.

Done, A. K.: Salicylate intoxication: Significance of measurements of salicylate in blood in cases of acute ingestion. Pediatrics, 26:800, 1960.

Etteldorf, J. N., Dobbins, W. T., Summitt, R. L., Rainwater, W. T., and Fischer, R. L.: Intermittent peritoneal dialysis using 5 per cent albumin in the treatment of salicylate intoxication in children. J. Pediat., 58:226, 1961.

Gleason, M., Gosselin, R., and Hodge, H.: Clinical Toxicology of Commercial Products. 3rd ed. Baltimore, Williams and Wilkins Company, 1969.

Holt, L. E., Jr., and Holz, P. H.: Activated Charcoal as an Antidote for Poisons. Nat. Clearinghouse Poison Control Cent. 1963, Jan.-Feb., pp. 1-3.

Meyer, R. J., Roelofs, H. A., Bluestone, J., and Redmond, S.: Accidental injury to the preschool child. J. Pediat., 63:95, 1963.

Robertson, W. O.: Syrup of ipecac—A slow or fast emetic? Amer. J. Dis. Child., 103:136, 1962.

Schertz, R. G., Latham, G. H., and Stracener, C. E.: Child-resistant containers can prevent poisonings. Pediatrics, 43:84, 1969.

Sobel, R., and Margolis, J. A.: Repetitive poisoning in children: A psychosocial study. Pediatrics, 35:641, 1965.

Vital Statistics of the United States, 1968. U.S. Dept. of Health, Education and Welfare. Public Health Service. National Center for Health Statistics.

VonOettingen, W. F.: Poisoning, A Guide to Clinical Diagnosis and Treatment. 2nd ed. Philadelphia, W. B. Saunders Company, 1958.

Wehrle, P. F., DeFreest, L., Penhollow, J., and Harris, V. G.: The epidemiology of accidental poisoning in an urban population. III. Pediatrics, 27.614, 1961.

HEAVY METAL POISONING
Edmund B. Flink

GENERAL CONSIDERATIONS

Many features of poisoning by the heavy metals are similar. The important metals from the standpoint of toxicology are arsenic, lead, mercury, antimony, cadmium, and thallium. The toxic and lethal doses of each metal are small. Antimony, arsenic, lead, mercury, and thallium all have effects on enzymes of the body. Antimony, arsenic, and mercury particularly poison sulfhydryl groups. Mercuric ions even in fairly dilute solutions denature proteins and cause protein precipitation. Thallium and cadmium have recently assumed importance industrially.

Other metals may be toxic also. *Beryllium* and *gold* intoxications are discussed elsewhere in this text. *Barium* ions cause epigastric pain, nausea, vomiting, diarrhea, chills, cramps, muscle contractions, and convulsions. Sodium sulfate or magnesium sulfate should be given immediately to precipitate the barium as sulfate. *Cobalt* was added to beer from 1957 to 1967. Ingestion of large volumes of this beer caused serious and often fatal myocardiopathy. Cobalt has been eliminated as an additive. *Manganese* poisoning occurs in mining and smelting of manganese ores. Damage to the basal ganglia of the brain occurs with attendant Parkinson-like symptoms. When symptoms begin, removal from exposure is mandatory. Proper ventilation of mines and processing plants will prevent intoxication.

Dubois, K. P., and Geiling, E. M. K.: Textbook of Toxicology. New York, Oxford University Press, 1959.

Fairhall, L. T.: Industrial Toxicology. 2nd ed. Baltimore, Williams & Wilkins Company, 1957.

Gleason, M. N., Gosselin, R. E., and Hodge, H. C.: Clinical Toxicology of Commercial Products. 3rd ed. Baltimore, Williams and Wilkins Company, 1969.

ARSENIC POISONING

Exposure. Many household and garden pesticides contain arsenous oxide, copper acetoarsenite (Paris green), or calcium or lead arsenate. Drugs that contain arsenic include sodium cacodylate, Fowler's solution, and the arsphenamines. Fowler's solution continues to be used in treatment of asthma in certain regions. Fruits sprayed with insecticides may contain enough arsenic to be toxic. Bootlegged whiskey has occasionally been contaminated with arsenicals. Arsenic trioxide (As_2O_3) or white arsenic has been a favorite for homicidal purposes.

Although toxic exposure occurs in a variety of industries, only a few cases are reported. Poisoning does occur among agricultural workers using insecticide sprays or dust. Accidental ingestion of arsenic-containing poison continues to be an important source of exposure for children especially.

Arsenic combines with sulfhydryl groups like mercury and antimony and thus interferes with vital enzymatic activity. It is stored in liver, nervous system, nails, hair, and other viscera and can be detected in them after excretion in urine has ceased. A single dose requires 10 to 70 days for excretion, so accumulation is possible from small daily doses.

The minimal lethal dose of arsenic trioxide (As_2O_3) is 60 to 180 mg., but there is a great variability in susceptibility. The lethal dose of arsine is smaller than this. The safe limit for arsenic particles in the atmosphere is 0.5 mg. per cubic meter of air and of arsine 0.05 parts of vapor per million parts of air.

Manifestations. *Acute poisoning* may be overwhelming and may produce shock and death within 20 minutes to 48 hours. Ingestion of smaller doses causes vomiting, diarrhea, abdominal pain, and muscle cramps but does not cause corrosion of mucous membranes. If the victim survives acute poisoning, he may recover without sequelae, or he may develop symptoms of chronic poisoning.

Arsine (AsH_3) is a very serious industrial hazard. It is produced accidentally by the exposure of nascent hydrogen to arsenic trioxide. It can occur in chemical laboratories and in metallic ore processing plants. Intravascular hemolysis and renal damage are characteristic, so hemoglobinuria, nausea, vomiting, and abdominal pain develop within six hours after exposure. This initial illness may be quickly fatal, or recovery may begin in a few days. Instances of chronic arsine poisoning have been reported.

Chronic poisoning results from repeated ingestion of small doses. This is the usual method for homicide, but it is less popular than formerly. Weight loss, diarrhea or constipation, nausea, anorexia, fatigue, pigmentation and scaling of the skin, peripheral neuropathy, headache, confusion, drowsiness, hyperkeratoses of palms and soles, and transverse striae of fingernails (Mee's lines) are the important symptoms and signs. Mee's lines appear as single solid transverse white bands 1 or 2 mm. in width completely crossing the nail and appearing in all fingers in the same relative position. Neuropathy may cause wrist drop or foot drop, or there may be numbness and paresthesias. Hyperkeratoses may go on to malignant changes in the form of multiple basal cell cancers. Perforation of the nasal septum is common.

Before penicillin became available in the early 1940's, syphilis was treated with intensive organic arsenical therapy, chiefly by means of oxophenarsine hydrochloride (Mapharsen) and neoarsphenamine. Many instances of acute, and sometimes fatal, poisoning occurred, with encephalopathy, liver damage, exfoliative dermatitis, nephropathy or pancytopenia. This has vanished as a problem.

Hematologic findings of chronic arsenic poisoning include anemia, leukopenia, thrombocytopenia, basophilic stippling, and disturbed erythropoiesis, and myelopoiesis.

Diagnosis. The differential diagnosis includes diabetes mellitus, chronic alcoholism, Guillain-Barré syndrome, other toxic states such as thallium and lead poisoning, and porphyria.

The diagnosis can be established by determining arsenic in the urine. Normal persons excrete an average of 0.015 mg. per day, with a range of 0.005 to 0.04 mg. Most patients with manifestations of arsenic poisoning excrete more than 0.1 mg. per day.

As in lead poisoning, urine coproporphyrin III excretion is increased markedly. Delta amino levulinic acid is not increased in experimental arsenic poisoning in rabbits and probably not in human intoxication. Coproporphyrin excretion should be determined in all instances of neuropathy of obscure origin.

Hair and nails store arsenic, so analysis of arsenic content may be of diagnostic value, particularly after removal of the patient from exposure. Hair and nail samples must be very carefully washed to exclude adhering dust and extraneous material. Normal values have ranged from 0.025 to 0.088 mg. per 100 grams of hair. Over 0.1 mg. per 100 grams is abnormal.

Treatment. When a poison has been ingested, immediate induction of emesis or gastric lavage is of prime importance. Dimercaprol (BAL) should be given immediately, using the same schedule as for mercury poisoning. BAL has not proved to be effective in arsine poisoning or in chronic poisoning, probably because the damage has already occurred. Removal from exposure in chronic poisoning usually suffices and, of course, is mandatory.

Acute anemia must be treated by transfusion. Treatment of acute renal insufficiency requires the same considerations as that due to a variety of causes.

Prevention. Proper storage and labeling of poisons in general should prevent accidental poisoning of children. Avoiding direct contact with insect sprays and wearing appropriate masks when using dusting powders will control this industrial exposure.

Heyman, A., Pfeiffer, J. B., Jr., Willet, R. W., and Taylor, H. M.: Peripheral neuropathy caused by arsenical intoxication: A study of 41 cases with observation of the effects of BAL. New Eng. J. Med., 254:401, 1956.

Kyle, R. A., and Pease, G. L.: Hematologic aspects of arsenic intoxication. New Eng. J. Med., 273:18, 1965.

Vallee, B. L., Ulmer, D. D., and Wacker, W. E. C.: Arsenic toxicology and biochemistry. AMA Arch. Industr. Health, 21:132, 1960.

LEAD POISONING

Etiology. Exposure to lead in the home is chiefly by ingestion of white lead paint by children, from new water systems in which white lead has been used in joints of pipes, by ingestion of soluble lead salts, and by use of tetraethyl lead gasoline for cleaning purposes. An outbreak of lead poisoning among 121 Gurkha soldiers in Hong Kong has recently been found to be due to curry powder contaminated with lead chromate. Drinking of "moonshine" whiskey distilled by use of an auto radiator as a condenser has resulted in epidemics of acute lead poisoning and constitutes an important cause of lead poisoning of adults in the United States. Lead is dissolved and absorbed from the gastrointestinal tract, deposited in the liver and then released into the systemic circulation. The respiratory tract epithelium may absorb lead fumes or may propel particles into the pharynx, where they are swallowed. Tetraethyl lead and related compounds may be absorbed through the skin. Soluble lead salts, such as lead acetate or lead carbonate, are readily absorbed and can cause acute poisoning when ingested.

Ingestion of lead paint scales by young children (pica) constitutes the greatest problem in the United States today. Sometimes emotional disturbances or mental retardation cause pica, which in turn results in serious sequelae. The recognized incidence in New York City rose from 1 in 1950 to 80 in 1955 because of increased interest and availability of appropriate tests. The incidence in areas of poor housing and crowding is much greater than in areas of good housing. The incidence in children is greatest in summer months and reaches a peak at the age of one to three years. Siblings of children with lead intoxication should be examined also, because about a third of them have been found to have serious exposure.

There are many industrial uses of lead and, therefore, many opportunities for exposure. In recent years the industrial consumption of lead in the United States has averaged about 1,110,000 tons a year. The industries using or producing lead are petroleum, mining and smelting, storage battery manufacture, printing, paint and pigment, ceramic and glass, construction (mainly plumbing and insulation), ammunition, wrecking and salvage (acetylene torch and electric arc volatilizing lead paints and alloys), and battery reclaiming. Any procedure that produces lead vapor, mist, or dust containing lead exposes workers to inhalation and absorption of lead from respiratory tract epithelium. Lead concentration in respired air should be below 0.15 mg. per cubic meter, and lead tetraethyl should be below 0.1 mg. per cubic meter. Some health authorities set the safe limit at 0.05 mg. per cubic meter. Lead concentration in air of heavily traveled freeways is as high as 0.018 mg. per cubic meter.

The lead-using trades have set up standards and checking procedures that have controlled industrial hazards well. Smoking and eating are restricted to uncontaminated areas. Washing hands and changing clothes before eating and leaving work are the most important personal preventive measures. The gasoline industry has rigid standards for tetraethyl lead workers, but exposure to dangerous amounts still occurs when there is a break in procedure. Cleaning and repairing large storage tanks pose a particular hazard.

Pathology. In chronic poisoning no gross or microscopic lesions are pathognomonic of lead poisoning. Lead is stored in an inert form in bone and is not harmful except when mobilized. Most of the remaining lead is found in the bone marrow, blood, liver, and kidneys. An increased amount of lead in tissues indicates exposure but not necessarily toxicity. Absence of an increased concentration of lead in tissues practically excludes lead poisoning.

In the encephalopathic type, small perivascular hemorrhages, necrosis of cells, and serous exudate around blood vessels may be found anywhere in the brain. In children with acute poisoning, nuclear inclusions are found in liver cells and renal tubular cells. Occasionally inclusions are found in renal tubule cells of lead workers. In Australia chronic lead exposure from the dust of white lead paint has been incriminated as a common cause of chronic renal failure in young adults.

Clinical Manifestations. Lead poisoning is usually divided into acute and chronic forms. Although "chronic poisoning" correctly describes prolonged exposure, manifestations often are acute. It is convenient for descriptive purposes to divide symptomatology into an alimentary form, a neuromuscular form, and an encephalopathic form.

There are symptoms and signs common to all three forms. Anemia and attendant pallor and weakness are present in most patients with chronic exposure, but not regularly among those with the acute encephalopathic form owing to tetraethyl lead poisoning or acute massive exposure to inorganic lead. Insomnia, headache, dizziness, and irritability are common symptoms without evidence of more serious encephalopathic disturbances. In a patient with poor oral hygiene lead sulfide is deposited along the gingival margin of some or all teeth and produces a blue-black "lead line." Stippling of the retina adjacent to the optic disc has recently been described as an early sign in lead poisoning. Chronic renal failure results from chronic lead intoxication. Saturnine gout is particularly common in lead poisoning from "moonshine" whiskey. The renal clearance of uric acid decreases.

Alimentary Form. Colicky pain (often called painter's or lead colic) is the cardinal feature and is the result of spasm of the bowel. Constipation is a natural consequence, and nausea, vomiting, and weight loss are common. As implied by the name, colic is intermittent and often severe enough to double the patient up. Between attacks there is merely a sense of pressure. Absence of tenderness differentiates the condition from appendicitis or other causes of peritoneal inflammation. Relief actually may be produced by pressure on the abdomen. Colic is not invariably present.

Neuromuscular Form. Weakness of a muscle group precedes actual paralysis. Extensor muscles of the upper extremities are more often paralyzed than flexors or lower extremity muscles. *Wrist drop* is a common and characteristic example. Muscle soreness and stiffness or hypertonus precede and accompany paralysis. The absence of sensory disturbance is important in differentiating this from other forms of peripheral neuropathy. Paralysis is confined to a functional muscle group and is not determined by the distribution of an entire motor nerve. Atrophy may occur after long-standing paralysis and may result in incomplete recovery of muscle function after termination of exposure.

Encephalopathic Form. At the present time this occurs primarily in children. The diagnosis is not suspected until a large amount of lead has been ingested. Because of the good safeguards in industry now, it rarely occurs in adults and then only following massive exposure to lead fumes or tetraethyl lead in a salvage operation, in cleaning large gasoline storage tanks, or in accidental breaks in techniques. Tetraethyl lead is lipid-soluble, so that exposure results almost exclusively in the encephalopathic form.

The presenting manifestations include *coma, convulsions, mania,* or *delirium.* There may be a history of antecedent behavioral changes such as irritability, insomnia, restlessness, loss of memory, hallucinations, and confusion.

Children may suddenly become very ill. Increased intracranial pressure may occur and is manifested by projectile vomiting, lethargy, convulsions, and coma. In very young children fontanelles bulge. The optic discs may not reflect increased pressure when the process is very acute in onset. Scattered neurologic findings indicate cerebral and cerebellar abnormalities. Blindness and deafness may occur and persist.

Laboratory Findings. The hematologic findings depend on the action of lead on hemoglobin synthesis. Lead interferes with the combination of glycine and succinic acid to form delta amino levulinic acid (ALA) and with the coupling of the two molecules of ALA to form porphobilinogen (PBG) by interference with enzymes ALA synthetase and ALA dehydrase, respectively. The intermediate steps are not affected, but lead also interferes with the incorporation of iron and protoporphyrin to form the heme molecule. Thus, lead interferes with at least three steps in the synthesis of hemoglobin, but the block at the ALA dehydrase step is most important quantitatively. ALA and coproporphyrin III accumulate and are excreted in the urine in excessive amounts, and protoporphyrin accumulates in erythrocytes as a result of the blocks in synthetic process. Normally 2 mg. of ALA or less is excreted per 24 hours. Lead poisoning results in a 20- to 200-fold increase in excretion of ALA. Excretion in-

creases before any other chemical or hematologic changes are manifest. In industrial workers exposed to lead, the ALA excretion is correlated better with lead concentrations in the blood than with any other test. ALA excretion, therefore, is the most sensitive indicator of lead intoxication available, and is more specific than coproporphyrin excretion, which increases in many other toxic states. ALA determinations on urine and serum now are relatively simple and are becoming the principal indicator of intoxication as well as a most useful tool in epidemiologic studies. Normally 60 to 280 mcg. of coproporphyrin is excreted per 24 hours. Lead poisoning results in a three- to tenfold increase in coproporphyrin excretion. There is general agreement that coproporphyrin excretion can be used as a sensitive measure of intoxication in workers exposed to lead. Normally isomers I and III are excreted in equal amounts, but in lead and other chemical poisoning the excess coproporphyrin is mostly type III. Urine specimens must be acidified if they are to be stored for any length of time before actual determination of ALA, and must be alkalinized with sodium carbonate for delayed coproporphyrin determination.

In experimental lead poisoning of rabbits the bone marrow contains a relatively large amount of coproporphyrin III, present probably as its porphyrinogen and converted to the prophyrin during extraction. The circulating erythrocytes in these rabbits contain a great excess of protoporphyrin but only relatively little coproporphyrin. Free erythrocyte coproporphyrin (FECP) serves as a chemical index of the number of reticulocytes normally, but when there is an interference with hemoglobin synthesis the FECP may be increased without parallel increase in reticulocytes.

Free erythrocyte protoporphyrin (FEPP) normally is 15 to 60 mcg. per 100 ml., and FECP normally is 0 to 2 mcg. per 100 ml. In lead poisoning FEPP ranges from 300 to 3000 mcg. per 100 ml., and FECP ranges from 1 to 20 mcg. per 100 ml. It is noteworthy that iron deficiency anemia and thalassemia result in FEPP values that overlap those of lead poisoning, but the range is not quite as great. If a fresh wet film of blood of a patient with lead poisoning is examined under ultraviolet light, 75 to 100 per cent of the erythrocytes have a red fluorescence. This fluorescence is the result of increased FEPP.

Lead poisoning and *hereditary acute intermittent porphyria* have manifestations that are similar. Both are characterized by colicky abdominal pain, mental symptoms, and paralysis. Acute intermittent porphyria regularly has a great increase in porphobilinogen excretion and uroporphyrin excretion, but lead poisoning usually does not result in excessive excretion of either substance.

Normochromic microcytic anemia, decreased red cell life span, decreased osmotic fragility, but increased mechanical fragility are found. Acute hemolytic anemia with hemoglobinemia, hemoglobinuria, and renal damage occur occasionally in acute poisoning. Death from shock may occur in two to three days. *Basophilic stippling* is non-specific, is rarely found in tetraethyl lead intoxication, is seldom found in acute poisoning of children, and cannot be relied on for screening purposes. Nevertheless, it frequently furnishes the initial clue for clinical recognition of chronic lead poisoning.

Aminoaciduria, renal glycosuria, fructosuria, hyperphosphaturia, and citraturia result from changes in the epithelium of the proximal convoluted tubules. Other toxins also cause these manifestations. The changes are usually reversible.

Diagnosis. Although clinical manifestations afford the clues, the laboratory must supply the definitive diagnostic information. Blood lead content and urine lead content should be increased above the empirically determined levels in normal healthy persons free from lead exposure (see the accompanying table of normal and abnormal values). In children, particularly, the normal level is low. If the higher range is used with the upper limit of 0.054 mg. per 100 grams, or, as recommended by some authors, 0.06 mg. per 100 grams, many children with serious acute poisoning will have normal levels. The lower value of 0.04 mg. per 100 grams is better. In adults the upper limits of normal coincide with the mean of "safe" exposure.

A diagnosis of tetraethyl lead intoxication is made on the basis of history of exposure. Urine lead determination is the most valuable test. Blood values usually are normal.

Because of the medicolegal implications, it is important to be certain that there is evidence of increased lead excretion. Detection of an earlier exposure may be accomplished by the use of calcium disodium edetate (CaEDTA). Striking augmentation of lead excretion occurs because of mobilization of lead from the skeletal stores. This proves previous exposure but not intoxication.

Collection of samples for analysis must be done with great care to avoid contamination. Pyrex

bottles or polyethylene flasks should be rinsed with nitric acid and distilled water. Urine should be collected directly in the flasks. Urinals or bed pans are usually contaminated and must not be used for collection of urine or stool.

Blood now can be collected in special vacutainer 20 ml. tubes (Becton, Dickinson Company) with pure gum rubber stoppers. These tubes have been chemically cleaned for lead analyses. The needle is a straight stainless steel tube. Duplicate samples are desirable.

Feces samples should be collected directly in a wide-mouth glass jar cleaned with citric acid and closed with a plastic stopper. Tissue specimens similarly should be placed directly into an acid-cleaned jar. The specimen should be handled as little as possible, should be stripped of fat and fibrous tissue, and should not be allowed to be in contact with intestinal contents. Air sampling is a responsibility of industrial engineers.

Lead determinations on blood and urine can now be performed quickly and accurately, using an atomic absorption spectrometer. All state and many large city departments of health have such facilities available.

Treatment. Cessation of exposure is of prime importance. A saline cathartic should be given to rid the gut of any unabsorbed lead before chelation of lead is attempted, especially in the encephalopathic form in children.

Colic may be controlled temporarily by intravenous infusion of 1.0 gram of calcium gluconate. The infusion may be repeated as needed.

Fluid intake should be high unless there is increased intracranial pressure. Electrolyte concentrations should be determined and corrected if abnormal.

Chelation of lead by the calcium salt of ethylene diamine tetra-acetic acid, by calcium disodium edetate, U.S.P. (CaEDTA), or by penicillamine is now the treatment of choice for inorganic lead and tetraethyl lead intoxication and is much more effective than any previous method. The chelated lead is excreted in the urine. CaEDTA in doses of 1 to 2 grams per day for an adult and not more than 75 mg. per kilogram for a child is given in six to twelve hours intravenously. This dose is repeated for two to three days with a five- to ten-day rest period between courses. Nephropathy has resulted rarely from therapy, but this usually has occurred with larger doses than those outlined above. CaEDTA usually increases strikingly the lead excretion in a person with excessive lead stores. If symptoms are severe, treatment should not be delayed to obtain results of lead analyses. Lead excretion should be determined during as well as before treatment.

Penicillamine not only chelates lead but also supplies sulfhydryl groups. A dose of 30 mg. per kilogram up to a total of 2.0 grams per day in four divided doses given orally is satisfactory. It has the additional advantages that it can be given orally continuously, and that it is much less toxic than CaEDTA. For moderate lead intoxication, penicillamine is the agent of choice. Successful

NORMAL AND ABNORMAL VALUES IN EXPOSURE TO LEAD

	Adults		
	Normal Industrial Exposure	"Safe" Industrial Exposure	Dangerous Industrial Exposure
Urine mg. per liter	Range: 0.00 to 0.06 Mean: 0.03	0.01 to 0.15 0.08	0.08 to 0.4 0.2
Blood mg. per 100 grams	Range: 0.01 to 0.05 Mean: 0.03	0.01 to 0.07 0.06	0.07 to 0.2 0.09
Feces mg. per specimen	0.25	0.6 to 1.0	1.1+
	Children		
		Normal Range	Poisoning
Blood mg. per 100 grams	British series	0 to 0.04	0.04 to 0.4
	American series	0.003 to 0.055	0.06+

treatment with CaEDTA or penicillamine results in a return of ALA and coproporphyrin excretion to normal. Erythrocyte protoporphyrin declines very slowly after successful treatment.

The most serious manifestation is lead encephalopathy, which requires prompt and skillful treatment. Increased intracranial pressure may occur suddenly and must be treated vigorously. Infusion of urea solution in a dose of 100 mg. per kilogram to 1000 mg. per kilogram as 30 per cent urea in 10 per cent glucose solution or of mannitol solution (20 per cent) in a dose of 7 to 10 ml. per kilogram can alleviate increased pressure effectively, but the benefit may last only a day or two, and repetition may be necessary. Craniotomy may even be required for relief of pressure. Chelation of lead with CaEDTA must be started immediately for patients who are gravely ill.

Physiotherapy is important for patients with neuropathy. Splinting to support the weak extremity prevents overstretching of muscles; otherwise, permanent disability can follow.

Prognosis. In the gastrointestinal form the outlook is good for complete recovery after adequate treatment and prevention of re-exposure. Recovery from paralysis is usually complete even after many months of paralysis.

Encephalopathy is very serious. It causes a mortality rate of 25 per cent or more, and often leaves mental retardation and various permanent neurologic lesions in those who survive. In adults permanent blindness, extraocular muscle paralysis or other lesions may result. The acute form caused by tetraethyl lead either is fatal or is followed by complete recovery. There is great urgency in treatment of this form. One cannot wait to get results of lead analysis before starting treatment.

Ball, G. V., and Sorensen, L. B.: Pathogenesis of hyperuricemia in saturnine gout. New Eng. J. Med., 280:1199, 1969.

Byers, R. K.: Lead poisoning. Review of literature and report on 45 cases. Pediatrics, 23:585, 1959.

Einarsson, O., and Lindstedt, G.: Nonextraction atomic absorption method for the determination of lead. Scand. J. Clin. Lab. Invest., 23:367, 1969.

Feldman, F., Lichtman, H. C., Oransky, S., Ana, E. S., Reiser, L., and Malemud, C. J.: Serum delta aminolevulinic acid in plumbism. J. Pediat., 74:917, 1969.

Fleming, A. J.: Industrial hygiene and medical control procedures. Arch. Environ. Health (Chicago), 8:266, 1964.

Haeger-Aronson, B.: Studies on urinary excretion of delta aminolaevulic acid and other haem precursors in lead workers and lead-intoxicated rabbits. Scand. J. Clin. Lab. Invest., 12: Supp. 47, 1960.

Moncrieff, A. A., Koumides, O. P., Clayton, B. E., Patrick, A. D., Renwick, A. G. C., and Roberts, G. E.: Lead poisoning in children. Arch. Dis. Child., 39:1, 1964.

Sonkin, N.: Stippling of the retina. A new physical sign in the early diagnosis of lead poisoning. New Eng. J. Med., 269: 779, 1963.

Watson, C. J.: Porphyrin metabolism. In G. Duncan (ed.): Diseases of Metabolism. Philadelphia, W. B. Saunders Company, 1964.

MERCURY POISONING

Etiology. Acute mercury poisoning results from accidental or intentional ingestion of soluble mercuric salts such as mercuric chloride ($HgCl_2$, corrosive sublimate) and is characterized by very serious corrosive effects on the entire gastrointestinal tract and serious renal tubular cell damage.

Chronic mercury poisoning results from inhalation of mercury vapor or ingestion of small amounts of mercuric nitrate, used in making felt, or other salts, and is characterized by mental symptoms and stomatitis.

Mercury is a liquid and is highly volatile at room temperature. In 1957 over 4 million pounds of mercury were used in the United States. It is used widely in medical research and clinical pathology laboratories, as well as in the manufacture of scientific instruments, electric meters, mercury vapor lamps, amalgams with copper, tin, silver or gold, in solders, and in the production of organic mercurial compounds. Mining cinnabar (HgS), refining mercury from it, and cleaning mercury distilling apparatus involve substantial hazards. Photoengraving, bronzing, and the production of certain paint colors such as vermilion and antifouling agents for hulls of ships all use mercury compounds.

As little as 0.1 gram of $HgCl_2$ may cause poisoning, but fatal doses are usually in excess of 1.0 gram. It is caustic and produces cell destruction by protein precipitation on direct contact. In more dilute solutions, such as concentrations effected by absorption from the intestinal tract after ingestion of a toxic dose, its effect is primarily due to selective affinity for sulfhydryl (-SH) groups of organic compounds, especially of enzymes. This property is counteracted by dimercaprol. Mercury also has an affinity for amino, carbonyl, and hydroxyl groups.

ACUTE POISONING

Symptoms. Acute poisoning usually results from accidental or intentional (suicidal) ingestion of $HgCl_2$. Symptoms include severe abdominal pain, a metallic taste, vomiting, and bloody diarrhea. Shreds of mucosa appear in the liquid stools. Depending on the dose, severe oliguria or anuria develops almost immediately or as late as two weeks after ingestion. Death usually is due to uremia, but a large dose can cause shock and death in a few hours. Ulceration of mouth and pharynx may be extensive and foul. The urine contains protein, erythrocytes, and casts. Fever develops, and a leukocytosis of over 20,000 is usually found. Electrolyte disturbances such as lowering of sodium, chloride, and bicarbonate are related to complex factors, including diarrhea, edema, and anuria.

Pathology. Extensive corrosion and ulceration of the entire digestive tract are found. Mercury is deposited in the kidney, liver, and brain. The kidneys are the principal site of damage and are swollen. Mercury localizes in and damages severely the proximal convoluted tubules and, to a lesser extent, the rest of the nephron.

Diagnosis. The first vomitus or the material

obtained by lavage should be saved for analysis. The characteristic symptoms and the history of ingestion of the poison usually make the diagnosis easy.

Treatment. Feeding of milk or egg whites in order to precipitate mercuric ions and the induction of vomiting will reduce the effective dose and may be life-saving. Gastric lavage is indicated. Sodium formaldehyde sulfoxylate reduces Hg^{++} to Hg^+, and, thus, makes it less toxic; a 5 per cent solution in a dose of 250 ml. is used for lavage, and 250 ml. is left in the stomach. Plain water should be used for lavage if sodium formaldehyde sulfoxylate is not available.

Dimercaprol (BAL: British antilewisite, 2,3-dimercaptopropanol) should be given immediately. BAL should be available in every hospital. It is available as 10 per cent suspension in oil with 20 per cent benzyl benzoate. It forms inactive mercaptides that are excreted by the kidney. The initial dose is 5 mg. per kilogram of body weight by intramuscular injection, then 2.5 mg. per kilogram is given every four hours for three doses, followed by 2.5 mg. per kilogram every six hours for six injections. Toxic reactions to BAL include nausea, vomiting, diarrhea, headaches, and burning sensation of mouth, throat, and eyes with tearing and blepharospasm. A dose of 30 mg. of ephedrine sulfate will lessen these symptoms. More severe symptoms include nervousness, muscle twitching, hyperreflexia, and convulsions. Calcium disodium edetate (CaEDTA) should not be used because of its nephrotoxic action.

The use of plasma volume expanders and other measures to support the circulation is indicated when shock is present. The measurement and replacement of fluid and electrolytes lost by vomiting and diarrhea are important. The management of acute renal failure includes water restriction and extracorporeal dialysis as in any case of acute renal failure.

Prognosis. The prognosis depends on the retained dose and the prompt administration of appropriate treatment. Mortality rates exceeded 30 per cent before effective treatment became available, but if BAL treatment can be begun within three hours the mortality rate can be reduced appreciably. Early deaths are due to shock, and late deaths are usually due to uremia.

CHRONIC POISONING

Clinical Manifestations. *Stomatitis.* Excessive salivation and a metallic taste are common. A blue line develops along the gingival margin. Gums become hypertrophied, bleed easily, and are sore. The teeth become loose.

Erethism. The term "erethism" is applied to the psychic disturbance characterized by irritability, shyness, and deterioration of family and social activities, suggesting hyperthyroidism. Since felt hat makers formerly used mercury salts in the manufacturing process and often became "mad," these symptoms gave rise to the phrase "mad as a hatter."

Tremors. Tremors of the eyelids, lips, tongue, fingers and extremities are characteristic of chronic poisoning. Coarse jerky movements and gross incoordination interfere with fine movements such as writing and eating. Atrophy of the cerebellar cortex and, to a lesser extent, of the cerebral cortex occurs. Microscopic changes occur in the granular layer of the cerebellum, ganglion cells, and posterior columns.

Nephrotic Syndrome. Contact with ammoniated mercury and other compounds has caused proteinuria and frank nephrotic syndrome. Removal from exposure is mandatory, so a careful history of medicinal or occupational exposure is needed.

ORGANIC MERCURIAL INTOXICATION

Ethyl and methyl compounds of mercury are used for fungal diseases of cereals and grain. These compounds have an affinity for the central nervous system and produce generalized ataxia, deafness, dysarthria, progressive visual deterioration, dysphagia, and, occasionally, coma and death. Changes in the central nervous system similar to the lesions of chronic mercury poisoning are found.

HYPERSENSITIVITY

Hypersensitivity reactions to mercurial diuretic agents include asthma, urticaria, exfoliative dermatitis, and sudden death. Fatal accidents can be prevented by avoiding intravenous injections. Death usually is due to ventricular fibrillation.

Hypersensitivity to calomel (HgCl) results from long-term ingestion of HgCl. Hypersensitivity to ammoniated mercury or other compounds results from topical application. Fever, morbilliform rash, leukopenia, eosinophilia, and enlargement of the spleen and lymph nodes characterize this condition. Mercury fulminate used in percussion caps and detonators may cause dermatitis of exposed parts, with pruritus, papules, vesicles, and pustules.

ACRODYNIA OR "PINK DISEASE"

This disorder of infants and young children is characterized by irritability, insomnia, stomatitis, loss of teeth, hypertension, erythema of fingers, toes, nose, cheeks, and buttocks and even acral gangrene. Fever, leukocytosis, and albuminuria occur. In 1948 Warkany and Hubbard suggested that sensitivity to mercury may be the cause, and that hypothesis is now fairly generally accepted. The diagnosis is established by finding excretion of more than 0.1 mg. of mercury per day in the urine. An organic mercury compound, phenyl mercuric propionate, has been incorporated into house paint to prevent growth of mold. This paint has been incriminated as a source of toxic exposure.

Diagnosis. Industrial exposure and characteristic symptoms usually make recognition of chronic mercury poisoning relatively straightforward, but, in the absence of known exposure, the diagnosis may be elusive. Patients with chronic mercury poisoning excrete in excess of 0.3 mg. of Hg per liter of urine. Normal values range from 0.0001 to 0.001 mg. per liter, but an excretion of 0.1 mg. per liter is considered evidence of toxic exposure. In instances of exposure to metallic mercury for more than five years a brown reflex from the anterior lens capsule can be seen by slit lamp. Some observers consider it an early sign of mercury poisoning. Albuminuria and hematuria are common findings in chronic poisoning.

Treatment. Removal of the patient from all possible exposure is of paramount importance. The use of BAL in chronic poisoning has not been established as effective treatment. However, the enhancement of mercury excretion and quick recovery by a patient with acrodynia by the use of n-acetyl-DL-penicillamine makes trial of this agent in chronic poisoning a reasonable procedure.

Prognosis. Recovery is slow even after removal from exposure. Patients with advanced intoxication fare poorly. Only 15 per cent of the more severely involved patients recovered completely in one series. Signs of cerebellar and cerebral damage persisted and prevented return to normal activities.

Prevention. Removal of $HgCl_2$, calomel, and mercury ointments from the market would eliminate acute poisoning and many instances of chronic poisoning. Good safe substitutes are available for each compound. Elimination of mercuric nitrate from the felt-processing industry has already occurred. Mercury salts for fingerprinting by police departments have been replaced by barium, zinc, or bismuth. Silver has replaced mercury in the manufacture of mirrors.

Mercury-containing paints should have a warning label "For Outside Use Only." Mercury cannot be replaced in many electrical apparatuses and scientific instruments. Proper exhaust ventilation, scrupulous avoidance of any exposed metallic mercury, and good personal hygiene are necessary precautions. The maximal allowable concentration of Hg has been set at 0.1 mg. per cubic meter of air. Medical supervision is necessary wherever potential exposure exists. Neurologic signs and especially visual field changes, tremor, ataxia, and dysarthria are serious danger signals.

Battigelli, M. C.: Mercury toxicity from industrial exposure. A critical review of the literature. J. Occup. Med., 2:337, 1960.

Hirschman, S. Z., Feingold, M., and Boylen, G.: Mercury in house paint as a cause of acrodynia. New Eng. J. Med., 269:889, 1963.

Longcope, W. T., and Luetscher, J. A., Jr.: Clinical uses of 2,3-dimercaptopropanol (B.A.L.). The treatment of acute mercury poisoning by B.A.L. J. Clin. Invest., 25:557, 1946.

ANTIMONY POISONING

Antimony and potassium tartrate (tartar emetic) is used for emetic purposes, and other organic antimony compounds are used in treatment of schistosomiasis, filariasis, and certain fungal infections. Antimony is encountered in metallurgic processes, mining and smelting, and in rubber manufacturing, but industrial poisoning is rare. Finely divided antimony is more toxic than compounds of antimony. Trivalent antimony combines with sulfhydryl groups of enzymes. The symptoms of acute poisoning are similar to those of acute arsenic poisoning. Vomiting is a prominent symptom. Dimercaprol (BAL) is an effective agent for treatment of antimony poisoning, and the regimen is like that for mercury. Dermatitis and conjunctivitis occur from exposure to dust in the smelting process. Stibine (SbH_3) is more volatile than arsine but is very toxic also. It attacks the central nervous system and causes acute hemolysis. Death occurs when there is a 0.01 per cent concentration in the air. The chemical process of formation and the effects are like those of arsine.

CADMIUM POISONING

Cadmium sulfide is associated with zinc minerals and particularly with zinc sulfide. Cadmium exposure can occur in the manufacture of alloys, vapor lamps, and storage batteries, grinding and polishing alloys, cadmium plating, welding, zinc ore smelting, and glass blowing. Inhalation of cadmium fumes results in pulmonary edema, followed in two to three days by proliferative interstitial pneumonia. Various degrees of permanent lung damage and fibrosis occur. Cadmium can be inhaled in fatal concentrations without enough discomfort to warn the worker. The inhalation of fumes with cadmium produces dryness of throat, cough, headache, vomiting, sensation of constriction in the chest, severe dyspnea, and prostration. There is no effective treatment except symptomatic treatment of pulmonary edema. Foods prepared and stored in cadmium-plated containers may be contaminated sufficiently to cause poisoning. Cadmium ingestion usually does not produce fatal poisoning, but causes rather violent gastrointestinal symptoms, with sudden onset 20 to 30 minutes after eating.

THALLIUM POISONING

Thallium (as thallium acetate) has been used a great deal as a depilatory agent in the treatment of ringworm in children. The sulfate is a potent rat poison. Over 1000 instances of thallium poisoning have been recorded. The lethal dose of thallium sulfate in man is from 0.2 to 1.0 gram. Liver radiopacity increases in some patients. Alopecia is a very important and unique sign. Neurologic and psychic symptoms include ataxia, vomiting, restlessness, delirium with hallucinations, delusions, and semicoma. Blindness due to retrobulbar neuritis, paralysis of other special sense functions, and facial paralysis also occur. Central lobular necrosis of the liver and renal damage occur. Treatment with BAL in small doses has been found to be ineffective by some, but large doses such as those used for mercury poisoning have been effective. Gastric lavage should be performed immediately after exposure. CaEDTA, thioacetamide, and beta-mercaptoethylamine have also been used with some success. Potassium chloride enhances excretion of thallium and has been used with success. During maximal thallium mobilization increased symptoms may occur.

Grunfeld, O.: Thallium poisoning treated with BAL. New Eng. J. Med., 269:1138, 1963.

Papp, J. P., Gay, P. C., Dodson, V. N., and Pollard, H. M.: Potassium chloride treatment in thallitoxicosis. Ann. Intern. Med., 71:119, 1969.

CARBON MONOXIDE POISONING

David H. Goldstein

Definition. Carbon monoxide is an asphyxiant gas capable of producing disease and death in man as a result of its ready capacity to induce severe hypoxia. The most vulnerable organs are the brain and the heart. The danger of this gas derives from its affinity for the hemoglobin of human red blood cells, which is 300 times that of oxygen; furthermore, the oxyhemoglobin dissociation curve is shifted to the left so that tissue oxygen tensions must fall to much lower levels before the oxyhemoglobin that remains can give up its oxygen. The hazard to the body of exposure to carbon monoxide is compounded by the insidiousness with which high concentrations of carboxyhemoglobin can be attained without ringing the physiologic alarm bell of dyspnea. Consciousness, of course, is dulled by anoxia.

When carbon monoxide is breathed, the absorption of the gas is rapid until an equilibrium is reached, provided an immediately fatal concentration is not inhaled. The reaction is reversible upon removal from exposure, the gas being excreted unchanged through the expired air in a matter of hours. The reversal is expedited by breathing oxygen–carbon dioxide mixtures or pure oxygen, still more if the oxygen is under pressure. Ledingham reports 100 per cent recovery in 32 patients treated with oxygen at two atmospheres of pressure (absolute). There is danger in exceeding two atmospheres of pressure. Recovery of consciousness can be expected within 30 to 90 minutes with this regimen.

Epidemiology. Carbon monoxide is colorless, odorless, and slightly lighter than air. It is produced whenever incomplete combustion of carbon or carbon-containing compounds occurs. Poisoning may occur by accident, at home or at work, or by suicidal intent. Rarely, carbon monoxide has been a homicidal weapon. Natural gas, predominantly methane and free of carbon monoxide, has largely replaced manufactured gas (20 to 40 per cent CO) in the United States. With this change a significant decline has occurred in accidental deaths from illuminating gas. Nonetheless, faulty gas refrigerators and heaters fueled by gas, coal, oil, or kerosene continue to cause accidental poisoning and death in houses and in trailer homes. The combination of incomplete combustion and inadequate venting provides the exposure. Picnic grilles brought indoors and the use of gasoline-powered machinery inside the home are often unsuspected hazards. The exhaust from gasoline internal combustion engines contains, on the average, 7 per cent carbon monoxide. It is generally held that so long as the carbon monoxide content of inhaled air does not exceed 0.01 per cent (100 ppm), it can be breathed for eight hours without ill effects. An air concentration of 1 per cent (10,000 ppm) produces a 50 per cent saturation of the hemoglobin in 15 minutes. Haldane extrapolated the rise in saturation in 23 minutes to be 80 per cent at this concentration in the air; this is a fatal level of carboxyhemoglobin. The blood of heavy cigarette smokers may contain as much as 10 per cent carboxyhemoglobin. A blood saturation of 20 per cent is a fair bench mark beyond which symptoms can be expected.

A running automobile engine in an enclosed garage is an increasingly common cause of death by accident and suicide. In 1967 in the United States, 1,417 deaths caused by accidental carbon monoxide poisoning were recorded, whereas 2,191 deaths were attributed to suicide resulting predominantly from exposure to motor vehicle exhaust gas.

In industry, sources of poisoning are charcoal ovens, kilns, blast furnaces, blasting with high explosives, mine explosions, and combustion engines. Much carbon monoxide is produced during fires, a hazard recognized by professional firemen.

Pathology. The skin of victims of carbon monoxide poisoning may be pink; in addition there may be areas of trophic erythema, blister formation, and decubital ulcers. The blood may be cherry red, as may the viscera. A variety of lesions are encountered, all attributed to anoxia. They are usually seen when unconsciousness has been prolonged or death delayed. The brain is often the site of hyperemia, edema, hemorrhage, and local or diffuse degeneration. Symmetrical softening in the lenticular nucleus in the globus pallidus is regarded as the most typical pathologic change. The heart may show necrosis of the papillary muscles or gross myocardial infarction, and the kidney may exhibit tubular degeneration.

Clinical Manifestations. The disease is best described as an acute poisoning with all degrees of severity. Chronic exposure does not produce chronic poisoning but, rather, repeated episodes of mild acute poisoning. Intermittent day-to-day exposures are not cumulative in effect. However, the higher morbidity and mortality from coronary heart disease among cigarette smokers has prompted some epidemiologists to suggest an association with chronic exposure to carbon monoxide in the air stream of cigarette smoke, which is considerably higher than community pollution by carbon monoxide.

In general, symptoms occur more acutely with higher air concentrations of carbon monoxide. Severity is increased by exercise and in the presence of anemia. With concentrations in the air higher than 1.5 per cent, unconsciousness, apnea, and death will occur in several minutes. However, protracted exposures to lower concentrations can be ultimately disastrous. Symptoms develop with a progression that roughly parallels the rise in concentration of carboxyhemoglobin. Victims become unconscious at about 60 per cent saturation, and fatal cases show saturations in the range of 60 to 80 per cent. Haldane, using himself as an experimental subject, displayed such incoordination and confusion at 40 per cent saturation as to be incapable of driving an automobile.

Meigs and Hughes analyzed the records of 105 patients admitted to the Yale–New Haven Hospital. In declining order of frequency, they recorded the following findings: abnormal mental state, neurologic abnormalities, abnormal skin color, suffused mucous membranes, abnormal chest signs, vomiting, headache, skin lesions, excessive sweating, palpable liver, localized pains in the chest or extremities, localized edema, evidence of bleeding and "pseudorecovery." The pulse, respiratory rate, and temperature may be elevated and there may be protein, sugar, casts, and erythrocytes in the urine. Leukocytosis with increase in neutrophils and decrease in lymphocytes and eosinophils, when present, is of serious prognostic import, as are temperature elevations above 102° F., neurologic abnormalities, relapse after the second day, irregularities of cardiac rhythm, tachycardia, and the presence of skin lesions.

Recovery without permanent sequelae is usual in nonfatal cases, and recovery of consciousness usually occurs over a period of several hours. However, unconsciousness may persist for days after relief of anoxia and may be followed by parkinsonism, peripheral neuritis, or a confusional psychosis. Recovery from psychosis may occur up to two years from onset. Cerebral hemorrhage has been observed some days after apparent recovery. Increasingly, electrocardiographic abnormalities, some reversible, and acute myocardial infarction have been reported, even in the absence of coma.

Diagnosis. Identification and quantitation of carboxyhemoglobin is decisive in diagnosis, but is not a requisite for the institution of treatment. Blood should be collected early if it is to reflect the degree of saturation.

Treatment. Removal of the patient from the contaminated atmosphere is the first and obvious indication. In mild cases without loss of consciousness, fresh air and absolute rest for four hours will probably suffice. The patient should not be allowed to go home without an escort. Treatment in a hospital is indicated when there has been even transient loss of consciousness. If the patient is found unconscious, emergency treatment is called for. If respiration has ceased, artificial respiration is instituted at once along with administration of 100 per cent oxygen. Since the concentration of carboxyhemoglobin is halved in about 40 minutes under conditions of adequate ventilatory exchange with pure oxygen, two to three hours of continuous oxygen therapy should suffice for the control of anoxia. Most police emergency squads are trained to use a positive pressure face mask respirator with an automatic cycling valve. The British Medical Research Council recommends use of 95 per cent oxygen and 5 per cent carbon dioxide.

Rapid recovery from profound coma by treatment in a pressure chamber with oxygen under two atmospheres of pressure has been reported. Persistent coma, after anoxia has cleared, calls for the usual treatment of the comatose patient. In the presence of temperature elevation over 102° F. or serious neurologic disorder appearing on the first day, induction of hypothermia should be considered.

Anderson, R. F., Allensworth, D. C., and De Groot, W. J.: Myocardial toxicity from carbon monoxide poisoning. Ann. Intern. Med., 67:1172, 1967.

Bour, H., and Ledingham, I. McA. (eds.): Carbon Monoxide Poisoning. Amsterdam, London, New York, Elsevier Publishing Company, 1967. (Progress in Brain Research Vol. 24).

Craig, T. V., Hunt, W. A., and Atkinson, R.: Hypothermia—Its use in severe carbon monoxide poisoning. New Eng. J. Med., 261:854, 1959.

Forbes, W. H.: Carbon monoxide. In Whittenberger, J. L. (ed.): Artificial Respiration, Theory and Application. New York, Harper & Row, Publishers, 1962, Chap. 12, p. 194.

Garland, H., and Pearce, J.: Neurological complications of carbon monoxide poisoning. Quart. J. Med., 36:445, 1967.

Goldsmith, J. R.: Carbon monoxide and coronary heart disease. Ann. Intern. Med., 71:199, 1969.

Meigs, J. W.: Acute carbon monoxide poisoning. An analysis of one hundred five cases. Arch. Industr. Hyg. (Chicago), 6:344, 1952.

Stewart, R. D., Peterson, J. E., Baretta, E. D., Bachand, R. T., Hosko, M. J., and Herrmann, A. A.: Experimental human exposure to carbon monoxide. Arch. Environ. Health (Chicago), 21:154, 1970.

Food Poisoning

M. Glenn Koenig

Foods may produce illness in three ways: They may become contaminated with micro-organisms or their products, they may themselves be poisonous, or they may contain noxious chemicals. The diagnosis of food poisoning should be considered whenever persons who shared in a common meal develop an acute gastrointestinal illness or an illness in which neurologic signs and symptoms are accompanied by intestinal complaints.

BACTERIAL FOOD POISONING

Bacteria or their products are responsible for most instances of food poisoning. Two general varieties of bacterial food poisoning are recognized: those that are actually intoxications, caused by the ingestion of preformed toxins produced by micro-organisms growing in contaminated foods; and those that are true infections, requiring the ingestion of large numbers of viable bacteria to produce illness.

PREFORMED TOXINS

Staphylococcal Food Poisoning

Definition. Staphylococcal food poisoning is the most common bacterial food poisoning observed in the United States. It is caused by the ingestion of a preformed exotoxin produced in contaminated food. Because it characteristically produces only brief illness, staphylococcal food poisoning often goes unnoticed and is brought to the attention of public health authorities only when it occurs in outbreaks involving large numbers of people. Most people on some occasion are victims of this intoxication.

Etiology and Pathogenesis. Only certain strains of coagulase-positive staphylococci produce the extracellular enterotoxin responsible for food poisoning. Most enterotoxigenic strains belong to phage groups III and IV and particularly to phage types 42D or 6/47. Coagulase-negative strains do not elaborate enterotoxin. The toxin itself is a protein of low molecular weight, and four types, A, B, C, and D, are currently recognized. The toxin is relatively heat-stable and has produced symptoms of food poisoning after exposure to a temperature equivalent to that of boiling water.

Foods are generally contaminated with enterotoxigenic strains of staphylococci from the hands of workers preparing them. Often the responsible individual has only a minor skin infection or is simply found to be a nasal carrier of an enterotoxigenic strain. Occasionally, a cow or goat with mastitis is the source of contaminated milk. In the United States, custard- or cream-filled bakery goods are the foods most commonly responsible for staphylococcal food poisoning. Ham, tongue, and other processed meats, cheese, ice cream, potato salad, hollandaise sauce, chicken salad, and human and goat's milk are foods often implicated. Foods containing enterotoxin have normal appearance, odor, and taste.

Enterotoxin has been produced by viable staphylococci in contaminated foods after only four to five hours' incubation at a temperature of 86° F., but it is not formed at refrigerator temperatures (38° to 42° F.).

Clinical Manifestations. Symptoms characteristically appear one to six hours after the ingestion of the contaminated food. The illness may have a sudden onset, with severe, cramping abdominal pain, nausea, retching, vomiting, and diarrhea. Sweating, increased salivation, and headache are sometimes seen. Fever is not a common feature. In some cases prostration may be severe, and shock may occur. However, recovery is generally rapid, symptoms usually disappearing within six to eight hours and rarely lasting longer than 24 hours. Both the incubation period and the severity of symptoms may be influenced by the amount of enterotoxin ingested, but individuals vary considerably in susceptibility to staphylococcal enterotoxin.

Diagnosis. The short incubation period and the presence of similar illness in others who have eaten the same food usually make the clinical diagnosis of staphylococcal food poisoning relatively straightforward. It must be differentiated from other bacterial food poisonings, and an isolated case must be differentiated from acute cholecystitis, appendicitis, and other intra-abdominal surgical emergencies. The rapid onset and absence of high fever are helpful clues. The neurologic symptoms noted with botulism help differentiate it from staphylococcal food poisoning. Poisonings caused by other foods and chemical agents usually cause symptoms within an hour and are often accompanied by neurologic signs that are absent in staphylococcal food poisoning.

By taking a careful food history it is often possible to decide which food was implicated in the poisoning. If possible, portions of it should be obtained for bacteriologic examination. Gram stains and cultures should be performed. Cultures may yield few staphylococci because the food may have been heated sufficiently to kill the micro-organisms but not to destroy the enterotoxin. In such cases the Gram stain may still show clumps of gram-positive cocci. Definitive diagnosis rests on the demonstration of enterotoxin in the suspected food or the production of enterotoxin by strains isolated from the food. This has proved to be a difficult task, for most laboratory animals are quite insensitive to enterotoxin; the most reliable test must be performed on either human volunteers or monkeys. Recently, immunologic assays utilizing gel diffusion techniques have shown promise for demonstrating enterotoxin in contaminated foods.

Treatment and Prognosis. In most cases no specific treatment is needed. Occasionally, a patient with severe vomiting and diarrhea becomes dangerously dehydrated and requires intravenous replacement of fluids containing sodium chloride and potassium. Antimicrobial therapy is not indicated.

Elderly, debilitated persons or young infants may die; otherwise, the prognosis is excellent.

Prevention. Prevention measures must be directed against heavy contamination of foods with staphylococci. Food handlers should be trained to observe strict personal hygiene and should be forbidden to work when they have active staphylococcal lesions. Because enterotoxin is not produced at temperatures below 42.8° F. (6° C.), the best preventive measure is careful refrigeration of all perishable foods. Foods should be reheated immediately before serving and should not be allowed to stand for long periods at room temperature.

Botulism

Definition. Botulism is a specific and often fatal type of food poisoning that results from ingestion of toxin produced by *Clostridium botulinum.* The clinical illness is characterized by variable gastrointestinal complaints, dilated and nonreactive pupils, dryness of the oral mucous membranes, and progressive muscle weakness.

Etiology. Six strains of *C. botulinum,* designated types A, B, C, D, E, and F, have been described. Each type produces an antigenically distinct toxin. Types A, B, and E are responsible for most human disease. Only two outbreaks of type F botulism have been reported, one in Denmark and one in California. Types C and D produce disease limited almost entirely to animals.

Botulinum spores are distributed in soil throughout the world. Type A spores are common in the western United States, whereas B spores are found in the eastern United States and in Europe. Type E spores are associated with northern latitudes, often being isolated from lake-shore mud, coastal sand, and sea-bottom silt. The intestinal tracts of fish are often contaminated with type E spores, accounting for the high incidence of type E strains observed in fish-borne botulism. Type F spores have been found in marine sediments off the California and Oregon coasts and in salmon from the Columbia River. The spores are heat-resistant and have remained viable after exposure to 100° C. for several hours. However, exposure to moist heat at 120° C. for 30 minutes will kill spores of all six types.

Botulinum toxins have been identified as proteins and are the most potent poisons known. They are less heat-stable than the spores, all toxins being destroyed by boiling for 10 minutes or by exposure to 80° C. for 30 minutes.

Pathogenesis. Human botulism results from ingestion of preformed botulinum toxin in contaminated foods. A large variety of home-processed foods have been implicated in outbreaks of botulism in the United States. Commercially processed products have been involved on only a few occasions.

Relatively anaerobic environments and temperatures above 80° F. provide the best conditions for toxin production. However, a strictly anaerobic atmosphere is not necessary, and some type E strains have produced toxin at temperatures as low as 6° C. (42.8° F.). Food contaminated with A and B botulinum strains may often appear spoiled because of the proteolytic enzymes produced by these micro-organisms. However, many type E strains do not elaborate these enzymes, so that foods containing type E toxin may appear and taste perfectly normal.

Botulinum toxin is primarily absorbed from the upper gastrointestinal tract, but toxin reaching the lower small bowel and colon may be slowly absorbed, thus perhaps accounting for the delayed onset and prolonged duration of symptoms seen in many patients with clinical botulism.

Botulinum toxins block transmission in cholinergic nerve fibers. Neural impulses are interrupted close to the terminations of nerve fibrils, but short of the motor end plate, thus preventing acetylcholine release. Muscle reactivity to acetylcholine remains intact. The toxins may have some effect on the central nervous system.

Clinical Manifestations. Clinical illness may vary from mild indisposition that requires no medical attention to rapidly fatal disease terminating in death within 24 hours. Characteristically, symptoms begin 12 to 36 hours after ingestion of the contaminated food. Nausea and vomiting may be severe with type E disease, but are less frequently observed in patients with type A or B intoxication. Weakness, lassitude, and dizziness are often early complaints. Severe dryness of the mouth and pharynx, occasionally associated with pharyngeal pain, is also noted. Neurologic symptoms may occur early in the course or may be delayed for 12 to 72 hours. These include blurred vision, diplopia, dysphonia, dysphagia, and muscle weakness. Difficulty in breathing accompanies respiratory muscle involvement. Constipation and abdominal distention may be prominent complaints.

Mentation remains intact and fever is not observed in uncomplicated cases. Difficulties in articulation and swallowing are often seen; the pupils are dilated and fixed; and extraocular palsies may be observed. The mucous membranes of the mouth and pharynx are often dry, crusted, and erythematous. Weakness of muscle groups, particularly of the neck, proximal extremities, and respiratory musculature, is often observed as the disease progresses, but superficial and deep tendon reflexes remain intact. Abdominal distention and absence of bowel sounds may be noted, and urinary retention may occur. Sudden respiratory paralysis and airway obstruction may develop, and, together with secondary infection, these are the major causes of death.

Diagnosis. The full-blown clinical syndrome of botulism in a group of people having ingested a home-canned product is readily recognized; on the other hand, diagnosis in an isolated case may be extremely difficult. The neurologic diseases most frequently confused with botulism are myasthenia gravis, acute poliomyelitis, Guillain-Barré syndrome, and stroke. A negative Tensilon test for myasthenia gravis, normal cerebrospinal fluid, absence of sensory involvement, preservation of deep tendon reflexes, mentative clarity, and absence of corticospinal tract signs in patients with botulism help in the differential diagnosis.

Other non-neurologic disorders have been confused with botulism. Pharyngeal pain, erythema, and dysphagia have sometimes suggested streptococcal or viral pharyngitis. The dry mouth and mucous membranes and dilated pupils resemble signs observed in atropine, belladonna, or jimson weed poisoning. The mentative clarity, absence of central nervous system excitement, and the delay in appearance of symptoms observed in botulism help exclude these possibilities. Nausea, vomiting, and abdominal distention, together with constipation and ileus, have led to the mistaken diagnosis of intestinal obstruction. The neurologic signs observed in botulism should help exclude this diagnosis.

Circulating toxin may occasionally be detected by injecting the patient's serum into mice. Fresh serum should be injected intraperitoneally in 1 ml. amounts, with and without the addition of types A, B, E, and F antisera. If toxin is present animals injected with serum alone may die, although mice protected with specific antiserum will survive. Portions of any suspected food should be suspended in saline and injected into mice in the same fashion, and should be cultured for anaerobic bacilli.

Treatment. Most patients with botulism die of respiratory failure; thus, early tracheostomy and utilization of a tank respirator or other mechanical aid to respiration may be life-saving. Cleansing enemas should be given to remove any unabsorbed toxin from the colon. As soon as the clinical diagnosis of botulism has been made, patients should be skin-tested for serum sensitivity. If they are negative, two vials of trivalent A, B, E botulinus antitoxin should be administered. This dose may be repeated in two to four hours. This preparation of antitoxin can be obtained from the U.S. National Communicable Disease Center by calling 404-633-3311 by day or 404-634-2561 by night. Bivalent A, B antitoxin, manufactured by Lederle Laboratories, is still available but should be given only to patients known to have type A or B botulism, or if a considerable delay in obtaining the trivalent preparation is anticipated. A small supply of type F antitoxin is also available from the National Communicable Disease Center. No cross protection between antitoxins exists. Patients sensitive to horse serum should be desensitized before antitoxin is given. If available, antitoxin in one third to one half the therapeutic dose may be given prophylactically to those who are known to have eaten the contaminated food but who have not yet developed symptoms.

Although many reports in the literature have indicated that antitoxin does not alter the course of type A botulism once symptoms have developed, reduction in mortality in several type E outbreaks by utilization of antiserum has been impressive. This suggests that the efficacy of antitoxin in all types of botulism be re-evaluated.

Prognosis. Mortality from type A botulism has generally been high, running between 60 and 70 per cent. The fatality rate with type B disease has been lower, ranging between 10 and 30 per cent. Type E botulism has produced mortality rates ranging from 30 to 50 per cent in large series. With prompt diagnosis, vigorous management of respiratory paralysis, and prompt administration of polyvalent antitoxin, it is likely that these mortality figures can be considerably improved. If a patient survives the severe paralytic illness, recovery is usually rapid, and complete return to health can be anticipated.

LIVING MICRO-ORGANISMS AS CAUSES OF FOOD POISONING

Salmonella Food Poisoning

Salmonellae are important causes of bacterial food poisoning. Large numbers of viable microorganisms must be ingested to produce symptoms. The resulting illness can be differentiated from staphylococcal food poisoning because its incubation period is longer, symptoms usually begin 8 to 24 hours after ingestion of contaminated food, and chills and high fever are an important part of the clinical syndrome. Nausea, vomiting, diarrhea, and severe prostration may occur. Salmonella food poisoning and gastroenteritis are discussed in detail elsewhere in this book.

Clostridium Perfringens Food Poisoning

Clostridium perfringens has been recognized as an important cause of food poisoning in Great Britain and, to a lesser extent, in the United States. Type A strains have usually been implicated. Reheated meats, which provide an anaerobic environment and appropriate temperatures for growth, have been implicated in most cases. Symptoms usually begin 8 to 24 hours after the ingestion of contaminated food. Diarrhea and cramping abdominal pain are prominent, but fever, chills, headache, and other signs of infection are inconspicuous. Some nausea may be observed, but vomiting occurs infrequently. Symptoms generally disappear within 8 hours and rarely persist more than 24 hours. Treatment should be symptomatic. No specific therapy is indicated.

A rare type of clostridial food poisoning termed *enteritis necroticans* has been described following ingestion of foods heavily contaminated with type F strains of *Clostridium perfringens.* This illness is characterized by acute onset, severe abdominal pain, vomiting, diarrhea, prostration, and shock, and may be rapidly fatal. Postmortem examination reveals a diffuse necrotizing enteritis of the jejunum, ileum, and colon.

Clostridium perfringens food poisoning is best prevented by avoiding lengthy periods of warming or cooling of foods that have already been cooked. If foods are to stand more than one and a half hours before serving, they should be stored at temperatures above 60° C. (140° F.) or below 15° C. (59° F.).

Shigella Food Poisoning

Shigella strains were reported to be responsible for 25 foodborne or waterborne outbreaks of shigellosis in the five year period 1964–1968. The source of infection almost always has been traced to a human carrier, who, through poor personal hygiene, contaminated foods which required extensive handling, such as salads and, in particular, potato salads. Incubation periods may vary from six hours to nine days. The illness resembles acute shigellosis described elsewhere in this book.

Enterococcal Food Poisoning

Species of enterococci (Lancefield group D streptococci) have been implicated in several food poisoning outbreaks, but a definite etiologic relationship to food poisoning has not been established. Symptoms have generally occurred 8 to 20 hours after ingestion of the food. The illness produced is similar to that observed with *clostridium perfringens* food poisoning and is self-limited. No specific therapy is required.

Bacillus Cereus Food Poisoning

Several outbreaks of food poisoning have been attributed to *Bacillus cereus,* a spore-forming, gram-positive aerobic bacillus. The incubation period has usually been 12 hours, and the symptoms observed have included nausea, occasional vomiting, and severe, colicky abdominal pains. Watery diarrhea may be noted. The illness rarely persists longer than 6 to 12 hours and is not accompanied by fever or severe prostration. No specific therapy is indicated.

A variety of micro-organisms have been isolated from foods that have caused symptoms of food poisoning. These include *E. coli,* paracolon bacilli, Proteus species, and *Alkaligenes faecalis.* There is no convincing evidence that any of these microorganisms can in fact produce the clinical syndrome of food poisoning, and further studies must be performed before they can be accepted as causes of such illness.

POISONOUS PLANTS AND ANIMALS

MUSHROOM POISONING

Most cases of serious mushroom poisoning in North America are caused by members of the genus Amanita, which contain five potent cyclopeptide toxins. *Amanita verna* and its subspecies and American phenotypes of *Amanita phalloides* produce most of the fatal intoxications, and the ingestion of only two or three of these mushrooms may be fatal. *Amanita muscaria* and *Amanita pantherina,* two species that contain the alkaloid muscarine, generally cause a less severe illness.

The clinical course of mushroom poisoning may pass through three phases. Nausea, vomiting, abdominal pain, and severe diarrhea initiate the illness, usually 6 to 12 hours after ingestion of the poisonous mushrooms. With those species that contain muscarine, symptoms may begin earlier — some two to three hours after ingestion — and abdominal cramping, salivation, sweating, miosis, and bradycardia may be prominent features.

Patients surviving the severe gastrointestinal illness may then appear to improve for 48 hours. However, tests of hepatic and renal function may disclose abnormalities during this period. The third stage of illness is ushered in by signs of severe hepatic, renal, and central nervous system damage. Hepatic necrosis may occur, and initial hyperglycemia is often followed by terminal hypoglycemia. Severe metabolic acidosis and oliguria may develop, and lactic acidosis has been noted. Myocardial conduction defects and arrhythmias have been described. Mental confusion, coma, and weakness, and paralysis of the extremities have been observed.

There is no effective specific treatment for mushroom poisoning. A vigorous attempt should be made to identify the species of mushroom ingested. If vomiting has not begun, the stomach should be emptied by inducing vomiting or by gastric lavage. If diarrhea has not occurred, a cathartic and high colonic enemas should be administered. If muscarinic effects are noted, atropine should be given cautiously. Careful electrolyte replacement and correction of the acidosis and hypoglycemia that may accompany hepatic necrosis are of great importance. Peritoneal dialysis or hemodialysis may be of aid in managing the oliguric phase of renal failure.

The mortality rate from severe Amanita poisoning may be high, over 50 per cent in some series. If the patient survives the acute hepatic and renal injury, however, the prognosis for complete recovery is excellent.

Mushroom poisoning can be prevented only by avoiding ingestion of wild mushrooms. Only an expert mycologist can differentiate edible species from poisonous ones, and, despite much folklore to the contrary, there is no safe method of detoxifying poisonous mushrooms.

SNAKEROOT POISONING
(Milk Sickness)

Snakeroot *(Eupatorium urticoefolium)*, a plant common in the midwestern United States, contains the poisonous alcohol *tremetol.* When natural food is scarce, cattle may feed on snakeroot and develop an illness called *trembles.* Human beings become ill after ingesting milk from an animal with trembles. The illness in man is characterized by anorexia, listlessness, weakness, abdominal discomfort, vomiting, constipation, ketosis, acidosis, occasional hypoglycemia, and, finally, coma. Treatment should be aimed at correcting the severe ketoacidosis; large doses of alkali may be required.

JIMSON WEED POISONING

Jimson weed *(Datura stramonium)* contains the stramonium alkaloids, hyoscyamine, scopolamine and atropine. Poisoning has been reported after ingestion of its seeds, of tea made from its leaves (a folk remedy reportedly effective in asthma), and of tomatoes grafted to a host jimson weed.

Symptoms often begin within several minutes of ingestion and consist of visual hallucinations, disorientation, weakness, blurred vision, thirst, vertigo, and nausea. On examination the oral mucous membranes are dry and the pupils are dilated and slowly reactive. There is no specific therapy, but some of the troublesome symptoms may be controlled by pilocarpine.

SHELLFISH POISONING

The ingestion of certain mussels and clams along the Pacific coast and along the shores of the Bay of Fundy in New Brunswick and Nova Scotia has led to severe illness. Such poisoning has usually been observed between May and October and has been traced to the plankton upon which the shellfish feed during that time of the year, *Gonyaulax catanella* in the Pacific and *Gonyaulax tamarensis* in the Atlantic.

Symptoms often begin within ten minutes after eating the shellfish. Initially, tingling and numbness about the lips are noted, followed by paresthesias about the fingertips. The throat is often dry. Staggering, giddiness, and ataxia may appear, and speech is often incoherent. In severe cases respiratory paralysis and death soon follow. No specific therapy is available, but in severe intoxications mechanical respiratory aids and tracheostomy may be life-saving. If patients survive the first twelve hours of illness the prognosis for complete recovery is good.

FISH POISONING
(Ichthyosarcotoxism)

Three varieties of fish poisoning deserve mention:

1. *Ciguatera poisoning.* This is one of the most common forms of fish poisoning in Caribbean waters and is caused by fish that in other parts of the world are considered to be excellent food items. Sea bass, grouper, barracuda, and snapper are some of the species involved. The conditions under which these fish become toxic are not known. Symptoms may develop immediately after ingestion or may be delayed as much as 30 hours. Tingling about the lips, tongue, and throat, nausea, vomiting, diarrhea, weakness and numbness, muscle pain, and generalized pruritus may be noted. The mortality rate is less than 10 per cent; death is caused by respiratory paralysis.

2. *Tetraodon poisoning.* This most lethal fish poisoning is produced by ingestion of puffer-like fish found in Far Eastern waters. The flesh of these fish may contain a potent neurotoxin, with both central and peripheral effects. Symptoms usually occur within minutes. Malaise, dizziness, and tingling about the lips and tongue may soon be followed by ataxia, convulsions, respiratory paralysis, and death. Japanese statistics indicate that the mortality rate is more than 60 per cent. Death usually occurs within six hours; survival for more than 24 hours is a good prognostic sign.

3. *Scromboid poisoning.* If scromboid fish (tuna, skip jack, bonito, and others in the mackerel family) are poorly preserved, a toxic "histamine-like" substance may be produced by the action of bacteria on histidine, a normal component of fish flesh. If this toxin is ingested, an illness characterized by nausea, vomiting, headache, epigastric pain, dysphagia, thirst, pruritus, and urticaria may be produced. Symptoms usually subside within 12 hours.

There is no specific treatment for any form of fish poisoning. Gastric lavage should be instituted if vomiting has not occurred. Mechanical respiratory aids and tracheostomy may be necessary. Antihistaminic drugs are sometimes helpful in scromboid poisoning.

CHEMICAL FOOD POISONING

A number of chemical agents have been known to contaminate food and produce illness. *Antimony* and *cadmium* are still responsible for sporadic outbreaks of food poisoning in the United States.

Antimony is often contained in the binding between the enamel and metal of old, cheap cooking utensils. A few cadmium-lined containers are still in use in the United States. The addition of acid foods or liquids (such as lemonade) to such containers may dissolve sufficient antimony or cadmium to produce acute illness. Symptoms usually begin 15 to 45 minutes after ingestion and are characterized by nausea, vomiting, cramping abdominal pain, and varying degrees of prostration. In mild intoxications recovery is usually prompt, and no specific therapy is necessary. In more serious poisonings BAL may be used to remove antimony, but should not be used in a case of cadmium intoxication, for the BAL-cadmium complex is nephrotoxic.

The *Chinese-restaurant syndrome* has been attributed to the ingestion of *monosodium glutamate* used to season foods in certain Chinese restaurants. In susceptible persons, symptoms begin 10 to 20 minutes after ingestion of food containing large amounts of monosodium glutamate (5 grams will produce the reaction in susceptible individuals), and consist of burning and tingling sensations in the back of the neck, upper back, arms, and anterior thorax. Pain in the infraorbital and temporal areas may be severe, and palpitations have been reported. Symptoms may fluctuate in intensity and usually disappear with-

in 45 minutes. No permanent sequelae have been noted.

Dack, G. M.: Food Poisoning. 3rd ed. Chicago, The University of Chicago Press, 1956.
Halstead, B. W.: Fish poisonings—Their diagnosis, pharmacology, and treatment. Clin. Pharmacol. Ther., 5:615, 1964.
Harrison, D. C., Coggins, C. H., Welland, F. H., and Nelson, S.: Mushroom poisoning in five patients. Amer. J. Med., 38:787, 1965.
Koenig, M. G., Drutz, D. J., Mushlin, A. I., Schaffner, W., and Rogers, D. E.: Type B botulism in man. Amer. J. Med., 42:208, 1967.
Koenig, M. G., Spickard, A., Cardella, M. A., and Rogers, D. E.: Clinical and laboratory observations on type E botulism in man. Medicine, 43:517, 1964.
Meyers, K. F.: Food poisoning. New Eng. J. Med., 249:765, 804, 843, 1953.

Venom Diseases
Sherman A. Minton, Jr.

SNAKEBITE

Identification, Distribution, and Classification of Venomous Reptiles. Recognition of venomous snakes is difficult, for the only character common to all species is the presence of venom-conducting maxillary fangs. Handbooks for identification of snakes of most geographic areas are available from natural history museums or government agencies. Local information about reptiles is often untrustworthy, and erroneous beliefs are widespread even among educated and professional persons. Harmless reptiles are often believed dangerous; dangerous species may sometimes be considered innocuous. The number of species of poisonous snakes is nearly always greater in tropical countries; nevertheless, certain species may be abundant in temperate regions, e.g., the prairie rattlesnake in the northern Great Plains of the United States. Even in the tropics it is unusual for more than three or four species to be important in a given area.

Following is a brief classification of venomous reptiles:

Lizards. *Family Helodermatidae.* Two species known as Gila monsters are restricted to parts of Mexico and the southwestern United States. There are venom-conducting teeth in the lower jaw; the venom has local irritant and neurotoxic effects.

Snakes. *Family Colubridae.* This family includes most of the world's snakes, about 2500 species. A few hundred, mostly tropical and subtropical, have grooved fangs on the posterior maxillae. The fangs frequently are not engaged in defensive biting. Little is known concerning the venoms, but some are powerfully hemorrhagic. Nearly all rear-fanged snakes are harmless for practical purposes, but bites of the African boom-

slang (*Dispholidus typus*) and bird snakes (*Thelotornis kirtlandii*) have caused deaths.

Family Elapidae. These snakes have fixed fangs on the anterior ends of the maxillae; the fangs may be followed by solid teeth. The venoms are predominantly neurotoxic and often very potent. About 120 species are confined to the Old World, and almost 50 species of coral snakes inhabit tropical and subtropical America.

Family Hydrophidae. These are marine or brackish water snakes characterized by laterally flattened tails and, in nearly all species, by great reduction or absence of enlarged ventral scales. They have fixed, short fangs followed by solid teeth. Their venoms act primarily on skeletal muscle, and are often extremely potent but small in quantity. About 50 species inhabit the coastal waters of south Asia, northern Australia, and islands of the southwest Pacific; one species reaches the western coasts of tropical America.

Family Viperidae. Single, large fangs on short and otherwise toothless maxillae rotate, permitting the fangs to be erected or folded against the roof of the mouth. Venoms usually cause local necrosis and hemorrhage, but some are predominantly neurotoxic. One subfamily, *Crotalinae* or pit vipers, is characterized by a deep pit lined with sensitive heat receptors situated between the eye and nostril. There are about 100 species of pit vipers, mostly in the Americas and southeast Asia. *All dangerous snakes of the Americas except the coral snakes belong in this group.* The other subfamily, *Viperinae*, lacks the sensory pit. There are about 50 species confined to Africa, Asia, and Europe.

Epidemiology. World mortality from snakebite is estimated as 20,000 to 25,000 annually. The greatest number of reported snakebite deaths occur in the Indian subcontinent (10,000 to 12,000 annually); high figures are also reported from Burma, Ceylon, Thailand and other southeast

Asian countries, Brazil, and other countries in the American tropics. Mortality is believed moderately high in tropical Africa, although reliable figures are not available. Moderate to low incidence is reported from southern Europe, the Middle East, Australia, and New Guinea, the temperate regions of Africa and South America, Japan and associated islands, and the United States (fewer than 20 deaths annually in recent years). Snakebite mortality is very low to nil in northern Europe and Asia, Canada, the West Indies (exclusive of Trinidad), New Zealand, the Malagasy Republic, and Oceania.

High snakebite mortality and morbidity are seen in localities where a dense human population lives in close proximity to dangerous snakes. Some southeast Asian venomous snakes (Indian cobra, kraits, bamboo vipers) are singularly adapted to life in local villages and even in suburbs of large, modern cities. Dangerous pit vipers of the genus Bothrops in Latin America are plentiful in sugar cane and banana plantations; Russell's viper in southeast Asia often frequents cultivated fields. Local practices in agriculture, irrigation, and construction may provide good refuges for snakes, or may bring about increase in the rodents and lizards that are the food of many venomous snakes.

Snakebite is most common in adult males. The incidence is next highest in children because of their carelessness and curiosity. Adult females are the least frequently bitten. Persons at greatest risk from snakebite are those who deliberately handle or work with venomous snakes, be they scientists, entertainers, or religious zealots. If this small, high-risk group is excluded, snakebite is chiefly a hazard to farmers who till their land by primitive methods, plantation laborers, and those engaged in construction work or brush-clearing by largely manual methods. Practices of fish netting and trapping sometimes expose fishermen to bites by sea snakes and other aquatic species. Recent studies indicate that snakebites in the eastern United States are usually sustained near the victim's home, and involve persons in the 5- to 19-year age group predominantly.

Ethnic factors increasing the incidence of snakebite include types of dress that do not protect the legs and feet, sleeping outdoors on mats on the ground, and religious protection of venomous snakes or their use in rituals.

Control of snakes is best accomplished by indirect means: better construction of dwellings, disposal of rubbish, and control of rodents. Direct control campaigns have not been successful, except in small areas, and may be undesirable as many beneficial snakes are also destroyed.

Properties of Snake Venoms. Snake venoms are slightly viscid fluids, usually pale yellow to amber, occasionally white or colorless. Most medically important species yield 0.1 to 1.5 ml. of fluid venom; yields of 5 ml. have been reported for large vipers. Snakes may inject the entire content of their venom glands in biting, but usually do not do so. It has been shown experimentally that the Palestine viper injects about 15 per cent of its venom in an average strike, but in some cases may inject up to half the contents of its glands. Sometimes snakes bite without injecting venom.

Venoms dry as platelets, representing 15 to 45 per cent of the original weight of the sample. In this form they are stable for years if kept in sealed vials at cool to moderate temperature.

Average venom yields from representative species of snakes and the estimated fatal doses for man are given in the accompanying table. It should be emphasized that both the amount of venom and its toxicity are subject to wide variation, according to geographic distribution, age, season, and other factors.

Numerous enzymes have been identified in snake venoms. Hyaluronidases, present in most venoms, account for the rapidity of absorption. Proteases cause local inflammation, necrosis, and damage to vascular epithelium. Phospholipase A alters membrane permeability and releases histamine, thus contributing to hemorrhage and shock. Phosphodiesterase may be responsible for some of the hypotensive effect of venoms. Esterases in some pit viper venoms liberate bradykinin. Mamba venoms are high in acetylcholine.

Snake venoms in vitro display both coagulant and anticoagulant activity depending upon experimental conditions. Clinically, anticoagulant activity is more important, and may result from destruction of fibrinogen or prothrombin, inhibition of thrombin formation, destruction of platelets, or in vivo defibrination with formation of minute fibrin emboli.

Relatively pure toxins have been isolated from snake venoms. Crotactin from the tropical rattlesnake (*Crotalus durissus*) and viperatoxin from the Palestine viper (*Vipera xanthina*) are low molecular weight proteins. Cobra cardiotoxin, cobra neurotoxin, crotamine from some populations of the tropical rattlesnake, bungarotoxins from krait venom, and erabutoxins from sea snakes of the genus Laticauda are all basic polypeptides with molecular weights of about 7000. None of these toxins have enzyme activity.

Immunodiffusion techniques indicate that snake venoms contain 6 to 16 antigens. Venoms of vipers and pit vipers are antigenically more complex than those of elapids and they in turn are more complex than those of sea snakes and colubrids. With some exceptions, venoms of phylogenetically related snakes have similar antigenic makeup, a matter of practical importance in production and use of therapeutic antisera.

Clinical Manifestations. The clinical picture in snakebite is difficult to summarize briefly. Several syndromes are seen.

In the United States, most snakebites are characterized by severe local pain, edema spreading from the bite, painful lymphadenopathy, and local ecchymosis, often with serum-filled blebs. Systemic manifestations include nausea and vomiting, thirst, sweating, and fever rarely exceeding 101° F. If no additional symptoms develop, the

Snake Species	Geographic Distribution	Venom Yield* (mg.)	Lethal Dose for Man† (mg.)
Beaked seasnake, *Enhydrina schistosa*	Coastal waters southern Asia and northern Australia	10–15	1.5
ELAPIDAE			
North American coral snake, *Micrurus fulvius*	Southern United States	3–5	5
Indian krait, *Bungarus caeruleus*	Most of India and Pakistan	8–12	2
Tiger snake, *Notechis scutatus*	Australia	35–45	3
Mamba, *Dendroaspis angusticeps*	East Africa	75–100	15
Death adder, *Acanthophis antarcticus*	Australia and New Guinea	70–100	10
Indian cobra, *Naja naja*	Southeast Asia to Indonesia and Formosa	150–200	20
Ringhals, *Hemachatus haemachatus*	South Africa	80–120	60
VIPERINAE			
Puff adder, *Bitis arietans*	Most of Africa; southern Arabia	160–200	100
Saw-scaled viper, *Echis carinatus*	Northern and western Africa to northern India and Ceylon	20–35	5
Russell's viper, *Vipera russelli*	West Pakistan to Formosa	150–250	70
Palestine viper, *Vipera xanthina*	Middle East	90–140	75
CROTALINAE			
Cottonmouth moccasin, *Agkistrodon piscivorus*	Southern United States	100–150	150
Fer-de-lance, *Bothrops atrox*	Mexico to Argentina	100–160	50
Jararaca, *Bothrops jararaca*	Tropical South America	40–70	40
Bushmaster, *Lachesis muta*	Costa Rica to Brazil	300–500	150
Western diamondback rattlesnake, *Crotalus atrox*	Southwestern United States and northern Mexico	200–300	100
Neotropical rattlesnake, *Crotalus durissus*	Southern Mexico to Argentina	25–40	10
Western rattlesnake, *Crotalus viridis*‡	Western United States and southwestern Canada	90–130	70

*Venom extractions from adult snakes of average size; maximal yields may be two to four times the upper limit of the average range.

†Estimated for an adult of 70 kilograms.

‡There are 13 other species of rattlesnakes in the United States. At least one species occurs in every state except Maine, Delaware, Alaska, and Hawaii.

prognosis is excellent, although there may be local necrosis occasionally severe enough to require skin grafting. Danger signs include numbness and tingling of the face, pronounced drop in blood pressure, violent muscle spasms or convulsions, hematuria, hematemesis, cyanosis, and difficulty in breathing. Increased clotting time and a drop in hemoglobin indicate severe envenomation. This syndrome is seen following bites of most rattlesnakes, the copperhead and cottonmouth moccasin, and a number of Old World vipers.

Hemorrhagic manifestations dominate the picture in bites by certain Latin American lancehead vipers (Bothrops), *some African and Asian vipers*, particularly the saw-scales (Echis), a few elapids such as the Australian genus Pseudechis, and the rear-fanged boomslang (Dispholidus). Local symptoms resemble those listed in the previous paragraph, but there is usually less edema. Persistent oozing of blood from fang punctures, bleeding gums, fever, and headache are prominent even in mild cases. Ecchymoses may be seen anywhere, particularly at sites of mild trauma. Gross hematuria, hematemesis, hemoptysis, and blood in the feces are common. Prothrombin time and sometimes clotting time are greatly prolonged; return

to normal is a favorable prognostic sign. The usual cause of death is massive cerebral, retroperitoneal, or intestinal hemorrhage that may occur as much as 12 days after the bite. Some patients die of anemia and exhaustion, particularly when there is associated scurvy, malnutrition, hookworn disease, or malaria.

Elapid neurotoxins rapidly involve the bulbar centers, causing ptosis, strabismus, slurred speech, and dysphagia with drooling of saliva. Other early symptoms are vomiting, giddiness, muscular weakness, and drowsiness. Respiration is labored; the patient may complain of a sensation of weight on the chest. The temperature is normal or subnormal. Violent abdominal pain sometimes occurs after krait and coral snake bites. General symptoms usually begin within 30 minutes after the bite; sometimes there is a latent period of several hours. Local symptoms vary. Cobra bites usually cause considerable pain and swelling, occasionally followed by necrosis. Bites by many types of elapids cause little immediate local reaction, but pain radiating from the bite may begin after an hour or more. Hemoglobinuria and albuminuria are common. Death usually occurs within 15 hours after onset of systemic symptoms; patients surviving longer generally recover. Despite severe nervous system involvement, permanent neurologic sequelae do not occur.

A *somewhat different neurotoxic syndrome accompanies bites by crotamine-secreting tropical rattlesnakes.* Local pain and swelling are slight to moderate. The outstanding symptoms are dizziness, intense headache, impairment of vision that may progress to blindness, paralysis of the neck muscles, and respiratory depression. Albuminuria and hematuria are seen, and suppression of urine flow may supervene. The prognosis is poor.

Seasnake bites show little or no local symptoms. After a latent period of 30 minutes to a few hours, the patient complains of muscular pain, stiffness, and progressive weakness. Trismus, ptosis, and loss of tendon reflexes are seen. In severe cases blurring of vision, thirst, vomiting, and difficulty in breathing occur. The urine contains myoglobin, albumin, and erythrocytes, although gross hematuria is rare. Tubular necrosis may be followed by acute renal failure. When symptoms are severe the prognosis is grave, but many seasnake bites are mild, probably because of the small amount of venom injected.

A *singular type of envenomation is ophthalmia,* caused by the so-called spitting cobras, of which there are two species in Africa and one in Malaysia. Venom is ejected in a fine spray through an opening on the anterior aspect of the fang. On contact with mucous membranes of the eye, it produces violent pain and sometimes temporary blindness. Permanent ocular damage is rare, and systemic symptoms do not occur. Prompt washing with water or other nonirritant fluids is usually adequate therapy; local use of dilute antivenin has been recommended. Venoms of these snakes have the same effect as other cobra venoms if the snake bites rather than spits.

Diagnosis. The diagnosis of snakebite is materially simplified if the snake has been captured or killed and correctly identified. Differential diagnosis involves distinction between (1) snakebite and other injuries, (2) bites of poisonous and nonpoisonous snakes, and (3) minimal envenomation, in which conservative management is indicated, and severe envenomation, which demands more active therapy.

Injuries by objects such as thorns and spines of plants must occasionally be distinguished from snakebite. Usually these are recognized readily by the nature of the wound and lack of progressive symptoms. Differentiation between snakebite and injuries by other venomous animals may be difficult if the patient did not see the animal that injured him, or is too young to give a reliable history. Wounds inflicted by arthropods such as scorpions, centipedes, spiders, and insects are usually smaller than those caused by fangs of snakes. Fish spines and teeth of small mammals usually cause deeper, more ragged wounds.

The pattern of puncture wounds will not reliably differentiate bites of poisonous snakes from those of nonpoisonous species. The writer has been bitten hundreds of times by many species of non-poisonous snakes and sustained injuries ranging from single punctures to six rows of multiple punctures. Bites by poisonous snakes showing a single fang puncture are not rare, and may terminate fatally. Bites in which the palatine and mandibular teeth cause wounds in addition to those made by the fangs are also seen. Nonpoisonous snakebites show very little local swelling, usually bleed freely, and cause little pain. Unfortunately, bites of some dangerous snakes also show little local reaction.

In North American pit viper (rattlesnake, moccasin) bites, the development of more than 30 cm. of edema and erythema in the first 12 hours plus any of the more serious symptoms mentioned in the paragraph on clinical manifestations calls for administration of antivenin and supportive measures. Cases with less edema and mildness or absence of systemic symptoms need only observation and symptomatic therapy. In bites by snakes with hemorrhagic venom, hemoptysis, hematuria, and increased prothrombin time are early evidences of serious poisoning. Early clinical signs of severe neurotoxic poisoning are impaired vision, ptosis, slurred speech, and drowsiness. The presence of trismus, muscle pain on passive movement, and myoglobinuria differentiates severe seasnake bites from mild ones and from injuries by other venomous marine organisms.

Treatment. Therapy in snakebite has four aims: (1) retarding absorption of venom and removing as much as possible by mechanical means, (2) neutralization of venom by immune serum, (3) counteracting specific pharmacologic activities of the venom, and (4) relief of symptoms and prevention of complications.

Local Treatment. Clinical and experimental evidence indicates that appreciable amounts of rattlesnake and other viperine venoms may be removed by incision and suction. A ligature should be applied immediately and tightly a few centimeters proximal to the fang wounds and released for 90 seconds every 15 minutes. It may be moved proximally as swelling increases. Two to four incisions about 1 cm. long are made completely through the skin through or near the fang wounds. Suction is applied intermittently over the incisions for approximately one hour after the bite. A breast pump, modified plastic syringe, or the devices in commercial snakebite kits may be used; oral suction should not be used if other means are available. Bracelet or multiple incisions are not advised. If circulation distal to the bite becomes badly impaired, fasciotomy may be necessary.

Incision and suction increase the danger of infection, and oozing of blood from incisions may be a problem following bites by snakes with powerfully anticoagulant venoms. Absorption of some highly neurotoxic venoms is so rapid that local measures must be begun within a matter of seconds following the bite to be effective.

After the first hour, the ligature is released. The bitten part should be immobilized 24 to 96 hours.

After acute symptoms of poisoning have subsided, treatment of vesicles and necrotic areas is similar to that advocated for severe burns.

Serum Therapy. Snake venom antisera or antivenins are prepared by hyperimmunization of animals (usually horses) against one or more snake venoms. The antibody-containing fraction of the serum is concentrated by methods used in preparation of bacterial antitoxins. Sometimes the product is lyophilized for greater stability. Antivenins are prepared by approximately 30 laboratories in various parts of the world. Most are intended for treatment of bites by the important venomous snakes of a particular geographic area. Some success has been achieved in preparation of antivenins against entire phylogenetic groups of venoms; e.g., polyvalent Crotalidae antivenin appears to be effective against venoms of most medically important species of pit vipers. There are no international standards for preparation and assay of antivenins. Products differ widely in potency and stability. The toxin-neutralizing capacity is low in comparison with bacterial antitoxins, and large doses are required. An initial dose of 20 to 50 ml. diluted with five times its volume of physiologic saline should be given by intravenous drip over a 30 to 45 minute period. More antivenin should be given as the patient's condition dictates. A total of 100 to 150 ml. in the first 24 hours may be required in a severe bite. If intravenous injection is not practicable, undiluted antivenin should be given intramuscularly. Infiltration of the bitten area with antivenin gives no advantage, and is contraindicated on fingers and toes. Allergic reactions to antivenin are common, and fatal anaphylaxis has been reported. A skin test for hypersensitivity should be done before administering serum; a positive reaction is contraindication to its use except in very severe cases. In bites by snakes known to be not highly dangerous (the copperhead in the United States, the European viper) or in bites by small snakes of more dangerous species, antivenin should be withheld unless the patient is a small child or there are signs of severe intoxication.

Supportive and Symptomatic Treatment. Except when it is obvious that only a minimal amount of venom has been injected, snakebite victims should be hospitalized at least 12 hours and kept in bed.

Blood transfusion is valuable therapy for bites by snakes with strongly hematotoxic venom. Blood typing should be done at the earliest opportunity, since the action of some venoms may make the procedure difficult. Adjustment of fluid and electrolyte balance is indicated in presence of shock, severe vomiting, hematuria, and albuminuria.

Oxygen is helpful in cases of hypoxia from blood destruction or respiratory impairment from the action of neurotoxins. In the latter, aspiration of secretions from the throat and trachea may be necessary, and the use of a respirator may be advisable. A tracheostomy may be required.

The presence of necrotic tissue, interference with local blood supply, and the toxic action of venoms on leukocytes and other phagocytic cells increase the hazard of infection even in relatively mild snakebites. Antimicrobial therapy should be instituted in most cases. Tetanus prophylaxis with toxoid or antitoxin is advisable; gas gangrene antitoxin is not recommended as a regular measure.

The necrotizing action of some snake venoms is greatly reduced by local infiltration of tissue with 20 to 100 ml. of 0.1 M ethylenediamine tetraacetic acid (EDTA). This must be done as soon as possible after the bite. Lethal factors of the venom are *not* neutralized by EDTA.

Although corticosteroids have been reported to be useful in snake envenomation, no clear rules for their administration can be laid down at present. Despite the histamine-like action of many snake venoms, antihistaminics have not proved effective in snakebite treatment.

Pain is often severe in viper bites, and may require codeine or meperidine. Anxiety and fear, sometimes to the point of hysteria, commonly accompany snakebite. Verbal reassurance and a confident attitude on the part of the physician are often more helpful than any medication; nevertheless, light barbiturate sedation is often advisable. An old and much maligned remedy, an ounce or so of whiskey or brandy, may accomplish the same purpose.

Nonpoisonous snakebites generally require no treatment unless the snake was a python or other large species. Precautions against infection should be taken. The snake's teeth frequently break off in the wound and should be removed. No specific diseases are transmitted by snakes in biting.

Behringwerk Mitteilungen: Die Giftschlangen der Erde, Wirkung und Antigenitat der Gifte. Therapie von Giftschlangenbissen. Marburg-Lahn, N. G. Elwert., 1963.

Kaiser, E., and Michl, H.: Die Biochemie der tierischen Gifte. Wien, Franz Deuticke, 1958.

Reid, H. A.: Snake-bite in the tropics. Brit. Med. J., 3:359, 1968.

Russell, F. E.: Clinical aspects of snake venom poisoning in North America. Toxicon, 7:33, 1969.

U.S. Navy Bureau of Medicine and Surgery: Poisonous Snakes of the World. Washington, D.C., U.S. Government Printing Office, 1968.

MARINE VENOMS

Venomous species occur in most phyla of marine animals. Their relative medical importance is increasing with the growing popularity of travel and of aquatic sports and with expanding exploitation of marine resources. Recognition of these animals and knowledge of their habits minimize opportunities for injury.

Most marine animal venoms appear to be proteins; however, quaternary ammonium compounds, epinephrine, 5-hydroxytryptamine, histamine, and other pharmacologically active compounds have been detected. Zootoxicologic properties of these venoms are too diverse for brief summary. Mechanisms of action for most species are poorly understood.

Jellyfish Stings. The pelagic coelenterates known as jellyfish belong to two main groups, the

Portuguese men-of-war or bluebottles of the class Hydrozoa and the "true" jellyfish of the class Scyphozoa. Medically important species occur in all oceans; however, more serious stings are reported from Australian and south Asian waters. The venom apparatus consists of tentacles that may be up to 30 meters long and are thickly studded with highly specialized stinging capsules or nematocysts. Their primary function is capture and immobilization of food. Coelenterates never *attack* man; indeed, they are physically incapable of doing so. Injuries usually occur through contact with floating or stranded coelenterates or their detached tentacles. Such contact is followed by intense burning pain and development of linear, erythematous wheals that may progress to vesiculation. Muscular cramps, dyspnea, and nausea may be seen. Local necrosis may follow severe jellyfish stings. A systemic reaction clinically similar to anaphylactic shock may follow stings by sea wasps (*Chiropsalmus* and *Chironex*); death has occurred three to four minutes after contact. Irukandji sting, caused by the Australian jellyfish *Carukia barnesi*, is characterized by a mild nettling rash followed after 10 to 60 minutes by sweating, cramps, severe myalgia, vomiting and, sometimes, cough with hemoptysis. Recovery occurs within a day or two.

If tentacles are clinging to the skin, they should not be pulled or rubbed off, as this may discharge additional nematocysts. Prompt application of alcohol to the tentacle will inactivate the nematocysts. If alcohol is not available, the tentacles should be covered with sugar, salt, or dry sand and left alone 15 to 20 minutes before being scraped off. Local application of analgesic cream or ointment, preferably one containing an antihistaminic, may give some relief. Systemic reactions have been successfully counteracted by epinephrine (0.5 to 1 ml. subcutaneously) plus 10 ml. intravenously of calcium gluconate, antihistaminics, artificial respiration, and oxygen. Morphine or meperidine may be required to control pain.

Cone Shell Stings. Large marine snails of the genus *Conus* inflict injury with a harpoon-like tooth that can be rapidly extruded and is used for capture of prey as well as defense. Nearly all injuries are seen in shell collectors. Mild cases show only local symptoms resembling those of wasp stings. In severe cases, initial pain is followed by numbness, paresthesia, paresis beginning in the region of the injury and occasionally spreading to involve the entire skeletal musculature, sensation of constriction of the chest, dysphagia, visual disturbances, and collapse. Fatalities are on record, nearly all of them ascribed to the large species, *C. geographus*, widely distributed in the warmer parts of the Pacific and Indian Oceans.

The active principle of cone shell venom has not been identified, and treatment of stings is symptomatic.

Miscellaneous Venomous Invertebrates. Spines of sea urchins cause painful injuries, occasionally accompanied by giddiness and muscular palsies

lasting several hours. A species of spiny Australian starfish inflicts a wound followed by bouts of vomiting lasting several days. Various sessile coelenterates such as hydroids, sea anemones, and stinging corals cause nettle-like stinging, sometimes with zosteriform hemorrhagic lesions and necrosis. Abdominal cramps, chills, diarrhea, and leukocytosis with eosinophilia may accompany severe stings. There is no specific treatment for any of these envenomations.

Venomous Fishes. Stonefish (Synanceja), scorpionfish (Scorpaena), lionfish (Pterois), weeverfish (Trachinus), and related species have venom glands associated with spines, especially those of the dorsal fin. Except for the greater weever, these are shallow-water fish particularly common about reefs, where they lie partly buried or concealed in crevices. Here they are apt to be accidentally touched or trodden upon. In open water the fish may adopt a more active defense, swimming so that the venomous spines are presented to an enemy. Skin divers and aquarium keepers have been injured under such circumstances. Fishermen may be injured when removing the fish from nets or traps. Similarity of symptoms and of venom activity in laboratory animals suggests common or similar active principles in their venoms. *Synanceja verrucosa*, found from Oceania to the east coast of Africa, appears to be the most dangerous member of this group.

Following injury by spines of these fishes, there is local pain that tends to spread and is often followed by hypesthesia or paresthesia at the site of puncture. Victims invariably describe the pain as almost unbearable, and it is regularly accompanied by hyperactivity often manifest by rolling about on the ground. There is severe local swelling, sometimes with formation of blisters and sloughing. Profuse sweating, dyspnea, hypotension, cyanosis, and collapse are seen especially with Synanceja stings; death may occur within an hour. Those who survive a severe sting may complain of weakness, dyspnea, and muscular aches for several weeks.

Ligature, incision, and suction as recommended for snakebite have some value as first aid if done within 15 minutes. Immersion of the injured site in hot water helps relieve pain.

Antivenin for Synanceja is available from Commonwealth Serum Laboratories of Australia; it may be expected to have some effect in stings by related species of fishes. The initial intramuscular or intravenous dose of 2 ml. may be repeated in severe cases. Infiltration of the wound with emetine hydrochloride solution (65 mg. per milliliter) is recommended if antivenin is not available.

Stingrays are widely distributed in warm coastal waters, including mouths of rivers; one genus is restricted to fresh water. There are about 30 medically important species; the larger ones are 8 to 10 feet long, and weigh more than 100 pounds. Venom-secreting tissue is in the grooves and sheaths of barbed bony spines on the dorsum of the tail; in large species of rays, the spine may be 35 to 40 cm. long. Stingrays typically bury themselves in sand or mud, where they may be stepped upon or grazed by persons diving. The fish lashes with its tail, driving the sting into its victim. Stings of large rays can readily penetrate the abdominal or thoracic wall. The wound is a puncture or laceration often surrounded by a zone of blanching for the first 30 minutes or so; later the area becomes hyperemic and edematous. Pain is severe, and sweating, nausea, weakness, and syncope are common. Muscular twitching, convulsions, irregular respiration, and cardiac arrhythmia indicate severe poisoning. Of 1097 stingray injuries reported in the United States during a five-year period, 62 patients required hospitalization, and two deaths resulted.

First aid for stingray injuries is immediate irrigation with salt water and removal of any fragments of the sting sheath that can be seen. This is followed by soaking in hot water for 30 to 90 minutes, administration of analgesics, and tetanus prophylaxis. Injuries by large rays, particularly when the chest or abdomen has been penetrated, require surgical management. There are no specific pharmacologic antagonists to stingray venom, nor is antivenim available.

Keegan, H. L., and Macfarlane, W. V. (eds.): Venomous and Poisonous Animals and Noxious Plants of the Pacific Region. New York, Pergamon Press, 1963.

Nigrelli, R. F. (ed.): Biochemistry and pharmacology of compounds derived from marine organisms. Ann. N. Y. Acad. Sci., 90:615, 1960.

Russell, F. E.: Marine toxins and venomous and poisonous marine animals. Advances Marine Biol., 3:255, 1965.

DISORDERS OF THE NERVOUS SYSTEM AND BEHAVIOR

Introduction

Fred Plum

Almost all diseases use the nervous system to express themselves and it is this fact that often makes neurology seem complex and difficult to the physician. Pain, sensory loss, weakness, disturbed thinking, and impaired mood or alertness are not specific indicators of specific diseases. To be sure, in many instances, they are symptoms of primary disease of the nervous system. Even more often, however, they reflect disease in some other system or organ of the body. Finally, and perhaps most frequently, these symptoms derive from man's faulty adjustment to his environment. Symptoms are error signals, and the nervous system is as sensitive to symbolic threats as to physical ones.

Based on the above concepts, the goals of the section that follows are to present neurologic disease as a problem to be approached logically and for which certain principles repeatedly provide the key for diagnosis and treatment. These principles are based on our current knowledge of how the brain functions as an adaptive organ, adjusting man to his external as well as to his internal environment.

The section is organized in two main parts. In the first the more general functions of the nervous system are considered: how it is organized, how it handles certain normal activities, and how it expresses psychologic and somatic symptoms in response to both real and symbolic threat or injury. In the second part the more traditional approach is taken, and neurologic diseases are discussed according to anatomic and causative categories. Heavy emphasis is placed on the biochemistry of disease and the specific physiology of signs and symptoms. It must be recognized, however, that this century's revolution in biologic science is just beginning to attack effectively the problems involved in understanding brain function, behavior, and neurologic disease. Thus, these pages often expose our ignorance as much as they do our knowledge.

A word about treatment. Man's brain is his uniquely human organ. Damage it and life loses its meaning in direct proportion, no matter what other physiologic benefits may accrue in the process. The brain cannot be regenerated, repaired, or homotransplanted. It accumulates no metabolic debts and, unless supplied continuously by an effective circulation carrying large amounts of oxygen and glucose, it digests itself irreparably. This means that one cannot "let the brain go" while solving other medical problems. For example, if an elderly man with severe anemia suffers an ischemic stroke while awaiting accurate blood studies, there is no satisfaction later in a correct hematologic diagnosis. If an adolescent girl suffers permanent dementia from hypoglycemia while having her diabetes regulated, the perfect control of glycosuria seems hardly worth it. The integrity of the nervous system must be the first goal in therapeutics.

Consciousness and Its Disturbances

GENERAL CONSIDERATIONS
Fred Plum

William James remarked that everyone knows what consciousness is until he tries to define it. Full consciousness is generally taken to imply not only wakefulness but the total complement of human mental faculties: complete awareness of self and environment. In clinical medicine, when one speaks of consciousness as opposed to unconsciousness or coma, a less encompassing state is usually meant, consisting of behavioral wakefulness plus the capacity to respond appropriately to at least a limited number of external stimuli. *Dementia, apathy, amnesia,* or *aphasia* may impair the content of consciousness, but as long as enough appropriate responses remain in other behavioral functions, consciousness is considered to be preserved. *Obtundation* and *drowsiness* describe states of dull behavior with blunted alertness in which part of the content of consciousness is lost, often with an excessive tendency to sleep. *Stupor* is a state wherein subjects respond when vigorously stimulated, but immediately sink back again as soon as external stimuli are withdrawn. *Coma* is complete unresponsiveness. In light coma, semi-appropriate movements occur in response to noxious stimuli, but in deep coma, subjects retain only primitive reflexes or no responses at all.

The present physiologic concept of consciousness is that it depends upon close interaction between the intact cerebral hemispheres and the upper brainstem. The hemispheres contribute most of the specific components of consciousness, including language, memory, intellect, and learned responses to sensory stimuli. But, in order to function effectively, the cerebrum must be aroused or activated by more caudally placed mechanisms that originate in the thalamus, hypothalamus, midbrain, and upper pons. An important component of this arousal mechanism is located within what Magoun and his colleagues called the ascending reticular activating system; other brainstem systems also influence cerebral cortical activity and the state of consciousness.

The relation of the cerebral cortex to consciousness is more quantitative than qualitative: All hemispheric lesions undoubtedly reduce, at least to some degree, the content of man's consciousness, and the total loss of the cortex causes coma even if the brainstem is left intact. Between the extremes of an injury so small that it is clinically almost undetectable and so large that it causes coma lies a continuum along which the size of the lesion and the impairment of mind, memory, wit, and personality are roughly proportional.

THE PATHOGENESIS OF STUPOR AND COMA
Fred Plum

The preceding paragraphs have described how stupor or coma results when a disease process either diffusely and bilaterally ·blots out the function of the cerebral hemispheres or blocks brainstem-activating structures so that the cortex cannot be aroused. A potentially bewildering series of individual maladies can have one or both of these effects, as may be seen in the accompanying table. However, if one examines the mechanisms by which neurologic diseases cause coma, all these maladies fall into three categories that can be distinguished by their signs and symptoms: (1) supratentorial mass lesions, (2) subtentorial compressive or destructive lesions, and (3) metabolic brain diseases.

Supratentorial Mass Lesions. Supratentorial masses are rarely so large that they produce coma by directly destroying or replacing the cerebral

THE COMMON CAUSES OF STUPOR AND COMA

Supratentorial Lesions (Causing Upper Brainstem Dysfunction)
      Cerebral hemorrhage
      Large cerebral infarction
      Subdural hematoma
      Epidural hematoma
      Brain tumor
      Brain abscess (rare)

Subtentorial Lesions (Compressing or Destroying the Reticular Formation)
      Pontine or cerebellar hemorrhage
      Infarction
      Tumor
      Cerebellar abscess

Metabolic and Diffuse Lesions (see also Table 1 in the article on Delirium)
      Anoxia or ischemia
      Hypoglycemia
      Nutritional deficiency
      Endogenous organ failure or deficiency
      Ionic and electrolyte disorders
      Exogenous poison
      Infections
          Meningitis
          Encephalitis
      Concussion and postictal states

hemispheres. Rather, they interfere with consciousness because they shift and squeeze the contents of the supratentorial compartment and, in so doing, compress the diencephalon. The expanding process can originate anywhere in the hemisphere and ultimately will produce this reaction because the fibrous tentorium and the bones of the base of the skull resist movement except toward the tentorial opening. As a result, when supratentorial masses demand room for expansion, the diencephalic tectum and adjacent midbrain are particularly likely to be compressed, and sometimes the diencephalon is even displaced downward through the tentorial notch (transtentorial herniation).

How do supratentorial masses progress so that these reactions occur? The brain has certain common responses to injury, including edema, vascular dilatation, and the invasion of leukocytes and proliferation of glial cells. The intensity, tempo, and exact contribution of each of these responses varies according to the nature of the original lesion and the rate at which it appears, but each shares in the brain's defenses against neoplasms, infections, infarcts, and irritants. Thus, the original lesion gradually enlarges and tends to impair structures ever more remote from itself in the inexpansible intracranial cavity. The remote effects are due partly to edema spreading away from the edges of the primary lesion and partly to an actual shift of the brain within the skull, compressing normal tissues and blood vessels against rigid structures such as the falx cerebri and the tentorium. At this stage, clinical signs of increased intracranial pressure are common and imply that an intracranial lesion is already exerting generalized deleterious effects.

The clinical picture of supratentorial mass

lesions producing stupor or coma has several distinctive features. If a history is available, localizing symptoms such as frontal headache, focal seizures, or other changes consistent with hemispheric disease will usually be found to have preceded unconsciousness. Physically, most patients demonstrate a combination of *focal* hemispheral signs, e.g., sensorimotor defect, aphasia, and visual field defect, reflecting the site of the original pathologic process, plus *diffuse* signs of supratentorial dysfunction, indicating that the lesion is exerting remote effects on the opposite hemisphere and the deep diencephalon. An important negative finding is that, unless the patient is in the terminal stages of illness, no evidence of direct subtentorial brainstem dysfunction can be found: pupillary and oculovestibular reflexes remain intact. If a patient with a supratentorial lesion progresses in his illness, the neurologic signs and symptoms evolve in a characteristic, orderly, rostral-caudal pattern. The more rostrally located neurologic functions first disappear, followed by more caudal impairment, first in the diencephalon and then down the brainstem almost as if the structures were being progressively transected from above downward, each plane of function being removed almost completely before the next is impaired.

The above description needs amplification to be complete. Some supratentorial masses begin and enlarge in neurologically silent areas such as the frontal lobes or the subdural space and lack a focal signature. Lesions of this type may be revealed only when the patient develops signs of diffuse forebrain dysfunction plus, perhaps, headache and evidence of increased intracranial pressure.

Stupor or coma with supratentorial lesions is ominous because it implies that the deeply located upper brainstem is already compressed or distorted and that the much more serious complication of herniation of the forebrain downward into the tentorial notch is about to occur. Such herniation begins either with direct downward displacement of the diencephalon (central herniation) or with the uncus of the temporal lobe squeezing into the tentorial notch and against the midbrain (uncal herniation). Either way, if the hernia develops fully, it usually impacts the midbrain and nearly always results in permanent brain damage or death. A characteristic constellation of symptoms heralds each of these patterns of transtentorial herniation. With impending *central* herniation, stupor becomes gradually deeper, and the subjects sigh, yawn, or develop periodic respirations. The pupils shrink to as little as 1 to 2 mm. in diameter, but retain their light reflexes. Oculovestibular reflexes are brisk, and the extremities stiffen into bilateral rigidity or spasticity, combined with extensor plantar responses. With *uncal* herniation, signs are in many ways similar to the above except that as the uncus slides over the tentorial edge, it often compresses the third nerve ahead of it, even before the diencephalon is com-

pressed. The result is that the pupil on the side of the herniation begins to dilate more than its fellow. Eventually, the pupil dilates widely and becomes light-fixed, and the patient becomes stuporous. Shortly afterward, oculomotor functions of the third nerve are usually impaired, and the involved eye turns outward. If the herniating process continues, the opposite third nerve becomes involved as well, and then the brainstem. To initiate effective treatment one must recognize the process before this advanced stage and halt it with osmotic decompressing agents or surgical treatment. Otherwise, when conditions progress this far, few subjects recover without substantial, permanent neurologic injury.

Subtentorial Mass or Destructive Lesions. These conditions cause stupor or coma if they destroy or compress the centrally located activating systems in the brainstem anywhere above approximately the midpons. Expanding lesions of the posterior fossa have the same effect if they compress the midbrain upward. Compression against the medulla oblongata with an ensuing cerebellar pressure cone produces stiff neck, along with respiratory and cardiac irregularities, but does not directly cause loss of consciousness.

The characteristic clinical feature of subtentorial destruction or compression causing coma is the presence of restricted and usually asymmetrical signs of focal brainstem dysfunction, which frequently can be anatomically pinpointed to a single locus by the clinical findings. Seldom do the signs indicate complete brainstem transection. This restricted, discrete localization is unlike metabolic lesions causing coma in which the signs commonly indicate incomplete dysfunction at several different levels of the brain, and also is unlike the secondary brainstem dysfunction and coma that follow supratentorial herniation, in which *all* function at any given level tends to be lost as the process progresses from rostral to caudal along the neuraxis.

Purely compressive lesions of the posterior fossa rarely cause coma until late in their course when the patient is near death. The pathologic process is usually a hemorrhage, abscess, or tumor of the cerebellum or fourth ventricle, and occipital headache, nystagmus, diplopia, nausea, vomiting, cranial nerve signs, and ataxia usually precede unconsciousness. Important points in distinguishing both destructive and compressive posterior fossa lesions from metabolic depression of the brainstem are that in metabolic depression oculovestibular responses are generally preserved until the advanced stages, and pupillary light reflexes are nearly always preserved. By contrast, structural brainstem lesions causing coma always disrupt the oculovestibular responses, and those involving the midbrain also interrupt the pupillary reflexes.

Metabolic Depression of the Brain Causing Coma. *Endogenous,* or primary, metabolic encephalopathies are intrinsic to the neuron, the glial cell, or the white matter, respectively. They often produce dementia, but rarely cause coma except terminally. *Exogenous,* or secondary, metabolic encephalopathies are those in which brain function is disrupted either because the brain is not supplied with a required substance, e.g., thiamine, oxygen, or glucose, or because it is poisoned by an ingested or endogenous toxin, e.g., depressant drugs or the products of uremia. The secondary metabolic encephalopathies are frequent causes of delirium as well as of stupor and coma; their relationship to the normal metabolism of the brain is discussed in detail elsewhere in this section.

Experimental evidence conflicts as to whether most metabolic agents causing coma depress mainly the brainstem reticular formation or the cerebral cortex. Clinically, most patients with metabolic encephalopathy appear to suffer more depression of the forebrain than of the brainstem. However, the striking finding with most metabolic agents is that they selectively depress certain susceptible functions at several different brain levels, but at the same time spare other functions that emanate from identical levels. For example, most metabolic poisons depress the reticular and motor functions of the midbrain, yet nearly all of them spare the pupillary light reflex so that reactive pupils persist into the deepest stages of metabolic coma until asphyxia intervenes. (Poisoning with glutethimide or parasympathomimetics provides the only exception to this rule, both drugs blocking the light reflex in large, coma-causing doses.) Most of the metabolic encephalopathies cause delirium before stupor or coma, and many of them are accompanied in their early stages by asterixis, a flapping irregular tremor of the outstretched hands, or by random myoclonic muscle twitches. Although the metabolic encephalopathies occasionally produce asymmetrical motor signs, they more characteristically impair body movement symmetrically, and they never impair central sensory pathways except as an accompaniment to the over-all depression of the sensorium.

To epitomize, diseases causing stupor or coma fall into three categories:

1. Supratentorial mass lesions, which present with asymmetrical neurologic signs of hemispheral dysfunction combined with evidence of intact subtentorial brainstem function. As supratentorial lesions evolve, the signs indicate progressive rostral-caudal neurologic deterioration, almost as if the brain were being serially sectioned from top to bottom.

2. Subtentorial compressive and destructive lesions, which present from the outset with either cranial nerve abnormalities or other focal brainstem signs, including pupillary and oculovestibular reflex abnormalities. Long tract motor signs are usually present and asymmetrical.

3. Metabolic brain diseases, which present a picture of either diffuse cortical depression or, more often, of impaired function in both the hemispheres and the brainstem accompanied by retained pupillary light reflexes. The multifocal distribution of metabolic encephalopathy is usually symmetrical and not accompanied by sensory impairments.

Approach to the Patient in Stupor or Coma. The physician must ensure that the brain and other vital organs receive no further injury while he obtains whatever additional history, examinations, and laboratory data are required. Before anything else he must provide a free and open airway and determine that the subject is breathing deeply enough to oxygenate his lungs and eliminate carbon dioxide. The techniques employed are the same as those for managing drug-induced coma described under Management of Acute Depressive Drug Poisoning (*vide infra*). Next, the heart and blood pressure should be examined, and possible sources of bleeding checked to be certain that cardiac output and blood volume are sufficient to supply the metabolic needs of the brain and kidney. In all patients in coma an intravenous infusion should be started, using a large-bore needle. Blood samples for typing and cross-matching, as well as for other appropriate laboratory determinations, can be obtained at this time. Whenever the cause of coma is doubtful, and particularly when the clinical signs suggest a metabolic disease as a possible cause, blood should be taken for sugar determination, and then 50 ml. of 50 per cent glucose should be given intravenously. Hypoglycemic encephalopathy can take many forms, some of which mimic other diseases. If glucose is given promptly, no further cerebral damage occurs while the doctor awaits definitive laboratory diagnosis. Intravenous sugar harms nothing if the coma has another cause.

Beyond these immediate, life-saving measures, it requires considerable restraint to approach a patient in a coma methodically, for the urge to act without delay is understandably strong, but potentially dangerous. Inquiry into both the past medical history and the circumstances under which the patient lost consciousness generally discloses more of diagnostic value than any other maneuver. Is there any suggestion that head trauma could have occurred recently? Has there been renal, hepatic, or myocardial disease? Could a seizure have preceded the present unconsciousness? Has the subject been taking insulin? Have there been recent changes in mood, behavior, or neurologic function to suggest an evolving intracranial process? Was the subject "blue," depressed, or moody, and did he have access to depressant drugs? Is he a "spree" drinker? These, and other, questions must be covered comprehensively with relatives, past physicians, friends, police, or ambulance personnel.

One must perform both a meticulous neurologic examination and a thoughtful physical review of every body system, because disease in remote organs often causes or accentuates dysfunction in the brain.

Fever implies infection, or, less often, lymphomatous neoplasm. On the other hand, hypothermia (30° to 36° C. [86° to 96.8° F.]) in a patient not severely exposed to cold suggests depressant drug poisoning, hypoglycemia, or severe lower brainstem injury, as by infarction. Hypertension may be the cause of hypertensive encephalopathy or the underlying cause of cerebral hemorrhage. Conversely, an elevated blood pressure can be a symptom of subarachnoid hemorrhage in a subject not previously hypertensive. Hypotension in a supine patient implies low blood volume (hemorrhagic or traumatic shock; severe nutritional and fluid depletion), low cardiac output (myocardial infarction), or low peripheral resistance (depressant drug poisoning). Tachycardia (over 160 per minute) can mean that unconsciousness is the result of lowered cardiac output from a supraventricular cardiac arrhythmia. Bradycardia suggests heart block and the Adams-Stokes syndrome or a myocardial infarct.

The pattern and depth of respiration are often informative in evaluating both neurologic function and acid-base balance, so much so that the evaluation of breathing is discussed more fully in the article on Delirium.

The skin should be searched for petechiae (thrombocytopenic or nonthrombocytopenic purpura, meningococcemia, and bacterial endocarditis), bruises, evidence of nutritional deficiency, icterus, angiomatous spiders, and the bright pinkness of carbon monoxide poisoning. Fleshy or clubbed fingertips suggest carcinoma of the lung, or, less often, lung abscess or congenital heart disease (with brain embolism or abscess). A meticulous examination of the optic fundi is imperative but should be completed without cycloplegics, the use of which destroys the potential diagnostic value of pupillary reactions in coma. In the fundus oculi, the pathologic changes of many diseases causing coma can be viewed directly: increased intracranial pressure, hypertensive vascular disease, diabetes, blood dyscrasia, tuberculosis, sarcoidosis, bacterial endocarditis, cryptococcosis, collagen vascular disease, and even subarachnoid hemorrhage producing subhyaloid bleeding.

Chest examination has two potentially rewarding findings: cardiac murmurs suggest bacterial endocarditis with consequent focal, embolic encephalitis; the wheezes and obstructive sounds of the pulmonary cripple suggest CO_2 retention causing narcosis. In the abdominal examination, the presence of masses suggesting polycystic kidneys increases the chances that subarachnoid hemorrhage has occurred, whereas liver enlargement (hepatic coma is common with hepatomas) or splenic enlargement (both blood dyscrasias and infectious mononucleosis can cause encephalitis-like illnesses) can provide valuable leads.

During the neurologic examination, certain potentially informative steps are sometimes overlooked. The skull should always be palpated and inspected meticulously. Edema of the scalp commonly overlies fresh fracture lines, and basal skull fractures predispose to blood pigment stains behind the ear (Battle's sign) and about the orbit (raccoon eyes). Blood also may escape from basal fractures into the ear canals, the middle ears, or the nostrils. The skull should be percussed since focal or unilateral skull tenderness, manifested by grimacing or withdrawal in a stuporous subject, often overlies an intracranial mass lesion. The neck should be tested carefully: stiff neck can reflect meningitis, cerebellar tonsillar herniation, or, occasionally, simply skeletal muscle spasticity. The stiff neck of acute bacterial meningitis is rarely equivocal; that of impending herniation is commonly less severe and lacks accompanying signs of infection or a prominent Kernig sign. It usually requires several hours or a day or more for stiff neck to develop after subarachnoid bleeding.

It is useful to watch the unconscious patient for a time, observing whether or not the extremities move equally and whether tremor, myoclonus, or single or repetitive seizures involve any part of the body. Status epilepticus with focal continuous epilepsy is not uncommon, but is often overlooked.

Laboratory Examination of the Patient in Coma. Patients should be subjected to a skull roentgenogram (looking for fracture lines, densities, and pineal shifts), a blood count and smear, and a urinalysis. When the clinical findings are consistent with metabolic encephalopathy but the cause is uncertain, the blood glucose and serum sodium, potassium, and bicarbonate should be obtained promptly. Knowledge of the arterial pH often can be almost diagnostic of the cause of metabolic coma (see Table 2 in the article on Delirium).

When to do a lumbar puncture is always a serious question. All physicians are aware that in patients with increased intracranial pressure the procedure sometimes induces fatal herniation of the brain through the tentorium or foramen magnum. For this reason, lumbar puncture is best avoided by the general physician who strongly suspects his patient of having an expanding intracranial mass, particularly in the posterior fossa. However, there are certain treatable diseases such as meningitis that can be diagnosed only by lumbar puncture, and many others in which the procedure yields valuable preliminary diagnostic information. When the advice of neurologic specialists is unavailable, the doctor has no choice but to proceed with lumbar puncture if the diagnosis is in doubt and he believes the procedure has a reasonable chance of offering valuable information. Certain steps minimize the risk. One is to use a small (No. 20), sharp needle. Another is to fill the manometer with saline and attach it to the needle before releasing fluid, a technique that prevents sudden subarachnoid pressure shifts. Finally, jugular manometrics should *never* be performed, for they offer little useful data and increase the risk of impacting potential herniations.

Magoun, H. W.: The Waking Brain. 2nd ed. Springfield, Ill., Charles C Thomas, 1963.
Plum, F., and Posner, J. B.: The Diagnosis of Stupor and Coma. Philadelphia, F. A. Davis Company, 1966.

DELIRIUM AND EXOGENOUS METABOLIC BRAIN DISEASE

Jerome B. Posner

INTRODUCTION

Metabolic encephalopathy is brain dysfunction due to diffuse or widespread multifocal failure of neuronal metabolism. When the cerebral disorder arises from an intrinsic failure of neuronal or glial metabolism, it is referred to as *primary or endogenous metabolic encephalopathy*. The primary disorders usually begin insidiously, progress inexorably, and produce a clinical picture of dementia, as discussed under that heading. When the encephalopathy results from interference with brain metabolism by extracerebral disease, it is called *secondary or exogenous metabolic encephalopathy*. The secondary encephalopathies usually begin acutely or subacutely and often subside with time and treatment. They produce a clinical picture in which confusion, thinking errors, behavioral abnormalities, disorders of consciousness, and abnormal motor activity predominate. The causes of secondary metabolic encephalopathy are as many and varied as the illnesses that disturb body chemistry. Some examples are listed in Table 1.

Metabolic brain disease is both common and often misdiagnosed. When early and mild, it often produces intellectual dullness, social indifference, and vague perplexity, called by some an *acute or subacute confusional state* and easily mistaken by observers for psychogenic depression or simply low intelligence. More severe degrees may elicit a florid picture, with tremulous agitation, rich and frightening hallucinations, and periods of seemingly complete loss of contact with the environment. This state, often called *delirium* or *toxic psychosis*, must be distinguished from a "functional" psychosis. Prolonged or severe metabolic dysfunction may lead to stupor or coma and then is likely to be mistaken for gross structural brain disease. Although certain specific systemic disorders characteristically cause one or another of the above syndromes, each can occur with any of the metabolic brain diseases; thus, the terms "delirium," "toxic psychosis," and "confusional state" are used interchangeably in this article to describe the wakeful stage of exogenous metabolic encephalopathy. An insidiously developing, quiet delirium may be clinically indistinguishable from the early stages of dementia.

PATHOLOGY

The gross and microscopic pathologic changes in patients with metabolic brain disease depend upon the nature and severity of their illness. The brains of some patients delirious during life are entirely normal at postmortem examination. In most cases, however, at least microscopic patho-

TABLE 1.   CAUSES OF METABOLIC BRAIN DISEASE

I. Deprivation of Oxygen, Substrate, or Metabolic Cofactors
   *A. Hypoxia (interference with oxygen supply to the entire brain—cerebral blood flow normal)
      1. Decreased oxygen tension and content of blood
         Pulmonary disease
         Alveolar hypoventilation
         Decreased atmospheric oxygen tension
      2. Decreased oxygen content of blood—normal tension
         Anemia
         Carbon monoxide poisoning
         Methemoglobinemia
   *B. Ischemia (diffuse or widespread multifocal interference with blood supply to brain)
      1. Decreased cerebral blood flow resulting from decreased cardiac output
         Stokes-Adams syndrome, cardiac arrest, cardiac arrhythmias
         Myocardial infarction
         Congestive heart failure
         Aortic stenosis
      2. Decreased cerebral blood flow resulting from decreased peripheral resistance in systemic circulation
         Syncope: orthostatic, vasovagal
         Carotid sinus hypersensitivity
         Low blood volume
      3. Decreased cerebral blood flow due to generalized increase in cerebrovascular resistance
         Hypertensive encephalopathy
         Hyperventilation syndrome
         Increased blood viscosity (polycythemia), cryo- and macroglobinemia
      4. Decreased local cerebral blood flow due to widespread small vessel occlusion
         Disseminated intravascular coagulation
         Systemic lupus erythematosus
         Subacute bacterial endocarditis
   *C. Hypoglycemia
      Resulting from exogenous insulin
      Spontaneous (endogenous insulin, liver disease, etc.)
   D. Cofactor deficiency
      Thiamin (Wernicke's encephalopathy)
      Niacin
      Pyridoxine
      B_{12}

II. Diseases of Organs Other than Brain
   *A. Diseases of nonendocrine organs
      Liver (hepatic coma)
      Kidney (uremic coma)
      Lung (CO_2 narcosis)
   *B. Hyper- and/or hypofunction of endocrine organs
      Pituitary
      Thyroid (myxedema-thyrotoxicosis)
      Parathyroid (hyper- and hypoparathyroidism)
      Adrenal (Addison's disease, Cushing's disease, pheochromocytoma)
      Pancreas (diabetes, hypoglycemia)
   C. Water and electrolyte imbalance
      Hypo-osmolality (water intoxication)
      Hyperosmolality (nonketotic diabetic coma)
      Hyper- and hypocalcemia

III. Exogenous Poisons
   *A. Sedative drugs
   B. Acid poisons or poisons with acidic breakdown products
      Paraldehyde
      Methyl alcohol
      Ethylene glycol
   C. Other enzyme inhibitors
      Heavy metals
      Organic phosphates
      Cyanide
      Salicylates
   D. Others
      Penicillin
      Anticonvulsants
      Steroids
      Cardiac glycosides

TABLE 1.   CAUSES OF METABOLIC BRAIN
DISEASE *(Continued)*

IV. Diseases Producing Toxins or Enzyme Inhibition in CNS
    A. Meningitis
    B. Encephalitis
    C. Subarachnoid hemorrhage

V. Abnormalities of Ionic or Acid Base Environment of CNS
    A. Water and sodium (hyper- and hyponatremia)
    B. Acidosis (metabolic and respiratory)
    C. Alkalosis (metabolic and respiratory)
    D. Potassium (hyper- and hypokalemia)
    E. Magnesium (hyper- and hypomagnesemia)
    F. Calcium (hyper- and hypocalcemia)

VI. Miscellaneous Diseases of Unknown Cause
    A. Sepsis
    B. Febrile states
    C. Seizures and postictal states
    D. "Postoperative" delirium
    E. Concussion

---

*Alone or in combination, the most common causes of delirium
seen on general medical wards.

logic changes can be identified if the process
causing delirium has lasted for some hours or days
prior to death. The pathologic changes are bilateral, symmetrical, and usually diffusely distributed
in the cerebral hemispheres. Lesions may be
present in the neurons, the glial cells, or the white
matter, depending on the nature of the primary
illness.

Perhaps the most common pathologic cerebral
changes are observed following anoxia, ischemia,
or hypoglycemia. The mildest abnormalities are
visible only microscopically and consist of swelling
of neurons of the cerebral cortex and hippocampus,
with dissolution of the Nissl granules (particles
of ribonucleic acid) and generalized pallor of
staining. Such changes are probably reversible.
After more severe insults, the nuclei shrink and
become hyperchromatic, and irregular basophilic
rings and granules appear in the swollen cytoplasm. These changes are not reversible. After
severe and prolonged insults, all neurons in the
cerebral cortex may disappear, and the third layer
of the cortex may completely degenerate so that
the naked eye detects a thin line of spongy necrosis
(laminar necrosis). Anoxic changes also affect the
basal ganglia to cause grossly visible focal necrosis
of the globus pallidus. Occasionally, there may be
diffuse demyelination of the subcortical white
matter. Characteristically, the brainstem and
spinal cord are spared unless the process has been
overwhelmingly severe.

Although the milder cell changes described
above are characteristic of deficiency of metabolic
substrate, they may be seen in patients with any
of the metabolic encephalopathies and are thus
nonspecific. Also nonspecific but common in
patients who have died with uremia, hyponatremia,
or CO_2 narcosis, is cerebral swelling, recognized
grossly by flattened gyri, obliterated sulci, and
small ventricles. The cut brain may appear either
"wet" or "dry," but, microscopically, large perivascular and perineuronal spaces attest to the
presence of edema.

Unusual glial cells with ballooned, lobulated

nuclei are found in the cortex and basal ganglia
of patients who die in hepatic coma, and are relatively specific for this disorder. Widespread perivascular "cuffs" of lymphocytes or polymorphonuclear leukocytes indicate an inflammatory
lesion of the brain and meninges from viral or
bacterial invasion.

BIOCHEMICAL ABNORMALITIES IN
METABOLIC BRAIN DISEASE

In all cases of metabolic brain disease, the
cerebral oxygen uptake declines in rough proportion to the degree of brain dysfunction as manifested clinically. So far, we understand in only a
few instances how systemic illnesses interfere with
cerebral oxidative metabolism, but these few serve
as models to suggest the possible mechanisms for
the others as well. The following material outlines
some of our knowledge of normal and abnormal
cerebral metabolism.

Glucose is the brain's only substrate under
physiologic conditions, and is transferred across
the blood-brain barrier by active or facilitated
transport. Other substances can serve as substrates of brain in vitro but do not cross the blood-
brain barrier rapidly enough to maintain metabolism in vivo. Under normal circumstances, each
100 grams of brain utilizes about 5.5 mg. of glucose per minute, which represents almost the
body's basal glucose consumption. Eighty-five per
cent of brain glucose uptake reacts with oxygen
to form CO_2, water, and energy; the pathway taken
by the remainder is presently unknown, although
some glucose metabolism may be accounted for
by lactic acid production even in the presence of
ample oxygen supplies. Under anaerobic conditions, lactic acid is the end product of glucose
metabolism, but the energy so produced is insufficient to maintain neuronal function. There
are about 2 grams of reserve glucose (as such and
as glycogen) in the brain, an amount that allows a
hypoglycemic patient to survive (although not to
function at a normal metabolic rate) for about
90 minutes without suffering irreversible damage.

Oxygen, the other substance vital for normal
cerebral function, is not stored by the brain, and
a mere six seconds of anoxia is sufficient to cause
coma. Four minutes of absolute anoxia irreversibly damages cortical neurons, and 15 to 20
minutes destroys virtually all nerve cells of the
brain, brainstem, and spinal cord. The normal
brain consumes about 3.3 ml. of oxygen per 100
grams per minute and produces an equal amount
of carbon dioxide (R.Q. = 1). Cerebral oxygen
consumption represents 15 to 20 per cent of the
total body oxygen consumption at rest and is
remarkably constant in normal man, whether
awake or sleeping. However, significant deviations
in oxygen consumption occur with brain dysfunction. Clinically, delirium usually accompanies
oxygen uptakes below 2.5 ml., and when the
uptake falls below 2.0 ml. per 100 grams per
minute, most patients are unconscious.

Blood brings both glucose and oxygen to the brain. Under resting conditions, the brain receives 55 ml. of blood each minute, about 15 per cent of the cardiac output. If the flow falls, the brain compensates by extracting more oxygen and more glucose from each volume of blood it receives. Increased extraction of oxygen maintains normal metabolism in the face of a decreased cerebral blood flow up to the point where so much oxygen has been extracted that the oxygen tension of the brain's venous blood falls to about 20 mm. of mercury (a level at which hemoglobin is about 35 per cent saturated). At this point, which is reached when cerebral blood flow falls to about half of normal, the oxygen tension of the cerebral tissues drops below 4 mm. of mercury, a value too low to maintain normal metabolism, and the patient loses consciousness.

In addition to glucose and oxygen, the brain requires *enzymes and cofactors* (vitamins and electrolytes) to maintain both oxidative metabolism and other systems that produce transmitter substances, preserve cellular structure, and maintain membrane potentials.

The above explains why deprivation of substrate should be an important cause of metabolic brain disease, and, indeed, hypoxia, ischemia, and hypoglycemia are the metabolic brain disorders in which the pathologic biochemistry is most clearly understood. Absence or inhibition of enzymes or cofactors might also be expected to interfere with cerebral metabolism, and these are the presumed mechanisms by which vitamin deficiency, electrolyte disturbances, and toxins produce brain dysfunction. The exact pathways that are disrupted or the exact substances that interfere with metabolism in toxic disorders, such as uremia and hepatic coma, are not known.

We have seen that the biochemical common denominator of metabolic brain disease is decreased oxygen uptake: Is there an anatomic common denominator? Two concepts have arisen delineating a principal locus of metabolic brain disease. One is that the neurons of the cerebral cortex are affected first and, as the process becomes more severe, subcortical structures are affected from the rostral end downward, the phylogenetically oldest and most caudal structures resisting most strongly. This view is supported by the pathologic distribution of cerebral anoxic and hypoglycemic changes and by physiologic studies of hypoglycemic animals in which abnormal electrical activity was recorded from the cortex before it appeared in the hypothalamus.

The second concept is that the neurons of the brainstem reticular formation are the most susceptible to metabolic change and, at least at first, the cortical neurons cease to function only because they lose their reticular stimulation. This concept is supported by physiologic experiments on animals, demonstrating that moderate degrees of hypoxia, hypoglycemia, anesthesia, and cyanide poisoning all block electrical conduction through the reticular formation before they block the ability of cortical neurons to receive messages via other afferent pathways (the lemniscal system).

Neither of these experimental concepts fully explains the several human disease states in which metabolic lesions clinically affect several different levels of the neuraxis simultaneously, the major locus of early dysfunction differing not only from patient to patient but sometimes from one attack to the next in the same patient. This phenomenon is exemplified by the varied picture of hypoglycemia: Some patients first suffer loss of consciousness and have bilaterally synchronous slow waves in the EEG, suggesting an initial reticular involvement. Others first experience restricted cerebral motor or sensory signs unaccompanied by either EEG abnormalities or impaired consciousness. Still other patients convulse with one attack of hypoglycemia but suffer only quiet coma in the next. It appears that in the clinical situation, regional cerebral factors such as blood flow and energy requirements must vary from moment to moment to predispose first one part of the brain and then another to metabolic insult.

CLINICAL FEATURES OF METABOLIC BRAIN DISEASE

Abnormalities in behavior, intellect, and orientation to the environment are the earliest manifestation of metabolic encephalopathy, and reflect the diffuse, nonfocal nature of the cerebral process. The range of symptoms is wide and extends from the one extreme of mild memory loss, with a minimal intellectual decline, through states of agitated hallucinating disorientation to the other extreme of unresponsive unconsciousness. Particularly prominent and sometimes characteristic abnormalities affect the respective functions of consciousness and behavior, motor activity, autonomic activity, and the electroencephalogram. A search for these changes deserves special effort.

State of Consciousness and Mental Content. Mental changes are the earliest and most subtle signs of metabolic brain disease. Altered awareness occurs first so that a previously interested person becomes less cognizant of his environment and appears preoccupied or bored. He lies quietly or sleeps when left alone and rarely reads or attends to the world around him. With more severe metabolic disturbances, patients become drowsy and finally stuporous or comatose. Disturbances in cognition appear along with the decreased alertness and awareness, and are revealed by an inability to handle specific problems, e.g., to subtract sevens or threes serially, to recall digits in forward and reverse direction, and to detect similarity between objects. Normal subjects readily subtract sevens serially from 100 to 0 in one minute, repeat 6 or 7 digits forward and 5 or 6 backward, and identify the common denominator between such pairs as an apple and an orange, a fly and a tree. However, innate intelligence and education also determine cognitive abilities and, unless the physician has examined the patient previously, it is difficult to attribute mild disturbances to a metabolic defect. An early sign of delirium, although usually not as early a sign as altered alertness and cognition, is impairment of memory and orientation. Loss of memory for recent events with relative preservation of remote memory is a hallmark of metabolic and other organic brain disease and is tested by asking the patient about the names of his doctors, some important current events, and his recent activities. Orientation to place and time should be specifically tested by asking the date and year, the day of the week, and the present location. Orientation for time is lost early in patients with delirium and orientation for place a little later.

Behavior is always abnormal in patients with metabolic brain disease, who may be either quiet, withdrawn, and apathetic or, conversely, anxious, agitated, tremulous, and hyperactive. The particular affect that prevails depends partly on the nature of the illness and partly on the rapidity of its development; previous personality often has surprisingly little influence. Thus, barbiturate- or alcohol-withdrawal syndromes, acute liver necrosis, and porphyria often cause an agitated delirium, whereas uremia, pulmonary encephalopathy, and anoxia usually produce a more quiet illness. Rapidly occurring metabolic processes are more likely to produce agitated delirium than those that develop slowly.

Perceptual errors, e.g., mistaking the physician for an old friend or family member, illusions, and hallucinations are common accompaniments of delirium. They frighten and agitate some patients, but are quietly tolerated by others. The nature of the illusions and hallucinations seems to be a property of the individual's personality, and often the same hallucinations accompany separate episodes of delirium. A quiet, withdrawn patient must be specifically asked about hallucinations since he often fails either to volunteer the information or to behave as if he is hallucinating.

Motor Activity. Tremor, asterixis, and multifocal myoclonus are the characteristic motor abnormalities of metabolic brain disease, and the specificity of the latter two makes them the most important physical signs that distinguish metabolic encephalopathy from psychiatric illness or from structural brain disease.

The *tremor* of delirious patients is coarse and irregular at a rate of about eight to ten per second. It is usually absent at complete rest. It is best seen in the fingers of the outstretched hands. It is less specific than asterixis and multifocal myoclonus, and may be seen in patients with psychiatric disease as well as systemic illness not associated with delirium.

Asterixis is an abnormal, involuntary jerking movement elicited in the hands by asking patients to dorsiflex the wrist and spread the extended fingers. In its mildest form there are irregular random lateral jerking movements of the fingers at the metacarpal phalangeal joints. With fully developed asterixis there is sudden palmar flexion of the fingers at the metacarpal phalangeal joint and of the wrist. The movements are asynchronous in the two hands, occur every 2 to 30 seconds, recover quickly, and cannot be controlled by the patient, even when he is aware of their presence. Asterixis may also involve the feet and tongue. In the lightly unconscious patient the same movement can sometimes be evoked by passively dorsiflexing the wrist. Bilateral asterixis almost universally accompanies metabolic encephalopathy at some stage of the illness. It is absent in patients with psychiatric disorders unless they are taking large amounts of drugs, and is encountered extremely rarely, and then unilaterally, in patients with gross structural brain disease such as decompensating subdural hematoma or deep hemispheral infarcts encroaching on the diencephalon.

Multifocal myoclonus consists of sudden nonrhythmic, nonpatterned gross muscle contractions in a resting person. The movements are most common in the face and shoulders but occur anywhere in the body. Multifocal myoclonus can often be elicited, if not present at rest, by passive movements of the shoulder and upper arm. It occurs in a later and more severe stage of metabolic illness than does asterixis, and may physiologically represent a more intense and widespread manifestation of that abnormal movement. Multifocal myoclonus makes its most frequent appearance in uremia, hypercarbic-anoxic encephalopathy, and penicillin overdose, but can occur in virtually all metabolic encephalopathies.

Seizures, weakness, and *hyperactive stretch reflexes* frequently accompany severe metabolic brain disease. The seizures are usually generalized, and the motor abnormalities are usually symmetrical. Focal paresis and focal seizures are by no means rare, however, especially with anoxia or hypoglycemia. Signs of focal disturbance make it more difficult to distinguish between metabolic and structural brain disease. However, in metabolic brain disease the focal signs are usually less severe and more fleeting, and they are accompanied by more widespread neurologic dysfunction than in gross structural disease.

Autonomic Activity. Pupillary light reactions are always preserved in metabolic coma with the few exceptions to be mentioned, and absence of the pupillary light reaction strongly suggests a structural lesion. The exceptions are glutethimide intoxication, which may produce mid-position or slightly dilated fixed pupils; anticholinergic drug administration, which produces fixed, dilated pupils; and exposure to severe anoxia, or asphyxia, which produces fixed dilated pupils and, if sustained, probably implies irreversible brain damage.

Hypothermia is common in delirious patients with myxedema, hypoglycemia, and barbiturate intoxication. Hyperthermia with profuse perspiration and tachycardia accompanies most agitated deliria and is especially common with delirium tremens. Hyperthermia without perspiration suggests anticholinergic drug ingestion or infection. Hyperthermia also marks salicylate and occasionally phenothiazine overdosage.

Ventilation. The clinical features of delirium that have been described are common to many metabolic disorders and aid little in the differential diagnosis of specific types of metabolic coma. Ventilation is an exception. A rapid evaluation of the patient's ventilatory status, coupled with an estimate of blood acid-base balance, frequently narrows the range of possible causes of metabolic coma. Some causes of metabolic brain disease associated with ventilatory abnormalities are listed in Table 2. A careful clinical examination of the respiratory rate and depth usually allows the physician to estimate whether his patient is hyperventilating, eupneic, or hypoventilating.

Caution must be exercised in evaluating patients with severe emphysema whose respiratory effort is increased and who may be tachypneic but nevertheless hypoventilating because of ineffective lungs. Caution must also be used in evaluating patients poisoned with depressant drugs who appear to be hypoventilating but are actually eupneic because their metabolic needs are so low. Unexplained abnormalities in the respiratory pattern demand rapid determination of blood gas and acid-base status, preferably by pH, Pco_2 and Po_2 measurements but, if these are unavailable, by serum bicarbonate determination. As may be seen in Table 2, a delirious and clinically *hyperventilating* adult with a low serum pH or a bicarbonate below 10 mEq. per liter probably has dia-

TABLE 2. A DIFFERENTIAL ANALYSIS OF HYPERVENTILATION AND HYPOVENTILATION IN DELIRIOUS PATIENTS

Clinical and Laboratory Findings	Probable Diagnosis
I. Hyperventilation:	
A. Metabolic acidosis	
(arterial pH < 7.30, Pco_2 < 35, HCO_3^- < 10 mEq. per liter)	
1. BUN > 60 mg. per 100 ml.	Uremic encephalopathy
2. Hyperglycemia (blood sugar > 250 mg. per 100 ml.)	Diabetic coma
a. 4+ Serum acetone	Diabetic ketoacidosis
b. No acetonemia	Diabetic lactic acidosis
3. Cyanosis (Po_2 < 50 mm. Hg) – shock	Anoxic lactic acidosis
4. History: diarrhea; hyperchloremia, ± hypokalemia	Diarrheal acidosis
5. Hyponatremia, hyperkalemia, ± hypoglycemia	Addison's disease
6. BUN, sugar, oxygen, blood pressure – normal	Exogenous poisoning
a. Paraldehyde odor on breath	Acidosis secondary to paraldehyde ingestion
b. Hyperemic optic discs, dilated sluggish pupils	Methyl alcohol poisoning
c. Oxalate crystals in urine	Ethylene glycol poisoning
7. None of the abnormal findings above	Spontaneous lactic acidosis
B. Respiratory alkalosis	
(arterial pH > 7.45, Pco_2 < 35, HCO_3^- > 15 mEq. per liter)	
1. Po_2 > 50, hepatomegaly, serum NH_3 elevated	Hepatic encephalopathy
2. Po_2 < 50, cyanosis	Cardiopulmonary disease
a. Rales, elevated venous pressure, cardiomegaly	Pulmonary edema
b. No heart disease	Pneumonia, alveolar-capillary block, pulmonary emboli
3. Absent pupillary and oculovestibular responses, decerebrate rigidity	Central neurogenic hyperventilation
4. Nystagmus on caloric testing, normal examination	Psychogenic hyperventilation
C. Mixed respiratory alkalosis and metabolic acidosis	
(arterial pH > 7.35, Pco_2 < 35, HCO_3^- < 15 mEq. per liter)	
1. Fever, tachycardia, hypotension	Gram-negative sepsis
2. Hyperthermia, positive urine $FeCl_3$ test	Salicylate poisoning
II. Hypoventilation:	
A. Respiratory acidosis	
(arterial pH < 7.30, Pco_2 > 45, HCO_3^- > 20 mEq. per liter)	
1. Serum HCO_3^- > 20 mEq. per liter but < 30 mEq. per liter	
a. Normal lungs	Depressant drug poisoning
b. Rales, emphysema, Po_2 < 40 mm. Hg	Chronic pulmonary disease with acute CO_2 retention
2. Serum HCO_3^- > 35 mEq. per liter	
a. Normal lungs	
(1) Obesity	Pickwickian syndrome
(2) Not obese	"Central alveolar hypoventilation"
b. Rales, emphysema, Po_2 < 40 mm. Hg	Chronic pulmonary disease with slowly developing CO_2 retention
B. Metabolic alkalosis	
(arterial pH > 7.45, Pco_2 < 55, HCO_3^- > 35 mEq. per liter)	
a. Alkali ingestion	
History of peptic ulcer	$NaHCO_3$ ingestion alkalosis
b. Gastric acid losses	
Vomiting, hypotension, hypovolemia	Gastric HCl depletion
c. Renal acid losses	
(1) Edema, heart disease	Diuretic therapy
(2) Hypokalemia, moon face, truncal obesity	Cushing's syndrome secondary to adrenal hyperfunction, steroid therapy, hormone-secreting lung neoplasms
(3) Hypertension, hypokalemia	Primary hyperaldosteronism

betic ketosis, uremia, lactic acidosis, or poisoning with an acidic product. Severe metabolic acidosis, if not treated, is rapidly lethal. Diabetes, uremia, and Addison's disease can be treated specifically (see Diabetes Mellitus, Chronic Renal Insufficiency, Uremia, and Acute Adrenal Insufficiency), and the others often respond to prompt and urgent treatment of the acidosis by infusion of bicarbonate. If, however, the serum pH is elevated in the delirious and hyperventilating adult or the bicarbonate is normal, pulmonary disease, cardiac disease, hepatic coma, or neurogenic hyperventilation are the possible causes. Pneumonia is probably the most common cause of mild respiratory alkalosis in unconscious patients; the others can be evaluated by appropriate laboratory tests. When the serum pH is elevated and the bicarbonate is between 10 and 15 mEq. per liter (mixed respiratory alkalosis and metabolic acidosis), sepsis, especially with gram-negative organisms, salicylism (which causes acidosis in children, alkalosis in adults), and severe hepatic coma are the probable causes.

A similar analysis can be applied to *hypoventilating* patients. In these, the severe problems are depressant drug poisoning, which produces a low serum pH with a normal bicarbonate, and chronic pulmonary failure, which produces a low serum pH and usually a high serum bicarbonate. (The serum bicarbonate level indicates the duration of hypoventilation.) Both situations demand ventilatory support.

Electroencephalogram (EEG). The EEG is useful in evaluating patients with metabolic brain disease because it is slower than in normal subjects and because it is symmetrical. The slowing indicates that there is neural dysfunction, and the bilateral symmetry suggests a diffuse process. The degree of slowing roughly parallels the severity of the encephalopathy. The normal EEG has a basic frequency of 8 to 13 per second. In metabolic disease, bilateral, synchronous, paroxysmal bursts of 1 to 3 per second activity are frequently superimposed upon a background of mildly slow 5 to 7 cps activity. A normal EEG is incompatible with severe delirium, and an EEG with focal or unilateral slow activity strongly suggests a structural and not a metabolic brain disorder.

DIAGNOSIS OF METABOLIC ENCEPHALOPATHY

Delirium due to metabolic encephalopathy is neither a difficult nor a rare diagnosis, yet the variety of its forms and the anxieties and resentments it induces in its witnesses often invite diagnostic errors or delays. Errors usually arise with two types of patients. One is the fearful, uncooperative, combative person who thrashes about in bed and either cries for help or shouts loud, obscene, or plaintive imprecations, meanwhile resisting or actually striking out at all who try to help him. It takes a remarkably clear clinical head to resist meeting such obstreperousness

immediately with sedation and incarceration and to consider that grave metabolic disease may be the cause, not just "schizophrenia," "hysteria," or plain "cussedness." Parenthetically, such unfortunate patients often inadvertently abet the misdiagnosis by expressing fears of "going crazy," a frequent delusion of metabolic brain disease. The other frequent error occurs in the unconscious patient with metabolic encephalopathy who receives trephination or cerebral roentgenographic contrast studies before metabolic coma is considered, and before such simple tests are carried out as a blood sugar, a serum sodium determination, or a toxicologic analysis. With both types of error, the delay can be fatal.

The physician should consider metabolic encephalopathy as the possible diagnosis for every patient whose thinking, behavior, or state of consciousness has recently become disordered. The diagnosis requires, first, that one establish that metabolic encephalopathy rather than psychiatric disease or a structural brain lesion is causing the abnormal behavior and, second, that one identify the specific metabolic illness responsible.

Psychiatric disease is distinguished in the awake patient by examination of the mental status and the motor function. Occasionally, patients with psychogenic amnesia are disoriented, but will also claim to be confused about who they are as well as to the place and time; patients with metabolic brain disorders are lethargic and disoriented, but know who they are. Hallucinations in psychiatric illness are usually auditory; in metabolic illness they are usually visual. Recent memory and cognitive abilities are generally preserved in psychiatric patients but are lost early in patients with metabolic illness. Tremor plagues anxious patients, and occasionally generalized seizures wrack those with catatonic schizophrenia, but asterixis and multifocal myoclonus are never present in psychiatric disease. Asterixis, if carefully searched for, is present in most patients with metabolic brain disease. Rarely, a patient with "hysterical coma" will present a diagnostic problem. Such patients are quietly unresponsive, and all their limbs are flaccid, but they often strongly resist passive eye opening. If the diagnosis is doubtful, irrigating the tympanum with 50 ml. of cold water is informative; this procedure produces nystagmus in the patient with "hysterical coma," but only tonic eye deviation in the comatose patient with metabolic disease. The EEG in "hysterical coma" shows a normal awake record; it is always abnormal in metabolic coma.

Supratentorial mass lesions that encroach on the diencephalon produce diffuse brain dysfunction (see article on Brain Function and Consciousness). However, supratentorial lesions produce focal motor and/or sensory signs early in the illness, often before mental changes, and these focal signs either persist or grow worse. Hemiparesis or hemisensory defects, although occasionally present in metabolic disease, are usually mild, often fleeting, and generally appear only after consciousness is lost. Late in the course of mass lesions, when transtentorial herniation has impaired midbrain function, bilateral decorticate or decerebrate rigidity usually replaces unilateral motor signs. These motor signs of midbrain dysfunction may also be present in metabolic coma, but in metabolic coma the pupillary light reflexes are retained, thereby ruling out a structural lesion. The EEG of a patient with a supratentorial mass lesion is usually slow either focally in one area or laterally over one hemisphere; that of a patient with metabolic brain disease, even when focal neurologic abnormalities are present, is symmetrically slow. Skull roentgenograms of patients with structural lesions reveal shift of the pineal gland (if calcified) away from the side of the mass, but the pineal is midline in metabolic disease. Injection of radiopaque dye into the carotid artery (cerebral arteriography) outlines the vascular pattern of that hemisphere and reveals displacement of cerebral vessels from their normal positions if a supratentorial lesion is large enough to interfere with consciousness.

Subtentorial structural lesions are distinguished from metabolic brain disease by the presence in the former of signs of cranial nerve and focal brainstem dysfunction. In patients with subtentorial lesions causing changes in consciousness, the pupils are almost always abnormal, either because pontine and medullary sympathetic pathways are involved or because the third nerve nuclei or fibers are destroyed. Both pupillary light reflexes and the ciliospinal reflex (pupillary dilatation to noxious cutaneous stimuli) are preserved in metabolic disease. Dysconjugate eye movements are common with subtentorial lesions, rare with metabolic disease. Unilateral facial weakness involving both the brow and lower face, unilateral facial anesthesia, absent caloric responses to one side, or eye deviation toward a paralyzed arm and leg all suggest a subtentorial lesion and are against the diagnosis of metabolic disease.

Dementia, as defined here, is really the expression of irreversible metabolic brain disease in which the primary metabolic error resides in the brain rather than affects the brain secondarily. For this reason, the incipient signs of dementia closely resemble certain forms of delirium, and distinction may sometimes be difficult. In general, dementia begins gradually, whereas delirium begins either acutely or subacutely. Recent memory loss, cognitive difficulties, and disorientation to place occur early in dementia and precede any change in consciousness, whereas lethargy, apathy, decreased awareness, and disorientation in time are early marks of delirium. Tremor, asterixis, and myoclonus are rare in dementia (except myoclonus in Jakob-Creutzfeldt disease). Mild or moderate dementia reduces the brain's defenses against metabolic insults, and thus it is common for a fully reversible delirium to complicate mild systemic illnesses in demented patients. In these cases only treatment of the systemic

disorders will separate the delirious component from the dementia (see Dementia).

Differential Diagnosis. Delirium means that a metabolic illness is so advanced that it not only threatens brain function but may threaten life itself unless promptly diagnosed and reversed by treatment. Since the neurologic manifestations of the various metabolic encephalopathies are often similar, specific diagnosis by physical examination is often impossible, so some systematic approach to the problem is needed.

In Table 1 are listed all of the common and many of the less frequent causes of metabolic brain disease. Those marked with an asterisk either alone or in combination account for most of the delirium encountered on general medical wards. The table is designed as a checklist; the specific symptoms, signs, and management of each of the systemic disorders causing delirium can be found elsewhere in this book.

When the cause of delirium is unclear, the first conditions to consider are *hypoxia, hypoglycemia,* and *metabolic acidosis.* Unless promptly treated, all three are potentially rapidly lethal, and the first two very quickly damage the brain irreversibly.

Hypoxia. A diagnosis of severe hypoxic delirium is easily made if the patient is still anoxic when seen by the physician. Cyanosis, shock, and skin pallor (anemia), or the characteristic cherry red color that carbon monoxyhemoglobin imparts to the skin, suggest hypoxia severe enough to cause delirium. An arterial blood oxygen tension below 40 mm. of mercury, a hemoglobin less than 70 per cent saturated with oxygen, or severe anemia (hemoglobin less than 7 grams) supports the diagnosis. If the hypoxia is no longer present but the patient remains delirious from its effects, the diagnosis can only be inferred from a careful history.

Hypoglycemia. Hypoglycemic encephalopathy may be a particularly difficult diagnosis because the clinical picture is so variable. Focal motor weakness, seizures, agitated delirium, or simply coma with decerebrate rigidity and reactive pupils may predominate. If the patient is a diabetic receiving insulin, the diagnosis of hypoglycemia is immediately suggested, but if no history is available, a confident clinical diagnosis is sometimes almost impossible because there are no physical or neurologic signs that specifically indicate hypoglycemia. Therefore, to prevent irreversible hypoglycemic brain damage, after blood for glucose determination is drawn, 50 ml. of 50 per cent dextrose should be injected intravenously; this should be done for every delirious patient in whom the cause is unknown. Even though immediate awakening may not follow profound hypoglycemia, further glucose treatment can safely await the laboratory report of the blood sugar.

Metabolic Acidosis. Hyperpnea suggests severe metabolic acidosis, a diagnosis that is confirmed by laboratory testing. The specific causes and steps in laboratory diagnosis of metabolic acidosis are listed in Table 2.

Certain physical signs, such as respiratory abnormalities, convulsions, and fever, suggest specific diagnoses. The examination of respiration aids in the diagnosis of pulmonary encephalopathy, sedative drug poisoning, gram-negative sepsis, and hepatic coma (Table 2). Often an early clue to the diagnosis of hepatic coma is the presence of respiratory alkalosis, which then prompts liver function tests or a blood ammonia determination to support the diagnosis. *Generalized convulsions* occur in many metabolic brain disorders, especially with hypoxia and hypoglycemia. Repeated seizures are dangerous since they create the risk of brain damage and should be treated even before their cause is clear. If hypoxia and hypoglycemia are not the cause, repeated seizures suggest sedative drug withdrawal, uremia, hyponatremia, or hypocalcemia.

Agitated delirium accompanied by fever prompts immediate consideration of intracranial infection. Often the patient with meningitis is so combative that nuchal rigidity cannot adequately be assessed, and only lumbar puncture confirms the diagnosis. A lumbar puncture should be performed on any patient who is delirious without obvious cause and who lacks evidence of sustained increased intracranial pressure. Encephalitis and subarachnoid hemorrhage often present initially with delirium accompanied by little or no fever and no nuchal rigidity, and may not be diagnosed unless the cerebrospinal fluid is examined. In any delirious patient with nystagmus or ocular palsies, thiamin deficiency encephalopathy (see Nutritional Disorders of the Nervous System) should be immediately considered because if this condition is untreated, cardiovascular collapse and death may follow.

Once the dangerous and potentially lethal illnesses detailed above are excluded, there is time to consider the many other causes of metabolic brain disease and to make the tests appropriate to their diagnosis. Often no single metabolic abnormality is severe enough to be held responsible for delirium; especially in elderly patients, a combination of minor insults may be responsible. A common example of this occurs with the decreased cardiac output of mild heart failure: mild cerebral anoxia, plus sedative drugs, plus a moderate electrolyte imbalance induced by diuretics become more than the aging brain can tolerate, and delirium results.

PROGNOSIS AND TREATMENT OF METABOLIC BRAIN DISEASE

Metabolic brain disease can be definitively treated only by correcting the systemic disorder responsible for the delirium, and the effectiveness of this correction, in turn, determines the prognosis of the delirium. With the exception of severe hypoxia, hypoglycemia, or thiamin deficiency, all of which can cause neuronal death, delirium clears as the systemic disorder causing it improves. Often, however, the encephalopathy improves much more slowly than the systemic illness so that severe encephalopathy may persist four to five days or more after the systemic disorder has been fully reversed. Such a delay need not portend an unfavorable outcome, and vigorous efforts to prevent infections and other complications of delirium and coma are indicated during this period, for full recovery of cerebral function still is possible.

Certain general therapeutic measures apply to all delirious patients. The awake, delirious patient should, preferably, be kept in a quiet room, away from the noise and bustle of the general ward. The room should be well lighted, and a light should be kept burning at night, since darkness accentuates disorientation and hallucinations. Physicians and nurses can reassure the patient by introducing themselves at each contact and quietly apprising him of his whereabouts. All procedures must be carefully and often repetitively explained before they are done. Drugs not essential for treatment of the patient's systemic illness should be withdrawn. This applies particularly to sedatives, narcotics, and tranquilizers, all of which commonly cause or accentuate delirium; it also applies to extensive use of diuretics, antihypertensive drugs, anticonvulsants, and even digitalis, medications that are less widely recognized to cause or accentuate delirium. If the patient is agitated and hyperactive, small doses of paraldehyde (5 to 10 ml. orally) or chlordiazepoxide (starting with 10 to 25 mg. orally or parenterally and increasing if necessary to 50 to 100 mg.) can be given to quiet him but not to render him unresponsive.

Careful attention is required to other systemic disorders that, although not of themselves sufficiently severe to cause delirium, may increase an already present encephalopathy. Oxygen should be given to mildly hypoxic patients, and transfusions should be administered to those with significant anemia. Mild electrolyte disorders such as hypokalemia and hyponatremia are diagnosed by periodic serum electrolyte determinations and are corrected by appropriate fluid control. Such measures often improve a patient's delirium considerably, even if the primary cause cannot be treated. Fluid losses should be routinely measured and replaced parenterally if the patient is not eating. Vital signs and the state of consciousness must be checked frequently to ensure that sudden worsening does not go undetected.

Engel, G. L., and Romano, J.: Delirium, a syndrome of cerebral insufficiency. J. Chronic Dis., 9:260, 1959.

Plum, F., and Posner, J. B.: The Diagnosis of Stupor and Coma. Philadelphia, F. A. Davis Company, 1966.

Sokoloff, L.: Metabolism of the central nervous system in vivo. *In* Field, J., Magoun, H. W., and Hall, V. E. (eds.): Handbook of Physiology. Section I: Neurophysiology. Washington, D.C., American Physiological Society, 1960, Vol. 3, Chap. 77, pp. 1843-1864.

SLEEP AND ITS DISORDERS
Fred Plum

DEFINITION

Adult man spends one third of each day asleep. Yet why he sleeps and what "rest" does for his tissues are questions for which we have no answer so far.

Sleep is a recurrent state of relative inactivity of mind and body movement, readily interrupted by external stimuli but largely preventing any awareness of self or environment while it exists. The mere physiologic ability to cycle in and out of sleep requires relatively little brain, although the amount of brain present modifies the cyclic pattern. Newborn babies, in whom the cerebral hemispheres are still little developed, sleep two thirds of each 24 hours in a series of cycles interrupted by several brief awakenings; anencephalic infants, whose brain stops at the midbrain, tend to do the same, as do adults who have been decorticated by injury. Paralleling the evolving functional development of the hemispheres in older children, periods of continuous wakefulness become longer and longer until at about the age of six the adult diurnal pattern of sleep is established. Children up to about the age of 13 sleep more than adults, and women sleep more than men. Data reviewed by Kleitman indicate a mean duration of sleep in healthy adults of about eight hours, with little difference among subjects of different ethnic groups, occupations, or intelligence.

THE PHYSIOLOGY OF SLEEP

Just what puts a man to sleep or wakens him again spontaneously after a fairly regular number of hours is unknown. For many years, workers have unsuccessfully sought metabolic sleep-inducing products of fatigue; nor have they found reproducible biochemical differences that distinguish sleep-deprived subjects from those fully refreshed. During the earlier part of the century, Piéron, a French worker, believed he had found a substance in the blood or cerebrospinal fluid of fatigued animals that induced sleep in others, and Pappenheimer et al. have reported somewhat similar results. One thing is clear, however: Sleep and coma are clearly different metabolically, since cerebral oxygen metabolism is always depressed with coma or anesthesia but remains equivalent to waking levels during natural sleep.

The anatomy of the reticular formation of the brainstem and its close interrelationship with the cerebral cortex have been discussed above under the subjects of consciousness and coma. When the important effects of the ascending reticular formation on arousal and wakefulness were first discovered, it was widely assumed that sleep was largely a passive phenomenon associated with reticular inactivity. More recently, however, sleep has been found to be associated with increased rather than decreased activity in certain reticular neurons. Recent work demonstrates that distinct areas in the hypothalamus, midbrain, anterior pons, posterior pons, and medulla influence various stages of sleep and are closely related to the associated changes in the electroencephalogram (EEG).

Sleep is marked by four stages. As normal subjects drift off, the normal 9 to 12 per second alpha rhythm of the EEG at first slows, then gives way to a lower-voltage, desynchronized, faster rhythm. This is *stage 1*. Within a few minutes, *stage 2* appears: The EEG slows again, its voltage increases, and quick, spindle-like bursts appear. The eyes may rove slowly and the subject is unmistakably, although still lightly, asleep. As sleep continues, it deepens into *stage 3*, in which large, one-per-second waves develop in the EEG. The muscles relax, the heart slows, and the blood pressure and temperature begin to decline. Subjects in stage 3 are largely unaffected by randomly occurring sensory stimuli and, if left alone, gradually sink into *stage 4*, from which they can be externally aroused only by vigorous stimulation. In stage 4, the EEG is continuously slow, and it is during this deep, insensate phase that somnambulism and bedwetting occur.

During a night's natural sleep, subjects drift up from the deepest stages approximately every 90 minutes to re-enter a stage that, on the EEG, looks like the low-voltage desynchronized activity of stage 1. The eyes move rapidly about (this stage has been called rapid eye movement, or REM, sleep), the respiration, pulse, and blood pressure quicken, and it is during this phase that most dreaming occurs. Paradoxically, instead of being easy to arouse as are subjects in stage 1 just going to sleep, those in subsequent stage 1 can be as difficult or more difficult to awaken than in stage 4. Presently, on the basis of experiments in animals, the REM, or "activated sleep," as it is sometimes called, is believed to be regulated by neural structures lying in the caudal pons. The close relationships between stage 1 sleep, dreaming, and autonomic activity have made it a subject of intense scrutiny by behavioral scientists who hope that within its physiology may lie some answers to the frequent, but unexplained, association of sleep disturbances and mental disorders.

DISORDERS OF THE QUALITY OF SLEEP

Too little sleep is known as *insomnia* or hyposomnia, and too much as *hypersomnia*. Insomnia most frequently results from something other than structural disease of the nervous system, whereas hypersomnia is often, but not invariably, a sign of organic neurologic disease.

Insomnia. Insomnia has three patterns: difficulty in falling asleep after retiring, intermittent waking throughout the period of attempted sleep, and early awakening. Direct observations on patients suffering from insomnia almost always reveal that they are less wakeful than they think, and there is little evidence that chronic insomnia takes any physical toll. Nevertheless, even brief difficulties in falling or staying asleep cause great subjective distress and lead to a large annual consumption of sedatives in the United States.

Physical causes of insomnia are comparatively few. Patients with chronic pain often suffer more at night, which keeps them awake. Those with unrecognized orthopnea due to heart disease sometimes translate their difficulties into a primary complaint of sleeplessness; the same is true of patients with marginal pulmonary insufficiency, in whom inability to sleep may be the first sign of respiratory decompensation. Insomnia can be an early symptom of acute infectious illness and is common in Sydenham's chorea and in bulbar poliomyelitis. Aside from these occasional associations with physical illness, difficulty in sleeping results mainly from the self-stimulation engendered by anxiety, worry, or depression. Early morning awakening has sometimes been said to be typical of depression, but this rule is undependable. The pattern of insomnia helps relatively little in estimating its seriousness as a symptom.

To treat insomnia requires understanding, patience, a close attention to its accompaniments, and a willingness to discuss psychologic issues. Patients with difficulty in sleeping should be advised to eat light evening meals and to avoid stimulants such as coffee or tea after midday. Early morning awakening in the elderly most frequently reflects a declining need for sleep, and is best met by having the subject plan his day better and avoid afternoon naps. All patients are reassured by knowing that sleeplessness will not harm their bodies, and many regain the ability to sleep after a sympathetic physician has taken the time to discuss with them the issues that keep them awake. Patients with insomnia should always be asked sympathetically but directly if they are depressed and particularly if they have considered suicide. Drugs to treat insomnia should be used sparingly. All sedatives are potentially addicting, and most subjects with severe insomnia rapidly tolerate the soporific effects of these agents. Alcoholic nightcaps are not particularly advisable; the sedative effect is moderate and the temptation to "drown" anxiety is great. Secobarbital or pentobarbital sodium are effective mild sedatives in doses of either 50 or 100 mg. For agitated patients a combination of chlordiazepoxide HCl, 10 mg., plus chloral hydrate, 1 to 1.5 grams, is generally satisfactory. When insomnia is associated with mild depression, amitriptyline, 25 to 100 mg., is useful; the entire dose should be given at bedtime, starting at the lower dose and increasing. Insomnia coupled with more severe symptoms of depression demands close supervision and skilled psychologic management.

Hypersomnia. Hypersomnia occasionally signifies nothing more serious than boredom and mild depression, particularly among adolescents and young adults. Young women sometimes develop transient hypersomnia during menstruation. Occasionally one encounters hysterical hypersomnia, with which patients may claim to sleep for days at a time, then awaken fully. More often, however, excessive sleepiness signifies either narcolepsy or structural nervous system disease; among patients with the latter, the dividing line between prolonged hypersomnia and coma may be difficult to establish. Many neurologic conditions prolong or excessively deepen sleep. These include increased intracranial pressure, neoplasms around the third ventricle or in the posterior fossa, head trauma, encephalitis, and many metabolic disorders, including carbon dioxide retention, hepatic encephalopathy, uremia, pituitary insufficiency, and the surreptitious taking of drugs. With so many potential causes, the approach to hypersomnia of unknown cause resembles that employed to evaluate undiagnosed coma.

A rare condition of recurrent hypersomnia combined with excessive eating is sometimes observed in adolescent males, and is known as the *Kleine-Levin syndrome*. The cause is unknown, but the attacks last several days to a week or more, during which the patient eats voraciously and often develops disturbed behavior. Intervals of months to years of normal behavior separate the attacks. There is no treatment, and the attacks tend to disappear as the patient reaches adulthood.

Narcolepsy. *Definition and Etiology.* Narcolepsy is a chronic disorder characterized by recurrent and excessive drowsiness or sleepiness from which subjects are readily awakened. It is frequently accompanied by cataplexy, sleep paralysis, and, less often, hypnagogic hallucinations. Some workers divide narcolepsy into primary and secondary forms, the latter representing symptomatic hypersomnia from structural lesions. In this text, the term narcolepsy is reserved for the primary syndrome because the symptoms of the idiopathic disorder are so consistent from one case to the next. As with most illnesses of unknown origin, many causes have been suggested. Some observers postulate a defect in the reticular formation of the brainstem, particularly since the REM stage tends to appear at the onset of narcoleptic sleep rather than approximately 90 minutes later, as with normal sleep. Other workers have been struck with the high incidence of psychologic disturbances (about 10 per cent of narcoleptics go on to develop schizophrenic reactions), and have tended to regard this as the cause rather than an associated symptom of the illness. A high familial incidence of narcolepsy has been invoked as indirect evidence that the syndrome has a constitutional basis.

Clinical Findings. Narcolepsy is uncommon but not rare. Both men and women are affected, and there appears to be no ethnic predilection. The onset is usually insidious during adolescence or young adulthood. Once the predisposition to excessive sleepiness starts, it is likely to last a lifetime if not treated. The symptoms range from mild drowsiness, which marks itself as abnormal only because it intrudes upon lecture hours, social events, or after-dinner conversations, to severe sleepiness in which subjects spend nearly the entire day drifting in and out of sleep, unable to work, play, or supervise the home. The sensation is reported as ordinary, uncontrollable drowsiness, perhaps with diplopia, but indistinguishable from that which normally follows severe fatigue. As witnessed by others, the sleep looks natural and is readily interrupted by stimuli. The naps refresh, but only briefly, and somnolence quickly recurs.

Cataplexy affects about three quarters of narcoleptic patients and consists of abrupt muscular weakness associated with emotion. In general, the stronger the emotion the greater the muscular paresis, and patients relate that laughter, anger, or surprise "turns them to jelly" and induces collapse or aphonia without impaired consciousness. *Sleep paralysis* is a sensation of being unable to move while drifting into sleep or, less often, just upon awakening. Usually, brief contact with another person or strong effort interrupts the sensation, which lasts only a few seconds anyway. *Hypnagogic hallucinations* principally coincide with the early drifting phase of sleep when sleep paralysis occurs. Their intensity, the completeness of the visual or auditory recollections, and the time of onset distinguish them from dreams.

Physical abnormalities are lacking in primary narcolepsy. Laboratory studies are similarly normal. Neither hypothyroidism, hypoglycemia, nor any other endocrine abnormality has been substantiated in these patients, although the basal metabolic rate is low in many, reflecting their tendency to sleep through the test. The blood gases, and particularly the arterial carbon dioxide tension, are normal if obtained while the subject is awake, and no higher than in sleeping normal persons if drawn during drowsiness. The EEG contains normal patterns but a high percentage of sleep frequencies.

Differential Diagnosis. Narcolepsy must be distinguished from psychogenic hypersomnia on the one hand, and occult central nervous system lesions on the other. Narcoleptic-cataplectic symptoms are intensifications of experiences known in a minor way to nearly everybody, and the exact point where excessive drowsiness, weakness during emotion, and sleep paralysis become a syndrome rather than a psychologic reaction to the environment can be difficult to decide. Narcolepsy is favored if the symptoms date back to adolescence or have been present for several years, if the drowsiness appears as a primary complaint interfering with other activities, and if other members of the family have similar difficulties.

Hypersomnia caused by central nervous system lesions usually resembles narcolepsy very little. Its onset is generally recent and fairly sharply identified in time. Also, the sleep is commonly deep, arousal is difficult, and the patients are slow and apathetic when awake in contrast to narcoleptic patients, who are alert as long as stimulated into wakefulness. Brain lesions causing hypersomnia often produce dementia and headache, neither of which complicates primary narcolepsy. Finally, structural brain lesions causing hypersomnia usually either are large or are situated near the deep midline structures of the third ventricle, and in both cases almost always result in oculomotor, skeletal motor, or sensory changes in the physical examination. In doubtful cases, lumbar puncture should be obtained as well as an electroencephalogram, which is almost always abnormal when a structural lesion produces hypersomnia.

Treatment. The treatment of narcolepsy is symptomatic and consists of stimulants. General measures include drinking coffee or tea with meals and otherwise increasing everyday stimuli to a maximum. Most patients can continue to drive automobiles, for enough warning is experienced for them to pull off the road to sleep. Narcolepsy has no relation to epilepsy, and anticonvulsants have no place in treatment. Many individual stimulants have been tried, ephedrine, dextroamphetamine (Dexedrine), and methyl phenidate (Ritalin) being most successful. Ephedrine cannot usually be tolerated comfortably in doses greater than 25 mg. four times daily and must be supplemented by another stimulant. Dextroamphetamine is usually initiated with doses of 10 mg. three times daily. If patients require much larger doses, slow-release capsules yield sustained effects. Methyl phenidate is the present drug of choice and is initiated in doses of 5 to 10 mg. three times daily, then gradually increased until it either relieves drowsiness or produces unwanted nervousness and irritability. All these drugs cause anorexia, and subjects must prevent weight loss by making conscious efforts to eat. Serious blood dyscrasias have not been reported. Occasionally the drugs produce excessive excitement or disturbed behavior, and must be discontinued.

Critchley, M.: Periodic hypersomnia and megaphagia in adolescent males. Brain, 62:627, 1962.

Kety, S. S., Evarts, E. V., and Williams, H. L. (eds.): Sleep and Altered States of Consciousness. Res. Publ. Ass. Res. Nerv. Ment. Dis., Vol. 55, 1967.

Kleitman, N.: Sleep and Wakefulness (revised and enlarged edition). Chicago, University of Chicago Press, 1963.

Moruzzi, G.: Active processes in the brain stem during sleeping. Harvey Lecture Series, 58:233, 1963.

Pappenheimer, J. R., Miller, T. B., and Goodrich, C. A.: Sleep-promoting effects of cerebrospinal fluid from sleep-deprived goats. Proc. Nat. Acad. Sci. U.S.A., 58:513, 1967.

Sours, J. A.: Narcolepsy and other disturbances in the sleeping-waking rhythm. J. Nerv. Ment. Dis., 137:525, 1963.

Focal Disturbances of Higher Nervous Function

Norman Geschwind

LANGUAGE, APHASIA, AND RELATED DISORDERS

Most investigators agree that although forms of communication exist among lower animals, only man has language. As a result the experimental studies in animals which have advanced our knowledge of many other types of disordered physiology are not available for the study of disturbances of language. Most of our knowledge of the relationship of the brain to language has been based on detailed postmortem study of brains of patients who had been carefully studied in life. A second technique has been that of stimulating portions of the surface of the brain exposed at operation, or stimulating deeper structures by means of stereotaxically placed electrodes.

A striking feature of the human brain is *dominance,* i.e., the superiority of one hemisphere in the performance of certain functions. Dominance appears in our present state of knowledge to be exclusively a human attribute. About 93 per cent of people are right-handed, and at least 99 per cent of right handers have left hemisphere dominance for speech. Among the non-right-handed, i.e., the frankly left-handed and those with varying degrees of ambidexterity, the situation is more complex, and not yet fully defined. A rough rule of thumb is that about 60 per cent of non-right handers suffering from language disorders have left hemisphere lesions, whereas 40 per cent have right hemisphere lesions. A third group should be mentioned, the *pathologic left handers,* those who are left-handed because of injury in early childhood to the left hemisphere. These are usually right-brained for speech.

The cause of dominance was in dispute for many years. Present evidence indicates that it is based on the larger size of the speech regions on the left side than of the corresponding regions on the right. Although language develops on the dominant side, the nondominant side is endowed genetically with the capacity to develop language (although almost certainly not to the same degree of refinement as the dominant hemisphere). If the dominant hemisphere is seriously damaged in childhood, language usually develops on the other side, although in such cases the over-all degree of intellectual development is lower than in a control group. This capacity to shift diminishes through childhood and is meager after the age of 12. Dominance in the intact human can be studied by two recently developed techniques. The *Wada test* consists of the injection of sodium amytal into the internal carotid artery. This causes a transient hemiplegia on the side opposite the injection, but aphasia results only from injection on the dominant side. This test is especially useful to neurosurgeons to ascertain the dominant side, especially in non-right-handed patients. Another technique, the *Kimura test,* is that of dichotic listening, in which different words are simultaneously presented to the two ears. Normal individuals tend to report the words presented to the ear opposite the dominant hemisphere.

APHASIA

The aphasias may be defined as disorders of language secondary to lesions of the brain. In most cases there is disorder of the output of speech. In the experience of the author aphasia in spoken speech is invariably accompanied by similar abnormalities in writing. Aphasia in spoken language is of two major types: (1) Non-fluent aphasia, in which few words are produced slowly and with great effort, and sounds are incorrectly articulated. Production of grammatical words is relatively more affected so that sentences tend to be ungrammatical, e.g., "Weather sunny." (2) Fluent aphasia, in the more extreme forms of which the patient produces runs of well-articulated speech, which has the rhythm and melody of normal language and a basically normal grammatical structure, but which tends to convey little information, e.g., "I was at the other one and then I was at this one," a fluent aphasic's circumlocutory manner of explaining that he was in another hospital previously. The speech of these patients usually contains many incorrect words, called *paraphasias. Literal* (or phonemic) *paraphasias* are substitutions of well-articulated but incorrect sounds, e.g., "spoot" for "spoon," and *verbal paraphasias* are incorrect usages of words, e.g., "knife" for "fork," or "department" for "hospital."

In differential diagnosis, one must be wary of describing *mutism* as aphasia, since even severe aphasics are usually not mute. Causes of mutism are (1) uncooperativeness, (2) psychiatric disorders, e.g., severe depression or schizophrenia, (3) widespread disorders of brain, such as trauma, subarachnoid hemorrhage, or metabolic disorders, (4) lesions of mesencephalic and pontine tegmentum, and (5) bilateral lesions of the cranial nerves serving the speech organs, their nuclei, or their supranuclear pathways.

Dysarthria should not be confused with aphasia. Dysarthric speech is incorrectly articulated, but if transcribed shows correct grammar and word usage. A helpful clue is that if a patient with disorder in speech writes correctly (or produces correct language on a typewriter), he is almost certainly not aphasic.

A common error is to misdiagnose a fluent aphasia as schizophrenic word-salad. Several clues help to make the differential diagnosis. Fluent aphasia is much more common than schizophrenic word-salad. The schizophrenic speech disorder usually develops in chronic "back ward" schizophrenics. By contrast fluent aphasia may come on abruptly as the result of a stroke in a previously well person. Finally fluent aphasia from vascular disease usually occurs in older people, whereas schizophrenia almost always is manifest before the age of 30.

Aphasic Syndromes and Their Localizations. *Broca's aphasia* is the result of a lesion of Broca's area, i.e., the portion of the frontal lobe just anterior to the face, lip, tongue, and mouth area of the motor cortex. This produces a nonfluent aphasia, and writing is also involved. Comprehension of language is intact. There is nearly always a right hemiplegia. *Wernicke's aphasia* results from a lesion of Wernicke's area, the posterior portion of the superior temporal gyrus. The aphasia is typically fluent. Written language is equally impaired. Comprehension of spoken and written language is severely impaired. Repetition of spoken language is poor. There is usually no hemiplegia, and other elementary neurologic signs are usually lacking. *Conduction aphasia* results from a lesion of the parietal operculum, i.e., the region lying above the sylvian fissure. There is fluent aphasia involving speech and writing, with severely impaired repetition but intact comprehension. Elementary neurologic signs are usually absent, with the occasional exception of cortical sensory loss on the opposite side. *Anomic aphasia* is characterized by fluent aphasia in speech and impairment of written language, but with intact comprehension and repetition. The components of the Gerstmann syndrome (discussed subsequently) are often present. In this syndrome the lesion, if focal, is at the region of the parietotemporal junction, but a similar syndrome is produced in nonfocal widespread disease of the brain, such as is caused by metabolic disease or by large tumors with raised intracranial pressure.

These four syndromes are the most common, and although overlapping forms are common, relatively pure forms are not rare. Certain other syndromes are much less common.

In *isolation of the speech area* there is a large lesion involving the cortex and underlying white matter in a **C**-shaped configuration that spares Broca's area, Wernicke's area, and their interconnections, but destroys the cortex and underlying white matter that surround the speech region. These patients either may show little spontaneous speech or may have fluent abnormal speech. The most striking characteristic of this disorder is that despite an almost total lack of comprehension, the patient can repeat well without dysarthria. This lesion is usually the result of anoxia or of carotid insufficiency. *Alexia without*

agraphia is a syndrome in which the patient speaks and writes normally but cannot comprehend written language. The lesion, almost always the result of infarction in the distribution of the left posterior cerebral artery, consists of destruction of the left visual cortex and the splenium, i.e., the posterior portion, of the corpus callosum. In *alexia with agraphia* the patient can neither write nor comprehend written language, but other language functions are normal. Other components of the Gerstmann syndrome (see below) may be present. The lesion involves a portion of the left angular gyrus. A right visual field defect may occur if the lesion extends deeply into the white matter but is often absent. *Pure word-deafness* describes a syndrome in which there is dense incomprehension of language in the presence of intact hearing, although other language functions are intact. Two types of lesion produce this: either a single lesion lying subcortically in the posterior temporal lobe or bilateral lesions of the middle portion of the first temporal gyrus. *Pure agraphia* is extremely rare. It has been said that the responsible lesion lies in the posterior portion of the second frontal gyrus, but there are few convincing cases.

OTHER DISORDERS OF THE HIGHER FUNCTIONS

Apraxia. Apraxia is the inability to perform a learned act in response to a stimulus which would normally elicit it, and which cannot be accounted for by weakness, incoordination, reflex change, sensory loss, incomprehension, inattention, or uncooperativeness. Three lesions may produce apraxia. With lesions of the corpus callosum there will be apraxia of the left side of the body, but not of the right or of the face. Patients with Broca's aphasia (who usually have a right hemiplegia) will show apraxia that is usually most marked in the face and is also often present in the left limbs. With lesions in the left parietal operculum, producing a conduction aphasia, there is usually apraxia in the face (where it is most marked) and in the limbs of both sides of the body. In all forms of apraxia whole-body movements, e.g., "stand up," "sit down," "turn around," and movements of eye-closing and eye-opening are best preserved. In all forms of apraxia the defect is most marked to verbal command (although the patient comprehends), usually somewhat less marked on imitation of the examiner, and least marked in the handling of objects, although in some patients even this latter category is impaired.

Agnosia. Agnosia is a failure of recognition of complex stimuli in the face of preserved elementary perception. The most common form is visual agnosia, in which there are usually bilateral posterior occipital lobe lesions. The agnosias are less well understood than the aphasias or apraxias.

Callosal Syndromes. These were first brilliantly described by Hugo Liepmann in the early 1900's, but have been rediscovered only in recent years. In some cases of anterior cerebral artery occlusion there is infarction of the anterior four fifths of the corpus callosum. The patient will carry out verbal commands with the right hand but not the left. He will name objects held (concealed from vision) in the right hand but not the left. He can, however, with the left hand draw or select from a group of objects the one previously held in the left hand. He manifests, in brief, inability to transfer information between the two hemispheres. Involvement of the splenium of the corpus callosum plays a role in alexia without agraphia (see Aphasia).

Gerstmann Syndrome. This consists of agraphia, right-left disorientation, acalculia (difficulty in carrying out calculations), and finger agnosia (inability to name fingers or to identify them). The patient almost invariably also shows constructional disorder, i.e., a difficulty in drawing or copying designs, especially three-dimensional ones. When all the components of this syndrome are present, the lesion almost invariably lies in the left posterior parietal region. It should, however, be kept in mind that a single component has little localizing value. Thus constructional difficulty without the other components may result from lesions in many locations.

Right Hemisphere Syndrome. Lesions of the right parietal region produce constructional difficulty that is more severe on the average than that produced from any other site. Patients with lesions in this location may also show a dressing disorder manifested by great difficulty in putting on clothes. Milder degrees of the difficulty may be brought out by such maneuvers as putting one sleeve of the bathrobe inside out; the patient may be unable to get the bathrobe on properly.

A striking feature of acute lesions of the right hemisphere is *anosognosia,* i.e., a tendency to deny or neglect disability, or when admitting its presence, to be unconcerned with it. It is a common experience that the patient with an acute left hemiplegia will show this type of behavior, although by contrast the patient with an acute right hemiplegia will, even if aphasic, show appropriate awareness of disability and will be depressed. These disorders in right hemisphere lesions are usually accompanied by a curious mental state, in which the patient shows apathy, poor attention, and often jocularity. These states (and the accompanying unconcern with illness) are usually transient, but are sometimes permanent in cases of large right parietal lesions. Patients with transient cases, however, do not necessarily have parietal lesions.

It should be noted that not all patients who deny illness suffer from right hemisphere disease. Weinstein has shown that a patient with any disability may deny illness if he is sufficiently obtunded. Thus a patient may deny blindness resulting even from disease of the eyes if he develops a confusional state from metabolic disorder or drugs.

MEMORY

Memory describes the processes by which past experience is stored and retrieved. Disorders of memory include *anterograde amnesia,* i.e., the failure to store new memories, or *retrograde amnesia,* i.e., disorders of storage or retrieval of memories laid down in the past.

Certain separable stages in memory storage have become clear from clinical observation. There is a stage of *immediate* memory, which is the ability to retain material presented as long as attention is not distracted. This is examined by such tests as digit span, i.e., the ability to repeat a series of digits spoken by the examiner. Most normal persons can immediately repeat a series of seven such digits. The next step is *transfer* to the long-term memory store. The first step in this is *intermediate memory storage,* and the later step is called *remote memory.* The reasons for separating these steps will become clear when we discuss the clinical syndromes.

ANATOMY OF MEMORY

Memories are probably held in short-term store simply by continuation of nervous activity. The transfer to the long-term store probably involves some molecular change either in the nerve membrane or in the intracellular organelles. The structures most involved appear to lie in the inner ring of the limbic system, including the hippocampus, fornix, mammillary body, mammillothalamic tract (or bundle of Vicq d'Azyr) anteroventral thalamic nucleus, and cingulate gyrus. The most important structures appear to be the hippocampus and mammillary bodies. The intactness of these structures appears to be important, in some as yet undefined way, in the transfer of memories from the immediate to the long-term stores. The memories are probably not laid down in these limbic structures since their destruction does not lead to loss of remote memories. They must therefore act on the structures which are the sites of storage. The limbic structures are also important, as will be seen below, in retrieval from the intermediate store.

CLINICAL DISORDERS OF MEMORY

Memory disorder may be evident in widespread disorder of the brain such as may be produced by drugs or metabolic disorders. On the other hand, memory may be relatively or dramatically spared in many of the dementias. Thus memory is much less impaired than such functions as calculation and abstraction in general paresis or Huntington's chorea. By contrast, in Alzheimer's disease, in which involvement of hippocampus is prominent, memory disorder is a salient feature of the initial stages.

Disease processes predominantly affecting the

hippocampal-mammillary system will produce significant memory disorder with little or no effect on other intellectual functions. This clinical state is called *Korsakoff's syndrome*. When due to thiamine deficiency, the most striking lesions are in the mammillary bodies. The hippocampus may be involved in Alzheimer's disease, head injury, or tumors. Disease of the posterior cerebral artery may cause infarction of the hippocampus. Herpes simplex encephalitis has a predilection for all the structures of the limbic system. Occasional cases of severe memory loss have been reported following bilateral removal of the medial temporal structures surgically.

In order to produce a permanent memory deficit, bilateral lesions of the mammillo-hippocampal system are required. However, a unilateral lesion of the *left* hippocampus will produce a transient memory disorder, which may last as long as three months.

The memory disorder that sometimes follows head injury illustrates well the different states of the memory process outlined above. A patient who shows this disorder let us say a week after the episode may exhibit the following picture. He will be alert, awake, and cooperative and may, on a standard IQ test, score in a normal or even superior range. In addition his immediate memory, as shown, for example, by digit span, will be normal. By contrast he shows an anterograde amnesia, i.e., an inability to learn new material. He also shows a retrograde amnesia extending back from 3 to 20 years. More remote memories, in particular most of what was learned before the age of 12, are much better preserved. Over the next two or three months the condition improves. The ability to learn new material reappears (but the patient will have a permanent gap in his memory for the period in which he lacked this ability). The retrograde amnesia gradually shrinks until it reaches its permanent form, with a duration of

seconds to minutes. The long retrograde amnesia must therefore have been a disorder of retrieval, rather than storage. It thus appears that the integrity of the limbic structures is necessary for the retrieval from intermediate, but not remote memory. In cases of persistent Korsakoff's syndrome, such as occur frequently with other forms of disorders that produce permanent bilateral limbic system damage, the retrograde amnesia does not improve significantly.

A prominent feature of many but not all cases of Korsakoff's syndrome, especially in the early stages, is confabulation, i.e., the tendency of the patient to invent fanciful replies to questions whose answers he doesn't know.

Functional amnesia occurs in hysteria (usually young women) or in older patients who are depressed. A similar clinical picture seen in malingerers is usually easy to recognize. The patient may show either a highly selective memory disorder, e.g., denying that he is married, although all other recent and remote facts are preserved, or a global disorder, e.g., professing total amnesia for all events of his life. Failure of a patient without aphasia to state his own name is invariably not organic in origin. Another common syndrome is the fugue state in which the patient denies any memory of his activities for a period of time ranging from hours to weeks, during which his external activities appeared normal or during which he disappeared and traveled extensively. Although some short-lasting fugue states may occasionally be the result of temporal lobe epilepsy, the author's experience has been that these are nearly all functional in origin.

Geschwind, N.: Disconnexion syndromes in animals and man. Brain, 88:237, 1965.

Talland, G. A., and Waugh, N. C.: The Pathology of Memory. New York, Academic Press, Inc., 1969.

Zangwill, O. L.: Cerebral Dominance and Its Relation to Psychological Function. Springfield, Ill., Charles C Thomas, 1960.

Dementia
Paul R. McHugh

Introduction. Dementia means deterioration in intellectual capacity. The condition is distinguished from mental retardation, in which subnormal intellectual ability has been lifelong and may or may not be caused by brain injury; and from aphasia and Korsakoff's psychosis, in which specific intellectual skills (language and memory, respectively) have deteriorated without a proportional disturbance in other cognitive functions.

Dementia is a clinical entity. Any pathologic process affecting the cerebral hemispheres can lead to an impairment in intellectual capacity. The extent of the brain injury and not the location of injury or the nature of the neuropathology determines its severity. The diagnostic task is twofold:

first, the physician must recognize the symptoms of dementia; then, he must identify the cerebral pathology producing it. The first aspect of diagnosis requires skill in testing mental function; the second, knowledge of the mode of onset of different pathologic conditions and of the associated neurologic signs and laboratory data.

Clinical Manifestations. The earliest symptoms of dementia can pass almost unrecognized. They may be merely a slight loss of mental quickness, spontaneity, and initiative. Symptoms are hard to differentiate from fatigue or boredom. The patient is vaguely changed. He has lost his sparkle, and seems slow and lacking in energy. It is usually a close family member who first recognizes these changes. But as the dementia progresses, symptoms become obvious to all. Difficulties in recent memory are often the first tangible symptom. The patient can't remember immediate happenings, although his remote memories remain. He overlooks appointments, forgets a recent conversation, becomes lost in familiar surroundings. Also, it becomes difficult for him to think through new tasks, and he cannot comprehend complex commands. He fails to follow the gist of conversations or to interpret the activities of other people correctly. His judgment is poor, and decisions are difficult. Language may be employed with less direction, pertinence, and nimbleness as the patient falls on clichés and habitual observations rather than choosing words with imagination and precision. At this time in the progress of a dementing illness a patient may maintain a façade of normality by comporting himself with his customary manners and employing his habitual modes of speech. But his social stance merely covers over his analytic and integrative failings, which are revealed when conversation or inquiry is carried beyond the stage of casual interchanges.

The demented patient may suffer also from depression, anxiety, or easy irritability. These symptoms may be the outcome of the difficulty he appreciates in accomplishing tasks that were previously easy, or may represent changes in emotional control owing to injury to significant cerebral tissue.

Finally, with worsening, the patient can lose all his mental efficiency. His behavior deteriorates badly as he fails to care for himself or appreciate his surroundings. He loses his remote memories, now failing to recognize his closest relatives. He eventually cannot care for himself, and becomes bedridden and totally unaware of his surroundings. At this time his duration of life is dependent upon the nursing care he receives.

Dementia, thus, is a decline in all intellectual functions, and is reflected in every aspect of behavior.

Diagnosis. It is not difficult to recognize intellectual impairment in individuals late in the course of a cerebral disease. The more taxing problem is the recognition of the intellectual impairment when it is slight and potentially reversible. The tests of cognitive function that are part of the neurologic examination of every patient are intended to accomplish this. But they must be interpreted with care.

It is customary to test (1) orientation to time, place, and person; (2) language skills, by naming common objects and comprehending commands; (3) fund of knowledge, such as the names of some capital cities and of presidents; (4) recent memory, by setting three objects to be remembered for 5, 10, and 30 minutes; (5) attention span, by asking for a serial subtraction of 7 from 100 or any other arithmetic task that requires "carrying over"; (6) abstract reasoning power, by asking for definitions of proverbs or the similarity of words such as apple-orange, ear-eye, poem-statue; and (7) constructional capacity, by asking the patient to draw simple objects such as a clock or to copy an abstract design.

The results of these tests must be interpreted in the light of other knowledge about the patient. If the patient was a gifted professional person whose family has noted a decline in his judgment and an increasing forgetfulness, the discovery that he cannot hold three names in mind for five minutes and that he interprets proverbs clumsily provides some evidence that he is suffering from a disturbance to his intellectual power. On the other hand, if the patient was not a person with intellectual achievements in the past and has received a poor education, difficulties in proverb interpretation or fund of knowledge are less likely to represent brain disease. Although it is possible to find all the intellectual functions disturbed in dementia, the tests for recent memory, for attention, and for constructional capacity are most useful. Deficiencies here are easy to document; these functions are affected early in the course of many brain diseases and they are little dependent on education. Also, tests for recent memory are useful in differentiating a patient with mental retardation from an individual of limited intelligence who is developing a brain disease, since memory function is intact in the mildly retarded individual.

It is important to differentiate Korsakoff's syndrome and aphasia. The patient with Korsakoff's syndrome will fail the tests of recent memory. He will be disoriented to time and place, but he will be able to name objects, obey commands, and accomplish tasks of abstract reasoning and drawing if he can hold the question in mind. His disorder is in memory. The rest of his intellectual function is relatively spared. The aphasic patient will have severe problems in naming objects and comprehending words. But if this difficulty can be surmounted, it will be evident that it is language specifically that is disturbed, and other mental functions such as memory, orientation, and the capacity to draw are relatively intact.

It is often useful to supplement the bedside tests of mental function with standardized examination of intellectual skills. The Wechsler Adult Intelligence Scale (WAIS) is most often employed. Nothing about this psychologic examination is different in concept from the bedside tests. It measures the intellectual performance of a patient by asking him to attempt problems in several different areas. Since a mathematical score is given, it is possible to compare his performance with other individuals objectively. Although the WAIS includes problems similar to those given at the bedside, it adds several "performance" tests which are actually unfamiliar tasks, such as recognition of errors in pictures, design of patterns from colored blocks, and assembly of parts of puzzles. These tests most specifically examine the ability of a patient to put his mind to an unfamiliar situation and solve it. They are less dependent on learning and in fact decline early in a dementia and so produce a discrepancy between these "performance scores" and the "verbal scores" which tend to remain intact for a longer period.

Diagnostic Issues in Dementia. As mentioned in the introduction, the symptoms of dementia appear with an injury to the cerebral hemispheres, and are not specific for a particular pathology. It is the course of their development, the associated neurologic signs, and the laboratory findings that permit diagnosis of the pathologic entities producing the dementia.

Since the same symptoms can be produced by curable, reversible pathology as by incurable and progressive disorders, the first diagnostic consideration should reflect a search for the treatable pathologic entities. Each of the following conditions should be considered in every patient with the symptoms of dementia: general paresis, myxedema, neoplasms and other chronic intracerebral lesions, hepatolenticular degeneration (Wilson's disease), avitaminosis B_{12}, folic acid deficiency, and occult hydrocephalus. Many of these conditions can be diagnosed by evidence derived from the clinical examination; others demand clinical laboratory studies. Thus the Argyll Robinson pupil of cerebral syphilis, lateralized motor-sensory signs of neoplasm, the Kayser-Fleischer ring of Wilson's disease, and a gait disorder caused by a spastic weakness of legs in hydrocephalus should all be sought in the physical examination of the demented patient. A group of laboratory tests are required in the diagnostic evaluation. As a routine, all patients should have a lumbar puncture to measure intracerebral pressure and to obtain a sample of cerebrospinal fluid for analysis. Cell count, protein content, and a test for the syphilitic precipitants will be needed in cerebrospinal fluid. An analysis of gastric contents for acidity is required to exclude B_{12} deficiency. Blood serologic examination and analysis for protein-bound iodine are also indicated. An electroencephalogram is useful, as it may reveal a local lesion or a severe generalized slowing of the rhythms characteristic of intoxication. Skull roentgenograms can also reveal a local lesion. In many patients it is necessary to proceed to a pneumoencephalogram in order to exclude some of the rarer but curable forms of dementia such as occult hydrocephalus.

The onset and course of a dementing disorder must be carefully analyzed when considering the likely pathologic entities. Particularly, has the decline been acute (a week or less), subacute (a week to eight weeks), or chronic (more than two months)? Was the onset abrupt or insidious, was the subsequent course a gradual and relentless loss of mental faculties, or was it a series of sudden losses producing a steplike decline in the mental faculties? Different pathologic entities produce different clinical histories in these respects. Thus the dementia associated with vascular disease of the brain will have a sudden onset and increase in an intermittent and variable fashion. The dementia of general paresis tends to be subacute and steadily progressive; that of degenerative disease is more insidious in onset and slow in development.

The characteristics of four known cerebral de-generations will be reviewed as they exemplify some of these general statements about dementia. These conditions are Alzheimer's disease, Pick's disease, Creutzfeldt-Jakob disease, and Huntington's chorea.

ALZHEIMER'S DISEASE

Alzheimer's disease is a degenerative disorder of the cerebral cortex that produces a dementia in middle to late life. It is a pathologic entity in that its ultimate defining characteristics are in neuropathology.

The brain in Alzheimer's disease gradually atrophies, nerve cells disappearing from the cortex. The major brunt of the atrophic process appears to be in the frontal and occipital regions of the brain, but microscopic examinations will demonstrate pathologic changes throughout the cortex. Many of the neurons that remain show a peculiar alteration of their neurofibrils. These become thick and twist into distinctive "neurofibrillary tangles." Within the atrophic cortex there are many "senile plaques." These are microscopic collections of granular argyrophilic particles which tend to form in a halo around an indefinite center containing sudanophilic fat or an amyloid-like substance. Exactly what these plaques are is uncertain, but they appear to represent collections of degenerating brain substance.

The dementia that accompanies Alzheimer's disease has few distinctive characteristics. All the symptoms and signs enumerated above for dementia eventually appear. Onset is insidious and progress slow. A disturbance in recent memory is usually the first symptom. Affective disturbances such as depression or anxiety and disorientation in time and place appear soon after. Often there is a considerable emotional unrest in these patients, with some 30 to 40 per cent suffering at some time from distressing false beliefs of a delusionary character. A sizable fraction of patients also has hallucinations during illness. Focal neurologic signs are rare early in the course of the disease, but with progression of the illness, focal cortical symptoms of aphasia, apraxia, and agnosia can become prominent. Seizures, both focal and generalized, are common only in far-advanced instances. With these intellectual and emotional disturbances there is the development of a disorder of gait. This takes the form of difficulty in starting the rhythmical movements of walking. A synchronous activation of agonist and antagonist muscles results in a locking of the legs and a hesitant shuffle.

The progress of all these symptoms is much the same in all patients. It is slow, but usually within five to eight years of the onset of symptoms the patient reaches a terminal stage. Here there is a profound dementia and a decerebrate physical state with flexion contractures of all limbs. Death comes from an intercurrent infection or some other complication of the bedfast condition.

The age of onset varies. Because this disorder

was first recognized among relatively young people, the term "presenile dementia" has been applied to Alzheimer's disease. This implies a distinction in kind between this condition and "senile dementia" that appears when many other changes of aging are evident. But the cerebral pathology and the clinical course of patients who develop symptoms before or after age 65 are the same. Alzheimer's disease, defined as it is by the cerebral pathology of atrophy with senile plaques and neurofibrillary tangles, is a disorder appearing with increasing frequency as people age.

Alzheimer's disease is not an uncommon disorder, but it is more common in females than in males. Autopsy diagnoses vary from 1 to 10 per cent in mental hospitals, the particular figure depending on whether the observers make a distinction between Alzheimer's disease and senile dementia.

The etiology of Alzheimer's disease is unknown. Most examples occur sporadically, but a few patients have a family history of dementia. It is not even certain whether Alzheimer's disease is a specific response to one noxious biologic process or whether it is a more general response of the brain to injurious processes. The latter possibility is suggested by the occasional appearance of Alzheimer pathology in such different situations as the punchdrunk syndrome of boxers, Down's syndrome (trisomy 21), and postencephalitic parkinsonism.

The diagnosis of Alzheimer's disease is made most often by exclusion. An individual who has a slowly progressive dementia without prominent neurologic signs and without any of the clinical and laboratory findings of the treatable conditions mentioned, as well as a pneumoencephalogram demonstrating a moderate dilation of the cerebral ventricles with some atrophy of cortex, is most likely to be suffering from Alzheimer's disease. Only by cerebral biopsy can more conclusive evidence for diagnosis be found, and this cannot be recommended in the usual clinical situation.

PICK'S DISEASE

Pick's disease is also a degenerative disorder of the cerebral cortex that produces dementia in middle and late life. It is distinguished from Alzheimer's disease by its morbid anatomy.

In contrast to Alzheimer's disease, in which cerebral atrophy is diffuse, in Pick's disease the atrophy is relatively circumscribed and confined to the frontal and temporal lobes. Here the atrophy is severe. The microscopic pathology is also distinct in Pick's disease. There is a particular degenerating neuron characterized by the accumulation close to the nucleus of a globular argyrophilic mass that distends the neuron into a swollen ballooned form. This is the *Pick cell* and it is usually found widespread in the atrophying areas of cortex. There are usually neurofibrillary tangles and senile plaques as well in the atrophic parts of brain.

It has proved impossible to distinguish Pick's disease from Alzheimer's disease on the basis of onset, progression, duration, or clinical symptoms. Patients with Pick's disease may have less difficulty in gait than patients with Alzheimer's disease. Otherwise, the conditions seem clinically identical. Pick's disease is considerably less common than Alzheimer's disease, but, as in that condition, no definite etiology has been identified. Some examples of Pick's disease appear to be transmitted by a dominant gene in a family, but many examples are without a family history.

CREUTZFELDT-JAKOB DISEASE

The dementia in Creutzfeldt-Jakob disease is also due to degeneration of the cerebral cortex, but the clinical manifestations are much more distinctive than in Alzheimer's and Pick's diseases, and a possible etiologic agent is presently under investigation.

In this disorder the clinical disturbance is often ushered in by motor or sensory symptoms. Any patient may notice a varied combination of difficulty in vision, hearing, motor strength, or coordinated movements. These symptoms may progress in the course of weeks to blindness, deafness, and hemiplegia, and will often be associated with abnormal myoclonic jerks and tremors. Simultaneously the patient loses intellectual capacity. All the signs and symptoms of dementia are seen, but they develop rapidly over the course of a few weeks. Within four to eight months of the onset of symptoms, the patient has lost all cognitive function and is bedridden and decerebrate, with severe total body and limb myoclonic jerking.

The EEG is helpful in the diagnosis of this condition because it is diffusely and severely abnormal quite early in the disease. The normal rhythms of the EEG are lost and replaced with slow activity, often interrupted with high amplitude sharp wave complexes that may be synchronous with the myoclonic jerks.

The cerebral pathology of Creutzfeldt-Jakob disease is distinctive. It consists of a severe degeneration of the cerebral cortex. In the most affected parts of the cortex there is a total obliteration of the cytoarchitecture. The normal appearance of cortical layers and columnar organization of neurons is lost and is replaced by a disorganized glial overgrowth. This most severely affected region may take on a peculiar sponge-like appearance because of vacuoles that occur in both neuronal and astrocytic processes (status spongiosus). The basal ganglia and cerebellum can also degenerate in this disease. The variety of clinical manifestations seen in patients with this disorder can be explained by variation in the sites of maximal pathologic disorder. If this is the occipital cortex, visual disturbances leading to blindness will be prominent; if the temporal cortex is affected early, then aphasia and deafness can be expected; if the cerebellum, then ataxia will characterize the early course. With the advance of the pathologic condition the decerebrate condition is an inevitable outcome.

Creutzfeldt-Jakob disease is an uncommon disorder. Most examples have occurred in middle-aged persons, but it has been described as early as age 20. There is no special sex incidence. Etiology has been as obscure as for the other dementias. However, an important discovery has been made that may have far-ranging implications for the other cerebral degenerations. It has proved possible to transmit a condition identical in clinical manifestations and in cerebral pathologic symptoms to the chimpanzee by injecting into that animal tissue from the brain of patients with Creutzfeldt-Jakob disease. It takes several months for the disorder to manifest itself in the animal. But once seen, the symptoms advance rapidly, as in the human. This evidence suggests some transmissible agent as a cause of Creutzfeldt-Jakob disease. In this respect it resembles the neurologic condition kuru discovered among New Guinea aboriginals and scrapie, a disease of sheep. Whatever the nature of these transmissible agents (they have been called slow viruses), they represent a new territory in the biology of neurologic disease, and may come to explain many other clinical and pathologic entities.

HUNTINGTON'S CHOREA

Huntington's chorea is a distinctive disease entity in which a dementia associated with chorea appears usually in the fourth or fifth decade of life. Its neuropathology is characteristic, and the disease is transmitted as an autosomal dominant.

The dementia of Huntington's chorea appears insidiously as a decline in intellectual efficiency. There is nothing unique about the intellectual impairment. There may be prominent affective symptoms, such as depression taking on suicidal proportions, severe irritability, and personality change. These may be the first signs of the disorder. The clinical diagnosis does not rest on a distinctive feature of the dementia but on the choreiform movements that appear usually prior to the dementia or simultaneously with it. Other characteristics of this disorder are given elsewhere (see Extrapyramidal Disorders).

TREATMENT OF THE DEMENTED PATIENT

With the obvious exception of the specific treatments for curable clinical conditions, the issue of treatment of the demented patient is most often the issue of management of particular symptoms rather than reversal of a pathologic process. Often, a treatment based on some research finding is proposed for the degenerative disorders only to prove of little value when employed in a clinical trial. Thus the discovery that cerebral oxygen consumption is reduced in Alzheimer's disease led to treatments with both oxygen inhalation and hyperbaric chambers. But these treatments failed to produce significant improvement, almost certainly because the observed reduction in oxygen consumption is due to a reduction in the number of viable neurons rather than to an inadequate oxygen supply. Any treatment that is proposed for these distressing conditions is liable to be uncritically acclaimed, with eventual disappointment. The importance of the clinical trial with double-blind technique in assessing these treatments cannot be exaggerated.

Some general principles of management of the demented patient can be emphasized. First, complicating medical conditions such as congestive heart failure, dehydration, iron deficiency anemia, infections, and electrolyte imbalance can, even if not severe in themselves, make the mental condition of a patient with degenerative brain disease much worse. A meticulous correction of all medical complications will do much to aid in management. Second, much of the emotional unrest in demented patients is caused by fear produced by their disorientation, misidentifications, and misinterpretations of their situation. Great relief of these symptoms can come from a willingness of nurses and doctors to explain repeatedly to the patient his surroundings and the proper interpretation of what is happening. Changes in surroundings and in nursing personnel should be minimized, distracting shadows should be avoided, well lighted rooms, preferably with familiar possessions, serve best, and an attitude toward the patient that demonstrates an appreciation of his personal style will do much to assist him. Third, considerable help for individual symptoms can be gained by the use of pharmacologic measures. Sleep disturbances in demented patients are best treated with chloral hydrate, up to 1.0 to 1.5 grams at night. Acute confusional aggression or agitation can be relieved by phenothiazine medication, and thioridazine in doses of 50 to 100 mg. three or four times daily has been effective. Depressive symptoms can respond to antidepressant medication (imipramine, 50 mg. three times to four times per day).

All these drugs should be used sparingly, as the patient with cerebral degeneration may demonstrate toxic signs at much lower doses than normal patients. Drug toxicity can worsen the condition severely.

In general, the management of the demented patient rests on an appreciation of the nature of his difficulties and the application of medical and nursing principles. The response to this management is often gratifying.

Beck, E., Daniel, P. M., Matthews, W. B., Stevens, D. L., Alpers, M. P., Asher, D. M., Gajdusek, D. C., and Gibbs, C. J.: Creutzfeldt-Jakob disease — The neuropathology of a transmission experiment. Brain, 92:699, 1969.

Corsellis, J. A. N.: Mental Illness and the Ageing Brain. London, Oxford University Press, 1962.

McHugh, P. R.: Occult hydrocephalus. Quart. J. Med., 33:297, 1964.

Post, F.: Clinical Psychiatry of Late Life. New York, Pergamon Press, 1965.

Sjogren, T., Sjogren, H., and Lindgren, A. G. H.: Morbus Alzheimer and morbus Pick: A genetic, clinical and pathological study. Acta Psychiat. Neur. Scand. (Suppl. 82), 1952.

Strachan, R. W., and Henderson, J. G.: Psychiatric syndromes due to avitominosis B$_{12}$ with normal blood and marrow. Quart. J. Med., 34:303, 1965.

Strachan, R. W., and Henderson, J. G.: Dementia and folate deficiency. Quart. J. Med., 36:189, 1967.

Terry, R. D., Gonatas, N. K., and Weiss, M.: Ultrastructural studies in Alzheimer's presenile dementia. Amer. J. Path., 44:269, 1964.

Psychologic Illness in Medical Practice

Paul R. McHugh

THE CONCEPT OF DISEASE IN PSYCHIATRY

Any general hospital can provide an experience in psychiatry, because an example of every psychologic disorder will eventually appear among patients admitted to its services. However, many skilled physicians feel unsure of their ability to manage these disorders. They are apt to contrast their knowledge of somatic illness founded firmly in morbid anatomy and pathophysiology with their understanding of psychologic medicine in which classifications seem based on confusing mixtures of symptomatology and speculative theories, and the most effective treatments are empirical. Such physicians will continue uncertain until they grasp how the basic concept of disease can bring order to psychiatry as it does in all of medicine. This they must accomplish before they can profit from a review of the clinical facts of particular psychiatric conditions; hence this article.

The term "disease" is difficult to define, because it is a concept and not something concrete or given in nature. It is intended to convey the idea that among all the morbid changes in physical and mental health it is possible to recognize groups of abnormalities as distinct entities or syndromes separable from one another and from the normal and that these separations will prove to have some biologic explanation when the entities have been thoroughly investigated.

All abnormalities can logically be viewed as quantitative changes merging imperceptibly into one another and into the normal, and can then be explained as consequences of disturbed interactions of a few vital processes. The Hippocratic concept of "humors" is just such a view. In fact the concept of disease based on qualitatively distinct syndromes is a convention proposed first by Sydenham, and remains but a convention today. But this has been the most useful convention in the natural sciences. It has become so indispensable in medical thinking that it is taken for granted in most discussions. Neglect of this convention explains much of the difficulty faced by students in psychiatry. Its logic thus needs review here.

The concept of any given disease passes through several stages as knowledge increases. At each stage attention focuses on certain features of the condition which are the "defining characteristics." At the first stage a "clinical disease entity" is recognized and defined as a constellation of symptoms and physical signs running a more or less predictable course or natural history. Dropsy, hemophilia, and epilepsy are typical clinical disease entities. But these entities are not pure species. Each can be the expression of any one of several different pathologic conditions. Dropsy, for example, is found with different pathologic conditions: glomerulonephritis, congestive heart failure, constrictive pericarditis. Thus, the second stage is the division of the clinical disease entity into several "pathologic disease entities." When a disease can be conceived as a pathologic entity, the defining characteristics on which concept and diagnosis rest are results of laboratory tests that reveal pathologic function or morbid anatomy. Again, by way of example, the demonstration of an elevated blood urea nitrogen and albumin and casts in the urine of a patient with dropsy leads to a presumptive opinion that the pathologic disease entity responsible for his condition is glomerulonephritis. This presumptive diagnosis is confirmed by studying the histopathology of the kidney. The third and final stage in the concept of a disease is the recognition of a particular etiologic agency. Recognition of an etiologic agent can derive from any of the biologic subspecialties: Genetics, microbiology, and biochemistry have all made their contributions. For glomerulonephritis the etiologic agency is the phenomenon of autoimmunity, and it will be from investigations of this phenomenon that physicians can expect to gain a complete understanding of glomerulonephritis and a treatment that can cure it.

For many medical diseases the mark of the twentieth century has been the discovery of etiologic agencies and their action. Not so for psychiatry. For most psychiatric disorders knowledge has not passed the first stage on the traditional path. For many even the hold on this stage is insecure. This insecurity arises in part from the difficulty of the subject matter, but also from a neglect of the standards of observation and history-taking that are required in defining a clinical disease entity.

This neglect has been defended by a prevailing opinion in psychiatry that all psychologic disturbances are to be viewed as emotional reactions to some form of environmental distress, and thus are quantitative abnormalities differing from normal in a continuous and smooth fashion rather than grouping into qualitatively distinct entities with separable pathologies and etiologies.

One objection to this view has to be the practical one that it discards for no obvious advantage a convention that has ordered other abnormalities successfully. Another is that it oversimplifies mental disturbances to make them all expressions of a few psychologic mechanisms. A consideration of the forms of disorder for which psychiatry assumes responsibility will demonstrate the utility found in the concept of disease for some of them.

Three groups of disturbances fall into manageable psychiatric categories. The first holds all those disturbances in mind and behavior that are a result of observable brain pathology. Represented here are the clinical disease entities of delirium, dementia, and mental retardation. The conceptual and investigative approach to these conditions is indistinguishable from that for other somatic diseases. Such pathologic disease entities as Alzheimer's disease and such etiologic agencies as perinatal hypoxia, infections, and metabolic changes have been discerned.

The second group holds the two functional psychoses in which no obvious brain pathology is evident: schizophrenia and manic-depressive disorder. That these conditions are not unlike somatic disorders and should be conceived as clinical disease entities defined by symptoms and course is impossible to prove at this time. But this view was first prompted by the alien character of the symptoms that seem unaccountable from an empathic understanding of the patient's temperament and his recent life experiences. It has been strengthened by the discovery of pharmacologic treatments specific to each entity and by the recognition of a few brain disturbances leading to identical clinical conditions—temporal lobe epilepsy, amphetamine toxicity leading to a schizophrenia-like disorder, and reserpine administration to a depressive disorder. It is now more conceivable that we are on the threshold of discoveries that will provide pathologic disease entities and etiologic agencies for these conditions than that they will be explained as quantitative exaggerations of emotional reactions.

The third group of disturbances in mind and behavior are the personality disorders and neurotic symptoms. The concept of disease does not fit these conditions. They seem to be quantitative rather than qualitative abnormalities in psychologic functions. It is difficult to say for these where normal leaves off and abnormal begins since they do seem to be extremes of normal variation. Personality disorders seem no more diseases than are shortness of stature, plainness of face, and dullness of wit. Neurotic symptoms such as anxiety or hysteria, like any symptoms of disturbance, can be evoked by many causes, including somatic or psychiatric diseases, but they most commonly appear as understandable reactions of an individual with a disordered personality faced with an environment that strikes at his special vulnerability.

Thus the concept of disease does provide in psychiatry a means for organizing clinical material that is similar to that used in general medicine. In the following articles its application in the detailed consideration of the separate conditions will be attempted.

Jaspers, K.: General Psychopathology. Translated by J. Hoenig and M. Hamilton. Manchester, Manchester University Press, 1963.
Scadding, J. G.: Diagnosis: The clinician and the computer. Lancet, 2:877, 1967.
Taylor, F. K.: Psychopathology. Its Causes and Symptoms. London, Butterworth and Co., Ltd., 1966.

FUNCTIONAL PSYCHOSES

Introduction. The psychoses form a loose category that gathers together several different clinical entities. To be placed within the category an entity must produce disturbances in thinking and perception that are inexplicable solely as responses to experience and are severe enough to distort the patient's appreciation of the real world and the relationship of events within it. The category, psychosis, has no uniform foundation as in somatic pathology nor any more objective aspects of psychopathology to mark its distinction from other collections of psychiatric symptoms. It is thus a term difficult to use with precision. Sometimes psychosis is used as a euphemism for insanity, sometimes as a synonym for schizophrenia, one of the entities within the category, and sometimes to draw an elusive and dubious distinction as between neurotic and psychotic depression.

The unmodified term can be qualified by a differentiation into organic psychoses and functional psychoses. Here the term psychosis means only severe mental illness. The organic psychoses, delirium, dementia, and Korsakoff's syndrome, are produced by a variety of cerebral pathologies. The functional psychoses, schizophrenia and manic-depressive disorder, lack a recognizable neuropathology.

This differentiation is practical. It draws a distinction in kind that affects treatment and prognosis, and it indicates the character of the clinical problem. For the organic psychoses the central problem is the etiology of the pathologic changes. For the functional psychoses the central problem is consistent diagnosis.

Schizophrenia and manic-depressive disorder are clinical disease entities. The criteria for their diagnosis are their symptoms alone. There are no objective tests verifying a diagnosis. Only the running out of the natural history or response to empirically discovered treatments can confirm a diagnostic opinion. Since they lack a neuropathology and are by definition inexplicable as responses to experience, there are no comprehensive etiologic explanations for these disorders. Treatment therefore is symptomatic rather than fundamental. Both prevention and radical cure await a chance discovery or a major scientific advance in understanding the biologic foundations of human behavior.

SCHIZOPHRENIA

Schizophrenia, a most devastating mental illness, is as well the most overdiagnosed entity in medicine, at least by North American physicians. It is a disturbance of mind and personality appearing in clear consciousness and characterized by several distinctive alterations in mental experiences, thinking capacity, and mood that are seldom completely resolved. The most characteristic features occur during the active phases of the disturbance, and take the form of hallucinations, delusions, and altered behavior toward others. Specific intellectual and affective disabilities varying from minimal to severe can develop insidiously or remain after an attack. A crucial element of the definition is that all these symptoms occur in a patient free of any relevant and discernible pathologic change in his nervous system.

Clinical Manifestations. The symptoms of schizophrenia can begin at almost any stage in life, but most commonly occur during adolescence and early adulthood and then either insidiously or as an acute attack followed by a series of attacks, each leaving behind personality defects of increasing severity.

In some patients it is possible to recognize a particular premorbid personality. They may have seemed more timid, shy, or seclusive than others. They may have been bookish, unsociable, and preoccupied with philosophic and religious ideas to the exclusion of friendships and community experiences. But this so-called *schizoid personality* is not found in most patients who develop schizophrenia. At least half of schizophrenic patients had premorbid personalities indistinguishable from normal.

Among the mental changes that mark the onset of a schizophrenic illness, only some are specific to this disorder. Emotional unrest, uncertainty, perplexity, and confusion can be found in many disorders other than schizophrenia, and therefore a diagnosis of schizophrenia cannot rest on them. There are, however, a number of mental changes that are more or less diagnostic. These can be usefully divided into abnormal mental experiences and disturbed modes of expression. The abnormal mental experiences are somewhat more reliable evidence of the illness simply because they are easier to elicit with confidence and less dependent upon interpretation than disturbances in expression.

Hallucinations and delusions are the outstanding schizophrenic mental experiences. Although hallucinations can arise in any sensory system, auditory hallucinations are the most common, and certain forms of auditory hallucinations are almost diagnostic. Thus, hearing one's own thoughts, hearing voices commenting about one's every action, or several voices engaged in a conversation about one in which derogatory and praising remarks are passed with the patient discussed in the third person are the most typical schizophrenic experiences.

Although delusions, i.e., false beliefs that are incorrigible, idiosyncratic, and preoccupying, can be found in many disorders other than schizophrenia, in this illness delusional experiences are dramatic and well developed. They can begin as vague, fearful interpretations and "half-beliefs" and develop into firm incorrigible convictions. A delusion coming on suddenly, not prompted by any hallucination or previous delusion, nor related in any obvious way to the patient's mood, is called a "primary delusion" and is highly suggestive of schizophrenia. Many other schizophrenic experiences are of delusional form, but have such individual characteristics that they have been named for themselves.

Common schizophrenic symptoms are the so-called passivity experiences or delusions of bodily control. The patient feels as though he were under the control of some outside force or power making him behave as an automaton without a will of his own. He may feel hypnotized and feel forced to make particular movements, speak with a special voice, or walk to certain areas. The patient may believe these feelings come to him as penetrating waves from electronic or telephonic equipment.

The schizophrenic patient may experience changes in his thinking. Particularly he may feel that his thoughts are disrupted by some outside agency, that his thoughts are withdrawn from his mind, or that other thoughts are inserted into it. He may believe that people can hear his thoughts, which are leaving his mind as waves broadcast to others.

In contrast to these abnormalities of experience are the disturbances in the patient's mode of expression. Particularly noticeable is his abnormal language. Characteristically, he is difficult to understand. His thinking is expressed in a vague and awkward fashion with words poorly chosen and ideas poorly related to one another. Strikingly, the patient makes no effort to correct the vagueness of his thinking or to improve the clarity of his talk. Often, asking a question of the patient, the examiner receives a reply that is off the point and that goes into unnecessary details. Although the questions of the interview seem to start the patient toward a particular answer, it is never reached, but the patient takes up abstract and unnecessary ideas and must be redirected toward his goal. The examiner, laying the responsibility for the confusion on himself, may work to express himself more clearly, and only after considerable effort recognize that the difficulty in communication rests with the odd replies from the patient.

Another prominent disturbance is emotional expression of these patients. They seem distant, unresponsive, and cold. On some occasions the patient's emotional attitude seems incongruous, particularly for the thoughts he is expressing. Thus, he may laugh while saying that he is in mortal danger. This cold or incongruous attitude and manner give the schizophrenic patient his most striking features, and even when at their mildest can be baffling and distressing symptoms to his family.

Other abnormal modes of expression of the schizophrenic patient are disturbances in stance and mobility called catatonic symptoms. Gestures may seem stiff, slow, and mannered. Some schizophrenic patients make repetitive movements or facial grimaces. Others may become totally immobile and mute. Still others may assume unnatural postures and hold them for long periods.

During the active phases of the schizophrenic illness the flamboyant subjective experiences are most prominent. During the chronic phase of schizophrenic illness expressive disturbances in thought and emotion are more evident, varying from mild to severe. Although at times some patients seem free of residual symptoms, usually a careful examination will reveal mild disturbances in thinking and emotional responsiveness.

Diagnosis. The diagnosis of schizophrenia rests on recognition of the distinctive clinical symptoms of this disorder and the exclusion of other conditions which may produce similar symptoms.

Many disorders of brain function can imitate schizophrenic symptoms; but with the exception of the three schizophrenia-like disorders to be discussed, the other brain disturbances also manifest disturbed consciousness, disorientation, and disruption of cognitive abilities, particularly recent memory function, that are not found in schizophrenia.

Mania or depression can be confused with schizophrenia (to the considerable embarrassment of the diagnostician when the patient recovers completely on receiving the treatment appropriate for these conditions). A source of difficulty is the occurrence of delusions, which are common enough but usually spring directly from the attitudes of self-confidence or self-blame that are so prominent in mania or depression.

In schizophrenia disturbances in experience, including the auditory hallucinations and delusions just described, form the most secure basis for diagnosis. Thus, in a person free of brain disease or drug intoxication, recognition of formed auditory hallucinations, primary delusional experiences, passivity experiences, or disturbances in "thought control" permit the diagnosis of schizophrenia to be made with some confidence.

If these symptoms cannot be found, then diagnosis must rest upon recognition of manifest disturbances in thought and emotional expression. It should be pointed out, however, that opinion holding a person's thought to be illogical and vague, or his affective responses to be inadequate or incongruous, is an evaluative judgment and must be held with somewhat less confidence than opinion resting on recognition of delusions and hallucinations.

Catatonic symptoms of immobility, posturing, and grimacing, along with the disturbances in behavior described as negativism or reluctance to cooperate, must be carefully interpreted. Only in those patients in whom no evidence of a prominent mood change can be found should a diagnosis of schizophrenia be made. Motility changes in the direction of psychomotor retardation are prominent features of depressive disorder, a condition as common as schizophrenia and more common than the catatonic variety of schizophrenia. As a rule of thumb, it can be stated that four of five patients who have psychomotor retardation as a prominent symptom suffer from depression.

Symptoms of emotional unrest, anxiety, withdrawal, hostility, and hyperactivity can be found in schizophrenic patients, but these are common to many other psychiatric disorders, and therefore can never form the basis for a secure diagnosis of schizophrenia. However, that diagnosis is rendered more likely if it can be established that the patient was developing normally without an apparently vulnerable personality, and if these symptoms appeared without a change in the patient's mood or the pattern of his life. Karl Jaspers made this important point first when he pointed out the distinction between a paranoid illness disrupting a life course without obvious predispositions and the development of jealousy and suspiciousness in an individual who had always been insecure, sensitive, and irritable. Since these more general symptoms can be found in both schizophrenia and many other psychiatric disturbances, it is important to search carefully for the more basic symptoms of hallucinations and delusions from which emotional unrest and unpredictable behavior may stem. Often repeated efforts are required to gain cooperation of the patient so that he will divulge the existence of those basic symptoms that make a diagnosis of schizophrenia certain.

Etiology. There is no neuropathology or consistent pathophysiology that can be observed to develop with the progress of the disorder and that might give some hint of causation. An approach to a consideration of etiology has to be more circuitous and the opinions derived held with somewhat less assurance than is true of other clinical entities. Two aspects of etiology can be conveniently separated for the purpose of organizing the information we have. One aspect is "causes proper," that is, the apparent prerequisite elements needed to set in motion a train of events leading to the symptoms defining the entity. The other is "mediation," that is, the particular nature of the train of events, be they psychologic, neurologic, or biochemical, that lead to the symptoms. For schizophrenia there is some information relating to "causes proper" and also to "mediation," but it is far from conclusive.

"Causes Proper" or Prerequisite Elements in Schizophrenia. The genetic constitution has been decisively demonstrated to be one of the "causes proper" in schizophrenia. The risk of schizophrenia increases with the closeness of blood relationship to a schizophrenic patient. Thus only 1 per cent of very distant relatives of a schizophrenic patient will themselves suffer from the disorder. This is no higher than the risk in the general population. But 5 to 6 per cent of siblings and 40 to 50 per cent of monozygotic twins of schizophrenic patients will have schizophrenia.

The possible objection that these data merely reflect the increasingly common environment of progressively closer relatives has been refuted by observations on monozygotic twins brought up apart who continue to show an identical high risk. Heston made the same point in a different fashion by studying a group of offspring of schizophrenic mothers. These particular children were raised from earliest infancy in foster homes by normal, nonschizophrenic mothers and fathers. The incidence of schizophrenia in these children was exactly the same as that reported for children raised by a schizophrenic parent. They thus resembled their biologic mother although reared apart from her.

It has nevertheless been impossible to fit schizophrenia into a clear mendelian pattern of dominant or recessive inheritance. Some students of the disease would describe the hereditary contribution to schizophrenia as polygenic, i.e., the sum of a number of contributions from the genes no one of which is solely responsible. The polygenic concept might permit environmental factors to play a larger role in causation. Thus a mild genetic vulnerability might express itself in a schizophrenic phenotype only in those who face stressful environments, whereas those carrying a more severe genetic vulnerability might show the disorder in any environment. It is difficult at the moment to propose a test that would exclude a polygenic hypothesis as a possibility.

Some studies that have established a genetic contribution to the etiology of schizophrenia have also given evidence of the inadequacy of genetics as a sufficient cause for the disorder. That 50 per cent of monozygotic twins of schizophrenic patients are free of this illness means one of the following: (1) Although the genetic constitution is necessary and sufficient to produce schizophrenia, the symptoms employed to define a case fail to provide an adequate means of recognizing all examples of the disorder, and 50 per cent are mistakenly called normal. (2) The defining symptoms encompass a mixed group of disorders, and in only 50 per cent of these disorders are genetic features necessary and sufficient causes for the symptoms. (3) A genetic vulnerability for schizophrenia is necessary but not sufficient. It must be combined with certain life experiences that need not be common for genetically identical individuals.

The present inadequacy of the genetic hypothesis to provide a complete description of the "causes proper" for schizophrenia reinforces a search for environmental and experiential causes. It has proved just as difficult to determine an environmental contribution as to define the genetic contribution. Thus the experiences of being raised by a cold and distant mother, or of receiving insistent, simultaneous, but incompatible directions from the parents, or of simply living in a disharmonious family incapable of providing a healthy environment for psychologic growth have all been considered causes of schizophrenia.

Such disturbed experiences have been found in the lives of schizophrenic patients when viewed retrospectively after the onset of the illness. But none has proved to be a common experience in all schizophrenic people. Nor has it been possible to predict an increased incidence of schizophrenia among other individuals living in comparably disturbed situations. Presently the most economical view of the role of life experiences in the "causes proper" of schizophrenia holds that *any* adversity, be it a psychologic shock, abnormality in critical relationships, or physical injury, may provide a partial contribution to the causes of schizophrenia, but that any given adversity must be acting upon a genetically vulnerable individual.

Mediation of the Schizophrenic Syndrome. This is the other aspect of etiology. Given that some combination of genetic and environmental attributes may be needed to produce this illness, how does this mediate its development? Does it do so by altering some psychological capacity or by producing some particular change in the nervous system, or still more remotely by altering some vital chemistry of the body that itself can act on the brain? There have been proposals for each of these mediations.

Many distinguished psychiatric studies have proposed that the mediation of the disturbance has been through the production of a particular psychologic change fundamental to the whole syndrome and from which all the symptoms can be explained. Thus Federn has proposed a "loosening of ego boundaries" as the essential feature mediating this illness, whereas Bleuler proposed a basic disturbance in associational thinking. A crisis of identity has been proposed by exponents of existential psychiatry. These views have a ring of plausibility perhaps derived from their resemblance to experiences common to all men, part of which can seem to be reflected in the behavior of schizophrenic patients. But they depend on concepts that are difficult to define except in terms of what they purport to explain.

Other psychiatric studies have attempted to demonstrate the possibility that the mediation of the causal formula is through some change in the central nervous system. The main problem for this approach lies in our ignorance of the physiology of that part of the nervous system related to emotional life. How then to explain the way the brain might be disturbed to produce schizophrenia, a clinical condition without a known pathologic substrate? A promising approach has been derived from the recognition that there are certain brain disorders that can produce a *"schizophrenia-like syndrome."* A consideration of the common features of the mediation of these conditions might shed light on the mediation of "true" schizophrenia.

Three well documented conditions affecting the brain can give rise to a mental disturbance resembling schizophrenia. The most familiar is the syndrome found with *amphetamine intoxication*. In this condition the patient is alert and oriented but preoccupied by auditory hallucinations and delusional ideas indistinguishable from those seen in schizophrenia. The disturbance may last from several days to a few weeks, but disappears eventually after the withdrawal of the stimulant.

Slater, Beard, and Glithero have demonstrated that among patients suffering from *psychomotor epilepsy,* caused by an irritative lesion in the limbic portions of the temporal lobe, a certain number develop a paranoid schizophrenia-like syndrome after 10 to 15 years of epilepsy. This condition displays all the classic delusional and hallucinatory symptoms of schizophrenia, but there is less tendency toward deterioration of thinking and personality.

Finally, certain patients, *withdrawing from excessive alcohol ingestion,* suffer from a period of auditory hallucinations. Although in most of these patients the hallucinatory experience clears within 24 to 48 hours, in a small proportion a chronic condition of persisting auditory hallucinations associated with delusional beliefs, incongruous affect, and disturbed thought develops. This chronic condition may be indistinguishable from the schizophrenic syndrome, and may persist for many years.

For all these schizophrenia-like conditions the possibility exists that the pertinent features might be the expression of a latent predisposition for schizophrenia in the affected individuals. This would reduce the value of these disorders as models for the possible mediation of the causal elements of schizophrenia. However, study of many of these individuals and their families failed to demonstrate an increased incidence of schizophrenic illness among the relatives; nor were schizoid traits found in the premorbid personalities of these subjects. This is fair evidence that they are not schizophrenic but have their symptoms because of the particular mediating conditions.

The common theme to these disorders is some extraexcitatory arousal of the brain, particularly of the reticular formation and limbic system, either directly via amphetamine or epileptic discharge or in rebound from long-continuing action of the depressant ethanol. It may be that the condition of schizophrenia itself is thus produced by some stimulatory action on these same regions

evoked by the genetic-environmental "causes proper" discussed above.

A third possible mediation of the "causes proper" in producing schizophrenia is through some change in body metabolism or chemistry that could itself alter cerebral and psychologic functions. Many students have been prompted to consider this alternative because of the remarkable growth in biochemical methodology. In fact the difficulties in establishing a role for biochemistry in the etiology of schizophrenia rest not with the chemical methodology but with such issues as defining the group being studied, avoiding chemical artifacts related to dietary habits or medications given chronically hospitalized people, and deciding what biochemical change to look for with little knowledge of what kinds of change might be instrumental in the symptoms. The papers of Kety should be consulted for a more thorough discussion of these difficulties.

Gjessing, in a work that is a model of its kind, was able to demonstrate a consistent relationship between a biochemical change, i.e., nitrogen balance, and one form of schizophrenic illness, periodic catatonia. Crucial to his study was his ability to isolate this homogeneous group of patients from other schizophrenic patients. Gjessing demonstrated that the phasic catatonic disturbances are associated with a phasic change in the total nitrogen balance of the body. That it is not a trivial relationship is suggested by his demonstration that protein restriction and thyroid medication interfering with the cyclical nitrogen changes also lengthen the interval between attacks of the illness.

Another study in the realm of biochemical mediation of schizophrenia sprang from a hypothesis on the action of a chemical on the brain. Hoffer and Smythies observed that the hallucinogenic drug mescaline has a chemical structure that resembles epinephrine. They proposed that the genetic predisposition for schizophrenia expressed itself in an abnormal metabolic path for epinephrine, so that a toxic agent similar to mescaline was produced when epinephrine was metabolized. Since epinephrine is released in excess during such stressful states as fright, this hypothesis proposed that the extra accumulation of the toxic metabolite could explain the precipitation of schizophrenia by a period of emotional distress. Intriguing as this hypothesis was, it has been impossible to demonstrate increased quantities of an abnormal metabolite of epinephrine in the circulation of schizophrenic individuals. In fact, biochemical investigations demonstrated that methylation of epinephrine, the means proposed for the production of the toxic product, was the normal and usual pathway for the metabolic inactivation of epinephrine.

This blow to the hypothesis was not decisive, since excessive methylation of epinephrine could be occurring in schizophrenic patients. In order to test this possibility Kety gave the methyl donor, methionine, to schizophrenic patients, which seemed to worsen the symptoms in some of them. This was the first example of a biochemical hypothesis generating a particular test and leading to the predicted results in schizophrenia. The observations have been duplicated by other workers. The crucial issue is how methionine can alter brain function to produce further symptoms. Does its action fall specifically on the reticular activating system and limbic regions that from the schizophrenia-like syndromes appeared important for schizophrenic activation? As yet we do not know.

Treatment. The treatment for any schizophrenic patient is complex and should not be attempted by the inexperienced. A period of hospitalization will usually be required. There a program to include drug therapy, psychologic treatment, and social evaluation can be planned.

The sheet anchor of treatment now for schizophrenia is the *phenothiazine* drugs, discovered in the 1950's almost by accident. To date there is no good explanation for their effectiveness. Clearly they are not simply acting by virtue of their sedative effect, since their remarkable action is not mimicked by other sedatives. They can remove the symptoms of schizophrenia, including the delusions, hallucinations, and disordered thought, and are not restricted to relieving excitement or anxiety as the term tranquilizer might imply.

The most versatile phenothiazine preparation is the original, chlorpromazine, effective in amounts from 200 to 1000 mg. per day. Usually 300 to 400 mg. is an effective range, although at first larger amounts may be needed. A maintenance dosage of 200 to 300 mg. per day should be continued indefinitely for every patient who has had a diagnosis of schizophrenia, since cessation of treatment results in the reappearance of symptoms in 60 to 70 per cent of patients within six months.

The *psychotherapy* suitable for the schizophrenic patient has been a subject of intense controversy. The more radical approaches based on psychologic and particularly psychoanalytic views of the genesis of schizophrenia have not achieved their optimistic goals of curing the patient by relieving some basic psychologic conflict. More modest psychotherapy is indispensable when it is intended to help the patient in his everyday affairs, taking advantage of those personal assets that persist despite his illness, and establishing a relationship of friendly rapport in order to guide him in his management of personal and social issues, which, if mishandled, can lead to distress and further illness. A particularly pressing issue for the schizophrenic patient is the social situation into which he is placed after hospitalization. His psychiatrist, usually at first with the help of a psychiatric social worker, must strive to find a job that is regular and well within the patient's power but not excessively challenging, a domestic arrangement that is calm and supportive but not too emotionally demanding, and a daily routine that combats the tendency to withdraw from all social contacts into an isolated and perhaps fantasy-ridden existence. To accomplish these goals is one of the most challenging exercises in medical treatment. The growth of "halfway houses" as residences for previously hospitalized schizophrenic patients has been prompted by recognition of the need for stable and structured social environments for schizophrenic patients once they have improved enough to leave the hospital.

Prognosis. Prognosis for any patient diagnosed as schizophrenic is always guarded. Before the advent of pharmacologic treatment only 20 to 25 per cent of patients could be expected to recover completely from an attack of schizophrenia, and such patients were always vulnerable to further difficulties later. The other 75 per cent did not recover completely, 50 per cent showing residual signs from mild to severe, and 25 per cent becoming severely and chronically deteriorated in thought and mood. The phenothiazines have considerably reduced the morbidity in schizophrenic patients, but the exact degree is not clear.

Certain features carry a rather good prognosis. Thus, if a patient had an apparently normal personality prior to the illness, his prognosis is better than one with a schizoid personality. If the illness came on acutely and dramatically, prognosis is better than if the illness began insidiously. If catatonic features are prominent, the prognosis is better than if disturbances in thinking and affect are the more prominent symptoms. Finally, if the patient has a family history not of schizophrenic illness but of a manic-depressive illness, or if his particular attack has prominent depressive or manic symptoms, his prognosis is better than that for individuals without these features.

Connell, P. H.: Amphetamine Psychosis. Maudsley Monographs, No. 5. London, Chapman and Hall, Ltd., 1958.

Fish, F. J.: Schizophrenia. Bristol, John Wright & Sons, 1962.

Heston, L. L.: Psychiatric disorders in foster home reared children of schizophrenic mothers. Brit. J. Psychiat., 112:819, 1966.

Kety, S. S.: Biochemical theories of schizophrenia, I and II. Science, 129:1528, 1590, 1959, 1969.

Klein, D. F., and Davis, J. M.: Diagnosis and Drug Treatment of Psychiatric Disorders. Baltimore, Williams and Wilkins Company, 1969.

Schneider, K.: Clinical Psychopathology. Translated by M. W. Hamilton. New York, Grune & Stratton, Inc., 1959.

Shields, J.: The Genetics of schizophrenia in historical context. In Coppen, A. J., and Walk, A. (eds.): Recent Developments in Schizophrenia. Brit. J. Psychiat., Special Publication No. 1, pp. 25-41, Ashford Kent, 1968.

Slater, E., Beard, A. W., and Glithero, E.: The schizophrenia-like psychoses of epilepsy. Brit. J. Psychiat., 109:95, 1963.

Victor, M., and Hope, J. M.: The phenomenon of auditory hallucinations in chronic alcoholism. J. Nerv. Ment. Dis., 126:451, 1958.

MANIC-DEPRESSIVE PSYCHOSIS

The essential feature of this psychosis is an excessive disturbance of mood and self-appraisal from which its other mental symptoms seem to arise. This disturbance can be in the direction of elation and self-confidence or sadness and self-blame. The course tends to be unpredictable, remitting, and relapsing, with attacks of elation (mania) or sadness (depression) interspersed with periods of apparent mental health varying in length from weeks to years. Individual patients may suffer attacks of only one kind throughout their lifetime. Single or repetitive attacks of depression seem to be the most common manifestation, but attacks alternately manic and then depressive or even repetitively manic are not unusual.

Clinical Manifestations. *Depression.* During an attack of depression the patient complains of feeling miserable and uncertain of himself. He may give evidence of his sadness by a dejected appearance and by restlessness and distractibility. Some patients are slowed in their activity, and this can progress to a psychomotor retardation of such severity that the patient seems totally unresponsive.

Mental examination of the depressed patient usually brings to light not only his feelings of sadness or misery but also an attitude of poor self-regard that can vary in intensity from feelings of inadequacy and incompetence to convictions of personal worthlessness, blameworthiness, and evil. This combination of depressed mood with self-despising blameworthiness is the diagnostic sign of this condition. It will also explain most of the other symptoms, modes of behavior, and dangers faced by the depressed patient.

Other symptoms include delusional extrapolations of the attitudes of self-blame. These can increase to a belief that the patient's guilt is notorious, that he is to be arrested, and that he will be condemned to die or to suffer some extraordinary punishment either in this world or the next. Suspiciousness and fear of mistreatment based on these delusional beliefs may be difficult to distinguish from similar attitudes in the paranoid schizophrenic patient. A useful if not cast-iron distinction is the depressive's belief that the suspected ill treatment comes as a justified punishment and not, as with the schizophrenic, as an undeserved persecution.

In some severely depressed patients delusional ideas can become bizarre and even grandiose in concept. Thus they come to believe that they have been the cause of cosmic disasters, that the sun is darkened by them, that whole cities have been deserted because of their presence, or that they and their progeny are accursed in the sight of the Divinity. Delusions of bodily change may take the form that their brains are rotting, their bowels totally blocked, or their bones fractured and dislocated.

Delusional ideas may concern the relationship of the patient to the world and to others. He may believe that he has lost all his money, that he has become a burden to others, that he is universally despised, or even that he gives off such a bad odor that people cannot stand his presence. Again, the beliefs even in these far-fetched delusional examples are usually reflective of the patient's inner attitude of self-blame, self-contempt, and hopelessness.

The point about these opinions is that they are delusional and not just false. They are unshakable opinions held in the face of all contrary evidence. Only treatment of the depressive disorder will remove them.

The most worrisome symptom of the depressed patient is *inclination to suicide*. It is easily appreciated that attitudes of such hopelessness and despair as have been described could prompt self-destruction. But it is not necessary to have such exaggerated delusions for suicide to be a distinct risk. Vigilance for suicidal intentions must be maintained throughout the course of the depressive disturbance. There is nothing to prevent a physician's asking any depressed patient about thoughts of self-injury. Often this simple action will reveal both the severity of the mood disturbance and the need to bring the patient into hospital for his own protection.

Homicide is also a possibility for the depressed patient, and is particularly likely in those who harbor beliefs that their family shares in their guilt and accursed characteristics. Any suggestions by the patient that he might prefer death should be most seriously believed.

Along with these psychologic symptoms the depressed patient will often suffer from disturbances in his sleep, particularly waking early in the morning and being unable to return to sleep. Other physical disturbances include bodily aches and pains, loss of appetite, constipation, and weight loss. These features may combine with the retardation to give the appearance of chronic physical ill health. In fact, many depressed patients will first consult internists complaining of such physical symptoms. Helpful to the differentiation of the patient whose somatic symptoms are part of a depressive illness is a discovery of the features of depressed mood, and attitudes of self-blame or hopelessness when these features are combined with complaints of poorly localized pains, with loss of appetite or weight loss, or even with preoccupations about the state of the inner organs.

Mania. Symptoms that are almost the exact opposite of those seen during an attack of depression appear during an attack of mania. Now the patient says that he is in excellent spirits, that he feels well, and in fact has never felt better. He is active and restless, and appears energetic, confident, and quick-witted. These characteristics tend to worsen, and it is in their more extreme form that they become recognized as symptoms. The restlessness and energy become overactivity, with the patient moving constantly and planning progressively less plausible projects. His speech becomes incessant, rapid, and disjointed, one idea following another with little connection between them. His attitude of confidence is that of grandiose self-satisfaction. He may be overbearing and pompous. He often will be irritated by his surroundings, easy to anger, and perhaps suspicious that the efforts being made to control him are unjust.

Although a manic patient can usually be recognized by his overactivity, ebullience, and great self-confidence, he can develop as well ideas of resentment and feelings that he is being in some way unfairly noticed or persecuted. These ideas, on investigation, are found to derive from his own delusional opinion that he is so important that he must be under scrutiny by forces such as foreign powers. Occasionally, these persecutory ideas are so prominent that a diagnosis of schizophrenia is entertained. It is, however, the direct connection of these ideas to the attitude of self-confidence that allows a diagnosis of mania to be made.

With the mental changes manic patients exhibit disturbed social behavior. They may have increased sexual interest and may become promiscuous. They tend to overspend and be reckless with money. They may insult their employers and so be fired from their jobs. In the first attack of mania and before the severe restlessness and disorganization of thought appear, these activities may not be recognized as the products of mental illness, but may be construed as actions for which the patient can be held accountable. Thus the patient can be subjected to severe losses, to legal actions, or to moral criticism that can hamper his life long after his manic attack is over. To protect him from these consequences hospitalization of the manic patient may be required.

Etiology. "Causes Proper" or Prerequisite Elements in Manic-Depressive Disorder. As with schizophrenia, an important genetic contribution to the etiology of the manic-depressive disorder seems certain. As with schizophrenia, there is a progressive frequency of incidence with increasing blood relatedness so that with monozygotic twins the concordance rate is over 50 per cent. It is likely that genetic constitution is a necessary but not sufficient cause for this disorder. Certain other features of the illness require consideration. First, the illness does appear in attacks interspersed with periods in which the person appears to be normal. Second, the attacks are somewhat seasonal, appearing more frequently in the spring and fall than in summer and winter. Third, although many attacks occur spontaneously, many seem to be precipitated by some disturbing event. Presumably some other elements must combine with the genetic vulnerability to explain these features. Again, the most easily defended position would hold that a necessary cause for manic depressive disorder is the genetic constitution of the patient, but that any of a large number of environmental disturbances can bring out the disorder.

Mediation of Manic-Depressive Disorder. Whatever the prerequisite ingredients of the manic-depressive disorder, much recent interest has been found in the possible neuronal changes that might produce these symptoms. A major source of relevant observations has been supplied by the response of depressed patients to certain classes of pharmacologic agents. Monoamine oxidase inhibitors and the tricyclic compounds of which imipramine is the prototype are effective antidepressant medications. These drugs affect the metabolism of biogenic amines in the brain, particularly norepinephrine and serotonin. Hence comes the hypothesis that depression results from an inadequate amount of norepinephrine at active synaptic sites in the brain. This hypothesis is overly specific in its exclusive consideration of norepinephrine as the responsible chemical.

Treatment. The first rule in managing either manic or depressed patients is that most of them should be in hospital. Their conditions can bring catastrophe to themselves and their families in the form of financial mismanagement in mania and suicide in depression. If these diagnoses are strongly suspected, then psychiatric opinion should be immediately sought so as to determine whether hospitalization should be imposed. It is critical to have expert help, because the patient can often hide the severity of the disorder in a mass of explanations which may appear quite plausible.

It is crucial to diagnose these patients and separate them from those with other conditions, because new drug treatments have proved effective for them and are specific to the affective disorders. Two classes of pharmacologic agents are effective in *depression*. Seemingly more effective are the so-called *tricyclic antidepressants,* the prototype of which is imipramine. This drug, given in doses of from 75 to 200 mg. per day, has been helpful in treatment of 50 per cent of depressive patients. If it is ineffective, the logical practice should be to switch to the other class, which includes the drugs that have as their primary action the capacity to inhibit the enzyme monoamine oxidase. These drugs, in doses of 45 to 75 mg. per day, have also proved useful in depression.

If *monoamine oxidase inhibitors* are used, the patient must be warned to avoid foodstuffs such as cheese, broad beans, and some yeast extracts, which have pressor amines of the phenyl-ethylamine group that includes tyramine. If absorbed by patients whose monoamine oxidase enzyme is depleted, they can cause sudden elevation of blood pressure with headache, blurred vision, and even cerebrovascular hemorrhage.

The mainstay of treatment for severe depression is *electroconvulsive treatment* (ECT). In contrast to the drugs which relieve the symptoms of depression, ECT will terminate an attack of depression usually in four to eight treatments. This treatment can produce the most dramatic and quick recovery from the depths of a life-threatening depression, and should not be withheld too long from a seriously depressed patient while drug treatments are being attempted.

The *treatment of mania* is often very difficult, particularly if the patient is suspicious about medicines. Haloperidol in doses of 1 to 4 mg. thrice daily taken orally has proved effective. This compound is liable to produce severe extrapyramidal side effects which can be combated with antiparkinsonian drugs and with Benadryl, 50 mg. three times daily.

A recent and effective measure for controlling

mania has been the use of lithium ion in the form of lithium carbonate. This compound is available in 250 mg. tablets. Dosage of 500 mg. to 1000 mg. per day can relieve manic excitement. It is, however, essential to follow plasma lithium concentration in these patients, because toxic signs of disorientation, tremor, anorexia, and diarrhea can appear if plasma lithium concentration rises above 2 mEq. per liter.

Prognosis. The prognosis for a single attack of mania or depression is excellent. Even without treatment patients tend to recover completely within six months. With drug treatment the medication can be withdrawn after six months with fair assurance that symptoms will not recur at this time.

The longer-range prognosis is not so favorable. Eighty per cent of people who have suffered one attack of affective disturbance will have another at some time in their lives, but this may not be for many years. Some patients, however, will have recurrent attacks of mania or depression interrupted by only brief intervals of normal behavior.

The best advice to give patients who have suffered from their first affective attack is that they will very likely be quite well for years, but that they and their family should be considered aware that their mood changes are to be considered seriously, and they should seek psychiatric attention promptly if such a mood change tends to persist or worsen.

Astrup, C., Fossum, A., and Holmboe, R.: A follow-up study of 270 patients with acute affective psychoses. Acta Psychiat. Scand. (Suppl. 135), 1959.

Lewis, A.: Melancholia. J. Ment. Sci., 80:277, 1934.

Schildkraut, J. J.: The catecholamine hypothesis of affective disorders: A review of supporting evidence. Amer. J. Psychiat. 122:509, 1965.

PERSONALITY DISORDERS AND NEUROTIC SYMPTOMS

GENERAL CONSIDERATIONS

When considering the issues of personality disorder and neurotic symptoms, a physician is often without a secure conceptual foundation. He may recognize that the concept of disease is not useful here, because for personalities the distinction of abnormal from normal seems arbitrary, and he may notice that the term "neurosis" refers not to disease entities but to symptoms that are qualitatively similar to the emotional responses of all people to many circumstances. His manuals of classification demand that he place patients into "personality types," but the concept of "types" ignores the graded character of human variation. The interpretations of neurotic symptoms offered to him are usually limited to explanations derived

from the instincts of sexuality and aggression, but such neurotic symptoms as anxiety or depression can appear in many circumstances unrelated to sexual or aggressive activities. To help him with these issues, several emotional disturbances seen in patients will be considered in this article. A conceptual approach will be provided that is generally applicable and that can offer a rational basis for treatment.

Personality disorders and neurotic symptoms indicate modes of human behavior expressed in terms of potential and response. Personality is the potential. It describes the abiding and distinctive traits or tendencies of an individual to react to circumstances in a particular fashion. Thus by optimistic personality is meant an individual who will tend to respond with confidence and optimism in situations in which others would be less likely to do so.

A comparison with others is implicit in personality description. Thus each trait of personality is a dimension along which humans vary probably in much the same fashion that they vary in other characteristics, such as height or intelligence. An individual's personality is the sum of numerous traits. For each trait an individual has a place along its range of variation. An individual can be said to have a disorder of personality if he deviates to such an extreme from the norm along the range of variation for that trait that he is prone to show distressing symptoms in circumstances in which others do not.

Circumstances are also implied in the term personality. Life situations, both external and internal, are always changing. Personality describes how a person will tend to respond to situations; personality disorder implies that he may be vulnerable to disruptive emotional behavior. The disorders of personality are but potentials and may never produce symptoms if the particular circumstances do not appear. Thus paranoid personality describes individuals who tend to show attitudes of suspiciousness and feelings of persecution in settings so minimally threatening that they will seldom provoke such attitudes in others. If the settings of their lives are relatively free from threatening features, these feelings will be diminished.

Whereas personality indicates potential, neurotic symptoms are emotional *responses* displayed when an individual is troubled by environmental circumstances. In everyone certain environments are conducive to anxiety, others to depression, and still others to suspiciousness. People with the personality potential to respond with particular neurotic symptoms are provoked by less extreme circumstances and less specific stimuli. Thus to comprehend and to manage a patient with neurotic symptoms it is necessary to gather information on his personal potentials and his past and present environment. It is usually easy to find this information. The patient can tell some of the facts of his past history and present concerns when his physical and his mental states are evaluated. His relatives can describe his previous personality, habitual ways of responding, and more recent changes in his behavior. A social worker can confirm these and discover additional facts from other acquaintances and employers, or by visiting the patient's home. Once known, an appraisal of these provoking elements is facilitated by organizing them into predisposing factors and precipitating factors, and considering the roles of these factors in the cause and formation of the particular emotional disturbance.

Predisposing Factors. Predisposing factors are those features special to an individual that make him vulnerable to an emotional disturbance or liable to react in a disturbed way to experiences that other men would find less troublesome.

First among the predisposing factors is the state of health, particularly the health of the central nervous system. Any physical illness or even severe fatigue interferes with a person's powers of analysis and integration and predisposes toward exaggerated and inappropriate emotional responses. Next are qualities of a patient's personality: his temperament, habitual responses, and special views. Personality develops from the hereditary genetic constitution, the intellectual endowment, and the lifetime experiences of the individual, and each of these is a predisposing factor in itself. Predisposing factors often overlooked are the patient's social status and cultural situation that derive from his race, social class, age, sex, and occupation. A young physician, coming from a comfortable, middle class background, may fail to appreciate the special experiences and vulnerabilities to emotional disturbance that poverty, racial discrimination, and cultural isolation bring to his patients. The scholarly study of Dr. Beatrice Berle, *80 Puerto Rican Families in New York City*, the more general *Beyond the Melting Pot* by Nathan Glazer and D. P. Moynihan, and the investigations of Dr. Robert Coles can be recommended for vivid descriptions of these predispositions.

Precipitating Factors. Precipitating factors are those events or experiences that have more immediately disturbed the emotional equilibrium and aroused the disturbed behavior.

Physical illness may precipitate a psychologic disturbance, either through the suffering produced or by its threatening implications to future happiness and success. Emotional conflict is a frequent precipitating factor, and can arise from hated but required activities or jobs that demand a high standard of performance close to the limits of a person's abilities. Some psychologic precipitants are more recondite, as they depend on a symbolic meaning that derives from attitudes of guilt and resentment developed in the past life of the patient. Before emphasizing these more abstruse psychologic precipitants, however, it is usually valuable for a physician to consider more proximate and obvious ones.

The factors of *predisposition* and *precipitation* must finally be assessed for their relative importance and particular contribution in any given emotional disturbance. Since an apparently similar experience may produce an anxiety state in one person, a depressive reaction in another, and a hysterical response in a third, any emotional disturbance can be comprehended as a meaningful reaction only when the individual elements of predisposition and precipitation are properly weighed, arranged in some hierarchy of importance, and their interactions considered.

A helpful distinction, discussed by Birnbaum, should always be made between those elements termed pathogenic that seem to be essential to the production of symptoms and those features termed pathoplastic that may provide form and some content to the reaction. Thus the adolescent may exhibit rudeness and aggressiveness in circumstances in which an older person would show fearfulness and insecurity.

Treatment is considerably easier to plan when an attempt is made to collect and study the predisposing and precipitating factors in the fashion suggested. Ideally, the aim of any treatment is to remove the cause of the disturbance. Thus, an attack on the major pathogenic elements is usually more appealing than one on the pathoplastic. Sometimes such a relatively simple measure as a clear explanation of his symptoms to a sick patient may relieve an anxiety aroused by symptoms that he has misconstrued as more serious than they are. In other patients, however, prolonged consideration of established habits of disturbed emotional response would be necessary in order to remove the cause of symptoms. For a given person, this may or may not be advisable. When the precipitating event is a social or legal problem, its resolution can be facilitated with the help of a social worker.

Often a doctor is defeated in his attempt to remove the primary cause of disturbed behavior. The disturbance may depend on an intractable disorder of personality, upon some incurable somatic illness, or upon social injustices that the physician cannot correct. Nevertheless, by identifying contributory or secondary elements, he can aid such patients by instruction in the avoidance of behavior that aggravates their difficulty. Also, he can appropriately turn to treatments that modify the neurophysiologic mechanisms elaborating emotional symptoms. The new pharmacologic treatments for anxiety or depression are extremely useful in restoring emotional equilibrium, but they are not used often enough for emotionally distressed, physically ill patients.

It can never be overemphasized that a doctor can give considerable help to an emotionally disturbed patient by providing psychologic support and human companionship. To accomplish this, the doctor must understand the somatic, psychologic, and social aspects of his patient's difficulties and must show a willingness to spend some unhurried time listening. He is then prepared to do everything possible to help or, at the very least, to bring vital comfort to his patient by sharing in some of the distress when nothing more can be done.

With this approach in mind, we shall now

consider three specific psychologic disturbances in detail: *anxiety,* because it is common; *depression,* because it is so frequently distressing for doctors to witness; and *hysteria,* because it is so problematic.

ANXIETY

Definition. Anxiety is an unpleasant mood of tension and apprehension. It is fear's first cousin and, like fear, has prominent autonomic effects when severe. But fear is an emotion sharply focused on immediate dangers, whereas anxiety is usually imposed by the anticipation of future danger, distress, or difficulties. As an emotional response common to all men, anxiety is useful. Activities that arouse it are avoided and those that diminish it are sustained. Although anxiety may spur people to perform difficult tasks skillfully and admirably, when excessive it is a hindrance, as some well prepared students demonstrate when facing a critical examination. *Anxiety is a medical problem when it is excessive, inappropriate, or without obvious cause.*

Predisposing and Precipitating Factors. Anxiety is the psychologic response to anticipated troubles, real or imagined, dimly or accurately perceived. But men and troubles vary. Some persons, the timid, the inexperienced, the excessively conscientious, are frequently anxious over trivia. Other men seem unaffected by the same experiences. Most people are at least mildly anxious whenever they seek medical advice, and when threatening dangers are intense or prolonged, as in chronic painful illness or in battle, even the most resistant individuals can develop incapacitating anxiety.

Resistance to anxiety varies with physical condition. When tired, sick, or injured, people are more easily threatened than when fresh. Also, they are more vulnerable to anxiety when their powers of analysis and discrimination are failing or underdeveloped. Thus, because of inadequate comprehension or imprecise perception, the immature, the elderly, or the person with brain damage may become anxious in situations in which a person with a healthy, mature brain is comfortable. In fact, one of the first indications of a beginning dementia can be an attack of severe anxiety without obvious provocation.

Common precipitants of anxiety in daily life are circumstances of conflict in which an action is demanded but the correct action may be difficult to discern. Thus, a person may be anxious over difficult decisions on which rest his economic and social success or because the decisions produce an unpredictable response in an inconsistent superior. Laboratory models for this kind of situation and its effects on the emotional state have been easy to produce. Pavlov trained dogs to respond to the picture of a circle by rewarding such responses with food. He did not reward responses to an ellipse. Then, by simply compressing the ellipse so that it gradually approached a circle in shape, he made the discrimination progressively more difficult. The emotional response of these dogs was remarkable. They became ferocious and violent when put into harness for the experiment. They tore at their restraints, barked uncontrollably, and refused to attempt the discrimination. In this state, not only did they make many mistakes, but they became unable to make discriminations that had previously been easy. It is not difficult to see analogies in both situation and behavior between Pavlov's dogs and men with emotional conflicts.

An emotional state of anxiety can be produced in other ways than as an understandable response to anticipated difficulties. An intractable anxiety state can follow a severe head injury as one of the symptoms of the so-called *post-concussional syndrome.* Similarly, a mood of tension and agitation with tremulousness can occur in the delirious states, such as those that follow withdrawal of alcohol or barbiturates and are sometimes produced by the hallucinogenic drugs such as LSD-25. In these situations, it may be disturbed perceptions and misinterpretations that arouse anxiety, but often the anxiety is independent of anything that the patient definitely experiences or understands. Roth describes a peculiar and chronic anxiety state that can follow a calamitous emotional experience. This condition, referred to as the *phobic anxiety syndrome,* occurs in mildly obsessional persons after a severe fright. The disturbance can last for many months. These patients are in a state of considerable anxiety, mostly unformulated, and, associated with this, they have an unwillingness to leave their homes because of vague fears. The peculiar psychologic response of *depersonalization,* which is a change in the awareness of self such that the person feels unreal, is present in many of these patients. In the phobic anxiety syndrome the mood of anxiety follows rather than precedes difficulty, demonstrating that anxiety, normally an anticipatory psychologic response, may take on a self-sustained activity after certain experiences such as severe frights or sudden disasters.

The role of learning and of conditioning has too often been neglected in considerations of anxiety. This probably derived from attempts to explain all anxiety in terms of basic instinctive drives. That a fear-provoking situation could train an individual to experience symptoms of anxiety in circumstances that resembled these situations is very likely, and is indicated by research on emotion in animals. The capacity to develop anxiety via conditioning mechanisms seems the probable explanation for certain cases of phobic anxiety focused on specific objects.

Manifestations of Anxiety. The manifestations of anxiety are divisible into three groups. *First* are the inner feelings of tension, apprehension, and dread that form the anxious mood itself. *Second* are disturbances of the intellectual power of the anxious patient. He is unable to think clearly, to use proper judgment, to learn efficiently, or to remember accurately. *Third* are the autonomic, visceral, and endocrine changes that have been analyzed by Walter B. Cannon and his followers as the constant companions of emotional excitement and particularly of anxiety or fear. These include tremor, tachycardia, hypertension, increased perspiration, dilated pupils, and reduced salivation and gastric secretion. Increased activity of the sympathetic nervous system and of the adrenal medulla mediates the majority of these visceral responses to anxiety.

A model anxiety state is to be seen among front-line soldiers. The infantryman is a prepared subject for anxiety. He is always threatened with death or mutilation. He must go without sleep, remain exposed to the weather, and often be hungry. He is usually unable to understand what is happening around him. He is repeatedly frightened by gun fire and distressed by the death of comrades. If he is exposed long enough, he develops a severe and persisting anxiety state sometimes called "battle fatigue." He becomes tense and easily startled. His judgment is poor, and he cannot efficiently sustain a complex offensive action. Among other physical complaints, he suffers from headache, anorexia, and diarrhea. He is usually convinced that death is imminent. Almost all men develop this condition if exposed to battle long enough. Wolff reports that the average man in the army of the United States reached this point after 85 days of combat; 75 per cent could be expected to break down by combat day 140, and 90 per cent by combat day 210. These figures vary little among nations, although few are willing to publish them. They make the point that, in his resistance to crippling anxiety, even the bravest man has a "breaking point." On reaching it, he does not betray his group or run from the enemy, but rather he becomes less efficient in protecting himself and runs a high risk of death.

The symptoms of anxiety that physicians see in patients are not different. The patients all have the same three groups of symptoms, but, depending in part on the cause, these symptoms can appear as a relatively brief attack or as a more prolonged, chronic disturbance of mood.

Anxiety attacks may be single episodes occurring in response to some acute threat, or may be periods of exacerbation in a chronic state of tension. They are short periods of tension, varying in severity from mild apprehension to severe panic. An anxiety attack can occur at any time. A curiously favored time is when the patient is traveling in a plane or fast train. Most commonly, though, an attack develops at night when, with the disappearance of daytime distractions, a patient begins to ruminate on his troubles. The apprehensions grow to preoccupy his thoughts, and he develops visceral responses to fear. Clear thinking becomes impossible, as does sleep. The heart pounds. A common complaint in an anxiety attack is the sensation of tightness in the chest as though the lungs could not be adequately filled. The patient responds to this sensation by deep and sighing respirations. Sometimes he may

produce in this way a respiratory alkalosis with feelings of giddiness and vertigo, tingling of his fingertips, and even tetany with carpopedal spasm. This is the *hyperventilation syndrome,* and the resulting symptoms may add to anxiety.

Full-blown anxiety attacks have an hysterical flavor and may, in part, depend on personal tendencies to self-dramatization and suggestibility. But they also can be the results of a psychic chain reaction, the initial apprehensions and anxiety stirring up cardiac and respiratory changes that are themselves frightening. Granville-Grossman and Turner have provided more evidence that visceral responses to anxiety can increase the subjective symptoms of anxiety by demonstrating that these latter symptoms are improved when an anxious patient is treated with propranolol, a drug that blocks the adrenergic beta-receptors of the sympathetic nervous system and slows the heart rate.

Chronic anxiety may be punctuated by or may begin with an acute attack, but it may be just a steady and distressingly prolonged disturbance of mood. The symptoms are less intense although not different in quality from those of acute anxiety. The patient is tense and "on edge." He may also report some feelings of sadness or hopelessness along with his anxiety. It can be difficult to differentiate his condition from an agitated depression. His intellectual powers are diminished, and he has considerable difficulty in concentration and in thinking. He will score poorly on intelligence tests, particularly on the performance subtests, just as does a patient with dementia. He will have a number of somatic complaints: frontal or occipital headache, anorexia, diarrhea, and weight loss, among other things. On examination, he may have the physical signs of tension, a fine tremor of the extended arms and brisk tendon reflexes, rapid heart beat, increased blood pressure, and pupillary dilatation. More extensive laboratory studies may reveal other visceral and endocrine disturbances, such as reduced gastric acid secretion or increased adrenocortical activity.

Diagnosis. Usually diagnosis is not difficult. In both acute and chronic anxiety, the patient's major complaint is the distressing emotional state. Associated disturbances in thinking and autonomic function serve to confirm the diagnostic impression. For these patients, the major issue is not the diagnosis of anxiety, but rather the question of why they have become anxious now. This question must be answered from knowledge of the circumstances and personality of the patient.

An occasional patient focuses his complaints on his physical symptoms, such as irregularities in the beat of his heart, the change in bowel habits, weight loss, anorexia, or easy fatigability. From these symptoms a more severe illness such as a hidden malignancy, a chronic infection, or some endocrine disorder like hyperthyroidism or Addison's disease may be suspected. Although these conditions are usually seen to be only remote possibilities, laboratory studies may be required to exclude them. As with all psychologically disturbed patients, laboratory studies should not be delayed or protracted but should be decided upon, and this phase of the examination should be finished as promptly as possible.

Treatment. Treatment will vary with the cause and severity of anxiety. Many mildly anxious patients can be helped by a physician who is willing to listen carefully to their difficulties and offer some support and occasional advice. Most patients with anxiety have this mild type. Their disturbances are transient and are based on some particular problem or self-doubt that has developed acutely and is eventually resolved.

Those with more severe anxiety can be aided by a combination of pharmacologic treatment and repeated compassionate discussions of their troubles. Barbiturates have been the preferred agents for relief of anxiety in the past. However, barbiturates can be addictive, and there is the ever-present danger that they may be used in a suicide attempt by an anxious patient who is also depressed. In several double-blind clinical trials, chlordiazepoxide (Librium) has been found as effective as barbiturates for treating anxiety, and can be recommended. Dosage of 10 mg. three to four times a day is usually effective. Up to 20 to 25 mg. three times daily can be given to severely disturbed patients.

Patients with persisting anxiety can be referred with some confidence to specialists in psychotherapy. The effectiveness of psychotherapy seems to depend on the comfort provided by frequent sympathetic discussions and an increased recognition by the patient of the irrational aspects of his anxiety. The particular school of psychotherapeutic theory subscribed to by the therapist seems less important.

Only the most severely anxious patients need hospitalization and then usually only for an acute attack of anxiety. They are treated best with sedation, and often heavy sedation is necessary. Sodium amytal, in doses of 200 to 300 mg. every four to six hours, is the sedative of choice. The somatic symptoms from the respiratory alkalosis of the hyperventilation syndrome can be treated by placing a bag over the nose and mouth that will retain the expired CO_2 for rebreathing.

Careful consideration should be given to any evidence that the anxious patient may be depressed. Agitated depression, as has been stated, can be easily confused with simple anxiety. If depression is thought to be an important feature, then antidepressant medication, such as imipramine, 25 to 50 mg. three to four times a day, should be given rather than tranquilizers.

For those individuals with restricted anxieties prompted by particular stimuli, i.e., phobias, there is growing evidence that deconditioning techniques based on learning theory may have an important place in therapy. Certainly some impressive controlled trials have been published indicating a faster response to this mode of management than to interpretive therapy for individuals suffering from a single phobia. This treatment, like any other, should not be attempted without experience and guidance.

A few chronically anxious patients do not improve despite years of psychologic and pharmacologic treatment.

DEPRESSION

Definition. Depression is an unpleasant experience of sadness and misery, accompanied by a loss of interest and a decreased capacity for enjoyment or productive work. The depressed patient appears gloomy. He may be tearful and may have difficulty sleeping. He reports that he has little appetite and has lost weight. His behavior reflects his pervading gloom. He may be preoccupied with feelings of guilt based on trivial transgressions. He may attempt suicide.

Predisposing and Precipitating Factors. The mood of depression, like that of anxiety, is an experience known to everyone as the accompaniment of unhappy events like the death of cherished relatives. Depression in such circumstances takes a rather predictable course, the intense feelings of loss and misery gradually lessening with time. Although depression can be a natural response, it may appear in an intensity that seems exaggerated and prolonged, or it may occur without obvious immediate precipitation. Explanations for more unusual depressive reactions must be sought by a closer examination of the patient and his situation.

Some people with a pessimistic cast of personality have a tendency to react in a depressed way to any disruptive difficulty. Certain physical illnesses frequently are accompanied by mild to severe depressive states. Common among these are influenza, hepatitis, and the endocrine disturbances, particularly hyperadrenocorticism, hyperparathyroidism, and the postpartum state. A depression can be the first manifestation of certain diseases of the brain, such as the cerebral atrophies or brain tumors, particularly brain tumors situated in the frontal area. Depression is the outstanding feature of the depressive psychosis (see the article on Psychoses).

Depression in the Dying Patient. Depression is a frequent emotional response in patients with a fatal disease. The impressive study of Hinton revealed that almost 50 per cent of a large group of fatally ill patients were experiencing a distressing degree of depression. Depression was directly correlated with the duration of illness, the degree of physical distress suffered, and awareness by the patient of the possibility that he might die. Although depression is common and distressfully severe in such ill patients, it may be overlooked by physicians because a depressed patient may be quiet and unobtrusive. His depression may not be distinguished from the general exhaustion of his illness.

Since the knowledge that one is dying commonly produces a depression, what should dying people be told? This question has no easy answer and remains a perennial problem. It does lose some of its force from Hinton's data demonstrating that three fourths of his patients were already aware of the probability that they had a fatal illness, although no specific information had been given them. Thus, the problem of what to tell a patient resolves itself into discovering just how much the patient already knows and how much more he actually wants to know.

It is not wise to supply gratuitous information by rushing into a full definition of the disease and its inevitable outcome in response to rather vague inquiries by the patient about himself. This action is often regretted by both patient and doctor because it almost always produces emotional distress that might at least be postponed. Most persons do not ask delving questions about their chances of survival. There are, however, some patients who are able to formulate specific and searching questions about the nature of their illness and its prognosis. For such people, to be answered by prevarication or an empty reassurance will only increase feelings of anxiety, distrust, and isolation. An honest answer, particularly if it can be given along with a description of the plan of treatment that can hold the patient's attention, usually will not increase his distress, but may aid him as he finds in the physician a friend with whom to face the future. An excellent paper by Abrams (see references) provides a more detailed consideration of this problem.

Diagnosis. Depression is easily recognized. The symptoms of sadness and misery are usually unmistakable. The patient looks sad and complains that he is "blue" and has lost his interest and energy. The major issue is not the diagnosis but the estimate of how severe the depression is and, particularly, whether it is so severe as to carry a risk of suicide. Although suicide is usually the act of a severely depressed person, there can be no certain estimate of the suicide risk in any one case. All depressed patients, regardless of the cause of their depression, should be specifically asked about suicidal thoughts; any evasiveness in reply is cause for concern and calls for increased supervision of the patient. Many suicides appear to be sudden and impulsive rather than well-planned and organized acts. Therefore, lethal instruments, drugs, or open windows should not be accessible to the patient. Imposed obstacles to finding a method for self-destruction often block the intention.

Management and Treatment of Depression. Direct treatment of depression in sick and dying patients is possible but often neglected. Considerable emotional and psychologic support can be given to these patients by just allowing them to talk with a sympathetic listener who need do no more than accept and understand. Late in the course of a terminal illness, patients often are overcome with a feeling of loneliness and abandonment. Physicians can give great help at this time by simply continuing to visit these patients regularly. The patients come to depend on the physician as their link with the living, and a failure by the physician to see these patients because "I have nothing further to offer" will add considerable suffering to their final days. Similarly, physicians should encourage visitors to such patients in an effort to combat this loneliness.

The observation that a significant number of mortally ill patients consider suicide indicates that vigorous treatment of symptoms of depression is needed for the sick. Since physical discomfort is an important cause of depression, a meticulous effort to keep the patient free of pain should always be made. All physicians need skill in the use of opium derivatives. These medicines are remarkable for their control of pain and simultaneous reduction of anxiety and depression. Any program intended to control pain and bring comfort to a patient must be carefully attended, repeatedly scrutinized, and revised to meet changing conditions. Also, direct pharmacotherapy of the depressive symptoms should not be neglected for patients who are sick or dying. Often they can be comforted with imipramine, 25 to 50 mg. three times a day.

HYSTERIA

Definition. Hysteria is a disturbance of behavior in which symptoms and signs of physical ill health are imitated more or less unconsciously for some personal advantage. As the phrase "more or less unconsciously" implies, hysteria may be hard to distinguish from "malingering," in which the imitation of illness is a well-appreciated fraud. Frank malingering is rare, though, because the power of human self-deception is usually adequate to persuade a person of the validity of his own symptoms. The only ones who can be called malingerers with any confidence are some self-mutilating patients and the remarkable pathologic liars, picturesquely called examples of the *Münchhausen syndrome,* who travel from hospital to hospital gaining admission by means of dramatic acts of illness.

Predisposing and Precipitating Factors. Hysterical symptoms are to be seen as responses to distressing experiences. They can occur in almost any person facing danger or difficulty, especially if, as with soldiers in battle or jailed prisoners, the distress is intense and prolonged and physical symptoms can provide a viable escape. Dull-witted or immature persons with inadequate powers of introspection and self-control may produce transparently hysterical symptoms in response to milder distress, such as school difficulties or family problems. Some of the exaggerations and elaborations of medical symptoms common in hospitalized, sick patients may be similarly interpreted as responses to the distress of illness by persons whose capacity for self-control has been weakened by somatic illness. Hysterical symptoms can be the first manifestations of a dementing illness or of a depressive or schizophrenic psychosis, and these disorders must be considered when a previously well balanced adult develops a suspiciously hysterical symptom.

Commonly, though, hysteria is a disturbance in the behavior of a person predisposed by an attention-seeking, emotionally unstable, and egocentric personality. In fact, these characteristics form what has become known as the "hysterical personality" even though hysteria can occur in other types of people, and these characteristics do not invariably produce hysterical symptoms. Most easily recognized in these people is their flair for the dramatic. They show this tendency in flamboyant dress and in exaggerated, even melodramatic, responses to questions about their symptoms. They are never so happy as when they are the center of attention. They often work in occupations such as modeling or acting that put them in the public eye. Although hysterical personality seems more frequent in women, it is found in men, and Dr. MacDonald Critchley points to Oscar Wilde as an example. The zeal of these patients for exaggeration and drama renders them liable to hysterical behavior in response to what seem trivial difficulties or even when simply unable to attract attention to themselves in other ways.

Symptoms and Signs. Many of the phenomena of somatic illness can be imitated by hysteria. The accuracy of the imitation depends on the medical sophistication of the patient. A doctor or nurse is more likely to produce a convincing imitation than is an unqualified person.

Common hysterical symptoms are vague subjective disorders, such as generalized weakness, dizziness, indigestion, or pain. Hysterical pain can occur in any part of the body, but the head and neck, the region over the heart, and the low back are particularly favored. Hysterical pain can be of any character, from dull aching to sharp and stabbing pain, but it is often described by the patient in vivid similes such as "like a bullet," "like a bolt of lightning," "aches like an abscessed tooth," or "sore as a hot boil." Usually, hysterical pain is not confined to a local area as around a pathologic lesion, nor is it referred into the distribution of a particular nerve or dermatome. Rather, hysterical pain is felt in a general region of the body and spreads, sometimes in bizarre ways, into contiguous areas without regard to neuroanatomic boundaries. Thus, pain beginning in the face may spread along the side of the head and into the back, crossing from the region of the trigeminal nerve into the upper cervical nerve regions. Hysterical pain often varies in its character, intensity, and distribution, changing considerably with attention or suggestion. Occasionally it can be remarkably improved by a small amount of intravenous amobarbital sodium when analgesics do not help. Characteristically, the tests of sensation often reveal that the cutaneous sensibility in a region of hysterical pain is heightened. The patient claims that light touches or pin pricks are not changed in character but are felt more acutely or sharply as though more pressure had been exerted by the examiner. This is hyperesthesia, and it is likely to be hysterical. It should be differentiated from hyperpathia, the sensory change associated with nerve injury in which sensory thresholds are raised so that light stimuli are not perceived, but stimuli exceeding the threshold produce a disagreeable and prolonged pain.

Although vague symptoms of a subjective kind such as pain or dizziness are the present vogue in hysteria, crude and gross symptoms are still seen. These may be psychologic, such as the amnesia or fugue states, in which, in the setting of some trouble that the patient would like to avoid or forget, his memory is partially lost. Amnesias are particularly common in soldiers in wartime. *Ganser's syndrome* is an hysterical twilight state and pseudodementia, first described in prisoners by a Dresden prison doctor. It consists of a mild disturbance of consciousness and an associated behavior that seems intended to represent madness. Particularly characteristic of the Ganser syndrome are replies to questions indicating that a correct answer is known but a wrong answer chosen. On being asked how many legs a cat has, the patient answers three or five, never four.

Motor disturbances in the form of abnormal movement, disturbed gaits, seizures, or paralyses are occasionally hysterical symptoms. Hysterical seizures can usually be distinguished from epileptic ones. The patients generally do not hurt themselves, bite their tongues, or lose their urine. They do not have the typical tonic and then clonic phases of a seizure, but tend to show a dramatic flailing of the limbs. Consciousness is usually retained, and seizures hardly ever occur when the patient is alone. The EEG is normal.

Sensory disturbances are particularly favored hysterical symptoms. Thus, *blindness* or *deafness* is common, often developing dramatically and conveniently to spare the patient embarrassment or other discomfort. Loss of sensation over one side of the body to pin prick or light touch is frequently found after a susceptible patient has been examined by a neurologist.

Diagnosis. Diagnosis of hysteria is seldom easy and never popular. Ideally, it should rest on three supports: first, the *form* of the hysterical manifestation; second, the *personality* of the patient; and third, the *setting* in which the symptoms developed. Often it is not possible to find all three supports to a diagnosis, but all should be sought.

Commonly, hysterical symptoms are vague and variable. In fact, the more definite and consistent a patient's description of the onset, location, nature, and duration of his symptoms, the less likely the symptoms are to be hysterical. Hysterical symptoms and signs are also usually incompatible with what is known of anatomy and physiology. Thus, sensory losses do not conform to patterns of nerve distribution; reflexes remain intact and unchanged in the palsies of arm and leg; seizures of the entire body do not disturb consciousness; total blindness appears without a disturbance of pupillary reflex or of opticokinetic nystagmus. The hysterically mute person can phonate on coughing. The hysterically deaf person speaks louder to be heard over increased ambient noises. Many other hysterical symptoms have been analyzed for such inconsistencies by Head.

Knowledge of the personality and past history of the patient is helpful to a diagnosis of hysteria. The recognition that the symptoms are occurring in an hysterical personality should prompt an observer to look very closely at the symptoms before embarking on extensive laboratory tests or upon surgery. Similarly, knowledge of a previous vague and poorly understood medical disturbance can lend weight to an opinion that a new symptom that has eluded diagnosis is occurring in an individual prone to hysteria. Conversely, hysteria can usually be eliminated as an explanation for symptoms in a responsible, stable, middle-aged person. People who have passed through adolescence and young adulthood without resorting to hysterical behavior are unlikely to employ it when older.

The setting in which the symptoms develop should be carefully scrutinized, and a search made for a distressing event that may have provoked an hysterical reaction or for any purpose that the hysterical symptoms may serve. Occasionally, a clear association between the symptoms chosen and a particular recent disturbance in the life of the subject can be found, such as an amnesia developing in a person who has done something shameful or criminal, or weakness and pain persisting in a person who is seeking financial compensation for an injury. Often, though, motivations behind hysterical symptoms are vague and uncertain. They may depend only upon a generally unhappy life situation in a person who employs hysterical symptoms to call attention and bring sympathy to himself and his present state. Also, it may be possible to demonstrate that the development of particular symptoms has been prompted by suggestion: weakness of legs, for example, developing in a nurse caring for a paraplegic patient, or peculiar falling attacks after the patient has witnessed an epileptic seizure.

A careful study of the symptoms, the personality, and the life setting of a patient usually allows a reasonably certain differentiation of hysterical symptoms from those of a medical illness. There are, however, certain medical problems that are notoriously easily confused with hysteria. These are the diseases that produce vague and changing symptoms that seem to vary with the patient's motivation and, at least in their early phases, lack convincing physical signs. If such an illness occurs in a patient who has features of the hysterical personality and who will therefore describe the symptoms in a dramatic and flamboyant fashion, physicians may be even more persuaded to believe that the illness is only deceptively physical. Examples of diseases frequently confused with hysteria because of their subtle clinical features are the first attack of multiple sclerosis, particularly if sensory changes alone are produced; the weakness of arms and legs seen early in acute idiopathic polyneuritis of the Guillain-Barré type; the difficulty in swallowing of bulbar myasthenia gravis; the attacks of muscular weakness in periodic paralysis; the tonic posturings and oculogyric crises of postencephalitic parkinsonism; the pain of a cauda equina tumor; and the abdominal pain of acute intermittent porphyria.

Management of Hysteria. The management of hysterical patients is difficult. No one method can be recommended unqualifiedly. But there are certain principles that can be followed. To help hysterical patients it is essential to have sympathy for them. Many doctors find these patients irritating. It is just as possible to see them as individuals displaying an intriguing aspect of human behavior that could be almost comical if it did not have such tragic implications in their lives. It is pointless to argue with these patients about the validity of their symptoms. A useful approach is to agree that they have had an illness producing their symptoms, but that they are now improving even though total recovery has not arrived.

It is important to diagnose hysteria promptly. Hesitation in diagnosis leading to several hospital admissions for extensive laboratory investigations is a good way to solidify hysterical symptoms in a patient. Among other things, the uncertainty of doctors helps persuade a patient that the symptoms are real. Repeated examinations increase the consistency with which symptoms are reported. Long hospitalization, mounting bills, and the inconvenience caused to others make it difficult for a patient to abandon symptoms without embarrassment. The gratifying attention given to the patient in the hospital, perhaps as an example of an intriguing diagnostic problem, can feed the self-dramatizing tendencies and so encourage the behavior.

There is always risk in any diagnosis since diagnosis is only a weighing of probabilities. The diagnosis of hysteria, though, depends purely on a physician's judgment and, before relief of symptoms is accomplished, can be confirmed in the laboratory only by evidence of health. Physicians, for obvious reasons, fear more the error of calling a physically sick patient hysterical than the error of mishandling hysteria. They often prefer to exclude, by laboratory examination, progressively more unlikely diseases than to study carefully the symptoms and the individual who has produced them, even though this would lead more directly to a definite diagnosis as well as an understanding of the response. It may be unwise to counsel too strongly against this behavior because medical diagnosis is never easy. A compromise can be found in the admonition to perform immediately the laboratory tests that seem necessary for a patient, but when hysteria is suspected, to bring the period of investigation as quickly as possible to a close so that management of the specific symptom can be begun.

Treatment of the specific symptoms rests basically upon persuasion. The doctor is persuading the patient to perform the functions that the patient claims are disabled. Intravenous amobarbital sodium given to the point where the patient is mildly intoxicated and his speech slurred is particularly helpful in making and establishing a persuasion. Usually, some ingenuity is required for success. The hysterically blind person can, for example, be persuaded first that he can distinguish light from dark and then gradually to distinguish forms, to read large print, and, finally, small newsprint. The person who claims he cannot walk can be encouraged first to move his legs in bed, and then to stand, to make a few tentative shuffles, and finally to stride out. The hysterically deaf person can be persuaded to hear through a stethoscope and then gradually that he can hear without it. A dramatic show of some kind is often helpful in removing these symptoms. If a physician has success in partially removing hysterical symptoms, he should persist in his treatment without interruption in order to bring about as much improvement as possible and even to restore full function. When there is recovery of function, the patient should perform his recovered skills in public—before his family, other patients and several doctors—to prevent his relapsing immediately into his former state.

The fear that sudden removal of hysterical symptoms will result in a disastrous psychologic collapse is exaggerated. Rarely, a depressed patient with hysterical symptoms has an increase in depression, but it is clear that in those situations a depression was overlooked and the more secondary hysterical symptoms were emphasized.

Some hysterical disorders are refractory to treatment. Among these are the disorders assumed for some material gain, such as compensation. They usually are not improved until some settlement is made. Episodic disorders such as hysterical seizures can be hard to control. Sometimes, however, a statement to the patient that they will not recur, given with full authority by a physician whom the patient trusts and respects, may eliminate these symptoms. The longer the patient has hysterical symptoms, the harder they are to remove. This is a corollary to the above observation that hysterical symptoms produced for transparent reasons and bordering on malingering are more difficult to eliminate than are the ones produced for more vague reasons by an attention-seeking personality. Symptoms held for a long time cannot be easily abandoned without embarrassing the patient.

Simultaneously with treatment of the specific symptoms, the present life of the patient should be studied to discover any distress that may have precipitated the illness and to understand the particular advantage that might be gained by means of the symptoms chosen. Then advice, instruction, social assistance, or moral guidance can be offered logically to aid the patient in disposing with the need for symptoms.

Long-term management of hysterical patients is much more difficult than treatment of individual symptoms. It is not wise to have the average hysterical patient embark on depth psychotherapy since he tends to produce more symptoms and to recount involved sexual and other fantasies in order to maintain the interest of his doctor. If possible, these patients should be followed by one physician who understands them and the behavior that they are liable to produce and is also competent to recognize physical illness should it arise. This physician can save these patients from needless surgery and long hospitalization. He can remove hysterical symptoms promptly by being alert to the diagnosis and providing help for the difficulties that precipitate them. Although such a physician can provide great help to an hysterical patient, the more severely disturbed individuals seldom stay with one physician. They wish to roam around to many doctors, gaining the satisfaction of being studied by a number of different men. A firm discussion of what they are doing may sometimes be helpful, but too often their condition is intractable.

Abrams, R. D.: The patient with cancer—His changing pattern of communication. New Eng. J. Med., 274:317, 1966.

Berle, B. B.: 80 Puerto Rican Families in New York City. New York, Columbia University Press, 1958.

Birnbaum, K.: In O. Bumke (ed.): Handbuch der Geisteskrankheiten. Berlin, Julius Springer, 1928.

Coles, R.: Southern children under desegregation. Amer. J. Psychiat. 120:332, 1963.

Glazer, N., and Moynihan, D. P.: Beyond the Melting Pot. Cambridge, Mass., M.I.T. Press, 1963.

Granville-Grossman, K. L., and Turner, P.: The effect of propranolol on anxiety. Lancet 1:788, 1966.

Head, H.: The diagnosis of hysteria. Brit. Med. J., 1:827, 1922.

Hinton, J. M.: Physical and mental distress of the dying. Quart. J. Med., 32:1, 1963.

Roth, M.: The phobic anxiety-depersonalization syndrome and some general aetiological problems in psychiatry. J. Neuropsychiat., 1:293, 1960.

Walters, A.: Psychogenic regional pain alias hysterical pain. Brain, 84:1, 1961.

Wolff, H. G.: Every man has his "breaking point." Milit. Med., 125:85, 1960.

PSYCHOLOGIC TESTING IN CLINICAL MEDICINE

The intent of this article is to describe some methods of psychologic testing that have proved helpful in clinical settings. The goal is to provide some capacity to evaluate critically any psychologic test instrument, whether presently in use or likely to be devised in the foreseeable future.

Psychologic tests are intended to assist clinical evaluation of behavioral disorders by bringing accurate measurement to the mental examination. Physicians are familiar with instruments that bring accurate measurement to observations in the physical examination; the clinical thermometer and sphygmomanometer give information in numerical form about body temperature and blood pressure that cannot be collected with such accuracy without their assistance. They are so easy to employ that knowledge of the normal readings in the human population and implications of deviations from normal have been established. Although psychologic tests are aimed at more abstract phenomena such as intelligence or personality, they similarly attempt to bring precision through numerical or graphic measurements and provide a means by which an individual can be compared in these features with the normal population.

The mere provision of a numerical expression does not prove a test useful, as the numbers may not be meaningful. Often in our fascination with a new test and its intriguingly plausible scales for measurement, we overlook its failure to satisfy the criteria of *reliability* and *validity*.

The reliability of a measuring instrument, whether it be for a physical or a psychologic phenomenon, is an expression of the accuracy and reproducibility of its findings. No instrument is perfectly reliable, but the range within which it is unreliable must be a small fraction of the potential range of measurement if it is to be capable of detecting a genuine deviation in the variable under study.

The validity of a measuring instrument is an expression of its capacity to measure what it claims to measure. The clinical thermometer does measure body temperature. How can we be sure that psychologic tests are actually measuring the psychologic variables that they claim to measure? How can we be sure that intelligence tests, for example, measure intelligence? The only proof that a test is valid is the demonstration that scores on it predict behavior in life thought to be the expression of the trait it claims to measure. For example, results on a valid intelligence test should correlate to some extent with scholastic performance.*

INTELLIGENCE

The quantitative measurement of the mental attribute, intelligence, was first attempted by Binet at the turn of the century. His success and the Stanford-Binet battery of tests developed from his work brought such predictive power to the study of intelligence that they provide an impetus to the development of tests to examine other mental functions. But the tests of intelligence have through their revisions, particularly the *Wechsler Bellevue Intelligence Scale* published in 1939 and the *Wechsler Adult Intelligence Scale (WAIS)* of

*The issues of reliability and validity can perhaps be made clearer with a homely example. The common ruler is an instrument designed to measure distances. It is a reliable instrument in that repeated measurements of the same object, say a cube one foot to a side, will give the same results. It is also a valid instrument for the measurement of the cube's dimensions. It is not, however, a valid instrument for measuring the cube's weight. This is determined by the material of the cube, and no number of repeated measurements with the reliable ruler will make it give a valid measure of weight.

1955, remained the most secure and useful tests of mental function.

Intelligence is difficult to define. It is the abstract concept used to explain the observation that individuals vary in the skill and effectiveness with which they employ their mental faculties. Intelligence is more easily defined in practice by pointing to instances of its action. This way is in fact used in our daily life. We judge a man's intelligence by observing his bearing, his speech, his apparent grasp of situations, his judgments, and his emotional control. Then in the light of our past experience of watching other men, we call an individual bright or dull. We are doing nothing conceptually different when we estimate intelligence at the bedside or by means of psychologic tests. We organize the testing so that a series of observations can be made within a reasonable period of time. We add scope to our examination by asking for performance in several different kinds of mental activity. We bring accuracy to the observations by scoring the performance.

The questions on orientation, memory, attention and concentration, fund of knowledge, and capacity to reason abstractly that constitute the tests of cognition routinely carried out at the bedside in the course of the physical and mental examination of a patient provide a doctor an estimate of his patient's intellectual functioning. In the light of knowledge of the patient's past life and demonstrated abilities, the doctor makes a judgment whether there has been damage to intellectual functioning. Psychologic testing should be able to give a more accurate estimate of the intelligence of a patient at the moment of testing than do these bedside examinations if the tests available are reliable and valid. The considerable experience of this century has provided such evidence.

The *Wechsler Adult Intelligence Scale* is the most reliable and valid test we have at the moment for measuring the intellectual function of the adult. Its reliability has been demonstrated by the close correlation of test scores given on separate occasions to the same individuals and by the similarity of scores when one half of a test is compared with another half (split-half method). Its validity has been demonstrated by its correlation with life performances of individuals it scores as intelligent or dull.

In its present form the WAIS consists of 11 subtests of mental skill. Six of these subtests are "verbal tests." In these the patient is requested to define words, to recognize similarities between words, to do arithmetic, to remember numbers forward and backward, to answer questions on his fund of knowledge, and to judge and interpret proverbs. These tests are followed by five "performance tests," in which a patient is asked to work with rather unfamiliar material and solve problems set to him by that material. Tests here include the putting together of puzzles, work with symbols, the setting out of logical stories from pictures disorganized for the test, construction of patterns from multicolored blocks, and the recognition of things missing from drawings. The performance tests seem somewhat less related to the education of a person than are the verbal tests. All the subtests that have been chosen for the WAIS have a long history of investigation. They are combined together to produce a thorough and accurate instrument.

The scoring of the WAIS is in the form of the *Intelligence Quotient (I.Q.)*. In fact, the WAIS derives a verbal I.Q. from the verbal tests and a performance I.Q. from the performance tests. A full-scale I.Q. is derived from the combination of all 11 subtests.

The I.Q. compares an individual with others. Historically it was developed for children. I.Q. then was the ratio of mental age over chronologic age times 100 when mental age was defined in terms of a child's ability to succeed on tests which the average child of a given age could do. Thus a child solving problems which the average nine-year-old could solve had a mental age of nine. If he, himself, was nine years old at the time of the test, he had an average ability and an I.Q. of $9/9 \times 100$, or 100; if his chronologic age was six, he would be an advanced child with an I.Q. of $9/6 \times 100$, or 150. Terman demonstrated the constancy of I.Q. in the growing child.

But a ratio of mental to chronologic age is unlikely to be useful in adults because tested intelligence does not increase after the late teens. The WAIS and many other tests for adult intelligence continue to use the term I.Q. This is possible because of the fact that tests of intelligence appear to distribute individuals in a gaussian fashion. This curve has a mean at I.Q. 100 and a standard deviation of ± 15 I.Q. points. It is possible to divide the curve into percentiles of the population. The WAIS score of any person places him in the percentile of the population with similar scores, and his I.Q. can be extrapolated from percentile by means of the distribution curve. Thus an individual whose performance on the WAIS is equal to 50 per cent of the population is said to have an I.Q. of 100, whereas individuals whose test performances exceeded 98 per cent of the population will be said to have an I.Q. of 135 or above.

The WAIS has found its greatest clinical utility in the study of patients with brain disease. Any damage to the cerebral hemispheres will injure intellectual ability and disturb the scores on the WAIS. An intriguing observation is that early in the course of brain disease performance tests are disturbed before the verbal tests scores change. This may indicate that verbal tests measure more what an individual has learned and practiced, whereas performance tests measure his capacity to meet new problems. Intelligence is required for success in both. The verbal and performance scores of normal individuals are usually comparable. The discrepancy between verbal and performance scores found with brain disease reflects a resistance of the verbal tasks to injury. The verbal I.Q. can be considered a fair estimate of the original intellectual endowment of an individual suffering from a brain injury. The decline of the performance I.Q. is a useful measure of the degree of injury to the cerebral tissue the patient has endured. With an advancing brain disease verbal I.Q. will fall eventually, but a patient will usually continue to demonstrate higher verbal than performance scores.

Emotional unrest such as anxiety or depression will also interfere with WAIS scores. Here, as with cerebral disease, the performance I.Q. will fall below the verbal I.Q., demonstrating that the capacity to work with unfamiliar material is disturbed more than tests of what has been well learned. But because these findings are identical to those in persons with brain disease, the differentiation of an emotional disturbance from dementia cannot come from WAIS results. It must rest on other information such as is derived from the history, physical examination, and mental status.

The WAIS is useful not only in demonstrating deterioration of intellectual function but also when done serially can document recovery of function with treatment. Since it is so simple to employ, its increasing utility in clinical research is assured.

PERSONALITY

By personality is meant all the abiding traits of character that constitute an individual's potential to respond in particular ways to circumstances. All physicians are aware of how much information they must acquire through several interviews with the patient and from independent sources before they can have much confidence in their diagnostic opinion on personality. Tests that could elucidate personality more accurately and more rapidly would be useful. Two alternative approaches have been developed, "projective" tests and questionnaires. Each approach has raised particular problems.

In the so-called projective tests of personality ambiguous situations are set before the patient, and his responses are recorded. Thus he is presented with sentences to complete, a picture to interpret, or in the most well known projective test, he is presented with a standardized set of ink blots and he is asked to describe the forms that he can recognize within them. Since there is nothing in the situations themselves that force any particular response, the responses of the patient are thought to derive from his personal predilections and inner needs, drives, and conflicts. This seems logical. But logic is not the essential criterion for a test intended to aid the clinical examination. It must be demonstrated that the responses on projective tests provide a measurement with sufficient reliability to make these tests valid instruments for the study of personality. This remains to be done.

Certain features of a patient can be expected

to be seen in any set of his responses. For instance, overly conscientious persons will tend to be fixed on details, the schizophrenic patient with his disordered thought will demonstrate this feature in distorted expression, and the depressed patient will speak of unhappy themes as he discusses any matter. These features will appear whether the patient is being examined by his doctor or doing a projective test. Until the reliability and validity of projective tests can be demonstrated, it cannot be known whether they are superior to the clinical examination. If they are not superior to the clinical examination, they are of doubtful utility to the physician, and the question of their value is shrouded in controversy.

The other approach to personality measurement is the questionnaire. This was developed from the clinical examination. Since questions are used there to gain information from the patient, it seemed logical that a questionnaire including these and many other questions with answers assessed precisely would improve on the clinical examination. It came as a surprise when tests developed in this fashion proved to be unreliable and invalid. This was demonstrated when different questionnaires intended to probe similar features of personality, such as introversion, did not correlate well with one another, and in fact could give quite opposite impressions of the same person. Questionnaires developed in this fashion proved so misleading that the method fell into disrepute. It was, however, eventually recognized that these early tests gratuitously assumed that questions would be accurately answered by patients. Consider the question, do you lack self-confidence, yes or no? To presume that a person will understand this question exactly the same way as the examiner intends and that his criterion for a yes or no answer is the same as that of all other people is to presume too much. Also these early tests failed to consider that many individuals might attempt to show themselves in some more favorable light and therefore not answer questions truthfully.

The most intriguing conceptual advance in the study of personality was the recognition that an objectively truthful answer to questions was not needed for a valid, useful test. In fact, more information can be obtained from observing the patient's replies to questions than from any belief that the statements they agree to or reject are in themselves accurate descriptions of their personality. The task of building questionnaires changed from finding questions that would display the inner feelings of people to finding questions that would be answered differently by different personality types.

To build such a questionnaire the first step was to gather specific groups of patients together, a group of normal people, a group of anxious patients, a group of hysterical patients, a group of depressed patients, for as many groups as could be differentiated. These patients, the criterion groups, were asked a large number of questions and the replies were compared from group to group. The questions which differentiated the groups best would then be collected for the questionnaire. This questionnaire then given to an individual was interpreted not from the content of questions rejected or affirmed but from the number of questions replied to in the same fashion as was followed by one or more of the criterion groups.

The most useful questionnaire that has been developed is the *Minnesota Multiphasic Personality Inventory (MMPI)*. The questions in that test have been carefully studied and chosen so that they differentiate to the greatest degree possible with it. Because of the complexity of issues of personality, the numbers of questions needed to derive a profile with this test is 550. It was possible in the MMPI to fit in many questions that give an indication of the tendency of the patient to lie, exaggerate, or misunderstand questions.

The results of the MMPI are expressed as a series of nine scales or dimensions along each of which an individual is placed by means of his responses that correspond to responses of nine criterion groups. These scales were originally derived from clinical groups and given clinical names, i.e., hypochondriasis, depression, hysteria, psychopathic, masculine-feminine dimension, paranoid, psychaesthenic, schizophrenic, and manic. Three so-called lie scales are also scored for each test.

The MMPI is a reliable instrument, the accuracy and reproducibility of its readings having been demonstrated in repeated testing of individuals over many years. The validity of its scales varies. Some of the scales measure the personality characteristics for which they are titled. Scores on the psychopathic and manic scales do correlate with the clinical features intended by these terms. Scores on the schizophrenic and hysterical scales do not correlate well with these clinical disorders but with aspects of bizarreness and self-dramatization, respectively. These features are not specific to schizophrenic or hysteria. In an effort to avoid these invalid implications, the MMPI scales are no longer referred to by clinical titles, but by letters derived from the original names.

The tendency to look at specific scales for diagnostic impressions has been replaced by consideration of the "profile," or pattern of the several scales together, hoping to derive in this way a more global view of personality structure. This approach emphasizes the multidimensional character of personality. It takes advantage of the features of reliability found in this test. But, once again, the establishment of validity for these profiles must be accomplished. This is being attempted by matching the life course of individuals with predictions from the profiles, but work is still in progress.

Current practice is to find the MMPI useful as a screening and probing instrument that often suggests aspects of personality difficulty that might well be more carefully studied. If knowledge of its validity increases, the MMPI may take a still more important role in clinical medicine.

Butcher, H. J.: Human Intelligence, Its Nature and Assessment. London, Methuen & Co., Ltd., 1968.

Penrose, L. S.: The Biology of Mental Defect. London, Sidgwick and Jackson, Ltd., 1963.

Terman, L. M., and Oden, M.: The Gifted Group at Mid-Life. Genetic Studies of Genius, Vol. V. Stanford, California, Stanford University Press, 1959.

Welsh, G. S., and Dahlstrom, W. G.: Basic Readings on the MMPI. Minneapolis, University of Minnesota Press, 1956.

Williams, M.: Mental Testing in Clinical Practice. London, Pergamon Press, 1965.

Medical Aspects of Sexuality

Harold I. Lief

The Physician's Role. Once almost completely neglected in medical education, sex counseling is now included in the curriculum of the majority of the medical schools in the United States. Physicians now recognize the frequency and importance of sexual problems in medical practice. Forty-two per cent of the emotional problems for which patients ask their doctors for help are related to marriage, and the most frequent marital difficulties, as perceived by a representative sample of physicians surveyed by Herndon and Nash, are problems of sexual adjustment. (In the Marriage Council of Philadelphia clinic about 75 per cent of couples report some sexual maladjustment, including 15 per cent for whom a sexual problem is a major problem and a primary cause of marital difficulty.)

The frequency with which sexual problems arise in practice varies with three factors: speciality, whether the physician routinely asks about sex problems, and the comfort of the physician in discussing sex with the patient. The highest frequencies according to Burnap and Golden are found in the practice of psychiatry, obstetrics-gynecology, urology, and in general practice. If the physician routinely asks about sex problems, the average frequency of patients with sexual problems is 14 per cent, whereas it drops to 7.9 per cent among the physicians who inquire about sexual matters "only when indicated." Among the group of physicians who inferentially displayed discomfort with sexuality, the frequency of sexual problems reported in their practices was only 2.7 per cent, as compared with an average of 15 per cent among those physicians who were reasonably comfortable.

Most sexual problems presented to physicians are in the context of a marital relationship, as either primary causes of marital dysfunction or as consequences of other areas of marital discord, but which, nevertheless, augment and maintain marital unhappiness. It seems reasonable, then, to make sex and marriage counseling a "package" in the training of the physician and in the delivery of medical care. Even in the case of the pediatrician, it is still logical, for he soon comes to recognize the direct connection between the marital relationship of the parents and the sexual problems of the child.

The busy physician or the physician who shies away from marital therapy may have to treat the couple by dealing with one patient only. And many situations can be handled adequately in this fashion, e.g., the urologist who cures male dyspareunia by clearing up the patient's prostatitis, the internist who helps restore his patient's potency by reassuring him that sexual activity will not give him another coronary occlusion, the gynecologist who reassures his patient that she will suffer no loss of sexual drive after hysterectomy. Yet, sexual behavior involves a relationship, and hence, in most instances, therapy should also be directed toward the relationship.

Not only are marital and sexual problems in medical practice frequent, but they are often overlooked or avoided — either because of the physician's lack of training and his feeling of incompetence in this area or because these problems impinge on his own marital and sexual conflicts or values and make him uncomfortable. Even if he consciously or unconsciously ducks the issue by failing to follow cues, changing the subject by responding with a trite and stereotyped form of reassurance, e.g., "this is just a phase — your problem will disappear in time," he is carrying out counseling of sorts. Vincent has stated it well:

> The theoretical position that the physician cannot or should not engage in any marriage or sexual counseling becomes meaningless when the patients expect this role of their physician and when their illnesses have sexual and marital implications — if not origins. The majority of physicians literally have no choice; even to do and say nothing in response to the patient's questions and/or presentation of symptoms in the sexual and marital areas is, by default, one form of counseling.

In dealing with sexual and marital problems, the physician has an unequaled opportunity to practice preventive as well as therapeutic medicine. By aiding patients to obtain greater sexual satisfaction, he may prevent the escalation of marital discord and consequent family disorganization through emotional conflict with or without divorce. Anything that seems to strengthen family life has positive repercussions on the next generation as well. Early intervention can occur in a number of clinical situations, e.g., premarital counseling, family planning services, during pregnancy, postpartum care, early marriage, as well as through family life education for teenagers and young adults. The pediatrician and obstetrician have especially significant points of entrance into the system of health care, enabling these specialists to practice effective prevention.

To be competent in handling the therapeutic and preventive aspects of the sexual, marital, and family problems he sees almost daily in his practice, the physician must not only have a store of *information*, but must also develop a set of *skills* and *attitudes* that facilitate his making optimal use of his information. Surely the key factor in competent sex and marital counseling is the degree of comfort of the counselor. His skill in interviewing, in eliciting salient data about the most intimate, personal dimension of patients' lives, will depend directly on his capacity to react, not with anxiety, anger, or self-righteousness, but with openness, ease, and a clear desire to achieve an atmosphere of genuine communication—of feelings as well as thoughts. In the absence of these skills and attitudes, his quantity of information, even if vast, is of little use.

Sexuality. Sexuality refers to the totality of one's sexual being, of which physical sex is only a part. In this sense, our sexuality is what we "are" rather than what we "do." One's sense of being male and masculine, female and feminine, and the various roles these self-perceptions engender or affect are important ingredients of sexuality. Cognitive, emotional, and physical sex all contribute to the totality.

Sexuality may be described in terms of a system analogous to the circulatory or respiratory system. The components of the sexual system are set forth in the accompanying table.

Abnormalities in biologic sex may be minor or major. Major abnormalities create problems of intersexuality, which may, if not corrected early in life, lead to conflicts in sexual or gender identity. The sex assigned is, with rare exceptions, more important in determining gender identity than is biologic sex, and change in sex is usually unwise after puberty. Some of these patients and some without evident biologic defect have grave difficulties in developing a core gender identity of the same biologic sex. These are transsexuals, mostly biologic males who think of themselves as "a female trapped in a male body."

With these relatively rare exceptions, development of sexuality leads to a secure sense of maleness or femaleness, which is generally complete by the age of three. However, in our culture, doubts and conflicts about masculinity and femininity are ubiquitous. Serious disturbances lead to such sex deviations as transvestitism, fetishism, voyeurism, and exhibitionism. Homosexuality is a special

SEXUAL SYSTEM (SEXUALITY)

1. Biological sex—chromosomes, hormones, primary and secondary sex characteristics, etc.
2. Sexual identity (sometimes called core gender identity)—sense of maleness and femaleness
3. Gender identity—sense of masculinity and femininity
4. Sexual role behavior: (a) sex behavior—behavior motivated by desire for orgasm (physical sex); (b) gender behavior—behavior with masculine and feminine connotations

case of disorder of gender identity. Parenthetically, homosexuals do not have doubts about their maleness or femaleness (core gender identity). Although the etiology of homosexuality is still in doubt, as long as one retains the perspective of masculine-feminine polarity as being indubitably related to the normal development of the sexual system, one has to regard exclusive or preferred homosexuality as a deviation from the norm.

Far more commonly, the physician is called upon to deal with less overt conflicts about gender identity that create significant marital problems with sexual connotations, examples of which are the Don Juan who has to prove his masculinity by sexual conquests; the promiscuous housewife who tries to prove to herself her femininity by finding the elusive orgasm, or by demonstrating her attractiveness; the woman who cannot respond sexually because she is afraid of being completely dominated or possessed by a male; and the husband who cannot have sexual intercourse with his wife on top, because it seems unmanly. The "battle of the sexes" is carried out not only in bed, but in every area of marital interaction, generally by people who are uncertain of their masculinity or femininity and who fight to gain self-respect by derogating the partner. Several generations ago, these sexually related social roles were handed down or "assigned" by tradition; today, roles are negotiable, and problems become serious when negotiation is impossible to attain because of faulty communication, or when it breaks down because of disturbed perception or the fear of compromise.

The sexual system develops as such an integral part of personality development that sexuality and personality are inseparably interwoven. The physician who wishes to be an effective sex counselor, therefore, must deal with sexual relations in the context of human, especially marital, relations.

Problem Areas. Sexual disturbances in marriage may be the result of (1) sufficient psychopathology on the part of one or both spouses, (2) a poor relationship or "fit" between the spouses, or (3) relative ignorance of one or both partners. An example of the first category is the wife whose life experience taught her that sex is nasty and sinful and who cannot experience sexual pleasure, for the pleasure would increase her guilt inordinately. Patients in this category with long-standing sexual dysfunction are generally referred to psychiatrists. Patients whose difficulties stem largely from a poor marital relationship or from lack of information may be seen by the nonpsychiatric physician, who, unless he has had special training in sex and marriage counseling, must be mindful of his own capacities and limitations.

In evaluating any sexual problem it is necessary to determine how much weight to attach to the three factors contributing to the problem. Often, all three are represented. The woman who has the concept of sex as a sinful activity and who inhibits her responsivity may have only a hazy idea of what pattern of stimulation (called by

Masters and Johnson "sensate focus") is best suited to increase her sexual excitement, and may make all sorts of excuses to her husband ("I'm tired"; "I have a headache"; "It's my period") to avoid sex, or she may grant or withhold sex as a weapon to punish her husband or in bargaining for something she wants.

Some of the more frequent problem areas are:

1. Sexual drive or interest.
2. Sexual responsivity, including premature ejaculation, impotence, and "frigidity."
3. Premarital and extramarital coitus.
4. Request for abortion.
5. Bodily complaints masking sexual and marital problems.
6. Sexual problems consequent to physical illness.
7. Concerns about masturbation and sex play among children.
8. Confusion about what constitutes normal or abnormal sex practices.

Patients frequently misperceive the spouse's desired frequency of intercourse; most often the wife overestimates her husband's desired frequency. In one sixth of the cases studied, there was a gross underestimation of the wife's desires. The *perception* of the problem is usually more significant than the *reality*. The physician can often help by asking each spouse separately how often he wants intercourse and his perception of his spouse's desires. Better communication is the first step toward relieving this problem, and in many instances may be all that is required. The physician also has to bear in mind that the sex drive in the male is at a peak between the ages of 15 and 25, whereas in the female it peaks a decade later.

Inadequate responsivity in the female is due either to faulty preparation or to the inhibiting influence of emergency emotions—fear, anger, and guilt. Faulty preparation may be due to ignorance or unconcern of the husband or the inability of the wife to communicate her needs and preferences to her husband. The physician should try to clear away areas of ignorance before tackling the more difficult problems of inhibition caused by emotions designed for emergency "survival" rather than for pleasure. The long-range goal of therapy is to substitute the welfare emotions—love, pride, hope, and joy—for the emergency emotions. Newer techniques of sexual education and re-education, increasing the couple's awareness of the "sensate focus" and increasing each spouse's positive regard for his own body, have been developed by Masters and Johnson.

Premature ejaculation is again either due to a faulty perception of the bodily cues signaling impending ejaculation or to the influence of emergency emotions. Unless the patient is diabetic, impotence is generally related to a fear of failing in penetration, superimposed on emergency emotions related to his feelings about his partner. The vast majority of men with this disorder can be helped by removing the fear of performance, as John Hunter discovered two hundred years ago. He counseled his patients to avoid coitus "in six consecutive amatory experiences" and reported signal success.

The problem of premarital coitus is characteristically presented by the unmarried girl who asks her physician for the "pill." If the freedom of the physician is not restricted by his own set of values, this provides him with an opportunity to discuss with the young patient her feelings and expectations about her relationship with her actual or intended partner. (More frequently the young woman asks *after* rather than *before* the initial coital experience.) Whether the doctor indeed prescribes contraception is determined by the entire set of circumstances, and whether he sees a possible unwanted pregnancy as a greater problem then premarital intercourse.

Extramarital intercourse is sometimes dealt with more easily by marital partners than one might think. If, however, it threatens to have a destructive effect on the marriage, referral to an experienced marriage counselor is appropriate.

Requests for abortion often create acute conflict in physicians who are torn between the patient's wishes, which make a great deal of sense, and the legal and medical sanctions of his state and community.* Refusal may drive the patient to undertake an illegal abortion with all the perils this entails, although acquiesence may be difficult or impossible. The buck is often passed to the psychiatrist, who, except in rare cases in which there is no doubt about the psychiatric indications, either must be a party to deceit or must refuse.

The astute physician has to be on the lookout for the presence of sexual or marital problems that lie behind a host of physical symptoms—headache, backache, fatigue, menstrual irregularities, or dysmenorrhea. Osler said of syphilis that it was "the great imitator" of other disease states. It may be said more accurately that sexual dissatisfaction plays that role today.

Chronic illness often has sexual connotations. Most physicians do not even discuss sex with their postcoronary patients, and when they do they may offer vague and uncertain advice, such as "take it easy." Patients who have chronic illness, or who have had organ ablation such as hysterectomy *are* concerned about their sexual function: How often? Under what circumstances? Am I still virile or attractive? are questions many patients are too embarrassed to ask.

Whereas childhood sex play and masturbation are now recognized as part of normal psychosexual development, many patients still have doubts and anxieties about these forms of sexual behavior. Unless there is a compulsive pattern to these sexual activities, a signal to the physician that there is an underlying problem requiring his attention, reassurance of the parent or teenager is called for.

Many patients are in doubt about what constitutes normal sexual behavior. These include questions about masturbation, oral-genital sex, sexual

*In the United States the legal and medical sanctions vary considerably by state; there is currently a strong trend toward liberalization or abolition of all legal restraints on abortion.

positions, coital frequency, sex during menstruation, pregnancy, or in the postpartum period, and sex in mid-life or later. The well-informed physician will be able to deal effectively with these concerns if he takes the trouble to inquire about the patient's sex life or is alert to cues that the patient wishes to discuss this area. History taking should utilize open-ended questions that preclude a yes or no answer and that go from less sensitive areas to ones of greater potential discomfort to the patient, e.g., from a discussion of marital relations to sex, or from menarche to petting to coitus, or from frequency to foreplay to coital positions.

Doctor-Patient Relationship. If the physician is interested in this area, if he is reasonably comfortable and tactful, and has an appreciation of the role his own feelings and attitudes play in his interviewing and management of his patients' sexual problems, he will be able to establish a feeling of confidence and hope in his patient. This emphatic relationship coupled with the physician's growing fund of information and skills in interviewing makes possible the competent management of marital and sexual problems that heretofore have been either neglected or mishandled. In no other area of his practice can the physician derive greater reward and satisfaction from his efforts.

Burnap, D. N., and Golden, J. S.: Sexual problems in medical practice. J. Med. Educ., 42:673, 1967.

Calderone, M. S.: Manual of Family Planning and Contraceptive Practice. 2nd ed. Baltimore, Williams & Wilkins Company, 1970.

Herndon, C. N., and Nash, E. M.: Premarriage and marriage counseling: A study of North Carolina physicians. J.A.M.A., 180:395, 1962.

Kinsey, A. C., Pomeroy, W. B., and Martin, C. E.: Sexual Behavior in The Human Male. Philadelphia, W. B. Saunders Company, 1948.

Kinsey, A. C., Pomeroy, W. B., Martin, C. E., and Gebhard, P. H.: Sexual Behavior in The Human Female. Philadelphia, W. B. Saunders Company, 1953.

Klemer, R. H.: Counseling in Marital and Sexual Problems: A Physician's Handbook. Baltimore, Williams & Wilkins Company, 1965.

Lief, H. I.: Preparing the physician to become a sex counselor and educator. Pediat. Clin. N. Amer., 16:44, 1969.

Lief, H. I.: New developments in the sex education of the physician. J.A.M.A., 212:1864, 1970.

Lloyd, C. W.: Human Reproduction and Sexual Behavior. Philadelphia, Lea & Febiger, 1964.

Masters, W. H., and Johnson, V. E.: Human Sexual Response. Boston, Little, Brown and Company, 1966.

Masters, W. H., and Johnson, V. E.: Human Sexual Inadequacy. Boston, Little, Brown and Company, 1970.

Nash, E. M., Jessner, L., and Abse, D. W.: Marriage Counseling in Medical Practice. Chapel Hill, The University of North Carolina Press, 1964.

Trainer, J. B.: Physiologic Foundation for Marriage Counseling. St. Louis, C. V. Mosby Company, 1965.

Vincent, C. E.: Human Sexuality in Medical Education and Practice. Springfield, Ill., Charles C Thomas, 1968.

Drug Dependence, Addiction, and Intoxication

DRUG DEPENDENCE
(Addiction)

Harris Isbell

The World Health Organization and the Committee on Drug Addiction and Narcotics of the U.S. National Research Council have recommended that the term "addiction" be replaced with "drug dependence." The latter term implies that abuse of a drug threatens physical health, psychologic functioning, or ability to adapt to the demands of society. The characteristics vary with the drug involved, which, in each case, must be specified—drug dependence of the morphine type, of the barbiturate type, and so forth.

All drugs that cause dependence act on the central nervous system, but not all drugs that affect the central nervous system produce dependence. Those that do (set forth in the accompanying table) usually cause one or more of the following effects: They reduce anxiety and tension; they produce elation and feelings of increased mental or physical ability; they reduce controls of behavior; they alter sensory perception; they increase or depress sexual drives. In addition, drugs may serve as psychologic symbols that permit aberrant fulfillment of psychic needs.

Definitions. *Psychic Dependence.* Psychic dependence is common to all drug dependence. The person is obsessed with obtaining the drug and persists in taking it despite conscious realization that it harms him physically, psychologically, or socially. Relapse after withdrawal is characteristic.

Physical Dependence. Repeated administration of a drug creates an altered physiologic state in the central nervous system that requires continuance of the drug to prevent a characteristic physical illness called an abstinence syndrome. Two types of physical dependence (I-A, opiate type, and I-B, alcohol-barbiturate type) are reasonably well understood. Type I-C, opiate agonist-antagonist type, is new, and less is known about its pathophysiology. The existence of type I-D, the amphetamine type, is still somewhat controversial.

The characteristic abstinence symptoms in dependence of the opiate type include signs of autonomic dysfunction and central nervous system irritability on withdrawal. Convulsions and delirium are not present. The alcohol-barbiturate type is manifested by convulsions and delirium following withdrawal. Physical dependence of

CLASSIFICATION OF DEPENDENCE-PRODUCING DRUGS

Class I—Drugs that produce both psychic and physical dependence

  A. Opiate (opioid) type

    1. Morphine group: opium, preparations containing opium (tr. opium, camphorated tr. opium), morphine, diacetylmorphine (heroin), dihydromorphinone (Dilaudid), dihydrohydroxymorphinone (Numorphan), methyldihydromorphinone (metopon), pantopon, codeine, dihydrocodeine, dihydrocodeinone (Hycodan), dihydrohydroxycodeinone (Percodan)

    2. Morphinans: levorphan (Levo-Dromoran), racemorphan (Dromoran)

    3. Benzomorphans: phenazocine (Prinadol)

    4. Meperidine group: meperidine (Demerol), alphaprodine (Nisentil), anilerdine (Leritine), piminodine (Alvodine)

    5. Methadone group: methadone (d-propoxyphene, or Darvon, has definite dependence liability but of such low degree that U.S. narcotic law controls are not applied)

  B. Alcohol-barbiturate type

    1. Ethyl alcohol: beer, wine, whiskey, etc.

    2. Barbiturates: all those sold in the United States for sedation and hypnosis

    3. Paraldehyde

    4. Chloral hydrate

    5. Meprobamate (Miltown, Equanil)

    6. Piperidinediones: glutethimide (Doriden), methprylon (Nodular)

    7. Benzodiazepines: chlordiazepoxide (Librium), diazepam (Valium)

    8. Tertiary carbinols: methylpentynol (Dormison), ethchlorvynol (Placidyl), ethinamate (Valmid)

  C. Opiate agonist-antagonist type

    1. Nalorphine

    2. Levallorphan

    3. Cyclazocine

    4. Pentazocine (Talwin)

  D. Amphetamine type

    1. dl-Amphetamine (Benzedrine), dextro-amphetamine (Dexedrine), methamphetamine (Desoxyn)

    2. Phenmetrazine (Preludin)

    3. Methylphenidate (Ritalin)

    4. Diethylpropion (Tenuate)

    5. Pipradol (Meratran)

Class II—Drugs that produce psychic but not physical dependence

  A. Cocaine type: coca leaf, cocaine

  B. Hallucinogens

    1. Lysergic acid diethylamide (LSD, LSD-25) and derivatives

    2. Mescaline (including peyote, or mescal buttons)

    3. Tryptamines

      a. Psilocybin and psilocin (including the mushroom *Psilocybe mexicana*)

      b. Dimethyl- and diethyltryptamines and related compounds

    4. Hallucinogenic amphetamines: 2,5-dimethoxy-4-methylamphetamine (STP, DOM)

  C. Cannabis type

    1. Crude drugs: Cannabis leaf (marihuana); hashish

    2. Tetrahydrocannabinols

  D. Bromides

---

the opiate-antagonist type is similar to, but quantitatively much milder than, the opiate type. Qualitative differences also exist. Physical dependence of the amphetamine type is manifest by an increase in sleep (and in rapid-eye-movement sleep—REM sleep) increased appetite, and psychologic depression.

The phenothiazine (chlorpromazine), reserpine, and butyrophenone tranquilizers are not included, as these classes of drugs do not produce either psychic or physical dependence.

Tolerance develops to most dependence-producing drugs, and refers to a declining effect from repeated administration or to a need for increased amounts to sustain the initial effect. Tolerance to one drug frequently confers cross-tolerance to others with similar characteristics. Tolerance may be either "metabolic"—enhanced detoxification—or "cellular"—adaptation of neurons to continued high drug concentrations. Both may occur with the same drug.

All drugs of class I-A (see table) show cross-tolerance and will completely or partially suppress symptoms of abstinence within the same group. Class I-B drugs do the same within their group. Drugs of the opiate type will not suppress abstinence symptoms of the alcohol-barbiturate type and vice versa. Abrupt withdrawal is contraindicated in both classes I-A and I-B. Abstinence from drugs of type I-C and I-D and all type II drugs requires no withdrawal treatment.

Etiology. Drug dependence most commonly begins during adolescent or involutional periods, and has several interacting causes.

Chronic Disease. Chronic painful disease may be inadvisedly treated with dependence-producing drugs over long periods of time. The patients are frequently referred to as "medical addicts." Diseases such as rheumatoid arthritis, asthma, and thromboangiitis obliterans are particularly likely to invite drug dependence. If one excludes terminal conditions, most drug-dependent persons with chronic painful disease also have severe neurotic traits that may be even more important in the genesis of their drug dependence.

Social Factors. Social attitudes have marked effects. In Western society, the moderate use of alcohol is almost a normal part of the culture, and its availability leads to widespread abuse. On the other hand, use of opiates is strongly condemned and is repressed legally, the result being that hostile, rebellious, immature persons may use drugs to flout social authority and custom. Adverse social conditions, including poverty, slum living, weak family structures, and discrimination are associated with a high incidence of drug dependence of the opiate type.

In contrast, young persons from middle-class backgrounds who are dissatisfied with what they believe are the purely materialistic views of their parents and with the policies of the government have been attracted to the "mind-expanding" (psychedelic) drugs such as LSD and marihuana. Young people have created drug-using subcultures—"hippies" and the like—which are currently of great social concern around the world. Thus the social factors associated with drug dependence vary with the drugs, the time, and the political circumstances, and are not specific.

Personality Factors. Most drug-dependent persons have personality or character disorders that antedate drug dependence and contribute to relapse after withdrawal. The most common psychiatric patterns are a mixture of neurotic traits (anxiety, conversion, compulsive-obsessive, depressive reactions) and character disorders.

Three important psychologic hypotheses of the processes leading to drug dependence have been formulated. The *psychobiologic hypothesis* holds that drug-dependent persons suffer from physical or psychologic discomfort, the latter arising from unresolved conflicts in life situations. The drug relieves the distress, and the relief leads to repetition of drug taking, with consequent development of tolerance and physical dependence.

The *psychoanalytic hypothesis* holds that addicts have arrested at, or regressed to, the oral stage of psychosexual development. In infancy and childhood, a strong father figure has consistently been lacking, whereas the mother has been inconsistently indulgent and rejecting. Because of faulty psychosexual development, the individual comes to regard other persons, particularly the mother, as objects for self-gratification. Since all his needs cannot be fulfilled in reality, he reacts with hostility to others, often to the mother or other women, and takes drugs to ameliorate the conflict.

Neither the psychobiologic nor the psychoanalytic hypothesis satisfactorily explains why, with similar personalities and equal exposure, some persons choose alcohol, others opiates, and still others neither. Another hypothesis, the *pharmacodynamic hypothesis*, has therefore been developed. This relates the choice to specific drug actions. Opiates depress pain, sexual drive, hunger, and thirst. Individuals in whom the main sources of anxiety are related to these drives find great relief from opiates. Alcohol and barbiturate drugs impair control of behavior, and permit direct aggressive acting out of conflicts, thus satisfying persons with this kind of emotional need.

Persons who become physically dependent on opiates, hypnotics, or alcohol experience abstinence symptoms in a variety of situations. If abstinence occurs frequently enough in the same situation, the abstinence symptoms become conditioned, and may recur after withdrawal and ostensible physiologic recovery under appropriate environmental conditional stimuli (seeing people who are intoxicated with the drug of addiction, stressful situations, and so on). Since the user has to seek the drug to relieve symptoms of abstinence, drug-seeking behavior is constantly reinforced and induces relapse.

DEPENDENCE OF THE OPIATE TYPE

Incidence and Epidemiology. Dependence on opiates has been widespread in Oriental countries, where opium eating or smoking is, or has been, a normal part of the culture. It has never been a large problem in Britain or in western Europe. In the United States, little is known about the incidence of medically induced opiate dependence. Excluding that in terminal cancer, the incidence is probably not high. Dependence of the opiate type occurs more frequently among physicians and nurses than among others. According to the Federal Bureau of Narcotics, there are about 125,000 "active" illicit opiate dependents in the United States, with some 6000 to 10,000 new cases annually. Most cases are in certain slum areas of large cities, particularly New York, Chicago, and Los Angeles, but heroin abuse is now spreading outside the slums to involve young people in middle-class areas. Most illicit opiate users are males between the ages of 20 and 30; experimentation usually begins at about age 15 or 16. About half the known illicit addicts are Negroes, and about 20 per cent are Mexicans or Puerto Ricans. The role of drug peddlers in spreading dependence has been exaggerated; practically all young opiate dependents are introduced to drugs by other addicts.

Drugs and Mode of Use. The main drug in the illicit traffic in the United States is heroin, which, most frequently, is taken intravenously ("mainlined") and is usually highly diluted with lactose, quinine, or other chemicals. The illicit drugs are also heavily contaminated with bacteria, fungi, yeast, and spores. There is considerable fluctuation in intake from day to day. Most illicit users obtain less than 50 mg. of heroin daily, but frequently take other drugs, including cocaine, amphetamines, marihuana, barbiturates, and other hypnotics. Abuse of alcohol may precede the abuse of opiates, but is seldom concomitant.

Patients who obtain their drugs through legal sources most commonly use morphine or meperidine (Demerol) and employ the subcutaneous route. Dependence on codeine or its congeners, dihydrocodeinone (Hycodan) and dihydrohydroxycodeinone (Percodan), sometimes occurs when the drug is taken orally, frequently in a cough syrup.

Pathology. Dependence causes no direct pathologic changes, although skin infections or tetanus may follow subcutaneous administration, and serum hepatitis is frequent in addicts who use the intravenous route. Sudden death is frequent among intravenous abusers of heroin. About 400 to 600 such deaths occur yearly in New York City. The pathologic picture is that of massive pulmonary edema. The condition has been attributed to cardiac arrhythmias due to quinine and other chemical contaminants with which the illicit heroin is diluted or to anaphylaxis from other materials. The same syndrome, however, has been reported in England in addicts taking pure heroin obtained from legal sources, so death is likely due to direct toxic effects of heroin, possibly respiratory arrest, convulsions, or both.

Distribution and Metabolism. Opiates and opioids are readily absorbed and are distributed throughout the body. Only small amounts reach the central nervous system. The opiates are metabolized in the liver and are excreted either in bile or in urine. Morphine is conjugated with glucuronic acid and is N-demethylated. Meperidine is both de-esterified and demethylated. One of the products of the metabolism of meperidine, normeperidine, is a convulsant and accounts for the high incidence of convulsions in meperidine abusers. Neither metabolites nor changes in drug distribution account for tolerance or physical dependence.

Biochemical Changes in Chronic Intoxication. Opiates and opioids stimulate the posterior pituitary through the hypothalamus, with consequent secretion of antidiuretic hormone and water retention. Tolerance to this action develops rapidly. Chronic intoxication depresses the adrenal cortices by inhibiting ACTH release. Gonadal function is depressed, with a decline in libido and the cessation of menses in women. Brain catecholamine levels are elevated in laboratory animals and decline to normal when the drugs are withdrawn.

Abrupt opiate withdrawal activates the adrenal cortices and elevates serum corticoids. Diminished intake and increased water loss from perspiration, hyperpnea, vomiting, and diarrhea increase the hematocrit, diminish the blood volume, and decrease extracellular fluid volume. Normal serum electrolyte concentrations are maintained. The blood sugar and metabolic rate are elevated.

Physiologic Changes in Maintained Addiction. The important changes are limited to the central nervous system. Opiates depress or stimulate polysynaptic reflexes at all levels of the central nervous system. Tolerance develops rapidly to the depressant action but more slowly to the stimulant actions. Responses mediated through two neuron arcs are little affected.

Following abrupt withdrawal, the changes seen in the central nervous system are opposite in direction to the acute effects of the opiates. Reflexes formerly depressed become hyperactive, and reflexes stimulated by the drug disappear. In man, about 60 days is required for restoration of normal central nervous system functioning.

Theories of Tolerance and Dependence. Currently, the adaptive or homeostatic theory is most widely accepted. It is believed that the neurons develop responses that oppose the actions of the opiates. These responses persist following withdrawal of drugs; hence, symptoms opposite to the acute effects of the drugs appear. Recently water-soluble substances of small molecular weight have been extracted from the brain of tolerant rats that confer tolerance when injected into other animals.

Clinical Manifestations. The symptoms and signs of opiate dependence vary with the dose and the degree of tolerance. The initial dose usually evokes nausea and vomiting. Tolerance develops rapidly and, on repeated trial, the potential addict begins to have experiences that he regards as pleasant, such as a feeling of increased ability to perform, reduction of anxiety, fantasies, and sedation, which, in severe states of intoxication, lead to alternating somnolence and wakefulness ("nodding"). There is little impairment of psychomotor coordination. Initially, respiratory rate and minute volume decline, temperature drops slightly, pulse rate slows, blood pressure falls, the pupils shrink, and constipation occurs. Intravenous injection creates a sudden flushing, dizziness, itching over the entire body, and rumbling of the stomach. Addicts compare this sensation to sexual orgasm.

Most of the effects of morphine disappear as tolerance develops, and the users may appear normal mentally and physically except for miotic pupils and chronic constipation. The only significant findings may be needle marks on the skin, abscess scars, and tattooing over the veins. An enormous tolerance can develop to morphine. Cases are on record of patients taking as much as 5 grams intravenously in 16 to 24 hours without harmful effect. Tolerance to any drug in Group I-A confers tolerance to any other drug in the group (crossed tolerance). This is the basis for the methadone maintenance treatment (see below) of opiate dependence, in which crossed tolerance is termed "narcotic blockade."

Morphine Abstinence Syndrome. The morphine abstinence syndrome is stereotyped, self-limited, and not dangerous to life in persons who have no serious physical disease. About 40 to 80 mg. (or the equivalent in class I-A) of morphine has to be taken daily for at least a month for detectable signs of abstinence to occur, and the intensity with doses of this order is so slight as to require no treatment. The abstinence syndrome is moderate after doses of 120 mg. daily for a month, marked with 180 to 240 mg. daily, and severe with 240 mg. daily or more. There is little increase in severity with doses higher than 360 mg. daily. Abstinence signs and symptoms are more severe the longer a drug has been used and more intense after regular administration. The abstinence syndrome comes on more quickly with short-acting than with long-acting drugs. Thus, abstinence from agents such as heroin and Dilaudid produces signs and symptoms after about eight hours, which become maximal at 24 hours, and largely subside after five days.

If morphine is abruptly withdrawn from a patient taking 240 mg. or more daily, symptoms develop after about 10 or 16 hours; the first to occur are restlessness and an abnormal, tossing sleep ("sleepy yen"). After 16 to 24 hours, yawning, tearing, rhinorrhea, sweating, dilatation of the pupils, and waves of gooseflesh appear. After 24 hours, the person is restless, cannot sleep, and complains of muscle cramps and chills. The temperature is elevated to 38 to 39.5° C. (100.4 to 103.3° F.). Blood pressure increases by 15 mm. of mercury or more. Respiratory rate and minute volume increase. Patients may vomit, have diarrhea, and lose 5 to 15 pounds in 24 hours. The acute symptoms are maximal between the thirty-sixth and seventy-second hour after the last dose. Thereafter, they decline rapidly, and most disappear by the fifth to fourteenth day.

The chronic phase of abstinence lasts for two to four months and is characterized by gradually decreasing insomnia, irritability, and muscular aches and pains.

Diagnosis. Diagnosis is usually made through the history. Objective findings are meager. Miosis, needle marks, abscess scars, and tattooing are suggestive but not conclusive. The diagnosis is usually confirmed by withholding drugs and allowing signs of abstinence to appear.

Physical dependence of the opiate type can also be demonstrated by rapidly precipitating abstinence with the morphine antagonist, nalorphine. The initial dose of nalorphine should be 3 mg. or less, subcutaneously, since large doses can precipitate fatal abstinence effects in a strongly physically dependent addict. The nalorphine test is performed by observing for signs of abstinence prior to administration of nalorphine; then 3 mg. of nalorphine is injected subcutaneously, and the observations are repeated at 15-minute intervals. If there is significant physical dependence, the pupils dilate 0.5 mm. or more within 30 minutes, the patient sweats and shows gooseflesh, and the respiratory rate increases. If no evidence of abstinence is observed after 30 minutes, an additional 5 mg. of nalorphine may be given. If physical dependence has not developed, signs of direct nalorphine effect—miosis and respiratory depression—will occur. The nalorphine test is unreliable in dependence on meperidine.

Tests for opiates in urine are reliable but difficult, and frequently are unavailable.

Dependence of the opiate type is frequently complicated by other types of drug dependence (usually on barbiturates, cocaine, or amphetamines). Infectious complications are frequent and may be serious. Viral hepatitis, bacterial and mycotic endocarditis, tetanus, thrombophlebitis, and subcutaneous abscesses all occur.

Treatment. The American Medical Association has issued a statement, approved by the Federal Bureau of Narcotics, that clarifies the role of physicians in the treatment of opiate dependence. Physicians prescribing opiates must minimize iatrogenic opiate dependence and, in addition, have both the right and the ethical responsibility to treat opiate-dependent persons. In some states (New York, California, Illinois) physicians must report opiate abusers to the Health Department. A physician may prescribe opiates for aged, debilitated, or severely ill addicts if withdrawal is dangerous to life. Withdrawal of opiates should usually be carried out in a hospital or other secure, drug-free setting, but physicians with special skill and experience may attempt ambulatory withdrawal. Physicians may administer narcotics for dependent patients awaiting admission to inpatient facilities. In general, such patients should receive only one day's supply of the drug at a time, should be seen daily, and should not be allowed to temporize about seeking admission.

Most physicians are well advised to refer drug-dependent patients to special institutions, such as private or state psychiatric hospitals and special state facilities in New York and California. The Federal Hospitals at Fort Worth, Texas, and Lexington, Kentucky, accept patients committed under the Narcotic Addict Rehabilitation Act. Information should be obtained by writing these institutions.

Goals of Treatment. The goal of standard or traditional treatment has been and is total abstinence from drugs plus social rehabilitation. Dis-satisfaction with the results of the standard treatment has led to experimentation with maintenance of addicts on methadone, the goal being social rehabilitation and not abstinence, at least in the initial period of treatment.

Standard treatment consists of three phases: withdrawal, rehabilitation, and postinstitutional supervision.

Withdrawal of opiates requires only an environment guaranteed to be drug-free. Any of the opiates may be used in withdrawal; methadone has special advantages because of its long action and good oral efficacy. The proper dose permits the appearance of mild signs of abstinence, e.g., sweating, yawning, but prevents severe effects of abstinence (insomnia, nausea, vomiting) and is determined by trial and error. Ordinarily, 5 to 30 mg. of methadone twice daily will suffice. After the initial dose, it should be reduced each day by one third to one tenth of the total daily amount. Withdrawal should usually be completed in 3 to 14 days, but may require up to 30 days in cases complicated by serious organic disease. Toward the end of withdrawal, a mild hypnotic may be needed, such as 0.5 to 1.0 gram of chloral hydrate at night. Withdrawal of hypnotics, if necessary, can be carried out concurrently.

The physician must adopt a kind but unyielding attitude to neurotic and psychopathic attempts to obtain additional drugs. Massive sedation, tranquilizers, scopolamine, exhausting physiotherapy, or insulin should be avoided.

Following completion of withdrawal, rehabilitation is undertaken. Any physical disease must be treated. If chronic pain is an important factor, neurosurgical procedures may be considered. If the patient is willing to participate and is a suitable candidate, group or individual psychotherapy should be provided. Patients should be given vocational and educational training to equip them with skills to earn a living.

Postinstitutional care is critical. Ideally, it should last for several years. Every drug-dependent patient should be assisted in finding work, and should be referred to local agencies for psychiatric care and social assistance. Testing with nalorphine or testing urine samples for opiates is required in some states and is said to reduce the frequency of relapse. Participation in the activities of Alcoholics Anonymous or Addicts Anonymous has helped some addicts.

Outcome of the Traditional Treatment. About 90 per cent of treated opiate dependents relapse within one year after discharge from an institution. The long-range results are better; about 30 per cent of patients become abstinent and adjust socially after about ten years. The mortality rate is approximately ten times that expected in the same age group of nondrug users and is due to overdoses, infections, suicide, and murder. Prognosis varies markedly with the social group. It is worst (90 per cent relapse) in psychopathic persons who come from, and return to, big city slums. Fifty per cent of addicts returning to rural environments successfully remain abstinent. In contrast to psychopathic patients, 90 per cent of physician addicts remain abstinent after one treatment.

The *Synanon program* is also based on total abstinence, but is a nonmedical program based on mutual help and "assaultive therapy" in a communal living situation. Synanon has been helpful to many but not all of a highly selected population of addicts.

The use of the narcotic antagonist cyclazocine as an aid to maintaining abstinence is an experimental treatment which involves withdrawal of opiates and maintenance of the patient on cyclazocine, an orally effective opiate antagonist with a duration of action of about 12 hours. The dose of cyclazocine must be elevated gradually to 2.0 to 3.0 mg. twice daily to avoid psychotomimetic effects. If the patient continues to take this dose, the euphoric effects of heroin are effectively blocked and nonrewarding. The cyclazocine treatment obviously requires the cooperation of the patient, as he has only to skip one dose in order to experience the euphoric effects of heroin again.

Methadone maintenance is an experimental treatment in which the goal, at least initially, is acceptable social adjustment and not total abstinence. It is based on the fact that tolerance to most effects of opiates is very complete so that a tolerant addict can function well socially, provided he is motivated and receives his drug, and on the fact that tolerance to one drug in group I-A confers crossed tolerance to any other drug in the group ("narcotic blockade"). Methadone has two properties which make it the drug of choice for this treatment: good oral efficacy and long length of action. These two advantages mean that one dose of methadone can be given orally in orange juice once daily by a clinic, and obviates the risk of diversion inherent in treatments (such as the "British system" and the clinics operated in the United States between 1918 and 1921) in which morphine or heroin is supplied to the addict for self-administration.

In methadone maintenance the patient is admitted to a special open ward. Heroin or other opiates are discontinued, and the patient is given methadone in orange juice. The dosage of methadone is gradually elevated to 120 to 180 mg. in one dose daily. Patients tolerant to this dose of methadone will be cross-tolerant to as much as 30 mg. of heroin intravenously, and they soon learn that there is no point in buying illicit heroin. They are encouraged to find work or to return to school, and are given social assistance.

The social results have been promising. Seventy per cent of the patients are working or going to school and refraining from criminal activities.

Methadone treatment is still experimental and should not be attempted by the ordinary practitioner. If methadone maintenance continues to be used, it will probably always have to be carried out by special clinics.

Several things should be remembered: Patients maintained on methadone are strongly dependent physically and psychically. Possible long-term toxic effects of methadone are still unknown. Finally, opiate dependence is the only form of dependence in which maintenance on the drug is pharmacologically rational, since tolerance to other types of drugs is not sufficiently complete to eliminate the toxic effects on tissue and on behavior.

DEPENDENCE OF THE OPIATE AGONIST-ANTAGONIST TYPE

Originally it was thought that the opiate antagonists would not cause either psychic or physical dependence. Later it was shown that these drugs were not pure antagonists (opposing the effects of morphine) but also had morphine-like (agonistic) actions which accounted for their analgesic properties. Finally it was found that chronic administration of these drugs leads to tolerance to some of their actions, notably the dysphoric and hallucinogenic effects, and to a mild type of physical dependence qualitatively different from that of morphine. In an effort to develop an analgesic drug that could not cause physical dependence, many compounds with varying ratios of agonistic-antagonistic activity were synthesized and tested. One of these, the injectable form of pentazocine (Talwin), a drug with weak opiate-antagonist but moderate opiate-agonist activity, became available without narcotic law controls. Unfortunately, cases of dependence on pentazocine soon appeared, and now over 55 such cases have been found. In nontolerant patients, pentazocine has morphine-like euphoric effects in doses of 40 mg. or less, intramuscularly or intravenously. The effects become dysphoric in doses of 60 mg. or more. Tolerance to the dysphoric and other effects develops on chronic administration, with consequent need to increase the dose. Pentazocine cannot be substituted for morphine in dependent patients, since it precipitates rather than suppresses abstinence from morphine. Abrupt withdrawal of pentazocine from persons taking 500 to 700 mg. daily results in mild abstinence characterized by nervousness, insomnia, sensations of electric shocks, perspiration, and aches and pains. Although the syndrome is mild, it leads to drug-seeking behavior. Most cases of pentazocine dependence have occurred in patients who were and had been dependent on other drugs. In addition, the large doses of pentazocine taken by dependent patients caused marked chemical inflammation of the skin, with fibrosis and ulcerations.

Accordingly, the same precautions should be followed in prescribing or dispensing pentazocine as are used with morphine and other opiates and opioids.

DEPENDENCE ON HYPNOTICS

Incidence. The incidence of dependence on hypnotic drugs in the United States has been estimated to be as high as 500,000 cases, and 12 per cent of psychiatric admissions to the University of Kentucky Hospital were for dependence on hypnotic drugs. Dependence on hypnotics and barbiturates commonly complicates alcohol and opiate abuse, and occurs in all social classes. There is an active illicit market, and in the state of California more arrests are made for possession of hypnotics and amphetamines than for possession of heroin.

Etiology. Hypnotics reduce tension and anxiety, induce sleep, and in large doses, cause drunkenness and resultant impairment of behavioral controls. There are no specifically susceptible personality patterns, but most patients are either markedly neurotic or have a character disorder, or a mixture of both. Depressive reactions may predispose to hypnotic dependence because of the associated insomnia, and dependence frequently results from medical prescription. Alcoholics and opiate abusers frequently become dependent on hypnotics in attempts to supplement the effects of their usual drugs.

Drugs and Mode of Use. Hypnotics (class I-B in the table) generally are taken orally. Occasionally, opiate abusers will take them intravenously. The amounts range from 4 to 50 hypnotic doses daily, frequently including several different drugs. Drugs are often obtained by prescription from different physicians, none of whom realizes that the patient has more than one source.

Distribution and Metabolism. All the hypnotics are well absorbed when taken orally and are generally distributed throughout the body. Only small amounts reach the central nervous system. Most of the drugs are metabolized in the liver by hydroxylation, dealkalization, and conjugation (barbital is an exception) and are excreted in the urine or bile. The metabolites of the drugs do not account for tolerance or physical dependence. The barbiturates that are metabolized in the liver stimulate induction of enzymes concerned with oxidation and hydroxylation, so that the metabolic degradation of barbiturates proceeds more rapidly, and the increased rate of transformation partly accounts for tolerance.

Physiologic Changes. Hypnotics elevate the threshold for excitation of all types of neurons and depress all kinds of central reflexes. Cortical neurons and those of the reticular activating system are the most sensitive. Neurons of the cerebellar-vestibular system are the next most sensitive, followed by the spinal neurons. Midbrain centers are the most resistant. In sufficient dose, all drugs of this type cause respiratory and cardiovascular depression.

During addiction partial tolerance develops that is never as complete as tolerance to opiates. Tolerance is due partly to increased metabolic degradation of the drugs and partly to adaptive cellular changes in the central nervous system. As with the opiates, the adaptive changes oppose and outlast drug action so that abstinence manifestations are opposite to acute drug effects. Early in chronic intoxication, thresholds for electrical induction of convulsions are increased. As tolerance develops, the electroconvulsive threshold declines to normal levels. When the drugs are abruptly withdrawn, the convulsive threshold falls below normal.

Theories of Tolerance and Dependence. Cellular tolerance (adaptive) develops by unknown mechanisms so that neurons function almost normally in the presence of high blood concentrations of drugs. Changes in the level of gamma aminobutyric acid in the brain may play a role.

Clinical Manifestations. The manifestations of chronic hypnotic intoxication resemble those of alcoholic intoxication, and include lethargy, ataxia, nystagmus, slurred speech, impaired judgment, and emotional lability. As chronic intoxication proceeds, partial tolerance develops, and the symptoms on a particular dose become less noticeable. However, tolerance is limited and, if it is exceeded by even a small amount, signs and symptoms of intoxication reappear. Behavioral disturbances range from simple confusion and increased emotional lability to paranoid psychotic states. Patients become untidy and disheveled, neglect their work, suffer from disturbed judgment, and exhibit impulsive behavior.

Abstinence Syndrome. When hypnotics are abruptly discontinued following long-continued ingestion, a stereotyped, self-limited illness occurs. "Minor" symptoms include anxiety, tremors, restlessness, insomnia, postural hypotension, nausea, and vomiting. "Major" symptoms include convulsions, delirium, and high fever. *In contrast to opiate abstinence, that from hypnotics is dangerous to life.*

Several factors affect the severity of abstinence. Significant dependence usually occurs only in patients taking three to four hypnotic doses daily in whom minor symptoms and, occasionally, a convulsion appear upon withdrawal. When five to six hypnotic doses are taken daily, half the patients convulse, and a third suffer delirium upon withdrawal. If eight doses or more are taken daily, convulsions occur in 75 per cent and delirium in 60 per cent. To produce abstinence signs and symptoms requires at least a month of continuous use; the longer the use, the more severe the abstinence syndrome. Signs and symptoms appear quickly following withdrawal of short-acting drugs such as meprobamate, pentobarbital, or chloral hydrate, but develop more slowly and persist longer after withdrawal from barbital, phenobarbital, and glutethimide. Recovery is usually complete in two to three weeks.

When hypnotics are abruptly withdrawn, the patient first "sobers up" and appears to improve. He then complains of nervousness, tremulousness, weakness, and insomnia. Startle responses, muscle twitching, hyperactive stretch reflexes, weakness, and postural hypotension emerge. Epileptic-like electroencephalographic abnormalities appear within 48 hours, and seizures, potentially leading to status epilepticus, delirium, and agitation may occur between the first and seventh days. Body temperature above 101° F. is ominous and requires vigorous treatment. The syndrome usually terminates in one to five days, either suddenly after a "critical" sleep or gradually. Recovery is complete and without permanent brain damage.

Diagnosis. Diagnosis of dependence is usually made from the history, and should always be suggested by signs of drunkenness without the odor of alcohol. Tests are available for some of the drugs and their metabolites in blood and urine. Abstinence from hypnotics is too dangerous to warrant establishing the diagnosis by withholding drugs, and thus is best established by determining tolerance to test doses of hypnotic drugs (*vide infra*).

Treatment. Treatment includes withdrawal, rehabilitation, and aftercare. Withdrawal must be conducted in a hospital, nursing home, or other institution. Since abstinence from hypnotics is dangerous to life, it should be prevented if possible and, if present, should be treated vigorously. As mentioned above, the drugs in group I-B are all partially equivalent so that any of them can be used in conducting withdrawal. Pentobarbital is as effective, flexible, and safe as any other member of the group. If the diagnosis is established before signs of abstinence have appeared, the patient is given no drugs until he is sober. Next, the least amount of pentobarbital that just maintains a mild but manageable degree of intoxication—the "stabilization dose"—must be established by trial and error. After the patient has become sober he is given a test dose of 0.2 gram of pentobarbital orally and is examined one and a half hours later. The desired effect is mild intoxication manifested by inconstant slow nystagmus on lateral gaze, slight dysarthria, and swaying, but not falling, on the Romberg test. If the desired endpoint is attained on the first test, 0.2 gram of pentobarbital is given orally every six hours, but the patient must be re-examined one and a half hours after each dose, since pentobarbital effects may cumulate.

If the patient is tremulous, agitated, and twitchy one and a half hours after the first test, the dose was insufficient and should be immediately reinforced with an additional 0.1 gram of pentobarbital, which may be repeated at hourly intervals until the desired effect has been attained, after which the patient can be placed on a regular schedule. If the patient becomes grossly ataxic, has constant nystagmus, dysarthria, and emotional lability after the test dose or any subsequent dose, too much pentobarbital has been given and the next scheduled dose should be reduced. In this way, the amount of drug required is titrated to the individual's requirements. The stabilization dose is diagnostic as well as therapeutic. If the patient can take 0.4 gram of pentobarbital daily without gross intoxication, he is tolerant to, and mildly dependent on, drugs of type I-B. If he

requires 0.6 to 0.8 gram daily, he is strongly dependent; and if he requires more than 0.8 gram daily, he is severely dependent. After the stabilization dose is known, the patient is maintained on that dose for a day or two while necessary examinations are being obtained. The dose of pentobarbital is then reduced progressively by 0.1 gram or less daily. Withdrawal is usually complete in 4 to 14 days. If the patient cannot or will not take pentobarbital orally, it may be given by intramuscular injection initially in the same fashion as described for oral use. Generally, patients can be switched to oral drugs after a few intramuscular doses.

Convulsions, delirium, or fever should be treated as emergencies. The patient should be given 0.2 gram of pentobarbital intramuscularly at once and additional doses of 0.1 gram at hourly intervals until asleep; additional doses should be given as required to maintain sleep for 8 to 12 hours. He is then allowed to awaken and to become sober, after which the stabilization dose is determined as described above.

Fluid and electrolyte losses must be replaced and complicating medical or surgical conditions treated. Increasing fever without evidence of infection requires additional sedation, antipyretics, sponging, or cooling blankets.

The same system of stabilization on pentobarbital to maintain slight drunkenness followed by progressive daily reduction of the pentobarbital can be used in treating abstinence from alcohol (see below).

The phenothiazines, reserpine, and the butyrophenones and diphenylhydantoin are ineffective, and should be avoided.

After withdrawal the patient needs two to three weeks for convalescence, during which institution of psychiatric treatment is desirable. Following discharge, the patient should be supervised, preferably for years. Participation in Alcoholics Anonymous may help. Prognosis is guarded and relapse is frequent. Depression and suicide attempts may follow withdrawal.

ALCOHOL PROBLEMS AND ALCOHOLISM
Harris Isbell

Incidence and Epidemiology. Dependence on alcohol exists when that drug is taken in amounts sufficient to interfere with interpersonal relationships, psychologic functioning, or physical health. Some 10 million Americans are dependent on alcohol and 1 to 2 million suffer from one of the organic complications. Dependence on alcohol occurs in all social classes and in all geographic locations. It is more common in large cities and affects more men than women.

Etiology. Most persons take alcohol to relieve

anxiety, to facilitate social interaction, or to produce sleep or unconsciousness. Cultural patterns may either increase or decrease the incidence. Dependence is hardly less frequent in cultures in which alcohol is taken with meals as wine or beer; the incidence in France is the world's highest.

Pharmacology and Physiology. Alcohol is absorbed chiefly from the duodenum and jejunum and is distributed in body tissues in proportion to their water content. Ninety per cent is metabolized, and less than 10 per cent is excreted in the breath or urine. Alcohol is first oxidized to acetaldehyde in the liver. The acetaldehyde is converted to acetate by aldehyde dehydrogenase in most tissues. The acetate enters the citric acid cycle, where it is oxidized to CO_2 and water, or is used for synthesis of fat or protein. A nontolerant person can metabolize 7 to 20 ml. of absolute alcohol per hour. Some chronic drinkers can oxidize as much as 25 ml. of alcohol (50 ml. of whiskey) per hour.

Alcohol's most important pharmacologic action is to depress the central nervous system, and its toxicity is increased by other depressants. Neurons of the cerebral cortex and the reticular formation are more sensitive than those of the spinal cord. Medullary centers are least sensitive, being seriously depressed only in overwhelmingly heavy, potentially fatal intoxication. The most important non-CNS actions of alcohol are on fat metabolism. Alcohol is a food that supplies no vitamins, proteins, or minerals, and excessive intake may cause both obesity and nutritional deficiency. Alcohol increases the amount of fat in liver cells, and large doses can produce massive fat deposition. This liver fat can resemble adipose tissue fat, dietary fat, or endogenously synthesized fat, depending on conditions of diet and nutrition. The deposition of excessive fat in the liver of human beings is followed in some cases (estimated at 10 per cent of chronic drinkers) by periportal necrosis and fibrous repair, though the exact role of alcohol and preceding fatty liver in the development of cirrhosis remains unclear. Less important actions of alcohol include depression of release of antidiuretic hormone, peripheral vasodilatation, increased pulse rate, and increased blood pressure. Alcohol stimulates production of gastrin, with a resultant increase in gastric acid and pepsin secretion. Alcohol recently has been shown to interfere with leukocyte mobilization in normal persons, which may help to explain the alcoholic's increased susceptibility to infection. Chronic alcoholics may be unable to mobilize leukocytes because of a deficiency in folic acid.

Acute Alcoholic Intoxication. Rapid ingestion of concentrated alcohol on an empty stomach causes more drunkenness than the slow ingestion of a similar amount with meals. The signs and symptoms of intoxication correlate reasonably well with the blood or breath levels. No clinical signs of drunkenness usually accompany a blood alcohol level of less than 50 mg. per 100 ml. Overt signs of intoxication may or may not accompany blood alcohol levels between 50 and 100 mg. per 100 ml. Above 100 mg. per 100 ml., close examination almost always reveals garrulousness, euphoria, lability in mood, occasionally excitement, increased aggressiveness, moderate pupillary dilatation, inconstant nystagmus on lateral gaze, dysarthria, and ataxia. With levels greater than 150 mg. per 100 ml., there is usually gross evidence of intoxication. The subject is excited, noisy, and aggressive. His pupils dilate, nystagmus becomes constant, strabismus may occur, and dysarthria and ataxia increase. With levels above 200 mg. per 100 ml., stumbling and falling are likely. When the blood alcohol reaches 250 mg. per 100 ml., sedation and sleep frequently ensue. Concentrations of 300 ml. or more per 100 ml. cause stupor, and those of 400 mg. per 100 ml. or more cause coma and general anesthesia. Levels over 600 mg. per 100 ml. are usually fatal.

Some unstable psychopaths and patients with brain injury suddenly develop irrational, combative, and destructive behavior after ingesting small or moderate amounts of alcohol, a condition termed *pathologic intoxication.* The patient may be confused and disoriented and may have hallucinations. The episode may last for moments or days, and usually terminates with deep sleep or stupor with amnesia.

The postalcoholic state—the "hangover"—follows excessive indulgence in alcohol with a severity proportional to the amount and duration of drinking. The symptoms include malaise, nausea, vomiting, weakness, headache, nervousness, difficulty in thinking, pallor, sweating, tachycardia, tremor, and nystagmus. The condition is self-limited and clears in hours to a day or so, depending on the severity of the debauch. All the symptoms are relieved by more alcohol.

Diagnosis. The diagnosis of acute alcoholic intoxication is made from the history, symptoms, and signs, and is confirmed by the blood alcohol. If the patient is stuporous or comatose, careful examination must exclude other causes of coma, such as head injury or pneumonia. Stupor or coma with blood alcohol levels of less than 250 mg. per 100 ml. suggests the ingestion of other central nervous system depressants.

Treatment. Acute alcoholic intoxication usually requires no more than withholding alcohol and protecting the patient. Excited, noisy, or combative patients are best managed by isolation and persuasion rather than by drugs, for these may be dangerous. If drugs are required, 4 to 8 ml. of paraldehyde or 10 mg. of chlorpromazine is suitable, but even these small amounts should be avoided if the blood alcohol level is over 250 mg. per 100 ml.

Patients in stupor or coma should be handled as emergencies and closely monitored. Gastric lavage or emetics increase the risk and are to be avoided. Deeply poisoned patients are managed like those with any other acute depressant drug poisoning (see Management of Acute Depressive Drug Poisoning). No drugs or other agents are available that antagonize alcohol or increase its metabolism. Since alcohol is a freely diffusible water-soluble substance, either peritoneal dialysis or hemodialysis can be used in severely depressed patients to reduce the blood alcohol level rapidly.

Hangovers require little treatment other than abstention. Bland liquids may be prescribed, and aluminum hydroxide gel may be given for gastric discomfort and aspirin for headache. It is unwise to prescribe sedatives or hypnotics because they may lead to dependence.

DEPENDENCE OF THE ALCOHOL TYPE (ALCOHOLISM)

Two kinds of abnormal drinking are frequently described: "addictive" and "nonaddictive." The nonaddictive alcoholic retains the ability to stop whenever he desires; high grades of tolerance and severe abstinence syndromes are unusual. In contrast, the addictive drinker continues until stopped by poverty, nausea, or illness, and develops high grades of tolerance, serious physical dependence, and severe organic complications.

Pathogenesis. The metabolism of alcohol is similar in periodic and chronic drinkers. Cellular tolerance develops in chronic drinkers so that only mild or moderate intoxication accompanies blood levels that initially were associated with stupor. Chronic alcoholics also become able to compensate for, or to conceal, the signs of drunkenness.

Protracted heavy drinking causes physical dependence manifested by tremors, convulsions, hallucinations, and delirium when the intake of alcohol is abruptly decreased or stopped. Abstinence symptoms depend more on a decline in blood alcohol than on absolute cessation of the drinking. This being the case, a chronic drinker who ordinarily ingests 600 ml. of alcohol (1200 ml. of whiskey) daily may develop abstinence symptoms if he reduces his intake to 480 ml. of alcohol (equivalent to a quart of whiskey) daily. Alcohol abstinence syndromes are not due to nutritional deficiencies or to liver damage. Like other abstinence syndromes, the symptoms are opposite to the acute effects of alcohol. Partial cross-tolerance and dose dependence occur between alcohol and the drugs listed in class I-B.

Clinical Manifestations. The incipient alcoholic simply drinks more than his peers. The wine drinker is no longer content with a glass at meals but drinks an entire bottle. Such drinking may persist for years, but gradually the pattern becomes exaggerated. The alcoholic continues to drink after the party is over and to the point of stupor. The wine drinker sips between and before meals and drifts into a constant alcoholic haze. Some go on binges of two or three days' duration; others begin to drink alone at night. Eventually, the alcoholic's family and associates realize the problem. Generally, their remonstrances and advice are rejected. Drinking becomes daily rather than periodic. The person is "hung over" each morning and begins to drink to alleviate the hangover, presaging the development of addiction. Personality deterioration sets in. The alco-

holic becomes resentful of advice, blames his drinking on others, is forgetful, unreliable, and quarrelsome. He loses his job, his social position, and his family. He becomes obsessed with obtaining and maintaining his supply, hiding bottles in various places against the time when he needs them. At this stage many patients experience alcoholic amnesia, remembering nothing after one or two drinks, awakening hours or days later in an unfamiliar place ("blackouts"). Many turn to poorer forms of alcohol: cheap wine, hair tonic, or lotions. At this stage, the alcoholic is likely to reinforce or replace alcohol, thereafter oscillating between alcohol and drugs. Finally, the alcoholic develops coma, pneumonia, or cirrhosis, and dies.

The progressive course just described varies greatly and may be arrested at any stage. Many alcoholics are unhappy, would prefer not to drink, and some succeed in stopping.

The objective signs of excessive protracted drinking include obesity, flabbiness, dilatation of peripheral blood vessels around the nose and eyes, reddened conjunctivae, tremors, evidence of hepatic dysfunction or nutritional deficiency, and poor personal hygiene.

Abstinence Syndromes. A number of tremulous, agitated, hallucinated, convulsive, and delirious states occur after cessation of drinking or after reduction in alcohol intake, and have been described as distinct clinical entities. All these states, however, are merely quantitative and qualitative variants of the same underlying disorder. The alcoholic abstinence syndromes vary in intensity in proportion to the amount and duration of excessive drinking. They occur in lesser degrees after debauches of a week or two. The more severe forms follow heavy drinking of 400 to 600 ml. of alcohol daily for a month or more.

Alcoholic Tremulousness. After the alcoholic first sobers up, he is alert, startles easily, and has difficulty in sleeping, anorexia, weakness, tachycardia, and tremulousness. The tremors vary from the barely perceptible to so strong that the patient cannot stand. The tremulous state may be the only overt abstinence manifestation, and may clear in a few days without treatment.

Alcoholic Hallucinosis. The next stage is alcoholic hallucinosis, in which the patient experiences "nightmares," misinterprets sounds or shadows, and has disturbances in perception of form and color. Most frequently the hallucinations are visual and animate and involve humans, insects, or animal life. Alcoholic hallucinosis is distinguished from delirium tremens by the fact that the patient is not markedly agitated, is not disoriented, and realizes that his experiences are unreal. The condition usually clears in a few days.

Acute Auditory Hallucinosis. Acute auditory hallucinosis usually includes accusing voices, but without confusion or disorientation. However, insight is lost, and the patient generally reacts inappropriately. For example, he may notify the police, barricade himself, or commit suicide. Recovery usually occurs in days. A small proportion of such patients develop a chronic auditory hallucinosis in which the voices persist for months or years. Such cases may represent the triggering of a schizophrenic psychosis by alcohol or abstinence from it.

Alcoholic Epilepsy or "Rum Fits." These often precede the development of delirium tremens. Major motor seizures occur in the first (18) hours after alcohol is stopped or reduced. The number of seizures varies greatly, but generally there are fewer than occur in abstinence from barbiturates.

Delirium Tremens. Delirium tremens is the most dramatic and dangerous form of reaction to abstinence from alcohol. It is characterized by agitation, increased autonomic activity, disorientation, confusion, and disordered sensory perception. Delirium tremens is frequently precipitated by a head injury, an infection, or a surgical operation. The condition begins about the third or fourth night after withdrawal, frequently following a seizure. Rarely, a quiet delirium is encountered, but usually the patient is agitated, constantly in motion, muttering, picking at the bed clothes, screaming, or wandering about the halls. He misidentifies people and objects and does not know the time or date. He suffers with vivid and frightening visual hallucinations, frequently of animals or insects. He is drenched with sweat, and has tachycardia and fever. The symptoms are worse at night.

Delirium tremens frequently terminates after three to five days with a sudden sleep from which the patient awakens clear and lucid and with only partial memory of the episode. There is a 20 per cent mortality in cases complicated by infection, head injury, or other serious disease. Steadily rising temperature without infection is ominous.

Diagnosis. The diagnosis of the alcoholic abstinence syndrome is based on signs, symptoms, and history. The chief conditions to be excluded are abstinence from hypnotics or convulsions and delirium due to other causes. The differential diagnosis between impending hepatic coma and delirium tremens may be difficult, but it is important since hypnotic drugs are contraindicated in hepatic coma. Advanced liver disease, gastrointestinal bleeding, lack of agitation, lack of vivid hallucinations, and the presence of asterixis all favor hepatic coma rather than delirium tremens.

Treatment. If the patient is a nonaddictive periodic drinker who has been drinking for less than a week, withdrawal treatment is usually unnecessary. If the patient is an addict who has been consuming a quart of whiskey or more daily for more than a week, withdrawal treatment in an institution is required.

The principles used in withdrawing alcohol are the same as those used in withdrawing hypnotics (see above). If possible, severe symptoms of abstinence should be avoided. Alcohol itself is unsatisfactory for conducting withdrawal because of its small margin of safety and because of its toxic effects on fat metabolism. Alcohol is stopped and one of the hypnotics listed in class 1-B is substituted in sufficient dose to cause mild drunkenness, after which the dosage of the hypnotic is reduced over a period of days.

Paraldehyde is a classic drug for this purpose, but has the disadvantage of unpleasant odor, gastric irritation, and insuitability for injection. Meprobamate, chlordiazepoxide, and diazepam are currently popular and effective if the principles of giving enough to induce initially sustained mild intoxication followed by gradual reduction of the daily dosage are followed.

Controlled clinical trials and experimental studies have shown that reserpine and the phenothiazine tranquilizers (chlorpromazine, proniazine, perphenazine) are not effective and that they actually increase mortality.

Pentobarbital is a very effective and flexible drug and can be used in withdrawing alcohol in exactly the same way as it is used in withdrawing hypnotics. The steps are (1) stop the intake of alcohol; (2) after the patient is sober, give a test dose of 0.2 gram of pentobarbital; (3) examine the patient one and a half hours later; if he shows no evidence of abstinence, has slow inconstant nystagmus, and sways slightly, the dose is right and may be repeated in six hours; if he is still tremulous, has no nystagmus or dysarthria, and does not sway, the initial test dose should be reinforced with an additional 0.1 gram of pentobarbital which may be repeated at hourly intervals until the desired degree of sedation is present; if, on the other hand, he has fine nystagmus, fails on the Romberg test, and is grossly ataxic, the dose was too large, and no more should be given for six hours when a smaller (0.1 gram) dose is given; (4) establish by titration the amount of pentobarbital required daily—"stabilization dose" —to maintain the desired degree of effect; (5) maintain this dosage for one to two days while completing necessary examinations and beginning treatment of other complicating conditions; and (6) reduce the daily stabilization dosage by no more than 0.1 gram daily. If the patient cannot or will not take the drug orally, treatment may be initiated intramuscularly.

If serious symptoms of abstinence—convulsions, hallucinosis, or delirium—are present, the patient should be reintoxicated rapidly, using an initial dose of 0.2 gram of pentobarbital intramuscularly followed by reinforcing doses of 0.1 gram intramuscularly hourly until the patient is asleep. After he has slept for 8 to 12 hours, he is allowed to awaken, the stabilization dose is determined, and gradual withdrawal is performed as described above. Complicating medical or surgical conditions—gastritis, pneumonia, head injuries—are frequently the precipitating causes of stopping alcohol intake, and must be treated appropriately.

Fluid and electrolyte losses may be extreme. Delirious, perspiring, vomiting patients may require as much as 6 liters of saline and dextrose plus vitamins and potassium in the first 24 hours. Hyperthermia requires, in addition to hypnotic drugs, reduction of temperature with alcohol sponges or cooling blankets.

Vitamins will not have any effect on abstinence, but they will correct complicating deficiencies.

Physical and Psychiatric Rehabilitation. Physical and psychiatric rehabilitation begin during withdrawal of alcohol. The physician must adopt a neutral attitude about the patient's drinking; he should neither condemn nor condone it. The patient must be told firmly, however, that he reacts differently to alcohol than do other people, that he can never drink socially, and that if he wishes to be cured, absolute and total abstinence is necessary. The patient must realize that he has a problem that he cannot manage alone, that he needs help, and that he must cooperate and contribute to his own treatment. If this hurdle is surmounted, psychotherapy, either individual or group, is carried out along customary lines. The patient should, if willing, be put in touch with Alcoholics Anonymous. It is generally best to avoid dependence-producing central nervous system depressants following completion of withdrawal. If drugs are used at all, hydroxyzine and chlorpromazine are best, for they do not cause dependence.

Disulfiram (Antabuse) and citrated calcium carbide block the oxidation of alcohol at the acetaldehyde stage so that a person who takes alcohol while ingesting these drugs will have nausea, vomiting, vasodilatation, and even cardiovascular collapse because of accumulation of acetaldehyde. These drugs are effective only as long as the patient continues to take them. Since they have not been especially successful, and the alcohol-disulfiram reaction can be severe or fatal, these drugs are used very little in the United States.

Prognosis.   Perhaps 15 to 20 per cent of patients manage to abstain permanently. Others abstain for months or years, only to relapse during a period of stress. However, many patients have long intervals of productive and apparently fulfilling lives between relapses of this naturally chronic illness.

AMPHETAMINE TYPE OF DEPENDENCE

Harris Isbell

The abuse of amphetamine and related central stimulant drugs has become widespread around the world and has involved Japan, Australia, the United States, Canada, Great Britain, and Sweden. All the drugs listed in type I-D in the table have been abused, but amphetamine, dextroamphetamines, methamphetamine, and phenmetrazine have been involved to a greater extent than the others.

Dependence of the amphetamine type is characterized by strong psychic dependence, marked tolerance, and mild physical dependence characterized by an increase in REM sleep, hunger, apathy, and depression. Harm to the individual and society includes occasional, acute psychotic reactions after single doses, the development of a

paranoid psychosis following chronic ingestion, senseless perseverative activity, alterations in judgment and mood, loss of weight, infections from intravenous injections, sudden death, and suicide.

There is a wide quantitative spectrum of abuse ranging from the student who may take one amphetamine tablet or so orally daily to the psychopathic "speed freak" who injects massive amounts of the drugs intravenously. Obese, mildly depressed women may become psychically dependent on amphetamines that have been prescribed as anorexiants, and feel that they cannot get along without their 10 mg. of sustained release dextroamphetamine each morning. Truck drivers may take the drugs orally in fairly large amounts to stay awake to drive. Alcoholics and hypnotic abusers may take them as antidotes for alcohol and hypnotic drugs and to combat psychic depression, thus creating mixed forms of dependence. Tolerance develops rapidly but is never entirely complete. Habitual users take as much as 100 therapeutic doses daily. Intravenous abuse is the most severe form, and is complicated by infections (hepatitis, endocarditis, tetanus) and pulmonary emboli. The death rate among intravenous abusers is 20 times the expected death rate.

Pharmacology.   All the drugs listed in type I-D are sympathomimetic amines, and have peripheral adrenergic effects as well as strong central stimulant effects. Some are direct adrenergic agonists that act by combining with adrenergic receptors. Others are indirect agonists that act by releasing, preventing reuptake, or blocking storage of norepinephrine by adrenergic nerve endings and by slow degradation of catecholamines by monoamine oxidase. Their central stimulant effects may depend on similar biochemical mechanisms. The threshold for stimulation of the midbrain reticular activating system is lowered, accounting for wakefulness, nervousness, and the sense of enhanced intellectual and physical ability. REM sleep is reduced or abolished. Anorexia is due to direct hypothalamic effects.

Clinical Manifestations.   The symptoms and signs vary with the dose, the length of time, and the continuity of use. Small oral doses (5 to 10 mg. of dextroamphetamine or equivalent) generally cause only mild elation, slight nervousness, anorexia, insomnia, relief of fatigue, and euphoric sensations of enhanced physical and mental efficiency. With doses of this order, signs of adrenergic stimulation are slight. The euphoric sensations last only about four hours and are succeeded by unpleasant dysphoric feelings of fatigue and a desire to sleep complicated by continuing anxiety or nervousness. Occasionally, even small doses may precipitate an acute psychotic state that clears in a few hours. If small doses are taken daily, tolerance to the anorexia, nervousness, and euphoria develops rapidly, so the dose must be increased to obtain the initial degree of effect. Continuous use of the drug can induce a paranoid psychosis occurring in a setting of clear consciousness. The amount of drug and the length of time for the psychosis to appear vary widely, and the mental changes can range from being mild and difficult to detect to bizarre or assaultive behavior. Generally, the psychosis disappears in less than three weeks when the drug is stopped, although occasional patients remain permanently psychotic.

The most serious form of amphetamine abuse is self-administration intravenously. In the United States most intravenous abusers are young adult males with marked psychopathic traits who are termed "speed freaks" by their peers. Such persons generally have used other drugs and are introduced to intravenous amphetamines by their friends. Not infrequently they may be members of fighting gangs. The main drug used is methamphetamine, termed "speed," "crystal," or "meth." An active illicit synthesis and market in this drug has sprung up. The drug is usually taken intravenously in binge fashion. This is called "firing." The intravenous injection, which may be repeated as often as every two hours, causes a strong, orgasm-like sensation termed a "rush." Tolerance develops rapidly, so the dose is rapidly increased. Signs of peripheral adrenergic stimulation become evident with pupillary dilatation, elevation of blood pressure, and enhanced tendon reflexes. The user walks about aimlessly or engages in senseless perseverative activity, and neither eats nor sleeps. As the user continues to take the drug (called a "run") he develops paranoid ideas, and may apply to the police for protection or be brought to a hospital by friends. Assaults on others can occur. Eventually, the "run" stops because of exhaustion, the mental symptoms, or lack of drugs. Stopping is called "crashing."

When amphetamines are discontinued, a train of symptoms ensues which may represent an abstinence syndrome. The amphetamine-dependent goes to sleep, and electroencephalograms show a marked increase (rebound) in REM sleep. Severe nightmares may occur. After sleeping for as much as 48 hours, the patient awakens ravenously hungry and eats voraciously. The paranoid psychosis usually clears rapidly, but is replaced by apathy and psychic depression which may lead to "refiring" and repetition of the cycle.

Many intravenous amphetamine abusers have been found dead with a needle in their veins. Such sudden deaths are believed to be due to cardiac arrhythmias. Infections, particularly serum hepatitis and bacterial endocarditis, are frequent and add to the death toll. Suicide is frequent.

Diagnosis. Diagnosis is usually made by the history, and is particularly suggested by a person who presents with a paranoid psychosis that clears in a few days following a period of sleep. Dilated pupils, increased blood pressure, and increased reflexes are helpful but not diagnostic. If these symptoms are present in a young person with numerous fresh needle marks over the veins, the diagnosis is likely. Cocaine induces a clinically indistinguishable illness. Differentiation from paranoid schizophrenia is usually easy because of the rapid clearing of the psychosis following hospitalization. Amphetamines can be detected chemically in body fluids.

Treatment. The milder forms of amphetamine dependence require little more than stopping the drug and supportive psychotherapy. Mixed intoxication must be detected and treated appropriately. Symptoms of depression should be sought for and, if need be, psychiatric consultation obtained. Persons with the amphetamine psychosis must be hospitalized and protected until the psychotic state has cleared. Agitation and hyperactive action behavior are treated by administering chlorpromazine orally or intramuscularly. After the patient has slept and eaten, precautions against relapse or suicide are required, and patients should be hospitalized or closely supervised until the period of depression has passed. A long period of aftercare with psychiatric and social rehabilitation is necessary.

COCAINE DEPENDENCE
Harris Isbell

Dependence of the cocaine type is clinically strikingly similar to amphetamine dependence but, although a strong psychic dependence on cocaine occurs, neither tolerance to, nor physical dependence on, cocaine develops. Cocaine sensitizes adrenergic receptors by preventing the uptake of the catecholamines by the adrenergic nerves and by interfering with the degradation of the catecholamines by monoamine oxidase. Intoxication with cocaine causes signs of marked adrenergic stimulation. Cocaine has powerful excitant effects in the central nervous system that may also depend on changes in catecholamines.

There are two kinds of abuse of cocaine: the chewing of the coca leaf and the use of the pure alkaloid. Chewing of coca is limited to South America, where the coca leaves are masticated with lime. In the United States, the pure drug is used as a snuff or, more frequently, is taken intravenously in combination with heroin or morphine ("the speed ball").

Clinical Manifestations. Two kinds of signs and symptoms occur: those attributable to peripheral adrenergic stimulation include pupillary dilatation, sweating, tachycardia, gooseflesh, hypertension, and increased temperature. The central nervous system manifestations are particularly marked if cocaine is taken intravenously. The users experience short-lived ecstatic sensations and take injections at short intervals until their supply is exhausted or a toxic psychosis supervenes. As the dose is repeated, insomnia, anxiety, increased startle responses, and increased muscle stretch reflexes appear. Finally, a paranoid psychosis with delusions and optical hallucinations ensues. Cocaine users frequently think that they are being watched by the police ("bull horrors") and, in this state, are dangerous. When the effects become too frightening, users frequently take heroin or morphine as an antidote to the cocaine.

Treatment. Cocaine does not cause physical dependence, and withdrawal treatment is unnecessary. The patient should be protected until the psychosis has cleared.

HALLUCINOGENIC DEPENDENCE (LSD TYPE)

Harris Isbell

A list of hallucinogens is shown in the table (class II-A, 2). These drugs induce changes in mood and sensory perception and vivid hallucinations, chiefly optical. They have proved especially attractive to young persons of bohemian habits who have rejected the accepted social values and are in passive rebellion against society and their elders. Pseudoreligious cults have sprung up that use these drugs to "expand consciousness" in the hope of attaining insight into personal emotional problems.

Hallucinogenic dependence is characterized by moderate psychic dependence, marked tolerance if the drugs are taken daily, and no physical dependence. The harm caused includes withdrawal from society, adoption of drug-seeking as a mode of life with resultant multiple drug use, triggering of acute and chronic psychoses, and infections resulting from unsanitary living habits.

Pharmacology. Most of these drugs are taken orally, but they can be injected. Dimethyl- and diethyltryptamine must be injected or smoked. The drugs differ chiefly in potency and length of action. Tolerance to any of the drugs of this type confers crossed tolerance to the others. All cause central adrenergic (hypothalamic) stimulation with resultant pupillary dilatation, elevated body temperature and blood pressure, and sweating. All spinal reflexes are enhanced. The threshold for stimulation of the reticular activating system is lowered, with resultant increased alertness, insomnia, and nervousness. Axodendritic synaptic transmission in the cerebral cortex is depressed. Filtering mechanisms that normally enable one to suppress most of the flood of sensory stimuli that are constantly impinging on the brain and to concentrate on only the stimuli of importance in the immediate situation are depressed so that the individual is inundated by a torrent of sensations that he cannot ignore.

Clinical Manifestations. The symptoms are dependent on the dose; 0.05 mg. of LSD (or equivalent doses of the other drugs) primarily causes changes in mood, chiefly euphoric, and enhancement of sensations. Colors appear brighter, sounds are clearer. With doses of 0.1 mg. of LSD (or 5 mg. of DOM, 5 mg. of psilocybin, 35 mg. of dimethyltryptamine, or 500 mg. of mescaline) anxiety and sensory distortion ensue. Walls pulsate, people appear strange, and flickering lights and colors are seen with the eyes closed. With doses of 2.0 μg. per kilogram all symptoms are more intense, and formed hallucinations, chiefly visual, and sensations of depersonalization occur. With such hallucinations the individual feels that his body is altered. He may feel huge and may feel that his hands have changed to animal paws; he believes he can see the blood and bones through the flesh; people appear old and gargoyle-like. Consciousness and orientation are maintained, and the person usually retains insight and realizes that the effects are due to the drug. With doses greater than 2.0 μg. per kilogram, insight may be lost and the subject may appear dazed and mute. Suicide or psychotic attacks on others may occur.

The pupils dilate but react to light. Temperature and blood pressure are slightly elevated. Sweating and gooseflesh may occur. The deep tendon reflexes become hyperactive. Coordination is not impaired.

The time course of the reaction varies with the drug. The action of dimethyl- and diethyltryptamine persists for two hours, that of psilocybin for 4 to 6 hours, that of LSD 8 to 12 hours, and that of mescaline and DOM 12 to 16 hours.

The complications are primarily psychiatric. Some persons may have panic reactions, with fears of becoming insane or dying, that disappear as the drug effects dissipate. Some persons develop a schizophreniform state that lasts days or weeks; a few have remained permanently psychotic. Others may have momentary returns of the symptoms experienced under the drug ("flashbacks") for weeks or months after the drug action has terminated. All these prolonged psychiatric states occur chiefly in persons who are only marginally adjusted emotionally.

Diagnosis. Diagnosis is usually made by the history. Persons who take hallucinogens do not ordinarily seek medical help unless they have one of the psychiatric complications described above and are brought to physicians by a friend or the police. The diagnosis should be suspected in any young person, particularly of bohemian habit, who presents with dilated pupils, elevated blood pressure, and hyperactive tendon reflexes and complains of kaleidoscopic optical hallucinations, sensory distortion, and depersonalization. Chemical tests are not generally available.

Treatment. The acute psychotic state caused by LSD and complicated by panic requires protection until the panic state has passed. The patient should be placed in a quiet, dimly lighted room that provides as few sensory stimuli as possible. Someone in constant attendance should give quiet reassurance and support. Chlorpromazine should be given orally or intramuscularly to especially agitated patients. Protracted reactions may require hospitalization for days or weeks, but the "flashback" states do not require hospitalization. Mild sedation and reassurance that the flashbacks are drug-related usually suffice. Social and rehabilitative treatment should be attempted, but may be disappointing because of the immaturity of most users of hallucinogens.

DEPENDENCE ON CANNABIS (MARIHUANA, HASHISH)

Harris Isbell

Abuse of the hemp plant, *Cannabis sativa,* is one of the oldest and most widespread intoxications in the world and involves millions of people in many parts of the world. For the last ten years the use of marihuana has been spreading rapidly in drug-using subcultures and among college and high school students in the United States and in Western Europe, causing a great deal of public concern and argument over the legal controls imposed on cannabis.

The hemp plant produces a complex resinous substance which is most abundant in the leaves and flowering tops at the time of flowering. The dried leaves and tops are marihuana (pot, grass, tea, reefers, muggles). If the resin is concentrated mechanically and compressed into cakes, it is termed hashish (ganja, charas). The most active materials in the resin are the *1-Δ⁸-* and *1-Δ⁹-trans*-tetrahydrocannabinols (TIIC's). The compounds are not water-soluble and do not crystallize; hence absolute chemical identification was not accomplished until 1965 and total synthesis until 1967. The extraordinarily difficult chemistry of cannabis accounts for our relative ignorance about this ancient intoxicant. The tetrahydrocannabinol content of the plant varies with the variety of the weed, the soil, the temperature, the rainfall, and other factors. Most of the marihuana available in the United States is either grown wild or illicitly produced from seeds from varieties that were developed for fiber rather than for the resin and, therefore, have relatively low THC contents (usually less than 0.2 per cent). This probably accounts for the mildness of the intoxication as usually observed in this country. Imported leaf sometimes contains more than 1 per cent tetrahydrocannabinol, and hashish may assay as high as 8 per cent.

Dependence on cannabis is characterized by moderate psychic dependence, little tolerance, and no known physical dependence. In the United States most of the drug is consumed as marihuana. Use is generally periodic and in the company of others. High level continuous use of potent material is practically nonexistent in the United States, but is common in India, the Middle East, and North Africa. The chief dangers in the United States appear to be alterations in mood, judgment, and perception and the precipitation of temporary psychotic states. In other parts of the world, heavy abuse of potent material is said to lead to social deterioration similar to that seen in chronic alcoholics and to chronic mental deterioration ("cannabis psychoses"). Scientific proof that hashish causes chronic psychotic states is lacking.

The *1-Δ⁹*-tetrahydrocannabinol, the active isomer that is most abundant in marihuana, is three times as active when smoked as when taken orally.

Doses of 7.0 mg. or less in one cigarette cause euphoria, silly behavior, and mild sensory distortion. Colors appear brighter, music more beautiful, and touch more sensitive. Time seems to pass slowly. The appetite is increased. The effects last two to four hours, after which the individual becomes drowsy and sleeps. Doses of 14 to 20 mg. cause, in addition to the symptoms described above, anxiety, marked sensory distortion, depersonalization, and optical hallucinations.

Tachycardia, which is proportional to the dose, occurs uniformly. Blood pressure and pupillary size are not altered. There is no gross impairment of coordination. The conjunctivae are frequently reddened.

The effects of smoking crude marihuana are usually mild. Experienced smokers are said to be able to titrate the potency of the marihuana and to avoid doses that cause unpleasant psychotic reactions. Marihuana affects tests of cognitive and psychomotor ability very little, the major effects being impairment of recent memory and the ability to concentrate. Persons under the influence of marihuana are usually well behaved and not assaultive, but marihuana occasionally triggers panic and schizophreniform reactions in susceptible persons. "Flashbacks" have also been described.

Diagnosis. Usually the diagnosis depends on the history. Marihuana users are not likely to seek medical help unless they are having or have had a panic or schizophreniform episode and are brought to the hospital by friends or the police. The diagnosis should be suggested by euphoria, bizarre behavior, reddened conjunctivae, tachycardia, and an odor similar to that of burned hay on the breath. A schizophreniform episode that clears rapidly is suggestive. There are no objective chemical tests available.

Treatment. No treatment is required for the usual acute intoxication. The person who has a panic reaction or a schizophreniform episode should be hospitalized and protected until the episode is over. The phenothiazine and reserpine tranquilizers should be avoided because they may add to the postural tachycardia. Barbiturates and other sedatives may be used for agitation. Social rehabilitative and long-term psychotherapy should be tried, but are usually unrewarding.

BROMIDES

Harris Isbell

Poisoning with bromides was once common and accounted for as many as 2 per cent of patients admitted to mental hospitals. Since the bromides have been replaced with other sedative drugs and since headache remedies that are sold without prescription can no longer contain bromide, the condition is now less frequent. The cause is self-medication. The half-life of bromide in the blood is about 12 days, so the drug accumulates if taken daily with the slow appearance of poisoning over a period of weeks. Symptoms are referable to the central nervous system, but acneiform eruptions and other skin lesions occur in 20 per cent of cases. Mental disturbances consist of headache, drowsiness, impaired memory and cognition, irritability, and emotional lability. Agitation may lead to taking even more bromide in the hope of alleviating the symptoms. In more severe grades of poisoning, delusions, hallucinations, lethargy, or coma may occur. The EEG is slowed when poisoning is sufficient to cause drowsiness or delirium. Neurologic disturbances include a notable carelessness in personal dress and toilet, tremors, dysarthria, decreased cutaneous reflexes, and extensor plantar responses.

The serum bromide concentration correlates only roughly with central nervous system symptoms. No symptoms usually accompany serum bromide levels below 6 mEq. per liter (50 mg. per 100 ml.), whereas most patients with levels over 25 mEq. have typical symptoms.

The *diagnosis* of bromide poisoning should be considered in any person presenting clouded consciousness and psychotic symptoms without demonstrable cause. A high serum bromide level establishes the diagnosis.

Treatment. Since tolerance and physical dependence do not occur, withdrawal treatment is not necessary. Treatment is based on hastening the removal of bromide ion. Since bromide is more effectively resorbed in the renal tubule than chloride, it "replaces" chloride in body fluid. Measures that increase the excretion of chloride also increase excretion of bromide. Ingestion of bromide should be stopped and, unless contraindicated by cardiac or renal disease, 200 mEq. of chloride should be given daily as sodium or ammonium chloride together with sufficient fluid to provide a large urine output. This reduces the half-life of bromide to three or four days. If more rapid removal of bromide is desirable, daily injection of meralluride can be added to chloride treatment. Hemodialysis rapidly clears bromides, and is indicated when massive doses cause coma.

including those in proprietary remedies for the common cold. Susceptible persons occasionally develop poisoning after taking only one or two cold capsules.

Poisoning is due to peripheral and central blockade of acetylcholine. The mental symptoms include drowsiness, confusion, disorientation, and vivid optical hallucinations, and frequently are accompanied by dilated and fixed pupils, dry skin and mouth, flush, fever, and urinary retention.

Diagnosis is made by history and the characteristic clinical picture. *Treatment* is symptomatic and consists of protecting the patient, supplying ample fluids, and reducing fever. Attempts to antidote the effects of the cholinergic blockers by administering cholinesterase inhibitors, such as eserine, are unnecessary and complicate management.

Since the effects of these drugs are unpleasant, they are seldom taken voluntarily more than once and, accordingly, are not drugs of dependence.

Cohen, S.: The Beyond Within. The LSD Story. New York, Atheneum Publishers, 1965.

Eddy, N. B., Halbach, H., Isbell, H., and Seevers, M. H.: Drug dependence: Its significance and characteristics. Bull. W.H.O., 32:721, 1965.

Eddy, N. B., and Martin, W. R.: Drug dependence of specific opiate antagonist type. Pharmacopsychiat. Psychopharmacol., 3:73, 1970.

Essig, C. F.: Addiction to non-barbiturate sedative and tranquilizing drugs. Clin. Pharmacol. Ther., 5:334, 1964.

Essig, C. F., Jones, B. E., and Lam, R. C.: The effect of pentobarbital on alcohol withdrawal in dogs. Arch. Neurol. (Chicago), 20:554, 1969.

Isbell, H., Altschul, S., Eisenman, A. S., Flannary, H. G., and Fraser, H. F.: Chronic barbiturate intoxication: An experimental study. Arch. Neurol. Psychiat., 64:1, 1950.

Isbell, H., Fraser, H. F., Wikler, A., Belleville, R. E., and Eisenman, A. J.: An experimental study of the etiology of "rum fits" and delirium tremens. Quart. J. Stud. Alcohol, 16:1, 1955.

Isbell, H., Gorodetsky, C. W., Jasinski, F. J., Claussen, U., v. Spulak, F., and Korte, F.: Effects of (-)-Δ⁹-*trans*-tetrahydrocannabinol in man. Psychopharmacologia (Berlin), 11:184, 1967.

Kalant, H.: The pharmacology of alcohol intoxication. Quart. J. Stud. Alcohol (Supp. 1:1), 1961.

Sapira, J.: The narcotic addict as a medical patient. Amer. J. Med., 45:555, 1968.

Sjöqvist, F., and Tottie, M. (eds.): Abuse of Central Stimulants. Stockholm, Almqvist and Wiksell, 1969.

Wikler, A.: On the nature of addiction and habituation. Brit. J. Addict., 57:73, 1961.

POISONING OF THE ATROPINE TYPE

Harris Isbell

Poisoning of the atropine type may be due to accidental ingestion of atropine, scopolamine, hyoscyamine, or of the plants or crude drugs (belladonna, stramonium) containing these alkaloids. Young persons sometimes smoke stramonium or inhale scopolamine snuff and develop an atropine type of poisoning. In addition, such intoxication may occur after ingestion of excessive amounts of antihistamines with cholinergic blocking effects,

THE MANAGEMENT OF ACUTE DEPRESSIVE DRUG POISONING

Fred Plum

Etiology. Many different drugs are taken in efforts to commit suicide. The most important ones causing stupor or coma are the sedatives, including the barbiturates, glutethimide, meprobamate, and, occasionally, bromides. Phenothiazine overdosage is sometimes encountered, but such patients are usually only lightly stuporous and require no special treatment. Alcohol ingestion accompanies many serious suicidal attempts and intensifies the central nervous system depression. Opiate overdosage is usually an accident rather than a conscious effort at self-destruction and is discussed elsewhere.

Pathogenesis. All these drugs depress the central nervous system, although not equally on a gram-molecular weight basis, and not to the same degree so far as different central structures are concerned. The duration of action varies widely and depends largely on how the particular drug is detoxified or eliminated. The short-acting barbiturates, pentobarbital, secobarbital, and amobarbital, are detoxified by the liver. They exert their maximal effects promptly after being absorbed and, even in huge doses, seldom cause neurologic depression lasting longer than three to five days. Barbital and phenobarbital are partially detoxified by the liver and partially excreted in the urine. Severe poisoning with the latter agent can cause coma lasting 10 to 14 days. Glutethimide has a short duration of action comparable to that of secobarbital, but it is poorly absorbed from the gut. This can prolong the effect of an ingested dose. Meprobamate has an intermediate duration of effect lasting for days. Bromide rarely causes full coma, but, once it reaches high levels, it displaces chloride in the blood and tissues, and persists to cause symptoms for weeks without further ingestion.

Although the sedatives have few important effects outside the nervous system, glutethimide and meprobamate in toxic doses tend to produce hypotension. Also, glutethimide possesses unique anticholinergic properties and is the only sedative that predictably produces light-fixed pupils in toxic doses.

Clinical Manifestations. Stupor or coma due to depressant drug poisoning presents the classic picture of severe metabolic brain disease. The depression of the central nervous system tends to be bilateral and symmetrical, and the drug affects simultaneously many levels, including the spinal cord. Respiratory and circulatory controlling mechanisms in the lower brainstem are affected late or not at all, and, except with glutethimide, the pupillary light reflexes are preserved. Early in the course of poisoning, patients can demonstrate muscular hypertonus or even spasticity as the result of uneven depression of different neurologic levels. Within a short time, usually an hour or less, flaccidity supervenes, and the stretch reflexes tend to disappear. Even moderate degrees of drug depression depress or block the oculovestibular reflexes.

Four grades of coma have been described in order to aid in estimating the severity of poisoning and the effects of treatment. *Grade I* is light coma in which vigorous noxious stimulation evokes withdrawal or groaning. *Grade II* is deep coma in which only minimal grimacing or reflex responsiveness can be evoked by a noxious stimulus. In *grade III* subjects fail to respond in any way to a noxious stimulus. In *grade IV* unresponsive patients remain in deep coma for over 36 hours or have serious respiratory or circulatory depression. A relationship between the blood level of a sedative drug and the depth of coma is only approximate because tolerance from previous drug exposure, alcohol ingestion, aspiration into the lungs, and exposure to the elements all influence the degree of CNS depression. Generally speaking, however, blood levels of short-acting barbiturates of more than 2.5 mg. per 100 ml. and phenobarbital blood levels of more than 12 mg. per 100 ml. are associated with grades III and IV coma.

Management of Coma. There are no specific antidotes for the sedative drugs. Treatment consists of keeping the patient alive and as free as possible of complications until the drug is detoxified and is either naturally or artificially excreted. Proper management saves all but a very few patients if they survive to reach the hospital. Among the writer's series of 356 consecutive patients in coma, 11 or 3.1 per cent died, all but three of whom were older than 45 years. To achieve this low rate required meticulous attention to the airway and ventilation, to the circulation, and to the potential complications of the comatose state. In laboratory animals, the fatal dose of barbiturates is seven times that required to produce apnea and almost twice that which first produces circulatory shock. Similar actions by the drugs in man guide the treatment of poisoning.

Airway and Ventilation. Several mechanisms threaten to obstruct the airway of patients in coma from sedative drugs. If the subject lies on his back, the tongue and pooled secretions occlude the hypopharynx, with the result that secretions are aspirated into the lungs. The cough reflex and the ciliary action of the tracheobronchial mucosa are depressed. Many subjects aspirate stomach contents into the lungs, particularly if gastric lavage is attempted before tracheal intubation.

Because of these potentially fatal complications, the first step is to secure the airway. An oropharyngeal airway is sufficient to manage patients in light coma who cough when the larynx is stimulated. A cuffed endotracheal tube should be placed in more deeply anesthetized patients who lack a cough reflex. It is wise to precede intubation with atropine, 0.0008 gram intravenously, to reduce the danger of cardiac arrest. How long to leave the endotracheal tube in place in an unresponsive subject is often a difficult question. One practice is to deflate the cuff hourly for 5 minutes, to replace the tube at 24 hours, and to perform a tracheostomy at somewhere between 36 and 48 hours if the cough reflex has not returned or if no other signs indicate a lessening of coma.

Patients should be suctioned gently through the endotracheal tube at least every half hour or oftener if pulmonary secretions accumulate. It is desirable to administer low concentrations

(25 per cent) of moistened oxygen, but not to occlude the tube with a large catheter. Tubes are removed when active coughing or bucking returns.

Hypoventilation should be treated with artificial respiration. Shallow breathing in a deeply comatose patient frequently reflects no more than the subject's depressed metabolism, but if the rate falls below 12 per minute or if the physician entertains serious doubts as to the adequacy of ventilation, artificial respiration is indicated. Ideally, arterial blood gases should be measured in deeply comatose patients and artificial respiration initiated if the arterial P_{CO_2} climbs above 45 mm. of mercury. High concentration (>30 per cent) oxygen therapy should be avoided for patients not receiving artificial respiration, for its use increases the risk of hypoventilation and CO_2 retention.

Circulation. Severe shock is rare with depressant drug poisoning unless the patient has been asphyxiated. However, moderate hypotension is common and significantly reduces glomerular filtration and renal clearance of the barbiturates. Fluids should be given liberally to restore blood volume and promote urine flow, and pressor agents, such as metaraminol or levarterenol, are indicated to keep the diastolic blood pressure above 60 mm. of mercury and the systolic above 90 mm. of mercury. Digitalis or similar compounds are useful only in patients with heart disease. Corticosteroids are unnecessary.

Prevention of Complications. Once a patent airway and effective ventilation are assured, patients should be placed semiprone with one hip elevated and the bed raised in the middle (see figure in Management of Severe Neurologic Disability). This enhances airway drainage and minimizes stasis. During coma, the patient is changed from side to side in the semiprone position, but is not placed on his back. Since the duration of unconsciousness is to be measured in days, the emergence of drug-resistance bacteria is of less concern than is pneumonia due to already aspirated material. Thus, it is useful to administer penicillin or tetracycline.

The blood pressure, pulse, and respiration should be recorded each half hour, and any abnormalities should be met appropriately. Body temperature elevations imply an infection if stimulants have not been given. To evaluate the rate of urine flow, most physicians prefer to insert an indwelling catheter.

Other Measures. *Gastric lavage* is desirable for any patient who has ingested depressant drugs within the preceding few hours. The procedure carries the risk of producing pulmonary aspiration, and is best preceded by tracheal intubation in deeply comatose subjects. Subjects too lightly anesthetized to tolerate intubation should be turned prone before being lavaged. Great care is required to avoid misplacing the tube and irrigating the lungs.

Forced diuresis and alkalinization of the urine have been recommended as adjuncts in treating barbiturate poisoning. Forced diuresis increases the renal clearance of both short- and long-acting barbiturates, and the quantity cleared increases proportionately to the volume of urine. Phenobarbital has a relatively high pK value, and raising the urine pH appears to increase its dissociation and excretion. Several programs have been employed to achieve diuresis. The first step is to assure an adequate blood pressure; the second, to infuse a hypotonic electrolyte solution. The infusions are given at hourly rates up to 600 ml., depending upon urine flow. Close attention must be given to hour-by-hour fluid balance and 12-hour electrolyte balance. If urine flow does not match the infusion rate by the second or third hour, infusions should be slowed and more attention given to raising the blood pressure. Chemical and osmotic diuretics are contraindicated. Hypokalemia is a greater risk than hyperkalemia.

For treating bromide intoxication, diuresis should be combined with a high intake of sodium chloride to displace bromide from blood and tissues.

Hemodialysis has been used by several centers to clear barbiturates, glutethimide, or bromides from the blood and tissues of severely poisoned patients. Among patients poisoned with short-acting barbiturate or glutethimide, the published results present no evidence that hemodialysis improves mortality beyond that achieved by the program of care outlined above. However, hemodialysis is indicated for patients who have ingested large amounts of long-acting barbiturates such as barbital or phenobarbital as well as for patients who have severe bromide poisoning. In these instances, dialysis can shorten into a day or less a period of coma or stupor that otherwise would last a week or more.

Analeptics and pharmacologic stimulants are not indicated for coma due to depressant drug poisoning. Most carry the risk of overstimulating or producing convulsions in lightly poisoned patients.

Recovery and Prognosis. Patients recovering from coma require close medical supervision. Severe pneumonitis can develop as late as three to four days after recovery. If antimicrobial drugs were started during coma, they are best continued for at least 48 hours thereafter. Permanent physical sequelae to coma are extremely rare. Among 356 cases, residual brain injury was observed only once (in a patient who suffered an acute cardiac arrest). Peripheral nerve injuries from pressure developed in 6 subjects, and 14 subjects had pressure skin lesions leaving scars. There were no other residua.

Later management varies according to the patient's underlying psychiatric disorder and his attitudes upon recovery. Serious suicide attempts are never accidents, and reports of near-fatal ingestion due to misunderstanding the dose or forgetting previous doses carry little validity. The expert opinion of a psychiatrist should be sought before deciding whether to release a patient or to institutionalize him. The immediate prognosis is good, but long-term results are less encouraging, and there is a high incidence of recurrent attempts at self destruction over the years.

Lavenson, G. S., Plum, F., and Swanson, A. G.: Physiological management compared with pharmacological and electrical stimulation in barbiturate poisoning. J. Pharmacol Exp Ther., 122:271, 1958.

Myschetzky, A., and Lassen, N. A.: Urea-induced osmotic diuresis and alkalinization of urine in acute barbiturate intoxication. J.A.M.A., 185:936, 1963.

Nilsson, E.: Treatment of barbiturate intoxication. Acta Med. Scand., 139(Supp. 253) 1951.

PHENOTHIAZINE TOXICITY

Fred Plum

The phenothiazine derivatives have a wide margin of safety, and relatively huge amounts can be taken without producing anything more serious than hypotension or akinesia. A few persons develop hypersensitive reactions to the drugs, including intrahepatic obstructive jaundice, rare agranulocytosis, and skin disorders with urticaria, contact dermatitis, photosensitivity, or slate-gray pigmentation.

Direct pharmacologic side effects include (1) transient orthostatic hypotension, (2) seizures, particularly following parenteral injections of promazine, and (3) extrapyramidal disorders. The last mentioned take the form of parkinsonism in adults and in the aged, and disappear if the drug is discontinued or the dosage reduced.

In children and young adults, the extrapyramidal reactions are more dramatic and include acute dystonia and various dyskinesias. There may be torticollis, retrocollis, facial tic, or even repeated oculogyric crises. Trismus may be so severe as to be mistaken for tetanus. The patients are restless, agitated, and usually exceedingly anxious. These disorders commonly disappear promptly and respond dramatically to intramuscular scopolamine injections (0.4 mg. for an adult). A few patients who have received several years of phenothiazine treatment develop facial grimacing and sucking movements that persist when the drug is discontinued; no satisfactory treatment exists for this sequel.

Prominent Neurologic Symptoms and Their Management

PAIN

August G. Swanson

Pain is a personal experience, and communication about it depends upon the experience and vocabulary of the sufferer, just as its interpretation depends upon the experience and bias of the listener. The physician, charged with alleviating suffering, must necessarily be concerned with pain. Being human, the physician experiences pain, and his attitudes toward it may modify his judgment. He may be incuriously sympathetic, too anxious to relieve pain without understanding its nature or source. He may too quickly dismiss the complaint, not recognizing its importance as a manifestation of disease. He may also fail to recognize that pain may be the manifestation of complex and stressful problems that face the patient. Ultimately, it is the physician who must determine the source of pain and select a means of relieving it.

Pain may produce suffering, but all suffering is not pain. A person may suffer from loneliness, fear, anxiety, or other emotional responses to stress. However, pain also produces fear, anxiety, and loneliness; for pain is the signal that warns of a threat to the integrity of the organism. This threat may alter the life pattern of a person and so color his interpretation of what he is experiencing that the exact nature of his problem is obscured. The skilled physician must learn to separate the patient's reaction to pain from his perception of pain; and, in obtaining this separation, he must view the patient in the setting of his past, his family, and his community.

The vocabulary for describing pain is limited. When interviewing, it is best to begin by asking the patient to describe what he feels without suggesting adjectives. Avoid leading questions, but direct the interview as necessary by asking such questions as: Where is the pain? Does it go anywhere else? Is it continuous? How does this pain interfere with your life? When the patient's descriptive resources are exhausted, directed questions regarding quality, radiation, and temporal phasing may be used to round out the description. Generally, the history alone distinguishes the variety of pain, its likely source, and its cause. Examination provides corroborative data.

The alleviation of pain not only is dependent upon correction of its cause but also may require modification of the patient's attitude toward himself, his life situation, and his disease. The approaches to treatment of pain will be dealt with after consideration of the anatomy and physiology of pain.

Pain Pathways. Until the late nineteenth century, pain was not included among the primary sensations, but was considered to arise from the intense stimulation of any afferent nerve or its terminals. The demonstration in a human that interruption of the spinothalamic tract stopped pain sensation below the level of the lesion proved that within the neuraxis the sensation of pain is conducted along a specific pathway. The exact pathways for pain conduction in the peripheral nervous system have remained open to question. However, most workers now believe that the small, finely myelinated fibers that occupy the lateral portion of the dorsal root and enter Lissauer's tract to synapse in the substantia gelatinosa and other nuclei of the dorsal gray horn are the fibers that subserve pain peripherally.

The means of transmission of the many shadings and gradations of pain remains to be clarified. Currently, it appears that pain is conducted over specific pathways, but complex integration of signals occurs at several levels. The first level is at the end organ. Finely branched, undifferentiated endings subserve pain. In skin these form an intricate, interlacing network. Partial denervation of an area of skin alters the quality of pain elicited from that site because of the interruption of the normal patterns of firing of several axons when that particular area of skin is stimulated.

Experimental and clinical evidence now suggests that the long, fast-conducting fibers in peripheral nerves serve to modulate the input from the small, slow-conducting fibers. This modulation occurs segmentally in the dorsal horn, and may be mediated through the small polysynaptic neurons in the substantia gelatinosa. If the faster conducting fibers are interrupted by compression-ischemic block, the pain produced by stimulating the affected part is more intense and uncomfortable. This type of response is also seen in patients with peripheral neuritis. A scratch on the sole of the foot produces immediate mild discomfort, followed within one to one and a half seconds by intense and prolonged discomfort. Histologic studies demonstrate that peripheral neuritis affects the larger fibers to a greater degree than the smaller. *Thus, in the peripheral nervous system, pain signals may be encoded by the geographic pattern of the interlacing nerve endings and by the differential conduction times of afferent axons.*

Upon entering the spinal cord, the pain-conducting fibers synapse in the *dorsal gray horn.* This is the first site within the neuraxis where integration of peripheral sensory impulses may occur. There are rich interconnections within the dorsal horn at each segment and between segments. The spreading zone of hyperalgesia, which may be demonstrated around a site of intense stimulation in skin, is due to facilitation of adjacent neurons in the dorsal horn. This site of integration also accounts for referred pain from deep sites and for hyperalgesia projected to skin from deeper sources of pain.

From the dorsal gray horn secondary neurons project cephalad in the contralateral *spinothalamic tract.* There are fewer fibers in the spinothalamic tract than the total aggregate of the entering primary pain fibers from the periphery. This is another indication of integration of this afferent system at the segmental level.

The spinothalamic tracts ascend through the brainstem, giving off fibers to the nonspecific reticular system. Relatively few fibers finally arrive at the posterior ventral nucleus of the thalamus. Tertiary neurons then project to the sensory cortex. These are the highest levels of integration. Disruption of the thalamic nucleus results in diminished pain sensation of the contralateral side. Following a lesion in the posterior ventral nucleus, spontaneous pain may develop on the opposite side of the body, referred to as "thalamic pain." Characteristically, the pain is severe and excruciating. A light touch to the involved part is felt as pain.

The conscious perception of pain appears to be localized to the upper brainstem and thalamus, but its localization and the recognition of the nature of the noxious stimulus is dependent upon projections to the parietal cortex from the thalamus. This is apparent when a patient with a parietal lobe lesion is stimulated with a pin or by hard pressure. The reaction is one of intense discomfort accompanied by dismayed concern about the nature and site of the discomfort. The patient complains of pain, but cannot identify the nature of the stimulus or its site.

Although the autonomic nervous system is an efferent system, fibers mediating pain signals from viscera and deep structures course with autonomic nerves and enter the central nervous system by way of the dorsal roots.

Painful Stimuli. Tissue injury is the adequate stimulus for pain. This is evident when skin is pierced, abraded, or burned and when deeper tissues are compressed and bruised. When tissue is injured, the release of various chemical products serves to excite pain. Pain may also be elicited by stretching hollow viscera or by tugging on omentum or distorting the vessels at the base of the brain. This type of pain less clearly results from tissue injury. Among the possible chemical exciters of pain are hydrogen ions, potassium ions, 5-hydroxytryptamine, histamine, polypeptides from protein breakdown (kinins), and acetylcholine. It is not proper to refer to these as chemical mediators of pain, for this implies a specific response between the end organ and the substance. A specific chemical mediator analogous to synaptic transmitter substances has not been identified for sensory end organs. The local release of these chemical products of tissue injury modifies the sensitivity of the pain endings. Thus, pressure over an inflamed joint or a light touch applied to a burned area produces pain. The prolonged pain from a first-degree burn results from the accumulation of these products of tissue injury.

Altered Pain Perception. The perception of pain results from stimuli that damage tissue and the transmission of this signal along the complex pathways already described. This concept is clear when simple cutaneous pain, as from a pin prick or a burn, is considered; but analysis of pain perception becomes more complex when the source of painful stimulus is from deeper sites and from diseased or partially denervated organs and structures. In these more complex problems, consideration must be given to reaction to pain both at the segmental level and suprasegmentally. *Hyperesthesia, hyperalgesia,* and *dysesthesia* are terms that must be examined and their meanings understood.

Hyperalgesia and *hyperesthesia* denote an intensification of the perception of the stimulus once the threshold is reached, but lowering of the threshold is not necessarily a part of hyperalgesia or hyperesthesia. Both may coexist. If touch or noxious stimuli induce pain of an aberrant and unnatural variety, the term *dysesthesia* applies.

Hyperalgesia can be viewed as primary or secondary. Primary hyperalgesia refers to a lowered pain threshold related to accumulation of chemical pain stimulants in the hyperalgesic tissue. Secondary hyperalgesia refers to a change in the central excitatory state at the segmental and suprasegmental levels. The hyperalgesia of a first-degree burn is a good example of simple primary hyperalgesia. The hyperalgesia developing in skin overlying a source of deep pain is secondary hyperalgesia. Here an increased central excitatory state probably accounts for the greater intensity of painful stimulation and the hyperesthetic qualities of touch stimuli. *Dysesthesia,* as the term implies, is an abnormal pain. This sensation results from disease of neural pathways at all levels. Peripheral neuritis with delayed or "C fiber" pain is an example of dysesthesia. Thalamic pain and the pain of causalgia are dysesthetic.

Another aspect of hyperalgesia is the development of pain within muscles sharing a closely adjacent innervation with the primary source of painful stimulation. Prolonged, painful stimulation results in tonic contraction of muscle. As this contraction persists, the muscles themselves become tender and painful. The pain arising from sustained muscle contraction is probably due to the local release of chemical excitants such as potassium ions and more complex substances. Even as the primary source of painful stimulation subsides, the pain arising from tonically contracting muscles may perpetuate the pain.

Referred Pain. The referral of pain from the primary locus of stimulation to another site may occur with awareness of the primary site—for example, in a toothache, pain may be referred to the temporomandibular region—or without awareness of the primary site, as in referral of pain from a subdiaphragmatic abscess to the posterior shoulder region of the same side. Deep structures such as the heart and hollow viscera are not specifically recognized as being painfully stimulated, the pain being referred to somatic areas that are more clearly recognized by the patient as a part of himself. An exhaustive catalogue of all the combinations of referred pain from deep structures is not within the scope of this article. However, there are common sites of pain referral worthy of consideration.

Referred pain in the head is discussed in the article on Headache. In the trunk, painful stimuli arising in the middle third of the esophagus are referred substernally. In the lower third of the esophagus, the stomach, the duodenum, and the remainder of the small intestine, pain is referred to the epigastric region. Pain arising from the large bowel is referred to the hypogastric region. Thus, the pain of duodenal ulcer is perceived as in the epigastrium, whereas the pain of appendicitis is periumbilical and in the lower abdomen. The spread of referred pain depends upon the duration and intensity of the painful stimulus. High intensity afferent input over a prolonged period results in spreading hyperexcitability in the segment of the cord that the afferent fibers enter and to adjacent segments. Disease processes may spread from viscera to involve the abdominal wall. When the parietal peritoneum is thus stimulated, pain may become more localized to the somatic region supplied by the segment involved. Hence, a posteriorly perforating duodenal ulcer causes pain radiating into the back, and acute pancreatitis localizes to the back close to the anatomic location of the pancreas.

Pain from the genitourinary tract is referred to the hypogastric area and the flanks. Ureteral colic causes pain along the border of the rectus abdominis spreading into the flank and groin. Bladder distention causes pain in the suprapubic area. Pain from the urethra is referred directly to the penis and perineum. Testicular pain is referred to the suprapubic area.

Insensitivity to Pain. In normal persons, pain serves to protect the body from exogenous injury and internal disease. Pain demands attention; persistent pain causes withdrawal of the organism, rest of the injured part, and avoidance of further injury. These are normal reactions that protect the injured tissue and promote healing. The importance of these reactions is dramatized in patients who are insensitive or indifferent to pain. The complete absence of any reaction to pain has been described in about 65 persons.

This rare lack of response to pain has been termed "indifference" by some and "insensitivity" by others. Both terms are probably correct. The clinical descriptions of many of the cases suggest that the patients are extraordinarily stoic and can endure remarkable pain without apparent awareness. In other cases, particularly those recognized in infancy, a true insensitivity seems more likely. These infants cut and burn themselves without notice. Bones are broken and go unheeded. The major weight-bearing joints are destroyed by the uncommon degree of trauma that they sustain. The utter disregard for the integrity of their bodies is dramatic proof of the importance of pain as a warning of tissue injury. Only two autopsies have been reported, and in one no anatomic explanation for insensitivity to pain could be identified. In the other, Lissauer's tract was absent, and there were no small, finely myelinated fibers in the dorsal roots.

Treatment of Pain. Insensitivity or indifference to pain is not the common human experience. During a lifetime, man is exposed to a multitude of pain-inducing injuries and diseases. When pain is persistent, overwhelming, or frightening, he turns to the physician for help. To the patient and to the physician, pain signifies an unnatural state that warns of tissue injury and disease. The primary attention is directed toward determining the source of the pain and correcting the cause. Generally, relief follows. However, pain may occur as a result of disease that cannot be eradicated, as in widespread carcinoma. Pain may also be the primary manifestation of diseases of the central and peripheral nervous system, such as tic douloureux, postherpetic neuralgia, and causalgia. Finally, pain may be a manifestation of reaction to life stresses, as in migraine headache, tension headache, and myalgias that can involve the entire musculoskeletal system. Alleviating pain requires that the physician utilize his knowledge of the origin and transmission of pain and that he understand the complex interactions between perception and reaction to pain. No drug or operation is a panacea for all pain.

TRIGEMINAL NEURALGIA

Trigeminal neuralgia, or tic douloureux, is a disease of unknown cause in which the principal manifestation is pain. The only other manifestation may be brief contractions of the facial musculature as the pain stabs in lightning-like paroxysms. Hence, the term "tic." The disease is rare in those younger than 50, but similar pain may occur in younger persons as a symptom of multiple sclerosis or of tumor impinging on the trigeminal nerve.

The patient's spontaneous description of the pain serves to distinguish trigeminal neuralgia from other pains in the face. It is a searing, agonizing stab clearly localized to a division of the fifth nerve. Each stab is momentary, but stabs may occur repetitively over periods lasting as long as 20 seconds. Often, but not always, the stabs are initiated by touching a trigger point, which may be on the skin or lips or in the buccal cavity. Even a slight breath of air across the trigger zone may initiate the paroxysm. If the trigger zone is in the mouth, the jaw may hang slack and speech may be slurred to avoid stimulation. Eating may be difficult or impossible. The episodes vary in frequency, often occurring many times an hour and then subsiding, with complete remissions lasting weeks or months. The spring and autumn are particularly likely times for exacerbations.

There is no interruption of sensory or motor function in trigeminal neuralgia. The corneal reflex is normal, and sensation over the face and within the mouth is normal. The cerebrospinal fluid is normal. *If abnormalities of sensation are found or if motor function of the fifth nerve is impaired, a careful search for disease impinging on the fifth nerve must be initiated.*

Medical treatment of trigeminal neuralgia should be attempted before turning to surgical treatment. Diphenylhydantoin in doses of 300 to 400 mg. per day has aborted exacerbations of the pain, but it is a common experience that the pain may recur while the patient is still taking the drug. Carbamazepine is the drug of choice if diphenylhydantoin fails. The initial dose is 400 mg. per day, and the maintenance dose is 400 to 800 mg. per day. Bone marrow depression is a hazard. Initial blood studies should be followed by regular follow-up studies. Injection of various branches of the fifth nerve with alcohol has been a popular form of treatment in the past, but relief is not often permanent. Section of the nerve root proximal to the ganglion is the surgical approach most likely to afford permanent relief.

GLOSSOPHARYNGEAL NEURALGIA

Glossopharyngeal neuralgia is characterized by pain that is similar in quality to that of trigeminal neuralgia. The trigger zone is in the posterior pharynx or tonsillar fossa, and the pain spreads toward the angle of the jaw and the ear. Syncope may occur during the attacks as a result of intense cardiac slowing and even arrest. The condition is much more rare than trigeminal neuralgia. Pontocaine spray to the trigger zone may afford temporary relief, but complete relief requires section of the glossopharyngeal nerve roots.

ATYPICAL FACE PAIN

The term "atypical face pain" serves to distinguish pain in the face with qualities quite different from trigeminal or glossopharyngeal neuralgia. The major distinguishing features are differences in the qualitative description of the pain by the patient and its course. The clear paroxysms of stabbing pain are lacking, and more indefinite and vague descriptions are given. "Aching" or "deep throbbing" are common terms. The patient claims few moments of relief. The pain usually goes on for days, or even months, and examinations of teeth, sinuses, nose, ears, and temporomandibular joints are unsuccessful in delineating a cause. Indeed, the pain frequently begins following dental work or sinus manipulation. As the pain becomes established, it spreads into the region of the ear and down the neck. The personalities of these patients and their reactions to life stress strongly suggest that atypical face pain is psychogenic. Treatment should be directed toward adjustment of life patterns. Nerve section is of no value, and opiates should never be used.

PAIN FROM PERIPHERAL NERVES AND ROOTS

Pain arising from injury to a peripheral nerve is common, and its incidence increases with age. Minor traumatic neuropathies occur after unusual exercise or postures in older folk, and often are not brought to the attention of a physician. When traumatic neuropathies become chronically painful or impair function, initial treatment is directed toward modifying postures and movements that aggravate trauma. If conservative measures fail, surgical excision of painful neuromas or nerve transplantation may be required.

Pain arising from cervical or lumbosacral roots is often described as "searing" or "stabbing," but other patients may experience only tingling paresthesias. The pain is in the distribution of the involved root, but as the process continues, prolonged muscle contraction in the paraspinous groups leads to aching pain in the neck, shoulders or low back. Changes in sensory threshold may be prominent or completely absent, and the appropriate segmental reflex may be normal, reduced, or absent. Root pain is frequently due to posterolateral protrusion of the intervertebral disc with impingement of the root at the intervertebral foramen. However, extramedullary spinal tumors and neuromas of the nerve root may first present with root pain. The pain from suspected disc protrusion is first treated by minimizing movement, reducing weight-bearing, and giving analgesics. When pain persists or recurs and signs of altered nerve function persist or progress, diagnostic myelography followed by surgery may be indicated.

CAUSALGIA

Causalgia is a specific syndrome that occurs after direct, partial injury to peripheral nerves, particularly of the sciatic or median nerves. It is distinguished from other painful neuropathies by the history of acute trauma, the dysesthetic quality of the pain, and the trophic changes that occur in the involved extremity. The involved limb is cool and hairless, and the skin is thin, shiny, and smooth. There is profuse sweating not only in the affected part, but over the entire body. The pain is almost continuous and usually is described as having a burning quality. It is worsened by stimulation of the part and by emotion or anxiety. This syndrome is most common in wartime injuries in young males.

Painful peripheral neuropathy is common in diabetes, dietary deficiency, pernicious anemia, periarteritis nodosa, and following the administration of toxic drugs. Pain may be almost continuous, but the patient particularly complains of pain when the skin over the involved part is stimulated. Even the weight of bedclothes may be intolerable. Although thresholds to pain, touch, and vibration are elevated in the distal parts of the extremities, once the threshold is reached, the patient experiences both hyperalgesia and dysesthesia. Pain is worse distally and lessens or disappears proximally. Delayed or "C fiber" pain is common. The painful neuropathies associated with vitamin deficiency diseases slowly subside once replacement therapy is started. Diabetic neuropathy may improve to some degree with careful control of the diabetes, but often is intractable. Large doses of vitamin B, including B_{12}, have been tried but with little benefit. General measures include gentle heat, a cradle for protection of the extremity, warm packs and meticulous attention to skin care.

POSTHERPETIC NEURALGIA

A few patients suffer severe and prolonged pain in the involved dermatome following an attack of herpes zoster. The pain is usually described as a constant, burning ache, but sharp stabs may occur spontaneously, and there are severe hyperalgesia and dysesthesia. Treatment is directed toward altering the abnormal pain by increasing the sensory input to the involved area. Brisk massage with a terry-cloth towel several times a day gradually brings relief, but may require several weeks or months. Surgical treatment gives uncertain results. Undercutting the skin of the involved area may afford temporary or permanent relief. Dorsal root section rarely helps. If undercutting fails, high thoracic spinothalamic tractotomy may give permanent relief when the site of the pain is below the upper six cervical segments. Some writers have advocated high doses of adrenal corticosteroids for this condition, but thus far there has been only limited experience with such therapy.

MUSCLE PAIN

Pain from skeletal muscle is common. Strenuous exertion by an untrained person may result in severe muscle soreness and pain on moving. Pain arising from prolonged tonic contraction of muscle is less conspicuous in its onset, and the cause of the pain may be obscure. Prolonged contraction may arise from tension and anxiety. The tension headache, which begins in the paraspinous muscles at the base of the skull, is an example. Muscle pain may arise from prolonged fixed and stressful postures. The pain in neck muscles that develops in neophyte typists and the pain of writer's cramp are examples. Muscle pain may develop from splinting the lower spine. The paraspinous muscle pain extending from lumbar into the thoracic region in patients with lumbar root compression is an example. Finally, muscle pain may arise from the tonic contraction of muscle secondary to pain from deep structures.

Although requiring experience, palpation of the involved muscles demonstrates unusual firmness, suggesting a contracted state. The muscles are tender, sometimes exquisitely so, but usually only moderately to mildly. The pain is deep and aching in quality, often accentuated by movement.

Acute muscle pain is treated with rest, local hot compresses, and aspirin. A degree of relief is afforded by enhancing the sensory input from the overlying skin, which explains the success of liniments containing methyl salicylate. Spraying the skin of the involved area with ethyl chloride sufficiently to lightly frost the hair affords similar relief. When a particularly tender point is found on palpation, infiltration of the tender point with 1 per cent procaine may afford dramatic relief. Because the pain of tonic muscle contraction is self-propagating, once the cycle is broken relaxation may be followed by sustained relief.

INTRACTABLE PAIN

When pain is severe and chronic and not amenable to relief by treating its source, the physician is forced to make choices between various means of decreasing the perception of pain or modifying the patient's reaction to pain. If pain accompanies a fatal disease and the *life expectancy is measured in days or weeks,* opiates in sufficient doses are best. Opiates modify reaction to pain more than perception of it and thus provide the dual advantage of easing anxiety as well as pain. However, it is tragic when a patient with *chronic pain and a normal life expectancy is provided opiates.* Although temporary relief for both the physician and the patient may ensue, the problems of addiction inevitably complicate management and aggravate morbidity. Patients with tension headache, frequent vascular headache, atypical face pain, and chronic low-back pain need attention to their life-adjustment patterns. Reassurance, empathy, and a willingness to help the patient understand his reaction to difficulties are combined with non-narcotic analgesics and sedatives.

The most vexing problems of intractable pain are presented by patients for whom pain fulfills an emotional need. These pain-prone patients often have pain that is bizarre, defying rational explanation. The physical findings are seldom commensurate with the pain described. The physician, frustrated by repeated efforts to relieve the pain, may unwisely undertake operative exploration. This approach may be repeated many times, resulting in multiple surgical efforts to no avail. Psychiatric treatment, though quite obviously necessary, is frequently rejected by such patients.

Intractable pain may also be perpetuated when disability may provide some gain. Pending litigation for damages resulting from injury may so magnify a patient's reaction to pain that effective treatment is impossible until the legal proceedings are concluded.

When a severe, intractable, and disabling pain has a specific identifiable source and the outlook for life is measured in months and years, relief by interrupting pain pathways to reduce or eliminate pain perception is worthwhile. Operative approaches for the trunk and lower limbs include section of multiple dorsal roots and spinothalamic tractotomy. Both procedures require major surgery. The relief of pain by tractotomy is generally more satisfactory than by root section.

When the source of pain is in the upper cervical segments or in the head, tract section is hazardous. Some surgeons meet this problem by modifying the patient's reaction to pain by bilateral frontal lobotomy or cingulomotomy. These operations inevitably modify *affect,* so the undesirability of changing the personality must be weighed against the need for relief from pain.

Buytendjik, F. J. J.: Pain; Its Mode and Functions. Chicago, University of Chicago Press, 1962.

Engel, G. L.: "Psychogenic" pain and the pain-prone patients. Amer. J. Med., 26:899, 1959.

Hardy, J. D., Wolff, H. G., and Goodell, H.: Pain Sensations and Reactions. Baltimore, Williams & Wilkins Company, 1952.

Killian, J. M., and Fromm, G. H.: Carbamazepine in the Treatment of Neuralgia. Arch. Neurol. (Chicago), 19:129, 1968.

Lewis, T.: Pain. New York, The Macmillan Company, 1942.

Melzack, R., and Wall, P. D.: Pain mechanisms; A new theory, Science, 150:971, 1965.

Rockliff, B. W., and Davis, E. H.: Controlled sequential trials of carbamazepine in trigeminal neuralgia. Arch. Neurol. (Chicago), 15:129, 1966.

Swanson, A. G., Buchan, G. C., and Alvord, Jr., E. C.: Anatomic changes in congenital insensitivity to pain. Arch. Neurol. (Chicago), 12:12, 1965.

White, J. C., and Sweet, W. H.: Pain. Springfield, Ill., Charles C Thomas, 1955.

HEADACHE
Fred Plum

INTRODUCTION

Headache is man's most common pain; in one form or another it affects an estimated 90 per cent of the population. The following is an outline of the principal types:

A. Extracranial headache:

1. Vascular headaches of the migraine type are recurrent and vary widely in intensity, duration, and frequency. The following subtypes are recognized:

a. *Classic migraine,* with sharply defined, transient visual, other sensory and/or motor prodromes.

b. *Hemiplegic or ophthalmoplegic migraine,* featured by sensory and motor phenomena that persist during and after the headache.

c. *Common migraine,* without striking prodromes and less often unilateral than (a) and (d). Synonyms are "atypical migraine" and "sick headache."

d. *Cluster headache,* predominantly unilateral, associated with flushing, sweating, rhinorrhea, and increased lacrimation, brief in duration and usually occurring in close-packed groups separated by long remissions. Identical or closely allied are histaminic cephalgia (Horton), and petrosal neuralgia (Gardner et al.).

e. *Lower half headache,* of possible vascular mechanism, centered primarily in the lower face. In this group are some instances of atypical facial neuralgia, sphenopalatine ganglion neuralgia (Sluder), and vidian neuralgia (Vail).

2. Muscle contraction headaches are occipitofrontal pains or sensations of tightness, pressure, or constriction associated with sustained skeletal muscle contraction and no permanent structural change. The ambiguous and unsatisfactory terms

"tension," "psychogenic," and "nervous" headache refer largely to this group.

3. Combinations of vascular headache of the migraine type and muscle contraction headache.

4. Anterior headache and nasal discomfort (nasal obstruction, rhinorrhea, tightness, or burning) can result from congestion, edema, and inflammation of nasal and paranasal mucous membranes. This is "sinus" headache.

5. Nonmigrainous vascular headaches associated with generally nonrecurrent dilatation of intracranial arteries.

6. Ocular headache due to spread of effects of noxious stimulation, as by increased intraocular pressure, excessive contraction of ocular muscles, trauma, new growth, or inflammation.

7. Aural headache due to spread of effects of noxious stimulation, as by trauma, new growth, or inflammation.

8. Dental headache.

9. Headache due to spread of pain from noxious stimulation of other structures of the cranium and neck (periosteum, joints, ligaments, and muscles or cervical nerve roots).

10. Cranial neuritides (caused by trauma, new growth, or infection).

11. Extracranial arteritis.

B. Intracranial headache:

1. Traction headache. Headache resulting from traction on intracranial structures, mainly vascular, by masses:

   a. Primary or metastatic tumors of meninges, vessels, or brain.

   b. Hematomas (epidural, subdural, or parenchymal).

   c. Abscesses (epidural, subdural, or parenchymal).

   d. Headache following puncture ("leakage" headache).

   e. Pseudotumor cerebri and various causes of brain swelling.

2. Headache due to overt inflammation of cranial structures resulting from usually nonrecurrent inflammation, sterile or infectious.

Intracranial disorders: infectious, chemical, or allergic meningitis, subarachnoid hemorrhage, post-pneumoencephalographic reaction, arteritis, and phlebitis.

C. Cranial neuralgias: trigeminal (tic douloureux) and glossopharyngeal (see preceding article on Pain). Trigeminal neuralgia must be distinguished in particular from the brief vascular headache of 1 c, with which it is often confused.

D. Headaches of a delusional or conversion reaction are those in which a peripheral pain mechanism is nonexistent. The diagnosis is rare and must be made cautiously. Closely allied are hypochondriacal and depressive reactions in which peripheral disturbances relevant to headache are minimal.

Pathogenesis of Headache. Wolff and his colleagues identified the principal pain-sensitive structures of the head as: (1) *extracranial*: all the tissues, especially the arteries; (2) *intracranial*: a very limited group of tissues, including the great venous sinuses and their venous tributaries from the surface of the brain, parts of the dura at the base, the dural arteries and the cerebral arteries at the base of the brain, the fifth, seventh, ninth, and tenth cranial nerves, and the upper three cervical nerves.

The cranium (including the diploic and emissary veins), the parenchyma of the brain, most of the dura, most of the pia-arachnoid, and the ependymal lining of the ventricles and the choroid plexuses are not sensitive to pain.

The fifth cranial nerve contains the pathways for pain from sensitive intracranial structures located on or above the superior surface of the tentorium cerebelli. Pain from these structures is experienced in various regions in front of a line drawn coronally joining the ears across the top of the head.

The ninth and tenth cranial nerves and the upper two or possibly three cervical nerves contain the pathways for pain from pain-sensitive structures on or below the inferior surface of the tentorium cerebelli. Pain from these structures is experienced in various parieto-occipital and upper cervical regions behind the line just described.

HEADACHE FROM INTRACRANIAL SOURCES

Six basic mechanisms of headache from intracranial sources have been formulated: (1) traction on and displacement of the great venous sinuses or of the veins that pass to them from the surface of the brain; (2) traction on and displacement of the middle meningeal arteries; (3) traction on and displacement of the large arteries at the base of the brain and their main branches; (4) dilatation and distention of intracranial arteries; (5) inflammation in or about any of the pain-sensitive structures of the head and portions of the pia and dura at the base of the skull; and (6) direct pressure by tumors on pain-sensitive cranial and cervical nerves. Intracranial diseases commonly cause headaches through more than one mechanism and may also cause secondary extracranial muscle-contraction headache, usually at the occiput, but often elsewhere.

The head pain associated with fever, bacteremia, sepsis, nitrite and foreign protein administration, carbon monoxide inhalation, hypoxia, and asphyxia is due principally to dilatation and distention of intracranial arterial structures. A similar vascular mechanism is the probable basis for the headaches following epileptic seizures (with or without convulsions) and certain "hangover headaches," and is a component of many migraine headaches and those associated with arterial hypertension and Meniere's disease. Painful distention of intracranial arteries is likewise responsible for the headaches that accompany sudden brisk rises in the arterial blood pressure, such as occurs with distention of the rectum or urinary bladder in paraplegics, rapid intravenous infusion of epinephrine, and the hypertensive crises occurring with pheochromocytoma.

The headache of meningitis is primarily related to the lowered pain threshold of inflamed tissues. The inflammatory changes are usually most noticeable in the basal dura and pia, and in adjacent blood vessels and nerves at the base of the brain. Under these circumstances, even the slight, usually painless arterial dilatation and distention during each cardiac systole becomes painful; hence, the characteristic throbbing headache.

Lumbar Puncture Headache

Dull, usually pulsating, headache develops in the occipital region of about one fifth of patients having lumbar puncture, particularly for the first time. The headache usually begins 12 to 24 hours after the puncture, comes on in the erect position, and subsides if the subject lies flat. The headache usually disappears spontaneously in a day or so, and in most patients is made tolerable by routine analgesics. Occasionally, patients develop more prostrating symptoms that sometimes last as long as 10 to 14 days, accompanied by secondary muscle-contraction headache as well as nausea and vomiting. Vigorous reassurance and sedatives added to the analgesics may help shorten the course.

The cause of post-lumbar puncture headache is unknown. Because of its relationship to position and the observation that replacing the removed cerebrospinal fluid with saline temporarily relieves the pain, it has been postulated that a CSF leak through the dura permits downward traction on unsupported, pain-sensitive posterior fossa tissues, particularly the veins. The headaches can often be avoided by using No. 20 caliber sharp spinal puncture needles, which are believed to minimize drainage through the dural needle wound.

Headache With Brain Tumor: With or Without Increased Intracranial Pressure

The headache with space-occupying lesions is deep, aching, steady, dull, and seldom rhythmic or throbbing. The pain is continuous in one tenth of the patients and is generally more intense in the morning. Aspirin, 0.3 gram, and local application of cold packs usually diminish the pain, and coughing or straining at stool may aggravate it. Some patients prefer the recumbent to the erect position. The headache is rarely as intense as that associated with migraine, ruptured cerebral aneurysm, or meningitis, and seldom interferes with sleep. Even when the tumor directly compresses and displaces pain-sensitive cranial nerves, headache may be absent or slight, and rarely is it as intense as the pain of tic douloureux, unless the tumor intermittently obstructs the cerebral ventricular system. In this instance, pain is excruciating, generalized, and may last 30 seconds to a half hour and then disappear as quickly as it commenced. During such an attack the sudden intracranial pressure shifts can be fatal.

Severe brain tumor headache is associated with nausea and vomiting. However, vomiting due to new growth may occur with neither nausea nor headache, and is then usually the result of medullary compression. Being unexpected, such vomiting may be projectile.

When the headache is occipital or suboccipital, it is often associated with "stiffness" or aching of the muscles of the neck and tilting of the head toward the side of the lesion.

Pathogenesis. Increased intracranial pressure, per se, is not necessarily associated with headache. The headache with brain tumor results from traction-displacement of intracranial pain-sensitive structures, chiefly the large arteries, veins, venous sinuses, and the cranial and somatic nerves mentioned.

Local traction and direct pressure may be exerted by the tumor upon adjacent pain-sensitive structures. Extensive displacement of the brain evokes pain from structures remote from, as well as adjacent to, the tumor.

Localizing Value. When the site of the headache is interpreted in terms of the following principles of intracranial pain production and pain reference, it may aid significantly in localization of a brain tumor:

(1) About one third of all headaches approximately overlie the tumor. (2) In the absence of increased intracranial pressure, two thirds of headaches are near or immediately over the tumor, and when unilateral are on the same side. (3) Occipital headache is almost always present and is the first symptom of posterior fossa tumors, except cerebellopontine angle tumors. When headache occurs with cerebellopontine angle tumors, it is frequently and sometimes solely postauricular. (4) Frontal headache is a first symptom in about one third of supratentorial tumors. Occipital headache rarely occurs with such growths unless associated with increased intracranial pressure or early tonsillar herniation. (5) A generalized headache with brain tumor signifies extensive displacement of the brain, usually with increased intracranial pressure, and has little localizing value.

Management. The most effective treatment for brain tumor headache is surgical removal of the mass. Measures that internally decompress the brain may be employed briefly while awaiting surgery. Effective but transient decompression can be achieved by the intravenous infusion of either 500 ml. of a 20 per cent sodium mannitol solution or 250 ml. of a solution containing 30 per cent urea in 10 per cent invert sugar. Adrenal corticosteroids in high doses also have been employed to reduce brain edema and transiently decompress the mass. Lumbar drainage is contraindicated, nor does it predictably reduce headache of meningitis or subarachnoid hemorrhage. Sudden changes in position from recumbent to sitting should be avoided since they augment headache.

If an irremovable tumor causing headache is above the tentorium, subtemporal decompression may diminish the intensity of the headache. If such a tumor is in the posterior fossa, occipital decompression may be tried. However, such drastic measures are rarely required if proper ventricular drainage and analgesics are employed.

Sometimes x-radiation or surgical procedures are justified in attempts to reduce headache due to clearly defined metastatic disease. Headache resulting from craniopharyngioma or pituitary tumors does not in itself constitute an indication for surgical procedures. Such tumors are difficult to remove, and removal or creating a bony defect is no assurance that headache will be diminished or eliminated.

HEADACHES FROM EXTRACRANIAL STRUCTURES

Six main categories of head and face pain from extracranial tissues and related structures can be distinguished: (1) headaches due to painful dilatation and distention of cranial arteries; (2) headaches due to sustained contraction of skeletal muscle about the face, scalp, and neck; (3) headache from disease of the nose, paranasal spaces, eyes, ears, and teeth; (4) craniofacial pain of the major neuralgias and the postinfectious neuralgias and postinfectious neuritides; (5) headache due to nonspecific inflammation of cranial arteries ("cranial arteritis," "temporal arteritis"); and (6) head pain due to trauma, infection, or new growth involving extracranial tissues.

More than 90 per cent of all headaches are in the first two of these categories and occur in a life setting that engenders frustration, resentment, anxiety, emotional tension, and fatigue.

Vascular Headaches

Vascular headaches are principally due to painful dilatation and distention of one or more of the extracranial and, probably, intracranial, i.e., dural, branches of the external carotid artery, with associated edema of adjacent tissues. The most common site of vascular headaches of the migraine type is the temple or the forehead, and one or both frontal, supraorbital, and superficial temporal arteries are most frequently involved. Many headaches at the back of the head and neck are associated with painful dilatation and distention of the postauricular and/or occipital arteries, and comprise one type of "occipital neuralgia."

Finally, the lower half of the head and face and the upper jaw in the vicinity of the back teeth may all be the site of pain of vascular origin, with spread to the neck and even the shoulder. Such headaches may be accompanied by the awareness of unusually forceful throbbing in the neck. "Atypical facial neuralgia" is but one of many designations applied to such headaches, which very probably result in good part from dilatation and distention of the extracranial portion of the middle meningeal artery, of the internal maxillary artery, and of the other branches and the trunks of the external and the common carotid arteries.

Migraine Syndrome

Clinical Features. The migraine syndrome is a pattern of dysfunction integrated within the central nervous system and manifested as widespread bodily disturbances, both nonpainful and painful. The outstanding feature is periodic headache, usually unilateral in onset but at times becoming bilateral or generalized. The attacks may vary in duration from a few minutes to several days and, in severity, from trifling symptoms to prolonged disabling illness. The headaches are associated with "irritability," nausea, and often photophobia, vomiting, constipation, or diarrhea. Although most common in the temple, headaches may be experienced anywhere in the head, face, and neck. The syndrome runs in families.

For a period of several hours to several days preceding the headache, the cranial arteries undergo a variable contractile state indicated by a facial flushing or pallor and by other transient cranial vasomotor phenomena such as vertigo. In the hour preceding the headache, a variety of visual and other neurologic abnormalities due to transient local constriction of cerebral or retinal arteries occur in about 10 to 15 per cent of the instances. These prodromes may take the form of scintillating scotomas, visual field defects such as unilateral or homonymous hemianopsia, and, occasionally, hemiplegia. More sustained neurologic defects and even cerebral infarction have rarely occurred. As the vasoconstrictor phenomena recede, vasodilator headache commences, sometimes overlapping, sometimes beginning after a short symptom-free interval. The pain is throbbing and aching, is appreciably reduced by pressure on the common carotid and the affected superficial artery, and is characteristically eliminated or reduced by vasoconstrictor agents, particularly ergotamine tartrate. The walls of the dilated cranial arteries and the adjacent tissues become edematous and tender. With sustained vasodilatation for several hours, the easily compressible arteries become rigid and relatively noncompressible, and the pulsatile pain becomes a steady ache. Redness and swelling of the eye with excessive tearing, and redness and swelling of the nasal mucosa with or without epistaxis, may occur along with the headache. A secondary muscle contraction component of the headache may outlast the vascular pain and will not be modified by vasoconstrictor agents.

One variety of headache closely related to migraine syndrome is the *cluster headache*. This head pain affects men much more than women, usually beginning between the third and sixth decade. Attacks come on abruptly with intense throbbing pain arising high in the nostril and spreading to involve the region behind the homolateral eye and sometimes the forehead as well. During the attacks, which last up to two hours, seldom more, the nose and eye water. The skin reddens and a homolateral Horner's syndrome with pupillary constriction and ptosis may develop. The attacks tend to occur from once to several times daily, in clusters lasting weeks or, less often, months. Without apparent reason, the cluster subsides as suddenly as it began, and the patient commonly remains free of headache for weeks or months until another cluster begins. During a cluster period, but not between, alcohol is likely to induce attacks. When headaches recur in close succession, the Horner's syndrome may outlast the headache.

Pathogenesis. Before the onset of migraine headache a generalized accumulation of fluid may occur as part of a nonspecific disturbance in fluid and electrolytes that is found in many persons with and without the migraine syndrome during periods of stress. There is evidence of a general abnormality of vascular behavior in many migraine subjects, and the extracranial vessels of such subjects show more variability in their contractile patterns than those of normal subjects even during headache-free periods. Sympathetic nerve stimulation or section has little effect on these vessels or on the migraine attack, and humoral agents have long been sought as the basis of the migraine syndrome. Local fluid collected from sites of swelling at the point of maximal headache and tenderness during an attack contains a vasodilator polypeptide of the bradykinin type that lowers pain thresholds and may be a factor in a local sterile inflammation. However, neither kinins, histamine, nor substances such as acetylcholine satisfactorily explain the generalized manifestations of the disorder. Several lines of evidence suggest that abnormalities in the metabolism of serotonin may play a role in the migraine syndrome. Reserpine, which induces a drop in serum serotonin levels, will often induce a migraine attack, and serum levels of serotonin have been found to drop spontaneously just before migraine attacks. During migraine attacks, an increased quantity of serotonin metabolites has been found in the urine. Methysergide, a powerful serotonin antagonist, prevents or reduces the frequency of migraine attacks in most subjects. How methysergide works is unclear. D'Alessio et al. suggested that it acts centrally on the brain to modify vasomotor regulation and peripherally to potentiate the vasoconstrictive responses of the cranial blood vessels to catecholamines. Curran and co-workers speculate that methysergide is a competitive antagonist to serotonin, occupying similar receptor sites in pain-sensitive vessels.

Management. Headaches of low intensity are usually eliminated by 0.3 to 0.6 gram of aspirin, but sometimes require 60 mg. of codeine phosphate as well.

For severe vascular headache, the restoration of the painfully dilated vessels to a nonpainful constricted state and the restoration of pain threshold to normal are accomplished best by the intramuscular administration of 0.25 to 0.5 mg. of ergotamine tartrate, not to exceed 0.5 mg. in any one week. If the agent is administered in amounts of 1.0 to 2.0 mg. by suppository, the side effects of nausea, vomiting, and elevated blood pressure are diminished. Ergotamine tartrate may also be given by mouth in 3.0 mg. amounts, to be swallowed or absorbed sublingually. This first dose may be repeated in 30 minutes, and a third given in another 30 minutes if the headache persists. Ergotamine tartrate, 1 mg., can also be given in tablets in combination with caffeine, 100 mg., up to 8 tablets for any single headache attack. The amount of ergotamine so administered should not exceed 10 mg. in any one week. Administration by mouth or by suppository is less predictably effective than intramuscular administration.

Prevention. Of utmost importance in the prevention of attacks is a consideration of the personal problems of the patient. Patients with migraine headaches are anxious, striving, perfectionistic, order-loving, rigid persons who, during periods of threat or conflict, become progressively more tense, resentful, and fatigued. The person with migraine often attempts to gain approval by doing more and better than his fellows and to gain

security by holding to a stable environment and a given system of excellent performance, even at a high cost of energy. This pattern brings increasing responsibility and admiration, but little love, so that he feels greater and greater resentment at the pace he feels obliged to maintain. Then tension associated with repeated frustration, sustained resentment and anxiety, often followed by fatigue and prostration, become the setting in which the migraine attack occurs. Treatment is best if it allows the patient free and repeated expression of his conflicts, resentments, and dissatisfactions, enables him to recognize the nature of his dilemma and its relationship to the physiologic basis of his pain, guides him toward accepting a more realistic appraisal of his needs, and establishes a more efficient regimen compatible with his individual equipment. About two of three patients can be appreciably helped by such aid.

For patients in whom attention to psychological attitudes and adjustment of life situations fail to bring significant relief, two forms of long-term pharmacotherapy have been useful. One is the monoamine oxidase inhibitor phenelzine sulfate, 45 mg. daily, which induces a significant reduction in headache frequency in most patients with migraine, and can be given indefinitely. The other is the serotonin antagonist methysergide, which in doses of 2 mg. three to four times daily is effective in about two of three cases in preventing headache of the migraine type. However, methysergide must be used with great caution. Both ergotamine tartrate and methysergide possess the ability to induce profound vasoconstriction and are contraindicated in pregnancy, peripheral vascular disturbance, severe hypertension, coronary artery disease, thrombophlebitis, and renal disease. Serious and unexpected vasospastic and psychic reactions have occasionally occurred with methysergide. Retroperitoneal fibrosis producing back pain and ureteral obstruction has been reported. Any of these serious complications necessitate prompt discontinuance of methysergide, and any single course of the drug should not outlast three months.

Muscle-Contraction Headaches

The pain of a muscle-contracting headache is a steady, nonpulsatile ache, unilateral or bilateral, in the temporal, occipital, parietal, or frontal regions. Additional descriptive terms include tightness bitemporally or at the occiput, bandlike sensations about the head, which may become caplike in distribution, viselike ache, weight, pressure, drawing, or soreness. Cramplike head pains and "feeling as if the neck and upper back were in a cast" are described by some patients. Pain may be fleeting, with frequent changes in the site and intensity of recurrences, or localized in one region. The headache may last for weeks, months, or even years.

Pathogenesis. Muscle contraction headaches are due to long-sustained contraction of skeletal muscle about the face, scalp, and neck. Concurrent vasodilatation of the associated cranial arteries frequently contributes to the irritability of the involved muscles and to the headache.

With prolonged sustained contraction, the muscles of the head, jaws, neck, and upper back become tender, causing the patient to limit their motion. Palpation may reveal sharply localized painful areas or nodules. Commonly, it hurts to comb or brush the hair or to don a hat. Exposure to cold, with shivering, may precipitate or aggravate the headache. Pressure on the contracted, tender muscles may augment the intensity and may elicit tinnitus, dizziness, and lacrimation — features that also occur spontaneously.

Sustained muscle contraction giving rise to headache often is secondary to noxious stimuli from other cranial tissues and structures, e.g., from distended arteries in vascular headache, inflammation or other disease in the eye, ear, nose, paranasal spaces, teeth, or scalp, and from brain tumor. Painful, sustained muscle contraction is also the primary source of many headaches associated with emotional tension states, especially in the adverse life situation of tense, aggressive, frustrated, anxious, or depressed persons.

Management. Reassurance, massage, manipulation, and manual stretching of the nuchal and occipital muscles, aspirin, and phenobarbital (30 mg. three times a day) reduce or eliminate most such headaches. Bed rest, local heat, warm baths, and the passage of time are important adjuvants. Removal of the primary source of noxious stimuli may eliminate the headaches secondary to disease of the eye, ear, nose, and sinuses or teeth.

Headaches due to sustained muscle contraction associated with life stress and emotional tension are only temporarily modified by sedatives or analgesics. Treatment should be directed at improving the patient's adjustment, as outlined under the management and prevention of migraine headache. Particularly among patients susceptible to recurrent headache of this type, the antidepressant amitriptyline in doses of 25 to 75 mg. daily may bring considerable relief.

Other Types of Extracranial Headache

Recurrent ("Chronic") Post-traumatic Headache. Head injury may rarely be followed by headaches that stem from intracranial sources such as subdural hematomas or subarachnoid hemorrhages. However, post-traumatic headaches more frequently stem from nonintracranial sources, four types being most common: (1) pain or tenderness due to local tissue damage in a scar or at a site of impact, (2) muscle-contraction headache, (3) attacks of throbbing and aching vascular headache, (4) infrequently, delusional headaches for which no tissue abnormality exists. The first two varieties are most common and are sometimes accompanied by fleeting vertigo with sudden

movement or rotation of the head, nausea, irritability, and insomnia.

Many injured patients harbor resentment related to the circumstances of their accident or fear that they have sustained permanent brain injury. These reactions and attitudes are intimately related to the pathophysiology and "chronicity" of post-traumatic headaches, and the headache often fails to subside completely as long as compensation claims remain unsettled.

Headaches Associated with Arterial Hypertension. When otherwise symptom-free and in the absence of hypertensive encephalopathy or pheochromocytoma, about 10 per cent of persons with arterial hypertension may experience severe, even disabling, headaches. Recent studies show that these are principally vascular and muscle-contraction headaches. Daily fluctuations in elevated blood pressure correlate only poorly with the headaches, nor is the extent of the elevation directly related to the severity of the attacks. However, headache attacks tend to be less frequent when the blood pressure is least elevated.

The headache associated with arterial hypertension resembles the vascular headaches of migraine and muscle tension and often regresses spontaneously with reassurance, bed rest, sedative medication, and the passage of time, especially when the patient is hospitalized. Ergotamine tartrate and methysergide are contraindicated in headaches associated with arterial hypertension.

Nasal and Paranasal Structures as Sources of Headache. It is likely that most of the discomfort from sinus infection comes from the ostia, which are many times more sensitive than the relatively insensitive walls of the sinuses. Typically, "sinus" headache commences in the morning (frontal) or early afternoon (maxillary) and subsides in the early or late evening. The pain is dull and aching, is made worse by changing head position, and seldom is associated with nausea and vomiting. It is due to mucosal inflammation and/or engorged turbinates, ostia, nasofrontal ducts and superior nasal spaces. Headache not associated with turbinate engorgement and inflammation is probably not due to sinus or nose disease. Nor is disease of these structures commonly the cause of frontal, temporal, zygomatic, or vertex headache, if the intensity of the pain is not greatly reduced or eliminated by intranasal application of vasoconstrictor agents or topical anesthetics, especially about the ostia to the sinuses. Suppurative disease in the frontal, ethmoid, and sphenoid sinuses, or in the mastoid air cells may result in osteomyelitis and inflammation of adjacent cranial tissues. Headache persisting following surgical drainage of the diseased sinus is evidence for extradural and possibly subdural infection.

Head Pain and Disease of the Teeth. Noxious stimuli in a tooth usually evoke local toothache, but pain can be referred to tissues remote from a diseased tooth. Afferent fibers for sensation in the teeth are contained in the second and third divisions of the fifth cranial nerve. Headache in the areas supplied by the latter is, in rare instances, associated with prolonged, intense toothache, or follows a tooth extraction. More commonly, in association with toothache, tooth extraction or a tender, diseased tooth, distant tissues exhibit surface hyperalgesia, tenderness, and vasomotor reactions, such as tender eyeballs, reddening of the conjunctivae, and tenderness of the auricular and temporal tissues. Because of secondary muscle contraction, other sites of tenderness and pain may be noted behind the ears, behind the lower border of the mastoid process, and in the muscles of the occiput, neck, and shoulders.

The teeth in the upper jaw are frequently the site of tenderness and pain in association with disease of the nasal and paranasal structures. Occasionally, in coronary insufficiency, pain is experienced in the lower jaw because of the close approximation of the fifth cranial and upper cervical neural segments in the cord. The teeth rarely cause craniofacial pains or "neuralgias" in the absence of toothache. Headache may not be attributed to a diseased tooth unless the injection of procaine into the tissues about the suspected tooth greatly reduces the intensity of, or eliminates, such headache.

Head Pain and Disease of the Ear. The fifth, seventh, ninth, and tenth cranial nerves contribute to the sensory innervation of the ear, and branches from the upper cervical roots supply the immediately adjacent scalp and muscles. Severe pain in the vicinity of the ear can be caused by disease of the teeth, acute tonsillitis, inflammatory and neoplastic disease of the larynx and nasopharynx, temporomandibular joint disorders, tumors, and inflammation in the posterior fossa and disease of the cervical spine and its soft tissues. Pain in the ear is also associated with vascular headaches and atypical facial neuralgias as well as herpes zoster of the fifth and seventh cranial nerves and, rarely, the glossopharyngeal nerve. True glossopharyngeal neuralgia causes severe pain radiating from the tonsil into the ear. It has the usual timing features of "tic."

Primary ear disease is relatively infrequent— but important—as a source of headache since it almost always indicates inflammation or destructive disease. Acute otitis media (purulent or nonpurulent), furunculosis of the ear canal, traumatic rupture of the tympanum, and fracture of the anterior wall of the bony canal all cause pain in the ear associated with sustained tender contraction of adjacent skeletal muscles. Osteomyelitis of the mastoid bone may be associated with inflammation of the nearby periosteum as well as dura and adjacent tissues (epidural abscess)—both sources of pain in or behind the ear. Pain in this region also accompanies tumors of the acoustic nerve and inflammation and thrombosis of the lateral sinus.

The Eye as a Source of Headache. Errors of refraction (hypermetropia, astigmatism, anomalies of accommodation), disturbances of ocular muscle equilibrium, and glaucoma are universally described as causing headache. Refractive errors are also said to give origin to such other symptoms as aching of the eyes, "sandy" feeling in the eyes, pulling sensations in and about the orbit, and conjunctival congestion. Headache usually starts around and over the eyes and subsequently radiates to the occiput and back of the head.

The pain of increased intraocular pressure at first remains localized in the eyeball, then extends along the rim of the orbit and, finally, throughout most of the area supplied by the ophthalmic division of the trigeminal nerve. Nausea and vomiting sometimes accompany such headaches.

Headache accompanying various ocular disturbances is regarded as secondary to (1) sustained contraction of the intraocular muscles, which is associated with excessive accommodation effort, or (2) sustained contraction of the extraocular muscles, resulting from the effort to produce distinct retinal images, and single binocular vision with fusion. Simple myopia, per se, in contrast to the aforementioned ocular defects, does not evoke headache because the myope, in attempting to improve his vision by the contraction of his eye muscles, actually makes his vision worse and soon abandons the attempt.

With inflammation of the iris and ciliary body, light may cause intense pain in the eye and adjacent areas when the light stimulus is accompanied by movement of the inflamed iris. When the iris is immobilized, pain is allayed.

Anthony, M., Hinterberger, H., and Lance, J. W.: The possible relationship of serotonin to the migraine syndrome. Res. Clin. Stud. Headache, 2:29, 1968.

Anthony, M., and Lance, J. W.: Monoamine oxidase inhibition in the treatment of migraine. Arch. Neurol. (Chicago), 21:263, 1969.

Bradshaw, P., and Parsons, M.: Hemiplegic migraine, a clinical study. Quart. J. Med., 34:65, 1965.

D'Alessio, D. J., et al.: Studies on headache: The relevance of the prophylactic action of UML-491 in vascular headache of the migraine type to the pathophysiology of this syndrome. World Neurol., 3:66, 1962.

Friedman, A. P. (ed.): Treatment of headache. Mod. Treatm., 1:1361, 1964.

Wolff, H. G.: Headache and Other Head Pain. 2nd ed. New York, Oxford University Press, 1963.

HEARING LOSS
J. R. Nelson

Approximately 3 per cent of the population suffer from hearing loss sufficiently severe to impair the understanding of speech. A new era of treatment of conductive hearing losses has recently begun with excellent surgical results from use of the operating microscope and new microsurgical techniques. Considerable help is available even to those with hereditary or congenital sensorineural losses through improved audiometric detection methods and rehabilitation programs.

Definition. The two major types of hearing loss are *conductive* losses, usually resulting from involvement of the mechanical sound transmission apparatus in the middle ear, and *sensorineural* losses, in which the cochlea, the cochlear nerve, or more central pathways are affected.

Conductive losses gradually reduce the difference in the hearing of air-conducted sounds and those produced by direct vibration of the skull (bone conduction). Discrimination of test words presented above threshold is not disturbed by conductive losses. The proper timing and phase relationships of various sound wave frequencies are maintained even though the mechanical oscillations from ear drum to oval window are dampened by disease processes. Simple tests for conductive hearing loss include the *Rinne test*, in which a 512 c.p.s. fork is first held against the mastoid process until the sound fades and then is placed 1 inch from the ear. With 20 to 25 db or more of conductive loss, bone conduction is superior to air conduction. A more sensitive test is the *Bing test,* in which a finger is placed in the ear just as the sound from a fork on the mastoid bone fades away. If the sound then reappears, a normal conductive mechanism is likely. The Bing phenomenon may be absent with as little as 5 db of conductive impairment. The *Weber test* involves the lateralization of sound to the diseased ear when a fork is held at midforehead or on a central incisor. Both the Bing and Weber phenomena are due to a paradoxical increased resonance of middle ear structures to bone-conducted sound even though air conduction is impaired.

Sensorineural deafness characteristically impairs discrimination of speech to a severe degree because of disruption of the neural coding mechanism. With cochlear pathology there is also paradoxically increased response to successive increments of sound intensity. One test of this is the *recruitment* phenomenon, in which the poorest hearing ear is first determined with a low intensity tone. If a second, higher intensity sound is presented to each ear quickly and the previously poorer ear now appreciates sound best, an abnormal loudness-to-intensity gradient has been demonstrated. A similar phenomenon underlies the short increment sensitivity index test (SISI), in which, in normal hearing, small 1 db pips of sound added to a steady tone 20 db above threshold are not heard; but with cochlear damage a near-perfect reception score of such small increments is found. With auditory nerve lesions, a phenomenon of nerve fatigue occurs whereby a steady tone gradually seems to fade in loudness. More than 20 to 30 db of such "tone decay" is suggestive of a sensorineural loss of retrocochlear (nerve) type. The *Bekesy test* involves presentation of continuous tones and interrupted tones at various frequencies. Because of tone decay, with nerve lesions the audiometric graph for continuous tones will show a greater loss than with interrupted tones when the nerve recovers between stimuli. Such recordings are rated type III or IV in contrast to the normal type I or type II response that occurs in cochlear lesions and in some normal ears. The Rinne test is normal with sensorineural loss, and the Weber test lateralizes toward the normal ear, contrasting with conductive losses.

A battery of simple audiometric tests now can differentiate the various types of deafness. Sensorineural losses can be subcategorized into cochlear and retrocochlear types with about 70 per cent or more accuracy. The idealized findings with various sites of pathology are shown in the accompanying table.

Etiology and Clinical Manifestations. *Hereditary deafness* accounts for up to half of childhood cases and up to a third of adult cases. It is usually of a sensorineural type with either dominant (10 per cent) or recessive inheritance (90 per cent). Onset is usually in childhood with bilateral involvement, but families with adult onset, mostly unilateral findings, or frequency-specific bands of loss are described. Such entities suggest selective abiotrophy ("early aging") of the cochlear neurons. In many cases there are other metabolic defects or malformations of the ear, eye, integument, skeleton, or nervous system (Konigsmark; Proctor and Proctor).

Nonfamilial *congenital deafness* syndromes with varying degrees of hypoplasia of the inner ear include complete failure of development of the inner ear (Michel), cochleosaccular dysgenesis (Scheibe), the most common cause, and subtotal development of either the membranous labyrinth (Alexander) or the entire osseous and membranous labyrinth (Mondini), both of which may show incomplete hearing loss. These deformities may show characteristic changes on temporal bone laminagrams.

Neurotropic Infections. Both viral and bacterial infections may seriously threaten hearing from embryonic life to adulthood. Maternal German measles (rubella) accounts for at least 20 per cent of congenital deafness and produces a severe

TYPES OF HEARING LOSS

	Conductive	Cochlear	Nerve	Pontine
Air>bone conduction	Reversed*	Normal	Normal	Normal
Recruitment	Absent	Present	Absent	Often present
SISI Score†	0–20%	80–100%	0–20%	0–20%
Tone decay	None	None	Present	Present
Bekesy (type)	I	I, II	III, IV	III, IV
Speech discrimination	Normal	Fair to good	Poor	Fair

*Except early, then use Bing test.
†SISI—short increment sensitivity index test (% of pips heard).

bilateral sensorineural impairment in addition to its other teratogenic effects. Reduction of this cause awaits widespread release of a newly developed vaccine. Only slightly less prevalent are cases of severe postmeningitic hearing loss. The incidence has decreased since the antimicrobial era, but unfortunately it is still all too common in infants and young children. Prematurity probably predisposes to this cause and is an important, poorly understood cause of deafness itself.

Certain cases of sudden, unilateral sensorineural hearing loss are associated with viral upper respiratory infections and produce "cochleitis" with a profound loss, which may be due to direct inflammation or vascular involvement. Some otologists advocate emergency treatment with intravenous histamine for vasodilatation and low molecular weight dextran to reduce blood viscosity. The rate of recovery may be enhanced, but controlled studies are still needed to clarify this point. Mumps is a well recognized cause of unilateral sensorineural deafness, and vestibular involvement may also occur. Other common childhood viral illnesses may occasionally produce hearing loss. Herpes zoster may simultaneously affect the eighth nerve and geniculate ganglion to produce deafness, vertigo, and facial palsy (Ramsay-Hunt syndrome) in addition to ear or throat pain and vesicles. Some of these patients may benefit from facial nerve decompression if nerve excitability tests suggest severe nerve damage from swelling of the nerve within its bony canal.

Otologic syphilis deserves special mention because it remains an enigma as to why a young adult who may have been sucessfully treated for congenital syphilis still develops late inflammatory changes of recurrent interstitial keratitis, joint effusion (Clutton's joints), and fluctuating progressive sensorineural hearing loss and vertigo. Eventual total deafness is the rule. A low-tone hearing loss is common early, as with Meniere's disease, but explosive total deafness in one ear suggestive of internal auditory artery occlusion may occur. Such inner ear manifestations may appear even in the absence of a positive VDRL in the blood or serum, and more sensitive tests such as the FTA-ABS test may be required. Some authorities believe that all cases of "bilateral Meniere's" should be considered syphilitic until proved otherwise. Softening of the capsular bone about the oval window occurs so that the stapes moves excessively, but only in an outward direction. This provides the basis for *Hennebert's sign,* which is a positive fistula test (vertigo with middle-ear pressure changes) that occurs only with negative suction applied with a pneumatic otoscope. Fistulas between the middle and inner ear usually give symptoms only when positive pressure is applied to the otoscope. Inner ear damage occurring long after "successful" treatment for syphilis raises the possibility that such cases represent treatment failures rather than autoimmune responses or late fibrotic reactions. The diagnosis is important because recent evidence suggests that long-term cortisone treatment

may partially reverse or halt the progression of deafness and vertigo. Some authorities also recommend intensive retreatment with oral ampicillin, 1.5 grams, and probenecid, 0.5 gram, four times per day for up to four to five weeks.

Otosclerosis. Otosclerosis is a very common cause of hearing loss in Caucasian adults, and is usually inherited as a dominant trait with up to 40 per cent penetrance. Pathologically, the process consists of an overgrowth of labyrinthine capsular bone around the oval window which leads to progressive fixation of the stapes. A poorly understood sensorineural component often is seen in long-standing cases. Hearing loss begins insidiously in early adult life, with slow progression. Pregnancy may accelerate the condition in females. The audiometric findings in far-advanced cases may be misleading with poor reliability about the amount of sensorineural loss. Careful correlation with tuning fork results is essential, as at high output levels, the audiometer may transmit energy throughout the entire skull in such a way as to give confusing results. Some patients with no measurable hearing loss by audiometry may still have partial recovery after surgery to the point where use of an aid allows serviceable hearing. The surgical treatment of otosclerosis has developed rapidly in the past 15 years with successive adoption of horizontal canal fenestration, stapes mobilization by fracture, and finally stapedectomy with replacement by Teflon plugs, steel pistons, or wire prostheses that bridge the gap between the incus and a new membrane on the oval window that forms over a fascia or gelfoam graft. Good to excellent long-lasting results occur in over 90 per cent of cases.

Middle Ear Infections. Antimicrobial drugs have not entirely eliminated suppurative otitis media, particularly chronic forms, although acute attacks usually respond to the drugs and to myringotomy. Once chronic drainage and infection have been arrested, several reconstructive surgical procedures are possible even though extensive destruction of middle ear structures has occurred. Modified radical mastoidectomy with tympanoplasty may improve function of the middle ear conductive mechanism. Numerous grafting and artificial prosthetic replacement techniques are available. Recurrent cholesteatoma formation represents a special challenge, as these imbedded epithelial fragments may grow to cause extensive destruction of the middle ear and temporal bone.

Chronic serous otitis media is the most common cause of chronic conductive hearing loss in children. A predisposing factor may be poor eustachian tube function from edema secondary to allergy, inflammation, large lymphoid follicles, large adenoids, or a congenitally small lumen. Insertion of a polyethylene tube in the tympanic membrane for several weeks may allow external drainage, equalize the middle ear pressure, and restore hearing while the eustachian tube hopefully regains its patency.

Traumatic Hearing Loss. There are two major types of temporal bone fractures that may be associated with hearing loss. With a longitudinal fracture along the axis of the petrous pyramid, damage to the inner ear is usually slight, but bleeding from the ear and disruption of the middle ear bones is common and may require surgical repair at a later date. In contrast, transverse fractures perpendicular to the petrous pyramid may cause severe inner ear damage and facial palsy. If facial paralysis is immediate, surgical exploration is mandatory.

Noise-induced acoustic trauma is an important cause of hearing loss in industrial settings, but exposure to gun blasts, airplane engines, and even rock and roll music may cause progressive high tone sensorineural hearing loss. Certain individuals are much more sensitive to acoustic trauma and must be protected with ear molds or protective ear covers if it is necessary to work in high noise levels. The magnitude of this problem is great, and has been often neglected in spite of advances in prevention.

Meniere's Disease. Although the episodic attacks of vertigo are more disabling, a fluctuating low-tone "cochlear" hearing loss with eventual involvement of other frequencies is common. This condition and acoustic neuroma, which also produces tinnitus, deafness, and vertigo, are more fully discussed in the article on Vertigo.

Ototoxic Drugs. Many antimicrobials, mostly when administered by injection, may cause severe cochlear damage. Dihydrostreptomycin fortunately has been removed from use; streptomycin causes semicircular canal and utricular damage with relative sparing of the cochlea and saccule. Other drugs which may cause deafness when blood concentration is high because of large dosage or renal failure are neomycin, kanamycin, vancomycin, gentamycin, ristocetin, ethacrynic acid, and quinine. Use of such drugs should be carefully considered, particularly in patients with renal failure.

Central Causes of Deafness. In order to markedly raise the threshold for hearing with central involvement, bilateral damage of the pontine projections or higher centers is required. A moderate impairment on specialized speech reception tests is the rule with near-normal pure tone thresholds, the presence of tone decay, and recruitment. Other signs of cranial nerve involvement, sensory and motor pathway damage should be sought. Lesions at the cortical level produce complex dysphasic impairments, and are beyond the scope of this article.

Hough, J. V. D.: Restoration of hearing loss after head trauma. Ann. Otol., 78:210, 1969.

Jaffe, B. F.: Sudden deafness. Arch. Otolaryng. (Chicago), 86:81, 1967.

Jerger, J.: Review of diagnostic audiometry. Ann. Otol., 77:1042, 1968.

Konigsmark, B. W.: Hereditary deafness in man. New Eng. J. Med., 281:713, 1969.

Patterson, M. E.: Congenital luetic hearing impairment. Arch. Otolaryng. (Chicago), 87:70, 1968.

Proctor, C. A., and Proctor, B.: Understanding hereditary nerve deafness. Arch. Otolaryng. (Chicago), 85:23, 1967.

Pulec, J. L. (ed.): Meniere's Disease. Philadelphia, W. B. Saunders Company, 1968.

Schuknecht, J. F., and Applebaum, E. J.: Surgery for hearing loss. New Eng. J. Med., 280:1154, 1969.

Shambaugh, G. E., Jr. (ed.): Third workshop on microsurgery of the ear. Arch. Otolaryng. (Chicago), 89:1, 1969.

Vernon, McC.: Current etiological factors in deafness. Amer. Ann. Deaf, 113:106, 1968.

VERTIGO
J. R. Nelson

The term *vertigo* strictly refers to an illusion of bodily movement involving either the person or the environment. It does not include the more prevalent but nonrotatory sensations of lightheadedness or giddiness. The term is often misused. For example, "aviator's vertigo" is a spatial disorientation without an illusion of movement, and "laryngeal vertigo" is cough syncope. True vertigo is a common complaint and may occur in any disease that involves the neural mechanisms that integrate vestibular, visual, and proprioceptive sensations. However, about 70 per cent of cases are due to peripheral labyrinthine disorders. Peripheral vertigo characteristically is of sudden onset and short duration, and the patient has a strong illusion of movement. Vertigo of central nervous system origin usually is a vague, prolonged disorientation without a prominent directional component. Both the common and unusual causes of vertigo are described here to encompass most of the pathophysiologic disturbances of the labyrinth or its central connections.

MENIERE'S DISEASE

Meniere's disease is the most common cause of true vertigo. In 1861 Prosper Meniere first described the triad of explosive vertigo, fluctuating hearing loss, and tinnitus. The disease begins in middle life, although patients younger than age ten and in late years have been reported. It affects both sexes about equally, and, rarely, may be a familial condition. The same perfectionistic, striving tendencies that characterize migrainous persons are often present in those with Meniere's disease, and appear to intensify the expression of the illness. Many variations in the order of appearance of the classic symptom triad have been described. *Pseudo-Meniere's syndrome* refers to explosive attacks of vertigo without hearing loss or tinnitus. However, most patients eventually develop the complete symptom triad. *Lermoyez' syndrome* consists of gradual, progressive hearing loss that strangely remits after the first attack of recurrent vertigo.

Clinical Manifestations. Intermittent, explosive attacks of vertigo lasting minutes to hours are the hallmark of Meniere's disease. The vertigo is of the peripheral type with sudden onset and an illusion of movement so violent that the patient cannot walk. The attacks may occur several times weekly, but long remissions of several years' duration are frequent. Between attacks, the patient has no disorder of equilibrium or nystagmus. During the attack, there is nystagmus with the slow phase usually toward the involved ear. Severe nausea, vomiting, and pallor are frequent because of involvement of the vagal and vasomotor areas of the brainstem that receive vestibular inputs. Loss of consciousness occurs occasionally, perhaps because the vestibular disturbance is transmitted to the brainstem reticular activating network that maintains consciousness. Half of the patients notice a feeling of fullness in the ear or head during attacks. Cold and warm water irrigation of the ear canal reveals in over half the patients at least a partial loss of thermal-induced nystagmus on the involved side.

The hearing loss with Meniere's disease starts either before or after the onset of vertigo and initially usually affects the low tones. Commonly, there is a decrement in hearing during an attack of vertigo, and recovery is incomplete so that progressive stepwise unilateral hearing loss occurs. The vertigo often ceases when hearing loss is complete. Total unilateral deafness occurs in only 10 per cent of patients, and the disease is bilateral in only 12 per cent. Associated auditory phenomena are sound distortion, diplacusis, and recruitment. Diplacusis is the hearing of a pure tone at a different pitch in the involved ear. Recruitment is an abnormal increase in loudness evoked by a very slight increase in sound intensity. Audiometry reveals a "perceptive" (sensorineural) deafness, with air and bone conduction equally depressed on the involved side. Speech reception is impaired to a degree appropriate for the severity of hearing loss. Refined testing reveals the deafness to be more typical of sense organ (cochlear) damage than of nerve trunk (retrocochlear) damage with: (1) hearing thresholds that are nearly similar on the continuous and interrupted tone audiogram (Bekesy type I or II), (2) no decay in loudness (adaptation) during prolonged pure tone stimulation, (3) an enhancement of ability to judge small changes in sound intensity during the short increment sensitivity index (SISI) test, and (4) loudness recruitment. Tinnitus persists between attacks and most commonly is a roaring noise, but higher pitched types may occur. It usually predominates in the involved ear and is not abolished by carotid artery compression.

Pathology. The few reports on Meniere's disease confirm the original findings of Hallpike and Cairns in 1938 of dilatation of the membranous sacs of the labyrinth and cochlea. Rupture of the sacs and degeneration of the sensory elements are seen occasionally. The abnormalities suggest a chronic elevation in intraluminal endolymphatic pressure. The postulated pressure increase may produce the sensation of fullness noted during attacks. The acute hearing loss and vertigo could result from sudden rupture of the membranes after a prolonged increase in pressure, but some investigators believe that sudden rupture of the sac may actually terminate the attack. Lesser fluctuations in hearing could result from small fluctuations in endolymphatic pressure without rupture. Studies of cochlear models subjected to increased fluid pressure reveal changes in basilar membrane elasticity that would explain the major audiologic findings in Meniere's disease except for recruitment, which may be related to sensory hair-cell degeneration. Autonomic or vascular theories of symptom production have also been popular, but remain unproved.

Treatment. The medical therapy of Meniere's disease consists of antivertiginous agents (Dramamine, Bonamine) every four hours during the acute attack and for several days thereafter. Sedatives or tranquilizers may be added. Nicotinic acid, 50 to 100 mg. four times daily, is recommended by many for acute attacks and for chronic usage, in an attempt to dilate the vessels of the inner ear. A low-salt diet with or without diuretics is often prescribed in an attempt to increase endolymph fluid absorption. Many authorities prohibit smoking. No single medical regimen has been uniformly successful. In those patients with severe vertigo, surgical intervention should be considered. If hearing on the involved side has deteriorated severely, labyrinthectomy is preferable. If useful hearing remains, various endolymphatic drainage procedures such as sacculotomy or shunts to the CSF have been employed. Selective vestibular nerve section may be advisable in some cases.

VESTIBULAR NEURONITIS

Vestibular neuronitis is an acute illness characterized by signs of sudden, unilateral vestibular failure with no tinnitus or hearing loss. Such cases have been called *acute labyrinthitis* in the past, and an infectious labyrinthine cause cannot be entirely excluded. However, etiologic theories favor a viral neuronitis or postinfectious demyelinating reaction. The illness occurs mainly in adults but occasionally in children.

Vestibular neuronitis often begins during or several days after an acute viral respiratory or gastrointestinal infection. The patient often awakens one morning with severe vertigo, nausea, and ataxia, with veering toward the involved side. He must remain perfectly still in bed since head movements markedly exaggerate the vertigo. The symptoms greatly lessen in two to three days but persist up to three weeks. Attacks of mild vertigo evoked by sudden positional changes may occur infrequently in the future. During the acute illness, brisk nystagmus is usually seen, with the slow component toward the involved side. Caloric responses are hypoactive on one or both sides. The abnormalities usually regress slowly, but may persist indefinitely. The treatment of acute vestibular neuronitis consists of bed rest, antivertiginous agents, and adequate hydration. Fortunately, the illness is short-lived, and only a minority have residual positional vertigo.

The term *epidemic vertigo* has been given to clusters of cases of a clinical entity which resembles the foregoing description of vestibular neuronitis. Details of examinations of vestibular function are insufficient to permit conclusions regarding their pathogenesis.

PAROXYSMAL POSITIONAL VERTIGO

Paroxysmal positional vertigo was first described by Bárány in 1921. It may occur after diverse labyrinthine damage from trauma, infection, or vascular occlusion, during prolonged systemic illness, or after exposure to toxins. No definite cause can be established in many patients. The attacks occur almost exclusively when the patient assumes certain positions, regardless of the speed of head or bodily movements involved. Assuming the supine position, turning over in bed or tilting the head backward while erect may evoke moderately severe vertigo and nausea, but rarely vomiting. The symptoms and associated nystagmus may be reproduced by a test procedure elaborated by Dix and Hallpike. With the patient sitting on a table and facing the examiner, his head is grasped firmly and then head and body are quickly guided to a position in which the patient is supine with his head tilted 30 degrees over the end of the table and 30 to 45 degrees to one side. A positive response may occur only when the affected ear is placed undermost. The response begins after a measurable delay, often up to five seconds. A period of intense distress then ensues and the patient often cries out and struggles to free himself. A chiefly rotatory nystagmus with or without a horizontal component is observed. The fast phase of the 12 o'clock portion of the globe rotates toward the undermost ear. The symptoms and nystagmus last only a few seconds and become progressively more difficult to elicit upon immediate retesting.

Pathologically, there is atrophy of the superior division of the vestibular nerve and its sense organs, the macula of the utricle, and cristae of the horizontal and superior semicircular canals. These structures are all nourished by the anterior vestibular artery, which has been postulated but not proved to have been occluded in patients presenting with this syndrome. Any pathophysiologic theory must explain the latent period before symptom production, the brief but severe vertigo, and the fatigability of the phenomenon. Schuknecht believes that crystalline calcium carbonate statoconia released from the damaged utricle fall slowly through the endolymph into the posterior canal ampulla and displace its cupula. However, the induced nystagmus often is inconsistent with an origin solely from posterior canal stimulation.

Paroxysmal positional vertigo is not always a benign end organ disorder. Positional vertigo or nystagmus of central origin has been described with cerebellar or temporal lobe tumors and after brainstem damage. Central positional nystagmus characteristically occurs in more than one position, has a rapid onset and does not fatigue with repeated testing. The nystagmus either beats away from the undermost ear (convergent type),

toward the undermost ear (divergent type), or resembles the peripheral form (Dix and Hallpike). Caloric tests are normal in less than half of either the peripheral or central types of positional nystagmus.

Vestibular nerve section should be considered for the peripheral variety when vertigo is very frequent, disabling, or refractory to antivertiginous drugs. Successful results have been reported in several cases.

VERTIGO WITH A CEREBELLOPONTINE ANGLE TUMOR

This is perhaps the most important entity to consider in the differential diagnosis of the symptom. Several tumor types can grow in the compact space lateral to the pontomedullary junction and ventral to the cerebellum. Cysts, aneurysms, cholesteatomas, and other rare tumors are found, but about 80 per cent are acoustic neuromas. Acoustic neuromas are benign growths, but cause death from brainstem compression if untreated. The neuroma begins its growth well out on the vestibular nerve within the internal acoustic meatus, gradually compressing or invading the canal contents, which are the acoustic nerve, the internal auditory artery, and the facial nerve. The tumor usually extrudes medially into the cerebellopontine angle before completely destroying the facial nerve. Pressure on the internal auditory artery or degenerative changes in the neoplasm may account for the sudden or fluctuating symptoms in some cases. Bilateral tumors occur rarely, especially with generalized neurofibromatosis.

Symptomatically, a Meniere-like triad of progressive hearing loss, tinnitus, and vertigo is the rule. However, important differences in the rate of onset and type of symptomatology exist in the tumor cases. Explosive attacks of vertigo are very unusual. More often, there are long periods of unsteadiness aggravated by positional changes, and continuous nystagmus may be seen. Caloric testing shows either partial or total unreactivity on the involved side in more than 95 per cent of patients. The hearing loss is usually slowly and steadily progressive over 1 to 20 years. A retrocochlear pattern of deafness is found with (1) greater hearing loss during continuous tone testing than during interrupted tone testing (Bekesy type III or IV), (2) pathologic tone decay, (3) a low SISI score, and (4) no recruitment. Speech discrimination often is affected much more than expected from the pure tone responses. Many patients show atypical audiologic features, including the "cochlear" pattern of hearing loss. The tinnitus often has a high-pitched metallic quality. Other neurologic abnormalities eventually appear, first in the facial nerve but careful testing of facial strength, taste, and tearing is required to detect early abnormalities. The fifth cranial nerve is next involved as the tumor spreads toward the pons, producing a reduction in corneal and facial sensation and finally, the ninth, tenth, and eleventh nerves and brainstem may be compressed.

Three roentgenographic views of the skull — the anteroposterior (Caldwell), the 30-degree fronto-occipital (Towne), and the right angle view (Stenver) — should be examined to detect erosion of the internal auditory meatus. A 1 mm. enlargement of the canal orifice may be significant. The cerebrospinal fluid protein is elevated in at least 75 per cent of the cases. An acoustic neuroma is unlikely if the cerebrospinal fluid, caloric tests, and good quality roentgenograms are *all* normal. In doubtful cases, 1 to 2 ml. of radiopaque dye can be fluoroscopically guided through the CSF to show nonfilling of the acoustic canal, even with very small tumors. At least three surgical approaches to cerebellopontine angle tumors are currently used; the choice depends on the magnitude and direction of tumor growth.

VERTIGO WITH CEREBROVASCULAR INSUFFICIENCY

Vertigo with cerebrovascular insufficiency occurs in diseases in which blood flow to the labyrinth or its central connections is impaired. Reduced flow through the vestibular artery may cause vertigo without auditory symptoms. The internal auditory artery irrigates both the cochlea and labyrinth, and sudden occlusion is manifested by a single attack of vertigo, tinnitus, and hearing loss. This usually occurs in subjects after the age of 50 who have evident vascular disease elsewhere in the body. Partial vertebrobasilar artery stenosis can reduce the blood flow to the brainstem vestibular connections as well as to the labyrinth. In such subjects, vertigo may occur spontaneously or during head rotation if bony projections from degenerated vertebrae partially compress the vertebral canals. Fluctuations in blood pressure or blood viscosity also predispose to attacks. Although vertigo is the most common symptom of vertebrobasilar insufficiency, it is usually accompanied by other symptoms of brainstem ischemia, including hemianopic visual loss, diplopia, hemiparesis, hemifacial and contralateral bodily sensory loss, dysarthria, or loss of consciousness. The complete syndrome can be seriously disabling, especially if the patient suffers unexpected falls. The management of vertebrobasilar insufficiency is discussed more fully in the article on Cerebrovascular Diseases.

CONVULSIVE DISORDERS

Convulsive disorders are rare causes of vertigo, but may involve the vestibular connections in at least two ways. Cortical epileptic discharges arising from the vestibular sensory projection area in the superior temporal gyrus often start with tinnitus followed by severe vertigo that strongly resembles the labyrinthine type. A major attack also includes sensory and psychic symptoms, twitching of the body contralateral to the involved cortex, and brief unconsciousness. There is no postictal vertigo. During attacks, the electroencephalogram shows an asymmetrical, diffuse electrical discharge, most prominent over the involved hemisphere. Between attacks the patient has no vestibular symptoms, and caloric tests are normal.

A second type of paroxysmal electrical disturbance is postulated to arise from stimulation of hyperexcitable neurons of the reticular formation of the brainstem region by inputs from the vestibular nerve. Such "vestibulogenic seizures" are not preceded by tinnitus, and the vertigo is more variable in intensity than that of cortical origin. Motor symptoms and unconsciousness occur frequently. The attacks may be precipitated by caloric labyrinthine stimulation. The electroencephalogram shows a posterior, bilaterally synchronous slow discharge during the attacks.

VERTIGO OF CERVICAL ORIGIN

Vertigo of cervical origin is common and is physiologically explained by the powerful inputs from the cervical muscles that convey information about the position of the head and neck in space. Cervical muscle spasm, neck trauma, or upper cervical sensory root irritation can produce asymmetrical spinovestibular stimulation and thus evoke prolonged mild vertigo and disequilibrium. The vertigo is often aggravated by neck movement, and may be accompanied by moderately severe nuchal spasm and headache. Relief can be obtained with a regimen designed to combat muscle tension, consisting of moist heat, muscle relaxants, and cervical traction. Antivertiginous agents are ineffective.

MISCELLANEOUS CAUSES OF VERTIGO

In addition to diseases of the labyrinth or its immediate central connections, ocular disease may cause mild vertigo when binocular gaze is disturbed so that visual fixation shifts from one eye to the other. Disease of the external and middle ear may cause vertigo because of pressure effects transmitted through the oval and round windows. For example, manipulation of impacted cerumen in the external canal or probing the bony ossicles during middle ear surgery may provoke vertigo. Vertigo may occur during air travel or underwater diving if the pressure between the middle ear and the atmosphere is not equalized because of blocked eustachian tubes. Bacterial infections of the middle ear may erode into the labyrinth and evoke vertigo. Such inward extension requires immediate surgery to establish external drainage. Toxic vertigo due to labyrinthine injury can appear during many prolonged illnesses, as a permanent side effect of kanamycin, neomycin, or streptomycin therapy, and after excessive use of alcohol, tobacco, or salicylates.

Although vertigo is common to a multitude of illnesses, a careful history and a thorough general otologic and neurologic examination should elucidate the cause in most cases. A simple screening test of vestibular function uses small amounts of ice water (0.2 ml.) instilled in the ear canal. Nystagmus is observed behind +20 lenses. The amount of water is progressively doubled if no reaction is obtained. All normal persons react to 0.4 ml. or less. More sophisticated methods use bi-thermal (30° and 44° C.) stimulation of each ear and electrical recording of eye movements. Vestibulospinal and otolith tests are under development.

Barac, B.: Vertiginous epileptic attacks and so-called "vestibulogenic seizures." Epilepsia (Amst.), 9:137, 1968.
Biemond, A., and DeJong, J. M. B. V.: On cervical nystagmus and related disorders. Brain, 92:437, 1969.
Coats, A. C.: Vestibular neuronitis. Acta Otolaryng. (Stockholm), (Suppl. 251), 1969.
Dix, M. R.: Modern tests of vestibular function, with special reference to their value in clinical practice. Brit. Med. J., 3:317, 1969.
Harrison, M. D.: "Epidemic vertigo"—"vestibular neuronitis." Brain, 85:613, 1962.
House, W. F. (ed.): Acoustic neuroma. Monograph II. Arch. Otolaryng. (Chicago), 88:575, 1968.
Jongkees, L. B. W.: Cervical vertigo. Laryngoscope, 79:1473, 1969.
Nelson, J. R.: The minimal ice water caloric test. Neurology, 19:577, 1969.
Pulec, J. L.: The surgical treatment of vertigo. Laryngoscope, 79:1783, 1969.
Schuknecht, H. F.: Positional vertigo: Clinical and experimental observations. Trans. Amer. Acad. Ophthal. Otolaryng., 66:319, 1962.
Stahle, J., and Terins, J.: Paroxysmal positional nystagmus. Ann. Otol., 74:69, 1965.
Williams, D., and Wilson, T. G.: The diagnosis of the major and minor symptoms of basilar insufficiency. Brain, 85:741, 1962.

SYNCOPE AND HYPERVENTILATION

Albert Heyman

Definition. Syncope is the cutting off or transient loss of consciousness. Although the term is usually applied to unconsciousness caused by a temporary decrease in cerebral blood flow, in this discussion a broader definition is employed that includes the brief disturbances in consciousness due to changes in the chemical composition of the blood as in hyperventilation or hypoglycemia. Syncope is extremely common; in fact, it has been found to occur in as many as 25 to 30 per cent of young, healthy adult males. It should be carefully differentiated from such disorders as epilepsy, vertigo, cataplexy, and strokes, all of which may produce transient disturbances in consciousness, generalized weakness, or inability to stand erect. The loss of consciousness in syncope may not be complete, but may consist of varying degrees of impaired sensorium with transient blurring of vision, weakness, and loss of postural tone. Such attacks may be described by the patient as dizziness, faintness, light-headedness, or a "drunk feeling." These partial manifestations have the rapid onset, brief duration, and complete recovery characteristic of the fully developed faint.

Pathogenesis. Syncope is most frequently caused by a reduction in cerebral blood flow below a critical level and is usually associated with a sharp fall in blood pressure. This, in turn, is the result of either a loss of peripheral resistance, as seen in vasodepressor faint and in orthostatic hypotension, or a decrease in cardiac output, as in Adams-Stokes attacks. In many patients, however, loss of consciousness is not caused by reduction of blood pressure but by a decrease in such essential blood components as glucose, carbon dioxide, or oxygen. In other instances, as in micturition syncope and cough syncope, the faint seems to result from cerebral ischemia caused by extracardiac disturbances.

There are several features common to almost all types of syncope. Electroencephalographic changes usually appear, and consist of high voltage, 2- to 4-cycle per second slow waves that promptly return to normal after consciousness is regained. Convulsive movements, such as tonic or clonic contractions of the arms or turning of the head, can occur in all types of fainting, depending on the degree and duration of the cerebral ischemia. Fully developed seizures with tongue biting and urinary incontinence, however, are unusual. Recovery is usually hastened in the recumbent posture, which helps to restore the normal cerebral circulation. The critical level of cerebral blood flow necessary to maintain consciousness has been estimated to be about 30 ml. per 100 grams of brain per minute. (Normal value is 50 to 55 ml.) The duration of asystole or the degree of hypotension necessary to produce critical levels of cerebral ischemia varies, depending upon the posture of the patient, the ability of the cerebral vessels to dilate, and other factors. In normal subjects in the erect posture, a mean arterial blood pressure as low as 20 to 30 mm. of mercury or an asystole of four or five seconds' duration is necessary to produce syncope. In the recumbent position, longer periods of asystole may occur before loss of consciousness develops.

Clinical Manifestations. *Chronic Orthostatic Hypotension.* Chronic orthostatic hypotension is a disorder of the autonomic nervous system in which syncope occurs when the patient assumes the upright posture. The condition is sometimes seen in diabetic neuropathy and in tabes dorsalis, but in many patients the site or nature of the neurologic lesion is unknown. These people have an abnormality in the baroreceptor reflexes that ordinarily compensates for the pooling of blood in the lower extremities and viscera. When an attempt is made to stand upright, there is an inadequate degree of reflex arteriolar constriction, with a subsequent reduction in venous return. This is associated with an immediate and sharp fall in arterial blood pressure, followed by syncope. The pulse rate remains unchanged during the episode, and there are none of the usual prodromal symptoms of pallor, sweating, and nausea seen in vasodepressor faint. These patients may have other aspects of autonomic dysfunction, such as impotence, bladder disturbances, and loss of sweating in the lower trunk. There is said to be a reduction in the 24-hour urinary excretion of norepinephrine and possibly of epinephrine as well.

Orthostatic hypotension has also been associated with a rare form of Parkinson-like syndrome in which tremor, rigidity, muscular wasting, iris atrophy, and ocular palsies are prominent manifestations. This condition is sometimes referred to as the Shy-Drager syndrome.

Failure of postural adaptation also appears following extensive sympathectomy for hypertension or during administration of vasodilating agents and ganglionic blocking medications. Patients recovering from chronic wasting illnesses associated with prolonged bed rest may experience syncope when they attempt to assume the upright position.

Vasodepressor Syncope (the Common Faint). Vasodepressor syncope is by far the most frequent cause of transient loss of consciousness. The term *vasovagal attack* has also been applied to this type of fainting. The condition is characterized by a fall in blood pressure associated with the development of a variety of autonomic manifestations. In the early presyncopal period, there may be pallor, nausea, and sweating; in later stages pupillary dilatation, yawning, hyperpnea, and bradycardia appear. When the mean arterial pressure falls below critical levels, loss of consciousness and characteristic electroencephalographic changes occur. Bradycardia is often severe at the onset of unconsciousness, and pulse rates of 50 to 60 per minute may be observed even after recovery. The duration of syncope is brief, ranging from a few seconds to several minutes. In the postsyncopal period the patient may complain of headaches, weakness, nervousness, and slight confusion. Vasodepressor faint is most often evoked by sudden emotional stress associated with fear, anxiety, or pain. Hypodermic injections, trauma, minor surgery, and the sight of or withdrawal of blood are common precipitating events. Attacks usually occur in the standing or upright posture, and consciousness returns quickly once the patient is recumbent.

The initial event in this complex vascular and neurogenic reaction is dilatation of the vascular bed throughout the body, particularly in peripheral muscles. Vasodilatation in the limb muscles is a normal response to emotional stimuli, and is thought to represent preparation for "fight or flight." The absence of immediate muscle activity, however, and the fall in peripheral resistance are not compensated for by an increase in cardiac output, and as a result there is a reduction in cerebral blood flow.

Adams-Stokes Syndrome. In the early nineteenth century Morgagni, Adams, and Stokes separately observed and described fainting associated with a persistently slow pulse in the range of 40 per minute. A patient with this syndrome has a disordered atrioventricular conduction system, usually secondary to coronary atherosclerosis. In most instances, the loss of consciousness occurs during the changes in rhythm when there may be asystole, ventricular fibrillation, or tachycardia, or a combination of these arrhythmias. The diagnosis can be made by the electrocardiographic changes of A-V block and by the characteristic clinical picture of syncope. Loss of consciousness is abrupt; prodromal signs are not usually present. On regaining consciousness, the patient usually shows little confusion or postsyncopal residua. The attacks may occur several times a day and have no relation to posture or activity. Only a brief period of asystole of four or five seconds' duration will produce loss of consciousness in the erect position, but longer periods of systole are not uncommon. In such instances, neurologic manifestations such as convulsive movements, pupillary dilatation, and prolonged confusion may be observed. Occasionally sudden death results from the cardiac standstill. The use of new radiotelemetered electrocardiographic tape systems has led to more accurate diagnosis of syncope caused by Adams-Stokes attacks. Such monitoring systems record the frequency and nature of the cardiac arrhythmia during the patient's hospitalization and provide a firm basis for definitive treatment such as implantation of an intracardiac pacemaker.

Reflex Cardiac Standstill. Persons without evidence of heart disease may have syncopal attacks as a result of cessation of cardiac action. In a few authenticated cases, dilatation of an esophageal diverticulum by food or by experimental inflation with a balloon has induced complete atrioventricular block and syncope. The alterations in consciousness and electrocardiographic changes disappear when the pressure within the diverticulum is relieved or after administration of atropine. A similar mechanism for cardiac standstill may also rise from vagal reflex activity following orthostatic stress, breath-holding, or distention of the duodenum, pleura, or bronchi. The syncopal episode occasionally seen during thoracentesis or bronchoscopic examination (so-called pleural shock) may be due to such a reflex mechanism. Rarely, syncope due to cardiac arrest has been observed in patients with glossopharyngeal neuralgia.

Carotid Sinus Syncope. In relatively few patients this is the mechanism of syncope. Many persons, particularly those more than 60 years of age, show reflex slowing of the heart and fall of blood pressure during massage of one or both carotid sinuses. Such responses are also seen frequently in patients with cardiac disorders, hypertension, or diseases of the carotid vessels such as atherosclerotic thrombosis or stenosis. The most common response to carotid sinus massage is either sinus bradycardia or sino-atrial block, both of which may be abolished by administration of atropine. Much less frequently, there may be a pure vasodepressor response without slowing of the heart. In a third but rare type of carotid response, fainting may appear in a few seconds without significant changes in either blood pressure or pulse; such instances probably occur only with vigorous pressure and when the opposite carotid is already thrombosed. Carotid sinus syncope is not accompanied by the prodromal symptoms seen in the common faint (nausea, sweating, pallor, etc.). It is more frequent in men, and usually occurs in the erect posture. It sometimes follows sudden head turning or pressure of a tight collar.

Only very few of the patients who exhibit asystole or a reduction in blood pressure on carotid massage experience loss of consciousness due to these factors. In eliciting carotid sinus responses, care should be taken to avoid obstructing blood flow to the brain by compression of the carotid vessels. Cerebral infarction and even death have been reported following carotid compression and massage. Massage of both carotid sinuses simultaneously may be hazardous.

Organic Heart Disease. Patients with myocardial infarction or valvular lesions may also have transient periods of unconsciousness. The mechanism of syncope in these disorders is not altogether clear, but may be related to a reduction in cardiac output with inadequate cerebral blood flow. In acute myocardial infarction, fainting probably results from decrease in stroke volume due to a weakened myocardium. Transient arrhythmias, such as ventricular tachycardia, fibrillation, or heart block, may contribute to the syncopal reaction. Transient loss of consciousness may occur during attacks of angina pectoris, and is probably caused by ventricular fibrillation or various types of heart block associated with temporary periods of myocardial ischemia. Syncope also appears during paroxysmal tachycardia even in the absence of structural heart disease. In such cases the loss of consciousness usually occurs at the onset or at the end of the attack, at which time there may be a brief period of cardiac standstill.

Approximately 10 per cent of patients with aortic stenosis have syncope, usually associated with physical exertion. The loss of consciousness may be due to shunting of blood to the peripheral muscles, but other factors such as inadequate cardiac output may also be present. Syncope is not common in other valvular lesions; occasionally, however, it is seen in patients with pulmonary hypertension and in patent ductus arteriosus.

Hyperventilation Syndrome. The hyperventilation syndrome is one of the most frequent causes of impaired consciousness, usually producing "faintness" and "light-headedness" without actual syncope. It is almost always a manifestation of acute anxiety. At the onset of an attack, the patient may complain of tightness of the chest and a feeling of suffocation. He may not be aware of overbreathing but usually recalls excessive deep sighing. Later, a sense of unreality develops accompanied by feelings of apprehension and sometimes panic. Symptoms related to the heart and gastrointestinal tract often appear. These consist of palpitations or pounding of the heart, precordial oppression, fullness in the throat, and epigastric discomfort. The syndrome may last for as long as a half hour or more and may recur several times a day. Sensations of "numbness" and "coldness" of the hands, feet, and perioral areas often develop, and in prolonged attacks tetany with carpopedal spasm may be noted.

The pathogenesis of the individual symptoms of this disorder is not altogether clear. With normal subjects, hyperventilation in the recumbent posture for as long as an hour will not produce loss of consciousness. They may, however, have sensations of decreased awareness, lightheadedness, and blurring of vision, but do not have the trembling, sweating, palpitations, or precordial distress frequently seen in patients with spontaneous overventilation. The high voltage slow wave activity in the electroencephalogram produced by hyperventilation can be prevented by hyperbaric oxygenation, suggesting that these EEG changes, and probably the alterations in consciousness as well, are due to cerebral hypoxia. The serum calcium level remains normal, but there is often a decrease in serum phosphate within 15 minutes after hyperventilation begins. The hypocapnia caused by overventilation causes cerebral anoxia. In addition, there may be fall in blood pressure due probably to muscle vasodilatation and increase in peripheral blood flow. These factors alone are usually insufficient to produce syncope, and the occasional loss of consciousness with this syndrome is probably due to vasodepressor mechanisms as in the common faint.

The hyperventilation syndrome is most common in nervous, anxious women who have other functional disturbances related to tension. The syndrome can often be reproduced by having the patient hyperventilate voluntarily for two or three minutes. Although the patient is often reassured by the fact that he can control the attack somewhat by breath-holding or breathing in a paper bag, therapy directed at the underlying emotional disturbance is warranted.

Cough Syncope. Cough syncope usually follows a paroxysm of explosive and vigorous coughing. It is commonly observed in men but rarely in women. In adults, the condition is often associated with chronic lung disease or bronchitis; in children, it may occur during severe pertussis. The syncope is brief, and there are no postsyncopal residua. The condition has also been described following hearty laughter. The loss of consciousness has been attributed to an increase in the intrathoracic and intra-abdominal pressure caused by vigorous coughing. This, in turn, is thought to produce a sudden sharp elevation in cerebrospinal fluid pressure, thereby "squeezing" blood from the intracranial and cerebral vessels. Other theories maintain that the condition is due to a Valsalva effect with reduction in cardiac output or to cerebral "concussive effect" caused by rapid rise in the cerebrospinal fluid pressure. There is clinical evidence to suggest that the presence of an intracerebral lesion such as brain tumor or stenosis of a major cerebral artery may produce increased susceptibility to syncope following paroxysms of cough. Such cases may have focal neurologic symptoms such as paresthesias or clonic movements of one limb prior to loss of consciousness.

"Fainting Lark." This trick, often indulged in by school boys, consists of sudden manual compression of the chest of the victim after he has been hyperventilating for about a minute. Loss of consciousness also occurs in a similar prank in which the individual hyperventilates in the squatting position, quickly stands, and then performs the Valsalva maneuver. The increase in intrathoracic pressure in both tricks interferes with the flow of blood in the heart and lungs and further reduces the cerebral blood flow and arterial blood pressure, which have already been impaired by hyperventilation. Voluntary syncope has also been observed in muscular teenage boys who can maintain a prolonged Valsalva maneuver by vigorous stretching of the trunk and back muscles. Such instances of "stretch syncope" are often self-induced to provide a curiously satisfying experience.

Micturition Syncope. This form of syncope is most often seen during or immediately after micturition in adult men who rise in the middle of the night to void. The loss of consciousness is brief and there is no postsyncopal confusion or weakness. Many such people give a history of drinking large quantities of beer before retiring, and considerable bladder deflation may take place during micturition. A similar fainting may be observed following drainage of a distended bladder in urinary retention or after removal of a large quantity of ascitic fluid by abdominal paracentesis. Sharpey-Shafer suggested that the loss of consciousness may be due to a reflex vasodilatation of the peripheral vascular system, a situation thought to be the converse of the paroxysmal hypertension seen in paraplegics during bladder distention. Others have attributed the syncope to a Valsalva maneuver during micturition or to peripheral vasodilation associated with a warm bed and perhaps the recent consumption of alcohol.

Hysterical Fainting. Hysterical fainting is seen almost entirely in young women with emotional illness. It differs from the vasodepressor faint and the hyperventilation syndrome in that the patient is relatively free of anxiety and shows little concern regarding the fainting episodes. The attack usually occurs in the presence of others. The patient generally slumps to the floor gracefully, sometimes dramatically, without injury or awkwardness. It thus resembles the mid-Victorian drawing-room swoon. In the present era, hysterical fainting often occurs in groups of young women during mass excitement, particularly that caused by the presence of screen or television idols.

During the attack the patient may be motionless or may show bizarre resisting movements. The attack may last from several minutes to as long as an hour or more, with fluctuations of responsiveness. There are no abnormalities in pulse, blood pressure, or skin color. The electroencephalogram is normal during the attack, indicating that there may be no actual loss of consciousness. The diagnosis can usually be made without difficulty on the basis of the setting of the episode, the patient's underlying emotional disturbance, and the absence of physical abnormalities.

Cerebral Arterial Occlusive Disease. Patients with generalized atherosclerosis may have frequent episodes of loss of consciousness over a period of days or weeks. In most instances the attack is accompanied by signs of focal neurologic deficits such as motor weakness, sensory loss, or cranial nerve disorders. In such cases the diagnosis can be made without difficulty. Occasionally, however, the patient has no localizing symptoms, and complains of vague dizziness, weakness, and visual disturbances. Many such patients are in the older age group and have evidence of hypertensive disease with coronary or cerebrovascular involvement. These cases of "blind staggers" are difficult to categorize, and a definite diagnosis often cannot be made. The symptoms are probably related to postural disturbances associated with vascular or labyrinthine disease.

Hypoglycemia. Hypoglycemia often produces weakness, faintness, and confused behavior but usually not loss of consciousness. Reactive hypoglycemia may appear in emotionally tense persons a few hours after ingestion of a high carbohydrate meal. It sometimes follows extensive gastric resection in association with the dumping syndrome. Hypoglycemia may also be due to islet cell adenoma of the pancreas. In this condition, nervousness, weakness, trembling, and sometimes convulsions occur after fasting and exercise. The fasting morning blood sugar level may be low, in contrast to that of patients with reactive hypoglycemia, in whom this determination is usually normal. The diagnosis can usually be made by observing the prompt recovery following administration of carbohydrates by mouth or glucose intravenously. Other conditions such as pituitary insufficiency, Addison's disease, and large sarcomas may also produce hypoglycemia.

Diagnosis. The diagnosis of syncope depends almost entirely upon a careful history of the attack and the setting in which it occurs. Differentiation of syncope from an akinetic epileptic seizure, such as a petit mal or psychomotor attack, may be difficult. Careful evaluation of the electroencephalographic findings, the onset and duration of the attack, and the postsyncopal manifestations can usually distinguish these conditions. These factors are also helpful in differentiating the various types of syncope. In vasodepressor faint, the patient usually has prodromal signs of autonomic hyperactivity such as pallor, sweating, salivation, and bradycardia. In cardiac arrest, orthostatic hypotension, and carotid sinus syncope, loss of consciousness occurs abruptly, and prodromal symptoms are not usually present. Postsyncopal confusion, headache, and weakness often follow vasodepressor faint and the hyperventilation syndrome. In chronic orthostatic hypotension and Adams-Stokes attacks, recovery of consciousness is rapid and complete without postsyncopal symptoms. Most types of fainting occur in the erect or upright position, but in cardiac arrest syncope may appear while the patient is recumbent. The duration of syncope is brief in postural hypotension but prolonged in hyperventilation and hypoglycemia. Most of these differentiating manifestations can be determined by careful history, but special methods of examination may be necessary. These consist of voluntary hyperventilation for approximately two minutes, massage of the carotid sinuses, and observations of pulse and blood pressure during change in posture from recumbency to erect position. Laboratory examinations, such as electrocardiogram or electroencephalogram, and blood sugar studies may also be necessary to arrive at a correct diagnosis.

Treatment. Therapy in syncope consists primarily of treatment of the underlying disorder. In all types of fainting, recovery is usually aided by maintaining the patient in a recumbent position with elevation of the lower extremities. Application of cold water to the face and head and inhalation of spirits of ammonia or other pungent aromatics are time-honored and certainly do no harm.

Ebert, R. V.: Syncope. Circulation, 27:1148, 1963.

Engel, G. L.: Fainting. 2nd ed. Springfield, Ill., Charles C Thomas, 1962.

Karp, H. R., Weissler, A. M., and Heyman, A.: Vasodepressor syncope: EEG and circulatory changes. Arch Neurol. (Chicago), 5:106, 1961.

Pedersen, A., Sandoe, E., Hvidberg, E., and Schwartz, M.: Studies on the mechanism of tussive syncope. Acta Med. Scand., 179:653, 1966.

Thomas, J. E.: Hyperactive carotid sinus reflex and carotid sinus syncope. Mayo Clin. Proc., 44:127, 1969.

Wayne, H. H.: Syncope: Physiological considerations and an analysis of the clinical characteristics in 510 patients. Amer. J. Med., 30:418, 1961.

THE MANAGEMENT OF SEVERE NEUROLOGIC DISABILITY

Fred Plum

Patients with severe neurologic injury or with depressed consciousness need special management lest their inabilities to feel or move lead to serious complications caused by infection, pressure, and immobilization. The general care of such patients is much the same whether their illness be head injury, encephalitis, stroke, polyneuropathy, poliomyelitis, or other.

Pulmonary Care. The lungs and airway are particularly vulnerable to complications in paralyzed patients. The body's inertness leads to dependent pulmonary congestion and this, in turn, predisposes to pneumonitis. If either a depressed cough reflex or paralysis of the swallowing or coughing mechanisms is added, the natural secretions of the mouth and tracheobronchial tree accumulate and obstruct the airway. Both congestion and obstruction can be prevented by proper *positioning and turning.* Patients who are obtunded or who have swallowing paralysis are best placed semiprone so that secretions drain spontaneously from the mouth, pharynx, and airway. Drainage is enhanced by raising the hips as in the accompanying figure. Patients who are alert and able to swallow can safely be placed supine, but they must turn or be turned regularly to the full side or semiprone position to drain their lungs. Many physicians recommend chest massage and squeezing to aid the drainage process.

Airways should be placed in obtunded or stuporous patients to prevent the tongue from occluding the pharynx. Oral airways are satisfactory except when patients are deeply comatose and need deep chest suctioning, in which case endotracheal tubes must be passed. When the process causing respiratory obstruction is expected to last more than a few days or when conscious patients are unable to clear the airway, tracheostomy must be performed.

Appropriate *suctioning* of the pharynx and upper airway greatly benefits the patients with excessive secretion. Catheters should be kept scrupulously clean, and the suction should be applied gently with a side arm release on the suction assembly so that the pressure can be released if the catheter "grabs" against mucous membranes. Excessively vigorous suctioning dangerously traumatizes the tissues and must be avoided.

Several principles guide the use of *antimicrobial drugs.* There is a widespread and understandable urge to treat unconscious or paralyzed patients to protect against future infection. When natural defenses are but briefly set aside, as in the short comas of drug poisoning, chemoprophylaxis appears to reduce the incidence of pneumonia during convalescence, although this point has not been carefully studied. However, with more prolonged coma (or, by inference, with prolonged immobilization), prophylactic antimicrobial drugs are followed by an increase rather than a decrease in the number of lung and bladder infections, and they accelerate the emergence of drug-resistant bacterial strains. Thus, in obtunded, paralyzed,

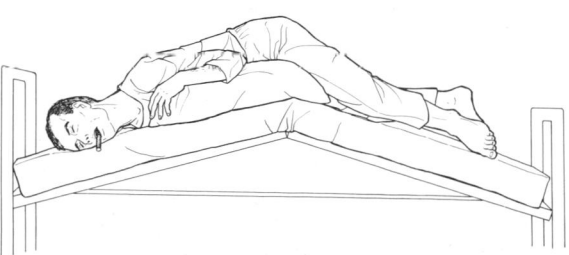

or immobilized patients, antimicrobials should be reserved for the vigorous and specific treatment of bacteriologically identified infections *after* the infection has appeared.

Skin. Decubitus ulcers are easier to prevent than to cure. The heels, the trochanteric prominences, and the sacral and scapular surfaces must be kept dry and clean. These prominences cannot safely be exposed to prolonged compression, and every effort should be given to turning patients at intervals of no longer than two to four hours. In seriously paralyzed, inert subjects, almost no amount of turning seems enough to prevent skin lesions; alternating pressure or "floating" sponge mattresses are particularly helpful in such severe problems. On exposed surfaces, circumscribed reddening or blistering precedes ulceration and is a signal that all pressure must be kept away from that point. Some authorities recommended dry heat from a lamp to accelerate healing of such early lesions. Painting the surface with lotions or creams has no value.

Extremities. To prevent contractures as well as pressure lesions of skin and nerves, the paralyzed members need to be supported against gravity and protected from the weight of the bedding. Gauze rolls may be placed in the palms, and the lower extremities should be protected against excessive outward rotation at the hip as well as posterior displacement at the knee. Foot boards, pressed flat against the plantar surfaces, counteract ankle tendon shortening and keep the sheets and blankets from deforming the toes. Joints that are partially or completely immobilized by muscle paralysis need to be limbered up at least three times each day by slowly passing the involved member through its full range of motion. A word of caution: Nurses and attendants must be warned against exerting heavy traction on the shoulder girdle when moving or turning paralyzed or insensate patients, for these maneuvers sometimes produce brachial plexus injuries.

Nutrition and Fluids. Impaired swallowing as well as nausea and vomiting accompany many neurologic illnesses and can lead to pulmonary aspiration. Hence, it is best not to feed neurologic patients until after examining them to be sure that their illness has not impaired the mechanics of swallowing and that their stomachs are not distended. During the illness, soft, low-calcium diets are most desirable, 1200 to 1500 calories daily being sufficient for most bed patients. If tube feedings are used, mixtures of a regular diet blended with water combine the best nutrition with the least gastrointestinal irritation. The stomach should be aspirated before each feeding to preclude overdistention and regurgitation.

Fluid and electrolyte replacement for neurologic patients is similar to that employed for others requiring parenteral feeding. Ideally, fluid intake should be kept high enough to provide 1500 ml. or more of urine daily. However, both hyper- and hypo-osmolality syndromes complicate neurologic disease, so that close attention must be given to laboratory determination of the BUN and serum sodium as well as to urine volume. *Hyperosmolality* (water depletion) appears in stuporous or comatose patients who are unable to express thirst and receive concentrated tube feedings in which the amount of water is too little to carry the ingested solute through the kidneys. As a result, some of the body's water stores are used to excrete the administered solute; the patient becomes dehydrated, and his serum sodium and BUN rise. The diagnosis is made by finding hypernatremia (serum sodium greater than 150 mEq. per liter). The treatment is administration of water. *Hypo-osmolality* (water intoxication) accompanies many neurologic disorders and develops as readily in patients who are awake and eating as in those receiving parenteral fluids. The condition has been attributed to an inappropriate and excessive secretion of antidiuretic hormone so that a normal water intake cannot be excreted. The diagnosis is made when serum sodium and osmolality are low but urine sodium and osmolality are high. The treatment is water restriction until osmolar balance is restored.

Hypokalemia is common in many elderly patients with stroke, particularly those who have received diuretics chronically; it contributes to delirium and weakness and can be corrected by adding potassium chloride to infusions or to the diet.

Gastrointestinal Problems. Gastrointestinal atony occurs acutely with many neurologic disorders, and constipation plagues most paralyzed patients. The degree of gastric dilatation sometimes can be extraordinary: We have removed 1800 ml. of gastric contents from one of our patients with poliomyelitis whose stomach bubble was so big that it encroached on his breathing. Such large accumulations require drainage by stomach tube, but smaller degrees usually subside spontaneously if feedings are stopped. For constipation, many clinicians employ stool softeners such as dioctyl sodium sulfosuccinate as soon as patients begin to eat. Others prefer to depend upon natural peristalsis and rely on enemas for whatever assistance is needed to empty the colon. Whatever method is preferred, it requires constant attention to prevent fecal impaction.

Severe diseases affecting the meninges and brainstem predispose to malacia, ulceration, and bleeding of the esophagus, stomach, and upper duodenum. Therefore, stools of recently paralyzed patients should be analyzed twice weekly for blood. Such hemorrhages *can* be fatal; at the least, they are a cause of blood-loss anemia. Blood replacement and bland antacids usually are sufficient to treat moderate degrees of bleeding, but severe hemorrhage may require gastric resection.

Urinary Bladder. *Incontinence* creates both social and practical problems that usually outweigh one's reluctance to manipulate the urinary tract. Incontinent males can be connected via a condom tube to bedside drainage, but incontinent females usually require catheters. *Urinary re-*

tention in either males or females requires catheterization. If the retention is unlikely to recur or is only episodic, as in some patients with acute poliomyelitis or multiple sclerosis, single catheterization may suffice. Chronic retention requires an indwelling tube, most often a Foley catheter.

Although it is probably impossible in chronically catheterized patients to avoid urinary tract infections completely, certain steps reduce their incidence and intensity. Catheters should be removed weekly and clean ones inserted aseptically. The tube should be taped to the thigh to prevent its weight from pulling the Foley bulb against the bladder base. The bladder should be irrigated twice daily, using 300 ml. of sterile saline solution (antimicrobial drugs probably have little value) to remove detritus and prevent progressive bladder contractures. A high urinary output (over 1500 ml.) reduces the incidence and extent of both infection and calcium phosphate calculi. High-calcium diets are contraindicated because they also contribute to urinary tract stone formation. Prophylactic antimicrobial drugs are contraindicated for patients with catheters because they do not suppress all infection and thus facilitate the emergence of drug-resistant bacteria. However, once an infection has begun, as indicated by pyuria, the urine should be cultured promptly and the offending organism combated with the appropriate antimicrobial drug.

Psychologic Management. To be paralyzed is a terrifying experience. Even confused patients often recognize that they cannot escape from their beds. Humane, sympathetic discussion by physicians can soften many of these blows, as can efforts by nurses and ancillary staff to provide a cheerful and diverting environment. Such patients should not be isolated in single rooms. Careful explanations of all procedures to be done reduce both the apprehension and confusion of these patients. More specific suggestions for managing patients with delirium are given in the article on Delirium.

Petersdorf, R. G., Curtin, J. A., Hoeprich, P. D., Peeler, R. N., and Bennett, I. L.: A study of antibiotic prophylaxis in unconscious patients. New Eng. J. Med., 257:1001, 1957.
Plum, F.: Disturbances of bladder function. *In* Williams, D. (ed.): Modern Trends in Neurology. London, Butterworth, 1961.
Plum, F., and Dunning, M. F.: Technics for minimizing trauma to the tracheobronchial tree after tracheotomy. New Eng. J. Med., 254:193, 1956.

Neurologic Diagnostic Procedures

Richard P. Schmidt

Many special tests and procedures are used to supplement the clinical examination in the establishment of a neurologic diagnosis. These may add precision to the localization and characterization of a disease process, or may record parameters of functional alteration as reflected in electrical activity of brain, nerve, or muscle. Their value is related directly to the judgment with which they are used and to the skill of their performance and interpretation. Some of the tests outlined below are relatively simple procedures which cause little discomfort, whereas others may be dangerous and must be used only by physicians skilled in the techniques and with full knowledge of potential complications and their treatment. The number of available tests is expanding rapidly, and it has become increasingly important for these to be selectively used and individualized. Those least dangerous and causing least discomfort are to be used first. Careful clinical examinations may obviate the need of a battery of expensive and time-consuming procedures.

In this article brief descriptions of the useful diagnostic procedures are given. Details of techniques and of interpretations may be found in definitive and specialized monographs.

ROENTGENOLOGIC EXAMINATIONS

Roentgenograms of the skull or spine may reveal evidence of disease by deformation or involvement of bony structures, by displacement of normal radiopaque structures such as the pineal body, or by abnormal opacification such as may be seen with calcification of a tumor, vascular malformation, infectious granuloma, or hematoma. Maximal information should always be obtained from plain roentgenograms prior to the institution of more complex studies. Such studies may not only permit a more satisfactory choice, but also may obviate the need for contrast studies such as arteriography or pneumoencephalography. Brain shift may be evident by displacement of a normally calcified pineal body. Increased intracranial pressure over a long period of time characteristically causes demineralization of the dorsum sellae by pressure from an expanded third ventricle or a beaten silver appearance to the inner table of the skull from pressure of the gyri of the cerebral cortex. Diagnosis of some diseases can be confirmed without further examination. For example, pituitary tumors usually cause enlargement of the sella turcica. Meningiomas are often associated with thickening of bone at the site from which they arise.

Patterns of calcification as seen roentgenographically may be highly specific in diagnosis of disease. Examples include arcuate densities in the wall of an aneurysm, calcification in the pattern of the cerebral cortex in Sturge-Weber syndrome, and diffuse nodular calcification in congenital toxoplasmosis. Amorphous calcification with or without erosion of the pituitary fossa is typical in craniopharyngioma, and the basal ganglia may be calcified symmetrically in hypoparathyroidism.

Lesions of the skull or spine occur frequently in neoplastic diseases. In some instances the appearance is quite characteristic, as is seen in the "punched-out" rarefactions of multiple myeloma. Special attention may be directed to the foramina at the base of the skull through which nasopharyngeal cancer may invade and cause cranial nerve paralysis. Axial projections of the base of the skull may reveal enlargement of these foramina with special advantage. Acoustic neurinoma characteristically enlarges the internal auditory meatus as shown in special projection.

Diagnosis of congenital malformations of the skull and spine usually can be made without contrast material. In platybasia there is flattening of the basal angle, frequently associated with malformation of the foramen magnum and cervical spine and with hydrocephalus. Injury to the brain in early life may be associated with asymmetric skull growth. Premature closure of the sutures results in microcephaly or in asymmetric growth in the direction of those sutures which remain open.

In examination of the spine special attention should be given to alignment, integrity of the intervertebral disc space, bony excrescences, and evidences of bone destruction. Intraspinal neoplasms commonly erode and cause increased separation of the vertebral pedicles. Characteristic patterns are seen in such diseases as tuberculosis of the spine, osteoporosis, metastatic carcinoma, and vertebral hemangioma. Oblique views are especially useful for demonstrating intervertebral foramina which may be enlarged in tumors such as neurofibromas or compromised by osteophytic spurs causing radicular syndromes.

Laminagraphic section roentgenography may be used for visualization of abnormalities of skull or spine which are otherwise obscure. This procedure has special value in demonstrating changes near the midline or base of the skull, and may also be used to advantage in intraspinal lesions.

Further stages of neuroradiologic diagnosis depend upon heightening contrast by use of radiopaque substances injected into arteries or the subarachnoid space, or by gas (usually air or oxygen) to provide increased radiolucency in cerebrospinal-fluid containing compartments. With increasing sophistication of instrumentation, the techniques of performing such studies are evolving rapidly, demanding high degrees of skill for their performance and interpretation.

Myelography is used when mass impingement upon spinal neural structures or nerve roots is suspected, and usually when surgical treatment appears probably to be required. It is usually done using iodized oil, which is heavier than the cerebrospinal fluid, injected into the subarachnoid space at a reasonable distance away from the suspected lesion. Oil is manipulated up and down by tilting the patient on a table under fluoroscopic control. Care is taken to prevent introduction of oil into the cranial cavity and to remove the oil after completing the procedure. Adequate myelography with fluoroscopy and spot films at various angles is usually satisfactory for demonstrating mass lesions within or impinging upon the spinal subarachnoid space. It has its greatest usefulness in outlining neoplasms, herniations of the nucleus pulposus, or impingements by spondylotic lesions. At times manipulation of fluid pressure may cause acute exacerbation of the patient's symptoms, and if a tumor is present this may call for urgent surgical intervention. The test is to be avoided unless there is strong and sufficient reason to suspect a mass lesion. There may, for example, be exacerbation of multiple sclerosis by the procedure. Iodized oil is a foreign substance to the subarachnoid space, and may initiate a sterile meningeal reaction or, rarely, a progressive adhesive arachnoiditis. For these reasons, in some centers myelography is performed using air-contrast or, less commonly, absorbable water-soluble radiopaque material. When more satisfactory, less irritating agents are found, they will probably replace oil.

In *pneumoencephalography,* oxygen or air is introduced in increments into the lumbar subarachnoid space from which it ascends into the basal cisterns and enters the ventricular cavities. By proper positioning, the entire ventricular system can be visualized, as can the basal cisterns and subarachnoid spaces over the cerebral cortex. *Ventriculography* may be used in the presence of increased intracranial pressure or when a tumor is suspected, because of lessened danger of initiating herniation as compared with pneumoencephalography. It is performed by introducing gas directly into the lateral ventricle by a needle introduced through a trephine opening in the skull. It has the disadvantage of limiting the examination to the ventricular system because of failure to fill the subarachnoid spaces. In these tests, atrophic processes or obstructions of fluid paths are reflected by enlargement of the ventricles. In the former, there may be concomitant enlargement of the basal cisterns and of the sulci over the convexity of the brain. Space-taking lesions such as neoplasms may obstruct with "upstream" dilatation appropriate to the site or, as is characteristic, may deform and shift the ventricles.

When appropriately used, pneumoencephalography is a safe procedure; however, it is usually distressing to the patient, as it causes severe headache.

The uses of *angiography* are increasing rapidly.

By the injection of appropriate root arteries, positioning of the patient, and timing of serial films, it is now possible to demonstrate practically all the intracranial arterial and venous systems and also to study parent vessels from the aorta upward. Techniques for performance vary, but increasing proportions of these examinations are being done by selective catheterization through the brachial, axillary, subclavian, or femoral arteries, and fewer by direct puncture of carotid or vertebral arteries in the neck.

Cerebral angiography has certain advantages over gas contrast studies. Pathologic processes of blood vessels such as aneurysms or malformations may be demonstrated. Complete or partial occlusions at any site from the level of the aortic arch to the intracranial vascular tree may be visualized. If surgery for occlusive disease is contemplated, all major vessels should be studied. Angiography is frequently the procedure of choice in delineating neoplasms or other space-occupying lesions. Masses may be localized by displacement of arteries or veins from normal positions and by the filling of abnormal vessels within a neoplasm (tumor stain). It is sometimes possible to predict the histologic type of a tumor from its blood supply and vascular pattern. Subdural hematoma is demonstrated to particular advantage by displacement of superficial blood vessels away from the inner surface of the skull, and is seen best on anteroposterior projections. Angiography may have an added advantage for patients with increased intracranial pressure in that it is less likely to cause herniation and brain shift than pneumoencephalography. Patients tolerate the procedure well, and do not have the headache, nausea, and vomiting associated with gas insufflation. Complications may occur, however, especially in older patients and in those with vascular disease. These range from transient dysfunction such as hemiparesis or confusion to more unusual permanent neurologic injuries or even death. Puncture of an artery can cause intraluminal rupture of an intimal atherosclerotic plaque or subintimal dissection. Embolization or thrombosis may occur from the site of puncture.

RADIOISOTOPE PROCEDURES

Isotope brain scanning depends upon the ability of certain radioactive substances to localize selectively in neoplasms or in injured tissues (such as infarctions) which damage the normally impermeable blood-brain barrier. Isotopes of short half-life, such as technetium^{99m} pertechnetate are now preferred because they permit a higher level of radioactivity and a much shorter elapsed time to the completion of the procedure. The scan may be recorded with multiple crystals in a scintillation camera or by more conventional scintillation scanners moving across the head and recording the scanning image instrumentally on paper or film. Several projections are used to "view" the head

from different directions. With the scintillation camera dynamic scans may be obtained, giving some evidence of blood circulation or demonstrating large vascular anomalies. Scans are of special worth for locating lesions relatively near the surface, and may be confusing or "negative" with deep or midline lesions. Artifacts may be produced by bruises of the scalp or such simple processes as contamination by saliva in which the isotope has been secreted. Scans are convenient because of safety and lack of discomfort or serious inconvenience.

ELECTRODIAGNOSTIC EXAMINATIONS

Functions of the brain, nerves, and neuromuscular apparatus may be examined by appropriate measurements of electrical activity.

The *electroencephalogram* (EEG) is the recording of amplified potentials generated by the brain by means of electrodes applied to the scalp. Recordings directly from the surface or from the depths of the brain may have application in selected instances such as the surgical treatment of foci generating epileptic partial seizures. An adequate routine examination includes the application of 18 or more electrodes on the scalp and observation of the EEG under conditions of nonattentive wakefulness, in response to overbreathing, and during the course of natural sleep. The instruments now used consist of eight or more matched channels for simultaneous recordings, and by convention the record is written in ink or paper moving beneath galvanometer pens. Variation in rhythm occurs with respect to normal processes such as sleep, and there are marked differences between the EEG of the child and the adult. Although the processes that generate the brain waves are largely unknown, normal or usual patterns and deviation from normal are well recognized and may be highly useful in clinical diagnosis. Deviation from normal may be termed a dysrhythmia, and the type of dysrhythmia and its distribution or localization may correlate with the type of the underlying disease. A normal EEG does not preclude the presence of serious disease. Mild deviations from normal may be observed in persons with no evidence of cerebral disease. Intelligence cannot be measured and psychologic diagnoses cannot be made by the EEG. The EEG can be properly interpreted only in concert with clinical data, and it cannot provide precise diagnosis in and of itself.

The EEG may provide evidence for diagnosis and localization of structural lesions such as neoplasms, infarcts, hematomas, and infections. The tool has the great advantage of relative simplicity of application and harmlessness to the patient. If the brain is infarcted, compressed, or disrupted by neoplasms or hemorrhage, slower than normal (delta) waves are observed and may be localized to areas overlying the pathologic processes. Serial or sequential examinations reflect changes of improvement or worsening in the pathologic process, and thus help to delineate the nature of the underlying disorder. Metabolic abnormalities affecting the brain may be followed by the EEG to ascertain the direction of improvement or worsening.

The *electromyogram* (EMG) records the electrical activity in muscle. Detailed diagnostic examination requires use of needle electrodes inserted into the muscles under study. Instrumentation is analogous to that used for the EEG, except that a cathode ray oscilloscope is necessary because of more rapid potential change. Permanent records may be made on photographic film or magnetic type. Records are obtained during rest, needle insertion, voluntary contraction, and in response to physical or electrical stimulation. Auditory monitoring with a loudspeaker is customary in many laboratories. The EMG is most helpful in the diagnosis of disease of the motor unit, which includes the ventral horn cell, ventral nerve root, motor nerve, myoneural junction, and muscle. Neuropathic disorders, such as amyotrophic lateral sclerosis or poliomyelitis, produce signs of muscle denervation, including increased insertion activity, fibrillation potentials at rest, and reduced, altered or absent normal muscle action potentials. Primary muscle disease (myopathy) frequently reduces the amplitude and duration of the muscle action potentials and increases the complexity of their wave form, although the number of potentials is little changed. Myotonia produces a highly characteristic repetitive pattern. Segmental investigation of muscle innervation may be of use in localization and diagnosis of spinal root compression, such as that caused by intervertebral disc protrusion.

Estimates of motor nerve conduction velocity are made by electrically stimulating the nerve, recording electromyographically from the muscle that it innervates, and measuring the latency. Slowing of conduction is observed in a wide variety of peripheral neuropathies and in many instances of neurologically asymptomatic diabetes mellitus. The site of local nerve compression or conduction block can be demonstrated, an example being the local block of median nerve conduction that is found in the carpal tunnel syndrome. Sensory nerve conduction velocity may be measured by recording nerve action potentials following digital nerve stimulation. Sensory neuropathy may produce slowing of conduction or inability to record the nerve potential.

ECHOENCEPHALOGRAPHY

High frequency (ultrasonic) sound pulses produced by an electrically activated crystal and conducted in a fluid or solid medium reflect or echo at physical interfaces, and their reflection can, in turn, be detected and recorded. This phenomenon may detect shifts or alterations of structures within the cranial cavity. Present application makes it possible to obtain a rapid, painless, and harmless estimate of the position of midline structures (third ventricle) in the intact cranium. Pulses of ultrasound are delivered to the head through a probe held firmly to the scalp and with liquid or jelly at the interface. A detector may be physically located in the same probe. Proper amplification and display with a cathode ray oscilloscope permit recognition of reflected pulse from skin, ventricle, skull, and other structures. By calibrating the sweep speed of the oscilloscope beam, the distance from the probe to the reflecting surface can be measured in millimeters. Measurement of the position of the midline third ventricle is particularly reliable. This is useful as a screening test for hemispheric mass lesions causing brain shift, and is well adapted to use in emergency hospital services for appraising patients with suspected subdural or epidural hemorrhage. Echoencephalography may also be used to estimate ventricular size and at times to demonstrate abnormal structures such as tumors.

Toole, J. F. (ed.): Contemporary Neurology Series, Vol. 3. Special Techniques in Neurologic Diagnosis. Philadelphia, F. A. Davis Company, 1969.

The Extrapyramidal Disorders

INTRODUCTION
Melvin D. Yahr

The basal ganglia or extrapyramidal diseases comprise a complex group of clinical disorders characterized by abnormal involuntary movements (dyskinesias) alterations in muscle tone, and disturbances in bodily posture. The major clinical states included under this title are parkinsonism, chorea, athetosis, dystonia, and hemiballism. These terms not only are used to denote particular disease entities, but in a descriptive sense refer to a constellation of symptoms that may occur in a variety of central nervous system disorders involving the basal ganglia and/or their connections. They are recognizable, one from the other, by the degree, form, and combination of the triad of symptoms noted above and distinguishable as disease entities by the age and mode of onset, identification of particular etiologic and genetic factors, as well as the rate and manner of progression of symptoms. Although much is known about the clinical aspects of extrapyramidal disorders, our information is deficient in regard to their fundamental anatomic, physiologic, and pathogenic bases.

The conventional anatomic concept of the basal ganglia as a group of nuclear masses in the forebrain has not proved adequate in explaining the clinical manifestations or what is known about the physiologic or pathologic aspects of these conditions. In consequence, neurologists have devised a functional anatomic approach that includes not only the basal ganglia nuclei, but also related structures in the brainstem as well as a neural network of connections with other parts of the nervous system. The structures of importance in this system are the caudate nucleus and putamen, which, because of their similarities in appearance, cellular structure, and phylogenetic development, are collectively known as the striatum; the globus pallidus or pallidum, an older structure but one in which many nonpyramidal pathways converge; the thalamus, another important way station and integrative region; and the subthalamic nucleus, red nucleus and substantia nigra, all brainstem centers with important connections to the basal ganglia. These nuclear masses, along with their connections with each other and with certain parts of the reticular formation, cerebellum, and cerebrum, make up an anatomic-physiologic unit that collectively has been termed "the extrapyramidal system." The role of this system in maintaining normal motor activity in man is not definitely known, and has only been inferred from studies of animals, in which it is more highly developed and not dominated by the cerebral cortex. In submammalian forms in which motor activities are stereotyped and resemble patterned reflexes, this system appears essential for maintaining normal locomotion, feeding, etc. In higher animals, except man, its integrity is necessary for the production of automatic movements and postural adjustments. Some believe that this same function is carried over to man and that coarse, gross automatic movements are mediated by the extrapyramidal system. Others have implied a more secondary role in which this system is incapable of initiating movements but provides a re-enforcing and modulating influence on movements of cortical origin. The latter thesis seems more in keeping with our present knowledge of the integrative function of the nervous system; hence it is best to view the pyramidal and extrapyramidal systems as operating in unison and constant balance. Movements having their origin in the cerebral cortex are mediated through the pyramidal tract but are influenced by reflex regulating mechanisms from various components of the extrapyramidal system. In this context, the prime role of the extrapyramidal system is automatic sensorimotor integration, which can be explained in terms of inhibition and facilitation of motor responses to appropriate stimuli. Hence dysfunction within this system results in motor responses that are delayed, slow, and incomplete and especially affect automatic or involuntary movements.

The manifestations of basal ganglia disorders previously noted fall into two general categories: those of a *positive* nature, such as abnormal movements, tremor and chorea, and those of a *negative* nature, such as postural changes, and loss of associated movements. The positive disturbances arise from an excess of neural activity, and as such cannot derive from destruction of neural elements but must represent the function of surviving structures. They are often termed release phenomena, in that a lesion in one structure removes the controlling or regulating influence on another, with the result that the latter becomes overactive. The negative symptoms, on the other hand, are considered to result from the direct loss or destruction of neural elements. Unfortunately, because of the nature of the disease processes affecting this region it has not been possible to correlate intimately the clinical symptoms with structural changes. Further, there are no naturally occurring animal counterparts to the disturbances of upright posture and of movements that occur in human diseases of the extrapyramidal system. Pathologic studies of most of these diseases show widespread neuropathologic changes throughout the cerebrum, although the basal ganglia and brainstem nuclei suffer the brunt of the damage. In some instances, however, the functional impairment is far more than that expected from the changes found on routine autopsy examination. There is a growing body of information that suggests that the abnormalities in such cases may be chemical rather than morphologic. The content of monoamines, such as dopamine and serotonin, is particularly high in structures such as the caudate nucleus, putamen, and substantia nigra. In at least one disease affecting this system, parkinsonism, the level of dopamine has been shown to be markedly decreased. Experimental lesions in the region of the substantia nigra and the pallidum produce similar effects. Since in many instances the chemical abnormalities do not follow the presumed anatomic connections, a neurochemical network is postulated for this system. In such a neural system chemical transmitter substances, such as dopamine, may be stored in nerve endings of axons whose somata or cell bodies are located in distant areas. The observed chemical changes may reflect injury or damage to a specific chemical system in these instances (a dopaminergic neuronal system) and may be similar regardless of the pathologic process. Extrapyramidal structures have other unique biochemical characteristics as indicated by high levels of acetylcholine as well as the enzymes responsible for its synthesis and degradation. All these findings suggest that better understanding of the extrapyramidal system and its diseases may be derived from intensive study of its chemical topography.

In the clinical evaluation of extrapyramidal disorders it is essential to have a clear understanding of the many and varied symptoms encountered.

Those of major significance are abnormal involuntary movements, alterations in muscle tone, and disturbances in bodily posture.

Abnormal Involuntary Movements. *Tremor* is a rhythmic involuntary alternating contraction of opposing muscle groups, fairly uniform in frequency and amplitude. It may involve a limited segment such as fingers or lips, or may be widespread. Characteristically, tremor of extrapyramidal origin is augmented when the part is at rest and diminished or abolished during voluntary movements and sleep. It differs from that of anxiety, thyrotoxicosis, and those due to intoxications by being slower, of greater amplitude, and more rhythmic. Its occurrence at rest and suppression during voluntary movements and sleep distinguishes it from the so-called "action" tremor of cerebellar involvement. Conclusive evidence regarding the anatomic site of origin of tremor is as yet unavailable. Pathologic changes are frequently found in the substantia nigra and globus pallidus in patients with tremor, but such lesions may also be found when tremor does not exist. Recent electrical recordings from the ventral anterior nucleus of the thalamus have revealed discharges synchronous with the tremor frequency. These findings suggest derangement of a rather complex sensorimotor mechanism with possible multiple pathologic sites.

Athetosis denotes an involuntary movement that results from instability of posture combined with voluntary movement. The result is a slow, writhing, wormlike movement usually most prominent in the fingers and hand, but the face, neck, and feet may also be involved. Multiple areas of the extrapyramidal system, particularly the globus pallidus and striatum as well as the cerebral cortex, have shown pathologic changes when this type of dyskinesia is encountered.

Chorea refers to brief, distal, rapid, explosive movements which at first glance appear to be purposeful and coordinated but on closer inspection are aimless and uncoordinated. They involve upper and lower limbs, face, trunk, and head, and may occur with such rapidity that the individual appears in constant motion. Choreiform movements are accentuated by movement and environmental stimulation, and interfere with normal voluntary function. They are differentiated from tics by being unpatterned, unpredictable, and nonreproducible. Athetosis and chorea may coexist in such a pattern that they are indistinguishable from one another. Pathologic changes accompanying chorea have been found in many areas of the nervous system but especially in the striatum.

Dystonia is a term applied to an abnormally maintained posture resulting from a twisting, turning movement that usually involves the limbs, neck, or trunk. Although there is no specific pattern or posture that describes this disorder, the usual appearance is one of marked distortion of the affected part. The movements appear readily induced by ordinary stimuli, such

as walking, talking, or light touch to the skin. The involved muscles appear to be alternately in a state of increased and decreased tone and, usually as the movement starts, the muscles involved appear to gradually build up tone. Patients with this type of movement cannot inhibit, modify, or terminate the posture, and voluntary movements become seriously impaired. In some instances the movements clear, but the abnormal postures become fixed with resultant torticollis, tortipelvis, and deformities of the limbs. Neither the pathologic nor physiologic substrate for this movement disorder has been fully defined. Some have considered it akin to athetosis but different because of the inherent peculiarities of the axial and appendicular musculature that is primarily affected.

Ballism is a violent dyskinesia consisting of forceful, flinging movements of the limbs. The muscles involved are in the shoulder and pelvic girdle, and usually only one side of the body or even one limb is affected. Of all the abnormal movements ballism is the one that appears to be due to a discrete lesion, usually in the subthalamic nucleus of Luys or its immediate connections.

Alterations in Muscle Tone. A wide range of degrees of tension in muscles is to be found in these disorders. Although it is common to associate heightened muscle tonus (rigidity) with extrapyramidal disorders, some, such as chorea and athetosis, may show normal tone or hypotonus of the musculature. Rigidity, which is most commonly encountered in parkinsonism, must be differentiated from spasticity. The former is identifiable by passively flexing and extending the muscles of an extremity or rotating the hand on the wrist. The movement obtained is one of a series of interrupted jerks at regular intervals, the so called cog-wheel effect. Terms such as "plastic" or "lead pipe" are utilized to describe the homogeneous degree of rigidity. Rigidity may be limited to groups of muscles and may be evident only at some joints, or it may be generalized, affecting the entire musculature. The mechanism underlying the rigidity appears to be impairment of reciprocal inhibition of agonist and antagonistic muscle groups. Electromyographic analysis of these muscles shows continuing activity in both groups throughout a movement such as flexion of the forearm. Rigidity reduces muscle power and velocity of movement to some degree, and also contributes to the production of deformities.

Disturbances in Bodily Posture. Patients with extrapyramidal disease in general, and those with parkinsonism in particular, have difficulty in preserving their equilibrium in the erect as well as the sitting position. They also have difficulty in changing from the horizontal to the upright position or in rolling over from back to front. The most profound difficulties are noted in walking, when tendencies to propulsive or retropulsive gait are evident as well as shuffling and festination. Careful analysis of these defects has indicated that the subjects have loss of control of their center of gravity in both sagittal and coronal planes. There are also tendencies to assume abnormal postures such as a flexion of the trunk on standing. There is a notable lack of normal and appropriate use of defense mechanisms, such as putting out the arms when falling. These abnormalities are thought to be due to disturbances in righting reflexes, impairment of vestibular reflexes, and release of proprioceptor mechanisms subsequent to degeneration in the pallidum. They form a distressing and disabling group of symptoms that to date have not been thoroughly investigated.

THE PARKINSONIAN SYNDROME
(Paralysis Agitans, Shaking Palsy)
Melvin D. Yahr

James Parkinson first described the major manifestations of this syndrome, which is characterized by tremor, muscular rigidity, and loss of postural reflexes. Not only is it one of the most frequently encountered of all the basal ganglia disorders, but parkinsonism is a prominent cause of disability due to diseases of all types. Its prevalence has been placed at close to one million patients in the United States, with the addition of 50,000 new cases each year. As a symptom complex its occurrence has been noted in a number of disease processes either as the sole manifestation or in association with other symptoms. However, in the vast majority of cases no definable cause has as yet been found; since the latter seem to have many features in common, particularly in regard to evolution, they have been designated as Parkinson's disease, paralysis agitans, or primary parkinsonism. The cases in which definable processes are found are best classified as secondary or symptomatic parkinsonism. This separation into clinical groups cannot be construed as indicative of a difference in pathophysiology or even pathogenic mechanisms for the production of symptoms, for all parkinsonism may well have a common origin. In some instances of parkinsonism, regardless of cause, cell loss is consistently found in the substantia nigra in association with other changes diffusely distributed in the corpus striatum and cortex.

PARALYSIS AGITANS
(Parkinson's Disease)

The largest number of cases of parkinsonism fall into this category. The disease most frequently makes its onset between the ages of 50 and 65 years. A rarely encountered juvenile form has been described. The disease affects both sexes and all races, and there is no evidence to indicate a hereditary factor, although a familial incidence is claimed by some authorities.

The disease begins insidiously with any of its three cardinal manifestations either alone or in combination. Tremor usually in one or sometimes in both hands, involving the fingers in a pill-rolling motion, is the most common initial symptom. This is often followed by stiffness in the limbs, general slowing of movements and inability to carry out normal and routine daily functions with ease. As the disease progresses the face becomes "masklike," with a loss of eye blinking and failure to express emotional feeling; the body becomes stooped, and the gait becomes shuffling with loss of arm swing; and the patient is unable to readily gain and maintain an erect posture. Speech becomes slow and monotonous. There is a tendency to drool. The skin takes on an oily quality, and there is a tendency to seborrheic dermatitis. Although paralysis agitans is invariably progressive, the rate at which symptoms develop and disability ensues is extremely variable. On only rare occasions is the disease so rapidly progressive that the patient becomes disabled within five years of onset. In the majority, intervals of 10 to 20 years elapse before symptoms cause incapacity.

The major neurologic findings are: (1) *Lack of facial expression*, with diminished eye blinking but ready induction of blepharospasm when the frontalis muscle is tapped (Myerson's sign). (2) *Tremor* of the distal segments of the limbs at rest, accentuated by suspension but decreased during active movements and eliminated in sleep. The tremor is rhythmical, alternately affecting flexor and extensor muscles, and may involve upper or lower limbs, mouth, or head. (3) *Muscular rigidity* is readily evident on passive movement of a joint, and is manifested by a series of interrupted jerks (cog-wheel phenomenon) rather than a smooth flowing, easy motion. (4) *Akinesia* is the tendency to slowness in the initiation of movement and sudden unexpected arrests of volitional movements while carrying out purposeful acts. The parkinsonian patient appears disinclined to move, and in the midst of performing a routine function suddenly finds himself "frozen" and unable to move through the sequence of motion necessary to complete the action. This is especially evident in writing or feeding and can be striking when, in attempting to walk, the patient finds that his feet are suddenly "frozen to the ground." (5) *Postural abnormalities* are most evident in the erect and sitting positions. The patient has a tendency to let his head fall forward on the trunk, and his body tends to fall forward or backward when seated on a stool unless supported; when pushed either from in front or behind in the erect position he falls, making no effort to catch himself with either a step or by movement of his arms. There is a tendency to deformities of the trunk, hands, and feet. Kyphotic deformity of the spine, causing a stooped posture is a hallmark. There are ulnar deviation of the hand, flexion contractures of the fingers, and an equinovarus posture of the foot.

SECONDARY OR SYMPTOMATIC PARKINSONISM

In a long list of diseases and conditions of the nervous system parkinsonism has occurred as the predominant manifestation. These include poisoning with carbon monoxide, manganese, or other metals; brain tumors in the region of the basal ganglia; cerebral trauma; degenerative diseases; intoxications, particularly with the phenothiazine group of drugs; and infectious processes, such as encephalitis. Cerebral arteriosclerosis has been implicated by some authorities who have even designated a special form of arteriosclerotic parkinsonism. However, it is exceedingly doubtful that such a disorder exists, and pathologic studies to date have not confirmed a vascular basis for the Parkinson syndrome. In most instances of secondary parkinsonism, neurologic abnormalities involving other areas of the nervous system are found, and the parkinsonism itself may show variations from the usual picture. Of all the conditions noted, only two are frequently encountered: postencephalitic and drug-induced parkinsonism.

Postencephalitic Parkinsonism

One of the most prominent sequelae of the epidemic of encephalitis lethargica (von Economo's disease) that occurred between 1919 and 1926 was the parkinsonian syndrome. The syndrome developed after mild as well as severe encephalitis lethargica, and, although in most instances they immediately followed the acute infectious process, in some patients prominent symptoms were not evident for intervals of up to ten years. Parkinsonism appears to have been a unique sequela of this form of encephalitis because it has rarely followed any other known viral encephalitides. There are still a significant number of survivors of encephalitis lethargica, and the evolution and consequences of this form of parkinsonism differ from others, so its clinical recognition is of importance.

Postencephalitic parkinsonism has a number of distinctive or unique features, including the following: (1) A history of encephalitis lethargica during the epidemic period 1918--1919. Since the pandemic of influenza occurred concurrently with encephalitis, it is essential that careful documentation be undertaken in differentiating these two infectious processes. (2) In addition to any or all of the parkinsonian symptoms indicated above, one or more of the following neurologic deficits may be found: hemiplegia, bulbar or ocular palsies, dystonic phenomena, tics, or behavioral disorders. (3) The parkinsonism itself is as a rule incompletely developed and has been static or slowly progressive over a period of years. (4) Episodes that have been termed oculogyric crises. These consist of attacks in which spasms of conjugate eye muscles occur so that the eyes are deviated upward, downward, or to one side for minutes or hours at a time.

Drug-Induced Parkinsonism

The use of phenothiazine derivatives as psychotherapeutic or antiemetic agents has resulted in the occurrence of a number of extrapyramidal syndromes. These reactions are in some instances dose-dependent, and in others they are related to individual susceptibility. They occur with increasing incidence in lower dosage and earlier after administration in direct relation to their potency and alterations in chemical structure from piperidines to piperazines. The reactions cover the entire gamut of extrapyramidal manifestations, but most frequently a Parkinson-like picture is seen. It primarily affects adults and is characterized by varying degrees of akinesia, rigidity, and tremor, which is rarely of the classic pill-rolling variety. In children dyskinetic movements, such as torticollis, facial grimacing, and choreoathetosis predominate. The symptoms disappear when the drugs are withdrawn, usually within days, but on occasion they have persisted for months. In some subjects permanent remnants of parkinsonian symptoms have been found years after elimination of the drugs. In most instances the occurrence of basal ganglia symptoms can be prevented or minimized by the simultaneous administration of one of the centrally active anticholinergic agents, such as Cogentin or Artane.

Treatment. General Principles. Until such time as the etiology and pathogenesis of parkinsonism are defined, its treatment must be considered as symptomatic, supportive, and palliative. It is only in the exceptional case of symptomatic parkinsonism resulting from the use of drugs or occurring in association with specific disease processes that treatment of the causative factor may result in total eradication of symptoms. The more frequently encountered patient will require lifelong treatment consisting of the administration of specific medications, supportive psychotherapeutic measures, physical therapy, and in rare instances surgical intervention. Judiciously employed combined treatment of this sort may control the symptoms of parkinsonism in a large proportion of patients for extended periods of time. In fact, in most it will allow for relatively normal activities of living during most of the phases of this disorder. Further, the introduction of new therapeutic approaches holds promise of forestalling or preventing the progressive disabling nature of this disorder and the appearance of new symptoms. However, at the time of this writing, the use of these new agents provides insufficient experience from which firm conclusions can be drawn.

Supportive Psychotherapy. The major symptoms of parkinsonism are markedly influenced by psychic factors, and a patient's outlook and motivation will affect the extent to which he can overcome disability. It is important for the physician to provide reassurance, encouragement, and sympathetic understanding to the patient and family so that they may meet the numerous difficulties to be encountered at various stages of the illness. To allay anxieties both should be counseled regarding the meaning of various symptoms, the nature of the disease in terms of its long and variable course, and the potential that most patients can lead active and productive lives for long periods after symptoms begin.

Physical Therapy. Simple measures such as heat and massage will alleviate painful muscle cramps and the muscle contraction headache that often accompanies pronounced rigidity of the cervical musculature. Exercises help in preventing flexion contractures. Gait training, walking exercises, and minor rehabilitative measures may enable the patient to maintain his independence with regard to personal hygiene and daily living activities for many more years than his disabilities might otherwise allow. Physical therapy in parkinsonism need not be elaborate, but when indicated should be done frequently and for an indefinite period. The patient should be instructed in simple home exercises and encouraged to develop a program of physical activity. Most patients in the earlier stages like to take long walks and should be encouraged to continue this habit as long as reasonably possible. Every effort should be made to keep them gainfully employed and to adjust their occupations as indicated by their symptoms.

Drug Therapy. The standard agents used for the treatment of parkinsonism are those capable of producing central anticholinergic effects. Those initially introduced for this condition were largely derived from the naturally occurring belladonna alkaloids and included stramonium (hyoscyamus) and scopolamine (hyoscine). Although still occasionally useful in some cases, they have generally been replaced by a number of synthetic agents. The first of these to be developed was trihexyphenidyl hydrochloride (Artane), and it is the initial drug of choice. Treatment is begun in low dosage of 2 mg. three times daily and is gradually increased to the level of tolerance, which may be as high as 20 mg. or more daily in some patients. Congeners of this compound—procyclidine (Kemadrin), cycrimine (Pagitane), and biperiden (Akineton)—differ by minor molecular alteration, but are clinically indistinguishable in their effects and may be used in equivalent dosage. They are useful for certain patients who seem better able to tolerate one or another. Benztropine methanesulfonate (Cogentin), a potent analogue of atropine, is an effective agent given alone or in combination with trihexyphenidyl hydrochloride. When given alone it is begun in a dosage of 2 mg. a day and is gradually increased to a total dose of 6 to 8 mg. Lower dosages of 1 to 4 mg. are used when benztropine methanesulfonate is combined with other drugs. Because of its relatively long duration of action it is often employed as a bedtime medication for patients having particular difficulty in the early morning. It is also available as a parenteral preparation, and can be used to counteract rapidly the effects of phenothiazine-induced extrapyramidal states.

There is little reason aside from convenience of dosage form for choosing one of these drugs over another. At present they may be used as the basic drugs in the treatment of parkinsonism, especially in its earlier stages.

As anticholinergic agents, they are capable of producing undesirable side effects such as dryness of the mouth, blurred vision, constipation, and psychic phenomena such as confusion and hallucinations. These are related to dosage and duration of treatment in most instances, but aged and infirm patients are more liable to side effects than are younger ones. Administration of these agents requires constant supervision by the physician, with readjustment of dosage, shifting of agents since some are more tolerable than others, and constant re-examination for evidence of toxicity. In most instances it is possible to achieve a beneficial effect by beginning treatment in low dosage and gradually increasing to a level of tolerance. After serial use of a number of these agents, the program most appropriate for the individual can be found.

A degree of tolerance for side effects may develop with continual use, and certain measures may be employed to render them more tolerable. Bitter hard candy makes the dryness of the mouth less disagreeable. Laxatives may be required to overcome constipation. Some atropic effects, however, are more serious. Urinary retention is a real danger in patients with prostatism. Glaucoma is a feared but somewhat overexaggerated contraindication. Adequately managed, glaucoma patients who also have parkinsonism may safely be given the standard antiparkinson drugs.

More serious toxic psychic effects frequently limit their use and prevent effective treatment. Impairment of memory occurs commonly, even at low dosages, and proves troublesome to patients in their jobs and in other requirements of daily living. Higher dosages, especially in some sensitive persons, often produce mental confusion and even audiovisual hallucinations. Typical atropine psychosis occurs more frequently in parkinsonian patients than is generally appreciated. Sometimes it is erroneously ascribed to the disease. The occurrence of psychic symptoms requires prompt withdrawal of the medication. In occasional patients, parkinsonism seems to be actually aggravated by the use of drugs. They may become more rigid and akinetic and their gait may be more severely disturbed. In such cases, a smaller daily dose may provide some benefit.

In most cases the maximal tolerable dosage does not provide satisfactory relief, and indeed may not be more helpful than a somewhat lower dosage. Rarely will more than 20 mg. of one of the trihexyphenidyl group or 8 mg. of benztropine daily be tolerated. In such instances one of a number of secondary drugs may then be added in an attempt to achieve additional benefit. Four antihistamines—diphenhydramine (Benadryl), orphenadrine hydrochloride (Disipal), chlorphenoxamine (Phenoxene), and orphenadrine citrate (Norflex)—are commonly used for this purpose. Individuals vary in their tolerance to the side effects of these drugs (drowsiness is the most troublesome), but there is no other reason for preferring one over another. Other antihistamines may be equally helpful, but some, notably tripelennamine (Pyribenzamine), do not seem to have any antiparkinson activity. Again, it is best to begin at lower dosages and gradually build up to tolerance. One may, for example, start the patient on diphenhydramine, 25 mg. twice daily, and with gradual increases it may be possible to reach a dosage of 50 mg. four times daily.

A number of phenothiazine derivatives have been found to have a degree of antiparkinson activity, and have proved useful as secondary agents. These include promethazine (Phenergan), ethopropazine (Parsidol), and diethazine (Diparcol). Some patients tolerate these well in moderate dosages, and additional relief of symptoms occurs. Unfortunately, their use has occasionally produced agranulocytic reactions, and they must be administered with caution.

Amphetamine is often helpful in combating lethargy, but has little, if any, antiparkinson effect and does not influence bradykinesia. It has been especially helpful in the postencephalitic cases for the control of oculogyric crises and relief of drowsiness, which is a frequent occurrence in this form of parkinsonism. Dextroamphetamine sulfate (Dexedrine) in doses up to 50 mg. a day may reduce the frequency of oculogyria.

Considerable interest exists in a new approach to the treatment of parkinsonism based on the depletion of striatal dopamine in this disorder. Since dopamine itself does not cross the blood-brain barrier, attention has been directed to its immediate precursor, levodopa, which readily penetrates the brain.

Several investigators have reported marked and sustained alleviation of all the symptoms of parkinsonism following the daily administration of levodopa in oral dosage of 3 to 10 grams per day. As this large daily dosage is not readily tolerable, it is necessary to commence therapy with smaller doses of 250 mg. given three or four times daily. The dose is then increased by small increments of 250 to 500 mg. every 48 hours until an effective total daily dosage is achieved. Anorexia, nausea, and vomiting are the chief side effects encountered during the early phases of treatment, but these appear to be self-limited and subside over a period of time. Cardiac arrhythmia, particularly paroxysmal tachycardia, hypotension with orthostatic syncope insomnia agitation, and occasional mental disturbances have been encountered at higher dosage level. Decrease in the dose usually alleviates these side effects. Involuntary movements of the choreatic and athetotic variety tend to appear in a significant number of patients on long-term treatment, but are well tolerated in most and are preferred to the parkinsonian symptoms. These movements can also be diminished by careful adjustment of the dosage of levodopa. Many patients experience synergistic effects when levodopa is combined with one of the anticholinergic agents and, in fact,

the combination of the two may prove to be the optimal form of therapy at the present time. It can be anticipated that further derivatives of the catecholamines will be developed which will significantly improve their effectiveness in controlling parkinsonism.

Surgical Measures. Surgical attempts to alleviate parkinsonism are primarily directed to the interruption of one or more neural pathways, the integrity of which appears essential for the production of symptoms, and at a site where normal sensory and motor functions will not be affected. Lesions produced by electrocoagulation or freezing in the ventrolateral nucleus of the thalamus have relieved contralateral tremor and rigidity in the limbs. However, akinesia and disturbances in gait, posture, and voice are not appreciably improved, and multiple lesions are necessary to relieve cervical, truncal, and bilateral limb symptoms. Since in most cases tremor and rigidity are bilateral, a good result on one side often encourages an attempt to do the same for the other. Most surgeons prefer to wait six months to one year before operating on the second side to minimize the complications that are apt to occur with bilateral procedures. Even so, the bilateral procedure frequently produces adverse effects on speech and, though recovery usually occurs, the patient may retain some degree of dysarthria and hypophonia. Since in most cases the manifestations become bilateral within a year or two of the onset, and disability is eventually due not so much to tremor or rigidity but to akinesia and postural abnormalities, stereotactic surgery benefits only a limited number of patients. The best candidate for surgery is the patient whose chief manifestation is unilateral tremor and rigidity, preferably in the upper extremity, and whose disease seems to progress slowly. These characteristics represent an early stage of the disease, and usually the patient is not yet seriously disabled. Thus, proponents of stereotactic surgery urge that thalamotomy be considered early in the course of Parkinson's disease, although its critics have pointed out that surgery does not benefit the more advanced patients who most need help, nor does it prevent progression of the disease. The introduction of more effective pharmacologic therapy with its potential of completely controlling parkinsonian symptoms has diminished the enthusiasm for surgical intervention. A balanced judgment would be that thalamotomy be reserved for cases resistant to other forms of therapy and in which relief of upper limb tremor is desired.

ESSENTIAL TREMOR
(Familial Tremor)
Melvin D. Yahr

This is a monosymptomatic condition in which tremor involves the hands and/or head and face. The tremor is usually more rapid than that encountered in parkinsonism, is accentuated by emotional factors, may be worsened by volitional movement, and is usually suppressed by the use of alcohol. The age of onset is variable, but in most cases the disorder begins prior to the age of 25 years and tends to persist throughout life. Some minor progression of the intensity of tremor and spread to other bodily parts usually occur over the years. There is a strong familial incidence, with occurrence in several successive generations and members of the same family, but the genetic pattern of inheritance has not been determined. To date no specific pathologic lesion has been reported in the nervous system of people with this condition. It has been suggested that the condition is an abortive form of parkinsonism, but this concept does not appear justifiable at present. There is no specific effective therapy for controlling the tremor, although sedatives such as phenobarbital, in dosage of 15 mg. three times a day, may reduce its intensity. It is of utmost importance to differentiate essential tremor from parkinsonism. By and large, the distinguishing characteristics are earlier age of onset; lack of severe progression, akinesia, rigidity, or postural abnormalities; and the strong family history of tremor.

SENILE TREMOR
Melvin D. Yahr

Tremor is a frequent finding in the elderly, most often involving the upper limbs and head. It differs from parkinsonian tremor in that it is finer and more rapid and at first occurs only with voluntary movements. As time goes on it becomes more constant and is also present while the limbs are at rest. There is no associated weakness or alteration in muscle tone. These features differentiate this form of tremor from parkinsonism. The cause is unknown. Since senile tremor has both cerebellar and extrapyramidal features, in that it occurs at rest and with movement, the assumption is that some critical pathway linking these systems has undergone degeneration. There is no effective treatment. Most patients accept it as another of the many changes that come with advancing years. Occasional patients have to be reassured that they do not have parkinsonism or some other progressive neurologic disorder.

THE CHOREAS
Melvin D. Yahr

There are a number of disease entities that, though wholly unrelated etiologically, have choreiform movements as their major manifestation. In some, intimate relationships with infectious processes have been found, whereas in others familial tendencies have pointed to a strong genetic component. In the light of newer concepts of inheritance, a common pathogenesis

for all may be found. Although controversy exists as to the exact anatomic site from which movements of this type may derive, pathologic changes are commonly found in the striatum, particularly in the small cell components of the caudate nucleus and putamen. The classification of chorea into separate entities is at present somewhat arbitrary and is based on age of onset, association with identifiable disease processes or familial tendency, and occurrence of other neurologic abnormalities.

ACUTE CHOREA
(Sydenham's or Infectious Chorea, St. Vitus' Dance)

Acute chorea is a movement disorder encountered primarily during childhood and having its greatest incidence between the ages of 5 and 15 years. Occurrence beyond this age is uncommon, and then is usually in association with pregnancy or in persons who have had symptoms earlier in life. Females manifest these symptoms at least twice as often as males. Acute chorea has been reported in people of all races.

Considered as a symptom complex rather than as a specific disease entity, acute chorieform movements have been encountered as initial manifestations of a variety of conditions. They have been reported in epidemic encephalitis, in the encephalopathies occurring with exanthema, with pertussis and diphtheria, in idiopathic hypocalcemia, hyperthyroidism, systemic lupus erythematosus, carbon monoxide poisoning, vascular disease, tumors, and degenerative processes of the basal ganglia. These instances, however, account for only a small percentage of cases. The closest relationship appears to be with rheumatic fever. In more than half of the cases, rheumatic manifestations consisting of carditis, valvular heart disease, or arthritis occur prior to, coincident with, or following an attack of chorea.

There are no specific pathologic changes or anatomic sites of involvement that can be correlated with acute chorea. In fact, because acute uncomplicated chorea is rarely fatal, there has been a paucity of detailed pathologic studies. Cases that have come to autopsy have shown scattered changes in the cortex, basal ganglia, cerebellum, and brainstem. These have consisted of varying degrees of arteritis combined with cellular degeneration.

The outstanding clinical features of chorea are involuntary movements, incoordination, muscle weakness, and emotional lability. Although the onset of symptoms may be abrupt and obvious, it is more often insidious and subtle. The most frequent initial complaints include clumsiness of the limbs, evidenced by dropping objects from the hands or an awkward gait, particularly during emotionally tense situations. When these are coupled with irritability, poor performance in school, and generally fidgety behavior, frequently a hasty conclusion is reached, blaming the child or implying a psychiatric disorder. The typical choreatic movements may be noted in any part of the body, limbs, face, hands, tongue, or trunk. They may at first appear to be a part of the natural pattern of coordinated movements but are soon noted to be completely random, jerking, aimless, and purposeless. They occur at rest, are accentuated by any attempt at volitional movement, and disappear in sleep. They may be very mild and may minimally affect normal function or may be so forceful and frequent as to be totally disabling. Facial grimacing and difficulty in speech, chewing, and swallowing occur when the muscles subserving these functions are involved. Interruption of voluntary movements by involuntary ones leads to incoordination so that the person drops objects, walks in an awkward, ungainly fashion and, in general, appears uncoordinated. Attempts to maintain forceful muscular contraction are similarly interrupted, and the resultant "waxing and waning" of motor power results in a relative degree of motor weakness. Although actual paralysis is rare, there is a disinclination to use a part of the body that is severely affected by involuntary movements of this type. Generalized reduction of muscle tone is an invariable feature of chorea and is readily demonstrable by hyperextensibility at finger, wrist, and ankle joints. In almost all choreatic children some degree of emotional lability is evident. It varies from total apathy to irritability, restlessness, and, infrequently, wild, inappropriate behavior.

Certain cardinal features can be found in almost all patients. These include (1) pronation of the forearm when the upper limbs are raised and extended; (2) inability to sustain muscle contraction when the examiner grasps the patient's hand or when the patient protrudes his tongue so that it darts rapidly in and out of the mouth; and (3) abnormal posturing of hands in which the wrist is noted to be sharply flexed and the fingers hyperextended at the metacarpal pharyngeal joints.

There are no specific laboratory tests for chorea. The cerebrospinal fluid is normal. The electroencephalogram may or may not show diffuse abnormalities correlated with the severity of the disease. Unless there are associated disease processes that manifest themselves in abnormalities of blood count, chemistry, or sedimentation rate, these studies are normal.

The age of onset and the distinctive involuntary movements readily differentiate acute chorea from other disorders of the basal ganglia. Tics and habit spasms may be confused with mild cases, but their movements are quite different, being stereotyped repetitive patterns localized to a single group of muscles. Huntington's chorea rarely begins in childhood and, in addition, there is a strong familial tendency with associated dementia. Movement disorders associated with cerebral palsy occur in infancy but have an athetoid element. The use of phenothiazines may induce abnormal movements, but the history of drug ingestion will differentiate these.

Acute chorea is a self-limited disease, recovery occurring in two to six months. Recurrence, with as many as two or three attacks over a period of years, appears in almost one third of the cases. There is no specific therapy. Bed rest and reduction of external stimuli to a minimum, combined with sedative drugs such as phenobarbital or chloral hydrate, are beneficial in controlling the severity of the movements. Paradoxically, the phenothiazines, such as thorazine and chlorpromazine, as well as reserpine in doses commensurate with individual tolerance, although capable of inducing chorea, have also been shown to be effective in its control. Because of the high incidence of rheumatic valvular heart disease complicating acute chorea, prophylaxis with antimicrobial drugs over a long interval of time similar to that utilized in acute rheumatic fever is now recommended. If emotional symptoms are intense, psychotherapy may be in order. When specific abnormalities of calcium metabolism or thyroid dysfunction are found, their correction may completely ameliorate the symptoms. With recovery most patients show few, if any, neurologic sequelae.

HEREDITARY CHOREA
(Chronic Progressive Chorea, Huntington's Chorea)

Hereditary chorea is a progressive degenerative disease of the basal ganglia and cerebral cortex, beginning in adult life and characterized by choreiform movements and mental deterioration. The inheritance of the disease is based on a single dominant autosomal gene. It may be transmitted by either sex, and both sexes are affected in equal numbers. The trait is transmitted from affected individual to affected individual so that those who escape rarely transmit the disease. Only about 50 per cent of the offspring are affected. The disease is relatively rare, although its incidence may be high in geographic regions where affected families have resided for many generations.

Although the pattern of inheritance suggests a disturbance in one of the enzyme systems of the brain, to date this defect has not been elucidated. Pathologically, widespread degenerative changes with cell loss and reactive gliosis are found, primarily in the cerebral cortex and caudate nucleus.

The clinical manifestations consist of choreatic movements, emotional disturbance, and intellectual deterioration in varying degrees, rate of appearance, and progression. The disease usually makes its appearance between the ages of 35 and 50 years, rather insidiously with any of the above symptoms, but as a rule with abnormal movements. The movements, though similar to acute chorea, are usually more jerky though less lightning-like and primarily involve the trunk and shoulder girdle and more often the lower limbs than the upper. This pattern of involvement tends to produce a dancing sort of gait, which is a prominent feature of the disease. In rare instances a Parkinson-like rigidity is encountered as the major manifestation rather than involuntary movements. The mental deterioration is similar to that of any organic dementia, with progressive impairment of memory and of intellectual capacity, and inattention to personal hygiene. Emotional disturbances include heightened irritability, bouts of depression, and fits of violent behavior.

With the typical triad of choreiform movements, dementia in adult life, and documentation of similar symptoms in family members, the diagnosis is readily evident. However, there is a tendency for families to deny the existence of mental disease, and it is sometimes difficult to obtain corroborative data even when the diagnosis is strongly suspected. Little difficulty occurs in differentiating hereditary chorea from acute chorea, but senile chorea may raise a problem. The latter, which comes on late in life, involves few mental changes, if any, lacks a familial history, and is usually benign in comparison. Other diseases such as the presenile psychoses, Alzheimer's and Pick's, because of their dementia and similarity in age of onset, may offer some difficulty, especially in instances in which choreiform movements are inconspicuous. Pneumoencephalography demonstrating selective atrophy of the caudate nucleus may help to establish the correct diagnosis in such instances. There is a tendency to overdiagnose hereditary chorea, applying it to diverse neurologic disorders such as cerebellar degenerations and familial tremors. The dire implications of this form of chorea require strict adherence to the diagnostic criteria.

There is no effective therapy. Huntington's chorea is relentlessly progressive, leading to total incapacity and inevitably death, usually within 15 years of onset. In the early stages the patient can be managed at home with supervision and the use of phenothiazines or reserpine to reduce the intensity of the movements and to control the behavior to some extent. As the disease advances, confinement to a psychiatric facility becomes necessary.

SENILE CHOREA

Infrequently, choreiform movements are encountered as an isolated symptom in persons above 60 years of age. As a rule, the movements are mild and may involve the limbs on one side of the body or bilaterally, with choreiform movements in both lower extremities. No associated mental disturbance occurs in such patients, and no family history indicative of Huntington's chorea can be obtained. In many instances the symptoms come on abruptly, are unilateral, and show little, if any, progression. This has suggested an underlying vascular lesion, which may be found in an exceptional case. More often than not the pathologic findings are similar to those of Huntington's chorea insofar as involvement of the caudate

nucleus is concerned, but the cerebral cortex is spared. This has led to the contrary consideration that these cases are a variant of Huntington's chorea occurring sporadically. Probably this form of chorea has several causes. As a rule, the symptoms are mild and the course benign so that therapeutic considerations are unimportant.

TICS
(Habit Spasms)
Melvin D. Yahr

A tic is a sudden, abrupt, rapid, purposeless, involuntary contraction of a muscle or group of functionally related muscles. Usually an irregular sequence of such contractions occurs that may result in eye blinking, head shaking, shrugging of the shoulder, or any sudden gesture of limbs or face. Tics may be voluntarily controlled for brief intervals, but such a conscious effort is usually followed by more intense and frequent contractions. Many persons experience minor transitory tic phenomena under periods of stress that are of no consequence. More persistent, sustained, and gross movements may be related to particular personality disturbances, and may be amenable to psychotherapy. In some instances tics have occurred during the acute phase of encephalitis; these are thought to be an expression of extrapyramidal dysfunction. Tics in younger patients must be differentiated from chorea. Their patterned, predictable, and stereotyped character makes this distinction.

An unusual form of generalized tic (*maladie des tics, Gilles de la Tourette's disease*) involving facial twitching, continuous gestures associated with echolalia, foul language, and obsessional ideas is occasionally encountered in childhood. The disorder is progressive, and sometimes associated with marked personality changes. Recently, however, a number of reports have appeared suggesting that haloperidol (Haldol) in divided dosage of 6 to 20 mg. a day may be effective both in reducing the movement disorder and in overcoming the unfortunate verbal outbursts.

ATHETOSIS
(Mobile Spasms)
Melvin D. Yahr

This involuntary movement disorder is most frequently encountered in early infancy. Although in some respects it resembles chorea and although there are, in fact, transitional forms (so-called choreo-athetosis), the athetotic movements are distinguishable by being slower, coarser, and more writhing. They occur when pathologic conditions involve the basal ganglia, primarily the pallidum, as well as additional motor pathways such as the corticospinal tract. Athetosis is most often found in the heterogeneous group of conditions now lumped together under the term "cerebral palsy." Congenital defects, anoxia, or trauma at birth and other degenerative conditions have all been implicated. Some attempt has been made to identify specific entities based on clinicopathologic correlations. One such is athetosis simplex or status marmoratus. Cases of this disorder, which exemplifies all of the features of athetosis, show at autopsy a distinctive marbled appearance of the basal ganglia, the result of an abnormal overgrowth of myelin sheaths and increased numbers of glial cells. The cause of this morphologic abnormality is unknown. Other cases have been grouped together in which the prime pathologic change is cell loss and failure of myelin sheath formation in the region of the basal ganglia—so-called status dysmyelination. Still other cases have been encountered in which abnormal deposits of pigments occur or one of the lipoidoses or other storage diseases is found with the predominant clinical picture of athetotic movements. Athetosis is infrequently encountered in adult life, but when it is, tumors, vascular insufficiency, or malformations and the effects of toxic agents have been found in the region of the basal ganglia.

Typical athetosis possesses the following features in varying degrees. One or both sides of the body are involved. The movements involve the upper limbs to a greater extent than the lower and primarily in their distal segments. The muscles innervated by the cranial nerves are invariably involved so that facial grimacing, writhing movements of the tongue, and disturbances in articulation and swallowing are encountered. Abnormal postures of the limbs are assumed. In the upper extremities, these consist of adduction and internal rotation at the shoulder, semiflexion at the elbow, flexion of wrist and metacarpal phalangeal joints, and extension at interphalangeal joints. In the lower limbs the foot is maintained in internal rotation and plantar flexion with dorsiflexion of the toes. Superimposed on these abnormal postures are the athetotic movements described above. Muscle tone is increased during movement but is hypotonic during relaxation, and some degree of weakness is usually found. The reflexes may be hyperactive, with abnormal toe responses. In many instances some degree of intellectual impairment may be found.

The abnormal movements and postural abnormalities are distinctive enough to make this condition readily recognizable. The age at onset, the admixture of other neurologic abnormalities, and the manner in which the symptoms progress identify the disease. Since most instances of athetosis appear in early infancy, before one year of age, diseases of the perinatal period are considered primarily. Athetosis occurring in later childhood or adult life may be a part of other extrapyramidal disorders, such as dystonia, chorea, or hepatolenticular degeneration. Less frequently athetosis is a manifestation of a wide spectrum of neurologic disorders already mentioned in which the pallidum is coincidentally involved.

There is no specific therapy for the relief of athetosis. The use of anticholinergic agents as previously indicated under the treatment of parkinsonism may decrease the intensity of the movements. Thalamotomy has on occasion afforded some degree of relief, but one is hesitant to advocate this surgical procedure on a nervous system already extensively damaged by a variety of pathologic processes.

DYSTONIA MUSCULORUM DEFORMANS
(Torsion Dystonia)
Melvin D. Yahr

This is a rare disease characterized by intense sustained torsion spasms of the musculature with resultant marked abnormalities of bodily posture. The dystonic movements may involve any or all of the musculature, but have a predilection for the trunk and shoulder and pelvic girdles. Although dystonic movements occur with hepatolenticular degeneration, postencephalitic Parkinson's, and tumors or other diseases involving the basal ganglia, dystonia musculorum deformans is a distinct clinical entity. The cause and morbid anatomy of this condition are unknown. A hereditary basis has been suggested for some forms of this disorder. Glial scarring in the basal ganglia, thalamus, and cortex has been described in some cases, and some have been associated with status marmoratus and dysmyelination, as indicated in the article on Athetosis.

The onset of the disease is variable and gradual, and usually occurs between the ages of 5 and 15 years. Most frequently it begins with intermittent spasmodic inversion of the foot, so that on walking the child finds difficulty in placing the heel on the ground. Bizarre stepping or a bowing gait may be noted when the dystonic movements affect the more proximal muscles of the leg or the spine. As the movements become more intense and the proximal musculature is more prominently involved, lordosis and tortipelvis appear. If the muscles of the neck and shoulder girdle are involved, torticollis is an early finding. Facial grimacing and difficulties in speech become evident as the muscles subserving these functions become involved. The continuous spasms over a period of time result in marked distortions of the body of a degree rarely seen in any other disease process. Although muscle tone and power appear to be normal, the involuntary movements interfere with function to such a degree as to make them useless. No changes in the deep tendon reflexes occur, and mentation remains normal.

In its early stages dystonia musculorum deformans must be differentiated from other movement disorders in which dystonic phenomena may occur. The history and physical findings rule out hepatolenticular degeneration and epidemic encephalitis. The age at onset and the involvement of proximal musculature in the movements are enough to differentiate it from athetosis. Chorea is characterized by movements more rapid and of shorter duration than those of dystonia. Hysteria is often a consideration; if it is not positively established by the personality characteristics of the patient, the course of the disease will soon suggest the correct diagnosis.

There is extreme variability in the rate of progression and eventual disability. In its early phases there may be complete remission of symptoms or lack of progression of initial symptoms for intervals of up to five years. Because the natural history is subject to wide variations, evaluation of the effects of treatment is difficult. Dystonic movements have been effectively controlled for varying periods of time by both drugs and surgical intervention. The medicines effective are anticholinergic agents such as those indicated for the treatment of parkinsonism, combined with sedative agents such as phenobarbital. In mild cases a combination of these drugs with some general supportive psychotherapy may be enough to control the patient's symptoms for years. In more serious cases thalamotomy has produced encouraging results. However, because rather extensive lesions must be placed in the thalamic nuclei, multiple operative procedures are required to produce the desired effect. Although the operations are well tolerated by most patients, they do carry an element of risk, and are indicated only in selective cases. Levodopa has been reported as being effective in selected cases. In general a lower daily dose (3 grams per day) than that used in parkinsonism has been required.

SPASMODIC TORTICOLLIS
Melvin D. Yahr

The restriction of dyskinetic movements to neck muscles so that abnormal postures of the head result is the distinguishing characteristic of this symptom complex. Involuntary activity involves the sternocleidomastoids, trapezius, and scalenus muscles in sustained contractions that result in slow, twisting, turning movements of the head (torticollis) or less often forward flexion (anterocollis) or forceful extension (retrocollis). In most instances there is bilateral involvement, and the resultant postural deformity is maintained for varying lengths of time. The muscles of the neck appear under tension, and the continual muscular activity may lead to some degree of hypertrophy, especially evident in the sternocleidomastoid. Similar activity may spread to facial and brachial musculature. The amount of active motion or static postural deformity is extremely variable.

Spasmodic torticollis has variably been described as a psychogenic disorder, a fragment of dystonia musculorum deformans, a compensatory postural defect in persons with congenital ocular muscle imbalance or defects of the cervical spine or musculature. In some instances it has occurred as part of a wide spectrum of extrapyramidal disorders following encephalitis lethargica. There is no information at present regarding either its pathophysiology or pathology.

The disorder has been encountered at all ages, but most frequently makes its appearance during the third to sixth decades of life. The course is extremely variable, being transitory and remitting after a few months in some patients and relentlessly progressive and leading to incapacity in others. Some cases reach a static phase in which movements cease or are minimal, and a minor postural deformity of the head persists.

The evaluation of this condition includes a search for ocular and vertebral signs, major psychiatric disturbances, and other neurologic conditions with which it may be associated. Definable conditions account for only a small percentage of cases. In most, no known cause is uncovered.

There is no specific therapy for torticollis except when an underlying correctible disease process is found. Many measures have been recommended to ameliorate the symptoms. In mild cases or in the initial stages, a combination of drugs previously discussed under the treatment of parkinsonism has proved useful. Symptoms may be reduced to a tolerable degree, and it can be hoped that spontaneous remission will intervene. In those more severely affected a variety of surgical measures have been attempted with inconsistent results. Denervation of the affected muscles by section of the anterior cervical roots and/or the spinal accessory nerve has been utilized. Although the movements decrease on the operated side, they frequently recur in the contralateral group of muscles. Bilateral procedures may result in extensive disability. Recently thalamotomy has been performed with encouraging results. One is hesitant, however, to recommend a procedure of this magnitude except in extreme situations.

HEMIBALLISM
Melvin D. Yahr

This rather violent involuntary movement occurs when lesions involve the contralateral subthalamic nucleus, the corpus Luysii. Although a variety of pathologic processes such as tumor and infectious diseases have been found as underlying causes, most are a result of vascular lesions, either hemorrhagic or occlusive. In consequence, they are encountered in older patients, sometimes after a transitory hemiparesis. The event leading to the onset of this movement disorder often is an acute cerebrovascular accident with weakness and/or sensory deficit. As the neurologic signs clear or at a variable interval afterward, the ballistic movements begin. The movements do not occur during sleep, are localized to one side of the body and involve the limbs in a forceful throwing movement, a result of almost continuous activity of the proximal musculature. Their violence exhausts and incapacitates the patient to such an extent that death may ensue. In some persons, the initial intensity decreases gradually so that they become tolerable, and in approximately half such patients the movements stop spontaneously. Surgical measures, such as thalamotomy, are rarely needed for control. In this regard, it is interesting to note that hemiballismus has followed attempted thalamotomy for other extrapyramidal disorders when poor localization for lesion placement has occurred. In such instances, the surgeon has inadvertently placed a lesion in the region of the corpus Luysii.

Aron, A., Freeman, J., and Carter, S.: The natural history of Sydenham's chorea. Amer. J. Med., 38:83, 1965.

Bucy, P. C., and Buchanan, D. N.: Athetosis. Brain, 55:479, 1932.

Carpenter, M. B.: Ballism associated with partial destruction of the subthalamic nucleus of Luys. Neurology, 5:479, 1955.

Chandler, J. H., Reed, T. E., and DeJong, R. N.: Huntington's chorea in Michigan. Neurology, 10:148, 1960.

Cooper, I. S.: Thalamic surgery for dystonia and torticollis. Bull. N. Y. Acad. Med., 41:870, 1965.

Costa, E., Cote, L., and Yahr, M. D.: Biochemistry and Pharmacology of the Basal Ganglia. Hewlett, New York, Raven Press, 1966.

Cotzias, G. C.: VanWoert, M. H., and Schiffer, L. M.: Aromatic amino acids and modification of parkinsonism. New Eng. J. Med., 276:374, 1967.

Courville, C. B.: Structural basis of athetosis in cerebral palsied children. Arch. Pediat., 78:461, 1961.

Critchley, M.: Observations on essential (heredofamilial) tremor. Brain, 22:113, 1949.

Denny-Brown, D.: The Cerebral Control of Movement. Springfield, Ill., 1966. Charles C Thomas.

Denny-Brown, D. E.: The nature of dystonia. Bull. N. Y. Acad. Med., 41:858, 1965.

Duvoisin, R. C., and Yahr, M. D.: Encephalitis and parkinsonism. Arch. Neurol. (Chicago), 12:227, 1965.

Fields, W. S. (ed.): Pathogenesis and Treatment of Parkinsonism. Springfield, Ill., Charles C Thomas, 1958.

Herz, E.: Dystonia. Arch. Neurol. Psychiat., 51:305, 319, 1944; 52:20, 1944.

Herz, E., and Glaser, G. H.: Spasmodic torticollis. Clinical evaluation. Arch. Neurol. Psychiat., 61:227, 1949.

Jager, B. V.: Hereditary tremor. Arch. Intern. Med. (Chicago), 95:778, 1953.

Lyon, R. L.: Huntington's chorea. Brit. Med. J., 1:1306, 1962.

Markham, C. H., Brown, W. J., and Rand, R. W.: Stereotaxic lesions in Parkinson's disease. Arch. Neurol. 15:480, 1966.

Marshall, J.: Observations on essential tremor. J. Neurol. Neurosurg. Psychiat., 25:122, 1962.

Martin, J. P.: Hemichorea resulting from local lesions of the brain. Brain, 50:637, 1927.

Martin, P. J., and McCaul, I. R.: Acute hemiballism treated by ventrolateral thalamolysis. Brain, 82:104, 1959.

McDowell, F. H., et al.: Treatment of Parkinson's syndrome with L-dihydroxyphenylalanine (levodopa). Ann. Intern. Med., 72:29, 1970.

Mettler, F. A., and Stern, G.: On the pathophysiology of athetosis. J. Nerv. Ment. Dis., 135:138, 1962.

Onuaguluchi, G.: Parkinsonism. London, Butterworth, 1964.

Patterson, R. M., and Little, S. C.: Spasmodic torticollis. J. Nerv. & Mental Dis., 98:571, 1943.

Schwartzman, J.: Chorea minor. Review of 175 cases with reference to etiology, treatment and sequelae. Rheumatism, 6:89, 1950.

Shapiro, A., and Shapiro, E.: Treatment of Gilles de la Tourette's syndrome with haloperidol. Brit. J. Psychiat., 114:345, 1968.

Yahr, M. D. (ed.): Symposium on Basal Ganglia Diseases. Bull. New York Acad. Med., 41:855, 1965.

Yahr, M. D., Duvoisin, R. C., Schear, M. J., Barrett, R. E., and Hoehn, M. M.: Treatment of parkinsonism with levodopa. Arch. Neurol. (Chicago), 21:343, 1969.

IDIOPATHIC AUTONOMIC INSUFFICIENCY
(Idiopathic Orthostatic Hypotension)
Fred Plum

Definition.   This is an uncommon disorder first clearly described by Bradbury and Eggleston in 1925 as idiopathic orthostatic hypotension; it has been more recently emphasized as including more generalized autonomic and nervous system defects. The cause is unknown and the course progressive, disability or death usually occurring within five to ten years after onset.

Pathology and Pathogenesis.   Only a limited number of patients have received detailed examination of the central and peripheral nervous system at autopsy, not always with consistent findings. Degenerative changes have been found involving the autonomic ganglia, the intermediolateral and ventral neurons of the spinal cord, as well as various nuclear structures in the brainstem, the cerebellum, and the basal ganglia. However in some patients with apparently typical clinical disease, any or all of these structures have also been found to be histologically normal, leading to the hypothesis that a defect in autonomic transmitter function precedes any morphologic changes. Suggestions that the neuropathologic changes are anoxic and secondary to recurrent hypotension are unlikely to be correct, since the lesions lack the appearance and distribution of those caused by well documented anoxia.

Several observations support the idea of a defect in transmitter function. Most of the patients demonstrate a blood pressure hypersensitivity to injected levarterenol, implying the absence of the humoral agent in the sympathetic ganglia. Also, patients with neurogenic orthostatic hypotension have been found not to synthesize norepinephrine and its metabolic products in normal amounts and to have below normal urinary catecholamine levels. Since the drug tyramine, which acts to release norepinephrine from peripheral autonomic nerve terminals, is effective in elevating the blood pressure, at least some epinephrine synthesis must be going on in postganglionic peripheral nerve terminals, but whether this is of a normal or reduced amount is unknown.

Clinical Manifestations.   Symptoms of autonomic insufficiency predominate initially. These include impotence in males, constipation, heat intolerance with anhidrosis, and above all, weakness or faintness on rising to an erect position or during quiet standing. Urinary urgency or retention is common. As the disease progresses, symptoms of more generalized neurologic dysfunction appear. Some patients develop a Parkinson-like illness with hypokinesia, rhythmic postural tremor, and mild to moderate rigidity. Others develop a cerebellar type of incoordination plus a gross rhythmic tremor in the lower extremities. The mind remains clear.

Physical signs include prominent evidence of autonomic insufficiency. Pupillary abnormalities with Horner's syndrome can alternate from side to side. Even with a high environmental temperature there is diffuse anhidrosis of the trunk and extremities. The blood pressure is normal when the subject lies supine, but when he stands, systolic and diastolic pressures drop 20 to 40 mm. Hg or more but the pulse fails to accelerate. In the early stage of illness the blood pressure can gradually climb during continued standing, but as the disease advances, autonomic compensation decreases then fails altogether, and syncope with unobtainable blood pressure tends to interrupt any sustained effort to be erect. By this time, many patients have associated signs of generalized neurologic dysfunction, including the Parkinson-like signs mentioned above as well as a cerebellar type of incoordination, muscle wasting and fasciculations, coarse tremors, and extensor plantar responses. Signs of peripheral neuropathy are notably lacking in the idiopathic disease.

Laboratory tests of the usual type are valueless except to exclude other disorders, but confirmation of the autonomic insufficiency makes the diagnosis.

Birchfield has presented a useful approach to evaluating autonomic insufficiency. Briefly, the evaluation investigates the blood pressure response to tilting and quiet standing, the patient's ability to sweat when heated, a cold pressor test (the response is absent), the blood pressure response to injected levarterenol and sublingual nitroglycerin (the responses are hyperactive), and the response to the Valsalva maneuver (the normal blood pressure overshoot with its accompanying tachycardia fail to occur).

Differential Diagnosis. Orthostatic hypotension can accompany acute cardiac failure (as with myocardial infarction or severe aortic stenosis), blood volume depletion (as with gastrointestinal or other massive hemorrhage), or vasodepressor syncope, but in all these conditions other signs of autonomic activity such as tachycardia and sweating are present and signs of diffuse neurologic illness are absent. Autonomic insufficiency also accompanies some clearly identifiable neurologic diseases, including central thiamin deficiency (Wernicke's encephalopathy), tabes dorsalis,

syringomyelia, surgical sympathectomy, the neuropathies of diabetes, amyloidosis, and the Guillain-Barré syndrome, and a small fraction of patients who have vascular occlusive disease producing infarction or ischemia of brainstem autonomic centers. The differentiation from most of these illnesses is readily made by the typical signs, symptoms, and laboratory findings of each, and particularly by the fact that most of them produce sensory impairments in the extremities and other peripheral nerve abnormalities which are altogether lacking in idiopathic autonomic insufficiency.

Course and Treatment. Although treatment is rarely completely satisfactory and does not affect the disease itself, much can be done to help these patients symptomatically, particularly during the early phase of the illness. Nine-α-fluorohydrocortisone given regularly by mouth is often effective in counteracting the orthostatic hypotension; it presumably operates partly by increasing the blood volume. Elastic bandages on the legs may help by reducing venous pooling. Placing the head of the bed on six-inch blocks for sleeping has been found to lessen the next day's degree of orthostatic hypotension. Pressor agents have generally been useless because of their short, intense action and undesirable side effects. However, a combination of monoamine oxidase inhibitors (which prevent the breakdown of tyramine in the liver) and tyramine (which in the United States must presently be given in the form of New York State cheddar cheese, since the drug is not approved by the United States Food and Drug Adminstration) has been found effective in maintaining the erect blood pressure of some patients previously bedridden from their illness.

Bannister, R., Ardill, L., and Fentem, P.: An assessment of various methods of treatment of idiopathic orthostatic hypotension. Quart. J. Med., 38:377, 1969.

Birchfield, R. G.: Postural hypotension in Wernicke's disease. Amer. J. Med., 36:404, 1964.

Bradbury, S., and Eggleston, C.: Postural hypotension: Report of 3 cases. Amer. Heart J., 1:73, 1925.

Diamond, M. A., Murray, R. H., and Schmid, P.: Idiopathic postural hypotension: Physiologic observations and report of a new mode of therapy. J. Clin. Invest., 49:1341, 1970.

Diamond, M. A., Murray, R. H., and Schmid, P.: Treatment of idiopathic postural hypotension with oral tyramine and monoamine oxidase inhibitor. Clin. Res., 17:237, 1969.

Shy, R. M., and Drager, G. A.: A neurological syndrome associated with orthostatic hypotension. Arch. Neurol. (Chicago), 2:511, 1960.

Stead, E. A., Jr., and Ebert, R. V.: Postural hypotension: Disease of sympathetic nervous system. Arch. Intern. Med., 67:546, 1941.

Cerebrovascular Diseases
Fletcher H. McDowell

It is estimated that there are 2 million persons alive today who have neurologic manifestations of cerebrovascular disease and that cerebrovascular disease of all varieties is annually respon-

sible for approximately 200,000 deaths in the United States. Fully a half million Americans each year suffer a new, acute cerebrovascular attack. The over-all problem is even more imposing than the annual incidence and mortality figures. Recurrent vascular accidents are common in nearly all forms of cerebrovascular disease, each recurrence carrying a high risk of mortality. For the survivors, disability and dependency are the usual result. The need for medical care and hospital facilities for these patients is enormous and is an imposing challenge to medical and social service agencies alike.

In the following discussion, the cerebral vascular diseases are divided into two general groups, those producing ischemic *cerebral infarction* and those producing *intracranial hemorrhage*. Much of the material is derived from observations on 966 patients with clinically diagnosed cerebral vascular disease undergoing long-term study at the Cornell Division of Bellevue Hospital in New York City. As a rough index of the frequency of the different types of cerebral vascular accident or "stroke," 88 per cent of these patients had acute infarction or less severe cerebral ischemic attacks, and 12 per cent had intracranial hemorrhage. Of the infarctions, about one in eight was attributed to cerebral embolism.

CEREBRAL ISCHEMIA AND INFARCTION

DEFINITION AND ETIOLOGY

Cerebral thrombosis and cerebral emboli produce clinical symptoms by causing cerebral infarction, which means neural death from ischemia. Cerebral ischemia is the result of either a generalized or a localized prolonged reduction of blood flow to the brain. If ischemia is transient, less than 10 to 15 minutes, usually no discernible neurologic deficit remains. If it lasts longer than that, neural damage results, producing neurologic dysfunction, disability, and death.

The causes of cerebral infarction are numerous. The following are the most common ones:

1. Atherosclerotic disease of the intra- and extracranial arteries
2. Cerebral emboli with: (a) rheumatic heart disease, (b) myocardial infarction, (c) cardiac disease and atrial fibrillation, (d) subacute bacterial endocarditis, (e) nonbacterial thrombotic endocarditis
3. Reduced cerebral blood flow from severe hypotension or dysrhythmia of cardiac disease
4. Cerebral arterial spasm following subarachnoid hemorrhage
5. Generalized cerebral hypoxia from (a) cardiopulmonary insufficiency, (b) pulmonary emboli, (c) carbon monoxide poisoning
6. Cerebral thrombosis due to arteritis: (a) collagen vascular disease, (b) giant cell arteritis, (c) bacterial arteritis, including syphilis
7. Cerebral thrombosis due to polycythemia or ischemia caused by severe anemia
8. Cerebral thrombosis adjacent to intracerebral hemorrhage
9. Cerebral arterial vasoconstriction associated with migraine
10. Dissecting aneurysm of the aorta or great vessels in the neck

INCIDENCE AND EPIDEMIOLOGY

Cerebral infarction is most commonly the result of cerebral atherosclerosis and cerebral emboli. In the Cornell-Bellevue series of 873 cases with nonhemorrhagic stroke, 92 per cent were clinically related to cerebral atherosclerosis and 8 per cent to cerebral emboli. In the group with cerebral emboli 20 per cent occurred in association with myocardial infarction, 26 per cent with rheumatic heart disease and atrial fibrillation, and the remainder in patients with atrial fibrillation associated with other varieties of heart disease.

Cerebral infarction is almost twice as frequent in males as in females. The peak age period is 60 to 69 years, but the incidence of stroke rises linearly with increasing age. In the Cornell-Bellevue study, stroke occurred earlier than the age of 50 in only 8 per cent of the patients.

NEUROPATHOLOGY

The brain is exquisitely dependent on its oxygen supply. There is no reserve of oxygen in cerebral tissue to sustain cerebral metabolism during periods of reduced or absent cerebral blood flow. When the brain is acutely and completely deprived of oxygen generally or locally, the electroencephalogram changes within 10 to 20 seconds, and irreversible and extensive neural damage occurs in the cerebral hemispheres after 3 to 10 minutes. When ischemia is prolonged, the ischemic tissue softens, and the usually distinct margins between gray and white matter become unclear and occasionally hemorrhagic. Under the microscope, neurons are seen to be necrotic and shrunken, i.e., infarcted.

Cerebral infarctions following ischemia may be "pale" (nonhemorrhagic) or hemorrhagic. The extravasation of blood into tissues more commonly follows an embolic arterial obstruction, and pale infarcts more frequently follow atherosclerotic or thrombotic arterial obstruction. Often the two varieties of infarction blend together, and there is little advantage in extensively weighing the difference of causation.

A variable amount of *cerebral edema* accompanies cerebral infarction. With large infarctions the edema may be so extensive that portions of the swollen hemisphere shift under the falx or down through the tentorium cerebelli. This change in intracranial space relationships further impairs the flow of blood and cerebrospinal fluid, thus increasing the ischemia and neurologic deficit. This is often followed by secondary congestion and ischemia of the upper brainstem, which is almost invariably fatal.

It is common to find numerous old, small cerebral infarctions in patients dying from other causes, indicating that cerebral infarctions need not always give rise to symptoms. Old infarctions that have been hemorrhagic are identified at postmortem examination by the presence of hemosiderin in the wall of the infarct. As the infarct ages, the necrotic area breaks down, is absorbed, and eventually may be replaced by a fluid-filled cavity lined with glial and fibrovascular tissue.

MECHANISMS

Cerebral infarction usually involves abnormalities in: the state of the conducting system, i.e., the arterial system from the heart to the brain and the venous system draining the brain; the efficiency of the heart as a pump in producing a constant blood flow at a sufficient arterial pressure; and the character of the circulating medium (blood), its viscosity, its oxygen-carrying capacity, and its capacity to change from a colloidal suspension to a gel. Most cerebral infarctions are due to simultaneous changes in several of these factors.

The arterial conducting system is most often altered by atherosclerotic disease. In the third decade of life atherosclerosis is usually evident in the arteries leading to the brain, particularly in the larger cerebral arteries. Sites of predilection for plaques (Fig. 1) are: the origins of the common carotid artery; just above the common carotid bifurcation; the internal carotid in its siphonous portion; the origin of the middle cerebral artery; and the vertebral arteries just after they enter the skull and the basilar artery. The atheromatous process in cerebral arteries is the same as that found elsewhere in the body, with lipid deposition in the intima, fibrous tissue overgrowth, hemorrhage into the plaques, ulceration of the plaques, and vessel obstruction.

Although atheromatous vascular disease begins early, it is a silent process for most of the life of the patient, and rarely produces symptoms until the middle years, when myocardial infarction, cerebral infarction, and lower extremity infarction

occur. Most postmortem studies show that 80 to 90 per cent of all adult patients examined at autopsy have significant atheromatous disease. Since by no means all of these had experienced adverse clinical effects, the factors determining symptomatic complications assume major importance.

The first factor of importance is the degree and extent of atheromatous vascular disease, both in the arteries in the neck leading to the head and in the intracranial cerebral arteries. In general, persons who have cerebral infarctions have the most extensive cerebrovascular disease in the arteries in the neck and in the head. However, the pathogenesis of infarction depends on several mechanisms, and patients with only small or moderate amounts of vascular disease sometimes suffer serious cerebral infarcts. Conversely, extensive atheromatous disease can be found in large and small intracranial and extracranial cerebral arteries in patients without cerebral infarction.

Diabetes or *hypertension* can be detected in over two thirds of patients who have had cerebrovascular accidents. Patients with either diabetes or hypertension develop atherosclerosis at an earlier age, and the process develops more rapidly than in patients without these complicating illnesses. The atherosclerotic disease is extensive and is found in the smaller intracranial arteries.

The condition of the *cerebral collateral circulation* influences the development of cerebral infarction in persons with atherosclerosis. Most collateral circulation from one major intracerebral

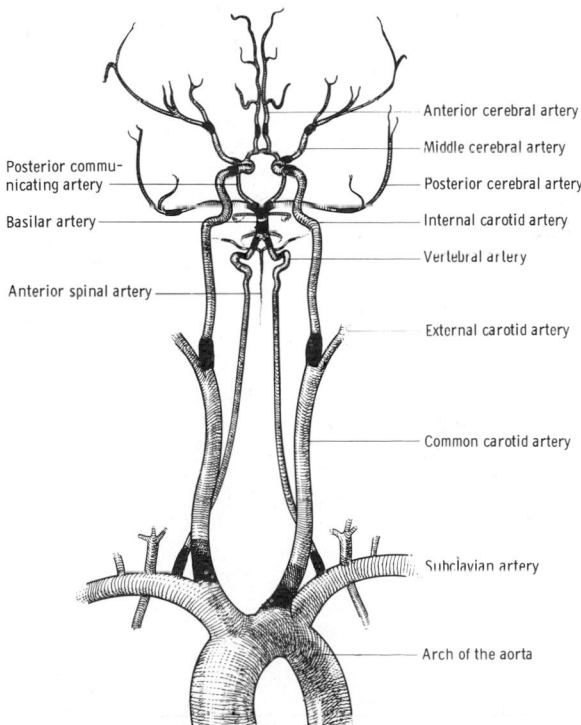

FIGURE 1. The darkened areas on the arterial diagram show the common sites of atherosclerosis and obstruction in the cerebral vessels.

arterial system to another is through the circle of Willis via the posterior communicating arteries or the anterior communicating artery. Other sites of collateral circulation include the interconnections of the pial arteries on the cerebral surface between the anterior, middle, and posterior cerebral arteries. Sites of collateral circulation that become functional only when circulation through other routes is impaired are also found between the external and the internal carotid artery system, via the ophthalmic artery, and through muscular branches between the vertebral arteries and the external carotid artery in the neck.

Anomalies of the circle of Willis occur in nearly half the population. The most common is atresia of the posterior communicating artery, which tends to isolate the anterior (carotid system) circulation from the posterior (vertebral basilar) circulation. Anomalies in the circle of Willis are even more common in patients with cerebral infarction, and thus are believed to increase the chances of stroke in patients with cerebral atherosclerosis.

Inflammatory states involving the cerebral arteries are another cause of cerebral infarction. Inflammation produces edema and fibrosis of the vascular wall, which reduces the carrying capacity of the vessel and causes a decrease in cerebral blood flow distally. Collagen-vascular disease is the most common vascular inflammation causing cerebral infarction. Syphilis was formerly the most common inflammation of cerebral arteries and a frequent cause of cerebral infarction, especially in young persons. Rarely, acute bacterial infections of the pharynx have been followed by vasculitis of the carotid arteries and cerebral infarction. Another uncommon illness is Takayasu's disease, which affects the origin of the cerebral arteries from the aortic arch and its branches, and often results in infarction, especially in young to middle-aged women.

CEREBRAL EMBOLI

Cerebral infarction can occur without intrinsic arterial disease when emboli block arteries and impair blood flow. The most common cause of cerebral emboli in patients under 50 is rheumatic heart disease with mitral stenosis and atrial fibrillation. Other conditions associated with embolus formation are myocardial infarction with mural thrombi, atrial fibrillation of unknown cause, subacute bacterial endocarditis, thyrotoxicosis with atrial fibrillation, and nonbacterial thrombotic endocarditis. Fat emboli are rare. Paradoxical emboli have been reported as a cause of cerebral infarction. These arise in distal veins, and are shunted through the heart to the brain through a patent foramen ovale.

The neuropathologic changes in the brain that follow embolic infarction are not different from those found with infarction from other causes except that hemorrhage into the infarct is found more often with emboli than with vascular occlu-

sion from atherosclerotic disease. The actual embolic material is often not retrieved from the cerebral vessels at autopsy unless the embolus is large, presumably because most small emboli are lysed. This evanescence means that many instances of embolic cerebral infarction must be inferred by finding a source of emboli in other sites. Multiple small areas of cerebral infarction are commonly found at autopsy in patients with embolic disease.

Cerebral emboli that originate from infected material with bacterial endocarditis or pulmonary infections may cause local inflammation as well as infarction. Infected emboli produce cerebral abscess, local encephalitis, or mycotic aneurysm.

Recurrent emboli have been postulated as a cause for the transient attacks of neurologic dysfunction often seen in patients with cerebrovascular disease (*vide infra*). The surface of atheromatous plaques in the internal carotid artery is frequently ulcerated. A granular lipid debris is present on the ulcer, and the surface of some plaques has been noted to be covered with collections of platelets or organizing blood clot. It is believed that some of the granular or thrombotic material on the surface breaks off, is carried into and obstructs small cerebral vessels, and produces small areas of ischemia. Because only minute vessels are occluded, infarction usually does not occur. In support of this concept is the observation in the optic fundi of some patients having transient ischemic attacks of small white or yellow refractile bodies moving through or blocking the retinal arteries. These emboli have been identified as platelet collections or cholesterol crystals; it is believed that they represent atherosclerotic debris from plaques in proximal vessels and that similar emboli go to brain vessels causing transient occlusion without necrosis. Embolic material from ulcerated atherosclerotic plaques can cause transient ischemic attacks in the absence of significant vascular obstruction.

Cerebral Venous Inflammation and Thrombosis

Cerebral infarction can result from thrombosis of one of the major venous sinuses, i.e., the superior sagittal sinus, the lateral sinus, or the cavernous sinus, or it can follow extensive thrombotic occlusion of cortical veins. The causes of cerebral venous thrombosis include dehydration, head injury, intracerebral hemorrhage, polycythemia vera, leukemia, infection, and the puerperal state. The most common cause is infection of the mastoid, the frontal sinus, or the subdural space. If the superior sagittal sinus is thrombosed anteriorly, both cerebral hemispheres become markedly congested, swollen, and hemorrhagic. The cerebral white matter may be involved, with small hemorrhages and edema. The surface veins become distended and filled with clot.

Thrombosis of surface veins is usually associated with cerebral or subdural abscess. The histologic picture is that of an acute inflammatory reaction with vascular congestion, edema, and neuronal loss.

Cavernous sinus thrombosis usually follows infection of the eye, face, or nose, and in many instances the thrombus extends through the perihypophyseal veins to involve the opposite cavernous sinus as well. Meningitis may follow spread of the infectious process through the sinus to the subarachnoid space.

Cardiac Disease

HYPOTENSION AND HYPERTENSION

Cardiac disease contributes to infarction in patients with cerebral atherosclerosis as the result of periods of hypotension following myocardial infarction, congestive failure, and cardiac arrhythmia. In the Cornell-Bellevue series, clinical heart disease not only preceded cerebral infarction in half the patients, but was the actual cause of at least half the deaths following cerebral infarction.

Hypotension. Both hypotension and hypertension have been implicated in the production of cerebral ischemia and infarction. Although cerebral blood flow in the normal person is relatively independent of the systemic blood pressure down to levels of 50 to 60 mm. of mercury, it has been suggested that a lesser drop in blood pressure may produce cerebral ischemia when a significant obstruction is present in a vessel leading to the brain. A localized obstruction must reduce the vessel lumen by nearly 80 per cent to produce a significant distal drop in pressure, but luminal encroachment that extends over long distances theoretically could significantly decrease the distal arterial pressure with less severe grades of obstruction. However, the contribution to cerebral infarction of obstruction and distal decreases in blood pressure and flow is still an unsettled matter. Thus, Marshall has reported that when patients with transient ischemic attacks were made briefly hypotensive with hexamethonium and tilting, nearly one half showed evidence of generalized cerebral ischemia only, and another one fourth developed evidence of generalized cerebral ischemia before any focal ischemia.

Failure to maintain the blood pressure may occur with cardiac arrhythmias and following myocardial infarction. The asystole that occurs in Stokes-Adams attacks, if prolonged, can reduce the cerebral blood flow so markedly that cerebral ischemia or infarction results.

Hypertension. The place of hypertension in the production of cerebral ischemia and infarction is less clear than that of hypotension. Rapid elevations of blood pressure evoke an increase in cerebrovascular resistance, and model experiments have demonstrated that stenosis coupled with this increased resistance significantly reduces blood flow. In animal experiments, marked hypertension causes constriction in small cerebral vessels leading, in turn, to areas of cerebral infarction. The clinical evidence is less clear, although bedside experience suggests that transient increases of blood pressure at the time of a cerebral ischemic attack may contribute to cerebral infarction.

Other physiologic changes in cerebral hemodynamics may contribute to cerebral ischemia. Osteoarthritis in the cervical spine may compress the vertebral arteries so that extension, flexion, or rotation of the head can reduce vertebral artery blood flow to the point that ischemic symptoms occur. Cerebral ischemia will be augmented in these instances if anomalies or extensive atherosclerotic deposits compromise the circle of Willis.

Changes in Blood: Clotting, Viscosity, and Anemia

A variety of blood changes have been linked to cerebral infarction. The most frequent is *thrombus formation*, although in many instances it is unclear whether this is primary or secondary to the ischemic process. Thus, infarction is not invariably associated with clot-filled vessels, and when thrombi do occur, they arise most commonly in association with ulcerated atherosclerotic lesions or atherosclerotic plaques, which by themselves produce a marked degree of vessel obstruction. In vessels with greatly reduced or absent flow, clots form readily, and long, wormlike clots have been removed from the distal segment of a partially or completely obstructed internal carotid artery shortly after the development of symptoms and signs of cerebral ischemia. A plausible reconstruction of this sequence suggests that marked stenosis was present first and was suddenly increased by hemorrhage into the atherosclerotic plaque, after which clotting occurred distally to the occlusion.

Alterations in blood clotting suggesting hypercoagulability have been described in patients with cerebral infarctions. However, a state of altered clotting has not been observed before an infarction, and some evidence suggests that hypercoagulability is an epiphenomenon that follows, rather than precedes, infarction.

Other potentially deleterious changes in blood include *increased viscosity* with polycythemia and *decreased oxygen-carrying capacity* with anemia. About 15 per cent of patients with polycythemia die from thromboembolism in the brain. Transient ischemic attacks that occur in patients with polycythemia are believed to result from the increase in blood viscosity that occurs when the hematocrit rises above 55.

Severe *anemia* sometimes precipitates cerebral ischemia, particularly if the hematocrit falls below 20, i.e., if the oxygen-carrying capacity drops more than half. Any degree of anemia may supplement severe atherosclerosis, cardiac disease, or hypotension in causing cerebral ischemia.

THE PATHOGENESIS OF SYMPTOMS AND SIGNS IN CEREBROVASCULAR DISEASE

To make accurate clinical diagnoses in patients suspected of having cerebrovascular disease, the clinician requires an effective working knowledge of the structural and vascular anatomy of the brain. This is presented in the following paragraphs and diagrams, reference to which will explain why patterns of neurologic dysfunction following infarction or ischemia are related more to arterial territories than to specific neuroanatomic systems.

The brain is supplied by four large arteries, the two common carotids and the two vertebrals. One common carotid artery arises from the aortic arch and the other from the innominate artery in the upper thorax. The two vertebral arteries originate from the right and left subclavian artery. The common carotid artery bifurcates in the neck, forming the internal and external carotid arteries. Each internal carotid artery enters the skull through the homolateral foramen lacerum, passes through the cavernous sinus, and gives off branches in the following order: ophthalmic, anterior choroidal, and posterior communicating. It then bifurcates into the anterior and middle cerebral arteries.

The Anterior Cerebral Artery

As may be seen in Figures 2 and 3, the anterior cerebral artery supplies the medial and superior surfaces of the cerebral hemisphere and the whole of the most anterior portion of the frontal lobes. This area contains the motor and sensory cortex for the foot and leg and the supplementary motor cortex. The anterior cerebral artery also supplies several deep structures of importance, including the anterior nucleus of the thalamus and a portion of the anterior limb of the internal capsule.

The Middle Cerebral Artery

The middle cerebral artery (Figs. 3 and 4) supplies the lateral surface of the cerebral hemisphere with the exception of the occipital and frontal poles. The cortex supplied includes the primary motor and sensory area for the face, hand, and arm, the optic radiations, and, in the dominant hemisphere, the cortical areas for speech. The perforating branches of the middle cerebral artery reach the center of the cerebral hemisphere supplying the internal capsule and basal ganglia.

The Posterior Cerebral Artery

As shown in Figures 2 and 3, the posterior cerebral artery supplies the posterior pole of the lateral surface of the cerebral hemisphere and the posterior portion of the medial and inferior surfaces of the hemispheres. This area contains the calcarine cortex or the primary visual receptive area. The short perforating branches of the posterior cerebral artery supply the thalamus, part of the optic pathways, and other diencephalic structures including the midbrain.

The Vertebral and Basilar Arteries

The vertebral arteries reach the head via a bony canal in the transverse processes of the sixth through the second cervical vertebrae and enter the skull through the foramen magnum. Immediately after entering the skull each vertebral artery gives off a medial branch (these unite to form the anterior spinal artery) and, just distal to this, the posterior inferior cerebellar artery. At all levels along the brainstem, the ventral medial portion is supplied by short paramedian vessels. The ventrolateral portion of the brainstem is supplied by short circumferential branches from the vertebrals or basilar artery. The dorsal lateral portion and cerebellum are supplied by long circumferential branches: the posterior inferior, the anterior inferior, and the superior cerebellar arteries.

The vertebral artery lies on the ventral lateral surface of the medulla oblongata, and from it and the anterior spinal artery short paramedian branches supply the pyramids, the inferior olives

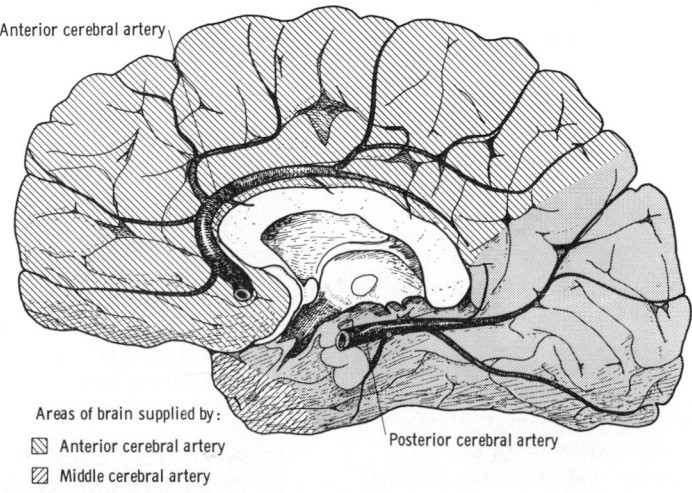

Anterior cerebral artery

Areas of brain supplied by:

╲╲ Anterior cerebral artery

╱╱ Middle cerebral artery

▩ Posterior cerebral artery

Posterior cerebral artery

FIGURE 2. The medial surface of the cerebral hemisphere, showing the course of the anterior and posterior cerebral arteries and the area of brain supplied by each.

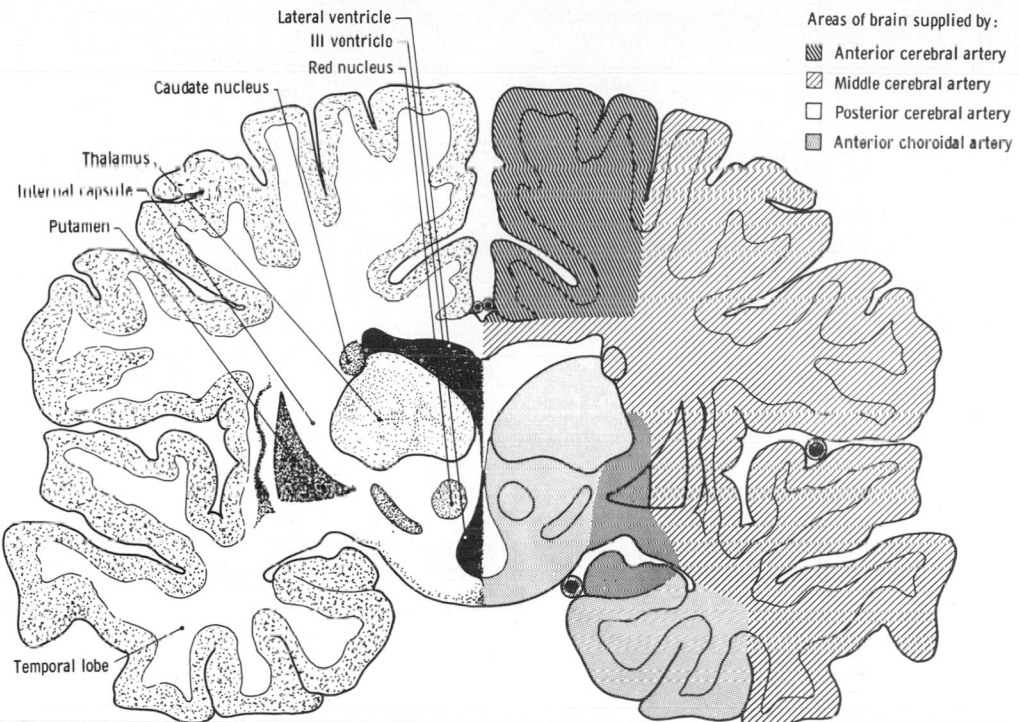

Areas of brain supplied by:

- ⬛ Anterior cerebral artery
- ⬛ Middle cerebral artery
- ⬜ Posterior cerebral artery
- ⬛ Anterior choroidal artery

Lateral ventricle
III ventricle
Red nucleus
Caudate nucleus
Thalamus
Internal capsule
Putamen
Temporal lobe

FIGURE 3. The cerebral hemispheres and the vascular supply, in coronal section.

and medial lemniscus, the medial longitudinal fasciculus, and the emerging fibers of the hypoglossal nerve as shown in Figure 5.

The more dorsal portion of the medulla includes the spinothalamic tract, the vestibular nuclei, the sensory nucleus of the fifth cranial nerve, the restiform body, and the emerging fibers of the vagus and glossopharyngeal nerves, and is supplied by longer branches from the vertebral artery and branches from the posterior inferior cerebellar artery. The most cephalad and dorsal segment of the medulla includes the vestibular and cochlear nuclei, and it and the posterior portion of the cerebellum are supplied by the posterior inferior cerebellar artery.

At the lower border of the pons, the two vertebral arteries unite to form the basilar artery. From this artery in the pons, short perpendicular branches enter the brainstem to supply paramedian structures including the corticospinal tracts, the pontine nuclei, the medial lemniscus, the medial longitudinal fasciculus, and the pontine reticular nuclei (Fig. 6). Circumferential branches supply the lateral portion of the pons, which includes the emerging seventh and eighth cranial nerves, the trigeminal nerve root, the vestibular

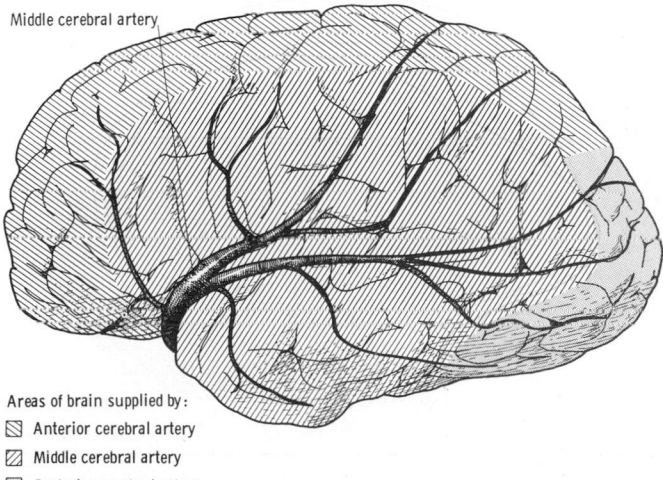

Middle cerebral artery

Areas of brain supplied by:

- ⬛ Anterior cerebral artery
- ⬛ Middle cerebral artery
- ⬛ Posterior cerebral artery

FIGURE 4. The lateral surface of the cerebral hemisphere and the course of the middle cerebral artery. The sylvian fissure has been opened to better illustrate the course of the vessel.

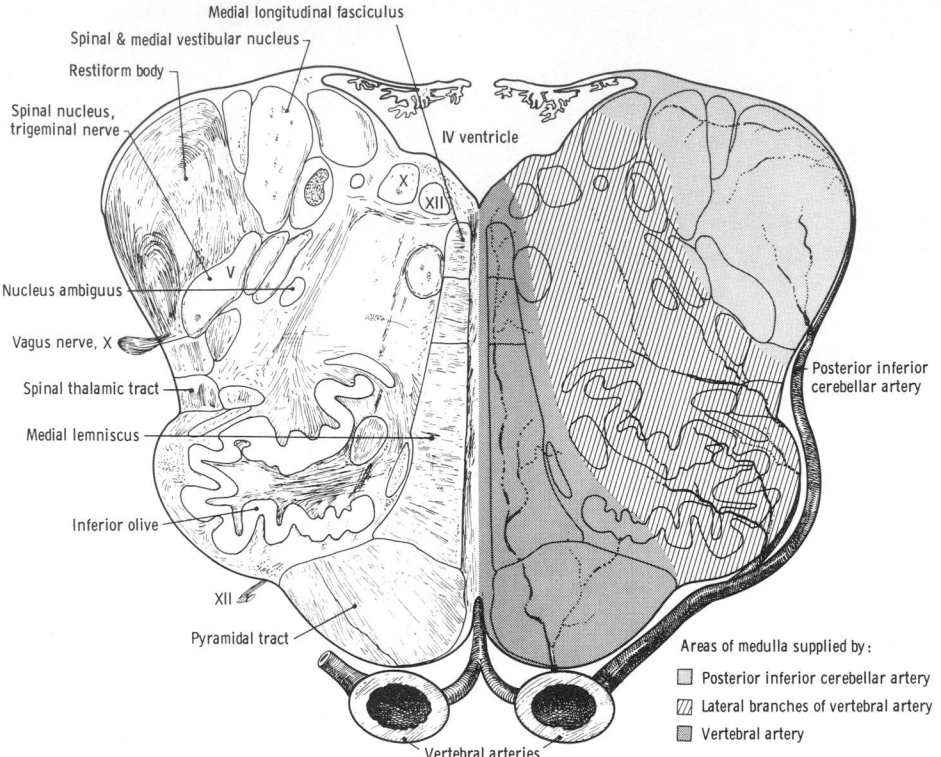

FIGURE 5.   Cross section of the medulla oblongata seen from above at the level of the hypoglossal nuclei. The medial structures are supplied by short branches arising from the vertebral arteries and anterior spinal arteries. The lateral portions are supplied by longer branches and the dorsal and lateral areas by long circumferential branches, at this level called the posterior inferior cerebellar artery.

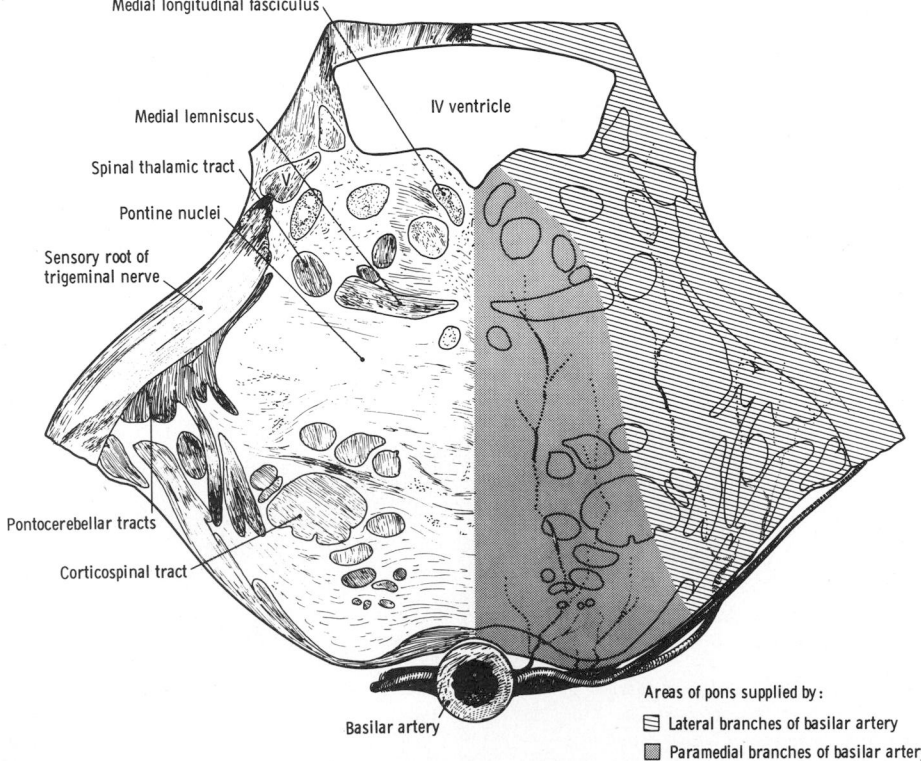

FIGURE 6.   Cross section of the midpons. The most medial regions are supplied by short perforating branches from the basilar artery. The more lateral regions are supplied by lateral branches of the basilar artery. At this level, the more dorsal structures are supplied by the long circumferential branch, the anterior inferior cerebellar artery.

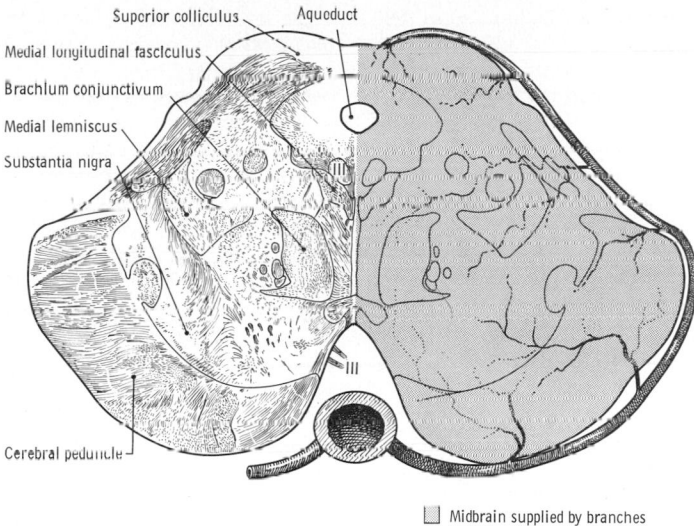

Superior colliculus   Aquoduct
Medial longitudinal fasciculus
Brachium conjunctivum
Medial lemniscus
Substantia nigra
III
III
Cerebral peduncle

Midbrain supplied by branches
of the posterior cerebral artery

FIGURE 7. Cross section of the midbrain seen from below. The medial, lateral, and dorsal regions are supplied by short branches from the posterior cerebral artery as it passes around the midbrain.

and cochlear nuclei, and the spinothalamic tracts. The anterior inferior cerebellar artery, the long circumferential branch at this level, also gives branches to the most dorsal and lateral of these structures as it runs dorsally to the cerebellum.

At the level of the midbrain the basilar artery lies in the interpeduncular fossa (Fig. 7). Short branches pass laterally and dorsally to both sides to supply the cerebral peduncles, the emerging third nerve roots, the medial portions of the red nuclei, the medial longitudinal fasciculus, oculomotor nuclei, and the midbrain reticulum. Branches of the posterior cerebral artery supply the lateral portions of the peduncles, the red nuclei, and the medial lemnisci. The superior cerebellar arteries supply some of the dorsal portions of the midbrain, including the colliculi and the anterior portion of the cerebellum on each side.

It will be clear from this review of neurologic and vascular anatomy that infarction can produce a large variety of clinical pictures, depending on the vessels involved. The pattern of most syndromes is helpful in localizing the area of the nervous system damaged by infarction, but only a few reliably indicate exactly which portion of the vascular tree is involved. As an example, diagnoses are often made of middle cerebral artery occlusion, but a review of the vascular anatomy of the brain quickly reveals why an identical clinical picture can be associated with occlusion of the internal carotid artery at any point along its course.

SIGNS AND SYMPTOMS IN CEREBRAL VASCULAR DISEASE: STROKE SYNDROMES

An adequate exposition of the symptoms and signs of cerebrovascular disease requires a classification of the various clinical entities that make up the stroke syndrome.

Cerebrovascular accidents are classified on the basis of the anatomic site of ischemia or infarction, the cerebral vessels occluded or obstructed, and the temporal character of the entire clinical episode. The latter is clinically the most valuable in that the indicated therapy is often different for the three kinds of temporal profiles found. The three profiles have been defined as *transient ischemic attack, stroke-in-evolution* or *progressive stroke,* and *completed stroke.*

The term *transient ischemic attack* or incipient stroke refers to transient episodes of neurologic dysfunction due to cerebrovascular disease. The attacks are believed to be caused by cerebral ischemia, and consist of fleeting, 5- to 30-minute disturbances in neurologic function that leave no permanent residue.

Stroke-in-evolution or progressive stroke refers to increasing neurologic dysfunction due to cerebral ischemia over a period of minutes, hours, or, rarely, days.

Completed stroke refers to the clinical picture seen in patients who have ceased to show further progression in neurologic deficit or in those who have developed a neurologic deficit earlier that is now stable or improving. *Cerebral embolism* is one cause of completed stroke in which the onset is an abrupt monophasic event, and there is clinically a demonstrable source of emboli.

Cerebral Transient Ischemic Attacks

The symptoms vary depending upon which area of the brain is ischemic, but there are two main types: those associated with ischemia of parts or the whole of a cerebral hemisphere and those associated with ischemia of the brainstem. The symptoms most often include transient contralateral weakness of the lower face, fingers, hand, arm, or leg, but such patients may also experience fleeting sensory symptoms such as tingling, "pins and needles," or numbness in parts of the body contralateral to the ischemia. Ischemia in the dominant hemisphere may cause dysphasia, with impairment in the context of speech and, at times, a transient lack of understanding.

Patients with ischemia in the portion of the brain supplied by the posterior cerebral artery may suffer blurred vision, or may notice transient hemianopic or altitudinal visual field defects or impairment of visual acuity.

Ischemia or insufficiency due to internal carotid artery stenosis often produces transient retinal ischemia, resulting in monocular blindness or reduced acuity on the side of the stenosis, combined with contralateral weakness of the face, arm, or leg.

Ischemic attacks which result from involvement of the brain supplied by the vertebral and basilar arteries have an extremely wide range of symptoms. Common symptoms include vertigo, tinnitus, diplopia, dysarthria, dysphagia, and dysphonia. Patients may complain of unilateral or bilateral face, arm, and leg weakness and unilateral or bilateral sensations of numbness and tingling in the face, arms, or leg. There may be tinnitus, hearing loss, and ataxia. In addition, patients with brainstem ischemia may experience "drop attacks," in which they suddenly lose postural tone and fall to the ground without losing consciousness, then immediately regain postural control and rise quickly. The most common complaint with transient ischemic attacks from vertebrobasilar insufficiency is dizziness. However, dizziness is commonly associated with other physiologic disturbances and is rarely the only symptom of brainstem ischemia.

Symptoms of vertebral basilar artery ischemia, although variable, tend to occur in combinations that aid in their diagnosis. Vertigo, ataxia, dysarthria, paresthesia, diplopia, tinnitus, dysphagia, and focal weakness in the face, jaw, or pharynx tend to coexist, although not always in the same sequence or combination. Another grouping of symptoms is that of unilateral or bilateral weakness of the extremities with drop attacks, and diplopia. The reason for these differences in symptom combinations can be found by referring to the diagrams of the blood supply to the brainstem. Ischemia of the dorsal and lateral portions of the brainstem supplied by the circumferential arteries produces the first group of symptoms. Ischemia of the more ventral portions supplied by the medial perforating arteries causes the second group.

Symptomatic vertebral basilar artery ischemia may occur with stenosis of the subclavian artery proximal to the origin of the vertebral artery. The arm on the side of the stenosis may be supplied by retrograde flow in the ipsilateral vertebral and, during exercise, enough blood can be diverted from the vertebral system to the arm to cause symptoms of brainstem ischemia. This mechanism of producing brainstem ischemia has been called the *subclavian steal syndrome*. However, most instances of reversed vertebral artery flow with subclavian artery stenosis or occlusion are asymptomatic.

Ischemic attacks may occur many times a day or at weekly or monthly intervals. They may be intermittently present over several months or several years. Some patients with internal carotid artery occlusion have transient ischemic attacks for as long as two years before cerebral infarction occurs. Others have clusters of attacks lasting only a few hours or days before carotid occlusion becomes complete and causes infarction. *The major importance of transient ischemic attacks is that they signal the existence of significant cerebrovascular disease and clearly indicate the potential danger of cerebral infarction.* It cannot always be predicted which patients with cerebral ischemia will develop cerebral infarction or even when it will occur. Some varieties of cerebral ischemic attacks carry a better prognosis than others. Thus, symptoms suggesting involvement of the dorsal and lateral portion to the brainstem, the lateral medullary area, imply the best prognosis. Attacks suggesting ventral brainstem involvement, such as bilateral paresis or unilateral transient paresis or drop attacks, connote a considerably poorer prognosis. Carotid ischemic attacks that occur close together in clusters carry a poor prognosis, for in a large percentage of such patients cerebral infarction rapidly follows.

In the interval between transient ischemic attacks, the neurologic examination is usually entirely normal. During a transient ischemic attack, patients commonly have neurologic deficits corresponding to their symptoms. Thus, with ischemia of a cerebral hemisphere, there may be a hemiparesis with reflex asymmetry and an extensor plantar response, or a mild hemisensory or visual field deficit. If the dominant hemisphere is affected, dysphasia may be noted: the patient has difficulty in naming and recognizing objects. Patients examined during a brainstem ischemic attack often exhibit nystagmus, complete facial weakness, palate and tongue weakness, and deviation, dysconjugate eye movements, sensory defects, and weakness on one side or on both sides of the body.

Consciousness is usually unimpaired during transient ischemic attacks, although thinking is sometimes slowed. This lack of alteration of consciousness coupled with the absence of either aura or convulsive movements helps to distinguish these attacks from convulsive seizures. Other conditions that must be considered in the differential diagnosis are Meniere's syndrome (which is rare in the elderly), migraine headache, cerebral emboli, or the progressive neurologic deficits caused by cerebral neoplasm.

Stroke-in-Evolution
(Progressive Stroke)

The evolving stroke is characterized by the gradual development of paralysis and sensory impairment over a period of several hours and, at times, one to two days. The symptoms and signs may develop as a series of steplike changes or as an unbroken continuum of worsening. When first examined, a patient may have mild weakness which, as the hours pass, is found to be more and more marked and to involve more and more of the body. The symptoms and signs found are identical to those of completed stroke; only the time course of the onset is different. This course also occurs with subdural hematoma and brain tumor, but, for these disorders, the duration usually extends over several days or weeks.

Cerebral Infarction
(Completed Stroke)

Cerebral infarctions resulting from cerebral emboli or from cerebral atherosclerosis and thrombosis, respectively, cannot be distinguished by the neurologic disorders they produce. Differences between these two causes of infarction do exist, however, in the mode of onset of symptoms and in the general physical evaluation.

The pattern of onset of neurologic symptoms and signs in cerebral infarction often suggests the cause. Cerebral embolism causes an abrupt onset of symptoms, and headache often precedes other neurologic symptoms by several hours. Cerebral infarction due to atherosclerotic vascular obstruction or occlusion often has a less sudden onset. There may be a distinct series of steplike increases in neurologic symptoms and signs, or infarction may be preceded by a series of transient ischemic attacks. A gradual onset with increasing neurologic deficit over several (one to five) hours is characteristic of the progressing stroke. A gradual onset of symptoms and signs over two days or, occasionally, one week, does occur but is uncommon. The frequency of these different patterns can be inferred from the experience of one large series of patients with ischemic infarction; about one third had a sudden onset of symptoms, about one fifth had symptoms that progressively increased over one to 12 hours, and only about one in 20 had symptoms that progressed for as long as 12 to 24 hours. One fifth of the patients with occlusive vascular disease and cerebral embolism had the onset of neurologic signs during sleep.

Headache is present in many patients with embolic or atherosclerotic infarction. The headache is usually mild and localized to the side of the infarction. Headache is believed to be caused by vasodilation of unoccluded vessels near the infarcted area, and is most common when vessels near the base of the brain are occluded.

Consciousness is usually not lost at the onset of infarction of the cerebral hemispheres, but may be reduced, particularly when large infarcts strike the dominant hemisphere. When unconsciousness is present from the onset or is the initial symptom, brainstem infarction is the most likely cause. When large hemispheric infarctions are complicated by rapidly developing and severe brain edema, loss of consciousness due to diencephalic and upper brainstem compression may occur shortly after the onset of symptoms. This may give the false impression of loss of consciousness from the onset unless a careful history documents

a lucid period at the very beginning of symptoms. Convulsive seizures are rare at the onset of cerebral infarction, but they occur in about 8 per cent of patients sometime in the course of the acute or convalescent phase of the illness. They are usually focal, but may be generalized.

When infarction is limited to the cerebral hemisphere, there is weakness or paralysis in the extremities contralateral to the infarction. Patients may also be aware that sensory perception on the side of weakness is impaired and may complain of heaviness or numbness in the arm or leg. They rarely have other sensory symptoms such as pain or paresthesias. Defects in visual fields are common but often escape the patient's notice. The defect is suspected when patients pay little attention to visual stimuli on one side of the body. At times, the eyes may be constantly deviated to the side away from the neurologic deficits.

The most serious consequence of infarction in the dominant hemisphere is dysphasia, which can range from a mild deficit of expression to aphonic mutism. The dysphasia is almost invariably a mixture of difficulty with expression (expressive dysphasia) and difficulty in understanding what is said, written, or indicated by gesture (receptive dysphasia); one or the other may predominate. In patients who have infarction in the nondominant hemisphere, lack of awareness or concern about paralysis of the contralateral side is often evident. Such subjects may, at times, be so completely unaware of their neurologic disabilities that they are hospitalized only after family or friends notice their disabilities. This phenomenon, *anosognosia,* is most common when a patient is obtunded and when there is a significant sensory deficit on the paretic side as a result of infarction of the parietal lobe. It accompanies nearly one fourth of all large strokes, but usually persists only if the patient remains obtunded or confused or has little return of sensation.

Infarctions in the brainstem produce a wide variety of symptoms. Among the most conspicuous are vertigo, diplopia, dysarthria, dysphagia, and ataxia. In addition, the patient may note unilateral or bilateral sensory impairment or weakness. Often patients note clumsiness and difficulty in performing skilled acts without paresis.

Specific Vascular Syndromes

INTERNAL CAROTID ARTERY OCCLUSION

Occlusion of the internal carotid artery at its origin from the common carotid or intracranially is the site of the major vascular lesion in nearly 20 per cent of strokes. The usual lesion is atherosclerotic with, at first, partial obstruction and, finally, occlusion with a thrombus. Occasionally the internal carotid artery is obstructed by a large embolus.

Symptoms and signs specific for internal carotid artery occlusion in the neck are intermittent visual impairment or blindness in the eye on the side of the occlusion (retinal artery insufficiency) combined with a contralateral hemiparesis and sensory loss (middle cerebral artery insufficiency). This clinical picture often begins with a series of transient ischemic attacks and only later causes permanent weakness and sensory loss. Unless the history of intermittent blindness can be obtained, it is difficult, on clinical grounds alone, to distinguish occlusion of the internal carotid artery from middle cerebral artery occlusion.

On neurologic examination, patients with cerebral infarction due to internal carotid artery occlusion have paresis of voluntary movement, with weakness most noticeable in the contralateral face and upper extremity. Infarcts usually produce motility defects as their main manifestations, but there is usually some impairment of sensory perception and, at times, visual field impairment as well.

In the paretic extremities, deep tendon reflexes are hyperactive, and pathologic reflexes such as the Babinski sign (extensor plantar response) are found. Muscle tone becomes increased on the weakened side, and spasticity may be so marked that early contracture is evident. Sensory impairment is most evident in modalities such as position sense, vibration sense, two-point discrimination, and tactile perception of shape and texture. Touch and pain perception may be moderately impaired, and extinction of stimuli on the involved side may be evident on double simultaneous stimulation. The size of the cerebral infarction produced by internal carotid occlusion is extremely variable. When there is no collateral circulation through the anterior communicating, posterior communicating, ophthalmic, or surface collateral arteries, the infarct can involve nearly the whole cerebral hemisphere, both lateral and medial surfaces. With a richer collateral circulation, smaller infarcts and proportionately fewer neurologic defects result. Occasionally occlusion of the internal carotid is asymptomatic, and is discovered only as an incidental finding at autopsy or when cerebral angiograms are done.

Internal carotid artery occlusion or stenosis sometimes causes a partial Horner's syndrome (slight ptosis and miosis) on the side opposite the paresis. The eye changes have been attributed to ischemia of the sympathetic fibers that lie in the adventitia of the arterial wall adjacent to the occlusion, but are more probably due to direct hypothalamic damage, for they can also be observed in patients with similar infarcts who do not have occlusion of the carotid arteries. An audible bruit in the neck at the angle of the mandible is a helpful indicator of stenosis of the internal carotid artery at that site. Occlusion of the internal carotid artery is also suggested when the retinal artery pressure on the affected side, as measured with an ophthalmodynamometer, decreases 25 per cent or more below the arterial pressure in the other eye. Some physicians find that palpation of the internal carotid artery in the pharynx behind the posterior tonsillar pillar is helpful in the diagnosis of carotid artery disease, as the pulse is absent when the artery is occluded.

However, patients are often unable to cooperate for the examination, so that the usefulness of the test is limited.

MIDDLE CEREBRAL ARTERY OCCLUSION

The cerebral tissue supplied by the middle cerebral artery is the most common area for infarction from emboli or vascular insufficiency, and the neurologic picture produced by either is the same.

When a middle cerebral artery is occluded, infarction occurs in the lateral portion of the hemisphere and produces varying degrees of contralateral paresis and sensory loss, mainly in the face, the upper extremities and the hand, and often blindness in the contralateral, homonymous visual field. Occlusions at the origin of the middle cerebral artery produce extensive neurologic disturbance with profound contralateral hemiplegia and sensory loss. Occlusions in branches of the middle cerebral artery may produce a variable clinical picture. At times, only paresis is evident in the arm and face. In some patients, sensory impairment is the dominant and occasionally the only neurologic abnormality, and some patients have only dysphasia.

ANTERIOR CEREBRAL ARTERY OCCLUSION

Anterior cerebral artery occlusion causes infarction in the cortical areas that control motor and sensory functions of the contralateral lower extremity, and impairs voluntary movement and sensory perception of that leg. The upper extremity and face are spared. Cerebral infarction caused by occlusion of the anterior cerebral artery is uncommon because collateral circulation through the anterior communicating artery is usually adequate to supply both hemispheres.

POSTERIOR CEREBRAL ARTERY OCCLUSION

Posterior cerebral artery occlusion causes infarction of the posterior lateral and posterior medial surfaces of the cerebral hemisphere, including the calcarine cortex. Proximal occlusions of the artery result in infarction of the thalamus and upper brainstem as well. Extensive infarctions in the occipital cortex cause homonymous hemianopic field defects, and those involving the dominant hemisphere may produce disturbances in reading, visual learning, visual recognition, and visual spatial orientation.

Infarction of both occipital poles can follow basilar artery stenosis or occlusion. The result is a double hemianopia and cortical blindness, a striking feature of which is that the patient is usually unaware that he is blind and may vigorously deny it (Anton's syndrome).

BRAINSTEM INFARCTION

Brainstem infarction, although not as common as hemisphere infarction, produces several distinct clinical syndromes, best categorized by noting whether the clinical picture suggests involvement of ventral paramedian, ventrolateral, or dorsal brainstem structures. As noted in the discussion of neurovascular anatomy, these three areas receive blood supply through different groups of arteries.

MIDBRAIN INFARCTIONS

Occlusion of the paramedian branches from the apex of the basilar artery or of the proximal posterior cerebral arteries causes infarction of portions of one or both cerebral peduncles, the oculomotor nerves, the oculomotor nuclei, the brachia conjunctivae, the red nuclei, and the midbrain reticular formation. The resulting symptoms and signs may be unilateral or bilateral, depending on the extent of the infarction. Unilateral signs include (1) ipsilateral oculomotor palsy and contralateral hemiparesis (Weber's syndrome), (2) ipsilateral oculomotor palsy, ipsilateral ataxia of gait, and poorly coordinated arm and hand movements (Nothnagel's syndrome). Bilateral signs include impaired consciousness, quadriparesis, divergent gaze, impaired vertical eye movements and midposition, or dilated pupils unresponsive to light. Purposeless, flail-like, involuntary movements (hemiballismus) may occur, and usually involve the upper extremity more than the lower. Patients in coma due to infarction of the midbrain often have an unusual appearance, seeming to be almost awake although unable to communicate in any manner. This state has been called *coma vigil* or *akinetic mutism*. Such patients, although unresponsive, may exhibit a sleep-waking cycle.

When the dorsal area, supplied by the posterior cerebral artery, is ischemic or infarcted, the spinothalamic tract, the red nucleus, the descending sympathetic tracts, and the medial lemniscus are involved. The clinical picture consists of slight ptosis and miosis (Horner's syndrome), ipsilateral ataxia, and choreiform adventitious movements and contralateral impairment of all modalities of sensory perception of the entire body, including the face. This clinical picture is often called the superior cerebellar artery syndrome.

PONTINE INFARCTION

Infarction in the pons is usually associated with basilar artery obstruction. Occlusion of the paramedian branches of the basilar artery causes necrosis of the corticospinal tracts, the pontine nuclei, the medial lemniscus, the medial longitudinal fasciculus, the abducens nucleus, the pontocerebellar tracts, and the pontine reticulum. Ipsilateral abducens palsy, facial weakness, and contralateral corticospinal tract dysfunction (Millard-Gubler syndrome) and the same findings with lateral conjugate gaze palsy (Foville's syndrome) are two unilateral syndromes that occur with occlusion in the paramedian arteries to the pons.

Bilateral signs include quadriparesis, reduced reaction to noxious stimuli, and abducens paresis. Other signs include coma, hyperventilation, apneustic or ataxic breathing, small pupils, and internuclear ophthalmoplegia. If only the most ventral portion of the pons is damaged, awareness may be maintained even though the patient is quadriparetic.

With occlusion of arteries to the lateral pons, the signs and symptoms are unilateral and include tinnitus, deafness, nausea, vertigo, impairment of facial sensation, complete ipsilateral facial paralysis, nystagmus, miosis and ptosis (partial Horner's syndrome), and impaired conjugate gaze toward the side of the lesion. Impaired pain and temperature perception of one half the contralateral body below the face is usually found. This clinical picture is often referred to as the syndrome of anterior inferior cerebellar artery occlusion.

MEDULLARY INFARCTION

Occlusion of the paramedian branches of the vertebral artery in the medulla causes contralateral paresis of the arm and leg, contralateral impaired sensory perception to touch, position sense and vibration sense in the arm, trunk, and leg, and ipsilateral tongue paralysis. With occlusion of arterial branches to the lateral medulla, the clinical picture includes vertigo, nausea, vomiting, dysarthria, dysphagia, nystagmus, ipsilateral Horner's syndrome, ipsilateral vocal cord paralysis, and impaired ipsilateral facial sensory perception to pain with impairment of pain sensation on the contralateral half of the body below the face. This clinical picture is referred to as the syndrome of posterior inferior cerebellar artery occlusion or Wallenberg's syndrome. It results as much or more frequently from occlusion of the vertebral artery itself as it does from occlusion of its branches.

BASILAR ARTERY OCCLUSION

When the basilar artery is completely occluded, infarction is found mainly in the ventral pons, midbrain, and occipital lobes. The clinical picture is like that seen with occlusion of the paramedian midbrain or pontine branches, but may include various defects in the visual fields and, at times, cortical blindness in addition. The brainstem tegmentum is almost invariably involved, causing major disturbances in consciousness.

Many of the particular groupings of symptoms and signs associated with various brainstem infarctions that have been given eponyms are believed to be common occurrences with brainstem infarction. However, in an analysis of 50 patients with brainstem infarction from the Cornell-Bellevue series, only two clearly fitted into these syndromes as originally described. The remaining 48 had an extensive mixture of symptoms and signs indicating an overlap in the areas believed to be infarcted with occlusions in specific arteries.

CEREBRAL EMBOLISM

The diagnosis of cerebral embolization is usually not difficult when it is remembered that the onset of neurologic symptoms and signs is abrupt, that they are often preceded by headache for a few hours before paresis is evident, and that a potential source for emboli is usually found on physical examination. Convulsive seizures occur at the onset, but they are uncommon. They are at first focal and later generalized in most patients. Loss of consciousness occurs in nearly one fourth of patients and is usually present for only a few minutes, but, after onset, patients may be confused. The neurologic signs depend upon which artery is occluded; the most common clinical picture is that of middle cerebral artery occlusion. Cerebral emboli can lodge in any major cerebral artery, and emboli commonly recur, often to the same artery. The cerebrospinal fluid is usually clear and without cells. When protein elevation and cells are found, subacute bacterial endocarditis should be suspected. Mitral stenosis with atrial fibrillation, myocardial infarction with mural thrombus, and subacute bacterial endocarditis are the cardiac disorders most commonly found. Normal sinus rhythm does not exclude the diagnosis of cerebral emboli, for it may be found in more than one third of such patients, particularly with a "tight" mitral stenosis or with past myocardial infarcts, respectively. Evidence of embolization to other sites strengthens the supposition that the cause of cerebral infarction is embolic.

CEREBRAL VENOUS THROMBOSIS

The symptoms of local cerebral venous thrombosis are headache, delirium, drowsiness, diplopia, and convulsions. The signs are usually those of increased intracranial pressure with papilledema and focal neurologic abnormalities. Focal fits are common, as are paresis and hemisensory loss. Such patients are restless, confused, and obtunded.

Superior sagittal sinus occlusion produces a somewhat similar clinical picture. At the New York Hospital, 21 patients with noninfective sagittal sinus thrombosis have been studied. Nine had terminal disease and marasmus, six had cyanotic congenital heart disease, and four had other, unexplained episodes of venous or arterial thromboses. Eleven of the 21 patients were children. Below the age of 10, cerebral infarction is more often due to venous than to arterial occlusion. Nearly all patients had fever, and their cerebrospinal fluids were under increased pressure, averaging 260 mm. of fluid, and contained more than 10 red blood cells. Neurologic symptoms appeared abruptly or progressed rapidly to a maximum, usually within 36 hours. Most patients were obtunded or confused and had headache. The white blood count was elevated in 10 patients; in 7 it was over 20,000. Nuchal rigidity was common, and papilledema, hemiparesis, and focal epileptic seizures occurred in about half the cases. Two patients presented later with signs of pseudotumor cerebri. The occurrence of hemiparesis or focal epilepsy was usually associated with cortical venous thromboses in addition to the sinus occlusion.

Cavernous sinus occlusion, usually a complication of sinus or paranasal skin infection, is characterized by proptosis, orbital chemosis, and edema, pain around the eye, papilledema, retinal hemorrhages, and fever. Extraocular palsy may be present. The disease carries a high risk of spread to the opposite cavernous sinus. Complications include meningitis and brain abscess.

Transverse or lateral sinus thrombosis, usually secondary to mastoiditis, is now uncommon with the decline in the incidence of that disease. When it does occur, it is usually manifested by headache, tenderness over the mastoid process, and, occasionally, paresis of the structures supplied by the glossopharyngeal and accessory nerve, with dysphagia, dysphonia, and weakness of the ipsilateral sternomastoid and trapezius muscle.

In all varieties of cerebral venous thrombosis, there is usually some evidence of sepsis with fever, malaise, headache, and leukocytosis.

Although the condition is uncommon, a diagnosis of cerebral venous thrombosis should be kept in mind for patients with evidence of cerebral infarction who have focal seizures, increased intracranial pressure, or evidence of infection. Cerebral venous thrombosis is particularly likely as a cause of postpartum cerebral infarction.

PHYSICAL AND LABORATORY FINDINGS

The general evaluation of the patient with cerebral infarction usually reveals evidence of vascular disease at other sites as well as a variety of associated diseases. About one fifth of patients with atherosclerotic cerebral infarction in the Cornell-Bellevue series had previous strokes, half of which had occurred in the preceding year. Another fifth had had myocardial infarction, usually within the previous year. Over one half of the patients were hypertensive, but the diastolic pressure was above 100 mm. of mercury in only one third of the patients. Nearly one fifth of the patients had diabetes mellitus, and one in ten gave a history of peripheral vascular occlusive disease.

Physical Examination. The physical examination of most patients with cerebral infarction discloses a normal or slightly elevated body temperature. Careful examination of the heart should never be overlooked because the presence of cardiac enlargement, atrial fibrillation, and cardiac murmurs, suggesting rheumatic heart disease with mitral stenosis, aids in detecting the presence of cerebral emboli. Patients with cerebral infarction often have atherosclerotic coronary heart disease, and perhaps one fifth have had recent or associated myocardial infarcts.

Palpation may reveal absence of pulsation in easily felt peripheral arteries. In the lower extremities, this is indicative of atherosclerotic vascular disease in the aorta, iliac, femoral or popliteal arteries. In the upper extremities, it may indicate occlusions in the major branches of the aorta, such as the innominate or subclavian arteries. Absence of pulses in one or both upper extremities should alert the physician to such diagnoses as "pulseless disease" (Takayasu's syndrome) or the "subclavian steal syndrome."

Auscultation for bruit over the neck is helpful in identifying sites of extracranial stenosis. A bruit heard in the neck under the angle of the mandible suggests atherosclerotic disease of the carotid artery, and bruit heard just above the clavicles is associated with vertebral or subclavian artery stenosis. Bruit, when loud and localized, is associated with atherosclerotic obstruction at that site in more than three fourths of patients.

Laboratory Examinations. Laboratory tests are aimed at both confirming the diagnosis and identifying complications. Every patient suspected of stroke should have a lumbar puncture and skull roentgenograms, and, if there are any unusual features at all about the illness, an electroencephalogram (EEG) should be obtained.

The cerebrospinal fluid should be examined promptly, for there is no other way to determine the presence of intracranial bleeding or an unsuspected infection. The lumbar puncture must be approached cautiously, however, when patients are in stupor or coma or when it is uncertain whether the illness is caused by stroke or by brain tumor, with increased intracranial pressure. In such instances, it is preferable to proceed with roentgenograms, electroencephalogram, radioactive brain scan, or an arteriogram, since lumbar puncture can inadvertently precipitate tentorial or foraminal herniation when there is an expanding intracranial mass.

The cerebrospinal fluid pressure is rarely over 200 mm. of CSF in cerebral infarction. The fluid is usually clear and colorless, but bleeding and xanthochromia from hemorrhagic infarction may be found. The CSF protein level is usually normal although slight elevations to 60 to 75 mg. per 100 ml. are found in perhaps one fifth of the patients. Elevations to 80 mg. per 100 ml. or above are found in less than 10 per cent, but particularly in those with basilar artery disease. With massive cerebral infarction, the protein may be raised to values of nearly 100 mg. per 100 ml. Although diabetes occasionally accounts for pronounced CSF protein elevations with stroke, patients with high values should always be carefully reviewed for the possibility of brain tumor.

Skull roentgenograms should be examined for evidence of fracture, erosion of the posterior clinoids (suggesting chronically increased intracranial pressure), abnormal calcification, and pineal shift.

The *electroencephalogram* (EEG) offers potential help both in differential diagnosis and in distinguishing infarction of the brainstem from that of the hemispheres. The EEG is usually abnormal in patients with cerebral infarction, and the degree of abnormality generally parallels the size of the lesion and the severity of the neurologic deficit. With hemispheric lesions, the abnormality is focal and the normal frequency of brain waves is slowed, so that, acutely at least, the records may resemble those found with brain tumor. In infarction, however, a decrease in the EEG abnormality is expected in serial recordings as the patient improves. With brainstem infarction, the EEG may be entirely normal, paroxysmally abnormal, or generally and diffusely abnormal.

The general evaluation of patients with cerebral infarction should include an electrocardiogram (ECG) and a chest roentgenogram. The ECG may confirm the presence of an arrhythmia or may disclose a silent myocardial infarction. (A potentially confusing point is that the ECG may show minor T wave and S-T segment changes caused by cerebral infarction and not by primary cardiac disease.)

Special Investigations

ARTERIOGRAPHY

Since the introduction of arteriography, its considerable potential in the diagnosis and management of cerebrovascular disease has been apparent. At first, its use was hampered by a high incidence of complications including transient or permanent worsening of neurologic defects, transient delirium, convulsions, hypotension, and, occasionally, death. The incidence of these adverse reactions has declined sharply in recent years as a result of improved contrast media, improved skill in cannulating arteries, and the use of techniques in which the contrast medium is injected peripherally. With these advances, transient complications develop in about 1 to 2 per cent of patients with cerebrovascular disease, and permanent worsening and death follow arteriography in less than 1 per cent of patients.

Cerebral angiography is indicated only for certain patients with cerebrovascular disease and has two main values. The first is in differential diagnosis. For the patient with an atypical history and findings, or who is unable to give an accurate history because of dysphasia or depressed consciousness, cerebral angiograms help to exclude remediable causes of illness, such as subdural hematoma or brain tumor. In the author's series of patients with suspected cerebrovascular disease, angiograms changed the clinical diagnosis of cerebrovascular accident in about 5 per cent of patients, particularly among those unable to give a history. The lesions most frequently revealed were subdural hematoma, brain tumor, and, less often, arteriovenous anomaly.

The second and more important value of cerebral angiograms is the accurate demonstration of the site, extent, and incidence of arterial obstructions that might be susceptible to surgical correction. Patients with such lesions include predominantly those who suffer transient ischemic attacks or incomplete strokes from which recovery has been substantial. In such cases, evaluation must include a complete angiographic study of the extracranial and intracranial vessels, for it is necessary to outline both the neck vessels and the nature and extent of the intracranial collateral circulation and the collateral channels from extracranial to intracranial vessels. Radiopaque contrast media are now introduced intra-arterially in a variety of sites, including the brachial, the subclavian, and the femoral arteries in addition to the carotid arteries. In some techniques, catheters are introduced and threaded up the vessel to the desired site before injection. In others, the contrast materials are injected under a pressure high enough to cause retrograde flow into the aortic arch or innominate artery. They are then caught in the anterograde physiologic flow and taken up the desired carotid or vertebral vessel.

Rapid roentgenographic exposures have clarified some aspects of the physiology of cerebral blood flow in patients with cerebrovascular disease. Cerebral angiography may identify unusual patterns of blood flow in cerebral vessels, such as regrograde flow down one vertebral artery with proximal subclavian artery stenosis (subclavian steal).

Brain scanning, using radiomercury-chlormerodrin or Tc^{99m} Pertechnetate shows a high uptake of radioactive material in the area of a cerebral infarction. This technique may aid in accurate localization of the infarcted area, but an identical picture can result from brain tumor, thereby limiting its usefulness in differential diagnosis. A normal brain scan during the first few days after the onset of symptoms suggesting a stroke, followed by a positive brain scan, is highly suggestive of cerebral infarction.

Echoencephalography is often helpful in the diagnosis of cerebral infarction. Reflected ultrasound waves are recorded to demonstrate whether midline structures are shifted. Shift of midline structures is uncommon immediately after cerebral infarction, although cerebral edema occurring 24 to 48 hours later can be responsible for a considerable shift. Acutely, at least, a midline shift of more than 2 mm. should make one suspect brain tumor or subdural hematoma.

DIFFERENTIAL DIAGNOSIS

The most common sources of error in the diagnosis of cerebral infarction are brain tumors, subdural hematomas, intracerebral hemorrhages, cerebral traumatic lesions, and cerebral infections.

When a clear history of the onset is available, cerebral infarction is seldom confused with other disorders. Stroke caused by cerebral emboli or cerebral thrombosis characteristically produces a maximal neurologic deficit initially, with gradual improvement in function over days, weeks, or months. The first symptoms of brain tumor and subdural hematoma occasionally are mistaken for stroke, but the general tendency is for these two disorders to cause gradually progressive worsening, even though the first symptoms may seem to begin suddenly. In addition, both brain tumor and hematoma tend to produce disturbances in consciousness that are as prominent as or more prominent than focal neurologic defects, which helps in their differentiation from cerebrovascular disease. Often the problem in differential diagnosis is reversed in that the onset of stroke may include a gradual steady progression of symptoms and signs of focal neurologic defects, making the physician think first of tumor and only later of cerebral infarction. When doubt occurs about the diagnoses of infarction, subdural hematoma, and neoplasm, cerebral angiograms and other tests should be done.

Clinically, it is easier to confuse cerebral infarction with intracranial hemorrhage, for the onset is often similar. The cerebrospinal fluid examination usually helps, but blood can be found in both states—although considerably less often in cerebral infarction. Large amounts of blood in a CSF under increased pressure is always caused by intracranial hemorrhage. Angiography helps to settle the problem by demonstrating aneurysm, A-V anomaly, or intracerebral hematoma.

When it is not known whether the patient could have suffered head trauma, it is often impossible to eliminate this as a cause of clinical states resembling cerebral infarction. Careful inspection for scalp lacerations and localized scalp edema and good quality skull roentgenograms identify most instances of trauma if it has been severe enough to cause neurologic injury. If trauma cannot be eliminated and the patient becomes progressively worse, angiography must be done to eliminate consideration of subdural or epidural hematomas. Angiography is preferable to exploratory burr holes, for it will not only indicate a hematoma but will also define other causes of illness such as tumor, intracerebral hemorrhage, or vascular occlusion.

Among the forms of intracranial sepsis only brain abscess is likely to be confused with cerebral infarction. The points that should alert the physician to the possibility of an abscess are a source of infection elsewhere in the body such as an ear, sinus, or chest infection; persistent headache; persistent low-grade fever; white cells, especially polymorphonuclear leukocytes, that persist more than 24 hours in the cerebrospinal fluid; a focal, highly abnormal EEG; and worsening of the clinical state. If abscess is suspected, angiograms performed on the side opposite to the paresis will demonstrate the presence or absence of an intracerebral mass, which, if present, then must be surgically explored and drained to prove the diagnosis.

COURSE

Some improvement in function following the initial neurologic deficit can be expected after almost every cerebral infarction. During the first 72 hours, however, gradual worsening of neurologic deficits and increasing or beginning impairment of consciousness are frequent. This change may indicate extension of the cerebral infarction, but usually is associated with cerebral edema in and around the necrotic area. *Some degree of cerebral edema complicates every infarct.* It appears almost immediately, and with large infarctions may be so extensive as to shift the brain laterally and downward to produce herniation through the tentorium cerebelli and subsequent brainstem compression. This course of events, with its associated impairment of consciousness and other vital functions, is a common cause of death in patients with extensive infarction. The diagnosis of cerebral edema is especially likely when a patient shows a decline in awareness without a significant increase in focal neurologic deficits. Other causes of lethargy and stupor in patients with cerebral infarction are fever, electrolyte imbalance, the injudicious use of sedatives, tranquilizers or narcotics, and malnutrition.

In patients whose course is not complicated by severe cerebral edema, there is usually an early improvement in neurologic function. If some voluntary movement is preserved, there is a good chance for return of more. When function improves rapidly after the onset, the outlook for a good recovery is excellent. A slow return of function over weeks or months is associated with a less complete recovery. If flaccid paralysis is present from the onset with no return of increased muscle tonus over 30 to 60 days, the outlook for recovery is poor, since a gradual change from flaccidity to spasticity always precedes the advent of voluntary movement. Significant sensory loss impairs the chances of recovery of motor function. With brainstem infarction, the course is usually one of gradual improvement if the infarct is localized in the lateral medullary area. Symptoms of nausea, diplopia, and ataxia lessen and eventually disappear. Although some residual impairment of eye and extremity movement may be detected on examination, such patients often have little physical limitation. It is important to realize that recovery from cerebral infarction with impaired neurologic function may continue for as long as one to two years.

PROGNOSIS

About one fourth to one fifth of patients with either thrombotic or embolic cerebral infarction die with their first attack. This figure varies somewhat with the cause of the infarction and especially with other factors such as age, cardiac status, and the degree of neurologic disability. The mortality rises sharply with increasing age; for patients over the age of 70 with cerebral infarction from atherosclerotic thrombosis or emboli the initial mortality is nearer 50 per cent. Patients with marked neurologic defects, coma, or extensive vascular disease elsewhere have an initial mortality of nearly 50 per cent. Infarction of the ventral portions of the brainstem following basilar artery occlusion, especially with quadriplegia, carries a poor outlook, although good medical and good nursing care may preserve a vegetative existence for long periods.

The prognosis with cerebral infarction is better in younger patients, in those with the least evidence of vascular disease at other sites, especially cardiovascular disease, and in those who do not have hypertension, diabetes, or severe neurologic defects.

About one fifth of patients who survive a cerebral infarction from atherosclerotic vascular disease suffer another cerebrovascular accident within the next 12 to 24 months. However, the most significant limiting factor on survival is not recurrent stroke but cardiovascular disease. Thus in the Cornell-Bellevue series, fully half of the patients who survived the initial cerebral infarction died at a later date from myocardial infarction or cardiac failure.

Recurrence of cerebral infarction is common with cerebral emboli. In the New York Hospital series about 22 per cent of patients with cerebral emboli suffered recurrences, and nearly all the patients had more than one embolus if extracerebral sites were included. There is a strong chance that each cerebral recurrence will cause death or further neurologic disability.

TREATMENT

General. Treatment of cerebral infarction has four goals: to preserve life, to limit the amount of brain damage, to lessen disability and deformity, and to prevent recurrences.

The treatment program designed to preserve life is similar to that outlined for all seriously ill patients with neurologic illness. Efforts are directed toward maintaining a clear airway, an adequate fluid, electrolyte, and caloric intake, and an adequate urine output. Constant care is required to protect the skin from ischemia and necrosis resulting from pressure. Such a program is necessary for the obtunded or comatose patient, and must often be continued for the remainder of his life.

In patients with hemispheric infarction *cerebral edema* can impair consciousness and vital function early in the course of the illness. When cerebral edema subsides, the patient may again be able to cough, swallow, and voluntarily move paretic parts. A variety of measures can often temporarily reduce the brain swelling and carry the patient through a period of severe difficulty. Hypertonic urea solution, 1 to 1.5 grams per kilogram of body weight given intravenously, rapidly reduces cerebral edema and causes a marked diuresis. The effect is transient, and a rebound effect attributed to recurrence of swelling has been reported. Hypertonic invert sugar, mannitol, has been used with similar results except that less rebound has been reported. One and one half to 2 grams per kilogram of body weight is given intravenously in a 20 per cent solution. In patients with cerebral infarction and brain edema this therapy is reserved until there is a serious threat to life with declining brainstem function, for the benefits are transient, and most patients can be carried through periods of depressed consciousness with careful nursing care alone. Although glucocorticoids such as methylprednisolone are often dramatically effective in improving patients with brain edema from primary and metastatic brain tumor, they have been found to be ineffective and therefore are contraindicated for reducing cerebral edema following infarction.

Several agents have been utilized to increase cerebral blood flow in an effort to decrease the amount of ischemic tissue and limit the extent of cerebral infarction. Nearly all known agents that produce vasodilatation, including aminophylline, papaverine, tolazoline hydrochloride, nicotinic acid, and histamine, have been used without clear evidence of success in cerebrovascular disease. The only agent that produces effective vasodilatation in cerebral vessels is carbon dioxide. Although it has been used to treat acute stroke, there is no evidence that it reduces the neurologic defects. Stellate ganglion block has also been employed in an effort to increase cerebral blood flow in patients with stroke. There is no evidence that it does this or that it reduces the neurologic deficits.

Treatment for the late acute and convalescent phase of a stroke is directed toward lessening deformity and disability, a goal that requires daily passive exercise of paretic parts to prevent joint fixation and to maintain normal muscle and tendon length. Some increase in muscle tone with spasticity invariably accompanies hemiplegia and tends to be most marked in the flexor muscles in the upper extremities and in the extensor muscles in the lower extremities. If this increase in tone in one muscle group over another persists and cannot be overcome by voluntary movement, daily passive movement of weakened or paralyzed parts through the full range of motion must be carried out by a nurse, physician, physiotherapist, or member of the family to prevent muscle and tendon contracture that may be nearly impossible to correct later on.

Rehabilitation. Following cerebral infarction, *programs of retraining and rehabilitation should begin as soon as there is no longer evidence of increasing infarction.* Stabilization of the neurologic findings for 12 to 24 hours with some evidence of improvement is usually sufficient evidence to permit a start. Rehabilitation programs have as their goal the retraining of the remaining functions for maximal effectiveness. Although a few patients do require and benefit from special hospital facilities for rehabilitation, most such programs can be carried out on medical services without the aid of extensive equipment. An internist or general physician who is interested in rehabilitation can direct programs of activity and exercise, and can achieve results in rehabilitating hemiplegic patients, that are nearly as effective as those of specialized centers.

An active program of rehabilitation begins by increasing the patient's tolerance to sitting and standing, which is impaired both by weakness and by changes in the sense of balance. Patients are allowed to sit up and then stand for increasingly long periods beginning with 5 to 10 minutes. During this period daily active and passive exercises of weakened extremities are carried out. When patients begin standing they need firm support and often splinting or bracing of the knee on the weakened side; marked quadriceps weakness may even demand a long leg brace. Ambulation is one of the main goals of rehabilitation. Gait training should begin when the patient can comfortably stand for 15 to 20 minutes without fatigue, and the support of parallel bars or a walker should be depended upon at first. After ambulation has started, it may be necessary to brace the foot to avoid the foot drop and supination that commonly occur following hemiplegia. At the same time that the patient is relearning to walk he should be trained in developing new skills with his unaffected arm and improving the strength and function in the paretic arm. This is done by an active program of exercise and by observing and retraining the patient in the activities of daily living such as eating, dressing and undressing, and personal hygiene. More complete details of programs of rehabilitation are outlined in other sources such as Covalt and can be followed by patients and their families under the direction of the physician. Usually, the maximal effect is gained in six to eight months, but some patients continue to show improvement over periods lasting as long as two years. Passive exercise must be continued indefinitely for severely paralyzed patients if contractures are to be avoided.

For patients with cerebral infarction who have mild to moderate dysphasia, speech therapy may be helpful. With severe dysphasia, therapy is rarely able to restore usable speech.

PREVENTION

Prevention of recurrent attacks and of cerebral infarction in patients with transient ischemic attacks and prevention of recurrent infarction in patients with cerebral atherosclerosis and cerebral emboli are the goals of much of the currently recommended treatment for stroke. Two methods to achieve this have been extensively evaluated, anticoagulation and surgical correction of arterial obstruction.

Anticoagulant Drugs or Surgery in Transient Ischemic Attacks. *Anticoagulant therapy* was introduced to treat transient ischemic attacks after its use in myocardial infarction suggested a beneficial action. A controlled study of anticoagulants in transient ischemic attacks indicates that as long as patients receive anticoagulants and their prothrombin times are kept at two to two and a half times the normal value, they have fewer ischemic attacks and less chance of having a cerebral infarction. As a result, anticoagulants are now generally accepted as effective in treating patients with transient ischemic attacks. The question is, which patients should receive the anticoagulants and for how long? The natural history of attacks is variable; attacks often stop spontaneously; some varieties carry a better prognosis than others. Even admitting these differences, anticoagulants should be given to the patients with transient ischemic attacks who do not have contraindications to their use. They should be continued for six months to one year and then gradually discontinued. If transient ischemic attacks recur, they should be given again. The management of patients on anticoagulants will be discussed below.

Surgical correction of extracranial arterial obstruction has been extensively tried in the United States in treating patients with transient ischemic attacks. Most carefully evaluated surgical series show that patients with significant extracranial arterial obstructions who have transient ischemic attacks are relieved after surgical removal of the obstruction and that chances of cerebral infarction are reduced. This conclusion has been supported by the results of the National Cooperative Study of Extracranial Arterial Occlusion which has conducted a large controlled surgical treatment trial. Where experienced vascular surgeons are carrying out such surgery frequently, surgical correction of obstruction should be offered to patients. If skilled, experienced surgeons are unavailable or referral is impossible for other reasons, anticoagulants are the treatment of choice. Patients with transient ischemic attacks in whom arteriography demonstrates no surgically correctable lesion are best treated with anticoagulants.

Anticoagulant Drugs or Surgery in Progressing Stroke or Stroke-in-Evolution. Anticoagulants have been shown by Carter to significantly reduce mortality and morbidity among patients with stroke-in-evolution. Such situations are emergencies and, unless specifically contraindicated, anticoagulation must begin with heparin and must be continued with coumarin derivatives. Anticoagulants are usually given for four to six weeks. Surgical correction of an arterial obstruction for the patient with progressing stroke has been recommended as a means of reducing neurologic disability. This form of treatment has been widely tried with uniformly poor results. Therefore, in view of the evidence that anticoagulants are beneficial, they are the treatment of choice.

Anticoagulant Drugs or Surgery in Completed Stroke. For the patient with an already completed stroke, there is no clear treatment of choice for preventing recurrences. Most series of patients with completed stroke studied by angiograms illustrate the widespread nature of atherosclerotic obstructive vascular disease. Intra- and extracranial vessels are commonly affected simultaneously and impose limiting factors on the successful outcome of surgical correction of extracranial arterial defects. A controlled evaluation of surgical therapy in this group of patients has been carried out and shows that surgical correction of an isolated carotid stenosis in patients with a mild neurologic defect is effective in reducing future mortality and morbidity. Surgical correction of arterial obstruction in patients with severe neurologic defects or with evidence of extensive atherosclerotic disease and occlusion does not reduce future mortality or morbidity and is therefore contraindicated.

Anticoagulants, given for one to four months, are useful during the acute and early convalescent period following a cerebrovascular accident to prevent pulmonary emboli in paralyzed, bedridden patients. The use of anticoagulants has also been recommended on a long-term basis for prevention of recurrent stroke. However, most studies of this problem indicate that there is no benefit from this form of treatment given routinely and that the complication rate from long-term treatment is too high to warrant its use. Anticoagulation, therefore, can be recommended only for highly selected patients after cerebral infarction.

Anticoagulant Drugs in Cerebral Embolization. Anticoagulants greatly reduce the mortality and morbidity associated with recurrent embolization, and patients with a well established diagnosis of cerebral embolus should be placed on these drugs if there are no contraindications. If the source of emboli is rheumatic heart disease, anticoagulants are given continuously. When emboli follow myocardial infarction, treatment is usually given for one year. Coumarin anticoagulants are used and should be started immediately after the diagnosis has been made and the lumbar puncture has revealed bloodless cerebrospinal fluid.

Patients with cerebral emboli who have atrial fibrillation are often considered for conversion to normal sinus rhythm. This may be valuable in increasing cardiac output, but does not clearly reduce the chance of recurrent cerebral emboli.

General Management of Anticoagulant Therapy. Anticoagulation therapy is carried out with oral coumarin derivatives, regulating the daily dosage so that the prothrombin time is maintained at two to two and a half times the control value. This treatment is never started without prior examination of the cerebrospinal fluid to exclude the presence of intracranial hemorrhage. Treatment is best begun in the hospital so that daily prothrombin determinations can be done and the patient's response to medication carefully followed. Following discharge from the hospital patients should be seen weekly at first. The interval between visits can be extended to as long as three weeks if the prothrombin time remains steady on a given dosage of Coumadin.

The *contraindications to long-term anticoagulant treatment* include blood in the cerebrospinal fluid, severe renal disease, peptic ulcer, bleeding diathesis, a blood pressure of more than 170/110 mm. of mercury, severe liver disease, inadequate laboratory facilities for the control of anticoagulants, and unreliable patients. The *contraindications for short-term anticoagulants* are less stringent but always include bleeding in the intracranial cavity and bleeding elsewhere.

Hemorrhagic complications from anticoagulants are serious in about 2 to 4 per cent of patients and fatal in 2 per cent. Minor bleeding does not require that the medication be discontinued, but with serious bleeding it should be. Minor surgical procedures can be undertaken safely in most patients on anticoagulants if the prothrombin time is slightly lowered.

Bleeding rarely occurs spontaneously in patients on coumarin compounds unless prothrombin times become prolonged to four or five times the control value. Each episode of bleeding must be thoroughly investigated, for there is frequently an underlying cause such as gastrointestinal or genitourinary malignant disease. When it is necessary to return prothrombin times rapidly to normal, vitamin K_1 is the most effective antidote: 5 mg. given orally or intravenously usually returns the prothrombin time to normal or nearly normal. Larger amounts of vitamin K cause refractoriness to coumarin compounds for several days.

Heparin is the anticoagulant of choice for the initial treatment of patients with progressing stroke. It is given intravenously in amounts sufficient to prolong the clotting time to two or two and a half times the normal value. The clotting time is determined before each dose, and dosages of 5000 units usually are required every three to four hours. If the clotting time is longer than 20 minutes, the dose is omitted, and the clotting time is checked in one hour; if it is less than 20 minutes, heparin is given, and the interval is shortened accordingly. At the time heparin is begun, a coumarin anticoagulant is started by mouth. When the prothrombin time reaches two to two and a half times normal, heparin is discontinued.

Patients with transient ischemic attacks, progressing strokes, or established strokes who also have hypertension should be treated with antihypertensive medication. Studies of patients with atherosclerotic cerebrovascular disease and hypertension show that when the blood pressure is returned to normal or nearly normal levels the recurrence rate and mortality rate of stroke are reduced. Hypertension, depending on its severity, should be continuously treated with reserpine, chlorothiazide, or hexamethonium, and the blood pressure should be maintained as nearly normal as possible.

To sum up the prophylaxis of strokes: Patients with transient ischemic attacks should be treated with anticoagulants. If arteriography indicates significant extracranial vascular disease and experienced surgical care is available, the patient should be offered this form of treatment. Patients with completed strokes are not likely to benefit from any prophylactic treatment. If they are to remain bedridden for long periods, anticoagulants help to reduce the chances of pulmonary embolism.

HYPERTENSIVE ENCEPHALOPATHY

Hypertensive encephalopathy is an uncommon, acute neurologic syndrome characterized by headache, nausea and vomiting, convulsive seizures, transient focal neurologic defects, retinal artery spasm, papilledema, stupor, and coma. The cerebrospinal fluid pressure and protein content are commonly elevated. The syndrome is encountered in patients with long-standing hypertension, and its occurrence is associated with sudden marked increases in blood pressure. There are various underlying causes of hypertension, including malignant hypertension, eclampsia, and glomerulonephritis.

The mechanism by which hypertension causes neurologic dysfunction is believed to be acute cerebral vasospasm causing cerebral ischemia and edema. Similar changes have been observed in hypertensive rats.

Mild transient focal neurologic defects can be encountered in this syndrome. When neurologic defects are severe and sustained, the correct diagnosis is more likely to be cerebral ischemia or cerebral hemorrhage. When the blood urea nitrogen is above 100 mg. per 100 ml., hypertensive encephalopathy can be difficult to distinguish from uremia, or can blend into that state.

The outlook for patients with hypertensive encephalopathy has been greatly improved with the use of antihypertensive medication, and temporary recovery is now frequent. The appearance of the syndrome, however, is usually associated with the end-state phases of advanced hypertensive vascular disease.

Treatment should be given to lower the blood pressure, for this is the only effective way to eliminate the symptoms. Initial treatment should be intramuscular reserpine, 2 to 5 mg. per day. Blood pressure will begin to fall in two to three hours after adminstration of reserpine, and it can be maintained at desired levels with daily injections. Care must be exercised to avoid cerebral ischemia from hypotension. Permanent medical therapy must be instituted to maintain the blood pressure at more nearly normal levels, utilizing hydrochlorothiazide, reserpine, or alpha methyldopa. (See article on Arterial Hypertension.)

PROGRESSIVE SUBCORTICAL ENCEPHALOPATHY

Progressive subcortical encephalopathy, described by Binswanger, is a rare disorder that occurs in patients with hypertension and atherosclerotic vascular disease. Progressive dementia, seizures, and focal neurologic signs characterize the clinical picture. The diagnosis is usually made at necropsy; the brain shows atrophy mainly in the temporal and occipital regions and patchy demyelination in the white matter of the hemispheres.

Baker, R. N., et al.: Anticoagulant therapy in cerebral infarction. Report on cooperative study. Neurology, 12:823, 1962.

Bauer, R. B., Meyer, J. S., Fields, W. S., Remington, R., Mac-Donald, M. C., and Callen, P.: Joint study of extracranial arterial occlusion. J. A. M. A., 208:509, 1969.

Carter, A. B.: Cerebral Infarction. New York, Pergamon Press and The Macmillan Company, 1964.

Marshall, J.: The Management of Cerebrovascular Disease. Boston, Little, Brown and Company, 1965.

McDowell, F. H. (ed.): Treatment of strokes. In Modern Treatment. New York, Harper & Row, 1965, pp. 15-24, 84-92.

Millikan, C. H., Siebert, R. G., and Whisnant, J. P.: Cerebral Vascular Diseases. Trans. Fourth Princeton Conference, January 8-10, 1964. New York, Grune and Stratton, Inc., 1965.

INTRACRANIAL HEMORRHAGE

DEFINITION

Intracranial hemorrhage, or apoplexy, comprises about one tenth of all acute cerebral vascular illness. Regardless of cause, intracranial hemorrhage is a serious illness with a high rate of mortality. At the bedside the physician can only suspect the diagnosis, which must be confirmed by finding blood in the cerebrospinal fluid or by the demonstration of a hematoma at surgery. The causes of intracranial hemorrhage are numerous, and the clinical pictures are similar regardless of the cause. It helps one to understand the clinical problem better if one remembers that nontraumatic bleeding within the cranium takes one of four separate anatomic courses and that these produce three relatively distinct clinical pictures:

1. Bleeding emanating from vessels on the surface of the brain and limited to the cerebrospinal fluid-filled space between the pial and arachnoid membranes is called *subarachnoid hemorrhage*.

2. *Subarachnoid hemorrhage with intracerebral extension* occurs when the sudden force of bleeding from a surface vessel also penetrates into the brain itself; signs and symptoms of both the subarachnoid and the parenchymal lesions result.

3. Bleeding from ruptured vessels within the substance of the brain is called *intracerebral hemorrhage*. This may remain isolated therein as a *cerebral hematoma*.

4. Intracerebral hemorrhage may extend through brain tissue to the ventricles or subarachnoid space, causing signs and symptoms of both the parenchymal and the subarachnoid lesions.

ETIOLOGY

Bleeding from ruptured arteries is the usual source of intracranial hemorrhage although veins also may bleed. The accompanying table lists the common causes.

Arterial Aneurysms

Berry Aneurysms. These are small, round, or saccular, berry-shaped dilatations that form characteristically at arterial bifurcations at or near the circle of Willis. Their cause is uncertain, for aneurysms are not familial and they are rarely found in infants. They arise, however, from what are thought to be congenital defects in the media of cerebral vessels. The wall of an

CAUSES OF INTRACRANIAL HEMORRHAGE

1. Arterial aneurysms
   a. *"Congenital" berry aneurysms*
   b. *Acquired arterial aneurysms*
      (1) Fusiform aneurysms
      (2) Mycotic aneurysms
2. Arteriovenous (A-V) anomalies
3. Hypertensive vascular disease
4. Vascular lesions associated with primary or metastatic brain tumors
5. Systemic bleeding diatheses
6. Undetermined and miscellaneous causes

aneurysm is thin, composed usually only of intima and subintimal connective tissue. Muscle or elastic tissues may be evident at the origin of the aneurysmal sac from its parent vessel, but these tissues thin out and disappear as the sac enlarges. Most aneurysms are less than 1 cm. in diameter; a few, however, dilate to as much as 2 to 5 cm. As the aneurysm enlarges, it may develop a narrow neck or may remain broadly attached to the vessel wall.

Most berry aneurysms, approximately 85 per cent, develop around the anterior portion of the circle of Willis, arising from the internal carotid, the posterior communicating, the middle cerebral, the anterior communicating, or the anterior cerebral artery, as shown in Figure 8. The most common site is the point of junction of the posterior communicating artery and the internal carotid. About 15 per cent of aneurysms arise from the vertebral-basilar artery system. Multiple aneurysms are found in about one of every six patients. Not all aneurysms bleed, and some are found incidentally at postmortem examination. Occasionally, they become so large that they compress adjacent cerebral tissue or cranial nerves, and, rarely, they enlarge sufficiently to cause a clinical state that simulates brain tumor.

What makes an aneurysm rupture at any given

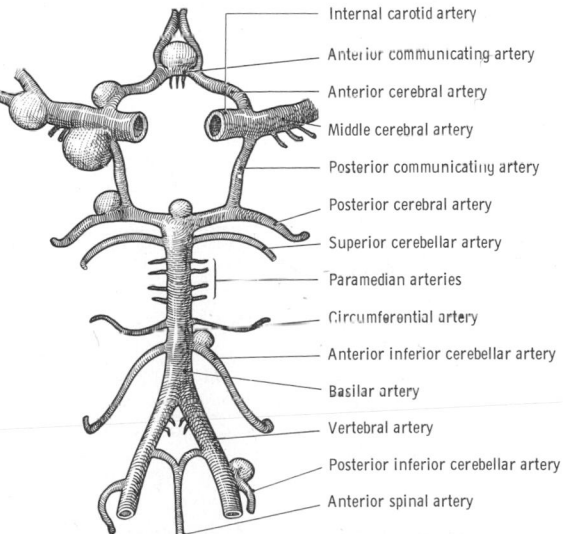

Internal carotid artery
Anterior communicating artery
Anterior cerebral artery
Middle cerebral artery
Posterior communicating artery
Posterior cerebral artery
Superior cerebellar artery
Paramedian arteries
Circumferential artery
Anterior inferior cerebellar artery
Basilar artery
Vertebral artery
Posterior inferior cerebellar artery
Anterior spinal artery

FIGURE 8. The more common sites of berry aneurysm. The size of the aneurysm at the various sites is directly proportional to the frequency at that site.

instant is not clear, although several factors seem important. These lesions gradually enlarge with time under the stress of the arterial blood pressure. They are more frequent in patients who are hypertensive, and their incidence is high in subjects with coarctation of the aorta and polycystic renal disease, both of which cause early hypertension. Atheromatous plaques form in their walls, and clots line the aneurysms, but whether either of these conditions increases the chance of rupture is problematic. Probably a change in the blood pressure is the single final event that precipitates perforation of the sac.

Fusiform Aneurysms. These spindle-shaped dilatations along the course of an artery, usually the basilar, sometimes the carotid artery in the cavernous sinus, are due to atherosclerosis. The resulting elongated and tortuous dilatation may be large enough to compress adjacent cranial nerves of the brain itself. Hemorrhage from such an aneurysm is unusual, but characteristically damages the brain fatally when it does occur.

Mycotic Aneurysms. Mycotic aneurysms are produced by septic emboli associated with bacterial endocarditis. A local necrotic vasculitis occurs at the site where the embolus lodges and results in thinning and dilatation of the vessel wall, which may eventually rupture. Such lesions tend to be multiple and they are the only aneurysms found distally in the smaller branches of the middle cerebral artery.

Arteriovenous Anomalies or Cavernous Angiomas

Arteriovenous anomalies or cavernous angiomas are tangled interconnected networks of vessels in which arterial blood passes directly to venous drainage without intervening capillaries. These lesions tend to be supplied by more than one parent cerebral artery, and they range in size from the microscopic to a huge cavernous network large enough to cover most of one cerebral hemisphere or to occupy an entire lobe of the cerebellum. The vessels in an A-V anomaly are themselves malformed so that some structurally resemble arteries, others veins. Since these vessels are usually thin-walled, circulating blood at arterial pressure distends and often eventually ruptures them, with a resultant subarachnoid hemorrhage, intracerebral hemorrhage, or both. Even without hemorrhage, large A-V malformations expand, and the neural tissue adjacent to the anomaly characteristically suffers an uneven pressure necrosis, causing progressively more abnormal neurologic signs or epilepsy. Hemorrhage can destroy all clinical evidence of a malformation of microscopic size and make antemortem diagnosis impossible.

Hypertensive Vascular Disease

Hypertension causes thickening and fibrinoid degeneration of the cerebral arterioles. Red cells can be found free in the perivascular spaces around many of the vessels, and microaneurysms have been described along the arteries since the time of Bouchard and Charcot in the nineteenth century. What part each of these abnormalities contributes to the eventual necrosis and rupture is still debated, although most contemporary pathologists view the fibrinoid degeneration as most important.

When hemorrhage occurs, it usually results from rupture of small arteries in the substance of the brain. This may occur anywhere; it is most common in the cerebrum and least common in the cerebellum and brainstem. In the cerebral hemispheres, small branches of the middle cerebral artery penetrating the region of the basal ganglia are most susceptible, and the lenticulostriate artery has even been termed "the artery of cerebral hemorrhage." In the brainstem, hemorrhages arise from paramedian perforating branches of the basilar more often than they do from the long circumferential branches of either the basilar or the vertebral arteries.

Hemorrhage in Brain Tumors

Hemorrhage may occur in either primary or metastatic lesions, usually in rapidly growing tumors with a large amount of vascular overgrowth. This complication is perhaps most common in glioblastoma multiforme and metastatic neoplasms from the lung. Among the more benign tumors pituitary adenomas have a tendency to cause apoplexy. Of the total number of cerebral hemorrhages, however, those from tumor contribute but a small fraction.

Bleeding Diatheses and Miscellaneous Causes

Leukemia, thrombocytopenia, and the ingestion of excessive amounts of anticoagulants all predispose to cerebral hemorrhage. In some patients it is difficult or impossible to establish what caused a cerebral hemorrhage. As mentioned, in some cases the hemorrhage may have erased the malformation. A hemorrhagic cerebral infarct can be so liquefied that it resembles a primary hemorrhage. However, with the increasing use of cerebral angiography, more and more intracranial aneurysms and malformations are being demonstrated in all age groups as the cause of intracranial hemorrhage.

PATHOLOGY AND PATHOGENESIS

Subarachnoid Hemorrhage. Subarachnoid hemorrhage most commonly comes from rupture of a berry aneurysm, less commonly from an A-V anomaly, a mycotic or a fusiform aneurysm. Blood suddenly released in this manner has several deleterious effects, each contributing to the seriousness of the disease. The sudden high pressure jet raises the intracranial pressure and sometimes acts like an acute concussion, causing sudden unconsciousness or, occasionally, rapid brain displacement and death. Blood is also a noxious agent, particularly as it hemolyzes and breaks down into its pigments. It irritates blood vessels, meninges, and the brain itself. Meningeal irritation causes the characteristic headache of subarachnoid hemorrhage, and later, within hours or days, the blood produces a sterile meningitis. This hemogenic meningitis itself becomes a source of considerable disability, for it not only causes subjective discomfort and systemic toxicity but leads to meningeal exudation, thickening, and scarring that can impair cerebrospinal fluid absorption and cause subacute or chronic communicating hydrocephalus. Moreover, the blood may irritate the underlying brain so as to evoke adverse descending autonomic discharges, causing hypertension and cardiac arrhythmias.

In addition to the brain destruction caused by the physical action of the hemorrhage, ischemic changes and infarction of brain tissue are found in as many as two thirds of patients dying from subarachnoid hemorrhage. The ischemia and infarction have been attributed to vascular spasm or vessel wall edema, and they are encountered most commonly in the area of the brain supplied by the artery with the ruptured aneurysm. Evidence for arterial spasm in subarachnoid hemorrhage comes from angiographic studies showing segmental vessel narrowing that correlates with a high incidence of clinical and pathologic evidence of cerebral infarction. The causative mechanism is believed to be a combination of the irritating effect of free blood plus vessel injury. During surgery, mechanical stimulation of cerebral arteries causes significant and sustained vessel narrowing. Presumably, vascular spasm has a potentially protective action in reducing the amount of bleeding from a ruptured artery. Why in some instances it lasts long enough and is severe enough to reduce distal cerebral blood flow to the point of ischemia and neural death is unknown. The possibility that persistent vessel narrowing may be due to edema of the vessel wall and not spasm needs consideration.

Extension of bleeding into the brain occurs in about half of all surface aneurysms and in nearly all A-V anomalies. The complication is particularly likely when the bleeding site lies close to cerebral tissue, as is true with aneurysms of the anterior communicating or anterior cerebral arteries, which are interposed between the frontal lobes, or of branches of the middle cerebral artery, which are buried within the sylvian fissure. Rupture from the anterior communicating vessel tends to damage one or both frontal lobes, and rupture of middle cerebral artery aneurysms tends to lacerate the temporoparietal or posterior frontal lobes.

Intracerebral Hemorrhage. Intracerebral hemorrhage is most often caused by hypertensive vascular disease or ruptured aneurysm, less often by a bleeding arteriovenous malformation. The path that the blood takes with these lesions and the amount of bleeding are somewhat unpredictable. Some hemorrhages dissect the brain along fiber tracts, destroying relatively little brain tissue along the way. Others damage considerable amounts of neural tissue in the region of bleeding. All hemorrhages enlarge the brain and evoke cerebral edema. When the enlargement occurs rapidly, it displaces cerebral structures laterally across the midline under the falx and downward through the tentorium cerebelli, with resulting brainstem compression. Such a course of events is often fatal; at postmortem examination smaller areas of bleeding are found in the midbrain and pons in addition to the massive intracerebral hemorrhage. These secondary brainstem lesions have been attributed to venous obstruction and ischemia from transtentorial herniation.

Small intracerebral hemorrhages can remain entirely confined within the brain substance. Occasionally, the hematoma absorbs fluid, and this plus the surrounding edema can create the clinical picture of an expanding new growth. More often, however, the fluid is resorbed, and the remaining cavity shrinks almost to the point of disappearance.

Most large cerebral hemorrhages rupture into the subarachnoid space, the ventricular system, or both. Although serious consequences have been attributed to this course of events, it is likely that the large size of the hemorrhage causes the disastrous clinical effects rather than the fact that bleeding penetrated into the cerebrospinal fluid spaces.

CLINICAL MANIFESTATIONS OF INTRACRANIAL BLEEDING

Subarachnoid Hemorrhage. Subarachnoid hemorrhage has as its most common initial symptom a sudden violent headache. Initially the headache is usually described as an excruciating, intense, aching pain. Later it becomes dull and throbbing but remains severe, and most patients describe it as the most intense headache they have ever experienced. Even if it is at first localized, it soon becomes generalized, and frequently patients complain of severe neck and back pain. The initial localized headache is due to vascular distortion and injury. The later generalized headache is due to meningeal irritation from blood in the subarachnoid space.

Localization of headache at the onset is helpful in determining the site of the bleeding. Headache that begins in the back of the head suggests a posterior fossa origin of bleeding, and headache that begins in the anterior part of the head suggests a supratentorial bleeding source. If the initial headache is localized to one side, bleeding usually has occurred from a vessel on that side.

Other symptoms include dizziness, vertigo, vomiting, drowsiness, sweating and chills, stupor, and loss of consciousness.

Shortly after the onset of symptoms, the patient may lose consciousness for a few moments. With massive subarachnoid hemorrhage and intracerebral extension, the patient may lapse into and remain in coma until death. In some instances of subarachnoid hemorrhage death may be sudden and is related to intraventricular hemorrhage and sudden intense transtentorial herniation and brainstem compression. When hemorrhage is confined to the subarachnoid space or when intracerebral extension of bleeding is minor, consciousness is regained in a few minutes to a few hours. Delirium and lethargy often follow and may persist for as long as two weeks; severe mental clouding, delirium or coma, usually indicates severe bleeding and brain damage.

Patients with subarachnoid hemorrhage usually complain of neck stiffness; this does not appear immediately in most patients but begins with the onset of the meningeal inflammatory reaction 6 to 12 hours after. When neck stiffness is evident shortly after the onset of symptoms, it is ominous and suggests that the meninges in the posterior fossa are stretched by beginning herniation of the cerebellar tonsils into the foramen magnum.

Although subarachnoid hemorrhage does occur during sleep, it most commonly occurs when patients are engaged in their usual activities. Many patients have reported that headache began during activity such as straining at stool, heavy lifting, or coitus.

Convulsions may occur, usually at onset, but sometimes during the acute phase of the illness. When present, they almost invariably indicate that the site of bleeding is in the anterior or middle fossa.

On examination the most conspicuous sign is marked neck rigidity and pain on attempting head movement. The most common localizing neurologic abnormality is the pupillary inequality or paresis of vertical and medial movements of one eye that follows oculomotor nerve compression by aneurysms of the internal carotid artery.

Lateralizing neurologic signs, such as hemiparesis or hemiplegia, hemisensory defects or hemianopia, indicate either an intracerebral extension of bleeding or vascular spasm. The distribution of signs of neurologic dysfunction, particularly at onset, may be helpful in localizing the site of bleeding. Marked hemiparesis and severe hemisensory defects suggest bleeding from an aneurysm on the middle cerebral artery in the sylvian fissure. Unilateral oculomotor paresis with ptosis, diplopia, and mydriasis suggests that the bleeding source is from the region of the posterior communicating artery where it joins the internal carotid artery. This junction lies in close approximation to the oculomotor nerve as it passes from the posterior to the middle fossa. Bilateral paresis of the extremities suggests that the bleeding site is near the anterior cerebral-anterior communicating artery junction and suggests extension of bleeding into both frontal lobes. Paresis or sensory impairment present from onset are most likely to be caused by intracerebral extension of bleeding, whereas neurologic signs developing later are more often due to arterial spasm.

Examination of the optic fundi in patients with subarachnoid hemorrhage may reveal smooth rounded hemorrhages near the optic nerve head, "subhyaloid hemorrhages." They are often unilateral and, when present on one side, indicate the side of the bleeding. They are venous in origin and result from sudden increase in intracranial venous pressure at the time of the intracranial bleeding.

Fever caused by the hemogenic aseptic meningitis is common in patients with subarachnoid hemorrhage, appearing usually one to three days after onset and reaching 38° to 39° C. (100.4° to 102.2° F.). Greater elevations of body temperature usually suggest intraventricular or intracerebral extension of bleeding. Subsequent elevations of temperature during the course of the illness may suggest recurrent bleeding, but they are more often related to intercurrent infections.

Rupture of an Arteriovenous Anomaly. The symptoms and signs of a subarachnoid hemorrhage from a ruptured A-V anomaly are identical to those from a ruptured aneurysm, because both bleed into the subarachnoid space or into the brain tissues. Bleeding into surrounding brain is common for a ruptured A-V anomaly, and symptoms and signs are like those of intracerebral hemorrhage from other causes. Seizures may occur at the onset of bleeding and are nearly always focal in pattern. The diagnosis of arteriovenous anomaly is suggested by a history of pre-existing focal seizures or focal neurologic signs and of recurrent, always unilateral, vascular headache, each of which occurs in about a third of the patients. Rupture of arteriovenous anomalies is more frequent at a younger age than is rupture of aneurysms, so that a history of focal seizures in a young patient with subarachnoid hemorrhage makes the diagnosis of arteriovenous anomaly particularly likely.

When the patient with an arteriovenous malformation is examined, in addition to signs of meningeal irritation and focal neurologic defects, careful auscultation may disclose an audible bruit over the eyes or skull. Although bruits may be present with either arteriovenous anomalies or aneurysms, they are more common with the former.

Intracerebral Hemorrhage. When intracranial hemorrhage occurs directly into the substance of the brain, the onset of symptoms is usually abrupt. Severe headache, nausea, and vomiting occur and sometimes precede other signs of a neurologic deficit or loss of consciousness by several hours. These early symptoms are the result of an acute increase in intracranial pressure. Focal neurologic dysfunction follows, with hemiplegia or hemisensory defects; this results from disruption or distortion of the main motor and sensory pathways in the cerebrum. Loss of consciousness within minutes after the onset occurs in more than one third of patients and indicates a large hemorrhage, intraventricular bleeding, or both. Among patients who are not initially in coma, half deteriorate with decline of awareness and eventually lapse into coma. With the progressive decline in consciousness, patients may show neurologic signs at first, indicating functional decortication and later indicating decerebration. This sequence follows herniation of the brain through the tentorial space with secondary brainstem compression.

In patients who retain consciousness but have motor or sensory deficits, it can be difficult to differentiate intracerebral hemorrhage from cerebral infarction until the cerebrospinal fluid is examined and found to be bloody. In about 20 per cent of patients, the intracerebral hemorrhage is circumscribed, and the fluid never becomes bloody. In these instances, except for the higher incidence of headache with intracerebral hemorrhage, it may be impossible to differentiate intracerebral hemorrhage from cerebral infarction.

The clinical picture produced by intracerebral hemorrhages at various sites is often characteristic and may enable an accurate localization of bleeding.

Capsular or Putamen Hemorrhage. Intracerebral bleeding into the region of the internal capsule causes abrupt flaccid hemiplegia, loss of sensory perception, and homonymous hemianopia. Capsular hemorrhages in the dominant hemisphere produce aphasia. When the hemorrhage is large, loss of consciousness promptly follows. With small hemorrhages changes are less severe. Paralysis is usually more prominent than sensory impairment, and paralysis of gaze to the side opposite the hemorrhage may be found.

Thalamic Hemorrhages. Hemorrhage into the thalamus also produces abrupt motor deficits, but in addition an impairment of all modalities of sensory perception is common and more prominent than deficits in motility or the visual fields. Consciousness is less likely to be lost with a thalamic than with a capsular hemorrhage. Thalamic hemorrhages are associated with distinct disturbances in eye movements. Patients commonly show paralysis of upward gaze. At rest, their eyes deviate downward and laterally and they are unable to look up on command or reflex. The pupils may be unequal and react poorly to light. There may be partial oculomotor palsy with ptosis and loss of convergence. The mechanism that causes the gaze palsy is compression of the region of the posterior commissure and the adjacent upper brainstem nuclei. Because the disturbances in gaze gradually clear, actual tissue destruction from extension of the hemorrhage into this area is probably not the cause of the defect.

Cerebellar and Brainstem Hemorrhage. Parenchymal hemorrhage in the posterior fossa can occur either in the cerebellar hemispheres or in the brainstem (usually pons). With intracerebellar hemorrhage, the patient may experience sudden severe occipital headache, diplopia, nystagmus, and ataxia. Examination reveals miosis, conjugate gaze palsy, and irregular respiration. In some subjects, these symptoms and signs may be present for several hours before any loss of consciousness; in others, loss of consciousness is immediate. When warning symptoms occur, the diagnosis can often be made from the clinical

examination alone, and prompt evacuation of the hematoma can be life-saving. Hemorrhage into the brainstem causes immediate impairment of consciousness, irregular breathing, pin-point pupils, and quadriplegia followed by a rapid decline to death.

LABORATORY FINDINGS IN INTRACRANIAL BLEEDING

Cerebrospinal Fluid Examination. Intracranial hemorrhage can be diagnosed ante mortem with certainty only when blood is found in the cerebrospinal fluid or in the brain substance at operation. Lumbar puncture can be safely carried out on most patients suspected of having intracranial hemorrhage, but should be done with caution when there is evidence of impaired consciousness or a progressive decline in awareness and focal neurologic defects. These signs indicate both extensive brain damage and the possibility of brainstem compression. With suspected intracerebral hemorrhages and hematoma, there is always the possibility of tentorial herniation, which may be precipitated or accentuated by changes in cerebrospinal fluid pressure after puncture. In such instances lumbar puncture is best postponed until after other studies have been carried out.

Examination of the cerebrospinal fluid shortly after the onset of intracranial bleeding (1 to 24 hours) reveals red cells with a constant red cell count in sequential samples. The supernatant fluid of a centrifuged specimen will have a pink color due to the presence of oxyhemoglobin. The fluid reacts positively with benzidine. Cerebrospinal fluid examined after 24 hours will begin to show, in addition, a yellowish coloration (xanthochromia) due to the degradation of oxyhemoglobin to bilirubin. This intensifies over a period of several days and usually reaches peak intensity at 36 to 48 hours after the onset of bleeding.

Bloody fluid due to a traumatic lumbar puncture is indicated by the absence of pink or yellow discoloration of the centrifuged supernatant cerebrospinal fluid, i.e., not xanthochromic, by failure to obtain a positive benzidine test for hemoglobin in the supernatant fluid and by a decreasing red cell count in sequential samples of the fluid.

The white cell count in the CSF, when determined shortly after bleeding, will be commensurate with the amount of bleeding — usually one white cell for every 1000 red cells. When the white cell count is made on specimens collected 12 hours or more after the onset of bleeding, it may be elevated. This increase in white cells is caused by the inflammatory reaction in the meninges and may reach levels as high as 500 per cubic millimeter. Early in the course of the inflammatory reaction the cells may be polymorphonuclear leukocytes and lymphocytes; later, the cells are all lymphocytes.

An exudative reaction accompanies intracranial hemorrhage, and the cerebrospinal fluid protein is usually elevated to levels around 100 mg. per 100 ml. or more. During fresh bleeding, for each

10,000 red cells in the fluid, the protein is said to rise 15 mg. per 100 ml. Protein elevations are maximal 8 to 10 days after bleeding and decline thereafter. The cerebrospinal fluid pressure is often elevated to levels of 200 to 300 mm. (of CSF) with subarachnoid hemorrhage. Elevations may be much higher, 300 to 500 mm. with large intracerebral hemorrhages. The white count in the peripheral blood can be elevated to levels up to 15,000 and some patients have a transient albuminuria and glycosuria.

Arteriography. It is often impossible on clinical grounds alone to distinguish between a bleeding aneurysm, a bleeding A-V anomaly, or intracerebral bleeding of unknown cause. Once the clinical diagnosis of intracranial hemorrhage has been made, cerebral arteriography is necessary to demonstrate the cause and site of bleeding. Thus, if the patient is a satisfactory operative risk, arteriography should be performed as soon as possible with the hope that specific treatment can be instituted.

Arteriography is most useful in demonstrating aneurysms and A-V anomalies. In patients with suspected ruptured aneurysm, cerebral angiograms will demonstrate the aneurysm in over 80 per cent of instances. They may also indicate whether the aneurysm can be approached surgically. In addition to the aneurysm, the angiogram may reveal distortion of the usual vessel patterns near the aneurysm, indicating a hematoma, and frequently there will be arterial narrowing. The technical details of arteriography are discussed elsewhere; however, the physician should see to it that the intracranial branches of both the right and left carotid arteries are visualized to determine whether more than one aneurysm is present. When more than one aneurysm is present, it is often difficult to determine which one ruptured. Points that are helpful are that the bleeding aneurysm is often irregular in outline and, in the surrounding area, there may be distortion of other vessels, suggesting a local hematoma, or the nearby vessels may show narrowing. Local hematoma is the most reliable evidence of bleeding. If an aneurysm is not seen in the carotid arterial tree, the vertebral and basilar arteries and their branches should be visualized. The demonstration of an aneurysm on the distal branches of the middle or anterior cerebral arteries is almost diagnostic of mycotic aneurysm.

Arteriovenous anomalies are readily demonstrated in cerebral angiograms, as the usually large flow of blood through these structures produces a characteristic picture of early arterial filling and venous drainage of the anomalous vessels.

Intracerebral hemorrhage often can be visualized on cerebral angiograms. Shift of midline vessels, widening of the space between the anterior and middle cerebral arteries, and downward or upward displacement of the middle cerebral branches are helpful evidence. However, roughly a quarter of small hematomas (20 to 30 per cent) escape detection by angiograms.

When hemorrhage has occurred into a cerebral neoplasm, angiograms help in demonstrating vascular changes suggestive of tumor. In addition to vessel distortion and shift of midline vessels, abnormal vessels in the tumor may fill with contrast media and produce a so-called "tumor stain."

PROGNOSIS

Ruptured Aneurysm. Subarachnoid bleeding from a ruptured aneurysm is extremely serious; the mortality rate is 45 per cent for each major attack, and there is a high risk of recurrence. Among those who succumb to bleeding, about one third do so within the first 48 hours, another one third within the next month, and the remainder from late major recurrences. Recurrence strikes about one patient in three, with the maximal danger during the first two weeks after the initial bleeding, when about 60 per cent of all rebleeding occurs. However, some patients bleed during the third and fourth weeks, and about 20 per cent have late recurrences, most of which are within the first six months after leaving the hospital. Fatal recurrences have been reported as long as 20 years after the initial bleeding, and there is no way to predict which patient will have a recurrence of bleeding or when he is likely to have it. The high mortality and the frequency of recurrence make accurate statements of prognosis impossible for individual patients. In general, the longer a patient survives after the initial bleeding, the less are his chances of recurrence. Data submitted to the National Co-operative Study of Subarachnoid Hemorrhage indicate that if a patient with subarachnoid hemorrhage is alive one week after onset, the chance of his surviving five more weeks is 65 per cent. If he lives two weeks without recurrence, he has a 76 per cent chance of living four more weeks. Patients 20 to 50 years of age have a better chance of survival than those over 60. As might be expected, patients with the least neural damage and the least impairment of consciousness have the best chance of survival.

Ruptured A-V Anomaly. The prognosis for bleeding from arteriovenous anomalies is better than for aneurysm. The initial mortality is about 25 per cent and the possibility of recurrence less than that. Because of their location and the tendency to bleed into brain tissue, the neurologic disability among survivors of bleeding A-V anomalies tends to be high. Seizures with A-V anomalies are common before bleeding, and patients who do not have seizures often develop them after bleeding.

Hypertensive Vascular Disease. The prognosis for intracerebral hemorrhage from hypertensive vascular disease is poor; the over-all mortality is more than 50 per cent. Mortality is highest with hemorrhage into the ventricle or when severe brain edema causes temporal lobe herniation with resultant compression of the midbrain. The initial mortality rises with the age of the patient. It is about 40 per cent for patients in the 40 to 60 age range, 50 per cent in patients over 60, and 80 per cent in patients over 70. Patients who are in coma when first seen have a mortality rate of 70 to 100 per cent. Recurrence of intracerebral hemorrhage is uncommon, but tissue destruction and displacement at the time of bleeding cause serious neural damage and residual neurologic dysfunction. Patients with small intracerebral hemorrhages usually are left with only slight disability.

TREATMENT

The treatment of intracranial hemorrhage has three goals: preserving life, reducing disability, and preventing recurrence. Treatment directed toward preservation of life is similar for all causes of intracranial hemorrhage and for most other life-threatening neurologic illnesses. During the acute phase of intracranial hemorrhage, the patient should be in bed for as long as the symptoms of headache, stiff neck, and prostration require. Rebleeding is unlikely with ruptured A-V anomaly and hypertensive vascular disease, and a patient with one of these disorders need not be kept in bed for a long period once he feels well enough to get up. Just when to mobilize the patient with subarachnoid hemorrhage from intracranial aneurysm is a question more difficult to answer. Four to six weeks of bed rest is usually recommended, because this is the period of maximal danger from rebleeding. Recurrent hemorrhage has been noted to occur with straining at stool and with other activity, and rest in bed is believed to lessen the chances for potentially dangerous activity.

When the patient is in coma or has impaired consciousness following intracranial hemorrhage, meticulous care must be taken to maintain an adequate airway, blood pressure, and fluid and electrolyte balance. The skin and eyes must be protected from pressure and irritation. The urinary bladder should not be allowed to become distended from urinary retention. These are common problems for all patients with neurologic illness and depressed consciousness; they are discussed more fully elsewhere.

Patients with intracranial hemorrhage who are conscious usually complain of severe headache and stiff neck. They also frequently are restless and delirious. Analgesics such as codeine sulfate by mouth or codeine phosphate intramuscularly in doses of 60 mg. may be needed as often as every two hours to relieve headache; in most instances this also relieves restlessness. Other narcotics for analgesia should be avoided because they depress respiration. *Delirium may persist for as long as two weeks.* No specific treatment is indicated, but having a member of the family present at all times and reducing examinations and procedures to a minimum greatly reduce the patient's anxiety and restlessness.

Initially, patients with intracranial hemorrhage should not take fluid or food by mouth for 24 to 48 hours because of the danger of vomiting and aspiration. Subsequently, it is best to give clear fluids for another 24 to 48 hours and then a soft diet. During the period of restricted fluid and food intake, intravenous fluids should be given in the usual physiologic quantities.

Constipation must be avoided. When patients require codeine for relief of pain, mild laxatives or stool softeners should be given if the patient is able to take medication by mouth. Otherwise, small enemas should be given every other day.

When the blood pressure is elevated, it should be returned to nearly normal levels, particularly in patients with bleeding from intracranial aneurysms. This should not be done rapidly, however, because of the risk of precipitating a hypotension-induced cerebral ischemic infarct. Methyldopa or reserpine orally or parenterally is usually an effective antihypertensive.

Ruptured Aneurysm. Prevention of recurrent bleeding from aneurysms is the primary goal of treatment and, in view of the close approximation of recurrent bleeding to the initial hemorrhage, should be attempted as soon as possible. Thus, angiograms to identify the source and site of bleeding should be made as soon as practicable, once the diagnosis of intracranial hemorrhage has been made. Similarly, if the aneurysm is believed to be amenable to surgical therapy, this is performed as soon as the patient's condition allows. Patients with no depression of consciousness, who are under 60 and normotensive, who have no evidence of arterial spasm on angiograms, and who have minimal neurologic deficits are considered good surgical risks and can be treated surgically immediately if this form of therapy is indicated for the particular aneurysm. Patients with depressed levels of consciousness or coma or with major neurologic deficits are very poor candidates for surgery; operative mortality in this group is extremely high; operation, if indicated, should be postponed until improvement occurs. Patients over the age of 60 who are hypertensive and who have arterial spasm on angiograms also are poor operative risks, and surgery should be delayed until their condition improves.

Surgical therapy is directed toward removal of the aneurysm or control of the bleeding by a direct surgical attack or toward decreasing the blood pressure in the feeding arterial tree by ligation of a proximal artery. Not all aneurysms can be treated surgically.

Some forms of surgical therapy are more suitable than others. In the past six years, several clinics and hospitals have worked together in a cooperative study to determine the type of surgery most suitable for a particular bleeding lesion. It has been concluded, through carefully controlled studies in England, that aneurysms arising from the internal carotid artery at the junction with the posterior communicating artery should be treated surgically, the procedure of choice being ligation of the common carotid artery in the neck or direct surgical attack on the aneurysm in good-risk patients.

The controlled studies indicate that patients with anterior cerebral artery aneurysms probably do not benefit from surgery and may actually do worse. However, some surgeons still believe that, in properly selected patients, surgical correction of an aneurysm of the anterior cerebral or anterior communicating artery is beneficial.

The outcome of surgical treatment of middle cerebral artery aneurysms is more uncertain. In the controlled treatment series, direct surgical attack provided better results in male patients, whereas women with middle cerebral aneurysms fared less well with surgery than when treated conservatively. The explanation of this difference appears to be that women are more prone to cerebral infarction after surgery than men. In addition, women have smaller, more fragile, aneurysms that make surgery more difficult.

Aneurysms on the vertebral basilar vascular tree are difficult to reach surgically. The most successful surgery reported has been for aneurysms arising from the vertebral artery near the branching of the posterior inferior cerebellar artery.

Current surgical techniques include a large number of methods for dealing with ruptured aneurysms. Most of the carefully controlled treatment trials have utilized either common carotid ligation or clipping or tying of the neck of the aneurysm or its feeding vessels. To reinforce the aneurysm and prevent recurrent bleeding, plastic coating and gauze wrapping have been utilized, but their superiority over other methods of surgical treatment has yet to be proved.

If the patient is not suitable for surgical treatment or if surgery must be delayed, a program of medical treatment should be instituted as outlined above.

Arteriovenous Anomaly. Surgery for A-V anomalies requires the tying of feeding vessels or the amputation of a portion of the brain containing the anomaly. The latter treatment is curative if the whole A-V malformation can be removed, but it is limited to those instances in which the anomaly lies entirely in or on the occipital pole or the frontal pole. The chance of neurologic disability associated with removal of A-V anomalies in other sites is usually too great to justify surgical therapy unless major disability had been present before bleeding.

Ligation of vessels feeding the anomaly has been recommended, but no carefully controlled evaluation of this form of surgical therapy has been done. Carotid ligation to reduce the blood pressure in the anomaly is also believed to reduce the chance of recurrent bleeding. Recently, artificial embolization with plastic spheres introduced into the feeding arteries has been reported to be successful in obliterating the anomaly.

Fortunately, the chance of recurrent bleeding with arteriovenous anomalies is less than with aneurysm. Also, bleeding carries a relatively low mortality, so that for most patients with arteriovenous anomaly and intracranial hemorrhage, medical management identical to that described for ruptured aneurysm is the treatment of choice. The frequency of disability and mortality associated with surgical treatment are too high to justify its use except in highly special instances. Convulsive seizures are common with arteriovenous anomalies and should be treated with anticonvulsants as outlined in the article on Epilepsy.

Intracerebral Hemorrhage. Cerebral hemorrhage is a severe disease and one for which there is no satisfactory form of treatment. The immediate medical treatment was outlined in the introduction to this article. It must include meticulous attention to the problems imposed by impaired consciousness and abrupt neurologic disability.

Whether and when to operate on cerebral hemorrhage is a recurrent question, and efforts have been made in this direction for years, although generally with poor results. Recently, McKissock and his colleagues in England carried out a carefully controlled evaluation of surgical treatment of acute cerebral hemorrhage due to hypertensive disease, in which they showed that patients treated surgically fared less well than those treated conservatively. No matter what the treatment, patients in deep stupor or coma from intracerebral hemorrhage rarely survive. For patients who survive the initial cerebral insult and become stable clinically, removal of a persistent encapsulated hematoma may lessen neurologic disability and hasten improvement.

Surgical removal of an intracerebral hematoma caused by bleeding from a ruptured aneurysm has been no more encouraging than when hypertensive vascular disease causes the hemorrhage. Patients with intracerebral hematoma from ruptured aneurysm are usually in coma and have severe neurologic dysfunction; survival in these circumstances is unlikely.

Removal of an intracerebral hematoma caused by bleeding from a ruptured A-V anomaly has been recommended for patients with neurologic disability. The results are difficult to appraise objectively, but surgical treatment has its best chance of offering relief if the patients have become stable clinically and have a well localized, encapsulated hematoma causing symptoms and signs of a mass lesion.

Patients who recover from intracerebral hemorrhage should begin programs of rehabilitation as soon as the effects of acute brain damage have subsided. Such a program begins with passive exercise of the paretic extremities to help avoid contractures and progresses to active exercises as voluntary movement returns. The program is as outlined in the discussion of cerebral infarction.

Dinsdale, H. B.: Spontaneous hemorrhage in the posterior fossa. Arch. Neurol. (Chicago), 10:200, 1964.

Fields, W. S., and Sahs, A. L.: Intracranial Aneurysm and Subarachnoid Hemorrhage. Springfield, Ill., Charles C Thomas, 1965.

McKissock, W., Richardson, A., and Taylor, J.: Primary intracerebral hemorrhage. A controlled trial of surgical and conservative treatment in 180 unselected cases. Lancet, 2:221, 1961.

McKissock, W., Richardson, A., and Walsh, L.: Anterior communicating aneurysms. A trial of conservative and surgical treatment. Lancet, 1:873, 1965.

McKissock, W., Richardson, A., and Walsh, L.: Middle-cerebral aneurysms. Further results in the controlled trial of conservative and surgical treatment of ruptured intracranial aneurysm. Lancet, 2:417, 1962.

Pool, J. L., and Potts, D. G.: Aneurysms and Arteriovenous Anomalies of the Brain; Diagnosis and Treatment. New York, Hoeber Medical Division, Harper & Row, 1965.

Report on the Cooperative Study of Intracranial Aneurysms and Subarachnoid Hemorrhage. J. Neurosurg., 24:779, 922, 1034; 25:98, 219, 321, 467, 547, 1966.

Walton, J. N.: Subarachnoid Hemorrhage. London, E. & S. Livingstone, Ltd., 1956.

Infections and Inflammatory Diseases of the Central Nervous System and Its Coverings

INTRODUCTION

Philip R. Dodge

The seriously ill patient with symptoms and signs of disease of the central nervous system and evidence of leptomeningeal inflammation presents a challenging diagnostic and therapeutic problem. Of crucial clinical significance is the determination of whether the involvement of meninges is primary, as in bacterial meningitis, or secondary, as in a variety of parenchymatous and parameningeal infections (encephalitis, brain abscess, subdural empyema, etc.). Central to this clinical problem is some degree of pleocytosis. Various bacteria, fungi, rickettsiae, viruses, and parasites may excite such a cerebrospinal fluid response. In addition, a similar reaction may be produced by a variety of noninfectious processes, including chemical irritation, hypersensitivity responses, and, occasionally, tumors. Elsewhere in this text many of the specific diseases that evoke an inflammatory response in the central nervous system and meninges are discussed. In this section emphasis will be placed on a systematic clinical approach to differential diagnosis and on the manner in which functions of the nervous system are deranged by such inflammatory processes.

AIDS TO DIAGNOSIS IN INTRACRANIAL AND INTRASPINAL INFLAMMATORY DISEASE

Philip R. Dodge

CEREBROSPINAL FLUID EXAMINATION

Because diagnosis rests in many instances on the cerebrospinal fluid findings, the importance of a carefully performed lumbar puncture and of meticulous study of the cerebrospinal fluid cannot be overstressed. The cerebrospinal fluid findings characteristic of various inflammatory diseases of the central nervous system and meninges are outlined in Tables 1 and 2. Measurement of the initial pressure should be part of every cerebrospinal fluid examination. In the presence of high pressure, just enough fluid should be removed slowly to allow for an adequate examination. Jugular compression (Queckenstedt's test) should be avoided except in cases of suspected spinal cord compression. Deeply yellow (xanthochromic) fluid derives its color primarily from bilirubin pigment. In the absence of prior hemorrhage, this is most frequently associated with high concentrations of protein, and is often seen with impaired cerebrospinal fluid circulation. Intense bilirubin staining of the cerebrospinal fluid may also occur in jaundiced patients with meningitis (as in Weil's disease).

As few as 200 to 300 leukocytes per cubic millimeter will impart an opalescence to the fluid, and fluid containing thousands of cells will be turbid. The fluid should be examined promptly for cells in a counting chamber, and an accurate differential count should be performed on a stained smear of the sediment after centrifugation. In the event of a traumatic lumbar puncture, care must be exercised to ensure that an underlying pleocytosis is not missed. A gram-stained smear for bacteria should be studied. Quellung and agglutination reactions with type-specific antisera may provide an almost certain, immediate etiologic diagnosis when *D. pneumoniae, N. meningitidis, or H. influenzae* organisms are responsible for meningitis. Whenever tuberculous meningitis is a consideration, a Ziehl-Neelsen stain should be performed on the sediment and on the protein coagulum or pellicle that frequently forms on standing. The India ink technique will usually outline *C. neoformans* in cases of crytococcal meningitis (torulosis). The finding of budding forms of the yeast in cerebrospinal fluid will help distinguish cryptococci from lymphoctyes with which they may be confused.

The cerebrospinal fluid should be cultured whenever leukocytes are found or when an inflammatory process is suspected. A variety of media (blood agar, chocolate agar, thioglycollate broth)

TABLE 1. INITIAL CEREBROSPINAL FLUID FINDINGS IN SUPPURATIVE DISEASES OF THE CENTRAL NERVOUS SYSTEM AND MENINGES

	Pressure (mm. H$_2$O)	Leukocytes per cu. mm.	Protein (mg. per 100 ml.)	Sugar (mg. per 100 ml.)	Specific Findings
Acute bacterial meningitis	Usually elevated; average, 300	Several hundred to more than 60,000; usually few thousand; occasionally less than 100 (especially meningococcal or early in disease); polymorphonuclears predominate	Usually 100 to 500, occasionally more than 1000	Less than 40 in more than half the cases	Organism seen on smear usually; recovered on culture in more than 90% of cases
Subdural empyema	Usually elevated; average 300	Less than 100 to few thousand; polymorphonuclears predominate	Usually 100 to 500	Normal	No organisms on smear or by culture unless concurrent meningitis
Brain abscess	Usually elevated	Usually 10 to 200; rarely fluid is acellular; lymphocytes predominate	Usually 75 to 400	Normal	No organisms on smear or by culture
Ventricular empyema (rupture of brain abscess)	Considerably elevated	Several thousand to 100,000; usually more than 90% polymorphonuclears	Usually several hundred	Usually less than 40	Organism may be cultured or seen on smear
Cerebral epidural abscess	Slight to modest elevation	Few to several hundred or more cells; lymphocytes predominate	Usually 50 to 200	Normal	No organisms on smear or by culture
Spinal epidural abscess	Usually reduced with spinal block	Usually 10 to 100; lymphocytes predominate	Usually several hundred	Normal	No organisms on smear or by culture; may enter abscess on L.P. and get pus
Thrombophlebitis (often associated with subdural empyema)	Often elevated	Few to several hundred; polymorphonuclears and lymphocytes	Slightly to moderately elevated	Normal	No organisms on smear or by culture
Bacterial endocarditis (with embolism)	Normal or slightly elevated	Few to less than 100; lymphocytes and polymorphonuclears	Slightly elevated	Normal	No organisms on smear or by culture
Acute hemorrhagic encephalitis	Usually elevated	Few to more than 1000; polymorphonuclears predominate	Moderately elevated	Normal	No organisms on smear or by culture

TABLE 2.   COMPARATIVE CEREBROSPINAL FLUID FINDINGS IN NONSUPPURATIVE MENINGITIS

	Pressure (mm. H$_2$O)	Leukocytes per cu. mm.	Protein (mg. per 100 ml.)	Sugar (mg. per 100 ml.)	Specific Findings
Tuberculous	Usually elevated; may be low with dynamic block in advanced stages	Usually 25 to 100, rarely more than 500; lymphocytes predominate except in early stages when polymorphonuclears may account for 80% of cells	Nearly always elevated, usually 100 to 200; may be much higher if dynamic block	Usually reduced; less than 50 in ¾ of the cases	Acid-fast organisms may be seen on smear of protein coagulum (pellicle) or recovered from inoculated guinea pig or by culture
Cryptococcal	Usually elevated; average, 225	0 to 800; average, 50; lymphocytes predominate	Usually 20 to 500; average, 100	Reduced in more than half of cases; average, 30; often higher in patients with concomitant diabetes mellitus	Organisms may be seen in India ink preparation and on culture (Sabouraud's medium); will usually grow on blood agar; may produce alcohol in CSF from fermentation of glucose
Syphilitic (acute)	Usually elevated	Average 500; usually lymphocytes; rarely polymorphonuclears	Average, 100; gamma globulin often high with abnormal colloidal gold curve	Normal (reduced rarely)	Positive reagin test for syphilis; spirochete not demonstrable by usual techniques of smear or by culture
Sarcoid	Normal to considerably elevated	0 to less than 100 mononuclear cells	Slight to moderate elevation	Normal	No specific findings
Tumor	Usually elevated; may be considerably so	0 to several hundred mononuclears	Elevated often to high levels	Normal or greatly reduced; low in ¾ of carcinomatous meningitis cases)	Neoplastic cells may be identified on smear, by Millepore filter technique or by tissue block
Viral	Normal to moderately elevated	5 to few hundred; but may be more than 1000, particularly with mumps or echovirus 9; lymphocytes predominate but may be more than 80% polymorphonuclears in first few days	Frequently normal or slightly elevated; less than 100; may show greater elevation in recovering stages (particularly poliomyelitis)	Normal (reduced rarely)	Viral agent may be recovered in tissue culture embryonated egg or animal inoculation

and various environmental conditions (reduced oxygen tension, increased CO_2 tension) are used routinely. Special media should be employed for the recovery of fungi. *M. tuberculosis* may be isolated on culture and from inoculation of guinea pigs. Tissue culture techniques and inoculation of mice and embryonated eggs are used for virus isolation.

The concentration of protein in the cerebrospinal fluid increases whenever there is interference with the blood-CSF barrier, as occurs with inflammation. In bacterial, tuberculous, mycotic, and carcinomatous meningitis the glucose concentration in the cerebrospinal fluid is commonly reduced (hypoglycorrhachia). Although the mechanism of hypoglycorrhachia is incompletely understood, the high metabolic activity of rapidly growing cells, phagocytosis, and impaired glucose transport may be involved. The gamma globulin concentration may be disproportionately increased, compared with other protein constituents, in certain inflammatory disorders such as syphilis, subacute inclusion body encephalitis, and certain demyelinating disorders (postinfectious encephalomyelitis, multiple sclerosis). A first zone colloidal gold sol (Lange) test will reflect this globulin increase. The only immunologic tests commonly applied to cerebrospinal fluid are those for the syphilis reagin.

RELATIONSHIP OF CEREBROSPINAL FLUID FINDINGS TO ANCILLARY CLINICAL AND LABORATORY DATA

An immediate etiologic diagnosis is possible only when the responsible agent is identified. However, the clinical and cerebrospinal fluid data can help to exclude certain clinical entities early in the diagnostic study. For example, when the symptoms and signs reflect involvement of the meninges and there is no evidence of cerebral or spinal cord disease, primary meningitis is probable. If, in addition, the cerebrospinal fluid contains about 100 or so lymphocytes, a normal quantity of sugar, and an only slightly elevated protein concentration, then bacterial, tuberculous, and cryptococcal meningitis are less likely, and some form of aseptic meningitis should be suspected. (However, it should be emphasized that the cerebrospinal fluid sugar may be normal on initial examination of patients with tuberculous meningitis and may be reduced in samples obtained subsequently.) A history of exposure to mumps and manifest parotitis make a diagnosis of mumps meningitis probable. On the other hand, the same findings in the CSF in a patient recovering from varicella, especially if there are symptoms and signs of cerebellar ataxia, suggest a diagnosis of postinfectious (varicella) encephalitis. In addition to primary meningeal disease, parameningeal infections can produce cerebrospinal fluid abnormalities similar to those just described. The coexistence of a progressive dysphasia, superior quadrantanopsia, and hemiparesis on the right side and a history of a chronic draining left ear should immediately direct the physician's attention to the diagnosis of a left temporal lobe abscess. Unfortunately, however, a definite diagnosis cannot be made from either the initial clinical or cerebrospinal fluid findings in many cases. Every attempt should be made to amplify the immediate and remote history, including epidemiologic data. One should search for foci of infection adjacent to or remote from the meninges. The extent of the dysfunction of the nervous system should be defined by repeated neurologic examinations and by laboratory studies. In addition to culturing the cerebrospinal fluid, blood cultures should be obtained, because bacteremia is present in about half the cases of primary bacterial meningitis, and similar cerebrospinal fluid changes may occur in bacterial endocarditis. Secretions of the upper and lower respiratory tracts should also be cultured for bacteria and fungi. Enteroviruses cause aseptic meningitis and encephalitis, and recovery of these agents from the stools of patients may aid in establishing the diagnosis. The development of specific neutralizing and complement-fixing antibodies will help confirm the diagnosis. Acute phase sera should be obtained on admission, and a convalescent serum sample obtained two to three weeks later. A fourfold rise in complement-fixing or neutralizing antibody titer is usually evidence of a recent infection with that agent.

Roentgenograms of the skull, sinuses, chest, or spine may be helpful in establishing a diagnosis by disclosing a related focus of disease. An electroencephalogram or isotope scan may direct attention to a region of the brain that clinically is relatively silent. Roentgenographic contrast studies (myelography, pneumoencephalography, ventriculography, and angiography) have their place in diagnosis, but are reserved for the more precise localization of a focal mass lesion that has already been suspected on clinical grounds. Occasionally the clinician must resort to a tissue biopsy; for example, the granulomatous lesions of sarcoidosis may be demonstrated in a lymph node or liver biopsy, and trichina, toxoplasma, or an unusual arteritis may be identified in microscopic sections of muscle tissue. Biopsy of the meninges or brain should be resorted to only rarely, but will at times help to establish the diagnosis in an obscure case. The pathologic findings in herpes, subacute sclerosing panencephalitis, and acute necrotizing hemorrhagic encephalitis are histologically specific enough to permit an exact diagnosis. Whenever tissue is obtained for routine histologic study, appropriate methods for the recovery of an infective agent should also be employed.

NEUROLOGIC ASPECTS OF MENINGITIS

Philip R. Dodge

Elsewhere in this textbook the meningitides are broadly considered as important problems in infectious disease. (See articles on Meningococcal Disease and Bacterial Meningitis other than That Caused by Meningococci and Mycobacteria) In the present article the effects of meningitis on the nervous system will be emphasized and the relationship of meningitis to other intracranial inflammatory diseases will be considered. Although the types of meningitis caused by various infective agents share much in common, the differences dictate that they be considered separately.

ACUTE BACTERIAL MENINGITIS

Pathology. The brains of patients dying during the early days of meningitis are frequently swollen, and temporal lobe or cerebellar herniations are found in more than 25 per cent of cases. The purulent subarachnoid exudate may be several millimeters in thickness or barely visible. It accumulates in sulci, along major veins and venous sinuses, in basal cisterns about the cerebellum, and over the dorsal aspect of the spinal cord. The ventricular walls are lined or flecked with pus in about half the cases. There is polymorphonuclear infiltration of small arteries and veins in about a third and thrombosis of vessels (usually veins) in 10 per cent of cases. An occluded venous sinus is found rarely. Infarction (frequently hemorrhagic) of cerebral tissue is a common consequence of thrombosis of vessels. Necrosis of cerebral cortex in the absence of demonstrated vascular occlusions is also seen, particularly beneath major accumulations of exudate. In such areas there is a diffuse polymorphonuclear infiltration of the tissue; damaged neurons, increased numbers of activated microglia (histiocytes) and astrocytes are also found. The pathogenesis of these cortical changes is uncertain, but toxic bacterial effects have been postulated. Similar changes are seen in the ventricular walls, often denuded of ependymal cells. A granular ependymitis may result from an abundant proliferation of subependymal astrocytes and, together with fibrosis of the leptomeninges, it may persist as the major residual finding in meningitis; hydrocephalus is a well recognized complication of such changes. It should be noted that a postmortem examination performed many weeks to years after recovery from meningitis often reveals no residual abnormalities.

Clinical Neurologic Manifestations. *Acute Stage.* The symptoms and signs of meningitis may develop explosively de novo or may appear in the waning stages of an infection localized elsewhere e.g., respiratory tract. (See articles on Meningococcal Disease and Bacterial Meningitis other than That Caused by Meningococci and Mycobacteria.) Headache, backache, nausea, and vomiting are common symptoms, and nuchal rigidity occurs in more than 80 per cent of cases. Kernig and Brudzinski signs are frequently present. Only in the neonate and very young infant is meningitis often unattended by evidence of increased pressure and meningeal irritation. Even fever may be absent at this age. Photophobia may be a prominent early symptom and is related in some way to the meningeal inflammation (it occurs also in subarachnoid hemorrhage).

Disturbances in mental status occur in nearly every case of acute bacterial meningitis. Irritability, confusion, delirium, and stupor are common; coma occurs in about 10 per cent of cases and indicates a poor prognosis. Focal or generalized seizures occur in about a fourth of all patients with meningitis, being encountered much more frequently in infants, who have a greater susceptibility to seizures. Signs of cerebral dysfunction, other than altered consciousness and seizures, are infrequent in acute bacterial meningitis and appear most often when treatment has been delayed. They include disturbed conjugate gaze, dysphagia, paresis of extremities, and visual field defects. When transitory they may represent postictal phenomena. Striking and persisting signs are usually due to bacterial encephalopathy or to infarction of tissue due to cortical venous thrombosis (see Cortical Thrombophlebitis). The latter complication commonly develops during the second week of disease when signs of infection and meningeal irritation are subsiding. Bilateral neurologic signs and convulsions occurring first on one side and then on the other always suggest an associated thrombosis of the superior sagittal sinus. Prominent and slowly progressive focal signs appearing early in the course of meningitis should bring to mind the possibility of an associated focus of sepsis such as subdural empyema, brain abscess, or bacterial endocarditis with cerebral embolism.

Perhaps 5 to 20 per cent of patients develop cranial nerve palsies during the acute stage of bacterial meningitis. Impaired ocular movement, deafness, and labyrinthine dysfunction are most frequently seen, but blindness and facial paralysis also occur. Most cranial nerve palsies are probably attributable to the meningeal exudate, but the eighth nerve complex may be damaged by bacteria or their toxins acting directly on the inner ear. Despite the fact that the cerebrospinal fluid pressure is usually elevated, papilledema is rare and more characteristic of brain abscess, subdural empyema, or venous-sinus thrombosis. The infrequent occurrence of papilledema in uncomplicated meningitis is probably explained by the short duration of increased pressure. Nevertheless, the heightened intracranial pressure, when present, is a disturbing finding, for death may result from the syndrome of transtentorial or foramen magnum herniation. Administration of excessive amounts of hypotonic fluids during treatment of meningitis should be avoided, for water intoxication may further elevate the intracranial pressure.

Collections of xanthochromic fluid containing a high concentration of protein (200 to more than 1000 mg. per 100 ml.) and, at times, inflammatory cells and bacteria may be recovered from the subdural space in up to 50 per cent of infants during the course of acute bacterial meningitis, but this complication is not recognized in adults.

Late Neurologic Sequelae. Neurologic sequelae are found in about 5 per cent of adults and 20 per cent of infants and children surviving an attack of acute bacterial meningitis. One of the more serious complications of meningitis is hydrocephalus, which develops in about 2 per cent of patients (usually infants). This is most often attributable to fibrosis of the meninges and consequent obliteration of the major basilar cisterns. Less often a noncommunicating hydrocephalus results from obliteration of the foramina of Magendie and Luschka, and rarely from ependymitis and narrowing of the aqueduct. Aside from monocular blindness and permanent deafness, which complicate meningitis in 3 to 5 per cent of cases, enduring dysfunction of cranial nerves is unusual. Residual parenchymatous damage following meningitis causes epilepsy in 4 per cent, impaired mental functions or retardation in 3 per cent, and hemiplegia or bilateral hemiplegia in 2 per cent of patients.

NONSUPPURATIVE MENINGITIS

Tuberculous Meningitis. Initial involvement of the central nervous system in tuberculosis usually occurs during a period of transient hematogenous dissemination. Tubercles of macroscopic or microscopic size can be demonstrated in the meninges in virtually every case of tuberculous meningitis. Tuberculomas of the central nervous system and of the meninges do not necessarily lead to frank meningitis, however. This subject is discussed in the articles on Tuberculous Meningitis and Tuberculomas.

Mycotic Meningitis. Fungi, although ubiquitous in nature, cause human disease infrequently and rarely involve the nervous system. Impairment of host defenses, as in leukemia, lymphomas, diabetes, and with immunosuppressive treatment, often predisposes to the development of mycotic infections. The possible coexistence of two disease processes, therefore, demands consideration whenever the physician is confronted by a patient with meningitis due to a fungus. A chronic granulomatous meningitis with mononuclear inflammatory cells and giant cells of the Langhans type is produced by most of the fungi pathogenic to man; torulosis, caused by *Cryptococcus neoformans,* is the most frequently encountered type of mycotic meningitis. The illness may be protracted, relapsing, and remitting over many years; less often it is subacute or acute. The reactive fibrosis of the meninges in infections due to *Aspergillus fumigatus* may be extreme, and occasionally may produce symptoms of a meningeal mass lesion. Involvement of small meningeal vessels, at times producing a necrotizing angiitis, is a feature of *Histoplasma capsulatum* meningitis but this rarely leads to hemorrhage from or thrombosis of the vessel. By contrast, in mucormycosis large veins and arteries are frequently occluded by extension of the infection into their walls and lumina. The infection commonly arises in the ancillary air sinuses in patients with diabetes mellitus and extends in a retrograde manner to

involve the sagittal sinus and carotid artery. A diffuse encephalitis, solitary granuloma, or true cerebral abscess may also develop in the course of a mycotic infection in man. The symptoms and signs of brain tumor may be simulated by a mycotic abscess. Although treatment of intracranial fungal infections with amphotericin B has brightened the therapeutic possibilities considerably, the mortality rate remains high.

Syphilitic Meningitis. See article on Syphilitic Infections of the Central Nervous System.

Sarcoidosis. Involvement of the nervous system occurs in about 3 per cent of cases of Boeck's sarcoid, but sarcoidosis is a rare cause of aseptic meningitis. The granulomatous lesions of this disease tend to accumulate about blood vessels, particularly at the base of the brain. Infiltration of the optic chiasm and hypothalamus can result in amblyopia and diabetes insipidus. Hydrocephalus and increased intracranial pressure may develop. Diagnosis depends upon ancillary clinical data or upon a histologically typical lesion obtained from tissue biopsy (see article on Sarcoidosis). The mortality rate is high when symptoms and signs of intracranial disease develop.

Neoplastic Meningitis. Diffuse infiltration of the leptomeninges by primary intracranial or metastatic malignant tumors may produce symptoms and signs of meningitis. The cerebrospinal fluid findings can include pleocytosis, elevated protein, and greatly reduced glucose concentrations. Recognition of neoplastic cells in the fluid will permit accurate diagnosis.

Viral Meningitis. A table listing the viral agents that may produce meningitis is included in the discussion of Viral Meningitis in the section on Microbial Diseases. Aseptic meningitis caused by *Leptospira* is easily confused with that caused by viral agents, and must be considered in any differential diagnosis. In viral meningitis variable numbers of mononuclear cells are found in the leptomeninges and about blood vessels in Virchow-Robin spaces. The process usually excites minimal reactions of meningeal fibroblasts. Typically, the induced illness is acute, mild, of brief duration, and is followed by complete recovery. Fever, malaise, headache, vomiting, and meningeal symptoms and signs can be expected, and seizures may occur in young children. When consciousness is significantly impaired or there are other prominent focal or generalized signs of involvement of the central nervous system, the term viral meningitis is inappropriate, and the designation meningoencephalitis or encephalitis should be employed. In these cases the prognosis must be more guarded.

Other Rare Forms of Meningitis. Several unusual types of meningitis may pose a significant problem in differential diagnosis. Although the meninges are rarely implicated in a hypersensitivity reaction, such involvement can occur in serum sickness and in sensitivity to certain sulfonamide drugs. A possible sensitivity to the rat lung worm, *Angiostrongylus cantonensis,* has been the suggested cause of eosinophilic meningitis.

Aseptic meningitis may result from the rupture of an intracranial epidermoid cyst or may follow the instillation of chemicals, e.g., iophendylate (Pantopaque) into the spinal subarachnoid space. Meningitis may complicate spinal anesthesia, and, rarely, a progressive adhesive arachnoiditis ensues. Pain, pareses, and impaired sensation from involvements of the spinal cord and roots are common; rarely, the arachnoiditis extends intracranially, producing cranial nerve damage and hydrocephalus. The cause of adhesive arachnoiditis following spinal anesthesia is unknown, but contamination of the anesthetic agent with phenol or a detergent has been suggested.

Butler, W. T., Alling, D. W., Spickard, A., and Utz, J. P.: Diagnostic and prognostic value of clinical and laboratory findings in cryptococcal meningitis. New Eng. J. Med., 270:59, 1964.

Camp, W. A.: Sarcoidosis of the central nervous system. A case with postmortem studies. Arch. Neurol. (Chicago), 7:432, 1962.

Dodge, P. R., and Swartz, M. N.: Bacterial meningitis. II. Special neurologic problems, postmeningitic complications and clinicopathologic correlations. New Eng. J. Med., 272:954, 1003, 1965.

Lorber, J.: Long-term follow up of 100 children who recovered from tuberculous meningitis. Pediatrics, 28:778, 1961.

Meyer, H. M., Jr., Johnson, R. T., Crawford, I. P., Dascomb, H. E., and Rogers, N. G.: Central nervous system syndromes of "viral" etiology—a study of 713 cases. Amer. J. Med., 29:334, 1960.

Swartz, M. N., and Dodge, P. R.: Bacterial meningitis. I. General clinical features, special problems and unusual meningeal reactions mimicking bacterial meningitis. New Eng. J. Med., 272:725, 779, 842, 898, 1965.

Weiss, W., and Flippen, H. J.: The changing incidence and prognosis of tuberculous meningitis. Amer. J. Med. Science, 250:46, 1965.

PARAMENINGEAL INFECTIONS
Morton N. Swartz

The three major localized intracranial suppurative lesions are *cerebral abscess, subdural empyema,* and *cerebral extradural abscess.* Of paramount importance in their early recognition and subsequent management is an understanding of the nature of the predisposing suppurative conditions and of the portals by which infection has spread intracranially. Not only must these conditions be distinguished from one another but they must also, from a therapeutic viewpoint, be clearly distinguished from meningitis due to bacteria or other infective agents.

CEREBRAL ABSCESS

Definition. Brain abscess represents a poorly or sharply delineated suppurative process of brain substance, resulting from extension from adjacent foci or from hematogenous spread.

Incidence. Despite the introduction of effective antibacterial therapy, the over-all incidence of brain abscess has not changed significantly over the past two decades (about 7 per 1000 neuro-surgical operations). It is seen approximately one fifth as frequently as bacterial meningitis in a large general hospital.

Predisposing Factors. Intracerebral infections are usually a consequence of an adjacent primary focus of infection: middle ear, mastoid, paranasal sinuses, face or scalp and skull (osteomyelitis, compound fracture with wound contamination, or craniotomy wound infection). Bronchiectasis, lung abscess, empyema, skin infections, and acute bacterial endocarditis may be the source of hematogenous brain abscess; congenital heart disease with right-to-left shunt is an important predisposing factor. In approximately 10 per cent of brain abscesses an underlying cause cannot be determined.

Subacute and Chronic Middle Ear Infection and Mastoiditis. Over one third of all brain abscesses stem from otitic infection. Infection usually spreads from the ear by either of two routes: direct extension to the roof of the tympanic cavity or mastoid bone (osteomyelitis) and then through the meningeal covering of the brain, or by extension along veins of the inner ear through diploic vessels of the skull and through intracranial venous channels into the substance of the brain. Thrombophlebitis of the pial vessels and dural sinuses, by impairing cerebral circulation, may cause infarction of brain tissue and facilitate development of local infection. The temporal lobe and cerebellum adjacent to the ear and mastoid, are the most common sites of otogenic abscess.

Infections of the Paranasal Sinuses. Frontal and sphenoid sinuses are most frequently implicated in "rhinogenic" brain abscess of the frontal and temporal lobes, respectively. Infection may erode the sinus wall and invade the brain directly or, as with otogenic infection, may spread by way of veins communicating with the cavernous sinus and brain.

Infections of the Face and Skull. Intracranial spread of infection from the face or nose to the frontal lobe occurs by way of a septic thrombophlebitis. Compound fractures of the skull may result in brain abscess, particularly when the dura and brain are lacerated leaving a nidus of bone or foreign body in the devitalized tissue. Occasionally the original traumatic episode has seemed trivial and has been overlooked. Several cases of brain abscess due to a pencil point introduced through the orbit have been reported. Brain abscess may complicate stereotactic surgery and ventriculovascular shunts.

Etiology. A wide variety of micro-organisms cause brain abscesses, and a careful attempt to establish a bacteriologic diagnosis should be made in every case. A Gram-stained smear of purulent material should be studied at the time of surgery, and aerobic and anaerobic cultures, as well as cultures for fungi, should be obtained. In about 20 per cent of brain abscesses cultures are sterile. In about 25 per cent, most often when there is a contiguous extracerebral focus, two or more microbial species are isolated.

Staphylococcus aureus and various streptococci

(either anaerobic or non-group A strains) are the most frequently isolated organisms. Pneumococcus, formerly a leading cause of brain abscess, is only rarely incriminated today. Species of the Enterobacteriaceae (*E. coli*, Proteus, Klebsiella) are sometimes isolated, particularly from otogenic brain abscesses. Anaerobic bacteria (particularly streptococci and Bacteroides) may have a more prominent role in brain abscess than heretofore appreciated. Rarely Actinomyces, *Nocardia asteroides* and other fungi may be recovered from an abscess cavity. Of interest is the frequent association of pulmonary alveolar proteinosis with pulmonary and occasionally cerebral nocardiosis. *Hemophilus aphrophilus* and the fungus *Cladosporium trichoides* rarely infect human beings, but when they do, they show a curious affinity for the central nervous system.

When *Entamoeba histolytica* causes brain abscess, there are associated lesions of the liver or lung in virtually every case. In Central and South America and parts of Europe and Asia cerebral cysticercosis (usually solitary cysts containing the larval form of the pork tapeworm *Taenia solium*) should be considered in patients presenting with symptoms of brain tumor. In the racemose form of disease, obstructive hydrocephalus results from the growth of cysts in the third or fourth ventricle. The clinical picture may suggest a diagnosis of pseudotumor cerebri. Very rarely the brain is the site of echinococcal cysts and the solitary or multiple granulomas of schistosomiasis.

Pathology. Abscesses resulting from direct spread of infection are found in the brain adjacent to the primary extracerebral site; those resulting from retrograde venous propagation are often located at some distance from the primary focus in the distribution of the nearest venous sinus. Thus, for example, cerebellar abscess from otitis media is the result of spread of infection from the middle ear to its deep venous drainage into the transverse sinus, and thence medially into the veins draining the anterior superior portion of the ipsilateral cerebellar hemisphere. Metastatic abscesses are usually found in the distribution of the middle cerebral artery.

Initially, the site is edematous and infiltrated with polymorphonuclear leukocytes. The lesion is poorly demarcated at this stage and represents a local suppurative encephalitis. Usually within two weeks of onset the center undergoes liquefaction necrosis. The surrounding zone of fibroblasts becomes progressively thicker and contains more collagen; this constitutes the wall of the abscess, and astrocytes proliferate in the adjacent cerebral tissue. Multiple satellite abscesses may develop and frequently communicate with the principal cavity. Since abscess cavities usually spread through the central white matter, they often extend to and through the ventricular wall, producing the dire complications of ventricular empyema and meningitis. Brain abscess seldom, if ever, results from primary bacterial meningitis. Coincidental occurrence of brain abscess and meningitis is usually related to intraventricular

leakage of the abscess. In support of this view, the three most common organisms in primary pyogenic meningitis (pneumococcus, *H. influenzae*, and *N. meningitidis*) occur only rarely as the cause of brain abscess.

Clinical Manifestations. *Age Incidence.* Brain abscesses are most common in the second to fifth decades, but may occur at any age. They are rare in infancy, even in patients with congenital heart disease.

General Features. A history of fever at the time of invasion of the brain by the infective agent may be elicited; but a third of patients will lack a history of fever and remain afebrile under observation. Blood cultures are usually sterile except in those with an underlying acute bacterial endocarditis.

Headache, the most frequent initial symptom of brain abscess, may develop suddenly or insidiously while the attention of the patient and physician is directed toward the primary infection of ear, sinus, or lung or to the congenital cyanotic heart disease. The headache may be localized to the side of the abscess, but it is often generalized and increases in severity as the infection progresses. Heightened intracranial pressure, manifested by nausea, vomiting, drowsiness, bradycardia, confusion, and stupor, is common. Papilledema is a relatively late finding that is recognized in a minority of cases. The increased intracranial pressure may result in signs of sixth- and, less often, in those of third-nerve palsy. They are often false localizing signs since the abscess may be remote from the cranial nerves. Although pathologically brain abscess progresses through several phases, there is no clear correlation with the clinical course of most patients. In some patients, usually those with metastatic brain abscesses, the illness runs a fulminating course, ending fatally in 5 to 15 days. In most, however, the course is considerably prolonged, and a diagnosis of cerebral neoplasm is often suspected.

Specific Neurologic Syndromes. *Temporal Lobe Abscess.* Most temporal lobe abscesses are secondary to ear infection. Involvement of the dominant temporal lobe may produce a nominal (inability to name objects) or Wernicke's (inability to read, write, or understand spoken words) aphasia. Personality changes with bizarre psychotic behavior, including uncontrolled rage, may occur. Commonly, homonymous upper quadrantic field defect results from dysfunction of the inferior fibers of the optic radiation that course about the inferior horn of the lateral ventricle in the temporal lobe. Involvement of the pyramidal tracts is not common, and the only motor deficit may be a slight contralateral faciobrachial monoparesis. Herniation of the temporal lobe through the tentorium may develop precipitously and cause a homolateral third-nerve paralysis, coma, and bilateral pyramidal tract signs.

Cerebellar Abscess. Cerebellar abscesses are almost exclusively otogenic. Increased intracranial pressure, suboccipital headache, and stiff neck may be the only manifestations. The patient may stagger and veer to the side of the lesion. Impaired coordination of extremities on the same side, with poor performance of rapid, alternating movements and with intention tremor, may be present. Nystagmus is frequent and usually coarser when the gaze is directed to the side of the inner ear. Associated diseases of the inner ear may contribute to the unsteady gait and nystagmus, and may produce vertigo. Seizures do not occur with abscesses restricted to the cerebellum.

Frontal Lobe Abscess. Frontal lobe abscesses are most commonly associated with disease of the frontal or, less frequently, the ethmoid sinuses. Drowsiness, inattention, disturbed judgment, and impaired intellectual functions are common; the findings may suggest a psychiatric diagnosis. Mutism and increased grasp, suck, and snout reflexes are often present. In about a fourth of cases focal or generalized convulsions occur; deviation of the head and eyes to the side opposite the lesion is a common pattern of seizure. When the abscess is large or in the posterior frontal region, a contralateral hemiparesis usually develops. Rarely, dysphasia results from a lesion on the dominant side.

Parietal Lobe Abscess. Parietal lobe abscesses are usually hematogenous but large otogenic temporal lobe abscesses may extend to the parietal lobe. Impaired position sense, two-point discrimination, and stereognosis are characteristic signs of an anterior parietal lobe abscess. Focal sensory and motor seizures occur. Homonymous hemianopia, visual inattention (often demonstrated by bilateral simultaneous stimulation of visual fields), and impaired opticokinetic nystagmus are encountered with more posterior and deep lesions. Dysphasia is a feature of inferior parietal lobe abscess on the dominant side. When the posterior parieto-temporo-occipital region is affected, there may be impaired recognition of fingers, difficulty in differentiating left from right, acalculia, and agraphia (Gerstmann's syndrome).

Brain Abscess Presenting as "Acute Meningitis." Occasionally patients with brain abscess present signs of meningitis, including fever, headache, stiff neck, and pleocytosis; focal neurologic signs are usually in evidence also. The syndrome is most often due to leaking of the abscess into the lateral ventricle. Massive rupture into the ventricle is a catastrophic event, with high fever, shock, and coma, and should be easily recognized. Pleocytosis with cell counts of more than 30,000 per cubic millimeter and reduced sugar concentrations are usual. Bacteria can often be seen on Gram stain and can be grown on culture.

In some patients with a similar clinical picture organisms are not found, and the syndrome may represent the phase of "bacterial encephalitis." The important point to be stressed is that one should be alert to the possibility of a brain abscess in any patients with chronic ear or sinus disease who develop meningitis. These patients often improve on treatment of the meningitis only to develop evidence of an intracranial mass lesion

one or two weeks later as encapsulation of the abscess progresses.

Laboratory Diagnosis. Cerebrospinal fluid pressure is commonly 200 to 300 mm. H_2O, but may be considerably higher, particularly in the presence of intraventricular rupture. The cell count varies from a few to several hundred, with lymphocytes predominating. In cases of intraventricular rupture of the abscess, cell counts may be in excess of 50,000 or 100,000 (mainly neutrophils). Also, cell counts of several thousand, with neutrophils predominating, may occur during the early phase of brain abscess ("bacterial encephalitis"). The sugar level is not reduced unless there is a simultaneous suppurative meningitis. The protein may be increased up to several hundred milligrams per 100 ml.

Roentgenograms of the chest, mastoid, and sinuses may identify the original focus. Displacement of the pineal or, very rarely, an air-fluid level in the lesion will be demonstrated by roentgenograms of the skull. A focus of high-voltage slow-wave activity on the side of the abscess, and maximal over the area of the lesion, characterizes the typical electroencephalogram. Localization of the abscess may also be obtained by scanning the brain after intravenous injection of an isotope, by arteriography, or by pneumography.

Treatment. Early diagnosis and prompt antimicrobial treatment are crucial. Surgery is employed once acute cerebral inflammation and edema are brought under control, and consists of initial aspiration of the abscess cavity, followed in some cases by excision at a later time, or primary total excision of the abscess. The method employed depends, to some extent, on the site of the lesion, but whenever feasible, primary excision is probably preferable.

Since in brain abscesses penicillin-susceptible organisms predominate, 10 million to 20 million units of penicillin per day intravenously should be started prior to operation. If there is reason to suspect an organism not susceptible to penicillin, e.g., gram-negative bacilli from a chronic ear infection, then chloramphenicol or similar drugs should be given concurrently. One of the semisynthetic penicillins, e.g., oxacillin, should be used if a penicillin-resistant Staphylococcus is suspected. The antimicrobial therapy should be modified as necessary at the time of operation, based on examination of a Gram-stained smear and culture of the abscess.

SUBDURAL EMPYEMA

Definition. The designation subdural empyema (less accurately termed a subdural abscess) refers to a collection of pus in the potential space between the dura and the arachnoid. It usually results from extension of infection from primary foci in the ears or sinuses. It is an infrequent complication of intracranial surgery, and may rarely represent a metastatic infection from a remote focus.

Incidence. Subdural empyema is about one fifth as common as brain abscess. Its prevalance has not changed in the past two decades.

Predisposing Factors and Pathologic Features. More than half of the cases of subdural empyema develop in patients with chronic paranasal sinus infection, usually frontal. An acute exacerbation of the sinusitis just prior to the development of the subdural infection is common. Osteomyelitis of the frontal bone and an epidural abscess often accompany subdural empyema. Chronic otitis media and mastoiditis result in subdural empyema less often than formerly. Postoperative infection, penetrating wounds, infection in subdural hematomas, bacteremia, pulmonary infection, and (very rarely) bacterial meningitis are other sources of subdural empyema.

Infection spreads from the sinuses or mastoid by direct erosion of bone and dura or through infected veins. Thrombosis of cortical veins is observed in 90 per cent of fatal cases. Once pus forms in the subdural space it spreads widely over the convexity of the hemisphere and mesially along the falx. Rarely, the exudate extends beneath the falx to the opposite side. Purulent subarachnoid exudate is usually present immediately subjacent to the subdural exudate.

Etiology. Streptococci, often non-group A or anaerobic strains, are implicated most commonly, but a wide variety of gram-negative organisms are also found. Postoperative infections are usually due to *Staphylococcus aureus.*

Clinical Manifestations. The symptoms and signs of antecedent sinusitis, otitis, or osteomyelitis often blend into those of subdural empyema. Swelling and erythema of the tissues overlying the primary infection may be prominent, and percussion of the underlying bone may evoke considerable pain. In the early stages, pain or headache is mild and is limited to the area over the subdural infection. As the illness progresses, headache becomes generalized and severe; concomitantly high fever, chills, vomiting, and nuchal rigidity develop. Progressive obtundation, culminating in coma within 48 to 72 hours, occurs in untreated cases. Focal or generalized seizures and hemiparesis are common. Sensory deficits and visual field defects and dysphasia also occur. Although these signs are in part attributable to the compressive effects of a mass lesion, the associated thrombophlebitis of cortical veins and the consequent infarction of cerebral tissue are probably of equal importance. In the late stages, the intracranial pressure is severely increased, but papilledema is rare except in chronic cases in which the clinical course has been modified by antimicrobial therapy. Without treatment, death usually occurs within a few days of onset of focal neurologic signs.

Laboratory Diagnosis. The cerebrospinal fluid pressure is elevated, and the fluid characteristically contains a few hundred to a thousand or more neutrophils, a normal amount of sugar, and no organisms. Roentgenograms of the skull may show destructive changes in the frontal or mastoid bones. Carotid angiography and diagnostic burr hole examination help to distinguish subdural empyema from brain abscess.

Treatment. The patient with a subdural empyema requires prompt and adequate surgical drainage by multiple burr holes or craniotomy. Surgical treatment of the accompanying sinusitis, frontal osteomyelitis, or mastoiditis is a secondary consideration and is usually postponed until the acute intracranial infection has subsided. Vigorous systemic therapy with penicillin (10 million to 20 million units daily) and/or other antimicrobials, depending on the background of the case, is begun before surgery and continued until the infection has been completely controlled. The results of smear and culture of pus obtained at the time of operation may dictate changes in the antimicrobial regimen. Bacitracin or other antimicrobial drugs are commonly instilled into the subdural space at the time of operation and for a variable period thereafter.

CEREBRAL EPIDURAL ABSCESS

Epidural abscess is usually secondary to mastoiditis, sinus infection, osteomyelitis of the skull, skull fracture, or infection of an operative wound. Etiologic and pathogenetic considerations are identical to those described for subdural empyema. The close adherence of the dura to bone limits the size of the epidural abscess. It often represents granulations rather than a frankly purulent collection. Rarely, an extensive destructive osteomyelitis of the frontal bone ("Pott's puffy tumor") may be associated with an epidural abscess.

Diagnosis may be difficult. The patient is not as ill as with a subdural empyema, and the size of the collection is rarely sufficient to produce focal neurologic signs or increased intracranial pressure. Fever, pain, and tenderness over the affected area are the common manifestations. In most cases the cerebrospinal fluid is sterile, and contains few cells (lymphocytes predominating) and a normal concentration of sugar. Many times the diagnosis is made incidentally at the time of sinus or mastoid surgery or when intracranial surgery is performed for an associated subdural empyema or brain abscess. Some cases of epidural abscess are probably cured by antimicrobial therapy alone. Spread of infection from the mastoid along the ridge of the petrous bone may result in a small epidural granuloma or abscess that gives rise to a homolateral sixth-nerve palsy and temporoparietal pain from involvement of the sensory fibers of the fifth nerve (Gradenigo's syndrome).

THROMBOPHLEBITIS AND THROMBOSIS OF MAJOR VENOUS SINUSES

Cortical Thrombophlebitis. The syndrome of cortical thrombophlebitis characteristically appears some three to ten days after the onset of bacterial meningitis. The signs include a secondary rise in temperature, focal or generalized seizures, and focal neurologic deficits, such as a hemiparesis. In some instances at least, the underlying phlebitis has its inception earlier and is the basis for many of the seizures and signs of focal cortical disease encountered in the early stages of meningitis. Treatment includes continuation of the antimicrobial therapy and anticonvulsants. Anticoagulant drugs have no established place in therapy. In most cases the process is limited in extent and the patient recovers, but, when the process is widespread, substantial neurologic deficits and death may result.

MAJOR DURAL SINUS THROMBOSIS

Thrombosis of the large dural sinuses may occur in meningitis, may complicate epidural or subdural abscesses, or may develop during the intracranial spread of infection from extracerebral veins. The thrombotic process may spread to connecting sinuses and cortical veins. Abscess formation within the thrombosed vessel may result in septicemia and infected emboli that travel to distant sites. The cavernous, lateral, and superior sagittal sinuses are most frequently involved.

Cavernous Sinus Thrombosis. Infection can spread to the cavernous sinus through venous channels by three routes: (1) from lesions of the upper half of the face through the facial veins communicating with the angular and superior ophthalmic veins, (2) from infections of the sphenoid and posterior ethmoid sinuses, inferiorly, and (3) from the ear, posteriorly. The initiating infection is usually an intranasal or facial furuncle, acute sinusitis, or an infection of the ear or mastoid. The widespread use of antimicrobial drugs in the treatment of superficial infections has markedly reduced the incidence of this disease. The majority of infections are due to *Staphylococcus aureus,* particularly in the presence of nasal furuncles.

Clinical Manifestations. The general clinical features are those of severe systemic infection: chills, fever, headache, nausea, lethargy, marked polymorphonuclear leukocytosis, and bacteremia. The specific findings are unilateral initially but become bilateral as the process extends to the opposite cavernous sinus via the connecting circular sinus. They include, in the case of infections about the face, unilateral edema of the forehead, eyelids, and base of the nose, as well as proptosis and chemosis — all due to obstruction of the ophthalmic vein as it enters the cavernous sinus. The superficial veins over the forehead may be distended. The retinal veins become engorged or even thrombosed. Retinal hemorrhages and papilledema occur but may be late manifestations. Involvement of the ophthalmic branch of the fifth nerve produces pain in the eye, photophobia, and hyperesthesia of the forehead. Partial or even complete paralysis of the ocular muscles develops as a result of involvement of the third, fourth, and sixth cranial nerves as they pass through the sinus. The pupils are usually dilated but may be small; the pupillary reactions are often lost.

In infection spreading by the inferior route (sphenoid sinusitis, etc.) the process may be less acute initially. A meningeal reaction commonly occurs, usually without organisms in the cerebrospinal fluid, but pyogenic meningitis sometimes occurs. Rarely, infarction and abscess of the pituitary complicate septic cavernous sinus thrombosis.

Differential diagnosis includes other causes of proptosis, especially orbital cellulitis, abscess, or acute carotid-cavernous fistula. Retinal hemorrhages, papilledema, and palsies of cranial nerves innervating extraocular muscles rather than general restriction of ocular movement from the mechanical effects of orbital swelling are useful differential points.

Lateral Sinus Thrombosis. Thrombosis of the lateral sinus is almost always a complication of acute or chronic otitis media, mastoiditis, or of cholesteatoma formation. Rarely, infection may spread in a retrograde fashion from a focus in the neck or from a tonsillar abscess. Streptococci, predominantly group A, and staphylococci have been implicated most frequently. The clinical manifestations include chills, fever, and signs of increased intracranial pressure. Pain, venous engorgement, and edema behind the ear may result from associated involvement of the mastoid emissary vein and may extend into the neck over the jugular vein. Papilledema is common; it may be unilateral as a consequence of extension to the cavernous sinus on that side. A generalized increase in intracranial pressure is more frequent with occlusions of the right lateral sinus, which is commonly larger and more important for venous drainage than the left. Convulsive seizures and obtundation occur, but focal neurologic findings are rare except when the thrombophlebitis extends into cortical veins over the convexity of the hemisphere. Rarely, ninth-, tenth- and eleventh-nerve palsies develop, presumably due to involvement of the jugular bulb and related venous channels.

Cerebrospinal fluid pressure is elevated, and the fluid contains several to many hundred leukocytes (lymphocytes predominating) but no bacteria.

Superior Sagittal Sinus Thrombosis. The superior sagittal sinus is less commonly involved in septic thrombosis than are the lateral and cavernous sinuses. Infection may spread from the lateral or cavernous sinuses, from the pelvis by way of the vertebral veins, from a primary meningitis, or from a contiguous osteomyelitis and peridural infection. If thrombosis is restricted to that portion of the sinus anterior to the rolandic veins, and there is no associated involvement of cortical veins, then the process is usually asymptomatic. Thrombosis of the posterior portion of the sinus results in increased intracranial pressure; at times there are engorgement of scalp veins and edema of the forehead. Extension of the inflammatory process into the cortical veins results in infarction of the underlying cortex. Focal seizures, which alternately involve one and then the other side of the body, are characteristic. Because the superior and mesial surfaces of the cerebral hemispheres are particularly liable to infarction, weakness and sensory changes are frequently more prominent in the legs. However, hemiparesis, homonymous hemianopia, aphasia, and paresis, or conjugate deviation of the eyes may occur.

The cerebrospinal fluid findings are similar to those in lateral sinus thrombosis. A suspected diagnosis of major venous sinus thrombosis can often be confirmed by angiographic study.

Treatment of Dural Sinus Thrombophlebitis. Appropriate antimicrobial drugs in high dosage and surgical drainage, with removal of infected bone and extradural or intrasinus abscess, constitute proper treatment for major sinus thromboses. Ligation of the jugular vein in lateral sinus thrombosis to prevent spread of infected emboli is usually not necessary. Because of the frequent involvement of penicillinase-producing staphylococci, the use of semisynthetic penicillins (nafcillin, oxacillin), cephalothin, or the combination of penicillin and methicillin is warranted until cultures are reported. Since infarction of cerebral tissue from venous thromboses tends to be hemorrhagic, anticoagulants are not employed. The prognosis for recovery is reasonably good when optimal treatment is given, although there are frequently residual neurologic symptoms and signs.

CEREBRAL MANIFESTATIONS OF BACTERIAL ENDOCARDITIS

Neurologic symptoms or signs occur in about 30 per cent of patients with bacterial endocarditis, and a patient may present as a diagnostic neurologic problem. The neuropathologic findings of subacute bacterial endocarditis (usually due to *Streptococcus viridans*) are distinct from those of acute bacterial endocarditis. (See Bacterial Endocarditis in section on Diseases of the Cardiovascular System.) Diffuse embolic infarctions, with a variable and usually limited inflammatory response about involved blood vessels and adjacent meninges, constitute the major neurologic findings in subacute bacterial endocarditis. Pyogenic brain abscess and purulent meningitis do not occur. The clinical picture can resemble that of diffuse encephalitis, or there may be focal signs such as hemiplegia and hemianopia. The cerebrospinal fluid contains modest numbers of polymorphonuclear leukocytes (sometimes red cells as well) and a normal concentration of sugar; bacteria are absent. Subarachnoid hemorrhage may result from rupture of a mycotic aneurysm.

In acute bacterial endocarditis due to invasive pyogenic organisms (usually *Staphylococcus*

aureus), brain abscess (usually small and multiple), acute purulent meningitis, and embolic infarction of cerebral tissue may occur.

Cerebral Abscess

Ballantine, H. T., Jr., and Shealy, C. N.: The role of radical surgery in the treatment of abscess of the brain. Surg. Gynec. Obstet., 109:370, 1959.
Gates, E. M., Kernohan, J. W., and Craig, W. M.: Metastatic brain abscess. Medicine, 29:71, 1950.
Heineman, H. S., and Braude, A. I.: Anaerobic infection of the brain. Amer. J. Med., 35:682, 1963.
Loeser, E., Jr., and Scheinberg, L.: Brain abscesses: A review of ninety-nine cases. Neurology, 7:601, 1957.
Matson, D. D., and Salam, M.: Brain abscess in congenital heart disease. Pediatrics, 27:772, 1961.
Victor, M., and Banker, B. Q.: Brain abscess. Med. Clin. N. Amer., 47:1355, 1963.

Subdural Empyema

Hitchcock, E., and Andreadis, A.: Subdural empyema: A review of 29 cases. J. Neurol. Neurosurg. Psychiat., 27:422, 1964.
Kubik, C. S., and Adams, R. D.: Subdural empyema. Brain, 66:18 1943.

Cerebral Manifestations of Bacterial Endocarditis

Jones, H. R., Siekert, R. E., and Geraci, J. E.: Neurologic Manifestations of bacterial endocarditis. Ann. Intern. Med., 71:21, 1969.
Kerr, A., Jr.: Subacute Bacterial Endocarditis. Springfield, Ill., Charles C Thomas, 1955, Chap. V. p. 92.
Ziment, I.: Nervous system complications in bacterial endocarditis. Amer. J. Med., 47:593, 1969.

Thrombophlebitis and Thrombosis of Major Venous Sinuses

Bailey, O. T.: Results of long survival after thrombosis of the superior sagittal sinus. Neurology, 9:741, 1959.
Brown, P.: Septic cavernous sinus thrombosis. Bull. Hopkins Hosp., 109:68, 1961.
Greer, M.: Benign intracranial hypertension. I. Mastoiditis and lateral sinus obstruction. Neurology, 12:472, 1962.
Kinal, M. E., and Jaeger, R. M.: Thrombophlebitis of dural venous sinuses following otitis media. J. Neurosurg., 17:81, 1960.
Ray, B. S., and Dunbar, H. S.: Thrombosis of the superior sagittal sinus as a cause of pseudotumor cerebri: Methods of diagnosis and treatment. Trans. Amer. Neurol. Ass., 75:12, 1950.

SPINAL EPIDURAL INFECTIONS
Philip R. Dodge

Definition. Spinal epidural infections consist of purulent or granulomatous collections contained within the spinal epidural space and overlying or encircling the spinal cord, roots, and nerves. Infection may be localized or may extend widely, at times involving the length of the spinal canal. In one large series an average extent of 4.3 bony segments was reported.

Incidence. This is a rare type of infection—one twentieth as common as bacterial meningitis, in our experience. Although persons of any age are susceptible, it occurs more frequently in young adults.

Etiology and Pathogenesis. *Staphylococcus aureus* is involved in more than 90 per cent of cases, but group A streptococci, other streptococci, pneumococci, Brucella, Salmonella, and various other gram-negative organisms may be responsible. *M. tuberculosis* is an important cause of chronic epidural infections in areas where tuberculosis is prevalent; occasionally fungi and parasites may be recovered from epidural granulomas. There is a primary infective site remote from the spine in most cases. This usually involves the skin, and furuncles, boils, and cellulitis are the common underlying infections. Less often infections of the upper respiratory tract, genitourinary system, or bone may be responsible. Hematogenous or lymphatic spread of infection to the highly vascular epidural space is postulated. Occasionally the responsible organism may be cultured from the blood. Minor injury to the back frequently antedates the symptoms of epidural abscess, and trauma may in some way determine the site of infection. The lack of restraining fibrous tissue in the epidural fat allows the infection to spread caudally and rostrally, and epidural abscesses may extend into the extraspinal tissues; in contrast, the dura is rarely penetrated. In less than half the cases the spine and adjacent soft tissues are primarily affected, and the infection spreads secondarily to the epidural space. Only in tuberculous infections is primary osteomyelitis the rule. Epidural abscess may rarely complicate a lumbar puncture, myelogram, or spinal operation.

Pathology. The purulent material or granulomatous tissue is usually most abundant over the posterior aspect of the spinal cord. When the primary lesion is in a vertebral body, intervertebral disc, or some other anterior structure, the abscess may be predominantly ventral. Epidural abscess occurs most commonly in the thoracic region, but may develop at any level of the spinal axis. The lesion may be purulent or granulomatous.

The mechanism of neural dysfunction in spinal epidural abscess is uncertain. Since the lesion occupies space, direct compression of spinal cord, roots, and nerves is a prime consideration, but the small size of many epidural abscesses, in association with severe impairment of neural function, demands consideration of other possibilities. The most plausible of these and the one for which there are some supporting facts is a vasculitis with secondary venous and arterial occlusions resulting in infarction of neural tissues.

Clinical Manifestations. Heusner has divided the clinical picture into four phases: spinal ache, root pain, weaknesses (voluntary muscles, sphincters, sensibilities), and paralyses.

Spinal Ache. The spinal ache, characteristically maximal at the level of the major pathologic process, soon spreads axially and may also include the paravertebral regions. Restricted movement of the spine, especially in the anteroposterior plane, is common. A functional or even a structural scoliosis may develop. The spines overlying the disease process are tender to percussion; pain so induced may be exquisite, particularly when there is vertebral caries. Signs of sepsis (fever, leukocytosis) are prominent, except in the more chronic cases. The diagnosis is rarely made at this stage.

Root Pain. Within two or three days (acute cases) nerve roots inevitably become encased by the purulent material, and radicular pains develop. Meningeal signs are present in most cases, and headache is a common symptom. At times reflex activity at the level of the involved segment may be depressed. An erroneous diagnosis of "neuritis" or "shingles" is frequently made, but at this stage of illness the combination of clinical symptoms and signs should permit an accurate diagnosis.

Weaknesses. The characteristic feature of this phase of the illness is progressive impairment of neural functions below the level of the lesion, the exact syndrome depending upon the site of maximal damage. If the abscess overlies the spinal cord, spastic weakness, heightened reflexes, and a sensory level over the trunk are to be expected. There may be urinary urgency and incontinence. Abscesses in the lumbosacral region exert their effects on spinal roots and nerves, giving rise to dysesthesias in dermatomes supplied by the implicated nerves, along with appropriate pareses and depressed stretch reflexes. Pain is usually excruciating and nuchal rigidity extreme. The skin and soft tissues overlying the abscess may be swollen, warm, and red. High fever and signs of systemic toxicity are often present.

The diagnosis may be made as late as this with reasonable anticipation that prompt laminectomy and drainage of pus or removal of granulomatous tissue will effect considerable if not total recovery.

Paralyses. Within hours or at most a few days, severe or even total paralysis of nervous functions below the site of the lesion supervenes. Immediate surgical treatment is mandatory at this stage. Procrastination may vitiate the effect of any subsequent therapeutic measures, for enduring paralyses are usual if the patient remains paraplegic for more than a few hours. When an epidural abscess remains unrecognized and untreated, death occurs in 25 to 33 per cent of cases.

It is axiomatic that the foregoing analysis of the clinical features of subdural abscess is arbitrary and somewhat artificial, since the various stages may merge one into the other. Yet, considered in this way the early stages are stressed and the importance of prompt diagnosis and treatment is underscored.

Differential Diagnosis. Spinal epidural abscess demands consideration in the patient with sepsis, back pain, and even minimal neurologic symptoms and signs. Confirmatory evidence may be obtained by tapping the epidural space with an ordinary spinal needle. This is most safely done in the lumbar area. Gentle suction is applied with a small (2 ml.) syringe while slowly advancing the needle. If no purulent material is obtained, the stylet should be replaced in the needle and the subarachnoid space entered. The cerebrospinal fluid is characteristically clear and xanthochromic. It may be acellular, but more often a few cells or a moderate pleocytosis (lymphocytes predominating) will be found. Normal sugar content and elevated cerebrospinal fluid protein are the rule (several hundred to more than 2000 mg. per 100 ml.). A partial or complete manometric block below the lesion is found in most cases.

An acute viral, postinfectious, syphilitic, or necrotizing myelitis may produce a neurologic syndrome similar to that seen in stage 4 of a spinal epidural abscess, and may be associated with symptoms and signs of infection and cerebrospinal fluid pleocytosis. There may be back pain in acute myelitis, but the duration of illness is compressed in time. Futhermore, xanthochromic cerebrospinal fluid and manometric block are unusual in myelitis. They are seen, however, in progressive adhesive arachnoiditis, which may be confused with subacute or chronic epidural infections. Spinal caries, demonstrable by roentgenography in less than 20 per cent of cases of spinal epidural abscess, suggests the correct diagnosis. In questionable cases a myelographic study will confirm the presence of a space-occupying intraspinal lesion. Rarely, malignant tumors, especially lymphomas that lodge in the epidural space, may present with fever, backache, neurologic signs, and spinal block. Chronic epidural abscess in which evidence of an inflammatory disease is meager or wanting will, on occasions, be confused with the more benign intraspinal tumors.

Treatment. Prompt laminectomy with drainage of purulent material or removal of granulomatous tissue and the administration of appropriate antimicrobial drugs constitute proper therapy. The antimicrobials must be continued in high doses for a minimum of six weeks when pyogenic osteomyelitis is present.

Heusner, A. P.: Nontuberculous spinal epidural infections. New Eng. J. Med., 239:845, 1948.
Hulme, A., and Dott, N. M.: Spinal epidural abscess. Brit. Med. J., 1:64, 1954.

DIFFUSE INFLAMMATORY DISEASES OF THE BRAIN AND SPINAL CORD (ENCEPHALITIS, MYELITIS, AND ENCEPHALOMYELITIS)

Philip R. Dodge

The terms encephalitis, myelitis, and encephalomyelitis designate diseases in which there is inflammation of the brain or of the spinal cord, or both. In classification, the term is modified by reference to the etiologic agent or pathogenetic mechanism whenever possible: e.g., Japanese B encephalitis, syphilitic myelitis, or postmeasles encephalomyelitis. Frequently, however, the clinician is unable to identify the specific cause, even after extensive clinical and laboratory study, and he must be content to indicate the extent and anatomic distribution of the disease process: e.g., myeloradiculitis, leukoencephalitis (white matter of brain), poliomyelitis (gray matter of cord), or disseminated encephalomyelitis. The almost uni-

versal involvement of the meninges in these inflammatory diseases of the brain and spinal cord was emphasized earlier; the prefix "meningo," e.g., meningomyelitis, is often used to indicate this fact. The rate of evolution of the disease (acute, subacute, or chronic) and certain characteristics of the pathologic process (inclusion body encephalitis, necrotizing hemorrhagic encephalitis, or subacute sclerosing panencephalitis, may help to describe a given illness better. A classification of the encephalitides and of the myelitides based on etiology whenever possible is presented in Tables 1 and 2, and the reader should refer to other sections in this text where various specific entities are discussed. The presentation here of an example

---

TABLE 1. CLASSIFICATION OF DIFFUSE INFLAMMATORY DISEASES OF THE BRAIN (ENCEPHALITIS)

I. Encephalitis due to bacteria (cerebral abscess, early stage; meningitis)

II. Encephalitis due to viruses
    A. Arthropod-borne (arbor-) viruses
        1. Eastern equine
        2. Western equine
        3. St. Louis
        4. Russian spring-summer
        5. Japanese B.
        6. Venezuela
        7. California
        8. Powassan
        9. W. Nile
    B. Enteroviruses
        1. Echo
        2. Coxsackie
        3. Poliomyelitis
    C. Other viruses
        1. Mumps
        2. Salivary gland viruses (cytomegalic inclusion disease)
        3. Herpes simplex (acute inclusion body, acute necrotizing encephalitis)
        4. Herpes zoster — varicella
        5. Rabies
        6. Rubeola, subacute sclerosing panencephalitis (SSPE)
        7. Rubella
    D. Probable viral diseases
        1. Infectious mononucleosis (E.B. virus)
    E. Postinfectious or postvaccinal encephalitis

III. Encephalitis due to spirochetes
        1. Syphilis
        2. Leptospiroses

IV. Encephalitis due to protozoa
        1. Toxoplasmosis
        2. Malaria (falciparum)
        3. Trypanosomiasis
        4. Amebiasis

V. Encephalitis due to metazoa
        1. Trichinosis
        2. Echinococcosis
        3. Schistosomiasis
        4. Cysticercosis

VI. Encephalitis due to fungi
        1. Cryptococcosis
        2. Aspergillosis
        3. Histoplasmosis
        4. Mucormycosis

VII. Noninfective encephalitis
        1. Lead poisoning (inflammatory reaction in cerebrospinal fluid)

TABLE 2.   CLASSIFICATION OF INFLAMMATORY
DISEASES OF THE SPINAL CORD (MYELITIS)

I. Myelitis due to viruses
   A. Poliomyelitis
   B. Coxsackie
   C. Herpes zoster
   D. Rabies
   E. B. virus myelitis

II. Myelitis of unknown etiology
   A. Demyelinative myelitis (acute multiple sclerosis)
   B. Postinfectious or postvaccinal myelitis
   C. Necrotizing myelitis (? myelopathy)

III. Myelitis secondary to inflammatory diseases of the meninges
   A. Syphilitic myelitis
      1. Acute meningitis
      2. Meningovascular spinal syphilis
      3. Tabes dorsalis
      4. Gummatous meningitis, including chronic spinal
         pachymeningitis
   B. Pyogenic or suppurative myelitis
      1. Subacute or chronic meningomyelitis
      2. Abscess of the spinal cord
      3. Subdural abscess
      4. Acute epidural spinal abscess or granuloma
   C. Tuberculous myelitis
      1. Pott's disease with spinal cord compression
      2. Tuberculous meningomyelitis
      3. Tuberculoma of the spinal cord
   D. Miscellaneous
      1. Parasitic and fungal infections producing an
         epidural granuloma, localized meningitis, or
         meningomyelitis
      2. Idiopathic meningomyelitis (chronic adhesive
         arachnoiditis)

of an acute form of encephalitis will serve to highlight certain neurologic aspects of this class of disease. Elsewhere, subacute sclerosing panencephalitis (SSPE) is discussed as a form of chronic encephalitis.

ACUTE INCLUSION BODY ENCEPHALITIS: ACUTE NECROTIZING ENCEPHALITIS, HERPES SIMPLEX ENCEPHALITIS (PROBABLE)

Definition. Acute inclusion body encephalitis is clinically and pathologically indistinguishable from encephalitis due to the herpes simplex virus. In all probability they represent a single disease, but the term acute inclusion body encephalitis is applied to those cases in which viral studies have not been done or are inconclusive. The disease occurs at all ages, but most cases occur in the second to fourth decades. Acute inclusion body encephalitis occurs sporadically in all parts of the world. There are no well defined seasonal or climatic determinants.

Pathology. Although hemorrhagic necrosis and associated swelling of gray and white matter may be widespread, the disease shows a striking predilection for the orbital surfaces of the frontal and inferior surfaces of the temporal lobes. Asymmetrical involvement is not uncommon, and may be reflected clinically by predominantly unilateral symptoms and signs. In addition to areas of frank hemorrhagic necrosis, histologic findings include infiltration of leptomeninges and perivascular

regions with leukocytes (mononuclear cells predominating), microglial nodules, and Cowdry type A inclusions within nerve cells, oligodendroglia, and, rarely, astrocytes. The numbers of inclusions vary considerably from case to case; in some cases they may not be found, especially late in the disease.

Clinical Manifestations. The illness has an abrupt or explosive onset, with high fever, headache, nausea, vomiting, and meningeal signs. In 25 to 30 per cent of cases the disease develops on the background of a minor upper respiratory or gastrointestinal infection. Mucocutaneous lesions (cold sores) are unusual during the course of acute inclusion body encephalitis, but a history of recurrent herpes labialis can be obtained in about 25 per cent of cases. Recently, the genital strain of herpes simplex virus has been incriminated as the prime source of encephalitis. Confusion, delirium, hallucinations, and delusions are early symptoms, and obtundation progressing to stupor and coma characterizes the later stages. Seizures, either focal or generalized, occur in more than half, and dysphasic difficulties in about a fourth of cases. Papilledema has been described in 10 per cent. Impaired motility is common, hemipareses being the usual pattern in adults and older children, whereas infants are more prone to develop bilateral, spastic weakness. Exaggerated stretch reflexes and Babinski signs are found. Choreoathetoid movements have been described rarely, but cerebellar symptoms and signs are absent.

The cerebrospinal fluid usually contains a few to several hundred leukocytes (polymorphonuclears may predominate in the early stages), a modest increase in protein, and a normal concentration of glucose. The cerebrospinal fluid pressure may be normal but is often elevated.

Slow waves (1 to 3 per second) of high amplitude characterize the electroencephalogram. These changes are usually generalized but may be focal, and indicate the areas of brain most affected by the encephalitic process. Radioactivity may be prominent in these same regions when radioisotopes are used to localize the disease process. Displacement of the swollen brain on pneumographic or arteriographic studies may mislead the clinician into considering the diagnosis of an abscess or, rarely, a tumor.

Differential Diagnosis. When evidence of cerebral dysfunction is prominent in a patient with fever, meningeal signs, and seizures, the diagnosis of meningoencephalitis should be seriously considered. Acute bacterial meningitis can usually be excluded by the lower polymorphonuclear leukocyte counts, the normal concentration of sugar, and the absence of bacteria in the cerebrospinal fluid. When the patient with bacterial meningitis has been partially treated, less reliance can be placed on the cerebrospinal fluid findings. In typical cases the rapid progression of bilateral signs of central nervous system dysfunction should add substance to the diagnosis of a diffuse parenchymatous disease. Highly malignant tumors and parameningeal infections always demand consideration but, with the exception of subdural empyema, the tempo of illness in a necrotizing encephalitis is more rapid. A compressive mass lesion is likely to produce early depression in the state of consciousness without delirium, hallucinations, and other mental aberrations. Evidence of diffuse slowing on the electroencephalogram should also direct attention toward an encephalitic process. But when there is a marked preponderance of signs pointing toward one or the other hemisphere, the diagnosis may be resolved only by surgical exploration and biopsy of the brain. Development of coma and signs of impending herniation of the temporal lobe through the incisura of the tentorium may necessitate surgical treatment. Epidemiologic and virologic studies will help exclude other causes of necrotizing encephalitis and incriminate the virus of herpes simplex. Acute necrotizing hemorrhagic encephalitis, a presumed immunologic disease, may so mimic acute inclusion body encephalitis that differential diagnosis during life is impossible (see article on Encephalomyelitis and Other Neurologic Lesions as Sequelae to Viral Infections and Viral Vaccines).

Treatment. Although specific antiviral therapy is not yet available, supportive measures directed at controlling seizures and reducing increased intracranial pressure and preventing incisural herniation may be life-saving and may lessen the morbidity.

Prognosis. In a recent series of verified cases of herpes simplex encephalitis, nearly a third of the patients died, and there were permanent neurologic sequelae in 40 per cent. Severe memory impairment, the most frequent residual finding, is explained by damage to the mesial temporal lobes.

Drachman, D. A., and Adams, R. D.: Herpes simplex and acute inclusion-body encephalitis. Arch. Neurol. (Chicago), 7:45, 1962.

Haymaker, W., Smith, M. G., Van Bogaert, L., and de Chenar, C.: Pathology of viral disease in man characterized by nuclear inclusions with emphasis on herpes simplex and subacute inclusion encephalitis. In Fields, W. S., and Blattner, R. J., (eds.): Viral Encephalitis. Springfield, Ill., Charles C Thomas, 1958, p. 95.

Lieder, W., Magoffin, R. L., Lennette, E. H., and Leonards, L. N. R.: Herpes simplex virus encephalitis. Its possible association with reactivated latent infection. New Eng. J. Med., 273:341, 1965.

ENCEPHALOMYELITIS AND OTHER NEUROLOGIC LESIONS AS SEQUELAE TO VIRAL INFECTIONS AND VIRAL VACCINES

Byron H. Waksman

Definition. Postinfectious or postvaccinal encephalomyelitis is an acute or subacute disease of the central and/or peripheral nervous system, characterized by focal, perivenous, demyelinative lesions that are particularly prominent in white matter and meninges. The disease occurs most frequently as a "postinfectious" complication of viral diseases that do not normally affect nervous tissue, but it may also occur as a complication of rabies vaccination, and sometimes without any obvious precipitating cause. It may take the form of acute aseptic meningitis or meningo-encephalitis, encephalitis, acute hemorrhagic leukoencephalitis, disseminated encephalomyelitis, transverse and ascending myelitis, optic neuritis, and polyradiculitis or polyneuritis.

Etiology and Pathogenesis. Essentially identical lesions are found following smallpox, measles, varicella, rubella, infectious mononucleosis, and poorly characterized upper respiratory diseases or influenza. Lesions may also develop following vaccination for smallpox or rabies, or without preceding infection. Lesions of the same type occur infrequently with poliomyelitis, and are reported to occur as rare complications of various bacterial infections (with streptococci, staphylococci) and injection of bacterial vaccines or foreign serum.

In laboratory animals, immunization with autologous or homologous nervous tissue gives rise to the production of "auto-allergic" meningoencephalitis, encephalomyelitis, myelitis, or polyradiculitis with lesions indistinguishable from those of the human diseases under consideration. Since the experimental lesions have been clearly shown to be based on an immune (allergic) reaction to an antigenic component of myelin, it is inferred that the human lesions have a similar allergic character. *Encephalomyelitis following rabies vaccination,* in which the patient is given repeated injections of nervous tissue, is almost certainly auto-allergic like the experimental process. In *postvaccinal encephalomyelitis,* however, Siegert has shown that vaccinia virus can be isolated from the brain and cerebrospinal fluid during the first five days of the disease, whereas virus is not found there in vaccinated persons who fail to get neurologic disease. This fact and the coincidence of the onset of postvaccinal encephalomyelitis with the allergic response to virus at the inoculation site make it highly probable that this disease is an immunologic reaction to viral antigen in the nervous system. The close similarity of the lesions to those of auto-allergic neurologic disease is determined by the fact that a single type of allergic response, though to different antigens, is concerned in lesion formation. In disease with other viruses, the relationships are probably the same as in disease with vaccinia. However, in only one case of *measles encephalitis* has virus been sucessfully isolated from the brain.

Meningitis and meningoencephalitis due to mumps, lymphocytic choriomeningitis, and various enteric viruses are not ordinarily regarded as "postinfectious" since parenchymal findings are usually overshadowed by the meningitis and since virus is easily identified in the cerebrospinal fluid. However, there is good evidence to suggest that the characteristic meningitis is also an allergic response to virus. In these diseases, especially mumps, characteristic "postinfectious" encephalomyelitis or polyradiculitis may also occur (rare), with or without the meningitis.

Within recent years simplified in vitro techniques have been developed for detecting and measuring the immune responses underlying experimental auto-allergic lesions of the nervous system: specific antigenic stimulation of blood lymphocytes in culture to undergo mitosis and blast transformation, specific inhibition by antigen of mononuclear cell migration, and myelin destruction by "sensitized" lymphocytes in cultures of nervous tissue. One may anticipate that these will soon permit an unequivocal demonstration of the allergic mechanism underlying postinfectious and postvaccinal nervous system lesions and will identify the responsible antigen(s).

Incidence and Prevalence. The incidence of "postinfectious" neurologic disease accompanying measles (in 911 cases collected by Miller et al.) varied from 0.001 to 0.36 per cent in different series, with an over-all incidence of approximately 1:1000. A similar range of incidence figures is found for disease accompanying other exanthemas and vaccination for smallpox. Following rabies vaccination, neurologic complications occur with a reported incidence varying from 0.02 to 0.13 per cent. In up to 1 per cent of cases of infectious mononucleosis, patients may show neurologic involvement. With all these diseases, males are affected somewhat more frequently than females, in many series in a ratio of approximately 2:1. Infants younger than one to two years and old people are unaffected, and the age incidence reflects the age incidence of the precipitating disease. Thus, 50 per cent of cases of measles encephalitis occur between 5 and 9 years of age, and more than 95 per cent between 1 and 25; postvaccinial encephalomyelitis is most common at 4 to 16, rare after 30. The neurologic complications of rabies vaccination occur usually between 20 and 40; since many children receive rabies vaccine, the significance of the age onset is unclear. Mumps meningitis and meningoencephalitis occur almost entirely before the age of 15. Disease may occur following a second smallpox vaccination if there is a primary take, i.e., little or no immunity to the virus. Conversely, disease occurs more frequently following a second course of rabies vaccination than a first. In general, it is rare following measles modified by the use of gamma globulin. In no instance does the incidence or severity of the "postinfectious" complication reflect the severity of the antecedent illness.

Encephalitis and encephalomyelitis make up more than 90 per cent of the cases following various exanthematic viruses, the remaining cases being about equally divided between myelitic forms and polyradiculitis (polyneuritis). Hemorrhagic leukoencephalitis appears to represent merely a more intense form of encephalitis, being found in 5 of 62 postvaccinal cases in one series. Following rabies vaccination, cases of encephalitis, myelitis, polyradiculitis, and mononeuritis (or plexitis) are almost equally common. With foreign serum, most of the cases observed are of the mononeuritic type, and less than one fourth fall into the other categories. The different types of disease overlap, central and peripheral involvement being present frequently in the same patient. Of patients with mumps meningitis, one third have cerebral involvement and one of 50, typical encephalomyelitis, myelitis, optic neuritis, or polyradiculitis.

Incubation. Neurologic complications commonly begin several days after the onset of an exanthem (or the parotitis of mumps). Miller's data, shown in the accompanying table, imply that myelitis and polyradiculitis occur later than encephalitis or encephalomyelitis. However, after measles, three fourths of the cases of encephalitis began at two to six days, and half the polyradiculitis cases at four to five days. Half of the meningoencephalitis seen after mumps begins at three to six days. Cases following smallpox usually begin slightly later, on the seventh or eighth day of the rash. The onset, with all these diseases, may also be simultaneous with the appearance of the rash or may precede it by several days (2.4 per cent of Miller's measles cases, 8 per cent of rubella). One fourth of mumps cases occur simultaneously with the parotitis, and another fourth precede it. After smallpox vaccination neurologic disease begins mostly on the tenth, eleventh, and twelfth days. After rabies vaccination, the usual onset is at 10 to 15 days, almost never less than 5 or more than 35.

Pathology. "Postinfectious" neurologic disease presents essentially constant histopathologic features with all types of precipitating illness, including mumps. Encephalomyelitis involves the white matter, and, to a much lesser degree, gray matter, of the hemispheres, cerebellum, brainstem, and spinal cord and may predominate in any one of these regions. Polyradiculitis affects the junction of anterior and posterior spinal roots and the adjacent sensory ganglia. The lesions are perivenous infiltrates of histiocytes (interpreted by many writers as microglia) with demyelination in the infiltrated zone and a relative sparing of axis cylinders (see accompanying figure). Neutral fat is found in infiltrating cells, and there may be an increase of astrocytes and glial fibers. Early lesions may show some polymorphonuclear infiltration and occasional erythrocytes. There are also perivascular cuffs of lymphocytes and histiocytes and a similar reaction about veins in the meninges (meningitis). The lesions are numerous, all at the same stage of development, and micro-

AVERAGE ONSET (DAYS) AFTER ONSET OF RASH OR PAROTITIS

	Encephalitis	Myelitis	Polyradiculitis
Measles	4.7	5.5	9
Varicella	6.3	8.3	11.3
Rubella	3.8	–	–
Mumps	7.2*	10.2	11.3

*Meningoencephalitis.

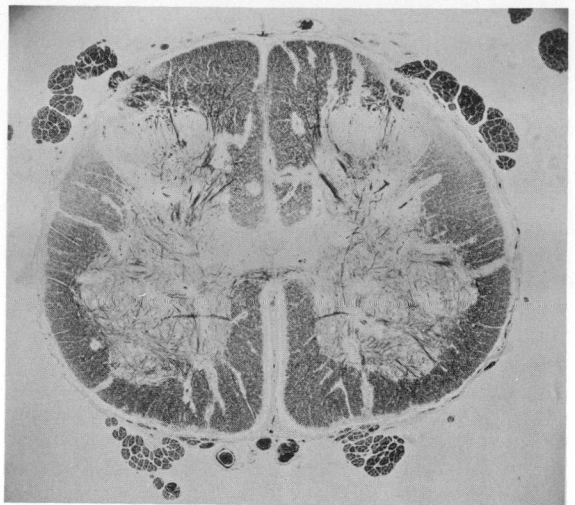

Characteristic demyelination about small veins in the spinal cord in acute postinfectious encephalomyelitis. Myelin stain, × 12.

scopic in size. Rarely, they may coalesce to give large lesions, even complete softening. In very intense lesions, there may be destruction of axons, nerve cells, and other tissue elements with or without "capillary" hemorrhages, serous exudation, fibrin impregnation of vessel walls, and polymorphonuclear infiltration (hemorrhagic leukoencephalitis). Varicella tends to produce greater involvement of cortical gray matter and basal nuclei; mumps and lymphocytic choriomeningitis, relatively more involvement of meninges, choroid plexuses, and ependyma. Smallpox vaccination in infants and in revaccinated adults with partial immunity produces atypical lesions with less microglial reaction and demyelination. Rabies vaccination is apt to produce recurrent crops of lesions, some of which may become confluent and resemble the plaques of multiple sclerosis. There is involvement of the neuraxis in about one fourth of the cases of polyradiculitis (Landry-Guillain-Barré syndrome) and meningitis somewhat more frequently.

"Postinfectious" encephalomyelitis is to be distinguished from encephalopathic reactions occurring, e.g., after vaccination. These are characterized by edema of the brain, degeneration of nerve cells, minimal cell reaction in the meninges and vascular sheaths, and complete absence of the characteristic perivenous infiltrative and demyelinative lesions.

Clinical Manifestations. In postinfectious or postvaccinal neurologic disease, one may distinguish encephalitic syndromes, with evidence of diffuse, transient brain involvement; single focal cerebral lesions, or multiple focal or diffuse lesions of the neuraxis; cerebellar syndromes; spinal syndromes; and polyradiculitis or polyneuritis. *Encephalitis cases* may start (1) abruptly with convulsions followed by coma, (2) with the gradual development of stupor, (3) with headache, vomiting, and signs of meningeal irritation, or (4) with behavior disturbances, restlessness, and

irritability leading to delirium and coma. Fever, drowsiness, headache, and vomiting are the most constant features. Convulsions, meningeal signs, ataxia, paralysis (mono-, hemi- and paraplegias), visual impairment, and involuntary movements are common. In severe cases, encephalography reveals diffuse, slow, high-voltage waves. Relatively pure cerebellar involvement may be seen, especially in cases following varicella. Symptoms of spinal cord disease may predominate. *Myelitis* may be transverse or of the acute ascending type. The latter may have an acute onset with backache, urinary retention, and progressive weakness of the legs leading to flaccid paraplegia; in some instances it progresses to involve the cervical cord and medulla oblongata with tetraplegia and bulbar signs. Perhaps half of those afflicted show a level of sensory loss. *Polyradiculitis* presents most frequently as an acute ascending, i.e., involving first the legs, then the trunk and arms, flaccid paralysis. A few cases have a more gradual onset or are descending. The disease may affect cranial or spinal nerves or both, may be circumscribed or widespread, and may involve sensory or motor functions or both. It may rarely occur in combination with brain and spinal cord lesions or with meningitis. Paralysis of the limbs is frequently accompanied by painful paresthesias, deep muscle pain, urinary retention, difficulty in breathing, and bulbar symptoms (dysphagia, dysarthria).

The cerebrospinal fluid may be normal or may show increased pressure and pleocytosis up to 1000 cells per cubic millimeter. The usual cell count ranges from 25 to 250; the majority are mononuclears, although polymorphonuclears predominate in occasional cases during the first days of illness. The protein is less frequently increased (usual range, 50 to 150 mg. per 100 ml.). In cases of polyradiculitis, the cell count frequently is normal, whereas the protein is elevated—the so-called "albumin-cytologic dissociation." The sugar and chloride are normal.

In cases of mumps and lymphocytic choriomeningitis the clinical picture tends to be dominated by signs of meningitis (severe headache, vomiting, and stiff neck) together with ocular nerve palsies and signs of brain involvement, less commonly with signs of myelitis or polyradiculitis. The mononuclear cells in the cerebrospinal fluid may reach 3000 per cubic millimeter, whereas the protein is normal or slightly elevated.

Diagnosis. The clinical picture of polyradiculitis is distinctive, and diagnosis presents no difficulty. "Postinfectious" encephalomyelitis may at times be difficult to distinguish clinically from direct viral infections of the central nervous system. When neurologic symptoms are preceded by exanthematic viral disease, infectious mononucleosis or mumps, or by vaccination for smallpox or rabies, diagnosis is based on the presence of the precipitating illness and its relation in time to the onset of neurologic disease. In the absence of precipitating illness, exact diagnosis may in the end depend on the isolation of virus or on postmortem examination. Failure to identify poliomyelitis, equine encephalomyelitis, and similar infections by direct virus isolation and by antibody titrations may point to the correct diagnosis. "Postinfectious" disease must be distinguished from direct invasion of the central nervous system by pyogenic organisms, as may occur in smallpox with meningitis and abscess formation, and from encephalopathic reactions ("*toxic encephalopathy*"). The latter is a common complication of measles and other acute illnesses. Its recognition is assisted by the finding of a normal cerebrospinal fluid in the presence of rapidly evolving cerebral symptoms (convulsions, coma, decerebrate rigidity, etc.). Meningoencephalitis due to mumps is easily identified in patients with accompanying parotitis or orchitis. Otherwise it may be distinguished from lymphocytic choriomeningitis and from infection with Coxsackie or echoviruses only by viral isolation from the cerebrospinal fluid, by rise in specific antibody titers, and by the appearance of specific skin reactivity.

Prognosis. The over-all mortality figures for postinfectious and postvaccinal neurologic disease vary in different series and from year to year. "Postinfectious" encephalomyelitis with smallpox or following vaccination for smallpox or for rabies may have a case mortality as high as 50 per cent. With measles, varicella, rubella, infectious mononucleosis, and mumps (encephalitis), the average mortality figures are 10 to 20 per cent. Encephalitic cases have a higher mortality than other types, and hemorrhagic leukoencephalitis is almost uniformly fatal. Uncomplicated meningitis is rarely fatal. Death occurs almost invariably within the first week of disease, usually in patients presenting with convulsions, coma, or hemiplegia. In nonfatal cases, disease may progress for one to two weeks and remain static for days or weeks. Recovery may be complete within two weeks of onset in mild cases (frequently with rubella) or may take several months. One third to one half of the survivors of measles encephalomyelitis show residual damage in the form of mental changes (decreased intelligence, irritability of mood), mild spastic paraplegia, or cerebellar ataxia. After varicella, such changes are seen in 20 per cent of survivors, and after mumps encephalitis they may be seen in approximately 30 per cent of cases. With other precipitating illnesses, sequelae are rare (less than 10 per cent). A small number of patients with polyradiculitis may show residual damage.

Treatment. Corticosteroid therapy, if started within 48 hours of onset of the disease, appears to produce dramatic improvement within a few hours in up to half of the patients so treated and may arrest the progress of disease in others. In some cases the disease recurs when treatment is stopped. The available evidence suggests that administration of gamma globulin, even early in the course of disease, is without therapeutic effect. Proper symptomatic measures include the use of aspirin, repeated lumbar puncture, and intravenous mannitol, dexamethasone (Decadron),

or methylprednisolone sodium succinate (Solu-Medrol) to relieve headache, anticonvulsant therapy and oxygen, antimicrobial drugs for pneumonia, and the control of fluid and electrolyte balance.

Prevention. Smallpox vaccination during infancy avoids the danger of postvaccinal disease in persons vaccinated later in life. Rabies vaccination should be undertaken only when it is certain or highly probable that there has been a bite by a rabid dog. If possible, the newer rabies vaccine, prepared in eggs, should be used. (See Rabies.) Modification of measles and mumps by injection of gamma globulin during the latent period is an important measure resulting in a diminished incidence of "postinfectious" complications. Still better is the use of mumps and measles vaccines to induce active immunity to these diseases.

Adams, R. D., and Kubik, C. S.: Morbid anatomy of the demyelinative diseases. Amer. J. Med., 12:510, 1952.
Asbury, A. K., Arnason, B. G., and Adams, R. D.: The inflammatory lesion in idiopathic polyneuritis: Its role in pathogenesis. Medicine, 48:173, 1969.
Behan, P. O., Geschwind, N., Lamarche, J. B., Lisak, R. P., and Kies, N. W.: Delayed hypersensitivity to encephalitogenic protein in disseminated encephalomyelitis. Lancet, 2:1009, 1968.
De Vries, E.: Postvaccinial Perivenous Encephalitis. Amsterdam, Elsevier Publishing Co., 1960.
Hurst, E. W.: Experimental demyelination in relation to human and animal disease. Amer. J. Med., 12:547, 1952.
Miller, H. G., Stanton, J. B., and Gibbons, J. L.: Para-infectious encephalomyelitis and related syndromes. Quart. J. Med., 25:427, 1956.
Paterson, P. Y.: Experimental autoimmune (allergic) encephalomyelitis. *In* Miescher, P. A., and Muller-Eberhard, H. J. (eds.): Textbook of Immunopathology. New York, Grune and Stratton, Inc., 1968, p. 132.
Pollard, M. (ed.): Virus-Induced Immunopathology. New York, Academic Press, Inc., 1968.
Siegert, R.: Das Verhalten des Vakzinevirus im Organismus bei zentralnervösen Impfschäden, Deutsch. Med. Wschr., 82: 2021, 2061, 1957.

SYPHILITIC INFECTIONS OF THE CENTRAL NERVOUS SYSTEM

Philip R. Dodge

A general exposition of *T. pallidum* infection is presented in the section on Microbial Diseases. The following presentation is restricted to a discussion of neurosyphilis.

Although the spirochete invades the nervous system and its coverings during the early weeks of infection in nearly every case, neurosyphilis develops in less than 10 per cent of untreated cases.

Pathology. Involvement of the leptomeninges is an essential feature of all forms of neurosyphilis. A meningitis of varying severity and extent is present in every case of active neurosyphilis regardless of the neurologic syndrome. The cerebrospinal fluid reflects this involvement. Even in cases of *asymptomatic neurosyphilis*, in which the presence of syphilis reagin constitutes the sole abnormality, rare postmortem examinations have disclosed definite meningeal inflammation and ependymal granulations. Similarly, in chronic tabes dorsalis with negative cerebrospinal fluid examination, evidence of prior active meningeal disease will be revealed by pathologic study.

Postmortem study of a few cases of acute syphilitic meningitis has shown a meningeal inflammatory reaction in which lymphocytes and plasma cells predominate. Cellular aggregates collect about blood vessels, and evidence of early arteritis may be found. Reactive fibrosis of the leptomeninges, especially about the base of the brain, is also seen. This accounts for the cranial nerve palsies and for impaired cerebrospinal fluid circulation that can result in increased intracranial pressure. A granular ependymitis is commonly present, and, rarely, this may obstruct cerebrospinal fluid flow through the aqueduct.

In so-called meningovascular syphilis, which is typically a more chronic disorder occurring months or a few years after the primary lesion, the inflammatory response is usually less acute and meningeal fibrosis more prominent. As the name suggests, there is an associated arteritis (usually small vessels) that predisposes to arterial occlusion and consequent infarction of neural tissue. When larger arteries become occluded, infarction of brain or spinal cord may be extensive. In some cases damage to regions of neural tissue adjacent to meninges occurs without obvious vascular occlusions.

The neurologic syndromes of so-called parenchymatous syphilis (tabes dorsalis, optic atrophy, general paresis) also are due in part to this meningeal affection and in part to the direct invasion of neural tissue by the spirochete. In tabes dorsalis extension of the meningeal inflammatory reaction to the dorsal roots leads ultimately to their destruction and to secondary atrophy of sensory nerve fibers that ascend in the dorsal funiculi of the spinal cord. On gross inspection the dorsal roots appear gray and atrophic, and the dorsal aspect of the spinal cord appears wasted. Myelin sheaths are damaged as well, and demyelination of dorsal columns is easily demonstrated by appropriate stains. Involvement of anterior roots with resultant amyotrophy occurs also but is exceedingly rare. Why the syphilitic process shows a predilection for dorsal roots is unknown.

Treponema pallidum has been demonstrated only rarely in the spinal cords of patients with tabes dorsalis, and direct invasion by the spirochete is probably of little clinical and pathologic importance. In optic atrophy, also, it is probably the contiguous leptomeningitis that is primarily responsible for damage to visual fibers, and those in the periphery of the nerve are most often affected. Direct invasion of the optic nerve by the spirochete may produce additional damage, but the spirochete has been demonstrated in the optic nerve very infrequently.

In general paresis there are, on gross examination, meningeal thickening, atrophy of cerebral tissue (especially of frontal and temporal lobes), and enlargement of ventricles; a granularity

of the ependymal surface is consistently present. Microscopically, diffuse destruction and loss of neurons, especially in the cortex, are found, and special stains may demonstrate a heavy infestation with Treponema pallidum. Reactive gliosis is often extreme, pleomorphic microglia being characteristically abundant. Inflammation of the meninges is prominent, and varying degrees of arteritis can be anticipated. Collections of subependymal astroglia account for the granularity noted grossly.

Focal granulomatous accumulations (gummas) are rare, but may occur in the meninges and extend into the parenchyma of the central nervous system. More diffuse granulomas of the dura (hypertrophic pachymeningitis) assume significance when they compress neural structures, especially the spinal cord.

CLINICAL SYNDROMES IN NEUROSYPHILIS

Asymptomatic Neurosyphilis. As the term suggests, the patient lacks symptoms or signs of neurologic disease, although pathologic involvement of the meninges and possibly of the nervous system parenchyma is implied. The diagnosis rests on the finding of cellular, chemical, or immunologic abnormalities of the cerebrospinal fluid. This is the most common form of neurosyphilis and constituted about 30 per cent of cases in one large neurosyphilis clinic. With adequate treatment (see Treatment) the development of neurologic symptoms can be prevented in most cases.

Symptomatic Neurosyphillis. Meningitis. Symptoms and signs of an acute meningitis are encountered only rarely by physicians, an incidence of less than 2 per cent among syphilitic patients being reported from one general hospital series. It seems likely that some patients with mild or even moderate symptoms go unnoticed. Symptomatic syphilitic meningitis usually occurs during the early weeks or months of infection, often during the period of the secondary rash or concurrently with a mucocutaneous relapse in a patient previously but inadequately treated. The illness is usually of less than a month's duration, but symptoms may persist for longer periods. Headache, vomiting, malaise, and irritability are prominent symptoms. Kernig and Brudzinski signs develop. Occasionally, confusion, delirium, seizures, and cranial nerve palsies (seventh and eighth nerves most common) occur. Argyll Robertson pupils are not part of the constellation of findings in acute syphilitic meningitis. Acute syphilitic hydrocephalus with evidence of increased intracranial pressure, including papilledema, may lead to confusion with other inflammatory and neoplastic conditions. But the diagnosis should not be difficult if the physician considers the possibility of syphilis. The cerebrospinal fluid will always contain an increased number of white blood cells (average about 500 per cubic millimeter—usually mononuclear, rarely polymorphonuclear) elevated total protein (average, about 100 mg. per 100 ml.), normal sugar concentrations (reduced rarely), and syphilitic reagins. An abnormal gold-sol (Lange) curve will be found in 70 per cent of cases. The serologic tests for syphilis are usually but not always positive.

The response to therapy is generally prompt and gratifying, although an occasional patient will subsequently develop some other form of neurosyphilis.

Meningovascular Syphilis. Although the incidence of this form of neurosyphilis is difficult to ascertain, a figure of 3 per cent of syphilitic patients has been recorded. As with the other forms of neurosyphilis, men are more often affected than women (3:1). Patients with meningovascular syphilis present most commonly from two to ten years after the primary lesion. Symptoms and signs of meningitis are lacking although headache is a frequent complaint. The major neurologic abnormalities result from the arteritis and consequent arterial thromboses. The neurologic deficits may develop slowly as the circulation through small vessels becomes compromised, or there may be an abrupt loss of function consequent upon occlusion of a major vessel. The specific syndromes depend upon the distribution of infarction within the brain or spinal cord. The patient may develop hemiplegia, hemisensory defect, dysphasia, or homonymous hemianopia. Involvement of the cortex accounts for seizures in a small percentage of cases. Various spinal cord syndromes have been described. A transverse myelopathy can be expected to produce varying degrees of paraparesis, sensory loss, and impaired function of bladder and bowel. Infarction of the anterior two thirds of the cord, with resultant paraplegia and loss of pain sensation below the lesion, follows occlusion of the anterior spinal artery. Sensory functions subserved by the posterior columns are usually preserved. Asymmetric infarction of one half of the spinal cord will result in weakness and impairment of light touch and position sense on that side and diminished pain and temperature sensation on the opposite side below the anatomic lesion (Brown-Sequard syndrome).

Some abnormality of the cerebrospinal fluid is always found in meningovascular syphilis. A lymphocytic pleocytosis (few to 100 cells per cubic millimeter) and/or an elevated protein concentration is characteristic. The globulin content is often elevated; this is reflected in an abnormal Lange curve. Syphilitic reagins are nearly always present in the cerebrospinal fluid as well as in the blood.

The progress of meningovascular syphilis can usually be halted by specific treatment, but the degree of functional recovery depends upon the extent and location of the infarcts and upon the many complex physiologic factors that condition recovery in cerebrovascular disease of any type.

General Paresis (Dementia Paralytica, General Paralysis of the Insane). This dread complication of syphilis makes its appearance from 2 to 30 (usually 10 to 25) years after the primary lesion. It occurs more often in men than in women (3:1), and 89 per cent of cases occur between the ages of 30 and 60 years. In one large series about 60 per cent of patients presented with simple dementia, and less than 20 per cent displayed manic symptoms and megalomania. Often faulty judgment, impaired memory (recent memory affected first), disturbed affect (depression or euphoria), or paranoia suggests the presence of a serious mental disturbance. Delusions and hallucinations occur less often, but when present prompt a quick referral to the physician. The patient himself may complain of "nervousness," but characteristically lacks insight into the nature of his difficulty. Fine or coarse tremors, often affecting facial muscles and tongue, are present in about two thirds of the patients with fully developed general paresis. Abnormal pupillary responses, including Argyll Robertson pupil (see Tabes Dorsalis), impassive facies, slurred or dysarthric speech, exaggerated stretch reflexes, and extensor plantar responses are additional neurologic signs. Convulsions occur in 10 per cent of patients, and strokes secondary to vasculitis are also seen. When symptoms and signs of tabes dorsalis accompany those of paresis, the designation taboparesis is used.

The cerebrospinal fluid is always abnormal, containing in excess of 5 white blood cells per cubic millimeter (mononuclear) in 85 per cent of untreated cases, and more than 30 cells per cubic millimeter in about a fourth of cases. An elevated total protein concentration (greater than 50 mg. per 100 ml.) of cerebrospinal fluid can be anticipated in 75 per cent, and a level of 100 mg. per 100 ml. or higher in about 20 per cent of cases. An elevated gamma globulin level accounts for the first zone colloidal gold (Lange) curve, e.g., 5554433211, which is frequently found in general paresis. Nearly every patient will have a positive reagin test for syphilis in the cerebrospinal fluid, and in more than 90 per cent of cases the blood serologic test will also be positive. Incomplete, prior treatment may modify but will not restore to normal the cerebrospinal fluid.

General paresis, once established, evolves rapidly, and patients soon become disabled mentally, socially, and, in the late stage, physically. The term general paralysis of the insane derived from observations of patients helpless and bedridden in the terminal stages of the disease. Untreated general paresis is universally fatal, usually within three years.

If the disease is recognized early and treated vigorously, about 80 per cent of patients will return to some form of work, but only in about one half will complete recovery be achieved. There is little hope of a satisfactory result when treatment is delayed until the patient is demented, incontinent, and bedridden.

Tabes Dorsalis (Locomotor Ataxia). Tabes dorsalis develops in less than 5 per cent of patients with untreated syphilis, and symptoms usually become manifest 10 to 20 years after the primary infection. Rarely, there is a latent period of 30 or more years. Men are more often affected than women.

Dysfunction of affected posterior roots accrues slowly, and symptoms develop insidiously. Impaired joint position sense frequently results in stumbling and difficulty in walking, especially in the dark when visual compensation is imperfect. As the disease progresses, this sensory ataxia worsens, and a broad-based gait is assumed. Profound hypotonia, secondary to a lack of modulation of muscle tension by afferent fibers, is expressed frequently in a slapping gait. Paresthesias usually appear early in the disease but may be ignored by the patient until the appearance of lightning pains. These pains are characteristic of tabes dorsalis but are in no way specific since they occur in other diseases affecting dorsal roots, e.g., diabetic neuropathy. Lightning pains develop in at least 75 per cent of patients and may appear in any area of the body, although they are most common in the lower extremities. Some patients insist that they are more troublesome when the barometric pressure is low. They may be described as sharp, burning, or aching. However, sharp jabs of pain are characteristic. These may be mild or excruciating, and frequently flit from one region to another. At times they are so transitory that by the time the patient has made the natural move to rub or massage the involved part, pain has disappeared. For a period of hours or days one spot will seem particularly vulnerable, but then the site of attack shifts to another place. Involvement of thoraco-abdominal nerve roots gives rise to visceral pains (gastric or visceral crises), which may simulate intrinsic visceral disease and may lead to unnecessary surgery; in one series an estimated 25 per cent of tabetic patients had undergone operation for tabetic pain. The converse is also true: on rare occasions visceral pain has been ascribed to tabes dorsalis and suppurative appendicitis, or a ruptured peptic ulcer has gone undiagnosed. As the disease advances, pain sensation may be so dulled that recurrent trauma is unnoticed by the patient and indolent ulcers of the skin develop; the toes and balls of the feet are especially vulnerable. Weight-bearing joints and adjacent bone, deprived of pain sensation, are destroyed by the constant trauma of use in 5 to 10 per cent of tabetic patients (Charcot joints).

Unless general paresis coexists, as it does in a small percentage of cases (taboparesis), tabetic patients are mentally normal. Optic atrophy complicates tabes dorsalis in about 10 per cent of cases or occurs as an isolated disorder. Pupillary abnormalities, including meiosis, irregularity, poor responsiveness to light and mydriatics, but retained reaction in accommodation (Argyll Robertson pupils), are present in most cases of tabes dorsalis. Involvement of other oculomotor functions is occasionally seen. Hypotonia, ataxia, and broad-based gait can usually be demonstrated. Affection of the sensory arc of the myotatic reflexes accounts for the greatly diminished or absent stretch reflexes. The Achilles reflex is affected most constantly. The plantar responses are normal in most cases of uncomplicated tabes dorsalis. Loss or diminution of position and vibratory sensation is found in every case. Increased swaying when the eyes are closed and the patient is standing with feet together (Romberg's sign) results from the impaired position sense. Variable degrees of hypesthesia and hypalgesia in a root distribution can be anticipated but may be difficult to plot. Isolated areas of hypalgesia (Hitzig zones) are sometimes found. Delayed perception of a pain stimulus (from one to several seconds) often can be demonstrated. Impaired deep pain sensation may account for a dramatic lack of responsiveness to squeezing of the Achilles tendon or testicles. Because of involvement of sacral nerve roots, functions of the urinary bladder and bowel are impaired in up to one third of cases; overflow incontinence and constipation develop. Impotence is a major complaint in the male. Characteristically a cystometrogram shows an absence of, or reduction in, the normal muscular contractions of the bladder in response to filling; the patient may be unaware of a volume in excess of 500 ml. Hydronephrosis and pyogenic infection are common complications of a hypotonic bladder.

Early in the course of tabes dorsalis the serologic tests for syphilis, are, as a rule, strongly positive. The cerebrospinal fluid may reflect the meningeal inflammatory process with pleocytosis, an elevated total protein, and a positive reagin test. Late in the disease, especially after some antisyphilitic treatment, the serologic tests may be negative (in 25 to 50 per cent of cases), and even the cerebrospinal fluid is negative in up to 20 per cent of cases.

The course of tabes dorsalis is unpredictable, and the response to antisyphilitic therapy is variable. In general, patients who have had symptoms for a few months or at the most a few years, with significant cerebrospinal fluid abnormalities and no prior therapy, are most likely to improve with treatment. Patients with far-advanced disease and severe degeneration of dorsal roots will not benefit significantly from antisyphilitic therapy. At least partial relief of pain may be achieved by analgesics, but when narcotics are used the risk of addiction is significant. Recently, some benefit has been reported with diphenylhydantoin (Dilantin) treatment (200 mg. per square meter per day). Recourse to spinal cordotomy and other surgical measures to relieve pain should be deferred until all medical measures have failed. Urologic assistance may be required to deal effectively with the tabetic uropathies, and surgery may be required for management of penetrating ulcers of the skin and Charcot joints.

Optic Atrophy. Visual impairment in syphilis may result from iritis, choreoretinitis, increased intracranial pressure (consecutive optic atrophy), or primary optic atrophy. Optic atrophy occurs in 1 per cent of patients with untreated syphilis and is five times more common in males than in females. It is stated that Negroes are more prone than Caucasians to optic atrophy, whereas the reverse is reported in other forms of neurosyphilis.

Because the outer portions of the optic nerve are first affected, the visual impairment tends to be peripheral in the early stages. Ultimately, however, the papillomacular bundle lying in the center of the nerve becomes involved, and impaired visual acuity, and central and paracentral scotomas develop. It has been estimated that, without treatment, 50 per cent of patients will be blind in two years and 90 per cent in ten years. One eye is typically affected before the other. Optic pallor is usually present by the time symptoms appear, but in the early stages it is recognizable only by the reduced vascularity. A chalk-white disc with sharp margins and prominent lamina cribrosa constitute the fully developed appearance of optic atrophy. The optic atrophy of syphilis is indistinguishable from that due to other diseases of the optic nerve in which there has been no antecedent papillitis or papilledema. The cerebrospinal fluid is abnormal in most patients with active disease of the optic nerve. Intensive antisyphilitic therapy may arrest the disease process and preserve what vision remains, but return of vision already lost should not be anticipated.

Gumma. This rare complication of syphilis usually declares itself as an intracranial or intraspinal mass lesion and behaves in every way as a slowly growing neoplasm. The correct diagnosis may be suspected from a positive serologic test for syphilis or from cerebrospinal fluid abnormalities. Frequently, however, the diagnosis is not made until the patient is operated upon, and histopathologic studies are made. Removal of the tumor mass, supplemented by antimicrobial therapy (see Treatment), should alleviate symptoms and prevent spread of the disease.

CONGENITAL NEUROSYPHILIS

Syphilis acquired by the fetus from an infected mother after the first trimester of pregnancy tends to be a fulminant disease. Miscarriages and stillbirths are common, and a wide spectrum of clinical manifestations may be recognized in the infant or child who survives. Neurosyphilis develops in an estimated 10 to 20 per cent of infants and children with congenital syphilis. Asymptomatic neurosyphilis may be diagnosed in the early months or years of life by doing routine cerebrospinal fluid examinations on children of syphilitic mothers. But, as with acquired neurosyphilis, symptoms and signs develop only after a latent period that, in the case of juvenile paresis, may be as long as 20 years. More often symptoms first appear late in the first decade or during adolescence. Clinical syndromes and cerebro-spinal fluid findings mirror those found with the acquired disease except that tabes dorsalis is exceedingly rare and choreoretinitis more common. Hydrocephalus, cranial nerve palsies (eighth cranial nerve especially) and seizures may complicate congenital syphilitic meningitis, and syphilis should be remembered as a cause of cerebrovascular accidents in children. Previous studies emphasize that more than a third of all children presenting with juvenile paresis have been retarded mentally since early life. Although mental retardation is very likely due to other factors in some cases, such statistics emphasize the vulnerability of the developing nervous system to syphilitic infection.

Other non-neurologic stigmata of congenital syphilis include dental deformities (Hutchinson's teeth), saddle nose, frontal bossing of the skull, saber shins, and interstitial keratitis (usually developing during the second decade). These signs are never seen with acquired syphilis. Fortunately, the current practice of doing routine serologic tests on all pregnant women and on infants of syphilitic mothers has all but eliminated congenital neurosyphilis in many areas of the world.

Early and intensive treatment of infants with congenital syphilis materially reduces the morbidity (see Treatment) from neurologic complications. Unhappily, results from even optimal treatment of patients with juvenile paresis remain poor.

TREATMENT

Penicillin is the preferred drug for treating neurosyphilis. Reasonable therapy for adults with all forms of neurosyphilis, except general paresis, is a total dose of procaine penicillin G of 9 to 12 million units given over two to three weeks. A total dose of 18 to 24 million units administered over the same period of time is used to treat patients with general paresis. For children, approximately one half of the adult dose is employed, and one quarter of the adult dose is given to infants. We prefer to treat patients with active neurosyphilis in hospital (mandatory in general paresis), but this is not always feasible. When outpatient treatment is necessary, an initial dose of 3 million units of long-acting penicillin (benzathine penicillin G, Bicillin) should be given. The sole use of benzathine penicillin G at weekly intervals in doses equivalent to those presented above has been advocated by some in the treatment of neurosyphilis.

Alternative drugs include the tetracyclines and chloramphenicol (3 to 4 grams per day for 15 days), but they should be reserved for cases in which there is a proved allergy to penicillin. Sensitivity to penicillin should not be confused with the Jarisch-Herxheimer reaction, which occurs within a few hours of the first injection of the drug in 50 per cent or more of patients (see the major discussion of Syphilis elsewhere in this book). During therapy neurologic symptoms and signs may exacerbate temporarily, probably because of the Jarisch-Herxheimer reaction.

Clark, E. G., and Danbolt, N.: The Oslo study of the natural history of untreated syphilis. J. Chronic Dis., 2:311, 1955.

Fiumara, N. J.: The treatment of syphilis. New Eng. J. Med., 270:1185, 1964.

Green, J. B.: Dilantin in the treatment of lightning pains. Neurology, 11:257, 1961.

Hahn, R. D., et al.: Penicillin treatment of general paresis (dementia paralytica) — Results of treatment in 1086 patients, the majority of whom were followed for more than 5 years. Arch. Neurol. Psychiat., 81:557, 1959.

Merritt, H. H., Adams, R. D., and Solomon, H.: Neurosyphilis. New York, Oxford University Press, 1946.

Montgomery, C. H., and Knox, J. M.: Antibiotics other than penicillin in the treatment of syphilis. New Eng. J. Med., 261: 277, 1961.

Slow and Latent Viral Infections and Neurologic Diseases

Richard T. Johnson

Traditionally, viral infections of the nervous system have been associated with acute diseases characterized by inflammatory changes in the cerebrospinal fluid and brain. Recently, however, viruses have been related to several subacute and chronic neurologic diseases in which inflammatory changes are lacking and in which pathologic changes suggest a degenerative or demyelinative process. Experimental transmission of these diseases has shown that the incubation period may extend for months or even years, followed by protracted clinical disease usually ending in death. These infections have been called "slow" to differentiate them from latent infections, such as recurrent herpes labialis (cold sores) or herpes zoster (shingles), in which a relapsing acute disease develops. Similarly, slow infections have been differentiated from chronic infections, such as tuberculosis, syphilis, or malaria, in which the clinical course tends to be irregular and unpredictable. The predictable progressive course of slow infections has been likened to a "slow-motion picture of the chain of events occurring in the acute infection."

The term slow infection was originally coined in the veterinary literature to describe several transmissible diseases of sheep. Two of these slow infections of sheep are of particular interest in that they cause chronic, progressive neurologic diseases with very unusual neuropathologic changes. *Scrapie,* long believed to be genetically determined, is a transmissible disease of sheep having an incubation period of nine months to four years. The disease has an insidious onset and an afebrile course characterized by ataxia, tremor, hyperexcitability, and weakness in which the disease progresses over many months, leading invariably to death. The cerebrospinal fluid remains normal. Pathologic changes are limited to the central nervous system and suggest a degenerative process. Although the brains are grossly normal, histologically there is hypertrophy and proliferation of astrocytes, degeneration and vacuolizations of neu-

rons, and striking absence of inflammation. Scrapie has been transmitted experimentally to goats and a variety of rodents, but the agent has not been visualized with the electron microscope or grown in tissue cultures. The transmissible agent passes through filters with pore sizes below 100 mμ, but has extraordinary stability to temperature, pH changes, formalin, and other treatments which inactivate most viruses. No antibody response to the scrapie agent has been demonstrated.

Visna is a nervous system disease of sheep found only in Iceland. It has an incubation period of several years, followed by slowly progressive paralysis often beginning as paraparesis. The clinical course leads relentlessly to death after several months. Unlike scrapie, the cerebrospinal fluid shows inflammatory changes with an increase in leukocytes and protein; and this reaction develops early in the one to four-year incubation period. Antibody against the agent also develops long before the onset of disease. Pathologic changes are limited to the central nervous system, but these changes are inflammatory, characterized by perivascular infiltration of mononuclear cells. The unusual pathologic feature is that the white matter is predominantly involved, giving features of a demyelinating process. The virus of visna has not been transmitted to other animals, but has been grown and studied in tissue cultures.

KURU

Kuru is an endemic disease of Melanesian tribal people inhabiting a remote area of the eastern highlands of central New Guinea. The disease has been seen only among the Fore linguistic group and several neighboring groups with whom the Fore have intermarried. However, within this limited area, kuru has been the most common cause of death, affecting predominantly adult women and children of both sexes. The disease begins insidiously with unsteadiness of stance and gait, followed by progressive disabling cerebellar ataxia. Late in the course, abnormalities of extraocular movement and mental changes develop. The disease leads to death in three to six months. Remissions or recovery have not been seen. Extensive laboratory examinations have failed to show any abnormalities limited to kuru victims, and the cerebrospinal fluid remains normal. Pathologic changes are confined to the brain, in which a marked increase of astrocytes and degeneration of neurons is found. The brain is diffusely affected, but the findings are most prominent in the cerebellum and pons, and, to a lesser degree, in the hypothalamus and basal ganglia. Inflammation is not found.

Because of similarities in the epidemiology, clinical progression, and pathologic changes found in kuru and scrapie, brain tissue from patients dying of kuru was inoculated into a variety of primates for long-term observations. After incubation periods of 18 months to 4 years, a similar disease developed in chimpanzees, and this disease subsequently was transmitted from chimpanzee to chimpanzee. The nature of the transmissible agent of kuru is still unclear, but studies thus far suggest that it is similar to the agent of scrapie, even though they are clearly not the same agent.

In recent years, there has been a striking decline in the incidence of kuru, particularly among children, in whom the disease has essentially disappeared. This decreasing incidence has been coincident with suppression of cannibalism in this primitive culture, and there is considerable circumstantial evidence indicating that kuru may have been transmitted by the widespread practice of ritual cannibalism.

CREUTZFELDT-JAKOB DISEASE
(Jakob-Creutzfeldt Disease)

These eponyms have been applied to a variety of subacute dementias of middle life. Whether they represent a single disease or multiple disease entities is unclear. The term generally is used to designate an uncommon, nonfamilial dementia accompanied by myoclonus. The dementia develops rapidly so that deterioration from day to day or week to week is evident. Myoclonic jerks develop early in the disease, and often massive symmetrical myoclonus of the limbs occurs when the patient is startled by unexpected light or sounds. Cerebellar ataxia and wasting of muscles with fasciculations are inconstant features. The disease is inexorably progressive, usually reducing the patient from good health to total helplessness or death in

less than a year. The cerebrospinal fluid shows no abnormality, but the electroencephalogram becomes abnormal early in the disease, showing diffuse slowing with superimposed sharp waves.

Neuropathologic findings include diffuse loss of cortical neurons with remarkable increase in fibrous astrocytes. In some cases, a spongiform state is prominent in the cerebral cortex. Inflammatory reactions and inclusion bodies are absent, as are neurofibrillary changes and senile plaques.

Since the subacute course and neuropathologic findings resembled kuru and scrapie, attempts to transmit the disease to chimpanzees were also undertaken. A similar disease developed in chimpanzees inoculated with brains of patients with Creutzfeldt-Jakob disease after an incubation period of about one year. The chimpanzees developed somnolence, ataxia, tremor, fasciculations, and intermittent jerking of the extremities. The pathologic changes in the brains resembled those of Creutzfeldt-Jakob disease.

Thus, scrapie in sheep and kuru and Cruetzfeldt-Jakob disease in man share a similar afebrile, relentlessly progressive course, singularly lacking in any clinical clues of infection. Neither the cerebrospinal fluid nor histologic changes within the nervous system show evidence of inflammation. Indeed, the pathologic changes in each of these transmissible diseases are those of a degenerative process.

SUBACUTE SCLEROSING PANENCEPHALITIS
(Dawson's Encephalitis, Subacute Inclusion Body Encephalitis)

This is an uncommon, subacute encephalitis usually occurring between the ages of 4 and 20 years. The onset is insidious, and is characterized by deterioration in school work and behavioral disorders. This is followed in weeks or months by overt mental deterioration and neurologic signs, the most characteristic of which is myoclonus. The disease usually terminates after a third stage of stupor, blindness, dementia, and decorticate rigidity, which may last months to several years. Characteristically, the cerebrospinal fluid is under normal pressure and acellular, but shows an increased concentration in gamma globulin, resulting in a first zone colloidal gold curve. During the stage of active myoclonus, the electroencephalogram usually shows general suppression of activity with periodic (8 to 15 seconds) synchronous bursts of high-voltage slow and sharp waves. Although the clinical course is usually characterized by progressive deterioration, occasionally an apparent arrest of the disease process or even transient clinical improvement is seen.

A viral etiology has long been suspected because of the pathologic changes. Perivascular infiltrates of mononuclear cells are characteristic, and eosinophilic intranuclear inclusion bodies are found in neurons and glial cells. Because of these inclusions, the herpes simplex virus was long suspected of being the etiologic agent. Recently, however, virus-like particles resembling the virions of the measles-distemper group of paramyxoviruses were found in cerebral biopsies, and astonishingly high levels of antibodies against measles virus were demonstrated in the serums of most patients. These studies led to the search for, and eventual isolation of, measles virus from brain biopsies from several patients.

This disease bears little resemblence clinically or pathologically to even the most fulminating acute measles virus infections, in which virus dissemination may lead to giant-cell pneumonia. Furthermore, it is quite distinct from the parainfectious encephalomyelitis that occasionally complicates measles virus infections and produces neurologic disease with perivascular demyelination of the brain and spinal cord. The pathogenesis of subacute sclerosing panencephalitis is obscure. Most of the patients with this disease give a history of uncomplicated measles infection years past. Just how measles virus leads to this subacute disease in the rare patient is unknown.

Treatment of patients with antiviral agents and synthetic interferon inducers has been attempted, but without definite beneficial effects.

PROGRESSIVE MULTIFOCAL LEUKOENCEPHALOPATHY

This is a rare, demyelinating disease of the central nervous system. It usually occurs in elderly patients against a background of leukemia, lymphoma, or other debilitating disease such as carcinoma, tuberculosis, or sarcoidosis. Although the pre-existing systemic disease may be longstanding, the neurologic abnormalities develop rather suddenly and follow a subacute progressive course until death. The signs are usually bilateral and asymmetrical, consisting of gross abnormalities of motor function, vision, or speech. Dementia frequently develops. Headache is not a common feature of the disease. The cerebrospinal fluid shows little, if any, abnormality, and the electroencephalogram shows only diffuse slowing. The pathologic picture is unique. Multiple foci of cerebral demyelination are found in various stages of evolution. Surrounding these foci are bizarre, distorted oligodendroglia as well as giant cells with multiple nuclei, mitotic figures, and eosinophilic intranuclear inclusions. However, inflammatory cells are not found.

The presence of the inclusion bodies and the association with diseases in which there is often altered immunologic activity led to speculation that a viral infection might be implicated. In the past several years, brains of over 20 cases of progressive multifocal leukoencephalopathy have been examined by electron microscopy, and in almost every case virus-like particles have been found in the glial cells. The particles, often forming crystalloid arrays, resemble the virions of the papova viruses, a group including polyoma virus of mice, vacuolating agents of monkeys, and papilloma (warts) virus of man. Although attempts to isolate or otherwise biologically characterize these particles have been unsuccessful, this repeated observation supports the idea that some virus is involved in the pathogenesis of this disease. It is not known, however, whether this disease represents a primary infection with a normally nonpathogenic agent or whether it represents reactivation or dissemination of a latent or noninvasive agent, such as warts virus or an unknown human polyoma virus. No treatment is known.

OTHER NEUROLOGIC DISEASES

Since viruses can cause disease with a long incubation period, can produce disease with a subacute or relapsing course, and can give rise to noninflammatory pathologic changes, the possible role of slow or latent viral infection in a variety of neurologic diseases has been entertained.

In several chronic or relapsing inflammatory diseases of the nervous system, a viral etiology has been suspected. *Chronic focal epilepsy* (epilepsia partialis continua, Kozhevnikov's epilepsy) is, in some cases, associated with a chronic focal inflammatory process in the brain. In the Soviet Union, this has been thought to represent a persistent focal infection with tick-borne viruses following acute encephalitis, and in several Soviet laboratories, tick-borne encephalitis virus has been isolated from surgically removed cerebral epileptogenic foci. No viruses have been isolated from similar cases in other countries. Chronic focal epilepsy can be a manifestation of focal disease processes such as neoplastic, vascular, or traumatic lesions, but chronic infection may play a role in some cases.

Recurrent acute meningitis or encephalitis occurs in three clinical syndromes of unknown etiology in which a latent viral infection has been suspected. *Mollaret's meningitis* is a rare, recurrent meningitis characterized by repeated attacks of headache, fever, and nuchal rigidity. Each attack is abrupt in onset and lasts for two to three days; the patient is entirely well between episodes. During attacks the cerebrospinal fluid may contain large numbers of both polymorphonuclear and mononuclear cells and also large, poorly staining "epithelial cells," characteristic but not pathognomonic of this disease. More severe recurrent neurologic involvement can occur in *Behçet's syndrome* and in the *Vogt-Koyanagi-Harada syndrome.* Behçet's syndrome is characterized by recurrent oral and genital ulcers and inflammatory ocular lesions, usually taking the form of acute recurrent iritis. In about one quarter of the patients neurologic episodes develop, consisting of cranial nerve palsies, focal seizures, hemiparesis, or other focal signs. Severe depression of consciousness, coma, or meningeal signs suggesting more diffuse involvement also occur. Neurologic deficits usually remit and relapse but may be progressive. Pathologic findings include meningeal inflammatory reactions, perivascular inflammation, and focal areas of necrosis. The Vogt-Koyanagi-Harada or uveo-encephalitic syndrome is characterized by depigmentation of skin and hair, inflammatory ocular lesions (usually consisting of iridocyclitis or exudative retinal detachment), and meningitis. In this syndrome, unlike Behçet's, neurologic involvement occurs in all cases, often precedes the ocular inflammation, and usually consists only of headache, nuchal rigidity, and a mononuclear cell pleocytosis. However, a transient decrease in hearing and tinnitus may accompany the meningitis, or a severe encephalitis may develop leaving permanent neurologic deficits. Neuropathologic findings have consisted only of chronic arachnoiditis.

Reports have been made of isolations of unidentified viruses from patients with Mollaret's, Behçet's, and Vogt-Koyanagi-Harada syndromes; but none of these claims has been entirely convincing. An allergic etiology has also been postulated, and consequently treatment with corticosteroids has been advocated.

A notion that *Parkinson's disease* might have a viral etiology has been entertained ever since the observation was made that a form of parkinsonism was a frequent sequela of encephalitis lethargica (von Economo's disease). Similarly, the possible role of a slow infection in *multiple sclerosis, amyotrophic lateral sclerosis,* and a variety of other demyelinating and degenerative diseases has also been postulated. Although the spectrum of neurologic disease that can be potentially attributed to slow, latent, or chronic viral infections has greatly broadened in recent years, evidence is still scant for incriminating a transmissible agent in these chronic neurologic diseases.

Dean, G.: The multiple sclerosis problem. Scientific American, 223:40, 1970.

Gajdusek, D. C.: Kuru. Trans. Roy. Soc. Trop. Med. Hyg., 57:151, 1963.

Gibbs, C. J., and Gajdusek, D. C.: Infection as the etiology of spongiform encephalopathy (Creutzfeldt-Jakob disease). Science, 165:1023, 1969.

Johnson, R. T., and Johnson, K. P.: Slow and chronic virus infections of the nervous system. *In* Plum, F. (ed.): Recent Advances in Neurology. Philadelphia, F. A. Davis Company, 1969.

Zu Rhein, G. M.: Association of papova virions with a human demyelinating disease (progressive multifocal leukoencephalopathy). Progr. Med. Virol., 11:185, 1969.

Nutritional Disorders of the Nervous System

Pierre M. Dreyfus

INTRODUCTION

A number of vitamins, trace minerals, and amino acids are indispensable to the normal metabolic activity of the nervous system. A severe deficiency of these fundamental nutrients leads to the improper function of one or more enzyme systems, resulting either in the inadequate production of other important substances or in the abnormal accumulation of potentially toxic metabolites or substrates that may interfere with normal development, growth, and function of the nervous system.

Among the vitamins, several are of particular importance to the metabolism of the nervous system. Whereas the role played by these vitamins in general metabolism is becoming increasingly clear, the specific mechanisms by which a deficiency state affects the nervous system remain to be discovered. Vitamin depletion can occur in a number of different ways, the most obvious being a *primary* or *dietary* deficiency resulting from inadequate quantities of the vitamins in the diet. A *secondary* or *conditioned* deficiency arises when increased metabolic demands are placed on the organism in states of stress, such as growth, pregnancy, exercise, debilitating illness, or chronic alcoholism. The limited absorption of vitamins by the gastrointestinal tract resulting from disease, surgery, or an absence of gastric intrinsic factor is another important cause of deficiency. In order to be metabolically active, vitamins must be converted into their corresponding cofactors. Pathologic states in which this conversion is faulty have recently been identified. Finally, the deficiency of one vitamin can result in faulty synthesis of another.

Nutritional disorders of the nervous system are associated with one or more biochemical lesions which invariably antedate the appearance of symptoms and signs and histopathologic alterations. The specific biochemical lesions responsible for the neurologic manifestations have not been clearly defined for each B vitamin deficiency. In most instances, speculations are based on fragmentary clinical and experimental observations.

Of all the vitamin and cofactor deficiencies known to affect animals and man, only those of vitamins B_6 and B_{12}, of thiamin, nicotinic acid, pantothenic acid, and perhaps of riboflavin can be readily associated with neurologic syndromes. In general, experimentally induced deficiencies of single vitamins have shed relatively little light on the naturally occurring nutritional disorders, which for the most part are the result of multiple deficiencies.

Thiamin (vitamin B_1) in its phosphorylated form, cocarboxylase, acts as cofactor in two major enzyme systems: alpha-keto acid decarboxylase and transketolase. Both participate in carbohydrate metabolism of the nervous system. The first of these two systems is essential to glycolysis, more specifically, to the oxidative decarboxylation of pyruvic and alpha-ketoglutaric acid. The second system involves two steps of the hexose-monophosphate shunt, an alternate route of carbohydrate metabolism. In experimentally induced thiamin deprivation, the activity of these enzymes within the nervous system is reduced before signs and symptoms of deficiency become manifest. Although all parts of the nervous system are affected, the biochemical lesion is most striking in the regions where histologic changes ultimately occur. In the rat, for instance, the lateral pontine tegmentum is the area of the brain in which enzymatic activity is most rapidly and drastically reduced during progressive vitamin depletion. Transketolase activity seems to be more severely affected than does pyruvate decarboxylase activity. In man, evidence of this biochemical lesion can be elicited by simple biochemical measurements of blood. Determinations of blood pyruvate levels before and after the administration of glucose, for many years the standard method of estimating thiamin deficiency, have proved to lack specificity. Other dysmetabolic states such as liver disease, diabetes, anemia, fever, states of agitation, and delirium tremens can cause an elevation of blood pyruvate levels. More recently, blood transketolase determinations have been found to reflect, in a highly sensitive and specific manner, the state of thiamin nutrition in man. Transketolase assays not only reveal the levels of available coenzymes, i.e., thiamin pyrophosphate, but also differentiate an acute from a chronic deficiency by reflecting the levels of available apoenzyme.

Vitamin B_6, in the form of pyridoxal phosphate, is an essential coenzyme for many enzymatic reactions. In animals, pyridoxine deficiency results in a lowered threshold to seizures induced by electroshock and in a reduction of cerebral glutamic and gamma-aminobutyric acid levels. Pyridoxal phosphate is necessary for a variety of transaminases and decarboxylases, some of which are involved in the "gamma-aminobutyric acid shunt," in which alpha-ketoglutaric acid is transformed into succinate by way of glutamic and gamma-aminobutyric acid. The latter, generally regarded as an inhibitory substance, has been found to exist exclusively in the nervous system. It has been speculated that the decreased seizure threshold seen in pyridoxine-deficient animals and in human infants following the inadvertent administration of a pyridoxine analogue is due to a failure of glutamic decarboxylase, a neuronal enzyme that regulates the production of gamma-aminobutyric acid from glutamic acid. It is also well established that pyridoxine is essential for tryptophan metabolism. In animals and humans, vitamin B_6 deficiency can be reflected by increased urinary excretion of the tryptophan metabolites, xanthurenic and kynurenic acid, after a tryptophan load. This is but one of many possible biochemical lesions and is not thought to be a sensitive index of deficiency so far as the nervous system is concerned. Another metabolic step of potential importance to normal neural activity involves the pyridoxine-dependent synthesis of serotonin from 5-hydroxytryptophan. High levels of this neurotransmitter substance are located in the synaptic vesicles of certain neurons in the midbrain and hypothalamus. In pyridoxine dependency, a familial disorder of infants characterized by seizures and a high daily vitamin B_6 requirement (10 mg. a day), no specific metabolic defect has yet been demonstrated. Although the seizures respond promptly to the administration of pyridoxine, biochemical evidence of vitamin deficiency is lacking. An abnormality of the glutamic decarboxylase system has been postulated.

The role of *pantothenic acid* in normal brain and peripheral nerve metabolism is poorly defined. As part of coenzyme A, pantothenic acid participates in important energy-yielding reactions and acetylations, such as the synthesis of acetylcholine and steroids. Pantothenic acid is also essential to the formation of certain amide and peptide linkages. Relatively high concentrations of this vitamin exist in the brain, which does not readily yield its stores. Peripheral nerve lesions develop in experimentally induced pantothenic acid deficiency in animals and man, but no associated biochemical lesion has yet been demonstrated.

Many of the syndromes to be discussed here are commonly associated with chronic alcoholism. The same disease states have also been described in cases of malnutrition in which alcohol played no role. The prolonged and abusive intake of alcohol, together with an inadequate diet, leads to a somewhat unusual and extreme state of nutritional imbalance characterized by an excess of carbohydrate, fatty acid, cholesterol, glycerol, glycogen, and calories, and by a severe deficiency of B vitamins and other essential nutrients. These dietary factors may explain in part why the alcoholic patient is so frequently subject to the most extreme and florid types of nutritional disorders. Patients afflicted with chronic debilitating illnesses, prisoners of war, and other undernourished persons suffer from a different type of malnutrition. Their caloric intake, although generally low, has a different composition and may have a higher ratio of vitamins to calories. Some syndromes are decidedly more common than others, and it cannot be stated why, under presumably similar circumstances, patients develop different types of disease. The various nutritional disorders affecting the nervous system can exist separately, in relatively pure form, but more frequently they combine with each other or with other nutritional diseases.

NUTRITIONAL POLYNEUROPATHY
(Dry Beriberi, Alcoholic Neuropathy)

Clinical Manifestations. Nutritional polyneuropathy, the most common of all the nutritional diseases of the nervous system, is characterized by progressive weakness and muscle wasting of varying degrees, involving, symmetrically, the legs more than the arms and the distal muscles more than the proximal ones. Weakness may be almost imperceptible or so severe that the legs are virtually paralyzed and the hands useless. Motor signs and sensory manifestations most frequently occur concomitantly. Abnormalities of sensation are usually striking. Patients complain of aching, coldness, hotness, deadness, numbness, prickliness, and tenderness, most commonly in the calves, on the plantar surfaces of the feet, and in the fingers. Deep pressure or light touch may be extremely unpleasant. In the most severe cases, the muscles become wasted, atrophic, flabby, and tender, and the skin may be dry, red, and shiny. Excessive perspiration of feet and hands is occasionally noted. The deep tendon reflexes, which may be exaggerated in some patients at the onset of the illness, are usually greatly diminished or totally abolished. The sensory loss is symmetrical, most severe distally, and diminishes gradually over more proximal parts; all modalities are involved, some more than others. On rare occasions, severe burning, shooting, lightning, or "electric" types of pain can occur in the absence of clear-cut signs of neuropathy. The term "burning feet syndrome" has been applied to this variety of neuropathic disorder. This syndrome has been encountered in inmates of prison camps, chronic alcoholics, and patients undergoing dialysis for chronic renal failure. In rare instances, nutritional polyneuropathy may be accompanied by vertigo, deafness, aphonia, and amblyopia.

The mode of evolution and the severity of nutritional polyneuropathy can be quite variable. Usually the onset is insidious, and the progression is slow. Sometimes the course is rapid and abrupt, crippling the patient in a matter of weeks. Recovery requires months and is sometimes incomplete.

A temporary worsening of paresthesias and of weakness may follow the start of therapy. In early or mild cases, a prolonged nerve conduction velocity may be the only objective manifestation of the disease. Examination of the cerebrospinal fluid reveals a normal level or a very slight elevation of the protein content.

Pathology. The salient pathologic changes suggest segmental demyelination of peripheral nerves involving distal parts to a greater degree than proximal ones. Occasionally dorsal root ganglia reveal a loss of nerve cells, and axonal reaction may be seen in some of the anterior horn cells of the spinal cord. It has been speculated that in nutritional polyneuropathy, primary axonal degeneration or a process of "dying back" results in destruction of both the axon and myelin sheaths in the periphery of the largest and longest nerve fibers.

Pathogenesis and Treatment. Nutritional depletion probably alters the normal metabolism of peripheral nerves in several different ways. Both experimental and clinical studies support the view that a deficiency of several of the B vitamins can result in neuropathy. Certain neuropathies respond to the administration of thiamin alone. Recent studies have shown decreased levels of thiamin in the blood, urine, and muscles of patients afflicted with alcoholic neuropathy. Prior to nutritional replenishment, the activity of blood transketolase is usually reduced, and blood pyruvate levels, measured before and after the administration of glucose, may be elevated. The fact that biochemical evidence of thiamin deficiency in nutritional polyneuropathy cannot always be obtained is explained by the slow evolution of this disorder. Whereas the biochemical lesion antedates all clinical manifestations of neuropathy, the latter linger on for many months after the metabolic insult has been removed. A deficiency of pyridoxine has also been blamed for nutritional polyneuropathy. A neuropathic disorder has been observed in patients who were given desoxypyridoxine, a metabolic antagonist of vitamin B_6. The neuropathy that develops in the course of isoniazid (isonicotinic acid hydrazide, INH) therapy can be reversed by pyridoxine alone. Isoniazid causes a deficiency of the essential cofactor pyridoxal phosphate by interfering with phosphorylation of the vitamin. Pyridoxal phosphate is an essential cofactor for a number of enzymatic reactions known to participate in protein metabolism. The specific role of these enzymatic reactions in the metabolism of peripheral nerves remains to be defined. A deficiency of pyridoxal phosphate results in the inadequate synthesis of nicotinic acid from tryptophan. Reduced blood levels of nicotinic acid and nicotinamide have been measured in some patients with nutritional polyneuropathy. Pantothenic acid deficiency may also be involved in the production of some forms of nutritional polyneuropathy. It has been claimed that the administration of pantothenic acid relieves the burning feet syndrome, regardless of its cause.

THE WERNICKE-KORSAKOFF SYNDROME

Of all the disorders of the central nervous system associated with the protracted and abusive intake of alcohol and nutritional depletion, Wernicke's disease and Korsakoff's psychosis are the most frequent. The term "cerebral beriberi" has sometimes been applied to these conditions.

Clinical Manifestation. *Wernicke's disease* is characterized by disturbed ocular motility, ataxia, impaired mentation, and, occasionally, polyneuropathy. The patient may complain of diplopia and unsteadiness of gait, but is usually unaware of his deficit. On examination, bilateral weakness or paralysis of the external recti muscles and paralysis of lateral conjugate gaze are common. Horizontal nystagmus is almost always present, although it sometimes cannot be elicited until abducens function has improved. Vertical nystagmus, particularly on upward gaze, is frequently present. Occasionally there are ptosis, complete paralysis of eye movements, miosis and, very rarely, unreactive pupils. The ataxia, which is almost always present, affects stance and gait primarily. It may be so slight that only special tests for cerebellar function betray its existence. When it is severe, the patient cannot stand or walk without help. Advanced polyneuropathy usually masks cerebellar ataxia. Intention tremor is less common and tends to affect the legs more than the arms. Scanning speech is a rarity. A mild to severe mixed sensory-motor polyneuropathy exists in at least 50 per cent of cases. When first seen, the patient with Wernicke's disease may display symptoms and signs attributable to alcohol withdrawal: i.e., delirium, tremulousness, confusion, agitation, hallucinosis, altered sense perception, and autonomic overactivity. More often, he lacks spontaneity, is apathetic, listless, indifferent, disoriented in time and place, and tends to misidentify objects and people around him. Dull mentation, impaired retentive memory, and general lack of grasp are more common than drowsiness or unconsciousness. With improved nutrition and supplemental thiamin the patient becomes more alert, more attentive, and more readily testable. He may then display a characteristic amnestic confabulatory syndrome known as *Korsakoff's psychosis.* In addition, the patient with Korsakoff's psychosis reveals a number of abnormalities of cognitive function. He may have a great deal of difficulty in forming visual and verbal abstractions. His capacity to shift from one mental set to another and his ability to learn are defective. Perceptual function and concept formation are affected. However, the most prominent and serious mental abnormality seen in Korsakoff's psychosis is the disordered memory function that renders some patients incapable of performing any but the simplest tasks. Recent retentive memory and the ability to learn newly presented material are strikingly impaired. An extensive retrograde amnesia covering a variable period of time is also

common. Finally, the patient confabulates and fabricates fictitious stories. Confabulation is by no means unique to Korsakoff's psychosis and tends to disappear in the chronic stages of the illness.

Features of Wernicke's disease and Korsakoff's psychosis are frequently encountered in the same patient. In many instances of Korsakoff's psychosis, slight, residual nystagmus and ataxia may be detected years later. The Wernicke-Korsakoff syndrome may be complicated by other stigmata of chronic malnutrition, including cirrhosis of the liver, anemia, and mucocutaneous lesions of various types. Many patients suffer from postural hypotension, dyspnea, and tachycardia, but full-blown beriberi heart disease is rare. The Wernicke-Korsakoff syndrome usually begins abruptly. Some degree of recovery is the rule, except in the most advanced cases and in those complicated by other illnesses. During the acute stage of the disease the mortality may be as high as 17 per cent. The ocular manifestations, except for nystagmus, respond promptly and dramatically to vitamin therapy. Ataxia improves more slowly. Korsakoff's psychosis tends to be irreversible if well established.

Pathology. The pathologic alterations that affect the cerebrum and the brainstem are remarkably constant. They almost always involve structures in a bilaterally symmetrical manner. Lesions are invariably seen in the mammillary bodies and the terminal fornices. Lesions in the periaqueductal region of the midbrain, in the floor of the fourth ventricle, in the vicinity of the dorsal motor nucleus of the vagus, and in the anterior superior parts of the cerebellar vermis probably account for the paralysis of gaze, nystagmus, and ataxia. The lesions involving thalamic nuclei (anteromedial, lateral dorsal, and pulvinar) and the hypothalamus and those seen in the mammillary bodies and fornices may underlie some of the psychologic abnormalities, particularly the amnestic syndrome. Microscopically, the lesions consist of necrosis of both nerve cells and myelinated structures. A striking glial reaction involves the center of the lesion. Both endothelial proliferation and hemorrhages are found, but the latter are usually fresh and may represent a nonspecific, terminal change. In the vermis of the cerebellum the principal changes consist of a loss of Purkinje cells and gliosis of the molecular layer of the cortex.

Pathogenesis. There is now an overwhelming body of evidence that favors a specific lack of vitamin B_1 (cocarboxylase) as the main nutritional factor in the Wernicke-Korsakoff syndrome. Most patients give a history of inadequate nutrition and weight loss. Other stigmata of malnutrition, such as loss of subcutaneous fat and skin turgor, mucocutaneous manifestations, and an enlarged liver are frequent. Clinical studies have shown that the continued intake of alcohol is not followed by aggravation of symptoms, provided adequate nutritional repletion is undertaken promptly. Thiamin alone, given orally or parenterally, can dramatically reverse some of the symptoms and signs. Victor and Adams maintained patients with Wernicke's disease on either glucose or a boiled rice diet containing no vitamins for brief periods, then gave them B vitamins selectively. Ophthalmoplegia, apathy, listlessness, and inattentiveness began to improve within a few hours and cleared completely within a few days after thiamin had been added to the regimen. Nystagmus and ataxia diminished, but Korsakoff's psychosis did not improve significantly. Other B vitamins were ineffective. The improvement of neurologic signs can be closely correlated with levels of blood transketolase activity, which are reduced prior to thiamin administration and increase toward normal with clinical improvement, sometimes within four to five hours after the injection of 25 to 50 mg. of thiamin.

NUTRITIONAL AMBLYOPIA
(Tobacco-Alcohol Amblyopia, Nutritional Retrobulbar Neuropathy)

Clinical Manifestations. A remarkably uniform and stereotyped disorder of vision is encountered occasionally in persons who are chronically undernourished. Characteristically it evolves slowly and subacutely, the mode of onset of symptoms being much the same from patient to patient. Visual impairment usually starts insidiously and reaches a maximum in several weeks to months. Blurred or dim vision, difficulty in reading, photophobia, and retrobulbar discomfort on moving the eyes are the common presenting complaints. On examination, the patient has bilaterally symmetrical central, centrocecal, or paracentral scotomata. Ophthalmoscopic changes are restricted at first to slight redness of the temporal margins of the optic discs; minimal pallor is observed at a later stage. Often, no abnormality is visible. The peripheral visual fields are usually intact. The visual disorder is, to a large extent, reversible with improvement of nutrition.

Pathology. The pathologic change in nutritional amblyopia consists of bilaterally symmetrical loss of myelinated fibers in the central parts of the optic nerves, chiasm, and optic tracts, corresponding in location to the papillomacular bundle. In severe cases, the retina loses macular ganglion cells, probably secondary to the "zonal" destruction of medullated fibers in the retrobulbar parts of the optic nerve.

Pathogenesis. This type of visual disturbance has been encountered in undernourished populations all over the world. It is commonly seen during famine, and among civilian and military prisoners of war. It is endemic in certain parts of Africa, Asia, and South America. Among the more privileged populations in the western world, the syndrome is seen in persons chronically addicted to alcohol or, occasionally, to tobacco, who neglect their nutrition. A similar syndrome also occurs as a complication of vitamin B_{12} deficiency and diabetes mellitus, as well as in patients treated with isoniazid for tuberculosis. This visual disorder accompanies other neurologic syndromes believed to have a nutritional cause, such as *Strachan's syndrome*, in which amblyopia is combined with paresthesias of the feet, hands, trunk, and, occasionally, face, loss of reflexes, dizziness, deafness, hoarseness, spasticity, ataxia, and a variety of mucocutaneous lesions (genital dermatitis, corneal degeneration, glossitis, and stomatitis). In the chronic alcoholic patient, amblyopia may occur in conjunction with Wernicke's disease, cerebellar degeneration, Marchiafava-Bignami's disease, and peripheral neuropathy. In recent years, a nutritional deficiency rather than a toxicity has been held responsible for so-called tobacco-alcohol amblyopia. Detailed clinical and pathologic studies fail to distinguish this type of amblyopia from nutritional amblyopia. In clinical experiments, patients with amblyopia continued their usual consumption of alcohol and tobacco, but ate an adequate diet supplemented by B vitamins. All showed some recovery of visual acuity and a reduction in the size of the scotomata. As yet, the metabolic aberration or specific vitamin deficiency responsible for the development of amblyopia has not been defined. A lack of vitamin B_{12}, thiamin, riboflavin, and pyridoxine or a failure in the detoxification of cyanide present in tobacco smoke, have been implicated in the genesis of the syndrome. Except for isolated findings of reduced serum vitamin B_{12} levels, the abnormal urinary excretion of methylmalonic acid and low levels of blood transketolase activity, no specific biochemical abnormalities have been reported in cases of amblyopia.

Treatment. Treatment with oral or parenteral B vitamins and improved nutrition are usually followed by improvement, depending upon the severity of the amblyopia and its duration before therapy is instituted.

CEREBELLAR CORTICAL DEGENERATION

Cerebellar cortical degeneration, or parenchymatous cerebellar degeneration, has often been referred to as alcoholic cerebellar degeneration, although well documented instances of cerebellar cortical degeneration have occurred as a result of chronic nutritional depletion not attributable to alcohol. This disorder can be set apart from all other known forms of acquired or familial cerebellar degeneration because of the uniformity of the clinical and pathologic manifestations. The clinical and pathologic findings are discussed in Degenerative and Heredofamilial Diseases of the Central Nervous System.

A substantial body of evidence favors the contention that cerebellar degeneration is due to nutritional factors. The history of chronic alcoholic patients is admittedly unreliable, yet most admit improper eating habits. Many patients with cortical cerebellar degeneration give a history of progressive weight loss before the onset of their symptoms. Signs of malnutrition are common, and the cerebellar syndrome frequently occurs in conjunction with cirrhosis and other nutritional complications of alcoholism. Furthermore, a number of nonalcoholic patients develop cortical cerebellar degeneration in the setting of other diseases associated with nutritional depletion, such as pellagra, amebiasis, and protracted vomiting. In general, improved nutrition and supplementary B vitamins result in some degree of improvement of ataxia.

CENTRAL PONTINE MYELINOLYSIS

Central pontine myelinolysis is a relatively rare disease characterized by demyelination of the central portion of the pons. It was described originally in patients afflicted with chronic alcoholism and malnutrition but has since been encountered in nonalcoholic patients who were nutritionally deprived. The illness affects adults mainly, but has been reported in children; males and females are equally afflicted. Although the precise clinical course has not yet been defined, the principal neurologic abnormalities are progressive weakness of facial muscles and tongue, causing severe impairment of speech and deglutition. In a number of cases, pseudobulbar phenomena such as emotional lability and pathologic crying have been noted. Quadriparesis at the onset of the illness usually leads to a flaccid and areflexic quadriplegia with Babinski signs. Lack of response to painful stimuli and absence of corneal reflexes are said to be common. Urinary incontinence, decerebrate posture, and respiratory paralysis have been reported in isolated cases. The illness evolves rapidly over a period of two to three weeks, ending in coma and eventual death. Examination of the cerebrospinal fluid is unremarkable.

Pathologic examination reveals a focus of demyelination, variable in size and extent, involving the center of the basal portion of the mid and upper pons. Axis cylinders, nerve cells, and blood vessels are relatively well preserved. An appropriate glial and phagocytic reaction is seen within the lesions. Vascular or inflammatory changes are absent. The clinical symptoms and signs depend upon the size of the lesion and, in general, correlate with its anatomic localization.

The pathogenesis of this curious disorder has been much debated, toxic and nutritional factors being the causes most frequently cited. The lesion has been found at postmortem examination in patients suffering from alcoholism, other forms of chronic malnutrition, neoplasia, renal disease, hepatic insufficiency, and a variety of infectious processes. To date, no biochemical data have been obtained.

MARCHIAFAVA-BIGNAMI DISEASE

Marchiafava-Bignami disease is among the rarest disorders complicating chronic alcoholism. Few cases have been examined in detail, and it is difficult to state the precise nature of the clinical manifestations. The disease affects males of middle age predominantly. The course is variable; it may evolve over a period of a few days or several months. Complete recovery, although rare, occurs. The patients are agitated, confused, and have hallucinations (visual, auditory, and gustatory), disturbance of memory, negativism, impaired judgment, and progressive dementia. Neurologic symptoms and signs suggest bilateral involvement of frontal lobes and include disturbance of language, gait and motor skills, seizures, incontinence, rooting, grasping, sucking, and delayed initiation of action. Tremulousness of the hands and dysarthria have been reported.

Pathologically, Marchiafava-Bignami disease is characterized by symmetrical zones of demyelination affecting the central parts of the corpus callosum, beginning in the most anterior parts and extending caudally. Similar changes affect the central parts of the anterior commissure, the optic chiasm and tracts, and, in severe cases, the central white matter of the frontal lobes. In zones of demyelination, axis cylinders tend to be preserved. Occasionally, there are extensive tissue destruction and cavitation. The degree of glial reaction in these areas depends on the chronicity of the process.

Originally, it was assumed that the disease occurred exclusively in males of Italian descent who consumed excessive amounts of crude red wine. The illness has since been encountered in patients of varied ancestry, some of whom were addicted to other types of alcoholic beverages. The characteristic pathologic changes of Marchiafava-Bignami disease have been encountered in conjunction with Wernicke's disease and nutritional amblyopia as well as in malnourished, nonalcoholic patients. It is probable that Marchiafava-Bignami disease is yet another example of a nutritionally determined disease entity characterized by symmetrical and zonal demyelination.

VITAMIN B$_{12}$ DEFICIENCY

Definition. Insufficient absorption of vitamin B$_{12}$ from the gastrointestinal tract can result in a subacute degeneration of the spinal cord, optic nerves, cerebral white matter, and peripheral nerves. Although the neurologic manifestations of vitamin B$_{12}$ deficiency are frequently associated with a macrocytic anemia (pernicious anemia), the latter is not always present. Neurologic symptoms develop in approximately 80 per cent of patients between the ages of 25 and 75 years afflicted with pernicious anemia. They rarely occur as a result of secondary vitamin B_{12} deficiency complicating fish tapeworm (*Diphyllobothrium latum*) infestation, sprue, vegetarianism, or gastrointestinal surgery. (This subject is also dealt with in the discussion of Megaloblastic Anemia.)

Clinical Manifestations. Symptoms and signs of spinal cord involvement (*combined system disease*) constitute the most common neurologic manifestations, and their mode of onset and progression is remarkably uniform. Symmetrical progressive paresthesias of the feet or hands in the form of numbness, tingling, burning, tightness and stiffness, and a feeling of generalized weakness constitute the most frequent initial symptoms. Vague asthenia and lameness progress to a measurable weakness and stiffness of the legs and an unsteadiness of gait that tends to be worse in the dark. The lower limbs may give way unexpectedly. The hands may be stiff and clumsy. When untreated, the illness progresses slowly and relentlessly. Spasticity, ataxia, and paraplegia ensue, often followed by bowel and bladder dysfunction. In the early stages of the disease, examination of the patient often reveals few objective changes, but eventually signs of disturbed peripheral nerve and posterior and lateral column function become readily apparent. Diminution or loss of position and vibratory sense involves the legs, the hands, and, occasionally, the trunk, and tends to be pronounced. Pain, temperature, and tactile sensation sometimes are blunted over the distal parts of the legs in a pattern suggestive of peripheral nerve involvement. The motor examination reveals weak and, later, spastic legs and extensor plantar responses. The activity of the deep tendon reflexes is variable and appears to depend upon the severity of the illness. The knee jerks are often hyperactive and the ankle jerks absent. In advanced cases, all stretch reflexes may be diminished or absent, but may return when vitamin therapy has been promptly instituted. Psychologic symptoms range from apathy, irritability, and suspiciousness to confusion and dementia, and at times are the presenting neurologic abnormality. On rare occasions, failing vision due to symmetrical centrocecal scotomata may be the presenting neurologic symptom of vitamin B_{12} deficiency.

Pathology. The lesions associated with subacute combined degeneration involve in sequence the posterior columns, the lateral columns, and the cerebral white matter. The earliest visible change consists of swelling of individual myelinated nerve fibers in small foci. These lesions subsequently coalesce into large, irregular, spongy, honeycomb-like zones of demyelination. Fibers with the largest diameter are predominantly affected. Axis cylinders tend to be spared. Myelin destruction frequently begins in the cervical and upper thoracic segments of the cord, spreading axially to involve other segments. The cerebral white matter is affected last. The large fibers of the peripheral nerves may show minimal loss of myelin.

Diagnosis. A number of diseases other than vitamin B_{12} deficiency affect the posterior and lateral columns of the spinal cord, the most important being multiple sclerosis, tumors, cervical spondylosis, syphilitic meningomyelitis, and familial spastic paraplegia. These entities can usually be differentiated from one another clinically, but ancillary examinations such as myelography and special tests involving the cerebrospinal fluid may be necessary to establish a correct diagnosis. In B_{12} deficiency of the nervous system, the cerebrospinal fluid is usually normal. The electroencephalogram is often abnormal. The serum vitamin B_{12} content correlates well with the severity of the neurologic impairment and is invariably low in untreated cases. The "Schilling test" using radioactive cyanocobalamin is always positive, and gastric achlorhydria can be demonstrated in almost every instance. Blood and bone marrow examinations are of limited value, particularly when the patient has been treated with folic acid, which corrects the anemia but not the neurologic manifestations. The urinary excretion of methylmalonic acid, an intermediary metabolite in the conversion of propionic acid to succinic acid, is a sensitive indicator of vitamin B_{12} deficiency, but its relation to the lesions in the nervous system is as yet unknown.

Pathogenesis. The pathogenesis of the neurologic manifestations of vitamin B_{12} deficiency is unknown, although it probably differs from the biochemical lesion affecting the hematopoietic system, since the neurologic manifestations are independent of the anemia and may appear when folic acid corrects the anemia. The specific biochemical role of vitamin B_{12} in the nervous system has not yet been elucidated. It is an essential cofactor for at least two enzyme systems which exist in mammalian tissue, including brain: (1) methylmalonyl-CoA isomerase, which converts methylmalonyl-CoA to succinyl-CoA, a step in the utilization of propionic acid, and (2) methylfolate-H_4 methyltransferase, which is responsible for the synthesis of methionine from homocysteine. In experimentally induced vitamin B_{12} deficiency, the activity of both of these enzyme systems is reduced in brain. These enzymes may be essential to the maintenance of the myelin sheath. An experimental approach to the pathogenesis of the neurologic manifestations of vitamin B_{12} deficiency in animals has been hampered by the absence of white-matter lesions in deficient animals.

Treatment. Prompt initiation of therapy is of the utmost importance, because the early neurologic manifestations can be rapidly and completely reversed. The greatest degree of improvement is achieved in patients treated within three months of onset of symptoms, although variable degrees of amelioration can be attained after longer untreated periods (six to twelve months). In the first two weeks, daily intramuscular injections of 50 mcg. of cyanocobalamin, or an equivalent amount of liver USP, should be administered. During the next two months, 100 mcg. of cyanocobalamin should be injected twice a week. For the remainder of his life, the patient should receive a minimum of 100 mcg. intramuscularly every month to prevent a relapse that might be caused by metabolic stress such as systemic illness or surgery. The administration of oral vitamin preparations containing folic acid must be avoided for patients with pernicious anemia since folic acid may actually precipitate neurologic complications.

PELLAGRA

This disease is described elsewhere in this book. The neurologic manifestations take the form of an encephalopathy frequently associated with signs of peripheral nerve and spinal cord involvement. Psychologic symptoms often precede the skin changes, which require exposure to sunlight for their development. In the early stages, the patient is depressed, apathetic, apprehensive, and morbidly fearful. He complains of insomnia, dizziness, and headaches. As the illness progresses, a florid psychosis characterized by confusion, delusions, disorientation, hallucinations, and delirium develops. In the end, the patient may become comatose. Spasticity of legs and ataxia of gait observed in some of the patients are indicative of spinal cord affliction. The neurologic symptoms and signs respond promptly and dramatically to the administration of niacin.

The neuropathologic changes associated with pellagra consist of a characteristic degeneration known as "central neuritis," which affects the large pyramidal cells (Betz cells) of the motor cortex. These neurons become pale, swollen, and round as though their axons had been severed. In the spinal cord, the posterior and the lateral columns may show varying degrees of demyelination. In the brain, as in other tissues, nicotinic acid is a constituent of the two hydrogen-transferring coenzymes (formerly DPN and TPN), nicotinamide-adenine-dinucleotide (NAD), and nicotinamide-adenine-dinucleotide-phosphate (NADP). Both participate in a number of important enzymatic reactions. In patients with pellagra, red blood cell NAD levels are reduced, and the urinary excretion of n-methylnicotinamide is diminished. In nicotinic acid-deficient rats, nucleotide levels are reduced in the blood and in various organs, including the brain. The administration of nicotinic acid to pellagrins and to deficient animals causes the nucleotide content of the blood and the tissues to rise temporarily above normal levels.

PROTEIN-CALORIE DEFICIENCY
(Kwashiorkor and Marasmus)

This disease is discussed elsewhere in this book. The effect of deficiency of proteins and calories on the nervous system has not yet been defined. Infants who suffer from protein-calorie deficiency are less easily conditioned, their performance on standard psychologic tests is often impaired and they commonly exhibit less curiosity and exploratory behavior, being apathetic, irritable, and drowsy. Weakness, hypotonia, diminished to absent deep tendon reflexes, seizures, and coarse tremor of the extremities have been described in kwashiorkor. The electroencephalogram is said to be abnormal in 40 per cent of severely afflicted children. There have been few critical neuropathologic studies.

Experimentally induced protein-calorie malnutrition in newborn pigs causes retardation of gait development. The learning ability of weanling rats fed a diet devoid of protein is markedly impaired and, in addition, spasmodic trembling of the head and forepaws may develop. Neurologic signs are said to be striking in puppies born of malnourished bitches. Neonatal death occurs in 50 per cent of the pups, and the development of the survivors is retarded. Athetoid movements of the head and neck, ataxia of gait, and seizures may develop after weaning.

Few of the large number of biochemical investigations in laboratory animals and in patients suffering from protein-calorie deficiency have dealt with the nervous system. Protein and amino acid metabolism is generally impaired; the levels of free essential amino acids are reduced in the plasma, and an adaptive reduction in enzyme activity ensues. The brains of rats fed a low-protein diet have shown a decrease in the content of gamma-aminobutyric acid, and the activity of enzymes concerned with its formation is reduced. The levels of alanine, glutamic acid, glutamine and aspartic acid are decreased.

Severe malnutrition during fetal growth and in early infancy affects the normal structural and biochemical development of the nervous system in an irreversible manner. Intrauterine malnutrition influences the rate of cell division, resulting in decreased brain size and cellularity. Severe malnutrition in the immediate neonatal period retards the growth of the brain as well as the metabolism of cerebral DNA, RNA, and protein, and has a marked influence on the rate of synthesis of myelin lipids. Cerebrosides, plasmalogens, sulfatides, cholesterol, and proteolipids are significantly decreased in the white matter of malnourished infants. In the cortex the content of RNA and protein per cell is normal, yet the total number and size of cells are reduced. The younger the child, the more marked is the abnormality. Evidence gleaned from the study of laboratory animals suggests that the deficit persists despite adequate nutritional replenishment. Thus profound nutritional deprivation occurring at a particularly vulnerable period of brain development permanently and adversely affects ultimate intellectual development and behavior.

Denny-Brown, D.: Neurological conditions resulting from prolonged and severe dietary restriction. Medicine, 26:41, 1947.

Lopez, R. J., and Collins, G. H.: Wernicke's encephalopathy—a complication of chronic hemodialysis. Arch. Neurol., (Chicago), 18:248, 1968.

Pant, S. S., Asbury, A. K., and Richardson, E. P., Jr.: The myelo-

pathy of pernicious anemia—a neuropathological reap
praisal. Acta Neurol. Scand., 44(Suppl. 35), 1968.
Scrimshaw, N. S., and Gordon, J. E. (eds.); Malnutrition, Learn-
ing and Behavior. Cambridge, Mass., M.I.T. Press, 1968.
Spillane, J. D.: Nutritional Disorders of the Nervous System.
Edinburgh, E. and S. Livingstone, Ltd., 1947.
Victor, M.: The effects of nutritional deficiency on the nervous
system. A comparison with the effects of carcinoma. In
Brain, R. L., and Norris, F. H. (eds.): The Remote Effects of

Cancer on the Nervous System. New York, Grune & Stratton,
Inc., 1965.
Victor, M., and Adams, R. D.: The effect of alcohol upon the
nervous system. A. Res. Ment. Dis. Proc., 32:526, 1953.
Wagner, A. F., and Folkers, K.: Vitamins and Coenzymes. New
York, Interscience Publications, John Wiley and Sons, 1964.
Wolstenholme, G. E. W.: Thiamine Deficiency: Biochemical
Lesions and Their Clinical Significance. Boston, Little,
Brown and Company, 1967.

The Demyelinating Diseases

Labe C. Scheinberg

INTRODUCTION: THE BIOLOGY OF MYELIN

Demyelination or myelin breakdown may be a secondary feature of many disorders of the nervous system such as infections, intoxications, degenerations or deficiency states. However, what concerns us here are the demyelinating diseases, in which the myelin is primarily affected. These have as a common feature the selective involvement of the myelin sheaths with relative sparing of the axons. The distribution of the lesions is random and the cause is unknown. Electrophysiologic studies of the axon have not been made in these diseases; the criteria for the functional and structural integrity of the axon are usually those established by light microscopy. Recently biopsy material of chronic areas of demyelination in the cerebral cortex and subcortical white matter has been studied by means of electron microscopy. These areas reveal denuded axons, vacuolization of the endoplasmic reticulum of oligodendrocytes, fibrous astrocytosis, and evidence of remyelination.

The devastating consequences of myelin breakdown indicate the vital importance of this structure. Recent work has provided much new information about the formation, structure, chemistry, and metabolism of myelin. There is also much new information about its pathology, and many studies have been made of experimental demyelinating disorders.

The neuroglia, namely the oligodendrocyte and astrocyte, are now recognized as more than supporting elements in the brain. They appear to participate in myelin formation, transport of material to the neurons, and the maintenance of the neurons' ionic environment.

The formation of myelin in both the central and peripheral nervous systems follows a similar pattern. Central myelin is formed by an exten-

sion of the external plasma membrane of the oligodendrocyte wrapping the axon, whereas peripheral myelin is formed by the extension of the Schwann cell membrane. This wrapping produces a structure comprised of layers of concentric, tightly packed membranes of uniform thickness. If one examines the C fibers of the peripheral nerve with the electron microscope, one sees the axon-myelin relationship in its simplest form. The individual membranes of the Schwann cell and the axon membrane of the C fiber each represent "unit membranes," which are equivalent to the plasma membranes of the cells. The unit membrane of the Schwann cell or oligodendrocyte closes upon itself to form the major and minor period lines of myelin. The internal surface becomes apposed to form the dark major line, and the external surfaces give rise to the intraperiod line. The results of studies employing x-ray diffraction, electron microscopy, and lipid analyses suggest that each unit membrane consists of a sandwich of a bimolecular lipid leaflet between parallel layers of hydrated protein, in close contact with the polar groups of the lipids. The lipids that make up this leaflet appear to be interdigitated molecules of cerebroside, phospholipid, and cholesterol. Detailed chemical analysis of myelin reveals protein (primarily proteolipid protein) 22 per cent of dry weight, and lipid 78 per cent of dry weight. The lipids are in approximately equal molar ratios of cholesterol and phospholipids with about one half as much galactolipid. The lipids in the myelin sheath, once deposited at the time of its formation, undergo little subsequent turnover.

The myelin sheath is a compact, highly organized membrane structure that must be regarded as one of the more permanent tissue elements of the body. However, myelin should not be considered as metabolically inactive since white matter accounts for about 30 per cent of total cerebral oxygen consumption and the glial cells utilize about two thirds of this.

THE DEMYELINATING DISORDERS

INTRODUCTION

The foregoing considerations suggest that demyelination must be considered as a basic disorder of the oligodendrocyte or the Schwann cell. To consider demyelination solely as myelin breakdown, ignoring the fact that the myelin lamellae are an integral part of the parent glial cell, may be contradictory to the pathogenesis. The etiologic agent may attack either the perikaryon of the glial cell or its plasma membrane to produce demyelination.

Prior to a consideration of the pathogenesis of demyelinative disorders, one must make some attempt to classify the varied primary disorders of myelin. In 1957 Poser suggested classification into two basic types. One, a so-called "myelinoclastic" or demyelinating type, includes disorders in which myelin forms normally to a certain age and then for unknown reasons breaks down. This includes the most common demyelinating disease, multiple sclerosis, and also acute disseminated encephalomyelitis and certain other disorders. The other, the "dysmyelinative" type, includes disorders in which a presumed inborn error of metabolism results in defective myelin formation. The category includes the so-called leukodystrophies or some of the diffuse scleroses and lipidoses of the nervous system and the aminoacidurias.

Pathogenesis. In most demyelinating disorders, the cause remains unknown. Demyelinization is the typical response of white matter to noxious stimuli not severe enough to cause complete necrosis of the tissue, and almost any infectious, nutritional, vascular, or toxic disorder can result in demyelinization. At present there is insufficient evidence to incriminate any one cause. However, the majority of workers interpret present evidence as supporting most strongly an allergic basis for most of the primary demyelinating disorders, with genetic and geographic factors influencing susceptibility. Autoradiographic studies in experimental allergic encephalomyelitis using tritiated precursors of DNA, RNA, and protein have shown a rise in circulating plasma-like cells prior to onset of neurologic signs. Supernatant from cultures of these cells produces demyelination in tissue culture of rat cerebellum similar to that produced by serum from multiple sclerosis patients.

Because of the wide divergence in their symptoms, the demyelinating disorders are grouped according to pathologic similarities that have been previously described. Within this framework further similarities have emerged between certain demyelinating disorders. The pathologic pictures of rabies postvaccinal encephalomyelitis and parainfectious encephalomyelitis are almost indistinguishable. This resemblance has stimulated many experimental studies and has provided a starting point for investigation.

It has long been known that a certain fraction of patients who receive antirabies treatment develop a neurologic syndrome called rabies postvaccinal encephalomyelitis (postimmunization encephalomyelitis). In the immunization therapy of rabies, the patient usually receives 14 daily subcutaneous injections of killed rabies virus in a suspension of rabbit brain tissue. Encephalitis, or paralysis, if it occurs, develops any time from a week after the first inoculation to two weeks after the last. There was much speculation that this complication was due to the virus until Rivers and co-workers in 1933 showed that multiple injections of normal rabbit brain tissue in monkeys resulted in encephalomyelitis with lesions similar to those seen in rabies postvaccinal encephalomyelitis. This was followed by the extensive investigations of Kabat, Wolf, and co-workers in the 1940's, who demonstrated that experimental allergic encephalomyelitis (EAE) could be produced in monkeys by a few injections of adult homologous, heterologous, or autologous central nervous system tissue mixed with paraffin oil and killed mycobacteria (Freund's adjuvant.) White matter appeared more encephalitogenic than gray, whereas peripheral nerve and fetal (unmyelinated) brain were ineffectual as encephalitogens. The encephalitogen is stable to heat and other physical treatments, indicating that it is probably not a transmissible infectious agent. EAE is not

TABLE 1. PRIMARY DISORDERS OF MYELIN

A. Demyelinating (myelinoclastic or leukoencephalopathic): breakdown of normally constituted myelin
  1. Postimmunization encephalomyelitis (smallpox and rabies vaccination, other immunizations)
  2. Parainfectious encephalomyelitis (postinfectious, postexanthematous, etc.)
  3. Acute necrotizing hemorrhagic encephalomyelitis (rare)
  4. Multiple sclerosis (disseminated sclerosis) and possible variants, including:
    a. Acute disseminated encephalomyelitis
    b. Optic and retrobulbar neuritis
    c. Transverse myelitis, including necrotizing myelopathy
    d. Neuromyelitis optica (Devic's)
    e. Transitional sclerosis
  5. Diffuse sclerosis (Schilder's cerebral sclerosis)
  6. Concentric sclerosis (Balo's) (rare)
  7. Progressive multifocal leukoencephalopathy (viral?)
  8. Subacute sclerosing leukoencephalitis (viral?) (see Encephalomyelitis)
  9. Central pontine myelinolysis (nutritional deficiency?) (see Nutrient Deficiency and Deficiency Diseases)
  10. Progressive subcortical encephalopathy (Binswanger's disease)
B. Dysmyelinating (leukodystrophic): Failure to form normally constituted myelin, possibly secondary to genetically determined errors of myelin anabolism
  1. Simple storage type (metachromatic leukodystrophy, glial insufficiency type or sulfatidosis)
  2. Sudanophilic type (Pelizaeus-Merzbacher disease)
  3. Globoid cell type (Krabbe's disease)
  4. Spongy degeneration of white matter (spongy sclerosis or Canavan's disease)
  5. Other lipidoses (Tay-Sachs disease, Gaucher's disease, gargoylism, etc.)
  6. Aminoacidurias (phenylketonuria, maple syrup urine disease, etc.)

transferable to other animals by serum, although the serum contains complement-fixing antibodies to brain. The pathologic change is primarily in the white matter of the central nervous system, with perivascular and meningeal inflammation and demyelination. These findings are in many instances indistinguishable from those in certain human demyelinating disorders. The cerebrospinal fluid in acute EAE shows pleocytosis with elevation of gamma globulin content similar to the changes in many cases of demyelinating disorders in humans. Finally it has been demonstrated that cortisone administered prior to immunization prevents the development of EAE.

This classic pioneering work has been followed by genetic, immunologic, biochemical, and ultrastructural investigations. It has been shown that there are variations in susceptibility to EAE among various species and strains within species. One inbred strain of mice was shown to be 100 per cent susceptible to induction of EAE, and another strain was shown to be 100 per cent resistant. A genetic analysis revealed that resistance was due to two pairs of resistance-conferring genetic factors. Other workers have successfully transferred EAE by means of sensitized lymphoid cells in isologous (inbred) strains. Finally, workers have found that serum from EAE animals or from some patients with multiple sclerosis causes destruction of myelin in cultures of transplanted brain tissue.

The nature of the encephalitogen in EAE has been extensively studied, and most work indicates that it is a basic protein of myelin (Kies and Alvord, 1965). Specifically sensitized lymphocytes are found in immunofluorescence studies to take up this myelin protein. Other investigators showed that the delayed type of skin reactivity to the myelin protein correlates well with the onset and severity of EAE. Drugs other than cortisone (6-mercaptopurine or methotrexate), which depress lymphoid activity, and irradiation of draining lymph nodes prevent the development of EAE. Serum from animals that have recovered from EAE has been shown to contain IgM antibody, which when transferred to recently sensitized animals prevents the development of EAE. The demyelination in EAE has recently been shown in electron microscopic studies to be a result of the phagocytosis of oligodendroglial cells and dissolution of the myelin lamellae by mononuclear cells.

The relationship of EAE to the spontaneous demyelinating disorders is still conjectural. Since the brain lacks a lymphatic drainage, myelin antigens are inaccessible to the body's reticuloendothelial system. It is plausible to assume that in certain situations the body could produce myelin autoantibodies (cellular or humoral) that would react with central nervous system myelin and produce demyelinating lesions. How the normally inaccessible myelin autoantigens reach the antibody-forming site and under what circumstances this occurs are still unknown.

POSTVACCINAL AND PARAINFECTIOUS ENCEPHALOMYELITIS

Postvaccinal or parainfectious encephalomyelitis is an acute disorder of the nervous system that may occur following immunizations or certain viral infections. Occasionally the preceding infection may be inapparent or nonspecific (see Acute Disseminated Encephalomyelitis). The clinical picture is dependent on the location of the lesions in each disorder, and there may be a spectrum of syndromes that include the signs and symptoms of meningitis, encephalitis, myelitis, or polyneuritis. The disorder is discussed in greater detail elsewhere, but it concerns us here because some cases of acute disseminated encephalomyelitis blend indistinguishably into acute multiple sclerosis. The history of vaccination or an exanthem may be helpful. Other clinical observations, such as the rarity of retrobulbar neuritis in acute disseminated encephalomyelitis or the paucity of radicular pains, seizures, or coma in multiple sclerosis, may aid in the differential diagnosis. However, often only prolonged follow-up with a recurrence of neurologic symptoms can enable one to diagnose multiple sclerosis and exclude acute disseminated encephalomyelitis.

ACUTE NECROTIZING HEMORRHAGIC ENCEPHALOMYELITIS

This is a rare and fulminant variant of demyelinating disease that often progresses to death in days or weeks. The disease is characterized by a rapid course, fever, headache, convulsions, progressive change in state of consciousness from drowsiness to coma, nuchal rigidity, and hemiplegia or quadriplegia. The cerebrospinal fluid examination reveals a pleocytosis up to several thousand white blood cells that are predominantly polymorphonuclear leukocytes, and an elevated protein content. On pathologic examination, there are large foci of hemorrhagic necrosis of white matter. Although most patients succumb within a few weeks, there are rare alleged reports of recovery. There appears to be an experimental allergic model of this disorder with similarities on histologic examination. The only therapy that can be offered is supportive, though ACTH and corticosteroids should be tried.

MULTIPLE SCLEROSIS

Definition. Multiple or disseminated sclerosis is the most common demyelinating disorder. It is usually pleomorphic and difficult to define completely in the absence of specific diagnostic tests.

There are a number of well recognized and readily diagnosed syndromes, but borderline cases may be difficult to categorize clinically and pathologically. Generally it is chronic and relapsing, but fulminating attacks occur and as many as 30 per cent of patients tend to progress steadily from the onset. The symptoms and signs reflect involvement of central myelin, but occasionally symptoms are typical of neuronal or gray-matter involvement. Multiple sclerosis is a disease of the central white matter with "lesions separated in time and space."

Incidence. The prevalence of multiple sclerosis in the United States varies from about 10 per 100,000 in the South to 60 per 100,000 in the North, with similar prevalence and distribution in Europe. The disease affects males and females about equally. About 67 per cent of cases begin between the ages of 20 and 40 years and 95 per cent between 10 and 25 years.

Populations residing between latitudes 40° N. and 40° S. (tropical and subtropical zones) have a low risk of multiple sclerosis. With a few notable exceptions, all populations residing north of this latitude in North America and Europe are at higher risk. Other exceptions to these generalizations are found in other parts of the world; e.g., a low incidence is reported in the Union of South Africa and in Japan. Efforts have been made to correlate these geographic variations with dietary intake, temperature, solar radiation, and geomagnetic latitude, without success. Racial factors seem to play little part in the United States since the incidence in Negroes is almost the same as in Caucasians.

Genetic studies have not elucidated the cause of multiple sclerosis. There are occasional reports of a greater family incidence than could be expected by chance, but these fail to exclude the common effects of environmental factors. A purely hereditary basis seems to be excluded by concordance studies in identical twins.

Pathology. The external surface of the brain and cord generally shows no abnormality. Occasionally there is atrophy of the optic nerves and rarely focal or generalized atrophy of the cerebral hemispheres. Acute large lesions may cause swelling of the cord. Rarely there may be sufficient focal swelling of the cerebrum to give the appearance of a neoplasm in roentgenologic contrast studies.

Cut sections of the brain or spinal cord reveal numerous scattered, grayish, well defined lesions that are slightly depressed and vary in diameter from a few millimeters to a few centimeters. These are found throughout the white matter of the brain, optic nerves, and spinal cord and occasionally extend into gray matter. The number of lesions is usually greater than would be expected from the clinical picture.

Microscopic abnormalities depend on the age of the lesion. Acute lesions show an infiltration of microglial phagocytes and mononuclear cells about vessels, as well as scattered in the lesion itself. The myelin sheaths are affected to varying

degrees, from partial to complete destruction, with relative sparing of axons, glia, and other structures. In more severe lesions there may be total destruction of tissue and cyst formation. As the lesions become chronic, there is a proliferation of glial cells and fibers to give the typical "sclerotic plaque." The axons in these areas may be preserved or destroyed.

Aggravating Factors. An infective process (upper respiratory infection, "influenza," urinary tract infection, gastroenteritis, etc.) is said to precede the initial attack or a relapse of multiple sclerosis in 10 to 40 per cent. Immunizations are without apparent effect on the course of the disease, and any exacerbations seen following these are probably coincidental.

Many workers have stated that pregnancy aggravates the disease, but this is open to question. The disease and pregnancy occur in the same age group, and although some studies show a higher incidence in married child-bearing women, more attacks occur during the puerperium than during pregnancy itself. The physician must consider many nonmedical factors when advising on this problem. Pregnancy is generally considered nondeleterious to the course of multiple sclerosis in any patient who has not had an attack in two years.

There seems to be no clear-cut association of attack or relapse with surgical procedures, and indications for surgery in patients with multiple sclerosis should be judged solely on their own merit.

Trauma has likewise been incriminated in an almost anecdotal manner, but there is no statistical evidence to support a relationship between peripheral trauma and the onset or relapses of multiple sclerosis. There is a tendency for patients to associate trauma with the onset of an attack or relapse, but in many cases it is more likely that the trauma resulted from the disability of multiple sclerosis. Similarly, emotional stress has been incriminated as a precipitant of attacks or relapses of multiple sclerosis. This is difficult to substantiate, but it is reasonable to assume that the cerebral changes in multiple sclerosis make it more difficult for the patient to cope with emotional stress.

Certain diagnostic procedures such as lumbar puncture, pneumoencephalography, cerebral angiography, and myelography have been implicated in the worsening of symptoms in multiple sclerosis. However, these procedures are performed usually in patients whose disease is progressing or soon after an attack or relapse. They should be performed in cases in which there are serious questions whether a neoplasm exists in the nervous system, and not simply in frustration because "there's nothing else that can be done."

Clinical Manifestations. The clinical picture of multiple sclerosis is pleomorphic, but there are usually sufficient typical features to enable one to diagnose the disorder in the absence of a specific diagnostic test or without extensive "excluding" other factors. This is particularly important in relation to pregnancy. The route of delivery is an obstetrical decision.

One must encourage and support the patient to remain active and yet protect him from constantly seeking untried and potentially harmful therapies or unnecessary diagnostic tests and operations.

Prognosis. In the early stages of the disease it is not possible accurately to predict the course, although certain symptoms seem to indicate a better prognosis. Monosymptomatic and acute symptoms lasting hours to weeks tend to give a better prognosis than polysymptomatic or slowly progressive manifestations. Cranial nerve, visual, and sensory symptoms carry a better prognosis for remission or a benign course than do motor or cerebellar symptoms. More than half the cases remit following an initial attack, but one cannot predict the next attack. The remission of certain symptoms, e.g., retrobulbar neuritis, may be so complete as to make the clinician doubt the history.

Within the first five years after onset, about 70 per cent of patients are able to be employed, although with occasional interruptions in some cases. By the end of ten years this drops off to 50 per cent. At the end of 20 years 35 per cent are still employed, with minor interruptions, and about 20 per cent of patients succumb to complications of the disease by this time. The major disabilities are spasticity, disturbances of coordination, and disturbance in bladder and bowel function.

Life expectancy varies considerably, ranging from a few weeks to over 50 years regardless of whether one considers hospitalized, severe cases or the more benign forms. The average life expectancy is from 13 to more than 25 years after onset. The cause of death is often an intercurrent infection, usually respiratory or genitourinary.

POSSIBLE MULTIPLE SCLEROSIS VARIANTS

Optic and Retrobulbar Neuritis

Optic or retrobulbar neuritis, an inflammatory condition of the optic nerve, is a frequent finding in multiple sclerosis. There are many known causes of optic and retrobulbar neuritis such as chronic alcoholism, toxins, local inflammatory conditions, heredo-degenerative disorders, etc., but once these have been excluded, demyelinating disease must be considered as a likely cause. In several large series of patients who presented with retrobulbar neuritis and were followed for many years, 13 to 50 per cent later developed other manifestations of multiple sclerosis.

Both optic and retrobulbar neuritis are characterized by an abrupt or progressive loss of vision that is rarely total and usually is unilateral. Associated with the visual loss may be pain in and around the eye that is accentuated by ocular movement. There may be tenderness on palpation of the eyeball. Visual testing reveals decreased acuity and central or paracentral scotomas. In optic neuritis the optic disc appears inflamed, and there may be hyperemia, blurred margins, and even elevation. A few hemorrhages may be seen in the retina adjacent to the disc. In retrobulbar neuritis the ophthalmoscopic picture is normal, but the features are otherwise similar to those of optic neuritis.

It is essential to differentiate optic neuritis from papilledema associated with increased intracranial pressure or other conditions. Papilledema is almost always bilateral, and vision is usually well preserved until late in the course. The disc elevation is usually greater in papilledema, and the only visual field defect is an enlarged blind spot. In optic neuritis the cerebrospinal fluid pressure is almost always normal, and there may be other findings indicative of multiple sclerosis.

Optic and retrobulbar neuritis may be treated with ACTH or corticosteroids. However, almost complete spontaneous recovery often occurs, and the benefits of therapy are difficult to assess.

The prognosis in a single attack of optic or retrobulbar neuritis is usually good. There may be complete recovery, or there may be residual visual field defects, temporal pallor of the discs, or optic atrophy. The visual acuity may be further impaired with subsequent attacks, but complete visual loss is rare.

Acute Transverse Myelitis

Myelitis is defined as an inflammation of the spinal cord, whereas the term myelopathy includes the noninflammatory disorders. However, the terms are often used interchangeably. Transverse myelitis is the usual term employed to describe partial or complete involvement of the spinal cord in a transverse fashion and extending only a few segments longitudinally. It may be caused by a viral or bacterial infection, toxin, nutritional deficiency, neoplasm, vascular disease, or cervical spondylosis. It may occur in association with exanthemas or nonspecific infections. Acute transverse myelitis may appear as the initial event in a subsequently typical form of multiple sclerosis, or it may develop during the course of the disease. The findings include complete or partial paralysis of both legs or of all four limbs, variable sensory loss, and bladder and bowel involvement. The symptoms are related to the lesions in the ascending and descending tracts of the spinal cord. The motor disorder is supranuclear in type, whereas the sensory loss is mainly for proprioceptive and vibratory sensation.

The onset may be abrupt or insidious, and the course is variable. There may be complete recovery or residual spastic weakness with quadriplegia or paraplegia. Severe sensory loss and loss of bowel and bladder control may also persist.

Subacute necrotizing myelopathy is often associated with vascular malformations of the spinal cord or thrombophlebitis (Foix-Alajouanine syndrome). In acute necrotizing myelopathy there

---

diagnostic procedures. The disease is chronic, often characterized by exacerbations and remissions, with evidence of multiple lesions in central white matter occurring in young adults without other systemic disorders. The symptoms of central white matter involvement are usually those of supranuclear weakness, incoordination, paresthesias, and visual complaints. Other symptoms and signs that are more characteristic of lesions in gray matter, e.g. aphasia, seizures, fasciculations, and neurogenic atrophy, are rare. Mental changes have an intermediate incidence and affect perhaps 30 per cent of patients.

The onset may be acute, with symptoms appearing within minutes to hours, or it may be insidious, with gradual, slow progression of symptoms over a period of months.

The frequency of occurrence of the first symptom of multiple sclerosis is given in Table 2.

The weakness usually begins or is most prominent in the lower extremities, but the upper extremities may be involved. When both lower extremities are involved, there are usually accompanying urinary complaints such as urgency or frequency. The weakness may be minimal, or there may be a total paralysis. There are usually upper motor neuron signs such as spasticity, hyperreflexia, and pathologic reflexes.

Visual complaints include blurring of vision with a central scotoma and decreased visual acuity or diplopia with extraocular paresis and nystagmus.

The incoordination is seen as ataxia or clumsiness and intention tremor of the upper extremities. Often a combination of spastic-ataxic gait is seen.

The paresthesias may involve any or all of the extremities. Usually there is impairment of vibratory sense and position sense in the lower extremities, whereas cutaneous sensation is relatively spared.

The typical clinical course of multiple sclerosis is one of exacerbations and remissions over a period of years, with increasing neurologic deficits due to an increasing number of disseminated lesions. Less frequent are (1) an acute, severe course progressing to death in a few days or weeks; (2) a chronic, progressive course over a period of years; and (3) a benign form with relatively few presenting symptoms and signs and long-lasting remissions. In middle age the insidious onset of a progressive spastic paraparesis is often seen as the major clinical manifestation, particularly in women.

Multiple sclerosis is sometimes divided into clinical types depending upon which portion of the neuraxis is most involved, e.g., spinal, cerebral, brainstem-cerebellar, or mixed. The most common form is spinal with prominent features of spastic paraparesis, lower extremity paresthesias, and urinary complaints. The brainstem-cerebellar variety with prominent visual complaints, cranial nerve signs, nystagmus, vertigo, and incoordination is also common, but the cerebral form with mental changes and hemiparesis and hemisensory changes is uncommon.

Although most cases may be classified as one of these forms early in the course, almost all patients appear to have a mixed type of involvement after about 15 years.

In Table 3 may be noted the frequency of various symptoms and signs of multiple sclerosis in clinical and autopsy series reported by Carter et al. and by Poser.

Certain uncommon symptoms and signs such as nausea, vomiting, facial pain, seizures, dysphagia, atrophy, hearing loss, tinnitus, and changes in states of consciousness occur in 2 to 10 per cent cases. Signs such as internuclear ophthalmoplegia are highly characteristic of multiple sclerosis; headache and aphasia are rare.

Laboratory Data. Abnormal findings in multiple sclerosis are usually confined to the cerebrospinal fluid. In the acute disease, there may be a mild mononuclear pleocytosis of as much as 200 to 300 cells per cubic millimeter, but usually less than 40. The protein content is usually normal or slightly elevated (50 to 100 mg. per 100 ml.); values higher than this are rare. The gamma globulin content is elevated in about two thirds of the cases and, correspondingly, there is often an abnormal colloidal gold curve (first or second zone) accompanied by a negative serologic test for syphilis.

TABLE 2. FREQUENCY OF OCCURRENCE OF FIRST SYMPTOM OF MULTIPLE SCLEROSIS IN CASES PROVED BY CLINICAL STUDY AND AUTOPSY

Symptom	Autopsy (Carter et al.) (46 cases) Per Cent	Autopsy (Poser) (111 cases) Per Cent	Clinical Diagnosis (Carter et al.) (539 cases) Range	Average
Weakness	42	39	40–68	54
Diplopia, impaired vision	35	32	9–39	21
Tremor, ataxia, incoordination	20	6	4–39	19
Paresthesias	13	16	14–46	32
Pain	11	1	2–13	7
Sphincter impairment	11	1	5–11	8
Dizziness or vertigo	7	1	–	–
Changes in muscle tone	7	–	–	–
Facial pain	2	–	–	–
Mental changes	2	2	–	3
Seizures	–	–	–	–

TABLE 3. FREQUENCY OF OCCURRENCE OF SYMPTOMS AND SIGNS IN COURSE OF MULTIPLE SCLEROSIS

	Carter et al. (46 cases)	Poser (111 cases)
	Per Cent	Per Cent
Weakness (symptom or sign)	89	96
Abnormal movements	67	
Abnormal reflexes (absent superficials, Babinski signs, or hyperreflexia)	99	95
Sphincter and genital difficulties	78	82
Visual disturbance (symptom or sign)	100	85
Nystagmus (any type)	85	70
Disc pallor, atrophy, decreased acuity	75	85
Third nerve impairment (and internuclear ophthalmoplegia)	67	
Tremor, ataxia	93	79
Impaired vibration and position sense	81	58
Impaired touch, pain, temperature sense	35	35
Mental changes (symptom or sign)	61	45
Paresthesias	44	65
Pain	42	19
Vertigo or dizziness	18	15

The electroencephalogram may be mildly abnormal in about two thirds of cases revealing either focal or generalized abnormalities.

Diagnosis. Because of the pleomorphic nature of the disease, it is often necessary to exclude many other neurologic disorders. Most often one must consider spinal cord, brainstem or cerebellar tumors, degenerative diseases such as the spinocerebellar degenerations, and combined system disease.

The fact that multiple sclerosis has a remitting nature in many instances and the dissemination of symptoms and signs should indicate that one is not dealing with an expanding lesion involving the nervous system. If all the symptoms and signs can be explained by a single lesion, then one should assume that the condition is not multiple sclerosis. If the patient complains of headache, seizures, or progressive focal neurologic signs, which are uncommon in multiple sclerosis, and if these are accompanied by abnormalities such as increased cerebrospinal fluid pressure, roentgenographic changes in the skull or spine, marked elevation of cerebrospinal fluid protein, etc., then one must proceed further to exclude a neoplasm. This can be done in most cases by a neuroroentgenologic procedure such as myelography, pneumoencephalography, or cerebral angiography. Vascular disease, particularly that involving the brainstem, can be confused with multiple sclerosis in middle-aged patients. In some of these cases only prolonged follow-up reveals the true diagnosis.

Certain degenerative disorders of the nervous system can be confused with multiple sclerosis. However, the former tend to have a family history, to be slowly progressive without remission, and to confine themselves to systems, e.g., cerebellar, extrapyramidal, or motor system. In the differential diagnosis of spastic paraparesis of middle age, one should consider, respectively, amyotrophic lateral sclerosis, cervical spondylosis, or spinal cord tumor. The first has no sensory abnormalities, and the latter two both have characteristic roentgenologic abnormalities. Combined system disease can be excluded in most cases by hematologic studies and gastric analysis.

Treatment. There are several aspects to the management of multiple sclerosis. The first is the possible benefit to be gained from ACTH or corticosteroids during acute exacerbations. Many authorities advise a course of three to four weeks of therapy with suitable precautions against complications, and some recent controlled studies have shown that this treatment has some benefit in the acute symptom complex. There are no indications for long-term maintenance therapy on ACTH or corticosteroids, and the risks outweigh any possible benefit. Preliminary studies with other immunosuppressive agents indicate that the course of the disease may be stabilized with fewer exacerbations. From a consideration of the pathology, it is unreasonable to expect alleviation of symptoms that have been static for many months.

The second aspect is the general management of the patient. During acute exacerbations, especially severe ones, there may be some benefit from bed rest, though the demoralizing effects of prolonged immobilization must be avoided. The prevention of complications, especially genitourinary infections, bedsores, contractures, and flexor spasms, requires adequate nursing care, physiotherapy, and occasionally more specific measures such as rhizotomy, tenotomy, antimicrobials, and other indicated measures. Exhausting physiotherapy with active exercises offers no benefit and may even be harmful. Certain other measures such as unnecessary catheterization have serious consequences and should be avoided.

The third aspect of patient care is the management of long-term disabling illness with an unpredictable course. Initially there arises the question of informing the patient, and this must be dealt with on an individual basis after considering the emotional makeup of the patient and his family, the patient's responsibilities, and

---

is hemorrhagic necrosis of the spinal cord without any associated vascular malformation. Such cases, which are rare, show a rapidly ascending motor and sensory paralysis with a polymorphonuclear pleocytosis of the cerebrospinal fluid, and death occurs in days or weeks.

Neuromyelitis Optica (Devic's Disease)

This clinical syndrome is characterized by acute transverse myelitis and optic neuritis. It may be considered to be a variant of multiple sclerosis and may occur as the initial illness or later during the course of the disease. There may be sudden loss of vision in both eyes, with central scotoma or sudden onset of paraplegia with sensory loss. The ocular involvement may be due to optic or retrobulbar neuritis, and the transverse myelitis may be partial or complete. Days or weeks may elapse between the onsets of the two symptom complexes. In severe cases the motor symptoms tend to be permanent, but otherwise the course, laboratory data, and treatment are similar to those of multiple sclerosis.

Transitional Sclerosis

Transitional sclerosis is probably a pathologic variant of multiple sclerosis in which the disseminated plaques tend to become confluent, creating large areas of myelin loss. Clinically these cases are indistinguishable from cases of typical multiple sclerosis. Transitional sclerosis probably represents an intermediate pathologic form between multiple sclerosis and Schilder's cerebral sclerosis.

DIFFUSE SCLEROSIS

There is a group of progressive neurologic disorders of young patients who manifest severe neurologic deficits of various types and progressive visual and mental deterioration. In three publications from 1912 to 1924, Schilder described three cases of diffuse disease of white matter that he proposed grouping under the name *encephalitis periaxialis diffusa* (now called Schilder's disease). Actually, Schilder had described three distinct entities, and these, plus cases subsequently described, are of three types: (1) the myelinoclastic group, closely related to multiple sclerosis, referred to hereafter as Schilder's cerebral sclerosis; (2) the leukoencephalitides, which are probably of viral origin; and (3) the dysmyelinating group or leukodystrophies, which are probably due to genetically determined enzymatic defects.

Schilder's Cerebral Sclerosis

The demyelinative disorders in this group are related pathologically to multiple sclerosis. The characteristic lesions are large, bilateral areas of demyelination in the cerebral hemispheres with preservation of the subcortical "U" fibers, a relative sparing of the axons, and a replacement gliosis. Recent lesions show a perivascular inflammatory reaction. Swelling of the cerebral hemispheres in acute, fulminant cases may rarely cause increased intracranial pressure and may mimic brain tumor. In more chronic lesions there is a suggestion of confluence of smaller plaques to make the large areas of demyelination. In some cases there are, in addition, randomly scattered small lesions in other areas of the central nervous system, and these have been called "diffuse-disseminated sclerosis" or transitional sclerosis. These cases may represent an intermediate form of the same process, diffuse sclerosis representing one extreme whereas multiple sclerosis represents the other.

The disease may occur at any age, but unlike multiple sclerosis the majority of cases begin in childhood. About half the cases begin prior to the age of 10 years, and three fourths begin before the age of 20. The disease is relatively rare; fewer than 50 autopsied cases have been reported. Both sexes are equally involved.

The onset is usually insidious but may be acute. It is usually slowly progressive, but there may be successive bursts to simulate the course of multiple sclerosis. A typical presenting picture is of insidious mental deterioration with loss of recently acquired intellectual achievements, and this progresses slowly to dementia. Many patients develop aphasia, apraxia, and dysarthria. Various psychiatric syndromes may be manifested. Visual loss with cortical blindness is characteristic, and auditory complaints with cortical deafness may follow involvement of the cortical radiations. Motor symptoms such as hemiparesis may be prominent, and seizures of various types tend to appear during the course. Other neurologic symptoms and signs such as vertigo, ataxia, nystagmus, paraplegia, or extraocular palsies are less frequent.

The course varies from days to many years, with an average duration of about three years. Terminally patients are severely demented and often in a decerebrate state.

Laboratory findings are usually abnormal only in the cerebrospinal fluid and electroencephalogram. The CSF pressure may be elevated, and there may be mild pleocytosis and elevation of protein content. The gamma globulin content is usually abnormal. The EEG findings vary from paroxysmal discharges to focal slowing. Patients with increased intracranial pressure may have misleading indications of a mass lesion in encephalographic or angiographic studies. There is no specific therapy.

Balo's Concentric Sclerosis

Some cases of demyelinating disease have an unusual concentric arrangement of the demyelinating lesions of the cerebrum. Balo gave these the name *encephalitis periaxialis concentrica*. This rare entity probably represents a variant of Schilder's cerebral sclerosis.

THE DYSMYELINATING DISORDERS (LEUKODYSTROPHIES)

This group includes heredofamilial diseases in which normal myelin is probably not formed because of some genetically determined enzymatic defect. The classification is not completely satisfactory; the group tends to merge with the lipidoses of the nervous system, so that authorities differ in their classifications. Only further elucidation of the enzymatic defects of myelin metabolism in these disorders will lead to a satisfactory classification.

SIMPLE STORAGE TYPE
(Metachromatic Leukoencephalopathy)

These are otherwise known as the glial insufficiency forms or the sulfatide lipidoses. This group includes those cases in which large amounts of metachromatic material accumulate in the central nervous system. The disease is inherited as an autosomal recessive and begins in the first ten years of life, usually with gait disturbances, convulsions of various types, hypotonia, ocular palsies, and dysarthria. There are coarse tremors of the extremities and, terminally, severe mental deterioration and spasticity or rigidity.

The cerebrospinal fluid protein is usually elevated (100 to 200 mg. per 100 ml.), and metachromatic material (staining red with toluidine blue) can be found in the urinary sediment. The metachromatic material also collects in the kidney, liver, gallbladder, spleen, or peripheral nerves, and biopsy confirms the diagnosis. Gallbladder function studies may be abnormal. The course is one of progressive neurologic deterioration leading to death in one to four years, although some patients have survived 10 to 20 years. Some cases may begin later in childhood and run a more protracted course. The disorder is one of the more common leukodystrophies and can often be diagnosed in life.

SUDANOPHILIC LEUKODYSTROPHY
(Pelizaeus-Merzbacher Disease)

This is a very rare, familial leukodystrophy, predominantly of males. The pathologic changes consist of extensive diffuse demyelination in the cerebral hemispheres and cerebellum. The disease appears to be transmitted as a sex-linked recessive and begins in early life with a slowly progressive course. Disturbances of coordination such as intention tremor, gait disturbances, dysarthria, spas-

ticity, abnormal movements and mental deterioration occur. The illness lacks pathognomonic features, but the predominant progressive cerebellar symptoms in a male with a positive family history should make one suspect the entity. It runs a course of several years or more before fatal termination. There is no therapy.

GLOBOID CELL LEUKODYSTROPHY
(Krabbe's Disease)

This rare familial type of leukodystrophy begins in infancy and rapidly progresses to death. The typical pathologic feature is the deposition of cerebrosides in globoid cells of the brain. These may be glial or another type of macrophage. The cases described by Krabbe began at about four months of age with seizures, spastic quadriplegia, abnormal startle responses, cortical blindness, and optic atrophy, and progressed rapidly to death in one or two years. The protein in the cerebrospinal fluid is usually elevated. There is no therapy.

SPONGY DEGENERATION OF WHITE MATTER
(Canavan's Disease)

In this rare familial leukodystrophy there is widespread demyelination accompanied by microscopic vacuolation that gives rise to a spongy appearance. It appears to be transmitted as an autosomal recessive and seems to be more common among Jews. Usually it begins early in infancy with atonia of the neck muscles, spastic paraplegia, severe mental retardation, optic atrophy, abnormal reflexes, and enlargement of the head. Laboratory studies except for skull roentgenograms showing enlargement are usually normal. Death usually occurs at about 18 months of age. There is no therapy.

LIPIDOSES OF THE CENTRAL NERVOUS SYSTEM

These comprise disturbances of metabolism that result in an increase of lipids in the brain. Included are amaurotic idiocy, or Tay-Sachs disease (gangliosides); Niemann-Pick disease (sphingomyelin); Gaucher's disease (cerebrosides); and Hurler's disease (mucopolysaccharides). All but the first are discussed elsewhere in this text.

The dividing line is by no means sharp between the dysmyelinating diseases, characterized by faulty myelin formation, and the lipid storage diseases, characterized by the accumulation of lipid-staining materials within nerve cell bodies. The distinction is further blurred by the fact that demyelination also occurs in many of the lipidoses, particularly amaurotic idiocy.

Amaurotic idiocy, or cerebromacular degeneration, can have an infantile (Tay-Sachs), late infantile (Bielschowsky), or juvenile (Batten-Spielmeyer-Vogt) onset. The Tay-Sachs variety is found chiefly among children of Jewish descent and has a recessive genetic pattern. The incidence of the other forms is genetic recessive and non-racial. All three are characterized by a progressive decrease in vision leading to complete blindness within one to two years. Concomitantly, there is a progressive and usually severe dementia combined with convulsions and advancing weakness, leading eventually to being bedridden with paralysis. Diagnosis in all three forms depends upon the characteristic clinical combination of dementia and blindness plus, in the Tay-Sachs and Batten-Spielmeyer-Vogt varieties, either a cherry-red or red-purple discoloration, respectively, marking the area of macular degeneration in the retina. An adult form (Kuf's) has also been recognized. This group of late onset neuronal storage disorders without organomegaly is characterized by seizures, pigmentary degeneration, or cherry-red spot changes in the retina, pyramidal signs, basal ganglia signs, cerebellar signs, and demen-

tia. The problem remains whether these disorders are examples of identical or different genetically determined enzymatic defects of the nervous system. Clinicopathologic changes are not diagnostic. Rectal biopsy disclosing fat-packed ganglion cells in Meissner's plexus provides morphologic confirmation of the diagnosis.

Carter, S., Sciarra, D., and Merrit, H. H.: The course of multiple sclerosis as determined by autopsy proven cases. A. Res. Nerv. & Ment. Dis. Proc., 28:471, 1950.

McAlpine, D., Lumsden, C. E., and Acheson, E. D.: Multiple Sclerosis. A Reappraisal. London, E. & S. Livingstone, Ltd., 1965.

Miller, H. G., Stanton, J. B., and Gibbons, J. L.: Parainfectious encephalomyelitis and related syndromes. Quart. J. Med., 25:427, 1956.

Poser, C. M.: Diseases of the myelin sheath. In Minckler and Neuberger (eds.): Pathology of the Nervous System. New York, McGraw-Hill Book Co., Inc., 1966.

Poser, C. M., et al.: Clinical characteristics of autopsy proven multiple sclerosis: A review of English, Norwegian and American cases. Neurology (Minneap.), 16:791, 1966.

Rapin, I., and Scheinberg, L. C.: Neuronal storage disorders starting in childhood. Trans. Amer. Neurol. Ass., 93:145, 1968.

Rose, A. S., and Pearson, C. M. (eds.): Mechanisms of Demyelination. New York, McGraw-Hill Book Co., Inc., 1963.

Scheinberg, L. C., Kies, M. W., and Alvord, E. C., Jr. (eds.): Research in demyelinating diseases. Ann. N.Y. Acad. Sci., 122:1, 1965.

Scheinberg, L. C., and Korey, S. R.: Multiple sclerosis. Ann. Rev. Med., 13:411, 1962.

The Epilepsies

Gilbert H. Glaser

Definition and Prevalence. Epilepsy is derived from the Greek *epilepsia* meaning a "taking hold of" or "a seizing." It refers to the many types of recurrent seizures produced by paroxysmal excessive neuronal discharges in different parts of the brain that can be due to a variety of cerebral and general bodily disorders. Designation of "the epilepsies" as symptom complexes, therefore, is more appropriate, and the term encompasses convulsions or convulsive disorders with loss of consciousness as well as nonconvulsive seizures with only slight changes in conscious awareness.

An accurate epidemiology of the epilepsies is difficult but various studies indicate an over-all incidence of 0.5 per cent in general populations involving all age groups. The experience of a single seizure is more common, especially in early childhood, but recurrence is necessary for the diagnosis of an epilepsy.

Descriptions of the epilepsies have been recorded for at least 2500 years, since the Hippocratic writings. Yet, it has been mainly since the mid-nineteenth century that the condition has received extensive anatomic, physiologic, and humanistic consideration, gradually diminishing the medieval conception and stigma of the epi-

leptic as being "possessed." Historical material is available in *The Falling Sickness* by Temkin (1945), and in the works of Penfield and Jasper (1954) and Lennox (1960).

Pathogenesis. Basic Mechanisms of Epileptic Discharge. Given the sufficient and proper electrical and chemical stimuli, abnormal discharges and seizures can arise in even the normal brain. Certain regions of the brain are particularly sensitive to seizures, having a low threshold and a high susceptibility. These include particularly the regions related to motor and autonomic functions, i.e., the motor cortex and the structures within the limbic system. The temporal lobe and its deeper nuclear aggregates, the amygdala and hippocampus, are especially susceptible; their vascularity is vulnerable to compression, and the tissues themselves are sensitive to biochemical disturbances such as are produced when hypoxia or antimetabolites block various phases of the oxidative metabolic cycle. It sometimes is difficult to separate cause from effect in temporal lobe lesions, since morphologic abnormalities in these regions may result when a severe seizure produces secondary vascular insufficiency and hypoxia.

Factors related to age and development are

important in the genesis of the epilepsies, and brain lesions acquired during the perinatal period often mature and produce clinical epileptic phenomena only years later. Certain seizure types such as massive spasms are more common in infants; petit mal seizures appear in childhood rather than later in life. This is reflected by different electroencephalographic patterns associated with seizures in infancy and childhood, compared with those in older age groups. The immature brain also is more susceptible than that of the adult to biochemical disturbances such as hypocalcemia, hypoglycemia, and hyponatremia. The occurrence of seizures with high fever is almost confined to early childhood. Otherwise, the periodicity of epilepsy is unpredictable except that it correlates with sleep or menstrual cycles in some patients.

Seizures may be *focal*, arising from an abnormal focus or a number of foci, or *generalized from the onset*, seemingly without focal origin. However, generalization throughout the brain of an initially focal paroxysmal discharge may occur so rapidly that the focal origin can be obscured, and the attacks of many patients with fixed cerebral lesions and *secondary or symptomatic seizures* are in this category. It is still uncertain whether generalized seizures, such as some idiopathic grand mal convulsions and the brief seizures of petit mal absence (see below), develop immediately as generalized cerebral discharges involving specific pathways, or whether initially a localized discharge occurs. Convulsions caused by metabolic disturbances such as water intoxication, hypocalcemia, or hypoglycemia may be considered examples of those generalized from the onset. In these instances, the initial detonation starting the seizure is believed to be in the subcortical mesodiencephalic nonspecific reticular systems, with diffuse propagation bilaterally into the cerebral cortex. The rapid loss of consciousness that first occurs and the marked memory disturbance after the seizure can be related to this spread.

Hughlings Jackson concluded many years ago from clinical observations that most seizures develop from a focus or aggregate of abnormally excitable neurons, and many studies since his time have supported this hypothesis. It is postulated that the nerve cells of patients with epilepsy contain intrinsic intra- and extracellular metabolic disturbances which produce excessive and prolonged depolarizations of the membrane, producing a defect in the recovery process following excitation. In experimental epilepsy, both the excitatory and inhibitory presynaptic potentials of the nerve cell have been found to be abnormal. The cortical regions containing such cells generate shifts in slow or standing wave potentials as a result of abnormal electrical activity arising in the region of neuronal dendrites. The neurons in the abnormal, epileptic focus are a hyperexcitable aggregate, and they tend to discharge paroxysmally. Clinical seizures develop if the discharge propagates along neural pathways or if sufficient local recruitment occurs. The abnormal discharges, once initiated, spread through essentially normal brain; the manifestations of the particular seizure then depend upon both the focus of origin and the region of the brain subsequently involved in the propagated discharge. In certain cases, seizures may be provoked by various sensory stimuli ("reflex" or sensory-induced epilepsy), especially flickering light or visual patterns and sound. At other times, peripheral sensory stimulation has been found to arrest the development of a seizure.

The metabolic environment of epileptogenic neurons is most important in the genesis of attacks, and many metabolic disturbances may be associated with seizures. For example, a balance of electrolytes is required to maintain resting potential of the neuronal membrane. An alteration in membrane permeability with an increased, intraneuronal sodium content could be a significant change preceding seizure discharge. Initiation and maintenance of neuronal hyperexcitability have been related to increases in extraneuronal potassium. Depletion of available calcium ions upsets membrane stability and causes oscillations. Both hypoxia and hypoglycemia deprive neurons of basic substrates, allowing insufficient energy for the maintenance of appropriate ionic gradients. However, if effects of excessive muscle metabolism and apnea during generalized convulsive seizure activity are eliminated, such seizures do not induce cerebral hypoxia; actually, cerebral blood flow increases to meet cerebral oxygen demands in this state.

An excess of excitatory transmitter, such as acetylcholine, produces repetitive discharges and seizure activity. This may be induced experimentally by anticholinesterase drugs, but it is not found significantly in naturally occurring epilepsy.

The coenzyme function of pyridoxal phosphate is directly involved in the metabolic pathway of gamma-aminobutyric acid, which has neuronal inhibitory activity. Experimental alterations of this system can be produced by such substances as the antimetabolite methoxypyridoxine and the hydrazides, but pyridoxine deficiency seizures occur only rarely and in infants. Isoniazid toxicity occurs with an overdosage by this mechanism.

Etiology. It is customary to divide epilepsy into two categories, *idiopathic* and *symptomatic or acquired*. A diagnosis of idiopathic epilepsy is made when no specific cause is found; in acquired epilepsy the cause can be determined by available diagnostic procedures. Present techniques fail to uncover a specific structural or biochemical cause of epilepsy in up to 75 per cent of patients.

Idiopathic Epilepsy. Idiopathic epilepsy has been designated as *genetic*, with the implication that a transmitted predisposition for seizures is present. There is no doubt that a family history of seizures exists in high incidence for some groups of cases, particularly those with an onset of seizure in early life. It has been determined that the relatives of patients with idiopathic epilepsy have a 3 to 5 per cent incidence of epilepsy, six to ten times that in the ordinary population. There is also an increased incidence of electroencephalographic abnormality in the relatives of seizure patients, particularly in monozygotic twins, in whom the incidence of concordant abnormalities may exceed 20 per cent. Since epilepsy may be but a symptom associated with other neurologic abnormalities, an inheritance pattern for a specific cerebral disease must be considered in some cases. There are also a number of indirect factors, such as cerebral birth trauma due to a narrow maternal pelvis, that tend to produce seizures in families.

Acquired Epilepsy. Most diseases or structural abnormalities of the brain may be associated with seizures. *Congenital malformations* induced chromosomally or otherwise, such as microgyria, porencephaly, and hemangiomas, have a varying incidence of associated epilepsy, depending upon the intensity of the abnormality and possibly on more general genetic factors. Maternal infection, as by rubella, can produce multiple cerebral abnormalities, and severe toxemia of pregnancy also can affect the fetus. Perinatal difficulties causing *birth trauma* and *asphyxia* are relatively common causes of cerebral damage and later epilepsy.

Acute, subacute, and chronic infections of the brain and its coverings, such as meningitis, encephalitis, and abscess, cause seizures, both during the active process and later as healing leaves cerebral scars. The prevalence of cerebral neurosyphilis has decreased, but there is still a significant incidence of bacterial meningitis with all its complications. Uncontrolled ear and sinus infections still produce meningitis, subdural empyema, brain abscess, and cerebral venous thrombosis, all associated with seizures. Acute viral encephalitis often causes seizures, and convulsions due to cerebral tuberculomas (more often to tuberculous meningitis) remain common in certain countries such as India. Cysticercosis and schistosomiasis have specific geographic distributions and are frequent causes of seizures in highly endemic areas.

Febrile convulsions commonly accompany nonspecific infections in infants and young children and are to be distinguished from direct infection of the nervous system. The seizure usually accompanies a high rise in fever in an otherwise neurologically normal child. However, at least 30 per cent of these children may develop epilepsy later without fever. Sometimes febrile convulsions precipitate status epilepticus and contribute to permanent cerebral damage.

Head injury is a major cause of acquired epilepsy, the seizures occurring both in the acute phase and as a chronic residual. The incidence of epilepsy after head injury is difficult to determine, because of the great variability of injury. General surveys report an incidence of up to 10 per cent following closed-head injury and between 30 and 40 per cent after open-head injuries, seizures developing in most cases within three years.

The seizure incidence is highest when the wound is severe, when the dura is penetrated, and when the injury involves the rolandic or parietal regions.

Brain tumors are an important cause of seizures, particularly in adults, but it has been difficult to ascertain the relative incidence of brain tumor within the large population of epileptics. Between 30 and 40 per cent of all patients with cerebral tumors have seizures, especially if the tumor is supratentorial. The seizure is apt to be focal and, in 15 to 20 per cent of cases, is the first symptom. The brain tumors most likely to cause seizure are astrocytomas, meningiomas, and metastatic neoplasms, especially those from the lung.

Cerebral vascular disease is a relatively common cause of seizures, particularly in the older age groups. The attacks may result from either localized vascular insufficiency and secondary ischemic hypoxia or from a chronic residual scar, left after thrombosis, embolism, or hemorrhage. Episodes of loss of consciousness due to diminished cerebral blood flow may progress into seizures, as in severe states of carotid sinus sensitivity and Adams-Stokes syndrome due to heart block. Seizures appear in up to 20 per cent of patients with the various collagen disorders, i.e., systemic lupus erythematosus and periarteritis nodosa, and are the result of small vascular lesions involving the brain.

Various *allergic reactions* may be related to single seizures, but usually not recurrent epilepsy. Convulsions have been reported after immunizations, in drug sensitivity reactions, and after insect bites.

Certain generalized *cerebral degenerative and demyelinating diseases* carry a significant incidence of seizures; in multiple sclerosis this is 5 per cent, and patients with Alzheimer-Pick dementia may experience generalized and myoclonic seizures. The complex cerebral lesions of tuberous sclerosis often produce seizures, including infantile massive spasms. The cerebral lipidoses, such as Tay-Sachs disease, may cause generalized and myoclonic seizures.

Toxic and metabolic disorders are an important cause of seizures since treatment may be directed quite specifically. Seizures are prominent during withdrawal from chronic drug intoxications, particularly from barbiturates (and other sedatives and tranquilizers), and from alcohol. Seizures developing in association with alcoholism usually appear within 48 hours after cessation of drinking and may precede delirium tremens. Carbon monoxide intoxication and other forms of hypoxia may cause seizures. Lead poisoning has been a common cause of convulsions in young children. Water intoxication or excessive hydration, with hemodilution, can produce seizures, again especially in the young. Other pertinent metabolic causes are pyridoxine deficiency, phenylketonuria, hypocalcemia (with or without hypoparathyroidism), porphyria, and hypoglycemia. Hypoglycemia may be a complication of the treatment of diabetes or may accompany islet cell tumors of the pancreas and other endocrine disturbances such as hypopituitarism. Seizures are common in acute and chronic renal insufficiency but are relatively unusual in hepatic failure. Secondarily induced magnesium deficiency, such as that following severe gastrointestinal fluid loss, has been implicated in the production of seizures.

It is likely that, in many patients, several factors combine to produce attacks: a genetically determined predisposition, an increased cerebral excitability related to a general metabolic disturbance, the presence of a focal brain lesion or a tendency to vascular insufficiency, and a triggering disturbance such as an emotional crisis or an excessively flickering light. Each patient, therefore, must be evaluated from many different aspects in order to establish causation on different levels and to develop appropriate total therapy.

Clinical Manifestations. The classification of seizures employed here is based, whenever possible, on a combination of clinical manifestations and electroencephalographic correlates.

Generalized Seizures (Grand Mal or Major Convulsions). The major generalized convulsions or grand mal (tonic-clonic) seizures have many causes and arise in all age groups. These seizures usually have a pattern or sequence starting with a *prodromal phase* that lasts minutes or even hours, with a change in emotional reactivity or affective responses, such as increasing anxiety or depression, often difficult to recognize. More commonly, the specific onset of the seizure is the *aura*, usually a brief sensory experience directly related to the locus of origin of the seizure. Frequently experienced auras are a sense of fear, a peculiar epigastric sensation welling up into the throat, an unpleasant odor, various visual and auditory hallucinations, and strange sensations in an arm or leg. At times, localized movements of an extremity or portions of the face precede the onset of the general convulsion. The *convulsion* itself occurs with sudden vocalization (the "epileptic cry"), loss of consciousness, tonic extensor rigidity of the trunk and extremities, then clonic movements, impaired breathing with brief cessation of respiration, cyanosis, and then heavy, stertorous breathing. Incontinence of urine and feces occurs; there is often biting of the tongue and the inside of the cheeks in the clonic phase. After some minutes, the excessive motor activity ceases, breathing becomes more normal, and consciousness gradually returns. Frequently, a *postictal state* appears characterized by confusion, general fatigue, headache, and, at times, certain specific, residual neurologic signs such as hemiparesis or monoparesis, sensory disturbances, and dysphasia. Automatic behavior may be present as well. As with the aura, these postictal phenomena have significance with regard to possible focal origins of the generalized seizure. The postictal paralysis, sometimes called "Todd's paralysis," ordinarily lasts for several minutes to hours after

the seizure. In general, there is a complete amnesia for a generalized seizure with the exception of possible recollections of the prodromal phase or the aura.

The designation *fragmentary seizure* is given to the occurrence of brief components of the generalized complex. For example, only auras may appear and may or may not be followed by abortive tonic movements or loss of consciousness. Such fragments occur particularly during therapy with anticonvulsant drugs and reflect incomplete control.

Grand mal seizures vary in their frequency from once or twice yearly to many times daily; 20 per cent of patients may have only nocturnal seizures. In females, the seizures may appear cyclically with or immediately before the menstrual periods, and the incidence may increase or decrease with pregnancy, being increased by toxemia and water retention.

The *electroencephalographic (EEG) patterns associated with generalized seizures* during the attack are difficult to distinguish from movement artifact. Between attacks, the EEG often contains paroxysms of bilateral, essentially synchronous, 4- to 7-cycle-per-second discharges from all areas, interspersed with nonspecific patterns of high amplitude spikes and slow waves. A paroxysmal or slow wave discharge localized to one region of the scalp suggests that a focal cerebral lesion may be present. Between seizures up to 25 per cent of patients have an electroencephalogram within the normal range.

Petit Mal (Absence Attack). The petit mal seizure is a specific form of minor epilepsy, consisting of a sudden brief lapse of consciousness, usually lasting no longer than 30 seconds, more commonly 5 to 10 seconds. Petit mal almost always appears in childhood, with onset usually between the ages of 3 and 10. Its incidence diminishes during postpuberty, and persistence into adult life after the age of 30 is extremely rare. Usually, no specific cause is found; this form of epilepsy is regarded as idiopathic. In rare instances a specific brain lesion such as a vascular calcified tumor of the frontal lobe or diffuse cerebral lipidosis has been reported with petit mal seizures, but the EEG was seldom entirely characteristic.

Clinically, the patient with petit mal has a sudden cessation of activity and stares blankly, making no movements, except at times a 3 per second blinking of the eyelids, a slight deviation of the eyes and head, or brief minor movements of the lips and hands. The end of the spell is equally abrupt. More complex behavioral disturbances or postictal confusion or drowsiness suggest the presence of another type of minor seizure such as psychomotor automatism rather than petit mal. The attacks of petit mal can be as few as a flurry every several days to as many as 100 or more per day. As the frequency increases, the repeated absences sometimes produce difficulties in continuing motor tasks and in learning. The designation *petit mal status* or absence state refers to many attacks occurring close together for minutes to hours and producing confusion and disorientation.

The *electroencephalographic correlate of the petit mal or absence seizure* is a rhythmic 3-cycle-per-second spike and wave discharge appearing synchronously from all scalp regions both during and between seizures. Usually, a discharge of more than a few seconds' duration is associated with a clinical absence. The characteristics of the seizure and the typical electroencephalographic discharge have led to these seizures being designated as "centrencephalic," implying an origin in the centrally placed, "integrating," mesodiencephalic regions of the brain. Experimentally, there is evidence to support this hypothesis, although direct confirmation in the human is inconclusive.

Akinetic Seizure. The term akinetic attack is applied to a generalized seizure associated with loss of consciousness and simple falling. It may be accompanied by an absence and minor movements, but generally there is a marked diminution of postural tone with falling and, often, self-injury. Afterward, the reappearance of normal posture and mental clarity is common although there may be a brief period of confusion. Electroencephalographically, there is a diffuse abnormality with slow wave discharges or atypical spike waves, often slower than 3 per second.

Myoclonic Seizures. These are characterized by sudden involuntary contractions involving an integrated response of a single muscle or several muscle groups, producing relatively simple arrhythmic jerking movements about a single joint or several joints, or of a segment of the body. The jerks may exist as an independent entity, as a phenomenon preceding and building up to a generalized grand mal convulsion or as an accompaniment to petit mal absences in children. Myoclonic attacks are often sensitive to sensory stimulation and may be precipitated or accentuated by sound or light, by change in posture, by movement of an extremity, by drowsiness, or by an emotional upset. Myoclonic jerks occur as a normal phenomenon in normal subjects during drowsiness.

Myoclonus Epilepsy. The myoclonus epilepsy of Unverricht refers to generalized myoclonus and mental deterioration secondary to a diffuse degenerative metabolic disorder of undetermined origin. Other forms of myoclonus appear in diseases of cerebral lipid metabolism, in subacute encephalitis, and with rare forms of cerebellar disease. A severe myoclonus appearing in the first 18 months of life and associated with general cerebral deterioration is called *infantile massive spasms* or jackknife seizures. In this condition, the infant develops severe flexion spasms of the head, neck, and trunk and extension of the legs and arms. Some known causes of this disorder are phenylketonuria, tuberous sclerosis, and Down's syndrome, but in most instances neither a biochemical nor anatomic abnormality can be found.

The *electroencephalographic correlates of the myoclonic seizure* are variable depending on the severity of the seizure state; in mild instances, generalized, synchronous slow spike and wave complexes or sharp and slow wave elements occur intermittently with relatively clear electroencephalographic patterns interspersed. Infantile massive spasms are commonly associated with *hypsarhythmia,* which consists of more or less continuous, nonsynchronous, asymmetric discharges of spike and sharp wave elements along with slow waves from all regions.

Focal or Partial Seizures. Involvement of a specific region of the brain may be manifested by characteristic signs and symptoms. They are typical of acquired epilepsy, although occasionally no definite morphologic lesion is found. As indicated above, a focal onset seizure can occasionally spread extremely rapidly to become generalized, but in seizure states specifically classified as focal or partial, the attack usually remains limited. There often is a disturbance of consciousness or awareness with varying degrees of amnesia, but total loss of consciousness occurs only with general spread.

Lesions involving any of the motor regions of the brain, but particularly the so-called motor cortex, produce focal motor seizures. The classic *jacksonian motor seizure,* due to a lesion sharply localized in a specific region of the motor cortex, begins as a repetitive movement of a distal portion of an extremity, such as the fingers or toes, and then spreads by a march of the clonic contractions up the extremity toward the trunk. Such a seizure usually remains limited to the extremity, but it may spread to the rest of the ipsilateral side, the face, and the contralateral side. Occasionally, these seizures begin at the corner of the mouth and are associated with masticatory movements and speech disturbances. Other focal motor seizures involve gross movements of the arms or legs without the classic jacksonian march. *Adversive seizures* produce turning movements of the head, eyes, and trunk toward the side opposite the cerebral lesion, which is usually in the prefrontal cortex.

Focal seizures originating from the *supplementary motor area* of the mesial frontal supracingulate cortex are not common; they are characterized by gross body movements, especially raising of the contralateral arm with the head turning toward that arm, rhythmic bilateral arm and leg movements, and repetitive speech, usually of syllables, not words. Occasionally, speech is slowed or totally inhibited during such a seizure. Other experiences are peculiar sensations in the abdomen, generalized flushing, and palpitations.

Focal sensory seizures caused by a lesion involving the sensory cortex may be jacksonian with a march of abnormal sensations such as numbness and tingling spreading up an extremity. Other sensory areas of the cerebral cortex produce more complex seizures with paroxysmal visual, auditory, olfactory, gustatory, and vertiginous components in varying degrees of organization.

As with other types of focal attacks, the pattern of onset is often the most accurate guide to the locus of an abnormal cerebral lesion.

Autonomic seizures are produced by focal lesions in the regions of the brain associated with autonomic representation, namely, the deep temporal, limbic, and diencephalic (hypothalamic) areas. Many autonomic symptoms are associated with other focal or generalized seizures, but they also appear in attacks more or less by themselves, as paroxysms of abdominal pain, sweating, piloerection, incontinence, salivation, and, rarely, fever.

Psychomotor (temporal lobe, limbic system) epilepsy is due to seizure activity involving the temporal lobe, its deeper nuclear masses (the amygdala and hippocampus), and their associated limbic system structures. Psychomotor epilepsy is common in both children and adults and occasionally coexists with grand mal seizures. Evidence of an acquired lesion is found in more than half the patients, with a frequent history of trauma at birth or, later, encephalitis or neoplasm. Some patients with psychomotor seizures are found to have focal frontal or occipital lobe lesions, but even with these there is evidence that the discharges produce their eventual manifestations by propagation through temporal-limbic lobe structures.

Psychomotor-temporal-limbic seizures are manifested by an initial aura of anxiety and visceral symptoms, especially by a peculiar epigastric sensation welling up into the throat. An alteration in consciousness follows, associated with many varied, complex feeling and thinking states, as well as automatic somatic and autonomic motor behavior. Activity is first arrested or suspended, then simple movements ensue, such as chewing, swallowing, sucking, lip smacking, and aimless twistings of the arms and legs. Automatisms then appear which are of varying complexity and involve either partially purposeful or inappropriate and bizarre behavior. Usually, the automatism is stereotyped, but, despite this, the movements usually interplay with the environment and, occasionally, they appear to be determined in part by psychologic factors. The activities in this phase of the seizure may merge into normal behavior. The complex attack beginning with unpleasant olfactory hallucinations due to lesions of the mesial portions of the temporal lobe, the uncus, was specifically called an uncinate seizure by Jackson, who also described the "dreamy" and confused state of the patient. Visceral manifestations are common in young patients, who experience hunger, nausea, vomiting, and abdominal pain as well as urinary incontinence. Destructive, aggressive behavior occasionally occurs but usually is not goal-directed. Affective disturbances may be present, particularly expressions of fear, anger, and depression. Occasionally, prolonged fuguelike states with running or wandering may last many minutes. During some psychomotor-temporal lobe seizures, patients are involved in experiential hallucinations, both visual and auditory, as well as interpretive illusions involving their own bodies or the immediate environment. These symptoms frequently are associated with ideational blocking and forced thinking as well as peculiar feelings of familiarity called "déjà vu" and déjà pensée." Amnesia is usually present for the events of the seizure.

Electroencephalographic Concomitants of Focal Seizures. These are represented by discharges of slow waves, spikes, and sharp and slow complexes localized over the particular cerebral region involved. Frequently, the abnormalities are bilateral but asynchronous, representing transmission and diffusion of the abnormal discharge from one hemisphere to its mirror point on the other. At times, deeply situated lesions produce only minimal or no significant alteration in the ordinary electroencephalogram recorded from the scalp.

Status Epilepticus. The rapid repetitive recurrence of any type of seizure without recovery between attacks is called status epilepticus. The term is usually applied to attacks of grand mal or generalized epilepsy in which the patient remains unconscious and in continuous seizures, with tonic and clonic fluctuations, incontinence, severely disturbed breathing, high fever, excessive sweating, and elevation of blood pressure. Such status may last for hours, even days, and requires emergency medical treatment because of the possible dangers of cerebral damage, thought to be due to ischemic anoxia and cardiac and renal failure. The onset of status epilepticus can be spontaneous, but frequently withdrawal from anticonvulsant medication or a too rapid shift of medication is the precipitating cause.

Focal motor seizures may appear in continuous fashion lasting many hours; this state has been called *epilepsia partialis continua*.

Petit mal status is associated with sustained 3-cycle-per-second spike-wave discharges in the electroencephalogram. The patient is in a state of confusion, has a continuously dazed expression, and has minor movements around the lips or in the arms and legs. *Psychomotor* or *temporal lobe status* also occurs, but less frequently. Such patients are found in a confused state with persistent, inappropriate, bizarre complex behavior patterns lasting over many hours, occasionally associated with fluctuating visceral symptoms.

The Interseizure State. The intellectual performance, character, and behavior of a patient with epilepsy, between obvious clinical attacks, whatever the type, is referred to as the interseizure state. A patient with a progressive cerebral degenerative disease, an extensive cerebral malformation, a severe encephalitis, or an expanding brain tumor may develop changes in behavior and intellectual functioning, primarily because of the underlying structural lesions and not directly because of any seizures that might be present. However, in the past much attention has been paid to the possibility of a specific personality distortion in epileptic patients. Most patients subject to seizures have normal behavior and intellectual functions, and are capable of appropriate productive adjustments in society. The literature is replete with descriptions of such people contributing to our civilization, culture, and history in all walks of life. In some instances, however, severe emotional problems do develop, usually in response to environmental restrictions. *Neurotic, maladjusted behavior* occurs, along with obsessional, particularly religious, preoccupations. Often, under these circumstances, the seizures increase and become more difficult to control.

An undetermined number of patients with frequent recurrent generalized seizures, especially status epilepticus, or with recurrent psychomotor temporal-limbic seizures, develop continuing *defects in intellectual function.* Psychologic tests reveal persistent impairments of concentration and attention, memory lapses, word-finding distortions, subtle losses in the ability to associate, and perceptual difficulties. It is possible that prolonged subclinical seizure activity contributes to these disturbances.

More severe personality disturbances ranging all the way to *psychosis with schizophrenic manifestations* complicate the interseizure course of a few patients with either psychomotor or severe grand mal epilepsy. The psychotic reactions often have psychologic precipitating factors; occasionally, they follow control of the actual seizures by medication, and these instances may be related, in part, to a reaction to the drug. The symptoms include paranoid, depressive, and hallucinatory reactions, catatonic disorders, flattening of the affect, and severe obsessional states. The patients suffer marked difficulty in concentration and disorientation of time sequences. Defects in memory are present and are accompanied by abnormalities in perception as well as difficulties in word finding, in calculating, and in analyzing the thought content of written material. However, the patients usually attempt to maintain contacts with reality, and major withdrawal is not present in contrast to most examples of spontaneous schizophrenic illnesses. Diffuse electroencephalographic abnormality, with either bilateral temporal lobe involvement or diffuse spike wave paroxysms, accompany some of these clinical phases, but with others, the electroencephalogram remains normal.

Diagnosis in Epilepsy. The patient with epilepsy should receive a thorough diagnostic evaluation to determine causative factors and precipitating circumstances. This requires a thorough history, a detailed medical and neurologic physical examination, and selected laboratory investigations, with particular reference to blood chemistry tests, cerebrospinal fluid analysis, electroencephalography, and special roentgenologic studies. Every effort should be made to identify a specific medical illness or a focal cerebral lesion.

History. The history must contain a detailed description of the attacks to help establish the fact of recurrent seizures. As much recollection as possible should be obtained from the patient, particularly of experiences of the aura and the onset of the seizure. The patterning or course of events during and after the seizure should be documented, especially by eye-witness accounts, with special attention to any phenomena that might possess localizing significance. Information should be sought as to the various circumstances under which seizures occur, such as the time of day or night, the frequency of attacks and how medication influences them, their relationship to the menstrual cycle, pregnancy, food intake, sound or light stimulation, intake of alcoholic drinks, or psychologic stresses. All symptoms of neurologic disturbances should be described, such as headache, hemiparesis, hemisensory disturbances, dysphasia, visual difficulties, or vertigo.

The *past medical and developmental history* is of great aid in establishing the cause. Information should be obtained concerning pregnancy, delivery, the neonatal period, the developmental neurologic milestones, head injuries, and reactions to immunizations and the various childhood illnesses such as measles, mumps, and chickenpox. The occurrence of any severe illness with delirium or coma that might be considered an encephalitis should be inquired about as well as any exposure to toxic substances. Drug intake needs particular investigation, particularly with adults suspected of taking barbiturates or tranquilizer drugs. One must inquire into the patient's social development and behavior in and out of the family setting, his intellectual performance at school, and his vocational adjustments and performance. Any alteration in these phases of existence should be related to seizure occurrence, to the interseizure state, and to the possible effects of medication.

A *family history* of susceptibility to seizures may delineate a significant number with a history of febrile seizures in early childhood as well as of generalized and focal seizures extending into later life. The family history may reveal not only genetically determined cerebral disorders associated with seizures but also other neurologic abnormalities as well.

The *general medical history* can reveal evidence of pertinent cardiovascular disease, blood dyscrasias, and metabolic and endocrine disorders; a seizure may be the first manifestation of a cerebral metastasis or of a generalized vascular disease.

Clinical Examination. In most patients with seizures, physical examination fails to disclose significant physical or neurologic abnormalities. Nevertheless, a thorough general examination is warranted; careful examination of the skin, for example, may produce the diagnosis in cases of tuberous sclerosis, neurofibromatosis, or cerebral hemangioma. Examination of the lungs provides evidence for consideration of metastatic tumor or abscess; evaluation of the peripheral circulation and blood pressure gives an indication of the possibility of the various types of cerebral vascular lesions or aids in differentiating between syncope and seizure.

The *neurologic examination* serves two purposes: to elicit signs of any general neurologic disorder and determine whether or not focal signs of a localized cerebral lesion are present. A neurologic examination is particularly valuable at the time of, or shortly after, a seizure if it reveals a transitory hemiparesis or related signs.

A battery of *psychologic tests* can aid the evaluation of both intellectual capabilities and psychologic adjustments. Simple tests of memory and perception are part of the regular neurologic examination. For more complete studies, the most useful tests include the Wechsler Intelligence Scale (especially the Kohs block test), the memory scales, the Bender-Gestalt, the Rorschach, and the Thematic Apperception tests. Attention should be paid to the patient's performance during these tests as well as to the actual scores.

Laboratory Investigations. Each patient with recurrent seizures, no matter the age, should be examined with certain laboratory investigations at least once and probably at additional times, particularly if changes develop in seizure patterns or neurologic signs. There are no routines, but at different ages certain tests are more apt to produce results leading to specific etiologic diagnosis. Additional studies are necessary to evaluate the general health of the patient and to follow the potentially toxic effects of medication.

There are no abnormal laboratory findings associated directly with seizure activity except electroencephalographic discharges. Urine analysis is necessary to determine the state of kidney function; if abnormal, a specific renal disorder may be present, and certain drugs cannot be administered. Similarly, a complete blood count is necessary. It should be noted that severe seizure states such as status epilepticus may be associated with proteinuria, leukocytosis, and fever as secondary manifestations. In certain instances, special blood chemistry studies are warranted, such as the blood sugar and glucose tolerance test for the diagnosis of suspected hypoglycemia and in the evaluation of a diabetic with epilepsy, and the serum calcium determination for infants and young children with seizure states. Evaluation of fluctuations in serum electrolytes and acid base balance is necessary to study both children and adults with disorders of the kidney, liver, heart, and lungs. Serologic tests help to diagnose past infections.

The *cerebrospinal fluid* is apt to be normal in all constituents and pressures, except in the minority of patients who have specific neurologic disease. Following severe seizures, there may be a slight increase in the cerebrospinal fluid protein and white cell count. In structural neurologic disorders with concomitant seizures, the protein and/or pressure may be elevated persistently, and the specific diagnosis then depends on other tests, such as contrast roentgenologic studies. Chronic nervous system infection can be associated with an increase in the white cell count of the cerebrospinal fluid; occasionally, a cerebral tumor may be revealed by neoplastic cells in the fluid.

Roentgenograms of the skull and chest must be taken of all patients. The film of the skull may reveal asymmetry due to early injury or maldevelopment, abnormal calcifications, shift of the calcified pineal, or signs of increased intracranial pressure. The chest film potentially detects pulmonary infection or tumor and aids in evaluating the cardiac status. Roentgenologic studies of the intracranial contents employing contrast media are extremely useful diagnostic procedures if employed at the proper time, but must be selected with care because of their morbid potential. Such procedures are considered when a focal intracranial lesion is suspected. *Ventriculography* is the procedure of choice when there is increased intracranial pressure, particularly when a lesion is suspected in the posterior fossa. Ordinarily, when the pressure is normal, a fractional *pneumoencephalogram* gives more information about a lesion occupying space within the skull or distorting the ventricular or subarachnoid systems. Pneumoencephalography also discloses focal brain atrophy as reflected by selective enlargements of important specific space such as the temporal horns. *Cerebral arteriography* is useful for patients with or without evidence of increased pressure and can demonstrate localized abnormal vascular patterns in neoplasms as well as intracranial hematomas, vascular malformations, and the location of vascular occlusions.

Radioactive isotopic brain scanning may be of use. There is increasing regard for such procedures as a means of determining the presence of certain types of tumors and vascular lesions. A negative brain scan often eliminates the immediate necessity for performing a contrast roentgenologic procedure. A significant lateralized pickup in scanning helps to indicate the side upon which to perform an arteriogram in a patient suspected of neoplasm in whom neurologic evaluation and electroencephalogram do not offer localizing signs.

Electroencephalography. The various electroencephalographic correlates of the different types of seizures have been described. The electroencephalogram is an indicator of a certain kind of cerebral activity determined by recording electrodes upon the scalp. This is important to realize, since electroencephalograms from up to 25 per cent of patients with seizures are normal; yet, abnormal discharges are disclosed in many of these same patients by depth electrodes recording from deeper cerebral structures such as the amygdala and hippocampus. The electroencephalogram, therefore, has limited diagnostic applications and must be correlated with other information from the various physical and neurologic examinations. It can be utilized to confirm the presence of a seizure disturbance, particularly if paroxysmal discharges are recorded during and correlated with a seizure. An example of this specificity is that up to 85 per cent of children with petit mal will have the typical three-cycle-per-second spike and wave discharges both during and between seizures and, in many instances, these discharges can be precipitated during the recording by over-ventilation and light stimulation.

In other instances of epilepsy, the electroen-cephalogram contains generalized, nonspecific slow wave discharges that merely indicate the presence of cerebral dysfunction, but not a definite seizure disorder. Focal slow wave abnormalities in the electroencephalogram suggest a localized structural lesion and ordinarily lead to further investigations. Finally, in certain forms of focal epilepsy, the electroencephalogram may show focal discharges of spikes, sharp waves and com-plex components indicative of the epileptogenic nature of the focus. Yet, in some of these instances, such an abnormality might be transmitted, the basic discharging focus being elsewhere.

In most laboratories of electroencephalography the test procedure involves recording in the waking state and during voluntary overventila-tion. Additional attempts usually are made to provoke generalized and focal paroxysmal dis-charges by means of sleep, sensory stimulation with light and occasionally sound, and sometimes by utilizing certain metabolic and pharmacologic adjuvants.

The recording of the electroencephalogram during sleep is useful in the attempt to demon-strate focal temporal lobe discharges in patients with psychomotor-temporal lobe epilepsy. In adults, such discharges are increased during sleep in up to 75 per cent of patients, but the results in children are less definitive, the increase oc-curring in only 30 per cent. In many patients, sleep produces increased bilateral appearance of abnormal temporal discharges. The use of sphenoi-dal electrodes is occasionally of some help in lateralizing temporal lobe discharge, particularly when patients are being evaluated for surgical therapy. At times, barbiturate-induced fast-wave activity is found to be diminished on the side of the involved temporal lobe. Photic stimulation identifies patients with light-sensitive epilepsy and, occasionally, produces lateralized discharges in patients with a sensitive focus. There have been many attempts to alter the electrical activity of the brain in susceptible patients by inducing metabolic changes, such as hydration following an injection of Pitressin. Various stimulant drugs have been used, such as Metrazol and Megimide. All of these methods, particularly the use of the drugs, may produce paroxysmal discharges as well as clinical seizures, usually generalized. However, attempts to measure seizure discharge threshold have been unsuccessful because of great variability, and many normal subjects respond with seizures to these procedures. Accordingly, these methods are not recommended for general use in the diagnosis of epilepsy. Occasionally, it may be important in the evaluation of a specific patient to study in detail the phenomena of the seizure and to determine focal components either in the electroencephalogram or clinically. In selected cases, this can be accomplished by the administration of a controlled dose of a seizure-producing drug.

The intensity of electroencephalographic abnor-mality, especially its paroxysmal characteristics, has sometimes been regarded as an objective in-dicator of the severity of a particular seizure dis-order. However, the use of the electroencephalo-gram in following patients with epilepsy is limited since, in many instances, some degree of electro-encephalographic abnormality persists even though seizures are controlled. This is most often the case in patients with psychomotor-temporal lobe epilepsy and least often in children with petit mal and myoclonic seizures.

Differential Diagnosis. The diagnosis of epi-lepsy has profound implications, medically and psychologically, as it affects the total life situa-tion of the patient and his family. Consequently, careful attention must be given to make this diagnosis positively and specifically, and to dif-ferentiate it from other disturbances that produce somewhat similar abnormalities of neurologic function that are not seizures.

Consciousness may be disturbed episodically by inadequate cerebral blood flow in attacks of *cere-bral vascular insufficiency* or of *syncope* of various types, particularly the vasodepressor form. Dis-turbances of cerebral circulation affect older per-sons especially, and such patients generally suffer other evidence of hypertension and cerebral arteriosclerosis. Periodic blackouts and recurrent confusional states are manifestations of basilar artery insufficiency as are other episodic signs of brainstem and cerebellar dysfunction. Patients with carotid arterial insufficiency characteris-tically experience transitory hemiparesis and hemisensory disturbances along with dysphasia, but the clonic movements of a paroxysmal disorder usually are absent. The electroencephalographic findings of paroxysmal discharge do not occur with cerebrovascular disease although, at times, bi-lateral rhythmic discharges are observed related to vascular lesions of the upper brainstem. The differential diagnosis is sometimes difficult and may require arteriographic confirmation of a vascular lesion as well as the usual evaluation of the history and general medical state of the patient.

Syncopal episodes may resemble akinetic or brief motor seizures; prolonged syncope can pro-gress into a convulsion due to the persistence of cerebral ischemia and hypoxia. The patient with syncope usually has indications of disturbed vasomotor reactivity with excessive sweating, pallor, and tachycardia. Specific precipitating factors often are present such as fear or other psychologic upset. The confusion, headache, and drowsiness that occur after a generalized seizure usually do not appear in syncope. The electro-encephalogram during simple syncope consists of diffuse asynchronous slow waves without paroxys-mal or focal discharges.

Certain *psychogenic disorders* resemble epileptic states and can be difficult to differentiate. Hysterical "seizures" occur not only as independent problems, but also complicate the course of a limited number of patients with known seizures, the combination being called "hysteroepilepsy." The clinical problem is difficult to unravel because of the inter-relationships between the actual seizure and the reactive psychologic disturbance. The hysterical seizure is not associated with neurologic signs of reflex abnormality and, during it, the electroencephalogram contains no paroxysmal discharges. The pattern of hysterical seizures is often bizarre and not a stereotyped tonic-clonic movement sequence. Self-injury is an unusual result of the seizure, and the postictal states of confusion, headache, and drowsiness are absent. Hysterical or psychotic fugue disturbances and dissociative reactions need to be distinguished from psychomotor-temporal lobe seizures. The diagnosis of an hysterical seizure state requires careful psychiatric evaluation because of the severe neurotic process involved.

Treatment. Treatment of the epilepsies must take into account not only the patient and his disorder, but his family and general life situation. Much depends on the diagnostic evaluation and the finding of specific causes whenever possible that can be treated directly. This is clearly defined in instances in which metabolic disturbance is obvious, such as hypoglycemia and hypocalcemia, or when an operable cerebral tumor is found. However, in many cases of acquired epilepsy, the basic cause of the seizure cannot be treated directly. Seizures may continue in patients even after removal of a brain tumor because of scarring, or when the tumor is found to be inoperable or incompletely removable. The diagnosis of an acquired epilepsy following head injury or encephalitis usually does not lead to specific therapy. Only a limited number of patients with post-traumatic epilepsy are satisfactory candidates for surgical removal of a localized meningocerebral scar. The administration of anticonvulsant drugs is necessary, therefore, for the majority of patients.

Medical Therapy. There are many available anticonvulsant drugs, as shown in the accompanying table. None is capable of achieving total seizure control in all patients, but careful selection and utilization in each case often leads to optimal results. Each physician should learn to use a number of these drugs well and to recognize disturbing side effects as early as possible. Periodic blood counts, urinalyses, and liver function tests are necessary with certain drugs.

The basic mechanisms of anticonvulsant drugs are not definitely known. Most of the drugs are neuronal depressants with certain variations in action. The hydantoin drugs reduce the synaptic activity of post-tetanic potentiation; the oxazolidine (methadione) drugs decrease nerve transmission during repetitive stimulation. The drugs are believed to increase the stability of excitable neuronal membranes by acting upon electrochemical characteristics involved in ion permeability and membrane polarization. Such stabilizing effects would decrease the activity of the hyperexcitable neuronal aggregates in an epileptogenic focus and prevent the spread of discharge through normal neuronal circuits.

The anticonvulsant drugs are administered to achieve the desired effect of seizure control and must be built up in dosage while not producing untoward toxic reactions. It is best to start with one drug of choice, but usually a single drug is not totally effective, and a second is necessary. Two drugs might be needed initially for patients with two different types of seizure such as grand mal and petit mal. This occurs fairly frequently (from 25 to 50 per cent in some series, especially in adolescents [statistics available in Lennox]). The process may require weeks of adjustment and, during this time, the patient's or parent's cooperation in reporting effects on seizure frequency or side-reactions is most important. Determination of anticonvulsant blood levels, i.e., diphenylhydantoin, phenobarbital, primidone, may be very helpful in identifying patients who are obtaining unsatisfactory control because they either fail to take the drug or metabolize it abnormally. Frequent and rapid shifting or replacement of drugs is to be avoided.

A specific anticonvulsant drug for each type of seizure is not available. However, there is one major therapeutic division; petit mal absences respond best to either succinimide or oxazolidines (methadiones). These drugs are not effective in the treatment of major generalized (grand mal) or focal cerebral seizures, nor are the hydantoins (used in grand mal and other seizures) effective in petit mal. It is stated that the drugs used in the therapy of petit mal may worsen a generalized seizure state, but this has not been proved.

Generalized grand mal and focal motor seizures are best treated by diphenylhydantoin sodium and phenobarbital. Initially, either drug may be administered to patients who have infrequent attacks, but generally the combination of diphenylhydantoin and phenobarbital produces the most effective seizure control. The average dose of diphenylhydantoin is 0.3 to 0.4 gram per day, usually administered as 0.2 gram in the morning after breakfast and 0.2 gram after dinner. The dosage of phenobarbital is initially 60 mg. at bedtime, with 30 mg. increments over the day, if necessary, limited by the unwanted sedative effect.

Patients with psychomotor-temporal lobe epilepsy are often more difficult to control. Many trials of different agents and different doses may be necessary in these cases; the best results are to be expected with diphenylhydantoin and either phenobarbital or primidone. Although in some clinics the two latter drugs are used together, primidone is partially converted to phenobarbital, and their sedative effects combine to make such administration difficult. It is most important with primidone to start therapy with small doses, such as 125 mg., increased at weekly intervals to reach a maximal dosage of 0.75 gram for children or

1.0 to 2.0 grams per day for adults. If untoward side effects to diphenylhydantoin occur, substitution with the less reactive Peganone is sometimes successful, although this drug has less anticonvulsant effect. Mesantoin and phenacemide are used only for the most difficult cases and even then with extreme care because of their high degree of toxicity.

Acetazolamide is an adjuvant to the treatment of any type of seizure. It seems to have a general effect upon hyperexcitable cerebral neurons because of its properties of inhibition of carbonic anhydrase and production of acidosis. ·Because tolerance develops, the drug should be administered intermittently. It is occasionally useful, for example, in helping to control seizures appearing periodically in females at the time of the menstrual cycle. Under these circumstances, acetazolamide is administered for a week prior to and during menses.

The *results of drug therapy* are difficult to predict. With careful attention to individual details and general management, most patients with occasional generalized and psychomotor seizures achieve either complete or nearly complete reduction of seizures. Satisfactory or complete control can be achieved in most children with petit mal absences. However, each group of patients, especially those with grand mal and psychomotor epilepsy, contains a refractory number who suffer from troublesome side effects of drugs and from increasing psychologic and sociologic difficulties as the years go by.

When to stop drugs for a patient whose seizures are completely controlled is a recurrent question. Some authorities recommend cautiously withdrawing anticonvulsants if patients have been free of attacks for two years, but in relatively few cases can drugs be withdrawn without seizures recurring even after symptom-free periods of three to five years. Thus, continued treatment is indicated for most adults with grand mal and psychomotor epilepsy. The electroencephalogram may remain abnormal in clinically seizure-free patients, indicating persistent seizure potentiality, but even in patients with normal electroencephalograms drug withdrawal may be unsuccessful. Yet, in the management of some patients, it is understandable that a calculated risk of drug withdrawal be considered if this represents a psychologic achievement of great magnitude. Under these circumstances, the drug should be withdrawn carefully with small decrements over many weeks. Drug elimination may be carried out more successfully in children with controlled petit mal, particularly since there is a natural tendency for the absences to diminish with age and maturity.

A presentation of drugs used in the medical treatment of epilepsy is given in the accompanying table in alphabetical order with statements concerning dose administration, indications for different seizure types, and toxic effects.

Adrenocorticotrophic hormone (ACTH) and adrenocortical steroids are now used in the treat-

ANTICONVULSANT DRUGS: DOSAGE, INDICATIONS, AND TOXIC EFFECTS

Bromides
Daily dosage:	1.0 to 3.0 grams for adults; not recommended for children
Indications:	All types of seizures, especially grand mal and psychomotor; may be combined with hydantoins
Toxic effects:	Drowsiness, dulling, rash, psychosis; rarely used now

Celontin
Dose:	0.3 gram capsules
Daily dosage:	Children: 0.6 gram; adults: to 1.5 gram
Indications:	Petit mal, psychomotor seizures, myoclonic seizures, massive spasms
Toxic effects:	• Ataxia, drowsiness; rarely, • blood dyscrasias

Dexedrine (dextroamphetamine)
Dose:	5 mg. tablets; 5 mg., 10 mg., and 15 mg. long-acting Spansules
Daily dosage:	Children: 5 to 15 mg.; adults: 15 to 30 mg.
Indications:	To counteract sedative effects, hyperkinetic behavioral disturbances in children, narcolepsy
Toxic effects:	Anorexia, irritability, sleeplessness

Diamox (acetazolamide)
Dose:	250 mg. tablets
Daily dosage:	Children: 0.75 to 1.0 gram; adults: 1.0 to 1.5 grams. Use intermittently; tolerance occurs.
Indications:	As an adjuvant in all types of seizures, especially those in females related to menstrual cycles
Toxic effects:	Anorexia, acidosis, drowsiness, numbness of extremities; rarely, blood dyscrasias

Dilantin (diphenylhydantoin)
Dose:	0.03 gram and 0.1 gram capsules; 0.05 gram tablets; 0.1 gram delayed action capsules; 0.025 gram per ml. suspension; 0.1 gram in oil, capsules; 0.25 gram ampules for parenteral use
Daily dosage:	Children: 0.15 to 0.3 gram; adults: 0.3 to 0.6 gram
Indications:	Grand mal, psychomotor and focal seizures, most useful in combination with phenobarbital or primidone
Toxic effects:	Rash, fever, gum hypertrophy, gastric distress, diplopia, ataxia, hirsutism (young females); drowsiness, uncommon; megaloblastic anemia (due to secondary folic acid deficiency); lymphadenopathy

Mebaral (mephobarbital)
Dose:	0.03 gram, 0.1 gram tablets
Daily dosage:	Children: 0.06 to 0.3 gram; adults: 0.3 to 0.6 gram
Indications:	Grand mal, petit mal, psychomotor, focal seizures; similar to phenobarbital; most useful in combination with hydantoins
Toxic effects:	Drowsiness, irritability, rash

Mesantoin (methylphenylethylhydantoin)
Dose:	0.1 gram tablets
Daily dosage:	Children: 0.1 to 0.4 gram; adults: 0.4 to 0.8 gram
Indications:	Grand mal, psychomotor, and focal seizures
Toxic effects:	Rash, fever, drowsiness, ataxia, gum hypertrophy (less than Dilantin), neutropenia, agranulocytosis

Milontin (methylphenylsuccinimide)
Dose:	0.5 gram capsules; 250 mg. per 4 ml. suspension
Daily dosage:	Children: 0.25 gram to 1.5 grams; adults: 2.0 to 4.0 grams
Indications:	Petit mal, myoclonic and akinetic seizures; occasionally psychomotor seizures
Toxic effects:	Nausea, dizziness, rash, hematuria (may be nephrotoxic)

Mysoline (primidone)
Dose:	0.05 gram, 0.25 gram tablets; 250 mg. per 5 ml. suspension

Daily dosage: Children: 0.25 gram; adults: 0.75 to 2.0 grams. The daily dosage should be built up very slowly.

Indications: Grand mal, psychomotor and focal seizures; occasionally, petit mal; useful in combination with Dilantin

Toxic effects: Drowsiness, ataxia, dizziness, rash, nausea

Paradione (paramethadione)

Dose: 0.15 gram, 0.3 gram capsules; 0.3 gram per ml. solution

Daily dosage: Children: 0.3 gram to 1.8 grams; adults: 1.2 grams to 2.4 grams

Indications: Petit mal, myoclonic and akinetic seizures, massive spasms, occasionally psychomotor seizures (in children); often useful in combination with Dilantin and phenobarbital; somewhat less effective and less toxic than Tridione.

Toxic effects: Rash, gastric distress, visual symptoms (glare, photophobia), neutropenia, agranulocytosis

Peganone (ethylphenylhydantoin)

Dose: 0.25 gram, 0.5 gram tablets

Daily dosage: Children: 0.5 gram to 1.5 grams; adults: 2.0 to 3.0 grams

Indications: Grand mal, psychomotor and focal seizures

Toxic effects: Similar to those of Dilantin but less frequent; may be substituted for Dilantin, but is generally less effective

Phenobarbital

Dose: 0.015 gram, 0.030 gram, 0.060 gram, 0.1 gram tablets; 4 mg. per ml. elixir

Daily dosage: Children: 0.045 gram to 0.1 gram; adults: 0.1 gram to 0.3 gram

Indications: All seizure states: grand mal, petit mal, psychomotor and other focal; most useful in limited dosage in combination with other drugs such as Dilantin

Toxic effects: Drowsiness, dulling, rash, fever; irritability, and hyperactivity in some children

Phenurone (phenacemide)

Dose: 0.5 gram tablets; 0.3 gram enteric-coated tablets

Daily dosage: Children: 0.5 gram to 2.0 grams; adults: 1.5 grams to 3.0 grams

Indications: May be effective in all types of seizures, especially psychomotor-temporal lobe seizures; should be used only in very resistant cases

Toxic effects: A highly toxic drug, producing liver damage, agranulocytosis, psychotic reactions, and rashes

Tridione (trimethadione)

Dose: 0.15 gram tablets; 0.3 gram capsules; 0.15 gram per 4 ml. solution

Daily dosage: Children: 0.3 gram to 1.8 grams; adults: 1.2 grams to 2.4 grams

Indications: Petit mal, myoclonic and akinetic seizures, massive spasms; occasionally, psychomotor seizures (in children); often useful in combination with Dilantin and phenobarbital

Toxic effects: Rash, gastric distress, visual symptoms (glare, photophobia) neutropenia, agranulocytosis, nephrosis

Zarontin (ethosuximide)

Dose: 0.25 gram capsules

Daily dosage: Children: to 0.75 to 1.0 gram; adults: 1.5 grams

Indications: Petit mal seizures (now the drug of choice); used with Dilantin in mixed seizure states

Toxic effects: Blood dyscrasias (pancytopenia, leukopenia) unusual; dermatitis, anorexia, nausea, drowsiness, dizziness

The following drugs may be used in the emergency treatment of status epilepticus:

Diazepam (Valium): 2.5 to 10 mg. intravenously
Sodium phenobarbital: 0.25 to 0.50 gram intravenously
Sodium amytal: 0.25 to 0.50 gram intravenously
Paraldehyde: 3.0 to 5.0 ml. intravenously or 10 to 20 ml. intramuscularly

Dilantin sodium (parenteral): 0.25 gram intravenously or intramuscularly (to 0.5 gram per 24 hours in patients previously receiving this drug or as much as 1.0 to 1.5 in previously untreated patients); *caution:* dilantin intravenously must be given slowly in 0.05 gram increments to avoid vasodepression

General anesthetics such as ether, Avertin, and zylocaine have a limited usefulness in the treatment of status epilepticus. Careful nursing and attention to fluid and electrolyte balance, airway, cardiac and renal functions, and temperature control are essential in the over-all management of status epilepticus.

ment of massive spasms in infancy associated with the "hypsarhythmic" electroencephalogram. Such therapy is administered after primary causes of massive spasms, such as phenylketonuria, have been ruled out. Although initial improvements in the spasms and the electroencephalogram may occur, the prognosis is poor, particularly with regard to the mental deterioration accompanying this condition. Nothing is known about the mechanism of action of the hormones in this disorder; this is somewhat paradoxical since these hormones are known to raise cerebral excitability and precipitate seizures in older persons and in experimental situations.

Dietary Treatment. In general, there are no dietary restrictions for the patient with epilepsy, nor is there a specific diet capable of aiding most patients. However, a diet high in fat content producing significant ketosis, the *ketogenic diet*, occasionally is helpful in treating young children, particularly those with intractable petit mal and generalized motor seizures. Anticonvulsant drugs usually have to be continued, and the diet is difficult to maintain because it is unpleasant.

Psychologic Therapy and Sociologic Management. Many basic problems in the over-all life adjustments of the patient need additional management even though drugs can achieve significant control of seizures. In many cases, the coexistence of seizures and personality problems requires a combination of medical anticonvulsant therapy and psychologically oriented management.

The sedative properties of anticonvulsant drugs usually are not used directly. The so-called tranquilizing drugs have limited usefulness in the management of seizure patients; chlordiazepoxide (Librium) and diazepam (Valium) may reduce disturbed behavior, particularly in children. The phenothiazine drugs have variable effects; an alerting phenothiazine, fluphenazine, is of some use in controlling abnormal behavior in certain patients with psychomotor seizures. However, other drugs in the chlorpromazine group are known to provoke seizures and paroxysmal discharges in the electroencephalogram.

There is often a direct interplay between emotional disturbances and clinical seizure activity. Some patients in a state of psychologic turmoil experience increased seizures and require greater amounts of anticonvulsant drugs. The subsequent achievement of psychologic adjustment decreases the frequency of seizures and lessens the drug requirement. This needs to be developed in various ways, depending on the patient's age and his family and social circumstances. Family understanding is of primary importance, because the child with seizures has to live, insofar as possible, as a normal person within home and school settings. A great problem, still to be overcome, is the stigma attached by society to the diagnosis of epilepsy, and the lack of understanding that not only exists among people in general but is reflected by various restrictive legal practices. Most children with seizures are able to attend schools and vocational programs successfully; most adults with controlled seizures are capable of developing productive careers and engaging in the activities that are so much a part of our culture, such as marriage, childbearing, obtaining an education, driving an automobile, traveling from country to country, and working with appropriate safeguards, protected by insurance and workers' compensation programs. Only a relatively small number of patients require a protected environment, such as that in schools or colonies specifically developed for epileptic patients. Even these no longer should be institutions where many hundreds or thousands of epileptic patients are kept in essentially custodial care. "Colonies" with schools, homelike units, and small villages exist in Great Britain, Holland, and Denmark and take care of relatively small numbers of patients (up to a few hundred at most in each), involved in intensive programs of medical therapy, psychologic management, education, and vocational training. From these places increasing numbers of adequately controlled patients are sent out into the general community, where they live well adjusted and productive lives.

Only a few occupations are contraindicated for patients with seizures. These include activities of potential danger to either the patient or others, such as work requiring unprotected climbing to great heights and utilizing heavy power equipment or dangerous chemical substances.

Informal and formal psychotherapeutic measures can be undertaken in order to reduce emotional disturbances. The role of the family physician is all-important in these considerations. Often he alone can judge the problems that exist in a family, school, or social setting. His understanding and guidance help both the patient and his family to overcome the feelings of despair, anxiety, fear, and self-consciousness that otherwise interfere with the normal adjustments of everyone involved. It is only when anxieties and depressive tendencies develop into more severe reactions, associated with paranoid states, increased withdrawal, and excessive obsessional tendencies, that more intensive psychiatric treatment becomes necessary. Occasionally, brief periods of hospitalization help in the evaluation of the intensity of the psychologic disturbance and any associated intellectual difficulties that may interfere with the patient's performance. Drug schedules may be revised at the same time, under controlled conditions.

Even the child with epilepsy and behavioral disorder can be cared for best if he attends a regular school in an understanding environment and is associated with a clinical outpatient service in which the physician and social service department work together with both the child and the family. It is becoming less necessary to arrange for either home tutoring or the placement of such children into schools or other facilities for the maladjusted.

Surgical Therapy. The patient with a potentially remediable lesion, such as a brain tumor, usually is considered for operation, whatever the state of the seizures. Surgical intervention for the removal of a focus of abnormal discharge is appropriate only for selected patients who have focal epilepsy that remains intractable after intensive medical therapy. A constant focally discharging area should be confirmed by serial electroencephalographic studies, and the region of brain considered for excision must be such that the patient will not be left afterward with a severe speech, memory, or other disabling neurologic deficit.

Patients so evaluated usually do not have gross space-occupying lesions, but the epileptogenic region eventually excised may contain a small tumor, a vascular lesion, or a scar secondary to trauma or previous encephalitis. The surgical approach has been utilized particularly for patients with focal motor and psychomotor-temporal lobe seizures. Even though many patients are considered for surgical therapy, relatively few are chosen, and the numbers of patients so treated are still only in the hundreds the world over. In carefully selected series, about half the patients enjoy significantly improved control of seizures postoperatively, although this sometimes merely represents less anticonvulsant drug requirement. In some patients, generalized seizures appear instead of previous psychomotor-temporal lobe attacks. A small number experience relief from severe personality disturbances, particularly aggressive psychotic behavior, but this is an uncertain effect, and surgical intervention usually is not primarily directed toward this. Bilateral operations on the temporal lobe have been of limited success and have produced severe memory disturbances.

Cerebral hemispherectomy has been accomplished in a small number of carefully selected children with severe infantile hemiplegia, intractable convulsions, and behavior disturbances. Improvement in the seizures and behavior has occurred despite the persistence of motor and sensory neurologic disability.

Much more must be learned about the natural history of the epilepsies in order to evaluate thoroughly the different therapies. Adequate seizure control can be achieved now for most patients. The drugs involved are increasingly less toxic, but anticonvulsant medication remains essentially nonspecific and is directed against mechanisms of neuronal hyperexcitability that are little understood. A relatively small number of cases not responding to other management can be selected for surgical intervention. It is hoped that combined physiologic and biochemical studies of disturbed cerebral and bodily functions in the epilepsies will lead eventually to more rational and effective therapy.

Epilepsia (Journal of the International League Against Epilepsy), H. Gastaut, G. H. Glaser, M. Lennox-Buchthal (eds.). Elsevier Press. Amsterdam.

Gowers, W. R.: Epilepsy and Other Chronic Convulsive Disorders: Their Causes, Symptoms and Treatment. London, J. & A. Churchill, 1881. Reprinted by Dover Publications, New York, 1964.

Jasper, H. H., Ward, A. A., and Pope, A.: Basic Mechanisms of the Epilepsies. Boston, Little, Brown and Company, 1969.

Lennox, W. G.: Epilepsy and Related Disorders. Boston, Little, Brown and Company, 1960.

Penfield, W. G., and Jasper, H. H.: Epilepsy and the Functional Anatomy of the Human Brain. Boston, Little, Brown and Company, 1954.

Schmidt, R. P., and Wilder, B. J.: Epilepsy. Contemporary Neurology Series Monograph No. 2. Philadelphia, F. A. Davis Company, 1968.

Tower, D. B.: Neurochemistry of Epilepsy. Springfield, Ill, Charles C Thomas, 1960.

Intracranial Tumors and States Causing Increased Intracranial Pressure

Robert A. Fishman

INTRACRANIAL TUMORS

Intracranial tumors include neoplasms, both benign and malignant, and other space-taking lesions of chronic inflammatory origin that develop in brain, meninges, or skull. Their clinical manifestations are diverse and vary greatly according to tumor type and location. Errors in diagnosis are relatively common because the clinical manifestations of tumor may simulate a variety of neurologic disorders. Brain tumors occur at any age; they are common in children under ten, but have their peak incidence in the fifth and sixth decades of life. Race, occupation, and history of trauma have not been established as predisposing factors in the occurrence of intracranial tumors. Genetic factors are relevant, however, to the occurrence of a few tumor types, e.g. hemangioblastoma and neurofibromatosis.

Classification and Pathology. A great number of tumor types have been variously classified. Most classifications include (a) primary tumors originating in brain, (b) meningeal tumors, (c) vascular tumors, (d) pituitary tumors, (e) congenital tumors, (f) adnexal tumors, (g) metastatic tumors, and (h) granulomas and parasitic cysts.

Primary Brain Tumors. The largest group of primary brain tumors are the gliomas, composed of malignant glial cells. These include the following:

Glioblastoma Multiforme. These most malignant gliomas are composed of very undifferentiated cells. Complete surgical removal is impossible. The average life expectancy is 12 months. They have a very rapid growth rate and are characterized by much tissue necrosis and brain edema.

Astrocytoma. Astrocytomas are composed of astrocytes that infiltrate the brain and are often associated with cysts of varying size. They are generally slow-growing and may occasionally run a course of many years or even decades. They may infiltrate normal brain widely but with relatively little effect on brain function early in the illness. Complete surgical excision of cystic astrocytomas of the cerebellum may be possible, particularly in children, but in most other instances their marked invasiveness of brain prevents complete removal. Astrocytomas may undergo malignant change, and a highly malignant glioblastoma may develop within a relatively benign astrocytoma.

Oligodendroglioma. Oligodendrogliomas, composed of oligodendroglial cells, are similar in behavior to astrocytomas and are distinguishable only on histologic study.

Ependymoma. Ependymomas are derived from ependymal cells. They arise from the walls of the ventricular system, filling or obstructing the ventricles and invading adjacent tissues. They are malignant and cause death in about three years.

Medulloblastoma. Medulloblastomas develop from a primitive cell within the cerebellum. They are chiefly tumors of childhood but can occur in older patients. They are highly malignant and frequently metastasize throughout the subarachnoid space to involve the cerebrum or spinal cord.

Meningeal Tumors. The most important tumor arising in the meninges is the *meningioma*, which may invade the adjacent bone as well as compressing and distorting the brain. It is slow-growing, well circumscribed, often highly vascular, and may be calcified. It is benign, and complete removal is often possible unless the tumor involves critical structures.

Vascular Tumors. Tumors composed of vascular elements include the arteriovenous malformations (angiomas) and hemangioblastomas. The angiomas are congenital malformations composed of an abnormal collection of blood vessels of adult structure. They are present from birth but slowly enlarge and may not cause symptoms for many years. They may compress normal brain, may bleed intracerebrally or into the subarachnoid space, may be manifest only as a source of seizures, or may be an incidental finding at autopsy. Hemangioblastomas are true neoplasms composed of primitive vascular elements that may be quiescent for many years or may enlarge very slowly. They are most commonly found in the cerebellum but occur also in the cerebrum. Cerebellar hemangioblastoma may be associated with angiomatosis of the retina and cysts of the kidney and pancreas (the von Hippel–Lindau syndrome).

Pituitary Tumors. Pituitary tumors may arise from chromophobe, eosinophil, or basophil cells of the anterior pituitary. Of these, chromophobe adenomas are the most common. Chromophobe adenomas are nonfunctioning tumors that give symptoms by compression of the normal pituitary gland as well as the optic chiasm, the hypothalamus, and the adjacent brain with their suprasellar growth. Eosinophilic adenomas give rise to hyperpituitarism, acromegaly in adults, and gigantism in children, but do not generally compress suprasellar structures unless the tumor is mixed with chromophobe elements. Basophil adenomas are small and, although associated with Cushing's syndrome, are not responsible for symptoms by compression of adjacent tissues. *Cranio-pharyngiomas* derived from Rathke's pouch may be intrasellar or suprasellar in location, may compress the pituitary and optic chiasm, and are similar in effect to the chromophobe adenoma. They are frequently calcified and often contain cysts filled with thick, lipid-laden fluid.

Congenital Tumors. These tumors develop from congenital rests and include craniopharyngiomas of the pituitary, chordomas, dermoids, and teratomas. Chordomas are composed of cells derived from the embryonic notochord. They are midline and usually arise on the clivus, posterior to the sella. They grow slowly, but are highly invasive, and their total extirpation can seldom be accomplished. Dermoids and teratomas may occur anywhere in the central nervous system, particularly near the midline, adjacent to the ventricular system, or at the distal end of the cord. They tend to become symptomatic during the first decade of life, but may be silent for many years.

Adnexal Tumors. These tumors include those originating within the pineal body and those derived from the choroid plexus, the choroid papilloma. Pinealomas are rare tumors that cause symptoms by compressing the aqueduct, resulting in obstructive hydrocephalus and giving paralysis of vertical gaze by involvement of the pretectum of the midbrain. They may compress the hypothalamus and give rise to precocious puberty, diabetes insipidus, etc. Choroid plexus papillomas are

benign lesions that may cause intraventricular bleeding. They may cause increased intracranial pressure by obstructing the ventricular system or, it has been suggested, by excessive formation of cerebrospinal fluid.

Metastatic Tumors. Metastatic tumors constitute 10 to 25 per cent of brain tumors. They may originate from almost any primary tumor, most commonly those of breast and lung, but also from neoplasms of the gastrointestinal and genitourinary tracts, bone, thyroid, nasal sinuses, etc. They may be single or multiple, well encapsulated or diffuse, spread by extension from adjacent tissues or hematogenously. They may occur as a late manifestation in widespread carcinomatosis or as the first manifestation of an unrecognized primary visceral malignancy.

Granulomas and Parasitic Cysts. Granulomas affecting the nervous system include those associated with tuberculosis, mycotic infection, sarcoidosis, parasitic infestation, and syphilis. *Tuberculoma* may present as a solitary mass lesion with the brain; although rare in the United States, it is common in some areas, including Central and South America. Tuberculoma usually develops without evidence of tuberculous meningitis, although evidence of pulmonary tuberculosis is common. Favorable results with surgical excision and antituberculosis therapy have been reported. *Toruloma* is the most common mycotic granuloma affecting brain. This is usually associated with some evidence of meningeal involvement as well. The *granulomas of sarcoidosis* have been reported to occur in the brain; there is usually evidence of meningeal or posterior pituitary involvement, although the evidence for systemic sarcoid may be minimal. *Cysticercosis*, due to the larvae of *Taenia solium* or *Taenia saginata*, may be responsible for single or multiple cerebral masses. This is seen chiefly in South America and in the Middle East and India. *Syphilitic gummas* are extremely rare, but have been reported, presenting like slow-growing cerebral gliomas.

Pathophysiology. Intracranial tumors give rise to focal disturbances in brain function and to increased intracranial pressure. Focal manifestations occur because brain is compressed or infiltrated by tumor, because the blood supply of the region is compromised, resulting in tissue necrosis, and because of cerebral edema. Tumors may be located either within or outside brain parenchyma, i.e., intra-axial or extra-axial in location. Brain dysfunction is generally greatest with rapidly growing, infiltrative intra-axial tumors, e.g., glioblastoma, because of marked infiltration, compression, and necrosis of brain. Cyst formation within tumors also compresses adjacent normal brain. Cerebral edema about tumors increases the neurologic deficit. In edema, the water and sodium content of the brain are increased due to their accumulation in the extracellular space and in glial cells. Extra-axial tumors, e.g., meningioma, which slowly compress brain, may reach great size with few, if any, clinical signs.

Tumors cause a generalized increase in intracranial pressure when they reach sufficient mass, because of the fixed volume of the intracranial cavity. Obstruction of the ventricular system also increases intracranial pressure and causes hydrocephalic dilatation of the proximal ventricles and thinning of the cerebral hemispheres. Tumors that obstruct the intracranial venous sinuses also cause increased intracranial pressure. Complete compensation with very little or even no rise in pressure can occur with slowly growing neoplasms, but with rapidly growing malignant tumors, increased intracranial pressure is an early sign. Increased intracranial pressure becomes life-threatening when there is sufficient displacement of brain to cause herniation of the uncus or cerebellum. In *uncal herniation*, the most medial gyrus of the temporal lobe, the uncus, is displaced inferiorly by a hemispheric mass through the tentorial notch, thus causing compression of the midbrain, which results in depression of consciousness and ipsilateral or bilateral dilated and fixed pupils due to compression of the third nerve. In *cerebellar herniation*, the tonsils are displaced downward through the foramen magnum by a posterior fossa mass, causing compression of the medulla and respiratory arrest. Characteristic vasomotor changes ensue with increased intracranial pressure, only if rapid or severe. These include *progressive bradycardia* due to vagal slowing of the heart, *systemic hypertension*, which occurs as the intracranial pressure begins to approach arterial diastolic pressure, inducing medullary ischemia, and compensatory systemic vasoconstriction and, finally, central respiratory failure. Any degree of CO_2 retention will further increase intracranial pressure because of its cerebrovasodilator effects and, therefore, adequate ventilation with maintenance of a clear airway is essential for the patient with increased intracranial pressure. (Drugs like morphine, which depress respiration sufficiently to raise arterial CO_2 levels, are therefore contraindicated.)

Clinical Manifestations. The natural history of intracranial tumor is characterized by insidious onset and progression of focal or general neurologic deficits, or both. Many tumors have rather characteristic manifestations that point to the diagnosis (*vide infra*). There is great variation, depending upon location and rate of growth. Occasionally symptoms may be explosive in onset, suggesting a vascular lesion, and there may also be variations in course, suggestive of a remission. The symptoms and signs of intracranial tumor are discussed below.

Headache. Headache is a major but not invariable symptom of intracranial tumor. Patients with extensive tumors may not complain of headache, particularly if they have slowly growing infiltrative tumors (astrocytoma) or slowly growing extra-axial tumors (such as meningiomas, acoustic neuromas, or pituitary tumors). Similarly, when tumors interfere with the higher intellectual functions, headache may not be reported. Tumors give rise to headache by displacement of the pain-sensitive structures within the cranial cavity. Rarely, tumors give rise to a chronic meningeal inflammatory response that also may be responsible for pain. The problem of headache with brain tumor is discussed more extensively in the article on Headache.

Mental Changes. Mental changes may occur either early or late in the history of brain tumor, depending upon tumor location. Subtle evidence of personality change may be the first manifestation of a mass in the cerebral hemispheres, particularly involving the frontal lobes. This may take several forms. The symptoms may be chiefly affective, simulating an involutional depression. Some patients develop confusional states, at times associated with episodes of bizarre behavior. The most common mental change is characterized by progressive impairment of abstraction, recent memory and judgment, and a shortened attention span. (See Dementia.) However, some patients, particularly those with slowly growing neoplasms in the right (nondominant) hemisphere, may harbor huge tumors with only minimal impairment of intellect. Drowsiness progressing to stupor and coma accompanies severely increased intracranial pressure.

Disturbances of Speech. Various forms of aphasia occur with neoplastic involvement of the dominant hemisphere. The aphasic disorders are insidious in their development, and minor disturbances may be overlooked or erroneously attributed to psychologic factors. The various discrete forms of apraxia and agnosia may occur in evolution of the tumor syndrome, and may be the initial symptom in otherwise well persons.

Papilledema and Vision. The presence of the characteristic ophthalmoscopic appearance of papilledema suggests increased intracranial pressure; however, the funduscopic findings may be indistinguishable from those of optic neuritis or pseudopapilledema. Differential points include the late loss of visual acuity in increased intracranial pressure as opposed to early and more severe visual loss in optic neuritis. Visual acuity is generally unaffected in pseudopapilledema. Episodes of *amaurosis fugax*, fleeting moments of dimming vision, may be associated with a marked degree of papilledema and are a dangerous warning sign of potential loss of vision. The visual fields in true papilledema or pseudopapilledema may show enlargement of the blind spots. Disturbance of vision in patients with intracranial tumor also can be caused by extraocular muscle palsies, disturbances of the central visual pathways (*vide infra*), and disorders of visual interpretation, as in the alexias and visual agnosias. Uniocular papilledema with contralateral optic atrophy occurs characteristically, with subfrontal tumors that cause optic atrophy by direct involvement of the nerve and papilledema in the opposite eye due to increased intracranial pressure. The fundi may not reveal papilledema despite very elevated intracranial pressure; this may be attributable to glaucoma when present, but may also occur for unexplained reasons.

Diplopia and Hemianopia. Diplopia with brain tumors is due to involvement of either or both sixth cranial nerves, either directly by the tumor or, more commonly, indirectly due to generalized increase in intracranial pressure (see False Localizing Signs, *infra*). Third-nerve palsy may be due to involvement of the superior orbital fissure by meningioma, although the nerve may be involved by a variety of other lesions anywhere along its course. Hemianopias result from involvement of the visual pathways. Lesions affecting the optic chiasm, most notably originating in or near the pituitary, give rise to bitemporal hemianopia. Lesions of the optic tract, optic radiation, or occipital cortex give rise to contralateral homonymous hemianopias. Lesions of the anterior temporal pole characteristically cause a contralateral homonymous, superior quadrantopsia.

Ataxia and Hemiplegia. Unsteadiness in walking may occur with tumor in various intracranial sites. Lesions affecting the midline cerebellum cause a characteristic truncal ataxia with lateralized ataxia of the extremities if the cerebellar hemispheres are also involved. Disease in the frontal lobes may give rise to unsteadiness in walking, an apraxia of gait, which may simulate cerebellar truncal ataxia. Drug intoxication due to diphenlhydantoin or barbiturates may potentiate ataxia. Tumors of the hemisphere characteristically cause contralateral spastic hemiparesis; initially the signs may be so minimal as to be easily overlooked.

Sensory Disturbances. Hemisensory defects occur with intracranial tumors affecting the contralateral sensory pathways. The primary sensory modalities of touch, pain, temperature, and proprioception are impaired when the thalamus or the ascending spinothalamic pathways are involved. Tumors of the parietal sensory cortex cause loss of cortical sensory functions that results in impairment of sensory localization, two-point discrimination, graphesthesia, stereognosia, and position sense. Tumors of the thalamus may be manifested by episodes of pain affecting the contralateral side of the face or body. Tumors of the cortex may cause focal sensory seizures with a jacksonian march; these may be reported as an aura before a grand mal seizure. Pain in the face occurs with tumors affecting the base of the skull, particularly those arising in the nasopharynx and paranasal sinuses. Tumors affecting the trigeminal nerve may give rise to paroxysms of pain in the face simulating trigeminal neuralgia (tic douloureux), but unlike the latter there is also some loss of facial sensation.

Seizures. Seizures may serve as the first clinical manifestation of brain tumor, or may occur at any time in the course of the illness. The types include classic grand mal seizures and various forms of focal seizures. Typical petit mal is probably never due to neoplasm; minor seizures with brain tumor that at first may resemble petit mal generally are, in fact, either fragmentary grand mal seizures or a variety of psychomotor attack. With any cerebral seizure, it is extremely important to note its aura or the pattern of its onset, for this often provides a reliable indicator of the location of the neoplasm. Focal motor and sensory seizures may be limited to one region of the body or may progress (jacksonian seizures) to involve the entire body. Lesions in the temporal lobe characteristically give rise to psychomotor seizures. These may be associated with olfactory hallucinations (uncinate fits), disorders of visual or auditory perception, experiential attacks such as déjà vu and various types of automatic behavior, for which the patient is generally amnesic. (See article on the Epilepsies.) The onset of convulsions in an otherwise healthy subject over the age of 20 without history of convulsions raises the possibility of an expanding lesion. This possibility is greater in such patients if any focal quality can be detected in the neurologic examination; if such focal changes are found, additional specialized neurologic diagnostic studies are warranted.

Nausea and Vomiting. Nausea and vomiting occur as a result of direct or reflex stimulation of the emetic center of the medulla. This is most likely to occur in association with increased intracranial pressure, particularly with displacement of the brainstem due to herniation or the presence of bleeding into the cerebrospinal fluid. In either instance the vomiting may occur without preceding nausea and may be projectile. Brain tumor is not suggested by the occurrence of nausea and vomiting alone, i.e., there are invariably other clinical manifestations of the tumor. Antiemetic drugs, e.g., the phenothiazines, inhibit this type of centrally induced vomiting.

Stiff Neck. Signs of meningeal irritation may occur in brain tumor as a manifestation of cerebellar herniation through the foramen magnum, because of the effects of bleeding into the subarachnoid space, or with meningeal involvement. Cervical rigidity may be striking but Kernig's sign is generally absent (see Tumors of the Cerebellum, *infra*).

Vasomotor and Autonomic Changes. These occur as ominous late signs. They include bradycardia and hypertension, as described above. Apnea generally precedes cardiac arrest in fatal cases. Autonomic manifestations of brain tumor include gastric ulceration (Cushing's ulcer), which may present as a massive gastrointestinal hemorrhage. This may occur with mass lesions anywhere in the intracranial cavity. (The use of adrenocortical steroids in the management of patients with brain tumor may further increase this hazard.) Fever may also occur in patients with mass lesions in the absence of pulmonary, urinary, or other infection, because of a central disturbance, presumably of hypothalamic origin. Hyperthermia is not uncommon just prior to death, but hypothermia may also occur. Fever commonly accompanies the presence of blood in the subarachnoid space. This may occur with rapidly growing neoplasms or as a result of surgery. Disturbances of sweating may occur, lesions of hypothalamus and brainstem giving rise to contralateral signs of sympathectomy.

Metabolic Manifestations. The complex interrelationships between the hypothalamus and the anterior and posterior pituitary may be deranged with intracranial tumors, giving rise to various systemic metabolic disorders. These include diabetes insipidus, inappropriate secretion of antidiuretic hormone, hypopituitarism, and precocious puberty. (See articles dealing with these problems elsewhere in the text.)

False Localizing Signs. These may occur with increased intracranial pressure or with shift of intracranial structures. The most common such sign is unilateral or bilateral lateral rectus palsy due to sixth-nerve compression. This need not imply neoplastic involvement of the nerve, for it frequently occurs as a pressure palsy of the nerve resulting from increased intracranial pressure itself. Signs of hemiplegia can occur ipsilateral to the tumor due to compression of the opposite cerebral peduncle on the tentorium; i.e., hemiplegia need not be contralateral to the mass. There are relatively silent areas in brain, wherein tumors reach large size with relatively little clinical deficit; these are the right frontal and temporal lobes. This must be considered in evaluating patients with the syndrome of increased intracranial pressure without localizing signs (*vide infra*).

Diagnosis. Patients suspected of having an intracranial tumor require complete medical evaluation to establish the relationship of the neurologic findings to possible coexisting systemic disease. Appropriate laboratory studies should be obtained to search for a primary systemic neoplasm, e.g., lung, breast, gastrointestinal, genitourinary, thyroid malignancies, etc. The major neurologic diagnostic techniques are described below.

Skull Roentgenograms. The films should be examined for the following: (a) changes suggestive of increased intracranial pressure, (b) bone destruction, (c) bony thickening or hyperostosis, (d) abnormal vascular channels, (e) abnormal calcifications, (f) the shape of the sella turcica, (g) the position of the pineal if calcified, and (h) the relationship of the skull to the cervical spine in suspected platybasia, basilar impression, and related disorders (see Anomalies of the Craniovertebral Junction).

Characteristic roentgenographic changes may occur with chronically increased intracranial pressure as a result of pressure atrophy of bone, which produces a beaten-silver appearance in the cranial vault, decalcification of the clinoid processes, and separation of the sutures in children. Bone destruction is characteristic of metastatic neoplasms arising from distant organs and of directly invasive tumors that arise in the paranasal sinuses and nasopharynx. Focal hyperostosis of the skull, i.e., thickening of the inner or outer tables of the skull, or both, with increased calcification, is characteristic of meningioma. Generalized thickening of the skull occurs with Paget's disease. Hyperostosis frontalis interna, localized bilateral thickenings

of the inner table of the skull, is generally considered an incidental finding without clinical significance. The vascular markings of the skull, which accompany arterial and venous channels, vary greatly in the normal subject. Focal enlargements of the markings occur characteristically with meningioma involving adjacent meninges and skull. Abnormal calcifications characteristically occur in very slowly growing primary neoplasms (astrocytoma, oligodendroglioma, craniopharyngioma, meningioma), in arteriovenous malformations, in aneurysmal walls, and in the glial nodules associated with tuberous sclerosis. Calcifications may also occur in the gliotic walls of old abscesses, in hemorrhagic cavities, and in granulomas of cerebral toxoplasmosis. Displacement of the pineal laterally more than 2 mm. is pathologic, and this or a shift superiorly or inferiorly suggests the presence of a space-taking lesion.

Electroencephalography. The electroencephalogram is useful in screening for possible brain tumor. Focal changes, particularly slowing in frequency of the record, are significant indications of neoplasm in the cerebral hemispheres. Rapidly growing tumors with adjacent cerebral edema are more likely to evoke focal changes than are slowly progressive tumors with only minimal clinical manifestations, and with the latter the record may be entirely normal. The electroencephalogram is often normal with posterior fossa neoplasms.

Cerebrospinal Fluid. Examination of the cerebrospinal fluid (CSF) for pressure, protein, sugar, cell count, cultures, serologic tests, and cytologic analysis is very helpful in diagnosis of intracranial tumor. The incidence of abnormalities varies with the stage of the illness and the site and nature of the neoplasm. The fluid is crystal clear unless the protein exceeds about 120 mg. per 100 ml. or unless bleeding has occurred. With slowly growing neoplasms the intracranial pressure will remain normal, less than 200 mm., until late in the illness, whereas in rapidly growing tumors increased pressure may be an early manifestation. Jugular compression for the Queckenstedt test is contraindicated in patients who are suspected of having brain tumor. A protein content greater than 100 mg. per 100 ml. is frequently associated with rapidly growing tumors near the ventricles or subarachnoid space. With slowly growing tumors, the protein may be normal despite the presence of a huge mass. Of the posterior fossa neoplasms, acoustic neuroma commonly results in marked elevation of the protein, 100 to 500 mg. per 100 ml. The fluid is normal in most patients with brainstem gliomas. The cell count is elevated from 5 to 100 white cells per cubic millimeter in about one third of the cases, and may exceed 1000 white cells, particularly when the tumor involves the ventricular wall and has undergone necrosis. Malignant cells may be detected with suitable techniques. The sugar content is normal with brain tumor, apart from patients with diffuse neoplastic involvement of the meninges, when it is characteristically reduced to levels below 40 mg. per 100 ml.; in some cases this may be the sole abnormality, although commonly 10 to 100 mononuclear cells are seen, and with special cytologic techniques malignant cells may be detected.

Lumbar puncture is contraindicated in critically ill patients with clinical signs of incipient herniation because the removal of fluid from the lumbar sac may increase the degree of *pre-existing* herniation of the temporal lobe or of the cerebellar tonsils.

Roentgenographic Contrast Studies. *Pneumoencephalography* by the lumbar route, *ventriculography*, and *arteriography* are of major importance in the diagnosis and localization of brain tumor. Lumbar pneumography delineates the ventricular system and the subarachnoid space and thus may reveal the presence of a mass lesion. In ventriculography, air is injected via burr holes in the skull directly into the lateral cerebral ventricles; this may prove necessary for patients with increased intracranial pressure, in whom the lumbar route is deemed hazardous, and for patients in whom there is nonfilling of the ventricular system by the lumbar route. Cerebral angiography, via the carotid, vertebral, or brachial arteries, may yield much information concerning the location and size of a tumor. The vascular patterns of the tumor, arterial, capillary, and venous, may give indications of its histology. The decision as to which contrast technique is most likely to give maximal information in any patient depends upon the specific circumstances of the diagnostic problem in question and must be resolved individually. Some patients need more than one such study.

Isotopic Localization. Various scanning techniques have become available that permit the recording of the radioactivity present over regions of the skull after intravenous administration of radioiodinated human serum albumin and other gamma emitters. The isotope may enter more rapidly and in greater concentration into the tumor and its adjacent area of edema because of the greater permeability of the capillaries and adjacent cellular membranes. The isotope scan does not readily differentiate between focal changes due to neoplasm, sepsis, or infarction, and is often negative with slowly growing tumors that do not greatly disrupt normal structural relationships. Further improvements should make isotopic localization techniques of greater use in the future.

Echoencephalography. This technique is useful in determining the position of midline structures, i.e., whether there is a shift of the intracranial contents. This is particularly valuable in patients without a calcified pineal. Although the technique gives no information regarding the cause of a shift, it is a useful screening device for patients with suspected mass lesions.

Ancillary Laboratory Tests. Audiometry and vestibular tests are necessary in evaluating patients with suspected tumor of the eighth nerve,

and visual fields are valuable in assessing lesions of the visual system.

Tumor Syndromes. *Tumors of the Skull.* Benign osteomas rarely reach a size sufficient to compress underlying brain; generally these can be extirpated. Malignant tumors arising in the paranasal sinuses or nasopharynx directly invade the base of the skull and cause chronic facial pain and multiple cranial nerve involvement. Tumors of the glomus jugulare (nonchromaffin paraganglioma) arise near the jugular bulb and often lead to progressive deafness and a bloody discharge in the external auditory canal. Other lesions that give roentgenographic evidence of bone destruction and that must be differentiated include Paget's disease, Hand-Schüller-Christian disease, eosinophilic granuloma, and cholesteatoma (epidermoids).

Diffuse Meningeal Neoplasia (Neoplastic Meningitis). Carcinomas, gliomas, sarcomas, melanomas, and lymphomas may diffusely infiltrate the leptomeninges and subarachnoid space to produce a syndrome of chronic meningitis, which may simulate chronic meningitis due to fungi, tuberculosis, sarcoidosis, and meningovascular syphilis. Common manifestations include headache, mental changes, cranial nerve palsies, areflexia, and minimal, if any, signs of meningeal irritation. The cerebrospinal fluid findings generally will establish the diagnosis. The pressure is usually normal; sugar content may be below 45 mg. per 100 ml. and as low as 10 mg. per 100 ml.; protein content is normal or elevated; cell count reveals from 5 to several hundred mononuclear cells; cultures are negative; cytologic studies may reveal malignant cells. The diagnosis may not be apparent at autopsy because gross lesions are generally absent, and microscopic sections are needed to verify the diagnosis.

Tumors of the Cerebral Hemispheres. Tumors affecting the cerebral hemispheres are characterized by progressive focal neurologic deficits and, commonly, by generalized or focal convulsive seizures. Hemispheric tumors involving any lobe may be associated with contralateral hemiplegia; when located in the parasagittal region the paralysis is greater in the leg than in the arm. Tumors of the frontal lobes are also characterized by early impairment of intellectual function. Tumors in the parietal region cause contralateral cortical (interpretive) sensory deficits, impairment of primary sensation, and homonymous hemianopia. Tumors in the occipital region also cause contralateral homonymous hemianopia plus disorders of visual interpretation. Tumors in the temporal lobe, in the nondominant hemisphere, are relatively silent apart from contralateral superior quadrantopsia. Tumors of regions adjacent to the sylvian fissure of the dominant hemisphere give rise to aphasic disorders; anterior lesions in the frontal lobe cause expressive aphasia, posterior lesions in the parietal region cause the receptive aphasias, and lesions in the superior temporal gyrus cause anomic aphasia.

Tumors of the Cerebellum. The common

tumors of the cerebellum include medulloblastomas, which affect the midline vermis most commonly in childhood, and tumors of the cerebellar hemisphere, chiefly gliomas and metastatic tumors. Early manifestations of tumor of the midline vermis include truncal ataxia on tandem walking and symptoms of increased intracranial pressure. Tumors of the cerebellar hemisphere cause ipsilateral limb ataxia as an early manifestation. Tilting of the head to one side may be an early sign as well. Stiffness of the neck is often seen in posterior fossa neoplasms as an early sign of herniation.

Brainstem Tumors. These intrinsic tumors of midbrain, pons, and medulla are most commonly gliomas. The initial symptoms are those of cranial nerve dysfunction, most commonly affecting the extraocular muscles (nuclear or internuclear ophthalmoplegia), chewing and swallowing, as well as the long tracts, ascending and descending. Headache and other manifestations of increased intracranial pressure occur late in the course. The cerebrospinal fluid is often normal.

Pituitary Tumors. The earliest symptoms may be those of endocrine disturbance (*vide supra*) or may be due to effects on the visual system. Frontal headache may be an early symptom, as well as progressive bitemporal hemianopia due to chiasmatic involvement. Pituitary tumors may invade the sphenoid sinus and thus permit the development of bacterial meningitis. The cysts associated with craniopharyngioma may release lipid-laden fluid into the subarachnoid space, thus causing bouts of sterile meningitis.

Optic Nerve Glioma. Gliomas may develop in the intraorbital, retro-orbital, or chiasmatic region of the optic nerve, the first of these being the most common location. These tumors usually occur in early childhood with uniocular loss of vision as the most common presenting symptom. Proptosis is seen in about one third of cases. Uniocular optic atrophy or papilledema may be noted. Roentgenographic evidence of enlargement of the optic foramen is common. The tumor is most often a slowly growing astrocytoma and may be associated with neurofibromatosis.

Acoustic Neuroma (Cerebellopontine Angle Tumor). These neurofibromas (schwannomas) of the eighth nerve begin within the auditory canal or in the subarachnoid space. They are slowly growing and characteristically cause progressive tinnitus and nerve deafness. The vestibular portion is more seriously involved than the acoustic portion, and in patients who do not have a dead labyrinth on caloric testing, the diagnosis is suspect. There are few symptoms referable to loss of vestibular function. A mild sensation of giddiness or unsteadiness is common, but recurrent episodes of vertigo are very rare in acoustic tumors. Adjacent cranial nerves are also commonly involved, particularly the fifth, sixth, and seventh nerves. Large tumors cause ipsilateral cerebellar signs and manifestations of increased intracranial pressure. Meningiomas of the cerebellopontine angle may give a similar clinical picture without, however, enlargement of the auditory canal on roentgenograms of the skull.

Metastatic Tumors. The clinical pictures that result from metastatic neoplasms are very variable, depending on the site and number of metastases and their rate of growth. The diagnosis is readily made in patients with evidence of widespread metastatic disease who then develop focal neurologic signs. However, frequently the metastatic tumor may become symptomatic in brain with few, if any, manifestations of systemic malignant disease. Therefore, patients with an apparently single intracranial mass lesion should be studied for a hidden neoplasm.

Differential Diagnosis A wide variety of neurologic diseases may simulate brain tumor because they are also characterized by progressive focal neurologic signs or signs of increased intracranial pressure. Some of the more common problems in differential diagnosis are considered in the following paragraphs.

Syndrome of Increased Intracranial Pressure Without Localizing Signs. A major diagnostic problem is seen in the patient who presents with increased intracranial pressure manifested by headache and papilledema and who is otherwise apparently normal. The many diagnostic possibilities (see Benign Intracranial Hypertension) include extra-axial neoplasms that obstruct the ventricular system, such as tentorial meningioma and pinealoma, and intraventricular tumors like ependymoma and glioma. Some patients have the syndrome of aqueduct stenosis, generally a manifestation of congenital forking (see Hydrocephalus). Tumors of relatively silent areas like the right frontal and temporal lobes must be excluded. Arteriography and ventriculography and/or lumbar pneumography are generally required to establish the diagnosis.

Tumor vs. Vascular Disease. The differential diagnosis between tumor and vascular disease is generally made on the basis of history: most tumors have an insidious onset and progress slowly, but most vascular lesions characteristically have an abrupt onset. However, some neoplasms such as glioblastoma or metastatic tumors may have a very abrupt onset, most often due to bleeding into the tumor. Also, the stepwise progression ("stuttering onset") of hemiplegia in some patients with vascular disease of the extracranial portions of the internal carotid and vertebral arteries and, at times, of the intracranial arteries, may pose diagnostic uncertainty. Careful analysis of the history, the laboratory studies, and observation of the patient's course will clarify the diagnosis.

Tumor vs. Chronic Subdural Hematoma. The clinical picture in these patients simulates an expanding hemispheric mass: headache, drowsiness, papilledema, hemiparesis, etc. About one third of patients with chronic subdural hematoma provide no significant history of head injury. The differential diagnosis can be made almost always with arteriography.

Tumor vs. Demyelinating Diseases, Multifocal

Leukoencephalopathy. The more common forms of multiple sclerosis do not usually simulate expanding intracranial lesions. There are occasional cases of acute multiple sclerosis or Schilder's disease that may simulate a progressive hemispheric deficit. Diagnostic difficulty also may be encountered in patients with another disorder of white matter, multifocal leukoencephalopathy, which has been reported in association with the lymphomas and malignant disease arising in lung and other organs. In this disorder, multiple foci of demyelination are associated with electron microscopic evidence of viral infection. Clinically, there are signs of multiple lesions in the brain that can simulate metastatic disease. However, despite clinical evidence of multiple lesions and rapid progression, signs of increased intracranial pressure are absent. Although the diagnosis may be suspected, pathologic confirmation is necessary and usually comes only after death.

Tumor vs. Presenile Dementia. Progressive development of an organic dementia in middle age may be caused by many diseases, including frontal or bifrontal neoplasms. Tumors most likely to present with dementia include frontal and subfrontal tumors (olfactory groove meningioma and tumors of the corpus callosum, "butterfly glioma"). Roentgenographic contrast studies may be necessary to establish the diagnosis. A CSF protein greater than 100 mg. per 100 ml. favors tumor over the degenerative dementias.

Tumor vs. Abscess, Granuloma. Encapsulated brain abscess and the granulomas associated with cysticercosis may simulate brain tumor. Cysticercosis must be considered in any patient in an endemic area having signs of a cerebral mass lesion. Differentiation between tumor and abscess may be particularly difficult because patients with encapsulated brain abscess generally do not have systemic manifestations of infection (fever, leukocytosis), and the primary source of infection may be obscure. The cerebrospinal fluid may show little, if any, inflammatory change. The correct diagnosis of abscess or granuloma may not be made until surgery is performed.

Tumor vs. Epilepsy. The common occurrence of convulsive seizures with intracranial tumors requires consideration of this diagnosis when patients develop seizures (apart from true petit mal, which is never due to brain tumor). This is particularly true of patients in whom seizures first develop after the age of 20. The occurrence of transient focal neurologic signs in the postictal state (Todd's paralysis) favors the presence of a structural lesion as basis for the attacks. It is estimated that about 20 per cent of patients who develop seizures after the age of 20, who do not have post-traumatic seizures, will in time be shown to have intracranial tumors. The likelihood of a brain tumor diminishes with the passage of years if focal signs do not appear. There are differences of opinion as to how far one should proceed with diagnostic tests in a patient otherwise normal, with onset of seizures after the age of 20, particularly with regard to the indications for contrast studies. The occurrence of focal seizures, a focal neurologic deficit on clinical examination, or focal EEG slowing all increase the likelihood of the presence of tumor; in the absence of any of these, air study or arteriography is generally unrewarding.

Treatment. *Surgical Therapy.* Total surgical removal without sacrifice of normal cerebral tissue is possible only with tumors that are extra-axial in location, such as some meningiomas, osteomas, neurofibromas, and pituitary tumors. Total surgical extirpation of the primary tumors of brain, glioblastomas and the less malignant gliomas, is seldom possible, although there are rare exceptions, e.g., cystic astrocytomas of the cerebellar hemisphere. Complete surgical removal of angiomas may be possible. Therefore, it is essential to establish the precise location and tumor type to allow optimal therapy. Surgical attack on primary brain tumors may be very helpful as palliative therapy, i.e., internal decompression or partial removal of tumor and edematous brain may relieve headaches and prolong useful life, particularly if the tumor is cystic and in the nondominant frontal or temporal lobes. There is no absolute rule for the surgical treatment of metastatic tumors. In some patients with major symptoms due to an apparent single brain tumor without widespread systemic disease, surgical excision may offer useful palliation.

Radiotherapy. The gliomas may have a high degree of radiosensitivity, and x-ray therapy is generally indicated for palliation. Although biopsy and tissue diagnosis are highly desirable prior to instituting radiotherapy, a specimen is not always obtainable, particularly when the tumor is located in an inaccessible area like the brainstem. In such cases, diagnosis must be made on clinical and roentgenographic grounds. Unfortunately, the response of the gliomas to radiation is often brief, and recurrent growth supervenes. Chromophobe adenomas of the pituitary are generally radiosensitive, and radiotherapy is often the treatment of choice unless there is a rapidly progressive threat to vision, in which case surgical therapy is indicated.

Supportive Measures. Anticonvulsant drugs are indicated for patients with a history of convulsive seizures and for patients who have had intracranial surgery. Diphenylhydantoin, 300 to 500 mg. per day, and phenobarbital, 30 to 60 mg. three times a day, are common dosages. Higher dosages of these and other anticonvulsant drugs may be necessary for seizure control. The use of hypertonic intravenous solutions such as 30 per cent urea or 25 per cent mannitol to lower intracranial pressure has a limited place in management of patients with increased intracranial pressure. This is chiefly for very acute situations while the patient awaits neurosurgical intervention. Adrenal corticosteroids, such as dexamethasone, in high dosages help to reduce cerebral edema associated with brain tumors, particularly in the postoperative period and during radiotherapy; gastrointestinal bleeding, however, is a potential complication. The administration of parenteral fluids must be planned carefully when hydrating patients with increased intracranial pressure since intravenous infusion of 5 per cent glucose in water is dangerous and can result in a significant increase in intracranial pressure. This danger can be avoided by use of normal saline, 5 per cent glucose in saline, or 5 per cent glucose in 0.42 per cent saline. The phenothiazines may be used as antiemetic agents for patients with severe vomiting. These drugs are depressants and must be used cautiously. Parenteral administration of caffeine transiently reduces intracranial pressure (it causes cerebral vasoconstriction and reduces cerebral blood flow) and may be useful in controlling brain tumor headaches. Specific chemotherapeutic agents have not yet been developed to treat the primary brain tumors.

Brain, Lord, and Norris, F. H., Jr.: The Remote Effects of Cancer on the Nervous System. New York, Grune & Stratton, Inc., 1965.

Dastur, H. M., and Desai, A. D.: A comparative study of brain tuberculomas and gliomas based upon 107 case records of each. Brain, 88:375, 1965.

Dixon, H. B. F., and Lipscomb, F. M.: Cysticercosis: An Analysis and Follow-up of 450 Cases. Medical Research Council Special Report, Series No. 299. London, Her Majesty's Stationery Office, 1961.

Fields, W. S., and Sharkey, P. C. (eds.): The Biology and Treatment of Intracranial Tumors. Springfield, Ill. Charles C Thomas, 1962.

Jelsma, R., and Bucy, P. C.: The treatment of glioblastoma multiforme of the brain. J. Neurosurg., 27:388, 1967.

Russell, D. S., and Rubinstein, L. J.: Pathology of Tumors of the Nervous System. 2nd ed. London, Edward Arnold, 1963.

Zulch, K. J.: Brain Tumors. Their Biology and Pathology. 2nd ed. New York, Springer Publishing Company, 1965.

RADIATION INJURY OF THE NERVOUS SYSTEM

Radiation injury of the nervous system occurs as a complication of x-ray therapy wherein tissue dosage has been excessive. Signs of injury may appear within hours or days of high-dosage irradiation in laboratory animals; in man, with the doses used therapeutically, the onset is delayed. Characteristically, a progressive neurologic deficit develops following a latent period of many months or years after the termination of radiotherapy. This complication occurs when irradiation has been directed at neoplasms of the brain or at other tumors in the head and neck. The spinal cord is also subject to injury from excessive radiation, whether directed at a primary cord tumor or at tumors overlying the spine and paraspinal regions, e.g., tumors of the thyroid or mediastinum. Peripheral nerves are relatively radio resistant but are injured also by high doses.

Pathology. The response of the central nervous system to ionizing radiation can be recognized in three phases: an acute phase of meningoencephalitis, a period of apparent normalcy, and a period of late nerve cell damage, demyelination, and vascular change. The lesions in the nervous system attributed to irradiation are extensive in both white and gray matter. There are hyaline thickenings in the walls of blood vessels that may partially or completely occlude the lumen. There is a variable degree of cellular necrosis and degeneration of myelin. Astrocytosis and thickening of the leptomeninges are common. The long latent period between the time of irradiation and the onset of progressive signs is poorly understood; it has been attributed to progressive ischemia due to gradual narrowing of the vascular lumen. Latent radiation effects in skin are readily attributable to vascular and connective tissue damage; this lends weight to the primary importance of the vascular injury in the brain, although it is likely that neuronal degeneration is not due to progressive ischemia alone. It has been suggested that autoimmune mechanisms play a role in the tissue damage that develops after a latent period.

Dosages. The precise tissue dosage that will induce radiation injury is uncertain. The minimal dose in Lindgren's series of 71 cases that produced pathologic evidence of brain necrosis was 4500 to 5000 roentgens, with delivery through medium-sized fields over a period of 30 days. The spinal cord is vulnerable to somewhat lower doses; radiation myelopathy has been reported following 4000 r in 28 days directed toward the mediastinum. Boden has defined the tolerance of the brainstem and spinal cord from a review of his own material. With small treatment fields of 10 by 7 cm. or less, tissue doses up to 4500 r in 17 days or their biologic equivalent seem to be tolerated by the cord and brainstem. With large fields, a tissue dose of 3500 r is considered as the maximal tolerance dose to the brainstem and cord. There is considerable biologic variation in susceptibility of normal tissue to radiation damage, and precise definition of the effects of various dosages on normal tissue is difficult.

Clinical Manifestations. When radiotherapy has been administered to tumors close to, but sparing, the brain and spinal cord, the development of a focal neurologic deficit after a latent period raises the possibility of radiation injury. Following radiotherapy to brain or spinal cord tumors, clinical improvement that persists for one to five years with subsequent regression suggests the possibility of late radiation damage to normal nervous tissue. Symptoms most often appear about a year after irradiation. The onset is insidious, and the rate of subsequent progress is unpredictable. The process may become arrested or may progress to cause a major cerebral hemispheric deficit or complete functional spinal cord transection. The clinical differentiation between radiation injury and recurrent tumor growth may be very difficult and uncertain pending pathologic confirmation at autopsy, and both may be coexistent. A repeated roentgenographic contrast study may help in differentiation. There is no specific therapy for radiation injury of the nervous system.

Boden, G.: Radiation myelitis of the brain-stem. J. Fac. Radiol., 2:79, 1950.

Haley, T. J., and Snider, R. S. (eds.): Response of the Nervous System to Ionizing Radiation. New York, Academic Press, Inc.,1962.

Jonis, A.: Transient radiation myelopathy. Brit. J. Radiol., 37: 724, 1964.

Lindgren, M.: On tolerance of brain tissue and sensitivity of brain tumours to irradiation. Acta Radiol. (Stockholm), (Suppl. 170):1, 1958.

Pallis, C. A., Louis, S., and Morgan, R. L.: Radiation myelopathy. Brain, 84:460, 1961.

Reagan, T. J., et al.: Chronic progressive radiation myelopathy. J.A.M.A.,203:106, 1968.

Van Cleave, C. D.: Irradiation and the Nervous System. New York, Rowman and Littlefield, Inc., 1963.

BENIGN INTRACRANIAL HYPERTENSION
(Pseudotumor Cerebri)

Definition. Benign intracranial hypertension (B.I.H.) describes the syndrome of increased intracranial pressure in which intracranial mass lesions, obstruction of the cerebral ventricles, intracranial infection, hypertensive encephalopathy, and chronic retention of carbon dioxide (pulmonary encephalopathy) have been excluded. It has also been termed pseudotumor cerebri, serous meningitis, and otitic hydrocephalus. B.I.H. includes a heterogenous group of disorders in which a number of different etiologic factors have been identified, although in most cases the cause and pathogenesis of these syndromes are poorly understood. They are termed "benign" because spontaneous recovery generally occurs; however, serious threats to vision may occur.

Clinical Manifestations. The presenting symptoms are headache and disturbance of vision. The headache is often worse on awakening and is aggravated by coughing and straining. It is often relatively mild and may be entirely absent. The most common ocular complaint is visual blurring, a manifestation of papilledema. Some patients complain of brief, fleeting movements of dimming or complete loss of vision, occurring many times during the day (amaurosis fugax), at times accentuated or precipitated by coughing and straining. This ominous symptom indicates that the patient's vision is in serious jeopardy. Visual loss may be minimal despite severe chronic papilledema, including retinal hemorrhages; however, blindness rarely may develop very rapidly—in less than 24 hours. Visual fields characteristically show enlargement of the blind spots, and may show constriction of the peripheral fields and central or paracentral scotoma. Diplopia due to unilateral or bilateral sixth nerve palsy may develop as a result of increased intracranial pressure. The neurologic examination is otherwise normal. A major clinical point is that patients with B.I.H. commonly look well; that is, their appearance and apparent well-being belie the ominous appearance of the papilledema.

Pathophysiology. The signs and symptoms of B.I.H. are due to the effects of increased intracranial pressure; pressures between 300 and 600 mm. are frequent. The intracranial pressure is normally between 50 and 180 to 200 mm. of water as measured in the lumbar sac or ventricles with the patient in the lateral recumbent position. This pressure is dependent upon the pressure-volume relationships within the intracranial and spinal cavities. The intracranial cavity contains about 1400 ml. of brain, 75 ml. of blood, and 75 ml. of CSF, and an additional 75 ml. in the spinal subarachnoid space. The CSF pressure is directly dependent upon the intracranial venous pressure; changes in the latter pressure are readily transmitted to the CSF, and thus a sustained increase in intracranial venous pressure may result in the syndrome of chronically increased intracranial pressure. The intracranial pressure is largely independent of the systemic arterial pressure, and it is normal in essential hypertension; however, it falls with acute systemic hypotension and rises acutely with very acute increases in systemic blood pressure, e.g., with the administration of vasopressor drugs or in the syndrome of acute hypertensive encephalopathy. Increased intracranial pressure also accompanies increased cerebral blood flow resulting from CO_2 retention, as in acute asphyxia or with chronic pulmonary insufficiency. In patients with B.I.H., apart from those with obstruction of the intracranial venous system, the mechanism of the increase in intracranial pressure is unknown. Two different kinds of changes have been noted on pneumoencephalography. The first has been normal air studies except for narrowed, slitlike ventricles and little air in the cortical subarachnoid space, which has been interpreted to mean that the brain volume is increased due to "edema." The second has been normal air studies apart from normal or enlarged ventricles with an excessive amount of air in the cortical subarachnoid spaces, implying an increased volume of CSF. It is not clear whether these differences represent separate entities or whether the differences can be attributed to variation in time, i.e., the first type may develop into the second type after sufficient time has elapsed. Although cerebral edema has been suspected, there are few clinical manifestations of cerebral dysfunction in these patients to denote any functional changes as a result of the edema.

There are new methods available that permit measurement of the rates of formation and of removal of CSF in man, but to date these have not been applied to patients with this syndrome. (The only disease in which there is any evidence in favor of a pathologic increase in CSF formation is papilloma of the choroid plexus). The calculation of the Ayala Index at lumbar puncture, an old clinical guide to the volume of CSF, favors an increased CSF volume in many patients with B.I.H. (Ayala Index $= \dfrac{\text{Final pressure}}{\text{Initial pressure}} \times 10$ ml. removed.

5.0 to 7.0 is normal. Values greater than 7.0 denote increased CSF volume; values less than 5.0 denote decreased CSF volume). The index is almost always increased in patients with benign intracranial hypertension. Although there are clinical correlations between various endocrinopathies (*vide infra*) the mechanism wherein the adrenal, parathyroids, ovaries, or anterior pituitary might affect brain or CSF volumes is obscure.

Etiologic Factors and Associated Disorders. *Intracranial Venous Occlusion with Relation to Infection, Trauma, and Pregnancy.* Increased intracranial pressure as a result of occlusion of the intracranial venous sinuses occurs most commonly as a consequence of otitis media with extension of the infection into the petrous bone and to the wall of the lateral sinus. This syndrome has been termed otitic hydrocephalus. It occurs as a complication of both acute or chronic infection; at times the evidence for otitis media is minimal and readily overlooked. The sixth cranial nerve may also be involved, giving rise to diplopia on lateral gaze. Thrombosis of the superior longitudinal sinus may occur as a consequence of relatively mild closed head injury and may give rise to a pseudotumor syndrome. (Occlusion of this sinus that drains both cerebral hemispheres is more likely to result in hemorrhagic infarction in the cerebrum as the thrombosis extends into the cerebral veins, giving rise to bilateral signs. In such cases, the course is frequently fulminant and the prognosis guarded, although occasionally complete recovery may occur.) Aseptic or primary thrombosis of the superior longitudinal sinus may also be responsible for a pseudotumor syndrome. This develops as a complication of pregnancy and has been reported to occur during the first two to three weeks post partum and also at the end of the first trimester of pregnancy. A disorder of the blood-clotting mechanism has been suggested as basis for these events during the postpartum period, although this has not been substantiated.

Menstrual Dysfunction. A common association is the occurrence of B.I.H. in women with a history of menstrual dysfunction. The women are frequently moderately to markedly overweight (without evidence of alveolar hypoventilation). Menstrual irregularity is common, often with amenorrhea. Galactorrhea is an uncommon associated symptom. The histories usually emphasize excessive premenstrual weight gain. Endocrine studies thus far have not revealed any abnormality of urinary gonadotrophins or estrogens in these patients, and the pathogenesis is unknown.

Hypoadrenalism. B.I.H. has been reported as a complication of Addison's disease, improvement occurring with replacement therapy. The mechanism is obscure.

Adrenal Corticosteroid Therapy. B.I.H. has been reported to have developed in patients treated with adrenal corticosteroids for prolonged periods. Many of the patients have been children with allergic skin disorders or asthma. There has been some suggestion that the syndrome is more likely to occur when the steroid dosage is reduced,

suggesting that relative adrenal insufficiency might have been present in some cases, but this has not been substantiated.

Hypoparathyroidism. Hypoparathyroidism may present with evidence of increased intracranial pressure. The presence of hypocalcemic seizures or cerebral calcifications roentgenographically may further complicate the clinical picture. Increased intracranial pressure disappears with replacement therapy.

Vitamin A Intoxication. B.I.H. has been reported in otherwise healthy adolescents taking huge doses of vitamin A for the treatment of acne. Doses in the range of 250,000 units per day, orally, have been noted to cause headache and papilledema; there is rapid improvement after cessation of the therapy. The syndrome is said to have occurred in Arctic explorers who consumed polar bear liver, a great source of the vitamin.

Tetracycline Administration. A few cases have been reported in very young children of increased intracranial pressure, manifested by a bulging fontanelle, following the administration of tetracycline. These cases have not been thoroughly studied, and it is possible that the bulging fontanelle was related to the infection for which the tetracycline was prescribed, generally respiratory or ear infections, or perhaps it was a manifestation of transient hypo-osmolarity. Spontaneous rapid recovery has been the rule.

Idiopathic. One of the most common forms of B.I.H. is its occurrence in otherwise healthy subjects in the absence of any of the etiologic factors described above. Both sexes are involved and the occurrence is most often between the ages of 10 and 50 years. These cases represent the idiopathic form of B.I.H.; its pathogenesis is a mystery.

Diagnosis. The patient with headache and papilledema without other neurologic signs must be considered to have an intracranial mass, ventricular obstruction, or intracranial infection until proved otherwise. Although the diagnosis of B.I.H. may be suspected by the appearance of apparent well-being and by the history of some of the associated features listed above, the diagnosis is essentially one of exclusion dependent upon ruling out the more common causes of increased intracranial pressure. Brain tumor, particularly when located in relatively silent areas such as the frontal lobes or right temporal lobe or when obstructing the ventricular system, may be manifest only by headache and papilledema. Patients with chronic subdural hematoma, without history of significant trauma, may present in the same way. Diagnostic evaluation requires skull films, electroencephalography, and arteriography and/or air studies (see Intracranial Tumors). Lumbar puncture is necessary in these patients, but is generally deferred until arteriography has revealed that the ventricular system is normal in size and location. Laboratory studies regarding possible hypoadrenalism or hypoparathyroidism may be rewarding in rare cases of these disorders that present with the pseudotumor syndrome. The cerebrospinal fluid pressure is elevated, between

250 and 600 mm., but the fluid is otherwise normal. The protein content is generally low normal, and lumbar CSF protein levels below 15 mg. per 100 ml. are common. The electroencephalogram is normal in B.I.H. Pseudopapilledema may be a source of diagnostic confusion. It is a developmental anomaly of the fundus wherein the ophthalmologic appearance may be indistinguishable from that of the true papilledema; there is elevation of the optic disc, but exudates or hemorrhages are absent. The visual acuity is normal although visual fields may show some enlargement of the blind spots. The unchanging appearance of the fundus in subsequent examinations favors the diagnosis of pseudopapilledema, as does the finding of normal CSF pressure on lumbar puncture.

Treatment. In patients with lateral sinus thrombosis due to chronic infection in the petrous bone, surgical decompression is often indicated. When the pseudotumor syndrome is a manifestation of hypoadrenalism or hypoparathyroidism, replacement therapy is indicated. Vitamin A intoxication disappears when administration of the vitamin is stopped. Anticoagulation therapy has been recommended for patients with dural sinus thrombosis; however, for patients with extension of the clot into cerebral veins with infarction of tissue, anticoagulation is hazardous because it increases the likelihood of hemorrhagic infarction.

The idiopathic form of B.I.H. and its occurrence in patients with menstrual disorders and obesity require individualized management. This syndrome is self-limited in most cases, and after some weeks or months spontaneous remissions occur, making evaluation of therapy difficult. In rare instances, the illness may last as long as two years. In the very obese, weight reduction is recommended. The use of daily lumbar punctures has been advocated to lower pressure to normal levels by removing sufficient fluid; 15 to 50 ml. of fluid may be required. Subtemporal decompression has been widely used in the past. This procedure may be necessary for patients with serious threat to vision due to pressure, although its efficacy has been questioned in a number of reports. The use of adrenal corticosteroids has been advocated because these drugs minimize cerebral edema of diverse causes. However, many patients with B.I.H. appear to have a large volume of CSF, and adrenal steroids have not been shown to affect CSF volume or the rate of CSF formation. Acetazolamide has been used because this carbonic anhydrase inhibitor has been shown to reduce CSF formation in animals, but there are no convincing data that this drug influences B.I.H. It should not be given intravenously because this results in an acute increase in CSF pressure. Hypertonic intravenous solutions (20 per cent urea or 25 per cent mannitol) to lower intracranial pressure can be used in acute situations when there is rapidly failing vision, while one awaits neurosurgical intervention; however, prolonged dehydration therapy is impossible because of its deleterious systemic effects. Management of these patients is difficult and requires the attention of neurologists and neurosurgeons experienced in these problems.

Feldman, M. H., and Schlezinger, N. S.: Benign intracranial hypertension associated with hypervitaminosis A. Arch. Neurol. (Chicago), 22:1, 1970.

Greer, M.: Benign intracranial hypertension. I. Mastoiditis and lateral sinus obstruction. II. Following corticosteroid therapy. III. Pregnancy. IV. Menarche. V. Menstrual dysfunction. Neurology, 12:472, 1962; 13:439, 1963; 13:670, 1963; 14:569, 1964; 14:668, 1964.

Lysak, W. R., and Svien, H. J.: Long-term follow-up on patients with diagnosis of pseudotumor cerebri. J. Neurosurg., 25: 284, 1966.

Paterson, R., De Pasquale, N., and Mann, S.: Pseudotumor cerebri. Medicine, 40:85, 1961.

Walker, A. E., and Adamkiewicz, J. J.: Pseudotumor cerebri associated with prolonged corticosteroid therapy. J.A.M.A., 188:779, 1964.

HYDROCEPHALUS

Definitions. Hydrocephalus is a pathologic state characterized by dilatation of the cerebral ventricles with an increase in volume of cerebrospinal fluid (CSF) almost always caused by an obstruction in the circulation of this fluid. In children, prior to fusion of the cranial sutures, there is enlargement of the skull. Hydrocephalus must be distinguished from other causes of macrocephaly in infancy, including subdural hematoma. In older subjects, cranial enlargement cannot occur. Hydrocephalus is termed "active," i.e., progressive and associated with increased intraventricular pressure, or "arrested" when the intraventricular pressure has returned to normal and is no longer a stimulus for ventricular enlargement. These forms of hydrocephalus are distinguished from hydrocephalus *ex vacuo*, which is characterized by an increase in the volume of CSF under normal pressure that is compensatory to a primary atrophy of the brain. "Normal" pressure occult hydrocephalus refers to the syndrome of ventricular dilatation associated with inadequacy of the subarachnoid spaces without evidence of increased intracranial pressure (*vide infra*).

Etiology and Pathophysiology. There are three possible mechanisms for the development of hydrocephalus: overproduction of CSF, defective absorption of CSF, and obstruction of the CSF pathways. *Overproduction* of the fluid has not been documented, although it may occur with the rare papilloma of the choroid plexus. *Defective absorption* of the CSF at the arachnoid villi, where the fluid passes through valvelike structures to enter the venous sinuses, may occur with subarachnoid hemorrhage, meningitis, and with a very high CSF protein. *Obstruction* of the CSF pathways, which results in dilatation of the channels proximal to the site of obstruction, is the most common underlying mechanism in both the hydrocephalus of infancy and in adults. When the block is within the ventricular system, the process is termed *non-communicating* hydrocephalus, whereas *communicating hydrocephalus* describes ventricular dilatation in which there is free flow of fluid and air between the ventricular system and the spinal subarachnoid space. Communicating hydrocephalus is characterized by extraventricular obstruction of the CSF pathways, most commonly in the subarachnoid spaces about the brainstem at the incisura of the tentorium or in the subarachnoid spaces about the cerebral hemispheres, or both. Ventricular dilatation develops in hydrocephalus because the intraventricular pressures (both the mean pressure and the pulsatile pressures, synchronous with cardiac systole) are pathologically increased; these give rise to a transmural pressure gradient across the cerebral mantle sufficient to cause characteristic compression of the adjacent white matter that has a loss of protein and lipid but an increase in water and sodium content. The magnitude and duration of the transmural pressure gradient necessary to induce ventricular dilatation have not been well defined. These changes may be reversible if surgical therapy can successfully relieve the increased intraventricular pressure (*vide infra*).

The major causes of obstruction in the CSF pathways that produce hydrocephalus are neoplasms, congenital malformations, and post-traumatic and postinflammatory lesions.

Neoplasms most likely to give rise to hydrocephalus are those that arise within or adjacent to the ventricular system and obstruct the flow of CSF. These include gliomas and ependymomas of the third and fourth ventricles and of the aqueduct (see Intracranial Tumors). Congenital malformations give rise to hydrocephalus by causing a variety of obstruction, the most common being "forking" or stenosis of the aqueduct. This may give rise to symptoms early in life, or manifestations may be absent until adulthood. Congenital malformations of the craniovertebral junction also may be associated with hydrocephalus (see Arnold-Chiari Malformation). Most frequently, hydrocephalus is related to postinflammatory or post-traumatic obstruction of the basilar cisterns, particularly in the region of the tentorium. In infancy, this follows intracranial bleeding at the time of birth, at times unrecognized, or episodes of bacterial meningitis or toxoplasmosis. These processes lead to progressive fibrosis of the subarachnoid pathways at the base of the brain, with subsequent obstruction. In adults, postinflammatory hydrocephalus may develop with or after purulent, tuberculous and mycotic meningitis or with cysticercosis, and also may follow subarachnoid hemorrhage due to trauma or ruptured congenital aneurysm.

Clinical Manifestations. The major signs and symptoms of hydrocephalus are those of increased intracranial pressure (see Intracranial Tumors). In infancy, this is manifest by a greater than normal growth rate and size of the head and by distended scalp veins; in severe cases there is downward displacement of the eyes and mental retardation. Although the head size (occipito-bregmatic circumference) in comparison with the chest circumference is of importance, repeated observations of the rate of head growth are more significant. Additional information can be obtained from measurements of the anterior fontanelle, as active hydrocephalus does not occur in conjunction with a closing fontanelle. On the other hand, a fontanelle enlarging from month to month is evidence for increased intracranial pressure, and further investigations are warranted.

In older children and adults, the major manifestations include headache, vomiting, diplopia due to sixth nerve palsy, papilledema, visual blurring, nausea, and vomiting. Thus, occult hydrocephalus due to a benign process must be differentiated from intracranial mass lesions, including tumor without localizing signs and chronic subdural hematoma, as well as from the various forms of benign intracranial hypertension and the chronic meningitides, including fungal meningitis, sarcoidosis, and diffuse meningeal neoplasia (carcinomatous meningitis).

"Normal" Pressure–Occult Hydrocephalus. In recent years, a new syndrome has been delineated as "normal" pressure–occult hydrocephalus. Typically, there is a gradual development over weeks or months of a mild impairment of memory with mental and physical slowness which progresses insidiously to a severe dementia with unsteady gait and urinary incontinence. The patients are usually headache-free and have no signs of increased intracranial pressure, e.g., they have normal fundi and normal CSF pressure at lumbar puncture. Pneumoencephalography reveals enlarged ventricles and a lack of filling of the subarachnoid space over the hemispheres. Isotope cisternography (intraspinal injection of RISA with serial scanning of the skull) has revealed a pathologic reflux of the isotope into the ventricular system with delayed and inadequate visualization of the cortical subarachnoid space. Some patients have a previous history of head injury or subarachnoid bleeding; in others, the etiology is obscure. Striking improvement in the mental state and gait has been noted to follow ventriculoatrial or other shunting procedures. This treatable syndrome is uncommon but must be differentiated from the more frequent forms of organic dementia as discussed in the article on Dementia.

Diagnosis. Detailed neurologic study is necessary to determine the cause of increased intracranial pressure and ventricular dilatation. Skull films show characteristic signs of increased intracranial pressure in young children; the signs in adults are generally less striking and may be absent. Electroencephalograms may be normal or may demonstrate bilateral slowing of nonspecific nature. Carotid angiography will show displacement of the arteries and veins characteristic of ventricular enlargement. Air contrast studies are essential to establish the diagnosis of hydrocephalus in most cases. Ventriculography via a parietal burr-hole or lumbar pneumoencephalography, or both, will reveal the degree of ventricular enlargement, the presence of obstructive lesions in the cerebrospinal fluid pathways, and the adequacy of the subarachnoid spaces about the brainstem, base, and cerebrum. Precise neuroradiologic analysis is essential to establish the diagnosis. The cerebrospinal fluid pressure is characteristically, but not invariably, increased in the cerebral ventricles and lumbar sac. The protein content is generally normal; elevated protein levels favor an underlying neoplastic process in the absence of bleeding or chronic meningitis.

Treatment. The treatment of hydrocephalus is surgical; it is directed toward reducing the volume and pressure of cerebrospinal fluid by bypassing obstruction. A wide variety of shunting procedures has been used. The choice of procedure will depend upon technical factors and the skill and experience of the operating surgeon. If the block exists in the third ventricle, aqueduct, or fourth ventricle (as with intraventricular tumors or with "aqueduct stenosis"), the Torkildsen procedure is often employed (ventriculocisternal shunt), wherein a catheter is placed from one or both lateral ventricles over the occiput into the cisterna magna to enable normal CSF reabsorption into the intracranial venous sinuses. In patients with communicating hydrocephalus, direct shunting of the ventricular fluid into the venous system is generally used, particularly the ventriculoatrial shunt wherein the fluid exits from the ventricle through a valved tube, which extends into the superior vena cava and right atrium of the heart. There are many variations of these procedures in use, including shunting to other body cavities, e.g., ventriculopleural, ventriculoureteral, and ventriculoabdominal shunts. Infections and recurrent obstruction of the shunt are common complications of the various shunting procedures, and the results of treatment particularly in young children are frequently discouraging. Acetazolamide, a carbonic anhydrase inhibitor, reduces the rate of formation of CSF in laboratory animals, but there is no convincing evidence that it is useful in the management of the various forms of hydrocephalus. Some hydrocephalic children will have spontaneous arrest and may function within the normal range with only a prominent forehead and large hat size as residual defects.

Allen, N.: Hydrocephalies. *In* Farmer, T. (ed.): Pediatric Neurology. Harper & Row, New York, 1964.
Foltz, E. L., and Shurtleff, D. B.: Five-year comparative study of hydrocephalus in children with and without operation (113 cases). J. Neurosurg., 20:1064, 1963.
Kibler, R. F., Couch, R. S. C., and Crompton, M. R.: Hydrocephalus in the adult following spontaneous subarachnoid haemorrhage. Brain, 84:45, 1961.
Matson, D. D.: Neurosurgery of Infancy and Childhood. 2nd ed. Springfield, Ill., Charles C Thomas, 1969.
Ojemann, R. G., Fisher, C. M., Adams, R. D., Sweet, W. H., and New, F. P. J.: Further experience with the syndrome of "normal" pressure hydrocephalus. J. Neurosurg., 31:279, 1969.

Russell, D. A.: Observations on the Pathology of Hydrocephalus. Special Report Series. Medical Research Council, No. 265. London, Her Majesty's Stationery Office, 1949.

ANOMALIES OF THE CRANIOVERTEBRAL JUNCTION, SPINE, AND MENINGES

A wide variety of neurologic syndromes are associated with morphologic anomalies in the region of the foramen magnum of the skull due to distortion of the brainstem, cervical cord, and cerebellum. The most common of these are: (1) Arnold-Chiari malformation, (2) fusion of the cervical vertebrae (Klippel-Feil syndrome), (3) basilar impression and platybasia, and (4) spina bifida and meningocele. These defects may occur singly or together, with or without clinical symptoms. Symptoms result from compression, distortion, or malformation of adjacent neural structures. These are most often congenital lesions, but acquired defects due to bone disease or neoplasms of this region may give rise to similar syndromes.

ARNOLD-CHIARI MALFORMATION

This congenital anomaly is characterized by downward displacement of the cerebellum through the foramen magnum of the skull and by similar caudal elongation of the medulla. These cases can be divided into two major types, the infantile and the adult.

Infantile Form. The infantile form is commonly associated with other midline defects such as spina bifida and meningocele, hydrocephalus due to aqueductal or fourth ventricular obstruction, and other congenital malformations of the brain and cord. The infantile form of the Arnold-Chiari malformation usually presents itself because of hydrocephalus in the early months of life, with evidence of spina bifida or frank paraparesis due to myelomeningocele. Therapy is directed toward surgical relief of the hydrocephalus with a ventricular shunting procedure and repair of the meningomyelocele. Prognosis is poor for patients with extensive defects.

Adult Form. The malformation may be asymptomatic until adult life, when there is the onset of symptoms and signs of damage to the cerebellum, lower cranial nerves, pyramidal tracts, and posterior columns. The presenting signs may be due to hydrocephalus secondary to obstruction of the cerebrospinal fluid pathways or to coexisting syringomyelia of the cervical spinal cord and medulla (see Hydrocephalus and Spinal Cord Tumors). Commonly, there is evidence, clinical or

roentgenographic, of fusion of the cervical vertebrae, platybasia, or basilar impression. The
Arnold-Chiari malformation in adults may simulate syndromes produced by tumors near the
foramen magnum and by multiple sclerosis. Surgical enlargement of the foramen magnum and decompression of the cervicomedullary junction are
beneficial in selected cases.

CONGENITAL FUSION OF CERVICAL VERTEBRAE
(Klippel-Feil Syndrome)

Fusion of one or more of the cervical vertebrae
is a congenital malformation that may be an
asymptomatic finding, detected only with roentgenograms of the cervical spine; malformation
of the atlas and axis may coexist. Multiple fusions
and condensation of vertebrae result in shortening
of the cervical spine, which produces a characteristic appearance of a short, thick neck, head set
low on the shoulders, and limitation of neck movements.

Coexisting abnormalities are common, including
undescended scapula (Sprengel's deformity), platybasia, basilar impression, Arnold-Chiari malformation, and other "dysrhaphic" disorders such as
syringomyelia and meningomyelocele. Clinical
evidence of spinal cord involvement is most likely
to be due to coexisting syringomyelia. "Mirror
movements" may occur with the Klippel-Feil syndrome, and other anomalies of the craniovertebral
junction and high cervical cord, in which voluntary
movements of one upper extremity are involun-
tarily imitated by the other upper extremity.
Surgical decompression may be indicated if there
is evidence of spinal cord compression.

BASILAR IMPRESSION AND PLATYBASIA

Basilar impression refers to abnormal invagination of the cervical spine into the base of the posterior fossa of the skull. The diagnosis is made from
lateral roentgenograms of the skull when there is
excessive protrusion of the tip of the odontoid
process of the axis above Chamberlain's line, that
is, a line drawn from the back of the hard palate
to the posterior margin of the foramen magnum.
Other radiologic criteria are also useful. *Platybasia* refers to flattening of the base of the skull,
wherein lateral roentgenograms of the skull reveal flattening of the angle between the orbital
plates of the anterior fossa and the clivus, the
sloping anterior floor of the posterior fossa. The
angle is normally 135 degrees, and becomes 145
degrees or more in platybasia. Platybasia alone is
asymptomatic.

These malformations, which commonly coexist
or may exist alone, are usually developmental in

origin, and there may be hereditary transmission.
Occasionally, these deformations of the base of the
skull may result from metabolic bone diseases
such as rickets, osteitis deformans, osteomalacia,
or osteogenesis imperfecta. The congenital form
may be associated with the Klippel-Feil syndrome, Arnold-Chiari malformation, and other
congenital malformations of the atlas and axis,
such as fusion of the atlas to the base of the skull
or malpositioning of the odontoid process. Minor
degrees of deformity of the base of the skull give
rise to no symptoms. The neck appears shortened,
and its movements may be limited. With more
severe invagination, there may be signs of impaired function of the cerebellum, lower cranial
nerves, pyramidal tracts, and posterior columns.
Syringomyelia and syringobulbia may also be
present. Increased intracranial pressure may
develop due to obstruction of the foramina of the
fourth ventricle and the basal cisterns. The clinical manifestations must be differentiated from
those due to neoplasms in the region of the foramen magnum and multiple sclerosis. When neurologic signs are progressive, surgical decompression
of the posterior fossa and upper cervical cord may
be indicated.

SPINA BIFIDA AND MENINGOCELE

Various malformations of the meninges and
spinal cord result from developmental defects in
the closure of the bony canal. Whereas many of
these are obvious at birth, some may not be
symptomatic until adult life. The classification of
these defects would include the following: (1)
Complete rachischisis, in which the bony vertebral
arches are missing in the lumbar region, the cord
is undeveloped or aplastic, and the nerve elements
have no covering. (2) *Meningomyelocele*, an obvious soft tissue saccular mass which extends over
the lumbosacral spine. The cerebrospinal fluid
may leak from a defect which may be responsible
for bacterial meningitis. (3) *Meningocele*, a bony
defect in the spine associated with a meningeal
diverticulum covered by atrophic skin. The spinal
cord and roots are generally not involved and
there may be no associated neurologic defect. (4)
Spina bifida occulta, a defect in the bony arches in
the lumbar region often discovered incidentally
on roentgenographic examination. In most cases,
neither cord nor roots are involved. The overlying
skin may be the site of a tuft of hair, a pilonidal
dimple, or a dermal sinus, which is continuous
with the subarachnoid space. The latter may serve
as a portal of entry for recurrent bouts of meningitis. It should be sought in all patients presenting
with bacterial meningitis. These malformations
may be associated with Arnold-Chiari malformation and with hydrocephalus. There may also be
evidence of syringomyelia. The neurologic deficit
varies with the degree of involvement of the spinal

cord, conus medullaris, and cauda equina. In adults the chief manifestation may be a neurogenic bladder and defective anal sphincter. Asymptomatic spina bifida requires no therapy. Dermal sinuses, when responsible for bacterial meningitis, require surgical excision. In patients with neurologic deficits, attempts at surgical correction may be indicated.

Bharucha, E. P., and Dastur, H. M.: Craniovertebral anomalies (a report on 40 cases). Brain, 87:469, 1964.

Bull, J., Nixon, W. L. B., and Pratt, R. T. C.: The radiological criteria and familial occurrence of primary basilar impression. Brain, 78:229, 1955.

Matson, D. D.: Neurosurgery of Infancy and Childhood. 2nd ed. Springfield, Ill., Charles C Thomas, 1969.

McRae, D. L.: Bony abnormalities at the cranio-spinal junction. Clin. Neurosurg., 16:356, 1969.

Peach, B.: The Arnold-Chiari malformation: Anatomic features of 20 cases. Arch. Neurol. (Chicago), 12:613, 1965.

Smith, E. D.: Spina Bifida and the Total Care of Spinal Myelomeningocele. Springfield, Ill., Charles C Thomas, 1965.

Spillane, J. D., Pallis, C., and Jonas, A. M.: Developmental abnormalities in the region of the foramen magnum. Brain, 80:11, 1957.

Nonmetastatic Effects of Cancer on the Nervous System

Jerome B. Posner

If patients with systemic cancer develop nervous system dysfunction, metastasis is usually suspected. However, cancer can also exert deleterious effects on the nervous system in the complete absence of any direct metastatic involvement. Recognition of these nonmetastatic neurologic complications can prevent inappropriate and perhaps harmful therapy directed at a nonexistent metastasis and also can suggest the presence of an occult neoplasm when the nervous system symptoms precede the symptoms of the cancer.

An almost bewildering variety of neurologic disorders has been ascribed to effects of systemic cancer, as shown in the accompanying table. Many of these bear only an indirect nutritional or metabolic (e.g., hepatic coma) relationship to cancer and are discussed elsewhere in this book. The term "remote effects of cancer on the nervous system" as used in this article applies to nervous system dysfunction of unknown cause specifically occurring in association with cancer (see table). The classification is similar to that of Brain and Adams (see Brain and Norris), but progressive multifocal leukoencephalopathy is not included because its cause is probably a slow virus.

The incidence of remote neurologic effects in most series of patients with cancer is 1 to 4 per cent. Croft and Wilkinson found remote effects in 96 of 1465 patients, an incidence of 6.6 per cent. The incidence varied according to the type of cancer, with ovary (16.4 per cent) and lung (14.2 per cent) leading the list. Rectal (0.5 per cent) and uterine (1.3 per cent) cancer rarely caused remote effects. Shy and Silverstein found a 3.5 per cent incidence of "neuromyopathy" in 1500 patients with cancer.

The pathogenesis of these disorders is unknown; suggestions have included autoimmune reactions, viral infections, toxins secreted by the tumor, and nutritional deprivation. It is possible that different mechanisms are responsible for the several types of remote effects. Although the neurologic disorders described below are separated into anatomic categories, there is some overlap in practice. This is particularly true of the dementias, which are often lumped together with brainstem, cerebellar, and spinal cord lesions as "carcinomatous encephalomyelitis," and of myopathy and peripheral neuropathy associated with cancer, often called "carcinomatous neuromyopathy." The latter term has also been applied by Brain to all the remote effects of cancer on the nervous system.

BRAIN AND CRANIAL NERVES

Cerebrum. Dementia, with or without other neurologic signs, characterizes about 40 per cent of patients with remote effects of carcinoma. The dementia is insidious in onset and progressive. There is usually a striking loss of recent memory and an alteration of the affect, manifested either by anxiety or depression. Generalized seizures occur in some patients, and others can have a fluctuating confusional state mimicking metabolic encephalopathy. When other abnormal neurologic signs are present, they usually point to brainstem, cerebellar, or peripheral nerve involvement (see below). The electroencephalogram in the demented patients is diffusely slow, and there is often a cerebrospinal fluid pleocytosis of 10 to 40 lymphocytes with a slightly elevated protein concentration.

NONMETASTATIC EFFECTS OF SYSTEMIC CANCER ON THE NERVOUS SYSTEM

I. *"Remote Effects," Etiology Unknown*
  A. Brain and cranial nerves
    1. Dementia
    2. Bulbar encephalitis
    3. Subacute cerebellar degeneration
    4. Optic neuritis
  B. Spinal cord
    1. Chronic myelopathy
      a. "Amyotrophic lateral sclerosis"
      b. "Long tract" degeneration
    2. Subacute necrotic myelopathy
  C. Peripheral nerves and roots
    1. Ganglioradiculitis
    2. Sensorimotor peripheral neuropathy
    3. Acute polyneuropathy, "Guillain-Barré" type
  D. Neuromuscular junction and muscle
    1. Polymyositis and dermatomyositis
    2. "Myasthenic" syndrome
    3. Myasthenia gravis
II. *Metabolic Encephalopathy*
  A. Destruction of vital organs
    1. Liver (hepatic coma)
    2. Lung (pulmonary encephalopathy)
    3. Kidney (uremia)
    4. Bone (hypercalcemia)
  B. Elaboration of hormonal substances by tumor
    1. "Parathormone" (hypercalcemia)
    2. "Corticotrophin" (Cushing's syndrome)
    3. Antidiuretic hormone (water intoxication)
  C. Competition between tumor and brain for essential substrates
    1. Hypoglycemia (large retroperitoneal tumors)
    2. Tryptophan (carcinoid)
III. *Infections* (usually associated with lymphomas)
  A. Parasites
    1. Toxoplasma cerebral abscess
  B. Fungi
    1. Meningitis (cryptococcosis)
    2. Encephalitis (cryptococcosis, mucormycosis)
  C. Bacteria
    1. Meningitis (*Listeria monocytogenes*)
  D. Viruses
    1. Herpes zoster (radiculitis, myelitis, encephalitis)
    2. Progressive multifocal leukoencephalopathy
IV. *Vascular Disease*
  A. Intracranial hemorrhage (secondary to bleeding disorders)
    1. Subdural hematoma
    2. Subarachnoid hemorrhage
    3. Intracerebral hemorrhage
  B. Cerebral infarction
    1. Thrombotic (due to "disseminated intravascular coagulation")
    2. Embolic (tumor emboli, marantic endocarditis)
V. *Effects of Therapy*
  A. Steroids
    1. Myopathy
    2. Psychosis
  B. Chemotherapy
    1. Central effects (asparaginase encephalopathy)
    2. Peripheral effects (vinca alkaloid neuropathy)
  C. Radiation
    1. Encephalopathy
    2. Myelopathy
    3. Neuropathy

Pathologically, there are two groups: In some patients, particularly those who also have subacute cerebellar degeneration, bulbar encephalitis, or carcinomatous neuropathy (q.v.), no significant pathologic changes can be found in the cerebrum. Other patients demonstrate widespread cerebral neuronal loss, particularly in the temporal lobes or the thalamus, with perivascular collections of lymphocytes suggesting inflammation. The etiology of the dementing illnesses is unknown, but the inflammatory changes have led some to propose that a viral illness is responsible. The differential diagnosis includes metastatic disease of the brain or meninges, fungal or parasitic infections of the brain, a metabolic encephalopathy, and multifocal leukoencephalopathy. In the first three, focal cerebral signs other than dementia are present, and appropriate contrast and cerebrospinal fluid studies support the diagnosis of infectious or metastatic disease of the brain. Metabolic encephalopathy can usually be diagnosed by appropriate laboratory tests, as indicated in the article on that subject. The presence of a progressive dementia in middle age accompanied by cerebellar, brainstem, or peripheral nerve dysfunction but no other focal cerebral signs suggests carcinomatous dementia. There is no treatment for the dementias associated with carcinoma.

Bulbar Encephalitis. Henson et al. have reported a series of patients in whom dementia usually coexisted with signs of brainstem dysfunction. The brainstem signs and symptoms included vertigo, nystagmus, dysphagia, ophthalmoplegia, and at times ataxia and extensor plantar reflexes. The onset of such illnesses is subacute or insidious and the course is progressive. The pathologic changes are predominantly found in the lower pons and medulla, particularly involving the nuclei of the floor of the fourth ventricle and the inferior oliva. There is both neuronal loss and perivascular lymphocytic cuffing in the involved areas. The lymphocytic infiltration is responsible for the term encephalitis. The etiology is not known and there is no effective treatment.

Cerebellum. Subacute cerebellar degeneration occurs in about 3 per cent of patients with cancer, according to Brain, and has a clinical picture sufficiently characteristic to suggest that cancer is present even when the tumor has not yet directly manifested itself. There is a subacute onset of bilateral and symmetrical cerebellar dysfunction, the patient being equally ataxic in arms and legs. Severe dysarthria is usually present, but nystagmus is generally absent or mild. Many patients have neurologic signs pointing to disease outside the cerebellum: extensor plantar responses are common; tendon reflexes may be either diminished or exaggerated; and dementia occurs in about half. The cerebrospinal fluid is usually normal, but there may be as many as 40 lymphocytes and an elevated protein content. The disease, which is usually associated with either carcinoma of the lung or of the ovary, precedes the discovery of the neoplasm by periods of from weeks to three years in more than half the patients, and it tends to run a progressive course over six to eight weeks, rendering the patient severely disabled. Characteristic pathologic changes consist of diffuse loss of Purkinje cells in all areas of the cerebellum with lymphocytic cuffs around blood vessels. There is often additional neuronal degeneration of brainstem nuclei and subthalamic structures as well. This illness can be distinguished from cerebellar metastases by the symmetry of its signs and the absence of increased intracranial pressure, and from alcoholic-nutritional cerebellar degeneration because dysarthria and ataxia in the upper extremities are prominent in the carcinomatous cerebellar degenerations, and are usually absent in the alcoholic variety. The hereditary cerebellar degenerations rarely run so rapid a course. There is no treatment for this disorder, and its etiology is unknown. There is no evidence that treatment of the tumor reverses the neurologic disability.

Optic Nerves. Acute optic neuritis is a rare remote effect of cancer which may precede the discovery of the cancer by months or years. The disease is bilateral, acute or subacute in its onset, and associated with decreased vision, central scotomas, and papilledema. The cerebrospinal fluid is normal, and vision usually does not improve. Pathologically, there is widespread demyelination of the optic nerves with relative preservation of the axis cylinders and occasional perivascular cuffing with lymphocytes. The illness cannot be distinguished from the optic involvement which is a common accompaniment of meningeal carcinomatosis. In the latter instance, papilledema and central scotomas may be similar to those of optic neuritis, but examination of the cerebrospinal fluid usually reveals increased protein and decreased glucose concentrations and the presence of malignant cells. Treatment of the acute neuritis with corticosteroids is rarely helpful.

SPINAL CORD

Two distinct myelopathies complicate carcinoma. The first has clinical and pathologic findings indistinguishable from amyotrophic lateral sclerosis except that the course appears to be somewhat more indolent in the patients with cancer. Norris and Engel reported that 10 per cent of 130 consecutive patients with amyotrophic lateral sclerosis developed carcinoma at various sites. This high percentage has not been verified by other series. However, Brain, Croft, and Wilkinson collected 11 cases of patients with cancer who also had amyotrophic lateral sclerosis; 5 of these patients presented with neurologic symptoms, and 3 were alive more than three years after neurologic symptoms began. The second myelopathy is that of a subacute necrotic destruction of the spinal cord in which both gray and white matter are affected to an equal degree. Clinically, there is a rapidly ascending sensory and motor loss, usually to midthoracic levels, the patient becoming paraplegic within hours or days of the onset of symptoms. The neurologic symptoms often precede the discovery of the neoplasm, and the illness is clinically and pathologically indistinguishable from idiopathic subacute necrotic myelopathy. Since epidural spinal cord compression from metastatic tumor or arteriovenous spinal cord

anomalies may present similar clinical signs, a myelogram is essential to the diagnosis. In addition to the above two entities, many patients with carcinomatous cerebellar degeneration develop extensor plantar responses, mild sensory changes, and reflex asymmetries associated with degenerations of long tracts of the spinal cord. However, spinal cord symptoms do not predominate in these patients.

PERIPHERAL NERVES

Three types of peripheral nerve disorders occur in association with cancer. Characteristic of carcinoma is a subacute sensory neuropathy (ganglioradiculitis) marked by distal loss of proprioception and cutaneous sensory modalities with relative preservation of motor power. The illness usually precedes the appearance of the carcinoma and progresses over a few months, leaving the patient with a moderate or severe disability. The cerebrospinal fluid protein is usually elevated. Pathologically, there is destruction of posterior root ganglia, perivascular lymphocytic cuffing, and wallerian degeneration of sensory nerves. Most of the patients have degenerative changes in brain and spinal cord as well. This almost pure sensory neuropathy is rare; in one series no examples were found on examination of 1476 patients with cancer. The illness is of interest, however, both because it is a relatively characteristic remote effect of cancer and because four such patients have been reported to have complement-fixing antibodies to brain tissue in their plasma. These findings suggest an autoimmune disorder, but the exact pathogenesis is unknown. There is no treatment.

More common than sensory neuropathy is a sensorimotor distal peripheral neuropathy characterized by motor weakness, sensory loss, and reflex absence distally in the extremities. This disorder tends to be less severe than the purely sensory types, and often undergoes spontaneous remission even when the underlying cancer goes untreated. The illness is pathologically characterized by both segmental demyelination and wallerian degeneration of sensory and motor peripheral nerves. Dorsal root ganglia are never involved to the same degree that they are in the purely sensory neuropathy. Pathologically and clinically, the sensorimotor neuropathy is indistinguishable from nutritional polyneuropathies as well as those associated with uremia and other metabolic defects. Indeed, some have suggested that this neuropathy may be due to nutritional deprivation associated with cancer. Its etiology, however, is not clear, and it rarely responds to treatment with vitamins and other nutritional supplements.

A polyneuritis clinically and pathologically indistinguishable from acute postinfectious polyneuropathy (Guillain-Barré syndrome) also complicates cancer, but the association may be coincidental because both acute polyneuropathy and carcinoma are common illnesses.

NEUROMUSCULAR JUNCTION AND MUSCLES

Neuromuscular Junction. Myasthenia gravis has been associated with thymomas but not with other systemic tumors. However, Lambert and Eaton described a "myasthenic syndrome" associated with small cell carcinoma of the lung (see Brain and Norris). The neuromuscular defect appears to result from decreased release of acetylcholine at the neuromuscular junction. Approximately 70 per cent of the patients reported with this syndrome either had at the time of diagnosis or eventually developed intrathoracic tumors. Clinically, the patients complain of weakness and fatigability of proximal muscles, particularly of the pelvic girdle and thighs. The cranial nerves and respiratory muscles are involved less commonly. In addition, patients complain of dryness of the mouth, impotence, pain in the thighs, and peripheral paresthesias. This disease occurs predominantly in men over 40 years of age. On examination there is weakness of the proximal muscles without muscle wasting and with a peculiar tendency of strength to increase over several seconds of a sustained contraction. The diagnosis is made by electromyographic studies in which repeated nerve stimulations at rates above ten per second cause a progressive increase in the size of the muscle action potential (exactly the opposite of the effect of myasthenia gravis). The illness responds poorly to anticholinesterase drugs, but does respond to guanidine hydrochloride given in doses of 35 to 50 mg. per kilogram per day. There is no direct relationship between treatment of the tumor and change in the myasthenic syndrome.

Muscle. Typical *polymyositis* and/or *dermatomyositis* may appear as a remote effect of cancer. About 20 per cent of patients with this disorder have cancer, and although polymyositis is considerably more common in women, the illness is more commonly associated with cancer in men over the age of 50. Thus, in 75 to 80 per cent of males over 50 with polymyositis, a cancer either can be found when the disease develops or will appear within a few months or years. The clinical and pathologic picture is indistinguishable from that of dermatomyositis or polymyositis. The patients respond somewhat less well to corticosteroid therapy than do those with dermatomyositis and no cancer, although improvement with steroid treatment does occur in some.

Brain, R., and Norris, F. H., Jr.: The Remote Effects of Cancer on the Nervous System. New York, Grune & Stratton, Inc., 1965.

Croft, P. B., and Wilkinson, M.: The incidence of carcinomatous neuromyopathy in patients with various types of carcinoma. Brain, 88:427, 1965.

Henson, R. A., Hoffman, H. L., and Urich, H.: Encephalomyelitis with carcinoma. Brain, 88:449, 1965.

Hildebrand, J., and Coers, C.: The neuromuscular junction in patients with malignant tumours. Brain, 90:67, 1967.

Shy, G. M., and Silverstein, I.: A study of the effects upon the motor unit by remote malignancy. Brain, 88:515, 1965.

Injuries of the Head and Spine

Russel H. Patterson, Jr.

INJURIES OF THE HEAD

Trauma claims over 110,000 lives each year in the United States and ranks in frequency as a cause of death after heart disease, cancer, and stroke. Head injury accounts for death in 70 per cent of cases and surpasses all other causes in persons between the ages of 1 and 35. Good management can benefit many of these patients, but often responsibility for their care falls first on someone who lacks formal training in the field of cerebral trauma. This need not be a disadvantage if the physician follows a few simple principles of management based on an understanding of the pathophysiology of the injury. Properly prepared, he can recognize the indications for specialized diagnostic procedures and possible surgery.

Pathophysiology. The scalp, hair, skull, and bones of the face protect the brain from trauma by absorbing energy from blows to the head. When struck by a blow of moderate velocity, the calvaria bends inward, but a few centimeters away the skull bends outward, and linear fractures radiate toward and away from the point of impact. A blow of higher kinetic energy may comminute or penetrate the skull to cause a depressed fracture.

Beneath the point of impact intracranial pressure may increase for a few milliseconds to as much as 5000 mm. Hg, and low or even negative pressure can be recorded simultaneously in the brain at the opposite side of the skull. Cavitation occurs in the brain in regions of low pressure, which accounts for many contrecoup injuries. The pressure gradients distort the brain which attempts to flow toward the foramen magnum, inducing shear stresses in the brainstem and upper cervical spinal cord. Other shearing forces, induced by rapid acceleration and deceleration of the head, tear axonal processes; this is manifest pathologically by chromatolysis in the cell body of the neuron and microglial proliferation in the white matter associated with abnormalities of the myelin sheath. These changes may not be visible macroscopically at autopsy but account for widespread dysfunction in the cerebral hemispheres, basal ganglia, and brainstem.

The brain and skull respond at different rates to forces of acceleration and deceleration produced by a blow which results in mass movements of the brain. Sharp and irregular surfaces inside the cranial cavity such as the orbital surface of the frontal fossa, the sphenoid ridge, the falx, and the tentorium lacerate and contuse the moving brain. Rotational forces shear nervous tissue around arterioles and result in parenchymal hemorrhages; fragile cerebral veins draining into the dural venous sinuses may tear and fill the subdural space with blood. Fractures that divide meningeal arteries or major venous sinuses commonly cause bleeding in the epidural space.

Cerebral blood flow increases markedly immediately after a head injury as the result of cerebrovascular dilation and loss of the normal autoregulatory mechanisms. Increased blood flow is associated with increased cerebral blood volume, which causes increased intracranial pressure. If systemic arterial pressure stays high, fluid shifts out of the vascular compartment of the brain into the extracellular space, and cerebral edema results.

Cerebral contusions and lacerations accompany 90 per cent of severe nonpenetrating injuries. Blood stains the cortical surface and subarachnoid space over both cerebral hemispheres, areas of hemorrhage are found in the brain parenchyma, and clots form in the subdural and epidural spaces. Edema further crowds the contents of an unyielding cranium. The swollen cerebrum displaces the uncus of the temporal lobe through the tentorial notch to compress the oculomotor nerve and the midbrain. Continued pressure obstructs the posterior cerebral artery and basilar vein, inducing ischemia and augmenting edema.

The supratentorial structures generally are most susceptible to damage from head trauma because a heavy layer of muscle protects the contents of the posterior fossa. But should the effects of an injury swell the cerebellum, the tonsils herniate downward through the foramen magnum to compress the medulla while the vermis pushes upward through the apex of the tentorial notch to squeeze the vein of Galen against the corpus callosum, which is backed by the rigid falx.

Increased intracranial pressure causes constriction of the peripheral vascular bed, bradycardia, and increased return of venous blood to the heart. The left ventricle of the heart may be unable to increase cardiac output sufficiently to prevent the development of high pressure in the left atrium and pulmonary edema. Even in the absence of pulmonary edema, pulmonary arteriovenous shunts may open in response to both the increased blood flow in the pulmonary artery and increased sympathetic tone in the pulmonary vascular bed. The consequence is frequently arterial hypoxemia even if the patient's ventilation is adequate to maintain normocapnia or hypocapnia. If the tongue or secretions obstruct the airway, hypoxia develops in association with hypercapnia. Hypercapnia augments cerebrovasodilatation and causes a further increase in intracranial pressure with the grave consequences outlined above. In addition, increased blood flow in the entire brain may shunt blood preferentially to a dilated vascular bed of low resistance and thereby deprive an injured area which is relatively ischemic.

Hemorrhages are found about the pituitary gland and hypophyseal stalk in about two thirds of patients dying of craniocerebral trauma. Necrosis of the anterior lobe is present in more than a fifth of cases and has been attributed to shock, swelling of the gland, and obstruction of the portal vessels. The consequence may be some combination of diabetes insipidus, absence of thirst, and hypoadrenalism producing a varied picture of abnormal fluid and electrolyte metabolism which can range from hypernatremia to water intoxication.

Concussion. Concussion is a clinical term that may be defined as loss of consciousness following an injury to the head without macroscopic damage to nervous tissue. Recovery is usually prompt after less severe injuries, but long periods of unconsciousness or death may occur, and amnesia for events before and after the accident is common. Concussion implies that contusions and lacerations of the brain have not accounted for the symptoms, but the diagnosis must be presumptive except in occasional fatal cases studied at autopsy. Information about the pathophysiology of concussion therefore is derived largely from experiments with animals.

How an injury to the head causes unconsciousness is not entirely clear. Transmitted pressure gradients and rotational forces distort the brainstem, but bilateral injury to the cerebral hemispheres may be equally important. Changes in the brainstem probably account for the apnea and bradycardia that immediately follow the blow as well as for the unsteadiness and giddiness with change in position of which patients often complain for a time. Amnesia, forgetfulness, irritability, fatigue, and impaired memory are attributed to neuronal damage in the cerebrum, although long persistence of these vague symptoms after cerebral trauma may be hard to evaluate, particularly if a lawsuit is unsettled.

Microscopic changes in the brain after a concussive blow are observed in the neurons and glia within a few hours. Some cells may recover, but others do not, and thus permanent damage to the nervous system occurs. Psychologic tests and neurologic examination may not reveal evidence for the loss of a relatively few neurons, but the effects of repeated small injuries are cumulative as the dull, querulous behavior of the punch-drunk fighter testifies.

Evaluation of the Acute Head Injury. The diagnosis of an intracranial clot may be difficult and often depends on the demonstration of an increasing neurologic deficit. Consequently, the initial examination of the patient assumes importance as a baseline for subsequent observations.

Details of the accident suggest what parts of the brain may be injured. The duration of unconsciousness is a rough index to the severity of the injury; even brief unconsciousness is evidence of enough damage to merit hospitalization and careful observation. The neurologic examination is repeated at intervals to detect any change in consciousness, breathing, pupillary diameter, motor strength, speech, or vision, which may signal the presence of an expanding intracranial mass.

The blood pressure, pulse, respirations, and temperature should be recorded frequently after an injury to the head. However, the classic response to increasing intracranial pressure of bradycardia and arterial hypertension may not occur, and any instability of vital signs implies a change in intracranial homeostasis.

As death after trauma is usually due to failure of the respiratory and circulatory centers, the physician must be particularly alert to the early signs of damage to the brainstem. Coma may result from extensive injury to both cerebral hemispheres, but stupor that progressively deepens usually results from distortion of the brainstem due to an enlarging clot or progressively edematous brain. The evolution of these signs of dangerous rostral-caudal deterioration is emphasized later in this discussion. Grave signs, however, are fixed pupils, impaired oculovestibular responses, and decerebrate posturing.

If edema or a clot herniates the temporal lobe through the tentorial notch, the uncus compresses the ipsilateral third cranial nerve, and the pupil first dilates, then fixes to light. Occasionally the contralateral third nerve is first affected, but eventually both nerves are paralyzed, and both pupils dilate. Later, when sympathetic centers in the midbrain are damaged, the pupils may contract to become fixed in midposition. Treatment, to be fully effective, must reverse the process before this advanced stage.

Sometimes retinal hemorrhages follow intracranial bleeding, or an occluded venous sinus causes papilledema, but mydriatics alter pupillary responses and for this reason should not be used to obtain a better view of the ocular fundus.

Diagnostic Procedures. Roentgenograms. Roentgenographic examination of the skull should be performed without undue delay in all cases of injury to the head. Fractures of the calvaria are generally visible, but most basilar fractures are obscured in the bony detail. The presence of skull fracture is reason enough to admit a patient to the hospital following an injury even if he appears to have sustained no brain damage. Roentgenograms perhaps will reveal an indriven fragment of bone, a displaced pineal gland, or intracranial air if a fracture through a paranasal sinus tears the dura and arachnoid. The patient is a likely candidate for an intracranial blood clot if fracture is found which crosses a venous sinus or meningeal artery.

Lumbar Puncture. Lumbar puncture is helpful in the differential diagnosis of coma because the cerebrospinal fluid is commonly xanthochromic after being centrifuged in cases of trauma. However, if a good history is available, lumbar puncture is better avoided because in a patient with an edematous brain or an intracranial clot the withdrawal of fluid can precipitate transtentorial or foramen magnum herniation. A measurement of cerebrospinal fluid pressure is not ordinarily helpful, for it can be either high or low after a severe injury.

Echoencephalography. A shift of the midline structures of the brain owing to edema or hematoma can be identified by a displaced pineal gland on roentgenograms of the skull or by echoencephalography if the gland is uncalcified. Following evacuation of a clot, the displaced midline structures return to their normal position unless the clot reaccumulates. The absence of a shift does not necessarily mean that an intracranial clot is not present; bilateral subdural hematomas are common and may cause transtentorial herniation of the temporal lobes without shift of the midline structures.

Electroencephalography. The electroencephalogram is rarely helpful in the management of acute injury to the head. An abnormal tracing is common immediately after the trauma and tends to improve as recovery takes place. In cases of chronic subdural hematoma the electroencephalogram may be of value if low voltages and abnormal wave forms are recorded from the scalp overlying the hematoma.

Radioactive Scan. Chronic subdural hematomas are often well demonstrated by the radioactive scan technique. In acute injuries a scan is less helpful because the study does not differentiate space-occupying lesions from contused areas of brain.

Cerebral Angiography. Angiography is widely used in evaluating trauma to the head, and in some cases, such as subdural hematoma, the films are almost diagnostic. The procedure is not without danger, particularly when the circulation to a region of the brain is already impaired by an injury. Consequently, angiography is best reserved for patients in whom progressive deterioration or focal signs such as hemiparesis raise suspicion that a blood clot may be present.

Burr Holes. Burr holes placed in the skull can be used to diagnose and treat subdural and epidural hematoma. The advantages of the procedure lie in low risk and speedy evacuation of the clot if the patient's condition is rapidly worsening. Unfortunately, a subdural hematoma in an unusual location may escape detection unless the burr holes are judiciously placed, and a parenchymal hematoma will not be revealed by inspection of the surface of the brain. Angiography remains the most useful diagnostic tool in head trauma; diagnostic burr holes are reserved for emergencies, occasions when angiography is not available, and when the risk of angiography may be high, as in the differential diagnosis of ischemic stroke and chronic subdural hematoma in the elderly.

Air Encephalography. Air encephalography carries more risk than angiography for patients with trauma because a change in pressure relationships in the head may precipitate an unfavorable shift in the brain with serious consequences. Nevertheless, a ventriculogram is sometimes helpful and is conveniently performed at the time of skull trephination if a clot is suspected but not readily located.

Management of Acute Head Injury. Bleeding from lacerations of the scalp is rarely sufficient by itself to cause hypovolemic shock. Consequently a patient with a head injury who is in shock is likely to have occult hemorrhage elsewhere, such as in the abdomen or retroperitoneal space. Scalp lacerations are best repaired in the emergency room before roentgenograms are obtained in order to control bleeding and to prevent infection. This is the time to initiate baseline observations of vital signs and neurologic status and to examine the patient for associated injuries of the skeleton, viscera, and soft tissues. Prophylaxis against tetanus is administered, as are antimicrobial agents if open fractures are present.

Respiration. A number of steps may be taken to reduce edema in the brain after an injury. The most important is the establishment of an adequate airway. Hypoxia and hypocarbia have grave consequences on cerebral homeostasis as outlined earlier. If a stuporous patient is unable to clear his own airway, the simple procedure of tracheostomy is often life-saving and should be performed promptly.

Blood gases should be monitored even in patients who appear to be respiring adequately, because pulmonary edema and shunting in the lung, described above, may result in low values of arterial Po_2 that the administration of oxygen can correct. When spontaneous respirations cease, even if cardiac action continues, death is inevitable, and mechanical ventilation is unavailing.

Opiates and sedatives are avoided for patients with injuries to the head. These drugs further depress an already damaged nervous system, impair respirations, and increase stupor. Urinary retention often accounts for restlessness in drowsy patients and is readily treated by catheterization.

Blood and Fluid Replacement. Motor vehicle accidents commonly result in multiple injuries. Hypovolemic shock occurs and is best treated by the ordinary measures except that the head-low position is avoided if the brain is damaged. Elevation of the extremities increases the return of blood to the heart without contributing to cerebral edema.

Cerebral swelling is increased when hypotonic fluids are administered. Fiver per cent dextrose in water becomes hypotonic as the sugar is metabolized, and therefore should not be given in large quantities. Isotonic saline is less hazardous because sodium chloride passes the blood-brain barrier poorly. Consequently, fluids are mildly restricted for patients with brain injury, and more saline is employed than in ordinary practice.

Patients with head injury sometimes develop inappropriate secretions of antidiuretic hormone with consequent water intoxication, even if fluids are replaced with care. The resulting symptoms of stupor and seizures are often mistakenly attributed to extensive parenchymal damage. Water intoxication is confirmed by demonstrating a serum sodium of 120 mEq. per liter or less. Hypertonic saline quickly improves the condition, but water may also have to be restricted if the abnormal secretion of antidiuretic hormone continues.

Occasionally trauma damages homeostatic centers in the hypothalamus so that diabetes insipidus results. A patient who is alert ordinarily will drink enough to prevent dehydration. However, if osmoreceptor mechanisms are also disturbed or the subject is in stupor with a lack of thirst, serum hyperosmolarity with high electrolyte levels occurs if adequate fluids are not administered. Replacement of water, restriction of salt, and administration of Pitressin are indicated until the condition corrects itself, as it usually does.

Severe injuries to the brain are sometimes associated with impaired renal function despite the absence of shock, or a reaction to blood transfusion, or other common causes of damage to the renal tubules. Characteristically the output of urine remains good, but the specific gravity is fixed at 1.010, albuminuria is present, and the sediment contains red cells, white cells, and casts. Death from renal failure may occur in spite of treatment. The mechanism of the renal damage is not entirely clear, but stimulation of certain cortical areas and destructive lesions in the hypothalamus cause similar renal lesions in laboratory animals.

Osmotic Diuretics. By administering a hypertonic solution it is possible to establish an osmotic gradient across the blood-brain barrier that removes water from the brain and reduces cerebral edema. Drugs that penetrate the brain slowly are employed, such as a 30 per cent solution of urea in 10 per cent invert sugar or 20 per cent mannitol given intravenously or glycerin given by mouth.

Osmotic diuretics are avoided if possible in acute injuries because a swollen brain may tamponade torn vessels and prevent a large clot from developing. Unfortunately, even after the risk of active bleeding is passed, hypertonic solutions are rarely of benefit if substantial damage to the parenchyma has occurred. If the brain is relatively intact but is compressed by a hematoma, transient improvement is often observed. Osmotic diuretics are of value in operations for chronic intracranial hematomas; occasionally rapidly developing edema in brain following removal of a compressing hematoma precipitates transtentorial herniation. Increasing the osmolarity of the blood can prevent this dangerous sequence of events.

Steroids. Steroids effectively reduce cerebral edema and are used when intracranial pressure persists for several days, a circumstance that limits the utility of the osmotic diuretics. Doses equivalent to more than 1000 mg. of cortisone daily are employed; dexamethasone, which has less salt-retaining property, is frequently prescribed in doses of 16 to 40 mg. daily. The substantial incidence of pituitary necrosis in severe head injury is an additional reason to administer steroids. However, the hoped-for benefits are often unrealized if structural damage to the brain is extensive.

Hypothermia. Hypothermia is sometimes used to treat cerebral edema and to diminish the oxygen requirement of the brain after an injury. Experience has shown that life is prolonged for a time by hypothermia, but the ultimate mortality is not reduced nor is the extent of the neurologic deficit lessened. Therefore, cooling is ordinarily used only to correct a fever that has resulted from intracranial bleeding, infection, or injury to temperature regulatory centers.

COMPLICATIONS OF HEAD INJURY

Cranial Nerve Injury. Damage may occur to the cranial nerves as they exit from the skull. Among the more common complications, anosmia and blindness are often permanent in contrast to extraocular palsies and facial paralysis, which usually improve.

Depressed Fractures. The incidence of epilepsy is 30 per cent or more after depressed fractures and penetrating wounds, but the risk is reduced if the fracture is elevated, and fragments of bone and other foreign bodies are promptly removed. As seizures may occur even if the site of fracture is remote from the motor areas of the cerebral cortex, all depressed fractures should be elevated except possibly a small depression over a major venous sinus. If a laceration of the scalp overlies a depressed fracture, antimicrobial agents are administered to prevent the occurrence of osteomyelitis and intracranial infection.

Debridement of a depressed fracture or penetrating missile wound often leaves an unsightly cranial defect that a properly executed cranioplasty will correct. The current use of synthetic materials such as tantalum, acrylic plastic, and stainless steel has simplified this operation and improved its cosmetic results. Some have thought that cranioplasty both ameliorates such subjective symptoms as headache and giddiness and reduces the frequency of convulsive seizures, but properly controlled studies do not bear this out.

Basilar Skull Fracture and Cerebrospinal Fluid Fistula. Because they are often not visible on skull roentgenograms, basilar fractures are usually diagnosed by clinical signs such as anosmia, Battle's sign, bilateral periorbital ecchymoses, and the drainage of blood or cerebrospinal fluid from the nose or ears. Cerebrospinal fluid can be distinguished from a mucoid nasal discharge by testing for sugar, which can be done conveniently with the paper test strips used in urine analysis. Patients with cerebrospinal fluid fistulas should be treated prophylactically with antimicrobial agents to prevent meningitis until the leak stops, as it does in 75 per cent of cases of rhinorrhea and almost all cases of otorrhea. The ear or nose should not be probed or packed, and sealing of the leak may be hastened by repeated lumbar punctures in which 30 ml. or more of cerebrospinal fluid is withdrawn. A fistula which persists more than 10 to 14 days demands surgical repair.

Epilepsy. The incidence of epilepsy after head injury varies with the severity of the injury to the brain. Seizures occur in 40 per cent of patients who sustain penetrating missile wounds, but follow only 10 per cent of the blunt injuries characteristic of civilian life. Depressed skull fracture is associated with an increased incidence of epilepsy, which reaches 40 per cent if accompanied by evidence of severe brain damage such as traumatic amnesia lasting more than 24 hours. Elevation of the depressed fracture, debridement of the wound, and prevention of the infection can reduce this toll.

The first convulsive seizure occurs within the first week following injury in 95 per cent of cases. These early seizures are typically focal motor in type and many do not recur. Late epilepsy, meaning seizures which occur after the first week, has a more ominous prognosis. It is treated by anticonvulsants. Fortunately in many patients the attacks decrease in frequency as the years pass and ultimately stop in one half of cases. A persistent, debilitating convulsive disorder can sometimes be improved by surgical excision of the epileptogenic focus.

Intracranial Hematomas. Both increasing edema and an enlarging hematoma cause neurologic signs that progress. As the two are difficult to distinguish, progressive signs are a justifiable reason in any patient to search for a clot by angiography or trephination of the skull.

Epidural Hematoma. Although small amounts of blood are often found in extradural space after fracture of the skull, large hematomas are uncommon, occurring in only 1 or 2 per cent of injuries to the head. Despite their rarity, epidural hematomas are important because they are potentially fatal, yet proper treatment is followed by recovery with little or no neurologic deficit if the brain has not sustained other injuries.

Epidural hematomas most frequently occur in the temporal region from a tear in the middle meningeal artery but are sometimes found in the frontal parietal, occipital, and suboccipital areas. Typically, a patient receives a blow on the temple that results in transitory unconsciousness. After a lucid interval of a few minutes or hours the expanding clot causes headache, drowsiness, contralateral hemiparesis, and paralysis of the ipsilateral third cranial nerve. Signs of decompensation of the brainstem soon follow, and death results.

The classic case is easily recognized but not often encountered. The patient may relate that the blow was light and unconsciousness brief. His prompt recovery and normal roentgenograms apparently substantiate the unimportance of the injury. Yet, an epidural hematoma may be present, may reach a critical size some hours later, and death may ensue if the patient has been sent home with inadequate observation.

Variations from the typical pattern are common. An associated serious brain injury may cause the patient to remain stuporous without the lucid interval, or symptoms may be delayed several days if the bleeding is slow or intermittent. Progressive coma without localizing signs is the rule with clots over the cerebellum, and occasionally occurs with supratentorial clots. At times a hematoma is missed at operation, especially in children in whom the dura adheres to the suture lines of the skull and restricts the spread of blood over the convexity.

About 40 per cent of patients with epidural hematoma die or are permanently incapacitated. Because the hematoma often occurs in patients with other severe injuries to the brain, some morbidity doubtless is inevitable. But the gratifying recovery that may follow surgery justifies a meticulous evaluation of every patient with severe head injury in a search for this infrequently occurring intracranial clot.

Subdural Hematoma. Subdural hematomas are conveniently divided into categories of acute, subacute, and chronic, which differ in both symptomatology and prognosis. A subdural hematoma is called acute when a rapid progression of symptoms leads to its discovery within hours or a day or two after the injury. Prospects for recovery depend on the severity of the associated brain damage. The fatality rate is 90 per cent in patients whose symptoms warrant operation within 12 hours of injury, but the outlook is much improved if the need for surgery is evident only after several days have passed.

Chronic Subdural Hematoma. Chronic subdural hematoma in adults usually occurs after the age of 50 and often in alcoholics because of their unsteadiness and frequent falls. With age the brain shrinks away from the dural lining of the skull and leaves a space that can fill with blood if a fragile vein should tear. The trauma that initiates the bleeding is often trivial and even forgotten when symptoms commence several weeks later. Headache occurs in 90 per cent of cases. Even if a confused patient denies it, the family may testify to his earlier complaints of pain or to his increased consumption of aspirin. Fatigue and irritability are insidiously followed by drowsiness, urinary incontinence, and stupor, which may be erroneously attributed to a natural deterioration in senescence. Hemianopsia, hemiparesis, or pupillary abnormality are observed in less than half the cases. Lumbar puncture usually reveals normal pressure, but in 50 per cent of cases the fluid is xanthochromic. Bruises about the head are frequently present, but a fracture of the skull is identified in only one third of cases, and a calcified pineal is displaced in only one fifth.

The patient usually deteriorates at an irregular rate. Intervals of substantial improvement interrupt the gradual decline and give hope of recovery, but sudden decompensation and unexpected death may occur.

Small clots may be tolerated or occasionally resorbed, but a persistent mass causes edema and irreversible anoxic-ischemic demyelination of the underlying brain. Subdural hematomas are therefore best treated by surgical drainage. The diagnosis, when suspected, is readily confirmed by arteriography or trephination. The results of treatment are good except that irreversible effects of pressure on the brain may leave a noticeable defect in mentation after recovery, particularly in elderly patients. If treatment is delayed until stupor signals dysfunction of the brainstem, evacuation of the clot and the administration of steroids and osmotic diuretics may be unable to reverse progressive transtentorial herniation which results in death.

Intracerebral Hematoma. Scattered petechial hemorrhages are commonly observed in fatal injuries to the brain, but large parenchymal hematomas occur in only 1 to 2 per cent of cases and are usually located in the frontal or temporal lobes or, less frequently, in the occipito-parietal region or cerebellum. The diagnosis is difficult because stupor from associated concussion or contusions may mask the focal neurologic signs produced by the hematoma. The mass is best demonstrated by arteriography, following which it can be removed through a small craniotomy. The results of surgery are often disappointing because the hemorrhage has destroyed sufficient cerebral tissue to leave a substantial neurologic deficit.

Vascular Complications. A blow to the head may rupture the carotid artery within the cavernous sinus and establish a *carotid-cavernous sinus fistula*. The arterial pressure dilates the tributaries of the sinus such as the orbital veins, with the result that the eye protrudes and pulsates, a bruit is usually heard, and chemosis and extraocular palsies occur. Altered arterial circulation to the eye causes loss of vision and, eventually, blindness. If the fistula is small, the symptoms may progress slowly, but spontaneous cure is uncommon. Repair by a direct approach through the cavernous sinus is not often attempted because of the threat of serious bleeding and injury to the nerves supplying the extraocular muscles. Ligation of the carotid artery in the neck or trapping of the fistula by proximal and distal ligation of the carotid artery are sometimes successful. Good results have been obtained by occluding the carotid artery distal to the cavernous sinus and then floating fragments of muscle up the artery to plug the fistula.

Trauma about the head occasionally leads to *thrombosis of the internal carotid artery* in the neck, resulting in hemiplegia. Less frequently, *thrombosis of the middle cerebral artery* by a dissecting aneurysm accounts for an unexpected paralysis several days after the injury.

Depressed fractures may cause *occlusion of the superior longitudinal sinus*, blocking venous drainage from the cerebral hemispheres and thereby raising intracranial pressure and causing the rapid appearance of papilledema and hemorrhages in the ocular fundus. Patients display paralysis of both lower limbs and often of one or both upper limbs.

Infection. Osteomyelitis of the skull, meningitis, and abscesses of the brain occasionally complicate open injuries of the head, and may recur for years after the injury. Antimicrobial therapy and proper debridement of the wound greatly reduce the incidence of these infectious complications.

Cerebral Swelling. From time to time aggressive surgery has been proposed to treat patients with serious injuries to the head. Some have reasoned that removal of large areas of the skull or resection of an edematous, contused temporal lobe might allow room for swelling and thus tide the patient over the acute effects of the trauma. Others have recommended that the tentorium be sectioned to relieve pressure on the brainstem by a temporal lobe that has herniated through the tentorial notch. Occasionally a patient seems to benefit from one of these procedures, but the general experience has been that they reduce neither morbidity nor mortality.

Cerebral Fat Embolism. Fat embolism is an infrequent complication observed after severe trauma in which a long bone is fractured, or occurs occasionally with just extensive soft tissue injury. Symptoms start between 12 and 48 hours after the accident, a frequent history is that a patient has remained comatose after general anesthesia to reduce a fractured extremity. Cerebral symptoms and signs consist of rapidly progressive stupor often associated with extensor plantar responses and decerebrate posturing but with preservation of pupillary responses. Petechiae may appear on the chest and in the conjunctivae; dyspnea, tachypnea, and cyanosis are evidence that the lungs are affected. The diagnosis is best made by bedside examination, but the finding of fat globules in urine and sputum can lend laboratory support to the clinical impression.

Although cerebral fat embolism has an ominous prognosis, some patients recover even after long periods of coma. Treatment consists of the usual measures to reduce cerebral edema; recently the use of low molecular weight dextran and alpha adrenergic blockade has been suggested.

Prognosis in Severe Head Injuries. The young tolerate severe head trauma better than the elderly. One study showed that patients over 50 years of age failed to recover satisfactorily from traumatic coma of more than 5 days' duration; those between 20 and 50 years were unlikely to be restituted after coma of 13 days' duration; but patients less than age 20 sometimes recovered from coma lasting several weeks.

Some patients remain in the unresponsive but alert-appearing state termed *coma vigil* or *akinetic mutism;* at autopsy multiple lesions are likely to be present in the cerebral white matter, basal ganglia, corpus callosum, hippocampus and limbic system, but the most characteristic pathologic changes are found in the periaqueductal gray matter of the rostral brainstem.

Less severely damaged patients profit from intensive care in a rehabilitation center where their physical, emotional, and social disabilities receive appropriate attention. Recovery from the injury continues for a long time, even several years. Ultimately 80 per cent can be returned to work, but others remain handicapped by permanent neurologic defects. Even some who appear to make a good recovery have subtle defects in memory, concentration, and comprehension which prevent their achieving their expected potential at work. Others manifest distressing psychopathology ranging from mildly asocial behavior through psychosis or dementia.

INJURIES OF THE SPINE

The Cervical Spine. Forced flexion of the cervical spine often compresses the vertebral bodies, dislocates a vertebra forward on the one below, and interlocks the articular facets. Either the squeeze between the upper lamina and the lower body or displaced fragments of bone or intervertebral disc then compress the spinal cord. A prolapsed intervertebral disc does not usually damage the cord in a flexion injury unless the force is sufficient to cause a fracture-dislocation as well.

Flexion injuries tend to block circulation in the branches of the anterior spinal artery as the result of either direct pressure or injury to the radicular or vertebral arteries in the intervertebral foramen. The resulting ischemic injury is most severe in the central portion of the spinal cord. Actual thrombosis of the anterior spinal artery is rarely observed.

Hyperextension of the neck, on the other hand, buckles the ligamentum flavum forward, pinching the cord, especially if an arthritic spur bridges the interspace anteriorly. Several centimeters of the central portion of the cord can be damaged by such an injury even though roentgenograms of the spine remain normal. The upper limbs are left weaker than the lower, and a variable loss of sensation occurs with relative sparing of touch, position, and vibration sense. Bleeding into the central cord (hematomyelia) may complicate the injury and has similar clinical effects.

Patients with injury to the cervical spine must

be handled carefully to prevent an unfavorable shift of the fracture-dislocation from further damaging the spinal cord. A conscious patient usually gives warning of his plight, but the possibility of an unstable spine is easily overlooked if the patient is unconscious. A gentle pull on the head in line with the spine is advisable to keep traction on the neck whenever the patient is moved. Spine boards to which the head and trunk can be strapped commonly are used to protect the spinal cord when removing a patient from a wrecked automobile. If one is not available, a bulky wrapping about the neck which supports the chin and occiput will help reduce motion that might be dangerous. A firm board or a door makes a better litter than a sagging canvas stretcher that flexes the neck. Roentgenograms are best obtained on the litter to avoid the manipulation of a transfer to the x-ray table.

The primary treatment of fracture-dislocation of the cervical spine is traction with tongs or wires inserted in the skull to achieve and maintain the reduction. The pull should be in the line of the spine, and weights exceeding 30 pounds should be avoided to prevent a sudden shift from causing further damage.

After reduction is obtained, traction can be continued for six weeks, following which the patient is ambulated in a collar that is worn for three months. An acceptable alternative that shortens the period of immobilization is to perform an operation at which loose fragments of bone and disc are removed and the vertebral bodies fused anteriorly. Atlantoaxial dislocations are characteristically unstable and are appropriately treated by early fusion of the first three cervical vertebrae.

The Thoracolumbar Spine. Hyperflexion in a fall characteristically causes compression of one or more vertebral bodies between T-12 and L-3. Unless neoplasm or osteoporosis has softened the bone, a heavy direct blow is needed to fracture the midthoracic vertebrae.

Hyperextension, plaster jackets, and operation were formerly used in an often futile effort to restore a normal roentgenographic appearance to the fractured spine. At present the deformity of a stable fracture is accepted and treated by bed rest until the pain subsides; this is followed by progressive ambulation. The occasional unstable fracture-dislocation requires open reduction and fusion.

Surgical Decompression. Whether surgical decompression restores function to a traumatized spinal cord is a matter of controversy. Almost no patient with a complete loss of motor power and sensation that persists more than 24 hours ever regains much useful function regardless of treatment. On the other hand, if a trace of motion or persistent sensation confirms that the cord has been only partially interrupted, surprising improvement may take place and may continue as long as two years, even without surgery.

All agree that the rare patient who shows progression of the neurologic defect after an injury should have a decompressive operation. Surgical debridement and closure prevent a spinal fluid fistula in open fractures, and possibly damaged nerve roots of the cauda equina benefit from decompression. At the present time many patients with fracture dislocation of the cervical spine are operated upon by the anterior approach to achieve decompression of the cord and fusion of the vertebral bodies. The results are difficult to assess because of the relatively good prognosis without surgery when the damage to the cord is incomplete, and a conservative approach is usually justified.

Brawley, B. W., and Kelly, W. A.: Treatment of basal skull fracture with and without cerebrospinal fluid fistulae. J. Neurosurg., 26:57, 1967.

Carlsson, C. A., von Essen, C., and Lofgren, J.: Factors affecting the clinical course of patients with severe head injury. Part 1: Influence of biological factors. Part 2: Significance of post traumatic coma. J. Neurosurg., 29:242, 1968.

Drake, C. G.: Cervical spinal-cord injury. J. Neurosurg., 19:487, 1962.

Ducker, T. B., Simmons, R. L., and Anderson, R. W.: Increased intracranial pressure and pulmonary edema. Part 3: The effect of increased intracranial pressure on the cardiovascular hemodynamics of chimpanzees. J. Neurosurg., 29:475, 1968.

Froman, C.: Alterations of respiratory function in patients with severe head injuries. Brit. J. Anaesth., 40:354, 1968.

Kornblum, R. N., and Fisher, R. S.: Pituitary lesions in craniocerebral injuries. Arch. Path. (Chicago), 88:242, 1969.

Lewin, W.: Vascular lesions in head injuries. Brit. J. Surg., 55:321, 1968.

Marshall, W. J. S., Jackson, J. L. F., and Langfitt, T. W.: Brain swelling caused by trauma and arterial hypertension: Hemodynamic aspects. Arch. Neurol. (Chicago), 21:545, 1969.

Perret, G.: Anterior interbody fusion in the treatment of cervical fracture dislocation. Arch. Surg. (Chicago), 96:530, 1968.

Stuteville, P., and Welch, K.: Subdural hematoma in the elderly person. J.A.M.A., 168:1445, 1958.

Symonds, C.: Concussion and its sequelae. Lancet, 1:1, 1962.

Walker, A. E., Caveness, W. F., and Critchley, M.: The Late Effects of Head Injury. Conference Proceedings. Springfield, Ill., Charles C Thomas, 1969.

White, R. J., Vedura, J., and Locke, G. E.: Emergency cerebral angiography in acute head injury. Angiology, 17:72, 1966.

SEVERE SPINAL CORD DYSFUNCTION AND PARAPLEGIA

Many disorders, including spinal trauma, neoplasms, acute myelitis, poliomyelitis, and multiple sclerosis, can result in extensive spinal paralysis and cause similar problems in care and in the management of complications.

Antimicrobial agents and improved medical care have greatly reduced the mortality among patients with paraplegia or other forms of extensive spinal paralysis. Life expectancy is related to the severity of the neurologic deficit. Patients who are partially paraplegic have a mortality which approaches the normal population; partial quadriplegia carries a mortality twice normal, complete paraplegia four times the normal, and complete quadriplegia twelve times the normal.

Prognosis. The degree of independence that a paraplegic achieves largely depends on how many muscle groups escape paralysis. The lower the spinal level of the injury or disease, the more skills a well motivated patient can develop if good care prevents the complications of muscle spasm, decubitus ulcers, and infection of the urinary tract.

An understanding of how much recovery is possible sets goals and supplies a yardstick with which to measure progress during rehabilitation. The patient with a complete or extensive lesion of the spinal cord just below C-5 retains innervation of the neck musculature and some of the shoulder girdle. He is unable to move in bed, and becomes easily fatigued because of poor respiratory reserve, but he may be able to feed himself with special equipment. With lesions of the lower cervical cord, function of more muscles of the upper limb is preserved; thus, the patient is able to roll over, sit up, propel a wheelchair and possibly learn a job at home that does not require strength and dexterity of the hands. He depends upon an attendant for most of his needs.

High levels of thoracic spinal cord injury leave a functional upper limb, but the trunk is unstable, and intercostal breathing is not possible. The patient can transfer to and from a wheelchair, but even with bracing cannot develop a useful gait. Lower thoracic injuries, which leave a strong pectoral girdle and good respiratory reserve, permit the patient to be independent in all his daily activities. Bracing is still cumbersome, and ambulation is generally not practical.

Patients with lesions at T-12 to L-3 can usually walk in long leg braces and even negotiate stairs, but depend heavily on wheelchairs. Even with an injury below L-3 a patient may sometimes use a wheelchair because such acts as arising from the sitting position, climbing steps, and standing for prolonged periods are difficult.

Emotional Aspects. Severe depression may accompany the realization that paralysis and partial dependency are permanent. Progress in rehabilitation is slowed, and recently learned skills may be temporarily lost, but emotional support from the hospital staff does much to reduce the depth and length of the depression. The environment of a center where others face and overcome similar hurdles also bolsters the morale of the paraplegic.

Cardiorespiratory System. Injuries in the cervical region paralyze the intercostal muscles and leave only diaphragmatic respiration. Exercise quickly results in dyspnea, so that the usefulness of a hand-driven wheelchair or braces for walking is limited.

Interruption of motor pathways in the cervical spinal cord isolates the thoracic sympathetic centers from higher control. Consequently, the patient cannot constrict peripheral arteries when he sits or stands. Blood pools in the limbs and viscera, thus reducing venous return to the heart, and even elastic supports cannot adequately compensate.

Venostasis in the lower limbs also accounts for a higher incidence of pulmonary embolus in paraplegics who are confined to bed.

Gastrointestinal System and Nutrition. Paralytic ileus commonly follows spinal injury or acute poliomyelitis for a few days. In treatment oral feedings should be omitted until bowel activity returns. If abdominal distention occurs, a nasogastric tube is advisable to decompress the intestinal tract.

Most paraplegics eventually begin to defecate without an enema. However, fecal impactions are frequent in patients with acute spinal paralysis, so that stool softeners, gentle laxatives, or low enemas may be needed at first. As recovery progresses a regular dietary schedule and adequate fluids are important to achieve spontaneous evacuation. Some patients initiate reflex evacuation by abdominal massage or digital stimulation of the rectum.

Adequate nutrition is imperative for recovery but is difficult to attain, particularly for patients confined to bed. A diet high in protein and calories helps repair injured tissue and prevent bedsores. A reasonable goal at first is 2000 to 2500 calories daily, although this may have to be lowered later to avoid obesity. During the early months the daily calcium intake should be kept below 0.5 gram to minimize the likelihood of urinary calculus. Transfusions to correct anemia and low blood volume in poorly nourished patients are often beneficial.

Skin. Decubitus ulcers are a serious problem for paraplegics and can occur in any paralyzed, immobilized patient who is neglected. The danger of an anesthetic region is that it tolerates continuous pressure without the pain that ordinarily prompts a shift in position. After about two hours of immobility ischemic changes begin in the subcutaneous tissue and are manifested by erythema of the overlying skin. Repeated ischemic insults are followed by ulceration.

Bedsores can be prevented by turning the patient at least every two hours, protecting reddened skin from further pressure, and maintaining adequate nutrition. Alternating air mattresses and rotating frame beds help to vary pressure points but are not by themselves guarantees against ulcers forming over the occiput, heels, trochanters, and sacrum. The weight of bedding is sometimes sufficient to erode the tips of the toes. Plaster casts over anesthetic areas may ulcerate the skin, and even supporting braces are dangerous.

Bedsores that heal with scar tissue remain particularly vulnerable to pressure. Therefore, the most satisfactory coverage of a sizable decubitis ulcer is obtained by rotating pedicle tissue into the defect after trimming off any underlying bony prominence.

Musculoskeletal System. Many operations and mechanical devices have been used to compensate for paralyzed muscles. Crutches, braces, or wheelchairs restore mobility. An automatic lift enables anyone to transfer a patient from bed to chair. Bracing or surgery can reconstruct the loss of pinch between the thumb and index finger and thus allow the patient to feed and shave himself.

Kyphosis or lordosis is a grave consequence of the unequal pull of partially paralyzed muscles that distorts the growing spine of a child. Spinal fusion halts progression of such deformity, and often can correct a moderate curvature. Good results have been reported with internal fixation of the spine to avoid the complications of plaster immobilization.

Although a certain amount of muscle spasm may help a paraplegic to support the trunk or to position an extremity, painful or recurrent spasms that forcibly flex or adduct the lower limbs interfere with sitting and ambulation and thus prevent rehabilitation. As flexor spasms are reflex responses, the first step is to remove sources of noxious, afferent stimuli such as infection of the bladder and bedsores. If these measures plus physical therapy fail, more drastic procedures may be required, such as myelotomy, excision of the distal end of the spinal cord, anterior rhizotomy, subthecal injections, peripheral neurotomy, or division of muscles and tendons. Any procedure that increases the neurologic deficit of an already paralyzed subject is undesirable. Accordingly, patients with flexor spasm who have residual motor or sensory function in the lower limbs are best treated by division of spastic muscle and tendons. Subthecal injections of alcohol or phenol are easily performed, but their neurologic effects are unpredictable, and relief may be inadequate or short-lasting. Myelotomy efficiently stops flexor spasms but increases the extent of the neurologic deficit, and removal of the spinal cord or anterior rhizotomy leaves all muscle groups flaccid, which is more suited for bedridden patients than for those who attempt ambulation.

Urinary Tract. Renal calculi, pyelonephritis, and hydronephrosis are the major causes of death in paraplegics and are sources of considerable disability in patients with lesser paralysis. These renal complications follow incomplete emptying of the bladder, which initially necessitates catheterization. Secondary infection and vesicoureteral reflux follow. These complications can be minimized by providing a low calcium diet, intermittently turning patients soon after the onset of paralysis, forcing fluids to achieve 1500 to 2000 ml. of daily urine output, and treating culturally proved urinary tract infections promptly — but not prophylactically — with antimicrobial drugs. During recovery, nearly all patients with poliomyelitis and about 80 per cent of paraplegics become able to void without catheterization. Patients with poliomyelitis regain essentially normal bladder function. In paraplegics with high lesions of the spinal cord, reflex micturition occurs, mediated through the distal spinal segments. If an injury has destroyed sacral roots, suprapubic pressure may be necessary to empty the bladder.

Regaining spontaneous voiding after spinal injury is always difficult. In many patients a fluid intake of 3000 to 4000 ml. daily and either intermittent catheterization or intermittent clamping of an indwelling catheter may establish spontaneous, automatic voiding. Intermittent catheterization using aseptic technique has given the best results as the urine remains sterile in three quarters of patients; if a catheter is left indwelling, one of the Gibbon type is preferred to the more irritating Foley. Some may need a transurethral resection of obstructing tissue at the bladder neck. If there is spastic hypertrophy of the bladder, especially with vesicoureteral reflux, satisfactory voiding usually cannot be obtained without partially interrupting the reflex arc. If there are no undesirable muscle spasms of the lower limbs, graded sacral rhizotomy is the most satisfactory procedure for enabling some patients to master bladder training. Anterior rhizotomy of the lumbar roots or excision of the conus is reserved for patients with disabling spasticity of both the bladder and lower limbs. The more extensive procedures will also relieve autonomic hyperreflexia manifested by unpleasant episodes of sweating, hypertension, and headache triggered by contraction of bladder, bowel, or skeletal muscle.

Even patients who have apparently established satisfactory micturition may have slowly progressive hydronephrosis that, if unrecognized, will eventually cause death. Consequently, all patients should be evaluated periodically by intravenous pyelography. Progressive renal damage is an indication for urinary diversion, usually by implantation of the ureters into an ilial conduit.

Garrett, A. L., Perry, J., and Nickel, V. L.: Traumatic quadriplegia. J.A.M.A., 187:7, 1964.

Kilfoyle, R. M., Foley, J. J., and Norton, P. L.: Spine and pelvic deformity in childhood and adolescent paraplegia. J. Bone Joint Surg. [Amer.], 47-A:659, 1965.

Kottke, F. J., Kubicek, W. G., Olson, M. E., and Hastings, R. H.: Studies on the parameters of cardiovascular performance of quadriplegic patients. Arch. Phys. Med., 44:635, 1963.

Long, C., II, and Lawton, E. B.: Functional significance of spinal cord lesion level. Arch. Phys. Med., 6:249, 1965.

Misak, S. J., Bunts, R. E., Ulmer, J. L., and Eagles, W. M.: Nerve interruption procedures in the urologic management of paraplegic patients. J. Urol., 88:392, 1962.

Moyes, P. D.: Longitudinal myelotomy for spasticity. J. Neurosurg., 31:615, 1969.

Proceedings of the Sixteenth Annual Clinical Spinal Cord Injury Conference, September 27–29, 1967. Veterans Administration Hospital, Long Beach, California. Washington, D.C., U.S. Government Printing Office.

Degenerative and Heredofamilial Diseases of the Central Nervous System

Donald J. Reis

MOTOR NEURON DISEASE

The motor neuron diseases are a group of disorders of the motor system of unknown etiology whose principal pathology is a degeneration of lower motor neurons in spinal cord and brainstem. Clinically, several distinctive syndromes can be recognized on the basis of heredity, age of onset, and course and associated signs, particularly of upper motor neuron dysfunction. These syndromes are amyotrophic lateral sclerosis, progressive muscular atrophy, including the infantile, juvenile, and adult forms, and the Mariana type of amyotrophic lateral sclerosis. In the absence of any knowledge of the etiology of the disorders, a clinical classification is useful, particularly because each nosologic entity tends to be true to type. However, cases intermediate to the major groups are occasionally found so that in "atypical" cases classification may be difficult.

AMYOTROPHIC LATERAL SCLEROSIS

Definition. Amyotrophic lateral sclerosis is a chronic progressive disease of the nervous system of unknown etiology. It is usually sporadic but rarely familial, and is characterized pathologically by degeneration of motor neurons in the spinal cord and the lower brainstem, and often of Betz cells in the motor cortex. Clinically, it appears in its usual form as a disturbance in motility, reflecting dysfunction of both lower and upper motor neurons.

Pathology. On gross inspection, the most obvious abnormality of the spinal cord is thinning of the ventral roots and reduction of the size of the cervical enlargement. In the brain, atrophy of the hypoglossal nerve and occasionally of the precentral gyrus is evident. Microscopically, there is a diffuse pallor of myelin staining, most noticeable in the lateral columns of the spinal cord, the bulbar pyramids, and the anterior limb of the internal capsule. Loss or degeneration of neurons occurs in the ventral horns and in the nuclei of some cranial nerves. The motor nucleus of the trigeminal nerve and nuclei of the facial and hypoglossal nerves are particularly involved. Affected muscles show the typical features of neurogenic atrophy with intermingling of small, atrophic muscle fibers and fibers of normal size. The structure and staining of the affected fibers are preserved until late in the disease when they finally disappear, leaving residual clumps of hyperchromatic sarcolemmal nuclei.

Clinical Manifestations. Amyotrophic lateral sclerosis is a disorder of later life with a peak incidence in the fifth and sixth decades. It is slightly more common in men than in women and is found in all races and on all continents. It has been estimated that in the United States there are about 3000 new cases occurring annually and a total of about 8000 to 10,000 persons afflicted with the disease at any given time. The clinical picture of the disorder reflects the underlying pathologic changes of the lower and upper motor neurons. Lower motor neuron dysfunction causes weakness and wasting of the afflicted muscles. An additional consequence of the disease process may be a spontaneous irregular discharge of motor neurons, reflected peripherally by irregular twitchings in the distribution of one or several motor units. This is termed fasciculation. Fasciculations may be observed as continuous movements of portions of muscles anywhere in the body and may be perceived by the patient. Characteristically, fasciculations are widely distributed, extending beyond the territory of a single nerve root or peripheral nerve, and are ominous when associated with weakness. Involvement of the upper motor neuron leads to spastic rigidity, augmented deep tendon reflexes, and extensor plantar responses. When the corticobulbar tracts are involved bilaterally, the syndrome of *pseudobulbar palsy* may ensue. In this state, voluntary swallowing, tongue movements, or facial mimicry may be impaired. In addition, the patient may have episodes of inappropriate crying or laughing which are often provoked by an innocuous stimulus and are dissociated from feelings of excessive sadness or mirth.

There are several clinical variations of the disease that depend upon the regional distribution and the relative involvement of lower and upper motor neurons. Most commonly the disease presents in the distal muscles of the upper limb. The anterior horn cells in the cervical region are the first affected, and this leads to the appearance of wasting and fasciculation in the upper limbs which is particularly obvious in the small muscles of the hand. Involvement of both lateral and medial thenar groups leads to the thumb falling into the plane of the palm of the hand—the "simian hand." Although bilaterally symmetrical in later stages, the disease may be unilateral or even hemiparetic early in its course. As the disease progresses, proximal muscles and then muscles of the trunk and bulb become weak. In some cases involvement of motor units in the leg may be the earliest sign of the disease. The disease may present as footdrop, which is confused in its earliest stage with palsy of the lateral peroneal nerve. As the signs of lower motor neuron dysfunction are progressing, some associated signs of upper motor neuron disease become evident, particularly in the lower extremities.

Less commonly, bulbar signs may predominate in the early stages of the disease, producing the syndrome of *progressive bulbar palsy*. The muscles of the palate, pharynx, and tongue are most commonly affected. Jaw movement and facial expression are impaired somewhat later. Extraocular movements are rarely involved in the disease. Involvement of the hypoglossal nucleus is an early sign, resulting in a slurring dysarthria and weakness of tongue movements. As the disease progresses, the tongue, small and shriveled, lies immobile but fasciculating in the floor of the mouth. The palatal and pharyngeal musculature becomes weak, and aphagia, nasal speech, and regurgitation of liquids result. Later there is often wasting of the facial muscles, especially the orbicularis oris, which may be coupled with the signs of pseudobulbar palsy. Usually some signs of involvement of upper or lower motor neuron innervation of the trunk and limbs are evident in later stages of the disease.

Rarely, the disease may present as a progressive spastic paraparesis in which the evident signs of the disorder can be attributed to dysfunction of the upper motor neuron. This form of the disease has sometimes been called *primary lateral sclerosis*. At this stage it is not possible to make the diagnosis of amyotrophic lateral sclerosis, and full investigation, particularly to exclude spinal cord compression, is mandatory. If there is no evidence of denervation, it is probably not amyotrophic lateral sclerosis. Only the subsequent development—perhaps a number of years later—of fasciculations, of electromyographic evidence of denervation, or of the characteristic pattern on muscle biopsy permits the proper diagnosis to be made with certainty. By then, the disease is no longer confined to the upper motor neuron.

Despite the massive involvement of upper and lower neurons of the cortical spinal system, there are no adventitious movements, signs of cerebellar dysfunction, sensory disturbances, or involvement of sphincteric function. In a few patients dementia may occur.

Diagnosis. In making the diagnosis of amyotrophic lateral sclerosis the only laboratory test of value is electromyography. A sampling of affected muscles will reveal a reduction in the number of motor units active on contraction, as well as fasciculations and fibrillation potentials which represent the electrophysiologic consequence of denervation. Nerve conduction velocities are normal until advanced stages of the disease. There are no characteristic changes in the blood chemistry or the cerebrospinal fluid. A muscle biopsy is useful in distinguishing between a neurogenic and myopathic process. However, the histologic findings in muscle are nonspecific for any neurogenic atrophy.

Differential Diagnosis. Because of the bleak prognosis of amyotrophic lateral sclerosis, it is imperative that all efforts be made to establish with certainty the diagnosis of the disease. The disease can be diagnosed without difficulty when presenting in its most typical form as progressive, painless, diffuse muscle weakness with atrophy, fasciculations, and an associated spasticity, enhanced stretch reflexes, and extensor plantar responses. In the earlier stages, when presenting as a more localized disease, it is necessary to distinguish amyotrophic lateral sclerosis from other conditions which may produce lower motor neuron dysfunction, particularly when signs of corticospinal tract involvement are evident. When presenting as localized wasting of muscles, particularly in the hand, the disease must be distinguished from *lesions of peripheral nerves*. Mononeuritis or multiple mononeuritis will have a distribution characteristic of the involved nerve or nerves, reduced or absent deep tendon reflexes, and sensory abnormalities in the territory of the sensory innervation of the nerve. The metabolic polyneuritides, such as diabetic polyneuritis, tend to involve the feet before the hands, and sensory abnormalities are common. Conduction velocity in those peripheral nerves that can be tested is commonly abnormal in these conditions. Polyneuritis of the Guillain-Barré variety will have a more rapid onset; it is unassociated with fasciculations and is usually accompanied by elevation of the cerebrospinal fluid protein. *Compression of the brachial plexus by cervical rib* may present itself with weakness and wasting of intrinsic muscles of the hand. The relatively static and localized nature of the disease, the presence of pain, and confirmatory roentgenographic evidence of bony abnormalities will establish the diagnosis. Compression of cervical or lumbar *nerve roots* by osteoarthritic spurs or a herniated intravertebral disc may result in painless wasting, and in limb muscles is often associated with fasciculations. A differential diagnosis from amyotrophic lateral sclerosis in this condition may be further complicated by evidence of spasticity in the extremities, occurring as a result of extradural compression of the spinal cord by bony ridges of the vertebra. Pain, sensory abnormalities, a fixed location of the defect, and localized EMG abnormalities, as well as the characteristic roentgenographic changes of the vertebral column, may help to establish this diagnosis. However, in some cases the differential diagnosis may be extremely difficult and may only be resolved by following the evolution of the disease. *Epidural compression* of the spinal cord by tumor, by arachnoidal thickening secondary to syphilis or other infectious processes of the meninges, or in cervical spondylosis may lead to segmental weakness, atrophy, and long tract signs in the legs. Most such lesions cause pain, and the fixed nature of the lower motor neuron disorder and the evidence on myelography of a compressive lesion of the cord can usually establish the diagnosis. *Intramedullary* lesions of the spinal cord, including tumors or syringomyelia, usually interrupt segmental reflex arcs and also produce sensory signs. The sensory loss may occasionally be of the dissociated type with selective loss of pain sensation and preservation of touch and deep sensibilities over several segments. When presenting as *bulbar palsy*, myasthenia gravis can be diagnosed by appropriate pharmacologic tests. The syndrome of *primary lateral sclerosis* is most commonly due not to amyotrophic lateral sclerosis, but to multiple sclerosis or spinal cord compression. Investigation of such a case must include careful cerebrospinal fluid examination and myelography. The diagnosis of motor neuron disease becomes established only when signs of lower motor neuron involvement are unequivocally demonstrated. *Benign fasciculations* or myokymia is a troublesome but innocuous syndrome of migrating or static fasciculations of skeletal muscles. It may be localized, often to one eyelid, or it can be more generalized. It is common in younger patients. The distinguishing feature in the differential diagnosis is that weakness or wasting of muscles does not occur with benign fasciculations. However, the overt fasciculations may alarm both the patient and unwary physicians, and may sometimes lead to a misguided clinical diagnosis of amyotrophic lateral sclerosis. However, such patients lack EMG evidence of muscle denervation. Degeneration of the lower motor neuron may occasionally occur as a remote effect of cancer on the nervous system, and is discussed under that topic.

Course and Prognosis. Amyotrophic lateral sclerosis almost always has a dismal prognosis. In most cases death occurs within three to four years after the onset of symptoms. There are atypical cases in which the condition may appear to become arrested with little or no progression of symptoms over many years. In general the prognosis is worse when the initial symptoms are bulbar; survival in these cases seldom exceeds two years. Inability to handle secretions and weakness of the respiratory muscles are the predisposing causes of the usual terminal event, bronchopneumonia.

Treatment. The absence of any treatment that could influence the course of motor neuron disease only increases the physician's responsibility for the symptomatic care of these patients. In advanced cases tracheostomy, may be indicated to prevent the patient from drowning in his own secretions. Tube feeding or gastrostomy may prolong survival.

THE MARIANA FORM OF AMYOTROPHIC LATERAL SCLEROSIS

In the early 1950's it was discovered that the Chamorro Indians in the Mariana Islands had an unusually high incidence of a disease very similar in both its clinical and pathologic features to amyotrophic lateral sclerosis. Subsequent studies have demonstrated that this disease deviates from the classic form of amyotrophic lateral sclerosis (1) clinically, by its appearance at a generally younger age, and (2) pathologically, by the presence, in most cases, of neurofibrillary changes and granulovacuolar bodies, an uncommon finding in sporadic cases. Of particular interest is the fact that 10 per cent of patients with the Mariana form of amyotrophic lateral sclerosis show evidence, in the course of the disease, of either dementia or extrapyramidal types of motor dysfunction, particularly parkinsonism. At present it has not been conclusively determined whether the disease is truly genetic or is caused by environmental factors. The clinical features of the disease and its prognosis are indistinguishable from the usual cases of amyotrophic lateral sclerosis.

THE PROGRESSIVE MUSCULAR ATROPHIES

PROGRESSIVE MUSCULAR ATROPHY OF INFANCY
(Werdnig-Hoffmann Disease)

Definition. Infantile progressive muscular atrophy is a heredofamilial disorder of early onset and progressive course, characterized pathologically by degeneration of anterior horn cells and bulbar motor nuclei, and clinically by signs of disease of the lower motor neuron.

Etiology. The etiology is unknown. It is, however, genetically determined and transmitted as an autosomal recessive trait.

Clinical Manifestations. The disease may begin in utero or in early or even late infancy. The features that draw attention to the disease are profound hypotonia and absence of volitional movements in an infant. An observant mother may note a lack of intrauterine movements, and soon after birth the infant, though bright and alert, is seen to lie immobile. The legs lie abducted and externally rotated at the hips and flexed at the knees. The arms hang limply at the sides. A few feeble movements may occur in the distal parts of the extremities. With handling the hypotonia is revealed. It may be so marked that when supported under the arms, the infant tends to slip through the examiner's hands. Painful stimuli are clearly appreciated, but there is little, if any, movement of withdrawal. The deep tendon and superficial reflexes are uniformly absent as a consequence of denervation. The limbs do not appear unduly thin, because the wasting of the muscles may be obscured by normal infant fat. Within a few months, weakness of the respiratory muscles leads to a characteristic retraction of the ribs on inspiration, and such accessory muscles as remain are brought into play. The disease spreads to involve the hypoglossal nuclei, and typical fasciculations of the tongue are observed. If life is prolonged beyond a year, contractures may occur, but death often supervenes before their advent. Less commonly, the paucity of movement is noted toward the end of the first year of life or even later when the child fails to stand or to talk at a normal age. In these cases the disease may be limited to the lower limbs, and the course may be slow. In general, the older the child at the onset of the disease, the more gradual its evolution. The natural rate of maturation of movement patterns may exceed the rate of destruction of anterior horn cells, so that apparent improvement occurs. Rarely, after development of paralysis, contractures, and wasting, the progress of the disease is apparently arrested for years. The occurrence of anterior horn cell disease during intrauterine life may result in *arthrogryposis multiplex congenita*, a clinical syndrome of multiple congenital contractures of the extremities that may also be caused by congenital muscular dystrophy, developmental defects of the spinal cord, intrauterine polyneuritis, or any disease which produces joint immobilization prenatally.

Differential Diagnosis. The diagnosis of the infantile form of progressive muscular atrophy is made on the basis of muscle biopsy and electromyographic findings, in addition to the clinical features of the disease. Generalized hypotonia may occur in a number of other disorders of infancy and lead to the syndrome of the "floppy infant." Malnutrition, chronic diseases, and lipidosis may all manifest hypotonia, which is also occasionally seen in retarded children. A small number of cases may be due to congenital myopathy, central core disease of muscle, or polyneuritis. In *benign congenital hypotonia*, unlike progressive muscular atrophy, there are spontaneous movements of the limb and reflexes that may be preserved. Recovery or improvement is the rule, and muscle biopsy shows no abnormality.

JUVENILE FORM OF PROGRESSIVE MUSCULAR ATROPHY
(Kugelberg-Welander Disease)

The juvenile form of progressive muscular atrophy may be inherited as an autosomal recessive or an autosomal dominant trait, and it has pathologic features similar to infantile spinal muscular atrophy. Indeed the presence of both diseases in members of a single family suggests that they may be variants on a continuum of motor neuron diseases.

Clinical Manifestations. The onset of the disease usually occurs in two peaks, in the preschool years or in adolescence. With an early onset there is no clear distinction from cases of infantile spinal muscular atrophy of late onset. When appearing in adolescence the clinical manifestations of the disease can be strikingly similar to those of the limb girdle form of muscular dystrophy. The initial complaint is usually clumsiness in walking. The gait is waddling and lordotic, and the child has

difficulty rising from the lying position. There is weakness and wasting of the proximal muscles of the legs and pelvic girdle, with relative preservation of the distal musculature. Weakness of the arms usually does not appear until several years later and is also proximal. Muscles innervated by the cranial nerves are often spared, with the exception of the sternomastoid. Fasciculations, when evident, help to establish the diagnosis as neurogenic. Deep tendon reflexes are impaired or lost in proportion to the muscular atrophy. Mental and sensory functions are unimpaired. Skeletal abnormalities, such as scoliosis, a high arched palate, or pes cavus, are sometimes seen. The course is long, and a number of patients are still able to walk more than 20 years after the onset of the disease. Many patients enjoy a normal life span despite this ailment.

Diagnosis. The diagnosis of neurogenic atrophy rather than muscular dystrophy can be made on the basis of the clinical history and of electromyographic and muscle biopsy findings characteristic of disease of the lower motor neuron.

ADULT FORMS OF PROGRESSIVE MUSCULAR ATROPHY

A number of patients have been described with progressive muscular atrophy with onset in adult life. The disorder may occur spontaneously or can be inherited as an autosomal dominant, recessive, or sex-linked trait.

Clinical Manifestations. In the familial form there is some interfamilial variation in the disease. In general, the disorder presents as progressive weakness, which may begin either proximally or distally, or rarely with preponderant involvement of the scapuloperoneal muscle groups. Bulbar involvement is variable. Weakness, atrophy, fasciculations, reduction or disappearance of deep tendon reflexes in the affected muscles, and the preservation of sensation are characteristic in this disorder as in other progressive muscular atrophies. Unlike amyotrophic lateral sclerosis, the course is prolonged and the prognosis generally favorable.

Diagnosis. The diagnosis of progressive muscular atrophy in the adult is clearly established when it presents as a familial disorder with clinical, electromyographic, and biopsy evidence of lower motor neuron disease. It is distinguished from rare familial forms of amyotrophic lateral sclerosis by the absence of any evidence of corticospinal tract disease, specifically spasticity, enhanced deep tendon reflexes, and extensor plantar responses. Sporadic cases of progressive muscular atrophy occur, although uncommonly, and present difficult diagnostic distinctions from amyotrophic lateral sclerosis early in the disease. The absence of both upper motor neuron dysfunction and a prolonged course marks these cases as different from that of the typical patient with amyotrophic lateral sclerosis. However, until a cause is found, it will not be possible to know whether such cases represent a separate disease or cases of amyotrophic lateral sclerosis with an uncommonly prolonged course.

Brody, J. A., and Chen, K.: Changing epidemiologic patterns of amyotrophic lateral sclerosis and parkinsonism-dementia on Guam. *In* Norris, F. H., Jr., and Kurland, L. T. (eds.): Motor Neuron Diseases. New York, Grune and Stratton, Inc., 1969, p. 61.

Dubowitz, V.: Infantile muscular atrophy, a prospective study with particular reference to a slowly progressive variety. Brain, 87:707, 1964.

Fenichel, G. M.: The spinal muscular atrophies. *In* Norris, F. H. Jr., and Kurland, L. T. (eds.): Motor Neuron Diseases. New York, Grune and Stratton, Inc., 1969, p. 122.

Kugelberg, E., and Welander, L.: Heredofamilial juvenile muscular atrophy. Arch. Neurol. Psychiat., 75:509, 1956.

Kurland, L. T., Choi, N. W., and Sayre, G. P.: Implications of incidence and geographic patterns on the classification of amyotrophic lateral sclerosis. *In* Norris, F. H., Jr., and Kurland, L. T. (eds.): Motor Neuron Diseases. New York, Grune and Stratton, Inc., 1969, p. 28.

THE SPINOCEREBELLAR DEGENERATIONS

The spinocerebellar degenerations are a group of closely related neurologic disorders, usually heredofamilial, but not infrequently sporadic, which manifest themselves clinically as progressive disorders of gait, posture, equilibrium, and movement. Pathologically they are characterized by a simple neuronal atrophy, affecting primarily the cerebellar cortex and peduncles, the inferior olivary nuclei, and the long motor and proprioceptive tracts of the spinal cord. Degeneration of the cerebral cortex, basal ganglia, anterior horn cells, and optic and peripheral nerves are sometimes associated, producing appropriate symptoms. The rich variety of signs and symptoms in this heterogeneous collection of disorders — over 50 "syndromes" may be found in the literature — reflect differences in the regional patterns of distribution of lesions as well as in age of onset and course. Certain neuropathologic and clinical forms of spinocerebellar degeneration are found more commonly than others. These have been recognized as single disease entities. However, even in families with the purest of clinical syndromes, some members may have a clinical disorder typical of another symptom complex. Because of intrafamilial variations in the clinical and pathologic manifestations, the spinocerebellar degenerations have been viewed as a continuum of inherited diseases linking the degenerative disorders of peripheral nerve at one extreme to those of the cerebral cortex at the other. The etiology of this group of diseases is unknown. In the absence of any identifiable biochemical defects it is not possible to state whether the varying clinical pictures are due to different biochemical abnormalities

THE SPINOCEREBELLAR DEGENERATIONS*

A. Spinal forms
  1. Friedreich's ataxia
  2. Roussy-Levy syndrome
  3. Hereditary spastic paraplegia
  4. Bassen-Kornzweig syndrome

B. Spinocerebellar forms
  1. Hereditary spastic ataxia
  2. Subacute spino-cerebellar degeneration (carcinogenic)

C. Cerebellar forms
  1. Olivopontocerebellar atrophy
  2. Cerebello-olivary degeneration
  3. Parenchymatous cerebellar degeneration (nutritional-toxic)
  4. Dyssynergia cerebellaris myoclonica

*Modified from Greenfield.

or just represent different expression of a common metabolic defect. A useful clinicopathologic classification of the spinocerebellar degeneration, modified from Greenfield, is presented in the accompanying table.

FRIEDREICH'S ATAXIA

Definition. Friedreich's ataxia is a heredofamilial disease of early onset. It is characterized pathologically by degeneration of the lateral corticospinal tract and the posterior columns and the spinocerebellar pathways in the spinal cord, and clinically by progressive ataxia, nystagmus, absent or diminished deep tendon reflexes, and extensor plantar responses.

Etiology. The disease is transmitted as an autosomal recessive, and rarely as a dominant trait, with equal incidence in both sexes.

Pathology. The disease predominantly affects the posterior columns and peripheral nerves, where there is a selective degeneration of the large primary sensory neurons, the spinocerebellar tracts, and the lateral corticospinal tracts. Degeneration of the axis cylinders and their myelin sheaths with gliosis occurs. In the posterior columns, the degeneration is most obvious in the middle root zone. There may be associated loss of nerve cells in the dorsal root ganglia, and less commonly in the retinal ganglion cell layer. There is often diffuse fibrosis and focal degeneration of the myocardium.

Clinical Manifestations. Friedreich's ataxia usually presents in the first decade of life as an abnormality of gait. At first, stumbling and awkwardness are seen, but as the disease progresses, the gait becomes markedly ataxic, with superimposed truncal titubation. Unsteadiness remains the most prominent and disabling symptom throughout the course of the disease. Later, ataxia in the arms and a progressive ataxic disorder of speech become evident. Words are unevenly scanned and syllables explosively uttered. As the disease progresses, the patient becomes confined to a chair and is unable to feed himself, and speech becomes unintelligible. Examination discloses signs referable to the three primary neuronal systems involved. Degeneration of the spinocerebellar pathways results in a profound ataxia of all extremities. Until its final stages, the disease is most pronounced in the lower limbs. Impairment of function of the posterior columns leads to a loss of position sense, particularly in the lower extremities, which may further aggravate the ataxia. Corticospinal tract dysfunction is indicated by extensor plantar responses. Spasticity is not a feature of the disease. Weakness, as a consequence of combined cerebellar and pyramidal tract dysfunction, is evident. Deep tendon reflexes at the ankle are usually lost; those in the arms are diminished, but those of the knees may be retained for considerable periods. Choreic and pseudoathetoid movements are sometimes observed. Nystagmus is almost invariably present and is usually horizontal, but vertical nystagmus is occasionally seen. Involvement of other neuronal symptoms occurs rather commonly. Primary optic atrophy and, rarely, retinitis pigmentosa are sometimes seen in afflicted members of some families. Intellectual impairment is not uncommon and can be progressive. Loss of anterior horn cells in cervical and lumbar enlargements of the spinal cord may, in rare cases, lead to distal wasting of the extremities, suggesting a link to familial amyotrophic lateral sclerosis. Conduction velocity measurements of motor fibers fall within the range of normal. Skeletal defects are commonly associated. Pes cavus with clawing of the toes may be evident before ataxia develops, and is thought by some to be caused by muscle imbalance. Kyphoscoliosis is usual as the disease develops. Cardiac abnormalities, including cardiac enlargement, murmurs, and congestive failure, are well recognized and may cause the patient's death. Bundle branch block, complete heart block, and inversion of the T-wave are the common electrocardiographic abnormalities. Patients with this disease have an unusually high incidence of diabetes mellitus.

Course and Prognosis. The usual course of Friedreich's ataxia is steadily progressive. Although some patients with mild forms of the disease may live a normal life span, it is more common for the disease to run a progressive, downhill course. Total disability occurs within five to ten years in most cases, and death from intercurrent infection, cardiac failure, or, rarely, from complications of associated diabetes, usually occurs sometime in the third or early part of the fourth decade. There is no specific treatment, and therapy is primarily effected through symptomatic treatment of the cardiac or metabolic abnormalities. However, in patients with very slowly evolving disease, physical therapy may offer useful training to help the patient compensate for his progressive motor impairment.

Laboratory tests are of little specific value in establishing the diagnosis. The cerebrospinal fluid, on examination, is usually normal. Electromyography may demonstrate signs of denervation in patients in whom anterior horn cell disease is evident. Nerve conduction velocity may be impaired. The differential diagnosis between Friedreich's ataxia and multiple sclerosis must be made in patients with a sporadic form of the disease characterized by late onset and minimal skeletal abnormalities. The principal features by which the two diseases may be distinguished are the progressive course and the absence of deep tendon reflexes in Friedreich's ataxia.

THE ROUSSY-LEVY SYNDROME
(Hereditary Areflexic Dystaxia; Hereditary Ataxia with Muscular Atrophy)

This disease is transmitted as an autosomal dominant trait. It is characterized by the development in childhood of an unsteadiness of station and gait, associated with a general loss of deep tendon reflexes, club foot, and kyphoscoliosis. A static tremor of the hands may be a prominent sign. There is occasionally some evidence of wasting of muscles of the legs and small muscles of the hand. Nerve conduction velocities may be reduced. It differs from Friedreich's ataxia in that nystagmus and dysarthria are absent, sensation is usually preserved, and there is a tendency for this syndrome to remain static or evolve slowly throughout life. However, since this particular combination of symptoms has been reported in relatives of patients with pure forms of both Friedreich's ataxia and peroneal muscular atrophy, some have considered the disease an intermediate between these two disorders.

HEREDITARY SPASTIC PARAPLEGIA

Definition. This is a rare, genetically determined disease transmitted as an autosomal dominant, and, less commonly, as an autosomal recessive or sex-linked recessive trait. It is characterized pathologically by degeneration in the spinal cord of the corticospinal tracts and dorsal columns, and occasionally of other spinal tracts as well, and clinically by the onset in early life of progressive spasticity.

Clinical Manifestations. The disease is more common in males than in females. Its onset is gradual and usually occurs in the first decade of life, but may occur later. The disease is characterized by a progressive bilateral and symmetrical spastic impairment of gait. Weakness of dorsiflexion of the feet results in the toes being dragged along the ground in a scissor gait. The patient has difficulty in climbing stairs because of weakness and rigidity of hip flexors. There is evident spasticity in extensor muscles with increased deep tendon reflexes and extensor plantar responses. Sensory disturbances are absent. Involvement of the bladder, upper limb, and bulbar musculature, when present, occurs late. The course may extend over many decades. Rarely, families have been described in which affected members, although presenting in early life with spastic paraplegia, have later developed wasting of the small muscles of the hand with lesser involvement of the peripheral musculature of the legs. Additionally such subjects usually have mild sensory loss of the modalities of touch-pressure, vibration, and joint position. The characteristics of the EMG in such patients suggest an axonal degenerative process. The distribution of this wasting, so suggestive of that of peroneal muscular atrophy, and the occasional association of pes cavus, scoliosis, and nystagmus indicate the close tie of this syndrome to the other spinal cerebellar degenerations. In the sporadic case the disease must be distinguished from multiple sclerosis and progressive muscular atrophy.

HEREDITARY SPASTIC ATAXIA
(Sanger-Brown's and Marie's Ataxia)

Definition.   Hereditary spastic ataxia, a usually heredofamilial disease, is characterized pathologically by atrophy of the cerebellum, cell loss in the dentate and olivary nuclei, and degeneration of the spinocerebellar tracts, and clinically by progressive ataxia associated with spasticity.

Clinical Features.   This is an uncommon form of spinocerebellar degeneration. It is usually hereditary with several clinical and pathologic variants. Clinically and pathologically, these variants represent an intermediate between Friedreich's ataxia, which is principally spinal, and olivopontocerebellar degeneration, primarily a cerebellar disease. The age of onset varies according to the pedigree, and often may not occur until the fifth and sixth decades of life. The disease consists of a mixture of ataxia and spasticity. The onset is most usually characterized by ataxia of gait, which may progress to incoordination of the upper extremities. There may be associated optic atrophy, ptosis, diplopia, and extraocular muscle palsies. Deep tendon reflexes are preserved and are often hyperactive, and ankle clonus and extensor plantar responses are frequently seen. In some patients spasticity may be the prominent finding. Unlike Friedreich's ataxia, nystagmus and abnormalities of the skeleton are usually absent. Dementia may sometimes be prominent. Phenotypic variation of the disease within a family may be striking.

Course and Prognosis.   The course, although progressive, is often slow so that impairment may be delayed over many years. There is no specific therapy.

OLIVOPONTOCEREBELLAR ATROPHY

This disorder, first described by Dejerine and Thomas in 1900, is usually sporadic, and is characterized by the onset in late life of a progressive disorder of cerebellar function. The disease is inherited as an autosomal dominant trait.

Pathology.   There is loss of the Purkinje cell layer, which may be limited to the lateral lobes of the cerebellum or may involve the vermis only slightly. In addition, there is atrophy of the middle cerebellar peduncle and pontine nuclei. In a number of cases loss of pigmented cells in the substantia nigra has been seen. In rare cases, there is degeneration of the corticospinal and spinocerebellar pathways in the spinal cord.

Clinical Manifestations.   The clinical syndrome is characterized by the development in late middle life of slowly progressive cerebellar deficiency. This includes a cerebellar ataxia of trunk and limbs, dysmetria, action tremor, impairment of rapid rhythmic alternating movements, dysarthria, and sometimes a static tremor of the head and trunk. Nystagmus is usually absent. Volitional movements are usually unimpaired, and the deep tendon reflexes are usually normal, although loss of ankle jerks and an occasional extensor plantar response are sometimes seen. A number of patients may display signs of an extrapyramidal nature, including rigidity, bradykinesia, and a parkinsonian tremor. A progressive dementia may also be associated. The diagnosis is made clinically, laboratory findings usually being normal. The course of the disease is progressive, incapacitation usually occurring within five to ten years after the onset of clinical signs. There is no specific therapy.

CEREBELLO-OLIVARY DEGENERATION
(Holmes Type of Hereditary Ataxia; Late Corticocerebellar Atrophy)

Cerebello-olivary degeneration is a rare form of spinocerebellar degeneration, characterized pathologically by atrophy of the cerebellum and shrinkage of the medulla and pons, and histologically by the almost complete disappearance of Purkinje cells diffusely throughout the cerebellum, with atrophy of the inferior and accessory olivary nuclei. The disorder is usually familial and inherited as an autosomal dominant trait. It is characterized by the onset, in early middle life or even later, of a progressive cerebellar syndrome, with gait ataxia, action tremor, dysmetria, dysarthria, and static tremor of the trunk and head. Deep tendon reflexes are normal, and the plantar responses are flexor. Nystagmus may occur late in the course of the disease. There are no visual, sensory, or skeletal disturbances. The diagnosis is made clinically. There is no specific therapy.

BASSEN-KORNZWEIG SYNDROME
(Acanthocytosis, A-beta-lipoproteinemia)

In 1950, Bassen and Kornzweig described a heredofamilial disease inherited as a recessive trait, in which a progressive ataxic disturbance of gait in childhood (similar in its clinical symptoms to Friedreich's ataxia) was associated with thorny erythrocytes (acanthocytes) and a marked diminution in the serum β-lipoproteins. These children usually first develop celiac disease with fatty stools as the presenting symptom. Somewhat later the patient becomes progressively more unsteady. The neurologic abnormalities include kyphoscoliosis, cerebellar ataxia, and distal sensory loss, involving especially dorsal column functions. Bilateral ptosis, paresis of extraocular muscles, and retinitis pigmentosa have been reported. The relationship among the abnormal erythrocytes, the absence of β-lipoprotein, and the neurologic syndrome remains to be determined. This disorder is also discussed in the article on Disorders of Lipid Metabolism.

PARENCHYMATOUS CEREBELLAR DEGENERATION

Degeneration of cerebellar neurons, particularly of the Purkinje cells, may result in an acute, subacute, or chronic cerebellar syndrome. The disease usually occurs in late middle life, and is sporadic. Pathologically, there is atrophy of the cerebellum which can be demonstrated microscopically to be due to disappearance of Purkinje cells in atrophic areas, to the reduction of the granular and molecular cells, and to some reduction of the white matter. No changes in the brainstem nuclei are seen. The etiology of the syndrome is multiple, the most common cause being prolonged and excessive intake of alcohol. This form of cerebellar degeneration occurs in chronic alcoholics, and its onset is usually subacute. Maximal disability is reached over weeks or months, and if the patient is abstinent the disorder may stabilize. The usual symptom is unsteadiness, which on examination may be demonstrated to be due to severe cerebellar impairment of the lower extremities. The gait is slow and lurching, and on heel-knee-shin tests, there is an evident ataxia of the legs. The arms are usually mildly affected, if at all, and nystagmus and dysarthria are usually mild or absent. Pure cerebellar degeneration may sometimes occur in association with carcinoma of ovary or lung. Heat strokes and intoxication with some heavy metals, particularly with organic mercuric compounds and lead, may also result in isolated degeneration of the cerebellum.

DYSSYNERGIA CEREBELLARIS MYOCLONICA
(Ramsay Hunt Syndrome, Familial Myoclonus and Ataxia)

This rare disease of children and young adults is both sporadic and familial and is characterized by myoclonic jerks, epilepsy, and progressive cerebellar ataxia. Postmortem examination has shown degeneration of the dorsal columns and atrophy of the dentate nucleus and the superior cerebellar peduncle. When familial, the inheritance appears to be by an autosomal dominant with incomplete penetrance.

Bell, J.: Hereditary ataxia and spastic paraplegia. Treasury of Human Inheritance. Vol. IV, Part 3. London, Cambridge University Press, 1939.

Boyer, S. H., Chisholm, A. W., and McKusick, V. A.: Cardiac aspects of Friedreich's ataxia. Circulation, 25:493, 1962.

Critchley, M., and Greenfield, J. G.: Olivo-ponto-cerebellar, atrophy. Brain, 71:343, 1948.

Gilbert, G. J., McEntee, W. J., and Glaser, G. H.: Familial myoclonus and ataxia. Neurology, 13:365, 1963.

Greenfield, J. G.: The Spino-cerebellar Degenerations Springfield, Ill., Charles C Thomas, 1954.

Schwartz, J. F., Rowland, L. P., Eder, H., Marks, P. A., Osserman, E. F., Hirschberg, E., and Anderson, H.: Bassen-Kornzweig syndrome: deficiency of serum β-lipoprotein. Arch. Neurol. (Chicago), 8:438, 1963.

Spillane, J. D.: Familial pes cavus and absent tendon jerks. Its relationship with Friedreich's disease and peroneal muscular atrophy. Brain, 63:275, 1940.

Victor, M., Adams, R. D., and Mancall, E. L.: A restricted form of cerebellar cortical degeneration occurring in alcoholic patients. Arch. Neurol. (Chicago), 1:579, 1959.

SYRINGOMYELIA

Definition. Syringomyelia is a chronic disease of the spinal cord, characterized pathologically by cavitation of the spinal cord with gliosis and clinically by a mixture of segmental and supra-segmental motor and sensory abnormalities and trophic disturbances. When a syrinx occurs in the brainstem, the disease is called *syringobulbia*.

Etiology. The cause of syringomyelia is unknown. Several theories have been proposed to explain its pathogenesis, but none are entirely satisfactory. Because of the common association of syringomyelia with other congenital abnormalities of the neuraxis and skeleton, the most popular hypotheses have attributed the disease to developmental anomalies. One hypothesis has suggested that the disease is due to abnormal closure of the neural tube; another, that it results from the persistence of ependymal cell rests which later proliferate and cavitate. A third, proposed by Gardner, suggests that the cavitation is caused by distention of the central canal by ventricular fluid displaced caudally from the fourth ventricle as a consequence of atresia of the foramina of Luschka and Magendie. The frequent association of intramedullary vascular malformations, vascular neoplasms, and gliomas with syrinxes has led Netsky to suggest that focal ischemia within the spinal cord caused by an abnormal vascular supply is pathogenic.

Pathology. On gross inspection the spinal cord may appear normal, enlarged, or flattened in its anteroposterior axis, depending upon the size and state of the syrinx. The syrinx itself, when intact, is filled with clear, slightly yellow serous fluid. The walls of the cavity are irregular, and consist of degenerated neural and neuroglial elements. The cavity is usually surrounded by gliosis, composed for the most part of glial fibers. Abnormal blood vessels with hyalinized walls may sometimes be seen. There is usually secondary degeneration and demyelination of long ascending and descending tracts of the spinal cord and brainstem as a result of extension of the syrinx. The syrinx most commonly runs over several segments in the cervical cord. It may extend into thoracic segments for a varying distance and may even terminate at lumbar levels. The cavity often begins in the gray matter adjacent to the central canal, and tends, as it enlarges, to interrupt the decussating fibers and destroy neurons in the dorsal and ventral horns. Within the thoracic cord, the cavity is commonly seen in the dorsal horns, and may affect the intermediolateral cell column, producing autonomic deficiencies. Syrinxes of the lumbar cord are uncommon. *Syringobulbia* is associated with cavitation that is usually slitlike and often in communication with the fourth ventricle. Bulbar syrinxes commonly involve several cranial nerve nuclei, notably the descending root of the trigeminal nerve, and the solitary, ambiguous, and hypoglossal nuclei. They also may involve the medial longitudinal fasciculus, the pyramidal tract, and the medial lemniscus. Extensions into the pons are rare. A *secondary syrinx* consisting of central cavitation of the spinal cord and sometimes associated with gliosis may occur as a result of chronic arachnoiditis, spinal tuberculosis, or meningeal or vascular syphilis.

Clinical Manifestations. The clinical manifestations of syringomyelia depend upon the localization and size of the lesion. The disease most commonly presents in the second decade, but sometimes the onset may be delayed until the patient is in his sixties or seventies. In its most usual form the signs and symptoms of the disease are referable to a *syrinx in the cervical cord*. The presenting symptoms often are wasting and weakness in the muscles of the upper extremity, associated with mild burning dysesthesias and loss of pain sensation distally in the arms. There are sometimes complaints of weakness of the legs, and bowel and bladder symptoms. On examination the patient may have Horner's syndrome as a consequence of interruption of the sympathetic pathways in the spinal cord. Nystagmus resulting from damage to the spinal projections of the medial longitudinal fasciculus may also be seen.

Muscle weakness in the upper extremity is usually associated with obvious atrophy, and frequently involves the small muscles of the hand. If the syrinx has extended into the corticospinal tract, weakness and spasticity in the lower extremities are evident. At the level of the lesion, the deep tendon reflexes may be absent or reduced. Because of the interruption of the second order afferent fibers arising from cells in the dorsal horn and crossing to the contralateral ventrolateral spinothalamic tracts, there may be a dissociated segmental type of sensory loss, often in a shawl or capelike distribution over the shoulders, upper trunk, and arms. In this zone, light touch, vibration, and deep sensibility are preserved with a striking absence of pain and temperature sensation. When the lesion has extended to include the dorsal columns or the spinothalamic pathways, there are appropriate sensory abnormalities in the trunk and lower extremities. Trophic changes, particularly involving the hands, are common. Their pathogenesis is not known, but may in part be related to the absence of pain sensation and to the interruption of vasomotor outflow to the limb. Unfelt burns from cigarettes or light bulbs may lead to tissue destruction and severe scarring. Cyanosis, hyperkeratosis, and thickening of subcutaneous tissues may result in puffy, swollen fingers. True hypertrophy of body parts may occur. Traumatic osteoarthropathy (Charcot's joint) is common. Sometimes the distal phalanges may atrophy and be lost painlessly, a condition known as Morvan's disease. The common clinical features of *lumbosacral syrinxes* are atrophic weakness of the lower limbs, loss of deep tendon reflexes, dissociated anesthesia, and fecal and urinary incontinence. If the lesion lies high in the lumbar cord, it may be associated with an extensor plantar response. Trophic changes of the lower extremity, particularly club foot deformities, are common. In *syringobulbia* the syrinx formation in the medulla may be unassociated with the syrinx in the cervical cord. Common findings in this disorder are atrophy of the tongue, nystagmus, impairment of pain and temperature sensation on one side of the face, dysphonia, and respiratory stridor. In addition, sensory and spastic motor abnormalities of the extremities may be seen.

There are many associated findings in syringomyelia. Papilledema may result from an associated hydrocephalus. Skeletal abnormalities are common and include cervical rib, spina bifida, premature closures of the skull, Klippel-Feil syndrome, basilar impression, and kyphoscoliosis. The association of syringomyelia with intramedullary gliomas or vascular tumors has long been recognized.

Diagnosis. The diagnosis may often be made clinically by the observation of muscular atrophy and weakness, dissociated sensory loss, trophic changes, and long tract signs attributable to a lesion in the cervical cord. The laboratory findings in this disorder are nonspecific. The cerebrospinal fluid may be under increased pressure as a result of an associated hydrocephalus. A mild pleocytosis or increased protein in the cerebrospinal fluid may sometimes be seen. Electromyography may reveal evidence of denervation in affected muscles. Roentgenographic evidence of bony deformities may be helpful. Pantopaque x-ray myelography may sometimes give evidence of a swollen syrinx.

Differential Diagnosis. Syringomyelia must be differentiated from tumors of the spinal cord or cervical ribs, other bony anomalies, amyotrophic lateral sclerosis, multiple sclerosis, and tabes dorsalis. Intramedullary tumors of the cord, which produce comparable symptomatology because of a similar location, and extramedullary tumors, which can sometimes simulate an intramedullary lesion by compressing the anterior spinal artery, can often be differentiated from syringomyelia by myelography. Cervical rib may be identified roentgenographically, although the fact that this abnormality may be associated with a syrinx sometimes complicates the differential diagnosis. Amyotrophic lateral sclerosis is never associated with sensory abnormalities. Multiple sclerosis can be differentiated by its remitting course and by the fact that muscular wasting, trophic changes, and dissociated sensory abnormalities are uncommon. Tabes dorsalis can be differentiated by the serology and by a different pattern of sensory loss.

Course and Prognosis. The course of syringomyelia is variable, but is usually protracted over many years. In some patients there may be gradual deterioration; in others, changes may occur in a stepwise fashion. In some patients, after an initial attack, the disease may appear to have become arrested. In syringobulbia, death from respiratory paralysis may sometimes occur.

Treatment. At present there is no satisfactory treatment for syringomyelia. X-irradiation or surgical decompression of the syrinx has been attempted in the past, but the therapeutic results have been at best doubtful.

Gardner, W. J.: Hydrodynamic mechanism of syringomyelia: its relationship to myelocele. J. Neurol. Neurosurg. Psychiat., 28:247, 1965.
McIlroy, W. J., and Richardson, J. C.: Syringomyelia. A clinical review of 75 cases. Canad. Med. Ass. J., 93:731, 1965.
Netsky, M. G.: Syringomyelia. A clinicopathological study. Arch. Neurol. (Chicago), 70:741, 1953.

NEUROCUTANEOUS SYNDROMES

MULTIPLE NEUROFIBROMATOSIS
(Von Recklinghausen's Disease)

Definition. Multiple neurofibromatosis is a congenital defect of the ectoderm characterized by cutaneous pigmentation and multiple tumors of the spinal and cranial nerves and skin.

Etiology. The disease is usually heredofamilial and is transmitted as an autosomal dominant trait with variable penetrance. It may be sporadic.

Clinical Manifestations. Cutaneous tumors in this disease are known as *fibromata mollusca*. These are multiple, pigmented, sessile or pedunculated tumors that arise from the neurilemma of cutaneous nerves. Tumors of the peripheral nerve are most characteristic, and occur as nodules along the course of the nerve or nerve roots, usually without interfering with nerve conduction. Occasionally diffuse involvement of the nerve trunk in its distal branches produces a plexiform neuroma which, when it occurs, is particularly common in the cervical and occipital regions. Other tumors of the nervous system, particularly meningiomas and gliomas, are often associated. Neurofibromas may undergo sarcomatous degeneration. The signs and symptoms of neurofibromatosis depend upon the localization and rate of growth of the tumors. When lying within the spinal canal, they may produce a syndrome of spinal cord compression. Cranial nerve tumors are often found. When tumors of the eighth nerve are bilateral, they are almost invariably a manifestation of neurofibromatosis, and optic nerve gliomas are frequently associated with that disease. Tumors of other cranial nerves may occur, particularly the trigeminal, vagus, and hypoglossal. The presence of von Recklinghausen's disease has been noted in about 10 per cent of pheochromocytomas. Intracerebral tumors may produce symptoms by compression or destruction, depending upon their location and cell type. The cutaneous and osseous manifestations of the disease are described in appropriate sections of the book.

TUBEROUS SCLEROSIS
(Epiloia, Bourneville's Disease)

Definition. Tuberous sclerosis is a congenital disease characterized by the presence of congenital tumors and malformations of the brain, skin, and viscera, and clinically by epilepsy and mental retardation.

Etiology. The disease is both sporadic and heredofamilial and is probably inherited through a single dominant trait.

Pathology. The brain, although usually normal in size, is studded by many small nodules or tubers. These are firm, and occasionally calcified. Sometimes they distort the normal configuration of gyri and may project into the cerebral ventricles, where they present as characteristic "candle gutterings." Microscopically, the tubers are composed of nests of glial fibers and abnormal ganglion cells. They may undergo gliomatous degeneration or develop into meningiomas. Glial tumors of the retina (phakomas) and gliomatous tumors of the nerve head and optic tract are also found in some cases. Adenoma sebaceum, the characteristic skin lesion, is a small firm tubercle often found over the nose and cheeks. These nevi arise from nerve fibers combined with hyperplasia of blood vessels and connective tissue. They are rarely present at birth, but usually develop during the first decade toward puberty. Although tending to cluster over the bridge of the nose and the cheeks, they may be found elsewhere over the head. In addition, a variety of other polyps, subcutaneous nodules, pigmented warts, and café-au-lait spots similar to those of von Recklinghausen's disease are found along with tumors of the kidney, liver, pancreas, and thyroid gland. Of particular importance is the association of a rhabdomyoma of the heart.

Clinical Manifestations. The presenting symptom of this disease is usually epilepsy, which appears in the first few years of life. The attacks may present as minor or focal seizures, but in time generally progress to major motor convulsions. Mental retardation is usually noticed during the early years of life and may vary in degree, differing in no way from mental retardation from any other cause. Some patients, however, may have normal I.Q.'s. The adenoma sebaceum usually appears toward the end of the second or the beginning of the third year of life as small lightly pigmented shiny papules that appear vascular. They may first appear on the malar areas, but as they proliferate they become confluent, more deeply pigmented, and extend in a butterfly distribution over the nose and cheeks. The retinal lesions are flat, white or gray, round or oval areas, and are present in almost half the patients. Subungual fibromas on the toes or fingers may be seen but most commonly not until after puberty. Patients with mild or partial forms of the disease are not uncommon.

Diagnosis. The clinical triad of seizures, mental retardation, and adenoma sebaceum will establish the diagnosis. Roentgenographic examination of the skull may often reveal scattered calcifications in areas of increased or decreased density in the skull vault. Pneumoencephalography may sometimes demonstrate the tubers projecting into the ventricles.

Course and Prognosis. The disease is usually progressive. The outlook in individual cases, however, depends on the severity of the mental impairment and the frequency and intensity of seizures. It must be emphasized that the three cardinal features of the disease may occur singly or in any combination with varying degrees of severity in members of the same family. Often the defects are progressive, and death occurs in the second decade of life. The development of gliomatous changes in the brain may also shorten the course of the disease. Sudden death from rhabdomyoma of the heart may occur.

Treatment. The treatment is the same as that for epilepsy with appropriate measures for the mental retardation. Institutionalization is sometimes indicated.

STURGE-WEBER-DIMITRI DISEASE
(Encephalotrigeminal Angiomatosis)

The Sturge-Weber-Dimitri disease is characterized by a unilateral, port-wine, facial nevus usually confined to the distribution of the first and occasionally the other divisions of the trigeminal nerve, together with a capillary hemangioma of the ipsilateral cerebral cortex. The full clinical picture consists of the nevus, a contralateral hemiparesis, smallness of the affected limbs, epilepsy—often consisting of jacksonian seizures beginning in the paralyzed limbs— ipsilateral exophthalmos, angiomas of the retina, and some degree of mental retardation. Incomplete manifestations of the disease may be observed, and there is great variability in the severity of the retardation, the frequency of the seizures, the profoundness of the hemiplegia, and the extent of the cutaneous abnormalities. Extensive linear calcification of the cortex often occurs in parallel lines, and, when visible roentgenographically, may help to establish the diagnosis. The films may also show hemiatrophy of the skull reflecting the maldevelopment of the underlying cerebral hemisphere. The cause of the disease is unknown, and there is no evidence of hereditary transmission. The diagnosis can be made clinically without difficulty.

VON HIPPEL–LINDAU DISEASE

This is a rare, usually heredofamilial disease, consisting of a hemangioblastoma of the brain (usually in cerebellum, but occasionally elsewhere) in association with an angioma of the retina and, less commonly cysts of the pancreas, kidneys, and other viscera. The disease is inherited as an autosomal dominant trait, probably with incomplete penetrance. Its onset usually occurs in the third decade of life with symptoms referable to the retinal or cerebral tumors. The angioma of the retina (von Hippel) is usually peripheral, and is supplied by a large, entering artery and drained by a single vein. Hemorrhages, exudates, and papilledema may occur in association with the lesion. The hemangioblastoma is usually a solitary cystic vascular tumor. It is most commonly localized to the cerebellum, but may occur in the medulla, brainstem, or spinal cord. The hemangioblastoma of the cerebellum presents with the usual signs of cerebellar deficiency. The protein content of the cerebrospinal fluid tends to be unusually high, and a polycythemia of unknown cause is commonly associated. However, it should be emphasized that the majority of cases of proved cerebellar hemangioblastoma present no evidence of von Hippel–Lindau disease. The diagnosis is established in patients with a positive family history by the onset of retinal or brainstem symptoms. Diagnosis of a tumor in the brainstem is made by the usual roentgenographic methods of pneumoencephalography or angiography. Early recognition of cerebellar tumors in afflicted members of the family is important, for early surgical resection may effect a cure.

ATAXIA TELANGIECTASIA
(Louis-Bar Syndrome)

Definition. Ataxia telangiectasia is a heredofamilial disease manifested by ocular and cutaneous telangiectasia, a progressive cerebellar ataxia, and recurrent sinopulmonary infections.

Etiology. The disease is transmitted as an autosomal recessive trait.

Pathology. The neuropathologic changes of the disease consist of widespread atrophy of the cerebellar cortex, with loss of Purkinje cells and thinning of the internal granular layer. There is chronic neuronal degeneration of the dentate and inferior olivary nuclei, and demyelination affecting particularly the posterior columns of the spinal cord. In addition, there are absence or atrophy of the thymus, hypoplasia of lymphoid tissue, acute and chronic bronchopulmonary inflammation sometimes associated with reticuloendothelial malignancies, and abnormalities of cells in liver, lungs, kidneys, and other viscera.

Clinical Manifestations. This rare disease is linked clinically and pathologically with both the neurocutaneous syndromes and the hereditary ataxias. The onset of the disease is usually marked by the appearance in infancy of the cerebellar ataxia first noted as the child begins to walk. The gait is reeling, and wide based. The loss of equilibrium persists, and is later aggravated by the onset of limb ataxia. At about the age of four, telangiectasia appears, first being noted in the bulbar conjunctiva and then spreading over the malar surfaces in a butterfly distribution, on the ears, the palate, along the neck, and in the antecubital and popliteal fossae. Occasionally, café-au-lait spots are seen. Patients also suffer from sinusitus and frequent pulmonary infections. As the disease progresses, other neurologic signs, including choreoathetoid movements and, rarely, myoclonic jerks may be observed. The disease is slowly progressive, and patients rarely live beyond the age of 25. The disease is associated with a deficiency of IgA immunoglobulins and a defect in the establishment of delayed hypersensitivity; the condition is discussed from that standpoint in the article on Immunologic Deficiency Syndromes.

Aguliar, M. J., Kamoshita, S., Landing, B. H., Boder, E., and Sedgwick, R. P.: Pathological changes in ataxia-telangiectasia. J. Neuropath. Exp. Neurol., 27:659, 1968.

Canale, D., Bebin, J., and Knighton, R. S.: Neurologic manifestations of von Recklinghausen's disease of the nervous system. Confin. Neurol., 24:359, 1964.

Chao, D. H.: Congenital neurocutaneous syndromes of childhood. III. Sturge-Weber disease. J. Pediat., 55:635, 1959.

Critchley, M., and Earl, C. J. C.: Tuberose sclerosis and allied conditions. Brain, 55:311, 1932.

Crowe, F. W., Schull, W. J., and Neel, J. V.: A Clinical Pathological, and Genetic Study of Multiple Neurofibromatosis. Springfield, Ill., Charles C Thomas, 1956, p. 181.

Gutmann, L., and Lemli, L.: Ataxia-telangiectasia associated with hypogammaglobulinemia. Arch. Neurol. (Chicago), 8:318, 1963.

Lagos, J. C., and Gomez, M. R.: Tuberous sclerosis: Reappraisal of a clinical entity. Mayo Clin. Proc., 42:26, 1967.

Melmon, F. L., and Rosen, S. W.: Lindau's disease: A review of the literature and study of a large kindred. Amer. J. Med., 36:595, 1964.

Penfield, W., and Young, A. W.: The nature of von Recklinghausen's disease and the tumors associated with it. Arch. Neurol. Psychiat., 23:320, 1930.

Peterman, A. F., Hayles, A. B., Dockerty, M. B., and Love, J. G.: Encephalotrigeminal angiomatosis (Sturge-Weber disease). J.A.M.A., 167:2169, 1958.

South, M. A., Cooper, M. D., Wollheim, F. A., and Good, R. A.: IgA system. II. Clinical significance of IgA deficiency: Studies in patients with agammaglobulinemia and ataxia-telangiectasia. Amer. J. Med., 44:168, 1968.

Mechanical Lesions of the Spinal Cord and Roots

GENERAL CONSIDERATIONS OF THE ARCHITECTURE OF THE SPINAL CORD, ROOTS, AND SPINE

Albert Aguayo

The *spinal cord* occupies the upper two thirds of the vertebral canal, extending from the superior border of the atlas to the upper border of the second lumbar vertebra, at which level the conus medullaris ends. It is continued as a delicate filament called the filum terminale which is attached to the coccyx. The cord is oval and flattened dorsoventrally, and in the adult measures about 10 mm. in anteroposterior diameter and 15 mm. in the transverse plane. Two enlargements are present, corresponding to the sites where the roots supplying the nerves to the limbs arise. The cervical enlargement usually extends from the third cervical to the second thoracic vertebral level, and the lumbar one from the ninth to the twelfth thoracic vertebrae.

Thirty-one pairs of *spinal roots* arise from the spinal cord: 8 cervical, 12 thoracic, 5 lumbar, 5 sacral, and 1 coccygeal. The cervical roots are short (2.5 cm. at the seventh cervical level) and run transversely, whereas those in the lumbosacral region are six to eight times longer (17 cm. at the fifth lumbar segment) and are directed almost vertically with a long intradural course. Their appearance in the lumbosacral region is such that these nerve roots have been named the cauda equina.

The first seven cervical nerve roots leave the spinal canal above the pedicle or arch of the vertebra of the same number. The eighth exists between C-7 and T-1, and following roots exit below the pedicles of the similarly numbered vetebrae.

The posterior nerve roots with their cell bodies in the dorsal root ganglion form a continuous series down the cord; the anterior ones with cells in the ventral horns of the spinal cord are more irregularly distributed. The rootlets are gathered in bundles. Anterior and posterior roots unite distal to the dorsal root ganglia, and together with the radicular and lymphatic vessels pass through a firm and narrow dural ostium. At this point, as age advances, they may become relatively fixed to the root sleeve by fibrosis and are more liable to damage. The posterior roots are thicker than the anterior ones in a proportion of 3 to 1 at the cervical level. They also have a longer segment of glial tissue. Both anterior and posterior roots contain myelinated and unmyelinated fibers. The latter amount to approximately 50 per cent of all afferent fibers in the dorsal roots. Nerve roots lack the large amount of perineurium that is characteristic of a peripheral nerve, and their endoneurium is scanty. This probably contributes to some extent to their elastic properties and their limited responses to traction and compression.

The *spine* is composed of the anteriorly situated vetebral bodies and discs whose main function is support. Posteriorly the pedicles and lamina protectively enclose the spinal cord and roots. The intervertebral discs consist of a nucleus pul posus, constituting 15 per cent of the total size of the disc. It is placed slightly more posteriorly and within a fibrocartilage ring called the anulus fibrosus. It is customary to give a disc the number of the vertebra situated above; for instance, the C-5 disc is between C-5 and C-6.

The interpedicular or apophyseal joints are formed by the adjacent superior and inferior facets of the vertebral pedicles. The uncovertebral joints of Luschka are found at the posterolateral aspects of the lower five cervical vertebrae. In the vicinity of these uncovertebral joints osteophytes may protrude into the intervertebral foramen and compress the exiting nerve root. The intervertebral foramen is bounded anteriorly by the vertebral bodies and discs and posteriorly by the ligamentum flavum and the corresponding superior and inferior articular facets, with the pedicles lying above and below. In the cervical spine when the neck is flexed, the intervertebral foramen is oval in shape and quite large, but on extension the size is considerably reduced. Such reduction may amount to 25 per cent, and this can be greater when pathologic changes in the surrounding tissues are present. The spinal nerves occupy one sixth to one fourth of the foraminal space, the rest being filled by vessels, lymphatics, and adipose tissue.

Some of the ligaments attached to the vertebral bodies are worth considering in some detail. The posterior longitudinal ligament is firmly adherent to the discs and margins of the joints but less so to the bodies. When bone changes occur it is raised up in ridges owing to the lipping of the vertebral bodies. The ligamenta flava, so called because of their content of yellow elastic tissue, are bilateral and attached to the lamina of the vertebrae situated above and below. These ligaments bulge into the canal during extension and flatten during flexion. Studies have shown that during extension the transverse area of the cervical canal from C-3 to C-7 diminishes by 11 to 16 per cent, owing to unfolding of the ligamenta flava, the anulus fibrosus, and the dura mater. The dentate ligaments extend from both sides of the cord as thin, longitudinally arranged septa originating from slight thickening of the pia mater. At one time the dentate ligaments were believed to be important in restraining movements of the cord, thereby contributing to the pathologic changes induced by trauma and displacement caused by compression. Such theories presently receive less support.

The diameters of the *spinal canal* are important in evaluating both congenital and acquired abnormalities compressing the spinal cord.

The normal anteroposterior diameters of the spinal canal are:

15 to 22 mm. at C-2 to C-7
17 to 22 mm. at the thoracic level
15 to 23 mm. from L-1 to L-3
16 to 27 mm. below L-3

The transverse or interpedicular diameters of the spinal canal have been charted by Elsberg and Dyke, and their figures are often consulted in evaluating roentgenograms of the canal.

Studies of the biomechanics of the human spinal cord during movement have shown that, rather than an up and down displacement, there is a uniform plastic elongation of the brainstem, cord, and roots, between the points of fixation in the mesencephalon and in the lumbosacral region.

ARTERIAL SUPPLY OF THE SPINAL CORD

The major sources of blood to the spinal cord are: (1) Vessels originating from the subclavian artery, among which the vertebrals are the most important to the cervical cord. The latter give rise to the anterior spinal arteries in their intracranial portion. The posterior spinal arteries originate from the vertebrals and occasionally from the posteroinferior cerebellar arteries. From the subclavian artery also arise the ascending cervical branches of the inferior thyroid, the deep cervical branches of the costocervical trunk, and the superior intercostal arteries that also supply the spinal cord. (2) The intercostal and lumbar arteries originating from the aorta. (3) The iliolumbar and lateral sacral arteries from the internal iliac. An important artery in the lower part of the cord is the anterior radicular artery of Adamkiewicz which often is found at the second lumbar level originating from the left side of the aorta.

The spinal radicular arteries enter the intervertebral foramina, reaching the cord by traveling on anterior and posterior roots to join the anterior spinal and posterior spinal arteries, respectively. From the anterior spinal artery a sulcal branch is given off into the anterior median sulcus, which, passing backward conveys blood to the central part of the cord. A plexus of small arteries interconnects the anterior and posterior spinal arteries while surrounding the cord in the pia mater. Branches from it penetrate the substance of the cord and form the peripheral cord circulation. The anterior spinal artery supplies the anterior two thirds of the transverse area of a cord segment, and the posterior spinal artery, the rest. Much of the border region of the gray and white matter receives its blood supply from central and peripheral branches.

Certain segments of the cord are particularly susceptible to ischemia, for example, the fourth thoracic segment, perhaps because the main radicular arteries are located some distance away at the cervical and lower thoracic segments.

Brieg, A.: Biomechanics of the Central Nervous System. Stockholm, Almqvist and Wiksell, 1960.

Elsberg, C. A., and Dyke, C. G.: Diagnosis and localization of tumours of the spinal cord by means of measurements made on x-ray films of vertebrae and the correlation of clinical and x-ray findings. Bull. Neurol. Inst., 3:359, 1934.

Sunderland, S., and Bradley, K. C.: Stress strain phenomena in human spinal nerve roots. Brain, 84:120, 1961.

Turnbull, I., Brieg, A., and Hassler, O.: Blood supply of cervical spinal cord in man. A microangiographic cadaver study. J. Neurosurg., 24:951, 1966.

Waltz, T. A.: Physical factors in the myelopathy of cervical spondylosis. Brain, 90:395, 1967.

SYMPTOMS OF COMPRESSION OF THE NERVE ROOTS AND SPINAL CORD

Albert Aguayo

Within the spinal canal the structures affected by pressure are the nerve roots and the spinal cord. The resulting symptoms can be radicular, spinal, or a combination of both.

Radicular Syndrome. Compression of nerve roots produces paresthesias, sensory loss, motor symptoms, and reflex changes which correspond to the segmental distribution of the lesion. A single nerve root may be affected, as in cases of intervertebral disc protrusion, or many roots can be involved in conditions such as spinal arachnoiditis or neoplastic intraspinal invasion.

The pain of nerve root compression may be projected to the overlying spine, to neighboring tissues, or to the cutaneous distribution of the root. Dorsally situated intraspinal lesions sometimes cause bilateral posterior radicular symptoms, with pain extending across the thorax or abdomen in a girdle distribution.

The sensory loss that results from interruption of a single root may give rise to sensory changes; it often is detectable only by careful testing of the patient's responses to pinprick (see accompanying figure). Impairment of touch sensation is less pronounced, a finding explained by a more complete overlapping of the neighboring cutaneous dermatomes.

The muscles supplied by a single spinal root constitute a myotome. Most muscles are supplied

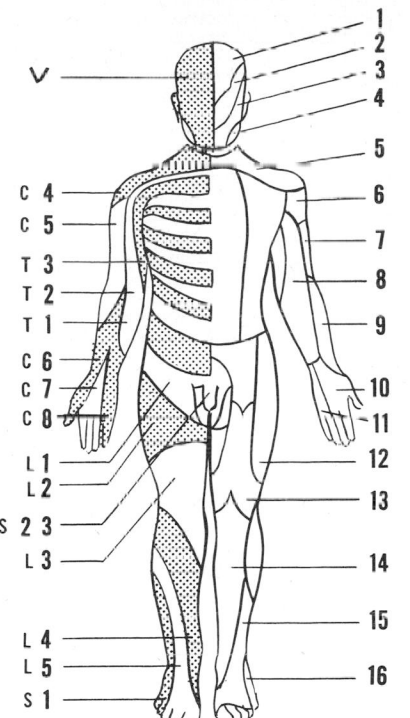

Schematic representation of dermatomes and peripheral nerve sensory areas:

1. Trigeminal 1st division
2. Trigeminal 2nd division
3. Trigeminal 3rd division
4. Greater auricular nerve
5. Branches from cervical plexus
6. Axillary nerve
7. Radial nerve
8. Medial brachial cutaneous nerve
9. Musculocutaneous nerve
10. Median nerve
11. Ulnar nerve
12. Lateral femoral cutaneous nerve
13. Femoral nerve
14. Saphenous nerve
15. Peroneal nerve
16. Sural nerve

by several adjacent nerve roots. Single nerve root lesions will cause variable degrees of muscle weakness and wasting according to the degree of dependence that each muscle has on the involved root. With some single nerve root lesions weakness is negligible because of the existence of more important innervation by other spinal segments. With other root lesions specific muscles will be affected to a greater degree, serving as clinical indicators of the involved level. For example, although the L-5 motor root provides some innervation to approximately 30 different muscles in the lower limb, the most severe weakness caused by lesions of this root can be demonstrated in the extensor hallucis longus and extensor digitorum brevis.

Muscle stretch reflexes can be diminished or absent at the levels where the reflex arcs are affected. The pathways of the various reflexes and the localizing value of their changes are well known. Because the second or terminal sympathetic neurons lie outside the spinal canal, auto-nomic fibers usually escape compression in most of the nerve root lesions referred to in this article. No demonstrable loss of sweating and preservation of piloerection is usually seen in such instances. Total anhydrosis, unresponsive to pilocarpine stimulation, and lack of histamine-induced flare favors a lesion of the peripheral nerve or spinal cord rather than of nerve roots.

The clinical distinction between lesions affecting nerve roots and those affecting peripheral nerves can be difficult, but is usually made by anatomic guides. Nerve root lesions (radiculopathy) are suggested by associated spinal cord signs, by spinal or paraspinal pain influenced by certain spine movements and straining, or by pain radiating along the peripheral distribution of the roots with paresthesias in a segmental distribution. With radiculopathy motor signs are present in muscles supplied by different nerves but belonging to a single myotome (see accompanying table). If weakness and reflex changes are confined to the territory of a certain nerve and the sensory loss involves all modalities and is sharply delineated, extending beyond the boundaries of a dermatome, a peripheral nerve lesion is favored. Autonomic and electrophysiologic testing assist the differentiation.

Spinal Cord Compression. The clinical symptoms of compressive spinal cord lesions depend on the rate at which the pressure develops, the nature of the pathologic process, the transverse and longitudinal extent of the lesion, and the functional importance of the affected levels of the cord.

The spinal cord accommodates considerably to slow forms of compression such as those caused by meningiomas and neurofibromas, but an acute hematomyelia or a rapid severe cord compression usually causes marked functional impairment. Infiltrating neoplasms or interference with the spinal cord blood supply by invasion or pressure also causes symptoms to develop rapidly. An acute intervertebral disc protrusion may be responsible for sudden partial cord compression.

The mechanical effects of compression may be limited to one portion of the transverse area of the cord. When a lesion affects only *one half of the spinal cord* above the tenth thoracic level, the resulting symptoms and signs are of a partial or complete *Brown-Sequard syndrome.* It is characterized by ipsilateral spastic weakness below the level of the lesion, combined with exaggerated stretch reflexes and an extensor plantar response (Babinski sign). Joint position sense and vibration sense are impaired on the same side of the lesion owing to posterior column involvement. Pain and temperature sensations are impaired on the opposite side because of the crossing of the responsible fibers. The upper limit of the thermoanesthesia is somewhat below the level of the actual compression, as fibers do not cross to join the opposite anterolateral columns for several segments. The main fibers conveying pain and temperature are arranged in the spinal cord in medial to lateral laminations, those originating at lower levels lying most laterally. As a result

PERIPHERAL NERVE AND RADICULAR INNERVATION OF MUSCLES

Upper Limb:

Nerves	Radicular Innervation					
	C-4	*C-5*	*C-6*	*C-7*	*C-8*	*T-1*
Suprascapular	— —Supraspinatus— —					
Circumflex		— — Deltoid — — — — —				
Musculocutaneous		— — Biceps — — — — — — —				
Median			— —Flexor carpi radialis— —			
				— — — — Flexor pollicis longus — —		
				— —Flexor digitorum— —		
				— — Abductor pollicis longus — —		
					— — Opponens pollicis — — — —	
Ulnar				— — Flexor carpi ulnaris — — — —		
				— —Opponens digiti quinti — —		
					— — Abductor digiti quinti — — — —	
					— — Interossei — — — — —	
Radial				— — Triceps brachialis — — — — —		
		— —Brachioradialis— —				
			— —Extensor carpi radialis— —			
				— —Extensor carpi ulnaris— —		
				— —Extensor digitorum longus— —		

Lower Limb:

Nerves	Radicular Innervation						
	L-1	*L-2*	*L-3*	*L-4*	*L-5*	*S-1*	*S-2*
		— — Iliopsoas — — — — —					
Gluteal					— — Gluteus maximus — — — — —		
Femoral		— — — — — — — — Quadriceps femoris — —					
Obturator			— — Adductors — — — — —				
Sciatic					— — — — Hamstrings — — — — —		
C. Peroneal				— —Tibialis anterior— —			
				— —Extensor digitorum brevis— —			
Tibial					— — — — — Gastrocnemius — —		
				— —Abductor hallucis brevis			
					— — Abductor digiti quinti — —		

extrinsic compressions may first produce symptoms well below the site of the lesion, with the level of sensory impairment gradually ascending as compression encroaches deeper into the cord. This laminated fiber arrangement explains the sparing of the sacral fibers in some intramedullary lesions. By their central position *intramedullary lesions* characteristically interrupt the decussating fibers carrying pain and temperature sensation and selectively impair such modalities while sparing touch and proprioception. This sensory dissociation, characteristic of syringomyelia, may also be present in cases of intramedullary tumors, vascular malformations, and spinal arachnoiditis. *Posterior spinal cord compression* can disturb dorsal column function, impairing postural sensibility and causing ataxia. Loss of joint position sense and vibration sense will be demonstrable clinically, and a level of sensory impairment may be detected by applying a tuning fork over the spinous processes.

Levels of Spinal Cord Compression. *Foramen Magnum and Upper Cervical Spine.* Compressive lesions in the foramen magnum and upper cervical spine are characterized by pain in the neck that radiates to the occipital area and is made worse by head movement. Motor signs usually follow, and weakness and wasting of the neck and at times of the upper limb muscles develop in association with spasticity of the lower limbs. Lateral extrinsic compression at this level may present with signs in the ipsilateral arm, followed by spasticity in the leg on the same side and involvement of the contralateral leg and arm as the compression increases. Spasms of the neck muscles and even contractures have been described. Paresthesias and sensory impairment may be present in the occipital region and in the hands, and if posterior compression is predominant, loss of proprioception may cause spastic ataxia easily confused with that caused by multiple sclerosis or subacute combined degeneration. Tumors in this region may extend intracranially to produce cerebellar dysfunction, nystagmus, trigeminal sensory impairment, wasting of the tongue, and increased intracranial pressure.

The lesions which most commonly affect the cranial-cervical junction are tumors such as meningiomas, ependymomas, and teratomas, vascular malformations, and particularly congenital bony abnormalities such as basilar invagination, and occipito-odontoid dislocations.

Cervical Region. Spinal cord compression in the cervical region produces a combination of segmental or radicular dysfunction in the upper limbs and altered motor and sensory tract function in the lower. Variable loss of power and bulk together with fasciculations may be seen in the muscles of the neck, shoulder girdle, and upper limbs. Sensory loss will be predominantly distal and unilateral when roots have been affected, but bilateral and asymmetrical when the cord is involved. If caused by an intramedullary lesion, sensory dissociation may be encountered. Sensory symptoms involving the radial border of the forearm and thumb suggest a lesion affecting the C-6 segment or root. Those in the index and middle fingers point to C-7, and those in the ring and little ones together with Horner's syndrome incriminate C-8. The presence of spinal cord signs such as spasticity in the legs helps differentiate the sensory changes from those of purely peripheral nerve or root origin. Of value are certain changes in the deep tendon reflexes such as inversion of the bicipital and radial jerks. The biceps reflex is said to be inverted when by stretching its tendon only contraction of the triceps muscle follows. When stretch of the tendon of the brachioradialis fails to induce its reflex contraction but causes only a flexion of the fingers, the radial reflex is inverted. Such signs indicate that a lesion at the C-5 or C-6 segment has interrupted the normal reflex arc at that level with exaggeration of the lower reflexes owing to coexistent compression of the corticospinal tract. Loss of sphincter control is rare in early cervical cord compression.

The most common conditions affecting this region are cervical spondylosis and intervertebral disc protrusions. Tumors, arachnoiditis, and syringomyelia comprise the differential diagnosis.

Thoracic Region. This is suggested by the presence of spasticity involving the lower limbs combined with normal upper limbs. When thoracic radicular symptoms precede or accompany the spasticity, a more precise topographic diagnosis can be made. It is useful to remember that the projection of the thoracic segments coincides with that of the intercostal nerves (See accompanying table). Important landmarks are the fourth thoracic extending to the level of the nipples, the seventh reaching the epigastrium, the tenth reaching the umbilicus, and the twelfth, the groin. Patients will often complain of a tight, "bound" feeling at the affected level. The intercostal muscles may be wasted, and in lower thoracic lesions the abdominal reflexes will be absent. *Beevor's sign* consists of an elevation of the umbilicus when the patient raises his head against resistance, and is found with lesions at the low thoracic level. The most important causes of thoracic spinal cord compression are meningiomas, metastatic tumors, neurofibromas, vascular malformations, epidural hematomas, and abscesses. Compression can rarely arise from a protruded intervertebral disc.

Lumbosacral Region. The close spatial relationship between the functionally important lumbar and sacral cord segments and the elements of the cauda equina often yields mixed symptoms combining pain, lower and upper motor neuron signs, and sphincter disturbances. When the spinal cord itself is involved at the first lumbar level, pain is referred to the groin and is accompanied by loss of cremasteric reflexes, weakness of hip flexion, and spasticity in the lower limbs. Lesions affecting the second and third lumbar levels cause weakness of the quadriceps and adductors associated with absent knee jerks, brisk ankle reflexes with clonus of the foot, and Babinski signs. In lesions of the L-5 and S-1 segments, the ankle jerk is lost, and weakness and wasting predominate in the peroneal calf, and small muscles of the foot. No extensor plantar responses can then be elicited. Normal power in the legs and preservation of the stretch reflexes characterize lesions involving the lower sacral segments, and care must be taken to examine the perianal-genital region for the typical saddle anesthesia. Impotence in the male, along with loss of sphincter control and of the anal and bulbocavernous reflexes may be noted. Pain in the low back with radiation to the anteromedial aspect of the thighs is usually associated with involvement of the first three lumbar segments, whereas the fifth lumbar and sacral segments produce a pain distribution that mimics that of the sciatic nerve.

Cauda Equina. Lesions of the cauda equina alone are difficult to differentiate from those of the conus. They are characterized by the early onset of pain of a dull and aching character mainly felt in the perineum, bladder, and sacrum, and commonly radiating in a sciatic fashion. The symptoms depend on the site of the lesion and the number of motor and sensory roots affected. Often, there is atrophic areflexic paralysis combined with asymmetrical radicular sensory impairment, but dissociated anesthesia does not occur. Progression is commonly slow, and bladder and rectal disturbances, late.

The most important cause of single or multiple root involvement at the low lumbar and sacral vertebral levels is an intervertebral disc protrusion. Spinal arachnoiditis, angiomas, ependymomas, lipomas, teratomas, neurofibromas, or neoplasms arising from the lumbar vertebrae or sacrum such as chordomas, osteomas, and parasitic cysts also affect this region. Tabes dorsalis, diabetes mellitus, and lesions affecting the lumbosacral plexus or the peripheral nerves to the legs enter the differential diagnosis.

Guttman, L.: Clinical symptomatology of spinal cord lesions. *In* Vinken, P. J., and Bruyn, G. W. (eds.): Handbook of Clinical Neurology. Vol. 2. Amsterdam, North Holland Publishing Company, 1969, pp. 178-216.
Haymaker, W.: Bing's Local Diagnosis in Neurological Diseases. St. Louis, C. V. Mosby Company, 1969.
Schliak, H.: Segmental innervation and the clinical aspects of spinal nerve root syndrome. *In* Vinken, P. J., and Bruyn, G. W. (eds.): Handbook of Clinical Neurology. Vol. 2. Amsterdam, North Holland Publishing Company, 1969, pp. 157-177.

LABORATORY AIDS TO INVESTIGATION

Albert Aguayo

To establish the location and nature of pathologic changes affecting the spinal cord and nerve roots one commonly employs auxiliary investigations, including cerebrospinal fluid examination, radiologic techniques, radioisotopic scanning, and electrophysiologic testing.

Manometric studies of the cerebrospinal fluid may indicate the presence of a partial or total block of circulation within the canal, but the dangers of irreparable damage to the cord by displacement of an intraspinal space-occupying lesion make the Queckenstedt test a risky one. Xanthochromia may result from a marked elevation of protein below a spinal block caused by tumors. Hemorrhagic or xanthochromic cerebrospinal fluid often accompanies bleeding from a spinal vascular malformation or tumors such as ependymomas or melanomas. Inflammatory cells may be found with infection or chronic arachnoiditis, and malignant cells may point to neoplastic invasion of the cord or nerve roots.

Certain teratomas spill ciliated cells, mucin, or keratin into the subarachnoid space, and meningitis may follow.

Roentgenographic investigations begin with plain films of the suspected spinal segments. A routine investigation should include anteroposterior, lateral, and oblique views. Lateral films in flexion and extension and tomograms may be helpful when investigating the cervical spine. Bone destruction can be demonstrated by roentgenograms if the area involved is at least 1.5 cm. Dumbbell neurofibromas can enlarge the intervertebral foramen without visible bone destruction. Occasionally a meningioma can be identified by the presence of calcification. Congenital anomalies of the vertebral bodies accompany teratomatous and arachnoidal cysts. Bone caries may be identified in the spine with Pott's disease, typhoid, and brucellosis.

The spinal canal diameter can be either narrowed or widened by disease. A sagittal diameter of 10 mm. at any level of the cervical spine almost always means cord compression. With a diameter of 10 to 13 mm. compression is possible, and with more than 13 mm., improbable. Thinning of the pedicles with widening of the transverse diameter of the canal is caused by intramedullary tumors, including ependymomas, lipomas, and syringomyelia, and occasionally by teratomatous and arachnoid cysts. Paget's disease causes a focal or general reduction of the lumen of the spinal canal. Narrowing of a disc space in a patient with corresponding radicular symptoms suggests an intervertebral disc protrusion. Myelography with radiopaque dye is usually required to identify mechanical spinal lesions when surgery is considered. Characteristic deformations of the oil column accompany intramedullary or extramedullary tumors and vascular malformations. Air myelography is useful in assessing congenital malformations and atrophy. Discography with radiopaque material is favored by some for the investigation of intervertebral disc disease.

Radioisotope studies using strontium 85 have received considerable attention in recent years for the investigation of benign and malignant neoplasms, fractures, osteomyelitis, and Paget's disease. They may demonstrate the presence of skeletal changes before roentgenographic visualization is possible, but a number of other conditions that induce an increased calcium accretion rate cause a high strontium 85 uptake, including degenerative arthritis, ankylosing spondylitis, and fibrous dysplasia.

Electromyography can be of value in the localization of lesions involving the motor unit at the anterior horn cell or peripheral level, as noted in the article on Diagnostic Techniques in Neurology.

ARTERIOVENOUS MALFORMATIONS AND OTHER VASCULAR LESIONS OF THE SPINAL CORD

Albert Aguayo

Arteriovenous malformations can involve the surface of the spinal cord or develop within its substance. They may thus present with the picture of spinal subarachnoid hemorrhage or with acute or chronic symptoms arising from involvement of the spinal cord elements.

The acute onset of a partial or complete transverse myelopathy is the most common form of onset. The legs may be initially flaccid and paralyzed with sensory impairment below the level of the lesion. Sphincter control is usually lost. When subarachnoid bleeding has occurred, back and neck pain along with spinal rigidity are among the earliest symptoms. Symptoms may be more severe at the level of the lesion, but headaches and nuchal rigidity can make differentiation from intracranial hemorrhages difficult. It may be possible at times to detect bruits on auscultation of the suspected spinal area. Exaggeration of symptoms during pregnancy has been reported. The gradual expansion of spinal vascular malformation also may compress the cord or give rise to hemodynamic alterations and ischemic spinal symptoms. Such lesions can present with slowly progressive motor and sensory changes, interrupted by transient exacerbations caused by ischemia or small hemorrhages, often with complete or partial recovery.

The focal repetitious character of the attacks and the prominence of pain helps differentiate them from other recurrent diseases such as multiple sclerosis. The cerebrospinal fluid commonly contains an elevation of protein content and at times a lymphocytic pleocytosis or xanthochromia.

Cavernous angiomas of the spinal cord are more restricted vascular hamartomas and may be associated with cysts and tumors in other organs such as the kidneys and pancreas, and with hemangioblastomas of the cerebellum. Retinal changes (*von Hippel–Lindau syndrome*) and cutaneous vascular nevi in a segmental distribution which corresponds to that of the spinal angioma may be present. The ischemic and hemorrhagic changes induced in the spinal cord by collagen disorders such as polyarteritis nodosa may resemble those of arteriovenous malformations, but provide more diffuse vascular symptoms.

Radiologic examination of the spine of patients with arteriovenous malformations may demonstrate bone erosion, a coexistent vertebral hemangioma or, occasionally, calcifications within the spinal canal. When myelography is performed, large amounts of contrast medium may be necessary for the demonstration of small anomalies. The oil breaks up into drops and serpentine streaks at the level of the lesion. Such an appearance may resemble spinal arachnoiditis, which may indeed coexist as a result of repeated hemorrhages. Angiography with catheterization of the feeding vessels demonstrates the vascular changes and is a necessary preliminary to successful surgical treatment.

Antoni, N.: Spinal vascular malformations (angiomas) and myelomalacia. Neurology, 12:795, 1962.

Henson, R. A., and Parsons, M.: Ischaemic lesions of the spinal cord: an illustrated review. Quart. J. Med., 36:205, 1967.

Hughes, J. T.: Pathology of the Spinal Cord. Chicago, Year Book Medical Publishers, 1966, pp. 38-57.

Russell, D. S., and Rubinstein, L. J.: Tumors of the Nervous System. London, Edward Arnold, 1959, pp. 72-92.

Taylor, J. R., and Van Allen, M. W.: Vascular malformation of the cord with transient ischaemic attacks. J. Neurosurg., 31:576, 1969.

SPINAL EPIDURAL HEMATOMA

Albert Aguayo

Bleeding into the spinal epidural space can occur spontaneously or in association with hypertension, trauma, or vascular malformations. It is a particular risk in patients receiving anticoagulants. The bleeding usually develops over the dorsal aspect of the thoracic cord, but other localizations are not uncommon. The resulting hematomas vary in size from a few millimeters to many cord segments in length. Epidural hematomas may originate in the epidural venous plexus, but the exact mechanism is obscure. Some follow minor trauma, but frequently no precipitating factor can be found.

The clinical picture is characterized by the sudden onset of pain over the affected area, often associated with corresponding radicular symptoms and a sensory loss to a level on the trunk. Weakness in the limbs and loss of sphincter control usually develop rapidly. The development of these signs in a patient on anticoagulants should allow few doubts regarding the nature of his neurologic disorder.

The cerebrospinal fluid may be clear or xanthrochromic. Although myelography is of great help in the diagnosis and localization of an epidural hematoma, this and other investigations can be omitted when the diagnosis appears highly likely, for urgent surgical intervention is required to avoid irreversible spinal cord damage.

Acute transverse myelitis, epidural abscess, hemorrhage from a vascular malformation, and anterior spinal artery occlusion, must be considered in the differential diagnosis.

Jacobson, I., MacCabe, J. J., Harris, P., and Dott, N. M.: Spontaneous spinal epidural haemorrhage during anticoagulant therapy. Brit. Med. J., 1:522, 1966.

Schultz, E. C., Johnson, A. C., Brown, C. A., and Mosberg, W. H., Jr.: Paraplegia caused by spontaneous spinal epidural Haemorrhage. J. Neurosurg., 10:608, 1953.

SPINAL ARACHNOIDITIS

Albert Aguayo

This condition is caused by a low-grade inflammatory process that leads to the formation of fibrous adhesions and loculated cysts that compress nerve roots or the spinal cord. In many instances the condition follows the introduction of noxious material by hemorrhage, lumbar puncture, myelography, or surgery; but in others no definite cause can be found. Syphilis, tuberculosis, and fungal and parasitic infections all can cause a chronic arachnoiditis. The thickened meningeal changes may be diffuse or restricted to certain segments of the spinal canal such as the lumbosacral or cervical region.

The clinical picture usually begins insidiously with intermittent radicular pains in the neck or low back that spread to involve the limbs bilaterally and asymmetrically in areas supplied by more than one root. The pain is often persistent and unrelated to movement or strain, and sensory symptoms exceed motor changes, although atrophy, weakness, and fasciculations can appear in the corresponding myotomes. Radicular symptoms may precede signs of cord involvement by months or years, but sooner or later are followed by loss of bladder and rectal sphincter control and spastic paralysis of the legs with sensory changes. Occasionally signs of cord involvement precede radicular changes so that the patient presents with paraplegia. In spinal arachnoiditis the disability may arrest and remit, but as a rule the condition is progressive and at times can resemble syringomyelia or spinal neoplasm.

The diagnosis of spinal arachnoiditis is facilitated by examination of the cerebrospinal fluid and by myelography. The fluid usually has a high protein content and a moderate number of inflammatory cells. Bacterial, fungal, or parasitic agents can sometimes be identified, and serologic tests for syphilis should be performed. Myelography, if characteristic, outlines spotty, irregularly loculated patterns and delays in the flow of contrast medium.

Laminectomy is usually performed for diagnosis, some improvement occasionally being reported after decompression and removal of thickened membranes. When a specific infective agent is identified, chemotherapy may arrest the progression of symptoms.

Cruickshank, E. K.: Neurologic Disorders in the Tropics. In Williams, D. (ed.): Modern Trends in Neurology. London, Butterworth and Co., Ltd., 1963, pp. 214-217.
Davidson, S.: Cryptococcal spinal arachnoiditis. J. Neurol. Neurosurg. Psychiat., 31:76, 1968.
Elkington, J.: Arachnoiditis. In Feiling, A. (ed.): Modern Trends in Neurology. London, Butterworth and Co., Ltd., 1951, pp. 149-161.
Guidetti, B., and LaTorre, E.: Hypertrophic spinal pachymeningitis. J. Neurosurg., 26:496, 1967.
Wise, B. L., and Smith, M.: Spinal arachnoiditis ossificans. Arch. Neurol. (Chicago), 13:391, 1965.

HERPES ZOSTER
(Shingles)
Albert Aguayo

Herpes zoster is an acute illness caused by a virus related or identical to that causing chickenpox. Pathologically, there is inflammation of the dorsal root ganglion of the involved segment and often of the immediately adjacent spinal segments as well. The disease is discussed elsewhere in this book. (See Viral Diseases.)

Denny-Brown, D., Adams, R. D., and Fitzgerald, P. J.: Pathologic features of herpes zoster. Arch. Neurol. Psychiat., 51:216, 1944.
Editorial: Amyotrophy and herpes zoster. J.A.M.A., 180:405, 1962.
McCormick, W. F., Rodnitzky, R. L., Schoshet, S. S., Jr., and McKee, A. P.: Varicella-zoster encephalomyelitis. Arch. Neurol. (Chicago), 21:559, 1969.

SPINAL CORD TUMORS
Albert Aguayo

According to the main localization of the tumors that affect the spinal cord, it is useful to divide them into three groups: *extradural tumors*, which usually arise in the bones of the spinal column or in the extradural space; *intradural extramedullary tumors*, which lie within the dura mater but outside the spinal cord; and *intramedullary tumors*, originating within the substance of the cord. Their comparative incidence in a general hospital has been estimated at 50, 40, and 10 per cent, respectively.

Extradural Tumors. Although mention should be made of osteomas, chondromas, and chordomas, the most important sources of these tumors are metastatic carcinomas from lung, breast, and kidney, lymphomas, multiple myeloma, sarcomas, prostatic carcinoma, and cancer of the gastrointestinal tract, uterus, and thyroid, in order of importance. Focal spinal compression is the rule, although some of these neoplasms, particularly those from the reticuloendothelial system, may ensheath the cord by extensive infiltration of the extradural space.

Although the manifestations of extradural tumors depend on their localization, type, and size, their onset and progression is usually rapid because of their malignant nature. The patient will usually present weeks or months after the onset of symptoms. However, an acute onset with cord compression and prominent radicular symptoms can follow either the collapse of an involved vertebra or neoplastic invasion of the spinal vessels, producing infarction or hemorrhage within the tumor. Severe pain from bone or nerve involvement is an early sign that can be accentuated by pressure over the corresponding vertebral spinous process. Occasionally a palpable spinal deformity will be encountered. The radicular symptoms are commonly bilateral and asymmetric. Spastic weakness below the lesion often precedes sensory symptoms. Disturbed function of bladder and rectal sphincters generally occurs late in extramedullary tumors.

In diagnosis, particular care should be given to the examination of the lungs and breast when searching for a primary neoplasm. Anemia, bone pain, radiologic enlargement of the mediastinal shadow, hepatomegaly, or splenomegaly suggests widespread metastatic disease or lymphoma. Skeletal changes, Bence Jones protein in the urine, morphologic examination of bone marrow, and serum electrophoresis help diagnose multiple myeloma. Bony changes will be present in 50 per cent of spinal roentgenograms taken at the time of onset of symptoms. The earliest signs of vertebral involvement may be a slight decrease in density together with changes in the radiologic configuration of the body, transverse processes, arches, or pedicles. When plain roentgenograms are negative, evidence of bone involvement may be obtained by radioiosotopic scanning with strontium 85. Elevation of the cerebrospinal fluid protein and spinal blockage are often found on lumbar puncture. Myelography usually demonstrates the presence of an extradural mass which occasionally may be found somewhat distant from the site of visible bone destruction.

Radiotherapy, hormones, and chemotherapy may assist in controlling the skeletal lesions and prevent or reduce their compressive effects on the spinal cord. Surgical decompression is indicated for radio-resistant lesions or rapidly developing cord compression.

Extramedullary, Intradural Tumors. These are commonly benign and present with a long history of unilateral radicular pain that precedes any signs of cord compression. Some tenderness on percussion of the neighboring vertebrae may be present. The two most important tumors in this group are meningiomas and neurofibromas, which account for almost two thirds of all primary intraspinal neoplasms. Rarer tumors are the teratomatous and arachnoid cysts, some lipomas, and meningeal carcinoma.

Meningiomas are found mainly in middle-aged women, about 90 per cent occurring in the thoracic region. They are usually single, relatively small, and located posterior or lateral to the spinal cord. Because of this position, meningiomas may produce an ataxic spastic syndrome which superficially resembles subacute combined degeneration. Pain is not usually prominent. Erosion of the pedicles and occasionally calcification of the tumor may be found on radiologic examination, but contrast myelography is required for accurate diagnosis.

Neurofibromas arise from the nerve roots, may develop at any age, and affect both sexes equally. They show no particular preference for any site within the spinal canal. In cases of neurofibromatosis of von Recklinghausen the typical skin pigmentation and the presence of multiple tumors along the peripheral nerves are diagnostic. A small percentage show sarcomatous degeneration. Occasionally a neurofibroma may arise within the substance of the spinal cord and behave as an intramedullary space-occupying lesion.

Plain roentgenograms may demonstrate widening of the intervertebral foramen with dumbbell tumors. The radiologic changes may be out of proportion to the presenting symptoms because of an asymmetric development of the tumor, the intraspinal portion being relatively small in comparison to the extraspinal, which can grow to a considerable size and even be palpable. Myelography, as in all cases of intradural extramedullary tumors, is diagnostic. The cerebrospinal fluid shows an early elevation of protein content. Complete neurological recovery usually follows the surgical removal of meningiomas and neurofibromas.

Intramedullary Tumors. The same histologic types of tumors that occur in the brain can involve the spinal cord, but with a different relative incidence. Ependymomas are most frequent, followed by astrocytomas, glioblastomas, oligodendrogliomas, vascular tumors, lipomas, and metastases.

Ependymomas can develop at any level but have a preference for the caudal region. They represent more than two thirds of the tumors that involve the conus medullaris, and are even more common in the filum terminale where they originate from its ependymal layer. Ependymomas may affect one or several segments of the spinal cord, and in rare instances they extend throughout the entire length of the cord. These neoplasms often produce an associated syringomyelia, making the clinical and radiologic findings more difficult to interpret. Although they occasionally bleed and give rise to acute, painful symptoms, the usual clinical course of intramedullary tumors is one of slow progression over several years. Pain at the level of the tumor is present, but usually is less severe and well localized than with extramedullary tumors. Impotence in males and sphincter disturbances in both sexes may be early symptoms, but the most common finding is that of a syringomyelic syndrome with muscle wasting and dissociated sensory loss. Anogenital or saddle anesthesia occurs when the lower spinal cord and cauda equina are involved.

Intramedullary tumors do not induce any radiographically visible changes in the walls of the spinal canal until fairly late in their course, at which time enlargement can be demonstrated by measurements of the width of the canal and identifying thinning of the pedicles. Contrast myelography usually demonstrates a typical spindle-shaped widening of the cord prior to any such bony changes. Surgical removal of some ependymomas is possible, whereas decompressive measures and radiotherapy may benefit others.

Hughes, J. T.: Pathology of the Spinal Cord. Chicago, Year Book Medical Publishers, 1966, pp. 160-180.

Rand, R. W., and Rand, C. W.: Intraspinal Tumours of Childhood, Springfield, Ill., Charles C Thomas, 1960.

Russell, D. S., and Rubinstein, L. J.: Pathology of Tumours of the Nervous System. London, Edward Arnold, 1959.

Slooff, J. L., Kernohan, J. W., and MacCarthy, C. S.: Primary Intramedullary Tumours of the Spinal Cord and Filum Terminale. Philadelphia, W. B. Saunders Company, 1964.

Wyburn-Mason, R.: Vascular Abnormalities and Tumours of the Spinal Cord. London, Kimpton, 1943.

ACUTE SPINAL INTERVERTEBRAL DISC DISEASE

John F. Sullivan

LUMBAR REGION

Herniation of lumbar intervertebral discs is the most common cause of pain of sciatic distribution. Herniation of the nucleus pulposus through the anulus fibrosus occurs most frequently at the lumbosacral interspace, somewhat less often at the interspace above, and, with diminishing frequency, at higher levels. Younger patients commonly give a history of flexion injury, but in older persons degenerative changes occur in the anulus fibrosus and the posterior longitudinal ligament so that trauma as trivial as a sneeze or a misstep may be sufficient to precipitate symptoms.

Clinical Manifestations. Herniation at the lumbosacral level compresses the first sacral root, causing pain in the buttock, posterior thigh, calf, and lateral aspect of the foot. At the L-4–L-5 interspace, the pain is distributed to the hip, the lateral aspect of thigh and calf, and the dorsum of the foot. At higher levels, L-2–L-3 and L-3–L4, the pain is referred to the anterior thigh and groin. (A diagram of these and other dermatomal patterns appears in the article on Symptoms of Compression of Nerve Roots and Spinal Cord.) The pain may be felt throughout these areas or may be confined to a smaller area. Straining, coughing, lifting, and bending tend to cause jolts of pain that may be associated with paresthesias in the more distal distribution. Back pain may be severe and associated with spasms or, especially in older patients, may be absent or relatively minor in degree. Signs include restricted movement of the lumbar spine, often with scoliosis, and tenderness over the appropriate interspinous space. Straight leg raising is limited on the affected side with both L-5 and S-1 root compression. An increase of pain on hyperextension of the hip suggests a rupture at L-1–L-2 or L-2–L-3. The ankle jerk may be diminished or lost with S-1 compression; there is usually no change in reflexes with L-5 root compression; the knee jerk is suppressed with L-4 or L-3 root involvement. Motor loss varies greatly from case to case but conforms to the involved root when present. Mild hypalgesia may be demonstrable on the lateral aspect of the foot with S-1 involvement and on the dorsum of the foot and great toe with L-5 root lesions.

The pain is usually unilateral. Occasionally, extrusion of a large disc fragment causes bilateral pain, perianal numbness, and disturbance of bladder function, usually with retention.

An unusual symptom complex that sometimes occurs in patients with significant canal narrowing caused by lumbar disc disease or certain congenital lesions is *the syndrome of intermittent claudication of the cauda equina.* Walking, running, or climbing induces an increase in sciatic pain or in other motor or sensory abnormalities in the lower extremities, but all the increased abnormalities subside promptly with brief rest. The absence of peripheral vascular insufficiency and the pre-existing neurologic abnormalities suggest the diagnosis.

Diagnosis. Although the diagnosis is easily made on the basis of typical back and leg symptoms and signs, there are many variations from the average. Roentgenograms of the lumbar spine may show narrowing of the interspace and loss of the lordotic curve. If surgery is contemplated, myelography is usually necessary and may show a filling defect at the interspace or a deformity of the involved root sleeve. Since the lumbar sac may be small, it is sometimes necessary to use large amounts of Pantopaque and to stand the patient upright to distend the sac and demonstrate small or lateral filling defects. Even then, myelography may not demonstrate the disc herniation.

The differential diagnosis includes root irritation due to lumbar spondylosis, which may exactly simulate an acute disc protrusion but which is often identified by the older age of the patient, the tendency to multiple root involvement, and the finding of advanced changes of spondylosis on roentgenographic examination. Femoral mononeuropathy associated with diabetes can be distinguished by its nonradicular distribution as well as by the absence of back signs, by severe aching, burning pain of the anterior thigh, and the rapid development of weakness and atrophy of the quadriceps muscle. The knee jerk is depressed, and sensory findings are minor in femoral neuropathy. A neurofibroma of the cauda equina or of a lumbar root develops gradually and is less likely to be accentuated by alterations in posture or by straining and coughing. Compression of the lumbosacral plexus by a malignant process may cause severe pain of femoral or sciatic distribution long before there are objective signs. Back pain is absent, and pain is usually increased by strongly flexing the thigh on the abdomen (iliopsoas contraction). Pelvic and rectal examination may reveal evidence of a pelvic neoplasm. Both cauda equina and plexus lesions generally cause signs of multiple rather than single root impairment.

Treatment. Acute disc herniation is best treated by complete bed rest, without even toilet privileges. Appropriate exercises designed to strengthen pelvic and back musculature should be initiated as soon as pain subsides, and preferably before ambulation. At times a lumbosacral corset is necessary. Operation is reserved for those who fail to respond to bedrest, have repeated relapses, or are unable to pursue their work because its physical nature induces further trouble. Severe motor loss or the loss of bladder function requires prompt surgery.

CERVICAL REGION

Herniation of a disc occurs less frequently in the cervical region than in the lumbar region. Acute disc protrusion occurs with about equal frequency at C-5–C-6 and C-6–C-7 levels, less frequently at C-4–C-5 and C-8–T-1. As in the lumbar region, trauma usually plays a significant role, although the event can be as apparently insignificant as a cough, a sneeze, or a misstep.

Clinical Manifestations. At the C-5–C6 interspace, the C-6 root is involved, and there is pain along the upper border of the trapezius, over the biceps, and along the radial side of the forearm to the thumb. Paresthesias may be felt in the same distribution but chiefly in the thumb. The biceps muscle is weakened, and the radial and biceps reflexes may be diminished. Involvement of the C-7 root at C-6–C-7 interspace causes pain referred to the scapula, the pectoral region, the posterior aspect of the upper arm, and the dorsal surface of the forearm to the thumb and index finger. Paresthesias are more prominent in the index finger and may spread to the thumb and middle finger. The triceps muscle is weak, and its reflex diminished.

Cough or strain causes a sharp, shooting increase of the pain of cervical root compression. The cervical spine is straightened, and pain is increased on tipping the head to the side of pain. Larger lateral and central protrusions may cause spinal cord compression. Roentgenograms may show narrowing of the disc space and straightening of the cervical spine. In the absence of signs of cord compression, myelography may be deferred until the patient has had a trial of conservative treatment. If this fails and surgery is contemplated, myelography is performed, seeking a filling defect at the corresponding level. Central protrusions may simulate intramedullary tumors on myelography.

Treatment. Conservative treatment consists of analgesics, bedrest, and immobilizing the neck in a slightly anteflexed position, particularly at night. A Thomas collar or a more comfortable equivalent may be used. Intermittent cervical traction with the head slightly anteflexed is indicated to treat more severe pain. There is much variation in the manner in which traction is used. Most commonly, traction of 15 to 20 pounds for periods of 20 minutes to one hour is used several times a day with the patient in a sitting position. The severity of the pain may be such that more constant traction is necessary. In this instance, 8 to 12 pounds of traction, with the patient reclining, may be employed as often as every other hour. Approximately 90 per cent of patients with acute cervical radiculopathy owing to disc protrusion recover with conservative treatment. Surgery is reserved for those who fail to respond or who have evidence of spinal cord compression.

Ehni, G., et al.: Significance of the small lumbar spinal canal: Cauda equina compression syndromes due to spondylosis (Parts I to V). J. Neurosurg., 31:490, 1969.
Rabinovitch, R.: Diseases of the Intervertebral Disc and Its Surrounding Tissues. Springfield, Ill., Charles C Thomas, 1961.
Spanos, N. C., and Andrew, J.: Intermittent claudication and lateral lumbar disc protrusions. J. Neurol. Neurosurg. Psychiat., 29:273, 1966.
Spurling, R. G.: Lesions of the Lumbar Intervertebral Disc. Springfield, Ill., Charles C Thomas, 1953.
Spurling, R. G.: Lesions of the Cervical Intervertebral Disc. Springfield, Ill., Charles C Thomas, 1956.

CHRONIC SPINAL INTERVERTEBRAL DISC DISEASE
John F. Sullivan

CERVICAL SPONDYLOSIS

Definition. Cervical spondylosis is a chronic degenerative disease of the cervical spine and intervertebral discs akin to osteoarthritis. Loss of elasticity of the disc owing to aging and trauma causes the intervertebral disc space to narrow. The anulus fibrosus consequently bulges, and may calcify to form osteophytes. Transverse osteophytic ridges diminish the anteroposterior diameter of the spinal canal, and spurs protrude more laterally into the spinal canal or encroach upon the intervertebral foramina, where they compress nerve roots or the spinal cord's blood supply. Spondylosis is present in most persons by middle age, but spinal cord and nerve root compression occurs in only a few. More severe degrees of the arthropathy, repeated trauma, a smaller than normal anteroposterior diameter of the cervical canal, and fibrosis of the adjacent root sleeves limiting mobility of the spinal cord are all factors that hasten the development of symptoms.

Clinical Manifestations. Almost all patients are 45 years old or more. The incipient symptoms include mild restriction of neck movement or aching discomfort and paresthesias in the C-6 or C-7 distribution, often accentuated by posture and movement and difficult to distinguish from symptoms arising from muscle tension or neurovascular compression at the thoracic outlet. In more advanced stages of the disease, laterally placed osteophytes are likely to cause root pain and paresthesias, segmental weakness, and atrophy and fasciculations in one or both upper extremities. The earliest signs of spinal cord compression may consist of a reduced perception of vibration sense in the lower extremities. Later, the stretch reflexes are increased, and extensor plantar responses emerge. With advanced spinal cord involvement, the legs become spastic and weak; paresthesias extend up the legs in socklike distribution, and loss of position sense is added to the vibratory impairment. A sensory level with change to pain and temperature sensibilities may develop on the trunk. Unless acute trauma is superimposed, the process follows an irregular course with long periods of lack of progression. Serious sphincter involvement almost never occurs.

Laboratory findings are only of partial help in diagnosis. Many patients have the roentgenographic changes of cervical spondylosis, so that correlation with the neurologic changes must be made cautiously. The cerebrospinal fluid is usually normal in spondylosis, although the protein content may be raised modestly, and some patients have a partial manometric block. Pantopaque myelography establishes the diagnosis in doubtful cases by demonstrating encroachment of the osteophytes on the spinal canal.

Differential diagnosis includes the subacute combined degeneration of pernicious anemia, spinal cord tumor, motor system disease, and syringomyelia.

Treatment. Treatment of cervical spondylosis is unsatisfactory in general. Most patients progress extremely slowly, and their neurologic deterioration halts if they are no longer exposed to trauma and if moderate traction and partial immobilization with a collar are intermittently employed. If paraplegia progresses despite these measures, surgical laminectomy, decompression, and section of the dentate ligaments may be needed.

THORACIC INTERVERTEBRAL DISC PROTRUSION

Thoracic intervertebral disc protrusion is a rare condition causing segmental pain in the thoracic segments associated with spastic weakness of one or both legs. Calcification in the intervertebral disc space may be present, but its absence does not exclude disc herniation. Erosion of the dura is said to occur in a significant proportion of cases. Infarction of the cord is a frequent and disastrous occurrence, and the results of surgery are unpredictable and often poor.

SUBLUXATION

Idiopathic, transient subluxation of a cervical vertebra is an uncommon condition that causes fleeting, shocklike sensations into the arms, or back, and legs associated with weakness of legs and falling. The symptoms recur when the patient loses his balance or stumbles and persist but a few seconds or minutes. Diagnosis is made by plain roentgenograms taken with the neck flexed and extended or by cineroentgenographic examination that shows a slipping of the vertebra on forward flexion.

Patients with rheumatoid arthritis may develop *atlanto-axial dislocation* caused by laxity of the transverse ligament. The condition is sometimes asymptomatic, but more often is discovered as a cause of neck pain or high spinal cord compression.

Atlanto-axial dislocations and transient recurrent dislocations causing intermittent spinal cord compression require spinal fusion.

Auld, A. W., and Buerman, A.: Metastatic spinal epidural tumors. Arch. Neurol. (Chicago), 15:100, 1966.
Brain, W. R., Northfield, D., and Wilkinson, M.: The neurological manifestations of cervical spondylosis. Brain, 75: 187, 1952.
Crandall, P. H., and Batzdorf, U.: Cervical spondylotic myelopathy. J. Neurosurg., 25:57, 1966.
Russell, D. S., and Rubenstein, L. J.: Pathology of Tumors of the Nervous System. 2nd ed. Baltimore, Williams & Wilkins Company, 1963.
Slooff, J. L., Kernohan, J. W., and MacCarty, C. S.: Primary Intramedullary Tumors of the Spinal Cord and Filum Terminale. Philadelphia, W. B. Saunders Company, 1964.
Sparling, H. J., Adams, R. D., and Parker, F., Jr.: Involvement of the nervous system by malignant lymphomas. Medicine, 26:285, 1947.
Stoltmann, H. F., and Blackwood, W.: The role of the ligamentum flavum in the pathogenesis of myelopathy in cervical spondylosis. Brain, 87:717, 1964.
Williams, H. M., Diamond, H. D., Craver, L. F., and Parsons, H. F.: Neurological Complications of Lymphomas and Leukemia. Springfield, Ill., Charles C Thomas, 1959.

Diseases of Nerve Roots, Plexuses, and Peripheral Nerves

Peter James Dyck

BIOLOGY OF THE PERIPHERAL NERVOUS SYSTEM

Peripheral nerves are made up of bundles of nerve fibers whose cell bodies lie within the ventral gray horn of the spinal cord (motor fibers), within the dorsal root ganglion (sensory fibers), and within autonomic ganglia. Myelinated and unmyelinated fibers are surrounded by longitudinally directed collagen fibrils (endoneurium). A bundle of fibers (a fascicle) is surrounded by a tough sheath (the perineurium) made up of neuroepithelial cells and collagen. Between the fascicles and surrounding them is the epineurium.

Peripheral nerves receive their blood supply along their length from various regional blood vessels. An anastomotic artery, which lies in the epineurium, is formed by the branches from regional arteries. Only the arterioles penetrating the perineurium are thought to be end-arteries. Because of the nature of the blood supply, large-artery disease unless extensive does not usually cause infarction within the nerve, but small-artery and arteriolar disease may cause extensive punctate infarctions. The collateral blood supply also explains why a peripheral nerve may be undercut for long distances and placed into a new bed without becoming infarcted. A schematic view of the morphology of a peripheral nerve and its blood supply is shown in the accompanying figure.

The peripheral nervous system includes all the cranial nerves (except the olfactory and the ocular) from their point of exit from the brainstem to their termination. It further includes all segmental nerve roots from their point of exit from the spinal cord; dorsal root ganglia; autonomic ganglia; mixed spinal nerves; brachial, lumbar, and sacral plexuses; and peripheral nerves. A description of the anatomic arrangement of these structures is beyond the scope of this article. However, such knowledge is necessary for adequately assessing the signs of motor, sensory, and autonomic dysfunction in disease of the peripheral nervous system. Since portions of both motor and sensory neurons lie within the spinal cord, it is apparent

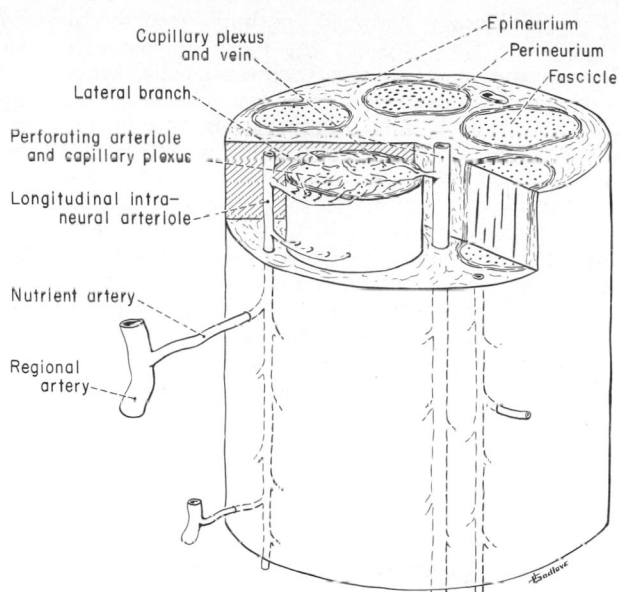

Schematic view of blood supply to a peripheral nerve trunk.

that diseases of these neurons may affect both the central and the peripheral nervous systems.

With the electron microscope, the nature of the structure of myelinated and unmyelinated fibers has been clarified. Both myelinated and unmyelinated fibers are clothed along their length by a series of Schwann cells of neuroectodermal origin. Unmyelinated fibers, first described by Remak, usually occur in clusters. In transverse sections, individual fibers may be seen occupying invaginations of the Schwann cell cytoplasm; but they remain extracellular. Myelinated fibers in their development also extend into invaginations of Schwann cell cytoplasm, but in addition—either by rotation of Schwann cells, or by differential growth—wrap Schwann cell membrane around themselves to form myelin. Especially from the x-ray diffraction and electron microscopic studies of nerve, it is now known that myelin is layered Schwann cell membrane and that nodes of Ranvier are constituted by abutment of two Schwann cells along a fiber.

There is evidence that certain proteins are synthesized in the cell body and flow down the axis cylinder. In addition, Schwann cells have a trophic influence on the axis cylinder.

A lower motor unit is the anterior horn cell (including its axon and terminal branches) and the muscle fibers innervated. Primary sensory units might be thought of as the nerve cell within the dorsal root ganglion which innervates a small region of skin by its peripheral axon and terminal branches. Its central axon makes connections within the spinal cord.

From the work of Gasser and Erlanger, it is known that if a peripheral nerve is laid on a series of electrodes in the appropriate environment, a rapidly conducted wave (usually called the A-α potential) evoked by low-voltage stimulation of large myelinated fibers can be detected.

As the voltage is increased, other deflections appear that correspond to groups of smaller myelinated fibers and finally of unmyelinated fibers (C fiber potential). The modality of sensation lost in diseases of primary sensory neurons usually falls into one of three types: (1) selective decrease or loss of touch-pressure, two-point discrimination, and perception of joint position and motion, with preservation of pain and temperature sensation, owing to selective loss of large myelinated fibers; (2) sensory loss inverse to that just mentioned, owing to loss of unmyelinated and small myelinated fibers; and (3) loss of all sensory modalities, owing to loss of all groups of fibers.

Myelinated nerve fibers undergo at least three types of degeneration. The first, *wallerian degeneration*, occurs in the distal segment after the fiber has been transected. Degeneration of the axis cylinder occurs first, and subsequently the myelin sheath collapses at nodes of Ranvier and at Schmidt-Lanterman incisures. Progressively, the size of the myelin breakdown products diminishes, and their staining characteristics change. In disease, nerve fibers may be focally destroyed and distal portions undergo wallerian degeneration. The second type of myelinated fiber degeneration has been called *"simple atrophy."* Probably a better term would be "axonal dystrophy." An error in metabolism affects certain populations of fibers, particularly in their distal portions (dying-back phenomenon). Probably if the process is rapid, a histologic pattern resembling wallerian degeneration may be seen; but if the development is slow, the visible pattern may resemble that of segmental demyelination. The third process is *segmental demyelination*. Although it is seldom pure (the axis cylinders often being affected also), the primary abnormality is that of demyelination, with portions or entire internodes of myelin breaking down but the axis cylinders remaining intact.

It is sometimes assumed, perhaps incorrectly, that when this happens the basic abnormality lies in the metabolism of Schwann cells. Since various neuropathies have been characterized by their type of fiber degeneration, recognition of the type provides some help in differential diagnosis. Furthermore, the loss of certain populations of nerve fibers may also be characteristic for certain disease processes—for example, selective loss of unmyelinated and small myelinated fibers in dominantly inherited amyloidosis and loss of large myelinated fibers in Friedreich's ataxia.

Pathologic alterations in peripheral nerve disease are seldom specific except in vasculitis, amyloidosis, leprosy, sarcoidosis, embolic disease, and infection. It is now thought that hypertrophic neuropathy is not a disease entity but occurs in any disorder in which there is repeated segmental demyelination and remyelination.

MANIFESTATIONS OF PERIPHERAL NEUROPATHY

The hallmarks of peripheral neuropathy are muscle weakness with or without atrophy, sensory changes, autonomic manifestations, or mixtures of these, all in the appropriate anatomic distribution. Conventionally, peripheral neuropathy is considered to be a disorder of the peripheral nerves that affects predominantly the distal muscles of the extremity, and is associated with sensory loss of all modalities, which also is greatest distally and shades off to normal in more proximal regions of extremities. Although this is a common clinical pattern, not all neuropathies conform to it. Some myelopolyradiculoneuropathies (for example, the Guillain-Barré syndrome) affect the spinal cord and mainly the motor roots, producing weakness in axial and proximal limb muscles as well as in the distal limb muscles. In other diseases such as Friedreich's ataxia or in subacute combined degeneration, the dorsal root ganglia neurons (in addition to other CNS structures) are particularly affected. In some maladies such as metachromatic leukodystrophy or Krabbe's disease, the central nervous system manifestations so dominate the clinical pattern that the disorder in nerve may be overlooked unless one subjects the nerve to histologic examination or measures its conduction velocity.

Patients with neuropathy may not have symptoms or may attribute them to other disease. Commonly the patient with an inherited neuropathy or a chronic neuropathy has no symptoms, or attributes them to a past accident or poliomyelitis. The insidious development of many neuropathies allows for accommodation to the disease. Motor symptoms in such patients are usually described as clumsiness of gait, difficulty in picking up the toes in walking, frequent tripping or stumbling, or inability to perform some ordinary act such as combing the hair, turning a key in a lock, or fastening a safety pin. Some patients notice muscle atrophy, but in chronic neuropathy many of them do not—presumably because the development is so gradual.

Patients with sensory nerve involvement may have symptoms of tightness, burning, jabbing, searing, pricking, tingling, and numbness. These are particularly common in the neuropathies associated with diabetes mellitus, vitamin deficiency, vasculitis, arsenic intoxication, and sprue. In other neuropathies, the predominant symptoms are not of pain or discomfort but rather of a decrease or loss of function, evident as inability to locate a pill in the mouth or to recognize a comb in the pocket, or as unsteadiness in walking owing to kinesthetic loss. Patients with a very slow course tend to have fewer symptoms. Patients with multiple nerve infarcts and acute degeneration of small and large fibers tend to have discomfort, whereas those with segmental demyelination usually have little if any. Loss of sympathetic nerve function, such as occurs in such diseases as diabetes mellitus and amyloidosis, results in postural hypotension, loss of sweating, and bladder and bowel incontinence.

DIFFERENTIAL DIAGNOSIS AND CLASSIFICATION OF PERIPHERAL NEUROPATHY

In evaluating a patient with possible peripheral nerve disease, it is first necessary to establish that there is disease of the peripheral nerves. In some cases the clinical symptoms, the diffuse muscle weakness and atrophy, and the sensory loss may unequivocally suggest a disorder of peripheral nerves. In patients with only muscle weakness and atrophy with either no or equivocal sensory loss, it may be difficult to decide whether the disease is neurogenic or myogenic, but there are three types of study that may help. (1) Concentrations of such serum enzymes as phosphocreatine kinase and the transaminases often are elevated in muscle disease but are usually normal or only slightly elevated in neurogenic muscular atrophy. (2) A particularly helpful study is determination of the conduction velocity of nerves and electromyography. In disease of muscle, conduction velocity of nerves should be normal, unless spuriously decreased by low temperature or by pressure palsies from the patient's remaining in bed for a long time. Conduction velocities may be normal in neurogenic muscle atrophy as well, but in this situation the characteristics of the electromyographic examination may be distinguishing. (See article on Neurologic Diagnostic Procedures.) (3) Biopsy of muscle or nerve. The diagnostic usefulness of these methods of examination varies considerably in different clinics, primarily because of differences in the experience of the persons doing the studies. Neither enzyme tests nor electrophysiologic studies ever provide a specific diagnosis, and the muscle and nerve biopsies do so only infrequently.

A second differential to be made is between disorders of peripheral nerve and disorders of central nervous system disease. In peripheral disorders, muscle weakness is usually associated with atrophy, denervation in electromyographic studies, decrease or absence of the tendon reflexes, and a pattern of sensory loss compatible with disease of multiple nerves. In central lesions muscle weakness is usually unaccompanied by atrophy, tendon reflexes are hyperactive with corticospinal and corticobulbar tract signs, and sensory loss is of the type seen in spinal cord or cerebral hemisphere disease.

Probably the most satisfactory method of classifying the peripheral neuropathies would be based on etiology. Unfortunately, however, the precise etiologic factors for most neuropathies are unknown. Additionally, the diagnosis of many other neuropathies depends entirely on an association with a disease, such as diabetes mellitus, carcinoma, or uremia.

Neuropathies may also be classified by the anatomic site of involvement: cranial neuropathy and peripheral neuropathy, mononeuropathy (single nerves) and multiple neuropathy (multiple nerves), radiculopathy (roots), and plexus neuropathy (brachial, lumbar, or sacral plexus). They may be classified as motor, sensory, and autonomic neuropathy, depending on the predominant type of fiber involvement. On the basis of their rate of progression, neuropathies may be divided into acute, subacute, and chronic categories. In general, they may further be divided into those associated with diffuse low conduction velocity of peripheral nerves (a velocity less than 60 per cent of the mean for normal nerves probably signifies a demyelinating type of fiber degeneration), and those in which the conduction velocities are borderline or only slightly reduced but in which there is other electrophysiologic evidence of fiber degeneration (probably an axonal type of fiber degeneration). Another classification is based on the nature of the sensory loss: in one type there is a selective loss of touch-pressure, two-point discrimination, and joint position, indicating involvement of large myelinated fibers; in another type there is a selective loss of pain and temperature sensation and of autonomic function, indicating loss of unmyelinated fibers; and in a third type there is loss of all sensory modalities, indicating loss of all groups of fibers. Pathologic classifications are based on the nature of the fiber degeneration (wallerian, axonal dystrophy, segmental demyelination) or site of pathologic changes, as well as on the specific histologic pattern (vasculitis, granulomatous reaction, hypertrophic neuropathy, amyloidosis, and specific infective organism).

Although these several ways of classifying the neuropathies may appear to be academic, they are not, for characterization of an unknown case by the criteria listed here will greatly reduce the number of diagnostic possibilities (see accompanying table).

CLASSIFICATION OF PERIPHERAL NEUROPATHY

I. *Mononeuropathy and Plexus Neuropathies*
   A. Cranial nerves
   B. Peripheral nerves
      1. Physical injury
      2. Entrapment neuropathies
         a. Carpal tunnel syndrome
         b. Tardy ulnar nerve palsy
         c. Acute radial nerve palsy
         d. Acute and tardy peroneal nerve palsy
         e. Tarsal tunnel syndrome
         f. Meralgia paresthetica
         g. Thoracic outlet syndrome
      3. Mononeuropathy multiplex
      4. Plexus neuropathy
         a. Brachial plexus neuropathy
         b. Lumbar and sacral plexus neuropathy

II. *Multiple Neuropathy*
   A. Associated with malnutrition and vitamin deficiency
      1. In alcoholism
      2. In malnutrition
      3. In pellagra
      4. In celiac disease
      5. In pernicious anemia
      6. In postgastrectomy condition
   B. Associated with carcinoma and other malignancy
      1. Primary sensory neuropathy with carcinoma
      2. Mixed neuropathy with carcinoma
      3. Peripheral neuropathy with lymphoma
   C. Associated with mesenchymal disease and with necrotizing arteritis
   D. Associated with diabetes mellitus
   E. Associated with drugs and toxins
      1. Heavy metals
         a. Lead
         b. Arsenic
         c. Thallium
         d. Mercury
         e. Copper, antimony, and zinc
      2. Organophosphate compounds (TOCP)
      3. Industrial poisons
      4. Drugs
   F. Neuropathy associated with hormonal disturbances
   G. Neuropathy associated with possible immunologic disorders
      1. Acute segmentally demyelinating polyradiculoneuropathy of the Guillain-Barré-Strohl type
      2. Chronic progressive segmentally demyelinating neuropathy
      3. Chronic relapsing demyelinating neuropathy
      4. Serum neuropathy
   II. Neuropathy associated with infection
      1. Diphtheria
      2. Leprosy
   I. Neuropathy associated with inborn errors of metabolism (hereditary disorders)
      1. Predominant involvement of lower motor neurons
         a. Infantile proximal muscular atrophy (Werdnig-Hoffman)
         b. Progressive bulbar paralysis of childhood (Fazio Londe)
         c. Neural type of arthrogryposis multiplex congenita
         d. Juvenile and late-onset proximal muscular atrophy (Wohlfart, Kugelberg, and Welander)
         e. Progressive spinal muscular atrophy of the Charcot-Marie-Tooth type
         f. Scapulo-peroneal muscular atrophy
         g. Amyotrophic lateral sclerosis (Duchenne and Aran)
      2. Predominant involvement of primary sensory neurons
         a. Hereditary sensory radicular neuropathy (Hicks, Thevenard, and Denny-Brown)
         b. Hereditary sensory neuropathy (Swanson, Buchan, and Alvord)
         c. Angiokeratoma corporis diffusum (Fabry's)
      3. Involvement of lower motor or primary sensory neurons and other systems
         a. Neuronal Charcot-Marie-Tooth disease

MONONEUROPATHY AND PLEXUS NEUROPATHIES

CRANIAL NERVES

Olfactory. Anosmia is most often the result of local disease in the nasal passageways, skull fracture, or brain tumor and is usually reported by the patient as a defect in taste.

Optic. Any visual field defect is a serious matter and demands thorough investigation. Permanent visual impairment or blindness can occur because of unnecessary delay in the diagnosis and treatment of benign and removable compressive lesions such as meningiomas, craniopharyngiomas, cholesteatomas, and chromophobe adenomas. Intrinsic lesions of the optic nerves, such as occur in multiple sclerosis, tend to produce scotomas, whereas compressive lesions like tumors and carotid aneurysms predispose to monocular and binasal or bitemporal visual field defects. Homonymous field defects are usually the result of lesions of the optic pathways posterior to the chiasm, generally as the result of lesions involving the brain itself.

Oculomotor, Trochlear and Abducens. The motor nerves to the eye may be damaged by a variety of diseases anywhere in their long course from brainstem to orbit. Tumor, aneurysm, and temporal lobe herniation often cause oculomotor palsy, usually with pupillary involvement. A slightly dilated pupil and sluggish response to light may be early, subtle signs of third-nerve compression. Either purulent or granulomatous meningitis may impair third- or, more commonly, sixth-nerve function. Increased intracranial pressure may cause unilateral or, especially, bilateral abducens palsy.

Loss of normal eye movement can be a difficult diagnostic problem. The rapid onset of oculomotor palsy associated with pain around or behind the eye immediately suggests diabetic mononeuropathy, migraine, or intracranial aneurysm. However, in as many as one third of such cases no satisfactory cause is found. The pupil usually is dilated with aneurysm and migraine, but not in diabetes or in the idiopathic types. Aneurysm is frequently, but not always, accompanied by hypertension and subarachnoid hemorrhage. A history

of typical headache, previous ocular palsy, and occurrence in childhood favors migraine. Diabetic ophthalmoplegia occasionally also includes the sixth nerve and may occur with only mild glucose intolerance; improvement usually begins within three to five weeks, though diplopia persists until motor balance is nearly perfect. Occurrence of other neurologic deficits, along with impaired ocular motility, is common with aneurysm or tumor, and is expected with a midbrain infarct. Myasthenia gravis can affect extraocular muscles as an isolated symptom and should be considered, especially when the weakness differs from typical cranial nerve patterns, is inconstant, includes eye opening and closing, does not involve the pupil, and is bilateral.

Abnormalities of pupillary size, shape, and reaction are not confined to third-nerve injuries. The *Argyll Robertson pupil* is small, irregular, usually bilateral, responds to convergence accommodation but not to light, and responds poorly to mydriatics; it is common with neurosyphilis and rare with diabetes. The pupils of diabetics are often unequal and may be completely nonreactive. *Adie's myotonic pupil* may cause confusion. It reacts only slowly to light or accommodation convergence, but constricts to fresh 2.5 per cent mecholyl instilled in the conjunctival sac, whereas a normal pupil does not.

Bilateral external ophthalmoplegia of rapid or sudden onset occurs with four diseases, all of which are potentially serious and demand prompt treatment: acute myasthenia gravis, acute thiamin deficiency with Wernicke's syndrome, botulism, and acute idiopathic cranial polyneuropathy.

Trigeminal. Impairment of function peripherally in the sensory components of the trigeminal nerve may result from a variety of neoplastic and inflammatory processes. Divergence of the third division from the first and second, which pass forward through the cavernous sinus, frequently allows precise localization.

Trigeminal neuralgia is described elsewhere in this book.

Facial. Brain injury above the facial nucleus usually spares the brow and forehead muscles because they are bilaterally represented at higher nervous levels; injury to the facial nerve at, or peripheral to, its nucleus paralyzes all the ipsilateral facial muscles. An intrapontine lesion causing facial weakness usually also affects abducens nerve function. As the facial nerve leaves the pons and enters the internal auditory meatus along with the acoustic nerve, it also carries fibers for lacrimation, salivation, and taste. As the nerve descends through the petrous bone, fibers to the lacrimal glands branch off first, then salivary and taste fibers depart in the chorda tympani and cross the middle ear. Only motor fibers to the face emerge from the stylomastoid foramen. Thus the syndrome of seventh nerve damage varies according to the site of injury. Acoustic neurinomas and other tumors of the cerebello-pontine angle often involve the facial nerves, as do infections and neoplasms of the meninges.

Bell's palsy is a peripheral facial weakness of

unknown cause and rapid onset, occasionally attended by aching pain about the angle of the jaw or behind the ear. Retraction of the angle of the mouth and eye closure are impaired, and the forehead is smooth on the affected side. Taste perception on the anterior part of the involved half of the tongue may be distorted. Rarely, hyperacusis results from paralysis of the stapedius muscle. Recovery usually begins within a week, and three of four patients fully recover over a period of several weeks. Occasionally, some permanent deficit remains after a protracted course. In these cases, distressing facial spasms may accompany voluntary facial movement. Adrenal corticosteroids begun near the onset of the illness and continued for seven to ten days may favor a more rapid and complete recovery.

Herpes zoster affecting the geniculate ganglion produces a severe facial paralysis that is associated with a painful eruption within the external ear canal. This, often referred to as the *Ramsay-Hunt syndrome,* may also involve the auditory nerve.

Chronic facial hemispasm affects middle-aged or older women somewhat more commonly than men, with spontaneous, unilateral, frequent, sudden, strong, brief contractions of part or all of the facial musculature. The condition usually begins with the orbicularis oculi muscle and, over many years, spreads to involve more of the face. The cause is not known, but a slowly progressive, degenerative condition of the facial nucleus in the pons has been postulated. Relief can be obtained by alcohol injection or section of the facial nerve, but it must be weighed against the facial paralysis necessarily produced.

Auditory. Disturbances of eighth nerve function are discussed in the articles on Vertigo and Deafness.

Glossopharyngeal, Vagus, and Spinal Accessory. The glossopharyngeal and vagus nerves supply sensory and motor innervation to the pharynx. They may be involved by tumor or aneurysm along with the spinal accessory nerves in their common exit through the jugular foramen. Hoarseness and asymmetric elevation of the soft palate result from lesions of the vagus nerve, and weakness and atrophy of sternocleidomastoid and superior trapezoid muscles result from disruption of the spinal accessory.

Glossopharyngeal neuralgia is described elsewhere in this book.

Hypoglossal. This motor nerve to the tongue is rarely involved in its peripheral course. Atrophy and fasciculation of the ipsilateral half of the tongue are seen, and the tongue deviates toward the affected side upon protrusion.

PERIPHERAL NERVES

Physical Injury

Spinal nerves, plexuses, and peripheral nerve trunks may be injured by traction, compression, contusion, and laceration. Nerves may be damaged be electricity and radiation. Fractured bones may lacerate or compress nerves. Excessively tight casts or tourniquets may damage nerves by direct compression or by ischemia. Injection of penicillin or other medications into the sciatic nerve can cause serious injury. The text by Sunderland gives details on these and other nerve injuries.

Entrapment Neuropathies

Peripheral nerves may be injured by compression or ischemia at points where they pass through rigid anatomic canals or beneath tight fascial bands. Such injury occurs more readily when inflammation or degeneration develops in adjacent joints and tendons (as may happen in rheumatoid arthritis, myxedema, and acromegaly), and when the nerves lie in shallow grooves allowing them to be compressed or repeatedly traumatized.

CARPAL TUNNEL SYNDROME

In the carpal tunnel syndrome the median nerve is compressed as it passes through the canal made by the carpal bones and ligament. Some cases are idiopathic, and, in these, surgeons report a flattening of the median nerve just distal to the crease of the wrist and either thickening of the ligament or, more commonly, noninflammatory thickening of the synovia of the flexor tendons. The median nerve may be compressed within the carpal tunnel by a ganglion or by degenerative joint and synovial changes from rheumatoid arthritis, myxedema, and acromegaly.

This common disorder affects women especially. Pricking numbness and pain in the fingers and hands, coming on especially during the night and relieved by changing the position of the hands (shaking them), are characteristic. It is uncommon for patients to localize the numbness to the exact cutaneous distribution of the median nerve. Furthermore, the aching discomfort that may accompany the numbness may extend up the arm. Atrophy of the muscles innervated by the median nerve (for example, the thenar muscles) is not an early sign. In many cases it is possible to reproduce the painful numbness by holding the wrist in extreme flexion for a short period (*Phalen's sign).* Also a burst of tingling may occur when the skin over the nerve at the wrist is percussed. (*Tinel's sign).* There may be sensory loss in the distribution of the median nerve, though more frequently none is detected.

An important confirmatory test can now be done in most electromyographic laboratories. It consists in determining the time from stimulation of the median nerve at a point above the carpal ligament to the appearance of the thenar muscle action potential. Similarly, one can determine the time from stimulation of digital fibers to the obtaining of an action potential in electrodes overlying the median nerve above the carpal ligament. In the carpal tunnel syndrome, the latency of both responses usually is prolonged.

Since the carpal tunnel syndrome may be

brought on by an excess of gardening, ironing, sewing, crocheting, or similar activity, relief may follow their discontinuance. Immobilization of the wrist during the hours of sleep with a posterior splint of forearm and hand may give relief. Injections of corticosteroid preparations beneath the carpal ligament sometimes help. Treatment for an associated disease (myxedema, rheumatoid arthritis, acromegaly) may effect an improvement. However, in most instances the treatment of choice is surgical section of the carpal ligament which usually provides almost immediate relief.

TARDY ULNAR NERVE PALSY

The ulnar nerve may be injured at the elbow, especially in persons with a shallow ulnar groove, those who rest their weight on their elbows excessively, and those who are cachectic and lie in bed.

Contrary to the finding in the carpal tunnel syndrome, muscle weakness and atrophy characteristically predominate over sensory symptoms and signs, possibly because the ulnar nerve at the elbow has relatively fewer sensory fibers than the median nerve at the wrist. Characteristically, the patient notices atrophy of the first dorsal interosseous muscle or difficulty in performing fine manipulations. There may be numbness of the small finger and contiguous half of the proximal and middle phalanges of the ring finger and ulnar border of the hand. Treatment consists in prevention of further injury. A doughnut cushion for the elbow may be helpful. Mobilizing and transplanting the nerve to a position in front of the median epicondyle may prevent further progression of the disorder.

ACUTE RADIAL NERVE PALSY

The radial nerve may be compressed against a hard edge or surface after digesting an excess of alcohol or sedatives (Saturday night palsy) or may be compressed for excessive periods by the weight of the head of another (bridegroom's palsy). With time, complete recovery may be expected.

ACUTE AND TARDY PERONEAL NERVE PALSY

The common peroneal nerve is vulnerable where it crosses the head of the fibula, and can be injured when a person falls asleep in the sitting position with the knees crossed. A more chronic form occurs in cachectic patients who lie for prolonged periods with the legs externally rotated. In this disorder, dorsiflexion of the foot at the ankle and extension of the toes are weak, but usually little or no sensory loss is found over the lateral surface of the leg and on the dorsum of the foot.

TARSAL TUNNEL SYNDROME

In fractures of the ankle, compression of the posterior tibial nerve may occur, resulting in pain and numbness of the sole of the foot.

MERALGIA PARESTHETICA

Fat people wearing tight corsets, people wearing gun belts, and people with pendulous abdomens may develop superficial paresthesia and burning discomfort in the distribution of the lateral cutaneous nerve of the thigh. Presumably the trouble results from compression of this nerve as it passes beneath the inguinal ligament.

THORACIC OUTLET SYNDROME

Formerly, paresthesias of the fingers were frequently attributed to compression of the brachial plexus by a cervical rib or a tight scalene anterior muscle. However, most such patients prove to have either a cervical disc or carpal tunnel syndrome.

Mononeuropathy Multiplex

The term "mononeuropathy multiplex" implies that a process involves several different peripheral nerves in different regions of the body. Characteristically, the disorder begins with pain, paresthesias, or weakness in the distribution of a peripheral nerve which progresses to a maximal deficit within a few hours to several days. Other nerves become affected within days. The nerves of the lower extremities are affected more often than the upper, and signs are usually asymmetric. After the initial involvement the disorder may improve, relapse, or deteriorate. This type of neuropathy is a common manifestation of polyarteritis nodosa, but is also encountered in diabetes mellitus, rheumatoid arthritis, disseminated lupus erythematosus, and scleroderma.

The pathologic changes in most instances affect the interfascicular arteries of nerves, which may show degeneration of the media, fragmentation of the internal elastic lamina, thickening of the intima, and infiltration of the media and adventitia by mononuclear cells and polymorphonuclear cells (especially eosinophils). Occlusion of an interfascicular artery produces a pie-shaped infarct with its arc along the perineurium and the apex toward the center of the fascicle. Because of separation and recombination of fascicles at more distal levels of the nerve, degenerating fibers in a section from the nerve taken distal to the infarct may contain in many of its fascicles degenerating fibers that come from the same circumsected origin.

Plexus Neuropathy

BRACHIAL PLEXUS

The brachial plexus can be injured by traction, penetrating wounds, or compression. *Acute nontraumatic brachial plexus neuropathy* is a disorder of unknown cause. Antecedent needle injections into shoulder muscles, intercurrent infections, and an allergic basis have been suggested as possible etiologic factors. Typically this disorder begins with aching pain in the lateral aspect of the shoulder or, less often, in the region of the elbow or arm. Muscle weakness develops within a few hours or days, and atrophy follows; sensory loss is usually minimal and is restricted to a small patch in the cutaneous distribution of the axillary nerve. The upper brachial plexus is much more commonly affected than the lower, and therefore the weakness and atrophy are more often located in the region of the shoulder. In mild cases, improvement begins in a few weeks, and clinical recovery is complete within months. More characteristically, improvement does not begin for several months and may not be complete for years. Recently it has been shown that the likelihood of eventual complete or almost complete recovery is good. Sometimes, as improvement on one side occurs, the other brachial plexus becomes affected. Careful examination by electromyography may reveal much more extensive involvement of nerves as expected from the clinical examination. The cerebrospinal fluid is usually normal. There is no known treatment.

LUMBAR AND SACRAL PLEXUS AND ROOTS

Under the term *femoral neuropathy*, a disorder has been described which in many cases arises from the lumbar plexus. Most such cases occur in association with diabetes, but occasionally no associated illness is found. Pain centered in the thigh and extending to the medial side of the leg may herald the onset of muscle weakness and atrophy, which usually develops rather rapidly over the next week. If the onset is abrupt and the neurologic signs are restricted to the distribution of the femoral nerve, an infarction of that nerve is a possibility. Careful examination and electromyography, however, often indicate that the condition is more widespread. Such studies often indicate that multiple lumbar and sacral roots are affected with or without involvement of lumbar and sacral plexuses (in reality a lumbosacral radiculoplexus neuropathy). Furthermore, the cerebrospinal fluid protein may be elevated. Although recovery may not occur before months or years have passed, the prognosis is good.

MULTIPLE NEUROPATHY

NEUROPATHY ASSOCIATED WITH MALNUTRITION AND VITAMIN DEFICIENCY

The common feature of these disorders is deficiency of one or more essentials in the diet owing either to inadequate intake (as in alcoholism, hyperemesis of pregnancy, food fads, and starvation) or failure of absorption (as in pernicious anemia, sprue, or gastrointestinal cancer). The pathologic changes in the peripheral nerves are similar in that distal axons of large fibers are affected first and more severely than proximal parts. Rows of myelin breakdown products are seen along peripheral nerves. At the dorsal root ganglion level there may be some slight decrease in the number of neurons. The posterior columns

may show some demyelination. Ordinarily the conduction velocities of the nerves are not markedly abnormal. These disorders are discussed fully under Nutritional Disorders of the Nervous System.

NEUROPATHY ASSOCIATED WITH CARCINOMA AND OTHER MALIGNANCY

In malignancy, peripheral nerves may be affected by direct implantation, by compression against bony structures, and by remote unknown mechanisms. (See article on Nonmetastatic Effects of Cancer). Sites at which peripheral nerves may be compressed are the foramina of exit of the segmental nerves, the retroperitoneal space, and the nasopharynx. Neuropathy in a patient with malignancy may also develop from drugs used in treatment, as from vinca alkaloids in treatment of lymphoma.

Mixed Neuropathy with Carcinoma

Mixed sensory motor neuropathies have been found in association with carcinoma of the bronchus, gastrointestinal tract, thyroid, ovary, and other organs. Whether this is a specific association or is due to nutritional effects is still unknown.

Peripheral Neuropathy with Lymphoma

Peripheral neuropathies have been found in association with multiple myeloma and various leukemias and lymphomas. The lack of pain and the symmetry of the disorder are usually interpreted as indicating that the peripheral nerve involvement is a remote effect and not due to direct invasion. However, such invasion has been demonstrated in a few cases, particularly when meticulously searched for. The treatment for the neuropathy is the treatment for the primary tumor.

NEUROPATHY ASSOCIATED WITH MESENCHYMAL DISEASE AND NECROTIZING ANGIITIS

The neuropathy associated with these disorders is usually a mononeuropathy multiplex as described above. However, in a small percentage of cases the onset is that of a symmetrical multiple neuropathy. With the latter presentation, the correct category of disease is suggested by the painful nature of sensory symptoms and the associated signs of multiple tissue involvement.

NEUROPATHY ASSOCIATED WITH DIABETES MELLITUS

It is now known that most patients with diabetes mellitus have some dysfunction of the peripheral nerves, and that even those who are asymptomatic may have an abnormality of conduction velocity. The neuropathies fall into two types: mononeuropathy, involving single cranial nerves such as the oculomotor or large single peripheral nerves and plexuses as described above, and polyneuropathy, as described in this section.

Pathology. Neither the pathogenesis nor the pathology of diabetic neuropathy is fully understood. The greater amount of atherosclerosis of limb vessels of diabetic patients probably does not account for the neuropathy. If the polyneuropathy is due to ischemia, it is more likely to be due to a specific angiopathy involving small arteries or arterioles. Thickening of the basement membranes of such vessels has been described. It is not clear whether the observed segmental demyelination is due to ischemia, to deranged metabolism selectively affecting Schwann cells, or is secondary to nerve fiber change.

Clinical Manifestations. Presumably most diabetics have asymptomatic polyneuropathy. Symptomatic polyneuropathy is typically a symmetric, distal sensorimotor neuropathy occurring in elderly patients with mild diabetes. Sensory symptoms in the toes and feet predominate and include numbness, burning paresthesia, and stabbing pains. The soles of the feet are often excessively sensitive to tactile or painful stimuli, rendering walking unpleasant. In the majority of patients with diabetic neuropathy, touch-pressure, vibration, and joint position sensations are predominantly affected, presumably because of a greater involvement of large myelinated fibers. If the loss of position sensation is severe, locomotor ataxia develops (pseudotabes diabetica). This ataxia is worse in the dark. Those patients with much discomfort are usually found to have loss of pain sensation, temperature sensation, and autonomic function, presumably owing to loss of small myelinated and of unmyelinated fibers. The disorder usually develops insidiously and may remain static or progress over the course of many years. It is unlikely to remit, as are the femoral, lumbosacral, radiculoplexus, and oculomotor neuropathies. It has not been established that good control of the blood sugar with insulin or with oral hypoglycemic agents prevents the development or results in improvement of symptomatic neuropathy. Charcot joints, although rare, do occur. Disturbances of intestinal motility, loss of hair, and shiny tight dry skin are attributable to autonomic nerve damage.

One clinical variant of the neurologic complications of diabetes has been called diabetic amyotrophy. Older males with recent substantial weight loss are said to be predominantly affected. Bilateral asymmetric proximal weakness of the lower limbs, with anterior thigh pain, myalgia, and muscle wasting, is seen. Some have extensor plantar responses. Based on the characteristics of the electromyographic examination, patients with the aforementioned symptoms usually can be shown to have involvement of multiple lumbar nerve roots or of the lumbar or sacral plexus. The relatively abrupt onset and good prognosis rule out spondylosis as a cause. Most of the cases described under this term would probably fall under the previously described category of femoral neuropathy, which in reality is a lumbosacral radiculoplexus neuropathy.

The protein concentration of the cerebrospinal fluid in diabetic neuropathy is often elevated from 50 to 400 mg. per 100 ml.

Treatment. It is the current practice to maintain good control of the blood sugar in order to prevent or improve neuropathy in spite of the lack of evidence of such prevention or improvement. There is a suggestion from some reports that repeated hypoglycemic attacks may hasten the onset or worsen the existing neuropathic state. To prevent trophic ulcers of the feet in patients with loss of pain and temperature sensation, good foot care and special shoes are needed.

NEUROPATHY ASSOCIATED WITH DRUGS AND TOXINS

Many drugs and toxins can damage peripheral nerves, and new agents constantly join the list. Publicity, legislation, and education have reduced the frequency of poisoning by some of the older chemicals.

Heavy Metals

Peripheral neuropathy has been reported in association with lead, arsenic, thallium, mercury, copper, antimony, and zinc. However, only the first two occur with any frequency.

Lead poisoning was formerly a common occurrence, but is becoming rare. Lead ingestion or inhalation may occur among farm workers using insecticides (for example, arsenate of lead), among painters using lead paint, among children who chew lead-containing paint from cribs and walls, among factory workers burning batteries or working with white lead, and among persons who drink beer or water stored in leadlined containers or run through lead pipes. Upper abdominal colic, joint pain, peripheral neuropathy, and encephalopathy develop. The encephalopathy is particularly characteristic of toxicity in children. The neuropathy is mainly motor and asymmetric, beginning in the upper extremity with wrist drop and weakness of the extensor muscles of fingers.

The peripheral nerves in lead neuropathy undergo segmental demyelination. The normal amount of lead in a 24-hour urine specimen is less than 80 μg. For a diagnosis of lead poisoning the value should be at least twice this. The treatment is discussed in the article on Lead Poisoning.

Arsenic has been a favorite choice for homicide. Arsenic poisoning has also resulted from drinking illegal alcohol ("moonshine") and from eating food sprayed with insecticides. It is manifested by vomiting and other gastrointestinal symptoms, a scaly exfoliating rash, and evidences of neuropathy. White lines in the fingernails (Aldrich-Mees lines) may provide a diagnostic clue.

Arsenic poisoning produces a mixed motor and sensory neuropathy which is symmetric and distal and affects the lower extremities preferentially. The nerve fibers undergo an axonal type of degeneration. Diagnosis is made by identifying increased levels of arsenic in the nails, hair, or urine. (See article on Arsenic Poisoning.)

Organophosphate (Triorthocresylphosphate) Compounds

Widespread ingestion of fluid extract of ginger in the United States in 1930 was followed by thousands of cases of severe polyneuropathy, mostly motor and distal in distribution. It was established that adulteration with triorthocresylphosphate was responsible and, since that time, periodic outbreaks have occurred traceable to adulterated cooking oil, the most recent being in Italy where used motor oil was sold for cooking purposes. The neuropathy is delayed 10 to 14 days after poisoning. Imperfect recovery is the rule. Years after the acute poisoning, spastic paraparesis emerges, indicating that damage to the spinal cord occurs but is not immediately apparent because of the severe neuropathy. There is no effective treatment.

Industrial Poisons

Trichlorethylene, an anesthetic agent, is also a powerful solvent used in industry. In toxic amounts, it produces multiple cranial nerve palsies and trigeminal nerve analgesia. Particularly in Japan, n-hexane an organic solvent used in printing, extraction of vegetable oil, and cleaning, has been associated with peripheral neuropathy. Acrylamide is a chemical that is pumped into soil to render it waterproof. In both man and animals, it produces peripheral neuropathy by an axonal type of degeneration of myelinated fibers.

Drugs

Many medicaments can produce numbness in distal extremities and neurogenic weakness, including isoniazid, diphenylhydantoin sodium, nitrofurantoin, and the vinca alkaloids. Arsenic in Fowler's solution, mercury in various antisyphilitic preparations, and gold in treatment for rheumatoid arthritis also can produce peripheral neuropathy.

NEUROPATHY ASSOCIATED WITH HORMONAL DISTURBANCES

Myxedema and acromegaly both predispose to the syndrome of the carpal tunnel. In myxedema a more diffuse peripheral neuropathy may occur.

NEUROPATHY ASSOCIATED WITH POSSIBLE IMMUNOLOGIC DISORDERS

Acute Segmentally Demyelinating Polyradiculoneuropathy

(Infectious Polyneuritis, Acute Polyneuritis with Facial Diplegia, Acute Polyradiculitis, Guillain-Barré-Strohl Syndrome)

Etiology. The cause is unknown, although a similar illness has been produced in animals by inoculating extracts of peripheral nerve plus adjuvants. This, plus the characteristic postinfectious timing has led many workers to postulate an autoimmune mechanism.

Pathology. The pathologic changes bear some resemblance to those of experimental allergic neuritis. There are foci of mononuclear cells in the roots and in the peripheral nerves, and these are associated with segmental demyelination. Proximal slowing of conduction velocity may be seen in about a third of the cases. In others the low conduction velocities are more generalized.

Clinical Manifestations. Most, but not all, patients give a history of a banal, nonspecific, febrile illness, usually respiratory, preceding the neurologic disorder by 10 to 21 days. The polyneuropathy usually begins insidiously and without fever, malaise, nausea, or prostration. A few patients suffer muscle pain or, occasionally, stiff neck. Weakness may start in the face or hands but is most common in the lower extremities, and always is bilateral, though sometimes asymmetrical. The motor paralysis is flaccid and has a considerable tendency to ascend the body (*Landry's ascending paralysis*) and to involve both the trunk and upper limbs. Less frequently, paralysis affects the face, the muscles of swallowing, or the oculomotor muscles. About 5 per cent of patients develop urinary retention. Sensory symptoms and signs affect 90 per cent of patients. Paresthesias usually begin in the toes and fingers, and may spread proximally, but demonstrable sensory deficits are usually modest. Variant onsets are common, and weakness may begin in the upper limbs or even in the oculomotor muscles. Progression may cease at any point in the course. Once weakness reaches its maximum, a plateau occurs that lasts for several days to several weeks, depending on the individual. Following this, improvement begins and continues for weeks or, rarely, many months. About one patient in 20 develops papilledema.

The classic cerebrospinal fluid findings are of a normal pressure with an elevated protein concentration but without increased numbers of leukocytes. However, many exceptions exist, and the protein concentration may be normal at any time in the course of the illness, particularly at the onset. Rarely, a mild lymphocytosis is discovered in the cerebrospinal fluid at the outset of the disease.

The prognosis for full recovery from paralysis is good but not invariable, and perhaps one of ten patients is left with muscle weakness of some degree. Without mechanical ventilation, there is 10 to 20 per cent mortality, the result of respiratory and vasomotor failure. Thus, upon first encounter with the patient, even one in whom weakness may be slight and distal, the physician must anticipate a possible need for a respirator and vasopressor agents within a day or so.

Treatment. Adrenal steroids have been widely used to treat severe cases, but there are no controlled studies by which to judge their effectiveness, and it is difficult to know whether they are beneficial. Skilled nursing care is imperative as is the availability of an intensive care unit to manage potential respiratory insufficiency. Full convalescence may require months, and a few patients suffer recurrent bouts of weakness and a relapsing course that may go on for years.

Chronic Progressive Segmentally Demyelinating Neuropathy

This disorder may be the same as the preceding one, except that possibly the pathogenic mechanisms persist, and so the disorder continues. Typically, the onset is much more protracted, and the disease is more prolonged; but the symptoms are symmetric and predominantly motor. When sensory loss is present, it affects the modalities of touch-pressure, joint position, and vibration. Occasionally papilledema develops, but without headaches or focal cerebral disorders. In addition, a tremor with the features of essential tremor may develop. Conduction velocities are usually diffusely low. In nerve biopsies, segmental demyelination and remyelination are evident. A few patients seem to respond favorably to corticosteroids.

Chronic Relapsing Demyelinating Neuropathy

This disorder is probably a variant of the Guillain-Barré syndrome and of chronic progressive segmentally demyelinating neuropathy. However, the course is different in that spontaneous remissions and relapses occur. Also, the stage of greatest deficit may be slower in development than the Guillain-Barré syndrome. In some cases, corticosteroids bring a remission; in others they worsen the disorder. The cerebrospinal fluid protein is elevated and without cells. Conduction velocities of nerves are diffusely low. Nerve biopsy discloses segmental demyelination and remyelination adjacent to foci of mononuclear cells. In cases responsive to corticosteroids, the aim of treatment is to produce a remission and then to decrease the dosage of the drug slowly so that exacerbation does not occur.

Serum Neuropathy

The use of antitetanus serum is sometimes associated with a diffuse and severe peripheral neuropathy.

NEUROPATHY ASSOCIATED WITH INFECTION

Diphtheria

Corynebacterium diphtheriae elaborates a protein neuro-exotoxin that particularly affects cranial nerves in nasopharyngeal diphtheria. With pharyngeal membranous diphtheria, the palate is first paralyzed, producing a nasal quality to the voice and an increasing tendency for nasal regurgitation of fluids between the fifth and twelfth days. Further spread of the effects may paralyze vagal motor filaments, causing difficulty in swallowing and hoarseness or aphonia. Because of sensory loss, sore throat is minimal or absent, and, despite its firm attachment, the membrane can be pulled away, leaving a painless bleeding bed. Improvement usually begins after about 10 to 14 days, and these local effects may be all that occur in mild cases.

In others, usually during the third week of illness, near vision becomes indistinct due to paralysis of the ciliary muscle of the eye and failure of accommodation. Rarely, paralysis occurs in structures innervated by the oculomotor, abducens, facial, or hypoglossal nerves.

Polyneuropathy can also develop in the extremities in diphtheria during the second month of illness at a time when weakness of the palate and pharynx may have subsided. It is believed that the polyneuropathy results from circulating exotoxin. The involvement is more severe distally in the extremities, and weakness usually exceeds sensory loss. The distribution is typically symmetrical and often affects the lower limbs earlier than the upper. Reflexes are lost early and often disproportionately to demonstrable weakness. Touch and pain sense are moderately reduced, and proprioception may be severely affected, producing ataxia of gait and clumsiness of the hands out of proportion to the degree of weakness. The proximal muscles are involved in severe cases, causing head drop and, occasionally, respiratory involvement so severe as to require mechanical assistance. The cerebrospinal fluid protein is usually elevated, but there is no increase in cell content.

Diphtheritic infections in tissues other than the pharynx are also potential causes of neuropathy. Infection has been discovered in the cervix uteri of adults, in the umbilical stump of infants and in skin wounds of both adults and children. In such cases, the first presentation can be the peripheral neuropathy leading to an erroneous diagnosis of acute segmentally demyelinating polyradiculoneuropathy of the Gullain-Barré-Strohl type.

Treatment is supportive once polyneuropathy has developed, because antitoxin is ineffective. Recovery from the peripheral neuropathy usually begins between one and three months after onset and continues over several months to a year. Complete recovery is the rule. Fatalities usually are the result of respiratory paralysis or myocarditis.

Leprosy

Mycobacterium leprae (Hansen) frequently invades peripheral nerves as well as the skin, and the two structures are characteristically involved together in the macular leprides. Small numbers of the bacteria may be distributed widely in the peripheral nerves, evoking chronic inflammatory responses, thickening, fibrosis, and distal degeneration. Less often, nodular swellings packed with mycobacteria are encountered along the nerve.

The earliest and most common peripheral lesion is the anesthetic, atrophic, and depigmented macular lepride which is classic for the disease. These lesions gradually enlarge and may cover large parts of the body. Neuritic pains are sometimes a prominent early feature. The nerves also can be involved in a more diffuse and less obviously leprous fashion, producing a distal and roughly symmetrical polyneuropathy in which pain and temperature sensation is selectively impaired far more than other modalities. Autonomic changes can be prominent, and the condition at this stage closely resembles the dissociated sensory loss and other changes of syringomyelia.

Inspection alone establishes the diagnosis of classic examples. Otherwise, leprosy should be suspected in a subject who has lived in an endemic area before the age of 25 and who develops a dissociated sensory loss in adult life accompanied by macular, atrophic skin lesions. Nerve biopsy in an anesthetic region usually reveals the mycobacteria.

NEUROPATHY ASSOCIATED WITH INBORN ERRORS OF METABOLISM

Predominant Involvement of Lower Motor Neurons

In these anterior horn cell disorders, symmetric muscle weakness and atrophy with fasciculations but without sensory loss are found. It often is impossible from the clinical examination alone to determine whether these patients have myopathic or neuropathic disease. Electromyography and muscle or nerve biopsy studies may be needed for differentiation. Electromyographic signs of denervation and alteration of motor unit potentials are characteristic of an anterior horn cell disorder and quite distinct from myopathic change. In biopsied motor nerves, linear rows of myelin breakdown products are seen. Cutaneous nerves are without abnormality. In muscle sections, a pattern characteristic of neurogenic atrophy is seen. The motor neuron diseases are discussed under Degenerative and Heredofamilial Diseases of the Central Nervous System.

Predominant Involvement of Primary Sensory Neurons

In several disorders losses of myelinated fibers in the posterior columns and peripheral nerves are common manifestations of degeneration of the entire neuron. Disease of these neurons can even show functional and structural alterations only at the extremities of their processes, such as the rostral extremity of fibers near the upper end of the posterior columns of the spinal cord and the distal process of fibers in cutaneous nerves. When the syndrome is present in pure form, there may be no evidence of muscle weakness and atrophy. Conduction velocity studies may be helpful in establishing the validity of the sensory symptoms. Typically, the amplitude of the potential from A-α fibers of cutaneous nerves will be too small for recording through the skin by the conventional methods that detect these potentials in normal individuals.

HEREDITARY SENSORY RADICULAR NEUROPATHY (HICKS, THEVENARD, AND DENNY-BROWN)

This dominantly inherited disorder usually begins in the second or third decade with symptoms due to sensory loss in the feet or lower legs, sometimes accompanied by lancinating pain. Sensory loss in the hands usually begins at a later age and is less severe. The loss is greatest distally and shades off to normal proximally. All modalities of sensation are markedly abnormal. Pain and temperature sensation may be absent in the skin of the foot and distal leg. (This pattern corresponds reasonably well to the type of nerve fiber degeneration; there is a greater loss of unmyelinated than of myelinated fibers.) Tendon reflexes are usually decreased. Muscle strength is usually normal, although kinships have been described with associated peroneal muscular atrophy. Trophic ulcers of the feet occur frequently, especially at such weight-bearing points as the head of metatarsal bones. If foot ulcers are neglected, cellulitis, lymphangitis, and osteomyelitis develop. Although no specific treatment is available, these patients should inspect their feet daily, avoid foot injuries, have special foot hygiene and shoes, and be required to stay in bed when foot ulcers develop.

HEREDITARY SENSORY NEUROPATHY (SWANSON, BUCHAN, AND ALVORD)

Siblings have been reported with mental retardation, insensitivity to pain, and lack of ability to sweat. Small dorsal ganglion neurons, Lissauer's tract, and small fibers of the peripheral nerves are lacking. A similar peripheral nerve defect might underlie the insensitivity to pain demonstrated by some children with familial dysautonomia.

ANGIOKERATOMA CORPORIS DIFFUSUM (FABRY'S)

This rare disorder, described elsewhere, is characterized by angiokeratomas, impaired renal function, and small purple to black spots distributed especially over the lower trunk and buttocks along segmental lines. Typically, patients have pain and numbness in the limbs but no motor symptoms.

Involvement of Lower Motor and Primary Sensory Neurons and Other Systems

In this group of disorders, lower motor and primary sensory neurons and other tract systems may be affected to varying degrees. Although not adequately studied or understood, it is thought that various neurons degenerate by a process which affects their extremities first, producing changes in the peripheral nerves and also in spinal cord tracts. This group of disorders is different from the preceding group in that there is clinical, electrophysiologic, and morphologic evidence of involvement of primary sensory neurons.

Peroneal muscular atrophy (Charcot-Marie-Tooth disease) was formerly considered to be a single disorder that was inherited and characterized by weakness and wasting of the distal parts of the limbs. It is now known that this clinical picture includes several distinct disorders that should be separated on the basis of their pattern of inheritance, natural history, and electrophysiologic and morphologic characteristics. The view that all disorders characterized by high arches and hammer toes of the feet and by distal atrophy with varying degrees of involvement of other systems are etiologically related is untenable. There are at least three types of neurogenic peroneal muscular atrophy. The first type is the progressive muscular atrophy form of Charcot-Marie-Tooth disease. The disorder occurs sporadically; it usually begins in the second decade, the muscle weakness and atrophy result in the typical stork-leg configuration, and the course is slowly progressive over many years. There is no sensory loss or electrophysiologic or morphologic evidence of disease of cutaneous nerves. The second type, neuronal Charcot-Marie-Tooth disease, will be discussed here. The third type, hypertrophic neuropathy of the Charcot-Marie-Tooth type, will be discussed below.

NEURONAL CHARCOT-MARIE-TOOTH DISEASE

This dominantly inherited disorder begins in the second decade of life or later. Not uncommonly it begins in the fifth or sixth decade. Symmetric muscle weakness with atrophy begins in small foot muscles, peroneal, long toe extensor, and ankle dorsiflexor muscles. Pes cavus and hammer toes may or may not be associated with the weakness. Initial symptoms include inability to pick up the toes in walking, instability of the ankle, difficulty in standing still in one position, and visible atrophy of muscles. These patients tend to stand with their feet spread apart, and shift their position constantly to maintain balance. Others tend to stand with their knees bent to lock the ankles. Later weakness of small hand muscles may make such acts as unlocking a door with a key, unscrewing the top of a glass jar, or buttoning

difficult. The muscle atrophy of the lower limbs may be typical of peroneal muscular atrophy, with a greater degree of atrophy in the distal aspect of thigh muscles and with much atrophy of leg muscles. Most frequently tendon reflexes are diminished or absent in the lower limbs. Touch-pressure, joint position, and vibration sensation are mildly decreased distally in lower limbs. Conduction velocities of motor fibers are within the limits of normal in upper limbs and only slightly reduced in lower limbs.

Sporadic cases similar in every way to the above are seen. These cases may be a different disorder or the same disorder in which the inherited nature has not been detected. However, Charcot-Marie-Tooth disease is genetically and morphologically entirely distinct from either Friedreich's ataxia or spastic paraplegia with peroneal muscular atrophy, disorders discussed with the Spinocerebellar Degenerations.

These patients can often be helped significantly by leg braces that stabilize the ankle joint. Their use permits these patients to stand still without losing their balance for such acts as shaving.

Predominant Involvement of Peripheral Nerves

HYPERTROPHIC NEUROPATHY OF CHARCOT-MARIE-TOOTH TYPE

This is a fairly common, mild, dominantly inherited variant of peroneal muscular atrophy described above. Affected persons may have no symptoms or signs, but yet be known to have the disorder by their position in the kinship and from characteristic low conduction velocities of all nerves.

Pathologically the disorder affects myelinated fibers only, producing segmental demyelination and remyelination and varying degrees of onion-bulb formation (the hallmark of hypertrophic neuropathy). An actual loss of myelinated fibers probably occurs.

In kinships with the disease an affected person may be recognized by high arches of the feet, hammer toes, curled-up toes (with convexity upward), frequent corns or calluses, and a high-stepping, awkward gait caused by paresis of the dorsiflexor muscles of the ankle and instability of the ankle joint. Persons with greater weakness may have weakness and wasting of the intrinsic hand muscles and weakness of the plantar flexor muscles of the ankles. Ankle-joint instability makes it difficult for such persons to stand still. The amount of muscle atrophy is usually not great. Typically, the tendon reflexes are reduced or absent, disappearing successively from the Achilles tendon, the quadriceps, and the upper extremity. Sensory loss is mild, affecting the modalities of touch-pressure, two-point discrimination, and joint position and motion in the distal parts of the extremities. Clinical enlargement of peripheral nerves may be detected in about one fourth of the cases. Some members of kinships have, in addition to the clinical features mentioned, a tremor of the head and outstretched hands which is indistinguishable from essential tremor (Roussy-Levy syndrome). Foot ulcers occur in occasional persons with this disorder. Osteomyelitis and mutilation of the feet develop only if the ulcers are neglected. There is no specific treatment. Corrective surgery should be reserved for those affected persons who develop ulcers at pressure points owing to excessively high arches and for those with excessive inversion of the foot. Foot-drop springs or braces may be used to elevate the toes in walking and to stabilize the ankle. When foot ulcers develop, a program of ulcer debridement and rest in bed should be begun immediately. Weight-bearing should not be resumed until the ulcer is completely healed. Then shoes should be fitted which have sufficient width, an adequate arch support, and a fit that distributes the weight to all parts of the foot.

HYPERTROPHIC NEUROPATHY OF DÉJÉRINE-SOTTAS TYPE

This is a rare disorder transmitted as an autosomal recessive trait and beginning in infancy. The children learn to walk late, have great difficulty in walking even at their best point of neuromuscular development (ages 8 to 12), and are usually in wheelchairs by the age of 20 years. The patients are usually short, and most have a severe, symmetrical, sensory motor neuropathy affecting predominantly the distal extremities with enlarged peripheral nerves. Some weakness of proximal muscles of the extremities usually is present also. Sometimes there are associated miosis and nystagmus. The conduction velocity of motor and sensory fibers of peripheral nerves is among the lowest determined in electromyographic laboratories. Pathologically, marked segmental demyelination and remyelination are found in myelinated fibers; unmyelinated fibers are probably not affected. A systemic biochemical abnormality involving ceramide hexoses and their sulfates has been found. No specific treatment is available.

HYPERTROPHIC NEUROPATHY OF REFSUM TYPE

This rare progressive or relapsing disorder is inherited as an autosomal recessive trait and is due to the inability of affected subjects to alpha-oxidize ingested phytanic acid. Clinical manifestations usually begin in the second decade with night blindness and constriction of the visual fields owing to an atypical retinitis pigmentosa. Additionally, symptoms caused by a distal sensorimotor neuropathy develop, as well as an ataxia which is thought to be greater than that accounted for by kinesthetic loss. Ichthyosis, skeletal abnormalities, and sudden death in the third or fourth decade from involvement of the heart all provide evidence of systemic extraneural involvement. The cerebrospinal fluid protein is usually markedly elevated. Pathologically, the peripheral nerves contain evidence of segmental demyelina-

tion and remyelination and onion-bulb formation. Pathognomonic is the occurrence of 3,7,11,15-tetramethylhexadecenoic acid (phytanic acid) in the serum, red blood cells, liver, heart, kidneys, and skeletal muscles. Treatment consists of withholding dietary phytols (chlorophyll-free diet); if begun early it can result in dramatic improvement.

DOMINANTLY INHERITED AMYLOIDOSIS (ANDRADE TYPE)

Amyloid neuropathy has been noted most often in countries surrounding the Mediterranean Sea, although kinships are sometimes encountered in the United States, Japan, and other countries. The disorder usually begins in the late second or third decade with loss of the sensations of pain, cold, and heat in the lower extremities accompanied by anhydrosis and, sooner or later, loss of spincter control. Males become impotent. Nerve biopsy studies disclose selective loss of small myelinated and unmyelinated fibers, accounting for the selective sensory loss. Subsequently other fibers are also affected so that sensory loss becomes more generalized, and motor weakness and atrophy develop. The disorder progresses relentlessly to death, usually in the fourth or fifth decade. Amyloid deposits may be found in many tissues, including peripheral nerve, muscle, vitreous of the eye, and many other organs.

DOMINANTLY INHERITED AMYLOIDOSIS (RUKAVINA TYPE)

In contradistinction to the Andrade type of dominantly inherited amyloidosis, the symptoms of the Rukavina type usually begin in the upper extremities, and may suggest the diagnosis of carpal tunnel syndrome. Eventually, a more generalized neuropathy develops.

NEUROPATHY ASSOCIATED WITH PERIPHERAL VASCULAR DISEASE

Besides the vasculitis previously described in polyarteritis nodosa and other collagen diseases, there are alterations produced in the peripheral nerves by atherosclerosis of larger vessels. Patients who experience claudication when walking or who have evidence of peripheral gangrene may also have a distal sensory and motor neuropathy that appears to be due to inadequate blood supply and infarction of nerves. All sensory modalities are affected, and there may be burning, pricking, and jabbing pains in the feet. Depending on the site and distribution of vascular involvement, the neuropathy may be symmetric or asymmetric.

NEUROPATHY ASSOCIATED WITH UREMIA

Particularly since the development of dialysis programs for the treatment of chronic renal disease, severe peripheral neuropathy has appeared in many patients with uremia, affecting approximately one half of the patients receiving dialysis. This neuropathy is mixed motor and sensory, symmetric, and more severe in the distal parts. Bladder and bowel disturbances are unusual. The pathogenesis is unknown. Frequent and apparently adequate dialysis does not always produce a remission, but with successful kidney transplantation the peripheral nerve function returns toward normal.

Asbury, A., Victor, M., and Adams, R.: Uremic polyneuropathy. Arch. Neurol. (Chicago), 8:413, 1963.

Austin, J.: Recurrent polyneuropathies and their corticosteroid treatment. Brain, 81:157, 1958.

Cooke, W., and Smith, W.: Neurological disorders associated with coeliac disease. Brain, 89:683, 1966.

Croft, P., Urich, H., and Wilkinson, M.: Peripheral neuropathy of sensorimotor type associated with malignant disease. Brain, 90:31, 1967.

Denny-Brown, D.: Primary sensory neuropathy with muscular changes associated with carcinoma. J. Neurol. Neurosurg. Psychiat, 11:73, 1948.

Dyck, P., and Lambert, E.: Lower motor and primary sensory neuron diseases with peroneal muscular atrophy. I. Neurologic, genetic, and electrophysiologic findings in hereditary polyneuropathies. Arch. Neurol. (Chicago), 18:603, 1968.

Dyck, P., and Lambert, E.: Lower motor and primary sensory neuron disease with peroneal muscular atrophy. II. Neurologic, genetic, and electrophysiologic findings in various neuronal degenerations. Arch. Neurol. (Chicago), 18:619, 1968.

Dyck, P., and Lambert, E.: Dissociated sensation in amyloidosis. Compound action potential, quantitative histologic and teased-fiber, and electron microscopic studies of sural nerve biopsies. Arch. Neurol. (Chicago), 20:490, 1969.

Dyck, P., Lambert, E., Nichols, P., Auger, R., and Taylor, W.: Quantitative measurement of sensation related to compound action potential and number and sizes of myelinated and unmyelinated fibers of sural nerve in health, Freidreich's ataxia, hereditary sensory neuropathy and tabes dorsalis. Electroenceph. Clin. Neurophysiol., 1970 (in press).

Engel. W., Dorman, J., Levy, R., and Fredrickson, D.: Neuropathy in Tangier disease. Arch. Neurol. (Chicago), 17:1, 1967.

Lovelace, R., and Horwitz, S.: Peripheral neuropathy in long-term diphenylhydantoin therapy. Arch. Neurol. (Chicago), 18:69, 1968.

Moress, G., D'Agostino, A., and Jarcho, L.: Neuropathy in lymphoblastic leukemia treated with vincristine. Arch. Neurol. (Chicago), 16:377, 1967.

Nickel, S., et al.: Myxedema neuropathy and myopathy. A clinical and pathological study. Neurology (Minneap.), 11:125, 1961.

Raff, M., Sangalang, V., and Asbury, A.: Ischemic mononeuropathy multiplex associated with diabetes mellitus. Arch. Neurol. (Chicago), 18:497, 1968.

Refsum, S.: Heredopathia atactica polyneuritiformis. Acta Psychiat. Scand., Suppl. 38:1, 1946.

Steinberg, D., Mize, C. E., Herndon, J. H., Fales, H. M., Engel, W. K., and Vroom, F. O.: Phytanic acid in patients with Refsum's syndrome and response to dietary treatment. Arch. Intern. Med. (Chicago), 125:75, 1970.

Sunderland, S.: Nerves and Nerve Injuries. Edinburgh and London, E. and S. Livingstone Ltd., 1968.

Swanson, A. G., Buchan, G. C., and Alvord, E. C., Jr.: Anatomic changes in congenital insensitivity to pain. Arch. Neurol. (Chicago), 12:12, 1965.

Thomas, P., and Lascelles, R.: The pathology of diabetic neuropathy. Quart. J. Med., 35:489, 1966.

Tyler, H.: Neurological complications of dialysis, transplantation and other forms of treatment in chronic uremia. Neurology (Minneap.), 15:1081, 1965.

Victor, M., Banker, B., and Adams, R.: The neuropathy of multiple myeloma. J. Neurol. Neurosurg. Psychiat., 21:73, 1958.

Wells, C., and Silver, R.: The neurologic manifestations of the acute leukemias. A clinical study. Ann. Intern. Med., 46:439, 1957.

Wiederholdt, W., Mulder, D., and Lambert, E.: The Landry-Guillain-Barré-Strohl syndrome or polyradiculoneuropathy. Historical review, report on 97 patients, and present concepts. Mayo Clin. Proc., 39:427, 1964.

Diseases of Muscle and Neuromuscular Junction

Lewis P. Rowland

INTRODUCTION

Definitions. Probably because there are so many unanswered questions involved, important concepts of neuromuscular disease are ill defined. An air of vagueness pervades the very language used, and the same words have different meanings to different authorities. It is not mere nit-picking to attempt definitions; the concepts are important. In this article, therefore, some of the prevalent words are defined before use.

The word *atrophy* means, literally, "lack of nourishment." It has come to mean wasting of muscle, or loss of muscle bulk from any cause, and it is also used to denote single muscle fibers that are smaller than normal when viewed microscopically. But when used in the name of a disease, it always implies that the muscle wasting is secondary to a neural disorder, e.g., infantile spinal muscular atrophy, progressive spinal muscular atrophy, or peroneal muscular atrophy. To avoid ambiguity, it is therefore appropriate in examining patients to use "wasting" rather than "atrophy" to describe diminution in muscle bulk unless the cause is known to be neurogenic. *Myopathies* include disorders characterized by weakness that is not due to emotional or neurogenic cause. Some authors speak of "primary" or "secondary" myopathies, but there is little evidence that any muscle disease is really "primary," in the sense that there is an abnormality in muscle and nowhere else. In some myopathies, as in thyrotoxic myopathy, the fundamental disorder is elsewhere, and this could be true even in genetically determined diseases. The *dystrophies* are a subgroup of myopathy with two special characteristics: they are genetically determined, and the weakness is progressive. There are other genetic disorders of muscle in which the weakness seems to be stationary, and some in which progressive weakness is not the dominant symptom (transient attacks of weakness in periodic paralysis, cramps, and myoglobinuria in some glycogen diseases, or myotonia); other names are given to these conditions individually.

DIFFERENTIATION OF NEUROPATHIC AND MYOPATHIC DISEASE

When muscles are sick, they are usually weak. Few other symptoms result; sometimes muscles ache (myalgia); sometimes they relax with difficulty (myotonia); sometimes they shorten abruptly and painfully (cramp or contracture). Weakness is the most common symptom of muscle disease, but it is also the symptom that results from neurogenic diseases affecting corticospinal pathways, motor neurons, or peripheral nerves. The differential diagnosis of muscle disease is therefore a problem in distinguishing myogenic from neurogenic causes. Corticospinal disorders have characteristic signs that immediately identify them, and therefore they do not often enter into this differential diagnosis. Disorders of the lower motor neuron or peripheral nerve may be difficult and sometimes impossible to separate from muscle disease. In this kind of neurogenic disorder and in myopathies, weakness, wasting, and depression of myotatic reflexes are common to both groups. Neurogenic disorders are apt to affect distal muscles primarily, whereas myopathic disorders are more likely to affect proximal muscle, but there are so many exceptions that this is an unreliable guide. (Distal myopathy is rare but does occur; proximal weakness is not so rare in motor neuron disease or peripheral neuropathy.) Twitching of muscle is probably a reliable guide to motor neuron disease, but it is not yet definitely excluded as a myopathic sign. The combination of active reflexes in a limb with weak, wasted, and twitching muscles is almost pathognomonic of amyotrophic lateral sclerosis, especially if there are also Babinski signs. Sensory loss and an increased protein content of the cerebrospinal fluid are reliable guides to peripheral neuropathy, but once it is established that there is a peripheral neuropathy, it may be difficult or impossible to state whether there is also a concomitant myopathy. Because of these ambiguities in diagnosis, increasing attention has been directed to three laboratory aids: serum enzymes, electromyography and nerve conduction velocities, and muscle biopsy. Two syndromes are virtually defined in terms of these tests: distal myopathy and "juvenile muscular atrophy simulating muscular dystrophy."

Serum Enzymes. Several different enzyme activities are increased in the serum of patients with X-linked dystrophies and polymyositis, whereas they are not increased in neurogenic diseases. It is often stated that determination of creatine phosphokinase (CPK) activity is the "best" because it is the most sensitive. This enzyme is significantly increased in almost all muscle diseases, but it is, if anything, too sensitive: it picks up all the myopathic cases, but it is sometimes also increased in neurogenic disease. Other serum enzyme levels, e.g., SGOT or lactate dehydrogenase, LDH, and others, do not rise so in myopathies, but do not give falsely positive reactions in neurogenic disorders either. For this reason, it it useful to couple determinations of CPK with SGOT or LDH in evaluating individual cases. CPK has one other considerable advantage: it is not present in erythrocytes or liver and is therefore normal in serum contaminated by hemolysis or in patients with liver disease.

Electromyography. Needle electromyography, the amplification of action potentials from muscle, has been refined to a very useful technique. Normal muscle is electrically silent at rest, and patterns of potentials evoked by voluntary contraction have been analyzed in terms of frequency, duration, and amplitude of individual motor unit potentials. In denervated muscle, there is spontaneous activity (fibrillations from single muscle fibers or fasciculations from motor units), the number of potentials during a voluntary contraction is reduced, and the duration of potentials is increased. In myopathic disorders, there is usually no spontaneous activity, there is no reduction in the number of potentials under voluntary control, and the potentials are reduced in duration. These signs are usually reliable, but in some cases the results are equivocal, and there may be features of both a neurogenic and myopathic disorder.

Nerve Conduction Velocities. The speed of conduction along motor nerves can be recorded accurately, and slowing of conduction is a reliable guide to neuropathy. A normal conduction velocity, however, does not exclude a nerve lesion.

Muscle Biopsy. The features of neurogenic and myopathic diseases can usually be differentiated in a muscle biopsy, especially when one utilizes the new techniques of the rapid examination of frozen tissue and the application of histochemical methods. The electron microscope has opened new approaches that are still in the process of refinement. Only a few diseases can be definitively identified by muscle biopsy: periarteritis nodosa, trichinosis, sarcoidosis, and most (but not all) cases of glycogen storage disease. The congenital myopathies are best identified by histochemical and other special procedures.

In most cases, the results of all these special studies are consistent, one with the other. In some cases, however, the results are conflicting, and problems of classification remain.

INHERITED DISEASES

MUSCULAR DYSTROPHIES

Definition. Muscular dystrophies are inherited myopathies, characterized primarily by progressively more severe weakness.

Etiology. Although it is generally believed that inherited diseases must be due to a missing or structurally abnormal protein (either an enzyme or a structural protein), this abnormality has not been identified in any form of dystrophy. Indirect evidence implicates the muscle membranes in several forms, but this hypothesis cannot now be put to direct test. Pathologic and biochemical abnormalities can be detected in muscle, and there is no clear evidence of neural abnormality, but it is possible that the fundamental abnormality is in another organ (such as the liver or bowel) and that the muscular abnormalities are secondary.

Classification. No classification of the muscular dystrophies is entirely satisfactory, but the application of clinical and genetic analysis provides the best approach at present. The classification in the accompanying table is based upon the clearly identifiable features of Duchenne dystrophy, facioscapulohumeral dystrophy, and myotonic muscular dystrophy. Limb girdle dystrophy is probably not a single disease, but merely encompasses cases that do not fall into the other categories.

Incidence. None of the muscular dystrophies are common. Incidence rates vary from 5 per million births for facioscapulohumeral dystrophy to about 250 per million births for Duchenne dystrophy. Many cases seem to be sporadic; the mutation rate of Duchenne dystrophy is high, 7×10^{-5} and about two thirds of the cases appear sporadically, with no other affected individual in the family.

Pathology. Pathologic abnormalities are restricted to skeletal muscle, and sometimes to cardiac muscle. The brain, spinal cord, and peripheral nerves are devoid of histologic change, although some authors have implicated the brain because of a seemingly high incidence of mental retardation in children with Duchenne dystrophy. Terminal pneumonia may cause changes in the lungs, and there may be a variety of associated diseases not directly linked to the dystrophy. In myotonic muscular dystrophy, however, baldness and testicular atrophy are integral parts of the disease in men, and corneal opacities affect both sexes.

The abnormalities in muscle seem to involve

CLASSIFICATION OF HUMAN MUSCULAR DYSTROPHIES

	Duchenne Dystrophy	Facioscapulohumeral Dystrophy	Limb Girdle Dystrophy	Myotonic Dystrophy
Genetic pattern	X-linked, recessive	Autosomal, dominant	Autosomal, recessive	Autosomal, dominant
Age at onset	Before age 5	Adolescence	Adolescence	Early or late
First symptoms	Pelvic	Shoulders	Pelvic	Distal; hands or feet
Pseudohypertrophy	+	0	0	0
Predominant weakness, early	Proximal	Proximal	Proximal	Distal
Progression	Relatively rapid; incapacitated in adolescence	Slow	Variable	Slow
Facial weakness	0	+	0	Occasional
Ocular, oropharyngeal weakness	0	0	0	Occasional
Myotonia	0	0	0	+
Cardiomyopathy	0 or late	0	0	Arrhythmia, conduction block
Associated disorders	None (?mental retardation)	None	None	Cataracts; testicular atrophy and baldness in men
Serum enzymes	Very high	Slight or no increase	Slight or no increase	Slight or no increase
Prevalence (per million population)	38	5	20	25
Incidence (per million births)	251	5	47	—
Mutation rate	9×10^{-5}	5×10^{-7}	3×10^{-5}	10×10^{-6}

all fibers in random fashion. Early, there is scattered evidence of necrosis and regeneration, with prominent variation in fiber size, including many fibers much larger than normal. Later, fibers disappear, to be replaced by fibrous connective tissue and fat. "Pseudohypertrophy" is probably due to both "true" hypertrophy (large fibers) and increased accumulations of fat and connective tissue. In myotonic dystrophy, unusual figures form "ring fibers" (with one fiber running at right angles, encircling the other fibers in the same bundle) and "sarcoplasmic masses," or accumulations of sarcoplasm that are free of myofilaments. However, these abnormalities occur occasionally in other diseases and are not pathognomonic of myotonic dystrophy. In Duchenne dystrophy, the myocardium may be affected by similar changes at autopsy, but cardiac symptoms are rarely evident in life, a discrepancy that has been attributed to the sedentary life imposed upon the patients by advanced muscular weakness. Myopathic changes in the heart are common in myotonic dystrophy. There is no good evidence that smooth muscle is affected in any form of dystrophy.

Clinical Manifestations. The symptoms and signs of all forms of the muscular dystrophies are related to weakness alone, except that additional systems are involved in myotonic dystrophy. In other forms, the symptoms depend upon the distribution of weakness and the age at onset. In *Duchenne dystrophy* weakness is primarily proximal at onset, and symptoms begin early. By definition, girls are not affected. There are no symptoms in the first year of life, but walking may be somewhat delayed beyond 18 months. Once the child walks, some abnormality is usually evident to an experienced observer (either a parent with a previously affected child or a skilled physician). The boys tend to waddle when they walk, or walk on their toes, or fall frequently and have difficulty rising. They are probably never able to run, because they have difficulty raising their knees. These symptoms become more evident as the children grow older, and even the most unsuspecting parent becomes aware of some abnormality by age five, or teachers sometimes may be the first to recognize the difficulty when the child starts school. Some cases are averred to start between ages five and ten, but these must be exceptional. It is difficult to examine individual muscles of a young child, but the waddling gait, the typical method of rising from the ground by "climbing up" himself (Gowers' sign), enlargement of calf or other muscles, and inability to run are characteristic. Myotatic reflexes may be normal at first, but by three years the knee jerks are usually lost, and later the ankle jerks disappear. As the child grows there are two countervailing influences; increased growth and coordination may compensate temporarily for the concurrent progressive weakness and wasting, but the disease always wins. There is increased difficulty walking. Going up grades or stairs first requires aid, then becomes impossible. Weak-

ness of the trunk muscles leads to increased lordosis and a protuberant abdomen. Then the arms become weak. Finally, in early adolescence, the child becomes unable to walk. This is inevitable, but may be accelerated by a period of inactivity after an injury or an orthopedic operation. Contractures appear, at first in the feet, as the gastrocnemius muscles tighten. When the child stops walking, flexion contractures limit motion of the knees, and scoliosis becomes more a problem with prolonged sitting. Ultimately respiration becomes shallow and the child is increasingly subject to pulmonary infection. Sooner or later, one of these infections is fatal, usually in the third decade. Although muscles are ravaged from the neck down, the cranial muscles are entirely spared, an important clue that is presently uninterpretable. Congestive heart failure and abnormalities of cardiac rhythm are rare.

Becker's dystrophy has manifestations similar to those of Duchenne dystrophy, but the onset is later in childhood or in adolescence, and the tempo is slower and more variable. This form may also be devastating, but some patients are able to function, albeit with limitations, well into adult life. The clinical similarities include pseudohypertrophy of calf muscles. However, it is clear that although the two forms are similar, they are genetically separate; there are no mildly affected individuals in typical Duchenne families, nor are children affected severely in Becker families.

The manifestations of *limb girdle dystrophy* are also similar because weakness of muscles of the pelvic girdle usually initiates the syndrome, but symptoms start in late childhood or adolescence. Girls are affected as often as boys, and pseudohypertrophy is rare. Waddling gait, difficulty in walking and climbing, and frequent falls are common. Occasionally, symptoms may begin in the shoulder girdle. In either case, there is usually weakness in all four limbs by the time the patient seeks medical attention. The severity, age at onset, and rate of progression vary considerably, suggesting that this category contains more than one disease.

Facioscapulohumeral dystrophy is distinct. Symptoms vary in severity so that some affected individuals never have any disability (but can be recognized by the signs), whereas others become incapacitated early; there are all grades in between. The first symptoms are apt to be related to difficulty in raising the arms or to prominence of the scapulae. Weakness of the legs may affect pelvic girdle muscles, or equally prominent weakness of the anterior tibial muscles may lead to a steppage gait. Truncal weakness may lead to prominent scoliosis. The face is always involved on examination; the perioral muscles may be more affected than those of the upper face, but ultimately patients develop difficulty in closing the eyes. The sternal head of the pectoral muscle is affected earlier than the clavicular head, a selectivity that can be detected on testing the individual muscles, and leads to a peculiar appearance of the axillary folds when the arms are dependent, because the anterior axillary fold of normal people is formed by the sternal portion of the pectoral muscle. Winging of the scapulae can be seen when the patient leans against a wall with the arms extended, and the weakness of shoulder girdle muscles leads to an unusual appearance because, viewed from the front, the superior margin of the scapula is higher than the clavicle.

Myotonic muscular dystrophy diverges from the preceding types in several respects. (1) The distribution of weakness differs in that cranial muscles are often affected and limb weakness is initially more marked in distal muscles. Thus weakness of the hands (as in twisting bottle caps or using tools) precedes shoulder weakness, and footdrop and a steppage gait precede symptoms of pelvic muscle weakness. Ptosis, facial weakness, and dysarthria are signs not seen in the other forms of dystrophy. Moreover, there is almost always selective weakness of the sternomastoids. The masticatory muscles either are poorly developed or waste early (even when not symptomatically weak), causing a characteristic facial appearance. The long, lean look has led physicians to use several callous descriptive phrases that are best not perpetuated. (Among the more foolish designations is "myopathic facies," but the facial appearance of a patient with myotonic dystrophy differs from facioscapulohumeral dystrophy or from myasthenia gravis.) (2) Myotonia, or difficulty in relaxation, may be symptomatic, and after a firm grip the patient may have difficulty letting go. Myotonia may cause other symptoms in patients with myotonia cogenita (see below), but in the dystrophy only the hands are affected by this kind of stiffness. Myotonia of grip may be evident on examination, and can also be elicited by percussing the thenar eminence. In normal persons this evokes a rapid twitch, whereas in patients with myotonia, a sustained contraction of the adductor pollicis muscle persists for several seconds, only gradually relaxing. Similar responses to percussion may be elicited uncommonly in other limb muscles, but can often be seen in the tongue. Although myotonia is a dramatic sign and a symptom that can be relieved by drugs, it is not the symptom that causes the major disability in myotonic dystrophy; weakness is the problem. (3) Other systems are involved in this pleomorphic disorder; cataracts appear sooner or later in all patients, and are sometimes the only signs of the disease; most of the men (but not the women) have frontal baldness; testicular atrophy affects most of the men, but often after they have sired children to perpetuate the disease (there is no definite evidence of gonadal insufficiency in affected women); the basal metabolic rate is often low, but other tests of thyroid function are normal (extrathyroidal hypometabolism). The incidence of diabetes mellitus may be increased. (4) Conduction defects are common in the electrocardiogram, and may lead to clinically significant arrhythmia or congestive heart failure.

Certain rare forms of muscular dystrophy are named after the prominent manifestations.

Ocular dystrophy is a slowly progressive disorder in which ptosis of the eyelids and progressive immobility of the eyes are the cardinal features. The pupils are spared, and both eyes are usually affected symmetrically so that diplopia is uncommon (but may occur). Other muscles of the head, neck, and limbs may also be affected, varying from family to family. This syndrome raises problems of definition; some cases probably are myopathic in origin, but this kind of ophthalmoplegia is often associated with other manifestations that are clearly neurogenic (such as spinocerebellar degeneration or peripheral neuropathy). The final distinction as to the origin of the ophthalmoplegia is often difficult or impossible to make because the ocular muscles normally differ so much from limb muscles that signs of myopathy in muscle biopsy or electromyography are not valid in studying them.

Distal myopathy, as the name implies, affects distal leg and hand muscles first. It is probably the rarest form of dystrophy, and can be identified only by characteristic signs of myopathy in electromyography and muscle biopsy.

In the *scapuloperoneal syndrome* distal weakness in the legs resembles that of neurogenic peroneal muscular atrophy, but sensory loss is lacking, and there is proximal weakness in the shoulder girdle very similar to that of facioscapulohumeral dystrophy. Some of these cases are myopathic and some seem to be neurogenic as distinguished by electromyography, muscle biopsy, and serum enzymes. In either case, an autosomal dominant inheritance and a relatively slow progression seem characteristic.

Diagnosis. The clinical picture of Duchenne dystrophy is so characteristic that it entails little diagnostic confusion. In its first stages, some children are merely regarded as clumsy, and some receive orthopedic care because of toe-walking; otherwise the diagnosis becomes obvious. As noted, the trait is transmitted as a sex-linked recessive, and once a case is recognized, members of the family rapidly detect the signs in subsequently affected youngsters. And once a family is known, affected individuals can be identified in the neonatal period because the serum enzymes are already markedly abnormal. Limb girdle and facioscapulohumeral dystrophy must be differentiated from neurogenic diseases, from congenital myopathies and from polymyositis, as will be discussed below. Myotonic dystrophy may be confused with endocrine disorders or, because of the distal weakness, with neuropathy or amyotrophy, or with hypothyroidism or gonadal disorders. Ocular myopathy must be differentiated from myasthenia gravis; this is usually not a problem because there is no fluctuation of symptoms in the myopathy, and the weakness does not respond to cholinergic drugs. The differential diagnosis of the dystrophies depends also upon the age of the patient. In childhood and adolescence, the major problems involve peroneal muscular atrophy (Charcot-Marie-Tooth) and "muscular atrophy simulating muscular dystrophy" (Wohlfart-

Kugelberg-Welander). In adults, amyotrophic lateral sclerosis is the major problem. At all ages, polyneuritis must be considered.

Treatment. There is no specific treatment for the weakness of any form of dystrophy. Physical medicine, exercises, splints, braces, and corrective orthopedic surgery are applied in different centers with varying degrees of enthusiasm. Some activists claim that walking can be prolonged into late adolescence in Duchenne dystrophy. They may be correct, but it is difficult to prove, and, in the end, all lose. The myotonia of myotonic dystrophy can be relieved by diphenylhydantoin (0.3 to 0.6 gram daily), quinidine (0.3 to 1.5 grams daily) or procaine amide (4 to 6 grams daily), but this is rarely the problem, and nothing can be done for the weakness. Cataracts are treated surgically upon appropriate indication, and cardiac arrhythmias or congestive heart failure are managed accordingly.

Prophylaxis. Genetic manipulation offers the only possibility to control muscular dystrophy at present. Carriers of Duchenne dystrophy may often but not always be identified by abnormally increased serum enzyme activity (higher than normal, but not as high as in affected boys). In some centers, antenatal detection of sex allows selective prophylactic abortion. There is no way to determine whether a male fetus is affected, however. Birth control ought to be effective in dominantly inherited diseases such as facio-scapulohumeral and myotonic dystrophy, but since many cases are mild, the families go on interminably. The high rates of mutation do not encourage optimism that genetic restriction can be the ultimate goal.

Caughey, J. E., and Myrianthopoulous, N. C.: Dystrophia Myotonica and Related Disorders. Springfield, Ill., Charles C Thomas, 1963.

Milhorat, A. T. (ed.): Exploratory Concepts in Muscular Dystrophy. New York, Excerpta Medica, 1967.

Research Committee, Muscular Dystrophy Group (eds.): Research in Muscular Dystrophy. London, Sir Isaac Pitman & Sons, Ltd., 1969.

Walton, J. N.: Disorders of Voluntary Muscle. 2nd ed. Boston, Little, Brown and Company, 1969.

Zundel, W. S., and Tyler, F. M.: The muscular dystrophies. New Eng. J. Med., 273:537, 1965.

CONGENITAL MYOPATHIES

Definition. These are rare diseases characterized by weakness that is usually relatively mild but persists throughout life, either slowly progressing or remaining stationary.

Etiology. The cause is not known. A few of these disorders are familial and are suspected of having a genetic basis, but so many cases are sporadic that other causes are not excluded, and there are no clear clues.

Pathology. These diseases are defined in terms of pathology, and most of them have been delineated within the past decade since the introduction of histochemical techniques to study muscle biopsy. The names of the diseases reflect the predominant anatomic disorder. In *central core disease*, the central portion of the muscle fiber appears rather amorphous, in contrast to the fibrillar appearance of the surrounding normal portion. In cross section, the central portion appears blue when stained with Gomori's trichrome, in striking contrast to the red periphery. The central areas lack all oxidative enzyme activity, and there are no mitochondria in this region. In *nemaline myopathy* or *rod myopathy*, small threadlike or rod bodies are scattered throughout the fiber. The rods are barely visible in conventional hematoxylin and eosin stains, but can be seen readily in phase contrast or with the trichrome stain. In electron microscopy the structures seem to originate in the Z-band, and circumstantial evidence suggests that they are composed of tropomyosin. *Myotubular myopathy* designates the appearance of myofibers that resemble a stage in the early development of fetal muscle, with nuclei located centrally rather than at the periphery and surrounded by a halo of apparently empty space. Because the pathogenesis of this appearance is uncertain, some investigators prefer the name *centronuclear myopathy*. In other disorders mitochondria have appeared abnormal, either in number (too many) or size (too large), often associated with accumulations of lipid droplets.

Clinical Manifestations. Although designated "congenital," these disorders are only exceptionally symptomatic in the first year of life, except that the onset of walking may be delayed. Later, the symptoms of proximal limb weakness become evident: waddling gait, difficulty in climbing stairs, frequent falls, and scoliosis. Later, there may be weakness of the arms. There are few clinical clues to each specific histologic abnormality. Among the nemaline cases there have been skeletal abnormalities (kyphoscoliosis, pigeon breast, pes cavus, high palate, and an unusually elongated face). In two families with myotubular disease, ophthalmoplegia was present as well as limb weakness. Central core and mitochondrial disorders have not been associated with distinctive clinical signs other than proximal limb weakness.

Diagnosis. Proximal limb weakness in a young child is usually myopathic in origin, but must be distinguished from the neurogenic Wohlfart-Kugelberg-Welander syndrome and from polyneuritis. Myopathic abnormalities in the EMG, an abnormal family history, an incidence in girls, and especially the histologic abnormalities define the individual entities. The serum enzymes may be normal or slightly increased. In some clinics most cases of apparently congenital myopathy fail to meet the specific histologic criteria, showing only nonspecific myopathic changes in biopsy. There is no better designation for these cases than "congenital myopathy," but it is likely that there is more than one cause.

Treatment and Prognosis. There is no specific treatment for any of these disorders. Physical therapy and orthopedic corrective measures are of value. There are too few cases to generalize about the course of these illnesses; most seem to be mild and nonprogressive, but occasional cases are more severe.

Dubowitz, V.: The Floppy Infant. London, Spastics International Medical Publications, 1969.

Hefferman, L. P., Rewcastle, N. B., and Humphrey, J. G.: The spectrum of rod myopathies. Arch. Neurol. (Chicago), 18:529, 1968.

Kinoshita, M., and Cadman, T. E.: Myotubular myopathy. Arch. Neurol. (Chicago), 18:265, 1968.

Shy, G. M., Engel, W. K., Somers, J. E., and Wanko, T.: Nemalino myopathy. Brain, 86:793, 1963.

Shy, G. M., Engel, W. K., and Wanko, T.: Central core disease. Arch. Intern. Med. (Chicago), 56:511, 1962.

MYOTONIA CONGENITA
(Thomsen's Disease)

Definition. Myotonia congenita is a disorder characterized by difficulty in relaxation of skeletal muscle after forceful contraction, present from early childhood.

Incidence. This is one of the rarest of all muscular disorders.

Etiology. There are occasional sporadic cases, but most are inherited in a pattern corresponding to an autosomal dominant trait. The biochemical fault is not known, but the muscle membrane is electrically unstable and tends to fire repetitively. The abnormality must be inherent within the muscle, because myotonic phenomena may be elicited after all neural influences are abolished by spinal anesthesia, block of motor nerves by local anesthesia, or blockade of the neuromuscular junction by intra-arterial injection of d-tubocurarine. Myotonia is abolished, however, by the intramuscular administration of procaine. That the membrane is abnormal is suggested by the myotonia that occurs in otherwise normal individuals taking diazacholesterol, a substance that interferes with the biosynthesis of cholesterol. How this affects the membrane, however, is not known, and membranes of other organs are not functionally altered.

Clinical Manifestations. The difficulty in relaxation in this disorder, in contrast to that in myotonic dystrophy, is widespread. Difficulty in relaxing the grip may lead to prominent and sometimes embarrassing symptoms. Ocular muscles may also be affected, so that the eyes seem momentarily "stuck" in one position, or the eyelids may remain closed after forceful closure. Sometimes oropharyngeal muscles are affected, with difficulty in speaking or swallowing. Startle reactions may induce stiffness of the legs, thwarting sudden attempts to catch a bus or run from home plate. There is no weakness, and one unexplained characteristic is the unusual muscular development of many patients, causing a Herculean appearance, and perhaps related to involuntary and repeated isometric exercise. The myotonia can be elicited by tapping any muscle in severely affected cases. Reflexes are unaltered.

Diagnosis. The major problem is in distinguishing these patients from those with myotonic mus-

cular dystrophy. Here the only symptoms and signs are related to myotonia. There is no weakness, no cataract, no baldness, no gonadal atrophy. Some authors have described "transitional cases," but these are probably patients in families with myotonic muscular dystrophy who are only mildly affected and show only myotonia before the other manifestations. In general, families with myotonia congenita breed true.

Treatment. Drug therapy is effective. For many years, quinine was the staple treatment in doses of 0.3 to 1.5 grams daily. Recently, diphenylhydantoin has proved equally effective and less apt to cause disagreeable side effects in therapeutic doses of 0.3 to 0.6 gram daily. Should this fail, procaine amide may also be used, in doses of 4 to 6 grams daily.

Landau, W. M.: The essential mechanism in myotonia. Neurology, 2:369, 1952.

Munsat, T.: Therapy of myotonia: A double-blind evaluation of diphenylhydantoin, procainamide and placebo. Neurology, 17:359, 1967.

FAMILIAL MYOGLOBINURIA

Most cases of myoglobinuria are sporadic, and they will be described below. Some individuals, however, have repeated attacks from early childhood, suggesting some genetic fault, and sometimes more than one individual in a family is affected. Some of these familial cases are due to lack of muscle phosphorylase or phosphofructokinase. They can be recognized by the ischemic work test in which contracture is induced and venous lactate fails to rise. (See Glycogen Storage Diseases.) Several families have been studied, however, in which glycogen metabolism was normal, and contracture could not be induced. The genetic abnormality in these patients has not been identified.

FAMILIAL PERIODIC PARALYSIS

Definition. Periodic paralysis is characterized by recurrent attacks of flaccid weakness usually associated with abnormally high or low serum potassium concentrations. Many cases are familial. In sporadic cases the abnormality may be secondary to identifiable aberrations of potassium metabolism.

Etiology and Pathogenesis. Familial cases are distributed in a pattern consistent with autosomal dominant inheritance. Hypokalemia during attacks was the first metabolic abnormality to be recognized, with no loss of potassium in urine. It was therefore presumed that potassium shifted from extracellular to intracellular compartments, especially muscle. This has been difficult to prove, and the anticipated hyperpolarization of the muscle membrane potential has not been substantiated by direct measurement with intracellular electrodes. Abnormalities of glucose metabolism have been suspected, because attacks can be precipitated by infusions of glucose and insulin, by eating a large meal, or by administration of epinephrine. However, biochemical studies have failed to pinpoint the abnormality.

During the past decade it has been recognized that the serum potassium tends to rise in some patients, and attacks in these individuals are induced by the ingestion of potassium. This variety is therefore called "hyperkalemic periodic paralysis," and is generally considered to be the mirror image of the hypokalemic type, with potassium presumably shifting out of muscle and into blood during attacks. Why this should happen is not clear, but at least in the hyperkalemic type there are alterations of the intracellular potential in the direction required by theory. There are clinical differences between the two forms of periodic paralysis, but there are so many areas of overlap and so many common features that it is difficult to decide just how many genetically distinct forms there really are.

Pathology. In both forms of periodic paralysis there may be vacuoles within muscle fibers. These may be numerous or scanty, and it is not clear that they are more frequent in paralyzed muscle. Most electron microscopists believe that the vacuoles are derived from the sarcoplasmic reticulum, but others think they originate in the T-system in areas of necrotic muscle. Glycogen seems to be increased in amount in ultrastructural studies, but the results of biochemical analysis have been inconsistent. There is no evidence that other organs are affected in either form of the disease. The heart is usually spared pathologically.

Clinical Manifestations. There are clinical differences between the two forms. In the hypokalemic variety attacks tend to start in late childhood or adolescence, frequently occur at night, are apt to be severe, and last for a day or more. In the hyperkalemic variety attacks start at an early age occur much more frequently tend to be milder, and may last minutes or hours. Moreover, patients with hyperkalemic periodic paralysis usually have some evidence of myotonia, which is rarely symptomatic and often limited to percussion myotonia of the tongue. Lid-lag and Chvostek's sign are identified with the hyperkalemic type. These clinical distinctions may break down in application to individual cases and are therefore only crude guides. Moreover, many features are common to both types: a dominant pattern of inheritance, a susceptibility to attacks during periods of rest after vigorous exercise, the ability to ward off attacks by mild exercise after a mild attack has begun, persistent weakness between attacks, vacuoles in muscle, a lack of clear relation between the serum potassium concentration and the severity of paresis, the induction of local weakness by cooling, and protection against attacks by acetazolamide. Some patients are affected by attacks in which the serum potassium may be either high or low.

Typical attacks start with weakness of the legs that ascends to the arms. Cranial muscles are affected in severe attacks only, and respiratory insufficiency is exceptional. The attacks may be mild and brief, or severe and prolonged, with all gradations in between. During severe attacks, the myotatic reflexes are lost, and the muscles are electrically inexcitable. Attacks are rarely apoplectic in onset and usually take an hour or more to develop, except that attacks beginning in sleep may be fully developed when the patient awakes. Paresthesias and myalgia may be prominent at the onset, or may be completely lacking. Some patients are aware of oliguria during the attack and of diuresis afterward.

The serum potassium is in the range of 2.5 to 3.5 mEq. per liter in hypokalemic attacks, and 5.0 to 7.0 mEq. per liter in the hyperkalemic type. Between attacks serum potassium values may be normal. The electrocardiogram is altered as would be predicted from the serum values, with low T waves in hypokalemia and peaked T-waves in hyperkalemia.

Patients with hyperkalemic periodic paralysis may have mild symptoms attributable to myotonia, especially of the hands. When individuals in a family are studied, some may be found to have myotonia without any history of periodic paralysis.

In both types of the disease, there may be persistent weakness between attacks, most often proximal, sometimes distal. In the past this has been attributed to a permanent "myopathy," but experience with acetazolamide therapy indicates that even long-lasting weakness may be reversible, regardless of pathologic changes in muscle. A few patients with intermittent normokalemic or hyperkalemic paralysis have had persistent cardiac arrhythmia, especially bigeminy, and bouts of ventricular tachycardia. The cardiac disorder is neither temporally related to attacks of limb weakness nor related to serum potassium content.

Diagnosis. Periodic paralysis can be recognized by the history of typical attacks; no other disease causes this pattern of recurrent weakness. In myasthenia gravis, weakness may come and go, but less abruptly and with a duration of weeks rather than hours or days; remissions are less frequent so that it is less "periodic." Polymyositis may be transient, but episodes are rarely shorter than several weeks or months. Attacks of myoglobinuric weakness could conceivably be confusing if the pigmenturia were not recognized, but myalgia and malaise are so prominent that it is rarely confused with periodic paralysis. Hysterical attacks might be confusing.

If the patient is seen during the attack and the serum potassium is abnormal, other causes of hypo- or hyperkalemia must be considered. Low serum potassium concentrations with paralysis are also encountered in hyperaldosteronism, potassium-losing nephritis, potassium depletion caused by laxative abuse or diarrhea, and thyrotoxicosis. Hyperkalemia is most often due to renal insufficiency, but may also occur in adrenal insufficiency, after administration of spironolactone, or as a manifestation of aldosterone deficiency.

or Raynaud's syndrome. The muscle biopsy ought to be crucial, but inflammatory lesions may be lacking in dermatomyositis, and may occasionally be seen in dystrophies; severe inflammation, of course, supports the diagnosis of polymyositis. The electromyogram is helpful, but, again, not distinctive; there are the usual features of myopathy with the additional evidence of irritable muscle (increased insertional activity and some spontaneous activity). Serum enzymes tend to be high. There may also be an increased erythrocyte sedimentation rate, increased serum gamma globulin concentration, or a positive latex fixation test for rheumatoid factor. But there are no antibodies to muscle.

The problem of diagnosis is best exemplified by a patient with limb weakness commencing at age 40 and evidence of myopathic disease in muscle biopsy and EMG. Search must be made for the known causes of muscle disease, to be discussed below. If none is found, the diagnosis of exclusion is polymyositis, no matter what the laboratory data show or do not show. That this residual group is all due to one disease seems unlikely, not only because there is clinical heterogeneity, but also because if there are so many known causes of the syndrome, there are some others still to be recognized. Because inflammatory cells are not always seen in the muscle biopsy, some authorities eschew the word "polymyositis" and prefer "myopathy of unknown cause." This, at least, identifies the problem, but for the present "polymyositis" seems to be entrenched. Clinicians should recognize, however, that "polymyositis" is no more a specific diagnosis than "headache," "polyneuritis," or "convulsive disorder," terms that also imply inadequately defined syndromes of diverse etiology.

Treatment. The problem of nomenclature is not merely academic, because a decision must be made whether to use potentially hazardous drugs. No one has ever conducted a well-controlled clinical trial of the effects of steroids, and it now seems unlikely that this will ever be done because it has become routine to treat patients with large amounts of prednisone, starting with 60 to 80 mg. daily for adults. In all clinics there have been dramatic results in isolated cases, usually ameliorating skin lesions more than the weakness. But it has not been shown that prednisone truly affects the long-range prognosis. Be that as it may, prednisone is certainly used universally. The initial dose is continued for several weeks. In some clinics it is continued until there is a distinct fall in serum enzyme activity; in other centers, the clinical response is given more weight. In either case, after some response the drug is gradually reduced, by 5 mg. every other day, until either enzyme activity or clinical signs appear again, thus adjusting the maintenance dose according to response. If there is no response at all after several weeks of high dosage, the drug may be withdrawn as a therapeutic failure. Therefore, whether or not there is a beneficial response, high-dose

therapy is continued for only a few weeks. Despite this, the incidence of complications of therapy may be considerable, because drugs are often administered for prolonged periods. Decisions about terminating prednisone therapy are based upon imprecise clinical criteria that vary with individual physicians. When steroid therapy fails, immunosuppressive therapy with azathioprine may be considered, but this is probably best left to investigators who see enough cases to evaluate therapy. A significant problem in evaluating treatment regimens is created by the natural tendency of the disease to be self-limited. About two thirds of the patients seem to show some response to treatment.

Pearson, C. M.: Patterns of polymyositis and their responses to treatment. Ann. Intern. Med., 59:827, 1963.

Rose, A. L., and Walton, J. N.: Polymyositis: A survey of 89 cases with particular reference to treatment and prognosis. Brain, 89:747, 1966.

Rowland, L. P., Sagman, D., and Schotland, D. H.: Polymyositis: A conceptual problem. Trans. Amer. Neurol. Ass., 91:332, 1966.

Winkelman, R. K., Mulder, D. W., Lambert, E. H., Howard, F. M., Jr., and Dressner, G. R.: Dermatomyositis-polymyositis: Comparison of untreated and cortisone-treated patients. Mayo Clin. Proc., 43:545, 1968.

OTHER ACQUIRED MYOPATHIES

Proximal limb weakness in patients with no rash, with or without inflammatory lesions in muscle, and with or without increased serum enzyme activity, occurs in several disorders. These may be considered diseases associated with polymyositis or causes of polymyositis. To identify these disorders, appropriate diagnostic tools must be utilized.

Carcinomatous Myopathy. Muscle weakness may occur in patients with carcinoma of the lung or of any other primary site. Myeloma and other gammopathies may also be associated with myopathy. The tumor itself may or may not be symptomatic, and treatment of the tumor may or may not affect the muscular symptoms.

Collagen Diseases. Proximal limb weakness may occur in the course of systemic lupus erythematosus, progressive systemic sclerosis, rheumatoid arthritis, and, rarely, periarteritis nodosa or giant cell arteritis.

Endocrine Disease. Thyrotoxic myopathy is a well-recognized syndrome. Usually there is clinical evidence of hyperthyroidism, but not always ("apathetic hyperthyroidism"). Signs of hypermetabolism are especially apt to be lacking in elderly patients. This myopathy always disappears when the patient is rendered euthyroid by treatment. Similarly, weakness may complicate hypothyroidism. Another muscle syndrome of hypothyroidism is Hofmann's syndrome, a peculiar difficulty in relaxing muscles that lacks the characteristic electromyographic abnormalities of myotonia and is therefore called "pseudomyotonia," but may appear similar clinically. This, too, disappears with appropriate replacement therapy. Infants with cretinism may have unusually well-developed muscles but not the disorder of relaxation.

Hyperparathyroidism and hyperadrenacorticism may also be responsible for weakness that looks like any other proximal myopathy. Surprisingly, because asthenia has so long been regarded as prominent, Addison's disease seems not to be a cause of this syndrome. Weakness may be part of hyperpituitarism, but acromegalic features always overshadow the myopathy.

Infections. Muscle may be affected by a variety of organisms, but the only one of practical importance in the differential diagnosis of acute or subacute myopathy is trichinosis. Toxoplasmosis may affect muscle in the course of a syndrome that looks like severe infectious mononucleosis with adenopathy, rash, mucosal lesions, and hepatomegaly. In tropical countries, trypanosomiasis and schistosomiasis are important.

Sarcoidosis. In muscle clinics, sarcoidosis is recognized as a significant cause of polymyositis. Usually there is other evidence of the disease, but sometimes the first symptoms are due to weakness, and in a few cases only muscle seems to be involved. Myalgia may be severe in these patients.

Drugs. A variety of drugs used to treat more common disorders may themselves cause muscular weakness, especially triamcinolone and other fluorinated adrenal steroids (but probably all steroids), vincristine, and chloroquine.

Alcoholic Myopathy. The clearest myopathic disorder in alcoholic persons is acute myoglobinuria. Some of these individuals are acute, and some who never have an attack of pigmenturia, also suffer from proximal limb weakness, especially affecting the legs. The serum creatine phosphokinase is often elevated. The problem in some of these patients, however, is that they also suffer from the typical polyneuritis of alcoholism, and it then becomes difficult to prove that the muscular weakness is not also secondary to a neurogenic disorder. Too few patients have been evaluated to know whether abstinence and a good diet will reverse the persistent weakness.

Byers, R. K., Bergman, A. B., and Joseph, M. C.: Steroid myopathy. Report of five cases occurring during treatment of rheumatic fever. Pediatrics, 29:26, 1962.

Frame, B., Heize, E. G., Block, M. A., and Manson, G. A.: Myopathy in primary hyperparathyroidism. Ann. Intern. Med. 68:1022, 1968.

Hall, W. H.: Proximal muscle atrophy in adult celiac disease. Amer. J. Dig. Dis., 13:697, 1968.

Harvard, C. W. H., Campbell, E. D. R., Ross, H. B., and Spence, A. W.: Electromyographic and histological findings in the muscles of patients with thyrotoxicosis. Quart. J. Med., 32:145, 1963.

Perkoff, G. T., Dioso, M. M., Bleisch, V., and Klinkerfuss, G.: A spectrum of myopathy associated with alcoholism. Ann. Intern. Med., 67:481, 1967.

Silberberg, D. H., and Drachman, D. B.: Late-life myopathy associated with Sjögren's syndrome. Arch. Neurol. (Chicago), 6:428, 1962.

Silverstein, A., and Siltzbach, L. E.: Muscle involvement in sarcoidosis. Arch. Neurol. (Chicago), 21:235, 1969.

Trojaborg, W., Frantzen, E., and Andersen, I.: Peripheral neuropathy and myopathy associated with carcinoma of the lung. Brain, 92:71, 1969.

Wilson, J., and Walton, J. N.: Some muscular manifestations of hypothyroidism. J. Neurol. Neurosurg. Psychiat., 22:320, 1959.

SPORADIC MYOGLOBINURIA

Definition. Sporadic myoglobinuria is a group of disorders characterized by injury of muscle and excretion of myoglobin in the urine. ("Rhabdomyolysis" has been proposed as a more precise term, focusing attention upon muscle rather than urine, but this is the kind of "progress" that is achieved by changing a name. It is more difficult to say, somewhat pompous sounding, no more revealing or scientific, and has gained favor for reasons which are difficult to fathom.)

Pathogenesis. Myoglobin may be released from muscle whenever there is extensive and rapid destruction. Sometimes, the cause is evident, as in the *crush injuries* of World War II when individuals were pinned beneath the timbers of buildings destroyed in bombing raids. Similar pressure injuries may occur in comatose persons who lie on one side without moving for prolonged periods. This kind of injury is perhaps more apt to occur when there are other causes of *metabolic depression;* for instance, in coma after suicidal ingestion of barbiturates or carbon monoxide intoxication, or prolonged unconsciousness in the snow. A similar effect may be induced by *arterial occlusion* by tourniquet or embolism, or even by prolonged knee-chest posture under anesthesia.

In other patients, the cause is less discernible. In every series of patients with myoglobinuria, a disproportionate number are *alcoholics*, but why this should occur is not known. Sometimes there has been exposure to a known *membrane toxin*, such as the bite of the Malayan sea snake. Or there may be *metabolic alterations* that do not ordinarily cause this kind of trouble, such as diarrhea with hypokalemia, diabetic acidosis, or systemic infection with fever. In many attacks, however, not even these clues prevail.

The most common cause of myoglobinuria is probably unusually *vigorous exercise* by an otherwise normal person. Most cases have been reported by military physicians, and local designations include such titles as the "squat-jump syndrome." Some cases are attributed to "march hemoglobinuria." When large numbers of recruits perform these tortures, a certain number will have attacks of myalgia followed by pigmenturia. Why these individuals have attacks and others are spared is not clear, but this seems to be a "normal" variation. In civilians cases have been caused by the excess muscular activity of an initiation rite into a club or fraternity, and isolated attacks have occurred after the vigorous muscular activity induced by succinylcholine before it achieves relaxation. Spontaneous convulsions and electroconvulsive therapy have been followed by myoglobinuria. If an individual is subject to repeated attacks, it may be suspected that there is some kind of undiscovered genetic defect, although the only ones recognized now are deficiencies of phosphorylase or phosphofructokinase.

Clinical Manifestations. In attacks other than those caused by local crushing or arterial occlusion, the clinical picture is similar. Affected muscles are apt to be the ones subject to greatest physical strain (the legs in squat-thrusts, the arms after chinning or push-ups, the arms and legs after wrestling matches). The muscles ache, may be swollen, and are weak. Sometimes there is so much edema that local vascular abnormalities are suspected. There may be fever and considerable malaise. Symptoms persist for several days even though pigmenturia rarely lasts more than 48 hours. Recovery may be gradual. Cranial muscles are rarely involved, and although respiratory failure is uncommon it is a hazard. The most important threat to life is renal injury secondary to excretion of heme. There may be red cells or myoglobin in the urine as well as casts. Oliguria is followed by azotemia and hyperkalemia. This may be treated by appropriate measures.

Diagnosis. The diagnosis of myoglobinuria can be made on clinical grounds and with relatively simple tests, but precise identification of the pigment depends upon biochemical analysis. The urine may appear red-brown because of hemoglobin, myoglobin, or porphyrins. The latter would not give a positive test with benzidine (or other heme-reacting reagents), and would not give a positive Watson-Schwartz test for porphobilinogen. Besides, the neurologic disorder of porphyria is neuropathy, not an acute myopathy. If the urine gives a positive test for heme and contains no or few erythrocytes, the pigment is either myoglobin or hemoglobin. If it is hemoglobin, the serum would be pink (after a hemolytic reaction), whereas the color of the serum in myoglobinuria is normal. (This distinction depends upon the affinity of serum haptoglobin for hemoglobin and not for myoglobin. Hemoglobin is not excreted until haptoglobin is saturated by visible amounts of the pigment, whereas myoglobin is excreted at much lower concentrations.) Furthermore, in attacks of myoglobinuria, the muscular weakness and myalgia are distinctive, and serum enzymes are greatly increased, whereas they are not in hemolysis. Positive identification of myoglobin can be achieved by several tests: absorption spectrophotometry is direct and simple, but in many laboratories the most convenient method is electrophoresis on starch gel or cellulose acetate. In the future, immunochemical methods are apt to gain favor.

Treatment. If there is no renal injury, myoglobinuria is not threatening. The hazards of renal injury are not directly correlated to the amount of pigment excreted, and other factors are probably involved. Once an attack starts, it is useful to encourage excretion of dilute urine, and some authorities still favor alkalinizing agents although it has not been clearly demonstrated that these treatments protect the kidneys. Few patients are left with residual weakness, but in some the syndrome is characterized by prolonged weakness punctuated by attacks of myoglobinuria.

Denborough, M. A., Ebeling, P., King, J. O., and Zapf, P.: Myopathy and malignant hyperpyrexia. Lancet, 1:1138, 1970.

Greenberg, J., and Arneson, L.: Exertional rhabdomyolysis with myoglobinuria in a large group of military trainees. Neurology, 17:216, 1967.

Kagen, L. J.: Immunologic detection of myoglobinuria after cardiac surgery. Ann. Intern. Med., 67:1183, 1967.

Rowland, L. P., Fahn, S., Hirschberg, E., and Harter, D. H.: Myoglobinuria. Arch. Neurol. (Chicago), 10:537, 1964.

Vertel, R. M., and Knochel, J. P.: Acute renal failure due to heat injury: An analysis of ten cases with a high incidence of myoglobinuria. Amer. J. Med., 43:435, 1967.

MYASTHENIA GRAVIS

Definition. Myasthenia gravis is usually defined as a state of abnormal fatigability. This definition has the merit of being consistent with the characteristic electrophysiologic disorder found in patients with this condition, but there are serious disadvantages. "Normal" fatigue is not defined, muscles weakened from any cause are apt to fatigue more readily than normal, and myasthenic muscle may be completely paralyzed (especially ocular muscles), with no signs of fatigue. Moreover, emphasis on fatigue has led to the treatment of many psychoneurotic patients with cholinergic drugs. An alternative definition has therefore been proposed: "Myasthenia gravis is a disease characterized by weakness that has special characteristics: predilection for ocular and other cranial muscles; tendency to fluctuate during brief periods of observation (in the course of a single day) or for longer periods (remissions and exacerbations); with no signs of neural lesion, and partial reversibility by the administration of cholinergic drugs."

Etiology. The cause of myasthenia gravis is not known. Several disorders tend to occur more frequently in patients with myasthenia gravis, such as hyperthyroidism or other thyroidal disorders, and a significant number of patients with myasthenia gravis have thymomas. But in neither of these situations, nor in others, has a causal relationship been proved. Whether or not there is a significant association with "autoimmune" diseases remains to be proved; rheumatoid arthritis and systemic lupus erythematosus have been reported in patients with myasthenia gravis, but the statistical significance of these associations is uncertain.

Several lines of evidence suggest an immunologic disorder in myasthenia gravis. Thymomas occur in about 15 per cent of all patients, more often in patients older than 40 years. Germinal centers are seen frequently in the thymus glands of patients who have no tumor. Infiltration of muscle by monocytes is characteristic, especially in perivascular collections called lymphorrhages.

Antibodies to muscle can be demonstrated by immunofluorescent techniques in approximately a third of all patients with myasthenia, and in almost all patients with concomitant myasthenia and thymoma. However, the nature of the antigen that elicits these antibodies is uncertain, and it seems quite clear that the antibodies are not responsible for the symptoms of myasthenia. Thus, antibodies may be present in patients with thymoma who have no evidence of myasthenia. There is no correlation between the presence of antibodies in serum and the appearance of transient neonatal myasthenia, and the concentration of serum antibodies does not correlate with the severity of symptoms. Finally, physiologic evidence indicates a disorder of neuromuscular transmission in myasthenia, and the antibodies react with proteins in the myofiber, but not at the neuromuscular junction. The significance of these human antibodies is therefore uncertain. Moreover, no one has yet succeeded in designing a reproducible experimental model of the disease by immunologic techniques or by any other method.

Neuromuscular Disorder. The symptoms of myasthenia gravis resemble those of curare intoxication. This observation led to the use of curare antagonists in the treatment of myasthenia gravis. All effective therapies have been derived from this initial observation, and all drugs currently in use are inhibitors of the enzyme cholinesterase. These drugs also partially repair a physiologic defect that can be detected in patients by relatively simple techniques. When the ulnar nerve of normal individuals is stimulated at rates of 25 per second or less, the action potential of the hypothenar muscles is sustained at a constant amplitude. In patients with myasthenia, however, there is a rapid decline in the height of the evoked potentials. If the patient is then given neostigmine, the amplitude of the evoked potentials is restored to normal. This pattern could be consistent with either excessive cholinesterase activity, inadequate release of acetylcholine, or blockade of the junction by some curare-like compound. Microelectrode studies have been performed upon intercostal muscle fibers of patients with myasthenia (after excision of these muscles, they can be studied in vitro with the most advanced techniques). Investigations of this nature suggest that the basic defect is a reduced amount of acetylcholine released in each quantum from the motor nerve terminal. This could be caused by either some defect in the binding of acetylcholine or the presence of a "false transmitter," but how the defect comes about is not known.

Incidence and Prevalence. The prevalence of myasthenia gravis is about 33 per million population and the annual incidence about 2 to 5 per million. Translated into the experience of a busy 1000-bed general hospital, about 20 new cases are encountered each year, or about the same incidence as for lupus erythematosus. Cases occur in all decades of life, most frequently at about age 40. Among young adults, the disease affects women about three times more frequently than

man. Among children and older persons, however, there is no sexual predilection.

Pathology. Pathological changes in myasthenia gravis are limited to muscle and thymus. Skeletal muscles may appear completely normal, but there are often collections of lymphocytes around blood vessels. In some cases there is evidence of degeneration of muscle fibers, and the inflammatory cellular response may be more extensive. Rarely, similar lesions are encountered in the myocardium. The thymus gland is often abnormal. Encapsulated tumors (thymoma) occur in about 15 per cent of the cases, almost all after age 30. In about 25 per cent of these tumors there is evidence of local invasion, but distant metastases are virtually unknown in patients with myasthenia, and the local invasiveness is not a cause of symptoms. Lymphocytic proliferation, in the form of germinal centers, is seen in the thymus glands of almost all other patients, but sometimes the gland appears normal, and in some older individuals the gland is so involuted that it cannot be found. Patients dying of this disease usually have some pulmonary disorder (edema, atelectasis, infection) but this is secondary to the terminal events. Patients with myasthenia may live long enough to develop a carcinoma of any organ, but it has not been shown that myasthenia occurs more frequently in patients with cancer than might be expected on the basis of chance.

Clinical Manifestations. The symptoms of myasthenia gravis are all due to weakness. The most common presenting symptoms relate to weakness of eye muscles, ptosis, or diplopia. At the onset these symptoms may last only a few days, then disappear, only to return weeks or months later. Ptosis frequently varies even in the course of a single day. Diplopia may be noted in particular directions of gaze. Difficulty in chewing, dysarthria, and dysphagia are other common initial symptoms. Limb weakness is perhaps more often proximal in accentuation, so that patients have difficulty climbing stairs or rising from chairs, or have difficulty lifting heavy objects or raising the arms overhead. However, distal weakness is not uncommon, and the initial symptoms may be related to the strength of the hands or fingers. Selective respiratory weakness is most unusual. There is no alteration of consciousness, no pain, and in untreated patients, no cramps or muscular twitching. Difficulty in eating and swallowing may lead to considerable loss of weight, but there is no specific wasting of muscle except in patients with severe chronic weakness.

On examination, evidence of weakness of the appropriate muscle groups is found. If any sensory abnormality is found, there must be some other disorder, alone or in combination with myasthenia. Similarly, hyperactive reflexes and Babinski signs imply some other disorder, as does the complete loss of reflexes. Weakness is responsible for all the signs of myasthenia. Ptosis may be unilateral or bilateral. The patient may experience diplopia even when there is no obvious weakness of the ocular muscles; more often, there is weakness of several muscles in a pattern that cannot be explained by disorder of a particular ocular motor nerve and is not usually symmetrical in the two eyes. In addition, there is frequently weakness of eye closure because of paresis of the orbicularis oculi. Muscles of the lower face are involved later. Lingual and palatal weakness are evident in patients with dysarthria. A nasal twang and indistinct speech imply that dysarthria has facial, lingual, palatal, and, sometimes, respiratory components. In advanced cases, patients support the chin with one hand to help them talk, a maneuver that seems almost pathognomonic of myasthenia. Neck weakness may be mild or severe enough to cause difficulty in holding the head erect. Limb weakness may be mild or so severe that the patient cannot walk or even turn in bed. Respiratory weakness does not occur alone; ventilatory insufficiency occurs only in severely affected patients and usually in generalized disease, but some patients with oropharyngeal weakness may be unable to breathe unassisted even though limb muscles are strong. Even though weakness fluctuates, a normal neurologic examination is inconsistent with the diagnosis of myasthenia gravis if the patient is symptomatic at the time.

SPECIAL FORMS OF MYASTHENIA

Neonatal Myasthenia. Infants born to myasthenic women may have a transient syndrome of weakness. The most prominent symptom is difficulty in sucking and swallowing. This may be the sole manifestation, or there may also be noticeable reduction in spontaneous movement and in the vigor of the baby's cry. Only rarely is there respiratory difficulty, but unrecognized neonatal myasthenia has been fatal in exceptional cases. The condition can be identified by the intramuscular injection of neostigmine (0.1 to 0.25 mg.), followed by improved sucking, a louder cry, better response to the Moro reflex, and stronger spontaneous movements. Small doses of cholinergic drugs may be administered therapeutically, but more often all that is needed is a nasogastric tube to insure adequate nutrition. Symptoms subside within a week, or at most, a month.

Congenital Myasthenia. Myasthenia gravis may commence at any age. But there are some children who seem to have had ophthalmoplegia from birth, with or without other signs of myasthenia. Although presumably congenital, this disorder rarely causes concern in the first year of life. It is only later, when the ophthalmoplegia is recognized, that the parents state the child's eyes have always been that way. There may be a disproportionate number of familial cases among children with congenital myasthenia; ophthalmoplegia occurs in almost all of them, and there may be somewhat less tendency for crisis and remission. Otherwise, there are no characteristics that distinguish this syndrome from myasthenia at any other age.

Thyrotoxicosis. About 5 per cent of patients with myasthenia have thyrotoxicosis at some time. Usually the two disorders occur simultaneously, but sometimes hyperthyroidism is evident for weeks or months before there are myasthenic symptoms. Only rarely does myasthenia come first, long before the thyrotoxicosis, and patients who appear euthyroid do not ordinarily have laboratory evidence of thyroid overactivity. Treatment of the two disorders is directed according to the usual indications for each. (There is still talk of a "see-saw" relationship, the myasthenia worsening if the patient is rendered euthyroid; this may have been a consideration years ago when surgery was the only treatment for hyperthyroidism, but it is not important now.)

Diagnosis. In almost all cases the diagnosis of myasthenia is obvious from the history and examination. The diagnosis is immediately confirmed by the response to cholinergic drugs. For adults, 1 ml. of edrophonium (10 mg.) is given intermittently; after injection of 2 to 3 mg., specific muscle groups are evaluated. If there is no response within 30 seconds, the injection is continued to a total of 6 mg. and the patient is evaluated once again. If there is still no response, the remainder is given, a total of 10 mg. This drug is preferred when cranial muscles are being tested because the response is prompt and dramatic. Cranial weakness cannot be simulated voluntarily, and placebo injections are therefore not necessary. If it is desired to evaluate limb strength, the injection of neostigmine has advantages because the effect lasts longer, permitting more leisurely testing. The adult dose is 1.5 mg. intramuscularly, and it is usually combined with atropine, 0.5 mg., to avoid the muscarinic symptoms of abdominal cramps and sweating. When limb strength is evaluated, it is sometimes advisable to evaluate placebo responses by giving the atropine 30 minutes before the neostigmine. In all cases of myasthenia gravis there is some response to these drugs, but the response is sometimes slight, and the test may have to be repeated on several occasions to provide convincing evidence.

To provide confirmatory evidence in some cases, the electromyographic response to ulnar nerve stimulation may be studied. The characteristic decline in amplitude of the evoked potential is usually seen in affected muscles, but the response may be normal when the disease is restricted to the eyes. Rarely, it is desirable to administer d-tubocurarine, a drug to which myasthenics are unusually sensitive. There are hazards in the administration of this drug, however, and it should probably be left to research centers; d-tubocurarine should never be given without appropriate precautions to support respiration.

No other laboratory tests provide diagnostic information, but it is useful to perform a standard series of studies. Laminagrams of the mediastinum are necessary to identify thymomas. Thyroid function should be tested in all myasthenics, and it is useful to evaluate immunologic disorders by serum protein electrophoresis, LE cell preparation, latex fixation test for rheumatoid factor, and anti-nuclear antibodies. Tests for muscle antibodies are performed in special centers.

The differential diagnosis of myasthenia includes most of neurology, but a few conditions require special consideration. Probably the most frequent error in diagnosis concerns patients with emotional fatigue states and hysterical weakness. There are no cranial muscle symptoms in these patients (except globus hystericus), whereas cranial muscles are involved in virtually all myasthenics. Their symptoms are not those of weakness but of exhaustion, and in tests of strength against resistance there is apt to be marked variation in effort, or dramatic giving way. Amyotrophic lateral sclerosis and peripheral neuropathy may be confused when these disorders affect cranial muscles, but signs indicative of a neurogenic disorder distinguish them from myasthenia. Polymyositis may be confusing, but ocular muscle paresis is not found. There is some debate about the specificity of the therapeutic effect of cholinergic drugs, but for practical purposes it may be taken that an authentic (not placebo), convincing (not equivocal), and reproducible (not seen by one examiner only) effect is found only in myasthenia gravis.

Treatment. *Drug Therapy.* The major drugs used to treat myasthenia gravis are inhibitors of cholinesterase, neostigmine, and pyridostigmine. Another drug, ambenonium, is also used in some clinics, but has no special advantages. It is best to use only one drug; there is no benefit from combinations of two or more. Neostigmine is provided in 15 mg. tablets, and pyridostigmine in 60 mg. tablets; these are essentially interchangeable. The choice of drug is arbitrary because there is no evidence that the maximal benefit achieved by one is more than that of the other. Most patients, but not all, prefer pyridostigmine because it is less apt to cause abdominal cramps and diarrhea, and it is less apt to cause noticeable peaks and valleys of strength. But these advantages have never been proved objectively, and some patients do very well with neostigmine. Pyridostigmine is also provided in a slow-release capsule (Timespan) of 180 mg., said to provide 60 mg. immediately and the remainder in 8 to 12 hours. Some clinicians use the prolonged-action preparation throughout the day, but because of uncertainties of release, it seems advisable to use this only at bedtime for patients who would otherwise have to awaken at night or who are very weak on waking in the morning. (For patients who cannot swallow pills, both drugs may be administered parenterally, and pyridostigmine may be given as a syrup. The intramuscular dose is about one tenth of the oral dose, and the intravenous dose is one thirtieth of the oral dose.) Decisions about optimal dosage are sometimes difficult. Some authorities advocate the use of edrophonium to evaluate oral drug therapy; a test dose of 2 mg. is given intravenously. If the patient improves, oral therapy has been too little. If there is aggravation of weakness, oral therapy has been too much. If there is no change,

oral therapy has been just right. But other authorities find this test an unreliable guide. If edrophonium is not used, there is nothing but clinical observation to guide the therapist. For mild cases, two tablets of either neostigmine or pyridostigmine three times daily, with meals, is useful. If there is inadequate response, the dose may be increased, first by shortening the interval between doses, then by increasing the quantity of drug with each dose. Problems arise because these drugs never completely reverse symptoms. Therefore, the dose should be increased only so long as there is clear-cut response, and it should not be increased beyond the amount giving some perceptible benefit.

The question of proper dosage is important because overtreatment itself can cause weakness; cholinesterase inhibitors may cause a depolarizing block at the neuromuscular junction. How often this happens is a matter of debate among experts, but that it can happen is unquestionable.

Because drugs currently available have limited effect, the search for better agents continues. Germine diacetate, a derivative of veratrine, seems promising, but is available for investigative use only. Steroid therapy is best reserved for the management of patients in crisis (*vide infra*), and immunosuppressive therapy is still to be evaluated. Drugs advocated as "adjuvants" include potassium chloride, ephedrine, and guanidine; they may have some effect in individual patients, but their true value is unproved.

Surgical Treatment. Thymectomy is followed by significant improvement in about two thirds of patients with myasthenia and no tumor. Patients with thymoma fare worse whether the tumor is excised or not. Chest surgeons, anesthesiologists, and respirator units for postoperative care are now so skillful that the risks of operation are almost negligible, and recent attempts to remove the gland through an incision in the neck rather than by splitting the sternum should reduce the morbidity considerably. Because not all patients improve, and because it is difficult to predict which patients will benefit, there is still some uncertainty in the selection of patients. Some recommend the operation for all patients who are incapacitated in daily living for more than six months despite adequate drug therapy. In preparing patients for operation, their usual oral dosage is continued until the day of operation, then stopped. Tracheostomy is performed for all patients with oropharyngeal weakness, and intermittent positive pressure breathing is used in the postoperative period. Specific drug therapy is withheld for several days, until fever subsides, and then started again at a level of one half or less of the preoperative dose.

Crisis. Patients with myasthenia gravis may suddenly have difficulty breathing, severe enough to require artificial ventilation. This may be induced by systemic infection or major surgical procedures, but often there is no apparent cause. Patients with oropharyngeal weakness are especially liable to this threat, perhaps because of aspiration. Whenever there is doubt about the need for a tracheostomy, it is best to err on the side of caution and perform it. The insertion of a cuffed tracheostomy tube makes intermittent positive pressure breathing feasible, and also reduces the hazard of aspiration. Patients are best transferred to a respirator intensive care unit. Cholinergic drugs are stopped. After several days, usually after fever (an almost inevitable concomitant of crisis and tracheostomy) has started to subside, drugs may be started once again, at half the pre-crisis dosage. The cause of crisis is not clear, but it is usually transient, and will subside if the patient can be kept alive. The mortality rate of crisis was formerly about 50 per cent, but since the advent of intensive care units, only about 10 per cent die, and these are mostly elderly patients with complicating cardiac and renal disease.

Some patients require assisted ventilation for prolonged periods, some longer than one year. For these patients, the use of ACTH seems advisable, and this form of steroid therapy has also been used in massive doses in other severely affected patients, 1000 units total in seven to ten days. Because worsening myasthenia precedes the improvement induced by ACTH, this treatment should be reserved for patients with tracheostomy and in centers with respirator units.

Prognosis. The course of myasthenia is variable. The disease may be restricted to ocular muscles for many years, with no threat to life. Other patients are disabled to a variable degree by oropharyngeal or limb weakness, and a few are crippled. Crisis occurs in about 25 per cent of the cases. The over-all mortality is probably about 15 per cent, and although myasthenia itself was formerly the main hazard, intercurrent and unrelated disease is now more often the cause of death.

Elmqvist, D., Hofmann, W. W., Kugelberg, J., and Quastel, D. M. J.: An electrophysiological investigation of neuromuscular transmission in myasthenia gravis. J. Physiol., 174:417, 1964.

Goldstein, G.: The thymus and neuromuscular function: A substance in thymus which causes myositis and myasthenic neuromuscular block in guinea pigs. Lancet, 2:119, 1968.

Greene, R. D. (ed.): Myasthenia Gravis. Philadelphia, J. B. Lippincott Company, 1969.

Osserman, K. E.: Myasthenia Gravis. New York, Grune and Stratton, Inc., 1958.

Osserman, K. E., and Whipple, H. E. (eds.): Myasthenia gravis. Ann. N. Y. Acad. Sci., 135:1, 1966.

Strauss, A. J. L.: Myasthenia gravis, autoimmunity, and the thymus. Advances Intern. Med., 14:241, 1968.

EATON-LAMBERT SYNDROME
(Myasthenic Syndrome)

Definition. Eponyms are in disfavor these days, but they are still useful when there is no other satisfactory name for a syndrome and when the eponym pays homage appropriately, without arguments of priority. This syndrome qualifies on both counts. The originators regarded it as "myasthenic" because of a disorder of neuromuscular function, but there are so many important differences from myasthenia gravis that this term

may be confusing. The syndrome is defined essentially in terms of electromyography. In the Eaton-Lambert syndrome, the amplitude of the muscle action potential evoked by stimulation of its nerve is markedly reduced, and with repetitive stimulation the action potential is augmented.

Pathogenesis. The first cases were all associated with oat-cell carcinoma of the lung, but cases have been found with other tumors, other diseases, and sometimes with no complicating disorder. Microelectrode studies indicate that the defect is due to impaired release of acetylcholine at the nerve terminals. How the tumor affects this syndrome is not known.

Clinical Manifestations. The first evidence of the Eaton-Lambert syndrome may be prolonged apnea after curarization for surgery. Formal testing with d-tubocurarine also indicates that patients are unduly sensitive. Other patients may have symptoms of limb weakness, but cranial muscle weakness is never prominent. The response to cholinergic drugs is usually equivocal at best. Pain in the limbs may be prominent. Movements may be peculiarly slow. In tests of strength it may seem as though the patient gets stronger with continued effort. Myotatic reflexes are frequently depressed.

Diagnosis. The signs listed above diverge sufficiently from myasthenia to avoid confusion; only limb weakness and curare sensitivity are similar. The remainder of the syndrome resembles polymyositis, and polyneuritis would also have to be considered. The diagnosis is made by electromyography.

Treatment. Under a variety of experimental conditions, guanidine promotes the release of acetylcholine. It was therefore a logical choice to treat this rare syndrome, and the drug is effective in daily doses of 35 mg. per kilogram of body weight, given orally.

Eaton, L. M., and Lambert, E. H.: Electromyography and electric stimulation of nerves in diseases of motor unit: Observations in myasthenic syndrome associated with malignant tumors. J.A.M.A., 163:1117, 1957.

Elmqvist, D., and Lambert, E. H.: Detailed analysis of neuromuscular transmission in a patient with myasthenic syndrome sometimes associated with brochogenic carcinoma. Mayo Clin. Proc., 43:689, 1968.

UNUSUAL CAUSES OF NEUROMUSCULAR BLOCK

Botulism and *tick paralysis* are described elsewhere. Both cause a syndrome of flaccid quadriplegia with paresis of cranial muscles, and must be differentiated from polyneuritis, myasthenia gravis, and periodic paralysis. In neither is there a sensory disorder, but autonomic fibers may be affected in botulism, especially pupilloconstrictor fibers (resulting in a dilated, fixed pupil). The physiologic disorder in both syndromes is impaired release of acetylcholine from motor nerve terminals. Guanidine has been used with benefit to treat botulism and might also be effective in tick paralysis. Supportive therapy (tracheostomy and assisted respiration) is mandatory in severe cases. Tick paralysis is reversed by removal of the organism.

Several *antimicrobial drugs* interfere with the release of acetylcholine, and may cause clinical syndromes in man. The offending drugs include neomycin, streptomycin, colistin, polymyxin, and kanamycin. The most common manifestation is postoperative apnea without other evidence of paralysis. This is most apt to occur in patients with renal failure, presumably with unusually high blood levels of the antimicrobial drug. In occasional cases, however, there may be flaccid quadriplegia. Administration of calcium and guanidine may be helpful, but the essence of management is supportive treatment and use of a safer antimicrobial.

Cherington, M., and Ryan, D. W.: Botulism and guanidine. New Eng. J. Med., 278:931, 1968.

McQuillen, M. P., Cantor, H. E., and O'Rourke, J. R.: Myasthenic syndrome associated with antibiotics. Arch. Neurol. (Chicago), 18:402, 1968.

SYNDROMES OF JUNCTIONAL OVERACTIVITY: CRAMPS AND RELATED DISORDERS

Cramps, due to painful, abrupt shortening of muscle, affect almost everyone at some time or other. Electromyographic investigation indicates that motor units fire at a rate of about 300 per second, much higher than the most vigorous voluntary contraction. It is presumably the high rate of discharge that causes the palpable muscle tautness and the pain. Anyone who has had more than one cramp knows that the pain can be relieved by stretching the affected muscle, or by massage. The stimulus responsible for cramps is not known; relief by stretching suggests that some central mechanism is involved, since this is the stimulus for receptors in muscle that inhibit discharge of the motor neuron to the same muscle. Certain conditions are known to be associated with a propensity to cramps: denervation (especially amyotrophic lateral sclerosis), pregnancy, and electrolyte disorders (especially water intoxication and hyponatremia). Some people are more susceptible than others for reasons which are not known. Sometimes cramps occur only at night, and can be prevented by quinine sulfate, 0.3 gram orally at bedtime. Sometimes cramps occur frequently during the day, occasionally so often that the individual is effectively crippled. Diphenylhydantoin, 0.3 to 0.6 gram daily, may be helpful to these patients, but some are resistant to this

and to other drugs that may be tried, including diazepam and procaine amide.

Tetany is a special form of cramp, identified by its predilection for flexor muscles of the hand and fingers, its association with laryngospasm, and its relationship to hypocalcemia. Tetany can be painful. It differs from other cramps electromyographically because of the characteristic rhythmic grouping of discharging potentials.

Contracture is reserved for the painful shortening of muscles in glycogen storage diseases, in which the muscles are electrically silent although maximally shortened.

Myokymia has been used to describe a variety of apparently different disorders characterized by cramps in association with spontaneous twitching of muscle. In some cases there are prolonged trains of spontaneous potentials, whereas in others there is grouping of potentials. Some of these patients have difficulty in relaxing grip, but, unlike myotonia, the muscular activity is abolished by neuromuscular blocking agents, indicating a neural rather than a muscular origin. Hyperhidrosis is prominent in some patients and is secondary to the increased muscular activity.

Continuous shortening of muscle would lead to abnormal postures and abnormally increased resistance to passive movement. These abnormalities, of course, are often due to central neurologic disorders. In recent years, however, an increasing number of patients have been described because of fluctuating rigidity of axial and limb muscles. For want of a better name, and lacking understanding of the pathogenesis, this has been called the *stiff man syndrome.* The diagnosis requires that there be no signs of cerebral or spinal cord disease, and there must be continuous electromyographic activity despite authentic attempts to relax. Ordinary cramps may be superimposed upon the persistent stiffness. Diazepam, 30 to 60 mg. daily, may bring dramatic relief.

A variety of other names have been applied to these syndromes, including *quantal squander, armadillo disease, neuromyotonia,* and *continuous muscle fiber activity.* Some cases of brief duration may be related to mild cases of tetanus. It will take some time to sort out the variety of causes. If these unusual forms can be analyzed, we may yet understand why an otherwise normal individual occasionally has a cramp.

Feldman, R. G., and Granger, C. V.: Electromyography and latent tetany. New Eng. J. Med., 269:1064, 1963.

Garner-Medwin, D., and Walton, J. N.: Myokymia with impaired muscular relaxation. Lancet, 1:127, 1969.

Geschwind, N.: Skeletal muscle cramps. J. Clin. Pharm. Therap., 5:859, 1964.

Gordon, E. E., Januszko, D. M., and Kaufman, L.: A critical survey of stiff man syndrome. Amer. J. Med., 42:582, 1967.

Wallis, W. E., Van Poznak, A., and Plum, F.: Generalized muscular stiffness, fasciculations and myokymia of peripheral nerve origin. Arch Neurol (Chicago), 22:430, 1970.

The recent direct demonstration of a measles-like virus in patients with subacute sclerosing panencephalitis suggests the awesome potential of common agents of acute infection.

In contrast to the bacterial diseases of man, the viral diseases are relatively insusceptible at present to chemotherapy, but the efficient immunity of natural viral infection can be duplicated with vaccines. The coat proteins of all viruses are antigenic, and it is reasonable to conclude that vaccines could be made for all viruses that can be cultivated in the laboratory. The great number of viral pathogens limits the feasibility of this approach, however, as does our uncertain knowledge of the ultimate potential of these viruses for good or evil. The vaccine itself may be a two-edged sword: if a living virus, it may be contaminated with alien viruses or nucleic acid; if inactivated, it may be poorly antigenic. At its best, however, the vaccine may be the ultimate weapon if eradication of the virus can be effected by substitution in the community of vaccine virus for wild type. A trend in this direction is evident with poliomyelitis.

The intractability of viral infections to chemotherapy is a corollary of the intimacy of virus-host association. To the extent that the viral parasite subverts the host's cellular machinery to its own synthesis, it cannot be interrupted without compromising the host as well. But the recent discovery of new, virus-coded enzymes in infected but not in normal cells suggests the possibility of employing highly selective antimetabolites specifically directed against virus synthesis. Indeed, this effect has already been realized in vitro, and in man limited success in arresting the progression of recurrent herpes simplex keratitis has been achieved even with antimetabolites not specific for virus. Chemoprophylaxis of smallpox and effective therapy of progressive vaccinia have attended the semi-empiric use of isatin β-thio-semicarbazone.

Man may never be free of viruses, but, hopefully, he may gradually replace the plagues of the past with more peaceful coexistence in the future.

VIRAL (AND FILTER-PASSING MICROBIAL) INFECTIONS OF THE RESPIRATORY TRACT

THE COMMON COLD

(Acute Coryza)

George Gee Jackson

Definition. The common cold is a symptom complex caused by viral infection of the upper respiratory passages. Most precisely, the term applies to afebrile, acute coryza of viral origin. In the broadest sense, the common cold refers to any undifferentiated upper respiratory infection. The terms rhinitis, pharyngitis, laryngitis, and "chest cold" are sometimes used to designate the principal anatomic site of infection. The main difference between the common cold and other viral or bacterial respiratory infections is the absence of fever and the relatively milder constitutional symptoms and signs.

Etiology. Many viruses and some nonviral filter-passing agents can cause the common cold. No single strain of virus accounts for more than a small proportion of the illnesses. Among the viruses recently identified, rhinoviruses comprise the largest single etiologic group. Isolates have been made from about 50 per cent of acute coryzal illnesses in young adults and about 25 per cent of common colds in children. All the viruses listed in Table 1 have been etiologically related to the common cold in some persons. (The Coxsackie and echoviruses listed therein are also considered separately in the articles on these two viral groups.)

The increasing ability to recover viruses and better serologic means for the diagnosis of viral infections have shown that 5 to 10 per cent of common colds are associated with more than one virus, and definite evidence of simultaneous dual infection is not rare. The causative agents of some of the infections have not been revealed by tissue culture methods currently in use. Certain of the more labile or fastidious viruses have been grown only in unusual cultures of human cell strains or in organ cultures of human embryonic trachea. Other viruses can be shown only by the transmission of illness to volunteers. It is estimated that more than 90 antigenically different strains of known types of respiratory viruses cause the common cold syndrome. The unknown viruses still to be isolated from infectious secretions suggest that there may be well over 100 viruses that can cause mild respiratory illnesses in man.

Incidence and Prevalence. The incidence of common colds is related to age and environment. Preschool children have an average of six to twelve respiratory illnesses per year, most of which are common colds. Parents with young children have approximately six viral respiratory illnesses per year, and older adults have two to three per year. Statistics gathered by the United States Public Health Service show that in the winter quarter of the year at least one half of all

TABLE 1. VIRUSES SOMETIMES ASSOCIATED WITH THE COMMON COLD

Myxoviruses
Influenza A, B, C
Parainfluenza 1, 2, 3, 4
Respiratory syncytial
Coronaviruses
Reovirus 1
Adenoviruses 1, 2, 3, 4, 5, 7, 14, 21
Picornaviruses
Coxsackie A 21, 24
Coxsackie B 4, 5
Echo 4, 7, 8, 9, 11, 20, 25
Rhinovirus ± 60 types

persons acquire a common cold; 20 per cent of persons have a similar illness in the summer quarter.

The prevalence of common colds is approximately 15 per cent of persons per week during the winter months. Surveillance of a group of student nurses during one winter revealed common cold symptoms on 10 per cent of the days. Among industrial employees in the United States, common colds accounted for nearly one million person-years lost from work among an industrial force of 60 million. This amounts to one half of all absences and one quarter of the total time lost. Similarly, acute respiratory illness is highly prevalent among military forces, especially recruits, and is a major cause of disability.

Epidemiology. The common cold is spread by direct person-to-person contact. Under conditions of household association, 10 per cent of adults acquired the disease from an index case. From studies in volunteers, it was shown that some persons became infected and shed virus without having symptoms. This could be the way in which the viruses persist during the nonepidemic season.

It is a common observation that an increase in the frequency of colds occurs in the winter. Sometimes this has been correlated with sharp changes in the temperature, humidity, or pollution of the air, but the popular belief that cold weather causes common colds cannot be substantiated from epidemiologic observations in the Arctic or tropics or from studies in volunteers. Exposure of volunteer subjects to cold did not activate latent respiratory viruses. The reason for the apparent relation between the season and common colds remains unclear. In the United States, it is usual to observe three waves of common colds per year. One occurs in the autumn a few weeks after the opening of schools, another in midwinter, and a third wave in the spring. The separate epidemics have usually been shown to be due to different viruses, each of which may have its own seasonal epidemiology.

Pathology. The pathologic changes in the mucous membranes of the respiratory passages are edema, hyperemia, transudation, and exudation. The severity of the cytopathic effect is related to the type and virulence of the infecting virus and the extent of infection. Picornaviruses (rhinoviruses and enteroviruses) have been observed to cause more metaplasia and degeneration in smears of exfoliated cells from the nasal turbinates than the myxoviruses. This generalization does not hold for infections of the lower respiratory tract. During the acute phase of infection, protein components of the respiratory secretions are altered, and serum globulins become more abundant. Abnormal soluble substances of cellular origin also can be found. The secretion is rich in glycoprotein. Repair is relatively rapid and, insofar as is known, occurs without residual pathologic damage. Recently, however, inquiry has been made regarding the role of repeated viral respiratory infections in the pathogenesis of later degenerative diseases, such as bronchitis and emphysema.

Viral infection induces swelling and some exudation, but it causes no significant change in the bacterial flora of the nasopharynx. When the inflammatory changes are of sufficient magnitude, channels connecting the paranasal sinuses and middle ear to the airway become obstructed. Suppuration can develop from secondary bacterial growth under these conditions.

Mechanisms of Infection and Immunity. Viruses from infected persons are airborne in droplet spray that is emitted during respiration, talking, sneezing, and coughing. Particles in the size range of 5 to 50 μ are probably the most infectious. The nasopharynx is the portal of infection. The incubation period is short, usually one to four days. Proliferation of virus can often be demonstrated within 24 hours after the infection of volunteers. Virus shedding usually precedes the onset of symptoms by one to two days, and the peak excretion occurs a few days later, during the symptomatic phase of the illness. Virus excretion ceases after several days, and symptoms decrease concomitantly. Later studies from the same person as well as attempts to recover viruses from well persons indicate that the carrier state after infection is transient, and the prevalence of asymptomatic carriers is not great. Rhinoviruses have not been recovered from more than 1 to 2 per cent of well persons.

Host susceptibility or resistance to infection is determined primarily by the immunologic status resulting from recent previous infection with the same or related viruses. Some physiologic functions, such as menses and fatigue, and constitutional factors, such as an allergic diathesis and vasomotor rhinitis, are secondary determinants of host susceptibility. Emotional distress and overconcern with personal health increase symptoms, whereas stoical and ascetic personality traits decrease overt susceptibility. In controlled studies, chilling did not increase the susceptibility of volunteers to infection nor did ventilation with frigid air.

The nasal secretion is the first barrier against infection of the epithelial cells of the respiratory tract. In addition to the mechanical movement of mucus, the secretion contains glycoprotein inhibitors for some myxoviruses that can compete with cell receptors for the virus. Because virus union with inhibitors is reversible whereas cellular infection is not, these inhibitors probably do no more than delay and decrease the multiplicity of infection. Specific gamma globulins of low molecular weight, principally IgA and IgG, also are contained in nasal secretion. In the non-infected person, these antibodies are present in low concentrations, but nasal washings from immune subjects neutralize the infectivity of specific viruses to a variable degree. The activity is related to, but poorly correlated with, the height of specific antibody in the plasma. In one study, the gradient between nasal and serum antibody was 1 to 30. During the early stages of infection, before symptoms have begun, there is an easily demonstrable increase of globulins in nasal washings. Infection with some respiratory viruses stimulates the local production of a protein or proteins referred to as interferon. Noninfected cells exposed to interferon are protected against viral infection. The mechanism offers an attractive thesis for the termination of infection and repair of the mucosa before specific antibody is formed.

A response in serum-neutralizing antibody against the infecting virus is not always sufficiently prompt or of great enough magnitude to permit diagnosis of the causative role of a virus in the infection. Specific immunity against illness from reinfection with the same strain of virus, however, is readily demonstrable in volunteers. This clinical immunity is apparent for the period between one month to one to two years after infection. Asymptomatic infections are not entirely prevented. Reinfection in the presence of serum antibody usually results in a modified illness. The specificity of the antibody and its concentration at the site of infection on the surface of the mucosa appear to be critical factors.

Clinical Manifestations. The common cold is in large part a subjective symptomatic diagnosis. The major symptoms for any individual tend to be repetitive, but they differ appreciably from person to person. Some persons have only "head colds," whereas others complain regularly of pharyngitis or cough as characteristic principal symptoms of their colds. The occurrence of symptoms that 100 young adults described as characteristic of a naturally acquired common cold is shown in Table 2.

The same symptoms occur in volunteers challenged with an infectious virus, and their time of occurrence and duration have been observed. Sneezing, headache, and malaise are the initial symptoms, followed by chilly sensations, sore throat, rhinorrhea, and nasal congestion. The chilly sensations may be associated with some lowering of oral temperature that is sometimes interpreted as the initiating cause in natural colds. Fever of any significant degree is absent. The constitutional symptoms usually are transient, lasting only one or two days. There is sometimes a lull for a day between the early symptoms and the development of characteristic nasopharyngeal symptoms of a full-blown cold. The

TABLE 2. THE SYNDROME OF THE COMMON COLD

Symptoms	Frequency
Severe:	
Nasal discharge	100
Nasal obstruction	99
Moderate:	
Sore or dry throat	96
Malaise	81
Postnasal discharge	79
Headache	78
Cough	76
Mild:	
Sneezing	97
Feverishness	49
Chilliness	43
Burning eyes and mucous membranes	28
Muscle aching	22

dry or sore throat tends to recede as the cold progresses. Nasal discharge is the hallmark of the common cold. At the onset, the secretion is clear, watery, and often profuse. Later, secretions thicken, become mucopurulent, yellow-green, and tenacious. Nasal obstruction is at first an intermittent symptom associated with an exaggeration of the rhythmic physiologic turgescence of the nasal turbinates. Later, the turbinates become swollen and boggy, encroaching on the nasal lumen, which contains increased secretions. These symptoms ordinarily run their course within a week. As the illness progresses, cough may appear as an increasingly prominent symptom, and may persist for one to two weeks. It may be dry or productive of a variable amount of mucoid sputum.

Physical signs are limited to the nasopharynx, the surrounding sinuses, and middle ears. Usually, mild hyperemia, congestion, or both, are all that can be seen, and the deviation from normal may be insufficient to recognize as pathologic.

Hematologic changes have been observed in association with infection in volunteers when the initial blood values and the time sequence of infection were known. Mild leukopenia with relative lymphocytosis is often the initial response, followed after a day or two by a slight leukocytosis with some increase in polymorphonuclear leukocytes. A fall in the hematocrit and rise in the erythrocyte sedimentation rate also can occur. Although the aforementioned changes can be shown to be related to the infection in volunteers, their deviation from normal is not great enough to be useful in isolated cases.

Complications of a cold are usually bacterial in origin. They are infrequent and consist of suppuration in the nasopharynx and its contiguous passages. Serous effusion, however, may appear in the middle ear and perhaps in the sinuses.

Diagnosis. The diagnosis of a common cold is made almost entirely on the basis of history and symptoms. At the peak of the illness, signs of the infection also are apparent. Examination is important for the recognition or exclusion of illnesses of more severe nature that patients may be prone to designate as a cold. The differential diagnosis includes prodromes of other infections and infectious, vascular, allergic, and neoplastic processes in the nose, pharynx, sinuses, or ears. Other serious diseases, such as bacterial endocarditis, tuberculosis, bronchitis, bronchiectasis, and lung abscess might masquerade as common colds because of lack of characteristic symptoms and incomplete examination of the patient by a physician. The diagnosis of common cold, therefore, should be avoided as a designation for a broad category of respiratory symptoms of diverse causes.

The clinical symptoms do not permit discrimination with regard to the specific viral cause of a cold. The overlap in the symptoms produced by infection with any one of many viruses that cause the common cold is so great as to preclude more than a judgment regarding the general group of viruses to which the etiologic agent might belong. Under the controlled conditions of studies in volunteers, different viruses cause appreciably different syndromes. For each, the clinical manifestations are also related to the dose, size of particle inhaled, and modifications by the host. The diagnosis of the specific viral cause of a common cold, therefore, is based on laboratory procedures.

Treatment and Prevention. In considering treatment and prevention of the common cold, the following factors that have been discussed must be kept in mind: (1) The number of antigenically distinct viruses that cause the common cold is large. (2) Except for the time and economic loss, the infection is benign and the duration of severe symptoms is brief. (3) Viral infection does not significantly change the bacterial flora of the nasopharynx, and bacterial complications are infrequent. (4) Infection initiates production of interferon and antibodies that naturally limit the infection. (5) Specific immunity to illness with the same virus exists for one to two years after infection. (6) Reinfection can occur in the presence of antibody in the plasma.

At present there are no antimicrobial drugs that are effective in man against the viruses responsible for the common cold; hence the use of such drugs is not recommended. Suppurative complications are caused by obstruction more often than by the virulence of local bacteria. Routine chemoprophylaxis selects resistant bacterial strains rather than prevents the suppurative complications.

Supportive treatment is desirable and helpful. Additional rest in bed, warm clothing, and prevention of chilling increase the patient's comfort. If ventilatory insufficiency, stridor, and anoxemia that may accompany a cold are present, steam inhalation, a decongestant, a bronchodilator, or an expectorant may be indicated. Postural changes can help in the drainage of secretions and the raising of sputum. Because of the diverse causes and syndromes, there is no one regimen to be recommended. Aspirin in a dose of 0.6 gram for an adult or 10 mg. per kilogram of body weight for children, one to four times daily, can reduce headache and malaise. Oral phenylpropanolamine hydrochloride (15 to 50 mg.), inhalation of hexamine vapor, or nose drops with 0.5 per cent ephedrine or phenylephrine shrink the vascular bed of the mucosa and assist in nasal decongestion. Nose drops in any oily vehicle should be avoided, and potent vasoconstrictors with transient action and physiologic rebound, such as epinephrine, are not desirable. Increased fluids or hard candy lozenges may be adequate for control of coughing. Cough syrups, such as elixir of terpin hydrate with codeine (64 mg. per 30 ml.) may be more effective if necessary. Antihistamines have no effect on the common cold, except possibly that a person prone to severe inhalant allergy may experience some reduction in the volume of nasal secretion. The numerous compounded remedies, including those with vitamins, bioflavonoids, quinine, alkalinizers, multiple analgesics, antihistamines, decongestants, and tranquilizers, are developed for sales profit in a large market of uninformed and uncritical people and are not for the benefit of the patient or his physician. Their widespread and repeated use invariably leads to cases of fatal hematologic disorders, eruptive or exfoliative dermatitis, and anaphylaxis or other severe idiosyncratic reaction.

Prevention of common colds by quarantine or isolation of cases is without effect because of the number of infected but asymptomatic persons and because virus excretion usually precedes the symptoms. The hygienic collection and disposal of respiratory secretions to reduce air-borne dissemination from coughing and sneezing should be encouraged as common courtesies. Interruption of the air-borne phase of transmission by increasing space, higher rates of air ventilation, alterations in temperature and humidity, vaporization of disinfectants, and ultraviolet irradiation of overhead air all have been given trials without clearly significant results.

Vaccines for protection against the common cold are not available. Former "cold vaccines" were bacterial suspensions and have no basis for effectiveness except as a placebo. The large number of antigenically distinct viruses augurs numerous difficulties in the production of an effective vaccine. Nevertheless, promising vaccines are being developed for specific groups of viruses.

Andrewes, H. H.: Rhinoviruses and common cold. Ann. Rev. Med., 17:361, 1966.

Badger, G. F., Dingle, J. H., Feller, A. E., Hodges, R. G., Jordan, W. S., Jr., and Rammelkamp, C. H., Jr.: A study of illness in a group of Cleveland families. II. Incidence of the common respiratory diseases. Amer. J. Hyg., 58:31, 1953.

Hendley, J. O., Gwaltney, J. M., Jr., and Jordan, W. S., Jr.: Rhinovirus infections in an industrial population: IV. Infections within families of employees during two fall peaks of respiratory illness. Amer. J. Epidem., 89:184, 1969.

Jackson, G. G., and Dowling, H. F.: Transmission of the common cold to volunteers under controlled conditions: IV. Specific immunity to the common cold. J. Clin. Invest., 38:762, 1959.

Jackson, G. G., Dowling, H. F., Anderson, T. O., Riff, L., Saporta, J., and Turck, M.: Susceptibility and immunity to common upper respiratory viral infections—The common cold. Ann. Intern. Med., 53:719, 1960.

Jackson, G. G., Dowling, H. F., Spiesman, I. G., and Boand, A. V.: Transmission of the common cold to volunteers under controlled conditions. I. The common cold as a clinical entity. Arch. Intern. Med. (Chicago), 101:267, 1958.

Kapikian, A. Z., et al.: Isolation from man of "avian infectious bronchitis virus-like" viruses (coronaviruses) similar to 229E virus, with some epidemiological observations. J. Infect. Dis., 119:282, 1969.

Paul, J. H., and Freese, H. L.: An epidemiological and bacteriological study of the "common cold" in an isolated arctic community (Spitzbergen). Amer. J. Hyg., 17:517, 1933.

Scientific Committee on Common Cold Vaccines: Prevention of colds by vaccination against a rhinovirus. Brit. Med. J., 2:1344, 1965.

Tyrrell, D. A. J.: Common Colds and Related Diseases. Baltimore, Williams & Wilkins Company, 1965.

NONBACTERIAL PHARYNGITIS, LARYNGITIS, AND BRONCHITIS

George Gee Jackson

The same viruses that sometimes cause the common cold also cause other syndromes of respiratory illness that may be even more characteristic of the infection than acute afebrile coryza. These are

TABLE 3. CLINICAL SYNDROMES

Virus	Coryza	Pharyngitis (Conjunctivitis) (Otitis)	Croup	Bronchitis	Pneumonia or Systemic Disease
Influenza A, B	++			++	++++
Influenza C	++			+	
Parainfluenza 1, 3	+++	++	+++	+	+++
Parainfluenza 2	+		++++		
Parainfluenza 4	++++				
Respiratory syncytial	+++		++	++++	+
Coronavirus	++++	+		+	
Reovirus 1	+				
Adenovirus 1, 2, 5	+	++			+
Adenovirus 3, 4, 7, 14, 21	++	++++		+	+
Coxsackie A 2, 3, 4, 6, 8, 10	+	++++	+		++
A 21, 24	++++	+			
Coxsackie B 2, 3, 4, 5	+	+	+	+	++++
Echo 4, 5, 7, 8, 9, 11, 19, 20, 25	++	++	+		++
Rhinoviruses	++++	+		+	
Mycoplasma		+			+++

commonly classified by the anatomic site giving rise to the predominant symptoms. The mildest infections are limited to the upper respiratory tract. As progressively more distal sites are involved, the infections are more severe and cause more constitutional symptoms. Acute rhinitis nearly always occurs without fever (the common cold), whereas exudative or nonexudative viral pharyngitis usually produces fever. When adenovirus is the cause, conjunctivitis may be a prominent part of the syndrome. The viruses causing pharyngitis also may cause primary or secondary otitis media and cervical adenitis. Croup is a distinctive clinical syndrome produced by laryngeal stridor, and is especially common in children. Bronchitis, bronchiolitis, and bronchopneumonia are relatively severe manifestations of viral respiratory infection that are nearly always associated with fever and constitutional symptoms. The relative frequency of these different clinical syndromes resulting from infection with some of the different viruses responsible for the common respiratory infections is indicated by + to ++++ in Table 3.

Children are more disposed to croup, febrile lower respiratory tract disease, and constitutional manifestations of infection than adults, who more often have only coryza from infection with the same viruses. In part, this may be an effect of the changing size of the airway, decreased lymphoid tissue, and maturation of the respiratory mucosa. A stronger effect on the amelioration of viral respiratory illness in the adult is exerted by the immunologic responses of the host to previous infection. The resolution of the initial infection and the capacity of the virus to cause reinfection have now been recognized as quite different for different viruses. This negates the validity of any simple statement about immunity or nonimmunity after infection except by specific reference to a particular virus.

Pathogenic Factors Related to the Manifestations and Prevalence of Viral Respiratory Infections. In order for a viral infection to maintain a high prevalence of infection, one or more of several epidemiologic conditions are required. The causative virus may produce a latent infection that can be activated by factors adverse to the host cell but favorable for the growth of virus. There may be multiple distinct types of virus, or the prevalent strain may undergo a series of distinct antigenic mutations. Reinfection of persons can occur if the natural infection does not elicit an adequate antibody response or if the virus at the site of infection is not neutralized by antibody in the plasma. Some viral infections produce only transient immunity,

TABLE 4. MECHANISMS THAT CONTRIBUTE TO THE HIGH PREVALENCE OF VIRAL RESPIRATORY INFECTION

Production of latent infection
    Adenovirus 1, 2, 3, 5
    Herpes hominis
Multiple distinct types of virus simultaneously present
    Rhinoviruses
Mutagenic variations in the prevalent strains of virus
    Influenza A, B
Inadequate antibody response from natural infection (children)
    Respiratory syncytial
    Rhinoviruses
Reinfection and illness in the presence of circulating antibody
    Parainfluenza 3, 1
    Respiratory syncytial
Transient specific immunity
    Rhinoviruses
Lasting immunity but epidemic disease among susceptibles
    Adenovirus 4, 7
    Measles
    Mumps

and thus there is always a large population of susceptible people. Others produce solid immunity in the host, but the viruses perpetuate themselves at high rates of prevalence by causing epidemic disease in selected groups of susceptible persons. All these mechanisms are found in the case of one or another of the different viruses that cause common respiratory infections. An appreciation of these factors is essential to the understanding of the problem of viral respiratory infections, their treatment and control. In Table 4 the behavior of some different respiratory viruses with regard to these viral and immunologic mechanisms is noted.

Chanock, R. M., Mufson, M. A., and Johnson, K. M.: Comparative biology and ecology of human virus and mycoplasma respiratory pathogens. Prog. Med. Virol., 7:208, 1965.

Chanock, R. M., and Parrott, R. H.: Acute respiratory disease in infancy and childhood: Present understanding and prospects for prevention. Pediatrics, 36:21, 1965.

Hamre, D., Connelly, A. P., Jr., and Procknow, J. J.: Virologic studies of acute respiratory disease in young adults: IV. Virus isolation during four years of surveillance. Amer. J. Epidem., 83:238, 1966.

Hilleman, M. R., Hamparian, V. V., Ketler, A., Reilly, C. M., McClelland, L., Dornfield, D., and Stokes, J., Jr.: Acute respiratory illnesses among children and adults. Field study of contemporary importance of several viruses and appraisal of the literature. J.A.M.A., 180:445, 1962.

Mufson, M. A., Webb, P. A., Kennedy, H., Gill, V., and Chanock, R. M.: Etiology of upper respiratory tract illnesses among civilian adults. J.A.M.A., 195:1, 1966.

INFECTIONS WITH RHINOVIRUSES

George Gee Jackson

Etiology. For many decades, attempts have been made to isolate the common cold virus. On some occasions, propagation of infectious material was accomplished for a brief period, but the viruses could not be sustained, and they were not characterized. In 1954, the virus known as 2060 and the closely related JH strain were isolated from adults with acute coryza. These viruses were believed to be enteroviruses and were designated echovirus 28. Soon thereafter, several different workers isolated similar viruses that were designated in the earlier literature as Salisbury agents, ERC viruses, entero-like viruses, coryzaviruses, muriviruses, and unclassified common cold viruses. Because of common biologic properties, these are all designated now as rhinoviruses. They comprise a subclass in the family of picornaviruses, which also include the Coxsackie, polio-, entero- and echoviruses. These are all small viruses (10 to 30 mμ) of the ribonucleic acid type that are not inactivated by ether. There appear to be approximately 60 different serotypes of rhinoviruses capable of infecting man. Their acid lability (pH 3) is probably the reason for their absence from the intestine, and is the major property that distinguishes them from the enteroviruses. Rhinoviruses characteristically grow best in tissue cultures held at a reduced temperature (33° C.)

similar to that found in the nose of man. Some authors have designated M and H strains according to whether the viruses will grow in cultures of monkey tissues (M strains) or only in human cell strains (H strains). This classification has no importance for infections in man.

Prevalence and Epidemiology. Rhinoviruses have been isolated from man in the United States, Great Britain, and Sweden. It is likely that they infect persons in all countries and climates. Similar viruses have been recovered from cattle, but transfer from other animals to man has not been shown. In human infections, some serotypes may occur annually, but in studies performed to date, the occurrence of different serotypes has been haphazard. Infection with rhinoviruses is more prevalent among adults than among children. About one third of adults with colds and 10 to 15 per cent of children have had rhinovirus recovered from the nasal secretion. Infection with these viruses is relatively more frequent in summer and in midwinter. Rhinoviruses have been recovered in 1 to 3 per cent of well adults observed in the winter months.

Clinical Manifestations and Diagnosis. Rhinovirus infections nearly always present with rhinitis, sore throat, dry cough, and malaise. Fever is absent or of slight degree and transient. No pharyngeal exudate is observed, but cervical adenopathy can occur. In children, rhinoviruses sometimes cause croup or lower respiratory tract disease, but most of the infections produce a typical common cold. The incubation period is one to three days, and the course of illness is about one week. Rhinovirus appears in the nasal secretion a day or two before the onset of nasal symptoms, and is shed during the period of illness. The pathologic findings and pathogenesis are described under the Common Cold. A rise in neutralizing antibody in the convalescent serum occurs in only about one half of the infections.

Treatment. There is no specific treatment; the supportive measures are the same as those given under treatment of the common cold. Quarantine is not necessary. No polyvalent vaccine is available, but experimental vaccines have been effective against a single type of rhinovirus. The large number of distinct serotypes is discouraging to the prospects of developing an effective vaccine unless strains that cause heterotypic responses are found. Immunity to reinfection is quite specific and probably lasts only several months to two years after most infections, although detectable serum antibody may persist longer. Investigational new drugs have shown a prophylactic effect against rhinovirus infection in volunteers. This is a promising omen for the future, but no chemotherapeutic remedy is presently available.

Bloom, H. H., Forsyth, B. R., Johnson, K. M., and Chanock, R. M.: Relationship of rhinovirus infection to mild upper respiratory disease. J.A.M.A., 186:38, 1963.

Cate, T. R., Couch, R. B., Fleet, W. F., Griffith, W. R., Gerone, P. J., and Knight, V.: Production of tracheobronchitis in volunteers with rhinovirus in a small particle aerosol. Amer. J. Epidem., 81:95, 1965.

Gwaltney, J. M., Jr., Hendley, J. O., Simon, G., and Jordan, W. S., Jr.: Rhinovirus infections in an industrial population: I. The occurrence of illness. New Eng. J. Med., 275:1261, 1966.

Gwaltney, J. M., Jr., and Jordan, W. S., Jr.: Rhinoviruses and respiratory illnesses in university students. Amer. Rev. Resp. Dis., 93:363, 1966.

Hamparian, V. V., Leagus, M. B., Hilleman, M. R., and Stokes, J.: Epidemiologic investigation of rhinovirus infections. Proc. Soc. Exp. Biol. Med., 117:469, 1964.

Reilly, C. M., Hock, S. M., Stokes, J., Jr., McClelland, L., Hamparian, V. V., Ketler, A., and Hilleman, M. R.: Clinical and laboratory findings in cases of respiratory illness caused by coryzaviruses. Ann. Intern. Med., 57:515, 1962.

ADENOVIRAL INFECTIONS OF THE RESPIRATORY TRACT

George Gee Jackson

Definition and Etiology. The adenoviruses comprise a distinct group of viruses of the deoxyribose nucleic acid variety. They have group antigen and certain biologic characteristics that are shared by all members of the group. There are more than 31 specific serotypes among the strains of human origin. Only a few of these cause infections of the respiratory tract. The common types involved are 1, 2, 3, 4, 5, and 7. Types 14 and 21 also have caused acute respiratory illness. Type 8 is the principal cause of epidemic keratoconjunctivitis.

Some early isolates were recovered from surgically removed adenoids grown as tissue culture explants. These were reported as adenoidal degenerative or AD agents. The first strains from respiratory illnesses were designated RI agents. A later name, used briefly, was adenoidal-pharyngeal-conjunctival or APC agents. All the strains are now included under the term adenoviruses.

Incidence and Prevalence. Adenoviruses types 1, 2, and 5 infect virtually all persons early in childhood. Whether these infections are important as a cause of respiratory disease is uncertain. In older children and adolescents, adenoviruses, predominantly types 3 and 7 in the United States and 3, 4, 7, 14, and 21 in Europe, cause about 5 per cent of the viral respiratory illnesses. The incidence among college students may be as great as 8 per cent. At military recruit camps, infection with adenovirus types 4 and 7 is highly prevalent. It is often the predominant cause of respiratory illness, and 70 to 80 per cent of all incoming recruits become infected. Among civilian adults, adenoviruses cause only 1 to 3 per cent of respiratory illness.

Epidemiology. Adenoviruses occur in all parts of the world. Man is the principal reservoir of infection. Many species of animals also are infected with adenoviruses, but these are of different serotypes, and cross infection between man and animals either does not occur or is rare. Transmission is by person-to-person contact, but spread occurs only when the contact with an infected person is close or prolonged. The incubation period is from three to eight days. Swimming pools have been an effective vehicle for the transmission of adenovirus type 3 induced conjunctivitis. Such epidemics occur in the summer and have been referred to as Greeley disease and pseudomembranous conjunctivitis. During the acute infection and for a period of one to three weeks, virus is excreted in the respiratory secretions or in those of the eye, or in both. A high proportion of infected persons have virus in the stool, which may be a source for the spread of infection. Viruria also has been observed during the acute respiratory illness.

Pathogenic Mechanisms. A most remarkable aspect of adenoviral infections with types 1, 2, 3, and 5 is the capacity of the virus to persist as a latent infection in lymphoid tissue for years after the initial infection. Fifty to 90 per cent of surgically removed adenoids yield adenovirus of one of these types. Whether this provides a source for infection of others or any harm to the host is unknown.

Some of the adenoviruses are capable of producing tumors when injected into newborn hamsters. Among the respiratory strains, some isolates of type 7 and type 3 have been oncogenic in baby hamsters. These studies on the tumorigenicity of adenoviruses also have shown the capacity of adenoviruses to combine within the same envelope (capsid) the oncogenic genome of some other tumor-producing viruses of DNA type, specifically the simian virus, SV-40. Thus, under defined experimental conditions, adenoviruses can be oncogenic in their own right or act as a carrier for oncogenic material. There is no evidence that these properties give the virus any oncogenic capacity in man, but the phenomena are of basic biologic importance.

Recently some adenoviruses have been found to be associated with smaller virus-like particles for which the adenovirus serves as a "helper." The significance of this adenovirus-associated virus in the pathogenesis of adenoviral infections is not known.

Clinical Manifestations and Differential Diagnosis. Different clinical syndromes produced by adenoviral infections in older children and adults are characteristic. Fever and pharyngitis are the hallmarks; catarrhal otitis occurs frequently, cervical adenopathy is common, conjunctivitis may be present, and a few patients develop pneumonia. The syndromes have been given descriptive names, as follows: (1) acute febrile pharyngitis, (2) nonstreptococcal exudative pharyngitis, (3) acute respiratory disease of recruits, (4) pharyngoconjunctival fever, and (5) adenoviral pneumonia. Any single type of virus among those that cause natural respiratory infections in man can produce the entire spectrum of these clinical manifestations and also the common cold. The age of the patient and the route of inoculation are important. In newborn infants, giant cell pneumonia, myocarditis, and encephalitis have been described. In young children, mesenteric adenitis and intussusception have been reported. Infection with adenovirus types 1,

2, 5, and 6 may occur in the preschool child without any overt illness, whereas type 7 causes severe illness in this age group, with 5 per cent fatality. The former types infect nearly all children, but type 7 infections are uncommon.

Conjunctivitis, when present, is an acute follicular lesion, often unilateral, with marked erythema, suffusion, and narrowing of the palpebral fissure. Keratoconjunctivitis, caused by adenovirus type 8, is a serious infection of the eye with corneal infiltrates; it rarely occurs in pharyngoconjunctival fever. Pharyngeal exudate, if present, is more likely to appear on the pharyngeal wall than as follicular tonsillitis. Cervical lymph nodes are enlarged and firm but less tender than with streptococcal infections. A maculopapular rash that is difficult to distinguish from rubella has been described in a few cases. The leukocyte count is normal or slightly elevated. A prompt antibody response usually accompanies the infection. It can be measured in the serum by complement fixation or virus neutralization tests.

Treatment and Prevention. Treatment is supportive and with few exceptions recovery occurs without sequelae, excluding those of type 8 keratoconjunctivitis. Immunity to reinfection is demonstrable, but second infections have been observed with types 1, 2, 3, and 5. These types cause latent infections, and it is possible that later episodes represent an activation or recrudescence of the latent infection. Reinfection, if it occurs, usually causes mild illness.

Vaccine administration can elicit protective antibody and effectively prevent specific adenovirus infections. An effective live, enteric-coated, oral adenovirus type 4 vaccine has been extensively evaluated in military recruits at stations where the incidence of infection and disease is high. Given prophylactically, it stimulates antibody, prevents specific adenovirus type 4 illness, and reduces pharyngeal infection after natural exposure by about two thirds. In epidemic situations mass immunization with live virus vaccine promptly interrupts the epidemic. Use of the vaccine is not recommended for civilians because of the low incidence and sporadic occurrence of infection with adenovirus type 4 among them.

No adenovirus vaccines are available commercially.

Bell, J. A., Rowe, W. T., Engler, J. I., Parrott, R. H., and Huebner, R. J.: Pharyngoconjunctival fever. Epidemiological studies of a recently recognized disease entity. J.A.M.A., 157:1083, 1955.

Buescher, E. L.: Respiratory disease and the adenoviruses. Med. Clin. N. Amer., 51:769, 1967.

Couch, R. B., Chanock, R. M., Cate, T. R., Long, D. J., Knight, V., and Huebner, R. J.: Immunization with types 4 and 7 adenovirus by selective infection of the intestinal tract. Amer. Rev. Resp. Dis., 88:394, 1963.

Ginsberg, H. S.: Identification and classification of adenoviruses. Virology, 18:312, 1962.

Hilleman, M. R., and Werner, J. H.: Recovery of new agent from patients with acute respiratory illness. Proc. Soc. Exp. Biol. Med., 85:183, 1954.

Huebner, R. J., Rowe, W. P., Ward, T. G., Parrott, R. H., and Bell, J. A.: Adenoidal-pharyngeal-conjunctival agents. New Eng. J. Med., 251:1077, 1954.

Jordan, W. S., Jr.: Occurrence of adenovirus infections in civilian populations. Arch. Intern. Med. (Chicago), 101:54, 1958.

Peckinpaugh, R. O., Pierce, W. E., Rosenbaum, M. J., Edwards, E. A., and Jackson, G. G.: Mass enteric live adenovirus vaccination during epidemic ARD. J.A.M.A., 205:5, 1968.

Van der Veen, J.: The role of adenoviruses in respiratory disease. Amer. Rev. Resp. Dis., 88:160, 1963.

INFECTIONS WITH PARAINFLUENZA VIRUSES
George Gee Jackson

Definition. Infection with parainfluenza viruses is a common and recurrent cause of respiratory illness. Croup is a prominent syndrome in children, but the spectrum of illness varies from the common cold to pneumonia and systemic illness.

Etiology. Parainfluenza viruses are members of the myxovirus family. They closely resemble influenza virus but differ from it serologically and in some biologic respects. Four distinct types of parainfluenza viruses are recognized that cause infections in man. They are closely related to one another and have some characteristics in common with mumps, measles, and respiratory syncytial virus. Types 2 and 4 differ somewhat from types 1 and 3 in the clinical illnesses produced and in their epidemiology.

Parainfluenza viruses were first designated as hemadsorption or HA viruses, owing to their property of causing erythrocytes to adsorb and stick to infected cells in tissue cultures. In early nomenclature, type 1 was identified as HA 2 and type 3 as HA 1. Type 2 was recovered from cases of croup and was called the "croup-associated" or CA virus.

A parainfluenza type 1, the Sendai virus, was first isolated in mice. It was also called influenza D. Mice and other rodents were then recognized to have natural infection with parainfluenza viruses. The Sendai and other animal strains of parainfluenza type 1 have some slight serologic differences from strains of human origin. A simian myxovirus (SV-5) is commonly found in monkey kidney tissue cultures, occasionally in eggs and other tissues. It resembles parainfluenza type 2; virus isolates from cattle with shipping fever (SF-4) were found to be parainfluenza type 3.

Incidence and Epidemiology. Few, if any, persons escape infection and reinfection with the different types of parainfluenza viruses. Most children develop antibody from infection with parainfluenza type 3 before the age of four years. By the time they enter school, 70 per cent of children have antibody against more than one type. Among older children and adults, nasopharyngeal reinfection with types 1 and 3 is common regardless of the presence of serum antibody. Reinfection with parainfluenza viruses accounts for an appreciable proportion of common colds and upper respiratory illnesses in adults.

Parainfluenza types 1 and 3 are endemic and cause illness in all seasons of the year. They also cause epidemics of respiratory disease in the winter season. Type 3 virus spreads easily from person to person. It infects virtually all contacts who have no antibody and reinfects many persons with a demonstrable level of antibody in the serum. Type 1 virus does not spread as efficiently as type 3, but is nevertheless highly transmissible. Type 2 infection has been less prevalent and more episodic in its occurrence than either types 1 or 3. Only about one half of susceptible persons become infected, and reinfection is not common. Infections caused by type 4 have been entirely sporadic.

Although many animal species have a high incidence of infection with the parainfluenza viruses, spread to man from these sources has not been well established.

Clinical Manifestations. The clinical syndrome of croup in children is the most common characteristic of infection with parainfluenza virus. Types 1 and 2 cause croup in a greater proportion of the infections than parainfluenza 3. The latter infections may be symptomatically more severe and cause more lower respiratory tract disease. Together the parainfluenza viruses account for one third to one half of the cases of severe croup in children. Although croup is the most distinctive syndrome, parainfluenza virus infections cause rhinitis or pharyngitis about twice as often as croup, and bronchitis, bronchiolitis, or pneumonia about as frequently as croup.

The initial infection with parainfluenza viruses produces more severe disease than reinfection. Among adults, parainfluenza viruses cause upper respiratory tract disease, predominantly the common cold. In dual viral infections, a parainfluenza virus has been recognized as a common member of the pair, with a resultant increase in the severity of the symptoms.

Diagnosis. Clinical differentiation of the type of parainfluenza viral infection and even the differentiation from other viral infections of the respiratory tract cannot be made with confidence. The virus can be isolated from nasopharyngeal secretions during the illness and for a brief period thereafter. This is the most certain and may be the only way to identify the specific type of parainfluenza virus involved. Serologic responses are often heterotypic owing to the nearly universal infection of persons with type 3 early in life and the common infection with types 1, 2, and mumps viruses. A rise in antibody against one of these viruses does not permit confidence in a strain-specific diagnosis.

Treatment. The treatment is supportive, as described for the common cold. The croup syndrome may be very acute, and may cause respiratory insufficiency requiring urgent and decisive management. A comfortably warm, draft-free environment with high humidity (steam) may be successful in reducing laryngeal stridor. Vaccines have been produced for types 1, 2, and 3, and their antigenicity has been shown. Studies of the effectiveness of the vaccines in the prevention of natural infection are being made.

Banatvala, J. E., Anderson, T. B., and Hocking, E. D.: Parainfluenza infections in the community. Brit. Med. J., 1:537, 1964.

Bloom, H. H., Johnson, K. M., Jacobsen, R., and Chanock, R. M.: Recovery of parainfluenza viruses from adults with upper respiratory illnesses. Amer. J. Hyg., 74:50, 1961.

Chanock, R. M., Parrott, R. H., Johnson, K. M., Kapikian, A. Z., and Bell, J. A.: Myxoviruses: Parainfluenza. Amer. Rev. Resp. Dis., 88:152, 1963.

Fulginiti, V. A., Amer, J., Eller, J. J., Joyner, J. W., and Askin, P.: Para-influenza virus immunization: IV. Simultaneous immunization with parainfluenza types 1, 2, and 3 aqueous vaccines. Amer. J. Dis. Child., 114:1, 1967.

LaPlaca, M., and Moscovici, C.: Distribution of parainfluenza antibodies in different groups of population. J. Immunol., 88:72, 1962.

McLean D. M., Roy, T. E., O'Brien, M. J., Wylie, J. C., and McQueen, E. J.: Parainfluenza viruses in association with acute laryngotracheobronchitis in Toronto (1960–1961). Canad. Med. Ass. J., 85:290, 1961.

Smith, C. B., Purcell, R. H., Bellanti, J. A., and Chanock, R. M.: The relative protective effect of antibody to parainfluenza Type I virus in serum and nasal secretions. New Eng. J. Med., 275:1145, 1966.

Tremonti, L., Lin, J. S., and Jackson, G. G.: Neutralizing activity in nasal secretions and serum in resistance of volunteers to parainfluenza Type 2. J. Immun., 101:572, 1968.

Von Euler, L., Kantor, F. S., Hsuing, G. D., Isaacson, P., and Tucker, G.: Studies of parainfluenza viruses: I. Clinical, pathological, and virological observations. Yale J. Biol. Med., 35:523, 1963.

INFECTIONS WITH RESPIRATORY SYNCYTIAL VIRUS

George Gee Jackson

Definition and Etiology. Infection with respiratory syncytial virus (RS) causes epidemic acute respiratory disease. The illnesses are rather acute in onset and may be mild or severe. Since its recognition in 1956 as an infection of man, RS has produced regular epidemics of respiratory disease.

Respiratory syncytial virus is a myxovirus that resembles influenza and parainfluenza viruses in its structure and many biologic characteristics. It is serologically distinct from them, does not agglutinate erythrocytes as they do, and does not cause lesions in eggs or common laboratory animals. The virus was first isolated from chimpanzees and was designated chimpanzee coryza agent (CCA). The name respiratory syncytial virus is descriptive of the cytopathic effect of the virus in infected tissue cultures. Only one type of the virus is known; some isolates have shown minor differences when tested against specific immune serum, but these appear clinically insignificant with regard to man.

Epidemiology. Respiratory syncytial virus has been recovered at several locations in the United States and elsewhere; it is likely that it has worldwide distribution. The epidemiologic pattern of infection lies somewhere between the epidemicity of influenza A and the endemicity of the parainfluenza viruses. Usually there are sharp, well defined limits to each epidemic. In the interepidemic period, the virus is detected much less frequently, but RS virus has been isolated from illnesses in every month of the year. Epidemics recur at intervals of 8 to 16 months. These have appeared simultaneously in geographically widely separated locations. During an epidemic, a large proportion of the population may experience infection, even persons who have had prior infection and have residual serum antibody. The pattern of the epidemic spread is characteristic of airborne or direct contact transmission. The incubation period is three to seven days.

Incidence and Prevalence. The high incidence of infection is indicated by the fact that 70 per cent of infants at birth have appreciable amounts of maternal antibody against RS virus. During the first few months of life this declines, and between 3 and 12 months about 35 per cent develop antibody as a result of natural infection. By five years of age, 95 per cent of children have been infected. The prevalence of RS virus varies because of its epidemicity, but it makes a significant contribution in the production of serious respiratory diseases of children. Among hospitalized pediatric cases, RS infection has been found to be etiologic in approximately 20 per cent. In this respect, it ranks ahead of the parainfluenza viruses or adenoviruses and is much more prevalent than influenza. In the first year of life, RS virus is the single most prevalent clinical infection causing lower respiratory illness. Among adults, the prevalence is less well documented because of the milder nature of the disease, but it appears to be proportionately of less importance, compared to the rhinoviruses, influenza, and Mycoplasma.

Pathogenesis. The annual epidemiologic recurrences of disease, the reisolation of virus from the same children in successive years, and investigations in adult volunteers have all emphasized the importance of reinfections with respiratory syncytial virus. If the pathogenesis of the reinfections were antigenic differences among strains of RS virus, as with major epidemics of influenza A, the demonstration of such difference should be made easily. So far, differences in neutralization of virus isolates by human sera have been slight. The studies in volunteers show convincingly that the presence in the serum of neutralizing antibody against the challenge strain does not prevent reinfection or illness. The high prevalence and importance of RS virus in the causation of respiratory disease appears to reside in this capacity to produce successive infections with clinical symptoms.

Clinical Manifestations. Fever and bronchiolitis are the characteristics of infection in children. Rhinitis and pharyngitis are usually present. In one study, pneumonia was shown roentgenographically in more than two-thirds of the cases. Croup may develop, but it is relatively infrequent. The average maximal temperature is 102° F., but in individual patients it may reach 105° F. Ordinarily, fever lasts for three days. Dyspnea, cough, and wheezing are obvious symptoms. Tachypnea,

rhonchi, and crepitant rales are present on examination. A few of the patients are cyanotic. The leukocyte count is elevated to between 10,000 and 20,000 per cubic millimeter in many cases. This clinical syndrome cannot be distinguished with certainty from epidemic influenza. Ordinarily, there is more rhinitis, and the onset is less abrupt. A fatality rate of 2.5 per cent has been estimated for hospitalized cases. Sudden death of infants and young children in their cribs at home following mild respiratory symptoms has been suspected by epidemiologic association to be of RS etiology.

In about two thirds of the documented cases there is a less severe syndrome, which has been diagnosed in outpatient clinics. These patients have fever, but they have fewer constitutional symptoms than those who are hospitalized. Rhinitis and pharyngitis are relatively more prominent. Cough is frequent, but rales and rhonchi are scarce.

Among adults with prechallenge antibody, the clinical manifestation of infection is acute coryza. At least, this is the conclusion reached from studies in volunteers and by isolation of RS virus from patients with common colds. An analysis of proved cases in adults admitted to a hospital in one study, however, indicated that persons with chronic bronchitis (one half of the cases studied) had an acute exacerbation of bronchitis; in one fourth of them infection caused bronchopneumonia, and in one fourth it produced the influenza syndrome with severe constitutional symptoms. Thus, the entire spectrum of viral respiratory illness is produced in adults by RS virus. In persons with chronic pulmonary diseases, the infection may be severe.

Diagnosis. The suspicion of RS virus infection is based upon clinical and epidemiologic observations. The diagnosis can be made by virus isolation from the respiratory secretions or by serologic tests. Respiratory syncytial virus is recovered by the inoculation of secretions into cultures of one of several human cell lines or diploid cell strains. The specimens must be fresh or collected and frozen in a stabilizing medium, because of the extreme sensitivity of the virus to freezing and thawing. Two or three weeks may be required before the virus becomes apparent in the tissue culture and can be identified; hence virus isolation is not of immediate value in the diagnosis of an ill patient.

Serodiagnosis can be made by either complement-fixation (CF) or neutralization tests using paired sera collected as early as possible after the onset of illness and again after two to three weeks. A fourfold or greater rise in the serum antibody titer is regarded as diagnostic of infection.

Treatment and Prevention. Careful assessment of respiratory competence, close observation, and supportive care are important, especially in children, in view of the relative severity of the involvement of the lower respiratory tract. Anticipation of the possible need for tracheostomy (to reduce respiratory dead air space and assist in the removal of secretions) and mechanical assistance with ventilation in occasional patients is wise. Antimicrobial drugs have no effect on the RS virus or on the outcome of the usual infection. Isolation of the patient from other susceptible contacts should be done during hospitalization, but the spread of infection in the community is not controlled by isolation procedures.

The annual occurrence of epidemic infection and the clear demonstration of reinfections, often with equally severe second episodes, might suggest that immunoprophylaxis would have little effect on the infection. On the other hand, the mildness and lower frequency of infections in adults are circumstantial support for immunity. The antigens of the RS virus are labile and poorly antigenic. Use of investigational inactivated vaccines has not been protective. Paradoxically, nonprotective levels of serum antibody acquired either from transplacental passage or killed vaccines may augment the clinical severity of the infection. Attenuated live virus preparations that can be given into the respiratory passages are being developed. Perhaps the larger amount of viral antigen and repeated doses that can be given in this way will induce protection.

Beem, M., Wright, F. H., Hamre, D., Egerer, R., and Oehme, M.: Association of chimpanzee coryza agent with acute respiratory disease in children. New Eng. J. Med., 263:523, 1960.

Hilleman, M. R.: Respiratory syncytial virus. Amer. Rev. Resp. Dis., 88:181, 1963.

Holzel, A., Parker, L., Patterson, W. H., White, L. L. R., Tompson, K. M., and Tobin, J. O.: The isolation of respiratory syncytial virus from children with acute respiratory disease. Lancet, 1:295, 1963.

Hornsleth, A., and Volkeit, M.: The incidence of complement-fixing antibodies to the respiratory syncytial virus in sera from Danish population groups aged 9–19 years. Acta Path. Microbiol. Scand., 62:421, 1964.

Johnson, K. M., Bloom, H. H., Mufson, M. A., and Chanock, R. M.: Natural reinfection of adults by respiratory syncytial virus. New Eng. J. Med., 267:68, 1962.

Parrott, R. H., Vargosko, A. J., Kim, H. W., Cumming, C., Turner, H., Huebner, R. J., and Chanock, R. M.: Respiratory syncytial virus: II. Serologic studies over a 34-month period of children with bronchiolitis, pneumonia, and minor respiratory diseases. J.A.M.A., 176:653, 1961.

Reilly, C. M., Stokes, J., Jr., McClelland, L., Cornfeld, D., Hamparian, V. V., Ketler, A., and Hilleman, M. R.: Studies of acute respiratory illnesses caused by respiratory syncytial virus: 3. Clinical and laboratory findings. New Eng. J. Med., 264:1176, 1961.

Sandiford, B. R., and Spencer, B.: Respiratory syncytial virus in epidemic bronchiolitis of infants. Brit. Med. J., 2:881, 1962.

Sommerville, R. G.: Respiratory syncytial virus in acute exacerbations of chronic bronchitis. Lancet, 2:1247, 1963.

INFLUENZA
Edwin D. Kilbourne

Definition. Influenza is an acute, contagious disease that is usually attended by fever and prostration and is ordinarily benign in outcome. The headache, myalgia, and asthenia that characterize the disease are severe out of proportion to the symptoms originating from involvement of the respiratory tract—the primary, and perhaps exclusive site of infection with the causative virus.

History. Epidemics of respiratory disease similar to modern influenza have been recorded through the centuries. Since the year 1510 there have been 31 pandemics described. The calamitous nature of these epidemics may have led to the naming of the disease by the Italians as an "influenza" or influence of the heavenly bodies or perhaps as an "influenza di freddo" (influence of the cold).

In 1933 the isolation of a virus in ferrets by Smith, Andrewes, and Laidlaw established the specific infectious etiology of the disease, and led rapidly to accurate definition of its epidemiology and clinical variations. The virus isolated in 1933 is now known as influenza A virus.

A second type of virus was isolated independently in 1940 by Francis and by Magill (influenza B virus). In 1950 influenza C was isolated from a patient in nonepidemic circumstances by Taylor, and later was shown by Francis and his associates to be the cause of epidemic disease.

The discovery by Burnet (1940) that the influenza viruses could be cultivated readily in the chick embryo led directly to simplified methods of studying influenza and to the development of an inactivated viral vaccine. Hirst's discovery (1941) that the virus could agglutinate erythrocytes in vitro (hemagglutination) (also noted by McClelland and Hare in 1941) provided not only a new technique for basic virology but a practical method for the precise measurement of virus and antibody.

In 1941 Horsfall and associates published the first evidence of protection of man against influenza by a vaccine containing inactivated influenza A virus. The Commission on Influenza of the Armed Forces Epidemiological Board has demonstrated the feasibility of mass immunization, and has developed the vaccines now in standard use.

Etiology. Influenza is a consequence of infection with certain *myxoviruses* that have common physical, chemical and biologic properties. These viruses comprise three groups (A, B, and C), which are completely unrelated antigenically, do not induce cross-immunity to one another, and have different epidemiologic characteristics. Four major subgroups of influenza A viruses have been identified since discovery of the virus in 1933, one having replaced the other in chronologic succession (Fig. 1). Three well-characterized subgroups are termed A_0, A_1 and A_2 (formerly Asian), whereas, classification of the recent Hong Kong mutant is presently undecided. However, the major (hemagglutinin) antigen which is the primary determinant of immunity is clearly different from earlier strains, and the minor (neuraminidase) antigen is indistinguishable from that of recent A_2 strains. The initial appearance of each subtype has been followed by global (pandemic) dissemination of virus and disease and the *disappearance of the immediately prevalent strain.* These varieties of influenza A viruses are classified together on the basis that they possess in common a "soluble" nucleoprotein antigen detectable by the complement-fixation reaction. Yet the other antigens (contained in the outer viral envelope) possessed by these strains are so different that they induce little cross-immunity. Thus, influenza A virus is perhaps unique among infectious agents of man in its capacity to mutate sufficiently under natural conditions to circumvent host immunity.

Only two major variants of influenza B virus have been noted (1940, 1954); these subgroups have not been named. Influenza B strains isolated since 1962 have shown considerable antigenic

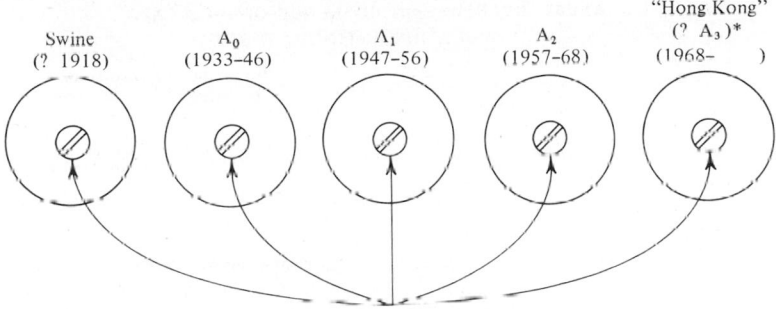

| Swine (? 1918) | A_0 (1933–46) | A_1 (1947–56) | A_2 (1957–68) | "Hong Kong" (? A_3)* (1968–   ) |

All share in common a "CORE" nucleoprotein antigen (not involved in immunity) that identifies these variants as influenza A viruses

*Note: A minor (neuraminidase) antigen of the Hong Kong virus is similar to the neuraminidase of recent A_2 strains. Therefore some cross immunity may be expected.

Influenza A & B are complete distinct from (i.e. share no antigens with) influenza C viruses.

FIGURE 1. Shifting antigenic nature of human influenza A viruses. (From Kilbourne, E. D., and Smillie, W. G. (eds.): Human Ecology and Public Health, The Macmillan Company, 1969.)

variation from both the 1940 and 1954 prototypes. Major antigenic variation of influenza C virus has not been described.

The etiologic agent of the notorious 1918 pandemic was never isolated, but serologic evidence suggests that it was closely related to the virus isolated from swine influenza by Shope (1931). The swine virus, like other animal influenza viruses, possesses the nucleoprotein antigen of the type A virus.

The influenza viruses are of medium size (approximately 850 Å. in diameter) and by conventional electron microscopy appear spherical or filamentous in form, with spike-like projections. The nucleic acid of the virus is ribonucleic acid (RNA).

Epidemiology. The arbitrary designation of the three types of influenza virus as A, B, and C coincides fortuitously with their relative rank as causes of severe epidemic disease. Influenza B and C viruses have been associated chiefly with sporadic epidemics in children and young adults, notably in school or other institutional populations. Most adults carry antibodies to these viruses, probably as the result of recurrent subclinical infection. There is no evidence that pandemics of influenza B or C have occurred.

Discussions of influenza are usually concerned with the influenza A viruses, for these are the important and apparently more mutable viruses that cause widespread epidemic and pandemic disease. The complicated and still puzzling epidemiology of influenza A is most conveniently considered by separate discussions of the *pandemic, epidemic,* and *endemic* infections—all attributable to the same virus under different conditions.

Pandemic Influenza. The isolation of a virus of the influenza A group from the pandemic of 1957 established that pandemic influenza was etiologically linked with the less extensive epidemic disease from which viruses had been recovered during the 1933-1956 period.

Influenza A virus is an obligate human parasite which is transmitted directly from man to man under conditions of close interhuman contact, presumably via the respiratory tract. Animal reservoirs of infection have not been demonstrated (although animal and avian influenza A viruses exist in nature), and the virus cannot persist in the environment. Survival of the virus thus depends on its serial transmission from man to man.

When an antigenic change in the virus occurs—perhaps as a reciprocal of high immunity in the general population—this mutation may be so extreme that acquired immunity in the population to previously existing influenza A viruses is inadequate to prevent infection or disease initiated by the new virus, which replaces the older virus completely. Under these conditions, people of all ages and in all places are susceptible to influenza, and a worldwide epidemic or pandemic may ensue (Fig. 2).

The incubation period of influenza is only 24 to 48 hours, so that, once progressive spread begins, the impact on the community is sudden and devastating. Both the incidence and the severity of illness are highly variable and are influenced by age, pregnancy, and pre-existing chronic disease and by such environmental factors as crowding and season of the year. Morbidity is usually first noted among schoolchildren, then in young adults, and finally in older, less active and presumably less exposed members of the community. Infection of the aged is more frequently followed by bacterial pneumonia. As a consequence, a "second wave" of increased community mortality may coincide with the delayed appearance of influenza in this age group—*at a time when*

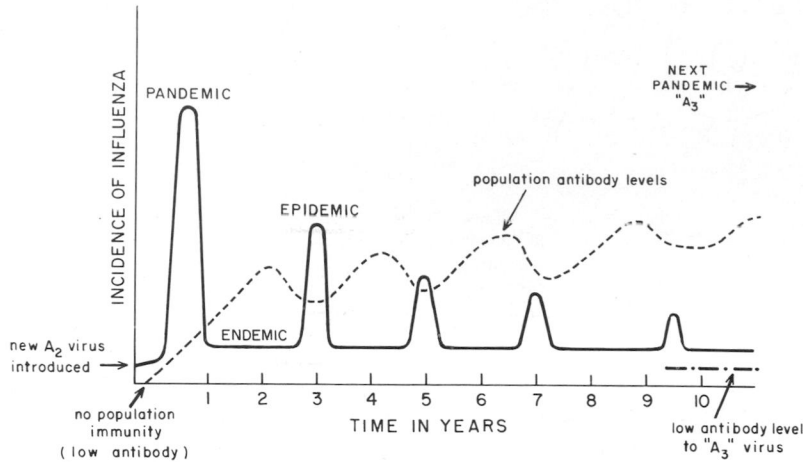

FIGURE 2. Schematic representation of the correlation of influenza incidence and mean population antibody levels after introduction of a new influenza virus variant. (From Kilbourne, E. D.: Sandoz Panorama, 6:7, 1968.)

influenza is no longer apparent in the community by the usual criteria of absenteeism from school or industry.

Specific immunity to influenza develops rapidly following infection, but it may decline within one or two years so that recurrence of infection and disease from the same antigenic type of virus may occur *under conditions of heavy exposure,* as in military barracks or boarding schools. On the other hand, the steady decline in community morbidity after the initial pandemic wave obviously points to the acquisition of immunity of some durability by most of the population.

Epidemic Influenza. Influenza occurs in its characteristic acute epidemics in the early months of the year in the north temperate zone. In a particular community the epidemic usually comes and goes within a month, rising to a peak in 12 to 14 days, and subsiding almost as rapidly. Although the case fatality rate is less than 1 per cent, the presence of influenza may be detected by a sudden increase in unspecified total mortality in the community. This mortality occurs at both extremes of age, and is occasioned principally by the bacterial pneumonias that may complicate influenza in the very young and very old.

Epidemics of influenza A have been demonstrated to occur every year since discovery of the virus, but communities are usually spared recurrence for two or more years after an epidemic.

Following a pandemic, the frequency and extent of epidemics gradually abates with the development of population immunity to the new virus. Minor antigenic variations of the virus may be detected during this time, but at least a decade seems to be required for change sufficient to establish a truly "new" subtype.

Endemic Influenza. The interepidemic survival of influenza virus has long been a puzzle in view of the fragility of the virus and its apparently obligate restriction to human hosts. It has become increasingly clear, however, that influenza virus infections may occur continuously within the population, either as sporadic instances of disease that are not recognized as influenza or as clinically inapparent infections. As more and more members of the population develop immunity, infections without disease become more and more frequent and serve to maintain the virus in the community. Such infections are recognized by serologic studies.

Pathology and Pathogenesis. The primary lesion of influenza is a necrosis of the ciliated epithelium of the respiratory tract. In the uncomplicated infection epithelial damage is probably confined to the upper and middle portion of the respiratory tract, the trachea being the most strikingly involved. Early in infection the necrotic ciliated cells are desquamated, leaving intact the basal cell layer. On about the fifth day of illness regeneration begins in the basal layer with the development of undifferentiated "transitional" epithelium, which may simulate metaplasia. After two weeks ciliated cells may again be seen.

When influenza is complicated by bacterial pneumonia, the pathologic findings are variable and depend on the nature of the secondary invader. However, *primary influenza virus pneumonia* presents a characteristic picture. The lungs are dark red, heavy, and edematous. The trachea and bronchi contain bloody fluid, and the mucosa is hyperemic. Microscopy shows ciliated epithelium to have been lost from the trachea, bronchi, and bronchioles, but evidence of epithelial regeneration may be seen. In the submucosa, focal hemorrhage, edema, and slight leukocytic infiltration may occur. Capillary thrombosis with focal leukocytic exudate has been described. The alveolar spaces contain neutrophilic and mononuclear cells admixed with fibrin and edema fluid. Intra-alveolar hemorrhage is common in the lower lobes.

The alveolar septa may be thickened, and acellular hyaline membranes may line alveolar ducts and alveoli.

Pathologic changes attributable to influenza occur only rarely outside the respiratory tract. There are no physiologic or biochemical changes in the patient that are pathognomonic of influenza. Although "leukopenia" is often stated to be characteristic, total leukocytic counts in the uncomplicated disease may vary from 2000 to 14,000 cells per cubic millimeter, and are usually in the normal range. However, *lymphocytopenia* is commonly detectable, especially in the first four days of illness. The erythrocyte sedimentation rate may be moderately elevated or normal. No characteristic changes occur in the bacterial flora of the respiratory tract.

The Complicated Disease. In primary influenza viral pneumonia, *leukocytosis* is the rule, even in the absence of bacterial pathogens, although the erythrocyte sedimentation rate may not be elevated. *Serum glutamic oxaloacetic transaminase concentrations* are elevated in proportion to the severity of pulmonary involvement and may exceed 60 units per milliliter. *Oxyhemoglobin saturation* is reduced to 46 to 85 per cent. *Partial pressure of CO_2* is elevated, and the *pH of arterial blood* is lowered. The *proteinuria* and elevated *blood urea nitrogen* concentrations that may be noted are the results of fever and dehydration and do not reflect primary renal damage. No notable changes in *serum electrolytes* or in *blood clotting* occur.

Clinical Manifestations. Infection with influenza virus may be asymptomatic, may be attended only by slight fever, or may result in the "typical" prostrating disease that identifies epidemics. This disease is remarkably constant in its expression from year to year, and the uncomplicated case of pandemic influenza does not differ from the "three-day fever" of nonpandemic outbreaks. The higher fatality rates associated with the 1918 pandemic were usually attributable to secondary bacterial pneumonia. Significant variations in the disease caused by any of the A or B subtypes of virus have not occurred. Influenza C appears to be a less severe disease, but it has not yet received adequate study.

Patients with influenza almost invariably *cough,* although this symptom may not be bothersome or even noted by the patient. The cough is brief and spasmodic, and usually not productive of sputum. Other symptoms related to the destruction of respiratory epithelium are *substernal burning pain* (from the trachea), *dryness or soreness of the throat,* and *nasal obstruction and discharge.* Neither sore throat nor evidence of rhinitis is particularly prominent in influenza. Slight *pharyngeal injection* may be noted. *Epistaxis* is rare, but is valuable diagnostically when it occurs. *Conjunctival burning and injection* are common.

In 5 to 10 per cent of patients with uncomplicated disease, crepitant or musical *rales,* roughened breath sounds, or *pleural friction rub* may be detected. Such signs rarely persist for more than one or two days. *Chest pain* may accompany the friction rub, or more often is substernal and referable to the trachea.

The prostrating effects of influenza are associated with *fever, chilly sensations* (seldom with rigors), *headache,* and *myalgia. Fever* usually exceeds 101° F. and may reach 106° F. It is usually abrupt in its onset and decline and lasts for only two to five days in the absence of complications. *Headache* is often frontal and is of the throbbing sort associated with fever; its severity is proportional to the degree of fever. *Extraocular myalgia* is a characteristic but not universal complaint that may be elicited only by examination. *Myalgia* may be generalized or confined to the back or lower extremities. *Gastrointestinal symptoms* are uncommon, and occur more often in patients with pre-existing gastrointestinal disease.

In sum, the picture of uncomplicated influenza is that of a patient with flushed face and reddened eyes who lies flat in bed and coughs occasionally with a dry spasmodic cough. He moves about fitfully, complaining of headache or backache. By contrast, the rare patient with influenza virus pneumonia *(vide infra)* sits erect, is extremely anxious and agitated, gasps for breath, and manifests *cyanosis* of the lips and nailbeds.

Course and Complications. In both pandemic and epidemic influenza the disease, although acute and prostrating, is brief, so that it is uncommon for any symptom to last beyond seven to ten days, and fever usually subsides earlier (Fig. 3). A protracted *postinfluenzal asthenia* has been emphasized in some reports. It is not clear to what extent secondary bacterial infections or psychogenic factors contribute to the state. Nevertheless, the alerting of the patient to the possibility may

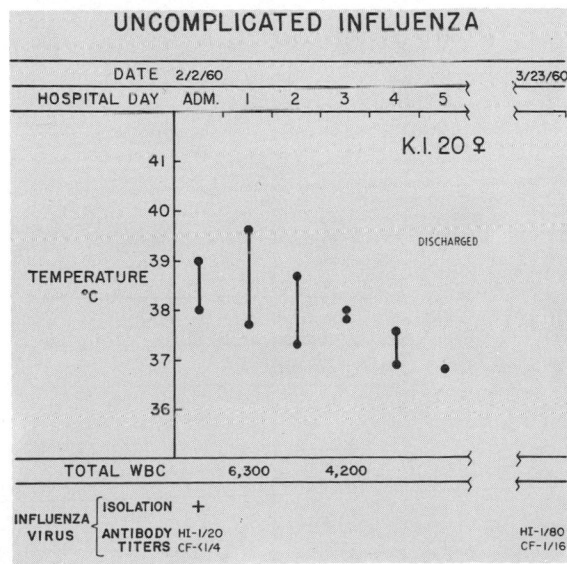

FIGURE 3. (From Kaye, D., et al.: Amer. Rev. Resp. Dis., 85:9, 1962.)

save some apprehension during the convalescent period. *Encephalitis* and *myocarditis* have been described infrequently as complications of influenza, and have rarely been well documented or associated with virus isolation from the brain or heart.

The important and potentially lethal complications of influenza derive from infection of the lung, either with the influenza virus itself or with bacterial pathogens. The pulmonary complications of influenza may be considered as (1) *primary influenza virus pneumonia,* (2) *combined influenza virus and bacterial pneumonia,* and (3) *influenza complicated by secondary bacterial pneumonia.* All three types of complication are more frequent in patients with pre-existing cardiac or pulmonary disease or in women late in pregnancy. The aged, in whom apparent or inapparent chronic disease is more frequent, are also understandably more vulnerable to pulmonary complications of influenza.

Primary Influenza Virus Pneumonia. Primary influenza virus pneumonia is a severe disease that is usually fatal. Within 24 hours of the onset of typical symptoms of influenza, the patient experiences high fever (103 to 104° F.), a cough productive of bloody sputum, and profound dyspnea and anxiety. Cyanosis is notable, and poor air exchange is indicated by the generalized pulmonary findings, which include suppression of breath sounds, expiratory wheezing, and diffuse, moist rales. Signs of consolidation are absent. Chest roentgenograms disclose diffuse bilateral nodular infiltrates that radiate outward from the hilum, sparing the lung periphery.

The patient almost always dies within five to ten days of the onset of illness after a course characterized by unremitting fever, progressive pulmonary involvement and terminal vascular collapse (Fig. 4). Antibacterial drugs, oxygen, bronchodilators and corticosteroids are usually unavailing.

Pathogenic bacteria are not recoverable from the sputum, blood, or lung during life or post mortem, and influenza virus is demonstrable in high concentrations in the lung.

Primary influenza virus pneumonia is restricted almost invariably to patients with pre-existing cardiac or pulmonary disease or pregnancy. Still more specifically, the victim usually has rheumatic cardiovascular disease and mitral stenosis. The predilection of this complication for the patient with mitral stenosis suggests that hemodynamic factors such as pulmonary hypertension are more important in its pathogenesis than general debility or the absence of specific immune mechanisms.

There appears to be a graded spectrum of severity of the disease caused by influenza virus, so that, intermediate between the uncomplicated case with transient rales and the fatal virus pneumonia, occasional instances of "mild segmental influenza virus pneumonia" have been described.

Combined Influenza Virus and Bacterial Pneumonia. In patients with primary influenza virus pneumonia, infection with bacterial pathogens may supervene. In such patients the characteristic and dramatic onset of the virus pneumonia may be attended or closely followed by such

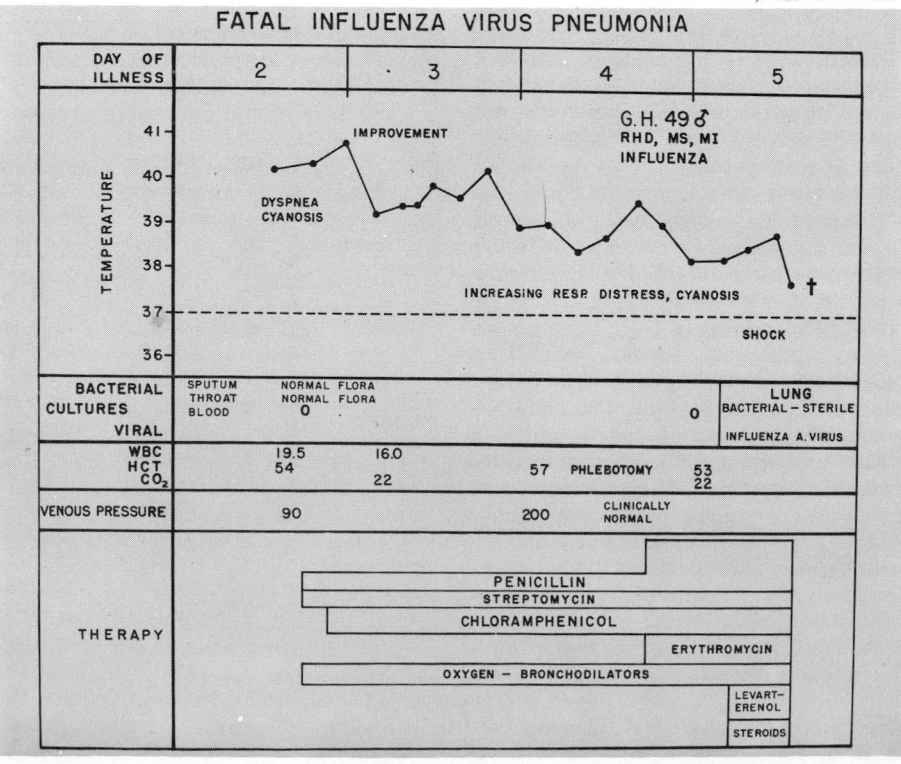

FIGURE 4. (From Kaye, D., et al.: Amer. Rev. Resp. Dis., 85:9, 1962.)

symptoms of bacterial pneumonia as *productive cough, shaking chills,* or *pleuritic pain.* Signs of focal consolidation may be engrafted upon the diffuse pulmonary findings of the viral infection. Pneumococcus, Staphylococcus, *Haemophilus influenzae,* or, more rarely, group A streptococci may be demonstrated by culture of lung, blood, or sputum. In 1957-1958, pneumococcus and Staphylococcus were the most frequent bacterial invaders.

The host setting and course of the combined infection are basically the same as in the pneumonia associated with influenza virus infection alone.

Influenza Complicated by Secondary Bacterial Pneumonia. Bacterial pneumonia, characterized by focal consolidation, may occur after influenza in previously healthy persons as well as in the ill and infirm. This complication is further distinguished from influenza virus pneumonia by (1) the lag between influenzal symptoms and the appearance of pneumonia, sometimes with brief interval of freedom from symptoms; (2) the presence of focal and not diffuse pulmonary involvement; and (3) the absence of influenza virus in throat washings, but the presence of bacterial pathogens in the sputum. This "late" type of pulmonary complication is by far the most common.

Diagnosis. In the context of an epidemic, influenza may easily be distinguished from other acute respiratory diseases, although diagnosis of the isolated case may be difficult. In its typical form influenza is characterized by relatively high fever, which sets it apart from the syndrome of the *common cold.* With the common cold, nasal symptoms predominate, but they are usually minor in influenza. *Adenoviral infections* are the most difficult to distinguish from influenza, but, in general, fever and prostration are less, onset is less sudden, and sore throat and laryngitis are more prominent in adenoviral disease. One of the clinical forms of respiratory syncytial viral disease may closely mimic influenza. The aching, febrile, minor illnesses associated with infection by various arbor- or enteroviruses may also simulate influenza but are notably unattended by cough, although sore throat may occur. In *streptococcal pharyngitis,* the greater frequency of vomiting, the predominance of sore throat, and the occurrence of cervical adenitis and leukocytosis are helpful in differential diagnosis. *Primary atypical pneumonia* is usually distinguishable clinically from influenza virus pneumonia by its more gradual onset, purulent sputum, and indolent, ordinarily benign course.

The *definitive diagnosis* of influenza depends upon isolation of the virus from throat washings or sputum and the demonstration of an increase in specific humoral antibodies. Viral isolation is most successful in the first two to three days of illness and is best accomplished by the intraamniotic inoculation of chick embryos. Primary cultures of mammalian cells may also be used but are less satisfactory. If virus grows to high enough titer on the first passage, isolation and identification of the agent may be accomplished within 48 to 72 hours of inoculation of the specimen. Recently, fluorescent antibody staining of exfoliated nasal epithelial cells has been applied as a quick and specific diagnostic test.

Antibody may be detected in the patient's serum by neutralization, hemagglutination-inhibition or complement-fixation tests as early as eight to nine days after the onset of illness, but maximal response is evident only after 14 days. The diagnosis cannot be made with a single serum specimen because of the prevalence of antibody in the population; rather an *increase* in antibody titer of fourfold or more must be demonstrated by the study of two or more serum specimens obtained early in illness and in convalescence.

Prognosis. The prognosis is ordinarily favorable in this brief and self-limited disease. However, the severity of the disease is a reciprocal of host susceptibility, and the outcome may be fatal in those with prior cardiac or pulmonary disease. The prognosis is also influenced by the prevalence of potential respiratory bacterial invaders in the community and the prospects for their control.

Treatment. There is no specific treatment for influenza. The general measures used in the symptomatic treatment of other infections are useful, including especially aspirin (0.3 to 0.6 gram) for the headache, malaise, and myalgia, and codeine sulfate (0.016 to 0.064 gram) for irritability, cough, and substernal pain. Diet may be regulated by the patient with the warning that high fat foods are not well tolerated. Fluids should be given in abundance.

Routine antibacterial prophylaxis is unnecessary and inadvisable, but may be considered for those with chronic disease with the view of forestalling the sequel of pneumococcal pneumonia. In this case, full therapeutic doses of penicillin should be given.

Treatment of primary influenza viral pneumonia is highly unsatisfactory, but oxygen therapy with positive pressure breathing devices has shown some promise.

Prevention. Influenza may be prevented by the parenteral injection of vaccines of influenza viruses that have been produced in the chick embryo and rendered noninfective (inactivated) by formalin or ultraviolet irradiation. The duration of protection probably does not exceed one year under conditions of epidemic exposure. Present vaccines are principally *monovalent* in that they contain only the contemporary influenza A virus (Hong Kong) component, but some contain also lesser amounts of influenza B antigen. These newer vaccines have been purified by density gradient centrifugation, and are far less toxic than preparations of the past. A so-called "hemagglutinin" vaccine contains antigens of the disrupted virus. It is also of low reactogenicity, but is correspondingly less immunogenic (especially in children) than vaccines made from whole virus.

In experimental field trials amantadine hydrochloride has had a chemoprophylactic effect in influenza, as evidenced by lower infection rates and less severe illness in subjects who received the drug shortly before exposure to the infection. Following infection, antibody titers were lower in drug-treated subjects, presumably reflecting a decreased antigenic stimulation from reduced viral replication. The drug is presumed to act by inhibiting virus penetration and not intracellularly on virus replication. Some evidence suggests that amantadine may have a slight therapeutic effect if given soon after the initiation of infection. Central nervous system toxicity may limit the usefulness of this compound in older people.

Because protection provided by influenza vaccine is transient, immunization of the general population is not feasible. The vaccine is useful in three special situations: (1) to reduce *morbidity* in groups essential for the community life, such as policemen, physicians, and the military; (2) to reduce *morbidity* in groups particularly subject to the occurrence of epidemics, as in boarding schools, institutions, and military camps; and (3) to prevent disease and hence reduce *mortality* in those peculiarly vulnerable to the effects of infection, especially those with chronic cardiac and pulmonary disease. In these groups, especially the latter, vaccine should be administered annually in the autumn in a dosage of 1.0 ml.

Live virus vaccines for influenza are in use in the Soviet Union, but have not received adequate evaluation in the United States.

International Conference on Hong Kong Influenza. Bull. W. H. O., 41:335, 1969.

Kilbourne, E. D.: The severity of influenza as a reciprocal of host susceptibility. *In* Wolstenholme, G.E.W., and O'Connor, C. M. (eds.): Ciba Foundations Study Group No. 4, Virus Virulence and Pathogenicity. Boston, Little, Brown and Company, 1960, pp. 58–77.

Louria, D. B., Blumenfeld, H. L., Ellis, J. T., Kilbourne, E. D., and Rogers, D. E.: Studies on influenza in the pandemic of 1957-1958. II. Pulmonary complications of influenza. J. Clin. Invest., 38:213, 1959.

Smith, W., Andrewes, C. H., and Laidlaw, P. P.: A virus obtained from influenzal patients. Lancet, 2:66, 1933.

PSITTACOSIS
(Ornithosis; Bedsonia Pneumonia)
David E. Rogers

Definition. Psittacosis is a specific infection of birds produced by a microbial agent whose precise classification is currently in question. When transmitted to man this agent can produce asymptomatic infection, a transient influenza-like illness, or serious pneumonic disease characterized by high fever, headache, cough, myalgia, pulmonary infiltrates, and a significant mortality. Because it is now recognized that many species of birds other than the order Psittaciformes transmit psittacosis or "Bedsonia" agent, *ornithosis* has been suggested as a more accurate title. Usage has made psittacosis the accepted term for the human disease.

History. In 1879, Ritter, a Swiss physician, described seven cases of an unusual pneumonia that occurred after contact with tropical birds. Morange, in 1894, established the parrot as a vector and termed the disease *psittacosis* after the Greek *psittakos* (the parrot). During the year 1929–1930 a serious epidemic of pneumonia occurred in Europe, America, and Asia following shipments of infected South American parrots. This epidemic led to clearer recognition of psittacosis as a human disease. The etiologic agent was demonstrated to be a filterable agent by Bedson, Western, and Simpson in 1930. Subsequent studies have shown that over 90 species of birds can harbor the agent, and its worldwide distribution has been documented. Since the lifting of quarantine restrictions on the importation of psittacine birds in 1951, there has been a significant increase in cases in the United States.

Etiology. The psittacosis agent is an obligate intracellular parasite. It is morphologically and serologically related to lymphogranuloma venereum and to a number of mammalian agents producing pneumonitis, meningoencephalitis, and abortion in their native hosts. To date, these agents have not been shown to produce human disease. Because of their large size (250 to 400 mμ), possession of both RNA and DNA, a demonstrable cell wall containing muramic acid, division by binary fission, and their susceptibility to chemotherapeutic agents known to inhibit bacterial enzyme systems, these agents more closely resemble Rickettsia or bacteria than true viruses. Parrots and parakeets are the most common carriers and until recently represented the major source of human infection. With better control of psittacine disease in aviaries, other birds now contribute more human infections with psittacosis, and cases have resulted from contacts with turkeys, pigeons, ducks, chickens, pheasants, finches, and other fowl. Although individuals of both sexes and all ages are susceptible, overt clinical infections in children are uncommon. Persons working with birds are at greatest risk of infection, and there is an increased incidence of psittacosis in pet shop employees, pigeon handlers, and poultry workers.

The agent is present in the blood, tissue, and discharges of infected birds. It is hardy and can withstand drying. Although the avian disease can be fatal, infected birds frequently show only minimal evidence of illness, such as ruffled feathers, lethargy, and failure to eat. Birds having active infections are most likely to transmit the disease, but asymptomatic carriers are common, and birds that recover can shed transmissible agent for many months. In general, human psittacosis acquired from psittacine birds or turkeys has been more severe than that acquired from pigeons, ducks, chickens, or pheasants. Bird ectoparasites can harbor the agent and may serve as a source of reinfection for domestic flocks. Antimicrobials incorporated in bird foodstuffs have not eradicated psittacosis from infected parrots or parakeets.

Psittacosis is generally acquired by the respiratory route through inhalation of infected dried bird excreta, more rarely by handling the feathers and the tissues of infected birds. On rare occasion the disease may be acquired through an open lesion or the bite of a bird. Small epidemics have been attributed to aerosols of dust laden with dried excreta. Cases have been reported after only brief exposure to birds. There is some evidence that the incubation period may be shortened by a large inoculum. Person to person transmission of psittacosis, although rare, has been documented. These cases of "human" strain psittacosis have been severe, with high mortality.

Pathology. In birds, the principal sites of disease are the liver, spleen, and pericardium. In man, the lung is most commonly involved. Although the psittacosis agent generally gains access to the human body via the respiratory route, there is clear evidence that it rapidly enters the blood and produces systemic disease involving the lungs and the reticuloendothelial tissues. The agent can be isolated from the blood of infected humans during the first two weeks of illness, and has been found in the spleen in fatal cases. The mature pulmonary lesion is a lobular pneumonitis. The process is initiated by inflammation and progressive edema of the alveolar cells. Exudation is often accompanied by small hemorrhages. Polymorphonuclear leukocytes appear early in the process. Later inflammatory exudates show lymphocytes and large numbers of mononuclear leukocytes within the alveoli and interstitial spaces. The mucosa of the trachea and bronchi generally remains intact but is edematous and invaded with mononuclear cells. Thick, gelatinous plugs of mucus may fill major and minor bronchi and may account for the severe cyanosis, and progressive anoxia seen in fatal cases. Foci of necrosis may occur in more severely affected areas of the lung and are sometimes associated with capillary thrombi. The process is generally most severe in dependent bronchopulmonary segments. Large monocytes and macrophages containing cytoplasmic inclusion bodies, which may represent the agent (L.C.L. bodies), are characteristic of psittacosis infection. Vasculitis and thrombosis may account for many findings. Hyperplasia and monocytic infiltration of pulmonary and hilar lymph nodes and splenic enlargement with occasional areas of focal necrosis may occur. Rarely the liver may show intralobular focal necrosis and swollen Kupffer cells containing the psittacosis elementary bodies. Changes in the myocardium, pericardium, meninges, brain, adrenals, and kidneys have been reported.

Clinical Manifestations. Wide variations can occur in the clinical picture. The incubation period ranges from 7 to 15 days but may occasionally be longer. Probably asymptomatic infection or mild influenza-like infections are the rule. Moderate or severe infections, although less frequent, are more commonly diagnosed. The onset of illness may be insidious, but it often starts with chills and a fever that rises slowly from initial levels of 101 or 102 to 103 to 105° F. during the first week of illness. Headache is severe. Malaise, anorexia, severe myalgias, particularly in the neck and back, and arthralgias are common. Cough is generally prominent but may be delayed until late in the first week. Small amounts of mucoid sputum with occasional blood streaking are the rule, and pleuritic pain is rare. Changes in mentation are often seen. Delirium or stupor may occur in severe cases toward the end of the first week, and is usually associated with severe pulmonary involvement, cyanosis, and other evidences of anoxia. Other neurologic manifestations are uncommon. Nausea and vomiting are frequent. Epistaxis may occur early in the course of the illness. A macular rash resembling that seen in typhoid has occasionally been described. Jaundice and progressive nitrogen retention have been reported in severe cases. Severe dyspnea, tachypnea, tachycardia, cyanosis, jaundice, delirium, and stupor are all poor prognostic signs.

The physical findings of pneumonia are often sparse. Chest roentgenograms may reveal evidence of infiltrates not detected at the bedside. Examination may reveal only fever, painful muscle groups, an elevated respiratory rate, and a relative bradycardia. Fine, crepitant rales may be heard in localized areas over the lungs. Frank percussion or auscultatory changes suggestive of true consolidation are less common. Pleurisy with effusion can occur but is unusual. Mild hepatomegaly is frequent. A palpable spleen has been reported in 5 to 70 per cent of patients. An erythematous pharynx may be noted. In rare instances there may be signs of pericarditis or myocarditis. In prolonged, severe illness, thrombophlebitis and pulmonary infarction have been reported as late complications.

Patients with mild cases may recover in 7 to 8 days. More severe infections may last 12 to 21 days without specific treatment. Fever is ordinarily sustained or remittent, and when accompanied by bradycardia, resembles the fever seen in untreated typhoid infections. Defervescence is generally slow, and prolonged convalescence is common. Secondary bacterial infections are rare.

Laboratory Findings. Simple laboratory studies are not helpful in establishing a diagnosis. The leukocyte count is usually normal, but leukopenia or low-grade leukocytosis ranging to over 20,000 cells per cubic millimeter may occur. The erythrocyte sedimentation rate is generally elevated. Proteinuria is common during the febrile period. Chest roentgenograms generally show soft patchy infiltrates radiating outward from the hilum, which tend to be more prominent in dependent lobes or segments. Occasionally diffuse miliary, nodular, or frank lobar distribution of infiltrates is seen.

A specific diagnosis can be made only by isolation of the agent or by serologic studies. The agent is present in the blood and sputum during the first two to three weeks, but isolation is hazardous, and should not be attempted except in special laboratories. Diagnosis is generally made by a diagnostic rise in complement-fixing antibodies against a heat-stable group antigen prepared from psittacosis agent grown in eggs. Paired acute and convalescent sera should always be tested. A significant change in antibody titers is generally present by the twelfth to fourteenth day of disease; the titers are usually maximal by 30 days, then slowly disappear. Treatment can delay or suppress antibody response. There is considerable cross reaction between antigens prepared from psittacosis and lymphogranuloma venereum viruses. False positive complement-fixation tests may occur with Q fever or brucellosis. Cutaneous hypersensitivity to the Frei antigen may develop during psittacosis.

Differential Diagnosis. Specific diagnosis of psittacosis is of extreme importance because of its potential severity (reported fatality rates range from 5 to 40 per cent), its response to antimicrobials, and the public health significance of psittacosis infection. The syndrome of viral pneumonia accompanied by protracted high fever, unusually severe headache, and relative bradycardia should suggest psittacosis. Often a history of contact with birds is the only clue to diagnosis. When pneumonic symptoms are prominent, psittacosis must be differentiated from viral pneumonias, mycoplasmal pneumonia, influenza, Q fever, tuberculosis, histoplasmosis, coccidioidomycosis, bacterial pneumonia, and other processes that produce pulmonary infiltrates. If pneumonic symptoms are not prominent, psittacosis can be confused with other systemic febrile illnesses such as typhoid fever, brucellosis, infectious mononucleosis, infectious hepatitis, miliary tuberculosis, or the viral meningoencephalitides.

Treatment. The tetracyclines are the drugs of choice, and early diagnosis and initiation of treatment may be life-saving. Following institution of therapy with 2 to 3 grams daily, both fever and symptoms are generally controlled within 48 to 72 hours. Chloramphenicol appears to be less effective. Although the disease apparently responds to penicillin in doses above 2 million units daily, tetracycline remains the drug of choice. Treatment should be continued for at least 10 days. The high fever and progressive anoxia secondary to extensive pulmonary involvement in severe cases may require appropriate measures directed at these problems.

Favour, C. B.: Ornithosis (psittacosis). Amer. J. Med. Sci., 205: 162, 1943.

Meyer, K. F.: The ecology of psittacosis and ornithosis. Medicine, 21:175, 1942.

Meyer, K. F.: Psittacosis-lymphogranuloma venereum agents. In Horsfall, F. L., and Tamm, I. (eds.): Viral and Rickettsial Infections of Man. 4th ed. Philadelphia, J. B. Lippincott Co., 1965, pp. 1006-1041.

Schaffner, W., Drutz, D. J., Duncan, G. W., and Koenig, M. G.: The clinical spectrum of endemic psittacosis. Arch. Intern. Med. (Chicago), 119:433, 1967.

Wilson, G. S., and Miles, A. A.: The psittacosis-lymphogranuloma group. In Wilson, G. S., and Miles, A. A. (eds.): Topley and Wilson's Principles of Bacteriology and Immunity. 4th ed. Baltimore, Williams & Wilkins Co., 1964, vol. 2, pp. 2246-2259.

OTHER DISEASES CAUSED BY FILTER-PASSING AGENTS

LYMPHOGRANULOMA VENEREUM
Albert Heyman

Definition. Lymphogranuloma venereum is a systemic infectious disease caused by a filter-passing agent and transmitted by sexual contact. The disease is characterized by the appearance of a small genital ulceration followed by suppuration of the regional lymph nodes, mild constitutional symptoms, and, occasionally, inflammatory lesions in various tissues of the body. Late manifestations of the disease consist of chronic ulcerative lesions and fibrotic changes in the genital tract and rectum.

Etiology. The agent causing lymphogranuloma venereum is a member of the psittacosis-lymphogranuloma group of filter-passing agents. These agents have common morphologic and immunologic characteristics that include large particle size, susceptibility to antimicrobial drugs, and cross reactivity in serologic tests. Strictly speaking, these filter-passing agents are not true viruses, but for convenience the terms *virus* and *agent* are used interchangeably here (see Psittacosis, Trachoma). The virus of lymphogranuloma produces meningoencephalitis in mice following intracerebral inoculation. It can be cultured in the yolk sac of the chick embryo, in which viral particles subjected to special staining methods can be seen with an ordinary microscope. Antigens prepared from the infected yolk material have been used for intradermal diagnostic (Frei) tests and for complement-fixation tests.

Prevalence and Incidence. Lymphogranuloma venereum is widely distributed throughout the world, but it is probably most prevalent in the tropics. Once a frequent cause of venereal disease among Negroes in the southern United States, the disease now appears less frequently. Surveys based on serologic methods during World War II showed a prevalence as high as one third of the adult southern Negro population, but in 1966 only 625 new cases were reported in all of the country. There is evidence to indicate that the incidence of the disease in the United States may increase because of spread of the infection by American soldiers returning from Southeast Asia. The illness has been described throughout the world under various names, such as *tropical bubo,* climatic bubo, lymphogranuloma inguinale, and lymphopathia venereum.

Pathogenesis. Approximately three to thirty days after sexual exposure, a small transient ulceration usually appears at the site of inoculation. This is followed within a few days by enlargement and suppuration of the regional lymph nodes, the so-called bubo. The virus is disseminated at this time throughout the body, and has been recovered from the blood and cerebrospinal fluid as well as from the lymph nodes draining the primary lesion. Systemic lesions consisting of arthritis, cutaneous lesions, and ocular manifestations (iritis and keratitis) may develop in the early stages of the illness. These initial symptoms may disappear spontaneously, and the patient may become asymptomatic for many years. A small but undetermined percentage of patients later develop chronic ulcerative lesions about the rectum and genitalia.

Shortly after the onset of lymphadenitis, complement-fixing humoral antibodies, skin reactivity to the viral antigen, and elevation of the serum globulin develop. These immune reactions may persist for many years.

Clinical Manifestations. The primary lesion of lymphogranuloma consists of a shallow, painless ulceration a few millimeters in diameter. It is often inconspicuous, and may pass unnoticed by the patient. In such cases the regional lymphadenitis may be the first evidence of the disease. Occasionally a pea-sized nodule, called a bubonulus, may develop in the lymphatics draining the primary lesion.

The painful enlargement and inflammation of the lymph nodes in one or both inguinal areas are the most conspicuous early features of the disease. The lymph nodes often become matted together to form conglomerate tender masses above and below the inguinal ligament. Within a few days suppuration develops and the overlying skin may ulcerate, with the formation of multiple chronic draining sinuses. The lymphadenitis is often accompanied by systemic manifestations of malaise, myalgia, and fever, and occasionally by arthritis or conjunctivitis. In rare instances, meningitis and pericarditis have been observed. In untreated cases, suppuration and drainage of the lymph nodes may persist for several weeks or months, but eventually spontaneous healing takes place. After a few years, however, chronic ulcerative lesions and fibrotic changes may develop on the external genitalia. In women, dense fibrous strictures of the rectum and purulent proctitis are not uncommon and may be associated with destructive lesions in the vaginal tissues. Another late manifestation is elephantiasis of the external genitalia, which is caused by obstruction of lymphatic channels. Proctitis and its sequelae may also be observed in homosexual men. These late complications are sometimes associated with a profound anemia, loss of weight, and severe cachexia. In a few instances death results.

Diagnosis. The diagnosis of lymphogranuloma is usually made on the basis of its clinical manifestations, but the demonstration of specific skin reactivity and complement-fixing antibodies may be needed to confirm the diagnosis.

Differentiation from chancroid infection may be difficult, as the genital ulceration and regional lymph node involvement in both diseases may be similar. The etiologic agent of chancroid, the Ducrey bacillus, is often found in stained smears or cultures of the purulent exudate in the undermined edges of the genital lesion. The inguinal nodes in both illnesses may enlarge to form a painful suppurative mass which, in chancroid infection, may rupture to form a single large ulceration, whereas, in lymphogranuloma venereum, the lymph nodes have multilocular areas of fluctuation that rupture to form multiple draining fistulas. Lymphogranuloma must also be differentiated from other conditions producing lymphadenopathy in the inguinal area such as syphilis, pyogenic infections, and neoplasms. Isolation of the virus is not practicable except perhaps in selected cases of meningitis, arthritis, or iritis. In such patients, an attempt should be made to obtain the virus from the involved tissues or from enlarged lymph nodes. A positive reaction to the commercial skin test antigen (Lygranum) will appear in a week or two in practically every patient with the disease. The skin test to this antigen as well as that made from the Ducrey bacillus must be interpreted with caution, because positive reactions may persist for many years after a previous infection. A two- or threefold change in titer of complement-fixing antibodies, however, is usually considered diagnostic of an active infection. Hyperglobulinemia is a common finding, and may at times be helpful in the diagnosis. The diagnosis can also be made by biopsy of the primary lesion or enlarged lymph nodes. The histologic appearance of lymphogranuloma venereum consists of a rather characteristic granuloma with abscess formation that can usually be differentiated from chancroid and other infections.

Treatment. The virus of lymphogranuloma venereum is susceptible to sulfonamide therapy, and the early manifestations of the disease usually respond well to sulfisoxazole in dosages of 4 grams daily for two to three weeks. The tetracyclines are also useful in the early stages of the illness as well as for the late complications of proctitis and chronic ulcerations of the genital tract. It is uncertain whether these medications produce complete eradication of the virus within the body, and there is evidence that the organism may persist in a subclinical state after prolonged sulfonamide therapy. Surgical treatment is usually necessary for the late manifestations of the disease such as rectal stricture and elephantiasis. No attempt should be made, however, to excise the inguinal buboes, but repeated aspirations of the suppurating lymph nodes may be necessary to prevent the formation of chronic draining sinuses.

Prevention. There is no specific vaccine against lymphogranuloma venereum. There is some reason to believe that careful washing of the genitalia with soap and water following intercourse is a preventive measure of some effectiveness.

Abrams, A. J.: Lymphogranuloma venereum. J.A.M.A., 205:199, 1968.
Favre, M., and Hellerstrom, S.: The epidemiology, aetiology and prophylaxis of lymphogranuloma inguinale. Acta Dermatovener. (Stockh.), 34-Suppl. 30:1, 1954.
Heyman, A.: The clinical and laboratory differentiation between chancroid and lymphogranuloma venereum. Amer. J. Syph., 30:279, 1946.
Koteen, H.: Lymphogranuloma venereum. Medicine, 24:1, 1945.
Sigel, M. M.: Lymphogranuloma Venereum. Coral Gables, University of Miami Press, 1962.

TRACHOMA AND INCLUSION CONJUNCTIVITIS

Ernest Jawetz

Definition. Trachoma and inclusion conjunctivitis are chronic infectious diseases of the eye and genital tract, caused by closely related microorganisms and exhibiting overlapping spectra of clinical manifestations and epidemiologic patterns. These range from mild and self-limited to severe and blinding eye disease, with or without involvement of the genital tract.

Etiology. The agents of *trachoma and inclusion conjunctivitis* (TRIC agents) are members of the psittacosis–lymphogranuloma venereum–trachoma group. Formerly these agents were considered viruses; now they are called *chlamydiae*. They are nonmotile, gram-negative, obligate intracellular parasites which multiply in the cytoplasm of their host cells by a distinctive developmental cycle. Chlamydiae differ from viruses in many important respects: they possess both RNA and DNA; they multiply by binary fission; they possess bacterial types of cell walls and ribosomes; they produce a variety of metabolically active enzymes; and their growth can be inhibited by several antibacterial drugs. It is probable that chlamydiae are closely related to gram-negative bacteria, but lack some significant mechanism for the production of metabolic energy so that they are restricted to an intracellular existence.

TRIC agents can infect epithelial cells of conjunctiva, cornea, urethra, and cervix of man and monkey, but do not replicate in most other tissues of the body. The infective particle ("elementary body") is a sphere with a diameter of 250 nanometers (millimicrons) and stains purple with Giemsa's or red with Macchiavello's stain. The infective particle is taken into the host cell by phagocytosis and, after replication, results in the development of an inclusion body. This is an oval or crescent-shaped mass of "elementary bodies" embedded in a matrix of glycogen, lying in the cytoplasm of an epithelial cell often adjacent to the nucleus. Inclusion bodies can be stained brightly with specific immunofluorescence.

TRIC agents can be grown in the yolk sac of embryonated eggs and in X-irradiated cells in culture. Only a few laboratory strains replicate freely in cell cultures. The growth of TRIC agents is markedly inhibited by tetracyclines, sulfonamides, erythromycins, penicillins, and chloramphenicol, but not by aminoglycosides. Therefore streptomycin or neomycin can be used to suppress bacterial contaminants in clinical specimens and to aid in isolation of TRIC agents in the laboratory.

TRIC agents share with other chlamydiae a heat-stable group antigen. In addition, species- or strain-specific antigens have been detected in the cell wall. Infected persons may develop antibodies to both types of antigens. TRIC agents, like other chlamydiae, contain a toxin which kills mice within a few hours after intravenous injection. Repeated injection of chlamydial suspensions can protect mice against the homologous toxin. Such toxin-protection tests indicate the presence of several antigenic types among TRIC agents, and provide the main available method for antigenic classification of new isolates. Thus, genital TRIC isolates often fall within certain antigenic groups, whereas ocular TRIC isolates from endemic trachoma areas often fall within other groups. Antigenic classification of strains is also being attempted with fluorescent antibody methods. However, to date there is no specific laboratory characteristic that can always differentiate isolates of trachoma from isolates of inclusion conjunctivitis agents.

TRIC agents can persist in man for years, with or without symptoms and signs of infection. Subclinical infection can be activated by trauma, corticosteroid administration, and perhaps bacterial superinfection. The development of scarring and blindness in some endemic trachoma regions is attributable to a large extent to recurrent bacterial infections of the eye, especially with Hemophilus or Neisseria.

Prevalence and Epidemiology. Since antiquity, trachomatous infection was recognized in the Mediterranean basin and in the Orient. Today, trachomatous eye disease is very prevalent in Africa and Asia. It has been estimated that up to 400 million persons may be infected with TRIC agents, and up to 20 million may be economically blinded as a result. Trachoma flourishes in areas that are hot and dry, and that have a shortage of available water and poor hygienic customs. In such areas endemic levels are high, and initial infection commonly occurs in early childhood. In certain parts of the world, e.g., in North Africa, virtually the entire population is infected with TRIC agents before reaching adulthood. The high prevalence of bacterial superinfection in such populations undoubtedly contributes to the severity of eye disease and to its causing widespread blindness. In parts of the United States, e.g., Indian reservations of the Southwest, endemic TRIC infection is relatively common, but it rarely leads to major visual impairment, perhaps because bacterial superinfection is infrequent. Throughout the world sporadic cases of ocular

TRIC infection occur, often with a clinical picture resembling trachoma. It is probable that some of these originate in genital infections rather than in contact with ocular trachoma.

Active cases of ocular TRIC infection shed the infective agent in desquamated conjunctival cells, conjunctival exudate, or tears. The infectious agent may be transmitted by fingers, fomites, and perhaps flies. Patients with early active cases probably shed more infective TRIC agent, and thus are more infectious for contacts than are those with chronic cases. However, even patients with long-standing scarred eye disease, and without signs of current activity, may shed TRIC agent and thus serve as a source of infection.

These comments concern ocular TRIC infection, particularly typical endemic trachoma. *Typical inclusion conjunctivitis* has a radically different epidemiologic pattern. Inclusion conjunctivitis is fundamentally an infection of the adult human genital tract, transmitted as a venereal disease. In the female the TRIC agent grows mainly in the transitional epithelium of the cervix. These cells may contain typical inclusions, and occasionally a mild cervicitis is present. In the male, genital infection may produce *urethritis,* as the TRIC agent replicates in urethral epithelium. In both sexes, adult genital tract infection is often asymptomatic. Adults may transfer genital secretions to their own or other eyes by fingers, by fomites, and—occasionally—in swimming pools. The infection may pass from the cervix of the infected mother to the eye of her newborn during passage through the birth canal. The newborn infant may then develop eye disease between 6 and 14 days after birth.

The epidemiologic patterns described for typical trachoma and typical inclusion conjunctivitis may be mixed. Thus, the genital tract of women in endemic trachoma regions may harbor TRIC agents, and these may produce either inclusion conjunctivitis or clinically typical trachoma in the offspring. Genital isolates from adults in non-endemic areas may, upon inoculation into the eye, give rise to disease resembling either inclusion conjunctivitis or trachoma.

Pathology and Pathogenesis. TRIC agents invade mainly the epithelium of the conjunctiva, cervix, and urethra. The earliest sign of infection is the appearance of inclusion bodies within epithelial cells and neutrophil infiltration of the epithelium of mucous membranes. Subepithelial infiltration with plasma cells and lymphocytes and the development of lymphoid follicles then follow. In the cornea, epithelial keratitis is often accompanied by the formation of subepithelial opacities. Blood vessels from the limbus, accompanied by fibroblasts, may invade the cornea to form a pannus. Progression of the inflammatory process leads to necrosis and scar formation in the conjunctiva. In classic trachoma, these changes occur more markedly in the upper half of the conjunctival sac and cornea; in inclusion conjunctivitis, more markedly in the lower conjunctiva.

Inflammatory changes, lymphoid infiltration, necrosis, and scar formation have also been observed in TRIC agent infection of cervix and urethra.

Classic inclusion conjunctivitis of the newborn is an acute purulent conjunctivitis; in the adult it is a follicular conjunctivitis. However, all pathologic changes from limited follicular conjunctivitis to full-blown "trachoma" with scars and pannus may follow inoculation of genital isolates into the adult eye.

Classic, chronic, severe trachoma in hyperendemic areas progresses to marked lid deformation and loss of vision. As a result of cellular infiltration and scarring near the lid margins, the tarsal plate is bowed and the lid margins inverted (entropion), and some eyelashes turn inward (trichiasis), rubbing against the cornea with each lid movement, and aggravating corneal opacification. The scarring may destroy tear function, with resulting keratinization of corneal epithelium.

TRIC agents exhibit a pronounced tendency to persist in infected tissues for years even in the absence of signs of active disease, and this predisposes to relapses and to chronicity.

Clinical Manifestations. In experimental human infection with TRIC agents the incubation period is from two to seven days. Inclusion conjunctivitis of the newborn usually begins between the fifth and fourteenth days of life (whereas gonococcal ophthalmia usually begins two days after birth). The incubation period of naturally occurring trachoma is uncertain because the onset is often insidious, particularly in children. Early symptoms of TRIC infection are those of irritation, lacrimation, and mucopurulent discharge. The earliest physical signs are conjunctival hyperemia, mucopurulent discharge, papillary hypertrophy in infants, and follicular hypertrophy in adults.

Typical *trachoma* in children and adults begins as a follicular conjunctivitis, most noticeable in the conjunctiva of the upper lid and the tarsal plate. There are epithelial keratitis and subepithelial corneal infiltration, followed by gradual corneal vascularization from the upper limbus downward. This evolves into a dense fibrovascular pannus extending over part, or all, of the cornea, grossly impairing vision. Linear or stellate scars appear on the conjunctiva. Progressive scarring of the subepithelial tissues leads to deformation of the tarsal plate, resulting in entropion, trichiasis, and further corneal damage. These changes often follow secondary bacterial infection, which may also produce corneal ulceration and accelerate loss of vision. Typically there are no systemic symptoms or signs of infection, and the eye is the sole involved organ.

Typical *inclusion conjunctivitis* of the newborn presents as an acute purulent conjunctivitis with papillary hypertrophy but little involvement of the cornea. Over a period of weeks or months this tends to regress spontaneously and eventually heal without any scars or with only fine linear conjunctival and corneal scars and minimal, if any, pannus. In the adult, inclusion conjunctivitis is an acute mucopurulent conjunctivitis, often accompanied by preauricular adenopathy. Follicular hypertrophy is most noticeable in the conjunctiva of the lower lid, and tends to persist for weeks or months, occasionally accompanied by epithelial keratitis and subepithelial corneal infiltrates. Some adults with chronic inclusion conjunctivitis develop a limited pannus and a few scars of conjunctiva and cornea. Adult genital TRIC infection usually precedes the eye involvement. Adult cervicitis and urethritis are either asymptomatic or produce only slight discharge and discomfort.

All intermediate stages between minimal self-limited inclusion conjunctivitis and typical progressive trachoma can occur as a result of infection with TRIC agents of either ocular or genital origin. The typical, severe trachoma that leads to blindness and is seen in hyperendemic areas occurs probably as a result of long-standing infection with many relapses of TRIC agent activity, hypersensitivity reactions, and repeated bacterial superinfections. Conversely, the self-limited inclusion conjunctivitis of the newborn may be characteristic of a first infection, without hypersensitivity reaction, and without bacterial complications in an immunologically immature host. The basis for different clinical patterns of mild or severe disease seen in different areas of the world is not clearly understood.

Diagnosis. The traditional criteria for the diagnosis of trachoma are the triad of follicular hypertrophy, most prominent on the upper tarsal conjunctiva, pannus, and conjunctival scars. The last two signs may be detected only by biomicroscopic examination.

The diagnosis of inclusion conjunctivitis rests on finding typical inclusions in a purulent conjunctivitis of the newborn or in a follicular conjunctivitis of the adult. There should be only minimal vascular invasion of the cornea. Examination of the adult genital tract may reveal cervicitis and urethritis with moderate discharge and inclusions in epithelial cells.

Among laboratory tests for TRIC infections, the demonstration of typical intracytoplasmic inclusions in conjunctival or genital cells is most widely used. Specific immunofluorescent stain is more sensitive than Giemsa stain. Polymorphonuclear leukocytes are often prominent in scrapings that contain TRIC inclusions. Isolation of TRIC agents in embryonated eggs or in irradiated cell cultures remains a specialized laboratory procedure. Serologic tests can support the diagnosis only if a rise in complement-fixing antibodies occurs during acute disease. The cytologic appearance of expressed follicular material may be helpful. Among follicular diseases of the conjunctiva, only TRIC infections (especially trachoma) produce the necrotic changes in follicles that are evidenced by the presence of many macrophages engorged with cell fragments.

Differential Diagnosis. In differential diagnosis of ocular TRIC infections, adenovirus infections, herpetic keratoconjunctivitis, folliculosis of children, chronic follicular conjunctivitis (Axenfeld type), reactions to allergens and irritating chemicals, and certain bacterial infections must be considered. Some of these entities may coexist with TRIC infections, and repeated competent ophthalmologic examinations and elaborate laboratory assistance may be required to establish a correct diagnosis. The demonstration of morphologically typical inclusions by immunofluorescent or Giemsa stain is most helpful in the diagnosis of TRIC infections, when combined with efforts to isolate viruses or bacteria of possible etiologic significance.

The single most difficult differential diagnosis may be between ocular trachoma and oculogenital inclusion conjunctivitis, as described above. This differentiation requires epidemiologic considerations, clinical and laboratory examination of the genital tract, and—if a TRIC agent has been grown—a "typing" of the isolate by mouse toxin protection tests. At times the eye lesions of trachoma and of oculogenital inclusion conjunctivitis in the adult cannot be distinguished. The most important differential diagnosis of inclusion conjunctivitis of the newborn is chemical or bacterial conjunctivitis.

Treatment and Prognosis. TRIC agents are susceptible to several antibacterial drugs. Tetracyclines and sulfonamides have been most widely used in treatment. Tetracycline suspensions or ointments can cling to the conjunctiva for prolonged effect. Ophthalmic topical tetracycline preparations have been administered in various dosage schedules for several months in chronic endemic trachoma. Sometimes there was clinical improvement, but often active disease recurred, and the over-all efficacy of topical tetracyclines in chronic TRIC infections is being questioned. In inclusion conjunctivitis of the newborn, there is a strong natural tendency toward healing. The administration of topical tetracycline two to four times daily for three weeks further accelerates healing.

Oral tetracycline hydrochloride, 1 to 2 grams daily, or oral trisulfapyrimidines, 4 grams daily for three to six weeks, often suppress signs of activity in chronic trachoma of adults. However, these treatment regimens often fail to eradicate the infectious agent. By contrast, in acute TRIC infections these oral drug regimens alone, or combined with topical tetracycline, may result in permanent cure. This is probably true for both eye infections and genital tract infections, providing that they are of short duration.

In areas of hyperendemic trachoma, mass treatment must be applied to early infection of children and must be repeated at intervals in order to control TRIC infection before scarring occurs. No conclusive evidence exists that mass drug treatment can eradicate trachoma from a population, but repeated courses of drug treatment are probably beneficial by reducing the reservoir of infection, by temporarily suppressing TRIC agent and clinical activity in the patient, and by controlling bacterial superinfection.

Drug therapy has no influence on established scars or pannus. Surgical correction is required in serious entropion or trichiasis. Topical corticosteroids and caustics have no place in therapy.

Prevention. Endemic trachoma is favored by ignorance, poverty, and cultural patterns that oppose hygienic improvement and medical treatment. In addition, the sheer lack of water available for washing seems to be important.

The most potent preventive measures include efforts to increase the total supply of water, simple cleanliness such as frequent hand washing, avoidance of common towel or common eye pencil, and measures to reduce flies. It is also important to detect mild, early infection in young children in endemic areas and to apply effective drug treatment repeatedly. This prevents the blinding progression of the disease, and probably reduces the infective reservoir. Detection and treatment of adults who already suffer visual impairment can probably reduce the source of infection for children.

Prevention of genital TRIC infections requires the control of sexual promiscuity, early diagnosis and effective treatment of cases and sexual contacts, and prolonged follow-up to establish that the genital or ocular infection is not relapsing. Effective treatment of pregnant women with genital TRIC infection can prevent inclusion conjunctivitis in the newborn. The usual instillations into the eye of the newborn (silver nitrate or penicillin) do not prevent inclusion conjunctivitis. A newborn baby with inclusion conjunctivitis should be isolated to prevent spread to others.

Experimental vaccines against TRIC infections have been prepared. In field tests no vaccine has given unequivocal protection against infection, or against progression of disease. Work is continuing in the hope of developing preparations of greater immunogenicity.

However, natural infection engenders only minimal protection against reinfection. The most that could be expected of artificial immunization is an attenuation of the disease resulting from infection. The best current hope for control of TRIC infections rests on a combination of public health measures and drug treatment.

Alexander, E. R., Wang, S. P., and Grayston, J. T.: Further classification of TRIC agents from ocular trachoma and other sources by the mouse toxicity prevention test. Amer. J. Ophthal., 63:1469, 1967.

Jawetz, E.: Chemotherapy of chlamydial infections. *In* Garattini, S., Hawking, F., and Kopin, I. J. (eds.): Advances in Pharmacology and Chemotherapy. Vol. 7. New York, Academic Press, 1969, pp. 253-282.

Jawetz, E., Hanna, L., Dawson, C., Wood, R., and Briones, O.: Subclinical infections with TRIC agents. Amer. J. Ophthal., 63:1413, 1967.

Jones, B. R.: Ocular syndromes of TRIC virus infection and their possible genital significance. Brit. J. Vener. Dis., 40:3, 1964.

Moulder, J. W.: The relation of the psittacosis group (Chlamydiae) to bacteria and viruses. Ann. Rev. Microbiol., 20:107, 1966.

Thygeson, P.: Trachoma Manual and Atlas. U. S. Department of Health, Education and Welfare, U.S. Public Health Service Publication No. 541, Revised 1960.

FOOT-AND-MOUTH DISEASE
(Aphthous Fever)
Walsh McDermott

Foot-and-mouth disease is a viral infection of animals, chiefly cattle, which occurs in man only with great rarity. Infection, when it does occur in man, presumably results from direct contact with the agent either in the laboratory or from handling the tissues or body fluids of infected animals. The disease in man is characterized by a short incubation period followed by the appearance of a febrile illness with vesicular lesions of palms, soles, and the oropharyngeal mucosa. Neurologic involvement has not been reported, and the disease is self-limited. There is no treatment of established value; the tetracycline drugs have yielded inconclusive results in the treatment of laboratory animals. Prevention of the disease in man has not been extensively studied, for man generally has a high degree of resistance to the infection. Spread among cattle is presumably by the air-borne route. An effective vaccine for use in cattle has been developed. As in influenza, however, there are many types and subtypes of foot-and-mouth (FMD) virus, and it is believed that for optimal effectiveness the homologous viral strain, i.e., the "epidemic" strain, should be present in the vaccine.

Annotations: Spread of foot-and-mouth disease. Lancet, 2:580, 1969.

Flaum, A.: Foot-and-mouth disease in man. Acta Path. Microbiol. Scand., 16:197, 1939.

Hyslop, N. St.G., Davie, J., and Carter, S. P.: Antigenic differences between strains of foot-and-mouth disease virus of type SAT 1. J. Hyg. (Camb.), 61:217, 1963.

VIRAL DISEASES CHARACTERIZED BY CUTANEOUS LESIONS

MEASLES
(Moribilli, Rubeola)
Edwin D. Kilbourne

Definition. Measles is an extremely contagious, febrile disease of high morbidity characterized by rash and catarrhal inflammation of the eyes and respiratory tract. It is principally a benign disease of children, but may afflict with equal frequency persons of any age not previously attacked by its virus.

Etiology. Measles is caused by a medium-sized RNA *paramyxovirus* approximately 1400 Å. in diameter. The virus is thermolabile, having a half-life of two hours at 37° C.; it is also inactivated rapidly below pH 4.5. Measles virus induces apparent infection with exanthem only in man and monkey. It has been found that tissue cultures derived from nonprimates, as well as from primates and chick embryos, will support propagation of the virus, as originally described by Enders and Peebles in 1954. The virus is structurally and biologically similar to the larger myxoviruses and agglutinates erythrocytes of the rhesus monkey and baboon in vitro and may thus be quantitated; inhibition of this reaction affords a method for titrating specific antibody in serum.

Prevalence and Epidemiology. Measles is a disease of cosmopolitan distribution, endemic in all but isolated populations. It may occur at any time of the year, but most outbreaks are in the late winter and early spring, with a peak at the end of April. The disease recurs in epidemic cycles at two- to three-year intervals in most civilized communities that have been studied. This epidemic periodicity is best explained as a result of the introduction of new susceptibles into the population by birth or ingress from other areas. When the proportion of nonimmunes reaches a certain crucial concentration (45 to 50 per cent), disease and coincident dissemination of virus may occur to produce an epidemic. It is likely that virus is introduced from sources external to the involved population, probably by incoming susceptibles; there is no solid evidence of subclinical infection or a postinfection carrier state with unmodified measles to suggest local persistence of virus in interepidemic periods. Isolated communities such as the Faröe Islands (Panum) are infrequently attacked by measles, at which times manifest illness appears in virtually all persons not previously infected. In Greenland, a country not known to have been invaded previously by the disease, an epidemic resulted in overt measles in 99.9 per cent of the indigenous population (Christiansen and others).

Throughout most of the world, measles is a disease of children; most adults possess acquired immunity. Beyond the age of ten more than 90 per cent of the population have specific antibody. Although the peak attack rate coincides with the beginning of school (age six) in technologically advanced societies, it occurs between the ages of two and three in most underdeveloped countries. Morbidity and mortality rates do not appear to be influenced by sex or race. Case fatality rates are highest in children less than five years of age, and are also relatively high in the aged. Congenital infection has occurred.

There is no evidence that the virus may vary in virulence in nature. The oft-cited and notorious virulence of the disease in primitive, isolated, or crowded populations may be explained as a corollary of (1) more prevalent infection of feeble and aged adults, (2) poor environmental conditions, (3) inadequate medical care, and (4) secondary bacterial infections. A strikingly increased mortality rate is observed in areas such as West Africa in which protein-calorie malnutrition is prevalent.

Because measles virus per se rarely induces fatal disease, it is evident that fatalities attributable to measles may vary in incidence according to the prevalence of bacterial pathogens and the resistance of the population to their presence.

Communicability. Measles is one of the most contagious of infections. Demonstration of virus in nasopharyngeal secretions is in accord with epidemiologic evidence that infection is disseminated and acquired by the respiratory tract. Close physical proximity or direct person-to-person contact is the usual requisite for infection.

Immunity. An unmodified attack of measles usually confers lifelong immunity. This observation is in accord with the observed persistence of both complement-fixing and neutralizing antibodies after infection and the relatively high titer of antibodies present even in older persons. Able observers have described apparently authentic instances of second or even multiple infections. Definitive proof of recurrent infection with measles virus is lacking, however, because specific diagnostic laboratory tests have only recently become available. Detailed study of a family subject to recurrent attacks suggests an hereditary defect in the capacity to develop immunity in certain cases. One such patient was found to be capable of antibody formation, and electrophoretic analysis of the serum showed no deficit of gamma globulin. Temporary immunity may be passively acquired by receipt of convalescent serum or gamma globulin derived from the pooled serums of human adults (see Treatment). Humoral antibody is demonstrable in patients convalescent from measles modified by gamma globulin. The low incidence of measles in early infancy (first six months) is attributed to transient protection by placentally transferred maternal antibody.

Pathology and Physiologic Responses. Pathologic changes in fatal measles usually represent the compound effect of viral and secondary bacterial infection. Pneumonia is almost invariably present; it is most frequently interstitial, but may produce purulent exudate within the alveoli. More representative are changes of the uncomplicated viral disease within the tonsillar, nasopharyngeal, and appendiceal tissue removed during the prodrome. These changes consist of subepithelial round cell infiltration and the presence of multinucleated giant cells. The latter are so characteristic that skilled pathologists have predicted the development of rash from their presence in surgical specimens. Similar cells are commonly observed in tissue cultures infected with measles virus. Cytoplasmic and nuclear inclusions may be seen in epithelial cells. The lesions clinically apparent as Koplik's spots derive from inflammatory mononuclear cell infiltration of buccal submucous glands and necrosis of focal vesicular lesions of the mucosa. Rash is the result of proliferation of capillary endothelial cells in the corium and the coincident exudation of serum, and occasionally erythrocytes, into the epidermis.

No consistent or characteristic physiologic aberrations are observed with measles. The transient hemoconcentration and albuminuria found with other febrile diseases may occur. A normal total leukocyte count or leukopenia is observed throughout the febrile period. Initially, the leukopenia is occasioned by a decline in lymphocytes on the first day of fever; subsequently, granulocytopenia ensues as well. The incubation period is characterized by neutrophilia, and convalescence by a relative lymphocytosis. Measles virus has been isolated from the leukocytic fraction of blood, and is propagable in suspensions of leukocytes in vitro. A false-positive serologic test for syphilis may be observed.

Hormone-like Effects of Measles Infection. Several striking physiologic effects of measles, although poorly understood, mimic the influence of corticotrophin or the adrenal corticosteroids. These are transient suppression of the tuberculin reaction (observed also with measles vaccines), improvement in eczema and allergic asthma, delay in wound healing, and the induction of remissions in leukemia, Hodgkin's disease, and lipoid nephrosis. Whether these effects are directly attributable to the virus or are hormonally mediated is not known.

Clinical Manifestations. Following an incubation period that averages 11 days, measles becomes clinically manifest with symptoms of fever, malaise, myalgia, and headache. Within hours *ocular symptoms* of photophobia and burning pain are evidenced by conjunctival injection, tearing, and exudate in the conjunctival sac. Concomitantly, or soon thereafter, *catarrhal inflammation of the respiratory tract* is manifested by sneezing, coughing, and nasal discharge. Less commonly, hoarseness and aphonia may reflect laryngeal involvement. In this prodromal stage of one to four days' duration, petechial lesions of the palate and pharynx or tiny white spots on the buccal mucosa (*Koplik's spots*) may herald the appearance of skin rash. The white lesions described by Koplik characteristically occur lateral to the molar teeth, and typically are mounted on red areolae of injected mucosa, which may coalesce to form a diffuse red background. Not invariably present, they constitute a valuable, if not pathognomonic, diagnostic sign. The enanthem may involve other mucous membranes such as the vaginal lining. It may "overlap" the subsequent appearance of the cutaneous rash by one to three days. Rarely, a transient, erythematous exanthema may occur in the prodromal period.

The *rash* of measles follows the prodromal symptoms by two to four days, occasionally as late as seven days. It first appears behind the ears or on the face as a blotchy erythema, spreads downward to cover the trunk, and finally is manifest on the extremities. The hands and feet may escape involvement. Initially, the eruption consists of discrete, reddish-brown macules that blanch with pressure. Subsequently, these lesions become slightly elevated, tend to coalesce, and may develop a hemorrhagic, nonblanching component. Rash is sometimes very extensive in children with protein-calorie malnutrition, and skin

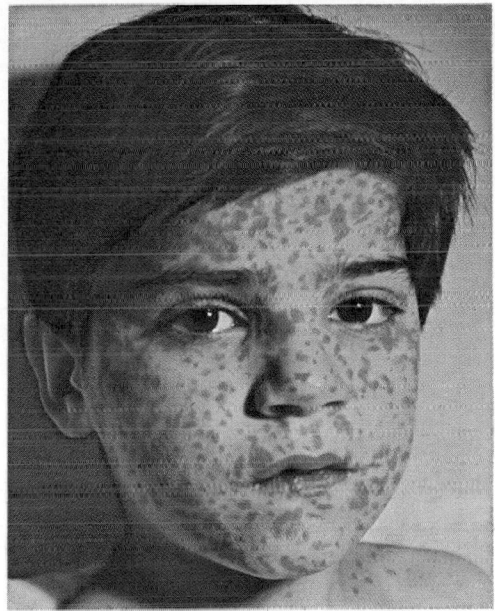

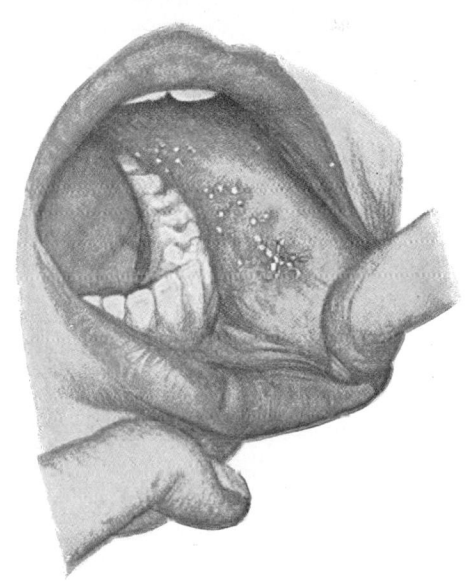

Upper: Early measles eruption. (Reproduction from Therapeutic Notes, by Courtesy of Parke, Davis & Company.) *Lower:* Koplik's spots in measles (Hecker, Trumpp, and Abt).

lesions associated with kwashiorkor may develop at the site of the exanthem. The rash fades in the order of its appearance; its disappearance about five days after onset is attended by a fine, powdery desquamation that spares the hands and feet. At its maximum the exanthema usually marks the termination of malaise and fever in the uncomplicated illness.

The *fever* of measles is commonly of the typhoidal, progressively rising type, and falls by lysis. It persists for about six days, and frequently reaches 103° F. In the adult, fever may follow rather than antedate the catarrhal symptoms. Throughout the febrile period, productive *cough* and auscultatory evidence of bronchiolitis may be evident. These manifestations may persist after defervescence, and cough is often the last symptom to disappear. It is probable that bronchopulmonary symptomatology is an integral part of the primary viral infection; roentgenographic evidence of pulmonary involvement is frequently seen in the uncomplicated disease in the absence of leukocytosis and obvious bacterial infection.

Complications. It is difficult to distinguish between those complications directly attributable to the virus of measles and those resulting from secondary bacterial infections. The persistence or recurrence of fever and the occurrence of leukocytosis are presumptive evidence of the usual bacterial sequelae of *otitis media* or *pneumonia*. The pneumonia resembles other forms of viral pneumonia and is often caused solely by a specific reaction to the measles virus. Superimposed bacterial infection is common, however, and accounts for most of the severe or fatal cases. Pneumococcus, *Streptococcus hemolyticus, Staphylococcus aureus,* and *Haemophilus influenzae* are the usual secondary invaders. The incidence of bacterial complications is increased by crowding, debility, and the prevalence of bacterial pathogens in the population. Bacterially engendered sequelae may be unduly frequent in crowded contagious disease hospitals.

Serious complications directly related to the measles virus are rare. *Laryngitis* of sufficient severity to embarrass respiration has been observed, and may warrant tracheostomy. *Electrocardiographic abnormalities* may be found in as many as 30 per cent of children, but clinical evidence of cardiac disease is meager in such cases. *Abdominal pain* or *diarrhea* may be related to invasion of lymphoid tissue of the appendix or Peyer's patches. These symptoms may lead to unnecessary surgery before the appearance of the typical rash. The frequency of stomatitis and gastrointestinal symptoms is greater in malnourished children in tropical areas and may reflect coincident bacterial and parasitic infection.

Encephalomyelitis. A rare (0.01 to 0.5 per cent) but serious consequence of measles is a demyelinating encephalomyelitis that may appear from one to fourteen days after the onset of infection. This complication is associated with a recurrence of fever, and headache, vomiting, and stiff neck. Stupor and convulsions occasionally follow. Localizing neurologic symptoms may or may not be present. Death ensues in about 10 per cent of patients; about half of survivors suffer permanent residuals of varying severity. Recently, abnormal electroencephalograms were recorded in 51 per cent of children with measles *without evidence of encephalitis.* In some of the children the abnormal encephalographic findings were persistent. The presence of a measles-like virus has been demonstrated in patients with subacute sclerosing panencephalitis (see Neurologic Diseases and Behavior).

Other late sequelae of measles are thrombocytopenic purpura and exacerbation or activation of pre-existing pulmonary tuberculosis.

Giant-Cell Pneumonia. In children with severe disease involving the recticuloendothelial system (especially leukemia), measles virus may induce an interstitial pneumonia characterized by giant cells and intracellular inclusion bodies. The disease is usually fatal; if the patient survives, persistence of virus and poor antibody formation are evident in convalescence. The pneumonia may occur in the absence of rash so that its etiologic relation to measles may be unsuspected.

Measles Modified by Vaccine or Antibody Administration. Attenuation of the natural disease by antibody prophylaxis may result in an illness of lessened severity comparable with the milder infection of the maternally immunized newborn. Fever alone may be observed, but some degree of exanthema is usually apparent. Koplik's spots may not appear. In general, the course is truncated and relatively uncomplicated. Similar attenuated disease may occur in children partially immunized with inactivated viral vaccine.

Unfavorably Modified Measles—A New Disease. Following administration of inactivated measles vaccine (no longer in general use), infection of vaccinees with either live measles vaccine or wild-type natural measles virus led to the development of a new syndrome characterized by dermal hypersensitivity to measles virus and an atypical (petechial, vesicular, or urticarial) rash atypical in distribution. In some cases pulmonary complications occurred. The exact mechanism of this reaction is unknown, but it is almost certainly a manifestation of delayed hypersensitivity to the viral proteins engendered by alum-precipitated inactivated viral vaccine. No such sequelae have followed use of live virus vaccine (see below).

Diagnosis. The experienced layman can diagnose typical measles. The querulous, bleary-eyed child, his face blotched and his nose crusted with exudate, presents a characteristic, if miserable, picture as he breathes open-mouthed between paroxysms of sneezing and coughing. The severity of the catarrhal symptoms distinguishes the disease from other eruptive fevers. In the prodromal period the diagnosis should be suggested by (1) fever higher than that of the usual common cold, (2) known measles in the community, and (3) Koplik's spots on the buccal mucosa.

Differential diagnosis (see accompanying table) includes consideration of rubella, scarlet fever, exanthema subitum, infectious mononucleosis, secondary syphilis, drug eruptions, and infection with certain Coxsackie and echoviruses. Of value in excluding these possibilities are the milder course and pinker rash of rubella, the sore throat and leukocytosis of scarlet fever, and serologic tests for infectious mononucleosis and syphilis. The rash of exanthema subitum does not appear until the termination of fever. Fever, enanthema, and catarrh are uncommon with the cutaneous manifestations of drug hypersensitivity.

Specific Diagnosis. Specific diagnosis de-

A GUIDE TO THE DIFFERENTIAL DIAGNOSIS OF MEASLES

	Conjunctivitis	Rhinitis	Sore Throat	Enanthem	Leukocytosis	Specific Laboratory Tests Available
Measles	++	+	0	+	0	+
Rubella	±	±	±	±	0	+
Exanthema subitum	±	±	0	0	0	0
Enterovirus infection	0	±	±	0	±	+
Scarlet fever	±	⊥	++	0	+	+
Infectious mononucleosis	0	0	+	0	±	+
Drug rash	0	0	0	0	0	0

0 not usually present; no test available   + present; test available
± variable in occurrence   ++ present and severe

pends on the isolation of measles virus from throat washings, blood, or urine by inoculation of various types of tissue culture with materials obtained during the first five days of illness. Increase in specific antibody may be detected as early as the first or second day of rash by the complement-fixation test. Antibody is also demonstrable by neutralization and hemagglutination-inhibition procedures.

Presumptive diagnosis may be made if giant cells are detected in stained smears of nasal exudate in the pre-eruptive period.

Prognosis. Uncomplicated measles is rarely fatal, and complete recovery from the disease is the rule. Fatalities are almost always the result of secondary streptococcal or pneumococcal pneumonia, occurring principally in children below the age of five who become infected after the dissipation of passive neonatal immunity. Mortality in underdeveloped countries may be 250 times that observed in the United States or northern Europe. Case fatality rates are also high in elderly and tuberculous patients. Congestive cardiac failure is a common cause of death in patients over 50 years old.

Antimicrobial drugs effective against the usual secondary invaders have reduced the case fatality rate of measles sharply. The incidence of otitis media and pneumonia may be lowered by the prophylactic use of penicillin or a tetracycline early in illness.

Encephalitis occurs as frequently in mild as in severe measles. However, modification of measles by gamma globulin prophylaxis *(vide infra)* affords an improved prognosis with reference to the encephalitic complication.

Treatment. There is no specific treatment for measles.

Symptomatic Therapy. In the absence of complications, bed rest is the essence of treatment in this usually benign, self-limited disease. Codeine sulfate (0.015 to 0.06 gram) is useful in the amelioration of headache and myalgia and is effective in the management of cough. Aspirin (0.3 to 0.6 gram) may be employed for its analgesic and antipyretic actions. Diet should be unrestricted. Bright light is not an ocular hazard, but photophobia may require darkening of the patient's room.

Antimicrobial Prophylaxis. The course of uncomplicated measles is not influenced by antimicrobial therapy. In common practice the incidence of serious bacterial infections is not sufficient to justify the routine prophylactic use of antimicrobials. Certain special circumstances may warrant full therapeutic dosage with penicillin or the tetracyclines in anticipation of the potentially fatal sequelae of pneumococcal or beta hemolytic streptococcal infections. These circumstances include treatment of the chronically ill, the very young, or the aged, and the treatment of patients under crowded conditions that foster the increase and dissemination of pathogenic bacteria, as may occur in contagious disease hospitals. If careful observation of the patient is possible, rational therapy is based on the prompt recognition and etiologic definition of complications, followed by initiation of the appropriate antimicrobial drug in proper dosage.

Prevention. The administration of convalescent serum or gamma globulin during the period of incubation may prevent or modify the manifestations of illness. The degree of modification obtained is dependent upon the quantity of antibody given and the time of its administration. In children of less than six years, the intramuscular injection of 0.025 ml. of gamma globulin per pound in the first half of the incubation period results in disease of lessened severity. Two to four times this amount will prevent disease in nearly 80 per cent of children. In older children and adults, one and one-half to two times as much globulin is recommended. In young or debilitated children the aim is complete prevention of disease. In children over five, less subject to complications, the goal of prophylaxis is attenuation of the infection sufficient to lessen symptoms but not the development of effective immunity.

Vaccination. Highly effective vaccines are now available for the prevention of measles. Most are derived from the Edmonston strain of measles virus isolated in the laboratory of Dr. John Enders. This strain, although it proved very effective in early trials as a live virus vaccine, produced febrile and other reactions (attenuated measles) with such high frequency that it is now usually administered concomitantly with *measles immune globulin* (injected at a different site). Further tissue culture passage has led to the development of *"further attenuated"* (*live virus*) *vaccines* that are apparently as effective as the original vaccine in inducing immunity but that may be given without gamma globulin. These live virus vaccines produce immunity by infection, and therefore need be given only as a single injection. They induce antibody response comparable to that following natural infection, and the persistence of antibody also seems to be comparable, although observations have been limited. Immunity to infection also appears to persist undiminished in parallel with the presence of antibody for at least five years. It is assumed (but not yet established) that immunity following live virus vaccine is permanent. The vaccine virus is not contagious.

Live virus vaccine is given as a single parenteral injection to persons more than one year of age. The coincident injection of standardized *measles immune globulin* (0.01 ml. per pound of body weight) at a different site will greatly reduce the incidence of fever and other symptoms. If *live "further attenuated" vaccine* is used under the same conditions, gamma globulin is unnecessary.

Contraindications to live virus vaccine include pregnancy, leukemia, and other systemic malignant diseases, active tuberculosis, and administration of resistance-depressing drugs such as corticosteroids and antimetabolites.

Inactivated vaccine produces impermanent immunity and unfavorably alters response to later infection. It therefore is no longer recommended (see Complications, above).

Eradication of measles through administration of live virus vaccines is a reasonable possibility. The introduction of immunization in the United States in 1963 led to a decrease in annual incidence of from 4,000,000 to 250,000 cases in five years.

Axnick, N. W., Shavell, S. M., and Witte, J. J.: Benefits due to immunization against measles. Public Health Rep., 84:673, 1969.

Christiansen, P. E., et al.: An epidemic of measles in southern Greenland, 1951. Acta Med. Scand., 144:313, 430, 450, 1952–53.

Enders, J. F., Katz, S. L., Milovanovic, M. V., and Holloway, A.: Studies on an attenuated measles-virus vaccine. I. Development and preparation of the vaccine: Technics for assay of effects of vaccination. New Eng. J. Med., 263:153, 1960.

Koplik, H.: The diagnosis of the invasion of measles from a study of the exanthema as it appears on the buccal mucous membrane. Arch. Pediat., 13:918, 1896.

Panum, P. L.: Observations Made during the Epidemic of Measles on the Faröe Islands, Delta Omega Society, 1940.

Tyler, H. R.: Neurological complications of rubeola (measles). Medicine, 36:147, 1957.

RUBELLA

(German Measles)

Edwin D. Kilbourne

Definition. Rubella is an acute, benign, contagious disease of children and young adults. The cardinal manifestations of the illness are a pale pink rash and posterior cervical lymphadeni-tis. Paradoxically, this mild disease is one of the few viral infections convincingly associated with the genesis of fetal abnormalities. When infection is acquired in utero, it often results in generalized disease of the infant and protracted excretion of virus after birth. Accordingly, recognition and prevention of the disease are matters of far reaching consequence.

Etiology. Rubella virus is a small, spherical RNA virus with a mean diameter of 550 to 600 Å. The particle is ether sensitive—an attribute of lipid-containing enveloped viruses. The virus develops by budding from marginal and intracytoplasmic membranes. Classification of the virus is uncertain at present, but similarities of structure and development to certain group A arboviruses have been noted. (There is no evidence of arthropod transmission.)

The virus agglutinates the erythrocytes of newly hatched chicks—a characteristic that permits measurement of both virus and antibody. Rubella virus replicates with the production of cytopathic effects in a number of commonly employed cell culture systems, including African green monkey and human diploid cells. Virus replication and production of embryopathic effects similar to those in humans have been experimentally induced in rats.

Incidence and Epidemiology. Accurate information on the incidence of rubella is not available. The mildness and brevity of its clinical signs may confound the diagnosis and reporting of many instances of infection. Studies of the experimental disease lend support to prior clinical evidence that infection may occur without rash, and indicate a further diagnostic pitfall. It can be said, however, that the disease is seen on every continent, may occur in epidemic form, and has its highest incidence in the early spring. The disease is less frequently acquired in childhood than measles, as is attested by serologic studies and by the fact that rubella is more common than measles in young adults. The higher incidence of infection in younger age groups in institutional outbreaks argues against a greater susceptibility of the adult. It is probable that rubella is spread by the respiratory route by close and sustained personal contact. The infection is contagious during the period of prodromal symptoms and the first day of rash. Only recently it has been recognized that the infant with congenitally acquired infection may excrete virus for months after birth and is contagious during this time. The epidemiologic implications of this fact—first established in the large epidemic of 1963–1964—are yet to be determined. There is evidence that the newborn may be unusually contagious, and that although he may have no obvious stigmata of infection, yet he may be shedding virus.

Immunity is lasting. Authenticated second attacks are rare, and are virtually unprovable because of the nebulous nature of the clinical syndrome. Passive immunity of variable efficacy may be conferred by the injection of gamma globulin from the serum of patients convalescent from the disease (see Prevention). Rubella has no immunologic relationship to measles.

Pathology. Death from uncomplicated postnatally acquired rubella is unknown. Histologic changes characteristic of the disease have not been demonstrated. The onset of disease is attended by leukopenia resulting from a decrease in both lymphocytes and neutrophils. After five days, absolute lymphocytosis is manifest. The total leukocyte count is normal at the tenth day.

Congenital Rubella. Necropsies of fetal and infantile victims of maternal infection have shown a variety of embryonal defects related to developmental arrest involving all three germ layers. Those defects most consistently associated with maternal rubella are microcephaly, cataract, patency of the ductus arteriosus, and defects of the interventricular septum. However, recent studies have revealed a wide spectrum of tissue damage in association with virologically proved disease of varying severity. In some infants hepatic and renal degeneration and myocardial necrosis without inflammation have been noted, whereas in others thrombocytopenia and purpura may be the sole abnormality. It has been proposed that the generalized visceral involvement and characteristic residua of the disease may result from a sequence of platelet damage, intravascular coagulation, and thrombosis (Bayer et al.). Another theory holds that the smaller size of the rubella-infected infant and some abnormalities may reflect inhibition of multiplication of embryonic cells by the virus.

Clinical Manifestations. *Postnatally Acquired Rubella.* Fourteen to twenty-one days after exposure to the infection, the onset of rubella is evidenced by symptoms variable in their occurrence and severity. Cough, sore throat, and coryza may initiate the illness, but are often absent; headache, malaise, and myalgia may precede the eruption, especially in young adults. Commonly, fever and obvious enlargement of posterior cervical nodes antedate the appearance of the rash. Fever, when present, rarely exceeds 101° F. and seldom persists beyond 48 hours. Injection of the bulbar conjunctivae may be noted. Palpable, tender, and occasionally visible lymphadenopathy involves postauricular and suboccipital nodes with sufficient frequency to be an important diagnostic sign. Generalized peripheral lymphadenitis, and, more rarely, splenomegaly, may occur.

The exanthema of rubella is usually apparent within 24 hours of the first symptoms as a faint macular erythema that first involves the face and neck. Characterized by its brevity and evanescence, it spreads rapidly to the trunk and extremities, sometimes leaving one site even as it appears at the next. The pink macules that constitute the rash blanch with pressure and rarely stain the skin. Diffuse erythema on the second day of rash may closely simulate scarlet fever. The eruption has vanished by the third day. Rubella may occur without rash. An enanthema has been described that is inconstant in form and

occurrence, and lacks the premonitory significance of the Koplik spots of measles. The lesions consist of red macules that usually involve the soft palate.

Complications. Recovery is almost always prompt and uneventful, although relapse occurs with greater frequency than with most viral diseases (5 to 8 per cent). Secondary bacterial infections rarely occur. Rare complications are arthralgia, neuritis, gingivitis, thrombocytopenic purpura, and increased capillary fragility. Heart block has been described. A *meningoencephalitis* of short duration may occur one to six days after the appearance of rash. Its incidence is estimated at 1 in 6000 cases, and it is fatal in approximately 20 per cent of those afflicted. Rubella encephalopathy is not associated with demyelinization (in contrast to other postviral encephalitides). Survivors may have electroencephalographic abnormalities, but intellectual function seems to be preserved.

Congenital Rubella. The fortuitous coincidence of the development of cell culture systems for the isolation of rubella virus and the occurrence of a global epidemic of rubella (in 1963–1964) has demonstrated that the classic ocular and cardiac "teratogenic" effects of rubella are but isolated manifestations of a continuing and persisting fetal infection. It is now clear that congenital transplacental infection of the fetus occurs as a consequence of maternal infection (which may or may not be clinically evident) usually in the first trimester of pregnancy. Virus is demonstrable in placental and fetal tissues obtained by therapeutic abortion at that time. If pregnancy is not interrupted (and spontaneous abortion is uncommon), fetal infection persists, and upon delivery of the infant, virus is recoverable from the throat, urine, feces, conjunctivae, bone marrow, and cerebrospinal fluid of the living infant and from most organs at autopsy. About 10 to 15 per cent of infants born to mothers infected in the first trimester of pregnancy have stigmata of infection readily recognizable in the first year of life. These include *cardiac lesions, cataracts, glaucoma, microphthalmia,* and *esophageal atresia.* Most infants in whom virus is detectable do not have evidence of disease at birth or may simply have a lower than normal birth weight. In others, disease of intermediate severity has been recently recognized. Most prominent of the newly observed manifestations is *thrombocytopenic purpura,* which disappears soon after birth. *Hepatosplenomegaly* may persist for months. Other signs include *corneal clouding, fullness of the fontanels, lesions of the long bones,* and *electroencephalographic abnormalities.*

A most striking finding has been the persistence of virus in the pharynx, gastrointestinal tract, and cerebrospinal fluid for as long as one year after birth (9 per cent). Infective virus was present in the lenses of 7 of 15 patients as old as 18 months. This evidence of continuing viral synthesis occurs coincidentally with circulating antibody (initially of maternal origin) and has suggested a form of "immunologic tolerance" to the virus. However, it has been shown that the character of the antibody changes during the first year from IgG (presumably maternal) to IgM, indicating a primary response of the infant to the persisting viral antigen. Studies of older infants and children with stigmata of congenital rubella show them to be free of demonstrable virus and to possess the IgG immunoglobulins that characteristically persist after other viral infections.

Diagnosis. Rubella may be diagnosed clinically with assurance only during an epidemic. It may be difficult to distinguish from mild or modified measles, infectious mononucleosis, or scarlet fever. Distinction from measles may be made on the basis of the pinker, nonstaining rash, the milder course, and the lesser catarrh of rubella. Sore throat is a more prominent complaint in scarlet fever; the course of infectious mononucleosis is often more protracted, and splenomegaly is more frequent than in rubella. Specific diagnosis of rubella may now be made by isolation of the virus in any of several cell culture systems, or by demonstration of neutralizing hemagglutination-inhibiting or complement-fixing antibody response during infection. The high incidence of dermatoglyphic abnormalities (50 per cent) and increased percentage of chromosome breaks described in patients following congenital rubella may prove to have diagnostic value when studied further.

Prognosis. Complete recovery from postnatally acquired rubella is almost invariable. The rare deaths attributable to rubella follow the infrequent complication of meningoencephalitis. Infection in pregnancy constitutes a hazard to the fetus but not to the mother.

Treatment. There is no specific treatment for the disease. Few patients suffer discomfort severe enough to warrant symptomatic medication. Headache and myalgia may be controlled by aspirin; bed rest is advisable for the duration of the fever.

Prevention. *Passive Immunization.* In contrast to measles, current evidence is conflicting with regard to the prophylaxis of rubella with convalescent serum and gamma globulin. Various lots of gamma globulin appear to vary in prophylactic potency, some being completely ineffective. However, the virus has been neutralized in vitro in human volunteer experiments by human gamma globulin or convalescent serum (Krugman and Ward, 1953). *Administration of gamma globulin to the pregnant woman may only mask her symptoms of infection yet not protect the fetus from viral invasion.* Its use may thus only obscure the picture and confound decision about the need for therapeutic abortion. Hence the practice seems inadvisable.

Active Immunization. Rubella may be prevented in children and adults by the parenteral administration of an attenuated live virus vaccine produced in duck embryo cell cultures and derived from passage of virus in African green monkey kidney cells. Seroconversion rates after immunization are approximately 95 per cent. As with other live virus vaccines, serum antibody titers are lower than those following natural infection. However, antibody persists for at least three years following vaccination, but the permanence of vaccine-induced immunity still must be established by further observation. In children, vaccination is attended by little, if any, reaction; but in women, rash, malaise, arthralgia, and mild, acute arthritis occur frequently, the incidence being directly related to age. For this reason, it is currently recommended that immunization be carried out principally in childhood. However, since the epidemic threshold—at least in semiclosed populations—is low (between 4.7 and 8.4 per cent), containment of the disease by mass immunization may prove difficult. Therefore, despite the higher reaction rates in adults, it seems advisable to immunize women of childbearing age for whose unborn children rubella may have tragic consequences.

Alford, C. A., Jr., Neva, F. A., and Weller, T. H.: Virologic and serologic studies on human products of conception after maternal rubella. New Eng. J. Med., 271:1275, 1964.

Bayer, W. L., Sherman, F. E., Michaels, R. H., Szeto, I. L. F., and Lewis, J. H.: Purpura in congenital and acquired rubella. New Eng. J. Med., 273:1362, 1965.

Cooper, L. Z.: Rubella: A preventable cause of birth defects. *In* Bergsma, D. (ed.): Birth Defects: Original Article Series, Vol. IV, No. 7, Intrauterine Infections, The National Foundation, December, 1968, pp. 23-35.

Gregg, N. M.: Congenital cataract following German measles in the mother. Trans. Ophthal. Soc. Austral., 3:35, 1941.

Rubella Symposium. Amer. J. Dis. Child., 110:345-476, 1965.

EXANTHEMATA ASSOCIATED WITH ENTEROVIRAL INFECTIONS

Edwin D. Kilbourne

Infection with any of a number of enteroviruses may be associated with erythematous, macular eruptions. In some patients occipital and cervical lymphadenopathy may be noted, so that the infection may closely simulate rubella. However, differential diagnosis is aided by the frequency of a vesicular ulcerative enanthem and aseptic meningitis in patients with enteroviral disease and also by its summertime occurrence. Those enteroviruses most frequently associated with rash are the Coxsackie group A viruses 9 and 16, and (quite fortuitously) echoviruses bearing the same numerical designations, i.e., echovirus 9 and echovirus 16). The eruptions associated with the Coxsackie viruses may include small vesicles, especially notable with Coxsackie A16 (hand, foot, and mouth disease). Echovirus 16 and Coxsackie virus B5 produce eruptions that mimic roseola infantum. Rash seems to be more common in children than in adults.

Lerner, M. A., Klein, J. O., Cherry, J. D., and Finland, M.: New viral exanthems. New Eng. J. Med., 269:678, 1963.

Wenner, H. A., and Lou, T. Y.: Virus diseases associated with cutaneous eruptions. Progr. Med. Virol., 5:219, 1963.

VARIOLA AND VACCINIA: INTRODUCTION AND HISTORY

C. Henry Kempe

Immunization against the dread disease of smallpox is perhaps the most widely applied immunization procedure currently in use. Over the past 150 years it has demonstrated its effectiveness beyond question. The vaccinia virus (*Poxvirus officinale*), which is in effect a laboratory strain carried for many generations in a variety of laboratory animals, differs from the newly isolated virus of cowpox (*Poxvirus bovis*), which was originally employed by Jenner (1798) and his predecessors for the immunization of man against the smallpox virus (*Poxvirus variolae*).

Smallpox was described in detail by Rhazes in the tenth century, and had been described previously by Galen in the second century. Spread from Asia to Europe and North Africa occurred in the Middle Ages, and the disease was prevalent in the sixteenth century. At approximately the same time the disease was introduced into the West Indies by African slaves and from there into Mexico and South America. The best studied epidemics are those in the eighteenth century in England when over 90 per cent of the cases occurred in children under ten years of age and when smallpox accounted for one third of all deaths in children. Smallpox occurred in epidemic form less frequently in North America until 1752 when over 30 per cent of the inhabitants of Boston, Massachusetts, were affected and the mortality rate was over 30 per cent (Creighton, 1894). In 1721 deliberate inoculation of smallpox as protection against the natural disease was introduced in England. It consisted of the inoculation of pustular material by puncturing the skin. This resulted in a febrile disease following an eight-day incubation and a general eruption on the ninth day. The mortality rate from this procedure was 1 to 2 per cent, and it is stated that 17 of 897 inoculated persons died from the disease (Woodville, 1796). Needless to say, modified infection did give rise to highly virulent natural disease in susceptible contacts. In 1738 variolation was successfully used in Charleston, South Carolina, with material that had been allowed to dry. With better care of the patients, the death rate from smallpox was somewhat reduced; it was thought to be about one or two out of 500, whereas the mortality from the naturally acquired smallpox was 10 to 20 per cent. Variolation was followed by inoculation of cowpox following widespread acceptance of Jenner's studies published in 1798. In truth, this practice had been current among a number of colleagues of Jenner's at a previous time, and he made no claim to originality. Jenner, however, did play a decisive role in popularizing this method of protection against smallpox, and variolation was outlawed in England in 1840. It is possible that the endemism of smallpox in England during the eighteenth century was due to the practice of variolation rather than to natural epidemic occurrence.

VARIOLA
(Smallpox)

C. Henry Kempe

Etiology. Smallpox virus is readily visible with any microscope equipped with darkfield illumination or by phase contrast microscopy. With electron microscopy, the smallpox virus resembles elementary bodies of vaccinia virus. The elementary bodies are small, brick-shaped structures with a diameter of about 200 mμ. They can be demonstrated by direct examination of smears of early skin lesions. The virus is very resistant to drying, and living virus can be demonstrated from scabs kept at room temperature for over three years. Virulent virus has survived on clothing of patients and on bedclothes of hospitalized patients, and has caused the disease in laundry workers who were not protected.

Incidence. Approximately 75,000 cases of smallpox were reported to the World Health Organization in 1966, principally from Asia and Africa. The last major importation of smallpox into western Europe occured in 1963, when the four original cases resulted in 141 secondary cases and 11 deaths. The United States of America has not had an importation since 1949. The control of smallpox by mass vaccination campaigns supported by the World Health Organization is currently under way in many parts of the world where endemic smallpox persists.

Epidemiology. The principal natural reservoir of smallpox is thought to be the patient suffering from the disease. It is true that smallpox affects monkeys and that there may be other animal reservoirs, but they have not been demonstrated to date as an important source of virus in the absence of human cases. Spread may be direct or, quite often, indirect through clothing or utensils infected by the patient. The patient is not infective until the third day of the clinical disease, that is, one day before the macular-papular phase of the skin eruption is noted. Contacts may be allowed at large until they actually become ill because they are not infective during the early pre-eruptive febrile disease.

Pathology and Pathogenesis. It is likely that the site of entry of the smallpox virus is the upper respiratory tract. In the 12-day incubation period the virus probably multiplies in the regional lymphoid tissues. The fact that no patient is infectious during the incubation period suggests that in this interval an open lesion does not exist in the respiratory mucosa. In the unmodified case, a massive viremia occurs at the onset of the fever, and remains during the first two or three days of the pre-eruptive phase. In this way the virus localizes in the mucous membranes and in the skin as well as in the internal tissues. After the virus disappears from the blood and the skin eruption appears, the patient feels better, and the temperature tends to decrease. Antibodies are noted in the blood as early as the fourth day of the disease. The virus multiplies in the epithelial cells of the skin while being relatively protected from the action of circulating antibody so that cell destruction continues for some time. When pustulation occurs, the temperature tends to rise again, probably because of the absorption of the toxic products of cell necrosis. It is of interest that patients become infectious on the third day of the disease, probably because saliva has been contaminated through the early mucosal lesions noted in the pharynx and mouth. Skin lesions become infective after the superficial corneal layer has been severely damaged. Scabs remain infectious throughout the illness and until their separation during the third to fourth week of illness. The pitting is generally confined to the face, even in severe cases, and is due to destruction of sebaceous glands followed by organization and subsequent shrinking of granulation tissue and fibrosis. In cases of hemorrhagic smallpox numerous blood cells are present in the corium. *Cytoplasmic inclusions* are characteristic of infection with the vaccinia-variola group of viruses. Inclusion bodies can be shown best in epithelial cells, particularly of the involved skin and mucous membranes. Skin scrapings stained with hematoxylin and eosin show the inclusion to be round or oval homogeneous masses, either basophilic or acidophilic, located in the cytoplasm fairly close to the nucleus. The appearance of the inclusion bodies varies with the stage of infection but also with the method of fixation and staining, and this suggests that they consist of masses of elementary bodies. Intranuclear inclusions have also been described but these are not invariably seen. With antimicrobial therapy, pathologic changes from bacterial complications are not found, and bacterial cultures, in this situation, are usually sterile.

Clinical Manifestations. The incubation period of smallpox is generally 12 days. The illness begins with intense malaise and high fever lasting for four to six days. There is intense prostration, and the clinical impression is often that of dengue. Severe headache, photophobia, and, occasionally, vomiting are noted. A small number of patients show a prodromal or "toxemic" rash, most easily noted in the groins, the axillae, and the flanks. On the fourth day the *focal rash* occurs, the fever diminishes slightly, and the patient feels much better, just at a time when the first macular skin lesions begin to form. The focal rash usually occurs first on the mucosa of the mouth and pharynx, the face, or the forearms, and it then spreads to the trunk and legs. A feature of variola is the fact that lesions in any one area are all at the same stage of development, whereas in varicella they are in all stages. The initial rash is macular and quickly becomes papular. Within two days the papules have developed into vesicles and these, within a few hours, become cloudy and pustular. On the eighth or ninth day from the beginning of the rash, drying and crusting begin. From three to four weeks from the onset of the disease, scabs have generally fallen off, leaving pigment-free skin, frequently with some scarring or pitting. The eruption is characteristically more severe on the face and the distal parts of the arms and legs, and least severe over the trunk and abdomen. The groins and axillae may be entirely spared. This centrifugal distribution is distinct from the characteristic rash of varicella, which tends to be centripetal. Lesions are generally found on the palms of the hands and the soles of the feet, a situation uncommonly seen in varicella of childhood, although these parts are often involved in the adult form. Fever generally recurs during the pustular stage, but the temperature returns to normal as the lesions become crusted. The characteristic pustular lesions of smallpox are round, raised, and tense with a tendency to central de-

pression as they begin to dry out. Clinical classification of disease from the mildest form (variola sine eruptione) to *modified,* to *confluent,* to *malignant confluent,* to *hemorrhagic* indicates degrees of severity of smallpox influenced in part by age, state of immunity, and state of hormonal balance. It is of great interest that women within a short time of term, either before or after delivery, tend to have a much more severe disease than those not pregnant.

In cases modified by vaccination or transplacental immunity in the first few months of life, the rash may be scant and the evolution of lesions may be very quick. Regardless of how mild an index case of smallpox may be, the susceptible infected contacts suffer *unmodified* disease, and overlooked early cases are frequently the cause of severe epidemics. Permanent scarring or pitting may result even in the absence of purulent infection of lesions with secondary bacterial pathogens (staphylococci and streptococci) in patients who have deep lesions and serious disease.

In previous years, the bacterial complications were incriminated as the principal cause of death, particularly after the pustular phase had commenced. It is now known that the mortality rate is chiefly related to the amount of virus present in the blood during the viremic phase that occurs in the first two days of the disease before any eruption is noted. It has been shown that if the amount of virus in the blood is so great that the whole blood of the patient in the viremic pre-eruptive phase can be used as the antigen in the complement-fixation test, the patient will surely die, although death may be delayed for nine or ten days. Patients who do die in the first week of illness often show evidence of heart failure and terminal pneumonia. Even in the absence of any antimicrobial therapy, the lungs are often sterile, indicating that the pneumonia is caused by the smallpox virus itself. The majority of deaths occur, however, in the pustular stage toward the end of the second week of the disease. Occasionally an encephalitis has been described that is indistinguishable from that associated with measles, varicella, or smallpox vaccination and tends to occur between the eighth and sixteenth day of disease.

Infection in Utero. No congenital anomalies have been described in infants of mothers infected with smallpox, but abortion is common because of the frequent bleeding that occurs during the toxemic phase. Infection of the fetus in utero may occur during the viremic phase in the mother; if this occurs near the end of pregnancy, the child will show clinical disease within a few days after birth. Infection has also been shown to occur at the time of birth if the disease is still active in the mother. There are two reports of smallpox in babies infected in utero a few days before birth, although the mother showed no signs of the disease (Bancroft, 1904; Lynch, 1932).

Variola Minor. Another form of smallpox, currently of great importance, particularly in South America, is alastrim or variola minor, a mild form of smallpox with a very low mortality rate (Marsden, 1948). Although the virus appears identical in size, by the measurements now available, to that of variola major, the mild clinical course tends to breed true, so that for practical purposes alastrim is a distinct clinical entity. There is complete cross protection for these two infections as there is from vaccinia. The *clinical picture* is similar in the prodromal or pre-eruptive phase to that of variola major, but hemorrhagic and toxic cases are almost never seen. The lesions tend to be more superficial and develop more rapidly; the total illness is shorter than in classic variola major. There may be no secondary fever during the pustular stage and the mortality rate for variola major is about 30 per cent. For example, in 1966, India reported 32,616 cases of the major disease with 9600 deaths.

Differential Diagnosis. Smallpox is easily diagnosed, particularly during an epidemic period. More difficult to diagnose is the first and unsuspected case in those countries where smallpox is not endemic. This is particularly true if the first case is hemorrhagic. In this situation meningococcemia, a bleeding diathesis as a part of a blood dyscrasia, or typhus may be the suspected diagnosis. Very mild smallpox, modified by previous vaccination or alastrim, may be thought to be varicella, a drug eruption, or erythema multiforme. Except after known exposure, the clinical diagnosis cannot be made with certainty during the febrile phase, because the picture is indistinguishable from that of dengue, enteroviral infections and other febrile diseases. In the eruptive phase, the most useful clinical points to remember are (1) the centrifugal distribution of lesions; (2) the fact that in a given area all the lesions are at the same stage of development; (3) the fact that there is a relative progression of eruptions from the face and arms to more recent lesions on the arms or legs; (4) the presence of a severe, febrile, three-day pre-eruptive disease; and, on occasion, (5) a known contact at least 12 days previously.

Laboratory Tests. Laboratory diagnostic procedures are of great value in firmly establishing the diagnosis of smallpox in the first case that appears in a community. These consist of (1) light microscopic or electron microscopic demonstration of viral particles in stained smears of vesicular fluid, (2) serologic demonstration of viral antigen in materials from cutaneous lesions, (3) isolation of virus from such materials, and (4) detection of antibodies in the serum early in the eruptive phase. The results of such tests are particularly helpful in differentiating varioloid from varicella and the hemorrhagic forms of the disease from other conditions (see articles on Varicella and Herpes Zoster). A detailed description of these procedures may be found in the 1969 article by Downie and Kempe.

Treatment. No specific treatment for smallpox is currently available, although a number of promising antiviral drugs are under study. Penicillin and broader-spectrum antimicrobials have been used in the prevention and treatment of bacterial complications. There is suggestive clinical evidence that secondary late bacterial complications, including pneumonia and staphylococcal involvement of skin and bones, are decreased by the use of antimicrobial therapy. But even with such therapy the mortality rates have not been reduced below 25 per cent in most outbreaks of variola major. Good nursing care and maintenance of fluid and electrolyte balance are essential. Convalescent smallpox serum and vaccinia-immune gamma globulin have been used in the treatment of severe cases without any evidence of success. It is possible that in the particular trials made such therapy may have been instituted too late.

Prevention of Smallpox. *Management of Recently Exposed Persons.* The use of vaccinia-immune gamma globulin has been successful in the prophylaxis of smallpox and has reduced the incidence after known contact by 75 per cent in controlled trials (Kempe et al., 1956, 1961). Thiosemicarbazone preparations have shown much greater and more practical promise in prophylaxis (Bauer, 1955, 1967). In the initial large-scale trial over 1100 household contacts were given B-isatin-thiosemicarbazone by mouth, and only three mild cases of smallpox occurred. In a comparable group of contacts who did not receive the drug there were 78 cases of smallpox and 12 deaths. The drug was effective even when given more than six days after exposure and was equally effective in either unvaccinated or previously vaccinated patients. Data from Brazil on prophylaxis of variola minor have confirmed the earlier findings of the efficacy of this drug.

Community Control. The American Public Health Association and the United States Public Health Service have approved steps for the control of smallpox under the following four preventive measures: (1) routine vaccination in infancy, with revaccination at school entry and/or exposure to risk of infection; (2) ensuring available supply of potent vaccine kept below freezing to maintain potency; (3) vaccination with multiple pressure on small area of skin, the deltoid being preferred (no dressing need be applied); and (4) prevention of vaccination of children with eczema, who also should not be allowed to come into contact with recently vaccinated persons.

After revaccination an examination should be made after one week to determine whether the reaction is of a major type (primary or vaccinoid) or equivocal (early or immediate). If the latter, the patient should be revaccinated. If there is no reaction the patient should always be revaccinated.

Control of Infected Persons, Contacts, and Environment. All cases should be reported to the local health authority and patients should be isolated in a hospital until all crusts have disappeared. All oral, nasal, fecal, and urinary discharges and articles associated with patients should be disinfected by burning, high-pressure steam, or boiling. All contacts at home, place of work, or elsewhere should be vaccinated or re-vaccinated with potent lymph and kept under surveillance for 16 days from the time of last contact. Any fever during surveillance calls for prompt isolation until smallpox can be excluded. The patient's source case should be sought assiduously. Adults with chickenpox or patients with hemorrhagic or pustular lesions of the skin need careful review for possible errors in diagnosis.

Epidemic Measures. In an epidemic the measures to be taken are as follows: (1) All cases and suspects should be isolated in hospital until they are no longer infectious. (2) All contacts should be carefully listed, vaccinated, and kept under surveillance for 16 days. (3) By all available methods, there should be a public statement of the situation and all possible contacts should be urged to be vaccinated. Potent vaccine should be provided and arrangements made for early vaccination of inner ring and outer ring contacts. (4) Chemoprophylaxis of contacts with N-methylisatin B-thiosemicarbazone has specific value in decreasing the number of secondary cases. (5) Mass immunization of the entire population of a community or larger area is an emergency measure to be used only when an outbreak has given evidence of material spread.

International Measures. The World Health Organization and countries adjacent to the one in which an outbreak occurs should be notified by telegram of the existence of *any* cases of smallpox. At all times the measures should be enforced that are applicable to ships, aircraft, and land transport arriving from smallpox areas, as specified in International Sanitary Regulations. It should be noted that evidence of a previous attack of smallpox or protection by successful vaccination or revaccination (within a period of three years) is a widely enforced requirement for entry to the United States.

Vaccination versus Chemoprophylaxis. Vaccination remains the best method of prevention for any individual likely to be exposed through travel in smallpox-endemic regions of Asia, Africa, or South America. To be fully effective, successful revaccination every three years, or, better, each year is recommended.

Upon exposure to a case of smallpox, vaccination and revaccination should be supplemented by chemoprophylaxis with methisazone, 3 grams given twice only 12 hours apart. For children three to ten years, 1.5 grams twice only should be given, and for infants under three years, 0.75 grams twice only. Vaccination *after* exposure is generally inadequate to prevent disease, but should be done because subsequent repeat exposures may occur in an epidemic situation. The use of vaccinia-immune gamma globulin also markedly reduces clinical incidence and severity when used in full doses of 10 ml. intramuscularly once for adults, and 5 ml. intramuscularly once for children under 12 years. Vaccinia-immune globulin and methisazone can and should both be given, when available, for a limited number of known contacts, such as may occur in aircraft exposures. A common but harmless side effect of methisazone is emesis. If vomiting occurs less than one hour after the dose, the full dose should be repeated with an antiemetic such as Mavezine or Dramamine. Alcohol is strictly contraindicated because of the similar structure of methisazone and of the antialcoholic Antabuse.

No clinical experience utilizing methisazone as a major antiepidemic chemoprophylactic agent has yet been gained, and primary reliance of WHO and health agencies of member countries in which there is endemic smallpox continues to lie with the mass vaccination programs designed to eliminate the last human reservoir of the disease. When an importation into a smallpox-free country occurs, however, widespread use of simple chemoprophylaxis and, in selected situations, the additional use of vaccinia-immune gamma globulin are indicated. Both agents are effective if given on the last few days of the 12-day inoculation period of smallpox, although vaccination, if effective, must be accomplished almost at once upon known exposure. This is a situation which rarely exists in clinical experience, as the index case is usually infective three to four days before the clinical illness is correctly diagnosed by clinical or laboratory means. This situation holds especially in the occasional imported case into a smallpox-free country.

VACCINIA
(Vaccination)
C. Henry Kempe

Smallpox vaccine commonly in use is prepared from the vaccinia lesions on the skin of inoculated calves or sheep or from the allantoic membranes of chick embryos. All currently used smallpox vaccine contains infective virus, and all successful vaccinations are deliberately induced mild viral infections. It is thought that within one year after primary vaccination the chance of an attack is reduced to one-one thousandth of that in the unvaccinated; within three years, to one-two hundredth; within ten years, to one-eighth; within twenty years, to one-half; and after twenty years there is little if any protection against infection. However, the mortality in smallpox patients successfully vaccinated many years before is less than in the unvaccinated. There is no question that regular revaccination induces a high degree of immunity even to very massive exposure to the disease. Mass vaccination in the remaining endemic areas in Asia, Africa, and South America will, in time, reduce the susceptible population below that necessary to permit the survival of the pathogenic virus.

Recommended Program for Vaccinations in the United States. The situation with regard to smallpox control can be visualized in three time periods. Sometime in the future, perhaps ten years from now, we can look forward to the time when the present eradication program will have eliminated smallpox as a threat to man. At that time, vaccination will no longer be necessary, and jennerian vaccinations will then be a matter of historical importance only. Until this is achieved, however, smallpox vaccination will continue to be necessary for those at risk, namely, travelers to endemic areas and those who by their occupation are likely to come into contact with such travelers. These include hospital personnel and those involved with transportation services, as well as those in the armed forces. Current research efforts are expected to make available new preparations that would confer protection with less danger to the recipient. The most likely approach will be by the use of attenuated strains of vaccinia in a prevaccination procedure.

The author believes that for a child raised in the United States, the use of routine vaccination now far outstrips the risk of future exposure to smallpox, and he favors discontinuation of routine smallpox vaccination in this country. Others believe that the continued increase of travel between the United States and areas of high endemicity requires continuing vaccination. It is realized that the old techniques may have to be changed to compensate for the higher vaccine potency.

Many of the important complications of vaccination occur in those with pre-existing abnormalities; identification of those persons who are most likely to develop significant reactions will eliminate much of the hazard that exists with the present program. As medical contraindications to vaccination are more sharply defined, they should be accepted as legal justifications for nonvaccination. Early treatment of complications with vaccinia-immune gamma globulin in sufficient quantity and with methisazone must be encouraged.

Contraindications to Vaccination. Primary routine vaccination is generally contraindicated in infant patients who fail to thrive, in persons with dysgammaglobulinemia, blood dyscrasias, eczema or other dermatitides, in the presence of radiation or other immunosuppressant therapy, as well as in those exposed to infectious diseases, or in unvaccinated siblings of children with eczema. In the eczematous child, vaccination can be performed safely with attenuated vaccine or under the cover of vaccinia-immune gamma globulin during a period when the skin is relatively clear. If vaccination is performed under these circumstances, it will spare the child the danger of acquiring accidental infection from a sibling or playmate at a time when he is not properly protected.

Vaccination or revaccination is fraught with danger for adult patients with *neoplastic diseases*, including *Hodgkin's disease*, *lymphomas,* and other conditions involving the prolonged use of corticosteroids, nitrogen mustard, or radiation therapy.

When travel outside the limits of the United States to nonendemic areas is contemplated by a person who has an absolute contraindication such as the neoplastic diseases mentioned above, a written statement from a physician indicating why vaccination should not be performed will be considered on return to the United States by the Quarantine Service of the United States Public Health Service. At most, telephonic health surveillance for 14 days after re-entry to the United States may be required. This is much to be preferred to life-threatening disease from vaccination. Vaccination has not been carried out by the Quarantine Service when the patient's physician has presented written evidence that the procedure should not be performed. If such a person must travel to an endemic area, the use of vaccinia-immune gamma globulin or chemoprophylaxis with N-methylisatin beta-thiosemicarbazone should be considered so as to provide temporary protection and act as a substitute for the use of vaccination with live vaccinia virus.

Recommended Vaccination Techniques. To minimize the risk of unnecessary complications, the following practices are recommended:

Age for Primary Vaccination. In nonendemic areas, primary vaccination is either not routinely done or is performed when the child is over two years of age. There are no conclusive data indicating the exact period when complication rates are minimal. The presence of some transplacental maternal immunity, provided that the mother has been vaccinated, may be desirable in modifying the primary vaccination reaction, and vaccination may be carried out in the first months of life. Vaccination of newborn infants has been done without complications (Kempe et al., 1952). However, in such cases in endemic areas, revaccination should be performed after an interval of six months. If primary vaccination is delayed for several months, children who are at increased risk, such as those suffering from the Swiss type of agammaglobulinemia, will have been readily identified by their clinical course and will, therefore, not become casualties of smallpox vaccination. The 1966 experience in the United States fails to show a higher risk of postvaccinia encephalitis for the two to ten age group (Neff et al., 1968), but some European authors have stressed that the first years of life may be a safer period. The case mortality for encephalitis is certainly highest among the youngest children (Berger, 1964; Coneybeare, 1948, 1964; Muller, 1946; Neff, 1968).

Site for Vaccination. Primary vaccination and revaccination are best performed on the outer aspects of the upper arm, over the insertion of the deltoid muscle or behind the midline. Reactions are less likely to be severe on the upper arm than on the lower extremity or other parts of the body. With proper technique, resultant scars are small and unobtrusive.

Preparation of the Vaccination Site. With a clean skin, the best preparation is none at all.

The use of chemical skin cleaners may leave a residue that contains virus-inactivating material, and vigorous physical cleansing of the site may create minute abrasions that then can become sites of secondary vaccinia eruptions, with resultant involvement of a comparatively large skin area.

Vaccination Technique. Regardless of age, routine primary vaccination should be performed with no more than two or three pressures with the side of a needle. These pressure points should be as close together as possible, and should be made only at one site. With the highly potent vaccines currently in use, more numerous pressure points are not necessary and certainly should not be utilized for a nonimmune person. When children or adults are to be revaccinated after a lapse of more than five years, the same small number of pressure points should be used. For revaccination within a five-year period of those persons known to have had a major reaction, the full complement of 30 strokes can safely be used (Leake, 1946).

Vaccination Reaction. The description of the reactions after vaccination or revaccination should follow the criteria recommended by the Expert Committee on Smallpox of the World Health Organization. A successful primary vaccination is one that on examination after seven to ten days presents a typical jennerian vesicle. If this is not present, vaccination must be repeated with fresh vaccine and a few more strokes of the needle. The successful revaccination is one that on examination one week (six to ten days) later shows a vesicular or pustular lesion or an area of definite palpable induration and congestion surrounding a central lesion; this lesion may be a scab or an ulcer. These reactions are termed *major reactions;* all others should be called *equivocal reactions.*

A major reaction indicates virus multiplication with consequent development of immunity. An equivocal reaction may merely represent an allergic response, which could be elicited by inactive vaccine or poor technique in someone who had been sensitized by earlier vaccination; or the equivocal reaction may result from sufficient immunity to prevent virus multiplication. Since the allergic response cannot be readily differentiated from the one caused by true immunity another vaccination should be performed using a different lot of vaccine if there is the possibility that the first was of weak potency, and the procedure should be completed with an additional number of pressures. The site should be examined one week later; if the result is again equivocal, revaccination should be repeated using a full 30 pressures, as recommended by Leake. For the sake of expediency, an equivocal reaction to revaccination with a minimal insertion may be followed by vaccination at two sites, not less than two inches apart, using known potent vaccine. This method will make a third return unnecessary in almost all instances.

In summary, successful smallpox vaccination consists of the production of a major reaction. When potent vaccine and good technique are used, repeated inability to produce a major reaction can be assumed to be due to solid immunity from previous immunization.

Frequency of Vaccination. Revaccination is essential to reinforce the immunity conferred by previous vaccination. This not only maintains a high level of immunity against smallpox, but minimizes the risk of complications on revaccination. To maintain adequate immunity against smallpox, revaccination should be carried out at approximately five-year intervals. Those persons at some increased risk, such as hospital personnel and public health personnel, members of the armed forces, and those working at port or airline offices as well as shipping personnel should be revaccinated at least once every three years. When exposure to smallpox is probable, by travel or residence in a smallpox-endemic area, annual revaccination is desirable.

Complications of Vaccination. The true state of complications in the United States is not known and is confused by the inclusion of more severe primary reactions among the complications. Complications are not reportable diseases through any of the usual state health department methods. Life-threatening complications of primary vaccination include eczema vaccinatum, postvaccinial encephalitis, and vaccinia gangrenosa (progressive vaccinia). The prinicpal danger after revaccination is *vaccinia gangrenosa*, a condition in which the impairment of the patient's immune mechanism permits the continuing multiplication of the vaccinia virus. Vaccinia gangrenosa is seen in seemingly normal subjects as well as in those suffering from dysgammaglobulinemia, Hodgkin's disease, leukemia, blood dyscrasias, and other conditions in which corticosteroid therapy or ionized irradiation have been administered therapeutically. The presence of these conditions is an absolute contraindication to vaccination. Human vaccinia-immune globulin, readily available on telephone request to the American Red Cross, has frequently been shown to be effective in the prevention and treatment of eczema vaccinatum and has also been used extensively in the treatment of other complications in which it also produces a significant reduction in mortality. Vaccinia-immune globulin reduces the incidence of postvaccinial encephalitis. In the Royal Netherland Army 53,630 of 106,174 recruits received hyperimmune vaccinia-immune gamma globulin, and the remaining 52,544 recruits received placebo. In the group treated with gamma globulin, 3 cases of postvaccinial encephalitis occurred in contrast to 13 cases in the control group. There was one fatality in each group. Gamma globulin failed to have a major effect on the severity and duration of the encephalitis produced by the vaccination, and it was not effective in treatment. There is evidence that transplacental maternal immunity is also effective in modifying the course of primary vaccination;

significant reactions are rarely reported in very young infants whose mothers have been vaccinated in the past. In cases of vaccinia gangrenosa, the simultaneous use of vaccinia-immune globulin and N-methylisatin beta-thiosemicarbazone appears to be of value. The therapeutic dose of the drug is 200 mg. per kilogram orally initially, followed by 50 mg. per kilogram every six hours for three days. After a rest of three days, another three-day course may be required.

Adequate early treatment of the complications of smallpox vaccination can materially reduce the morbidity and mortality. Through the American Red Cross a group of experts is available for telephone consultation. When such consultation is used in conjunction with vaccinia-immune globulin and chemotherapeutic agents, effective diagnostic and therapeutic aids are available for all.

We in the United States are now in an interim period with regard to smallpox prophylaxis. The areas of the globe where the smallpox is endemic are gradually being diminished. A number of changes in vaccination practice are indicated to avoid unnecessary complications. The risk of vaccinia complications can be reduced by a more gentle vaccination technique, and by the recognition (and legal acceptance) of additional medical contraindications that will help to eliminate many of the opportunities for development of complications. It is likely that an attenuated live vaccinia virus will soon be available for prevaccination in an effort to make possible safe immunization for those who require it. For the rest, as indicated above, in the writer's judgment, routine primary vaccination could be discontinued.

Bauer, D. J., St. Vincent, L., Kempe, C. H., Young, P. A., and Downie, A. W.: Prophylaxis of smallpox with methisazone. Amer. J. Epidem., 90:130, 1969.

Downie, A. W., and Kemp, C. H.: Variola and vaccinia viruses. In Lennette, E. H. (ed.): Diagnostic Procedures for Viral and Rickettsial Diseases. New York, American Public Health Association, 1969, Chap. 25.

Do Valle, L. A. R., De Melo, P. R., De Salles Gomes, L. F., and Proença, I. M.: Methisazone in prevention of variola minor among contacts. Lancet, 2:976, 1965.

Kempe, C. H., et al.: The use of vaccinia hyperimmune gamma globulin in the prophylaxis of smallpox. Bull. WHO, 25:41, 1961.

Kempe, C. H., et al.: Smallpox vaccination of eczema patients with a strain of attenuated live vaccinia (CVI-78). Pediatrics 42:980, 1968.

Neff, J. M., Lane, J. M., Pert, J. H., Moore, R., Miller, J. D., and Henderson, D. A.: Complications of smallpox vaccination. I. National Survey in the United States, 1963. New Eng. J. Med., 276:125, 1967.

WHO Expert Committee on Smallpox: Second Report, Publication 393, World Health Organization Technical Report Series. Geneva, World Health Organization, 1968.

For more detailed lists of references, see the following:

Dixon, C. W.: Smallpox, London, J. & A. Churchill, Ltd., 1962.

Downie, A. W.: Smallpox. In Horsfall, F. L., Jr., and Tamm, I. (eds.): Viral and Rickettsial Infections of Man. 4th ed. Philadelphia, J. B. Lippincott Company, 1965.

ORF

(Ecthyma Contagiosum, Contagious Pustular Dermatitis)

Clayton E. Wheeler

Orf is a worldwide viral infection of sheep and goats that is occasionally transmitted to the skin of man. The disorder occurs most often in sheepherders and shearers, meat porters, butchers, veterinarians, technicians engaged in vaccine manufacture, and children or adults caring for pet lambs.

The virus is a round-ended, brick-shaped particle that measures 260 by 160 mμ and is classified with the paravaccinia viruses. Inoculation into the glabrous skin of sheep produces erythematous macules in three or four days, followed by pustular, granulomatous, papillomatous, and crusted phases. Healing occurs in four to six weeks. Infected animals show crusted, warty, or granulomatous lesions about the lips, nose, and eyelids that have occasioned the term "scabby mouth." The agent proliferates in primary tissue cultures of human amnion, monkey kidney, and bovine testis, in which a characteristic appearance is produced. Neutralizing and complement-fixing antibodies have been demonstrated in the blood of recovered animals and man.

Human lesions are usually single and appear most often on the hands, fingers, forearms, or face. There is often a history of trauma at the site of the lesion, followed in four to eleven days by the appearance of a red macule or papule. In a week or two this becomes a multiloculated vesicle from which little fluid can be expressed upon incision. In the next two weeks the surface becomes white and sodden, a crust usually forms, and a granulomatous reaction often develops. Healing takes place with little or no scar formation in four to six weeks. Mature lesions are 1 to 4 cm. in diameter, elevated, dome-shaped, plateau or tumor-like, and well-demarcated from normal skin. Regional lymphangitis or lymphadenopathy may occur as part of the viral infection or as a result of secondary bacterial involvement. Erythema multiforme is an uncommon complication.

Microscopically, proliferation, ballooning, and reticular degeneration of epidermal cells, multilocular vesiculation, and pseudoepitheliomatous hyperplasia may be found. A granulomatous reaction is present in the dermis.

Treatment is symptomatic and directed toward prevention or cure of secondary bacterial infection. Vaccination with live virus provides effective control in animals but it is not practicable in man.

Leavell, U. W., Jr., McNamara, M. J., Muelling, R., Talbert, W. M., Rucker, R. C., and Dalton, A. J.: Orf: Report of 19 human cases. J.A.M.A., 204:657, 1968.

Nagington, J., Newton, A. A., and Horne, R. W.: The structure of orf virus. Virology, 23:461, 1964.

Nagington, J., and Whittle, C. H.: Human orf. Isolation of the virus by tissue culture. Brit. Med. J., 2:1324, 1961.
Peters, D., Müller, G., and Büttner, D.: The fine structure of paravaccinia viruses. Virology, 23:609, 1964.

MOLLUSCUM CONTAGIOSUM
Clayton E. Wheeler

Molluscum contagiosum is an infection of the skin, and occasionally of the conjunctiva, with the largest of the true animal viruses. The viral particle is oval or brick-shaped and measures approximately 300 by 220 mμ. It does not grow in the skin or cornea of animals or in tissues of the chick embryo, and its growth in tissue culture is questionable, although a cytopathic effect occurs, and interferon production is induced. Experimental inoculation of ground, filtered molluscum material into human skin is followed by a new lesion at the inoculation site in 14 to 50 days. Studies of immunity are fragmentary, although there is suggestive evidence for the development of complement-fixing antibodies and cutaneous sensitivity of the delayed type.

The pathologic change is confined to the epidermis, which grows into the dermis as multiple, closely packed, pear-shaped globules. Epidermal cells undergo characteristic degeneration as they progress from the basal layer to the surface, where they form a cavity at the center of the growth. Cellular degeneration is produced by intracytoplasmic growth of viral particles that form huge inclusions. These enlarge and distort the cell and crowd the nucleus to one side. Inclusions contain large amounts of deoxyribonucleic acid and stain deeply with hematoxylin and eosin.

This common disorder is worldwide and usually affects children. The disease is autoinoculable and mildly contagious, but the source of the infection and method of spread are often unknown.

Lesions are most often seen on the trunk, face, arms, or genital areas, although they occur almost anywhere. Conjunctival infection may result in epiphora, discharge, conjunctivitis, or keratitis. Lesions may be solitary, few and localized, numerous and generalized, or eruptive in association with atopic dermatitis or immunosuppressive therapy. They vary in size from barely visible to 0.5 cm. or larger. They are usually discrete, but they may be grouped or form plaques or tumor-like masses. Characteristic papules are skin-colored or slightly pink, pearly, circumscribed, elevated, firm, rounded, or semiglobular, and present central umbilication from which a curdlike material can be expressed. Inflammation is usually absent, but it may develop from irritation or secondary infection. Systemic infection with the virus is unknown.

The clinical appearance of the papules and the expression of a gelatinous central core usually suffice for diagnosis. The microscopic picture is diagnostic. Molluscum contagiosum is most often confused with nevi, warts, epithelioma, pyogenic granuloma, folliculitis, and other forms of pyo-

derma. Cure can usually be accomplished by curettage or light electrodesiccation. Spontaneous involution is not uncommon.

Blattner, R. J., Jr.: Molluscum contagiosum: Eruptive infection in atopic dermatitis. J. Pediat., 70:997, 1967.
Friedman-Kien, A. E., and Vilček, J.: Induction of interference and interferon synthesis by non-replicating molluscum contagiosum virus. J. Immun., 99:1092, 1967.
Sutton, J. S., and Burnett, J. W.: Ultrastructural changes in dermal and epidermal cells of skin infected with molluscum contagiosum virus. J. Ultrastruct. Res., 26:177, 1969.

WARTS

See Certain Cutaneous Diseases with Significant Systemic Manifestations.

VIRAL DISEASES THAT MAY INVOLVE THE CENTRAL NERVOUS SYSTEM

RABIES
(Hydrophobia, Lyssa)
Hilary Koprowski

Definition. Rabies is an acute infectious disease of the central nervous system to which all warm-blooded animals and man are susceptible. The virus, frequently present in the saliva of an infected host, is usually transmitted by bites or licks. The disease is characterized by a profound dysfunction of the central nervous system and ends almost invariably in death.

History. Rabies is one of the oldest diseases of man. First mention of it dates to the twenty-third century B.C., when it was referred to in the pre-Mosaic Eshunna Code. Democritus and Aristotle recognized rabies as a disease of animals, and Celsus described the transmissibility of the disease to man. Rabies, as a disease of wild animals, was known in Europe as early as the thirteenth century. In the eighteenth century epizootics among domestic animals were noted in urban centers. The earliest report of rabies in the Americas dates back to the sixteenth century when Petrus Martyr Angelicus, the first Bishop of the New World, observed rabies as a bat-transmitted disease fatal to man. Descriptions of the disease were also recorded in the Colony of Virginia in 1753. Since that time, its presence has been evidenced throughout the North and South American continents.

The transmission of rabies from the saliva of a rabid dog to a normal dog was first recounted by Zinke in 1809; in 1879 Galtier described the susceptibility of rabbits to rabies and their use for diagnostic purposes. The modern concept of the disease was developed by Pasteur and his associates (1881). They not only identified the causative agent, but also were able to adapt it to laboratory animals, and thereby modified the pathogenic properties of the virus (1884).

Etiology, Host Range, and Experimental Infection. Virus recovered in nature, the so-called *street virus*, is characterized by extremely variable, usually long incubation periods and by its ability to invade salivary glands as well as central nervous tissue. The term *fixed virus* is used for strains of rabies that have been adapted to laboratory animals by means of serial intracerebral passages. Fixed virus is characterized by a short incubation period (usually four to six days) and by its apparent inability to multiply in salivary glands. Prolonged cultivation of some strains of rabies virus in the developing chick embryo or in tissue culture has resulted in modification to the point of complete loss of pathogenicity for animals injected extraneurally.

The physicochemical properties of the virus are shown in Table 1. In addition, the virus is readily inactivated by sunlight, ultraviolet irradiation, formalin, 50 to 70 per cent alcohol, and 0.1 to 1.0 per cent quaternary ammonium compounds, bichloride of mercury, and strong acids. It is relatively resistant to phenol. In aqueous solution, its thermal death point is reached at 56° C. after an exposure of one hour. It survives desiccation from the frozen state, and rabies-infected tissue may be stored successfully at 4° C. in 50 per cent glycerol saline or kept frozen at temperatures below 20° C.

All warm-blooded animals are susceptible to rabies. It is principally a disease of mammals, including bats. The virus is also pathogenic for birds, but to a lesser degree than for mammals. As far as we know, the disease is not transmissible by insects or arthropods. It has been found in all parts of the world, in all climates and seasons. The virus cannot invade the body through intact skin, and is apparently harmless when ingested; however, infection through unabraded mucosa seems possible. An air-borne infection occurring in caves inhabited by rabid bats has been described.

Rabbits, guinea pigs, mice, and hamsters are most commonly employed for experimental infection. Hamsters are remarkably susceptible to intramuscular infection with street virus, but intracerebral injection of mice is usually employed for diagnostic purposes.

Epidemiology and Epizootiology. Rabies is enzootic in many areas of the world in such wild animals as wolves (Arctic regions of Canada, Eastern Europe, Turkey, Iran); mongooses (South Africa, the Caribbean); bats (Central and South America, the United States and Europe); and foxes, coyotes, and skunks (United States). In the urban type, a number of domestic animals, including cows and cats, may become involved, but the propagation of the virus in dogs is mostly responsible for the epizootics. After the elimination of canine rabies, the disease rarely persists in urban areas.

Epizootics of rabies occur in any climate during any season of the year. Wars and mass movements of men and animals favor the geographic spread of the disease. Man becomes an accidental host upon exposure to the infected saliva of the biting animal, and although wild animals are often sources of human rabies, dogs are mostly responsible for human infection. The attack rate in man, following exposure, depends to a certain extent on the location and on the severity of the inflicted wounds. Head and neck bites lead to a higher incidence of infection than bites on other parts of the body. The bites of rabid wolves are apparently very dangerous; an attack rate of 47 per cent was observed in 32 persons who were bitten by the same animal and did not receive antirabies treatment.

Pathology. At autopsy, the brain is friable, edematous, and congested; the convolutions are broad and flattened. Severe vascular congestion of the white and gray matter may extend to the medulla and the spinal cord. Virus-infected salivary glands are usually soft and swollen. On microscopic examination of the central nervous system, the nonspecific findings consist of hyperemia, perivascular and perineuronal infiltration with mononuclear cells, and considerable neuronal degeneration. Mononuclear cell infiltration of periacinal interstitial tissue accompanied by degeneration of acinar cells may be observed in the parotid and sublingual and submaxillary salivary glands.

If proper staining technique, such as Sellers' method, is applied, intracytoplasmic inclusion bodies can be demonstrated in the neurons of the majority of rabies cases. These so-called *Negri bodies* are ribonucleoproteins, pathognomonic for rabies encephalitis. In the absence of Negri bodies, the lesions are indistinguishable from those observed in other viral encephalitides.

In experimental infection of animals or tissue culture cells, lysis of the infected cells is generally *not* observed. Thus the nature of rabies virus-host cell interaction remains obscure.

Incubation. The incubation period in man varies from ten days to over twelve months. As minor and seemingly insignificant contacts with rabies virus in the saliva of an animal not obviously sick at the time of exposure are sometimes forgotten, claims of extended incubation periods (one to two years) have to be critically evaluated. In dogs, signs of rabies may appear after an incubation period of ten days to several months.

The length of the incubation period is related to the amount of virus introduced at the time of exposure and to the severity of the laceration. The site of the original exposure does not seem to affect the duration of the incubation period.

TABLE 1. PHYSICOCHEMICAL PROPERTIES OF RABIES VIRUS

Shape and size	Bullet-shaped; 180 × 75 m. (some particles are shorter)
Sedimentation coefficient	600 S
Buoyant density in sucrose solution	1.17
Chemical composition	Ribonucleoprotein; the viral coat contains lipids
Specific activities	PFU*/mg. protein: 1×10^{10} HAU†/mg. protein: 1×10^4 CFU‡/mg. protein: 5×10^3
Viral RNA	Sedimentation coefficient 50 S, corresponding to molecular weight of 6×10^6 daltons; single-stranded
Viral protein	Seven major and five minor polypeptide components

*PFU = Plaque-forming units.
†HAU = Hemagglutinating units.
‡CFU = Complement-fixing units.

Clinical Manifestations. *Dogs.* In dogs the prodromal phase of the disease lasts two to three days and consists of fever, anorexia, and, very frequently, a change in the tone of the bark. However, these signs are often so slight that only a trained observer may note them. The animal's disposition is altered, and symptoms give way to the excitation phase, usually lasting three to seven days, during which time the animal grows unnaturally restless and agitated. General tremor owing to stimulation of the muscular system appears frequently. In the furious type of the disease, agitation intensifies as the illness progresses. The animal, erratic and aggressive, growls and barks constantly. It will grab viciously at any object or animal encountered. At this stage, an unrestrained animal sometimes leaves home and travels great distances, inflicting damage on other animals and humans along the way. Convulsive seizures are often observed, and the animal may become completely paralyzed. In many cases, however, the excitation phase predominates until the time of death.

In the paralytic type of rabies, the excitation phase may be slight or totally absent, and the disease is characterized only by the paralytic syndrome. Paralysis of the lower jaw, accompanied by excessive salivation, appears as an early symptom, and the animal acts as though it is choking on a foreign body. Paralysis of the muscles of phonation may lead to loss of the bark. As the disease progresses, paralysis of the posterior extremities sets in, followed by general paralysis and death. The time from the onset of the disease to the death of the animal ranges from one to eleven days. On the other hand, dogs may die suddenly without noticeable signs of illness.

Man. In man, the prodromal phase is marked by fever, anorexia, headache, malaise, nausea, and sore throat. *Abnormal sensations around the site of infection,* such as intermittent pain, tingling, or burning, are of diagnostic significance. Extreme stimulation of the general sensory system is manifested by hyperesthesia of the skin to temperature changes and to drafts, and by acute sensitiveness to sound and light. Other symptoms include increased muscular tonus, prompt gag and corneal reflexes, dilation of pupils, and increased salivation.

As the disease progresses, spasmodic contractions of the muscles of the mouth, pharynx, and larynx on drinking — and later at the mere sight of fluid — are observed in the majority of cases. This dysfunction of deglutition gave the disease its common name, *hydrophobia,* or fear of water. Spasms of respiratory muscles and convulsive seizures leading to opisthotonos also may occur. The pulse is very rapid. Periods of irrational and often maniacal behavior are interspersed with those of alertness and responsiveness. Paralysis of the muscles of phonation may lead to hoarseness or loss of voice.

The excitation phase may remain predominant until the time of death. However, in many cases it gives way shortly before death to cessation of muscle spasms, hyporeflexia or areflexia, and to general paralysis of the flaccid type.

In rabies in man *resulting from vampire bat infection,* the excitation phase is almost totally absent, and the disease is characterized by ascending paralysis without hydrophobia. Without an adequate history of exposure, this type is indistinguishable from other viral encephalitides, and the diagnosis may be overlooked.

Diagnosis. Profound dysfunction of the central nervous system accompanied by impairment in deglutition, following a history of exposure to a bite or lick of an animal, or any type of exposure to bats, facilitates the clinical diagnosis. Isolation of virus from saliva obtained in the course of the disease and from brain tissue obtained at autopsy, followed by proper identification of the agent by means of neutralization test, will confirm the diagnosis. Syrian hamsters, rabbits, guinea pigs, and mice are used for diagnostic purposes. Demonstration of rabies virus particles in brain tissue smears by means of specific staining with antibody coupled with fluorescein isothiocyanate is of diagnostic significance. The presence of Negri bodies is pathognomonic, but their absence does not exclude the diagnosis of rabies encephalitis, as the presence of virus may be demonstrated by other means.

Prognosis. Although inapparent infection with street virus may be induced artificially in laboratory animals, and although animals have recovered completely after exhibiting signs of the disease, *there is no proved instance of the recovery of man from rabies.*

Postexposure Treatment. A treatment for rabies does not exist in the strict sense of the word, for there are no therapeutic measures available that would save the life of a person exhibiting symptoms of the disease. *A protective type of treatment* can be used following exposure to the virus and prior to the development of the disease. The protective treatment, particularly in a rabies endemic area and adjacent territory, has to be based on the assumption that every animal inflicting a wound on a human may be rabid, until proved otherwise by clinical observation or by failure to discover virus in its tissues after death.

Local Treatment of Wounds. All bite wounds, as well as scratches and other skin abrasions exposed to licks of animals, should be treated immediately by thorough cleansing and adequate mechanical flushing of the wound with soap solution or with cationic detergents such as benzalkonium chloride (Zephiran Bayer) or cetrimonium bromide (Cetavlon ICI) in 1 per cent solution. Other rabicidal quaternary ammonium compounds or 50 to 70 per cent solution of alcohol are also effective in the local treatment. If debridement is necessary, infiltration with local anesthetics is not contraindicated. Bite wounds should *not* be sutured immediately.

Preliminary application of antimicrobial drugs is of no value as a prophylactic measure. However, antitetanus treatment and local application of antiseptics and antimicrobials should be instituted if indicated.

Indications for Specific Treatment. These are summarized in Table 2, prepared by the Expert Committee on Rabies of the World Health Organization. Emphasis is placed on the condition of the biting animal at the time of the exposure and during the ensuing ten days. It is assumed that the saliva of an animal that is not obviously ill at the time of exposure may be infectious during a maximal period of five days preceding the appearance of clinical signs of the disease.

Passive-Active Immunization. Passive-active immunization by the administration of antirabies serum and immunogenically potent vaccine in repeated doses is the most effective protective treatment of the exposed human being. Because of the existence of various vaccine preparations, no emphasis is placed on the use of any special type of vaccine, provided it meets the standard potency requirement.

Administration of Preventive Treatment. The administration of preventive treatment may give rise to local allergic reactions, to serum sickness (if combined serum-vaccine therapy was used), and to nervous system reactions caused by the presence of nervous tissue in most of the vaccines. These occur most frequently during a repeated course of protective treatment. Treatment should be interrupted if signs of dysfunction of the central or peripheral nervous system are observed. *Avian embryo vaccines* and vaccines prepared from brains of suckling mice, rats, or rabbits apparently free of paralysis-inducing properties have recently been used for preventive treatment in man. Many problems can be avoided if treatment is given only when specifically indicated (Table 2). All courses of vaccine should include booster doses at 10 *and* 20 or more days after the regular course of vaccine.

Prevention. Effective immunization, preferably with avian embryo vaccine, is important for persons engaged in veterinary practice, experimental surgery involving handling of dogs and cats, spelunking, dog catching, or any activity involving unusually high risk of exposure.

Control Measures. Although the presence of rabies-infected bats in the United States introduces new problems, most human exposures can

TABLE 2. GUIDE FOR SPECIFIC POSTEXPOSURE TREATMENT OF RABIES

Nature of Exposure	Biting Animal*		Recommended Treatment† (In Addition to Local Treatment)
	At Time of Exposure	During Observation Period of Ten Days	
I. No lesion; indirect contact	Rabid	—	None
II. Licks:			
(1) Unabraded skin	Rabid	—	None
(2) Abraded skin, scratches, and unabraded or abraded mucosa	(a) Healthy	Clinical signs of rabies or proved rabid (laboratory)	Start vaccine[1] at first signs of rabies in the biting animal
	(b) Signs suggestive of rabies	Healthy	Start vaccine immediately; stop treatment if animal is normal on fifth day after exposure
	(c) Rabid, escaped, killed, or unknown	—	Start vaccine[1] immediately
III. Bites:			
(1) Mild exposure	(a) Healthy	Clinical signs of rabies or proven rabid (laboratory)	Start vaccine[1,2] at first signs of rabies in the biting animal
	(b) Signs suggestive of rabies	Healthy	Start vaccine immediately; stop treatment if animal is normal on fifth day after exposure
	(c) Rabid, escaped, killed, or unknown	—	Start vaccine[1,2] immediately
	(d) Wild (wolf, jackal, fox, bat, etc.)	—	Serum[2] immediately, followed by a course of vaccine‡
(2) Severe exposure (multiple, or face, head, finger, or neck bites)	(a) Healthy	Clinical signs of rabies or proven rabid (laboratory)	Serum[2] immediately; start vaccine‡ at first sign of rabies in the biting animal
	(b) Signs suggestive of rabies	Healthy	Serum[2] immediately, followed by vaccine; vaccine may be stopped if animal is normal on fifth day after exposure
	(c) Rabid, escaped, killed or unknown	—	Serum[2] immediately; followed by vaccine‡
	(d) Wild (wolf, jackal, fox, bat, pariah dog, etc.)		

*This schedule applies equally whether or not the biting animal has been previously vaccinated.

†See Explanatory Notes.

‡Course of vaccine to be followed by supplemental doses of vaccine of non-nervous tissue if possible, 10 and 20 days after the last usual dose.

be prevented by the use of control measures that will rid an area of enzootics or epizootics of rabies.

The following measures should be applied in an efficiently organized rabies control program conducted by public health authorities: control of the canine population (registration, restraint, elimination of stray dogs), reduction in number of susceptible dogs by mass vaccination, reduction in number of wildlife species that are a reservoir of the virus, and continuous educational campaigns for the general public.

Explanatory Notes to the Guide. 1. *Vaccine.* Practice varies concerning the volume of vaccine per dose and the number of doses recommended in a given situation. In general, the equivalent of at least 2 ml. of a 5 per cent tissue emulsion should be given subcutaneously daily for 14 consecutive days. Many laboratories use 20 to 30 doses in severe exposures. The Committee feels so strongly concerning the effect of booster doses in producing and maintaining high levels of serum-neutralizing antibodies that it now recommends booster doses at 10 days and 20 or more days following the last daily dose of vaccine in *all* cases. This is especially important in order to overcome the interference effect if antirabies serum has been used. (See Expert Committee on Rabies, section 6.4.)

2. *Antirabies serum or its globulin fractions.* In all severe exposures and in all cases of unprovoked wild animal bites, antirabies serum or its globulin fractions together with vaccine should be employed. This is considered by the Committee as the *best* specific treatment available for the postexposure prophylaxis of rabies in man. Although experience indicates that vaccine alone is sufficient for mild exposures, there is no doubt that here also the combined serum-vaccine treatment will give the best protection. However, both the serum and the vaccine can cause deleterious reactions and the combined therapy is more expensive, so its use in mild exposures is considered optional. As with vaccine alone, it is important to start combined serum and vaccine treatment as early as possible after exposure, but serum should still be used regardless of the time interval. Serum should be given in a single dose (40 International Units per kilogram of body weight), and the first dose of vaccine should be inoculated at the same time. Sensitivity to the serum must be determined before its administration.

3. *Special situations.* It is fully recognized that Table 2 is only a guide and in certain situations specific conditions may warrant modifications, e.g., exposure, especially in young children or when a reliable history cannot be obtained, and particularly in areas where rabies is known to be enzootic even though the animal at the time of exposure is considered to be healthy. Such cases may justify treatment immediately in a modified way. Possible modifications would be that, following local treatment of the wound as described above, a single dose of serum or three doses of vaccine at daily intervals be given and no further

vaccine be administered as long as the animal stays healthy for 10 days following exposure.

Another example of a local situation in which a modified interpretation of these recommendations may be indicated is that of rabies-free areas where frequent exposures to animal bites are encountered. In areas where rabies is endemic, adequate laboratory and field experience indicating no infection in the species involved may justify the local health authorities in recommending no specific antirabies treatment.

Expert Committee on Rabies, Fifth Report. WHO Techn. Rep. Ser., No. 321, 1966.

Johnson, H. N.: Rabies. *In* Horsfall, F. L., Jr., and Tamm, I. (eds.): Viral and Rickettsial Infections of Man. 4th ed. Philadelphia, J. B. Lippincott Company, 1965.

Hummeler, K., and Koprowski, H.: Investigating the rabies virus. Nature, 221:418, 1969.

Laboratory Techniques in Rabies. 2nd ed. Geneva, World Health Organization, 1966.

Tierkel, E. S.: Rabies. *In* Advances in Veterinary Science, Vol. 5. New York, Academic Press. Inc., 1959, p. 183.

MUMPS
Dorothy M. Horstmann

Definition. Mumps is an acute contagious viral infection, most commonly manifested by nonsuppurative swelling of the parotid glands. Other salivary glands, the testes, pancreas, and central nervous system are among the various organs that may also be involved.

Historical Note. Hippocrates described mumps in the fifth century B.C. Because of its characteristic manifestations, it was one of the earliest diseases to be recognized as a clinical entity. A classic description was written by Hamilton (1790), who was the first to stress the importance of orchitis as a complication. He also noted that central nervous system signs sometimes accompany the parotitis, but it was early in the twentieth century before clinicians recognized meningoencephalitis as a relatively frequent manifestation. In 1940 Wesselhoeft called attention to the occurrence of oophoritis and pancreatitis, and later others reported involvement of many organs and tissues. Not until 1934 did Johnson and Goodpasture prove the viral etiology of mumps by reproducing the disease in monkeys inoculated with filtrates of infective human saliva. The virus was adapted to growth in hens' eggs in 1945 by Habel, and by Levens and Enders, who demonstrated its hemagglutinating properties. Enders and his associates also described the appearance of dermal hypersensitivity and of complement-fixing (CF) antibodies following mumps. The availability of a skin test and of serologic tools allowed the demonstration that infection with mumps virus can occur without parotitis and not infrequently without any signs at all. Immunization with a killed virus vaccine was tried in the 1950's with limited success. In 1966 Bunyak and Hilleman developed a highly effective live attenuated mumps virus vaccine, prepared in chick embryo tissue culture, which is currently widely used.

Etiology. Mumps is an RNA virus, a member of the myxovirus family that includes the influenza and parainfluenza viruses. These agents all have the property of agglutinating chicken, human, and other erythrocytes. In monkeys, mumps virus induces parotitis, and in suckling mice or hamsters it may cause fatal meningoencephalitis. The virus multiplies in embryonated chick embryos and in a variety of tissue culture cells. For primary isolation (usually from saliva), eggs or preferably cell cultures derived from monkeys or humans are used. In tissue cultures the presence of the virus is recognized either by the appearance of cytopathic changes or by means of the hemadsorption test, which depends on the ability of the virus-infected cells to adsorb guinea pig erythrocytes. In infected cultures these are seen firmly attached to the cell sheet, whereas in control tubes the erythrocytes float in the media. The specificity of the reaction is established serologically, using the hemadsorption inhibition test. Mumps virus is associated with soluble (S) and viral (V) complement-fixing (CF) antigens and a skin test antigen. Infection induces CF, hemagglutination-inhibiting, and neutralizing antibodies.

Epidemiology. Mumps is a common disease, endemic all over the world. It occurs throughout the year, but there is a seasonal prevalence, with a regular increase in cases in winter and spring. Epidemics are frequent, large outbreaks tending to have a seven- or eight-year cycle. The disease incidence is the same in both sexes, but males are more prone to develop central nervous system complications. Most cases occur between the ages of 5 and 15 years; young adults are nevertheless sometimes susceptible, as evidenced by epidemics in military camps and schools.

The only known reservoir of infection is man. In experiments in volunteers, Henle et al. showed that the virus may be present in the saliva from two to six days before the occurrence of parotid swelling, and as long as seven to nine days after onset. *Transmission* is thought to be by direct contact, air-suspended droplets, or fomites contaminated with saliva. Rather more solid contact appears to be necessary for transmission of mumps than is the case with measles or chickenpox.

Although it is a common disease, only about 60 per cent of the adult population gives a positive history, in contrast to more than 90 per cent for measles. The difference is due in part to the frequency of inapparent infection with mumps virus. About 50 per cent of those with a negative history give a positive serologic test, indicating previous silent infection. One experience with mumps virus appears to confer lifelong immunity.

Pathogenesis and Pathology. The widespread involvement of glandular and other tissues in the body indicates that mumps is a systemic infection. The virus apparently enters and multiplies first in the upper respiratory tract; it then invades the blood stream, localizes in the salivary as well as other glands, and in the central nervous system. The parotids are one of many target organs, the greater frequency with which they are involved being simply a reflection of greater sensitivity.

Limited observations on pathologic specimens indicate that the reaction in the parotid gland is a nonspecific inflammatory one, which is not extensive. The testes and pancreas also demonstrate inflammatory and degenerative changes. Lesions induced by the virus in the central nervous system are uncertain, because in the few cases that have terminated fatally the findings have been those of postinfectious encephalomyelitis.

Clinical Manifestations. The incubation period is 17 to 21 days, usually 18; extremes of 12 and 35 days have been reported. In most cases, pain and swelling in the parotid region are the first signs of the disease, although occasionally in adults pain in the testicle may be the initial symptom. Rarely, meningitis appears first, followed later by parotitis. In more severe cases, there is often a prodromal period, sometimes lasting as long as two or three days, with fever, malaise, headache, chills, sore throat, earache, and tenderness along the region of the parotid ducts.

Parotid swelling is first observed below the ear, usually obliterating the hollow between the mastoid process and the ascending ramus of the lower jaw. The gland increases in size over a two- to three-day period, but there is great variation in the degree of swelling; in mild cases it may be scarcely apparent, but in severe ones the associated edema may eventually spread superiorly to the eyes, posteriorly to the mastoid region, and inferiorly below the chin and over the anterior aspect of the neck. For the first two days, unilateral involvement is the rule, but eventually both glands are affected in about 70 per cent of cases. The skin over the swollen parotids is not usually reddened, but is tense and tender on pressure. Not infrequently the submaxillary and sublingual glands are also affected. Involvement of the sublingual glands can result in swelling of the tongue, with attendent painful swallowing. Presternal pitting edema is also occasionally present, apparently because of obstruction of the lymphatics by the enlarged salivary glands.

The patient seldom suffers severe pain except on movement of the jaws, e.g., in talking or chewing. If Stensen's duct becomes partially occluded as the gland swells, there is sharp pain on taking food or an acid drink, which stimulates the secretory mechanism. Because this occurs only with partial occlusion of the duct, it is not a constant sign. The papillae at the opening of Stensen's or Wharton's duct may be reddened, but this also is inconstant.

Constitutional symptoms vary greatly and may be virtually absent. They are especially mild in children, but tend to be more severe in adults, in whom the incidence of extraparotid lesions is higher. Fever varies with the extent of involvement, ranging between 101 and 103° F. in full blown, uncomplicated cases, but going as high as 105 and 106° F. if orchitis, meningoencephalitis, or both develop.

The duration of parotid swelling and fever is dependent upon the extent and severity of the process. Usually the temperature is normal within five days, and swelling has disappeared by seven to ten days. A peculiar tendency to relapse with recurrence of parotid swelling has been noted in buglers, horn players, and others whose occupations involve similar exertion.

Neurologic Manifestations. The incidence of

aseptic meningitis varies widely in different epidemics, but can be as high as 25 per cent. Serial examination of the cerebrospinal fluid indicates that the cell count is elevated in approximately one half of all cases of mumps. Clinically evident neurologic involvement may occur preceding, simultaneously with, or following parotitis. It affects males three to five times more commonly than females, and may be the only manifestation of the infection. The clinical picture of headache, fever, stiff neck, and lethargy is similar to that in other forms of viral meningitis, but the cerebrospinal fluid findings differ in several respects. Thus cell counts tend to be higher; 500 to 1000 cells, predominantly lymphocytes, are common, and occasionally even several thousand are present. The pleocytosis in mumps is also more prolonged, and may persist for several weeks. Glucose levels below 40 mg. per 100 ml. have recently been reported in 10 to 20 per cent of cases. The protein levels are moderately elevated. *Encephalomyelitis,* whether resulting from mumps virus or occurring as postinfectious encephalitis, is rare. The pathologic picture of the postinfectious type is predominantly one of perivascular demyelinization typical of this syndrome.

Other rare neurologic complications include permanent nerve deafness, either unilateral or bilateral; labyrinthitis; polyneuritis, sometimes affecting the facial or trigeminal nerves; disturbances in accommodation; and optic neuritis, iritis and iridocyclitis.

Orchitis. Orchitis is rare before puberty. After puberty, its incidence varies, but is usually about 25 per cent; there is considerable variation in different epidemics. Testicular involvement is most often unilateral, but may be bilateral, one following the other by one to nine days. The onset is commonly between the fifth and tenth days of illness, as the parotid swelling is subsiding. In mild cases there may be nothing more than discomfort, with tenderness and slight fever. In others, onset is abrupt, with a chill, fever to 104° F. or higher, nausea, vomiting, sweats, backache, prostration, and severe testicular pain. Swelling of the testicle may be moderate, or the gland may rapidly reach three to four times normal size, in which case it is excessively hard, tender, and so painful that even 0.030 gram of morphine is not always effective. In severe cases, the epididymis, spermatic cord, or tunica vaginalis may be involved, and straw-colored hydrocele fluid sometimes collects.

In mild cases the testicle may be normal in four days, although in the most severe, it may require three or four weeks before all evidence of inflammation has disappeared. Some degree of atrophy, apparently caused by pressure necrosis, occurs in about a third to a half of all cases of orchitis, *but in most instances it is unilateral. Even when both testes are involved, the distribution of the inflammatory reaction and loss of functional tissue are apt to be spotty, and seldom result in sterility.*

Oophoritis. Oophoritis occurs occasionally in adult females, but it may be more frequent than suspected, as mild forms are difficult to recognize. High fever, chills, lower quadrant or back pain, and palpable ovarian enlargement have been described. Sterility resulting from mumps oophoritis is unknown.

Pancreatitis. Pancreatitis has been estimated to occur in less than 10 per cent of cases. Severe epigastric pain, vomiting, diarrhea or constipation, and fever are characteristic; abdominal tenderness and muscle spasm may be marked.

Other Organs. More rarely, other glands or organs are involved, particularly in adults. The following have been reported as complications of mumps: prostatitis, bartholinitis, and mastitis (in both male and female); involvement of the thyroid, thymus, and lacrimal glands; splenomegaly; and hepatitis. Transient abnormalities of renal function occur frequently, but persistent nephritis is unusual, although fatal cases have been reported. Polyarthritis, occuring ten days to two weeks after onset, is a rare complication. Myocarditis, accompanied by precordial pain or heart block, has been described. Serial electrocardiograms on patients with mumps have revealed some abnormality in as high as 15 per cent, although very few patients show clinical evidence of myocarditis.

Diagnosis. Sudden onset of parotitis in a previously healthy patient with a negative history of mumps presents no diagnostic problem. Other causes of parotid swelling are suppurative parotitis, an acute bacterial infection in which there is marked tenderness, the skin over the gland is red and hot, and pus can often be expressed from the duct; preauricular and anterior cervical lymphadenopathy; and salivary calculi obstructing the duct and giving rise to recurrent parotitis. Chronic enlargement of the gland occurs with tumors, Mikulicz's disease, and uveoparotid fever of sarcoidosis.

Mumps infection in the absence of parotitis is often difficult to recognize. Orchitis can be due in rare instances to infection with other viruses such as Coxsackie B, echo-, and lymphocytic choriomeningitis virus. A variety of viral agents cause aseptic meningitis or meningoencephalitis that cannot be distinguished clinically from central nervous system involvement caused by mumps. In such situations specific laboratory tests are necessary to establish the etiology. Mumps virus can be isolated from saliva, urine, and, in meningitis, from the cerebrospinal fluid. More commonly, confirmation of the diagnosis is based on the demonstration of a significant rise in antibody titer (either complement-fixing, or hemagglutination-inhibiting) when acute and convalescent serum samples are tested. If only a single convalescent specimen is available, the presence of a high titer is suggestive of recent infection. The *skin test* is of no value in diagnosis, because dermal hypersensitivity usually does not develop until three to four weeks after onset; it is less reliable than serologic tests in determining immune status.

Routine laboratory tests frequently indicate a

relative lymphocytosis in uncomplicated parotitis; with orchitis, pancreatitis, or aseptic meningitis, the total leukocyte count often reaches 15,000 to 20,000, with a high percentage of polymorphonuclear cells. The blood amylase is usually elevated as a result of parotitis and is therefore not a reliable indication of pancreatic involvement.

Prognosis. Complete recovery is the rule, and mortality is virtually nil. A few fatal cases of postinfectious encephalitis have been reported; bilateral testicular atrophy with resultant sterility (vide supra) and permanent nerve deafness are rare residua.

Treatment. Bed rest and symptomatic therapy are all that can be offered. For parotid pain, aspirin or codeine is effective. Some patients find an ice bag applied to the parotid region comforting, but others prefer heat. The headache associated with meningitis may be relieved by lumbar puncture. If orchitis is mild, no special treatment is required; if severe, meperidine (Demerol) (0.05 to 0.1 gram) or morphine (0.01 to 0.015 gram) may be necessary to control the pain. Local support and provision of warmth by means of a nest of absorbent cotton are more effective than an ice bag to the scrotum. Corticosteroids relieve the pain but do not appear to alter the duration of illness, nor do they protect against the subsequent development of atrophy. They are not indicated in mild cases, but in severe ones hydrocortisone, 10 mg. per kilogram per day, may be given for three to four days.

Prevention. A live attenuated mumps virus vaccine, grown in tissue cultures of chick embryo cells, was licensed in 1968. To date, some 4 million persons have been immunized in the United States. The vaccine, given subcutaneously in a 0.5-ml. dose, causes virtually no clinical reaction, and induces antibody conversions in more than 95 per cent of susceptibles. The serum titers are lower than those following natural infection, but they have persisted satisfactorily for the four-year period over which antibodies have been tested. Vaccinees have been shown to be resistant to mumps when subsequently exposed to siblings with the disease.

Until there is further evidence of the long-term duration of protection induced by the vaccine, immunization is indicated primarily for (1) susceptible children, especially boys approaching puberty; and (2) adolescents and adults (males particularly) with a negative history of the disease. If the vaccine is given after exposure, it is unlikely that it will protect. However, it may be given under these circumstances so that if contact infection failed to develop in a susceptible subject who was exposed, he will be protected when he next meets the virus.

Mumps vaccine should not be given to persons with allergies to egg proteins or to neomycin. It is contraindicated for those with any disease that results in compromised immune mechanisms and for patients on immunosuppressive therapy.

Henle, W., and Enders, J. F.: Mumps virus. *In* Horsfall, F. L., Jr., and Tamm, I. (eds.): Viral and Rickettsial Infections of

Man. 4th ed. Philadelphia, J. B. Lippincott Company, 1965, pp. 755–768.
Johnson, C. D., and Goodpasture, E. W.: An investigation of the etiology of mumps. J. Exp. Med., 59:1, 1934.
Reed, D., Brown, G., Merrick, R., Sever, J., and Feltz, E.: A mumps epidemic on St. George Island, Alaska. J.A.M.A., 199:113, 1967.
Russell, R. R., and Donald, J. C.: The neurologic complications of mumps. Brit. Med. J., 2:27, 1958.
Weibel, R. E., Buynak, E. B., Stokes, J., Jr., and Hilleman, M. R.: Persistence of immunity four years following Jeryl Lynn strain live virus vaccine. Pediatrics, 45:821, 1970.

ENCEPHALOMYELITIS AND OTHER NEUROLOGIC LESIONS AS SEQUELAE TO VIRAL INFECTIONS AS VIRAL VACCINES

See Disorders of the Nervous System and Behavior.

VIRAL MENINGITIS
(Nonpurulent Meningitis; Aseptic Meningitis)
Dorothy M. Horstmann

Definition. The term "viral meningitis" is used to describe a syndrome characteristic of acute viral infections of the central nervous sytem manifested by signs of meningeal irritation, cerebrospinal fluid pleocytosis (predominantly lymphocytic), and a short uncomplicated course. The syndrome can be induced by a variety of different viruses.

Etiology. At present a specific cause can be established in approximately two thirds of the cases of presumed viral origin. The relative frequency and importance of the many agents that have been implicated vary in different parts of the world. In the United States and in temperate climates generally, the enteroviruses and mumps virus are the most common causes. More than 60 enteroviruses have been identified; not all have yet been associated with meningitis, but in view of the frequent additions from among previously known and newly recognized members of this family of agents, the list can be expected to grow. Herpes simplex and lymphocytic choriomeningitis viruses are less frequently responsible for viral meningitis; rarely, the syndrome may be seen as a complication of adenovirus infections, infectious mononucleosis, viral hepatitis, and herpes zoster. Aseptic meningitis associated with the arthropod-borne group of viruses follows the geographic distribution of these agents, which is dependent upon specific arthropod vectors.

Viral Etiology of the Aseptic Meningitis Syndrome
Enteroviruses
    Polioviruses (types 1, 2, 3)
    Coxsackie A (types 1, 2, 4-11, 14; 16-18, 22, 24)
    Coxsackie B (types 1-6)
    Echoviruses (types 1-9, 11-24, 25, 30, 31)

Mumps virus
Herpes simplex (*Herpesvirus hominis*)
Varicella-zoster (*Herpesvirus varicellae*)
Arthropod-borne encephalitis (arboviruses)
Lymphocytic choriomeningitis virus
Encephalomyocarditis virus
Infectious mononucleosis (presumed viral)
Viral hepatitis
Adenoviruses

Epidemiology. In temperate climates, aseptic meningitis resulting from *enteroviruses* occurs most characteristically in small or large outbreaks during the summer and autumn, whereas in tropical and semitropical areas there is no striking seasonal incidence. Children are more frequently affected than adults, but in some epidemics as many as 50 per cent of cases occur in persons over 15 years of age. The agents are often widely disseminated in the population, giving rise chiefly to inapparent infections or minor febrile illnesses. Spread is primarily by contact with an infected person, and the healthy transient carrier is as infectious as the frank case. Dissemination is greatest in areas of poor sanitation with a high density of young preschool children, who are the most frequent carriers. Although one virus tends to be dominant and to account for the bulk of illness at any given time and place, it is not unusual during epidemic or endemic periods to find several agents circulating at the same time, causing similar illnesses, including meningitis. *Mumps meningitis* follows the epidemiologic pattern of mumps infections generally, with a peak seasonal incidence in winter and spring. On rare occasions, it appears in epidemic form, without accompanying parotitis. *Lymphocytic choriomeningitis* is an uncommon disease, occurring in the late autumn and winter. The infection is endemic in the common house mouse, *Mus musculus,* and is probably spread to man through dust or food contaminated by mouse excreta. Wild rodents are also the probable source of infections with *encephalomyocarditis virus,* which may rarely be associated with typical aseptic meningitis. *Herpes simplex meningitis* occurs sporadically, either as a primary herpetic infection spread by contact, or in some instances as a result of reactivation of a latent infection. It has no seasonal distribution.

Aseptic meningitis owing to infection with one of the *arthropod-borne viruses* (arboviruses) occurs usually during an epidemic in which most of the cases have the more characteristic encephalitic picture. However, St. Louis and western equine in the United States and Murray Valley encephalitis virus in Australia often may induce a milder disease with aseptic meningitis as a common form.

Pathogenesis. Like the epidemiology, the pathogenesis of the syndrome varies with the nature of the infecting agent. The general pattern for enteroviruses is thought to be similar, the sequence being primary multiplication in the alimentary tract, spread to regional lymph nodes, a viremic phase, and eventually invasion of the central nervous system. There is evidence that in enteroviral infections in humans, as well as in experimentally infected primates, viremia precedes the onset of illness by several days and has usually disappeared by the time neurologic signs appear. Mumps, lymphocytic choriomeningitis, herpes, and the arthropod-borne viruses probably reach the central nervous system mainly via the blood stream. There is experimental evidence that herpes virus is also capable of traveling by neural spread. In the central nervous system, the lesion of aseptic meningitis is apparently limited to an inflammatory response in the meninges, although in nonparalytic poliovirus infections in monkeys scattered anterior horn cell involvement also occurs.

Clinical Manifestations. Whatever the specific viral cause, the symptoms and signs are similar and not readily distinguishable from the pattern of aseptic meningitis from other causes. The onset is commonly abrupt. The most constant features are severe headache, fever, and stiff neck; other symptoms that may occur are sore throat, nausea and vomiting, listlessness, drowsiness, vertigo, pain in the back and neck, photophobia, paresthesias, myalgias, abdominal pain, and chills or chilly sensations. With certain Coxsackie and echovirus infections a striking skin eruption may appear. In general, the severity of symptoms increases with the age of the patient. Although sudden onset is characteristic, in some patients there is a prodromal nonspecific "minor illness" followed by several days of well-being before the reappearance of fever and the development of signs of central nervous system involvement. This occurs most commonly with poliovirus infections in young children, but may be associated with other enteroviruses and with lymphocytic choriomeningitis.

On *physical examination* there are few findings. The temperature is elevated (100 to 104° F.), but the patient does not appear as ill as one with bacterial meningitis. Neck and back stiffness are the only neurologic signs in the typical case; Kernig and Brudzinski signs are sometimes positive. Nuchal rigidity may be minimal and apparent only in the last degrees of neck flexion. The deep tendon reflexes are normal or hyperactive. Transient weakness (rarely frank paralysis) has been noted with the Coxsackie B group, Coxsackie A7, and echoviruses 6 and 9. *Rash* is encountered chiefly in young children. It has been a prominent feature in certain epidemics in which aseptic meningitis has also occurred, including outbreaks associated with echoviruses 4, 6, 9, and 16, and Coxsackie A9 and 16; rash has also been observed occasionally with many other enterovirus types. The eruption usually appears with the fever and lasts four to five days, in severe cases eight or nine days. Characteristically it is maculopapular, discrete, erythematous and nonpruritic. The lesions may be confined to the face and neck, or may spread over the chest and extremities and sometimes involve the palms and soles. At times the rash is petechial (echo-9) or vesicular (Coxsackie A9 and A16), but the character is not constant, and a single virus type may induce any of the various forms of eruption even during the same epidemic. An *enanthem* consisting of grayish white dots on the buccal mucosa has been described in as many as one third of the patients in certain outbreaks caused by echo-9, but only occasionally with other types (echo-6 and 16).

Laboratory Findings. The *blood count,* regardless of the etiology, is commonly within normal range, but leukopenia or moderate leukocytosis without marked shift to the left may be present. The *cerebrospinal fluid* findings are diagnostic: the fluid is usually clear, with a cell count ranging from 10 to 3000 or more cells per cubic millimeter, most frequently 30 to 300, and no organisms are seen when the stained sediment is examined microscopically. Very early in the disease, the cells may be predominantly polymorphonuclear, but within a few hours there is a shift to the characteristic pattern, more than 90 per cent being lymphocytes. In contrast to bacterial meningitis, the glucose content is normal, although transient depression below 40 mg. per 100 ml. may be encountered occasionally, particularly in mumps meningitis. The protein level is normal or moderately elevated. The height of the cell count bears no fixed relation to the severity of the disease or to signs of meningeal irritation such as neck stiffness. The number of cells tends to return to normal within a few days, except in mumps and echo-9 meningitis, in which pleocytosis may persist for seven to ten days or more, often after nuchal rigidity has disappeared.

Diagnosis and Differential Diagnosis. Recognition of the aseptic meningitis syndrome is not difficult except in young infants, who frequently do not have the classic signs of meningeal irritation. There are a number of clinical and epidemiologic features that may suggest the viral agent involved, but specific etiologic diagnosis can be established only in the laboratory. With enteroviral infections, virus isolation is the usual means of accomplishing this; serologic identification based on antibody rises is impracticable because of the multiplicity of virus types. Enteroviruses are readily isolated from fecal specimens and throat swabs, and Coxsackie and echoviruses (in contrast to polioviruses) may be found in the cerebrospinal fluid in 50 per cent or more of cases associated with these agents. Adenoviruses and herpes simplex virus can be recovered from the same sources as enteroviruses, except that herpes is very rarely found in the cerebrospinal fluid. Both blood and cerebrospinal fluid are sources of lymphocytic choriomeningitis virus. Infections caused by mumps, lymphocytic choriomeningitis, and the arthropod-borne viruses are usually diagnosed serologically (rising titers of complement-fixing, neutralizing or hemagglutination-inhibiting antibodies), although virus isolation is also possible, if more difficult.

Differential Diagnosis on Clinical Evidence. A careful analysis of the history is most likely to suggest the correct etiologic diagnosis. The season of the year, the presence or absence of an epidemic, and the geographic location (particularly with respect to the arthropod-borne viruses) should be considered. In the United States, epidemics are more often associated with enteroviruses, whereas sporadic cases are likely to be induced by mumps, herpes simplex virus, or other agents. In the summer and autumn, leptospiral meningitis enters in the differential diagnosis, for it has the same seasonal incidence as enterovirus infections. In an epidemic in which there are many patients with paralysis, a relatively high percentage of aseptic meningitis cases will be due to polioviruses. In family epidemics caused by Coxsackie and polioviruses, most infections are inapparent, usually only a single member exhibiting overt illness such as meningitis; in contrast, with certain echoviruses (particularly echo-4, 6, and 9) it is common to find that all members of the family have recently experienced some febrile episode with or without meningeal signs.

The age and sex of the patient are also helpful. Mumps meningitis is much more common in males than in females (at least 3 to 1), and a similar but smaller difference has been noted in meningitis caused by enteroviruses in persons under 20 years of age. Lymphocytic choriomeningitis occurs in the 20- to 40-year age group; mumps, herpes, and enteroviral meningitis affect chiefly children and young adults.

The appearance of parotitis, salivary gland enlargement, or orchitis in patients with aseptic meningitis strongly suggests mumps, but occasionally orchitis has been noted with Coxsackie B infections and infectious mononucleosis. Lymphocytic choriomeningitis virus has been isolated from a patient with meningitis, orchitis, and parotitis. The presence of pleurodynia (with or without orchitis) in a patient with aseptic meningitis is characteristic of Coxsackie B virus infection, but pleurodynia occurs on rare occasions with echovirus infections also.

Cerebrospinal Fluid Findings. An immediate practical problem in dealing with a patient who is thought to have viral meningitis is to exclude the presence of leptospirosis or a bacterial infection that might be susceptible to antimicrobial therapy. A stained smear of the cerebrospinal fluid sediment should be examined carefully for micro-organisms, which can usually be detected if the infection is a bacterial one. The question of a bacterial etiology arises particularly in cases in which polymorphonuclear leukocytes are predominant in the cerebrospinal fluid and especially if the total count is high, i.e., more than 1000. In enteroviral infections, if the cerebrospinal fluid is examined within a few hours of onset, the finding that 60 to 90 per cent of cells are polymorphonuclears is not unusual; but the pattern then shifts rapidly to more than 90 per cent lymphocytes. In meningitis resulting from echo-9 virus, however, predominance of polymorphonuclears may persist for a week or more. Echo-9 viral meningitis has been associated with unusually high cell counts (occasionally 6000 to 8000) in the cerebrospinal fluid. Relatively high counts, i.e., between 500 and 1000 cells, are also characteristic of mumps and lymphocytic choriomeningitis.

Simulation of Brain Abscess or Bacterial Meningitis. Confusion with meningococcal and other bacterial meningitis may also arise in echo-9 or other enterovirus infections with petechial rash. The milder clinical course, the lower cerebrospinal fluid cell count and normal glucose, and the peripheral blood picture usually indicate a viral infection. If reasonable doubt exists, however, the case should be treated as one of purulent meningitis until this has been excluded by appropriate cultures. *Inadequately treated bacterial meningitis* and mechanical irritation of the meninges owing to *brain abscess* (or other intracranial lesions) may also produce an aseptic meningitis syndrome. The possibility of a silent brain abscess is suggested by a history of recent pneumonia, chronic pulmonary infection, congenital heart disease, bacterial endocarditis, otitis media, or infection of the paranasal sinuses. *Tuberculous meningitis* in its early stages is another remote possibility. Aseptic meningitis owing to *neurosyphilis* may present as an acute illness, although the course is more typically subacute, with papilledema, cranial nerve palsies, and little or no fever.

Other Forms of Aseptic Meningitis. Among other causes of aseptic meningitis, the presence of severe sore throat, generalized lymph node enlargement, mild icterus, and a transient rash are compatible with *infectious mononucleosis*. *Leptospirosis* is to be considered seriously in areas where the infection is common and when there is a history of exposure to dogs, cattle, swine, or rats, which excrete the agent in their urine. *Mycoplasma pneumoniae* infections may be complicated by aseptic meningitis or meningoencephalitis, with cerebrospinal fluid findings as in viral meningitis. The presence of respiratory symptoms and central nervous system signs suggests the possibility of infection with this agent; a significant titer of cold agglutinins in the serum supoorts the diagnosis.

Treatment. There is no specific therapy for the syndrome of aseptic meningitis. Bed rest, adequate fluid intake, and symptomatic treatment are indicated as in any acute febrile illness.

Prognosis. Aseptic meningitis caused by viruses is a self-limited disease, complete recovery occurring in three to five days in mild cases, and in seven to fourteen days in the more severe ones.

Adair, C. V., Gauld, R. L., and Smadel, J. E.: Aseptic meningitis, a disease of diverse etiology: Clinical and etiologic studies on 854 cases. Ann. Intern. Med., 39:675, 1953.
Buescher, E. L., Artenstein, M. S., and Olson, L.: Central nervous system infections of viral origin: The changing pattern. *In* Proceedings of the Association for Research in Nervous and Mental Disease (Infections of the Nervous System), Vol. 44. Baltimore, Williams & Wilkins Company, 1968, p. 147.
Jamieson, W. M., Kerr, M., and Sommerville, R. G.: Echo type-9 meningitis in East Scotland. Lancet, 1:581, 1958.
Lepow, M. L., Coyne, N., Thompson, L. B., Carver, D. H., and Robbins, F. C.: A clinical, epidemiologic and laboratory investigation of aseptic meningitis during the four-year period 1955-1958. I. Observations concerning etiology and epidemiology. New Eng. J. Med., 266:1181, 1962. II. The clinical disease and its sequelae. Ibid., 266:1188, 1962.
Sköldenberg, B.: Aseptic meningitis and meningoencephalitis in cold-agglutinin positive infections. Brit. Med. J., 1:100, 1965.
Wenner, H. A.: The benign aseptic meningitides. Med. Clin. N. Amer., 43:1451, 1959.

ENTEROVIRAL DISEASES

MENINGITIS DUE TO ENTEROVIRUSES

See Viral Meningitis.

POLIOMYELITIS
Louis Weinstein

Definition. Poliomyelitis is a common acute viral infection. It occurs naturally only in man. Various parts of the central nervous system, especially lower motor neurons, cranial nerves, the medulla, autonomic nervous system, cerebral cortex, and posterior columns of the spinal cord are involved in the most severe form. Nervous system invasion does not occur in most instances. Infection may produce no apparent illness, nonspecific syndromes, or disease of the nervous system in which evidence of neurologic dysfunction, notably motor paralysis, may or may not be present.

History. Poliomyelitis has unquestionably been known since ancient times. It was not until 1789, however, that an English physician, Underwood, first recorded a description of this disease in the medical literature. A German orthopedist, Heine, discussed the deformities resulting from this infection and their therapy in a monograph published in 1840. The latter part of the nineteenth century witnessed a number of epidemics; the contagious character of poliomyelitis was established during this period, especially by the work of Medin, a Swedish physician, who described the epidemic form of the disease in 1890. Two important discoveries were made in 1908: Wickman established the basic epidemiologic principles, and Landsteiner isolated the responsible virus in monkeys. The twentieth century has seen an increasing number of epidemics of poliomyelitis in various areas of the world. The most significant advance in recent years in the field of poliomyelitis was the development of a method for growing the virus in tissue culture by Enders, Weller, and Robbins in 1949. This made it possible, for the first time, to make vaccines of predictable antigenic potency and minimal danger. The preparation of formalin-inactivated virus suspensions by Salk, and later of "live virus" vaccines by Sabin, by Cox, and by Koprowski in the latter half of the 1950's, has made the greatly reduced incidence or even eradication of poliomyelitis a realistic goal.

Etiology. The causative agent of poliomyelitis is a virus that ranges from 8 to 30 mμ in diameter and is pathogenic for man, monkeys, and chimpanzees. Three antigenically distinct types have been defined: Type I, Type II, and Type III. Although some degree of cross-neutralization is demonstrable in highly immunized laboratory animals, infection in man with one type does not protect against invasion by another. Poliomyelitis virus has been cultivated in human and monkey kidney cells, HeLa cells, and human amnion; characteristic cytopathic changes neutralizable by type-specific antiserum are produced.

Poliomyelitis virus remains viable in water or sewage, under proper conditions, for as long as four months. It is not killed by ether, merthiolate, tincture of Zephiran, ethyl alcohol, or low concentrations of phenol, but it is inactivated by heat, bichloride of mercury, oxidizing agents, 2 per cent tincture of iodine, ultraviolet light, and 10 minutes' exposure to chlorine concentration of 0.05 part per million.

Epidemiology. Poliomyelitis is worldwide in distribution, but epidemics have been limited to a relatively small number of areas. That it has been much more prevalent than it would appear to be on the basis of the number of clinically obvious cases is proved by the widespread distribution of neutralizing antibody to the virus in population groups in which the disease is recognized only rarely. Even in outbreaks in which infection with involvement of the nervous system is present, as many as 95 per cent of the cases may be clinically inapparent. The highest frequency of poliomyelitis is from July through September in the temperate zone, although it may appear as early as April or as late as December. In tropical or subtropical regions, the "season" may be prolonged.

Certain environmental factors may play a role in conditioning the risk of exposure to poliomyelitis virus and the development of infection. Most persons who live in areas of poor sanitation develop neutralizing antibodies in early childhood; the peak of population immunity is not reached until 15 years of age or older, however, in those who reside in localities where sanitation is good. In regions with a relatively high level of sanitation, urban dwellers are apt to become immune earlier than those who live in rural areas, probably as a result of the relative crowding. Evidence of contact with poliomyelitis virus appears at a younger age in low income groups than in those whose financial status is good; this may merely reflect differences in crowding and sanitation. In some but not all parts of the world, certain racial groups appear to be more susceptible to the disease than others.

Until about 30 years ago, poliomyelitis was most common in preschool children. Since then, however, it has been occurring more frequently in older age groups; in some recent epidemics, 25 to 30 per cent of the patients have been older than 15 years. This increased incidence in adults is not due merely to aging of the population or increased reporting of paralytic and nonparalytic cases, but is probably related to a decreasing rate of exposure to virus, associated with general improvement in socioeconomic status. Young children are still affected more often than adults. Paralytic disease has been described in the neonatal period and late in the sixth decade of life, but it is very uncommon at these age extremes.

Man is the sole reservoir of poliomyelitis virus. Human carriers, especially those with inapparent infection or healthy carriers rather than clinically recognizable patients, are the usual sources from which virus is transmitted to susceptible contacts. Milk has been incriminated in the transmission of virus in one epidemic.

Virus is present in the stool and oropharynx of patients with all types of poliomyelitis. It is recoverable from pharyngeal secretions for only a few days, but is demonstrable in the feces for several weeks. The weight of opinion at present favors the intestinal tract as the main source from which dissemination occurs. The mode of infection is, therefore, mainly fecal-oral. Very small quantities of stool contain thousands of infective doses of poliomyelitis virus. The role of the fly in the transmission of the disease is not settled. Flies trapped close to areas in which there are active cases may carry the virus. Food exposed to flies from homes in which poliomyelitis was present has produced the disease when fed to monkeys. Attempts to contain the spread of epidemics by eradication of the fly population have not been successful. Spread of disease in families is very uncommon. Multiple cases in a household are usually due to simultaneous exposure. Poliomyelitis is as highly communicable as measles or varicella; in persons less than 15 years of age, infection, most often without neurologic or other manifestations (proved serologically), is said to occur in 100 per cent of household and 87 per cent of daily contacts.

Pathogenesis. The older concept that poliomyelitis virus multiplies only in nervous tissue and reaches the central nervous system only by way of peripheral nerves from the pharynx or intestinal tract is now open to serious question because of the demonstration of viremia prior to the onset of clinical manifestations.

The following sequence of events is thought to be involved in the pathogenesis of poliomyelitis: (1) The virus enters by way of the mouth and multiplies in the oropharynx and lower intestinal tract. It escapes from both areas; there is, however, no conclusive evidence as to which is more important in transmission. The main site of viral growth is probably extraneural. Virus is present in pharyngeal secretions and stool during the incubation period; it is recoverable from the feces as early as 19 days prior to onset of the disease. (2) The prodromal phase or "minor illness" (described later) develops in association with the presence of the virus in the blood, throat, and feces. The viremia persists for only a few days because antibodies develop early. The following pathway for migration of the infectious agent has been suggested: Virus in the intestinal tract first enters the lymphatic channels and then the blood stream, from which it is disseminated into the interstitial tissue spaces; from here it gains access to the lymph nodes, in which it may be detected for some time after the viremic stage has ended. There is still some question whether viremia is the primary event in infection of the nervous system or whether it is merely a manifestation of "spill-over" from already infected neural tissues. (3) The final stage in the pathogenesis of poliomyelitis is invasion by and multiplication of the virus in the nervous system. It has been suggested that the area postrema in the medulla oblongata is the site at which the virus leaves the blood and enters the brain. There is evidence, however, that virus may penetrate the nervous system at many points by direct passage from capillaries to neurons rather than at a single area of specialized vascular permeability. Spread of the infectious agent takes place along nerve fibers.

Two groups of factors determine susceptibility and reaction to invasion of the central nervous system by poliomyelitis virus: those associated with the host, and those related to the virus. Strains of the infecting agent vary greatly in their ability to invade nervous tissue and to destroy neurons. Repeated passage in animals or tissue cultures may induce changes in invasive capacity without affecting the basic antigenic character of the virus. One of the host factors of importance in determining whether or not involvement of nervous tissue occurs is circulating type-specific neutralizing antibody; this is very often detectable before manifestations of disease appear. The presence of "immunity" early is in favor of multiplication of virus in non-nervous tissue and accounts for the short-lived persistence of the agent in the pharynx and blood, sites in which antibody is demonstrable. The fact that the virus remains in the nervous system and intestine for relatively long periods is probably related to the difficulty with which antibody reaches these areas.

Inapparent infection and illness without invasion of the nervous system are common in areas where paralytic poliomyelitis occurs; these and clinically recognizable forms of the disease lead to the development of type-specific antibody and resistance to reinvasion by the same serotype, usually for life. Many children and most adults possess antibody to all three types of virus; this probably accounts for the relative infrequency of infection in older age groups. Infants less than three to six months old rarely get poliomyelitis because of immunity passively transferred from the mother. Babies born to women in the acute phase of poliomyelitis may develop the disease shortly after birth, indicating in utero infection or exposure during delivery. Sex plays a role in determining susceptibility. Among children, males are affected more often than females; the opposite is true in adults. Pregnancy increases the risk of clinically apparent poliomyelitis. Multiparous females are more susceptible than primiparas. The disease is somewhat more frequent in the second than in the first or third trimesters. Menstruation or ovulation appears to heighten susceptibility. Absence of the tonsils and adenoids, regardless of the time of their removal, is associated with an increased incidence of bulbar poliomyelitis. Chilling or physical exertion of moderate to severe degree after invasion by the virus leads to more frequent development of paralytic poliomyelitis, especially in adults.

Pathology. The anterior horn cells of the spinal cord bear the brunt of the damage produced by the poliomyelitis virus. Although any segment of the cord may be affected, the cervical and lumbar areas are the ones in which damage is most frequent. Disease of the motor nuclei of the medulla and midbrain is not uncommon. In addition, the vestibular nuclei in the medulla, the reticular formation, and the cerebellar roof nuclei are often involved. Although the gray matter is almost exclusively attacked, extension into the white matter with destruction of long-fiber pathways may take place, especially when the brainstem is injured. The lesions are not limited to the anterior gray region of the spinal cord; the posterior and lateral columns as well as the dorsal root ganglia are often affected. Gross examination of the cord reveals hyperemia owing to engorgement of the pial vessels with blood. As the disease progresses, the spinal cord becomes edematous, and softening of the gray matter leads to a change in color to yellow-gray.

Microscopic study reveals intense infiltration of the perivascular spaces with leukocytes, dilatation of and inflammatory reactions in the blood vessels, and small hemorrhages; these are noted throughout the spinal cord but are least evident in the white matter. Parenchymatous degeneration is most severe in the areas of greatest infiltration. The cellular response becomes primarily lymphocytic in the later stages of the disease. Large numbers of granulocytes and lymphocytes are present in the meninges; this response is secondary to the inflammatory reaction within the tissue. The diseased ganglion cells are swollen, show chromatolysis of the Nissl substance and pyknosis and eccentric location of the nuclei, and eventually are completely degenerated; the involved area is softened and the glial stroma edematous. Mobilization of the microglia that rounds up into phagocytic gitter cells filled with neutral fat results in an increase in glial fibrillae and subsequent scar formation.

As the disease activity comes to a halt, the hyperemia, edema, and mild ganglion cell changes in the areas adjacent to degenerated foci gradually recede. As the cells resume function, paralysis of muscles may disappear.

Clinical Manifestations and Laboratory Findings. The incubation period of poliomyelitis varies from 3 to 35 days; about 80 per cent of cases occur within 6 to 20 days after contact with the virus. Four types of clinical picture may develop: *inapparent infection, "minor illness," nonparalytic poliomyelitis,* and *paralytic poliomyelitis.*

Inapparent Infection. In families in which a clinically recognized case of poliomyelitis appears, inapparent infection usually develops in other susceptible members. Most poliomyelitis (probably 95 per cent or more) occurs in this form. Although there are no manifestations of illness, virus is recoverable from the pharynx and intestine. It is also present in the blood in some instances. Type-specific neutralizing antibody usually develops.

"Minor Illness." The entire course of poliomyelitis may consist of a minor nonspecific illness that lasts for several days and in which clinical and laboratory evidence of central nervous system invasion is absent; this is "abortive" poliomyelitis. Three syndromes have been observed: *upper respiratory*—fever of varying degree, pharyngeal discomfort, with or without coryza, and reddening and swelling of the lymphoid tissues of the throat; *gastrointestinal*—nausea, vomiting, diarrhea or constipation, and abdominal discomfort, accompanied by a moderate elevation of temperature; and *"grippe"-like disease*—fever and generalized aching of muscles, bones, and joints resembling mild to moderately severe influenza. Virus can be demonstrated in the pharynx, feces, and blood in the early stages of these "minor" illnesses. Type-specific neutralizing and complement-fixing antibodies are present in the convalescent phase.

Nonparalytic Poliomyelitis. Nonparalytic poliomyelitis is a syndrome composed of prodromal manifestations, signs of meningeal irritation, and abnormalities of the cerebrospinal fluid. The prodrome is one of the "minor illnesses." It is usually present for several days before the onset of other signs, but it may be entirely absent. Varying degrees of stiffness of the neck and back, positive Kernig signs, and, with severe meningeal irritation, leg and neck Brudzinski signs are present. The tripod (patient extends arms behind back with hands on bed for support when sitting up) and Hoyne's signs (head falls back when, with patient in supine position, shoulders are elevated) can be elicited in paralytic or nonparalytic poliomyelitis. These signs are not pathognomonic because they are demonstrable in any type of meningeal irritation. The cerebrospinal fluid usually contains between 25 and 500 cells, rarely as many as 1000 to 2000. Very early in the disease, there is often a preponderance of neutrophils (up to 80 per cent); within a few days, however, lymphocytes become predominant. The protein is usually normal or only slightly elevated at the beginning of the illness, but may increase to between 50 and 100 mg. per 100 ml. The sugar content is normal or moderately elevated. The cerebrospinal fluid chloride reflects the plasma chloride level. These findings indicate an inflammatory reaction of the meninges and are not specifically diagnostic of poliomyelitis.

The course of nonparalytic poliomyelitis is entirely benign. Defervescence usually occurs in three to five days, but meningeal irritation may persist for as long as two weeks beyond this. No changes in reflexes or muscle or cranial nerve function are detectable. The leukocyte count may be elevated to 10,000 to 15,000 per cubic millimeter in the early stage of the disease, but usually returns to normal within one week. The cerebrospinal fluid often contains an increased number of cells (predominantly lymphocytes) and ele-

vated protein for two to three or more weeks after the onset of the disease.

Paralytic Poliomyelitis. The syndrome of paralytic poliomyelitis is made up of prodromal manifestations ("minor illness"), signs of meningeal irritation, abnormal cerebrospinal fluid, and dysfunction of various areas of the spinal cord, brain, or cranial nerve nuclei that leads to paresis or paralysis of muscles. Parts of the nervous system other than anterior horn cells may be involved: the precentral gyrus, reticular formation in the medulla, roof nuclei, and vermis of the cerebellum; Auerbach's and Meissner's plexuses and sympathetic ganglia may be affected. Frequently, there is a lack of correlation between the anatomic changes and the clinical findings. "Skip" areas are common in spinal paralytic disease; for example, the cervical and lumbar cord may be involved but the thoracic portion is spared.

Paralytic poliomyelitis is subdivided into the following types:

I. *Spinal*
   (1) Cervical
   (2) Thoracic
   (3) Lumbar
   (4) Any combination of (1), (2), and (3)
II. *Bulbar*
   (1) Upper cranial nerve involvement— N 3, 4, 5, 6, 7, 8
   (2) Lower cranial nerve involvement— N 9, 10, 12
   (3) Autonomic center involvement
      (a) Respiratory center
      (b) Circulatory center
      (c) Combinations of (a) and (b)
III. *Bulbospinal*
IV. *Polioencephalitis*—paralytic or nonparalytic
   (1) Diffuse encephalitis
   (2) Focal encephalitis
   (3) ? Cerebellar involvement
   (4) Bulbo-encephalitic disease
   (5) Spinal-encephalitic disease

A prodromal period may be absent in any type of paralytic poliomyelitis. In some cases, the disease is biphasic. In these, it starts with a varying degree of temperature elevation and the manifestations of one of the "minor illnesses." After several days, all symptoms disappear. In five to ten days there are recrudescence of fever, development of signs of meningeal irritation, and appearance of paralysis. In adults, the most common prodromal symptoms are generalized muscle and bone discomfort. In children, upper respiratory tract syndromes are most frequent. All the signs of meningeal irritation are usually present. In some cases, however, they are incomplete; stiffness of the neck and back may be minimal and the Kernig sign strongly positive, or the neck may be very stiff and the back and hamstring muscles exhibit little "spasm." The cerebrospinal fluid findings in paralytic poliomyelitis are identical with those in the nonparalytic infection; the number of cells and quantity of protein bear no relationship to the severity of involvement or prognosis. The fluid is said to be completely normal in about 10 per cent of cases. This incidence is probably much too high because of the inclusion of cases of "nonparalytic poliomyelitis," many of which are instances of a variety of other diseases (see Differential Diagnosis). The cerebrospinal fluid may be entirely normal throughout the course of paralytic poliomyelitis, but I have personally noted this in no more than 0.2 per cent of cases. In some patients, the decrease in the number of cells in the cerebrospinal fluid is accompanied by a progressive rise in protein, which may reach relatively high levels and cause confusion with the cyto-albuminologic dissociation noted in some cases of "infectious" polyneuritis. The peripheral leukocyte count in paralytic poliomyelitis may be normal or elevated, with a relative increase in neutrophils.

Spinal Paralytic Poliomyelitis. Cramping pain in the muscles innervated by the affected neurons and hyperesthesia of the skin overlying them are striking features of the early stage of spinal paralytic poliomyelitis. The discomfort may be very severe; muscle "spasm," the exact mechanism of which is not clear, and fine, rapid fasciculations are usually detectable. Paralysis may not appear for some time after the onset of nervous system manifestations. In some instances, increase in muscle weakness is very slow; in others, it proceeds with moderate speed; in still others, it becomes widespread within 48 hours. Rarely, a rapidly ascending paralysis of the Landry type may develop. Age is important in conditioning the extent of involvement. In children less than 5 years old, paresis of one leg is most common; in patients between 5 and 15 years of age, weakness of one arm or paraplegia is most frequent; in adults (16 to 65 years old), quadriplegia is observed most often. Dysfunction of the urinary bladder is at least ten times more frequent in adults than in children. Paralysis of the muscles of respiration is most common in those older than 16 years. Infants younger than 1 year are subject to very extensive involvement. Among adults, men develop quadriplegia, respiratory paralysis, and loss of bladder function more frequently than women. Pregnancy does not increase the severity of the disease unless parturition takes place during the acute phase. There is a definite association of inoculation of antigenic materials ("triple vaccine," for example) with an increased risk of involvement of the muscles around the site of injection.

The location of muscle weakness depends on the portion of the spinal cord involved. Isolated infection of the cervical, thoracic, or lumbar areas may be present, or two or more parts of the cord may be affected simultaneously. The lumbar area is the one most frequently damaged. "Skip" areas, with disease of isolated segments of the various divisions of the cord, are often observed.

When the cervical portion of the spinal cord is involved there is paresis or paralysis of the muscles of the shoulders, arms, neck, and diaphragm. Very early in the disease, the reflexes in the arms may be exaggerated; they diminish rapidly in intensity, however, and are usually absent when paralysis becomes established. Fasciculation of the affected shoulder or arm muscles is common. With cervical cord disease, there is a constant threat of spread of the infection to the cranial nerves, medulla, or phrenic nerve nuclei.

Weakness of the muscles of the chest, upper portion of the abdomen, and spine follows involvement of the thoracic portion of the spinal cord. Difficulty in breathing results from dysfunction of the intercostal and other thoracic muscles. The chest wall may be in "spasm," appearing rigid and immovable despite the presence of only a minor degree of paresis. Fasciculation of the thoracic, abdominal, or spine-supporting muscles may sometimes be noted. This form of respiratory paralysis is characterized by progressive failure of the chest muscles or diaphragms or both to move air in and out of the lungs. The outstanding manifestation is a slow-to-rapid decrease in vital capacity. Breathing becomes rapid and shallow, but is not irregular as when the respiratory center is involved.

Disease of the lumbar portion of the spinal cord produces weakness of the upper and lower legs and inferior portions of the abdomen and back. Pain, tenderness, "spasm," and fasciculation of the affected muscles are often detectable early. The reflexes in the legs are decreased and disappear when flaccid paralysis becomes established. Dysfunction of the iliopsoas muscles leads to inability to sit up from a lying position. Varying degrees of paresis of the hip muscles, quadriceps, femoris, hamstrings, gastrocnemii, peroneals, anterior tibials, tensor fasciae latae, glutei, and sartorius may be present. In some cases, especially in adults, complete paraplegia develops. Paralysis of the urinary bladder occurs in about one third of patients more than 16 years of age, but is rarely observed in the absence of weakness of the legs.

The abdominal and cremasteric reflexes usually disappear before severe muscle weakness occurs in paralytic poliomyelitis and may be absent during the entire course of the disease. An extensor plantar response (positive Babinski) is not uncommon during the first one or two days; persistence or late development of this reflex is incompatible with poliomyelitis. Hyperesthesia of the skin is frequent; increased vibratory sensation may be detected by special techniques. Sensory loss is extremely rare. Constipation, abdominal cramps, and meteorism are common and are due to partial ileus resulting from involvement of the autonomic nervous system and weakness of the abdominal muscles. When the disease is severe, sympathetic nervous system disturbances with tachycardia, hypertension, abnormal sweating, and cyanosis and coldness of the involved extremities, not owing to superficial vasospasm, are present.

Fever is usually present for the first few days of spinal paralytic poliomyelitis and disappears by gradual lysis. In about 90 per cent of cases, there is little or no extension of paralysis after defervescence has been established for about 48 hours. In about 10 per cent, however, progression of weakness to a notable degree may continue for as long as a week after the temperature has returned to normal.

Bulbar Poliomyelitis. The incidence of bulbar poliomyelitis differs from one epidemic to another and varies between 6 and 25 per cent. In patients subjected to tonsillo-adenoidectomy within 30 days of onset of the disease and in those in whom the operation was performed years before, the bulbar form of infection occurs in about 85 per cent. Pure bulbar dysfunction (without any signs of spinal cord involvement) is most common in children; adults with this type of involvement usually have associated spinal cord disease. The prodromal manifestations of bulbar poliomyelitis are the same as in the spinal form. The syndromes that develop depend on the area of the brainstem involved and result from damage to the medulla, pons, and midbrain. Signs and symptoms are produced by (1) dysfunction of the upper cranial nerve nuclei, (2) damage to the lower cranial nerve nuclei, and (3) disturbances of the respiratory and vasomotor regulating centers in the medulla. Combined bulbar and diffuse or focal encephalitic or spinal involvement may occur.

Upper cranial nerve nuclei—N 3, 4, 5, 6, 7, 8. Isolated ocular nerve palsies, total external ophthalmoplegia, pupillary disturbances, Horner's syndrome, and hippus occur. There may be unilateral or bilateral involvement of the fifth nerve with difficulty in chewing and closing the mouth, as well as deviation of the jaws. Paralysis of the seventh cranial nerve is common and usually unilateral. It is most often of the central type; the entire face or only the upper or lower parts may be affected. Disturbances of vestibular function and deafness result from damage to the nucleus of the eighth nerve; this is rare.

Lower cranial nerve nuclei—N 9, 10, 12. Life may be endangered when function of the tenth nerve is impaired because swallowing is controlled by the combined action of N 9, 10, and 12. When these are involved, the voice has a nasal quality, and movement of one or both halves of the soft palate is decreased or absent. Saliva collects in the hypopharynx because of difficulty in swallowing and not because of excessive secretion. Hoarseness and laryngeal stridor follow weakness or paralysis of the vocal cords. Unilateral or bilateral weakness of the tongue, sternocleidomastoid, and trapezius muscles may be present. Inability to swallow results in pooling of saliva and food in the pharynx with obstruction to the airway. Aspiration of fluid into the larynx, reflex spasm of the glottis, and bilateral abductor paralysis of the vocal cords constitute very serious threats to life.

Disease of the medullary respiratory center produces irregularity of the rhythm, depth, and rate of breathing (*Biot respiration*). Respirations are shallow and, as the disease progresses, are interrupted by longer and longer periods of apnea until breathing stops completely. Function of the thoracic muscles and diaphragm is normal, unless spinal involvement is present. Hiccups are frequent in the early phase of respiratory center dysfunction. Hypoxia, without visible cyanosis, is common and contributes to nervous tissue damage and the intensity of the manifestations. In the late stages, cyanosis, unresponsive to oxygen administration, is usual, and the temperature, pulse rate, and blood pressure are elevated. The final event is usually severe hypotension and clinical shock, which are irreversible despite use of the most heroic measures in practically all cases.

A deep cherry red color of the lips, flushed florid appearance of the skin, a very rapid, irregular pulse, small pulse pressure, and moderate to severe hypotension characterize involvement of the circulatory-regulating center. Hyperthermia, mottled cold and clammy skin, shallow respiration, anxiety, restlessness, and confusion appear as the circulatory mechanism becomes progressively more impaired; irreversible shock is usually the terminal event.

Polioencephalitis. Encephalitis resulting from poliomyelitis virus occurs as an isolated syndrome or in company with bulbar or spinal involvement. The incidence of polioencephalitis is variable; one small epidemic has been described in which most of the patients had this type of illness. Symptoms of diffuse or focal involvement of the brain may be present. The outstanding features of the diffuse form are anxiety, apprehension, a feeling of impending doom, and a sensation of ideas racing through the mind. Quivering, trembling, twitching, and jerking of the facial muscles and extremities, flushing of the face, tremor of the hands, and extremely rapid movements occur. Insomnia may be severe. In fatal cases, severe confusion progresses to lethargy, coma, and death. Somnolence may be the outstanding feature and may continue throughout the course of the disease.

There may be clinical evidence of brain damage, or the lesions may be silent and demonstrable only at necropsy in cases of focal polioencephalitis. Visual-verbal agnosia, myoclonic jerks, grand mal convulsions that occasionally persist for a long time after recovery, spastic hemiparesis, ataxia of one arm or leg, and increased intracranial pressure with papilledema have been reported.

Diagnosis. The diagnosis of poliomyelitis is more commonly suspected than it is established. The clinical features of the acute phase, the course of the more severe types of infection, and the final outcome, although highly suggestive in some instances, are not sufficiently characteristic in others to be diagnostic. The form of the disease that appears as a "minor illness" is so nonspecific that its etiology is usually completely overlooked except in the presence of an epidemic, when it is often considered but infrequently proved. The physical findings and cerebrospinal fluid abnormalities observed in nonparalytic poliomyelitis are also present in a large variety of infectious and noninfectious disorders of the nervous system (*vide infra*) and are, therefore, diagnostically useless. The paralytic types of the disease, if studied carefully over a sufficient length of time, are more readily recognizable on clinical grounds. Even these, however, may be mimicked by a number of unrelated illnesses.

The only firm basis on which the diagnosis of any type of poliomyelitis can be established during life is the demonstration of a significant rise in titer of neutralizing antibody in the serum (at least fourfold) when blood specimens drawn in the acute and convalescent stages of illness are studied. The serologic determinations may be carried out with virus isolated from a patient's stool or pharyngeal secretions or, if this is not available, with type strains maintained in tissue culture. Recovery of poliomyelitis virus from the bowel or throat is of no diagnostic help because this may merely reflect the carrier state. Isolation of virus from cerebrospinal fluid is usually not possible. The agent can be cultured in many instances, however, from spinal cord or brain at necropsy.

Differential Diagnosis. Nonparalytic poliomyelitis may be confused with any disorder in which fever, signs of meningeal irritation, and abnormalities of the cerebrospinal fluid of the type described above are present. In essence, the differential diagnosis of this type of disease includes all the causes of so-called aseptic or nonpurulent meningitis. These include partially treated or healing bacterial infections of the meninges, tuberculous meningitis, the serous meningitis of scarlet fever, pertussis encephalopathy, leptospiral meningitis, mumps meningitis, Coxsackie and echovirus infections of the meninges, brain abscess, lymphocytic choriomeningitis, meningeal involvement in infectious mononucleosis, chemical irritation of the meninges following intrathecal administration of anesthetics, antimicrobial drugs or roentgenographic contrast media, allergic reactions involving the nervous system, and syphilitic meningitis, in which there is no evidence of brain or spinal cord involvement. This syndrome of aseptic meningitis is considered in greater detail in the preceding article (Viral Meningitis). The difficulty of making an exact diagnosis of nonparalytic poliomyelitis is emphasized by the fact that studies of cases diagnosed as nonparalytic poliomyelitis have indicated that, in general, not more than 40 per cent are actual instances of this disease.

The differential diagnosis of paralytic poliomyelitis may be difficult because the same manifestations, including cranial nerve or muscle dysfunction or the picture of encephalitis, may be characteristic of a number of other disorders. Some of these, as has been noted, usually are not accompanied by paralysis but, in uncommon instances, may exhibit striking degrees of nervous system disturbance. In others, there is practically always evidence of involvement of brain, spinal cord, or cranial nerves. Diseases that, especially in their early stages, may be confused with para-

lytic poliomyelitis are trichinosis, acute rheumatic fever with encephalitis, cerebrovascular accidents with paralysis, acute syphilitic meningitis (frequent cranial nerve palsies), postinfectious encephalitis (rubeola, rubella, varicella), meningomyeloencephalitis following sensitization to foreign proteins (horse serum, tetanus toxoid, rabies or pertussis vaccine), acute multiple sclerosis, pseudobulbar palsy, myalgic meningoencephalitis (Iceland, Tallahassee, or Coventry disease, epidemic neuromyasthenia), spinal epidural abscess or tumor, neoplasms of the brain, Coxsackie and echovirus infections, the encephalitides caused by a variety of viruses, including those in the arthropod-borne (arbor) group, the encephalitis in the pre-icteric phase of viral hepatitis, leptospiral meningoencephalitis, lymphocytic choriomeningitis with encephalitic manifestations, mumps meningoencephalitis, encephalomyelitis of infectious mononucleosis, toxic, "infectious," or idiopathic polyneuritis, focal embolic encephalitis associated with subacute bacterial endocarditis, brain abscess (with cranial nerve palsy), and tuberculous meningitis with hemiplegia or cranial nerve (especially sixth nerve) dysfunction.

Study of these diseases over a period of a few days to a week or more clarifies the situation on clinical grounds alone in many instances; occasionally, however, the diagnosis is not established until serologic determinations have been carried out. Points that may be of help in distinguishing paralytic poliomyelitis are that the paralysis in this disease is always of the lower motor neuron type, that sensory loss does not occur, and that extensor plantar responses are not demonstrable for longer than the first one or two days after neurologic dysfunction first appears. In its earliest clinical stages botulism can be confused with bulbar poliomyelitis, but can be distinguished from it by the history and the absence of signs of infection.

Complications of Paralytic Poliomyelitis. Paralytic poliomyelitis may present a number of serious and potentially lethal complications, especially in adults. These occur most often when the respiratory muscles are involved or when the disease is bulbar or bulbospinal; frequently these complications are the direct cause of death.

Disturbances in water and electrolyte balance are common in patients receiving continuous artificial respiration. The fever and sweating that follow enclosure in a tank during the summer months, together with vomiting, diarrhea, inability to take food, and disturbances in carbon dioxide related to improperly regulated ventilation, produce a series of chemical disturbances, the repair of which taxes the ingenuity of the physician. Edema and low electrolyte levels often follow overenthusiastic hydration and have been misinterpreted as evidence of a salt-wasting syndrome.

Myocarditis is common in poliomyelitis; it is probably due to direct viral invasion. Electrocardiographic changes, mainly T, ST-T and P-R abnormalities, are present in 10 to 20 per cent of cases. Interstitial infiltration of the myocardium with round cells and mild muscle changes are frequent, but acute necrotizing myocarditis is rare. Verrucous endocarditis involving the mitral valve has been described. Severe myocarditis has been thought to be responsible for death in some cases. Hypertension may develop; it is most often transient and due to hypoxia. Less frequently, hypothalamic involvement leads to the appearance of persistent hypertension that may become "malignant"; unless this is treated, it may produce severe retinopathy, convulsions, and mental deterioration. Pulmonary edema and shock, the exact pathogenesis of which is not known, are usually the terminal events in most fatal cases of poliomyelitis. Although relatively young adults are involved, phlebothrombosis of the legs, most commonly the left, with or without pulmonary embolism, is common. All methods of artificial respiration produce hemodynamic disturbances that are countered, in healthy persons, by reflex mechanisms acting to maintain normal blood pressure and cardiac output. When patients in impending shock or those with established hypotension are placed in respirators under negative tank pressure (positive intratracheal pressure), these reactions cannot be called into play, and peripheral vascular collapse develops or, if already present, is made worse.

Acute and severe dilatation of the stomach and large bowel, perforation of the cecum, acute ulcers of the duodenum, stomach, and esophagus, multiple erosions of the entire gastrointestinal tract with considerable bleeding, and severe ileus have been observed. Depression of prothrombin and massive spontaneous hemorrhage from the intestine may develop in patients with severe poliomyelitis, especially if they are receiving large oral doses of "broad-spectrum" antimicrobial drugs.

Severe bulbar or bulbospinal disease with paralysis of swallowing and breathing muscles is accompanied by the risk of *major pulmonary atelectases* and *bacterial pneumonia*, one of the most dangerous complications. The incidence of pulmonary infection is greatly increased by tracheostomy and is highest in patients who have had this operation and are undergoing artificial respiration. The organisms involved most often are *Staphylococcus aureus* and gram-negative bacteria such as Proteus, *Ps. aeruginosa*, *E. coli* and *K. pneumoniae;* many strains of these are not susceptible to the commonly used antimicrobial agents. Chemoprophylaxis is without value in preventing secondary bronchopulmonary bacterial invasion.

A common site of infection in paralytic poliomyelitis is the urinary tract because of the frequent necessity for chronic catheterization in adult patients, in whom bladder dysfunction is most common; chemoprophylaxis, even when given together with tidal drainage, is usually ineffective. Although the symptoms may suggest only cystitis, involvement of the kidney is practically always present. The responsible organisms are those that are usually found in urinary tract infections; they are often insusceptible to the antimicrobial drugs. The renal problem is complicated by the frequency of stone formation, which may be responsible for renal colic, obstruction of the pelves and pyonephrosis, increase in severity of pyelonephritis, renal decompensation, hypertension, and vascular disease. The factors that contribute to renal lithiasis in these cases are immobility leading to calcium mobilization, infection, stasis, dehydration, and calcium intake. Attempts to control this problem consist of the liberal administration of fluids, decrease of calcium ingestion, acidification of the urine, administration of salicylate, and mobilization as early as possible.

A syndrome resembling rheumatoid arthritis, with redness, swelling, pain, and tenderness of the larger joints is observed rarely in the convalescent phase of paralytic poliomyelitis. A variety of skin rashes may occur; these include miliaria, seborrhea, and purpuric, morbilliform, or exfoliative eruptions usually the result of drug sensitization. Bed sores are common in respirator patients because of the difficulty in moving them about. Severely paralyzed patients, especially those whose life is threatened by respiratory difficulty, frequently experience very difficult emotional problems. Disorientation, acute panic states, Korsakoff-like syndromes, and acute psychoses, the type depending on the basic personality, have been noted. Chronic anxiety and depression are almost universal in severely damaged adults and probably are the result of the sudden impact of a crippling disease, with its serious social and economic implications, on the breadwinner or homemaker of a family, rather than of brain damage caused by viral invasion.

Treatment. Cases of "abortive" poliomyelitis require no therapy except for "symptomatic" relief of the manifestations of the "minor" illnesses. Antimicrobial drugs are without value.

The management of nonparalytic poliomyelitis involves primarily the relief of the headache, pain in the back, and "spasm" of the legs, associated with meningeal irritation. Rest in bed, with the mattress supported by a board, is helpful in reducing the back discomfort. The application of wet heat in the form of "hot packs" to the neck, back, and thighs produces considerable relief. Analgesics such as meperidine (Demerol) and codeine are very useful. It is best not to administer morphine derivatives. Antimicrobial agents are useless because they have no effect on the primary disease and do not decrease the risk of secondary bacterial infection. Neuromuscular examination should not be carried out more often than every three to four days. Bed rest is terminated as soon as severe discomfort is absent, in order to reduce the risk of phlebothrombosis and pulmonary embolism. Every patient thought to have nonparalytic poliomyelitis should have orthopedic follow-up study for two to three months after recovery in order to detect and correct minor degrees of weakness, which may become apparent only when muscles that appear normal at rest are taxed by the exertion of normal physical activity.

Treatment of Paralytic Poliomyelitis. The treatment of paralytic poliomyelitis involves (1) the use of all measures to spare the life of the patient threatened by involvement of vital areas, (2) relief of discomfort, (3) maintenance of weak muscles in as good a condition as possible until normal neuronal function has sufficient time to return, (4) immediate recognition and treatment of complications, (5) efforts to prevent or ameliorate emotional disorders, (6) surgical treatment of correctable defects, and (7) social, economic, occupational, and physical rehabilitation.

Patients with paralysis of swallowing, loss of function of the breathing muscles, pulmonary edema, or shock are in great danger of death.

The Question of Tracheostomy. Difficulty in deglutition, although it leads to the development of complex problems of infection and regulation of caloric, water, and electrolyte balance, is most important because of the danger of lethal obstruction of the airway. For this reason, it has been suggested that tracheostomy be performed in all such cases. However, this operation is followed by a high incidence of bronchopulmonary infections owing to drug-resistant organisms. The preferred initial management of swallowing difficulty involves postural drainage, suction to keep the hypopharynx as free of fluids as possible, and maintenance of adequate intake of food and water by nasogastric intubation. The prone position takes advantage of the normal forward inclination of the trachea as an aid to drainage. Elevation of the foot of the bed 2 to 3 feet from the floor also helps to keep fluids out of the lower respiratory tract. Most important is judicious suctioning of the throat by an experienced physician or nurse. If, in addition, fluids and electrolytes are administered parenterally at first and later by gavage, most patients have little or no trouble. In some cases, however, tracheostomy becomes necessary, despite the risks. The indications for this operation are (1) abductor paralysis of the vocal cords confirmed by indirect or direct laryngoscopy — *this makes the operation mandatory;* (2) pneumonia with inability to clear the lungs of exudate — the opening in the trachea permits easy toilet of the lower airway; (3) repeated bouts of major degrees of pulmonary atelectasis requiring repeated tracheal catheterization or bronchoscopy; and (4) inability to keep the airway relatively free of secretions — this is often simply a matter of availability of a sufficient complement of experienced personnel.

Respiratory Difficulty. The development of difficulty in respiration demands immediate recognition of its presence and the application of therapeutic measures based on the pathogenesis of the mechanisms involved. It is mandatory that respiratory insufficiency resulting from weakness or paralysis of the chest muscles or diaphragms or both be differentiated from that owing to occlusion of the upper airway or that resulting from dysfunction of the respiratory center. The mode of treatment effective in one of these is not only of no help in the others, but often is actually dangerous because it increases rather than alleviates the difficulty. The characteristics of each of these forms of respiratory problem have been discussed above. The therapy of choice for weakness of the chest muscles or diaphragm is the respirator tank, chest cuirass, or rocking bed, in this order of preference; some clinicians prefer tracheal intubation plus positive pressure breathing in this situation; the writer has used this approach only as a last resort. For respiratory impairment caused by accumulation of fluids in the upper airway, properly performed suction or tracheostomy is the treatment of choice (see above). When the respiratory center is involved but skeletal muscles and swallowing mechanisms are not affected, indicated therapy is the use of the electrophrenic respirator. Tank, cuirass, and positive pressure breathing are contraindicated when swallowing mechanisms or respiratory center dysfunction is the problem because it tends to aggravate these situations and may even lead to a fatal outcome. (The specific details of each of these forms of treatment are presented in the article on Respiratory Failure in the section on Disorders of the Nervous System and Behavior). The use of antimicrobial agents to prevent secondary bacterial infections in patients with respiratory difficulty of any type is not only not beneficial, but may be dangerous because of an increased risk of superinfection by organisms that may be difficult to eradicate.

Infection. The treatment of infections of the lungs and urinary tract that complicate paralytic poliomyelitis is the same as that employed in these types of disease without nervous system infection. The frequency of involvement by drug-resistant organisms necessitates determination of resistance of the isolated bacteria to a variety of antimicrobial drugs. The specific details of the therapy of these types of disease are discussed elsewhere in this book.

Circulatory Failure. There is no specific treatment for poliomyocarditis. When pulmonary edema supervenes in patients receiving artificial respiration, the use of positive intratank pressure or positive pressure breathing through a cuffed tracheostomy tube may be helpful. Shock is easier to prevent than to treat. Assurance of adequate oxygen saturation, prevention of dehydration, and early treatment of superimposed bacterial infection are of prophylactic value. When serious hypotension develops, a central venous catheter should be inserted and, depending on the level of venous pressure, plasma, whole blood, isoproterenol, or digitalis should be administered. Very large doses of corticosteroids have been recommended as a last resort. Tissue perfusion should not be sacrificed to maintain a "normal" blood pressure. More important indications of effective management are the absence of clinical manifestations of this syndrome and the presence of adequate urine secretion. (Details of the therapy of the shock of infection are discussed elsewhere in this book.) Hypotension appearing during artificial respiration may respond to alternating positive and negative tank pressures of approximately the same degree.

Relief of Muscle Discomfort. The relief of discomfort is one of the most important problems in the treatment of paralytic poliomyelitis. Hot wet packs, diathermy, warm baths, or dry heat may reduce pain caused by muscle "spasm." Analgesic drugs should be used whenever necessary; morphine derivatives are *not* given. Changing the position of paralyzed limbs and moving the patient about in bed are very effective in reducing the frequency and intensity of pain.

Physiotherapy. Weak muscles must be maintained in as good condition as possible until neuronal function returns; the time, degree, and extent of resumption of function is unpredictable, but treatment should be continued for at least two years. This aspect of therapy is best managed by a physiotherapist with broad experience with poliomyelitis. Muscle examinations should be carried out infrequently in the acute phases of the disease and should never be too strenuous, in order to minimize the possible effect of exercise in increasing the degree of paralysis. Daily physiotherapy is usually started three to four days after complete defervescence has occurred and extension of weakness has stopped. Exercise against resistance, even that of gravity, is thought to be most beneficial by some clinicians. In many clinics, exercise in water to remove the effects of gravity is standard practice.

Prevention and Treatment of Emotional Disorders. The physician must be constantly aware of the complications of paralytic poliomyelitis that have been described above, because their immediate recognition and treatment are often life-saving. The prevention and therapy of the emotional disorders that accompany severe paralytic poliomyelitis are often best achieved by the attending physicians and nurses. The help of a psychiatrist may be necessary, especially for difficult situations.

Return of Muscle Function. Maximal return of muscle function usually is established at the end of two years following the onset of paralytic poliomyelitis. The aid of an orthopedic surgeon should be enlisted after this time, and a program of surgical rehabilitation should be started. Persistent coldness and cyanosis of the lower extremities suggests consideration of lumbar sympathectomy.

Rehabilitation. The social and economic impact of paralytic poliomyelitis on adults is often very severe. Every effort must be made to enlist the cooperation of social service agencies to minimize the disruptive effects of the disease. Many patients require occupational rehabilitation because of inability to perform the work in which they were engaged prior to being crippled. For others, the use of devices such as movable splints or hooks is very helpful if physical rehabilitation cannot be accomplished surgically.

Prognosis. The over-all case mortality rate for poliomyelitis is about 5 per cent. Patients with "abortive" and nonparalytic disease recover completely. About 2 to 5 per cent of children and 15 to 30 per cent of adults (the rate increases with age) with paralyzing infection die. When bulbospinal involvement, especially with medullary or phrenic and intercostal nerve dysfunction, is present, the fatality rate varies between 25 and 75 per cent; in these cases, it is greatly influenced by age and the presence of shock, pulmonary edema, superimposed infection, or other complications.

Many patients with paralytic poliomyelitis recover completely. In a considerable number, there is return of some degree of muscle function. Very few remain totally paralyzed. It is striking, though paradoxical, that the more life-threatening the disease is in the acute stage, the more frequently complete functional recovery takes place if the patient survives. Thus, paralysis of the respiratory center usually disappears completely. Dysfunction of swallowing is followed by total recovery in most instances, although mild palatopharyngeal weakness may occasionally persist for life. Paralysis of the muscles of respiration often disappears completely. In some cases, the final vital capacity, although reduced, is adequate to maintain ventilation, even with moderate physical exertion. In very few instances is chronic respirator care necessary. Weak extremities regain about 60 per cent of the total strength that they will ever recover within three months and 80 per cent within six months. Improvement may continue for as long as two years. The final degree of functional return depends on the number of neurons totally destroyed, and varies from as low as zero to 10 per cent to as high as 100 per cent.

Immunity. One attack of poliomyelitis usually confers immunity for life against reinvasion by the same serotype. Both neutralizing and complement-fixing antibodies appear early in the disease; the latter persist for only several years after infection, but the former are detectable throughout life. Theoretically, a person may suffer three episodes of the disease because immunity is strictly type-specific. Most adults and many children have poliomyelitis, without paralysis or even nervous system invasion, two or three times, as shown by the presence in their serums of neutralizing antibody for more than one virus type. This probably accounts for the decreasing frequency of the disease with increasing age. There are, however, well-documented instances of two episodes of paralyzing infection separated by a number of years in the same patient. Infants may be protected against infection during the first three to six months of life by antibody passively transferred from the mother.

Prevention. Because 90 to 95 per cent of cases of poliomyelitis are inapparent or "minor" infections and are not diagnosed, the prevention of the disease by isolation is very difficult. The common practice of isolating clinically evident cases is of much greater benefit to the ill patient than to the public health. The usual period of isolation is about two weeks, although virus may be present in the feces for a much longer period. Contact with known cases should be avoided. Restriction of community activities such as swimming, gatherings of people, and so forth is not necessary except during large epidemics when it is more effective in allaying panic than in reducing the incidence of disease. Pregnant women should take special precaution because of their heightened susceptibility to poliomyelitis. Tonsillectomy is contraindicated in areas where this infection is present. All persons with "minor" illnesses during the poliomyelitis season should limit their physical activity and avoid becoming chilled until all symptoms have disappeared.

Vaccines. *Killed Virus Vaccine.* Active immunization against paralytic poliomyelitis has been successfully produced by parenteral administration of formalin-inactivated strains of the three viral serotypes grown in monkey kidney tissue cultures—the Salk vaccine. This vaccine is said to be about 60 to 70 per cent effective against Type I and 85 to 90 per cent against Types II and III. It has been suggested that two doses of vaccine be given one month apart, a third injection seven to twelve months later, and a fourth dose one to two years after the third. Booster doses should be given bienially thereafter. During the initial period of the widespread use of Salk vaccine, it was noted that from 20 to 45 per cent of persons with paralytic poliomyelitis in various areas of the United States had been immunized with this agent. This apparent relative ineffectiveness of the vaccine probably did not indicate a lack of value but rather a relatively low antigenic potency of some of the preparations. The commercial vaccines presently available have been improved in quality so that the expected high level of protection can probably now be attained. The most recently developed vaccine is said to be about five times more potent antigenically than earlier preparations, contains a Type I strain that is basically less virulent than the one first used, and is almost free of kidney protein and antimicrobial drug. No antibody is demonstrable in about 20 per cent of patients after the first injection of vaccine. In most persons without immunity prior to vaccination, a neutralizing capacity of low degree appears in about four to six weeks after the first dose of vaccine but falls gradually over the next few months. Increase in the level of immunity follows the administration of booster doses. Another type of killed poliomyelitis virus vaccine has been used extensively in Sweden. Only one case of the disease was observed in 5,400,000 people (75 per cent of the population) who received this preparation from 1963 to 1967. During this period, 15 to 20 million doses were given; no nervous system complications were observed.

The vaccine does not appear to decrease the incidence of nonparalytic poliomyelitis. It prevents viremia and invasion of the nervous system, but has no effect on the intestinal phase of the disease and fails, therefore, to interrupt the spread of "wild" virus from one vaccinated person to another. Another disadvantage of the formalin-inactivated vaccine is the necessity for repeated "booster" doses for the maintenance of a protective level of antibody. Reactions to the vaccine are uncommon; headache, stiffness of the neck, arms, and legs that may be accompanied by pain, skin hypersensitivity, fever, sore throat, vomiting, and pain at the site of injection have been noted. Untoward allergic effects owing to the antimicrobial drugs contained in the vaccine have been observed and may be severe. Killed poliomyelitis vaccine is now used very infrequently. It should be pointed out, however, that both short and long-term immunity follow its use and, when its effects are measured by the degree of serologic response, it is as good or better than attenuated vaccine. It has been suggested that the killed preparation may be of value in areas of the world where the efficacy of attenuated live vaccine is suboptimal. This is particularly a problem in the warm climates because of the high level of prevalence of enteroviruses which may interfere with the establishment of the vaccine strains of poliomyelitis virus in the intestine. It is common practice at present to administer live vaccine to individuals who, in the past, have received only the killed virus.

Live Virus Vaccines; Oral Poliomyelitis Vaccine (OPV). Immunization with orally administered living poliomyelitis virus produces neutralizing antibodies and protection against infection. The virus strains are prepared by isolation of a single virus particle that has low virulence and a high degree of antigenicity. The vaccine may be given in a capsule, in milk, in candy, or by medicine dropper. It is stable in a deep-freeze for many months, in an ordinary refrigerator for one month, and at room temperature for three to five days. After oral administration, vaccine virus multiplies in the intestinal tract and remains at this site. Viremia occurs very rarely, and then only with some strains. Live vaccine virus spreads and infects unvaccinated persons, but more than three consecutive transmissions do not occur among close contacts. The incidence of spread is lowest in high income groups (about 9 per cent), is higher in families living under relatively poor conditions (about 53 per cent), and is highest (40 to 80 per cent) following feeding to infants. Three months after oral administration to large groups, vaccine virus disappears almost completely from a community. The widespread use of this type of immunization in the presence of epidemic poliomyelitis may lead to replacement of the "wild" paralytogenic strain by the one in the vaccine.

The degree of antibody response varies, to some extent, with the strain in the "live" vaccine. Ingestion of the Sabin "triple" vaccine, for example, produces a good response to Type II and a relatively poor one to Types I and III. The serologic response depends on whether single types are given separately or are administered simultaneously. In general, the effect is best with monovalent and least with trivalent preparations. An adequate antibody response is produced, however, by giving "triple" vaccine twice. Significant levels of antibody develop in 90 to 100 per cent of persons receiving "live virus" vaccine; they develop more rapidly and persist longer than those that follow the use of formalinized vaccines. Intestinal immunity is present after feeding of the "live" preparations so that minimal or no multiplication in the bowel occurs on exposure to "wild" strains of virus. Because both intestinal immunity and circulating neutralizing antibody are present after immunization with the "live virus" vaccine, the degree of protection against infection is superior to that produced by the parenteral administration of formalinized vaccine. Coproantibody (IgA) for poliomyelitis virus is present in the stools of persons receiving live attenuated vaccines but not in those given killed vaccines. Excretion of this type of antibody over a period of three months is 100 per cent for Types I and II and 40 per cent for Type III virus; it may be detected for months to years in an appreciable number of immunized individuals. Antibodies (IgA) to the virus are demonstrable in the nasal and duodenal secretions of individuals receiving the live attenuated vaccine; they are absent in those given killed preparations.

Live poliomyelitis virus vaccine has been administered to millions of people. Its effectiveness in controlling the spread of this disease and in preventing infection has been completely established. The incidence of the paralytic form of this disorder fell from an annual level of 14.6 per 100,000 over the period 1950 to 1954 to about 1.8 cases per 100,000 in 1961; this decline has been attributed to the widespread use of the formalin-inactivated vaccine. Since the introduction of OPV, the incidence of paralytic poliomyelitis declined to a very low level. In 1965, poliomyelitis was the lowest in incidence in the United States since records of the disease have been kept. There were only 61 cases in that year and 5 deaths. More than 50 per cent of the patients were less than five years old; 70 per cent had received no vaccine. In 1966, there were 103, and in 1967, 40 cases of paralytic poliomyelitis reported in the United States; 3 persons in each of these groups had received what appeared to be adequate immunization.

Live poliomyelitis virus vaccines possess a high degree of safety; significant reactions have not been observed. However, the possibility that paralytic poliomyelitis may follow the administration of these preparations has been raised. In 1964, a Special Advisory Committee to the Surgeon General of the United States Public Health Service analyzed 57 cases of paralytic disease that developed within 30 days of the ingestion of OPV that they considered as "compatible" with infection by vaccine strains; of these, 15 subjects had received Type I, 2 had been given Type II, 36 had been treated with Type III, and 4 had taken trivalent preparations. Disease was observed primarily in adults and more often in males than females. On the basis of estimated total number of doses of OPV administered and the number of "compatible" infections, the Committee suggested the following incidence of paralytic poliomyelitis associated with specific types of vaccine virus: Type I, 0.16; Type II, 0.02; and Type III, 0.4 per million doses of vaccine; the risk was considered to be greatest in persons 30 years of age or older. Sabin expressed doubt of the significance of the very small number of cases of vaccine-associated paralytic disease, questioned the fact that these occurred largely among adults, and did not agree that unvaccinated adults in rural areas and upper socioeconomic groups were, as suggested by the Committee, at greater risk.

All infants should receive monovalent live poliomyelitis vaccine during the first year; OPV is distinctly superior to formalin-inactivated preparations during this period of life. A "booster" of trivalent OPV should be given at the time youngsters first enter school; if they have not been immunized previously, the primary series of monovalent vaccines must be administered. All communities that have not been thoroughly immunized should be given the benefit of widespread vaccine ingestion. Although it has been suggested that the risk of infection by vaccine strains, especially Type III, is highest in adults, this does not mean that such persons should not receive OPV. In fact, the greater frequency of extensive paralysis and death in patients over the age of 16, especially those 30 or older, indicates an even greater need for immunization in this age group than in young children, in whom poliomyelitis is generally less severe and the fatality rate low (2.5 per cent of paralytic cases). Persons at high risk, such as those living in or traveling to areas of the world where the disease may be still present, should receive OPV.

Monovalent vaccines are preferred to trivalent preparations. Although the conventional order of administration of the monovalent vaccines has been Type I followed by Type III and then Type II, it has recently been recommended that this be changed to the following: Type II followed no earlier than eight weeks later by Type I and then Type III six or more weeks later. It is thought that Type II infection may confer heterologous immunity against Types I and III. The necessity for and advantages of this order of administering monovalent preparations of OPV have been questioned.

Although passage of vaccine virus from one person to another leads to some increase of pathogenicity, as determined by assessment of neurovirulence in monkeys, the heightened invasive capacity quickly reaches a plateau and becomes stabilized at a level below that thought to be dangerous for man. There is presently no evidence that viral agents that may be present in the monkey kidney tissue, the culture medium for the vaccine virus, will infect man when given orally. The presence of other enteroviruses in the intestinal tracts of those given OPV may "interfere" with implantation of the vaccine strains, leading to failure of immunity to develop. That this is so has been demonstrated in the tropics, where many people carry enteroviruses and where the rate of successful immunization has been only around 60 per cent. This points up the fact that immunization with OPV should be carried out in the cooler months of the year, a period when the intestinal carriage of enteroviruses is at a low level. More than 70 million doses of all types of attenuated oral poliomyelitis vaccine were administered in the United States from 1965 to 1967. Among the people who had received these preparations, there were only 8 cases of the disease that appeared to be related to the vaccine. There were 16 other cases involving individuals with family or other close contacts of those who had been immunized. The highest risk seemed to be associated with the administration of monovalent Type III vaccine.

Experiences with the use of live poliomyelitis virus vaccine indicate that its widespread application to persons of all age groups and saturation, especially of children of the preschool age, may come very near to eradicating poliomyelitis. Its administration in the face of a threatened epidemic of the disease is highly effective in limiting spread of infection and preventing the large epidemics that not long ago were the scourge of populations in various parts of the world. Although the necessity for booster doses is still in question, it is relatively common practice to administer a single dose of trivalent vaccine one year after completion of immunization with the monovalent preparations. The administration of a second dose of "triple vaccine" one year later has been recommended by some. "Booster" doses may be of special value in those instances in which the efficacy of the primary immunization may have been reduced because of the prevalence of "interfering" viruses in the intestinal tract.

Beale, A. J.: Immunization against poliomyelitis. Brit. Med. Bull., 25:148, 1969.

Katsuro, K., Tatsumi, H., Tatsumi, M., and Reisaku, K.: Studies on poliovirus coproantibody. I. Neutralizing antibodies in feces of children following Sabin oral poliovirus vaccination. Amer. J. Epidemiol., 83:1, 1966.

Lepow, M. L., Serfling, R. R., and Sherman, I. L.: A survey of immunization levels after an oral poliovaccine program in Cleveland. J.A.M.A., 187:749, 1964.

Ogra, P. L., Karzon, D. T., Righthand, F., and MacGillivray, M.: Immunoglobulin response in serum and secretions after immunization with live and inactivated poliovaccine and natural infection. New Eng. J. Med., 279:893, 1968.

Sabin, A. B.: Oral poliomyelitis vaccine: History of its development and prospects for eradication of poliomyelitis. J.A.M.A., 194:130, 1965.

Special Advisory Committee on Oral Poliomyelitis Vaccines to the Surgeon General of the Public Health Service: Oral poliomyelitis vaccines. J.A.M.A., 190:49, 1964.

Weinstein, L.: Cardiovascular disturbances in poliomyelitis. Circulation, 15:735, 1957.

Weinstein, L.: Influence of age and sex on susceptibility and clinical manifestations in poliomyelitis. New Eng. J. Med., 257:47, 1957.

Weinstein, L.: The influence of muscular fatigue, tonsilloadenoidectomy and antigen injections on the clinical course of poliomyelitis. Boston Med. Quart., 3:11, 1952.

COXSACKIE AND ECHOVIRUSES: GENERAL CONSIDERATIONS
Albert Z. Kapikian

The Coxsackie viruses A and B, echoviruses, and polioviruses comprise the enterovirus subgroup of the human picornaviruses. In addition to the enterovirus subgroup, the human picornaviruses include two other subgroups, the rhinoviruses (described in a preceding article), and the unclassified picornaviruses representing those viruses that cannot be classified with certainty into the proper subgroup. The picornaviruses are grouped on the basis of certain common biochemical and biophysical properties, such as small size (15 to 30 nm.), ribonucleic acid (RNA) core, and resistance to inactivation by ether. The term picornavirus was chosen to signify two of these properties: "pico" implying small, and "rna" referring to the nucleic acid type.

COXSACKIE VIRUSES

The isolation of the first of the Coxsackie A viruses during a study of a small poliomyelitis outbreak was reported by Dalldorf and Sickles in 1948. Suspensions of fecal specimens from two patients with paralytic poliomyelitis were found to cause paralysis in suckling mice, with widespread degeneration of the skeletal musculature. Since polioviruses were not known to cause illness in suckling mice and since these newly recovered agents (unlike the polioviruses) produced no illness in monkeys, it was assumed that a new agent distinct from the polioviruses had been isolated. As neither the anatomic lesions nor the range of symptoms induced by infection with this agent in man was known, it was suggested that the virus be called "Coxsackie virus" because the first strains were isolated from residents of Coxsackie, New York. The following year additional types, including the first of the Coxsackie B viruses, were isolated. In the ensuing years numerous other Coxsackie A and B viruses were isolated; at this writing, there are 23 Coxsackie A viruses (numbered A1 to A22 and A24) and 6 Coxsackie B viruses (numbered B1 to B6). Coxsackie A23 is omitted because it is currently classified as echovirus type 9.

The Coxsackie viruses are divided into groups A and B on the basis of differences in lesions induced in suckling mice. In this animal the group A viruses characteristically produce flaccid paralysis with widespread degeneration of skeletal musculature and no other lesions, whereas the group B viruses produce fewer and less severe skeletal muscle lesions, but produce in addition encephalitis, fat necrosis, pancreatitis, hepatitis, and myocarditis; clinically, group B-infected suckling mice develop tremors, spasticity, and spastic paralysis. All Coxsackie B viruses (and echo- and polioviruses) grow readily in monkey kidney tissue cultures, but none of the Coxsackie A viruses (with the exception of A9) are capable of consistently growing in this tissue.

ECHOVIRUSES

The first echoviruses were isolated in the early 1950's as a result of the introduction of tissue culture techniques as an efficient tool for the isolation and study of polioviruses. During the course of studies attempting to isolate poliovirus in tissue cultures from fecal specimens, agents were found that not only were not neutralized by either poliovirus or Coxsackie virus antisera but also were incapable of inducing illness in suckling mice or in monkeys. These new "enteric viruses" were later termed enteric cytopathogenic human orphan viruses (echo), because they were isolated predominantly from the lower alimentary tract, caused cytopathogenic changes in monkey and human cell cultures, were not pathogenic in any laboratory animal, and were human in origin. The term "orphan" was suggested because these viruses had not been associated etiologically with any disease.

At this writing 31 echovirus types are known and are numbered 1 to 33, types 10 and 28 being omitted. Type 10 was found to be considerably larger in size than other echoviruses and is now classified as reovirus type 1; type 28 was found to possess certain properties (such as inactivation at pH 3) not shared by other echoviruses and is now classified as rhinovirus 1A.

DISEASES DUE TO COXSACKIE AND ECHOVIRUSES

A definitive presentation of diseases caused by Coxsackie and echoviruses is difficult, because these agents have been isolated from an ever increasing list of specific diseases and clinical syndromes. The mere isolation of the virus from a patient's throat or anal swab and/or the demonstration of serologic evidence of infection is not sufficient evidence to establish an etiologic relationship between the virus and the patient's illness. Isolation of the virus from blood, cerebrospinal fluid (CSF), or diseased tissue is more meaningful evidence for an etiologic association than the above, but even more meaningful evidence may be obtained from controlled epidemiologic studies. The establishment of an etiologic association is especially difficult with the Coxsackie and echoviruses. These viruses not only commonly cause subclinical infections but are also frequently shed in the stools for several weeks after either subclinical or clinically apparent infection. Therefore an isolation could occur by chance during various periods of illness or well-being. Only those specific diseases or clinical syndromes in which either satisfactorily controlled

epidemiologic studies have established the etiologic relationship between Coxsackie or echovirus infections and an illness, or in which virus isolations have been made from blood, CSF, or diseased tissue will be presented in the following discussions (see accompanying table).

Epidemiology. Coxsackie and echoviruses are widely distributed throughout the world. They are found most commonly in human feces, but may also be found in the oropharynx or in nasopharyngeal washings; in patients with aseptic meningitis these agents may also be recovered from the CSF. They are resistant not only to the common antimicrobial drugs such as penicillin, streptomycin, and the tetracyclines, but also to many of the commonly used antiseptics such as 70 per cent alcohol, 5 per cent Lysol, and 1 per cent quaternary ammonium compounds. The occurrence of these infections is not influenced by sex or race. They have been isolated from all age groups, but it is apparent that infants and children are most susceptible to infection. The prevalence of these agents in surveys of presumably normal infants and children has ranged from less than 5 per cent to 50 per cent, depending on the location of the survey. Season appears to be an important factor in the epidemiology of Coxsackie and echovirus infections, for the majority of infections occur during the summer and early autumn months. The incubation period may vary widely, but usually ranges from 2 to 15 days.

These viruses produce a broad spectrum of clinical manifestations, ranging from inapparent infection and mild undifferentiated respiratory or nonrespiratory illnesses to severe illnesses with varying involvement of the central nervous system. Illnesses associated with one or both of these agents are described in the next series of articles below (see table).

DISEASES CAUSED BY COXSACKIE AND ECHOVIRUSES

Coxsackie viruses group A, types 1–22, 24:
  Herpangina (types 2, 3, 4, 5, 6, 8, 10, 22)
  "Hand, foot and mouth disease" (types 5, 16)
  Acute lymphonodular pharyngitis (type 10)
  Aseptic meningitis (types 1, 2, 4, 5, 7, 9, 10, 14, 16, 22, 24)
  Epidemic exanthemata (type 9)
  "Common-cold like" (type 21)
  Acute undifferentiated respiratory or nonrespiratory illnesses (all types listed above)
Coxsackie viruses group B, types 1–6:
  Epidemic pleurodynia or Bornholm disease (types 1–5)
  Aseptic meningitis (types 1–6)
  Myocarditis of newborn infants (types 1–5)
  Myocarditis and pericarditis of infants beyond newborn period, children, and adults (types 1–5)
  Orchitis (types 1–5)
  Acute undifferentiated respiratory or nonrespiratory illnesses (types 1–6)
Echovirus types 1–9, 10–27, 29–33:
  Aseptic meningitis (types 1–9, 11, 12, 14–19, 21, 22, 25, 30, 31, 33)
  Epidemic exanthemata (types 9, 16)
  Diarrhea (type 18, possibly types 6, 7, 14, 19)
  Acute undifferentiated respiratory or nonrespiratory illnesses (all types listed above plus type 20)

PREVENTION OF COXSACKIE AND ECHOVIRUS INFECTIONS

The ability to produce effective inactivated and live poliovirus vaccines offers hope that such vaccines can also be produced for the Coxsackie and echoviruses. However, at the present time, the need and demand for such vaccines have not been determined.

HERPANGINA
Albert Z. Kapikian

Definition. Herpangina is a specific infectious disease characterized by the presence of small papulovesicular lesions on the anterior pillars of the tonsillar fauces and the soft palate; it occurs frequently in outbreaks among infants and children during the summer and early autumn.

History. It was first described in 1920 as a distinct clinical syndrome by Zahorsky in a report of 82 cases of "herpetic sore throat"; he subsequently suggested that this "peculiar throat disease . . . the clinical features of which are sufficiently clear to separate . . . from other diseases of the mouth and throat" be named "herpangina." Two other outbreaks of illness resembling herpangina were reported in 1939 and 1941.

Etiology. Herpangina was not described again until 1950 when Huebner et al. described studies in which certain group A Coxsackie viruses were recovered from 32 of 37 herpangina patients, and on the basis of epidemiologic evidence an etiologic association was suggested. Numerous clinical and epidemiologic reports from many parts of the world have confirmed an etiologic relationship between certain group A Coxsackie viruses and herpangina (see table). Reports have appeared recently relating certain Coxsackie B and echovirus infections temporally with herpangina-like syndromes; further epidemiologic studies are needed to elucidate the role of the Coxsackie B and echoviruses in the pathogenesis of herpangina-like syndromes.

Epidemiology. Herpangina is a common infectious disease occurring frequently in outbreaks, but also sporadically, in most parts of the world predominantly during the summer and early autumn. Although it occasionally occurs in adults, the highest incidence is found in infants and young children. Multiple cases in a family are frequently observed. Spread is from person to person with an incubation period of about four days. Subclinical infections as well as illnesses without the characteristic herpanginal lesions commonly occur in family members infected with the same serotype as that recovered from the herpangina case. Immunity to the infecting type appears permanent, but recurrent attacks occur as a result of infection with a different serotype.

Pathology. The pathologic process of herpangina in man is not known, as no deaths have been reported.

Clinical Manifestations. The illness is characterized by a sudden elevation of temperature (101 to 105° F.) and the development of the characteristic throat lesions in association with variable systemic signs and symptoms. In a study of 69 Coxsackie A virus-positive infants and children with herpangina, 89 per cent developed a fever which lasted an average of two days with a range of one to four days; 5 per cent of patients with temperature elevations developed febrile convulsions. Anorexia, dysphagia, or sore throat was evident in 70 per cent, vomiting in 38 per cent, abdominal pain in 21 per cent, and headache in 16 per cent (Parrott and Cramblett, 1957). The disease is characterized by the presence of discrete 1 to 2-mm. grayish papulovesicular pharyngeal lesions on an erythematous base. These lesions, which gradually progress to slightly larger ulcers, may appear on the anterior pillars of the tonsillar fauces, the soft palate, the uvula, and the tonsils, and are usually present for four to six days after the onset of illness. In one herpangina case in a seven-year-old girl, small ulcers were also observed on the labia and skin near the genital region (Mitchell and Dempster, 1955). White blood cell counts usually reveal no characteristic abnormality; cerebrospinal fluid examinations have been normal.

Diagnosis. In a typical case, careful, repeated examination of the oral cavity and pharynx should facilitate the diagnosis. Herpangina can be differentiated from acute infectious gingivostomatitis resulting from herpes simplex virus, because the lesions in the latter disease are located on the gums, lips, tongue, or buccal mucuous membrane; lesions may also be found on the anterior pillars of the faucial tonsils or soft palate (as in herpangina), but almost always they occur in association with similar lesions in the anterior portions of the mouth. In addition, herpetic gingivostomatitis occurs sporadically in all seasons of the year. In recurrent aphthosis the lesions do not usually occur in the pharynx and are not generally accompanied by fever. Herpangina should also be differentiated from "hand, foot, and mouth disease" and acute lymphonodular pharyngitis, both of which are described below.

Prognosis and Treatment. Herpangina is a self-limited disease, with complete recovery occurring usually within four to six days. There is no specific therapy for the Coxsackie virus infection. Treatment is supportive and symptomatic.

HAND, FOOT, AND MOUTH DISEASE
(Vesicular Stomatitis and Exanthem)
Albert Z. Kapikian

An outbreak in Toronto of a new clinical syndrome caused by Coxsackie A16 virus was reported in 1958 (Robinson et al.). Observed chiefly in infants and children, and occasionally in young adults, the new syndrome was characterized by vesicular and ulcerative lesions of the mouth and oropharynx or fauces and a vesicular eruption involving the hands, feet, and legs. In 1960 the term "hand, foot, and mouth disease" was first used to describe a similar outbreak in England (Alsop et al.). Coxsackie A5 virus has also been found to be associated with sporadic cases (Flewett, et al., 1963).

ACUTE LYMPHONODULAR PHARYNGITIS
Albert Z. Kapikian

An outbreak in Kentucky of a new clinical syndrome caused by Coxsackie A10 virus was reported in 1962 (Steigman et al.). Observed chiefly in children, the illness was characterized by lesions on the uvula, anterior pillars, and posterior pharynx. The lesions were raised and discrete, whitish to yellowish in color, solid and not vesicular, and surrounded by a 3 to 6 mm. zone of erythema. Patients experienced fever, headache, and sore throat, with symptoms lasting 4 to 14 days. Incubation period was estimated at 5 days.

EPIDEMIC PLEURODYNIA OR BORNHOLM DISEASE
(Epidemic Myalgia, Devil's Grip)
Albert Z. Kapikian

Definition. Epidemic pleurodynia or Bornholm disease is a specific acute infectious disease of viral etiology, characterized by the sudden onset of severe abdominal and/or chest pain, fever, and headache. It occurs most often in the summer or early autumn, frequently in outbreaks, but may also occur sporadically.

History. Numerous outbreaks of this disease were described in early medical literature. Windorfer relates that Hannaeus described an outbreak occurring in Schleswig-Holstein in 1732. In 1872, Daae and Homann each reported an epidemic in Drangedal, Norway. Two years later Finsen, using the term pleurodynia, described outbreaks in 1856 and 1865 in Iceland. In 1888, Dabney provided the first description of such an outbreak in the United States; a patient described the severe chest pain as the "devil's grip" — a term subsequently applied on occasion to designate this disease. Hanger, McCoy, and Frantz reported 16 cases in 1923 and called the syndrome epidemic pleurodynia. Sylvest in 1930 described an outbreak on Bornholm, a Danish island in the Baltic; in 1933 he wrote a classic monograph "Epidemic Myalgia," in which he reviewed the world literature and presented detailed case histories of 93 patients with the disease in Bornholm and Copenhagen; the designation Bornholm disease was frequently applied following Sylvest's descriptions.

Etiology. The Coxsackie B viruses are recognized as the etiologic agents of epidemic pleurodynia or Bornholm disease. In 1949 Curnen, Shaw, and Melnick recovered a Coxsackie B virus from the feces of a 14-year-old boy with acute pleurodynia; in addition, they reported the occurrence of illnesses resembling pleurodynia in several laboratory personnel working with this virus.

Subsequently, numerous studies appeared relating temporally epidemic pleurodynia and Coxsackie B virus infections (see table).

Epidemiology. Outbreaks of Bornholm disease have been reported from most parts of the world. It is noteworthy that they generally occur in the summer and early autumn. Although all age groups can be affected, children and young adults experience the highest incidence. Intrafamilial spread is common, multiple cases in a single family being observed frequently; however, absence of intrafamilial spread should not exclude the diagnosis. In one large study, about one third of the patients developed the illness as single cases in a household (Warin et al., 1953). Although both large outbreaks and sporadic cases have been described, epidemic pleurodynia is not a common disease in that it is not generally prevalent each summer and early fall, but rather occurs in sharp outbreaks confined to geographically limited areas. The mode of transmission is probably by person-to-person contact, with an incubation period of about two to five days.

Pathology. The specific pathologic manifestations in humans are unknown as no deaths have been reported.

Clinical Manifestations. Epidemic pleurodynia is characterized typically by the sudden onset of abdominal and/or chest pain, fever, and headache. The spasmodic abdominal or chest pain which may range from mild to extremely severe and which is often aggravated by respiration and movement is the most characteristic feature. In a report on 22 patients with epidemic pleurodynia who had a mean age of 25 years, Huebner et al. described the sensation of difficult breathing as particularly striking, and cited some characteristic descriptions of this symptom: "I can't breathe," "pain cut off my breath," "can't get a real long breath," and "it hurts to breathe." In a study of 114 patients hospitalized with epidemic pleurodynia in Boston, Finn et al. reported that the typical severe paroxysmal pleuritic type of pain was often described as "smothering," "stabbing," "knifelike," "catching," and "like a vise around the lower ribs." It is noteworthy that, although the onset of pain is typically the initial symptom, in the Boston study about one quarter of the patients had prodromal symptoms one to ten days before the onset of pain — symptoms such as "head cold," headache, anorexia, and myalgia.

Review of several outbreaks reveals that the location of the characteristic pain in infants and young children tends to be more abdominal than thoracic, whereas in older children and adults it tends to be more thoracic than abdominal. For example, in the 1949 Boston study in which almost three quarters of the patients were between 10 and 30 years of age, the characteristic pain was located in the chest alone in 48 per cent, in the chest and abdomen in 37 per cent, and in the abdomen alone in 14 per cent. In contrast, in a 1953 Birmingham, England, study of 104 hospitalized children whose average age was 5½ years, the characteristic pain was located in the abdomen alone in 81 per cent, in the abdomen and chest in 11 per cent, and in the chest alone in 9 per cent (Disney et al.). Similar findings were reported in a South African outbreak in which 32 (80 per cent) of 40 children had abdominal pain alone, 4 both abdominal and chest pain, and 4 chest pain alone (Patz et al., 1953).

In the Boston study the chest pain was located "over the lower ribs and for varying distances up the chest, usually on the lateral aspect but not infrequently over the front and back" except in six patients whose thoracic pain was limited to the substernal region only; about one third of patients with chest pain experienced referral of such pain to one or both shoulders, one or both scapulae, the interscapular region, or the neck. Among those with abdominal pain, approximately three quarters experienced epigastric or upper abdominal pain; it was noteworthy that in two patients the site of pain was in the right lower quadrant. Other symptoms among the total group included moderately severe or severe headache (44 per cent), cough (33 per cent), anorexia (26 per cent), nausea (24 per cent), chilly sensations (21 per cent), chills (18 per cent), "head cold" (16 per cent), vomiting (16 per cent), sore throat (12 per cent), and diarrhea (7 per cent). Physical examination revealed that 95 per cent were febrile (99 to 104° F.) with a mean temperature of 101° F.; the fever lasted a mean of 3½ days with a range of 1 to 14 days. Recrudescences of fever after the temperature had returned to normal or nearly normal were common. The pulse rate was proportional to the temperature. Visible splinting of the chest was observed commonly, especially during paroxysms of pain. In addition, a pleural friction rub confined to the lower half of the chest was heard in about one quarter of all cases. Localized tenderness to pressure was found in about one quarter of cases and was usually confined to those areas of the chest where pain was present. Tenderness confined to the abdomen (in 29 per cent), or tenderness in both abdomen and chest (in 9 per cent) were the most common abdominal findings, although "splinting and rigidity of the upper abdominal area were not infrequently present, especially when the pain was severe" (Finn et al.). In the Birmingham children's study, generalized abdominal tenderness was present in 34 per cent and right iliac fossa tenderness in 13 per cent (Disney et al., 1953). Roentgenographic examinations of the chest have revealed no characteristic abnormalities. The white blood cell count is usually within normal limits; occasionally a moderate leukopenia, leukocytosis, or eosinophilia may be present. The majority of patients are well within one week of onset, but longer periods of illness are not unusual. It is noteworthy that not infrequently relapses may occur a few days or more than one month after recovery.

Complications. Complications of epidemic pleurodynia occur relatively infrequently and include orchitis, aseptic meningitis, and pericarditis. Cases of Coxsackie B myocarditis of new-

born infants have occasionally been reported during outbreaks of epidemic pleurodynia. It is noteworthy, however, that myocarditis has only very rarely been reported as a complication in a patient with epidemic pleurodynia; however, the possibility should be borne in mind.

Diagnosis. A clinical diagnosis is usually not difficult once the presence of an epidemic is known. However, during the early stages of an outbreak or when a sporadic case is encountered, it may be quite difficult, if not impossible, to make the correct diagnosis. A vivid illustration of this difficulty is provided by a children's hospital study in which it was found that, until the house staff and other medical personnel in the community became aware that a pleurodynia outbreak was occurring, admission diagnoses on children eventually shown to have epidemic pleurodynia included the following: acute abdomen, possible appendicitis, possible duodenal ulcer, pyelonephritis, pneumonia, pleurisy with pneumonia, rheumatic fever, pain of unknown origin, trauma (fractured rib), myositis (influenzal), collagen disease, tuberculosis, and intussusception (Bain et al., 1961). Symptoms of common duct obstruction, pancreatitis, coronary occlusion, and intestinal infections may also be mimicked by epidemic pleurodynia.

Laboratory Findings. Laboratory diagnosis of Coxsackie B infection is made by isolation of the virus from throat washings or stools during the early phase of illness and by demonstrating a rise in neutralizing antibody against one of the Coxsackie B viruses in acute and convalescent phase sera. Unfortunately results of such tests become available too late to be of assistance in making a diagnosis in the acute case.

Treatment and Prognosis. There is no specific therapy for the Coxsackie virus infection. Treatment is supportive and symptomatic. Recovery is usually complete and follows after variable periods as noted above. However, some patients may experience lingering after effects of tiredness and weakness, with a gradual return to normal health.

CARDIAC MANIFESTATIONS OF COXSACKIE VIRUS INFECTIONS
Albert Z. Kapikian

MYOCARDITIS NEONATORUM
(Epidemic Myocarditis of Newborn; "Acute Aseptic Myocarditis")

Coxsackie B viruses were first recognized as a cause of severe, often fatal myocarditis in the newborn infant in the mid-1950's when investigators in South Africa, the Netherlands, and the United States reported 14 fatalities among 20 newborns who developed the disease from 3 to 21 days after birth (Montgomery et al., 1955; Javett et al., 1956; van Creveld and De Jager, 1956; Verlinde et al.,

1956; Kibrick and Benirschke, 1956). Isolation of a Coxsackie B virus from the myocardium of six fatal cases provided firm evidence of an etiologic association. In most cases infection undoubtedly occurred soon after birth; however, in several it may have occurred in utero. It was noteworthy that outbreaks of other syndromes etiologically associated with Coxsackie B viruses (such as Bornholm disease, "summer grippe," and aseptic meningitis) were occurring concurrently in the general population.

The onset of the disease is typically acute and is characterized by dyspnea, cyanosis, pallor, and tachycardia. Some patients may have a fever, and in others the temperature may be subnormal. Vomiting and coughing attacks may also be present. Initially the disease may be mistaken for pneumonia, but symptoms of cardiac decompensation with enlargement of the heart and liver soon appear. Significant cardiac murmurs are not usually present. The electrocardiogram shows evidence of severe damage to the myocardium. In fatal cases the infant rapidly develops severe prostration and circulatory collapse. Pathologic examination of the heart reveals both a diffuse and focal infiltration of lymphocytes, polymorphonuclear leukocytes, plasma cells, and reticulum cells. In some areas the striations of the myocardial fibers are distinct but in others degeneration and necrosis may be present. Encephalitis, aseptic meningitis, and hepatic and adrenal lesions have also been observed in newborns with myocarditis. There is no specific therapy for Coxsackie virus infections. Treatment is supportive and symptomatic. (See later article on Myocarditis.) Individuals suspected of having Coxsackie B virus infections (based on epidemiologic, clinical, or other evidence) should, of course, be restricted from visiting maternity and nursery units; in addition, appropriate quarantine measures should be taken if a patient in a maternity or nursery unit develops an illness suggestive of a Coxsackie B virus infection.

MYOCARDITIS AND PERICARDITIS IN INFANTS BEYOND THE NEWBORN PERIOD, IN CHILDREN, AND IN ADULTS

Cases of myocarditis and pericarditis in infants beyond the newborn period, in children, and in adults have also been found to be associated with Coxsackie B virus infections. In addition to occurring as a distinct clinical entity, pericarditis may also occur as a complication of Bornholm disease. Myocarditis has only rarely been reported as a direct complication of Bornholm disease, but the possibility should be borne in mind.

It is not possible at this time to estimate the relative importance of the Coxsackie viruses in the over-all etiology of myocarditis or pericarditis; epidemiologic and laboratory studies are needed to answer this important question. (See articles on Myocarditis and Pericarditis.)

"ASEPTIC MENINGITIS" DUE TO COXSACKIE AND ECHOVIRUSES
Albert Z. Kapikian

Coxsackie and echoviruses are important causes of aseptic meningitis in infants and children, as numerous serotypes have been implicated etiologically with this syndrome (see table). The epidemiology, clinical manifestations, and diagnosis of aseptic meningitis caused by Coxsackie and echoviruses (and other agents as well) are presented in a preceding article on Viral Meningitis.

It is noteworthy that sporadic cases of paralytic illness resembling paralytic poliomyelitis have been associated temporally with certain Coxsackie and echovirus strains (especially Coxsackie A7, which also causes neuronal lesions in monkeys); in addition, sporadic cases of encephalitis have been associated with these viruses as well. Further epidemiologic studies are needed to elucidate the role of these viruses in the pathogenesis of such illnesses.

EXANTHEMATA AND "ASEPTIC MENINGITIS WITH RASH" DUE TO COXSACKIE AND ECHOVIRUSES
Albert Z. Kapikian

In 1954 Neva et al. described the isolation of a new virus, later classified as echovirus 16, from patients with a mild exanthematous illness. The same virus was recovered during a similar outbreak occurring three years later, and it was suggested that the disease be called "Boston exanthem," because the first outbreak had occurred in and around that city. The illness, which affected infants and children, and adults as well, was characterized by several days of fever and a macular or maculopapular rash which usually appeared soon after the fever and other signs and symptoms had subsided; no central nervous system (CNS) manifestations were observed. It is noteworthy, however, that echovirus 16 was also recovered during the Boston outbreak from hospitalized patients with aseptic meningitis without rash (Kibrick et al., 1957).

In the mid and late 1950's numerous outbreaks of aseptic meningitis with rash caused by echovirus type 9 were observed in many parts of the world; in a few of the outbreaks an exanthem was not present. In typical outbreaks the clinical manifestations may vary widely from a very mild illness to the classic aseptic meningitis syndrome with or without rash. The eruption, which is characteristically macular or maculopapular, usually appears during the febrile period and occurs most often in infants and young children.

Coxsackie A9 virus has also been found to be a cause of an illness characterized by fever and a maculopapular or vesicular eruption with or without signs of CNS involvement; CNS involvement without rash may also occur. "Hand, foot, and mouth disease" has been associated etiologically with Coxsackie A16 and A5 virus infections and is discussed above. In addition, it is noteworthy that various other Coxsackie and echovirus serotypes have been associated with sporadic cases or small outbreaks of exanthematous illnesses.

ACUTE UNDIFFERENTIATED RESPIRATORY AND NON-RESPIRATORY ILLNESS DUE TO COXSACKIE AND ECHO-VIRUSES

Albert Z. Kapikian

Most of the Coxsackie and echovirus serotypes that are etiologically related to specific or severe illnesses such as aseptic meningitis, epidemic pleurodynia, herpangina, various exanthemata, myocarditis, and pericarditis have also been shown to be capable of producing mild acute undifferentiated febrile or afebrile respiratory or non-respiratory illnesses that are indistinguishable from such illnesses caused by many other agents. (see table). These mild illnesses are the most common clinical manifestations of Coxsackie and echovirus infections in infants and children, and are frequently described as "summer grippe." It is of interest that these nonspecific illnesses occur with greater frequency than the specific ones and often in the total absence of any concomitant occurrence of the more specific illness usually regarded as characteristic of these viruses.

Coxsackie A21 (Coe) virus has been shown to be the etiologic agent of an upper respiratory illness in an outbreak in a military population in which the agent was shed by 32 (26 per cent) of 122 patients with respiratory illness and by only 6 (6 per cent) of 108 of the controls (Bloom et al., 1962). A "common cold syndrome" was the most frequent illness observed, a fever of at least 100° F. occurring in 14 of the virus-positive patients; fever in 5 of the 14 patients reached 102° F. Studies of this agent with volunteer subjects have also shown its ability to induce a characteristic upper respiratory illness (Parsons et al., 1960). It is of interest that Coxsackie A21 virus was isolated much more frequently from throat swabs than from anal swabs in both the naturally occurring and artificially induced illnesses. Coxsackie A21 virus does not appear to be a major cause of upper respiratory infections in civilian populations. In volunteer studies, echovirus types 11 and 20 have been shown to be capable of inducing mild undifferentiated illnesses in adults (Philipson, 1958; Buckland et al., 1959, 1961).

COXSACKIE AND ECHOVIRUSES IN DIARRHEAL DISEASES OF INFANTS

Albert Z. Kapikian

The relative importance of the Coxsackie and echoviruses in the etiology of gastroenteritis and epidemic diarrhea in infants and young children is difficult to determine at this time and awaits further epidemiologic studies. However, evidence has accumulated that indicates that echoviruses are capable of causing outbreaks of mild diarrheal syndromes in infants and young children. In 1958 conclusive epidemiologic data were presented on the etiologic association of echovirus type 18 in an epidemic of summer diarrhea occurring in 12 premature and 5 older full-term infants in a hospital in New York City (Eichenwald et al.). Echovirus 18 was isolated from 15 of the 17 infants; in addition, all 17 demonstrated serologic evidence of infection. Clinically this disease was not severe. No significant temperature elevations or hypothermia was seen. The infants passed five or six fairly large watery greenish stools each day, for one to five days, with a mean duration of three days. No mucus or pus cells were seen.

Controlled studies among infants and young children under four years of age conducted in Cincinnati demonstrated that enteroviruses were recovered 2.5 times more frequently from patients with diarrhea than from controls (48 per cent versus 20 per cent) (Ramos-Alvarez and Sabin, 1958). Echoviruses were recovered six times more often from children with diarrhea than from controls (31 per cent versus 5 per cent), whereas the recovery of polioviruses and Coxsackie viruses was about the same in the diarrhea and control groups. Echovirus types 6, 7, and 14 were isolated from the majority of echovirus-positive children. In a controlled study of infants and children with diarrhea in the summer and fall in Mexico, it was found that echovirus infections occurred 8.5 times more often in diarrheal patients than in controls (Ramos-Alvarez and Olarte, 1964). Two other controlled studies (one in Texas, the other in Scotland) have failed to demonstrate statistically significant differences in the recovery rate of enteroviruses from infants and children with and without diarrhea (Yow et al., 1963; Sommerville, 1958). It was noteworthy, however, that the recovery rate of echoviruses was greater in the diarrheal patients than in the controls in both studies, although the difference was not sufficiently great to be of significance.

Dalldorf, G., and Melnick, J. L.: Coxsackie viruses. *In* Horsfall, F. L., Jr., and Tamm, I. (eds.): Viral and Rickettsial Infections of Man. 4th ed. Philadelphia, J. B. Lippincott Company, 1965, p. 474.

Finn, J. J. Jr., Weller, T. H., and Morgan, H. R.: Epidemic pleurodynia; Clinical and etiologic studies based on one hundred and fourteen cases. Arch. Intern. Med. (Chicago), 83:305, 1949.

Horstmann, D. H.: Viral exanthems and enanthems. Pediatrics, 41:867, 1968.

Huebner, R. J., Beeman, E. A., Cole, R. M., Beigelman, P. M., and Bell, J. A.: The importance of Coxsackie viruses in human disease, particularly herpangina and epidemic pleurodynia. New Eng. J. Med., 247:249, 1952.

Kibrick, S.: Current status of Coxsackie and echoviruses in human disease. Progr. Med. Virol. 6:27, 1964.

Melnick, J. L.: Echoviruses. In Horsfall, F. L., Jr., and Tamm, I. (eds.): Viral and Rickettsial Infections of Man. 4th ed. Philadelphia, J. B. Lippincott Company, 1965, p. 513.

Weller, T. H., Enders, J. F., Buckingham, M., and Finn, J. J., Jr.: The etiology of epidemic pleurodynia: A study of two viruses isolated from a typical outbreak. J. Immun., 65:337, 1950.

ARTHROPOD-BORNE VIRAL FEVERS, ARTHROPOD-BORNE VIRAL ENCEPHALITIDES, AND ARTHROPOD-BORNE VIRAL HEMORRHAGIC FEVERS (ARBOVIRUSES)

GENERAL CONSIDERATIONS
Karl M. Johnson

Arthropod-borne viruses (arboviruses) are defined on an epidemiologic basis. Thus any virus is an arbovirus if it actually multiplies in one or more arthropods and if it is biologically transmitted to vertebrates with sufficient frequency by arthropods to make this an important means of virus survival. More than 220 distinguishable agents have been tentatively so classified. Many have similar physical and chemical properties and could reasonably be placed within families on this basis as well; others have fundamental properties relating them to animal virus groups not generally associated with recognized arthropod transmission.

Immunologic properties are currently used to cluster individual arboviruses. Viruses having such relationships are included in groups that historically began with A and B (still the largest), and then C; thereafter, the name of the first virus to be discovered was used to designate the group. In the beginning virus names were derived from antecedent diseases, e.g., yellow fever, dengue, equine encephalitides. Later, geography in combination with disease syndrome was favored, providing names such as St. Louis encephalitis and Colorado tick fever. Finally, there are many geographically named arboviruses for which no clinical syndromes have been defined, either because they rarely infect man or because they have not been associated with morbidity of dramatic proportions.

About 80 arboviruses are known to infect man, and most of these have been shown to produce illness. With rare exceptions, such as dengue and

urban yellow fever, these are zoonoses in which man is an accidental host of no apparent importance in the fundamental natural history of the virus.

Clinical syndromes produced by arboviruses share the common properties of fever and myalgia accompanied by viremia. Beyond that, classification is inevitably arbitrary, as the same virus can induce a wide variety of patterns in different patients, and different viruses have been linked to remarkably similar syndromes. Emphasis here is given to the often infrequent but spectacular severe diseases some of the agents evoke. Thus individual descriptions are placed in one of the following groups: (1) fevers of a relatively undifferentiated type, with or without rashes, usually benign; (2) *encephalitides*, often severe and with significant case fatality rates; and (3) *hemorrhagic fevers*, also frequently severe and fatal.

The largest number of viruses has been associated with milder, undifferentiated disease. The majority of these have been encountered most commonly in tropical and semitropical countries, and prior to specific etiologic work were clinically known as three-, four-, or seven-day fevers, jungle fever, sandfly fever, and so on. The classic clinical prototype is dengue. Those to be described represent but a small sample. Of these *Semliki Forest* and *Mayaro* are group A viruses, *dengue* and *West Nile* belong to group B, and the remainder are unclassified or are in the sandfly fever group. Although each gained entry to this book because of its proved epidemic disease potential for man, clinical differentiation even during epidemics is generally difficult; epidemiologic and laboratory methods are more important. When more than one such virus is simultaneously *endemic*, the latter techniques are essential.

All arboviruses conspicuously associated with encephalitis and hemorrhagic fever are included. In the case of the latter syndrome, each virus is antigenically a group B agent even though important epidemiologic and clinicopathologic features of the respective syndromes may be widely different. Yellow fever is listed among the hemorrhagic fevers because many cases do not display the "classic" picture of jaundice, but manifest gastrointestinal hemorrhage (black vomit), epistaxis, and melena with fatal shock and thus fit this description better than either of the other two arbovirus clinical syndromes.

DENGUE*
(Break-Bone Fever, Dandy Fever, Seven-Day Fever, etc.)
Karl M. Johnson

Definition. Dengue is an acute, febrile, infectious disease, Aedes mosquito-borne and caused by

*In previous editions the article on Dengue was written by Dr. William McD. Hammon. Significant portions of that article are included in the present version prepared by Dr. Johnson, who joins with the Editors in expressing indebtedness to Dr. Hammon.

a dengue virus. Typically it has an abrupt onset associated with malaise and severe prostration, pain of muscles and joints, one or two episodes of exanthems, lymphadenopathy, leukopenia, and duration of about a week followed by severe depression and weakness. It is observed most frequently in epidemic form.

Etiology. Four distinct immunologic subtypes of dengue virus have been isolated from patients during epidemics. These viruses produce only partial cross-immunity. A primary infection wth one will protect against another subtype only for a few months, although homologous immunity lasts many years. There is accumulating evidence, however, to indicate that sequential infection with any two subtypes produces long-lasting protection against subsequent infection with disease by any of the remaining two subtypes.

Incidence and Prevalence. The distribution of the viruses is only partially known, but it appears that all continents and many islands are or have been involved. The size of human populations and the ecologic factors affecting the mosquito vector and virus multiplication in that host seem to be of principal importance. Thus, dengue fever occurs only in "summer-like" temperatures, and only where there are large numbers of Aedes aegypti, Aedes albopictus, or some of the Aedes scutellaris complex mosquitoes, the only recognized natural vectors.

Most primary infections produce clinically apparent disease. Thus, there is a strong correlation between morbidity and infection rates, the latter measured during epidemics by serologic methods. In contrast, conditions favorable to endemic transmission of the virus, e.g., large human populations, perpetual "summer" with continuous mosquito breeding, lead to a smoldering situation in which age-specific acquisition of dengue virus immunity is high in the absence of clinically apparent clustering of dengue fever disease. In specific circumstances, often associated with insular ecology, introduction of dengue virus at intervals measured in decades may produce morbidity rates as high as 50 to 80 per cent within a few months.

Epidemiology. Man and certain Aedes mosquitoes are both essential links in the recognized natural epidemiologic cycle. Viremia adequate for mosquito infection is present for the first three to five days of illness. A mosquito of a suitable species feeding on a patient during this period requires about eight to twelve days at summer temperatures to become infective. It is then capable of initiating infection in one or a series of susceptible persons it may feed on or probe. The mosquito remains infectious as long as it lives. Transovarian infection has not been demonstrated. The incubation period and interval until viremia occurs in man is about five to six days. Aedes aegypti, the common urban vector, usually breeds only in and near human habitations, rests and feeds ordinarily only in the house, and is primarily attracted to man. It is a daylight and twilight feeder. These qualities make it an ideal epidemic vector. Multiple cases occur within a house, and daytime visitors carry the infection to other domiciles, where another group of mosquitoes acquires infection.

No jungle reservoir has been discovered, but monkeys and forest mosquitoes are suspected of playing such a role, as in jungle yellow fever.

The virus is frequently transported over great distances when infected human travelers carry it during the incubation period or when infected mosquitoes are carried by land, sea, or air vehicles.

In rural areas, Aedes albopictus or other Aedes species may serve as vectors, but their habits and the more sparsely distributed human hosts render severe, explosive epidemics less likely.

Pathology. Because dengue fever is rarely, if ever, fatal, the pathologic processes are unknown except as revealed by biopsy of the skin rash. In this regard Sabin states that "the chief abnormality occurred in and about small blood vessels and consisted of endothelial swelling, perivascular edema and infiltration with mononuclear cells. In the petechial lesions extensive extravasation of blood, without appreciable inflammatory reaction, was observed." Pathologic findings have been reported in fatal cases, but as none was of confirmed origin, the diagnosis is very much open to question. The various stages in the pathogenesis of the disease are unknown.

Clinical Manifestations. As described by Hammon in previous editions of this text, the "classic" case of dengue from etiologically identified epidemics and inoculation of volunteers has a sudden onset marked by rapidly rising temperature, usually without a shaking chill, but almost always associated with some chilliness. Headache and fatigue are severe. By the second day the temperature is 103 to 105° F., the headache is still very severe, and the patient complains of severe ocular or retrobulbar pain, particularly on moving the eyes. There are excruciating back pain and generalized aching of various muscles, frequently involving joints. In walking this results in a stiffness of the joints and the mincing gait of a "dandy," from which the disease is said by some to have received its name. A fleeting *erythematous macular or pinpoint rash* may be noted during the first or second day, particularly on the limbs, but more frequently the only skin manifestation is a diffuse blushing, particularly of the face, neck, and chest. Anorexia is severe. Pulse and temperature at this stage are roughly proportionate. General lymphadenopathy is usually apparent, but hepatomegaly and splenomegaly are seldom present. The leukocyte count at this early stage is likely to be essentially normal.

Beginning about the third or fourth day, a rather conspicuous *maculopapular* or *scarletiniform rash* appears. It usually starts on the trunk and spreads to the face and extremities. This generally lasts three or more days and may be conspicuous even after the temperature is normal. The fever generally lasts for five to seven days, frequently with a fall on about the fourth day, giving a saddle-back type of curve. The final bout of fever may be the most severe. Occasionally on about the last day of illness, a few petechiae appear, usually about the ankles.

The total leukocyte count falls considerably as the disease progresses and by the fourth or fifth day may be extremely low. The number of segmented leukocytes is greatly reduced, but the more immature or nonsegmented polymorphonuclear cells typically show an absolute increase in number. Monocytes and lymphocytes decrease in absolute numbers.

A relative or even absolute bradycardia may exist during the last phase of the illness and during early convalescence. The fading rash is frequently itchy but rarely desquamates. During convalescence extreme weakness, anorexia, and mental depression form an important part of the disease pattern. The patient may not feel able or may not desire to resume normal activity for two weeks or more following return of the temperature to normal.

As children have not been reported in volunteer studies with known viruses and have not been referred to in detail in authenticated outbreaks, the widely varying clinical responses attributed to them in epidemics of undetermined cause lead to uncertain interpretation. The disease is generally described as much milder and frequently unrecognized in the very young, and it is probable that many infections in children go undiagnosed because of their mildness. This appears to account for the absence of recognized dengue among natives in endemic areas, where only children are susceptible to primary infection.

Diagnosis. In the presence of a sharp epidemic with many "classic" cases, compatible environmental temperatures, and heavy exposure to bites of recognized vector species of mosquitoes, the diagnosis of many cases with average severity will usually be correct. However, it must be recalled that chikungunya, also known to be transmitted by *Aedes aegypti,* and probably other viruses may also be the cause. Thus, laboratory confirmation of a *few* cases during every epidemic becomes important. When cases occur *sporadically,* the cause of *each one* must be determined in the laboratory.

During the period of viremia, virus may be isolated from blood or serum by intracerebral inoculation of suckling mice or by certain types of tissue culture. Isolation of virus provides the most convincing proof of the cause. Serologic diagnosis is less satisfactory. In areas where several group B arthropod-borne viruses are present, if the patient has been infected previously with one or more of these (the usual finding in tropical and subtropical areas), it is not usually possible by presently available serologic methods to distinguish the particular group B virus responsible for the current infection. It may not be possible even to determine whether the infecting virus is

in the dengue subgroup. Serologic tests performed on an acute and a convalescent phase serum sample from a patient not previously infected with a related group B agent, using any dengue virus as an antigen, will usually demonstrate a titer rise; but the titer will be highest when the infecting type of dengue virus is used. Complement fixation, neutralization and hemagglutination-inhibition tests are all of use. Their relative ability to differentiate specifically between dengue types is approximately in the order listed.

In differential diagnosis, without the assistance of a virus laboratory, careful attention must be paid to clinical symptoms, the presence or absence of other similar cases in the area, the ambient climatic temperature, and exposure to and bites from known vector species. Travel in a known endemic or epidemic area five to eight days prior to onset may be an important part of the history of a sporadic case encountered in a region where the disease is not ordinarily seen.

Treatment. There is no specific therapy. The nonspecific therapy should include bed rest, if possible, maintenance of fluid and electrolyte balance, and alleviation of discomfort. Aspirin, 0.3 to 0.6 gram, alone or in suitable combination with phenacetin and caffeine, should be given every three to four hours. (Salicylates may produce aberrations from the typical fever chart.) Severe pains may necessitate oral or subcutaneous administration of codeine sulfate, 30 to 60 mg. Other therapeutic measures should be designed to keep the patient as comfortable as possible. Complications should be anticipated, recognized, and treated as indicated. Resumption of normal activities should not be rushed; a two-week period of convalescence is desirable and often needed.

Prognosis. Except in severely debilitated persons the prognosis is excellent. The case fatality rate in etiologically proved cases is zero except for patients concurrently suffering from another relatively severe disease. Final recovery is usually complete, although temporary emotional disturbances, usually depression, are not uncommon during convalescence.

Prevention. No vaccine is available from commercial sources, but experimental attenuated mouse-brain (live) vaccine for both types 1 and 2 has been produced and tested in volunteers. This gives rise to a relatively mild febrile disease with rash, and apparently affords solid immunity to experimental inoculation with virulent virus.

Community protection is possible only through eradication or effective control of the appropriate Aedes vector. Bed nets are essentially useless for individual protection of older children and adults, because biting by the specific vectors does not occur at night. Mosquito repellents have limited usefulness.

Patients during the febrile stage (first four or five days) must be kept in mosquito-free quarters or under a bed net to prevent infection of more mosquitoes. All mosquitoes in the home or building in which a patient has resided or visited during the onset or early phase of disease should be killed by space spraying, as viremia has usually been present before the diagnosis can be made.

Hotta, S.: Twenty years of laboratory experience with dengue virus. I. Epidemiology—past and present. *In* Sanders, M., and Lennette, E. H. (eds.): Applied Virology. Sheboygan, Wis., Ellis Corporation, 1965, pp. 228-256.
Sabin, A. B.: Dengue. *In* Rivers, T. M., and Horsfall, F. L., Jr. (eds.): Viral and Rickettsial Infections of Man. 3rd ed. Philadelphia, J. B. Lippincott Company, 1959.
Siler, J. F., Hall, M. W., and Hitchins, A. P.: Dengue, its history, epidemiology, mechanism of transmission, etiology, clinical manifestations, immunity and prevention. Philipp. J. Sci., 29:1, 1926.
Simmons, J. S., St. John, J. H., and Reynolds, F. H. K.: Experimental studies of dengue. Philipp. J. Sci., 44:1, 1931.
Wisseman, C. L., Jr.: The ecology of dengue. *In* May, J. M. (ed.): Studies in Disease Ecology. New York, Hafner Publishing Company, Inc., 1961, Chap. 2, p. 15.

SEMLIKI FOREST–MAYARO VIRUS DISEASE
Telford H. Work

Definition. *Semliki Forest virus infection* is an uncharacterized nonfatal disease, probably mildly febrile and of short duration, in tropical Africa. *Mayaro virus disease* of the New World tropics is characterized by fever, headache, photophobia, conjunctival injection, generalized aches and pains, occasional nausea, and slight icterus with mild leukopenia for a period averaging three days. The infection is induced by bites of culicine mosquitoes infected with these antigenically very closely related viruses of the Semliki-Mayaro complex of Casals' arbovirus group A.

Etiology. Semliki Forest virus was first isolated in a locality of the same name in Uganda in 1944 from *Aedes abnormalis* mosquitoes. A strain known as Kumba, isolated from *Eretmapodites* mosquitoes in the West African Cameroons, has been shown to be antigenically the same. Recently the virus has been isolated in Mozambique. Infection with this virus has been recognized in man only by serologic survey studies that demonstrated development of specific neutralizing antibodies in blood sera of substantial numbers of native residents of West and East Africa. A specific human infection is known by accidental infection of a laboratory worker (Shope).

The virus is small, being in the range of 15 to 30 mμ, and is unusually resistant to heat, 60° C. for one hour being required for inactivation. It is neurotropically pathogenic for mice by intracerebral and intraperitoneal inoculation; a variety of other laboratory animals, including guinea pigs, rabbits, and certain monkeys, are susceptible only by intracerebral inoculation. It also infects and grows in hamsters, embryonated eggs, and several tissue culture cell systems.

Mayaro virus was isolated on five occasions from blood of acutely ill residents of Trinidad in 1954 by intracerebral inoculation of suckling mice. It does not produce disease in adult mice. By means of cross complement-fixation and hemagglutination-inhibition tests, Casals (1957) demonstrated antigenic distinctness—but very close relationship—of neotropical American Mayaro virus with African Semliki Forest virus. Contrary to virologic custom, the differences that were evident by in vitro serologic tests could not be distinguished in mouse neutralization tests that are usually applied to show distinctive differences between arboviruses.

Semliki Forest and Mayaro viruses of Casals' group A are most closely related to *chikungunya virus*, which is discussed in another part of this section. Mayaro may be identical with *Uruma virus*, isolated from sick human beings observed in a Bolivian jungle.

Epidemiology. By serologic surveys and outbreaks of disease in Trinidad and Brazil, it is apparent that Semliki Forest–Mayaro virus diseases are widespread arbovirus infections in tropical Africa and South America. The slight but distinct antigenic differences between the two etiologic agents may reflect discontinuous evolution from a prototype virus owing to geographic isolation in ecologic situations differing slightly from the old to the new world. A similar phenomenon has been demonstrated between African and American strains of yellow fever virus.

The nonhuman vertebrate blood source of Semliki Forest and Mayaro viruses for mosquito vectors is unknown. Their appearance repeatedly in human infections over long time periods in many tropical countries indicates that they are geographically and endemically widespread, producing in newly exposed nonimmune persons epidemics such as occurred in the Guama River region, 100 miles east of Belem in the Amazon Basin of Brazil in 1955. The cases in this epidemic have provided the most comprehensive and detailed characterization of the human disease to date.

Clinical Manifestations. After an incubation period believed not to exceed seven days, which is important in establishing possible exposure to infected mosquito bite, the disease begins with the onset of fever associated with headache, usually most severe in the frontal region. There follows the development of generalized aches and pains with severe myalgia in the back and occasional arthralgia. Photophobia is associated with conjunctival injection. Careful examination may reveal slight icterus without other skin manifestations. The patient may complain of epigastric pain and nausea and may have a bout or two of diarrhea and vertigo. Blood count reveals a slight leukopenia ranging from 5000 to 6000 cells. The disease is self-limited, with no sequelae or mortality. The average duration is three days, although fever has continued for as long as five days in some cases.

Diagnosis. Because the clinical symptoms and signs are like those of many infections, specific diagnosis rests on positive results from laboratory examinations. Blood should be collected as soon as possible after onset of fever for inoculation of serum intracerebrally into suckling mice. Saline or buffered borate saline suspension of brain material harvested from the inoculated mice when they appear sick or moribund can be used as antigen for preliminary identification by complement-fixation test. In lieu of virus isolation from acute blood, paired sera can be used in complement-fixation and hemagglutination tests to detect a significant rise in titer against group or homologous serum antigens.

Treatment. The patient should be put to bed and treated symptomatically with antipyretics and analgesics for the fever and pain. No known therapy will shorten the course of the infection, so the problem is that of keeping the patient as comfortable as possible while the disease runs its self-limited course.

Prevention. There is no specific prophylaxis other than control of the specific mosquito vector or avoidance of bite by mosquitoes in an area where control measures are not effective. Avoidance consists of the usual sleeping under mosquito nets, screening of houses, wearing appropriate clothing, application of repellents, and restricted movement during hours of mosquito activity. No vaccine is available for specific immunization.

Anderson, C. R., Downs, W. G., Wattley, G. H., Akin, N. W., and Reese, A. A.: Mayaro virus: A new human disease agent. II. Isolation from blood of patients in Trinidad, B.W.I. Amer. J. Trop. Med., 6:1012, 1957.

Downs, W. G., and Anderson, C. R.: Distribution of immunity to Mayaro virus infection in the West Indies. W. Indian Med. J., 7:190, 1958.

WEST NILE FEVER
Telford H. Work

Definition. West Nile fever is an acute febrile illness of sudden onset often associated with severe headache, generalized lymphadenopathy, and macular skin eruption. It is a self-limited disease with a febrile phase usually of less than one week followed by relatively slow convalescence of one to two weeks. Low mortality owing to encephalitis occurs in the aged. This is the only age group in which overt central nervous system disease has been observed. The disease results from infection by mosquito-borne virus of the Japanese B–West Nile complex of Casals' arbovirus group B.

Etiology. West Nile virus is one of the smaller arboviruses, measuring 20 to 30 mμ in size. Its name derives from isolation of the first strain in 1937 in the West Nile province of Uganda from the blood of a native woman suffering a febrile illness that first implicated it as a human pathogen. Philip and Smadel in 1942 demonstrated its propagation in and experimental transmission by culicine mosquitoes. Hurlbut, Whitman, and Aitken (1960) have demonstrated propagation and transmission of the virus in hard and soft ticks.

West Nile virus is closely related antigenically to Japanese B encephalitis, Murray Valley encephalitis, St. Louis encephalitis, and Ilheus viruses that constitute the Japanese B–West Nile complex of arbovirus group B. These mosquito-borne viruses of this complex are regionally widespread, covering most of the inhabited temperate and tropical areas of the earth. It is worthy of note that, although the concept of antigenic regionalization and mutual exclusion is generally applicable within such antigenic complexes or subgroups, both West Nile and Japanese B encephalitis viruses have repeatedly been isolated from the same mosquito species in the same localities in southeastern India.

The usual infection of man occurs by bite of infected culicine mosquitoes. The virus rapidly multiplies and reaches titer of 3000 LD$_{50}$ per milliliter of blood and is recoverable up to four days after onset of disease. The virus produces infection (viremia and antibody response) in a variety of vertebrates, and is neurotropic on intracerebral inoculation into white mice or peripheral inoculation of suckling mice, producing paralytic and fatal encephalitis. This is the routine laboratory method for its isolation. As with all members of arbovirus group B, JBE–WN complex viruses, saline suspensions, and sucrose-acetone or acetone-ether extractions of West Nile virus infected mouse brain provide high titer complement-fixing and hemagglutinating antigens.

West Nile virus has been shown to have an oncolytic effect on certain types of tumor cells, and has produced palliative but not permanent regression of tumor tissue in patients who also suffered encephalitis as a result of the experimentally induced massive infection.

West Nile virus is also highly infectious by unnatural routes of exposure during laboratory manipulation of fluid or dried materials containing the agent. Many laboratory infections have occurred, ranging from inapparent to the fully characterized clinical course.

Epidemiology. It is probable that millions of people have suffered infection with West Nile virus. It is known to be endemic in many inhabited areas of Africa, the Middle East, and southwest Asia, including peninsular India, by detection of specific antibodies in serologic surveys and by virus isolations from man, birds, and mosquitoes. However, the general outline of West Nile virus epidemiology is derived from clinical and immunologic studies in Israel and a classic study of the ecology of the virus in Egypt. Epidemics have afflicted all ages of new nonimmune immigrants into Israel from temperate European countries, where no mosquito transmission of group B arboviruses is known. West Nile virus isolations and epidemiologic association implicate *Culex molestus* as the primary vector in Israel.

In contrast, West Nile fever is a childhood disease in Egypt, where the virus is endemic. Epidemic transmission occurs every summer primarily by *Culex univittatus* mosquitoes, which serve as key vectors in the natural bird-mosquito-bird cycle. The annual spring hatch of new nonimmune wild birds, such as the hooded crow and rock pigeon, following infection, provides a pool of virus that ultimately reaches human beings by the bites of mosquitoes infected by feeding on the viremic birds. Experimental work has demonstrated that many avian species circulate West Nile virus at high titer for many days.

In the Nile Delta, mosquito transmission of the virus is so common and extensive that even immune residents are apparently repeatedly infected subclinically almost every year. Thus, evaluation of virus transmission to all ages of the Egyptian population can uniquely be accomplished by in vitro testing for short-duration complement-fixing antibody as well as by more orthodox testing for lifelong neutralizing antibody. Although West Nile virus has been experimentally propagated in and transmitted by ticks, their role in the overwintering or dissemination of the virus has not been established.

Even though no virus isolations from mosquitoes or human patients have been made during winter months, serologic conversion of Egyptian children to West Nile immune status during all seasons of the year indicates a low level of continuous virus transmission during the nonepidemic months, possibly by *Culex pipiens*, the predominant mosquito in cool weather. The disease contributes significantly to the etiology of fevers of obscure origin in Egyptian children just as two thirds or more of the summer fevers of Israel are now considered to result from West Nile virus infection.

Clinical Manifestations. West Nile fever, as the terminology implies, is a disease that is essentially febrile in its clinical appearance. Although inapparent and subclinical infections have been documented, most human infections result in clinically recognizable symptoms and signs of disease. The most detailed clinical descriptions derive from the epidemic cases in Israel, where thousands of cases have occurred.

After an incubation period of three to six days, there is sudden onset of fever associated with severe headache and malaise. The febrile phase is of three to six days' duration, occasionally with a "saddle back" temperature curve. Fever has been known to last as long as twelve days, but such cases are rare. Chills, photophobia, and dispersed myalgia may accompany the fever. Gastrointestinal disturbances, anorexia, and nausea have occurred in some patients.

An exanthem occurs in most pediatric patients and is commonly, but not so frequently, seen in adults. It is a *maculopapular rash* found usually on the trunk but sometimes also on the face and extremities, often so vague as to require pressure or chilling for detection. It lasts 24 to 72 hours, is not irritating, and fades without desquamation. Lymphadenopathy is commonly found on examination, but there is no regular localization, distribution, or character of lymph node enlargement. Blood examination almost always shows a decided leukopenia with relative lymphocytosis in the febrile phase.

Meningismus occurs and cerebrospinal fluid examination has shown increase in cells and protein. However, it is to be stressed that, contrary to the clinical picture of disease caused by antigenically closely related viruses (Japanese B encephalitis, Murray Valley encephalitis, St. Louis encephalitis) of this arbovirus subgroup, this is not clinically a neurologic disease except very rarely in the aged, who may succumb from encephalitis. These are the only fatalities attributed to this infection. Because West Nile fever is a self-limited nonfatal disease, the histopathology in humans has not been studied.

The older the patient, the slower the recovery, sometimes requiring several weeks of convalescence, weakness being the main complaint. There are no sequelae.

Diagnosis. An acute febrile illness of sudden onset associated with severe headache, lymphadenopathy, macular rash, and leukopenia in a tropical or subtropical area of Africa, the Middle East, or South Asia, or following laboratory exposure to the virus, suggests West Nile fever. Clinically, it is so similar to a dengue syndrome that it has actually been termed by some clinicians "Mediterranean dengue." A definite diagnosis is therefore a virologic diagnosis, which can be accomplished only by examination of appropriate specimens in the laboratory.

Because of prolonged viremia, an acute-phase blood specimen can hopefully be expected to yield a virus on intracerebral inoculation into suckling mice or yolk sac inoculation of embryonated eggs. Acute-phase blood collected as late as the fourth day after acute onset is worth inoculating for virus isolation. With or without isolation of virus, testing of paired or sequential acute and convalescent sera is mandatory by complement-fixation, hemagglutination-inhibition and neutralization tests. The hemagglutination-inhibition screening against any of a number of the mosquito-transmitted arbovirus group B antigens will orient further complement-fixation and neutralization testing with specific antigens. The complement-fixation test will give the most expeditious presumptive etiologic diagnosis, which must be confirmed for specificity by neutralization test using the homologous isolate and several other Japanese B encephalitis–West Nile complex viruses to determine specificity by maximal neutralization index.

High-titer complement-fixation and hemagglutination-inhibition test results with particular antigens may lead to misinterpretation of what specific etiologic agent is involved, particularly in patients with demonstrable antibody to previous exposure to group B viruses as, for instance, by 17D yellow fever vaccination or tropical exposure to one of the dengue viruses. Without a test against a homologous virus isolated from the patient during the acute illness, a report of laboratory diagnosis based exclusively on serology must be qualified.

Treatment. The treatment is exclusively symptomatic. In a self-limited viral disease for which there is no specific therapy, antipyretics and analgesics are indicated for relief of discomfort. Bed rest, maintenance of hydration, and controlled ambulation during convalescence are the extent of medical management beyond a special effort to collect required specimens for laboratory diagnosis. The resulting immunity is probably lifelong, preventing clinical recurrence when the person is exposed to later reinfection under normal environmental circumstances.

Prevention. There is some clinical impression that antibody to other arbovirus group B agents by vaccination or natural infection mitigates the severity of illness. There is no specific vaccine for West Nile fever. Killed and attenuated strains of West Nile virus have been used in various combinations in investigational procedures for production of broad-spectrum group B arbovirus antibody resulting from active immunization, but are not available for clinical use.

The only specific preventive measures consist of environmental control of vector mosquitoes or prevention of exposure to mosquito bite through the use of mosquito nets, wearing appropriate clothing, household screens, and application of repellents during periods of outdoor exposure.

Goldblum, N., Sterk, V. V., and Paderski, B.: West Nile fever: The clinical features of the disease and the isolation of West Nile virus from the blood of nine human cases. Amer. J. Hyg., 59:89, 1954.

Philip, C. B., and Smadel, J. E.: Transmission of West Nile virus by infected *Aedes albopictus*. Proc. Soc. Exp. Biol. Med., 53:49, 1943.

Taylor, R. M., Work, T. H., Hurlbut, H. S., and Rizk, F.: Study of ecology of West Nile virus in Egypt. Amer. J. Trop. Med., 5:579, 1956.

RIFT VALLEY FEVER
Telford H. Work

Definition. Rift Valley fever is a toxic generalized febrile illness of short duration, accompanied by headache, photophobia, myalgia, anorexia, prostration, and leukopenia. It is caused by a mosquito-borne pantropic virus that is epizootic in domestic animals and enzootic in wild game, restricted, as its name implies, to East and South Africa.

Etiology. Rift Valley fever virus ranks second only to yellow fever virus in historic order of isolation as a filterable arthropod-borne cause of disease. Although first isolated from blood and tissues of diseased sheep and cattle in 1930 in East Africa, it was not isolated from wild mosquitoes until 1944. In propagation in and experimental transmission by mosquitoes, Rift Valley fever virus is species-selective.

Like the other arboviruses, Rift Valley fever virus is small, in the 23 to 50 mμ range. It can be preserved indefinitely in the lyophilized state. Appropriately prepared suspensions of infected material contain complement-fixing and hemagglutinating antigens. Very high titer antigens can be prepared by extraction of infected brain material by organic solvents.

Human infection results not only from mosquito transmission but from contact with tissues and secretions of sick animals and especially from handling the virus in the laboratory. Because of its high infectivity for man and widespread endemic and epidemic involvement of domestic and wild animal populations of Africa, to which its apparent natural range is limited, it is one of the few viruses prohibited in the United States, even for experimental work.

Epidemiology. The investigations that led to the isolation of Rift Valley fever virus in 1930 as a cause of disease in domestic animals and associated human beings in East Africa are classic in veterinary medicine. By moving afflicted flocks of sheep from mosquito-infested environments to higher elevations where mosquitoes were few, and by experimentally holding susceptible sheep under mosquito nets in perfect health while adjacent freely exposed pasture animals fell victims to the infection, indirect evidence accumulated that implicated mosquitoes as Rift Valley fever virus vectors. The geographic association of outbreaks of this disease and its elucidation in naturally exposed animals in the great Rift Valley of East Africa have given the virus and the resulting disease its name. Isolation of the virus from wild mosquitoes was not achieved

until fourteen years after its recovery from blood and tissues of infected vertebrates.

Rift Valley fever virus has been isolated from a number of species of naturally infected *Aedes, Culex,* and *Eretmapodites* mosquitoes, including *A. tarsalis, A. caballus, Culex theileri,* and *A. circumluteolus.* The variety of species and their distribution indicate that the virus is enzootic in wild game and other animals that abound in the zone of incidence. Following unusually heavy rains, which promote excessive mosquito production, the virus spills over from its wild reservoir into domestic herds and flocks, and the associated mosquito transmission results in epizootics that have been recorded many times in East and South Africa.

The first outbreak of Rift Valley fever recognized in South Africa occurred in 1951. Several have occurred since that time. Although livestock was affected primarily, associated cases resulted in persons who handled sick animals or their flesh. Antibody surveys indicate that virus activity is widely dispersed in East and South Africa, where natural human exposure seems to be uncommon.

Histopathology. The characteristic macroscopic and microscopic pathologic changes of this disease in sheep led veterinarians to label it initially as enzootic hepatitis. It was its nonfatal occurrence in man, in whom the pathologic processes are obscure because of the paucity of postmortem tissue, that caused adoption of the geographic term.

The pathognomonic lesion is necrosis in the liver, which in lambs, calves, and inoculated mice may be so extensive that even lobular architecture is lost. The process involves focal hyaline degeneration of the cell cytoplasm that ultimately results in development of cytoplasmic inclusion. Nuclei of hepatic cells are also attacked, and acidophilic intranuclear inclusions appear. As necrosis proceeds, there is massive accumulation of polymorphonuclear leukocytes around cell detritus, and erythrocytes may pack the sinusoids. Toxic degeneration, such as sloughing of the tubular epithelium in the kidneys and erythrocytic extravasation in the viscera, even with hemorrhagic enteritis, may occur. The pathologic process in Rift Valley fever in sheep and cattle is very similar to that seen in yellow fever and Kyasanur Forest disease in man, the two latter being respectively mosquito-borne and tick-borne group B arbovirus infections in man. Despite similarities that have been noted, lesions of yellow fever and Rift Valley fever can be readily differentiated in sections of liver tissue.

Clinical Manifestations. The numerous laboratory infections that have occurred provide the most detailed information about the disease in man. However, the patient's history may include association, in East and South Africa, with sick domestic animals, postmortem examination of domestic or game animals, or exposure to forest mosquitoes. Whatever the mode of virus transmission may be, it appears that some degree of overt disease occurs in most human infections.

The onset may be gradual over a number of hours, but it is usually sudden with high fever, photophobia, and intractable headache after an incubation period ranging from three to six days. In severe disease there are extreme prostration and generalized shifting myalgia, which may be most painful in the back and extremities. Anorexia is common. Pain occurs in the epigastrium. Nausea and vomiting may also occur.

The temperature ranges from 101 to 104° F. and often presents a "saddle back" curve in the course of acute illness, which lasts from two to six days, averaging something more than three days. Bradycardia relative to the level of fever is commonly observed as it is in a number of other pantropic toxic arbovirus infections, such as yellow fever. Leukopenia in the range of 4000 cells per cubic millimeter is characteristic and parallels the duration of the fever. It should be remembered that malaria parasites have appeared during the febrile phase in patients with Rift Valley fever. There is no response to antimalarial drugs, and the fever does not subside until shortly after viremia ceases.

Convalescence from Rift Valley fever usually progresses rapidly to complete recovery, although severe prostration during the acute illness may require prolonged convalescence of ten days or more. Vascular changes and hemorrhage may also result from infection with this virus.

Complications. The complication most frequently reported in man is a *central serous retinopathy* with associated *central scotomata*. Examination of the fundus shows exudative areas of variable size involving the macula that may result from thrombosis of the vessels. These exudative areas may last for several weeks, changing from a white mass to crenated shrinkage and ultimate disappearance. Although most patients recover completely and have a return of normal vision, *retinal detachment* has occurred. This is the most serious sequel to Rift Valley fever. In Africa any sudden visual defect following an acute febrile illness should suggest the possibility of Rift Valley fever complicated by serous retinopathy.

Diagnosis. Occupational or recreational exposure in potentially infected areas of Africa, association with diseased animals or their tissues, and laboratory exposure to the virus are the only leads to a tentative clinical diagnosis in a patient with an acute fever, myalgia, and leukopenia. Isolation of the virus by intracerebral inoculation of suckling or weanling mice with blood collected during the first three days of illness is the most certain way to establish a diagnosis. Rift Valley fever virus has a short incubation period, so the mice should sicken within three days after inoculation. Identification, using immune reference serum, can be accomplished by complement-fixation, hemagglutination-inhibition, or neutralization tests.

To date, Rift Valley fever virus has not been found to be related to any other virus. Therefore, a rise in specific antibody titer in paired acute and convalescent sera by complement-fixation or hemagglutination-inhibition test with Rift Valley fever virus antigen provides a definite diagnosis.

Treatment. There is no specific therapy for the arthropod-borne viral fevers. Management of the patient requires antipyretics and analgesics to relieve the discomfort of the acute illness. Blood examination may show, in addition to leukopenia, malarial parasites that do require administration of antimalarial drugs. The fever will not respond, however, until the viral infection has run its course. The serous retinopathy that may be detected on careful examination in the later phase of the illness is not amenable to specific treatment beyond continued rest for the patient.

Prevention. The original animal experiments that implicated mosquitoes as the vector demonstrate the value of elimination of exposure to mosquito bite in potentially infected areas by use of mosquito nets, screening, and repellents. This should be kept in mind by anyone in pursuit of game animals in East and South Africa.

Serial intracerebral passage of one strain of Rift Valley fever virus in mice has increased neurotropism at the expense of hepatotropism. This attenuated strain is now effectively used to immunize sheep, cattle, and other susceptible animals. No evaluation of the vaccine has been reported in man. A formalin-killed virus vaccine for human prophylaxis is presently under study.

Schrire, L.: Macular changes in Rift Valley fever. South African Med. J., 25:926, 1951.
Smithburn, K. C., Mahaffy, A. F., Haddow, A. J., Kitchen, S. F., and Smith, J. F.: Rift Valley fever. Accidental infections among laboratory workers. J. Immun., 62:213, 1949.

COLORADO TICK FEVER
Gordon Meiklejohn

Definition. Colorado tick fever is an acute, tick-transmitted viral disease that occurs throughout the Rocky Mountain area, and is characterized by a biphasic febrile course and profound leukopenia.

Etiology. Colorado tick fever virus is a member of the arbovirus group. The virus contains RNA, is small in size, and has not yet been shown to be related to other members of the arbovirus group. The virus is readily isolated from the blood in suckling mice or tissue culture. The virus has been isolated from a wide range of ticks and from a number of species of small mammals in the Rocky Mountain area. It appears, however, that only the wood tick, *Dermacentor andersoni*, is important in human transmission, because human cases are limited to the geographic distribution of this vector. All the states in the Rocky Mountain area have reported cases, the largest number occurring in Colorado. Cases also occur along the eastern border of California and in the western Canadian provinces.

Epidemiology. The disease occurs in the spring and summer, when tick exposure is common. At lower elevations, cases are observed from March onward; at higher altitudes, they occur late into the summer, reflecting the slower emergence of ticks at the higher altitudes. The reservoir of the disease is probably in numerous small mammalian hosts, particularly ground squirrels and chipmunks, which have a prolonged viremia and infect larvae or nymphs. The latter maintain the virus over the winter months, and the adult tick then transmits the virus to another small mammalian host or to man. In the majority of patients, tick attachment has been observed, and the tick may be present at the time of examination. Other patients, however, state that they have seen ticks on themselves or in their clothes, but that the ticks have not become attached. In a few instances, the ticks have been transported in bedding to distant locations and have caused disease outside the endemic area. Patients usually develop symptoms of illness three to seven days after tick exposure.

Pathogenesis. Viremia can be detected at the time of onset of fever, and persists throughout the febrile course. The virus may persist in or in association with the red blood cells long after it has disappeared from the serum. This has been shown, in both experimentally infected rodents and man. Red cells from human patients, presumably washed free of antibody, were found to contain virus as long as 39 days after the onset of illness.

The disease is characterized by a profound leukopenia, which is usually greatest during the second febrile episode. The most striking decrease is found in the granulocytes, but there is also frequently a marked thrombocytopenia and some anemia. Pathologic data on the disease in man are meager, because there has been only one reported fatal case. In this instance, the pathologic changes were those of an extensive hemorrhagic diathesis and encephalitis.

Symptoms and Clinical Course. The onset is usually sudden with chilly sensations, malaise, and fever. Muscle aching and pain about the joints are common manifestations, along with headache and backache. In children, anorexia, nausea, and vomiting are common. The disease is characteristically biphasic. The first episode of fever usually lasts two or three days, following which the temperature returns to normal. After a day of normal temperature, the fever again rises, and the second cycle usually approximates the first in length. Occasionally, there may be only a single febrile bout, or there may be three febrile episodes. The height of fever is extremely variable, ranging from 99.6 up to 105° F. Rashes are uncommon, but a small proportion of patients have petechial or macular rashes. Involvement of the central nervous system, especially in children, is an uncommon but more serious manifestation. In such patients, headache is frequently more severe. Signs of meningeal irritation are present, and the cerebrospinal fluid may show a pleocytosis. Patients who develop encephalitis have findings similar to those infected with other arboviruses such as disorientation, coma, and convulsions. Hemorrhagic manifestations, including epistaxis and gastrointestinal bleeding, occur very infrequently and are most commonly seen in patients with encephalitis.

Diagnosis. The diagnosis is based on a history of tick exposure during the preceding three to seven days, followed by a biphasic course with leukopenia. The initial febrile episode cannot be readily differentiated from many other acute febrile illnesses. However, by the time the second cycle has started, after an afebrile day during which the patient has felt moderately well, it becomes apparent that the illness is different. At this time, the peripheral blood count shows a profound leukopenia. The physical findings are not specific. A rash may be present that suggests an enterovirus infection. Moderate lymphadenopathy may be observed, and splenomegaly of mild degree is often present.

The diagnosis is confirmed by isolation of the virus from either serum or whole blood by the inoculation of suckling mice. These are still more sensitive indicators of the presence of virus than available tissue culture systems. The examination of acute and convalescent sera will also usually reveal the development of both neutralizing and complement-fixing antibodies.

The most difficult point in differential diagnosis arises from the fact that both Colorado tick fever and Rocky Mountain spotted fever are transmitted by Dermacentor andersoni. Rocky Mountain spotted fever may resemble Colorado tick fever during the first day or two before a rash becomes obvious. This differentiation is extremely important, because the early treatment of Rocky Mountain spotted fever with tetracycline will abort the illness and cure the patient.

Prevention. Protection against ticks by appropriate clothing or repellents is possible in tick-infested areas, but is rarely carried out. Frequent inspection for ticks and their removal may be helpful, but it has been noted earlier that prolonged tick attachment does not appear to be necessary for transmission of the disease.

Vaccines have been prepared from purified, infected suckling mouse brains. Repeated injections of these vaccines produce neutralizing antibody titer in recipients at levels that would probably provide a high degree of protection. These vaccines, however, have not been tested under field conditions.

Prognosis. The disease almost invariably runs a benign course, and the patient recovers in a relatively short period after defervesence. The rare exception is the patient who develops either an encephalitic or hemorrhagic tendency. Immunity is long lasting, and second infections in later life have not been reported.

Treatment. Treatment is symptomatic. Analgesic drugs such as salicylates are usually adequate to control the myalgia and headache. When the patient appears seriously ill and the diagnosis of Rocky Mountain spotted fever is seriously entertained, it is advisable to give tetracycline in doses of 2.0 grams per day. If the patient has Rocky Mountain spotted fever, the temperature usually falls to normal within 48 hours, whereas the course of Colorado tick fever is not altered by this regimen.

Eklund, C. M.: Natural history of Colorado tick fever virus. J. Lancet, 82:172, 1962.

Emmons, R. W., and Lennette, E. H.: Immunofluorescent staining in the diagnosis of Colorado tick fever. J. Lab. Clin. Med., 68:923, 1966.

Florio, L., Stewart, M. O., and Mugrage, E. R.: The etiology of Colorado tick fever. J. Exp. Med., 83:1, 1946.

Silver, H. K., Meiklejohn, G., and Kempe, C. H.: Colorado tick fever. Amer. J. Dis. Child., 101:30, 1961.

SANDFLY FEVER
(Phlebotomus Fever, Pappataci Fever)
John P. Fox

Definition. Sandfly fever is a viral disease characterized by fever, headache, ocular pain, conjunctival injection, and malaise followed by complete recovery. It occurs during the hot, dry season in parts of the European and African littoral of the Mediterranean, Asia Minor, the Russian shores of the Black Sea, Pakistan, and northwest and central India, where the vector fly, *Phlebotomus papatasii*, exists.

Etiology. The disease is caused by two small (about 25 mμ) antigenically unrelated viruses (Sicilian and Neapolitan) with closely similar properties, including a common, restricted host range (man, newborn mice, or, after adaptation, intracerebrally inoculated weaned mice). Both types can be propagated with cytopathic effect in several cell cultures, primary mouse (best) or human kidney and HeLa. Complement-fixing and hemagglutinating antigens can be prepared from brain tissue of infected newborn mice. Strains of both types, adapted to adult mice by Sabin, produce immunizing infections in man with no disease (Sicilian type) or negligible disease (Neapolitan type). Several viruses newly isolated from Brazil, Panama, Iran, and Pakistan, including some from febrile patients, are antigenically related to the Neapolitan type, which, thus, becomes the prototype of a new arbovirus group.

Epidemiology. The only known mechanism for virus maintenance is the man-vector (*Phlebotomus papatasii* female) cycle. The vector has a flight range of up to 200 yards, tends to stay close to ground level, and, because of its small size, readily penetrates conventional screens and mosquito netting. It thrives best in hot, dry periods, breeding in organic debris beneath stones and in cracks in masonry or other equivalent sites. Its life span is short, perhaps no more than two to three weeks. Recovery of Neapolitan group viruses from females of the phlebotomus subgenus, Sergentomyia, suggests a possible new vector.

The basic reservoir mechanism remains undetermined. Viral persistence in the hot, dry season is adequately explained by serial transmissions between susceptible humans via the vector. Recovery of a virus from phlebotomus males (Barnett and Suyemoto) supports the earlier disputed observation of transovarial transmission as a possible mechanism of virus overwintering.

Geographic distribution and seasonal occurrence are determined by the distribution and activity of the vector. In endemic areas, the majority of the inhabitants presumably experience unrecognized immunizing infections in infancy or early childhood, and disease is virtually restricted to newcomers. Large outbreaks require substantial immigration, such as troop movements.

Pathogenesis and Pathology. Because fatalities do not occur, the pathologic processes are unknown. However, extensive experimental infection of man during World War II (Sabin, Philip, and Paul) has provided much data on pathogenesis. Regular induction of disease requires use of the intracutaneous or intravenous rather than the subcutaneous or intramuscular paths for infection. The usual incubation period is three to six days. Viremia begins 24 hours before onset and endures only about two days. Postinfection immunity to homologous challenge lasts at least two years and is evidenced by low-level antibody response that is best shown by the neutralization test. There appears to be no postinfection immunity to heterologous challenge.

Clinical Manifestations. The experimental infections of man permitted close scrutiny of etiologically certain disease. Inapparent infections were rare. Onset typically is sudden, with fever reaching its peak (not more than 104.5° F.) in 24 to 48 hours and subsiding usually in two to four days. In relation to the temperature, the pulse is disproportionately rapid early in the illness but slow later. Other common signs and symptoms are frontal headache, photophobia, ocular pain, severe conjunctival injection, erythema of the face and neck (but no true rash), aches or pains in the back and extremities, stiffness in the neck, various gastrointestinal manifestations including constipation early and diarrhea later, sore throat, and chilliness. Moderate leukopenia is usual. The cerebrospinal fluid is unchanged. In about 5 per cent of patients, fever and symptoms recur after five to seven days of convalescence.

Diagnosis and Treatment. The differential diagnosis includes malaria, preicteric viral hepatitis, influenza, and dengue. Recognition of the disease is usually based on clinical and epidemiologic grounds, i.e., outbreaks of brief febrile illness in the hot, dry season among tourists or other immigrant groups. Although recovery of blood-borne virus in suckling mice and detection of neutralizing antibody response are possible, exclusion of other viral infections is the usual role of the viral laboratory. Only symptomatic treatment is available.

Prognosis. In addition to occasional recurrence of febrile disease, as already noted, convalescence is characterized by weakness and sweating and, occasionally, by severe but transitory mental depression. Full recovery is apparently invariable.

Prevention. No vaccine of established value is generally available. Effective vector control is feasible, using residual DDT or other insecticidal sprays for dwellings and nearby breeding sites, supplemented by repellents such as dimethylphthalate to guard against possible attack after sundown.

Barnett, H. C., and Suyemoto, W.: Field studies on sandfly fever and kala-azar in Pakistan, in Iran, and in Baltistan (Little Tibet). Trans. N.Y. Acad. Sci., Ser. II, 23:609, 1961.

Casals, J., and Clarke, D. H.: Arboviruses other than groups A and B. *In* Horsfall, F. L., Jr., and Tamm, I. (eds.). Viral and Rickettsial Infections in Man, 4th ed. Philadelphia, J. B. Lippincott Company, 1965, ch. 28.

Henderson, J. R., and Taylor, R. M.: Phlebotomus (sandfly) fever viruses in tissue culture. Amer. J. Trop. Med., 9:32, 1960.

Sabin, A. B., Philip, C. B., and Paul, J. R.: Phlebotomus (pappataci or sandfly) fever. A disease of military importance. Summary of existing knowledge and preliminary report of original investigations. J.A.M.A., 125:603; 693, 1944.

Taylor, R. M.: Phlebotomus (sandfly) fever in the middle east. Proc. 6th International Congress on Tropical Medicine and Malaria, Lisbon, 1958, 5:149, 1959.

ARTHROPOD-BORNE VIRAL ENCEPHALITIDES: GENERAL CONSIDERATIONS
Telford H. Work

Any brief exposition presenting the most important features and essential concepts of the arthropod-borne viral encephalitides must necessarily be somewhat arbitrary. This one is intended to provide key clues to the physician who must sift so many variables against a background choice of so many possibilities in selecting a rational course, for he must strive to establish a diagnosis, not just for proper management of the patient, but for responsible guidance of control and preventive measures in a potentially threatened community.

The arthropod-borne viral encephalitides form a complex of clinically similar diseases induced by hematophagous arthropod injection of viruses with proclivities for invasion of the central nervous system (CNS), and producing transient affliction or irreversible destruction of nerve cells. The salivary glands and other mouth parts of the arthropod become infectious only after an extrinsic incubation period, usually ten days or more, following ingestion of blood from a reservoir vertebrate in which virus was circulating. Infectivity persists for the life of the arthropod.

On occasion, infection occurs by mucous membrane contamination, inhalation, ingestion or artificial injection during laboratory exposure, or ingestion of physiologically contaminated dairy products such as unpasteurized goats' milk, as documented in outbreaks of the European form of tick-borne encephalitis.

The arthropod-borne viral encephalitides can be classified and subdivided in a number of different ways. Virologically distinct, they can be antigenically grouped into several different complexes, which is important in laboratory diagnosis. With so many common clinical characteristics, epidemiologic manifestations provide another basis for subdivision. Epizootic maintenance and vector transmission to man display still a different series of characteristics that are important for the physician to understand.

The Equine Encephalitides. This group of diseases includes *western equine encephalitis (WEE)*, *eastern equine encephalitis (EEE)*, and *Venezuelan equine encephalitis (VEE)*. The distinctly different but antigenically related viruses of Casals arbovirus group A are all transmitted by culicine mosquitoes from a wild vertebrate-mosquito reservoir cycle. Although it is now evident that the same mosquito-transmitted viral encephalitis of horses rarely has any *direct* connection with the causation of similar disease in man, the inclusion of the term "equine" in the nomenclature of the human disease remains important because (1) the simultaneous or recent occurrence of equine disease may be the essential fact in a clinical history or the only forewarning that an epizootic condition exists that may foster transmission of virus to man, and (2) effective reference to the extensive clinical, virologic, and epidemiologic literature on these diseases requires inclusion of the term. In fact, a veterinary report of one or more cases of the "staggers" often precedes the appearance of human cases of these encephalitides, preparing the physician to include the possibility in the differential diagnosis of his earliest case.

Overt febrile and severe CNS disease of man in the equine group of viral encephalitides appears to be more common in children, but for different reasons. Western equine encephalitis afflicts very young children because of their immobility in rural and semirural conditions of exposure in the west. Eastern equine encephalitic viral infection induces severe and frequently fatal disease in the young because of an apparent age-related susceptibility of the central nervous system. Attack rates for Venezuelan equine encephalitis in the areas where it occurs reflect a periodic epidemic wave through an indigenous population, the older members of which have been immunized by previous epidemic waves.

Encephalitides of the Japanese B–West Nile Virus Complex. Equine epizootics like those that have been observed in southeast Asia may result from infection with *Japanese B encephalitis (JBE)* virus of the Japanese B–West Nile antigenic complex of arbovirus group B, which also includes *St. Louis encephalitis (SLE)* and *Murray Valley encephalitis (MVE)* viruses. All have been etiologically involved in remarkably similar cases of arboviral encephalitis.

Although SLE virus has never been etiologically associated with an equine epizootic, SLE viral infection of man can, in many respects, be considered the New World form of Japanese B encephalitis because of clinical, virologic Culex vector–avian reservoir epizootology, and latitud-

therefore, as soon as a diagnosis is suspected, collection of these specimens and immediate dispatch to the virus laboratory may establish a diagnosis soon enough for mosquito control measures to cause a dramatic and abrupt cessation of occurrence of new cases in humans.

Serologic diagnosis in cases seen too late for virus isolation, or to confirm the preliminary finding of VEE virus, is accomplished by demonstrating a fourfold rise or fall in CF and/or HI antibodies in two or more sequential serum specimens. Although there is accumulating evidence that there are antigenically detectable geographic differences in strains of VEE virus, some giving rise to two separate types (Mucambo and Pixuna of Brazilian Amazonia), the strains are similar and sensitive enough for any type to produce diagnostic antigen that in a serologic test will establish an etiologic diagnosis in a human case.

Treatment. There is no specific treatment, although considerable relief of discomfort can be accomplished by intelligent use of analgesics and antipyretics. Neurologic complications require appropriate nursing care, with maintenance of fluid and electrolytes to avoid further CNS damage. In such cases the temperature should be taken every one or two hours because of the possibility of hyperthermia. If the temperature rises to 104° F., every external means to reduce it should be applied because loss of heat regulation may result in death.

Prophylaxis. An experimental vaccine has been produced that is useful for protection of laboratory workers who must work with VEE virus. It is an attenuated live virus derived from an equine strain isolated in Trinidad. Reactions are frequent and severe enough to militate against general use of the vaccine for all but the most highly exposed, for whom the probability of accidental infection is great. There are several reports of VEE infection in vaccinated persons containing significant titers of neutralizing antibody against VEE virus; therefore, successful vaccination should not be considered an excuse not to continue exercise of intelligent preventive measures.

For rural residents of regions where recognized VEE virus is known to be prevalent, personal protection from mosquito bites through use of mosquito nets and screened windows at home and protective clothing outside is the most reasonable measure. This can be augmented by application of repellents to exposed skin surfaces, particularly after reports of epidemic or sporadic VEE cases in the region.

In a situation in which VEE cases are known to occur, it is important to establish the mosquito vector through special field studies. Subsequent mosquito control measures can then be intelligently planned for dealing with that particular vector. If an epidemic occurs before the identity of the vector species can be established, adjunct agents for mosquito control by fogging and residual spraying around human premises are essential.

Because of the frequency with which VEE virus has been recovered from the nasopharynx of patients and reports of medical personnel suffering the disease following intimate association with infected patients, isolation of the acutely ill and adherence to a medical regimen for isolation by medical personnel are strongly recommended.

Castillo, E.: Informe sobre una reciente epidemia de encefalitis equina Venezolana en la Zona norte del estado Zulia. Rev. Venez. Sanid. Asist. So., 29:325, 1964.

McKinney, R. W., Berge, T. O., Sawyer, W. D., Tigertt, W. D., and Crozier, D.: Use of an attenuated strain of Venezuelan equine encephalomyelitis virus for immunization in man. Amer. J. Trop. Med., 12:597, 1963.

Tigertt, W. D., and Downs, W. G.: Studies on the virus of Venezuelan equine encephalomyelitis in Trinidad, W.I. I. The 1943–1944 epizootic. Amer. J. Trop. Med., 11:822, 1962.

Work, T. H.: Serological evidence of arbovirus infection in the Seminole Indians of southern Florida. Science, 145:270, 1964.

CALIFORNIA ENCEPHALITIS
Telford H. Work

Etiology. The BFS-283 prototype and two other strains of what is now known as the California encephalitis virus complex were isolated in the San Joaquin Valley of California from *Aedes dorsalis* and *Culex tarsalis* mosquitoes in 1943 and 1944. First known as the Hammon-Reeves virus, and subsequently given the geographic name according to the accepted practice for naming new arboviruses, it was found serologically to be etiologically associated with CNS disease that previously had been suspected to be due to WEE and SLE viruses but that had proved serologically negative for these strains. Although serologic surveys in the central valleys of California showed rather widespread infection, there was little evidence that it was the cause of much serious CNS disease.

In 1960 a six-year-old child died of acute viral encephalitis in La Crosse, Wisconsin. Brain tissue collected post mortem and processed in suckling mice in 1962 by Thompson yielded a virus antigenically similar to but not identical with the prototype California strain. Additional strains of related but antigenically separable strains were isolated from mosquitoes in New Jersey, Alabama, Texas, Florida, New Mexico, Utah, and Ohio (1965). These constitute one of the most perplexing arbovirus complexes yet to come under laboratory scrutiny, because the disease potential associated with so many different definable antigenic characteristics is unknown.

Whereas the occurrence of detectable disease in California has been negligible, it is now apparent that frequent, perhaps annual, epidemics of California encephalitis have occurred in Wisconsin, Indiana, and Ohio for a number of years.

Epidemiology. California encephalitis has been recognized as a geographically extensive, annual, warm-season, epidemic, febrile central nervous system disease only since a sensitive CF antigen for the La Crosse strain was recently made available for routine serologic study of sera collected from patients who suffered febrile CNS signs that were demonstrated not to be due to WEE, EEE, and SLE or some enterovirus. From west of the Appalachians to the midwest, many general practitioners call the syndrome farm encephalitis.

Studies of 1964 and 1965 epidemics in Indiana and Ohio, supported by characterization of sporadic cases in Florida and North Carolina, establish that more than 90 per cent of the recognized cases were in persons under 16 years of age, the highest incidence being in those who were 5 to 7 years old.

Almost all cases can be associated with rural or sylvan exposure, primarily in recreational pursuits of picnicking, camping, fishing, or hunting in or adjacent to woods or the subtropical vegetation characteristic of Florida. These habitats breed an abundance of a variety of man-biting mosquitoes, mostly Aedes species, from which numerous strains of California encephalitis virus have been isolated.

California complex viruses have been isolated from *Aedes atlanticus-tormentor* and *A. infirmatus* in Florida and Georgia, *A. taentorhynchus* in Florida, *A. atlanticus* in North Carolina, Virginia, and Maryland, *A. canadensis* in Maryland and Ohio, *A. triseriatus* in Ohio, *Culiseta inornata* in Colorado, *A. dorsalis* in a number of western states, and *Anopheles crucians* in several southeastern states. It is obvious from the plethora of mosquito species that bite man and that have been found infected with these viruses that greater recognition of widespread occurrence of this disease is imminent.

Mammalian species found to contain neutralizing antibody to these viruses also demonstrate the complicated zoonotic maintenance cycle that supports such a variety of ecologic situations in which man can be infected. These include chipmunks, tree squirrels, and rabbits. A type of California encephalitis virus has been isolated from a snowshoe hare in Montana. This evidence of mammalian rather than avian vertebrate hosts helps explain the widespread focal nature of California encephalitis virus activity as well as why there appear to be so many antigenically distinct types.

At least six antigenically different types of virus of the California complex have been characterized in different regions of the United States. The La Crosse strain, which produces the most sensitive CF antigen for the cases diagnosed in the Ohio Valley, is the only strain of human origin. Related viruses of the California group have been isolated in tropical America, Europe, Africa, and Asia. Whether all varieties of the California complex in the United States or others of the group active in other continents will cause the disease described here as California encephalitis is not yet known. It is therefore extremely important for the clinician who suspects this as the cause of a febrile CNS syndrome to collect appropriate serum specimens for dispatch to a capable arbovirus laboratory for examination.

An accurate mortality rate has not yet been established. It is not more than 5 per cent and is probably less, although sequelae of mental deterioration and emotional instability may be more common.

Clinical Characteristics. Limited circumstantial evidence suggests that the incubation period is between five and ten days. The time of the first symptoms is often difficult to establish because this is primarily a disease of young children and because California encephalitis usually has a more gradual and insidious onset than the other North American arboviral encephalitides. Mild fever and headache are often the only signs of illness for several days. The patient may then recover fully, the physician noting only a diagnosis of "summer fever."

More severe cases are marked by gradual rise of the temperature over several days, the headache localizing and becoming severe in the frontal region. As primary complaints, the fever and headache are often attributed to some traumatic incident that the patient or parent remembers as having occurred within the previous few days. The fever and headache are frequently accompanied by vomiting.

Mental confusion and lassitude may or may not precede sudden occurrence of convulsions. These have occurred spontaneously in a febrile child riding in a car, and have been so violent as to dislodge a reclining child from bed. Convulsive seizures may be the only overt sign of CNS involvement, but are often only a prelude to coma. Either may be the presenting condition for hospital admission.

In rural areas where the physician is called to see a feverish, confused, somnolent, convulsive, or comatose child, the condition is often diagnosed as "farm encephalitis." It is well known by many general practitioners, who associate this children's disease with summer or early autumn. In such environmental situations the most difficult differential diagnosis is from western equine and St. Louis encephalitis. Only appropriate laboratory examination can establish the diagnosis with certainty.

Meningeal signs occur but are uncommon. In contrast to the transient neurologic signs, such as changes in reflexes and shifting flaccid and spastic paralyses seen in the other encephalitides, these signs are not characteristic of California encephalitis. This may indicate localization of the neuropathologic process in the cortex more than involvement of the motor centers.

Lumbar puncture following recognition of overt CNS signs yields clear cerebrospinal fluid under pressure, with a marked pleocytosis consisting of polymorphonuclear leukocytes and increase in lymphocytes as the disease progresses. A mild to severe leukocytosis in an otherwise normal blood picture is characteristic of this stage, an increase in lymphocytes being associated with high counts that may reach 30,000 per cubic millimeter.

Fever continues to increase. This and dehydration are the two clinical conditions requiring close attention and immediate treatment. Although death may occur suddenly, within a few hours, it may come only after several days' progression of high fever, convulsions, coma, and respiratory difficulty that requires oxygen and a respirator. Upper respiratory signs are negligible.

Fever falls by lysis, and the convalescence is prolonged, weakness and lassitude continuing for some time. Although paralytic sequelae have not been observed, emotional lability at home and difficulty in learning at school have been noted in children following California encephalitis. Not enough cases have been studied to establish whether this is a permanent change.

Diagnosis. During the summer or early autumn, severe frontal headache associated with gradually rising temperature over several days, leading to somnolence, irritability, disorientation, vomiting, convulsions, and coma, should stimulate consideration of California encephalitis. A history of exposure to mosquito bites in rural or wooded areas strengthens the suspicion.

Mild leukocytosis, which may be lymphocytic, and significant polymorphonuclear or lymphocytic pleocytosis in the cerebrospinal fluid, with or without abnormal increase in protein, further support the clinical diagnosis.

No virus has yet been isolated from the blood of an acutely ill patient. Virus has been recovered from brain tissue of a fatal case, but most patients survive. The laboratory diagnosis is therefore serologic. Because antibody levels tend to vary widely in residents of areas where California encephalitis occurs most commonly, at least a fourfold rise in titer of CF or HI antibody is required to establish the diagnosis. A high titer of CF antibody in a single specimen of convalescent serum from a characteristic clinical case provides important circumstantial evidence of the possible cause.

Treatment. There being no specific antiviral therapy available, the treatment is symptomatic. The severe frontal headache may require powerful analgesics for relief. The fever will respond somewhat to antipyretics, but resolution of the fever is usually by lysis over a period of several days. The more severe cases of somnolence and coma require closest attention and constant nursing to ameliorate hyperthermia and to watch for respiratory difficulty that may require a respirator.

Relatively slow convalescence is associated with malaise that may require environmental change as well as supportive treatment for recovery from depression. How much of this is due to CNS affliction is as yet unknown.

Prophylaxis. Although there has been no attempt to develop a vaccine, accumulating epidemiologic evidence increasingly focuses on a rural transmission of the virus by the Aedes mosquito. Protection against such sylvan mosquito attack is the most difficult mosquito control measure known. When children congregate in summer camps, extensive and frequent use of insecticides in the camp and at the periphery will destroy mosquitoes that otherwise might bite during periods of rest or outdoor activities. Beyond the immediate environs of camping or picnic sites, personal protection from mosquito bite by use of protective clothing and application of repellents to exposed skin surfaces is recommended. The tree-hole breeding proclivity of sylvan Aedes complicates elimination of these mosquitoes immensely. In suburban areas, where people are constantly or repeatedly enveloped by a sylvan environment, the expensive elimination of tree-hole breeding by drainage and filling holes in trees may prove to be the only practical Aedes control measure.

Cramblett, H. G., Stegmiller, H., and Spencer, C.: California encephalitis virus infections in children. J.A.M.A., 198:108, 1966.

Quick, D. T., Smith, A. G., Lewis, A. L., Sather, G. E., and Hammon, W. M.: California encephalitis virus infection: A case report. Amer. J. Trop. Med., 14:456, 1965.

Thompson, W. H., and Evans, A. S.: California encephalitis virus studies in Wisconsin. Amer. J. Epidem., 81:230, 1965.

Thompson, W. H., Kalfayan, B., and Anslow, R. O.: Isolation of California encephalitis group virus from a fatal human illness. Amer. J. Epidem., 81:245, 1965.

ST. LOUIS ENCEPHALITIS
John P. Fox

Definition. St. Louis encephalitis (SLE) is the most important arbovirus disease in the continental United States and is associated with signs and symptoms of viral infection of the brain and meninges. It occurs sporadically and in outbreaks in the late summer and fall, typically afflicting rural populations in the far West and urban-suburban residents elsewhere in the country.

Etiology. The causative agent is a small spherical virus of 20 to 30 mμ in diameter that antigenically belongs to the B group of arthropod-borne viruses. It is most closely related to the viruses of Japanese B and Murray Valley encephalitis and West Nile fever. Like other arboviruses, the virus of SLE is thermolabile, readily inactivated by ether and bile salts, and is associated with complement-fixing (CF) antigen and a hemagglutinin (HA) for chick and goose erythrocytes.

The virus multiplies in chick embryos and various cell cultures, including hamster and chick kidney, in which cytopathic effect results, and in duck kidney monolayers, in which plaques form under agar. However, maximal virus yields are from brains of suckling mice, which are highly susceptible to extraneural infection. Mice of all ages, rhesus monkeys, hamsters, and suckling rats develop encephalitis after cerebral infection. Inapparent but immunizing infections occur or can be produced in many domestic and wild vertebrate species, including horses, wild birds and chickens, certain bats, and wild rodents. Such infections in nature are of great epidemiologic importance when, as with avian species and bats, the blood contains sufficient virus to infect arthropod vectors, and when, as with bats, infection persists during hibernation and may be transmitted transplacentally.

Epidemiology. St. Louis encephalitis apparently was a disease truly new to man in 1932, when a few cases recognized in retrospect occurred in Paris, Illinois. In 1933, just across the Mississippi river, the St. Louis metropolitan area experienced a major epidemic involving 1130 reported cases. The causative virus was first isolated from fatal cases in 1933. Since then, sporadic cases and small to major outbreaks have occurred in the late summer and autumn in rural portions of Washington and California and in suburban and urban areas in Texas, the lower Ohio Valley, Florida, Pennsylvania, and New Jersey. Disease incidence rises sharply with age but does not vary with sex except in rural areas, where the disease is more common in males. Viral presence is indicated by serology in Mexico, Panama, Colombia, Brazil, and Argentina and by virus isolation in the West Indies, but only in Jamaica has disease been recognized.

The work of many investigators, including particularly Reeves and Hammon, suggests a basic sylvatic transmission cycle in avian species and certain Culex mosquitoes. Possible overwintering mechanisms include reintroduction by migrant birds and bats, hibernation of infected adult mosquitoes (probable in California), recrudescent infection in birds, and persistence of infection in bats during hibernation (demonstrated in Texas following the 1964 Houston and 1966 Corpus Christi epidemics). In the far West the principal vector is *C. tarsalis,* which is abundant in irrigated areas. Elsewhere the urban-suburban outbreaks have been associated with domestic species, *C. pipiens, C. quinquefasciatus* and, in Florida, *C. nigrapalpus,* and have followed conditions unusually favorable for mosquito breeding. Presumably introduced from the sylvatic cycle, virus is amplified locally by domestic and resident wild avian species. Neither horses nor human beings serve as sources for mosquito infection.

Although the distribution of SLE virus in the United States overlaps extensively with that of both Western and Eastern equine encephalomyelitis, certain differences in epidemiologic features should be stressed. First, all three agents "spill over" into horses, but only the latter two cause equine disease. Second, the extrinsic incubation period of SLE virus in the mosquito is longer than that of the equine viruses. Presumably because of this, the latter viruses cause disease distinctly earlier in the summer and also occur in northern areas (including Canada), where SLE virus is absent.

Pathogenesis and Pathology. Virus is introduced through the skin by the bite of a mosquito. Lack of a suitable laboratory model has precluded careful studies of pathogenesis, but the basic process in man probably resembles that described by Theiler for neurotropic yellow fever virus infection in the rhesus monkey. If so, following intradermal inoculation, virus is transported via lymph channels to regional lymph nodes, where multiplication results in wide seeding via the blood stream of various systemic sites of multiplication. Similar wide seeding would occur more directly if, as well may occur, the infecting mosquito introduced the virus into small blood vessels. However it is achieved, such seeding is followed by major viremia that endures for several days until terminated by the development of neutralizing antibody. During this viremic phase, virus may localize in the central nervous system. Incubation, from exposure to onset of encephalitis disease, probably does not exceed 21 days.

Pathologic examination in fatal cases reveals grossly evident edema, vascular congestion, and tiny hemorrhages throughout the central nervous system and the meninges. Microscopic findings occur throughout the brain but are most common in the midbrain and brain stem. They include diffuse and focal (often perivascular) infiltration of lymphocytes, focal glial proliferation, degeneration and necrosis of neurons, but no demyelination. Focal necroses are relatively uncommon, perhaps explaining the rarity of permanent neurologic sequelae.

Clinical Manifestations. Recognized disease occurs in only 1 of 50 to 200 infections and usually runs a fairly benign course, consisting of a few days of febrile illness with severe headache followed by rapid and complete recovery. In more severe illness, the course varies widely, partly according to age. Abrupt onset with high fever, severe generalized or occipital headache, stiff neck, nausea, and vomiting are common. Children are restless and irritable and may develop convulsions; adults tend toward lethargy and disorientation. Muscular weakness, tremors, and speech difficulties also are observed. Fever lasts for three to ten days or, in older persons, up to three weeks, declining gradually.

The leukocyte count varies between mild leukopenia and moderate leukocytosis. Cerebrospinal fluid examination reveals slightly increased pressure, 50 to 500 cells, which may be largely polymorphonuclear in the early stages, elevated protein, and normal sugar.

Diagnosis. St. Louis encephalitis does not differ clinically from encephalitis or aseptic meningitis of many other causes and its inclusion in the differential diagnosis is governed by the epidemiologic setting. Specific diagnosis comes only from the virus laboratory. Virus is no longer in the blood at disease onset, is not present in the cerebrospinal fluid, and has been isolated from the brain only in rapidly fatal cases. Thus, diagnosis largely depends on demonstrating significant increases in specific antibody in paired acute and convalescent phase sera. This may be done by hemagglutination-inhibition (HI), complement-fixation (CF) or neutralization tests (listed in order of increasing specificity). Tests for neutralizing antibody can now be done conveniently in suitable cell cultures (see Etiology). Where other group B viruses are rare, as in the United States, the group-specific HI test is useful. However, the CF test is the method of choice since CF antibody develops slowly, and a rise in titer usually can be detected.

Treatment. Treatment can only be symptomatic and should be aimed principally at relieving headache.

Prognosis. The mortality rate in St. Louis encephalitis among reported cases averages about 20 per cent, being higher among the very young and the elderly. The occurrence of convulsions suggests a poor prognosis. Severe but nonfatal disease results in prolonged convalescence during much of which weakness, tremors, and mental dullness may persist, but complete recovery is usual. The rare permanent sequelae include muscular weakness or paralysis, personality changes, and mental deterioration.

Prevention. Since no effective vaccine is available, vector control is the only method for prevention. Based on thorough knowledge of the *C. tarsalis* vector, this has been proved effective in California. Elsewhere in the United States, effective control depends on early recognition of impending epidemics. For this, surveillance of mosquitoes for virus is best, but early specific diagnosis of cases is valuable. The usual vectors are readily attacked because of their domestic nature.

JAPANESE B ENCEPHALITIS
(Russian Autumnal Encephalitis, Japanese Encephalitis or Summer Encephalitis)
John P. Fox

Definition. Japanese B encephalitis is one of the most serious of the arbovirus encephalitides. It occurs in eastern Asia from Siberia to southeast India and on the offshore islands, including Japan, Okinawa, Guam, Taiwan, the Philippines, and the East Indies. Two cases have occurred in the United States in persons returning from Korea and Japan.

Etiology. The causative agent, a group B arbovirus, is closely related to Murray Valley, West Nile, and St. Louis viruses. At least two distinct immunotypes have been recognized. These differ from St. Louis virus antigenically and in behavior in various hosts. Infection of porcine kidney cell cultures results in clear cytopathic effect. Cerebral infection of rhesus or cynomolgus monkeys usually induces fatal encephalitis. Naturally infected horses often develop encephalitis, and infection of sows early in pregnancy results in abnormal or stillborn offspring. Swine and many birds including waterfowl experience silent infections with viremia sufficient to infect feeding mosquitoes.

Epidemiology. The designation "Japanese B encephalitis" dates from an epidemic of more than 6000 cases in 1924, which were recognized as different from encephalitis A or Von Economo's disease. However, the disease probably has existed in Japan at least since 1871. The virus was first recovered in monkeys from a fatal case in 1934.

In temperate zones disease occurs only in the warmer months, and large epidemics with high case fatality may occur at irregular intervals; in tropical areas cases are sporadic and unrelated to season. In Japan some 10 per cent of children are infected annually, but only about one in 500 develops disease (in Korea, one case develops among 25 infected U.S. troops). Because of this extensive early immunization, disease is largely restricted to children, adults recently entering the country (U.S. military included), and native adults 60 years or older. The incidence is unrelated to sex.

Present epidemiologic knowledge derives largely from the long-continued efforts of Japanese workers and American teams working with U.S. military support. The basic cycle is mosquito–lower vertebrate–mosquito, the particular species differing with locale. Principal vectors are *C. annulirostris* on Guam, *C. gelidus* in Malaya, and *C. tritaeniorhynchus* in most other areas including

Japan. Important amplifying hosts are herons and egrets in Japan and swine throughout the Far East, where pork is popular and pig populations turn over rapidly. Thus, as noted in Japan, a high prevalence of antibody in pigs coming to slaughter portends an epidemic in man. Human infection occurs only after a high density of infected mosquitos is attained. Overwintering mechanisms for the virus in temperate zones remain to be determined.

Pathogenesis and Pathology. Pathogenesis presumably is similar to that described previously for St. Louis encephalitis. Incubation time is undetermined. The morbid anatomy also resembles that of St. Louis encephalitis but involves a generally greater neuronal destruction in many vital areas and extensive destruction of the Purkinje cells in the cerebellum.

Clinical Manifestations. Japanese B infection of man parallels that with St. Louis virus in the high frequency of inapparent infection or abortive illness and in the general nature of the onset, signs, and symptoms of true central nervous system disease. However, such disease resulting from Japanese B infection is of much greater overall severity. Facial paralysis or paralysis of extremities is common in children, whereas symmetrical paresis without corresponding sensory changes occurs in adults. Other findings may include signs of cerebellar involvement, sensorial changes, general spastic rigidity, and coma. Fever, with a relative bradycardia, reaches its peak in two to four days and then subsides gradually. Duration of the acute illness is variable and is usually followed by prolonged convalescence. A transient leukocytosis, averaging about 14,000 leukocytes per cubic millimeter, occurs early. The cerebrospinal fluid shows some increase in pressure, a pleocytosis ranging up to 400 or more, an elevated protein, and normal sugar.

Diagnosis. Although time, place, and clinical picture may strongly suggest it, the specific diagnosis of Japanese B encephalitis requires virologic procedures similar to those described for St. Louis encephalitis. Virus can be recovered, rarely, from early blood specimens and from brains of rapidly fatal cases. However, viral antigen can be demonstrated by fluorescent antibody methods in a high proportion of brains examined post mortem. Early (IgG) antibody possesses neutralizing and hemagglutination-inhibiting (HI) reactivity, but only the later (IgM) antibody fixes complement. Hence, the HI test is useful when the acute phase serum is taken very early; otherwise, the complement-fixation (CF) test is more reliable. Use of both HI and CF tests yields 15 to 25 per cent more diagnoses than either alone, and when both are negative the neutralization test may still prove positive. Where other group B arboviruses abound, as in India, use of a battery of group B antigens may be necessary.

Treatment. Although no specific treatment exists, control of hyperpyrexia is important (tepid sponges, ice packs, artificial hibernation), and for severe convulsions anticonvulsants may be necessary. Intensive supportive and nursing care with prolonged hospitalization are required with severe disease.

Prognosis. The mortality rate for encephalitis varies with age from 30 per cent for those under age 20 to 80 per cent in older age groups. Prognosis in nonfatal cases must be guarded, because slow improvement is possible over a lengthy period. Permanent sequelae are most common under age ten and most severe in infants. They include, in approximate order of frequency, mental deterioration and personality changes, upper or lower motor neuron types of paralysis, aphasia, cerebellar syndromes, organic psychoses, and decerebrate rigidity.

Prevention. Vector control is not usually practicable because of the habits and extensive breeding area of the vector. Vaccine prepared from formalinized mouse brain is widely used with children in Japan and is credited with significant effect, but it is not available in the United States. Formol-inactivated vaccines produced from virus grown in cell culture have given promising results in pilot studies. Because proved potential vectors and vertebrate hosts abound on the West Coast, prevention of importation of the virus into the U.S. is vitally important.

MURRAY VALLEY ENCEPHALITIS
(Australian X Disease)
John P. Fox

Murray Valley encephalitis, in its clinical manifestations, pathogenesis, and morbid anatomy in man, is very similar to Japanese B encephalitis and is caused by a very closely related virus. Specific diagnosis requires essentially similar laboratory studies.

The disease almost certainly has occurred intermittently in Victoria and New South Wales, Australia, in the valleys of the Murray and Darling rivers, since 1917–1918 when an epidemic of 134 cases, then referred to as *Australian X disease*, took place. More than half of those afflicted were less than five years of age, and the disease was fatal in 70 per cent. Viral strains isolated then were soon lost. The present designation derives from an epidemic of at least 40 cases in 1951, from some of which viral strains were again recovered and were thoroughly characterized. Endemic infection is maintained in a bird-mosquito cycle in New Guinea and Northern Australia and escapes south intermittently, via migratory birds, to more populous areas where domestic fowl and waterbirds amplify the infection via *C. annulirostris*, and epidemics result. Excessive rainfall in the endemic areas may aid but is not essential to the southward migration of the virus.

RUSSIAN SPRING-SUMMER ENCEPHALITIS AND LOUPING ILL
(Central European Encephalitis, Biundulant Meningoencephalitis)
John P. Fox

Definition. Except for two viruses (Omsk hemorrhagic fever and Kyasanur Forest disease, described in a following article), members of the tick-borne complex of group B arboviruses cause mild to severe febrile illness often accompanied by neurologic manifestations. These are widely distributed throughout Eurasia (Russian spring-summer encephalitis) and the British Isles (louping ill), and one member (Powassan virus, so far only once related to human disease) occurs in Canada and the western United States.

Etiology. The group B tick-borne viruses constitute an antigenic complex within which by careful serologic methods Clarke has distinguished several antigenic subtypes, including Far Eastern and Central European tick-borne encephalitis, louping ill (limited to the British Isles), Omsk hemorrhagic fever, Kyasanur Forest disease, and Powassan virus (Canada and U.S.). These agents share many properties with other group B arboviruses, including production of complement-fixing (CF) and hemagglutinating (HA) antigens and ability to produce well defined cytopathic effect (CPE) or plaques in a variety of cell cultures. The tick-borne encephalitis viruses in milk are very stable, and high temperatures are needed to ensure inactivation. Virus isolation is best achieved in suckling mice, but mice of all ages develop encephalitis, even after extraneural inoculation. Alimentary infection is followed by shedding of virus in feces and in the milk of lactating mice. In rhesus and cynomolgus monkeys, goats, and sheep cerebral inoculation leads to variable encephalitis that is most severe with Far East strains. Louping ill virus inoculated peripherally in sheep may cause encephalitis associated with the staggering gait responsible for the disease name. The natural occurrence of disease in sheep is favored by coincidental infection with the rickettsial agent of the tick-borne fever.

Of known or potential epidemiologic importance are inapparent infections in many vertebrate species that follow peripheral inoculations or tick-bite. Such infection in goats (and also, in cows and sheep with Central European virus) results not only in viremia *but also in viral shedding in milk*. Significant viremia also occurs in some birds and various wild rodents, and may persist for prolonged periods during hibernation in hedgehogs, dormice, and bats. Transovarial transmission has been demonstrated in the natural tick vectors after experimental infection.

Epidemiology. The viruses persist in natural foci by means of interchange between lower vertebrate hosts and the principal tick vectors,

Ixodes persulcatus and *I. ricinus*, the latter serving also in the British Isles as the vector of louping ill. Viral perpetuation, especially over the winter, presumably is facilitated by transovarial transmission in the vector and by the ability of the viruses to persist during hibernation of both ticks and vertebrate hosts (see Etiology).

Human infections directly caused by tick bite vary with tick exposure, which may result from residence, occupation, or recreation. Residents of rural, forested areas, especially agricultural and forest workers, are at highest risk. Ingestion of raw milk (so far only from goats) is an important indirect means of human infection, especially in central Europe and Russia, which reaches urban-suburban residents, with high attack rates in children and familial clustering of cases. Louping ill attacks chiefly sheep farmers, veterinarians, and abattoir workers handling tick-infested sheep. Sero-epidemiologic studies indicate that a high proportion of human infections are inapparent.

Seasonal disease patterns reflect temperature-dependent tick activity, disease occurring during spring and early summer in Siberia and continuing into early autumn in central Europe. Large epidemics have occurred in years following a peak in the vole population.

Pathogenesis and Pathology. Pathogenesis of infection owing to tick-bite presumably resembles that for other arboviruses (see St. Louis encephalitis). Existence of an alimentary portal of entry is indicated by milk-transmitted infections. Incubation time to the systemic phase of illness is seven to ten days. Histopathology in fatal encephalitis resembles that described for St. Louis encephalitis but frequently includes neuronal damage in the cervical cord similar to that seen in poliomyelitis.

Clinical Manifestations. When infection is not silent, onset of disease is usually abrupt and its course is typically diphasic, although in individual cases only one phase may materialize. The initial phase is often described as influenza-like with fever, headache, generalized aching, and gastrointestinal disturbances. A leukopenia is common. This phase may subside in five to ten days.

The second phase in neurotropic infection follows in four to ten days and usually begins with high fever and severe headache. Very roughly, the severity of the disease and the fatality rate increase as one moves eastward from the United Kingdom, where louping ill virus usually causes mild to moderately severe meningoencephalitis, with full recovery. In central Europe, Russia, and Siberia, serous meningitis and mild meningo-encephalitis are the most common types of disease over all, but true encephalomyelitis becomes increasingly common as one approaches the far eastern Soviet Union. This is frequently associated with transient or permanent flaccid paralysis, nystagmus, visual disturbances, deafness, vertigo, somnolence, and, in severe cases, delirium and coma. Bulbospinal disease is the most serious, and may result in paralysis of the neck and shoulder muscles. Moderate leukocytosis usually occurs, and the cerebrospinal fluid constantly shows pleocytosis and elevated protein. This second phase usually lasts for eight to twelve days and is followed by prolonged convalescence.

Diagnosis. Although history of tick exposure or ingestion of goat milk may be suggestive, specific diagnosis is virologic. Virus can be recovered from acute phase blood and from the brain in rapidly fatal cases. Because CF antibody may not develop in mild infections and both neutralizing and HI antibody may appear so rapidly that a diagnostic rise cannot be shown, serodiagnosis may require tests for all three types of antibody. Interpretation of serologic results is not usually complicated by antibody to other group B viruses as these are uncommon in most of the affected areas.

Treatment. In general, treatment is symptomatic. According to Chumakov, convalescent human or hyperimmune animal serum may be helpful if given prior to neurologic involvement.

Prognosis. Infections with louping ill virus have led to no recognized sequelae or fatalities. Mild disease caused by the other neurotropic viruses also has a good prognosis. However, paralytic disease, particularly if bulbospinal, may lead to death or permanent sequelae. A fatality rate of up to 28 per cent was reported in early Far East outbreaks. The most common sequela is persistent paralysis, and shoulder girdle paralysis is usual among survivors of bulbospinal disease. Also, Russian sources report a chronic progressive course in 3 to 5 per cent of paralytic patients that may develop into Kozhevnikov's epilepsy. This takes the form of clonic spasms of certain muscle groups that periodically increase in extent to result in epileptic attack.

Prevention. Russian reports claim favorable results for a formolized mouse brain vaccine against Russian spring-summer encephalitis. For nonimmune persons subjected to tick bite in endemic areas or exposed in the laboratory, immune serum prophylaxis is recommended. Otherwise, repellents, protective clothing and efforts to control ticks are advised. Suspect goat milk should be boiled.

A cooperative study: Epidemic St. Louis encephalitis in Houston, 1964. J.A.M.A., 193:139, 1965.

Anderson, S. G., et al.: Murray Valley encephalitis in the Murray Valley, 1956 and 1957. Med. J. Aust., 2:15, 1958.

Clarke, D. H., and Casals, J.: Arboviruses: Group B. *In* Horsfall, F. L., Jr., and Tamm, I. (eds.): Viral and Rickettsial Infections in Man, 4th ed. Philadelphia, J. B. Lippincott Company, 1965, chap. 27.

Drozdov, S. G.: The role of domestic animals in the epidemiology of biphasic milk fever. J. Microbial. Epidem. Immun., 30:4, 103, 1959.

Gordon, W. S., et al.: The epizootiology of louping ill and tick-borne fever with observations on the control of these sheep diseases. *In*: Aspects of Disease Transmission by Ticks. London, Zoological Society of London, 1, 1962.

Ishii, K., Matsunaga, Y., and Kono, R.: Immunoglobulins produced in response to Japanese encephalitis virus infections of man. J. Immun., 101:770, 1968.

Kimoto, T., Yamada, T., Ueba, N., Kunita, N., Kawai, A., Yamagami, S., Nakajima K., Akao, M., and Sugiyama, S.: Laboratory diagnosis of Japanese encephalitis: Comparison of the fluorescent antibody technique with virus isolation and serologic tests. Biken J., 11:157, 1968.

Konno, J., Endo, K., Agatsuma, H., and Ishida, N.: Cyclic outbreaks of Japanese encephalitis among pigs and humans. Amer. J. Epidem., 84:292, 1966.

Kuznetsova, R. I., Sukhomlinova, O. I., and Churilova, A. A.: The character of biphasic meningoencephalitis in the Leningrad Oblast. J. Microbial. Epidem. Immun., 21:262, 1960.

Luby, J. P., Sulkin, S. E., and Sanford, J. P.: The epidemiology of St. Louis encephalitis. A review. Ann. Rev. Med., 20:329, 1969.

McLean, D. M., and Larke, R. P. B.: Powassan and Silverwater viruses: Ecology of two Ontario arboviruses. Canad. Med. Ass. J., 88:182, 1963.

Okuno, T., Okada, T., Kondo, A., Suzuki, M., Kobayashi, M., and Oya, A.: Immunotyping of different strains of Japanese encephalitis virus by antibody-absorption, haemagglutination-inhibition and complement-fixation tests. Bull. WHO, 38:547, 1968.

Reeves, W. C., and Hammon, W. M.: Epidemiology of the arthropod-borne viral encephalitides in Kern County, California, 1943–1952. Univ. Calif. Publ. Public Health, 4:1, 1962.

Scherer, W. F., Buescher, E. L., et al.: Ecologic studies of Japanese encephalitis virus in Japan, Parts I–IX Amer. J. Trop. Med., 8:644, 651; 665; 678; 689; 707; 716; 719, 1959.

Theiler, M.: The virus. In Strode, G. K. (ed.): Yellow Fever. 1st ed. New York, McGraw-Hill Book Co., Inc., 1951, Chap. 2 (esp. pp. 69–75).

YELLOW FEVER
Wilbur G. Downs

Definition. Yellow fever is an acute viral disease characterized by sudden onset, prostration, moderately high fever, and a pulse rate slow in relation to temperature. Severe cases are often characterized by vomiting of altered blood, albuminuria (sometimes massive), and jaundice, and may progress to collapse and death. The disease is endemic in tropical rain forest regions of Africa and South America; in the past, summer epidemics occurred sporadically in the temperate zone even in New York and Philadelphia, and persistent endemic foci existed in the larger coastal cities of South America, Africa, and the Caribbean region. There are two epidemiologic types of the disease. When the virus is transmitted from man to man by the domestic mosquito, *Aedes aegypti*, it is called *urban yellow fever*, but when it occurs in a forest environment and is transmitted to man by some forest mosquito, usually in the absence of *A. aegypti*, it is called *sylvan (or jungle) yellow fever*.

Etiology and Epidemiology. Yellow fever is a group B arbovirus, according to Casal's serologic classification of the arboviruses. Related viruses in group B include among others the causative agents of the dengues, Japanese B encephalitis, St. Louis encephalitis, and Russian spring-summer encephalitis. The virus is small, $38\mu \pm 5m\mu$ and readily passes Berkefeld V and N and Seitz filters. Unadapted virus exhibits both viscerotropic and neurotropic characteristics. Viscerotropism is manifested by involvement of liver, kidneys, and heart, and neurotropism by infection of cells of the central nervous system. By successive brain-to-brain passage in mice, the virus becomes adapted and manifests more neurotropism, losing its viscerotropic properties almost entirely. Prolonged passage of the virus in chick embryo tissue culture has produced an attenuated strain, 17D, widely used as a vaccine.

Man is universally susceptible to the virus, and characteristic symptoms and lesions of yellow fever in man are reflections of its viscerotropism. Certain monkey species, including *Macacus rhesus* and *Alouatta* species, are very susceptible to infection and usually die, whereas other species, for example, *Cebus* species, may be readily infected but usually recover. Albino mice, especially of the Swiss strain, are highly susceptible to the neurotropic element of virus strains recovered from nature, provided they are inoculated intracerebrally.

In urban yellow fever, the *A. aegypti* mosquito transmits the virus by biting a human host during his initial three-day period of viremia and later biting a susceptible person. An extrinsic incubation period of nine to twelve days in the mosquito must elapse before the mosquito can transmit infection by bite.

In sylvan yellow fever, man acquires his infection through the bite of some mosquito other than *A. aegypti*. In south and Central America the virus has been isolated from wild-caught mosquitoes of the genus *Haemagogus*, *Aedes leucocelaenus*, and *Sabethes chloropterus*. These are by far the most important vectors. In Africa virus has been recovered from wild-caught *Aedes simpsoni* and *A. africanus*. Haemagogus and *A. africanus* inhabit chiefly the forest canopy, which is also the habitat of monkeys, the most frequently infected wild hosts. *Aedes simpsoni* is found in areas of mixed cultivation and low secondary forest, often near human habitation, and bridges the gap between the deep forest and the primitive settlements and between forest monkeys (raiding crops near the settlements) and man. A cycle for virus maintenance in nature more basic than the mosquito-monkey-mosquito cycle has been diligently searched for but not found.

Since 1934 no large epidemics of urban yellow fever have been reported from the Western Hemisphere, and the few small *A. aegypti*-transmitted epidemics that have occurred, such as that in Trinidad in 1954, have been secondary to sylvan yellow fever. The announcement of urban yellow fever, *A. aegypti*-transmitted, in a seaport or airport brings strict international quarantine regulations into effect. The 1948–1957 epidemic of sylvan yellow fever in Panama and Central America has burned itself out after decimating the monkey populations. As the monkey populations are reestablishing themselves, however, repeated epidemic sweeps are a certainty. In Africa, in areas contiguous to the rain forest areas where sylvan yellow fever is endemic, there are still frequent epidemics of urban yellow fever. A large epidemic occurred in the Nuba mountains of Sudan in 1940, and others in Nigeria in 1946 and 1951–1952. A massive outbreak in southwestern Ethiopia in 1961–1962 caused an estimated 35,000 deaths.

Aedes simpsoni was demonstrated to have been an important vector in this epidemic. More recent epidemics have been reported from Portuguese Guinea in 1964–1965, from Senegal in 1965 and from Nigeria in 1969.

There is no evidence that yellow fever has ever been present in the Orient.

Using refined serologic techniques, it is possible to distinguish Old World strains of yellow fever virus from New World strains. The significance of this with regard to geographic epidemiology and relating to the original home of yellow fever is not settled.

Pathology. Yellow fever produces characteristic lesions in the liver of man. There are necrosis and necrobiosis of the parenchymal cells, most evident in the midzones of the lobules, with normal or much less involved cells around the central and portal veins. The necrosis is scattered and irregular rather than massive and uniform. Scattered among the necrotic cells are Councilman bodies, parenchymal cells that have undergone eosinophilic hyaline necrosis. There are also fatty changes in the parenchymal cells. The liver lobules are not collapsed. Pathologic changes in the kidneys are seen mainly in the tubules, with extensive damage to the epithelium and with lumina containing debris, casts, and basophilic concretions.

Clinical Manifestations. Most attacks of yellow fever are mild and show few if any of the classic symptoms. The only symptoms may be fever and headache, both of short duration. The epidemiologic implications of this disease make diagnosis of great importance, and it is essential to maintain a high index of suspicion with regard to undiagnosed fevers (vernacular terms: "P.U.O.," "F.U.O.," flu," etc.) in regions where yellow fever is known to be, or can be suspected of being, endemic.

The incubation period is from three to six days. The onset is sudden, often with a chill, and without prodromal symptoms. The first stage of the disease, which lasts about three days, is the *period of infection.* The symptoms are feverish feeling, severe headache, backache, pain in the legs, and prostration. The face is flushed, and the eyes are injected; there is photophobia. The tongue is bright red at the tip and edges. There is no jaundice at the onset of illness. The temperature rises abruptly to about 104° F., sometimes higher. The pulse rate may rise to 90 or 100 initially, only to become increasingly slow in relation to the temperature (Faget's sign). The pulse is strong and full during this stage. Nausea and vomiting are the rule, as are epigastric distress and tenderness. Constipation is to be expected. A progressive leukopenia, sometimes pronounced, has frequently been observed early in the disease. The sudden development of intense albuminuria about the third or fourth day is characteristic.

After a short remission, the *period of intoxication* begins about the fourth day. The remission in fever is often indefinite or absent, and it may be accompanied by a deceptive temporary improvement. In this period, lassitude and depression may replace restlessness and agitation. Headache may diminish, and jaundice gradually develops. Although jaundice is always present in severe cases, it is usually not so intense as the name of the disease would indicate. Various hemorrhagic manifestations are evident. The gums are swollen and bleed easily, either spontaneously or when pressed; the nose may bleed. There may be petechiae in the skin. Hemorrhages from the stomach, intestine, or uterus, or subcutaneously, may be massive. The pulse rate falls progressively and may go below 50 per minute. Even in otherwise mild cases there may be dilatation of the heart and low blood pressure as evidence of myocardial damage. Vomiting may be frequent and distressing, and the vomitus in this stage usually contains altered blood, whence the name "el vomito negro" often applied to the disease in Latin America. The amount of albumin in the urine rises, often to 3 to 5 grams per liter, sometimes much higher. Fatal cases often exhibit hiccup, copious vomiting of altered blood, tarry stools, and anuria. Coma may last two or three days, or death may be immediately preceded by a short period of wild delirium. Death occurs most frequently from the sixth to the ninth day.

When there is recovery from a severe case, the temperature is likely to reach normal by the seventh or eighth day. Convalescence begins then and progresses rapidly to complete recovery with rapid disappearance of the albuminuria. Relapses do not occur, and there are no sequelae. Complications are rare. A lifelong immunity follows the attack, whether it be mild or severe.

A feature of yellow fever is the great variation in the degree to which different organs are affected. With much renal involvement there may be no cardiac symptoms, and vice versa. In mild and moderate cases there is little or no albuminuria, jaundice, or hemorrhage.

Diagnosis. In a severe illness with "black vomit," intense albuminuria, jaundice, and melena, as a group or in combinations, yellow fever must be suspected. Diseases that must be differentiated from severe yellow fever include infectious and serum hepatitis, "acute yellow atrophy" of the liver, carbon tetrachloride poisoning, other jaundices, malaria, and typhoid. In mild cases, which have been confused with dengue and influenza, clinical diagnosis is notoriously inaccurate. The necessary laboratory procedures are highly specialized. The isolation of virus in mice, rhesus monkeys, or certain tissue cultures from serum of the acutely ill patient or from serum or liver of a deceased patient affords convincing diagnosis. Specialized procedures are needed for the identification of the isolate. Serologic tests on paired acute-phase and convalescent serums, using techniques of complement-fixation, hemagglutination-inhibition, and virus neutralization, can also give positive diagnosis. Although the tests must be done in a specialized laboratory, nevertheless under most primitive conditions the serum specimens can be collected and submitted to such laboratory.

For postmortem diagnosis, specimens of liver and other tissues should be preserved in 10 per cent formalin for histologic examination. Virus recovery can be attempted from such tissues if small pieces are placed in 50 per cent glycerol-saline and shipped, under refrigeration if possible, to a laboratory.

Prognosis. Early in the disease the prognosis should be guarded, because sudden changes for the worse may occur. If early symptoms are mild, rapid recovery is probable. Some patients with severe disease will recover, but symptoms of hiccups, copious black vomit, melena, and anuria imply a very grave prognosis.

The over-all average case fatality rate is less than 10 per cent, and rates of less than 5 per cent have been observed in epidemics involving completely susceptible populations. Rates as high as 85 per cent have been observed, but they are most exceptional. Even the often cited 50 per cent is misleading, since in earlier, and also in present day epidemics, large numbers of mild cases may go undiagnosed.

Treatment. There is no specific treatment. A patient should be moved as little as possible and should be kept quiet in bed. Heroic efforts to get a patient from some remote area to a district hospital should be discouraged. The severe headache and body aches may require relief with an analgesic. The heart should be watched carefully throughout the illness and into early convalescence.

Water should be given in adequate amounts, parenterally if necessary. Easily assimilated food should be given to the extent that the patient will tolerate. Milk in moderate quantities can be recommended. When vomiting has ceased and the temperature is down, full diet may be given. Full activity should be resumed only gradually.

Prevention. If a case of yellow fever is treated in a place in which vector mosquitoes exist, the patient must be kept under a bed net or in a mosquito-proof room during the first four days of illness.

Vaccination is essential for persons who intend to visit yellow fever endemic areas and for the people resident in such areas. Yellow fever is notorious for existence in endemic areas with no overt signs of its presence, and despite negative reports of the most recent weekly international epidemiologic bulletins relative to a given area, vaccination for persons going to an endemic area must be stressed. Two strains of living virus have been used extensively for human vaccination. The 17D vaccine is prepared in chick embryos and is given by subcutaneous inoculation. At the Pasteur Institute of Dakar, the technique of vaccination by scarification of the skin was developed, using the neurotropic French strain suspended in gum arabic solution. With either strain, an effective immunity to yellow fever is regularly pro-

duced, provided that viable vaccine is used. Severe reactions to the Dakar type of vaccine are more frequent than are reactions to 17D. Vaccination ordinarily gives protection in a week, and the consequent immunity has been shown to last at least ten years. An urban epidemic can be stopped by mass vaccination of the population combined with vigorous anti-aegypti measures.

Bergold, G. H., and Weibel, J.: Demonstration of yellow fever virus with the electron microscope. Virology, 17:554, 1962.

Groot, H., and Bahia Ribiero, R.: Neutralizing and hemagglutination-inhibiting antibodies to yellow fever 17 years after vaccination with 17D vaccine. Bull. WHO, 27:699, 1962.

Horsfall, F. L., Jr., and Tamm, I. (eds.): Viral and Rickettsial Infections of Man. 4th ed. Chapter 14 (Casals and Reeves: Arthropod-borne viruses) and Chapter 16 (Clarke and Casals: Arthropod-borne viruses: Group B). Philadelphia, J. B. Lippincott Company, 1965.

Serie, C. et al.: Études sur la fièvre jaune en Ethiopie. Parts 1–6. Bull. WHO, 38:835, 1968.

Smithburn, K. C., et al.: Yellow Fever Vaccination. Geneva, World Health Organization, 1956.

Strode, G. K.: Yellow Fever. New York, McGraw-Hill Book Co., 1951.

HEMORRHAGIC FEVER CAUSED BY DENGUE VIRUSES*

(Philippine Hemorrhagic Fever, Bangkok or Thai Hemorrhagic Fever, Singapore Hemorrhagic Fever, Southeast Asian Mosquito-Borne Hemorrhagic Fever)

Karl M. Johnson

Definition. These hemorrhagic fevers of Southeast Asia and India are acute, infectious, urban, mosquito-borne diseases caused by dengue viruses. Endoepidemic in pattern, they were first recognized less than 20 years ago. There is still much confusion regarding clinical definitions of various entities associated with dengue and chikungunya virus infection in this region. The following description is based on Halstead's definitions, which state that dengue hemorrhagic fever is a dengue disease that worsens two or more days after onset, and is characterized by hypoproteinemia and one or more hemostatic abnormalities, i.e., thrombocytopenia, prolonged bleeding time, or elevated prothrombin time. The dengue shock syndrome, frequently fatal, consists of hemorrhagic fever plus shock (hypotension or a pulse pressure of 20 mm. Hg or less) and hemoconcentration (hematocrit at least 20 per cent higher than convalescent value). Cases fulfilling these criteria are rarely associated with chikungunya virus infection.

Etiology. All evidence suggests that these diseases are caused by each of the four recognized dengue virus subtypes. How they produce such disease is still not clear. Although minor antigenic

*In previous editions the article on Hemorrhagic Fever Caused by Dengue Viruses was written by Dr. William McD. Hammon. Significant portions of that article are included in the present version prepared by Dr. Johnson, who joins with the Editors in expressing indebtedness to Dr. Hammon.

differences among virus strains have been detected, no consistent correlation between such properties and either of the severe dengue syndromes has been found. A current hypothesis is that severe dengue disease is produced by an immunologic reaction that occurs in some individuals experiencing a second dengue infection. Available evidence for this concept is summarized below.

Incidence and Prevalence. These hemorrhagic fevers were first seen in epidemic proportions in Manila and Bangkok (1954) and in Singapore (1960). Other outbreaks have been reported from Malaysia, South Vietnam, and India. The best data over the longest interval are from Bangkok, where rates for hospitalized cases have been as high as 1 to 2 per 1000 population and age-specific rates in children have reached 7 to 8 per 1000. In most outbreaks cases occur only in children, principally below the age of eight years. Numbers of young adults were affected in Singapore, and numerous adult cases were recorded in Calcutta. The occurrence of the severe shock syndrome was much less common in adults than in children. Almost without exception, cases have been limited to persons indigenous to the area.

Epidemiology. The epidemiology of *infection* leading to dengue hemorrhagic fever is basically similar to that associated with ordinary dengue fever; outbreaks occur during the rainy season in large urban centers where *Aedes aegypti* is well established. Several unique features associated with *severe dengue disease* eludicated over the past decade by workers at the SEATO laboratory in Bangkok deserve special mention. This is particularly the case because they also contribute to a basic hypothesis that may explain the etiology of these hemorrhagic fevers and orient future study of their pathogenesis. The main points are as follows: (1) dengue hemorrhagic fever is endemic with annual seasonal epidemics, and this pattern is associated with endemicity of all four dengue virus subtypes; (2) modal peak age-specific attack rates are between three and five years of age; (3) in children of more than one year of age, nearly all cases of hemorrhagic fever and shock are marked by a secondary type of dengue immune response; that is, antibody titers to all dengue subtypes are very high at the time of admission to hospital; (4) in children more than three years of age, females are attacked twice as often as males; (5) infants less than one year old display primary rather than secondary immune responses, and the modal peak within this age group occurs between six and nine months of age; (6) virus isolation rates are always lower from patients with secondary as compared to primary dengue infection, and virus or viral antigen has been but rarely detected in tissues of fatal cases. From these and other data Halstead has proposed that dengue hemorrhagic fever and the shock syndrome are immune diseases brought on usually by a second (but not a third) dengue virus infection in a previously sensitized host. In the case of infants, passively acquired immunity from the mother provides the sensitizing stimulus.

Pathology. Autopsy findings are compromised to a degree by the inability to restrict cases to those virologically confirmed. Again the Bangkok reports appear to provide the best data in terms of clinical, virologic, and immunologic control.

The chief abnormalities include generalized vascular congestion and dilatation with edema and multiple focal hemorrhages in most organs, mild to moderate pleural effusion and ascites; mononuclear cell infiltration of interstitial tissues and alveolar walls of lungs; focal myocardial congestion; and a decrease in mature lymphocytes with proliferation of mononuclear forms in the germinal centers of lymph follicles.

Necrosis is unusual, and no specific damage of the blood vessels has been observed. Perivascular infiltration by mononuclear cells is common, but there is no evidence for significant vasculitis or for platelet or thrombin thrombosis of vessel walls. About one third of cases show evidence of globulin on endothelial surfaces and the walls of arterioles. Bone marrows often show maturation arrest of megakaryocytes, and sometimes there is marked generalized cellular hypoplasia with rapid restoration to normal following emergence from shock.

Pathologic change in the liver, though generally inconspicuous, consists of focal lesions and varies greatly in degree of severity. These lesions are of particular interest, as occasionally Councilman bodies and other changes characteristic of yellow fever are observed. In two fatal cases of jaundice reported by Bhamarapravati, not diagnosed at the time as hemorrhagic fever but subsequently believed to be severe cases of this disease, there were similar but more extensive changes; the lesions in the two livers were entirely comparable with those of yellow fever. Thus, if these two cases are part of the spectrum of this hemorrhagic fever, the spectrum of pathologic change in the liver is from that of severe yellow fever to scattered and sparse, inconspicuous, focal, paracentral degeneration of liver cells. Usually, the pathologic findings have been insufficient to account for death.

Pathogenesis or Mechanism of Disease. The pathogenesis of the viral hemorrhagic fevers is as yet poorly understood. The vascular congestion, dilatation, and increased permeability lead to the extensive edema and hemorrhage observed in the gastrointestinal tract, the skin, and other tissues. The cause of these vascular changes is unknown, but they result in loss of plasma volume and associated electrolyte disturbances. Platelet deficiency probably plays a role in the hemorrhages. Bleeding time is usually prolonged, prothrombin times are somewhat prolonged, clot retraction is poor, and the blood fibrinogen is slightly reduced. None of these changes is very profound. The circulatory collapse and shock observed appear to be far in excess of what might be expected from the extent of loss of edema fluid and blood. The adrenal changes suggest exhaustion of steroid reserve. Death in some cases has been accompanied by severe hyperkalemia.

Clinical Manifestations. The diseases observed in different areas have not been identical clinically; however, many similarities have been noted. The common features are as follows. The onset is usually abrupt, with fever. Nausea and vomiting are common. The throat appears injected, and there may be a dry cough. About the second or third day petechiae appear, usually first on the face or distal portions of the extremities but sparing the axillae and chest. The tourniquet test may be conspicuously positive before petechiae appear. Purpura and large ecchymoses as well as other manifestations of bleeding tendency are occasionally prominent. There may be severe abdominal pain and tenderness. About the third or fourth day, vomiting may produce copious coffee-ground material. Melena also is not uncommon, but gross bleeding from the intestines is rare. *Shock* is likely to occur in severe cases about the fourth day, and this critical state lasts about 12 to 24 hours. At this time the temperature falls to normal, the blood pressure and pulse pressure are low or unmeasurable, and the limbs are cool and present a purple or brownish mottled appearance. Perspiration is frequently profuse. The face and hands appear edematous. Restlessness and apprehension are conspicuous as the patient enters shock. This state of shock is entirely out of proportion to the apparent loss of blood. Thrombocytopenia is noted during this period, and bleeding time is prolonged. Leukocytes remain at approximately normal levels but are elevated in number in serious cases more frequently than they are depressed. The total and differential leukocyte count are not those observed in dengue. Although the numbers of both immature and mature polymorphonuclear cells are decreased, there is an increase in lymphocytes and sometimes in monocytes.

In Bangkok several clinicopathologic parameters were found to be correlated with type and severity of dengue virus infection. About one fourth of patients with secondary infection had serum Na less than 135 mEq. per liter, CO_2 equal or less than 15 mM. per liter and SGOT levels of at least 150 S.F. units. Forty per cent had serum protein values less than 5.6 grams per 100 ml., and half had hemoconcentration as previously defined (*vide supra*). Such abnormalities were unusual in primary dengue infection (not hemorrhagic) among children more than one year old. When secondary infections with shock were examined, these abnormalities were found in 60 to 95 per cent. Serum urea nitrogen levels on admission to hospital were greater than 20 mg. per 100 ml. in two thirds of cases with shock syndrome.

Differences observed between the diseases seen in the Philippines in 1956 and in Bangkok in 1958 are as follows: (1) Hepatomegaly was common in Bangkok, absent in Manila. In Bangkok this was accompanied by an elevated serum glutamic oxaloacetic transaminase (SGOT). (2) A deep red-purplish blush of the skin that did not blanch on pressure and pale, normal colored skin in small blotchy irregular areas was common in Manila but rare in Bangkok. This phenomenon frequently was brought on by application of a tourniquet and remained conspicuous for several days. (3) Epistaxis was very common in Manila, rare in Bangkok. Fleeting, dengue-like early and late rashes were occasionally seen in Bangkok only, but these were missed unless searched for carefully. In Singapore in 1960 splenomegaly was a conspicuous part of the disease syndrome, but this did not occur in Manila or Bangkok.

Not observed or extremely rare in all outbreaks were hematuria, heavy albuminuria, oliguria or anuria, bleeding gums, uterine bleeding, jaundice, nuchal rigidity, paralysis, encephalitis, retro-orbital pain, joint pains, swelling of joints and general lymphadenopathy (exception, Singapore).

If the patient survives the shock, recovery is very prompt and ordinarily is not followed by a period of asthenia or depression. Total duration of fever and illness is usually five to seven days.

Milder cases without bleeding tendencies or shock and of shorter duration are frequently observed. These are characterized essentially by fever only, and may well represent the characteristic dengue fever manifestations of young children.

Diagnosis. As in dengue, association with other classic cases during an epidemic greatly facilitates the diagnosis of the hemorrhagic fevers in patients with epidemic disease of moderate or great severity. The diagnosis in a febrile child acutely ill for only two or three days is rendered highly probable by the presentation of petechiae, purpuric lesions, and unusual ecchymoses of the skin with most prominent distribution on the extremities and face, together with melena, thrombocytopenia, and a relatively normal leukocyte count. In a milder case or at an earlier stage, the tourniquet test may be of great assistance in detecting unusual capillary fragility. The rapid development of circulatory collapse and shock during the fourth to sixth day, associated with the above findings, differentiates this from most other exanthematous diseases. *Meningococcemia* and the *Waterhouse-Friderichsen syndrome* need careful consideration. The nephrosonephritis type of "epidemic hemorrhagic fever" has conspicuous hematuria and heavy albuminuria, generally absent in this disease. Other hemorrhagic fevers such as Omsk, Crimean, Argentinian, and Kyasanur Forest disease will probably occur only in those areas with essential vectors and reservoirs. All these other types of viral diseases have been of rural rather than urban origin. Thrombocytopenic purpura can be expected to have an entirely different onset and is usually not associated with fever.

Unquestionably, the viruses causing the hemorrhagic fevers of the tropical Orient produce also a mild, nonhemorrhagic form of illness that is much more difficult to diagnose. In the Philippines, for each severe case there are several diagnosed as "influenza." These actually resemble more closely the dengue syndrome, without rash and with fever of only three to five days' duration. Classic dengue fever is readily differentiated clinically from severe hemorrhagic fever, but the two syndromes overlap extensively in the milder and atypical manifestations and even laboratory tests cannot differentiate these, as the etiologic agents themselves cannot be differentiated as yet.

As in dengue, laboratory diagnosis is essential for at least a sample of cases in every epidemic, in all sporadic cases, and in all very mild, suspect fevers. Laboratory methods available are those described for dengue fever.

Treatment. Although there is no specific therapy, case fatality can be greatly reduced by skillful management. The administration of oxygen, correction of metabolic acidosis and hypovolemia by use of appropriate intravenous solutions, and reversal of hypoproteinemia with plasma are of fundamental importance. Great care is necessary, however, to ensure that too sudden or over-correction does not result in severe pulmonary edema and death. Pressor amines, alpha adrenergic blocking agents, and a variety of steroids have been used, but with no clear evidence of benefit. It has been suggested that infusions of calcium lactate may be of use in controlling hyperkalemia seen in a minority of severely ill patients.

Prognosis. Case fatality rates among hospitalized patients with hemorrhagic fever have ranged from 5 to 50 per cent, depending to a large extent on the severity of the disease and the facilities available for treatment. Although over-all mortality for those with shock approaches 50 per cent, workers in Bangkok demonstrated that careful management saved all but the 5 to 10 per cent of such cases admitted in a moribund state. Death is almost entirely associated with shock, and rarely occurs after the sixth day of illness. Residual effects have not been observed, and, in contrast to dengue, recovery is usually prompt and complete from seven to ten days after onset. Mental depression is seldom observed.

Prevention. The control of the hemorrhagic fevers is the same as that for dengue, and consists of mosquito control or protection from mosquito bites and isolation of the patient from mosquitoes. No vaccine is available, and if the immunologic theory of etiology is confirmed, vaccines as presently conceived would be specifically contraindicated.

Chew, A., Yuen, H., Kiat, L. Y., Leng, G. A., Teik, K. O., Hong, L. C., and Wells, R.: A haemorrhagic fever in Singapore. Lancet, 1:307, 1961.

Halstead, S. B., et al.: Observations related to pathogenesis of dengue hemorrhagic fever. Yale J. Biol. Med., 42:261, 1970.

Hammon, W. McD., Rudnick, A., Sather, G., Rogers, K. D., and Morse, L. J.: New hemorrhagic fevers of children in the Philippines and Thailand. Trans. Ass. Amer. Physicians, 73:140, 1960.

Nelson, E. R.: Hemorrhagic fever in children in Thailand. J. Pediat., 56:101, 1960.

Piyaratn, P.: Pathology of Thailand epidemic hemorrhagic fever. Amer. J. Trop. Med., 10:767, 1961.

Report of the WHO Seminar on Mosquito-borne Haemorrhagic Fevers in the South East Asia and Western Pacific Regions, Bangkok (Thailand), October 1964. New Delhi, World Health Organization, 1965.

Weiss, H. J., and Halstead, S. B.: Studies of hemostasis in Thai hemorrhagic fever. J. Pediat., 66:918, 1965.

OMSK HEMORRHAGIC FEVER AND KYASANUR FOREST DISEASE
John P. Fox

Definition. The tick-borne complex of group B arboviruses includes two agents causing severe febrile illnesses characterized by hemorrhagic manifestations, Omsk hemorrhagic fever (OHF) of western Siberia and Kyasanur Forest disease (KFD) of Mysore State, India.

Etiology. The viruses of Omsk hemorrhagic fever and Kyasanur Forest disease possess most of the properties of the group B tick-borne encephalitis group (see Russian Spring-Summer Encephalitis and Louping Ill). However, both are sufficiently different to have caused laboratory-acquired disease in persons with antibody to the encephalitis agents. OHF virus is pathogenic for field mice and causes hemorrhagic pneumonia in muskrats. Langur and bonnet monkeys infected with KFD virus develop occasionally lethal disease closely similar to that in man.

Epidemiology. Vectors of OHF virus include *Dermacentor pictus* and *D. marginatus.* Voles and muskrats have been implicated as vertebrate hosts. Human disease occurs in a spring-summer-autumn pattern paralleling the activity of the vectors. First described in the Omsk Oblast, its distribution may extend into northern Roumania.

KFD, first described in 1958, is still localized to one area in Mysore State. The principal vectors are two Ixodid ticks, *Haemaphysalis turturis* and *spinigera.* Presence of virus is signaled by disease in monkeys, which also are important amplifiers of virus among ticks. The role of small mammals which also become infected is uncertain. KFD occurs in the dry season and chiefly in forest workers.

Pathogenesis and Pathology. Infection is by tick bite, but respiratory infection may occur in laboratories. The incubation period is three to seven days. Accounts of morbid changes are scant. The basic pathologic lesion of OHF is vascular dilation and increased permeability, leading to gross alimentary hemorrhages and minute hemorrhages elsewhere. In KFD, focal necrosis of the liver, gastrointestinal and pulmonary hemorrhages, and acute tubular degeneration of the kidneys have been described.

Clinical Manifestations. Sudden onset with fever and headache occurs in both diseases. In Omsk hemorrhagic fever, there is moderate epistaxis, hematemesis, and a hemorrhagic enanthem but no profuse hemorrhage. Bronchopneumonia is common. KFD is characterized by similar, often more severe hemorrhagic manifestations, bronchiolar involvement, severe myalgia, and prostration. In many patients recurrent febrile illness may follow an afebrile period of 7 to 15 days. This second phase takes the form of a mild meningoencephalitis. Severe leukopenia and thrombocytopenia occur in both diseases and, in KFD, the urine often contains albumin, casts, and leuko-cytes.

Treatment and Prognosis. Treatment is supportive and includes analgesics for headache and myalgia and fluids or transfusions to combat dehydration and hemorrhage. There are no sequelae to either illness, but, especially in KFD, convalescence is prolonged. Case fatality is between 0.5 and 3 per cent for OHF and 5 per cent for KFD.

Prevention. A formol-inactivated mouse brain vaccine is said to be effective in protecting against both laboratory and natural OHF disease. There is no KFD vaccine. Proper clothing and repellents may reduce exposure to ticks.

Boshell-M, J., Rajagopalan, P. K., Patil, A. P., and Pavri, K. M.: Isolation of Kyasanur Forest disease virus from Ixodid ticks: 1961-1964. Indian J. Med. Res., 56:541, 1968.
Casals, J., Hoogstraal, H., Johnson, K. M., Shelokov, A., Wiebenga, N. H., and Work, T. H.: A current appraisal of hemorrhagic fevers in the U.S.S.R. Amer. J. Trop. Med., 16:751, 1966.
Clarke, D. H., and Casals, J.: Arboviruses: Group B. In Horsfall, F. L., Jr., and Tamm, I. (eds.): Viral and Rickettsial Infections in Man. 4th ed. Philadelphia, J. B. Lippincott Company, 1965, chap. 27.
Webb, H. E., and Rao, L.: Kyasanur Forest disease: A general clinical study in which some cases with neurological complications were observed. Trans. Roy Soc. Trop. Med. Hyg., 55:284, 1961.

HEMORRHAGIC FEVER, TRANSMISSION UNKNOWN

HEMORRHAGIC FEVER OF SOUTH AMERICA: ARGENTINE AND BOLIVIAN HEMORRHAGIC FEVER

Karl M. Johnson

Definition. Argentine and Bolivian hemorrhagic fevers are acute diseases caused by serologically related Junin and Machupo viruses. Clinically these diseases may be considered as a single entity characterized by fever, severe myalgia, leukopenia, hemorrhagic manifestations, shock, and acute neurologic abnormalities.

History. Hemorrhagic fever was recognized in Argentina in 1953. Since that time it has been reported annually in the form of seasonal outbreaks in the rich farming province of Buenos Aires northwest of the capital city. A similar disease was reported from the dry, tropical savannah province of Beni in northeastern Bolivia in 1959. Cases have been recorded from this region in each subsequent year without apparent spread to neighboring provinces.

Etiology. Argentine hemorrhagic fever is caused by an agent first isolated in 1958 and named Junin virus. The etiologic agent of the Bolivian disease is Machupo virus, a serologic relative. Both these viruses are members of the Tacaribe complex, a group of American viruses isolated from rodents and, in one case, bats. By definition, Tacaribe viruses share complement-fixing antigens but are distinct in neutralization tests. Tacaribe viruses are ether-sensitive and contain ribonucleic acid. Recent morphologic studies show Machupo virus to be indistinguishable from the virus of lymphocytic choriomeningitis virus of *Mus musculus*. These agents are pleomorphic, varying in size from 50 to 250 mμ, are formed by budding from cytoplasmic host-cell membrane, and contain one or more electron-dense bodies that resemble cellular ribosomes. An immunologic relationship between lymphocytic choriomeningitis virus and Tacaribe viruses also has been demonstrated by the indirect fluorescent antibody technique.

Incidence and Prevalence. Cases of Argentine hemorrhagic fever have been reported annually since 1955. Although precise attack rates have not been calculated, hundreds to several thousands of cases occur each year during the months of April through July. The disease is restricted to a slowly expanding area to the northwest of Buenos Aires, in recent years reaching the eastern margin of the Province of Córdoba. The recognized endemic area of Bolivian hemorrhagic fever consists of about 15,000 square miles of the sparsely populated province of Beni between the rivers Mamoré and Blanco. Here the disease appears to be less strongly seasonal, although the months of November and December mark an interepidemic trough between annual epidemics. Within the endemic area there are settlements that have never been attacked. In others, such as the town of San Joaquín, incidence of disease has reached values as high as 200 per 10,000 population per month. Serologic studies indicate that virus infection is usually manifested by clinical illness. Reinfection with disease has not been observed. Accuracy of mortality figures for both diseases suffers from serious deficiencies in specific etiologic diagnosis in both fatal and nonfatal illnesses. In Argentina the case fatality has been estimated as varying from about 30 per cent down to as low as 7 per cent. During a 16-month study in Bolivia, where the majority of cases were adequately diagnosed, mortality was 18 per cent, with higher incidence in both very young children and the aged.

Epidemiology and Probable Mode of Transmission. Both viruses have been repeatedly isolated from wild rodents: Junin virus from *Mus musculus, Akodon arenicola, and Calomys laucha, laucha;* and Machupo virus from *Calomys callosus.* Both diseases occur predominantly in populations having intimate, repeated contact with such rodents, particularly adult male migrants harvesting extensive fields of maize in Argentina, and farmers and their families raising maize, rice, yucca, and beans in Bolivia. The annual maize harvest appears to be a major factor in the seasonal pattern of Argentine hemorrhagic fever.

Isolation of Junin virus from mites parasitizing rodents has been reported, but is not regarded as definitive evidence that such arthropods represent biologic vectors of infection for humans. Machupo virus has been recovered from throat swabs in human disease, and, in unusual instances, direct human-to-human transmission has occurred. The principal mode of transmission of Bolivian hemorrhagic fever, however, is believed to be by direct contamination of the human environment by rodent excreta. In San Joaquín certain houses were "infected," giving rise to multiple cases of disease over irregular intervals often lasting several months. The disease spread through this town very slowly from house to house and block to block. Experimental studies showed that Machupo virus produced asymptomatic, *chronic* infection in both newborn and adult *Calomys callosus*. Infection of newborn animals resulted in immune tolerance, and tolerant infection was acquired through the milk by all babies born to viremic mothers. In all cases *viruria* was readily detectable in rodents for many months. Virus was subsequently recovered from urine of healthy Calomys trapped in houses where human disease had been reported. Finally, a human epidemic was abruptly halted 12 to 15 days (the estimated incubation period of human disease) after initiation of an intensive rodent control study that almost completely eliminated *C. callosus* from homes and gardens. Thus a current hypothesis is that Bolivian hemorrhagic fever, at least, is acquired by direct human contact (ingestion, inhalation, or entrance through mucous membranes or skin breaks) with virus-containing rodent excreta.

Pathology. Observations are based on a very small number of cases, not all of which were etiologically defined. The principal finding has been irregularly focal diapedesis and capillary hemorrhage without much evidence of associated inflammatory reaction. Gross hemorrhage was most common in mucosa of stomach and intestines and in the brain. Pulmonary infection, probably intercurrent, was frequently noted, but the pathognomonic lesion in the renal medulla and the large retroperitoneal accumulations of proteinaceous fluid so often seen in epidemic hemorrhagic fever of northeast Asia were conspicuously absent (see article on Nephroso-Nephritis, *infra*).

Clinical Manifestations. Although as many as half of all etiologically confirmed cases may best be described as acute undifferentiated fevers, the findings and clinical course of "full-blown" Argentine and Bolivian infections are so nearly identical as to warrant joint description. Onset is usually gradual, with increasing fever, headache, diffuse myalgia, and anorexia. By the third day, the temperature may be 103 to 105° F., with severe myalgia, particularly in the lumbar region. Conjunctival injection is present, a flush involving the upper trunk and face is frequently observed, and there may be a relative bradycardia. Beginning about the fourth day, scattered fine petechiae may appear on the face and neck, about the pec-

toral girdle, and/or in the buccal mucosa and palate. The Rumpel-Leeds test is frequently positive, and may then be followed by frank hemorrhages from one or more sites, including the stomach, intestines, nose, gums, and uterus, accompanied by microscopic hematuria. Although hemorrhage per se is rarely the precipitating cause, a hypotensive crisis frequently develops between the sixth and eighth days, coincident with a rapid return of temperature to normal after five or more days of sustained fever. Patients surviving this stress for 48 hours generally make slow but complete recovery.

Perhaps a fifth of the patients develop neurologic signs. These are quite characteristic, and begin about the fifth or sixth day with a fine intention tremor of the tongue. This may become so severe as to render speech unintelligible and preclude oral ingestion of solid or even liquid food. If so, gross intention tremors of the extremities usually appear, occasionally accompanied by an intermittent nystagmus. Such patients often become delirious, and may experience generalized clonic and tonic convulsions. The cerebrospinal fluid appears normal, however, and contains neither leukocytes nor virus. Convalescence is marked by weakness and signs of autonomic nervous system lability such as postural hypotension, spontaneous flushing and blanching of the skin, and precipitate episodes of diaphoresis. Transient loss of scalp hair and typical Beau's lines in the nails, particularly those of the fingers, are observed in a majority of cases several weeks after subsidence of the high, sustained fever. Many patients are not able to resume full activity for at least one month following illness.

Leukopenia is almost invariably present, and cell counts may be as low as 1000 per cubic millimeter by the fourth or fifth day. All elements are reduced nearly equally, and there is often a mild to moderate thrombocytopenia during the first week. Usually the peripheral blood picture returns to normal rapidly after defervescence, although there may be transient relative lymphocytosis and mild anemia. During the latter portion of the febrile period, progressive increase in hematocrit similar to, but usually milder than, that of hemorrhagic nephroso-nephritis (q.v.) is frequently observed. At about the same time, moderate proteinuria is common, although renal function is rarely compromised seriously, and frank azotemia and hyperkalemia are almost never present. Detailed systematic investigation of the abnormal physiology of the disease has not yet been done.

Diagnosis. The presence of high fever, severe myalgia, and leukopenia should arouse immediate suspicion of viral hemorrhagic fever within the known endemic areas of its occurrence. Potential intimate contact with wild rodents in a rural or semirural setting serves to strengthen the likelihood of this diagnosis. Since these findings and all others described can not be relied upon to differentiate the disease clinically from other infections of South America, such as yellow fever, typhoid and paratyphoid fevers, typhus, and lepto-spirosis, specific identification of cases depends upon laboratory confirmation. Virus can some-times be isolated by intracerebral inoculation of guinea pigs, infant hamsters, or infant mice with blood or throat washing, or both, during the febrile period. At autopsy splenic tissue almost always yields the agent. Serologic detection of infection is a reliable method if paired acute and convalescent serums are employed. Both group-reacting complement-fixing antibodies and virus type-specific neutralizing antibodies appear three to four weeks, and reach peak values seven to ten weeks, after the onset of illness.

Treatment. In the absence of any specific therapy, successful treatment presents an acute challenge in the science and art of physiologic management. Patients require complete rest and maximal comfort. Mild sedatives and analgesics should be judiciously used. Careful measurement of fluid intake and output is mandatory. The electrolyte balance should be checked regularly; marked underhydration and overhydration are to be avoided because these conditions appear to compromise the patient's ability to weather the hypotensive crisis. Daily hematocrit determina-tions and examinations of urine for protein are the most valuable tests for anticipating and managing this problem. Frequent measurement of blood pressure is also important because many patients enter the shock phase with persistent relative bradycardia and warm, dry skin. Raising the foot of the bed may suffice to stabilize the pres-sure at levels adequate to preserve vital urinary output. If not, careful administration of human plasma or concentrated albumin (not whole blood) is indicated. Great care should be exercised in administering plasma or other fluids intraven-ously during shock, since intractable pulmonary edema is readily induced. Complications, particu-larly bacterial infections, should be anticipated and promptly treated. Convalescence should never be hurried.

Prognosis. Although the case mortality may reach 20 per cent, there is no single finding early in the disease that aids prognosis in the individual case. In general, the very young and the very old as well as those who do not receive medical attention prior to the sixth day of disease are subject to the highest risk. The onset of severe shock and neurologic abnormalities are both ominous prog-nostic signs, and at least half the patients ex-hibiting these signs succumb.

Prevention. Effective elimination of intimate human contact with certain wild rodents repre-sents the only proved method for prevention of disease. This may be achieved by maintaining sound standards of personal and environmental hygiene. Campaigns to eliminate rodents, repair buildings, and clean rubbish near dwellings are highly successful when the disease is acquired mainly from peridomestic animals. There is insufficient evidence at present to warrant recom-mendation of systematic measures to control attacks by any potential arthropod vector.

Comision Nacional ad hoc para Estudiar el Brote de 1958: Virosis Hemorragica del Noreste Bonaerense (Endemo-Epidemica, Febril, Enantematica y Leucopenica). Talleres Graficos del Ministerio de Asistencia Social y Salud Publica, Buenos Aires, pp. 197, 1959.

Johnson, K. M., Halstead, S. B., and Cohen, S. N.: Hemorrhagic fevers of Southeast Asia and South America: A comparative appraisal. In Melnick, J. L. (ed.): Progress in Medical Virol-ogy, Vol. 9. Basel/New York, S. Karger, 1967, pp. 105-158.

Symposium on some aspects of hemorrhagic fevers in the Americas. Amer. J. Trop. Med., 14:789, 1965.

LASSA FEVER
Wilbur G. Downs

An acute febrile illness, with high mortality in recognized cases, was first noted in three American missionary nurses in Nigeria in early 1969. The first patient was infected in Lassa, and the two subsequent patients, in contact with the first, in Jos. From exposure to passage materials from these patients in a laboratory in the United States, two subsequent cases developed in 1969. Early in 1970, the disease was again seen in Jos, when some 30 patients were hospitalized in a two-month period. The mortality in hospitalized patients, in the limited experience to date, approaches 35 per cent. Epidemiologic studies of the 1970 Jos out-break indicate, on the basis of complement-fixation test serology, that mild cases of illness and even infections without recognized illness occur. The proportion of such cases to severe cases remains to be determined.

Clinically, the disease is characterized by gradual onset, increasing prostration, and un-remitting fever, progressing to extreme prostra-tion and death between 6 and 15 days of onset. Some patients have shown EKG evidence of myo-cardial involvement, and in late stages, blurring of the sensorium and a semicomatose state have been observed. Myalgia has been noted in some cases. A feature of several cases has been a diffuse oropharyngeal inflammation, sometimes with small white or hemorrhagic patches on the mucosa. In several patients accumulation of pleural or abdominal cavity fluid has been observed. Hemor-rhagic manifestations have been observed in several patients, but do not appear to be a constant feature of the disease. The disease picture in severe cases closely resembles that seen in severe lym-phocytic choriomeningitis virus infections, and possibly also in Junin (Argentine hemorrhagic fever) and Machupo (Bolivian hemorrhagic fever) infections.

Laboratory findings include a lowered WBC count (4000 to 5000) with no pronounced changes in the leukogram, and a drop in platelets (to approximately 100,000).

Lassa virus, which has been isolated from serum, pleural fluid, throat washings, and urine of pa-tients, closely resembles morphologically the viruses of lymphocytic choriomeningitis and the Tacaribe-Junin-Machupo group, and has a dis-tant relationship, demonstrable serologically, with these viruses.

No positive information is available yet to confirm epidemiologic conjectures. It is suspected that, in a fashion similar to lymphocytic choriomeningitis and the Tacaribe-Junin-Machupo group of viruses, rodents constitute a reservoir host and that transmission from rodent to rodent and rodent to man occurs through contact with materials contaminated by infected rodents. Human-to-human passage of virus occurs, again probably through exposure to contaminated fomites.

Treatment of the infection is poorly understood. In one instance, early administration of plasma from a recovered patient appeared to abort the illness.

Management of patients poses a particular problem. Those with suspected cases should be held under conditions of strictest isolation. In view of long-persisting viremia and protracted presence of virus in throat and urine, recovered patients should not be discharged until negative reports of laboratory examinations are at hand.

Laboratory infections already experienced indicate that laboratory work (virus isolation attempts in mice or tissue culture systems and serologic testing) should be attempted only in laboratories equipped to handle materials in special high-risk facilities (such as the National Center for Disease Control, Atlanta, Georgia).

Buckley, S. M., and Casals, J.: Lassa fever, a new virus disease of man from West Africa. III. Isolation and characterization of the virus. Amer. J. Trop. Med., 19:680, 1970.

Buckley, S. M., Casals, J., and Downs, W. G.: Isolation and antigenic characterization of Lassa virus. Nature, 222:174, 1970.

Frame, J. D., Baldwin, J. M., Jr., Gocke, D. J., and Troup, J. M.: Lassa fever, a new virus disease of man from West Africa. I. Clinical description and pathological findings. Amer. J. Trop. Med., 19:670, 1970.

Leifer, E., Gocke, D. J., and Bourne, H.: Lassa fever, a new virus disease of man from West Africa. II.: Report of a laboratory-acquired new infection treated with plasma from a person recently recovered from the disease. Amer. J. Trop. Med., 19:677, 1970.

Speir, R. W., Wood, O., Liebhaber, H., and Buckley, S. M.: Lassa fever, a new virus disease of man from West Africa. IV. Electron microscopy of Vero cell cultures infected with Lassa virus. Amer. J. Trop. Med., 19:692, 1970.

Troup, J. M., White, H. A., Fom, A. L. M. D., and Carey, D. E.: An outbreak of Lassa fever on the Jos Plateau, Nigeria, in January-February 1970. A Preliminary report. Amer. J. Trop. Med., 19:695, 1970.

EPIDEMIC HEMORRHAGIC FEVER: HEMORRHAGIC NEPHROSO-NEPHRITIS

Karl M. Johnson

Definition. Epidemic hemorrhagic fever is an acute disease of unknown cause that occurs during the spring and autumn in northeastern Asia. It is characterized by fever, prostration, vomiting, proteinuria, hemorrhagic manifestations, shock, and renal failure.

History. This disease was first described in the far east of the Soviet Union in the 1930's. Archives of the general hospital in Vladivostok, however, contain descriptions of classic cases as early as 1913. The Soviets call the disease hemorrhagic nephroso nephritis or hemorrhagic fever with renal syndrome, and 300 to 500 cases are still recorded annually from that region. Western physicians first encountered it in 1951 in the form of a seasonal epidemic occurring among UN troops in Korea. It was then learned that the Japanese had observed an identical clinical disease in eastern Manchuria, which they designated epidemic hemorrhagic fever.

Etiology. Soviet investigators reproduced the disease in human volunteers by the parenteral injection of serum or urine obtained prior to the fifth day of illness from patients with the naturally occurring disease. They further found that the disease agent was filterable through a Berkefeld filter (grade N), that the incubation period was usually 12 to 16 days, and that a single attack conferred immunity. After years of failure, Soviet virologists claim (1969) to have isolated the causative agent in human and porcine kidney cell cultures, using fluorescent antibody technique as marker of viral replication. Acute and convalescent human sera showed specific antibody increases to this agent, which is not yet available outside the Soviet Union for confirmatory study.

Epidemiology. The endemic area includes far eastern Siberia, parts of eastern Manchuria, and Korea north of Seoul. Sporadic cases occur throughout the year, but the large majority are recorded during late spring and autumn. All ages and races and both sexes are susceptible, but adult males usually experience the highest number of attacks. The disease is rural, and is characterized by isolated cases widely separated in place. Environmental exposure to forests or fields near forests is invariably noted. Person-to-person transmission does not occur.

Since World War II Soviet scientists have studied many outbreaks in forested regions west of the Ural Mountains of what they now believe to be an identical disease. Other reports of similar disease have been made from northern Scandinavia, Czechoslovakia, Rumania, and Bulgaria. Although the incidence and severity of hemorrhagic manifestations and mortality are lower than in northeast Asia, the renal lesion is apparently the same. The epidemiology is also similar, with one important difference. The largest epidemics were marked by a slowly accumulating number of cases beginning in late spring, culminating in an often explosive burst between November and January. In these remarkable outbreaks the peak of the epidemic was preceded by an eruption of cyclically large forest rodent populations (usually the red-backed vole *Clethrionomys glareolus*) into the fields, barns, and even houses of people living in or next to forests. These rodent "invasions" were probably precipitated by meteorologic conditions unfavorable for winter survival of the animals (rain and sleet instead of a snow blanket). Only under these conditions were multiple cases in the same family frequently observed. *On the basis of these data Soviet workers now believe that epidemic hemorrhagic fever is transmitted directly from asymptomatically infected rodents to man by means of virus-contaminated rodent excreta.*

Pathology. Profound, protein-rich retroperitoneal edema is characteristic of early death in shock, but not of later deaths. Changes in various organs apparently have a similar pathogenesis and consist of widespread, often focal, congestion and hemorrhage, sometimes accompanied by necrosis, without significant inflammatory response. The "pathognomonic" lesion is found in the kidneys, which appear swollen, and when incised exhibit extreme hemorrhagic congestion sharply localized to the medulla. Gross congestion or hemorrhage derived from dilated, congested small blood vessels is also found frequently in the right atrium, the pituitary, and the stomach; less often in intestines, adrenals, lungs, and central nervous system. Liver and spleen are usually not grossly involved. Petechial hemorrhages may occur in the skin, heart, adrenals, brain, and serous surfaces.

Clinical Course and Pathologic Physiology. The clinical and laboratory manifestations of hemorrhagic fever make up a confusing array of problems that occur in rapid sequence with considerable overlapping and variation in severity. However, many patients follow a fairly typical course that is conveniently considered in relation to several phases. Although all patients exhibit proteinuria and many have petechiae and some degree of hemoconcentration, the hypotension and renal failure, and such consequences as shock, serious hemorrhages, and fluid and electrolyte imbalances, occur in no more than 20 per cent.

The febrile phase lasts three to eight days and is characterized by fever, malaise, a flush of the face and neck, injection of the eyes and palate, and other nonspecific features. Evidence of widespread vascular dysfunction appears at this time. Toward the end of the febrile phase, petechiae occur, blood platelets decrease, the hematocrit begins to increase, and faint traces of protein appear in the urine.

The hypotensive phase develops suddenly during defervescence and generally lasts one to three days. Despite shock, which accounts for a third of all deaths, the extremities may remain warm, and arteriolar dysfunction may contribute to the hypotension. The dominant feature, however, is a reduction in blood volume owing to loss of plasma from the vascular system, as evidenced by a rapid increase in hematocrit to as high as 70 per cent and to trapping of erythrocytes in dilated capillaries. Heavy proteinuria, oliguria, acute renal failure, and hemorrhages of capillary origin associated with thrombocytopenia are prominent clinical features, whether or not hypotension develops. Nausea and vomiting are common. Backache and particularly abdominal pain resulting from localized edema have occasioned exploratory laparotomy in certain misdiagnosed instances. The leukocytes, which earlier were normal or reduced, now show a leukemoid reaction.

The oliguric phase begins as the hematocrit decreases and the sequestered plasma returns to the vascular system. It usually lasts for three to five days. Deaths in this phase are due to pulmonary edema, electrolyte abnormalities, and shock secondary to dehydration or pulmonary infections. This phase is one of increasing renal failure and nitrogen retention, continued vomiting, and dehydration. Hyperkalemia is common. Despite improvement in many of the earlier symptoms, increasing confusion and extreme restlessness are common, as is hypertension. Some patients exhibit a hypervolemic syndrome that may respond to phlebotomy. Hemorrhages into the skin, sclerae, gastrointestinal tract, lungs, and renal pelvis continue, but rarely are large in amount and generally decrease toward the end of the oliguric phase.

The diuretic phase, which may last for days or weeks, usually initiates clinical recovery and rapid improvement in renal function. However, a diuresis of 3 to 8 liters daily represents a hazard to patients who are already extremely dehydrated and who have had limited caloric intake for seven to ten days. These patients exhibit a brittle fluid volume homeostasis and may fluctuate rapidly between shock, on the one hand, and hypertension and pulmonary edema, on the other, depending on the state of the fluid balance. Serious potassium deficiency may occur, and hypernatremia can be troublesome. Deaths in this phase account for a third of the total, and are usually due to shock secondary to dehydration and to pulmonary complications, including bacterial infections. The diuresis characteristic of this phase does not represent mobilization of edema fluid, but is the result of residual renal tubular damage.

Convalescence requires three to twelve weeks and is characterized by gradual return to normal of appetite, strength, and urinary concentrating ability.

Diagnosis. In the absence of any specific test, the diagnosis must be made on clinical evidence and should be suspected when an acute febrile illness associated with the characteristic flush and petechiae occurs in a subject who has been in an endemic area. The subsequent developments such as hypotension or shock, increased hematocrit, thrombocytopenia, oliguria, and renal failure assist in establishing the diagnosis, but proteinuria and isohyposthenuria developing near the time of defervescence are the most useful diagnostic signs.

Prognosis. The case fatality rate, once techniques for prompt diagnosis and early, adequate treatment were developed, has been 5 per cent or less. No single finding is of great prognostic value in individual patients. However, prolonged high fever, protracted or recurrent shock, and persistent hemoconcentration are all ominous features. With rare exceptions, survivors who have not had central nervous system hemorrhages make apparently complete recoveries.

Treatment. Because antimicrobial drugs, convalescent serum, hormones, and other agents are entirely ineffective, the management of hemorrhagic fever must be supportive and based on an understanding of its physiologic and biochemical characteristics and on frequent clinical observations. Adequate sedation with barbiturates or opiates is frequently required for restlessness. *Contrary to the practice in other febrile diseases, fluid intake must be limited because any excess will simply leak out of damaged capillaries and increase edema and symptoms.* When intravenous fluid is required, it usually should be 10 per cent dextrose in water, and must be given very slowly. If shock fails to respond to simple measures such as shock blocks, then concentrated (salt-poor) human serum albumin to restore plasma volume and continuous intravenous infusion of pressor drugs such as norepinephrine may be required. Doses of the latter must be based on the response of the shock, blood pressure, and hematocrit. Occasionally, large doses of both albumin and pressor drugs are required. Treatment in the oliguric phase is that of acute renal failure, with careful control of electrolytes and particular attention to hyperkalemia. If oliguria persists, hemodialysis or peritoneal dialysis is indicated. Soviet workers have treated 60 severe cases with an "artificial kidney" and report only three deaths. Phlebotomy may be required for the fully developed hypervolemic syndrome. The chief problem of the diuretic phase is one of careful matching of fluid and electrolyte intake against the brisk urinary output, so as to avoid excessive dehydration and shock, on the one hand, and hypervolemia and pulmonary edema, on the other. Electrolyte abnormalities are still a problem, especially potassium deficiency.

Prevention. Preventive measures are based on the assumption that the disease is transmitted by rodents with or without the aid of an associated arthropod parasite. Vigorous rodent control measures, as well as dipping of clothing in acaracidal solutions and the individual use of insect repellents, are recommended in endemic areas during seasonal periods of disease activity.

Casals, J., Hoogstraal, H., Johnson, K. M., Shelokov, A., Wiebenga, N. H., and Work, T.: A current appraisal of hemorrhagic fevers in the U.S.S.R. Amer. J. Trop. Med., 15:751, 1966.
Entwisle, G., and Hale, E.: Hemodynamic alterations in hemorrhagic fever. Circulation, 15:414, 1957.
Hullinghorst, R. L., and Steer, A.: Pathology of epidemic hemorrhagic fever. Ann. Intern. Med., 38:77, 1953.
Oliver, J., and MacDowell, M.: The renal lesion in epidemic hemorrhagic fever. J. Clin. Invest., 36:99, 1957.
Smorodintsev, A. A., Kazbintsev, L. I., and Chudakov, V. G.: Virus Hemorrhagic Fevers (Y. Halperin, translator). Washington, D.C., Office of Technical Services, U.S. Department of Commerce, 1964.
Symposium on Epidemic Hemorrhagic Fever. Amer. J. Med., 16:617, 1954.

VIRAL DISEASES CHARACTERIZED BY PROTRACTED, RECURRENT, OR LATENT INFECTION

HERPESVIRUS INFECTIONS: GENERAL CONSIDERATIONS
Edwin D. Kilbourne

The long appreciated clinical similarities of the dermal and neurologic manifestations of herpes simplex and herpes zoster have often suggested a similarity of their causative viruses not verified by studies of their differing antigenicity. It is remarkable (and perhaps indicative of the value of clinico-pathologic observations) that the virus of varicella-zoster proves to be morphologically identical with the herpesviruses, with which it is now classified. Thus, to the common pathogenic attributes that suggested a common consideration of the viruses in the previous edition of this text as "latent DNA viruses" can now be added the important taxonomic criterion of viral structure.

Human cytomegalovirus (cytomegalic inclusion disease) and the *Epstein-Barr virus (EBV)* of cryptic potential are also now recognized as herpesviruses, so that four human herpesviruses—latent, persistent, and reactivable—must be reckoned with in any consideration of human disease. (See also Introduction to Viral Diseases.)

HERPES SIMPLEX
Robert R. Wagner

Definition. There are two stages of this disease, both of which are caused by the same virus. *Primary herpes simplex* is usually an asymptomatic infection but sometimes presents as a localized or systemic disease in susceptible children who are exposed to the virus from an outside source. *Recurrent herpes simplex* is a localized vesicular eruption caused by activation of virus that lies latent in the lips or other tissues of persons with circulating antibody.

Etiology. The virus of herpes simplex (*Herpesvirus hominis*) is the prototype of the Herpesvirus group, which range in size from 120 to 180 mμ and multiply primarily in cell nuclei. The infectious unit or virion is a three-layered structure consisting of a core of double-stranded DNA, a protein coat (capsid) made up of 162 capsomeric subunits arranged in icosahedral symmetry, and an outer lipid-containing envelope. There is one major antigenic type, but a minor antigenic variant, designated type 2, is associated with genital infections. Man is the only natural host, but similar viruses are found in many vertebrates, and the human virus can be propagated readily in chick embryos, mice, rabbits, and tissue cultures derived from almost all vertebrate species. Other members of the Herpesvirus group include the viruses of varicella-zoster (*H. varicellae*), monkey B disease (*H. simiae*), pseudorabies (*H. suis*), and cytomegalic inclusion disease. Herpeslike viruses are suspected to be causative agents of *Burkitt's lymphoma, infectious mononucleosis* and *carcinoma of the cervix.*

Incidence and Prevalence. Primary infection with herpes simplex virus usually occurs before the age of five years, but maternal antibodies often afford protection during the first six months of life. A higher infection rate at an earlier age is noted among children in lower socioeconomic groups. Serologic surveys have revealed the presence of herpes antibody in 90 per cent of adults. The virus is intermittently present in the mouths of healthy carriers. Epidemics are rare, but small outbreaks occur in nurseries and orphanages, and multiple cases of cutaneous herpes simplex have been noted among hospital personnel.

Pathogenesis. In primary herpes simplex the virus multiplies at the portal of entry in the oropharyngeal mucosa or, far less commonly, in the vagina, cornea, skin, or esophagus. Viremia sometimes occurs in nonimmune persons. After resolution of the primary infection and formation of antibody, intracellular virus apparently persists in the tissues throughout the life of each infected person. A great variety of stimuli can reactivate the latent virus and induce an attack of recurrent herpes simplex. Antibody prevents dissemination of virus to other tissues, but does not inhibit virus multiplication or evolution of local lesions. Tissue culture studies reveal that herpes simplex virus can spread from infected cells to contiguous uninfected cells by fusion and dissolution of adjacent cytoplasmic membranes.

The lesions of primary and secondary herpes simplex are indistinguishable microscopically, and can be differentiated from chickenpox and herpes zoster only by immunofluorescence. Vesicles or ulcerated areas contain degenerated epithelial cells with "ballooned" cytoplasm, multinucleated giant cells, and intranuclear eosinophilic inclusion bodies.

Clinical Manifestations. Primary herpes simplex is an inapparent infection in at least (90) per cent of persons exposed to the virus for the first time. However, mild or severe illness, which runs its course in one to three weeks, may result from initial contact with the virus. Fever and malaise are often prominent manifestations. Lesions can develop at single or multiple mucosal and cutaneous sites, depending on the portal of entry of the virus and local tissue resistance. In *herpetic gingivostomatitis,* white plaques and vesicles appear in the oral cavity and sometimes extend to the posterior pharynx. These soon ulcerate and leave a denuded mucosal surface, which accounts for the bleeding gums, severe pain, fetid breath, secondary bacterial infection, and cervical adenopathy. *Herpetic keratoconjunctivitis* usually involves one eye and the preauricular lymph node on the affected side. This disease is characterized by edema and inflammation of the cornea and extension of infection to the bulbar and palpebral conjunctivae. *Herpetic vulvovaginitis* occurs in susceptible infants and children who develop ulcerating and necrotizing lesions of the external genitalia similar to those of gingivostomatitis.

Abrasions of the skin or pre-existing dermatoses also predispose to primary herpetic infection. *Traumatic (inoculation) herpes simplex* is characterized by the appearance at the site of injury of large vesicles and pustules that sometimes assume a radicular distribution not unlike that of herpes zoster. *Eczema herpeticum* is a serious, sometimes fatal, form of primary herpes simplex that occurs as a generalized cutaneous eruption in children with chronic eczema. This disease is often mistakenly diagnosed as eczema vaccinatum; the confusion is compounded by application of the eponym "Kaposi's varicelliform eruption" to both disorders.

On occasion, the virus of herpes simplex invades internal organs of persons who lack circulating antibody. A relatively rare consequence of primary infection is *herpes meningoencephalitis,* which presents as either a severe encephalitis or a benign aseptic meningitis. Even more uncommon is *visceral herpes simplex,* a fatal disease of newborn infants who contract the infection from mothers with recurrent herpetic vulvovaginitis. In this generalized form of infection, necrotizing lesions are found in liver, spleen, lungs, adrenals, kidneys, and brain.

Recurrent herpes simplex is thought to occur at the same site as the primary subclinical or symptomatic infection. If the virus is introduced initially onto the vaginal mucosa or abraded skin, herpetiform lesions similar to those of fever blisters may recur periodically in these areas. There are also rare cases of recurrent generalized cutaneous eruptions in children who recover from eczema herpeticum, and even rarer instances of relapsing herpes meningoencephalitis. A serious and more frequent form of recurrent infection follows primary herpetic keratoconjunctivitis. This progressive disease is characterized by punctate lesions at the corneal margins that either heal or coalesce to form dendritic ulcers and corneal opacities.

In the vast majority of cases, reactivation of latent virus takes the form of *herpes labialis (fever blisters* or *cold sores)*. These lesions appear as superficial clear vesicles on an erythematous base, and are most frequently located at the mucocutaneous junction of the lips and face. In flagrant cases the vesicles extend from the lips to involve the skin of the chin, nose, cheeks, and ears. The fragile vesicles soon rupture, exude a sticky serous or serosanguineous fluid, and form a yellow crust. Unless secondarily infected with bacteria, the lesions heal without scarring in two to seven days. Individuals vary greatly in their susceptibility to recurrent herpes labialis. Some fair-skinned people, for example, may be unable to tolerate even short exposure to sunlight or heat. Others may be regularly afflicted with fever blisters following short febrile episodes, common respiratory infection, minor gastrointestinal disturbances, trauma, trigeminal neuralgia, or even physical exertion. Pregnancy, menstruation, or emotional strain may also precipitate attacks of herpes simplex in susceptible persons. However, if the stimulus is sufficiently intense, virtually every adult may be affected. Herpes simplex frequently follows severe pneumococcal pneumonia and bacterial meningitides.

Diagnosis. Virus isolation and serologic studies are chiefly of value in confirming the diagnosis of primary herpes simplex. Laboratory data in recurrent herpes simplex are more difficult to interpret because neutralizing and complement-fixing antibody titers do not rise consistently. Virus can also be isolated from the mouth, feces, and even the cerebrospinal fluid of healthy persons. Such studies have led to invalid assumptions that herpes simplex virus causes aphthous stomatitis ("canker sores"), erythema multiforme, and a host of other diseases. The various forms of herpes simplex must sometimes be differentiated from chickenpox, herpes zoster, herpangina, thrush, Vincent's angina, pyoderma, and eczema vaccinatum.

Treatment. Antimicrobial drugs do not affect the course of herpes simplex uncomplicated by secondary bacterial infection. Topical application of nucleoside analogues that inhibit DNA synthesis, particularly 5-iodo-2'-deoxyuridine (IUdR), may ameliorate the acute manifestations of ocular herpes and prevent the sequelae associated with herpetic corneal infections. IUdR is much less effective in recurrent herpetic keratitis, presumably because of emergence of drug-resistant mutant viruses. Corticosteroids are said to be contraindicated in herpetic keratoconjunctivitis because they appear to induce perforation of corneal ulcers. Soothing dressings and topical anesthetics are occasionally required to alleviate severe inflammation, pain, and itching. The common practice of using smallpox vaccine to prevent recurrent herpes labialis has no rationale, and is not more effective than placebos or simple reassurance.

Brain, R. T.: The clinical vagaries of the herpes simplex virus. Brit. Med. J., 1:1061, 1956.
Kaufman, H. E.: Treatment of herpes simplex and vaccinia keratitis with 5-iodo- and 5-bromo-2'-deoxyuridine. *In*
Pollard, M. (ed.): Perspectives in Virology III. New York, Hoeber Medical Division, Harper and Row, 1963.
Rawls, W. E., Tompkins, W. A. F., Figueroa, M. E., and Melnick, J. L.: Herpesvirus type 2: Association with carcinoma of the cervix. Science, 161:1255, 1968.
Roizman, B.: An inquiry into the mechanisms of recurrent herpes infections of man. *In* Pollard, M. (ed.): Perspectives in Virology IV. New York, Hoeber Medical Division. Harper and Row, 1965.
Scott, T. F. M., and Tokamaru, T.: The herpesvirus group. *In* Horsfall, F. L., Jr., and Tamm, I. (eds.): Viral and Rickettsial Infections of Man. 4th ed., Philadelphia, J. B. Lippincott Company, 1965.

VARICELLA; HERPES ZOSTER
(Chickenpox; Zona, Zoster, Shingles)

Thomas H. Weller

Introduction. Varicella and herpes zoster are now considered the consequence of the activity of a single virus and the dissimilarity of the clinical features of the two syndromes as a reflection of differences in the response of the human host to the same agent. Although the mechanism of pathogenesis is incompletely understood, varicella may constitute the response of the nonimmune host and herpes zoster that of the partially immune person.

Definition. *Varicella* is a highly contagious disease characterized by a generalized vesicular exanthem developing in crops over a period of a few days. Usually benign in children, in adults it may be accompanied by severe symptoms.

Herpes zoster is an infectious process associated with the appearance of a circumscribed vesicular eruption of the skin or mucous membranes. The localized eruption, often involving one or more dermatomes, reflects a concurrent inflammatory process in related dorsal root ganglia or extramedullary cranial nerve ganglia.

Although varicella and herpes zoster are usually considered as discrete syndromes, the patient with zoster not infrequently shows evidence of generalization of the cutaneous process, and rarely a zosteriform concentration of vesicular lesions occurs in the patient with varicella.

Etiology. The virus is highly host-specific and has been transmitted experimentally only to man. Electron microscopic examination of varicella or zoster vesicle fluid reveals the virus particles as round bodies 210 mμ in diameter. Isolation of virus from vesicular lesions of cases of varicella and zoster was accomplished by Weller (1953) in cultures of human tissues. Employing viruses thus grown in vitro, the similarity of agents recovered from the two clinical syndromes was established. Now commonly termed varicella-zoster virus or V-Z virus, the agent is classified in the herpes virus group, and contains nucleic acid of the deoxyribose type. *Varicella-zoster virus is distinct from, and not to be confused with, the herpes simplex viruses, although possessing a similar ultrastructure, and having minor antigens in common.* In tissue culture the virus produces a cytopathic effect comparable to that seen in vivo with the development of multinucleate giant cells and eosinophilic intranuclear inclusions.

Incidence and Epidemiology. Varicella occurs at any age. In temperate regions, the greatest prevalence is observed between the ages of two and eight years. Fortunately, relatively few cases occur in the adult population, which is generally immune. However, in some tropical areas varicella is primarily a disease of adults. Varicella in temperate areas commonly presents in epidemic form during the cooler months, whereas zoster is a sporadic disease occurring throughout the year. Although cases of zoster occasionally are seen in infants and children, zoster is characteristically a disease of adults, attack rates increasing with age. In England, a recent study indicates that approximately half of the people achieving age 85 will have experienced an attack of zoster (Hope-Simpson, 1965).

Varicella is the consequence of contact with a pre-existing case of varicella, or, as first reported by von Bokay (1909), of contact with a person with herpes zoster. Zoster, on the other hand, often appears in the absence of contact with an external source of virus, and is believed to be the result of reactivation of virus lying latent in the body. Careful investigation of zoster occurring in children yields a history of prior varicella in a high percentage, evidence consistent with the concept of viral latency. Occasional patients with zoster give a history of recent contact with an external source of virus; such contact is probably coincidental, for epidemiologic studies fail to reveal an increased prevalence of zoster during periods when varicella is epidemic.

Pathology and Pathogenesis. In varicella the initial site of viral replication is not known, but may be in the respiratory tract. Thereafter, viremia probably follows with the initiation of focal lesions that apparently enlarge by spread of virus from cell to contiguous cell. As described by Tyzzer (1906), the initial changes in the skin take place in the endothelium of capillaries in the corium. Cells in the basal and prickle layers undergo ballooning degeneration, and fluid accumulates, the intact stratum corneum forming the roof of the vesicle. Nuclear changes with margination of chromatin and the appearance of intranuclear inclusions are characteristic of the reaction of infected cells. In the skin, multinucleate giant cells appear, each nucleus containing an inclusion. Virus is present in large amounts in the clear fluid of the young vesicles; as the vesicle fluid becomes cloudy with accumulating inflammatory cells and debris, the viral content declines. In fatal cases, focal areas of necrosis with associated specific nuclear changes occur in many organs.

In zoster, the cutaneous lesion morphologically is like that of varicella. The posterior root ganglion corresponding to the cutaneous site is acutely involved, and intranuclear inclusions have been demonstrated in ganglion and in satellite cells. Extension of the inflammatory process to the posterior horns and less often to the anterior horns of the cord may occur; virus has been recovered from the cerebrospinal fluid, and a pleocytosis in the fluid is not unusual. Partial degeneration of the dermal nerve network occurs in the affected dermatome, and there may be loss of functional integrity of the sensory afferent nerves. Zoster most commonly involves areas of skin innervated by the thoracic ganglia (50 per cent), the cervical ganglia (15 per cent), and the ophthalmic branch of the gasserian ganglia (10 per cent). The pathogenesis of zoster is not understood; in the "idiopathic" type, no reason for activation is apparent. In other instances, a trigger mechanism in the form of trauma, injections of drugs such as arsenicals, or concomitant disease such as tuberculosis or malignancy (particularly lymphoma and chronic leukemia), may be evident. Zoster is a relatively common iatrogenic complication in the recipient of immunosuppressive therapy.

Clinical Manifestations. *Varicella.* After an incubation period that usually is between 12 and 17 days, the rash appears, either concurrently with the onset of malaise and fever or shortly thereafter. The lesions appear in crops over a one- to five-day period. They are numerous on the trunk and face and relatively sparse over the extremities; mucosal surfaces may also be involved. The typical lesion develops within a few hours from a small macule to a fragile, slightly elevated, dewdrop-like vesicle with a red areola. With involution, it becomes crusted, and frequently is secondarily infected. The vesicle is delicate and easily broken but is not unilocular as is sometimes stated. Pruritus may be severe. The duration and degree of fever parallel the severity of the eruptive process. Lesions are usually more numerous in regions of pre-existing inflammation.

Because of the appearance of new crops, the presence of lesions in various stages of development in a single area is characteristic. Those appearing in the final crop may not progress beyond the maculopapular stage.

In infants, in children with leukemia or on steroid therapy, and in adults, varicella may be serious and may have a fatal outcome. The rash may persist, may become more extensive and hemorrhagic, and a specific pneumonitis demonstrable roentgenographically as a bilateral nodular infiltration may develop. There may be a focal hepatitis. *Varicella pneumonia* occurs primarily in adults. After recovery, serial roentgenographic examinations may reveal the development of small nodular calcifications scattered throughout the lung fields. Postvaricella encephalitis is a rare and grave complication of mild as well as of severe cases. In a different category is the disturbing but transient cerebellar type of ataxia occasionally seen in children after varicella.

Herpes Zoster. Pain and paresthesia often precede the appearance of skin lesions by a few days. The individual lesions evolve as in varicella, singly or irregularly in almost confluent patches on an erythematous base, but are concentrated over the area of distribution of one or more spinal nerves or the sensory division of a cranial nerve; thus, a unilateral bandlike eruption is characteristic. However, in one third of cases scattered cutaneous lesions may appear on other areas of the body. (See also Disorders of the Nervous System and Behavior.) The regional nodes enlarge; rarely this enlargement may precede the pain and skin involvement by a few days. Systemic complaints in the form of malaise, headache, and fever are present in a small percentage of cases.

In the majority of patients with zoster, spontaneous resolution of the cutaneous lesions and disappearance of pain occur within two weeks. However, in a minority, postherpetic neuralgia persists as a distressing and refractory consequence of infection. Scarring of the cornea may result from ophthalmic zoster.

Diagnosis. Differentiation of varicella from mild smallpox on clinical grounds may be difficult; the demonstration of the characteristic multinucleate giant cells with intranuclear inclusions in stained scrapings of young vesicles or biopsy materials will establish the presence of either varicella-zoster or herpes simplex virus and will eliminate variola or vaccinia virus from consideration. Other entities with a generalized vesicular eruption to be considered in differential diagnosis include eczema vaccinatum and eczema herpeticum, rickettsialpox, and certain Coxsackie virus infections. An atypical zoster eruption may be clinically indistinguishable from the lesions of recurrent herpes simplex. Pain in the pre-eruptive stage of zoster may suggest a variety of conditions such as pleurisy or appendicitis. To establish a specific diagnosis, virus may be isolated by the inoculation of appropriate cell cultures with fluid from newly appearing vesicles; cutaneous lesions that are purulent or crusted are usually virologically negative. The demonstration of a rising titer of complement-fixing antibodies for varicella-zoster antigen is helpful, but must be interpreted with some caution owing to antigenic components shared with the herpes simplex viruses.

Treatment. There is no specific treatment for varicella or zoster. Therapy is symptomatic and is directed at relief of local discomfort and the control of secondary infection. Prolonged mechanical ventilation may be required to maintain oxygenation of the patient with varicella pneumonia. It is to be noted that critical evaluation of therapeutic approaches to the treatment of zoster is difficult because of the self-limited and variable nature of the acute process. Postherpetic pain may ultimately require neurosurgery.

Prevention. No vaccine exists. Ordinary human immune serum globulin administered to children exposed to varicella does not prevent infection, but may modify the severity of the illness. However, recently it has been established that immune globulin prepared from selected donors recovering from herpes zoster will prevent infection if administered to susceptible children within 72 hours of exposure.

Brunell, P. A., Ross, A., Miller, L. H., and Kuo, B.: Prevention of varicella by zoster immune globulin. New Eng. J. Med., 280:1191, 1969.

Brunton, F. J., and Moore, M. E.: A survey of pulmonary calcification following adult chickenpox. Brit. J. Radiol., 42:256, 1969.

Cimons, I. M., Lacher, M. J., LaMonte, C. S., Levitt, L., Cady, B., and Beattie, E. J., Jr.: Treatment of varicella pneumonia. J.A.M.A., 206:372, 1968.

Muller, S. A., and Winkelmann, R. K.: Cutaneous nerve changes in zoster. J. Invest. Derm., 52:71, 1969.

Öberg, G., and Svedmyr, A.: Varicelliform eruptions in herpes zoster — Some clinical and serological observations. Scand. J. Infect. Dis., 1:47, 1969.

Rifkind, D.: The activation of varicella-zoster virus infections by immunosuppressive therapy. J. Lab. Clin. Med., 68:463, 1966.

Schmidt, N. J., Lennette, E. H., and Magoffin, R. L.: Immunological relationship between herpes simplex and varicella-zoster viruses demonstrated by complement fixation, neutralization and fluorescent antibody tests. J. Gen. Virol., 4:321, 1969.

Weller, T. H.: Varicella-zoster virus. In Lennette, E. H. (ed.): Diagnostic Procedures for Viral and Rickettsial Infections. New York, American Public Health Association, 1969, pp. 733–754.

CYTOMEGALOVIRUS INFECTIONS
Edwin D. Kilbourne

Definition. Cytomegalovirus infection (cytomegalic inclusion disease; salivary gland virus disease) is manifest clinically in a number of guises, depending upon the age and physical condition of the host and whether the disease is associated with primary (initial) or reactivated infection. The disease was originally recognized as a pathologic entity associated with the postmortem finding of enlarged epithelial cells bearing intranuclear and cytoplasmic inclusions in salivary glands, liver, spleen, lungs, and other viscera. The disease has emerged to prominence in recent years as a legacy of iatrogenic impairment of host defenses in the course of surgery requiring extensive transfusion or immunosuppressive therapy. The cardinal manifestation of such cases is a mononucleosis without heterophil antibody (post-transfusion or post-perfusion mononucleosis).

Etiology. Human cytomegalovirus is less thoroughly characterized than other human herpesviruses but, like other members of the group, has a capsid with icosahedral symmetry containing 162 elongated hollow capsomers. The virion is 960 Å in diameter and contains double-stranded DNA with a molecular weight of 32×10^6 daltons. The capsid is enclosed in a lipid-containing envelope. The virus is relatively unstable, having a half-life of less than an hour at $37°$ C. Cytomegalovirus is highly specific in its cultural requirements so that viral replication and cytopathic effects occur only in human fibroblast cultures. For this reason, and because of the slow growth rate and low yield of virus in culture, some have suggested that cytomegalovirus be categorized as a subgroup separate from herpes simplex and herpes zoster–varicella viruses. At present, these minor biologic differences are outweighed by the chemical and structural similarities of the viruses.

Incidence, Prevalence, and Epidemiology. Cytomegalovirus infection is common. Incidence increases cumulatively with advancing age so that more than 80 per cent of those over 35 have serum-neutralizing antibodies as evidence of previous infection. As with herpes simplex, the presence of neutralizing antibody may be equated with persistence of the virus, although direct demonstration of infective virus or cytomegaly has been rare in asymptomatic "carriers" of the virus.

With rubella and toxoplasmosis, cytomegalo virus infection is one of the few proved congenital infections of man. As with rubella, virus may be excreted for months after birth. Postnatal infection occurs less frequently in infancy and early childhood than is the case with herpes simplex. The frequency of infection varies widely (7 to 50 per cent) with increased prevalence noted in lower socioeconomic groups or in institutionalized populations of children.

The mechanism of virus spread is unknown in the case of the naturally occurring disease. In some cases, transmission of infection has been plausibly associated with the transfusion of fresh blood — usually in large amounts. These observations are not surprising in view of the presumably persistent carriage of virus in most of the population of blood donor age.

The source of infection, whether exogenous or endogenous, is not easy to establish in many cases, as initial antibody titers may be low or equivocally positive, and because parenteral reinfection in the presence of antibody has been observed.

Pathogenesis and Pathology. The slow replication of cytomegalovirus in tissue culture is paralleled by a lag of a month or more from introduction of virus (probably by maternal contact in newborns or by transfusion in adults) and the appearance of disease. Intrauterine infection leads to hepatosplenomegaly with jaundice, microcephaly, mental retardation, and death. Postnatally acquired infection of the newborn is also serious and is characterized by generalized visceral involvement. Even the more common asymptomatic infections in infants and young children are attended by viremia and protracted excretion of virus in urine and sputum.

The characteristic cytopathology of the disease is denoted explicitly by the name *cytomegalic inclusion disease.* Infected cells may be greatly enlarged and contain eosinophilic, intranuclear, and basophilic cytoplasmic inclusion. These cells may be seen as part of a mononuclear cell infiltration in almost all viscera, but predominantly in salivary glands, lymph nodes, liver, spleen, and lungs. The interstitial "transplantation" pneumonia that follows renal allografting commonly causes death through respiratory insufficiency.

Clinical Manifestations. Clinical manifestations have been considered in part in previous sections of this article. In summary, the acute, initial (primary) stage of infection is more often than not asymptomatic in the infant or child, with hepatosplenomegaly (with hepatitis) more common in the neonatally or congenitally infected. A maculopapular erythematous rash is an inconstant occurrence in childhood infections. Primary infection in previously healthy young adults resembles the febrile or typhoidal type of infectious mononucleosis without exudative pharyngitis or lymphadenopathy. Fever in such cases usually lasts for three weeks, and is the principal clinical sign. Recovery is usually uneventful in such patients.

Post-transfusion mononucleosis related to cytomegalovirus infection may be either primary or reactivated. The febrile disease evoked may be very severe in the debilitated or immunosuppressed patients who require transfusion or extracorporeal circulation in the course of cardiac surgery or renal allotransplantation. As one would expect, the prior presence of specific antibody has a better prognostic augury. It is now clear that cytomegalovirus infections account for many cases of cryptic postoperative febrile syndromes. Infections associated with surgery and transfusion can be asymptomatic like the naturally occurring disease.

Diagnosis. Protracted fever with minimal clinical findings save for evidence of low-grade hepatitis and the presence of abnormal mononuclear cells in the blood in the absence of heterophil antibody suggest the diagnosis of cytomegalovirus infection. The demonstration of large inclusion-containing mononuclear cells in urinary sediment is strongly presumptive evidence of cytomegalovirus infection. Definitive diagnosis demands (1) recovery of virus from blood, urine, or biopsy material by inoculation of human fibroblast cultures, or (2) increase in specific complement fixing or neutralizing antibody during illness.

Other human herpesviruses, including the Epstein-Barr virus (EBV) and, rarely, herpes simplex virus, have been associated with mononucleosis. Current evidence favors the EBV as the cause of heterophil antibody-positive infectious mononucleosis.

Treatment. As with most virus diseases, treatment is supportive with an emphasis on antipyretics. The severe disease that may occur in leukemic children has been reported to respond to the DNA (thymidine) antagonist 2′-deoxy-5-fluorouridine (FUDR).

Prognosis. Except with congenital or neonatal infections the prognosis for complete recovery appears to be excellent. However, reactivated or primary infections as complications of cardiac or transplantation surgery may contribute to a fatal outcome, especially if interstitial pneumonia results. The full potential of this persistent latent virus is yet to be determined.

Editorial. The post-transfusion syndrome and cytomegalovirus. Lancet, 2:526, 1969.

Foster, K. M., and Jack, I.: A prospective study of the role of cytomegalovirus in post-transfusion mononucleosis. New Eng. J. Med., 280:1311, 1969.

Hanshaw, J. B.: Clinical significance of cytomegalovirus infection. Postgrad. Med., 35:472, 1964.

Klemola, E., vonEssen, R., Wager, O., Haltia, K., Koivuniemi, A., and Salmi, I.: Cytomegalovirus mononucleosis in previously healthy individuals. Ann. Intern, Med., 71:11, 1969.

Plummer, G.: Cytomegaloviruses. *In* Heath, R. B., and Waterson, A. P. (eds.): Modern Trends in Medical Virology. 1. London, Butterworth and Co., Ltd., 1967, pp. 182-206.

SLOW VIRUS
(Kuru)

See Slow and Latent Viral Infections and Neurologic Diseases.

VIRAL DISEASES (PRESUMPTIVE)
Paul B. Beeson

CAT SCRATCH DISEASE

The essential feature of cat scratch disease is lymphadenitis, usually limited to one anatomic region, developing as a sequel to accidental injury of the skin. In two thirds of the reported cases there has been a history of scratch or bite by a cat.

Epidemiology. The disease occurs in all parts of the world, most often in winter. Children are affected more frequently than adults. Although injuries by cat claws or teeth are the most common form of skin injury, other puncture wounds, by wood splinters, thorns, and metallic objects have appeared to be responsible at times. Cats thought to have caused human infection show no sign of illness, do not react to the cat-scratch antigen, and probably merely convey the causative agent on claws or teeth. "Epidemics" of cat scratch disease, though reported, are difficult to evaluate because they may simply reflect special interest and awareness of certain physicians. There are, however, several reports of more than one case developing in a family over a period of a few months.

Etiology. Although this disease has the features of a specific infection, efforts to demonstrate a causative bacterium, fungus, or filterable virus have met with failure. Perhaps the most impressive evidence for viral etiology is in a report of electron microscopic examination of affected lymphatic tissue, in which herpes-like viral particles were observed. The hypothesis has been offered that the clinical manifestations result from an immunologic reaction; hence the inciting agent may no longer be demonstrable at the time the patient seeks medical help. Several groups of workers have reported serologic evidence that the causative agent is related to viruses of the psittacosis–ornithosis–lymphogranuloma venereum–trachoma group, but the proportion of patients exhibiting such positive serologic reactions has varied considerably, and, furthermore, patients with cat scratch disease do not react to intradermal injection of antigens prepared from this group of viruses.

Pathogenesis. An indolent or subacute inflammatory lesion develops at the site of primary inoculation in approximately one third of cases. It becomes clinically evident one to several weeks after the injury. Lymphadenitis, the hallmark of the disease, appears a few days later. Initially this takes the form of a granulomatous inflammation, sometimes containing giant cells. In cases of some duration micro-abscesses can nearly always be found; in about one fourth of cases these coalesce to form a grossly evident abscess.

Clinical Manifestations. The site of inoculation is most likely to be on the hand, forearm, or face. It may exhibit one or more erythematous papules. Less frequently there is vesicle formation going on to rupture and production of a small eschar. The lesion usually heals without scar formation. The lymph nodes most frequently affected are in the epitrochlear, axillary, or cervical groups, but when the injury has been on the legs the inguinal nodes may be the site of the disease. The process varies in clinical severity and acuteness, sometimes smoldering for weeks with enlarged and tender nodes, at other times progressing more quickly to pronounced swelling, with redness and edema of the overlying skin. There may be fluctuation, and in rare instances the skin undergoes necrosis, permitting discharge of exudate. The usual course is for the swelling and tenderness gradually to subside in two to eight weeks. Systemic manifestations are not prominent, although young children sometimes have high fever for a few days. The erythrocyte sedimentation rate may be elevated; there is often a moderate leukocytosis, and sometimes mild eosinophilia. Transient morbilliform rashes may accompany the adenitis; occasionally lesions are developed which have the appearance of erythema nodosum. Pulmonary and arthritic manifestations are extremely rare, perhaps only coincidental. Development of osteolytic lesions near the adenitis has been described.

The most serious complication is *encephalitis*, evidenced by fever, delirium, cranial nerve palsies, and pleocytosis in the cerebrospinal fluid. The encephalitis usually subsides without residual damage. When the primary lesion affects the conjunctiva, the preauricular nodes are affected, giving the clinical picture of *Parinaud's oculoglandular syndrome.*

It has been suggested that cat scratch disease may present as *mesenteric lymphadenitis,* because positive skin tests have been associated with that clinical picture. The presumption is that the portal of entry in such cases is the intestine.

Diagnosis. The diagnosis is based largely on the clinical circumstances, i.e., a subacute lymphadenitis limited to one region with or without suppuration, with or without a primary skin lesion distal to the node, and history of cat scratch or bite or of some comparable trauma to the skin. Several other processes must be considered in the differential diagnosis. Among infections are tuberculosis, infectious mononucleosis, tularemia, lymphogranuloma venereum, and sporotrichosis. Hodgkin's disease may cause difficulty, because the granulomatous picture in the lymph node of cat scratch disease may bear some resemblance to that of Hodgkin's disease; but the presence of micro-abscesses usually serves to differentiate these.

The Hanger-Rose test appears to be relatively specific for cat scratch disease. This employs an "antigen" prepared from the purulent matter aspirated from nodes of other patients, in a manner comparable with that formerly employed for lymphogranuloma venereum (Frei test). The exudate is diluted 1 to 5 in saline, and sterilized by heating at 60° C. for one hour on two occasions. After intradermal injection of this material, the reaction is read at 24 to 48 hours. A positive result consists of induration 5 mm. or more and erythema 10 mm. or more in diameter. Unfortunately test material is not available commercially.

Treatment. There is no evidence that antimicrobial therapy, including tetracycline, is of value. Bed rest is advisable when fever and general malaise are present. If fluctuation becomes evident in the affected lymph node, it is recommended that the pus be aspirated (and used for the preparation of skin test antigen). Incision of an abscess is inadvisable, because sinus formation with prolonged drainage sometimes results, but biopsy of intact nodes seems safe in the pre-suppurative stage.

Daniels, W. B., and MacMurray, F. G.: Cat scratch disease. Report of one hundred sixty cases. J.A.M.A., 154:1247, 1954.
Kalter, S. S., Kim, C. S., and Heberling, R. L.: Herpes-like virus particles associated with cat scratch disease. Nature, 224: 190, 1969.
Spaulding, W. B., and Hennessy, J. N.: Cat scratch disease. Amer. J. Med., 28:504, 1960.
Warwick, W. J.: The cat scratch syndrome, many diseases or one disease? Progr. Med. Virol., 9:256, 1967 (This useful review lists nearly every publication up to 1966.)

NONBACTERIAL GASTROENTERITIS
(Epidemic Nausea, Epidemic Vomiting, Winter Vomiting Disease, Epidemic Diarrhea)

Acute illnesses characterized by nausea, vomiting, and diarrhea are among the most common of human ailments, especially in children of school or preschool age. This pattern of indisposition has many of the characteristics of infectious disease: occurrence in epidemics, short incubation period, sudden onset, fever, brief course, and complete recovery. Indeed, these features may also be manifestations of gastrointestinal infections by recognized pathogens: Salmonella, *Entamoeba histolytica*, Shigella, and the enteroviruses. Furthermore, especially in young children and in travelers, such illness may be attributed to colonization of the bowel by strains of "normal" gut flora, a mechanism thought by some to be involved in the extremely serious syndrome known as infant (or "weanling") diarrhea. There remains, however, a large residue of gastroenteritis in which no microbial etiologic agent can be indicted, and it is generally assumed that as yet unidentified viruses are responsible.

The presenting symptom may vary in different epidemics; this has given rise to reports of "epidemic nausea," "epidemic vomiting," and "epidemic diarrhea." Nevertheless in nearly all of them the clinical descriptions show that the allied symptoms were also present. In some epidemics, especially those affecting schoolchildren, hysteria appears to have played a role in determining the prominence of various symptoms.

The onset is abrupt, usually with nausea and vomiting, followed within a few hours by diarrhea. In young children there may be rise of body temperature, but fever is less common in older persons. The illness usually begins to subside within 24 hours, and recovery is established by the second to fourth day.

In the majority of cases the illness is easily dealt with at home; indeed, the best management could be characterized as masterful inactivity. Bed rest and sips of water or carbonated drinks are sensible therapy during the acute phase. Antimicrobial drugs should not be given. Codeine or paregoric may be used if diarrhea is exceptionally troublesome. In rare instances admission to hospital may be advisable so that fluids and electrolytes can be given parenterally.

Dingle, J. H., et al.: A study of illness in a group of Cleveland families. XIII. Clinical description of acute nonbacterial gastroenteritis. Amer. J. Hyg., 64:368, 1956.
Leading Article: Epidemic vomiting. Brit. Med. J., 1:327, 1969.
Webb, C. H., and Wallace, W. M.: Epidemic gastroenteritis, presumably viral. Pediatrics, 38:494, 1966.

EPIDEMIC NEUROMYASTHENIA
(Iceland Disease; Benign Myalgic Encephalomyelitis)

Since 1934 numerous epidemics have been recorded of a disease that, at the onset, may resemble poliomyelitis and may follow a prolonged course, punctuated by exacerbations, with headache, muscular weakness, fatigue, and mood depression.

Most outbreaks have occurred in summer, and about half of those reported have involved hospital personnel, especially student nurses. In all instances the attack rate has been much higher in women. Sporadic cases have been reported, but the diagnosis is difficult in the absence of an epidemic.

Severe generalized headache is nearly always a prominent complaint at the onset, and frequently there are pain and stiffness of the neck. Generalized tenderness of the muscles is common, and they frequently exhibit a characteristic of rapid fatigue and loss of motor power on repeated contraction. In perhaps 40 per cent of affected persons, areas of muscle weakness or paralysis appear during the first two weeks. These may be in the trunk or the extremities, and the pattern of involvement often changes from day to day. Cranial nerve signs, bladder dysfunction, and paresthesia may also be noted. In most cases complete recovery of neurologic function occurs within four to eight weeks, but relapses and exacerbations are common during the next few months.

Fever is inconspicuous or absent. The cerebrospinal fluid is usually normal, and routine tests of blood and urine reveal nothing of significance.

A striking feature of this illness is the prolonged period of disability after subsidence of the acute phase. Particularly troublesome are the behavioral manifestations of irritability and mood depression, which together with easy fatigue, may interfere with normal living for months and even years after the acute episode. In this stage the subject may present a picture of hysteria or of simple neurasthenia. (Although there is no specific treatment, there is value in warning the patient that this may lie ahead.)

Deaths have not been reported; therefore, nothing is known of the pathology.

Extensive laboratory investigations have failed to yield evidence of participation of any known pathogenic micro-organism; nevertheless, the presumption had seemed warranted that it is an infectious disease. However, McEvedy and Beard have cast doubt on the likelihood of an infectious etiology. They carefully reviewed the reports of 15 recorded outbreaks, with special attention to the well-documented epidemic among nurses at the Royal Free Hospital, London. They suggest alternatively that these epidemics represented psychosocial phenomena: either mass hysteria among the subjects or altered medical perception. Their analysis and argument are persuasive.

Acheson, E. D.: The clinical syndrome variously called benign myalgic encephalomyelitis, Iceland disease and epidemic neuromyasthenia. Amer. J. Med., 26:569, 1959.

McEvedy, C. P., and Beard, A. W.: Concept of benign myalgic encephalomyelitis. Brit. Med. J., 1:11, 1970.

EPIDEMIC CERVICAL MYALGIA
("Stiff Neck")

The entity described here has been reported mainly when it has occurred in epidemic form; probably, however, it is a relatively common disorder, to which most persons are subject one or more times before they attain middle age.

The typical illness has a sudden onset. Moderately severe, sharp pain is felt on one or both sides of the neck on movement. The sufferer tends to hold his head still and to turn his upper body in order to look to one side — the characteristic "stiff neck" posture. Aside from local pain, there are few other symptoms. Pyrexia is slight or lacking, and the appetite is not affected. The leukocyte picture and erythrocyte sedimentation rate are normal. Symptoms usually persist for one to three days, but may continue longer. Occasional patients seized acutely during epidemics have been reported to continue to suffer muscle pains for some months.

The usual site of pain is the area along the upper free margin of the trapezius muscle; this may be exquisitely tender to pressure. Other common areas of pain and tenderness are along the inner margins of the scapula, the insertion of the deltoid, and near the origins of the muscles of the forearm. The lower back and lower extremities are seldom affected.

The occurrence of this disorder in epidemics, together with its short, self-limited course, has led to the assumption that it is an infection, probably viral. Transmission of the disease to volunteer subjects by injection of whole blood has been described, but attempts to demonstrate an infectious agent by animal or tissue culture inoculation have so far been unsuccessful.

Davies, D. M.: Epidemic cervical myalgia. Lancet, 1:1275, 1960.

Rickettsial Diseases

INTRODUCTION
Edward S. Murray

The rickettsial diseases are caused by a family of micro-organisms (Rickettsiaceae) that have characteristics common to both bacteria and viruses. They are now considered to be more like bacteria, because among other characteristics they (1) possess metabolic enzymes, (2) have cell walls, (3) utilize oxygen, and (4) are susceptible to broad-spectrum antimicrobial drugs. They resemble viruses by virtue of the fact that they grow only within living cells. These micro-organisms were named "rickettsiae" to honor Dr. H. T. Ricketts

who died in 1910 while investigating the etiology of epidemic typhus and Rocky Mountain spotted fever.

The rickettsial diseases are grouped together because they possess a number of common characteristics. (1) The etiologic agents are similar in size and shape and can be seen as pleomorphic coccobacillary forms under the light microscope. (2) All rickettsial organisms occur under natural conditions in either fleas, lice, ticks, or mites, and these arthropods are in all cases except Q fever the primary means by which the diseases are transmitted to man. (3) All rickettsiae take on a characteristic red color with the Gimenez stain. (4) In all rickettsial infections except Q fever and rickettsialpox, agglutinins are produced to either the OX-19 or OX-K strains of the bacillus *Proteus vulgarus* (Weil-Felix reaction). (5) The characteristic pathologic lesion is a widespread peripheral vasculitis. (6) All are acute infectious diseases characterized clinically by fever, headache, and a rash (except Q fever, which has no rash). Finally, as previously noted, all rickettsial diseases in the early stages are readily susceptible to optimal doses of broad-spectrum antimicrobial drugs, e.g., chloramphenicol and the tetracyclines.

All rickettsial organisms, except the antigenically heterogenic strains of scrub typhus, produce complement-fixing antibodies. Data from these tests when combined with results of Weil-Felix reactions and clinical and epidemiologic features constitute definitive criteria for the diagnosis of each disease.

The immunity produced by any one of the rickettsial diseases is usually of long duration. Although the members of one group confer either partial or complete immunity to diseases caused by other members of the same group, there is, in general, no cross immunity between groups. A minor degree of cross immunity does exist, however, between some members of the typhus and spotted fever groups.

Since incubation periods for all the rickettsial diseases vary from 2 to 14 days, any of the rickettsial diseases can appear in air travelers reporting ill in any part of the world.

THE TYPHUS GROUP
Edward S. Murray

The typhus group is made up of three diseases: epidemic louse-borne typhus fever, Brill-Zinsser disease and murine flea-borne typhus fever. Clinically and pathologically, these three illnesses are nearly identical. Differences occur only in the intensity of the symptoms and signs, the severity of the course, and the case fatality rate. Epidemiologically, however, the three members of the typhus group are very different, and hence will be described under separate headings.

EPIDEMIC LOUSE-BORNE TYPHUS FEVER

(Classic, Historic, Human, European Typhus; Jail Fever, War Fever; Camp Fever; Fleckfieber [German]; Typhus Exanthematique [French]; Tifus Exantemático, Tabardillo [Spanish]; Dermotypho [Italian])

History. It is probable that typhus fever has afflicted mankind since ancient times. Although the plague of Athens in 430 B.C. is believed to have been epidemic typhus (MacArthur, 1954), the account of Fracastorius in 1546 is the earliest medical record that describes typhus fever with sufficient accuracy to permit its definite identification. Despite the work of Fracastorius, typhoid and typhus fevers were usually regarded as one entity by

TABLE 1. SUMMARY OF CERTAIN IMPORTANT EPIDEMIOLOGIC AND CLINICAL CHARACTERISTICS OF RICKETTSIAL DISEASES

| Disease | Epidemiologic Features | | | Usual Incubation Period (Days) | Rash | | |
	Geographic Occurrence	Usual Mode of Transmission to Man	Reservoir		Eschar	Distribution	Type
Typhus group Primary epidemic typhus	Worldwide	Infected louse feces rubbed into broken skin or as aerosol to mucous membranes	Man	12 (8-15)	None	Trunk to extremities	Macular, maculopapular
Brill-Zinsser disease	Worldwide	Recrudescence months or years after a primary attack of epidemic typhus		—	None	Trunk to extremities	Macular, maculopapular
Murine typhus	Scattered pockets, worldwide	Infected flea feces rubbed into broken skin or as aerosol to mucous membranes	Rodents	12 (6-14)	None	Trunk to extremities	Macular, maculopapular
Spotted fever group Rocky Mountain spotted fever	Western hemisphere	Tick bite	Ticks, rodents	6 (2-12)	None	Extremities to trunk; palms and soles	Macular, maculopapular, petechial
Tick typhus	Mediterranean littoral, Africa, Asia	Tick bite	Ticks, rodents	12 (7-18)	Frequent	Trunk, extremities, face, palms, soles	Macular, maculopapular, petechial
Rickettsialpox	USA, USSR, Korea	House mouse, mite bite	Mites, mice	12 (9-24)	Usually present	Trunk, face, extremities	Papular, vesicular
Scrub typhus	Japan, SW Asia, W and SW Pacific	Mite bite	Mites, rodents	11 (6-21)	Frequent	Trunk to extremities	Macular, maculopapular, evanescent
Q Fever	Worldwide	Inhalation of dried dusts from environment of infected animals	Ticks, mammals	14 (9-20)	None	None	None

physicians until 1837, when Gerhard in Philadelphia clearly differentiated the two disorders on the basis of the important clinical and pathologic differences. Even today, however, confusion in terminology persists in those parts of Europe where *typhoid* fever is called "typhus abdominalis."

Typhus fever has played a major role in the history of the past four centuries. It followed in the wake of wars, famines, and human misfortunes. It often has had a more decisive effect on military campaigns than the actual battles themselves, a subject admirably treated by Zinsser in his book, *Rats, Lice and History.* Typhus epidemics in eastern Europe and Russia between 1918 and 1922 are estimated to have caused 30,000,000 cases and at least 3,000,000 deaths. Millions of cases occurred again during World War II in Nazi prison camps, in the Eastern European combat zone, among Yugoslav partisan forces, and in North Africa.

Etiology. In 1916 da Rocha Lima showed that typhus was caused by the micro-organism that he named *Rickettsia prowazeki.* This organism has a protean morphology with coccobacillary forms predominating. However, the most typical form is a diplobacillus which has slightly pointed ends with a transparent band between the two bacilli. The organism takes on a characteristic red color when stained by the Gimenez method. *R. prowazeki* possesses a soluble antigenic moiety which is shared also by *Rickettsia mooseri,* the other member of the typhus group.

R. prowazeki is readily killed by common antiseptics and dies in a few hours if exposed to room temperature. It remains viable for several days in blood at +5° C. Hence, a specimen of blood from a suspected case of typhus can be held for a day or more in a refrigerator pending isolation procedures. Organisms remain viable for several months in dried louse feces, and have survived for over 20 years when quick-frozen in an alcohol bath and stored at −60° C.

Living *R. prowazeki* organisms contain a toxin that is lethal for mice as well as a substance that is hemolytic for the red blood cells of many animals.

Transmission. The role of the human body louse in the transmission of typhus was first demonstrated experimentally by Nicolle, Comte, and Conseil in 1909. A few years later mechanisms of transmission were precisely worked out by Wolbach, Todd, and Palfrey (1922) in their classic experiments in Poland on the etiology of typhus fever.

Man and the louse are the only known natural hosts of *R. prowazeki.* There is no passage of *R. prowazeki* organisms from one louse vector generation to the next via the egg. Furthermore, there is no confirmed evidence as yet of an animal reservoir. The chain of typhus infection starts when *R. prowazeki* appears in a patient's blood during the febrile period. A louse becomes infected during one of his frequent blood meals. The rickettsiae multiply in the cells lining the gut of the infected louse. First these cells become greatly distended and then burst, discharging myriads of micro-organisms into the gut where they invade other lining cells or pass out in the feces. The disease is invariably fatal to the louse owing to the ultimate complete destruction of its intestinal epithelium. Transmission of rickettsiae from an infected louse to a new human host can occur by several mechanisms. When a louse takes a blood meal, it makes a small puncture wound in the skin, defecating at the same time. The louse bite is irritating, causing the patient to scratch and thus rub infected feces into the wound. It is also possible for one to become infected if dried infected louse feces gain access to the mucous membranes of the eye or respiratory tract. In an epidemic the spread of typhus from patient to patient and community to community is clearly related to the temperature preferences of the louse. Lice choose a 29° C. environment which they find in the folds of the garments of a healthy man. Here they live and lay their eggs. Lice tend to leave a typhus patient when his temperature rises to 104° F. or higher. Also, they quickly abandon a corpse in search of a warm host. Transmission of typhus from man to man occurs only by means of the louse; hence, once deloused and bathed, a typhus patient cannot transmit the disease.

Pathology. The microscopic pathology of typhus is characteristic. Rickettsiae multiply in the endothelial cells lining the small blood vessels. Endothelial proliferation and perivascular infiltration lead to thrombosis and leakage. Such vascular lesions when they occur in the skin produce the rash, whereas lesions in the meninges most probably account for the highly characteristic rickettsial headache. The myocardium is also a frequent focus of vascular lesions. Gangrene is directly related to thrombosis of capillaries, small arteries, and veins in affected areas (McAllister).

Clinical Manifestations and Course. The incubation period is approximately ten days to two weeks. Prodromata of vague malaise and headache are not uncommon, especially in vaccinated individuals. The *onset* is usually abrupt, and the patient can frequently state the exact hour when his illness began. The major clinical signs and symptoms are fever, headache, and rash. The fever may rise to 102 to 104° F. (39 to 40° C.) the first day, or it may take two or three days to reach this level. However, once the temperature reaches 104° F. (40° C.) it tends to remain at this

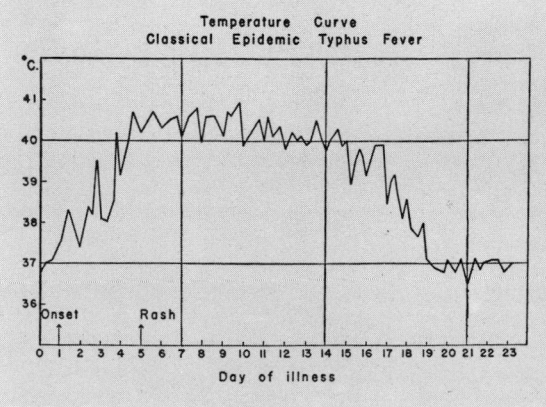

Temperature curve in a case of classic epidemic typhus. (From Horsfall, F. L., Jr., and Tamm, I. [eds.]: Viral and Rickettsial infections of Man, 4th Ed. J. B. Lippincott Company, 1965.)

level or higher with only slight fluctuations until altered by treatment or recovery. A remittent (or widely fluctuating) temperature is not characteristic of untreated typhus except very late in the disease or in vaccinated persons.

The headache is characteristic. It is intense, persists night and day, and is intractable to all efforts at alleviation. The rash makes its appearance on the fourth to seventh day of illness and consists at first of pinkish macules that fade on slight pressure. These discrete macules usually appear first on the upper trunk in the axillary area. In the course of one or two days the rash spreads over the entire body, usually sparing the face, palms, and soles which are involved only rarely. The macules soon become darker, fixed, and maculopapular. In severely ill patients the rash may progress to petechial, hemorrhagic, or confluent forms.

Patients often have a slight cough without sputum as in mycoplasmal pneumonia. An accompanying patchy pulmonary consolidation is more often diagnosed roentgenographically than by physical examination. Respirations may be increased out of all proportion to findings in the chest.

At first the pulse rate is slow in relation to the temperature, but by the end of the first week it becomes rapid (110 to 140), weak, and frequently undulating or irregular. The blood pressure is usually low, and there may be brief episodes of severe hypotension. Conjunctivitis and flushing of the face are frequent findings. The spleen is palpable in about half the cases. Renal insufficiency of varying degree is a common occurrence. During the acute phase, deafness and ringing in the ears are common complaints, as is also myalgia of the back and legs.

In fatal cases the terminal period is usually characterized by a profound stupor, peripheral vascular collapse, and severe renal failure. In cases without complications, the temperature begins to drop rapidly by lysis between the thirteenth and sixteenth days of illness. Recovery of normal mental and physical powers is remarkably rapid, although the patient may not regain his full strength for two to three months.

Typhus Fever in Previously Immunized Persons. The symptoms and clinical course of typhus are greatly modified as a consequence of prior active immunization. The illness may consist merely of a mild headache and fever of several days' duration. Most patients, however, go on to develop a transient macular rash and suffer from a relatively severe headache and fever for about a week. Complications are rare; mortality has not been reported, and the diagnosis can be established only by serologic or isolation studies.

Typhus Fever Modified by Specific Treatment. If specific treatment is begun early, the clinical course of typhus is usually arrested at whatever stage is present when treatment begins. The temperature usually drops to normal within 36 to 72 hours, and the major clinical signs and symptoms (including the rash) disappear soon there-

after. However, weakness of a greater or lesser extent almost always persists for days or weeks after recovery. On the other hand, if the disease is allowed to progress untreated beyond the eighth or ninth day, treatment becomes less and less effective. In such cases clinical recovery will depend largely upon the extent of vascular damage produced in the heart, brain, and kidneys before therapy was begun.

Diagnosis. **Clinical Diagnosis.** Before the characteristic rash appears, it is impossible to assert on clinical grounds alone that a patient is suffering from epidemic typhus. The early stages of a number of acute infectious diseases closely resemble the first few days of epidemic typhus—for example, smallpox, relapsing fever, malaria, typhoid fever, meningococcal infection, yellow fever, and several of the other rickettsial diseases. Of major help in the differential diagnosis is the characteristic maculopapular typhus rash that begins on the upper trunk and extends centrifugally to the extremities. The rash may be evanescent in children as well as in mildly ill adults. It is also difficult to recognize in dark-skinned subjects.

Laboratory Diagnosis. *Specific Serologic Tests.* Complement-fixing antibodies first appear in the serum of patients between the seventh and twelfth days of the disease. Soluble antigens that are commercially available detect group antibodies common to both murine and epidemic typhus. In most instances epidemiologic considerations such as geographic location and type of vector involved (flea or louse) will suffice to distinguish between these two diseases in the typhus group. When confusion in diagnosis arises, specific washed antigens (available in special rickettsial laboratories) can be used to differentiate between murine and epidemic typhus. In performing the complement-fixation test it is important to use 4 to 8 units of either type of antigen employed in order to detect the early IgM type of antibodies.

Other special serologic tests that can be used in laboratory diagnosis include immunofluorescence, mouse toxin neutralization, and rickettsial agglutination. Agglutination can also be carried out using sheep or human group O erythrocytes sensitized with a serologically active fraction derived from rickettsiae treated with ether, heat, and alkali (erythrocyte-sensitizing substance or ESS—Chang). These special tests are available in rickettsial research laboratories, but are rarely if ever needed to establish a diagnosis.

Persons recovered from typhus may show significant antibody titers in their sera for months or years after an attack of the disease. Hence for definitive diagnosis it is important to demonstrate a rise or fall in antibody titer related to the acute or convalescent period of the clinical disease.

Weil-Felix Test. The Weil-Felix reaction, although nonspecific, is of great value in indicating the strong probability of a typhus infection. The test is positive in over 90 per cent of bona fide cases of primary epidemic typhus. The basis for the Weil-Felix reaction is related to the fact that a certain antigenic component found in rickettsiae is shared by some strains of *Proteus vulgaris*. Thus *R. prowazeki* can stimulate antibodies that will agglutinate the OX-19 strain of Proteus. Since low levels of Proteus OX-19 antibody are present in many healthy individuals, diagnostic significance is only attached to titers of 1 to 160 or greater. Such titers are usually demonstrable between the seventh and eleventh days after onset of typhus. The rapid slide method which can be carried out in only three to five minutes is quite satisfactory when performed with controls. Occasionally agglutinins develop for the OX-2 Proteus strains but none for OX-K. Proteus OX-19 antibody titers also develop in other rickettsial diseases, notably murine typhus and Rocky Mountain spotted fever.

Isolation of Rickettsiae from the Patient. The laboratory diagnosis of typhus may be made by inoculating blood from a patient into a susceptible species such as the guinea pig or chick embryo if facilities are available for the further manipulations required to establish the identity of the micro-organisms thus obtained.

Prognosis. The prognosis in untreated cases is closely correlated with age. In children under ten years the disease is usually mild, and fatalities are uncommon. In adults the mortality ranges from 10 per cent in the second and third decades of life to more than 60 per cent in those over 50. However, active immunization and the use of specific therapy greatly affect mortality figures.

In the absence of specific treatment, the appearance of renal insufficiency is an early sign that a patient's illness will be severe or fatal. The extent and severity of the typhus rash is also roughly indicative of the severity of the disease. Complications such as pneumonia or gangrene of the skin are likewise serious prognostic signs. A fall in systolic blood pressure to values below 80 mm. of mercury for a few hours or longer may cause damage from which the patient may not recover, even though the blood pressure rises after the period of severe hypotension.

Treatment. Chloramphenicol or the tetracyclines are highly effective when given early and in adequate dosage. The clinician must decide on the basis of his own preference which drug he will use. Recent reports suggest that doxycycline is also an effective drug in the treatment of rickettsial infections.

Prompt and optimal specific therapy is urgent. A maximally effective rickettsiostatic blood level of drug should be obtained at the earliest possible moment. Since large doses of chloramphenicol are well absorbed from the gastrointestinal tract, this drug may be preferred in gravely ill patients. For chloramphenicol the following dosage schedule is considered optimal: Therapy is begun with an initial loading dose of 50 mg. per kilogram of body weight, followed by a daily dose of 50 mg. per kilogram of body weight divided into three or four equal doses during each 24-hour period. For an adult this schedule would amount to approximately 5 grams of chloramphenicol given over the first 24-hour period (an initial loading dose

of 3 grams followed by 0.5 gram every six hours). This dosage of chloramphenicol for the first 24 hours of illness is higher than that recommended in bacterial diseases. However, a large body of experience in using high initial doses of this drug in treating rickettsial diseases fully justifies such a schedule.

Since large single doses of tetracyclines are irregularly absorbed from the gastrointestinal tract, a loading dose of these drugs is not indicated. The daily recommended dose of the tetracyclines is calculated on the basis of 25 mg. per kilogram of body weight. Treatment is more effective if the daily dose is divided and administered at intervals of three or four hours rather than on a six- to eight-hour schedule.

As the temperature approaches normal, the daily dosage of the antimicrobial being administered can be cut in half and then continued for two or three more days. Relapses are uncommon even when treatment is begun as early as the first or second day of illness.

Intravenous preparations of chloramphenicol and tetracyclines are available, and should be used in critically ill patients when oral medication is not possible because of vomiting or uncooperativeness. For adults, 1 gram of chloramphenicol sodium succinate in glucose or saline solution can be given intravenously followed by 500 mg. every four to six hours. Recent reports suggest that intravenous tetracyclines may be superior to chloramphenicol sodium succinate. Intravenous tetracycline can be administered in glucose or saline solution, 1 gram initially, followed by 500 mg. every six hours. Intravenous therapy should be discontinued as soon as the patient is able to take the drug by mouth.

Penicillin and streptomycin have very little, if any, effect. Their use should be considered only when secondary bacterial infections develop for which they are specifically indicated. The sulfonamides may have a harmful effect, and are contraindicated. Steroid therapy has been used by some clinicians in severely ill patients. Carefully controlled hormone therapy may be of practical value in patients first seen late in the course of illness at a time when supplemental antitoxemia measures could be lifesaving.

Special nursing care is of utmost importance. Comatose patients should be turned frequently to prevent decubitus ulcers and hypostatic pneumonia. Vomiting necessitates small frequent feedings. Sedatives should be used with care so that the course of the disease is not obscured. Excessively high temperatures should be controlled by alcohol sponging.

It should be kept in mind that because of the widespread endothelial damage in epidemic typhus, as well as in all the other rickettsial diseases, a severely ill patient may be even more desperately ill than he appears. Therefore, all laboratory and other manipulative measures that disturb and exhaust him should be reduced to a minimum. The antimicrobial drugs are rickettsiostatic only; hence the patient's own defense and recuperative powers are major factors in his recovery.

Prevention. Two highly effective measures, immunization and louse control, are available for the prevention and control of typhus. Both are applicable to an individual as well as a community. For immunization, there are commercially available killed typhus vaccines produced from yolk sacs of infected chick embryos. Immunization with killed vaccines does not fully protect against infection. However, when vaccinated individuals do contract typhus, the course of illness is shorter and milder, and fatalities have not been reported. An experimental living attenuated "Strain E" typhus vaccine is under trial in the United States, the USSR, and Africa. Moderately severe illness has occurred in a small percentage of those inoculated with minimal immunizing doses of this vaccine. However, the prompt development and prolonged duration of the immunity resulting from a single dose of Strain E vaccine indicates that under certain circumstances this vaccine may be found to play a useful role in typhus control.

Louse control with DDT and the newer developed insecticides offers a powerful weapon against typhus epidemics. Both infected and noninfected lice can be eliminated almost completely by mass delousing of a population. A major factor in the efficacy of DDT is the persistence of its lethal effect on lice for two to four weeks after being dusted into garments.

Recent reports indicate that in several areas lice have become partially resistant to DDT. Other insecticides such as malathione or lindane may have to be used under these circumstances.

BRILL-ZINSSER DISEASE AND THE CARRIER STATE

History. In 1898 Nathan Brill in New York described sporadic cases of a typhus-like illness with fever, headache, and a maculopapular rash which occurred characteristically in immigrants from Russia and Poland. The disease was clearly distinguishable from typhoid, because the Widal test was negative. However, the illness was not typical of typhus, as all cases were sporadic with no spread to family or other contacts.

Over the next three decades many clinicians in the large cities of the eastern United States reported cases that were referred to as Brill's disease. In 1912 Anderson and Goldberger demonstrated by cross-immunity tests in monkeys that Brill's disease was a form of typhus, and for a period thereafter Brill's disease and murine typhus were confused with each other. However, by 1931 murine typhus was clearly defined as a flea-borne disease and Brill's disease remained an isolated syndrome of unknown etiology.

In 1934 Hans Zinsser carried out extensive epidemiologic studies on 538 cases of Brill's disease occurring in New York and Boston. Almost invariably patients were immigrants from eastern Europe where louse-borne typhus was prevalent. This led Zinsser to postulate that the syndrome represented a relapse of a prior typhus infection. He reasoned that man was a carrier and through the medium of recrudescent "Brill's disease" cases served to maintain the disease between epidemics. Over the next two decades Zinsser's hypothesis was widely accepted. To acknowledge the contributions of the two scientists whose observations revealed the interepidemic reservoir of typhus, the syndrome was renamed Brill-Zinsser disease.

Typhus, the Carrier State, and Recrudescence. Clinical and epidemiologic features of Brill-Zinsser disease are consistent with the view proposed by Zinsser that it represents a relapse or recrudescence of a primary epidemic typhus infection suffered at some time in the past. This makes Brill-Zinsser disease analogous in many ways to a relapse of malaria occurring years after an original malarial attack. Zinsser's hypothesis has received additional confirmation recently from laboratory studies in which normal lice were fed on patients during the acute phase of Brill-Zinsser disease. From these lice micro-organisms were isolated that proved to be *R. prowazeki* the etiologic agent of primary epidemic typhus.

Brill-Zinsser disease, however, differs from primary epidemic typhus in a number of respects. (1) Clinically the disease is shorter, milder, and frequently without a rash. This picture is consistent with the fact that the syndrome represents an *R. prowazeki* infection in an individual already partially immune. (2) No louse vector or exogenous source of the infection is apparent. (3) The majority of patients give a history of having suffered an attack of primary epidemic typhus in the past. But it is the serologic data that provide the most sharply distinguishing characteristics of these two disease entities caused by the same organism. In primary epidemic typhus the acute phase antibodies are IgM in type, whereas the antibodies in Brill-Zinsser disease are from their very earliest appearance of the IgG class. These differences are characteristic of the primary and secondary immune response.

An interesting feature of the Brill-Zinsser syndrome is the frequent absence of a significant Weil-Felix reaction. In fact the reaction is almost always negative when a Brill-Zinsser disease relapse occurs within the first few years following the primary attack at a time when immunity from the original illness is presumably still quite high. As the interval between the original attack and the recrudescence lengthens, positive Weil-Felix reactions occur more frequently. The Weil-Felix reaction is usually also negative in those who develop primary epidemic typhus after prophylactic vaccination, as well as in typhus patients who receive antimicrobial therapy very early in the course of their illness.*

Brill-Zinsser disease has now been reported from many parts of the world. Wherever it has been recognized, it has always occurred in individuals who were born or had lived for some time in an area where louse-borne typhus occurs in epidemic form—particularly the countries of eastern Europe. Brill-Zinsser disease also occurs

---

*Weil-Felix reactions are related to the fact that certain Proteus organisms share a common antigen with certain of the rickettsiae. Because the amount of this common antigen in each individual Rickettsia must be extremely minute, a relatively large mass of rickettsiae may be required to stimulate the Proteus agglutinins. The partially immune status of a Brill-Zinsser disease patient as well as that of a typhus-vaccinated individual may prevent the rickettsial mass in the blood and tissues from obtaining the necessary level to evoke a Proteus response. Likewise, early antimicrobial treatment may reduce the likelihood of a Proteus response by contributing to an early and rapid elimination of rickettsiae from the infected individual.

in eastern Europe itself. In this area, particularly in Bosnia, Yugoslavia, small family epidemics of primary epidemic typhus in children have been described in which a direct relationship could be traced from the children's infection to an adult recrudescent case of Brill-Zinsser disease that occurred several weeks earlier in the same family.

The epidemiologic significance of Brill-Zinsser disease cases is clear. They indicate the existence of carriers with latent infection who constitute the interepidemic reservoirs of typhus. Thus in a community where louse infestation is prevalent, when a latent carrier relapses and becomes an overt Brill-Zinsser disease case, the scene is then set for a possible epidemic of louse-borne typhus.

Pathology. The findings in Brill-Zinsser disease are the same as those described under Epidemic Typhus.

Diagnosis. The clinical diagnosis of Brill-Zinsser disease should be considered when a fever of unknown origin with an intense persistent headache occurs in a patient who has lived at some previous time in an area where louse-borne typhus occurs in epidemic form. A macular or maculo-papular rash, if present, is of additional help in diagnosis.

The diagnosis can be confirmed in the laboratory by employing the complement-fixation test. A negative Weil-Felix test in the presence of rising CF antibodies is highly suggestive of Brill-Zinsser disease rather than primary epidemic typhus, because more than 95 per cent of cases of the latter disease show a significant rise in Proteus OX-19 agglutinins. However, it should be kept in mind that the Weil-Felix test may be positive in Brill-Zinsser disease if the period elapsed between the original and the recrudescent attack is ten years or longer. The demonstration of the IgG class of antibodies in the early acute phase of illness is highly diagnostic of Brill-Zinsser disease.

Prognosis and Treatment. Statements in the paragraphs on Prognosis and Treatment of Epidemic Typhus apply to Brill-Zinsser disease as well.

Control of the Interepidemic Typhus Reservoir. The factors that precipitate an attack of Brill-Zinsser disease are unknown, and methods to prevent recrudescent attacks have not yet been discovered. However, the spread of infection from recrudescent Brill-Zinsser disease cases to non-immune contacts can be curtailed. When Brill-Zinsser disease occurs in an area such as the United States where louse infestation is extremely rare, no spread of the disease will occur, and no measures are required beyond treatment of the Brill-Zinsser disease itself. However, when Brill-Zinsser disease cases occur in a community where louse infestation is prevalent, one practical method of control is the "fire brigade" technique. This consists of a surveillance network throughout the community organized to report promptly the occurrence of a Brill-Zinsser disease case or the first ensuing cases of primary epidemic typhus. A centrally based control team should then be available to come in with insecticides to eliminate all lice in the environment, including lice on all contacts near and far.

MURINE FLEA-BORNE TYPHUS FEVER
(Endemic Typhus, Rat Typhus, Flea Typhus, Urban or Shop Typhus of Malaya)

History. Murine typhus fever probably has occurred for centuries as a sporadic or endemic disease, but only since 1931 has it been clearly distinguished from classic epidemic louse-borne typhus. During the early part of this century in the United States murine typhus was confused with Brill's disease. However, in 1926 Maxey, after extensive investigation, concluded that the typhus occurring in the southeastern United States must have a reservoir other than man, and he mentioned mice and rats specifically. He further suggested that fleas, mites, or ticks could be the vector. Mooser, in 1928, observed a basic difference in behavior of certain strains of typhus rickettsiae in the tissues of guinea pigs. Dyer and colleagues isolated typhus rickettsiae from rat fleas in Baltimore (1931), and Mooser, Zinsser, and Ruiz Castaneda found the agent in rats in Mexico City. Mooser subsequently named the disease "murine typhus" to indicate

TABLE 2. DISTINGUISHING CHARACTERISTICS OF PRIMARY EPIDEMIC TYPHUS AND BRILL-ZINSSER DISEASE

	Primary Epidemic Typhus	Brill-Zinsser Disease
Epidemiologic		
Past history of typhus	No	Yes
Occurrence of cases	Epidemic	Sporadic
Seasonal occurrence	Winter-spring	Year round
Transmission	By infected lice	Occurs in absence of lice
Clinical		
Duration of fever	12-18 days	7-11 days
Rash	Regularly present	Frequently absent or evanescent
Mortality	10-50% depending on age	Rare
Laboratory		
Specific antibody rise	Slow — begins 7th to 10th day, maximum 15th to 20th day	Rapid — begins 4th to 5th day, maximum 9th to 11th day
Type of immunoglobulin response during acute phase	Primary — IgM	Secondary — IgG
Weil-Felix reaction	Regularly present in titers of 1/160 or higher	Frequently absent (see text)
Cross-reacting specific *R. mooseri* antibodies	No	Yes

TABLE 3. COMPLEMENT FIXATION AND WEIL-FELIX REACTIONS IN RICKETTSIOSES

Group	Disease	Rickettsial Complement Fixation (CF)*			Weil-Felix (WF) Agglutination*		
		Group Antigen Type			Proteus Strain		
		Typhus	RMSF	Q Fever	OX-19	OX-2	OX-K
I	Primary epidemic typhus	+++	0	0	+++	+	0
	Brill-Zinsser disease	+++	0	0	0 or +++	0	0
	Murine typhus	+++	0	0	+++	+	0
II	RMSF	0	+++	0	+++†	+++†	0
	Tick typhus	0	+++	0	+++†	+++†	0
	Rickettsialpox	0	+++	0	0	0	0
III	Scrub typhus	0	0	0	0	0	+++
IV	Q fever	0	0	+++	0	0	0

*+++ = Strong reactions in CF 1:40 to 1:280.
   Strong reactions in WF 1:160 or greater.
  + = OX-2 reactions relatively weaker than OX-19.
  0 = Negative at 1:5 dilution in CF.
   Negative at 1:40 dilution in WF.
†In RMSF or tick typhus, agglutinins to either OX-19 or OX-2 or both can be present in either high or low titer.

its presence as a natural infection of rats. Reports showing the worldwide distribution of murine typhus rapidly accumulated. In the United States the incidence of the disease was increasing up to 1946. The rapid decrease in incidence since that time has been attributed, in part, to vigorously applied control measures.

Etiology. The etiologic agent, *Rickettsia mooseri* is similar to *Rickettsia prowazeki* in metabolic, biochemical, and staining characteristics; however, in size, *R. mooseri* is slightly smaller and more uniform. *R. mooseri* and *R. prowazeki* are classed together in the typhus group by virtue of the fact that they possess a common soluble antigenic moiety.

Epidemiology and Transmission. Rats infected with murine typhus are found scattered throughout the world in circumscribed areas. In the United States reservoirs of the disease are found along the southern Atlantic seaboard and in states bordering on the Gulf of Mexico. Other known areas of infection are Mexico, South America, the Mediterranean littoral, and Manchuria. However, the disease is widespread, occurring elsewhere in such areas as Ethiopia, Malaysia, and Australia.

Murine typhus is maintained in nature as a mild infection of rats, and is transmitted from rat to rat by the rat louse or by the rat flea, *Xenopsylla cheopis*. A flea becomes infected while feeding on a rat during the acute phase of an infection. The rickettsiae multiply in the flea without causing any damage to the host. Once infected the flea continues to discharge rickettsiae in its feces for the remainder of its life; however, infected female fleas do not transmit *R. mooseri* via their eggs to the next generation of fleas. Man usually acquires the disease when bitten by an infected flea. Rat fleas generally prefer to feed on rats, but they will attack man if rats become scarce. At the same time that an infected flea sucks blood it deposits feces that are teeming with rickettsiae. These may be rubbed into the flea bite wound or, as dried aerosol of feces and micro-organisms, they may gain access to the body through the mucous membranes of the conjunctivae or respiratory tract. Infection of man is an accidental occurrence and is not related to the maintenance of the disease in nature.

Pathology. Information on the pathology of murine typhus is limited. It is usually assumed that the lesions are essentially the same as those in epidemic typhus.

Clinical Manifestation and Course. The incubation period of murine typhus lasts from six to fourteen days. The symptoms are similar to those of epidemic typhus, the principal differences being that murine typhus is milder and shorter, the rash is less extensive and persists for shorter periods, there are fewer complications, and the case fatality rate is lower.

Diagnosis. *Clinical Diagnosis.* The diagnosis of murine typhus may be suspected when a patient has a sustained fever of several days' duration accompanied by headache, generalized aches and pains, and a macular or maculopapular rash appearing on the fifth or sixth day after onset of fever. The rash is first noted on the trunk and later spreads to the extremities; the face, palms, and soles are not involved. Since murine typhus is present in many of the areas where Rocky Mountain spotted fever (RMSF) occurs, it is helpful to remember that the rash of RMSF first appears on the wrists and ankles, rapidly spreads up the extremities to the trunk, and regularly involves the palms and soles. The patient with murine typhus usually gives a history of activities that have brought him into contact with places where rats are numerous. However, there is often no definite recollection of a flea bite.

It is impossible on clinical evidence alone to distinguish an ordinary case of murine typhus from a case of Brill-Zinsser disease or a mild case of epidemic typhus. Epidemiologic and laboratory data will almost always be required to arrive at a definitive diagnosis.

Laboratory Diagnosis. Both the complement-fixation and Weil-Felix tests are employed in the laboratory to confirm the clinical suspicion of a murine typhus infection. Rising antibodies to the commercially available soluble typhus group antigen indicate either a primary epidemic typhus, Brill-Zinsser disease, or murine typhus infection. From the time of onset Brill-Zinsser disease antibodies are IgG in type. In contrast, the antibodies produced in the acute phase of murine and epidemic typhus are characteristically IgM. One may have to resort to specific washed rickettsial antigens to distinguish between epidemic and murine typhus. In murine typhus as in primary epidemic typhus 4 to 8 units of antigen are required to obtain optimal fixation of complement during the acute phase of illness.

The Weil-Felix test employing Proteus OX-19 strains is regularly positive in murine typhus. Isolation of *R. mooseri* from patients may be accomplished early in the course of the disease by inoculating blood into guinea pigs, mice, or chick embryos. (See Laboratory Diagnosis in Epidemic Typhus.)

Prognosis. Even when untreated, murine typhus is usually a mild disease with fatalities occurring only in the elderly. The use of specific therapy further reduces the duration and severity of the disease.

Treatment. Treatment of murine typhus is similar to that for epidemic typhus. However, the usual mildness of murine typhus permits more leeway in a therapeutic regimen. For example, tetracycline can be used as the preferred drug, thus avoiding the greater potential toxicity of chloramphenicol.

Prevention and Control. Measures to prevent and control murine typhus depend upon limiting the rat population. The first step is to reduce the flea population of rat colonies by dusting rat runs with DDT or its equivalent. Following this, rat populations are reduced by poisoning, trapping, eliminating rat harborages, and rat-proofing buildings.

A vaccine has been produced and demonstrated to be effective. However, its use is hardly justified in view of the clinical mildness and sporadic nature of the disease.

Elisberg, B. L., and Bozeman, F. L.: Serologic diagnosis of rickettsial diseases by indirect immunofluorescence. Arch. Inst. Pasteur Tunis, 43:193, 1966.

Fox, J. P., Montoya, J. A., Jordan, M. D., Cornojo Ubillus, J. R., Garcia, J. L., Estrada, M. A., and Gelfand, H. M.: Immunization of man against epidemic typhus by infection with avirulent *Rickettsia prowazeki* (strain E). Arch. Inst. Pasteur Tunis, 36:449, 1959.

Gear, J. H. S.: Rickettsial vaccines. Brit. Med. Bull., 25:171, 1969.

Gimenez, D. F.: Staining rickettsiae in yolk sac cultures. Stain Tech., 39:135, 1964.

Loeffler, W., and Mooser, H.: Ein weiterer Fall von Brill-Zinsserscher Krankheit in Zurich. Schweiz. Med. Wschr., 82:493, 1952.

MacArthur, W. P.: The Athenian plague: A medical note. Classical Quarterly, 4:171, 1954.

McAllister, W. B.: The pathology of louse-borne typhus fever from the epidemic of 1943-5 in Egypt. Nav. Med. Res. Inst., Proj. NM 007 017 (X-696), Rep. No. 1, 25 January 1949.

Mooser, H.: Twenty years of research in typhus fever. Schweiz. Med. Wschr., 76:877, 1946.

Murray, E. S., O'Connor, J. M., and Gaon, J. A.: Differentiation of 19S and 7S complement-fixing antibodies in primary versus recrudescent typhus by either ethanethiol or heat. Proc. Soc. Exp. Biol. Med., 119:291, 1965.

Murray, E. S., and Snyder, J. C.: Brill-Zinsser disease: The interepidemic reservoir of epidemic louse-borne typhus fever. Proceedings Sixth International Congress of Microbiology, Rome. 4, Section 11, 31–44, 1953.

Smadel, J. E.: Status of the rickettsioses in the United States. Ann. Intern. Med., 51:421, 1959.

Snyder, J. C.: The typhus fevers. *In* Horsfall, F. L., Jr., and Tamm, I. (eds.): Viral and Rickettsial Infections of Man. 4th ed. Philadelphia, J. B. Lippincott Company, 1965, Chapter 50.

Wolbach, S. B., Todd, J. L., and Palfrey, F. W.: The Etiology and Pathology of Typhus. Cambridge, Mass., Harvard University Press, 1922.

Zdrodovskii, P. F., and Golinevich, H. M.: The Rickettsial Diseases. New York, Pergamon Press, 1960 (in English).

Zinsser, H.: Rats, Lice, and History. Boston, Little, Brown and Company, 1935.

ROCKY MOUNTAIN SPOTTED FEVER

(Spotted Fever, Tick Fever, Tick Typhus [England], Fiebre Manchada [Mexico], Fiebre Petequial [Colombia], Febere Maculosa [Brazil])

Herbert L. Ley, Jr.

Definition. Rocky Mountain spotted fever is a relatively severe, self-limited rickettsial infection transmitted to man by various species of hard ticks. The disease is characterized by fever, headache, bone and muscle pains, and a generalized rash that frequently may become petechial or hemorrhagic.

Etiology. The disease is caused by *Rickettsia rickettsi* (*Dermacentroxenus rickettsi*), the prototype rickettsia of the spotted fever group of organisms. These include, in addition to *R. rickettsi*, the agents of rickettsialpox, north Asian tick-borne rickettsiosis, and African and Queensland tick typhus, all of which are distinctive among rickettsiae in their ability to multiply in the nucleus as well as in the cytoplasm of mammalian and tick cells. All these agents share an antigen common to the group, and each possesses an individual species-specific antigen as well. Serologic differentiation among members of the group has been complicated by the shared antigen; specific antisera, prepared in mice, are useful in laboratory identification of the individual members of the group. All the tick-borne rickettsioses of the Western Hemisphere have proved, to date, to be caused by *R. rickettsi*, regardless of the country of origin or the local name given the disease. The incubation period of the disease may vary from 2 to 14 days; severe illnesses appear to be associated with short incubation periods.

Distribution and Incidence. Rocky Mountain spotted fever is limited in distribution to North and South America. The disease was first described in the United States in Montana at the turn of the century, and for some time was thought to be limited to that area. Beginning in the 1930's, the disease was recognized in the eastern United

States, Canada, Mexico, Brazil, and Colombia. Incidence and mortality data are difficult to obtain outside the United States, but in this country an average of 300 cases has been reported annually for the ten-year period from 1950 to 1959, with an average mortality rate of 6 per cent. During the 1960's about 300 cases have been reported annually in the United States, approximately half occurring in the Atlantic seaboard states from Delaware to Florida.*

Epidemiology. Rocky Mountain spotted fever is widely disseminated in nature and is principally a disease of ticks and small mammals. Man is rarely involved except when he intrudes into the "silent" wild cycle of disease. The hard ticks involved in transmission, the Ixodidae, feed on small mammals during their development through the larval and nymphal stages to tick adulthood. Once infected with *R. rickettsi* the tick may transmit the rickettsiae to its progeny transovarially or to man and other animals by feeding upon them. Thus the tick is both a vector and a reservoir of infection. The species of tick involved in the disease cycle varies according to geographic area. In the northern United States, the rabbit tick, *Haemaphysalis leporis-palustris*, rarely bites man, but appears to be responsible for maintaining the disease among rabbits and small mammals. Human infection in the United States is most commonly acquired in the West from *Dermacentor andersoni* (the wood tick), in the East from *Dermacentor variabilis* (the dog tick), and in the South from *Amblyomma americanum* (the Lone Star tick). Many other species of hard ticks have been implicated in transmission of the disease in Central and South America. Under laboratory conditions soft ticks of the genus Ornithodorus are also capable of transmitting the agent, but appear to be unimportant as vectors in nature. Among the animals believed to be involved in the natural cycle of disease are squirrels, rabbits, porcupines, chipmunks, weasels, several species of feral rats and mice, and, perhaps most important from the human viewpoint, dogs. All these animals have been shown to be susceptible to infection with *R. rickettsi;* the disease produced is usually mild and limited in duration but is associated with a rickettsemia sufficient to infect ticks feeding on the animal at the time.

Although it was once considered that the western form of the disease was more serious than the eastern, the higher mortality rates in the western United States appear to be a reflection of a much higher average age among patients. Formerly the disease was one of the adult male in the West and of children of both sexes in the eastern United States. In recent years more than half the patients reported nationally have been less than 15 years of age. As might be expected, the disease has a striking seasonal pattern in which nearly 90 per cent of all cases occur during the period from May through September.

---

*Source: Morbidity and Mortality Weekly Report, Communicable Disease Center, United States Public Health Service.

Pathology and Physiologic Responses. Histopathologically, the disease is an endangitis, starting in the endothelial cells and extending into the smooth muscle of the vessel walls. Rickettsiae may be demonstrated in the lesions by appropriate stains. Thrombi are formed at the points of inflammation and lead to areas of focal necrosis and hemorrhage. The major organ systems involved are the skin, subcutaneous tissues, and the central nervous system, although mononuclear cell infiltration may also be found in the lungs, heart, liver, and spleen. Except for the rash, gross findings at autopsy are minimal.

Clinical laboratory findings in the milder cases are usually limited to a moderate leukocytosis. Peripheral vascular collapse, the most serious consequence of the disease, may result from the pooling of blood in the damaged capillaries and from loss of water, electrolytes, and proteins into the extravascular space. Patients having this complication will show a decrease in hematocrit, blood chloride, and serum protein levels, and an increase in serum nonprotein nitrogen levels. Thrombocytopenia has also been observed in severe illnesses.

Clinical Manifestations. Headache and fever, frequently accompanied by mild chills, appear as initial symptoms of infection 2 to 14 days following contact with ticks. Within the first day of fever the patient usually complains of pains in the bones, joints, and muscles, photophobia, and increasing prostration. Initial physical examination usually reveals only flushing of the skin, conjunctival injection, and minor respiratory signs referable to a dry cough. By the second day the fever usually rises to 104° to 105° F. and stays at that level until the end of the second week. Between the second and sixth days of fever a generalized macular rash develops that resembles the eruption of measles. Initially the rash blanches with pressure, but after 24 to 48 hours the eruption frequently becomes petechial or, in the more severe cases, hemorrhagic. In mild illnesses, or in previously vaccinated persons, the rash may be minimal. Central nervous system symptoms in the form of agitation, insomnia, delirium, or coma usually appear by the end of the first week of fever. It is during the second week of fever that the most critical circulatory and pulmonary complications of the disease occur. Gangrene of the extremities or other dependent parts and pneumonia are sometimes seen in untreated patients. Fever usually abates by the end of the second week, and full recovery commonly takes several weeks or months in untreated patients.

Diagnosis. Rocky Mountain spotted fever should always be considered in the differential diagnosis of a febrile illness with rash occurring in the months of May through September in the United States. The most common initial diagnosis of illness for patients subsequently found to have Rocky Mountain spotted fever is measles, despite the fact that measles usually does not occur during the period when Rocky Mountain spotted fever is most common. As in all the rickettsial diseases, the initial diagnosis must be made solely on clinical grounds because confirmatory laboratory tests are of no assistance until relatively late in the illness. The symptoms, physical findings, and history of exposure in an area known to harbor ticks must be weighed carefully by the physician, and, if the diagnosis is considered probable, treatment should be initiated. Two other rickettsial diseases, rickettsialpox and murine typhus, may mimic mild cases of Rocky Mountain spotted fever. Fortunately, both respond equally well to treatment appropriate for Rocky Mountain spotted fever.

Laboratory confirmation of the clinical diagnosis may be obtained by isolation of R. rickettsi from the blood during the first week of illness. *Isolation studies in guinea pigs or embryonated eggs should be attempted only by laboratories equipped for such work because of the danger of infection of laboratory personnel.* More commonly, laboratory diagnosis depends upon serologic tests with paired serum samples, the first obtained as early as possible during illness and the second about the fifteenth to twenty-fifth day of disease. These tests utilize either the Weil-Felix Proteus OX-19 and OX-2 agglutination reactions or the complement-fixation test with yolk sac antigen. In the agglutination test, positive results may be obtained with either or both of the OX-19 or OX-2 antigens; approximately 15 per cent of patients may show no rise in Weil-Felix titers even though complement-fixation tests are positive.* A fourfold or greater rise in titer with the complement-fixation test is considered confirmatory.

Treatment and Prognosis. Until 1945 treatment of Rocky Mountain spotted fever was limited to supportive therapy; mortality rates were 20 per cent or greater. In 1945, para-aminobenzoic acid (PABA) was shown to be effective in treatment, producing defervescence in approximately three days and reducing mortality virtually to zero. By the early 1950's, chloramphenicol and the tetracyclines replaced PABA in the treatment of this disease because the newer antimicrobial drugs were equally effective as PABA and far better tolerated. In the majority of patients, headache and other symptoms abate within 24 to 48 hours, and fever disappears within three to four days after beginning therapy with 25 mg. per kilogram per day of the tetracyclines or 50 mg. per kilogram per day of chloramphenicol, given in four divided doses by mouth. With either regimen, treatment should be continued for 24 to 48 hours after the patient becomes afebrile. The physician must weigh the disadvantages of gastric irritation with the tetracyclines against the risks of blood dyscrasias with chloramphenicol. In general, because of the greater seriousness of the toxicity to chloramphenicol, tetracycline is the preferred therapy. For patients too ill to take oral medication,

parenteral preparations must be used; when these are necessary, the patient will also require intravenous fluids to correct electrolyte or fluid abnormalities. Corticosteroids may also be of help for severely ill patients.

The most important step in treatment is early diagnosis; no amount of drug therapy can modify the course of the disease in the patient who is admitted *in extremis.* Heroic measures such as corticosteroid therapy and parenteral administration of antimicrobials are completely unnecessary if the diagnosis is made and treatment begun early in the course of the disease. Early treatment will also prevent sequelae such as brain or heart damage, which have been observed in patients who have been treated late in their illness.

Prevention. Although protective vaccine is available, its use has decreased markedly in recent years, presumably because effective antimicrobial therapy is now available for treatment. Nevertheless, use of the vaccine is appropriate for selected persons who may be exposed to the danger of infection in remote areas in which medical treatment may be difficult or impossible to obtain.

Because ticks cannot transmit infection to man without having been attached for several hours, a degree of protection can be achieved by careful examination of one's person and careful removal of attached ticks on a twice daily schedule. Considerable difference of opinion exists regarding the safest method of removal. The use of a lighted cigarette or the application of kerosene, both highly regarded in some circles, appear to have the disadvantage that agonal responses of the tick may cause actual expression of rickettsiae into the wound. Another method appears to be preferable: the tick is grasped by the head and thorax with a pair of fine forceps and pulled gently but firmly until the mouth parts are extracted from the skin. The third category of control measures is directed against the tick vector of the disease. The use of clothing impregnated with tick repellents provides significant protection to those who must travel through tick-infested areas. When groups of people may be exposed to ticks in summer camps or recreational areas, the selective use of residual insecticides, such as DDT, dieldrin, or lindane, has proved effective in limited areas in reducing tick populations.

---

*See preceding article, The Typhus Group, for discussion of the Weil-Felix reaction.

Lackman, D. B., Bell, E. J., Stoenner, H. G., and Pickens, E. G.: The Rocky Mountain spotted fever group of rickettsias. Health Lab. Sci., 2:135, 1965.

Ricketts, H. T.: Contributions to Medical Science by Howard Taylor Ricketts, 1870–1910. Chicago, University of Chicago Press, 1911, p. 278.

Wisseman, C. L., Jr. (ed.): Symposium on the Spotted Fever Group of Rickettsiae. Medical Science Publication No. 7, Walter Reed Army Institute of Research. Washington, D.C., U.S. Government Printing Office, 1960.

Woodward, T. E., and Jackson, E. B.: Spotted fever rickettsiae. *In* Horsfall, F. L., Jr., and Tamm, I. (eds.): Viral and Rickettsial Infections of Man. 4th ed. Philadelphia, J. B. Lippincott Company, 1965, p. 1095.

Zdrodovskii, P. F., and Golinevich, H. M.: The Rickettsial Diseases. New York, Pergamon Press, 1960, p. 277.

TICK-BORNE RICKETTSIOSES OF THE EASTERN HEMISPHERE

Herbert L. Ley, Jr.*

Definition. The three diseases that constitute this group, i.e., *African tick typhus, North Asian tick-borne rickettsiosis,* and *Queensland tick typhus,* are caused by rickettsiae that are closely related to one another and to the agent of Rocky Mountain spotted fever. Each is transmitted by the bite of an ixodid tick.

African tick typhus (*Boutonneuse fever*) may be regarded as the prototype of the group. It is the most widely distributed geographically, occurring throughout the African continent, in those parts of Europe and the Middle East adjacent to the Mediterranean, Black and Caspian Seas, and in India. Boutonneuse fever is a mild to moderately severe febrile illness of a few days' to two weeks' duration. It is characterized by a primary lesion that develops at the site of the infected tick bite and a generalized maculopapular erythematous rash that appears about the fourth day. As in Rocky Mountain spotted fever, agglutinins against Proteus OX-19 (Weil-Felix reaction) usually appear during convalescence, as do specific complement-fixing antibodies against the rickettsial organisms.

History, Distribution, Etiology, and Epidemiology. Boutonneuse fever was first recognized in 1910 in Tunisia by Conor and Bruch. During the next several decades the occurrence of similar diseases was noted in Africa, Europe, and the Middle East; these were given various local names. However, it was not until modern serologic methods employing specific rickettsial antigens were applied that *Rickettsia conori* was shown to be the etiologic agent for a single widely disseminated disease, African tick typhus. Queensland tick typhus caused by *R. australis* was established as an entity during World War II. Although the rickettsial nature of North Asian tick-borne rickettsiosis was demonstrated in 1938, only in recent years has its etiologic agent, *R. siberica,* been clearly differentiated from other members of the spotted fever group of organisms.

The etiologic agents of the three diseases of the Eastern Hemisphere are all members of the spotted fever group of rickettsiae. Together with *R. rickettsi* and *R. akari* they possess common group antigens that are readily demonstrated by agglutination and complement-fixation procedures. In addition, type-specific antigens characterize each member of the spotted fever group; these are demonstrated by similar in vitro serologic procedures employing specially purified antigens. *Rickettsia conori, R. australis,* and *R. siberica* may be differentiated from one another and from *R. rickettsi* and *R. akari* by complement-fixation tests using antisera from mice, by cross-vaccination tests performed in guinea pigs, or by cross-neutralization tests using the mouse lethal toxin obtained from each agent and homologous antisera. Experimental infection of animals with one member of the spotted fever group of rickettsiae induces appreciable resistance to infection with other members.

For the most part, the *epidemiology* of the three tick-borne rickettsioses of the Eastern Hemisphere resembles that of spotted fever in the Western Hemisphere. Thus, the rickettsial agents are maintained in nature by cycles involving ixodid ticks and small wild animals; man, if he intrudes into the cycles, serves as a dead end in the chain of transmission. Boutonneuse fever in the Mediterranean area has a more domesticated and urbanized pattern. Here, another cycle is also involved with the brown dog tick as the vector and the dog as the animal host.

Pathology. In fatal cases, which are few and usually limited to the aged and debilitated, the findings are similar to those in Rocky Mountain spotted fever except for the presence of the *tâche noire,* the black button-like necrotic primary lesion that is generally found on the surface areas of the body ordinarily covered by clothing. The basic pathologic changes are found in the small blood vessels (see article on Rocky Mountain Spotted Fever).

Symptoms, Laboratory Findings, and Diagnosis. The three tick-borne rickettsioses that occur in different parts of the Eastern Hemisphere resemble one another closely. Following an incubation period of about five to seven days, the disease begins with fever, headache, malaise, and conjunctival injection. The primary lesion, which is present in most cases at the onset of fever, consists of a small ulcer 2 to 5 mm. in diameter with a black center and a red areola; the regional lymph nodes are enlarged. The generalized erythematous maculopapular rash appears about the fourth day and quickly involves most of the body, including the palms and soles and often the face. In severe cases the rash becomes hemorrhagic. Fever abates during the second week. The prognosis is good except in the aged and debilitated. Complications and sequelae are unusual.

The laboratory findings of greatest importance are those derived from the Weil-Felix and rickettsial complement-fixation tests. Agglutinins against Proteus OX-19 develop during the second week and complement-fixing antibodies appear shortly thereafter.

Diagnosis is established by the clinical picture including the *tâche noire,* the geographic location and positive serologic reactions. In the differential diagnosis the typhus fevers, meningococcal infections, and measles must be considered.

---

*The articles Rocky Mountain Spotted Fever to Q Fever, inclusive, have been written to replace articles on the same subjects prepared for previous editions by the author's former teacher and colleague, the late Dr. Joseph E. Smadel. Thus, Dr. Smadel's many contributions to these subjects understandably permeate the whole section. For this article on Tick-Borne Rickettsioses, however, the present author found it inadvisable to do more than make trivial changes and update the references so that, to all intents and purposes, it is as it was originally prepared by Dr. Smadel.

Treatment. Adequate information is available to indicate that treatment with the broad-spectrum antimicrobial drugs is as effective in patients with African tick typhus as in those with other rickettsioses (see article on Rocky Mountain spotted fever for details of therapy). Presumably, these measures are also applicable to the other two tick-borne rickettsioses of the Eastern Hemisphere.

Prophylaxis. Prevention of human disease is based on avoiding the bites of infected ticks. In the article on Rocky Mountain spotted fever are set forth details regarding personal prophylaxis, including the use of chemical insect repellents, and for reduction of tick populaton by measures involved in terrain control. Experimental vaccines prepared from formalin-treated yolk sac tissue infected with each of the Eastern Hemisphere rickettsiae under discussion are effective in animals, but commercial vaccines for human use are not available.

Bozeman, F. M., Humphries, J. W., Campbell, J. M., and O'Hara, P. L.: Laboratory studies of the spotted fever group of rickettsiae. *In* Wisseman, C. L., Jr. (ed.): Symposium on the Spotted Fever Group of Rickettsiae. Medical Science Publication No. 7, Walter Reed Army Institute of Research. Washington, D.C., U.S. Government Printing Office, 1960, p. 7.

Freyche, M. J., and Deutschman, Z.: Human rickettsioses in Africa. Epidemiol. Vital Stat. Rep., WHO 3:161, 1950.

Woodward, T. E., and Jackson, E. B.: Spotted fever rickettsiae. *In* Horsfall, F. L., Jr., and Tamm, I. (eds.): Viral and Rickettsial Infections of Man. 4th ed. Philadelphia, J. B. Lippincott Company, 1965, p. 1095.

Zdrodovskii, P. F., and Golinevich, H. M.: The Rickettsial Diseases. New York, Pergamon Press, 1960, p. 292.

RICKETTSIALPOX
Herbert L. Ley, Jr.

Definition. Rickettsialpox is a mite-borne rickettsial disease, mild and self-limited, which is characterized by an initial eschar-like lesion and a fever of a week's duration accompanied by headache, backache, and a generalized papulovesicular rash.

Etiology. The disease is caused by *Rickettsia akari,* a member of the spotted fever group of rickettsia. Although *R. akari* possesses an antigen in common with *Rickettsia rickettsi,* it is most closely related to *Rickettsia australis,* the agent of North Queensland tick typhus. The organism is transmitted to man, with an incubation period of 10 to 24 days, by the bite of the mouse mite, *Allodermanyssus sanguineus.*

Incidence and Distribution. The incidence of the disease is difficult to determine. In the first three years after the disease was described in 1946, 500 cases were reported in the United States, most of them from New York City. Reporting of the disease has decreased markedly since that time. It is likely that small numbers of cases continue to occur without being reported because the disease is one in which national reporting is not required. The disease has been reported from Boston, West Haven, Connecticut, New York, Philadelphia, Pittsburgh, and Cleveland in the United States, and from the U.S.S.R.

Epidemiology. When the disease was first described in 1946–1947, in a New York apartment housing project, the investigators demonstrated the presence of the agent in both the commensal mouse, *Mus musculus,* and its mite ectoparasite, *A. sanguineus,* both of which were present in large numbers. The single piece of information that was missing from the initial study was the manner in which the disease agent, *R. akari,* entered the mouse and mite populations. The subsequent isolation from a field mouse in Korea of a rickettsial agent indistinguishable from *R. akari* suggests that the agent may be widely distributed among feral rodents and their ectoparasites. If this view is correct, the disease may be expected to occur in areas of expanding suburbia where man and commensal populations of domestic mice come into contact with feral mice and their ectoparasites.

Pathology. Because rickettsialpox is a benign infection with no reported deaths, pathologic examination has been limited to biopsy material. The initial lesion or eschar resembles the eschars of scrub typhus and boutonneuse fever. The skin lesion of the early rash is characterized by perivascular infiltration with mononuclear cells. During the later stages of the rash when vesiculation occurs, the histologic changes are highly characteristic and consist of necrosis of the superficial epithelial cells leading to an intra-epidermal vesicle. Clinical laboratory findings are limited to a minimal leukopenia during the febrile period.

Clinical Manifestations. The first sign of infection is the initial lesion or eschar, which appears approximately a week before onset of fever. Most patients are unaware of the small papule that develops at the site of the infecting mite bite or, if they note it, they interpret it as a "pimple." The lesion begins as a small papule that enlarges slowly to 0.5 to 1.5 cm. in diameter, develops a central vesicle, and finally forms a dark crust without pustulation. Except for the lack of itching, tenderness, or pustulation, the lesion resembles that of a primary vaccinia reaction, and usually leaves a small scar. When searched for carefully, the initial lesion will be found in over 90 per cent of cases.

About a week after the appearance of the initial lesion, fever of an intermittent type develops, with chills or chilly sensations and drenching sweats. After approximately a week the fever gradually subsides. The early febrile period is characterized by headache, photophobia, marked lassitude, and muscle pains, including backache. Beginning on the first to fourth days of fever a maculopapular rash appears, which develops into a vesiculopapular rash. The vesicles are firm, sometimes surrounded by erythema, and on drying form a dark crust that falls off without leaving a scar. In contrast to chickenpox, the rash appears on many areas of the body at almost the same time and does not itch; it is absent from the palms and soles.

Physical examination during the febrile period yields little additional information. An enlarged spleen or lymphadenopathy will be found in only a few cases. The differential diagnosis very early in the disease should include measles, chickenpox, and smallpox; with the appearance of the vesicles only the latter two diseases need be considered. The presence of an initial lesion, the more superficial position of the vesicle, and the persistence of the papular base throughout the period of rash argue strongly for rickettsialpox rather than chickenpox. Smallpox lesions resemble those of rickettsialpox, but progress to pustules. In addition, the constitutional symptoms of most patients with smallpox are considerably more severe than those of patients with rickettsialpox.

Diagnosis. The clinical characteristics of the disease are so distinctive that in most patients a presumptive diagnosis may be made on clinical grounds. Chickenpox in adults poses the most difficult diagnostic problem. Laboratory confirmations of the diagnosis is possible by isolation of the agent from blood obtained during the acute phase of illness and also by complement-fixation tests on paired specimens of serum. Because the agent of rickettsialpox is closely related to that of Rocky Mountain spotted fever, complement-fixation tests may be performed with antigen prepared from either organism. A fourfold or greater rise in antibody titer may be expected in patients with rickettsialpox when the acute phase specimen is collected early in the febrile period and the convalescent specimen is collected three to four weeks after onset of disease. The Weil-Felix agglutination reaction is of no diagnostic value in rickettsialpox.

Treatment and Prognosis. The disease may be so mild in some patients that no specific treatment may be indicated. When therapy is desirable, the tetracyclines may be used in oral doses of 25 mg. per kilogram per day for three or four days. Response to treatment is rapid; most patients become afebrile in 24 to 36 hours. Relapses of infection have not been reported. The course of the disease is benign and the prognosis is excellent.

Control. The principal target of preventive measures is the mite vector of the disease, *A. sanguineus,* which may be controlled by the use of residual insecticides (DDT or dieldrin) in areas of mouse harborage. Vector control should be achieved prior to initiating mouse control measures to avoid further dispersal of the mites in their search for food. No vaccine is currently available.

Dolgopol, V. B.: Histologic changes in rickettsialpox. Amer. J. Path., 24:119, 1948.

Greenberg, M., Pelliteri, O., Klein, I. F., and Huebner, R. J.: Rickettsialpox — A newly recognized rickettsial disease. II. Clinical observations. J.A.M.A., 133:901, 1947.

Lackman, D. B.: A review of information on rickettsialpox in the United States. Clin. Pediat., 2:296, 1963.

Roueché, B.: The alerting of Mr. Pomerantz. *In* Roueché, B.: Eleven Blue Men. Boston, Little, Brown and Company, 1954, p. 48.

SCRUB TYPHUS
(Tsutsugamushi Disease, Mite-Borne Typhus, Japanese River Fever, Tropical Typhus, Rural Typhus)
Herbert L. Ley, Jr.

Definition. Scrub typhus is a mite-borne rickettsial disease that occurs in southeast Asia and adjacent areas and is characterized by fever, headache, lymphadenopathy, conjunctival injection, a maculopapular rash, and, in most patients, a distinctive eschar or skin lesion.

Etiology. The disease is caused by *Rickettsia tsutsugamushi (R. orientalis),* a group of rickettsial agents that produces a single distinctive clinical syndrome in man, but is characterized by extreme variation in antigenic composition of organisms isolated in different geographic areas and even in adjacent foci of the disease within the same country. All strains of *R. tsutsugamushi* can be propagated in mice and embryonated eggs; some strains will also produce disease in the guinea pig. Because of antigenic variation in the organisms, complement-fixing antibodies produced in response to infection in man appear to be specific only for the infecting or closely related strains. Nevertheless, all strains of *R. tsutsugamushi* have the potential of stimulating Weil-Felix Proteus OX-K agglutinins in man.

Distribution and Incidence. The disease occurs in a roughly triangular area of southeast Asia and adjacent countries approximately 5,000,000 square miles in extent. The western apex of the triangle is located in West Pakistan, the northern in north Japan, and the southern in the north coastal areas of Australia. It is impossible to obtain reliable data on the incidence of the disease among the indigenous populations of the area. However, World War II provided numerous examples of explosive outbreaks of the disease in military units in the Asiatic-Pacific area. In one such outbreak among British troops in Ceylon, 756 patients were hospitalized with scrub typhus as a result of a four-day jungle training exercise. American forces operating on the islands of Owi and Biak experienced over 1000 cases of the disease in less than two months. During the period from 1942 to 1945, nearly 16,000 cases of the disease occurred in American, British, and Australian troops alone. At present the disease is reported sporadically among the people of southeast Asia and becomes a major medical problem only when development projects or recreational activities bring groups of people into contact with foci of the disease in nature.

Epidemiology. Like Rocky Mountain spotted fever, scrub typhus is principally a disease of rodents and their ectoparasites that is propagated in a "silent" cycle in nature involving man only when he unwittingly comes into contact with the mites that transmit the disease. A variety of rodents, chiefly rats and feral mice, have been shown to be infected in nature. The disease in these animals is relatively mild but is associated with a rickettsemia that provides an opportunity to infect mites feeding on the animals during their illness. In some areas ground birds have also been implicated in the disease cycle in nature. The vector mite in most areas is a species of the genus Leptotrombiculidium highly adapted to the local ecology, although mites of the genus Schongastia have been shown to transmit the agent in the less important jungle cycle of the disease. The mite vectors are free-living, feeding upon vegetation and insect eggs, except in their larval stage, during which they must obtain a meal of tissue fluid from a vertebrate host in order to complete their maturation to the adult stage. The mites are not only capable of transmitting *R. tsutsugamushi* to their vertebrate host during this feeding but are also capable of transmitting the agent to their offspring transovarially. Thus, the mite is both a vector and a reservoir for scrub typhus, just as is the tick for Rocky Mountain spotted fever. The highly specific ecologic requirements for propagation of the mite in terms of temperature, humidity, and food sources, coupled with its limited range of locomotion, lead to the formation of "mite islands," highly localized in terms of both geographic and seasonal distributions. In some exceptional areas, such as Malaysia, the mite population is present throughout the year. More commonly, the mites are highly seasonal in appearance, and are most numerous during the warm, moist months of the year, although one focus of infection in southern Japan is characterized by a winter peak of mite population. The seasonal distribution of scrub typhus understandably parallels the distribution of the mite vector. Man exposes himself to infection by transferring mites from vegetation to his body; most infections have followed contact with grassy "scrub" areas or straw cut from them. The disease may occur elsewhere because infected mites have been found in other habitats.

Pathology. As with the other rickettsioses, the basic lesion is one of inflammation of the walls of the small blood vessels with perivascular infiltration of mononuclear cells. Pneumonitis and a diffuse myocarditis with mononuclear infiltration of the myocardium are frequently observed at autopsy. Gross pathologic findings are usually limited to enlargement of the spleen, lymphadenopathy and the cutaneous eschar of the disease.

Clinical Manifestations. The initial symptoms of the disease, frontal headache and temperature of 104 to 105° F., follow the infecting mite bite by 6 to 21 days. Physical examination at onset reveals only generalized lymphadenopathy, conjunctival injection, and, in most Caucasian patients, the developing eschar. This skin lesion, absent in most Asian patients, appears first as a small papule at the site of the mite bite and enlarges during the first few days of fever to approximately 1 cm. in size. On this papular base a multilocular vesicle develops that evolves into the flat, black eschar characteristic of the disease. Regional lymph nodes draining the area of the eschar may

become painful, and may enlarge to the size of an acorn. About the end of the first week of fever a generalized macular rash appears, which may last only a few hours or may develop to a livid maculopapular eruption of a week's duration. In untreated patients complications such as pneumonitis, encephalitis, and cardiac failure occur late in the second week of fever; if the patient survives, defervescence begins about the fifteenth day of fever.

Diagnosis. Early diagnosis of the disease must be based on the clinical findings and the history of exposure in an endemic area. Laboratory confirmation of the diagnosis is based on isolation from blood of the agent in mice or on a rise in Weil-Felix OX-K agglutinins in serum during the course of illness. If the acute specimen is obtained before the tenth day of fever and the late specimen is obtained during the third week of illness, fourfold or greater rises in Weil-Felix OX-K titers will be observed in almost all untreated patients and in three fourths of those receiving antimicrobial therapy. Because of strain variation in the etiologic agent, the complement-fixation test is unsatisfactory in the laboratory diagnosis of the disease. Clinical laboratory data are of little assistance in diagnosis; patients usually show only a moderate leukopenia. The differential diagnosis of the disease should include leptospirosis, typhoid fever, dengue, murine typhus, and malaria.

Treatment. The tetracyclines or chloramphenicol are the therapeutic agents of choice for scrub typhus at oral dosage levels of 25 and 50 mg. per kilogram per day, respectively. Drug therapy may be discontinued 24 hours after defervescence, which usually occurs within 36 hours after beginning therapy. Relapses have been observed in patients treated during the first week of fever; continuation of therapy through the fourteenth day of disease, or the administration of single 3.0 gram oral doses of drug on the seventh and fourteenth days following cessation of the initial course of antimicrobial therapy will prevent recrudescences of infection. The relapses occur because the antimicrobial drugs are not eradicative.

The choice between the tetracyclines and chloramphenicol is difficult. Chloramphenicol may infrequently produce a blood dyscrasia. The tetracyclines may cause severe nausea and vomiting, leading to significant problems of fluid and electrolyte balance in the acutely ill patient. The case for assuming the added risk of chloramphenicol is slightly stronger for scrub typhus than for other rickettsioses because of the severity of the disease and its relatively high fatality rate.

Prognosis and Mortality. Before effective treatment was available, mortality from scrub typhus was appreciable, varying from 5 to 40 per cent. Early antimicrobial therapy has essentially eliminated deaths from the disease. If the patient is treated in the first week of illness he is usually ready to resume full activity in several weeks.

Prevention. Preventive measures are directed at minimizing contact of man with the mites transmitting the disease. During periods of political stability, the application of residual miticides such as dieldrin or lindane to large areas of terrain will permit safe continuation of operations in rubber plantations and similar industrial activities that bring workers into contact with areas previously known to be the source of numerous infections. When area miticide application is impracticable, as in military operations, the use of clothing impregnated with mite repellents provides significant protection against infection. Under research conditions the intermittent use of chloramphenicol chemoprophylaxis has been shown to be effective in preventing clinical manifestations of infection. No protective vaccine is available.

Audy, J. R.: The ecology of scrub typhus. In May, J. M. (ed.): Studies in Disease Ecology. New York, Hafner Publishing Company, Inc., 1961, p. 389.
Smadel, J. E.: Influence of antibiotics on immunologic responses in scrub typhus. Amer. J. Med., 17:246, 1954.
Smadel, J. E., and Elisberg, B. L.: Scrub typhus rickettsia. In Horsfall, F. L., Jr., and Tamm, I. (eds.): Viral and Rickettsial Infections of Man. 4th ed. Philadelphia, J. B. Lippincott Company, 1965, p. 1130.
Tamiya, T. (ed.): Recent Advances in Studies of Tsutsugamushi Disease in Japan. Tokyo, Medical Culture Inc., 1962.
Traub, R., and Wisseman, C. L., Jr.: Ecological considerations in scrub typhus. Bull. WHO, 39:209, 1968.

TRENCH FEVER
(Five-Day or Quintana Fever, Shin Bone Fever, Volhynian Fever, etc.)

Herbert L. Ley, Jr.

Definition. Trench fever is a self-limited louse-borne rickettsial disease characterized by intermittent fever, generalized aches and pains, negligible mortality, and multiple relapses.

Etiology and Epidemiology. The disease is caused by *Rickettsia quintana,* a rickettsial agent that grows extracellularly in the louse intestine and is excreted in louse feces. Transmission takes place by rubbing louse feces into skin abrasions or into the bite wound left by the louse. The incubation period of the disease may vary from 5 to 38 days, but is usually two to four weeks. The disease was a major military problem during World War I, when an estimated 1,000,000 cases occurred in western Europe. It was not seen in epidemic form again until World War II when 80,000 cases were reported in eastern Europe. Recent studies have demonstrated the disease in endemic form in Mexico. During epidemics man is clearly the principal reservoir. He may also be the major long-term reservoir because the disease agent has been isolated from asymptomatic patients years after their initial infection.

Pathology and Clinical Manifestations. Because the disease has a negligible mortality, information on the histopathologic changes is limited. Biopsy studies reveal only perivascular inflammation, principally in the form of lymphocytic infiltrations. The presenting symptoms of the disease are recurrent fever, severe weakness, headache, dizziness, back and leg pains (particularly in the shins), and photophobia. Physical and laboratory examinations are not remarkable except for slight enlargement of the spleen and liver, areas of cutaneous tenderness distributed over the body, and a moderate leukocytosis. A transient rash of erythematous macules or papules occurs in about 70 per cent of patients. The patient's fever may rise as high as 105° F. in an irregular fashion with intervals of nearly normal temperature between peaks of fever. The fever may last for only four or five days in the more fortunate patients. In others, the initial pyrexia may be followed after five or six days of normal temperature by one to eight relapses of fever similar to the initial episode. In still other patients, the initial fever may decline, shading into relapses without a true afebrile period, producing a "saddle-back" or "typhoidal" fever curve.

Diagnosis. The most important fact supporting the diagnosis of trench fever is a history of contact with lice within the incubation period of the disease. Xenodiagnosis—the feeding of clean uninfected lice on a patient suspected of having the disease—is a useful diagnostic aid. The lice are examined a week after feeding on the patient for the presence of rickettsiae in the lumen of the gut. The technique of cultivation of *R. quintana* on blood agar containing 10 per cent of fresh blood has also been used diagnostically. Recently developed serologic tests appear promising in the diagnosis of the disease. The differential diagnosis of the disease should include leptospirosis, dengue, malaria, relapsing fever, and the typhus fevers.

Treatment and Prognosis. Although chloramphenicol and the tetracyclines may be expected to be as effective in the treatment of trench fever as in the treatment of the other rickettsial diseases, no reliable information regarding their efficacy is available in the absence of epidemics of trench fever. Because the disease has a negligible mortality, the long-term prognosis is excellent. Even without treatment the majority of patients are able to return to full activity within one to two months after onset, although a few continue to experience recurrences of the symptoms of infection for months or years.

Prevention. The only practicable method of control of trench fever is the elimination of the louse vector of the disease by dusting clothing with residual insecticides. Ten per cent DDT powders proved highly effective for louse control during the World War II period, but the development of DDT resistance in lice in many parts of the world has forced the use of 1 per cent lindane or 1 per cent malathion powders. For additional comments on louse control, see the section on The Typhus Group.

Trench Fever: Report of Commission on Trench Fever. American Red Cross Medical Research Committee. London, Oxford University Press, 1918.
Varela, G., Vinson, J. W., and Molina-Pasquel, C.: Trench fever. II. Propagation of *Rickettsia quintana* on cell-free medium

from the blood of two patients. Amer. J. Trop. Med., 18:708, 1969.

Vinson, J. W., Varela, G., and Molina-Pasquel, C.: Trench fever. III. Induction of clinical disease in volunteers inoculated with *Rickettsia quintana* propagated on blood agar. Amer. J. Trop. Med., 18:713, 1969.

Warren, J.: Trench fever rickettsia. *In* Horsfall, F. L., Jr., and Tamm, I. (eds.): Viral and Rickettsial Infections of Man. 4th ed. Philadelphia, J. B. Lippincott Company, 1965, p. 1161.

Q FEVER

Herbert L. Ley, Jr.

Definition. Q fever is a self-limited rickettsial infection characterized by fever, headache, and constitutional symptoms, associated, in approximately half the patients, with a pneumonitis. It is unique among the rickettsial diseases of man in that human infection is most commonly acquired by inhalation of the agent rather than by contact with an arthropod vector.

Etiology. The disease is caused by *Coxiella burnetii*, a rickettsial agent having the general biologic characteristics of this class of microorganisms but possessing, in addition, a resistance to desiccation and to exposure in dusts and soils that is unique among the rickettsiae. The organism may be propagated in embryonated eggs and in mice, hamsters, and guinea pigs, and has frequently infected laboratory personnel engaged in isolation studies on clinical material. Both patients and animals develop agglutinating and complement-fixing antibodies for the agent. On the other hand, *C. burnetii*, unlike most of the other rickettsiae, does not stimulate the production of Weil-Felix Proteus agglutinins in man.

Incidence and Distribution. The true incidence of the disease in the human population is impossible to determine because the majority of infections are undiagnosed. Isolated serologic surveys have revealed that many persons exposed to infection in sheep and cattle ranches, abattoirs, meat packing plants, wool processing plants, etc., present serologic evidence of past infection. More detailed investigation of animals and arthropods on a worldwide basis has shown *C. burnetii* to be ubiquitous in distribution except for the countries of Denmark, Finland, Ireland, the Netherlands, Norway, and Sweden. In the United States the disease, first recognized in the states of Montana and California, is now recognized as prevalent in most of the states in which sheep and cattle are produced. Small numbers of cases have been reported for most of the remaining states.

Epidemiology. The epidemiology of the disease is complex because it involves two major patterns of transmission. The first pattern, described in Australia, is a disease cycle in wild animals with transmission of the agent from animal to animal by a tick vector. Although the species of animal and arthropod vary from country to country, such a cycle has been demonstrated in Australia in two forms, bandicoot-tick-cattle and kangaroo-tick-sheep. In both these cycles the agent can be transmitted indefinitely as an inapparent infection in the wild reservoir (bandicoot or kangaroo) by ticks, but it may also be transmitted laterally by arthropod to a domestic animal in close contact with man. In these and similar cycles recognized in other parts of the world, *C. burnetti*, like the other rickettsial agents of human disease, is vector-transmitted.

However, Q fever patients rarely give a history of tick bite. Human infection with the agent has now been shown to occur almost exclusively by a second transmission pattern capable of sustaining itself independently of the wild animal cycle. The reservoirs of infection in the second pattern are animals domesticated by man, principally cattle, sheep, and goats, in which *C. burnetii* produces only an inapparent or mild infection. In sheep, Q fever organisms are excreted in very large numbers in placental tissue, and to a lesser degree in birth fluids, milk, and feces. In the cow, and probably the goat, excretion occurs mainly through the placenta and milk. *With all infected animals, the period of parturition is associated with the formation of a primary infectious aerosol, easily demonstrated by air-sampling studies.* Such aerosols infect other cattle in the herd and also the human population in direct contact with the animals. Further, because contaminated clothing, wool, hides, bedding, and soil may be the source of secondary aerosols, *the infections may be transmitted via these vehicles at considerable distances from the infected cattle;* in certain circumstances these distances are measurable in miles. The unique resistance of *C. burnetii* to prolonged exposure in nature contributes to the spread of the agent by such infectious microenvironments. Within California, where the local epidemiology of the disease has been studied in great detail, sheep are the major reservoir for human infection in the northern part of the state and cattle in the southern part. In the latter area milk may be a vehicle of infection if consumed raw. Although the pulmonary route is the most important portal of access of the agent to man, the transmission of the rickettsia from man to man by this method is rare, despite the occurrence of an infectious pneumonitis in some patients.

Pathology. Because the mortality rate is low, postmortem studies have been limited. In those patients having a pneumonitis, the histopathology is similar to that seen in the viral pneumonias and psittacosis. Recent studies in patients have directed attention to hepatic pathology during the acute phase of the disease, demonstrable both in biochemical abnormalities of liver function (elevated cephalin-cholesterol flocculation, alkaline phosphatase, and thymol turbidity tests) and in histologic abnormalities in biopsy specimens (focal inflammation and granulomas). Q fever endocarditis, producing valvular vegetations from which rickettsiae may be isolated, has also been described.

Clinical Manifestations. After an incubation period of 9 to 20 days following respiratory exposure, most patients complain of an abrupt onset of fever, headache, muscle pains, and severe malaise. The temperature may rise as high as 104° F. and remain elevated, with considerable fluctuation, for one to three weeks. Occasionally, patients may suffer a prolonged fever of several months' duration. In contrast to the other rickettsial infections, there is no rash. In approximately half the patients there is roentgenographic evidence of pneumonitis, manifested clinically as a slight, nonproductive cough developing in the second week of fever.

Diagnosis. Q fever should always be suspected in a patient having a febrile illness for which no obvious cause can be found. If the patient's occupation brings him into contact with sheep, cattle, or goats, or byproducts such as wool or hides, particular care should be exercised to exclude Q fever from consideration. The presence of Q fever should be suspected in any patient in whom the differential diagnosis includes viral pneumonia, psittacosis, primary atypical pneumonia, pulmonary mycotic disease, or comparable infections. Furthermore, recent data would also support consideration of Q fever in the differential diagnoses of endocarditis and of hepatitis with or without jaundice.

Diagnostic laboratory studies usually must be limited to serologic studies because of the extensive history of accidentally acquired laboratory infections resulting from attempts at isolation. Either complement-fixation or agglutination tests may be employed and with either test a fourfold or greater rise in titer of antibody may be expected to occur between the first and fourth weeks of illness. Recent reports have emphasized the importance of both strain and phase variation in the selection of antigens for diagnostic use.

Treatment and Prognosis. The tetracyclines or chloramphenicol are both effective in treatment of acute infections with *C. burnetii,* but because of the nature of chloramphenicol toxicity, the tetracyclines are definitely to be preferred. The dosage of antimicrobial given should be the same as that for epidemic typhus or Rocky Mountain spotted fever. The mortality is low (1 per cent or less), even in untreated patients, and is lower still in those treated with antimicrobial drugs. Therapy should be continued for approximately one week even though the patient usually becomes afebrile within 48 hours. Patients occasionally may experience relapses after treatment, and when this complication occurs additional drug therapy should be administered. Prognosis is less favorable for the rare patient in whom Q fever endocarditis develops. In some of these patients the disease has been reported to have been unresponsive to antimicrobial therapy.

Prevention. Experimental lots of yolk-sac vaccines have been effective in prevention of clinical disease in volunteers experimentally infected via the respiratory route. Because this vaccine is not commercially available, control measures are limited to minimizing exposure to the agent. In particular, milk from cattle, sheep, and goats in endemic areas should be pasteurized or boiled before use. Because rickettsiae are excreted in the sputum and urine of patients, these materials should be disinfected by autoclaving to prevent secondary infection in hospitals.

Grist, N. R.: Q fever endocarditis. Amer. Heart J., 75:846, 1968.

Johnson, J. E., and Kadull, P. J.: Laboratory-acquired Q fever: A report of fifty cases. Amer. J. Med., 41:391, 1966.

Ormsbee, R. A.: Q fever rickettsia. *In* Horsfall, F. L., Jr., and Tamm, I. (eds.): Viral and Rickettsial Infections of Man. 4th ed. Philadelphia, J. B. Lippincott Company, 1965, p. 1144.

Powell, O. W.: Liver involvement in "Q" fever. Aust. Ann. Med., 10:52, 1961.

Tigertt, W. D., and Benenson, A. S.: Studies on Q fever in man. Trans. Ass. Amer. Physicians, 69:98, 1956.

Bacterial Diseases

INTRODUCTION
Walsh McDermott

For the past few decades the problems presented by bacterial and mycotic diseases have been substantially different, depending upon the nature of the society. In the economically underdeveloped parts of the world, the individual diseases have presented in classic form, each occupying its traditional niche in the over-all pattern. By contrast, in nations with highly developed health services, the familiar bacterial diseases have by no means disappeared, but their menace has been largely nullified by vaccines and by prompt and appropriate antimicrobial therapy. For example, one hears that lobar pneumonia "has largely disappeared." In actuality it *has* become much less frequent, not because its major cause, pneumococcal infection, is any less frequent, but because with prompt chemotherapy the early pneumonic lesion is halted in its progress well short of the confines of the lobe. It is the same old pneumonia, but it is no longer "lobar." Expressed differently without any change in the annual incidence of pneumococcal infection or disease, the annual incidence of *serious problems* from this cause has substantially diminished. In place of such clinical problems there are now essentially new menaces in the serious systemic disease produced by *E. coli,* Proteus, Pseudomonas, Candida, and other microbes that were formerly regarded as essentially harmless inhabitants of man. The disease caused by staphylococci and tubercle bacilli is likewise of this character in that the microbes can subsist harmlessly in the tissues for considerable periods between eruptions as destructive disease.

In effect these new clinical patterns represent *endogenous microbial disease*—clinical entities that appear almost exclusively in people with some temporary or sustained lowering of local or general defenses. This new part of the situation represents the unsought-for consequence of practical therapeutic gains that in themselves represent great scientific achievements. What is happening was biologically predictable, and the changing nature of the situation may be expected to continue.

To be capable of staying with this change the physician must know considerably more about the behavior of microbes, as they cause disease and are exposed to drugs within a host, than he had to master only one or two decades ago. This knowledge is of two sorts: certain concepts and principles related to the microbe-drug-host interactions, and a body of knowledge sufficient to permit him to make microbiologically relevant diagnoses on clinical grounds.

For in choosing the initial therapy for a patient with a presumed microbial disease, the physician is confronted with a formidable dilemma. On the one hand, if therapy is to be maximally effective, the correct drug or drug-pairing must be chosen quickly so that it may be administered before significant tissue damage or irreversible physiologic changes have occurred. On the other hand, if the choice is to be made quickly, it is difficult to make it exactly; for there are only a few techniques by which the cause of an infection can be positively identified during the early hours of acute illness. Thus the physician is in the uncomfortable position of knowing that if he is to obtain the greatest advantages of antimicrobial therapy for his patient, he must make the correct choice of drugs one to five days before solid evidence of the identity of the infection will be forthcoming. An obvious way out of the dilemma would be by the introduction of rapid diagnostic methods such as can be provided by adaptations of the fluorescent antibody detection technique. Surprisingly little effort has been devoted, however, to this question of rationalizing drug choices by developing a better diagnostic technology. Given this situation, the physician has to rely on his *clinical* acumen and a full knowledge of all the microbial diseases that might reasonably be expected to institute threats to his patients. In actuality, to make this choice of the initial drug regimen from evidence obtained at the bedside is not as difficult as it sounds once the physician realizes what it is that he should be trying to do. While doing it, he can also be comforted by the thought that the expert consultant must go through exactly the same exercise; for he, too, seldom has any secret diagnostic weapons, and is equally hampered by the slowness of the available diagnostic tests. Attempts should be made to differentiate, on clinical grounds, those situations or syndromes that require immediate and intensive action from those that properly may be left to unfold until precise identification becomes possible. Moreover, when a choice of therapy is made it should be made on the basis of careful consideration of the most serious threats to the patient that could be considered reasonable possibilities. The drug or drugs chosen should be the ones that do most to protect the patient overnight or for a somewhat longer interval against the reasonably likely threats, while at the same time they would do the least to mask the identity of other infections that might conceivably be present. Above all, once the identity of the infecting microbe *is* established, the physician should be quick to discontinue all but the scientifically relevant therapy. The body of knowledge on which that selectivity can be based is presented in the articles on bacterial and mycotic diseases that follow.

The other sort of knowledge needed has to do with certain principles and concepts related to the reactions among microbes, drugs, and host systems. *Endogenous microbial disease* has already been mentioned. The disease-producing microbes are evoked from the dormant or latent state in response to changes in the tissue environment that can occur as a direct or indirect consequence of our modern therapies. Among these are the suppression of the customary microbial flora by drug therapy, i.e., the selective suppression of the host protective phenomenon known as *bacterial interference;* the use of drugs such as the corticosteroids or certain surgical procedures that tend to suppress previously acquired resistance to microbial proliferation; and the longer survival of many patients despite protracted, severe, and ultimately fatal illness. This increasing ability to alter man's internal environment has had the effect that virtually no microbial species today can be considered nonpathogenic, for in appropriate circumstances virtually any can give rise to disease.

All these mechanisms unleash what are, in effect, "new" microbial diseases (see Introduction to Microbial Diseases). There are other "new" diseases that either may have been similarly unleashed or may have merely become easier to recognize by virtue of the selectivity of drug action. The separation of "atypical" pneumonia from bacterial pneumonia by the introduction of sulfonamide and the growing prominence of the nontuberculous mycobacteria as disease agents are cases in point. Viewing the microbial world as a whole, these "new" diseases are a form of survival of drug challenge. For species survival itself there are two quite different patterns, *microbial persistence* and *microbial drug resistance.* The latter phenomenon, under the name "drug-fastness," had been recognized since the early days of this century. Microbial persistence, on the other hand, was not recognized—indeed could not be recognized—until the development of penicillin, because it was only then that a powerful antimicrobial drug could be given in virtually any dosage and thus permit exclusion of the obvious possibility that the microbial survival was only a consequence of underdosage. Microbial persistence can be defined as the phenomenon whereby a microbial strain that is susceptible to a drug in the test tube is nevertheless capable of surviving long-term exposure to that drug in the body. Persistence is thus sharply distinguished from drug resistance, which is a heritable property of a microbial strain and is demonstrable in the test tube as well as in the body. In numerical terms, microbial persistence is of the greater importance, as it is the phenomenon that is responsible for most instances of post-treatment relapse, that interferes with the effectiveness of chemoprophylaxis, and that balks attempts to use drugs for the "eradication" of microbes (see Introduction to Microbial Diseases). Once recognized and studied, it became clear that microbial persistence—the drug-related phenomenon—was only one aspect of the larger phenomenon of latent microbial infection with its potentiality for evocation as endogenous microbial disease. As our knowledge accumulates, it is likewise beginning to appear as if microbial persistence and genotypic drug resistance are veering toward each other, and may eventually come to overlap. Persistence thus serves as a link between the other two phenomena, and indeed all three may ultimately be seen to shade into each other. However, we are not yet at that point. Recognition of the present clearly visible difference among the three has been most valuable in that it has made it possible for each to be recognized, reasonably well defined, and isolated for study. For more detailed consideration of these phenomena, the reader is referred to the references at the end of this article. Certain aspects of microbial persistence and heritable drug resistance deserve mention at this point.

Until microbial persistence was recognized in the 1940's, the conceptual base of antimicrobial therapy was the *therapia sterilisans magna* as originally conceived by Ehrlich; namely, the goal was to effect a total eradication of the infecting microbes from the host. With penicillin and the subsequently introduced drugs it was discovered that such total eradication did not occur uniformly and predictably. In a significant number of cases of virtually any bacterial disease, drug-susceptible cells of the infecting strain could be isolated well after completion of drug therapy. At times these persisters would increase and produce clinical relapse, which was then easily treatable by the appropriate drug. At other times they would persist in the carrier state or might ultimately disappear either into latency or presumably by leaving the host altogether. Evidence was obtained that this microbial survival could not be explained by failure of drug delivery, namely, that the microbes were located in some sanctuary such as a body compartment, the center of a necrotic area, or the interior of a phagocyte where they could not be reached by the molecules of drug in the extracellular fluid;* nor could the phenomenon be explained on the basis that the drug molecules were

*Although one frequently reads that such and such a drug fails to "penetrate" the monocyte or some other host cell, *what has usually been observed* is that when introduced into the extracellular fluid, the drug exerts less complete inhibitory activity on bacteria subsisting intracellularly than on those in the extracellular fluid. To the extent drug transfer has been studied with isotopic or other labeling methods, substantial quantities of most antimicrobial drugs do in fact "penetrate."

deviated from making contact with the microbes because the inflammatory-necrotic lesion either chemically degraded the drug or wholly bound it in some way. On the contrary, convincing evidence exists that the capacity to persist is a nonheritable property of a minority of a microbial population, and it is mediated by the ability to assume a metabolic state that has been termed "drug indifference" or "physiologic" spore formation. To what extent bacterial pleomorphism, including such forms as protoplasts, plays a role in persistence is not known. It is clear, however, that such terms as *bactericidal* and *bacteriostatic* apply only to specialized sets of circumstances in the test tube. These terms fail to reflect what happens in the body in the sense that even the most "bactericidal" drugs are not uniformly or predictably eradicative. As mentioned above, it is this capacity of drug-susceptible bacteria to survive and outlast periods of drug administration that is responsible for most clinical relapse, failures to eliminate the carrier state, and certain failures of chemoprophylaxis. It is not generally known that Ehrlich in his late years came to perceive that *magna sterilisans* conceived as eradication was untenable. He then subtly changed the *concept* of the "sterilisans" without changing the *word*, and offered the idea that the bacteria in the tissues were in effect rendered sterile, i.e., incapable of having progeny. In the last analysis all that is added to this "latter-day Ehrlich" by the present concept of microbial persistence is the point that the sterile state is reversible.

Strictly speaking, any microbial strain that is unaffected by appropriate concentrations of a drug in vitro could be called drug resistant. In actual practice, however, the designation is reserved for the drug-resistant representatives of bacterial species that are customarily susceptible to the drug in question. *Primary resistance* refers to situations in which the infecting bacterial strain is already drug resistant at the time it initiates the infection. *Emergent resistance* refers to the emergence to predominance of a drug-resistant population during the treatment of a microbial disease that was drug susceptible when treatment was started.

All drug-susceptible bacterial species possess the capability to show emergent resistance—that is to say, to escape during therapy—to *some* drug or drugs. But *all drugs* are not associated with emergent resistance. Specifically, no instance of emergent resistance to penicillin has been observed, and all penicillin resistance is primary. Whether drug resistance can emerge or not thus *depends not on the bacterial species but on the drug*, and there exists a type of drug action on a microbe wherein the emergence to predominance of drug-resistant forms is not to be feared. The existence of this type of drug action is of obvious importance in considerations of the possible mechanisms involved in multiple drug regimens as discussed below.

The pluralistic nature of the broad phenomenon

called "drug resistance" can readily be seen by examining different drugs or drug-microbe pairings. At least four distinct forms are identifiable. There is the *sulfonamide-streptomycin form*, in which the resistant bacteria maintain full pathogenic potential and are otherwise altered little, if at all, except for their loss of susceptibility to the drug. There is *a major isoniazid form*, in which certain enzymes have been lost (catalase and peroxidase), and the pathogenicity for laboratory animals including primates has been drastically reduced. There is a form characterized by *episomal* or by *plasmid* transfer, exemplified by enteric bacteria but also by staphylococci. There is also a form seen most clearly with penicillin and staphylococci in which the critical element in producing the resistance, the formation of the enzyme penicillinase, is an *inducible* phenomena. Combinations of these various forms of phenomena occur. For example, some strains of isoniazid-resistant tubercle bacilli are of the sulfonamide-streptomycin form, although these are rare; the genetic capability of staphylococci to elaborate penicillinase can be passed from one cell to another by episomal transfer, and the actual enzymatic process of synthesizing penicillinase is induced by exposure to the substrate penicillin.

Episomal transfer is an example of nonchromosomal inheritance, for not only do bacteria have chromosomal genes, but they have what are in effect free-floating genes that can pass from one cell to another as if they were a virus. The particles are of two sorts: the episomes and the plasmid. The difference between them is that the plasmid does not attach itself to the chromosome at any time, whereas the episome can either exist freely in the cytoplasm or at times attach itself to the chromosome. Synergism between an episomal gene and a chromosomal gene can occur. In one such experiment, two genes, one present in the episomal factor and the other in the chromosomal, each of which singly conferred resistance to streptomycin concentrations of 25 μg. per milliliter, *co-operated* to yield organisms resistant to 1000 μg. per milliliter. It is believed that the synergism was acquired as a direct result of genetic recombination between the chromosome and the episomal factor. The "infection" of the strain of *E. coli* in the form of the episomal factor could be removed by treatment with an acridine dye—in effect, a form of drug therapy in vitro.

In what way is the clinician benefited by acquaintance with this expanding body of knowledge on the multiple forms of what can only loosely be called "drug resistance?" The principal gain—and it is by no means a minor one—is that he is able to perceive that the results of testing a microbial strain for drug susceptibility in vitro is only one bit of information, and one that is not always relevant to the therapeutic problem presented by his patient. The identity of the microbial species, its probable source, e.g., whether acquired in hospital or acquired from a drug-treated household contact, and the *history* of drugs received earlier in the illness and their observed effects

usually represent a body of evidence of greater reliability and predictive value than drug-susceptibility tests as they are frequently performed. Above all, the clinician should be very wary of abandoning a particular drug therapy that appears to be working satisfactorily and introducing a substitute *solely* on the basis of drug-susceptibility tests. Like many ancillary laboratory procedures, drug-susceptibility tests have a role, but it is usually more a confirming one than a determining one.

Consideration of the mechanisms of drug resistance leads to scrutiny of the use of two antimicrobial drugs together. One of the avowed goals of such multi-drug therapy is to postpone or prevent drug resistance of the emergent type; the other is to obtain greater antimicrobial effectiveness per unit of time. Conceivably the same process could be responsible for both effects, although this is not the customary way of looking at the matter. With respect to drug resistance, the orthodox explanation dates from Ehrlich's day and is based on the notion that emergent resistance is prevented or postponed because drug A is effective against those bacterial mutants that are resistant to drug B, and vice versa. By this concept it would be possible for a two-drug regimen to affect emergent resistance without exerting an enhanced antimicrobial effectiveness per unit of time. The latter phenomenon, as seen in the penicillin-streptomycin treatment of enterococcal endocarditis, presumably would have to be explained on some other basis. The issue here is not whether, in appropriate circumstances, two-drug therapy can affect emergent resistance or increase total antimicrobial effectiveness. The question is *how* are these phenomena brought about. If the combined drug action is exerted independently, with drug A acting on cells resistant to drug B, virtually any two-drug regimen would be expected to be effective. Contrariwise, if the respective drug actions are dependent, it would presumably represent a highly specialized phenomenon. To settle this issue would thus be a matter of considerable practical importance. Unfortunately, a reasonably complete and authoritative answer cannot be given at this time.

It can be said from the relatively few sets of observations available that enhancement of antimicrobial effectiveness by concurrent administration of two drugs appears to be a *dependent* phenomenon, with both drugs generally acting on the same microbial cell. The phenomenon seems to have considerable specificity in terms of drugs and microbial species involved; hence superior drug pairings are relatively rare, and are not to be expected with just any pairing and any drug-susceptible parasite. Whether the "dependent" mechanism is also the major way by which two-drug regimens influence emergent resistance is less clear. In the writer's judgment, there is considerable reason to believe that this is indeed the case and that when a drug pairing does exert an influence on emergent resistance, it does so by the action of both drugs on the microbes susceptible to both drugs. Hence in large measure the action would consist of both drugs acting on the same microbial cell. As in the situation with enhancement, such effective drug pairings would represent highly specialized sets of circumstances.

The indication that drug pairings superior to the more powerful drug alone are special affairs is in agreement with the rarity with which multiple drug regimens are of demonstrated value in clinical medicine. Indeed to all intents and purposes, the examples are largely limited to infections with enterococci or tubercle bacilli, and possibly to some infections caused by staphylococci. It is important for the physician to keep reminding himself that, except for these few microbial diseases, the justification for the use of more than one antimicrobial drug at a time is largely limited to situations in which an etiologic diagnosis is not available, notably during the early hours of treatment.

The day has gone by when the physician could prescribe all two or three of the available antimicrobial drugs to an acutely febrile patient and relax with the comforting thought that all that modern science could do was being done. With today's multiplicity of drugs, the emergence of "new" microbial diseases, and our considerably expanded knowledge about mechanisms of microbial survival, the physician must be highly selective in his drug choices, and hence must have mastery of a considerably greater body of clinical and laboratory-derived knowledge than was needed even a few decades ago. The physician's "comforting thought" today is of quite a different sort. It consists of the knowledge that, however difficult modern science is making things for *him* in the management of infections, it is making things ever so much better for his patients.

Dubos, R. J.: Man Adapting. New Haven, Yale University Press, 1965, pp. 1–527.
McDermott, W.: Inapparent infection. The Dyer Lecture. Public Health Report, 74:485, 1959.
McDermott, W.: Microbial Persistence. Harvey Lecture Series No. 63, 1969, pp. 1–31.
McDermott, W.: Microbial drug resistance. Barnwell Lecture. Amer. Rev. Resp. Dis., 102:855, 1970.

PNEUMONIA

GENERAL CONSIDERATIONS
Walsh McDermott

To discover that a pneumonia, i.e., an intrapulmonary process of some sort, is present in an adult patient is no very difficult feat; neither is the knowledge particularly helpful unless two further steps can be taken. These are detection of evidence that the disease is indeed microbial in origin and not an infarct or neoplasm, and identification of the specific microbe or kind of microbe

that is involved. Every aspect of management— the choice of treatment, the complications to be watched for, and the hour-by-hour prognosis— depends on the nature of this information. To obtain it accurately *and in proper time* requires that the physician be wholly familiar with the various ways in which each one of the microbial pneumonias expresses itself. Some of these—for example, plague pneumonia—he may never see. Yet he must know at least enough about plague pneumonia so that he could avert its terrible consequences for others should he ever encounter a case. Other forms of pneumonia encountered relatively rarely arise as complications of some familiar microbial disease such as measles or tuberculosis or streptococcal disease. Occasionally, well-known viruses such as influenza or chicken pox cause pneumonia, or the physician may be asked to see a patient with psittacosis. In the defenseless host, necrotizing pneumonias caused by Pseudomonas and other gram-negative bacilli are being recognized increasingly as one form of the endogenous microbial disease mentioned above. Most of the time, in an adult patient the physician is dealing with mycoplasmal pneumonia or with one of three bacterial pneumonias, pneumococcal, staphylococcal, or some other form of necrotizing pneumonia in an obviously altered host. This narrowing of the probabilities does not really lighten the seriousness of making the correct choice. The most effective treatment for pneumococcal pneumonia is utterly without value in klebsiella pneumonia; a choice of therapy based on a diagnosis of mycoplasmal pneumonia when the patient actually has staphylococcal pneumonia could result in a fatality.

Mycoplasmal pneumonia (as well as the pneumonias caused by the individual viruses, rickettsial and psittacine agents) is considered in an earlier section of the book. As staphylococcal pneumonia is so closely related to viral influenza, it is discussed both under staphylococcal disease and in the article on influenza. The other major bacterial pneumonias, pneumococcal, klebsiella, and the other necrotizing pneumonias, are presented immediately below. Klebsiella pneumonia, although infrequent, is of great importance because of its potential severity and the ease with which it can be misdiagnosed. Pneumococcal pneumonia is the most important of all pneumonias, not only in numerical terms, but because in large measure, and especially in its complications, it is the prototype of all the bacterial pneumonias.

MYCOPLASMAL PNEUMONIA
Robert B. Couch

Definition. Mycoplasmal pneumonia is the most severe manifestation of respiratory infection with *Mycoplasma pneumoniae.* Bronchitis, pharyngitis, and asymptomatic infections are frequently seen, particularly in young children; pneumonia occurs predominantly among older children and young adults. The disease responds to treatment with the tetracyclines and erythromycins.

History. A pneumonia that was unlike lobar pneumonia of *Diplococcus pneumoniae* was recognized in the 1930's. Extensive bacteriologic studies failed to reveal a specific etiology in many of these cases, and Dingle and Finland in 1942 applied the term primary atypical pneumonia to this group of nonbacterial pneumonias. In 1943 the discovery that cold hemagglutinins developed in the sera of many of the patients provided a useful diagnostic test. During World War II the Armed Forces Commission on Acute Respiratory Disease described many of the clinical and epidemiologic characteristics of an atypical pneumonia, retrospectively identified by serologic tests as caused by infection with *M. pneumoniae*.

The causative agent was first isolated by Eaton in cotton rats, and subsequently was shown to infect hamsters and chicken embryos. It is filterable and for this reason was considered to be a virus for many years. In 1957, Liu reported an immuno-fluorescent test for antibody, using sections of infected chicken embryo bronchi for antigen, and Chanock in 1961 reported that the organism was the cause of virtually all cases of pneumonia associated with the development of cold hemagglutinins. Subsequent to these studies and the demonstration that the organism was a Mycoplasma, it was given the name *Mycoplasma pneumoniae*.

Etiology. *Mycoplasma pneumoniae* is a member of the genus Mycoplasma and can readily be distinguished from five other known human species of Mycoplasma. *M. pneumoniae* is about 200 mμ in size and is thus the smallest known free-living organism that will produce disease in man. It will grow aerobically or anaerobically on artificial media, but the media must be enriched with 20 per cent horse serum and yeast extract. The small granular colonies grow embedded in the surface of the agar, and are best detected by microscopic examination. Tentative identification procedures utilize the fact that it ferments glucose, hemolyzes red blood cells in guinea pigs and sheep, and is resistant to methylene blue. Final identification requires serologic procedures.

Epidemiology. *M. pneumoniae* infection is endemic in large populations, but numerous localized outbreaks have occurred in schools and military populations. There is no periodicity such as occurs with influenza and no seasonal prevalence as with bacterial and viral respiratory illnesses.

The basic epidemiologic unit is the family, where the infection is often introduced by five- to nine-year-old schoolchildren. Infection spreads slowly but will ultimately involve 80 to 90 per cent of family members who are not immune. Though most common in young school-age children, the very young, adolescents, and young adults frequently acquire the infection. It is rare above age 50 when serum antibody is almost universally present.

Roentgenographic evidence of pneumonia occurs in 30 to 50 per cent of infected family members, but studies in the military have suggested that only about 10 per cent of infections result in pneumonia. This disparity may be accounted for by the finding that illness is more likely to occur and to be more severe with advancing age.

Pathogenesis. *M. pneumoniae* is a primary pathogen of the respiratory tract that is spread by close and frequent contact between infected and susceptible persons. The organism can be recovered from sputum and throat swab specimens two to three days prior to onset of illness. Thereafter, the concentration of organisms in secretions rises to the time of occurrence of illness and remains high for four to six days. After illness subsides, the agent may persist in respiratory secretions for several weeks in a considerable percentage of cases, and positive cultures frequently occur after antimicrobial treatment.

The organism grows on the ciliated border and between respiratory epithelial cells. All evidence indicates that it does not invade lung parenchyma. It has been suggested that the peroxide produced by the organism might produce cell damage; more recently it has been suggested that the illness may be a result of hypersensitivity to the organism or one or more of its products.

Resistance to infection has been shown to correlate with presence and magnitude of serum antibody, and this mechanism may also influence recovery from illness. Since *M. pneumoniae* initially deposits on the respiratory mucosa, it has been suggested that antibody in secretions may be of primary importance in resistance to infection, although attempts to demonstrate antibody in secretions have not been successful. The association between antibody and resistance probably accounts for prevalence of the infection in younger age groups, as most adults have detectable serum antibody. Nevertheless, reinfection with mild illness has been shown to occur.

Pathology. From the limited studies available, it is apparent that a great variety of pathologic findings may occur in pneumonia, including patchy or confluent bronchopneumonia, interstitial pneumonia, and lobar pneumonia. Pleuritis with a small pleural effusion may be present, but significant pleural effusion is rare. Gross pathology usually reveals patchy areas of lung infiltration and inflamed bronchial and bronchiolar lumina containing mucoid and occasionally purulent exudate. Microscopic sections reveal mononuclear peribronchial and peribronchiolar infiltrates with edema and mononuclear cell infiltration of neighboring alveolar septa. Mucosal cell lining of respiratory passages usually remains intact, and polymorphonuclear cell infiltration is prominent only if necrosis and sloughing of the mucosal cell lining occur. No pathologic alterations have been described in other areas of the body.

Clinical Manifestations. The incubation period to onset of illness is about three weeks, most cases occurring in 15 to 25 days. The onset is usually insidious, with malaise and headache as prominent symptoms. For a period of two to three days these symptoms increase in severity, and feverishness, myalgias, and sore throat may also occur. Cough is usually not prominent until two to three days after onset of illness. It is either nonproductive or productive of small amounts of mucoid sputum that occasionally contain flecks of blood. *Despite the delayed appearance of cough, it becomes the* *dominant respiratory symptom in mycoplasmal pneumonia, and its absence or the occurrence of only mild cough makes a clinical diagnosis questionable.* In some cases cough occurs early, and patients may exhibit the paroxysms, substernal discomfort, and tracheal tenderness characteristic of acute tracheobronchitis. Headache is commonly reported as the most distressing symptom in an adult. Ear discomfort, owing to myringitis, mild nasal symptoms, and prominent sore throat may also occur, especially in the younger age groups. Substernal or diffuse chest discomfort on inspiration is common, but typical pleuritic pain is rare.

Patients usually do not appear seriously ill. Tachypnea, dyspnea, and cyanosis are rare and are not seen unless pulmonary involvement is extensive or other disease is present. The degree of fever is variable but is present in virtually all cases of pneumonia.

Physical examination usually reveals mild nasal obstruction and discharge and mild to moderate injection of the posterior pharynx. Mild injection of the tympanic membranes is commonly seen, and about 15 per cent of patients will exhibit frank myringitis, some of whom will develop blebs or bullae. Hemorrhage into the blebs or bullae is common, and these patients usually complain of severe ear pain. Tender cervical lymphadenopathy is a common finding, particularly when pharyngitis is also present.

Findings on chest examination may be minimal, and roentgenographic findings that seem out of proportion to physical findings frequently occur. Auscultation of the chest may reveal rhonchi and wheezes over the involved area of the lung owing to mucus in large bronchi and bronchioles, and fine to medium moist rales may also be heard. In the occasional patient with more extensive disease, signs of consolidation may be detected.

Roentgenographic Findings. No roentgenographic changes can be considered typical of mycoplasmal pneumonia. Infiltrates are usually unilateral, confined to a lower lobe, and more prominent near the hilum. Frequently a single segment is involved, but on occasion the infiltrate may be extensive and lobar or may involve more than one lobe. Small pleural effusions are not uncommon.

Laboratory Findings. Peripheral leukocyte counts are within normal limits in about 50 per cent of cases and rarely exceed 10 to 15,000 per cubic millimeter in the remainder. Differential counts usually reveal slight neutrophilia with counts of 60 to 85 per cent neutrophils. During the period of acute illness lymphopenia may be seen. The erythrocyte sedimentation rate is usually elevated. Urinalysis is within normal limits except for occasional albuminuria, which may be attributed to fever. Gram stain and culture of sputum usually reveal normal flora.

Clinical Course and Complications. Illness on occasion may be severe, but very few deaths from mycoplasmal pneumonia have occurred. Fever is variable in duration, lasting from three days to two weeks. Fever usually subsides by lysis, and

when this occurs, slow but progressive improvement in the cough, malaise, and lethargy ensues. However, symptoms may persist for three to six weeks. Roentgenographic abnormalities frequently persist for two to four weeks.

The most common pulmonary complication is relapse soon after clinical recovery. This appears to occur in about 10 per cent of cases, and the disease may involve the same or a different lobe of the lung. Cases of residual pleural abnormality have also been reported. Clinically significant intravascular hemolysis in association with demonstrable cold hemagglutinins occurs in a small percentage of cases. Such patients exhibit cold hemagglutinin titers of 1:500 or greater and also have demonstrable hemagglutinins at room temperature. Hemolysis usually occurs when fever subsides or chilling of peripheral tissues occurs.

Recent reports have associated *M. pneumoniae* with central nervous system and cutaneous manifestations. The former patients have had meningitis, encephalitis, or both with a variable number and type of cells in the cerebrospinal fluid. Skin manifestations have included urticaria, vesiculopustular eruptions, maculopapular eruptions, erythema multiforme, and erythema nodosum, although many patients were simultaneously receiving drugs, so that causation is not certain. A reported association with Stevens-Johnson syndrome is perhaps of special significance as these cases are frequently preceded by respiratory symptoms and accompanied by pneumonia. Evidence of *M. pneumoniae* infection should be sought in such cases.

Hemorrhagic bullous myringitis (see Clinical Manifestations), bronchiectasis, pericarditis, myocarditis, Guillain-Barré syndrome, and thrombocytopenic purpura have also been reported as complications of mycoplasmal pneumonia.

Diagnosis. Early diagnosis can be made only by clinical means. The presence of marked headache, lassitude, myalgias, definite nasopharyngeal findings, and nonproductive cough suggests nonbacterial pneumonia. Absence of the usual features of bacterial pneumonia, such as sudden onset, shaking chills, pleuritic pain, and purulent or bloody sputum, offers important support for the diagnosis. Other causes of pulmonary infiltration such as tuberculosis, mycotic infection, pulmonary infarction, and malignancy must be considered.

Among the causes of non-bacterial pneumonia that may mimic mycoplasmal pneumonia are psittacosis and Q fever, for which an exposure history should be sought, and adenoviral and influenzal pneumonias, which are usually more acute in onset and occur primarily during recognizable epidemics. If the age of the patient is 5 to 30 years and other similar cases have occurred in a family, diagnosis is more certain, but the only clinical finding that makes mycoplasmal pneumonia almost a certain diagnosis is the additional presence of myringitis with a bleb or bulla on the tympanic membrane.

Isolation of *M. pneumoniae* may be accomplished

from sputum or throat swab specimens. Either enriched solid or special liquid medium may be used, although identifiable isolations are not usually detected for at least five days after inoculation, and 14 to 21 days of incubation may be required.

The cold hemagglutinin test is generally available and useful. Sera of about 50 per cent of patients with *M. pneumoniae* pneumonia will develop this autoantibody which agglutinates human red blood cells when reacted in the cold (4° C.). It is more likely to occur in more severely ill patients, and usually appears toward the end of the first week or the beginning of the second week of illness. *Serum for this test should be separated from red blood cells before refrigeration.* Positive direct Coombs tests and an occasional false positive serologic test for syphilis may occur.

A variety of serologic procedures have been described for detecting rise in specific serum antibody titer to *M. pneumoniae* between acute and convalescent sera. Complement fixation is the most available procedure and will demonstrate a rise in titer in 75 to 80 per cent of cases. Growth inhibition is a more sensitive and specific method and is preferred, but it requires experience with cultivation techniques which is not widely available.

Treatment. Tetracycline and its derivatives and erythromycin have been shown to hasten the disappearance of fever, rales, and cough in treated cases. Since definitive diagnosis is not possible within the first few days after onset of illness, decisions regarding administration of antimicrobials must be made on clinical grounds. Patients presumed to have mycoplasmal pneumonia should receive tetracycline or its equivalent in doses of 0.25 gram every six hours. Erythromycin in doses of 0.5 gram every eight hours appears to be an acceptable alternative. Incomplete relief of cough, occasional relapse, and continued shedding of the organism frequently follow six to eight-day courses of treatment with these antimicrobials. It is possible that continuing treatment for two to three weeks will provide more complete recovery, and therefore this duration of treatment is recommended. The additional use of antipyretics, antitussives, intermittent positive pressure breathing, oxygen, and the like is determined by individual needs.

Prevention. No established method is presently available to prevent mycoplasmal pneumonia. Patients in the acute stage of illness should probably be isolated and attempts made in the home to prevent close contact with ill individuals. There is no vaccine currently available.

Chanock, R.: Mycoplasma infections of man. New Eng. J. Med., 272:1257, 1965.

Dingle, J. H., and Langmuir, A. D.: Epidemiology of acute respiratory disease in military recruits. Amer. Rev. Resp. Dis., 97 (Supplement):1, 1968.

Hayflick, L. (ed.): The Mycoplasmatales and the L-phase of Bacteria. New York, Appleton-Century-Crofts, 1969.

Mufson, M., Manko, M., Kingston, J., and Chanock, R.: Eaton agent pneumonia: Clinical features. J.A.M.A., 178:369, 1961.

Rifkind, P., Chanock, R., Kravetz, H., Johnson, K., and Knight, V.: Ear involvement (myringitis) and primary atypical pneumonia following inoculation of volunteers with Eaton agent. Amer. Rev. Resp. Dis., 85:479, 1962.

PNEUMOCOCCAL PNEUMONIA
W. Barry Wood, Jr.*

Definition. Pneumococcal pneumonia is an acute bacterial infection of the lungs caused by pneumococcus and characterized clinically by an abrupt onset, with rigor, fever, chest pain, cough, and bloody sputum.

History. Although pneumonia was known to Hippocrates, its usual cause was not learned until late in the nineteenth century. Pneumococcus was first isolated from normal saliva in 1881 by Pasteur and by Sternberg. Several years later its causative role in pneumonia was demonstrated independently by Fränkel and Weichselbaum. Identification of different serologic types of pneumococci, which began with the studies of Neufeld in Germany and Dochez in this country, led eventually to serum therapy and to the highly significant observations of Avery, Enders, Heidelberger, and Goebel concerning the chemical nature of the capsular antigen and its relation to pathogenicity. In 1928 Griffith demonstrated that pneumococci of one type may be transformed into pneumococcal cells of another type. This remarkable transforming reaction was shown by Avery and his collaborators to depend upon the highly polymerized deoxyribonucleic acid of the bacterial cell, thus initiating the modern revolution in molecular biology. Present concepts of the pathogenesis of pneumococcal pneumonia derive from the systematic histologic investigations of Robertson and Loeschcke. The seriousness of the disease in man was drastically modified by the advent of sulfonamide therapy in the late 1930's, and later treatment was further improved by the introduction of penicillin and other antimicrobial drugs.

Bacteriology and Immunology. Bacterial pneumonias occurring in otherwise healthy persons are usually caused by *Diplococcus pneumoniae*. The somatic portion of the lancet-shaped pneumococcal cell is gram-positive. In its virulent form pneumococcus has an outer capsule consisting of a loosely packed gel containing a high molecular polysaccharide polymer that is specific for each serologic type. In addition to the type-specific capsular antigen, there is a species-specific carbohydrate in the cell wall, known as the "C" substance. A non-type-specific protein antigen can also be demonstrated in the somatic portion of the cell, and Austrian and MacLeod have identified a type-specific protein analogous to the M substance of beta-hemolytic streptococci. The capsule of pneumococcus acts as an armor against phagocytic cells and thus contributes significantly to the pathogenicity of the organism. Pneumococcal variants having no capsules (rough or R strains) are essentially avirulent. Antibody to the type-specific carbohydrate promotes phagocytosis by combining with the highly polymerized polysaccharide of the capsular gel. Antibodies to the other antigens have never been shown to affect significantly the invasive properties of the organism. The pneumococcal cell also produces hyaluronidase, a pneumolysin that causes hemolysis in blood agar, and autolytic enzymes that, when

*Deceased.

activated, render the organism gram-negative and eventually cause its dissolution.

Pneumococci can be grown on a variety of bacteriologic media. Blood agar and beef infusion broth containing 0.5 per cent dextrose and 5 to 10 per cent blood or serum are the media most commonly used. The *pH* of the medium should be approximately 7.5. In a suitable broth the organism grows rapidly, and on blood agar virulent (smooth, S) strains form circular, glistening, dome-shaped colonies that are alpha-hemolytic. Because of the great quantity of capsular polysaccharide formed by type III pneumococcus, its colonies are more mucoid and usually about twice as large (2 mm. in diameter) as those of other types. Unlike the alpha-hemolytic Streptococcus, pneumococcus is soluble in bile, sodium deoxycholate and other surface-active agents, is highly sensitive to optochin, and is mouse-virulent. Most strains are virulent for mice, rats, rabbits, dogs, and monkeys as well as for man.

The extraordinary virulence of pneumococci for mice may be made use of in isolating the organisms from sputum. The technique usually used consists in injecting intraperitoneally 0.5 ml. of sputum previously emulsified by having been drawn repeatedly into a tuberculin syringe. When virulent pneumococci are present, the mouse usually dies within 48 hours, and a pure culture of the organism can be isolated from the heart's blood. Since other bacteria in the sputum do not ordinarily produce fatal infections in mice, the animal serves as a convenient and highly sensitive differential "culture medium" for the isolation of pneumococci.

More than 82 different serologic types of pneumococci have been identified by agglutination tests with specific antiserums or by the quellung test. The latter is based upon the characteristic capsular "swelling" (quellung) caused by homologous type-specific antibody. Tests used for the identification of type-specific antibody in serums and other body fluids include, in addition to the agglutination and quellung methods, mouse protection tests, precipitin reactions, and opsonocytophagic and bactericidal tests.

Anticapsular antibody usually appears in the blood of patients with pneumococcal pneumonia between the fifth and tenth days of the disease. In some untreated patients its appearance coincides with recovery; in others no such relation is demonstrable. In severe pneumococcal infections, specific polysaccharide, which has diffused away from the multiplying bacteria, can often be identified in the urine by precipitin test and sometimes can even be detected in the blood. Patients frequently continue to excrete the capsular carbohydrate in the urine for days and even weeks after recovery.

Epidemiology. Pneumococcal pneumonia may occur at any season, but is most common during the winter and early spring, when viral respiratory infections are most prevalent (see Pathogenesis).

The types of pneumococci that most commonly cause pneumonia in adults are types I, III, IV, V, VII, VIII, XII, XIV, and XIX. Together, these nine types account for more than three quarters of all cases. The most common types encountered in childhood pneumonias are I, VI, XIV, and XIX.

Pneumococci, particularly of the higher types, are frequently present in the respiratory tracts of normal subjects. Ordinarily the prevalence of carriers of highly pathogenic types is relatively low, except for type III, which is a common inhabitant of the normal pharynx. Nevertheless, there is evidence that normal carriers play a more important role in the dissemination of infective types than do patients ill with pneumonia. Occasionally, in relatively closed communities, high carrier rates of pathogenic types are encountered. In such circumstances the occurrence of widespread viral disease of the respiratory tract may result in an epidemic of pneumococcal pneumonia. Except for these rare epidemics, most of which occur in hospitals or custodial institutions, the disease is sporadic. Pneumococcal pneumonia occurs frequently in patients with multiple myeloma or hypogammaglobulinemia.

Pathogenesis and Pathology. The lung is the only major viscus of the body exposed to air. As the atmosphere, particularly in congested places, contains many pathogenic bacteria, it is remarkable that pneumonia is not more common. The failure of normal subjects to acquire acute bacterial pneumonia as an air-borne infection is due to the efficient defense-barriers of the lower respiratory tract. These include (1) the epiglottal reflex, which prevents gross aspiration of infected secretions from the pharynx; (2) the sticky mucus that lines the bronchial tree and to which air-borne organisms adhere; (3) the cilia of the respiratory epithelium, which keep the infected mucus moving constantly upward toward the pharynx (at a rate of 1 to 3 cm. per hour); (4) the cough reflex, which serves to propel the mucus out of the lower tract; (5) the lymphatics that drain the terminal bronchi and bronchioles; and (6) the mononuclear phagocytes (dust cells) that are ever present in the normal alveoli. In addition, the alveoli themselves are relatively dry and thus offer a poor medium for growth to the few bacteria that succeed in reaching them. Only when the defense barriers of the normal respiratory tract are disturbed does acute bacterial pneumonia result.

The thesis that bacterial pneumonia usually results from aspiration of infected secretions from the upper respiratory tract is strongly supported by both experimental and clinical observations. Rats infected with pneumococci in the nasopharynx regularly exhibit pulmonary lesions only when subjected to experimental procedures involving chilling of the body, anesthesia, administration of morphine, or alcoholic intoxication, all of which are common predisposing factors in human pneumonia and have been shown in laboratory animals to slow the epiglottal reflex and thus to facilitate aspiration. Experimental pneumonia can best be produced by intrabronchial inoculation of organisms suspended in mixtures of gastric mucin or starch having viscosities similar to that of mucus. Viral infection of the upper respiratory tract in man usually precedes the onset of acute bacterial pneumonia by several days. Not only is the volume of secretion from the nasopharynx greater than normal during viral infections such as the common cold, but also the number of pathogenic micro-organisms in the secretions is significantly increased. Thus, the stage is set for aspiration of infected mucus. That such aspiration often occurs at the onset of human pneumonia is suggested by the usual sites of initial involvement of the lung. The earliest lesions of bacterial pneumonia usually appear in those parts of the lungs into which aspirated fluid is most likely to drain. Whereas most airborne bacteria are caught on the sticky surfaces of the bronchial tree and never reach the alveoli, organisms contained in thin nasopharyngeal secretions are readily carried into the alveoli by the liquid mucus. The latter, like Lipiodol, cannot all be ejected by ciliary action, and much of it penetrates to the farthest reaches of the bronchial tree, where it establishes the initial focus of infection.

Other factors known to predispose patients to acute bacterial pneumonia include exposure to noxious gases and anesthetics, cardiac failure, influenza viral infection of the lungs, trauma to the thorax, and pulmonary stasis resulting from prolonged bed rest. A feature common to all these conditions is the accumulation of fluid in the alveoli. Harford (1950) has shown that the dry lungs of normal mice are able to rid themselves of large numbers of inspired bacteria, whereas lungs containing fluid are readily infected. This observation suggests that pulmonary edema, by providing a suitable culture medium for the bacteria, may facilitate the establishment of active infection within the alveoli.

Occasionally the primary source of an acute pneumonic lesion is chronic pulmonary disease, such as bronchiectasis or lung abscess. Pneumococcal pneumonia may also occur as a complication of bronchogenic carcinoma.

Early Lesion. Once the infection has gained a foothold within the alveoli, the lesion evolves in a characteristic manner. The first response of the lung to bacterial invasion is an outpouring of edema fluid into the alveoli. This serous fluid not only serves as a suitable culture medium for the organisms but also "floats" them into new alveoli through the pores of Cohn and terminal bronchioles (see accompanying figure, *a*). Centrifugal spread of the alveolar fluid is enhanced by motion of the pulmonary parenchyma caused by respiration and cough. After the outpouring of edema fluid, polymorphonuclear leukocytes and some erythrocytes accumulate in the infected alveoli, first in small numbers (figure, *b*), but later in such quantities as to fill each alveolus and thus render the area completely consolidated (figure, *c*). Once the infected alveoli become crowded with leuko-

cytes, phagocytosis of bacteria takes place, and the invading organisms are destroyed. Macrophages appear in the exudate, and resolution begins only after most of the organisms have been ingested. The macrophages that accomplish the final clearing of cellular debris from the resolving lesion appear to be derived both from monocytes of the blood and from the septal cells of the alveolar walls, which become characteristically thickened during the process of resolution (figure, *d*).

Spreading Lesion. Three stages in the inflammatory reaction account for the distinguishing histologic features of the spreading pneumonic lesion. In the outermost portion there appears an "edema zone" in which the alveoli are filled with acellular serous fluid containing many bacteria. Inside the edema zone a second zone may be identified in which there are signs of early consolidation with leukocytes in most of the alveoli. Here phagocytosis is often noted. Still more centrally a third transition to a "zone of advanced consolidation" is noted where the alveoli are packed with cells and where beginning resolution may be evident. In the central zone of advanced consolidation fibrin is often noted in the alveolar exudate, the large fibrinogen molecules having passed through the injured walls of the alveolar capillaries along with erythrocytes.

From the foregoing description it is clear that all stages of inflammation can be found in a spreading lesion. In the most recently invaded areas at the periphery, edema and hemorrhage predominate, causing "red hepatization," whereas in the older, more central parts of the lesion, dense consolidation with leukocytes accounts for the characteristic color of "gray hepatization." Only if the infection has stopped spreading hours before necropsy will the entire lesion be in the stage of "gray hepatization." Thus, the spread of pneumococcal pneumonia may be likened to that of a grass fire, in which the flames, having spread centrifugally, are concentrated at the periphery, leaving behind a charred and burned-out center.

Not all pneumococcal pneumonia causes lobar consolidation. Less malignant lesions may be patchy in distribution and concentrated particularly about the bronchi. Because a clear-cut distinction between pneumococcal bronchopneumonia and lobar pneumonia cannot always be made even by the pathologist, and because management of the two conditions is essentially the same, it is rarely important for the clinician to differentiate them. The etiology rather than the anatomy of the lesion determines therapy.

Interlobar Spread. If the pneumonic process has involved all the parenchyma of a single lobe, its spread may be stopped by the pleural boundaries of the lobe, and spontaneous recovery may then ensue. Often, however, the infection spreads to other lobes of the lungs. Interlobar spread has been shown in experimental pneumonia to result from the flow of infected edema fluid (figure, *e*) from bronchi of the involved lung into the bronchial tree of a new lobe. Spread to a given lobe may be brought about by suspending the infected

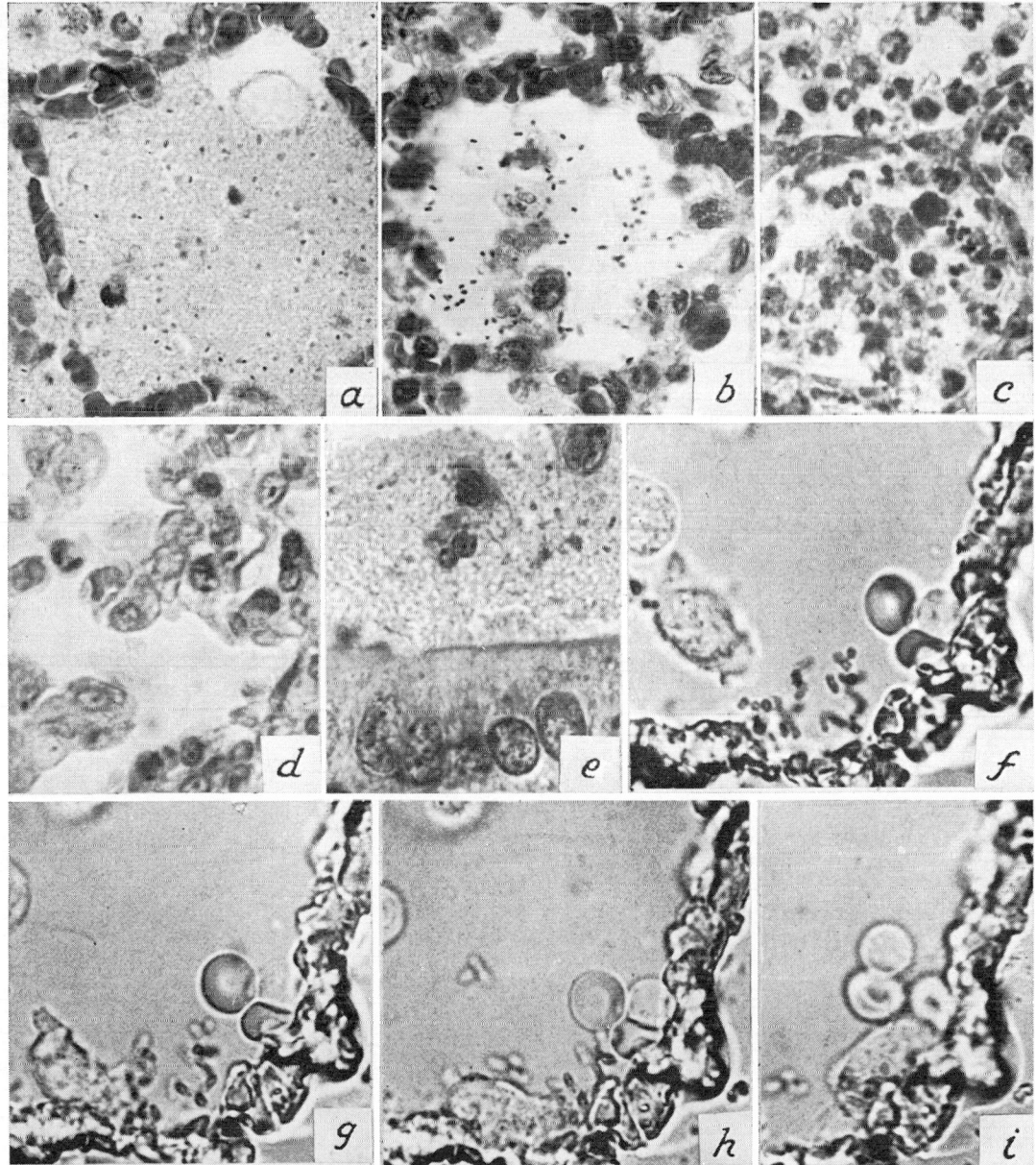

a, Pneumococci in edema-filled alveoli at margin of spreading pneumonic lesion (×800).

b, Beginning stage of polymorphonuclear exudation in zone of early consolidation. Note leukocytes in alveolar capillaries, some in process of diapedesis (×800).

c, Leukocytic exudate (still predominantly polymorphonuclear) in inner zone of advanced consolidation. Pneumococci have been phagocytized and destroyed (×800).

d, Alveolar macrophage reaction characteristic of late stage of resolution (×800).

e, Pneumococci in edema fluid contained within lumen of a large bronchus, Such infected bronchial fluid causes spread of pneumonia to other lobes of the lungs (×1250).

f–i, Surface phagocytosis of encapsulated micro-organisms in formalin-fixed rat lung (×1250). Bacteria shown in these photomicrographs are klebsiella, but same results have been obtained with pneumococci.

f, Polymorphonuclear leukocyte is seen approaching bacteria near alveolar wall. Time 12:30.

g, Leukocyte has reached alveolar wall and is about to trap organisms against the tissue surface. Time 12:31.

h, Cell has trapped some of the encapsulated bacteria against the wall and is in the process of phagocytizing them. Time 12:32.

i, Having ingested several of the organisms, the leukocyte is moving up the alveolar wall. Time 12:35.

(Photomicrographs from studies on experimental pneumonia. W. B. Wood et al.: J. Exp. Med., Vol. 73; and Smith and Wood: *ibid.,* Vol. 86.)

animal in such a way that gravity will carry the bronchial fluid into the desired lobe. It may be assumed that a similar mechanism operates in human patients with multilobar lesions. The fact that the most common spread in human pneumonia is from one lower lobe to another is in keeping with the assumption that organisms are carried to the new lobe by infected bronchial fluid, the flow of which is influenced by cough, respiration, and force of gravity.

Bacteremia. Bacteremia frequently occurs during the course of pneumococcal pneumonia, particularly when the infection is fulminating. The fact that organisms appear in the thoracic duct in experimental pneumonia before they appear in the systemic circulation suggests that most of them reach the blood stream via the lymphatics. (It is well known that particles introduced experimentally into the alveoli are cleared primarily by lymphatic drainage.)

To cause bacteremia the lymph-borne organisms must first traverse the cellular defenses of the regional (hilar) lymph nodes to reach the thoracic duct and enter the blood. Once there they must accumulate in sufficient numbers to overpower the combined cellular defenses of the reticuloendothelial system and circulating phagocytes of the blood stream. In other words, their rate of entrance into the circulation must exceed their rate of destruction. Hence, a positive blood culture in pneumococcal pneumonia indicates that the infection is out of control and that the patient's condition is therefore serious.

Invasion of Pleura and Pericardium. The exact mechanism whereby pneumococci invade the pleura or pericardium is not known. As the lymphatics at the periphery of the lung drain outward toward the pleura, it is possible that pleural invasion results from lymphangitic spread. On the other hand, it is also possible that organisms are carred through the visceral pleura along with edema fluid that accumulates in infected subpleural alveoli. When infection of a pleural or pericardial cavity occurs, there results an outpouring of serous fluid followed by the deposit of fibrin. Later, leukocytes accumulate in the infected cavity, and, if infection persists, a purulent focus results. The pus in such cavities is at first thin but later becomes thick and stringy as a result not only of fibrin formation but also of the precipitation of deoxyribonucleic acid derived from the nuclei of disintegrating leukocytes. Finally, the thick fibrinous pus becomes walled off, forming loculated foci of chronic suppuration.

Similar purulent foci may occur in the meninges, peritoneum, or joints, as a result of hematogenous spread. Acute vegetations on the endocardium of the heart valves are sometimes encountered, and acute splenic tumor indicative of systemic infection is a common finding in fatal cases observed at necropsy. Degeneration of renal tubules is also occasionally noted, and, as identical changes can be produced in the kidneys of laboratory animals by repeated injections of killed pneumococci, the lesions are assumed to be of pneumococcal origin.

Mechanism of Recovery. *Surface Phagocytosis.* Owing to the antiphagocytic properties of their capsules, fully encapsulated, virulent pneumococci are resistant to phagocytosis when suspended in a fluid medium devoid of opsonins. In the presence of relatively immovable cellular surfaces, however, as in the alveoli, leukocytes are able to trap the encapsulated organisms and ingest them without the aid of opsonizing anti-

body (see figure). The efficiency of "surface phagocytosis," which operates also in the interstices of fibrin clots, is greatly enhanced when the leukocytes have accumulated in sufficient numbers to utilize each others' surfaces in the trapping process.

Heat-Labile Opsonins. Leukocytes in vivo are also assisted, right from the start of infection, by heat-labile opsonins that are present in normal mammalian plasma. These opsonins, which gain access to acute inflammatory exudates, are immunologically polyspecific, i.e., they act on all sorts of bacteria, in contrast to the monospecific anticapsular antibody that is eventually generated in the infected host (see below). Their opsonizing action on pneumococci has recently been shown to involve multiple components of the complement system, including C3. Its cleavage product, C3b, appears to act as a ligand between the organism on which it is deposited and the surface of the phagocyte.

Anticapsular Opsonins. Most patients with pneumococcal pneumonia, who survive long enough, eventually generate an excess of monospecific anticapsular antibody. As already stated, the process usually takes five to ten days. These newly formed immunoglobulins, when present in sufficient quantity, not only agglutinate the pneumococci in the edema zone of the lesion and thereby inhibit their spread, but also act as potent accessory opsonins and further increase the efficiency of phagocytosis. Their opsonizing action involves at least two sets of ligands between the organism and the phagocyte. The first is provided by the Fc fragment of the antibody molecule itself; the second results from fixation of complement by the antigen-antibody reaction in the capsule and the generation of the C3b ligands already mentioned. The potentiating effect of the combined ligands can be readily demonstrated in vitro.

Stages of Immunity. It is thus evident that, in the early phases of pneumococcal pneumonia, pneumococci in the lesions are destroyed by surface phagocytosis and by phagocytosis resulting from the polyspecific action of heat-labile opsonins. Only after the patient has been ill for a number of days do monospecific anticapsular immunoglobulins, also acting synergistically with heat-labile opsonins, play a significant role in recovery. The efficiency of the early cellular defense accounts for the prompt destruction of bacteria that occurs even in spreading pneumonic lesions. It likewise helps to explain why patients treated with antimicrobial drugs that are merely bacteriostatic often recover many hours before anticapsular antibodies can be detected in their blood.

Macrophage Reaction. The exact role of the "macrophage reaction" in the recovery process is not entirely clear. Because the appearance of macrophages in the alveolar exudate coincides in general with the disappearance of organisms from the lesion, it has long been assumed that these large mononuclear phagocytes take an active part in destroying the bacteria, and in the final analysis tip the scales in favor of the cellular defenses of the host. Studies relating to experimental lymphadenitis cast some doubt upon this assumption. The "macrophage reaction" in a regional lymph node draining an area of active infection can be artificially initiated at any stage of the nodal inflammation by merely cutting the afferent lymph vessels bringing bacteria to the node. Thus it appears that macrophages accumulate in the exudate only when the active stimulus of direct bacterial invasion has been eliminated. If this interpretation is correct, the polymorphonuclear leukocytes may be looked upon as the "shock troops" that play the major role in controlling the infection, whereas the macrophages serve primarily to remove the particulate debris from the resolving exudate and thus promote clearing of the lesion.

Resolution. One of the most remarkable features of pneumococcal pneumonia is the completeness with which it resolves. Even when several lobes are completely consolidated at the height of the illness, recovery usually results in restoration of the entire pulmonary parenchyma to its normal state within a few weeks. Not all the processes that take part in this dramatic resolution have been identified, but they appear to include (1) the action of cytolytic enzymes upon disintegrating leukocytes; (2) increased acidity of the exudate; (3) transport of cells from the lesion via lymphatics; and (4) phagocytosis and digestion of cellular debris by macrophages. The rarity with which tissue necrosis occurs in pneumococcal pneumonia, despite the violence of the inflammatory response, appears to account for the completeness of the healing. Occasionally recovery proceeds more slowly than usual and leads to "delayed resolution." The factors responsible for delaying the removal of exudate from the lesion in such cases are not known. In rare instances, as the result of irreversible damage to the pulmonary parenchyma, resolution fails to take place altogether, and the lesion becomes the site of intense fibroblastic activity that leads to the permanent scarring of "organized pneumonia."

Although resolution is usually complete in pneumococcal pneumonia, infection with type III pneumococcus may occasionally lead to pulmonary suppuration. This particular type of pneumococcus, in its most virulent form, has a large capsular "slime layer" that interferes with phagocytosis and accounts, at least in part, for its extraordinary pathogenicity. Type III pneumococci may accumulate in huge numbers in infected alveoli and on occasion cause necrosis, not only of leukocytes, but also of the alveolar walls. If the necrosis is sufficiently widespread, chronic lung abscesses result.

Suppurative Extrapulmonary Foci. Suppurative pneumococcal lesions, which usually occur in such extrapulmonary sites as the pleura, pericardium, meninges, joints, mastoids, or accessory sinuses, resolve much less readily, even with intensive chemotherapy, than does uncomplicated pneumococcal pneumonia. In such areas of suppuration, phagocytosis is relatively inefficient because most of the leukocytes in the exudate are not viable. In addition, antimicrobial drugs administered systemically probably do not penetrate subacute or chronic suppurating lesions as readily as they do areas of acute pneumonia. But even when a drug like penicillin reaches the organisms in a purulent focus, it usually does not destroy them; for pneumococci do not multiply rapidly in pus of long standing, and "resting" bacteria are not susceptible to the bactericidal action of penicillin. In fact, most purulent pneumococcal lesions respond satisfactorily only when chemotherapy is combined with some form of drainage that removes the bulk of the necrotic exudate.

Clinical Manifestations. **Symptoms.** Victims of pneumococcal pneumonia are often seriously ill when first seen. The degree of prostration may be such that an adequate history can be obtained only from the family or some other close associate of the patient. The story of a mild *nasopharyngitis* preceding by several days the onset of major symptoms is frequently elicited by careful questioning. The first distressing symptom is usually a *shaking chill* lasting for several minutes to a half hour. More than 80 per cent of patients with pneumococcal pneumonia experience one or more chills during the earliest stages of the disease. The initial rigor is often so violent as to cause the bed to shake and the patient's teeth to chatter. It is followed in about one case in three by vomiting. The exact cause of the initial chill is not known, but it usually coincides with bacterial invasion of the lung and marks the onset of fever. Several chills may occur at the start of pneumococcal pneumonia, but repeated attacks of rigor late in the disease suggest an extrapulmonary complication such as endocarditis or empyema.

Chest Pain. In approximately 70 per cent of cases severe chest pain occurs at the onset and may even precede the rigor. The pain, which is "stabbing" in character and is exaggerated by cough and respiration, is caused by inflammation of the pleura resulting from the characteristically peripheral location of the initial lesion. There may be local tenderness in the chest wall at the site of the pleurisy. When the diaphragmatic surfaces of the pleura are affected, the pain is referred either to the corresponding side of the lower chest wall and upper abdomen or to the shoulder, depending upon whether the peripheral (intercostal innervation) or central (phrenic innervation) part of the diaphragm is involved. The patient may gain some relief from the knifelike pain by lying on the affected side, thereby partially splinting that half of the thorax.

Cough. A cough may be absent at the onset, but usually is a prominent symptom during the course of the disease. Stimulation of the cough reflex results from irritation of the lower respiratory tract and from accumulation of mucus and exudate within the bronchial tree. Approximately 75 per cent of patients raise diffusely bloody or "rusty" sputum in contrast to "blood-streaked" sputum. The thorough mixing of the blood and mucus appears to be due to the fact that bleeding occurs directly into the alveolar exudate and thus constitutes an integral part of the inflammatory response to the infection. When the sputum is particularly sticky or jelly-like, type III pneumococcus or Klebsiella should be suspected as the cause of the pneumonia, because both these organisms produce, during growth, an inordinate amount of capsular polysaccharide that causes the exudate to be highly viscous.

Fever and Toxemia. Constant features of the disease are fever and toxemia, with the temperature usually ranging between 103 and 106° F. During the febrile period complaints of malaise, anorexia, weakness, myalgia, and general prostration are extremely common.

Physical Signs. Since pneumococcal pneumonia may occasionally progress with great rapidity and the general condition of the patient may deteriorate alarmingly within a few hours, it is essential that the initial physical examination be as thorough as possible.

The temperature, pulse rate, and respiratory rate are usually elevated by the time the patient seeks the aid of a physician. The temperature should be taken by rectum, because oral measurement with the subject breathing rapidly through the mouth is likely to be inaccurate. The pulse pressure is characteristically widened, as in any high fever, and the pulse at the wrist may be collapsing in quality. Subnormal blood pressure indicates shock and a poor prognosis.

Patients with well established pneumococcal pneumonia appear acutely ill. There is moderate to severe respiratory distress. The nostrils dilate with each inspiration. Paroxysms of hacking cough, often productive of bloody or rusty sputum, occur during the examination. The chest pain, which is usually unilateral, may be so severe as to interfere with the patient's breathing and coughing; in these circumstances grunting expiration results. The location of the pain indicates immediately the approximate site of at least part of the lesion. The patient occasionally appears apprehensive and may even be delirious.

The skin is usually hot and moist with beads of perspiration visible on the face and forehead. Cold extremities may indicate impending shock. Herpetic blisters are frequently noted about the mouth. The lips, mucous membranes, and nail beds are often cyanotic as a result of blood passing through poorly aerated lung. The cyanosis may be exaggerated by lowered respiratory exchange associated with rapid shallow breathing, often resulting from pleural pain. Icterus of the sclerae should be carefully looked for because of the prognostic significance of overt jaundice in pneumonia (see below). Only rarely are petechiae found in the skin of patients suffering from complicating pneumococcal endocarditis.

The ears should always be examined with an otoscope to exclude the presence of active otitis.

Tenderness over a mastoid process or over an accessory nasal sinus should also be noted. The presence of exudate in the pharynx or over the tonsils suggests the possibility of streptococcal pneumonia. Definite nuchal rigidity is usually indicative of pneumococcal meningitis, a serious complication of pneumonia. The neck veins must be carefully examined to detect the presence of increased venous pressure caused by complicating congestive heart failure. Deviation of the trachea constitutes an important sign of either atelectasis (toward the involved side) or pleural effusion (away from the involved side).

Examination of the Chest. The thorax must be examined with the utmost care. Diminished respiratory excursion or a slight inspiratory lag of one side of the chest often reveals the site of the principal lesion. A localized area of tenderness in the chest wall, noted during percussion, may be one of the earliest signs of pleural invasion. The presence of large pleural effusion sometimes causes a noticeable fullness of intercostal spaces. Careful percussion and auscultation do not always reveal signs of consolidation. In early cases, particularly, there may be no conclusive physical signs. Lesions at a distance from the chest wall are difficult to outline by percussion. Breath sounds may be only slightly depressed if normal lung tissue separates the lesion from the large bronchi. When consolidation is extensive, the typical findings of dullness to percussion, bronchial or tubular breath sounds, and fine crackling rales are easily elicited, except in the presence of complicating bronchial obstruction or extensive pleural effusion. A coarse "leathery" friction rub is frequently audible in the region of consolidation.

Examination of the heart may be difficult because of loud respiratory sounds. Its position and size should be carefully determined by palpation and percussion. A later shift in the position of the left cardiac border may indicate any one of the following complications: cardiac enlargement from heart failure, invasion of the pericardial cavity, atelectasis, or pleural effusion. An apical systolic murmur is frequently heard during high fever and is often of no significance, although it may be due to bacterial vegetation. Diastolic murmurs, on the other hand, arising from either the mitral or aortic valve are usually indicative of underlying organic heart disease or complicating pneumococcal endocarditis. A pericardial friction rub often constitutes the first sign of spread of the pneumococcal infection to the pericardial cavity. Ventricular premature contractions are not uncommon in the presence of any moderate or severe infection.

Abdominal Distention. Distention of the abdomen is frequently encountered in advanced bacterial pneumonia. When tympany is noted in the left axilla and left upper quadrant, acute gastrectasia should be suspected. Occasionally, the examiner will note rigidity and even tenderness in one or both upper quadrants of the abdomen, suggesting a subdiaphragmatic lesion. This sign is usually due to referred pain resulting from involvement of the parietal pleura over the outer part of the diaphragm. The right upper quadrant should be carefully examined for signs of enlargement or tenderness of the liver resulting from congestive heart failure.

In addition to edema from heart failure, the most important physical signs to be detected in the extremities are those of phlebothrombosis. As pulmonary infarction may closely resemble acute bacterial pneumonia, it is of the utmost importance to look for evidence of venous thrombosis of the legs.

The neurologic examination is rarely abnormal in pneumococcal pneumonia except in the presence of meningitis or brain abscess. Digital examination of the rectum may be postponed if the patient is acutely ill, but in women a sufficiently complete pelvic examination should be performed to rule out the possibility of an infected abortion, which often leads to metastatic bacterial pneumonia.

Laboratory Findings. The most important laboratory findings in pneumococcal pneumonia may be grouped under the following headings:

Findings Indicating the Presence of an Acute Infection. As in most acute bacterial infections, the total leukocyte count in pneumococcal pneumonia is elevated, and there is a "shift to the left" in the differential count; the erythrocyte sedimentation rate is also increased. The number of leukocytes in the peripheral blood during the active infection usually ranges from 15,000 to 40,000 per cubic millimeter; counts above 40,000 are occasionally encountered. Leukopenia (with a "shift to the left") is observed in fulminating pneumococcal infections, particularly in the presence of bacteremia.

Findings Indicating Pulmonary Consolidation. Although the presence and location of the pulmonary lesion can usually be determined by physical examination, confirmatory roentgenographic evidence is often helpful. Both posteroanterior and lateral views of the chest should be taken. The lateral film may be of great value in (1) detecting retrocardiac consolidation in the left lower lobe, (2) indicating whether a lesion visible in the posteroanterior view is located anteriorly or posteriorly and thus in what lobe it is situated, and (3) identifying interlobar accumulations of fluid. If the patient is too ill to be subjected to such a complete examination, a portable chest film should be taken at the bedside. Proper management of pneumococcal pneumonia in the home does not necessarily require roentgenographic examination.

Findings Indicating Etiology. Whenever the diagnosis of pneumococcal pneumonia is suspected, the patient's blood should be cultured. Anaerobic (candle jar) as well as aerobic cultures are recommended, as many strains of pneumococci grow best at an elevated CO_2 tension. A positive blood culture provides important information regarding both etiology and prognosis. The physician should also make a real effort to obtain a suitable specimen of sputum. Whenever possible, the patient should be made to expectorate mucus raised directly from the bronchial tree; secretions from the nasopharynx may be unsatisfactory. The specimen should be taken to the laboratory immediately to be cultured and smeared for Gram stain. Alphahemolytic, gram-positive cocci isolated on a culture should be reported as pneumococci only if shown to be bile soluble or sensitive to optochin. Because of the scarcity of type-specific antisera and the effectiveness of modern antimicrobial therapy, typing of pneumococci is now rarely performed. Neglect of this relatively simple procedure, however, deprives the attending physician of important information regarding prognosis (see Prognosis). When no sputum specimen can be obtained, particularly from a child, a throat swab may be cultured. Although it is not a hazardous procedure, lung puncture is now rarely used to determine the etiology of acute bacterial pneumonia.

Other laboratory examinations that may be of value in the management of the patient include blood electrolyte and urea determinations.

Clinical Course. During the course of the disease the patient should be examined carefully once a day. More frequent physical examinations may unduly exhaust an acutely ill subject. The common complications of pneumococcal pneumonia should be specifically looked for during each examination, particularly when fever persists.

Defervescence. The fever of untreated pneumococcal pneumonia may either terminate abruptly by "crisis" five to ten days after onset or may gradually subside by lysis. When effective antibacterial therapy is used, a dramatic crisis may occur within 24 hours, or the fever may persist for several days (see Antibacterial Therapy). Sometimes a slight secondary rise in temperature occurs after the crisis. Not only does defervescence often begin promptly after effective therapy, but the patient may experience a striking relief of symptoms and exhibit a noticeable improvement in appearance. Physical signs in the chest may also change, coarse sticky rales of resolution replacing the fine crepitant rales and tubular breath sounds of consolidation. Complete clearing of the pulmonary lesion may occur within a few days, but usually the auscultatory signs of resolution persist for a week or more after defervescence. If resolution is not complete within 21 days, it is arbitrarily classified as delayed. The promptness of defervescence and the speed of resolution are in general inversely proportional to the age and extent of the lesion at the time treatment is begun.

Crisis marking the start of recovery must be differentiated from the "pseudocrisis" occasionally noted at the onset of shock or at the time of interlobar spread of the infection. Although the temperature may fall precipitously during a pseudocrisis, the pulse rate remains elevated, and the patient's general condition fails to improve.

Relapse. Relapse may occur in pneumococcal pneumonia when chemotherapy is discontinued too soon. If fever, tachycardia, and other signs of active infection recur while the patient is still receiving intensive penicillin therapy, it may usually be assumed that a previously unrecognized purulent complication of the pneumococcal infection (such as empyema) exists, that a drug-resistant secondary invader has gained a foothold in the lung, or that hypersensitivity of the patient to penicillin has caused the development of drug fever.

Complications. The most common specific complication of pneumococcal pneumonia is pleurisy with effusion. In somewhat less than 10 per cent of cases fluid can be demonstrated in the pleural cavity by either physical or roentgenographic examination. Such effusions are usually small, and, when sterile, are rarely of significance. They result from inflammation of the pleura overlying the lesion in the lung. Occasionally they may be of sufficient volume to cause respiratory embarrassment and necessitate thoracentesis. Whenever pleural effusion is detected in a patient who has failed to respond promptly to treatment, a thoracentesis should be performed in order to determine whether the fluid is infected and thus represents an early empyema. Samples of the fluid obtained should be examined directly with bacterial stains and cultured both aerobically and anaerobically.

Empyema. Empyema, though less common than sterile pleural effusion, is far more serious. Before the advent of chemotherapy the incidence of this complication was approximately 5 per cent. With the present widespread use of penicillin, empyema is much less common (less than 2 per cent). Its presence is indicated by continued fever (often irregular), persistent leukocytosis, repeated sweats, and signs of pleural effusion. Localized tenderness is frequently noted in the chest wall overlying the site of the lesion. The exudate in the pleural cavity may become loculated by thick, fibrinous adhesions. If it is present in sufficient quantity, it may cause fullness of intercostal spaces and a shift of the trachea and mediastinum away from the side of the lesion. When the lesion is confined to an interlobar fissure or is located in the thoracic "gutter" adjacent to the spine, it may be detectable only by roentgenographic methods. Repeated exploratory thoracenteses, done preferably with the help of fluoroscopy, may be required to prove the presence of empyema. Its detection is of the greatest importance, because, once discovered, it is amenable to proper therapy; whereas, if left untreated, it may eventually drain exteriorly through the chest wall (empyema necessitatis) or rupture into a bronchus and cause a bronchopleural fistula. Rarely, empyema heals spontaneously, causing calcification of the pleura.

The fluid contained within an empyema cavity is at first thin, but soon becomes so thick and "stringy" that aspiration through a needle is difficult. The initial sample of exudate obtained by thoracentesis should always be subjected to bacteriologic study (see under Pleural Effusion), as identification of the offending organism is essential for proper treatment.

Meningitis and Endocarditis. Two serious, but now comparatively rare, complications of pneumococcal pneumonia that are often associated with one another are endocarditis and meningitis. Eighteen of nineteen cases of *pneumococcal endocarditis* described by Ruegesegger (1958) were complicated by the presence of meningitis. Endocardial infection, which occurs most commonly on the aortic valve, may be suggested by repeated chills, persistent fever, and leukocytosis, and the presence of a cardiac murmur. The diagnosis is established by the demonstration of persistent bacteremia. Only rarely does recovery occur without treatment. Equally serious is *pneumococcal meningitis* resulting from blood-borne metastasis to the meninges. Its presence is indicated by the usual manifestations of meningitis (headache, nausea and vomiting, stiff neck, positive Kernig's sign, stupor, and so forth), and the diagnosis is established by the demonstration of purulent cerebrospinal fluid containing pneumococci. The meningitis is characterized by the presence in the pia-arachnoid of a heavily infected exudate, which may cause subarachnoid block or may lead to localized subarachnoid abscesses. Unless vigorous therapy is instituted promptly, the prognosis is hopeless. Even when treatment is intensive, the patient may fail to recover, or (particularly if a child) may sustain permanent damage to the brain.

Pericarditis. Like the other complications of pneumococcal pneumonia, pericarditis has also become relatively rare since the introduction of potent antimicrobial drugs. When the pericardium is invaded, the patient usually experiences precordial pain, and a leathery friction rub may be heard over the heart. Pericardial effusion usually results, causing a "dampening" of the heart sounds. If the fluid is sterile, the condition is benign, unless so large a volume accumulates as to cause cardiac tamponade. Empyema of the pericardium, on the other hand, is a serious complication requiring prompt and vigorous treatment. If it is allowed to persist untreated, purulent pericarditis may gradually heal, but will often lead to pericardial calcification. Years later, serious constriction of the heart may result from contraction of the healed lesion.

Other Specific Complications. Still rarer specific complications include peritonitis and pyogenic arthritis. Occasionally the pulmonary lesion of pneumococcal pneumonia fails to resolve even after many weeks, and finally is replaced by fibrous tissue. This complication (organized pneumonia) rarely causes serious disability unless accompanied by suppuration.

Nonspecific Complications. Four nonspecific complications of importance occur frequently during the acute phase of pneumococcal pneumonia: acute dilatation of the stomach (gastrectasia), paralytic ileus, shock, and congestive heart failure. *Gastrectasia* and *ileus* occur particularly in patients suffering from anoxia and severe toxemia and give rise to gaseous distention of the abdomen (tympanites) that causes discomfort and often increases respiratory embarrassment. *Shock*, likewise, is a complication of severe toxemia and indicates a serious prognosis. Its incidence is increased in the presence of acute gastrectasia. The circulatory disturbance is characterized by hemoconcentration, a depressed cardiac output, and elevated peripheral resistance. Whether "toxic myocarditis" plays a role in the diminished cardiac output is uncertain. The skin, particularly of the extremities, is cold and moist and exhibits a characteristic gray cyanosis. Shock, when present for a sufficient length of time, becomes irreversible, and the patient eventually dies even though the infection in the meantime may have been adequately controlled by antimicrobial therapy. *Congestive heart failure,* which also occurs frequently as a complication of severe pneumonia, particularly in patients with underlying heart disease, must be differentiated from shock, because the proper methods of treating the two conditions are different. As congestive heart failure is an important predisposing factor in bacterial pneumonia, it is not surprising that they are often associated, and obviously both must be treated. The diagnosis of congestive heart failure in the presence of pneumonia may at times be difficult, but should be considered in any patient with abnormal distention of neck veins, peripheral edema, an enlarged tender liver, elevated venous pressure, and a prolonged circulation time. Pulmonary signs of congestion may be unreliable, particularly if the pneumonia is bilateral.

Jaundice, the pathogenesis of which appears to be related to lysis of the erythrocytes in the pneumonic lesion and depressed liver function resulting from anoxia, occurs most often in patients who have severe pneumonia and have had a poor diet. The presence of prominent icterus usually indicates a poor prognosis, and may be associated with chronic liver disease, e.g., cirrhosis. As in any bedridden patient, *phlebothrombosis* may occur during pneumonia. Its early presence should suggest the possibility that the pulmonary lesion is due to infarction of the lung rather than to primary pneumonia. *Herpes labialis* occurs in at least 10 per cent of patients with pneumococcal pneumonia and constitutes an essentially benign complication. Occasionally the herpetic lesions become secondarily infected, causing mild pyoderma.

Differential Diagnosis. The symptoms and signs of pneumococcal pneumonia are usually so characteristic as to make the diagnosis relatively simple. Atypical cases occasionally occur in which a definitive diagnosis cannot be made and in which antimicrobial treatment on suspicion is justified. Sometimes the disease is mistaken for less serious forms of respiratory tract infection, such as acute tracheobronchitis or "grippe." This error can often be avoided if proper significance is attached to the history of chills, bloody sputum, and chest pain, if the lungs are carefully examined at frequent intervals for signs of pulmonary consolidation, and if posteroanterior and lateral roentgenograms are made of the chest.

Pneumonia resulting from organisms other than pneumococcus may at times be difficult to differentiate from pneumococcal pneumonia. Only by bacteriologic study of the sputum can pneumonia caused by *Klebsiella pneumoniae* (Friedländer's bacillus), *Staphylococcus aureus,* or group A beta-hemolytic Streptococcus be identified. Tuberculous pneumonia rarely causes the acute prostration characteristic of coccal infection. *Mycoplasmal pneumonia* and other nonbacterial infections of the lungs, such as psittacosis and Q fever, do not often cause shaking chills, diffusely bloody sputum, severe pleural pain, or a marked leukocytosis, although they may at times by confused with acute bacterial pneumonia. Tularemic pneumonia and pneumonia caused by *H. influenzae* in young children must also be considered. When the diagnosis is in doubt, repeated examinations of the sputum should be made, using both the Gram and Ziehl-Neelsen stains. Sputum specimens should not only be cultured but should be injected into mice. Specific diagnosis of pneumonia is of great practical importance, because of therapy. Whereas tuberculous, tularemic, Klebsiella and *H. influenzae* pneumonia often respond to streptomycin, and the course of mycoplasmal pneumonia is favorably influenced by tetracyclines, most other forms of acute pneumonia (except that caused by penicillin-resistant staphylococci) are best treated with penicillin.

Nonpulmonary Bacterial Infections. Bacterial infections other than pneumonia must be considered in the differential diagnosis. Pleurisy involving the outer part of the diaphragm and resulting from right lower lobe pneumonia often causes referred pain to the right side of the abdomen, thus simulating acute appendicitis. Subdiaphragmatic abscess arising from perforation of the appendix conversely may simulate pneumonia. Acute pyelonephritis with chills, fever, flank pain, and leukocytosis must not be confused with pneumonia; the diagnosis is usually established by examination of the urine and by the absence of signs of frank consolidation in the lungs. Differentiation of acute pyelonephritis from pneumococcal pneumonia is of primary importance, as most urinary tract infections are caused by organisms not susceptible to penicillin.

Noninfectious Diseases. Among the essentially noninfectious processes that must be differentiated from pneumococcal pneumonia are congestive heart failure, pulmonary infarction, and atelectasis. That congestive heart failure predisposes to acute bacterial pneumonia has already been emphasized. The two conditions frequently coexist, but occasionally congestive heart failure is mistaken for pneumococcal pneumonia. This error is most frequently made in patients with dyspnea, cough, blood-streaked sputum, and signs in the chest that simulate those of consolidation, but in reality are due to compressed lung under a pleural effusion. In such cases the absence of high fever and leukocytosis and the presence of distended neck veins and peripheral edema usually suggest the correct diagnosis.

Pulmonary infarction, on the other hand, is

more difficult to differentiate from pneumonia. The dyspnea, pleural pain, hemoptysis, fever, physical signs of pulmonary consolidation, roentgenographic findings, and leukocytosis are all in keeping with an acute infection of the lungs. Frequently, however, the initial symptom is intense pleural pain of sudden onset; shaking chills rarely occur; there is no preceding history of respiratory infection; the fever is usually not high; frank hemoptysis is common; pulmonary signs, when present, appear early; and the total leukocyte count rarely reaches 20,000 per cubic millimeter. When a pulmonary infarct becomes infected, as sometimes happens, differentiation from primary bacterial pneumonia may be extremely difficult. Although in such cases the patients should receive antimicrobial treatment as in pneumonia, recognition of the infarction is of importance because of the need for anticoagulant therapy.

Pulmonary atelectasis, resulting from bronchial obstruction, not only may simulate pneumonia but often leads to serious infection of the lung if the bronchial obstruction is not relieved. Aspiration of mucus during or after surgical anesthesia is a common cause of atelectasis. Dyspnea, cough, chest pain, splinting of one side of the thorax, dullness to percussion, and suppressed breath sounds may all suggest primary pneumonia. Fever and leukocytosis also are noted when infection is present. As pulmonary atelectasis may be relieved by forced coughing and postural drainage or, if necessary by bronchoscopy, it is important to differentiate it from primary pneumonia. Occasionally, sufficient shift of the mediastinum occurs to make the diagnosis obvious. Collapse of a segment of the lung may also result from chronic bronchial obstruction caused by bronchogenic carcinoma or aortic aneurysm.

Even when the diagnosis of pneumococcal pneumonia is established beyond doubt, the possibility of a second underlying lesion of the lung must be borne in mind. Chronic obstructive pulmonary disease or lung abscess may lead to repeated attacks of bacterial pneumonia and often becomes evident only after the pneumonic consolidation has resolved. Bronchogenic carcinoma, as well as pulmonary tuberculosis, must also be looked for in the follow-up examination.

Treatment. The treatment of pneumococcal pneumonia may best be discussed under three headings: (1) antibacterial therapy, (2) supportive measures, and (3) the treatment of complications. Before the advent of effective antibacterial therapy, supportive treatment was of the greatest importance. The introduction, first, of antipneumococcal serum and, later, of sulfonamides, penicillin, and the other antimicrobial drugs has so altered the management of pneumococcal pneumonia that today supportive treatment is rarely crucial, and serious complications are only occasionally encountered.

Antibacterial Therapy. *Penicillin.* Penicillin is at present the drug of choice in the treatment of pneumococcal pneumonia. All strains of the organism are extremely susceptible to penicillin, and most are inhibited in broth culture by concentrations of less than 0.01 unit per milliliter. No mutants significantly resistant to penicillin have ever been recovered from patients with pneumonia.

The effectiveness of antimicrobial treatment is due in part to the natural resistance of the host, which accounts for the destruction of a large proportion of the invading bacteria. Host resistance, which results primarily from the activity of phagocytic cells in the lung, when combined with the bacteriostatic and bactericidal effects of drug therapy, controls promptly all but the most malignant pneumonia. Even with no treatment at all, approximately seven of every ten patients with pneumococcal pneumonia eventually recover, but some will have experienced a very severe illness before recovery has occurred.

Antipneumococcal therapy should be initiated promptly, therefore, in order to halt the spread of the infection both locally and through the blood stream. The most effective way of doing this is to give aqueous penicillin G by the intramuscular route in a dosage of 300,000 to 600,000 units two to four times in the first 24-hour period, depending upon the severity of the infection. The subsequent therapy should consist of aqueous procaine penicillin intramuscularly in a dosage of 300,000 to 600,000 units at 12-hour intervals. In severe infections it is safest to continue administration of the aqueous penicillin for 6 to 12 hours after the start of the procaine penicillin, and in the presence of shock, the aqueous penicillin should be given intravenously. Treatment should be maintained for at least one week or until the temperature has been normal for 72 hours; if treatment is discontinued too soon, relapse of the infection occurs.

Penicillin may also be given by mouth. When oral penicillin V is used, it should be given in a dosage of at least 250 mg. every six hours.

Response to penicillin therapy is often dramatic. Bacteremia, when present at the start of treatment, clears within a few hours. A crisis, characterized by rapid defervescence and a striking subsidence of symptoms, occurs in less than 96 hours in approximately half the patients. The other half experience a more gradual recovery, the temperature falling by lysis over a period of four to seven days. Frequently a secondary rise in temperature occurs after the crisis. This elevation is usually low-grade and subsides spontaneously within a few hours, or at most a few days. Such secondary fever must be distinguished from that caused by complications or continued pulmonary infection, and can usually be recognized by the fact that it is accompanied neither by symptoms of continued toxemia nor by significant leukocytosis.

When a patient fails to respond satisfactorily to penicillin therapy, three possible explanations should be considered: (1) that the patient is suffering from a serious complication such as empyema, endocarditis, meningitis, or pulmonary suppuration (possibly secondary to bronchogenic carcinoma); (2) that the primary infection is of non-pneumococcal origin and is due to an agent that is resistant to the antimicrobial action of penicillin, e.g., a penicillin-resistant strain of Staphylococcus or Klebsiella; or (3) that drug fever has developed as a result of penicillin hypersensitivity. Lack of response to penicillin cannot be explained on the basis of a penicillin-resistant strain of pneumococcus, because no such strains have ever been encountered in human pneumonia. Occasionally, patients will respond initially to treatment only to have unmistakable signs of persistent pneumonia subsequently develop, in spite of continued therapy This sequence of events is usually due to the presence of a mixed infection, the initial response to treatment resulting from control of penicillin-susceptible organisms, and the relapse occurring as a result of persistence of a penicillin-resistant species. Re-examination of the sputum and modification of the antimicrobial therapy is immediately indicated. Patients with underlying chronic pulmonary disease are particularly prone to such mixed infections.

Toxic reactions to penicillin are rarely of sufficient severity to warrant discontinuation of treatment. Urticaria may be bothersome, and a combination of symptoms and signs suggesting "serum sickness" occasionally occurs. Patients with dermatophytosis may experience an exacerbation of the lesions during penicillin therapy. Persons giving a history of having had a severe penicillin reaction in the past should, of course, not be treated with penicillin.

Other Antimicrobial Drugs. The tetracycline drugs may be used in the treatment of acute bacterial pneumonia. When the diagnosis of pneumococcal pneumonia is not clearly established, it may be advisable to use one of the tetracyclines (0.5 gram by mouth every six hours) because of their broader antibacterial action and their beneficial effect in mycoplasmal pneumonia. However, it should be remembered that pneumococcal mutants resistant to tetracyclines (as well as to erythromycin and lincomycin) are being encountered with increasing frequency. Staphylococcal enteritis also may result from the use of "broad-spectrum" drugs such as the tetracyclines, and if not promptly treated may be fatal. Erythromycin is about as effective as penicillin and should be used (0.3 to 0.5 gram every six hours) to treat patients with a history of penicillin allergy or when the lesion is suspected of harboring penicillin-resistant staphylococci. In the latter situation, methicillin (1.0 gram intramuscularly every four hours), cloxacillin (0.25 to 0.50 gram intramuscularly every six hours), or cephalothin (1.0 to 2.0 grams intramuscularly or intravenously every four hours) may also be used.

Supportive Treatment. Patients suffering from pneumococcal pneumonia should be kept at bed rest, and visitors to the sick room should be limited to the immediate family. Pleural pain, if mild, may be treated with codeine sulfate (30 to 60 mg.) orally, and, if severe, with subcutaneous morphine sulfate (10 to 15 mg.), an equivalent analgesic such as methadone hydrochloride (5 to 10 mg., subcutaneously), or intercostal nerve block. A tight chest-binder is sometimes helpful in providing "something to cough against." Restlessness and insomnia, which are most commonly associated with delirium, are best controlled by chloral hydrate (1 to 1.5 grams by mouth) or by paraldehyde (4 to 12 ml. by mouth or 10 to 20 ml. in 20 to 30 ml. of olive oil by rectum). Dyspnea and cyanosis should be treated with oxygen, administered by tent (40 to 60 per cent oxygen) or by nasal catheter (35 to 50 per cent oxygen, when gas is delivered at 4 to 7 liters per minute). Oxygen masks are usually unsuitable because of the patient's cough and expectoration.

Fluid and Electrolytes. During the acute state of pneumococcal pneumonia considerable fluid is lost from the body, chiefly through the skin as the result of high fever. Dehydration may develop rapidly and, if severe, may become a contributing factor in the development of shock. Most patients require between 3 and 4 liters of fluid and 6 to 10 grams of sodium chloride a day when the fever is high. In the presence of congestive heart failure the use of supplementary sodium chloride is, of course, contraindicated. In the absence of renal disease, glycosuria or congestive heart failure, the patient's state of hydration may be estimated by the specific gravity of the urine. When hydration is adequate, the specific gravity should remain below 1.020.

Diet. Many patients with pneumococcal pneumonia are too ill to tolerate a full diet and should receive only liquids during the height of the fever. Fruit juices, ginger ale, and soups are well tolerated After the crisis a regular diet may be prescribed.

The patient should be kept in bed until the temperature is approximately normal and should be observed closely until the pneumonic lesion has resolved. As already emphasized, all patients should be subjected to a follow-up roentgenographic examination three to four weeks after recovery.

Treatment of Complications. *Shock.* Patients with peripheral vascular collapse (shock) resulting from severe pneumococcal pneumonia usually respond poorly to the accepted forms of antishock therapy. The prognosis is almost invariably grave when this complication develops. Oxygen therapy should be begun immediately, even if cyanosis is absent. Norepinephrine is one of the best drugs available for combating the hypotension of shock. It should be given continuously by intravenous drip in sufficient amounts to maintain the systolic pressure at levels between 100 and 110. Enough norepinephrine (one vial contains 4 mg.) must be added to each liter of salt solution so that the hypotension can be controlled by the administration of not more than 2000 to 3000 ml. of fluid in 24 hours. Aramine may be similarly employed. Hydrocortisone given intravenously is also of value (500 to 1000 mg. during the first 24 hours, with daily dose decreased thereafter to 50 or 100 mg.). These measures should be used only with the greatest caution if signs of congestive heart failure are also present. The treatment of congestive heart failure in patients with pneumococcal pneumonia is essentially the same as that of heart failure under other conditions (see Treatment of Congestive Heart Failure).

Abdominal Distention. Abdominal distention is best managed by the use of gastric suction, daily enemas, the insertion of a rectal tube, the administration of oxygen, and repeated hypodermic injections of Prostigmin methylsulfate (0.5 mg.). The Prostigmin injections should be repeated every hour until a definite effect is obtained; subsequent doses should be spaced at intervals of two to four hours and maintained as long as is necessary.

Delirium. Delirium may sometimes be difficult to control, particularly in patients with a history of chronic alcoholism. The use of 30 to 90 ml. of whiskey per day may quiet alcoholic patients during the acute phase of the disease. The safest hypnotic to use is paraldehyde. A restraining net over the bed is often required to prevent the patient from climbing out of bed and injuring himself.

Empyema and Pericarditis. For the reasons already discussed under Mechanisms of Recovery: Suppurative Extrapulmonary Foci, the treatment of established empyema and persistent pericarditis is primarily surgical. During World War I, Graham demonstrated (1918) that open thoracotomy must always be delayed until the pus aspirated from the chest is relatively thick and the area of infection is sufficiently well walled off to prevent marked shift of the mediastinum. Since the advent of penicillin, cases of both empyema and pericarditis have been successfully treated by repeated aspiration and injection of aqueous penicillin (50,000 to 200,000 units daily) through either a thoracentesis needle or a thoracotomy tube (closed drainage). When these measures are not effective, open surgical drainage with continued systemic antimicrobial therapy should be instituted.

The treatment of the remaining two major complications of pneumococcal pneumonia, namely, meningitis and endocarditis, are discussed elsewhere (see Meningitis and Bacterial Endocarditis).

Prognosis. The case fatality rate in untreated pneumococcal pneumonia ranges from 20 to 40 per cent. The widespread use of sulfonamide drugs in the late 1930's resulted in a lowering of the fatality rate among treated patients to approximately 10 per cent. Penicillin therapy has lowered the rate still further. At present approximately 95 per cent of patients with pneumococcal pneumonia recover when properly treated with penicillin.

The prognosis in pneumococcal pneumonia is influenced adversely by each of the following: (1) old age (and also infancy), (2) late treatment, (3) infection with certain types of pneumococci (particularly types II and III), (4) involvement of more than one lobe of the lung, (5) leukopenia, (6) occurrence of bacteremia, (7) jaundice, (8) the presence of complications (notably shock and meningitis), (9) pregnancy (particularly in the third trimester), (10) the presence of other disease such as heart disease or cirrhosis of the liver, and (11) alcoholic intoxication and delirium tremens. Through a consideration of these factors a rough estimate may be made of the severity of the infection in each case, and therapy may be modified accordingly.

Even with the most intensive penicillin treatment a significant number of patients will die of pneumococcal pneumonia. A recent study, for example, has revealed that in patients destined, at the onset of illness, to die within five days (because of complicating disease, old age, etc.) penicillin therapy has little, if any effect. Similarly, the case fatality rate in type III pneumococcal pneumonia with bacteremia still exceeds 50 per cent regardless of treatment.

Prevention. Because pneumococcal pneumonia is not highly contagious and usually responds promptly to early therapy, prophylaxis constitutes less of a problem than in many other infectious diseases. It is estimated that only one in every 500 persons of all ages in the United States may be expected to contract the disease in any one year. In certain closed communities, however, and in areas where the pneumococcal carrier rate is particularly high, epidemics occasionally occur. Under such conditions, immunization with pneumococcal polysaccharide may be indicated. During World War II, the effectiveness of polyvalent pneumococcal vaccine in preventing pneumonia and in lowering the pneumococcal carrier rate was clearly demonstrated in a controlled experiment on Army personnel. Although immunization may prove to be of value in military medicine, its application to the general population is not indicated because the incidence of the disease in ordinary circumstances is too low to justify vaccination. For persons at especially high risk, however, because of age or chronic systemic disease, particularly of the heart or lungs, its use would seem justified.

Although pneumococcal pneumonia can undoubtedly be prevented (or at least aborted) in many patients by the intensive treatment of every upper respiratory tract infection with antimicrobial drugs, their indiscriminate use for this purpose should be avoided. The possible inconvenience to the patient of hypersensitivity reactions and the theoretical danger of favoring drug-resistant strains of bacteria outweigh the advantages to be gained in preventing such a relatively uncommon and readily treatable disease as pneumococcal pneumonia. Such chemoprophylaxis during outbreaks of epidemic influenza, on the other hand, might conceivably be indicated (see Influenza).

Patient Isolation. The cross-infection rate in pneumococcal pneumonia is low and patients receiving chemotherapy are probably not highly infectious. The danger of cross-infection in a general hospital, particularly among patients with congestive heart failure, pulmonary edema, or other severe debilitating diseases, may be greater than in the general population, and care should be taken to protect them from exposure.

Austrian, C. R., and Austrian, R.: Pneumococcal pneumonia (lobar pneumonia). In: Tice's Practice of Medicine. Hagerstown, Md., W. F. Prior Co., Inc., 1959, vol. 1, p. 1.

Austrian, R., and Gold, J.: Pneumococcal bacteremia with especial reference to bacteremic pneumococcal pneumonia. Ann. Intern. Med., 60:759, 1964.

Heffron, R.: Pneumonia with Special Reference to Pneumococcus Lobar Pneumonia. New York, Commonwealth Fund, 1939.

Johnston, R. B., Klemperer, M. R., Alper, C. A., and Rosen, F. S.: The enhancement of bacterial phagocytosis by serum: The role of complement components and two co-factors. J. Exp. Med., 129:1275, 1969.

Shin, H. S., Smith, M. R., and Wood, W. B., Jr.: Heat labile opsonins to pneumococcus. II. Involvement of C3 and C5. J. Exp. Med., 130:1229, 1969.

Wood, W. B.: Studies on The Cellular Immunology of Acute Bacterial Infections. The Harvey Lectures, Series 47, 1951-52.

Wood, W. B., and Smith, M. R.: An experimental analysis of the curative action of penicillin. J. Exp. Med., 103:487, 1956.

KLEBSIELLA AND OTHER GRAM-NEGATIVE BACTERIAL PNEUMONIAS

Jay P. Sanford

The combination of improved identification of gram-negative bacilli by diagnostic laboratories and the increased frequency of their isolation from clinical specimens has resulted in a striking increase in recognition of various gram-negative bacilli as serious human pathogens. Previously, procedures for the identification of gram-negative bacilli were primarily designed to enable rapid detection of Salmonella and Shigella from fecal specimens and Klebsiella from sputum specimens, with a lumping of the remaining organisms as "coliforms." Today, members of three families of aerobic gram-negative bacteria (Enterobacteriaceae, Pseudomonaceae, and Achromobacteraceae) have been recognized as potential pulmonary pathogens. The family Enterobacteriaceae is composed of numerous interrelated bacilli, all of which are gram-negative, are nonsporing, grow on ordinary media, and rapidly ferment glucose. The following genera are included in the family: Shigella, Escherichia, Salmonella, Arizona, Citrobacter, Edwardsiella, Klebsiella, Enterobacter (formerly Aerobacter), Hafnia, Serratia, Proteus, and Providence. Whereas the Enterobacteriaceae have received considerable attention, the nonfermenting aerobic gram-negative bacilli are being recognized with increased frequency. Organisms that fall into this category include genera in the families Pseudomonadaceae and Achromobacteraceae. The following organisms are included in these families: Mima polymorpha, Herellea vaginicola (Bacterium anitratum), Flavobacterium spp., Alcaligenes spp., Pseudomonas aeruginosa, Pseudomonas pseudomallei, Pseudomonas maltophilia, Aeromonas hydrophilia, and organisms that are as yet unclassified but grouped together and designated by cultural characteristics, such as "eugonic oxidizer, Group 1 (EO-1)."

Pulmonary infections associated with the small aerobic gram-negative bacilli belonging to the genera Bordetella, Brucella, Hemophilus, and Pasteurella and nonsporulating anaerobic gram-negative bacilli, e.g., Bacteroides, Spherophorus, Dialister, will be discussed in other articles. Likewise, infections caused by Pseudomonas pseudomallei (melioidosis) are presented elsewhere (see Melioidosis).

PNEUMONIA DUE TO KLEBSIELLA PNEUMONIAE (FRIEDLÄNDER'S PNEUMONIA)

In 1882, Friedländer first cultivated the organism now designated as Klebsiella pneumoniae from the lungs of patients who had died of pneumonia. Although he considered it to be the etiologic agent in most cases of pneumonia, four years later the pneumococcus was described and established as the predominant etiologic agent in lobar pneumonia. Consequently for many years Klebsiella pneumoniae (Friedlander's bacillus) was thought to be only a secondary invader. It is now recognized that a small but definite percentage, 0.5 to 5.0 per cent, of primary pneumonias are due to Klebsiella pneumoniae. This historical background is of interest because it reflects the current disagreements regarding the role of other gram-negative bacilli as primary pulmonary pathogens.

Bacteriology. Klebsiella pneumoniae are encapsulated gram-negative bacilli that belong to the family Enterobacteriaceae. Members of the family can be readily differentiated by means feasible in clinical laboratories. The commonly used triple sugar agar slants, IMViC reactions, and urea or phenylalanine deaminase tests are adequate to place most cultures within a group; 99 per cent of Klebsiella ferment lactose and are typically citrate positive, indole and methyl red negative and usually Voges-Proskauer positive. Following these biochemical tests, which group Klebsiella-Enterobacter and Serratia, motility is an effective means of separating Klebsiella, which are nonmotile, from other members of the group, which are typically motile. Other useful tests include positive lysine and negative arginine and ornithine decarboxylase tests and inability to liquefy gelatin. Susceptibility to relatively high concentrations of cephalothin (50 μg. per milliliter) is seen with 90 per cent of Klebsiella, whereas most strains of Enterobacter and Serratia are resistant. Because drug-susceptibility patterns are subject to change with the use of different antimicrobial agents, this criterion is probably of less diagnostic value. Strains of Klebsiella can be further characterized by type-specific capsular antisera, with at least 77 capsular types described to date. Recent studies have demonstrated that types 1 through 6 are no more frequent in respiratory diseases than are the higher serotypes, in contrast to the older concept that most cases of primary Klebsiella pneumonia are due to type 1 Klebsiella. Capsular typing is not of aid in predicting virulence, but represents a valuable epidemiologic tool.

Pathogenicity. Klebsiella may persist in the oropharynx of normal persons, although the prevalence is low, 1 to 6 per cent. There is no tendency for contacts to acquire the organism from a carrier, and Bloomfield was unable to implant organisms in the pharynx of healthy volunteers. Yet the prevalence in pharyngeal cultures increases to 8 to 23 per cent in hospitalized subjects. Pulmonary infections arise most likely from the inhalation or aspiration of organisms from the oropharynx during circumstances when the major pulmonary antibacterial defense mechanisms, the mucociliary blanket, or alveolar macrophages are compromised.

The pathogenesis of experimental Klebsiella pneumonia is similar to that of encapsulated type 1 pneumococcal pneumonia. The outer margin of the spreading lesion is characterized by an edema zone in which the alveoli are filled with fluid containing many bacteria (see illustration in article immediately preceding). The organisms multiply freely in the fluid, and are carried mechanically into adjacent alveoli through the pores of Cohn. Phagocytosis is noticeable only in the central zone of consolidation where alveoli are packed with leukocytes, thus allowing "surface phagocytosis." Three differences in experimental Klebsiella pneumonia in comparison with type 1 pneumococcal pneumonia are (1) greater numbers of Klebsiella in the areas of consolidation, (2) destruction of alveolar walls, and (3) organization with fibroblastic activity.

Klebsiella pulmonary infections are usually classified as primary, i.e., infection developing in a patient without underlying disease, or secondary. The demarcation between primary and secondary is often indistinct, as classic primary Klebsiella pneumonia usually occurs in patients with underlying conditions such as alcoholism, chronic obstructive airway disease (emphysema-fibrosis), or diabetes mellitus. Operationally, infections may be considered as primary if Klebsiella are isolated from specimens obtained when the patient first seeks medical aid. The designation "secondary" is then applied to those infections that represent either superinfection of an underlying infection or are opportunistic in origin.

Predisposing Factors. In patients with primary pneumonia, males heavily predominate (80 to 90 per cent), most infections occurring in middle-aged and older patients (average age being the mid-50's). The most common co-existing disease is alcoholism (66 per cent). The few series in which alcoholism is not frequent are drawn from predominantly Negro populations. Both chronic bronchopulmonary disease and to a lesser extent diabetes mellitus appear to predispose patients to Klebsiella pneumonia.

Pathology. The involvement in fatal primary Klebsiella pneumonia is most often lobar, but may be lobular or a combination of the two. An upper lobe is most commonly involved. The pleural surface is covered by a fibrinous exudate and adhesions form early. Empyema is appreciably more frequent than in pneumococcal pneumonia, probably occurring in one fifth to one quarter of cases. Microscopically in the acute stage, the alveolar walls are congested. Usually the alveoli are filled with an exudate composed of a mixture of polymorphonuclear and mononuclear cells, with a predominance of the former. In rare cases, mononuclear cells may predominate. There is often necrosis of alveolar walls, with abscess formation. Other findings at autopsy may include extrapulmonary sites of dissemination, e.g. pericarditis or meningitis. Evidence of alcoholic hepatosis and alcoholic cirrhosis is common.

Clinical Manifestations and Course. Based upon clinicobacteriologic findings, Klebsiella infections can be classified as primary or secondary (as defined under Pathogenicity); pure or mixed, depending upon whether Klebsiella are isolated as the predominant organism or associated with other organisms, especially other gram-negative bacilli; and acute or chronic.

Primary Klebsiella Pneumonia. The "classic" clinical pattern is that of acute primary Klebsiella pneumonia. As with pneumococcal pneumonia, the onset is usually sudden (90 per cent), associated with cough productive of sputum (90 per cent), pleuritic chest pain (80 per cent), and true rigors (60 per cent). Early prostration is a usual feature. Occasionally the acute onset is preceded by an undifferentiated upper respiratory infection and cough. Rarely epigastric pain and vomiting are the initial symptoms. The characteristic sputum has been described as a nonputrid homogeneous thick mixture of blood and mucus, often brick red in color, which is sufficiently thick to be expectorated with difficulty. This typical sputum is seen in one quarter to three quarters of patients. In some patients the sputum is thin, resembling currant jelly, although in most it is either blood tinged or rusty. Frank hemoptysis may occur. On examination, patients appear acutely ill, febrile, dyspneic, and often cyanotic. Although temperatures are often said to be less than those observed with pneumococcal pneumonia, two thirds are between 102 and 104° F. Tachycardia coincides with the fever. Chest examination typically reveals signs of pulmonary consolidation; there may be loss of lung volume as manifested by decreased size and expansion of the involved hemithorax and diaphragmatic elevation. Auscultation may reveal suppressed breath sounds with few rales, even with advanced consolidation. Involvement of more than one lobe is frequent (in two thirds of patients) with a predilection for upper lobes.

Laboratory and Roentgenographic Findings. Peripheral leukocyte counts range from marked leukopenia to leukocytosis, leukopenia and neutropenia being poor prognostic signs. In one quarter of patients the total leukocyte count may be in the normal range. On sputum culture, either gram-negative bacilli other than Klebsiella or pneumococci often may be isolated. A mixed sputum flora containing other gram-negative bacilli such as *Pseudomonas spp.* is especially common in secondary infections. In the prechemotherapeutic era, blood cultures were positive in about 15 per cent of cases during the course of the illness. At present, a pulmonary source is still often incriminated in patients with Klebsiella bacteremia. This is unusual in other types of gram-negative bacillary bacteremia, in which the urinary tract usually represents the major primary source.

The roentgenographic features are variable, and include massive lobar consolidation, lobular involvement, lung abscess formation with either multiple small thin-walled or large abscess cavities, and residual parenchymal fibrosis. Bulging of a fissure, sharp advancing borders of the infiltrates, and abscess formation occur with greater frequency than in other types of pneumonia. The pneumonic infiltrate is relatively dense, but shadows of similar density are seen with other types of pneumonia. Bronchopneumonic distribution is less usual but can occur, and even bilateral perihilar infiltrates are reported. The diagnostic usefulness for any given roentgenographic configuration has been questioned; however, in many instances a correct diagnosis can be suggested from the roentgenogram.

Complications. Rapid destruction of pulmonary tissue with suppuration or residual fibrosis occurs in as many as half of the surviving patients. Necrosis may occur within 24 to 48 hours, and abscess formation may be recognized within four days. Other less common pulmonary complications include pleural effusion and pneumothorax. In the past, activation of quiescent pulmonary tuberculosis has been reported.

The course of illness is not marked by an unusual propensity for extrapulmonary manifestations, but they can occur, and include pericarditis, meningitis, gastroenteritis, erythematous skin rashes, and nonsuppurative polyarthritis.

Prognosis and Treatment. In the pre-antimicrobial era, the case mortality of Klebsiella pneumonia ranged from 51 to 97 per cent. With the advent of drug therapy, the various tetracycline derivatives, streptomycin, and chloramphenicol were found to have an excellent in vitro effect, and clinical use resulted in a marked decrease in mortality in most series. In some series, the mortality remains nearly 50 per cent; in these there has been a predominance of severely ill alcoholic patients, although good results have been reported even in this group. Analysis of the mode of death frequently reveals inadequate removal of tenacious pulmonary secretions to be a significant factor. The correlation of blood stream invasion and fatality is frequently close.

In vitro studies reveal the majority of strains of Klebsiella to be susceptible to cephalothin, chloramphenicol, colistimethate, gentamicin, kanamycin, and polymyxin B. The antimicrobial regimen of choice is often varied according to the gravity of the acute clinical situation and the extent of underlying problems. In less seriously ill patients, cephalothin or gentamicin is preferable, but in patients with life-threatening infections combination therapy, e.g., cephalothin and kanamycin or gentamicin, is usually employed. Meticulous measures directed at supportive care, maintenance of clear airways, adequate but not excessive ventilation and oxygenation, adequate fluid and electrolyte replacement, and often control of delirium tremens are essential.

PNEUMONIA DUE TO AEROBIC GRAM-NEGATIVE BACILLI OTHER THAN KLEBSIELLA PNEUMONIAE

The large number of bacterial species other than *Klebsiella pneumoniae* that belong to the families Enterobacteriaceae, Pseudomonaceae, and Achromobacteraceae are considered together because of the similarities in their abilities to produce pulmonary infection.

Until recently the over-all frequency of pneumonia caused by gram-negative bacilli other than Klebsiella received relatively little attention. The reports of Tillotson and Lerner constitute the best analyses of the over-all problem. Between 1963 and 1965, 4.3 per cent of all pneumonias of patients admitted to the Detroit General Hospital were considered to be caused by gram-negative bacilli (82 episodes, 78 of which were classified as primary). Among these gram-negative bacillary pneumonias, the following organisms were encountered: Klebsiella Enterobacter, *Escherichia coli*, *Pseudomonas spp.*, Bacteroides, Proteus, *H. influenzae*, and Achromobacter. In addition, in many hospitals other gram-negative organisms such as nonpigmented *Serratia marcescens* are being encountered, especially in hospital-associated secondary pneumonias. Thus, it appears that collectively gram-negative bacilli other than Klebsiella may be as prevalent as Klebsiella in causing primary pneumonia and even more common in secondary hospital-acquired pneumonias.

Predisposing Factors. As with primary Klebsiella pneumonia, in primary pneumonias caused by these other agents, older males are more often affected. Underlying disease conditions occur in almost all patients; these include renal disease, diabetes mellitus, and chronic bronchopulmonary disease.

Infections are most likely to occur in patients who are receiving inhalation therapy that incorporates reservoir nebulization and who are also receiving antimicrobial therapy. Adrenocortical steroids, immunosuppressive agents, and tracheostomy may also be predisposing factors. However, such infections may occur in patients who are not receiving inhalation therapy, as these organisms are ubiquitous and appear with increased frequency in seriously ill patients.

Pathology. On microscopic section, bronchopneumonia with confluent microabscesses is seen. The intra-alveolar inflammatory exudate is mixed polymorphonuclear leukocytic and mononuclear. With infection caused by *E. coli* and Pseudomonas, however, the cellular infiltrates may consist predominantly of mononuclear cells admixed with fragmented pyknotic nuclei of necrotic neutrophils. At a later stage, alveolar spaces are filled with a deeply basophilic granular material containing large macrophage-like cells and dense colonies of gram-negative bacilli.

When caused by Pseudomonas, in the areas of an abscess there is often focal hemorrhage. The dominant microscopic lesion is that of alveolar septal necrosis. In association with these necrotizing lesions, necrosis of arterial walls and secondary thrombosis of vessels have been encountered when the Pseudomonas pneumonia was of bacteremic origin or associated with nebulization therapy equipment. With the primary Pseudomonas pneumonia reported by Tillotson and Lerner, the vascular involvement was not a feature. The Pseudomonas "eugonic oxidizer, Group 1 (EO-1)" was also associated with a necrotizing granulomatous pneumonia. With the other non-Klebsiella gram-negative bacilli, alveolar septal necrosis is not a usual feature.

Clinical Features and Course. The clinical features are similar to those observed in patients with primary Klebsiella pneumonia, except that hemoptysis is unusual.

In patients with Pseudomonas pneumonia, apprehension, toxicity, confusion, and progressive cyanosis are characteristic. Relative bradycardia may occur. Alteration in diurnal temperature patterns with the peak temperature in early morning was noted by Tillotson and Lerner. The physical signs over the thorax are not characteristic. The development of empyema and bronchopleural fistulas is common (80 per cent). Roentgenograms reveal bilateral bronchopneumonic nodular infiltrates that may undergo necrosis.

Primary *E. coli* pneumonia tends to present as a bronchopneumonic process in the lower lobes. The pulse is proportional to the temperature. Early findings include rales without consolidation. Empyema formation is less common than with Klebsiella or Pseudomonas.

Proteus species also produce a clinical picture similar to Klebsiella, with fever, chills, dyspnea, pleuritic chest pain, and cough productive of purulent sputum. Signs of consolidation are usual. Roentgenograms reveal dense infiltrates in the posterior segment of an upper lobe or superior segment of the right lower lobe. Progression to lung abscess or empyema is common.

Serratia infections, which are almost always secondary, have been associated with the clinical oddity "pseudohemoptysis" owing to the red pigment prodigiosin produced by some strains of *Serratia marcescens*. Other features may include abscess formation or empyema, or both.

Clinical experience with the other bacterial genera such as Hafnia, Flavobacterium, Mima, and Herellea, is limited, but other characteristics suggest that their clinical features are similar to secondary Klebsiella infections.

Laboratory Findings. The usual laboratory findings such as leukocyte counts are of little help, being either normal or moderately increased. Cultures of sputum or even tracheal aspirations are only of moderate help, because these organisms are frequently present as commensals in patients who are receiving antimicrobial therapy or in those who are critically ill. Quantitative culture of sputum is of assistance; large numbers of bacteria are more suggestive of superinfection than colonization. With empyema, thoracentesis with staining and culture of the fluid will confirm the diagnosis and facilitate the selection of optimal therapy.

Prognosis and Treatment. Prognosis varies with the type of organism as well as with the underlying condition of the patient. Mortality rates in the range of 80 per cent are not uncommon with Pseudomonas pneumonia, whereas they are generally lower with the other organisms.

The antimicrobial regimen of choice must be selected according to antimicrobial susceptibilities anticipated in a given community. In general, *Pseudomonas aeruginosa* and *E. coli* are most susceptible to carbenicillin, colistimethate, gentamicin, and polymyxin B. *Serratia marcescens* and *Proteus spp.* are resistant to colistimethate and polymyxin B, and most susceptible to gentamicin and kanamycin. *Enterobacter spp.* are susceptible to colistimethate, kanamycin, gentamicin, and polymyxin B, but are resistant to cephalothin. Susceptibility of Enterobacter to carbenicillin is quite variable. As with Klebsiella pneumonia, in pneumonias caused by these other gram-negative bacilli, meticulous attention to supportive care is as important as the antimicrobial therapy.

Bloomfield, A. L.: The fate of bacteria introduced into the upper air passages. V. The Friedländer bacilli. Bull. Hopkins Hosp., 31:203, 1920.

Dailey, R. H., and Benner, E. J.: Necrotizing pneumonitis due to the pseudomonad "eugonic-oxidizer-group 1." New Eng. J. Med., 279:361, 1968.

Edmondson, E. B., and Sanford, J. P.: The klebsiella-enterobacter (aerobacter)-serratia group. Medicine, 46:323, 1967.

Felson, B., Rosenberg, L. S., and Hamburger, M. J.: Roentgen findings in acute Friedländer's pneumonia. Radiology, 53:559, 1949.

Hyde, L., and Hyde, B.: Primary Friedländer pneumonia. Amer. J. Med. Sci., 205:660, 1943.

Jervey, L. P., Jr., and Hamburger, M.: The treatment of acute Friedlaender's bacillus pneumonia. Arch. Intern. Med. (Chicago), 99:1, 1957.

Manfredi, F., Daly, W. J., and Behnke, R. H.: Clinical observations of acute Friedländer pneumonia. Ann. Intern. Med., 58:642, 1963.

Pierce, A. K., Edmondson, E. B., McGee, G., Ketchersid, J., Loudon, R. G., and Sanford, J. P.: An analysis of factors predisposing to gram-negative bacillary necrotizing pneumonia. Amer. Rev. Resp. Dis., 94:309, 1966.

Pierce, A. K., Sanford, J. P., Thomas, G. D., and Leonard, J. S.: Long-term evaluation of decontamination of inhalation-therapy equipment and the occurrence of necrotizing pneumonia. New Eng. J. Med., 282:528, 1970.

Tillotson, J. R., and Lerner, A. M.: Characteristics of pneumonia caused by *Escherichia coli*. New Eng. J. Med., 277:115, 1967.

Tillotson, J. R., and Lerner, A. M.: Characteristics of non-bacteremic pseudomonas pneumonia. Ann. Intern. Med., 68:295, 1968.

STREPTOCOCCAL DISEASES

GENERAL CONSIDERATIONS
Gene H. Stollerman

Streptococci constitute a large, heterogeneous group of bacteria that parasitize man. The most simple classification of these organisms, and the one most useful for clinical purposes, is based on their action on blood agar plates. *Beta* hemolytic streptococci are those that produce a completely clear zone around the colony as a result of the formation of either or both extracellular hemolysins, streptolysin O and streptolysin S. The *alpha* hemolytic streptococci produce a zone of incomplete hemolysis and green discoloration. This appearance characterizes the organisms known as *Streptococcus viridans*. Many streptococci are completely *nonhemolytic*. Enterococci, as described below, are the streptococci normally present in the human bowel.

A more definitive serologic classification of hemolytic streptococci is that developed by Lancefield, based upon antigenically distinct carbohydrates in the streptococcal cell wall and designated as groups A through N. The hemolytic streptococci pathogenic for man include Lancefield's groups A, C, and G, the first of which accounts for the vast majority of human infections. "Human" group C strains may occasionally cause illnesses that closely resemble those of group A, but such infections are relatively rare. Moreover, as far as is known, only group A organisms cause rheumatic fever. Group G organisms may occasionally cause mild infections, but these are relatively infrequent and are uncomplicated. All three serologic groups may elaborate, in vivo, antigenically similar streptolysin O, streptokinase, hyaluronidase, and erythrogenic toxin. Other serologic groups of streptococci rarely possess these capacities and are only occasionally pathogenic agents in human diseases, and then only as secondary invaders of devitalized tissues. Beta hemolytic streptococci of groups B and F, in addition to G, are sometimes carried rather persistently in the throats of some persons. These may cause unnecessary concern unless the identity of the serologic groups is determined.

The *alpha* hemolytic and nonhemolytic streptococci are normal inhabitants of the upper respiratory tract of man from a few hours after birth until death, and may also be recovered from the feces. Many require reduced oxygen tension for initial isolation. Infection by the several varieties of alpha and nonhemolytic streptococci is unusual except in bacterial endocarditis (see article on Bacterial Endocarditis) and in suppurative lesions arising by direct extension of organisms to traumatized or diseased structures from the upper respiratory tract, bowel, or female genital organs, or by contamination of skin wounds. Thus, these relatively avirulent streptococci may multiply and cause inflammation in obstructed sinuses, bronchi, urinary and biliary tracts, and abraded endometrium.

Enterococcal Infections. Enterococcal infections deserve special comment. The enterococci are the streptococci normally present in the human bowel and are members of Lancefield group D. Most strains belonging to this group produce no change on a blood-agar medium, although some may form alpha hemolytic or beta hemolytic colonies. The enterococci are further distinguished by their property of heat resistance (they can withstand a temperature of 60° C. for 30 minutes). They are often isolated from the blood in bacterial endocarditis and from the urine in urinary tract obstruction. The precise role of these organisms in the pathogenesis of acute and chronic pyelonephritis has not been fully evaluated. A significant portion of the mixed flora in cases of intra-abdominal sepsis is often composed of enterococci. Less frequently these organisms are responsible for puerperal sepsis and purulent meningitis (see Other Bacterial Meningitides).

The most important aspect of enterococcal infection arises from the fact that these streptococci are frequently penicillin-resistant, whereas no penicillin-resistant group A streptococci have ever been reported. Effective therapy of an enterococcal infection involves the use of penicillin in combination with streptomycin or kanamycin in endocarditis, and these and other broad-spectrum antimicrobials may have to be employed in the management of infections elsewhere. The tendency of enterococci to produce viable L-forms (spheroplasts or protoplasts) in vivo as well as in vitro has been noted and may explain why apparently penicillin-susceptible strains often relapse after therapy with this drug. It may also explain the adjuvant action of antimicrobials of the streptomycin-kanamycin type which interfere with protein synthesis rather than with cell wall metabolism. The role of so-called "aberrant" forms of enterococci in relapsing sepsis and in some cases of Whipple's disease is not yet clear, but has aroused much interest and deserves further study (see Whipple's Disease).

The failure of many laboratories to distinguish the enterococci from other streptococci often leads to inappropriate therapy in serious infections. These organisms may also be recovered from the respiratory tract and may be regarded mistakenly as penicillin-resistant hemolytic streptococci. This occurs most often during the post-treatment follow-up study of cases of group A streptococcal sore throat and may lead to needless overtreatment in an attempt to eradicate them from the pharynx. It cannot be emphasized too strongly that enterococci do *not* cause pharyngitis and tonsillitis.

GROUP A STREPTOCOCCAL INFECTION

Gene H. Stollerman

History. Many of the clinical syndromes caused by group A streptococcal infection were recognized for many years before the discovery of *Streptococcus pyogenes* by Rosenbach in 1884. Thus, Sydenham is often stated to have described scarlet fever, but the early accounts are inadequate and inexact. Certainly clinical recognition of scarlet fever, of tonsillitis and pharyngitis without a skin rash, of erysipelas, and of puerperal sepsis date back for many centuries before the modern era of bacteriology. Significant understanding of streptococcal infections, however, began with the discovery by Schottmüller, in 1903, that certain strains produce hemolysis on blood agar. Brown, in 1919, defined this reaction in greater detail and coined the descriptive terms that are still in use.

The streptococcal cause of scarlet fever and tonsillitis was known by 1895. The more modern work of the Dicks and of Dochez (1925) resolved the temporary issues raised concerning the possible role of other pharyngeal bacteria in scarlet fever, and Bloomfield clearly defined the streptococcal etiology of most cases of tonsillitis. The serologic classification of the organism into groups by Lancefield and into types by Lancefield and Griffith by 1935 and the introduction of the antistreptolysin O titer by Todd (1932) to identify streptococcal infection immunologically led to the modern era of the clinical bacteriology, immunology, and epidemiology of streptococcal infections and their nonsuppurative sequels, acute rheumatic fever (ARF) and acute glomerulonephritis (AGN).

The great epidemics of streptococcal disease in the armed forces in World War II supplied an enormous volume of clinical material for the clearer definition of the epidemiology of group A streptococcal disease and of the effect of penicillin therapy and prophylaxis upon the prevention of rheumatic fever and glomerulonephritis. The current era has been one of precise chemical definition of the structure and antigenic composition of Streptococcus and the pathophysiology of the cellular and extracellular antigenic and nonantigenic products it produces. Of particular interest has been the demonstration of immunologic cross-reactivity of streptococcal products with tissues of the heart and of the skin and the demonstration of complement-fixing immune complexes in the glomeruli of patients with acute nephritis.

The recent intensive studies of group A streptococcal skin infections have clarified the roles of these organisms in impetigo and secondary pyodermas and have pointed out the difference in the serotypes that produce such infections from those that produce pharyngitis alone. Such studies have sharpened the distinction between three populations of group A streptococci: (1) those that infect the throat but not the skin and that cause acute rheumatic fever (ARF) but not acute glomerulonephritis (AGN); (2) the streptococcal pharyngeal strains that cause AGN but not ARF; and (3) the pyoderma strains that primarily affect the skin but may also be found in the throat, and that cause AGN but apparently little or no ARF. The persistent enigma of the pathogenesis of ARF and of AGN continues to stimulate studies that unfold the remarkable complexity and variation of *Streptococcus pyogenes*.

Pathogenesis. The two most common sites of infection with streptococci in man are the nasopharynx and the skin. Most of our knowledge of the host-parasite relation is based on studies of the former, whereas streptococcal skin infection received little attention until recently. A growing interest in the role of streptococcal pyoderma in acute glomerulonephritis has led to increasing awareness of many distinctive features that set skin infections apart from those of the upper respiratory tract. In the ensuing discussion, some of these will be pointed out, and the specific clinical features of skin infections will be considered separately.

Strains of group A streptococci may vary greatly in infectivity or virulence. During epidemics of pharyngitis, most strains isolated from the throats of patients who are acutely ill contain relatively large amounts of the type-specific surface antigen, M-protein. At least 60 antigenically distinct types of M-protein have been differentiated so far. This substance has particular importance in the pathogenesis of group A streptococcal infection because immunity is type-specific, that is, dependent upon antibody to the homologous type of M-protein. Such antibodies tend to persist for many years after infection. For this reason, repeated infections with strains of different M-types occur during the lifetime of most persons, but reinfection with the same M-serotype is very rare unless the type-specific immune response is suppressed by penicillin therapy.

The production of large amounts of M-protein is correlated with the ability of Streptococcus to resist phagocytosis. A hyaluronic acid capsule, which may attain very large size in some epidemic strains and produce large mucoid colonies, also contributes to the organism's resistance to phagocytosis, particularly in certain laboratory animals such as mice. Rapid passage of group A streptococci through mice usually results in increase in M-protein production by group A strains and frequently in an increased size of the capsule. Interestingly, strains that form mucoid colonies (large capsules) are rarely, if ever, found in the skin. In the presence of homologous anti-M antibody, virulent group A streptococci are rapidly and efficiently destroyed by human blood phagocytes. This phenomenon forms the basis for the so-called bactericidal test for the presence of circulating type-specific anti-M antibody. It is not yet clear to what extent cross-immunity exists to strains of streptococci less virulent than those that are rich in M-protein and that are highly encapsulated. Strains of group A organisms lacking both these virulence factors are readily phagocytized and destroyed by human and animal blood. It is possible that with increasing age and number of previous streptococcal infections, the human host acquires greater resistance to all but the most virulent strains of group A streptococci. This may account, in part, for the striking age incidence in the epidemiology of human group A streptococcal pharyngitis and streptococcal pyoderma. It also may account for the progressive tendency, between infancy and childhood, for nasopharyngeal inflammatory reactions to become more and more focalized and intense. Certainly, immediate and delayed skin allergy to streptococcal products becomes increasingly frequent and severe during childhood and adolescence. Indeed, the widespread incidence of immediate and delayed allergy to streptococcal products has seriously hampered the development of effective vaccines against streptococcal M-protein preparations.

In the course of human infections, group A organisms produce a great variety of antigenic extracellular products, such as streptolysin O, streptokinase (fibrinolysin), hyaluronidase, diphosphopyridine nucleotidase (DPNase), several deoxyribonucleases (DNases), and proteinases. The antibody responses to many of these substances are useful in diagnosis (*vide infra*), and some of these products undoubtedly contribute to the pathologic features of streptococcal infection. For example, the breakdown of fibrin and nucleic acids by streptokinase and the DNases, respectively, produces the characteristic thin pus of streptococcal infections and, with hyaluronidase, may aid the organisms' rapid spread through tissues, as observed in streptococcal cellulitis and lymphangitis. The erythrogenic toxin causes the typical erythema of scarlet fever (*vide infra*). The pathogenic role of other toxins is not yet clearly understood.

With the virtual disappearance of diphtheria in the United States, the group A Streptococcus is the only significant bacterial organism that commonly causes primary sore throat, that is, that can invade the normal tissues of the pharynx. Because nasal and throat carriage of these organisms is very common, virulent streptococci may be inoculated into open wounds or skin abrasions, producing rapidly spreading *cellulitis* and *lymphangitis* or *erysipelas;* they may contaminate the denuded postpartum endometrium to produce puerperal sepsis; they may secondarily infect the lungs to produce a *streptococcal pneumonia* following viral respiratory diseases such as influenza. Therefore, group A streptococci have always been a major cause of sepsis and suppurative complications. In addition, certain so-called *nonsuppurative complications* such as *rheumatic fever*, *glomerulonephritis,* and *erythema nodosum* may follow streptoccal infection by pathogenic mechanisms that are not yet clear, although delayed allergy to bacterial antigens is the probable mechanism in erythema nodosum. In addition, anaphylactoid or Schönlein-Henoch purpura may follow streptococcal infection (in addition to other infectious agents), representing, presumably, another form of immunologic disorder to infection with this agent. The relation of streptococcal antigens to the pathogenesis of ARF and AGN is discussed elsewhere (see article on Rheumatic Fever, and article on Glomerulonephritis under Renal Diseases).

Epidemiology. Quantitatively, upper respiratory infections, including scarlet fever, pharyngitis, and tonsillitis, are the most important forms of group A streptococcal infection. Illness in these categories occurs most frequently in children from 5 to 15 years of age, but younger and older persons are also highly susceptible to infection. The key to the understanding of the epidemiology of streptococcal infection is an appreciation of its mode of transmission. Transmission of group A streptococcal infections occurs as a result of direct contact between infected persons or healthy carriers and susceptible persons. Significant extrahuman or animal reservoirs of these organisms do not exist, although occasional outbreaks due to contamination of an article of food, often milk, have occurred. In general, however, streptotocci dissociate rapidly outside the human host, and organisms recovered from clothing, bedding, or house dust, although identifiable as group A, have been found to be noninfective when inoculated into the throats of human volunteers. Children, among whom infection is commonplace and healthy carriers are abundant, are primarily responsible for the spread of streptococcal disease. The introduction of an untreated, infected five-year-old into a family will be followed by pharyngeal infection of more than half of his siblings and a significant number of adults in the household. The spread of an M-typable, virulent strain of group A Streptococcus through a family occurs much more readily than that of non-M-typable organisms. The problem of control of hemolytic streptococcal disease is complicated by the fact that a very large proportion of infections by these organisms is either exceedingly mild or completely inapparent. Persons with this type of "subclinical" infection are fully capable of disseminating the streptococci, but will not necessarily come under the care of a physician who could apply modern chemotherapy, eradicate streptococci from the pharyngeal tissues, and eliminate the possibility of transmission of the disease.

Epidemiologic factors such as climate, season, and geography are important primarily as they affect close contact of individuals. For example, military recruit populations, particularly when mobilized in large camps in cold climates and crowded housing conditions, provide the most ideal circumstances for the rapid passage of the organism from individual to individual, and such populations give rise to some of the most severe epidemics on record. Streptococcal disease is most severe in civilian populations when poverty and poor housing promote the most crowded living conditions.

In the temperate zones of the United States pharyngeal streptococcal infections vary strikingly with the season of the year. The peak incidence occurs between December and May, and only rare sporadic infections appear during the hot summer months. In recent family studies of a large metropolitan area in the northern part of the United States, it was estimated that a streptococcal infection occurs approximately once every three to four years during childhood and adolescence, and that in a middle class population in this metropolis only about 2 per cent of all respiratory illnesses that occurred were due to group A streptococcal infection.

The epidemiology of *scarlet fever* is the same as that of other group A streptococcal infections except that the strains producing the infection seem to be lysogenized by a bacteriophage that induces the production of erythrogenic toxin in a manner entirely analogous to diphtheria organisms that produce diphtheria toxin. Thus, the epidemiology of scarlet fever is essentially that of any other strain of group A Streptococcus that does not produce the erythrogenic toxin. This explains the mild sporadic cases of scarlet fever, the severe epidemics of streptococcal pharyngitis *without* any scarlet fever cases, and the localized outburst of scarlet fever in a single concentrated population such as a school or institution.

The epidemiology of streptococcal pyoderma is strikingly different from that of streptococcal pharyngitis in several respects. Seasonal occurrence of the two is quite disparate in temperate climates: pharyngitis is more common and intense in cold weather, whereas streptococcal pyoderma occurs often in the late summer and early fall. The close indoor contact during the colder months may facilitate respiratory spread, whereas increased exposure of the uncovered skin to minor trauma and insect bites may favor skin infection during the warmer months. Although, geographically, epidemic streptococcal pharyngitis is more common in temperate or cold climates and streptococcal pyoderma in hot or tropical climates, exceptions are not uncommon in both diseases.

Streptococcal pyoderma affects an even younger age group than pharyngitis, occurring most often in children of preschool age and in infants. Transmission of streptococcal pyoderma may be aided mechanically by insects, particularly flies, that are attracted to skin lesions. Poverty and filth, as well as crowding, are major predisposing factors. Patients with streptococcal pyoderma often harbor the same organisms in the throat that colonize the skin.

The Contrasting Epidemiology of Acute Rheumatic Fever and Acute Glomerulonephritis (see accompanying figure). Students of the suppurative sequels of group A streptococcal infection have long been impressed with the extreme rarity with which ARF and AGN occur in the same patient at the same time, and the antecedent infection is considered, therefore, to be due to a strain that is *either* "rheumatogenic" *or* "nephritogenic," but not both! Simultaneous appearance of both sequelae has not been a fea-

ture of the reported experience of large numbers of patients with either disease in severe epidemics in which a single streptococcal strain could be identified as the cause (Rammelkamp, 1953). The route of infection also seems to differentiate rheumatogenic from nephritogenic strains. Acute rheumatic fever seems to be almost always, if not exclusively, a complication of a pharyngeal infection. Acute glomerulonephritis occurs after *either* skin or pharyngeal infection. Although skin strains often parasitize the throat, the best known rheumatogenic pharyngeal strains do not seem to parasitize the skin.

The strains belonging to the M serotypes that have clearly caused pharyngitis followed by rheumatic fever are those commonly encountered in the throats of children in the cities of the temperate zones of the United States and western Europe and include, among others, 1, 3, 5, 6, 14, 18, 19 and 24. *All* strains containing these M antigens are not necessarily non-nephritogenic, and from time to time sporadic cases of AGN have appeared which seemed to be due to strains representing some of these serotypes (types 1, 3, and 6).

The identification of M type 12 organisms as the major pharyngeal serotype that has been associated with AGN (Rammelkamp et al., 1952) is of interest because this M serotype is perhaps the most common one encountered in the throats of schoolchildren, and yet AGN does not appear consistently in populations harboring this strain. Thus, all members of a given M serotype are not necessarily nephritogenic.

The recent attention to the bacteriology of skin strains of streptococci have revealed them to contain M and T proteins of types hitherto unrecognized (types 49 and 52 to 57). Although AGN has occurred in association with most of the strains in these categories, no specific M or T antigen per se has been related to this complication.

The factors of infection determining the attack rate of rheumatic fever are also quantitative. The attack rate may vary from as low as 0.3 per cent following very mild, sporadic streptococcal infections associated with strains of low virulence to as high as 3 per cent or greater following infections with highly virulent strains of group A streptococci. The two factors that appear to have most influence on the frequency with which rheumatic fever follows a streptococcal infection are (1) the duration of convalescent carriage of the strain following the infection, and (2) the magnitude of the immunologic response associated with the infection. Thus, patients with relatively feeble antistreptolysin O responses may show an attack rate of rheumatic fever of considerably less than 1 per cent, whereas those with the most vigorous streptococcal antistreptolysin O responses may suffer attack rates of rheumatic fever as high as 5 to 10 per cent. The acquisition of streptococci in the throat and their subsequent carriage *without* immunologic response has not been associated with reactivation of rheumatic fever in rheumatic subjects, nor do primary attacks of rheumatic fever occur very often without a well defined immune

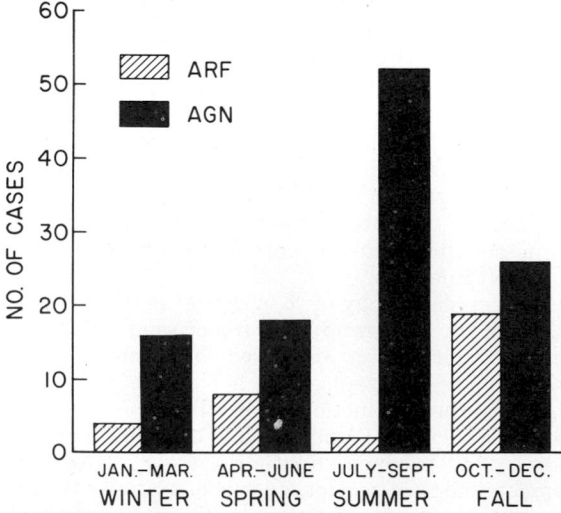

Seasonal distribution of acute rheumatic fever (ARF) and acute glomerulonephritis (AGN) admissions at City of Memphis Hospitals, September 1965–August 1968. (After Bisno, A. L., Pearce, I. A., Wall, H. P., Moody, M. D., and Stollerman, G. H.: New Eng. J. Med., 283:561, 1970.)

response. The epidemiology of rheumatic fever is, therefore, a reflection of the prevalence and severity of group A streptococcal pharyngitis.

CLINICAL SYNDROMES OF GROUP A STREPTOCOCCAL INFECTION
Gene H. Stollerman

STREPTOCOCCAL SORE THROAT

The general term "hemolytic streptococcal sore throat" is often used to describe the various forms of nonpneumonic group A streptococcal respiratory infection. The classic syndrome described as most typical of group A streptococcal infection in older children and adults is as follows:

Symptoms: sudden onset of sore throat, sometimes associated with abdominal pain and nausea, especially in children, and accompanied by constitutional symptoms of malaise, headache, and feverishness.

Signs: redness and edema of the throat, and particularly the presence of an *exudate* on the tonsils or tonsillar fossae; enlargement and particularly *tenderness* of the anterior cervical nodes, and fever of 38.2° C. (101° F.) or greater. Helpful laboratory data, other than results of throat culture, include leukocytosis greater than 12,000 leukocytes per cubic millimeter.

Although this classic syndrome is, indeed, associated with group A streptococcal infection, the full clinical picture develops in a minority of patients with pharyngitis, except during epidemics. Much more common in clinical practice is the patient with some, but not all, of the above signs and symptoms. It is not unusual for mild streptococcal disease to be associated with *nonexudative* pharyngitis, and, conversely, for viral infections, particularly adenovirus, to produce purulent tonsillar exudate and a syndrome indistinguishable from streptococcal tonsillitis (see Nonbacterial Pharyngitis, etc.). Hemolytic streptococci are the only significant *bacterial* cause of nonexudative pharyngitis. Many viral infections may mimic this clinical state, making the study of upper respiratory infection without bacteriologic control most difficult.

Streptococcal respiratory infection is not accompanied by significant cough or by coryza. The presence of either of these manifestations should suggest a different cause. Rhinorrhea does occur, especially in young children, who frequently develop suppurative sinusitis.

Scarlet Fever. The disease is clinically similar in almost all respects to tonsillitis and pharyngitis caused by nonscarlatinal strains of group A streptococci. Its name, however, comes from the presence of a skin rash caused by the erythrogenic toxin produced by scarlatinal strains. The erythrogenic effect of the toxin on the skin can be neutralized by antitoxin. This is the basis of the diagnostic *Schultz-Charlton reaction.* The injection of 0.1 ml. of scarlet fever antitoxin, or of 0.2 to 0.3 ml. of convalescent human serum, into an area where the rash is florid will be followed by blanching around the site of injection in 8 to 12 hours. Streptococcal antitoxin is no longer readily available, and usually clinical and bacteriologic studies suffice for diagnosis.

The enanthem of scarlet fever includes a tongue that may be bright red with large papillae (raspberry tongue) or coated with the red papillae protruding (strawberry tongue). These manifestations of the disease are rarely seen in adults. The rash usually appears on the second day of the disease. It consists of a diffuse, bright scarlet erythema with many points of deeper red. The distribution is variable, but the trunk and inner aspects of the arms and thighs are most often affected. In many cases the rash is clearly seen only in the axillae and groins. The face is flushed and red, but a pale area, the *circumoral pallor*, is often seen around the mouth. The palms and soles are not erythematous. Petechiae and occasionally ecchymoses are observed, especially in severely ill patients. The application of a tourniquet to the arm for five minutes will be associated with the appearance of large numbers of petechiae distal to the obstruction in nearly all cases. This is the *Rumpel-Leede* sign; it is not specific for scarlet fever. The erythema disappears usually by the sixth to the ninth day of the infection in association with the return of the temperature and the throat to normal. Desquamation of the skin is characteristic of scarlet fever, and it begins as a fine scaling of the face and body that is usually completed during the second week. About this time the extensive and characteristic desquamation of the palms and soles starts and continues for one to two weeks. Often the diagnosis is made retrospectively in patients who show this desquamation following a sore throat and in whom the scarlatinal rash may have been overlooked.

The course and clinical features of scarlet fever vary greatly with the severity of the disease. Many mild cases are observed in which constitutional symptoms and sore throat are minimal, fever is low-grade and of short duration, and the rash is evanescent. A florid eruption is sometimes seen in persons in whom all other evidences of the disease are slight, indicating that the reaction to the erythrogenic toxin per se is not primarily responsible for the systemic manifestations of scarlet fever. Again, the situation is comparable to that in diphtheria. A mild sore throat with a strain that is a potent toxin-producer may result in a clinical picture dominated by the effects of the exotoxin. Conversely, severe pharyngeal infection may be present with a strain that is a relatively mild toxin-producer, and the clinical manifestations resulting from the toxin may be slight.

Course of Streptococcal Pharyngitis. The course of untreated hemolytic streptococcal pharyngitis in older children and adults is benign. Seventy-five per cent of patients are afebrile within 72 hours after onset, but sore throat, abnormal signs in the pharynx, and tender adenitis may persist for two or three days after the return of the temperature to normal. Although the whole process is shortened by appropriate antimicrobial therapy by 24 to 48 hours, it is not always easy to distinguish the treated from the untreated patient. An acute pharyngitis that *fails to respond* to adequate penicillin therapy is virtually never due to group A streptococcal infection. On the other hand, the course of viral pharyngitis is often also very brief, and a spontaneous defervescence in 24 to 48 hours may mislead the clinician who has treated the patient into believing the patient has had a therapeutic response to penicillin therapy. In severe streptococcal infections, leukocytosis, when present in the acute stage, may persist in more than one half of untreated patients for a week or more, but this disappears more quickly after the institution of antimicrobial therapy. The erythrocyte sedimentation rate returns to normal in 80 per cent of patients by the third week.

Group A streptococci tend to persist in the pharynx for long periods after recovery if antimicrobial therapy has not been employed. In general, the more virulent the strain, the longer and more consistent is the duration of convalescent throat carriage. Under epidemic conditions, 80 per cent of untreated patients may carry the infecting strain for as long as four weeks. On the other hand, sporadic and mild streptococcal infections among schoolchildren studied in recent years are not as frequently associated with such prolonged throat carriage.

Streptococcal pharyngitis in infants and small children lacks an acute and well defined onset, has rhinorrhea as a dominant manifestation, is rarely associated with high fever, and runs a protracted and indeterminate course. The physical signs in the throat are nondescript, and usually do not permit an accurate clinical diagnosis. Suppurative complications such as otitis media and cervical lymphadenitis occur frequently.

The change of the pharyngeal response after the first few years of life to an explosive onset with fever, sore throat, and exudative pharyngitis may be a reflection of the sharp increase in delayed hypersensitivity (cellular immunity) that appears after the first or second year of life as a result of repeated infection with different types of group A streptococci. It is noteworthy that rheumatic fever is very rare before heightened cellular and humoral immunity to the Streptococcus occurs, whereas acute glomerulonephritis is common.

Diagnosis of Streptococcal Pharyngitis. Streptococcal tonsillitis and pharyngitis in its typical form needs to be differentiated from diphtheria, nonstreptococcal exudative pharyngitis (usually adenovirus), and infectious mononucleosis. When streptococcal infection is nonexudative, however, it cannot be differentiated (in the absence of scarlet fever) from a variety of viral agents producing an identical clinical picture. Cough, coryza, and rhinorrhea (in adults), make a nonbacterial disorder more likely. Unfortunately, therefore, the clinical diagnosis of the kind of streptococcal pharyngitis that now occurs most commonly as a sporadic infection in civilian communities is usually a crude guess. It is possible, however, to *exclude* the diagnosis of streptococcal disease in considerably more than half the patients studied for sporadic pharyngitis by the use of throat cultures. The incidence of throat cultures positive for beta hemolytic streptococci decreases progressively with age in patients with sporadic acute respiratory diseases in civilian communities. In several large cities in the northern sections of the United States, surveys have shown that less than 5 per cent of adults who had routine cultures for upper respiratory infections harbored group A streptococci in their throats. It is obvious, therefore, that without bacteriologic confirmation, the clinical diagnosis of viral versus streptococcal pharyngitis is quite unsatisfactory.

Before any antimicrobial therapy is administered swabs should be passed through the mouth under direct vision, using a good light, and rubbed over the tonsils and posterior pharynx. The swab should be streaked directly, with a minimum of delay, on sheep blood agar plates of low dextrose content. After incubation overnight, the number of hemolytic streptococci present should be recorded in a roughly quantitative manner. These organisms will be very numerous in nearly all cases if they are the cause of the infection. The presence of a few does not provide convincing evidence that they are responsible for the illness, because 5 to 10 per cent of the general population are nasopharyngeal carriers of these organisms. *Their absence may be regarded as excluding streptococcal disease.* Serologic grouping and typing of the isolated organisms is usually not necessary for routine clinical diagnosis. Because all group A streptococci are susceptible in vitro to discs containing no more than one to two units of bacitracin, some laboratories determine the bacitracin susceptibility of hemolytic streptococci routinely. A hemolytic Streptococcus resistant to such low concentrations of bacitracin is virtually never a group A Streptococcus. On the other hand approximately 5 per cent of non-group A hemolytic streptococci are also susceptible to this low concentration.

Immunologic Diagnosis of Streptococcal Pharyngitis. The immunologic diagnosis of group A streptococcal infection is of no value in the treatment of the acute illness, as an antibody response will not usually be detected until 10 to 20 days after the onset of the disease. Measurement of antistreptolysin O, antihyaluronidase, antistreptokinase, anti-DPNase (NADase), or anti-DNase B is of great value in determining whether or not there has been preceding streptococcal pharyngitis in patients with possible rheumatic fever or glomerulonephritis. The presence of low titers of such antibodies during convalescence virtually excludes recent streptococcal disease except in patients who have been intensively treated early in the illness. It should be noted that streptococcal pyoderma does not produce an equally strong immune response to all strepto-coccal antigens. In particular, antistreptolysin O and anti-DPNase are increased relatively infre-quently, whereas anti-DNase B and antihyaluron-idase, particularly the former, are far better indi-cators of recent streptococcal pyoderma. The clinician should be aware that elevated serum levels of streptococcal antibodies may persist for long periods of time after an immune response has occurred. Such elevated serum levels do not neces-sarily imply an unfavorable prognosis, and are not an indication for additional prolonged anti-microbial therapy.

The Value of Throat Cultures in Deciding When to Treat.
There may be some difficulty in inter-preting the significance of a throat culture weakly positive for hemolytic streptococci when strepto-coccal disease is mild and sporadic. Such a posi-tive culture may represent the acquisition of a strain temporarily in the pharynx that does not actually invade the deeper tissues of the host, does not produce a significant immune response, and does not lead to acute rheumatic fever. Such a positive culture may also represent the con-valescent carriage of an infection that occurred several weeks previously and may bear no rela-tion to subsequent acute symptoms of viral pharyngitis from which the patient may now be suffering. The physician's problem in deciding which patient with pharyngitis to treat with antimicrobial drugs will be clarified if he obtains throat cultures routinely in all such patients whom he examines. By doing this he becomes alert to the epidemiology of the infections he encounters. A throat culture negative for beta hemolytic streptococci will exclude a great many patients from unnecessary and promiscuous use of expensive antimicrobial drugs. In outbreaks of exudative pharyngitis, negative throat cultures in a succession of patients will immediately reveal the nonstreptococcal nature of the disease en-countered. Conversely, a succession of strongly positive cultures leaves little doubt that a local outbreak of streptococcal pharyngitis is in prog-ress.

When exudative pharyngitis is associated with a throat culture heavily seeded with beta hemo-lytic streptococci, there is little argument with the general recommendation for prompt and adequate antimicrobial therapy. Moreover, when a succession of such cases is observed, the prac-titioner is immediately alerted to the need to culture also material from the throats of asympto-matic contacts to prevent the spread of an epi-demic. It is with the sporadic cases of nonexudative pharyngitis that are associated with positive throat cultures that some argument has been raised as to the need to employ intensive penicillin therapy in the regimens recommended for the prevention of rheumatic fever (*vide infra*). In some populations and under some conditions, such intensive treatment may not be necessary. At present, however, these conditions have not yet been sufficiently defined to justify broad general-izations. Until further studies define more pre-cisely the risk of withholding or modifying chemo-therapy of such infections, it is safer to err on the side of overtreatment and thus to ensure the prevention of passage of streptococcal strains through a population. Indeed, with the assistance of the throat culture, all contacts of patients with well diagnosed exudative streptococcal pharyngitis may be studied for acquisition of potentially dangerous strains, and those identi-fied as carriers may be treated. The consequence of such practice would undoubtedly have a pro-found influence on the epidemiology of strepto-coccal infection and, therefore, upon the inci-dence of rheumatic fever and glomerulonephritis.

Complications of Pharyngitis. Suppurative and nonsuppurative complications may follow un-treated streptococcal tonsillitis and pharyngitis.

Suppurative Complications. Peritonsillar ab-scess or quinsy sore throat is an interesting and infrequent complication of streptococcal tonsil-litis. Its exact pathogenesis is unknown. Suppura-tion extends through the capsule of the palatine tonsil into the loose connective tissue of the neck. This is associated with formation of brawny edema of the affected side with movement of the tonsil toward the midline of the throat. An abscess eventually forms and drains in untreated cases, *but the pus does not regularly contain streptococci.* It is probable that the initial streptococcal infec-tion does not cause this lesion directly, but may permit other organisms such as anaerobic gram-negative bacilli of the Bacteroides group and anaerobic nonhemolytic streptococci to gain a foothold in the affected tissues. The onset of this complication is marked by an abrupt increase in soreness and swelling of the neck, and often by increased fever and malaise. The involved tonsil and anterior pillar are greatly swollen, the cervical nodes are large and tender, and eventually a fluctuant mass may be felt in the affected area with the gloved finger. Complications of periton-sillar abscess arise when the infection extends further into the neck or leads to the development of suppurative thrombophlebitis. Peritonsillar abscess is only rarely seen today because severe hemolytic streptococcal tonsillitis is often treated early in its course with effective antimicrobial agents.

Direct extension of hemolytic streptococci from the locus in the throat to the surrounding tissues may result in certain suppurative complications. Paranasal sinusitis, otitis media, mastoiditis, suppurative cervical adenitis, and impetigo are the most common, and will occur most frequently in untreated children less than four years old. It has been demonstrated that otitis media occurring early in the course of streptococcal respiratory infection is caused by the same serologic type that was present in the throat at the onset. A similar complication that develops after the first week is likely to be the result of a reinfection, and a different type will be recovered from the purulent exudate. Bacteremia was once observed rather frequently during the course of streptococcal respiratory infection and was often associated with metastatic lesions in the joints, bones, and elsewhere. Such cases are now almost unknown, even if antimicrobial therapy is withheld. Similarly, there has been a nearly complete disappearance of group A streptococcal meningitis. Pneumonia has always been a surprisingly uncommon complication of streptococcal upper respiratory infections. Tender cervical adenitis is regularly present and is not to be regarded as a complication unless the lymph nodes become very large and fluctuant. All the various suppurative streptococcal complications may be prevented by early and adequate antimicrobial therapy. Response to similar management is excellent if any such complications should develop in an untreated patient.

Nonsuppurative Complications. The principal nonsuppurative complications of streptococcal disease, acute rheumatic fever (ARF) and acute glomerulonephritis (AGN), are discussed in an article below (ARF) and in the section on Renal Diseases (AGN).

STREPTOCOCCAL SKIN INFECTIONS

Streptococcal Pyoderma

Clinical Features. Aside from secondary infections of wounds or burns, group A streptococci can cause at least two kinds of skin infection, *pyoderma* and *erysipelas*. These differ markedly in clinical appearance, in epidemiology, in pathogenesis, and perhaps in the strains of streptococci causing infection. The term streptococcal pyoderma includes all kinds of streptococcal skin infections, other than erysipelas, many of which are secondary infections. The term *impetigo*, or *impetigo contagiosa*, describes what often appears to be a *primary* infection, is initially and transiently vesicular, and presents as crusted, nonscarring lesions in its later stages.

The initial lesion of streptococcal impetigo is a papule that develops rapidly into a vesicle with a small surrounding area of erythema. The vesicles are often missed clinically because of their evanescence and rapid transformation into pustules with thick, amber-colored crusts that appear to be "stuck on" the skin. Aside from occasional itching and burning, the lesions are not painful unless they become deep seated. Regional lymph nodes are commonly involved even without extensive local cellulitis. Often an apparently innocuous lesion may yield large numbers of group A streptococci in cultures taken beneath dried crusts, and such indolent-appearing lesions can produce full-blown acute glomerulonephritis. Bacteremia, which is rare in streptococcal pharyngitis, occurs more frequently with skin and wound infections, and occasionally scarlet fever has been reported. Superficial streptococcal skin infections often pursue a chronic course of weeks or months, and their onset is often difficult to establish. A deeply ulcerated form is known as *ecthyma*.

Contagiousness of streptococcal skin infections is evident from the tendency of multiple cases to occur in a family and from their tendency to occur in epidemics. The importance of antecedent skin trauma is apparent in the epidemiology of streptococcal pyoderma (see above). Its preponderance in the summer when insect bites and trauma to exposed parts of children are most common, especially in populations in which poverty results in poor hygiene, neglect, flies, and crowding, suggests the conditions for maximal opportunity of invasion of the skin by virulent strains. Because of the frequency, especially in children, of such minor skin trauma as mosquito bites, abrasions, burns, eczema, dermatitis venenata, scabies, and pediculosis, it is often difficult to determine whether or not group A streptococci invade the unbroken skin. In epidemic conditions owing to particularly virulent strains, the clinical appearance of the lesions often suggests direct invasion, but it is virtually impossible to exclude minute and transient antecedent trauma.

Diagnosis. The frequency with which staphylococci colonize the skin makes contamination of skin lesions with these organisms almost the rule. Cultures of lesions more clearly considered streptococcal pyoderma are frequently also associated with staphylococci, and the relative role of each organism in the etiology of impetigo has caused much confusion and controversy. Although the issue is not entirely settled, current evidence suggests that impetigo can be divided on clinical, bacteriologic, and epidemiologic grounds into two basic forms: a bullous type, in infants, which forms thin, varnish-like crusts and is primarily staphylococcal in origin, and a vesicular type, which develops thick "stuck-on" crusts and is primarily streptococcal in etiology. Whereas the classic bullous impetigo caused by staphylococci yields a pure culture of phage Type 71 organisms, the early vesicular stage of streptococcal impetigo may yield pure cultures of group A streptococci, but in the purulent and crusted stages large numbers of staphylococci may be present also. The latter are of a variety of phage types suggesting secondary colonization.

Skin cultures of pyodermas should be made after careful cleansing of the surface of the lesions with gauze soaked in sterile warm water, avoiding antiseptics, soaps, and detergents that kill or suppress the more fastidious streptococci and favor the survival of the more adaptable Staphylococcus. Often the removal of crusts and careful culture of the serous exudate beneath will yield large numbers of hemolytic streptococci in almost pure culture. Sheep blood agar plates incubated anaerobically or in 10 per cent CO_2 favor the growth of streptococci.

The higher numbered M and T serotypes associated with pyoderma strains of group A streptococci set them apart from the primarily pharyngeal strains, although it should be noted that throat carriage of the "skin strains" may be high in populations in which much pyoderma is present, especially during the summer months.

The weak antistreptolysin O response to pyoderma strains should be borne in mind, and anti-

DNase B or antihyaluronidase titers should be measured when studies of the immune response to these streptococcal infections are indicated (see above), as in the diagnosis of post-streptococcal AGN.

Erysipelas

This form of group A streptococcal skin infection has special characteristics and may be considered in greater detail. Erysipelas usually involves the face and head, but may affect any area of the body. Other than an occasional case of a group C strain that has been recognized, erysipelas is caused by group A streptococci. The precise way in which the bacteria are introduced into the skin in primary facial erysipelas has not been determined. Large numbers of group A streptococci are fairly constantly present among the nasopharyngeal flora of patients with early erysipelas. It may be that the primary infection is a nasopharyngitis from which the organism is transferred to the skin.

After reaching the face, the streptococci may enter the skin through minute abrasions that are not recognizable after the disease is well established. In surgical and wound erysipelas, it is probable that streptococci are introduced into the traumatized areas from external sources, usually the nose and throat of attendants and other patients. The epidemiology of facial erysipelas differs somewhat from that of group A streptococcal infection in the affected age groups. This disease, when large numbers of cases were observed in the past, was rather common in infancy, rare between the ages of six and thirty, and was predominantly a disorder of middle age. There has been no explanation for this discrepancy in age distribution.

Erysipelas usually begins as an abrupt onset of fever with a shaking chill. A history of preceding acute or subacute upper respiratory infection is obtained in about one third of adult cases and more frequently in infants. Very early in the disease a definite zone of redness and edema of the skin appears most frequently around the bridge of the nose or around a surgical incision, traumatic wound, area of dermatitis, or the newly severed umbilical cord. Facial erysipelas is usually self-limited if no antibacterial therapy is administered. Under these circumstances, the temperature remains at a high level for four to ten days and then falls by lysis or crisis. During this interval a local process involves a large part of the face. As the lesion develops and spreads from the central focus, the skin is red, hot, edematous, and glistening. Blebs are frequently formed. The advancing edge of the lesion is sharply defined and slightly elevated. Great swelling occurs when the infection involves the eyelids.

The disease may involve one or both sides of the face, and usually remains active and spreading until the cheeks and eyelids are affected. Very often the inflammatory process does not extend over the bony prominences, and is limited to the area between the mandible, the malar eminence, and the hairline. In certain cases the ear is included, but spread to the scalp and trunk is rare except in infants.

Untreated *erysipelas of the trunk or extremities,* which usually occurs in infants or persons who have undergone surgery or have been injured, is a more malignant disease. Large areas of skin are often involved rapidly, prostration frequently occurs, and death is a common event. In this form of the disorder it is often possible to observe the characteristic recovery of the skin first affected while the process advances elsewhere. Healing of the skin requires one to two weeks after the temperature has returned to normal.

HEMOLYTIC STREPTOCOCCAL PNEUMONIA

Group A hemolytic streptococci were once responsible for 3 to 5 per cent of cases of bacterial pneumonia, but this form of the disease is now rarely seen. It usually appears as a complication of influenza or other viral respiratory infection or in persons with underlying pulmonary disease. It is almost never observed as a sequel to streptococcal tonsillitis and pharyngitis or scarlet fever.

The pneumonic process is lobular in distribution in the lung. Empyema develops in 30 to 40 per cent of untreated cases. It is present early in the illness and is characterized by the formation of large amounts of thin fluid. Bacteremia is demonstrable in 10 to 15 per cent of the cases of streptococcal pneumonia. The demonstration of large numbers of hemolytic streptococci in the sputum by cultural methods, or the isolation of these organisms from the blood or pleural fluid, is required for diagnosis.

TREATMENT OF GROUP A STREPTOCOCCAL INFECTION AND CHEMOPROPHYLAXIS OF NONSUPPURATIVE COMPLICATIONS

Gene H. Stollerman

The management of the various group A streptococcal illnesses should include those general measures that are applied in all acute infections. Bed rest, light or liquid diet if pharyngeal discomfort is present and severe, and adequate but not excessive fluid intake are indicated.

Most important is the prompt institution of appropriate antimicrobial therapy, which has four goals: (1) the prompt control of the acute suppurative process in the respiratory tract or elsewhere, (2) the prevention of suppurative complications, (3) the prevention of nonsuppurative complications, and (4) the elimination of the carrier state and the prevention of transmission of the organism to others. The third and fourth goals will be fully attained only if the organism is permanently eradicated from the tissues. This can best be accomplished by the administration of penicillin. Sulfonamides are not effective either in eradicating the carrier state or in preventing an immunologic response, and thus do not prevent nonsuppurative complications. Erythromycin is an acceptable second choice to penicillin in the presence of allergy to penicillin. Tetracycline-resistant group A streptococci have been described with increasing frequency, and this drug is therefore an unreliable choice. It is essential that treatment in full doses be given over a period of at least ten days, regardless which of the effective drugs is used.

Group A streptococci are among the most susceptible of all bacteria to the action of penicillin. The range of susceptibility for all strains of this serologic group is extremely narrow, between 0.01 and 0.04 unit per milliliter of culture. Moreover, no penicillin-resistant strains of group A streptococci have been demonstrated.

Duration of exposure to penicillin is the most important factor in therapy. Prolonged exposure to small concentrations of penicillin, therefore, is just as effective as a more intensive form of treatment of group A streptococcal pharyngitis. A single intramuscular injection of 600,000 units of benzathine penicillin provides blood levels that are barely detectable but that persist for about ten days; 1.2 million units results in levels that persist for at least two to four weeks or more. Such doses cure streptococcal pharyngitis, terminate carriage in the throat, and prevent rheumatic fever with optimal efficiency. Shorter-acting penicillin salts, such as aqueous procaine penicillin, must be administered still more often (usually daily for ten days) in a dose of 300,000 or 600,000 units intramuscularly to accomplish the same results. In the treatment of streptococcal pharyngitis, combinations of aqueous, procaine, and benzathine penicillin have no advantage over a single injection of benzathine penicillin G alone if a dose of at least 600,000 units or, preferably, 1.2 million units of the latter is employed.

If given orally, penicillin G must be administered in doses of 200,000 to 250,000 units four times daily for ten days. Thus, penicillinemia of about ten days' duration, regardless of the choice of preparation, is necessary to ensure bacteriologic cure. Sulfonamides are ineffective in preventing rheumatic fever when used to treat streptococcal pharyngitis. They do not suppress the immune response, do not terminate pharyngeal carriage of streptococci, and thus do not reduce the attack rate of subsequent rheumatic fever. They may be used, however, as continuous prophylaxis to *prevent* new infections *(vide infra)*.

Although the more promptly penicillin therapy is instituted, the more effective is prevention of subsequent rheumatic fever, there is no harm in delaying therapy for 24 hours to await report of a throat culture. It has been shown that the incidence of acute rheumatic fever can be partially reduced by treatment instituted as long as nine days after the onset of pharyngitis. When the patient has been seen within the first day or two of his infection, withholding treatment for one day more has not proved to constitute a risk. One exception to this statement involves the patient with a history of rheumatic fever. In such a patient, the prevention of rheumatic recurrence is not always possible unless treatment is instituted at the first clinical sign of streptococcal infection. In such a patient, any delay of therapy entails the risk of reactivation of the disease. Certain features of the chemoprophylaxis of rheumatic fever are also presented in the article on Rheumatic Fever.

Patients with more serious streptococcal infections, such as streptococcal pneumonia, severe wound infections with sepsis, or suppurative complications of ordinary respiratory infection, should receive 600,000 units of procaine penicillin G per day intramuscularly for several days until the illness is well controlled, when a shift to a single dose of benzathine penicillin or to oral penicillin may be made. The response of extrapharyngeal suppurative complications of streptococcal infection to penicillin is good, and recovery without surgical intervention is the rule, with one exception. Sterilization of abscesses in well-established suppurative cervical adenitis is most difficult. *Incision and drainage* are usually required in such cases unless spontaneous rupture occurs. As in all situations of antimicrobial therapy in the presence of pus and necrosis, prolonged therapy for as long as several weeks may be required when adequate debridement is not possible. For patients allergic to penicillin, erythromycin is recommended in doses of 1 gram per day, which may be given in four divided doses for a period of ten days. Severely ill patients may receive 500 mg. of erythromycin twice daily intravenously for a short time until they are able to accept the drug by mouth.

As in rheumatic fever, initial attacks of glomerulonephritis are preventable by prompt and adequate penicillin treatment of streptococcal pharyngitis. The latent period between streptococcal infection and glomerulonephritis is, however, generally shorter than for rheumatic fever. Therefore, glomerulonephritis is not as efficiently prevented by treatment of the antecedent streptococcal infection with penicillin as is rheumatic fever. When the clinician is aware of the appearance of other cases of acute glomerulonephritis or rheumatic fever in the population he attends, he should treat sore throat promptly and vigorously and should be more energetic than ever in obtaining throat cultures from the contacts of his patients.

The treatment of streptococcal pyoderma has been studied far less methodically than pharyngitis and has varied widely in practice. The principles guiding the treatment of pyoderma may be somewhat different from those of pharyngitis in which prevention of rheumatic fever requires thorough eradication of group A streptococci. Unlike pharyngeal infections, topical treatment of skin infections may be adequate for mild cases of impetigo. Whether or not parenteral antimicrobial drugs are used, the removal of crusts and cleansing of the affected skin surfaces with soap seems to be an important part of the treatment of streptococcal pyoderma. In patients with extensive, persistent, or recurring impetigo, intramuscular benzathine penicillin is the treatment of choice.

PROPHYLAXIS OF STREPTOCOCCAL INFECTION
Gene H. Stollerman

Mass Prophylaxis. Mass prophylaxis is the term applied to the treatment of an entire population, both healthy and affected persons, to interrupt or prevent an epidemic, impending or in progress. This has been done frequently in military populations when epidemic streptococcal pharyngitis and its aftermath of rheumatic fever or glomerulonephritis have appeared. Occasionally, similar measures have been taken against local epidemics in schools or institutions. A single injection of 1.2 million units of benzathine penicillin G intramuscularly has proved extremely effective for this purpose because it (1) is therapeutic in those actually infected, (2) terminates pharyngeal carriage, and (3) protects against the acquisition of new infections for four to five weeks.

Unfortunately, no form of immunization is of avail. However, alert medical practitioners who will promptly detect and adequately treat streptococcal infections, a good system of public health reporting of rheumatic fever and acute glomerulonephritis, and good facilities for routine use of throat cultures should reduce extensive epidemics of streptococcal disease to a rarity. This should so alter the spread of streptococcal infections as to diminish the virulence and epidemicity of the Streptococcus and thereby continue the present trend in the decline of nonsuppurative complications of streptococcal disease.

Tonsillectomy has been employed prophylactically in the past, but is now known to be useless for this purpose, as it does not prevent infection by hemolytic streptococci. Subsequently acquired streptococcal respiratory illnesses may be less severe, but the frequency of occurrence of nonsuppurative complications is not reduced.

Continuous Chemoprophylaxis. Continuous chemoprophylaxis against group A streptococci has proved to be highly effective in preventing recurrences of rheumatic fever (*vide infra*) and may be attained by one of three regimens listed here in order of their apparent efficacy and practicability:

1. Benzathine penicillin G in a single injection of 1.2 million units will provide protection for about 30 days. The disadvantages and discomfort of this regimen have to be weighed against the susceptibility to rheumatic recurrences of the individual patient. Those with rheumatic heart disease, those who have had a recent attack of rheumatic fever, and those exposed to an environment in which the incidence of streptococcal infection is frequent deserve the most effective protection. For such patients, benzathine penicillin by injection monthly is recommended.

2. Sulfonamide in daily administration by mouth of 1.0 gram of sulfadiazine or one of the other sulfapyrimidines provides satisfactory prophylaxis, but failures will occur. Toxic reactions may be observed during the first 60 days of continuous treatment. These have been rare, however, with the small doses of sulfadiazine that have been employed extensively.

3. Oral penicillin in doses of 200,000 (125 mg.) units of penicillin G has been employed widely for prevention of streptococcal infections. This regimen has not been any more effective, however, than the daily dose of 1.0 gram of sulfadiazine. Indeed, 200,000 units of penicillin *twice* daily has not proved as yet to be clearly superior to the single dose. It is possible that the oral dose of penicillin may have to be increased to nearly therapeutic proportions to be more effective than sulfonamides, and this would increase further its expense and impracticability.

Ayoub, E. M., and Wannamaker, L. W.: Evaluation of the streptococcal desoxyribonuclease B and diphosphopyridine nucleotidase antibody tests in acute rheumatic fever and acute glomerulonephritis. Pediatrics, 29:527, 1962.

Committee on Prevention of Rheumatic Fever and Bacterial Endocarditis (American Heart Association): Prevention of rheumatic fever. Circulation, 31:948, 1965.

Lancefield, R. C.: Current knowledge of type-specific M antigens of group A streptococci, J. Immun., 89:307, 1962.

Parker, M. T., Bassett, D. C. J., Maxted, W. R., and Arnaud, J. D.: Acute glomerulonephritis in Trinidad: Serological typing of group A streptococci. J. Hyg (Camb.), 66:657, 1968.

Rammelkamp, C. H., Jr.: Epidemiology of Streptococcal Infections. Harvey Lectures, Series 51, 1955–56. New York, Academic Press, Inc., 1957, p. 113.

Seegal, D., and Seegal, B. C.: Facial erysipelas: A study of 281 cases treated at the Massachusetts General Hospital from 1870–1927. J.A.M.A., 93:430, 1929.

Siegel, A. C., Johnson, E. E., and Stollerman, G. H.: Controlled studies of streptococcal pharyngitis in a pediatric population. I. Factors related to the attack rate of rheumatic fever. New Eng. J. Med., 265:559, 1961.

Stetson, C. A., Rammelkamp, C. H., Jr., Krause, R. M., Kohen, R. J., and Perry, W. D.: Epidemic acute nephritis: Studies on etiology, natural history, and prevention. Medicine, 34:431, 1955.

Stollerman, G. H.: Factors determining the attack rate of rheumatic fever. J.A.M.A., 177:823, 1961.

Stollerman, G. H.: Nephritogenic and rheumatogenic group A streptococci (editorial). J. Infect. Dis., 120:258, 1969.

Stollerman, G. H., and Pearce, I. A.: The changing epidemiology of rheumatic fever and acute glomerulonephritis. Advances Intern. Med., 14:201, 1968.

Uhr, J. W.: The Streptococcus, Rheumatic Fever and Glomerulonephritis. Baltimore, Williams & Wilkins Company, 1964.

Wannamaker, L. W.: Infections of the throat and skin. New Eng. J. Med., 282:23, 78, 1970.

Wood, H. F., Feinstein, A. R., Taranta, A., Epstein, J. A., and Simpson, R.: Rheumatic fever in children and adolescents. III. Comparative effectiveness of three prophylaxis regimens in preventing streptococcal infections and rheumatic occurrences. Ann. Intern. Med. (Suppl. 5), 60:31, 1964.

RHEUMATIC FEVER
Richard M. Krause

Definition. Rheumatic fever is an uncommon, but by no means rare, delayed sequel of an upper respiratory tract infection caused by Group A hemolytic streptococci. The pathogenesis remains obscure. Multiple focal aseptic inflammatory lesions are the basis for the acute manifestations, which may include migratory arthritis, carditis, chorea, erythema marginatum, and subcutaneous nodules, as well as a number of less prominent signs and symptoms. Recurrences of rheumatic fever are common following an untreated streptococcal infection in patients with a previous history of this disease. The acute disease is of limited duration, but the carditis may lead to permanent valvular damage. It is for this reason that extensive studies have been concerned with methods to prevent first attacks as well as recurrences of rheumatic fever. Prevention can be achieved only by the prompt detection, diagnosis, and treatment of streptococcal pharyngitis.

Etiology and Pathogenesis. Despite the decline in recent years in the incidence of rheumatic fever, interest in the disease is unabated because of its unique relationship to streptococcal infections. All the available evidence indicates that only Group A streptococcal infections of the upper respiratory tract lead to rheumatic fever. Further, the two episodes are separated by a latent period during which the signs and symptoms of either illness are commonly absent. Although streptococci may be present in the throat from the onset of pharyngitis to the onset of rheumatic fever, there is no satisfactory evidence that the localization of the rheumatic inflammatory lesions is determined by the presence of living streptococci in such areas. Thus, rheumatic fever is a reaction to the streptococcal infection, and not a continuation of the infectious process.

The epidemiologic, clinical, and laboratory evidence for the association between streptococcal infections and rheumatic fever deserves special comment. Numerous epidemiologic studies have described a temporal relationship between these two diseases. Prior to the days of penicillin, an epidemic of scarlet fever in a closed population, such as a boarding school, was followed in two to four weeks by an uncommonly high incidence of rheumatic fever. But the certain relationship between the two diseases was only established once there had been major advances in the bacteriology of streptococci. The advent of methods to delineate the antigenic structure of the Group A Streptococcus and the immune response to the various streptococcal antigens permitted the identification of the Group A Streptococcus as the only pathogen that causes the pharyngitis leading to rheumatic fever. The serologic methods to detect antibodies to streptococcal antigens played an especially important role in establishing this relationship. With such methods, it was possible to determine for the first time that nearly every patient with rheumatic fever had a preceding streptococcal sore throat. This was not always evident from the results of throat cultures taken at the onset of rheumatic fever. Although Group A streptococci may persist in the throat during the interval between streptococcal pharyngitis and rheumatic fever, it is not uncommon for repeated cultures of the pharynx to be negative for these organisms. The absence of consistent recovery of the Group A Streptococcus from the pharynx of patients with rheumatic fever was one of the factors that ruled against an association between these two illnesses.

The most persuasive argument in favor of a relationship between streptococcal pharyngitis and acute rheumatic fever stems from the treatment schedules that have been devised to prevent primary as well as recurrent attacks of rheumatic fever. In brief, it is clear that adequate antimicrobial therapy of streptococcal pharyngitis will prevent a subsequent attack of rheumatic fever.

Once the bacteriology of streptococcal pharyngitis was clarified, the recurrent nature of rheumatic fever was no longer a mystery. Almost all serologic types of Group A hemolytic streptococci are apparently capable of causing a pharyngitis that can lead to rheumatic fever (the possible exceptions to this rule are some of the recent new types of streptococci that have been most prominently isolated from skin lesions, and are associated with the occurrence of acute nephritis). Because immunity to streptococcal infections is type specific, infection with one type results in no significant protection against the many other types. Thus, it is common for a child to experience several different streptococcal infections during the school years, and this, in turn, makes possible repeated attacks of rheumatic fever. A child who has had an attack of rheumatic fever retains a special susceptibility to repeated attacks in subsequent years. However, the reason for this special susceptibility remains to be explained.

Although most, if not all, serologic M types of Group A streptococcal infections of the pharynx can lead to rheumatic fever, it should be stressed that only 3 per cent or less of all patients who do not receive adequate antimicrobial therapy for a streptococcal infection will develop subsequent rheumatic fever. Epidemiologic evidence indicates that rheumatic fever occurs only after streptococcal pharyngitis, but not in association with streptococcal skin infections, e.g., impetigo. It is conceivable that the response to the pharyngeal infection is qualitatively and quantitatively different from the response to skin infections. It is known, for example, that the antibody response to streptolysin O is more likely to be elevated after pharyngeal infections than after skin infections, whereas the antibody response to DNAse B is more likely to be elevated after skin infections than after throat infections. Thus, it is conceivable that the special consequences of a pharyngeal infection set the stage for the occurrence of rheumatic fever.

The selective occurrence of rheumatic fever in only a few people with pharyngitis argues for the importance of host factors in addition to the infectious process in the pathogenesis of rheumatic fever. It is possible that the accumulative effects of repetitive streptococcal infections in any one individual are a factor that increases the risk. Young children under the age of three have streptococcal pharyngitis, but rheumatic fever is uncommon in this age group. Throughout the remainder of childhood repetitive streptococcal infections lead to delayed hypersensitivity to streptococcal products, but such hypersensitivity is not commonly present in children less than three years of age. It is after the age of four that rheumatic fever is most common in children. The possible importance of genetic factors in predisposition has been suggested. Although it has been observed that rheumatic fever may occur in families, no clear-cut genetic pattern has been found. In a study of monozygotic twins, less than one fifth were concordant for rheumatic fever. Unsatisfactory and inconclusive though these studies are, the selective occurrence of rheumatic fever in only a few of all those infected with streptococci suggests that predisposing factors work in conjunction with the infectious process to produce rheumatic fever, but the nature of such contributory causes has remained obscure.

Although the central role of streptococcal infections in the etiology of rheumatic fever is now established beyond question, the mechanism by which the hemolytic streptococci initiate the disease process is unknown. For convenience, evidence can be marshaled for the support of three different theories of pathogenesis. Each of these theories is less than satisfactory.

The most currently attractive hypothesis is that rheumatic fever is a consequence of an immunologic response or hypersensitivity reaction, or both, to streptococcal antigens. An immunologic mechanism is suggested by the intriguing parallel between the latent period of serum sickness and rheumatic fever. Patients who develop rheumatic fever appear to have an exaggerated antibody response to streptococcal antigens. Such patients commonly, but not always, have a higher antistreptolysin O response than those who do not develop this complication after streptococcal pharyngitis.

The arguments suggesting that autoimmunity may be of importance in pathogenesis cannot be recorded in detail here. The occurrence of autoantibodies that react with mammalian muscle in the sera of patients with rheumatic fever in concentrations greater than in the sera of patients who do not develop this complication has been emphasized. What remains to be determined is the source of antigenic stimulus for this autoantibody and the pathologic significance of such autoantibody. Because this autoantibody cross-reacts with a streptococcal antigen, it has been argued that these antibodies are only another manifestation of the immune response to the preceding streptococcal infection. It is also possible, however, that the host's own tissues were so altered by the toxic processes at the time of the infection that altered tissue antigens became the stimulus for autoantibody production. In addition to the controversy over the the source of the stimulus that gives rise to these autoantibodies, there is the additional controversy over their pathologic significance. It is unknown if they participate in the genesis of the inflammatory lesions in a manner similar to the autoantibodies to nucleic acid which appear to be intimately associated with the inflammatory lesions of lupus erythematosus.

Another possible explanation for the pathogenesis of rheumatic fever is that the inflammation is a direct consequence of the deleterious effects of streptococcal toxins produced at the time of the infection. Despite the marked toxicity of certain streptococcal products, such as streptolysin O and S, there is little evidence for or against the importance of toxins in pathogenesis.

It remains to mention the possible role of persistent foci of the infecting Streptococcus in the pathogenesis of rheumatic fever. Aside from several earlier bacteriologic reports prior to the era of antimicrobial drugs, there is little bacteriologic evidence for a direct infection of the heart valves, the myocardium, or other organs involved in rheumatic fever. Nevertheless, because the prevention of rheumatic fever requires the successful and complete eradication of the infecting Streptococcus from the pharynx by drug therapy, the view lingers that persistence of the infecting Streptococcus in some form may be a factor in the disease process.

Epidemiology. It is obvious from what has been said that the epidemiology of acute rheumatic fever and the epidemiology of streptococcal pharyngitis are clearly interrelated. The incidence of the two diseases is parallel. Any environmental or host factor that enhances the occurrence of streptococcal pharyngitis will enhance the occurrence of rheumatic fever. Streptococcal disease is most common between the ages of five and fifteen years, with a peak incidence between six and eight years, and this is the age group with the highest attack rate of rheumatic fever. Although adults have fewer streptococcal infections than children because of acquired immunity and less exposure to streptococci, the special circumstances of military service or close association with children enhance the risk of higher attack rates for adults.

As is the case for most other respiratory diseases, the occurrence of streptococcal pharyngitis fluctuates widely with the seasons. The occurrence of acute rheumatic fever parallels such fluctuations. The peak occurrence falls in the late winter and early spring months, although not uncommonly the number of cases increases sharply for a brief period shortly after the onset of school in the early fall.

Classic epidemiologic studies indicate that rheumatic fever occurs most commonly in the temperate zones. But recent scattered reports from Africa, India, and countries of Southeast Asia suggest that rheumatic heart disease is by no means rare in these areas. Why acute rheumatic fever has been unrecognized in these regions remains to be determined, but it is conceivable that the disease is modified there so that the manifestations are less typical than the classic picture that defines the illness in the United States and Europe. In this connection it has been noted that the southern United States has had a low incidence of acute rheumatic fever, but at autopsy the population has a prevalence of rheumatic heart disease similar to that seen in the north. It is conceivable that, for unknown reasons, the manifestations of the acute disease are blunted in the south as well as in subtropical and tropical regions of the world.

From what has been said, it is obvious that all socioeconomic factors, such as overcrowding, either in tenement areas or in army barracks, that favor the spread of streptococcal disease, also favor the occurrence of rheumatic fever. There is no evidence for differences of susceptibility because of race or sex, although chorea and mitral stenosis are more common in females, and aortic insufficiency is more common in males.

A number of factors have undoubtedly been responsible for the decline in the occurrence of rheumatic fever and rheumatic heart disease in the past several decades. Not the least of these are improvements of socioeconomic conditions and the treatment of streptococcal infections with penicillin. Certainly antimicrobial therapy has had a major impact on the prevention of recurrent attacks of rheumatic fever, and such cases have shown a precipitous decline. Less well documented is the decline in first attacks. Indeed, long-time students of the disease have commented on the persistent occurrence of first attacks in the large cities of the United States, and suggest that the over-all decline in cases stems primarily from the prevention of recurrences and less from the prevention of first attacks. Recently it has been estimated, for example, that no less than 200 cases of acute rheumatic fever occurred in the city of Cleveland during on year.

For the United States at large, the yearly incidence of first attacks of rheumatic fever has been estimated at about 50,000 to 100,000 children, but for a variety of reasons such estimates are unsatisfactory. The disease is not reportable in all states and, in addition, without unequivocal pathognomonic signs and symptoms that clearly establish diagnosis, the disease is both over- and under-reported. Some idea of the continued occurrence of rheumatic fever in the population can be obtained by the examination of schoolchildren, college students, and military recruits for the prevalence of rheumatic heart disease. Among schoolchildren, the prevalence is between 0.7 and 1.6 per 1000. The prevalence for freshman college students and servicemen is between 6 and 9 per 1000.

Clinical Manifestations. The most striking clinical manifestations are due to arthritis, carditis, and chorea. Each sign and symptom of rheumatic fever may be either mild or severe, and the severity of each may vary independently. Thus, severe carditis may be associated with minimal or no evidence of arthritis, and vice versa. Because

the manifestations of rheumatic fever at first glance appear so variable, and because no single set of manifestations is typical for rheumatic fever, the Jones criteria have been devised as a guide to aid in the differential diagnosis. The signs and symptoms that comprise the Jones criteria are listed in the accompanying table. Use of these criteria for guidance in differential diagnosis will be discussed later.

Although a history of a preceding streptococcal pharyngitis is common, this infection may have been so mild as to have escaped medical attention. Indeed, a number of patients can recall no recent sore throat. The interval between the pharyngitis and the onset of rheumatic fever has been termed the latent period. This is a period of one to four weeks, and during this time the patient usually appears entirely well. On some occasions, however, laboratory examination will reveal evidence of disease activity.

The onset of rheumatic fever, with characteristic signs and symptoms, is usually sudden, but it may be insidious. In the latter case, diagnosis depends on observation of the clinical course and the interpretation of laboratory data. Usually the first symptoms are fever and joint pain. Fever may be high and sustained in severe cases, but more frequently it is moderate and often low grade. Sore throat is not uncommon, even though examination reveals minimal evidence of acute inflammation. Epistaxis occurs commonly both at the onset and throughout the acute stage of the disease, and in some cases results in serious loss of blood. In children, severe abdominal pain is not uncommon, and vomiting may occur. Localization of such pain in the right lower quadrant with fleeting signs of peritoneal inflammation may suggest the diagnosis of appendicitis.

CLINICAL AND LABORATORY MANIFESTATIONS OF ACUTE RHEUMATIC FEVER

Major Manifestations	Minor Manifestations
1. Carditis	1. Clinical
2. Polyarthritis	a. Previous rheumatic fever or rheumatic heart disease
3. Chorea	b. Arthralgia
4. Erythema marginatum	c. Fever
5. Subcutaneous nodules	2. Laboratory
	a. Acute phase reactions, erythrocyte sedimentation rate, C-reactive protein, leukocytosis
	b. Prolonged P-R interval
	plus

Supporting evidence of preceding streptococcal infection (increased ASO or other streptococcal antibodies, positive throat culture for Group A Streptococcus, recent scarlet fever)

The Jones criteria (revised) have been employed as a guide in the diagnosis of rheumatic fever, but this scheme has not received universal acceptance. The presence of two major manifestations, or of one major and two minor manifestations, indicates a high probability of the presence of rheumatic fever *if supported by evidence of a preceding streptococcal infection.* The absence of the latter should make the diagnosis doubtful, except in situations in which rheumatic fever is first discovered after a long, latent period from the antecedent infection, e.g., Sydenham's chorea or low-grade carditis.

Adapted from the recommendations of the Committee of The American Heart Association (Circulation, 32:664, 1965).

Arthritis. The arthritis in rheumatic fever may involve multiple joints, but a characteristic feature is that the inflammation occurs and subsides in the joints first affected, only to occur in others that were initially spared. This phenomenon has been termed migratory polyarthritis. The large joints of the extremities are most frequently affected, but all are potentially susceptible. Arthritis can occur in the hands, feet, or spine, or in such joints as the sternoclavicular and the temporomandibular.

The manifestations of arthritis may be either mild with vague discomfort in the joints of the extremities, or severe. Acutely inflamed and swollen joints are commonly very painful. In mild cases there may be no objective evidence of arthritis. When arthritis is severe, the skin over the joint shows local redness and heat, the joint is swollen, and fluid is obviously present within the joint cavity. Passive or active movement of the joint is extremely painful. The fluid in such cases is turbid and contains inflammatory leukocytes, but is sterile on bacteriologic culture.

Although uncommon, the arthritis may not affect multiple joints. Experienced clinicians have observed the occasional case in which arthritis may persist for prolonged periods in only one joint, with minimal evidence of arthritis in the others.

There is usually a difference between the pattern of arthritis in children and that in adults. Frank arthritis is less common in children between four and six years of age. Only mild joint pains may be noted, or merely vague localized aching in the extremities. It is this type of complaint that has been referred to in the past as "growing pains." Such symptoms and low-grade fever suggest a mild illness, but examination of the heart may reveal severe carditis. It bears repetition that rheumatic fever can occur without any evidence of joint involvement whatever.

Carditis. Palpitation and precordial chest pain or discomfort are common symptoms. If the carditis is severe symptoms of cardiac failure may occur in addition to those of rheumatic fever. The final and definitive diagnosis of carditis depends upon the physical, roentgenographic, and electrocardiographic examinations.

The carditis may be mild or severe. In mild cases, tachycardia, persistent during sleep, may be the only sign suggesting carditis. Persistent bradycardia has been well documented in rheumatic fever, but it is far less common than tachycardia. In the more severe cases generalized cardiac enlargement frequently occurs, often associated with a diffuse precordial impulse.

On auscultation, the heart sounds in the apical area may be muffled, indistinct, and of poor quality. The second sound in the pulmonic area is usually greatly accentuated in comparison with the second aortic sound. Gallop rhythm may occur, and is usually an indication of serious myocardial disease. The sounds may seem distant if precordial effusion is present, and the pericarditis may produce a to-and-fro friction rub (see article on Diseases of Pericardium).

The most common cardiac murmur during the acute phase of the initial attack of rheumatic fever is a blowing systolic murmur best heard in the apical area. Such murmurs are caused by dilatation of the valve rings as a result of general dilatation of the heart. Less commonly, soft diastolic murmurs are heard along the left sternal border in the third and fourth interspaces. It is difficult to determine whether inflammation of the valve leaflets contributes significantly to these murmurs in all cases. As the murmurs may disappear permanently on recovery, their final significance cannot be determined except by repeated examinations during and after convalescence. Mitral stenosis and aortic stenosis are late manifestations of cardiac damage that do not develop until months or years after the initial or repeated attacks.

Disturbances of the conduction system are a common feature of rheumatic carditis. Although certain irregularities, such as second-degree heart block, can be recognized clinically, the electrocardiogram is the best method to detect all potential conduction system disturbances. One of the most commonly observed electrocardiographic changes is the prolongation of the P-R interval. In some cases, the Wenckebach phenomenon is observed. Further delay in conduction may lead to drop beats, with the occurrence of couplets and triplets. Finally, complete dissociation is indicated by an independent rhythm for both the ventricles and the atria. Atrial fibrillation is uncommon during the acute attack.

In addition to these conduction abnormalities, the electrocardiogram may show T wave changes, such as inversion of the T wave in one or more leads. When pericarditis is present, elevation of the ST segment is observed initially. Late in the course, the configuration of the T wave simulates that seen in coronary disease.

Although cardiac enlargement, when present, is usually detectable on physical examination, the dilatation of the various chambers of the heart is more accurately determined by roentgenography of the chest. It is not uncommon for dilatation to arise rapidly when severe myocarditis is present.

The recurrence of active rheumatic fever should be suspected in patients with chronic rheumatic heart disease when the character of the murmurs changes over a short period of time. Cardiac failure may occur, but the carditis associated with recurrent rheumatic fever in such cases poses several diagnostic problems, because the manifestations of acute rheumatic carditis are superimposed on those of chronic valvular disease. Furthermore, the status of the pre-existing heart disease is often unknown. When there is evidence of advanced valvular deformity, any final assessment of the extent of cardiac damage must await convalescence from the acute attack.

Erythema Marginatum. *Erythema marginatum* or *circinatum* of the skin is one of the characteristic manifestations of acute rheumatic fever and occurs in 10 to 20 per cent of the childhood cases. It is a multiform type of erythema, and consists of roughly circular lesions that may be distributed over the extremities, the trunk, and sometimes the face, and that spread centrifugally, leaving a clear center. The lesions tend to coalesce so that, although individual areas are iris-like, the larger areas are serpiginous in outline. The erythema blanches on pressure and may be evanescent, disappearing and later reappearing at the same sites. The lesions are usually not elevated, although in some cases a slight papular quality may be detected. Most commonly, no discomfort is associated with the lesions. Erythema marginatum is uncommon in other diseases.

Subcutaneous Rheumatic Nodules. These lesions are one of the physical findings that lend strong support to the diagnosis of rheumatic fever, but in recent years they have occurred less commonly than was the case in the past. They are firm, insensitive nodules that occur over the bony prominences of the various joints and tendons of the extremities, the spine, and the back of the head. They are loosely attached to the underlying tissue, and the skin is freely movable over them. If the joint can be flexed without undue pain, the nodules are more readily apparent because of the tension of the skin. If nodules are numerous, they may occur in a symmetrical distribution. The nodules are more frequently encountered in the more severe cases of rheumatic fever with serious cardiac involvement.

Sydenham's Chorea. Chorea may occur in combination with other symptoms of rheumatic fever, but it is commonly seen as the sole manifestation of the disease. This phenomenon is explained by the fact that chorea tends to make its appearance late in the course of rheumatic fever. The onset may be delayed for as long as six months after the initiating streptococcal infection, although the delay is usually less than this. Patients with chorea may have had an easily recognizable preceding attack of arthritis and carditis, and, indeed, may have been hospitalized with it, only to have the chorea occur as a late manifestation at a time when all other evidence of any inflammatory process had disappeared. On the other hand, it is not uncommon for chorea to occur in patients who can recall no such earlier illness. It seems likely that such individuals had an attack of acute rheumatic fever in the recent past which was so mild that it escaped clinical detection. It is for this reason that patients with so-called "pure chorea" may develop rheumatic heart disease.

The onset of chorea is usually insidious and the parents of the child with chorea may first note increased awkwardness and a tendency to spill food or drop objects that is attributed to carelessness. Even the appearance of involuntary purposeless movements of the extremities may be discounted as nervousness. However, with further progression of the disease, the irregular and uncontrollable movements become obvious. They may become extensive, and may involve not only the hands, feet, arms, and legs, but the tongue and facial muscles. The severity may range from no more than minimal involuntary movements observed only by close inspection, to violent, continual activity, totally incapacitating the patient and requiring protection from self-injury. In moderate cases, interference with all coordinated activity, such as writing and eating, is common. On occasion, chorea may be limited to one side of the body. The disease appears to affect females somewhat more frequently than males.

Miscellaneous Clinical Manifestations. Rheumatic pneumonitis may occur, but this is difficult to detect clinically, particularly if there is superimposed heart failure. Rheumatic pneumonia has seldom been seen in recent years, probably because the disease process itself appears to be much more mild than in former times. Such few cases as do occur are in patients with severe rheumatic fever.

Erythema nodosum is less common than erythema marginatum. The dull, red nodular lesions occur most frequently on the extensor surfaces of the extremities in various sizes from less than 1 cm. to several centimeters in diameter. They are extremely tender on pressure, and the pain is aggravated by movements of the extremities. These lesions occur in patients in whom there is little or no other clinical evidence to suggest acute rheumatic fever. They have been seen in association with a number of infections, including tuberculosis, as well as streptococcal pharyngitis. For these reasons, the presence of erythema nodosum is not considered a major sign for the diagnosis of rheumatic fever.

Laboratory Findings. Hematology. There are no characteristic abnormalities of the leukocyte differential count that are indicative of rheumatic fever. Leukocytosis is common, but not always present, with a total count from 12,000 to 24,000 per cubic millimeter. This is associated with an increase in the percentage of polymorphonuclear cells.

A moderate degree of anemia is generally seen, which is normochromic with proportional decreases in the hemoglobin concentration and the erythrocyte count. The anemia usually persists for as long as the rheumatic process is active. The most severe anemias are obviously encountered in patients who have an associated blood loss owing to epistaxis.

Urinary Findings. Some proteinuria and an increase in the number of red and white cells in the urine are common during the acute phase of the disease. However, it is seldom that these abnormalities are as great as those characteristically encountered in acute glomerulonephritis. When this is the case, simultaneous acute nephritis and rheumatic fever must be considered, but such a combination is a most uncommon event.

Evidence for a Prior Streptococcal Infection. The most important laboratory information for establishing the diagnosis of rheumatic fever is data that substantiate the prior occurrence of streptococcal pharyngitis. The detection of Group A beta hemolytic streptococci by a throat culture is helpful in this regard, but of greater usefulness is the serologic detection of antibodies that are indicative of a previous streptococcal infection.

Because the streptococci that caused the initial infection may persist for many weeks in the pharynx in those instances in which antimicrobial therapy was not given or was inadequate, a throat culture may detect the infecting Group A streptococci at the time of the onset of rheumatic fever. But such a finding is only suggestive of a preceding streptococcal pharyngitis and is not an unambiguous indication of it. This stems from the fact that 5 to 30 per cent of the healthy population may carry Group A streptococci in the pharynx during the respiratory disease season. Thus, the recovery of this organism from a patient may be an inadvertent finding and not indicative of a preceding streptococcal sore throat. Nevertheless, the throat culture is helpful, and should be obtained in all cases. When the patient has a negative throat culture, it is frequently possible to isolate the Group A streptococci from other members of the family. Such a finding is indicative of a recent intrafamilial spread of streptococci.

The most helpful information that is indicative of a recent streptococcal infection is obtained with tests that detect serum antibodies to streptococcal antigens. The most widely employed test is the antistreptolysin O determination. As with all antibody tests, the detection of an antibody rise over a one- to three-week interval is the only unequivocal evidence for the recent occurrence of a streptococcal infection. If a patient is seen in the first few days after the onset of rheumatic fever, the antistreptolysin O titer at that time may be less than the titer seen several weeks after onset of rheumatic fever. Not uncommonly, however, the titer has reached a maximal plateau so that it is not possible to detect a progressive increase in titer. When this is the case, the antistreptolysin O titer should be at least 250 units in adults and at least 333 units in children over five years of age to be acceptable as an indication of a previous streptococcal infection. Obviously, a certain proportion of the individuals in the normal population have had a recent streptococcal infection at any one time, and they will have antistreptolysin O titers similar to these.

Approximately 15 to 20 per cent of the patients with rheumatic fever and nearly all patients who exhibit only chorea have a low or borderline low antistreptolysin O titer. In such instances, it is helpful to employ another antibody test. Although not commercially available at this time, the anti-DNAse B test is used in several medical centers, and it is a useful means to obtain additional evidence for the occurrence of a previous streptococcal infection. When both these antibody tests are used, it is possible to obtain antibody evidence for a preceding streptococcal infection in almost all cases of rheumatic fever.

One other serologic test should be mentioned because it may be used more widely in the future. It has been noted that nearly all patients with rheumatic fever have readily detectable serum autoantibodies that react with muscle tissue, including heart, whereas the concentration of these antibodies is very much less or absent in sera of patients with other rheumatic diseases. Such findings suggest that this antibody test may have clinical usefulness for the differential diagnosis of rheumatic fever.

Other Laboratory Tests. An elevated sedimentation rate and a positive C-reactive protein are present in rheumatic fever, but these findings are nonspecific indicators of inflammation, and they cannot be used to differentiate rheumatic fever from other diseases. However, a normal C-reactive protein and a normal sedimentation rate are helpful in excluding active rheumatic fever. In patients with mild symptoms, such as vague arthralgia and lassitude, if the sedimentation rate and the C-reactive protein are normal, active rheumatic fever is unlikely.

Diagnosis and Differential Diagnosis. A history of severe sore throat in the recent past, migrating polyarthritis, carditis, fever, and an elevated antistreptolysin O titer is such a classic combination of signs and symptoms that the diagnosis can seldom be questioned. But the problem is often not as straightforward as this. The various major manifestations of rheumatic fever that have been described above are considered to be part of the same disease because they occur together with a frequency that far exceeds chance. Because they may occur singly or in various combinations in any individual patient, the diagnostic criteria originally proposed by Jones have been suggested as a guide to diagnosis. These criteria are listed in the accompanying table. Any combination of these criteria can occur in patients with other disorders. It is for this reason that stress is placed on supporting evidence for a preceding streptococcal infection. When this is the case, the diagnosis is weighed in favor of rheumatic fever and against the other connective tissue disorders that may mimic it.

The designation major and minor for the various criteria are based on the diagnostic importance of the particular findings. The major ones are more indicative of rheumatic fever than the minor. The occurrence of two major manifestations is strong presumptive evidence for rheumatic fever. Only one major manifestation and any combination of the minor ones is generally observed. In any case, if evidence is lacking for a preceding streptococcal pharyngitis, the possibility of other diseases must be kept in mind.

In many ways the most useful purpose of the criteria is their value in reducing overdiagnosis. For example, not uncommonly, patients, after streptococcal infections, may have vague pains in the extremities, an increased sedimentation rate, and a borderline temperature elevation. Careful follow-up of such patients has not revealed the delayed occurrence of rheumatic heart disease. Therefore, the diagnosis of rheumatic fever should be made with caution and only with clear evidence of one or more of the major manifestations. When the diagnosis is in doubt, because the symptoms are of such a mild nature, treatment with aspirin and steroids should be withheld until the signs and symptoms are unmistakable. Early treatment of a questionable case may so depress the disease activity that clear-cut clinical signs and symptoms do not develop.

In the early stages, during the acute onset, *rheumatoid arthritis* and *systemic lupus erythematosus* may mimic rheumatic fever. Indeed, if the streptococcal antibody tests are elevated, the diagnosis may be in question unless the special diagnostic tests for the other diseases are clearly positive. Usually as time progresses, the special distinctive clinical features of rheumatoid arthritis and lupus serve to exclude the diagnosis of rheumatic fever. On occasion, at the onset, Still's disease may be confused with rheumatic fever, but again the clinical course will aid in differentiating the two.

Subacute bacterial endocarditis occurs most commonly in persons with valves previously damaged by rheumatic fever, and it often presents a clinical picture that is not readily distinguishable from a rheumatic recurrence. Vague pains in the extremities are more common than overt arthritis, but these symptoms together with fever and debility in a known rheumatic patient are sufficient to suggest a rheumatic recurrence. The difficulties are increased by the fact that in some cases it is not possible to recover the offending organism in a blood culture. The characteristic petechiae and painful septic emboli of endocarditis are helpful in differential diagnosis (see article on Bacterial Endocarditis, in section on Diseases of the Cardiovascular System).

The so-called *benign idiopathic pericarditis,* which is apparently not rheumatic in origin, is indistinguishable in the acute phase from those cases of rheumatic fever in which pericarditis is the major detectable manifestation. The diagnosis of idiopathic pericarditis is dependent primarily on elimination of other possibilities and on the subsequent course of the disease, which is characterized by complete recovery without residual damage. Thus, the final conclusion is often reached only in retrospect, and must remain somewhat uncertain because rheumatic pericarditis with minimal involvement of the myocardium and endocardium could conceivably behave in a similar fashion.

Fever, arthritis, and positive acute phase reactants may also occur in bacterial arthritis, serum sickness, subacute bacterial endocarditis, sickle cell anemia, and acute aleukemic leukemia. In such cases in which confusion exists, only a careful assessment of the clinical course, physical examination, and laboratory findings will exclude rheumatic fever.

Persistent monarticular arthritis, without other major manifestations of rheumatic fever, is usually not due to rheumatic fever, and osteomyelitis or local injury must be considered.

Therapy. There is no specific treatment for rheumatic fever. Therapeutic measures are devised to promote, or at least hopefully not to hinder, the natural healing processes. Bed rest is always prescribed, and most students agree that it should continue for as long as there is unequivocal evidence of disease activity. It is not at all clear that absolute bed rest without bath privileges is essential. Nevertheless, hospitalization has an advantage over home care because the degree of activity is more readily supervised. This is particularly true because aspirin and steroids will generally eliminate all painful manifestations, and the patient sees no necessity for remaining at rest and in bed. A program for a progressive increase in recreational and occupational therapy has important psychologic value and should be an integral part of the long-term bed rest management. Schooling should not be neglected during this time. Hospital or home visit teaching programs, or both, are available in many cities, and instruction should be begun as soon as the acute manifestations of the disease are brought under control by anti-inflammatory therapy.

After the first few weeks of bed rest in patients without carditis, gradual ambulation can be started. In patients with carditis, this is usually delayed until six to ten weeks after onset of the disease. As long as the presence of carditis is suspected, even though masked by treatment, ambulation should not be started. During the period of bed rest, the patient is permitted a number of activities in increasing amounts, such as sitting up in a chair, occupational therapy, and schoolwork.

The period of bed rest is a good time for patients of all ages to be informed about the nature of the illness and the optimistic prospects for an active, long life. The need for a continuous program to prevent streptococcal pharyngitis should be discussed in detail. It is at this time, also, that patients with more severe forms of heart disease should be advised that some curtailment of normal physical activity may be necessary during convalescence. But pessimism is not warranted. All too often, patients are left with the impression that their useful, active life is at an end. This is almost invariably not the case.

It is recommended that all patients with acute rheumatic fever be treated with a course of penicillin to eliminate the hemolytic Streptococcus from the pharynx. This is recommended even if the throat culture does not reveal Group A beta hemolytic streptococci, because these organisms may persist in areas where they remain undetected, such as the interior of the tonsils. Parenteral penicillin is the drug of choice unless there is a history of allergy to it. Three hundred thousand units of penicillin G once a day in children and twice a day in adults for ten days is an effective dose. A single dose of 1.2 million units of long-acting benzathine penicillin is preferred by many, as the one injection facilitates administration. Oral penicillin, 200,000 units four times a day, also for ten days, is acceptable therapy, but requires careful supervision in order to be sure that all doses are taken without fail. If there is a history of penicillin allergy, the drug of choice is erythromycin. The dose is 250 mg. four times a day for ten days. Sulfonamide in any form should never be used. After completion of the ten-day course of penicillin or erythromycin, a continuous prophylaxis regimen should be started to prevent reinfection with Group A streptococci and to reduce the risk of recurrent attacks of acute rheumatic fever (see previous article on Treatment of Group A Streptococcal Infection).

Aspirin and Steroid Therapy. Most patients respond rapidly to either steroid or aspirin therapy. After one or two weeks, arthritis and fever have disappeared, and the acute phase reactants frequently have returned to normal, or nearly so. On occasion, neither fever nor arthritis responds to full aspirin dosage, and steroids are required to control the disease. Most clinicians favor use of steroids in nearly all patients with carditis. It is certainly indicated in patients with severe carditis and pancarditis. Some prefer to withdraw the steroid treatment after several weeks and continue treatment by substituting aspirin. Others continue steroid therapy for the full course. The arthritis in nearly all patients responds readily to aspirin alone. The evidence remains equivocal for the beneficial effect of steroid therapy in preventing the development of permanent rheumatic heart disease, even though there is apparent clinical improvement in the acute carditis when steroids are used.

It should be stressed again that when full and adequate treatment eliminates all the clinical manifestations of the disease, including laboratory abnormalities, the underlying disease process is still continuing unabated for its natural course. If the drugs are withdrawn before the process is at an end, the disease with all its clinical manifestations will recur. Duration of therapy is discussed below.

The daily dose of aspirin is 60 mg. per pound of body weight. The actual total dose per day varies from 3 grams in young children to 10 grams in adults. It is preferable to give this total amount in at least six divided doses. Aspirin should be given throughout the 24-hour day, at least during the early stages of the disease. Individual variation in the efficacy of absorption or excretion of the drug and in its therapeutic effectiveness requires readjustment of the dose in many cases. The aim is to give the minimal dose that results in full control of symptoms and to avoid serious toxic side reactions because of overdosage. Studies on the concentration of salicylates in the blood have shown that optimal therapeutic effect usually requires at least 25 mg. per 100 ml. of serum. The optimal therapeutic range is between 25 and 35 mg. per 100 ml. of serum. Levels greater than the upper limit are associated with toxicity. When aspirin is given in conjunction with the prednisone, it is frequently necessary to give a daily dose of aspirin larger than that recommended above in order to achieve the therapeutic salicylate level. Furthermore, as aspirin is continued upon the withdrawal of prednisone, less aspirin is frequently required to maintain an adequate serum salicylate level.

The most common toxic manifestations of aspirin therapy are nausea, vomiting, and gastric distress. Tinnitus and partial but temporary impairment of hearing usually occur only at full therapeutic dosage. Hyperpnea frequently results from central stimulatory action in respiration and can lead to alkalosis. It is uncommon to see the more severe metabolic disturbances of acute salicylate toxicity.

In practice, nausea and vomiting are the most frequent complications that result from starting aspirin. This can be minimized if the initial daily dosage is below the optimum and is then gradually increased over a period of a few days. Attempts to achieve full and optimal salicylate levels within 24 hours often result in severe nausea and vomiting. In such cases it may be difficult to reach an effective therapeutic level of salicylate, and in such instances steroids afford an alternative therapeutic approach. The use of sodium bicarbonate to reduce gastric irritation is not recommended, as it increases the excretion of salicylate and interferes with the maintenance of an anti-inflammatory concentration of the drug in the blood. If a portion of the aspirin is given as enteric-coated pills, some degree of gastric irritation can be eliminated.

Prednisone is the recommended steroid because a low salt diet and added potassium are usually not required. There is no firm agreement on the dosage of this drug. The usual procedure is to begin with a relatively large daily dose until activity of the disease appears to be under control, and then to reduce the dosage to the minimal amount that will maintain the full effect. In the experience of many, the total daily dosage of 0.5 mg. per pound given in divided doses is adequate to bring the signs of inflammation, including fever, rapidly under control. Almost all signs and symptoms are suppressed in two or three days. It is at this point that the daily dose may be reduced. After two or three weeks of steroid therapy, some prefer to shift to aspirin, particularly for those patients without carditis. The advantage of this is that most side effects of prolonged steroid therapy, such as the mild manifestations of Cushing's disease, are avoided. Prolonged use of steroid therapy may lead to complications, such as infections, growth retardation, gastric ulcers, and toxic psychoses.

The treatment of chorea is symptomatic. There is no evidence that either steroids or aspirin have any influence on the symptoms of chorea. The usual case lasts from two weeks to several months, but in rare instances it may persist longer. Many patients show improvement when bright light, noise, and undue activity are eliminated from their bedroom. In some cases, measures must be taken to prevent self-injury due to violent chorea movements, including tongue-biting. Phenobarbital and other sedatives may be helpful.

Duration of Therapy. The duration of therapy bears some relationship to the severity of the acute manifestations. The disease process in the typical mild case without carditis subsides in three to four weeks. When severe arthritis and carditis are present, the natural course lasts two to three months. Such estimates for the duration of the disease can be used to determine the termination of therapy, recognizing, however, that disease activity in the occasional case may persist for many months.

Many clinicians prefer to withdraw either aspirin or steroid therapy gradually over a period of one or two weeks. After withdrawal, a clinical "rebound" is commonly seen. This may be so mild that only the acute phase reactants indicate its occurrence, but not uncommonly clinical manifestations are present. These may be mild or severe, and include fever, arthritis, and tachycardia. Usually the rebound subsides in five to ten days without use of anti-inflammatory drugs. But progressive clinical severity and particularly the emergence of severe carditis may require reinstitution of therapy. In such instances, it is assumed that the natural duration of the disease has yet to run its course. In practice, if therapy must be reinstated because of the emergence of carditis, the drugs are continued for another three to four weeks.

If no significant rebound occurs, ambulation should begin, and usually full activity, except vigorous exercise, may be permitted three to four weeks after the termination of therapy. If persistent rheumatic heart disease is present, the permissible level of physical activity is determined by an assessment of its severity.

Prevention. Prior to the days of antimicrobial drugs, measures were not available to prevent recurrences of rheumatic fever. Now properly supervised continuous chemoprophylaxis is effective in preventing these recurrences, and it should be employed for all patients with a well-documented history of rheumatic fever or unequivocal evidence of rheumatic heart disease. Prophylaxis prevents streptococcal pharyngitis and, therefore, the recurrences of rheumatic fever.

A detailed consideration of drug regimens for prophylaxis has been presented in the preceding article on the treatment of Group A streptococcal disease. Intramuscular benzathine penicillin, 1.2 million units each month, is the preferred drug and route of administration. Such a route of administration does not leave open to question the degree of patient compliance, as is the case with orally administered penicillin.

The duration of antimicrobial prophylaxis should be extended through childhood. In the case of adolescents and adults, it should not be terminated as long as the patient is associated with population groups that have high attack rates of streptococcal infections, such as military recruits, schoolchildren, medical personnel, and school teachers. Prophylaxis should be continued for life for all patients with rheumatic heart disease. Contrary to popular belief, people in late middle age can have a recurrence of rheumatic fever following streptococcal pharyngitis.

Epidemiologic studies clearly indicate that streptococcal disease spreads in the home and in the school. The physician must be alert to the occurrence of streptococcal pharyngitis in the family and the school of the patient on prophylaxis. This is a potential risk to the patient, and strict compliance with the prophylaxis must be urged. If streptococcal disease occurs in the family, it should be treated with adequate antimicrobial drugs.

For a number of reasons, the prevention of first attacks of rheumatic fever is difficult to achieve. Prompt recognition and treatment of streptococcal pharyngitis is hampered in a number of cases by the fact that the symptoms are so mild that the patient does not see a physician. Not uncommonly, when the patient is seen by a doctor, the disease is misdiagnosed or the antimicrobial therapy prescribed is inadequate. For example, the tetracyclines should never be used to treat streptococcal pharyngitis, because 25 to 40 per cent of all Group A streptococci are now resistant to this family of drugs.

The occasion arises when special measures are needed to control epidemics of streptococcal pharyngitis in a school or a community or in an army recruit camp. Several unexpected cases of rheumatic fever in a short period of time in a small population group should alert the physician to the possibility that there is a serious streptococcal epidemic in the community in question. Methods to curtail such epidemics have been described in an earlier article (Prophylaxis of Streptococcal Infections).

Prognosis. Recovery from the acute attack is the rule. Death at this stage is very rare, even in cases of severe carditis, because of the anti-inflammatory effects of steroid therapy. The disease process in mild cases of rheumatic fever without carditis usually subsides in two to four weeks, and the patient usually makes a complete recovery. When carditis is present, the disease usually persists for six weeks to three months. Patients with carditis during the acute attack may progress to valvular rheumatic heart disease. This is less common in patients without carditis, but absence of carditis during an acute attack is unfortunately not an absolute guarantee against the development of subsequent valvular deformity.

Chronic disability and death owing to rheumatic heart disease are related to recurrent attacks. In former years, before antimicrobial therapy, patients who had had rheumatic fever usually suffered recurrences. Additional valvular deformity was the frequent outcome of each recurrence. As a result, a progressive severity of rheumatic heart disease was common. In current times the prognosis is more optimistic. Although the epidemiologic data are difficult to assess without question, the general impression is that progressively severe valvular deformity after an initial attack, if recurrences are prevented, is now much less common than in former times. The efficacy of adequate chemoprophylaxis in the prevention of recurrences is clearly documented. In one study more than two thirds of the patients with a history of rheumatic fever who were not on prophylaxis had one or more recurrences over an eight-year follow-up period. If prophylaxis is adequately supervised and the drug is taken without fail, a recurrence is an extremely uncommon event.

Kuttner, A. G., and Mayer, F. E.: Carditis during second attacks of rheumatic fever: Its incidence in patients without clinical evidence of cardiac involvement in their initial rheumatic episode. New Eng. J. Med., 268:1259, 1963.
Lendrum, B. L., Simon, A. J., and Mack, I.: Relation of duration of bed rest in acute rheumatic fever to heart disease present 2 to 14 years later. Pediatrics, 24:389, 1959.
Markowitz, M., and Kuttner, A. G.: Rheumatic Fever—Diagnosis, Management and Prevention. Philadelphia, W. B. Saunders Company, 1965.
McCarty, M.: Missing links in the streptococcal chain leading to rheumatic fever: The T. Duckett Jones Memorial Lecture. Circulation, 24:488, 1964.
United Kingdom and United States Joint Report: The natural history of rheumatic fever and rheumatic heart disease: Ten-year report of a cooperative clinical trial of ACTH, cortisone, and aspirin. Circulation, 32:457, 1965.
Wood, H. F., and McCarty, M.: Laboratory aids in the diagnosis of rheumatic fever and in evaluation of disease activity. Amer. J. Med., 17:768, 1954.
Zabriskie, J. B.: Mimetic relationships between Group A streptococci and mammalian tissues. Advances Immun., 7:147, 1967.

STAPHYLOCOCCAL INFECTIONS

F. Robert Fekety, Jr.

GENERAL CONSIDERATIONS

Staphylococci are the most frequent cause of superficial suppurative infections of man, and they also cause serious infections of lungs, pleura, endocardium, bones, or deep soft tissues. These infections have become increasingly frequent and troublesome because pathogenic staphylococci are part of man's normal flora and ubiquitous in his environment; because many strains are resistant to antimicrobials and emerge when these drugs are used; and because hospitalized patients are particularly likely to develop these infections and to have difficulty in withstanding them.

Bacteriology. Staphylococci are spherical gram-positive cocci that grow well on simple laboratory media. Grapelike clusters of organisms are characteristic in stained smears. In smears of pus, small clusters, pairs, and short chains may also be seen, and the organisms may be found within leukocytes.

Staphylococci are the most important pathogens of the genus Micrococcus, which also includes many saprophytes. Pathogenic staphylococci (*Micrococcus pyogenes*) are noteworthy for their biochemical versatility. Two species can be tentatively identified by pigment production on agar: *S. aureus* (golden yellow) and *S. epidermidis* (white). Pathogenic staphylococci may produce toxins with hemolytic, necrotizing, leukocidal, or lethal properties. They are usually capable of fermenting mannitol. They also may produce an enterotoxin, fibrinolysin, hyaluronidase, lipase, and coagulase (a plasma-clotting substance). The role of these toxins in the infectious process is unclear, but coagulase production and mannitol fermentation are thought to correlate best with pathogenicity for man. By convention, coagulase-positive, mannitol-fermenting staphylococci are called *S. aureus* (without regard to pigment production). *S. aureus* is the most important pathogenic Staphylococcus. Those strains lacking both of these characteristics are called *S. epidermidis* (formerly *S. albus*). *S. epidermidis* rarely causes infection of man unless susceptibility is increased or there is a nidus of infected foreign material.

Pathogenesis and Epidemiology. Abscess formation is a characteristic feature of staphylococcal infection. When staphylococci gain access to susceptible tissues and local multiplication begins, there is an acute inflammatory response. Thrombosis of small blood vessels is seen, and fibrin is deposited at the periphery of the lesion, which becomes relatively avascular and necrotic. The tissues become congested, tense, and painful. The lesion gradually liquefies, and the characteristic thick, creamy yellow pus forms, surrounded by a fibroblastic wall. Further evolution of the lesion is slow unless it drains. Antimicrobial drugs influence bacteria within abscesses very little, either because the drugs may not diffuse into abscesses very well, because they may be destroyed or inactivated there, or because the organisms may be in a relatively insusceptible state. A granulomatous reaction is occasionally seen at the site of a chronic staphylococcal infection.

Very little is firmly established about the factors responsible for the pathogenicity of staphylococci. The dermonecrotic, lethal, and leukocidal toxins have obvious but unproved clinical implications. Factors that promote or impair phagocytosis and killing of the common strains are poorly understood. An effect of coagulase in helping to wall off the lesion and in protecting the organism from granulocytes has been proposed, but has not been established. One can only speculate about the importance of hyaluronidase, fibrinolysin, or hemolysins. Partly because so many poorly understood toxins are involved, immunization as a means of enhancing resistance to staphylococci has met with little success. Most adults possess serum antibodies to a variety of staphylococcal antigens, but these have not been correlated well with protection or with recovery from disease. Furthermore, there is evidence that hypersensitivity reactions to some of the products of the microorganism may contribute to the development of the lesion.

Pathogenic staphylococci are normally acquired by a high percentage of healthy infants within a few days or weeks after birth, and most healthy humans harbor them in their anterior nares or on the skin either for long periods or intermittently (asymptomatic carriage). Clinical disease may occur in exposed persons or carriers when local or general resistance is decreased or when exposure is heavy. Exposure of tissues to large numbers of staphylococci is probably an uncommon mechanism initiating disease. The evidence that some strains of pathogenic staphylococci are especially virulent is not conclusive. To produce experimental skin infections in healthy men, more than a million pathogenic staphylococci must be inoculated, and no significant difference between strains has been detected. Factors that increase host susceptibility thus seem of primary importance in explaining the frequency of staphylococcal disease.

Although certain conditions are known to predispose to staphylococcal disease, the associated mechanisms and abnormalities that permit the organism to become invasive are not well understood. Skin infections usually begin about hair follicles, sebaceous glands, or at sites of abrasion or foreign body penetration. Greasy substances, oils, and conditions causing obstruction of the ducts of cutaneous glands predispose to infection. Burns, surgical wounds, and areas of dermatitis commonly become infected with staphylococci. In some cases this is the result of massive multiplication of the organism within exudates or devitalized tissues. Sutures enhance susceptibility to staphylococcal infection, possibly because bacteria can multiply within their interstices or because a tight suture may reduce local blood flow and impair cellular or humoral defense mechanisms. These mechanisms may also help explain the predilection for infection at the site of other foreign bodies, such as prosthetic devices and intravenous catheters. Diabetics seem to have an increased frequency of cutaneous staphylococcal infections, possibly because their acute inflammatory response may be delayed and deficient (especially during ketoacidosis), because of vascular disease, or because of their frequent exposure to hospitals and medical procedures that increase the risk of infection. Malnutrition and a great variety of serious debilitating diseases also predispose to serious staphylococcal infection. In some cases this may occur following treatment with antimicrobial drugs that encourage implantation or overgrowth of pathogenic staphylococci. In others it may be a consequence of therapy or disease processes that adversely affect cellular or humoral defense mechanisms. Neoplasms, uremia, extensive operations, and treatment with adrenal steroids or immunosuppressive agents predispose to staphylococcal infection. Influenza, measles, and mucoviscidosis predispose to staphylococcal pneumonia. Infants are subject to primary staphylococcal pneumonia, mastitis, and skin infections.

Because of their ubiquity, versatility, and complexity, staphylococci have become a major cause of serious infections in those highly susceptible persons who tend to congregate in hospitals. Bacteriophage typing of staphylococci has contributed to understanding of the modes of transmission of these infections. Man is the major source of the organism. Patients and personnel in hospitals are more commonly carriers of the organism than are those without hospital contact. The organism is most easily found in the anterior nares, in intertriginous areas, and on the hands. Carriers readily contaminate their environment, and staphylococci can be isolated from air, dust, floors, blankets, clothing, dressing carts, floor mops, and other fomites in hospitals.

Studies in nurseries for the newborn have shown that transmission of the organism occurs primarily via the hands of personnel, either because they are carriers or because they have handled infected or colonized newborns. Most postoperative wound infections appear to be attributable to strains carried by the patient prior to operation. Infected patients or infected personnel are also important sources of strains causing wound infections; direct contact or transmission via hands is the usual mechanism. Transmission via air, environment, or fomites is a less common means of wound infection, but all these mechanisms contribute to the perpetuation of the reservoir of staphylococci in the hospital and to the spread to personnel and highly susceptible patients.

Most authorities believe that intensive efforts to prevent the spread of staphylococci within hospitals are worthwhile. Infected patients should be isolated. Personnel with clinical infections should avoid contact with susceptible patients. The indiscriminate use of antimicrobial drugs should be decreased, as the practice favors the transmission and perpetuation of drug-resistant strains. Because so many persons are asymptomatic carriers of pathogenic staphylococci, it is not practicable to exclude all of them from contact with susceptible persons in hospitals. However, carriers of dangerous strains, as demonstrated by bacteriophage typing and clinical experience, should be excluded from nurseries, delivery rooms, and operating rooms.

Treatment. Although antimicrobial therapy has markedly improved the prognosis of serious staphylococcal infections, it should be emphasized that surgical drainage of abscesses or removal of infected foreign bodies is not only equally important, but may be the only way to achieve a cure. Patients with staphylococcal infections usually respond slowly to drug therapy, and despite optimal treatment the mortality rate is very high in persons with compromised defense mechanisms.

Although many antimicrobial drugs are available, the often unpredictable susceptibility of the organism narrows the initial choice to only a few. A bactericidal, penicillin-like drug is preferred. Because most strains causing infection in the hospital and many in the community are resistant to penicillin, the initial choice should include drugs that are not significantly influenced by staphylococcal penicillinase. Methicillin, oxacillin, nafcillin, cloxacillin, dicloxacillin, cephalothin, and cephaloridine are in this category. Other than cost and ease of administration, there is little reason for selecting one of these preparations over another. Since these drugs are adequate for the treatment of infections caused by penicillin-susceptible staphylococci, pneumococci, and Group A beta streptococci in the dosages commonly recommended for staphylococcal disease, it is not necessary to add penicillin to the regimen if these organisms are also suspected of playing a role in the illness. However, if the organism is susceptible to penicillin, it is preferred because it is usually the most active drug and the most convenient and inexpensive one to administer. Cultures and drug-susceptibility tests should be performed so that therapy can be altered appropriately. If the patient is allergic to penicillin, none of the semisynthetic penicillins should be used. Vancomycin, lincomycin, or cephalothin is a suitable substitute. However, allergic cross-reactions between penicillin and cephalothin have been observed. Kanamycin, gentamicin, erythromycin, and bacitracin are also occasionally useful. Tetracyclines and chloramphenicol are less frequently employed because of drug resistance or fear of toxicity.

Because of the variety of antimicrobial agents and clinical situations, few specific guidelines for dosage and duration of treatment can be given here. In general, the more severe the infection, the larger the dose and the longer the agent is administered. In severe infections, parenteral therapy is preferred because of the desirability of maintaining high concentrations of the antimicrobial in blood and tissues. Relapses are common if therapy is terminated too early, especially if the lesion has not drained.

Although methicillin-resistant strains of *S. aureus* have been isolated frequently in Europe, they are fortunately less common in the United States. Such organisms may show multiple resistance to the other semisynthetic penicillins and cephalosporins. They may be recognizable only after prolonged incubation in the presence of methicillin or oxacillin, presumably because the isolates contain only a small proportion of highly resistant cells. These organisms have occasionally been of clinical importance and the cause of outbreaks in hospitals. Wide misuse of the new penicillins will probably result eventually in an increase in the prevalence and importance of these strains. Vancomycin or a combination of kanamycin with cephalothin or methicillin has been recommended for treatment of infections with these organisms.

FURUNCLES AND CARBUNCLES

A *furuncle* or boil is an acute circumscribed abscess of the skin and subcutaneous tissues. When such lesions involve only a hair gland, they are termed *folliculitis*. Folliculitis is more common in persons with oily or greasy skin, and frequently it is caused by *S. epidermidis*.

Furuncles are most common on the face, back of the neck, buttocks, thighs, perineum, or breasts, or in the axillae. Most furuncles begin at the base of a hair follicle and take three to five days to evolve. Itching may be prominent at the onset. As inflammation progresses, the lesion may become exquisitely tender, but there is usually little systemic reaction. As the center of the lesion becomes necrotic and hypertonic, fluid is drawn into the furuncle, and it swells, thinning the overlying skin. Spontaneous drainage of pus then occurs, and pain is relieved. A hard core of necrotic debris from the center of the abscess may be extruded. Spontaneous healing of the abscess is usually rapid and complete within a few days of drainage, although erythema may persist for several weeks. Patients with multiple or recurrent lesions are said to have *furunculosis*. It has been estimated that normal adults experience an average of five or six furuncles per year. Furuncles may regress without draining, forming a "blind boil" that is indolent and prone to exacerbation following minor local trauma.

If sebaceous glands of the face and upper back are extensively involved with furuncles, the condition known as *pustular acne vulgaris* may result. Although juvenile acne is not caused by staphylococci, these organisms may secondarily infect the lesions.

Furuncles involving sweat glands (*hydradenitis*) are extremely painful and troublesome. The infection tends to spread to other local sweat glands and hair follicles and to result in chronic infection and extensive scarring. Axillary hydradenitis is particularly common and difficult to cure.

Although bacteremia rarely occurs with an uncomplicated furuncle unless the lesion is manipulated, furuncles are extremely common, and they are believed to be important in the initiation of endocarditis, osteomyelitis, and pyarthrosis by causing transient bacteremia. Septic thrombophlebitis is another complication of furuncles. For this reason, furuncles in the middle third of the face are especially dangerous, because they may extend intracranially via veins and cause cavernous sinus thrombophlebitis.

Carbuncles are extensive furuncles or aggregates of interconnected furuncles which drain through multiple skin openings. Acute suppurative inflammation of subcutaneous tissues extending between hair follicles in clefts along fibrous and adipose tissue is characteristic of carbuncles. They usually occur where the skin is thick (such as the back of the neck), possibly because thick skin favors internal rather than external drainage and lateral extension. Carbuncles may attain the size of lemons, be extremely painful, and be associated with chills, fever, leukocytosis, malaise, prostration, bacteremia, and death.

Treatment. Some authorities believe that early furuncles may be aborted by the administration of an antimicrobial drug or by the local application of an antiseptic such as alcohol. Once drained, small lesions require no further therapy, but they should be kept covered to help prevent contamination of other sites. More severe lesions require local and systemic therapy. Rest, heat, and elevation of the affected site tend to relieve pain and minimize spread of the infection. Warm compresses favor maturation of the lesion, but care should be taken to ensure that they do not cause maceration of the skin. Incision should be delayed until frank suppuration and fluctuance are detectable, as early incision is ineffective and favors local extension.

Antimicrobial agents should be given if the furuncle is large, on the face or neck, or accompanied by lymphadenitis or systemic reaction. They should also be given if the patient has diabetes or an underlying disease predisposing to complications, or if surgical incision is to be performed. Oral therapy with penicillin, erythromycin, or lincomycin is usually satisfactory. Therapy should be continued until signs of active inflammation have disappeared; a week is usually sufficient. Gamma globulin, adrenal steroids, and bacteriophage preparations are of no value.

Prevention. Furuncles are difficult to prevent, because the patient usually continues to be susceptible and the organism is ubiquitous. However, measures that minimize contact with the organism are often worth the trouble they entail. Predisposing conditions should be treated or eliminated. Skin irritants and tight clothing should be avoided. The fingernails should be kept short, and frequent handwashing should be stressed. Draining lesions should be considered highly contaminated and kept covered. Daily bathing and shampooing with antiseptic soap may be useful. Very rarely it may be possible to eradicate the carrier state and thus prevent recurrences by administering antimicrobial drugs for several weeks or months. Antibiotic ointments may be applied frequently to susceptible areas or to the anteror nares to suppress the carrier state. It may be of help to interchange organisms by intentionally inducing nasal carriage with a relatively nonpathogenic species after the patient's Staphylococcus has been suppressed by drug therapy (bacterial interference). Staphylococcus vaccines, toxoids, or bacteriophages are of no proved value in prevention. Irradiation to produce glandular atrophy is not recommended.

PNEUMONIA

Except during influenza epidemics, staphylococci cause less than 5 per cent of all bacterial pneumonias, but the disease is especially important because of its high mortality rate. Staphylococcal pneumonia is most often seen in infants, in children with mucoviscidosis or measles, in adults with influenza, or in debilitated, hospitalized persons being treated with antimicrobials or immunosuppressants. Diagnosis and treatment of staphylococcal pneumonia in adults with predisposing diseases are often difficult. High spiking fever, multiple chills, cyanosis, rapidly progressive dyspnea, chest pain, and the production of thick creamy yellow or reddish-yellow sputum should lead to the suspicion of staphylococcal pneumonia. Peripheral vascular collapse and marked signs of toxicity should also cause one to suspect the diagnosis in patients with pulmonary infiltrates. In some patients, an unexplained abrupt and nondescript worsening of the general condition is the first clue to the diagnosis. Fever, cough, dyspnea, and chest pain may be minimal during early stages of staphylococcal pneumonia. Staphylococcal pneumonia developing in association with influenza characteristically begins with a sudden and marked worsening of the illness, accompanied by prostration, a peculiar reddish-blue (heliotrope) cyanosis, tachypnea, and high fever. In infants the sudden development of *pneumothorax, pneumatoceles, or empyema* is a characteristic feature.

The physical signs in patients with staphylococcal pneumonia are variable. A toxic appearance of the patient may be the only detectable manifestation. Patchy bronchopneumonia with multiple small abscesses is usual, and is detected by the presence of coarse or fine rales. Dullness to percussion is not an early sign. Signs of frank consolidation are rarely found. Because pleural effusion and empyema are common, signs of fluid may be found; however, the fluid is commonly loculated in intralobar fissures and is not easily detected.

The leukocyte count is usually elevated to between 15,000 and 25,000 per cubic millimeter. Chest roentgenograms show patchy infiltrates, most often near the hilum. Cavity formation and pleural effusion are common. The Gram-stained smear of the sputum shows polymorphonuclear leukocytes and large numbers of clustered gram-positive cocci. When cocci are seen within leukocytes in the sputum, staphylococcal pneumonia should be suspected. The blood culture is not often positive unless the pneumonia is secondary to staphylococcal bacteremia originating at some other site. As resistant staphylococci frequently colonize the respiratory tract soon after the administration of antimicrobial drugs, it is not proper to diagnose staphylococcal pneumonia solely on the basis of a sputum culture revealing rare or moderate numbers of the organism.

Differential Diagnosis. All other forms of pneumonia must be considered. The distinction from pneumonia caused by gram-negative organisms is especially important in patients developing pneumonia in the hospital. A carefully performed Gram stain of a good sample of sputum is the keystone of choosing initial therapy, and may be helpful in interpreting subsequent culture reports.

Prognosis. Even under the best of circumstances, the case mortality rate is 15 to 20 per cent. Higher fatality rates are seen in very young infants or in elderly debilitated patients. As this pneumonia is characterized by necrosis of lung parenchyma, recovery is gradual, and usually the illness lasts three to four weeks. Convalescence may be markedly prolonged when empyema is present. Bronchiectasis is sometimes a consequence of staphylococcal pneumonia.

Treatment. Once the diagnosis is tentatively established, vigorous antimicrobial therapy, including use of the parenteral route, should be initiated promptly. Methicillin, oxacillin, nafcillin, or cephalothin in doses of at least 1 gram every four to six hours are preferred and equally good. The organism should be considered resistant to penicillin and ampicillin until it is demonstrated to be otherwise. If the organism is susceptible, penicillin G (20 million units intravenously per day) is the drug of choice. If the patient is allergic to penicillin, vancomycin (0.5 gram intravenously every six to eight hours) may be used. Therapy should be continued for 10 to 14 days after the patient shows a definite clinical response. The clinical response is usually very gradual. Surgical drainage with a chest tube is usually required if empyema is present, because the pus is often loculated or too thick for needle aspiration. Proteolytic enzymes may be instilled into the pleural cavity to help thin the exudate. Oxygen, bronchodilators, expectorants, fluids, and other supportive measures are also of great importance.

OSTEOMYELITIS

Staphylococcus aureus is the most common cause of primary hematogenous osteomyelitis,* which is becoming a rare disease. Bacteremia from a minor skin infection is the usual inciting event, with organisms settling out in the diaphysis. Relatively minor antecedent trauma often appears responsible for localization at a particular site. Acute osteomyelitis is primarily a disease of children, and is more frequently seen in boys. The arterial blood supply of the diaphysis seldom crosses the epiphyses so that to a considerable extent when the epiphyses have closed, the circulation is terminal and hence subject to embolization. The infection tends to spread from the diaphysis along the marrow cavity or to the surface, forming a subperiosteal abscess. As necrosis of bone occurs, a *sequestra* may be formed, and new bone laid down by osteoblasts during healing forms an *involucrum*. If not treated early or adequately, the infection tends to become chronic and subclinical, with recurrent acute exacerbations and formation of chronic draining sinuses. Amyloidosis occasionally develops after extensive long-standing osteomyelitis.

High fever, chills, and pain in the bone are the early signs of osteomyelitis. Local muscle spasm and splinting are common. Redness, swelling, and warmth are seen later, and the patient may appear critically ill. Leukocytosis and positive blood cultures are usual. Anemia is common. Rarefaction of bone is the earliest radiologic sign, but may not appear until two weeks after onset. Later, periosteal reaction with new bone formation, dead bone, or sequestra may be seen. Frank infection only rarely extends to nearby joints, but sterile effusions are fairly common.

*Secondary osteomyelitis refers to infection of a bone as a consequence of trauma with contamination from the outside, e.g., a compound fracture.

Infections of vertebrae and intravertebral disks with staphylococci are being recognized more frequently. Paravertebral abscesses may be the first sign of the process, but usually the patient has back pain, pain radiating down the leg, or abdominal pain. The condition may be mistaken for tuberculous spondylitis. Bacteremia resulting in acute staphylococcal endocarditis is an important complication.

Rheumatic fever, traumatic lesions, leukemia, scurvy, pyogenic arthritis, and neoplasms should be considered in the differential diagnosis of osteomyelitis.

Treatment. If treatment is appropriate, death from acute osteomyelitis is rare, and progression to chronic osteomyelitis is not likely. Since early treatment is important, therapy directed against the Staphylococcus should be started as soon as cultures have been obtained when the diagnosis appears likely. Parenteral therapy should be given initially; one of the penicillins, cephalosporins, or lincomycin is recommended. Some clinical response should be noted within four days. Treatment should be continued for at least three weeks. Although small sequestra usually absorb, larger pieces of dead bone may require surgical removal, especially if there is a slow or incomplete clinical response.

With chronic osteomyelitis, antimicrobial therapy should be given, and sequestrectomy, saucerization of infected bone, and removal of sinus tracts should be performed. Only rarely will such patients respond to drug therapy alone.

BACTEREMIA AND ENDOCARDITIS

Bacteremia may occur with any localized staphylococcal infection. Skin infections, infected intravascular foreign bodies, operative wound infections, endocarditis, and osteomyelitis are the most common foci causing bacteremia. It is usually associated with hectic fever, with temperatures to 104° F. or more, repeated shaking chills, and marked systemic toxicity. Metastatic abscesses commonly develop in kidneys, lungs, bone, skin, brain, meninges, myocardium, and other tissues. The case mortality rate with staphylococcal bacteremia is 50 per cent when there is a predisposing underlying disease, and about 20 per cent when there is not. Staphylococcal bacteremia is frequent in patients with marked granulocytopenia. Bacteremia with coagulase-negative staphylococci may pursue an indolent course with remarkably few clinical manifestations for many weeks; blood stream infections with these organisms are fairly common following ventriculoatriostomy or cardiac surgery with insertion of prostheses.

Endocarditis may complicate staphylococcal bacteremia. The disease is usually of the acute, malignant, or ulcerative type, but a form indistinguishable from that caused by *S. viridans* is occasionally seen. The illness usually has an acute onset with shaking chills, high fever, rapidly progressive anemia, marked leukocytosis, changing cardiac murmurs, cutaneous pustules and petechiae, splinter hemorrhages, hematuria, and metastatic abscesses. This is usually a fulminating infection; normal heart valves may be destroyed in just a few days. Abscess of the myocardial valve ring is a common complication, and should be suspected when arrhythmias develop. The distinction between bacteremia from another focus and endocarditis may be difficult. Continuous bacteremia suggests endocarditis or other intravascular focus; intermittent bacteremia suggests an extravascular focus.

Even with appropriate therapy, staphylococcal bacteremia still has a very high mortality rate. Parenteral therapy is necessary, and the regimen *must* be bactericidal. Therapy for bacteremia should be continued for at least four weeks, and preferably eight weeks if it is believed that the patient has endocarditis as well as bacteremia. In doubtful cases, therapy should be prolonged. Surgical treatment of the focus of infection is important. When the site is an intravascular foreign body, the infection is rarely cured until the foreign material is removed.

GASTROENTERITIS AND ENTEROCOLITIS

The enterotoxins produced by staphylococci are an important cause of acute epidemic gastroenteritis. The toxin is formed prior to ingestion of contaminated and usually improperly refrigerated or stored food. Symptoms begin abruptly one to six hours after eating. Nausea, vomiting, cramping abdominal pain, prostration, and diarrhea may be severe. Fever is unusual, and the stools rarely contain blood, pus, or mucus. Only supportive treatment is needed. (See Staphylococcal Food Poisoning.)

Staphylococci are normal inhabitants of the intestines. Their numbers may increase during antimicrobial therapy, and the patient may experience diarrhea. Much more rarely they may cause *acute necrotizing pseudomembranous enterocolitis*. Most common following abdominal surgery, shock, or antimicrobial therapy, this condition has a high mortality rate. Symptoms include abdominal pain and distention, shock, fever, diarrhea, dehydration, and electrolyte depletion. Gram stain of the stool reveals large numbers of cocci in sheets and clumps, and establishes the diagnosis. Vancomycin (2.0 grams per day) given by mouth is the mainstay of treatment; parenteral therapy with another drug may also be given. Oral neomycin is not recommended, as so many staphylococci in hospitals are resistant to it. Shock and electrolyte imbalance should be treated vigorously.

MISCELLANEOUS INFECTIONS

Staphylococci are commonly found in throat cultures, but they do not cause pharyngitis or tonsillitis, except possibly in patients with agranulocytosis.

Staphylococcal pyarthrosis should be suspected in all patients with rheumatoid arthritis who show an apparent exacerbation of joint disease with fever, pain, effusion, and leukocytosis. Chills favor the diagnosis of septic arthritis over rheumatoid disease. Joint aspiration is essential for early diagnosis. Skin ulcers and intra-articular injections or aspirations are often important in pathogenesis. Immobilization, repeated aspirations, or surgical drainage and appropriate antimicrobial drugs are the treatment.

Staphylococcal meningitis is uncommon. It is usually the result of penetrating trauma, local surgery, or a manifestation of bacterial endocarditis.

Staphylococcal pericarditis usually occurs following bacteremia, often from an osteomyelitic focus, with formation of focal myocardial abscesses and spread to the pericardium. This organism is the most frequent cause of purulent pericarditis. Treatment consists of antimicrobial therapy and pericardiocentesis, but if rapid improvement is not noted open surgical drainage should be instituted.

Staphylococcal parotitis is usually seen in debilitated adults who become dehydrated and receive poor mouth care. Extensive edema, erythema, and tenderness are seen in the parotid area, and pus may be seen oozing from Stensen's duct. The patient usually has a high fever and disorientation. Shock and death are common. Irradiation of the gland may be a useful adjunct to therapy, but appropriate antimicrobial therapy and supportive care are far more important.

Barrett, F. F., McGehee, R. F., and Finland, M.: Methicillin-resistant *Staphylococcus aureus* at Boston City Hospital. New Eng. J. Med., 279:441, 1968.

Cluff, L. E., and Reynolds, R. J.: Management of staphylococcal infection. Amer. J. Med., 39:812, 1965.

Elek, S. D.: Staphylococcus Pyogenes. Edinburgh, E. and S. Livingstone, Ltd., 1959.

Fekety, F. R.: The epidemiology and prevention of staphylococcal infection. Medicine, 43:593, 1964.

Fisher, A. M., Trever, R. W., Curtin, J. A., Schultze, G., and Miller, D. F.: Staphylococcal pneumonia. New Eng. J. Med., 258:919, 1958.

Petersdorf, R. G., Forsyth, B. R., and Bernanke, D.: Staphylococcal parotitis. New Eng. J. Med., 259:1250, 1958.

Pollack, N., Spinner, M., and Richman, R.: Hematogenous pyogenic spondylitis. N.Y. J. Med., 64:2870, 1964.

Shinefield, H. R., Ribble, J. C., Boris, M., and Eichenwald, H.: Bacterial interference: Its effect on nursery acquired infection with *Staphylococcus aureus*. Amer. J. Dis. Child., 105:646, 1963.

DISEASES CAUSED BY NEISSERIA

GONOCOCCAL DISEASE
Donald Kaye

Definition. Gonorrhea is an infection of the mucous membrane of the urethra and genital tract caused by *Neisseria gonorrhoeae*. Infection is almost always the result of sexual contact. Following invasion of the genitourinary tract, gonococci may spread to extragenital sites and cause infections such as arthritis, tenosynovitis, perihepatitis, endocarditis, and meningitis. Since the advent of antimicrobial therapy, extragenital gonococcal infections have become rare.

Etiology. *N. gonorrhoeae* is a gram-negative coccus that was first described by Neisser in 1879 in exudates from patients with gonorrhea. In stained smears of exudates the organisms appear as diplococci with flattened or slightly concave adjacent sides and resemble a pair of kidney beans. A considerable portion of the organisms in exudates are within polymorphonuclear leukocytes. Gonococci grown in laboratory media assume an oval or spherical form, and single cocci and clumps of cocci may be found in addition to diplococci. *N. gonorrhoeae* can be distinguished from other Neisseria by its ability to ferment glucose but not maltose or sucrose.

Primary isolation of the gonococcus is difficult. The organism is fastidious in its growth requirements, and is susceptible to toxic substances that are present in many media. Blood, serum, ascitic fluid, or other agents must be added for enrichment, as growth will usually not occur on plain agar. Blood is commonly used, and the medium is heated (chocolate agar) to reduce the deleterious effect exerted by certain amino acids toxic to the gonococcus. Commerical media are available that satisfy the various growth requirements of *N. gonorrhoeae*. Most strains require an atmosphere of 2 to 10 per cent carbon dioxide. Colonies of *N. gonorrhoeae* are round, gray-white, and translucent. Overgrowth with other bacteria occasionally occurs in cultures of exudate from the urethra, vagina, and cervix and is frequent in cultures from the rectum if nonselective media are used.

All Neisseria produce an oxidase that can be used for tentative identification of colonies of *N. gonorrhoeae* (colonies turn purple on exposure to 1 per cent para-aminodimethylaniline monohydrochloride). With cultures from the genital tract, the combination of colonies of typical morphology composed of gram-negative diplococci and a positive oxidase test is strong presumptive evidence of the presence of *N. gonorrhoeae*. However, other Neisseria and members of the tribe Mimeae resemble *N. gonorrhoeae* both in colonial morphology and microscopic appearance and give a positive oxidase reaction (*Mima polymorpha* var. *oxidans* is the only Mimeae that is oxidase-positive). Therefore, cultures that are presumptively positive for *N. gonorrhoeae* should be confirmed by fermentation reactions or by fluorescent antibody techniques.

Thayer-Martin selective medium, containing vancomycin, sodium colistimethate, and nystatin, permits growth of *N. meningitidis* and *N. gonorrhoeae* but inhibits growth of many other bacteria frequently found in specimens from urethra, cervix, vagina, and rectum. Growth of other Neisseria and of *Mima polymorpha* var. *oxidans* is inhibited.

Incidence and Prevalence. There has been an increase in the reported incidence of gonococcal infections in recent years. However, the true incidence and prevalence of gonorrhea are unknown because of problems in diagnosis, antimicrobial therapy by nonmedical persons, incomplete reporting by physicians, and the presence of many undetected asymptomatic female carriers. It has been estimated that over 1.5 million new cases of gonorrhea occur annually in the United States. The magnitude of the problem of asymptomatic gonorrhea in females may be demonstrated by the results of one study which reported a 6 per cent incidence of asymptomatic gonorrhea in a large group of pregnant women.

Gonorrhea is a disease of the sexually active, and most cases occur in patients 15 to 24 years of age. Gonorrhea rates are higher among military personnel, migrant groups (such as itinerant laborers and seafarers), homosexuals, and prostitutes. In recent surveys 10 to 33 per cent of prostitutes had gonorrhea.

Epidemiology. *N. gonorrhoeae* is a parasite of man; it does not cause disease in animals. Gonorrhea is almost always acquired from sexual contact; exceptions are gonococcal conjunctivitis (which occurs primarily in infants) and vulvovaginitis. Conjunctivitis results either from passage of the infant through an infected genital tract (ophthalmia neonatorum) or from contamination after birth. Vulvovaginitis is an infection of the genital tract of infants and preadolescent girls that results from direct contact with infected adults or, rarely (in institutional outbreaks), is spread by contact with towels or linens contaminated with gonococci.

An episode of gonorrhea confers little or no immunity to subsequent infections, and repeated attacks are common. However, individual variation in susceptibility to infection has been demonstrated following inoculation of *N. gonorrhoeae* into the urethras of male volunteers. Trauma to the urethra probably increases susceptibility to gonorrhea. Following an episode of acute gonorrhea, *N. gonorrhoeae* may remain in the genital tract for months. Chronic asymptomatic carriers of the gonococcus (usually women) are important in the epidemiology of gonorrhea because they are difficult to detect and therefore are rarely treated.

Pathogenesis and Pathology. *N. gonorrhoeae* are unable to penetrate stratified squamous epithelium, but penetration and infection of columnar epithelium readily occurs. In males the urethra is attacked first, resulting in purulent urethritis and involvement of the urethral glands. Direct spread of infection may result in prostatitis, epididymitis, or seminal vesiculitis. During stages of healing, stricture formation may occur. Gonococcal proctitis in the male is almost always the result of rectal intercourse.

In the female, urethritis is mild and transient. Bartholin's and Skene's glands and glands of the cervix may become infected with or without involvement of the urethra. Contiguous spread of infection can cause salpingitis or proctitis. Gonococcal salpingitis is usually bilateral and may cause pyosalpinx and formation of a tubo-ovarian abscess. The inflammation tends to heal with fibrosis and adhesions that may produce obstruction of the fallopian tubes and sterility. Ascent of infection to the fallopian tubes often occurs during or just after menstruation. Although endometrial infection is usual when *N. gonorrhoeae* invades the fallopian tubes, it is not serious and tends to subside promptly. The vagina does not become infected in adults, probably because of the presence of squamous epithelium with many layers of cells and the lack of glands.

Conjunctivitis is the most common manifestation of gonococcal disease in infants. It is a destructive inflammation of the eye and before the use of antimicrobial agents frequently caused blindness. Between one year of age and pubescence, gonococcal infection is rare in males but causes vulvovaginitis in females. The increased susceptibility to gonococcal infection of the immature vaginal mucous membrane in contrast to the resistance of the mucosa of adults is probably explained by the thin mucous membrane present prior to adolescence.

Occasionally invasion of the blood occurs and *N. gonorrhoeae* may disseminate and produce infection at distant foci. Joints are the most frequent extragenital sites of localization, but tenosynovitis, endocarditis, meningitis, skin lesions, and infection at other foci may also occur.

Gonococcal pharyngitis has been reported to occasionally result from oral-genital contact.

Clinical Manifestations. Gonorrhea in the Male. The incubation period of gonococcal urethritis in the male is usually two to eight days. There is sudden onset of dysuria, urgency, and frequency associated with mucoid urethral discharge that rapidly becomes purulent and profuse. Gonococcal urethritis usually does not cause fever, but prostatitis, seminal vesiculitis, or epididymitis is frequently associated with fever. Acute urinary retention may result from involvement of the prostate. Rectal examination reveals tenderness of the affected organ in the presence of prostatitis or seminal vesiculitis. Epididymitis causes severe pain and tenderness of the epididymis.

Untreated gonorrhea subsides over a period of weeks, but a small amount of mucoid discharge from the urethra may continue to be found each morning for months. Gonococci may persist, usually in the prostate. Urethral stricture is a common sequela of untreated urethritis, especially after recurrent attacks of gonorrhea. Epididymitis can result in sterility.

Gonorrhea in the Female. In females the disease may begin with dysuria, urgency, and frequency after an incubation period of two to eight days. However, the urethritis is frequently of short duration and often is mild or completely asymptomatic. Cervicitis gives rise to a muco-

purulent discharge that varies from scant to profuse. Involvement of Skene's ducts or Bartholin's glands is common, and abscess formation may occur. Gonococci can be isolated from the rectum in 20 to 40 per cent of women with gonorrhea, and occasionally can produce symptomatic proctitis manifested by anal discharge, burning rectal pain, blood and pus in the stools, and pain on defecation. The duration of symptoms from an untreated infection that remains localized in the lower genital tract is usually no longer than a month or two. However, the patient may remain a carrier of the disease for many months.

Salpingitis is manifested by acute onset of fever and lower abdominal pain. Physical examination usually reveals lower abdominal tenderness, pain on movement of the cervix, and tenderness of the adnexa (with or without palpable masses). Acute pelvic inflammatory disease tends to recur, and pelvic pain and fever are present intermittently. Sterility is common.

Extragenital Gonococcal Infection. *Arthritis.* Arthritis is the most common form of extragenital gonorrhea and usually occurs within one to three weeks after initial infection in the genital tract. Onset may be gradual with migratory polyarthalgias leading to frank arthritis in one or more joints, or it may be sudden with hot, swollen, and extremely painful joints. Fever and leukocytosis are usually present. Over 75 per cent of patients have polyarthritis. The joints that are most commonly involved are the knees, ankles, and wrists, in that order, but any joint may be involved, including the spine and sternoclavicular and temporomandibular joints. *Tenosynovitis,* which is rarely observed in other types of pyogenic arthritis, is common in gonococcal arthritis and most often occurs about the wrists and ankles.

N. gonorrhoeae can be isolated from joint fluid in only 25 to 50 per cent of cases. The fluid ranges from serous to frankly purulent, has the protein content of an exudate and usually contains increased numbers of leukocytes that are mainly polymorphonuclear. Muscle wasting about the joint and permanent deformity may result. Some authorities believe that two types of arthritis are produced by the gonococcus, one with infection in the joint and the other related to a hypersensitivity reaction. Evidence in support of the existence of the hypersensitivity form is inconclusive. Other investigators believe that sterility of the joint fluid in some patients is due to taking cultures early in the disease, before micro-organisms in the joint have sufficient time to proliferate.

Ten to 20 per cent of patients with arthritis have conjunctivitis that is usually nonpurulent and sterile. Rarely, iridocyclitis occurs and can result in blindness. Keratodermia blennorrhagica occurs in association with Reiter's syndrome (abacterial urethritis, conjunctivitis, and arthritis), but may be a rare complication of gonococcal arthritis. Keratodermia blennorrhagica is a symmetrical eruption with a predilection for the soles, palms, and genitals. The lesions start as erythematous macules that vesiculate, become keratotic, and tend to become confluent. A rheumatoid syndrome may occasionally follow gonococcal arthritis. This association may be coincidental, or perhaps gonococcal arthritis provokes clinical rheumatoid arthritis in some predisposed people.

Gonococcal Bacteremia. Gonococcal bacteremia can produce a syndrome with recurrent episodes of fever, skin lesions, arthralgia or arthritis, mild to severe constitutional symptoms, and intermittently positive blood cultures. This syndrome is most common in females, occurs with acute or chronic genital tract infection, and can recur over a period of months or even years. The rash usually appears during the first day of symptoms and may recur with each episode of fever. The rash is found on the distal part of the extremities and consists of scanty pin-point erythematous macules that rapidly become maculopapular, vesiculopustular, and frequently hemorrhagic. Bullae can form. The mature lesion is elevated, has a dirty gray necrotic center, and is surrounded by erythema. It heals in three to four days. Gram-negative cocci can often be seen in stains of fluid from the lesions, and occasionally *N. gonorrhoeae* can be isolated from the fluid. Identical skin lesions may be seen in patients with meningococcemia, which can present an indistinguishable clinical syndrome.

Gonococcal Endocarditis. Gonococcal endocarditis is extremely rare at present. In most patients, previously normal valves are attacked. The valves on the left side of the heart are involved most often, but valves on the right side are affected with a higher frequency than with endocarditis caused by other bacteria. A double daily temperature elevation (double quotidian) is common in patients with gonococcal endocarditis, and jaundice occurs in a higher proportion of patients than with any other type of endocarditis.

Perihepatitis (Fitz-Hugh-Curtis Syndrome). Perihepatitis is a rare complication in women with gonococcal pelvic inflammatory disease and results from spread of gonococci from the pelvis to the upper abdomen. It is manifested by fever, upper quadrant pain (usually right upper quadrant), tenderness and spasm of the abdominal wall, and occasionally a friction rub over the liver. During the acute stage the gallbladder temporarily may not be visualized on cholecystography; this can lead to an erroneous diagnosis of cholecystitis. The patient often has a recent history of pelvic pain or vaginal discharge, and physical examination may reveal evidence of pelvic inflammatory disease. *N. gonorrhoeae* can frequently be demonstrated in the cervical or vaginal discharge.

The symptoms respond to antimicrobial therapy. The untreated disease subsides after one to four weeks of fever and abdominal pain, leaving "violin-string" adhesions between the anterior surface of the liver and the anterior abdominal wall.

Diagnosis. The combination of urethritis and the presence of intracellular gram-negative diplococci in smears of exudate from the urethra is strong presumptive evidence of gonorrhea. Confirmation is obtained by culture or, if available, fluorescent antibody studies. In the female, cultures of exudate from cervix, vagina, and rectum should be obtained in addition to cultures from the urethra. Members of the tribe Mimeae have been isolated from patients with syndromes resembling gonorrhea. The morphology of these organisms is very similar to that of *N. gonorrhoeae,* especially in exudates, and culture or fluorescent antibody studies are necessary for differentiation.

Gonorrhea is frequently asymptomatic in the female. The diagnosis should be suspected in any female contact of an infected male. Chronic carriers of *N. gonorrhoeae* are difficult to detect because cultures for gonococci are often negative (especially in females). In the suspected male carrier the yield of positive cultures can be increased by studying prostatic secretions.

Gonococci die within hours if allowed to dry. Therefore, exudates should be inoculated as soon as possible on a suitable medium for *N. gonorrhoeae* (Thayer-Martin selective medium is preferable for specimens from urethra, vagina, cervix, or rectum). With use of fluorescent antibody it is frequently possible to definitively identify *N. gonorrhoeae* in exudate within one hour of obtaining the specimen.

Acute salpingitis must be differentiated from appendicitis and tubal pregnancy. The presence of bilateral tenderness in the adnexa with or without masses, a history of recent sexual intercourse followed by urethritis or vaginal discharge, and demonstration of gonococci on cervical smear are strongly suggestive of gonococcal salpingitis. When it is impossible to differentiate acute salpingitis from appendicitis or tubal pregnancy, the diagnosis must be established at operation.

The diagnosis of gonococcal arthritis should be suspected in a patient with a recent history of urethritis, especially if *N. gonorrhoeae* can be isolated from the genital tract. The presence of tenosynovitis is very suggestive. Demonstration of gonococci in the joint fluid is confirmatory. The serum complement-fixation test for gonococci may be of aid in suggesting gonococcal arthritis, especially if titers are rising. However, this test is not well standardized.

When stains and cultures of joint fluid are negative for gonococci (50 to 75 per cent of cases), it is frequently difficult to differentiate gonococcal arthritis from Reiter's syndrome. The problem in differential diagnosis is compounded by the fact that patients with Reiter's syndrome may have concomitant gonococcal urethritis. Urethritis and arthritis in a female suggest gonococcal arthritis, as this disease is more common in females, whereas Reiter's syndrome is rare in females. The presence of tenosynovitis and response to antimicrobial therapy strongly imply gonococcal arthritis. Patients with Reiter's syndrome frequently have prolonged courses with recurrences and do not respond to antimicrobial therapy. Gonococcal arthritis can often be differentiated from acute rheumatic fever, rheumatoid arthritis, and gout by the absence of carditis, lack of rheumatoid factor in serum, and failure to respond to colchicine, respectively.

When *N. gonorrhoeae* cannot be isolated from the joint, the response to penicillin therapy is often the strongest confirmatory evidence of gonococcal arthritis.

Treatment and Prognosis. Penicillin is the drug of choice for all gonococcal infections. Prior to 1954 a single injection of 300,000 units of penicillin cured almost all cases of gonorrhea. In recent years gonococcal strains of increased resistance to penicillin (requiring 0.08 to 1.0 μg. per milliliter for inhibition) have constituted as much as 50 per cent of all isolates. Concomitantly there has been a striking increase in the incidence of failure of therapy with 600,000 to 1,200,000 units of penicillin. It must be stressed that penicillin remains the drug of choice for gonorrhea but that larger doses are required than in previous years. The current recommendations of the United States Public Health Service for treatment of uncomplicated gonorrhea are: for men, a single intramuscular injection of 2.4 million units of procaine penicillin; for women, 4.8 million units of procaine penicillin injected intramuscularly at one visit (two sites of injection are recommended). The cure rate with these regimens is over 90 per cent in the continental United States. However, it has become apparent that these doses of penicillin are inadequate for treatment of gonorrhea in certain areas of the Far East where more resistant gonococcal strains are found. The addition of 1 gram of probenecid one hour before the penicillin injection and 0.5 gram taken 6, 12, and 18 hours after the injection has given excellent results in the Far East, decreasing the failure rate from 29 to 2 per cent (Holmes et al.).

Urethritis should subside within two to three days after administration of penicillin. A watery urethral discharge may persist in males for weeks despite elimination of gonococci and usually requires no treatment (postgonococcal urethritis or nongonococcal urethritis). Several studies have demonstrated that postgonococcal urethritis can usually be prevented by use of tetracycline for therapy of gonorrhea and that postgonococcal urethritis will usually respond to tetracycline treatment.

Relapse of gonorrhea occurs most commonly during the first week after treatment. Therefore, to evaluate cure, a culture should be obtained one week after therapy and, if possible, at two more weekly intervals. If relapse occurs, the patient should be re-treated with double the original dose of penicillin over a period of one to two days or with tetracycline as detailed below.

Causes of failure of penicillin therapy, other than infection with gonococci relatively resistant to penicillin, are failure to distinguish between relapse and reinfection; failure to identify nongonococcal urethritis, e.g., Reiter's syndrome, Mimeae infection or mycoplasma infection (Csonka et al.), and possibly the presence of penicillinase-producing bacteria at the site of infection.

Patients with gonococcal prostatitis, seminal vesiculitis, epididymitis, salpingitis, or arthritis should be treated with bed rest and 4.8 million units of procaine penicillin intramuscularly each day for seven to ten days (two weeks for arthritis) or longer until signs of infection have subsided and cultures become negative. Response to therapy usually occurs within two to three days. However, arthritis frequently responds more slowly, and it may take seven to ten days for the patient to become afebrile.

In acute gonococcal disease in the genital tract, surgery is indicated only for drainage of abscesses. However, in the chronic stage in some female patients it may become necessary to remove involved pelvic organs. In gonococcal arthritis, pus should be aspirated by needle when possible, but occasionally surgical drainage of the joint becomes necessary. Injection of penicillin into the joint is not indicated. Physiotherapy should be started during the period of convalescence to promote return of function of the joint.

Patients who are allergic to penicillin may be treated with tetracycline. The regimen for urethritis or cervicitis is a single oral dose of 1.5 grams followed by 0.5 gram given orally every six hours for four days. For prostatitis, seminal vesiculitis, epididymitis, salpingitis, or arthritis, this drug may be administered in doses of 0.5 gram orally four times a day for one to two weeks.

For gonococcal endocarditis or meningitis, 20 million units of aqueous penicillin G should be administered parenterally each day (four to six weeks for endocarditis and two weeks for meningitis).

About 3 per cent of patients with gonorrhea may be in the incubation period of syphilis. The doses of penicillin suggested may abort syphilis or may just delay appearance of manifestations. Therefore, serologic tests for syphilis should be performed for all patients treated for gonococcal infections prior to therapy and periodically until six months after therapy.

Prevention. Use of a condom provides a high degree of protection for the uninfected partner. Past experience has indicated that prophylactic use of oral penicillin in a dose of 250,000 units within two to three hours after exposure markedly decreases the incidence of infection. Sexual partners of patients with gonorrhea should be identified and treated as quickly as possible to prevent further spread of disease.

The instillation of 1 per cent silver nitrate (Credé method) or an antimicrobial drug into the eyes of the newborn has largely eradicated gonococcal ophthalmia neonatorum.

Abu-Nassar, H., Hill, N., Fred, H. L., and Yow, E. M.: Cutaneous manifestations of gonococcemia. A review of 14 cases. Arch. Intern. Med. (Chicago), 112:731, 1963.
Csonka, G. W., Williams, R. E. O., and Corse, J.: T-strain mycoplasma in non-gonococcal urethritis. Lancet, 1:1292, 1966.
Holmes, K. K., et al.: Studies of venereal disease. J.A.M.A., 202:461, 467, 474, 1967.

Keiser, H., Ruben, F. L., Wolinsky, E., and Kushner, I.: Clinical forms of gonococcal arthritis. New Eng. J. Med., 279:234, 1968.

Thayer, J. D., and Garson, W.: The Gonococcus. *In* Dubos, R. J., and Hirsch, J. G. (eds.): Bacterial and Mycotic Infections of Man. 4th ed. Philadelphia, J. B. Lippincott Company, 1965.

Thayer, J. D., and Martin, J. E., Jr.: Improved medium selective for cultivation of *N. gonorrhoeae* and *N. meningitidis.* Public Health Rep., 81:559, 1966.

Thayer, J. D., Samuels, S. B., Martin, J. E., Jr., and Lucas, J. B.: Comparative antibiotic susceptibility of *Neisseria gonorrhoeae* from 1955 to 1964. *In* Antimicrobial Agents and Chemotherapy—1964. Ann Arbor, American Society for Microbiology, 1965.

Today's VD Control Problem. A Joint Statement by the American Public Health Association, American Social Health Association, and American Venereal Disease Association, New York, American Social Health Association, 1969.

Vickers, F. N., and Maloney, P. J.: Gonococcal perihepatitis. Report of three cases with comments on diagnosis and treatment. Arch. Intern. Med. (Chicago), 114:120, 1964.

Wright, V.: Arthritis associated with venereal disease. A comparative study of gonococcal arthritis and Reiter's syndrome. Ann. Rheum. Dis., 22:77, 1963.

MENINGOCOCCAL DISEASE

Harry A. Feldman

DEFINITION

Meningococcal infections may affect the upper and lower respiratory tracts, blood (meningococcemia), central nervous system (meningococcal meningitis, cerebrospinal fever, spotted fever, or epidemic cerebrospinal meningitis), joints (arthritis), heart, eyes, skin, and other organs, singly or in any combination in a given patient. First recognized in 1805 by Vieusseux in Geneva and in 1806 by Danielson and Mann in Massachusetts, meningococcal meningitis, the best known form, occurs sporadically and as localized or widespread epidemics.

ETIOLOGY

Neisseria meningitidis, a gram-negative coccus, variable in size and occurring singly or as biscuit-shaped diplococci, was established as the causative agent by Weichselbaum in 1887. A metabolically fastidious organism, it grows best on enriched laboratory media at body temperature in an atmosphere of increased CO_2. Suitable media are Mueller-Hinton or meat infusion broths or agar containing 10 per cent of blood (rabbit, sheep, or horse), or human ascitic fluid. Chocolate agar is especially good for initial isolation. Cultures incubated in an atmosphere of 5 to 10 per cent carbon dioxide will grow more luxuriantly. This also improves the isolation rate. Meningococci are very susceptible to chilling or drying, so all cultures should be inoculated and incubated promptly. Some meningococcal strains are exquisitely susceptible to sulfonamides, and as the patient may have received such drugs, para-aminobenzoic acid (5 mg. per 100 ml.) should be added to media to be inoculated with clinical specimens.

Identification of meningococci is based on morphology, Gram-staining, fermentation of glucose and maltose but not sucrose, and immunologic reactions. The four classic immunologic groups, A, B, C, and D, have been expanded to include X, Y, Z, Z', 29-E, and W-135. The most common are A, B, C, and Y. Group D is exceedingly rare. The groups are identified by their agglutination with specific antisera. The A and C strains are encapsulated and may be identified by quellung (capsular swelling) with specific antisera. This reaction is especially useful for the rapid, precise identification of organisms in cerebrospinal fluid.

Lipopolysaccharides or "endotoxins" in purified form have been prepared from meningococci. Although these are toxic for animals and probably play significant roles in the pathogenesis of human disease, much of this remains to be defined. A true, group-specific exotoxin has not been demonstrated.

EPIDEMIOLOGY

Any discussion of the epidemiology of meningococcal infections is complicated by the multiplicity of serogroups. Sporadic infections may be seen almost constantly in all areas. Major epidemics are generally caused by Group A organisms and seem to occur in approximately 20-year cycles. For example, during World Wars I and II massive outbreaks occurred which persisted for several years. Groups B and C produce lesser outbreaks, usually in the intervening years. Thus, the overall picture is that of high waves about every 20 to 25 years and lower ones in the interims. There are localized exceptions to this generalization. Detroit had a major Group A epidemic in 1929, with 724 cases reported in an eight-month period and a general mortality rate of 50 per cent. In infants, however, the mortality rate was 84 per cent and in those over 40 years, 72 per cent. Santiago, Chile, had a severe Group A epidemic in 1941 to 1942 with 5885 cases; of these, 15.9 per cent died. The contrasting mortality rates probably reflect the effectiveness of sulfonamide treatment.

In recent years the most devastated area has been that portion of Africa which lies below the Sahara and north of the Equator. This "meningitis belt" now averages about 10,000 cases per year with about 1200 deaths, but from 1939 to 1962 it reported 593,738 cases with 102,956 (17 per cent) deaths! In earlier outbreaks in the same area, as many as 85 per cent of cases were fatal. Here, as in South Africa, Group A organisms continue to predominate.

Infants and children are most frequently attacked, accounting for about half of all cases in the general population. Military recruits are especially vulnerable, for no known reason; about 80 to 85 per cent of their cases occur within the first 90 days of service, most often in the first month. The incidence of both cases and carriers is usually higher in males. Race and color do not seem to influence either incidence or susceptibility.

The higher rates reported among Negroes in certain urban areas have been attributed primarily to crowding. The exact incubation period is often nondeterminable, but the range is probably one to ten days. There are a few instances in which longer (about three weeks) such periods seem to have occurred.

The portal of entry of meningococci is the upper respiratory tract, and transmission from person to person occurs by direct or intimate contact, by air-borne droplets, or by articles contaminated with fresh secretions from the respiratory tract. Mouth-to-mouth resuscitation has resulted in several cases in physicians. Yet even during severe epidemics, the majority of clinical infections seem to be unrelated to others so that case-to-case spread is usually impossible to trace. Culture surveys during outbreaks may demonstrate as much as 90 per cent of the population to be nasopharyngeal carriers of meningococci, constantly or intermittently, without clinical evidence of disease. Although the carrier rate is usually less than 5 per cent during interepidemic periods, much of the population may harbor meningococci at some time, as the respiratory tract flora is constantly undergoing change.

Group A meningococci and, to a lesser extent, Groups B and C strains have been the usual causes of epidemics in the past. Organisms of these groups were highly susceptible to sulfonamides so that such drugs were exceedingly effective for both the treatment of cases and mass prophylaxis. In 1963, a significant increase in the prevalence of sulfonamide-resistant Group B meningococci was noted. Subsequently, markedly resistant Group C strains were detected, and more recently, and perhaps even more disturbing, sulfonamide-resistant Group A strains have been isolated from an epidemic in North Africa. The latter subsequently seems to have spread into the "belt" below the Sahara. Resistant A strains now have been found in Europe, Southeast Asia, South Africa, and Australia. This phenomenon is now so widespread that *all cases must be considered to be due to sulfonamide-resistant strains unless specifically proved to be otherwise.* The same holds for carrier strains as well. Many Group Y strains, although not yet a major cause of disease, are sulfonamide-resistant.

The physician is often concerned with the question of whether family members or other contacts of meningococcal cases are at excessive risk from this disease. Fortunately, secondary cases are unusual, but they do occur. In the Detroit epidemic of 1929, 4 per cent of cases were in affected households. In the Santiago epidemic of 1941–1942, the over-all secondary attack rate was 2.5 per cent. Household carrier rates, on the other hand, are high. In several studies of families of meningococcal patients, 45 to 50 per cent were found to be carrying organisms of the same type as the patient. These figures provide some justification for the anxieties of both families and physicians when cases occur. The solution was relatively simple when sulfonamide-susceptible strains were the rule. Since no suitable substitute drug is available at present, proper management requires culture and study to determine drug susceptibility. If the strain is resistant, then one can only search carefully for symptoms and institute immediate therapy should any appear. Hopefully, as will be seen below, this situation may change in the not too distant future.

PATHOGENESIS AND PATHOLOGY

In *meningococcemia* the essential lesion is vascular, with endothelial damage, inflammation of vessel walls with necrosis and thrombosis and focal hemorrhages into cutaneous, subcutaneous, submucosal, and synovial tissues. In rapidly extending meningococcemia the Waterhouse-Friderichsen syndrome is often present. This is usually accompanied by bilateral adrenal hemorrhage.

Involvement of the central nervous system is characterized by *acute purulent meningitis,* although, if suspected early, there may be only hyperemia. Some degree of encephalitis usually accompanies the meningitis. When treatment is delayed or ineffective, permanent damage to the cranial nerves is to be expected.

The pathogenesis of meningococcal infections is usually initiated by the colonization of the posterior nasopharynx and adjoining structures by bacteria entering through the upper respiratory passages. Symptoms and signs of an acute upper respiratory infection probably result, although this is not accepted by all observers. Invasion of the blood stream follows, but this may be relatively asymptomatic. The resulting dissemination of the meningococci leads to metastatic lesions in *skin, meninges, joints, eyes, ears, lungs, pericardium, urethra,* and in other organs and tissues. The sites of these localizations determine the symptoms and signs that follow.

We are totally at a loss to explain why meningococcal infections are so limited and innocuous in some individuals and so extensive and overwhelming in others. *No microbe can kill more quickly; deaths have been observed several hours after the onset of the first symptom.*

Chemical alterations reflecting the severity of the meningococcal infection may be profound. Their cause is not known, but it is assumed that they are endotoxic in origin. They may be furthered by the release of various substances from damaged tissue cells. Hemorrhagic manifestations may be owing to direct vascular damage because of a Shwartzman-like reaction, to thrombocytopenia, or to both. Other changes are those found in acute sepsis: fever, dehydration, reduction in blood volume, altered acid-base balance, and negative nitrogen balance. In severely ill patients, cyanosis, circulatory collapse, and other signs of shock appear, probably the result of the combined actions of bacterial endotoxins and tissue anoxia. Alterations suggestive of acute adrenal insufficiency, low serum sodium, elevated potassium, low chloride, and hypoglycemia, may be present and are consistent with absent or diminished cortical secretion by damaged adrenal glands. There is no evidence that adrenal insufficiency as judged by the degree of excretion of corticosteroids in fulminating infections per se occurs independently of glandular destruction.

CLINICAL MANIFESTATIONS

A sequential development of clinical manifestations of meningococcal infections can be discerned from a number of cases, but any one patient may present with symptoms and signs of advanced diffuse illness. The usual sequence consists of infection of the upper respiratory tract, bacteremia, septicemia, meningitis and/or other metastatic localization. One stage will appear to dominate, giving the appearance of mild illness, grave illness, or none.

Infection of the Upper Respiratory Tract

Infection of the upper respiratory tract numerically is the most common meningococcal infection. Most patients have no or inconsequential symptoms so that the infection is detectable only by culture of the posterior nasopharynx. Whether any symptoms ever result from such colonization is contested by many observers, because descriptions of this stage have usually been made in military recruits who are also subjected to many viral and mycoplasmal respiratory infections. On the other hand, many but not all patients with meningococcal illnesses give histories of preceding or concurrent nasopharyngitis.

Meningococcemia

Bacteremic meningococcal infections may vary from acute fulminating illnesses of a few hours' duration to indolent, chronic infections lasting days, weeks, or months. Symptoms may be relentlessly progressive or intermittent with relapses and recrudescences at different times.

Mild or Subacute Meningococcemia. The most common form of meningococcemia is that of a relatively mild, acute, or subacute infection. Prodromal symptoms are frequently absent except for those of a mild upper respiratory infection in some. Onset is usually sudden, with fever, chilliness or frank chills that may be recurrent, malaise, myalgia, and apathy. The presenting symptoms may be any combination of these, but frequently the initial complaints are those of recurrent fever, rash, arthralgia, acute mono- or polyarthritis, nausea and vomiting, and conjunctivitis. The symptoms may regress or persist if the disease progresses. Fever may be remittent and irregular with "spikes" to 102 or 103° F. The pulse rate is proportionate to the fever. Respirations are usually normal or only slightly increased except when there is pneumonia or pleurisy.

The most striking feature on physical examination is the rash that is present in many cases. It appears soon after onset, is variable (the severest is petechial or purpuric), measuring from 1 or 2 mm. to 1 cm. or more in diameter, and is pink to reddish blue (see accompanying figure). Early in the disease there may be a generalized, mottled erythema which appears dusky in slightly cyanotic patients. Light pink macules resembling the "rose spots" of typhoid, wheals, or nodules like erythema nodosum may appear before petechiae and ecchymoses. Careful search in good daylight may be necessary to detect early lesions. Occasionally,

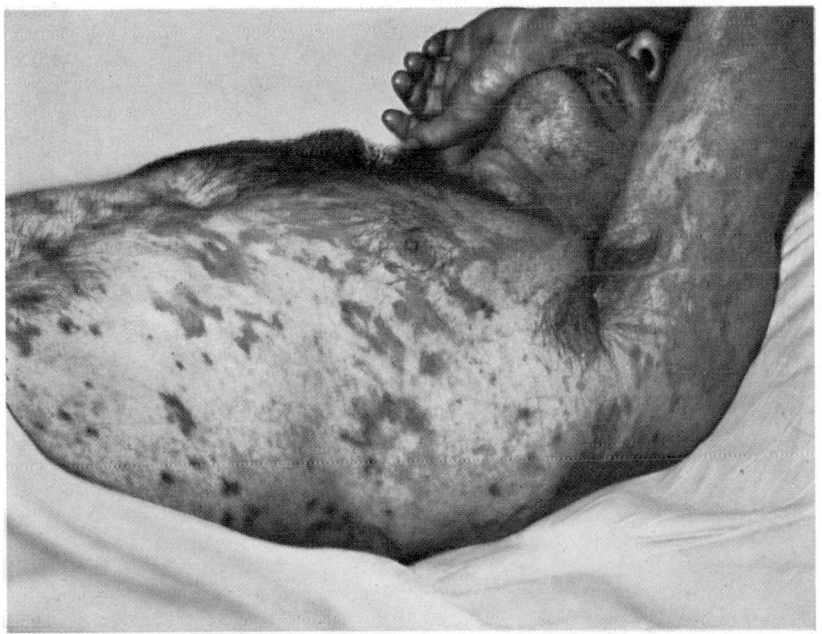

Skin lesions in fulminating meningococcemia. (Courtesy of Dr. Worth B. Daniels.)

vesicular, pustular, or bullous lesions are present. Superficial or deep ulcerations may result from petechiae. These are sometimes very extensive and may ultimately require grafting. The rash often appears first on the wrists and ankles, but any area may be involved, including the conjunctivae and the mucous membranes. Hemorrhagic lesions fade to a brown, rusty color three or four days after their appearance; if new crops appear, often after chills, multiple skin lesions may be present at the same time. This is likely if treatment is delayed or unsuccessful.

Other physical findings, including splenomegaly, are inconstant. Herpetic lesions of the lip are found in about 10 per cent of the cases. Unless meningismus develops, symptoms referable to the central nervous system are absent, although those resulting from metastatic localizations are usually self-evident, depending upon their site.

The firm diagnosis is established with laboratory aids. Leukocytosis up to 40,000 cells per cubic millimeter is almost always present. From 80 to 90 per cent are neutrophils. Occasionally, gram-negative intracellular diplococci are seen within leukocytes in stained smears from capillary blood, buffy coat, or directly from skin lesions. A blood culture positive for meningococci furnishes final etiologic proof. It should be emphasized that several cultures of the blood may be necessary to detect meningococci and that growth of the organism in liquid medium may be slow. Other laboratory examinations are either normal or compatible with any febrile illness.

The subsequent course is dependent on therapy, although some patients with very mild disease recover spontaneously after several weeks or months. Any of the complications and sequelae of meningococcal infections may develop.

Acute Fulminating Meningococcemia. Acute fulminating meningococcemia differs from the milder form in the rapidity with which it progresses and in its overwhelming character. The onset is usually abrupt and quite dramatic, with a shaking chill, severe headache, dizziness or vertigo, collapse, or unconsciousness. Patients with massive purpura, low blood pressure, rapid, quiet respiration and overwhelming bacteremia are said to have the Waterhouse-Friderichsen syndrome. They are often clear mentally. Their extensive rash (see figure) involves skin and mucous membranes as well as internal organs such as skeletal muscle and, classically, the adrenal glands. Body temperature may be subnormal, normal, or slightly elevated. Within a few hours there may be circulatory collapse with intravascular coagulation. There is often evidence for the presence of a consumptive coagulopathy.

Others may have the *encephalitic form*, which is characterized by rapidly developing coma, rapid stertorous breathing, a petechial but not massive purpuric rash, and normal blood pressure. Some may present with a combination of encephalitis and adrenal involvement with early deep coma, purpura, and low blood pressure. Occasionally, the pituitary gland, like the adrenals, is damaged by hemorrhage. These severe illnesses often are rapidly fatal. It is in the attempt to prevent this rapid course that so much emphasis is placed upon early, intensive treatment.

Chronic Meningococcemia. Chronic meningococcemia is an uncommon form of meningococcal disease in which episodes of fever of a few days' duration recur at intervals of days, weeks, or months. Chills and arthralgic symptoms are frequent, but rash may be absent or evanescent. Repeated cultures of the blood may be necessary before meningococci are recovered. Failure to suspect, recognize, and treat chronic meningococcemia may result in meningitis or endocarditis.

Meningitis

Although it constitutes only a relatively small percentage of the total number of meningococcal infections, meningitis is their most characteristic and important manifestation. The onset and symptoms are often indistinguishable from those of a generalized infection; in some, meningeal involvement seems to predominate. In others, both groups of symptoms appear almost simultaneously, but there may be great variations in their intensity and severity. In addition to the signs of sepsis and the rash, patients with meningitis have evidence of inflammation of the meninges: pain in the neck and back on forward flexion of the head, stiff neck, retraction of the head or severe opisthotonos, Kernig's and Brudzinski's signs, hyperesthesia, hyperirritability, and exaggerated reflexes. Unequal reflexes are unusual, but may be present. Involvement of the cranial nerves when present may result in strabismus and deafness. The increased intracranial pressure may lead to severe headache, nausea, vomiting, dilated or irregular pupils, engorgement of the fundal veins, choking of the disks, irregular slow pulse, and moderately elevated blood pressure. Cheyne-Stokes or Biot's respiration may appear. As the disease progresses, restlessness and irritability may be followed by delirium or by generalized or jacksonian type convulsions; the patient may become greatly depressed, somnolent, and finally stuporous and comatose. In infants the signs of meningitis may be no more than refusal of feedings, vomiting or regurgitation, diarrhea, irritability, and fever. Convulsions and bulging of the fontanelles, when present, are extremely useful signs.

Laboratory Findings in Meningitis. The cerebrospinal fluid is under increased pressure and varies from clear to frankly purulent. The cell count is elevated, often to thousands per cubic millimeter, mostly neutrophils. Gram-negative intra- and extracellular diplococci can be seen in variable numbers in stained smears of the sediment. The total protein in the cerebrospinal fluid is increased, and its sugar content is usually reduced. Meningococci may be grown from the fluid by proper cultural methods. Fluid obtained early in meningitis may have few or no cells and no reduction of its glucose content, but cultures nonetheless will often be positive.

Course of Meningitis. Extremely variable, the course is greatly influenced by therapy. In untreated cases the temperature is erratic and symptoms progress to early death or to chronic meningitis with severe sequelae or delayed death.

COMPLICATIONS

The complications of the different forms of meningococcal infections include intercurrent infections, metastatic localizations, and permanent damage to the central nervous system. These may appear during the acute stage or subsequently. Intercurrent infections of the respiratory tract with other agents may occur. Bacteremic or metastatic complications include *conjunctivitis, panophthalmitis, otitis, purulent mono- or polyarthritis, pneumonia, pleurisy, pericarditis, endocarditis, myocarditis, orchitis, epididymitis, jaundice, hepatorenal failure, transient albuminuria* and *hematuria,* and *adrenal hemorrhage with necrosis.* Infection of the central nervous system may produce transient or permanent *paralyses, hemiplegia, neuroradiculitis, encephalitis, encephalomyelitis, altered cerebration, convulsions, cranial nerve damage, cerebral thrombosis* and *brain abscess.* Organization of exudate in the ventricular channels and the subarachnoid space may mechanically obstruct the flow of cerebrospinal fluid, producing *hydrocephalus.* The accumulation of subdural fluid of high protein content, which when encapsulated resembles a subdural hematoma, is fairly frequent in infants and young children. Recurrent meningitis caused by meningococci or other bacteria is usually due to structural defects of bone resulting from trauma or other causes which sometimes require surgical repair. Complications resulting from therapy can be avoided or minimized, if anticipated.

Permanent sequelae may result from almost any complication; the most frequent are deafness, ocular palsies, blindness, changes in intellectual ability, psychoses, and hydrocephalus.

DIAGNOSIS

The specific diagnosis of meningococcal disease depends primarily upon differentiation from other acute systemic and meningococcal infections. Final confirmation of the diagnosis requires bacteriologic identification of the causative organism as a meningococcus. During an epidemic, *especially in a recruit military camp or a closed population, all cases of fever with abrupt onset,* of prostration with or without fever, of petechial or purpuric rash, of drowsiness or coma, and of meningitis should be treated vigorously as meningococcal infections whether or not organisms are found in initial smears and cultures.

Meningococcal infections in their early stages may resemble any acute systemic infection. In sepsis caused by pyogenic organisms such as staphylococci, streptococci, or pneumococci, there may be a preceding upper respiratory infection, recurrent fever, malaise, arthralgia, and leukocytosis. A rash similar to that of severe meningococcemia and even signs of the Waterhouse-Friderichsen syndrome, on rare occasions, may be present in such cases. Final proof is accomplished by isolation of the offending organisms from the blood, joint fluid, sputum, and so forth. Meningococcal infections must also be differentiated from the acute exanthemata, typhus (both endemic and epidemic) typhoid, and other enteric fevers, subacute bacterial endocarditis, rheumatic fever, brucellosis, and others.

Diagnosis of Meningitis. The diagnosis of meningococcal meningitis requires differentiation from meningismus, other bacterial meningitides, viral meningoencephalitis, myeloencephalitis resulting from bacterial toxins (tetanus, botulinus) or chemicals, and noninfectious problems such as subarachnoid or cerebral hemorrhages or thrombosis, diabetic coma, and uremia.

In most cases of meningococcal meningitis, the diagnosis is readily established by the specific identification of the organism; in others the etiology may not be determinable when the patient is first seen, but a number of helpful procedures can be carried out. The usual medical history should be obtained, but a careful inquiry should be made into recent localized infections, especially of the ear, and trauma to the head, as these predispose to secondary bacterial meningitides.

Physical examination should include a thorough search for diseases of the eyes and upper respiratory passages, sinuses, and ears, and for evidence of injury to the head, in addition to careful general and neurologic examinations. A complete blood count should be made and cultures of the blood obtained. Any suspected localized areas of infection should likewise be cultured. Urinalysis and determinations of serum electrolytes and the blood nonprotein nitrogen may aid in the differential diagnosis and help to indicate precautions to be observed in therapy. In seriously ill, if not all, patients, blood coagulation analyses should be performed to determine the presence of a consumptive coagulopathy.

Lumbar puncture should be made as soon as possible and before specific treatment is instituted. After determining the initial pressure, fluid should be removed slowly until the pressure is reduced to an approximately normal level. The dynamics of the cerebrospinal fluid then can be estimated by jugular compression for evidence of block or sinus thrombosis. *Examination of the cerebrospinal fluid* should include the following: gross appearance, total and differential cell counts, determination of sugar and protein, and cultures and examination of Gram-stained smears. If organisms are seen, they can often be identified in the cerebrospinal fluid quickly and precisely with proper antisera.

A tentative diagnosis can usually be made from the Gram-stained smear, the differential cell count, and the sugar content of the cerebrospinal fluid. Caution should be exercised in the interpretation of smears, as even experienced personnel may be misled by overdecolorized or dead gram-positive diplococci or other bacteria. Final diagnosis depends on typing or culture; with Groups A and C meningococci, a positive direct quellung test will give immediate identification. The leukocytes are almost entirely neutrophils in purulent meningitides, except syphilitic or tuberculous. In the latter, as well as in viral infections (mumps, herpes, Coxsackie and echoviruses and others), mononuclear cells predominate except in their early stages. The sugar content is usually low in bacterial meningitis and normal in viral infections. In meningismus the fluid is usually normal. The proportion of erythrocytes to leukocytes is similar to that in whole blood in cases of subarachnoid hemorrhage. The history, other physical findings, and special laboratory tests should help to differentiate myeloencephalitides resulting from toxins or chemicals.

TREATMENT

For the past 30 years, Groups A, B, and C meningococci have been responsible for almost all meningococcal infections regardless of their clinical forms. Practically all strains of these groups were exquisitely susceptible to the bacteriostatic and bactericidal actions of the sulfonamide drugs, whether in carriers or cases. For these reasons, the sulfonamides were the agents of choice, for both treatment and prophylaxis. They are still excellent, *providing that one is certain that the patient or carrier has a sulfonamide-susceptible organism.* Without suitable tests of the homologous strain, such an assumption is unwarranted in the present era.

Since sulfonamide-resistant Group A, B, C, and Y strains are now commonplace, the treatment of patients is based upon penicillin G in massive dosage. For adults, this means 20,000,000 units per day intravenously or 1,000,000 units every two hours intramuscularly. The latter should not be used for patients in, or on the verge of, shock. When the 20,000,000 unit dose is used intravenously, it is best to divide it into four or more doses per day rather than administering it by continuous drip. Doses in children should be reduced in accordance with pediatric therapeutic principles.

Ampicillin may be used as an alternate, although an occasional patient does not seem to respond adequately to this drug. Close observation of the patient's course will alert the physician to this problem, should it arise. The dose should be at least 150 mg. per kilogram per day for children and 10 to 12 grams per day for adults. These parenteral daily doses are divided into six to eight doses.

In patients known to be truly allergic to penicillin, chloramphenicol is the alternative drug of choice. The use of this drug imposes precautions of its own. These can be managed, but close watch should be kept on the hematopoietic system and the drug withdrawn if a complication appears. Thus far, no meningococci resistant to penicillin or chloramphenicol have been identified. If the patient's organism is identified and shown to be susceptible to sulfonamide, then the specific treatment can be altered accordingly.

Patients with meningococcal disease are usually more dehydrated than they appear. Care should be taken to ensure a daily urinary output of more than 1000 ml. Treatment should be continued at least until all signs and symptoms have been normal for a minimum of two days and preferably for five. It may be stopped abruptly. Relapse occurs occasionally and requires prompt retreatment.

Patients with fulminating meningococcemia or meningitis, or both, should be started on therapy as soon as the diagnosis is suspected and specimens obtained, without waiting for bacteriologic confirmation. Penicillin should be given by vein. The central venous pressure should be monitored and corrected as necessary. Heparin should be administered if there is any evidence or suspicion of intravascular coagulation. Norepinephrine, intravenously, may be required to maintain blood pressure. Steroids are clearly required if there is evidence of adrenal collapse; such patients are managed as are those with acute adrenal insufficiency. Otherwise, there is no good evidence that these agents are of any positive value. Intravenous infusions will be required to correct dehydration, but an excess should be avoided. Oxygen therapy should be instituted and maintained as long as cyanosis or dyspnea is present. Blood transfusions have not been shown to be of significant value in this type of circulatory failure.

Regardless of the clinical form of meningococcal infection, or of the drugs employed, therapy should be continued until clinical and bacteriologic recovery are assured.

Certain laboratory tests such as *hematologic examinations* should be repeated as aids in monitoring the patient's course. This is especially true for patients admitted with severe leukopenia or thrombocytopenia. Their reversal is of considerable prognostic importance. Blood cultures should be repeated if the fever persists or returns, for continued bacteremia suggests the presence of endocarditis or other metastatic localization. Additional lumbar punctures are indicated if there is persistent increased intracranial pressure, failure to respond to adequate therapy, or meningitic relapse.

Symptomatic and supportive treatment is essential for patients with meningococcal infections. Sedation should be minimal, yet sufficient to assure adequate rest but not to interfere with the assessment of the patient's course. Approximately one month of convalescence is required for complete recovery in most cases, and even more for those with severe illnesses.

The treatment of the complications of meningococcal infections is primarily that of the underlying disease. Should fever or signs of meningeal irritation recur, then the most probable causes are recurrence of infection with the meningococcus because of inadequate treatment, drug fever, or superinfection with another organism. In such circumstances, the cerebrospinal fluid and blood should be re-examined and cultured. If meningococcal infection has recurred, then intensive treatment should be reinstituted and maintained until the patient has fully recovered.

PROGNOSIS

The prognosis in meningococcal infections has improved enormously because of the efficacy of the sulfonamides, penicillin, and other antimicrobial drugs. In untreated cases of meningococcemia and meningitis the mortality formerly varied from 20 to 90 per cent, averaging about 70 per cent. The introduction of serum therapy reduced this to about 50 per cent. With the sulfonamides the case fatality rate has been reduced to 5 to 10 per cent, depending upon age and complicating conditions. The recent recognition of sulfonamide-resistant meningococci has not altered this significantly because cases can be treated so successfully with penicillin. Age is perhaps the most important factor in prognosis, for the greatest mortality, despite adequate therapy, occurs in those less than two or more than forty years old. In the U.S. Army during World War II, the over-all mortality was slightly less than 5 per cent and, in some series, even below 1 per cent. More than 90 per cent of these cases were caused by sulfonamide-susceptible Group A strains. In addition to a most favorable age distribution in the Army, the excellent physical condition of patients, early diagnosis, and the prompt institution of effective therapy were probably responsible for this remarkable recovery rate. The prognosis is still poor in fulminating cases with abrupt onset, extensive cutaneous lesions, and circulatory collapse. In spite of rapid, intensive therapy, such cases frequently terminate fatally. Relapses, recurrences, and complicatons have been greatly reduced by specific treatment so that the prognosis for total recovery is generally good. *The most frequent permanent sequelae despite adequate treatment* are deafness, cranial nerve paralyses, mental deficiency and, less frequently, blindness and hydrocephalus. These are all relatively uncommon, and usually result from treatment delays in the very young or elderly.

PREVENTION

Until recently epidemics of meningococcal infections in both open and closed populations were easily controlled by the mass administration of as little as 2 grams of sulfonamide daily for two days. This procedure is no longer recommended unless the epidemic is known to be caused by a sulfonamide-susceptible strain of meningococci. Even then, the procedure should be carefully monitored by examination of strains isolated from patients, for the mass administration of sulfonamides may eliminate susceptible meningococci

from the population, permitting resistant strains to become dominant. If this occurs, then the sulfonamides should be discontinued. Isolation of patients with meningococcal infections is not necessary after 24 to 48 hours of adequate therapy. Close contacts of patients should be observed for evidence of clinical disease. Appropriate drugs may then be given to the contacts, or they may simply be observed daily for several days and treated promptly if clinical illness occurs. If desired, posterior nasopharyngeal cultures may be obtained from contacts to detect carriers. As a single negative culture is not reliable for this purpose, several daily cultures are required to be reasonably certain that the contact has not acquired the organism.

These rather complicated suggestions result from the fact that the antimicrobial drugs that are so effective in treating cases are quite inadequate for eliminating the carrier state. There is no good explanation for this difference between sulfonamides and penicillins. Large doses of oral penicillin (5- to 6,000,000 units per day) will only temporarily eliminate meningococci from carriers. This is also borne out by patient experiences. Whereas the sulfonamide-treated patient rarely, if ever, leaves the hospital as a meningococcal carrier, many penicillin-treated patients do. Thus, there is no suitable substitute at present for sulfonamides in removing resistant strains from carriers.

Recently, it was suggested that rifampin be used for this purpose. It is effective in eliminating the carrier state, but some meningococci are resistant to this drug before exposure to it. Furthermore, resistance is rapidly induced in the laboratory and in carriers so that the future of this drug for this purpose is somewhat cloudy at this writing.

Prospects for an Effective Vaccine. There may be more reason for optimism from another direction. Group-specific polysaccharides have been prepared from Groups A and C, but not yet from B strains. The A and C preparations have been injected into humans without any apparent difficulties. The Group C polysaccharide preparation is currently under field trial in recruits as a vaccine. The results available at this time indicate that single subcutaneous injections of 50 µg. have decreased the number of cases by 87 per cent when compared with Group C cases in an uninoculated control population. If this encouraging early experience continues, and if similar responses to the other serogroups can be obtained, then the true solution to the meningococcal problem will most certainly have been achieved.

Artenstein, M. S., Gold, R., Zimmerly, J. G., Wyle, F. A., Schneider, H., and Harkins, C.: Prevention of meningococcal disease by Group C polysaccharide vaccine. New Eng. J. Med., 282:417, 1970.
Cerebrospinal meningitis in Africa. WHO Chronicle, 23:54, 1969.
Evans, R. W., Glick, B., Kimball, F., and Lobell, M.: Fatal intravascular consumption coagulopathy in meningococcal sepsis. Amer. J. Med., 46:910, 1969.
Feldman, H. A.: Recent developments in the therapy and control of meningococcal infections. Disease-a-Month, February 1966.

Feldman, H. A.: Neisseria infections other than gonococcal. *In* Diagnostic Procedures for Bacterial, Mycotic and Parasitic Infections. 5th ed. New York, American Public Health Association, Inc., 1970.

Gotschlich, E. E., Goldschneider, I., and Artenstein, M. S.: Human immunity to the meningococcus. V: The effect of immunization with meningococcal Group C polysaccharide on the carrier state. J. Exp. Med., 129:1385, 1969.

OTHER BACTERIAL MENINGITIDES

Robert G. Petersdorf

BACTERIAL MENINGITIS OTHER THAN THAT CAUSED BY MENINGOCOCCI AND MYCOBACTERIA

DEFINITION

Meningitis is an inflammatory process involving the coverings of the central nervous system. Bacteria, viruses, spirochetes, parasites, and fungi may be the offending pathogens. This article is concerned with meningitis caused by bacteria other than meningococci and mycobacteria; these are discussed in the preceding article and in Diseases Due to Mycobacteria.

ETIOLOGY

With the exception of *Mycobacterium tuberculosis,* the three most common micro-organisms causing meningitis are *Diplococcus pneumoniae, Neisseria meningitidis,* and *Hemophilus influenzae.** *H. influenzae* meningitis is usually of type B and occurs uncommonly after the age of 6 and rarely after 12. When it occurs in adults, a parameningeal focus, head trauma, or alcoholism should be suspected. Occasionally a deficiency in immune globulins predisposes to *H. influenzae* meningitis in adults. Meningococcal disease is found in both children and adults, but is rare after the age of 50. Pneumococcal meningitis is most common in infancy and old age. Other, less common pathogens are *Staphylococcus aureus,* which is usually found in association with epidural or brain abscess, thrombosis of the cavernous sinus, or following cranial trauma and neurosurgical procedures; *Escherichia coli,* a common offender in meningitis in newborns; and other enteric

---

*Another disease caused by Hemophilus is chancroid, which is a localized venereal disease caused by *H. ducreyi.* It is characterized by painful, nonindurated ulceration involving the genitalia, accompanied by enlargement and suppuration of regional lymph nodes. Early syphilis often occurs simultaneously with chancroid. Infection with *H. ducreyi* responds to sulfadiazine in dosage of 4.0 grams per day for seven to ten days.

organisms, including Proteus species, Klebsiella-Enterobacter, Paracolon, Salmonella, and Pseudomonas. Infection with Pseudomonas has followed lumbar puncture, spinal anesthesia, and the establishment of shunting procedures to relieve hydrocephalus. The group A hemolytic Streptococcus, formerly a common offender, is now a relatively rare cause of meningitis, although enterococci and anaerobic streptococci continue to be isolated, primarily from patients with brain abscess and meningitis. Rarer organisms include *Listeria monocytogenes,* a small gram-positive rod resembling nonpathogenic diphtheroids; *Mima polymorpha,* a pleomorphic gram-negative organism that is difficult to differentiate on Gram stain (but not culture) from *H. influenzae* and *N. meningitidis;* and *Cl. perfingens* and *Past. multocida.*

INCIDENCE

The precise incidence of bacterial meningitis is difficult to determine, in part because one of the major forms, meningococcal meningitis, tends to occur in epidemics widely separated in place and time. Nevertheless, there is some evidence that the number of patients with bacterial meningitis of all forms is declining. However, the mortality rate has remained relatively constant. This may reflect the susceptibility of aged or "poor risk" patients to meningeal infections.

PATHOLOGY

There is considerable variation in the pathologic picture, depending in part on the duration of the disease, the infecting organism, the resistance of the host, and the type and duration of therapy. Although bacterial meningitis is usually localized to the subarachnoid space, infections caused by viruses, spirochetes, parasites, and fungi are commonly complicated by cerebritis or encephalitis. In bacterial meningitis, grossly purulent exudate is present over the cortical and basal surfaces of the brain, and may invest the spinal cord as well. The pus is often localized to the cerebellopontine angles. Cortical phlebitis with its consequences of vascular congestion, thrombosis, and infarction may be prominent findings. Microscopically, exudate consisting of several hundred layers of polymorphonuclear leukocytes is present over the surface of the brain and in the ventricular system, where the pus may produce noncommunicating hydrocephalus. Occasionally, the exudate penetrates the arachnoid, forming a subdural empyema. Although migration of inflammatory cells into subjacent neuronal tissue and necrosis of nerve cells may occur, in general the meninges provide remarkable protection to the neurons, which are usually spared from the inflammatory process and invasion by bacteria.

PATHOGENESIS

The routes by which micro-organisms penetrate the blood–cerebrospinal fluid barrier and establish infection in the subarachnoid space have not been clearly defined. In a number of instances, bacterial meningitis follows infection of the middle ear, mastoid, paranasal sinuses, and trauma or surgery to the face and head. In these instances, it seems likely that bacteria enter through a rent in the leptomeninges or that infection in a neighboring focus may render the meninges more permeable to micro-organisms. Pneumococci, streptococci, staphylococci, and (more rarely) *H. influenzae* and gram-negative enteric bacilli have been implicated in this type of meningitis. Meningococci, which are usually carried in the nasopharynx, have been assumed to ascend to the meninges via the small venules and via arachnoid sheaths investing the olfactory nerves and accompanying them through the lamina cribrosa. However, there is no direct evidence for this route of infection in man. It has been postulated that infection emanating from distant foci, such as pneumococcal meningitis following pneumonia, or infection without a primary focus, is blood borne. In laboratory animals, bacteremia is not associated with meningitis unless the meninges are subjected to microtrauma (in the form of needle puncture) at the height of bacteremia. It is conceivable that this situation exists in man and that a microscopic defect in the meninges is a prerequisite for entry of bacteria from the blood. Occasionally, meningitis follows the rupture of a brain abscess. Anaerobic streptococci, enterococci, staphylococci, mixtures of bacteria, and actinomycetes may be isolated under these circumstances.

CLINICAL MANIFESTATIONS

History. Most patients with meningitis report fever, lethargy, confusion, headache, vomiting, or stiff neck. The mode of onset may vary. Some patients rapidly develop headache, confusion, and loss of consciousness within 24 hours; they usually do not have antecedent respiratory symptoms. Others complain of headache, fever, and stiff neck associated with otitis, rhinorrhea, sore throat, or cough for one to seven days prior to the appearance of the full clinical picture. Still others have symptoms referable to the respiratory tract for several weeks before meningitis sets in. *Cough* is a common symptom in meningococcal and pneumococcal infection; *earache* often antedates infection with *H. influenzae,* and a *sore throat* may precede neisserial meningitis. Other symptoms of bacterial meningitis include backache, weakness, dizziness, ataxia, photophobia, and generalized myalgias. Additional clues are a history of alcoholism, a common accompaniment of pneumococcal meningitis; previous or recent infection or surgery involving the nose, throat, or sinuses;

head trauma; recent lumbar puncture or spinal anesthesia; and close and intimate contact with a patient who has a meningococcal infection.

Physical Findings. Most patients demonstrate the signs of meningeal irritation, i.e., stiff neck and positive Kernig or Brudzinski signs. Patients without these signs are often very young, very old, or severely obtunded. A *petechial eruption* is relatively rare in meningitis owing to bacteria other than meningococci unless bacterial endocarditis is present. There may be physical signs of pneumonia, particularly in patients with pneumococcal meningitis, and evidence of aural infection may also be found. Often, however, a primary focus (otitis, mastoiditis, sinusitis, pneumonia, or empyema) is not apparent on physical examination and should be carefully sought by other means because failure to eradicate the primary focus may result in failure of therapy or post-treatment relapse. Although intracranial pressure is characteristically elevated, papilledema is rare. When it is encountered in the course of acute bacterial meningitis, it should call to mind the possibility of subdural empyema, brain abscess, or venous sinus thrombosis. The level of consciousness in patients with meningitis may vary from mild lethargy to deep coma. Most patients show some degree of confusion. In approximately 50 per cent, other signs of neurologic damage develop during the course of infection. These include major motor seizures, hemipareses, which are often transient and probably post-ictal, signs of diffuse central nervous system damage (bilateral Babinski signs and fixed, mid-stage pupils), or paresis of the second, third, sixth, seventh, and eighth cranial nerves.

Associated Disease. With the exception of epidemics of meningococcal meningitis, which are usually confined to closed environments such as army camps or schools, bacterial meningitis occurs sporadically, usually in a setting of some associated disease. Pharyngitis antedates meningitis in many patients with meningococcal and Hemophilus infection. Otitis with or without mastoiditis, although much rarer nowadays than 20 years ago, remains an important precursor of Hemophilus and pneumococcal meningitis, which is also frequently associated with pneumonia. Pneumonitis is also often present in meningitis caused by gram-negative pathogens. A number of patients with pneumococcal meningitis have multiple myeloma; patients with this neoplasm are generally prone to recurrent pneumococcal infections. In addition to the common meningeal pathogens, meningitis in patients with diabetes mellitus is likely to be caused by uncommon organisms such as Klebsiella Enterobacter, and *Staphylococcus aureus*. Cranial trauma may precede meningitis by several days and occasionally months or years; in such instances, *D. pneumoniae,* hemolytic *Staph. aureus* or coliform bacteria are usually the offending organisms. Cranial osteomyelitis may intervene between head trauma and the development of meningitis. Patients undergoing shunt procedures for relief of hydrocephalus tend to have infections with bacteria that are ordinarily not pathogenic such as *Staphylococcus epidermidis* or micrococci; gram-negative enteric bacterial and Pseudomonas meningitis also complicate shunting procedures. Occasionally, subcutaneous or mucosal infections such as furunculosis, decubitus ulcers, omphalitis in neonates, and endometritis precede leptomeningitis.

Rare Types of Meningitis. *Mima polymorpha* Meningitis. *Mima polymorpha* is a gram-negative pleomorphic bacillus that is easily confused on Gram stain with members of the Neisseria group and *H. influenzae.* It can be separated from these organisms, however, by cultural and serologic techniques. Meningitis caused by *Mima polymorpha* closely resembles meningitis caused by the more common pathogens and cannot be differentiated from them on clinical grounds. Separation of mimae from Neisseria is of more than academic importance because mimae may be resistant to penicillin and sulfonamides and respond only to the tetracyclines.

Listeria Meningitis. The most common clinical illness caused by Listeria is meningitis, and any patient with clinical and laboratory evidence of meningeal infection said to be caused by a diphtheroid should be assumed to harbor Listeria in the cerebrospinal fluid. Clinically, the illness cannot be distinguished from meningitis caused by other bacteria (see Listeriosis).

Other Organisms. Bacteria that have caused infections usually in patients with antecedent head trauma or neurosurgical procedures include *Cl. perfringens* and *Past. multocida,* although any organism can occasionally produce infection in this setting.

RECURRENT INFECTIONS

Recurrent bouts of meningitis are most frequently related to remote as well as to recent head trauma. The individual episodes are usually caused by the same bacterial species that are associated with meningitis occurring in the absence of trauma, except that pneumococci of higher serologic types are isolated more commonly than *H. influenzae* and Neisseria. Bouts of meningitis may be separated by an interval of several years. Cerebrospinal fluid rhinorrhea owing to a defect in the cribriform plate is often associated with recurrent meningeal infection. All patients with repeated bouts of meningitis should be subjected to vigorous search for a communication between the subarachnoid space and the nasopharynx, and if roentgenographic techniques fail to disclose the defect, craniotomy should be considered. Other situations predisposing to recurrent meningeal infections include chronic mastoiditis or petrositis, congenital abnormalities of the cranial vault, and congenital dermoid sinus tracts. Ventriculomastoid shunts aimed at relief of hydrocephalus are also complicated by recurrent infections, which are often heralded by otitis media. Recur-

rent bouts of meningitis have been reported in children who have undergone splenectomy; this does not appear to be true of adults. Nor is there evidence that the incidence of meningitis is increased in children with hypo- or dysgammaglobulinemia.

INFECTIONS WITH MULTIPLE ORGANISMS

Meningitis caused by two or more organisms occasionally occurs in infants, young children and neonates, who may develop brain abscesses following surgery or birth trauma. *H. influenzae* is usually one of the organisms, and has been found in conjunction with *N. meningitidis, D. pneumoniae,* group A Streptococcus and *E. coli.* In adults infections with multiple organisms most commonly follow rupture of a brain abscess into the subarachnoid space, and streptococci, staphylococci, and gram-negative enteric pathogens may all be isolated from the same specimen of cerebrospinal fluid.

COMPLICATIONS OF BACTERIAL MENINGITIS

Disseminated Intravascular Coagulation. This syndrome, which is also called consumptive coagulopathy, is manifested by multiple petechiae, ecchymoses, purpura, bleeding from other surfaces, hypotension progressing to shock, and gangrene of distal extremities (see Meningococcal Disease). It is almost always seen with meningococcal disease, and is unusual in meningitis caused by other bacteria.

Temporal and Cerebellar Herniation. These complications are commonly found in fatal meningitis, and may be recognized by distinct respiratory, ocular, and motor signs that indicate loss of diencephalic, mid-brain, pontine, and medullary function in an orderly rostral-caudal sequence. In the presence of these signs, repeated lumbar punctures should be avoided.

Endocarditis. Endocarditis, most often involving the aortic valve, is found in 10 to 15 per cent of fatal cases of pneumococcal meningitis. Pneumonia is also frequent in this setting. Rheumatic or congenital valvular disease may antedate development of endocarditis, but frequently normal valves are involved. Staphylococci and coliform organisms may also be the cause of the endocarditis-meningitis syndrome. Endocarditis may be difficult to detect clinically but should be seriously considered in patients with meningitis, pneumococcal, staphylococcal, and coliform bacteremia, and heart murmurs.

Purulent Arthritis. Purulent arthritis may complicate pneumococcal, meningococcal, and staphylococcal meningitis. In general, it responds to antimicrobials, although aspiration of synovial fluid may be necessary.

Subdural Effusions. Subdural effusions have been a frequently reported complication of Hemophilus meningitis, but may also follow other types of meningitis in children. Prolonged unexplained fever, confusion despite adequate antimicrobial therapy, and convulsions after the apparent subsidence of infection are classic manifestations of accumulating subdural fluid that is usually sterile. Aspiration of this fluid, which may need to be repeated, results in relief of symptoms.

Residual damage to the nervous system occurs in 10 to 20 per cent of patients, and is more common following pneumococcal meningitis than infection with *H. influenzae* and meningococci. *Deafness* remains the most common sequel of pyogenic meningitis; hemiparesis, convulsive disorders, and dementia are seen occasionally.

DIAGNOSIS

General Considerations. The diagnosis of bacterial meningitis is not difficult, providing that a high index of suspicion is maintained. Meningeal infection should be considered in every patient with a history of upper respiratory illness interrupted by vomiting, headache, lethargy, confusion, or stiff neck. When first seen, some of these patients present only with low-grade fever, mild headache, or occasional emesis. Nevertheless, the possibility of meningeal infection must be carefully considered. In patients with pneumonia it is particularly dangerous to ascribe confusion to age or "toxemic" depression. Meningitis may be present in addition to pulmonary infection, and the dosage of an antimicrobial drug used to treat pneumonia is often inadequate to control meningeal infection. The susceptibility of alcoholics to meningitis cannot be emphasized too strongly. Fever and confusion in these patients should not be attributed to alcoholic intoxication, delirium tremens, or hepatic encephalopathy unless the cerebrospinal fluid has been examined.

Two unusual types of recurrent meningitis may mimic bacterial infection, at least initially. *Mollaret's meningitis* consists of recurrent febrile attacks, malaise, headache, and meningeal signs accompanied by a marked polymorphonuclear inflammatory reaction in the CSF. Attacks last two to three days and subside spontaneously. *Behçet's syndrome* is characterized by recurrent oral and genital ulcerations and relapsing ocular lesions along with meningitis. Other neurologic abnormalities may include cranial nerve palsies, seizures, hemiparesis, extrapyramidal signs, and chronic brain syndromes.

Cerebrospinal Fluid. The cerebrospinal fluid should be examined in any patient with evidence of meningeal irritation. In patients with papilledema or other evidence of elevated cerebrospinal fluid pressure, lumbar puncture should be performed with care, employing a small-gauge needle. Papilledema does not constitute a contraindication to lumbar puncture in patients in whom the diagnosis of meningitis is suspected. The cerebrospinal fluid pressure is usually elevated, and the gross appearance of the fluid may vary from slight turbidity to gross pus. The fluid should be centrifuged immediately, and the sediment stained by Gram's method and cultured on blood and chocolate agar under increased CO_2 tension and anaerobically in thioglycollate. Some common pitfalls encountered in Gram staining include washing the organisms off the slide, decolorizing gram-positive bacteria, and interpreting particles of stain as bacteria. Nevertheless, carefully performed Gram stains are accurate in 90 per cent of cases in which organisms are seen. Pneumococci are more easily identified than meningococci. Although immunofluorescent techniques have been used to expedite the diagnosis in a variety of bacterial meningitides, they appear to be no more accurate than a well-performed Gram stain.

The number of cells in the cerebrospinal fluid is always elevated and varies between 100 and 100,000 per cubic millimeter. Initially, polymorphonuclear leukocytes predominate; these are replaced by lymphocytes as the inflammatory process progresses. Early in the infection one may find a plethora of bacteria with only a few cells. This is particularly true in pneumococcal and staphylococcal infections.

A low cerebrospinal fluid sugar is the hallmark of bacterial meningitis, and distinguishes it from the viral meningitides. Usually the value is below 40 mg. per 100 ml. and may be close to 0. Patients who have diabetes mellitus or who are receiving intravenous infusions of glucose may have falsely high glucose values. However, the ratio of blood to cerebrospinal fluid sugar in these patients is always higher than the normal value of 1.5 to 1. For example, a cerebrospinal fluid sugar of 150 mg. per 100 ml. in the presence of a blood sugar of 500 mg. per 100 ml. is highly significant. The information obtained from blood sugar, which should be obtained routinely at the time of initial lumbar puncture, is frequently critical.

The protein content of the cerebrospinal fluid is generally elevated and may be as high as 800 mg. per 100 ml. Higher values are usually obtained in pneumococcal meningitis than in infections with other pathogens. The development of subarachnoid block is usually heralded by very high CSF protein values (800 to 1500 mg. per 100 ml.).

Other Cultures. Blood cultures should be obtained routinely in patients suspected of having meningitis; they are positive in approximately 50 per cent of cases. Occasionally, when the cerebrospinal fluid cultures are negative, the blood cultures may provide the only clue to the etiologic agent. Nose, throat, and ear cultures may not reflect the meningeal pathogen and are misleading too often to be of more than ancillary value in diagnosis.

Roentgenographic Studies. All patients with meningitis should have roentgenograms of the chest, skull, mastoid, and paranasal sinuses as soon as their condition permits. Frequently these provide the clue to the portal of entry of the pathogen. Eradication of these foci with antimicrobial therapy or surgical drainage may be essential for control of the meningeal infection.

Other Laboratory Tests. Most patients with meningitis are sufficiently ill to warrant determination of blood urea nitrogen and serum electrolytes, particularly because water intoxication and severe hyponatremia are not uncommon. Blood sugar should be determined routinely (best in conjunction with determination of the cerebrospinal fluid sugar). Lactic dehydrogenase and its isozymes are elevated in bacterial meningitis. Most of this increase is due to a rise in fractions representing leukocytes, but a rise in LDH isozyme fractions emanating from brain occurs only in patients who die or who are destined to develop neurologic sequelae.

PROGNOSIS

Untreated meningitis is almost always fatal. Antimicrobial therapy has dramatically improved the outlook for patients with meningeal infections. Despite this, the mortality in adequately treated pneumococcal meningitis remains between 10 and 70 per cent, and 50 per cent of infections with staphylococci and gram-negative enteric bacilli are lethal. On the other hand, the mortality rate associated with meningococcal and *H. influenzae* meningitis is less than 10 per cent. In addition to the difference in prognosis engendered by different micro-organisms, factors that adversely influence outcome include (1) improper or delayed diagnosis, usually a consequence of falsely attributing confusion or delirium to "toxemic" depression of the central nervous system or hepatic encephalopathy; (2) fulminating infection with rapid loss of consciousness; (3) bacteremia; (4) old age or the neonatal period; (5) certain underlying and complicating illnesses, including bacterial endocarditis, brain abscess, diabetes mellitus, and pneumonia; and (6) development of coma, localizing neurologic signs, and convulsions.

TREATMENT

Choice of Therapy. Antimicrobials are the mainstay of therapy in bacterial meningitis and should be administered parenterally at the earliest possible moment. If the Gram stain of the cerebrospinal fluid reveals the causative micro-organism, specific treatment may be instituted from the beginning. However, if microscopy of the stained smear has been inconclusive, the initial therapy must be sufficiently broad to be fully effective against the most reasonable possibilities. For example, purulent meningitis in an adult without evidence of an overt portal of entry is most apt to be pneumococcal or meningococcal; in a young child, *H. influenzae* must also be considered. Primary staphylococcal meningitis would be rare in a previously healthy adult, but should be considered in a long-hospitalized patient, particularly if neurosurgery has been performed.

Penicillin is the drug of choice for pneumococcal and meningococcal meningitis, and should be administered parenterally in a dosage of 10 to 20 million units a day. For patients who are sensitive to penicillin, chloramphenicol in dosage of 4.0 to 6.0 grams per day should be used if Neisseria is the causative pathogen, although cephalothin, in dosage of 6.0 to 12.0 grams per day, or cephaloridine, in dosage of 4.0 grams per day, can be substituted for penicillin in pneumococcal meningitis. Chloramphenicol (2.0 to 4.0 grams a day) may be given in *H. influenzae* meningitis, but ampicillin in dosage of 6.0 to 12 grams a day is at least as effective and has the additional advantage of being bactericidal for pneumococci and meningococci. Use of this agent should, for all practical purposes, eliminate multiple drug therapy in "undiagnosed meningitis." A few "ampicillin failures" have been reported in children with *H. influenzae* meningitis. These were probably related to inadequate dosage or poor absorption of the drug. Staphylococcal meningitis should always be treated with one of the penicillinase-resistant penicillins, e.g., methicillin, oxacillin, or nafcillin in dosage of 6.0 to 12.0 grams parenterally, or with cephalothin in similar dosage. For the rare cases of meningitis caused by the Enterobacteriaceae, kanamycin in a dosage of 2.0 grams a day is probably the agent of choice until drug-susceptibility tests have been performed. If Pseudomonas meningitis is suspected, polymyxin B or colistin should be employed both parenterally and intrathecally. *Only the preparation free of dibucaine should be used for intrathecal therapy.* The dosage of colistin is 5 mg. per kilogram per day parenterally and 5 mg. daily intrathecally. Polymyxin B should be given in approximately half the dose of colistin. Gentamicin, in dosage of 5 mg. per kilogram daily in divided dosage may become the drug of choice in Pseudomonas meningitis, and its use may obviate intrathecal therapy.

In patients with mastoiditis, an infected ventriculomastoid shunt, or cranial osteomyelitis, surgical attack on these primary foci while the patient is receiving appropriate antimicrobial therapy is indicated, but may be postponed until the acute meningeal episode is over.

Duration of Therapy. The duration of antimicrobial therapy in meningitis cannot be prescribed categorically. The cerebrospinal fluid should be examined every 24 to 48 hours during the early days of therapy, but once the patient is recovering, the intervals between lumbar puncture may be as long as a week, and numerous examinations of the CSF are rarely necessary. In the absence of extrameningeal foci, a seven- to ten-day course of antimicrobial therapy should suffice.

Other Measures. If there is evidence of increased intracranial pressure, and supratentorial or cerebellar herniation, therapy with mannitol, urea, or dexamethasone should be instituted. Adrenal cortical hormones also have been used as an adjunct to antimicrobial therapy, but have not resulted in noteworthy improvement. They should never be used unless the etiologic organism has been clearly identified and the appropriate drug is being administered. There have been some enthusiastic reports about proteolytic enzymes in the treatment of pneumococcal meningitis, but these agents have not been evaluated in sufficient detail to recommend their general use.

Other supportive therapy includes administration of adequate but not excessive parenteral fluids and anticonvulsants when indicated. Sedation should be employed with caution, even for delirious patients; of the many agents available, paraldehyde continues to be safe and effective.

Beaty, H. N., and Oppenheimer, S.: CSF lactic dehydrogenase and its isoenzymes in infections of the central nervous system. New Eng. J. Med., 279:1197, 1968.

Boe, J., and Huseklapp, H.: Recurrent attacks of bacterial meningitis: A new clinical problem. Report of five cases. Amer. J. Med., 29:465, 1960.

Carpenter, R. R., and Petersdorf, R. G.: The clinical spectrum of bacterial meningitis. Amer. J. Med., 23:262, 1962.

Cherry, J. D., and Sheenan, C. P.: Bacteriologic relapse in Hemophilus influenzae meningitis. New Eng. J. Med., 278:1001, 1968.

Harter, D. H., and Petersdorf, R. G.: A consideration of the pathogenesis of bacterial meningitis. Review of experimental and clinical studies. Yale J. Biol. Med., 32:280, 1960.

Olafsson, M., Lee, Y. C., and Abernathy, T. J.: Mima polymorpha meningitis: Report of a case and review of the literature. New Eng. J. Med., 258:465, 1958.

Oppenheimer, S. J., O'Toole, R. D., and Petersdorf, R. G.: Bacterial meningitis: In Shy, G. M., Goldensohn, E. S., and Appel, S. H. (eds.): The Cellular and Molecular Basis of Neurological Disease. Philadelphia, Lea and Febiger, (in press).

Snyder, S. N., and Brunjes, S.: H. influenzae meningitis in adults. Amer. J. Med. Sci., 250:658, 1965.

Swartz, M. N., and Dodge, P. R.: Bacterial meningitis—A review of selected aspects. New Eng. J. Med., 272:725, 779, 842, 898, 954, 1003, 1965.

Welshimer, H. J., and Winglewish, N. G.: Listerosis—Summary of seven cases of listeria meningitis. J.A.M.A., 171:1319, 1959.

WHOOPING COUGH
(Pertussis)
Stephen I. Morse

Definition. Whooping cough is an acute respiratory illness that primarily affects infants and young children. The etiologic agent is usually Bordetella pertussis; occasionally B. parapertussis, and rarely B. bronchiseptica produce a similar syndrome. The descriptive name derives from a distressing, prolonged inspiratory effort that follows paroxysmal coughing. Although both morbidity and mortality have markedly declined, whooping cough is still responsible for a significant number of deaths in infants.

History. The disease was first recorded in the middle of the sixteenth century by Moulton and by DeBaillou. Whether whooping cough was indigenous to Europe or had been transported there in the preceding century is uncertain. Sydenham applied the name "pertussis" to any illness accompanied by violent coughing, but the term became restricted to the epidemic disease that was a well-recognized clinical entity by the middle of the eighteenth century. In 1900 Bordet and Gengou observed coccobacilli in the sputum of a child with whooping cough, but it was not until 1906 that they were able to culture the organism. Many years passed before the Bordet-Gengou bacillus was

universally accepted as the etiologic agent of whooping cough. Leslie and Gardner (1931) recognized that B. pertussis underwent marked biologic and morphologic changes on prolonged cultivation, thereby accounting for the difficulties in establishing the etiologic role of the agent and the inconstant protective effect of immunizing preparations. Although the mortality rate of whooping cough in the United States began to decline in the early part of this century, the incidence in young children did not significantly decrease until after the use of prophylactic vaccines became widespread 25 years ago.

Etiology. When first isolated, Bordetella pertussis is a minute, nonmotile, poorly staining, gram-negative coccobacillus, 0.5 μ to 1.0 μ in length. Capsules can be demonstrated by special procedures, and bipolar metachromatic granules are present. The complex medium containing blood originally employed by Bordet and Gengou is still often used for cultivation. Primary isolates, phase I organisms, will not grow on conventional laboratory media, but will do so after prolonged passage. At the same time colonial morphology changes, marked pleomorphism of individual cells is evident, and there is an alteration in antigenic composition. The change from phase I to phase IV has been likened to the smooth to rough transition of other microbes. Only phase I organisms are virulent, and only phase I organisms provide effective immunizing material.

Members of the Bordetella genus were formerly regarded as species of Hemophilus. However, the Bordetella group does not have the strict requirement for X and V growth factors, and they are antigenically distinct. Although the addition of blood to Bordet-Gengou medium is required for the growth of phase I organisms, the blood acts to neutralize bactericidal substances, probably fatty acids, rather than to provide nutrients. Media containing charcoal, starch, or ion exchange resins will support the growth of phase I bacteria.

B. pertussis produces a heat-stable toxin (endotoxin) and a heat-labile toxin. A role of toxins in the development of disease has not been demonstrated. A hemagglutinin has also been isolated. The capsular material does not swell in the presence of antiserum. A species agglutinogen has been recognized as well as agglutinating factors that differ between strains. Serotyping is therefore a useful epidemiologic tool. The role of the interaction between the organism and phagocytes has not been defined, although the presence of antisera appears to increase uptake of B. pertussis by leukocytes.

Remarkable biologic effects are induced in laboratory animals by the injection of killed phase I organisms. These include development of heightened sensitivity to histamine and serotonin; increased susceptibility to anaphylaxis and to experimental allergic encephalomyelitis; increased antibody production in response to heterologous antigens; and hyperleukocytosis and hyperlymphocytosis. The factors responsible for these reactions have not been characterized, and the relationship of any of these effects to the primary clinical expression of whooping cough is obscure.

It should be emphasized that none of the cellular components or products of B. pertussis has been shown to be of central importance in the pathogenesis of whooping cough.

Approximately 5 to 10 per cent of clinical whooping cough is caused by *B. parapertussis.* The animal pathogen *B. bronchiseptica* is responsible for a very minor percentage of cases. On primary isolation these organisms are indistinguishable from *B. pertussis,* but can be differentiated by further bacteriologic or serologic procedures.

Incidence and Epidemiology. In communities of susceptibles the family attack rate is 80 to 90 per cent, which is extremely high for a bacterial disease approaching that seen in varicella or measles. Transmission is by droplet infection. Carriers of *B. pertussis* are found infrequently, and the reservoir is therefore unknown. Disease usually occurs in late winter in the northern climates and in late spring in southern zones, but there is great variation.

The mortality rate from whooping cough fell markedly after the beginning of this century, before the advent of antimicrobial therapy and the general use of pertussis vaccine. In 1920 the mortality rate in the United States was 12.5 per 100,000; in 1930 it was 4.8 per 100,000. For more than the past decade the mortality rate has been below 1 per 100,000. Three fourths of the deaths occur in infants, i.e., persons under one year of age.

The *incidence* of whooping cough, however, did not change until after 1940, when immunization of young children became standard practice. Large epidemics among the very young are no longer seen except in areas where prophylactic immunization is not carried out. In 1957 there were some 28,000 cases; in 1966 approximately 8000 cases of pertussis were reported in the United States.

It is not generally appreciated that immunization against pertussis is not lifelong. Thus, approximately 10 to 20 per cent of immunized young children exposed to whooping cough will acquire the disease. It is also significant that the incidence of pertussis in children over ten years of age has not changed. Indeed, in local epidemics, the family attack rate among older children who have been immunized early in life is greater than 50 per cent.

Similarly, natural disease does not lead to protection for life. Second attacks or attacks occurring after primary immunization may not be diagnosed because they are often atypical and less severe than classic whooping cough in young children.

Pathology. Interpretation of pathologic material obtained at autopsy is difficult because of the common presence of complicating respiratory infections. Lesions caused by *B. pertussis* are found principally in the bronchi and bronchioles, but changes are also seen in the nasopharynx, larynx, and trachea. Masses of bacteria are intertwined with the cilia of the columnar epithelium together with mucopurulent exudate. There is also necrosis of the midzonal and basilar epithelium with infiltration of polymorphonuclear leu-

kocytes and macrophages. Peribronchial accumulation of lymphocytes and granulocytes produces the picture of interstitial pneumonitis. Secondary atelectasis and localized emphysema are common. The alveoli in uncomplicated whooping cough do not contain exudate.

Clinical Manifestations. Following an incubation period of 7 to 16 days, symptoms appear. It is customary to divide the clinical course into three stages, each of two weeks' duration, but variation is frequent, particularly in the immunized community.

Catarrhal Stage. Whooping cough begins with symptoms indistinguishable from those of a mild viral upper respiratory infection or common cold. Sneezing is frequent, the conjunctivae are injected, and a nocturnal cough appears. The temperature may be slightly elevated at this time. Infectivity is greatest during the catarrhal stage.

Paroxysmal Stage. Seven to 14 days after onset, the cough becomes more frequent, diurnal, and then paroxysmal. In a typical paroxysm there is a series of 15 to 20 short coughs of increasing intensity, and then with a deep inspiration the air is drawn into the lungs, making the "whoop." A tenacious mucus plug is usually expelled, and vomiting frequently follows the spasmodic episode. Paroxysms may occur as often as every half hour, and are accompanied by signs of increased venous pressure. The conjunctivae are deeply engorged; there is periorbital edema; and petechial hemorrhages, particularly about the forehead, as well as epistaxis are common. During the attack the infant may be cyanotic until the crowing whoop occurs. In between paroxysms the child usually feels well though justifiably apprehensive.

Physical examination of the chest is usually unremarkable, though scattered rhonchi may be heard. The chest roentgenogram sometimes reveals hilar and mediastinal nodal enlargement. The presence of fever immediately suggests the development of a secondary infectious process.

Convalescent Stage. Gradually the paroxysms become less frequent and less intense, vomiting ceases, and slow recovery ensues. Often for many months even a mild, unrelated respiratory infection will be manifested by a return of paroxysmal cough and whoop.

It is important to recognize those patients with whooping cough in whom variation from the pattern frequently occurs. In young infants the paroxysms and the whoop are often absent; instead, choking spells and apneic periods may be the major manifestations. Second attacks of whooping cough as well as disease occurring in older, previously immunized children are usually mild or abortive and difficult to recognize as clinical pertussis.

Complications. Complications may be related to the primary disease or to secondary events. Alterations in acid-base balance occur as a result of metabolic alkalosis when vomiting is severe. Recurrent vomiting can also lead to malnutrition. Anoxemic manifestations are seen when ventilation is markedly impaired. Central nervous system changes can result from cerebral anoxia or hemorrhages consequent to the elevated venous pressure. Rarely, cortical degeneration occurs, but the exact pathogenesis of the encephalopathy is unknown. A serous meningitis with lymphocytosis of the cerebrospinal fluid has been described. Localized areas of emphysema and atelectasis generally return to normal after the disease has run its course, and pneumothorax and interstitial emphysema are infrequently seen.

The major cause of death in whooping cough is complicating pneumonia or bronchopneumonia caused by other bacteria or viruses. In addition, secondary bacterial otitis media occurs frequently.

Diagnosis. There is little difficulty in making the clinical diagnosis of whooping cough in a patient who, after a variable period of coryzal symptoms, develops paroxysmal coughing with a terminal inspiratory whoop. Toward the end of the catarrhal stage, or early in the spasmodic phase, leukocytosis often occurs. In contrast to the leukocytosis found in most bacterial diseases, the predominating cell type is the mature small lymphocyte. Characteristically the leukocyte count ranges from 15,000 to 30,000 per cubic millimeter, and 80 per cent of the cells are small lymphocytes. However, the leukocyte count either may be normal or may reach a level greater than 100,000 per cubic millimeter. Polymorphonuclear leukocytosis suggests a secondary bacterial complication.

Difficulty in recognizing whooping cough occurs in the catarrhal stage, in abortive or mild cases, and in young infants. Epidemiologic awareness may suggest the possibility, but microbiologic identification of the organisms is required. During the early stages of whooping cough B. pertussis can be isolated from approximately 90 per cent of patients. By the third or fourth week of illness the organism can be recovered in only 50 per cent of cases, and in the convalescent stage it is unusual to obtain a positive culture.

Adequate specimens and appropriate media are essential if bacteriologic diagnosis is to be efficient. *Specimens are best obtained by pernasal swab rather than by the cough plate method.* A sterile cotton swab wrapped about a flexible copper wire is passed through the nares, and mucus is obtained from the posterior pharynx. The swab must not be allowed to dry out because B. pertussis is readily killed by desiccation. As quickly as possible the specimen is plated onto fresh Bordet-Gengou medium, to which penicillin has been added to prevent overgrowth of adventitious organisms. Incubation is at 35° C., and although the trained observer can recognize the small, bisected pearl colonies of B. pertussis within 48 hours, at least 72 hours of growth is usually required. Presumptive identification can be made by agglutination tests with appropriate antisera. It is virtually impossible to distinguish between Bordetella species on primary isolation except by serologic means.

A fluorescent antibody staining procedure that can be applied directly to clinical specimens as well as to organisms grown in culture is a rapid diagnostic technique which is finding more general use.

Serologic procedures are of little help in the diagnosis of whooping cough because a rise in titer of most antibodies does not occur until at least the third week of illness.

It is difficult to distinguish abortive or mild cases of pertussis from tracheobronchitis caused by other agents except by bacteriologic means. On the other hand, paroxysmal coughing may be associated with pulmonary lesions such as allergic bronchitis, atypical pneumonia, or cystic fibrosis. Pertussis-like illnesses, associated with lymphocytosis, have been reported in adenovirus infections.

Treatment. Mild cases of pertussis require only supportive treatment. Specific therapy of severe whooping cough has been disappointing despite the in vitro susceptibility of B. pertussis to various antimicrobial agents and the protective effect of passively administered antibody in experimental disease.

Antimicrobials. A number of antimicrobial drugs have significant in vitro activity against B. pertussis. Agents that readily eradicate the organisms in human disease may shorten the course of the illness if given in the catarrhal or early paroxysmal stages. In the established paroxysmal stage the organisms can also be readily eliminated by antimicrobials, but the course of the illness is unaltered. Even in the paroxysmal stage the use of drugs is justified in order to render the patient noninfectious.

In a recent study, erythromycin, oxytetracycline, and chloramphenicol were shown to be more effective in eliminating organisms than ampicillin, an often recommended agent. On the basis of drug safety and efficacy either erythromycin or tetracycline is the drug of choice. The daily dose for each is 50 mg. per kilogram of body weight given in four divided doses. The organism is eliminated after a few days of therapy, but because bacteriologic relapse may occur, treatment should be continued for ten to fourteen days.

Immunotherapy. Hyperimmune human gamma globulin is often used in therapy of unimmunized patients, particularly small infants. The usual dose is 1.25 or 2.5 ml. intramuscularly for three successive days.

Supportive Therapy. Particularly in the young infant, supportive measures combined with careful nursing care are of paramount importance. Specific attention must be devoted to the maintenance of proper water and electrolyte balance, adequate nutrition, and sufficient oxygenation. Constant alertness for the presence of secondary infectious complications such as pneumonia is required, and appropriate therapy should be promptly instituted upon discovery.

Prevention. The great communicability of whooping cough, particularly during the first few weeks of illness, makes it desirable to isolate the patient for four to six weeks, or, ideally, until cultures are negative. Unfortunately, the diagnosis is usually not made until the end of the catarrhal stage, and by then spread of the disease has already occurred. Exposed susceptibles should be isolated from social groups until it is determined whether disease is present. Unimmunized contacts, especially infants, should receive 2 to 4 ml. of hyperimmune gamma globulin intramuscularly, the dose to be repeated in five days. Those young children who have not received a booster dose of vaccine in more than a year should receive an injection upon exposure.

Recent studies have suggested that erythromycin may be effective in prophylaxis against pertussis in exposed, susceptible persons.

Active Immunization. There is little doubt that the fall in incidence of whooping cough in the very young is directly related to widespread immunization with suitable, killed suspensions of *B. pertussis.* The highest risk of serious morbidity and mortality is in the young infant. Women of child-bearing age generally do not have significant levels of protective antibody in their sera, and consequently the newborn are not protected by maternal antibodies. Therefore, active immunization is begun as early as is commensurate with the production of a satisfactory immune response. At the present time, it is recommended that the infant receive three injections of pertussis vaccine at one-month intervals beginning at 6 to 12 weeks of age. Each injection provides four NIH* units. The NIH unitage is based upon the ability of a vaccine to protect mice against a standard intracerebral infection. The pertussis suspension is usually incorporated into a triple vaccine with alum-precipitated diphtheria and tetanus toxoids (DPT). Booster injections are given one, three, and five years after completion of the initial course. Administration of pertussis vaccine to those over six years of age is not generally recommended because of an apparent increased incidence of untoward reactions. There is no protection against parapertussis.

It has become increasingly apparent that pertussis vaccine does not yield solid, lifelong protection. It is difficult to ascertain the exact duration of protection because there is variation between vaccines as well as in intimacy of exposure. In a recent epidemic only 20 per cent of those vaccinated within four years of exposure contracted whooping cough, whereas all of the unimmunized who had similar exposure acquired the disease. However, as the time between immunization and exposure increased, the incidence in both groups became equal. Thus, in the face of routine immunization, it is possible that pertussis will become primarily a disease of older children and adults.

Instances of "vaccine failure" have usually been shown to be due to the use of preparations of low potency. However, it has recently been suggested that a change in the dominant serotype causing

disease, unrepresented in vaccine preparations, may be of importance. This controversial point is under study.

Local reactions as well as fever may occur after injection of pertussis vaccine. The exact incidence of the more severe complication of encephalopathy is uncertain, but both fatalities and residua have been reported. The occurrence of neurotoxicity appears to be decreasing as more refined immunizing suspensions are used, and certain soluble extracts of *B. pertussis* may prove to be effective without engendering serious side effects. Despite the small, but real, incidence of neurologic complications of pertussis immunization, the risk still seems far less than the hazards of whooping cough in the young child, including whooping cough encephalopathy. Nevertheless, in infants with a personal or family history of convulsions or other neurologic disorders, pertussis immunization should be deferred, or very small doses should be cautiously administered. Care should also be exercised in the immunization of children with a family history of an allergic diathesis.

Bass, J. W., Klenk, E. L., Kotheimer, J. B., Linnemann, C. C., and Smith, M. H. D.: Antimicrobial treatment of pertussis. J. Pediat., 75:768, 1969.
Bradford, W. L.: The Bordetella group. *In* Dubos, R. J., and Hirsch, J. G. (eds.): Bacterial and Mycotic Infections of Man. 4th ed. Philadelphia, J. B. Lippincott Company, 1965.
Connor, J. D.: Evidence for an etiologic role of adenoviral infection in pertussis syndrome. New Eng. J. Med., 283:390, 1970.
Lambert, H. J.: Epidemiology of a small pertussis outbreak in Kent County, Michigan. Public Health Rep., 80:365, 1965.
Lapin, J. H.: Whooping Cough. Springfield, Ill., Charles C Thomas, 1943.
Medical Research Council, Great Britain: (a) Vaccination against whooping cough: Relation between protection in children and results of laboratory tests. Brit. Med. J., 2:454, 1956. (b) Final report. *ibid.*, 1:994, 1959.
Pittman, M.: *Bordetella pertussis* — bacterial and host factors in the pathogenesis and prevention of whooping cough. *In* Mudd, S. (ed.): Infectious Agents and Host Reactions. Philadelphia, W. B. Saunders Company, 1970.

GRANULOMA INGUINALE
Walsh McDermott

Granuloma inguinale is an indolent granulomatous and ulcerative disease usually localized to the genitalia and caused by a pleomorphic coccobacillus, *Donovania granulomatis,* the so-called "Donovan body." When grown on artificial medium, the organism develops a large capsule that reacts immunologically with klebsiella capsular material. *Donovania granulomatis* also resembles *K. pneumoniae* in morphology. Presumably, the infection is customarily transmitted during coitus or other close bodily contact, and the degree of communicability appears to be relatively low. The lesion tends to be single, and may rarely appear on surfaces of the body

---

*National Institutes of Health.

other than the genitalia. Systemic infection, notably with the production of arthritis or osteomyelitis, has been reported. Usually, the lesion appears on the genitalia or in the perianal area as a relatively painless nodular infiltration that soon breaks down, leaving a sharply demarcated ulcer with friable granulation tissue at the base. On histologic examination, the lesion appears well vascularized and is the site of considerable cellular infiltration, especially with polymorphonuclear leukocytes and monocytes. In appropriately stained tissue scrapings, the causative microbe, *Donovania granulomatis*, may be seen situated principally within the monocytes, although smaller numbers of extracellular micro-organisms can usually be identified. The lesion spreads by direct extension, is highly destructive to the skin and subcutaneous tissue, and secondary infection with other micro-organisms is common. Rarely, if sufficiently extensive, the process may cause elephantiasis of the genitalia.

There is nothing particularly characteristic about the lesions of granuloma inguinale, and the early lesion is indistinguishable from those produced by *T. pallidum, H. ducreyi*, or other processes that involve the genitalia. The diagnosis can be established only by appropriate microbiologic techniques, and these should be employed whenever the physician encounters a genital lesion (or an indolent ulceration elsewhere) that is not clearly caused by some other process. Microscopy of deep scrapings or impression smears from the lesion of granuloma inguinale stained by the Wright method usually reveals *Donovania granulomatis* within the monocytes. The ease with which the micro-organisms can be detected varies to some extent with the age of the lesion. In a relatively old lesion, the scrapings should be made from the depth of the lesion, and an extensive search of the smears may be necessary. The micro-organisms can also be cultured in medium containing chick embryo yolk by methods originally developed by Anderson and her associates. Antigen prepared from capsular material of *D. granulomatis* has been employed in a complement-fixation reaction and in a cutaneous reaction, but these have not yet been developed to the point of general application.

Granuloma inguinale has been successfully treated with streptomycin, the tetracyclines, and chloramphenicol. As initial therapy, tetracycline should be employed in a total daily dosage of 2.0 grams administered by mouth in divided doses for a two-week period. In unusually extensive lesions it may be necessary to continue the treatment for a longer period in order to attain complete healing. If relapse occurs or the lesions appear refractory to tetracycline treatment, streptomycin should be administered intramuscularly in a total daily dosage of 2.0 grams in divided doses for a two-week period.

No detailed studies are available concerning the prevention of granuloma inguinale. It seems likely, however, that thorough washing of the genitals with soap and water immediately after sexual intercourse has a significant influence in reducing the probability of infection.

Anderson, K., Goodpasture, E. W., and DeMonbreun, W. A.: Immunologic relationship of *Donovania granulomatis* to granuloma inguinale. J. Exp. Med., 81:41, 1945.

Davis, B. D., Dulbecco, R., Eisen, H. N., Ginsberg, H. S., and Wood, W. B., Jr.: Microbiology. New York, Hoeber Medical Division, Harper & Row, 1970, Chap. 36.

Sheldon, W. H., Thebaut, B. R., Heyman, A., and Wall, M. J.: Osteomyelitis caused by granuloma inguinale. Amer. J. Med. Sci., 210:237, 1945.

DIPHTHERIA
F. S. Cheever

Definition. Diphtheria is an acute infectious disease caused by a bacillus, *Corynebacterium diphtheriae*. The primary lesion is usually located in the pharyngeal area (fauces, nasopharynx, or larynx) and is characterized by the formation of a grayish pseudomembrane. The organism elaborates a specific soluble exotoxin, which is responsible for the local cellular injury and the systemic manifestations of the disease.

History. Although a diphtheria-like disease was described by medical writers as early as the second century A.D., diphtheria was first established as a clinical entity by the publication of Pierre Bretonneau's classic monograph in 1826. In 1883, Klebs described the diphtheria bacillus; a year later Löffler demonstrated its etiologic relationship to the disease, and in 1888 Roux and Yersin clarified the pathogenesis of the disease by their discovery of the specific exotoxin. The first effective antitoxin was produced by von Behring in 1890. Schick introduced his skin test for determining susceptibility in 1913. Active immunization, first introduced by Theobald Smith and by von Behring, received its greatest impetus from Ramon's demonstration, in 1923, that formalin-treated toxin, i.e., toxoid, represented a nontoxic, antigenically effective immunizing agent. Today the disease occurs throughout the world. In recent years morbidity and mortality rates have shown a significant decline in western Europe and North America. In the United States diphtheria occurs chiefly in the autumn and early winter months. The majority of severe and fatal cases occur among unimmunized children.

Etiology. The causative agent of diphtheria, *Corynebacterium diphtheriae,* is a gram-positive, nonmotile, nonsporulating bacillus that is characteristically club-shaped and frequently beaded in appearance. In stained smears the organisms are usually found arranged so as to form sharp angles with each other, giving the characteristic Chinese letter appearance. Diphtheria bacilli grow well on ordinary laboratory media containing "peptones" or tissue extracts. The most common media used are Löffler's coagulated blood serum and potassium tellurite agar. Virulent diphtheria bacilli are distinguished by the ability to elaborate and secrete a specific poisonous substance, diphtheria toxin, which is a true exotoxin. It is the cause of the tissue necrosis occurring in the course of the clinical disease. Chemically, it is a complex protein; the mechanism of its action remains unclear, although when applied to susceptible mammalian cells grown in tissue culture, it inhibits protein synthesis. So-called nonvirulent strains of *C. diphtheriae* fail to produce this toxin. Freeman (1951) and others have shown that the ability to produce toxin is frequently associated with infection of the bacterial cell with a lysogenic bacteriophage that under proper conditions can convert an avirulent non-toxin-producing strain into a fully virulent toxin-producing one. Three types of *C. diphtheriae* are recognized, largely on the basis of their characteristic colonial formation on potassium tellurite medium and their distinctive fermentation reactions. All three types, *gravis*, *mitis*, and *intermedius*, produce the same toxin and the same clinical picture. The original hypothesis that *gravis* strains were more frequently associated with epidemic diphtheria remains unproved.

Epidemiology and Immunity. *Corynebacterium diphtheriae* is essentially on obligate parasite of man; hence, the human host represents the only significant reservoir of diphtheritic infections. The organisms may be transmitted directly or indirectly from one person to another. As the usual habitat of the organism is the upper respiratory tract, droplet infection is probably the most common method of spread, although contamination of the hands, handkerchiefs, and similar objects may play an important role. Discharges from extrarespiratory sites of infection (such as superficial ulcers of the skin) are infectious. Although the organism may survive for a brief period outside the human body, spread of infection by contaminated dust appears to be a rare occurrence. A few milk-borne outbreaks have been reported.

Invasion and infection of the human body by the diphtheria bacillus is not always followed by the development of clinical disease. More frequently, the organism multiplies in the mucous membrane linings of the air passages for a shorter or longer period without causing signs of illness. Presumably, in such a case, the "carrier" possesses a pre-existing immunity of greater or lesser degree, which, although it does not prevent the actual implantation of the organism, does limit the amount of damage to the host's cell so that no clinical manifestations develop.

Immunity against the clinical disease depends primarily upon the presence of antitoxin in the blood of the infected person. Although it is probable that upon occasion antibacterial mechanisms play a role in preventing the diphtheria bacillus from actually establishing itself in the throat of the human subject, nothing is known concerning the nature or specificity of the reaction. On the other hand, recovery from an attack of clinical diphtheria is associated with the appearance of appreciable amounts of antitoxin in the blood.

This antitoxin is formed in response to the direct stimulation of diphtheria toxin. It has the characteristics of a true antibody: it may be formed in response to either clinical or subclinical infection or as a result of artificial active immunization. Although it is produced relatively slowly in response to the primary stimulation, it appears rapidly and in large amounts following secondary stimuli, even though little or no antitoxin can be demonstrated at the time of the secondary stimulation. The antibody may be transferred to other persons (naturally, by transplacental passage in utero; artificially, by transfusion), thereby conferring temporary passive immunity upon the recipient.

Schick Test. Although the accurate determination of anti-toxin levels is a laboratory procedure, the Schick test will usually yield valuable information concerning the immune status of a person. This test is performed by injecting into the skin of the forearm 0.1 ml. of diluted highly purified diphtheria toxin. A positive reaction is characterized by the development of a variable area of redness at the site of inoculation over a period of 72 to 120 hours. The reaction reaches its height about the fifth day; after this it gradually fades, leaving an area of brownish pigmentation that may persist for some weeks. Such a positive reaction is associated with an antitoxin level in the circulating blood of less than 0.03 unit of antitoxin per milliliter, and is interpreted to mean that the patient is susceptible to the clinical disease. A negative Schick reaction signifies that the blood antitoxin level exceeds 0.03 unit per milliliter and that the subject's chances of contracting clinical diphtheria are comparatively slight. The occasional negative reactor who does develop clinical illness usually has a mild attack.

In actual practice, the diluted toxin is injected in one forearm, while the other forearm is injected with a similar amount of the same material that, however, has been heated to 60° C. for 30 minutes in order to destroy the toxin. This control is necessary in order to detect *pseudo-Schick reactions*, reactions caused by products of growth of the diphtheria bacillus other than the toxin itself. Thus, some workers recommend the use of highly purified toxoid as control material. The pseudo-Schick reaction is characterized by the development of erythema at the site of inoculation about 18 hours after injection. This increases to reach its maximal intensity at 24 to 36 hours, and then fades gradually to disappear completely within the next 72 hours. Such a reaction connotes allergy to some component of the injected material rather than absence of circulating antitoxin in quantities adequate to confer immunity. Thus, four types of reaction are possible, as indicated in the accompanying table.

Babies born to immune mothers will give negative Schick reactions at birth, owing to the transplacental transfer of antitoxin. This passive immunity wears off rapidly, and by the sixth month, in the absence of artificial immunization, nearly all infants are susceptible to the disease as evidenced by the demonstration of a positive Schick reaction. From this point on there is a gradual rise in the proportion of persons giving Schick-negative reactions as a result of natural immunization, usually following subclinical infection. In the absence of continued contacts with the diphtheria bacillus, the antitoxin level gradually falls to a point where the person is again susceptible to the disease.

Pathogenesis. The usual habitat of the diphtheria bacillus is the upper respiratory tract of man. In a susceptible person, the organism multiplies on the superficial epithelial cells of the pharynx, elaborating and secreting the specific toxin in the process. The absorption of this toxin by neighboring cells initiates a process of tissue necrosis, which furnishes conditions favorable to the growth of the organism, which in turn produces more of the toxin. As the process continues, it stimulates an inflammatory reaction on the part of the body, leading to the formation of the typical diphtheritic membrane. The absorption of toxin into the general circulation results in a degree of prostration usually out of proportion to the relatively innocuous appearance of the local lesion at this stage. If the membrane involves the larynx and trachea, either primarily or secondarily, mechanical obstruction to the airway may develop,

REACTIONS TO SCHICK TEST

Type of Reaction	Observation				Interpretation	
	Test arm		Control arm		Immunity	Sensitivity
	36 hr.	120 hr.	36 hr.	120 hr.		
Positive	−	+	−	−	Absent	Absent
Negative	−	−	−	−	Present	Absent
Pseudo	+	−	+	−	Present	Present
Combined	+	+	+	−	Absent	Present

and death owing to suffocation may occur unless the oxygen lack is corrected by intubation or tracheotomy. The soluble toxin is carried in the general circulation to susceptible organs such as the heart and cranial or peripheral nerves. Cardiac failure may be the result of specific necrotic injury to the myocardium or it may be secondary to peripheral circulatory disturbances. The cranial or peripheral nerve involvement is presumably due to the direct action of the toxin on the nerve cells. The explanation of the relatively selective action of the toxin remains obscure.

Aside from the striking picture of the local lesion, the pathologic changes noted in fatal cases of diphtheria are relatively nonspecific. Grossly, the heart, liver, kidneys, and adrenal glands may show degenerative changes characterized microscopically by necrosis, fatty infiltration, and parenchymatous degeneration.

Clinical Manifestations. Diphtheria is characterized by a relatively short incubation period — one to four days on the average, with an outside limit of one week. The clinical manifestations depend, *first*, upon the severity of the process (which may show every gradation between a mild, nearly inapparent infection and a highly malignant progressive one), and, *second*, upon the anatomic location of the primary lesion. The more important clinical types are faucial (or tonsillar), nasopharyngeal, and laryngeal. Extra-respiratory forms of the disease such as ocular, aural, and cutaneous diphtheria do occur, but in general are of less importance.

In *faucial diphtheria* the process is limited essentially to the tonsillar area. The onset is abrupt and is characterized by moderate fever, chilliness, general malaise, and mild sore throat. Swallowing is relatively painless. The pharynx is moderately injected and dull red. The pseudomembrane first appears as a thick gelatinous exudate confined to one tonsil. This spreads to the other tonsil and thickens so as to give the typical dirty white or grayish-yellow diphtheritic membrane. If the pseudomembrane is forcibly removed, a raw, bleeding surface is exposed beneath, over which the membrane rapidly forms anew. Tonsillar swelling is usually present, and frequently there is some enlargement of the cervical lymph nodes. If the tonsils are absent, the membrane may be less characteristic. Often the process spreads to involve the uvula and soft palate, which become edematous. If the process remains limited to the tonsillar area, the clinical manifestations may be so mild that a definite diagnosis can be made only by isolation of the organism.

Nasopharyngeal diphtheria represents a spread of the original process from the faucial area to the uvula, soft palate, posterior pharyngeal wall, and nasal mucosa. The membrane covering these areas presents a dirty yellow appearance; in some instances it invades the anterior nares and actually protrudes through the external opening. Occasionally the middle ear may be invaded as well. There is considerable faucial edema and usually a serosanguineous nasal discharge. Enlargement of the cervical lymph nodes is almost invariably present; the swelling may be so severe as to deserve the name *bullneck*. A characteristic diphtheritic odor is usually present as well as pallor and cyanosis. Toxemia is the rule, and the patient is almost always prostrated. Oliguria, albuminuria, weak, rapid pulse, and high fever are prominent features. If recovery ensues, sequelae are common. This form of the disease should not be confused with *anterior nasal diphtheria*, in which the disease process is limited to the anterior nares, which is a relatively benign process with minimal toxicity, and which is important chiefly because of its epidemiologic implications.

Laryngeal diphtheria usually results from the spread of infection downward from the nasopharynx, although the primary lesion may be in the larynx itself. It is a particularly dangerous form of the disease, because the membrane and accompanying edema produce mechanical obstruction of the airway, giving rise to the classic diphtheria croup. The first symptoms are hoarseness, dyspnea, and a characteristic brassy cough. As the obstruction increases, dyspnea becomes more severe, and ultimately cyanosis appears together with aphonia and expiratory and inspiratory stridor. As bronchial secretions accumulate behind the obstruction, the accessory muscles of respiration are brought into play, and the spasmodic attacks of severe dyspnea gradually become frequent and persistent. Unless the airway is restored by intubation or tracheotomy, death by suffocation ensues. Rarely the process involves the bronchial tree as well.

Extrarespiratory diphtheria. Although diphtheria is usually a disease of the upper respiratory tract, other parts of the body may be the site of primary or secondary diphtheritic lesions. Thus, wounds, sores, and abrasions of the skin may become secondarily infected. During World War II a number of skin infections occurred among men serving in the tropics. These took the form of chronic, nonhealing ulcers that developed at the site of minor abrasions. In the course of time a dirty grayish membrane appeared. The majority of these infections yielded *mitis* strains on culture. The relatively low percentage of sequelae suggests that the absorption of toxin from such wounds was not great, although some were accompanied by polyneuritis (see below). The fact that antitoxin alone usually gave disappointing results in these cutaneous cases raises the possibility that many of these so-called "tropical sores" had a complex etiology.

Ocular diphtheria is a rare form of the disease; the conjunctivae are chiefly involved.

Diagnosis. The *presumptive diagnosis* of diphtheria must be made on clinical grounds without waiting for laboratory confirmation, since the early specific therapy of the disease is paramount. The cardinal features pointing to the diagnosis are (1) a comparatively painless pharyngitis involving the tonsils (or tonsillar beds) and frequently the uvula and soft palate as well; (2) a relative lack of redness in spite of the presence of a significant degree of edema; (3) the appearance of the characteristic membrane in the tonsillar area; and (4) moderate pyrexia. In severe cases, significant systemic manifestations occur; in mild cases, however, the patient may feel well throughout, and the throat may appear comparatively innocuous.

The *laboratory diagnosis* depends upon the isolation and identification of the causative organism from the lesion. The throat or wound swab should be taken by an experienced person and sent to the laboratory without delay. Here a Löffler's slant, a tellurite plate, and a blood agar plate should be inoculated promptly. Although experienced workers can recognize the organism in a fair percentage of cases by smears made directly from the wound or throat swab, this procedure is not recommended for the average laboratory. The inoculated cultures may be inspected at the end of 16 to 24 hours and a presumptive diagnosis made on the basis of characteristic colony formation and cellular morphology. Confirmatory evidence may be obtained by a study of fermentation reactions, and, whenever indicated, virulence tests should be carried out. Other laboratory findings include a moderate leukocytosis and a transient albuminuria in all but the mildest cases.

Streptococcal tonsillitis and pharyngitis are most often confused with diphtheria. In the former conditions the throat is usually a fiery red, the tonsillar exudate is thinner and lighter colored, the fever is higher, and swallowing is painful. Frequently the follicles in the faucial area are prominent. Upon occasion it may be impossible to differentiate the two infections without resort to laboratory means. Rarely a concomitant streptococcal infection may mask the underlying diphtheritic process. Other conditions that must be considered in the differential diagnosis are Vincent's angina, agranulocytic angina, infectious mononucleosis, post-tonsillectomy throat, and exudative pharyngitis caused by an adenovirus.

Complications. The most important complications are related to the *myocardium* and the *nervous system*. Signs of myocarditis may appear as early as the second week of the disease, although the usual time of onset is somewhat later. They are characteristically associated with the more severe forms of respiratory diphtheria. In general, those patients showing early myocardial involvement tend to run a graver course. The onset may be insidious, with rising pulse of poor quality, distant heart sounds, premature contractions and gradual cardiac enlargement. Less often, cardiac failure may appear with little warning. Pallor, epigastric pain, vomiting, and circulatory collapse are the usual signs and symptoms. Inversion of the T waves, delayed conduction time, bundle branch block, and terminally ventricular flutter or fibrillation are the most common electrocardiographic changes noted. Occasionally peripheral circulatory collapse occurs in the absence of demonstrable cardiac damage. Recovery, when it takes place, is usually complete.

Postdiphtheritic paralysis affecting the cranial or peripheral nerves is a relatively frequent complication. The most common form of cranial nerve palsy is *paralysis of the soft palate*. This makes its appearance in the third to fifth week of the disease, and is ushered in by the development of a nasal twang in the voice and regurgitation of fluid through the nose upon attempted swallowing. Although the course is usually mild, occasionally tube feeding may be required. The condition tends to clear up completely in the course of a week or ten days. *Ocular paralysis* may occur in the fourth to sixth week of the disease. The two most common types are *oculomotor*, affecting the external rectus muscle of one or both sides, thus resulting in a convergent squint, and *ciliary*, in which the power of accommodation is weakened or lost. Spontaneous recovery in the course of a week is the general rule. Rarer forms of cranial nerve palsies are *facial, pharyngeal*, and *laryngeal* paralysis. The prognosis in these forms is good unless there is concomitant involvement of the respiratory muscles.

Paralysis of the peripheral nerves appears somewhat later than do the cranial nerve palsies; the usual time of occurrence for the former is between the fifth and eighth week of the disease. The most common form is a polyneuritis of the lower extremities, as evidenced by weakness or paralysis of certain muscle groups. Total loss of function is rare, and sensation is unimpaired. Complete recovery over a period of a few weeks is the general rule. Less commonly, the upper extremities, the neck, and the trunk may be involved. Again, in general, the prognosis is good; if, however, the intercostal muscles are involved there is danger of serious respiratory embarrassment, particularly in the presence of diaphragmatic weakness or paralysis.

It must be emphasized that polyneuritis of diphtheritic origin may occur in the absence of faucial manifestations of the disease. For example, generalized polyneuritis can follow cutaneous diphtheria. During World War II, it represented the most important sequela of so-called "wound diphtheria."

Treatment. The prompt administration of diphtheria antitoxin in adequate amounts is the first and most important step. Laboratory studies and clinical experience have demonstrated the importance of administering antitoxin as early as possible in the course of the disease. Presumably, the union between toxin and cell is a stable one that cannot be broken down by any practicable amount of antitoxin; the role of the latter is confined therefore to neutralizing unbound toxin circulating in the blood and other body fluids, thereby protecting the undamaged cells that have not come into intimate contact with the toxin as yet. Antitoxin should be administered as soon as diphtheria is suspected on clinical grounds without waiting for confirmation from the laboratory. Assurance of prompt and vigorous treatment of the actual case of diphtheria is well worth the price of occasionally administering antitoxin unnecessarily. In a severe case of diphtheria the prognosis depends largely upon how early in the course of the disease an adequate amount of antitoxin can be administered.

There is no agreement among clinicians as to the amount of antitoxin that should be administered. A conservative scheme calls for 10,000 to 20,000 units for mild cases and 50,000 to 100,000 units for severe cases. These figures are for average adults, but in actual practice age and weight are not often taken into account except among the very young. The total dose required should be administered at one time if possible. The route of administration may be intramuscular or intravenous. The latter route has the advantage of speedier absorption but in theory gives a greater risk of an overwhelming anaphylactic reaction. In general, the intramuscular route is preferred for doses up to 20,000 units and the intravenous route for amounts above this. The subcutaneous route should not be used, because absorption is relatively slow.

As diphtheria antitoxin is a foreign protein (horse serum), precautions should be observed against the occurrence of hypersensitivity reactions, i.e., anaphylaxis. These are (1) inquiry of the patient or of his family concerning a history of sensitivity to horses (or equine products such as dander, etc.) or of previous exposure to horse serum, and (2) performance of ophthalmic and intradermal sensitivity tests. In both tests a 1:10 dilution of antitoxin in saline is used. In the first method, one drop of this dilution is dropped into the conjunctival sac, and the eye is observed for the development of redness during the next 30 minutes. In the second method, 0.1 ml. of the 1:10 dilution is injected intracutaneously in the forearm, and the area is observed for the development of erythema, wheals, and similar reactions for the next half hour. If a positive reaction is obtained by either method, it is *prima facie* evidence of sensitivity to the horse serum, and hence antitoxin should be administered with great caution. *Desensitization* is carried out by giving small doses of highly diluted antitoxin subcutaneously at first and then gradually working up to intramuscular and intravenous administration until the full dose has been given. Desensitization may be a tedious and nerve-racking task, but as antitoxin is the only specific therapeutic weapon available, it is a process that must be carried out in cases in which sensitivity exists. Epinephrine must be at hand before antitoxin is administered by any route.

Since it has been shown that the administration of certain antimicrobial drugs (notably penicillin, tetracycline, and erythromycin) helps to eliminate the causative organisms from the nasopharynx and the cutaneous lesions, there has been an understandable tendency toward the routine use of one or more of these drugs in the treatment of all cases of diphtheria. Although diphtheria bacilli are susceptible to the action of these drugs in vitro, the drugs have no neutralizing effect upon the toxin; thus, they cannot be substituted for antitoxin. They find their greatest usefulness in the prevention of secondary infections and in the treatment of chronic carriers. The real danger in the routine use of these antimicrobial drugs lies in their masking effect; the elimination or reduction of the infecting organisms may render a laboratory diagnosis impossible and hence may prevent the physician from administering the life-saving antitoxin.

General Management. Complete bed rest is the first requirement. The period over which this should be maintained depends upon the degree of toxicity and the presence or absence of cardiac complications. In any event, the return to activity should be gradual and guided by the careful observations of the physician. Local therapy of the throat is rarely needed in the absence of secondary infection, although hot saline irrigations may be comforting. Dehydration should be treated with parenteral fluids containing dextrose. Careful watch must be kept for signs of developing cardiac or neurologic complications. With these complications adequate rest is also the main feature of therapy. Digitalis appears to be without benefit in the treatment of cardiac complications. The patient should be kept isolated until two successive daily pharyngeal and nasal cultures are negative for the presence of virulent diphtheria bacilli.

Prevention. *Active immunization* represents the basic and practical means at hand with which to control the occurrence of clinical diphtheria. Of the various preparations available, fluid toxoid and adsorbed (aluminum phosphate, aluminum potassium sulfate, etc.) toxoid are the most widely used in the United States. Both preparations consist of a filtrate of a broth culture of diphtheria bacilli, i.e., diphtheria toxin, which has been treated with 0.3 to 0.5 per cent formalin at a temperature of 37° C. until toxicity has disappeared. The resulting fluid toxoid is given in a primary course, consisting of three injections (0.5 ml., 1.0 ml., 1.0 ml.) at weekly intervals. If suitable amounts of alum are added to the fluid toxoid, a precipitate forms. This alum-precipitated toxoid may be resuspended, giving a relatively purified immunizing preparation with a slightly superior antigenic potency because of a local stimulating effect of the alum on the tissues. A primary course consists of two 1 ml. injections spaced a month apart. Against the obvious advantage of the alum-precipitated toxoid must be weighed the fact that the greater sensitizing ability of this preparation may lead to unpleasant reactions upon subsequent reinjection. In addition, a sterile abscess occasionally develops at the inoculation site as a result of the irritating action of the alum. Both fluid and aluminum-adsorbed toxoid are excellent immunizing agents; at least 85 per cent of persons receiving a primary course may be expected to become Schick-negative.

The primary course of active immunization should be administered within the first year of life, preferably at about the third month. It may be combined with immunizations against tetanus, pertussis, and poliomyelitis. One stimulating dose should be administered two years later and another at the time the child enters school. In susceptible older children or adults, the possibility of a sensitivity reaction to the toxoid should be guarded against by the prior administration of 0.1 ml. of 1:10 dilution of fluid toxoid intradermally (the *Moloney test*). The development of a local reaction (best described as a severe pseudo-Schick reaction) is a warning that toxoid must be administered cautiously in multiple, small, suitably diluted doses. These reactions, fortunately almost unknown before adolescence, represent the great problem in immunizing adult population groups. Presumably they represent some degree of immunity, and the mere carrying out of a Moloney test in a person giving a positive reaction may serve as an adequate antigenic booster.

Passive immunization is possible because the administration of relatively small amounts of antitoxin (1000 units) will confer protection for a period of two to three weeks. Because of the danger of inducing sensitization or of eliciting anaphylactic shock in a person already sensitized to the foreign protein, its use should be limited to immunization of persons peculiarly at risk of infection, as, for example, nonimmunized children heavily exposed to virulent diphtheria bacilli. Inasmuch as the protection conferred by antitoxin is of such short duration, active immunization with one of the toxoid preparations should be carried out at the same time.

In the event of an outbreak of diphtheria in a closed community (such as a school), the exposed persons should be observed closely in order that antitoxin may be administered at the first sign of suspicious illness. Routine throat cultures usually yield little information of practical value. The exposed persons should be given Schick and Moloney tests, and those found susceptible and not sensitive should be immunized promptly with one of the toxoid preparations. Under special circumstances, the administration of prophylactic antitoxin may be indicated.

Belsey, M. A.: *Corynebacterium diphtheriae* skin infections in Alabama and Louisiana. A factor in the epidemiology of diphtheria. New Eng. J. Med., 280:135, 1969.

Davis, B. D., Dulbecco, R., Eisen, H. N., Ginsberg, H. S., and Wood, W. R., Jr.: Microbiology, 1st ed. New York, Paul B. Hoeber Inc., 1967.

Frost, W. H.: Infection, immunity and disease in the epidemiology of diphtheria, with special reference to some studies in Baltimore. J. Prev. Med., 2:325, 1928. (Reprinted in Maxcy, K. F. (ed.): Papers of Wade Hampton Frost, New York, The Commonwealth Fund., 1941, pp. 447-466.)

Greenberg, L.: The use and results of diphtheria immunization. Bull. WHO, 13:367, 1955.

Heath, C. W. Jr., and Zusman, J.: An outbreak of diphtheria among skid-row men. New Eng. J. Med., 267:809, 1962.

Semple, R. H. (translator): Memoirs on Diphtheria from the Writings of Bretonneau, Guersant, Trousseau, Bouchat, Emphis and Davoit. London, The New Sydenham Society, 1859.

Smith, J. W. G.: Diphtheria and tetanus toxoids. Brit. Med. Bull., 25:177, 1969.

Zalma, V. M., Older, J., and Brooks, G.: The Austin, Texas, diphtheria outbreak: Clinical and epidemiological aspects. J.A.M.A., 211:2125, 1970.

Zamiri, I.: Diphtheria today: Some experiences in Iran. Lancet, 1:1222, 1970.

CLOSTRIDIAL DISEASES

GENERAL CONSIDERATIONS
Emanuel Wolinsky

The clostridia are spore-forming anaerobic gram-positive bacilli that for the most part lead a saprophytic existence in nature. They may be found in large numbers in the intestinal tracts of humans and animals, and in the soil. They are capable of producing disease by virtue of their elaboration of powerful exotoxins, but special conditions must be present in the tissues to allow the organisms to germinate, proliferate, and elaborate toxins. The mere presence of clostridia in the wound or on the surface of the body is not significant. Most clostridial disease is caused by *C. perfringens,* although occasionally *C. novyi (oedematiens), septicum, sordelli (bifermentans), histolyticum,* and *fallax* may be human pathogens.

The pathologic states attributable to clostridial infection cover a wide range of severity and localization, from the relatively benign wound infection to the highly fatal gas gangrene; from transient bacteremia to life-threatening septicemia; from relatively mild food poisoning to necrotic enteritis; and from pleural empyema to purulent meningitis. The neurotoxic disease caused by *C. tetani* is discussed below, and that caused by *C. botulinum* is discussed in Bacterial Food Poisoning.

BACTERIOLOGY

All the clostridia owe their pathogenicity to the elaboration of exotoxins that have enzymatic activity. Four major toxins and eight minor ones have been described and given Greek letters. The most important of them is the alpha toxin, which is a lecithinase. Many of the species of clostridia have been separated into types according to their ability to elaborate specific exotoxins. *C. perfringens* may be divided into five or six toxigenic types; Type A elaborates more alpha toxin than any other type or species and is by far the most important variety of Clostridium in human disease, particularly gas gangrene.

CLOSTRIDIAL MYONECROSIS
(Gas Gangrene)
Emanuel Wolinsky

The clostridial gas gangrene is best called *clostridial myonecrosis* because the outstanding feature is rapidly progressive muscle necrosis with relatively little inflammatory reaction, and because other organisms can produce skin and subcutaneous gangrene with gas formation. The disease most often arises from traumatic or surgical wounds in which anoxic conditions prevail as a result of ischemia or crushed muscle. Battle wounds of World Wars I and II supplied plentiful case material for study; gas gangrene occurred in approximately 10 per cent of World War I wounds and in 1 per cent of those that occurred in World War II. In civilian practice the rate of gas gangrene among 188,000 major open wounds has been estimated to be 1.8 per cent. The rate of contamination or local infection of open wounds, on the other hand, amounts to 30 to 80 per cent. The soil is the usual source of the clostridia in exogenous infection, the intestine or biliary tract in autogenous infection.

Pathogenesis. The factors that predispose to the invasion of muscle by the bacilli with the subsequent elaboration of exotoxins are related to lack of oxygen and lowering of the oxidation-reduction potential of the tissues. These factors are (1) impaired local vascular supply owing to vessel trauma or pressure from foreign bodies, casts, or tourniquets; (2) presence of metallic bodies, clothing, or dirt in the wound; (3) presence of necrotic tissue or hemorrhage; and (4) growth of aerobic micro-organisms in the wound.

Under these circumstances the bacilli can multiply anaerobically and elaborate toxins, which diffuse out and damage surrounding muscle, which in turn becomes colonized with the bacilli. Thus, the disease spreads rapidly to surrounding muscles and gains momentum. The severe generalized toxemia remains poorly explained. Alpha toxin is not found in the blood, and it is postulated that a toxic factor that acts on certain vital centers or enzymes is produced by the interaction of clostridial toxin with infected muscle.

Clinical Manifestations. The clinical picture of gas gangrene is dominated by rapidly progressive toxemia and shock. After a relatively short incubation period of one to four days the patient suddenly exhibits restlessness and anxiety; the temperature and pulse rate begin to rise and the blood pressure to fall. He is noted to be pale and sweating. The wound becomes painful and markedly swollen. Some hours later, after progression of the signs and symptoms, a thin brownish exudate begins to ooze from the wound, and a small amount of crepitus may be noted in the surrounding tissues. A bronze discoloration starts at the edge of the wound and progresses outward. Blebs filled with purplish fluid may appear. An odor characterized as "mousy" or "sickly sweet" is described by many observers. By this time the patient may be anuric and in irreversible vascular collapse. When the muscle is exposed by incision, it appears to be "cooked" or dead—it does not bleed when cut or retract when pinched. Smears from *involved muscle* show many large gram-positive rods and no other organisms, but very few pus cells. Smears and cultures from the *wound exudate* at the surface may reveal other organisms in addition to the clostridia, especially in grossly contaminated wounds. Roentgenograms reveal the presence of gas in and around muscle bundles in the form of fernlike, lacy patterns. Untreated,

fully developed clostridial myonecrosis is almost always fatal.

Myonecrosis must be differentiated from clostridial and nonclostridial crepitant cellulitis, from anaerobic streptococcal myonecrosis, and from physical and chemical causes of gas in the tissues. *Clostridial cellulitis* (anaerobic cellulitis, local gas gangrene, epifascial gas gangrene, or gas-forming fasciitis) is a gas-forming infection of connective tissue mainly localized to subcutaneous areas with spread in fascial planes, but healthy muscle is not involved. It arises as a result of clostridial infection of tissue already necrotic from ischemia or trauma. The onset is gradual, and toxemia, pain, and swelling are less than in gas gangrene. A large amount of gas is distributed in the form of large bubbles along the fascial planes, but not in the muscle. Incision will show that the muscle is viable, and smears from muscle tissue away from the open wound will not reveal organisms.

Nonclostridial crepitant cellulitis is similar to clostridial cellulitis, except that the infection is associated with other organisms usually in a mixed flora consisting of two or more of the following: aerogenic coliforms (*E. coli, Klebsiella, Enterobacter*), anaerobic streptococci, *Bacteroides* and gamma streptococci. In many cases this mixed bacterial flora in gas-forming cellulitis includes clostridia; these cases do not appear to differ in prognosis from those in which clostridia are absent.

Anaerobic streptococcal myonecrosis was described by MacLennan in infected war wounds from the Middle East in 1948, but there have been few reports since then. Other organisms, especially group A streptococci and *Staph. aureus* were always found with the primary agent, and 3 of 19 patients had anaerobic streptococcal bacteremia.

Simple contamination of wounds with clostridia is not uncommon. The organisms, usually in association with a mixed flora, exist as saprophytes on necrotic tissue and debris and do not invade further. Clostridia may also be found in localized collections of purulent material in wounds, or in a collection of foul-smelling brownish fluid known as a "gas abscess" or a "Welch abscess." Drainage will usually suffice to bring these conditions under control. There is not always a clean-cut distinction among the various pathologic states described above, nor is it clear how often one can recognize an orderly progression in the severity of clostridial invasion from simple contamination to full-blown myonecrosis.

Diagnosis. The diagnosis of gas gangrene is essentially a clinical one. Upon first suspicion of the disease, dressings and casts must be removed and the wound or suspected area thoroughly inspected. Roentgenograms may help to show the fine bubbles of gas distributed in and around muscle bundles. Incision should be made into the muscle so that the characteristic appearance may be appreciated. At the same time a specimen of muscle may be examined by Gram stain and by anaerobic cultural techniques. Slides may also be made for staining by the fluorescent antibody technique (Clark et al., 1969). Smears and cultures from the exudate around the wound surface may be misleading. Tables 1 and 2 summarize the most important findings for the differential diagnosis.

Treatment. Treatment must be prompt and vigorous. Most important is thorough *debridement* and *excision* of all devitalized tissue and dead muscle. Hopelessly involved extremities usually need to be amputated except perhaps under the influence of hyperbaric oxygen. It is said that if any infected muscle is left behind, it will prevent cure. General *supportive measures* should include intravenous fluids and blood, other measures to combat vascular collapse and shock, and peritoneal dialysis when necessary. *Antimicrobial* treatment is given to prevent blood stream invasion and to suppress further spread of infection. Penicillin is the drug of choice given in large doses of 10 to 20 million units per day intravenously. Erythromycin may be substituted in patients allergic to penicillin. In a recent study it was found that 11 per cent of clostridial strains were resistant to tetracycline. *Antitoxin* is recommended in the hope of neutralizing any free toxin in the body fluids, although its usefulness is doubtful because the exotoxins are very rapidly bound to cells. The recommended dose is 40 thousand units of trivalent or pentavalent antitoxin intravenously at once and 20 to 40 thousand units repeated at four to six hour intervals. The usual precautions for horse serum must be observed. *Hyperbaric oxygen* at 3 atmospheres has been recommended by some as a dramatically successful mode of therapy that should take precedence over immediate surgical treatment and antitoxin. It is said that debridement may be deferred until systemic toxicity has been relieved and demarcation between necrotic and viable tissue is clear. In this way loss of tissue may be minimized and amputation sometimes avoided. If a suitable chamber is not available locally, it is probably unwise to delay surgical extirpation in favor of a long journey.

Treatment of "anaerobic" cellulitis and streptococcal myonecrosis need not be so radical. Usually wide excision and debridement along with supportive measures and appropriate antimicrobials will suffice. A Gram-stained smear of wound exudate and muscle aspirate will help one to decide whether penicillin alone should be given (for pure Clostridium or Streptococcus) or whether antistaphylococcal or anticoliform agents should be added or substituted. For the former, one should use a semisynthetic penicillinase-resistant penicillin (methicillin, nafcillin, or cephalothin) to initiate treatment; for the gram-negative bacilli one can add tetracycline, gentamicin, or kanamycin.

Prevention. The prophylactic use of antitoxin and antimicrobials at the time of injury does not prevent gas gangrene. Careful attention to good surgical technique is most important. All devitalized tissue must be excised and vascular supply left intact. Care must be taken with tourniquets and casts to prevent undue ischemia. Plaster of Paris itself may be contaminated with clostridia.

TABLE 1.   CLASSIFICATION OF HISTOTOXIC CLOSTRIDIAL DISEASE

Traumatic
  A. Wound infection (war and civilian)
    1. Simple contamination
    2. Localized (purulent or "gas abscess")
    3. Gas-forming cellulitis
    4. Myonecrosis
  B. Uterine infection (postabortion and postpartum)
  C. Burns, panophthalmitis, brain abscess, etc.

Nontraumatic
  A. Postoperative (abdominal, amputation)
  B. Postinjection
  C. Spontaneous
    1. Localized (pneumonia, empyema, cholecystitis, myonecrosis)
    2. Septicemic (malignant disease, intestinal lesion)
  D. Bacteremia without hemolysis or sepsis (from decubitus ulcer, gangrenous extremity, uterus)

TABLE 2.   GAS-FORMING SOFT TISSUE INFECTIONS

	Clostridial Myonecrosis	"Anaerobic" Cellulitis	Streptococcal Myositis
Onset	Sudden	Gradual	Gradual
Toxemia	Extreme	Slight	Slight
Pain	May be severe	Slight	Gradually increasing
Swelling	Marked	Slight	Marked
Skin color	Bronze	No change	Erythematous
Exudate	Thin, brown	Thin, bloody; later purulent	Profuse, thin seropurulent
Gas	Little, in muscle	Profuse, large bubbles in fascial planes	Little, in muscle
Muscle	Dead, "cooked," healthy muscle invaded	Not involved	Initially edematous, then hemorrhagic
Bacteriology	Mixed flora from exudate or open wound; from muscle aspirate pure gram-positive rods	May be pure clostridia or mixed flora from exudate or subcutaneous tissue; no organisms in muscle aspirate	Anaerobic streptococci, along with Group A Streptococcus, *Staph. aureus, etc.*, from exudate and muscle
Prognosis	Serious	Good	Good
Treatment	Radical surgery, penicillin, antitoxin, hyperbaric oxygen	Surgical drainage and debridement, appropriate antimicrobials	Surgical drainage and debridement, penicillin

UTERINE INFECTION

Postabortion and postpartum clostridial infections of the uterus are still important causes of serious disease in obstetrics. At least 5 per cent of women harbor clostridia in the vagina as simple contaminants. Fulminant infection usually follows criminal abortion or prolonged and difficult labor, and presents a clinical picture similar to that seen in traumatic gas gangrene. Unlike wound gas gangrene, however, uterine infection is frequently accompanied by clostridial sepsis leading to jaundice, hemolysis, hemoglobinemia, hemoglobinuria, and renal shutdown. As in wound infection, there may be various grades of clostridial involvement, from simple contamination to secondary invasion of necrotic matter in the uterus or a dead fetus to true invasion of intact uterine muscle producing myonecrosis or "physometra." Clostridial infection must be differentiated from the more slowly progressive uterine infection produced by anaerobic streptococci and Bacteroides which commonly leads to pelvic thrombophlebitis and septic pulmonary infarcts.

Treatment is essentially the same as that outlined above, except that a decision must be made quickly on whether to do a hysterectomy or merely to empty the uterus. Evidence for uterine perforation or necrosis will call for the more radical procedure. Antimicrobial therapy should probably include tetracycline or chloramphenicol in addition to penicillin to control Bacteroides.

POSTOPERATIVE GAS GANGRENE

Nontraumatic gas gangrene following surgical operations is probably the most common variety of the disease in civilian hospitals today. Of 42 cases of *C. perfringens* infection reported from a single hospital, 18 followed operations and 10 were secondary to trauma (Pyrtek and Bartus, 1962). Most of these infections involve the abdominal wall after biliary or intestinal surgery, or the leg or hip after amputation or correction of hip fractures, although the complication has been described following many other kinds of surgical procedures. Recent investigation in England indicated that most of these infections were sporadic and autogenous in origin, probably as a result of fecal contamination of the skin. Parker called attention to the importance of adequate preoperative sterilization of the skin with sporicidal agents and the advisability of giving prophylactic penicillin from a few hours before operation to one week after to those patients at greatest risk from postoperative clostridial infections—elderly patients who will have hip surgery or thigh amputations.

OTHER CLOSTRIDIAL DISEASES
Emanuel Wolinsky

SEPTICEMIA

Clostridial septicemia occurs rarely from traumatic wound gangrene, occasionally from postoperative gas gangrene, and commonly from uterine infection. In addition, nontraumatic or spontaneous clostridial septicemia has been described from such conditions as acute cholecystitis, perforated peptic ulcer, ulcerating carcinoma of the colon, acute pancreatitis, diverticulitis, appendiceal abscess, decubitus ulcer, and gangrenous limbs. Septicemia may occur in terminal cancer patients from portals of entry such as ulcerations of the respiratory or alimentary tracts. A recent report describes 21 patients suffering from various malignant diseases who had septicemia caused by *C. septicum* (Alpern and Dowell, 1969). As a result of septicemia, infection may localize in the pleura, myocardium, endocardium, and meninges. Benign clostridial bacteremia without hemolysis was recently described in a series of 20 patients, all of whom survived (Rathbun, 1968).

MISCELLANEOUS FORMS

Pneumonia and empyema may be associated with clostridial infection, usually as a result of aspiration of contaminated material from the mouth or the stomach, but occasionally by way of the blood stream. Penetrating injuries may lead to serious clostridial infections of the eye, brain, and meninges. Severe gas gangrene may result from injections into the buttock or thigh, presumably from inadequately sterilized skin. In at least one instance the organism was also isolated from the cotton sponges soaked in alcohol.

CLOSTRIDIAL GASTROENTERITIS
Emanuel Wolinsky

Clostridial food poisoning was the second most common variety reported to the Communicable Disease Center in 1968, representing 16 per cent of the total outbreaks and 34 per cent of the cases. There was no seasonal preference, and the most common vehicles were beef and turkey products. *C. prefringens* type A may be recovered from the stools of patients and from the suspected food product. The disease is characterized by a short incubation period, acute onset, absence of fever, and a relatively benign course. The outbreaks are self-limiting, and the disease is not spread to other people directly. Evidence points to an infection rather than an intoxication as the primary mechanism of the disease. *Enteritis necroticans* ("Darmbrand") was first described shortly after World War II in Germany. Other outbreaks occurred in North Germany and the Rhineland; then the disease apparently vanished. The disease was characterized by severe diarrhea, collapse, high mortality, and patchy hemorrhagic necrosis of the small bowel. It was originally attributed to a new type of *C. perfringens* called type F, but these organisms are now considered to be members of type C. It corresponds in many ways to certain clostridial enterotoxemias of animals.

Altemeier, W. A., and Culbertson, W. R.: Acute non-clostridial crepitant cellulitis. Surg. Gynec. Obstet, 87:206, 1948.

Ayliffe, G. A. J., and Lowbury, E. J. L.: Sources of gas gangrene in hospital. Brit. Med. J., 2:333, 1969.

Bentley, D. W., and Lepper, M. H.: Empyema caused by *Clostridium perfringens*. Amer. Rev. Resp. Dis., 100:706, 1969.

Bornstein, D. L., Weinberg, A. N., Swartz, M. N., and Kunz, L. J.: Anaerobic infections—Review of current experience. Medicine, 43:207, 1964.

Cabrera, A., Tsukada, Y., and Pickren, J. W.: Clostridial gas gangrene and septicemia in malignant disease. Cancer, 18:800, 1965.

MacLennan, J. D.: The histotoxic clostridial infections of man. Bact. Rev., 26:177, 1962.

Parker, M. T.: Postoperative clostridial infections in Britain. Brit. Med. J., 3:671, 1969.

Slack, W. K., Hanson, G. C., and Chew, H. E. R.: Hyperbaric oxygen in the treatment of gas gangrene and clostridial infection. A report of 40 patients treated in a single-person hyperbaric oxygen chamber. Brit. J. Surg., 56:505, 1969.

TETANUS

Alexander Crampton Smith

Tetanus, often called "lockjaw," is a disease of the nervous system characterized by intense activity of motor neurons resulting in severe muscle spasms. It is caused by an exotoxin of *Clostridium tetani*.

History. Tetanus has caught the imagination of physicians since Hippocrates, and this is probably in part due to the horrifying nature of the clinical picture in the established untreated case. The presence of the causative organism in soil was demonstrated by Nicolaier, who produced tetanus in animals by soil injections. The Clostridium was isolated in pure culture in 1899 by Kitasato, and in 1892, Nocard immunized horses by injections of antitoxic horse serum. Passive immunization after wounding saved many lives in World War I, and active immunization with toxoid almost eliminated tetanus in the allied armies in World War II. Curare was first suggested as having an application in the treatment of tetanus in 1811, but as curare in sufficient dosage to abolish the spasms of severe tetanus will certainly paralyze the muscles of ventilation, the large-scale use of curare had to wait almost 150 years until intermittent positive pressure ventilation (IPPV) through a cuffed tracheotomy tube was introduced into the treatment of tetanus in Denmark in 1953 (Bjørnboe et al.).

ETIOLOGY AND PATHOGENESIS

Clostridium tetani is a gram-positive, actively motile bacillus, which in its spore-bearing form has a characteristic "drumstick" appearance. Spores may develop at either end of the bacillus, giving a "dumbbell" appearance. It is a strict anaerobe, and spores will not germinate in the presence of even the smallest amount of oxygen. An oxidation-reduction potential of + 0.01 volt or less at pH 7 is required if germination is to take place. The Clostridium grows well on laboratory media at 37° C., and growth occurs slowly at 22° C. Vegetative bacilli are readily killed by antiseptics and by heat, but spores are highly resistant to antiseptics and, to a certain extent, are resistant to heat. To kill most spores, boiling for one hour is necessary, but the most resistant may require boiling for four hours. Autoclaving for ten minutes at 120° C. may, however, be relied on to sterilize contaminated objects. *Clostridium tetani* is commonly found in soil and in the feces of domestic animals and humans. Presumably by contamination with soil and feces, spores can be recovered from dust and clothing; in suitable surroundings like dried earth, spores will survive for many years.

Clostridium tetani produces two exotoxins, *tetanospasmin* and *tetanolysin*, and of these tetanospasmin is the neurotoxin which produces the typical muscle spasms of tetanus. It is extremely potent, each milligram of crystallized toxin containing 50 to 75 million mouse lethal doses. This extreme toxicity may be the reason why an attack of tetanus does not confer immunity, as it is postulated that the fatal dose of tetanus toxin is less than the amount required to provoke an immune response. Tetanolysin can cause hemolysis on blood agar plates, but does not seem to play any significant part in the pathologic process caused by the Clostridium.

There have been differences of opinion about the site of action of tetanospasmin and about the route by which it spreads, but it now seems firmly established that the toxin acts in the spinal cord and in the brain stem and that it spreads centrally along motor nerve trunks and up the spinal cord. Tetanus will follow the intravenous injection into animals, but the route by which toxin in the blood enters the nervous system is not clear. Toxin injected intramuscularly apparently spreads not only by passing up motor nerves but also by absorption into the blood, and it has been suggested that vascular spread is the more important route in generalized tetanus. Payling Wright surveyed the evidence for neural and vascular spread, but research, notably with radioactive isotopes (Fedenec, 1967), is continuing.

EPIDEMIOLOGY

The incidence of tetanus is difficult to establish because it is not a notifiable disease in many countries. The total world deaths each year, however, probably exceed 160,000, and if the average crude fatality rate is about 45 per cent (and it may be much higher) there must be more than 350,000 cases in the world every year. Tetanus is thus still a major public health problem in developing countries. The organism is found in soil and human and animal feces, and tetanus is common in warm climates and in rural areas that are highly cultivated and consequently have a large population of men and animals. Agricultural workers, in whom injuries may easily be contaminated with the Clostridium, are particularly at risk. *Clostridium tetani* can also be found in urban areas, but the degree of contamination is not high, and it is likely that the increased standard of living and hygiene which urbanization implies also contributes to a lower incidence of tetanus in cities. Further evidence of the importance of education and hygiene is the absence of neonatal tetanus in countries where obstetric hygiene is good, compared with the high incidence in countries where dung is sometimes used as a dressing for the umbilical stump.

PREVENTION OF TETANUS

Before Injury

Active Immunization. The U.S. Public Health Service Advisory Committee has stated that the need for active immunization against tetanus is universal and that such immunization is the only way by which tetanus may be eliminated as an important health problem. There is little doubt that active immunization with adsorbed tetanus toxoid will convey a remarkably high degree of immunity. In a recent paper, LaForce et al. (1969) calculated that the incidence of tetanus in the under-ten age group in the United States of America was about 3.8 per 100 million. This underscores the excellent results obtained by active immunization of American and British military personnel in World War II.

In the United Kingdom, the recommended course of injections is three doses of adsorbed toxoid in a mixed vaccine, one injection at six months of age, and two others, with six to eight weeks between first and second and six months between second and third. A "booster" is advised at school entry and another at 15 to 19. Thereafter, "booster" doses should be given at ten-year intervals. The American Academy of Pediatrics suggests three injections of toxoid no less than one month apart in infancy, a reinforcing dose about twelve months later, and a fifth or "booster" injection on entering school. Subsequent routine toxoid "boosters" should be administered at intervals of approximately ten years.

After Injury

Prevention of Contamination. Simple measures that prevent contamination can contribute significantly to the prevention of tetanus, and the effect of attention to treatment of the umbilical stump on the incidence of neonatal tetanus is a good example of the effectiveness of simple hygiene. The aim of surgery in prophylaxis is to remove all dead tissue and foreign bodies from a wound. This will not only remove spore-bearing material, but will also deny

the spores the anaerobic conditions necessary for their growth. As Adams et al. suggest, it is probably realistic to recognize a "tetanus-prone" wound. Such wounds include deep penetrating puncture wounds in which anaerobic conditions are likely to exist and surgical exposure is difficult or impossible. Tetanus-prone wounds also include wounds heavily contaminated with soil or manure, wounds with dead or devitalized tissue or retained foreign bodies, and wounds seen more than six to eight hours after infliction.

Active Immunization. In the United Kingdom a "booster" dose of toxoid is recommended if an injury occurs more than three years after the completion of the past course or more than three years after a "booster." If the wound is judged to be "tetanus prone," a "booster" should be given. The American Academy of Pediatrics recommends than an emergency injection of toxoid should be given if injury occurs more than one year after the last "booster." In spite of this, it has recently been suggested (Peebles et al., 1969) that if there is a valid history of an accepted immunization program, special tetanus boosters on admission to camps, schools, and colleges and emergency injections at times of injury are unnecessary and should be abandoned to minimize toxoid reactions. If a wounded patient's immune status is in doubt, he should be regarded as unimmunized, and other means of preventing tetanus should be used. If passive immunization with antitoxin is chosen, active immunization should be commenced at the same time with an injection of toxoid in another limb. Antitoxin will not influence active immunization conferred by a full course of adsorbed toxoid.

Passive Immunization. The use of passive immunization by means of antitoxin has probably resulted in the saving of many lives. The absence of a controlled trial precludes certainty, but circumstantial evidence is very strong. Animal experiments show that antitoxin given soon after inoculation with tetanus will protect against the disease, and Bruce (1920), reviewing 1458 cases of tetanus occurring in World War I showed that the incidence of tetanus, after prophylactic antitoxin was available in large quantities, fell from 9 per 1000 wounded to 1.4 per 1000 wounded. Other improvements in surgical care could have been contributory, but it seems likely that antitoxin was an important factor in the decrease in incidence.

Antitoxin has two disadvantages, both relative. The antitoxin commonly used is produced by the active immunization of horses, first with toxoid and then with tetanus toxin. If a patient has had a previous injection of horse serum, he may develop antibodies against horse serum proteins very soon after an injection of prophylactic equine antitoxin. This will result in immune elimination of the subsequently injected equine antitoxin so that protection is absent or incomplete. This elimination may be accompanied by sensitivity reactions, either local redness and swelling of the injected limb or generalized serum sickness.

If circulating antibodies are present, immune elimination may be very rapid and may be accompanied by fatal anaphylaxis. The dose of equine antitoxin for prophylaxis is 1500 units, but prophylactic antitoxin should not be given if either local or general reactions follow the subcutaneous injection of a test dose of 75 units. Epinephrine, 1 per 1000, should always be available whenever equine antitoxin is given; in cases in which antitoxin is indicated and either a history of previous injections of horse serum or a reaction to a test dose has been elicited, prophylaxis with human anti-tetanus immunoglobulin, 250 units, will be more effective and much safer.

Chemoprophylaxis. Antimicrobial drugs can inhibit the multiplication of *Clostridium tetani* and kill the vegetative form of the organism. By killing aerobic organisms coexisting with the Clostridium, antimicrobial drugs can prevent multiplication by denying the Clostridium the conditions favorable to its growth; they have no effect, however, on tetanus toxin. Because of the dangers of passive immunization, some centers in the United Kingdom have largely abandoned the use of antitoxin in favor of chemoprophylaxis, and at least one of these has provided data showing no increase in the incidence of the disease. Although the efficacy of chemoprophylaxis is not yet certain, it seems clear that in certain circumstances it may provide an alternative to prophylaxis by antitoxin.

For effective chemoprophylaxis certain criteria must be fulfilled: the organism must be susceptible to the drug chosen, and the patient must not be sensitive to the drug. *Clostridium tetani* is susceptible to a variety of drugs, including penicillin, tetracycline, and erythromycin so that it is probably not difficult to make a suitable choice for a particular patient. Chemoprophylaxis must be started early. Smith (1964) has shown that in mice inoculated with tetanus spores, chemoprophylaxis was effective if it was started four hours after inoculation but not if started eight hours after inoculation. The time interval in humans is not established, but it is suggested that in injuries seen later than six hours after infliction, some other form of prophylaxis should be chosen. Antimicrobial therapy must be continued for a sufficient time to ensure that tetanus spores cannot survive, and this means for at least five days.

PATHOGENESIS

If tetanus is to supervene, the Clostridium must be introduced into human tissue, and the disease may follow a trivial or a serious injury. In countries with good medical services, serious wounds receive effective treatment, and tetanus is usually avoided. Apparently minor wounds then become a common cause of the disease, but in quite a high proportion of cases no responsible injury can be identified. The site of action and method of spread of the exotoxin have been mentioned, but it is rather surprising that no unequivocal evidence of recognizable pathologic lesions caused by tetanus has yet been forthcoming even after careful postmortem studies.

CLINICAL FEATURES AND CRITERIA OF SEVERITY IN TETANUS

The criteria of severity may be established in two ways: from the history and from the symptoms and signs.

From the History. The severity of an attack of tetanus is related to the incubation period (the period from injury to the first sign of tetanus) and the onset period, described by Cole (1940) as the period from the first sign to the first generalized spasm. If the former is less than 9 days and the latter less than 48 hours, the attack of tetanus may be expected to be severe. The length of the onset period is, in general, the more reliable guide to the expected severity of the attack.

From the Symptoms and Signs. *The Mild Case.* Tetanus usually presents with rigidity of muscles, and this rigidity may be severe enough to cause pain. The patient with mild tetanus may have "local tetanus" in which rigidity affects only one limb, or the patient may have mild generalized rigidity. Stiffness of the jaw muscles causes trismus, and stiffness of the facial muscles may cause a change of expression. Stiffness of the muscles of the neck and back may cause discomfort or even pain on attempted flexion of the spine.

The Moderate Case. The patient has more severe generalized rigidity. Trismus is pronounced, the mouth can hardly be opened, and rigidity of the muscles of the face may cause the sneering "risus sardonicus." Opisthotonos may be pronounced, but more typically the stiffness of the antagonist muscles makes the patient lie "at attention" in bed, and the muscles of back and abdomen are hard to the touch. Patients with moderate tetanus may show mild exacerbations of this generalized rigidity as "reflex spasms." These spasms may arise spontaneously or more commonly as a result of stimuli. The important difference, however, between the patient with mild and the patient with moderate tetanus is the presence or absence of dysphagia. Spasm of the pharyngeal muscles makes swallowing difficult, and the patient coughs or splutters while drinking. This will predispose to the inhalation of pharyngeal contents and is the diagnostic characteristic of the moderate case.

The Severe Case. The patient who represents a severe case is distinguished from the patient with a moderate case by the presence of reflex spasms that may be of appalling intensity. If the spasms are untreated opisthotonos becomes extreme, and the intense muscle spasm may fracture vertebrae. Spasm of the laryngeal muscles, the diaphragm, and the intercostals prevents ventilation, and cyanosis occurs. The occurrence of reflex spasms that cause cyanosis and cannot be controlled except by powerful relaxants such as curare is the characteristic feature of the severe case of tetanus.

Patients with severe tetanus may also show a group of signs that have often been described but have recently been attributed by workers in Oxford to overactivity of the sympathetic nervous system (Kerr et al.). Many patients sweat profusely and, in some, oxygen uptake and carbon dioxide output are increased. In some patients most severely affected, extreme peripheral vasoconstriction develops with a glove-and-stocking distribution and a sharp line of demarcation between warm skin and cold skin. Hyperpyrexia may also develop, and probably reflects the inability of the vasoconstricted patient to lose heat. The most striking features of this syndrome, however, involve the cardiovascular system. Sinus tachycardia occurs and may progress to multifocal ventricular ectopic beats. The blood pressure is generally elevated, and superimposed on this elevation are peaks, often associated with spasms or stimuli, in which the systolic pressure may reach 300 mm. Hg, and the diastolic 150 mm. Hg. The syndrome may progress to hypotension that does not respond to pressor agents.

Perhaps fortunately, patients with severe tetanus often remember little of their illness and have failed to remember such bizarre incidents as a Union Jack being waved in the ward during the playing of "Rule Britannia." Electroencephalography shows a sleep pattern, with arousal during stimulation such as tracheal aspiration.

DIAGNOSIS

The diagnosis of the established case of tetanus is all too easy, and strychnine poisoning is the only condition which is truly similar to established tetanus. Trismus may occur from dental infections, and the author has seen one case of hysterical tetanus. More recently, overdose with the phenothiazine group of drugs has been confused with tetanus, but the movements in this condition usually include grimacing and jaw movements in which the jaw is opened widely.

CAUSES OF DEATH IN TETANUS

One of the most remarkable features of tetanus is that when patients recover, even from the most severe forms of the disease, they recover completely. It would therefore seem reasonable to study the causes of death carefully in tetanus so that by avoiding them the natural tendency of the disease toward recovery may be exploited. In a survey in Oxford, the causes of death in 18 of 82 patients were bronchopneumonia, 4; pulmonary embolus, 3; technical failure, 2; coincidental causes, 5; and no identifiable cause of death, 4.

Bronchopulmonary complications of tetanus are becoming less common now that the management of patients receiving IPPV through a tracheotomy tube is better understood, and it is likely that chest complications will become still less common in the future. In general on the writer's service, pulmonary embolus is not a common cause of death in patients with other diseases treated by tracheostomy and IPPV. However, the difference in the incidence of pulmonary embolus between *patients with tetanus* requiring treatment with curare and IPPV and patients *with other diseases similarly treated* is so striking that anticoagulants are now used in patients with tetanus severe enough to merit treatment in this way. The incidence of technical failure underlines the complexity of treating the fully paralyzed patient; the coincidental causes of death apparently had nothing to do with the main disease. No identifiable cause of death could be found in four patients who had all displayed a syndrome suggestive of sympathetic overactivity. Careful study of patients with similar symptoms and signs admitted subsequently has reinforced our belief that in some patients with severe tetanus the sympathetic nervous system is as grossly uninhibited as is the motor nervous system (Prys-Roberts et al.).

TREATMENT

There are certain forms of treatment required by all patients with tetanus.

Control of Rigidity and Reflex Spasms. Drugs to control rigidity vary with the severity of the case. *Barbiturates* have been used for many years, and in mild or even moderate cases are useful, but the amount of barbiturate necessary to obtund severe reflex spasms would cause coma. *Chlorpromazine* has proved antispasmodic properties in tetanus and is a sedative. It also is useful in mild and moderate cases, but has been shown by a clinical trial (Adams, 1958) to be no more effective than barbiturates, and like the barbiturates is inadequate to obtund the spasms in the severest cases. It may be used in doses of up to 50 mg. intramuscularly every four to six hours. *Mephenesin* is a centrally acting muscle relaxant that has been used extensively in the treatment of tetanus with good results, especially in moderate cases, but it must be given frequently and in large doses. The effect of a dose as large as 1 gram can be observed to have diminished significantly in one hour, and this dose, continued at hourly intervals, is close to that which will paralyze ventilation. If it becomes necessary to give paralyzing doses of mephenesin to control rigidity or reflex spasms, it is clearly not the drug of choice. Mephenesin is a local anesthetic and must be given by nasogastric tube. If given intravenously, except in extremely dilute solutions, it will cause hemolysis and hemoglobinuria. *Diazepam* is currently popular and has been used in mild and moderate cases in doses from 10 mg. every four hours intramuscularly, to 600 mg. intravenously per day. Like the other drugs mentioned above, it will not control the spasms of the severest case, and it is probably unwise to use very large doses. The severity of the case should be admitted and treatment changed to curare and IPPV. *Curare* and similar powerful relaxants will completely abolish the reflex spasms of the severest case of tetanus, but will also paralyze the muscles of ventilation. It is therefore necessary in addition to apply IPPV through a cuffed tracheotomy tube. Curare can be given intramuscularly in doses from 15 to 30 mg.

Wound Excision. Wound excision has been discussed under Prevention and seems a logical course of action if the causal injury can be identified. It has been suggested that excision of the wound is ineffectual in established tetanus because all the exotoxin produced by the organism has been fixed by the nervous system before symptoms and signs develop. Francis (1914) inoculated animals with tetanus and killed them when symptoms and signs began. He was able to recover many thousands of mouse lethal doses of toxin from the site of the inoculation, and this would seem to make the case for wound excision unassailable. A careful search should be made for foreign bodies in any wound excised, and excision should probably be conducted under cover of antitoxin.

Chemotherapy. Antimicrobial therapy has also been discussed under Prevention. As a therapeutic measure all patients with tetanus should have large doses of penicillin or another active antimicrobial for a sufficient time to ensure that the Clostridium cannot survive. This should be for at least five days.

Antitoxin. The advisability of using equine antitoxin as a therapeutic measure has been a controversial matter for many years. There is some, but not clear-cut evidence that the use of equine antitoxin reduces mortality in established tetanus. On general grounds, however, the work of Francis cited above suggests that toxin is still being produced at the time when symptoms and signs begin, and hence it would seem reasonable to neutralize any accessible toxin. Therapeutic antitoxin is subject to the same objections and hazards as prophylactic antitoxin, and its dangers must be balanced against the possible gain by its use. A suitable dosage regimen, including subcutaneous, intramuscular, and intravenous injections, should be designed to uncover sensitivity if present, and to avoid anaphylaxis. Ten thousand units intravenously is a suitable dose, but up to 100,000 units has been used. If a history of previous injections of horse serum can be obtained, or if a sensitivity reaction occurs, equine antitoxin should not be used. If available, human antitoxin in the same dose is more effective and much safer.

Mild Tetanus

The patient with mild tetanus needs only these general measures, including a relaxant and sedative such as diazepam. The patient should be encouraged to drink water under supervision every two hours in the early stage of the disease when it may be progressing. If a patient coughs or splutters while drinking, dysphagia is present, and the patient moves into the moderate group.

Moderate Tetanus

The patient with moderate tetanus differs from the mild case by the presence of dysphagia. He needs the general measures applicable to all patients with tetanus, but in addition he must have a tracheostomy and have a cuffed tracheostomy tube inserted into the trachea to make inhalation of pharyngeal contents impossible. The operation is performed under general anesthesia with a cuffed endotracheal tube in situ so that the operation may be careful and unhurried. A cuffed tracheostomy tube should be inserted through a high U-shaped incision into the trachea so that the tube lies easily in the trachea where it is approximately parallel to the skin. If the tracheostomy is high, there is sufficient distance between the tracheostome and the carina to make it unlikely that the tube will enter the right main bronchus. The wound should not be covered and should be cleaned frequently with a mild antiseptic. It is necessary to aspirate secretions from the trachea, and disposable gloves should be worn during this procedure, not only to prevent contamination of the trachea with organisms carried on the aspirating catheter, but also to avoid contamination of the tracheostomy wound. The patient with moderate tetanus must be fed by nasogastric tube, and may require large amounts of fluid to offset excessive sweating. A high calorie diet of about 3000 calories a day is necessary, but too much protein should not be given. Patients with moderate tetanus may have a considerable degree of muscle rigidity and may even have occasional mild reflex spasms. Diazepam in divided doses of up to 400 mg. intravenously per day has a considerable effect on the rigidity of tetanus without interfering with ventilation. In spite of treatment, muscular rigidity is painful and uncomfortable, and the patient should be turned every two hours to lessen this discomfort and avoid pressure sores.

Severe Tetanus

The patient with severe tetanus differs from the patient with moderate tetanus in that he has frequent reflex spasms that cannot be controlled by muscle relaxants other than curare, and needs to be paralyzed with curare or another powerful relaxant. Curare may be given by intramuscular injection of 15 to 30 mg.; if the patient must be paralyzed, there seems little to be gained by withholding the drug. At Oxford the nurses are instructed to give a further dose of curare when reflex spasms become obvious, and 400 mg. of curare per day has been necessary. The high incidence of pulmonary embolus in patients with severe tetanus has led to the use of anticoagulants in patients severely enough affected to require treatment with curare and IPPV. Anticoagulants are not, however, used within 24 hours of tracheostomy. The treatment of a paralyzed patient with IPPV is complex, and appropriate monographs should be consulted (Adams et al., 1969; Spalding and Crampton Smith, 1963). The patient cannot breathe, and IPPV must be applied through the cuffed tracheostomy tube. It has become common practice in recent years to ventilate with a large tidal volume at a slow rate, for example, with a tidal volume of 1 liter and a rate of 12 to 14 per minute. An artificial dead space is introduced between ventilator and patient so that rebreathing of expired air may bring the tension of carbon dioxide in the arterial blood to about 30 mm. Hg. Large tidal volumes seem to contribute to the health of the lungs, but the patient must also be turned every two hours to promote lung drainage, the inspired air must be fully humidified and at body temperature, and chest physiotherapy three times a day is indicated. Frequent chest films are necessary, and tracheal aspiration must be carried out with aseptic precautions. The patient cannot drink and must be fed by nasogastric tube or by vein if absorption fails. Patients with severe tetanus sweat profusely and may need large quantities of fluid, but the urine specific gravity is not always a good guide to hydration, and the patient should be weighed daily. It is not uncommon to observe a patient seriously ill with tetanus who is having a large fluid intake and gaining weight, but who still produces a high specific gravity urine. Later in the disease a diuresis may occur, and the patient may lose weight abruptly. A patient with severe tetanus needs 3000 calories per day, but too much protein is not advised, even though the patient, being functionally denervated by curare, may show muscle wasting. Urine is voided normally, but manual extraction of feces may be necessary. The patient cannot communicate, and sedation is probably indicated for patients paralyzed with curare. Withdrawal of sedation in severely ill patients may, however, disclose that the patient is unconscious.

Some patients most severely affected by tetanus develop a syndrome suggesting sympathetic overactivity. The cardiovascular component of this syndrome, tachycardia, arrhythmias, and hypertension, should be treated with beta and alpha adrenergic blockers (Prys-Roberts et al.). If it is thought necessary to administer a beta blocker intravenously, this should be done with great caution. Propranolol in 0.2 mg. aliquots to a total of 2 mg. has been successfully used to control arrhythmias and severe tachycardia. Control can sometimes be maintained by intragastric propranolol, 10 mg. every eight hours, but larger doses may be required. In some cases, when hypertension is not severe, control of the heart rate may be all that is necessary, but if the blood pressure is elevated, alpha adrenergic blockade is also indicated. Bethanidine, 5 mg. by nasogastric tube every two hours, has been used successfully, and as

this drug acts at postganglionic nerve endings, an overdose could be counteracted by pressor agents. The receptors, however, remain susceptible or perhaps hypersensitive to circulating catecholamines, and other combinations of antihypertensive drugs may be more effective. The author is aware of a patient successfully treated with propranolol, reserpine, and bethanidine. It is important not to reduce the heart rate to a point at which the cardiac output fails, because the depressed heart is working against an increased peripheral resistance. Moderate control of heart rate should be effected with a beta blocker, but hypertension when the heart rate is 100 or less must be controlled by alpha blockade.

In summary, in *a mild case* the patient needs (1) wound excision, (2) human or equine antitoxin, (3) penicillin or another appropriate antimicrobial drug, and (4) a centrally acting relaxant and sedative drug, such as diazepam.

In *the moderate case* the patient needs in addition (5) tracheostomy and the insertion of a cuffed rubber tracheostomy tube to separate the pharynx from the trachea and to make inhalation of foreign material impossible, and (6) nasogastric tube feeding.

In *the severe case* the patient needs in addition (7) virtually complete paralysis with curare or another powerful relaxant and IPPV, (8) anticoagulant drugs, and (9) if sympathetic overactivity is present, treatment with alpha and beta adrenergic blockers.

PROGNOSIS

The patient with mild tetanus will almost certainly survive whether treated or not. The patient with moderate tetanus, if untreated, is at risk from inhalation of foreign material. Repeated episodes of this kind may lead to fatal pneumonia. The patient with moderate tetanus, if treated, should not die except from causes unrelated to the primary disease. The patient with severe tetanus who is having reflex spasms severe enough to cause cyanosis will certainly die if untreated. Even with treatment, the severity of the illness and the complexity of the therapeutic regimen makes the outlook uncertain. In the United Kingdom in 1967, even in the best centers the mortality in patients with tetanus severe enough to indicate treatment with curare and IPPV varied between 10 and 40 per cent. Over-all mortality in the best hands is often still as high as 20 per cent, and at the extremes of age the mortality may be higher. It is paradoxical that in advanced countries where the immunization programs are efficient, mortality in the cases that do occur is high, not only because unimmunized patients are generally at the extremes of age, but also because patients who escape the immunization programs tend to have a poor physical status. Tetanus is becoming increasingly common among drug addicts.

Adams, E. B., Laurence, D. R., and Smith, J. W. G.: Tetanus. 1st ed. Oxford, Blackwell Scientific Publications, 1969.

Bjørnboe, M., Ibsen, B., and Johnson, S.: Et tilfaelde af tetanus behandlet med curarisering, tracheostomi of overtryksventilation med kvaelstofforilte og ilt. Ugeskr. Laeg., 115:1535, 1953.

Kerr, J. H., Corbett, J. L., Prys-Roberts, C., Smith, A. C., and Spalding, J. M. K.: Involvement of the sympathetic nervous system in tetanus. Brit. Med. J., 2:236, 1968.

Prys-Roberts, C., Corbett, J. L., Kerr, J. H., Smith, A. C., and Spalding, J. M. K.: Treatment of sympathetic overactivity in tetanus. Lancet, 1:542, 1969.

Wright, G. P.: Neurotoxins of *Clostridium botulinum* and *Clostridium tetani.* Pharmacol. Rev., 7:413, 1955.

BACTEROIDES, ANAEROBIC STREPTOCOCCAL, AND FUSOSPIROCHETAL DISEASE

Edward W. Hook

Etiology. Bacteroides species, anaerobic streptococci, *Fusobacterium fusiforme,* and a variety of spirochetes are members of the indigenous microbial flora of the mouth, intestinal tract, vagina, and mucous membranes of the external genitalia. *F. fusiforme* and the indigenous spirochetes are often present in large numbers in the gingival areas of the mouth, and Bacteroides usually outnumber *Escherichia coli* in the feces of man.

The Bacteroides are a group of gram-negative, non-spore-forming, nonmotile, strictly anaerobic bacilli. *Bacteroides funduliformis (B. necrophorus), B. fragilis,* and *B. nigrescens (B. melaninogenicum)* are the most common species associated with clinical infections of man. Anaerobic streptococci are gram-positive, grow in short or long chains, and, although varying considerably in size, are usually smaller than the common aerobic streptococci. These organisms comprise many different groups of species, but available information is too scant to permit systematic classification. Many, but not all, species of Bacteroides or strains of anaerobic streptococci form abundant gas and produce an extremely foul odor.

F. fusiforme is a gram-negative, anaerobic, nonmotile bacillus. The bacterial cells are small with tapered ends, may be evenly stained or granular, and often occur in roughly parallel bundles. *F. fusiforme* is closely related to Bacteroides but can be distinguished by certain biologic and biochemical reactions. Spirochetes are often found in association with *F. fusiforme.* Although "specific" designations, such as *Treponema microdentium, Borrelia vincenti,* or *Borrelia buccale,* have been applied to these spirochetes on the basis of differences in morphology, it is not certain whether these organisms belong to a single variable species or many separate groups.

Pathogenesis. Anaerobic streptococci and Bacteroides are not highly invasive organisms and usually initiate infection at sites of trauma or tissue necrosis where these organisms exist in large numbers. Local lesions are characterized by suppuration, abscess formation, and often a foul odor. Infection usually remains limited to one area, but blood invasion may occur and may lead to metastatic abscess formation at distant sites. The incidence of severe Bacteroides infections appears to be increased in patients with serious underlying diseases such as malignancy or diabetes mellitus, or in patients receiving therapy with multiple antimicrobials or corticosteroids. *Thrombophlebitis* occasionally develops adjacent to the site of initial infection, and may result in septic emboli. Thrombophlebitis is considered characteristic of Bacteroides infection, but is also observed occasionally in anaerobic streptococcal infections.

Although Bacteroides or anaerobic streptococci may be isolated in pure culture from local suppurative infections, an additional organism is present in most cases.

F. fusiforme and the indigenous spirochetes apparently act in concert to produce superficial inflammatory and ulceromembranous lesions of the gums, pharynx, and external genitalia. Local tissue damage, malnutrition, and a variety of debilitating diseases predispose to fusospirochetal infections.

Clinical Manifestations. *Bacteroides and Anaerobic Streptococcal Infections.* Bacteroides and anaerobic streptococci produce localized suppurative infections in many locations but most often in tissues liable to contamination with the flora of the intestinal tract or vagina. These organisms have been isolated from infected human bites, contaminated wounds, peritonsillar, appendiceal, ischiorectal and pelvic abscesses, exudate in localized or generalized peritonitis, and purulent discharges from patients with endometritis. The manifestations, course, and outcome of localized infection obviously depend on the site and extent of involvement.

Invasion of the blood by Bacteroides or anaerobic streptococci is usually secondary to infection of the peritoneum, female genital tract, or tonsils, but may be related to local infection at any site. The initial manifestations are determined by the portal of entry and may be symptoms of peritonsillar abscess, endometritis, appendicitis, etc. Gastrointestinal surgery is a frequent predisposing event. Patients with blood invasion are extremely ill and frequently have chills, hectic fever, and severe diaphoresis. The clinical picture of septic shock may be observed. A leukocytosis of 12,000 to 35,000 cells per cubic millimeter of blood is usually present. *Septic thrombophlebitis,* especially characteristic of Bacteroides infection, may extend from the area of the initial lesion and may lead to multiple septic pulmonary infarcts that are manifested by rales, dyspnea, cough, hemoptysis, pleurisy, lung abscess, or empyema. Metastatic infection may also occur in the brain, meninges, liver, bones, endocardium, or joints. A diffuse hepatitis occasionally develops in patients with Bacteroides septicemia, leading to icterus and enlargement and tenderness of the liver.

Anaerobic streptococci and Bacteroides often occur in the mixed bacterial flora found in the sputum of patients with aspiration pneumonia or lung abscess, and may be responsible for the spreading necrosis and foul pus encountered in these conditions. These organisms also occasionally produce acute otitis media, sinusitis, or mastoiditis.

Anaerobic streptococci and Bacteroides occur frequently in chronic suppuration of the ears, sinuses, or lungs; *brain abscess* may result from extension of infection from these sites. Anaerobic streptococci and Bacteroides are apparently the most common bacterial species isolated from brain abscesses.

Anaerobic streptococci also cause an *infection of muscle* that simulates clostridial myositis ("gas gangrene"). Infection begins insidiously two to nine days after an injury and is characterized by fever and severe pain, swelling, and erythema extending from the wound. Disorientation occurs in some cases. Gas formation is invariably present but is rarely pronounced. Smears of the profuse seropurulent exudate usually reveal enormous numbers of gram-positive cocci among masses of pus cells, and cultures show anaerobic streptococci mixed with *Streptococcus pyogenes* or *Staphylococcus aureus*.

Anaerobic streptococci in association with *Staphylococcus aureus, Streptococcus pyogenes,* or *Proteus* species may also cause a rather rare cutaneous infection known as *"progressive bacterial synergistic gangrene."* The infection usually begins after an operation on the thoracic or abdominal viscera. Erythema, edema, and finally gangrene and ulceration of the skin appear at the site of incision and extend peripherally. If infection is not controlled, enormous ulcers may form.

Fusospirochetal Infections. In gingivitis caused by *F. fusiforme* and spirochetes the free edges of the gums are reddened and swollen and bleed easily. Severe infections are characterized by painful, tender, extremely swollen and ulcerated gums, foul breath, and, rarely, fever and leukocytosis.

Manifestations of fusospirochetal pharyngitis (Vincent's angina) are sore throat and pharyngeal ulcers covered with a gray necrotic pseudomembrane, removal of which may cause bleeding. Fever and leukocytosis are observed occasionally. Infection may occasionally spread from gums or pharynx to the buccal mucosa and underlying tissues to produce an extensive necrotizing lesion of the cheek or lip (cancrum oris, noma).

Fusiform bacilli and indigenous spirochetes also produce vulvovaginitis and balanitis, and may on occasion contribute to the genesis of aspiration pneumonia, lung abscess, and necrotizing cellulitis complicating human bites.

Diagnosis. The presence of localized infection with foul pus or signs of systemic infection after manipulation of the gastrointestinal or female pelvic organs should suggest the possibility of infection with an anaerobic organism, but definitive diagnosis of Bacteroides or anaerobic streptococcal infection depends on isolation of the causative organism. Hectic fever and intense rigors occurring several days after onset of severe sore throat or peritonsillar abscess, especially if associated with a firm tender cord indicating a thrombus in the internal jugular vein, should suggest the possibility of Bacteroides septicemia originating in the oropharynx. Exudates or blood must be cultured under anaerobic conditions. The frequent association of aerobes with anaerobes in exudates may make recognition and isolation of the anaerobic organisms difficult. Bacteroides in blood may grow slowly, and blood cultures should be incubated for two to three weeks.

Diagnosis of fusospirochetal infections is based on the appearance of the lesions and smears of exudates showing a predominance of fusiform bacilli and spirochetes. Interpretation of smears is difficult because fusospirochetes are often present in scrapings of the gingivodental fold from normal persons.

Treatment. Therapy of Bacteroides or anaerobic streptococcal infections consists of drainage of collections of pus, removal of devitalized tissues and, if infection is not localized or if blood invasion is suspected, administration of an appropriate antimicrobial drug. The majority of strains are susceptible to tetracycline, and virtually all strains are susceptible to chloramphenicol. Patients with mild or moderate infections not threatening to life should be treated initially with tetracycline, 20 mg. per kilogram per day orally in divided doses. However, because tetracycline-resistant strains occur relatively often, chloramphenicol, 50 mg. per kilogram per day, should be used as initial therapy for patients with serious infections such as Bacteroides sepsis. Penicillin, ampicillin, erythromycin, kanamycin, colistin, or gentamicin cannot be relied upon in the therapy of Bacteroides infections unless the organism is known to be drug-susceptible.

Anaerobic streptococcal infections should be treated with benzyl penicillin (penicillin G), tetracycline, or chloramphenicol. Anaerobic streptococci are relatively resistant to penicillin and, if this drug is used, it should be administered parenterally in doses of 6 million or more units per day. Penicillin, tetracycline, and chloramphenicol alone are not active against all strains; in life-threatening infections, penicillin plus tetracycline or chloramphenicol should be used.

Mild cases of fusospirochetal gingivitis respond to irrigation with bland solutions and improvement in dental hygiene. Severe cases of gingivitis or pharyngitis should be treated with procaine penicillin, 600,000 units daily intramuscularly, or tetracycline, about 20 mg. per kilogram per day orally, for one week.

Bodner, S. J., Koenig, M. G., and Goodman, J. S.: Bacteremic Bacteroides infections. Ann. Intern. Med., 73:537, 1970.
Bornstein, D. L., Weinberg, A. N., Swartz, M. N., and Kunz,

L. J.: Anaerobic infections—Review of current experience. Medicine, 43:207, 1964.

Finegold, S. M., Harada, N. E., and Miller, L. G.: Antibiotic susceptibility patterns in classification and characterization of gram-negative anaerobic bacilli. J. Bact., 94:1443, 1967.

Goldsand, G., and Braude, A. I.: Anaerobic Infections. Disease-A-Month, November, 1966, pp. 1–62.

Heineman, H. S., and Braude, A. I.: Anaerobic infection of the brain. Observations on eighteen consecutive cases of brain abscess. Amer. J. Med., 35:682, 1963.

Moore, W. E. C., Cato, E. P., and Holdeman, L. V.: Anaerobic bacteria of the gastrointestinal flora and their occurrence in clinical infections. J. Infect. Dis., 119:641, 1969.

Rotheram, E. B., and Schick, S. F.: Nonclostridial anaerobic bacteria in septic abortion. Amer. J. Med., 46:80, 1969.

Tynes, B. S., and Frommeyer, W. B., Jr.: Bacteroides septicemia. Cultural, clinical, and therapeutic features in a series of twenty-five patients. Ann. Intern. Med., 56:12, 1962.

DISEASE CAUSED BY SALMONELLA

Edward W. Hook

GENERAL CONSIDERATIONS

The genus Salmonella consists of more than 1300 serologic types. The majority of serotypes are capable of producing disease in animals and man and should be considered as primary pathogens of animals that are readily transmitted to man. A few serotypes, among which *Salmonella typhosa* is the best example, exhibit marked host preference. *S. typhosa* is a parasite of man only, and does not cause disease in lower animals in nature.

Human infection with salmonellae may be expressed as *acute gastroenteritis* ("food poisoning"), *enteric fever* (typhoid or paratyphoid fever), or *bacteremia* with or without clinical evidence of localized infection. Asymptomatic transient infection of the intestinal tract is also common with certain species. A chronic carrier state may occur after infection with *S. typhosa* or occasionally other serologic types, and is characterized by prolonged excretion of salmonellae in feces or urine.

Typhoid fever is considered separately here because of its historical identity, the host specificity of the pathogen, and the wealth of data on basic and clinical aspects of the disease. This approach is unrealistic to the extent that an illness closely resembling typhoid fever can result from infection with other salmonellae, and *S. typhosa* can on occasion produce all of the clinical syndromes described for the other salmonella serotypes.

Etiology. Salmonellae are gram-negative, aerobic, nonsporing rods that are motile (with the exceptions of *S. pullorum* and *S. gallinarum*) and that grow readily on simple culture media. Presumptive identification of salmonellae involves relatively simple biochemical and agglutination reactions, but definitive identification of species depends on precise analysis of the somatic (O)

and flagellar (H) antigens of the organism. Subdivision of certain species, especially *S. typhosa* and *S. typhimurium,* can be achieved by bacteriophage typing. Specific identification of all isolates is desirable, especially for epidemiologic reasons, and can be obtained through local, state or federal health agencies.

Salmonella species most frequently isolated from human infections in the United States during 1968 are, in descending order of frequency, *S. typhimurium, S. enteritidis, S. heidelberg, S. newport, S. saint-paul, S. infantis, S. thompson, S. typhosa, S. javiana,* and *S. blockley.* These ten serotypes accounted for about 72 per cent of the total salmonellae isolates from man during 1968. *S. typhimurium* is the serotype most frequently isolated year after year, usually accounting for 20 to 30 per cent of the total.

TYPHOID FEVER

Definition. Typhoid fever is an acute, often severe illness caused by *S. typhosa* and characterized by fever, headache, apathy, cough, prostration, splenomegaly, maculopapular rash, and leukopenia. Typhoid fever is the classic example of enteric fever caused by salmonellae.

Incidence and Prevalence. Typhoid fever is a disease of major importance in areas of the world that have not attained high standards of public health. A progressive decrease in incidence of typhoid fever has occurred in the United States since 1900, but sporadic cases and limited outbreaks continue to occur. About 400 to 500 cases per year have been reported in recent years. Some of these infections were acquired in other areas of the world, but many were acquired in the United States from food contaminated by chronic typhoid carriers. In the United States more than 3000 chronic typhoid carriers are under supervision by health departments, but the actual number of chronic carriers is probably considerably higher. Typhoid fever will continue to occur on a limited scale in countries with high standards of public health because of the frequency of typhoid in other areas of the world, the magnitude of intercontinental travel, and the existence of reservoirs of chronic carriers.

Epidemiology. The ultimate source of infection with *S. typhosa* is a patient with typhoid fever or a typhoid carrier. Patients with typhoid fever excrete large numbers of *S. typhosa* in feces or urine, and viable bacilli may also be present in vomitus, respiratory secretions, or pus. Chronic enteric carriers, the most important source of infection, often excrete 10^6 or more viable bacilli per gram of feces. The typhoid bacillus can survive for weeks in water, ice, dust, and dried sewage. Water containing typhoid bacilli has been responsible for many outbreaks in the past; it may be contaminated directly by excreta containing *S. typhosa* or by excreta washed down from remote sites by rain or introduced by faulty sanitation or plumbing. Foods may be contaminated directly by excreta, by water containing *S. typhosa,* and occasionally by contaminated dust. Flies also have been implicated as mechanical vectors in the transmission of infection. Oysters and other shellfish may be infected in polluted tidal waters. In areas where typhoid fever is common the incidence of the disease increases during the summer.

Pathogenesis. The portal of entry of *S. typhosa* is almost always the gastrointestinal tract. The initial invasion is not associated with marked multiplication of *S. typhosa* in the intestine, although organisms are occasionally detected in stools for several days during this period. Bacilli apparently gain access to the blood through lymphatics in the small intestine and produce an initial transient bacteremia that is rapidly terminated as organisms are removed from the blood by reticuloendothelial cells in liver, spleen, bone marrow, and lymph nodes. Organisms multiply at these intracellular sites and are discharged into the blood for a period of days. The incubation period of typhoid fever may correspond to the phase of invasion from the intestine and intracellular multiplication in phagocytes; clinical manifestations of the disease may become evident as bacteria begin to re-enter the blood. During the phase of bacteremia, infection of the biliary tract regularly occurs, and multiplication of organisms in bile leads to seeding of the intestinal tract with millions of bacilli. The entry of infected bile into the intestine is responsible for the increase in number of organisms in stools during the second and third weeks of disease. Infection of the gallbladder is usually asymptomatic, although symptoms of cholecystitis occasionally develop.

The infective dose of *S. typhosa* for man is influenced by many factors. It has been assumed that a small number of bacilli, possibly 10 or 100, could initiate infection. This view is supported by studies of certain laboratory accidents and the occurrence of typhoid fever after exposure to water containing a small number of bacilli. Observations on volunteers infected orally with several strains of *S. typhosa* indicate that a dose of about 10^6 viable units is required to infect 50 per cent of a group. The applicability of these results in volunteers to naturally occurring typhoid infection is unknown. Variation in pathogenicity among different strains of *S. typhosa* is known to exist, and changes related to cultivation on artificial media cannot be excluded.

It has been suggested but not definitely established that the endotoxins of *S. typhosa* are responsible for some of the clinical manifestations of typhoid fever. This concept is based on the similarities of certain manifestations of typhoid fever and the events observed after injection of bacterial endotoxin. For example, both typhoid fever and injection of endotoxin are associated with headache, chills, fever, polymorphonuclear leukopenia, thrombocytopenia, and reticuloendothelial cell hyperplasia. It has been demonstrated in volunteers that tolerance to the pyrogenic action of endotoxin is present during the convalescent phase of typhoid fever and that vascular hyper-reactivity to epinephrine or norepinephrine appears during the febrile phase of the disease and persists into convalescence. Both of these phenomena – the development of tolerance and vascular hyperactivity – are considered to be indicators of endotoxin activity. However, volunteers made tolerant to endotoxin prior to challenge with *S. typhosa* develop typical typhoid fever, an observation apparently in conflict with the hypothesis that endotoxin released during infection is responsible for the fever and other manifestations.

Pathology. Proliferation of large mononuclear cells derived from reticuloendothelial tissue is the most prominent feature of the pathology of typhoid fever. Involvement of lymphoid tissue in the intestinal tract, principally Peyer's patches in the terminal ileum, leads to necrosis and ulceration. Erosion of blood vessels may give rise to intestinal hemorrhage. Intestinal lesions are usually confined to mucosa and submucosa but occasionally penetrate muscular and serosal layers and produce intestinal perforation. Healing of intestinal lesions does not give rise to appreciable scarring or stricture formation. The liver is enlarged and often shows cloudy swelling and focal areas of necrosis. The spleen and mesenteric lymph nodes are enlarged and show hyperplasia of reticuloendothelial cells. Bronchitis is common, and pneumonia is not unusual. Microscopic examination of the maculopapular skin lesions reveals round-cell infiltration and vascular congestion.

Clinical Manifestations. The incubation period usually is 8 to 14 days but varies from five days to five weeks. The duration of illness in a case of average severity is about four weeks. The onset is usually gradual and associated with anorexia, lethargy, malaise, headache, general aches and pains, and fever. During the first week there is a gradually increasing remittent fever. Dull, continuous headache is a prominent symptom in almost all cases. About two thirds of the patients have a nonproductive cough, and epistaxis occurs in about 10 per cent. The majority of patients have vague abdominal pain or discomfort. Constipation is frequent and more common than diarrhea, which occurs in only about 20 per cent of the patients. During the second week of illness the temperature shows less of a tendency to remit and is often sustained at around 40° C. During this phase patients are often severely ill with marked weakness, abdominal discomfort, and distention. Mental dullness is prominent, and delirium may occur. Diarrhea is more common during the second week than during the first, and stools may contain blood. As the illness extends into the third week, the patient continues to be febrile and becomes increasingly exhausted and weak. Patients without complications usually begin to improve during the third and fourth weeks. The temperature gradually begins to decline and may be normal by the end of the fourth week.

The physical signs vary with the stage of the disease. During the first week fever and slight abdominal tenderness may be the only findings.

However, during the second and third weeks findings characteristic of typhoid fever may develop. The patient appears acutely ill with a dull, expressionless, lethargic face. The mental state varies within wide limits from normal to frank mental confusion and delirium. The pulse is often not as fast as might be expected to accompany the degree of temperature present. Rhonchi or scattered moist rales may be present as a manifestation of bronchitis. The majority of patients have slight abdominal tenderness, most pronounced on the right side and in the upper abdomen. Abdominal distention may be severe. A soft spleen can be palpated in about three fourths of the patients. Maculopapular skin lesions appear during the second or third week of illness in about 80 to 90 per cent of patients with typhoid fever. These "rose-colored spots" are 2 to 5 mm. in diameter, blanch on pressure, are located predominantly on the upper abdomen or anterior chest, and are sparse, usually not exceeding 20 in number. The skin lesions last for two to four days and then disappear, but may be followed by fresh crops. Rose spots are difficult to see in highly pigmented patients. The signs of illness subside as fever diminishes. Convalescence is slow; a month or more is often required to regain normal status.

Variation in the typical course described in preceding paragraphs is common. The illness may be mild and last only a week or may be prolonged, with a febrile course as long as eight weeks.

Laboratory Findings. Normochromic anemia develops during the course of the disease. Anemia may be aggravated by blood loss in stools. Leukopenia is observed in many cases, and is characterized by a relative decrease in the number of polymorphonuclear leukocytes and an absence of eosinophils. Albuminuria is common during the febrile period of the disease. Feces often give a positive reaction for occult blood during the third and fourth weeks of illness.

S. typhosa can be isolated from the blood in about 90 per cent of patients during the first week of disease and in about 50 per cent at the end of the third week; positive blood cultures are infrequent after the fourth week. Typhoid bacilli can be cultured from rose spots, and may persist in the bone marrow after blood cultures are negative. S. typhosa can be isolated from feces at any stage of illness, but the greatest incidence of positive results is obtained during the third to fifth weeks when 85 per cent of the patients have positive cultures. Many reports indicate that typhoid bacilli can be cultured from the urine in about 25 per cent of those with typhoid fever during the third and fourth weeks of illness. Care should be taken in collection of urine to avoid contamination with feces containing typhoid bacilli.

The frequency of positive stool cultures begins to decrease rapidly about six weeks after onset of illness; two or three months after onset only 5 to 10 per cent of patients continue to excrete bacilli. Other patients become negative for typhoid bacilli during subsequent months, but 3 per cent continue to excrete organisms for periods in excess of one year. Persons with documented excretion of bacilli in feces for one or more years are termed *chronic enteric carriers*. Chronic carriers will continue to excrete organisms for many years, usually for life, unless means are taken to terminate the carrier state. Organisms persist in the gallbladder or biliary tract in chronic enteric carriers and enter the intestinal tract in large numbers in bile. The enteric carrier state is more frequent after typhoid fever in adults than in children, and women are much more likely to become carriers than men.

An increase in titer of agglutinins against the somatic (O) antigens and flagellar (H) antigens of *S. typhosa* (Widal reaction) usually occurs during the course of typhoid fever, reaching a peak during the third week of illness. A fourfold or greater increase in titer in the absence of typhoid immunization should be considered highly suggestive of infection. Interpretation of agglutination tests is often difficult because of cross-reactions with other enteric organisms and because agglutinins persist, sometimes in high titer, for many months or years after immunization. In occasional cases there is no increase in agglutinins during the course of typhoid fever. The use of the agglutination reaction as a diagnostic test should always be subordinated to direct cultural demonstration of the causative organism.

Complications. *Intestinal hemorrhage* and *perforation* may occur during the second or third week of illness. Severe hemorrhage occurs in about 2 per cent of patients, although gross blood in feces is present in 10 to 20 per cent of cases, and a positive test for occult blood is even more common. Intestinal perforation, usually in the lower ileum, develops in about 1 per cent of cases and is the most serious of all complications of typhoid fever. The first signs of hemorrhage or perforation may be a sudden drop in temperature and an increase in pulse rate. Often, however, one or more episodes of bleeding will precede a perforation. The perforation is usually associated with acute abdominal pain, tenderness, and rigidity, which are most marked in the right lower quadrant of the abdomen. Signs of peritonitis develop rapidly after perforation, and temperature returns to febrile levels. Thrombophlebitis, particularly of the femoral vein, pneumonia, and cholecystitis occur in a small proportion of patients. Other complications include osteomyelitis, meningitis, and localized infection of almost any organ. Alopecia was a well known sequela of typhoid fever in the pre-antimicrobial era. The incidence of abortion is increased when typhoid fever occurs during pregnancy, especially during the first trimester.

Relapse. One or two weeks after defervescence illness may recur with signs and symptoms similar to those during the initial illness. Relapse occurs in 8 to 10 per cent of patients with typhoid fever who do not receive antimicrobial therapy and in 10 to 20 per cent of patients treated with chloramphenicol. The relapse is usually milder than the initial episode but may be severe, even fatal. Manifestations may last as long as three weeks during a relapse. Second and third relapses have been described.

Diagnosis. The diagnosis of typhoid fever can often be suspected on the basis of the clinical picture. Definitive diagnosis is established by isolation of the organism from blood, feces, urine, or, occasionally, sputum or purulent exudates. A fourfold or greater increase in agglutinin titer, especially against the O antigen of *S. typhosa* and in the absence of recent immunization, provides confirmatory evidence of infection.

Since in the early stages the patient frequently appears ill, is highly febrile, has a leukopenia and no localizing signs, the differential diagnostic possibilities include many diseases. Prominent among these are systemic infections with other salmonellae, disseminated tuberculosis, malaria, brucellosis, shigellosis, murine typhus fever, tularemia, Rocky Mountain spotted fever, acute bronchitis, influenza, and pneumonia caused by viruses or *Mycoplasma pneumoniae*. Certain non-microbial diseases associated with fever and abdominal complaints, such as Hodgkin's disease, may also be confused with typhoid fever. Herpes labialis is rare in typhoid fever, and its presence should lead to a consideration of other diagnoses.

Prognosis. The fatality rate prior to effective antimicrobial therapy varied among different socioeconomic and age groups but was around 10 per cent. Death was usually associated with profound toxemia, intestinal perforation, intestinal hemorrhage, or intercurrent pneumonia. The fatality rate since the introduction of chloramphenicol is 1 or 2 per cent when facilities are available for appropriate supportive care.

Treatment. Chloramphenicol has been employed successfully in the management of typhoid fever since 1948 and is still the antimicrobial agent of choice. It is given orally in doses of approximately 50 mg. per kilogram per day in four divided doses until the temperature is normal; thereafter, the dose may be reduced to 30 mg. per kilogram per day. Chloramphenicol therapy should be continued for a total of two weeks. Response to treatment is not rapid. Patients usually show subjective improvement after one or two days, but the temperature does not return to normal until three to five days after the beginning of therapy. Hemorrhage and perforation may develop during chloramphenicol therapy, even in afebrile patients. Treatment of relapse is the same as for the initial episode. Chloramphenicol therapy does not alter the incidence of chronic carriers after typhoid fever. Chloramphenicol may result in suppression of agglutinin response in patients treated during the early phase of typhoid fever.

Ampicillin is also effective in the treatment of typhoid fever, but the response appears to be slower with ampicillin than with chloramphenicol. If ampicillin is used in the treatment of typhoid fever, it should be administered intramuscularly in a dose for adults of 1 gram every six or eight hours until the patient is afebrile, and should then be continued orally for a total of two weeks of therapy.

Occasional patients with typhoid fever without evidence of suppurative complications show no evidence of clinical response to chloramphenicol or ampicillin after six to eight days of therapy, although blood cultures may become negative. For these patients, and patients with severe toxemia during typhoid, the use of prednisone or drugs with similar activity should be considered. Prednisone should be given in a dose of 60 mg. per day in four divided doses for the first day, 40 mg. during the second day, and 20 mg. on the third day; corticosteroid therapy should be discontinued after the third day. In patients treated with prednisone, temperature returns to normal or occasionally decreases to hypothermic levels within hours, and the toxic state rapidly ameliorates. Prednisone should be administered only in conjunction with appropriate antimicrobial therapy, and under these conditions it does not increase the risk of complications.

Perforation, although previously managed by surgical means, is now usually treated conservatively without surgical intervention. When perforation occurs, chloramphenicol should be continued, and additional antimicrobial drugs should be administered to control multiplication of intestinal flora in the peritoneal space. Transfusion is required for large hemorrhages.

Patients with typhoid fever are unusually sensitive to the antipyretic effect of salicylates and may develop profound hypothermia after small doses. Tepid sponge baths are effective in lowering temperature and should be used instead of salicylates. Laxatives and enemas should not be used because of the danger of inciting intestinal perforation or hemorrhage.

Treatment of Carriers. Cholecystectomy results in termination of the chronic enteric carrier state in about 85 per cent of cases. Ampicillin in a total dose of 6 grams per day given orally in four equal doses for a period of six weeks combined with probenecid will apparently terminate the carrier state in most patients without gallstones and with normal gallbladder function as indicated by cholecystogram. Ampicillin occasionally terminates the carrier state in persons with evidence of gallbladder disease or gallstones, but the proportion of apparent cures is less than 25 per cent. Penicillin G in doses of 12 million units or more daily combined with probenecid for 14 days has also been successful in terminating the carrier state in some persons. Chloramphenicol has not been shown to be effective in the treatment of the chronic carrier state and should not be used in this situation.

Prophylaxis. Typhoid vaccine is effective in reducing the incidence of disease among properly immunized persons. Immunization should be considered for inhabitants of areas where the incidence of the disease is high, for travelers to these areas and for persons working with *S. typhosa*. A course of immunization consists of three subcutaneous injections of 0.5 ml. of vaccine at weekly intervals. Local discomfort and fever frequently follow administration of the vaccine. Vaccine can also be inoculated intracutaneously in doses of 0.1 ml.; the frequency of systemic reactions is less after this method of immunization than after administration of vaccine subcutaneously, but the local pain and tenderness may be severe and as uncomfortable as with the subcutaneous injection. To maintain optimal immunity it is necessary to repeat immunization with a booster injection of vaccine at intervals of one year. The degree of immunity conferred by typhoid vaccine is not strong and can be overcome by exposure to massive numbers of organisms.

Patients with typhoid fever should remain in isolation during hospitalization. Persons known to be carriers should not be permitted to work as food handlers, and members of their households should be immunized against the disease.

Second attacks of typhoid fever have been observed, but, as a general rule, one attack confers lifelong immunity.

Ashcroft, M. T., Ritchie, J. M., and Nicholson, C. C.: Controlled field trial in British Guiana school children of heat-killed-phenolized and acetone-killed lyophilized typhoid vaccines. Amer. J. Hyg., 79:196, 1964.

Dinbar, A., Altman, G., and Tulcinsky, D. B.: The treatment of chronic biliary Salmonella carriers. Amer. J. Med., 47:236, 1969.

Freitag, J. L.: Treatment of chronic typhoid carriers by cholecystectomy. Public Health Rep., 79:567, 1964.

Greisman, S. E., Hornick, R. B., Carozza, F. A., Jr., and Woodward, T. E.: The role of endotoxin during typhoid fever and tularemia in man. I. Acquisition of tolerance to endotoxin. II. Altered cardiovascular responses to catecholamines. III. Hyperreactivity to endotoxin during infection. J. Clin. Invest., 42:1064, 1963, and 43:986, 1774, 1964.

Huckstep, R. L.: Typhoid Fever and Other Salmonella Infections. Edinburgh, E. and S. Livingstone, Ltd., 1962.

Kaye, D., Merselis, J. G., Jr., Connolly, C. S., and Hook, E. W.: Treatment of chronic enteric carriers of Salmonella typhosa with ampicillin. Ann. N. Y. Acad. Sci., 145:429, 1967.

Merselis, J. G., Jr., Kaye, D., Connolly, C. S., and Hook, E. W.: Quantitative bacteriology of the typhoid carrier state. Amer. J. Trop. Med., 13:425, 1964.

Robertson, R. P., Wahab, M. F. A., and Raasch, F. O.: Evaluation of chloramphenicol and ampicillin in salmonella enteric fever. New Eng. J. Med. 278:171, 1968.

Stuart, B. M., and Pullen, R. L.: Typhoid: Clinical analysis of three hundred and sixty cases. Arch. Intern. Med. (Chicago), 78:629, 1946.

Typhoid Panel, U. K. Department of Technical Co-Operation: Controlled field trial of acetone-dried and inactivated and heat-phenol-inactivated typhoid vaccines in British Guiana. Bull. W.H.O., 30:631, 1964.

Woodward, T. E., and Smadel, J. E.: Management of typhoid fever and its complications. Ann. Intern. Med., 60:144, 1964.

SALMONELLA INFECTIONS OTHER THAN TYPHOID FEVER

Definition. Salmonella infection may be asymptomatic or manifested as acute gastroenteritis, bacteremia, or paratyphoid fever. The clinical syndromes resulting from Salmonella infection cannot always be sharply differentiated and sometimes overlap.

Incidence and Prevalence. Salmonellae, with the exception of a few serotypes, are widespread among members of the animal kingdom in all parts of the world. Virtually all domestic and wild animal species have been shown to harbor these organisms, and infection rates range from 1 per cent to more than 40 per cent. For example, in certain studies salmonellae have been isolated from 41 per cent of turkeys, 7 to 50 per cent of swine, and 24 per cent of apparently healthy cattle.

The true incidence of human salmonellosis is unknown, but it is probably much higher than the number of reported cases. Since 1963 the incidence of reported isolations of salmonellae from man in the United States has remained relatively constant at about 20,000 per year.

The incidence of asymptomatic human carriers of salmonellae in the general population has been estimated to be about 0.2 per cent. The carrier state in the vast majority of these people is transient and probably represents persistence of organisms in the stools after asymptomatic or mild intestinal infection. The transient carrier state is more frequent in persons whose occupations provide opportunity for contact with salmonellae in foods, such as professional food processors or abattoir workers, than in the general population.

Epidemiology. Man almost always acquires Salmonella infection by the oral route. Any item of food or drink can be contaminated directly or indirectly with viable bacilli from infected animals or men and can serve as a source of infection. Although the role of human carriers in the spread of salmonellosis must not be minimized, the majority of infections of man in the United States are related to the enormous reservoirs of salmonellae in lower animals.

The greatest single source of human disease is poultry products, including chickens, turkeys, ducks, and eggs. Other animal meats, especially pork, beef, and lamb, also serve as sources of infection. Salmonellae on meats or other foods contaminate utensils, tables, and other items in the processing plant, market, or kitchen, and may be transferred from these items to previously uninfected foods. A significant proportion (1 to 58 per cent) of raw meats purchased in retail markets is contaminated with salmonellae.

Eggs or egg products are very common sources of Salmonella infection. The bacilli may be found on the external surface of the egg shell, between the shell and the shell membranes, or in yolks of eggs from hens with ovarian infection. The incidence of infection of eggs is low, but pooling of large numbers for freezing or drying increases the possibility of contamination of large quantities of materials. Prepared food mixtures containing dried eggs have been implicated many times in outbreaks of Salmonella infection.

Sterilization of contaminated foods is not always achieved by cooking. Viable salmonellae contaminating large birds such as turkeys, especially if the fowl is stuffed, may persist despite the baking process, and organisms in eggs occasionally survive frying, scrambling, or boiling in the shell.

The numerous by-products of the meat-packing industry, such as bone meal, fertilizer, domestic animal food, and fish meal, often contain salmonellae and may serve as sources of infection, especially among lower animals. Finally, in considering potential sources of infection, household pets, including dogs, cats, birds, and turtles, should not be overlooked; all have been shown to harbor salmonellae.

Direct transmission from man to man without food as the intermediate source occurs occasionally. For example, a highly susceptible newborn may acquire infection at birth from an infected mother or in the neonatal period from a nursery attendant. Several nursery and hospital outbreaks have been described in which infection appeared to be perpetuated by air-borne spread of salmonellae.

Pathology. Death from Salmonella gastro enteritis occurs primarily in infants, the aged, and persons with underlying diseases. The intestinal mucosa is red and swollen and often shows petechial hemorrhages. The pathologic findings in paratyphoid fever are qualitatively similar to those of typhoid fever, although the involvement of Peyer's patches is less prominent and ulcerations are much less frequent. Intestinal lesions are usually absent in patients with Salmonella bacteremia, and the findings are similar to those of any acute generalized infection. Blood-borne salmonellae may localize in almost any organ, producing single or multiple suppurative lesions.

Pathogenesis. Multiplication of salmonellae in the intestinal tract may cause inflammation of the intestinal mucosa and symptoms of gastroenteritis. Gastroenteritis is a true infection of the mucosa; ingestion of a large number of dead bacilli will not produce the disease. Salmonellae multiplying in the intestinal tract occasionally gain access to the blood, producing transient bacteremia or localized infections that can serve as sources of persistent bacteremia. The pathogenesis of enteric or paratyphoid fever is similar to that of typhoid fever.

The prevalence of salmonellae in foods for human consumption makes it almost inevitable that man comes in contact with these organisms relatively frequently. The outcome of such exposures depends on the characteristics of the Salmonella species, the number of bacteria ingested, and the status of the host.

Every species of Salmonella has the capacity to produce asymptomatic infection, acute gastroenteritis, bacteremia with or without localized infection, or paratyphoid fever. However, some species are much more likely to produce certain of these clinical syndromes than others. For example, *S. anatum* usually produces inapparent infection or gastroenteritis and only rarely invades the blood. In contrast, *S. choleraesuis* only occasionally produces gastroenteritis or inapparent infec-

tion but is a common cause of bacteremia or metastatic infection. Differences in pathogenicity are observed not only between species, but also between strains of the same species.

Limited information is available on the number of organisms required to produce salmonellosis in man. Experiments in volunteers suggest that a large number (approximately 10^6) of viable salmonellae are usually required to produce gastroenteritis in normal adults. A transient carrier state may follow ingestion of inocula 10 or 100 times smaller than those required to produce disease.

The resistance of the host also plays a major role in determining the wide range of responses from no disease to rapidly fatal illness observed in human salmonellosis. Local factors in the stomach and intestine may be the first lines of defense. It has been established that major gastric surgery, including subtotal gastrectomy, gastroenterostomy, and/or vagotomy, predisposes to Salmonella gastroenteritis. The mechanism of this effect is unknown, but may be related to reduced bactericidal activity of gastric juice or altered intestinal flora. It has been shown in experimental Salmonella infections of mice that the microbial flora of the normal intestine exerts a protective action by suppressing multiplication of salmonellae. In these studies alteration of intestinal flora by antimicrobial drugs increased susceptibility to infection with *S. typhimurium* 100,000 times, and resistance was restored by re-establishing the normal enteric flora. Prior antimicrobial therapy also apparently enhances susceptibility of man to symptomatic intestinal infection with salmonellae.

The incidence of severe Salmonella infections is increased in patients with certain underlying diseases. Another process, such as hepatic cirrhosis, lupus erythematosus, leukemia, lymphoma, or neoplasm, is present in one third to one half of patients with Salmonella bacteremia. These conditions are associated with a general depression of resistance to microbial invasion, and secondary infection is not unexpected. However, in a few diseases—acute bartonellosis, sickle cell anemia, and, perhaps, malaria—there appears to be a predisposition to infection with salmonellae that exceeds any general susceptibility to other bacterial species. The acute hemolytic phase of bartonellosis is complicated by the development of Salmonella bacteremia in as many as 40 per cent of cases. Patients with sickle cell anemia and other sickle hemoglobinopathies are unusually susceptible to invasion of the blood by salmonellae, and there is a strong tendency for localization of infection in bone. In fact, Salmonella species, not staphylococci, account for the vast majority of instances of osteomyelitis in patients with sickle cell anemia. Osteomyelitis is probably related to the localization of organisms in the areas of ischemia and necrosis of bone so common in sickle cell anemia; this is but one example of the striking tendency of salmonellae to localize at sites of pre-existing disease. Localization of salmonellae has been reported in vascular aneurysms, bone compressed by aortic aneurysms, hematomas, areas of infarction, and a variety of cysts and neoplasms.

Clinical Manifestations. *Salmonella Gastroenteritis.* Symptoms of gastroenteritis develop 8 to 48 hours after ingestion of contaminated food. The relatively long incubation period represents the time required for multiplication and invasion by the organism. Nausea and vomiting are common initial manifestations and are rapidly followed by colicky abdominal pain and persistent diarrhea, occasionally with mucus or blood. An initial chill is not unusual, and fever of 38 to 39° C. is common. Symptoms usually subside in two to five days, and recovery is uneventful.

Considerable variation in the severity of Salmonella gastroenteritis is observed, even among patients infected at the same meal. Some patients have a mild afebrile disease with a few loose stools, whereas others have high fever and 30 to 40 liquid stools per day. Severe diarrhea occasionally occurs in an afebrile patient. Abdominal pain may be intense, localized, and associated with rebound tenderness, suggesting appendicitis or some other acute intra-abdominal process. Symptoms of gastroenteritis persist in some patients for as long as two weeks.

The leukocyte count is usually normal, and blood cultures are sterile in almost all cases. The causative organism can be isolated from the feces of almost all patients during the acute illness. About 50 per cent of the patients continue to have stool cultures positive for salmonellae at two weeks after onset of gastroenteritis, but only about 15 per cent remain positive at the end of the fourth week. A small proportion of patients continue to excrete organisms after two months, but in most of these the cultures become negative in the next six months. The period of excretion of organisms in stool tends to be longer in infants than in older children or adults. The term "chronic enteric carrier" should be reserved for the patient shown to have persistently positive stools with the same Salmonella species for one or more years.

Enteric or Paratyphoid Fever. Salmonellae other than *S. typhosa* may produce an illness with all of the features of typhoid fever, including prolonged sustained fever, respiratory and gastrointestinal symptoms, rose spots, leukopenia, and positive blood, stool, and urine cultures. Although paratyphoid fever may be clinically indistinguished from typhoid fever, it is usually milder with a shorter course and a lower mortality rate. The organisms most likely to produce this syndrome are *S. paratyphi A, S. paratyphi B,* and *S. choleraesuis.* Paratyphoid fever is occasionally preceded by manifestations of Salmonella gastroenteritis.

Bacteremia. Salmonellae also produce a clinical syndrome that is characterized by chills, prolonged intermittent fever, anorexia, and weight loss. The characteristic features of typhoid or paratyphoid fever, such as rose spots, sustained fever, and leukopenia, are absent. Patients with this form of illness usually have no gastrointestinal complaints and, indeed, stool cultures are usually negative for the causative organism despite its presence in blood. The leukocyte count is normal in most cases.

A prolonged febrile illness lasting weeks or months and characterized by weight loss, anemia, hepatosplenomegaly, and bacteremia with salmonellae including *S. typhosa* has been described in South America and the Middle East in patients with schistosomiasis.

Localized Disease. Signs of localized infection appear in many cases of Salmonella bacteremia. Abscess formation may occur at almost any site, or bronchopneumonia, empyema, endocarditis, pericarditis, pyelonephritis, osteomyelitis, or arthritis may develop. Meningitis is a focal manifestation more common in newborns and infants than in adults. Patients with localized infections usually have striking polymorphonuclear leukocytosis as high as 20,000 to 30,000 cells per cubic millimeter of blood.

Diagnosis. Salmonella gastroenteritis must be differentiated from other acute diarrheal diseases, especially shigellosis, staphylococcal food poisoning, and enteritis produced by viral agents. Differentiation on the basis of clinical information alone is difficult, especially in sporadic cases, and definitive diagnosis depends on isolation of the causative organism from the stool.

In patients with enteric fever, blood cultures are usually positive early in the course of the disease, and feces and urine become positive somewhat later. In patients with Salmonella bacteremia, the organisms can be isolated from blood, or in some cases from pus or exudate from localized infection.

Patients with salmonellosis may show during the course of illness a fourfold or greater increase in titer of agglutinins against the causative organism or closely related species. However, agglutination tests performed in the ordinary clinical laboratory are usually not helpful in diagnosis because only a limited number of Salmonella antigens are used.

Treatment. The most important aspect of the management of patients with Salmonella gastroenteritis is prompt correction of dehydration and electrolyte disturbances. Paregoric or small doses of morphine may be used to relieve abdominal cramps and diarrhea if contraindications do not exist. There is no convincing evidence that antimicrobial drugs, including chloramphenicol, reduce the duration of illness or the period of excretion of organisms in the stool. In fact, recent studies indicate that the period of excretion of salmonellae in the stool during convalescence after symptomatic intestinal infection is actually longer in patients who have been treated with antimicrobial drugs during the acute illness than in patients who have received no antimicrobial therapy.

In Salmonella bacteremia, paratyphoid fever or localized infections of bones, joints, meninges, and other sites, chloramphenicol is the drug of choice and should be administered in divided doses of about 50 mg. per kilogram per day for at least two weeks. Four to six days may be required for defervescence in favorable cases and even longer in patients with localized infection. In patients with localized infections, it may be necessary to continue antimicrobial therapy for four to six weeks, and surgical drainage of collections of pus may be required. Salmonellae persisting in tissues during chloramphenicol therapy may be responsible for relapse after the antimicrobial is discontinued. Relapse is not related to the emergence of chloramphenicol-resistant strains during therapy, and clinical response to a second or third course of therapy usually differs in no way from the first.

Ampicillin has also been shown to be effective in treating paratyphoid fever, but the response to ampicillin is slower than the response to chloramphenicol. Ampicillin is also often effective in the treatment of other systemic Salmonella infections if the causative organism is susceptible to this drug. Ampicillin is preferred over chloramphenicol for patients requiring prolonged therapy. Approximately 10 to 20 per cent of the *S. typhimurium* strains isolated in the United States and a somewhat higher proportion in England are resistant to ampicillin. Ampicillin resistance is mediated by transferable resistance determinants or R factors, and is uncommon among serologic types other than *S. typhimurium*. Very few strains of Salmonella are resistant to chloramphenicol in vitro.

Excretion of salmonellae in stool after clinical or subclinical infection ceases spontaneously in almost all patients; the convalescent carrier state is not an indication for antimicrobial therapy. Chronic enteric carriers of salmonellae other than *S. typhosa* are managed as are typhoid carriers.

Prognosis. The case fatality rate in Salmonella gastroenteritis rarely exceeds 1 or 2 per cent, and probably averages about 0.3 per cent. Fatalities occur almost entirely in infants, the aged, and persons with major underlying disease. The case fatality rate in the more serious systemic infections is high; it approaches 20 per cent in *S. choleraesuis* bacteremia.

Prevention. Every effort should be made to prevent the spread of salmonellae among the population by the excreta of clinical cases and convalescent or chronic carriers. Patients with acute illness should be isolated, and convalescent or chronic carriers should not be employed as food handlers and should practice strict personal hygiene.

The control of salmonellosis among animals and prevention of spread of infection to man present many problems. Progress is being made in developing methods of detection and control of salmonellosis in domestic animals and in improving hygienic conditions in food-processing and food-dispensing establishments.

An Evaluation of the Salmonella Problem. Prepared by the Committee on Salmonella, Division of Biology and Agriculture, National Research Council. National Academy of Sciences Publication No. 1683. Washington, D.C., Printing and Publishing Office, National Academy of Sciences, 1969.

Aserkoff, B., and Bennett, J. V.: Effect of therapy in acute salmonellosis on salmonellae in feces. New Eng. J. Med., 281: 636, 1969.
Bennett, I. L., Jr., and Hook, E. W.: Infectious diseases (some aspects of salmonellosis). Ann. Rev. Med., 10:1, 1959.
Black, P. H., Kunz, L. J., and Swartz, M. N.: Salmonellosis — A review of some unusual aspects. New Eng. J. Med., 262:811, 864, 921, 1960.
Gezon, H. M.: Salmonellosis. D. M., July, 1959.
Proceedings of the National Conference on Salmonellosis, March 11-13, 1964. Public Health Service Publication No. 1262, Washington, D.C., U.S. Government Printing Office, 1965.
Van Oye, E. (ed.): The World Problem of Salmonellosis. The Hague, Dr. W. Junk Publishers, 1964.
Wahab, M. F. A., Robertson, R. P., and Raasch, F. O.: Paratyphoid A fever. Ann. Intern. Med., 70:913, 1969.

ENTERIC BACTERIAL INFECTIONS (INCLUDING URINARY TRACT INFECTONS)

Calvin M. Kunin

Definition. The wide variety of micro-organisms commonly found in the gastrointestinal tract, particularly the gram-negative, nonsporulating bacilli, have become increasingly important in clinical medicine. They are the principal organisms found in infections of the abdominal viscera, peritoneum, and urinary tract, as well as being frequent secondary invaders of the respiratory tract, burned or traumatized skin, and sites of decreased host resistance and instrumentation. Currently, they are the most frequent cause of life-threatening bacteremia. Infections with these organisms will be considered together because of their common habitat in the gut and on mucous surfaces, the similarity of epidemiologic and pathogenic characteristics, and the common approach used in diagnosis, treatment, and prevention.

Bacteriology. The gastrointestinal flora is exceedingly complex. The large intestine contains about 10^{10} to 10^{11} organisms per gram of contents. Of these, 90 to 95 per cent are obligate anaerobes. Most common are the gram-negative bacilli, Bacteroides, and Fusobacterium, gram-positive bacilli including Bifidobacterium, Eubacterium, Corynebacterium species, and a wide variety of anaerobic streptococci. Other anaerobes include the gram-positive spore-forming rods of the Clostridia species and gram-negative cocci, Veillonella. Lactobacilli and enterococci are also present. The well-known aerobic gram-negative rods, which are members of the family Enterobacteriaceae account for only 5 to 10 per cent of the total flora. These include the most common, *E. coli*, as well as the Klebsiella-Enterobacter group, Proteus, Providencia, Edwardsiella, Serratia, and, under pathologic conditions, Salmonella and Shigella. Pseudomonas is an entirely unrelated species, and is usually found in only small numbers in the bowel. Various yeasts and related forms are also found in lesser numbers in the normal large intestine.

Although the human gastrointestinal tract is usually considered to be colonized in the anatomic regions proximal to the cardia of the stomach and distal to the ileocecal valve, recent studies have demonstrated organisms in the jejunum and almost always in the ileum. Moderate changes in the diet do not affect the ratio of predominant bacteria in the feces, but antimicrobial therapy has a strong selective effect and is the single most important reason for the increasing emergence in human infection of these heretofore unusual organisms.

All the micro-organisms of the gastrointestinal tract are potentially pathogenic under conditions of altered host resistance. The major diagnostic problem is to differentiate superficial colonization from actual tissue invasion.

Endotoxins. The gram-negative bacteria of the gastrointestinal tract produce disease by invasion of tissue and by release of a pharmacologically active lipopolysaccharide from the cell wall, known as endotoxin. Endotoxins from a wide variety of unrelated species behave quite similarly, regardless of the inherent pathogenicity of the micro-organism from which they are derived or their antigenic structure.

In the intact micro-organism they exist as complexes of lipid, polysaccharide, and protein. The biologic activity seems to be a property of the lipid and carbohydrate portions. When inoculated intravenously, the endotoxins cause fever, leukopenia, circulatory collapse, capillary hemorrhages, necrosis of tumors, and the Shwartzman phenomenon. Noteworthy is the remarkable tolerance that develops after repeated injections of endotoxin. For example, the first intravenous injection in man of as little as 0.01 ml. of typhoid vaccine will give rise to a violent response, with chill and high fever; yet after 10 to 14 daily injections of increasing quantities, the subject can accept 25 ml. or more without symptoms and with only a slight rise in temperature. This state of tolerance is not obviously dependent on specific antibodies; it extends to endotoxins of unrelated bacterial strains. The clinical features of gram-negative bacteremia (*vide infra*) resemble the reaction of laboratory animals or man to intravenous injection of purified endotoxic preparations, and may well represent a direct "pharmacologic" response to bacterial endotoxin. In other types of infectious process there is reason to doubt that such phenomena as fever, leukocytosis, and leukopenia are direct effects of endotoxin liberation.

The phenomenon of endotoxin tolerance may explain the remarkable tendency of the symptoms of pyelonephritis to subside spontaneously. By contrast, endotoxin tolerance is not a feature of experimental typhoid fever, but, rather, volunteers infected with this organism have been shown to be hypersensitive to its effects. Endotoxin toler-

ance is currently under intensive study because of the presumed important pathologic effect of this substance. Tolerance may be due to enhanced removal by the reticuloendothelial system, enzymatic degradation, cellular desensitization, a common immunologic factor, or combinations of these.

Antibodies. Antibodies reacting with most Enterobacteriaceae can be demonstrated in sera of normal animals and man, probably because of the continual production of antigen in the gastrointestinal tract. Antibodies to the O or somatic antigens of *E. coli* have been most extensively studied. Very low titers are present in human newborns, presumably because they are mostly of the high molecular weight IgM variety, and do not readily pass the placenta. Human colostrum is rich in O antibody, but this is not absorbed during breast feeding. Colonization of the digestive tract, however, is soon accompanied by appearance of a wide variety of antibodies in serum, which contains virtually all the *E. coli* O antibodies by one year of age. A serologic response to the specific O antigen of the invading strain of *E. coli* can be demonstrated in acute pyelonephritis. It is likely that the great susceptibility of the newborn to overwhelming gram-negative bacterial sepsis is related to lack of maternal antibodies.

As a rule, most strains are susceptible to opsonization and lysis by the combined effects of antibody and complement. Some strains, however, seem insusceptible to lysis in vitro. Nonetheless, this system may be of great importance in preventing strains from invading and persisting in the blood.

URINARY TRACT INFECTION

The phrase urinary tract infection is a broad term used to describe both bacterial colonization of the urine and invasion of structures in any part of the urinary tract. Colonization of the urine, that is, multiplication of large numbers of bacteria in the urine, is often difficult to distinguish from actual tissue invasion eliciting a host response, because of the frequent tendency of urinary tract infections to exhibit either few or no symptoms. This phenomenon is known as *asymptomatic bacteriuria*. At any given point in time, an individual may have bacteriuria alone, or bacteriuria with silent tissue invasion, or bacteriuria accompanied by signs of inflammation of the bladder (cystitis) or kidneys (pyelonephritis). Infections of the structures of the urinary tract are usually accompanied by colonization of the urine which bathes the kidney, ureter, bladder, and urethra. Thus, bacteriuria is the most common denominator of urinary tract infections. Bacteriuria may be absent, however, when the infected focus is not contiguous with the urine as in early lesions of hematogenous pyelonephritis, when there is marked obstruction of the affected portion of the tract or when it is masked by antimicrobial therapy. Bacteriuria does not necessarily indicate that the patient has pyelonephritis or cystitis. Rather, it is an important and generally reliable laboratory finding that indicates an abnormal situation, reflecting either the presence of, or potential for, infection of the urinary tract. It is an excellent guide to early diagnosis and evaluation of therapy, because signs and symptoms of infection may be absent or disappear without bacteriologic cure.

The normal urinary tract is free of bacteria except near the external urethral meatus. In both sexes, some organisms are normally present in the distal urethra. These are usually similar to the flora of the skin, and frequently consist of staphylococci and diphtheroids. Urine is a variable culture medium, depending upon pH, tonicity, and its constituents. High concentrations of urea, low pH, hyperosmolality, and products of dietary organic acids are generally unfavorable to bacteria. In addition, the dynamics of urine flow, or washout, and antibacterial properties of the lining membrane of the urinary tract appear to be important defense mechanisms.

The large bowel is considered to be the reservoir of most of the bacteria that invade the urinary tract because of the high frequency of aerobic coliforms found in urinary tract infection. Several possible pathways from the lumen of the intestine to the urinary passages and kidney can be postulated. There has been some dispute regarding their relative importance. The principal possibilities are the hematogenous, the lymphatic, and the "ascending" routes. The "ascending" pathway, involving migration of bacteria from the anus to the periurethral zone and through the urethra to the bladder, is the most favored at the present time. This route can be demonstrated experimentally, particularly in the presence of obstruction or of a foreign body. It also fits in well with the very much higher rate of urinary infections in the female, whose urethra is shorter than that of the male, and with the marked frequency of urinary infections associated with instrumentation of the urethra and bladder. Clear instances of the hematogenous origin of urinary infection have been demonstrated, particularly in the presence of staphylococcal or gram-negative bacteremia, but these are relatively less common.

Clinical Manifestations. The manifestations of pyelonephritis are discussed elsewhere (see Pyelonephritis). Symptoms of cystitis and urethritis include frequency of urination, burning pain on urination, and passage of cloudy, occasionally blood-tinged urine. The patient may complain of a foul odor to the urine, lassitude, and suprapubic discomfort. Fever and leukocytosis are rarely evident in urinary tract infection confined to the bladder and urethra; as a general rule, their presence should be looked upon as evidence of infection of the upper part of the tract. Nevertheless, absence of fever and leukocytosis does not by any means exclude the possibility of kidney involvement.

Course. The symptoms of inflammation of the lower urinary tract tend to disappear after several days even without bacteriologic cure. Recurrence of symptomatic infection is frequent in this group. Bacteriuria also tends to be highly recurrent. In the unobstructed patient, this is usually associated with reinfection with a new bacterial strain. Early recurrence, however, is frequently due to emergence of bacteria from a partially suppressed focus. Persistent infection with the same organisms should alert the physician to the presence of obstruction, calculus, or neurogenic lesions. Frequent follow-up examination of the patient's urine is essential to the management to be described below.

Concept of Significant Bacteriuria. Bacteriuria literally means the presence of bacteria in the urine. The concept of "significant bacteriuria" was introduced to distinguish between bacteria that are actually multiplying in the urine from contaminants in collection vessels, periurethral tissues, the urethra itself, and gross focal or vaginal contamination. This separation can be accomplished by knowledge of the site and manner in which the urine is collected from the patient and enumeration of the number of organisms present in the sample. The criterion of 100,000 or more organisms per milliliter of urine for diagnosis of significant bacteriuria is an excellent *operational definition* when the clean voided method is used to collect specimens. It is based on the finding that contaminants will usually be present at numbers ranging from 1000 to 10,000 per milliliter. Organisms found in urinary tract infections grow well in urine; they usually achieve concentrations of greater than 100,000, and are often in the range of 1 to 10 million per milliliter. With proper instruction and cleansing, and prompt processing or refrigeration of specimens, it is usually not difficult to obtain reliable results by the clean voided method in both males and females. It is emphasized that, because the reliability of the method will differ with experience and care, it is often wise to avoid overdiagnosis by obtaining multiple specimens, particularly in the asymptomatic patient. Thus, survey and screening procedures for bacteriuria generally require two or three consecutive positive specimens, indicating that the patient has "persistent significant bacteriuria." Bacterial counts lower than 100,000 per milliliter may occur in patients with true bacteriuria, but when the clean voided method is used, these counts can only be established as valid when shown to be persistent and when the same species of bacteria and preferably the same serotype can be repeatedly isolated. Bacterial counts are higher when urine is allowed to incubate for some time in the bladder. A first morning specimen is preferred, but is not essential. Low or borderline counts may be due to dilution in a well-hydrated patient.

Aseptic methods of collection of urine such as from the renal pelvis or ureter, or by bladder puncture, *permit the diagnosis of significant bac-*

teriuria regardless of the number of organisms found, providing that the specimen is not contaminated prior to culture.

Bacteriologic Findings. The species of bacteria most likely to be recovered in individuals with bacteriuria depends, for the most part, upon previous history of infection, receipt of antimicrobial therapy, hospitalization, and instrumentation of the urinary tract. In this respect, the bacterial flora found in individuals with asymptomatic bacteriuria is no different from that in cases of clinically obvious pyelonephritis. Enterobacteriaceae are by far the most common organisms identified. *E. coli* generally accounts for more than 80 per cent of all species recovered in so-called uncomplicated cases, whereas Proteus, Klebsiella, Enterobacter, *Pseudomonas aeruginosa,* enterococci, and *Staphylococcus aureus* are more likely to be found in patients who have had previous infection or instrumentation (the so-called complicated group). Occasionally, organisms such as *Serratia marcescens,* Mima-Herellea, *Candida albicans,* and even *Cryptococcus neoformans* may be significant and produce disease in diabetics and in patients treated with corticosteroids and immunosuppressive agents. Diphtheroids, *Staphylococcus epidermidis,* and microaerophilic streptococci are highly suspect as contaminants. They usually will not be isolated on repeated culture. They should not, however, be dismissed if repeatedly recovered under optimal conditions of collection.

Despite the abundance of anaerobic flora in the gut, they are actually rare in urinary infections, presumably owing to the poor growth of these organisms in urine.

Microscopic Methods. Rapid diagnostic methods are available by either preparation of a Gram stain of unsedimented urine and examination with an oil immersion lens, or by study of the centrifuged urinary sediment for bacteria, employing the high dry objective under reduced light with or without the addition of methylene blue. The Gram stain has been the most widely used of these methods and correlates about 80 to 90 per cent with quantitative culture. Examination of the unstained sediment as prepared for search for formed elements in the urine is very helpful. It is much less time consuming than preparation of a stained slide, and can be done in conjunction with the routine examination for formed elements. This method lends itself particularly well in office practice to assessing the presence of a urinary tract infection. The criterion for a positive sediment is the presence of many (preferably more than 20) obvious bacteria. The presence of marked pyuria can mask bacteria in the sediment. Fresh urine is required, because crystals will also obscure the bacteria. If crystals do form, the urine should be warmed until they dissolve.

Ten or more leukocytes per high-powered field in the centrifuged specimen is usually accepted as representing pyuria. When inflammation of the bladder mucosa is intense, there may be some erythrocytes in the urine, and gross hematuria sometimes occurs. *Proteinuria* is not common in urinary infections.

Epidemiology and Natural History. Extensive epidemiologic studies have provided information of the frequency of bacteriuria in various populations. Bacteriuria in the newborn period has been difficult to define because of problems inherent in collection, but information is being obtained with the widespread use of the bladder puncture method. Infection of the urinary tract in this age group appears to be part of a generalized, life-threatening gram-negative sepsis, and is more common in boys than girls. Symptomatic urinary infections, particularly among girls, are prominent in the preschool years, and are frequently associated with important obstructive or neurogenic lesions. Urologic investigation is extremely valuable in this age group. *It is mandatory in males of any age because of the high frequency of important structural abnormalities* found (valves, malformations, obstructive and neurogenic lesions). The prevalence of bacteriuria among schoolgirls is 1.2 per cent; it is only 0.03 per cent in boys of the same age. The incidence rate in girls is 0.3 per cent per year; it is linear with time throughout the school years and is unaffected by menarche. The cumulative frequency or urinary infection in girls occurring at one time or another during the school years exceeds 5 per cent. Bacteriuria in schoolgirls is independent of socioeconomic status and race, and is not increased in diabetic girls. The prevalence of bacteriuria rises with age, and is increased in lower socioeconomic groups, probably because of limited antimicrobial therapy delivered to this population. Urinary infection is common after marriage. The "honeymoon cystitis" syndrome may be due to either infection or local irritation, and these should be clearly differentiated by culture. Bacteriuria in pregnancy varies from 2 to 6 per cent, depending upon age, parity, and socioeconomic groups. Early detection and treatment of bacteriuria in this age group will prevent the emergence of symptomatic infection. Elderly women may have frequencies of bacteriuria as high as 10 per cent; this rate may rise even higher in hospitalized patients, particularly diabetics. Bacteriuria in the male begins to appear in the "prostate" years, and is often initiated by instrumentation.

Role of Instrumentation. Persistent bacteriuria follows single catheterizations at a frequency of 1 to 2 per cent and with open indwelling catheter drainage exceeds 90 per cent within three to four days. This may lead to life-threatening pyelonephritis and gram-negative sepsis. Fortunately, it is partially avoidable by (1) careful preselection of criteria for catheterization, and (2) use of aseptic closed drainage or antimicrobial bladder rinse during prolonged catheterization. The catheter should be removed as soon as it is no longer needed.

THE ROLE OF ENTERIC BACTERIA IN PYOGENIC INFECTIONS OF THE ABDOMINAL CAVITY

The mixed flora of the intestinal tract participate in infections that originate from lesions of the bowel, such as appendicitis, cholangitis, diverticulitis, and perforation (from ulcerative colitis, ileitis, or carcinoma). These may lead to subdiaphragmatic, hepatic, and pelvic abscesses, which are frequent causes of fever of unknown origin in the patient recovering from abdominal surgery or trauma to this region. Because enteric bacteria grow luxuriantly in both aerobic and anaerobic media and therefore are likely to predominate in cultures, their relative importance tends to be exaggerated. There is good reason to believe that anaerobic bacteria Bacteroides, Clostridia and anaerobic streptococci — play more important roles in this kind of process. It should be pointed out here that a "fecal" odor of pus, though often ascribed to coliforms is doubtless caused by associated anaerobic bacteria. Anaerobic bacteria are usually present as mixtures of two or more species. They should be suspected when there is foul pus and when organisms can be visualized microscopically but fail to grow under routine conditions.

OTHER INFECTIONS CAUSED BY THE ENTERIC BACTERIA

Gastroenteritis. A significant proportion of cases of gastroenteritis occurring in the neonatal period of life appear to be caused by enteric bacteria. About ten serologic strains of *E. coli* have been identified with this capability; they are spoken of as enteropathogenic strains. Certain strains of Proteus and Pseudomonas have at times also been held responsible for similar illness.

Meningitis and Brain Abscess. During the first four weeks of life, purulent meningitis is frequently caused by members of the enteric group of bacteria. Such cases occur sporadically in nurseries, and may be associated with infection of any other tissue of the body. Infants with meningoceles are especially liable to enteric bacterial meningitis. In adults, such infections are rare, but may occasionally be seen as complications of gram-negative bacteremia or in association with other diseases affecting host resistance, e.g., diabetes mellitus or lymphoma (see Meningitis Caused by Bacteria Other Than Meningococci). Nontraumatic brain abscess is frequently due to infection by multiple species of anaerobic organisms similar to those found in the gastrointestinal tract. The sites of origin include chronically infected ears, sinuses, lung, abdomen, and pelvis.

Bacteremia in Hepatic Cirrhosis. Occasionally persons with cirrhosis of the liver develop an acute febrile illness and are found to have bacteremia caused by one of the enteric organisms, usually *E. coli*. Occasionally these patients have signs of peritonitis, but in most of them the event comes "out of the blue" without evidence of localized sepsis anywhere. The illness is short and self-limited or responds to appropriate chemotherapy. Speculation as to its pathogenesis has included the possibility of shunting bacteria away from the filtering action of the liver, impairment of humoral or cellular defense mechanisms, or complement inactivation owing to high blood ammonia. In actuality a satisfactory explanation is lacking at present.

Surface Infection. Enteric bacteria, particularly Proteus and Pseudomonas, are commonly recovered from the surfaces of burns, varicose ulcers, decubitus ulcers, tracheostomy sites, and the like. Generally, these organisms appear to play no pathogenic role, and satisfactory healing may proceed regardless of their presence. They can at times result in fulminant gram-negative sepsis, particularly in the patient with severe burns. The exudate from the sinus of a chronic osteomyelitis or chronic otitis media often contains Proteus as the dominant organism. Otitis of the external auditory canal owing to Pseudomonas may give troublesome local symptoms, especially in swimmers.

Perirectal Abscess. This is an important complication in patients with marked granulocytopenia. Rectal examination should be carefully performed in such patients, particularly when they develop fever and perianal pain.

Abscesses at Sites of Subcutaneous Injections. Rarely, enteric bacilli cause abscesses in subcutaneous tissue at sites of hypodermic injections, notably in diabetic subjects who inject their own insulin. These are sometimes characterized by gas formation, and they thus arouse fear of more serious clostridial infection, whereas, in fact, they are usually of minor clinical importance.

Metastatic Infections. Despite the frequency with which enteric bacteria succeed in invading the blood, metastatic localization of infection is rare. There are, however, occasional instances of such suppurative lesions as arthritis and panophthalmitis in patients with bacteremia originating in acute pyelonephritis. Of special interest in this regard is osteomyelitis of the spine. This is usually seen in men with prostatic disease, chronic cystitis, and posterior urethritis. Possibly the method of spread here is by way of septic emboli to the spine through the vertebral venous plexus.

Superinfection. Enteric bacteria frequently predominate in the bronchial secretions of patients under treatment with large doses of penicillin or broad-spectrum antimicrobial agents. In most instances, this is not of significance and simply represents emergence of unaffected bacterial strains following the suppression of the primary pathogens. It is not an indication for cessation or change in antimicrobial therapy unless there is clinical evidence of tissue invasion by the newly emergent organism. Primary gram-negative bacterial pneumonia often superimposed on viral influenza, however, does occur and may be exceedingly difficult to manage.

GRAM-NEGATIVE BACTEREMIA

Bacteremia caused by gram-negative bacilli has become a problem of greater relative importance since the advent of penicillin and better control of gram-positive coccal infections. Urinary tract infection accounts for about two thirds of all cases of blood invasion by the enteric bacteria. Other causes include surgical disease of the gastrointestinal tract, infections developing at the site of "cut-downs" and "intracaths" for intravenous therapy, postpartum or postabortal sepsis (including the so-called "placental bacteremia"), and infection of wounds, ulcers, burns, and internal prosthetic devices such as heart valves. Sometimes there is a clearly apparent precipitating factor such as cystoscopy, surgical or obstetrical procedure, or manipulation of an infected wound.

These bacteremias have clinical characteristics closely resembling the recognized biologic effects of gram-negative bacterial endotoxins. Onset of symptoms may occur with a shaking chill and rise in temperature of 101 to 105° F. There is an initial leukopenia, but after 6 to 12 hours usually there is leukocytosis. An *important and highly significant accompaniment is circulatory embarrassment with lowering of the blood pressure.* This may be manifested only by some alteration in the patient's state of consciousness, and the skin may continue to feel warm, although sometimes the skin is cold and clammy. Occasionally patients slip into a shocklike state without much elevation of temperature; hence infection of this kind must always be taken into consideration in evaluation of peripheral circulatory failure. Petechial hemorrhages and purpura are not common. There are diminution in urine output, increase in proteinuria, and often a rise in nonprotein nitrogen of the blood. Some patients show shifts in acid-base balance in the direction of metabolic acidosis, whereas others have hyperventilation and respiratory alkalosis. Much depends on the nature of the underlying disease and the renal reserve. The outlook is grave, being influenced by age, associated disease, and evidence of shock. When obvious signs of circulatory collapse are present, the fatality rate may be as high as 75 per cent.

UNIQUE FEATURES OF PSEUDOMONAS INFECTIONS

Pseudomonas infections, although often similar to those caused by other gram-negative bacteria, sometimes have unique characteristics. As already mentioned, this organism frequently appears in necrotic tissue, as in ulcers, burns, or draining sinuses. Usually such colonization is of little clinical significance, and mere removal of necrotic tissue may cause it to disappear. Nevertheless, under certain circumstances, especially in chronically debilitated persons or in patients with agranulocytosis or acute leukemia, severe sepsis may be produced by this class of bacteria.

Pseudomonas is notoriously resistant to antimicrobial therapy; hence it tends to emerge as the dominant micro-organism following eradication of other bacteria by drugs, and it may then be responsible for the phenomenon of superinfection, as in the bronchopulmonary infections that may complicate prophylactic chemotherapy of chronic lung disease.

Because Pseudomonas commonly occurs in tap water, and because it may be resistant to antiseptics used in sterilizing instruments, it is likely to be carried into the body by such procedures as cystoscopy. Furthermore, most of the reported instances of meningitis following lumbar puncture have been associated with this organism.

Tissue invasion is characterized by necrotizing vasculitis with bacterial invasion of the walls of arteries and veins. This leads to a distinctive necrotic skin lesion (called ecthyma gangrenosa) that is found most commonly along the axillary folds or in the anogenital area, but may also develop on any part of the body. It may begin as a vesicle that later becomes necrotic. The typical lesion of ecthyma gangrenosa is a round, indurated ulcer with a black center that varies from a few millimeters to several centimeters in diameter.

TREATMENT OF ENTERIC BACTERIAL INFECTIONS

General Principles. The major clinical problems in management of enteric bacterial infections are (1) differentiation of superficial contamination that often requires no treatment from true or potential tissue invasion, (2) early recognition and drainage of abscesses, (3) anticipation of the role of anaerobic bacteria that cannot be readily cultured, and (4) early recognition of bacteremic shock. *Many of these infections are preventable,* particularly those arising from instrumentation of the urinary tract, intravenous catheters and contaminated fluids, suction, and ventilation equipment. *Every physician must consider elimination of such sources of contamination as one of his prime responsibilities.*

Gram-Negative Bacteremia. The presence of gram-negative organisms in the blood should alert the physician to search for a site of origin such as intravenous or urinary catheters and abdominal or perirectal abscesses. Removal of devices and drainage of abscesses should be done as soon as possible. Antimicrobial therapy should be guided as often as possible by in vitro drug-susceptibility tests because of the remarkable ability of enteric bacteria to develop resistant strains. Among the aminoglycoside antimicrobials, gentamicin and kanamycin are most reliable, followed by streptomycin. The so-called broad-spectrum drugs such as tetracycline and chloramphenicol are also useful against the Enterobacteriaceae. Large doses of penicillin G are effective against many of the gram-positive and some gram-negative anaerobes. Tetracycline and chloramphenicol are useful for Bacteroides, whereas Pseudomonas will generally respond only to drugs such as polymyxin B or colistin methane sulfonate (polymyxin E) and gentamicin. Carbenicillin is a new semisynthetic penicillin that may be of considerable value in treatment of Pseudomonas, Enterobacter and Proteus infections. The problems are the large doses required, development of resistance, tendency for sodium overload, and high cost. It should be reserved for clearly established infection caused by a susceptible organism. It is generally advisable to use two and sometimes more agents in severe gram-negative sepsis, particularly when bacteriologic identification is delayed. In general, this treatment would include an aminoglycoside drug, a broad-spectrum drug, and penicillin G. Ampicillin and cephalothin (or cephaloridine) are considered to have generally similar properties to penicillin G, and usually would not be used simultaneously. At times, they offer special advantages over penicillin, because both ampicillin and the cephalosporins are active against many gram-negative bacteria as well as gram-positive cocci. The cephalosporins are generally more active against Klebsiella than is ampicillin, but ampicillin is much more effective against enterococci. The cephalosporins are also useful in patients allergic to penicillin. The inherent toxicity of the polymyxins should restrict their use mainly to treatment of Pseudomonas. Satisfactory results have been achieved by combinations of large doses of penicillin-like drugs with tetracycline in mixed anaerobic infections such as peritonitis or brain abscess, but many other combinations appear to be good.

Management of bacteremic shock is complex, requiring corrective measures designed to improve cardiac function, tissue perfusion, and electrolyte imbalance, particularly acidosis. This requires monitoring of the central venous pressure by a well-placed catheter in the superior vena cava or right atrium in an attempt to achieve a pressure of about 8 to 12 cm. of water, and following the dynamics of pressure changes as fluid replacement is given. Replacement fluids include blood, dextran, and saline solutions. Drugs such as isoproterenol may be used to increase cardiac output and improve tissue perfusion; vasopressors such as metaraminol should be used sparingly except in severe shock. High doses of corticosteroids are widely used, but their efficacy has not been established by controlled studies.

Urinary Tract Infection. The therapeutic principles are similar for all urinary infections, including bacteriuria, cystitis, or pyelonephritis. *Recognition and relief of obstruction are essential.* Therapy is then directed to sterilization of the urine and careful follow-up to detect recurrence, using significant bacteriuria as a guide. Infections uncomplicated by obstruction or many previous episodes will generally respond to oral therapy with sulfonamides, tetracycline, ampicillin, chloramphenicol, nalidixic acid, or nitrofurantoin. The last-named drug is particularly useful in recurrent infections because of relatively less frequency of emergence of resistant strains. Drugs are selected on the basis of relative cost, side effects, and antimicrobial sensitivity, all of which may be highly variable. Bacteria should disappear within 24 to 48 hours even if pyuria and symptoms continue. It is important to recognize bacteriologic failure early and change to another drug. Generally, short courses of treatment, from 10 to 14 days, are quite adequate; short-term high-dose therapy, sometimes with the parenteral agents described above, may be required in some instances of failure with lower doses. Recurrence within a few weeks after treatment is usually due to persistance of the same focus, whereas later recurrence, particularly in females, is more often the result of reinfection. Highly recurrent infections may be managed by either very close follow-up and treatment of each episode or by prophylaxis with nitrofurantoin or urinary antiseptics such as methenamine mandelate or hippuric acid. *These agents require an acid urine,* preferably at pH 5.5. This may be achieved by addition of a high protein diet, ammonium chloride, or methionine. Methionine is a particularly effective acidifier, but it may have to be given in doses as high as 10 grams per day. The dose can be titrated downward by measuring urinary pH. Prophylaxis should not be given for more than three to six months if at all possible, and should be abandoned if bacteriuria persists or recurs.

Complex urinary infections, that is, those in the presence of obstructive uropathy, neurogenic bladders, or catheters, are exceedingly difficult to eradicate and may be managed by suppressive therapy with urinary antiseptics *if shown effective,* or simply left alone unless systemic complications develop. Sepsis in these cases is usually due to obstruction and should be promptly relieved. *Bacteriuria in the aged* is frequent, usually uncomplicated, and highly recurrent. It should not be overzealously treated if simple measures fail, because toxicity and expense of therapy may outweigh the risk of disease.

Curtin, J., Petersdorf, R. G., and Bennett, I. L., Jr.: Pseudomonas bacteremia: Report of ninety-one cases. Ann. Intern. Med., 54:1077, 1961.

Kass, E. H.: Chemotherapeutic and antibiotic drugs in the management of infections of the urinary tract. Amer. J. Med., 18:764, 1955.

Kunin, C. M., Deutscher, R., and Paquin, A. J., Jr.: Urinary tract infection in school children: An epidemiologic, clinical and laboratory study. Medicine, 43:2, 1964.

Maiztegui, J. I., Biegeleisen, J. Z., Jr., Cherry, W. B., and Kass, E. H.: Bacteremia due to gram-negative rods: A clinical, bacteriologic, serologic and immunofluorescent study. New Eng. J. Med., 272:222, 1965.

Moore, W. E. C., Cato, E. P., and Holdeman, L. V.: Anaerobic bacteria of the gastrointestinal flora and their occurrence in clinical infections. J. Infect. Dis., 119:641, 1969.

Steinhauer, B. W., Eickhoff, T. C., Kislak, J. W., and Finland, M.: The Klebsiella-Enterobacter-Serratia division. Clinical and epidemiologic characteristics. Ann. Intern. Med., 65:1180, 1966.

Tisdale, W. A.: Spontaneous colon bacillus bacteremia in Laennec's cirrhosis. Gastroenterology, 40:141, 1961.

Weinstein, L., and Klainer, A.S.: Management of emergencies: IV. Septic shock—Pathogenesis and treatment. New Eng. J. Med., 274:950, 1966.

SHIGELLOSIS

Leighton E. Cluff

Definition. Shigellosis is an enteric infection with one of the species of Shigella bacilli, which may be asymptomatic or may cause dysentery.

Bacillary dysentery is usually a self-limited, acute illness characterized by diarrhea with mucous-bloody feces, tenesmus, fever, and abdominal colic and tenderness. Symptomless infected persons and those convalescing from dysentery may harbor Shigella in the stool for several days, serving as a source of infection for others. The infection is worldwide and is most common among persons living in crowded unhygienic circumstances. Man is the principal host to the microorganism, and the infection is usually transmitted from person to person, directly or indirectly.

History. Dysentery has been recognized for centuries. Delineation of dysentery attributable to Shigella, however, was not possible until 1896, when epidemic diarrhea in Japan was shown by Shiga to be caused by a specific micro-organism.

Association of the bacillus isolated from feces of patients with the disease was possible by demonstration of rising titers of specific serum agglutinins in a significant proportion of patients. Subsequently, Flexner, Boyd, and Lentz identified other species of Shigella bacilli responsible for dysentery in man. From the beginning, dysentery has been a nemesis to encamped military troops, persons living in unhygienic conditions, and patients in mental institutions. It has occasionally caused epidemic disease in hospitals, nurseries, and schools. Currently, Shigella infection is responsible for a significant proportion of diarrheal disease particularly among children and older persons living in crowded urban areas. There was a progressive increase in the number of infections identified in England and Wales after 1940. Over 40,000 cases were noted in 1960.

Etiology. Strains of Shigella can be characterized antigenically, and there are four serologic groups responsible for disease in man. These are usually identified as serotypes of *Shigella dysenteriae* (shiga), *Shigella flexneri,* *Shigella boydii,* and *Shigella sonnei.* Another group, formerly referred to as *Shigella alkalescens,* may also produce enteric infection in man, but biochemically and antigenically it is more closely related to coliform bacilli.

The Shigella are gram-negative, slender, nonmotile, nonsporulating bacilli, which on primary isolation resemble coccobacilli. They are aerobic and facultative anaerobic, growing readily on relatively simple media at 37° C. They can be selectively grown in the presence of various bile salts (SS and desoxycholate media), thereby being distinguished from most coliform bacilli. Species and strains of Shigella can be identified by carbohydrate fermentation and antigenic analysis with specific antiserum. As with other enteric pathogens, Shigella bacilli do not ordinarily ferment lactose.

Epidemiology. Shigellosis is most common in tropical countries under unhygienic, crowded conditions, but is endemic throughout the world. Young children appear to be more susceptible than adults to bacillary dysentery, but the disease is less common in the first six months of life than in older infants and children. Eighty per cent of children under nine years of age infected with Shigella will develop dysentery, whereas only about 50 per cent of infected older persons develop illness. Under the age of 20 years the frequency of shigellosis in males is greater than in females, but over the age of 20 years the reverse is true. Nevertheless, the case fatality rate is higher in men at all ages. In some countries bacillary dysentery has its peak incidence in summer months, often following heavy rains, whereas in other areas, such as the United States, the highest incidence may be in winter, spring, or autumn. The months when shigellosis is particularly prevalent in tropical and semitropical countries corresponds with the time of year when flies are prevalent. Shigella may be found in the intestinal tracts of flies having contact with infected human feces, but carriage of the bacilli on the insect's feet is probably the means by which it may spread infection. In countries with a high standard of sanitation flies play an inconsequential role in transfer of infection.

Infection is usually transmitted by patients with dysentery, ambulatory persons convalescing from the disease, or asymptomatic carriers. Inadequately washed hands or contaminated inanimate articles are the principal means of transmission. The seats of toilets may become contaminated during flushing and serve as a source of infection. Epidemics of shigellosis have been related to milk, ice cream, and other foods and water contaminated by the hands or feces of infected persons. Shigella in dust has also been incriminated in outbreaks of bacillary dysentery. These sources of infection are also important in perpetuation of endemic infection. Outbreaks of shigellosis in winter usually spread from an infected person in a school or institution to other persons. Secondary cases may result in extension of the disease to other schools or institutions such as hospitals or nurseries. Relapsing disease, reinfection, and chronic infection may enable perpetuation of infection among patients in nursing homes and inmates of mental hospitals. In this setting, outbreaks are often not explosive.

Endemic and epidemic shigellosis is commonly characterized by isolation of several different serologic types of Shigella. Major outbreaks caused by a single serotype are rare, but small outbreaks may be attributable to a single serologic type. *Shigella dysenteriae* (shiga) is an uncommon cause of infection in Britain, Europe and North America, but is responsible for a significant proportion of cases in Asia. *Shigella sonnei* is the prominent cause of bacillary dysentery in countries where personal contact and endemic infection, rather than poor sanitation and unhygienic conditions, are responsible for spread of the disease.

Following infection, the bacilli may be isolated from feces or rectum for only a week or slightly longer. Rarely does carriage of the bacilli persist as long as three months. Carriage of *Shigella dysenteriae* (shiga), however, persists longer than with other species, and carriage of *Shigella flexneri* may be intermittent during convalescence from infection. Generally, however, persistent carriers of *Shigella dysenteriae* remain ill, whereas carriers of *Shigella flexneri* are well. Convalescence from infection owing to *Shigella sonnei* is not associated with prolonged excretion of the bacilli in feces except in the very young and very old.

Although Shigella infection is largely confined to human beings, primates have been shown occasionally to be a source of infection in man. Shigella survive in eggs, oysters, clams, and shrimp for many days, but these serve as sources of infection only when contaminated by infected persons and their excreta.

Pathogenesis and Pathology. Shigella species possess an endotoxin similar to that of other gram-negative bacteria, but it seems unlikely that it plays a significant role in the pathogenesis of bacillary dysentery. *Shigella dysenteriae* (shiga) produces an exotoxin that can exert a deleterious effect upon the nervous system. The occurrence of paralytic manifestations in dysentery produced by this species may be attributable to the exotoxin.

Bacillary dysentery is infrequently associated with bacteremia, and the infection is confined to the intestinal mucosa, occasionally invading mesenteric lymph nodes. Morphologic lesions are most frequently observed in the colon, occasionally involving the terminal ileum. Ulceration of the mucosa develops, with intervening inflamed membrane but no undermining of the ulcer edges as in amebic dysentery. The bowel wall is infiltrated with granulocytes, there is edema of the submucosa, and occasionally the involvement may extend to the serosa. If ulceration is not extensive, healing occurs without scarring, but when it is severe, fibrosis and even stenosis of the bowel may develop.

Clinical Manifestations. Patients with shigellosis may have simple self-limited diarrhea, acute gastroenteritis, true dysentery, or no symptoms of illness. It has been proposed that bacillary dysentery may occasionally be responsible for chronic colitis, but it has been difficult to establish this relationship with certainty.

The incubation period of dysentery is usually about 48 hours, but it may be shorter. The illness begins abruptly with abdominal cramps, pain relieved by defecation, and watery diarrhea. This is followed promptly by the development of tenesmus, feverishness, and passage of mucous stool, occasionally containing blood. Abdominal tenderness, most pronounced in the lower quadrants, is found, and the bowel is hyperactive on auscultation. The temperature rarely rises very high, except in children, in whom it may become 104° F. or more. Without treatment the illness persists for a few days and then subsides.

Acute gastroenteritis, associated with nausea, some vomiting, and diarrhea, is seen particularly in outbreaks of infection by *Shigella sonnei*.

Shigella dysenteriae (shiga) infection is often more severe than that caused by the other species. The fever may be higher, hypotension develops more frequently, and the intestinal symptoms are more intense. Recovery may be delayed, and debility may persist for several weeks. Peripheral neuritis more commonly complicates infection by *Shigella dysenteriae*.

Conjunctivitis, iritis, and nystagmus are occasional complications of bacillary dysentery, appearing between the first and second weeks of disease. Nonsuppurative arthritis may also develop. Fluid and electrolyte depletion may be considerable, particularly in infants and children, producing severe dehydration and acidosis. Potassium deficit may be recognized, particularly as the patient's fluids are replenished. Convulsions develop occasionally in children, but appear to be correlated to the degree of fever.

At times, bacillary dysentery seems to have been precipitated by onset of measles, and almost half the cases may be accompanied by infection with enteropathic viruses including adenovirus, echovirus, poliovirus, and Coxsackie virus. The association of a virus with the disease, however, does not influence its clinical manifestations. The frequency of serious underlying disease in persons with shigellosis is not as common as in salmonellosis. Massive intestinal bleeding occurs in severe bacillary dysentery when there is extensive intestinal necrosis and ulceration.

Diagnosis. Isolation and identification of Shigella in the stool or from swab culture of the rectal mucosa are the only means of establishing the diagnosis of shigellosis. The serum agglutinin titer will rise in about half the patients with bacillary dysentery, but it is not ordinarily useful for diagnostic purposes. Shigella survive in feces for only a short while. Therefore, feces should be promptly cultured, or the specimen should be collected in a 30 per cent glycerol-saline solution for preservation. Examination of the feces microscopically in bacillary dysentery will usually reveal a large number of granulocytes, comprising about 90 per cent of all cells, apart from erythrocytes. As convalescence begins, mononuclear cells become predominant. Specific immunofluorescence techniques have been developed for the rapid detection of Shigella in feces. This test agrees with cultural results in over 90 per cent of instances.

Viral enteritis caused by echovirus, Coxsackie, and poliomyelitis viruses may be epidemic and may be confused with shigellosis. Fever is uncommon, however, in viral enteritis unless there is severe dehydration, and the feces contain no blood or pus. *Staphylococcal enterocolitis* develops usually in hospitalized patients undergoing abdominal surgery who have received antimicrobial therapy. *Amebic dysentery* usually has a gradual onset, the diarrhea is ordinarily not severe, there is often little or no fever, and microscopic examination of the feces will reveal a predominance of mononuclear cells. Sigmoidoscopy reveals undermined ulcers with normal intervening mucosa. *Salmonellosis* is more often accompanied by nausea and vomiting at onset and occasionally by a chill and very high fever. Blood cultures are often positive. *Staphylococcal food poisoning* and many forms of viral gastroenteritis are more prominently associated with nausea and vomiting than with diarrhea.

Treatment. Sulfonamides were effective in treatment of shigellosis when they were first used. Resistant bacilli emerged, however, and sulfonamides are not now considered to be the most effective drugs for the infection. Resistance of Shigella to multiple antimicrobials has been induced by episomal transfer from other enteric bacilli. Conceivably, therefore, drug-susceptible Shigella may become drug-resistant from other drug-resistant bacilli in the intestinal tract.

Tetracycline has been an effective drug against Shigella, but resistant strains have been identified. A few strains of Shigella are resistant to chloramphenicol. Colimycin and neomycin are almost always effective in vitro, but a few strains resistant to ampicillin have been found. Streptomycin given orally has been used to treat shigellosis, but strains resistant to this drug have also been identified. Cephalothin and massive doses of penicillin G may be effective.

At present, ampicillin in a dosage of 2 or more grams orally each day in divided doses for five days is the preferred agent in treatment of shigellosis in adults. Chloramphenicol or tetracyline may be effective alternatives if either the micro-organism is resistant to ampicillin or the patient is allergic to the penicillins. Oral streptomycin, 0.5 gram twice daily, is also recommended in Great Britain.

Fluid and electrolyte replacement should be given to the patient who is in collapse or who is dehydrated. Opiates such as paregoric or morphine may alleviate the abdominal discomfort and tenesmus but should be used cautiously.

Prognosis. The mortality rate in untreated bacillary dysentery is about 0.1 per cent or less, but it may be higher during famine or starvation. In addition, the fatality rate with dysentery caused by *Shigella dysenteriae* (shiga) is higher than with that attributed to other Shigella. Death rarely occurs when appropriate treatment is prescribed.

Dammin, G. J.: The pathogenesis of acute diarrheal disease in early life. Bull. WHO, 31:29, 1964.

Gordon, J. E., Behar, M., and Scrimshaw, N. S.: Acute diarrheal disease in less developed countries: I. An epidemiological basis for control. Bull. WHO, 31:1, 1964.

Ramos-Alvarez, M., et al.: Diarrheal disease of children. The occurrence of enteropathogenic viruses and bacteria. Amer. J. Dis. Child., 107:218, 1964.

Reller, L. B., et al.: Shigellosis in the United States, 1964–1968. J. Infect. Dis., 120:393, 1969.

Watanabe, T.: Infective heredity of multiple drug resistance in bacteria, Bact. Rev., 27:87, 1963.

Wilson, G. S., and Miles, A. A.: Topley and Wilson's Principles of Bacteriology and Immunology. 5th ed. Baltimore, Williams and Wilkins Company, 1964, Vol. II. p. 1876.

CHOLERA
(Asiatic Cholera)
Leighton E. Cluff

Definition. Cholera is a specific infectious disease of man caused by *Vibrio cholerae*. It is characterized by severe diarrhea with fluid and electrolyte depletion, and now occurs endemically and epidemically in Asia.

Etiology. In a classic study in 1857, Snow described an outbreak of cholera in London and incriminated contaminated water as the source of disease. In 1883, Koch identified *Vibrio cholerae* in the feces of a large number of patients with cholera. The cholera vibrio is a comma-shaped, gram-negative, nonhemolytic, flagellated, and motile micro-organism that grows aerobically on nutrient media at 37° C., preferentially at an alkaline pH. *V. cholerae* can be characterized and differentated from noncholera vibrios by its fermentative, nonhemolytic, pathogenic, and antigenic reactions.

Incidence and Prevalence. Cholera is endemic in India, China, Burma, Pakistan, Thailand, and a few other areas in Asia. It has occurred in epidemics throughout the world. Prior to the nineteenth century, cholera was unknown outside India, but during that century it was observed sporadically and as an epidemic in Europe, England, Russia, and North America. In the twentieth century, cholera has largely disappeared from the Western Hemisphere and Europe but continues to occur endemically and epidemically in Asia, primarily along the Ganges River in India and in Pakistan. The last pandemic of cholera began in 1902. During the period 1898 to 1907 cholera was responsible for at least 370,000 deaths in India.

Epidemiology. Only man is naturally infected with *V. cholerae.* The infection is transmitted most commonly by contaminated water, but it can be transmitted by contamination of fresh leafy or root vegetables and fruit fertilized with human feces or contaminated with water containing the micro-organism. *V. cholerae* has been isolated from flies, roaches, and other insects, but these may be an unimportant source of contagion. Doctors and nurses caring for patients with cholera rarely contract the disease, suggesting that direct contact under hygienic conditions is an uncommon mode of transmission of the infection. Cholera is primarily a disease of persons who live in poverty or who have poor standards of living and sanitation.

Outbreaks of cholera usually appear during dry, hot weather preceding a rainy season. The reason for this seasonal occurrence of cholera is unexplained. Although sporadic cases may occur throughout the year, there are rare chronic carriers of *V. cholerae,* as there are of typhoid bacilli, and the principal reservoir of the organism in interepidemic periods is unclear. In endemic areas around river basins, *V. cholerae* can be isolated from the water throughout the year, although most cases of cholera occur seasonally.

Pathology and Pathogenesis. Recent studies of cholera indicate that the small intestine is most severely involved. There is an intact gastrointestinal epithelium, even in the acute phase of the disease, but there are mononuclear cell inflammation of the mucosa, vascular congestion, and goblet cell hyperplasia. This acute stage may be followed by increased "turnover" of the epithelial cells. These morphologic changes are similar to those seen in nonspecific diarrhea but do not explain the clinical features of the disease. Chronic atrophic enteritis may precede and persist after the infection. It is likely that nutritional and other chronic affections of the intestine and stomach are predisposing causes of cholera. Occurrence of the disease in impoverished and malnourished persons further suggests this possibility. A cholera-like disease has been produced in dogs by feeding vibrio cultures (10^{11} bacteria) in bicarbonate.

The cholera vibrio elaborates a substance altering sodium transport that produces intestinal intoxication, diarrhea, and fluid and electrolyte depletion. A mucolytic enzyme is also produced by the vibrio, and may participate in the pathogenesis of the disease. The essential mechanism producing cholera, however, remains unknown.

The primary difficulty in cholera is severe fluid and electrolyte depletion. The feces contain mucus, epithelial debris, large quantities of water, sodium, potassium, and bicarbonate, but little plasma protein. There is no significant loss of albumin into the intestines, as illustrated by the failure of intravenously injected Evans blue dye to appear in the feces.

V. cholerae infection does not extend beyond the intestinal tract but may invade, to a limited degree, the mucosa of the bowel and, rarely, the regional lymphatics.

Clinical Manifestations. Cholera begins as an acute diarrhea with abdominal pain. Vomiting may appear early, but is not prominent. Fever and chills are usually absent. The oral and axillary temperature may be depressed, whereas the rectal temperature may be elevated slightly above normal. It is of interest that there may be considerable postmortem elevation of temperature. Over a few hours the diarrhea increases in severity, and the volume of feces may be as great as 15 to 20 liters in 24 hours. Initially, the feces are bile-strained, but as the diarrhea worsens, the feces become watery, mucoid, and odorless, and occasionally may contain blood. The feces of patients with cholera may resemble rice water or starch water and may contain cellular debris and masses of cholera vibrios. The patient becomes rapidly dehydrated, the skin is cold and withered, and the face becomes drawn. As dehydration increases, the patient becomes stuporous, comatose, hypotensive, and cyanotic, and may die in shock. Urine output decreases, mouth and eyes become dry, but lacteal and sweat secretion may persist. Muscular cramps may be severe. Thirst is intense, and the

ingestion of fluid rarely induces vomiting. Recovery ordinarily is prompt after replacement of fluid and electrolyte, but the patient may continue to have anuria or oliguria and may die in renal failure. The renal insufficiency may be attributable to hypokalemia, shock, or reduced renal blood flow owing to dehydration.

With severe dehydration the hematocrit, leukocyte count, and specific gravity of the plasma rise. This plasma sodium chloride and total serum protein are increased above normal. The plasma potassium may be slightly elevated or normal, although potassium depletion is severe. Metabolic acidosis is usually severe.

In cholera the fecal sodium and chloride concentrations are increased above normal, as is fecal osmolarity, but these are consistently lower than the plasma values. Fecal potassium and carbonate concentrations, however, are higher than those of the plasma. These electrolyte changes in cholera resemble those in other diarrheal disease, but are more severe.

Many patients with cholera are anemic before onset of the disease; therefore, the rise in hematocrit with dehydration may not be demonstrable. The degree of dehydration in cholera can be clinically estimated, but is best measured by determination of plasma specific gravity and central venous pressure.

Diagnosis. In endemic areas and during epidemics, cholera is easily recognized clinically. Sporadic cases must be differentiated from other diarrheal diseases such as typhoid fever, bacillary dysentery, amebiasis, other forms of intestinal parasitism, viral enteritis, staphylococcal food poisoning, and chemical poisoning. The epidemiologic and fulminant characteristics of cholera, however, are helpful diagnostically. Bacteriologic and immunologic identification of *V. cholerae* from the feces is usually possible. Microscopic examination of the feces may reveal masses of the microorganism. *V. cholerae* may be cultured from the feces of patients convalescing from cholera, but ordinarily disappears within a few days or a few weeks.

Many patients with cholera will have a positive serologic test for *V. cholera* antibodies on the day of onset of disease. Serum antibody titers, measured by hemagglutination or vibriocidal assay, however, rise to maximal levels in about seven days after onset of cholera. Vibriocidal titers fall rapidly after illness.

Other Vibrio Infections. *V. cholerae* may be confused with El Tor vibrio, which may also produce diarrheal disease. El Tor vibrio, however, is hemolytic and can be differentiated from the cholera vibrio serologically. The noncholera vibrios are widespread in surface water throughout the world and have been associated with diarrheal disease. *Vibrio fetus* produces disease in human beings but is primarily an infection of cattle causing septic abortion, and can be differentiated serologically from *V. cholerae*. Man is infected following occupational exposure to diseased animals or animal products. *V. fetus* infection of man does not produce diarrhea, but is responsible for bacteremia, abortion, pneumonia, endocarditis, thrombophlebitis, and an illness resembling acute brucellosis.

Treatment. The treatment of cholera is replacement of the fluid and electrolyte depletion attributable to the severe diarrhea. Urine output is an index of hydration if the patient does not have renal failure, and administration of fluids sufficient to restore urine output to normal will often return the plasma specific gravity toward normal. The degree of hydration cannot be accurately estimated clinically, however, and is best measured by the degree of hemoconcentration. The hemoglobin or hematocrit determination may be misleading, because of pre-existing anemia. When the patient is first seen, the blood electrolyte determinations also may be unreliable as indices of the degree of electrolyte depletion and dehydration. Plasma protein concentration, and particularly plasma specific gravity, can usually serve as a reliable index for administration of fluids and electrolyte.

For the cholera patients, "normal" plasma specific gravity is considered to be 1.025. For each 0.001 increase in plasma specific gravity above 1.025, the patient requires 4 ml. of fluid per kilogram of body weight. This volume of fluid should be given promptly as isotonic (0.85 per cent) sodium chloride and 2 per cent sodium bicarbonate in a ratio of 2 or 3 to 1 by volume, adminstered intravenously. Giving fluids equal to 10 per cent of the patient's body weight (three quarters of this to be given rapidly) is usually adequate for initial treatment. After initial hydration, the fecal loss, measured hourly, should be replaced volume for volume with the same saline and alkali combination as given initially. The plasma specific gravity should be measured every eight hours, at least, during the first day and once daily thereafter until the patient has fully recovered. Many liters of fluid will be needed (25 or more) until the administration of fluid is no longer required. The cholera patient, even if in shock and comatose when first seen, will often be able to take oral feeding after four hours. At that time potassium, as juices or in other form, may be fed. Otherwise, if the diarrhea continues for more than 24 hours, the intravenous fluids should contain 10 mEq. of potassium chloride per liter.

Tetracycline in a dosage of 100 mg. per liter of intravenous fluid and administered in a total dosage of 250 to 500 mg. during the first day of treatment shortens the period of diarrhea, decreases the requirement for fluid replacement. This is associated with a hastening of the disappearance of *V. cholerae* from the feces.

Prognosis. The case mortality rate from untreated cholera in persons 10 to 20 years of age is 50 per cent; in persons over 50 it is 70 per cent. Death is more common among those less than 10 years of age than among patients between 10 and 20 years of age. Almost invariably, death can be prevented if the fluid, electrolyte, and alkali

therapy is begun early in the illness and if there is no serious associated disease or renal failure.

Prevention. Cholera can be eliminated by improved standards of living, public health, and sanitation. In those parts of the world where water supply and sewage disposal are controlled effectively, cholera no longer occurs.

There is a killed bacterial vaccine for immunization against cholera that provides some temporary protection. It may be useful in reducing the incidence of the disease in endemic areas.

Carpenter, C. C. J., et al.: Clinical studies in Asiatic cholera. Bull. Hopkins Hosp., 118:165, 1966.

Gangarosa, E. J., Beisel, W. R., Benyajati, C., Sprinz, H., and Piyaratn, P.: The nature of the gastrointestinal lesion in Asiatic cholera and its relation to pathogenesis: A biopsy study. Amer. J. Trop. Dis., 9:125, 1960.

McIntyre, O. R., Feeley, J. C., Greenough, W. B., III, Benenson, A. S., Hassam, S. I., and Saad, A.: Diarrhea caused by noncholera vibrios. Amer. J. Trop. Med., 14:412, 1966.

Oseasohn, R. O., Benenson, A. S., and Fahimuddin, M.: Field trial of cholera vaccine in rural East Pakistan. Lancet, 1:450, 1965.

Phillips, R. A.: Water and electrolyte losses in cholera. Fed. Proc., 23:705, 1964.

Phillips, R. A.: Asiatic cholera. Ann. Rev. Med., 19:69, 1968.

Snow, J.: Snow on Cholera. The Commonwealth Fund. London, Oxford University Press, 1936.

PLAGUE

Fred R. McCrumb, Jr.

Definition. Plague is an acute or chronic disease of wild and commensal rodents transmissible among these lower animal hosts and to man through the bite of infected ectoparasites. The infection in man is acute and frequently fulminant and usually is characterized by abrupt onset of high fever, lymphadenopathy near the site of exposure, bacteremia, and prostration. Secondary or embolic pneumonia may result in direct respiratory spread of the disease from man to man. Thus, two clinical types of human infection are recognized: *bubonic plague,* characterized by either regional lymphadenopathy or bacteremia wherein organisms invade the blood by way of the lymphatics and produce overwhelming sepsis, and *primary plague pneumonia.*

Etiology. *Pasteurella pestis* is a nonmotile, aerobic gram-negative bacillus that grows readily but slowly on artificial media. Small convex dewdrop colonies become grayish and present a surface appearance like that of beaten copper after 48 hours' incubation at 37° C. on blood agar. Virulent organisms are sticky because of the presence of a protein capsule. In liquid media, a surface pellicle and stalactites are characteristic. *P. pestis* is highly virulent for a variety of laboratory animals. The micro-organisms may be seen on microscopy of suitably stained node impressions, peritoneal exudate, and peripheral blood of these hosts as coccoid or large ovoid "safety-pin" bacilli.

This bipolar staining is best demonstrated with Giemsa or Wayson's stain, and may be conspicuous in lymph node aspirates and sputum of infected human beings. The organism is destroyed quickly by sunlight and common chemical disinfectants and is noninfectious after 15 minutes at 55° C. *P. pestis* may survive for several weeks in dry flea feces and human sputum, and may be kept viable and virulent in the frozen state for months. Although streptomycin-resistant mutants have been encountered in experimental plague infections, all naturally occurring human strains of *P. pestis* studied to date are inhibited *in vitro* by low concentrations of streptomycin, chloramphenicol, and the tetracyclines.

Incidence and Prevalence. The first adequate description of widespread disease deals with an outbreak of plague in the Egyptian port of Pelusium in 542 A.D. During the next 50 years, plague spread widely into Asia and Europe and it has been estimated that 100 million people perished at that time. Plague assumed catastrophic proportions again during the fourteenth century when it appeared not only in Europe and the Middle East but also in China and India. Pneumonic plague was prominent in this pandemic, which, for unclear reasons, became known as the "Black Death." In Europe alone, 25 million, or one fourth of the population, succumbed. The spread of plague resulted in the establishment of numerous widely distributed permanent foci among rodent populations.

During recent years, human plague has occurred in China, Vietnam, Burma, Indonesia, India, Iran, the Malagasy Republic, Central and South Africa, the United States, and several countries of South America. There has been a continuing decline in the incidence of human plague, however, and, in many instances, this decrease in incidence is unquestionably spontaneous. Certain endemic areas are characterized by a constant low human case rate resulting from sporadic infections that occur as a result of man's accidental contact with wild rodent foci. In the United States between 1908 and 1951, only 91 human plague infections associated with wild rodents were distributed over 15 western states.

Epidemiology. The ecology of plague varies from one region to another, and the extent to which man is affected by enzootic infections is determined in part by the proximity of human and rodent habitations and the bionomics of rodent ectoparasites. Although ticks and lice are capable of transmitting *P. pestis* to susceptible animals, practically speaking, the important vectors are fleas. Occasionally man contracts plague by handling the carcass of an infected animal. Epidemics of plague usually arise from infected commensal rats such as *Rattus rattus* and *Rattus norvegicus,* the causative organism being transmitted to man by *Xenopsylla cheopis,* the common rat flea. There is general agreement that sylvatic foci of plague infection among so-called wild rodents (mice, field rats, gerbils, ground squirrels) accounts for the persistence of this disease in endemic areas. In some instances, man's agricultural pursuits into sylvatic foci may result in outbreaks of human plague, and there is ample evidence of an interchange of fleas between commensal and wild rodent species. Flea-borne plague in man is usually of the bubonic variety, and as such does not represent a serious risk to other human beings. By contrast, plague pneumonia secondary to bacteremia may initiate a series of direct transmissions to susceptible contacts in whom the disease is manifest by a fulminant primary pneumonia. Primary pneumonic plague may spread among a susceptible human population with alarming rapidity.

Age and sex distribution of plague is dependent upon the nature of rodent foci and the habits of the human population at risk. Thus, domestic rat plague will be distributed evenly among both sexes of all ages when the home is infested with rat fleas. When field rodents constitute the source of infection, the disease will occur predominantly among field workers.

Pathology. Evidence of infection is usually not present at the portal of entry into the skin, although a small pustule is observed in a few patients with bubonic plague. Similarly, lymphatics leading to regional nodes are grossly normal. The primary bubo is usually enlarged, exquisitely tender, and surrounded by a broad zone of subcutaneous edema. There is an intense hemorrhagic inflammatory reaction with infiltration of polynuclear cells. As the inflammation progresses, necrosis and suppuration of the bubo occur. There is a characteristic gelatinous edema of contiguous connective tissue and dilatation of small blood vessels. Occasionally, infection of the oropharyngeal mucous membrane will lead to tonsillar or mediastinal reaction of the type seen in lymph nodes. Pathologic changes noted in other organ systems can be ascribed to small blood vessel disease, as evidenced by hemorrhages in serous membranes and gastrointestinal mucosa. In addition, degenerative changes of renal tubular epithelium and parenchymal cells of the liver are frequent. There may be slight enlargement of the liver and spleen. Vascular congestion of the meninges is accompanied by cerebral edema.

Secondary or embolic plague pneumonia is characterized by perivascular foci of inflammatory cells and colonies of *P. pestis.* As the disease progresses, distinction from primary plague infection of the lung is less obvious, and both may show gradation from lobular pneumonia to lobar consolidation. It is not unusual for several lobes to become involved within a period of 24 to 48 hours. In all instances, reaction in the lung is intense, there being cellular infiltration, gross hemorrhage, and copious exudation of watery sputum. There is overwhelming growth of plague bacilli in the lung that can be readily demonstrated in impression smears of cut lung surface. Bronchial lymph nodes are usually enlarged and hyperemic.

Pathogenesis. Following the ingestion of plague bacilli, the proximal digestive tract of the flea becomes obstructed as organisms multiply in the proventriculus. Refeeding results in regurgitation of the freshly ingested human blood as well as *P. pestis* into the feeding site. Organisms are then carried to regional lymph nodes, where a local inflammatory reaction leads to the formation of a bubo. In most instances, bacteremia occurs early in the disease and may assume enormous proportions in fulminant infections. Plague pneumonia is associated with the production of infectious droplets and respiratory spread of

P. pestis. Epidemiologic studies suggest that intimate contact is a prerequisite to successful respiratory transmission of this organism, and the nature of the primary lung lesion favors spread by particles of small size.

Although much has been said about intoxication in human plague infection, evidence of specific toxin activity in human beings is wanting. Extraction of virulent and attenuated strains of *P. pestis* has revealed the presence of a water-soluble toxic substance that is highly lethal for Swiss mice. Although this material is antigenic in laboratory animals and antibodies may be demonstrated in the sera of patients recovered from plague, its role in the pathogenesis of plague has not been established.

Clinical Manifestations. Most plague infections make their appearance abruptly with high fever, tachycardia, malaise, and aching of the extremities and back. Temperature usually rises to 103 or 104° F. within a few hours of onset, and the patient has the general appearance of profound illness, with flushed face and anxious expression. As the disease progresses, delirium may become a prominent feature of the clinical syndrome, and anxiety gives way to depression.

Bubonic Plague. The incubation period in bubonic plague varies from one to six days in most instances and progresses to fulminant bacteremia, death ensuing within three to five days of the onset of symptoms. The case fatality in untreated bubonic plague is variously estimated at 60 to 90 per cent. Regional lymphadenopathy or buboes of flea-borne plague are found in the groin in more than 50 per cent of patients with this form of the disease. Femoral and inguinal buboes are followed in frequency by axillary and cervical node involvement. The site of infection is influenced by the nature of exposure to vectors, there being a high frequency of lower extremity exposure among working adults and axillary and cervical buboes among children exposed as they sleep in a flea-infested dwelling. The involved node may not be greatly enlarged but is invariably painful and exquisitely tender. Within a few hours, there is periadenitis with edema of surrounding tissue. Buboes may involute slowly or suppurate with discharge of necrotic material in patients who survive the acute phase of infection. When bacteremia progresses relentlessly, the clinical picture is one of overwhelming sepsis, and death is associated with peripheral vascular collapse.

Plague Pneumonia. Plague pneumonia acquired as a result of respiratory spread of *P. pestis* is even more fulminant, untreated patients rarely surviving for more than three days. The disease is characterized by an explosive onset of high fever, tachycardia, tachypnea, and restlessness. Flushing of the skin, conjunctival suffusion, and anxious expression are common. Headache and myalgia may be severe, but are inconstant. During the early phases of illness, the paucity of signs is disproportionate to the obvious severity of the infection. Cough may be absent until six or more hours have passed. Subjective symptoms referable to the chest may be absent, or the patient may complain of pleural pain or dull substernal oppression. Physical signs of pneumonitis may be lacking at this time; however, as the disease progresses, rales, suppressed breathing, and impaired percussion appear. Signs of consolidation are not encountered frequently until after therapy has been instituted. The general clinical state rapidly deteriorates, and patients with this disease are gravely ill after 10 to 15 hours of fever. The patient may find it difficult to produce more than small amounts of sputum in the early hours of illness; however, blood-tinged sputum usually appears within the first 12 hours. Bloody, frothy, liquid sputum typical of plague pneumonia is produced in large quantities late in the disease at a time when the prognosis is uniformly poor.

Laboratory Findings. Peripheral blood leukocytosis with total counts of 12,000 to 15,000 and neutrophilia usually occur in both types of human plague. There is elevation of the erythrocyte sedimentation rate, but other hematologic abnormalities have not been observed. Proteinuria and mild hematuria may accompany the acute febrile phase of plague.

Diagnosis. The clinical diagnosis of plague is confirmed by conventional bacteriologic techniques and inoculation of susceptible laboratory animals. *P. pestis* may be isolated in pure culture after 48 to 96 hours from bubo aspirates, blood, and sputum, using blood agar and infusion broth. Inoculation of these materials into mice or guinea pigs produces bacteremia and death of the animal in two to five days. A smear of heart's blood of these animals will reveal numerous bipolar staining rods.

In all instances, however, a tentative diagnosis of plague must be made on clinical and epidemiologic grounds, there being dire consequences of a missed diagnosis, especially of plague pneumonia. Careful examination of stained smears of bubo aspirates or sputum will usually reveal the presence of small gram-negative bacilli, and proper isolation precautions and specific therapy must be based on the judgment of this examination. Stained smears from organs of cadavers in cases of sudden death in plague endemic areas should be examined with great diligence to avoid catastrophic spread of this disease.

Patients recovering from plague develop specific antibodies that may be demonstrated in convalescent-phase serum by bacterial agglutination, agglutination of erythrocytes sensitized with capsular antigen, complement-fixation, and mouse protection tests. Antibodies make their appearance early in the second week of disease and continue to rise up to the fourth or fifth week. In all cases, serodiagnosis is retrospective but of value in establishing the presence of infection with *P. pestis* as well as the immune status of a vaccinated population.

Plague infections in man must be differentiated from tularemia, lymphogranuloma venereum, and other causes of localized lymphadenopathy. The disease is frequently confused with malaria, influenza, enteric fevers, and various causes of acute pneumonia, among them Klebsiella, staphylococcal, tularemic, and viral infections of the lung. In the absence of buboes or pneumonia, bacteremia owing to a variety of gram-negative organisms may resemble acute septicemic plague.

Treatment. *P. pestis* is readily inhibited in vitro by relatively small concentrations of streptomycin, chloramphenicol, and the tetracyclines. The disease responds readily when antimicrobial therapy is started during the early phase of illness, but it rapidly becomes refractory to specific treatment as it progresses. In view of the ease and uniform success of early therapy, delay in diagnosis and administration of chemotherapy is a grave error in clinical judgment. Pneumonic plague is uniformly fatal, and becomes difficult to treat after the twelfth to fifteenth hour of fever. Bubonic plague is generally less severe, but may progress to death with equal swiftness.

Early studies with sulfonamides revealed that mortality from bubonic plague could be reduced to 5 to 20 per cent by the administration of sulfadiazine or sulfamerazine at the rate of 12 grams daily for four to seven days. These drugs were found to be ineffective in plague pneumonia.

Streptomycin or the broad-spectrum antimicrobials represent the therapy of choice in all plague infections. Streptomycin should be administered parenterally at the rate of 4 grams daily for two days followed by 8 to 10 grams given over a period of five additional days. Chloramphenicol should be administered at the rate of 6 to 8 grams daily for the first 48 hours followed by 3 grams (50 to 75 mg. per kilogram) daily for a total dosage of 20 to 25 grams. Chloramphenicol should be given intravenously and orally during the first 48 hours of therapy if the latter route of administration is feasible. Tetracyclines should be administered in a similar manner, large doses (4 to 6 grams daily) being given during the first 48 hours of therapy. Intravenous therapy during the first 24 hours is mandatory in severely ill patients but should be supplemented by oral administration of the drug if this is tolerated by the patient.

When specific therapy is not instituted within the first 15 hours of overt illness in plague pneumonia, antimicrobial therapy usually will not favorably alter the outcome of the disease.

Supportive care includes the use of intravenous fluid therapy, pressor drugs to support failing peripheral circulation, and oxygen therapy when respiratory function has been compromised by widespread pneumonitis. Tracheostomy frequently results in improved pulmonary function and facilitates care of patients severely ill with primary respiratory disease.

Prevention. Prevention of plague is best accomplished by eliminating endemic foci of rodent infection. Improvement in living standards is usually associated with spontaneous disappearance of this disease or at least its confinement to sylvatic foci. However, there are many areas where such an evolution is not likely to occur and sylvatic foci will probably always exist. Under such circumstances, three general approaches to plague control are available. In practice, rodent control has proved to be the least effective method in most endemic regions, primarily because human living standards cannot be sufficiently improved. Rodenticides in common use include sodium fluoroacetate (1080), arsenic trioxide, red squill, alphanaphthylthiourea (ANTU), and anticoagulants such as warfarin. In underdeveloped areas, vector control with dichlorodiphenyltrichloroethane (DDT) and other insecticides such as benzene hexachloride, chlordane, and dieldrin is probably the most effective single control method. The residual effect of 10 per cent DDT dust or 5 per cent spray dispersed around rat habitations and human dwellings is sufficient to reduce sharply the flea populations and thus eliminate large numbers of vectors. Finally, although millions of human beings have been inoculated with living, attenuated or formalin-killed plague vaccines, the protective effect of these immunoprophylactics has not been assessed adequately. However, there is evidence to support the concept that the production of specific antibodies in man is associated with a significant degree of resistance to plague infection. Protection of human populations against plague is best assured in endemic areas when all available control measures are employed.

Baltazard, M.: Déclin et destin d'une maladie infectieuse: la peste. Bull. WHO 23:247, 1960.
McCrumb, F. R., Jr. et al.: Chloramphenicol and Terramycin in the treatment of pneumonic plague. Amer. J. Med., 14:284, 1953.
Meyer, K. F.: Recent studies on the immunity response to administration of different plague vaccines. Bull. WHO, 9:619, 1953.
Politzer, R.: Plague. Geneva, World Health Organization Monograph Series No. 22, 1954.

TULAREMIA
Theodore E. Woodward

Definition. Most cases of tularemia are characterized by the formation of a focal ulcer at the site of entry of the causative bacillus, enlargement of regional lymph nodes, and a constitutional reaction of fever, prostration, myalgia, and headache. There may be pneumonia, which is occasionally accompanied by pleurisy or a typhoidal-like illness.

Franciscella tularensis, the microbial agent, is transmitted to humans by insect vectors such as ticks or deer flies, by the handling or ingestion of infected animal tissues, or by inhalation of infected aerosols. The clinical diagnosis is confirmed by demonstration of bacteremia, by isolation of the bacillus from the sputum, tissue exudates, or gastric washings, and by demonstration of serum agglutinins in early convalescence.

Historical Features. The knowledge of the ecology and clinical features of tularemia has been developed in the United States through the pioneering work of Francis and other Public Health

Service investigators. McCoy described the disease in 1911 while studying a plaguelike illness in ground squirrels in Tulare County, California. The first clinical description and bacteriologic proof of illness is attributed to Wherry and Lamb in 1914. In a series of studies conducted in Utah and elsewhere, Francis (1928) incriminated rabbits as important animal hosts and established the transmissibility of disease by deer flies.

Etiology, Specific Laboratory Diagnosis, and Epidemiology. Tularemia is of considerable interest because the causative micro-organism is a member of the important gram-negative group characterized by intracellular parasitism about which basic information on immunity mechanisms is incomplete. The bacillus is pleomorphic and non-motile, and propagates best on such artificial media as blood-glucose-cysteine agar or following inoculation of animals with suspensions of infected tissues.

Culture. During the early stages of illness, *F. tularensis* is isolated readily by direct culture in appropriate media or by the subcutaneous or intraperitoneal inoculation of exudate into mice or guinea pigs. Positive cultures are obtained from the local ulcer or regional lymph nodes during the first several weeks in patients with ulceroglandulary type of illness. Regardless of the clinical type of tularemia, viable organisms may be isolated from nasopharyngeal or gastric washings during the active systemic phases of illness. Pleural fluid and bronchial secretions are suitable for cultural purposes. Bacteremia may be demonstrated in all forms, although isolation from the blood by culture on an artificial medium is difficult because of the paucity of organisms present. Organisms have been isolated from cerebrospinal fluid or bone marrow, although such cultural procedures are rarely indicated. Under ideal conditions, if suitable media are inoculated with appropriate material, the organism may be identified within two to four days. Impression smears of splenic tissues often reveal the characteristic coccal or bacillary forms intracellularly following preparation with Giemsa or Wayson's plague stain.

Serologic Diagnosis. The conventional serum agglutination reaction is a very useful diagnostic test, because specific agglutinins appear within eight to ten days from the onset of illness. Maximal titers are reached in about four weeks. Demonstration of a rise in titer through examination of serial specimens is confirmatory evidence of infection, although single titers of 1:160 or more are usually significant. Sera from patients with brucellosis or tularemia may show cross-agglutination, although the titer is usually higher with the homologous antigen.

Cutaneous Test. Foshay described a diagnostic skin test that consists of the intradermal inoculation of a purified antigen consisting of a killed suspension of *F. tularensis*. The reaction is of the delayed tuberculin-type, becoming positive in 48 hours. The test is highly specific and becomes positive during the first week of tularemia either prior to or coincident with the development of agglutinins. The test remains positive for years.

Epidemiology. Tularemia has been detected in many countries of the Northern Hemisphere. *F. tularensis* has been found in practically all animal species. In much of North America cottontail rabbits are the most important animal host and were formerly a very common source of the ulceroglandular and typhoidal forms of tularemia. Restricted sale of wild rabbits in metropolitan areas resulted in a sharp decline of the disease.

The clinical infection develops following puncture wounds by bony spicules of infected rabbits or by the ingestion of improperly cooked food. Foxes, squirrels, rats, mice — indeed, all rodents — have been incriminated as sources of infection. Streams are contaminated for variable periods by infected animal carcasses (or by other less well understood routes), so that drinking the water or handling aquatic mammals such as muskrats may be hazardous.

Many cases have their origin from infected arthropods such as ticks, deer flies, or mosquitoes. In North America the ticks *Dermacentor andersoni*, *Dermacentor variabilis*, and the Lone Star tick are important reservoirs and vectors. Infected female ticks transmit *F. tularensis* transovarially. A primary ulcer often forms at the site of tick attachment.

Tularemia occurs in all seasons: among hunters and trappers in the fall and winter, and during the spring and summer when ticks and deer flies are active. All ages and both sexes are susceptible.

Mechanism of Infection and Pathology. The disease may present in a variety of forms with two major subdivisions, depending on whether or not the initial site of entry can be visualized. In all forms there is lymph node involvement. In most instances there is a primary ulcer, variable in size, which may be located on the skin (ulceroglandular), in the eye (oculoglandular), or in the nasopharynx with necrotizing lesions. Sometimes the cutaneous lesion may be insignificant, so that the picture is that of "glandular tularemia" without an overt primary lesion. The entry also may be through the intestinal tract (enteric or typhoidal) or via the lungs (pulmonary).

Following infection, *F. tularensis* reaches the blood via the lymphatics and nodes; the microbe, although phagocytized, resides intracellularly without loss of viability. Granulomatous lesions develop within the reticuloendothelial system, particularly in lymph nodes, liver, and spleen. These lesions, usually hyperplastic, bear some resemblance to tuberculosis and may caseate or form small local abscesses. The macrophage is the predominant cell type that surrounds an area of caseous necrosis. Langhans' cells are observed occasionally, and the larger lesions are liable to central abscess formation.

Bronchopneumonia is a common development in tularemia, occurring in approximately 30 per cent of patients who acquire the disease, regardless of the type of infection. Histologically, the early lesion is edematous, and consists of fibrin and leukocytes associated with necrosis of alveolar walls. In non-necrotic areas the exudate consists of the large mononuclear type. The gross lesions resemble the bronchopneumonia of tuberculosis, although histologically there is less epithelioid cell transformation. Tubercle-like nodules are more common in lymph nodes than in the lungs. Mediastinal nodes are involved frequently.

Clinical Manifestations. The incubation period of tularemia ranges from two to ten days. Headache, fever, and toxic signs characterize all forms of the illness and are in no way dissimilar to those in other infectious illnesses. The pertinent historic and epidemiologic features are often helpful clues, and in approximately three fourths of all patients there is a primary lesion associated with adenopathy.

Ulceroglandular Tularemia. The initial lesion begins as a reddish papule, which is often undermined and more extensive than the small area of superficial induration indicates. Neighboring and draining lymph nodes are enlarged, tender, and discrete. Fluctuation of these nodes occurs later in the illness, after two or more weeks, when other acute signs may have partially abated. Such diseased nodes may subsequently require incision and drainage. The lymph nodes during the early stages are laden with *F. tularensis* and, if incised, may provoke bacteremia and toxemia. Fluctuant buboes four or more weeks old are usually sterile. Generalized lymphadenopathy occurs. Systemic signs of toxemia may be severe in ulceroglandular tularemia, although most cases are mild or moderate in severity. Pneumonia of all gradations may accompany this type of infection.

Occasionally, tularemia referred to as the glandular type may occur as generalized adenopathy and toxemia but without cutaneous lesions.

Enteric Form of Tularemia (Typhoidal or Cryptogenic). Following ingestion of infected animal tissues or water, ulcerative lesions of the buccal mucosa, pharynx, and intestine, and subsequent involvement of cervical, pharyngeal, and mesenteric lymph nodes may occur. The course of illness may be fulminant and fatal unless the disease is recognized and treated properly. Certain of these patients manifest illness that is similar to various forms of gastroenteritis and typhoid fever. These patients may be severely ill with sustained high fever, profound toxicity, stupor, and delirium or coma. This typhoidal systemic reaction may typify any of the clinical varieties of tularemia regardless of the presence of a cutaneous lesion. The term "cryptogenic" has often been used to connote the absence of an obvious portal of entry.

Pulmonary Tularemia. Lung involvement occurs in all forms of tularemia, subsequent to the bacteremia. Available evidence suggests that primary tularemic pneumonia is an entity, particularly in those persons such as laboratory workers who are exposed to infected aerosols. The incubation period varies from two to five days, depending upon the number of viable bacteria inhaled. In addition to headache, fever, malaise, and prostration, there is a nonproductive harassing cough and a sensation of substernal discomfort. Later the sputum may be mucoid or bloody and, in severely ill patients, there are pleural pain, dyspnea, tachycardia, and cyanosis.

In spite of extensive pulmonary involvement, there may be a paucity of physical signs. The early roentgenographic signs, seldom evident before the second to the fourth day of fever, consist of small irregular oval lesions with hilar adenopathy. Later in the illness, the infiltrate may be annular. True abscess formation is rare, although during resolution and convalescence, which in untreated cases or in those treated late may be prolonged, shadows suggesting abscess formation may be noted. Pleuritis with effusion is not uncommon.

Oculoglandular Tularemia. Following ocular contamination there may be pain, photophobia, intense congestion, itching, lacrimation, chemosis, and a mucopurulent discharge. Small yellowish granulomatous lesions may appear on the palpebral conjunctivae or cornea and may eventually ulcerate. The preauricular and other regional lymph nodes may enlarge and ultimately suppurate. In untreated patients, serious ocular complications including corneal perforation or optic atrophy may ensue.

Other General Manifestations. Initially, in severely ill patients, there is a rigor followed by pyrexia that persists for a month or more. The fever may be continuously high or remittent, and defervescence is usually gradual. Hepatomegaly and splenomegaly with tenderness over the respective organs are relatively common. Toxic signs in all cases include fever, headache, myalgia, and nausea. Rashes are very uncommon; when present, they consist of localized papular lesions along the peripheral lymphatics or maculopapular body eruptions. In untreated patients or in those first given antimicrobial therapy late in the course of illness, convalescence may be prolonged with sporadic episodes of fever, weakness, muscular pains, and chronic respiratory signs.

Nonspecific Laboratory Findings. The erythrocyte sedimentation rate and C-reactive protein are elevated during the active stages. In contrast, the total blood leukocyte count is usually normal or low. Occasionally there may be moderate leukocytosis. Mild albuminuria may occur at the height of illness.

Differential Diagnosis. Ulceroglandular tularemia is recognized readily in endemic areas. Punctate lesions with surrounding erythema at the site of prior arthropod attachment suggest *Rocky Mountain spotted fever*, particularly when associated with fever, headache, and toxic signs. The absence of a rash would favor tularemia, because patients with rickettsial disease develop a characteristic exanthem. *Meningococcemia* is recognized by its fulminant character, the typical exanthem, leukocytosis, and the bacteriologic findings. Fever, toxic signs, pharyngitis, adenitis, hepatomegaly, and splenomegaly are common to tularemia and *infectious mononucleosis*. The hematologic and serologic findings are usually distinctive. *Cat scratch disease* is characterized by peripheral ulceration and regional adenopathy; a history of contact with cats, the cutaneous reaction to specific antigens, and the absence of agglutinins for *F. tularensis* are distinguishing features. *Ecthyma* and *furunculi* are similar in some respects to this form of tularemia, although lymphadenitis and systemic signs are less likely to develop.

The lesions of *sporotrichosis* are multiple, occur along the course of lymphatics, attach themselves firmly to the skin, and are freely movable.

Certain forms of tularemia may present with clinical features similar to those of psittacosis, Q fever, and mycoplasmal pneumonia. Broad-spectrum antimicrobial drugs are effective in each of these conditions. Appropriate serologic tests or viral isolation may be required to define the precise cause. Influenza with associated pneumonia is similar but does not respond to specific drugs, and its clinical course is short. Fungal diseases, such as *histoplasmosis* and *coccidioidomycosis,* may be acute and may simulate pulmonary tularemia. Consideration of the history, the epidemiologic data, and the cutaneous manifestations, as well as the bacteriologic and serologic findings, usually will permit proper identification.

The presence of unexplained pleural effusion, similar to tuberculous fibrinous pleurisy, requires differentiation. The results of cultural and serologic tests will aid in differentiation.

Complications. Pericarditis and meningitis are distinctive but unusual complications of tularemia. Pericardial involvement may develop by direct extension from the pulmonary lesions or lymph nodes, and is characterized by a fibrinous or fibrocaseous exudate. In untreated patients constrictive pericarditis may ensue. Tularemic meningitis is characterized by a lymphocytic pleocytosis in the cerebrospinal fluid, and was usually fatal prior to the availability of specific antimicrobial drugs. Rare instances of tularemic peritonitis, perisplenitis, osteomyelitis, and endocarditis have been reported.

Treatment. Specific Therapy. Tularemia is very amenable to treatment with antimicrobial drugs. Streptomycin is preferable, but the broad-spectrum antimicrobials are equally beneficial in ameliorating the active manifestations. They are less effective, however, in eradicating the organism, primarily because of their bacteriostatic mode of action. With the latter drugs, relapses are liable to occur if treatment is initiated within the first week of illness.

Streptomycin. Streptomycin, when given in doses of 1.0 gram daily to adults for about one week, results in prompt recovery. Most patients are improved within 24 hours, and are afebrile within 48 hours. Relapses are uncommon with streptomycin except when insufficient drug is given during the very early stages of illness. Strains resistant to streptomycin do appear, a fact

which is of no clinical significance when infection is acquired naturally.

Chloramphenicol and Tetracycline Treatment. Broad-spectrum antimicrobials are very effective in rendering the patient afebrile and free from toxicity witin 48 to 72 hours. Relapses are uncommon when therapy is initiated 10 to 12 days after the onset of illness, but are frequent if it is given during the first week. *F. tularensis* does not develop resistance to chloramphenicol or tetracycline; hence, re-treatment leads to prompt response. Tetracycline is the preferable drug solely because reactions to it are less potentially serious.

The following dosage schedule is considered optimal: for chloramphenicol, an initial oral dose of 50 mg. per kilogram of body weight, and for tetracycline, 25 mg. per kilogram of body weight. Subsequent daily doses are calculated on the same basis as the initial loading dose, dividing the requirement equally and giving it at six- to eight-hour intervals. Antimicrobial therapy is continued until the patient is improved and has been afebrile for about five to seven days. Any of the above three drug regimens is wholly satisfactory, and no supplementary chemotherapy is necessary.

General Management. An adequate diet with appropriate protein intake is advisable. Oxygen treatment is indicated for all severely ill patients with pneumonia whether or not cyanosis is present. Other supportive measures useful for treating patients with pneumonia, such as frequent turning and the performing of a tracheostomy to provide a proper airway, are indicated. Thoracentesis for removal of fluid will allay respiratory embarrassment. The presence of any superimposed infection is detected by appropriate examination of the sputum, blood, or tissues.

The local ulcer requires no special measures. During the early several weeks of illness, lymph nodes should not be manipulated unduly or incised. Later, fluctuant buboes, which are usually sterile, may require incision and drainage. Recovery ensues rapidly.

Prognosis and Postinfection Immunity. In untreated patients, the case fatality rate in ulceroglandular tularemia was formerly approximately 5 per cent. However, of those patients with typhoidal tularemia or with pulmonary manifestations, about 30 per cent succumbed. With the advent of streptomycin and later the broad-spectrum antimicrobials, death from tularemia has been virtually eliminated and the morbidity shortened drastically to several days after institution of treatment, even among severely ill patients.

Second attacks of tularemia with systemic complications are uncommon, because recovery from the initial episode usually confers immunity. However, it is not unusual for patients to develop primary lesions when reinfected long after the initial systemic infection. Viable *F. tularensis* may be isolated from such recurrent primary ulcers, which resemble a Koch reaction. Under these conditions, systemic manifestations are unusual.

Under test conditions in volunteers, when streptomycin is given soon after intradermal infection (before the onset of clinical illness), an attack may be aborted fully. Immunity does not develop, agglutinins fail to appear, and such subjects are prone to further infection. This phenomenon is of little practical significance, as patients are usually encountered after about a week of incubated disease. Partial to complete resistance to infection follows such antigenic stimulation.

Control Measures. General. In infected areas those measures designed to repel ticks, mosquitoes, or deer flies should be employed. Gloves should be used for handling all potentially infected animals, particularly rabbits, and animals to be consumed should be cooked thoroughly. Laboratory workers exposed to infected aerosols should exercise care by wearing suitable masks and utilizing other protective devices.

Vaccination. The available killed vaccines afford only partial protection to man against tularemia. Viable attenuated preparations have been used with considerable success in the Soviet Union. The vaccine is administered intradermally and provokes a reaction similar in severity to that following smallpox immunization. Significant protection has been demonstrated in volunteers in the United States vaccinated with a similar viable product and who subsequently were exposed to virulent strains of *F. tularensis* by the respiratory or cutaneous routes. In those subjects who have developed clinical illness after immunization, the disease has been mild.

Foshay, L.: Tularemia. Ann. Rev. Microbiol., 4:313, 1950.

McCrumb, F. R.: Aerosol infection of man with *Pasteurella tularensis.* Bact. Rev., 25:262, 1961.

Meyer, K. F.: Pasteurella and franciscella. *In* Dubos, R., and Hirsch, J. G. (eds.): Bacterial and Mycotic Infections of Man. 4th ed. Philadelphia, J. B. Lippincott Company, 1965, Chap. 27, p. 659.

DISEASES CAUSED BY MALLEOMYCES

Leighton E. Cluff

GLANDERS
(Farcy)

Definition. Glanders, or farcy, is an infectious disease of horses, mules, and donkeys caused by *Malleomyces mallei.* The infection is occasionally transmitted to man, and is characterized by an acute fulminant febrile illness or a chronic indolent disease with abscesses of the respiratory tract or skin. Farcy refers to the nodular abscesses observed in skin, lymphatics, and subcutaneous tissues.

Etiology. Glanders was described by Aristotle about 330 B.C., and the occurrence of the disease in horses was observed by Apeyrtos about 375 A.D.

Royer's (1837) monograph on glanders in man remains the classic description of the disease. The micro-organism responsible for glanders was isolated in 1882. It is a gram-negative bacillus culturable aerobically on ordinary nutrient media. It is variously called *Malleomyces mallei, Bacillus mallei,* or *Pfeiferella mallei. M. mallei* is nonmotile. It elaborates a specific antigen (mallein) upon lysis that is used as a skin test material for diagnostic purposes. The bacillus is antigenically separable from *M. pseudomallei,* which causes melioidosis. When grown on potato slices or potato infusion agar, *M. mallei* produces a brown pigment resembling that of *Pseudomonas aeruginosa.* The bacillus produces fatal infection experimentally in guinea pigs and hamsters but will not cause disease in rats, cattle, hogs, or fowl.

Incidence and Prevalence. Glanders has probably never been a common disease in man. It occurs almost exclusively in persons handling horses and, therefore, is an occupational disease. It has been reported from all parts of the world. It has been eradicated in the United States and the United Kingdom, but may still occur in Asia and South America.

Epidemiology. Glanders is a communicable disease among horses, and it may occur sporadically in other animal species in contact with horses. In horses, glanders is manifested by nasal symptoms and abscesses and by cutaneous nodules or abscesses (farcy). Glanders is transmitted to man by direct contact with infected horses, the bacillus preferentially invading areas of abraded or injured skin. Experimental infection can be induced in animals by inhalation of the bacillus, and certain laboratory-acquired infections indicate that infection may develop in man following inhalation of the micro-organism. *Unlike melioidosis, glanders can be transmitted from person to person.*

Pathology and Pathogenesis. Characteristically glanders is associated with cellulitis, necrosis, abscess, and thromboses with septic embolization. Healing occurs by fibrosis, and, rarely, by calcification.

Clinical Manifestations. Glanders may occur as a fulminant acute febrile disease, as a chronic indolent and relapsing disease, or as a subclinical occult infection detectable incidentally at postmortem examination or by serologic test. The two principal features of glanders are (1) nasal cellulitis and necrosis-producing septal perforation, palatal and pharyngeal ulceration; or (2) cutaneous cellulitis, vesiculation, and ulceration at the site of inoculation of the bacillus into the skin, followed by lymphangitis with nodular abscesses along the lymphatics and lymphadenopathy (farcy).

Pulmonary involvement is common in glanders, producing pneumonia, abscesses, pleural effusion, and empyema. Occasionally, in chronic indolent glanders, small nodular granulomatous lesions may be found in the lungs. Hilar lymph node enlargement is common in pulmonary glanders.

When glanders becomes disseminated, destructive polyarthritis, subcutaneous and muscular abscesses, osteomyelitis, meningitis, and pustular skin lesions, particularly over the joints and face, are seen. Prostration and stupor may develop, and are followed by death in two to three weeks.

Chronic glanders may be punctuated by recurrent acute relapses with bacteremia, often resulting in a fulminant course and death. Amyloidosis may be a complication of chronic glanders.

Fever and chills, headache, and backache are common in acute glanders. Leukopenia or a normal leukocyte count is the rule, but leukocytosis has been observed.

Diagnosis. There are no pathognomonic clinical features of glanders. The nodules along lymphatics resemble those seen in sporotrichosis. The respiratory lesions may be difficult to distinguish from other ulcerative infections of the nose and mouth. The cutaneous lesion often resembles streptococcal cellulitis. The multiple abscesses mimic many mycotic and staphylococcal infections and are difficult to distinguish from those of melioidosis. The acute fulminant illness may resemble typhoid fever or disseminated tuberculosis. The diagnosis of glanders can be established by combination of a history of exposure to horses, isolation of *M. mallei,* serologic tests (agglutination, complement-fixation), and skin test with sterile culture filtrate (mallein). Inoculation of infected material into guinea pigs may facilitate identification of the micro-organism.

Treatment. There are reports of successful treatment of glanders with sulfonamides. Tetracycline, chloramphenicol, and streptomycin may be useful, but there is little clinical experience with these drugs in glanders. Because of the serious prognosis and the lack of documented experience with drug therapy, it is advisable to administer daily streptomycin (1.0 gram) in association with a sulfonamide or a tetracycline until all evidences of disease have disappeared. Incision, drainage, and excision of abscesses must be done with caution, for the infection may be disseminated by such manipulation.

Prognosis. Although a few patients have been cured with chemotherapy, the effect of treatment on the mortality rate is not known. *More than 90 per cent of patients with glanders will die from the disease if untreated.* However, the frequency of occurrence of occult or subclinical glanders is not known.

Prevention. Infected horses have been identified by skin tests with mallein and by serologic tests. Destruction of infected animals has eliminated glanders as a public health problem in the United States and most other countries.

Eghbal, M., Rafyi, A., Chamey, H. M., and Farvar, B.: Development of bacterial resistance to sulfonamides during therapy of glanders in man. Presse Med., 61:1535, 1953.

Howe, C.: Glanders. *In* Christian, H. A. (ed.): Oxford Medicine, vol. 5 (part 1, pp. 185-202). New York, Oxford University Press, 1950.

Howe, C., and Miller W. R.: Human glanders. Report of six cases. Ann. Intern. Med., 26:115, 1947.

Mendelson, R. W.: Glanders. U.S. Armed Forces Med. J., 1:781, 1950.

MELIOIDOSIS

Definition. Melioidosis is a rare disease of man caused by *Malleomyces pseudomallei.* It has been observed most frequently in Malaysia, China, Burma, India, and other parts of the Far East, but rarely has been observed in North and South America. It is a disease of wild rodents and some domesticated animals, and probably is transmitted to man by contact with diseased animals or animal excreta and possibly by contact with contaminated soil. The disease in man appears in a subclinical (only positive serologic tests), pulmonary, septicemic, or extrapulmonary form. The septicemic and pulmonary disease may be acute and fatal. The pulmonary and extrapulmonary infection with abscesses may be chronic and debilitating.

Etiology. Melioidosis was first identified by Whitmore and Krishnaswami (1912) in Rangoon. The disease was recognized as similar to glanders and attributable to a gram-negative bacillus resembling but differing from *Malleomyces mallei.* The micro-organism causing melioidosis has been variously called *Malleomyces pseudomallei, Bacillus whitmori,* and *Pfeiferella whitmori.* It is a motile bacillus that grows aerobically on nutrient agar. Culturally it may resemble Klebsiella and *Pseudomonas aeruginosa. M. pseudomallei* is antigenically distinguishable from *M. mallei.* It produces fatal infection in guinea pigs, rabbits, and other laboratory animals.

Epidemiology. *M. pseudomallei* has been found to cause disease sporadically, endemically, and epidemically among a wide variety of animal species, including rats, rabbits, goats, hogs, dogs, cats, and horses. In addition, the bacillus has been found to be harbored by mosquitoes and fleas. Frequently, the initial manifestations of melioidosis in man are cutaneous abscesses, diarrhea, and pneumonia; therefore, it is probable that the disease is transmitted by direct contact with infected animals or by ingestion or inhalation of contaminated material. All these routes of inoculation can produce the disease experimentally in animals. It is unlikely that melioidosis is ever transmitted from man to man. Infection has been observed in narcotic addicts, and in infants, or in patients with diabetes mellitus, renal or liver disease, and pregnancy as predisposing factors.

Clinical Manifestations. Melioidosis may appear acutely or insidiously, and most often follows a fulminant course with septicemia or a chronic indolent course with multiple abscess formation. The incubation period of the disease is not known. The acute illness is often associated with fever, chills, cough, production of bloody and purulent sputum, diarrhea, or abdominal pain. Physical examination may reveal signs of pneumonia, empyema, lung abscess, hepatomegaly, jaundice, and splenomegaly. *A subacute or chronic illness may follow the acute disease or may develop in the absence of an acute illness.* In this situation the patient often has osteomyelitis, suppurating lymphadenopathy, subcutaneous abscesses, psoas abscess, lung abscess, pyelonephritis, or liver or spleen abscess. Bronchocutaneous and other types of fistulas may appear. Patients with this chronic illness may survive for many months, and occasionally may recover.

Diagnosis. Melioidosis may resemble typhoid fever, malaria, mycotic infection, and occasionally acute staphylococcal septicemia or staphylococcal pneumonia. The chronic pulmonary disease most resembles tuberculosis. Melioidosis can be differentiated from these diseases only by bacteriologic identification of the bacillus from blood, sputum, urine, or pus. Hemagglutination and complement fixation tests may be useful when acute and convalescent serologic titers are compared. A single positive test may only indicate previous clinical and subclinical infection.

The leukocyte count of the peripheral blood often is normal in melioidosis, but may rise to levels of 20,000 per cubic millimeter. Urinalysis may show pyuria and hematuria.

Treatment and Prevention. There is no available antigen for active immunization against melioidosis. Prevention of the disease is possible by controlled sanitation and improved standards of living. Patients have been successfully treated with chloramphenicol, sulfonamides, or tetracycline, given over long periods of time. The drug susceptibility of *M. pseudomallei*, however, is variable. In adults, 3 grams of tetracycline a day orally for 30 days, or, alternatively, in septicemia, large doses of chloramphenicol are preferred. Surgical drainage of abscesses is essential for proper management.

Khaira, B. S., Young, W. B., and Hart, P. DeV.: Melioidosis. Brit. Med. J., 1:949, 1959.
Prevatt, A. L., and Hunt, J. S.: Chronic systemic melioidosis. Review of literature. Amer. J. Med., 23:810, 1957.
Spotnitz, M., Rudnitsky, A., and Rambaud, J. J.: Melioidosis pneumonitis. J.A.M.A., 202:950, 1967.

ANTHRAX
Leighton E. Cluff

Definition. Anthrax is an infectious disease of wild and domesticated animals caused by *Bacillus anthracis*. Occasionally it is transmitted to man. A necrotic ulcer of the skin or mucous membranes is the most common feature of the disease, but hemorrhagic mediastinitis and disseminated infection with hemorrhagic meningitis may also develop. Depending upon the most prominent feature of the disease, anthrax has been variously referred to as *malignant pustule, splenic fever, woolsorters' disease, milzbrand,* and *charbon.*

Etiology. *Bacillus anthracis* was identified in 1849 by Davaine, and was further characterized by Koch in 1877. It is a gram-positive, spore-forming, encapsulated, hemolytic, aerobic micro-organism. It resembles *B. subtilis* and *B. cereus* but can be

differentiated from these organisms by its virulence for laboratory animals such as the mouse and rabbit, by its lack of hemolytic activity on blood agar, and by lysis of *B. anthracis* with specific bacteriophage. In broth, the bacillus elaborates an antigen that can be used for specific immunization ("protective antigen"). The spores of *B. anthracis* are killed by boiling for ten minutes but survive for long periods of time in soil, in animal carcasses, and following aerosolization.

Epidemiology. Anthrax has occurred sporadically and in epidemics throughout the world. Cattle, sheep, goats, horses, and swine are most commonly found to have anthrax; outbreaks of the disease in these animals rarely occur in the United States. Although the disease has been acquired by butchering, skinning, or dissecting infected carcasses, human infection in the United States is observed almost exclusively in persons handling imported contaminated hides, wool, goat hair, or other animal products. There has been a progressive decrease in anthrax in the United States in the past several years (17 cases from 1956 to 1964). The infection may be transmitted to man by direct contact, inhalation, and ingestion of infected material.

Pathology and Pathogenesis. Anthrax is characterized by edema, hemorrhage, necrosis, and various degrees of inflammation. *B. anthracis* possesses a glutamyl polypeptide capsule that interferes with phagocytosis, and this contributes to its pathogenicity. The gelatinous edema of anthrax infection contains large amounts of bacterial capsular material. The serum of many animals has lytic activity against the bacillus, but this anthracidal substance seems to bear little, if any, relationship to natural resistance. It is probable that *B. anthracis* initiates infection in the skin only through abrasions, cuts, or other types of injury. During the course of lethal anthrax infection in laboratory animals a bacterial toxin is produced that is responsible for death. This lethal toxin can be neutralized by specific antitoxin.

Clinical Manifestations. The skin lesion of anthrax usually begins as a small erythematous papule that becomes vesicular, necrotic, and covered with a dark crust or eschar. Intense nonpitting edema, which may not be erythematous, often surrounds and may extend a considerable distance from the eschar. Characteristically the lesion is pruritic but not very tender or hot. The skin lesion is commonly on exposed areas of hands, arms, neck, or face; and there may be mild regional lymph node enlargement. Lymphangitis is not usually observed. Constitutional symptoms and fever are frequently absent unless the skin disease is severe or the infection becomes disseminated, when high fever, prostration, and death may occur.

Infrequently anthrax may develop without a lesion, possibly following inoculation into the skin, but probably more commonly following inhalation of spores of the bacillus in contaminated air. Characteristically, this form of anthrax is severe and is associated with disseminated infection. *Hemorrhagic mediastinitis,* often without pneumonia, and *hemorrhagic meningitis* may occur. Death is common in this form of anthrax; the illness may begin abruptly, be of short duration, and terminate rapidly. Dyspnea and cyanosis are indicative of respiratory or ventilatory insufficiency. Roentgenographic examination of the chest in inhalation anthrax reveals widening of the mediastinum. Leukocytosis is ordinarily not pronounced. Pleural effusion may complicate pulmonary anthrax. Anthrax in man from ingestion of bacilli is rare.

Diagnosis. Anthrax is most readily diagnosed in persons known to have been exposed to animals or animal products potentially contaminated with *B. anthracis.* Cutaneous anthrax can be differentiated from many other bacterial infections of the skin by the insignificance of regional adenopathy, lymphangitis, and cellulitis in relation to the severity of the eschar and edema. Furthermore, pruritus, lack of tenderness, and intense nonpitting edema are characteristic of anthrax. Small skin lesions, however, may be more difficult to recognize. Pulmonary anthrax can be identified by a history of occupational exposure and acute widening of the mediastinum shown by roentgenographic examination. Anthrax meningitis is confused with subarachnoid hemorrhage or cerebrovascular accident, but is usually associated with prominent signs of infection, and gram-positive bacilli can be seen in the cerebrospinal fluid.

In disseminated anthrax infection, blood cultures are often positive. Occasionally, the bacilli may be identified in the centrifugal sediment of blood treated with 3 per cent acetic acid solution and stained with Wright's stain.

In cutaneous anthrax, the bacilli can usually be cultured from the lesions, or typical encapsulated bacilli will be seen when stained with a polychrome eosin–methylene blue stain (Wright or Giemsa). Their direct cultivation on peptone agar should always be attempted. If the specimen has to be shipped, the specimen should be dried on silk threads or on a sterile glass slide. In view

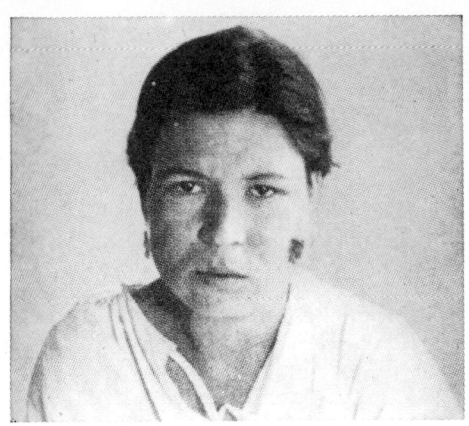

FIGURE 2. Same patient 72 hours after start of oxytetracycline therapy. Note virtually complete disappearance of edema. *B. anthracis* no longer demonstrable in stained smears of exudate. (Courtesy of Drs. Vernon Knight and A. Ruiz Sanchez.)

of the occurrence of anthrax-like bacilli on the skin, it is imperative that diagnoses be confirmed by animal inoculations, preferably in guinea pigs or mice or by specific bacteriophage lysis. In pulmonary anthrax, the bacillus has been found microscopically in the sputum and in the pleural exudate.

Prognosis. Cutaneous anthrax is often a self-limited disease, but dissemination of the infection and death may occur in 20 per cent of patients. A fatal outcome in cutaneous anthrax can be averted by appropriate treatment, but treatment of disseminated infection is often unsuccessful in preventing death.

Treatment. *B. anthracis* is susceptible to the action of penicillin and the tetracyclines. Penicillin G should be given in total daily doses of at least 1.2 million units, starting as soon as anthrax is diagnosed or seriously suspected. The effectiveness of the tetracyclines is probably not quite so great as that of penicillin; nevertheless, they are effective in cutaneous anthrax (Figs. 1 and 2), and may be administered in total daily dose of 2.0 grams. Therapy with penicillin or the tetracyclines should be continued for seven days. It should be emphasized that, in patients with disseminated anthrax, the progressive course may be so rapid that antimicrobial drugs may not save the patient's life.

Prevention. Anthrax can be prevented in man by control of infected animals or animal products. Sterilization of wool during manufacture is often impracticable, although this is the means employed to prevent infection from clothing and other products, such as shaving brushes, made of potentially infected materials. Vaccination with "protective antigen" is effective in preventing infection in persons likely to be occupationally exposed.

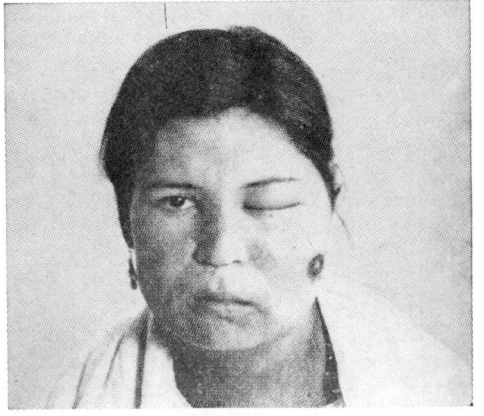

FIGURE 1. Cutaneous anthrax with facial and orbital edema immediately preceding oxytetracycline therapy. Innumerable *B. anthracis* visible on stained smear of material from lesion. (Courtesy of Drs. Vernon Knight and A. Ruiz Sanchez.)

Brachman, P. S.: Human anthrax in the United States. *In* Hobby, G. L. (ed.): Antimicrobial Agents and Chemotherapy. Baltimore, Williams and Wilkins Company, 1965.

Brachman, P. S., Plotkin, S. A., Bumford, F. H., and Atchison, M. M.: An epidemic of inhalation anthrax. II. Epidemiologic investigation. Amer. J. Hyg., 72:6, 1960.

Gold, H.: Anthrax: Report of 117 cases. Arch. Intern. Med. (Chicago), 96:387, 1955.

Plotkin, S. A., Brachman, P. S., Utell, M., Bumford, F. H., and Atchison, M. M.: Epidemic of inhalation anthrax, first in twentieth century. I. Clinical features. Amer. J. Med., 29:992, 1960.

Smith, H., and Keppie, J.: Studies on the chemical basis of pathogenicity of *Bacillus anthracis* using organisms grown in vivo. In Howie, J. W., and O'Hea, A. J. (eds.): Mechanisms of Microbial Pathogenicity. London, Cambridge University Press, 1955.

LISTERIOSIS
Leighton E. Cluff

Definition. Listeriosis is an infectious disease of animals and man with exceptionally protean manifestations, including meningitis, disseminated granulomas, lymphadenopathy, respiratory symptoms, and ill-defined acute febrile illness. It can produce abortion and fetal or neonatal death. The infection is caused by a gram-positive bacillus called *Listeria monocytogenes* and is world-wide in distribution.

Etiology. Infection of the human being with *Listeria monocytogenes* was identified in 1929 by Nyfeldt. The micro-organism was first characterized, however, by Murray, Webb, and Swann in 1926 during an epizootic among rabbits and guinea pigs. Subsequently the micro-organism has been identified as a cause of disease in fox, raccoon, goat, lemming, mouse, rat, hamster, pig, horse, cow, dog, domestic fowl and wild birds, and other animals. *L. monocytogenes* is a gram-positive, non-spore-forming, aerobic or microaerophilic, motile bacillus. It ferments a number of sugars, with formation of acid but no gas. It can be grown on nutrient agar or broth, preferably containing 1 per cent glucose, and produces beta hemolysis on blood agar. *L. monocytogenes* resembles *Erysipelothrix rhuziopathiae* and diphtheroids, but can be differentiated from these bacteria by its motility (best at 20 to 30° C.), its specific antigenicity, and its animal pathogenicity. Listeria regularly — and Erysipelothrix occasionally — produces purulent keratoconjunctivitis in rabbits following inoculation into the conjunctival space, whereas diphtheroids do not.

Incidence and Prevalence. Listeriosis in man and animals has been observed throughout the world. It has been recognized more frequently in humans in recent years, but its true incidence is not known. Confusion in bacteriologic differentiation accounts largely for inadequate recognition of listeriosis. In addition, the diverse manifestations of the disease render it difficult to identify clinically.

Epidemiology. Listeriosis may develop following inhalation, ingestion, or direct contact with contaminated food or animal products. The disease is more common in persons living in rural areas. Although infection with Listeria occurs in many domesticated and wild animals, there are only rare instances of epizootics or outbreaks in animals other than man. Transmission of infection from person to person probably does not occur. Women can carry Listeria in the vagina, and infection may be transmitted venereally. Whether or not man can be an asymptomatic carrier of Listeria under other conditions is not known.

Pathology and Pathogenesis. Human listeriosis is characterized by disseminated granulomas and focal necrosis or suppuration in involved tissues. Lesions may develop in liver, intestinal tract, skin, mucous membranes of the respiratory tract, lung, heart, spleen, lymph nodes, placenta, and brain. The fetus may be infected transplacentally through the umbilical vein, with production of septicemia. Debilitating diseases such as chronic infection and cancer predispose to the occurrence of listeriosis. Pregnancy may increase susceptibility to infection, but the disease in pregnant women may be less severe than in other persons. Administration of adrenal cortical steroids may also increase susceptibility to listeriosis.

Clinical Manifestations. *Meningitis* is the most commonly recognized form of listeriosis in the United States. It is characterized at onset by symptoms of headache, myalgia, fever, chills, nausea, vomiting, and photophobia, followed by the development of stiff neck, stupor, convulsions, somnolence, and, finally, death. The onset may be abrupt or gradual, and the initial symptoms may be those of gastrointestinal or respiratory illness. Examination reveals manifestations of meningitis or encephalitis in varying degrees of severity. There may be pharyngitis, rhinitis, otitis media, neck rigidity, ocular palsy, and signs of depressed cerebral function. Leukocytosis is the rule, with granulocytosis and, occasionally, monocytosis, in the early phase of the disease. The cerebrospinal fluid, with decreased sugar, elevated protein, and cell counts of 150 to 3000 per cubic millimeter, is indistinguishable from that in many purulent meningitides. Early, the cells in the fluid may be principally granulocytes, but later there may be a predominance of mononuclear cells.

Febrile pharyngitis with cervical and generalized lymphadenopathy can be caused by Listeria, and may be difficult to differentiate from infectious mononucleosis. Patients with this type of illness, however, may have an abrupt onset of fever, chills, headache, myalgia, conjunctivitis, macular rash, and sore throat. Lymph nodes in the neck and elsewhere may enlarge, and there may be hepatosplenomegaly. Blood leukocytes occasionally increase in number with a more or less pronounced monocytosis. The absorbed heterophil serologic test for infectious mononucleosis is negative, Listeria can be isolated from blood and pharynx, and there will be a rising serum agglutinin titer for Listeria.

Lymph node enlargement in the neck and elsewhere without respiratory symptoms may also be attributed to listeriosis. In addition, lymph node enlargement associated only with conjunctivitis may occur. Isolated acute upper respiratory illness may be attributable to listeriosis, although for obvious reasons this diagnosis is seldom established. Chronic urethritis in men has been described, and possibly may be responsible for subclinical or occult infection, demonstrable by culture of the bacillus from bone marrow.

Papular skin lesions associated with disseminated listeriosis have been seen in infants, but adults may acquire primary cutaneous infection after direct contact with infected animal tissues. *Disseminated listeriosis* in infants has been reported frequently in Europe, but infrequently in the United States. The disease may arise by transplacental infection of the fetus, causing abortion, fetal death, or serious illness within several days after birth. The disease is characterized by disseminated visceral granulomas and abscesses. When it manifests itself in infants a few weeks old, it often begins as a mild febrile illness with cough, coryza, gastrointestinal symptoms, and pneumonia. Granulomas may be formed on the posterior pharyngeal wall. Granulocytosis and occasionally mononucleosis are present. Pleural and pericardial effusions may develop. Listeriosis has been reported as a common cause of neonatal death and fetal damage in Europe.

Listeriosis in pregnancy may be subclinical or may be associated with an acute febrile illness resembling influenza and occasionally pyelonephritis; it is rarely severe. Its occurrence after the fifth month of pregnancy, however, is likely to affect the fetus seriously. A woman may become a vaginal carrier of Listeria and may possibly infect her infant at birth.

Disseminated listeriosis in adults has an abrupt onset with chill and fever. Meningitis can occur, as well as bacterial endocarditis. Blood cultures are usually positive, and there may be a consumptive coagulopathy. This type of listeriosis is observed most often in patients with carcinoma or debilitating disease, and its development may have been facilitated by adrenal steroid therapy.

Diagnosis. There are no pathognomonic clinical features of human listeriosis. The diagnosis rests on isolation of the micro-organism or rising agglutinin titers in the serum. It is likely that the recognition of listeriosis has been difficult because of the failure to differentiate Listeria from diphtheroid bacilli in culture. The isolation of micro-organisms resembling diphtheroids from infectious material or blood should alert one to the necessity for further bacteriologic characterization.

Listeriosis may resemble influenza, miliary tuberculosis, typhoid fever, mycotic infections, and several bacterial infections with septicemia. *Infectious mononucleosis* is most often confused with listeriosis in adults, for the two diseases may be clinically alike. However, listeriosis is infrequently associated with monocytosis, does not produce a positive absorbed heterophil serologic test, and in systemic disease the bacillus can be isolated from blood, bone marrow, urine, or upper respiratory tract.

Treatment. *Listeria monocytogenes* is susceptible in vitro to sulfonamides, penicillin, tetracycline, chloramphenicol, erythromycin, novobiocin, and occasionally streptomycin. Penicillin is the drug of choice, but the tetracyclines and erythromycin are also effective. Treatment should be continued for a period of several days, depending upon the characteristics of the disease.

Prognosis. Listeria meningitis has a fatality rate of 70 per cent in untreated patients. The fatality rate in treated patients has not been defined, but is considerably lower. The prognosis in adults with pharyngitis and lymph node enlargement is good, whether treated or not, but meningitis may supervene. Recovery from meningitis may leave residual symptoms of central nervous system damage. Infection of the newborn is very serious; the fatality rate and the incidence of congenital defects are high. Untreated, disseminated listeriosis is usually a fatal disease.

Prevention. Listeriosis must be regarded as a contagious disease of animals; prevention of human infection would require elimination of animal reservoirs. Pasteurization prevents transmission of the disease by contaminated milk. Animal products, including meat, should be declared unfit for consumption if the disease is found in slaughtered animals. Better recognition of the disease should clarify its epidemiology and indirectly facilitate control measures. There are no effective agents for immunization.

Gray, M. L., and Killinger, A. H.: *Listeria monocytogenes* and listeric infections. Bact. Rev., 30:309, 1966.

Hoeprich, P. D.: Infections due to *Listeria monocytogenes*. Medicine, 37:143, 1958.

Seeliger, H. P. R.: Listeriosis. New York, Hafner Publishing Company., 1961.

ERYSIPELOID OF ROSENBACH
Leighton E. Cluff

Erysipeloid of Rosenbach is a specific infectious disease attributable to *Erysipelothrix rhuziopathia*. It occurs in man following contact with infected animals or animal products, particularly swine, cattle, sheep, fish, birds, dogs, horses, reindeer, rabbits, mink, rats, and mice. The disease in man, therefore, usually arises in abattoir employees, butchers, kitchen workers, those handling fish, those handling animal hides and pelts, and those working with bone or bone meal. Most infections in human beings can be related to skin injury. The causative micro-organism is a gram-positive bacillus, non-spore-forming, that can be grown aerobically or anaerobically on nutrient broth containing 1 per cent glucose or upon blood agar. It produces death in laboratory animals, particularly mice, causing focal abscesses in the liver or cutaneous cellulitis. The bacillus is susceptible in vitro to tetracycline, penicillin, and chloramphenicol.

Erysipeloid in man occurs seasonally, usually in

summer and early fall, and is worldwide in distribution. Most commonly it is characterized by a nonsuppurative violaceous lesion of the hand or fingers that is swollen, very slightly tender, and has a sharply defined margin rarely extending above the wrist. In contrast to streptococcal cellulitis there are usually burning, tingling, and itching, but little pain in the involved area, rarely does the patient have systemic symptoms of fever, chills, malaise, or headache. Lymphangitis is infrequent, and when it develops it is often attributable to secondary infection with staphylococci or streptococci. The localized disease is self-limited, lasting a few days, and resolution is rapid, associated with brownish discoloration of the involved skin and rarely desquamation. A bacteriologic diagnosis can be made by culture of material aspirated or biopsied from the margin of the lesion, but isolation of the bacillus is not invariable. Ordinarily, the lesion is sufficiently distinctive to permit a clinical diagnosis when the microorganism is not cultured.

Infrequently Erysipelothrix infections may become disseminated, causing a diffuse involvement of skin. Rarely, bacteremia may develop, and bacterial endocarditis can occur.

Erysipeloid continues to occur frequently in exposed persons. The ubiquitousness of the bacillus has made it difficult to eradicate the disease. The ordinarily benign character of the infection, however, has made it an insignificant public health problem. Treatment of erysipeloid with penicillin has been shown to shorten the illness, but relapses of the disease have occurred in persons who are untreated or who receive inadequate treatment.

Ewing, M.: Erysipeloid. Med. J. Aust., 1:449, 1957.
Klauden, J. V.: Erysipeloid as an occupational disease. J.A.M.A., 111:1345, 1938.
Price, J. E. L., and Bennett, W. E. J.: The erysipeloid of Rosenbach. Brit. Med. J., 2:1060, 1951.
Sneath, P. H. A., Abbott, J. D., and Cunliffe, A. C.: The bacteriology of erysipeloid. Brit. Med. J., 2:1063, 1951.

BARTONELLOSIS
(Carrión's Disease, Oroya Fever, Verruga Peruana)
Herbert L. Ley, Jr.

Definition. Bartonellosis is an insect-borne bacterial disease limited to South America. It is characterized by two distinctive clinical stages. The first of these (Oroya fever) presents a severe febrile infection associated with a marked anemia, bone and joint pains, bacteremia, and an appreciable mortality. The second stage (verruga peruana) is more benign and is distinguished by the appearance of a generalized eruption of hemangiomatous papules and nodules.

Etiology. The disease is caused by *Bartonella bacilliformis,* a small gram-negative pleomorphic bacillus that may be cultivated readily in enriched

bacterioloic media. The disease is transmitted to man by the bite of sandflies of the genus *Phlebotomus,* with development of the characteristic symptoms of Oroya fever after an incubation period of two weeks to three months.

Prevalence and Distribution. Although a number of epidemics of the disease have been reported, it is more commonly seen as sporadic cases among populations of Peru, Colombia, and Ecuador, and is restricted within these countries to those who live at altitudes of 1500 to 9000 feet on both slopes of the Andes. In general, the distribution of the disease coincides with the ecologic zones supporting populations of *Phlebotomus.*

Epidemiology. In Peru the disease is transmitted by *Phlebotomus verrugarum,* a night-biting sandfly. The biting habits of the vectors in the other countries are similar, although the species of *Phlebotomus* involved in transmission in the other areas are not conclusively identified. The principal reservoir of the disease appears to be man; no additional animal reservoirs have as yet been implicated in nature. Reports of cultivation of the agent from apparently healthy persons suggest that as much as 10 per cent of infections may be subclinical. Persons convalescent from the disease are known to have a low-level bacteremia for months or years, providing frequent opportunities for infection of the disease vector.

Pathology and Physiologic Responses. In the Oroya fever stage of illness the causative organism may be found in peripheral blood smears stained with Giemsa or Wright's stain as well as in the reticuloendothelial cells of the viscera and lymphatics. In the blood the parasite is found both free in the plasma and adhering to the erythrocytes. The parasitization of the erythrocytes causes an increased mechanical fragility and also an increased sequestration of the cells in the spleen and the liver. A hypochromic and macrocytic anemia develops rapidly during the febrile period, erythrocyte counts decreasing within a period of only a few days to levels of one million to two million cells per cubic millimeter. The bone marrow is hyperplastic, with an abundance of nucleated erythrocytes. The pathologic findings secondary to the anemia are absent in the verruga stage of infection. The histopathology of the skin lesions is that of dilation of the capillaries and proliferation of the vascular endothelial cells that may be shown to contain the causative agent.

Clinical Manifestations. The presenting symptoms of patients with Oroya fever are intermittent high fever, painful muscles and joints, tender enlarged lymph nodes and the systemic symptoms and prostration of a severe anemia. These symptoms may persist from several weeks to several months in untreated patients, half of whom may die within the first three weeks of fever. If the patient survives, gradual convalescence is punctuated, after a few days to a month, by the appearance of the cutaneous lesions of the second phase of the disease. The verrugae may persist for a month to a year in untreated persons, but mortality is negligible. Occasional patients may experience only the fever and anemia without the skin manifestations, or only the cutaneous lesions without the initial fever. Although these two aspects of the infection were once thought to be different diseases, there is no doubt that both syndromes are manifestations of infection with the same organism. The current interpretation that the skin lesions are an expression of developing immunity in the patient is supported by the observation that second attacks of the disease are exceedingly rare even in highly endemic areas and that the attacks are almost always caused by verruga rather than by Oroya fever.

Diagnosis. In endemic areas the diagnosis can usually be made on the basis of clinical findings. In the acute stage of Oroya fever both blood smears and blood culture usually reveal the presence of the agent. As the patient progresses toward the verruga stage of infection, or with treatment, the organism becomes more difficult to demonstrate.

Treatment and Prognosis. The prognosis in the untreated patient depends upon both the nature and the severity of his infection. Mortality in the Oroya fever phase of the disease may exceed 50 per cent, particularly when the infection is complicated by concurrent attacks of malaria, amebiasis, tuberculosis, salmonellosis, or other diseases. The disease responds well to treatment with penicillin, streptomycin, chloramphenicol, and the tetracyclines. Chloramphenicol is favored by many South American clinicians because of the frequency of concurrent salmonella infections, but the risks of its potentially more serious toxicity must be weighed against the fact that the other drugs mentioned are therapeutically effective. In general, as in the rickettsial infections, the tetracyclines are the preferred form of antimicrobial therapy for bartonellosis. When the broad-spectrum antimicrobials have been used, oral doses of 1 to 2 grams per day have been used for a period of a week or more with excellent results. Patients become afebrile in 24 to 48 hours, and, if they receive transfusions, recover strength rapidly. Although the mortality of the verruga stage of infection is less than 5 per cent, antimicrobial therapy is desirable to hasten the disappearance of the skin lesions.

Prevention. Control measures are directed principally against the *Phlebotomus* vector. Because the insect is a night feeder and moves by a series of short "hops" between surfaces, the application of a residual insecticide, such as DDT, to the exterior and interior of doorways, windows, and other avenues of entry to human habitation is effective. Where insecticide application is impracticable, bed nets or insect repellents provide significant protection. Control of breeding of the vector is difficult, but may be undertaken when it is otherwise impossible to prevent contact of the vector with man. No protective vaccine is available. Patients need not be isolated in hospital wards if the vector is absent because the disease cannot be transmitted by person-to-person contact.

Reynafarje, C., and Ramos, J.: The hemolytic anemia of human bartonellosis. Blood, 17:562, 1961.
Urteaga, B. O., and Payne, E. H.: Treatment of the acute febrile phase of Carrión's disease with chloramphenicol. Amer. J. Trop. Med., 4:507, 1955.
Weinman, D.: The Bartonella Group. *In:* Dubos, R. J., and Hirsch, J. G. (eds.): Bacterial and Mycotic Infections of Man. 4th ed. Philadelphia, J. B. Lippincott Company, 1965, p. 775.

BRUCELLOSIS
(Undulant Fever, Malta Fever)
Vernon Knight

Definition. Brucellosis is an infectious disease caused by micro-organisms of the genus Brucella, transmitted to man from lower animals. The disease may be subclinical, subacute, acute, chronic, or relapsing, and infection may localize in various viscera and tissues, including the endocardium, bone marrow, biliary tract, liver, spleen, meninges, and eye.

Etiology. Brucellae are small, gram-negative, aerobic, nonmotile and non-spore-forming coccobacilli. Three species, characterized by their affinity for a particular animal host, account for most human infections: *Brucella abortus* (cattle), *Brucella melitensis* (sheep and goats), and *Brucella suis* (pigs). A newly described species, *Brucella canis,* causes abortion in beagles and has, on infrequent occasions, been transmitted to humans in contact with infected dogs.

History. Brucellae were first isolated by Bruce in 1887 from the spleens of British soldiers dying on the island of Malta. This disease, now known to have been caused by infection with *B. melitensis,* was contracted by drinking raw goat's milk. Bang, in 1897 in Denmark, isolated a strain of the species now designated *B. abortus* from cattle with infectious abortion. Traum in 1914 isolated the third species, *B. suis,* from an infected sow.

Epidemiology. Human brucellosis in the United States most commonly results from ingestion of raw milk or unpasteurized milk products from infected cattle. Infection also occurs in slaughterhouse workers, farmers, and veterinarians as a result of contact with infected meat or infected placentas of cattle, pigs, goats, and sheep. Although species affinities of brucellae are usually maintained, pigs may be infected with and spread *B. melitensis,* as well as *B. suis.*

Up to 5 per cent of cattle and 1 to 2 per cent of swine in this country are infected. In countries that utilize sheep and goats more extensively, these animals constitute the predominant sources of infection. In the case of ingested dairy products, the organism penetrates the gastrointestinal mucosa; with direct contact the organism enters through breaks in the skin or the conjunctiva. It presumably may also be inhaled, because brucellae have been isolated from the air of a slaughterhouse where infected animals were killed, and infection is readily transmitted to laboratory animals by aerosol. Many persons have become infected with the organism in the laboratory, and one laboratory accident involving apparent airborne spread has been described. Brucellae are destroyed in milk and milk products by pasteurization; otherwise, they may remain viable in refrigerated milk for 10 days and in cheese up to 90 days. They may persist in meat for several weeks.

Pathogenesis and Pathology. After penetration of skin or mucous membranes, the organisms spread via lymphatics to regional nodes and thence to thoracic duct and the blood stream. Hematogenous dissemination leads to localization in spleen, bone marrow, liver, kidneys, endocardium, and elsewhere. In cattle, swine, sheep, and goats, organisms also localize in mammary glands, male and female genital organs, and in the pregnant uterus, fetal fluids, and membranes, causing abortion. Correlated with genital, uterine, and fetal infection is the finding, in these tissues, of a 4-carbon, polyhydric alcohol, erythritol, which promotes the growth of brucellae. Although erythritol is apparently not present in the human testicle, orchitis is, paradoxically, a complication of human brucella infection. Erythritol is not present in human placentas, and brucellosis is not associated with abortions in humans.

Characteristically, Brucella infections are granulomas consisting of foci of lymphocytes, epithelioid cells, plasma cells, and multinucleated giant cells. In severe cases, caseation necrosis and abscess formation may occur, a finding most characteristic of infection with *B. suis*. The brucellae are found within monocytes. In this location they are apparently protected, to a degree, against bactericidal antibodies and are altered in their susceptibility to some antimicrobial drugs. This property may be related to the phenomenon of chronicity, yet monocytes in animals previously infected with Brucella have an increased capacity to destroy the organisms, presumably as an expression of "cellular" immunity.

Manifestations. The incubation period varies from a few days to a few weeks or even months. Onset may be insidious with nonspecific findings such as low-grade fever, headache, weakness, joint pains, insomnia, sweats, and low back pain. Less commonly, onset may be abrupt with high fever, chills, and prostration, but with few localizing signs. It is probable that fever and some of the other acute manifestations of infection are an effect, at least in part, of Brucella endotoxin, which resembles endotoxin from other gram-negative bacteria. Some lymphadenopathy occurs in about one half of cases, and splenomegaly occurs in about one third, usually in the more severely ill. Some exposed persons develop no detectable illness or mild symptoms not distinguishable from other common illnesses. Such patients usually develop agglutinins and, rarely, patients with few symptoms have been found to have positive blood cultures.

Brucellosis has been diagnosed occasionally in patients with Hodgkin's disease and other forms of reticuloendothelial neoplasia. Apparently, when such neoplastic processes affect patients with Brucella infection, the neoplasia may interfere with immunity and lead to dissemination of the organism from localized foci of infection.

Infrequent but severe *complications of brucellosis* include *meningoencephalitis*, *spondylitis*, *endocarditis*, *orchitis*, *pancytopenia*, *nephritis*, *hepatic* and *splenic suppuration*, *cholecystitis*, *arthritis*, and *uveitis*. When the complication is the presenting complaint, as is sometimes the case, the diagnosis of brucellosis may not be suggested. For that reason the varied involvement possible with this disease should be kept in mind. Careful questioning will usually elicit a history consistent with exposure to infection with this organism.

The initial illness may persist a few days or a few weeks, and improvement may be followed by one or more relapses. Renewed physical activity may provoke relapse. The accompanying figure illustrates the course of a patient with acute *B. melitensis* infection who responded to treatment with oxytetracycline. Her disease relapsed a few weeks later but was successfully re-treated with the same drug. In untreated cases, disability for a year or more is not unusual. A few patients may have low fever, weakness, joint pains, mental depression, and other vague complaints for up to several years, in association with serologic evidence of infection. Such patients, usually designated as having chronic brucellosis, may show little response to antimicrobial treatment, and the mechanism of their illness is unclear.

Instances of chronic, recurrent, suppurative disease of liver or spleen of many years' duration have also been described. The lesions often calcify with the passage of time, and calcific densities in roentgenograms of liver or spleen may be a clue to diagnosis. Such cases usually respond to treatment, although recovery is slow, and relapses may occur.

Diagnosis. Definitive diagnosis will depend upon isolation of the organism from blood, bone marrow, or local sites of involvement. Cultures should be examined for growth every four to five days, and not be discarded before six weeks of incubation.

The organisms may be isolated in trypticase soy or tryptose phosphate broth; the primary isolation of *B. abortus* requires the presence of 10 per cent carbon dioxide. Virulent organisms possess a capsule and grow as small, glistening translucent colonies on agar. This property is gradually lost by cultivation on artificial media (smooth → rough mutation). *B. abortus* is inhibited by thionine, whereas *B. suis* and *B. melitensis* are inhibited by basic fuchsin and crystal violet. *B. suis* may be distinguished from the other species by production of H_2S. Within species, patterns of metabolic activity and other characteristics permit the definition of several "biotypes," which may be of value in epidemiologic work.

Cross-reacting agglutinating antibodies are formed in response to two principal antigenic determinants common to virulent strains of the three major species. Studies suggest that the anti-

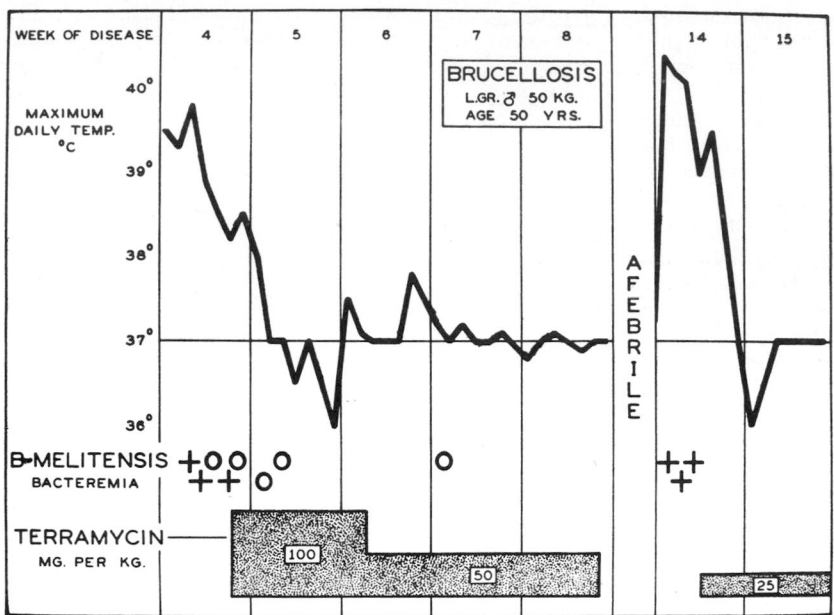

Bacteremic relapse in *B. melitensis* infection and successful re-treatment with oxytetracycline. (Case of Dr. F. Ruiz Sanchez, Guadalajara, Mexico; from Knight, V.: Ann. N.Y. Acad. Sci., 53:332, 1950.)

gens are specific, surface polysaccharides. They are designated M and A (M for *melitensis,* which predominates in this species, and A for *abortus,* which predominates in *B. abortus* and *B. suis*). These characteristics permit serologic differentiation of *B. melitensis* from the other two species.

Agglutinating antibody is usually present by the time the patients are first seen. Titers of 1:80 or greater are indicative of past or present infection. There is considerable variation in the titer of agglutinating antibody in both acute and chronic brucellosis; in addition, in some cases, lower dilutions of serologic tests will not show agglutination when higher dilutions are positive (prozone reaction). This reaction is caused by incomplete or blocking antibodies, and can be avoided by using 5 per cent sodium chloride or albumin solution as a diluent instead of physiologic saline.

An intradermal skin test is available utilizing several preparations of Brucella antigen. It is of the delayed hypersensitivity type, and has about the same significance as the tuberculin test. As positive skin tests are frequent in endemic areas, the test is of little value in diagnosis of individual cases; moreover, the test may elicit a low titer of circulating Brucella agglutinins.

Differential Diagnosis. Acute febrile brucellosis must be differentiated from diseases whose onset is associated with fever but without localizing signs. These include influenza, other viral respiratory infections, infectious mononucleosis, early stages of infectious hepatitis, malaria, typhoid, primary histoplasmosis, disseminated tuberculosis, and lymphoma.

Chronic brucellosis may simulate psychoneurosis, anxiety states, and mental depression. Except in infrequent cases when serum agglutinins are not detected because of prozone reactions and blood cultures are negative, it is usually possible to discover laboratory evidence of Brucella infection, and the diagnosis should not be made without such evidence. The skin test should not be depended upon for diagnosis of brucellosis.

Treatment. Tetracycline and its derivatives are usually effective in relieving the acute manifestations of the infection. Tetracycline, 0.5 gram four times daily for a period of 21 days, is recommended for uncomplicated Brucella infection in adults. Some patients in the first few hours of treatment will have a Herxheimer-like reaction characterized by increased fever, weakness, hypotension, and generalized discomfort. These clear spontaneously and, in the author's experience, have not been a serious problem. In more severe cases streptomycin, 0.5 gram twice daily, may be given during the first two weeks of tetracycline treatment. Relapses can be re-treated on the same regimen as was used initially. In patients with the rare but serious complication of pancytopenia, steroids, such as prednisone, 40 to 50 mg. per day, should be given for the first seven to ten days of antimicrobial treatment. Steroids may also be beneficial in relieving the prostration of more severely ill patients.

Prognosis. Most acute cases of brucellosis respond to a course of antimicrobial therapy with a prompt and lasting recovery. Relapse may occur one or more times in about 5 per cent of cases treated 21 days or longer, but responds to re-treatment. There is some evidence that there may be residual damage in patients with Brucella nephritis. In untreated brucellosis, the mortality is less than 2 per cent, and the majority of the patients make a complete recovery within three to six months. There remains a group, however, approximately one fifth of those infected, in whom relapsing disease is present for a year or more. As the individual episodes are usually acute, although milder than the original attacks, this protracted course of acute brucellosis is not easily confused with so-called "chronic brucellosis."

Chronic brucellosis is a syndrome that is not well understood, and its variable and relatively mild symptomatology may not respond to antimicrobial therapy. When a basis for treatment exists, i.e., history of possible exposure, symptomatology consistent with the infection, and serologic (or cultural) evidence of infection, it is reasonable to give antimicrobial treatment. If relapse occurs, re-treatment may be given once or twice. Thereafter, barring the presence of localized foci of infection, the illness is probably not related to brucellosis infection, and no more antimicrobial treatment should be given.

Prevention. There is a continuing and successful effort to reduce brucellosis in cattle and swine populations. The ultimate eradication of the disease in man depends upon the success of this effort. As the disease is spread principally through milk and milk products, it is essential that all milk be pasteurized not only for use in fluid form, but in cheese, creams, and other dairy products. At present there is no acceptable vaccine or other method to prevent infection in slaughterhouse workers, farmers, veterinarians, and laboratory workers dealing with this agent.

Knight, V.: Chemotherapy of brucellosis. Ann. N.Y. Acad. Sci., 53:332, 1950.

McCullough, N. B.: Microbial and host factors in the pathogenesis of brucellosis. In Mudd, S. (ed.): Infectious Agents and Host Reactions. Philadelphia, W. B. Saunders Company, 1970, Chapter 15, pp. 324-345.

Werner, C. A., and Knight, V.: The suppressive effect of antimicrobial drugs on *Brucella melitensis* infection in mice. J. Immun., 65:509, 1950.

DISEASES DUE TO MYCOBACTERIA

TUBERCULOSIS
Roger Des Prez

Definition. Tuberculosis is a chronic infection potentially of life-long duration, caused in humans by two species of mycobacteria, *M. tuberculosis* and rarely *M. bovis*. It is initiated almost always by inhalation of infectious material, producing a pneumonitis and a transient bacteremia that may seed other areas of the body. Infection may also be due to ingestion, particularly in areas in which bovine tuberculosis is common. Immediate progression to a severe and acute bacteremic or pneumonic illness may occur, but more often the infection assumes a latent form that may later progress to manifest chronic disease, usually in the lungs, but also in virtually any tissue in the body. It must be differentiated on bacteriologic grounds from chronic mycobacterial infections caused by so-called atypical mycobacteria, which may be clinically indistinguishable from tuberculosis but are very different in terms of treatment, epidemiology, and prognosis.

History. Skeletal remains from Neolithic times containing lesions very suggestive of tuberculosis of the spine illustrate that the association of man and tubercle bacilli is ancient. Earliest medical writings contain descriptions of persons ill with pulmonary symptoms and general wasting, to which condition the Greek word *phthisis,* meaning consumption of the flesh, came to be applied. However, tuberculosis did not assume epidemic proportions until conditions of crowding and poor nutrition attendant on the progressive urbanization and industrialization of Europe provided circumstances most favorable to its spread. It has been estimated that one fourth of the adult population of Europe in the mid-nineteenth century died of pulmonary tuberculosis, which had become "'The Great White Plague' threatening the very survival of the European race" (Dubos and Dubos).

In the nineteenth century three great strides led to an accurate conception of the disease and its cause. In earlier years the relationship between pulmonary and extrapulmonary tuberculosis had not been appreciated, and even pulmonary lesions of differing appearance were thought to represent different diseases. In 1804, Laennec, on the basis of anatomic and clinical studies of great insight, published the opinion that diverse forms of tuberculosis in the lungs and elsewhere were in fact different stages of the same basic pathologic process. This view was gradually accepted, and in 1839 the term tuberculosis first appeared in medical writing, coined because of the unifying anatomic feature of tubercle formation. During this period, the concept that tuberculosis was a contagion gained acceptance. In 1865, Villemin proved that disease could be produced in laboratory animals by injection of diseased tissues from pulmonary and extrapulmonary lesions of man and cow. With admirable precision he noted that human material caused less progressive disease in rabbits than did bovine material, one critical feature that Theobald Smith used to differentiate these two mycobacterial species four decades later. In 1882, Robert Koch reported isolation and culture of the tubercle bacillus, and successful production of disease in animals by these isolates. This outstanding accomplishment was balanced by two misconceptions of some importance. Koch shortly came to believe that tuberculin, which he had isolated from boiled cultures of the bacillus, had curative properties. He also maintained that mycobacteria from nonhuman sources, including cows, did not cause human illness. His justifiable eminence gave great weight to these opinions, resulting in many tuberculin-induced therapeutic misadventures and the slowing of public health efforts directed toward milk-borne tuberculosis. However, when the evidence implicating bovine mycobacteria in human disease became overwhelming, Koch's tuberculin provided the diagnostic tool that made possible detection and elimination of infected cows and led to the eventual disappearance of bovine tuberculosis as a significant human disease in much of the world. It has been estimated that half the population of sixteenth century England developed tuberculous cervical lymphadenitis (scrofula) caused by contaminated milk; so, indirectly, the therapeutic value of Koch's tuberculin was immense.

Because some populations seemed less afflicted by tuberculosis than others, physicians came to attribute healing properties to climate and environment, and affluent consumptives congregated in spas having favorable reputations. The sanatorium movement, which took its origins in part from this concern with climate, received further impetus from the demonstration of the infectious etiology of the disease. Originally sanatorium care consisted of good food and rest in salubrious environs. However, the importance of the pulmonary cavity in determining the outcome of phthisis soon became appreciated, and considerable expertise developed in different modes of collapse therapy, directed at reduction of cavity size and obstruction of the bronchocavitary junction. The introduction of air into the peritoneal cavity (pneumoperitoneum) or the pleural cavity (pneumothorax), separation of the periosteum and tissues from the ribs and insertion of inert materials between the denuded rib cage and the medially depressed chest wall (extraperiosteal plombage), and removal of the denuded ribs with construction of a smaller chest cage (thoracoplasty) required refined judgment in application, but were only modestly successful.

In 1945, streptomycin was established as the first effective antituberculous drug. This was most dramatically demonstrated in a small study of patients with meningeal tuberculosis, a previously fatal condition. It was also established that some patients relapsed after an initial favorable response owing to the appearance of drug-resistant organisms. A few years thereafter it was shown that administration of para-aminosalicylic acid (PAS) with streptomycin tended to prevent the emergence of drug resistance, establishing the principle of multiple drug therapy. The availability of streptomycin also made surgical removal of diseased lung possible, a procedure previously so often complicated by dissemination of infection that it was only rarely and unwisely attempted. During the era of surgical enthusiasm, which persisted up to 1960 and beyond, many persons with pulmonary tuberculosis came to pulmonary resection as a part of their treatment, often accelerating the development of respiratory insufficiency and cor pulmonale in the many predisposed to such problems.

In 1951, isoniazid was found to be an antituberculous drug of a different and higher order than streptomycin, and tuberculosis became a medically curable illness in most cases. Since patients on treatment often became promptly noninfectious and vigorous, the need for prolonged isolation and rest came into question, the usefulness of specialized sanatoriums largely disappeared, and completion of therapy at home or at work became possible. As a consequence, tuberculosis, long the province of specialized hospitals, returned to the mainstream of medicine and became the concern of general hospitals and general physicians. Further, the extraordinary effectiveness of isoniazid administered with other drugs over prolonged periods eventually made surgical resection uncommon. The safety and convenience of isoniazid also led to its wider application, not only for persons with manifest disease but also for those in whom disease was only likely to develop. Finally, more meticulous bacteriologic studies stimulated by an enlarged interest in drug susceptibility led to recognition and definition of the so-called atypical mycobacteria which are all resistant to isoniazid.

Bacteriology.   Mycobacteria are acid-fast nonmotile, nonsporulating, weakly gram-positive rods regarded as transitional forms between Eubacteria and Actinomycetes, and classified in the order Actinomycetales. Until the past two decades, only *M. tuberculosis,* the human tubercle bacillus, and *M. bovis* were regarded as pathogenic for man. *M. avium,* the species responsible for tuberculosis in poultry and swine, was thought to produce human disease only rarely, usually in persons with compromised host defense mechanisms. However, recent evidence suggests that one of the most important atypical mycobacteria, the Battey bacillus (*M. intracellulare**), may be very closely related to or identical with *M. avium,* and if this be the case infection with *M. avium* is very common indeed (*vide infra*). *Mycobacterium microti,* which causes disease in rodents and attenuated infections in other small mammals, is significant only in that a strain isolated from voles and naturally attenuated for man has been used as a vaccinating infection. *M. balnei,* the cause of superficial skin granulomas acquired in swimming pools, and *M. marinum,* originally isolated from marine fish, are now known to be the same and are designated by the latter term. *Mycobacterium ulcerans* is an uncommon cause of granulomatous skin ulcers, but does not cause systemic disease.

Atypical Mycobacteria.   Recently it has become clear that other mycobacteria, previously either unrecognized or regarded as saprophytes, cause human infection resembling pulmonary or lymph node tuberculosis. The clinical importance of these "atypical," "unclassified," or "anonymous" mycobacteria is discussed subsequently. However, some of their bacteriologic features will be mentioned here, because bacteriologic investigation of tuberculosis requires differentiation from these other organisms.

The lipid content of mycobacteria is quite high, comprising 20 to 40 per cent of total cell and 60 per cent of cell wall dry weight. Such distinguishing characteristics as slow growth rate, growth in adherent clumps producing pellicle formation in liquid media, resistance in high degree to chemical disinfectants, the ability to survive for long periods within phagocytic cells, resistance to stains, and, once stained, to decoloration are properties related in part to the lipid-rich relatively impermeable, and hydrophobic cell wall. Colonies of virulent tubercle bacilli may demonstrate a convoluted, cordlike appearance produced by parallel orientation and adhesion of individual cells. Because of the apparent relationship of this serpentine cording to virulence, considerable effort was made to isolate the responsible chemical moiety which is a specific mycocide. Another product of lipid fractionation, called Wax D, is a potent immunologic adjuvant. In combination with protein tuberculin, itself a poor immunogen, Wax D induces tuberculin hypersensitivity of the delayed type. Many other lipid fractions of uncertain functional significance have been isolated.

Mycobacteria are relatively impermeable to most stains. In the Ziehl-Neelsen method, staining with carbolfuchsin is enhanced by steaming the smear. Subsequent treatment with acid-alcohol elutes stain from other bacteria and organic material, but "acid-fast" mycobacteria resist decoloration. Stained bacilli from tissues or sputum appear as slender, slightly curved, often beaded red rods, at times lying side by side in sheafs. Mycobacteria can also be stained by fluorescent dyes (auramine and rhodamine), providing a useful but less specific screening procedure.

When pulmonary tuberculosis is sufficiently advanced to cause symptoms, most cases can be diagnosed by direct examination of the sputum smear. Slides should be examined for 15 minutes before discarding them as negative. Sputum for culture is best collected over a 24-hour period; the first sputum raised in the morning is an acceptable specimen as well. When sputum is not produced, the respiratory secretions raised and swallowed during sleep can be obtained by gastric aspiration, preferably soon after the patient has awakened and before he has left his bed. Induction of sputum by inhalation of heated, hypertonic aerosols (10 per cent saline) is superior to gastric aspiration, and is much more adaptable to office and clinic practice. The heated aerosol is inhaled for 15 minutes, and all sputum raised then and for a 15-minute period thereafter is collected and submitted for smear and culture. Sputum, gastric aspirates, and other materials containing pus and organic matter are liquefied and decontaminated by agitation with alkali prior to culture; mycobacteria, which resist this digestion to an appreciable degree, are concentrated by centrifugation, and the sediment is used for microscopic examination and culture. Positive smears from gastric aspirate digests may be due to saprophytic mycobacteria on foods or in the mouth; however, many will be due to legitimate tuberculous infection and should be regarded as presumptive evidence for such. Growth occurs on simple synthetic media but is enhanced by a source of lipid such as egg yolk. Antibacterial substances such as malachite green are included in most media.

Differentiation of Clinically Important Mycobacterial Species. Definitive identification of mycobacteria is usually accomplished by reference laboratories. However, in a practical sense good species identification can be achieved by a few fairly simple observations. Rate of growth and production of pigment were used by Runyon to classify the so-called atypical mycobacteria in four groups; Group I is characterized by formation of yellow colonies after brief exposure to light but not in the dark (photochromogens); Group II by production of yellow or orange colonies without light stimulation (scotochromogens); Group III, by nonpigmented colonies; and Group IV by the appearance of growth within seven days. These characteristics, together with susceptibility to isoniazid, production of niacin, and production of the enzyme catalase, suffice for tentative identification of those mycobacteria known to be of pathogenic importance in man, and should be within the capacity of laboratories responsible for tuberculosis diagnosis.

M. tuberculosis requires over ten days and usually two or three weeks for visible growth. Colonies are rough, cord formation is the rule, and no pigment is produced. It is the only species that produces niacin in quantities large enough to be detected by

---

*Species designation not formally recognized.

a simple chemical test. Isoniazid-susceptible strains of *M. tuberculosis* produce catalase which is inactivated by heating (68° C.). Isoniazid-resistant strains are usually catalase negative and also have decreased avidity for isotopically labeled isoniazid, which has led to the suggestion that this type of catalase activity is necessary for uptake of the drug by the organism. *M. tuberculosis* is virulent for guinea pig but not for rabbit or chicken.

M. bovis resembles *M. tuberculosis* but does not produce niacin, and is virulent in the rabbit as well as the guinea pig.

M. kansasii (Runyon Group I) was initially recognized by the production of yellow pigment after brief exposure of young, grouping colonies to light. This *photochromogenic* property remains its most distinguishing characteristic. Growth is slow, the colonies are either rough or smooth, isoniazid resistance in moderate degree is usual, catalase production is marked and usually not heat-labile, and niacin is not produced. The organism is not virulent for guinea pig, rabbit, or chicken but causes progressive disease in the mouse. *M. marinum*, also known as *M. balnei*, resembles *M. kansasii* except that growth is poor at 37° C. and good at room temperature. It is also placed in Runyon's Group I.

M. avium and *M. intracellulare** (the Battey bacillus) are identical-appearing organisms that grow slowly, produce smooth, thin, nonpigmented colonies, are highly resistant to isoniazid, produce heat-stable catalase in large quantities, and do not produce niacin. They are serologically closely related and regarded by many as the same. They are differentiated on the basis of good growth at 45° C. and production of progressive disease in the chicken, which characterizes *M. avium* but not *M. intracellulare.** However, these may be strain variations rather than species differences. They are classified in Runyon's Group III.

Scotochromogenic mycobacteria have been grouped (Runyon Group II) on the basis of yellow to orange pigment production not requiring light stimulation. The organism of most importance in human disease has been designated *M. scrofulaceum** and is a cause of cervical granulomatous lymphadenitis. Scotochromogens grow slowly, have smooth colonies, are highly resistant to isoniazid, produce heat-stable catalase activity, do not produce niacin, and are not virulent for laboratory animals.

Rapid growers (Runyon Group IV) produce good colonial growth within seven days. The most important of this group with respect to human disease is *M. fortuitum*. All produce heat-stable catalase, do not produce niacin, are very resistant to isoniazid, and are nonvirulent for laboratory animals.

Epidemiology. In many parts of the world, bovine tuberculosis remains a significant problem, and infection by the oral route is not infrequent. In the United States and western Europe, however, infection is almost always by inhalation, i.e., by the air-borne route. This means that the entire journey from the lesion in one host to the lodgment and beginning of a new lesion in another is made via the air. Moist drops of sputum are too large to be carried in this way because they cannot avoid entrapment by bronchial cilia and removal in the sputum. It is the dried residues of contaminated secretions, called *droplet nuclei*, that may remain suspended in air for prolonged periods and are sufficiently small to reach terminal air passages in which removal is difficult and bacterial multiplication can begin. Thus the area that an infectious person occupies may remain potentially contagious in his temporary absence. The urban poor have always borne the greatest part of the burden of tuberculosis. Although the prejudicial effects of poverty are many, crowded living conditions must be among the most significant, providing the greatest opportunity for infection to occur. Well-studied epidemics in certain closed environments such as naval vessels, boarding schools, and institutions indicate that one person with cavitary disease may infect virtually all susceptible persons in the same environment. A tuberculosis ward is probably not a great risk when care is taken. Instruction of patients to cough into disposable tissues will lessen aerosolization of infectious material. Considerable decontamination of patient areas has been achieved by ultraviolet light positioned so as to avoid exposure of the patient, but such arrangements are not usually practical. Surprisingly, persons excreting tubercle bacilli in the urine are contagious, especially for children using the same toilet facilities, presumably because of aerosolization of the urine. Transmission of tuberculosis by the genital route is quite rare. Inoculation of abraded skin by contaminated tissues at autopsy examination may produce a primary skin infection in tuberculin-negative individuals (prosector's wart). Fomites are probably not important in the spread of infection.

Incidence and Prevalence. The continual decline in tuberculosis mortality, which began in the middle of the last century, was probably due to improved housing, nutrition, and other benefits of increasing social awareness and concern. In the past two decades, the first in which drug treatment has been widely applied, mortality declined at a somewhat more rapid pace, but the incidence of new cases fell much less rapidly, suggesting a residue of infection not susceptible to further modification. This residue of infection is in older people infected in earlier years when the level of contagion was greater. When incidence of infection in the young is considered, as in tuberculin surveys, it is clear that this has continued to decline in urban United States (Table 1), and it can be anticipated that the incidence of new disease in older groups will eventually do likewise. Active tuberculosis in the United States is now most frequently seen in nonwhite older males (Figs. 1 and 2), reflecting both increased opportunity for infection during youth and factors of age and race favoring evolution of infection into disease.

Of 45,647 new active tuberculosis cases reported in the United States in 1967, nine tenths were pulmonary and one tenth extrapulmonary forms. Slightly over 10 per cent of the pulmonary cases were reported as primary infections. Some rural pockets of high prevalence existed in 1967, attributable to a high percentage of American Indian, Mexican, or Oriental persons in conditions of poverty; however, over-all the new case rate was higher in urban areas (41.4 per 100,000 in cities with populations over 500,000) than in rural areas

TABLE 1. TUBERCULIN REACTIVITY IN PHILADELPHIA SCHOOL CHILDREN*

	Age 6 %	Age 16 %
1928	25.0	52.7
1948	4.2	16.4
1958	1.9	5.9
1968	0.4	1.4

*Species designation not formally recognized.

*Data from Stein, S. C.: Amer. Rev. Resp. Dis., 99:298, 1969.

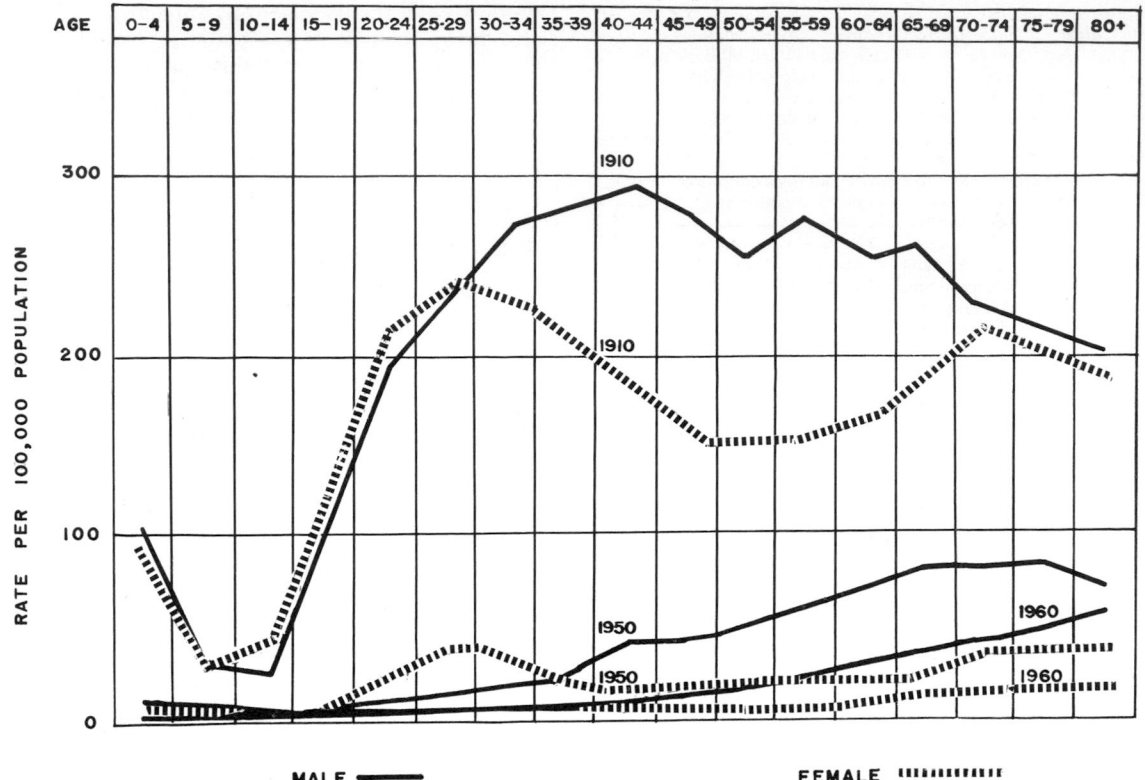

FIGURE 1. Tuberculosis death rate by years. (Modified from Lowell, A. M., Edwards, L. B., and Palmer, C. E.: Tuberculosis. Cambridge, Mass., Harvard University Press, 1969.)

(17.7 in areas with no cities with populations greater than 100,000).

The pattern of decreased childhood infection, decreased disease in the young adult, increasing involvement of older individuals, and a continuing fall in over-all mortality and morbidity is typical of advanced countries with predominantly white populations. In other countries, tuberculosis remains the leading cause of death in young adults (one quarter of all deaths in this age group in the Phillippines) or the leading cause of death excluding accidents, war, murder, suicide, and malignancies (Panama, Chile, Hong Kong, Portugal, Poland, Paraguay, Puerto Rico, Taiwan, Mexico, Japan). Although the incidence of childhood infection and disease remains high in economically underdeveloped nations, the increasing incidence of new cases and mortality in older males are very serious problems in these countries as well.

Immunologic Response to Infection. The previously uninfected host has no effective defense against tuberculous infection during the earliest phases of its evolution. The infecting inoculum multiplies without inhibition whether existing free in alveoli or within alveolar macrophages at the point of initial lodgment, in draining lymph nodes, or in sites seeded by silent bacteremia. In several weeks, however, tuberculin hypersensitivity develops, and the ability of the host to contain the infection is greatly enhanced. This phenomenon was first observed by Koch, who demonstrated that cutaneous inocula in previously noninfected guinea pigs caused an indolent local reaction with marked bacterial multiplication and systemic dissemination. In contrast, similar inocula in tuberculin-sensitive animals produced acute, exaggerated, and often necrotic local reactions, but bacillary multiplication and systemic dissemination were inhibited. The time between acquisition of infection and development of tuberculin hypersensitivity is longer with small inocula and shorter with large, but even when the challenge is so great as to eliminate the necessity of achieving a critical bacterial mass, at least several days elapse prior to the appearance of hypersensitivity during which multiplication is unimpeded.

Tuberculin hypersensitivity is the prototype of hypersensitive reactions of the delayed type. In contrast to immediate (Arthus) reactions these are not mediated by circulating antibody, cannot be passively transferred by serum, require 24 to 48 hours to develop, and produce an accumulation of macrophages and lymphocytes with little polymorphonuclear infiltrate or local edema. The basic event that results in tuberculin reactivity is the appearance of a population of lymphocytes specifically sensitive to antigens of the tubercle bacillus. Transfer of such lymphocytes from a positive donor to a negative recipient confers tuberculin reactivity and enhanced resistance on the recipient, a phenomenon termed *adoptive immunity* to distinguish it from the passive im-

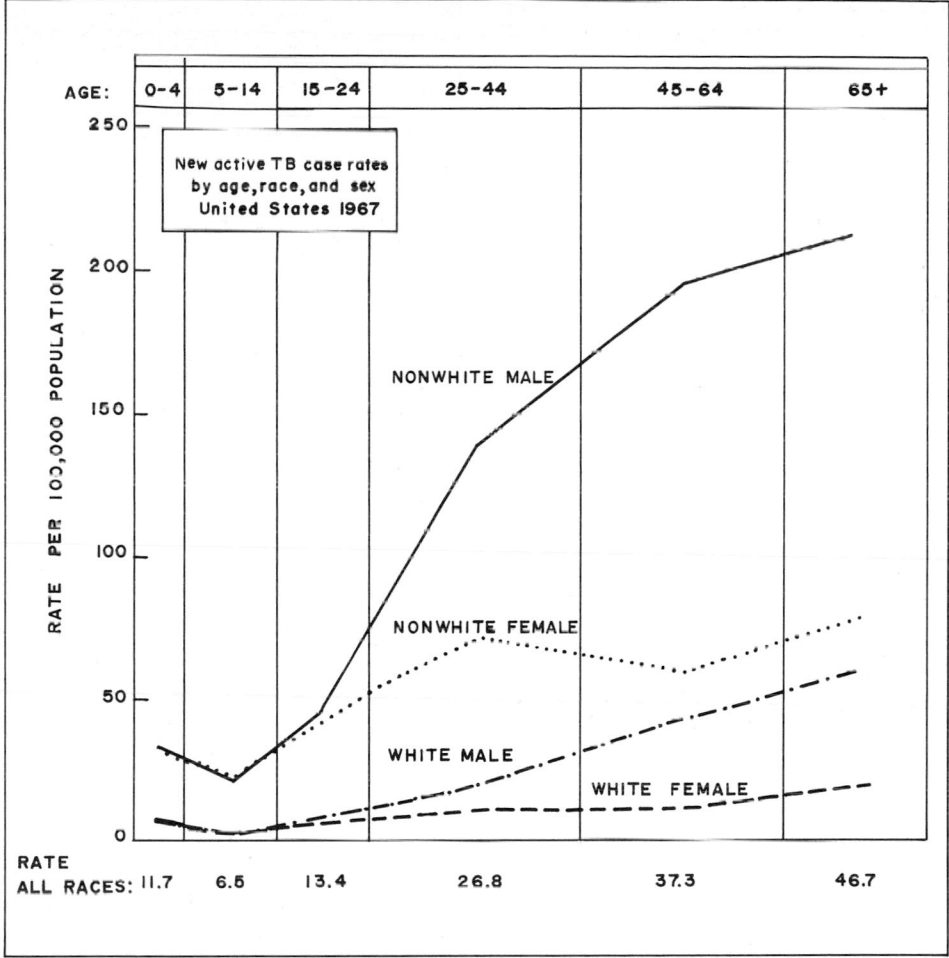

FIGURE 2. New active tuberculosis case rates by age, race, and sex. United States, 1967. (From Reported Tuberculosis Data, 1967, U.S. Department of Health, Education and Welfare, Public Health Service.)

munity produced by serum transfer. The mode of antigenic challenge probably has much to do with whether or not the response of the host is the production of circulating antibody only or both antibody and a specifically sensitized lymphocyte population. Antigens that are promptly removed from the circulation and degraded usually induce only circulating antibody, whereas those that persist for longer periods tend to induce tissue hypersensitivity as well. This latter situation is characteristic of the earliest phases of tuberculous infection because the microbe is very resistant to degradation by normal macrophages. Circulating antibodies reactive with the tubercle bacillus also appear, but their role in the control of infection, if any, is not known.

How lymphocytes are committed to reactivity with antigens of the tubercle bacillus is not known. The present hypothesis is that some lymphocytes contain genetically determined receptor material reactive with the antigens. When combination with antigen or with macrophage-processed antigen occurs, the lymphocyte is stimulated to divide and eventually produce a population of lymphocytes with similar reactivity distributed widely throughout the lymphatic system. The receptor

material on the lymphocyte is regarded as antibody-like, but is different from any immunoglobulin class now known.

One central consequence of the appearance of a specifically sensitized lymphocyte population is *macrophage activation* in a manner enhancing cellular bactericidal activity. Activated macrophages demonstrate accelerated metabolism, increased content of lysosomal granules and granule-associated hydrolases, enhanced bactericidal activity, and a tendency to aggregate with other macrophages and accumulate at antigenic foci; they are stimulated to cellular division and differentiation into epithelioid cells. All these macrophage changes may be secondary to interaction of sensitized lymphocytes and antigens of the tubercle bacillus, resulting in release of nonspecific effector substances, which in turn activate macrophages. Since lymphocytes and macrophages are intimately associated in tuberculous lesions, this notion fits histologic evidence as closely as does the concept that macrophages themselves are specifically sensitized.

Both macrophage activation and cellular immunity in tuberculosis are thought by some to be nonspecific consequences of the same specific immunologic stimulus. The evidence for non-specificity is based on two considerations: first, superficially similar macrophage changes can be produced by nonspecific stimuli such as phagocytosis of particulate debris; second, activated macrophages demonstrate enhanced bactericidal activity not only against the organisms of the activating infection but also against unrelated intracellular bacteria such as Listeria and Brucella (Mackaness, 1967). According to this view, cellular immunity in experimental tuberculosis is always preceded by and associated with tuberculin hypersensitivity. The difference between macrophage activation (cellular immunity) and tissue necrosis (caseation) is thought to be quantitative only, activation resulting when antigen concentration is small, and necrosis when antigen concentration is excessive. The opposing and more traditional view regards cellular immunity to tuberculosis as a more complex event resulting from a different type of antigenic stimulation or a different antigen than that producing hypersensitivity and the tendency to tissue necrosis. It has been shown that animals injected with a mixture of Wax D and tuberculoprotein are tuberculin-positive but not resistant to challenge tuberculous infection. Conversely, animals injected with a heat-labile RNA-protein complex, isolated by Youmans from disrupted tubercle bacilli, demonstrate greatly enhanced resistance to experimental tuberculous infection but no cutaneous tuberculin hypersensitivity. Furthermore, animals rendered resistant to tuberculosis in this fashion are not resistant to challenge with other facultative intracellular parasites, indicating that, in this specific experimental situation at least, cellular immunity in tuberculosis is specific.

The notion that tissue hypersensitivity and cellular immunity are separable phenomena caused by different chemical moieties of the tubercle bacillus or perhaps different populations of lymphocytes has theoretic importance; but from a clinical point of view, cellular immunity and tuberculin hypersensitivity are closely associated phenomena, and large concentrations of antigen tend to favor cell necrosis rather than successful cellular immunity. Thus in one part of the body, a small bacterial population may be dealt with successfully by macrophage proliferation and tubercle formation, whereas elsewhere, notably in the apices of the lung, larger bacterial populations may induce tissue necrosis and dissemination of infection via the bronchial tree.

Pathology. The pathologic response to tuberculous infection is determined in large part by interaction of two factors, the degree of hypersensitivity present in the host and *the mass of antigen present in the lesion,* as modified by structural characteristics of the tissue involved. Small numbers of bacilli in a host with well established hypersensitivity induce *tubercle formation,* characterized by central multinucleated giant cells surrounded by a cluster of epithelioid cells. More peripherally, lymphocytes are seen admixed with fibroblasts and, in older lesions, fibrosis. Visible bacilli are few or absent. Lesions of this histologic character are referred to as *productive,* and usually represent successful local containment of infection. When large bacterial concentrations coexist with good levels of hypersensitivity, injury to the vasculature leads to a nonspecific exudate rich in fibrin and containing polymorphonuclear leukocytes, monocytes, and small numbers of epithelioid and giant cells. Such lesions, which are termed *exudative,* may progress to *caseous necrosis.* In contrast to many other infections, tissue autolysis in tuberculosis is initially incomplete. The term caseous depicts its cheesy, semisolid, or solid consistency. In some tissues this appears microscopically as amorphous, homogeneous, eosinophilic material with no structural features. In the lung, in early stages, some suggestion of original architecture may persist. Primary infections in which large bacillary populations have been achieved at the time at which tuberculin hypersensitivity appears are usually associated with caseation. However, in contrast to apical pulmonary lesions, in which softening and liquefication of caseous tissue is prone to occur, the relatively uncommon caseous lesions in the lower lung fields usually remain in a solid state in which anaerobic conditions discourage bacterial multiplication, and eventually calcification ensues.

Tuberculous bacteremia may produce quite different histologic pictures, depending on the balance between bacterial population and tissue hypersensitivity. When hypersensitivity is present at high level and the bacteremia is minor in extent, hard tubercle formation predominates and necrosis is absent or minimal. Larger bacterial populations tend to produce necrotic miliary foci. When hypersensitivity has waned owing to intercurrent illness of a type that hampers immunologic responsiveness, and breakdown of a previously quiescent chronic focus leads to extensive bacteremia, the cellular response may be minimal or lacking entirely in the presence of large concentrations of multiplying bacteria in the miliary foci. This histologic picture has been termed *nonreactive tuberculosis.*

Because the histopathologic response is determined in part by local factors, it follows that quite different pictures may occur simultaneously in the same individual and even in different parts of the same lesion, some representing progression of infection and some its successful containment. In pulmonary caseous foci, for instance, the histologic response at increasing distances from the caseous center (where antigen concentration is greatest) comes more and more to resemble that associated with successful containment of infection, with tubercle formation and fibrosis predominating.

It is important to emphasize that these histologic features are not diagnostic of tuberculosis. Indistinguishable tubercle formation may be seen in a wide variety of conditions, including sarcoidosis, regional enteritis, berylliosis, fungal infections, lymphatic neoplasms, and even in lymph nodes draining neoplasms in which fat released from necrotic tumor may stimulate foreign body granulomas. Caseous necrosis is somewhat more specific than tubercle formation, but may be seen in some of the infectious processes enumerated above. Even the presence of stainable acid-fast organisms is not diagnostic, in that these may represent mycobacteria other than *M. tuberculosis* or *M. bovis. Accordingly, any material obtained at diagnostic biopsy should be submitted to culture as well as examined histologically.*

Pathogenesis. The tubercle bacillus requires ready access to oxygen for growth. Even under the most favorable circumstances, cell division occurs no more frequently than every 18 to 24 hours (Pneumococcus divides every 15 minutes), explaining the subacute character of advancing tuberculous disease. When circumstances become unfavorable for growth because of oxygen lack, drug treatment, or any other reason, the tubercle bacillus has a remarkable capacity to retreat into a metabolically dormant state and persist in necrotic tissue for years.

Infection occurs by either ingestion or inhalation. Transmission by ingestion probably requires relatively large numbers of organisms and results in infection of the pharyngeal lymphoid tissue and cervical lymph nodes or the intestine and abdominal nodes. This mode of transmission, still important in some parts of the world, has all but disappeared in areas in which pasteurization is employed and tuberculosis in cattle has been eradicated. Transmission by inhalation, i.e., by the air-borne route, is presumably the way the infection is usually spread, and in the lung very few infectious units may produce a colony of tubercle bacilli. The initial pulmonary infection is usually in the mid or lower lung field where increased air flow enhances the likelihood of lodgment of bacilli. Bacterial multiplication proceeds silently with little or no tissue reaction. The infection has ready access to lymphatic channels, spreads to regional nodes in the hilum of the lung, and thence gains access to the blood stream. *It is important to emphasize that asymptomatic blood stream dissemination of the primary infection before the acquisition of tuberculin hypersensitivity probably occurs in almost all instances; it is this event that sets the stage for the development of chronic pulmonary and extrapulmonary tuberculosis at a later time.* This preallergic bacteremia results in metastatic foci throughout the body which also multiply in unimpeded fashion. Circulating bacilli are most efficiently cleared from the blood stream by reticuloendothelial organs, but metastatic foci flourish and reach largest size in those areas known to be associated with clinical tuberculosis, notably the apices of the lungs, the kidneys, richly vascularized skeletal areas, and the central nervous system. High tissue oxygen tension is one factor favoring bacterial growth in these areas; in the apices of both upper and lower lobes, for instance, oxygen tension may reach 150 mm. Hg.

From two to ten weeks after initial infection, *tuberculin hypersensitivity* develops, and the subsequent appearance of *cellular immunity* greatly alters the balance in favor of the host. Activated macrophages reduce the bacterial population at both initial and metastatic foci, and further bacterial growth is inhibited. It is likely, however, that slowly metabolizing viable bacilli persist at most foci. As a result of this inflammatory reaction, the bronchial, hilar, and sometimes mediastinal lymph nodes become enlarged. In infants and young children particularly, massive enlargement may occur. When antigen concentration at the site of initial infection or in the regional lymph nodes is sufficiently large, cellular necrosis may develop and eventually calcify, a process requiring only months in young children but several years in adults. Calcific deposits in the mid or lower lung field together with calcified hilar nodes, the so-called *Ghon complex,* represent a common sequel of tuberculous infection with quantitative implications, because healing with visible residue implies a large bacillary population at the initial infection site and probably more advanced metastatic foci as well. For years this roentgenographic finding was considered pathognomonic of tuberculosis. It is now known that certain fungal infections, notably histoplasmosis and coccidioidomycosis, and other mycobacteria produce similar healed primary lesions.

Fate of the Primary Infection. In a majority of persons, possibly 99 per cent, the infection remains quiescent after the development of tuberculin hypersensitivity, and is of no further clinical significance. In the remainder, infection may evolve into clinical tuberculosis in a number of ways. In some, particularly the very young, the preallergic bacteremia (early hematogenous dissemination) may progress directly into generalized acute hematogenous tuberculosis. Initial metastatic foci in the area or within the walls of small blood vessels enlarge, undergo necrosis, and then discharge secondarily into the vessel lumen so as to progressively enhance the bacteremia. The gross pathologic resemblance of the resulting disseminated tubercles to millet seeds led to the designation *miliary tuberculosis.* At times it is the strategic location of miliary tubercles rather than progression of the bacteremia that is critical, particularly with respect to development of *tuberculous meningitis.* Rich established that the meninges, themselves quite resistant to infection by blood-borne inocula, become infected when subependymal foci in brain or spinal cord rupture into the subarachnoid space and produce spread of the infection via the subarachnoid fluid. Meningitis may occur in the setting of obvious, progressive blood stream infection, but may also be due to a nonprogressive and otherwise asymptomatic bacteremia.

Local rather than hematogenous events may also determine the outcome. The initial focus may directly evolve into progressive pneumonia (*progressive primary*); rarely cavitation may result. Large hilar nodes may become necrotic, liquefy, discharge into the bronchial tree, and produce tuberculous pneumonia in this fashion. Hilar lymph node enlargement in the young may partially compress the major bronchi with or without secondary granulomatous involvement of the bronchial wall, producing bronchial obstruction and collapse of a pulmonary segment or lobe.

When the site of the initial infection is subpleural in location, rupture into the pleural space may occur. This results in an outpouring of fluid that spreads the infection over the pleural surfaces and produces the clinical picture of *serofibrinous pleurisy with effusion*. A hematogenous focus located near the pleural surface may produce a similar clinical picture. It is likely that the occurrence of pleurisy with effusion indicates that an extensive initial infection has evolved, because more than three fourths of such cases will later demonstrate either pulmonary or extrapulmonary tuberculosis, usually with no direct anatomic relationship to the pleural disease and most often long after it has resolved.

In numerical terms, *the most frequent serious consequence of the preallergic bacteremia is chronic pulmonary tuberculosis.* Pulmonary sequestration of blood-borne bacteria occurs in a distribution proportional to blood flow, but, as mentioned, conditions in the superior and posterior aspects of the lungs greatly favor bacterial multiplication. Culture of small healed fibrocalcific foci in the apical and posterior areas of the upper lobes, so-called *Simon foci,* contain viable tubercle bacilli on culture more frequently and to a greater extent than the concomitant mid or lower lobe lesion representing the healed initial infection site (autopsy studies).

Over the past four decades it has been a matter of controversy whether chronic apical pulmonary tuberculosis of the so-called *reinfection type* results from breakdown of latent residua seeded at the time of the initial infection (*endogenous reinfection*) or from acquisition of new infection from the environment (*exogenous reinfection*). Many authorities assume that both can occur. However, it now seems likely that exogenous reinfection is considerably less important. Stead has convincingly supported this opinion in an analysis of a number of reports in which time of maximal exposure risk could be determined and the tuberculin reactivity of the population prior to the known exposure was known. Clinical tuberculosis occurred most frequently in those with negative tuberculin reactions at the outset, and for the most part this occurred within 24 months of exposure (Table 2). In these patients, it is likely that the initial metastatic apical focus or foci progressed without interruption while the initial mid or lower lung field focus was healing. In those with

positive tuberculin reactions at the outset, chronic pulmonary tuberculosis, when it occurred, developed in random fashion without any time relationship to the exposure period. In these patients it seems likely that both first infection and the apical foci were consequences of a more remote exposure.

Similar studies confirm that clinical disease is most apt to develop during the first 24 months after infection. Beyond that time quiescent foci in the lungs and elsewhere may evolve to produce clinical disease at random when a combination of local and systemic factors produces circumstances favoring activity. When infection in childhood was the rule, most pulmonary tuberculosis was observed in late adolescence and early adulthood. At present, when acquisition of infection is often delayed beyond this period, pulmonary tuberculosis is becoming a condition of elderly men, many of whom must have weathered the dangers of early adulthood with quiescent foci only to fall victim to conditions of old age favoring activation of latent infection.

The importance of local factors is emphasized by the frequency with which tuberculous arthritis is related to antecedent trauma and the occasional case in which nontuberculous pulmonary inflammation causes reactivation of latent pulmonary tuberculosis. The dissection of an indolent mediastinal node into the pericardium or an inapparent tubo-ovarian or retroperitoneal node into the peritoneal cavity is the usual mechanism by which *pericarditis* or *peritonitis* develops, often without clinically detectable tuberculosis elsewhere. Thus, any tuberculin-positive individual is at risk to develop any form of tuberculosis, often as a result of a remote and clinically undetectable primary infection.

Endobronchial Spread of Chronic Pulmonary Tuberculosis; the Importance of the Cavity. In contrast to the earliest stages of tuberculous infection in which lymphohematogenous dissemination is the rule, once chronic pulmonary tuberculosis has become established further spread occurs for the most part via the bronchial tree. A solid pulmonary focus contains relatively few bacteria whether or not caseation has occurred. However, such foci may at any time liquefy, spill infectious material into the bronchial tree, and contaminate other areas of the lung. Moreover, an open cavity, probably because of high oxygen tension, provides optimal conditions for bacterial multiplication, and very large populations are achieved. The pulmonary cavity, which is responsible for both progression of disease in the individual and infection of others, has provided the environment that has nurtured the tubercle bacillus through so many centuries of coexistence with the human species. *Especially in the era prior to the availability of effective drugs, cavity formation was the pivotal event in the course of pulmonary tuberculosis, to the prevention or treatment of which most forms of therapy were directed.*

Late Hematogenous Dissemination. Foci seeded at the time of the preallergic bacteremia may, after prolonged quiescent periods, break down and

TABLE 2. RELATIONSHIP OF EXPOSURE TO DEVELOPMENT OF CLINICAL TUBERCULOSIS ACCORDING TO ANTECEDENT TUBERCULIN STATUS*

	New Case Rate per 100 Person-years
Heavily exposed	
Tuberculin-negative	49.4
Tuberculin-positive	7.6
Not particularly exposed	
Tuberculin-negative	10.8
Tuberculin-positive	4.3

*Data from Stead, W. W.: Amer. Rev. Resp. Dis., 95:729, 1967.

liberate bacteria into the blood stream. Chronic pulmonary foci may cause late bacteremia in this manner, but extrapulmonary and often clinically inapparent foci, particularly in lymph nodes, bones, and the urogenital system, cause most instances of miliary and meningeal tuberculosis in adults. Host circumstances such as old age, malnutrition, and malignancy are important factors favoring this sequence of events; less commonly, trauma can be clearly implicated. Multiple episodes of bacteremia may occur from the same focus and produce relapse. Not only miliary and meningeal tuberculosis, but also some instances of disseminated tuberculous lymphadenitis and some uncommon and confusing hematologic syndromes based on marrow involvement may result.

The Tuberculin Test. Koch's tuberculin was essentially a filtrate of a boiled culture of tubercle bacilli. The preparation known as Old Tuberculin (OT) is still obtained in much the same fashion. Koch injected the material subcutaneously and measured both febrile response and local reaction. The scratch test (Pirquet) avoided the systemic reaction, but the amount of tuberculin absorbed was an unknown variable. The intracutaneous injection of tuberculin (Mantoux, 1908) permitted quantitative evaluation of reactivity for the first time, and this mode of administration is preferred. The multiple-puncture Tine and Heaf techniques are useful in surveys because of ease of administration, but are less accurate. The patch test may be of use in the pediatric age group for convenience and to avoid severe reactions, but it is not otherwise recommended.

Old Tuberculin is a crude mixture of materials, and dosage is expressed in terms of dilution. The isolation and partial purification of a protein fraction responsible for tuberculin reactivity (Long and Seibert, 1937) made it possible to express dosage of this purified protein derivative (PPD) in weight terms. For purposes of comparison, one lot of tuberculin (prepared by Dr. Siebert) has been adopted as the standard by which other lots may be assayed (PPD-S). In spite of its crude chemical nature, OT is a very constant and satisfactory preparation, still preferred in many parts of the world. To facilitate comparison, the dosages of OT and PPD possessing equivalent biologic activity (skin reactivity) have been carefully determined (Table 3). One should note that there is not a strict mathematical relationship between the two. It is

TABLE 3. COMPARABLE DOSES OF OT AND PPD*

Dilution of OT	Dilution of PPD (mg.)	Tuberculin Units	Strength of PPD
1-100,000	0.000002	0.1	
1-10,000	0.00002	1	First
1-2000	0.0001	5	Intermediate
1-1000	0.0002	10	
1-100	0.005	100	Second

*Adapted from Smith, D. T.: Ann. Intern. Med., 67:919, 1967.

now preferred to express dosage in terms of tuberculin units (one TU equals 0.00002 mg. PPD).

When infection was nearly universal, most persons reacted to small (1 or 5 TU) doses of tuberculin. As tuberculous infection gradually became exceptional, weak tuberculin reactions, i.e., those requiring large challenge doses, became the rule. Palmer postulated that the majority of those with weak tuberculin reactions were actually infected with mycobacteria other than tuberculosis, and then demonstrated this to be the case by use of PPD reagents prepared from these other organisms. Although varying widely in geographic incidence, most tuberculin reactivity in the United States is at present due to mycobacterial infections other than tuberculosis (Table 4).

The Mantoux test is performed by introducing 0.1 ml. of tuberculin intracutaneously into the volar aspect of the forearm, using a number 26 or 27 needle. Proper introduction is critical; if the injection is too deep, the antigen diffuses from the site; if it is too superficial, much may leak out and be lost. A raised, white wheal persisting for some minutes will indicate that proper positioning of antigen has been achieved. In adults, a 5-TU dosage is usually administered first. Production of *visible and palpable induration over 10 mm. in diameter after 48 or 72 hours is considered almost diagnostic of infection with M. tuberculosis. Erythema is not used as an index of positivity.* A zone of induration less than 10 mm. in diameter is read as doubtful, as it may be due to other mycobacterial infections. In those in whom hypersensitivity is suspected, particularly young children, or in persons with evidence of ocular involvement, it may be advisable to begin with 1 TU or less. Very extensive or necrotic reactions suggest that the infection is in a progressing phase. If the first test is negative, retesting with 100 or 250 TU is performed. A positive reaction to these larger doses

TABLE 4. FREQUENCY AND MEAN SIZE OF REACTIONS AMONG NAVY RECRUITS TO 0.0001 MG. OF PPD OF MYCOBACTERIA*

PPD Antigen	Prepared From	Number Tested	Reactions of 2 mm. or More	
			Percentage	Mean Size, mm.
PPD-S	*Mycobacterium tuberculosis*	212,462	8.6	10.3
PPD-F	*Mycobacterium fortuitum*	3,415	7.7	4.8
PPD-Y	*Mycobacterium kansasii*	13,913	13.1	6.2
PPD-A	*Mycobacterium avium*	10,060	30.5	6.7
PPD-B	Battey type	212,462	35.1	7.7
PPD-G	Scotochromogen	29,540	48.7	10.3

*From Smith, D. T.: Ann. Intern. Med., 67:919, 1967, after data from Edwards, L. B.: Ann. N. Y. Acad. Sci., 106:32, 1963. PPD= purified protein derivative.

has relatively little diagnostic importance, but a negative reaction in a *nonfebrile and relatively well individual* virtually excludes mycobacterial infection. By contrast, tuberculin reactivity is much less reliable in persons with constitutional symptoms. One study indicated that 31 per cent of patients with subsequently proved active tuberculosis failed to react to 5 TU on admission to the hospital and 15 per cent did not react to 100 TU. As general health improves and infection comes under control, tuberculin reactivity returns. False negative reactions may also be caused by associated illness such as sarcoidosis or Hodgkin's disease, less commonly by other neoplasms and acute infections, notably the viral exanthemas but also bacterial infections such as pneumonia, and by corticosteroid therapy. False positives are almost always due to infections with other mycobacterial species. It can be anticipated that present experimental interest in factors that modify antigen-induced lymphocyte transformation will provide some basic understanding of mechanisms producing false negative tuberculin reactions.

Factors Modifying the Course of Tuberculosis. Mortality statistics from urban populations in the early part of this century, when infection in childhood was the rule, clearly show the effect of age on the progression of tuberculosis. All mortality curves from this period demonstrate a peak in the first three years of life, owing to age-related factors favoring development of progressive hematogenous tuberculosis, particularly miliary and meningeal disease. The tendency to extensive lymphatic involvement, hematogenous spread, and progressive extrapulmonary disease are characteristics more related to the age of the host than to the duration of the infection. Primary infections that progress in adults, probably seldom seen or at least recognized in the epidemic era, in most instances produce chronic apical tuberculosis with much less prominent lymphatic involvement and less progressive extrapulmonary disease. As milk-borne infections usually occurred in early childhood, it is easy to see how the erroneous notion developed that bovine bacilli were especially prone to produce disease in lymph nodes or bone. Older prepuberal children (roughly between ages 5 and 15), although in no way resistant to *infection* in the epidemic era, very seldom manifested progressive *disease*. After puberty a second mortality peak was seen that continued through the second and into the third decade and was more pronounced in females than in males. Thereafter the death rate continued at a lower level until old age, when a third, less dramatic mortality peak was seen. At present, in countries with low prevalence, clinical tuberculosis is becoming more a disease of the elderly, particularly the older male, presumably owing in part to waning immunologic competence in old age.

Resistance to the development of tuberculous disease is less well demonstrated in nonwhite races. It is argued that the increased opportunity for infection owing to crowded conditions and the untoward effects of poor nutrition is responsible rather than any constitutional susceptibility. However, it is the opinion of most clinicians that tuberculosis in the nonwhite tends to assume a more progressive and florid character irrespective of socioeconomic factors, suggesting that genetic factors may play some role in the process. By the same token, antimicrobial therapy, which definitely requires host resistance to maintain its gains, seems equally effective among all races. This suggests that if any genetic factors are involved, their influence is slight. At the opposite pole, the Jewish people are thought to be relatively resistant to tuberculosis, presumably because of long exposure resulting in a relatively resistant population.

That nutritional status, mental and physical stress, and exhaustion modify the course of tuberculosis is well illustrated by the peak in mortality statistics observed during the major wars, in both belligerent and nonbelligerent nations. *Pregnancy, delivery, and the puerperium,* long regarded as risk periods, are probably prejudicial for the most part in that they may be associated with exhaustion, loss of sleep, and poor nutritional status.

Although statistical evidence is lacking, there is little doubt that *prolonged therapy with corticosteroids* predisposes to exacerbation of tuberculosis. It is very probable that *therapy with oncolytic or immunosuppressive agents* also favors progression. Clinical tuberculosis occurs in *diabetes* to a greater extent than in the general population, and the course of the disease is more fulminant, particularly in young, poorly controlled diabetics subject to episodes of ketoacidosis. *Silicosis or anthracosilicosis* alters host response to tuberculosis in important ways. Instances of infection with the usually nonpathogenic *M. avium* are observed in silicotics. Once established, tuberculosis in silicotics may produce massive conglomerate fibrosis with little potential for resolution and little response to antituberculous drugs. Moreover, this type of tissue reaction is often not associated with large bacterial populations, and bacteriologic diagnosis may be difficult. The association between tuberculosis and *sarcoidosis* is complex, in part because of the difficulty in differentiating these two conditions histologically. In times past, sarcoidosis was thought to predispose to the progression of tuberculosis, but this no longer appears to be the case. Hodgkin's disease, leukemia, and other lymphatic neoplasms are often both confused with and complicated by tuberculosis, owing presumably to their detrimental effect on tissue hypersensitivity and cellular immunity. *Carcinoma and destructive infections* such as histoplasmosis, other mycobacterial infections, and lung abscess may erode an old tuberculous focus, particularly when involving the apicoposterior areas of the lung, releasing tubercle bacilli that may or may not produce disease. *Severe viral illness,* notably rubella and influenza but others as well, may have detrimental effects on the course of tuberculosis. (Interestingly, these infections not only temporarily inhibit tuberculin skin reactivity but also depress in vitro lymphocyte transformation by both specific antigens and nonspecific mitogens.) *Gastric resection,* for reasons possibly related to nutritional status, may cause reactivation of previously quiescent but roentgenographically detectable pulmonary tuberculosis in as many as 20 per cent of patients with this combination of illnesses, and may be responsible for the appearance of overt pulmonary tuberculosis in 2 to 4 per cent of those who are merely tuberculin reactors without prior roentgenologic evidence of disease. *Pulmonary surgery* may also cause progression of quiescent pulmonary foci. Finally, the development of clinically manifest tuberculous arthritis or spondylitis after trauma, the appearance of miliary tuberculosis after injury or even after retrograde pyelography, and the development of tuberculous peritonitis after delivery or after diagnostic tubal insufflation illustrate the untoward effects that *physical injury* may have on latent tuberculous foci.

Prevention of Tuberculosis. Vaccination. BCG is a strain of originally virulent. *M. bovis* attenuated by Calmette and Guerin by serial passage on inhibitory media and maintained since. Several large studies in highly industrialized societies have established beyond question that vaccination of tuberculin-negative persons in populations with a high prevalence of tuberculosis will reduce the incidence of clinical disease to 20 per cent of what would otherwise be seen. Not only is the overall incidence of disease reduced, but also vaccinated persons who become ill develop less progressive forms of tuberculosis. The appearance of miliary and meningeal disease in young children, for instance, is rare after BCG vaccination, a considerable advantage because tuberculous meningitis in the very young may be neurologically disabling even with bacteriologic cure. Disseminated infection with BCG itself is so exquisitely rare as to be of no importance whatsoever. BCG vaccination programs have been carried out with substantial success in some European countries. Reluctance to do so in the United States has been largely based on the consideration that successful BCG vaccination induces tuberculin positivity and thus sacrifices the major method by which early infection may be diagnosed, a quite important consideration in the United States and other areas of low prevalence. Moreover, extensive BCG vaccination in areas of low prevalence would make epidemiologic studies based on tuberculin reactivity impossible. The success of isoniazid prophylaxis (see below) is another factor weighing against widespread vaccination. Above all, there is no satisfactory measure of the immunizing potency of an individual strain or lot of BCG unless it happens to have been employed in large studies, and different strains of BCG may vary widely in this respect. British investigators have demonstrated that a strain of *M. microti* (the vole bacillus), which is naturally attenuated for man, is of the same order of effectiveness as BCG, but this has not been widely used because of reactions at the site of injection.

Almost all authorities advise the use of BCG in tuberculin-negative children in areas in which the incidence of positive tuberculin reactions among secondary schoolchildren is as high as 20 per cent. (Vaccination is of no use in tuberculin-positive persons, who presumably are already infected.) Vaccination may also be appropriate for missionary or government personnel prior to assignment to areas of known high prevalence, in groups of health profession personnel in whom the incidence of infection is known to be high (over 20 per cent), and even in some military personnel. The usefulness of vaccination in infants born to mothers with tuberculosis, or who are to be returned to environments of known high risk, is compromised by the difficult requirement of keeping the infant apart from the suspicious environment for the four- to ten-week period required for development of tuberculin hypersensitivity in response to BCG infection. A strain of BCG resistant to isoniazid has been developed, use of which would allow chemoprophylaxis with isoniazid between vaccination and development of hypersensitivity. However, wide use of this strain would require documentation of its effectiveness as an immunizing agent, and this would require a large field trial.

Chemoprophylaxis. The term chemoprophylaxis has been applied in tuberculosis to two quite distinct situations: first, the treatment of tuberculin-negative individuals in the hope of preventing infection in situations in which infection would otherwise be likely; and second, treatment of tuberculin-positive individuals in the hope of preventing evolution of infection into disease. In a practical sense, it means treatment with isoniazid, first, because of its effectiveness and convenience, and second, because the toxicity and intolerance of any other drug or combination of drugs are too great to justify use in situations in which disease is not known to be progressive.

Circumstances in which *infection prophylaxis* (primary prophylaxis) is indicated are few. When an infant cannot be isolated from a mother with active tuberculosis long enough to establish tuberculin hypersensitivity with BCG, isoniazid may be administered to the child until and for a few months after the mother's sputum becomes negative for tubercle bacilli under treatment. When the period of risk cannot be defined, as in households with recalcitrant, "sputum-positive" patients, or in geographic pockets of known high risk, it may be useful to continue therapy for two years or more as the morbidity associated with meningitis is less in older children. Alternatively it may be reasonable to stop chemoprophylaxis at some point for a period long enough to achieve vaccination and tuberculin conversion, and then to resume therapy for another year, making the assumption that the conversion could be due either to vaccination or infection and that in either case protection would result. (Tuberculin reactivity owing to natural infection in young children is almost always marked and that owing to BCG less so, but this difference cannot be used with confidence in individual cases to decide whether reactivity is due to vaccination or infection.)

A definite exposure to highly contaminated material such as may occur in laboratory accidents or in mouth-to-mouth resuscitation of infectious patients may be covered with prophylactic isoniazid for a period of several months. In the latter situation, attention should be given to the possibility of isoniazid resistance, if these data are available, and therapy adjusted accordingly. The status of the tuberculin test during and after treatment should be monitored.

In certain conditions, notably sarcoidosis and Hodgkin's disease, cutaneous anergy may make it impossible to determine whether or not infection has occurred. Moreover, both roentgenographic and histologic abnormalities in sarcoidosis may resemble those produced by tuberculosis, further confusing the picture. This is true to a lesser extent in Hodgkin's disease. Further, both these conditions may require corticosteroid therapy (see below). For these reasons, many persons with sarcoidosis, Hodgkin's disease, and related lymphomas are treated with isoniazid without certain knowledge as to whether or not infection has in fact occurred. Similarly, corticosteroid therapy in gravely ill patients is ordinarily accompanied by isoniazid whether or not the status of the tuberculin test is known, because all debilitating conditions may produce cutaneous anergy, making it impossible to exclude either old or active tuberculosis.

By contrast, *disease prophylaxis* (secondary prophylaxis) is a frequently employed and well-established procedure. Its greatest use is in the recent tuberculin converter, which in point of fact represents treatment of an early and active infection. (Recent studies indicate that the majority of recent converters without roentgenographic evidence of disease will have cultures positive for tubercle bacilli if these are searched for assiduously.) Treatment of children under five with a positive reaction to a 5-TU dose of tuberculin is recommended without exception. This is also the case in older persons in whom tuberculin conversion is known to be a relatively recent (within two years) event. In a practical sense, in the United States and other areas of low prevalence, at present almost all positive reactions to 5 TU in persons under 30 can be assumed on statistical grounds to be due to recent infection, and treatment is advisable. The degree of tuberculin reactivity is important in reaching the decision to treat, because most weak tuberculin reactions have entirely different implications and do not require treatment (see above). A florid or necrotic reaction is regarded by most as an indication for therapy at any age. Although not yet established, it seems likely that the incidence of tuberculosis in later life will be substantially reduced by early treatment of the tuberculin converter.

In addition to treatment of the preclinical infection as defined above, a number of situations known to be prejudicial to the course of tuberculous infection constitute sufficient reason for chemoprophylaxis in tuberculin-positive persons. These include silicosis, severe diabetes, especially when control is poor, the post-gastrectomy state, and progressive neoplastic disease, especially of the myeloid or lymphatic systems and particularly when treatment with oncolytic agents is employed.

The occurrence of severe viral illness in a tuberculin-positive person is regarded by some as an indication for chemoprophylaxis.

Finally, persons with an undiagnosed pulmonary infiltrate and a positive tuberculin reaction in whom for one reason or another definitive diagnosis is not indicated, and persons with known and presumably arrested tuberculosis never treated with chemotherapy, should receive isoniazid. Often the previously stable infiltrates will regress under this therapy, demonstrating that the presumed inactivity was illusory.

Chemoprophylaxis in adults consists of isoniazid in dosage of 300 mg. daily for a period of a year or two, depending on the circumstances. In children, the dose is 6 to 8 mg. per kilogram. Although the risk of untoward reactions to isoniazid is perhaps greater than was thought to be the case in the past, it is not sufficient to compromise the usefulness of the drug in these situations.

PULMONARY TUBERCULOSIS
Robert Goodwin

It has been traditional to describe pulmonary tuberculosis as two different disease syndromes, *primary* or *childhood* tuberculosis, and *secondary* or *adult* or *reinfection* tuberculosis. The age-related terms have descriptive force because age is perhaps the most important factor modifying the clinical manifestations of tuberculous infection. The terms *primary, secondary,* and *reinfection type* have much less to recommend them because almost all clinical tuberculosis results from the evolution of the initial infection, either promptly or after variable periods of latency but without superimposition of new infection.

CHILDHOOD TUBERCULOSIS

In the majority of both children and adults, tuberculous infection runs its course without producing clinical illness. Infection is more often symptomatic in infants and young children than in adults, because of a tendency in the young to more extensive lymph node involvement and hematogenous spread. At the time at which hypersensitivity develops, a few may show varying degrees of fever and lassitude for a few days. Rarely will development of hypersensitivity be associated with *erythema nodosum* or symptomatic inflammation of the eye (*phlyctenular keratoconjunctivitis*), but these are nonspecific allergic reactions, caused more often by hypersensitivity states other than tuberculosis. Hilar lymph node enlargement in the young may partially compress the major bronchi, producing a brassy cough and occasionally sputum and clinical signs of localized bronchial obstruction. The chest roentgenogram will often reveal hilar adenopathy, usually unilateral, and less frequently a small parenchymal infiltrate in the mid or lower lung fields. Diagnosis is based on a positive tuberculin test, which is almost always marked in degree. Occasionally the sputum smear is positive for acid-fast bacilli on microscopy, and tubercle bacilli can probably be cultured from gastric aspirates if several specimens are obtained on different days. Although, as mentioned, symptoms are most often either lacking entirely or else evanescent and subtle, more advanced clinical syndromes based on hilar adenopathy, pleural effusion, and, rarely, direct progression of the initial pulmonary infiltrate may be seen. In the majority in whom tuberculosis produces symptoms, however, these result from either early or late progression of hematogenous foci in the apices of the lungs or elsewhere in the body (see Chronic Pulmonary Tuberculosis and Extrapulmonary Tuberculosis).

Hilar adenopathy may produce symptoms in the infant and young child owing to a tendency to massive enlargement of lymph nodes and the small size and relative flaccidity of the bronchi, which in combination favor compression and obstruction. Extrinsic compression may produce partial or complete bronchial obstruction, resulting in segmental or lobar collapse and obstructive pneumonitis. Involvement of the bronchial wall from contiguous tuberculous inflammation in the node may progress to produce granulation tissue within the bronchial lumen and seeding of tuberculous foci in the associated segment or lobe. Prolonged partial bronchial obstruction caused by enlarged nodes, cicatricial changes within the bronchus, or both, may result in bronchiectasis distally. Occasionally a node may dissect into the bronchus, emptying its highly antigenic contents and causing an intense bronchitis and pneumonitis or frank tuberculous pneumonia progressing to caseous necrosis. (At any time the node involvement may become quiescent and in later life dissect into the bronchus and produce symptoms of hemoptysis or segmental tuberculous pneumonitis.)

Tuberculous pleurisy and effusion (see Diseases of the Pleura) is an important and not uncommon complication occurring soon after infection both in children and young adults. A subpleural primary focus may either dissect into the pleural cavity or drain into pleural lymphatics. Less commonly, the hematogenous dissemination associated with the initial infection may produce secondary subpleural foci which dissect into the pleural cavity. Even though the effusion usually subsides spontaneously, a large percentage of patients will subsequently develop progressive pulmonary or extrapulmonary tuberculosis. Idiopathic pleurisy and effusion, especially in children or young adults with a positive tuberculin test, should be treated as active tuberculosis unless another diagnosis is established beyond doubt.

The term *progressive primary* is usually applied to direct evolution of a poorly contained initial infiltrate into a pneumonic and eventually caseous process. It may be differentiated from the usual case of chronic pulmonary tuberculosis by roentgenologic evidence of hilar adenopathy and by the more frequent nonapical position of the infiltrate. This term has also been used to describe all forms of pulmonary tuberculosis occurring soon after the initial infection, whether in the area of the initial infiltrate, secondary to lymph node disease, or in apical foci seeded at the time of initial tuberculous bacteremia. This broader definition is less helpful.

It should be emphasized that features characteristic of childhood tuberculosis may also be seen in groups with low genetic resistance to tuberculosis. Thus extensive hilar adenopathy apparently occurs more frequently in young black adults than in whites. Particularly in isolated populations into which tuberculous infection has only recently been introduced, clinical manifestations in adults take on many of the features ordinarily associated with disease in children, except, of course, those related to the size and compressibility of the bronchial tree.

Treatment of childhood tuberculosis varies little from treatment in the adult, except that isoniazid dosage is larger (10 to 15 mg. per kilogram). The risk of induction of pyridoxine deficiency and peripheral neuritis is negligible in the young. An identified but uncomplicated infection is usually treated with isoniazid alone, except when drug resistance seems likely on epidemiologic grounds (contact with a known drug-resistant patient). Limitation of activity and provision for added sleep and rest during the day are advisable for the first few weeks. Patients symptomatic because of bronchial compression by enlarged nodes may be benefited by a short course of corticosteroids (in dosage equivalent to prednisone, 20 to 40 mg. per day). It must be recognized that resolution of a tuberculous process under therapy may proceed less rapidly in a lymph node than in lung parenchyma. Hence, the roentgenologic density, which is due to lymph node compression and not to intrinsic disease, may not recede rapidly with drug therapy (see Extrapulmonary Tuberculosis). Treatment of progressive, caseous pulmonary parenchymal disease is the same for children as for adults, except for the higher isoniazid dosage.

CHRONIC PULMONARY TUBERCULOSIS

In contrast to that in children, tuberculosis in adults is predominantly a disease of the pulmonary parenchyma. As mentioned, most if not all chronic pulmonary tuberculosis in the adult is due to the evolution of foci seeded during the preallergic bacteremic phase of the initial infection. This evolution may occur either fairly promptly or after long periods of quiescence when subtle changes in the host resistance or other factors produce conditions favorable for this to occur. Whether or not a latent period intervenes, these foci gain largest size and, therefore, are most prone to reactivation in the apical posterior aspects of the lung, in which local factors are most favorable to bacterial growth.

The earliest infiltrate in chronic pulmonary tuberculosis appears most commonly in the posterior or apical segment of an upper lobe or the apical segment of a lower lobe, beginning as a small patch of bronchopneumonia surrounding a growing colony of tubercle bacilli. This inflammatory reaction in the hypersensitive host produces an alveolar exudate containing fibrin-rich fluid and a mixture of inflammatory cells. With increasing intensity of the inflammatory reaction, tissue necrosis of a type quite characteristic of tuberculosis and termed *caseous* (of a cheesy consistency) develops. As long as it persists intact, caseous necrosis is an effective mechanism of host defense, inhibiting bacterial growth and causing the death of most organisms, presumably because of low oxygen tension and probably other factors as well. (Invariably, however, a few metabolically dormant organisms persist.) The critical factors reversing this favorable trend are the tendency of the caseous material eventually to liquefy and the access of liquefied material to the bronchial tree. Bronchial drainage of liquefied material produces a *cavity* in open communication with inspired air, in which high oxygen tension enhances bacterial multiplication and from which secretions rich in bacteria are spread via the bronchi to other areas of the lung and to the outside environment. *Once reactivation occurs, the progressive nature of tuberculosis in the hypersensitive host is largely due to the combination of these three factors: the tendency of caseous necrosis to liquefy, the access of liquefied and infectious material to the bronchial tree, and the aerobic nature of the organisms, resulting in huge bacterial populations within open cavities.*

Organisms delivered to the draining bronchus expose other areas of the lung to infection. Bronchogenic spread may take place by simple spillage, but is enhanced by the cough mechanisms which, because of explosive expiration followed by deep inspiration, aerosolize infectious material and then distribute it widely throughout the lung. Sooner or later new foci of disease develop. Each in turn may undergo caseous necrosis and then heal, or liquefy, slough, and produce another cavity. New lesions usually appear first within other portions of the segment or lobe initially involved. Although contiguous spread may occur, bronchial spread is more frequent, producing scattered, patchy disease. The apical posterior areas of the contralateral lung are apt to become diseased, presumably again because of local factors intrinsic to these areas favoring growth of organisms spread via the bronchi. In addition to the exudative tissue response characteristic of progressive disease, there is usually also a productive tissue reaction characterized by giant cells and epithelioid cells forming tubercles and leading eventually to fibrosis and healing. This is particularly true in the anterior and basal portions of the lung which have a remarkable capacity to resist progressive infection. Continuing, heavy exposure to these areas from cavities above usually produces gradual destruction by scarring and fibrosis rather than new necrotic areas. Almost all lesions will show some mixture of exudative and productive tissue responses, with progressive disease in one area coexisting with regression in another. Moreover, the pace and tempo of progressive disease is highly variable from one patient to the next and in the same individual at different times. Lowered host resistance, owing to either intercurrent or genetic factors, vigorous hypersensitivity reactions, and large numbers of organisms favor acute inflammatory reactions and rapid progression, which may produce the clinical and roentgenographic picture of acute, confluent, bacterial pneumonia (*tuberculous pneumonia* or *phthisis florida*). At the other end of the spectrum, relatively effective immunity, limited hypersensitivity, and a low bacterial population favor predominantly productive lesions, slow progression, and a greater tendency to spontaneous healing. Large, thick-walled cavities in a shrunken, extensively carnified lobe (chronic fibroid tuberculosis) may persist for years without causing symptoms but serving as a constant source of contagion for susceptible persons in the environment.

Mechanisms of healing are basically the same whether they occur spontaneously, under the influence of rest therapy, or after drug treatment. The exudative component of the early bronchopneumonic infiltrate may resolve with preservation of normal lung architecture and function. More often the exudate organizes and is replaced with fibrous tissue. Caseous foci may remain solid and become encapsulated by fibrosis. The bronchus draining an open cavity occasionally becomes obstructed by granulation tissue and debris at the bronchocavitary junction. Such blocked cavities may become inspissated and encapsulated with fibrotic tissue and result in a tenuous form of healing. A cavity that remains open probably always remains infectious except under the influence of antimicrobial therapy of prolonged duration, which may produce elimination of all necrotic and infectious tissue and a clean fibrotic cavity wall. It must be remembered, however, that regardless of the type and extent of healing, viable though dormant organisms persist, which in favorable circumstances are capable of renewed growth and reactivation of disease.

Clinical Manifestations

Symptoms. Pulmonary tuberculosis in its incipiency is most often asymptomatic. Small apical infiltrates may persist for months or even years in tenuous balance, undergoing minor extensions and regressions and producing no indication by which their presence might be known unless fortuitously discovered by chest roentgenogram. When sufficient in amount, however, absorption of tuberculoprotein and other antigenic substances results in *constitutional or general symptoms* such as anorexia, weight loss, asthenia, lassitude and fatigue, fever, chilliness, rarely frank rigors, night sweats, and wasting. These are in no way specific, being produced in indistinguishable fashion by a wide variety of chronic, progressive infectious and neoplastic processes. However, in earlier years tuberculosis so greatly overshadowed all other causes alone or in combination of these constitutional symptoms that they were taken, with justification, as indicative of phthisis. In the majority, constitutional symptoms begin insidiously and progress gradually over so protracted a period that the patient may not realize that he is ill. Not infrequently the magnitude of the illness is recognized with surprise only when viewed retrospectively in comparison with the state of restored health effected by drug therapy. Weight loss and fatigue are more likely to lead to medical attention than is fever, which is often unappreciated by the patient although usually present in the later course of the illness, characteristically in the afternoon.

Symptoms related specifically to the local inflammatory reaction in the lung are also variable in degree and in time of onset, and although they tend to appear somewhat later, do in general parallel constitutional symptoms in onset and degree. *Cough* and *sputum* are the most consistent and predictable local symptoms. Both are due to bronchial involvement, which usually does not occur until parenchymal cavitation develops. Accordingly, their presence indicates an already advanced extent of disease. Bronchial irritation in the path of draining cavities with or without actual tuberculous bronchitis stimulates the cough reflex. Cavity drainage, together with bronchial secretions, results in sputum production. Depending upon the degree of bronchial reaction, the size of cavities, and the quantity of drainage, cough may vary from mild and unnoticed to paroxysmal and severe, and sputum may be scant and mucoid or copious and purulent. Usually cough and sputum appear gradually and progress slowly over months or years, varying with the tempo and destructiveness of the pulmonary process. Temporary improvement may dissuade the patient from seeking diagnostic attention, with tragic and, in earlier years, often mortal consequences.

Two symptoms which are fortuitous and unpredictable are *hemoptysis* and *chest pain*. Hemoptysis may be associated with rapid slough of a caseous lesion or may be due to ulceration in a draining bronchus. It usually presents as bloodstreaking or a small amount of fresh blood. It can occur early, but is usually a manifestation of advanced disease. Particularly in late chronic disease, bleeding may be copious and sudden, owing to involvement and necrosis of an artery within the fibrous wall of a cavity (Rasmussen aneurysm). Exsanguination is unusual, but particularly in advanced disease with compromised pulmonary function there may be a real threat of drowning, which requires prompt positioning for drainage (prone or Trendelenburg) and avoidance of reflex-dulling drugs. Hemoptysis of almost any degree is attended by great concern. Prior to the availability of effective chemotherapy, a large hemoptysis was often associated with extensive bronchogenic spread of infectious material. However, at present the fever and new basilar infiltrates caused by aspirated blood do not result in new tuberculous foci, being rapidly responsive to chemotherapy, and clearing in a few days or a week is the rule. A less startling symptom, but one also meriting concern, is pleural pain. This is usually due to extension of inflammation to the pleural surface with involvement of the parietal pleura without production of pleural fluid (*dry pleurisy*). Much less commonly, pleural pain will be associated with serofibrinous pleurisy with effusion (which ordinarily occurs earlier in the course of the infection than does established apical pulmonary tuberculosis), and rarely tuberculous empyema will be discovered. Like hemoptysis, chest pain is a seldom ignored symptom, and these two are the symptoms most likely to lead to a diagnosis of tuberculosis. Rarely, medical attention is not sought until manifestations of very advanced illness occur. These may be due to disease in other tissues bathed in the highly infectious pulmonary secretions. Painful mouth ulcers, hoarseness and dysphagia owing to laryngeal involvement, tuberculous otitis media, or anal pain caused by a tuberculous perirectal abscess may first bring the patient to the physician. Shortness of breath may accompany acute tuberculous pneumonia or indicate impending pulmonary insufficiency following extensive destructive disease.

Lower and Middle Lobe Tuberculosis in Older Persons. As the frequency of chronic pulmonary tuberculosis in young adults recedes, certain atypical presentations in older persons are being recognized with some frequency. A chronic and progressive infiltrate in the lower or mid lung field may be due to a recently acquired primary infection, with direct progression in an older person with the weakened immunologic responsiveness attendant on old age. Also, long quiescent tuberculous hilar lymph nodes may dissect into a bronchus, release infectious material into it, and cause tuberculous pneumonia in the associated lobe or segment. Particularly in older women, some instances of the "middle lobe syndrome," ordinarily caused by nontuberculous infection in an obstructed lobe, will be found to be due to tuberculosis activated in this manner.

Physical Examination. A complete physical examination is essential to the proper assessment of individuals with pulmonary tuberculosis and will provide valuable information regarding the degree of illness, the patient's tolerance to it, the presence of associated diseases, and the anatomic and functional changes in the lung. There are no physical findings per se that are diagnostic of tuberculosis. In the assessment of the pulmonary disease, it is important that information derived from the physical findings be evaluated in conjunction with the chest roentgenogram. *Both provide information unavailable from the other, and neither examination is adequate without the other.* It is as necessary to recognize the deficiencies of the physical examination as it is to appreciate its usefulness. The physical examination of the chest usually suggests less extensive disease than is found by roentgenogram, and may be entirely negative in the presence of advanced pulmonary tuberculosis. Negative findings should never be accepted as evidence that disease is not present.

In spite of these inadequacies, physical examination provides some information concerning the details of pulmonary involvement not obtainable in any other way. Careful inspection may reveal asymmetry in respiratory excursion, most easily appreciated by careful observation of the subclavicular areas tangentially viewed from the foot of the bed with the patient lying flat. The rate, depth, and effort associated with respiration will provide some index of ventilatory reserve, especially after light exertion. Advanced fibrotic lesions may produce contraction of the hemithorax and deviation of the trachea. Palpation and percussion will usually demonstrate dullness and increased tactile fremitus over the side of the lesion. Dullness associated with decreased rather than increased fremitus may be caused by either marked pleural thickening or, less commonly and generally over the lower lung fields only, pleural fluid. Auscultation may reveal obvious rales, but frequently these can be detected only during a quick inspiration following a short cough. Maneuvers to elicit these fine showers of *post-tussic rales* are essential for an adequate chest examination, even of normal individuals. (Interestingly, rales may persist for years after disease has become inactive, owing presumably to permanent distortion of small bronchial passages during healing.) Although large areas of infiltrate may occasionally produce decreased breath sounds, more commonly tuberculosis produces increased transmission of breath sounds originating in the larger air passages, as the bronchi characteristically remain patent. Bronchial or frankly tubular breath sounds, bronchophony, and, when the process is extensive, whispered pectoriloquy may be heard. The distant and hollow tubular breath sounds heard over a thick-walled cavity appropriately positioned in relation to a bronchus are termed *amphoric* to suggest their resemblance to the sounds made by blowing across the mouth of a large jar (amphora). Examination during forced hyperventilation may detect local stenosis and obstruction of a bronchus not appreciated during quiet breathing.

Usually examination of the remainder of the body provides little information pertaining to the pulmonary disease. Careful funduscopic examination in severely ill, febrile patients may reveal choroidal tubercles. Careful search for associated extrapulmonary tuberculosis in the central nervous system, spine, lymphatic system, and skeletal system should be carried out. Splenomegaly is unusual and when present may indicate associated secondary amyloidosis.

Roentgenologic Findings. The chest roentgenogram is critically important in the diagnosis of pulmonary tuberculosis, in evaluation of the character and course of the disease, and in follow-up studies. Although the diagnosis cannot be established on the basis of roentgenologic findings alone, the character and location of infiltrates may be strongly suggestive to the practiced eye. The lesions tend to be patchy and to be located primarily in the apical posterior areas. Gross cavities can usually be easily seen in the standard P-A chest roentgenogram, but may be missed entirely. Cavities are much more clearly seen with planigrams, which are very helpful both in initial assessment and in determining whether cavity closure has taken place during treatment. It is possible to a considerable extent to estimate certain histopathologic characteristics of the infiltrate seen on chest roentgenogram. Exudative lesions tend to have soft margins that shade off into the surrounding normal lung tissue. The presence of caseation is suggested by increased density. Productive lesions tend to be small and nodular and have hard or more sharply demarcated margins. Scar tissue has a particularly discrete and sharply defined margin against a background of normal lung, and tends to contract. Healing exudative lesions characteristically first decrease in size and density and later, as scarring develops, become more sharply defined. When these changes level off to the point of only slow further contraction, the lesion is said to be roentgenologically stable, providing one of the criteria by which achievement of quiescent or inactive status is determined. In follow-up studies unchanging shadows are taken as evidence of a healed lesion.

Other Laboratory Findings. The normocytic, normochromic anemia of chronic infection is usually present and may be severe. The white blood count is usually within normal limits; marked leukocytosis should suggest a complicating bacterial infection. A monocytosis of 8 to 15 per cent may be seen. The erythrocyte sedimentation rate is usually elevated. In prolonged and severe infection, hyperglobulinemia and hypoalbuminemia in some combination may be seen. Hematuria or pyuria may direct attention to coexisting renal tuberculosis. Marked albuminuria should suggest complicating amyloidosis. A low serum sodium is sometimes found in extensive chronic pulmonary tuberculosis owing to abnormal retention of water and is attributed to inappropriate secretion of antidiuretic hormone. Treatment is water restriction, and the problem disappears as the infection responds to drug therapy. It is important to exclude diabetes because of the higher incidence of tuberculosis in this disease.

Diagnosis. The diagnosis of tuberculosis is usually suggested by the clinical picture and roentgenographic findings. A strong presumptive diagnosis may often be made on the basis of roentgenographic characteristics alone. A *direct sputum smear* positive for acid-fast bacteria on microscopy will in the proper setting provide nearly conclusive evidence, and positive findings on microscopy are the rule in extensive or cavitary disease (see Bacteriology in previous article). However, even in advanced disease, failure to demonstrate bacilli on microscopy cannot be used as evidence excluding a diagnosis of tuberculosis. Rarely, acid-fast bacilli on microscopy will be misleading, as not all destructive mycobacterial pulmonary disease is tuberculosis, although the nontuberculous forms are certainly a small minority. Moreover, any destructive process in the lung, particularly in the apical posterior area, may erode an inactive focus and cause appearance of acid-fast bacilli in the sputum with or without the development of new, active tuberculosis. Acid-fast bacilli on microscopy of *a gastric concentrate* represent less strong presumptive evidence, but still, in cases in which tuberculosis is suspected, the majority of positive findings in gastric smears will be due to active infection with *M. tuberculosis. The tuberculin test,* although of great use in children and in adults who are not severely ill, is of much less crucial diagnostic importance in the seriously ill individual, particularly in the older age groups. The causes of false positive tuberculin reactions, quantitative aspects of tuberculin testing, and the techniques and dosage employed have been discussed in the previous article (see Tuberculin Test). However, it bears repeating that some patients with proved tuberculosis are negative reactors to high concentrations of tuberculin when first seen. In patients with pulmonary infiltrates but not otherwise ill, a negative reaction to high concentrations of tuberculin should exclude tuberculosis in 99 per cent. A positive tuberculin test at any strength is of limited diagnostic significance in the individual patient. *Histologic demonstration of granulomatous disease* is only presumptive evidence of tuberculosis, varying in its implications with the source of the specimen. Demonstration of typical histologic changes in a cervical lymph node carries less weight than in pulmonary tissue. (Diagnostic thoracotomy is usually employed to exclude neoplasm rather than to diagnose tuberculosis.) However, even demonstration of acid-fast bacteria in granulomatous or caseous tissue is not definitive in that they may represent mycobacteria other than *M. tuberculosis. Definitive diagnosis requires cultural identification of M. tuberculosis.* The techniques for obtaining and culturing specimens have been discussed in the preceding article (see Bacteriology). Although efforts to make a bacteriologic diagnosis should be assiduous, it is seldom justified to pursue them to lung biopsy, except when treatable neoplasm is a possibility. Accordingly, therapy with isoniazid may often be initiated with proof of diagnosis. The therapeutic response may leave little doubt as to diagnosis, but in any event, therapeutic trials of antituberculous drugs, once embarked upon, are usually continued for a period of time appropriate for treatment regardless of whether the diagnosis is eventually established by either culture or clinical response.

Differential Diagnosis. Although tuberculosis may be confused with virtually any intrathoracic condition, certain diseases are frequently considered in differential diagnosis. *Fungal disease,* particularly histoplasmosis, can be indistinguishable from chronic cavitary or fibroid tuberculosis. Moreover, coexistence of histoplasmosis and tuberculosis in the same person is not rare. *Disease caused by mycobacteria other than tubercle bacilli* is often indistinguishable from pulmonary tuberculosis in its more chronic forms. *Bronchiectasis* may present with hemoptysis or with symptoms of chronic infection, including cough, sputum, and chronic ill health, and bronchiectatic areas surrounded by infiltrate may suggest cavitation roentgenographically. Symptomatic bronchiectasis is more frequently located in a lower lobe, but upper lobe areas may be involved. Diagnosis is based on bronchography, failure to identify *M. tuberculosis,* and response to antimicrobial therapy. *Cavitary lung abscess* may be confused with cavitary tuberculosis. Again, location of disease is of some help, lung abscesses being more common in dependent portions of the lung. However, both tuberculosis and lung abscess may involve the dorsal segments of the lower lobes and posterior segments of the upper lobes, which are likely areas for lodgment of material aspirated during sleep or coma. A fluid level in a cavity is more suggestive of nonspecific lung abscess, in which intermittent obstruction of the bronchocavitary junction is common and secretions copious, than of cavitary tuberculosis in which secretions are less extensive and the bronchocavitary junction tends to remain patent. The tuberculous cavity, if properly located, transmits bronchial breath sounds well, and tubular breathing, often with amphoric character, may be heard. Auscultation over a lung abscess usually reveals markedly suppressed breath sounds with a few inspiratory rales. The presence of scattered infiltrates elsewhere in the lung suggests tuberculosis, because successful bronchogenic spread of disease caused by the less virulent organisms in a nonspecific lung abscess is unusual. *Acute bacterial pneumonias* may resemble florid tuberculosis in all particulars save for the absence of acid-fast bacilli on sputum microscopy and the response to antimicrobial agents. *Neoplasm* may closely resemble tuberculosis, as in an isolated coin lesion, a central obstructing and inconspicuous endobronchial tumor with distal chronic inflammation, or a neoplastic mass that has undergone necrosis and cavitation. The roentgenographic picture of a thickened cavity wall with irregular masses and nodules extending into the excavated center suggests necrotic neoplasm, but in some instances a thin and smooth-walled cavity will be found to be due to cancer. The association between neoplasm and tuberculosis is complex, first, because cancer may erode into and reactivate a latent tuberculous focus; second, because saprophytic mycobacteria may be found in association with a destructive neoplasm; and third, because chronic scarring in a tuberculous focus may induce neoplastic degeneration. Roentgenographic progression of a previously stable, fibrotic tuberculous focus may be due to "scar cancer" rather than progressive infection. Many other chronic pulmonary processes may be indistinguishable from tuberculosis. This confusion ordinarily leads either to diagnostic thoracotomy or, when the presence or absence of tuberculosis is the only consideration with important therapeutic implications, to therapy with isoniazid.

Classification of Pulmonary Tuberculosis. The American Thoracic Society has maintained an up-to-date classification of pulmonary tuberculosis, incorporating new principles and concepts as they have developed. The following classification and definitions are summarized from the 1969 *Diagnostic Standards and Classification of Tuberculosis.* The two main variables are extent of disease and status of clinical activity. By defining these variables in terms of time, it is possible to describe the course of each case from diagnosis to any point in time thereafter.

Extent of Disease. Minimal. The total area of disease, taken in the aggregate regardless of distribution, is less than the area from the second chondrocostal junction and the fifth vertebral body to the apex of the lung on one side, and no cavity is demonstrable (planigrams usually required).

Moderately Advanced. The aggregate total area of scattered, small lesions is less than one lung field, or of dense, confluent lesions less than the equivalent of one third of one lung field. The total diameter of cavitation, if present, is less than 4 cm.

Far Advanced. This term describes disease greater in extent than moderately advanced.

Status of Clinical Activity. The stages of activity are defined by roentgenographic changes and bacteriologic findings; the duration of each stage is given. The initial diagnosis is dependent upon the demonstration of *M. tuberculosis* on culture.

Active. The disease is considered to be active as long as, and for a three-month period after, either tubercle bacilli have been detected in the sputum (or gastric aspirate) or the chest roentgenogram shows serial changes of more than slight clearing or contraction of lesions. The duration of activity begins with date of diagnosis. Example: Active (since August 1969). After a period of observation, the terms "improved," "unimproved," or "worse" may be added.

Quiescent, Noncavitary. This status requires both negative bacteriologic findings (monthly examinations) and a stable roentgenogram (only slight clearing or contraction) without cavitation for three months or more, but less than six months. Duration of status should be given. Example: Quiescent, noncavitary (since October 1969).

Quiescent, Cavitary. The requirements are the same except that the presence of cavitation is permitted. The duration of this status should also be given. Example: Quiescent, cavitary (since October 1969).

Inactive, Noncavitary. Negative monthly bacteriologic findings and stable chest roentgenogram without cavitation for six months are required. The duration of inactivity should be given. Example: Inactive, noncavitary (since November 1969).

Inactive, Cavitary. The persistence of cavitation is permitted, but there must be negative bacteriologic findings (preferably at monthly, but at least at three-month intervals) and stable roentgenogram *for 18 months.* The duration of this status should be given. Example: Inactive, cavitary (since November 1969).

The terms "activity undetermined," "probably active," or "probably inactive" are useful in circumstances when there is inadequate bacteriologic or roentgenographic data. Chemotherapy and surgical procedures should be added to the description of the clinical status. Example: Quiescent, noncavitary (since November 1969), chemotherapy (since May 1969); inactive, noncavitary (since May 1968) (24 months' chemotherapy completed August 1969); quiescent, noncavitary (since November 1969), chemotherapy (since January 1969), (right upper lobectomy August 1969). Example of complete diagnosis: On admission: pulmonary tuberculosis, far advanced, active (since February 1969). At present: pulmonary tuberculosis, moderately advanced, quiescent, cavitary (since October 1969), chemotherapy (since May 1969).

Treatment of Pulmonary Tuberculosis

Prior to the demonstration of the antituberculous activity of streptomycin in 1945, the man-agement of pulmonary tuberculosis was based entirely upon efforts to bolster host resistance, mainly by bed rest and procedures to aid in cavity closure (pneumothorax, pneumoperitoneum, phreniclasia, and thorocoplasty). The development of effective antimicrobial drugs provided a much more effective means of management through direct attack upon the tubercle bacillus. However, the inherent characteristics of the tubercle bacillus and of the host response in humans have raised obstacles to the development of successful drug therapy. The capacity of the tubercle bacillus to retreat into a metabolically dormant state allows some viable cells to survive the bacteriostatic drugs presently available. The development of caseation also encourages the metabolically dormant state favoring persistence of infection. Therefore, although effective drug therapy may control the active phase of pulmonary tuberculosis, the slow processes of host-healing mechanisms are required for permanent control.

At the onset of the antimicrobial era, drugs were used as adjuncts to established treatment methods. It was quickly learned that drugs had to be administered for prolonged periods in order to avoid relapse and that use of more than one drug tended to prevent development of a drug-resistant infection, particularly in the case of the pulmonary cavity, in which the large bacterial population provides significant numbers of naturally occurring variants resistant to any presently available drug. The proper use of these two principles and the use of isoniazid as the main drug resulted in such effective treatment of tuberculosis that older methods became relatively insignificant and have been employed less and less. Collapse procedures gave way to resectional surgery in dealing with residual cavities, and more recently even the residual cavity has been shown in most cases to be safely managed by effective antimicrobial therapy without resection.

Pulmonary tuberculosis is a chronic disease, its course measured in months and years. The antimicrobial era has very gradually evolved over more than 25 years as new drugs and drug combinations appear and are evaluated by long-term clinical studies. Controlled clinical studies and trials have established certain basic principles of drug usage, but concepts gradually change as new data become available. Many of these changing concepts have not been fully evaluated and they, and the practices based upon them, are in some cases controversial. A textbook presentation must offer a definite and somewhat oversimplified plan of approach which in the author's judgment is the most reasonable at the time; it cannot include the discussion of both sides of all controversial points.

Effective use of presently available antimicrobial drugs is potentially capable of providing permanent healing in 95 to 100 per cent of cases of previously untreated pulmonary tuberculosis. In actual practice in many if not most areas, the figure falls far short of this value. In part, this represents poor medical direction, but in larger part, the often carefully concealed failure of the patient to take the drugs is responsible. The necessary prolonged use of drugs long after the patient feels normally well is difficult for even the most well informed and intelligent patient. Continued direction, encouragement, and support are important aspects.

There are presently nearly a dozen drugs with significant antituberculous activity and acceptable toxicity. Most of these are available for general use. *Isoniazid* (INH), the most potent and least toxic drug, is central to all plans of therapy. *Streptomycin* (SM) is presently second in degree of effectiveness (see rifampin below), but must be administered intramuscularly. *Para-aminosalicyclic acid* (PAS) has little antimicrobial activity itself, but has enjoyed a long and effective service as a companion drug. *Ethambutol* (EMB), relatively new on the scene, has considerable promise for general use if experience allays fears of potential optic nerve toxicity. *Ethionamide* (ETH) and *pyrazinamide* (PZA) are the best of those secondary drugs which are characterized by relatively low potency and high toxicity; these are useful in re-treatment cases in which resistance has developed to the more effective agents. *Cycloserine, viomycin,* and *kanamycin* also belong in this group. *Capreomycin,* close to streptomycin in therapeutic range and similar in toxicity, has not been released for general use. On the basis of the initial clinical experience, the orally administered drug *rifampin* appears to rival isoniazid in potency and low toxicity. If its early promise is fulfilled, it has attractive prospects as a powerful companion drug for INH in initial treatment. A more detailed description of these agents appears at the end of this article.

Principles of Drug Therapy. The Role of Isoniazid. Isoniazid is central to the treatment of virtually every case of tuberculosis (see detailed description below). Its effectiveness is of a higher order than that of any other agent. It is administered by mouth, is the least toxic antimicrobial of any sort now available, is very inexpensive, is specific for *M. tuberculosis* and *M. bovis,* and diffuses readily into tissues and body cavities. These characteristics make it an ideal drug not only for acute therapy but also for prolonged treatment. Also, in contrast to all other agents, most strains of isoniazid-resistant tubercle bacilli are less virulent than drug-susceptible organisms; for this and perhaps other reasons isoniazid seems to have at least suppressive effect even in infections caused by highly resistant organisms. *Accordingly, the chemotherapy of tuberculosis includes isoniazid in every case except for the exceptional patient in whom its use is associated with serious toxic reactions and desensitization procedures are ineffective or particularly dangerous.*

Drug Resistance and the Need for Combined Drug Therapy. Drug resistance is of two sorts: *primary resistance* discovered in previously untreated patients, and *resistance emerging during the course of treatment.* Although understandably a matter of great concern, primary resistance has not yet become a major problem in most areas.

Continuing surveys in the United States, Great Britain, and elsewhere indicate a rather stable level of 2 to 3 per cent of previously untreated infections primarily resistant to either isoniazid or streptomycin, and less than 1 per cent to both drugs at the same time. However, some careful studies have demonstrated a higher incidence of primary drug resistance in children in urban areas of known high prevalence. In many of these patients, however, response to isoniazid was good in spite of the demonstrated resistance to this drug. The incidence of resistance is much higher, perhaps as great as 20 per cent, in certain underdeveloped areas in Africa and elsewhere. The reliability of these figures has been questioned, and it is suspected that considerable numbers of previously treated patients with *emergent* resistance are included. It is possible that the full weight of primary drug resistance will not be felt for many years, because clinical tuberculosis often results from an infection remote in time. Accordingly, continuing studies of primary drug resistance in various locations are vital, and their recent results should be followed closely by all concerned with the treatment of tuberculosis.

Drug resistance incurred during treatment is a problem of major concern, recognized ever since the earliest studies with streptomycin. In any large bacterial population, naturally occurring mutants resistant to isoniazid appear at a predictable rate of one per 10^5 or 10^6 bacterial cells. This is true with respect to streptomycin and probably all other antituberculous drugs as well. Thus, when isoniazid is administered without a companion drug, drug-susceptible cells are killed or suppressed, and the resistant bacteria, if other circumstances allow, in time repopulate the site of infection. This is of little practical importance in closed lesions with a low bacterial population, but is extremely important in lesions associated with large bacterial populations, as is typically the case in the pulmonary cavity. The bacterial population in a cavity may be as large as 10^9 or 10^{10} organisms and, therefore, as many as 10^3 or more isoniazid-resistant bacteria might be present from the outset, providing an ample nidus for establishment of a drug-resistant infection once the larger susceptible population is suppressed. Under these circumstances, and with the continued discharge of culturable bacilli, significant numbers of resistant organisms appear in the sputum in a few weeks; after three to four months, the major portion of the bacterial population is converted to strains resistant to the drug in vitro. If two drugs to which the bacterial population are basically susceptible are used at the same time, and organisms resistant to each are present in a ratio of 1 to 10^5 bacterial cells, then the chance of a strain appearing resistant to both is in the range of 1 in 10^{10}, which is unlikely in even the largest bacterial populations. This is the basis of the principle of combined therapy in which two or more effective drugs are used, each active against the organisms resistant to the other. Although the purpose of combined therapy is primarily the prevention of the development of resistance to an effective drug, it may also be designed to increase drug effectiveness. It is important to accomplish either or both of these aims with the least hazard of drug toxicity. The character and severity of the disease should determine the drug combinations used. Cavities with thick necrotic walls and large areas of caseation provide both the greatest hazard of drug resistance and the severest test of drug therapy. Isoniazid and streptomycin represent the most effective combination. Each is more effective than any other drug in suppressing strains resistant to the other. Also there is reason to believe that the combined bacteriostatic effect is greater than that of isoniazid alone. This combination is, therefore, recommended for severe disease. Triple therapy (INH + SM + PAS) has long been advocated in severe disease as a further effort to avoid drug resistance, but there is no substantial evidence that it is better in this respect or has a greater bacteriostatic effect than isoniazid plus streptomycin, and it is clearly more subject to drug hypersensitivity reactions.

Prolonged Therapy. The principle of prolonged therapy was also firmly established early in the antimicrobial drug era by the observation that activity recurred if drug therapy was terminated too soon and that ordinarily this was due to organisms still susceptible to the agents administered. Since the antituberculous drugs were not eradicative for dormant organisms, it became evident that suppressive therapy must be continued until the slow processes of host-healing mechanisms secured control of residual infection. Strangely, there have been few controlled clinical studies designed to test the important question of how long is "prolonged," and what circumstances modify the duration of appropriate suppressive therapy. General experience indicates that for most diseases without residual cavity or large areas of caseation, two years of over-all drug treatment are usually adequate to secure permanent healing. For years persistent cavities were surgically excised when possible in order to diminish risk of relapse. As more prolonged periods of suppressive drug therapy came into use, it became apparent that the persistent "open negative" thin-walled cavity was not a serious threat, and with prolonged drug treatment most sloughed their necrotic lining, leaving a clean and sterile fibrous wall. For most thin-walled cavities, three to four years of drug therapy is usually indicated. For caseous "open negative" thick-walled cavities, even longer suppressive drug therapy is indicated, or surgical excision may be advisable. In some cases of advanced, extensive, necrotic disease, indefinite prolongation of isoniazid therapy is sometimes advisable.

Stages of Therapy. The drug treatment of pulmonary tuberculosis is best considered as consisting of an *active treatment phase* during which a combination of drugs is administered, and a *suppressive phase* during which isoniazid, usually as a single agent, is continued. These incorporate

the principles of combined and prolonged treatment. An effective combination of drugs, usually isoniazid and streptomycin in severe disease, and isoniazid and PAS in less severe disease, is continued until control of the active stage of the disease is assured. Definition of assured control has been neglected in clinical studies and trials, but general experience suggests that if there are no persistent cavities, drugs other than isoniazid can be discontinued at the point at which the particular disease is technically quiescent, that is, three months after the sputum shows no tubercle bacilli on microscopy and culture. Reversal of infectiousness (sputum conversion) is the most important assessment. In cases of residual cavitation, combined therapy should be continued for a longer period, usually at least 6 to 12 months after disappearance of tubercle bacilli from the sputum, as the few persistent resistant organisms are more apt to establish a relapse in the favorable environment of a cavity than in a closed lesion. A "rapid converter" (sputum negative for tubercle bacilli in two to three months) has a better prognosis than a "slow converter" (still discharging bacilli after four to six months). A "slow converter" with persistent cavitation on effective drugs should continue combined drug therapy for a year or longer after the sputum is noninfectious. In patients initially treated with isoniazid and streptomycin, PAS may be substituted for streptomycin during the latter part of this period to make treatment easier and more acceptable to the patient.

The suppressive phase of drug therapy begins when the active stage of the disease is controlled. Isoniazid alone is ordinarily used at this time, and continued in patients without infectious sputum or residual cavities for a total treatment period of two years. When thin-walled residual cavities persist, this period is prolonged to three to four years.

Patient Participation. The best laid plans for drug therapy are at the mercy of reasonable patient cooperation. Failure on the part of the patient to take the prescribed drugs is probably the most frequent and important cause of treatment failure. There are many reasons for lapses in drug self-administration such as simple forgetfulness, the illusion of health associated with disappearance of symptoms and the return of a sense of well-being, and the always underestimated reluctance of almost all individuals to subject themselves to any discipline for prolonged periods. Some overtly discontinue drugs, following the dictum: "If I feel well I must be well." Alcoholics engrossed in their activities frequently forget or don't care. Patients notoriously lapse or are irregular in taking PAS because of the unpleasant gastrointestinal distresses. There are many less obvious reasons for drug lapses, including imagined drug reactions, queer health ideas, and rumors of many sorts passed on by other patients. There is a strong tendency in many patients to cover up such lapses. Every physician who treats tuberculosis has often observed relapse in a patient who indignantly maintains that he has taken his drugs faithfully only to find that the infection is still drug-susceptible and that the disease promptly responds to the same drugs given under supervision. It is important that the physician remain constantly aware of this human element which cannot be dissociated from the drug therapy formula.

A Plan of Drug Therapy. Initial Treatment. *Active Phase of Therapy.* Under most circumstances treatment is best initiated in a hospital where full roentgenologic and laboratory studies can be made, the patient can be kept under close observation and at reduced activity during the early stages of treatment, and he can be isolated during the period of contagiousness. In ideal circumstances, these aims can be achieved in the home. But even under the worst circumstances, reasonably good results may be obtained if only the patient will take the drugs. The consideration of first importance in any event is the institution and maintenance of effective antimicrobial drug therapy.

In selecting drugs for initial therapy, it is reasonable to assume that the organism is susceptible to all the antituberculous drugs. As mentioned, current studies show that *primary resistance* to either isoniazid or streptomycin occurs in only 2 to 3 per cent of new cases. Primary resistance to PAS is less than 1 per cent. The chance of resistance to two or more drugs is very small. The first choice for the main drug is always isoniazid. The decision as to what companion drug to use must be based on the character and severity of the disease, determined primarily by the roentgenologic findings. In *severe cavitary disease*, isoniazid plus daily streptomycin provides maximal drug effectiveness and maximal protection against development of resistance. Some physicians prefer to add PAS to the two major drugs as a further precaution against drug resistance, but without solid justification and clearly at the price of increased drug toxicity. In *moderate cavitary* or *noncavitary disease*, PAS is usually chosen as the companion drug for reasons of convenience. The antimicrobial activity of isoniazid suffices, and PAS is adequate to prevent emergence of resistant strains. As this clinical category includes the major portion of pulmonary tuberculosis, isoniazid plus PAS is the most frequently used form of combined therapy. It is to be hoped that a substitute for PAS is close at hand. If circumstances permit (which usually means hospitalization), it is quite reasonable to start treatment in all patients having more than minimal disease with isoniazid plus daily streptomycin. In two or three months, granting satisfactory progress, the companion drug can be changed to PAS or to twice-weekly streptomycin. However, the elective use of streptomycin is generally avoided over age 50 because of the more severe consequences of vestibular toxicity in older patients (see Streptomycin).

In *minimal, noncavitary disease* with at most a very few organisms in the sputum, it is permissible to use isoniazid alone. The single drug is less toxic and has much greater patient acceptance than isoniazid plus PAS. When initial bacterial populations are small, the emergence of drug-resistance is usually no problem. Care must be exercised in following the presence of organisms in the sputum, and if they do not promptly disappear (within two months), a second drug should be added.

Drug dosage: Under usual circumstances isoniazid is given in a dose of 4 to 6 mg. per kilogram, which in adults is ordinarily 300 mg. in a single daily dose. In unusually severe disease, the dose may be increased to 10 mg. per kilogram given in a single daily dose or in two divided doses. Occasionally a dose of 15 to 16 mg. per kilogram is used, but this adds considerable hazard of toxicity with little increase in effectiveness. Any dosage of isoniazid greater than 300 mg. daily must be accompanied by pyridoxine (50 to 100 mg. daily). In patients unable to take oral drugs, isoniazid may be given intramuscularly. Streptomycin is administered in a single intramuscular dose of 1 gram daily during the active treatment phase, but may be reduced to twice-weekly dosage for suppressive effect once the disease is under control. The usual dosage of PAS is 4 grams three times a day (5 grams of NaPAS three times a day). It may be given in a single daily dose of 8 grams (10 grams of NaPAS). The incidence of gastric intolerance may be reduced by beginning at half dosage and increasing gradually to full dosage over several days.

Laboratory studies: Ordinarily a bacteriologic diagnosis is established at least by the demonstration of acid-fast bacilli on sputum microscopy before institution of drug therapy. If the microscopy is negative, at least five or six adequate sputum specimens should be submitted for culture before interfering with the chance of a bacteriologic diagnosis by giving drugs. In a severely ill patient, drugs should be started immediately. In cavitary pulmonary tuberculosis, a few days of antituberculous drugs will not seriously interfere with demonstration of tubercle bacilli in the sputum. Complete roentgenographic studies, including, if possible, planigrams, should be obtained to evaluate the character and severity of the disease at the outset and progress on treatment. In addition to routine laboratory studies, renal function should be evaluated and the possibility of diabetes investigated. During the early course of treatment, the hemogram and urinalysis should be repeated at weekly intervals. Throughout the active treatment phase, chest roentgenograms and sputum concentrates for smear and culture should be obtained at no less than monthly intervals.

Drug-susceptibility studies for the commonly used drugs should be obtained on a pre-treatment sputum specimen, and again in three or four months if tubercle bacilli persist in the sputum.

The most significant event in the course of the active treatment phase is the disappearance of culturable tubercle bacilli from the sputum. In noncavitary disease or in patients with small and thin-walled cavities, this frequently occurs within one or two months. In more extensive cavitary disease, the "rapid converters" cease discharging tubercle bacilli in about two months. This has important prognostic significance in patients with residual cavitation, as it is associated with lower relapse rates than is observed in "slow converters" (tubercle bacilli persisting in the sputum for four months or longer). This may be due to larger initial bacterial populations in the "slow converters" and, therefore, larger numbers of resistant organisms. There may be differences also in certain host factors. "Slow converters" who achieve noninfectious sputum in four months usually do well. The continued discharge of tubercle bacilli in the sputum after four months is associated with a rapidly rising incidence of drug resistance, and after six months it is likely that the infection has become drug-resistant. Between the four- and six-month period, therefore, there is need to consider strengthening the drug regimen. Early in the period, adding a more potent companion drug, such as substituting streptomycin for PAS, may suffice, particularly if there are relatively few organisms in the sputum. If there are many organisms still present in the sputum, two new drugs are needed. If the original regimen was isoniazid plus streptomycin, it is best to continue these drugs and add ethambutol and PAS, or ethambutol and ethionamide while awaiting drug-susceptibility studies. If these show a significant proportion of the population to be resistant to either of the major drugs, then a regimen should be designed that contains at least two drugs to which drug-resistant cells are known to be susceptible. Although isoniazid is always continued even with high degrees of in vitro resistance, other drugs to which significant resistance is demonstrated are usually discontinued.

When the absence of tubercle bacilli from the sputum has been demonstrated for three consecutive months under the primary drug regimen, appropriate roentgenologic improvement has occurred (much less important), and no cavities or large areas of caseation persist, the active treatment phase may be superseded by the suppressive phase of treatment (usually isoniazid alone). In the case of persistent cavities ("open negative"), combined therapy should be continued for a longer time because of the greater hazard of resistant persisters re-establishing disease when the companion drug is stopped. For thin-walled cavities the additional period of combined drug therapy should be at least six months. In the presence of thick-walled cavities that usually contain much necrotic material, combined drug therapy should be continued for at least a year and perhaps a good deal longer. Expert judgment is required in these cases. The advisability of surgical excision may need to be explored.

The continued discharge of tubercle bacilli in the sputum after six months of drug therapy ordinarily means either that the patient is not taking his drugs or that there is a drug-resistant infection. Drug-susceptibility studies will answer this question. If the presence of a resistant infec-

tion is established and there are relatively few organisms in the sputum, adding two new drugs may suffice. In patients with a larger resistant population and unfavorable residual disease such as a large necrotic-walled cavity, surgical excision before using up all effective drugs must be considered. If drug-susceptibility studies reveal resistance to the companion drug and the clinical course suggests continued normal drug effect, replacement of the companion drug with one to which the organism is susceptible should be adequate. If resistance to isoniazid is as great as growth in 1 μg. per milliliter of the drug, the course is variable. In some cases the infection will be controlled in spite of in vitro resistance (in approximately 60 per cent). In order to cover all eventualities, it is best to add another effective drug, preferably streptomycin if not already used, so that there are two drugs to which the organism is susceptible. Isoniazid is continued regardless of the degree of in vitro resistance.

Suppressive Phase of Therapy. Once control has been established during the active phase, combined therapy is usually discontinued, and a prolonged period of suppressive treatment is then begun. In all but the more severe cases, it is reasonable to allow the patient to return to work at the beginning of the suppressive period of treatment. Ordinarily, isoniazid alone in a single daily dose of 300 mg. is used. In disease without residual cavitation this is continued until a total treatment period of at least two years is reached. In circumstances in which there is residual cavitation, the suppressive phase is continued until the total treatment period reaches three to four years or longer. In those cases in which isoniazid resistance was present, whether primary or acquired, another drug to which the strain is susceptible should also be used during the suppressive treatment phase. This may be necessary for only a few months for those in whom the resistant strain was not clinically significant, but should be continued longer, perhaps throughout the suppressive phase, in instances in which a clinically significant infection existed, i.e., uncontrolled until new drugs were added.

Re-treatment. In most re-treatment circumstances it is very important that the patient be managed in a hospital equipped to deal with problems of tuberculosis. Expert judgment and experience are particularly important in drug-resistant tuberculosis in order to attain maximal effectiveness from the limited drug resources available. Bed rest and other measures designed to augment host resistance become increasingly important, and should be used to maximal advantage. Even though resistance to isoniazid is demonstrated or suspected, it is important to continue the use of this drug and usually in higher than normal doses (up to 10 to 15 mg. per kilogram). Although there is little information from controlled studies, the consensus of general experience indicates that isoniazid-resistant strains are less pathogenic in human disease in rough proportion to the degree of resistance. It is, therefore, a reasonable aim to encourage even more resistant strains by continuing to use the drug.

There are an infinite variety of circumstances attending each re-treatment case, and each must be handled individually on its own merits. The determination of the susceptibility of the organism to all available drugs is critical to the proper management of most re-treatment cases. Some circumstances and principles of re-treatment are listed below.

1. Relapse in a patient whose sputum had promptly become negative for tubercle bacilli under treatment results in almost all cases from premature discontinuation of drugs (usually on the part of the patient). If drugs are stopped completely, most such patients will harbor drug-susceptible strains and will respond again to the regimen initially employed.

2. If lapse in treatment is followed by a relapse of disease and then drugs are taken irregularly, organisms resistant to these drugs will probably be present.

3. A patient with continued infectious sputum for more than six months who has taken drugs regularly or irregularly is probably excreting organisms resistant to these drugs.

4. The patient who has had interrupted courses involving several drugs to which his disease has responded in the past is apt to have an infection that is resistant to some of the drugs and susceptible to others.

5. If resistance is suspected to one or more or all of the drugs previously administered to a patient with relapse, it is best to begin with all these drugs and add, if possible, two that have not been previously administered while awaiting drug susceptibility studies.

6. When complete drug-susceptibility studies are available and the organism is resistant only to isoniazid, this drug should be given and, in addition, two other drugs to which the organism is susceptible (one of these should be streptomycin).

7. If the organism is resistant to both isoniazid and streptomycin, isoniazid should be continued, and in addition ethambutol plus another drug, or capreomycin plus another drug, or ethambutol plus capreomycin should be employed.

8. If drug-susceptibility studies indicate that only the following drugs are still effective: pyrazinamide, ethionamide, cycloserine, viomycin, or kanamycin—the use of three is advisable in conjunction with isoniazid in high dosage.

9. There is some evidence favoring the use of one injectable drug in any re-treatment regimen. Preference is given in the following order: streptomycin; capreomycin, viomycin, and kanamycin.

10. Streptomycin, viomycin, kanamycin, and capreomycin have similar toxicities that are additive (renal, vestibular, and auditory), and no more than one should be used at the same time.

Other Forms of Treatment. The effectiveness of drug therapy in previously untreated disease has made most other forms of treatment largely unnecessary. Bed rest and surgery still have a place in many re-treatment cases and in treatment failures. Steroids are useful and occasionally critically important in certain types of severe disease.

Bed Rest. Strict bed rest, long the mainstay of treatment of pulmonary tuberculosis, was thought to improve host resistance, enhance healing mechanisms, and favor cavity closure. Combined with collapse procedures aimed at closing remaining cavities, bed rest, when used conscientiously and for sufficiently long periods (two to four years) could be expected to benefit the majority of cases without residual cavities. In the presence of effective antimicrobial drug therapy, the influence of bed rest is not detectable. Consequently, strict bed rest is no longer generally used in any circumstances. Modified bed rest might be advised during the symptomatic stage of the early treatment period in an overly fatigued patient. During the active treatment phase, ambulation is allowed, but full work activity is usually avoided, mainly to avoid exposure of others to potential infection. When the sputum is negative for tubercle bacilli at about the time the suppressive phase of therapy begins, the patient is usually allowed to return to work. In treatment failures resistant to all drugs, modified bed rest and continued use of isoniazid may together in time salvage many apparently hopeless cases. In re-treatment cases that have only the weakest drugs still available, it is important to add the support of modified bed rest in order to improve chances of success. In general, bed rest is unimportant in the face of effective drug therapy, might be helpful with weak drug therapy, and is essential for treatment of completely drug-resistant disease.

Surgery. In the pre-drug era, persistent cavitation was always associated with active infection, and collapse therapy to favor cavity closure was central to treatment. When effective chemotherapy became available, surgical resection became possible, and for many years residual cavities were resected whether or not the discharge of tubercle bacilli had stopped. Recently, surgery has been used less and less as more effective use of combined and prolonged drug therapy has demonstrated the relative innocuousness of the "open-negative" status. Surgery is no longer recommended for the thin-walled cavity when the sputum promptly becomes noninfectious. Surgical resection remains important and is advisable (1) in cases of drug treatment failure, providing that there is sufficient pulmonary reserve and sufficient drug coverage available to avoid complications; (2) in patients with a thick-walled cavity persisting after six months or more of effective drug therapy, particularly if the discharge of tubercle bacilli continues; and (3) in patients with any persistent cavity when lack of patient cooperation compromises the prospects of prolonged drug therapy. Expert judgment is required in making these decisions. When drug resistance is present, a lobectomy is less apt to lead to complications than a segmental resection.

Adjunctive Therapy with Corticosteroids. The demonstration that treatment with adrenal steroid therapy suppresses tuberculin hypersensitivity, of which caseation is one expression, understandably led to a clinical trial of adjunctive therapy in routine cases of pulmonary tuberculosis, in the hope that tissue destruction might be minimized thereby and prognosis improved. The results of this study indicated that clinical improvement and roentgenographic progress were enhanced in the steroid-treated group as compared to controls, but after six to eight months no persisting benefit of steroid therapy could be demonstrated. The safety with which corticosteroids could be administered to patients receiving effective antimicrobial therapy, long suspected to be the case on the basis of less rigorous observations, was definitely established by this study.

Corticosteroids will suppress hypersensitivity in tuberculosis at relatively low dosage (equivalent of 30 mg. daily of prednisone) and will abolish the constitutional symptoms. High dosages (60 to 80 mg. of prednisone) are required to block the local inflammatory reaction, and the cost in terms of side effects is usually greater than the benefit attained. Although not applicable to the ordinary case, steroid therapy may be of great benefit in certain specific situations in pulmonary tuberculosis (the usefulness of these agents in nonpulmonary tuberculosis is discussed in a later article). First, in life-threatening extensive disease in which hypersensitivity-induced debility and wasting may be fatal before the stores of absorbable antigen are significantly reduced (several weeks after control of bacterial growth by antimicrobial agents), the use of corticosteroids by abolishing these constitutional symptoms may tide the patient over this critical period. Second, in less serious disease in which fever, anorexia, and anemia of infection will be expected to lead to many weeks of serious morbidity, corticosteroids will lead to prompt symptomatic recovery and repair of the anemia. In these two circumstances a moderate dose of corticosteroids (approximately 10 mg. of prednisone three times daily) will suffice, and it is usually possible to diminish the dose by 2.5-mg. decrements every four or five days. In the rare instance of hypoxia caused by a diffusion defect, usually in severe miliary tuberculosis, a large dose of corticosteroids (60 to 80 mg. of prednisone daily) may be necessary for a few days before quickly decreasing to 30 mg. daily and then diminishing. The rare coexistence of Addison's disease and active pulmonary tuberculosis should be borne in mind and treated with steroid therapy in replacement rather than pharmacologic dosage.

The well-known adverse effect of steroids on latent tuberculous infection can be disregarded in the presence of effective antituberculous drug therapy. If long-term steroids are given for other reasons in a person with a positive tuberculin test, it is advisable to give isoniazid prophylactically throughout the treatment period and for two or three months thereafter (see Chemoprophylaxis).

Hospitalization. The classic reasons for hospitalization, provision of effective bed rest, and isolation of the patient from the community are no longer pertinent. Bed rest is no longer necessary in initial treatment, and effective drug therapy reduces the period of significant infectiousness to only a few weeks. Under the influence of effective drugs, organisms excreted in the sputum after two weeks are metabolically sluggish and less capable of inducing infection even though they can be encouraged to grow by laboratory methods. However, proper management of pulmonary tuberculosis requires a variety of services. These include facilities for frequent roentgenographic studies including planigrams, a bacteriologic laboratory competent to culture tubercle

bacilli and to determine drug resistance, availability of a variety of laboratory studies for evaluation of possible drug-susceptibility reactions, diagnostic facilities for evaluation of concomitant or associated disease, opportunity for frequent patient observation during the early stages of treatment, and, above all, the availability of expert judgment in severe or difficult cases. There is no question that home care is entirely adequate if these services are available, but in most circumstances they are best provided in the specialized tuberculosis hospital or service. Also, the advantages of isolation cannot be entirely denied. For re-treatment cases, hospitalization is more strongly indicated, because precise and frequent drug-susceptibility studies, the advice and skills of a thoracic surgical service with experience in tuberculosis, and expert medical judgment are critically important in cases in which drug resources are limited for reasons of drug resistance. The use of the less effective and more toxic drugs also requires careful observation for drug reactions, best carried out in a hospital setting.

The Antituberculous Drugs. *Isoniazid (INH).* Isoniazid (isonicotinic acid hydrazide, INH, INA, INAH), the best and by far the most valuable of the presently available antituberculous drugs, is the keystone of therapy in every case. It has all the properties of an ideal antimicrobial agent. It is highly effective; it is absorbed so rapidly and effectively through the gastrointestinal tract that there is no therapeutically significant difference in drug concentration following administration by mouth, by intramuscular injection, or by vein; it is distributed throughout body tissues and cavities in concentrations greater than required for antimicrobial activity; its toxicity is probably less than that of any other major drug of any purpose; and it is remarkably specific, being active only against *M. tuberculosis* and *M. bovis* and to a very limited extent some other mycobacteria, particularly *M. kansasii.* Furthermore, having been synthesized in 1912 and used as a dye mordant, it was not subject to patent protection when its antituberculous activity was discovered in 1950, and accordingly is very inexpensive. It is a stable, water-soluble, easily synthesized crystalline substance. Its low molecular weight contributes to its wide distribution throughout body tissues and fluids. It penetrates and is effective within phagocytic cells. Penetration of caseous tissue has been demonstrated in studies utilizing isotopically labeled drug. In normal persons, isoniazid concentration in the cerebrospinal fluid is approximately 20 per cent of serum concentration; when meningeal inflammation is present, even greater penetration is attained. It is secreted in milk and crosses the placental barrier. Isoniazid is partially conjugated in the liver to an acetylated derivative that is nontoxic and inactive. Both free, therapeutically active drug and the acetylated conjugate are excreted in the urine, mostly within 24 hours, but the presence of renal insufficiency does not require altered dosage. There is no accumulation in tissues with prolonged therapy. Individuals vary considerably in the rapidity and degree of acetylation of isoniazid, which is a genetically determined characteristic. This phenomenon has led to the designation of individuals as "rapid inactivators" or "slow inactivators." Clinical studies, however, have shown that there is no significant difference in therapeutic response in the two groups, and the phenomenon has no importance in clinical management. Because of this and the fact that isoniazid serum levels with usual dosage are much higher than the minimal inhibitory concentration, there is little use for serum concentration determinations.

The minimal inhibitory concentration of isoniazid for *M. tuberculosis* ranges from 0.02 to 0.05 μg. per milliliter. From twenty to one hundred times these concentrations are attained in serum following usual oral dosage. The mode of action of isoniazid is not yet well understood, but it is maximally effective against actively growing and metabolizing cells. Isoniazid, although highly effective in acute aspects of the disease, does not eradicate all tubercle bacilli from the lesion.

As is the case with all known antituberculous drugs, bacterial mutants resistant to the action of INH occur at a predictable rate (one per 10^5 or 10^6 bacterial cells) in large bacterial populations. Presumably these mutants existed prior to the use of isoniazid, and suppression of the more numerous drug-susceptible organisms by treatment with isoniazid merely favors their emergence as the predominant organism. In clear contrast to all other drug-resistant mutants, however, isoniazid-resistant tubercle bacilli differ from those susceptible to the drug in several important ways. The ability to take up neutral red stain and the microcolonial characteristic of serpentine cording, characteristics that have been associated with virulence, are both less marked. Individual bacterial cell morphology may be altered with the appearance of coccoid forms and other variants and some loss of acid-fastness. Resistant mutants are biochemically different in that production of certain enzymes, notably the heat-labile species of catalase characteristic of virulent *M. tuberculosis* and *M. bovis,* is either diminished or absent (see Bacteriology). Most important, there is clear evidence that isoniazid-resistant mutants cause less progressive disease in laboratory animals, and inferential evidence that they are less virulent for man as well. This phenomenon of decreased pathogenicity and altered bacterial physiology associated with isoniazid-resistant mutants has implications for therapy. Even infections subsequently demonstrated to have been due to primarily resistant organisms from the outset (2 to 3 per cent at present in the United States) have shown a favorable response to isoniazid administered as a single agent in about one fourth of the cases in which such observations have been possible. In cases in which isoniazid-resistant populations have emerged as the predominant infecting organism, some benefit is derived from continuing the suppression of the more virulent isoniazid-susceptible organisms in favor of the less virulent and less progressive isoniazid-resistant mutants, and there is suggestive evidence that isoniazid may have low-grade effectiveness in vivo against organisms highly resistant to its action in vitro. *Rapidly progressive, toxic disease* and the development of laryngeal, gastrointestinal miliary or meningeal tuberculosis are very rare in persons receiving only isoniazid and excreting large populations of resistant organisms. Such patients demonstrate slow progression and succumb to progressive respiratory insufficiency, or perhaps a terminal hemoptysis, rather than to progressive and uncontrolled infection. *For these reasons, isoniazid should be continued even when the infecting population demonstrates high-grade in vitro resistance to the drug. This is not the case with any other antituberculous agent now available, and is the reason that isoniazid remains a keystone of therapy in virtually every case of tuberculosis.*

The *toxicity* of isoniazid is remarkably low. When administered as a single agent, hypersensitivity reactions are rare (0.5 per cent). Hepatitis, agranulocytosis, vasculitis of the lupus erythematosus type, fever, and skin rash may be related to isoniazid sensitization, but these are far more frequently triggered by prior or concomitant sensitization to PAS. Because of the pivotal importance of isoniazid in every case, desensitization procedures are often attempted when the seriousness of the reaction would make this unwise with respect to other, less irreplaceable agents.

A fascinating and poorly understood property of isoniazid is the induction of *pyridoxine deficiency.* Administration of isoniazid results in prompt appearance of pyridoxine metabolites in the urine, as if the vitamin had been released or leached from body stores. Although biochemical evidence of relative pyridoxine deficiency (decrease in urinary excretion of kynurenic acid after a loading dose of tryptophane) is more frequent, the peripheral neuritis of pyridoxine deficiency occurs in only 1 to 3 per cent of patients receiving conventional (300 mg.) isoniazid dosage. At a 10 mg. per kilogram dose, the incidence is approximately 10 per cent, and almost half of one series of patients receiving 20 mg. per kilogram developed this complication. Children are quite resistant to the development of neuritis even at an isoniazid dosage of 10 to 15 mg. per kilogram. Signs and symptoms of neuritis usually do not appear until after several weeks or even months, and may occur at any time thereafter. If patients are made aware of the importance of paresthesias or numbness in the extremities, the problem can easily be handled by interruption of isoniazid for a few days and institution of pyridoxine (200 mg. per day for two weeks and 100 mg. per day thereafter). For this reason, and because of the expense involved, pyridoxine supplementation is not routinely advised, except when isoniazid dosage greater than 5 mg. per kilogram is employed in adults. Certain groups can be identified, however, in whom pyridoxine deficiency is more likely to be present. These include persons with poor nutrition, notably alcoholics, and pregnant women. In alcoholics especially, isoniazid has been noted to rapidly produce disabling and severe neuritis. In these circumstances, a four- or five-day period of repletion with pyridoxine (200 mg. per day) and other B vitamins is advisable before initiating isoniazid therapy along with maintenance (100 mg. per day) pyridoxine. Although peripheral neuritis is by far the most common neurologic consequence of pyridoxine deficiency, more rarely malfunction of other levels of the neural axis, such as long tract signs and symptoms, have been observed.

Isoniazid in large doses may produce central nervous system symptoms unrelated to pyridoxine deficiency. Disturbances in mood and mentation, euphoria, transient loss of memory, feelings of unreality, and rarely convulsions may be seen. These are more apt to occur in those who already have psychic disturbances or a disposition to convulsions. Severe and disabling confusion may be produced by isoniazid in some older persons with underlying cerebrovascular disease. Isoniazid given with Dilantin potentiates the effect of the latter drug; when given together, Dilantin dosage should be decreased. Isoniazid may produce elevated blood ammonia levels, particularly in "rapid converters." Some reports have suggested that isoniazid may rarely accentuate manifestations of rheumatoid disease and may cause or accentuate Dupuytren's contractures.

The drug is usually administered orally in a dose of 4 to 6 mg. per kilogram per day, generally rounded off to 300 mg. per day. In children a larger dose (10 to 15 mg. per kilogram) is generally recommended. For many years it has been given in divided dosage three times daily. Recently it has become customary to administer a single daily dose. The peak effect may be useful, and it is easier to remember one dose than three. Isoniazid may be given at unaltered dosage (usually three times daily) by intramuscular injection if the oral route is not possible. In vitro studies have demonstrated that a single dose of isoniazid exerts a suppressive effect on growth of tubercle bacilli for several days after the drug is washed out of the media. This, and the uncertainty of self-administration of drugs, has led to administration of isoniazid together with streptomycin on a twice-weekly basis to some clinic populations with acceptable though not ideal results. Given once weekly, the regimen is clearly not acceptably effective.

Rifampin. Rifampin is a new semisynthetic drug developed in Italy, which in early studies appears to hold great promise. Studies in laboratory animals reveal it to be approximately the equal of isoniazid. The development of resistant strains seems similar to that of isoniazid. Early reports indicate remarkably low toxicity in humans. Clinical studies and trials are under way all over the world. There is great hope that this drug will prove to be the long sought ideal companion to isoniazid in initial treatment of pulmonary tuberculosis.

Streptomycin (SM). Streptomycin, the first effective antituberculous drug, was discovered in 1944, and its effectiveness against the tubercle bacillus was demonstrated shortly thereafter. Its use in tuberculosis became widespread in 1947, and it continued as the only really effective agent until isoniazid became generally available in 1952. Much of what is known concerning its dosage and activity was determined in that five-year period, as it was quickly replaced and overshadowed by isoniazid. It is a product of *Streptomyces griseus.* It is provided as a hygroscopic, fairly stable, water-soluble powder, usually dispensed as the sulfate salt; the molecular weight is approximately 580. It is not absorbed from the gastrointestinal tract, and administration is by intramuscular injection. The drug is apparently not metabolized, and is excreted almost entirely by glomerular filtration, a small amount appearing in bile. Effective levels persist in the serum for six hours in normal persons, and there is no accumulation in the body. In anephric persons, in contrast, the half-life may be as long as 50 to 100 hours, and accumulation of drug will occur on daily dosage, producing toxic serum concentrations. Distribution is mainly in the extracellular fluid. The drug does not exert maximal effectiveness on tubercle bacilli subsisting within body cells. Diffusion into caseous tissue occurs, but may be limited by the size of the area. Streptomycin diffuses into pleural, pericardial, peritoneal, and synovial fluid, appears in saliva, bile, and milk, and passes the placental barrier. Significant concentrations do not appear in the cerebrospinal fluid of normal people, but in the presence of meningeal irritation the drug does pass the meningeal barrier but to a variable and unpredictable degree. Accordingly, it was often administered by intrathecal injection in cases of meningitis before isoniazid became available, but with such marked morbidity that it was justified only by the otherwise fatal course of illness. Except possibly for rifampin, streptomycin is second to isoniazid in effectiveness and is the second most valuable antituberculous drug. The minimal inhibitory concentration for susceptible organisms is 0.2 μg. per milliliter, which is 50 to 100 times less than the peak following the usual dosage. The mode of antibacterial action is thought to be the same with respect to M. tuberculosis as with other bacteria, involving inhibition of protein synthesis, possibly by inducing a misreading of the genetic code. It is maximally active against actively metabolizing cells; as with isoniazid, dormant cells persisting in diseased tissue are less affected by the drug action. In vitro, streptomycin is most effective at pH 7.8, and less effective in the more acidic environment of caseous tissue. It is effective against strains resistant to other antituberculous drugs.

Resistance to streptomycin develops through drug-induced selection of naturally occurring mutants in the same manner as described for isoniazid. Streptomycin-resistant strains are biologically stable, and, in contrast to the case of isoniazid-resistant mutants, do not differ from streptomycin-susceptible strains in any way other than resistance to the drug itself. Probably for this reason, streptomycin does not retain clinical effectiveness against cells shown to be resistant in vitro. Between 2 and 3 per cent of those with previously untreated tuberculosis in the United States will harbor strains of tubercle bacilli resistant to streptomycin.

Streptomycin is reasonably tolerated by most patients at the usual dose of 1 gram daily. Larger dosage administered for any but brief periods is associated with unacceptable vestibular or auditory toxicity, and smaller dosage is much less effective. In exceptional circumstances, increased dosage may be administered for no longer than a few weeks. Because of the prolonged half-life of streptomycin in renal insufficiency, the dosage should be decreased in proportion to the degree of functional compromise, and, ideally, should be monitored by determination of serum concentrations. When this is not feasible, frequency of administration may be decreased to every other day in mild renal insufficiency and to every third or fourth day in severe uremia. Intramuscular injection may cause local irritation and some pain in the first few injections. It is important to make the injection deep in muscle tissue, avoiding subcutaneous location which may be quite painful. It is good practice to rotate injection sites. Perioral paresthesias and paresthesias of the extremities may be disturbing but not serious.

The most common and troublesome untoward effect of streptomycin is a very specific toxic effect on the vestibular or auditory apparatus. With dosage of 2 grams daily or greater, loss of vestibular function will occur sooner or later in almost all patients. At a 1-gram daily dose, serious loss of function is uncommon. Perhaps 10 per cent of patients will complain of some dizziness or vertigo, and should be watched carefully for loss of function. A caloric stimulation is the optimal test to detect vestibular damage, but simpler maneuvers testing ability to maintain balance when the head is turned suddenly with eyes closed or when walking on a rough surface with eyes closed are also valuable. The young may compensate for vestibular loss by visual and proprioceptive mechanisms for the maintenance of balance, but may continue to experience some difficulty in the dark and on sudden head motion. In contrast, persons much over 50 may have already compromised proprioceptive mechanisms, and may be rendered permanently ataxic. Auditory damage is less common but may occur with dosage larger than 1 gram daily. It is more common in older persons and in those who already have some nerve deafness. For these reasons, some physicians hesitate to give streptomycin to persons over 50 if it can with justification be avoided, as is almost always the case. There are rare instances of deafness in the newborn following administration of streptomycin during pregnancy, and it would seem wise to avoid its use in this situation.

Hypersensitivity reactions of mild or severe degree may occur in up to 5 per cent of patients. Eosinophilia is fairly common but is not an indication for stopping treatment. Skin rashes are the most troublesome allergic reaction, and vary from a pruritic, fine, scaling skin eruption to urticaria and, rarely, exfoliative dermatitis. Skin rashes may be transient even with continued therapy, but if they persist or are severe, streptomycin should be discontinued. Drug fever is fairly uncommon but has been associated with the eventual development of vasculitis when therapy was not interrupted. Desensitization may be accomplished (see below) but is less often attempted than is the case with isoniazid because the less critical role of streptomycin may

make the risks and inconvenience of desensitizing procedures less desirable than alternative drug therapy. A contact type of dermatitis may develop in nurses and others who handle streptomycin. The use of gloves in such individuals becomes mandatory.

Para-Aminosalicylic Acid (PAS). The tuberculostatic effect of para-aminosalicylic acid (PAS) was first reported in 1946. Although a weak antimicrobial agent, PAS has been considered one of the major drugs because of its usefulness as a companion drug. It is a rather unstable, crystalline compound, slightly soluble in water. Because of its instability, it is usually dispensed as the sodium salt. It is readily absorbed from the gastrointestinal tract. Following an oral dose of 4 grams, a peak concentration of 5 to 10 mg. per 100 ml. of serum occurs in two hours. The drug is freely diffusible into caseous tissue; appears in the cerebrospinal fluid, although it is transferred less fully than INH; and does not exert its maximal activity on tubercle bacilli located within phagocytic cells. Hepatic conjugation into acetyl and glycine derivatives is rapid, and some protein binding occurs. It is excreted by the kidney, mostly in conjugated form.

The action of PAS is not understood. In some unexplained manner it increases the oxygen requirements of the tubercle bacillus, and in this and perhaps other ways produces a weak bacteriostatic effect. It has little value in its own right, but for years has been an important companion drug. In combination with isoniazid, it is quite effective in suppressing emergence of isoniazid resistance in all but the most serious infections. It has a minimal inhibitory concentration of 1 μg. per milliliter of medium. Resistance develops to PAS if it is not protected by another effective drug. Primary resistance is found in less than 1 per cent of patients who have not previously been treated with this drug. Intolerance and toxic reactions have made PAS far from a perfect companion drug, and it is hoped that it will be supplanted by a more effective and less toxic agent. There are two main types of reactions, intolerance related to gastric irritation and toxicity resulting from hypersensitivity. In the doses required, PAS has a direct irritant action on the gastric mucosa somewhat similar to aspirin. In at least 10 per cent of patients, anorexia, nausea and vomiting, diarrhea, bulky and more frequent stools, or crampy abdominal pain become so troublesome that either decreased dosage or discontinuance of the drug is required. It should always be given with food. Sometimes a pause of two or three days followed by gradual reinstitution of normal dosage over several days will result in better tolerance. A few patients find a different PAS salt more tolerable. It may, however, become necessary to use some other antituberculous drug such as cycloserine, ethionamide, or ethambutol as a companion drug. Deterioration products seem to increase this untoward manifestation of PAS, and a fresh supply of the drug protected from moisture and light should be assured.

Hypersensitivity reactions to PAS may be serious. They occur in approximately 7 per cent of patients and, although they may appear at any time, are more common in the fourth to fifth week after beginning treatment. These allergic reactions are protean in their manifestations. Fever, itching, and skin rashes, lymphadenopathy, eosinophilia, leukemoid reactions, granulocytopenia, exfoliative dermatitis, hepatitis, and encephalopathy are among them. If the drug is continued in the face of even the mildest reaction, there is a strong tendency for progression to more serious reactions. Occasionally fever, lymphadenopathy, and changes in the peripheral blood smear may suggest infectious mononucleosis. This form, if not recognized, may lead to potentially fatal hepatitis. Another serious problem of PAS hypersensitivity is the frequency with which co-sensitization to isoniazid and to other simultaneously administered drugs is observed. When allergic reactions occur in the presence of two or more antituberculous drugs, PAS is the most likely offender. It should be the first to be discontinued or the last to be reinstituted if all are discontinued. Desensitization programs have been developed and may be successful, but it is far better to discontinue PAS and substitute another drug than take a chance on renewal of sensitization. Mild antithyroid activity occasionally produces goiter. Rarely PAS may cause a significant prolongation of the prothrombin time.

The customary dosage of PAS is 12 grams daily of the acid, usually given in three divided doses. The dosage is given in acid equivalents, but if the drug is administered as one of the salts, dosage must be altered appropriately. The equivalent dose of the sodium salt is 15 grams daily (5 grams three times a day). When used with isoniazid, a single daily dose has been shown to be essentially as effective as thrice daily dosage. A single dose of 8 grams (10 grams NaPAS) seems to be effective, whereas a single dose of 6 grams of the acid is not adequate. In patients on restricted sodium diets, potassium PAS may be substituted. Other forms of PAS are the calcium salt, an organic acid resin complex, a buffered derivative, and PAS-C. Enteric-coated tablets or granules are not recommended because of unreliable absorption.

Ethambutol (EMB). Ethambutol is a relatively new drug and has not yet been subjected to extensive clinical trial. It is a water-soluble, heat-stable crystalline compound with very promising antituberculous activity which is limited in humans by drug toxicity. It is rapidly absorbed from the gastrointestinal tract. A dose of 25 mg. per kilogram results in a peak serum level of 5 μg. per milliliter, and a dose of 15 mg. per kilogram provides approximately 3 μg. per milliliter. The drug is excreted in the urine rapidly and principally in unchanged form. The minimal inhibitory concentration is in the range of 1 to 4 μg. per milliliter.

Studies in laboratory animals indicate that effectiveness is dose-related up to 100 mg. per kilogram. In humans, the threat of optic nerve toxicity has limited dosage to no more than 25 mg. per kilogram and for long-term treatment to no more than 15 mg. per kilogram. In preliminary clinical studies, it appears that ethambutol alone in this dosage is an effective drug, but definitely less effective than isoniazid. Resistance develops fairly early and EMB is not recommended for use as a single drug. Combined with other antituberculous drugs (PZA, CS, VM, KM) in re-treatment cases, EMB has proved to be effective. Preliminary studies in initial treatment cases in which EMB was used as a companion drug to INH are highly encouraging. Ethambutol may prove to be the first acceptable substitute for PAS in major drug combinations. There is some evidence that this drug may be effective against *M. kansasii*. Reports of primary resistance have ranged from 0.75 to 4.0 per cent.

In the limited dosage schedules, ethambutol has met with good patient acceptance. Symptoms of intolerance are minimal. There are rare reports of mild gastrointestinal disturbance and paresthesias of the extremities. In dosage of 50 mg. per kilogram or higher, there is an unacceptable incidence of optic nerve toxicity. In prolonged courses at a dosage of 25 mg. per kilogram, the incidence is approximately 2 per cent, but is negligible at a dose of 15 mg. per kilogram. Optic nerve toxicity is manifested by a gradual loss of visual acuity, usually with contraction of the visual fields and frequently with loss of the ability to perceive the color green. These disturbances are usually completely reversible if the drug is discontinued within a reasonable period of time after toxic manifestations occur. The problem of visual toxicity is largely a psychologic one. The threat of loss of sight has tremendous psychologic impact, and great care is being exercised to make sure that even the psychologic hazard is acceptable before recommending widespread use of the drug.

Ethionamide (ETH). Ethionamide is a derivative of isonicotinic acid chemically related to isoniazid. It is a crystalline compound with low solubility in water. It is absorbed slowly from the gastrointestinal tract, reaching a peak serum level in two or three hours. The drug is excreted by the kidneys in a metabolically inactive form. It is widely distributed in tissues, including the cerebrospinal fluid. The minimal inhibitory concentration is 0.6 μg. per milliliter of medium. Ethionamide is less effective than isoniazid and streptomycin. It is not used in initial treatment, but is one of the more useful drugs in re-treatment of patients resistant to isoniazid and streptomycin.

Symptoms of gastrointestinal intolerance, which occur in the majority, markedly limit the drug's clinical usefulness. Anorexia, nausea, vomiting, and diarrhea resulting from a central effect rather than direct gastric irritation frequently make it necessary to discontinue the drug (30 per cent of cases) or reduce dosage to ineffective levels. Rarely, mental confusion, peripheral neuritis, and convulsions occur. Gynecomastia has been described. The most serious toxic reaction is hepatitis. About 10 per cent of patients develop some evidence of abnormal liver function, and 1 per cent may develop overt jaundice. Frank hypersensitivity reactions are uncommon.

Ethionamide is given orally in a dose of 0.5 to 1.0 gram daily in either two or three divided doses. The aim is to administer as large a dose as the patient can tolerate up to 1 gram daily. Administration of a large part of the dose at night is sometimes helpful.

Pyrazinamide (PZA). Pyrazinamide is an effective antituberculous drug with the two major limitations of serious toxicity and rapid development of microbial resistance. It is a synthetic compound, readily absorbed from the gastrointestinal tract. When given alone, significant drug resistance develops in as little as eight weeks. It is an effective companion drug to isoniazid and streptomycin, but is too toxic to be used in initial therapy. Pyrazinamide is a relatively ineffective companion drug to cycloserine or to PAS. When given only with weak drugs, it is best to use three at a time.

Liver toxicity limits the drug's usefulness and requires careful observation, usually in a hospital. About 15 per cent of patients treated with PZA show some alteration in liver function tests, approximately 3 per cent develop jaundice, and in 1 per cent the toxic hepatitis reaches serious proportions. The hepatitis usually subsides with discontinuation of the drug. Death from liver necrosis has been reported. Liver toxicity is not dose related.

Patients receiving pyrazinamide should have weekly serum glutamic oxalacetic transaminase (SGOT) determinations. If significant elevation occurs, and BSP retention is demonstrated, the drug should be promptly discontinued. Pyrazinamide has a hyperuricemic effect, and serum uric acid levels of 10 to 16 mg. per 100 ml. are not uncommon. Rarely, clinical gout develops, but this can be controlled with colchicine while continuing the drug. Dosage is 40 to 50 mg. per kilogram per day, usually rounded to the closest 500 mg., and given in either two or three divided doses.

Cycloserine (CS). Cycloserine, a drug with considerable toxicity and relatively low effectiveness, is useful only when tubercle bacilli are resistant to the major drugs. It is soluble in water, rapidly absorbed from the gastrointestinal tract, and widely distributed within the body, including the cerebrospinal fluid. The drug has a moderate bacteriostatic effect in concentrations of 10 μg. per milliliter or higher, which are attained with usual dosage. Cycloserine is a reasonably good companion drug when used with one of the major drugs. When administered with other weak drugs, it is best to use three at a time.

Symptoms of central nervous system toxicity frequently accompany dosage of 1 gram daily or higher. Convulsions and paranoid psychoses are the most serious. When the highest dosage is given, anticonvulsant drugs and sedatives may be helpful. It has been a widespread practice to administer pyridoxine to counter neurotoxicity, but there is no good evidence that this is effective or appropriate. It is advisable not to use cycloserine in any patient with a history of epilepsy or psychosis. Other toxic neurologic manifestations include ataxia, slurred speech, blurred vision, tremors, and muscular weakness. Psychic effects include anxiety, inability to concentrate, impulsive behavior, nightmares, somnolence, lapses in memory, confusion, and rarely hallucinations. With serious reactions, it is best to discontinue the drug, but minor toxic effects may clear with decrease in dosage. The maximal dosage is 1 gram daily (250 mg. four times a day), which few patients will tolerate. The lowest effective dose is 250 mg. twice daily, which is tolerated fairly well by most patients. A medium dose of 250 mg. three times daily is reasonable to try in the average patient.

Viomycin (VM). Viomycin, an intramuscular drug, is considerably less effective than streptomycin and has similar toxic manifestations. It has no place in initial treatment of tuberculosis, but is useful in re-treatment of drug-resistant cases. It is effective against strains resistant to all other antituberculous drugs with the possible exception of kanamycin. It is frequently combined with one or two of the oral drugs in re-treatment cases. Toxicity for the vestibular and auditory apparatus is similar to that of streptomycin. It also produces renal irritation and may cause elevation of blood urea nitrogen. It should be given cautiously and in lower dosage to patients with renal disease. Viomycin frequently causes a depletion of serum electrolytes, and potassium chloride may have to be given in order to control hypokalemia. Allergic reactions similar to those caused by streptomycin are not uncommon. Many patients complain of pain at the site of injection. It is important that the injection be given deep in the muscle. Viomycin is commonly administered in a dosage of 2 grams (1 gram twice daily) twice a week, as there is some evidence that this schedule reduces toxic reactions. The drug may be given in a dosage of 1 gram daily, which is probably more effective. Viomycin is not ordinarily used with streptomycin, kanamycin, or capreomycin because of additive toxicities.

Kanamycin (KM). Kanamycin is a highly toxic drug when administered in effective dosage, and is seldom used in the treatment of tuberculosis except as a last resort in disease resistant to all the better drugs. It has a low order of effectiveness, similar to viomycin. It is effective against strains resistant to any of the antituberculous drugs with the possible exception of viomycin.

Kanamycin may be used in combination with one or two of the less effective oral drugs. The major toxic effect is on the auditory apparatus, and irreversible deafness may accompany use of the drug in therapeutic dosage. Hearing loss begins in the higher frequencies. Auditory loss is related to the serum level and to duration of treatment. In prolonged courses some loss of function can be expected, and great care must be exercised to prevent this. Frequent audiograms are necessary. Once hearing loss develops, the drug must be discontinued because toxicity is cumulative. Kanamycin is most hazardous in the presence of renal insufficiency, as it is normally excreted by the kidney. Kanamycin has a moderate nephrotoxic action and may itself cause renal insufficiency. The minimal effective dose is 1 gram three times weekly. The drug has been given in prolonged courses as frequently as 1 gram daily with acceptable toxicity, but very careful observation is necessary. It is reasonable to use a dosage between these ranges, that is, 3 to 7 grams a week.

Capreomycin (CM). Capreomycin is a promising drug which has not been released for general use. Preliminary animal and clinical studies indicate that its effectiveness and toxicity are within the range of streptomycin. It must be administered intramuscularly. There are no reports of primary resistance to this drug, and the development of acquired resistance is relatively slow. It is effective against strains resistant to the other antituberculous drugs, including streptomycin. Although it will probably not replace streptomycin in initial treatment, capreomycin should prove to be a valuable substitute for the potent drugs in infections resistant to isoniazid and streptomycin. Toxicity is relatively mild and limited almost entirely to nephrotoxicity and auditory and vestibular damage. Although uncommon, damage to the tubular epithelium may occur, and renal function tests (BUN, PSP, and urinalysis) should be followed at regular intervals. Capreomycin may cause hearing loss, but rarely vestibular damage. Hearing loss is permanent but not progressive if the drug is discontinued. Careful clinical observation and audiograms at regular intervals are important. Capreomycin is given by intramuscular injection in a dose of 1 gram daily.

Desensitization. Hypersensitivity reactions occur in up to 5 per cent of patients receiving streptomycin and in 7 per cent of patients receiving PAS. Hypersensitivity to isoniazid when used alone is very infrequent (less than 0.5 per cent). The types of reactions are described under the discussion of each drug. It should be remembered that PAS has an ability to induce cross-reactions to other drugs given at the same time. It is this phenomenon that accounts for most cases of isoniazid hypersensitivity.

When an allergic reaction occurs in the presence of two or more drugs, it is best to discontinue all drugs, and then after the reaction has subsided or in a few days to restart the drugs one at a time, with isoniazid first, streptomycin next, and PAS last. If it appears by the process of elimination that PAS is responsible, it is wise not to test then for susceptibility to this drug because of the chance of inducing cross-sensitization. Even though some allergic reactions may be tolerated well and even subside under continued use of these drugs, others may rapidly precipitate serious reactions and, therefore, the offending drug should be discontinued immediately and there should be as little future exposure as possible.

Desensitization can be carried out to any of the frequently used antituberculous drugs and probably to all of them. However, with the exception of isoniazid and possibly streptomycin, there seems little justification in risking the later return of the allergic state. For PAS and the other less effective drugs, it is best not to attempt desensitization but to choose a substitute from the list

SCHEDULE FOR DRUG DESENSITIZATION USING CORTICOSTEROIDS*

Day	Medication	Dosage	
1	Prednisone†	20 mg.	Each t.i.d.
	Isoniazid	25 mg.	
2	Prednisone	15 mg.	Each t.i.d.
	Isoniazid	50 mg.	
3	Prednisone	10 mg.	Each t.i.d.
	Isoniazid	75 mg.	
4	Prednisone	5 mg.	Each t.i.d.
	Isoniazid	100 mg.	
1	Prednisone†	20 mg.	Each t.i.d.
	Streptomycin	0.025 gram	
2	Prednisone	15 mg.	Each t.i.d.
	Streptomycin	0.05 gram	
3	Prednisone	10 mg.	Each t.i.d.
	Streptomycin	0.1 gram	
4	Prednisone	5 mg.	Each t.i.d.
	Streptomycin	0.2 gram	
5	Prednisone	5 mg.	Each b.i.d.
	Streptomycin	0.5 gram	

*Adapted from Simpson, D. G., and Hubaytar, R. T.: Amer. Rev. Res. Dis., 86:738, 1962.

†Prednisone given 1 hour before INH or 1.5 hours before STM.

of unused drugs. Each case must be decided on its own merits and needs. Because of the over-all importance of isoniazid, it is reasonable to consider desensitization if the reaction is not a serious one. This can be accomplished by beginning with a dose of 0.01 mg. and increasing gradually until a full dose is reached in approximately 30 days. Similarly, desensitization to streptomycin can be accomplished by starting with a dose of 0.01 gram. A successful rapid method using adrenal steroids has been advocated by Simpson and Hubaytar. With very slight modification, the method is given in the accompanying table.

EXTRAPULMONARY TUBERCULOSIS
Roger Des Prez

The extrapulmonary forms of tuberculosis fall into two groups with different pathogeneses, clinical settings, and levels of importance. The first is made up of conditions developing from foci seeded by *lymphohematogenous dissemination*, frequently at the time of the initial or primary infection. These include *miliary tuberculosis, tuberculosis of bones and joints, renal tuberculosis*, most cases of *tuberculous lymphadenitis, female genital tuberculosis, peritonitis, pericarditis, meningitis*, and some instances of *pleural effusion*. Although often associated with tuberculosis elsewhere, *these illnesses may present as isolated clinical manifestations*. They are now the most frequent and important forms of extrapulmonary tuberculosis in areas in which pulmonary tuberculosis is usually promptly detected and treated.

The second group comprises conditions that are essentially complications of active, chronic, and usually far advanced pulmonary tuberculosis. Tissues bathed in infectious pulmonary secretions for prolonged periods will eventually develop surface ulceration which may then progress to granulomatous change, hyperplasia, caseous necrosis, or cicatrization. Lesions caused by this *intracanalicular* mode of spread via the bronchial and gastrointestinal lumina were much the most frequent forms of extrapulmonary involvement encountered prior to the availability of drugs, and doubtless are still so in areas in which pulmonary tuberculosis may remain untreated. (Symptoms resulting from intracanalicular spread of renal tuberculosis to the ureters, bladder, and male genitalia are still important manifestations of genitourinary tuberculosis). Tuberculosis of the *bronchial mucosa, larynx, middle ear*, and *gastrointestinal tract* now rarely become clinically important because prolonged contact with infectious secretions is required for establishment and maintenance of such foci, and they are very responsive to chemotherapy. The importance of this group now lies in the rare instance in which a focus "downstream" leads to discovery of active pulmonary tuberculosis and the even more rare and poorly understood case in which oral, laryngeal, or gastrointestinal tuberculosis is found in the absence of demonstrable pulmonary disease.

Chronic pulmonary tuberculosis may also progress by direct extension, commonly to the pleura, and rarely to the pericardium, esophagus, and other intrathoracic structures.

Principles of Drug Therapy. Most extrapulmonary tuberculosis responds much more readily to drug treatment than does most pulmonary tuberculosis, in part because the area of necrosis is apt to be smaller, and hence the very large bacterial populations characteristic of the pulmonary cavity are lacking. The exception to this is cavitary renal tuberculosis in which both the necrosis and the bacterial population may be quite large and hence this form is always treated with combined drug therapy. In the remainder, the problem of drug resistance emerging during therapy, the chief reason for combined drug therapy in pulmonary tuberculosis, is usually not a consideration (see Treatment of Pulmonary Tuberculosis). The choice of drugs, therefore, depends on how life-threatening the illness seems to be. Those carrying a threat of early mortality, such as miliary and meningeal tuberculosis, and probably spondylitis and pericarditis as well, are always treated with maximal drug therapy (isoniazid and daily streptomycin) at least until a favorable response has been established. This both increases the antimicrobial effect and protects against the small possibility of a primary isoniazid-resistant infection. Those illnesses of less threatening character, such as serous membrane involvement, tuberculous lymphadenitis, bone and joint tuberculosis (excluding the spine), and genital tuberculosis, may be treated with isoniazid given as a single agent. When response is good, as it almost always is, only prolonged isoniazid therapy is required. When it is not, streptomycin and PAS may be added without significant loss.

TUBERCULOSIS OF THE PLEURA

Pulmonary tuberculosis commonly produces pleural involvement. When this occurs early after the initial infection, relatively large subpleural foci may have developed by the time hypersensitivity develops. Rupture of such a focus into the pleural space evokes a brisk allergic reaction and the clinical syndrome of *primary serofibrinous pleurisy with effusion*. This occurrence is important more in detecting individuals with flourishing initial infections and a proclivity to development of progressive tuberculosis at a later time than in its local manifestations, as spontaneous resolution is the rule (see Diseases of the Pleura). Pleural effusion may also occur as a complication of subpleural hematogenous foci, in association with pericardial and peritoneal tuberculosis (tuberculous polyserositis), or less commonly as a complication of established chronic pulmonary tuberculosis. Pleural involvement in the latter situation is usually dry, because small concentrations of antigen diffusing from an underlying chronic pulmonary focus to the pleural surface will ordinarily result in a local area of inflammation and pleural symphysis, precluding sudden delivery of large amounts of antigenic and infectious material into the pleural cavity. Rarely, rupture of a necrotic chronic focus into the pleural space may produce tuberculous empyema and secondary bronchopleural fistula (see Diseases of the Pleura).

ENDOBRONCHIAL TUBERCULOSIS

Some degree of tuberculous bronchial involvement invariably complicates cavitary tuberculosis. This results from surface infection, ulceration, and granuloma formation, most marked in the immediate vicinity of the cavity, but also occurring in spotty distribution any place in the path of the infectious secretions. Before the availability of drugs, such bronchial involvement at times constituted an important though tenuous healing mechanism, producing obstruction at the bronchocavitary junction or even obstruction of a whole segment or lobe, with subsequent inspissation, fibrosis, and contraction. Superficial bronchial lesions respond much more readily to chemotherapy than do parenchymal foci, and in most instances now require little attention. However, partial degrees of bronchial obstruction and cicatrization may persist after healing and give rise to nontuberculous complications such as atelectasis, obstructive pneumonitis, and suppurative lung disease. Some degree of permanent bronchial distortion probably occurs in every case of moderately extensive pulmonary tuberculosis, and may produce permanent rales or even frank bronchiectasis.

The frequency and consequences of bronchial involvement in childhood have been discussed elsewhere (see Pulmonary Tuberculosis).

Tuberculosis of the trachea essentially represents an extension of extensive endobronchial tuberculosis. It is now rare.

TUBERCULOSIS OF THE LARYNX

Tuberculosis of the larynx was previously one of the most common and dreaded complications of extensive and long-standing pulmonary tuberculosis, usually seen late in the course of uncontrolled pulmonary disease. The onset of hoarseness, pain on swallowing, and perhaps pain referred to the ear often ushered in a terminal downhill course, with inanition owing to dysphagia, and often with extensive further bronchogenic spread throughout both lung fields from copious, thin, laryngeal secretions. Involvement usually began in the area of the arytenoids and the posterior commissure and spread forward to the cords, the anterior aspects of the larynx, and even the epiglottis. Edema, ulceration, and granulomatous lesions developed. Scarring at times led to obstructive changes. This complication is now almost never seen, even in drug-resistant cases with heavily positive sputum, a further indication that isoniazid-resistant organisms have decreased virulence. However, rare cases occur in which the initial symptom of an active pulmonary lesion is laryngeal involvement, producing isolated ulcers or nodules with intact mucosa, resembling carcinoma and diagnosed either by biopsy or by the demonstration of associated active pulmonary tuberculosis. Exceedingly rare are cases in which tuberculous laryngeal lesions are discovered without roentgenographically demonstrable tuberculosis in the lung. The pathogenesis of such cases is not known. Response to drug therapy is excellent, and surgery is usually not required except for diagnosis.

GASTROINTESTINAL TUBERCULOSIS

In earlier times, gastrointestinal tuberculosis was a frequently observed complication of extensive and uncontrolled pulmonary tuberculosis. It was also caused by ingestion of contaminated milk. It is now rare, but occasional cases are still seen in which complaints related to a gastrointestinal focus lead to the diagnosis of pulmonary tuberculosis. Even more rarely, gastrointestinal tuberculosis may present without recognizable active pulmonary disease.

Tuberculosis of the tongue and mouth may present as painful, deep ulcerations or as a draining, nonhealing tooth socket after dental extraction. Local extension to bone occurs. Untreated, the process is indolently progressive, but response to chemotherapy is rapid. *Tuberculosis of the middle ear and mastoid bone* can occur as an extension of oropharyngeal disease spread via the eustachian tube. *Tuberculosis of the tonsil and pharyngeal lymphatic tissue* was common when contaminated milk was a major cause of infection with *M. bovis,* leading to regional tuberculous adenitis or *scrofula.* A similar sequence of events is now seen with some frequency in scrofula resulting from other mycobacteria (see following article). The tonsil involvement is usually unimpressive compared to the lymph node component, and removal is not indicated. *Tuberculosis of the esophagus* is a rarity even within the now rare category of gastrointestinal tuberculosis. Involvement can occur by perforation of an adjacent node leading to bronchoesophageal fistula formation or to ulcerative or hyperplastic disease of the esophageal wall. *Tuberculosis of the stomach* may resemble diffuse neoplastic involvement of the linitis plastica type or produce a nonhealing ulcer. Involvement may be due to surface infection or to extension from an adjacent lymph node focus, and accordingly may rarely present as a primary clinical manifestation. Hyperplastic or ulcerative *duodenal tuberculosis* may resemble peptic or neoplastic obstructive disease. Tuberculosis of the intestine may produce ulceration with bleeding and a tendency to perforation and fistula formation, hyperplasia with obstructive symptoms, or a combination of the two. *Tuberculosis of the small intestine is* more liable to produce perforation than disease elsewhere. *Ileocecal tuberculosis* was the most frequently observed form of bowel involvement, presumably because of cecal pooling of fecal material, providing an increased opportunity for surface contamination. The roentgenographic finding of cecal spasm, irritability, and rapid expulsion of contrast material was in times past regarded as relatively specific for tuberculosis. Iliocecal tuberculosis may produce occult bleeding, obstruction, or fistula formation. *Tuberculosis of the ascending and transverse colon* is much less common, and may present as a concentric, hyperplastic lesion producing obstruction. *Tuberculosis of the sigmoid colon* may resemble carcinoma, atypical ulcerative colitis, or diverticulitis. All these lesions may perforate and product *tuberculous perirectal and pelvic abscesses* associated with rectal pain, cutaneous fistula formation, or obstructive symptoms.

Diagnosis is now made at surgery in almost all instances, and is usually an unexpected finding. If diagnosed in the presence of obvious pulmonary tuberculosis, the effects of chemotherapy should be determined prior to resorting to surgery, as even the most advanced lesions may heal to such an extent that surgical intervention becomes unnecessary.

MILIARY TUBERCULOSIS

The term *miliary tuberculosis* was first used to described the postmortem appearance of the lungs and other organs from fatal cases of progressive tuberculous bacteremia in which the disseminated small tubercles were thought to resemble millet seeds. It is at present applied to any form of disseminated tuberculosis in which persistent or recurrent hematogenous dissemination is a major feature, a usage justified more by custom than descriptive force, because the pathologic changes produced may be quite variable.

In infants and very young children, the hematogenous phase of the primary infection is especially liable to evolve into miliary tuberculosis. Metastatic foci seeded during the pre-allergic bacteremia and lodged in the immediate vicinity of small blood vessels may enlarge and, with the development of tuberculin hypersensitivity, undergo necrosis, gain access to the vascular lumen, and re-seed the blood stream, progressively enhancing the level of bacteremia. Miliary tuberculosis and the associated meningitis account for most tuberculosis deaths in this age group.

In adults, miliary tuberculosis is usually due to old, chronic residua of more remote infections which for some reason become progressive, undergo further necrosis, and gain access to the circulation. Seeding of the blood stream from an active pulmonary lesion may occur as a terminal event in untreated cases, but is probably now rarely seen. Usually the initiating focus is extrapulmonary in location, in the lymphatic, genitourinary, or skeletal system, and often will have been previously undetected. These foci may cause multiple episodes of bacteremia, and the process may be protracted, intermittent, and low grade. Host factors known to favor activation of latent infectious foci, such as debility, advanced age, intercurrent therapy with oncolytic agents, immunosuppressives, or corticosteroid hormones, malignant disease, particularly of the lymphatic and hematopoietic systems, and occasionally local injury, are frequent underlying features.

Clinical Features and Diagnosis. In the very young, the illness is usually acute and severe, with high intermittent fevers, occasionally rigors, and severe night sweats. Complications such as pleurisy, peritonitis, or meningitis, which occurs in as many as two thirds, may be a part of the presenting picture, although usually these develop several weeks after the onset of constitutional symptoms. A similar acute illness is the usual picture in adults as well. However, in some adults, particularly the aged, miliary tuberculosis may be a covert and subtle illness with weeks or months of nonspecific, slowly progressive constitutional symptoms such as weight loss, weakness, and malaise, low-grade or absent fever, and usually no pulmonary symptoms. This clinical picture is usually ascribed to small and frequently intermittent episodes of bacteremia, and has been designated as *chronic hematogenous tuberculosis.* As in the more acute form, the presenting complaint may be due to serous membrane involvement, meningitis, or less commonly disseminated lymphatic involvement. Choroidal tubercles may be seen but are often absent. Splenomegaly is uncommon.

Studies resulting in diagnosis are usually initiated because of the appearance of a disseminated, fine, nodular, or linear infiltrate on the chest roentgenogram. It is important to emphasize, therefore, that *individuals may succumb to miliary tuberculosis before the miliary pulmonary infiltrate has developed enough to be roentgenographically detectable.* The tuberculin test is also of little help, because *as many as one fourth of proved cases may be nonreactors to tuberculin.* When treatment results in improvement, tuberculin reactivity returns. Anemia is frequent. The white blood count is usually normal or depressed initially (*vide infra*). Cultures of the gastric contents and urine are frequently positive, but this information is often no help to the problem of immediate diagnosis. Culture of the cerebrospinal fluid may be positive without pleocytosis or protein elevation, although usually other indications of meningitis are present. Evidence of associated tuberculosis is of obvious help, but is often lacking. In many, a tentative diagnosis is made when granulomatous lesions are discovered on bone marrow aspiration or in sections of liver obtained percutaneously or at diagnostic laparotomy. Both tissues should also be cultured, not only for confirmation but also because culture may be positive without histologic evidence of disease. Negative findings in either tissue do not exclude the diagnosis.

Primary Hepatic Tuberculosis. In rare cases the sole clinical manifestations of miliary tuberculosis may be hepatic dysfunction and fever. The hepatic functional derangement is similar to that produced by disseminated hepatic infiltrates of neoplastic or nontuberculous granulomatous origin, with elevation of serum alkaline phosphatase, much less elevation of serum bilirubin, and little indication of hepatocellular damage. The clinical picture may closely resemble extrahepatic obstruction with ascending cholangitis. Diagnosis is made by liver biopsy, but multiple sections of the specimen or occasionally several specimens may be required. The apparent location of disease only in the liver has been regarded by some as evidence of seeding from a focus discharging into the portal venous system.

Miliary Tuberculosis in the Aged. As mentioned above, miliary tuberculosis in older persons may be extremely subtle, presenting simply as a wasting illness with intermittent, low-grade fever or no fever at all, commonly misdiagnosed as neoplastic disease, and frequently discovered only at autopsy. In such cases, a therapeutic trial of isoniazid will often be unequivocally diagnostic, and may be a conservative alternative to diagnostic laparotomy, particularly in persons whose general condition increases the risk of surgery.

Miliary Tuberculosis Presenting as Hematologic Disease. A variety of hematologic illnesses may be mimicked by miliary tuberculosis. These include leukemoid reaction, leukopenia, thrombocytopenia, aregenerative anemia, hemolytic anemia, leukemia, myelofibrosis, and even polycythemia. This also is particularly true in older persons. The often associated histologic picture of caseous foci containing myriads of acid-fast organisms but very little cellular reaction, has been designated *nonreactive tuberculosis*. Many such cases are misdiagnosed as leukemia, a confusion compounded by the fact that miliary tuberculosis complicates as much as 2 per cent of cases of true leukemia. Further, steroid therapy administered for bona fide hematologic illness may be responsible for reactivation of a latent tuberculous focus, leading to secondary miliary tuberculosis. As steroid therapy is often indicated for serous hematologic disease, awareness of the possibility that the underlying cause may be cryptic miliary tuberculosis is critically important.

Treatment and Prognosis. Prior to the availability of streptomycin, miliary tuberculosis was almost invariably fatal, usually because of the development of meningitis. When streptomycin was used as the major drug, some of these patients were observed to relapse owing to drug resistance or to develop meningitis after an initial good response. In contrast, treatment of miliary tuberculosis with regimens containing isoniazid (including isoniazid given as a single agent) is *not* associated with relapse or the late appearance of meningitis, and, except for persons dying within the first few days, the cure rate of miliary disease uncomplicated by meningitis should approach 100 per cent. The prognosis with concurrent meningitis is less favorable. Maximal drug therapy with isoniazid and daily streptomycin is recommended. Once a good response has been established, streptomycin may be decreased to thrice weekly dosage for a total of six months or a year. Isoniazid should be continued for one or two more years. When a good response to isoniazid has been established in a therapeutic trial of unproved disease, there is little reason to add another drug. Response to treatment may be dramatic or may require some weeks. Adjunctive therapy with corticosteroids is advisable in severe cases with extensive pulmonary involvement, marked toxicity, hypoxemia, and respiratory distress. It may also be helpful in cases with poor response owing to severe debility and is mandatory in the very rare instance of coexistent adrenal insufficiency (see Treatment of Pulmonary Tuberculosis). Other causes for poor response to treatment, such as miliary disease resulting from mycobacteria other than *M. tuberculosis* or from isoniazid-resistant *M. tuberculosis*, are fortunately very rare, presumably because of the decreased virulence of these organisms.

TUBERCULOUS MENINGITIS

Tuberculous meningitis is the most serious form of tuberculous infection, invariably fatal when untreated, and responsible for a large portion of the tuberculosis deaths in infants. It was long regarded as primarily a disease of very young children, but at present half or more of the cases are observed in adults. It remains a dread disease because of the permanent and often incapacitating neurologic damage that may occur, particularly in the very young, even with prompt diagnosis and therapy.

Meningitis complicates miliary tuberculosis in the majority of untreated cases. This is not due to direct implantation, however, as the meninges are themselves quite resistant to blood-borne infection. Rather, the infection reaches the subarachnoid space by direct extension from a subjacent tuberculous focus, most frequently a small, subependymal tubercle at or near the surface of the brain. Less frequently, larger tuberculomas may reach the subarachnoid space. Direct extension from a larger parameningeal focus in the spine, middle ear, or elsewhere may also rarely occur. The fact that meningeal infection occurs by direct extension from adjacent foci explains the observation that meningitis may develop several weeks or months after overt miliary tuberculosis. Also, as the critical factor is location, the extent of the bacteremia merely enhances the probability of meningeal involvement, which may occur as a consequence of a small, transient, and otherwise inapparent hematogenous phase. As in miliary disease, the seeding focus in infants is usually the primary parenchymal–hilar node complex, and in adults a chronic, extrapulmonary, and often clinically latent focus is usually responsible.

Once infectious material gains access to the subarachnoid space in the hypersensitive host, an allergic inflammatory response develops, and the infection is spread via the cerebrospinal fluid, resulting in secondary implantation of bacilli elsewhere on the meningeal surfaces. Anatomic and physiologic factors concerning the flow and pooling of subarachnoid fluid result in maximal involvement at the base of the brain, where the exudate may become grossly thickened, collagenous, or caseous, assuming the characteristics of a space-occupying mass and causing pressure injury to neighboring cranial nerves and long tracts. Obstruction of the foramina at the base of the brain may produce obstruction to the flow of cerebrospinal fluid and hydrocephalus. Involvement of the vasculature often produces thrombosis and ischemic brain damage.

Clinical Features and Diagnosis. The course of the illness may vary from abrupt and severe, resembling acute bacterial meningitis, to subtle and chronic, extending over several months. In some instances slowly developing defects in mentation or affect may dominate the picture, with little to suggest either meningitis or infection. Active extrameningeal tuberculosis is clinically apparent in approximately half the patients and the tuberculin test is positive in over three fourths, *but the absence of both does not exclude the diagnosis.* A variety of neurologic abnormalities may be present or develop, including cranial nerve palsies, blindness, deafness, long tract signs, subarachnoid block, and disorders of consciousness ranging from mild confusion to dementia or coma.

Cerebrospinal fluid pleocytosis with over 50 per cent mononuclear cells is the rule. Cell counts are rarely over 1000 per cubic millimeter, more frequently in the 50 to 200 range, and may be as low as only a few lymphocytes. Patients with acute and severe symptoms may demonstrate a high and predominantly polymorphonuclear cerebrospinal fluid cell content early in the course, causing confusion with bacterial meningitis. The cerebrospinal fluid protein concentration is almost always elevated, and the glucose content is usually depressed in comparison with simultaneously determined blood glucose. Smears of the sediment will reveal acid-fast bacilli in less than 25 per cent; the productivity of such microscopy will be improved if the pellicle which often forms on the top of the cerebrospinal fluid specimen is stained and examined. Culture will eventually be positive for *M. tuberculosis* in 75 per cent. Of the cerebrospinal fluid abnormalities, only the degree of pressure elevation has prognostic import, higher pressures being associated with a tendency to early deterioration owing to brain stem herniation. Accordingly, the fluid should be removed cautiously and very slowly, especially when the pressure is over 300 mm. of water.

Treatment and Prognosis. Therapy should always include isoniazid and streptomycin except when coexisting renal insufficiency complicates the use of the latter. In this case, another effective drug, e.g., ethambutol or rifampin, may be substituted for streptomycin. Early in the course, isoniazid should be administered in larger than conventional dosage (8 to 12 mg. per kilogram in the adult, and 15 to 20 mg. per kilogram in children). If response is favorable, these dosages may be reduced, respectively, to 5 mg. per kilogram and 10 mg. per kilogram after four to eight weeks. Pyridoxine (100 mg. per day) should be administered during the period in which increased isoniazid dosage is administered. Isoniazid is usually given as a single oral daily dose, but this may be replaced by intramuscular administration of an equal total dose, usually in two or three divided doses, if oral therapy is not possible. The drug diffuses well into the subarachnoid space (see Chronic Pulmonary Tuberculosis – Isoniazid). Streptomycin dosage is 1 gram daily in adults and 40 mg. per kilogram in children, given as a single injection. Before isoniazid became available, streptomycin, which is transferred poorly across the blood-brain barrier, was often administered by intrathecal injection, but with such marked toxic effects, principally deafness, that this route is no longer acceptable or recommended. Streptomycin may be safely reduced to administration every other day or be replaced by PAS after three or four months of treatment with favorable response. When clinical symptoms have been absent and the cerebrospinal fluid normal for six months, it is reasonable to continue with isoniazid alone for a total course of two to three years.

Bacteriologic cure should be achieved in three fourths or more of the patients. However, this does not prevent the development of permanent neurologic residua such as weakness, paralysis, blindness, or deafness, other cranial nerve palsies, hydrocephalus, compromised intelligence, and, rarely, symptoms and signs of pituitary or hypothalamic dysfunction such as precocious puberty, obesity, diabetes insipidus, and panhypopituitarism. These complications are thought to be local consequences of the inflammatory response, and accordingly adjunctive therapy designed to alter this response might have great advantage. The use of intrathecal tuberculin in the hope of favoring the resolution of the basilar hyperplastic exudate has been tried, but this treatment has never been generally accepted. *Use of corticosteroid hormones or corticotrophin* has received much wider acceptance. Although evidence is conflicting, most studies reveal a slight but definite survival advantage in groups receiving adjunctive corticosteroid therapy, particularly in prevention of early deaths from brainstem herniation, presumably owing to the ameliorating effect of these agents on cerebral edema. The response to corticosteroid therapy is often dramatic, with rapid clearing of sensorium, regression to cerebrospinal fluid abnormalities, defervescence, and loss of headache. Even if the long-term beneficial effects are slight, this prompt symptomatic improvement is thought to justify corticosteroid therapy. Accordingly, prednisone in dosage of 60 to 80 mg. per day is recommended in all cases of tuberculous meningitis complicated by any alteration in sensorium, neurologic abnormality, evidence suggestive of subarachnoid block, or cerebrospinal fluid pressures in excess of 300 mm. of water. This will obviously include most cases. Therapy may be tapered rapidly in the second or third week to a level of 30 mg., and thereafter decreased at a slower rate every third or fourth day, using the signs and symptoms of meningeal inflammation as a guide in the dosage reduction. If these recur, dosage should be elevated again. Usually steroids can be entirely discontinued after six to eight weeks.

Recovery in patients treated with isoniazid-containing regimens should approach 75 per cent. Infancy, old age, associated active tuberculosis, severe neurologic abnormalities, and high (over 300 mm. of water) cerebrospinal fluid pressures are unfavorable prognostic factors. One quarter of cases will demonstrate some permanent neurologic residuum, although usually this will not be disabling.

Tuberculomas. Tuberculomas, once the most frequent cause of intracranial mass lesions in children, are now very rare. Except in cases in which meningitis develops because of extension to the subarachnoid space, the symptoms are those of an expanding cerebral or cerebellar mass. Diagnosis is usually made at surgery. Antimicrobial therapy should be administered when the diagnosis is made, both in the hope of some resolution and to prevent the development of meningitis after operation.

TUBERCULOUS PERICARDITIS

Tuberculous pericarditis usually results from direct extension of a contiguous caseous mediastinal lymph node and less commonly from an adjacent pulmonary focus. Pericarditis occurring in the setting of tuberculous bacillemia may be due to seeding of adjacent structures or to progression of subserosal hematogenous foci. As is the case in peritoneal and pleural effusion, contamination of the pericardial sac evokes an allergic effusion which then may disseminate the infection over the pericardial surface. Although always secondary to extrapericardial tuberculosis, pericarditis is quite frequently the only clinical manifestation of infection. The most frequent associated manifestation is simultaneous pleural effusion, present in approximately half the cases. Coincident peritonitis is less frequent. The simultaneous or sequential involvement of all major serous sacs has been designated as *tuberculous polyserositis*. Such cases may be due to poorly contained primary infections in which abdominal as well as thoracic lymph nodes become extensively involved, or to subserosal hematogenous tubercles.

Prior to the availability of effective antituberculous drugs, tuberculous pericarditis was usually fatal (90 per cent of cases), in half because of progressive tuberculosis and in the remainder as a result of acute or chronic cardiovascular effects such as cardiac tamponade, constrictive pericarditis, or involvement of the myocardium or coronary arteries in the inflammatory reaction.

Clinical Features and Diagnosis. The onset may be acute, with rapid development of fever, pericardial pain, and symptoms of cardiac compression. More often, however, the patient will have been ill for several weeks or more with nonspecific symptoms of weight loss, asthenia, malaise, and low-grade fever when complaints related to cardiac compression such as dyspnea and dependent edema lead to medical attention. At times the process may be so covert that illness is not recognized until constriction has already occurred.

Usually it is not difficult to suspect the presence of pericarditis with effusion. The physical signs and symptoms, discussed in detail elsewhere (see Pericarditis), are fairly characteristic. A pericardial rub is often heard, the chest roentgenogram is usually suggestive, and the electrocardiogram frequently, though by no means always, is confirmatory. However, it is important to emphasize that *similar signs and symptoms may be produced by cardiomegaly without effusion, and therefore establishment of the diagnosis of pericarditis with effusion requires special roentgenographic studies.* The simplest and safest of these is delineation of the right auricle by carbon dioxide (CO_2 contrast study), providing a measure of the distance between the endocardium and the outer border of the pericardium. When results are equivocal, much more information can be obtained, at the price of only slightly more morbidity, by *angiocardiography.*

In contrast to anatomic diagnosis, the etiologic diagnosis of tuberculous pericarditis is often very difficult. Approximately 10 per cent of patients with clinically apparent pericarditis with effusion will have tuberculosis, but the clinical picture produced is often indistinguishable from pericarditis caused by other infectious agents, particularly fungi, by occult hemopericardium, and by neoplasm. If present, recognition of associated neoplastic or tuberculous foci is obviously of great help. The white blood count is usually normal, and fever is low grade, in contrast to pyogenic pericarditis. Pericardial pain is the exception, occurring in about 10 per cent, in contrast to acute benign pericarditis. The tuberculin test is positive in the majority (90 per cent), but may be negative. *Pericardiocentesis* is often employed for both anatomic and etiologic diagnosis. It should be emphasized that *this procedure is associated with a significant morbidity and mortality. If done, it should always be preceded by unequivocal demonstration of pericardial fluid by contrast roentgenographic techniques*, as the majority of fatal consequences have been due to the misinterpretation of generalized cardiomegaly as pericarditis with effusion. Not only does pericardiocentesis carry substantial risk, but most often provides only meager information. The pericardial fluid in tuberculous disease is more frequently bloody than serous, and usually contains a moderate number of predominantly mononuclear inflammatory cells, findings of small differential diagnostic import. The appearance of the pericardium after instillation of air into the sac (shaggy or smooth) is likewise of no differential diagnostic import. Acid-fast bacilli are only rarely seen in the fluid sediment, and culture of the fluid, although eventually diagnostic in as many as 40 per cent, is of little help in the reaching of immediate therapeutic decisions. It is the writer's practice to advise pericardiocentesis only to relieve symptoms of developing tamponade (detected by careful monitoring of venous pressure, pulse pressure, and pulse rate) or to attempt to diagnose pyogenic pericarditis when the clinical features (the presence of sepsis, pneumonia, high spiking fevers, marked leukocytosis) make this a likely possibility. When indicated, the procedure should be performed by someone with more than casual experience with the technique. When immediate diagnosis is essential, a *small open biopsy of the pericardium* is diagnostically much more productive, carries no more and possibly less risk, and provides a more satisfactory approach to the problem of recurrent tamponade, though not the most satisfactory one.

Treatment and Prognosis. Although prompt antimicrobial treatment decreases the frequency with which constriction develops, this is still observed in an appreciable percentage of cases. The usefulness of *adjunctive corticosteroid therapy* in preventing constriction has never been rigorously demonstrated, although most clinicians think that it may be of some help. Its use is, of course, limited to those patients in whom the diagnosis of tuberculosis has been established. Because in most this means pericardial biopsy, the unproved advantage of corticosteroid therapy must be balanced against the morbidity of a surgical procedure that otherwise might be delayed or avoided.

In view of the unpredictable course of each patient, it is the writer's practice, in cases compatible with tuberculous pericarditis and not suggesting pyogenic disease, to initiate drug therapy with isoniazid and streptomycin or with isoniazid alone in conventional dosage (see Chronic Pulmonary Tuberculosis, Treatment) and not to administer corticosteroids. Pericardiocentesis is not routinely employed, but the presence and degree of cardiac compression is assessed more than daily to determine if pericardiocentesis is required. If treatment produces a favorable response, the cardiac shadow returns to normal size, and signs and symptoms disappear, treatment may be continued on an outpatient basis but with close attention to the possibility of developing constriction, which may supervene with little warning at any time. If tamponade persists and requires more than one or two pericardiocenteses, if signs of constriction develop, or if the general response casts suspicion on the diagnosis, thoracotomy with pericardiectomy is advised for both diagnosis and therapy. This decision is usually reached within a month or six weeks, while effusion persists, thus avoiding the increased risk of pericardiectomy at a time when fluid is no longer present and substantial myocardial involvement may have occurred. All patients should recover with appropriate medical and surgical therapy.

TUBERCULOUS PERITONITIS

Tuberculous peritonitis usually results from rupture of an adjacent caseous focus in a lymph node, fallopian tube, or subserosal tubercle, into the peritoneal cavity. It is often the only clinical manifestation of infection. Advanced tuberculous ulceration of the bowel may extend to the serosal surface and contaminate the peritoneum, but this form of tuberculous enteritis is now rare. Once contamination has occurred, the process may become loculated and limited in extent, or may involve the entire peritoneal surface. The inflammatory response varies from copious, thin ascitic fluid with few inflammatory cells to a hyperplastic reaction with gelatinous exudate, progressing eventually to fibrosis or to caseous necrosis.

The onset may resemble acute, pyogenic peritonitis with chills, fever, leukocytosis, ascites, and painful abdominal distention, or may be quite subtle, producing the picture of occult malignancy with unexplained debility, a fever of unknown origin, or complaints related to bowel obstruction. Fever may be absent, and the tuberculin test, although usually positive, is so often negative that it is of little diagnostic help. Recognition of tuberculous peritonitis in persons with cirrhosis may be very difficult, because the symptoms may closely resemble those of uncomplicated cirrhosis with ascites. However, the ascitic fluid in uncomplicated cirrhosis usually contains less than 200 cells per milliliter. When more than this number is found, the possibility of tuberculous, neoplastic, or pyogenic peritonitis should be considered.

Diagnosis is usually based on either laparotomy or response to specific antituberculous chemotherapy. Studies of peritoneal fluid usually reveal elevated protein concentration and mononuclear pleocytosis, resembling fluid obtained in tuberculous pleurisy with effusion, but also indistinguishable from that which may occur in peritoneal carcinomatosis. Acute cases may demonstrate a predominantly polymorphonuclear pleocytosis, suggesting a pyogenic process. Acid-fast stain of the fluid sediment is so rarely positive that it is of no importance in excluding the diagnosis, and tubercle bacilli can be cultured in less than 20 per cent of proved cases. Needle biopsy of the parietal peritoneum (Cope or Abrams needle) will yield the diagnosis in a high percentage of cases but is more dangerous than needle biopsy of the pleura and has resulted in death from occult intraperitoneal bleeding. Accordingly, if tissue is required, a limited exploratory laparotomy is preferable. When the therapeutic advantage gained by tissue diagnosis is limited to the question of whether or not to treat for tuberculosis, a trial of isoniazid is often an acceptable alternative, producing in some cases therapeutic results that leave no question as to the diagnosis. As a therapeutic trial, it is the writer's practice to employ isoniazid as a single agent, because it is vastly less toxic and better accepted than any multiple drug regimen. Multiple drug therapy is advised by some authorities, but single drug therapy with isoniazid for a period of 24 months has produced completely satisfactory responses in all cases known to the writer.

TUBERCULOUS LYMPHADENITIS

All foci of tuberculous infection involve the regional lymphatics, and so in that sense lymphadenitis is an invariable feature of tuberculosis. The involvement of the intrathoracic nodes in the primary infection, particularly in children, and the late complications of mediastinal lymphatic tuberculosis have been discussed elsewhere, as has the role of caseous lymph nodes in the production of pericardial, peritoneal, and, more rarely, pleural disease. Prior to the control of bovine tuberculosis, cervical tuberculous lymphadenitis, or *scrofula*, was commonplace, owing presumably to a local infection of the oropharynx and draining cervical lymphatics (see Tuberculosis, History). At present, this mode of acquisition of tuberculous cervical lymphadenitis must be extremely rare, at least in areas with no bovine tuberculosis problem. In contrast, cervical granulomatous lymphadenitis in children, caused by myobacteria other than *M. tuberculosis* and *M. bovis*, is almost certainly acquired by the oral route and represents a local infection.

The term "tuberculous lymphadenitis" is now best reserved for the rather unusual instance in which a generalized tuberculous infection manifests itself principally by the appearance of superficial lymph node involvement. This may occur because of extensive lymphatic spread from a primary pulmonary lesion or as a part of a generalized hematogenous dissemination. The apparently more frequent occurrence of this syndrome in nonwhite races suggests that it is associated with host factors favoring extensive lymphohematogenous spread. The cervical and mediastinal nodes are most frequently involved. Clinical evidence of associated tuberculosis in the lungs or elsewhere is lacking in more than half the cases. Painless or, less frequently, painful node enlargement is the usual presenting complaint, but a substantial minority of patients demonstrate associated symptoms of systemic infection such as fever, malaise, and weight loss. The nodes may become fluctuant and produce draining sinuses.

The effect of drug therapy should be assessed before surgery is resorted to, as often even large, necrotic, chronically draining nodes will resolve completely. In some instances, masses that are fluctuant, draining, or painful may require resection in addition to drug treatment, but this is the exception. Drug therapy should continue for at least a year and probably two. Most authorities recommend use of isoniazid and a companion drug, but isoniazid given as a single agent is adequate therapy in almost all instances. Prolonged rest or hospitalization is not necessary once a favorable response has been established, and relapse is very rare. Careful bacteriologic investigation of the responsible organism is particularly important in view of the frequency with which lymphadenitis in children is due to other mycobacterial species, most of which are indifferent to the effects of isoniazid and require a different therapeutic approach with more emphasis on surgical removal.

GENITOURINARY TUBERCULOSIS

Renal Tuberculosis. Renal tuberculosis develops from cortical foci seeded via the blood stream, usually at the time of the initial infection. Renal infection from a chronic pulmonary or extrapulmonary focus probably occurs much less frequently; such coexistent foci outside the genitourinary system are best regarded as parallel consequences of the initial infection. Although renal tuberculosis is usually unilateral when detected, 50 per cent will progress to bilateral involvement in the absence of treatment, presumably because of progression of contralateral hematogenous foci.

The bacilli lodge in the cortex, but infection does not become progressive until it reaches the medulla (via the renal tubules), where the environment is much more favorable to the progression of tuberculosis and all other types of renal bacterial infection. Progressive foci in the renal papillae may cause obstruction and retrograde involvement of the obstructed segment, or may undergo necrosis, excavate, and seed the ureteral and bladder mucosa. A combination of papillary obstruction and infection can progress to massive segmental renal destruction, scarring in the renal pelvis and ureters may result in total renal obstruction and hydronephrosis, and the contaminated urine may cause bladder irritability,

contracture, and scarring, as well as infection of the male genitalia.

Clinical Features and Diagnosis. Symptoms are usually subtle and quite often entirely lacking even with advanced, cavitary renal tuberculosis. Pyuria in the absence of culturable pyogenic organisms is suggestive of renal tuberculosis, especially when symptoms of an irritable bladder such as frequency and dysuria coexist. Pyuria may be intermittent and low grade (10 WBC per high-power field). Intermittent hematuria may also be seen. Fever and backache are uncommon and probably late symptoms. Male genital tuberculosis may be the first symptom suggesting renal involvement. History of prior tuberculous infection or coexistent extrarenal foci other than in the bladder and genitalia are more the exception than the rule. The importance of latent renal foci as a source of late tuberculous bacillemia bears re-emphasis.

Diagnosis is based on culture of first morning urine specimens. Demonstration of acid-fast bacilli by microscopy of urine concentrate may be due to contaminating mycobacteria, principally the smegma bacillus, but in some will represent *M. tuberculosis* and should be regarded with some suspicion. Intravenous or retrograde pyelography may provide the first evidence of disease and are necessary to assess the degree of involvement. However, unless calcification is present, the findings are nonspecific and similar to those produced by nontuberculous pyelonephritis.

Treatment and Prognosis. Treatment with a two-drug regimen, including isoniazid for a period of at least two years, will result in sterilization of the urine and arrest of disease in the majority of patients. When relapse does occur, drug resistance is usually found, and re-treatment with two drugs to which the infection is susceptible is advised. The progress of therapy should be followed by intravenous pyelograms obtained at three-month intervals in order to detect and treat ureteral strictures that may occur as a consequence of healing of the superficial ureteral mucosal lesions. Some authorities employ ureteral catheterization and dilatation to avoid this complication. Occasionally, obstruction with complicating pyogenic infection or pain may require removal of renal tissue or other surgical procedures. However, one major urologic service devoted to the study of renal tuberculosis has not found nephrectomy necessary in the past several years.

Male Genital Tuberculosis. Male genital tuberculosis affects the *prostate*, the *seminal vesicles*, the *epididymides,* and more rarely the *testes.* Prostatic infection is usually secondary to renal tuberculosis, although the responsible renal focus may have been remote. Contaminated urine initiates infection in the prostatic ducts, which then may spread retrograde to involve the gland, and, via the seminal fluid, the epididymides. Although prostatic and seminal vesicular involvement is pathologically more frequent, most instances of male genital tuberculosis present with an epididymal lesion, varying from a firm, painless, small nodule to an inflamed and draining mass.

Evidence of associated prostatitis and seminal vesiculitis may or may not be found. Diagnosis is usually made by prostatic or epididymal biopsy. Some instances of genital tuberculosis may be detected because of poor healing and fistula formation complicating prostatic or scrotal surgery. Diagnosis in such cases may require a therapeutic trial of isoniazid, as culture of the draining material is often unrevealing. Response to drug therapy is excellent in most patients, and surgery is usually not required for other than diagnostic purposes. Combined drug therapy is usually recommended, but in the absence of active renal disease isoniazid is also adequate therapy.

Female Genital Tuberculosis. Tuberculous infection of the female pelvic organs begins as a hematogenous focus in the endosalpinx. Infection may spread via the tubal lumen to the ovary, the endometrium, and rarely the cervix, producing an ulcerating granulomatous lesion resembling carcinoma. Spread may occur to the serosal tubal surface and result in peritonitis, either confined to the pelvis or generalized throughout the peritoneal cavity.

The most common symptoms are sterility, menstrual disorders, and abdominal pain, occasionally with distention. In most cases the patient will have never become pregnant, and sterility clinics frequently discover female genital tuberculosis that is otherwise asymptomatic. In a smaller number, pregnancy and delivery appear to activate a previously latent focus. When conception does occur, tubal disease favors ectopic pregnancy. The picture of pelvic inflammatory disease with poor response to antimicrobial therapy may lead to the recognition of tuberculosis. In the majority, however, local symptoms are mild or absent, and constitutional reaction is minimal. Diagnosis is made by histologic study and culture of endometrial scrapings, by culture of menstrual blood, and often by exploratory laparotomy. Response to a drug regimen containing isoniazid or to isoniazid alone is usually excellent, and surgery is necessary only in exceptional cases to remove large tubo-ovarian abscesses. Reconstructive tubal surgery to modify sterility has met with only limited success.

TUBERCULOSIS OF BONES AND JOINTS

Blood-borne tubercle bacilli tend to lodge in the anterior aspects of vertebral bodies and in the metaphyseal areas of long bones. Evolution of foci in bone may produce cystic areas of osteomyelitis without joint involvement, but often erode the end plate and involve the nearby joint space. Although it is difficult to establish, Rich believes that tuberculous arthritis is always secondary to adjacent bone disease, which itself may be quite inconspicuous. In years past, much skeletal tuberculosis was due to infection with *M. bovis*. At present, bone and joint tuberculosis is not common in the United States, but several cases are seen each year on most medical services. It remains a major problem in other areas of the world.

Tuberculous Spondylitis

The most frequent and severe form of skeletal tuberculosis is *tuberculous spondylitis* or *Pott's disease*. The originating focus is usually in the anterior aspect of the vertebral body near an intervertebral disc. The developing infection usually erodes through the cortex and into the intervertebral disc, destroying it and extending to involve the adjacent vertebral body. The resulting roentgenographic picture of rarefaction and destruction of the adjacent areas of two vertebral bodies, loss of the intervening disc space, and a tendency to anterior wedging or collapse is typical of tuberculous spondylitis but is also caused by other infectious processes. The anterior foreshortening and angulation of the spine may result in a visible posterior bony prominence or *gibbus* which may be tender. Less frequently, the infection may begin in the center or posterior aspect of the vertebral body. The thoracic, thoracolumbar, cervical, and lumbosacral areas are involved in order of decreasing frequency. More than one area may be involved with intervening normal vertebrae. Characteristically, the inflammatory process dissects anterolaterally from the vertebral body, producing a paraspinal abscess. In the thoracolumbar area, this may be seen as mediastinal widening or a pear-shaped retrocardiac density on chest roentgenogram. In the lumbar area, a flat plate of the abdomen may reveal obliteration of the psoas shadow. In the cervical area, the abscess may displace the esophagus and trachea anteriorly, and cause symptoms of respiratory obstruction or dysphagia. The constricting effect of the firm paraspinal ligamentous structures may result in high pressure in the abscess and produce ischemic changes in the subjacent spinal cord leading to paralysis. The pressure in the abscess may also cause it to dissect along ligamentous planes and present as a fluctuant or firm mass some distance from the initiating vertebral focus, such as in the groin, in the gluteal area, or in the supraclavicular space. The release of large quantities of pus following biopsy of such "masses" may lead to the discovery of unrecognized tuberculosis of the spine. The paraspinal abscess may spread the infection so that three or four adjacent vertebral bodies become involved.

Clinical Features and Diagnosis. Symptoms are usually insidious, prolonged, and not associated with fever, although weight loss and asthenia are common. Local back pain is frequent, and referred pain imitating renal colic or abdominal disorders occurs. Walking may be painful, and the gait may become stilted but go without notice because of the chronicity of the process. Acute back pain at night, presumed to be due to relaxation of paraspinal muscle spasm that protectively splints the involved area during the waking hours, is thought to be the mechanism of the "night cries" of children with tuberculous spondylitis. Miliary, meningeal, or pulmonary tuberculosis may develop and dominate the picture in the untreated case. Severe anterior angulation of the spine may eventually produce a hunchback deformity. Frequently, however, it is the development of *weakness or paralysis* that leads to medical attention. Paralysis, which is now the most serious consequence of Pott's disease, may develop owing to pressure from abscess fluid, to generalized inflammatory edema, or to intrusion of a bony sequestrum or granulation tissue on the anterior aspect of the cord. Paralysis owing to angulation and displacement is unusual, as the anatomic abnormality develops slowly, but violent movement rarely may produce cord transection when spine instability is marked.

In prior years most infectious spondylitis was tuberculous, and etiologic diagnosis was often based solely on the characteristic abnormality on a roentgenogram of the spine. However, it is now clear that entirely similar roentgenographic and clinical pictures can be produced by several other organisms, notably staphylococci, gram-negative enterobacteria, fungi, and rarely mycobacteria other than *M. tuberculosis.* Accordingly, in the absence of strong ancillary evidence for tuberculosis, aspiration or open biopsy of the vertebral body is indicated.

Treatment. Treatment of Pott's disease is based on antimicrobial therapy and immobilization. Usually therapy with isoniazid and streptomycin for a period of two years or more is recommended. The orthopedic approach is a matter of controversy. Most orthopedists advise some form of prompt surgical intervention such as debridement of the abscess cavity and spinal fusion, followed by a prolonged period of body casting. Others, particularly in areas in which surgical facilities are limited, have reported comparable results using just drug therapy and a brief period (two or three months) of bed rest without casting. When paralysis develops or fails to improve on therapy, surgery is required, and the procedure, whether abscess evacuation, debridement of granulation tissue, or removal of sequestra, is dictated by the findings at operation. Usually some form of spinal fusion will also be carried out. Although the course of therapy is usually decided by the responsible orthopedist, it is the writer's preference to assess the effects of drug therapy and bed rest while maintaining close surveillance of the neurologic status, as many patients will achieve stable spines and remission of neurologic symptoms without operative intervention or casting. The argument that diseased tissue must be removed lest relapse supervene is even less applicable to bony tuberculosis, in which the bacterial population is small, than to pulmonary tuberculosis, in which it is large. In the latter case, in spite of an environment much more conducive to bacillary multiplication, surgical removal of residual diseased tissue as a principle has largely been abandoned as the effects of adequate and prolonged chemotherapy have become more clear.

Tuberculous Arthritis

Clinical Findings and Diagnosis. Tuberculous arthritis involves the hips, knees, elbows, shoulders, and small joints of the hands and feet in roughly that order. The initial symptoms are pain on motion or weight-bearing, usually with some swelling. The process is usually monarticular, chronic, and associated eventually with considerable muscle wasting, pain, and stiffness. A history of trauma to the involved joint can frequently be obtained. As mentioned, overt or inapparent involvement of juxta-articular bone is probably always present and serves as the initiating focus. In the absence of proved associated tuberculosis, diagnosis requires biopsy, histologic study, and culture. The need for verification by culture has been emphasized by reports of cases of granulomatous arthritis caused by mycobacteria other than *M. tuberculosis (vide infra).*

Treatment. Most authorities recommend isoniazid and daily streptomycin; it is the writer's practice to utilize isoniazid alone. Intra-articular injection of drugs is not recommended, as isoniazid diffuses well into joint spaces. As with spondylitis, the orthopedic management of tuberculous arthritis is controversial. However, many and perhaps most instances of tuberculous arthritis will heal with preservation of joint function when treated with mild immobilization, bed rest in the case of weight-bearing joints, and chemotherapy, especially when treatment is begun promptly. When progress is not entirely satisfactory, joint exploration and removal of hypertrophied and fragmented synovial granulation tissue may be required. Casting and procedures to effect joint fusion are thought to be rarely necessary and at times detrimental, an opinion, it should be emphasized, that runs counter to much orthopedic advice. The argument that all residual disease must be surgically extirpated is not applicable for reasons discussed above and, in fact, is unrealistic in view of the multiple foci present in every case of tuberculosis.

Other Forms of Skeletal Tuberculosis

Cystic tuberculosis of bone (tuberculous caries) is a rare condition in which osteolytic cystic areas of long and flat bones and occasionally the tubular bones of the hands or feet are caused by tuberculosis. The term *osteitis tuberculosa multiplex cystica* has been applied. It is rare and mentioned only to point out that tuberculosis is one cause of cystic bony changes. *Tuberculosis of the costochondral junction* may present as a cold abscess overlying the area of involvement. *Tuberculosis of the tendon sheaths and bursae* is usually secondary to involvement of the adjacent joint. These are responsive to therapy either with isoniazid alone or combined with streptomycin.

RARE FORMS OF TUBERCULOSIS

Ocular tuberculosis is most frequently mentioned as one of the causes of *granulomatous intraocular infection.* Although usually described as more posterior (chorioretinitis) than anterior (iridocyclitis), either or both areas may be involved. Other causes (toxoplasmosis, syphilis, histoplasmosis, sarcoidosis) are probably much more common than tuberculosis. From a practical point of view, however, an etiologic diagnosis is usually impossible, and treatment with isoniazid is often administered if the tuberculin test is positive, especially, as is frequently the case, steroid therapy is used. It is thought to be due to the presence of organisms in the ocular tissues. *Phlyctenular keratoconjunctivitis is a rare allergic* external ocular inflammation observed in children at the time of the primary infection and characterized by small blisters (phlyctenules) at the junction of conjunctiva and cornea. It may be severely exacerbated by tuberculin testing and result in corneal injury. *Choroidal tubercles* will often provide a clue to the presence of disseminated tuberculosis. They produce no symptoms and are difficult to differentiate from other retinal exudates.

Cutaneous tuberculosis, once an important, but now only rarely seen, group of illnesses, is usually grouped into two categories. The first, caused by the presence of organisms in the skin, includes *lupus vulgaris* (a red-brown, thickened, slightly nodular, nonulcerated process, most frequently on the face), *tuberculosis verrucosa cutis* (anatomic or prosector's wart), *scrofuloderma* (the skin changes surrounding a draining tuberculous sinus or overlying a tuberculous node), and *tuberculosis orificialis* (nodular and ulcerated lesions around the mouth or other orifice through which highly infectious material passes). All these are granulomatous histologically, and are very responsive to isoniazid alone. The second group comprises the *tuberculids* (including *erythema induratum* or Bazin's disease). These reactions are thought to be based on allergy to a distant bacterial infection. They assume a wide variety of erythematous, papular, and ulcerative forms. Their relationship to tuberculosis is poorly understood. *Tuberculosis cutis miliaris, acuta disseminata* is a rare complication of overwhelming miliary tuberculosis, usually in children, presenting as a disseminated petechial or purpuric rash, at times with minute papule formation.

Tuberculosis of the adrenals is important only as an uncommon cause of adrenal insufficiency. Tuberculosis of the *spleen, thyroid, pancreas,* and *breast* may all occur, and suggest other infections or neoplastic change in these organs.

American Thoracic Society: Chemoprophylaxis for the prevention of tuberculosis. Amer. Rev. Resp. Dis., 96:558, 1967.

Bentley, G., and Webster, J. H. H.: Gastrointestinal tuberculosis. A 10-year review. Brit. J. Surg., 54:90, 1967.

Brown, A. B., Gilbert, R. A., and TeLinde, R. W.: Pelvic tuberculosis. Obstet. Gynec., 2:476, 1953.

Canetti, G.: Present aspects of bacterial resistance in tuberculosis. Amer. Rev. Resp. Dis., 92:687, 1965.

Diagnostic Standards and Classification of Tuberculosis. New York, National Tuberculosis and Respiratory Disease Association, 1969.

Dubos, R., and Dubos, J.: The White Plague. Boston, Little, Brown and Company, 1952.

Falk, A.: U.S. VA–Armed Forces cooperative study on the chemotherapy of tuberculosis. XII. Results of treatment in miliary tuberculosis: A follow-up study of 570 adult patients. Amer. Rev. Resp. Dis., 91:6, 1965.

Falk, A.: U.S. VA–Armed Forces cooperative study on the chemotherapy of tuberculosis. XIII. Tuberculous meningitis in adults, with special reference to survival, neurologic residuals, and work status. Amer. Rev. Resp. Dis., 91:823, 1965.

Friedman, B.: Chemotherapy of tuberculosis of the spine. J. Bone Joint Surg. (Amer.), 48-A:451, 1966.

Goyette, E. M.: Treatment of tuberculous pericarditis. Progr. Cardiov. Dis., 3:141, 1960.

Groth-Petersen, E., Knudsen, J., and Wilbek, E.: Epidemiological basis of tuberculosis eradication in an advanced country. Bull. WHO, 21:5, 1959.

Kaplan, C. J.: Conservative therapy in skeletal tuberculosis: An appraisal based on experience in South Africa. Tubercle (London), 40.355, 1959.

Kent, D. C.: Tuberculous lymphadenitis: Not a localized disease process. Amer. J. Med. Sci., 254, 866, 1967.

Konstam, P. G., and Blesovsky, A.: The ambulant treatment of spinal tuberculosis. Brit. J. Surg., 50:26, 1962.

Lattimer, J. K.: Renal tuberculosis. New Eng. J. Med., 273:208, 1965.

Lowell, A. M., Edwards, L. B., and Palmer, C. E.: Tuberculosis. Cambridge, Mass., Harvard University Press, 1969.

Mackaness, G. B.: The immunology of antituberculous immunity. Amer. Rev. Resp. Dis., 97:337, 1968.

Mitchison, D. A.: Chemotherapy of tuberculosis: A bacteriologist's viewpoint. Brit. Med. J., 1:1333, 1965.

Proudfoot, A. T., Akhtar, A. J., Douglas, A. C., and Horne, N. W.: Miliary tuberculosis in adults. Brit. Med. J., 2:273, 1969.

Rich, A.: The Pathogenesis of Tuberculosis. 2nd ed. Springfield, Ill., Charles C Thomas, 1952.

Smith, D. T.: Diagnostic and prognostic significance of the quantitative tuberculin tests. Ann. Intern. Med., 67:919, 1967.

Sochocky, S.: Tuberculous peritonitis: A review of 100 cases. Amer. Rev. Resp. Dis., 95:398, 1967.

Stead, W. W.: Pathogenesis of the sporadic case of tuberculosis. New Eng. J. Med., 277:1008, 1967.

Stead, W. W.: Pathogenesis of a first exposure of chronic pulmonary tuberculosis in man: Recrudescence of residuals of the primary infection or exogenous reinfection? Amer. Rev. Resp. Dis., 95:729, 1967.

Twomey, J. J., and Leavell, B. S.: Leukemoid reactions to tuberculosis. Arch. Intern. Med. (Chicago), 116:21, 1965.

Varma, B. N., and Smith, J. M.: Tuberculous pericarditis: A review of 17 recent cases. Tubercle (London), 48:160, 1967.

Youmans, G. P., and Youmans, A. S.: Recent studies on acquired immunity in tuberculosis. Curr. Top. Microbiol. Immun., 48:129, 1969.

DISEASES DUE TO MYCOBACTERIA OTHER THAN M. TUBERCULOSIS AND M. LEPRAE

Robert Goodwin

By tradition the term tuberculosis refers to infection and disease associated with *M. tuberculosis* (var. *hominis* and var. *bovis*). It has long been known that other mycobacterial species exist in nature, some of which cause disease in animals. For years, by arbitrary and, in retrospect, amusing definition, a mycobacterium was considered a human pathogen only if it produced disease in the guinea pig. This notion prevailed until modern culture methods demonstrated some of these guinea pig nonpathogens present in diseased human tissue. Several species of mycobacteria, some not previously known, have recently been identified as potential human pathogens. A few of these have received formal taxonomic designation, but others, including the most important, have not. Much of the most important bacteriologic work on these *"atypical," "anonymous,"* or *"unclassified"* mycobacteria has been carried out by Runyon, who classified them into four groups primarily on the basis of the presence and type of pigment production and growth rate. This tentative arrangement has been useful and widely accepted. (See Bacteriology in the article on Tuberculosis). More recently most of the known human pathogens have received tentative but widely accepted species designations, which will be employed herein. The relationship of these to the Runyon classification is as follows: *M. kansasii** and *M. marinum*—Runyon Group I (photochromogens); *M. scrofulaceum**—Runyon Group II (scotochromogens); *M. intracellulare** (Battey bacillus), *M. avium,* and *M. xenopei**—Runyon Group III (nonpigmented species); and *M. fortuitum*—Runyon Group IV (rapid growers).

The diseases produced by these organisms have roentgenologic, pathologic, and to a large extent clinical similarities to tuberculosis, but there are distinct differences in virulence, treatment, and prognosis. The term *mycobacteriosis* has been suggested for diseases produced by this group of infections to differentiate them from tuberculosis. However, species orientation is preferable, because there are differences in organ susceptibility, treatment, and prognosis within the group. It is convenient from a clinical standpoint to group these infections according to organ involvement. Pulmonary disease is the most common clinical manifestation. Lymphadenitis and granulomatous skin lesions are less frequent. The widespread tissue involvement that may be produced by the more virulent *M. tuberculosis* is not seen in mycobacteriosis save for rare instances of disseminated opportunistic infection in abnormal hosts, unusual skeletal involvement, and, occasionally, abscesses at injection sites.

PULMONARY DISEASE

M. kansasii and *M. intracellulare* (Battey bacilli), the most virulent of this group of organisms, may produce a tuberculosis-like pulmonary disease in susceptible individuals, as rarely may the less virulent *M. fortuitum, M. xenopei,* and *M. avium.*

Prevalence. In the United States and Europe, 1 to 2 per cent of hospital admissions for tuberculosis are due to infection with either *M. kansasii,* or *M. intracellulare.* There are geographic variations, particularly in the United States. The incidence of *M. intracellulare* infections is relatively high in Georgia and Florida, and *M. kansasii* infection is more frequent in Texas, Kansas, and Illinois. In some localities incidence is as high as 7 to 10 per cent of hospital admissions for tuberculosis.

Epidemiology. The epidemiology of these infections is obscure. *M. kansasii* and *M. intracellulare* have been demonstrated in soil. Both organisms have been found in throat swabs and saliva of healthy individuals (in one report from Florida the incidence was as high as 14 per cent). It is not known whether this transient carrier state is transmitted from man to man or from some other source; however, the person with clinical disease is not thought to transmit infection, as neither

overt disease nor the incidence of infection, determined by use of a PPD prepared from the organism in question, is increased in family contacts. Skin-testing surveys suggest a high incidence of subclinical infections in the endemic areas. Two thirds of naval recruits from Georgia and Florida reacted to a *M. intracellulare* PPD, whereas only 6 per cent were positive to PPD-S (*M. tuberculosis*). Cross reactions occur with PPD preparations from different mycobacteria, but are generally weaker than reactions to the homologous PPD. Accordingly simultaneous skin testing with several different PPD preparations can be used for diagnosis, assuming that the strongest reaction indicates the infecting organism. Data gathered in this fashion indicate a very high infection rate and low incidence of disease, illustrating the low virulence of these organisms for humans. Once disease develops, pathologic changes are essentially the same as those found in tuberculosis.

Clinical Manifestations. Pulmonary disease caused by *M. kansasii* and *M. intracellulare* is primarily a disease of white males over the age of 45; it is less frequent in females and in blacks of both sexes. Prior chronic bronchitis and emphysema have a definite predisposing influence, being present in 40 per cent of patients with disease due to *M. kansasii* and in 60 per cent of those with disease due to *M. intracellulare.* Pneumoconiosis may increase susceptibility. Although virulence is less, disease, once established, tends to become cavitary and progressive. The clinical picture at any given time is indistinguishable from chronic pulmonary tuberculosis. Although in general slower in tempo than untreated tuberculosis, these infections may produce relentless destruction of pulmonary tissue and may lead to death from respiratory insufficiency. Constitutional symptoms such as fever, anorexia, weight loss, and wasting are much less prominent. Local symptoms of cough and sputum are similar, and hemoptysis may occur somewhat more frequently than in tuberculosis. Roentgenographic studies usually reveal a process already far advanced at the time of discovery. Cavities are more frequently thin-walled and pneumonic lesions less prominent than in tuberculosis, but there is much overlap and roentgenographic differentiation is not possible in the individual case. Lesions have the apical posterior localization characteristic of tuberculosis. Pleural effusions are rare and pleural changes of any sort inconspicuous.

Diagnosis is dependent upon bacteriologic identification of the specific organism. As mycobacteria other than *M. tuberculosis* may be found as a carrier state in the saliva, diagnosis of disease requires repeated demonstration of the organism in the presence of compatible pulmonary disease. A tuberculosis-like disease that does not respond to antimicrobial therapy or the demonstration of a high order of primary drug resistance should suggest the possibility of one of the other mycobacterial species.

Treatment. Mycobacteriosis differs most strikingly from tuberculosis in the conspicuous lack of susceptibility to the antituberculous drugs

---

*Species designations not yet formally recognized.

Pulmonary disease caused by these less virulent agents is actually much more difficult to treat than drug-susceptible tuberculosis. In disease caused by *M. kansasii*, multiple drug therapy may be moderately helpful and is always used. In disease caused by *M. intracellulare*, the use of drugs is generally disappointing, and drugs are probably entirely ineffective against *M. fortuitum*. These organisms almost always show in vitro resistance to isoniazid. This drug is generally used, however. In disease caused by *M. kansasii*, a combination of isoniazid, ethionamide, ethambutol, and streptomycin has been reported to produce the best results. The susceptibilities of the organism to all drugs should be obtained and the most appropriate combination of several drugs continued. There is no established plan for drug management of disease caused by *M. intracellulare*. Although some strains are susceptible to some of the drugs, this is quite unpredictable. The most commonly useful drugs are ethambutol, ethionamide, pyrazinamide, and cycloserine (in addition to isoniazid). Multiple drugs increase the chance of success but at greater risk of drug toxicity. When thought effective, drugs are usually continued in both infections for one year after the organism has disappeared from the sputum. To the degree that drug therapy is less useful, other methods of treatment become more so. Most authors recommend hospitalization and a fairly confining type of rest therapy. Most agree that residual cavities should be resected if possible, whether or not the bacilli have disappeared from the sputum. This argument is stronger in the case of disease caused by *M. intracellulare* than that by *M. kansasii*, and is more compelling if the bacilli persist in the sputum despite nonsurgical treatment. The incidence of surgical complications is remarkably low even without effective drug coverage.

A statement of *prognosis* must be quite broad. Without treatment the prognosis is generally bad. In disease caused by *M. kansasii* the results are generally better in those without prior lung disease than in those with bronchitis and emphysema. Persistence of the bacilli in the sputum in the face of drug treatment indicates an unfavorable outlook. The presence of residual cavitation, even with "negative" sputum, carries a high risk of relapse. "Negative" sputum for a year with no residual cavity (with or without surgery) indicates a good prognosis, with a relapse rate perhaps no greater than 5 to 10 per cent. With vigorous treatment, the best success rates in pulmonary disease caused by *M. kansasii* are reported to be in the range of 85 per cent, and in disease caused by *M. intracellulare* a maximum of 75 per cent.

LYMPHADENITIS

Reports from the United States, Europe, and Australia in recent years have revealed the surprising finding that 75 per cent of granulomatous cervical adenitis suggestive of tuberculosis is actually caused by mycobacteria other than *M. tuberculosis*, explaining the fact that the incidence of tuberculosis-like cervical adenitis (scrofula) remains high in some areas in which most tuberculosis disease is declining rapidly. *M. scrofulaceum*, a scotochromogen found abundantly in nature and often in tap water, *M. intracellulare*, and less commonly *M. kansasii* are the responsible agents. Each of these may be the predominant cause of adenitis in certain geographic areas and not found at all in others. These organisms are found in the soil and transiently in the respiratory flora. In the vast majority the adenitis is cervical in location, but occasionally the inguinal, axillary, or epitrochlear nodes may be involved. The portal of entry in cervical adenitis is probably the tonsils or pharyngeal lymphoid tissue, presumably as a result of ingestion of materials contaminated with soil. In the extremities the infection usually follows a puncture wound. Cervical lymphadenitis occurs almost entirely in children, predominantly in infancy and early childhood. No other manifestation of disease elsewhere in the body has been reported. The pathologic findings of the lesion are similar to that of tuberculosis as are the clinical manifestations. An enlarged, firm, and nontender single node or group of nodes in the submandibular or upper cervical chains may appear and persist unchanged or progress to fluctuation, drainage, and sinus formation. Surgical excision is usually relied upon for both diagnosis and treatment as these organisms are notoriously drug resistant. However, isoniazid treatment of granulomatous cervical adenitis is indicated prior to cultural identification of the organism to cover the possibility that the infection is due to *M. tuberculosis*. If antigens are available, the demonstration of skin hypersensitivity to some other mycobacterial species and a negative or smaller reaction to PPD-S (*M. tuberculosis*) is regarded as diagnostic. Although recurrence may develop in an adjacent lymph node, surgical excision of grossly involved nodes is usually curative.

SUPERFICIAL SKIN DISEASE

In addition to *M. leprae* (leprosy) and *M. tuberculosis*, two other mycobacteria, *M. marinum* and *M. ulcerans* can produce an uncommon type of skin infection. Both these mycobacteria have temperature requirements below 37° C., accounting for limitation of infection to superficial areas of the skin, usually on the extremities. Visceral involvement does not occur.

M. marinum, frequently referred to as *M. balnei*, is a photochromogenic saprophyte first described as the cause of tuberculosis in marine fish. It is widely distributed in nature, occurring in soil and fresh water fish as well. The temperature for optimal growth is 30° C. to 32° C. It has been implicated in rare epidemics of granulomatous skin disease traced to infected swimming pools, beaches of several of the Hawaiian Islands, and, more rarely, tropical fish aquariums. The granulomas occur at the site of minor abrasions, most commonly on the elbows, but also on the knees, toes, fingers, dorsum of the feet, and bridge of the nose, appearing two to three weeks after infection as papules or nodules that slowly increase in size and may ulcerate. Spontaneous healing is to be expected after several months. Diagnosis may be established by culturing a biopsy of the lesion at 30° C. Histologically, the tissue usually suggests a tuberculosis-like granuloma, but may appear to be a nonspecific chronic inflammatory reaction. A weakly positive tuberculin test (cross-sensitivity) may be found. No treatment is recommended.

Disease resulting from *M. ulcerans* is quite rare. This agent, which grows best at 30 to 33° C., has been reported as the cause of indolent skin ulcerations in man. The lesions may be quite destructive and persistent, and may require surgical excision.

Bates, J. H.: A study of pulmonary disease associated with myco-bacteria other than *Mycobacterium tuberculosis:* Clinical characteristics. Amer. Rev. Resp. Dis., 96:1151, 1967.
Mackellar, A., Hilton, H. B., and Masters, P. L.: Mycobacterial lymphadenitis in childhood. Arch. Dis. Child., 42:70, 1967.
Schaefer, W. B., and Davis, C. L.: A bacteriologic and histo-pathologic study of skin granuloma due to *Mycobacterium balnei.* Amer. Rev. Resp. Dis., 84:837, 1961.
Selkon, J. B. "Atypical" mycobacteria: A review. Tubercle, 50(Supp.):70, 1969.

LEPROSY
(Hansen's Disease)
Harry L. Arnold, Jr.

Definition. Leprosy is a chronic disease caused by *Mycobacterium leprae.* Its principal clinical lesions occur in the cooler tissues of the body: skin, superficial nerves, nose, pharynx, and larynx. The distal portion of the eye and the testicles may also be damaged. Disfigurement and deformity owing to skin infiltration and peripheral nerve destruction in untreated patients may be extremely severe and conspicuous. The disfigurement is the principal reason for the fear and loathing historically — and tragically — attached to the disease.

Etiology. *Mycobacterium leprae,* the cause of leprosy, was discovered in 1873 by G. Armauer Hansen of Norway. It is an acid-fast rod about the same size as *M. tuberculosis,* from 1.5 to 6.0 μ long and 0.2 to 0.45 μ thick. It occurs in tissues singly, in "cigar-bundle" clusters, and in oval aggregates 15 to 25 μ in diameter called globi. Though many efforts have been made (notably by Danielssen in Norway and Mouritz in Hawaii) to infect humans by injecting bacillus-containing material into them, only one (by Arning, in Hawaii) has been successful, and in it the possibility of prior infection of the subject by ordinary means could not be excluded. Apparent accidental inoculation of two Marines by tattooing was reported during World War II. The successful inoculation of footpads of mice, achieved in 1960, has made it possible to identify sulfone-resistant strains of *M. leprae.*

Incidence and Epidemiology. Known of old throughout south Asia and Africa, and almost epidemic throughout Europe in the eleventh to thirteenth centuries, leprosy persists today in a patchy endemic zone encircling the world largely between the thirtieth parallels of latitude, but also including Japan, Korea, south China, and South Africa. Outside of these areas it does not appear to be communicable. Only a handful of cases remain in Scandinava and none in most European countries. In Spain and Portugal, it may be increasing in incidence. In the United States, leprosy is endemic in those states bordering on the Gulf of Mexico and in Hawaii.

The transmission of leprosy is mysterious. It is so difficult to acquire that it was believed for many decades to be hereditary rather than contagious. Yet, it is so easy to acquire that nearly half the patients with recently acquired disease are unaware of having had any contact with another diseased person. Perhaps this paradox can best be resolved by the view that leprosy is easily acquired by contact with lepromatous persons *during transient periods of increased susceptibility,* to which some persons are subject. Such susceptibility may be inherited, though this is unproved.

The determinants of susceptibility are not known. Hawaiians have seventy times the leprosy morbidity experienced by Caucasians in Hawaii, and similar racial differences are reported from many other areas. Children are more susceptible, other things being equal, than adults, though the difference is much less marked in nonendemic areas. A family history of leprosy probably means heightened susceptibility to infection, though it is not necessarily associated with low resistance to the established disease. Persons with a negative Mitsuda reaction to injected lepromin are more susceptible to leprosy, and they are more apt to have the lepromatous form of the disease if they do become infected than persons with a positive reaction. Diet is probably unimportant.

Pathogenesis and Clinical Manifestations. Leprosy involves principally the skin and subcutaneous nerves. It occurs in reasonably well-defined types, in both of which the disfigurement and deformity may be produced either by the disease process itself or by the consequences of the loss of sensation or motor or trophic innervation of an affected area or part. The clinical picture may also be significantly modified, in the lepromatous type, by the development of systemic amyloidosis or by associated infection with tubercle bacilli. Because of these very considerable differences between types and groups, no single clinical description will usefully depict leprosy. Consequently, in the present discussion, the principal attention will be devoted to defining the individual manifestations, in themselves quite recognizable, that serve to characterize the various forms of the disease.

Types and Groups of Disease. There are two principal types of leprosy: the *lepromatous* (formerly called cutaneous) type, in which the patient manifests no resistance to the disease, and the *tuberculoid* (formerly called neural) type, in which he manifests more or less vigorous resistance to it. Most cases of leprosy fall into one or the other of these two categories. Transition does occasionally occur from one to the other (most often from tuberculoid to lepromatous), and a patient undergoing such transition may present features of both types. Nevertheless, no "mixed" form of leprosy, as such, is recognized. In Mexico and Costa Rica, a variation of the lepromatous form known as the Lucio type is encountered. In this form of the disease, the involvement is diffuse, no lepromas occur, and acid-fast bacilli may be observed in fairly large numbers in serum obtained from scraping the side of an incision in what appears to be normal skin. The Lucio form has been observed only rarely outside the North American continent.

In addition to these two relatively stable "polar" types of leprosy, two "groups" of leprosy cases are recognized, the *indeterminate* (I) and the *borderline or dimorphous* (B). The types, subtypes, groups, and subgroups, are outlined in Table 1, and the principal distinctions among these types and groups are given in Table 2.

Definition of these types and groups adopted by the Sixth International Congress of Leprosy in Madrid in 1953 were as follows:

Lepromatous type (L). A malign type, especially stable, strongly positive on bacteriologic examination, presenting more or less infiltrated skin lesions, and negative to lepromin. The peripheral nerve trunks become manifestly involved as the disease progresses, habitually in symmetrical fashion and often with neural sequelae in advanced stages.

Tuberculoid type (T). Usually benign, very stable; generally negative on bacteriologic examination; presenting in most cases erythematous skin lesions which are elevated marginally or more extensively; positive to lepromin. Sequelae of peripheral nerve trunk involvement may develop in some cases, and this may give rise to serious and disabling deformity. This frequently appears to occur as a result of extension from or through cutaneous nerve branches, rather than of systemic dissemination, and consequently it is often asymmetrical and unilateral.

The tuberculoid type was subdivided (Table 1) into *macular* (T_m), *minor tuberculoid* (T_t), and *major tuberculoid* (T_T) subtypes, characterized by flat, pale anesthetic macules; pebbled, erythematous, slightly raised plaques; and decidedly elevated and thickened erythematous plaques, respectively. The T_m variety is precisely that orig-

inally known as "maculoanesthetic." Wade believed that it should still be so designated, on the ground that patients with such flat lesions have not developed enough resistance to warrant being classified as tuberculoid.

Indeterminate group (I). A benign form, relatively unstable, seldom bacteriologically positive, presenting flat skin lesions which may be hypopigmented or erythematous; the reaction to lepromin negative or positive. Neuritic manifestations, more or less extensive, may develop in some cases which have persisted as of this group for long periods. The indeterminate group consists essentially of "simple macular" cases. These cases may evolve toward the lepromatous type or the tuberculoid type, or may remain unchanged indefinitely.

Borderline (dimorphous) group (B). A malign form, very unstable, almost always strongly positive on bacteriologic examination, with the lepromin reaction generally negative. This group may arise from the tuberculoid type as a result of repeated reactions, and sometimes evolves to the lepromatous type. The nasal mucosa is generally negative for acid-fast bacilli. The skin lesions are usually seen as plaques, bands, nodules, etc., with a regional distribution similar to that of lepromatous leprosy, except for [usually but not always] conspicuous asymmetry. The ear lobes are likely to present the appearance of lepromatous infiltrate. The lesions frequently have a soft or succulent appearance, and their periphery slopes away from the center and

TABLE 1. TYPES AND GROUPS OF LEPROSY, WITH SUBTYPES AND SYMBOLS, AS APPROVED BY THE SIXTH INTERNATIONAL CONGRESS OF LEPROSY AT MADRID IN 1953, AND REAFFIRMED AT TOKYO IN 1963

Types	Groups
Lepromatous (L)	*Indeterminate* (I)
Macular	Macular (I_m)
Diffuse	Pure neuritic (I_n)
Infiltrated	
Nodular	
Pure neuritic (?)*	
Tuberculoid (T)	*Borderline* (dimorphous) (B)
Macular (T_m)	Infiltrated
Minor tuberculoid (T_t)	Macular (?)*
Major tuberculoid (T_T)	Pure neuritic (?)*

*The bracketed question marks, inserted by the Classification Committee of the Congress, indicate that the queried categories have not yet been described in the literature.

TABLE 2. FUNDAMENTAL DISTINCTIONS AMONG THE TWO TYPES AND TWO GROUPS OF LEPROSY CASES

	Lepromatous Type	Borderline Group	Indeterminate Group	Tuberculoid Type
Clinical Features				
Character and prognosis	Stable, malign, and progressive	Unstable, either progressive or regressive	Unstable, often regressive; may progress to either "polar" type	Stable, benign, usually regressive
Skin lesions	Lepromas, papular or nodular*	Plaques, often annular	Pale or pink macules	Pale macules or raised plaques, often annular
Nerve damage	Slow and symmetrical	Generally more rapid than in lepromatous; symmetrical	Usually only slight and symmetrical	Sudden, severe, asymmetrical
Bacterioscopy	Abundant bacilli	Many bacilli	Few bacilli, if any	Usually no bacilli except during reactions, and in nerves
Histology	Xanthoma-like	Sarcoid-like but with some lipid-filled cells: "dimorphous"	Banal round-cell infiltration	Sarcoid-like
Lepromin reaction	Negative	Negative or weakly positive	Negative or weakly positive	Positive, often strongly so

*Except in Lucio's "pure diffuse" lepromatous leprosy, in which no lepromas occur. This form is rare outside of Mexico and Costa Rica.

does not present the clear-cut, well-defined margins seen in the tuberculoid type; the lesions are therefore liable to be mistaken for lepromas. The surface of the lesions is generally smooth, with a shiny appearance and a violaceous hue, sometimes (in light skins) with a brownish (sepia) background.

A detailed catalogue of the many contrasts between the two "polar" types of leprosy—lepromatous and tuberculoid—is given in Table 3.

Reactions. More or less transitory states of exacerbation or reactivation known as reactions may occur once or repeatedly in all forms of leprosy. In lepromatous leprosy, these are known as "lepra reactions," and two principal forms are recognized. The ordinary lepra reaction consists of aggravation of existing skin lesions, development of new ones, and usually fever, neuralgia, and malaise or prostration lasting for hours, days, or weeks. This may or may not be accompanied by erythema multiforme of either the ordinary or bullous variety. The lepra reaction may take the form of an atypical, sparse, generalized erythema-

nodosum-like reaction, *erythema nodosum leprosum,* which characteristically occurs when the proportion of dead to living *M. leprae* rises above a critical ratio.

In tuberculoid or borderline leprosy, reactions, consist of aggravation of previous lesions or the appearance of succulent, elevated new plaques; painful swellings of nerves may occur; *M. leprae* may become numerous in the lesions; and the lepromin reaction may decrease in intensity. Fever and constitutional symptoms (including erythema multiforme) do not occur in tuberculoid cases.

Diagnosis. An advanced case of leprosy with the combination of skin lesions and obvious nerve lesions should be readily recognized by the reasonably alert physician. It is in the early cases, in which the nerve involvement is not readily apparent, that the diagnosis of leprosy may be missed. In certain forms of the disease, the diagnosis can be definitely established by demonstration of the presence of *M. leprae* in material obtained from the

TABLE 3. DETAILED COMPARISON OF THE TWO "POLAR" TYPES OF LEPROSY

	Lepromatous	Tuberculoid
Clinical Features		
Sites of election	Skin (and nerves)	Nerves (and skin)
Distribution	Generalized usually	Localized often
Type of lesion	Leproma or nodule	Macule and plaque
Visceral involvement	Widespread subclinical	Perhaps lymph nodes
Mucous membrane lesions	Regularly and early	Nose only; infrequently
Eye involvement	Often; late	Very rarely
Hypopigmented macules	Occasionally; early; many	Frequently; few
Annular plaques	Sometimes	Frequently
Erythema multiforme or nodosum	In reactions often	Not seen
Fever	In reactions usually	Rarely
Eyebrow alopecia	Often	Not seen
Gynecomastia	Sometimes; late	Not seen
Symmetry of involvement	Usual	Exceptional
Nerve enlargement	Slow and symmetrical	Rapid and asymmetrical
Nerve damage	Late; often partial	Early, often complete
Skin anesthesia	Late but inevitable; often on extremities	Early and coextensive with skin lesions
Visceral damage	Testicle only	Not seen
Histologic Features		
General pattern	Xanthoma-like; macrophages and histiocytes	Sarcoid-like: epithelioid cell tubercles and lymphocytes
Vacuolated lepra cells	Always	Rarely; in reacting cases only
Giant cells	Occasional; foreign body or Touton type	Often; Langhans' type
Lymphocytes	Few	Abundant
Lipoid	Abundant	Minimal
Necrosis	Rarely	Caseation: rare in skin, common in nerves
Nerve changes	Fibrosis: structure well preserved	Obliteration of normal architecture
Visceral amyloidosis	Common; late	Not seen
Bacterioscopy		
Acid-fast bacilli (*M. leprae*)	Abundant except in long-treated or burned-out cases	Rare or lacking except during reactions; never abundant
Special Tests		
Lepromin (Mitsuda) reaction	Negative	Positive
Serologic tests for syphilis	Biologic false positive in half of cases	No false positives
Hyperglobulinemia	Usual	Exceptional
Erythrocyte sedimentation rate	Elevated, especially during reactions	Usually normal
Clinical Course		
Course, untreated	Progression; fatal in 10 to 20 years usually	Spontaneous recovery as a rule in 1 to 3 years
Course, treated with sulfones	Slow regression (3 to 8 years)	More rapid regression
Intercurrent tuberculosis	Common in untreated cases	Rare
Transition to other type	Rare even under treatment	Occurs in some severe and reacting cases
Contagiousness for others	Definitely established	Slight or nil
Disposition of case	Hospitalization if illness requires it	Hospitalization if illness requires it

patient's lesions. It is important to realize, however, that a clinical impression or suspicion of leprosy, as such, cannot be *excluded* by any one diagnostic procedure. A suspicion of *lepromatous* leprosy can be excluded by finding no acid-fast bacilli in the lesions, but such a negative finding will not exclude the indeterminate or tuberculoid variety. A suspicion of *tuberculoid* leprosy can be eliminated by excluding all evidence of nerve damage in the lesions, but such a finding will not exclude the indeterminate or lepromatous type.

Nasal scrapings, though they will show acid-fast bacilli in perhaps one third of early lepromatous cases and in all advanced ones, may be either positive or negative in either type of leprosy, and cannot be relied upon either to confirm or to exclude the diagnosis. Nonpathogenic acid-fast diphtheroid bacilli indistinguishable from *M. leprae* may be found even in a normal nose.

A simple and trustworthy method of looking for bacilli in skin lesions is Wade's "scraped incision" procedure. The point of a scalpel, or, better still, the corner of a safety razor blade, is inserted 3 or 4 mm. deep into a pinched-up fold of involved skin, or even uninvolved skin, e.g., an ear lobe. It is then rotated about an axis perpendicular to the skin surface so that its edge scrapes the side of the cut, and a small drop of tissue pulp and lymph is obtained. Blood does not interfere seriously. This drop is spread in a dime-sized area on a clean slide, dried, and stained by the Ziehl-Neelsen method, destaining with, preferably, Gabbett's solution. The carbolfuchsin should be used cold, not warm, for fifteen minutes. The preparation should not be subjected to decolorization too long because *M. leprae* is much less acid-fast than *M. tuberculosis*. A count of bacilli may be made in high-power fields per bacillus (or bacilli per high-power field) for comparison with future counts.

The standard Ziehl-Neelsen staining procedure is not sensitive enough to be used on paraffin sections of tissue if bacilli are at all scarce. Wade's modification of the Fite-Faraco stain (Amer. J. Path., 28:157, 1952) should be used to prevent defatting the bacilli.

In the absence of bacilli, a suspicion of leprosy needs confirmation by demonstration of nerve damage. Such damage may consist of anesthesia or anhidrosis (usually coextensive with a skin lesion in tuberculoid cases, often on feet or hands in lepromatous disease), thickening of superficial nerves, muscular weakness or atrophy, especially in the face and hands, or histologic changes in a biopsy specimen.

Leprous neuritis often produces sensory dissociation similar to that seen in syringomyelia: sense of touch may be preserved, but that of heat and cold, or pain, or both, may be lost. Each should be tested separately. Palpation of the great auricular nerves where they cross the sternocleidomastoid muscles, of the ulnar nerves just above and behind the internal humeral epicondyles, or of the peroneal nerves behind the heads of the fibulas may reveal thickening, nodularity, stiffness, or tenderness, any or all of which cause suspicion of leprous neuritis. Drooping of one or both

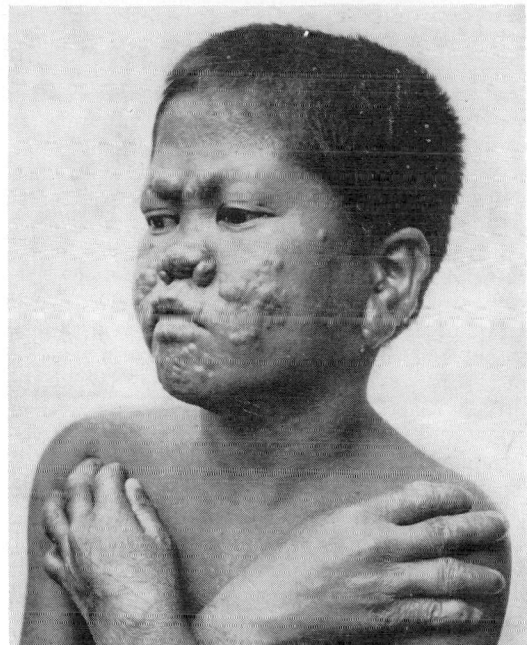

Lepromatous leprosy in a young boy. Note symmetrical involvement and predilection for cooler acral parts: brows, ears, nose, cheeks, chin, and fingers. Of interest also are madarosis (loss of eyebrows) and the burn scar on his anesthetic left hand. (From Arnold, H. L., Jr.. Modern Concepts of Leprosy Springfield, Illinois, Charles C Thomas, 1953.)

lower eyelids or oral commissures, or weakness of elevation of one eyebrow may disclose the patchy weakness of facial muscles, which Monrad-Krohn has said is the most distinctive single neurologic sign of leprosy. Contracture of a fifth finger, or flattening of a hypothenar or thenar eminence, or the grooving produced by atrophy of the interosseous muscles of the hands, may betray the presence of leprous ulnar or median neuritis. Actual "claw" hand deformity or foot drop may ultimately occur.

Biopsy of a thickened great auricular nerve or of other skin nerves that subserve no important motor function is a practicable procedure of value if a diagnostic biopsy of skin is not possible. The histologic changes are usually characteristic, and, in tuberculoid leprosy, bacilli are much more readily found in the nerves than in the skin.

Roentgenograms of hands and feet may show concentric absorption of phalangeal or metatarsal shafts, a characteristic "trophic" lesion that leads ultimately to loss of continuity of the bone and shortening of digits or of the whole foot. Rarely, diabetic peripheral neuritis may produce such changes, but without anesthesia. "Dropping off" of digits is a myth.

Painless trophic plantar ulceration, identical with that seen in tabes dorsalis and in syringomyelia, may also occur. Such ulcers are not primarily leprous, and no bacteriologic or histologic evidence of leprosy is to be found in them. They often lead to osteomyelitis of metatarsal bones.

Lepromin Test. The lepromin test is performed by the intradermal injection of 0.1 ml. of a boiled or autoclaved, gauze-filtered suspension of *M. leprae* and human tissue, prepared by grinding lepromatous granulation tissue in a mortar and suspending it in saline solution. Mitsuda reported in 1919 that such an injection was followed by no reaction in patients with lepromatous leprosy, but that in tuberculoid cases an inflammatory nodule resulted, reaching its height in about three weeks and sometimes ulcerating. Fernandez later described a 48-hour Mantoux-like reaction, fairly well correlated with the Mitsuda response. A positive lepromin reaction does *not* denote the presence of leprosy. It is positive in roughly half the population in many areas in which leprosy does not even occur. It apparently denotes resistance to leprosy. Its high correlation with a positive Mantoux reaction, especially in persons without leprosy, and the regularity with which BCG vaccine causes negative Mitsuda reactors to "convert" to positive suggest a relationship with exposure to tuberculosis that has not yet been explained or even fully evaluated. The use of BCG vaccine to protect susceptible contacts against leprosy is still undergoing extensive experimental testing, and its value is still moot.

Prognosis. Without treatment, patients with lepromatous leprosy tend to suffer steady progression of their disease and to die of tuberculosis, amyloid nephrosis, intercurrent infection, or leprosy. Patients with tuberculoid leprosy, untreated, tend to recover completely, except for residual nerve damage, within a year or two if only one or a few annular plaques are present. If their skin lesions are numerous and widespread, the disease may run a rather protracted course, with repeated relapses, but the patients still tend to recover completely if the lepromin reaction is strongly positive.

With chemotherapy, most patients experience immediate arrest of the disease and steady improvement. Recovery (except for residual nerve destruction) is usually complete in a year or two if bacilli were initially few or absent, or in three to perhaps six or eight years if bacilli were initially abundant and the lesions widespread. The problem of longer persistence of disease in some lepromatous cases remains unsolved.

Treatment. The sulfones are the major specific chemotherapy of leprosy. Diaminodiphenylsulfone (DDS, Avlosulfon, dapsone) has preempted the field. Many leprologists start with 25 mg. once a week and raise the dose to a 100 mg. daily maximum in weekly 25-mg. increments, although some start and continue with 50 or 100 mg. orally two days a week. The duration of treatment in tuberculoid cases is determined by the clinical response; as bacilli are usually lacking from the start, a clinically satisfactory result is likely to require a year or two. In lepromatous cases, treatment is continued until the skin lesions and nasal mucosa are healed and virtually devoid of acid-fast bacilli — usually at least two or three years in early cases, and perhaps as long as six or eight years in heavily involved cases. Maintenance therapy for prevention of relapse is necessary for many patients and advisable for most. Patients with a strongly positive reaction to lepro-

min, however, usually remain well indefinitely without maintenance therapy.

Reactions are mild and infrequent with small doses of sulfones. Moderate overdosage may cause headache, anorexia, nausea, dizziness, insomnia, or tachycardia. Anemia, which may occur at any dose level, is the most common potentially serious reaction, and should be watched for by hemoglobin determinations weekly and, later, monthly. Toxic psychosis, agranulocytosis, hematuria, or erythema nodosum may be seen with larger doses of any sulfone and require interruption of treatment or reduction of the dose.

In the event of complete intolerance for even small doses of sulfones, amithiozone is probably the best substitute. The dose is 25 mg. a day initially, increased slowly to a maximum of 100 to 150 mg. a day, by mouth. Dihydrostreptomycin, 1.0 gram intramuscularly three times a week, is much less effective, according to most observers, though controlled studies over short periods in the Philippines and South Africa under Doull's direction (1956) suggest that it is almost as good as the sulfones. (For discussion of dihydrostreptomycin toxicity, see Pulmonary Tuberculosis.) Isoniazid and para-aminosalicylic acid are not reliable in their effects upon the disease.

During lepra reactions, bed rest is indicated, and aspirin and antihistaminics may be helpful. The sulfone dosage may have to be reduced, but need not be if symptoms respond well to intramuscularly injected triamcinolone acetonide (Kenalog IM) suspension. Erythema multiforme, ordinary or bullous, or erythema nodosum may be controlled with steroids as a rule.

Keratitis, iritis, or iridocyclitis may occur in lepromatous cases and may require treatment with 1 per cent hydrocortisone drops or oral, or better, intramuscular triamcinolone. Atropinization is indicated for iridocyclitis. In advanced cases, eyelid paralysis may lead to exposure keratitis.

Although lepromatous neuritis is slowly progressive, tuberculoid leprous neuritis may cause rapid swelling of one or more nerve trunks, sometimes with such intense and persistent pain as to require surgical decortication of the nerve involved. Nerve abscesses, which occur rarely, may require incision and drainage.

Orthopedic procedures aimed at rehabilitation of patients with "claw" hand resulting from ulnar neuritis, or foot drop from peroneal palsy, differ in no essential respect from those devised for similar lesions due to other diseases.

Prevention. Prevention of leprosy is promoted best by protecting uninfected persons, especially children, from exposure to untreated, lepromatous patients. In nonendemic areas adults are probably as susceptible as children. Mouse footpad inoculation studies by Shepard (1960) and by Levy and Fasal (1968) suggest that infectivity of lepra bacilli is reduced to nearly zero after 60 to 90 days of sulfone therapy. A recent retrospective study of Hong Kong families by Worth (1968) showed that infection occurred in more than 10 per cent of children exposed to an untreated lepromatous parent, but none had been infected (up to seven years' observation) when exposure to such a parent had occurred after treatment had been started. Isolation is no longer regarded as playing a role of any importance—even in endemic areas—in the prevention of leprosy. The emphasis is all on early diagnosis and treatment. Hospitalization is desirable for initiation of treatment in most lepromatous cases, but it should be voluntary and usually need not exceed two or three months.

Cochrane, R. G., and Davey, T. F. (eds.): Leprosy in Theory and Practice. 2nd ed. Bristol, John Wright & Sons Ltd., 1964.

Spirochetal Diseases

TREPONEMAL DISEASES
Thorstein Guthe

SYPHILIS

Definition. Syphilis is a chronic infectious disease caused by *Treponema pallidum*. From the portal of entry—usually the genitals—there is lymphatic invasion and blood-borne spread (treponemia), and the infection is generalized from the beginning. Subsequently the disease becomes localized and dispersed. The early lesions are benign and the late manifestations destructive in character. Several organs of the body may be involved, but late treponemia and establishment of further lesions occur rarely in the acquired disease; this reflects the relative stability of the immunity that develops during the course of the disease. The host response includes specific humoral and cell-mediated immunity. Immune responses can be detected by serologic and other tests. Despite its slow evolution and remarkable immunologic features, syphilis will, if untreated, eventually incapacitate one of three and kill one of ten infected persons.

Treponema Pallidum. *T. pallidum*, discovered by Schaudinn and Hoffman in 1905, is a helical cell about 0.15 μ wide and 6 to 15 μ long. Around its central protoplasmic core is wound a bundle of three to four axial fibrils that provide the "muscle," giving *T. pallidum* a characteristic motility pattern. Treponemes undergo transverse fission. Multiplication time is 30 to 35 hours. *T. pallidum* has not been cultivated in vitro. It can remain viable for many hours on special media, or indefinitely if preserved at extremely low temperatures (carbon dioxide ice, liquid nitrogen).

Transmission. A few treponemes suffice to implant infection (Magnuson et al., 1956). Transmission is facilitated by moist conditions and congenial temperature, and occurs almost exclusively by direct contact with infectious lesions. Injured or inflamed areas will favor implantation.

Sexual transmission is the rule. Not infrequently genito-oral, genito-rectal or mouth-to-mouth transmission takes place. The chain of infection sometimes involves both heterosexual and homosexual practices. As many as 30 to 40 infected persons have been brought to treatment on the basis of a single index case. "Innocent" transmission by adults or children occasionally occurs. Contact between the infected host, the moist object, and the susceptible must be rapid to achieve indirect transmission. Inoculation into the skin or a vein has resulted from an accidental needle prick. An initial lesion does not arise in blood-borne transmission when it occurs in utero of pregnant syphilitic women (prenatal syphilis) or more rarely by blood transfusion from an infected blood donor (syphilis d'emblée). A macerated fetus and the mucocutaneous lesions of early prenatal syphilis are highly contagious. Infected individuals can pass asymptomatically through the early stages of syphilis for unknown reasons, as distinct from misinterpretation of early trivial symptoms or their being "masked" by treatment of other conditions, e.g., gonorrhea. Physiologic secretions (salivary, vaginal, seminal) may contain treponemes from contagious lesions. Direct intrauterine infection of the egg or the fetus from semen of a syphilitic male cannot arise.

Epidemiology. The health of the public is affected when syphilis spreads within and between countries. Propagation is facilitated by the properties of the agent, by its mode of transmission, and by behavioral, social, and several environmental factors. In recent years the climate of opinion concerning sexual behavior has become overtly permissive among the young. The pattern of promiscuity and of heterosexual and homosexual relations has altered. Industrialization, urbanization, migration, and unprecedented tourism have facilitated human contact and sexual encounters with concomitant risk of acquiring venereal disease. Paradoxically, medical advancements have contributed in the same direction. Thus fear of infection has been removed by easy and effective antimicrobial therapy and fear of pregnancy by oral contraceptives and intrauterine devices. Generally it has become clear that medical advancements have been to some extent outweighed by the complex ecologic forces in a rapidly changing environment. It has been recognized that new ways are

The author wishes to acknowledge the valuable advice, criticisms, and suggestions by his colleague Dr. O. Idsøe, Consultant on Treponematoses, World Health Organization, Geneva, concerning this article.

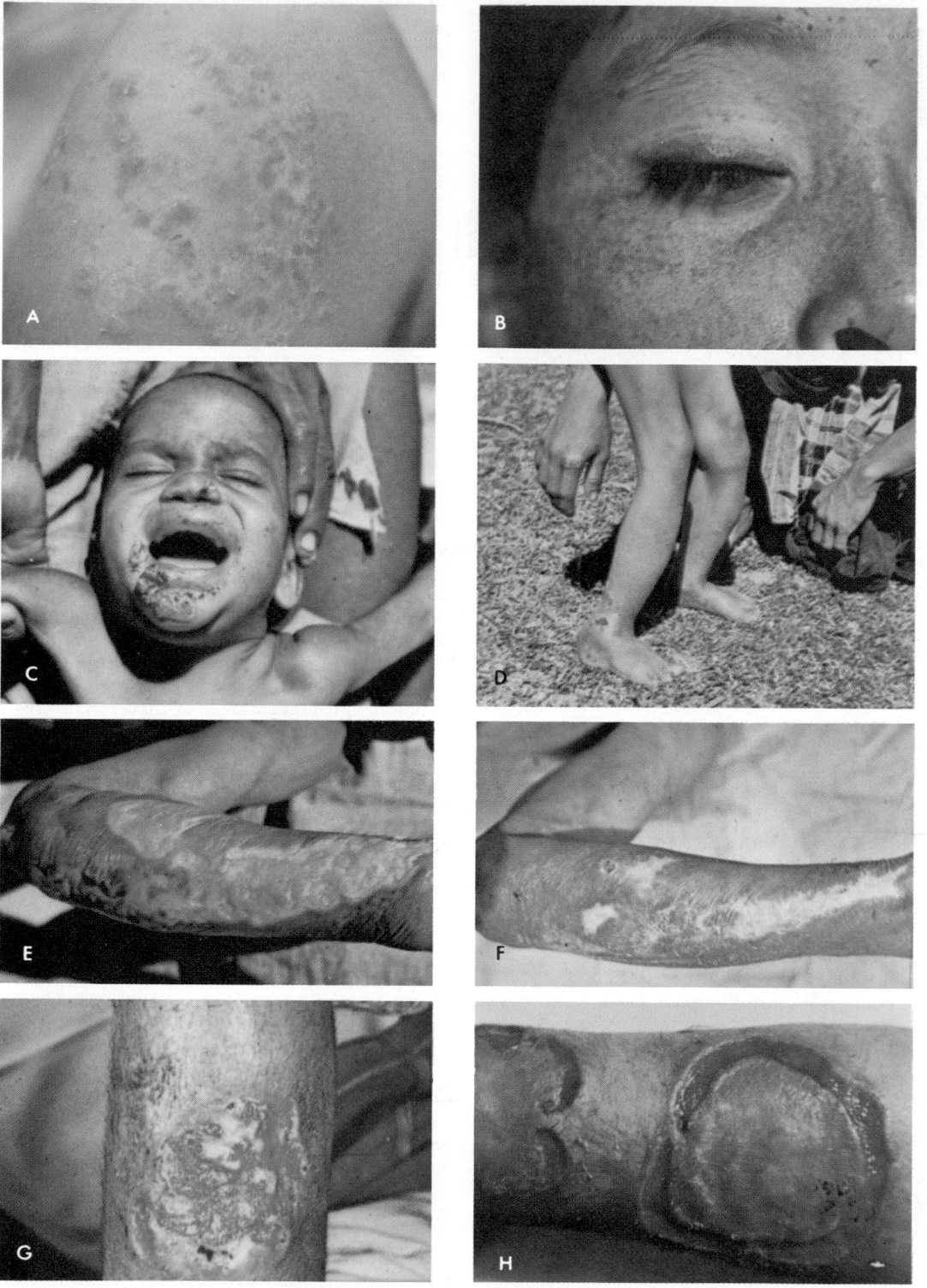

A, Inital lesions in early pinta. B, Late pigmented blue variety pinta. C, Early papillomatous yaws. D, Osteoperiostitis of yaws. E, Deep ulcerated late yaws of arm before therapy with long-acting penicillin. F, Same patient after treatment. G and H, Syphilitic tertiarisms.

needed to promote the mental and physical health of individuals and communities, e.g., health education, recreation, city planning.

The long-term trend of syphilis in the last 100 years has been downward. However, the epidemic outbreak of syphilis (and gonorrhea) during World War II was first followed by a rapidly declining incidence until 1958, since which time there has been a noticeable recrudescence of these conditions. Examples of reported incidence of *early syphilis* per 100,000 population are: United States, 3.8 in 1958 and 10.3 in 1968; Poland, 18.6 in 1958 and 53.8 in 1968; France, 3.3 in 1958 and 8.0 in 1968; greater Bombay, 177.7 in 1967. It has been shown (United States) that for each reported case of early infectious syphilis three additional cases are diagnosed and treated by private physicians but not reported to the health authorities. A decline in *late* cardiovascular and neurosyphilis and in *congenital syphilis* has been observed since the mid-1940's. This decline has occurred despite the experience that late syphilis can be expected to increase after periods of high incidence of early syphilis. *The prevention of the late forms of syphilis by the penicillin treatment of early syphilis is one of the great achievements of the chemotherapy era.*

Host-Treponeme Relationship. Man is the only natural host of *T. pallidum.* Hormonal and genetic factors may affect susceptibility to infection. The host-treponeme interaction is best portrayed by the rhythm and features of the development of lesions during the course of untreated syphilis.

Natural Course of Syphilis. Following implantation and local multiplication of *T. pallidum* and extension of the infection to lymph nodes, treponemes spread rapidly to all body tissues via venous blood, the pulmonary circulation, and the arterial system. Human syphilis therefore ceases rapidly to be a local disease (even incubating infection can cause blood-transfusion syphilis). The agent does not grow in the blood stream, but on passage through the small vessels, numerous metastatic foci are set up in the body, e.g., in the skin, mucous membranes, and nervous system. After the appearance of the initial lesion some three weeks following infection, multiplication continues for several weeks in these metastatic foci. Some eight to nine weeks after the original implantation the first generalized mucocutaneous outbreak occurs. The primary lesion heals spontaneously within a few weeks, and the secondary eruption within a few weeks or months. The treponemes in the metastatic foci of internal organs are presumably killed in most instances, but sometimes they become only temporarily inactivated (latent), giving rise to further manifestations. In the untreated disease further secondary episodes occur in 25 per cent of patients within the first four years, mostly within two years. With increasing duration of infection the hematogenous "showers" of treponemes generating these contagious episodes become less frequent and less rich in treponemes. The cutaneous lesions tend to group and localize, or may occur solitarily until the mucocutaneous system no longer responds to trepo-

nemes with pathologic changes. The further course of the untreated infection is illustrated by data from the University Clinic, Oslo, where by the turn of the century some 1100 patients with diagnosed early syphilis remained untreated under hospitalized conditions and were subjected to follow-up studies. In the last representative follow-up investigation 50 to 60 years after the original infection (Gjestland), late "benign" syphilis had occurred in 15 per cent, cardiovascular syphilis in 10 per cent, and neurosyphilis in 6.5 per cent of these patients. Ten per cent died as direct consequence of their disease. In about two thirds, latency continued indefinitely after subsidence of the secondary attacks. They went through life without major physical or mental consequences of their disease.

These features of the host-treponeme relationship in syphilis raise the question of the mechanisms concerned in the pathogenesis of lesions and their nature in both early and late disease, and point to the remarkable role of the defense forces of the host against the invading pathogen during the natural course of the infection.

Immunology. The immune response of the host directed against the pathogen is signaled by the modification of the natural course of syphilis as outlined above. The underlying waning treponemia, the decrease in demonstrable treponemes in late lesions, and the presence of presumed resistance to superinfection after the initial phase of the disease point in the same direction. Moreover, a varying degree of cross resistance to syphilis in persons infected with yaws and pinta suggests the broader role of immunity in treponematoses. Knowledge is, however, meager or absent concerning the effector mechanisms in the protective host responses and the role of humoral and cell-mediated immunity.

The humoral response involves formation of two main antibody types, reagin* and treponemal antibody.

Reagin develops early, four to five weeks after infection, and forms more rapidly than treponemal antibody described below. It declines when the disease moves toward latency, and may fall below detectable levels in late disease. It is affected considerably by therapy in the early phase of syphilis. A rising titer is a precursor of clinical outbreak, and reagin is therefore a useful gauge of disease activity, but of limited value as indicator of immunity. All evidence contradicts a protective role of reagin which is directed against cardiolipin present in the tissues of the antibody-producing host. Reagin is presumably an autoantibody formed in response to small amounts of cardiolipin "leaking" from host cells in the pathologic process (WHO, 1970). It is not known if reagin has a pathogenic significance.

---

*The term *reagin* is used throughout this article. It is widely accepted by physicians, clinicians, and epidemiologists to denote antibodies to cardiolipin-type antigens formed in syphilis and other treponematoses. Reagin is often referred to by immunologists and allergists to describe antibodies concerned in the immediate types of skin hypersensitivity and anaphylactic reactions.

Of the *treponemal antibodies* the immobilizin appears to be the more important. Fluorescent and agglutinating treponemal antibodies also appear. Immobilizin is operative in the treponemal antibody immobilization test (TPI). It appears late—two to three months after the infection. It is formed slowly but can persist for life as an indicator of infection. Immobilizin reflects roughly the development of host resistance, although the evidence is equivocal that it has a direct protective role.

As in most infections, the principal antibodies in syphilis belong either to immunoglobulins of the IgM class of high molecular weight or to those of the IgG class of lower molecular weight. The immunoglobulins are formed by different sets of antibody-producing cells, generally believed to be plasmocytes. In syphilis these are characteristically present in early lesions and in lymph nodes. Antibody demonstrated by reagin tests may belong to both IgM and IgG immunoglobulins. IgM is produced early in the infection. IgG exclusively forms the immobilizing antibody when it appears later in the infection. In immunofluorescent tests both IgM and IgG antibodies react with *T. pallidum*. Whether or not formation of antibody continues after treponemes have been eradicated by treatment—as well as the circumstances under which such eradication may take place—is not known (see Persistence of Treponemal Forms). IgG antibodies can pass the placenta, in contrast to IgM. The presence of IgM in the serum of newborns suggests local formation of antibodies and, therefore, prenatal active infection. IgG also passes the blood-brain barrier when the meninges are inflamed. This explains why serodiagnostic tests that mainly identify IgG antibody are preferred in examining the cerebrospinal fluid for syphilis of the nervous system.

Cell-mediated immunity manifests itself as delayed hypersensitivity demonstrable by the response to intradermally injected antigen after 12 to 48 hours. Interaction of antigen with specifically sensitized lymphocytes and cell structures is believed to be the underlying mechanism. Although knowledge is very limited, cell-mediated immunity apparently does not play a major role during the secondary eruptions of syphilis (Levene, 1969). However, delayed hypersensitivity is believed to be operative in gummatous lesions. Moreover, the striking clinical and histopathologic similarity of late destructive skin and bone lesions in venereal syphilis, bejel, and yaws suggests a common cell-mediated or other mechanism of the host response at this stage.

Immunopathologic mechanisms involving tissue damage are very little known in syphilis. Multiple humoral antibodies circulate in all phases of the disease, antigen is present, and antigen-antibody complexes may have pathogenic significance. Nevertheless a direct cytotoxic effect on host cells has not been established. Immunopathologic mechanisms have been suggested in a few and rare manifestations engendered by syphilitic infection, notably biphasic paroxysmatic cold hemaglobulinuria and membranous glomerulonephritis (syphilitic "nephrosis"). The occurrence of cryoglobulins in syphilis has also been reported.

In recent years there have been several important scientific developments in basic immunology concerning humoral and cellular immunity and immunopathology (WHO, 1964 and 1969), which may be expected to be applied also in syphilis and other treponematoses. *At present the clinical and laboratory findings can only illustrate the capacity of immunocompetent cell systems to react to antigenic stimuli in the early phase of syphilis, and to generate protection against further metastatic spread and superinfection with the pathogen. The human host can contain the infection at the time of latency by establishing a notable equilibrium between the pathogenic potential of treponemes and the immune forces, as evidenced by a relatively infrequent disturbance of this equilibirum resulting in occurrence of late injurious manifestations.*

Persistence of Treponemal Forms. Adequate penicillin therapy of early syphilis will usually heal lesions and prevent late manifestations in most instances. Symptomatic manifestations after penicillin therapy of latent syphilis are rare. When occurring, they signal survival of pathogenic treponemes notwithstanding the immune forces and therapy. When not occurring, e.g., late latency, the persistently positive serologic tests have sometimes in the past been considered to be due to persistent antibodies produced by "immunologic memory" rather than to treponemes persisting in the host. However, persistence of treponemal forms (treponeme-like structures) in host tissues has been observed in recent years. Thus in some instances of treated late syphilis treponemal forms were described in lymph nodes and cerebrospinal fluid (Collart et al., 1962, 1968), in aqueous humor of the eye (Smith and Israel), and in treated congenital syphilis, as well as in pathologic and nonpathologic ophthalmic situations apparently unrelated to syphilis. Rarely treponemal forms have also been found (lymph nodes) following treatment of early syphilis (Yobs et al.). The treponemal forms that have been demonstrated following treatment of early and late syphilis have only rarely been shown by animal infectivity tests to be viable (Turner). Others may be modified or "dormant" *T. pallidum,* acting as antigenic stimulus for continued treponemal antibody production, whereas others may be saprophytic organisms indigenous to the human host. In some instances these situations may coexist. Persistence of abated forms of micro-organisms in the face of normally effective drugs has already been studied in mycobacteria and corynebacteria, and is a phenomenon apart from true drug resistance (McDermott). There is no evidence that penicillinase-producing, resistant pathogenic treponeme strains have developed. Knowledge concerning immunologic tissue and humoral aspects of persistent treponemal forms is extremely limited, but regardless of the extent to which such forms are viable or modified pathogenic treponemes—or related indigenous organisms—their role may be significant in the immunologic life of the host. *For the physician it is important to realize that studies in this area are very few, that accepted treatment practices need not be reconsidered in early syphilis, and that in late syphilis special considerations continue to pertain.*

Pathology. The early treponemia and the resulting metastatic foci are reflected in the diversity of the body organs involved in the pathology of this chronic inflammation. The macroscopic characteristics of skin manifestations are described later. The histopathology of lesions is basically characterized by endarteritis and periarteritis of the small vessels and capillaries, which show infiltration of lymphocytes and plasmocytes and multiplication of histiocytes. Granulomatous inflammation is typical of the late stages of syphilis as of other chronic infections, e.g., tuberculosis.

In the *early skin lesions* in which many treponemes are present lymphocytosis and plasmacytosis are particularly marked, although varying in intensity. Acanthosis usually occurs. Many treponemes are present. *Lymph nodes* in the early disease show adenitis with prominent follicles, plasmacytosis, sometimes focal necrosis, fine fibrosis, and presence of treponemes. The histologic picture in lesions and lymph nodes is compatible with antibody production by stimulated cells (WHO, 1970). *Late nodular and gummatous lesions* (usually treponeme-free) show chronic granulomatous tissue with lymphocytes, epithelioid cells, and eventually giant cells in addition to the endovascular changes of early lesions. Coagulation necrosis occurs from obstruction endarteritis, possibly as a result of delayed hypersensitivity. In *cardiovascular syphilis* there is endarteritis of the vasa vasorum, particularly in the ascending aorta and arch. All layers of the large vessel are involved with destruction of elastic and muscle tissue, weakening the entire structure and predisposing to aneurysm. The aortic ring may also be weakened with shortening and thickening of valve leaflets leading to regurgitation. Coronary ostia may become narrowed, resulting in rare ischemic heart disease. *Central nervous system* syphilis is either meningovascular with inflammation of the pia-arachnoid and its vessels or parenchymatous with the nervous tissue attacked. The leptomeningitis may be acute or chronic. Infiltration of small meningeal vessels may cause thrombosis and local brain damage. The parenchymatous process may engender paresis if the brain is predominantly involved, or tabes dorsalis if the spinal cord is predominantly involved. Tabes begins as extradural leptomeningitis around the dorsal nerve roots, followed by degeneration of axis cylinders and demyelinization of posterior columns of the spinal cord. Optic atrophy may occur from basal meningitis or interstitial neuritis in the nerve or chiasma, or central gummatous lesions may affect the optic nerve directly. Involvement of afferent vessels to the spinal cord may lead to degeneration of pyramidal tracts and a rare condition known as Erb's spastic paraplegia.

Ophthalmic lesions include uveitis with serofibrinous exudate and synechiae in acquired syphilis, and interstitial keratitis with substantial lymphocytic infiltration in congenital syphilis. Rare membranous *glomerulonephritis* ("nephrosis") in early syphilis shows peculiar vascular or granulomatous tissue changes. Other forms of visceral syphilis, e.g., interstitial nephritis, may occur. In *prenatal syphilis* the placenta is often voluminous, thickened, and pale with enlarged cotyledons and perivascular fibrosis throughout the villi, such as can also be seen in erythroblastosis (Rh-negative mother). Fibrous proliferation and monocellular infiltrates characterize fetal tissues in congenital syphilis; but in addition to the placenta changes, the most characteristic findings are in the lungs (pneumonia alba) and the bones (osteochondritis and periostitis), the latter changes being diagnosable roentgenologically.

Notwithstanding the diversity of the organs affected and the multiformity of the lesions underlying the clinical picture, the elementary pathologic changes in all syphilitic processes are of vascular and inflammatory nature.

Clinical Manifestations and Diagnosis. Untreated acquired syphilis shows a great variety of clinical manifestations, depending *inter alia* on the duration of the infection and the immunologic state of the host. The accepted classification of syphilis into *early syphilis* of less than four years' duration, and *late syphilis* of more than four years' duration is based on these immunologic grounds, as well as on clinical and epidemiologic considerations rather than on definite "stages" of disease that may sometimes merge or overlap. In congenital syphilis, in which there is prenatal hematogenous transmission of *T. pallidum* to the fetus from the syphilitic mother, the disease is usually divided into *early congenital syphilis* in children less than two years old and *late congenital syphilis* in those who are older.

Early Syphilis. The incubation period, initial lesions, secondary manifestations, and early latent period are comprised by this designation.

The Initial Lesion (Primary Chancre). Following an incubation of two to six weeks after the original infection, the initial lesion appears at the site of implantation of *T. pallidum:* in males usually on the penile shaft, coronal sulcus, glans, or prepuce, and occasionally intraurethrally; and in females on the external genitalia and cervix. In 5 to 10 per cent of patients the initial lesions are extragenital (lips, tonsils, fingers, within the anus, but also anywhere else). The initial lesion is usually a painless lenticular papule, rapidly eroding and becoming a flat indurated infiltrate, usually with elastic consistency, 3 to 20 mm. in diameter, and of round or oval shape. However, lesions are frequently "atypical," modified by size, location, and the nature of underlying tissue, if not by treatment. Solitary chancres are usual. Multiple chancres may appear after manifold simultaneous implantation of *T. pallidum,* especially in women. Regardless of site, initial lesions are accompanied by moderate enlargement of regional lymph nodes, usually recognizable clinically within a week of their appearance. The nodes are firm, freely movable, and painless. The initial lesion heals slowly (two to six weeks), and may or may not leave an atrophic scar. Lymphadenopathy may last for several months. With approaching secondary manifestations metastatic lesions of skin and mucous membrane sometimes go unrecognized while the primary sore is still present. On the other hand, the initial lesion is occasionally absent from the beginning, the secondary lesions nevertheless developing in due course (syphilis d'emblée).

In diagnosis of a suspected solitary genital or other lesion, careful general clinical examination of the patient should be undertaken in addition to mandatory dark-field examination for *T. pallidum* in material from the sore and the repeated performance of serologic tests, e.g., VDRL. These may be reactive as early as four weeks after the infection and one week after the appearance of the lesion. If treponemes are not found but seroreactivity has been established, the diagnosis is made in conjunction with clinical and anamnestic data. The most common lesions to suggest, erroneously, syphilitic sores are *chancroid* (which may coexist with chancre) and *granuloma inguinale. Balanoposthitis, erosion and carcinoma of the cervix uteri, and lymphogranuloma venereum* should also be considered. Other conditions include *traumatic sore, herpes progenitalis, condylomata acuminata, lichen planus, scabies, fissura in ano,* and *Vincent's angina.* Differential diagnostic considerations may vary from one country to another, according to the prevalence of the various conditions.

From its earliest phases the incubation period of syphilis is one of considerable biologic activity. When the patient with an initial lesion is first seen by the physician, generalized infection has already occurred as a result of the early treponemia, although generalized symptoms may not as yet have appeared. Unless initial lesions give rise to suspicion of disease, the patient may not seek medical care during the early period of infectiousness. Local clinical genital lesions should therefore always be considered suspect of syphilis until proved otherwise.

Secondary Manifestations and Early Latency. About the sixth week of the infection there is generalized lymphadenitis with palpable superficial lymph nodes. Lymph nodes, otherwise seldom swollen, are involved, e.g., the pre- and postauricular, occipital, and supratrochlear lymph nodes. All nodes are firm, freely movable, and painless. *Cutaneous rashes,* notably the macular rash, appear six to eight weeks after the initial lesion, the vestiges of which remain in some patients. The macules are pale red, roundish patches 5 to 10 mm. in diameter, neither infiltrated nor scaling, and do not itch. They are usually bilateral, and are distributed to the trunk and proximal parts of extremities. On black skin, macules appear as darker patches. Macular rashes last one

to two months. *Papular lesions* often develop before disappearance of macules. The papules are coppery-red, round infiltrates 3 to 10 mm. in diameter, sometimes leaving pigmented patches on healing, e.g., "necklace of Venus." The papules are distributed anywhere, and include scalp, soles, and palms. The latter show up as flat, slightly scaly lesions or as a characteristic bluish-red rash covered by normal keratin. The papular rash may last two to four weeks.

In its further development and notably during relapses many varieties of papules may appear in syphilis. Large hypertrophic papules ("condylomata lata") are localized to skin folds, e.g., genitals, anus, axillae, under pendulous breasts, and elsewhere, and are often humid and eroded. Split papules at the oral angles resemble perlèche. On black skin circinate and arciform papules are common around the mouth and on the chin. Seborrheic, psoriasiform, and acneiform papules may occur. Varioliform papules are sometimes encountered in the tropics. They may give impression of smallpox, but the base of the latter is less infiltrated beneath the pustule which shows umbilical depression and later also characteristic crusts. Follicular and corymbiform grouped papules are late manifestations in secondary syphilis. Patchy loss of hair occurs three to eight months after infection and gives a motheaten appearance. It is evident from the above that polymorphism characterizes the early and particularly the subsequent relapsing lesions in secondary syphilis, even in the same person. *Mucous membranes,* notably in the mouth, vulva, and anus, may be involved separately or conjointly with skin manifestations. Erosive superficial mucosal patches are often covered by a thin gray membrane with a red halo. Ulceromembranous tonsillitis and pharyngitis may cause moderate symptoms (hoarseness). Mucous membrane lesions are very contagious. At least 20 per cent of patients with early syphilis will have transient *subacute meningitis* ("meningeal rash"), causing headache and increase of cells and protein in the cerebrospinal fluid. *Ophthalmic conditions* may occur, notably iritis with demonstrable synechiae, but seldom before six months after the infection. *Interstitial nephritis* may give minor or no symptoms. *Periostitis,* particularly of the long bones, is common and shows up as swelling, tenderness, and ostealgia (nocturnal pains).

Relapsing Syphilis. Condylomata lata are likely to recur. The skin manifestations tend to be unilateral, the eruptions more dense, marked, with fewer lesions, and sometimes solitary. They are also more infiltrated and of somewhat longer standing, and have some characteristics that resemble the skin lesions in late syphilis. This reflects the increasing immunity with the duration of the early disease. Neurorecurrences, as well as ophthalmic and other relapsing manifestations, may occur. If the patient has been inadequately treated, relapses may be delayed.

Diagnosis of Secondary Syphilis. The diagnosis of secondary syphilis is made on the basis of lymphadenopathy, mucocutaneous lesions, demonstration of *T. pallidum* by dark-field examination of lesion fluid or lymph node aspirate, and seroreactivity in reagin tests. The history may or may not be helpful. In the presence of mucocutaneous manifestations, the necessary serologic tests are usually obtained by the physician. Errors arise from a syphilitic lesion that is misinterpreted as representing some localized body lesion of nonmicrobial origin, e.g., an anal fissure, or from solitary lesions that may be considered "trivial." Close search for clinical manifestations other than the presenting symptom may well reveal lesions on other parts of the skin or simultaneously occurring mucosal eruption, e.g., oral or genital mucous patches, loss of hair, palmar or volar lesions, pointing to the serious systemic nature of the condition.

The most common eruptions that should be considered in differential diagnoses of early generalized secondary syphilitic rashes are *acute microbial disease, exanthemata,* and *drug eruptions.* In the later phase of secondary syphilis when lesions become more localized, the following conditions are of differential diagnostic importance: *pityriasis rosea, perlèche, psoriasis,* and *superficial fungus infections.* Also *lichen planus* and sometimes certain forms of *tuberculids, scabies, venereal warts,* and *Reiter's disease* may come into purview. *Aphthous stomatitis* and *Stevens-Johnson* syndrome are among oral cavity manifestations to be considered.

As a whole it is noted that manifestations of secondary syphilis have a very wide range; they involve the skin and other body systems, often extensively, but sometimes in a more limited way and discreetly, with corresponding variation of clinical symptomatology in patients who are usually not feeling subjectively ill. *Hardly in any other disease is it of such importance as in suspected syphilis to make a careful and complete examination of the entire skin, mucous membranes, and body systems. Laboratory examination should always be undertaken in suspected cases.*

Early Asymptomatic (Latent) Syphilis. This designation serves to identify seroreactive persons who have no signs and nonreactive cerebrospinal fluid within the first four years of infection. *In view of the tendency of early syphilis to contagious secondary relapses and the potential seriousness of neurosyphilis, which sometimes may develop after two years' duration of the infection, patients in whom a diagnosis of early latent syphilis is established should be treated and kept under surveillance by the physician in the same way as is done for symptomatic secondary syphilis.*

Late Syphilis. In the natural course of syphilis, further infectious mucocutaneous relapses seldom occur after the second, and hardly ever after the fourth year. Refractory immunity has then been established, and persists for life in two thirds of patients who remain asymptomatic. In the remainder, slow chronic destructive inflammation and fibrosis continue in various affected tissues, giving rise to late manifestations.

Late Asymptomatic (Latent) Syphilis. Latent syphilis has reactive serologic tests as its sole evidence. The cerebrospinal fluid is nonreactive, and there is absence of all manifestations at the time of diagnosis four years or more after the original infection. The history, antecedent treatment, and previous serologic tests are important in establishing the diagnosis. Confirmatory treponemal antibody tests (FTA/TPI) are essential to exclude biologically "false" seroreactivity. In addition to careful clinical examination of skin, mucous membranes, and eyes, examination of the cerebrospinal fluid and roentgenologic studies of the heart and aorta are mandatory.

Late Symptomatic Syphilis. Late symptomatic syphilis may cause inapparent to severe damage of body systems. *Late "benign" syphilis* may show mainly nodular or squamous skin lesions of destructive character, containing few or no treponemes, with tendency to peripheral extension, central healing, and scar formation, a pattern usually not encountered in other skin lesions except lupus vulgaris. Certain forms of *skin tuberculosis, deep mycosis,* and occasionally *cancer* are the main differential diagnostic problems. Serologic examination is obviously important. The typical lesion of late syphilis is the *gumma,* which can involve the skin, mucous membranes, skeletal system, and viscera. Nodular ulcerative lesions spread peripherally, the subcutaneous gumma infiltrating and later perforating the skin, creating a roundish ulcer with cutout, not undermined borders in contrast to tuberculous ulcerations. The hard and soft palate can be perforated. In rare instances the total anterior or central part of the palate and nose may be mutilated by gummatous and other involvement of skin and bones, a condition known as rhinopharyngitis mutilans ("gangosa"), which is also encountered in late yaws and bejel. *Skeletal lesions* involve mostly periosteum, more rarely cortex and medulla, and are of a diffuse or localized gummatous nature, particularly affecting the long bones, e.g., tibia, clavicle. Pain, swelling, and roentgenologic findings are diagnostic characteristics. Syphilitic joint lesions are less frequent. Charcot's joints, frequently associated with tabes dorsalis, are considered as a neuroarthropathy. *Nervous system syphilis* includes affliction of cranial nerves from basal syphilitic meningitis, giving symptoms according to the nerve involved, e.g., eighth-nerve deafness, diplopia. Damage to the central nervous system can otherwise give rise to a very wide range of neurologic and other signs and symptoms which characterize meningo-vascular and parenchymatous neurosyphilis, e.g., general paresis, tabes dorsalis. The latter is frequently associated with primary optic atrophy. *Cardiovascular syphilis* manifests itself primarily as aortitis of the ascending aorta and may lead to aortic insufficiency and aneurysm. Roentgenography is as essential as cerebrospinal fluid examination for the diagnosis of late syphilis. (See Syphilis of the Aorta and Syphilitic Infection of the Central Nervous System elsewhere in the text.)

A relatively frequent coexistence of cardiovascular syphilis with neurosyphilis (10 to 15 per cent), neurosyphilis with "benign" late syphilis (13 per cent), and the latter with cardiovascular syphilis (10 per cent) should be kept in mind by the physician. Almost all fatalities in syphilis result from neurosyphilis or syphilis of the heart or aorta. These most serious forms of the disease are discussed elsewhere in this text and in a monograph on venereology (Willcox).

Maternal and Prenatal ("Congenital") Syphilis.
The manifestations of maternal syphilis depend on the stage of disease; diagnosis is established on usual anamnestic, clinical, and serologic criteria. Serologic screening may detect pregnant women with no past history of disease. These should be investigated and treated as early latent syphilis. During the first years of infection most pregnancies will terminate in fetal death if the mother is left without treatment. Later in the course of the infection the risk decreases, and untreated syphilitic women may give birth to healthy children. Presumably this is related to the lessening likelihood of the occurrence of treponemia with time. Nevertheless, occasionally an untreated syphilitic woman may deliver a congenitally syphilitic child many years after infection.

Early Prenatal Syphilis. Early congenital syphilis is prenatally acquired infection diagnosed in children less than two years old. The fetus is infected after the fourth month of pregnancy. The lesions on delivery depend on the time of infection, and may vary from marasmic to apparently healthy infants. Fibrotic visceral lesions are characteristic. Osteochondritis is diagnosed by roentgenographic examination. The child may be born with "snuffles" from affliction of the nasopharynx with mucous and sometimes hemorrhagic discharge. The cutaneous rash after birth can be impressive papular and bullous eruptions in the palms and soles (exceptional in acquired syphilis), and tend characteristically to affect facial, circumoral, anogenital, and diaper areas, and palms and soles. Such lesions are highly contagious, and T. pallidum can easily be demonstrated. Infants without signs of disease, who are suspected of being infected by a seroreactive mother, should be clinically and serologically kept under surveillance for at least six months to establish active infection or passive reaginemia.

Late Prenatal Syphilis. Late congenital syphilis is a prenatally acquired infection that has persisted and developed in children over two years of age. On discovery the condition is often latent and should be confirmed by FTA/TPI tests. Residual manifestations of early lesions may be present, notably rhagades radiating from the prolabium and frontal bosses and saber tibia from periostitis of the shaft. There may be osseous destruction (saddle nose) and dental deformities, with wedge-shaped, widely spaced, often notched permanent upper central incisors (Hutchinson's teeth). Other "signs" include eighth nerve deafness and syphilitic synovitis in both knee joints

(Clutton's joints). The most common affliction is interstitial keratitis, usually appearing in late childhood and eventually becoming bilateral. There is photophobia, ground glass appearance of the cornea, and vascularization of adjacent sclera. Other late manifestations resemble those of acquired late adult syphilis of similar duration. Meningovascular syphilis, paresis, and tabes occur, but cardiovascular syphilis is rare.

The profound pathologic processes of prenatal syphilis and the personal and social limitations that they impose are preventable through routine serologic testing of all pregnant women and adequate treatment of those found infected.

Interpretation of Laboratory Findings.
In addition to clinical and anamnestic examination, the diagnosis of syphilis depends on laboratory findings. In early syphilis dark-field examination of lesions and serologic tests are indispensable; in late syphilis in addition to serologic tests examination of the cerebrospinal fluid is the most important laboratory procedure.

Dark-Field Examination. T. pallidum cannot be readily identified in dried, fixed fluid or tissue specimens by silver, chromatic, or fluorescent staining. Its presence can best be ascertained in the living state by microscopic dark-field examination which can be done by the trained physician. Material for examination includes tissue fluid from initial and secondary lesions after saline washing and gentle squeezing or an aspirate from an enlarged lymph node. Preferably, specimens should be examined on the spot. They can, however, be collected in a capillary tube, sealed with wax, and mailed to a competent laboratory. Care must be taken in interpreting the findings. T. pallidum may resemble spirochetes normally inhabiting genitalia and the oral cavity. The regular corkscrew-like coils, the slow, rotating, forward-backward motions, and graceful sideways bendings help in identification of T. pallidum. Repeated failures to demonstrate T. pallidum with adequate technique in a suspected lesion may mean that the lesion is healing, that the patient has received topical or systemic treatment, or that the lesion is nonsyphilitic. Before the lesion is diagnosed as nonsyphilitic, an examination of lymph node aspirate should be made.

Serologic Tests. Serologic tests are indispensable for individual diagnosis of syphilis, for following the effect of therapy, for routine screening of pregnant women, blood donors and other, "risk groups," and for case and contact finding in community, national, and international health programs. It is essential for the physician to utilize laboratories that employ standard reagents and methods and that partake in a proficiency testing program of sensitivity, specificity, and reproducibility in co-operation with a regional or national reference center. Serologic tests detect antibodies formed during the course of the syphilitic infection.

Reagin tests use cardiolipin antigen according to different methods. These may vary from one country to another, but are either based on complement fixation or flocculation techniques, e.g., VDRL.*

The pattern of antibody production has been outlined under "Immunology," indicating that treponemal antibody, notably the immobilizin, is specific and reflects roughly the immunity status of the patient, whereas reagin is rather an indicator of disease activity. *The use of quantitative reagin methods† is essential to permit the physician to assess the effect of treatment and compare antibody titers of periodically examined serum specimens in the post-treatment surveillance of the patient.*

Three types of *treponemal antibody tests* are in use: (1) The treponema immobilization test (TPI) uses live *T. pallidum* as antigen, immobilized by antibody in the presence of complement. It is the only test in which the biologic action of serum antibody can be determined directly under the microscope. (2) The fluorescent treponemal antibody test (FTA) uses killed treponemes as antigen. Syphilitic serum is bound to the surface of treponemes fixed onto a slide, and the antibody is made visible by use of fluorescein-tagged antiserum against human globulin. Nonspecific antibodies are removed either by dilution of serum (FTA$_{200}$ test) or "absorbed" (FTA/ABS test). (3) The passive treponemal hemagglutination test (TPHA) uses disrupted *T. pallidum* as antigen, coated onto tannin-treated sheep erythrocytes which are agglutinated in the presence of specific antibody.

"False" reaginemia occurs in certain pathologic conditions not caused by syphilis. Transient low-titer seroreactivity may, for example, arise from acute bacterial and viral infections, or following vaccinations, e.g., for smallpox. "False" seroreactivity occurs also from disease of connective tissue, e.g., disseminated lupus erythematosus, leprosy, and malaria; from the continued use of heroin; or from conditions affecting serum globulins, e.g., malnutrition. Moreover, both reagin and treponemal serologic tests for syphilis are also reactive by definition in other treponematoses (yaws, pinta, and bejel). *It should be realized, however, that syphilis remains the most common cause of reagin seroreactivity and that in screening examinations only one of ten VDRL seroreactive persons may be a problem case requiring confirmation with a specific treponemal test.* If TPI or FTA tests, or both, are needed and such tests are not undertaken by a local recognized laboratory, serum specimens can be mailed for examination to a laboratory of repute. If there is doubt about the interpretation of serologic tests, consultation should be arranged with a syphilologist.

Reagin tests may generally confirm a diagnosis of syphilis when a suspected initial lesion is present, although they are usually subordinate to dark-field findings of T. pallidum in the early stage. Reagin tests are reactive in all instances of secondary syphilis; they are important in the diagnosis of congenital syphilis, offer a clue in latent syphilis, and have supplementary value in late syphilis. Treponemal antibody tests are essential for diagnosis in patients with repeated low or fluctuating reagin titers, in patients without anamnestic and/ or clinical evidence, and in acquired and congenital disease, as well as in suspected late manifestations.

Cerebrospinal Fluid Examination. Lumbar puncture* can be undertaken at the physician's office or at a clinic. Examination of the cerebrospinal fluid serves to establish a diagnosis of latent syphilis by exclusion of asymptomatic neurosyphilis, aids in following the effect of therapy once such diagnosis has been made, and generally assures surveillance of patients in different phases of the disease. Syphilitic meningitis increases the permeability of the blood-brain barrier, causing increase of lymphocytes, proteins, and in some instances antibody. The first sign of asymptomatic neurosyphilis or meningitis arising from latency is pleocytosis of more than four cells per cubic milliliter, closely followed by an increase in protein to 40 mg. or more (depending on laboratory method) and reactive antibody tests. When progressing to parenchymatous neurosyphilis, 150 cells or more, marked protein increase (globulin) and strongly reactive antibody tests are encountered. Complement-fixation tests for reagin (Kolmer) and treponemal antibody tests (TPI/ FTA) are most suitable in cerebrospinal fluid examinations. When reactive they are pathognomonic of neurosyphilis; flocculation tests are sometimes nonreactive when antibody is present. Successful treatment leads to rapid regression of the cell count. Normalization of protein requires more time. Reversal of serologic tests may take several years.

Therapy. Mahoney and co-workers (1943) introduced penicillin therapy in syphilis, and this drug has replaced previous metal therapy in most countries of the world. Benzyl penicillin G preparations are more effective antitreponemal agents than the newer penicillins, e.g., ampicillin, methicillin. Injection therapy is preferred, and oral therapy is not recommended. Uninterrupted treponemicidal blood-tissue levels are more effective than intermittent penicillinemia, which may be sublethal to *T. pallidum* and allow growth of surviving treponemes, the multiplication time of which is 30 to 35 hours. Long-action procaine penicillin G in oil with aluminium monostearate (PAM) and benzathine penicillin G (DBED) and therefore preferred to short-acting aqueous preparations. The latter require frequent injections, higher

---

*Among the reagin tests, flocculation reactions, e.g., VDRL, Kline, Eagle, and complement fixation reaction, e.g., Kolmer, are used. In the present article the Venereal Disease Research Laboratory (VDRL) test is referred to as the prototype of reagin tests. It is subjected to national proficiency testing within and between laboratories in several countries and is based on the use of antigens referable to International Standard Preparations for the components used.

†In quantitative serologic tests a series of a progressively higher dilution of serum is made and each dilution is tested separately. The highest dilution that is reactive represents the titer.

*In some countries suboccipital puncture is preferred.

dosages, and more involved patient management, and have a lesser safety margin than long-acting preparations. As a whole, therapy is based on internationally known dose-time relationships. The characteristics of the penicillin preparation used is more important than number, frequency, and total dosages of treatment schedules of undefined preparations. The accompanying table shows the generally accepted treatment schedules.

Early Syphilis. Usually *T. pallidum* disappears from initial lesions within 24 hours, somewhat more slowly from secondary lesions. There is rapid involution of the lesion following adequate penicillin therapy, and the long-term outcome is highly satisfactory (Guthe and Idsøe). A co-operative international study of 688 serononreactive and 494 seroreactive patients with primary syphilis, adequately treated and followed up to 11 years, showed no clinical relapses. Among 499 adequately treated patients with secondary syphilis, also followed up to 11 years, less than 5 per cent were re-treated for clinical relapse, seroresistance, and—in most cases—reinfection. In 2485 patients with nonspecified "early syphilis" followed up to 12 years, re-treatment in different subseries of patients varied from 1 to 9 per cent with an average of 1.5 per cent re-treated for serorelapse, seroresistance, and clinical relapse, the remainder being reinfections (WHO, 1970). The few true failures may be due to abnormal penicillin metabolism, renal leakage, or other circumstances, as these patients usually react well to intensified re-treatment. *For the physician it is therefore unnecessary to subject all patients with early syphilis to the intensive treatment re-quired by the few patients who experience sero-resistance or relapses after currently accepted therapy schedules. But the need for proper post-treatment observation and surveillance of the patient is obvious. For community health reasons it is essential that a large "epidemiologic dose" of penicillin be administered immediately on diagnosis of infectious syphilis (see table), rendering the patient rapidly noninfectious and providing protection against spread of infection should the patient default from further treatment.*

After adequate penicillin treatment of *early syphilis*, the VDRL titers begin to descend, usually after two months, and a subsequent rapid fall is to be expected in most cases. As a whole, the time to reach seronegativity depends on the duration of infection when treatment was started, although in the majority of cases it is achieved within six months. At the ninth month 5 to 10 per cent may still be seroreactive at a low titer.

A few patients will retain seroreactivity at the end of the second year, mostly those treated in the late secondary and early latent phases. Fluctuations of titers during post-treatment surveillance examinations may occur. Only a persistent rise from nonreactivity or a fourfold titer increase from previous titer level should be considered as *serologic relapse*. Failures occur within one to two years, most of these within three to nine months. Serologic relapse usually precedes or accompanies infectious clinical relapse in which the mucocutaneous lesions are often localized. Cerebrospinal fluid examination is then essential, and retreatment should be provided at once. Occasionally, titers fail to decrease the first six to nine months

TABLE 1. PENICILLIN TREATMENT PRACTICES IN SYPHILIS

Indications for Syphilis Therapy†	Dosage and Administration*		
	N,N-Dibenzylethylenediamine Dipenicillin G (DBED) or Benzathine Penicillin G	Procaine Penicillin G in Aluminium Stereate Suspension (PAM)	Aqueous Benzyl Penicillin G or Procaine Penicillin G
Primary, secondary, and early latent syphilis with nonreactive cerebrospinal fluid and adequate opportunity for follow-up; epidemiological treatment	Total of 2.5 megaunits; single dose of two injections of 1.2 megaunits in one session	Total of 4.8–6.0 megaunits; first dose of 2.4 megaunits, and 1.2 megaunits at each of two subsequent injection 3 days apart, over 9 days	Total of 6.0 megaunits in dose 600,000 u. daily for 10 consecutive days
Late latent or when cerebrospinal fluid not examined in "latency": asymptomatic neurosyphilis, symptomatic neurosyphilis, cardiovascular syphilis, late benign (cutaneous, osseous, visceral gumma)	Total of 6 to 9 megaunits in doses of 3 megaunits at 7-day intervals, over 14–21 days	Total of 6 to 9 megaunits given in doses of 1.2 megaunits at 3-day intervals, over 15–21 days	Total of 9 megaunits in doses of 600,000 u. daily, over 15 days
Congenital Early Up to 2 years of age	Total of 50,000 u. per kg. in a single or divided dose at one session	Total of 100,000 u. per kg. given in three divided doses at 2- to 3-day intervals	Total of 100,000 u. per kg. as 10,000 u. per kg. per day for 10 consecutive days‡
Late 2 to 12 years, weight 32 kg. (71 lb.) or less	Same as early congenital syphilis	Same as early congenital syphilis	Same as early congenital syphilis
Over 12 years, or over 32 kg.	Same as adult latent syphilis	Same as adult latent syphilis	Same as adult latent syphilis

*Individual doses can be divided for injection in each buttock to minimize discomfort.
†In *pregnancy*, treatment is dependent on the stage of syphilis.
‡Preferable in very small children.

after therapy. Re-treatment is also then indicated. Re-treatment should be intensive, usually effected by doubling the previous dosage scheme. The few patients who retain a residual low reagin titer after the second year and who after CSF examination have no evidence of syphilis may safely be followed without further treatment. Both these as well as the reagin nonreactive patients can be considered as "cured" of syphilis when the surveillance scheme has been completed. Whether or not the last treponeme has been eliminated—or will eventually be eliminated by the immunity forces—is another matter. *Long-term practical experience shows no convincing evidence that late clinical manifestations occur following penicillin therapy of early syphilis, providing that it was adequate and that the exceptional early failures were re-treated; the assurance that can be given to the patient is thus of a high order.* Distinction between infectious relapse and reinfection is sometimes not possible except on epidemiologic grounds. If the patient is cured of his infection before his immunity defenses have been mobilized, reinfection may occur on renewed exposure to *T. pallidum.*

Late Syphilis. During the course of untreated late syphilis, regression or reaginemia as a rule takes place very slowly and may occasionally reach nondetectable levels by usual reagin tests. Such reagin nonreactivity may be encountered in parenchymatous or cardiovascular syphilis. Treatment does not substantially affect reagin reactivity, or serologic nonreactivity is reached only after many years. Treponemal antibody tests (TPI/FTA) are normally reactive in late syphilis, and despite treatment may remain so throughout life.

The considerable capacity of the immunity in untreated syphilis to prevent progression of late latent infection to symptomatic disease has already been emphasized. This function cannot, however, be accurately measured by serologic tests as distinct from the clinical effect of therapy, although the latter is convincing. It has been estimated by McDermott (1967) that probably less than 2 per cent of diagnosed late latent syphilitics may develop serious manifestations following proper penicillin therapy. Principally, these are older patients with pre-established unrecognizable manifestations, e.g., aortitis, at the time they are treated for their presumed late latent infection. In the treatment of actual late manifestations, the character, location, and extent of the latter dictate the amount of specific therapy; the indications given in the table—mainly based on the generally accepted schedules applied in the United States Public Health Service VD control program—should be considered only as norms in this respect. Functional and other damage caused by the syphilitic processes require supporting therapy and collateral medical care.

As gummatous lesions may coexist with or precede cardiovascular and/or neurosyphilis, routine physical examination, including roentgenologic examination of the cardiovascular system and examination of the cerebrospinal fluid should be made before treatment, which should be adjusted to the findings. Gummas resolve rapidly, but require several months to heal, depending on size and location.

Maternal and Prenatal ("Congenital") Syphilis. The provision of treatment in diagnosed maternal syphilis is often urgent. Even with diagnosis late in pregnancy, a normal infant can be expected after adequate penicillin therapy. Treatment of maternal syphilis depends on the stage of disease as in other infected persons. With solely anamnestic or serologic evidence of syphilis, the need for treatment should be evaluated at each pregnancy. Confirmation of past adequate therapy and subsequent absence of evidence of active syphilis justify withholding treatment unless reinfection occurs. *If doubt exists concerning diagnosis or previous therapy, pregnant women should be re treated adequately, regardless of reagin titer.*

Infants with manifest early congenital syphilis are often seriously ill and require treatment and medical care in hospital. Penicillin is provided by body weight of children and preadolescents. Patients with interstitial keratitis should be hospitalized for intensive treatment (0.3 megaunits of benzyl penicillin G daily for three weeks) and local hydrocortisone application. Treatment of ocular, aural, osseous, and late systemic manifestations requires consultation with specialists.

Prophylactic Treatment. In persons with suspected or known exposure to infectious syphilis lesions, it is fallacious to await development of clinical or serologic symptoms before treatment. If the chain of infection involves a pregnant woman, it is generally accepted that prophylactic treatment should be given immediately. However, prophylactic treatment is increasingly being accepted in other circumstances also, because considerations applicable in previous arsenical therapy (long-treatment courses and toxicity) do not apply to present-day antimicrobial drugs Syphilis is often acquired from promiscuous heterosexual or homosexual practices. Physicians cannot influence behavioral patterns of contacts. In individual cases, however, the physician can endeavor to elicit contact information comprising the three previous months in primary, six months in secondary, and twelve months in latent syphilis as a basis for epidemiologic action and treatment by a local clinic or health authorities.

When prophylactic treatment is given by the physician, it should be adequate, meaning curative for early syphilis, so as to prevent any larvated or asymptomatic infection from developing, and appropriate clinical and laboratory post-treatment surveillance should be arranged.

Patients Previously Treated. Older patients sometimes confront the physician with information concerning previous injections of arsenicals and/or bismuth or penicillin. Such patients may show low titer reagin tests and TPI/FTA seroreactivity. The physician is justified in treating these patients as newly discovered cases of late latent syphilis after exclusion of systemic involvement when adequate history of disease or therapy cannot be obtained.

Penicillin Side Reactions. An acute systemic febrile reaction – the Herxheimer reaction – with intensification of lesions occurs in about half the patients with early syphilis when treated with antitreponemal drugs, e.g., penicillin. It occurs within 12 to 24 hours, lasts for 6, seldom for 24 hours after the first injection. Corticosteroid preparations appear to attenuate Herxheimer symptoms. Reaction to subsequent penicillin injections signals intolerance to the antimicrobial drug in late syphilis, e.g., aortitis or paresis, the Herxheimer reaction can be severe, but does not – according to modern authorities – indicate interruption of therapy, gumma of larynx being among particular exceptions.

Penicillin may give rise to drug-induced hypersensitivity based on antigen-antibody reactions. The *immediate* or accelerated type shows urticaria, angioneurotic edema, and anaphylactic shock. It is common practice therefore for the patients to be observed for 20 to 30 minutes after penicillin administration, which should not be used in those with known or suspected penicillin hypersensitivity. Syphilis in allergic, e.g., asthmatic, or atopic patients should be managed with caution during treatment sessions. The physician should always have resuscitation remedies readily available, notably epinephrine (Adrenalin), 0.5 ml. subcutaneously, which may be lifesaving, aminophylline, and corticosteroids. The *late* or delayed penicillin hypersensitivity reaction causes dermatitis, various skin eruptions, and exfoliation, and occurs within days or weeks after challenge. The condition is successfully treated with corticosteroids and antihistamines. (See article on Drug Allergy.)

The true extent of penicillin hypersensitivity is unknown, but reactions appear to be relatively rare. The frequency varies from 0.07 to 10 per cent, depending on degree of selection in patient material studies in different countries. Fatality from anaphylactic shock is 15 to 20 per million treated patients (Idsøe et al.). Most deaths are preventable if resuscitation remedies are used immediately. Objective prediction of adverse reactions is not possible. Immunodiagnosis (skin testing, serohemagglutination) is not yet suitable for general practical use.

Alternatives to Penicillin. In persons with suspected or known penicillin hypersensitivity, other antimicrobial drugs must be used. None are as effective as penicillin in the treatment of syphilis. The experience with cephaloridines, for example, must be regarded as experimental; others have marked side effects. The usefulness of orally administered erythromycin and tetracycline, on the other hand, has been demonstrated. A total dose of 30 to 40 grams over 10 to 15 days (750 mg. four times daily) of both erythromycin and tetracycline is given. In pregnant women erythromycin and not tetracycline should be used. The latter in large dosages may cause serious conditions in the mother (pancreatitis, azotemia, fatty liver), and teratogenic effects, e.g., dental deformities, in the offspring. In indicated re-treatment of early syphilis and in late manifestations, the total dosage should be doubled or another drug used.

Surveillance. The short period of actual penicillin treatment is in contrast to the relatively long post-treatment surveillance required. The demonstrated persistence in host tissues of treponemal forms following presumably adequate therapy and the continued TPI reactivity that may signal presence of *T. pallidum* in host tissues suggests a prudent attitude to be justified in post-treatment surveillance of syphilis patients.

Early Syphilis. Quantitative reagin tests should be undertaken at 1, 2, 3, 4, 5, 6, 9, 12, 18, and 24 months after treatment, with FTA/TPI tests at 18 and 24 months; in addition to periodic clinical examinations, the cerebrospinal fluid should be examined at 24 months. (1) If all serologic tests are nonreactive and the cerebrospinal fluid normal at 24 months, the patient can be discharged. (2) If reagin titers are persistently low or nonreactive, the cerebrospinal fluid normal, and FTA/TPI tests reactive at 24 months, further six-monthly serologic follow-up examinations are indicated, with renewed cerebrospinal fluid examination four years after original treatment. (3) If the cerebrospinal fluid is reactive in (1) or (2), it is necessary to proceed as in neurosyphilis.

Late Latent Syphilis. Quantitative reagin tests should be undertaken at 3, 6, 9, 12, 18, and 24 months and FTA/TPI tests at 1, 12, and 24 months, with examination of the cerebrospinal fluid and radiologic examination of the heart and aorta *before* treatment. Unless there is roentgenographic or other evidence of cardiovascular syphilis, the patient can be discharged from observation.

Neurosyphilis. In asymptomatic neurosyphilis, clinical examination, quantitative reagin tests, FTA/TPI tests, and cerebrospinal fluid examination should be undertaken every six months for four years. If the cerebrospinal fluid becomes reactive, the patient should be re-treated, the cerebrospinal fluid examination repeated six months later, and the subsequent follow-up observations conducted as above. In symptomatic neurosyphilis, quantitative reagin tests, FTA/TPI tests, and cerebrospinal fluid examination should be obtained at six-month intervals for four years. If there is no improvement at six months, the patient should be re-treated and the surveillance continued. If two nonreactive cerebrospinal fluid tests are obtained a year apart, no further tests are necessary. (See Syphilitic Infections of the Central Nervous System.)

Cardiovascular Syphilis. In addition to clinical and roentgenographic surveillance, quantitative reagin tests and FTA/TPI tests should be undertaken every six months for four years, cerebrospinal fluid examination having been made before treatment. In cases of reactive fluid, the patient should be treated as in neurosyphilis (see Syphilis of the Aorta).

Late "Benign" Syphilis. The follow-up observations for late "benign" syphilis are the same as for late syphilis when cardiovascular and/or neurosyphilis present.

Maternal and Prenatal ("Congenital") Syphilis. In the first pregnancy clinical examination and quantitative reagin tests should be undertaken preferably at monthly intervals after treatment until term, and thereafter as appropriate for the stage of disease. In subsequent pregnancies in women with previously adequately treated syphilis, quantitative reagin tests should be undertaken at least on the initial visit and during the last month before delivery. Thereafter they should be obtained whenever appropriate in terms of the stage of disease. In *early prenatal syphilis* when lesions are present, the patient should be treated as in "early syphilis." If no lesions are apparent, quantitative reagin testing of child and mother should be carried out at one, two, three, four, five, and six months to ascertain possible differential titers. If reaginemia of the child is passive and no diagnosis of syphilis appears justified, this decision should be reconfirmed at 12 and 24 months. If disease is "active," the patient should be treated, as appropriate for early latent syphilis. In *late prenatal syphilis* (over two years) quantitative reagin tests should be obtained at three-month intervals in the first year, at six-month intervals in the second year, and thereafter at yearly intervals for four years. If the cerebrospinal fluid is reactive or if other late involvement is present the patient should be treated accordingly.

Aspects of Prevention. Efforts at containment of syphilis and other sexually transmitted diseases through broad social and educational prevention have apparently been outweighed by behavioral and environmental changes in a permissive society. Moreover, sex education—when undertaken in schools—does not always include sufficient information on venereal diseases. Even in enlightened community programs concerning sex and family-life education, the sexually transmitted diseases are often ignored. Although the physician can provide a measure of health education, prevention of disease ultimately depends on individual decisions influenced by knowledge, motivation, and convenience. These decisions concern protection from risk of infection by some (chemoprophylaxis, condoms, postexposure measures), while causing others to report for early treatment should symptoms occur.

The physician should take the *psychologic effect* of a diagnosis of syphilis into account and give the patient sufficient time to alleviate his anxiety, distress, and ignorance; on the other hand, the indispensability for the patient to provide contact information, to complete treatment, and accept post-treatment surveillance should be emphasized. The physician should put forward a balanced view concerning the communicability of the disease to others, risk of late manifestations, anticipated course of serologic tests, and similar matters. To patients contemplating marriage, inter-partner transmission of infection and the chances of having nonsyphilitic children are particularly important. The physician should advise against marriage until the danger of infectious relapse is minimal. Such advice has less meaning if the couple are already living together. Advice concerning pregnancy prevention may then be required, and the physician should specifically inquire as to the need. Late manifestations, e.g., neurosyphilis, should receive consideration similar to other physical handicaps. General paresis is a contraindication for marriage. A dilemma arises when syphilis has been acquired from an extramarital source. The patient must then be urged to arrange for examination of the spouse. Careful surveillance is obviously needed.

The early stages of syphilis and other sexually transmitted diseases are health problems for large numbers of people. The late stages are also chronic social and economic burdens of the individual and the community. To those not seeking the services of the private physician, the community should in its prevention program make available *treatment facilities free of charge* in addition to laboratory, case finding, and social services. In several countries these are provided by state or national public health services. Internationally, the Brussels Agreement administered by the World Health Organization provides these facilities to seafarers in major ports regardless of nationality. *It is important that the private practitioner and specialist diagnosing syphilis in any community take advantage of the epidemiologic facilities of the health authorities so as to have contacts of infectious cases and their associates brought for examination and treatment by him, by a colleague, or at a clinic.*

Collart, P., Borel, L. J., and Durel, E.: Étude de l'action de la pénicilline dans la syphilis tardive: persistance du tréponème pâle après traitement. Première partie: La syphilis tardive expérimentale. Seconde partie: La syphilis tardive humaine. Ann. Inst. Pasteur, 102:596, 692, 1962.

Gjestland, T.: The Oslo Study of untreated syphilis: An epidemiologic investigation of the natural course of the syphilitic infection based upon a re-study of the Boeck-Bruusgaard material. Acta Dermatovener. (Stockholm), 35, Suppl. 34, 1955.

Guthe, T., and Idsøe, O.: Antibiotic treatment of syphilis. *In* Current Problems in Dermatology. 2. Antibiotic Treatment of Venereal Diseases. Basel and New York, Karger, 1968, pp. 1–38.

Idsøe, O., Guthe, T., Willcox, R. R., and De Weck, A. L.: Nature and extent of penicillin side-reactions, with particular reference to fatalities from anaphylactic shock. Bull. WHO, 38:159, 1968.

McDermott, W.: Microbial persistence. Yale J. Biol. Med., 30:257, 1957/58.

Smith, J. L., and Israel, C. W.: The presence of spirochetes in late seronegative syphilis. J.A.M.A., 199:980, 1967.

Syphilis and other venereal diseases. Med. Clin. North America, 48:613, 1964.

Turner, T. B.: Syphilis and the treponematoses. *In* Mudd, S. (ed.): Infectious Agents and Host Reactions. Philadelphia, W. B. Saunders Company, 1969.

United States Department of Health, Education and Welfare: Syphilis: A Synopsis. Public Health Service publication No. 1660. Washington, D.C., U.S. Government Printing Office, 1968.

Willcox, R. R.: A Textbook of Venereal Diseases and Treponematoses. 2nd ed. Springfield, Ill., Charles C Thomas, 1964.

World Health Organization: Cell-mediated immunity responses. Report of a Scientific Group. WHO, Tech. Rep. Ser. 423, 1969.

World Health Organization: Report of a Scientific Group on Treponematoses Research. WHO, Tech. Rep. Ser. 455, 1970.

Yobs, A., Clark, J. W., Jr., Mothershed, S. E., Bullard, J. C., and Artley, C. W.: Further observations on the persistence of *Treponema pallidum* after treatment in rabbits and humans. Brit. J. Vener. Dis., 44:116, 1968.

NONSYPHILITIC TREPONEMATOSES

GENERAL CONSIDERATIONS

The course and manifestations of venereal syphilis include many of the features of other nonsyphilitic treponematoses endemic among children and adults in tropical, subtropical, or adjoining regions, where rural populations reside in unhygienic and poor socioeconomic conditions. Clinical features have given distinct names to each of these conditions: yaws, bejel, and pinta. Each is caused by treponemes morphologically indistinguishable from *T. pallidum,* and a scale of pathogenicity can be established based on the degree and type of tissue damage. *T. carateum (pinta)* is the least invasive, affecting only human skin. *T. pertenue (yaws)* affects both the cutaneous and osseous systems. The *treponeme of bejel* affects, in addition, mucous membranes. In contrast to venereal syphilis, there is as a rule no cardiovascular and nervous system involvement or congenital disease in the nonsyphilitis treponematoses.

All persons with nonsyphilitic treponematoses develop reagin and treponemal antibodies just as in venereal syphilis; there is a varying degree of cross immunity between all these conditions, and all respond to penicillin and other antisyphilitic drugs. This group of infections—including venereal syphilis—is therefore referred to as *Treponematoses,* notwithstanding individual clinical, biologic, and epidemiologic differences within the group, reflected in problems of diagnosis, treatment, prevention, and community control.

In addition to the treponemes causing the human infections, the related *T. cuniculi* is responsible for a naturally occurring venereally transmitted spirochetosis of rabbits. The organism is morphologically indistinguishable from pathogenic human treponemes and gives rise to the formation of reagin and treponemal antibodies; the condition responds to antisyphilitic drugs and shows some degree of reciprocal immunity to syphilis and yaws. Finally, cynomolgous monkeys in Africa sometimes have a naturally occurring, apparently asymptomatic treponematosis with significant treponemal serum antibody levels. When isolated and "reactivated" by experimental hamster passages, the treponemes found in lymph nodes are apparently closely related to *T. pertenue* of yaws (Fribourg-Blanc et al.; Sepetjian et al.).

In controlled laboratory experiments, each disease condition usually reproduces itself. However, long-term exposure of infected animals to different environmental conditions may, in some circumstances, modify the biologic characteristics of the particular treponemes. The extent to which this phenomenon occurs in nature has given rise to several speculations concerning the origin and phylogenesis of treponematoses through the ages (Hudson; Willcox; Hackett).

Fribourg-Blanc, A., Nicol, G., and Mollaret, H. H.: Note sur quelques aspects immunologiques du cynocéphale Africaine. Bull. Soc. Path. Etol., 56:474, 1963.
Hackett, C. J.: On the origin of the human treponematoses. Bull. WHO, 29:7, 1963.
Hudson, E. H.: *In* Christian, H. A. (ed.): Treponematosis. New York, Oxford University Press, 1946, p. 122.
Sepetjian, M., Tissot-Guerraz, F., Salussola, D., Thivolet, J. Z., and Mournier, C.: Contribution à l'étude du tréponème isolé du singe par A. Fribourg-Blanc. Bull. WHO, 40:141, 1969.
Willcox, R. R.: Evolutionary cycle of treponematoses. Brit. J. Vener. Dis., 36:78, 1960.

YAWS
(Frambesia Tropica, Pian, Bouba, Parangi, Patek)

Definition. Yaws is produced by a spirochetal microorganism, *T. pertenue,* which causes a chronic human infection, most often with onset in childhood. An initial cutaneous lesion usually appears, followed by relapsing infectious secondary nondestructive lesions of the skin, periosteum, and bones, frequently interspersed with symptom-free periods. Late manifestations include destructive and deforming lesions of skin, bones, and joints. Hyperkeratosis, notably of the soles, may develop in secondary and late yaws. There is no evidence of cardiac or nervous system involvement or of prenatal manifestations. Infected persons slowly develop relative immunity, and humoral antibodies can be detected by serologic tests reactive also in other treponematoses (syphilis, pinta).

History. Yaws probably existed in Africa from remote times. Early accounts suggest that it was brought to the West Indies with the slave trade in the sixteenth century. By the eighteenth century it had become a serious health problem of the Antilles, Central America, and South America, as well as in areas of Oceania and Southeast Asia. Sauvages (1778) proposed the name frambesia for the disease because of the raspberry-like appearance of its papillomatous secondary lesions. Moseley (1800) observed its clinical course, notably that yaws ends in shocking nodes and destructive lesions. Maxwell (1839) determined its incubation period to be three to four weeks following inoculation of lesion material into humans. Castellani (1905) identified *T. pertenue* as the causative micro-organism of yaws. Lambert (1923) first attempted community-wide treatment with arsenicals in the Pacific Isles. The advent of long-acting penicillin preparations and single injection therapy revolutionized case treatment and made possible important reduction of yaws by mass penicillin campaigns (World Health Organization, 1950–1970) in the tropics.

Etiology. The causative agent, *T. pertenue,* is a helical cell 8 to 12 μ in length, about 0.2 μ in diameter, with several closely set spirals. It resembles *T. pallidum* (syphilis) and *T. carateum* (pinta) morphologically in dark-field illumination and structurally in electron microphotographs. *T. pertenue* has not been grown in vitro, but will survive for several days without multiplication in

The author wishes to acknowledge the valuable advice, criticisms, and suggestions by his colleague Dr. J. Ridet, Medical Officer, Communicable Diseases Division, World Health Organization, Geneva, concerning this article.

special media. Strains stored in glycerin remain virulent for many years at $-70°$ C. (CO_2 ice) or lower temperatures, e.g., liquid nitrogen or helium. *T. pertenue* is pathogenic for the same animal species as *T. pallidum*. The latter causes subclinical "silent" infection in the hamster, whereas *T. pertenue* causes a specific dermatitis — a procedure sometimes used to differentiate between treponemes in the laboratory (Vaisman, 1969). Pathogenic treponemes closely resembling or identical with *T. pertenue* have been isolated from wild cynomolgous African monkeys (Fribourg-Blanc et al.; Sepetjian et al., 1968).

Epidemiology and Pathogenesis. Despite mass penicillin campaigns in recent years, yaws has remained a disease of many rural communities in the intertropical zone in Africa, the Americas, Southeast Asia, and Oceania. Areas of high prevalence of active yaws sometimes lie within a few miles of communities where the disease is rarely observed, depending on the ecologic situation, the evolutionary stage of endemicity, and the number of susceptibles at any given time. There is also a higher frequency of early yaws lesions in the rainy than in the dry season (Harding, 1947). Moreover, skin lesions are less frequent in cooler climates in mountainous tropical communities where they also become less moist and where papillomas tend to erupt in sweaty, mucocutaneous junctions and skin folds rather than involving the flat body surfaces (Ramsey, 1925). Furthermore, the occasional yaws lesions encountered following mass penicillin campaigns appear to be less extensive and less moist. In areas where no further lesions are encountered following such campaigns, continued specific seroreactivity (TPI) in a small proportion of children born after the campaigns has suggested the possibility of asymptomatic infection taking place in the new circumstances.

T. pertenue is incapable of penetrating unbroken skin. It is also unable to pass the placenta and cause congenital yaws. Transmission usually occurs through contact of skin abrasions, cuts, or lesions, e.g., trauma, injury, dermatoses, with infectious yaws lesions of another person. Indirect transmission via contaminated hands is believed to occur among children. Nursing mothers are sometimes infected directly by their infants. In addition to early infectious lesions, untreated latent yaws cases which are liable to relapse with active lesions — form an important part of the reservoir maintaining the disease in rural communities. Humidity, moisture-holding soil, and mean annual temperatures of $27°$ C. or more are also necessary for the spread of yaws. Moreover, transmission is favored by scant clothing, bare feet, crowded dwellings, and deficient personal hygiene. The gradual improvement of environmental and socioeconomic conditions will reduce the attack rate of yaws (Saxena and Prasad, 1963).

No true vector has been found in which *T. pertenue* actually multiplies, but it has been shown that disease can be transmitted by experimentally infected gnats. In some areas *Hippelates pallipes* may serve as mechanical carriers (Kumm and Tur-ner, 1936). Geographic coexistence of foci of human yaws and natural treponematoses of wild cynomolgous monkeys have been observed in Africa (Baylet et al., 1970).

The age distribution of yaws depends on the rate of transmission and level of endemicity. In hyperendemic communities, e.g., the former Netherlands New Guinea (Kranendonk), the highest relative frequency of infectious lesions was in the two- to five-year-olds, with a seroprevalence of more than 90 per cent at an early age, pointing to almost complete epidemic "saturation" of the community with yaws. In areas of moderate or low endemicity the highest seroprevalence is in older age groups. Following mass penicillin campaigns, maximal seroprevalence was in the 45- to 59-year-olds, e.g., Nigeria, signaling regression of a hyperendemic situation many years ago. In the latter instance many more young individuals are susceptible to yaws in the new generation, but there are also more barriers to impede renewed spread of the infection, e.g., education, health consciousness, chemotherapy, and health services. However, the greater number of serologically nonreactive young people in the new generation have, when reaching puberty, less protective cross immunity to infection with venereal syphilis. This has been reported to be among the reasons for the increased incidence of syphilis noted in tropical countries in the last decade.

Pathology. A main pathologic feature of yaws is the involvement of the skin. In early lesions the epidermis is thickened. There are cell infiltration ("plasmocytoma") of the dermis, hyperplasia, edema, and the presence of many treponemes. The papillae are elongated, often with thickening of the interpapillary pegs. Proliferation of vascular endothelium and obstruction of vessels are less characteristic of yaws than of syphilis. The epithelium may show hyperkeratosis, become superficially eroded, and be covered by dried exudate. The acanthotic epidermis and the papillary proliferation give rise to a fungating, frambesiform, crust-covered lesion. Diffuse periostitis and cortical rarefaction of the long bones are common in early yaws and are more marked than in venereal syphilis. The late lesions of yaws are due to a different tissue response, and endarteritis is observed histopathologically. Late lesions include ulcerating granulomatous nodules and gumma of the skin and bones. The gumma is built of elements similar to syphilitic lesions. Late skeletal affliction is mostly characterized by periosteal proliferation, rarefaction, or destruction of multiple areas of the long bones which can lead to extensive deformities.

Clinical Characteristics. At the site of entry of *T. pertenue* an initial lesion usually develops after an incubation period of three to four weeks. The implantation is facilitated by previous breaks in the skin (abrasion, injury, vaccination). The lesion is a papule situated on the legs in more than half the cases. In babies and toddlers it often appears on the buttocks or in the perineum. The papule grows into a round, broad-based granulomatous lesion ("mother yaw") covered by a serous crust from which *T. pertenue* can be recovered. The regional lymph nodes are frequently enlarged, not "shotty," and do not suppurate. An initial lesion will heal spontaneously within three to six months; ulcerating initial lesions require more time to heal.

As a result of early treponemia a generalized secondary eruption appears before or after the healing of the initial lesion. The most frequent and characteristic eruptions are roundish, raised, rough, granulomatous papules ("yaws" or frambesides), often covered by a brownish crust. These lesions appear anywhere on the skin, but rarely on the scalp. They sometimes show arciform arrangements. Secondary lesions may last for more than six months. A new crop may appear before the preceding lesions heal. Relapsing crops tend increasingly to become localized, e.g., to periaxillary, perianal, or circumoral areas. Sometimes the papilloma may be solitary. Plantar papules appear late, often after the generalized eruption, and are modified by the thick keratotic layer characteristic of barefoot people: a cherry-like granuloma appears in a well of cracked horny layer, frequently giving rise to painful disability ("crab yaws"). On the body, micropapular as well as various forms of macular or desquamative macular ("pian dartre") lesions may also appear. Lesions of mucous membranes are rare, but occur. Desquamatous macules can develop in the palms and notably on the soles, which are sometimes covered by a thick hyperkeratotic layer. In addition to skin eruptions in early yaws, there is superficial lymph node enlargement. In many cases there are pain and tenderness of the tibial shaft and other long bones owing to early periostitis. Such periostitis sometimes leads to saber tibia and polydactylitis. In many cases the general health of the patient appears little affected; in others there are systemic manifestations, with irregular fever, loss of appetite, and weight loss.

The secondary lesions begin to regress after several months, but relapses may occur on and off for four to five years before true latency is reached. The latter can be interrupted by late lesions of several types. (1) *Superficial ulcerations* of the skin with central healing tendency are observed, and *cutaneous and subcutaneous nodules* with ulceration and marginal healing may leave markedly dyspigmented atrophic scars, sometimes with deforming contractures. (2) *Diffuse or more localized hyperkeratosis* of the soles—less frequently of the palms—with fissuring and pitting can result in a characteristic mottled pattern, occasionally complicated by ulceration and sometimes developing more than 15 years after the infection. (3) *Osteal or periosteal gummatous lesions* of the tibia and other long bones may penetrate subcutaneous and cutaneous tissues, resulting in chronic ulcerations. These may also affect tarsal and carpal bones, the scapula, the sternum, and the skull. Affliction of palatonasal structures may lead to gangosa (rhinopharyngitis mutilans), a spectacular condition similar to that in syphilis. The osteitis and periostitis can occur both in association with generalized skin lesions and after these have receded.

Other yaws lesions are less common and include painless subcutaneous fibromatous juxta-articular nodes, paranasal egg-shaped swelling of the superior maxillary bone (goundou), chronic late macular or hyperkeratotic lesions of palmar surfaces, and volar aspects of wrists and insteps of soles, frequently followed by depigmentation.

Diagnosis. Typical early yaws lesions are generally not confused clinically with other conditions. Ulcerated initial leg lesions may sometimes be mistaken for other ulcerations, e.g., tropical ulcer. Also, spirochetes found in tropical ulcers resembling *Borrelia vincentii* may be mistaken for *T. pertenue*. Facial yaws papules may look like crusted impetigo. Individual lesions may resemble those of secondary syphilis or cutaneous leishmaniasis. Demonstration of treponemes by microscopic dark-field examination of exudate from the lesion and seroreactivity in reagin and treponemal antibody tests (VDRL, FTA, TPI) serve to distinguish yaws from other conditions except those of the treponematosis group. Reagin tests become positive in serum about a month after the initial lesion (Li and Soebekti, 1955), and TPI titers can be very high (1:2560) in early yaws (WHO, Eastern Nigeria, 1968). Ulcerating contractures and mutilating lesions may present differential diagnostic problems in relation notably to leprosy and tuberculosis. Hyperkeratosis of the soles is often confused with other plantar conditions, mainly keratoma plantare sulcatum, plantar pitting, and tropical hyperkeratotic conditions of unknown origin (Hackett and Lowenthal).

Prognosis. In infected persons the prognosis is favorable when early treatment is provided. Otherwise, periodic infectious recurrences over many years give rise to months of partial incapacity. An undetermined number of infected persons develop late lesions. Others go on to spontaneous clinical cure; some also become serologically nonreactive ("burnt-out yaws"). Among those developing late chronic lesions extensive incapacitation and deformities often result.

Treatment and Control. The aim of treatment of individual patients is cure of the early disease and prevention of late manifestations. Intramuscular injection of 1.2 megaunits of benzathine penicillin or 2.4 megaunits of PAM (procaine penicillin G in oil and 2 per cent monostearate) in adults and half doses for children suffices to cause disappearance of early lesions and prevent relapses. The response is dramatic. The early lesions usually become dark-field-negative within 48 hours, and healing takes place within 1 to 2 weeks. Serologic titers decline, but many retain low-titer reagin seroreactivity, depending on the duration of the infection (D'Mello and Krag, 1955). Penicillin sometimes causes a Herxheimer reaction. The usual safeguards against hypersensitivity reactions to penicillin should be taken (see Syphilis). Persons with late yaws lesions may require repeated therapy. Oxytetracycline and chlortetracycline are reported to be useful in cases of deforming osteoperiostitis, indolent gummas, or ulcerations. Two grams daily for five to ten days in adults and proportionately less for children are given. Ulcerations of late yaws may also require application of local antiseptic dressings. Deformities caused by chronic osteitis and contractures necessitate local surgery at times in addition to drug therapy.

In the efforts to achieve community-wide control of yaws, the previous work of the Jamaica Yaws Commission (1936) was in recent years extended under the auspices of the World Health Organization. Since 1950 some 200 million people in 45 countries were examined, and some 50 million treated with long-acting penicillin in large-scale control programs. The aim was (1) to survey entire area populations so as to control the reservoir of infection, (2) to interrupt the spread of yaws through mass treatment, rendering early cases noncontagious, preventing infectious recurrences, and aborting incubating disease, and (3) to undertake post-campaign yaws surveillance by periodic re-surveys to detect and promptly treat overlooked cases or new infections that might arise. Untreated early cases free of clinical symptoms between outbreaks form an important part of the reservoir of infection and contribute to maintain the disease in rural communities. Accordingly, mass treatment criteria in these campaigns were based on a certain association in the population between the occurrence of clinically active lesions and of seroprevalence owing both to such lesions and to clinically symptom-free infections (Hackett and Guthe, 1956). These criteria for mass treatment are: (1) When the prevalence of active yaws cases is 10 per cent or higher (hyperendemic areas), more than 50 per cent of the population is seroreactive, and all members of the community are to be treated. (2) When there are 5 to 10 per cent of active cases (mesoendemic area), all children and their obvious contacts are treated, as most contagious cases occur in the lower age groups. (3) When there are less than 5 per cent active cases (hypoendemic areas), solely case and contact treatment is provided. This wide use of penicillin results in rapid regression of active lesions. The prevalence thus has declined within a few years from more than 20 per cent to less than 1 per cent following mass campaigns in many areas. Examples of reduction in *infectious* yaws are: in N. Nigeria from 4.2 (1954) to 0.1 per cent (1964); in W. Samoa 3 per cent (1955) to nil (1965).

Indifference must be anticipated in rural populations toward long-term surveillance after mass campaigns following "disappearance" of community-wide diseases. In the case of yaws, seroepidemiologic studies have shown continued low-level transmission with tendency to focal outbreaks ten to fifteen years after mass-campaigns (Guthe). Using cardiolipin serology, 40 per cent of children in areas of Indonesia remained seroreactive four to eight years after treatment, and 13 per cent of the seroreactive children still had high seroreactivity titers. A potential for clinical relapses therefore remains. It is really not possible to drive a community disease out of existence by the use of a drug alone even if the population coverage in mass campaigns is nearly complete. Broader measures are needed, notably development of basic health services, into the functions of which the continued surveillance of communicable diseases can be integrated following mass campaigns (World Health Organization, 1965).

Prophylaxis. Prevention of yaws depends on avoidance of minor injuries to the skin, and of shielding of open wounds and abrasions from contamination by flies. Open infectious lesions should be protected. Health education should aim at improvement of personal hygiene (soap) and community hygiene (water). Children with infectious lesions should be treated and excluded from school until noninfectious. Mass therapy represents an important control measure. No method of artificial immunization is available.

Fribourg-Blanc, A., Niel, G., and Mollaret, H. H.: Confirmation sérologique et microscopique de la tréponématose du cynocéphale de Guinée. Bull. Soc. Path. Exot., 59:54 1966.

Furtado, T.: Manifestações tardias da framboesia. Belo Horizonte, Imprensa Oficial, 1955.

Guthe, T.: Clinical, serological and epidemiological features of framboesia tropica (yaws) and its control in rural communities. Acta Dermatovener. (Stockholm) 49:343, 1969.

Hackett, C. J., and Guthe, T.: Some important aspects of yaws eradication. Bull. WHO, 15:869, 1956.

Hackett, C. J., and Lowenthal, L. J. A.: Differential Diagnosis of Yaws. WHO Org. Monograph Series No. 45, Geneva, 1960.

Kranendonk, O. J. M.: Serological and Epidemiological Aspects in Yaws Control: Report on a Mass Treatment Campaign against Yaws in Netherlands New Guinea. Amsterdam, Academisch Proefschrift, 1958.

Turner, L. H.: Notes on the Treponematoses with an Illustrated Account of Yaws. Kuala Lumpur, Government Press (Institute for Medical Research, Federation of Malaya, Bulletin No. 9), 1959.

Turner, T. B., and Saunders, G. M.: Yaws in Jamaica: 1. An epidemiological study of two rural communities. Amer. J. Hyg., 21:483, 1935.

World Health Organization: Bibliography on Yaws 1905–1962. Geneva, 1963.

BEJEL

(Endemic Syphilis, Nonvenereal Childhood Syphilis, Belesh, Dichuchwa, Njovera, Skerljevo)

Definition. Bejel is a chronic, inflammatory childhood disease of the treponematosis group. The early disease is characterized by infectious mucocutaneous lesions and osseous manifestations resembling those of secondary syphilis. Following disappearance of early lesions and an undetermined latency period, late manifestations may develop. There are skin and bone lesions similar to those of late "benign" venereal syphilis. If they occur at all, cardiovascular, nervous system, and prenatally acquired manifestations are extremely rare.

Etiology. The bejel treponeme is morphologically indistinguishable from *T. pallidum*, *T. pertenue*, and *T. carateum*. It is present in early lesions or lymph node aspirate. The organism has not been cultivated in vitro. In laboratory animals Turner and Hollander showed consistent differences in clinical reaction as compared with that of yaws and venereal syphilis treponemes. The bejel treponeme is apparently an intermediate between the two (Paris-Hamelin et al., 1968). Like other treponematoses, bejel is accompanied by antibody formation with seroreactivity in reagin, e.g., VDRL, and treponemal antibody (TPI/FTA) tests. Childhood infection with bejel protects against later infection with syphilis.

Epidemiology. Humans are the reservoir of bejel. Treponemes are most likely transmitted directly among children by skin-to-skin contact, or by hands moistened with treponeme-containing saliva, or indirectly via drinking flasks, the spouts of which have been demonstrated to contain treponemes (Grin). Treponeme implantation is generally facilitated by labial and oral fissures, occurring in dry climates, or by small mucosal lesions. Bejel is a household disease. In some instances 60 to 70 per cent of rural community populations have been reported to be infected. Narrow huts, crowded dwellings, unhygienic living conditions, and low socioeconomic standards favor transmission.

There are many scattered endemic centers of bejel in backward rural areas north and south of the tropics. Bejel occurs along the Kalahari and Sahara deserts in Africa, in the countries of the Balkans and the Eastern Mediterranean region, on the Arabian peninsula, in central Asian countries, and in Australia. It prevails in arid areas in contrast to yaws, which is prevalent in moist, tropical jungle regions. Bejel was first described as a disease of nomadic people, subsequently to occur in settled rural populations, e.g., among the Dogons of Mali, the Islamic descendants of Bosnia, and the Bakwenas of Botswana. Previously it was widespread in the Middle East and Europe. Bejel has not been observed in the Western Hemisphere, where pinta and yaws are the prevailing childhood treponematoses. Bejel is in regression from its higher prevalence of two to three decades ago as a result of extensive mass penicillin campaigns and some improvement of health services. In certain areas the prevalence of bejel has remained higher than that of yaws because of occurrence in nomadic tribes, on account of geographic inaccessibility of endemic foci, and inadequacy of health services (Basset, 1963). It is likely to recur when mass treatment has been incomplete. Thus, in Niger infectious lesions (5 per cent) and seroreactivity (30 to 40 per cent) were found some years after a mass treatment campaign.

Clinical Manifestations and Diagnosis. The experimental incubation period is approximately three weeks. Initial lesions are rarely encountered. The earliest lesions are "mucous patches" of the secondary type localized to the oral and faucal mucosa. "Split papules" occur at the oral angles. Local papular condylomata lata or anal, genital, or other intertriginous skin areas were observed in 25 per cent of infected children in Iraq (Guthe

and Luger). Generalized secondary rashes and alopecia are relatively rare. Regional lymphadenopathy is common. Polyadenitis is rare. The early disease is followed by a latency period of undetermined duration, with seroreactivity as the sole sign of infection. Late "benign" manifestations of the skin develop in some patients. They do not differ in character from those in late venereal syphilis. Superficial tuberoulcerative skin lesions and characteristic serpiginous nodular ulcers occur. Nasopharyngeal ulcerations may occur and range from palate perforation to rhinopharyngitis mutilans as in yaws and syphilis (gangosa). Gummatous ulceration of the breast may occur in women previously infected with bejel who are suckling a child with oral lesions, a phenomenon which supports the concept that gumma may be delayed hypersensitivity reactions from repeated exposure (see Syphilis). Juxta-articular nodes have been described in some geographic areas.

Bone lesions are the most frequent manifestations of late bejel, affecting the clavicle, other long bones, and the frontal bones, giving rise to swelling, tenderness, and pain. There is periosteal endosteal proliferation, and deformities may result. Isolated cases of cardiovascular and neurologic system involvement have been described in Bosnia (Grin) and Botswana (Murray et al.). Incidental cases of prenatally acquired disease have also been reported. No case of prenatal or systemic disease was observed in several thousand examinations in a WHO project in Syria which included radiologic and cerebrospinal fluid examinations. When observed, the systemic manifestations may be due to the occurrence also of venereal syphilis in the geographic area concerned.

Diagnosis. The diagnosis of early bejel is established on epidemiologic and clinical grounds. It may be confirmed by dark-field demonstration of treponemes in the lesions or in node aspirate and by serologic tests (VDRL), reactive in nearly 100 per cent of cases. Serodiagnostic tests cannot differentiate latent bejel from latent yaws or syphilis. Because late clinical lesions are similar to those of yaws and syphilis, the local epidemiologic situation is an important diagnostic consideration. As distinct from the manifestations of late prenatal syphilis, dental deformities and interstitial keratitis are not observed in bejel.

Treatment and Prevention. Penicillin is as effective against bejel as it is against yaws, syphilis, and pinta. In the control campaigns initiated by the World Health Organization in several countries (1950 to 1960), one dose of 1.2 megaunits of long-acting penicillin PAM or benzathine penicillin G was given intramuscularly in early cases, with two further doses at three- to seven-day intervals to patients with late manifestations. Half doses are used for contacts. The longer acting benzathine penicillin is preferred in contact treatment among nomadic tribes. Rapid healing of early lesions was followed by seroreversal within a year in a large proportion of cases. Late destructive lesions required more time. Healing with scars progressed slowly but definitely and with some reduction in reaginemia, but with little or no effect on treponemal antibody tests (TPI/FTA), as in syphilis.

Seroepidemiologic studies undertaken in Bosnia, Yugoslavia, 20 years after the penicillin mass campaign — which was followed by systematic periodic surveillance over ten years — showed that childhood infection had been reduced to nil, the community seroimmunologic profiles indicating complete interruption of transmission. During this period adequate basic health services were provided, health education promoted, and general socioeconomic development took place. Bosnia remains the only example of eradication of endemic treponematoses. However, eradication of childhood infection has resulted in a population susceptible to venereal syphilis in later life. The absence of protective cross-immunity has thus created a new epidemiologic situation in which sporadic cases of the venereal treponematosis occurs.

Grin, E. I.: Epidemiology and control of endemic syphilis. Report on a mass treatment campaign in Bosnia. WHO Monograph, series no. 11, Geneva, 1953.

Guthe, T., and Luger, A.: Epidemiological aspects of non-venereal "endemic" syphilis. Dermatologia, 115:248, 1957.

Hudson, E. H.: Non-venereal Syphilis. Edinburgh and London, E. & S. Livingstone, Ltd., 1958.

Murray, J. F., Merriweather, A. M., Freedman, M. L., and de Villiers, D. J.: Endemic syphilis in the Bakwena reserve of the Bechuanaland Protectorate: A report on mass examination and treatment. Bull. WHO, 15:975, 1956.

Turner, T. B., and Hollander, D. H.: Biology of the Treponematoses. WHO Monograph series no. 35, Geneva, 1957.

PINTA
(Mal del Pinto, Carate)

Definition. Pinta is a chronic skin infection caused by *Treponema carateum*, giving rise to an initial lesion and a generalized secondary rash, both containing treponemes. Late skin manifestations comprise extensive dyschromic (treponeme-containing) and achromic (treponeme-free) conspicuous splotches. Antibodies are produced, detectable by serologic tests reactive also in syphilis and yaws. Organ systems are not involved, physical health is not impaired, and prenatal disease is not known.

History. Manifestations of pinta were described by Berochea and by Corona (1811). Frequent seroreactivity (Wassermann complement fixation test) in pinta patients led Menck (1926) to imply association with syphilis and made Herrejon (1927) assume a treponeme to be the causative micro-organism. Armenteros and Triana (1938) identified *T. carateum* in Cuban pinta. Leon Blanco (1939) obtained early generalized eruptions by self-inoculation of dark-field-controlled material from lesions. In therapy Corona (1811) showed the usefulness of mercury, Maria Graz (1913) of arsenobenzolos, and Varela (1944) of penicillin.

Etiology. The etiologic agent, *T. carateum*, is a slender helical cell, 8 to 35 μ long and 0.2 to 0.3 μ wide. It has regular spirals and performs charac-

The author wishes to acknowledge the valuable advice, criticisms, and suggestions by his colleague Dr. S. Christiansen, Scientific Adviser, WHO Reference Centre for Treponematoses, State Serum Institute, Copenhagen, Denmark, concerning this article.

teristic movements in microscopic dark-field examination and is morphologically indistinguishable from the treponemes causing syphilis and yaws. *T. carateum* has not been cultivated in vitro.

Epidemiology. Pinta is an endemic treponematosis of large rural populations in tropical forest and valley regions of Central and South America. For example, in rural areas of Mexico the prevalence of pinta varied from 1.3 to 9 per cent (1964) of the census population. Pinta cases occasionally reported from Pacific islands, India, Indonesia, and West Africa have not been verified and may have been "pintide" yaws. Unlike yaws, pinta is not a disease of earliest childhood. Community data (Mexico) indicate age-specific prevalences of early pinta lesions to be 2.5 per cent below 5 years of age, 8.8 per cent between five and ten years, and 12.2 per cent between ten and fifteen years. In later life some early lesions occur also after 40 years of age.

Transmission presumably takes place by person-to-person contact and is facilitated by poor hygiene, low economic standards, and limited health services. Treponemes are present in early lesions as well as in extensive late dyschromic lesions, where they can be found up to 40 years after the infection. Pinta does not appear to be very contagious, because an infected spouse with treponeme-containing lesions may sometimes not infect a serologically nonreactive partner or other family members. Scratches and insect bites may provide portals of entry for the agent. Blanco found 63 per cent of 257 initial lesions located on the legs and dorsum of feet. Arthropods (Simuliidae, Hippelates, or Ornithodorus) have not been convincingly demonstrated to be reservoirs of treponemes or biologic vectors, although mechanical transmission cannot be excluded.

Host-Treponeme Relationship. Experimental animal infection has only recently been achieved in the chimpanzee (Kuhn et al., 1968), and man is the only known natural host of *T. carateum*.

As in syphilis, two types of antibody are formed during the human infection: (1) *Reagin*, detectable by cardiolipin antigen tests (VDRL), appears two to six months after the infection. (2) *Treponemal antibody,* identified in treponemal tests (fluorescent [FTA] hemagglutinating [TPHA], and immobilizing [TPI] antibody tests) is produced notably during dyschromic late manifestations but possibly before this stage. In untreated pinta the antibodies persist for many years. Asymptomatic seroreactors in communities affected by pinta are rare or absent. Superinfection can be achieved experimentally during the early generalized erythrosquamous stage of disease, but not after establishment of dyschromic late lesions. Varying degrees of cross-immunity between pinta, syphilis, yaws, and bejel have been reported (Medina, 1965). However, knowledge of humoral and cell-mediated immunity mechanisms is lacking. The same applies to immunologic (immunopathologic) processes possibly concerned in the genesis of lesions. Related aspects are discussed in the article on Syphilis.

The histopathology of pinta is characterized by a perivascular infiltrate of inflammatory cells composed of lymphocytes, some plasma cells, histiocytes, and macrophages. Swollen endothelial cells show no proliferation, arterioles and capillaries are not obliterated (as is the case in syphilis), and granulomatous tuberculoid structure is not observed. In dyschromic lesions accumulation of melanin-filled chromatophores in the upper corium is characteristic, and is caused by pigment "fallout" from the epidermis. This might be a consequence of the primary process. In achromic lesions the picture is quite different — epidermis is atrophic with flattened rete pegs, melanocytes and melanin are lacking, elastic fibers are destroyed, and there is collagenic sclerosis, which explains the porcelain whiteness of achromic lesions. The pigment changes may result from direct action of *T. carateum* on the epidermal "melanin unit" (a melanocyte with a pool of associated malpighian cells [Duchon et al., 1968]). Pinta lesions are localized to skin areas exposed to sunlight. This is unrelated to the number and distribution of melanocytes. A photosensitization process is therefore unlikely.

Clinical Manifestations and Diganosis. The incubation period in experimental pinta is 7 to 21 days. In man, the initial manifestation is a small papule developing by extension or by coalescence with satellite lesions into a scaly maculopapular lesion. There is regional lymphadenopathy. A generalized erythrosquamous rash develops three to nine months after infection, and can be of the "wandering" type. Palpable polyadenitis is not a feature of secondary pinta in contrast to secondary syphilis. One to three years after the initial lesion, sizable dyschromic macules develop. These late lesions develop from secondary pintides or independently, and pass from slate blue through violet to brown and white — the final achromic phase of the pathogenic process. The time to pass these stages varies for different patches in the same individual, and the coexisting colored and white skin areas present a mottled appearance. Dyschromic lesions are usually located on frontal skin, cheeks, ears, forearms, back of hands, and dorsum of feet, but never the scalp. Blue lesions may be punctate, but most often appear as smudges on the brow, cheeks, and side of nose, and may last for one to two years. Brown lesions last much longer, and white elements are of lifelong duration. The achromic lesions are porcelain white, exhibit a "geographic coast" appearance; the skin is not supple and has no skin lines or lanugo. A different clinical course of pinta has been described in Cuba (Pardo-Castello, 1942), where the early phase is limited to palms and soles, with hyperpigmented spots turning into keratotic elements. The hyperpigmentation extends to the backs of hands and forearms. In Cuba implication of the cardiovascular and nervous systems has also been suggested. Such systemic involvement has not been verified in other pinta-affected areas of Central and South America. For instance Mazotti (1966) found nonreactive treponemal antibody tests (TPI) in the cerebrospinal fluid of a series of advanced pinta patients in Mexico.

Early pinta may be difficult to differentiate from *neurodermatitis* (dark-field examination is decisive even if there is seroreactivity); *trichophytosis of the glabrous skin* (pinta does not have vesicles or pustules); *pityriasis alba* (early pinta is more infiltrated); *tinea versicolor* (secondary pintides are more sharply delineated and infiltrated); or *psoriasis* (on removal of scales in pinta no bleeding points appear on a smooth surface). In *late pinta* the leukoderma may closely resemble similar lesions in *syphilis* and *yaws* (scarring); *vitiligo* (supple skin in scalp and perianal areas); *chloasma* (pregnancy and disorders of female genitals); *melanosis* (teleangiectasis and poikiloderma are not features of pinta); or *incontinentia pigmenti* (urticaria prior to spots in infancy, pattern of splotches different, concomitant retinal and organ disease).

Laboratory Methods. A diagnosis of pinta depends on microscopic dark-field demonstration of *T. carateum* in fluid from early initial and secondary generalized lesions and late dyschromic lesions, as well as on serological reagin and treponemal antibody tests. Methodologic considerations and interpretations concerning these are related to those in syphilis.

Treatment. The treatment of choice is repository, long-acting penicillin, notably procaine penicillin G in oil with aluminium monostearate (PAM) and benzathine penicillin G (DBED). The considerations regarding time-dose relationship, oral therapy, and alternative antimicrobial drugs in persons hypersensitive to penicillin are the same as are discussed in the article on Syphilis. Rein et al. (1952) obtained highly satisfactory treatment results with 2.4 to 4.8 megaunits of PAM in early and late pinta. Injections of 2.4 megaunits of the longer-acting benzathine penicillin G can be effectively applied in a single dose or two injections of 1.2 megaunits in each buttock in one session.

Prognosis. Pinta neither endangers life nor gives rise to prenatal disease. It has no appreciable effects on the general health of patients. Treatment causes treponemes to disappear rapidly from the lesions, which sometimes regress very slowly, depending on their extent. Achromic patches in which atrophy of the epidermis has occurred do not change. However, the disfigurement from pinta, notably of younger persons, is sometimes associated with psychologic misery and social ostracism. Freedom of choice of habitat, mate, and employment is curtailed.

Prevention. Pinta prevention consists in examination and treatment of all cases and their contacts with long-acting penicillin, improvement of rural health services, hygiene, and economic standards. In the frame of the international treponematoses program of the World Health Organization (WHO) and the Pan-American Health Organization (PAHO) extensive penicillin treatment campaigns have been undertaken in rural endemic pinta areas by several national health administrations in Central and South America during the last two decades. For instance, in Mexico an estimated 350,000 pinta patients and contacts have been treated since 1959. Prevalence was reduced from 5.9 to 0.4 per cent in five main states.

Christiansen, S.: A study of pinta in Mexico. Bull. WHO, 1970 (in press)

Mazotti, L.: Negatividad de la prueba de inmovilizaciom de treponemas (TPI) en el liquido cefalorraquideo de 10 enfermos de pinto (carate). Rev. Inst. Salubr. Enferm. Trop., 22: Nos. 1 and 2, 1962.

Medina, R.: El carate en Venezuela. Direc. Venezuele, 3;169, 1962-1963.

Osuna, G. G.: La endemia pintosa. Salud Publica Mex., 11:211, 1969.

Rein, C. R., Kitchen, D. K., Marquez, F. and Varela, G.: Repository penicillin therapy of pinta in the Mexican peasant. J. Invest. Derm., 18:137, 1952.

SPIRILLARY AND LEPTOSPIRAL DISEASES

RELAPSING FEVERS

(Recurrent Fever, Famine Fever, Tick Fever, Mianeh Fever, Carapate Disease, Kimputu)

Thorstein Guthe

Definition. Human relapsing fevers are acute arthropod-borne infections characterized by toxemia and febrile episodes that subside and recur over a period of weeks. They are caused by spirochetes of the genus Borrelia and occur in an epidemic form usually transmitted through the louse *Pediculus humanus,* and an endemic form transmitted through tick species of the genus Ornithodoros. The ecology and epidemiologic features are not alike. The clinical course and manifestations tend to be similar, although some characteristics are different.

History. Rutty (1739) first described the disease clinically. Henderson (1843) reported an epidemic in Edinburgh, differentiating the disease from typhus. Obermeier (1868) discovered spirochetes in the blood of relapsing fever patients. Munch (1874) and Motchoukoffski (1876) confirmed the etiology of the disease by self-inoculation of blood from relapsing fever patients. Flugge (1891) suggested the body louse to be a vector. Ross and Milne (1904) showed that "tick fever" mentioned by Livingstone in 1857 was caused by spirochetes in the peripheral blood. Dutton and Todd (1905) described the mechanism of infection in *Ornithodoros moubata* and the passing of the infection to its progeny. Koch (1906) confirmed the mechanism of ovarian transmission.

Etiology. Relapsing fever spirochetes are classified in the genus Borrelia. They are delicate helical organisms with length varying from 8 to 30 μ and width from 0.3 to 0.5 μ, with five to ten loosely wound irregular coils. These vary in different strains or in the same strain in varied conditions. The organism divides by transverse fission, is actively motile, and colors readily with usual blood stains.

Among numerous species of relapsing fever spirochetes, *B. recurrentis* (*B. obermeierei*) is generally accepted as the louse-borne species pathogenic for man. *B. carteri, B. berbera,* and *B. aegypti* — also louse-borne — may be subspecies or possibly only synonyms. Among tick-borne spirochetes *B. persica, B. hispanica, B. duttoni, B. turicatae,* and *B. venezuelensis* are strains with affiliation to natural transmitters of related tick species in different parts of the world. Morphologically the organisms do not differ significantly. They induce essentially the same clinical syndromes in humans. Based on animal experimentation and epidemiologic features, a distinction between louse-borne and tick-borne fevers is generally maintained. Staining methods, antigenic characteristics, serologic, and other methods have not shown consistent differences between strains as a basis for classification. Distinction of the tick-borne strains according to their *Ornithodoros* species vector has been attempted.

Borreliae cannot withstand desiccation and are susceptible to many chemical agents. They survive in citrated blood for three months at 0 to 2° C. When frozen at −72° C., strains are viable for long periods of time. Present culture methods on artificial media have maintained the organism alive for several months without multiplication. Borreliae multiply abundantly in developing chick embryos. Rodents can be used for maintenance of strains (rats, hamsters). The long life of ticks (*O. tholazani* can live for 25 years) makes these insects suitable for preservation of tick-borne strains.

Transmission. Under natural conditions relapsing fevers are transmitted by body lice and ticks, although head lice, bedbugs, and fleas have sometimes also been implicated as vectors. (1) When *lice* feed on patients during attacks of relapsing fever, borreliae enter the midgut. Within five to six days the organisms penetrate into the celomic cavity outside the gut, and feces do not contain Borrelia. These do not reach the salivary glands, ovaries, or eggs. Thus borreliae are not injected into humans when bitten by infected lice. Mutilation or crushing is necessary to transfer infection through abraded skin or by the hand to the conjunctiva, or to the gastrointestinal tract by ingestion. The louse remains infected during its short lifetime (27 to 50 days). Since transovarian transmission is not generally accepted, it is assumed that man is the only host. (2) The many *tick vectors* of relapsing fever — mainly belonging to genus Ornithodoros — attach themselves to the host for a short time, taking up blood. Several methods of infection have been reported, including infected saliva reaching capillaries opened by the bite, gut content being evacuated by the end of the meal and excreta being passed from the malpighian tubules, and infected coxal gland fluid being passed while feeding. Continued transovarian passage of Borrelia to the progeny takes place, and Ornithodoros are invertebrate hosts acting as chronic vectors in the transmission of relapsing fever to man.

Epidemiology. The epidemicity or endemicity of relapsing fevers is dependent on the biology of the vectors.

Louse-borne Relapsing Fever. Louse-borne relapsing fever is typically epidemic under conditions in which overcrowded poor populations live under unhygienic conditions that facilitate wide dissemination of body lice. Louse-borne fever has been the scourge of armies campaigning in the field, as with typhus, with which it is sometimes confused. Cold spells or climates and heavy clothing favor lousiness and transmission of infection. Louse-borne disease has occurred in sporadic outbreaks, spreading with great rapidity across whole continents, thereafter dying down and disappearing, often for long periods. Epidemics with extensive mortality include that in Russia and Central Europe (1919 to 1923), and in West Africa and French Equatorial Africa (1920 to 1930). In recent years a serious epidemic in North Africa (1942 to 1944) spread to the Eastern Mediterranean region and Europe. An estimated one million persons became ill, and some 50,000 died. Since then louse-borne relapsing fever has mainly been reported to occur in the cooler highlands of West, East, and Central Africa, representing possibly a transition from louse- to tick-borne disease. Cases of louse-borne disease have also been reported in the Far East and in several countries in the Americas.

Tick-borne Relapsing Fever. Tick-borne relapsing fever is endemic with many circumscribed centers in the Eastern and Western Hemispheres, and has been reported from the Far East, Africa, Central America, tropical and temperate South America, the United States (western and central western states), and Canada (British Columbia). Wild rodents and other small animals constitute the vertebrate reservoir for many Borrelia species (rats, foxes, weasels, jackals, chipmunks, squirrels, owls, marmosets, and bats). A variety of tick species of genus Ornithodoros are of ecologic importance. They feed on these animals as well as on man. The frequency of relapsing fever transmission by ticks to man depends on the contact opportunities with humans. Many small animals which are common hosts of ticks bring these into houses and dwellings.

Pathology. Borreliae circulate in the peripheral blood during the pyrexial attacks, disappear prior to the crisis, and are probably present in the internal organs during remissions. In autopsy material their presence can be demonstrated notably in the spleen and brain. The pyrexial attack, the intercalate period, and subsequent relapses probably reflect an immunity pattern in which antibody is first produced against the original Borrelia strain with subsequent formation, persistence, and multiplication of antigenic variants. These in turn give rise to further specific antibody varieties in a cyclical manner. Eventually lysins and immobilizins seem to be the most important antibodies in modifying and eliminating Borrelia from the body of animals and man (Felsenfeld). Knowledge of immunologic aspects is inadequate.

Clinical Characteristics. Variations occur in symptoms of toxemia, severity of clinical manifestations, and recurrence of febrile periods, not only between louse-borne and tick-borne fevers, but also within outbreaks of each of these varieties. Generally, louse-borne fever has a longer incubation (up to 15 days), fewer relapses (usually one or two), longer pyrexial episodes (four to seven days), and longer intercalate periods (seven to ten days) than tick-borne fever. The incubation of the latter has been reported as short as one day (*B. hispanica*). As many as 14 waning relapses with pyrexial periods of two days' duration have been described (*B. persica*).

In both types of fever the initial attack is ushered in with chills, nausea, vomiting, joint and muscle pain, photophobia, and fever. The temperature rises rapidly to 104 to 105° F. (40 to 40.5° C.), remains elevated during the attack, except for slight morning remissions, and usually falls by crisis. Cough and bronchitis are frequent. An erythematous, evanescent macular or petechial rash develops in some patients, notably in louse-borne fever. The rash involves the neck, shoulders, chest, and abdomen. There are abdominal pain, splenomegaly, hepatomegaly, and sometimes jaundice of varying intensity. Epistaxis, hemoptysis, hematuria, or hematemesis occurs. Uterine hemorrhages and abortion are not infrequent. Headache, delirium, and symptoms of meningeal irritation may occur; pleocytosis and Borrelia in the cerebrospinal fluid have been described. The initial attack ends with crisis. There are profuse sweating, sometimes prostration, and occasionally cardiac weakness or collapse. In the intercalate period there is usually noticeable clinical improvement. The relapse sets in acutely with remanifestation of previous symptoms, although milder with each subsequent attack. The pyrexial attacks become shorter and the intercalate period longer.

In tick-borne fever ophthalmic and neurologic manifestations are special features. Iritis, iridocyclitis, retinitis, choroiditis, and temporary blindness may occur. Cerebral involvement may generate coma, focal hemiplegia, meningitis, aphasia, and cranial nerve palsies. These may appear late and remain as sequelae.

Convalescence in both fevers is protracted. The mortality is reported at from 2 to 8 per cent. It can be much higher in epidemic outbreaks of louse-borne fever.

Diagnosis. Except in epidemic periods, definitive diagnosis of relapsing fever depends on demonstration of borreliae present in the peripheral blood, mostly in the early pyrexial period. Borrelia can sometimes also be found in the lesions of the rash. In wet blood films borreliae can be seen under the light microscope, but preferably by dark-field illumination. The organisms are diagnosed in Wright- or Giemsa-stained films. When these methods fail, intraperitoneal inoculation of infected whole or citrated blood (0.2 to 0.5 ml.) into young white mice or rats gives rise to detectable borrelemia within 24 to 48 hours.

From the onset there is a marked polymorphonuclear leukocytosis, 15,000 to 25,000 per cubic millimeter, with increase in immature forms. Blood sedimentation is accelerated. There are secondary anemia and urobilinuria, and sometimes also albuminuria and hematuria.

Agglutinating, complement-fixing, immobilizing and borrelicidal antibodies can readily be demonstrated in the serum of infected persons. Inconstant variations between species and strains and variability of antigen and antibodies, even during the fever attack in the same person, limit the usefulness of serodiagnostic procedures. Reagin tests, e.g., VDRL for syphilis are reactive in 10 to 20 per cent of cases. The Weil-Felix test is reactive in titers of 1:80 or higher. Lice removed from patients can be shown to contain borreliae after grinding, suspension, and inoculation of mice. Demonstration of borreliae in ticks in this way is only presumptive evidence, as some ticks carry the organism but are unable to transmit it to the human host. Chick embryos can be infected, and this is the basis for a method of detecting positive ticks collected in nature (Bairamova).

In the differential diagnosis of relapsing fever, confusion may arise with other acute infectious fevers, notably *malaria, typhus,* and *dengue,* but also *influenza* and *early smallpox.* When jaundice is present, *yellow fever* and *leptospirosis* should be considered. The differences emerge as the attack develops. However, definitive diagnosis depends on detection of Borrelia.

Treatment. The patient with relapsing fever is extremely ill. Bed rest, careful nursing, ample fluid, and careful diet are necessary. Antimicrobial drugs are therapeutically effective. One of the tetracyclines (tetracycline, oxytetracycline, or chlortetracycline) is the treatment of choice. Doses of 0.5 gram every six hours for five days, then 1 gram twice daily for another five days or higher are held to be curative and to prevent relapses. In children under ten years of age, half doses are used. Only rarely need treatment be repeated. Chloramphenicol, streptomycin, and novobiocin are also effective, but for various reasons are not the preferred treatment. Repository penicillin must be given in large doses to prevent failures, although it has been suggested that penicillin-resistant strains of Borrelia may have developed (Nauck). All borrelicidal drugs may give rise to initial exacerbation of symptoms in a Herxheimer type of reaction similar to that observed in treponematoses. Subsidiary treatment of the general and particular symptoms of the patient are required.

Prevention. No effective vaccine has been developed. Antimicrobial drugs, e.g., repository penicillin used prophylactically, have been described to be effective under epidemic conditions. Prevention of louse-borne relapsing fever is through avoiding exposure to body or head lice, notably by personal hygiene, cleanliness, and disinfestation of louse-infested clothing and persons. DDT-resistant louse strains have developed since World War II, and control may depend on the use of other insecticidal powders or residual sprays, e.g., the dimethyl-dithiophosphate group (Malathion).

Tick-borne relapsing fever is much more difficult to control, because the vectors do not live on the victim. The ticks inhabit cracks of walls and floors of houses, caves, burrows of small animals, and so forth. Some ticks are night feeders and require intensive search to be discovered. Newer insecticides have a high, but not complete, degree of success against ticks, e.g., benzene hexachloride (Lindane), dimethyl dithiophosphate (Malathion), naphthylmethylcarbamate (Carbaryl). In rural endemic relapsing fever areas, avoidance of ticks might mean a change in the domestic environment and habits of residents. Exclusion of animals, maintenance of smooth walls and floors, installation of windows, and upgrading of housing are generally necessary for long-term prevention.

Bairamova, R. A.: Experience in infecting chick embryos with tick spirochetes by means of infected Ornithodoros. Journal Microbial (Moscow), 40:83, 1963. (English summary).

Bryceson, A. D. M., Parry, E. H. O., Perrine, P. L., Warrell, D. A., Virkotich, D., and Leithead, C. S.: Louse-borne relapsing fever. Quart. J. Med., 39:130, 1970.

Coffey, E., and Eveland, W. C.: Experimental relapsing fever initiated by *B. hermsi.* J. Infect. Dis., 117:23, 28, 29, 1967.

Correa, P., Baylet, R. J., and Brougein, P.: A propos d'un cas de fièvre recurrent chez un nouveau-né ou l'infection par voie transplacentaire parait peu contestable. Bull. Soc. Med. Afr. Noire Lang. Franc., 9:215, 1964.

Felsenfeld, O.: Human relapsing fever, and parasite-vector-host relationships. Bact. Rev., 29:46, 1965.

Gefel, A., Anzarut, A., and Pruzanski, J.: Clinical picture and therapy of tickborne relapsing fever. Israel Med. J., 23:211, 1964.

Nauck, E. G.: Lehrbuch der Tropenkrankheiten. Stuttgart, G. Thieme Verlag, 1967, p. 249.

World Health Organization: Louseborne relapsing fever. Wkl. Epid. Rec., 44:425, 1969.

PHAGEDENIC TROPICAL ULCER
Thorstein Guthe

Ulcerative skin processes are often encountered in outpatient clinics and hospital practice in the intertropical zone. In addition to clinical types recognizable etiologically, as in treponematoses, leprosy, blastomycosis, and leishmaniasis, the phagedenic ulcer is sufficiently common and characteristic to be considered as a distinct entity. It prevails in tropical Africa, the West Indies, Central and South America, the Far East, and Oceania.

Repeated experimental ulcer production in human volunteers (Panja, 1951) supports attributing an *etiologic role* to spirochetes resembling *Borrelia vincentii* and/or fusiform bacilli which are present in sloughs and deep tissues of phagedenic tropical ulcers. Proteus, staphylococci, and hemolytic streptococci are invaders of ulcers of one week's duration. Hot, humid climate furthers the occurrence—sometimes epidemic—of phagedenic ulcers in the intertropical zone, notably in jungle-forest regions. Trauma is a precipitating factor, whether by excoriation, insect bite, or wound. They provide portals of entry for the infective agents on unprotected skin, usually of young males with an active occupation, rarely in females. Forest and plantation workers, labor gangs, campaigning soldiers, and similar workers, as well as individuals of all races, are attacked. Some 90 to 95 per cent of lesions occur on the lower third of the limbs. Deficiency of protein, vitamin A, and other nutrients may favor the occurrence of ulcers, if not their chronicity. The latter is also ascribed to impaired local circulation, anoxemia, and formation of arteriovenous shunts, as in varicose ulcers.

The *course* of phagedenic ulcers is characterized by an acute phase of one to ten days' duration. A papule rapidly develops into an angry hemorrhagic bulla with surrounding inflammation and necrotization, which leads to a round, cup-shaped, fetid, painful ulcer, 3 to 6 cm. in diameter, with ragged edges and a sloughing debris-covered base. The ulcer is usually single. In serious cases it may extend and affect deeper tissues, exposing muscle tendons and periosteum. Regional lymphadenopathy is usually absent; fever is moderate and inconsistent. In the later indolent phase the pain subsides and the ulcer base becomes cleaner, with hypertrophic edges owing to epithelial hyperplasia and dermal sclerosis. Ulcers may recur in the same or other areas (8 per cent), suggesting absence of immunity. Prior to penicillin therapy, ulcers sometimes required hospitalization and local treatment for many months. Acute complications are rare (septicemia, gangrene). Chronic complications include carcinomatous changes in ulcers of long duration (Serafino and Menye).

Diagnosis is established on the basis of anamnestic information and the characteristics of the lesion. Demonstration of fusospirochetal organisms is of relative value. Histopathologic characteristics are nonspecific unless malignant changes occur. Among early differential diagnostic considerations are ecthyma, boils, and gangrene, and later the ulcerations of leprosy and treponematoses (notably yaws), leishmaniasis ("oriental sore"), and septic sore ("desert sore"). Phagedenic ulcers may become papillomatous when *T. pertenue* of yaws is implanted. Varicose ulcers are rare in indigenous populations in the intertropical zones. Sickle cell anemia is a not uncommon cause of ulceration, and the presence of sickling should be excluded by appropriate hematologic examinations.

Treatment in the acute stage includes bed rest and local application of mild antiseptic dressings. Intramuscular injection of long-acting benzathine penicillin G, 1.2 megaunits a week apart with half doses for children (Basset), usually controls infection within a few days. Reinforcement of dietary proteins and vitamins has been recommended. In old chronic cases skin grafting is required.

Prevention of phagedenic ulcers is aided by improvement of rural sanitation, development of local health services, and health education. The latter is directed toward bodily cleanliness, protective clothing and footwear, prompt disinfection when injuries occur, and correction of dietary deficiencies.

Basset, A.: Tropical phagedenic ulcer. *In* Simons, P., and Marshall, J. (eds.): Essays on Tropical Dermatology. Amsterdam, Excerpta Medica Foundation, 1969, pp. 25–33.

Castellani, A.: The common ulcers of the leg, cosmopolitan and tropical. J. Trop. Med. Hyg., 60:55, 91, 1957.

Panja, G.: Tropical phagedenic ulcer (Vincent's ulcer). *In* Gradwohl, R. B. H., Soto, L. B., and Felsenfeld, O. (eds.): Clinical Tropical Medicine. St. Louis, C. V. Mosby Company, 1951, pp. 641–646.

Serafino, X., and Menye, P. A.: Les ulcères phagédéniques cancérisés de jambe. Bull. Cancer, 55:353, 1968.

THE RAT-BITE FEVERS
(Sodoku, Haverhill Fever)

Thorstein Guthe

Definition. Rats are sometimes infected with two independent agents, *Spirillum minus* and *Streptobacillus moniliformis*. Rat-bite fever in humans is a clinical syndrome characterized by local lesion, irregular septicemia, metastatic rash, and febrile episodes that commonly follow bites by infected rats, infrequently bites by some other rodents, and rarely bites by carnivores or other animal sources of infection. In humans both the spirillary fever (Sodoku) and streptobacillary fever (Haverhill fever) have similar clinical courses with certain differential characteristics. An etiologic diagnosis can be established only by laboratory means.

Etiology. *S. minus* is a short, thick spirillum 2 to 5 μ long and 0.2 μ wide with three to four regular coils and pointed extremities with tufts of flagella. It exhibits rapid, darting motions in the dark-field microscope. Cultivation in vitro has not been achieved. *Str. moniliformis* is a pleomorphic, nonmotile, gram-negative bacillus 2 to 15 μ long and 0.1 to 0.4 μ wide. It grows in liquid media showing single rods, chains, or long filamentous forms. On solid media symbiont microscopic colonies appear adjacent to or beneath other colonies, and are made up of pleuropneumonia-like stable L-form organisms. Serologic evidence suggests that *Str. moniliformis* may be an intermediate between Corynebacterium and its own L-form (Peace).

Epidemiology. The distribution of both rat-bite fevers is worldwide and coincidental with reservoirs of infected rats where these live in close association with man. Although the rat is the principal natural host, both agents may also inhabit other rodents, e.g., mice, squirrels, ferrets, weasels, and some higher species such as cats, dogs, and pigs. By bites or ingestion of infected cadavers animals infect each other and in turn infect humans. Infection with *S. minus* is usually inapparent in its natural hosts. The agent is mainly in the blood and lacrimal secretion in rodents transmitting infection. Traumatic bleeding of gums and mucosal lesions of the oral cavity may explain nasopharyngeal presence of the agent. Reported prevalence of *S. minus* in rats varies greatly, i.e., 25 per cent in London, 2 to 22 per cent in India, 6 to 14 per cent in Japan, and nil in Atlanta

(Brown and Nunomaker). *Str. moniliformis* is found in the saliva and nasopharynx of rodents with inapparent infection. The agent has also been reported to be associated etiologically with epizootics of septicemic infections of wild and laboratory rodents. Apart from bites, streptobacillary fever in humans can also occur by ingestion of food containing infected excreta. Epidemics caused by contaminated raw milk were reported in Haverhill, Massachusetts, and "Haverhill fever" has become synonymous with streptobacillary rat-bite fever in the literature (Place and Sutton). Sporadic cases, sometimes in the late stages, continue to be reported (Latrille et al., 1966; McCormack et al)

Pathology. In spirillary rat-bite fever there is at the bite site intense cellular infiltration, edema, and degeneration leading to necrosis. Degenerative changes occur in the liver and kidneys. Hyperemia of cerebral cortex has been noted. *S. minus* is present at the bite site, in regional lymph nodes, and sometimes in the blood, whereas *Str. moniliformis* can invariably be recovered from the blood as well as local tissues. The morbid anatomy and histopathology of the rat-bite fevers have not been thoroughly studied. This also applies to the possible role of humoral or cell-mediated immunity in the pathogenesis of the disease. Spirillolytic substances appear in the serum. Cardiolipin antigen tests for treponematoses can be reactive in spirillary infection. In the streptobacillary infection serum agglutinates antigens of the bacillus.

Clinical Manifestations. The clinical features are similar but not identical in both fevers. The incubation periods described vary with averages of two to three weeks in spirillary fever and three days to a week in streptobacillary fever. The onset is ushered in by chills, nausea, and fever. There is activation of the quiescent bite lesion in spirillary fever, with pain, swelling, edema, and sometimes ulceration of the site of the infecting bite. Regional lymph nodes are also swollen, firm, and nonadherent. This is not a prominent feature in streptobacillary fever. General symptoms include muscle pain, tenderness, and prostration. With each of several episodes of spirillary fever pain returns with exacerbation of local symptoms. In the streptobacillary variety there may be few fever episodes, even a single one. Migrating arthralgias are encountered in *S. minus* infections, whereas polyarthritis with fibrinous synovial fluid characterizes streptobacillary fever. In spirillary fever the temperature may rise to 104° F. and last for two to three days with abrupt fall. All symptoms fade and temperature returns to normal between pyrexial periods. There can be six to eight attacks separated by three to seven days. The attacks then get less frequent, shorter, and milder. The rash may develop with the first or a subsequent fever attack. It is macular or maculopapular in both fevers, and in the spirillary variety sometimes petechial. In spirillary fever the color is notably of a deep purplish shade. The rash is distributed to the trunk and extremities and is not associated with itch. It fades and disappears with the fall

of the temperature. It reappears in periods of remission. Endocarditis is reported as a late complication in both fevers; pericarditis has also been described in streptobacillary fever (Carbeck et al., 1967). Sometimes motor and sensory disturbances occur. Urticaria is occasionally observed. The fatality rate in the spirillary fever previously reported at 2 to 10 per cent is greatly reduced by antimicrobial therapy. Most untreated cases subside spontaneously, but others may go on indefinitely.

Diagnosis. A history of rat or other animal bite, infiltration at the bite site, the pattern of the fever, and the rash will in many instances justify a presumptive diagnosis by the physician. Differentiation from other relapsing or trench fevers may be difficult. Malaria may coexist. Weil's disease is rarely transmited by actual rat bite. The rash may be confused with secondary syphilis or yaws.

Dark-field examination of exudate from the bite site, serous fluid from rash, or aspirate from lymph nodes may confirm a diagnosis of suspected spirillary fever. It is difficult to demonstrate *S. minus* in thick blood drop preparations even at the height of fever attacks. The serum agglutinates spirillum in low dilutions. Reagin tests for treponematoses may be reactive in individuals known not to have had syphilis, yaws, pinta, or bejel. Diagnosis is best confirmed by inoculation of blood, lymph, or excised bite site into the scrotal skin of guinea pigs or intraperitonally in mice. In streptobacillary fever the micro-organism can readily be recovered by culture from the blood, wound serum, or synovial fluid. High serum agglutination titers after three to four weeks are considered of diagnostic value. Reagin tests for treponematoses are usually nonreactive.

Treatment. Lourie and Collier (1943) demonstrated the *spirillocidal* effect of penicillin. This drug is also effective against *Str. moniliformis*, although possibly less so. Time-dose relationship studies in rat-bite fevers concerning choice of short-acting or long-acting penicillin have not been published. Benzyl penicillin G structured preparations are preferable. The extensive appraisal of therapy in rat-bite fevers by Roughgarden emphasizes that intramuscular dosages of penicillin should (in both fevers) be no less than 0.4 to 0.6 megaunit daily for seven days in the early disease, and that the dosages should be doubled if little or no effect is observed. In endocarditis the dosages should be as in similar conditions of streptococcal origin: 10 to 15 megaunits daily for three to four weeks. Streptomycin, 0.5 gram twice daily for three to four days and half dose for children, and oxytetracycline, 0.5 gram initially and half-maintenance doses for several days, have been shown to be effective. These drugs are in reserve for use in penicillin-hypersensitive persons and in patients with streptobacillary infection attributed to persistence of penicillin-resistant L-forms of the organism.

Prevention. Prevention rests on rat destruction. Antiplague measures to extinguish rats also affect the distribution of rat-bite fever; as shown in

Manila. Rat-bite wounds in children and adults should be treated promptly with antiseptic dressing and a prophylactic dose of penicillin or other effective antimicrobial drug.

Brown, T. M., and Nunemaker, J. C.: Rat-bite fever: A review of the American cases with re-evaluation of etiology; report of cases. Bull. Hopkins Hosp., 70:201, 1942.
McCormack, R. C., Kaye, D., and Hook, E. W.: Endocarditis due to streptobacillus moniliformis. J.A.M.A., 200:77, 1967.
Mollaret, P.: Infektionen nach Katzen- oder Rattenbisse. Münch. Med. Wschr., 111:13, 1969.
Peace, P.: Evidence that *Streptobacillus moniliformis* is an intermediate stage between a corynebacterium and its L-form or derived PPLO. J. Gen. Microbiol., 29:91, 1962.
Place, E. H., and Sutton, L. E.: Erythema arthriticum epidemicum (Haverhill fever). Arch. Intern. Med. (Chicago), 54:659, 1934.
Roughgarden, J. W.: Antimicrobial therapy of rat-bite fever. Arch. Intern. Med. (Chicago), 116:39, 1965.

LEPTOSPIROSIS
Jay P. Sanford

Definition. Leptospirosis is a broad term applied to all infections due to leptospires regardless of specific serotype. Correlation of clinical syndromes with infection by specific serotypes leads to the conclusion that a single serotype of Leptospira may be responsible for a variety of clinical features; likewise, a single syndrome, e.g., aseptic meningitis, may be caused by multiple serotypes of leptospires. Hence, there is preference for the general term leptospirosis rather than the multiple synonyms such as Weil's disease, Canicola fever, etc.

Classification and Epidemiology. The genus Leptospira contains only one species, *L. interrogans,* which may be subdivided into two complexes, interrogans and biflexa. The interrogans complex includes most of the pathogenic strains, whereas the biflexa complex includes mainly saprophytic strains with no recognized hosts. Within each complex, strains are classified by agglutination reactions into serogroups and serotypes. Despite contrary common usage, an example of the correct designation of leptospira is as follows: pomona serogroup of *L. interrogans,* not *L. pomona.* The interrogans complex now contains about 130 serotypes arranged in 16 serogroups (the number in parentheses refers to number of serotypes within the serogroup): icterohemorrhagiae (13), hebdomadis (28), autumnalis (13), canicola (11), australis (10), tarassovi or hyos (10), pyrogenes (9), bataviae (8), javanica (6), pomona (6), ballum (3), cynopteri (3), celledoni (2), grippotyphosa (2), panama (2), and shermani (1). At least 22 serotypes of Leptospira occur naturally in the United States.

Infection in man is an incidental occurrence and is not essential to the maintenance of leptospirosis in nature. A wide range of domestic and wild animal hosts have been shown to have leptospirosis. In many species, such as opossums, skunks, raccoons, and foxes, infectivity ratios in the range of 10 to 50 per cent are not unusual. Interspecies spread of specific serotypes of leptospires between animal hosts is frequent, e.g., pomona, a serotype principally associated with livestock, has been demonstrated in dogs. The infection in animals may vary from inapparent illness to severe fatal disease. The carrier state may develop in many animals wherein the host may shed leptospires in its urine for months to years.

It has not been established that pathogenic leptospires are capable of multiplication outside a host. Survival in nature is governed by factors including pH of the urine of the host, pH of soil or water into which they are shed, and ambient temperature. Acid urine permits only limited survival; however, if the urine is neutral or alkaline and is shed into a similar moist environment which has low salinity and is not badly polluted with micro-organisms or detergents, and with a temperature above 22° C., leptospires may survive for several weeks. Human infections can occur either by direct contact with urine or tissue of an infected animal or indirectly through contaminated water or soil. The usual portals of entry in man are abraded skin, particularly about the feet, and exposed mucous membranes, conjunctival, nasal, and oral. The previously held concept that organisms could penetrate intact skin has been questioned. Although leptospires have been isolated from ticks, they appear to be unimportant in transmission.

With the ubiquitous infection of animals, leptospirosis in man can occur in all age groups, at all seasons, and in both sexes. However, it is primarily a disease of teen-age children and young to middle-aged adults (75 per cent of patients are between ages 10 and 50 years), occurs predominantly in males (90 per cent), and develops most frequently in hot weather (in the United States two thirds of infections occur from June to September). The wide spectrum of animal hosts results in both urban and rural human disease. Leptospirosis has been considered an occupational disease; although up to one third of patients have direct contact with animals, e.g., farmers, abattoir workers, and veterinarians, the majority of patients have incidental exposure. Swimming or partial immersion in contaminated water has been implicated in one fifth of patients.

Pathology. In patients who have died with either hepatic involvement (Weil's syndrome), renal involvement, or both, the significant gross changes include hemorrhages and bile-staining of tissues. The hemorrhages, which vary from petechial to ecchymotic, are widespread but are most prominent in skeletal muscle, kidneys, adrenals, liver, stomach, spleen, and lungs.

In skeletal muscle, focal necrotic and necrobiotic changes thought to be rather typical of leptospirosis occur. Biopsies early in the illness demonstrate swelling, vacuolation, and subsequently hyalinization. Leptospiral antigen has been demonstrated in these lesions by the fluorescent antibody technique. Healing ensues by the formation of new myofibrils with minimal fibrosis. Renal involvement consists of focal damage to tubular cells, characterized by loss of the brush border, disjunction of cellular limits, mitochondrial depletion, and a secondary interstitial inflammatory reaction. Hyaline and bile casts may be seen in the tubules. On electron microscopy, focal thickening of the glomerular basement membrane and fusion of the foot processes of the epithelial cells have been recognized. Microscopic alterations in the liver are not diagnostic, and correlate poorly with the degree of functional impairment. The changes include frequent double nuclei in hepatic cells, cloudy swelling of parenchymal cells, disruption of liver cords, enlargenent of Kupffer cells and bile stasis in biliary canaliculi. The changes in the brain and meninges are also minimal and are not diagnostic. Thickening of the meninges with a polymorphonuclear leukocytic infiltration has been observed. Rarely, parenchymal lesions consisting of perivascular round-cell infiltration may be encountered. Microscopic evidence of myocarditis, including focal hemorrhages, interstitial edema, and focal infiltration with lymphocytes and plasma cells, has been recorded. Pulmonary findings consist of a patchy, localized hemorrhagic pneumonitis. Special staining techniques utilizing silver impregnation methods have demonstrated organisms in the lumina of renal tubules but rarely in other organs.

Clinical Manifestations. General Features.

The incubation period for icterohemorrhagiae following immersion or accidental laboratory exposure has shown extremes of 2 to 20 days, the usual range being 7 to 13 days and the average, 10 days. This incubation period does not vary significantly with other serotypes.

Leptospirosis is typically a biphasic illness. The leptospiremic or first phase is characterized by manifestations of an acute infectious process. During this phase, leptospires are present in the blood and cerebrospinal fluid. The onset is typically abrupt (75 to 100 per cent of patients). Initial symptoms include headache, which is usually frontal, less often retro-orbital, but occasionally may be bitemporal or occipital. Severe muscle aching occurs in most patients, the muscles of the thighs and lumbar areas being most prominently involved. The myalgia may be accompanied by extreme cutaneous hyperesthesia. Chills followed by rapidly rising temperature are prominent. Following the abrupt onset, the leptospiremic phase typically lasts four to nine days. Features during this interval include recurrent chills, high spiking temperatures (usually 102° F. or greater), headache, and continued severe myalgia. Anorexia, nausea, and vomiting are encountered in one half or more of the patients. Pulmonary manifestations, usually either cough or chest pain, have varied in frequency of occurrence from less than 25 to 86 per cent. Hemoptysis occurs but is rare. Examination during this phase reveals an acutely ill febrile patient. A relative bradycardia may be noted. The blood pressure is usually normal, although European authors comment on early hypotension. Disturbances in sensorium may be encountered in up to 25 per cent of pa-

tients. The most characteristic physical sign is conjunctival suffusion. This may be associated with photophobia, but serous or purulent secretion is unusual. The redness of the eyes originates at the folds of the conjunctivae and usually first appears on the third or fourth day. Less common findings (in 25 to 50 per cent of patients) may include pharyngeal injection, nuchal rigidity, cutaneous hemorrhages, and skin rashes that are usually macular, maculopapular, or urticarial, and usually occur on the trunk. Uncommon findings (less than 10 per cent) are splenomegaly, hepatomegaly, lymphadenopathy, or jaundice. The first phase terminates after four to nine days, usually with defervescence and improvement in symptoms. This coincides with the disappearance of leptospires from the blood and cerebrospinal fluid.

The second phase has been characterized as the "immune" phase and correlates with the appearance of circulating antibodies. The clinical manifestations of this phase exhibit greater variability than those during the first phase. After a relatively asymptomatic period of one to three days, the fever and earlier symptoms recur and, meningismus, may develop. The fever rarely exceeds 102° F. and is usually of one to three days' duration. It is not uncommon for fever to be absent or quite transient. Even when symptoms or signs of meningeal irritation are absent, routine examination of cerebrospinal fluid after the seventh day has revealed pleocytosis in 80 to 90 per cent of patients. Less common features include iridocyclitis, optic neuritis, and other nervous system manifestations, including encephalitis, myelitis, and peripheral neuropathy.

Some clinicians recognize a third or convalescent phase. During this period and usually between the second and fourth weeks, both fever and aching may recur. The pathogenesis of this stage is poorly understood.

Leptospirosis during pregnancy may be associated with an increased risk of fetal loss.

Specific Features. Weil's Syndrome.

Weil's syndrome, which may be due to serotypes other than icterohemorrhagiae, is defined as severe leptospirosis with jaundice, usually accompanied by azotemia, hemorrhages, anemia, disturbances in consciousness, and continued fever. There is uncertainty as to the pathogenesis of the syndrome, i.e., whether it represents direct toxic damage caused by leptospires or whether it is the consequence of immune response to leptospiral antigens. The consensus favors toxic damage.

The onset and first stage are identical with the less severe forms of leptospirosis. The distinctive features of Weil's syndrome appear from the third to the sixth day but do not reach their peak until well into the second stage. As in the other forms of leptospirosis, there is a tendency for the fever to lyse about the seventh day; however, with its recurrence it is marked and may persist for several weeks. Either renal or hepatic manifestations may predominate. Hepatic disturbances include tenderness in the right upper quadrant and hepatic enlargement, both of which are common when jaundice is present. Abnormalities of liver function involve primarily tests of hepatocellular function such as the thymol turbidity or cephalin-cholesterol flocculation. Serum glutamic oxalo-acetic acid transaminase values are only moderately elevated.

Renal manifestations consist primarily of proteinuria, pyuria, hematuria, and azotemia. Dysuria is rare. Serious renal damage usually occurs in the form of acute tubular necrosis associated with oliguria. Hemorrhagic manifestations are most prevalent in this group of patients; epistaxis, hemoptysis, gastrointestinal bleeding, hemorrhage into the adrenal glands, hemorrhagic pneumonitis, and subarachnoid hemorrhage have all been described. These have been explained on the basis of capillary injury. In addition, in some patients hypoprothrombinemia and thrombocytopenia have been observed.

Aseptic Meningitis. The syndrome of aseptic meningitis, which is characterized by cerebrospinal fluid pleocytosis, usually with tens to hundred of leukocytes that are predominantly mononuclear cells, normal sugar, i.e., greater than 60 per cent of the concomitant blood sugar, and protein of less than 100 mg. per 100 ml., has been associated with leptospirosis. Meyer and associates incriminated a leptospiral etiology in 6 per cent of a group of sporadic cases of the aseptic meningitis syndrome. An observation causing difficulty in differential diagnosis has been the infrequent but definite demonstration of lowered cerebrospinal sugar levels. Xanthochromic cerebrospinal fluid has been observed in the presence of jaundice; although observed only infrequently, its occurrence is of suggestive diagnostic importance. Each of the serotypes of leptospires that are pathogenic for man is probably capable of association with this syndrome. The most prevalent serotypes have been icterohemorrhagiae, canicola, and pomona.

Pretibial (Fort Bragg) Fever. An illness was observed in the summer of 1942 that had an onset identical with that of the first phase of leptospirosis. The most distinctive feature was the development on about the fourth day of a rash, characterized by 2 to 5 cm. slightly raised erythematous lesions that were usually symmetrically distributed over the pretibial areas. In contrast to other leptospiral syndromes, splenomegaly occurred in 95 per cent of these patients. This outbreak was shown to be due to the autumnalis serogroup. Subsequently pomona has been observed in association with rashes, which are usually truncal in distribution but have also been pretibial in location.

Myocarditis. Cardiac arrhythmias, including paroxysmal atrial fibrillation, atrial flutter, ventricular tachycardia, and premature ventricular contractions, have been described, but are usually of little clinical significance. However, on rare occasions definite cardiac dilatation with acute left ventricular failure has been observed. Associated manifestations have included jaundice, pulmonary infiltrates, arthritis, and skin rashes.

The serogroups thus far incriminated have included icterohemorrhagiae and pomona.

Laboratory Features. Leukocyte counts vary from leukopenic levels to mild elevations in the anicteric patients. In patients with jaundice, leukocytosis as high as 50,000 per cubic millimeter may be present. However, regardless of the total leukocyte count, neutrophilia of greater than 70 per cent is very frequently encountered during the first stage.

Hemolytic substances have been demonstrated in cultures of pathogenic leptospires. In contrast to many hemolysins of bacterial origin, which are not hemolytic in vivo, the leptospiral hemolysins appear active in vivo. In patients with jaundice, anemia may be severe and is most characteristically due to intravascular hemolysis. Other mechanisms include azotemia and blood loss secondary to hemorrhage. Anemia owing to leptospirosis is unusual in anicteric patients.

Rarely thrombocytopenia sufficient in magnitude to be associated with bleeding is encountered. Additional hematologic abnormalities include almost uniform elevation of the erythrocyte sedimentation rate.

Urinalyses during the leptospiremic phase reveal a high frequency of abnormalities, including mild proteinuria, casts, and an increase in cellular elements. In anicteric infections, these abnormalities rapidly disappear after the beginning of illness. Proteinuria and abnormalities in urine sediment usually are not associated with elevations in blood urea nitrogen values. Since the anicteric form of the disease has often gone undiagnosed, estimates of the frequency of azotemia and jaundice are probably high. Azotemia has been reported in approximately one fourth of patients. In three fourths of these patients the blood urea nitrogen is less than 100 mg. per 100 ml. Azotemia is usually associated with the occurrence of jaundice. The serum bilirubin levels may reach 40 mg. per 100 ml.; however, in two thirds of patients the levels are less than 20 mg. per 100 ml.

Diagnosis. Diagnosis is based upon either cultural or serologic studies. Leptospires may be isolated quite readily during the first phase from blood and cerebrospinal fluid or during the second phase from the urine. Whole blood should be inoculated immediately into tubes containing semisolid medium, such as Fletcher's medium. If culture medium is not available, leptospires reportedly will remain viable up to 11 days in blood to which anticoagulants, preferably sodium oxalate, have been added. Animal inoculation (preferably of either suckling hamsters or guinea pigs) may also be used and is of particular value if specimens, e.g., urine, are contaminated. Direct examination of blood or urine by dark-field methods has been employed; *however, this method so frequently results in failure or misdiagnosis that it should not be employed as the only diagnostic test.* Serologic methods are applicable during the second phase, antibodies appearing from the sixth to the twelfth day of illness. Four serologic tests are available: the macroscopic plate agglutination test (the easiest to perform but a relatively insensitive technique), hemolytic test (complex in performance but requiring only a single antigen), microscopic agglutination test (complex in performance but most specific), and complement-fixation test. Serologic criteria for diagnosis include a fourfold or greater rise in titer during the course. Cross-agglutination reactions between various serotypes commonly occur so that the infecting serotype often cannot be determined with certainty without isolation of leptospires.

Prognosis and Sequelae. The prognosis is dependent upon both the virulence of the organism and the general condition of the patient. Age is the most significant host factor related to increased mortality. In a representative series, the mortality rose from 10 per cent in men less than 50 years of age to 56 per cent in those over 51 years of age. The virulence of the infecting leptospires correlates best with the development of jaundice. In anicteric patients, mortality is essentially unknown. With the occurrence of jaundice, mortality in various series has ranged from 15 to 40 per cent. The long-term prognosis following the acute renal lesion of leptospirosis is good.

Therapy and Management. A variety of antimicrobial drugs, including penicillin, streptomycin, the tetracycline congeners, chloramphenicol, erythromycin, and oleandomycin, have been effective in vitro and against experimental leptospiral infections. The data obtained from controlled observations in man are conflicting as to over-all efficacy. If antimicrobial drugs have any beneficial effect, they must be administered within four days, and preferably within two days, of the onset of illness. The agents most studied have been penicillin G and the various tetracycline congeners. Turner states that large doses of penicillin G or tetracycline are indeed advantageous. There is general agreement that antimicrobials administered after the fifth day have no beneficial effect. Since diagnosis within the first five days requires a very high index of suspicion, management is primarily supportive. The clinical impression exists that early bed rest may minimize the subsequent morbidity. The presence of azotemia and jaundice requires meticulous attention to fluid and electrolyte therapy.

Alston, J. M., and Broom, J. C.: Leptospirosis in man and animals. Edinburgh and London, E. S. Livingstone, Ltd., 1958.

DeBrito, T., Freymuller, E., Penna, D. O., Santos, H. S., Soares de Almeida, S., Ayroza Galvao, P. A., and Percira, V. G.: Electron microscopy of the biopsied kidney in human leptospirosis. Amer. J. Trop. Med., 14:397, 1965.

Edwards, G. A., and Domm, B. M.: Human leptospirosis. Medicine, 39:117, 1960.

Heath, C. W., Jr., Alexander, A. D., and Galton, M. M.: Leptospirosis in the United States. Analysis of 483 cases in man, 1949-1961. New Eng. J. Med., 273:857; 915; 1965.

Meyer, H. J., Jr., Johnson, R. T., Crawford, J. P., Dascomb, H. E., and Rogers, N. G.: Central nervous system syndromes of "viral" etiology; Study of 713 cases. Amer. J. Med., 29:334, 1960.

Turner, L. H.: Leptospirosis. Brit. Med. J., 1:231, 1969.

World Health Organization: Current problems in leptospirosis research. Report of WHO Expert Group. Techn. Rep. Ser. 380, Geneva, 1967.

The Mycoses

John P. Utz

Recent developments in epidemiology and histopathologic techniques and the emergence of amphotericin B as an effective antifungal drug have led to a great increase in awareness of the medical problem of systemic fungal disease. The fact that infection occurs with fungi that are free-living forms in soil, decaying vegetation, and bird excreta poses a difficult problem of control. The deliberate impairment of immune response, e.g., to decrease host versus graft reactions in patients with organ transplants, has created still another setting for infection by "opportunistic" fungi. It is a safe speculation that systemic mycotic infection will continue to be an increasing cause of human disease.

In addition to their point of origin in nature, the systemic mycoses have other important properties in common. With few exceptions, they are not contagious from animal-to-man or man-to-man, and epidemics or outbreaks arise from a common source. Infection is acquired by inhalation or, in a few instances, by traumatic implantation. The primary focus is usually the lung, and infection spreads hematogenously or, less commonly, by direct extension. The gross and microscopic appearance of infected tissue is that of a granulomatous process. The immunologic response is generally effective (reinfection is rare), and a delayed cutaneous hypersensitivity and circulating antibodies have been demonstrated.

HISTOPLASMOSIS

Definition. Histoplasmosis is a systemic fungal disease, respiratory in origin, that spreads to the pulmonary lymphatics and by the blood to the mediastinal lymph nodes, spleen, liver, adrenals, gastrointestinal tract, kidneys, skin, central nervous system, heart, and other organs. It may be asymptomatic, acute, and benign, or progressive and eventually fatal.

History. Darling in Panama in 1905 reported three fatal cases of disseminated disease, which he considered to be due to a *plasmo*dium" with a rigid wall or *"capsule,"* in *histiocytes* which he termed *Histoplasma capsulatum.* In a study of tissue section, da Rocha Lima concluded in 1913 that the agent was a fungus. In 1934 De Monbreun correctly identified the fungus in cultural and in laboratory animal studies. Ten years later Christie and Peterson recognized the benign form of human disease with pulmonary calcification and associated skin hypersensitivity to histoplasmin. Subsequently, Palmer showed widely varying rates of hypersensitivity according to geographic areas in this country.

Etiology. *H. capsulatum* has two morphologic forms, *yeast* and *hyphal*, dependent upon a variety of environmental factors. The yeast form seen in tissues measures 2 to 3 by 3 to 4 μ and has a clear area resulting from shrinkage of cytoplasm from the rigid cell wall. In artificial media or natural substrate the yeast form is converted readily at room temperatures to the hyphal form with the production on Sabouraud's glucose medium of a white to brown cottony mold. On microscopic examination this is composed of branched hyphae, characteristic spherical forms with spiny projections (tuberculate macroconidia) 8 to 14 μ in diameter, and smaller forms (microconidia) measuring 2 to 5 μ. Conversion of the hyphal to the yeast form occurs characteristically after inoculation into animals or less readily on enriched media at 37° C. Skin hypersensitivity, complement-fixing, and other antigens have been demonstrated. Mice and guinea pigs are susceptible to experimental infection.

Epidemiology. Histoplasmosis occurs with highest frequency in infancy and old age and equally in the sexes except more often in the male in old age. It has been reported in more than 30 countries in both temperate and tropical zones. Skin hypersensitivity rates are as high as 80 to 90 per cent in some parts of the eastern and midwestern United States. Rates of skin reactivity increase rapidly with age to young adulthood and then more slowly thereafter. Man and animals are infected by inhalation of the fungus in dust. Soil from chicken houses or from areas contaminated or composted by bat or bird dung is especially rich in organisms. Massive exposure through such activities as destruction of chicken houses or exploration of caves has resulted in outbreaks. Fifty per cent of dogs and cats in some areas and many species of wild animals are known to be infected. *Histoplasma duboisii*, a closely related fungus, produces in African patients a disease marked by lymphadenopathy and bone, joint, and skin involvement.

Pathology. The tissue reaction is characteristically engulfment of yeast forms by histiocytes or macrophages derived from organs of the reticuloendothelial system. Epithelioid or histiocytic granulomas are formed with tubercle-like nodules, caseation necrosis, and calcification in the lung, lymph nodes, liver, spleen, adrenals, and other organs. The organism can best be identified in tissues by culture or by use of special stains (periodic acid–Schiff, Gridley, or Gomori methenamine silver methods). However, fungal cells may be few, crowded, and not differentiated with certainty from those of *H. duboisii, Blastomyces dermatitidis, Torulopsis glabrata,* or *Candida albicans.*

Clinical Manifestations. On the basis of delayed cutaneous hypersensitivity studies, it appears that primary infection with *H. capsulatum* is usually asymptomatic or produces a respiratory illness that is not distinctive.

Primary Acute Form. The primary acute form is characterized by respiratory symptoms of cough, shortness of breath, pleuritic chest pain, hoarseness, hemoptysis, and cyanosis in that order. Associated generalized symptoms are commonly fever, chills, myalgia, malaise, and weight loss. In focal outbreaks where there is exposure to large numbers of spores, sudden onset and pleuritic pain are common. Pleural effusion, however, is rare. The chest film may show bilateral disease with the characteristic diffuse miliary type of lesion, or, more commonly, localized infiltrations, especially in the lower lobes. There may be hilar and peritracheal lymphadenopathy unaccompanied by other lesions. That infection is not localized to lungs alone is attested to by the frequent splenic calcification seen later and the occasional isolation of *H. capsulatum* from urine during the acute illness. In many patients lesions resolve completely, but in others calcification or fibrotic scarring persists. Calcified peribronchial nodes may compress the bronchus leading to bronchiectasis or may erode and result in broncholithiasis. A distinctive residue of primary infection is the solitary nodule of the lung, located just beneath the pleura, appearing roentgenographically as a "coin lesion."

Disseminated Forms. Rarely the disease progresses and resembles that form originally described by Darling. Pulmonary findings are often not prominent; illness is characterized instead by fever, enlargement of the liver and spleen, generalized lymphadenopathy, weight loss, anemia, and leukopenia. One particular feature may predominate, and illness then appears as endocarditis, pericarditis, meningitis, adrenal insufficiency, or multiple ulcerations of mouth, pharynx, larynx, stomach, or small or large bowel. Granulomatous uveitis has been considered, but not yet proved, to be due to *H. capsulatum.*

Chronic Cavitary Form. In older adult males especially, a chronic, cavitary pulmonary disease occurs that closely simulates and is often labeled tuberculosis. This form is characterized by cough, weight loss, dyspnea, low-grade fever, chest pain, and hemoptysis. This form is most likely a reactivation of a previously quiescent primary infection.

Diagnosis. The isolation in culture and microscopic identification of the fungus establish the diagnosis. In suspected cases of acute primary disease both sputum and urine should be cultured. In the widely disseminated forms, blood, bone marrow, cerebrospinal fluid, ulcer swabs, urine, sputum, lymph nodes, and material from liver biopsy may yield the fungus on culture. Conversion of a skin test from negative to positive and a titer of the complement-fixing antibodies that rises and falls or is in excess of 1:32 only support the clinical impression. A single positive histoplasmin skin test indicates only recent or remote exposure to this or related antigen. Frequently, both skin and complement-fixation tests will be negative in a patient with severe early disease.

Careful microscopic study of properly stained tissue sections may reveal characteristic fungal forms, providing additional supporting evidence for the clinical diagnosis (see Pathology).

Acute primary histoplasmosis should be considered in the differential diagnosis of any persistent febrile respiratory disease, especially those occurring after exposure to chicken or other bird excreta and in any pneumonia without appropriate bacterial organisms in sputum. Hepatosplenomegaly, lymphadenopathy, anemia, and leukopenia of the severe disseminated form may closely simulate Hodgkin's disease and leukemia. Mucosal alterations so closely resemble cancer that repeated biopsies for tissue studies have been performed, all with negative results, before cultures were done. As a general rule, histoplasmosis should be suspected in any patient with findings suggestive of tuberculosis but without supporting laboratory data.

Treatment. Amphotericin B is the most active presently available antifungal drug in the treatment of the disease in man. The drug is customarily given intravenously; a dose of 1.0 mg. dissolved in 500 ml. of a 5 per cent glucose solution is recommended as the first dose. Dosage should be increased daily by increments of 5 to 10 mg. At present there are many recommendations and no consensus as to optimal daily dosage (from 0.5 to 1.0 mg. per kilogram), duration of therapy (from 10 to 14 weeks), or total dosage (from irrelevant to at least 2 grams). Each infusion should be administered over at least a two-hour period. Such undesired side-effects as local thrombophlebitis, fever, chills, nausea, vomiting, anorexia, rise in serum urea nitrogen, hypokalemia, and anemia may occur in approximately 80 per cent of patients but should not require abandonment of the therapy. After treatment is stopped, most indices of renal function return toward normal, but in about 80 per cent of patients on higher drug doses values are never again the same as before treatment. Salicylates, antihistamines, and corticoids reduce the severity or frequency of such side-effects of treatment as nausea, chills, and fever.

A newer polypeptide drug, saramycetin (X-5079C) has striking antifungal activity in experimental mycoses in mice and appears, from early studies, to be effective in the natural disease in man. With doses of 4 to 10 mg. per kilogram per day administered subcutaneously, the drug improved patients, and the fungus could not be cultured from previously positive specimens. It was well tolerated, and side-effects were limited to a prompt retention of sulfobromophthalein and, to a lesser extent, direct reacting bilirubin. These laboratory values return to normal within a week of cessation of therapy.

A few patients with localized disease in the lungs have been helped by surgical excision of lesions.

Sulfonamides have a measurable benefit in infections in laboratory animals and a reported activity in disease in children.

Prognosis. Except in localized outbreaks with inhalation of large numbers of fungi, acute primary histoplasmosis is almost always a benign illness from which the patient recovers rapidly. Therapy usually has not been administered.

Since progressive disseminated disease is fatal in 80 to 90 per cent, and the chronic cavitary form in 30 per cent of cases, chemotherapy is indicated. The numbers of patients treated are generally small, and case fatality rates are only approximate. It is likely that 80 to 90 per cent of patients with severe disease have recovered with amphotericin B treatment.

Corticoid treatment has been associated with deleterious effects in experimental infections of animals and with relapse after amphotericin B therapy in man.

Butler, W. T.: Pharmacology, toxicity and therapeutic usefulness of amphotericin B. J.A.M.A., 195:371, 1966.
Drutz, D. J., Spickard, A., Rodgers, D. E., and Koenig, M. G.: Treatment of disseminated mycotic infections: A new approach to amphotericin B treatment. Amer. J. Med., 45:406, 1968.
Furcolow, M. L., Doto, I. L., Tosh, F. E., and Lynch, H. J., Jr.: Course and prognosis of untreated histoplasmosis. J.A.M.A., 177:292, 1961.
Witorsch, P., Andriole, V. T., Emmons, C. W., and Utz, J. P.: Antifungal agent X-5079C: Further studies in 39 patients. Amer. Rev. Resp. Dis., 93:876, 1966.

COCCIDIOIDOMYCOSIS
(Valley Fever)

Definition. Coccidioidomycosis is a systemic fungal disease, respiratory in origin, that spreads hematogenously to skin, subcutaneous tissues, bone, central nervous system, and other organs. Severity ranges from inapparent infection to fatal outcome.

History. In a series of papers between 1892 and 1898 Posadas and Wernicke described an illness characterized by severe skin lesions and widespread dissemination in a soldier from northern Argentina, hospitalized in Buenos Aires. The infection was caused by an organism they considered a protozoan. This misinterpretation was shared by Rixford and Gilchrist, who in 1894 and 1896 named the organism *Coccidioides* (considering it related to Coccidium) *immitis* Ophuls in 1900 correctly identified it as a fungus. Gifford and Dickson associated the disease they termed coccidioidomycosis with *San Joaquin Valley fever*, and mild disease in the majority of cases.

Etiology. *Coccidioides immitis* is a dimorphic fungus existing in either a tissue or a saprophytic form. Arthrospores from the saprophytic phase, when inhaled by man or inoculated into animals, germinate, with the formation of the distinctive spherule measuring from 10 to 70 μ in diameter. This ruptures, releasing 10 to 200 endospores that reinfect adjacent or remote tissue. Spherules or endospores on inoculation onto Sabouraud's glucose medium produce a cottony, aerial mycelium, composed of arthrospores (saprophytic form). Cutaneous hypersensitivity and complement-fixing antigens have been demonstrated. Mice and guinea pigs are susceptible to experimental infection.

Epidemiology. Coccidioidomycosis is endemic in desert areas of the United States (California, Arizona, New Mexico, Texas, southern Utah, Nevada), northern Mexico, and in northern Argentina and Paraguay. In parts of the western United States, 50 to 84 per cent of the population show delayed cutaneous hypersensitivity to coccidioidin. Disease in patients from other areas has been explained by infection from fomites. Infection is acquired by inhalation of dust from soil usually heavily infected with arthrospores. Both sexes are equally susceptible, and, although disease occurs in persons of all ages, it is most prevalent in those 25 to 55 years old. Laborers have increased risk of infection and of a large inoculum. Rodent burrows are important in protecting the fungus during the summer, and the rodents themselves are infected. The disease has been reported also in cows, dogs, gorillas, and apes. However, neither animal-to-man nor man-to-man contagion is known.

Pathology. In early lesions the reaction about endospores is pyogenic and similar to that in pneumonias of bacterial origin. Spherules, however, induce a histiocytic reaction with giant cells. Pulmonary lesions may progress with caseation, cavitation, pleuritis, and involvement of the peribronchial or peritracheal lymph nodes. As healing occurs, there is hyalinization of nonnecrotic granulomas. Solitary nodules resembling those of tuberculosis or histoplasmosis (q.v.) may result. Lesions of other organs are also both suppurative and granulomatous.

Clinical Manifestations. In 60 per cent of infections no illness suggestive of coccidioidomycosis can be identified. In the remaining 40 per cent an influenza-like illness can be diagnosed retrospectively (15 per cent), or a more severe illness causes the patient to see his physician at the time (25 per cent).

Primary Pulmonary Form. The incubation period varies from 7 to 28 days depending, probably, on the severity of exposure. The prototype of this illness, "valley fever," is well characterized by headache, backache, fever, malaise, cough, fatigue, and pleuritic pain, all resembling those of influenza. Valley fever differs, however, in the greater frequency of summer illness, erythema nodosum, arthritis, and eosinophilia. The appearance of the chest film is dependent on the severity of illness and may show peribronchial infiltration, patchy pneumonitis, thin-walled cavities, or hilar adenopathy. Laboratory studies reveal a leukocytosis, an increase of the erythrocyte sedimentation rate, and the transient appearance of circulating antibodies. Pleurisy with effusion and pericarditis are occasionally encountered.

Disseminated Form. Although more than 90 per cent of patients with primary pulmonary coccidioidomycosis recover completely, hematogenous dissemination may occur in a few cases either promptly or after a quiescent period. Characteristically there are burrowing abscesses and draining sinuses involving the skin, subcutaneous tissues, and bones. Meningitis and visceral organ involvement also are seen. The coccidioidin skin test is usually negative, whereas the complement-fixing antibody titer generally rises.

Benign Residual Form. Two to 8 per cent of patients are left with residual cavitary disease in the lungs. Hemoptysis, rupture with pneumothorax, and pleuritis with or without effusion are occasional complications. Solitary nodules (coccidioidomas) measuring from a few millimeters to 5 cm. in diameter resemble those of tuberculosis or histoplasmosis in the frequency of calcification, occasional excavation, and refilling. Diffuse pulmonary fibrosis is a common but not clinically important manifestation of residual disease. Bronchiectasis occurs with greater frequency in endemic areas and may be related to past infection with this fungus.

Primary Extrapulmonary Form. This is a rare form of disease that follows traumatic implantation of the skin or subcutaneous tissue. It is characterized by a local lesion with regional lymphadenopathy.

Diagnosis. The diagnosis of coccidioidomycosis is proved by the isolation of the fungus in culture or by the microscopic demonstration of characteristic spherules in properly stained tissue sections. Skin tests and serologic studies as described under Histoplasmosis (q.v.) have been more helpful in coccidioidomycosis, though often negative in early disease.

Coccidioidomycosis should be suspected as the cause of any febrile or pneumonic process in a patient living in or recently returned from an endemic area. Disseminated subcutaneous and osseous forms of the disease must be differentiated from bacterial cellulitis and osteomyelitis. All forms of the disease may resemble tuberculosis and other fungal infections, especially histoplasmosis.

Treatment. Amphotericin B, the only antifungal drug of demonstrated efficacy in coccidioidomycosis, is indicated in all cases of disseminated disease and should be administered as described for histoplasmosis (q.v.). In general, it is demonstrably less effective, but larger doses have been associated with dramatic responses in patients desperately ill with meningitis and osteomyelitis. In coccidioidal meningitis, intrathecal administration is necessary two to three times weekly in dosage of 0.5 to 1.0 mg. in 1 ml. of glucose solution, diluted with 5 to 10 ml. of cerebrospinal fluid and injected slowly. A cisternal rather than lumbar site of injection seems preferable. Even with these precautions, side effects of pain and paresthesias are not uncommon.

In benign residual coccidioidomycosis, complications of cavities are indications for pulmonary resection. Amphotericin B therapy pre- and post-operatively is a reasonable, though apparently not always necessary, adjunct to surgery. Coccidioidomas, rarely dangerous to the patient, cannot be distinguished beforehand from malignant lesions, and surgical excision is usually necessary.

Bed rest and supportive therapy are sufficient treatment for the influenza-like primary form of disease.

Prognosis. The disease is life-threatening in less than 1 in 1000 infections. A negative skin test and a continuing high, or rising, titer of circulating antibodies has been associated with disseminated disease and a poor prognosis. The case fatality rate in untreated meningitis has been virtually 100 per cent.

Ajello, L. (ed.): Coccidioidomycosis. Phoenix, University of Arizona Press, 1967.

Fiese, M. J.: Coccidioidomycosis. Springfield, Ill., Charles C Thomas, 1958.

Smith, C. E., Saito, M. T., and Simons, S. A.: Pattern of 39,500 serologic tests in coccidioidomycosis. J.A.M.A., 160:546, 1956.

BLASTOMYCOSIS
(North American)

Definition. Blastomycosis is a chronic systemic fungal disease, respiratory in origin, which, classically, disseminates to the skin and occasionally to subcutaneous tissue, bone, and other organs.

History. In 1894 Gilchrist and in 1898 Gilchrist and Stokes reported the first two cases and named the responsible fungus *Blastomyces dermatitidis.*

Etiology. *B. dermatitidis* is a dimorphic fungus existing in tissue as a yeastlike form (8 to 15 μ, rarely 30 μ), with a characteristic thick wall (0.5 to 0.75 μ). The yeast form reproduces by budding, and the typical bud is characterized by its large size and attachment to the parent cell by a persistent wall and a wide pore. On Sabouraud's glucose medium *B. dermatitidis* grows as a white mycelium composed of slender hyphae to which are attached, either directly or by lateral slender stalks (conidiophores), smooth spherical 2 to 10 μ forms (conidia). Skin hypersensitivity and complement-fixing antigens have been demonstrated. Mice and other laboratory animals are susceptible to experimental infection.

Epidemiology. Blastomycosis was at first exclusively American in distribution: Canada, Mexico, Central America, northern Latin America, and, in 98 per cent of reported cases, the United States. Recently, however, cases have been reported from widely separated sites in Africa. The disease affects all ages, but there is a slightly higher frequency in the third and fourth decades. Males are affected six to nine times more frequently than females. Man is infected by inhalation of conidia, but the saprophytic source of the fungus in nature is not known. Benign, subclinical cases have been reported, but skin test studies do not support a high incidence of infection in certain areas similar to that of histoplasmosis and coccidioidomycosis. Multiple cases in one small town have been reported.

Pathology. The characteristic tissue response to *B. dermatitidis* is a combination of suppuration and epitheloid and giant cell granulomas. In the lung the disease may be localized or may spread as a bronchopneumonia. Cavitation and circumscribed, calcific nodules are rarely encountered.

The skin lesions reveal characteristically pseudoepitheliomatous hyperplasia and micro-abscesses in which *B. dermatitidis* may be seen. In bone, subcutaneous tissue, meninges, prostate, epididymis, and other organs the histologic appearance is again a combination of suppuration and granulomas.

Clinical Manifestations. *Primary Pulmonary Form.* Primary pulmonary blastomycosis begins usually as a mild respiratory infection (rarely as a fulminant pneumonia) with cough, pleuritic chest pain and, occasionally, hemoptysis. As the disease progresses, generalized symptoms of fever, night sweats, anorexia, and weight loss appear. Physical signs may not be prominent. However, there may be dullness, decreased breath sounds, and rales. Roentgenographically, manifestations vary from those of a consolidated lobar pneumonia to multiple infiltrations. Hilar adenopathy is common, localized nodules are less so, and cavitation is rare. Although pleural disease is common, effusion is characteristically extremely rare.

Cutaneous Form. Although cutaneous blastomycosis represents spread from a primary pulmonary infection, the presenting complaint of many patients is a cutaneous lesion, either solitary or multiple. The initial papule or pustule progresses within weeks or months into an ulcerated or warty lesion. The advancing border of this lesion is serpiginous, dusky red, or violaceous, elevated 1 to 3 mm., and has an outer edge that slopes abruptly. The base of the lesion contains small abscesses, from which characteristic budding yeast cells can be demonstrated. The central area may become crusted or, in older lesions, may show a tendency to healing with a thin atrophic scar. In contrast to the skin lesion that follows accidental laboratory implantation, regional lymphadenopathy does not occur.

Other Systemic Forms. A subcutaneous form of the disease consists of single or more often multiple soft to firm nodules, palpable deep beneath the skin. These may enlarge to become bulging abscesses, but in various stages contain pus. The skin over the nodules may have a slightly reddish hue.

Osteomyelitis or periostitis of long bones or spine occurs frequently. The first manifestation of disease may be a psoas abscess. A septic arthritis may occur either alone or by extension from bone.

Genitourinary blastomycosis is frequently seen in men and is manifested by pain and swelling of the epididymis, prostate, or seminal vesicles.

There may also be involvement of the central nervous system, eye, adrenals, thyroid, and larynx. In contrast to paracoccidioidomycosis, the gastrointestinal tract is almost never involved.

Diagnosis. Although skin lesions may be strongly suggestive, the diagnosis of blastomycosis is confirmed by the finding of typical budding yeast cells in direct preparations or by the culture and identification of *B. dermatitidis* from pus or lesions. When appropriate, sputum, urine, cerebrospinal fluid, bone marrow, or other biopsy and autopsy tissue should also be cultured. Skin tests are almost always negative and, especially in earlier stages of the disease, serologic procedures may show a higher titer or a positive reaction only to *Histoplasma capsulatum*.

The pulmonary form of the disease is rarely diagnosed clinically or roentgenographically and is usually thought to be tuberculosis or, less frequently, sarcoidosis, acute bacterial pneumonia, malignancy, or other fungal infections more common in the geographic area. Skin lesions are suggestive of basal cell carcinoma, tuberculosis, nodulo-ulcerative syphilid, pyoderma, or other fungal infections. Other systemic manifestations mimic those of tuberculosis of staphylococcal infection.

Treatment. Amphotericin B has been used extensively for all forms of the disease. Details of administration are given under Histoplasmosis. Rather less drug is necessary, however, and for involvement of other organs and tissues than bones, 1 to 2 grams is usually sufficient.

2-Hydroxystilbamidine, administered intravenously, is probably less toxic than amphotericin B, and has been effective in many patients. The usual dosage has been 225 mg. per day and 8.0 grams per course of therapy.

A new antifungal agent, saramycetin (X-5079C), appears from early studies to be effective and well tolerated. Directions for its use may be found under Histoplasmosis.

Surgical drainage of abscesses is frequently indicated. Chemotherapy before and after surgery is advisable.

Prognosis. Pulmonary infection of an inapparent or benign form occurs only rarely. Blastomycosis is, if untreated, a chronic and usually progressive disease. Cutaneous and other disseminated disease is eventually fatal in 10 to 30 per cent of cases.

Except with moribund patients chemotherapy usually effects a prompt recovery. Relapse requiring additional therapy has occurred, however, in at least 10 to 15 per cent of patients.

Abernathy, R. S.: Clinical manifestations of pulmonary blastomycosis. Ann. Intern. Med., 51:707, 1959.

Busey, J. F.: Blastomycosis: A review of 198 collected cases in Veterans Administration Hospitals. Amer. Rev. Resp. Dis., 89:659, 1964.

Lockwood, W. R., Allison, F. L., Batson, B. E., and Busey, J. F.: The treatment of North American blastomycosis: Ten years' experience. Amer. Rev. Resp. Dis., 100:314, 1969.

CRYPTOCOCCOSIS
(European Blastomycosis, Torulosis)

Definition. Cryptococcosis is a chronic systemic fungal disease, respiratory in origin, which disseminates characteristically to the central nervous system and occasionally to the genitourinary tract, skin, bone, and other organs.

History. Sanfelice first isolated the fungus from peach juice in 1894. In the same year Busse and in 1895 Buschke described the first case of human disease. Von Hausemann in 1905 was apparently first to observe the fungus in meningitis, and in 1916 Stoddard and Cutler first isolated the fungus from the brain of man.

Etiology. Cryptococcosis is due to a thin-walled, spherical to oval fungus, *Cryptococcus neoformans*, measuring 4 to 20 μ in diameter. It is surrounded by a polysaccharide capsule, the size of which varies from strain to strain but which may equal in thickness the diameter of the cell. Reproduction is by budding, and the buds are attached to the parent cell by a thin wall and narrow pore. On Sabouraud's glucose medium, soft, mucoid, cream-colored colonies are formed. Recently a hyphal form of the fungus has been found on culture media, in human tissue, and in human specimens. The morphology and taxonomy of the fungus are currently undergoing re-evaluation. Mice and other laboratory animals can be infected. *C. neoformans* is a poor antigen, and no skin test or complement-fixing antigen is commercially available.

Epidemiology. The disease is worldwide in distribution, affects all ages (40 to 60 years more commonly), and males almost twice as frequently as females. The fungus has been shown by Emmons to be a saprophyte in excreta of pigeons, although the birds need not be infected systemically. Epidemics of mastitis in dairy cattle and spontaneous cryptococcosis in the cow, horse, dog, cat, leopard, and other animals have been reported. Animal-to-man or man-to-man contagion is unknown.

Pathology. The distinctive feature of cryptococcosis is the paucity of cellular reaction and the absence of suppuration, necrosis, caseation, infected abscesses, or hemorrhage. In early lesions the tissue granulomas are gelatinous (mucinous), and in older lesions these may be granulomas with tissue macrophages, giant cells, lymphocytes, and plasma cells.

Lung lesions may be single or multiple, but the most common is a subpleural nodule. In cases of meningitis there is thickening of the meninges, especially at the base, with exudation and occasionally hydrocephalus. Neural parenchyma, especially of the optic nerves, may be involved, and there may be compression of tissue by expanding masses of fungal cells.

Clinical Manifestations. *Pulmonary Form.* Cryptococcosis limited to the lungs is being recognized more frequently, and is only currently being characterized. Cough, sputum production, low-grade fever, malaise, and weight loss may be present. Pleural effusion rarely occurs. Physical findings when produced by infection are due to consolidation. The chest film shows, usually, a solitary nodule in the lower lung fields, less frequently localized, or bronchopneumonic infiltration and pleural effusion. Miliary lesions are rare except in patients with lymphomas. In many cases symptoms and physical and roentgenographic findings are those of the underlying disease, e.g., bronchitis, inactive tuberculosis, or bronchiectasis, to which the Cryptococcus is only an asymptomatic superinfection or a transitory, mild complicating pneumonia.

Central Nervous System Involvement. In cryptococcal meningitis the onset may be acute and the course fulminant, but more commonly begins insidiously. In about 10 per cent of patients infection is present without symptoms or findings suggestive of meningeal or nervous system disease. Intermittent and increasing headache, impairment of vision, and vertigo commonly occur. In nearly one fourth of the cases the clinical picture has been so suggestive of an expanding intracranial lesion that surgical procedures have been done. Characteristic cerebrospinal fluid findings are pleocytosis with lymphocytes predominating, low glucose, and high protein.

Other Disseminated Forms. Skin lesions in the form of ulcers, papules, pustules, mucosal ulcers, or nodules are seen in 10 per cent of cases. Bone lesions occur in 10 per cent of cases (and in the first case described by Busse-Buschke). Pain, swelling, and a slowly progressive course are suggestive of osteomyelitis. Periostitis, occasionally seen in actinomycosis, coccidioidomycosis, and blastomycosis, is rare in cryptococcosis. Septic arthritis occasionally occurs.

Lesions in the kidney, with perirenal abscess, in the prostate, adrenals, and endocardium are sometimes encountered. Recently typical acute pyelonephritis caused by *C. neoformans* has been described.

Diagnosis. The diagnosis is established by the isolation of *C. neoformans* in culture from cerebrospinal fluid, sputum, blood, pleural effusion, ascites, skin, or bone biopsy material. Occasionally, and even in cases of frank meningitis, fungus is cultured from cerebrospinal fluid only after many attempts. In these patients the fungus may be cultured from other specimens, especially urine. In partially treated cases the fungus cannot be cultured from cerebrospinal fluid, but may be clearly identified with India ink preparation.

Cryptococcosis should be suspected especially in patients with leukemia, Hodgkin's disease, sarcoidosis, or diabetes mellitus who develop fever or central nervous system manifestations.

Cryptococcal pulmonary disease must be distinguished from tuberculosis, other fungal infections and (less frequently) from bacterial pneumonia. Except for a more prolonged course, cryptococcal meningitis resembles that resulting from tuberculosis. Cryptococcal adrenal insufficiency, endocarditis, skin lesions, and pyelonephritis must be distinguished from identical disease caused by bacteria.

Treatment. Amphotericin B has been highly successful therapy in cryptococcal infections. The methods of intravenous treatment are described in the article on Histoplasmosis. Intrathecal therapy, described under Coccidioidomycosis, has been recommended for those patients with severe, life-threatening disease or for those whose disease has relapsed following intravenous therapy. 5-Fluorocytosine has appeared active in some patients, but it is too early to state its exact role, daily dose, duration of therapy, or toxicity.

Prognosis. Prior to amphotericin B therapy

there were no reported survivors of cryptococcal meningitis. In some patients, however, the course of disease was prolonged (up to 16 years) and was marked by occasional remissions. With amphotericin B therapy, survival rates approximate 85 per cent. Relapse occurs in approximately 15 per cent of treated patients.

Other forms of the disease have been reported in the past to be cured by surgical excision of lesions. With amphotericin B treatment more than 90 per cent of patients with non-central nervous system disease will survive.

Death from infection, despite treatment, is much more likely in those patients with underlying lymphoma, leukemia, or diabetes.

Butler, W. T., Alling, D. W., Spickard, A., and Utz, J. P.: The diagnostic and prognostic value of clinical and laboratory findings in cryptococcal meningitis: A follow-up of 40 patients. New Eng. J. Med., 270:59, 1964

Littman, M. L., and Zimmerman, L. E.: Cryptococcosis. New York, Grune and Stratton, Inc., 1956.

Tynes, B., Mason, K. N., Jennings, A. E., and Bennett, J. E.: Variant forms of pulmonary cryptococcosis. Ann. Intern. Med., 69:1117, 1968.

ACTINOMYCOSIS

Definition. Actinomycosis is a chronic, systemic disease characterized by multiple indurated abscesses and sinus tracts characteristically in the face, neck, chest, and abdomen.

History. Lebert is credited with the first report, in 1857, of actinomycosis in man. Bollinger described the disease in cattle in 1876. In 1877 Harz named the causative organism *Actinomyces bovis*. In 1878 Israel clearly defined the disease in man by a summary of the clinical and pathologic characteristics observed in 38 patients. The same author in collaboration with Wolff in 1891 succeeded in growing the micro-organism in anaerobic culture. In 1910 Lord observed *A. bovis* in and about carious teeth and tonsillar crypts in the mouths of otherwise normal persons.

Etiology. Actinomycosis in man is caused by *A. israelii* and in cattle by *A. bovis*, but species characteristics overlap. In the normal mouth *A. israelii* grows as a pleomorphic rod-shaped bacterial form and in tissues as a granule. In draining pus, mycelial clumps measuring 1 to 2 mm. in diameter and white to yellow in color have been termed "sulfur" granules. Microscopically these are composed of 0.5 to 1.0 μ hyphae which stain gram-positive. On agar media under strictly anaerobic conditions, *A. israelii* grows as a white spherical or lobulated colony. Laboratory animals are not, generally, susceptible to experimental infection.

Epidemiology. The disease is worldwide in distribution. During the first part of the twentieth century it was the most common of the systemic mycoses but has been decreasing lately. Males are affected almost twice as frequently as females, and illness seems more common among farmers and in rural areas. Disease is produced by direct invasion of contiguous tissues by *A. israelii* commonly present in the mouth or bowel. There is usually concurrent infection with anaerobic bacteria. Disease in the brain, heart valves, or extremities may be exceptional instances of hematogenous dissemination. Disease in cows, dogs, or swine has no contagious relation to that in man.

Pathology. In tissues the characteristic and classic findings are the actinomycotic granules. These are usually found in abscesses and are surrounded by polymorphonuclear leukocytes. Chronic granulomatous reactions are also seen with giant cells, especially about granules.

Clinical Manifestations. Cervicofacial Form. The cervicofacial form occurs in approximately half of all cases. Infection probably spreads secondarily to trauma or to carious teeth or infected tonsils. The subcutaneous tissues at the angle of the mandible and of the neck have a characteristic "woody" or indurated feeling, and the skin over these areas is reddened and may have single or multiple draining sinus tracts. Pain is seldom prominent even with osteomyelitic or periosteal lesions of bone.

Thoracic Form. In 15 per cent of cases disease arises from aspiration into the bronchi of *A. israelii* or in a few instances from extension of disease from the esophagus to mediastinal tissues and secondarily to pleura and lung. Fever and cough are minimal early in the illness. As disease progresses to consolidation, pleurisy, and draining sinuses, prominent symptoms are weight loss, night sweats, and high fever. Rib involvement occurs occasionally, pleural effusion rarely.

Abdominal Form. Actinomycosis of the abdomen generally follows appendicitis, appendiceal abscess, a perforating lesion of the stomach, or a diverticulum of the large bowel. An abdominal mass is usually palpable, and may be extensive; and there may be burrowing sinus tracts, some of which may open to the skin in the inguinal or other regions. Retroperitoneal and thoracic spread through the diaphragm are common.

Other Forms. Approximately 10 per cent of patients have lesions in the brain, heart valves, anorectal area, or subcutaneous tissue of the extremities. Rare instances of actinomycosis of the finger have been attributed to injury to the hand by an adversary's tooth.

Diagnosis. The diagnosis of actinomycosis is supported by the finding in pus of granules that microscopically are composed of gram-positive, branching, often beaded hyphae. It should be emphasized that granules may be expressed from otherwise normal tonsils and may not be found in cerebrospinal fluid in cases of central nervous system disease. The diagnosis is confirmed by the isolation of the micro-organism in anaerobic culture from a lesion.

Skin test and serologic methods of confirmation are unreliable and unavailable.

Cervicofacial forms of actinomycosis must be distinguished from Ludwig's angina, tuberculosis, osteomyelitis, and malignancy. The thoracic form of disease is suggestive of tuberculosis, other fungal infections, and malignancy. Abdominal actinomycosis is often suspected of being tuberculosis, malignant disease, and, occasionally, amebiasis.

Treatment. Penicillin, first used for actinomycosis in 1944, continues to be the best drug in treating all forms of the disease. Although most strains are inhibited in vitro by levels of 0.1 unit per milliliter, the nature of the pathologic process leads often to treatment failures and necessitates prolonged therapy. Doses of 1 to 20 million units daily for at least six weeks or until lesions have healed are recommended. Other antimicrobial drugs, especially tetracycline, chloramphenicol, and streptomycin, may be of supplemental benefit.

Surgical resection and incision and drainage of chronically infected tissues are important adjunctive therapeutic measures.

Prognosis. Prior to antimicrobial therapy, prognosis for life was poor in all forms. With penicillin therapy, the approximate recovery rates are: cervicofacial, 90 per cent; abdominal, 80 per cent; and thoracic, 40 per cent.

Cope, V. Z.: Actinomycosis. London, Oxford University Press, 1938.

Nichols, D. R., and Herrell, W. E.: Penicillin in the treatment of actinomycosis. J. Lab. Clin. Med., 32:1405, 1947.

Peabody, J. W., Jr., and Seabury, J. H.: Actinomycosis and nocardiosis. J. Chron. Dis., 5:374, 1957.

NOCARDIOSIS

Definition. Nocardiosis is a chronic systemic disease, respiratory in origin, that disseminates characteristically to the brain and occasionally to the kidney, heart, spleen, and other organs.

History. Nocard in 1889 described an acid-fast, aerobic actinomycete isolated from cattle on the island of Guadeloupe with a lymphatic disease called farcy. In 1890 Eppinger first reported human nocardiosis in a glass blower, characterized by pulmonary disease and metastatic brain abscesses. The subsequent history of this disease is marked by clinical and mycologic confusion with actinomycosis.

Etiology. Of the 35 species of nocardia, *N. asteroides* and *N. brasiliensis* are important pathogens for man; *N. brasiliensis* will be discussed under Maduromycosis.

N. asteroides in tissues appears as septate hyphae 0.5 to 1.0 μ in diameter, which may fragment into rod or coccoid forms that are gram-positive and partially acid-fast. In contrast to actinomycosis, granule formation is rare. In artificial media reproduction occurs by elongation, branching, and fragmentation. The micro-organism is aerobic and thermophilic but grows at room temperature as well. Colonies are pale yellow or creamy. Most strains in large inocula produce acute disease in guinea pigs and rabbits.

Epidemiology. The disease is world-wide in distribution without recognized increased incidence in any geographic area. It occurs more frequently in older adults and twice as often in males as in females. The micro-organism may be isolated from soil and from compost heaps. Mild or self-limited pulmonary nocardiosis may occur, but skin test surveys demonstrating widespread infection have not been done. Mastitis in dairy cattle and disease in dogs and other domestic animals have been recognized, but animal-to-man or man-to-man contagion is not known. The frequency of disease appears to be increasing.

Pathology. Suppuration and abscess formation are seen more often than granulomas. When the latter are present giant cells and caseation necrosis typical of tuberculosis are rare. The organism in tissue is stained well with Gram's stain by the Brown and Brenn method.

Clinical Manifestations. *Pulmonary Form.* In approximately 75 per cent of cases, frank pulmonary parenchymal disease is seen. The patient complains of cough productive of purulent and sometimes blood-tinged sputum. In 25 per cent of patients, pleurisy with effusion occurs, resulting occasionally in characteristic pleural-cutaneous fistulas. Fever and other systemic symptoms are common. Roentgenographically, the disease varies from localized nodules and infiltrations to dense lobular consolidation with abscess formation. However, cavitation is uncommon, and miliary lesions are rare.

Recently some cases of pulmonary alveolar proteinosis have been associated with concurrent Nocardia (and other microbial) infections, but causal relationships have not been established.

Disseminated Form. In contrast to actinomycosis, but like other systemic mycoses, *N. asteroides* infection spreads hematogenously. Brain abscess is an important feature historically and clinically. In contrast to cryptococcosis, fever is prominent and meningitis uncommon. The liver, kidney, spleen, subcutaneous tissue, and, rarely, adrenals, eyes, or other organs may be involved.

Diagnosis. The diagnosis of nocardiosis is confirmed by the culture and identification of the micro-organism. Despite occasional contrary opinions, *N. asteroides* is rarely a saprophyte in man, and isolation strongly suggests etiologic relationship to disease present. Diagnostic skin and serologic tests have not been generally available.

The pattern of lung and metastatic brain lesions is suggestive of malignancy and of suppurative disease caused by a variety of pyogenic organisms. The pulmonary form resembles an acute bacterial pneumonia or tuberculosis. Nocardiosis may coexist occasionally with tuberculosis or may be a complication of other disease, especially pemphigus, leukemia, and Hodgkin's disease.

Treatment. The sulfonamide drugs are the most effective therapeutic agents in experimental infection of laboratory animals and in human disease. Dosage should be adjusted to maintain a serum concentration of approximately 10 mg. per 100 ml., and treatment must be continued for at least two to three months. In some patients the infection does not respond to sulfonamide alone, and combination therapy with other antimicrobial drugs is necessary. Streptomycin and the tetracyclines are of demonstrated value in vitro and in experimental infections.

Incision and drainage of abscesses are necessary and helpful.

Prognosis. Man probably has a significant natural immunity to this micro-organism as indicated by the few cases of disease and the ubiquity of the organism in nature. Once active infection has occurred, however, disease is often progressive, resistant to treatment, and fatal. Even with treatment, probably not more than 50 per cent of patients recover.

Murray, J. F., Finegold, S. M., Froman, S., and Will, D. W.: The changing spectrum of nocardiosis. Amer. Rev. Resp. Dis., 83:315, 1961.

Peabody, J. W., Jr., and Seabury, J. H.: Actinomycosis and nocardiosis; A review of basic differences in therapy. Amer. J. Med., 28:99, 1960.

Weed, L. A., Andersen, H. A., Good, C. A., and Baggenstoss, A. H.: Nocardiosis: Clinical, bacteriologic and pathologic aspects. New Eng. J. Med., 253:1137, 1955.

Wilson, D. E., and Williams, T. W., Jr.: In vitro susceptibility of Nocardia to antimicrobial agents. In Hobby, G. L. (ed.): Antimicrobial Agents and Chemotherapy, Ann Arbor, American Society for Microbiology, 1965, p. 408, 1966.

SPOROTRICHOSIS

Definition. Sporotrichosis is a chronic systemic fungal disease, acquired usually by traumatic implantation and localized to cutaneous lymphatic tissues, or rarely by the respiratory route with dissemination throughout the body.

History. From a patient at Johns Hopkins Hospital, in 1896 Schenck isolated a fungus that was identified by E. F. Smith as Sporotrichum; it was called *Sporotrichum schenckii* by Hektoen and Perkins in 1900. A great number of cases were seen subsequently in France, and more than 2800 cases in a single epidemic in the gold mines of South Africa.

Etiology. *Sporotrichum schenckii*, a dimorphic fungus, is occasionally observed in tissues as round to cigar-shaped yeastlike forms. On Sabouraud glucose medium at room temperature, a white, cottony, aerial mycelium appears that in three to seven days becomes wrinkled and changes in color from cream to black. Microscopically, branching, septate hyphae are seen, 2 μ in width, bearing directly or on lateral branches ovoid to spherical bodies (conidia) measuring 2 to 4 by 2 to 6 μ in diameter. Mice are susceptible to experimental infection. Delayed cutaneous hypersensitivity and agglutinogen antigens have been demonstrated.

Epidemiology. The disease is world-wide in distribution; it has appeared epidemically in South Africa and in localized outbreaks in Mexico and Florida. It is more common in the male. It frequently affects laborers, farmers, and florists and is considered a true occupational disease. The fungus exists in its saprophytic form in soil, peat moss, decaying vegetation, and on thorns. In the cutaneous lymphatic forms, infection results from accidental implantation into the skin. In disseminated forms, the mode of entry is probably respiratory. Spontaneous sporotrichosis has been reported in dogs, horses, mules, cats, and other animals, and human disease has resulted from animal contact. Direct transfer from man to man is not known to occur.

Pathology. The histopathologic reaction to *S. schenckii* is varied, frequently acute and suppurative, but also subacute or chronic. In some instances granulomas are seen with epithelioid and giant cells either diffusely distributed or localized in a typical tubercle. Fungi may be seen more readily after staining with a modified Schiff-MacManus technique.

Clinical Forms. *Cutaneous Lymphatic Form.* The earliest lesion is a pustule, papule, or nodule of the skin appearing characteristically on a finger and at a site where the patient may recall an earlier, seemingly insignificant scratch or prick. The nodule enlarges, becomes red to violaceous, and is followed by a chain of subcutaneous nodules along regional lymphatics. These at first freely movable nodules may become attached to the skin, and may ulcerate and drain a thin gray to yellow pus. Streaking and pain characteristic of acute lymphangitis are not present. Generalized symptoms are rare.

Other Forms. Other forms may appear secondary to the cutaneous lymphatic lesion either by direct extension to contiguous subcutaneous tissue, bone, and joint or by hematogenous spread to distant sites. Sometimes the original site of infection is inapparent, and the disease presents as a septic arthritis or osteomyelitis. Less frequently, there may be involvement of the eye, lungs, gastrointestinal tract, central nervous system, or skin. In disseminated disease, systemic symptoms of fever, weight loss, inanition, malaise, pain at sites of lesion, anemia, and leukocytosis are commonly present. Disease limited to the lungs or localized there suggests that there is a respiratory form acquired by inhalation of the fungus. Too few cases have thus far been reported to characterize this form at present.

Diagnosis. Although the diagnosis may seem readily apparent in the cutaneous lymphatic form of disease, the clinical impression is confirmed by the culture and identification of the fungus. Agglutination or complement-fixation serologic and skin tests may be helpful, but are not generally available.

Cutaneous lymphatic sporotrichosis must be distinguished from tularemia, pyoderma of bacterial origin, and other fungal infections. Disseminated disease resembles tuberculosis, staphylococcal osteomyelitis, or neoplastic disease.

Treatment. The cutaneous lymphatic form of disease responds slowly but progressively to the oral administration of iodides in the form of a saturated solution (1 gram per milliliter) of potassium iodide given in dosage of 2 ml. four times daily. Treatment should be prolonged one to two months beyond the time of apparent healing.

Disseminated disease, especially of bone and joints, is frequently resistant to iodide therapy. Dramatic improvement has been seen in a few patients treated with amphotericin B and saramycetin (X-5079C) (see Histoplasmosis), and for this form of disease these drugs are recommended.

Prognosis. Untreated cutaneous lymphatic sporotrichosis may persist for many months to years. Treated lesions respond slowly but com-

pletely. Disseminated disease is progressive and usually fatal unless treated.

Baum, G. L., Donnerberg, R. L., Stewart, D., Mulligan, W. J., and Putnam, L. R.: Pulmonary sporotrichosis. New Eng. J. Med., 280:410, 1969.
Duran, R. J., Coventry, M. B., Weed, L. A., and Kierland, R. K.: Sporotrichosis: A report of twenty-three cases in the upper extremity. J. Bone Joint Surg. (Amer.), 39:1330, 1957.
Mikkelsen, W. M., Brandt, R. L., and Harrell, E. R.: Sporotrichosis: A report of 12 cases including two with skeletal involvement. Ann. Intern. Med., 47:435, 1957.

MUCORMYCOSIS*

Definition. Mucormycosis is an acute and usually fulminant systemic fungal disease originating in the paranasal sinuses, orbit, bronchi, or intestines and disseminating by the hematogenous route to the brain, kidney, heart, and other organs.

History. In 1876 Fürbringer reported the first documented case of human pulmonary mucormycosis. In 1884 Lichtheim demonstrated the pathogenicity of Mucorales in rabbits, and in 1885 Paltauf first described a case with central nervous system involvement. Baker, Bauer, and Sheldon have made important recent contributions to our knowledge of the pathogenesis of the disease.

Etiology. Mucormycosis is caused by species of three genera—Absidia, Rhizopus and Mucor—of the order Mucorales. In tissues fungi appear as broad (6 to 50 μ), nonseptate hyphae. On Sabouraud glucose medium at room temperature there is rapid growth of a large, aerial mycelium that microscopically consists of hyphae bearing large (100 μ) globular sacs (sporangia) containing small (6 to 8.5 μ) round to elliptical bodies (spores). Laboratory animals, especially those treated with steroids or made diabetic by alloxan, can be experimentally infected.

Epidemiology. The disease is worldwide in distribution. It occurs equally in all races and at all ages, but twice as often in males. A prominent feature of illness is the association with diabetes mellitus (40 per cent of cases) and less frequently with leukemia, lymphomas, tuberculosis and burns. Fungi of the order Mucorales readily colonize dead plant and animal tissues and are exceptionally widespread saprophytes in soil and fruits. They are commonly called "bread molds." Infection is exogenous. In experimental infections in laboratory animals, induction of diabetic acidosis by alloxan has been shown to impair tissue mast cells and the degranulation and migration of polymorphonuclear leukocytes to the site of infection. Naturally occurring disease has been reported in horses, dogs, cows, pigs, and birds. Animal-to-man or man-to-man spread is not known to occur.

Pathology. The histopathology of mucormycosis is characterized by necrosis, acute inflammation, and suppuration. An especially prominent feature is early invasion of blood vessels

---

*See also Phycomycosis.

with arteritis, thrombosis, and infarction. Giant cells are seen occasionally. Lesions may be found in the central nervous system, orbit, paranasal sinuses, lung, gastrointestinal tract, skin, heart, and kidneys.

Clinical Forms. Mucormycosis is an acute, inflammatory process either in the nose or paranasal sinuses with purulent nasal discharge and a characteristic gangrenous nasal mucosa, or unilaterally in the orbit with ophthalmoplegia, edema, proptosis, and chemosis. Disease may then spread to involve heart, kidneys, or brain (one third of cases).

Lung disease is that of a primary pneumonia followed by infarction and abscess formation. Myocardial infarction from mycotic occlusion of a coronary artery has been reported in three patients. In the gastrointestinal form ulcerations are produced, usually in the terminal ileum and large intestine or rarely in the esophagus and stomach. There is a preponderance of cerebral involvement in diabetic patients, of the pulmonary form in leukemic patients, and of more widespread disease in nonleukemic, nondiabetic patients.

Diagnosis. Although the large nonseptate hyphae are distinctive when seen in stained tissues, the diagnosis is confirmed and the genus of Mucorales identified only when the fungus is isolated in culture.

Mucormycosis must be distinguished from acute cellulitis and central nervous system infection owing to pyogenic bacteria, from tuberculosis or other fungal disease of the lung, and from ulcerative enteritis and colitis of other causes.

Treatment. Amphotericin B (see Histoplasmosis) is effective in experimental infection in the rat, has been used in a few patients, and deserves additional trial. The amount of drug necessary has not been determined.

A few patients have responded to control of the underlying diabetes and one at least to surgical resection of diseased tissue.

Prognosis. Until 1955 the patients in all cases reported had died. Recently a few patients have responded to control of the underlying diabetes, to resection of diseased tissue, and to amphotericin B treatment. The disease should be considered potentially and rather rapidly fatal if untreated.

Baker, R. D.: Pulmonary mucormycosis. Amer. J. Path., 32:287, 1956.

Bauer, H., Ajello, L., Adams, E., and Hernandez, D. U.: Cerebral mucormycosis: Pathogenesis of the disease. Amer. J. Med., 18:822, 1955.

Ferry, A. P.: Cerebral mucormycosis (phycomycosis). Ocular findings and review of the literature. Survey Ophthal., 6:1, 1961.

McBride, R. A., Corson, J. M., and Dammin, G. J.: Mucormycosis. Amer. J. Med., 28:832, 1960.

Sheldon, W. H., and Bauer, H.: The role of predisposing factors in experimental fungal infections. Lab. Invest., 11:1184, 1962.

PARACOCCIDIOIDOMYCOSIS
(South American Blastomycosis)

Definition. Paracoccidioidomycosis is a chronic systemic fungal disease, probably respiratory or gastrointestinal in origin, with dissemination to the lymph nodes, skin, lung, and other organs.

History. Lutz in 1908 first described the disease and the organism observed in tissues of a Brazilian patient. In 1909 and 1912, Splendore described more fully the characteristics of the disease and the fungus.

Etiology. The disease is caused by a dimorphic fungus, *Paracoccidioides brasiliensis*, which appears in tissues and exudates as a multiple-budding yeastlike organism 2 to 60 μ in diameter. The bud is characterized by a thin wall (0.2 to 1.0 μ) and narrow pore. At temperatures less than 30° C. on Sabouraud glucose medium, a white (later brown) membranous or wrinkled mycelium appears that microscopically is composed of branching hyphae and oval forms (conidia). Delayed cutaneous hypersensitivity and complement-fixing antigens have been demonstrated. Guinea pigs and mice can be experimentally infected.

Epidemiology. Except for a report of one patient from Oregon, the disease occurs exclusively in residents of Central and South America and is especially prevalent in Brazil. It is approximately ten times more frequent in males, and is slightly more frequent in persons 40 to 50 years of age. Manual laborers and farmers seem especially susceptible. Infection is considered to be exogenous, but a saprophytic, environmental source of fungi is not known. Disease in animals and animal-to-man or man-to-man spread are unknown. Widespread infection of a benign form has been suggested by skin test surveys.

Pathology. The histopathologic reaction to *P. brasiliensis* may be suppurative with abscess formation; in other sites it may be granulomatous with fibroblasts, macrophages, lymphocytes, caseation, and giant cells containing organisms. Lesions are seen in the mucosa of the gastrointestinal tract, lymph nodes, spleen, lungs, and liver.

Clinical Forms. *Primary.* The primary lesion is commonly on the oral or nasal mucosa. Rarely, the conjunctival or anorectal mucosa may be involved. The earliest lesion is a papule that ulcerates and spreads to adjacent tissue.

Cutaneous Form. A variety of skin lesions may be seen, most of which progress to an ulcerative, crusted form suggestive of blastomycosis. In contrast, however, regional lymphadenopathy frequently accompanies skin lesions only in paracoccidioidomycosis. A keloidal form (Lobo's disease) of milder nature, without lymphadenopathy and caused by a different species (*P. loboi*), may be another type of paracoccidioidomycosis.

Lymphangitic Form. In this form there are lymphangitis and enlargement of regional lymph nodes, which suppurate and drain. Cervical and submandibular nodes are most commonly affected.

Visceral Form. The gastrointestinal tract is frequently involved as a primary site of infection. The spleen, adrenals, lungs, and liver may be affected by hematogenous spread. Bone, myocardium, and central nervous system involvement are less frequently seen.

Diagnosis. The diagnosis is established by the culture and identification of *P. brasiliensis* and is only supported by positive skin and complement-fixation tests.

The disease must be differentiated from syphilis, tuberculous adenitis and skin disease, yaws, leishmaniasis, and other fungal infections.

Treatment. Amphotericin B (see Histoplasmosis) is the drug of choice. In the past, continuous sulfonamide therapy resulted in remission but not cure.

Prognosis. All forms of the disease are fatal if untreated. Over 90 per cent of cases are cured by amphotericin B.

Furtado, T. A., Wilson, J. W., and Plunkett, O. A.: South American blastomycosis or paracoccidioidomycosis. Arch. Derm. (Chicago), 70:166, 1954.

Hildick-Smith, G., Blank, H., and Sarkany, I.: Fungus Diseases and Their Treatment. Boston, Little, Brown and Company, 1964.

Jordan, J. W., and Weidman, F. D.: Coccidioidal granuloma: Comparison of the North and South American diseases, with special reference to *Paracoccidioides brasiliensis*. Arch. Dermat. & Syph., 33:31, 1936.

MADUROMYCOSIS
(Mycetoma, Madura Foot)

Definition. Maduromycosis is a chronic systemic fungal disease that follows traumatic or imperceptible implantation of the skin. It is characterized by swelling, induration, suppuration, and draining sinuses of the skin, subcutaneous tissue, and bone, typically of the foot.

History. The disease was first recognized and described in 1712 by Kaempfer in India, and was called Madura foot, after the city of that name. It has been suggested, however, that Madura foot was described by Sophocles in the hero of *Philoctetes*.

Etiology. Many species of ten genera have been reported as etiologic agents; the most common of these have been *Madurella mycetomi, Nocardia brasiliensis,* and, in the United States, *Allescheria boydii.* In tissues or pus these fungi, except for Nocardia (q.v.), are characterized by the appearance of "grains" of oval or irregular shape measuring 0.5 to 2.0 mm., and of white, red, black, or yellow color. Microscopically they are composed of 2 to 4 μ segmented, branched hyphae or round encysted forms (chlamydospores).

A. boydii grows rapidly on Sabouraud's glucose medium, forming a white (later gray or brown) cottony, aerial mycelium, which microscopically consists of thin hyphae to which are attached short or long stalks (conidiophores) bearing a single 8 to 10 by 5 to 7 μ pyriform or ovoid form (conidium). Large (50 to 200 μ) flask-shaped vessels containing asci and spores (4 to 7 μ) can be seen when material from the surface of agar is crushed and examined.

When inoculated intraperitoneally into mice, *A. boydii* is pathogenic, but progressive disease similar to that in humans has not been produced.

Epidemiology. Although occasionally reported from temperate areas, the disease is seen most often in those tropical zones where few people wear shoes. The disease occurs chiefly in adults and more often in males. Most causative organisms are saprophytes of soil or plants. The disease has been reported in the dog, cow, and horse, but animal-to-man or man-to-man spread has not been reported.

Pathology. The typical swollen foot of maduromycosis has numerous draining sinuses communicating with abscesses of the skin, subcutaneous tissue, or bone. Drainage sites have characteristic collars of fibrous or epithelial tissues. Suppuration with epithelioid, plasma, and giant cells is intermingled with areas of fibrosis, and one or the other reaction may predominate. With Gram, hematoxylin and eosin, or periodic acid–Schiff stains, fungal cells may be seen either in pus or within macrophages or giant cells.

Clinical Forms. Although lesions have been reported on the leg, trunk, hand, and face, the characteristic site of disease is the foot. The first manifestation consists of a papule, small nodule, indurated area with a vesicle, or an abscess that ruptures with sinus tract formation. Infection spreads and new nodules appear, leading to generalized swelling and distortion of the toes. Pain is infrequent, and there are few generalized symptoms. Roentgenographic examination may show lytic lesions with reaction and proliferation of the bone.

Diagnosis. Diagnosis is confirmed by the demonstration of granules in draining material, but the specific etiology is dependent on isolation of the fungus in culture. Serologic and skin tests have not been developed for most of the responsible fungi. Maduromycosis must be distinguished from other fungal infections and from tuberculosis, yaws, neoplasms, and elephantiasis.

Treatment. With the variety of antimicrobial agents available, each with specific activity, it is essential that definitive mycologic studies be done prior to treatment to determine the identity and, if feasible, the drug susceptibility of the causative fungus. The failure to do so in many past reports is undoubtedly a factor in the generally pessimistic attitude toward treatment and the early resort to amputation.

The drug of choice for infections caused by *Nocardia brasiliensis* is a sulfonamide (see Nocardiosis), whereas for those caused by Aspergillus, potassium iodide or amphotericin B is indicated (see Aspergillosis). Tetracycline and diaminodiphenyl-sulfone have been reported to be successful in a few cases of *M. mycetoma* infections, and saramycetin (X-5079C) (see Histoplasmosis) was active chemotherapeutically in an atypical case of *M. grisea* infection. Amphotericin B has been reported ineffective in two cases of *A. boydii* infection. Recently, there has been an intriguing case report of benefit in this latter infection related to menstrual periods, and estrogens have been shown to inhibit fungal growth in vitro.

Prognosis. The disease is usually progressive and rarely self-limited.

Carrion, A. L., Hutner, M. S., Nadal, H. M., and Belaval, M. F.: Maduromycosis: An unusual case with a description of the causative fungus. Arch. Derm. (Chicago), 82:371, 1960.

Mohr, J. A., and Muchmore, H. G.: Maduromycosis due to *Allescheria boydii.* J.A.M.A., 204:335, 1968.

Zeisler, E. B.: A case from Sophocles. Arch. Derm. (Chicago), 84:136, 1961.

CHROMOBLASTOMYCOSIS

Definition. Chromoblastomycosis is a chronic systemic fungal disease, acquired in the cutaneous form by traumatic or imperceptible implantation, and characterized by wartlike, ulcerated, crusted lesions of the skin and subcutaneous tissues.

History. Although rare in this country, chromoblastomycosis was first reported from Boston in 1915, separately by Lane and Medlar, and the organism responsible was named *Phialophora verrucosa* by Thaxter. Subsequently, cases owing to other genera of fungi were described by Brumpt and Carrion. The first case of cerebral disease was reported in 1948 by Bonne.

Etiology. A number of fungi have been incriminated, but chiefly *Phialophora verrucosa, P. pedrosoi, P. compactum,* and *Cladosporium carrionii*. In tissues these fungi resemble each other and appear as single or clustered, round, thick-walled, 6 to 12 μ budding cells of a striking brown color, from which the disease draws its name. On culture, mycelia are produced that vary according to genus and species. Skin hypersensitivity and complement-fixing antigens have been demonstrated in some fungal species. Laboratory animals are susceptible to experimental infection, but the equivalent of natural disease in man is not produced.

Epidemiology. The disease is seen more often in adult males in the rural areas of the tropics, especially in Brazil, Puerto Rico, and Cuba. The responsible fungi are saprophytes of soil, but are found more often in decaying wood and vegetation. Infection in animals has not been reported, and animal-to-man or man-to-man spread is unknown.

Pathology. Varying degrees of hyperkeratoses, acanthosis, and pseudo-epitheliomatous hyperplasia are seen. In the cutis the reaction may be granulomatous with mononuclear, epithelioid, and Langhans' giant cells. Fungal cells are seen readily with hematoxylin and eosin stains.

Clinical Forms. Chromoblastomycosis is a disease of the skin and subcutaneous tissue.

The first patient reported had lesions of the buttock. The most common site is the lower extremity. The disease appears also, in descending order of frequency, on the hand, forearm, arm, neck, and shoulders. The earliest lesion is a nodule or pustule that, over a period of weeks to months, ulcerates, drains, enlarges, dries, and becomes violaceous and wartlike. There is rarely pain, but itching is common. Lesions do not spread generally, but scratching results in autoinoculation and satellite or secondary distal lesions.

Diagnosis. Although older typical skin lesions may be clinically and histologically suggestive, the diagnosis is confirmed by the culture and identification of the causative organism.

Early lesions may be confused with blastomycosis, tuberculosis, leprosy, yaws, and syphilis.

Treatment. Surgical resection of early skin lesions has been the most common and efficacious therapy. Amputation has been required in a small number of cases. Most of the fungi causing chromoblastomycosis are resistant to amphotericin B, but successful treatment has been reported in two cases when the drug was injected locally into the skin. This drug needs further trial in this disease.

Prognosis. The cutaneous form of chromoblastomycosis is chronic and compatible with long life (in one case, 40 years).

Carrion, A. L.: Chromoblastomycosis. Ann. N. Y. Acad. Sci., 50:1255, 1950.

Costello, M. J., De Feo, C. P., Jr., and Littman, M. L.: Chromoblastomycosis treated with local infiltration of amphotericin B solution. Arch. Derm. (Chicago), 79:184, 1959.

Vanbreuseghem, R.: Mycoses of Man and Animals. London, Sir Isaac Pitman & Sons, 1958.

ASPERGILLOSIS

Definition. Aspergillosis is a fungal infection of the lung, from which site disease may disseminate to bone, meninges, heart, or other organs.

History. The disease was first reported by Bennett in 1842, and many cases thereafter were described by French workers.

Etiology. Among species of the genus Aspergillus, *A. fumigatus* is the most common pathogen that produces invasive disease. In tissues or secretions *A. fumigatus* appears as septate hyphae with oval forms measuring 2 to 4 μ in diameter (conidia). On Sabouraud glucose medium white feltlike mycelia appear that microscopically contain intertwined hyphae. Some hyphae enlarge and send up a stalk with swollen vesicle (conidiophore) from which shorter stalks (phialides) project. These in turn bear 2 to 4 μ oval bodies (conidia). Rabbits and mice may be experimentally infected, more readily after corticosteroid or antimicrobial medication. A hemolytic endotoxin is elaborated by *A. fumigatus,* and circulating antibodies to this have been produced. A skin test antigen has also been developed, but is not generally available.

Epidemiology. Aspergillosis is worldwide in distribution. Males are more often affected than females, and especially at risk are workers in contact with infected grains or dusts. The early French literature reported the disease to be an occupational illness of pigeon-feeders and wig-makers who used grain in their work. Any of a variety of species may be present in the oral cavity of otherwise normal persons. A variety of species are widespread as saprophytes in nature, and a few are pathogens for plants, insects, domestic animals, and birds, especially penguins. Animal-to-man or man-to-man contagion has not been reported.

Pathology. In ectatic bronchi, Aspergillus species may proliferate, forming a 2 to 6 cm. mass composed of hyphae, fibrin, and mucosal cells, a "fungus ball." With this form of disease, tissue invasion rarely occurs.

In relatively rare instances *A. fumigatus* invades normal lung and disseminates. Lesions may be present in lung, bone, meninges, heart, and other organs. The histologic picture is that of a combination of suppuration and granulomas.

Clinical Manifestations. *Localized Forms.* Under a variety of conditions in man species of Aspergillus have been cultured from skin, sputum, or mucous membranes, but the relationship of this isolation to disease in the patient is variable and difficult to establish. Many times the fungus is a saprophyte producing no illness or playing no etiologic role in disease that is present. In other patients an immediate reaction on skin testing may indicate that Aspergillus is an allergen in a pulmonary process characterized by asthmatic symptoms, transient migratory infiltration on chest film, a sputum containing Curschmann's spirals and Charcot-Leyden crystals, and a peripheral circulating eosinophilia. The fungus may colonize ectatic or tuberculous bronchi, especially after antimicrobial therapy. The "fungus ball" appears on the chest film as an opaque shadow capped by a thin meniscus of air in a dilated bronchus or cavity. Hemoptysis and increased sputum production are the only symptoms attributable to this lesion. In none of these situations is tissue invasion seen.

Invasive Forms. Under conditions of impaired host defenses, e.g., immunosuppressive therapy, leukemia, or lymphoma, *A. fumigatus* (and rarely other species) may invade tissue and disseminate hematogenously. Such infection is manifested as a septicemia with fever, chills, and shock. Occasionally, signs of localized disease predominate, as in endocarditis or meningitis.

Diagnosis. The ubiquitous occurrence of Aspergillus in the laboratory, in nature, or in the patient as a commensal growing luxuriantly on diseased tissue requires that the physician carefully interpret the results of a culture. Skin tests and serologic methods have given inconsistent results and are not generally available. Finding hyphal fragments and microconidia in direct examination of fresh sputum specimens from patients suggests that the fungus is multiplying in bronchi, but not necessarily invading tissue. A culture and a biopsy with microscopic demonstration of tissue invasion provide conclusive evidence of invasive disease. In patients with invasive disease, unfortunately, the fulminant course does not allow time for such diagnostic efforts or for their results.

Localized aspergillosis must be distinguished from bronchitis, allergic pulmonary disease, and lung abscess of other cause. Invasive pulmonary disease is usually diagnosed as tuberculosis and less frequently as possible neoplastic or other fungal infection. Widespread dissemination must be distinguished from septicemia of other cause.

Treatment. Amphotericin B and saramycetin (X-5079C) (see Histoplasmosis) have measurable antifungal effect in experimental infections in laboratory animals and have been of benefit in a few patients. Treatment should be administered until clinical improvement has resulted and until the fungus cannot be cultured from specimens previously positive. Surgical drainage of abscesses is advisable and helpful.

Prognosis. Prognosis is good in localized and poor in invasive disease. *A. fumigatus* is generally more resistant in vitro, and the course of illness is too fulminant to lead to much hope for better prognosis with available antifungal agents.

Emmons, C. W., Binford, C. H., and Utz, J. P.: Medical Mycology. 2nd ed. Philadelphia, Lea & Febiger, 1970.

Orie, N. G. M., de Vries, G. A., and Kikstra, A.: Growth of Aspergillus in the human lung. Amer. Rev. Resp. Dis., 82: 649, 1961.

Smith, D. T.: Miscellaneous fungus diseases. J. Chron. Dis., 5:528, 1957.

CANDIDOSIS
(Candidiasis, Moniliasis, Thrush)

Definition. Candidosis or thrush is an acute or chronic fungal disease involving superficial tissues of skin or mucous membrane or less frequently disseminating hematogenously to produce systemic disease, especially in kidneys, heart, and brain.

History. Oral candidosis or thrush was first described by the English physician Underwood in 1784. In 1839 von Langenbeck, a German surgeon, discovered *C. albicans*, and two years later Berg, a Swedish physician, demonstrated this fungus to be the cause of thrush. Systemic candidosis was first recognized in 1869 by Parrot, and in 1940 the first case proved by positive antemortem blood culture was reported by Joachim and Polages.

Etiology. Man may be infected by a variety of species of Candida, which in tissues or on direct examination of fresh material appear as 2 to 4 μ, budding, thin-walled, oval yeastlike forms, or occasionally as pseudo- or true hyphal forms. On Sabouraud glucose medium, moist, cream-colored colonies appear. Some Candida species can infect laboratory animals, especially those treated with corticoids or made diabetic with alloxan. In some patients especially prone to repeated or severe Candida infections, there has been absence of a leukocytic enzyme, myeloperoxidase, or of a serum candidicidal alpha (or beta, but not gamma) globulin. Delayed cutaneous hypersensitivity and agglutinogen antigens are produced.

Epidemiology. Candida organisms are commonly present in the mouth, vagina, sputum, and stools of otherwise normal persons. Candidosis in the form of oral thrush, skin lesions, or disseminated disease seems to arise in patients with other diseases or under special circumstances: infancy, diabetes, debilitated or dehydrated states, antibacterial or corticoid treatment, drug addiction, leukemia, and tuberculosis. Candidosis is also more frequent in occupational groups (housewives, fruit packers, bartenders) whose skin is frequently in water and macerated. Thrush may occur in epidemics. Birds more frequently, but other animals as well, may be naturally infected, but animal-to-man contagion is not important.

Pathology. The histopathologic lesion in candidosis may be variously acute and suppurative with multiple abscess formation, or chronic and inflammatory with giant cells and occasionally caseation. Either yeastlike or hyphal forms may be seen after hematoxylin and eosin or periodic acid-Schiff staining.

Candidosis of the skin and mucous membranes is superficial and epithelial. When dissemination occurs, kidneys, heart, brain, pancreas, lungs, adrenals, thyroid, liver or joints may be involved.

Clinical Forms. *Mucous Membrane Form (Thrush).* In infants or in older patients with debilitating, dehydrating disease, the classic lesion of thrush of the oral cavity appears as multiple, sometimes confluent, white to creamy patches of exudate on a fiery red and painful mucosa. The disease may spread to the pharynx and esophagus to produce dysphagia. Similar lesions and local irritation may occur also in the mucosa of the rectum or of the vagina and cervix.

Cutaneous Form. Skin lesions may be those of intertrigo with reddening, maceration, and weeping of contiguous folds of skin; onychia with

hardening, thickening, grooving, and loss of the nail; or paronychia with reddening, swelling, and pain of the skin about the nails. Candidid with multiple, grouped vesicles is another form of the skin disease.

Disseminated Form. From superficial and endogenous sites, Candida species may occasionally invade local tissue directly or distant tissues hematogenously under conditions listed earlier. Pulmonary disease may result as a spread from the oral cavity or bronchi with completely nonspecific lobular or patchy bronchopneumonia.

When Candida invades the blood stream, symptoms may be absent or transient and self-limited. Although such invasion may begin in the lung, no characteristic clinical disease has ever been defined in that organ.

Three distinctive forms are well accepted. Candida septicemia bears the earmarks of other bacterial disease: fever, chills, shock, oliguria, coma, and bleeding. Candida meningitis is usually less acute than bacterial disease, but is accompanied by headache, stiff neck, and delirium.

The third and striking form is an *endocarditis* with characteristically large vegetations and large artery embolism (see accompanying figure). Disease after vascular trauma, notably in heroin addicts and in patients who have had cardiac surgery. Antimicrobial therapy in man probably predisposes toward Candida superinfection at this site, and in animals is essential to the production of lesions.

Diagnosis. A typical clinical picture of thrush, vulvovaginitis, onychia, or skin lesions and the finding of organisms on direct examination or culture constitute the diagnosis in superficial infection. A biopsy demonstrating tissue invasion of

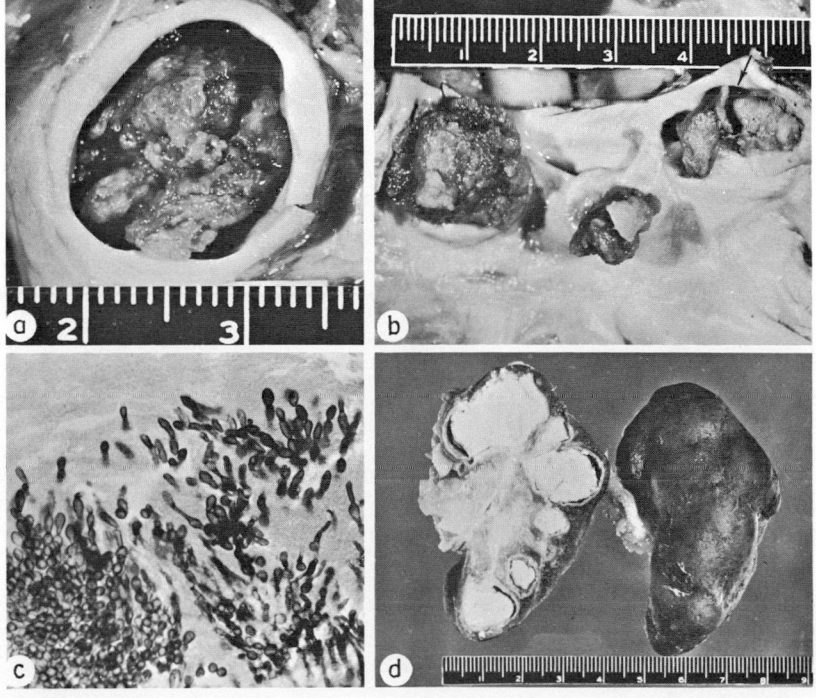

Candida endocarditis. *a,* Aortic valve viewed from above. Note almost complete occlusion of orifice. *b,* Aortic valve opened. Note vegetations on ventricular aspect. Arrow indicates ostium of the left coronary artery partially occluded by valvular vegetation. *c,* Gomori methenamine silver stain of Candida organisms (× 495) in vegetations. *d,* Right kidney (wt. 50 grams). Note large focal areas with caseous necrotic material that on microscopic examination showed Candida organisms.

typical fungal forms or a positive culture from blood, cerebrospinal fluid, or deep tissue is conclusive evidence of disseminated disease.

Candidosis of the skin must be distinguished from other dermatophytoses. Thrush may resemble exudative disease of bacterial (streptococcal or diphtherial) origin, infectious mononucleosis, or Koplik spots. Endocarditis meningitis, or septicemia caused by Candida resembles its bacterial equivalent.

Treatment. Local lesions of thrush respond to a variety of procedures, including hydration, better oral hygiene, and, as necessary, mouth washes four times a day with nystatin solution (2 ml. of 200,000 units per milliliter). Gastrointestinal or vulvovaginal thrush should be treated with oral tablets of nystatin, 1 million units four times daily by mouth. A suppository (100,000 units) may also be inserted intravaginally nightly. This drug in the form of cream should be applied locally to skin or nail lesions.

Candida fungemia may clear spontaneously. The factors, other than antibacterial therapy, are not well known or clinically recognizable that lead to implantation on heart valves or to multiple abscesses. For the latter complications amphotericin B is advisable (see Histoplasmosis). Nystatin is not absorbed from the gastrointestinal tract and is not available for parenteral use.

Prognosis. Untreated disease of the skin and mucous membranes may be chronic and respond poorly to therapy, but dissemination and fatal outcome are rare. Candida septicemia is a severe and usually fatal disease; survival time is often insufficient to achieve an effective concentration of drug in the blood and tissues. By contrast, Candida meningitis, curiously, can be less severe and spontaneous; recovery, (without appropriate antifungal therapy), ensues frequently. Candida endocarditis is a chronic and inexorably fatal disease in at least 90 per cent of patients, even when treated with amphotericin B.

Benham, R. W.: Species of Candida most frequently isolated from man: Methods and criteria for their identification. J. Chron. Dis., 5:460, 1957.

Braude, A. I., and Rock, J. A.: The syndrome of acute disseminated moniliasis in adults. Arch. Intern. Med. (Chicago), 104:91, 1959.

Utz, J. P.: Treatment of Candida infections. *In* Winner, H. I., and Hurley, R. (eds.): Candida Infections. Edinburgh, E. and S. Livingstone, Ltd., 1966.

Winner, H. I., and Hurley, R.: Candida Albicans. Boston, Little, Brown & Company, 1964.

RHINOSPORIDIOSIS

Rhinosporidiosis is a fungal infection localized to skin or mucous membranes or, in two reported cases, widely disseminated to liver, kidneys, spleen, brain, and other organs. It is caused by a fungus, *Rhinosporidium seeberi*, first described by Seeber in 1900, but never obtained in culture. Seen principally in Asia (15 cases only from the United States), the infection is acquired probably by traumatic implantation. The histopathologic lesion consists of granuloma formation with giant cells typically about the pathognomonic large (300 to 350 μ) vesicles (sporangia) containing many oval 7 to 8 μ bodies (spores). It is characterized by polypoid masses on the nose or nasal, conjunctival, pharyngeal, or other mucous membranes. Surgical resection has been the customary treatment, but a trial of amphotericin B (see Histoplasmosis) appears indicated.

Agrawal, S., Sharma, K. D., and Shrivastava, J. B.: Generalized rhinosporidiosis with visceral involvement. Arch. Derm. (Chicago), 80:22, 1959.

Allen, F. R., and Dave, M.: The treatment of rhinosporidiosis in man: Based on the study of 60 cases. Indian Med. Gaz., 71: 376, 1936.

PHYCOMYCOSIS

Phycomycosis is a broad term suggested for acute and chronic systemic fungal disease caused by members of the class Phycomycetes, which include genera of Mucor, Rhizopus, and Absidia (see Mucormycosis) and also Mortierella and Basidiobolus. The last named fungus has caused a characteristic localized, painless swelling of subcutaneous tissues of the arm, thigh, or back. The skin over the swelling is intact. The histopathologic picture is also distinctive in the number of eosinophils and the smudgy granular necrosis around the hyphae. In one case, the disease seemed to respond to iodide therapy. Infection is seen principally in Indonesia and Africa.

Joe, L. K., and Eng. N. I. T.: Subcutaneous phycomycosis: A new disease found in Indonesia. Ann. N.Y. Acad. Sci., 89:4, 1960.

MISCELLANEOUS MYCOSES

In one reported instance each, tissue invasion by *Geotrichum candidum* and *Penicillium commune* has been demonstrated. In patients with predisposing conditions or diseases, various other fungi, e.g., *Torulopsis glabrata, Rhodotorula saccharomyces,* are being reported in blood, abscess, or tissue specimens. Pneumonitis, pleuritis, and pericarditis have been ascribed to *Waksmania rosea* in one patient. Predominantly allergic pulmonary symptoms have followed exposure to *Thermopolyspora polyspora* (Farmer's lung, q.v.) or *Cryptostroma corticale* (maple bark disease).

PROTOZOAN AND HELMINTHIC DISEASES

Introduction

Philip D. Marsden

With rapid air travel, so-called parasitic infections are becoming more important in temperate climes. They have always been important in the tropics.

Parasitic disease is usually taken to imply infections caused by protozoa and helminths, although, in their relationship to the host, bacteria, viruses, and rickettsia equally fulfill the general criteria used to describe an organism as parasitic. The reason for this is historic; because they are bigger organisms, helminths and protozoa were discovered relatively early by medical investigators. Ascaris and tapeworms are dramatic enough to have been recognized in ancient times, and protozoa were seen with the first crude microscopes.

For the correct diagnosis of parasitic disease the physician must be as competent at the microscope and in using the laboratory procedures to find parasites as he is at defining the clinical presentation at the bedside and interpreting it. As with other infectious diseases, a firm diagnosis rests on finding the infectious agent. Recently serologic tests have been used much more to aid diagnosis, and, interpreted wisely, they are valuable. Broadly speaking, they mean that a patient has developed antibodies of a certain type to a parasitic antigen. Rarely do they give any confirmation about the status of the parasite in the body of man in terms of numbers present or whether they are multiplying. Positive serologic findings should often be an indication for redoubling one's efforts to find the parasite.

Whether a complement fixation test, hemagglutination test, fluorescent antibody test, or gel diffusion test is positive at a significant titer must be decided in the light of known facts about the specificity of the tests.

Many of the drugs used are toxic to man but more toxic to the parasites. We know little of the mechanism of drug action in many cases, e.g., Pentostam in leishmaniasis. With some drugs such as heavy metal containing compounds and emetine the toxic dose for man is near the therapeutic dose. Physicians should be especially careful to check their prescriptions of these drugs, especially if they are not used to prescribing them often.

The National Communicable Disease Center, Atlanta, Georgia, offers unique services to the physician in the United States for the management of parasitic disease. Not only is there a laboratory for diagnostic serology, but recently a number of rare drugs previously not available in the United States and mentioned in this book have become available through the Parasitic Disease Drug Service in the Epidemiology Program. These include drugs for the treatment of both types of human trypanosomiasis, leishmaniasis, amebiasis, pneumocystis infection, and schistosomiasis.

With regard to diagnostic serology, Dr. Irving G. Kagan has kindly provided the accompanying table of serologic tests available for parasitic diseases in the United States.

IMMUNODIAGNOSTIC TESTS FOR PARASITIC INFECTIONS

| | Complement Fixation | Precipitin | Particle Agglutination Tests | | | | Fluorescent Antibody | Methylene Blue Dye |
			Bentonite Flocculation	Hemagglutination	Latex Agglutination	Cholesterol Flocculation		
Trichinosis			+*	±*	+*	+*	+*	
Echinococcosis		±	+*	+*	+*		0	
Schistosomiasis	+*		±*	±*		+*	+*	
Ascariasis/toxocariasis			+*	+*				
Filariasis	±		+*	+*			0	
Cysticercosis	+			+*			0*	
Chagas' disease	+*			+*	0		0	
Leishmaniasis	±			±*			0	
Toxoplasmosis	+*			+*	0		+*	+*
Amebiasis	+*	+	±*	+*			±*	
Malaria				±*			+*	

* = Tests available in the U.S.
0 = Under experimental investigation.
± = Used for diagnosis, but requires further evaluation for routine use.
+ = Generally accepted useful routine diagnostic test.
Adapted from data supplied by Dr. Irving Kagan, National Communicable Disease Center.

Protozoan Diseases

GENERAL CONSIDERATIONS
Philip D. Marsden

Malaria remains the greatest challenge in parasitic disease both in terms of prevalence (1038 million people still live in malarious areas) and in the amount of morbidity and mortality caused by this infection. In many tropical countries, notably Africa, it has a profound influence on the pattern of clinical medicine.

Trypanosomiasis is a good example of geographically restricted disease. *Trypanosoma brucei* infections are restricted to Africa because tsetse flies (Glossina species) are not found elsewhere. African sleeping sickness demands attention because human infections once established are so frequently fatal. Also, this same group of trypanosomes are responsible for widespread fatal disease in cattle, profoundly influencing animal husbandry. South American trypanosomiasis (Chagas' disease) is restricted to the Americas because again the great majority of reduviid bugs occur in this location. The significance of this infection as a public health problem is a matter of current concern. One estimate suggests that 7 million people are infected and 30 million exposed to the risk of infection. Permanent cardiac damage often ensues, and at the time of writing there is no cure.

Also in the family Trypanosomidae, Leishmania is responsible for considerable human suffering. Visceral leishmaniasis is a debilitating infection, and without treatment the terminal event is usually a secondary bacterial infection, often a pneumonia. Cutaneous and mucocutaneous leishmaniasis can be disfiguring infections. Therapy is far from satisfactory.

Amebiasis ranks fourth in this consideration, because, although bowel infections are widely prevalent, invasive disease is less common. Then come a miscellany of rarer protozoal disease entities.

The reader will appreciate that the first three groups of diseases caused by protozoa all have arthropod vectors: Anopheles for malaria, Glossina and Reduviidae for trypanosomiasis, and Phlebotomus for leishmaniasis. It is relevant and important for medical men to have some knowledge of these vectors. A few examples of why this is so will suffice. At the time of writing there have been a few cases of indigenous vivax malaria recognized in the United States. Epidemiologic work has revealed vector Anopheles in the area. Xenodiagnosis using clean Reduviidae is the best way of finding *Trypanosoma cruzi* parasites in a patient with a chronic infection, and because of this these insects are most important, as they are used in diagnostic medicine. Phlebotomus remains very susceptible to DDT, and spraying of this

insect's habitats will result in the control of human leishmaniasis.

Another medical consideration worth emphasizing is that blood protozoa can be transmitted by blood transfusion. Particularly important in this respect are malaria and *Trypanosoma cruzi* infections. Suitable selection of donors in temperate countries is necessary to avoid this complication in nonimmune persons exposed to the risk of malaria parasites in transfused blood. *Trypanosoma cruzi* infections transmitted by blood transfusion are said to be particularly acute. It is of interest that recent advances in immunology enable us to screen blood donors for malaria with the indirect fluorescent antibody test, whereas for *Trypanosoma cruzi* the valuable and specific complement-fixation test is still used.

Belding, D. L.: Textbook of Parasitology. 3rd ed. New York, Appleton-Century-Crofts, Inc., 1965.

Faust, E. C., and Russell, P. F.: Clinical Parasitology. 8th ed. Philadelphia, Lea and Febiger, 1970.

Hunter, G. W., Frye, W. W., and Swartzwelder, J. C.: A Manual of Tropical Medicine. Philadelphia, W. B. Saunders Company, 1966.

Manson-Bahr, P. M.: Manson's Tropical Diseases. 16th ed. London, Baillière, Tindall & Cassell, Ltd., 1966.

MALARIA
L. J. Bruce-Chwatt

GENERAL CONSIDERATIONS

Malaria is an acute, often severe, and sometimes protracted disease caused by parasitic protozoa of the genus Plasmodium. Four species of this genus (*P. falciparum, P. malariae, P. ovale,* and *P. vivax*) infect man in natural conditions. The main symptoms of the disease comprise fever, anemia, and enlargement of the spleen. The febrile paroxysms, preceded by shivering and followed by sweating, often occur at regular intervals: on alternate days (tertian fever), with an interval of two days (quartan fever), or daily (quotidian fever). Falciparum malaria may be fatal if the treatment is delayed or inadequate; the infection with other plasmodial species is less severe and has a tendency to relapses, which are separated by periods of latency. The term "chronic malaria" is at times used to describe a special clinical type of recurring infection with severe anemia, malnutrition, and splenomegaly, found in underdeveloped areas of the world. Man is the only important source of human malaria; the malaria parasite can be transmitted from one subject to another naturally by the bite of an infected Anopheles mosquito or directly by accidental or intentional transfer of infected blood.

History. It is likely that the evolutionary history of mammalian plasmodia started with the adaptation of Coccidia of the intestinal epithelium to some tissues of the internal organs and then to life in the circulating cells of the blood, from which they could be transmitted by blood-sucking arthropods. The ancestry of primate malaria in the Old World is well established; it is probable that the disease originated in Africa, which is believed to be the cradle of the human species. It then spread to the Mediterranean shores, to Mesopotamia, the Indian peninsula, and Southeast Asia; the way of its spread to the New World is subject to speculation, as no reliable historical data are known on this point.

References to intermittent fevers exist in the ancient Assyrian, Chinese, and Indian medical texts, but the clinical entity of malaria was established in Greece by Hippocrates only in the fifth century B.C. The Romans knew it well, associated it with marshy areas, and attempted to control it by drainage. Subsequent historical milestones of the history of malaria were introduction of cinchona bark from Peru to Europe at the beginning of the seventeenth century; isolation of quinine and other alkaloids in 1820 by Pelletier and Caventou; discovery of the malaria parasites in the blood in 1880 by Laveran; discovery of malaria parasites of birds by Danielewski in 1885, followed by the discovery of the sexual stages of plasmodia in 1897 by MacCallum; discovery of mosquito transmission of malaria by Ronald Ross in 1897, and confirmation of the role of Anopheles by Bignami, Bastianelli, and Grassi in 1898.

The first large-scale demonstration of malaria control through antimosquito measures was made by Gorgas in Cuba and in the Panama Canal Zone during 1899 to 1914. The period 1924 to 1950 saw the development of the synthesis of several antimalarial drugs, started by Schulemann with plasmochin, and pursued by a number of German, American, British, and French workers. Following the discovery of insecticidal properties of DDT in 1939 the first nationwide malaria control projects took place during the next ten years, and many new insecticides were introduced in subsequent national control programs.

In 1948 the exo-erythrocytic stages of malaria parasites of primates were described by Shortt, Garnham, Bray, and others; in the same year *Plasmodium berghei*, the first malaria parasite of rodents, was discovered in the Congo by Vincke. In 1963 Eyles, Coatney, and their colleagues discovered a number of new parasites of monkey malaria in Malaya and indicated the possibility of natural transmission of some of these infections to man. The development of resistance of Anopheles to several insecticides during the 1950's and the discovery of resistance of plasmodia to synthetic drugs during the following decade has stimulated much research aimed at finding new and improved means to assist the global program of eradication of malaria.

EPIDEMIOLOGY

Malaria is one of the most widely spread communicable diseases; it is particularly common and severe in the tropics and subtropics but occurs also in some temperate regions. Falciparum malaria is generally found in hot and humid climates, although seasonal outbreaks may be seen outside the tropics. Vivax and quartan malaria are widespread, but the latter has a patchy distribution; ovale malaria exists mainly in West Africa.

It has been estimated that in the early 1950's there were throughout the world at least 250 million cases of malaria every year and 2.5 million deaths owing to this disease. Ten years later, the malaria eradication program (*vide infra*) had decreased the morbidity figure to less than 100 million, and endemic malaria had disappeared from many countries, thanks to modern methods of control.

A considerable proportion of malaria mortality falls on underdeveloped areas of the tropical world, where malaria remains the most prevalent disease of rural communities. It has been esti-mated that in some parts of Africa at least 10 per cent of all deaths in infants and children below three years of age are due to direct effects of malaria. The contributory effect of malaria infection to deaths from other diseases cannot be easily estimated, but it is certainly large; malaria has also some bearing on the frequency of abortions, stillbirths, and neonatal mortality. In tropical areas where socioeconomic levels are already low, endemic or epidemic malaria impedes the agricultural, industrial, and social progress of the newly independent countries.

Epidemics of malaria, so common in the past, are now exceptional. One of the greatest epidemics of malaria in modern times struck the Soviet Union after World War I; more than 5 million cases were reported in 1923, and there were at least 60,000 deaths. The Ceylon epidemic of 1934-1935 caused nearly 3 million cases of malaria and 82,000 deaths; in 1938 the invasion of Brazil by *A. gambiae* was followed by an epidemic with over 100,000 cases and at least 14,000 deaths; in 1942-1944 the same mosquito invaded lower Egypt and caused about 160,000 malaria cases and more than 12,000 deaths; in 1958 an epidemic of malaria in Ethiopia caused more than 3 million cases and 150,000 deaths; in 1963 there was an epidemic of malaria in Haiti, in the wake of hurricane Flora, with 75,000 cases. In 1967-1968 the malaria eradication program of Ceylon suffered a serious setback, and the island had an epidemic of *P. vivax* malaria with about one million cases but with very low mortality. An increase of malaria has also been reported from North and Central India and from some areas of Pakistan, but it would be unjustified to refer to these outbreaks as epidemics.

The assessment of the incidence of malaria in nonendemic areas is normally based on the official reporting of cases. From this the morbidity (and mortality) rate can be determined in relation to the given unit of the population and over a unit of time. In endemic malarious areas this is rarely possible, and the prevalence of malaria (relative frequency of disease or infection at any given time) can be estimated by finding the relative proportion of children with enlarged spleens (spleen rate) or the relative proportion of people of well-defined age groups having malaria parasites in a sample of blood examined under a microscope (parasite rate). Both rates are an index of the endemicity of malaria in the population.

In countries where, as a result of eradication activities, the incidence of malaria has greatly decreased, the malariometric surveys carried out on a sample of the population must be replaced by the screening of the whole community for individual case detection. This method forms the basis of the surveillance process that aims at the discovery, epidemiologic follow-up, and radical cure of remaining cases of malaria and the elimination of foci of transmission by application of insecticides and drug administration. Imported malaria has now become a serious public health problem in several countries. In the United States there were 2686 cases in 1968 and 3806 cases in 1969. This is due to the great increase of the speed and volume of international travel and to the return of military personnel from the tropical war areas.

Malaria may be described as sporadic, epidemic, or endemic. One refers to *sporadic malaria* when the cases of disease (seen as primary attacks or relapses) are very few and too scattered to have any appreciable effect on the community.

The term *epidemic malaria* indicates a seasonal or other periodic sharp rise of the number of cases affecting all age groups fairly equally; an epidemic may occur either in an area where this disease was previously unknown or in one where its incidence is low so that the resistance of the community is negligible.

Malaria is described as *endemic* when there is an obvious and fairly constant incidence of cases owing to natural transmission over a succession of years. Various degrees of endemicity have been described in relation to the duration of the transmission season. In areas where the high degree of transmission is nearly perennial without marked fluctuations over the years, malaria achieves a high degree of stability and is known as *hyperendemic* or *holoendemic*; the resulting collective immunity of the population is high. Actual epidemics of malaria are unlikely in these conditions, but a large proportion of infants and small children suffer and die from the direct effects of the disease and from concurrent illnesses.

Relation to the Environment. Physical, biologic, and socioeconomic environment has a potent effect on the transmission of malaria. Temperature, humidity, rainfall, water surface, and other factors determine the physical environment that acts on both the man and the mosquito. The presence of certain plants (in which mosquitoes may breed) or animals (on which mosquitoes may prefer to feed) affects the biologic environment. The occupations, habits, and various activities of people often have a decisive effect on the conditions of transmission of malaria.

Many epidemiologic variables determine the response of the human subject to the infection. Neither sex nor age plays any part in temperate climates, but age is an important factor in endemic areas where the longer duration of exposure of the adult makes him more resistant to the disease. Some genetic differences owing to evolutionary selection may be present; thus, Negroes appear to be less susceptible to *P. vivax* infection.

Relation to Hemoglobin Types. The high frequency of some "abnormal" hemoglobin types such as S, C, and E in certain populations in tropical Africa, Greece, parts of India, and Southeast Asia is positively correlated with distribution of endemic *P. falciparum* malaria. It now appears that this correlation is not fortuitous but is due to the relative biologic advantage conferred on individuals heterozygous for a genetic character of an "abnormal" hemoglobin. The selective survival and a high frequency of such a character is known in population genetics as "balanced polymorphism." This condition has been generally confirmed with regard to hemoglobin S (HbS) or sickle-cell hemoglobin, which has a certain protective effect against severe falciparum malaria. The biochemical mechanism of it may be due to the altered growth of malaria parasites in erythrocytes containing hemoglobin with a slightly different molecular structure. The possible selective advantage in other hemoglobinopathies (C and E) and inherited enzymatic defects such as β-thalassemia and glucose-6-phosphate dehydrogenase (G-6-PD) deficiency has been postulated because their geographic distribution is similar to that of *P. falciparum*. However, the evidence for the protective effect of these genetic traits is still incomplete.

The deficiency of G-6-PD affects the viability of the erythrocyte. Individuals with this sex-linked defect, which is fully expressed in the male sex, are particularly sensitive to certain antimalarial drugs (8-aminoquinolines), sulfones, and some other drugs, which produce a hemolysis of the affected cells.

Simian Malaria. It has been known for a long time that some human plasmodia are closely related to malaria parasites of higher apes (chimpanzees, gorillas). On the other hand, plasmodia of lower monkeys were not thought to be transmissible to man (with the exception of *P. knowlesi*, which can produce a mild blood-induced infection). Studies in Malaysia and the United States indicate that *P. brasilianum, P. cynomolgi, P. inui, P. knowlesi,* and *P. schwetzi* can be transmitted to humans not only by blood infection but also by bites of infected Anopheles mosquitoes. About 20 simian malaria parasites are known today, and

the question of human malaria with an animal reservoir has now been reopened by the discovery of a case of *P. knowlesi* naturally transmitted to man in Malaysia and a case of *P. simium* malaria found in a human subject in Brazil. Whether a natural monkey-to-man transmission (and vice versa) can easily take place in other parts of the world remains to be seen. However, it is not thought that simian malaria is an obstacle to the eradication of human disease.

THE PARASITE

Malaria parasites of the order Hemosporidia may be found in the blood of reptiles, birds, and various mammals. The pathogenic agents responsible for human malarial infections belong to the genus Plasmodium (which includes the subgenus Laverania) and comprise the parasites that undergo the asexual phase of development in the tissues and red blood cells of the mammalian host, and a sexual phase of development in the body of an Anopheles mosquito.

Some plasmodia of man can infect apes and monkeys. This applies particularly to *P. malariae*, which may be found in chimpanzees. Other species of human plasmodia have been experimentally transmitted to chimpanzees and gibbons; infections of some lower monkeys of Central America, e.g., Aotus, have also been successful. These investigations are of importance, as they greatly expand the possibilities of assessment of antimalarial drugs on primates other than man. Each species of the malaria parasites of man has a characteristic appearance; the amount of pigment it contains and some specific changes in the infected erythrocytes, such as enlargement, decolorization, and certain forms of granulations ("stippling"), allow for correct identification. Mixed infections with more than one species may occur.

The main features of the two phases of the life cycle of each of the four species of human malaria parasites are essentially the same (Fig. 1).

In man, sporozoites introduced into the blood during the bite of an infected female Anopheles disappear rapidly from the circulation, and invade the parenchymatous cells of the liver and perhaps other internal organs.

During the following one to two weeks of this pre-erythrocytic stage, the duration of which depends on the species of Plasmodium, the malaria parasites form tissue schizonts; their growth and segmentation are followed by the rupture of the tissue schizont containing several thousand merozoites. At the end of this period, merozoites are released into the blood, enter the red blood cells, and start the erythrocytic stage of the asexual phase.

Young parasites in the red blood cells are known as trophozoites and appear as small, comma- or ring-shaped lumps of cytoplasm with an undivided denser blob of nuclear chromatin. Older trophozoites are larger, often ameboid or band-shaped, and contain granules of characteristic pigment. They grow in size and divide, showing two, four, and more nuclei, and are then called schizonts. Mature schizonts are fully developed with divided

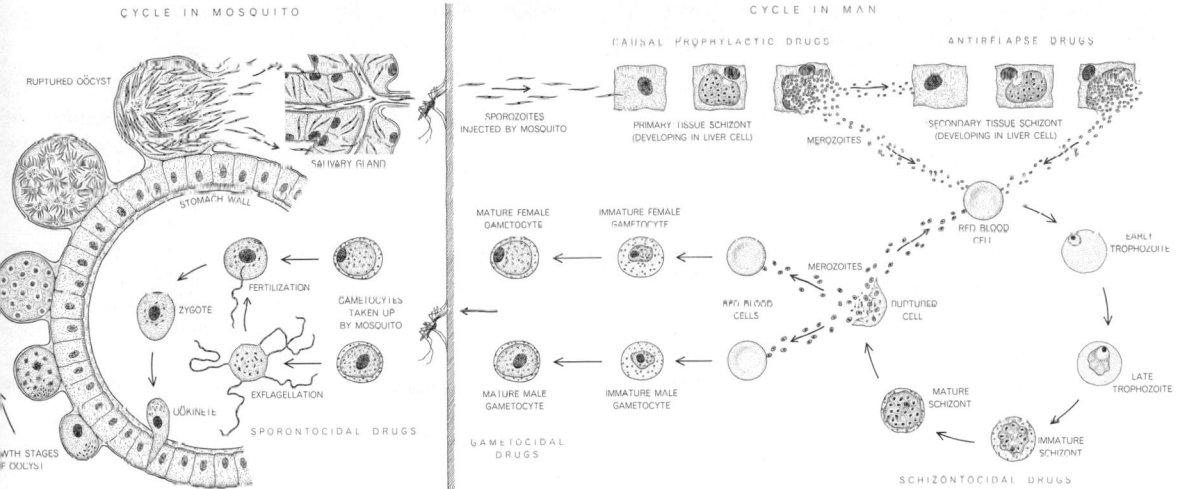

FIGURE 1. The life cycle of malaria parasites and action of antimalarial drugs. (Scientific American.)

nuclei and cytoplasmic segments, and each of these is known as a merozoite (also blood merozoite to distinguish from the tissue merozoite).

Groups of schizonts maturing and rupturing at the same time are released into the circulation at about the same time on successive days, and this characteristic periodicity of the asexual phase of the life cycle is related to the more or less regular appearance of clinical symptoms of the disease. Many merozoites are destroyed in the blood upon their release from the ruptured cell, but a proportion of them enter new erythrocytes and repeat again and again the asexual phase of the life cycle of the parasite.

Some merozoites upon their entry into the red blood cell develop into male and female cells (gametocytes). They are round in three species of human plasmodia, but have a half-moon appearance in *P. falciparum* so that in this case they are commonly called "crescents."

When ingested by the female Anopheles with the blood, gametocytes start the sexual phase of the life cycle of malaria parasites. In the stomach of the mosquito the male gametocyte extrudes several flagellum-like gametes (exflagellation) while the female gametocyte matures. The female gamete, after being fertilized by the motile male, undergoes further changes. The fertilized cell (oökinete) passes from the inside to the outside of the stomach wall of the mosquito and develops under its lining into an oöcyst within which many thousands of spindle-shaped sporozoites appear. After about one to four weeks (depending on the species of the Plasmodium and the temperature), the mature oöcyst ruptures; the free sporozoites are released into the body cavity of the mosquito, and eventually reach its salivary glands. Sporozoites penetrate into the blood of the new host when the mosquito injects the content of salivary glands under the skin during its next blood meal. This initiates the cycle of development in the human subject.

TRANSMISSION TO MAN

The source of natural malaria infection of man is nearly always a human subject, whether a sick person or a symptomless parasite carrier, and the infection is transmitted by an Anopheles. Such natural transmission requires not only the presence of suitable species of Anopheles but also certain appropriate environmental conditions of temperature and humidity.

However, malaria may be transmitted intentionally (induced) as a therapeutic measure (malaria therapy for neurosyphilis) or experimentally by injection of either sporozoites or infected blood. Malaria (especially quartan) may also be seen as an accidental disease following blood transfusion or (in drug addicts) the use of syringes containing small quantities of infected blood. Congenital malaria may occur when red blood cells containing parasites pass across the placenta and transmit the infection from the mother to the baby before its birth.

Various colloquial names applied to the infections caused by the few species of human plasmodia, e.g., "benign tertian fever" for *P. vivax* infections, "malignant tertian" for *P. falciparum*, "quartan fever" for *P. malariae,* are now obsolete. It is preferable to speak of "vivax malaria," "falciparum malaria," or "ovale malaria," but the term "quartan malaria" is acceptable.

IMMUNITY

Immunity to malaria is a state of relative resistance to the plasmodial infection or to the adverse effects caused by it. A degree of natural immunity, at least to certain species of malaria parasites, may be genetically determined, but generally the resistance is of the acquired kind subsequent to a previous infection. There is also evidence of the existence of passive immunity of short duration (congenital immunity) transmitted from the highly immune mother to the fetus through the placenta.

The degree of immunity depends on the physiologic condition of the human subject and on the activity of its humoral and cellular defense mechanism. The humoral factors are represented by various antibodies, whereas the cellular factors are the free and fixed cells of the lymphoid-macrophage (reticuloendothelial) system. All the processes involved in malaria immunity have a considerable degree of specificity and are related to the previous blood infection; there is no evidence that the exo-erythrocytic stages in the liver produce any significant degree of immunity. Permanent "sterile" immunity is rarely achieved, and small numbers of plasmodia may continue to survive in the immune host. This state has been named "premunition."

In the early stages of malarial infection the multiplication and pathogenic effects of the parasite are controlled by phagocytosis, which represents a natural defense mechanism of the host. As the infection develops, the lymphoid macrophage system is stimulated to further activity, the testimony of which is the hypertrophy of the spleen. Several types of antibodies neutralize the adverse effects of the parasite multiplication. As a result of the increasing efficiency of the defense mechanism, the infection subsides or becomes latent for various periods of time, but relapses are common in vivax or quartan malaria, presumably because of the persistence in the liver of the tissue phase of the relevant parasite.

The immunity acquired after many attacks of malaria protects the human subject against reinfection with the same parasites, but he remains susceptible to infections with other species of plasmodia.

In highly endemic malarious areas where the population is exposed to an intensive process of repeated infections, a degree of collective immunity may be observed. Although malaria attacks are common and may be severe in infants and young children, the disease is often mild and may be even asymptomatic in older children, adolescents, and adults. However, such a state of balance between the parasite and the host is often precarious, and may be upset by nutritional deficiencies or intercurrent diseases.

The high concentration of gamma globulins found in the serum of Africans living in highly malarious areas suggests that these substances are related to the presence of immune antibodies. An increase of immunoglobulin levels is always observed in malarial infections after the onset of parasitemia. Immunoglobulin G (IgG) and M (IgM) are higher, especially in repeated infections. There is less evidence that the changing level of IgA and IgD is related to malaria infection. Only a small proportion of the immunoglobulins thus produced (especially IgG) represents the specific protective antibody. Nevertheless the transfer of protective effect was achieved by injection of an isolated IgG fraction of immune serum.

Experimental development of a "malaria vaccine" has been attempted by immunizing animals with killed or variously attentuated plasmodia of birds, rodents, or monkeys, but the results have been only moderately successful. The practical difficulty stems from the complex and highly variable antigenic structure of plasmodia.

Modern immunologic techniques are increasingly used. Indirect fluorescent antibody test and hemagglutination test are of practical importance. Although they cannot yet be relied upon for diagnosis of acute malaria, they are of value for screening blood donors who might be carriers of malaria parasites, for investigations of some immunologic aspects of populations living in highly malarious areas, and for studies on various strains of plasmodia. Other methods such as gel precipitation and complement fixation may also become of value.

PATHOGENESIS AND PATHOLOGY

The pathologic processes in malaria are due to four main factors: (1) the degree of multiplication of parasites and their invasion of erythrocytes; (2) the general effects of the destruction of erythrocytes; (3) the physiologic consequence of high fever and of changes in the general circulation of the blood; and (4) the local circulatory or other changes in the internal organs. As with many microbial diseases, our knowledge of the exact relationship of the parasite to many of the symptoms is unclear.

Of the four species of malaria parasites, the invasive powers are greatest in *P. falciparum;* every tenth red blood cell may be parasitized, and aggregates of such cells may form in the capillaries of various organs. In *P. vivax* and *P. ovale* infections, more than 2 per cent of erythrocytes are seldom invaded, and in *P. malariae* 1 per cent is exceptional.

The destruction of red blood cells by rupture at the time of schizogony and perhaps also by some lytic processes leads to progressive anemia that can be very severe and rapid, especially in falciparum malaria. Together with the blockage of the capillaries, this may lead to local anoxia of various tissues, and particularly of the vascular endothelium, so that capillaries are distended and occluded. Such local circulatory changes occurring in the brain, liver, kidneys, and bone marrow may result in irreversible damage to these and other organs.

The lymphoid-macrophage system of the spleen, liver, and bone marrow responds by an intense phagocytic activity destroying large numbers of parasitized cells; this is shown as an enlargement of the respective organs. The malarial pigment of parasites (hemozoin), derived from hemoglobin of the destroyed erythrocytes, accumulates in the tissue spaces and in phagocytic cells.

All these processes can be related to the pathologic changes most obvious in fatal cases of falciparum malaria: hyperemia and diffuse brown or slate-gray coloration of the spleen and liver, with centrilobular degeneration and necrosis of hepatic cells; diffuse cellular hyperplasia of the spleen; congested medullary vessels and ischemic cortex of the kidneys; and similar but less pronounced changes of other organs. As mentioned above, patients with falciparum malaria develop generalized vasodilatation during the acute illness. This has been shown to result in a decrease in effective circulating blood volume, then secondary changes of increased plasma volume, hyponatremia, reversal of the urinary sodium to potassium ratio, and increased urinary aldosterone. Orthostatic hypotension is a primary manifestation of these circulatory changes. Severe complications of progressive organ impairment have been seen in patients shown also to have evidence of accelerated intravascular coagulation. Factors V, VII, VIII, and X, fibrinogen, and platelets are decreased, and prothrombin and partial thromboplastin times are prolonged. The mechanism producing these circulatory and coagulation abnormalities is not understood.

Recurring infections with *P. malariae* in children may produce a nephrotic syndrome.

A syndrome of tropical splenomegaly seen in some patients in endemic tropical areas is related to repeated malarial infections, but its pathogenesis is not fully understood (*vide infra*).

CLINICAL MANIFESTATIONS

Incubation Period. The incubation period in malaria covers the time between the infection and the first appearance of clinical signs, of which fever is the most common. For mosquito-transmitted infection, this period, during which the pre-erythrocytic stages of parasites develop in the liver, varies according to the species of the Plasmodium. Usually about 12 days are required for *P. falciparum* to develop, 13 to 15 days for *P. vivax* or *P. ovale,* and up to one month for *P. malariae.* With some strains of *P. vivax* the incubation period may be delayed for several weeks or months; this may also occur in persons who have been taking suppressive antimalarial drugs. Even before the onset of clinical symptoms, scanty parasites may appear in the blood because the duration of the primary tissue phase in the liver is shorter than the incubation period.

The Attack. Preceded by various premonitory signs such as headache, malaise, and nausea, an attack of malaria consists of several short febrile paroxysms recurring every second day (tertian or vivax malaria) or every third day (quartan malaria); falciparum malaria produces either daily or irregular fever.

A typical paroxysm starts with a feeling of chill accompanied by shivering (rigor), pallor, cyanosis, and, at times in children, by a convulsive seizure.

Other symptoms comprise severe frontal headache, myalgia of the lower back, neck, and legs, dizziness, and general malaise. The pulse is usually fast, but this is not constant. Many patients have hypotension and dry cough. Herpes on lips and nose may be seen. There is often a low leukocyte count, a hematocrit level less than 40 per cent, increased bilirubin in urine, and some proteinuria. During the "cold stage," lasting up to one hour, the temperature rises slowly, and in the subsequent "hot stage" may go up to 104 to 106° F., (40 to 41° C.) and higher. In this stage the patient feels very hot and restless, his respiration is fast, his skin is dry and flushed, his pulse is full and bounding, and headache, thirst, and vomiting are common. After two to four hours comes the "sweating stage": the patient breaks out in profuse perspiration, and his temperature falls to normal or below, at times with a suddenness that may lead to near collapse; later the pulse rate becomes normal, and the drowsy and weak patient usually falls asleep.

Variations of Clinical Course. Such classic paroxysms are far from being the rule; variations of the clinical course are common. *Intermittent fevers with periodic paroxysms are not frequent in P. falciparum infections,* the protean symptoms of which may be very misleading. This explains why falciparum malaria is always a potentially dangerous disease. Because of the high rate of multiplication of *P. falciparum,* its symptoms may appear with dramatic suddenness. Bloody diarrhea and respiratory, renal, and hepatic symptoms with jaundice and anemia may be present. The clinical picture of falciparum malaria may deteriorate rapidly, and "pernicious" complications may be fatal. Among these complications six groups are recognized: (1) *cerebral malaria* with headache, drowsiness, coma, or acute mental disturbances and other signs of the involvement of the central nervous system; (2) *gastrointestinal malaria* simulating acute dysentery or typhoid with subsequent renal failure; (3) *acute renal failure itself,* characterized by progressive oliguria, often in the absence of the rapid hemolysis associated with blackwater fever; (4) *acute pulmonary edema,* thought in the past to be secondary to vigorous fluid therapy, but observed recently (Vietnam) to occur in the absence of documented fluid overload; (5) *hyperpyrexia* with excitement, delirium, and convulsions that may be mistaken for heat stroke or intoxication; and (6) *algid malaria* with cold, clammy skin, shallow breathing, low blood pressure owing to generalized vasodilatation, and cardiovascular failure.

"Pernicious malaria" develops usually when the *P. falciparum* parasites are numerous in the blood but, exceptionally, also when they are scanty. Rapid diagnosis and immediate, adequate treatment are necessary in every case of falciparum malaria and especially in nonimmune persons.

In vivax, ovale, and quartan malaria, splenic enlargement is frequent and, although some anemia with mild leukopenia occurs, hepatic and renal complications are uncommon. The latter, if seen, are associated with quartan malaria. Malaria owing to these infections is rarely fatal by itself but can be serious, especially in children, as it undermines the physiologic defense mechanism of a growing organism exposed to intercurrent diseases.

Recurrence and Relapse. In untreated infections, malaria attacks may recur more or less regularly, but with decreasing severity, for several weeks or longer. *Relapses,* in which the clinical course of the first attack of tertian or quartan malaria repeats itself, usually in a milder form, may occur many months later (Fig. 2).

It is unusual for vivax and ovale malaria to relapse more than three years after the patient's first attack; on the other hand, quartan malaria is much more persistent, and relapses may be seen occasionally five, ten, or more years later. In fact some persons with untreated or poorly treated quartan malaria may become asymptomatic carriers of plasmodia, and can transmit the infection for many years whenever their blood is used for transfusion.

Recurrences of acute falciparum malaria are generally milder than the initial attack; they usually disappear within one year. However, in immune persons from highly malarious areas, parasites may persist in the blood much longer and often with very mild, if any, clinical symptoms.

Clinical Picture in Children. Acute malaria in children rarely presents a classic clinical picture. Its vague symptoms may simulate many diseases such as gatroenteritis, meningitis, and respiratory or urinary infections, as well as obscure surgical conditions.

The malarial infection in indigenous inhabitants of some highly malarious areas (especially in tropical Africa) is much modified by their acquired immunity.

In many young children repeated attacks of malaria are conducive to severe anemia, wasting, enlargement of spleen and liver, stunted growth, and nutritional disturbances. Although a proportion of older children and adolescents eventually achieve a degree of immunity to infection, malaria in infants and small children may be just as severe as in the nonimmune, so that full and prompt treatment must always be given.

DIAGNOSIS

The description of the clinical course of malaria indicates that the classic and prominent symptoms of the disease, namely, periodic fever with rigor, sweating, anemia, and enlarged spleen, may be absent at the beginning of tertian and quartan malaria *and are not constant in falciparum malaria.* Yet the last named infection not only can simulate a number of other diseases and surgical conditions, but also can be quickly fatal. *Thus an early and accurate diagnosis of malaria is of paramount importance today when travel to the farthest tropics is so rapid and easy.* As the only certain proof of the infection is the finding of malaria parasites in the peripheral blood, this examination should never be neglected. Malaria should be suspected in every patient with pyrexia who has ever been in a malarious area or who has ever had a blood transfusion. Precise information on the patient's travels and medical history and on the taking of protective drugs is of great value

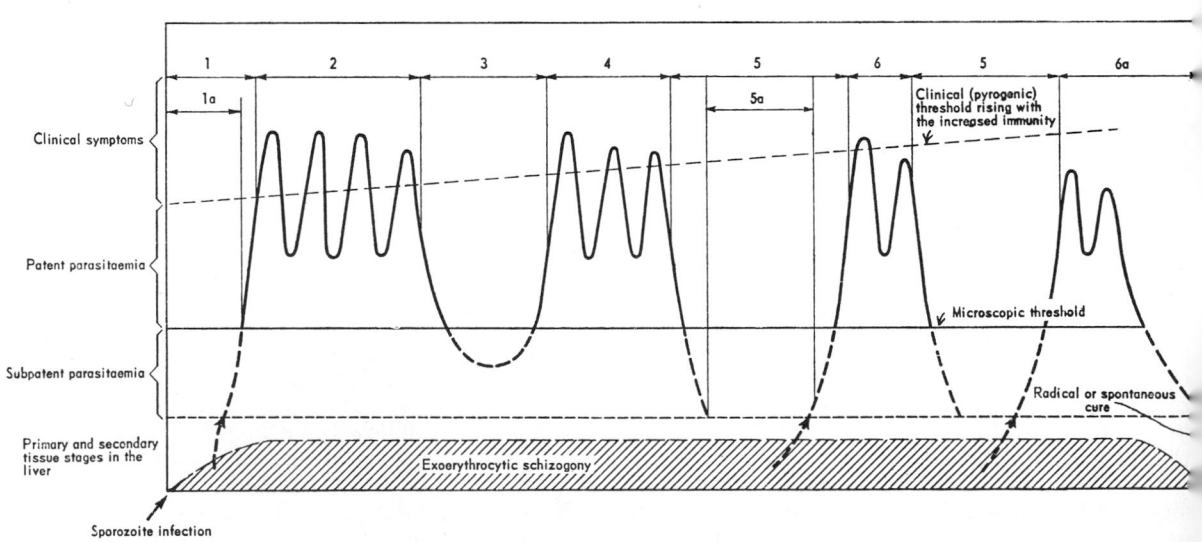

1 — Incubation period

1a— Pre-patent period

2 — Primary attack composed of paroxysms

3 — Latent period (clinical latency)

4 — Recrudescence (short-term relapse)

5 — Latent period

5a— Parasitic latency

6 — Clinical recurrence (long-term relapse) followed by parasitic recurrence

6a— Parasitic relapse

FIGURE 2. The course of a malaria infection. (World Health Organization, 1963.)

in this respect. Although the finding of parasites in the blood establishes the diagnosis, one or two negative reports are not sufficient to discard the possibility of this infection. Several thick blood films should be taken in any suspected case and examined as rapidly as possible by a competent microscopist. The correct identification of the species of the malaria parasite gives much guidance for the treatment of the patient. The parasites are usually in greatest numbers for a few hours after the rigor.

If rapid examination of blood films is not possible and the probability of malaria exists, adequate treatment may be instituted at once after taking the blood film but without waiting for the result of its examination. The prompt response of the disease to treatment may confirm the suspicion of malaria but should not be regarded as a definite proof of it.

Repeated examination of thick films from the peripheral blood is a reliable method of diagnosis. Sternal marrow puncture has no advantage whatever. Serologic methods of diagnosis are still uncertain, but may become more reliable in the future.

In the case of confirmed falciparum malaria the disappearance of parasites following treatment should be checked by several subsequent blood examinations so that records of parasite count per 100 fields of thick film or per 1000 red blood cells of the thin film should be kept. Rising falciparum parasitemia is a danger sign and demands emergency treatment.

The technique for taking the blood slide is as important as its subsequent staining. The correct result of the examination depends largely on the specimen, and this is related to the method of its collection. For the taking of the blood film the glass slide should be meticulously clean, free of dust, grease, and scratches; the ball of the middle finger (or the big toe in infants) must be wiped with an alcohol-soaked pledget of cotton wool and punctured with a needle or the tip of a lancet.

A large, free-flowing drop of blood is allowed to touch one third of the slide and is rapidly spread with the pricker to form a round or square thick smear about 1 cm. in diameter. This "thick film" should dry by itself, without exposure to any undue heat, and must be protected from dust, flies, ants, and cockroaches. It must be properly labeled on the clean part of the slide.

If possible a "thin film" should be prepared on the clean part of the slide. A small drop of blood is placed near the center of the slide, and the slide is laid on the table. The blood is touched with the narrow edge of another clean slide held at an angle. As soon as the blood spreads along the edge, this slide is pushed along the surface of the first slide to form a thin and even film. When such a "thin film" is dry, the date, name of the patient, and so forth can be written on it with a lead pencil.

It is desirable to have the "thick film" and the "thin film" on the same slide, as this allows for a better identification of some species of malaria parasites and minimizes various technical errors.

The detailed methods of staining with one of the variants of Romanovsky stains (Giemsa, Wright, Leishman, Field, and others) and the criteria for identification of species of malaria parasites are described in special manuals (see references). The standard practice is to examine thick films for five minutes, but at times longer examination may be necessary when the parasites are very scanty; taking several "thick films" may greatly increase the reliability of diagnosis. A number of artifacts in thick films may be confused with malaria parasites, and the advice of experienced workers should be sought when any doubts arise.

The diagnosis of malaria cannot depend solely on a laboratory report but requires sound clinical judgment. The finding of plasmodia in the blood film provides a criterion of paramount importance. However, parasites may be so scanty that they escape detection in the blood of a patient who took small doses of antimalarial drugs before the blood slide was taken.

A therapeutic test is of value, but must be interpreted with caution. If an adequate dose of an active antimalarial drug fails to reduce fever and other symptoms, the diagnosis of malaria is unlikely, unless one is dealing with a drug-resistant strain of the parasite.

TREATMENT OF INDIVIDUAL PATIENT

Chemotherapy and Prophylaxis

All antimalarial drugs may be considered under two main categories: protective, for the prevention of the disease, and therapeutic, for its treatment. There are several chemical groups of antimalarial compounds in general use. For practical purposes, the drugs belonging to the five most important groups are given here under their international nonproprietary names: (1) quinine, mepacrine (Atabrine), the latter now rarely used, chloroquine, and amodiaquine (the two latter drugs belong to the 4-amino quinoline group), (2) primaquine (a drug of the 8-amino quinoline group), (3) proguanil (chlorguanide), (4) pyrimethamine (and trimethoprim), and (5) sulfones and sulfonamides. The value of these drugs and their limitations can be fully understood if one realizes that they have different actions on the parasites in relation to their phase of the developmental cycle (Fig. 1).

The first two groups are essentially therapeutic drugs; primaquine is a radically curative drug as it has a specific action against the tissue forms of malaria parasites responsible for relapses of tertian and quartan malaria. Proguanil and pyrimethamine are essentially protective (prophylactic) compounds, although they have also a useful though slow therapeutic action and a sporontocidal action on the parasite developing in the mosquito. Sulfones and sulfonamides are slow-acting blood schizontocides, and their synergism with pyrimethamine is of particular value for treatment of chloroquine-resistant falciparum malaria.

All therapeutic drugs are also good protective drugs, but the reverse is not true. *For prevention of malaria in an individual visiting* or residing in malarious areas, one of the following drugs should be taken, preferably one week before arrival and then continuously and regularly during the possible exposure and also for one month after leaving the endemic area:

1. Pyrimethamine (Daraprim): 1 or 2 tablets (25 mg. each) once a week (preferably on Sundays, to assure regular taking).

2. Proguanil hydrochloride (Paludrine): 1 or 2 tablets (100 mg. each) every day.

3. Chloroquine diphosphate or sulfate (Aralen, Avloclor, Nivaquine, Resochin, etc.): 2 tablets (150 mg. base each) once a week, or 1 tablet twice a week.

4. Amodiaquine dihydrochloride dihydrate (Basoquin, Camoquin, Flavoquine, etc.): 2 or 3 tablets (200 mg. base each) once a week.

In areas where malaria is highly endemic and exposure to infection is high, once weekly administration of the two last-named drugs does not give a sufficiently wide margin of safety, and more frequent taking of these drugs, e.g., up to 600 mg. of chloroquine base over the week, is preferable. Proguanil (chlorguanide), 2 tablets daily, has also been widely used in these conditions.

As an alternative, quinine sulfate or dihydrochloride may be taken for suppression at the adult dose of 650 mg. daily if other drugs are not available.

In the war areas of Southeast Asia, the U.S. Army introduced a prophylactic regimen consisting of once weekly administration of 300 mg. base of chloroquine and 45 mg. of primaquine. In addition to that, diaphenyl sulfone (DDS) is taken daily in a dose of 25 mg. The British and Australian forces in Southeast Asia continue to rely on proguanil (chlorguanide), 1 to 2 tablets daily.

Some persons may have mild gastrointestinal or other symptoms with any of these drugs. A change to a different drug is then indicated.

Children should be given proportionately lower doses of drugs. A practical method of reckoning of dosages for children can be based on Table 1.

In modern pediatrics the calculation of drug dosage from the age of the child is increasingly avoided, as weight is more justified as a basis for determining dosage. However, it is recognized that this method also has disadvantages. Drug dosage is often calculated in relation to body surface area (BSA) according to the general rule: BSA of child divided by BSA of adult times dose for adult. Simple tables and nomograms for conversion of weight into BSA and giving the proportion of adult dose are available. Antimalarials should be kept out of children's reach; this applies particularly to tasteless or flavored and sweet preparations.

Treatment of Acute Malaria. *It should be noted that, except for some special circumstances outlined below, the initial chemotherapy of all acute malaria is the same irrespective of the species of Plasmodium. It is in the additional "follow-up" therapy that the chemotherapy of relapsing malaria is different.* For acute malaria the most active drugs are chloroquine and amodiaquine; quinine is still of value in some circumstances, e.g., resistance of parasites to other drugs, and for parenteral administration in very severe infections. The generally advocated oral treatment of moderately severe malaria in adults of average weight (70 kg.) is shown in Table 2.

It should be noted that the administration of chloroquine or amodiaquine indicated for days 4 to 7 is optional, and in many cases a three-day treatment may suffice. On the other hand, the "loading dose" on the first day is of utmost importance.

This treatment of tertian and quartan malaria effects a clinical cure, but usually relapses of malarial attacks occur several months later. Freedom from recrudescences of falciparum infection can be assured by a "follow-up" treatment of 300 mg. of chloroquine or amodiaquine, taken once a week for a month.

In Southeast Asia, where quinine has often been used for treatment of chloroquine-resistant malaria, the above quinine regimen was associated with the daily administration of 50 mg. of pyrimethamine during the first three days, followed by sulfone given at the prophylactic dose (25 mg. daily) for one month.

All these drugs are very bitter and must be given with a generous drink of milk, fruit juice, or other flavored fluid. Care must be taken to make certain that the patient swallows the tablets and does not later vomit. Proper nursing and relief of general symptoms are important in the treatment of malaria. Particular care must be taken to combat hyperpyrexia, dehydration, anemia, and renal and hepatic involvement.

Strains of malaria parasites from different

TABLE 1.

Age of Child	Fraction of Adult Dose	
Over 12 years	$^3/_4$–1	
6–12 years	$^1/_2$–$^3/_4$	Allowance to be made for size and weight of child
2–6 years	$^1/_4$–$^1/_2$	
Infants up to 2 years	$^1/_8$–$^1/_4$	

TABLE 2.

	Chloroquine*(base)		Amodiaquine* (base)		Quinine
Day 1 followed six hours later by:	600 mg.		600 mg.		650 mg. (10 grains)
	300 mg.	1500 mg.		1400 mg.	650 mg. and eight hours later again the same dose
Day 2	300 mg.		400 mg.		650 mg. three times a day
Day 3	300 mg.		400 mg.		650 mg. twice a day
Day 4	300 mg. (if necessary)		400 mg. (if necessary)		650 mg. twice a day
Days 5 to 7	300 mg. (if necessary)		400 mg. (if necessary)		650 mg. twice a day
Total dose	1500 to 2100 mg.		1400 to 1800 mg.		10,500 mg. (160 grains) over 7 days

*Synthetic antimalarials are usually prepared as salts of the basic compounds, but the dosage should always be expressed in terms of base, e.g., tablets of chloroquine *diphosphate* of 250 mg. contain 150 mg. of chloroquine *base*. The labels of available drug preparations refer normally to the content of base, but this should be checked to avoid confusion of dosage.

geographic areas may differ in their susceptibility to drugs. Consequently the therapeutic regimen should not be rigid. Some variation of the dosage of antimalarials is needed according to the weight of the patients and their condition. The judgment of the attending physician should be guided not only by the symptoms of the disease, but also by the results of frequent blood examinations, including parasite counts and hematologic data.

Relapsing Malaria. A radical cure for relapsing malaria can be obtained when the usual treatment by chloroquine or amodiaquine is followed by administration of primaquine at an adult dosage of 15 mg. of base every day for 14 days, or 30 mg. once a week for 8 weeks. Daily treatment may occasionally produce cyanosis, abdominal pain, and hemolytic symptoms in individuals whose erythrocytes are deficient in the enzyme glucose-6-phosphate dehydrogenase. Drug taking once a week does not normally produce such symptoms. Some degree of medical supervision is necessary when primaquine treatment is given.

Parenteral Route. Irrespective of the species of the parasite, any severe malarial infection with cerebral symptoms, vomiting, pronounced nausea, or defective absorption from the gastrointestinal tract requires parenteral administration of a rapidly acting antimalarial. Falciparum malaria, when over 5 per cent of erythrocytes are infected, even though clinical symptoms may not be very alarming, should always be treated as a medical emergency, and preferably the patient should be transferred to the hospital for dealing with any "pernicious" complications that may develop with dramatic suddenness.

Quinine and chloroquine are the best drugs for parenteral administration. Intravenous injection acts somewhat more rapidly than intramuscular injection but presents a relatively greater risk in some patients. For intravenous injection both quinine and chloroquine are almost equally acceptable. The first acts rather more quickly but (unless given very slowly) may cause a fall in blood pressure and, more exceptionally, other symptoms in patients with hypersensitivity to this drug. The consensus from past experience is that quinine should be withheld if there is any evidence of intravascular hemolysis or oliguria, but this position has recently been challenged.

Intravenous quinine or chloroquine must be given with caution and in high dilution. Quinine dihydrochloride solution may be given at the adult dose of 500 to 650 mg. (8 to 10 mg. per kilogram of body weight) diluted in 20 ml. of physiologic saline with 5 per cent glucose or in plasma. It should be injected *very slowly* (at least ten minutes) or, preferably, given as an intravenous drip in 0.5 liter of plasma or physiologic saline with glucose. This may be repeated, if necessary, after six to eight hours. The dose of 2000 mg. over 24 hours should not be exceeded.

Intravenous injections of chloroquine sulfate, diphosphate, or hydrochloride can be given at a single dose of 200 mg. base (4 ml. of 5 per cent solution) with the same precautions as with quinine.

Higher doses, but not exceeding 400 mg. of base, may be given, but it is preferable to give such a dose in 0.5 liter of physiologic solution or plasma over a period of one hour. This can be repeated, if necessary, after eight hours, but the parenteral dose of 800 mg. of chloroquine base over 24 hours should not be exceeded.

As with many other drugs, faulty technique of intravenous injection of quinine or chloroquine solutions may produce local necrosis of surrounding tissues; this risk is greater with quinine than with chloroquine.

Unless there are good clinical indications for intravenous administration of quinine or chloroquine, a safer alternative is intramuscular injection. For this, quinine hydrochloride can be given in a single adult dose of 500 to 650 mg. in 10 per cent neutralized solution. The total adult dosage over 24 hours should not exceed 2000 mg.

Intramuscular injections of chloroquine salts are given at the single dose of 200 to 400 mg. of base, a total dose not to exceed 800 to 1000 mg. spaced over 24 hours. In children the dose must not exceed 5 mg. per kilogram of base.

Proper technique of intramuscular injection, especially that of quinine, must be strictly observed. After a thorough cleaning of the skin, the drug should be given in the classic site of the upper external quadrant of the buttock deep into the gluteal tissue. Sterile precautions must be strictly observed to avoid accidental contamination. Quinine injections may produce local transient reactions, which occasionally leave long-lasting fibrotic indurations. This is exceptional with chloroquine.

Mepacrine (Atabrine) methane sulfonate may be given intramuscularly in a single adult dose not exceeding 300 mg. and not over 600 to 900 mg. in 24 hours. This drug should never be given by intravenous injection, and its intramuscular administration carries some small risk of toxic effects, with cerebral or cutaneous symptoms in certain patients and especially in children. Injectable preparations of amodiaquine are not available, but a similar compound (propoquine) has been used.

Intravenous injections of any antimalarial drugs in children below seven years of age may be dangerous and should be avoided if possible. Intramuscular injections should be given only when really necessary in severe infections requiring rapid treatment, and the dosage of the drug must be based on the weight of the child (*vide supra*). It is safer to give the drug in two halves separated by an interval of one to two hours. Oral treatment of all cases of malaria should be preferred and used whenever possible.

Toxic Effects of Antimalarial Drugs. Side effects of conventional antimalarial drugs taken by mouth are relatively few, provided that their dosage is related to the size and the condition of the patient. None of these drugs is contraindicated during pregnancy. Proguanil and pyrimethamine are usually better tolerated than mepacrine, the 4-aminoquinolines, or primaquine. Nevertheless, cases of accidental death of children have occurred after swallowing several pyrimethamine tablets at once; large doses of this compound given over a long time have a depressive effect on the bone marrow. Mepacrine taken prophylactically over a long period produces a yellow discoloration of the skin, nails, and mucous membranes, and occasionally lichenoid dermatitis; given in large doses, it may be responsible for transient mental disturbances. Quinine may cause tinnitus, tremor, and ocular symptoms. Chloroquine and amodiaquine may cause abdominal discomfort, vomiting, and other symptoms; administration of very large doses of these drugs over a long period may produce punctate keratitis and neuroretinitis. The dosage of these drugs in children must be adjusted to the weight and condition of the subject; when an appropriate and relatively large dose of these drugs must be given, it is preferable to divide it into two or three smaller ones adequately spaced. Primaquine and other 8-aminoquinolines, as well as the sulfones and sulfonamides, may cause nausea, vomiting, cyanosis, and other symptoms, especially in dark-skinned people. The hemolytic effect of these compounds in subjects with G-6-PD deficiency was mentioned earlier. Some long-acting sulfonamides taken at high doses may have serious toxic effects and should not be given for more than two or three days.

Drug-Resistant Plasmodia. In some parts of the world malaria parasites have developed resistance to antimalarial drugs and especially to the synthetic compounds that began to replace quinine during and soon after World War II. The term "resistance" has been defined as the ability of a parasite strain to survive or to multiply, or both, despite the administration and absorption of an active drug given in doses equal to or higher than those usually recommended but within the limits of tolerance of the subject.*

The observation of resistance to proguanil and pyrimethamine during the early 1950's was of limited importance because these drugs are not normally used for treatment of acute malaria. Whenever there is sufficient evidence that these two drugs fail to give the protective (prophylactic) effect, chloroquine or amodiaquine can be used. However, the reports on resistance of malaria parasites (mainly *P. falciparum*) to 4-aminoquinolines (chloroquine and amodiaquine) first observed in 1960–1961 in Colombia and in Brazil were of greater consequence, as together with quinine these are the most valuable drugs for treatment of acute malaria. Further reports on drug resistance came from Thailand, Malaysia, Cambodia, Vietnam, and recently from Laos and some Philippine islands. This presents a problem of great medical, military, and public health importance, especially if such strains should spread more widely.

In practice, drug resistance is suspected when

*It should be noted that this concept of drug resistance customarily used for malaria is considerably broader than the concept of drug resistance in the chemotherapy of bacterial and other microbial diseases.

cases of malaria (usually *P. falciparum*) do not fully and rapidly respond to "standard treatment" with 4-aminoquinolines or when recrudescence of symptoms and parasitemia are seen soon after their temporary disappearance subsequent to therapy. The first situation has greater validity, as recrudescence of the infection may be due to a number of causes. One should remember that there are strains of plasmodia with an inherent higher tolerance of specific compounds that therefore require somewhat larger doses of certain drugs to be given over a longer period. Moreover, there may be differences between individual patients in the way they absorb and metabolize drugs.

Some strains of *P. falciparum* resistant to 4-aminoquinolines have also proved to be resistant to mepacrine, and have shown variable patterns of response to proguanil and pyrimethamine, and a lessened susceptibility to quinine.

Any reports of apparent resistance of malaria parasites to 4-aminoquinolines should be based on a careful investigation of each case to exclude the possibility of the drug's not having been taken by the patient or having been vomited. Attention must be paid to the quality of the drug, and the dose should be adjusted to the weight of the patient. Accuracy of the blood examination following the administration of the drug is essential, and records of parasite counts should be kept.

Criteria for recognition of suspected resistance of malaria parasites to 4-aminoquinolines have been proposed, and a standard procedure for determining the response of malaria parasites to chloroquine in the field has been recommended (WHO, 1967). Final confirmation of drug resistance can be obtained from the study of the induced malaria infections on human volunteers in a special reference center.

Should the drugs of the 4-aminoquinoline group given at the adequate dosage fail to produce the desired therapeutic effect, quinine is still one of the more reliable alternative drugs.

Laboratory and field studies have stimulated much interest in the therapeutic value of certain sulfones and sulfonamides. It has been known for some time that 4,4'-diamino-diphenyl-sulfone (DDS) has a blood schizontocidal activity. These compounds have a relatively slow action when given to nonimmune individuals infected with chloroquine-resistant strains of *P. falciparum*. Some sulfonamides such as sulfadiazine, sulfadimethoxine, sulfalene, and sulphormethoxine (now known as sulfadoxine) have undergone a number of recent trials. The last-named compound, with a prolonged action owing to an extensive binding to plasma protein, appears to be of value for treatment of malaria caused by chloroquine-resistant strains. The treatment advocated on the basis of present experience is 1 gram of sulfadoxine and 50 mg. of pyrimethamine given as a single dose or, at most, for two days. Sulfalene with trimethoprim has also been used with good effect. Other sulfonamides (sulfadiazine) have been used, but these must be administered at 250 mg. daily for five days with one or two doses of pyrimethamine.

It should be noted, however, that the evaluation of the antimalarial value of sulfones and sulfonamides and their synergists is still in a relatively early stage. Some serious side effects owing to indiscriminate use of long-acting sulfonamides have been observed, and this indicates the need for caution in their use until more information becomes available. Various other compounds are now undergoing screening tests and many laboratory and clinical trials. Among these, one should mention pyrocatechol and acridin derivatives, diamidin ureas, various aminoquinolines, and antibacterial drugs such as lincomycin. New and better antimalarial drugs are urgently needed.

Multiple-Drug Regimens and Long-Acting Drugs. For both suppressive treatment and drug administration on a large scale, associations of drugs are often used. These consist mainly of chloroquine with pyrimethamine (150 mg. base plus 15 mg. base, respectively, per tablet), chloroquine with chlorproguanil (150 mg. base plus 20 mg., respectively, per tablet) and chloroquine or amodiaquine with primaquine (75 to 150 mg. base plus 15 mg., respectively, per tablet). The latter combination of drugs is useful in areas where *P. falciparum* and *P. vivax* are common.

Progress has been made in the development of a long-acting injectable prophylactic antimalarial. A dihydrotriazine (cycloguanil pamoate or Camolar) in a single dose of 5 to 10 mg. per kilogram has given full protection for three or more months against malarial infections with susceptible strains of plasmodia. Such protective action of dihydrotriazine can be enhanced by association with sulfone derivatives.

General Management of Complications

Treatment of patients with complications of falciparum malaria, such as involvement of the central nervous system, anemia, hyperpyrexia, dehydration, cardiovascular and gastrointestinal symptoms, and renal and hepatic failure, must be instituted rapidly and carried out concurrently with the specific antiplasmodial measures. Cautious administration of heparin (0.5 mg. per kilogram) has been advocated if there is some evidence of intravascular coagulation. Adrenal steroid therapy in the form of dexamethasone (10 mg.) has been found effective in cerebral malaria. (For the renal complications and their therapy, see Acute Renal Failure.)

Blackwater Fever. Blackwater fever is a syndrome of acute hemolysis and subsequent hemoglobinuria caused by *P. falciparum* infection. At one time, when quinine was widely used as a prophylactic drug, blackwater fever was very common, but the introduction of synthetic antimalarials decreased its incidence. *The clinical picture* is that of a severe attack of malaria, frequently but not always associated with high parasitemia and followed by the sudden passage of small amounts of dark red or black urine with a copious amorphous deposit containing albumin, hyaline and granular casts, epithelial cells, and blood pigments. In severe cases there are oxy- and methemoglobin, bile pigments, and red blood cells, with subsequent retention of urine and acidosis. The hemolysis may be so severe that the erythrocyte count may fall within one or two days to below 1 million per cubic millimeter. Vomiting, pain in the loins, dehydration, and jaundice are common, and the patient may present a state of shock with rapid and threadlike pulse. In mild cases the hemolytic crisis abates slowly, but in 25 to 50 per cent of patients there are progressive anemia, hepatic damage, and irreversible renal failure with death owing to cardiac failure or anemia. The pathologic picture is that of a renal ischemia followed by tubular necrosis. Mild hemoglobinuria induced by drugs in patients with G-6-PD deficiency should not be mistaken for blackwater fever.

Absolute rest is imperative unless the patient can be easily transferred to a well-equipped hospital. Blood transfusion may be a life-saving procedure, but careful cross matching of the blood must be assured; excessive transfusion may be harmful. Corticosteroids may prevent further hemolysis. When anuria develops, blood dialysis or peritoneal dialysis is needed (see Acute Renal Failure and Dialysis and Ultrafiltration Therapy). It should be emphasized that it is very worthwhile to persist in dialysis and the other filtration measures, as the anuria is usually the result of lower nephron necrosis, and spontaneous regeneration occurs.

Antimicrobial drugs may be given if necessary; quinine should be avoided or used with caution; slow intravenous infusion is the best method in this situation. Diuretics and alkalinization of the blood are harmful. In dehydrated patients restoration of body fluids is necessary, but care must be taken not to overload the circulation by excessive intravenous infusions. Perfect nursing care of the patient is particularly important.

GROUP PROTECTION

Chemoprophylaxis. General protection of groups of people residing temporarily in malarious areas and of populations living there permanently can be achieved by individual or collective chemotherapeutic measures based on prevention of the infection or on its suppression, although the last two effects often overlap.

Prevention of infection by the elimination of parasites from the organism before they start multiplying in the blood is possible with proguanil given at an adult dose of not less than 100 mg. daily, or with pyrimethamine at not less than 25 mg. once a week. These two drugs are safe and efficient prophylactics of *P. falciparum* unless the relevant strains of this species have become resistant to either or both drugs. They are less effective for prophylaxis of *P. vivax* and probably other species.

Suppressive treatment by repetitive drug administration aims at prevention of clinical symptoms and, possibly, elimination of some infections if given over a long period. Chloroquine and amodiaquine are excellent suppressants, and will achieve a radical cure of infections caused by *P. falciparum* susceptible to these drugs. Chloroquine should be given at the adult dosage of not less than 300 mg. base a week, although a double dosage may be needed for nonimmune persons exposed to the infection in highly malarious areas.

At the appropriate dosage none of these drugs taken for general protection has any serious side effects.

The suppressive treatment is usually reserved for more vulnerable groups such as children or pregnant women, but it may be given to the whole population. This mass drug administration can be achieved either by supervised distribution of tablets or by incorporation of the drug (chloroquine or amodiaquine) into common salt used for normal daily preparation of food. The latter form of indirect drug distribution is often referred to as Pinotti's method.

Environmental Control. Mosquito reduction measures such as filling, draining, and larvicides should be applied in a malarious area whenever possible to control the breeding of Anopheles. An effective method of malaria control in highly malarious countries consists of spraying all inhabited structures of entire communities within a determined area with a residual insecticide at the proper dosage (1 to 2 grams of DDT to each square meter of inside surface of walls and ceilings). This should be repeated twice a year, or more often if necessary. Other insecticides such as hexachlorocyclohexane (HCH), dieldrin, malathion, and carbamates may be preferable to DDT in some conditions, especially if the local malaria vector has developed resistance to DDT or other compounds. A degree of control of vectors can also be achieved by frequent indoor application of quick-acting preparations of pyrethrum as atomized spray; aerosol formulations for outdoor fogging or "space-spraying" are also used. Volatile dichlorvos compounds incorporated into synthetic wax strips may be useful.

In endemic malarious areas, all sleeping and living quarters should be mosquito-proofed, and mosquito nets should be used over the beds. Insect-repellent liquids such as dimethylphthalate applied to the exposed parts of the body of persons remaining out of doors after dark protect for three to four hours from bites of mosquitoes.

Malaria Eradication

The concept of malaria eradication on a global scale, advocated by the Fourteenth Pan-American Sanitary Conference in 1954, was supported by the Eighth World Health Assembly in Mexico in 1955. In 1957 the World Health Organization approved the principles and practice of malaria eradication activities.

In concept, malaria eradication means the extermination of the malaria parasites of man in the human population of a large area; it does not imply the eradication of the species of Anopheles that transmit the infection. The main conceptual differences between the eradication of malaria and its control is that control attempts only a reduction of the incidence of disease and is virtually a permanent commitment. An eradication program should be limited in time, and aims at the ending of transmission and the elimination of the reservoir of infected cases. A malaria eradication program has four phases: preparatory, attack, consolidation, and maintenance. The expected duration of the first three phases that lead to the entry into the maintenance phase is eight years, but this could take longer, as it depends on the epidemiologic features of the area concerned, on technical problems encountered, and on the socioeconomic conditions of the country (*vide infra*).

The operational methods of malaria eradication are based on an area-wide indoor spraying of dwellings with residual insecticides at the appropriate dosage and frequency. Antimalarial drugs are used either as a complementary method or for prevention of new cases and cure of remaining cases of malaria. Surveillance activities comprise prompt detection, radical treatment, reporting of cases of malaria, and focal spraying. By the end of 1968, of the estimated population of 1733 million people living in the originally malarious areas of the world, a total of 1353 million lived in areas in which eradication programs were in progress or from which malaria had apparently been eradicated. However, there remained 380 million people inhabiting areas of the globe (two thirds of them in tropical Africa) not covered by eradication programs.

In its initial stages, the general progress of the global malaria eradication program was satisfactory, but at the present time a number of biologic, technical, administrative, and other difficulties are hindering its early completion in developing countries and particularly in tropical Africa. Among the technical and biologic problems are the resistance of Anopheles to residual insecticides (DDT or dieldrin) and the high degree of exophily of certain malaria vectors. The type of housing that precludes the use of residual insecticides and mobility of certain human populations must be mentioned. Resistance of plasmodia to present antimalarial drugs is a potentially serious problem. The administrative obstacles are related to the shortages of trained staff, operational shortcomings, financial provision, and other similar problems bearing on the socioeconomic levels of the countries concerned.

The global strategy of malaria eradication was reviewed at the Twenty-Second World Health Assembly (Boston, 1969), and several important changes of policy were made so that control methods could be more widely used in countries where eradication of malaria proves difficult at present.

Adams, A. R. D., and Maegraith, B. G.: Clinical Tropical Diseases. 4th ed. Oxford, Blackwell Scientific Publications, 1966.

American Public Health Association: Control of Communicable Diseases in Man. 11th ed. A. S. Benenson (ed.), New York, American Public Health Association, 1970.

Boyd, M. (ed.): Malariology. Philadelphia, W. B. Saunders Company, 1949.

Covell, G., Coatney, G. R., Field, J. W., and Singh, J.: Chemotherapy of Malaria. WHO Monograph No. 27, Geneva, 1955.

Garnham, P. C. C.: Malaria Parasites and Other Hemosporidia. Oxford, Blackwell Scientific Publications, 1966.

Hunter, G. W., Frye, W W., and Swartzwelder, J. C.: A Manual of Tropical Medicine. 4th ed. Philadelphia, W. B. Saunders Company, 1966.

Macdonald, G.: The Epidemiology and Control of Malaria. London, Oxford University Press, 1957.

Manson-Bahr, P.: Manson's Tropical Diseases. 16th ed. London, Bailliere, Tindall & Cassell, Ltd., 1966.

Pampana, E.: A. Textbook of Malaria Eradication. 2nd ed. London, Oxford University Press, 1969.

Russell, P. F., West, L. S., Manwell, R. D., and Macdonald, G.: Practical Malariology. London, Oxford University Press, 1963.

Wilcox, A.: Manual for the Microscopical Diagnosis of Malaria in Man. 2nd ed. Washington, D. C., National Institutes of Health, Bull. No. 180, 1960.

World Health Organization: Terminology of Malaria and of Malaria Eradication. Geneva, 1963.

World Health Organization: Chemotherapy of Malaria. Technical Report Series No. 375. Geneva, 1967.

World Health Organization: Immunology of Malaria. Technical Report Series No. 396. Geneva, 1968.

SYNDROMES ASSOCIATED WITH MALARIA

Philip D. Marsden

In hyperendemic areas where transmission is intense and individuals may be bitten daily by malaria-carrying mosquitoes, it is not surprising that the clinical syndromes encountered may be quite different from those present in nonimmune persons. Much research is needed on the question of the effects of such frequent plasmodial challenge; but it has become clear in recent years that two clinical syndromes appear to be encountered with malaria, and these require mention here.

MALARIAL NEPHROSIS
(Quartan Nephrosis)

Malarial nephrosis can be defined as the association between a specific malaria parasite, namely, *Plasmodium malariae,* and the presence of the nephrotic syndrome. It occurs especially in children. Although it has been described from Guyana, Malaya, New Guinea, and many parts of Africa, the best studies come from Nigeria. Epidemiologic studies have shown that (1) the prevalence of *P. malariae* parasitemia is significantly higher in children with the nephrotic syndrome than in sick or healthy controls; (2) there is a high incidence of nephrotic syndrome in areas where *P. malariae* is common; and (3) the age of onset of childhood nephrosis is different in Africa from that in North America and Europe.

The histologic lesions in the glomeruli have been described as local, segmental, proliferative, and membranous glomerulonephritis. The prognosis is poor, most children appearing to have poorly selective proteinuria and to be steroid resistant. It has been suggested that repeated untreated attacks of *P. malariae* may promote an abnormal immunologic response in which the glomerular basement membrane is damaged by an antigen-antibody complex from which it has become sensitized. Fluorescent antibody studies have revealed heavy deposits of host gamma globulin in the glomerular basement membrane, suggesting an accumulation of immune complexes at this site.

Gilles, H. M., and Hendrickse, R. G.: Nephrosis in Nigerian children. Role of *Plasmodium malariae* and effect of antimalarial treatment. Brit. Med. J., 2:27, 1963.

Kibukamusoke, J. W., Hutt, M. S. R., and Wilks, N. E.: The nephrotic syndrome in Uganda and its association with quartan malaria. Quart. J. Med. (NS), 36:393:1967.

TROPICAL SPLENOMEGALY SYNDROME
(Big Spleen Disease)

It is well known that many patients are encountered in the tropics with marked splenomegaly for which no cause can be found. In the past this finding has been dismissed without any real evidence as being due to chronic malaria, as malaria parasites are not seen in the peripheral blood. Of recent years, however, evidence has accumulated to implicate malaria. Apart from marked splenomegaly and hepatomegaly, patients with the tropical splenomegaly syndrome frequently have hepatic sinusoidal lymphocytosis on liver biopsy. The coexistent anemia is a compound effect of an increased plasma volume, splenic pooling of red cells, and intrasplenic red cell destruction. The gamma globulin levels are above the normal for the area, with a marked increase in the IgM fraction. The principal evidences that malaria is implicated are (1) the occurrence of the syndrome in hyperendemic malarial areas and its disappearance when malaria is controlled, and (2) the presence of elevated fluorescent malarial antibody titers when compared with similar patient populations with and without splenomegaly. Prolonged treatment with antimalarials has resulted in resolution of the splenomegaly, and recently it has proved possible to induce hepatic sinusoidal lymphocytosis in some monkeys after frequent plasmodial challenge. At one time *P. malariae* was implicated in the etiology of this syndrome, but this is no longer thought to be the case. That only a proportion of patients in an hyperendemic area develop marked splenomegaly is thought to be an expression of an unusual host response to plasmodial antigen or the interaction of malaria with an unidentified virus.

Marsden, P. D., and Hamilton, P. J. S.: Splenomegaly in the tropics. Brit. Med. J., 1:99, 1969.

Pitney, W. R.: The tropical splenomegaly syndrome. Trans. Roy. Soc. Trop. Med. Hyg., 62:717, 1968.

TRYPANOSOMIASES

AFRICAN TRYPANOSOMIASIS
(African Sleeping Sickness, Maladie du Sommeil, Schlafkrankheit)
W. E. Ormerod

Definition and Etiology. African trypanosomiasis (sleeping sickness) is a disease of the central nervous system caused by the protozoan *Trypanosoma brucei* (Plimmer and Bradford, 1899). The disease occurs in several clinico-epidemiologic patterns. The two principal patterns are Rhodesian sleeping sickness, which is relatively acute, and Gambian sleeping sickness, which is chronic. Another form, Zambezi sleeping sickness, although chronic, is more like the acute (Rhodesian) form in its epidemiologic behavior. The terms "Rhodesian" and "Gambian" are used without geographic implication.

It was formerly believed that each type of the disease was caused by a sharply characterized species of trypanosome (*T. rhodesiense* and *T. gambiense*). Zoologists are tending to abandon this concept, because the strains involved are largely indistinguishable except for their behavior in man. As it is now realized that even in man there is no clear-cut distinction, there is little justification for retaining the terms *T. rhodesiense* and *T. gambiense* in the medical literature. The name of the "type species" *Trypanosoma (Trypanozoon) brucei* (previously restricted in its use to strains of animal trypanosomes that do not infect man) is now used for the various strains that cause disease either in man or in other animals.

T. brucei is variable in size; the first forms to appear are long and thin (approximately $20 \times 3\ \mu$), but by the time infection is established, short stumpy forms (approximately $10 \times 5\ \mu$) are present together with a full range of intermediate sizes. It was discovered in the 1890's by Sir David Bruce to be the cause of nagana in cattle in Zululand. The Gambian disease of man was first found in 1902 by Todd and the Rhodesian disease in 1910. *T. congolense* and *T. vivax* are important causes of trypanosomiasis in cattle, but, as they do not infect man, they are of no direct medical interest. Trypanosomiasis can cause serious losses in domestic cattle and where good husbandry is practiced can reduce the food supply, but in Africa where husbandry is usually bad, and the yields are negligible, the existence of cattle trypanosomiasis acts as an important restraint on overgrazing and consequent soil erosion.

The term "Zambezi sleeping sickness" describes the disease as it occurs today in the Zambezi-Okovango basin. It was previously ascribed to *T. rhodesiense;* indeed, the original strain of *T. rhodesiense* was described in this area, but there are now known to be significant differences between these strains and those in Tanzania, Uganda, and Kenya that are now said to cause "Rhodesian" sleeping sickness.

Prevalence. Although animal strains of *T. brucei* occur throughout the tsetse belt of Africa, that is to say, south of the Sahara and north of the Limpopo River and the Kalahari, human strains are not so widespread. The chronic (Gambian) form is to be found in West Africa from the Gambia to the Congo, penetrating inland to Lakes Tchad, Victoria, and Tanganyika. The chronic (Zambezi) form with similar pathology is also to be found in Botswana, Rhodesia, Zambia, and Portuguese East Africa but, as mentioned above, in its epidemiology it resembles the more acute (Rhodesian) form now found in Tanzania, Uganda, Kenya, and (most recently) Ethiopia. Distinction among these forms is not always useful to the clinician because today the treatment of all forms is the same. Nevertheless, there is some difference in the prognosis of the different forms, and to the epidemiologist the differences are of great importance.

Transmission. *T. brucei* is transmitted by several species of the tsetse fly Glossina. When the fly bites an infected host, if its feeding is interrupted it can pass the infection to a second host by regurgitating part of the first feed. This mode of infection may occur at the height of an epidemic when other biting flies such as Stomoxys or tabanid (horse) flies may also be involved. Usually, however, the trypanosomes develop in the tsetse into noninfective forms, and this process continues for about 20 days until infective trypanosomes are formed; these remain in the salivary gland of the fly until it dies from other causes. The duration of the developmental cycle in the fly varies with temperature and does not continue below 18° C. Thus, temperature and altitude form a limit on the cyclical transmission of trypanosomiasis.

Epidemiology. Rhodesian Sleeping Sickness. The Rhodesian strains of *T. brucei* are transmitted mainly by *G. morsitans.* This fly is associated with the edge of Brachistegia woodland (the miombo of Tanzania) and with the woodland that fringes watercourses in which, during the dry season, its habitat resembles that of *G. pallidipes,* also a transmitting agent. Although these flies feed on the blood of a wide range of species of game animals, *there is evidence that the only important wild animal reservoir of Rhodesian sleeping sickness* is the bushbuck *Tragelaphus scriptus.* This small antelope differs from other game in that it can live in close proximity to man, runs only a short distance when disturbed, and returns to its original "stand" in a thicket where it shares the same population of Glossina with man if he happens to be present. Zambezi and sporadic Rhodesian disease are spread by this means, but epidemic Rhodesian strains are spread by *G. morsitans,* ranging widely in or between scattered thickets at the edge of the miombo, and under these conditions direct "man-fly-man" transmission occurs. Recent evidence suggests that domestic cattle may also act as a reservoir (Onyango et al.).

Epidemic Rhodesian sleeping sickness occurred in Tanzania in the 1930's, and large areas remain depopulated, because the disease has become "enzootic" and is still liable to break out again and cause acute disease in man. To the north of Lake Victoria, where epidemics have occurred more recently, the disease is spread mainly by *G. pallidipes,* which ranges widely in the lakeside thickets. In Kenya a recent epidemic has been attributed to *G. fuscipes,* a fly related to *G. palpalis,* which has otherwise always been associated with Gambian sleeping sickness. This serves to emphasize the unstable and fluctuating epidemiology of the disease in this area.

Gambian Sleeping Sickness. Gambian sleeping sickness is transmitted mainly by *G. palpalis.* This fly obtains its blood meal from reptiles, birds, and man; it is a shade- and moisture-loving fly, and consequently transmission occurs most readily when a population of flies becomes isolated by unfavorable climate around a small woodland area. Frequently in West African savannah country such woodlands contain the water supply of a village. Here interchange of trypanosomes between fly and man takes place, and a focus of infection is built up. *G. tachinoides*, a fly associated with river thickets of West Africa, also transmits Gambian strains. This fly feeds on the blood of mammals other than man; *consequently it cannot be stated with confidence that there are no other animal reservoirs of Gambian sleeping sickness.* Indeed, the domestic pig has been shown to harbor strains, but there is no evidence that these are of epidemiologic importance.

Pathology. The extent of pathologic lesions depends on the duration of the disease. The most acute cases, those in which death occurs within two months, show little effect other than that associated with infectious disease generally. There are general wasting, hemorrhages into lung and bone marrow, and cellular proliferation in lymph nodes and in the malpighian bodies of the spleen. Acute myocarditis rarely occurs but is said to be the cause of death in some cases. Most cases of acute disease show some small round-cell infiltration of the meninges, but the brain appears normal. After about six months, the lymph nodes and malpighian bodies lose much of their cellularity, and fibrosis occurs in lymph nodes and vessels. At this stage the red bone marrow decreases, and a normocytic anemia and a leukopenia with a relative increase in lymphocytes occur. There is slight infiltration of the brain substance with small round cells, but heavy infiltration of the leptomeninges. Where the leptomeninges extend into the Aschoff-Robin space that surrounds meningeal vessels as they penetrate into the brain substance, the lesion known as *perivascular cuffing* is produced; this may vary from a single layer of infiltrating cells surrounding the vessel in cases lasting for about six months, to a depth of about 20 cells when the disease has continued for two or more years. The nature of the cellular reaction has not been studied in detail, but there is one type of cell, the large *morular cell* (Mott's cells) with loculated eosinophilic cytoplasm, that is present in the leptomeninges or the cuffing (rarely in the brain substance). The presence of this cell is considered pathognomonic of advanced sleeping sickness. Thrombosis is liable to occur in the cuffed vessels and gives rise to the cerebral degeneration that causes the progressive mental deterioration and coma from which the disease is named.

Pathogenesis. The tsetse fly feeds by rupturing small vessels and sucking from the subcutaneous pool that is formed. It may inject trypanosomes either into the blood stream or into the pool where they lodge and grow to form a *chancre*, a hard painful nodule that contains trypanosomes. Initial growth of the trypanosomes is in the blood and seldom reaches a level greater than one organism per cubic millimeter, probably because of the action of antibodies that are produced in response to an *exoantigen* secreted by the trypanosome. The antigenic nature of this exoantigen can change with remissions in the infection, thereby favoring the prolonged survival of the organism. The host responds by production of globulins in amounts sufficient to produce very high erythrocyte sedimentation rates; these globulins are in the IgM (19S) rather than in the IgG (7S) range, which is

normally associated with infectious disease. In the advanced disease, when lesions are maximal, the smallest numbers of trypanosomes are to be found in the blood. An occult stage of *T. brucei*, consisting of amastigotes (Leishman-Donovan bodies) has been found in the capillaries of the choroid plexus (Ormerod and Venhateran), but its full significance remains to be assessed.

Clinical Manifestations. The clinical diagnosis of sleeping sickness is usually difficult, for there are few reliable physical signs of the disease. A history of exposure to tsetse bite is essential. A chancre may develop at the site of the bite of the infected tsetse fly, although more frequently this passes unobserved or may be confused with the reaction to a normal tsetse bite, which is often very severe. The occurrence, site, and appearance of the chancre vary greatly between different areas and individual patients.

With typical *Rhodesian disease* the bite will have occurred about two weeks before the first symptoms. With the *Gambian* and *Zambezi* disease, however, the symptoms may be delayed for several years; the history of, or the scar from, a chancre may be useful in diagnosing the disease in a European.

Irrespective of the demonstration of a previous bite, the most important early symptom of sleeping sickness is the *severe headache*. This is associated with loss of nocturnal sleep and a *feeling of oppression* that African patients will often recognize, causing them to trek many miles to a sleeping sickness clinic. Wasting, mental disturbance, and drowsiness occur only when the disease is established in the central nervous system.

Physical signs in the early stages include fever, which may be high and fluctuating, especially in the Rhodesian disease. A fleeting circinate erythematous rash occurs on the chest and shoulders of some European patients, but is not seen in Africans. Enlarged lymph nodes are associated with Gambian disease and are found characteristically in the posterior triangle of the neck. Periostial tenderness is described as a diagnostic sign but is neither frequent nor specific; similarly, swelling of the dorsum of the foot is easily confused with famine edema, which may coexist in the type of population at greatest risk of acquiring trypanosomiasis.

Diagnosis. Because there is nothing conclusive about the clinical manifestations of trypanosomiasis, the diagnosis depends entirely on the demonstration of the presence of the organism. In the *Rhodesian disease* it is usually made by microscopic examination of a thick (unfixed) blood film stained with Giemsa, a tedious but fairly reliable procedure in the hands of a well trained microscopist. Injection of blood into rats or mice is of value in doubtful cases. Zambezi strains are more difficult to diagnose by microscopy but are very easily isolated in rats and mice.

Gambian disease cannot with certainty be diagnosed by microscopic examination of the blood or by injection of laboratory animals. Microscopic examination of the fluid obtained by puncture of swollen lymph nodes is the best method in early cases. In later cases microscopy of cerebrospinal fluid is preferable, although concentration of the trypanosomes by centrifugation is often necessary. Culture of the organism as a method of diagnosis is difficult as compared with culture of *T. cruzi*. Immunologic methods are not usually successful in the diagnosis of sleeping sickness, except for the fluorescent antibody test which shows some promise as a specific diagnostic method. A simple and promising method of selecting cases for further study is based on the formation of precipitin bands by the patient's serum or cerebrospinal fluid in a gel containing antiserum against IgM, β_2 macroglobulins, which are a feature of trypanosomal infections (Mattern et al.).

It is impossible at the present time to distinguish sleeping sickness from other febrile and wasting diseases without demonstrating trypanosomes. These organisms must be sought with care in any patient who has been exposed to tsetse bites in an area in which sleeping sickness has ever been known to occur.

Treatment. The two essential drugs for treatment of sleeping sickness are *suramin* (Bayer 205) and *melarsoprol* (Mel B). Suramin can be used in the early febrile stage of the disease but, because it is a large molecule unable to pass the blood-brain barrier, it becomes ineffective once the central nervous system has been invaded; consequently examination of the cerebrospinal fluid is of importance in deciding which drug to use. If the cerebrospinal fluid is normal, suramin alone may be used, but if trypanosomes, lymphocytes, or a raised protein is found, melarsoprol becomes the drug of choice either alone or after a preliminary course of suramin. Suramin is given intravenously in a course of five doses of 1.0 gram every second day, and this may be repeated after a week. Suramin produces some toxicity to the kidney, with the appearance of casts and albumin in the urine. It causes fetal abnormality in rats, but this has not been noted in man. In Nigeria 1 of 2000 patients has a dangerous sensitivity to suramin; this can be detected by giving a preliminary dose of 0.2 gram.

Melarsoprol is much more toxic than suramin, but it is effective in all stages of the disease and is active on most strains of *T. brucei*, including some that are tryparsamide-resistant. Doses are given intravenously as the 3.6 per cent solution; three doses of 0.5, 1.0, and 1.5 ml. are given at daily intervals, and after a week three more doses of 1.5, 2.0, and 2.5, and so on until a total of 35 ml. has been given. It must be emphasized, however, that this very high dosage should be reached only if the patient shows no signs of toxicity, notably of arsenic encephalopathy. Sudden death with encephalopathy may occur in the early stages of melarsoprol therapy, and it is believed that this may be due to the rapid liberation of trypanosomal antigen; it is therefore wise to begin therapy of the Rhodesian form with suramin to reduce the number of parasites before continuing with the larsoprol. The effect of melarsoprol therapy can be assessed by following the reduction

of protein levels in the cerebrospinal fluid, but it can only be a rough guide because melarsoprol will of itself raise the level of protein for periods up to six months after injection. Melansonyl Potassium (Mel W) may be given intramuscularly, but less experience has been acquired concerning its curative effect. Nitrofurazone, which can be given by mouth (0.5 gram three times a day for 15 days) is even more toxic, but it may be the drug of choice in cases in which the patient is known to be sensitive—or his trypanosomes resistant—to arsenic. It is likely to cause polyneuritis and cardiac arrhythmia, and in patients with hereditary glucose-6-phosphate dehydrogenase deficiency it can cause severe hemolytic anemia (a property which it shares with melarsoprol). Tryparsamide is also used in combination with suramin for mass therapy of Gambian disease; it is not suitable for patients treated individually and is ineffective in the Rhodesian disease. It can produce toxic ambylopia leading to optic atrophy in some patients.

Prognosis. Relapse may follow treatment, especially after suramin, when the central nervous system had been already involved at the time when the chemotherapy was started. Relapse may also occur because of drug resistance; in such a case the success of treatment depends on the use of a different and chemically unrelated drug. Recovery after treatment is usually complete when the disease is treated at an early stage. If treatment is first given late in the disease, the survivors are often mentally sluggish and sometimes obese. A patient from whom trypanosomes have been isolated will sooner or later be killed by the disease unless it is treated. With Rhodesian disease the patient dies fairly soon, but with both Zambezi and Gambian disease the patient may survive for several years. This is especially true in Zambezi disease, of which so-called "healthy carriers" occur. It is suggested that some patients may be able to overcome the infection by natural means. If this in fact occurs, it is so exceptional that adequate treatment of diagnosed cases should always be performed. The neglect of an outbreak of sleeping sickness may result in extermination of the human population of the locality.

Prevention. African sleeping sickness can be prevented by measures aimed at destroying the habitat of the vector, the shade trees, and the other vegetation upon which the tsetse flies rest. As individual communities become larger, and especially when water sources are provided inside the villages, the risk to the inhabitants is reduced. The use of insecticides may also supplement this process. Elimination of the blood meal of the fly by game destruction programs has no effect on human sleeping sickness.

Probably the most effective measures against the Rhodesian disease involve the isolation of human populations from areas known to harbor infective game and systematic search for and treatment of all infected humans. Search for and treatment of cases is even more important in Gambian disease, because man himself is the reservoir of infection.

Pentamidine, administered intramuscularly, is the only suitable drug for chemoprophylaxis, and is of established effectiveness only against the Gambian disease. Its use is limited to the protection of a controlled population, such as a labor force, exposed to the Gambian disease. Pentamidine should not be used for therapy of individual cases of the disease because, like suramin, it is not active within the nervous system. A single injection of 4 mg. per kilogram is believed to provide a preventive effect in the Gambian disease for at least six months.

Mattern, P., Masseyeff, R., Michel, R., and Peretti, P.: Étude immunochimique de la β2 macroglobuline des sérums de malades atteints de trypanosomiase Africaine à T. gambiense. Ann. Inst. Pasteur, 101:382, 1961.
Mulligan, H. W., and Potts, W. H. (eds.): The African Trypanosomiases. London, Allen and Unwin, 1970.
Onyango, R. J., van Hoeve, K., and De Raadt, P.: Evidence that cattle may act as reservoir hosts of trypanosomes infective to man. Trans. Roy. Soc. Trop. Med. Hyg., 60:175, 1966.
Ormerod, W. E., and Venhateran, S.: The choroid plexus in African sleeping sickness. Lancet, 2:777, 1970.
Robertson, D. H. H.: Chemotherapy of African trypanosomiasis. Practitioner, 188:80, 1962.

CHAGAS' DISEASE
Heonir Rocha

Definition. Chagas' disease is caused by an infection with a protozoan, *Trypanosoma cruzi*. It has a self-limited acute phase, detected only in a minority of infected persons. The disease usually presents as a chronic process, characterized by cardiac and digestive manifestations. In most cases there is no clinical evidence of the infection. Chagas' disease, however, is an important cause of morbidity and mortality in an endemic area.

Etiology. In the blood, *T. cruzi* is a spindle-shaped trypanosome showing a scanty undulating membrane and a large kinetoplast. Following penetration of tissue cells the parasite changes into Leishmania forms, which are round or ovoid bodies containing a large nucleus and a rodlike kinetoplast. Multiplication is cyclical and takes place intracellularly by binary fission. Within tissues there is production of intermediate forms, from which the circulating trypanosome forms are derived. There are strains of *T. cruzi* with widely different virulence for mice; also, great differences in tissue tropism have been documented. These variations have been considered of possible significance in clinical infections, and they could explain some of the diversity of the clinical picture of this disease in different geographic areas.

Epidemiology. Men and probably domestic animals (chiefly dogs and cats) infected with *T. cruzi* are the main reservoirs for contamination of the insect vectors. These vectors are winged but capable of only short flights, and are strictly hematophagous. They belong to the family Reduviidae, subfamily Triatominae, of which several dozen species have been found to be infected. However, only three species, *Triatoma infestans*, *Panstrongilus megistus*, and *Rhodnius prolixus*, well adapted to human dwellings, are major transmitters of the infection in large areas of South and Central America.

The insect vectors live in cracks and holes in walls and roofs, and in the thatch of primitive adobe houses. Their habits are very much like those of bedbugs; they feed at night or in the dark and seek shelter by day. The flagellate forms of *T. cruzi* are ingested with the blood meal by the insect, and after a series of changes and multiplications in the digestive tract of the vector, the metacyclic trypanosome forms are produced in large numbers and are discharged in the feces. The transmission of the disease usually results from contamination of mucous membranes or broken skin with feces containing the infective trypanosomes.

Occasionally man can be infected by blood transfusion or accidental laboratory contamination. Infection of the newborn via the placenta has also been documented. Transmission via breast milk and by eating infected meat is also possible.

Chagas' disease has been detected in a large area in the Western Hemisphere extending from the southern United States (Texas) to Argentina. In the United States several species of wild rats, opossums, armadillos, and house mice have been found to be infected; also, several species of triatomid bugs have been found to have *T. cruzi*. However, the disease in humans is practically nonexistent in the U. S. The major feature of the epidemiology of Chagas' disease is the association of infection in man and domestic animals with the presence of species of the insect vector in the domestic habitat. This intimate contact of man and vector is apparently lacking in the United States.

The incidence of Chagas' disease has been shown to be greatly variable, depending on the existence of favorable conditions for endemicity. Well conducted epidemiologic studies are certainly needed to give a better picture of its geographic distribution. So far the disease has been reported only in the Americas, where it has been estimated that at least 7 million people are infected.

Pathogenesis and Pathology The invading organism, after penetration through mucous membranes or skin, multiplies within cells of surrounding tissues or regional lymph nodes as Leishmania forms. These forms produce pseudocysts that eventually rupture, causing an inflammatory and lymphatic reaction. The liberated bodies either again penetrate adjacent tissue cells or invade the blood.

The lesions and clinical manifestations of the *acute stage* of the disease are mainly related to the destruction of cells by growth and multiplication of the parasite and the resulting inflammatory reaction. Practically every organ of the body may be invaded, but the reticuloendothelial system, muscle fibers (especially cardiac), and neuroglial cells of the central nervous system are more likely to be involved.

Inflammation is seen mainly around ruptured pseudocysts containing leishmania, particularly in muscles. In the cardiac muscle there is diffuse interstitial mononuclear cell infiltration and interfibrillar edema, with many pseudocysts of leishmania in the cardiac fibers; also, various degrees of muscle degeneration are seen, waxy and fatty degeneration predominating. In the brain and meninges there is frequently a mild mononuclear infiltration.

Parasitemia may persist for four to twelve weeks, after which the parasite remains quiescent in tissues as Leishmania forms with occasional transient blood invasion.

In the *chronic stage*, the main pathologic lesions are observed in the heart and digestive tract. The heart is dilated and hypertrophied, with no valvular or specific vascular lesions. There are frequent mural thrombi, particularly in the right atrium and at the apex of the left ventricle with thinning of this region. Although this thinning may be extreme, leading to aneurysm of the apex, it does not seem to lead to rupture of the ventricle. The myocardium shows a variable degree of mononuclear inflammatory reaction, degenerative changes, and a predominant diffuse interstitial fibrosis. Quantitative studies of the intrinsic nervous system of the heart have shown a pronounced reduction in the number of parasympathetic ganglion cells. The presence of leishmania within muscle fibers is detected in only about 30 per cent of chronic cases (Fig. 1). Embolic infarcts are frequently found in the lungs, spleen, kidneys, and, occasionally, in the brain of patients dying from this disease.

Frequently the patients with digestive tract involvement have megaesophagus and/or megacolon with only minor inflammatory reaction in

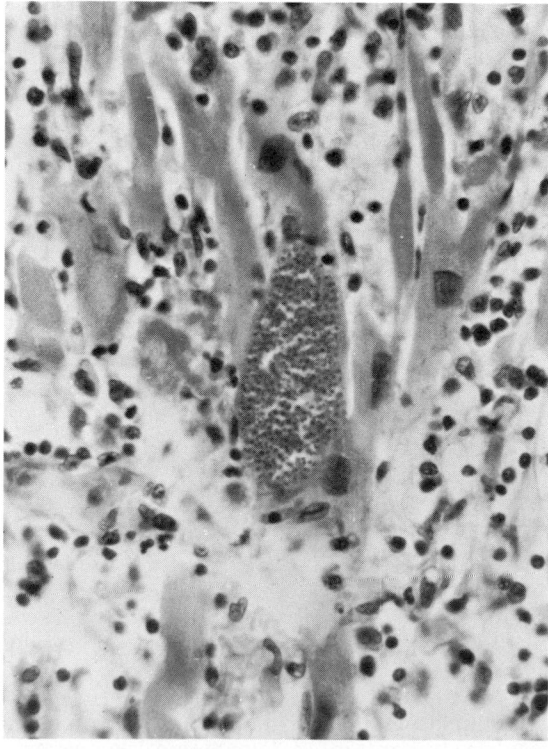

FIGURE 1. Leishmania bodies within myocardial fiber of a patient with chronic Chagas' heart disease. Note also the mononuclear inflammatory reaction and edema.

the myocardium; occasionally there also is severe diffuse myocarditis. In the esophagus and colon there is a marked decrease in the number of cells of the autonomic nervous system, and there are focal inflammatory lesions in the muscular layer. It is thought that megaesophagus and megacolon are the result of destruction of the intramural nervous system, probably related to the parasitic infection and to the secondary inflammatory and vascular lesions.

The detection of widespread inflammation in the myocardium, not associated with the presence of the parasite, the continuous destruction of muscle fibers, and the necrotizing arteriolar lesions described in muscular layers of the esophagus have suggested an immune allergic mechanism for lesions of the acute phase and particularly of the chronic phase of this disease. Furthermore, the reduction of the intrinsic nervous control of the heart and digestive tract has been taken as an important pathogenic mechanism in this parasitic infection.

Clinical Manifestations. In the course of Chagas' disease there are distinct phases with peculiar clinical features.

Acute Form. In an endemic area, the acute manifestations of Chagas' disease usually occur in the first decade of life, and are recognized in only a small minority of infected cases. The local signs at the portal of entry frequently call the attention of the physician to the condition. Characteristically there is *unilateral* painless periorbital edema with mild conjunctival reaction, a bluish or darkish discoloration of the skin, and satellite lymphadenopathy usually with enlarged preauricular lymph nodes. These physical findings are referred to as Romaña's sign (Fig. 2). The subsidence of the palpebral edema usually takes four to eight weeks.

In a minority of cases, the initial lesion occurs in other exposed areas of the skin. It is usually a lesion resembling a furuncle that increases to become a purplish indurated papule, 4 to 6 cm. in diameter, with regional adenopathy, leaving a pigmented scar when it subsides.

Concomitantly with the local signs the patient develops a variable clinical picture usually characterized by malaise, anorexia, remittent or continuous fever, mild generalized nontender lymphadenopathy, moderate hepatosplenomegaly, and, in some instances, peripheral edema or a generalized edema of varying degrees which supervenes later on in the course. In a few cases a morbilliform or maculopapular erythematous skin rash is present. The pulse is usually fast (even when fever is absent) and regular. In severe cases there may be marked cardiac dilatation, gallop rhythm, and signs of heart failure. Myocarditis of variable degree probably occurs in all cases, but it is severe only in a very small percentage. Laboratory findings include a moderate leukocytosis with lymphocytosis, increased sedimentation rate, increase in alpha-2 and gamma globulins, and decrease in serum albumin. The serum glutamic oxaloacetic transaminase (SGOT) has been

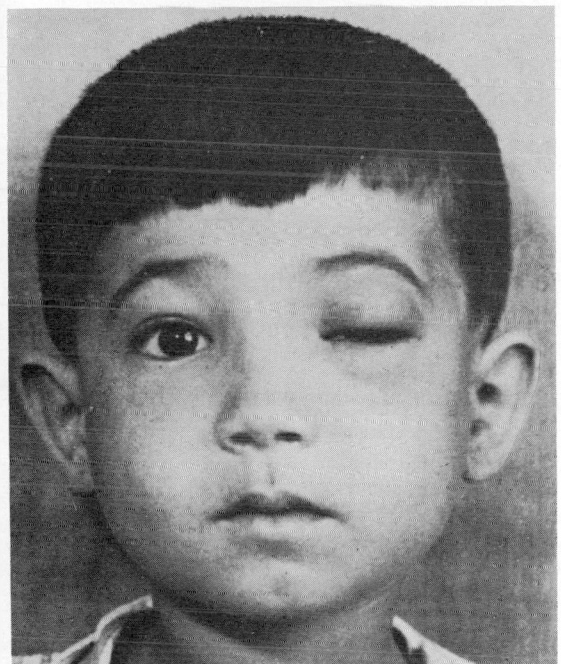

FIGURE 2. Romaña's sign in acute Chagas' disease. Note unilateral periorbital edema. (Courtesy of Professor Aluizio Prata, Salvador, Bahia, Brazil.)

found elevated in severe cases. Electrocardiographic (EKG) abnormalities are present in about 50 per cent of patients, commonly showing prolongation of P-R interval, low voltage of QRS, and primary T wave changes. These are more pronounced in the most severe cases. The presence of intraventricular block is a very ominous sign.

The disease subsides within two or three months in 90 to 95 per cent of cases. The 5 to 10 per cent fatality rate is usually related to severe myocarditis or acute meningoencephalitis (occurring in the newborn or in the very young). *In the great majority of patients with the chronic form of Chagas' disease there is no history of an acute phase.* It is thought that probably only 1 per cent of infected subjects have noticeable clinical signs following the initial contamination.

Indeterminate or Latent Phase. Patients who had acute manifestations of the disease, as well as those with inapparent infection, may remain asymptomatic for periods of 10 to 30 years, or for their whole lives. Those patients show only serologic evidence of the disease by complement-fixation (positive Machado-Guerreiro reaction), and occasionally the parasite can be recovered from their blood. This is actually the most common situation in an endemic area. Yet, there are few clinical and anatomic data available concerning this particular stage of the disease.

Chronic Form. The chronic manifestations of *T. cruzi* infection are primarily due to cardiac and digestive involvement.

Cardiac Manifestations. Approximately 20 to 40 per cent of patients with chronic *T. cruzi* infection in an endemic area exhibit evidence of chronic heart damage. This is the most important

finding in the chronic phase of this disease. Symptoms and signs are the result of a progressive diffuse chronic myocarditis.

In the early stages the patient may have no symptoms, and the diagnosis of heart disease rests on the electrocardiographic changes.

With advanced disease the patient may present a clinical picture of heart failure of gradual onset, with serious systemic congestion. Signs of right-sided heart failure usually predominate over those of left ventricular failure. The pulse is weak and irregular because of ventricular premature contractions. The heart is greatly enlarged, the heart sounds are muffled, and there is a systolic murmur of functional mitral insufficiency and sometimes one of tricuspid regurgitation. A widely split second pulmonic sound and an apical third heart sound are commonly heard. The heart shadow roentgenographically shows marked global enlargement, with clear pulmonary fields (Fig. 3). The course of these patients is usually complicated by pulmonary or systemic embolism arising from the frequently occurring mural thrombi. Occasionally, the episode of heart failure begins abruptly, without apparent precipitating cause, usually running a short fatal course; on other occasions it is brought on by pregnancy or delivery, severe pulmonary infection, or an associated severe chronic anemia.

In some instances the patient may complain only of palpitation or syncopal attacks resulting from disturbances in cardiac rhythm (ventricular premature contractions or atrioventricular block, Adams-Stokes attacks). In cases of complete atrioventricular block the patient may present with Adams-Stokes syndrome. Rarely, the first manifestation of chronic Chagas' disease is a

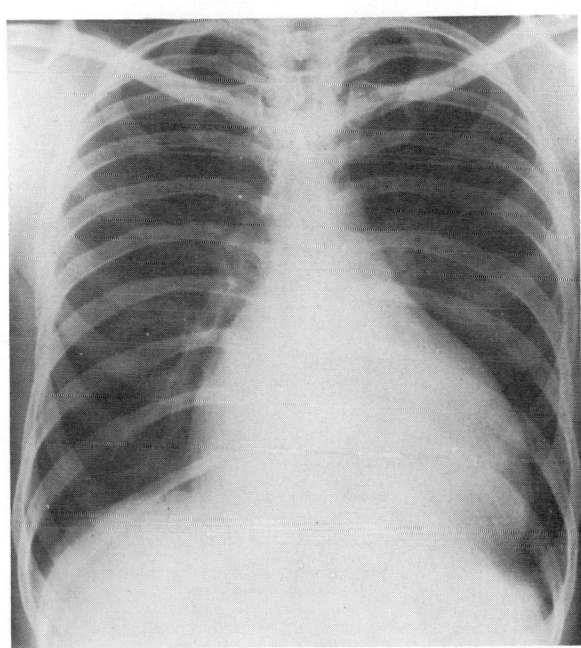

FIGURE 3. Chest film in a case of chronic Chagas' heart disease. Marked global enlargement of cardiac shadow, with clear pulmonary fields.

cerebral embolism owing to dislodgement of a thrombus located in the left ventricle.

A great variety of EKG abnormalities are detected in chronic Chagas' heart disease. Complete right bundle branch block is the most frequent conduction disturbance, occurring in about 50 per cent of cases; similarly, ventricular premature contractions (usually multifocal) are present in half the patients; also frequent are negative symmetric T waves. Atrioventricular block of variable degree occurs in one third of cases, but complete A-V block is detected in only about 10 per cent. Atrial fibrillation or flutter is relatively uncommon (about 10 per cent), and left bundle branch block is rare.

Digestive Manifestations. Mega-esophagus and megacolon are important manifestations of chronic *T. cruzi* infection. The evidence for the etiologic role of the parasite in these conditions is (1) the high incidence of these abnormalities in endemic areas of Chagas' disease; (2) the finding of a positive Machado-Guerreiro reaction in 85 per cent of patients with megacolon or mega-esophagus in endemic areas; when xenodiagnosis is also performed in these cases, the incidence of *T. cruzi* infection rises to 95 per cent, which is significantly higher than that in the general population of the same area; (3) the frequent detection of EKG changes (about 50 per cent), similar to those described in chronic Chagas' myocarditis, in patients with megacolon or mega-esophagus; and (4) the capability of reproducing these lesions in animals chronically infected with *T. cruzi*. This infection in animals and humans produces a marked decrease in the number of cells of the autonomic nervous system in esophagus and colon, even in the absence of anatomic changes of these organs.

Patients with mega-esophagus complain of long-standing progressive dysphagia, regurgitation, retrosternal discomfort, and sometimes paroxysmal attacks of night cough. They may get repeated respiratory infections as a result of aspirations of esophageal contents. The esophagus becomes enormously dilated, and in some cases it can be seen in a plain chest film as a right paramediastinal shadow.

Megacolon is characterized by persistent severe constipation of many years' duration. The incidence of fecal impaction and volvulus with intestinal obstruction is high in endemic areas of Chagas' disease.

The concomitance of mega-esophagus, megacolon, and heart failure is not common. Most frequently, patients with digestive involvement present only EKG abnormalities or a moderate enlargement of the heart.

Prenatal Chagas' Disease. Prenatal transmission of *T. cruzi* infection has been verified by clinical and experimental observations. The mother may be in the latent or indeterminate phase of the disease.

The infected newborn may present generalized edema, enlargement of liver and spleen, petechiae or purpuric manifestations, sometimes jaundice, and a picture of meningoencephalitis. The patho-logic findings are those of acute Chagas' disease. A microscopic picture of placentitis occurs in those instances. The characteristic feature is the finding of Leishmania within histiocytes of the inflammatory reaction. It has been shown that this infection may be responsible for premature birth or fetal death.

Diagnosis. In the acute stage, the diagnosis lies mainly in the demonstration of the parasite in the blood of the patient. *T. cruzi* may be seen in a fresh blood smear, in a thick-drop preparation of blood, or in a buffy coat smear up to three months after the onset of the disease. As the parasitemia decreases, or if blood preparations are negative, xenodiagnosis or animal inoculation of freshly drawn blood or blood culture can be used. Xenodiagnosis is a method of having laboratory-bred triatomid bugs feed on patients and examining the insects 40 days later for the presence of *T. cruzi* in the intestinal tract. The method is practical and is very sensitive in the detection of this stage of Chagas' disease. Blood culture in NNN media and inoculation of blood in young mice or guinea pigs require special laboratory facilities, but can be helpful particularly when xenodiagnosis is not available. A precipitin reaction using antigen obtained from *T. cruzi* culture gives positive results in almost every acute case.

The clinical diagnosis of chronic Chagas' heart disease is based on the following: (1) epidemiologic evidence (patient from endemic area, usually of poor socioeconomic group); (2) clinical picture of primary myocardial disease (enlarged heart, with no signs of valvular, coronary artery or any other cause of heart disease); (3) EKG changes of the types (previously mentioned) usually seen in Chagas' disease; and (4) serologic evidence of infection or isolation of *T. cruzi*.

The most valuable procedure in diagnosing chronic Chagas' disease is the complement-fixation test (Machado-Guerreiro reaction), which is positive in about 95 per cent of cases. Xenodiagnosis is positive in only about 20 per cent of chronic cases.

Differential diagnosis may include rheumatic heart disease, particularly when there is a loud systolic murmur simulating organic valvular disease, in patients under 30 years of age. Coronary heart disease may be another difficult problem in patients over 40. It is often impossible on clinical grounds to dissociate chronic myocarditis owing to Chagas' disease from certain cardiomyopathies of unknown cause. Besides the great help derived from careful evaluation of clinical and epidemiologic data, the Machado-Guerreiro reaction and xenodiagnosis are of major importance in making a definite diagnosis of Chagas' disease.

Clinical Course and Prognosis. Acute Chagas' disease is relatively benign, with subsidence of symptoms in 90 to 95 per cent of cases. The chronic form usually has a slowly progressive course. It is clear that by no means all of those infected ultimately develop the serious forms of the disease, but the exact proportion that do so is not known.

This important question could be settled only by a large-scale, long-term prospective epidemiologic study; the need for such a study is great.

Sudden and unexpected death is common in Chagas' disease. Complete A-V block, multifocal premature ventricular contractions, ventricular tachycardia, and marked enlargement of the heart with signs of heart failure are severe prognostic signs. Pulmonary embolism is a frequent terminal complication in patients with heart failure.

Treatment. There is no satisfactory treatment for *T. cruzi* infection. Several antimicrobial agents have been tried without success, including prima-quine, pyrimethamine, nitrofurans (levofuralta-done), aminopterin, intravenous gentian violet, amphotericin B, and puromycin, among others. These agents may cause transient disappearance of parasitemia, but follow-up studies usually show a relapse. This is probably related to the ineffec-tiveness of all those agents against the tissue forms of the parasite. Some of them (nitrofurans) may demonstrate great in vitro potency against *T. cruzi* in tissue cultures, and also in experimen-tal infection in mice. However, despite extensive killing of intracellular parasites, some intact leishmanial bodies can always be found in the tissues of the laboratory animal. None of the drugs commonly employed in the treatment of African trypanosomiasis have shown value in Chagas' disease (see preceding article).

After a certain degree of tissue damage has oc-curred, even the eradication of the parasite may not prevent the progression of the disease. In chronic cases, therapy is only symptomatic, com-prising the usual measures for heart failure, Adams-Stokes syndrome, mega-esophagus, mega-colon, or one of its complications. Digitalis prepa-rations should be managed with great care because of the unusual degree of sensitivity to toxic effects.

Prevention. Controlling the transmission of the disease is the most important preventive measure. This requires housing of satisfactory quality; more-over, it requires the repeated systematic applica-tion of residual insecticides (benzene hexachloride) effective against the triatomid bugs. For individual short-term protection, fine-mesh bed nets are use-ful.

Blood transfusion is a potential hazard in en-demic areas. The incidence of positive Machado-Guerreiro reactions among blood donors may be as high as 15 per cent. To prevent infection from transfusions, the addition of gentian or crystal violet to the blood has been used. Persons having a positive complement-fixation test should not be accepted as potential blood donors.

Köeberle, F.: Chagas' heart disease (pathology). Cardiologia (Basel), 52:82, 1969.

Laranja, F. S., Dias, E., Nobrega, G., and Miranda, A.: Chagas' disease. A clinical, epidemiologic and pathologic study. Circulation, 14:1035, 1956.

Resenbaum, M. B.: Chagasic myocardiopathy. Progr. Cardiov. Dis., 7:199, 1964.

Woody, N. C., and Woody, H. B.: American trypanosomiasis. I. Clinical and epidemiological background of Chagas' dis-ease in the United States. J. Pediat., 58:568, 1961.

World Health Organization: Chagas' Disease, Report of a Study Group. Technical Report Series No. 202, 1960.

LEISHMANIASIS
Harry Most

Leishmaniasis is infection with protozoan organ-isms of the genus Leishmania, which is trans-mitted by Phlebotomus sandflies. Many authorities today group all cases into two categories, visceral leishmaniasis, which is infection with *Leishmania donovani*, and cutaneous leishmaniasis, which is due to *Leishmania tropica* or *Leishmania brazili-ensis*. In man and the dog *Leishmania tropica* causes oriental sore. Susceptible mammals re-covered from *L. tropica* infection are resistant to reinfection, but can be infected with *L. donovani*. Recovery from *L. donovani* results in protection from reinfection and against infection with *L. tropica*. This evidence and the different geographic locations in which *L. tropica* and *L. donovani* infec-tions occur are the basis for the belief that these agents are not identical, although related. *L. donovani* is the cause of visceral leishmaniasis as observed in both infants and adults. Whereas cutaneous leishmaniasis usually involves only the skin and subcutaneous tissue and, in some cases, the nasopharyngeal mucosa and submucosa, visceral leishmaniasis always causes widespread lesions.

KALA-AZAR
(Visceral Leishmaniasis)

Definition. Kala-azar is a disease produced by a protozoan organism, *Leishmania donovani*. It is characterized by irregular fever of long duration, chronicity, enlargement of the spleen and often of the liver, emaciation, anemia, leukopenia, and hyperglobulinemia.

Etiologic Agent. *Leishmania donovani*, the causal organism of visceral leishmaniasis, is a protozoan parasite belonging to a group known as hemoflagellates, which inhabit the blood or other tissues of vertebrates. Two forms of *Leishmania donovani* are present in its life cycle, the Leish-mania form—a stage lacking a flagellum—which occurs in man or other mammalian hosts, and a leptomonad or flagellate form, which develops in the sandfly intermediate host and in artificial culture media.

The Leishmania forms, commonly referred to as Leishman-Donovan bodies, are small ovoid or round unicellular organisms measuring 2 to 4 μ in diameter that occur in reticuloendothelial cells and macrophages and are abundant in certain tissues, being present also in small numbers in peripherally circulating monocytes. With Giemsa or Wright's stain, the cytoplasm appears pale blue and the nucleus and kinetoplast red or reddish purple.

The leptomonad forms result from a transfor-mation that the Leishmania forms undergo in the digestive tract of sandfly vectors after they have

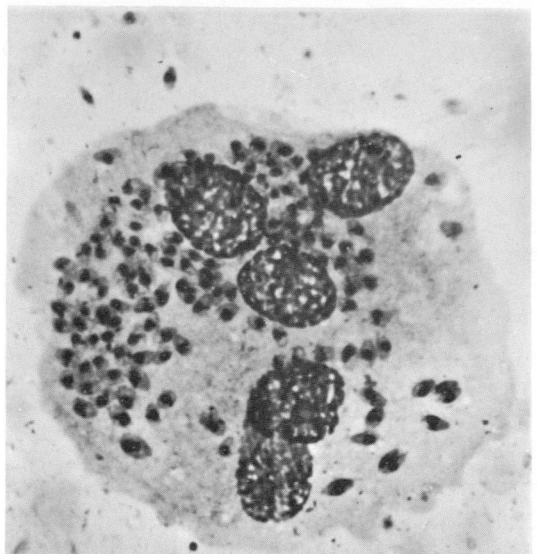

FIGURE 1.   Kala-azar. Leishman-Donovan bodies in macrophage cell, bone marrow (× 1500).

fed on an infected vertebrate host or in cultures when inoculated on suitable media. The leptomonad forms are spindle-shaped bodies 14 to 20 μ long by 1.5 to 3.5 μ broad, with a more or less centrally placed nucleus. The kinetoplast is at the anterior end and from it springs a flagellum. In cultures, the leptomonads frequently tend to agglomerate in rosette groups with their entangled flagella directed inward. The leptomonads are presumed to gain access to man when the flies subsequently feed. Inside the body they undergo transformation and multiply as intracellular Leishmania forms.

Epidemiology.   So far as is known, there is no natural immunity to kala-azar. Although the disease is uncommon in persons of Caucasian origin in India and mainland China, the low incidence is due apparently to infrequent exposure to the disease. Kala-azar is often sporadic in its occurrence, but it may appear in epidemic form. The disease is particularly common in villages, although it also occurs in cities. In India and mainland China there are particular villages and even individual houses that are known to be foci of kala-azar. Those infected belong predominantly to the lower socioeconomic groups of the population. Statistics show a higher incidence in males, but it is doubtful that the data are reliable, as far more males than females attend hospitals in the Orient. Kala-azar is predominantly a disease of childhood and youth, but it is also common in the third decade of life and may occur at any age. In the Mediterranean area the incidence in infants is said to be relatively higher than it is in other areas. Many animals, including especially the hamster, are susceptible to artificial infection, but the only animal found to be infected in nature is the dog.

Kala-azar is widespread, but the areas in which its existence is well known are discontinuous, and the importance of the disease varies greatly in

localities relatively near one another. The incidence is especially high in parts of China north of the Yangtse River and in parts of eastern India, particularly in Bihar, Bengal, and Assam. The disease is endemic in the region about Tashkent in southern Asiatic Russia, and occurs in Mesopotamia, Saudi Arabia, and Turkey. It is present in areas scattered all around the Mediterranean Sea and in a belt across Africa from Kenya through Ethiopia and equatorial Africa to Nigeria. Cases have been reported from Argentina, Paraguay, Bolivia, Brazil, Venezuela, and Colombia, but so far the disease does not seem to be very important on the South American continent. Autochthonous cases have not been found in the United States, but many imported cases have been reported, especially in soldiers previously stationed in endemic areas.

Sandflies of the genus Phlebotomus have been shown to be important vectors of kala-azar in India and mainland China. Since various species of Phlebotomus exist wherever the disease occurs, these insects may be vectors in other areas. In mainland China and elsewhere a natural reservoir host for Leishmania has been found in dogs, in addition to that in infected human beings. Visceral leishmaniasis has been found in a dog imported into the United States from Greece. In endemic areas in India, however, dogs apparently rarely

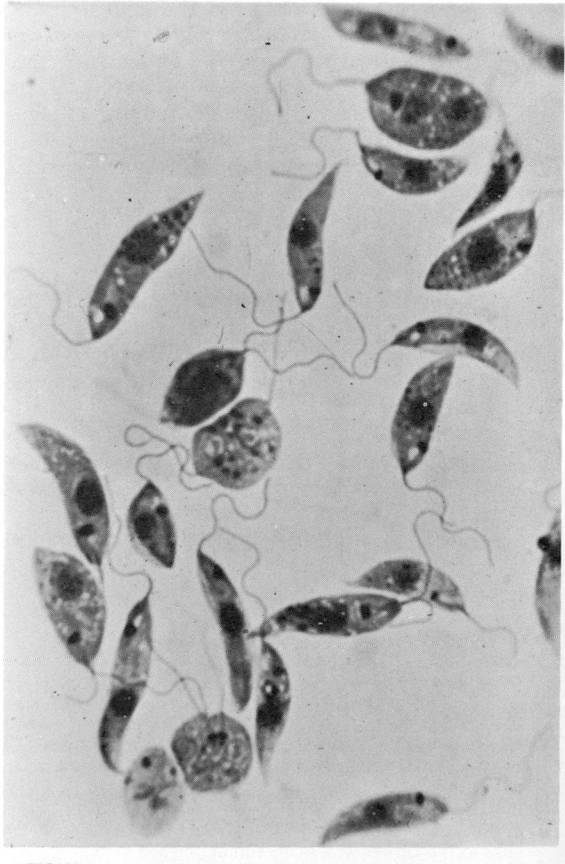

FIGURE 2.   Kala-azar. Leptomonad forms of *Leishmania donovani* in NNN culture of spleen puncture material (× 1200).

harbor the infection. It is generally assumed that in India kala-azar is transmitted by sandflies directly from patient to patient. This may be one of the methods of infection in all endemic areas. Although rarely parasites are present in the stools, urine, and nasopharyngeal secretions of patients, there is no evidence that infection arises from these sources. The disease has been inadvertently transmitted by blood transfusion.

Pathology. The chief lesion of kala-azar is essentially a hyperplasia of the cells of the reticuloendothelial system, particularly of the spleen and liver. The leishmania multiply within these cells, which ultimately rupture, releasing the parasites, which are then taken up by other reticuloendothelial cells. They are ingested to a lesser extent by leukocytes and monocytes, which occasionally may be found containing leishmania in films of the peripheral blood.

The spleen may be greatly enlarged, owing principally to the enormous increase of reticuloendothelial cells, many of which are parasitized. There is replacement of splenic pulp by these parasitized cells and often pressure atrophy of the malpighian bodies. There may be some fibrosis in advanced chronic cases.

The liver is usually, but not always, enlarged in kala-azar. There is a great proliferation of the Kupffer cells, which contain large numbers of leishmanial bodies. Pressure atrophy of the liver cords occurs, and both cloudy swelling and fatty degeneration may be observed. In advanced chronic cases there may be some fibrosis of the parenchyma.

The villi of the small intestine, especially the duodenum and jejunum, may be crowded with parasitized reticuloendothelial cells, and ulceration of the overlying mucosa occasionally occurs. Less often similar lesions are reported in the colon, and, rarely, cells containing parasites may be observed in the mucous membrane of the stomach.

In the bone marrow there is a progressive replacement of the hematopoietic tissue and the fatty marrow by masses of heavily parasitized reticuloendothelial cells. In experimental infections of animals amyloid disease of the kidneys may be found, and it is probable that similar changes occur in human infections.

There are no characteristic lesions of other organs. Scattered infected phagocytic cells may be observed. The lymph nodes are often enlarged owing to obstruction of the lymph sinuses by parasitized reticuloendothelial cells.

Laboratory Findings. The most important abnormalities are found in the blood. About 90 per cent of patients have leukopenia, which is largely due to reduction in the number of granulocytes. Leukopenia usually develops early. After the disease is established, counts of 3000 or less per cubic millimeter are common. There is usually a relative lymphocytosis; sometimes an absolute increase is seen. The same changes occur in the mononuclears. Occasionally (but usually with difficulty), parasitized macrophages or mononuclears are seen in blood smears, especially in Indian kala-azar. Anemia is also characteristic; it develops more slowly than leukopenia, and may be absent or trivial in early cases. As a rule, after the first month hemoglobin values are 40 to 60 per cent of normal, and erythrocyte counts are from 2 to 4 million per cubic millimeter. The serum bilirubin value is normal. Thrombocytopenia is regularly present. Serum proteins show an increase in globulin (chiefly in the gamma component, and mainly IgG), which may be so great that total globulin amounts to 8 or 9 grams per 100 ml. Serum albumin is usually decreased, especially in long-standing cases. A cold-precipitable protein has been found in some serums. Bromsulfalein tests give normal results, suggesting good hepatocellular function.

Patients with kala-azar have a decided lack of resistance to other infections. It is usually considered that those who have recovered are immune to further infection with kala-azar but not to other forms of leishmaniasis.

Clinical Manifestations. The incubation period is variable, extending from two weeks to eighteen months. In most cases, it is believed to be within two to six months, although cases have been described as having occurred three weeks to three years after exposure. The onset is also variable. Sometimes it is very slow and insidious, and sometimes it is well defined, with a gradual development of high fever over a period of five to seven days, as often happens in typhoid fever. The onset in most cases encountered in World War II was sudden and manifested by chills and high fever.

There is nothing characteristic about the symptoms of kala-azar. In many instances symptoms are of the vaguest sort, and patients feel well. In one large series of early cases, the symptoms in order of frequency were fever, chills, dizziness, headache, anorexia, cough, sweating, constipation, weakness, loss of weight, diarrhea, malaise, epistaxis, abdominal discomfort, nausea and vomiting, and bleeding gums. In rare instances, attacks of pain occur in the splenic region. In children irritability, mental clouding, and, rarely, convulsions may appear.

The temperature curve is variable, usually showing an irregular remittent or intermittent fever, occasionally reaching high levels and rarely subsiding for a week or more. The undulant pattern may resemble the fever of brucellosis.

Patients often do not appear as ill as the temperature would indicate, and in early cases the general examination may reveal little. Enlargement of the spleen is characteristic of established infections with kala-azar. It is an error to suppose that the spleen is necessarily huge, however, because the diagnosis may be made when the spleen is not palpable and is often made when it projects only slightly beyond the costal margin. It should be noted that when the spleen becomes very large it sometimes lies in a horizontal position and sometimes lies vertically. The liver is also enlarged, but the enlargement appears to take place somewhat later than that of the spleen. Tenderness of spleen or liver is unusual. Jaundice and ascites are rare, and, when present, are perhaps not directly due to kala-azar. An important finding in some cases is enlargement of lymph nodes (the enlargement has no characteristic distribution). Other physical signs are of less importance and are associated chiefly with progressive advance of the disease beyond the early stage. After kala-azar has been active for weeks or months, wasting appears. When blood changes are advanced, pallor and other signs of anemia may be seen. Among the incidental findings may be pulsations in the neck vessels, tachycardia, cardiac murmurs, and low blood pressure. Purpura is an occasional feature. Petechiae are rare, and rose spots do not occur. In time, the skin tends to acquire a dusky hue, especially in patients with a dark complexion, but the change is often difficult to distinguish. The skin may become coarse and dry, and the hair may become scanty.

In unusual instances, particularly among patients who have been treated inadequately, specific skin lesions may develop. These constitute the so-called *post-kala-azar dermal leishmanoid*. They occur occasionally on the trunk, but usually on the cheeks and nose (where they may assume a "butterfly" configuration), or on the lips. Such lesions are originally macular, but become raised and in time nodular. They are associated with depigmentation and do not break down. They may contain Leishman-Donovan bodies, but in depigmented and macular lesions parasites are very scanty.

Course and Complications. Patients with kala-azar appear to be peculiarly susceptible to other infections. Stomatitis is common in neglected children. Once established, oral infection may result in noma or cancrum oris, a well-nigh intractable condition. Bronchitis and pneumonia are the most common secondary infections. Nephrotic syndrome owing to secondary amyloidosis has been reported. In advanced cases, edema may be seen, usually because of plasma albumin deficiency.

The clinical manifestations usually develop slowly but progressively. Many patients have minor symptoms for weeks without reporting sick. Without treatment, the disease usually runs a course, with remissions and relapses, of two years or more. During remissions patients may feel, and appear to be, well. In some epidemics, especially in the Sudan, the course is fulminating.

Diagnosis. The diagnosis should always be confirmed by demonstration of the parasite. A "therapeutic test" is not considered satisfactory evidence of the disease. The outstanding considerations, apart from demonstration of the parasite, are exposure to the disease, the type of onset and temperature curve, palpable spleen and usually palpable liver, and the blood changes. The changes in the blood in kala-azar are extremely helpful in diagnosis. The profound leukopenia with a relative lymphocytosis and varying degrees of anemia and thrombocytopenia should suggest this disease. Very high IgG globulin values strongly support the diagnosis. Indeed, elevation of IgG values to such levels as are attained in kala-azar is not seen in any other disease.

Definitive diagnosis of visceral leishmaniasis should be based upon the demonstration of Leishmania forms in stained preparations or upon the growth of leptomonad forms in cultures inoculated with suspected blood or tissue. In rare instances, parasites may be found in monocytes in the circulating blood, but in general this method is not a practicable means of establishing the diagnosis. Leishmania infection may be established in hamsters by the intraperitoneal injection of blood or, preferably, tissue material. Tissue, not blood, is desired for examination. Sternal puncture is the diagnostic procedure of choice for finding the parasite. In 75 per cent of cases L.D. bodies will be found on Giemsa-stained films of the bone marrow aspirate by a skilled observer. Possible other sources of specimens in which organisms might be found include the spleen, liver, lymph nodes, and skin lesions. Liver puncture is not recommended. If enlarged lymph nodes are present and safely accessible, aspirated material or biopsy may show the parasite. Spleen puncture may furnish diagnostic material when other methods fail to do so. It is, therefore, the most reliable approach. Spleen puncture is not free from danger. It should never be attempted without careful study of the technique. If any difficulty is anticipated, lymph node puncture or biopsy or sternal puncture should be chosen for the first trial in diagnosis and *should be done only when the edge of the spleen is well below the costal margin.* The blood-clotting time and the bleeding time should be determined beforehand and, if significantly prolonged, whole blood should be transfused. Tissue puncture material should be spread as thin as possible, allowed to dry, and, after staining with Giemsa or Wright's stain, should be examined under an oil immersion lens. In the preparation of smears, large parasitized mononuclear cells are frequently broken and parasites liberated. As a result, free Leishman-Donovan bodies may be found. These must not be mistaken for platelets and hence disregarded; conversely, platelets should not be identified as Leishman-Donovan bodies. When doubtful objects are seen, further search should be made for parasites that show typical morphology and leave no doubt as to the identification. When parasites cannot be found by direct microscopic examination of tissue smears, they may be demonstrable in cultures of the tissue material but one to four weeks may elapse before the flagellates multiply sufficiently to be detected. However, they should be employed routinely whenever possible. With puncture material, after a smear is made, a few drops of sterile saline solution should be taken up into the syringe. The resulting mixture is then expelled onto the base of a slant of NNN medium. The NNN (Novy-MacNeal-Nicolle) medium containing defibrinated rabbit blood is the most satisfactory medium for cultures. Cultures for L. donovani should be kept as near 22° C. (71.6° F.) as possible. The cultures should be examined for parasites every few days and not discarded until at least a month has passed. If the examination is negative, a small amount of water of condensation in the culture may be obtained with a capillary pipette and examined in the same way. Morphologic detail may be observed in smears of culture material stained by Giemsa's or Wright's method. Recently complement-fixation and other serologic tests, including the fluorescent antibody test, have indicated reactivity in patients with proved leishmaniasis. If laboratories with suitable antigens and experience in performing such tests are accessible, sera from doubtful or early cases should be examined. In addition, the serologic pattern after definitive treatment may be helpful in a follow-up evaluation of its effectiveness.

Differential Diagnosis. Malaria is probably the most frequent source of diagnostic confusion. The two diseases should be separated by parasitologic studies. Other diseases that may need differentiation from kala-azar are schistosomiasis (eggs in stools or urine), relapsing fever (spirochetes in blood), leptospirosis, or Weil's disease (agglutination tests, spirochetes obtained by animal inoculation), typhoid fever (blood cultures, agglutination tests), undulant fever (blood cultures, agglutination tests), diseases such as bacterial endocarditis (blood cultures), pulmonary or abdominal tuberculosis, histoplasmosis, Hodgkin's disease, Banti's syndrome, blood diseases (especially aleukemic leukemia), and amebiasis with liver involvement.

Prognosis. In the absence of treatment, about 75 per cent of patients die, often with an intercurrent infection and usually within two or three years. Spontaneous recovery has been observed in rare proved cases. Good treatment ultimately cures about 98 per cent of patients (including patients with relapses who are retreated), except that this high cure rate has not been attained in the Sudan, where fulminating and drug-resistant cases are apparently numerous.

Treatment, General. Patients with fever, severe anemia, or leukopenia should be kept in bed. A well balanced and liberal diet should be given. Fluids should be given freely. Special attention should be paid to the care of the mouth in order to obtain and maintain cleanliness. Mouth washes should be bland and nonirritating, especially if any lesions are present. If severe anemia, leukopenia, or bleeding tendency exists, transfusions of blood should be given. In cases of secondary infection or cancrum oris, the use of penicillin or other antimicrobial substances is advised. In general, the chemotherapy of kala-azar takes precedence over the specific treatment of other concomitant infections. Splenectomy should never be performed for the initial treatment of this disease.

Chemotherapy. *General.* The early institution of chemotherapy for kala-azar is highly desirable. There are few contraindications to such treatment except serious disease of the lungs, heart, liver (aside from disease due to leishman-

iasis) and kidneys. The presence of the usual complications of kala-azar is only a further reason for pressing ahead with chemotherapy. At present, ethylstibamine (Neostibosan) or Pentostam ([Solustibosan] sodium antimony gluconate) is considered the drug of choice for general use. These are pentavalent antimicrobials and much less basic than the trivalent antimicrobials used for the treatment of schistosomiasis. Drugs such as Fuadin should not be used for the treatment of leishmaniasis. Pentostam is available from the Communicable Disease Center (C.D.C.) drug service (Atlanta, *vide supra*) for preventive disease. Infections acquired in the Sudan and the Mediterranean may be resistant to the drugs enumerated above and may require repeated courses of Pentostam or treatment with certain aromatic diamidine compounds. Patients who are under treatment should be kept in bed and should be observed closely.

Pentostam is given in an adult dose of 60 mg. slowly intravenously. This dose is given daily for seven to ten injections. After a week's rest, the course may be repeated, and some writers advocate a trial of 21 injections over six weeks, or even longer courses. Surprisingly few toxic effects occur from Pentostam in contrast to those from trivalent antimonials.

Ethylstibamine (Neostibosan). Ethylstibamine consists of para-aminophenylstibonic acid, para-acetyl-aminophenylstibonic acid, antimonic acid, and diethylamine, and contains 41 to 44 per cent antimony. The drug is relatively unstable in solution and should be given only when freshly prepared with sterile distilled water. The solution should not be boiled or heated and should be used as soon as possible. Ethylstibamine is administered intravenously in 5 per cent solution. For adults, the first dose is 0.2 gram and subsequent doses are 0.3 gram. The total dose is 5.0 grams (16 injections). A total of 5.0 grams of ethylstibamine should be administered to patients as initial treatment or in relapse following treatment with other drugs or following relapse from total amounts of ethylstibamine of less than 5.0 grams. Doses may be given daily, unless untoward effects appear. If untoward effects appear, the drug should be given on alternate days, the dosage should be reduced, or administration should be stopped, as the circumstances indicate. The most frequent toxic effects are nausea and vomiting. In rare instances, increased fever, dizziness, urticaria, abdominal and muscular pain, renal irritation, and increased bleeding may occur. It is said that bronchitis and pneumonia may be made worse. A few cases of anaphylactic reaction have been reported. Unfortunately, neostibosan or other effective pentavalent antimony compounds such as sodium antimony gluconate (Pentostam, Solustibosan, Stibanose) or urea stibamine (aminostiburea, carbostibamine) may not be easily available in North or South America.

Stilbamidine and Pentamidine. Certain aromatic diamidines have given better results than pentavalent antimonials in the treatment of kala-azar in the Sudan and in some resistant cases elsewhere, although they have not been found more satisfactory in general. However, these drugs have potentially great toxicity, and stilbamidine, in particular, is now generally avoided. Pentamidine isethionate is best not given intravenously, as it may cause hypoglycemia and vascular collapse. It can be given intramuscularly in doses of 2 to 4 mg. per kilogram daily for up to 15 doses. In North America, it is available from the C.D.C. (Atlanta).

Immediate Results of Treatment. The response to treatment may be dramatic, but it is usually slow. Reduction of temperature to normal values may take a week or more. When ethylstibamine is given in daily doses, the patient may show relatively little improvement until the course of treatment is nearly over. In the majority of cases, however, improvement is then steady. Frequently there are improvement in appetite and rapid gain in weight. The liver and spleen may recede rapidly, but in protracted cases the spleen may remain large for months. The return of the leukocyte count to normal values is an important criterion of progress, and as a rule it is restored to normal within a month after completion of treatment. Frequently there is an increase in the number of reticulocytes during or shortly after treatment, and gradually the erythrocyte count and hemoglobin return to normal. Serum proteins, however, may take three to six months to return to normal values. A sudden rise in the leukocyte count and recurrence of fever after a normal interval during treatment may be indicative of an intercurrent bacterial infection (otitis media, bronchitis and pneumonia, prostatitis). Specific treatment is not interrupted or discontinued. Antibacterial drugs may be given in addition to ethylstibamine to control intercurrent infection. Acute agranulocytosis has been described as a complication of both the disease and the treatment. Careful clinical observation and frequent leukocyte counts are indicated because of this rare complication. How frequently relapse occurs depends on the geographic origin of the parasite and how well the patient tolerates initial therapy, as well as on other factors.

Follow-up. The condition of the patient should be carefully appraised at the end of each week following treatment. As a rule, the minimal period of strict hospitalization should be 30 days from the end of treatment. A further convalescence of at least 30 days is necessary in most cases. At present, cure can be demonstrated only by adequate follow-up. Patients for whom a diagnosis of kala-azar has been established should be re-examined every month for six months after disposition, and again at the end of the year. If possible, they should be retained on patient status for at least four months, because most relapses appear within six months after treatment, although, rarely, they may appear as much as a year later. When relapses occur they are usually manifested by return of fever, loss of weight, enlarge-

ment of the spleen, return of leukopenia, and elevation of serum globulin. The occurrence of a relapse should be established by parasitologic study. However, the presence of parasites in suitable tissue four to eight weeks after completion of treatment does not in itself constitute failure of treatment or relapse. Many such patients progress to ultimate cure without additional treatment. If signs and symptoms persist that are not otherwise explained, another course of treatment should be given. Likewise, additional treatment should be instituted immediately in the face of definite clinical relapse substantiated by positive parasitologic findings. Relapse following 5.0 grams of Pentostam should be re-treated with a total of 10.0 grams (0.5 gram daily for 20 days). Rarely, repeated relapses may occur after several courses of apparently adequate amounts of Pentostam. Such patients should be re-treated with stilbamidine in a specialized treatment center. In a few instances splenectomy has resulted in cure of patients previously given several courses of unsuccessful treatment with proper doses of antimonials and diamidine drugs. Repeated relapse, hematologic evidence of hypersplenism, and persistence of parasites in tissue are reasons for considering splenectomy. The operation should be followed by a full course of chemotherapy. Post-kala-azar dermal leishmaniasis may be refractory, but the probability of terminating the infection is greatest following a full course of Pentostam, as outlined for the visceral stage.

Prevention. There are no specific prophylactic measures against kala-azar. The basic problem centers around the control of species of Phlebotomus that act as vectors. The sources of infection in patients should be eradicated by appropriate treatment and, in areas where dogs are infected, by suitable steps against such animals. Sandfly control measures, particularly against the adult form, by the use of residual sprays are very effective. Ordinary screens and sleeping nets do not exclude sandflies, but a barrier against them may be created by impregnation of clothing and bedding with insect repellants. Protective clothing is helpful. Effective adult control is easily accomplished with DDT. Effective repellents are dimethylphthalate and N,N-diethyl toluamide.

CUTANEOUS LEISHMANIASIS
(Oriental Sore)

Definition and Epidemiology. The term "oriental sore" has many synonyms, such as Aleppo, Bagdad, or Delhi boil; bouton d'Orient; bouton de Biskra; chiclero ulcer; forest yaws. It is applied to an infection characterized by cutaneous granulomas with a tendency to ulceration and chronicity.

Oriental sore is prevalent in many tropical and subtropical regions in both Eastern and Western Hemispheres. It occurs in Asia, especially in the Middle East, in the Mediterranean littoral, in southern Europe and the Mediterranean islands, in Africa, and in every country in Central and South America except Chile.

The agent is *Leishmania tropica*, which is morphologically identical with *L. donovani* and *L. brasiliensis*.

Experimental and epidemiologic evidence indicates that sandflies are natural vectors of the disease, particularly *Phlebotomus papatasii* and *P. sergenti* in the Near East and *P. macedonicum* in Italy. Successful inoculation of man by the bite of *P. papatasii* has been accomplished. In Central and South America *P. intermedius* is generally regarded as a vector, and several other species may be concerned. In central Asia, the gerbil, a rodent, is an important reservoir. Although infection by *L. tropica* occurs by direct inoculation, the parasites do not penetrate the unbroken skin.

Cutaneous leishmaniasis may occur in almost epidemic form. Children are more commonly affected than adults. There is no distinctive sex incidence. A fairly solid immunity follows infection in man. This has long been the basis for deliberate inoculation of children in endemic areas, the inhabitants knowing that the induced attack confers protection against naturally acquired infection. Sites are chosen where the resultant scar will be least disfiguring.

Pathology. Following inoculation of the skin either through the bite of an infected sandfly or by some other means, a nodule develops that is produced by infiltration of the corium with plasma cells, lymphocytes, and large endothelial macrophages. Thinning and atrophy of the overlying epidermis often occur. Perivascular infiltration then becomes prominent and inflammatory cells more numerous. Focal accumulations of endothelial phagocytes filled with leishmania are seen.

With further progression, an ulcer develops that has a granulation tissue base and a surrounding zone of inflammation. Infiltration extends into the subcutaneous connective tissue in which reticuloendothelial cells, plasma cells, and lymphocytes are prominent. Occasional giant cells are present.

The leishmania are often difficult to demonstrate in the fully developed ulcer and may be found only at the margin of the lesion or in scrapings from its floor. There is no general dissemination of the parasites. Ultimately the leishmania disappear, granulation tissue becomes more abundant, and healing occurs, leaving a depressed fibrous scar.

Clinical Manifestations. The incubation period of oriental sore may vary from a few weeks to several months. The lesions may be multiple. They appear first as slowly growing papules on an exposed skin area. As ulceration develops, they become covered with a crust that exudes a sticky secretion. On removal of the crusts, moist, freely bleeding ulcers are revealed. These ulcers are usually not deep and ordinarily vary from 1 to 3 cm. in diameter. Secondary infection is usual and, when severe, greater tissue destruction may result. After effective treatment, or after a number

of months if no treatment is given, healing occurs by granulation, and a lasting immunity is produced. In extensive multiple ulceration there may be numerous associated subcutaneous nodules that contain leishmania. A nodular or verrucose form affecting the limbs and face has been described, particularly for Venezuela and Ethiopia. It may closely resemble leprosy—many patients have been incarcerated in leprosariums—and is known as leishmaniasis tegumentoria diffusa. Numerous parasites are present in the nodule. It probably represents an unusual host response, as the leishmania skin test is negative.

Dry and moist types of cutaneous leishmaniasis have been described. In the dry type the incubation period and duration of the lesions are long; dry papules persist for months before ulcerating. The incubation period and duration of the moist lesions are shorter; they ulcerate rapidly. Vaccination with either type apparently does not provide cross-immunity.

Diagnosis. The development of one or more cutaneous ulcers on exposed skin areas of the body in a region where oriental sore is known to be endemic and where sandflies are present should arouse suspicion of this condition. Definitive diagnosis depends upon the demonstration of *L. tropica* obtained from the lesion. In general, the longer the lesion has been present, the more difficult it is to find parasites. Examination of the exudate will seldom be successful. Smears made from curettings of the base or the sides of the ulcer should be used, or a fine hypodermic needle introduced through normal skin may be inserted into the indurated margin of the lesion and material aspirated for preparation of a stained smear. Under sterile conditions, material aspirated from the margin of the lesion may be inoculated into NNN (Novy-MacNeal-Nicolle) medium and leptomonad forms recovered after incubation at 22° C. Bacterial contamination of cultures for leishmania may be prevented or controlled by the addition of penicillin and other suitable antimicrobials.

The other diagnostic procedures of value in kala-azar are not appropriate for oriental sore. Leishmania are not found in the blood, and anemia, leukopenia, and hyperglobulinemia are not features of this infection.

The differential diagnosis of cutaneous leishmaniasis must include blastomycosis, yaws, tertiary syphilis, and lupus of the discoid type. The leishmania test is usually positive.

Treatment. The tendency is for spontaneous cure with solid immunity against further challenge. Therefore, if the lesion is solitary and not on the face, all that is usually needed is the treatment of the secondary bacterial infection often found with the sore. If there are multiple lesions or if it is a disfiguring site, i.e., top of the nose, systemic Pentostam should be given in the aforementioned dose. A one-week course is usually sufficient. Infrared lamp exposure has been successful, as the organisms are very temperature dependent.

AMERICAN MUCOCUTANEOUS LEISHMANIASIS

Definition and Epidemiology. The American form of leishmaniasis is attributed to *Leishmania brasiliensis* and resembles the oriental cutaneous type in that it is characterized by skin granulomas; in addition many patients show ulcerative lesions of the nose, mouth, and pharynx.

Naso-oral or mucocutaneous leishmaniasis occurs predominantly in forest workers, and men are more frequently affected than women. This difference in sex incidence, therefore, is probably occupational. It is believed, on epidemiologic grounds, that various species of sandflies, Phlebotomus, are the vectors and that transmission from infected man or animals is accomplished by the bite of these insects. The spiny rats, *Proechimys semispinosus panamensis* and *Hoplomys gymnurus,* have been found naturally infected with *L. brasiliensis* in Panama. The disease has occurred in epidemic form in man in Paraguay.

Pathology. American leishmaniasis is distinguished from oriental sore primarily by the greater incidence of mucocutaneous involvement. In 10 to 20 per cent of cases in South America the mucous membranes are involved, leading to extensive ulceration and necrosis of the nose, mouth, and pharynx. During the period of active infection there is frequently profound cachexia, and healing is often accompanied by great deformity of the affected structures. The mucosae may be invaded by direct extension from an adjacent cutaneous lesion, or the nasopharyngeal process may be secondary to a distant primary focus, which in some cases has healed prior to the onset of the secondary development.

The development of the lesion is similar to that of oriental sore. It appears first as a small papule, later becoming crusted and exuding a sticky substance. Removal of the crust reveals a freely bleeding ulcer. This extends slowly into adjacent tissues, increasing both in size and depth as secondary infection is established. The cartilage and bony support of the nose are often destroyed, and the hard and soft palate and walls of the pharynx are sometimes similarly affected. Death occurs from sepsis or malnutrition.

Leishmania may be recovered from nodules and the indurated margins of ulcers. There is no general dissemination, although rarely they may be found in the regional lymph nodes adjacent to an active lesion.

Clinical Manifestations. The disease begins as a small papule appearing on an exposed skin surface, often on the margins of the ears. Ulcer formation follows, and the process at this stage does not differ from oriental sore. Later, ulcers develop about the margins of the nose and mouth and may extend, causing widespread destruction of tissue in the naso-oral region.

Diagnosis. In advanced cases with extensive secondary infection it may be impossible to demonstrate Leishmania organisms. Material for staining or culture should be obtained by curettage of the indurated margin of the lesion or by aspiration from this area. The Montenegro intradermal test is of considerable diagnostic value.

The differential diagnosis of this condition involves consideration of yaws, leprosy, tertiary syphilis, blastomycosis, lupus, and nasal myiasis.

Treatment. The prognosis in American leishmaniasis is much more serious than that in oriental sore because of the destructive mucocutaneous lesions. To prevent these serious complications, intensive treatment with Pentostam intravenously should be instituted at the earliest possible moment. This drug has not been evaluated in South American leishmaniasis, but another pentavalent antimonial, glucantine, has not been successful in most cases. Tartar emetic and amphotericin B have been used, with some favorable reports. This appears to be the form of human leishmaniasis that is most resistant to therapy. Treatment should be continued until apparent cure is obtained, and the patient should be observed for an extended period.

Additional or subsequent treatment, if required, consists of the administration of a course of tartar emetic intravenously. Secondary bacterial infection must be treated by the appropriate antimicrobial drugs. Recently, amphotericin B and cycloguanil pamoate have been found to have therapeutic efficacy in American leishmaniasis but have not displaced Pentostam as the drug of choice in primary therapy. Cycloguanil pamoate is given as a single dose of 350 mg. base intramuscularly, and if healing is not complete in six to ten weeks, it should be repeated.

Langsjoen, P. H.: Cutaneous leishmaniasis: Report of 10 cases. Ann. Intern. Med., 45:623, 1956.

Most, H., and Lavietes, P. H.: Kala-azar in American military personnel. Medicine, 26:221, 1947.

Napier, L. E.: Principles and Practice of Tropical Medicine. New York, The Macmillan Company, 1946.

Shanbrom, E., et. al.: Visceral manifestations of American mucocutaneous leishmaniasis. Amer. J. Med., 20:145, 1956.

Shortt, H. L.: Diagnosis of kala-azar. Trop. Dis. Bull., 44:145, 1947.

Stone, H. H., et al.: Kala-azar (visceral leishmaniasis): Report of case with 34-month incubation period. Ann. Intern. Med., 36:686, 1952.

AMEBIASIS
Philip D. Marsden

Definition. Amebiasis is the disease caused by infection with *Entamoeba histolytica.* The protozoan inhabits the large bowel where environmental conditions are suitable for its multiplication. It may either live as a commensal in the lumen or invade the bowel wall, causing symptoms. The most common organ to be secondarily involved is the liver by blood-borne embolism from the large bowel.

Etiology. *E. histolytica* may have evolved from

the free-living ameba *E. moshkovski*, which has an identical morphology. Man is infected by ingesting cysts of *E. histolytica*. The wall of the cyst is digested in the small intestine. A resultant multinucleated ameba divides into four or eight individuals. Thus the organism exists in two major forms: a relatively resistant cyst responsible for the transmission of the disease, and a trophozoite or ameba which survives poorly outside the body.

Trophozoites vary much in size (10 to 40 μ). In acute dysentery they are large and often contain red blood cells. They exhibit unidirectional movement, thrusting out clear pseudopodia of ectoplasm into which the granular endoplasm flows. There are a single nucleus and a number of food vacuoles. This trophozoite is the actively growing phase which divides by binary fission. Cysts are formed as the trophozoites move toward the rectum, but the exact stimulus to cyst formation is unknown. The mature trophozoite eliminates cytoplasmic inclusions, and, becoming a small precystic ameba (minuta form), secretes a cyst wall to form a uninucleate cyst. The nucleus then divides twice to form the mature cyst with four nuclei. Both mature and immature cysts are infectious.

The four nucleated cysts (10 to 20 μ) contain thick rods with rounded ends, the chromatoid bars believed to be a ribosome store. There is a food reserve in the form of a glycogen vacuole. The nuclear structure common to all forms has a central small karyosome and an even distribution of chromatin granules around the nuclear membrane.

Strains of amebae vary in their pathogenicity, and an attempt has been made to correlate this with morphology. A small ameba (5 to 14 μ) with a small nucleus and clumped peripheral nuclear chromatin has been given species status as *Entamoeba hartmanni*. The cysts are also smaller than *E. histolytica* (4 to 10 μ), and all intracystic structures are correspondingly reduced. These amebae are alleged to be nonhistolytic and consequently nonpathogenic.

E. histolytica and *E. hartmanni* must be differentiated particularly from the nonpathogenic *E. coli.* Both the trophozoite and the cyst of this species are larger than *E. histolytica*. The trophozoite is sluggish, contains bacteria, and has a coarse granular endoplasm. The ectoplasm is not as clearly defined as that of *E. histolytica*. The nucleus has an eccentric karyosome and coarse peripheral chromatin beading. The cyst has usually more than four nuclei, and up to 32 may be present.

At a time when macrophages are still being mistaken for *E. histolytica* trophozoites in some laboratories, the basic parasitology given above is highly relevant. It is important for the clinician to realize the difficulties facing the parasitologist. It is often necessary to examine a population of cysts before the morphologic criteria necessary to define a species can be recognized. An eyepiece micrometer for measuring the size of cysts is an essential piece of equipment for every diagnostic laboratory.

Epidemiology. Human *E. histolytica* infections have been found in all parts of the world, and it is estimated that 10 per cent of the world's population is infected. Incidence figures reported from the different parts of the United States vary considerably, but commonly average about 2 to 5 per cent. Much higher incidence figures occur in the tropics (25 to 45 per cent). These figures are based on detection of *E. histolytica* in the stool; a more accurate criterion for assessing the prevalence of pathogenic strains is the incidence of amebic liver abscess. There are many reports of liver abscess from the tropical zones of Asia, Africa, and South America. Mexico is an important focus in the Americas, and hundreds of cases have been reported from the United States. There are many areas of Southeast Asia where amebic liver abscesses are frequently seen. There is a high incidence on the west coast of Africa and in Natal.

Encystment seems primarily designed for meeting adverse conditions outside the host, and mature cysts can withstand the action of gastric juices. Cysts are killed by drying but can survive as long as a month in water. They are not destroyed by the concentration of chlorine usually used in water purification.

Usually the infection is acquired by ingesting cysts in fecally contaminated food and water. Several famous epidemics in the United States have been water borne, such as the Chicago epidemic in which there were 1400 known cases and more than 100 deaths. Uncooked foods such as salads and fruits are common vehicles, especially if night soil is used as fertilizer. *E. histolytica* cysts may be carried by house flies, and have been shown to survive for 48 hours in these insects. The infected carrier, passing a large number of cysts, is an important source of infection, especially if he is a food handler. The incidence is often determined by the sanitary conditions available, and a high incidence is found in some mental institutions.

Pathogenesis. Amebae thrive under conditions of low oxygen tension, and conditions in the large bowel are favorable because bacterial multiplication lowers the oxidation reduction potential and provides favorable growth factors. Recently *E. histolytica* has been grown in axenic culture. What part bacterial associates play in determining the pathogenicity of a strain of *E. histolytica* is still not clear. In one study in germ-free animals monocontaminated with different bacterial species, sterile amebae have shown different degrees of invasiveness, suggesting that the type of bacterial associate may be important.

In symptomless carriers as well as in latent periods of chronic infection the amebae probably live in the lumen of the gut and feed on fecal bacteria and other available nutrients. If one accepts that this organism is more commonly a commensal, the question arises as to why on occasion it invades the tissues of man and produces disease. The possible role of associated bacteria has already been mentioned, but there is good evidence to suggest that strains of *E. histolytica* vary in their capacity to produce disease in laboratory animals and man. Currently much work is being done on the characterization of strains of *E. histolytica,* utilizing criteria such as their drug resistance, their capacity to grow at low temperature, and the analysis of their antigens and enzymes. It may well be that the virulence of a strain depends on its capacity to produce proteolytic enzymes, that is, its histolytic effect, and a variety of such enzymes have been identified.

Undoubtedly host factors play a part in determining whether a patient will be a symptomless cyst passer or acquire invasive disease of the bowel. Virulence can be enhanced by rapid passage through susceptible hosts. Corticosteroids tend to exacerbate bowel amebiasis, and consequently stress is deleterious. The severe dysentery sometimes encountered in pregnant women could be a corticosteroid effect. High carbohydrate–low protein diets aggravate amebiasis in laboratory animals, and similar diets of Durban Africans may account in part for their high incidence of invasive amebiasis.

Penetration of the bowel wall by *E. histolytica* is associated with host cell necrosis but little inflammatory reaction. The degree of bowel wall invasion is very variable. The most frequent sites of ulceration are the cecum, splenic and hepatic flexures, descending colon, and rectum. The site and shape of the ulcers are variable, but they have undermined edges (the so-called flask-shaped ulcers). Sometimes in acute infections the muscularis mucosa is invaded, and histolysis, thrombosis of capillaries, and necrosis extend into the deeper layer of the bowel. The ulcers enlarge, and large areas of mucosa can be lost in a severe infection. Secondary bacterial infection of the ulcers produces purulent slough and sometimes a severe inflammatory reaction in the wall. This may be associated with a peripheral leukocytosis and the appearance of leukocytes in the stool, though seldom in the numbers found in shigellosis. In ordinary hematoxylin and eosin sections the internal structure of amebae is not well seen, but they shrink away from the host tissue, appearing as round, vacuolated bodies. Stained with periodic acid–Schiff stain, tissue amebae stand out as bright red bodies. A persistent bowel infection rarely promotes a localized fibrotic reaction in an area of marked ulceration, the granuloma so formed being called an ameboma.

Hepatic Amebiasis. Amebae probably reach the liver in every patient with invasive intestinal amebiasis, either by the lymphatics or more commonly by the portal vein. Yet only a small proportion (10 per cent) of patients with intestinal amebiasis develop a liver abscess. Many liver abscesses arise long after the acute intestinal phase of the disease, and we know little of the factors responsible for this variable pattern. Although amebic liver abscess is seen in children of both sexes with equal frequency, in adults the condition is far more common in males (70 to 90 per cent). Work in laboratory animals suggests that the blood level of sex hormones such as progesterone and testosterone may influence the development of liver abscess and account for this striking difference.

Every abscess must start on a small scale as one or more areas of localized liver necrosis associated with trophozoite multiplication by binary fission. Once outside the bowel *E. histolytica* cannot form cysts, so in a sense every extraluminal infection is disadvantageous to the parasite. Small microabscesses may coalesce, or a single one may grow to produce a clinically detectable lesion. The wall of the abscess consists of necrotic tissue and compressed liver parenchyma with a variable infiltrate of macrocytes, plasma cells, lymphocytes, and fibroblasts. It is not a true abscess in the sense of containing pus consisting of masses of polymorphonuclear leukocytes. The so called "anchovy sauce" pus is autolyzed liver, the result of amebal enzyme activity and perhaps released host cell enzymes. Approximately three quarters of abscesses are single, and rather more than this proportion occur in the right lobe. The abscesses are bacteriologically sterile, so in this situation the amebae do not seem to need bacteria. In animals it is easier to induce amebic liver abscesses in those animals which have active bowel amebiasis or previous bowel amebiasis. This is perhaps evidence of a hypersensitivity phenomenon.

E. histolytica prospers in a complex protein environment at 37° C., so it is not surprising that trophozoites will multiply in the lung, pericardium, pleura, or peritoneum if an amebic abscess ruptures into these sites. Similarly the environment of the cervix, uncircumcised penis, natal cleft, and covered colostomy is satisfactory. In all these sites only trophozoites are found, and fresh material must be searched diligently for them.

Clinical Manifestations. Intestinal Amebiasis. A wide spectrum of clinical manifestations are found in association with this infection. We have come to realize that most patients who have *E. histolytica* cysts in their stools have no current symptoms. On close questioning some of them will not admit to any bowel disorder in the past, whereas others have had a transient episode of diarrhea or an alteration in bowel habit. Often in retrospect it is difficult to evaluate the significance of such a history as there are many causes of diarrhea in the tropics. However, because such a patient could return in a few weeks with a liver abscess, his infection must be taken seriously and treated.

Other patients give a history of intermittent diarrhea and constipation, which is held to be more classic of amebiasis. They may have noticed mucus in the stools and an occasional fleck of blood. Flatulence and colonic pain may be prominent features. Occasionally in such patients trophozoites are found in the mucus flecks adherent to the outside of a relatively formed stool. On examination there may be a tender palpable cecum or descending colon; such symptoms may persist for many years with periodic exacerbations and remissions. The constitutional symptoms of fatigue, arthralgia, headache, and backache are attributed to such infections, but the mechanism is a difficult one to understand.

The bloody diarrhea of acute amebic dysentery is a relative rarity and is accompanied by fever and debility. The stools can resemble red currant jelly, being just blood and mucus, or else may be diarrheal and streaked with blood. Tenesmus and colicky abdominal pain may distress the patient. Warm fresh stools should be examined for trophozoites, and they are usually found. If such examinations are negative, however, it is worthwhile to do a gentle sigmoidoscopy. The risk of bowel perforation has been much exaggerated. After an initial rectal examination to determine that the rectum is empty, the sigmoidoscope is gently introduced and all further manipulation done under direct vision. A gentle scrape of an ulcerated area with a curette and examination of these scrapings immediately will often reveal amebae, and the physician should persist in his search for amebae if he suspects this diagnosis.

Complications. Strictures can be produced by excessive granulomatous tissue and are most common in the rectum and sigmoid. The patient may present with signs of partial intestinal obstruction, and a localized mass may be palpable in the colon. Amebic appendicitis has been described and intussusception and pseudopolyposis can occur. In cases in which there is severe damage to the bowel wall, perforation may lead to bacterial or amebic peritonitis. Rarely in such cases massive hemorrhage may result. A syndrome of postdysenteric ulcerative colitis is described with strongly positive serologic tests but no demonstrable amebae. Some of these patients ultimately develop the irritable colon syndrome.

Hepatic Amebiasis. Tender hepatomegaly occurs in association with acute amebic dysentery (about 50 per cent in one series), but this does not necessarily mean amebic involvement of the liver. Nevertheless, the tendency is quite rightly to protect the patient from developing a liver abscess by giving him a tissue amebicide.

There is no doubt that there is a clinical syndrome of fever, tender hepatomegaly, mild leukocytosis, and positive serologic findings for amebiasis, which responds dramatically to emetine therapy. Associated symptoms are nausea and right upper quadrant pain. Clinicians use the term *amebic hepatitis* to describe this syndrome, although pathologists are quick to point out that there is no evidence of diffuse involvement of the liver with amebae, but only infiltration of the portal tracts with chronic inflammatory cells and Kupffer cell hypertrophy.

In an established amebic liver abscess, intermittent fever, night sweats, and loss of weight are often prominent symptoms. There is a dull aching pain over the liver which may be referred to the tip of the right shoulder via the phrenic nerve. An abscess in the posterior part of the dome of the liver may force the diaphragm up, and abdominal hepatomegaly may be absent. Usually, however, the liver can be palpated, and there may be a localized swelling. Gentle compression of the ribs produces right hypochondrial pain or right shoulder tip pain. Fifty per cent of right lobe abscesses have signs at the right lung base, either a small effusion, collapse, or crepitations. Sometimes if an

abscess is "pointing," there may be a localized area of tenderness and edema. In tropical practice, owing to neglect, patients may present with a sinus discharging amebic pus in the liver area.

A polymorphonuclear leukocytosis is usually present and the blood sedimentation rate is increased. A normocytic normochromic anemia disappears with successful therapy. Serum transaminases and alkaline phosphatase may be raised, but liver function tests are of little diagnostic value. Jaundice is rare, and if present is usually associated with pressure of a large abscess on the biliary tree. Roentgenographic examination may show a raised right diaphragm with diminished movement on screening. Liver scans using radioactive labeled rose bengal or gold have helped considerably in defining sizable liver abscesses. Positive serologic tests for amebiasis occur in over 90 per cent of patients. With scanning techniques, blind aspiration of the liver is seldom necessary. A decision whether or not to aspirate the liver must be made in each case. However, if there is a visible site of "pointing" of the abscess, such as a localized bulging of the chest wall or a definite area of tenderness, aspiration relieves the patient's pain and the characteristic pus obtained is diagnostic. If characteristic pus is obtained, effective chemotherapy should be commenced immediately.

Complications. Apart from rupturing to the surface, amebic pus may gain access to any structure contiguous to the liver. Rupture through the diaphragm into the lung causes lung abscess, consolidation, and a bronchohepatic fistula so that the patient coughs up amebic pus. If the pus is localized to the pleura, the signs are those of empyema. Rupture into the pericardium of a liver abscess results in signs suggestive of a pericardial effusion. Pericardial aspiration relieves cardiac tamponade and reveals amebic pus.

Amebic peritonitis may arise as the result of a bowel perforation or rupture of a liver abscess. The clinical presentation may be deceptive in that all the signs of acute peritonitis are not necessarily present. Cerebral amebiasis presents with signs of a cerebral abscess and is invariably secondary to a liver abscess, in contrast to primary amebic meningoencephalitis owing to free-living amebae (see later).

Cutaneous amebiasis is often realized for what it is by its site of occurrence. It occurs around the anus or a colostomy in association with acute bowel infection, or on the surface of the abdomen. If an amebic liver abscess is discharging to the skin surface, it takes the form of a granulomatous ulceration of the skin. Cervical amebiasis is usually secondary to bowel disease, and the vulva and vagina may be involved. Primary amebiasis of the penis is probably the result of irregular sexual practices.

Differential Diagnosis. *Acute Intestinal Amebiasis.* In acute intestinal amebiasis the stool should be cultured for Salmonella and Shigella in any case, as sometimes amebic and bacillary dysentery coexist. Failure to demonstrate an infectious agent after repeated stool examination suggests nonspecific ulcerative colitis as the cause of the dysentery. Some clinicians recognize the entity of postdysenteric ulcerative colitis. Barium enema examination is valuable in selected cases in defining the extent of the inflammation, although it gives no clue as to the cause. Rarely, carcinoma of the colon can present as dysentery.

Chronic Intestinal Amebiasis. As well as the entities mentioned above, a presentation of intermittent diarrhea and constipation may be associated with diverticulitis, Crohn's disease, or the irritable colon syndrome. Just how frequently the latter syndrome complicates or is a sequel to intestinal amebiasis is not known. Amebomas are particularly worrisome for the clinician because they may be impossible to distinguish from a carcinoma of the bowel, both presenting as localized large bowel strictures. If amebae are found in the stool, treatment with emetine hydrochloride and a luminal amebicide should be tried; if an ameboma is the correct diagnosis, roentgenologic improvement may be noted in a few weeks. If amebae are not found, exploratory laparotomy is indicated. Rarely a carcinoma can be secondarily invaded by amebae.

Hepatic Amebiasis. Other space occupying lesions of the liver may mimic an amebic abscess. Hydatid cyst must always be considered in an endemic area. A large secondary carcinomatous deposit or a primary carcinoma of the liver is sometimes difficult to exclude. It must also be remembered that although the great majority of liver abscesses are amebic, primary bacterial abscesses can occur, as well as those secondary to suppurative disease of the bowel. Amebiasis of the cervix can resemble a cervical erosion. The granulomatous reaction of penile amebiasis has to be distinguished from chancroid, cancer of the penis, and granuloma inguinale.

Laboratory Diagnosis. Finding the Parasite. Stool or bowel scrapings should be examined immediately for trophozoites, preferably on a warm stage. A drop of buffered physiologic saline is often needed to dilute the material. A concentration technique is essential when looking for cysts, as it increases tenfold the chance of finding them. The formol ether concentration technique is satisfactory. A drop of Lugol's iodine run under the coverslip helps to define nuclear morphology. Stool smears stained with iron hematoxylin also permit evaluation of intracystic structures, but this is a lengthy procedure. Culture of such material at 37° C. in a protein-rich medium with added starch and a balanced salt solution overlay increases one's chances of finding amebae.

Even with a concentration technique, several specimens should be examined, for sometimes *E. histolytica* is only found on the third or even the fourth examination. The reason for the periodicity of cyst excretion is not fully understood but may depend on factors such as diet and bowel motility, as well as parasitic multiplication.

Ideally in all suspected amebic liver abscesses aspiration should be attempted, as the characteristic pus obtained is diagnostic. The pus should be discharged into a series of containers and the last examined for amebae; 1 ml. of tenacious pus incubated at 37° C. in a culture medium preconditioned with *Escherichia coli* or *Clostridium welchii* may facilitate detection of amebae. Aspiration of the left lobe abscess is hazardous because of the danger of peritoneal soiling. Open operation is sometimes necessary to establish the diagnosis and evacuate the pus.

Serologic Tests. The degree of tissue invasion probably determines antibody formation. IgG fraction of gamma globulin contains these antibodies, which can be detected by a variety of techniques using standardized antigens. The following tests, in order of decreasing sensitivity, have been useful: indirect hemagglutination, fluorescent antibody complement fixation, and gel diffusion precipitation. In endemic areas serologic tests must be interpreted in relation to the general pattern of antibody levels in the asymptomatic population.

Therapy. This is a most confusing aspect of the disease, because there are almost as many regimens advocated as there are experts. Many of the drugs are effective but none ideal, with the possible exception of metronidazole. This drug, first used for human trichomoniasis, appears to be very effective in most forms of amebiasis. In invasive amebiasis it is valuable especially in children, pregnant women, and patients with heart disease in whom emetine is contraindicated. As it is not approved in the United States for use in amebiasis, the older regimens are given first; but eventually metronidazole may supersede these. Often two or more drugs are used in combination or successively to cure the diease and minimize chances of a relapse. The therapeutic regimens given below are those that the writer has found to be effective.

Intestinal Amebiasis. *The Cyst Passer.* As there is no practical way of determining which strains of *E. histolytica* are potentially pathogenic, most physicians treat all cyst passers, whether symptomatic or not, especially in communities where the incidence is low. In this way the incidence of infection is kept down in countries such as the United States and England. In tropical areas where there is a high prevalence of carriers (25 to 50 per cent), the frequency of reinfection and the cost of therapy make such an approach impracticable. There are several poorly absorbed amebicides which act "intraluminally" and when given alone will eradicate the majority of such infections (adult doses are given). A drug is needed that is effective, has minor side effects, and can be given on an outpatient basis. Entamide furoate, 20 mg. per kilogram of body weight daily for ten days, is very satisfactory, having a high cure rate and only flatulence as a side effect, but it is not available in the United States. Paromomycin (Humatin), 500 mg. three times a day for seven days, is usually effective, and unlike other antimicrobial drugs has a direct amebicidal effect. Diodoquin (diiodohydroxyquin), in a dose of 650 mg. three times a day for 21 days, is still widely used in the United States, although it has a lower cure rate than the two drugs previously mentioned. Recent studies indicate that metronidazole (Flagyl) cures many cyst passers in a dose of 400 to 800 mg. three times a day for five days.

Invasive Bowel Amebiasis. This includes patients with acute and subacute amebiasis. The therapeutic choice will be determined partly by the patient's age and general condition. Acute amebic dysentery implies tissue invasion, and here the drugs mentioned above, with the possible exception of metronidazole, are not sufficient.

Emetine has been an important drug for acute amebiasis for more than half a century. No drug controls acute dysentery as quickly as emetine, which (being a tissue amebicide) protects against hepatic involvement. Unfortunately it is toxic to the patient as well as to the *E. histolytica* trophozoite. Side effects include weakness, headache and muscle pain, nausea and vomiting, diarrhea, and cardiotoxic effects. The last-named are accompanied by a fall in blood pressure, dyspnea, precordial pain, and tachycardia. ECG changes occur, in the form of T wave inversion, prolonged PR interval, widened QRS complex, and arrhythmias. Marked ECG changes are an indication for terminating emetine therapy. *Emetine hydrochloride should not be given to patients with evidence of cardiovascular disease.* Sterile intramuscular abscesses can develop if the site of infection is not varied. Dehydroemetine, a less toxic isomer, is being increasingly used. Both emetine and dehydroemetine should be given only to patients on bed rest. Severe intestinal amebiasis in young, otherwise healthy adults can be treated with emetine hydrochloride, 65 mg., or dehydroemetine, 80 mg., intramuscularly daily for five to ten days; oxytetracycline, 250 mg. every six hours for seven days; and Diodoquin, 650 mg. three times a day for 21 days. When oral therapy is not possible, oxytetracycline can be given in an intravenous drip. A regimen useful for patients who cannot be hospitalized or for those who have myocardial insufficiency is oxytetracycline, 250 mg. every six hours for seven days; chloroquine diphosphate, 150 mg. base twice daily for 21 days; and Diodoquin, 650 mg. thrice daily for 21 days. This second regimen can be scaled down for pediatric practice. Any of the luminal amebicides previously mentioned can be used in preference to Diodoquin. The action of oxytetracycline is to change the bacterial flora of the gut, creating an environment unfavorable to amebae. When used alone, however, there is a high relapse rate. Chloroquine is used in the second regimen to protect the liver.

Recent trials with metronidazole (Flagyl) in acute dysentery have suggested that the drug is highly effective when used alone in an oral dose of 800 mg. three times a day for five days. It is both a luminal and tissue amebicide. The dosage level is higher than that used for trichomoniasis. Side effects are nausea, dizziness, skin rashes, and an unpleasant taste in the mouth. Patients should be warned against drinking alcohol while on Flagyl therapy as an acute confusional state may ensue.

Hepatic Amebiasis. If hepatic amebiasis is suspected on the criteria previously discussed but there are no signs to localize an abscess or attempted aspiration has failed to reveal pus, drug treatment should be started and the patient's progress watched. An emetine derivative and chloroquine should be used together. They are both concentrated in the liver. A satisfactory regimen consists of dehydroemetine, 80 mg. daily by intramuscular injection for ten days, and chloroquine diphosphate, 900 mg. daily for two days, and then 450 mg. daily for 21 days. Established abscesses can disappear on this treatment without the necessity for further aspiration. If after such therapy the liver remains large or is enlarging, the diagnosis should be reconsidered. If the diagnosis of an amebic liver abscess is still favored, further aspiration is indicated. With secondarily infected amebic abscesses, correct therapy involves identification of the bacteria responsible and appropriate antimicrobial therapy. A luminal amebicide is also given to eradicate any coexistent bowel infection.

Metronidazole (Flagyl) in an oral dose similar to that already quoted has been successful in the treatment of amebic liver abscess. This can be considered an alternative or additional therapy. It has also proved effective in skin amebiasis and can be tried in other forms of extraintestinal amebiasis. Here emetine hydrochloride, 65 mg. intramuscularly for ten days, is effective therapy. With large amebic lung abscesses emetine therapy may have to be pushed to the limit of tolerance with careful electrocardiographic monitoring. Postural drainage is important, and drainage of the pericardium may be required to relieve cardiac tamponade. Skin amebiasis also responds dramatically to emetine.

Prognosis. Intestinal amebiasis usually responds well to adequate therapy. The more severe the form, the more difficult the cure, and relapses are common. Severe dysentery, especially when complicated by intestinal perforation and peritonitis, carries a grave prognosis. A fatal outcome is more often the result of a large liver abscess and its complications.

The use of hepatic scanning techniques has given us better information on how successful our therapy has been in amebic liver abscess. Most heal in two to four months, but occasionally resolution takes longer than one year. There is a poor correlation between size and the time of resolution. In the absence of secondary infection, little liver scarring results, but sometimes bizarre hepatic calcifications are seen years afterward. Multiple abscesses were present in less than 20 per cent of cases in one postmortem series. Wilmot gives a figure of 10 per cent mortality in his experience of amebic liver abscess in Durban.

Reasonable criteria of cure in amebiasis are resolution of symptoms and stool specimens repeatedly negative for *E. histolytica*. Ideally stools should be examined monthly for six months and again at one year. The relapsing nature of the infection makes follow-up very important. Repeat sigmoidoscopy and barium enema are required if abnormalities were found in the acute phase.

Prevention. Proper filtration rather than chlorination of water supplies is more reliable for removing *E. histolytica* cysts. The soaking of salads and vegetables in vinegar or potassium permanganate solution, as sometimes recommended, makes them inedible. A weak solution of iodine is more effective. Most residents in the tropics blithely consume salads, vegetables, and fruit without ill effects. It is wise to screen the stools of domestic staffs involved in food handling.

Chemoprophylaxis with entamide furoate has been successful in some studies. However, as many strains seem to be virtually nonpathogenic, it is doubtful whether this is justified. Perhaps the wisest course is to examine the stools of all persons returning from residence in endemic areas with a high prevalence rate, whether or not they have a suggestive history of amebic disease, with the intention of starting appropriate chemotherapy in the presence of any positive findings.

Amoebiasis: Report of a WHO Expert Committee. WHO Technical Report Series No. 421, 1-52, 1969.

Biagi, F. F., and Beltran, H. F.: The Challenge of Amoebiasis: Understanding Pathogenic Mechanisms. International Review of Tropical Medicine. New York, Academic Press Inc., 1969, Vol. 3, pp. 219-231.

Elsdon-Dew, R.: The epidemiology of amoebiasis. *In* Advances in Parasitology. New York, Academic Press, Inc., 1968, Vol. 6, p. 1.

Neal, R. A.: Experimental studies on Entamoeba with reference to speciation. *In* Advances in Parasitology. New York, Academic Press, Inc., 1966, Vol. 4, p. 1.

OTHER INTESTINAL PROTOZOA
Philip D. Marsden

Apart from *Entamoeba histolytica,* at least four genera and seven species of amebae have been established as living in man. Common stool amebae are *Entamoeba coli, Endolimax nana,* and *Iodameba buetschlii.* They are nonpathogenic, but such protozoa have a double importance. First, they must be distinguished from the pathogenic *E. histolytica* by the available clear morphologic criteria. Second, they provide an index of fecal contamination. If any stool protozoan is encountered, it is wise to examine a further specimen, for, because of the variable appearance of protozoa in the stool, the second specimen may reveal a pathogen. *Dientamoeba fragilis* is a delicate ameba without a cystic stage. Some clinicians believe it is a cause of mild diarrhea, but the evidence is not convincing.

Several flagellates are also found in the stool, among them the nonpathogenic *Trichomonas hominis* and *Chilomastix mesnili.* Information on the differential diagnosis of these intestinal protozoa can be found in texts of parasitology. Here we must consider briefly the clinical significance of three pathogenic protozoa: *Giardia lamblia* (a flagellate), *Balantidium coli* (a ciliate), and *Isospora belli* (a coccidium).

Marsden, P. D., and Hoskins, D. W.: Intestinal parasites. A progress report. Gastroenterology, 51:701, 1966.

GIARDIASIS

Abdominal pain, distention and flatulence, and recurrent diarrhea may be associated with *Giardia lamblia* infection, especially in children. Inhabiting the duodenum and upper jejunum, the parasite is a pear-shaped flagellate, anteriorly broad and rounded and tapering to a point not unlike a tennis racket. It is convex dorsally with a ventral attachment disc. There are sets of identical structures on either side of the median line. When stained, there are two nuclei, four pairs of flagela, and a parabasal body. In fresh stool this trophozoite is actively motile with an irregular characteristic progression. It reproduces by longitudinal binary fission.

The thick-walled cysts are 10 to 14 μ by 6 to 10 μ and have two to four nuclei with curved rods or axostyles. In some infections several million cysts per gram of feces may be passed. Only in patients with very rapid bowel transit times do trophozoites appear in the stool, although they may be found in duodenal aspirate. Cultivation of Giardia in vitro has recently been achieved.

The infective cysts are transmitted in food and drink, and the infection is cosmopolitan. The great majority of patients are asymptomatic, but there is no doubt that heavy infections are associated with symptoms. Diarrhea is the most common symptom, and the stools are pale and contain mucus. Giardia is in fact a cause of steatorrhea, and patients have abnormal fat balances and D-xylose tests which return to normal after successful treatment. The hypothesis that this malabsorption is the result of a mechanical barrier produced by large numbers of parasites attached to the microvillar surface is attractive, but effects on digestive enzyme activity and microvillar function are possible. Villous flattening with inflammatory infiltration has been demonstrated in one study.

Diarrhea may alternate with constipation, and apart from these symptoms epigastric pain resembling a peptic ulcer may be a disabling symptom. Anorexia, meat intolerance, and loss of weight may occur. Although Giardia may be found in the gallbladder, the evidence that it is responsible for cholecystitis is unsatisfactory. Giardiasis must be distinguished from other causes of malabsorption and peptic ulcer.

Giardiasis, symptomatic or not, should always be treated. Two drugs are equally effective. Quinacrine hydrochloride (Atabrine), in a dose of 100 mg. three times a day after food for seven days, is an established therapy, but the drug has a bitter taste, and nausea and vomiting may result. It may also stain the skin yellow, but psychosis does not occur at this dosage level. Metronidazole (Flagyl), 200 mg. three times a day after food for ten days, is equally effective with few side effects. Both drugs have about an 80 per cent cure rate, and in the event of failure of one drug the other can be tried. The follow-up procedures are similar to those in amebiasis.

Hoskins, L. C., Winawer, S. J., Broitman, S. A., Gottlieb, L. S., and Zamchek, N.: Clinical giardiasis and intestinal malabsorption. Gastroenterology, 53:265, 1967.

Yardley, J. H., Takano, J., and Hendrix, T. B.: Epithelial and other mucosal lesions of the jejunum in giardiasis: Jejunal biopsy studies. Bull. Hopkins Hosp., 115:389, 1964.

BALANTIDIASIS

Balantidium coli is the largest protozoon of man, measuring 50 to 70 μ in length by 30 to 60 μ in width. It infects the colon of man and may produce diarrhea and dysentery. When viewed under the low power of the microscope in a saline smear of stool, the grayish-green trophozoite can be seen gliding across the field powered by spiral longitudinal rows of cilia. There is a large oral macronucleus and a smaller micronucleus. A cytostome or mouth ingests organic matter that circulates as food vacuoles. Erythrophagocytosis has been observed. Reproduction is by binary fission or conjugation. A resistant cyst form is passed in formed stools, and this is the infective form. *Cosmopolitan in distribution, it is a rare infection of man although common in pigs.* When man and pig share shelter, human infections are common, and this accounts for the high incidence of human infection in parts of New Guinea (20 per cent) and Peru. *B. coli* of man can be transmitted to monkeys, cats, guinea pigs, and rats, but the importance of these animals as reservoirs is minor. Handling pigs in slaughterhouses may be an occupational risk.

This ciliate can be a tissue invader, and similar factors to those mentioned for *E. histolytica* may well determine this behavior. Proteolytic secretions produce necrosis and ulceration of the mucosa. Columns of balantidia may be seen lying in the submucosa. Secondary infection with bacteria results in an accompanying inflammatory reaction. The ulcers are often quite large and deep, with a broad, indurated base. A liver abscess with *B. coli* in situ has been described, and balantidia have been found in the lung and heart in isolated cases.

Less than one fifth of infected persons have symptoms. Severe infections are associated with diarrhea and the passage of blood and mucus in the stools. Constitutional symptoms of fever, nausea, vomiting, and asthenia are described. Examination of fresh stools reveals the trophozoite or cyst. Culture of the stools on media similar to those used for amebiasis may reveal an infection when conventional microscopy has failed; in symptomatic patients this is usually not necessary. Balantidiasis must be differentiated from amebic dysentery and ulcerative colitis. Although arsenical preparations have been used in the past, oxytetracycline is probably the drug of choice in an adult dose of 500 mg. three times a day for ten days. Paromomycin (Humatin) or metronidazole (Flagyl) is also effective. Spontaneous recovery has been noted. The infection may be fatal if bowel perforation occurs.

Arean, V. M., and Koppisch, E.: Balantidiasis: A review and report of cases. Amer. J. Path., 32:1089, 1956.

Van der Hoeven, J. A., and Rijpstra, A. C.: Intestinal parasites in the central mountain district of Netherlands, New Guinea. An important focus of *Balantidium coli*. Docum. Med. Geog. Trop., 9:225, 1957.

COCCIDIOSIS

Coccidia have alternate asexual and sexual generation in the same host, and the nature of the cycle is not dissimilar to plasmodia in the forms produced. There is probably only one human species, *Isospora belli,* which parasitizes the small intestinal epithelium. Since the parasite produces mild disease with no deaths, the stages in the small intestine have not been observed to date but must resemble closely related species studied in laboratory animals. The case for the pathogenicity of Isospora rests mainly on laboratory infections that have resulted in diarrhea lasting about three weeks, accompanied by the passage of the diagnostic form of the parasite in the stool. This is a thick-walled oocyst 25 to 35 $\mu \times$ 12 to 16 μ in size. Both ends are rounded, and one is contracted to form a neck. This stage is the zygote. Further development in two to four days results in the formation of two sporoblasts, which mature into oval sporocysts. Each sporocyst ultimately contains four sporozoites. These oocysts are very resistant to physical and chemical insult and will readily sporulate in potassium dichromate. Many instances of spurious parasitemia have been reported in man when oocysts of various animals and fish coccidia have passed unchanged through the bowel to appear in the stool and pose a diagnostic problem. The mild persistent diarrhea during the active phase of the infection is accompanied by nausea and abdominal discomfort. The infection is self-limiting; only rarely is blood noted in the stool.

Smitskamp, H., and Oey-Muller, E.: Geographical distribution and clinical significance of human coccidiosis. Trop. Geogr. Med., 18:133, 1966.

PRIMARY AMEBIC MENINGOENCEPHALITIS

Recently it has been realized that free-living amebae are capable of producing severe brain lesions in man. Now several species are implicated, but *Acanthamoeba castellani* was among the first to be recognised. An ameba 6 to 8 μ long, with foamy cytoplasm, a nucleus of $2\ \mu$, and a $1\ \mu$ darkly staining central karyosome, it is present as a commensal in human mouths and throats and was shown to be pathogenic for mice and monkeys before the first cases were reported in man. An initial report from Australia in 1965 described a rapidly progressive meningitis that proved fatal. There were lethargy and dulling of interest on the first day, followed by fever, headache, sore throat, and obstructed nostrils on the second day, vomiting and impaired consciousness on the third day, and deepening coma and death on the fourth day. At postmortem, destruction of the inferior surface of the frontal lobes and olfactory bulbs was seen, associated with a purulent exudate. Histologic examination revealed columns of amebae extending into the brain substance, especially via the perivascular spaces.

This clinical entity has now been reported from several parts of the United States (Florida, Virginia, Texas), Great Britain, and Czechoslovakia. It is usually found in children and young people, and is invariably fatal. It appears to be acquired by swimming, diving, or water skiing in lakes known to contain large numbers of free-living amebae. Pressure changes under water probably force the amebae through the cribriform plate. Naegleria, another genus of free-living amebae, has repeatedly been found in the cerebrospinal fluid of man. The CSF also shows an increased protein level, decreased sugar, neutrophils, and red cells, but is bacteriologically sterile. Most of the patients to date have died, usually because the diagnosis has been missed.

Emetine, arsenicals, sulfonamides, tetracyclines, and metronidazole have been used without much success. Amphotericin B therapy has resulted in recovery of a patient in whom Naegleria organisms were recovered from the CSF. In one recent fatal case *Naegleria gruberi* was recovered from the lungs, liver, spleen, and heart blood, as well as from the central nervous system.

Butt, C. G.: Primary amebic meningoencephalitis. New Eng. J. Med., 274:1473, 1966.
Culbertson, C. G.: Pathogenic acanthamoeba (Hartmannella). Amer. J. Clin. Path., 35:195, 1961.
Duma, R. J., Ferrell, M. W., Nelson, E. C., and Jones, M. M.: Primary amebic meningoencephalitis. New Eng. J. Med., 281:1316, 1969.
Fowler, M., and Carter, R. F.: Acute pyogenic meningitis probably due to Acanthamoeba sp.: A preliminary report. Brit. Med. J., 2:740, 1965.
Symmes, W. St.C.: Primary amoebic meningoencephalitis. Brit. Med. J., 2:449, 1969.

TOXOPLASMOSIS

Vernon Knight

Definition. Toxoplasmosis is a protozoan infection of man and animals. It occurs in man in a severe congenital form manifested by destructive lesions of the central nervous system, eyes, and viscera, or in acquired forms with (1) acute lym-

phadenopathy and illness resembling infectious mononucleosis; (2) dissemination and severe illness in which hepatitis, pneumonitis, myocarditis, or meningoencephalitis may predominate; and (3) ocular disease that occurs alone in a chronic form or, rarely, complicates acquired systemic disease.

Etiology. The disease is caused by *Toxoplasma gondii,* an intestinal coccidian (class Sporozoa) of the cat. The organism has evolved to multiply in extraintestinal sites in the cat and, presumably, by a similar mechanism to infect viscera, muscle, and nervous tissue in man and other susceptible animal species. Schizogonic stages and microgametocytes and macrogametocytes typical of coccidia are formed in the intestine of cats fed Toxoplasma. These stages are associated with the production of oocysts, which are infectious when shed in the feces. No other animal species has yet shown this characteristic of the infection. The trophozoite of Toxoplasma is crescent shaped and measures 3 by $6\ \mu$ in the fresh state. It multiplies intracellularly, and after a few days in animal tissues forms large cysts which contain 50 to 3000 organisms. Infection tends to continue in nervous tissue and in the eye; elsewhere it usually subsides gradually with the development of antibody.

Epidemiology. Congenital toxoplasmosis with neurologic disease occurs in the United States in about 1 per 1000 to 2000 live births. Congenital infection without detectable disease is considerably more frequent. In the general population, antibody surveys show the lowest rates of infection in the far north and the highest in the tropics. Children have the lowest rates, which increase progressively with age. There is considerable national and regional variation. In a serologic survey, U.S. military recruits from Appalachia had rates of infection greater than 25 per cent, although rates in those from Rocky Mountain states were less than 5 per cent. Negroes had higher rates than whites.

Lymphadenopathic toxoplasmosis, probably the most common clinical form of acquired infection, is being diagnosed with increasing frequency. Recently, an epidemic of this disease followed ingestion of raw hamburger, which presumably contained infected beef or was admixed with infected pork or mutton. Lymphadenopathic illness occurred in a pathologist following autopsy of a case of disseminated toxoplasmosis, and such illnesses are not infrequent among workers exposed to the parasite in the laboratory.

Severe visceral and central nervous system toxoplasmosis is increasingly recognized as a complication of malignant disease of the reticuloendothelial system and the immune suppressed state. Cytomegalovirus, herpesvirus, fungi, and gramnegative bacteria cause frequent additional complicating infections in these cases.

Natural infection has been found in a variety of mammals, including cats, swine, dogs, sheep, cattle, and rabbits. Several domestic birds were also infected. The cat alone, among 14 animal species tested, discharged infectious feces with oocysts; fecal infectivity persisted for at least four months in water or moist soil. In addition to congenital infection there is no doubt that ingestion of raw or undercooked meat from infected animals will infect man, but high rates of infection in some groups who do not eat meat suggests additional means of transmission. The persistent infectiousness of cat feces will require investigation in this regard.

Pathology. *Congenital Toxoplasmosis.* This is a disseminated infection, the most prominent lesions occurring in the brain and eyes. In the brain there are large areas of periventricular necrosis, and inflammatory reaction or disease may be confined to a single large spherical mass in which many parasites may be visualized. In some cases thrombotic vascular lesions may be observed that have preceded or followed the infectious lesions. Cerebral calcification occurs with healing and appears only in congenital infections. Congenital ocular disease is a severe form of that to be described under "acquired" ocular disease. Lesions in viscera and muscles resemble those to be described under "acquired" disease.

Acquired Form. The distinguishing feature of *acquired lymphadenopathic toxoplasmosis* is reticulum cell hyperplasia of affected lymph nodes, with formation of islands of eosinophilic cells. Parasites may occasionally be seen in the cytoplasm of macrophages. Muscle often shows areas of focal necrosis in which free and encysted parasites may occasionally be seen. Little other pathologic human tissue has been available for study, but chimpanzees sacrificed during acute lymphadenopathic illness had lesions in brain, myocardium, and other organs. It may be suspected that similar dissemination occurs in human cases.

The more severe *disseminated acquired disease* is characterized by lesions in many organs, especially lungs, liver, heart, skin, muscle, brain, and meninges. They consist of areas of focal or more extensive necrosis with inflammatory reaction. Parasites occasionally are visualized, but more often are demonstrable only by isolation techniques. Involvement is widespread in severe cases, and the clinical manifestations may indicate the viscera with the greatest damage. The organism has been isolated from the uterus of women with chronic asymptomatic toxoplasmosis and, rarely, from the products of conception of such patients.

Ocular Disease. Involvement of the eyes is usually bilateral in congenital cases and often unilateral in the acquired type. The definitive lesion consists of discrete patches of retinochoroiditis, often in the macular area. Within lesions the retina exhibits various degrees of coagulative necrosis. The retinal architecture is destroyed. Parasites may be seen free around karyolytic retinal cells. The adjacent choroid and sclera may show coagulative necrosis or thickening by proliferation of epithelioid cells, lymphocytes, and plasma cells. Margins of the lesions are sharp, and nonspecific inflammatory changes may be seen

elsewhere. On ophthalmoscopic examination the retinochoroiditis appears as yellowish to white, irregularly oval patches. The vitreous may be clouded with fibrinous and cellular exudate, and the anterior segment may show mononuclear cells adherent to the corneal endothelium and on the anterior surface of the iris or lens. The ciliary body may be inflamed.

Pathogenesis. *Congenital Toxoplasmosis.* This infection appears to result almost exclusively from primary maternal infections occurring during pregnancy. Whether or not primary maternal infections are symptomatic, up to 50 per cent of fetuses will be infected. Maternal infections with onset in the last trimester almost invariably lead to fetal infection. With chronic toxoplasmosis, as indicated by positive Toxoplasma serology before pregnancy, rare cases of congenital infection are thought possibly to occur. Toxoplasma organisms probably reach the placenta hematogenously where they cause widespread necrotic foci of infection. Organisms are more frequent on the fetal side of the placenta, perhaps indicating a lesser resistance of fetal tissues to infection. The fetus may become infected hematogenously or by ingestion of amniotic fluid. Other forms of fetal wastage, such as abortions and stillbirths, occur with unknown frequency, apparently with both primary and chronic maternal infections.

Acquired Form. After inoculation and regional lymph node invasion, the organisms appear to spread hematogenously to many organs and tissues where intracellular localization and proliferation occur. Parasites reproduce several times daily, with rupture of host cells and further dissemination. Parasitemia may persist for a week or two when first antibody response occurs, and at this time cysts may begin to form in various tissues. Late parasitemia in asymptomatic acquired infection has also been described. Proliferation of parasites in the brain and eye may continue, perhaps because of failure of antibody to penetrate to these areas, leading to persistence of infection or relapse. The severity depends upon the virulence of the strain, the dose, and the resistance of the host. Many observers believe that *relapsing retinochoroiditis* represents intermittent rupture of cysts with inflammatory reaction resulting from hypersensitivity of eye tissues to the organism.

Clinical Manifestations. Important signs of congenital toxoplasmosis are retinochoroiditis, microphthalmus, cerebral calcification, convulsions, hydrocephalus, and other neurologic abnormalities. In severe cases, they may be accompanied by evidence of visceral involvement, consisting of icterus and hepatomegaly, enlargement of spleen, pneumonitis, skin rash, and fever. Some patients with primarily neurologic disease are apparently well at birth, and the disease appears after a few weeks to many months. Congenital toxoplasmosis may be confused with congenital cytomegalovirus infection, which occurs with about the same frequency and is often manifested by brain destruction leading to microcephaly and mental retardation.

Acquired disease may vary from asymptomatic cases discovered in serologic surveys to the fulminating, often fatal, illness of patients with disseminated infection. The clinical picture of the latter is predominantly one of meningoencephalitis, hepatitis, myocarditis, or pneumonitis, often with maculopapular skin rash, high fever, and extreme prostration.

The more common acquired lymphadenopathic form usually presents with a picture of relatively painless cervical or axillary lymph node enlargement followed by malaise and muscle pain. Fever is low, intermittent or absent. The illness may persist for several weeks or a few months. There is usually a moderate anemia, normal leukocyte count, and some degree of lymphocytosis. Liver function may be slightly abnormal. The illness closely resembles infectious mononucleosis but lasts longer and is not associated with increase in heterophil antibody. A rather typical case of the lymphadenopathic form is illustrated in the accompanying figure. Acquired eye disease may be insidious in onset or marked by pain and progressive blindness.

Diagnosis. The indirect fluorescent antibody (IFA) test for toxoplasmosis is replacing the methylene blue dye test. Results with this test are almost identical with the dye test, and it is more rapid and convenient. The test is usually done in fourfold dilutions, and titers of 1:256 and greater are considered diagnostic of acute Toxoplasma infection. Titers of 1:1024 and greater are suggestive of active infection.* An indirect fluorescent antibody test using immunoglobulin M (IgM) has been developed to detect congenital infections. IgM antibody is formed by the fetus in utero, and

---

*In chronic infection, especially in retinochoroiditis, any measurable titer is significant, as there are no cross reactions with other parasites known in man.

the placenta is not normally permeable to this immunoglobulin; thus a positive test in a newborn should indicate congenital infection. This test has not been fully evaluated, but it is a promising procedure. An indirect hemagglutination test is available which gives results comparable to the IFA test. The complement-fixation (CF) test becomes positive late after onset of illness. Accordingly, a first positive or rising CF titer after the other kinds of tests have become positive may indicate primary infection.

As a result of wide prevalence of serum antibody in the general population, serologic tests may not always be adequate for diagnosis. Minimal evidence for diagnosis should consist of the demonstration of changing titers from negative to low, from low to high, or maintained high titers. In acquired ocular disease there may be little or no rise in serum antibody with onset of illness, and rises have been observed in the presence of eye disease from other causes. Diagnosis must, therefore, depend upon a careful evaluation of all the factors favoring toxoplasmosis and upon the exclusion of alternative causes of disease such as brucellosis, tuberculosis, cytomegalovirus infection, and syphilis. If the cause of retinochoroiditis remains uncertain after careful study, it is often decided to treat for toxoplasmosis.

The skin test is a delayed tuberculin type of reaction. It becomes positive not earlier than a few months after onset of infection. If the test is positive early in illness, acute Toxoplasma infection is excluded (see figure).

Isolation of the parasite by injection of suspected materials into mice has yielded positive results in acute cases with specimens of blood, cerebrospinal fluid, muscle, lymph nodes, and other materials, and in this situation is confirmatory of the diagnosis. Histologic studies give support to the diag-

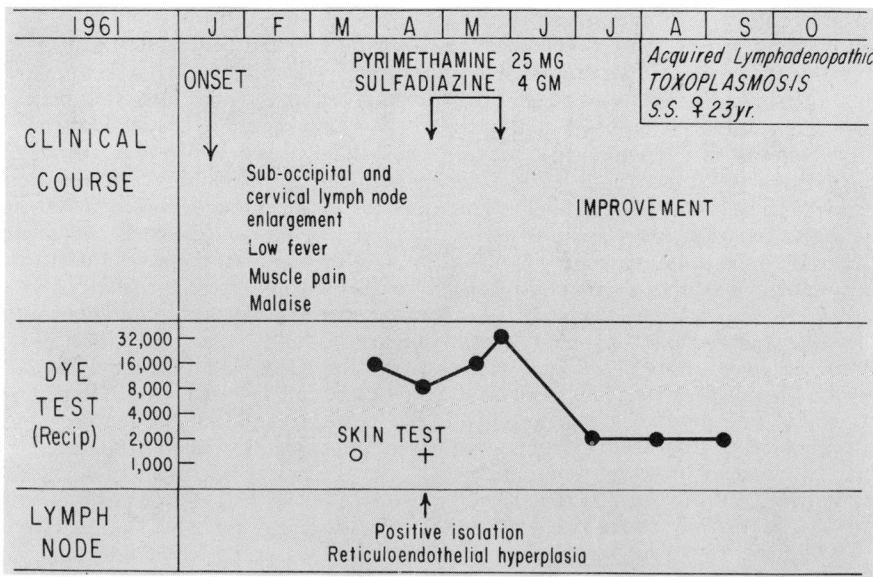

S.S., 23-year-old female. Acute acquired lymphadenopathic toxoplasmosis. Illness began in January 1961, and the dye test was found positive in high titer three months later. Skin test was negative at three months but was positive at four months. Lymph node biopsy revealed reticuloendothelial hyperplasia, and the parasite was isolated from material injected into mice. The patient improved after treatment, and the dye test titer dropped significantly. (Case of Dr. J. P. Utz.)

nosis because of reticuloendothelial cell proliferation and the occasional presence of parasites or
cysts. Biopsies have been positive many weeks
after subsidence of symptoms, however, and for
that reason great care must be taken in interpreting the significance of such results.

Treatment. All symptomatic forms of toxoplasmosis should be treated, but regimens should be
modified during pregnancy, as described below.
Pyrimethamine (Daraprim), 25 mg. twice daily
for one day followed by 25 mg. daily for one month,
and sulfadiazine, 4 grams daily for one month,
are currently recommended for the disease in
adults. Loading doses of 50 and 100 mg. of pyrimethamine have been used in treatment of ocular
disease. Triple sulfonamides (equal amounts of
sulfamethazine, sulfamerazine, and sulfadiazine) in a total daily dosage of 6 grams may be
substituted for the sulfadiazine. In infants and
children daily doses of pyrimethamine should be
given, 25 mg. per 30 kg. of body weight, up to
but not exceeding a total dose of 25 mg. per day.
Sulfadiazine may be given to infants in divided
doses of 100 mg. per kilogram of body weight per
day.

Failure of rapid response in cases of eye disease
has been considered evidence of hypersensitivity
to Toxoplasma, and steroids may be given during
the first course or during a second month in a daily
dose equivalent to 100 mg. of cortisone along with
continued antiparasitic treatment, as spread of
infection has been observed in mice treated with
cortisone alone.

Toxicity to pyrimethamine may occur, manifested by thrombocytopenia, agranulocytosis, or
megaloblastic anemia. If any of these occur, it
may be possible to reverse the effect by administration of folinic acid (leucovorin), 6 mg., and refrigerated baker's yeast, 5 to 10 grams, daily.
Infants should receive 1 mg. of folinic acid and 100
mg. of yeast daily. As folinic acid does not interfere
with the chemotherapeutic effect of pyrimethamine, folinic acid and brewer's yeast may be given
with the antiparasitic treatment, if desired. If
severe toxicity occurs, it is preferable to discontinue treatment and to await reversal of toxicity.
Re-treatment can often be tolerated without difficulty. The usual manifestations of toxicity to sulfonamides should be watched for and the use of
these agents stopped if toxic reactions occur.

*Treatment of primary infection in pregnant
women is probably indicated in an attempt to control fetal infection. However, it should be undertaken with an appreciation of the following limiting factors. Fetal damage from infection during
the first trimester is unlikely to be reversed by
treatment, and the potential teratogenic effects of*
pyrimethamine are greatest at this time. Sulfonamides are not contraindicated in pregnancy,
but they are probably less active against the infection than pyrimethamine. Tetracycline derivatives are active in experimental infections in
animals and may be used in pregnancy, 1.0 gram
daily orally for one month or longer. It should be
recalled, however, that the use of tetracycline
during tooth development in the last trimester or
given to infants during the early neonatal period
may result in yellow-brown discoloration of teeth.

There is much less evidence for response in congenital cases, but this might be anticipated from
the often appreciable destruction in the eye and
central nervous system before treatment is begun.
Nevertheless, early and vigorous treatment of
symptomatic and asymptomatic cases is advised.

The uncertain status of chronic maternal toxoplasmosis as a cause of abortions and stillbirths
provides an even less satisfactory basis for the use
of potentially toxic agents, especially pyrimethamine. Treatment of these patients has been carried out, however, in periods when the patients
were *not* pregnant with some evidence of a reduced frequency of fetal loss. Treatment should
consist of the regimen for adult systemic infection
plus folinic acid and brewer's yeast. A repeat
course may be given.

Prognosis. Acute acquired disease of moderate
severity, if untreated, may persist for many
months, but will usually subside without complications or unfavorable sequelae. In a limited experience, treatment appears to abbreviate this
course of events, although recurrent symptoms
and lymphadenopathy may require more than one
course of treatment. About half the cases of ocular toxoplasmosis respond to antiparasitic chemotherapy alone or supplemented with corticosteroids, but relapses or treatment failure may occur.
An extended trial of treatment is indicated in
those circumstances. Severe disseminated cases
appear to benefit from treatment if it is started
soon enough. The over-all mortality rate of congenital disease untreated is about 12 per cent,
although it is much higher in those patients with
obvious disseminated infection at birth.

Feldman, H. A.: Toxoplasmosis. New Eng. J. Med., 279:1370,
    1968.
Feldman, H. A.: Toxoplasmosis (concluded). New Eng. J. Med.,
    279:1431, 1968.
Frenkel, J. K.: Toxoplasmosis. In Benirschke, K. (ed.): Compara-
    tive Aspects of Reproductive Failure. New York, Springer-
    Verlag, Inc., 1966, pp. 296–321.
Frenkel, J. K., Dubey, J. P., and Miller, N. L.: *Toxoplasma gondii*
    in cats: Fecal stages identified as coccidian oocysts. Science,
    167:893, 1970.
Hutchison, W. M., Dunachie, J. F., Sim, J. Chr., and Work, K.
    Coccidian-like nature of *Toxoplasma gondii*. Brit. Med. J.,
    1:142, 1970.

Helminthic Diseases

GENERAL CONSIDERATIONS

Philip D. Marsden

Compared to protozoans, helminths are very large organisms with a complex cellular structure. As they feed on host tissue, their metabolism results in various protein secretions and excretions; and because they themselves largely consist of complex protein, it is not surprising that invasion of the body by worms is frequently associated with an eosinophilic response. Thus, in the invasive stage of schistosomes, hookworm, ascaris, and similar parasites, an eosinophilia is usual. Yet when these worms have matured and settled at their site of election, eosinophilia often is not found. It might be argued in the case of intestinal nematodes that this is because they are in the gut and in a strict sense outside the body, but because the phenomenon also occurs with schistosomiasis and tissue filariae this is too facile an explanation. At the present time the mechanisms and course of eosinophilia produced in a host in response to a foreign protein are not clearly understood.

With regard to immunology, understandably, complex helminths produce complex crude antigens of low specificity. At the moment, with a few exceptions, group-specific reactions with antigens for schistosomes, hermaphroditic flukes, nematodes, and cestodes are all that are available using tests such as complement-fixation or indirect hemagglutination. Skin tests on the whole are much less satisfactory than those based on serology. Many of these helminths are recognized by the presence of characteristic progeny in the form of either eggs in the stools, sputum, or urine, or larvae in the tissues.

The concept of the over-all population or load of worms is important in human disease, as *the parasitic load* is one of the factors determining the extent of pathology (another would be the host response). Today many helminthic infections can be quantitated, and these methods will be mentioned under diagnosis. Another important aspect of worm infections is their relatively long life. Many flukes live for decades after the infection has been acquired, and similarly many filarial species are long lived. This illustrates the importance of obtaining a very detailed history of the patient's movements around the world because a visit to an endemic area 20 years ago may be connected with a current clinical problem.

TABLE 1. PREVALENCE OF COMMON HELMINTH INFECTIONS IN MAN*

Parasite	Source of Infection	Approximate Locality	Estimated Incidence in U.S. and Canada	Estimated World Incidence
Trematodes (flukes):				
Schistosoma japonicum	Water through skin	Far East	–	46,000,000
Schistosoma haematobium	Water through skin	Africa, Middle East	–	39,200,000
Schistosoma mansoni	Water through skin	Africa, South America, Caribbean	–	29,200,000
Clonorchis sinensis	Fish	Far East	In Chinese immigrants	19,000,000
Opisthorcis felineus	Fish	Far East	–	1,100,000
Paragonimus westermani	Crabs, crayfish	Africa, South America	–	3,200,000
Fasciolopsis buski	Water nuts	Far East	–	10,000,000
Cestodes (tapeworms):				
Diphyllobothrium latum	Fish	Around Arctic Circle, N. Europe, Russia, America	†	10,400,000
Taenia saginata	Beef	Cosmopolitan	10,000	38,900,000
Taenia solium	Pork	Cosmopolitan	†	2,500,000
Echinococcus granulosus	Dog feces	Cosmopolitan	†	†
Nematodes (roundworms):				
Intestinal nematodes				
Strongyloides stercoralis	Human feces	Cosmopolitan	400,000	34,900,000
Hookworm	Human feces	Cosmopolitan	1,800,000	456,800,000
Ascaris lumbricoides	Human feces	Cosmopolitan	3,000,000	644,400,000
Trichuris trichuria	Human feces	Cosmopolitan	400,000	355,100,000
Enterobius vermicularis	Human feces	Cosmopolitan	18,000,000	208,800,000
Tissue Nematodes				
Trichinella spiralis	Pork	Cosmopolitan	21,100,000	27,800,000
Wuchereria bancrofti and Brugia malayi	Mosquitoes	Africa, South America, South Asia	–	189,000,000
Loa loa	Chrysops	Equatorial Africa	–	13,000,000
Acanthocheilonema perstans	Culicoides	Africa, South America	–	27,000,000
Mansonella ozzardi	Culicoides	South America	–	7,000,000
Onchocerca volvulus	Simulium	Equatorial Africa, Central America	–	19,800,000
Dracunculus medinensis	Cyclops	Middle East, India, Africa	–	48,300,000

*Based on data calculated by N. R. Stoll (J. Parasit., 33:1, 1947). Since the World population has increased by more than 50 per cent, all the figures given can be regarded as extremely conservative. For instance, it is said that 180 million people in the world are infected with one of the three species of schistosome that infect humans.

†Represents less than 100,000 infections.

It must be remembered that there are a large number of helminths that rarely infect man, and many cannot be mentioned in this book. For information on these a standard textbook on parasitology (see references in general introduction) should be consulted. An important topical point is that we are now beginning to realize that for every worm adapted to man there are many others which gain access to man's tissues but fail to mature because they are natural parasites of other mammals or birds. These may cause very puzzling clinical problems. An increasing proportion of unexplained eosinophilia encountered in clinical practice is being explained on a basis of invasion of the body by a worm that will not mature in man because he is not the definitive host.

By a simple classification, worms may be separated into trematodes or flukes, cestodes or tapeworms, and nematodes or roundworms. A check list adapted from H. W. Brown's table in the previous edition is given here in Table 1, together with information on the source of infection and the main areas of occurrence in the world. The most important helminthic infections in terms of disease in man and incidence are schistosomiasis, hookworm, and filariasis.

THE CESTODES
(Tapeworms)
Philip D. Marsden

GENERAL CONSIDERATIONS

The cestodes are endoparasitic flatworms, the hermaphroditic adults of which are flat and ribbon-like and inhabit the intestinal tract of vertebrates. The larval forms may require more than one intermediate host and develop in the tissues of vertebrates, and in some instances invertebrates. Most adult tapeworms consist of a scolex or head equipped for attachment with suckers, hooks, or grooves and a strobila or tapelike chain of progressively developing segments or proglottides. The neck is the site of segment generation, and mature segments are complete hermaphroditic units with both sets of sex organs. There is no digestive system, food being absorbed directly through the cuticle. There are longitudinal primitive excretory systems and a nervous system. In gravid segments the uterus is loaded with eggs, and these pass out of the bowel either in the segment or free in the stool. The delicate outer membrane of the eggs is often lost, but the thick-walled inner membrane contains a form infective for the intermediate host.

As might be expected, starving the host reduces the number of tapeworms, curtailing their growth and ova production. Overpopulation with tapeworms in the host results in stunting of the individuals. Although obviously dependent on what the host eats for its food supply, the beef tapeworm, for instance, appears to do little harm. Taenia species and the fish tapeworm may have a life of 25 to 30 years if left alone.

As Brown has pointed out, there are two types of tapeworm infection in man: those species in which man acts as the definitive host and harbors the adult in his bowel, and those for which he is the intermediate host, having an infective form in the tissues. In *Taenia solium* infections both situations occur. We will deal with the common human tapeworm of the 30 or more species that have been found in man according to the classification given in Table 2. There are thus three genera to be considered, and they will be taken up in the order given in the table.

DIPHYLLOBOTHRIUM LATUM
(The Fish Tapeworm)

Infection with the fish tapeworm is most common in temperate areas such as Scandinavia and around the Baltic Sea. It also occurs in the northern United States, Canada, and Alaska. Central Europe is an endemic focus. In the tropics relatively few reports have appeared from the Philippines, Madagascar, Botswana, Uganda, and Chile. Recently a new human parasite, *Diphyllobothrium pacificum*, has been described from Peru. The adult is the largest tapeworm of man, reaching 10 meters and having 4000 segments. (The spatulate head has two deep sucking grooves for attachment to the wall of the ileum.) The gravid segment disintegrates, and operculated ova are passed in the feces.

From the egg a ciliated embryo is eaten by a freshwater flea (Cyclops or Diaptomus species) in which it develops to a *procercoid*. When the infected flea is swallowed by freshwater fish, e.g., salmon, pike, further development takes place in the muscles of the fish to the *plerocercoid,* the form infective to man. The plerocercoid on being liberated into the small intestine grows to an adult in three to six weeks. Although the adult worm causes no pathologic lesion, there is a very important complication to this infection, namely a megaloblastic anemia. This appears to be due to the avidity of the worm for vitamin B_{12}, as 44 per cent of a single dose of Co^{60} labeled vitamin B_{12}

TABLE 2. COMMON IMPORTANT TAPEWORMS

Official Name	Intermediate Host(s)	Stage in Man
Diphyllobothrium latum	Water fleas, freshwater fish	Adult worm
Taenia saginata	Cattle (beef)	Adult worm
Taenia solium	Pigs (pork)	Adult worm and larval stage
Echinococcus granulosus	Man, sheep, cattle	Larval stage
Echinococcus multilocularis	Man, sheep, cattle	Larval stage

was absorbed by the worm, the radioactivity being concentrated in the proximal growing part. Also the nearer the worm is to the jejunum, the greater the chance of developing megaloblastic anemia. It is not clear why the worm needs so much vitamin B$_{12}$. The worm also appears to require folic acid in the same way. The full range of neurologic symptoms of subacute combined degeneration of the cord may appear, particularly in severe cases of multiple parasitism. Peripheral neuritis appears very early in the parasitism, and recently optic atrophy has been reported.

The *diagnosis* is made by direct examination of the stools, because the eggs are present in very large numbers. Yellowish-brown and operculated, they have to be distinguished from fluke eggs such as Paragonimus, but the large number in the stool favors the diagnosis of fish tapeworm even to the uninitiated. The operculum is actually less conspicuous in Diphyllobothrium, and there is a small knob at the anopercular end (mean size 70 by 45 μ). Because the treatment for the tapeworms of this group and of the Taenia genus is the same, they are considered together later.

Prophylaxis is readily accomplished by thoroughly cooking fish before consumption. Freezing of fish for 48 hours at −10° C. will also prevent infection. The infection is not uncommon in New York among Jewish housewives who make their own gefilte fish and sample it in the process.

SPARGANOSIS

This condition requires mention here, because it is the name of an infection caused by the migrating larvae or spargana of several species of tapeworm related to *D. latum* but requiring final hosts other than man. It presents as a migrating subcutaneous painful swelling suggesting a cellulitis. Marked eosinophilia is usually present. The eye may be involved with orbital swelling or even actual penetration of the globe. In China this results from applying infected frogs on poultices to the eye. Biopsy reveals inflammatory tissue reactions and an immature cestode, many of which are quite impossible to identify. *Diphyllobothrium mansonoides (Spirometra mansonoides)* is a common offender. So-called *Sparganum proliferum* is unknown in the adult stage, but may distribute thousands of larvae throughout the body, and in contrast to other forms carries a poorer prognosis. This type of infection is rare, but occurs in many tropical countries, diagnosis being made by finding the plerocercoid larvae in tissues.

TAENIA SAGINATA
(The Beef Tapeworm)

The beef tapeworm has a cosmopolitan distribution, being particularly common in the Middle East, Kenya, and Ethiopia. In the last-named country people habitually take a monthly purge of herbs to get rid of an impressive length of worm, but rarely get rid of the head. Beef tapeworm is also common in parts of South America, Mexico,

and Russia. In all these countries it is acquired by eating undercooked or raw beef—a delicacy in Ethiopia. In one series in the United Kingdom, fashion models seemed commonly infected because rare steaks were fashionable at the time. In spite of the harmless nature of the parasitism, a fastidious fashion model with a beef tapeworm can be a real problem in medical management. It is doubtful whether *T. saginata* causes any symptoms, although epigastric pain, appetite disturbances, and general malaise have been ascribed to the presence of the worm. It is possible that multiple worms may be associated with symptoms. Very rarely the worm may block the pancreatic or cystic duct or appendix, producing acute inflammation (16 such cases have been reported). The 5- to 10-meter adult worm has four suckers on the head to attach it to the wall of the small intestine. The gravid segments are usually recognized in the stool, but, being muscular, they can traverse the anal sphincter and appear in the underclothing. They contain more than 12 uterine branches, which distinguish them from *T. solium*. Characteristic Taenia eggs may be found in the stool or on the anal margin. When the eggs are swallowed by cattle, llamas, or buffaloes, the hatched embryos gain the skeletal muscles by the blood stream after bowel penetration and develop into the encysted bladder-like larval forms or cysticerci which are infective for man.

Man is the only definitive host in which the adult worm can develop. The larval cysticercus form has been reported only three times in man, so host specificity seems to be strict. Treatment will be discussed later; prevention consists in not ingesting beef containing cysticerci.

TAENIA SOLIUM
(The Pork Tapeworm Causing Human Cysticercosis Due to Cysticercus Cellulosae)

In contrast to *T. saginata,* both larval and adult forms of this species can develop in man. Again this worm is cosmopolitan in distribution although relatively rare in North America and western Europe; cysticercosis is the most common identifiable cause of epilepsy in the Durban African population and is a serious disease because of the frequency of brain involvement. Man, again the only definitive host of importance, acquires the infection by eating undercooked measly pork containing cysticerci. Pigs and wild boars are the usual intermediate hosts.

The adult worm usually causes no symptoms in the small intestine. For attachment the head has four suckers and two rows of hooklets on a prominent rostellum. It is smaller than *T. saginata* (2 to 4 meters). Its segments are more delicate than *T. saginata* and there are usually less than twelve branches to the uterus in the gravid segment. The eggs are indistinguishable from *T. saginata,* both being approximately 35 μ, thick-walled, brown, and containing an embryonic oncosphere with six hooklets. In *T. solium* infection, however, these eggs are infective to man, but must pass through the stomach and undergo tryptic digestion before hatching occurs. The usual way in which man is infected with eggs is by external autoinfection, transferring eggs from the anus to the mouth or to food fecally contaminated by a carrier of the worm. Internal autoinfection by regurgitating segments of the worm into the stomach is a theoretic possibility, but has not been recorded.

Once free from the egg in the intestine, the oncosphere penetrates the intestinal wall with its hooklets and, as in the pig, settles in the body tissues. The invaded organs in order of frequency are subcutaneous tissue, brain, eye, muscles, heart, liver, lung, and peritoneum. The cysticercus matures in four months to an ellipsoidal translucent cyst, 10 to 20 by 5 to 10 mm., with an opaque invaginated scolex with suckers and hooks. It is gradually surrounded by a thick fibrous capsule and may live for years. Death is frequently associated with calcification.

The invasive phase may be associated with fever, headache, muscle pains, and high eosinophilia. Usually years after this stage more serious symptoms occur owing to brain involvement, with the onset of epilepsy, personality changes, signs of raised intercranial pressure, or long tract signs. In every patient with epilepsy of late onset coming from an endemic area this possibility should be excluded by (1) taking a detailed history, especially in relation to a past history of tapeworm infection; the stool should be examined for Taenia eggs and segments, because rarely the worm may still be in situ; (2) having a full physical examination, especially for subcutaneous nodules containing cysticerci; biopsy will establish the diagnosis; (3) taking roentgenograms of the skull, buttocks, and thighs for calcified cysticerci which have a characteristic size and shape; and (4) performing either a complement-fixation test or an indirect hemagglutination test, using antigen from lyophilized pig cysticerci.

More rarely the globe of the eye is involved, as well as the heart and skeletal muscle. A cysticercus may be visible on the tongue. Sometimes the cysticerci become secondarily infected. In the brain, inflammation around them may produce internal hydrocephalus. Although the adult worm can be eradicated easily, there is no medical treatment for *Cysticercus cellulosae* save palliative anticonvulsants. Rarely surgical intervention may be necessary in cases of raised intracranial pressure. Again prophylaxis rests on avoiding opportunities of eating infected meat and the inspection and thorough cooking of pork.

TREATMENT OF INFECTIONS WITH ADULTS OF THE FISH, BEEF, AND PORK TAPEWORM

Quinacrine hydrochloride (Atabrine, Mepacrine) is an effective drug for treatment of all three species of adult worm. The rationale is that a single comparatively large dose of this drug causes the worm to release its hold and it can then be voided. The most successful technique for adults is as follows: Admit the patient to hospital and give only fluids for 36 to 48 hours. Then pass a tube into the duodenum and, with the patient resting quietly, inject 1 gram of quinacrine hydrochloride down the tube in 40 ml. of water, using a 20-ml. syringe. Half an hour later a saline purge is injected down the tube, and all feces saved for the next 24 hours. Long lengths of the worm stained yellow with the drug are passed, and the head should be identified. If the head is not dislodged, the worm will regenerate in two to three months, and segments will reappear in the stools. The duodenal tube reduces the chances of vomiting the drug which is a particular hazard with *T. solium* infections. (Obviously, in many endemic areas it will not be possible to get every patient into hospital.) If the head of the worm is found, one can usually reassure the patient that the worm is eliminated unless it is a rare case of multiple infection.

Niclosamide (hydroxychlorobenzamide) is a relatively new drug that may well replace Atabrine, as it is said to be safe, effective, and easy to administer. When the patient wakes in the morning, two tablets of 0.5 gram each are chewed thoroughly and swallowed with a little water. The same procedure is repeated one hour later. No fasting or purgation is necessary, and children receive a proportionately smaller dose. The worm disintegrates so that unfortunately the head cannot be sought as proof of cure. For this reason follow-up at six months is desirable. Although no report has appeared, some authorities believe that this drug should not be used in *T. solium* infection because worm disintegration may be followed by cysticercosis. It must be remembered that feces from patients harboring *T. solium* are an infectious risk. The patient should scrub his hands after defecation and pass his feces into disinfectant.

ECHINOCOCCOSIS
(Hydatid Disease)

There are two species of the genus Echinococcus which infect man, *Echinococcus granulosus* and *Echinococcus multilocularis*. They are the most important cestodes producing serious disease in man because of the size and location of their larval form, the hydatid cyst. Man is only one of a number of intermediate hosts, other important ones being sheep, cattle, and deer. The definitive hosts for these very small adult tapeworms are canines such as dogs, wolves, jackals, and foxes.

Hydatid disease is cosmopolitan because infected stock have been distributed all over the world for breeding purposes. The incidence of human infection is low in many countries, but where the triad of man, dog, and sheep or cattle is common, hydatid disease is relatively frequent. Examples are countries such as Australia, Argentina, Chile, Kenya, New Zealand, and Wales. It has been reported from 15 states in the United

States. Canada and Alaska seem to enjoy a distinct variant, *E. granulosus var. canadensis.*

Human infection follows ingestion of the eggs excreted by infected dogs. The adult tapeworm measures only 2.5 to 9.2 mm. and has a head with hooklets and suckers, a growing neck, and only three segments: immature, sexually mature, and gravid. Heavy infections of dogs are common, but the worm lives for only about six months in the upper jejunum. The eggs produced are indistinguishable from Taenia eggs and like them produce an oncosphere with six hooklets. On reaching the intestine of the intermediate host such as man, they pass through the intestinal wall and circulate in the blood and can develop in any body tissue. It may take 20 to 30 years before the slowly growing hydatid cyst causes symptoms. Often they remain small (less than 10 cm.), but they may grow as large as the human head. The host parasite factors determining growth are not clearly understood, but growth is variable from 0.25 to 1 cm. a year. The structure of a developed hydatid cyst is complex. Briefly it really consists of a whole colony of infective larval forms, for inside the laminated, defined cyst wall is a germinal layer that is constantly budding off new infective individuals. The cyst is filled with fluid, and second and third generation cysts containing thousands of infective forms or scolices are suspended in this fluid. There is little wonder that when a dog eats an infected sheep's liver he acquires many adult Echinococcus organisms.

When the infective embryo or oncosphere passes into the portal circulation of man, it is first held up in the liver where more than half of those that survive develop (59 per cent). Many are destroyed by phagocytic cells. The next tissue filter is the lungs, where 27 per cent lodge. Finally, 15 per cent escape into the general circulation to involve the abdominal cavity, muscle, kidney, spleen, bone, heart, and brain.

ECHINOCOCCUS GRANULOSUS

Echinococcus granulosus is the common species; there are several types of cysts, as follows: (1) The classic unilocular cyst is usually fertile and surrounded by a false capsule of host tissue fibrosis. Rupture of such a cyst will cause dissemination of daughter cysts with secondary hydatids. (2) Alveolar hydatids have a reticulated irregular outline and resemble those of *E. multilocularis,* but there is no metastatic growth. Owing to irregular growth of the germinal membrane, this cyst usually occurs in the liver and is difficult to remove. It is often sterile, and its contents degenerate. (3) Osseous hydatid. The nature of bone does not permit a host or parasite capsule to form. Daughter cysts form in the bone medulla, erode the cortex, and produce a pathologic fracture. If they escape from the bone, the cysts grow in their normal spherical shape with the usual capsules in the extraosseous tissues.

Clinically, the hydatid cysts may produce signs of a space-occupying lesion in relation to the organ in which it occurs. In the liver abdominal pain and vomiting may be presenting symptoms, a mass being visible or palpable. Usually the cysts are too tense to show fluctuation. In the lung they are usually detected on routine chest films as spherical, well-defined shadows. They are more common in the right lung, and rarely are associated with cough and hemoptysis. Those of the brain are indistinguishable from a cerebral tumor. In the kidney, hematuria or loin pain may be the first sign, whereas hydatid cyst of bone may present as a pathologic fracture.

The *complications* of hydatid disease are important. The most serious is rupture and dissemination of further infective larvae. Patients with suspected hydatid disease should always be gently palpated—a leaking cyst may present as anaphylactic shock with an urticarial rash and high eosinophilia. The cyst may become secondarily infected with bacteria and present similarly to a liver or lung abscess.

A suggestive tumor in a patient from an endemic area demands the following investigations. An eosinophilia may be present. Plain roentgenograms may show calcification in the cyst wall, although this does not mean that the cyst is not infective. An isotope scan of the liver reveals the extent of the tumor, but gives no clue as to its nature. In the chest film the round, uniformly dense shadow is suggestive. A fluid level with air in the cyst means communication with a bronchus and possibly secondary infection. A skin test using cyst fluid is positive in the majority of patients, but it has been shown that the reaction depends on the concentration (nitrogen content) of protein in the fluid injected. Until there is universal acceptance of a standard skin test antigen, a negative result is meaningless. Hydatid complement-fixation tests, hemagglutination tests, and bentonite flocculation tests are all practicable and are helpful. Rarely cyst fragments, such as scolices, may be found in the sputum or urine. It must be recalled that one in five patients have multiple cysts, so that if a cyst is located in one site, especially if it is not the liver, there may be others. A liver scan should be done in every patient with an extrahepatic cyst. Diagnostic aspiration is never indicated because of the risk of rupture. In the liver and lung, carcinoma and abscess are often difficult differential diagnoses.

It should be emphasized that many hydatid cysts never get very large (5 to 10 cm.) and never cause symptoms. There is no medical treatment. Surgery is only indicated in cysts that are enlarging, producing pressure symptoms, or developing complications. The physician should consult a surgeon who has experience with this problem. If possible the cyst should be removed entirely. To prevent spillage and dissemination, the cyst is usually aspirated at operation after packing off the site; 20 ml. of fluid is withdrawn, and an equal quantity of 2 per cent formalin, 1 per cent iodine or 30 per cent sodium chloride is introduced to kill the scolices. Injection of a 1 per cent aqueous solution of iodine in a volume amounting to one twentieth of the whole cyst volume is lethal to scolices within one minute. It is said to produce fewer complications than formalin. Anaphylactic reactions owing to spillage during operation may require corticosteroids.

E. granulosus var. canadensis is common in Alaska and Canada where it has a sylvatic cycle in deer and wolves. It produces smaller and more delicate cysts in man than the classic E. granulosus; the latter are more frequent in the lung, usually asymptomatic, and almost never cause serious complications so that the distinction is important.

ECHINOCOCCUS MULTILOCULARIS

The medical importance of distinguishing between these two species is that Echinococcus multilocularis does not produce large single cysts with endogenous growth and well-defined fibrous tissue encapsulation but rather an aggregate of innumerable small cysts that multiply by exogenous budding to produce the so-called alveolar or malignant hydatid. More than 90 per cent occur in liver, which is progressively honeycombed by a multitude of small cysts. They may become confluent and even metastasize like a malignancy. Intrahepatic or portal hypertension develops with splenomegaly, and biliary obstruction may produce icterus. The hepatic infection may be difficult to differentiate from a malignancy. This species of cestode occurs in south central Europe, Russia, and Alaska. Rarely cases have occurred in Australasia, England, and Argentina.

Prevention of infection with both these species entails elimination of the infection from dogs by worming with arecoline hydrobromide regularly and preventing their eating infected offal. Contamination of the hands, food, and drink with dog feces should be avoided.

OTHER TAPEWORMS

Three other species of adult tapeworms that parasitize the human intestine are usually mentioned, but in comparison with those discussed above they are of little importance in human disease. Dwarf tapeworm infection (Hymenolepis nana) is usually asymptomatic and requires no intermediate host, direct infection from man to man being possible. The rat tapeworm Hymenolepis diminuta is acquired by swallowing infected insects carrying the Taenia eggs from rats. Dipylidium caninum is the common tapeworm of cats and dogs throughout the world, and is transmitted by their fleas to children handling their pets. The gravid proglottids are shaped like melon seeds and may be seen in the stool. For all three of these parasites Niclosamide is usually used, although recently paromomycin has given high cure rates in most of the human intestinal cestodes.

More sinister but fortunately very rare is another tapeworm of the dog, Multiceps multiceps, which in 25 cases has infected man in the larval stage. The larva called Coenorus cerebralis has

occurred in the brain in 20 cases and in the eye in five. In structure it is not unlike a small hydatid. These larvae are commonly found in the brain of sheep, producing a fatal disease known as "gid," which is characterized by somnolence, loss of weight, visual disturbance, and ataxia.

Bjorkenheim, G.: Neurological changes in pernicious tapeworm anaemia. Acta Med. Scand., 140 (Supplement):260, 1961.

Dew, H. R.: Hydatid Disease. Sydney, Australian Publishing Co., Ltd., 1928.

Dixon, H. B. F., and Hargreaves, W. H.: Cysticercosis (T. solium). Quart J. Med., 13:107, 1944.

Echinococcosis. Bull. WHO, 39, No. 1, 1968.

Jalayer, T., and Askavi, I.: A study of the effect of aqueous iodine on hydatid cysts in vitro and in vivo. Ann. Trop. Med. Parasit., 60:169, 1966.

Katz, A. M., and Pan, C.: Echinococcus disease in the United States. Amer. J. Med., 25:759, 1958.

Keeling, J. E. D.: The chemotherapy of cestode infections. In Goldin, A., Hawking, F., and Schnitzer, R. J. (eds.) Advances in Chemotherapy. London and New York, Academic Press, Inc., 1968, Vol. 3, pp. 109–152.

Powell, S. J., Procter, E. M., Wilmot, A. J., and McLeod, I. N.: Cysticercosis and epilepsy in Africans: A clinical and serological study. Ann. Trop. Med. Parasit., 60:152, 1966.

Swartzwelder, J. C., Beaver, P. C., and Hood, M. W.: Sparganosis in the southern United States. Amer. J. Trop. Med., 13:43, 1964.

Vik, R.: The genus Diphyllobothrium. Exp. Parasit., 15:361, 1964.

Webbe, G.: The hatching and activation of Taeniid ova in relation to the development of cysticercosis in man. Z. Tropenmed. Parasit., 18:354, 1967.

Wilson, J. F., Diddams, A. C., and Rausch, R. L.: Cystic hydatid disease in Alaska: A review of 101 cases of Echinococcus granulosus infection. Amer. Rev. Resp. Dis., 98:1, 1967.

DISEASES CAUSED BY TREMATODES
(Flukes)

SCHISTOSOMIASIS
(Bilharziasis)

Kenneth S. Warren

DEFINITION

Schistosomiasis, a chronic infection of 180,000,-000 people in Asia, Africa, the Caribbean, and South America, is caused by three different worm species, Schistosoma mansoni, S. japonicum, and S. haematobium. Infection occurs during immersion in fresh water containing schistosome cercariae. These larval forms penetrate the skin and migrate via the lungs and liver to the final habitat of the half-inch-long adult worms: the veins of the intestines and urinary bladder. The worms themselves do not multiply within man, but produce large numbers of eggs, many of which remain in the body, damaging primarily the intestines, liver, and urinary tract. Eggs that are excreted in the urine and feces and that reach fresh water hatch into ciliated miracidia. These organisms penetrate into snails, multiply, and develop into cercariae, the infective form for man.

ETIOLOGY

Although the cercariae of many different schistosome species penetrate human skin, there are three major species that complete their life cycles in man and are thus capable of causing systemic disease: *Schistosoma mansoni, japonicum,* and *haematobium.* The life cycles of these schistosomes are essentially similar, all being digenetic trematodes alternating a sexual phase of reproduction in man (definitive host) with an asexual reproductive phase in snails (intermediate host). Nevertheless, at each phase of the life cycle there are differences among the species that play crucial roles in the epidemiology, pathogenesis, and clinical picture of the disease.

The adult worms or schistosomes are members of the class Trematoda of the phylum Platyhelminthes or flatworms. The male worms (10 to 20 × 0.5 to 1 mm.) have cleft bodies within which the longer and thinner females reside, *S. japonicum* being the largest of the three species. The worms may live in man for as long as 30 years, but epidemiologic evidence suggests that their mean life span is three to five years. The habitats of the adult *S. mansoni, japonicum,* and *haematobium* worms are, respectively, the veins of the large intestine, small intestine, and urinary bladder.

The worms absorb metabolites through both their intestines and integument. Their energy processes depend on anaerobic catabolism of carbohydrates; the schistosomes utilize an amount of glucose equivalent to one fifth of their dry body weight each hour and convert 80 per cent of it to lactic acid. In addition, the ingestion of red blood cells appears to be of nutritional significance as the worms contain a proteolytic enzyme that breaks down globin; the remaining insoluble hematin-like pigment is regurgitated, because the schistosome intestine terminates blindly. The rapid metabolic rate of these worms may in part be related to their continual output of large numbers of eggs, estimated at 1400 to 3000 per day for *S. japonicum* and one tenth that number for *S. mansoni.* The eggs of the last-named species are released singly, whereas those of the other two species are deposited in clutches of as many as ten. They embryonate over a period of six days and increase in size, reaching a mean of 60 × 140 μ for *S. mansoni* and *S. haematobium* and 35 × 97 μ for *S. japonicum.* The shape of the eggs is distinctive, *S. mansoni* being ellipsoidal and having a lateral spine; *S. haematobium,* also ellipsoidal but with a terminal spine; and *S. japonicum,* spheroidal with a tiny knob. The eggs remain viable for approximately 21 days after laying, during which time they must pass out of the body if their life cycle is to be completed. Passage from the blood vessels through the tissues and into the lumen of the excretory organs is apparently facilitated by enzymatic secretions of the eggs plus muscular movements of the gut or bladder. A large proportion of the eggs, however, either remain in the intestinal and vesical tissues or break free in the blood stream and are carried into the liver and lungs.

The eggs that pass out of the body in feces or urine and reach fresh water hatch rapidly into free-swimming ciliated miracidia. The miracidia of *S. mansoni* are negatively geotropic and positively phototropic, although those of *S. haematobium* appear to be the opposite. Their average life span is about six hours. If during this time a snail is encountered, the organisms may penetrate it, and if it is of the genus Biomphalaria for *S. mansoni,* Bulinus for *S. haematobium,* or Oncomelania for *S. japonicum,* the organism can complete its life cycle. The former two snail genera are aquatic, the latter amphibious. The miracidium remains close to the site of penetration, developing into a mother sporocyst. After about ten days daughter sporocysts begin to migrate into the digestive gland of the snail, and at about five weeks from the inception of the process cercariae produced from the daughter sporocysts begin to be shed by the snail. Maximal stimulus for shedding of *S. mansoni* and *haematobium* cercariae is provided by light, but darkness seems to favor the output of *S. japonicum* cercariae. The average daily output of *S. mansoni* and *S. haematobium* cercariae is about 700, but that of *S. japonicum* cercariae is only about two. These organisms may live for two to three days under ideal conditions, but their infectivity begins to decrease by 24 hours. The fork-tailed schistosome cercariae are about 125 to 200 μ in length by 50 to 75 μ in width. *S. mansoni* and *haematobium* cercariae alternate periods of rest during which they sink slowly with periods of movement in which they rise toward the surface of the water. In contrast, *S. japonicum* cercariae attach themselves to the surface film where they tend to remain at rest. When cercariae encounter mammalian skin, they attach themselves with suckers, and by mechanical means, aided by enzymatic secretions, the head penetrates, leaving the tail behind. This process occurs during immersion in water or while the skin remains moist (drying kills the organism), and takes four to ten minutes for *S. mansoni,* but only a few seconds to three minutes for *S. japonicum.*

As the worms do not multiply in the mammalian host, each cercaria that penetrates the skin can develop into only one worm. Many cercariae die in the skin, however, and in the best of experimental hosts only about 60 per cent of the *S. mansoni* organisms reach maturity. Within a few hours to days the schistosomula (the cercariae are completely changed both biochemically and physiologically immediately following penetration) migrate to the lungs by either the blood stream or lymphatics. After a few days in the pulmonary vessels the schistosomula migrate to the liver, either directly through the lungs and diaphragm or by the blood stream. This phase takes ten to twelve days for *S. mansoni,* a somewhat shorter period for *S. japonicum,* and a longer one for *S. haematobium.* Once in the intrahepatic portal venules the worms rapidly reach maturity, mate, and move against the blood flow to their final habitats. Egg output is detectable at five to six weeks for *S. japonicum,* seven to eight weeks for *S. mansoni*, and ten to twelve weeks for *S. haematobium*.

INCIDENCE AND PREVALENCE

Initial infection in schistosomiasis usually occurs in childhood, and reinfection may continue as long as there is contact with fresh water. It must be remembered that the worms do not multiply in the human body, that complete immunity apparently does not occur, and that the worms may live for decades. Therefore, although large worm burdens may develop following initial exposure, heavy infections are usually built up from multiple small exposures. Under these circumstances the incidence of schistosomiasis in endemic areas is low and occurs principally in children, but the prevalence of the disease may build up to massive proportions.

The worldwide prevalence of schistosomiasis is usually estimated at 180,000,000 cases, conservatively at 118,000,000. It is known to be endemic in 72 countries that have a total population of 1,348,000,000.

In Africa, *S. haematobium* and *S. mansoni* are widespread. Only the former species occurs in Tunisia, Algeria, Morocco, Mauritania, Portuguese Guinea, Niger, the Congo Republic (Brazzaville), Somalia, and the island of Mauritius. Both species are found in all other countries, including the Malagasy Republic. Of Africa's 302,000,000 total population, 188,000,000 are estimated to be exposed to infection and 75,000,000 to be infected.

In Southwest Asia, *S. haematobium* is endemic in Aden, Saudi Arabia, Yemen, Israel, Iraq, Iran, Syria, Turkey, and Lebanon. *S. mansoni* occurs in the first four of these countries, and is particularly prevalent in Yemen, where half the 3,500,000 population are thought to be infected. The highest prevalence rate for *S. haematobium* occurs in Iraq, where 20 per cent of the exposed population of 5,000,000 are infected. Of the 84,000,000 population of Southwest Asia an estimated 10,000,000 are exposed, and 3,000,000 are thought to be infected.

In the Orient, *S. japonicum* occurs in China, Japan, the Philippines, and the Celebes. The prevalence in China has been estimated at 32,000,000, but it is claimed that this number has been markedly reduced by a recent massive control campaign. Schistosomiasis is under control in Japan, but seems to be spreading in the Philippines. Small foci of schistosomiasis japonica have recently been discovered in Thailand and Laos. Of the 885,000,000 population of the Orient, 102,000,000 are estimated to be exposed, and 33,000,000 infected. A small focus of *S. haematobium* infection has been found in India, near Bombay.

In the New World, only *S. mansoni* is found. Brazil has the largest number of cases, estimated at 8,000,000, and the infection seems to be spreading. Schistosomiasis also occurs in Venezuela, where it is apparently on the wane, and in Surinam. It is endemic in the following Caribbean islands: Puerto Rico, Vieques, Dominican Republic, Antigua, Guadeloupe, Martinique, and St. Lucia. The parasite has not been found in any of the Central American countries.

The one tiny focus of schistosomiasis in Europe, *S. haematobium* in southern Portugal, has now been eliminated.

EPIDEMIOLOGY

The life cycle of schistosomiasis will become established only in areas where there is a susceptible snail species. Thus the infection is prevalent on the West Indian island of St. Lucia, although St. Vincent, 30 miles away, is completely free of the parasite. It is estimated that there are 100,000 Puerto Ricans with schistosomiasis in New York City alone, but the presence of susceptible snails in the continental United States has not been established. Prevalence rates within endemic areas may be exceedingly variable, ranging from close to 100 per cent in some localities to almost 0 in others. This is governed by the interaction of multiple local ecologic factors relating to both the snail and human populations. Another important factor in the epidemiology of schistosomiasis is the variation in geographic strains of the species; for example, *S. japonicum* on Formosa is highly infective to domestic and wild animals but not to man, and *S. mansoni* in Africa south of the Sahara appears to be relatively avirulent.

Animal reservoirs are undoubtedly of significance in maintaining the life cycle of *S. japonicum* — in particular, cows and dogs. Natural *S. mansoni* infections have been found in rodents, baboons, insectivores, and dogs in Africa, but it is generally believed that animal reservoirs do not play a significant role in the life cycle of this species. *S. haematobium* is rarely encountered in animals.

Although transmission patterns differ among the three species of schistosomes, *there is little question that for each species agricultural development, particularly irrigation, may lead to a marked increase in the prevalence of schistosomiasis.* A major epidemic occurred in Egypt following the construction of the low Aswan dam, and in Rhodesia after development of large scale irrigation schemes.

In regard to morbidity and mortality, reliable demographic figures are not available, particularly because schistosomiasis is such an insidious disease. The few investigations of morbidity now available show little or no effect of schistosomiasis on educational attainment or work capacity. There is no question, however, that in all its forms schistosomiasis is potentially lethal — Katayama fever in *S. japonicum* infections, portal hypertension with hematemesis in both schistosomiasis japonica and mansoni, uremia in *S. haematobium* infection, and cor pulmonale in all three. Schistosomiasis may also potentiate the development of other diseases such as hepatitis, hepatoma, cirrhosis, and cancer of the urinary bladder.

Several different approaches to the mathematical epidemiology of schistosomiasis have been tried. Most recently a modification of the Kermack-McKendrick theory of epidemics was applied to the problem. The level of the snail population appeared to play a critical role in the occurrence of epidemics, maintenance of endemic states, and disappearance of the disease, i.e., if the density of susceptible snails is above a critical level, an epidemic will occur; if the total number of snails is above the critical level but the number of susceptibles is at or below it, the process will be stable (endemic); and if the density of snails falls to or below the critical level, then a decline in the disease will ensue.

PATHOGENESIS AND CLINICAL MANIFESTATIONS

Basic to an understanding of the disease processes in schistosomiasis are these facts: the schistosomes do not multiply in man; complete immunity does not follow initial infection; repeated infections usually occur; the worms are long lived; large worm burdens may gradually accumulate; and a large proportion of schistosome eggs are not excreted but remain within the body. Disease is related not only to the presence of the various stages of the schistosomes in the body tissues and their secretions and excretions, but to the inflammatory responses of the host as well.

Clinically, three distinct syndromes occur at different stages of schistosome infection. Within one day of cercarial penetration, swimmer's itch, a pruritic papular rash, may appear. Several weeks later Katayama fever, a self-limited but possibly fatal illness resembling serum sickness, may develop. Finally, after many years, during which the infection may be either asymptomatic or associated with relatively mild intestinal or urinary tract symptoms, fibrosis of the liver may result in the signs and symptoms of portal hypertension in schistosomiasis mansoni and japonica; fibrosis of the ureters and bladder in schistosomiasis hematobia may result in changes associated with urinary tract obstruction.

Schistosome Dermatitis. Schistosomiasis begins with penetration of the skin by cercariae. These organisms are not discriminating and will penetrate the skin of most animals whether they are susceptible or insusceptible, living or dead. When nonhuman schistosomes, those that complete their life cycle in animals or birds, enter the skin of man, they die. Even in highly susceptible experimental hosts many S. mansoni cercariae die in the skin and perhaps in the lung; in the hamster almost 40 per cent are lost in this manner. In the highest primate thus far studied, the chimpanzee, only 4 to 8 per cent of S. mansoni cercariae and 14 to 40 per cent of S. haematobium cercariae were recovered as adult schistosomes. In most laboratory animals the recovery rate for S. japonicum is usually higher than that for the other two species.

The death of cercariae in the skin leads to the development of a pruritic papular rash known as swimmer's itch. This syndrome occurs in its most severe form following exposure to animal schistosomes, and has been shown to be a sensitization phenomenon, rarely occurring on primary exposure. Papules appear in sensitized persons at 5 to 15 hours, and there is massive round cell invasion of the dermis and epidermis, suggesting a delayed hypersensitivity response. Swimmer's itch has been demonstrated in infected patients experimentally re-exposed to S. mansoni and S. haematobium cercariae. A mild form of swimmer's itch appears to occur in patients exposed to S. japonicum cercariae, but the rice paddy dermatitis of the Far East is caused mainly by avian schistosomes.

Katayama Fever. The next clinical phase of schistosomiasis begins 20 to 60 days after exposure and has been known in Japan as Katayama fever since the mid-nineteenth century. This syndrome occurs most frequently and is most severe in S. japonicum infections; in schistosomiasis mansoni it is usually found only in patients with very heavy initial infection; it is rarely if ever seen in schistosomiasis hematobia. In addition to fever, the patient suffers from chills, sweating, anorexia, headache, diarrhea, and cough. Hepatosplenomegaly is frequent, and generalized lymphadenopathy and urticaria are often seen. Eosinophilia occurs in most cases, averaging about 40 per cent. The fever may last for several weeks; when it subsides the other signs and symptoms also disappear. Death may occur in the Katayama fever stage of schistosomiasis japonica, but rarely does so in S. mansoni infection. At autopsy, massive infection is almost invariably found, with large numbers of eggs in the liver and intestines; 1608 worm pairs were demonstrated at autopsy in a Brazilian child. Katayama fever, which usually appears on initial infection, begins at about the time of onset of egg-laying by the worms; thus large amounts of antigen are suddenly added to moderate levels of cross-reacting antibody formed in response to the developing worms. It is possible, therefore, that this serum sickness-like syndrome may be a form of immune-complex disease.

Chronic Schistosomiasis. A correlation between the number of worms and the development and extent of chronic disease (except for patients with advanced liver fibrosis) was recently demonstrated by techniques quantitating human worm burdens at surgery and at autopsy. Heavy worm burdens were apparently a prerequisite for the development of severe disease, whereas light infections appeared to be of little consequence pathologically. *Thus, patients with few worms may never show any signs or symptoms related to schistosome infection.*

The patient with chronic schistosomiasis mansoni or japonica may, however, complain of fatigue, abdominal pain, and intermittent diarrhea or dysentery; on sigmoidoscopy granulomatous nodules or polyps may be observed. In S. haematobium infection, hematuria, and, occasionally, dysuria and frequency are found. Mild chronic blood loss has been measured by radioisotope labeling in both S. mansoni and S. haematobium infections, but anemia is not usually seen in areas where there is normal iron intake. All of the aforementioned signs and symptoms are related to the passage of eggs through the mucosa of the intestine and the urinary bladder.

Many eggs do not, however, leave the body; in laboratory animals less than half of them are excreted. Over a period of 20 years, for each *S. mansoni* worm pair producing eggs at a rate of 300 per day, at least 1,000,000 eggs will remain in the body. This figure can be multiplied by 10 for each *S. japonicum* worm pair.

In *S. mansoni* and *S. japonicum* infections, some of the eggs remain in the intestinal walls, but many of them enter the circulation and are carried into the liver. In schistosomiasis hematobia many eggs remain in the tissues of the bladder and adjacent organs, but some (usually too few to cause significant disease) enter the lungs via the inferior vena cava as well as the liver via the portal system. Granulomatous inflammation develops around the eggs trapped in the tissues; in the case of *S. mansoni* this has been demonstrated to be an immunologic response of the delayed hypersensitivity type. Both the eggs and the reactions to them are being constantly resorbed, but if large numbers of eggs gather together, the fibrosis subsequent to inflammation may remain. In schistosomiasis mansoni and japonica this leads to hepatic portal fibrosis, and in schistosomiasis hematobia, to fibrosis of the ureters and bladder.

Hepatosplenic Schistosomiasis. As the liver parenchyma is relatively unharmed by the pathologic processes involved in hepatic schistosomiasis japonica and mansoni, the clinical consequences of the disease relate primarily to periportal fibrosis. Pathophysiologically this results in an intrahepatic block to portal blood flow and the development of portal hypertension and portal-systemic collateral circulation. The lesion is presinusoidal; thus intrasplenic and portal pressures are usually markedly elevated whereas wedged hepatic vein pressure is normal. Total liver blood flow tends to remain within normal limits owing to a compensatory increase in arterial flow.

Clinically, the earliest sign of significant liver involvement is hepatomegaly. With progression, the spleen enlarges and becomes firm in consistency. Eventually it may extend to well below the umbilicus. At this point the patient tends to be in good general health, but may consult a physician because of a dragging feeling in the left upper abdominal quadrant.

The other major factor bringing the patient to the physician is a sudden hematemesis because of bleeding esophageal varices. Such an episode may not reappear for many years or may recur at fairly frequent intervals. The consequences of hematemesis in schistosomiasis are very different from those in cirrhosis of the liver: the blood ammonia concentration tends to remain normal, hepatic coma rarely occurs, and mortality is very low, being primarily due to exsanguination. This is consistent with relatively normal liver function. Jaundice is almost never seen in uncomplicated

schistosomiasis, and the levels of both conjugated and unconjugated bilirubin are usually normal. Serum albumin concentration is normal or only slightly decreased, and globulin is somewhat elevated. As a consequence, ascites and edema are rarely encountered. Even sulfobromophthalein retention is often normal in these patients. Stigmata of chronic liver disease such as palmar erythema, spider angiomas, altered hair distribution, and gynecomastia are rare. Patients may suffer multiple severe hematemeses, but aside from temporary changes, liver function tends to remain relatively normal.

In spite of moderate chronic and occasional severe acute intestinal blood loss, a significant degree of anemia rarely occurs in uncomplicated schistosomiasis. The white blood count is usually within normal limits, but there is a moderate eosinophilia. Splenomegaly, however, may result in hypersplenism, the patient developing leukopenia, thrombocytopenia, and anemia with decreased red blood cell life span.

Patients with decompensated hepatic disease characterized by liver parenchymal malfunction and all the physical stigmata of this state, including jaundice and ascites, are seen in localities in which schistosomiasis is endemic. This is particularly common in the case of schistosomiasis japonica, and may, perhaps, be related to overwhelming embolization of the liver with the large numbers of eggs produced by this parasite. Pathologists have stated, however, that it has not been possible to prove the transformation of advanced schistosomal fibrosis into true cirrhosis. In Egypt it has been suggested that patients with schistosomiasis might concomitantly have other forms of liver disease. Finally, it must be recognized that all those infected with *S. mansoni* and *S. japonicum* perforce have some degree of liver involvement, and that the effect of malnutrition, hepatotoxins, and hepatitis may be potentiated; such interrelationships have been demonstrated in laboratory animals.

Pulmonary Schistosomiasis. Pulmonary schistosomiasis, which in its most severe state is characterized by signs and symptoms of cor pulmonale, is a complication of hepatosplenic schistosomiasis. Portal-systemic collateral circulation enables the eggs to bypass the liver, and they are trapped in the pulmonary capillary bed. Arteritis with angiomatoid formation occurs, and there is obstruction to pulmonary blood flow. Pulmonary hypertension is found in every case, but cardiac output usually remains within the normal range. Arterial oxygen saturation is usually normal, and cyanosis is rare. The lungs are often involved in schistosomiasis hematobia because of the passage of eggs from the vesical plexuses into the inferior vena cava, but egg embolization appears to be relatively light, and significant disease is uncommon.

Urinary Tract Schistosomiasis. Severe urinary tract disease may occur in both the early and late phases of *S. haematobium* infection. Initially there may be ureteral obstruction owing to florid granulomatous inflammatory reactions to the eggs in both the ureters and the bladder; these lesions appear to be highly reversible following anti-schistosomal therapy. Later in the course of the disease irreversible fibrosis may supervene. Bladder fibrosis and calcification lead to frequency and dysuria. On cystoscopy, so-called sandy patches may be seen on the bladder walls; these are made up of large numbers of schistosome eggs. The disease may progress through hydronephrosis, secondary infection, and finally uremia. An association between cancer of the bladder and urinary schistosomiasis has been demonstrated.

Central Nervous System Schistosomiasis. Schistosomiasis of the central nervous system, although relatively rare, is an important complication of the infection. *S. japonicum* usually involves the brain, whereas *S. mansoni* and *S. haematobium* tend to affect the spinal cord. Schistosomiasis japonica is reputed to be one of the important causes of focal epilepsy in the Far East. The disease may also present as a space-occupying lesion or occasionally as a generalized encephalitis. Cerebral schistosomiasis japonica may appear at any time in the course of infection from the first three weeks on. At autopsy the lesions almost always consist of large collections of eggs in the venous circulatory system, suggesting the presence of adult worms, although they have never been found. *S. mansoni* and *S. haematobium* may be associated with a transverse myelitis-like syndrome; at surgery or autopsy large granulomas made up of eggs are usually found.

DIAGNOSIS

When schistosomiasis is considered as a diagnosis in nonendemic areas, the first question that should be asked is: "Where have you been?" It must then be determined whether there was contact with fresh water, whether a rash was observed soon thereafter, and if there was a febrile episode several weeks later. For schistosomiasis mansoni and japonica, abdominal symptoms and signs should be considered, and for *S. haematobium* infection, hematuria, dysuria, and frequency are important. The presence of eosinophilia is a useful sign of schistosome infection. A wide variety of serologic tests (e.g., complement-fixation, flocculation, fluorescent antibody, and circumoval precipitin) and a skin test of the immediate type are available. *These immunologic methods, which are all based on detection of circulating antibody, essentially have no place in the diagnosis of the individual case,* as cross-reactions with other parasitic infections providing false positive results are relatively common; false negative reactions also occur.

Definitive diagnosis can be made only by finding schistosome eggs in the excreta feces or urine) or in a biopsy specimen—usually rectal. Eggs may not be present in the early stages of acute schistosomiasis. Schistosome eggs are relatively large, and are easy to identify because of their distinctive shape. Direct fecal smear is too insensitive, however, and a concentration technique should be utilized. The formol-ether method provides a 20- to 30-fold concentration and takes only five minutes: 1 gram of feces is emulsified in 7 ml. of 10 per cent formol-saline and strained through wire gauze (40 meshes per inch) into a centrifuge tube. Three milliliters of ether is added, and the tube is shaken for one minute and centrifuged for two minutes at 2000 r.p.m. The supernate is decanted, leaving 1 or 2 drops, which are shaken, poured on a slide, covered with a coverslip, and examined under low-power magnification. Rectal biopsy is a highly efficient method for the diagnosis of *S. mansoni* and *japonicum* infection, and will often pick up *S. haematobium* eggs. Through a proctoscope, snips are taken from the valves of Houston (8 to 10 cm. from the anus), pressed between glass slides, and examined immediately under a microscope. Sometimes only opaque dead eggs are observed, suggesting a burnt-out or successfully treated infection. Liver biopsy has been suggested as a means of diagnosis, but will only rarely detect an infection not revealed by the aforementioned methods.

For the diagnosis of schistosomiasis hematobia, urine is collected at midday, because a diurnal variation in egg output has been demonstrated. The urine specimen is centrifuged and the sediment examined. *S. mansoni* eggs are occasionally found in urine.

Quantitative egg-counting techniques are now available which seem to be a useful indicator of the severity of infection. The Bell method, which includes dilution, sieving onto filter paper, and ninhydrin staining, is effective for either urine or feces, and the Kato thick smear technique is excellent for the latter. Five- to 10-gram samples of feces appear to be sufficient, as recent studies indicate that eggs are uniformly distributed in the feces.

For determining the severity of intestinal disease, sigmoidoscopy and barium enema are of value. The extent of liver disease may be estimated by liver biopsy, barium swallow, esophagoscopy, and especially splenoportography with measurement of intrasplenic pressure. In schistosomiasis hematobia, cystoscopy and intravenous and retrograde pyelography are useful techniques.

TREATMENT

Antischistosomal treatment should never be instituted without proof of infection by the demonstration of living eggs in excreta or biopsy specimens. A positive serologic or skin test does not provide a definitive diagnosis. Complete cure is not necessary and indeed is not always desirable in schistosomiasis (particularly in endemic areas where reinfection may occur), as disease is related to intensity of infection, surviving worms do not multiply, and immunity may be premunitive, i.e., dependent on the presence of living organisms. The recent use of quantitative egg counts has shown that in cases in which cure is not achieved by the full course of treatment with an established drug, egg output is usually reduced by over 90 per cent. Thus striving for cure by increasing the drug dosage or repeating the course of treatment is rarely necessary and, because of the toxicity of the antischistosomal drugs, may actually be harmful.

The three schistosome species vary considerably in their response to drugs, S. japonicum being the most resistant and S. haematobium the most susceptible. Thus, it is still necessary to use the highly toxic antimony compounds for treating schistosomiasis japonica, although less toxic, more easily administered drugs may be used for the other two species.

During the early Katayama fever stage of S. japonicum infection, the parasite is relatively insusceptible to treatment. Antimony potassium tartrate (tartar emetic) is still the drug of choice. It should be made up fresh just prior to administration in an 0.5 per cent solution. It is injected intravenously (infiltration must be avoided as the drug is intensely irritating) at a slow rate not to exceed 4 ml. per minute. The patient must be at rest for at least one hour after injection. Injections are given every other day, beginning with 8 ml., increasing to 12, 16, 20, 24, and 28 ml., and continuing at the 28-ml. level for nine more doses for a total of 360 ml. containing 648 mg. of antimony. The drug is cardiotoxic and in addition causes coughing, vomiting, and muscle and joint stiffness. Hepatitis, nephritis, encephalitis, and exfoliative dermatitis are occasional complications. An intramuscularly administered preparation, sodium antimony dimercaptosuccinate (Astiban) has also been used for treating Schistosoma japonicum infections.

For schistosomiasis mansoni, an intramuscularly administered antimony preparation, stibophen (Fuadin), is widely used; the regimen is 4 ml. every other day for a total of 80 to 100 ml. The side effects of all the antimony preparations are similar, although Astiban and Fuadin tend to be less toxic than tartar emetic.

A new drug, hycanthone, administered in a single intramuscular injection of the methane sulfonate salt, 2.5 mg. per kilogram, is most promising. Recently, however, fatalities associated with hycanthone treatment have suggested that its use be deterred until more information is available.

For the treatment of schistosomiasis hematobia, niridazole (Ambilhar), which is both reasonably safe and effective, is presently the drug of choice, although it is not now available for use in the United States. It is administered orally in two divided daily doses totaling 25 mg. per kilogram for a period of seven days. Vomiting, diarrhea, cramps, and dizziness may occur. This drug is contraindicated in patients with liver or cerebral disease. Hycanthone and the antimony preparations, tartar emetic, Astiban, and Fuadin, may also be used to treat Schistosoma haematobium infections.

Based on the questionable theory that dead worms cause significant harm to the liver, a new method of treatment has recently been developed, extracorporeal hemofiltration. Utilizing a combination of surgery and a single dose of an antischistosomal drug, the worms are sieved out of the blood stream. Standard drug treatment, however, during which all the worms pass into the liver, is not followed by an exacerbation of disease. Furthermore, repeated infection and treatment of laboratory animals, causing vast numbers of dead worms to enter the liver, does not result in any significant pathophysiologic changes. Therefore, although extracorporeal hemofiltration is a valuable research tool, it should be used as a form of treatment only under special circumstances.

In general, the surgical treatment of schistosomiasis should be approached with caution. Many of the apparently irreversible lesions of urinary tract schistosomiasis will resolve completely following antischistosomal treatment, particularly in young patients. Cerebral schistosomiasis japonica is frequently cured or markedly ameliorated by drug therapy. Finally, prophylactic portacaval shunts should never be performed in hepatosplenic schistosomiasis, as hematemesis is not invariable, is unpredictable in onset, and, when it occurs, mortality is low. If the creation of shunt by surgery is necessitated by repeated bleeding episodes, splenorenal anastomosis is preferable to portacaval shunt because of a much lower incidence of chronic portal systemic encephalopathy. Prior to shunting, however, antischistosomal therapy is necessary to prevent prolonged passage of eggs into the lungs which may lead to the development of cor pulmonale.

PROGNOSIS

The prognosis is usually good. Many patients with schistosomiasis never have symptoms or signs of disease, or have only relatively mild ones. Epidemiologically, both the infection and the disease reach their peak in early adult life and decline with age. Disregarding the factor of death among heavily infected patients, this may be due to decreased exposure to infection, gradual death of the worms, slow development of immunity, and diminution in the inflammatory response to the parasite and its products.

The early stages of hepatic or urinary tract disease appear to be reversible following antischistosomal therapy. Although late disease seems relatively irreversible, progression may be halted and gradual improvement may follow drug therapy. In hepatosplenic schistosomiasis the prognosis in patients suffering a hematemesis is far better than in those with cirrhosis, as the former do not tend to go into hepatic coma. Patients with cerebral schistosomiasis japonica may show remarkable improvement following antischistosome therapy.

PREVENTION

On the individual level, schistosomiasis may be prevented by avoidance of contaminated waters. If this is not possible, boots should be worn; if contaminated water reaches the skin, rapid drying or rubbing with alcohol will prevent infection. Storage of water for several days will ensure the death of cercariae as will the boiling of drinking water. Sea water is safe for swimming, although the mouths of rivers and streams should be avoided; chlorination of swimming pools will prevent infection. Repellents are of no great value, and vaccines or prophylactic drugs are not available.

There are three approaches to the control of schistosomiasis on a mass basis: (1) destruction of the snail intermediate host, (2) prevention of snail infection by the treatment of human infection and the construction of privies, and (3) elimination of contact with contaminated water by the provision of safe water supplies. Destruction of the snail is primarily based on the use of molluscicides such as the various copper salts, sodium pentachlorophenate, Bayluscide, and n-trityl-morpholone. Molluscicides, however, are quickly inactivated by sunlight and adsorption to mud and organic matter; they pass rapidly through running water or are diluted in vast volumes of water, and they often destroy other aquatic fauna and flora. Also, although molluscicides may appear to be highly effective, only a few surviving snails can rapidly repopulate an area. Many biologic control measures have been advocated, including the use of nonsusceptible snail species which may compete for miracidia, food, and space; snail-eating fish and ducks; and snail pathogens. None of these measures has shown outstanding promise. Moreover, as the snails that transmit *S. japonicum* are amphibious and are frequently found along the banks of water courses, their eradication has necessitated the use of earth-moving equipment and flame throwers.

An attempt to break the life cycle at the stage of transmission from man to the snail has been hampered by the lack of practical mass therapy. The recent development of effective oral drugs and of a single-dose intramuscular drug offers great promise for the future. An important adjunct to this approach is the construction of privies. Breaking the cycle at the stage of transmission from the snail to man can be accomplished by the provision of safe water supplies for washing and recreational purposes.

Control measures based on the destruction of snails are an end in themselves, and in addition may be inimical to the environment. In contrast, mass antischistosomal treatment coupled with the construction of privies or the provision of safe water supplies should contribute greatly to the general health of the population.

Cort, W. W.: Studies on schistosome dermatitis. Status of knowledge after more than 20 years. Amer. J. Hyg., 52:251, 1950.

Díaz-Rivera, R. S., Ramos-Morales, F., Koppisch, E., García-Palmieri, M. R., Cintrón-Rivera, A. A., Marchand, E. J., González, O., and Torregrosa, M. V.: Acute Manson's schistosomiasis. Amer. J. Med., 21:918, 1956.

Hairston, N. G.: On the mathematical analysis of schistosome populations. Bull. WHO, 33:45, 1965.

Jordan, P.: Chemotherapy of schistosomiasis. Bull. N. Y. Acad. Med., 44:245, 1968.

Kane, C. A., and Most, H.: Schistosomiasis of the central nervous system. Experiences in World War II and a review of the literature. Arch. Neurol. Psychiat. (Chicago), 59:141, 1948.

Shaw, A. F. B., and Ghareeb, A. A.: The pathogenesis of pulmonary schistosomiasis in Egypt with special reference to Ayerza's disease. J. Path. Bact., 46:401, 1968.

Warren, K. S.: Pathophysiology and pathogenesis of hepatosplenic schistosomiasis mansoni. Bull. N. Y. Acad. Med., 44:280, 1968.

Wright, W. H.: Schistosomiasis as a world problem. Bull. N. Y. Acad. Med., 44:301, 1968.

THE HERMAPHRODITIC FLUKES
Philip D. Marsden

The hermaphroditic flukes, unlike Schistosoma flukes, have both sets of sex organs in the same worm, and frequently self-fertilization occurs. These flukes are flat leaflike worms with oral and ventral suckers. They have a complex life cycle. The egg hatches to produce a motile ciliated *miracidium,* which penetrates the soft tissue of a snail and undergoes a cycle of development similar to that in schistosomiasis. *Cercariae* are produced by the snail after a few weeks, but unlike schistosomes these cercariae encyst in a second intermediate host, either fish, crab, or plant. These encysted cercariae or *metacercariae* are a relatively resistant form which can survive adverse conditions. If the metacercaria is then ingested by man, it hatches to produce an immature fluke which migrates through the body tissues to gain its site of final development. This varies with the species concerned, being the liver for Clonorchis and Fasciola, the lung for Paragonimus, and the intestine for *Fasciolopsis buski.*

Initial invasion is often accompanied by eosinophilia, but it takes a month or longer before the characteristic eggs are produced. All the eggs have an operculum or lid through which the miracidia escape, unlike Schistosoma eggs. Some of these flukes live for a long time, producing progressive damage in the tissues of the host. When searching for the ova of trematodes in the biliary tree, duodenal aspiration may be more rewarding than stool examination. Therapy, especially in the hepatic hermaphroditic trematodes, is unsatisfactory.

HEPATIC HERMAPHRODITIC FLUKES

Clonorchiasis (Clonorchis sinensis). Man is infected by eating the flesh of undercooked or raw freshwater fish in which the metacercariae are encysted. More than 40 species of fish, mainly of the carp and salmon (cyprinoid) group, have been found to harbor metacercariae. The natural definitive hosts other than man are fish-eating mammals, including cats, dogs, mink, and rats. Widespread in the Far East, the main endemic areas of human infection are Japan, Korea, China, and Vietnam. As the flukes live for decades (20 to 30 years) in the biliary tree, immigrant Orientals have been found infected in many countries. A proportion of the Chinese in New York and San

Francisco are infected. Infections recorded in Hawaiians are attributed to imports of infected frozen, dried, or pickled fish from Japan.

It appears that most of the larval flukes ascend the biliary tree directly from the duodenum, but some may pass via the portal circulation to the liver. They mature in the bile ducts, and the grayish-brown adults, measuring 10 to 20 mm. by 2 to 4 mm., move sluggishly around by means of their suckers in the distal biliary passages. They feed on secretions from the mucosa of the bile duct and possibly also on cellular elements. Occasionally they gain access to the gallbladder and pancreatic ducts. In effect they cause a chronic cholangitis with inflammation of the biliary tree, proliferation of the biliary epithelium, and progressive portal fibrosis. The severity of these changes depends upon the load of flukes.

After ingesting the metacercariae, the patient may present with epigastric pain, malaise, and tender hepatomegaly. An eosinophilia is usually present in the early stages, but no eggs can be found until about one month has passed and the flukes have matured. Light infections are often asymptomatic, but a firm liver edge is often discovered within the costal margin on routine examination. In an Oriental this finding should prompt a careful search for ova in the stool. In heavy infections (10,000 to 20,000 flukes), more serious sequelae occur. The marked portal fibrosis may be associated with signs of portal hypertension. Extension of the fibrosis into the liver parenchyma may be associated with liver cell death and fatty change. Jaundice is more likely to be associated with biliary obstruction owing to a mass of flukes or stone formation. Cholangiocarcinoma is a late complication of severe clonorchiasis, a metaplastic change occurring in the irritated biliary epithelium. In Hong Kong there is a high incidence in males after the fourth decade, the adenocarcinomas showing varying degrees of differentiation. Suppurative cholangitis caused by superimposed bacterial infection may present as hypoglycemic coma. Chronic pancreatitis is a rare complication.

The diagnosis is made by finding the eggs in the stool. Unfortunately they are not characteristic and can be easily confused with a number of other trematodes producing small, similar eggs (Heterophyes, Opisthorcis, Metagonimus). The eggs average 29 by 16 μ; they are light brown and ovoid. There is a definite shoulder in a shell wall near the operculum and a boss at the anopercular end.

The invasive stage must be distinguished from that of other fluke infections, visceral larval migrans, and hepatic amebiasis. The last-named condition is not associated with eosinophilia. The late stages may resemble cirrhosis and uncomplicated cholecystitis. Hypoglycemic coma can also be a manifestation of a hepatocellular carcinoma. In the elderly, repeated nonparasitic cholangitis is sometimes a difficult diagnosis to establish in patients with pyrexia of unknown origin.

Treatment and Prevention. Most investigators agree that the drugs available for treating this infection are often ineffective and disappointing.

Prolonged chloroquine therapy is chiefly suppressive; however, it is still the drug of choice. Chloroquine diphosphate in a dose of 300 mg. base (two 250 mg. tablets) three times a day for three to six weeks is a standard course. Some workers have increased this dose or used it for periods of up to a year. Various percentages of cures are claimed, but it depends on the criteria used and especially on what stool concentration technique is employed and how frequently. At the higher dosage levels the more severe side effects of chloroquine toxicity may be seen, namely, corneal deposits and retinopathy, central nervous system changes (a parkinsonian-like syndrome), dyspigmentation, cardiac arrhythmias, and peripheral myopathy and neuropathy. A new compound, hexachloroparaxylol, proved effective, but alarming toxicity tests in recent animal studies have resulted in its withdrawal. Biliary obstruction may require surgical relief, and at surgery as many flukes as possible should be removed from the biliary tree. Prevention of this infection relates to the competent cooking of freshwater fish.

Opisthorchiasis (Opisthorchis viverrini and felineus). *Opisthorchis felineus* is prevalent in the Philippines, India, Japan, and Vietnam, as well as in the USSR and parts of Eastern Europe, whereas *Opisthorchis viverrini* is common in north Thailand and Laos. The life cycles of these flukes are similar to that of *Clonorchis sinensis* and are completed in about four months under favorable conditions. Snails are infected by fecal contaminants of water from infected persons or animal reservoirs, e.g., cats. In northeast Thailand 90 per cent of people more than ten years of age are infected with *O. viverrini,* and 3.5 million in the whole country. With all infections of this type, as might be expected, the incidence rises with age. The source of infection is a popular dish of raw fish, rice, vegetables, and spices.

The pathologic findings are similar to those in *Clonorchis sinensis,* although stone formation is said to be unusual. Cholangiocarcinoma has also been reported to be associated with this infection. The eggs are indistinguishable from Clonorchis. This emphasizes the importance of a geographic history, for the only other way of distinguishing the parasite would be by examination of the adult flukes. Percutaneous transhepatic cholangiography may reveal radiologic changes such as a single cystic cavity or mulberry-like dilatation of the intrahepatic bile ducts.

Dicrocoeliasis. *Dicrocoelium dendriticum* is acquired by eating ants in which the metacercariae have developed following ingestion by the ant of slime balls containing cercariae secreted by the snail. Infections are generally uncommon, but occur in Europe and Asia and around the Mediterranean basin. Being light infections, their main importance is for the physician to recognize the small, fully embryonated thick-shelled eggs ($40\mu \times 25\mu$) for what they are. Spurious parasitism, in which nonhuman species ingested in liver pass through the bowel unchanged, is well documented.

Fascioliasis (Fasciola hepatica). This is also a biliary fluke, but it is less well adapted to man than is *Clonorchis sinensis*. It is a common parasite of sheep, producing marked liver damage. Worldwide in distribution in sheep, it is prevalent in low wet pastures where suitable species of snails are indigenous. The metacercariae encyst on plants, and man is infected mainly as a result of eating wild watercress and other plants gathered in these pastures. Human infections are more common where such salad is favored, e.g., Europe, Cuba, and Chile. In England outbreaks are associated with particularly wet summers.

The adult fluke is large, 2 to 3 cm. in length by 0.8 to 1.3 cm. in breadth, and may occlude the *common bile duct*. Indeed, many human infections have been first recognized at surgery for bilary obstruction. Again an invasive stage of fever, eosinophilia, and hepatomegaly is associated with larval flukes moving through the liver substance to gain the biliary tract, for the larval flukes produced from the metacercariae in the jejunum pass across the peritoneal cavity to pierce Glisson's capsule and move through the liver substance. Far fewer flukes than Clonorchis are found in man, but again hyperplasia, necrosis, and cystic dilation of the biliary tract, accompanied by leukocytic infiltration and eventually periportal fibrosis, can ensue if the load of flukes is heavy enough. The differential diagnosis is similar to that of clonorchiasis.

The *diagnosis* depends on finding large yellowish operculate eggs 130 to 150μ in length in the feces or aspirated bile. Liver should be excluded from the patient's diet in areas where raw liver is eaten, because eggs in such livers will pass through the intestinal tract unchanged. A complement-fixation test using an extract of the adult fluke as antigen is a useful diagnostic aid, especially in infections in which the flukes are ectopic. A hemagglutination test has also been developed.

Unlike the other hepatic hermaphroditic flukes, *Fasciola hepatica* and the closely allied *Fasciola gigantica* are occasionally found in sites other than the liver. This could be related to man's being a relatively poor host species. Thus a migrating subcutaneous swelling associated with intense eosinophilia may contain such an immature fluke, and there are records of occurrences in many sites, including the brain.

A further oddity associated with *Fasciola hepatica* infection is the parasitization of the pharynx by young post-metacercarial flukes which are acquired by eating raw liver in which the young flukes are actively migrating. This occurs in Lebanon, where such raw sheep and goat livers are eaten; the patient complains of intense inflammation of the back of the throat. This syndrome of parasitic pharyngitis, known as halzoun, can also be produced by a leech or a pentosomid (a wormlike arthropod).

Emetine hydrochloride is still considered by many the most effective therapy in a dose of 65 mg. intramuscularly daily for ten days, but cure is rarely achieved. (For side effects see Amebiasis. It may be replaced by the less toxic dehydroemetine.) Some physicians give chloroquine concurrently, 300 mg. of base three times a day for a longer period, although chloroquine alone fails to cure. Bithionol has been shown to be effective in a dose of 50 mg. per kilogram on alternate days for 10 to 15 doses, and, being less toxic, may be used as an alternative. Ectopic flukes are removed surgically.

Clonorchiasis

Hou, P. C.: The relationship between primary carcinoma of the liver and infestation with *Clonorchis sinensis*. J. Path. Bact., 72:239, 1956.
Komiya, L.: Clonorchis and clonorchiasis. *In* Dawes, B. (ed.): Advances in Parasitology. London, Academic Press, 1966, Vol. 4, pp. 53–106.
McFadzean, A. J. S., and Yeing, R. T. T.: Acute pancreatitis due to *Clonorchis sinensis*. Trans. Roy. Soc. Trop. Med. Hyg., 60:466, 1966.
Weng, H. C., Chung, H. L., Ho, L. Y., and Hou, T. C.: Studies in *Clonorchis sinensis* in the past 10 years. Chin. Med. J. (Peking), 80:441, 1960.

Opisthorchiasis

Harinasuta, C., and Vajrasthira, S.: Opisthorchiasis in Thailand. Ann. Trop. Med. Parasit., 54:100, 1960.

Fascioliasis

Facey, R. V., and Marsden, P. D.: Fascioliasis in man. An outbreak in Hampshire. Brit. Med. J., 2:619, 1960.
Khalil, G. M., and Schacher, J. F.: *Linguatula serrata* in relation to halzoun and the Marrara syndrome. Amer. J. Trop. Med., 14:736, 1965.
Neghume, A., and Ossandan, M.: Ectopic and hepatic fascioliasis. Amer. J. Trop. Med., 23:545, 1943.
Pantelouris, E. M.: The Common Liver Fluke. Oxford, Pergamon Press, 1964.

PARAGONIMIASIS
(Paragonimus Westermani; The Lung Fluke)
Philip D. Marsden

Although *Paragonimus westermani* is the most common species of this group infecting man, recently a number of other human pathogens have been recognized in the genus Paragonimus, which to date numbers 31 species. These include *P. africanus* found in Nigeria, the Cameroons, and the Congo, and two new Chinese flukes, *P. skrjabini* and *P. heterotremus*. *P. westermani* is widely distributed in the Far East, occurring as an important human infection in China, Japan, Vietnam, Korea, Formosa, the Philippines, and Thailand. It also occurs in South America in Brazil, Peru, Ecuador, and Venezuela.

Paragonimiasis is a chronic lung infection of man caused by this group of flukes, the adults living in cystic spaces in the lung. Reddish-brown plump oval flukes, they resemble in size a coffee bean (0.8 to 1.6 cm. long by 0.4 to 0.8 cm. wide). They are covered with little spines and live singly or in pairs in the lung parenchyma, feeding on host exudates. They live five to six years usually. Oval yellowish-brown operculated ova (85 μ by 35 μ) are coughed up in thick, bloodstained sputum. These hatch to produce a miracidium which invades specific snails. The cercariae subsequently produced by these snails encyst as metacercariae in the muscles and viscera of freshwater crabs. Man acquires the infection by eating the crabs raw or partly cooked. The larval flukes released from the metacercariae usually migrate to the lung via the peritoneal cavity, penetrating the diaphragm, but may mature in the abdomen or brain.

For many species man is not the definitive host, felines being preferred. For instance, other hosts apart from man for *P. westermani* are cats, tigers, leopards, mink, badgers, dogs, lions, and rats. *P. westermani* was discovered by Westerman in 1877 in a tiger in the Amsterdam zoo.

Pathogenesis and Pathology. The larval fluke tunnels into the lung at the periphery. There is an inflammatory reaction around it with many eosinophils. Later it forms a cystic space with a fibrous tissue wall. These cysts usually communicate with a bronchus and often become secondarily infected with abscess formation. Death of the fluke is often followed by calcification. Ova may be reaspirated with an eosinophilic inflammatory response and the formation of small lung granulomas.

Although the target organ for Paragonimus is the lung, it must be realized that often adults go astray, and if the invading species is one less adapted to man, this is more liable to happen. Thus a characteristic feature of *P. skrjabini* infection is migrating subcutaneous nodules that contain active flukes. Such granulomas in the subcutaneous tissue may require excision as in fascioliasis.

In the brain the temporal and occipital lobes are occasionally the site of an eosinophilic granuloma containing flukes and, in a few cases, ova. A transverse myelitis is known. Flukes in the peritoneal cavity produce adhesions and abscesses, and ulceration of the intestine occurs with ova in the stool. Adult and mature flukes have been found in many other organs, including intestine, spermatic cord, testis and scrotum, vagina, and muscles.

Clinical Manifestations. Lung infections are encountered with symptoms of persistent hemoptysis, breathlessness on exertion, pleural pain, and recurrent pulmonary infections. The condition is known as endemic hemoptysis. Clubbing of the fingers is common, and persistent rales may be heard over the affected lung segments as in nonparasitic bronchiectasis. A lung abscess may be present. Pneumothorax, pleural effusion, and empyema are rarer complications. Chest films early in the disease show infiltrations, but later dense nodular opacities or ring shadows indicate the site of the cysts. Pleural adhesions and calcification are late signs. Coexistent pulmonary tuberculosis occurs in some patients. There are rarely more than 20 parasites in the lungs.

It has been estimated that there were 5000 cases of cerebral paragonimiasis in South Korea in January 1968. Cerebral paragonimiasis may present signs of a space-occupying lesion with epilepsy and paresis of varying degrees. Ophthalmic signs are optic atrophy associated with papilledema or direct involvement with the inflammatory process. The cerebrospinal fluid shows a raised protein, and eosinophils are present. There may be calcifications present on skull roentgenograms; pneumoencephalography may show the site of a pseudotumor. Abdominal paragonimiasis is a difficult condition to diagnose, but an abdominal mass in a patient with lung disease should raise this suspicion.

Diagnosis. This rests mainly on finding ova in the sputum. One third of patients also have ova in the stools because of swallowed sputum or a coincidental intestinal lesion. Complement-fixation tests are useful, and positive results correlate closely with an active infection. Yokogawa has treated patients on this basis alone. The intradermal test remains positive for a long while after active infection and is not a reliable guide. Work goes on defining the antigenic structure of the parasite. The extent to which the Paragonimus antigen cross-reacts with other flukes is not clear.

Pulmonary paragonimiasis may resemble bronchiectasis, lung abscess, bronchial carcinoma, or — most important of all — pulmonary tuberculosis. Cerebral paragonimiasis mimics other space-occupying lesions but especially other helminths in the brain. These include Fasciola, *Schistosoma japonicum, Angiostrongylus cantonensis,* and hydatid.

Prognosis. Fatalities are rare, and lung lesions resolve spontaneously in five to ten years. Cerebral involvement may be associated with persistent epilepsy. Two per cent of lung paragonimiasis is complicated by pulmonary tuberculosis.

Treatment. Bithionol (Actamer, Biton) is 2,2'-thiobis(4,6-dichlorophenol) and is given orally in a dose of 30 mg. per kilogram of body weight on alternate days for 20 days. Skin reactions and gastrointestinal irritation are rarely severe enough to interrupt treatment. Results are far superior to those obtained with chloroquine or emetine drugs used in the past. Granulomas containing Paragonimus adults and ova may require surgical removal from the skin, testis, abdominal organs, or brain.

Prevention. It might be thought that it would be a simple matter to dissuade people from eating raw, fresh salted, pickled, or imperfectly cooked crabs and crayfish, but such local delicacies are not easily relinquished. Drunken crab, a favorite dish, involves immersing live crabs in alcohol prior to consumption. In Korea fresh crab juice is used as a home remedy in the treatment of measles.

Chang, H. T., Wang, C. W., Yü, C. F., Hsü, C. F., and Fang, J. C.: Paragonimiasis, a clinical study of 200 adult cases. Chin. Med. J., 77:3, 1958.

Sadun, E. H., and Buck, A. A.: Paragonimiasis in South Korea: Immunodiagnostic, epidemiological, clinical, roentgenologic and therapeutic studies. Amer. J. Trop. Med., 9:562, 1960.

Yokogawa, M.: Paragonimus and paragonimiasis. In Dawes, B. (ed.): Advances in Parasitology. London, Academic Press, 1969, Vol. 7, pp. 375–387.

Yokogawa, M., Okwa, T., Tsuji, M., Iwasaki, M., and Shigeyasu, M.: Chemotherapy of paragonimiasis with bithionol. III. The follow-up studies for 1 year after treatment with bithionol. Jap. J. Parasit., 11:103, 1962.

Yokogawa, S., Cort, W. W., and Yokogawa, M.: Paragonimus and paragonimiasis. Exp. Parasit., 10:81, 139, 1960.

INTESTINAL FLUKES
Philip D. Marsden

FASCIOLOPSIASIS
(Fasciolopsis buski)

Fasciolopsis buski is a large fleshy fluke, 3 cm. long and 1.2 cm. wide. It is found mainly in China but also in India, Indonesia, Thailand, Malaya, and Taiwan, normally as an intestinal parasite of pigs. The eggs are passed in the feces, and miracidium is released to penetrate a snail. The cercariae subsequently produced encyst as metacercariae on edible water plants called water caltrop or water chestnuts. The tubers and fruits of these plants are eaten fresh and raw from July to September and as they are peeled with the teeth, people are easily infected. The ponds are often fertilized with night soil or contaminated by pigs.

Most infections are asymptomatic, but foci of inflammation may occur at the site of attachment of the worms in the small intestine. In heavy infections abdominal pain may simulate a peptic ulcer, and there may be alternating diarrhea and constipation. A recent investigation does not suggest that malabsorption occurs. Intestinal stasis, ulceration, and even obstruction have occurred. Several thousand worms may be harbored by the patient, and in severe cases, especially in children, edema of the face and trunk has been described. The mechanism of this edema may be complex, as anemia and hypoproteinemia from blood loss in the bowel are possible. Definite allergic edemas do not appear to be reported in the literature, but there is a variable eosinophilia with heavy loads. Brown, in the previous edition, suggested that an absorption of toxic metabolites may be responsible for this edema. Ascites and death from exhaustion are rare.

Diagnosis. Diagnosis depends on finding the characteristic eggs in the stool. These are large, 130 to 140 μ by 80 to 85 μ, yellowish, and rather similar to Fasciola but with a smaller operculum. Occasionally an adult fluke may be vomited or passed in the stool. Facial edema may raise the question of differential diagnosis from trichinosis or the nephrotic syndrome.

Therapy. Tetrachloroethylene is effective (see hookworm therapy). Some advocate hexylresorcinol in an adult dose of 1 gram. Either drug should be given on an empty stomach. Not all the flukes may be eradicated, but the therapy can be repeated after a few days. Prevention entails cooking the offending plants, eradicating snails with molluscacides, and preventing fecal contamination of ponds.

OTHER INTESTINAL FLUKES

Two very small intestinal flukes—*Heterophyes heterophyes* and *Metagonimus yokogawai*—deserve mention. The former is found in Egypt, Tunisia, South China, India, and the Philippines, and the latter occurs in the Far East and Indonesia. Both are acquired by eating raw or inadequately cooked fish that contain the respective metacercariae. The adult flukes, 2 to 3 mm. long, are attached to the mucosa of the small intestine and are alleged to produce superficial inflammation and ulceration. Usually they are not present in sufficient numbers to produce symptoms. Very rarely eggs may gain access to the circulation and be found in internal organs. Usually they are passed in the stool and closely resemble Clonorchis eggs, which is perhaps their main importance. Both species can be treated with tetrachloroethylene as used for hookworm. Many species of the genus Echinostoma can also infect man in the Far East, but again rarely produce symptoms. Their eggs resemble those of Fasciola but are smaller. *Gastrodiscoides hominis* is a fascinating fluke with a large ventral sucker. Like the others, it can produce diarrhea. It occurs in Assam, Indochina, India, and Malaya. In Canada the eggs of *Metorchis conjunctus* are occasionally found in the stools of man.

Barlow, C. H.: The life cycle of the human intestinal fluke *Fasciolopsis buski* (Lankester). Amer. J. Hyg., Monograph 4, 1925.

Plaut, A. G., Kampanort-Sanyakorn, C., and Manning, G. S.: A clinical study of *Fasciolopsis buski* in Thailand. Trans. Roy. Soc. Trop. Med. Hyg., 63:470, 1969.

THE NEMATODES
(Roundworms)
Philip D. Marsden

GENERAL CONSIDERATIONS

Roundworms have an intestinal tract and a large body cavity bordered by a complex cuticle and containing the reproductive, nervous, and excretory systems. They have elongated, cylindrical, bilaterally symmetrical, smooth, nonsegmented, translucent, flesh-colored bodies, often filiform, with a pointed posterior and rounded anterior end. The Nematoda constitute the second largest class in the Animal Kingdom with 500,000 species. Many are free living. They are unisexual, and the female is usually bigger than the male. There is a great variation in size among the common human species. For example, in the intestinal nematodes a female Ascaris may reach 18 cm. whereas a female Strongyloides is smaller than 1 mm. Their bodies are muscular and require high carbohydrate reserves.

The common human nematodes can be roughly

divided into the *intestinal nematodes*, of which the common ones in order of importance are hookworms, Ascaris, Strongyloides, Trichuris, and Oxyuris, and the *tissue nematodes*. The latter group includes Trichinella and the various filarial worms. Heyneman has suggested that the life cycles of the intestinal nematodes of man can be shown to demonstrate an increasing dependence upon the host and a decrease in the proportion of metabolically active time in the free-living stages if they are arranged in a certain sequence. This sequence reflects different degrees of adaption by the parasite to the host and is presented in Table 1.

Rhabditis, a free-living nematode which rarely infects man, is but one step away from the relatively common *Strongyloides stercoralis*. Strongyloides represent the first stage in parasitic adaption. Hookworms are obligate parasites with no free-living stage. Both these nematodes and Ascaris have a phase of lung migration by immature larvae in the host, the explanation of which is not known. Ascaris, Trichuris, and Enterobius have progressively shorter oval maturation times. *Trichinella spiralis* is viviparous; the intestinal phase is transient, and the larvae persist in the host muscle.

Although the adult Trichinella organisms are intestinal nematodes, from a clinical viewpoint trichinosis can be considered as a tissue parasitic infection, as it is the larvae that produce the disease syndrome. The final break from the free-living state is illustrated by the filariae, in which the adult worms live in the host tissue, specific arthropods serving as the intermediate hosts. Whether filariae evolved from insect parasites or arose by adaption of intestinal parasites to insects following ingestion of eggs by coprophagic insects is a matter for speculation.

As in schistosomiasis, the number of worms present in the host determines the clinical manifestations, and many mild infections are asymptomatic. Quantitative techniques to determine adult worm load are commonly used in some nematode infections. Among the intestinal nematodes,

Strongyloides and Oxyuris infections cannot be quantitated owing to the variability in excretion of progeny. Ascaris produces so many eggs that quantitative techniques are usually not worthwhile, but hookworms and Trichuris eggs can be quantitated by a stool-dilution technique. For example, in Stoll's method 3 grams of stool is emulsified in 42 ml. of water in a special flask. Tenth normal sodium hydroxide may be used to soften hard feces. Glass beads and shaking after standing produces a uniform fine emulsion; 0.15 ml. volume of this is pipetted onto a glass slide, and all the eggs counted in this volume are equivalent to 0.01 gram of feces. Knowing the number of eggs per gram of stool, the total volume of stool, the egg output per female worm, and the usual sex ratio of the species population, it is possible to calculate the approximate worm load. Tissue helminths can also be quantitated in terms of larval output by expressing results in *Trichinella spiralis* infections as the number of larvae per gram of skeletal muscle or the number of microfilariae per milliliter of blood at a certain time of day. Onchocerca infections are likewise expressed as number of microfilariae per milligram of skin.

Another important feature of nematode infections is the frequency with which infections with nonhuman parasites are encountered as abortive infections, with larvae only rarely maturing to adults, thus suggesting helminths in a process of adaption into man. A number of such parasites will be mentioned in the text that follows, including the genera Oesophagostomum, Toxocara, Anasakis, Angiostrongylus, Dirofilaria, and others of clinical importance.

Heyneman's sequence is followed in the present discussion of the nematodes, although it is important to point out that, in terms of human suffering, hookworm and Bancroftian filariasis are by far the most serious infections.

Beaver, P. C.: Wandering nematodes as a cause of disability and disease. Amer. J. Trop. Med., 6:433, 1957.

Beaver, P. C.: The nature of visceral larva migrans. J. Parasit., 55:3, 1969.

Heyneman, D.: The life cycle of the nematodes parasitic in man: An evolutionary sequence. Med. J. Malaya, 20:249, 1966.

Marsden, P. D., and Hoskin, D. W.: Intestinal parasites, a progress report. Gastroenterology, 51:701, 1966.

Marsden, P. D., and Schultz, M. G.: Intestinal parasites, a progress report. Gastroenterology, 57:724, 1969.

TABLE 1. SEQUENCE FOR COMMON HUMAN INTESTINAL NEMATODES (HEYNEMAN)

Species	Details of Life Cycle
Strongyloides stercoralis	Most primitive since parasitism is irregular and exists in free-living adult stage in soil
Necator americanus *Ancylostoma duodenale*	Regular parasitism; no free-living adults, only larvae in soil
Ascaris lumbricoides	All hatched larval stages as well as adults in host; only eggs in soil
Trichuris trichiura	Similar to Ascaris, but newly hatched larvae do not migrate through host's body; all development confined to the intestine
Enterobius vermicularis	Eggs infective shortly after being laid; soil phase for eggs rarely involved
Trichinella spiralis	No eggs laid; larvae hatch within female, are deposited in mucosa, which they penetrate, and migrate via blood stream to encyst in tissues

INTESTINAL NEMATODES

STRONGYLOIDIASIS
(Cochin-China Diarrhea)

Definition. Strongyloidiasis is an infection of the small intestine with the invasive small nematode *Strongyloides stercoralis*. Most infections are asymptomatic, but a few can be life threatening; because of this, treatment is always necessary.

Etiology and Transmission. The parasitic female worm is small (2.2 mm. long) and lives in the mucosa of the intestinal villi. The parasitic male has rarely been observed, and experimental work suggests that parthenogenesis is the rule. The eggs produced by the female hatch rapidly, producing larvae in the small intestine, and these may reinvade the bowel mucosa before being voided in the feces (internal autoinfection). On the other hand, they may invade immediately after voiding via the perianal skin (external autoinfection). Other larvae become infective within hours of contact with the soil, and invasion of a fresh host occurs via the skin. Alternatively, voided larvae may develop into *free-living adults in the soil* (hence the necessity above to talk about adult parasites). These adults produce further generations of infective larvae in the soil. These alternative cycles make the life history of Strongyloides the most difficult one to grasp.

After skin penetration, the infective larvae undergo the same curious migration as hookworms via the venous system to the lungs (in 24 to 48 hours). Autoinfective forms may take a peritoneal or lymphatic route to the same site. From the lungs the developing larvae ascend the trachea, drop down into the stomach, and mature in the small intestine. Because of the frequency of autoinfection this nematode is self-perpetuating, and infections can last for 30 to 40 years. Man is the only common host, although primates and dogs can be experimentally infected.

Distribution. The parasite is cosmopolitan, but it is more frequent in the tropics. Local habitats where warmth, moisture, and lack of sanitation favor the free-living existence are endemic sites. Curiously enough in nearly all populations, however, the infection seems to be sporadic and an incidence comparable with that seen in hookworm infection is not encountered. Conceivably, however, this may be due to diagnostic difficulties, as mentioned below. This infection, like all intestinal parasitic infections, has been reported in high incidence from some mental institutions. Resistance to reinfection has been suggested by animal studies.

Pathology and Pathogenesis. The adult female worms burrow through the intestinal submucosa above the muscularis mucosa, depositing eggs as they go. They cause a chronic inflammatory cell infiltrate with many eosinophils. The rapidly hatching larvae are responsible for most of the pathologic findings, and their powers of penetration are such they can be distributed widely throughout the body. For reasons not clearly understood, the whole process may be accelerated (the so-called hyperinfective syndrome). Debility on the part of the host, malnutrition, or corticoid administration favors the development of this syndrome. Obviously prolonged bowel transit time would increase the possibility of internal autoinfection. Inflammation of the small bowel may be so intense as to cause malabsorption, thickening, and edema visible roentgenographically. The mesenteric lymph nodes enlarge, and ulceration and necrosis of the mucosa may occur. The lungs and liver may also show abscess formation,

and fatty changes in the liver may indicate primary or secondary malnutrition. In recent years several series of fatal cases have been described from the West Indies, Brazil, and Africa. Acute small bowel obstruction has been described, as well as *E. coli* bacteremia with meningitis, the latter perhaps arising from bacteria being introduced from the bowel on migrating larvae. The gut may be invaded at any level by larvae, and gastric and colonic involvement are well documented. Rarely larvae are found in other abdominal organs. Involvement of the kidney, heart, and endocrine glands is described.

Clinical Manifestations. Dermal invasion, either as a result of primary exposure or by external autoinfection, may be characterized by linear, erythematous, urticarial wheals, which are the sites of migrating larvae. Particularly common around the buttocks, they may occur anywhere, and are often recognized for what they are, as they are relatively fast moving. It is a form of cutaneous larva migrans (see Hookworm Disease). Lung invasion may be associated with signs of bronchospasm or bronchopneumonia. These may be short-lived or recurrent if several waves of larvae arrive in the lung. Hemoptysis is not uncommon as the larvae burst through the pulmonary alveoli. They may be found in the sputum, and there is usually a marked eosinophilia. Bowel involvement may give rise to a variety of clinical manifestations, but again it must be stressed that many light infections are asymptomatic. The most common gastrointestinal symptom is epigastric pain, which is often to the right of the midline, constant, and of a dull, aching character. Tenderness may be present on abdominal palpation over the duodenum. In heavy infections diarrhea is common; it may not be just the result of inflammation but may also reflect the coexistent malabsorption. Upper abdominal pain and vomiting from the involved upper gut are frequent, but intestinal obstruction is rare. Marked large bowel involvement may resemble ulcerative colitis. In the hyperinfective syndrome death may result from disseminated inflammatory lesions, often with superimposed bacterial infection.

Diagnosis. Strongyloidiasis must always be thought of in patients with unexplained eosinophilia. In an unpublished series of patients with obscure eosinophilia in a New York hospital this was the second most common cause after drug reactions. The high eosinophilia is probably associated with recurrent larval invasion. The diagnosis is made by finding the larvae in the stool, preferably by using a concentration technique. Unfortunately there are a number of difficulties. In warm climates fresh stool should be examined, as hookworm larvae hatch quickly from the eggs; they can be differentiated, but only by an expert. The excretion of larvae in strongyloidiasis is intermittent, and several stool specimens should be examined. The Baermann funnel technique and filter paper culture technique have facilitated diagnosis. Sometimes larvae are demonstrated in the duodenal aspirate or sputum when other techniques have failed. Jejunal biopsy may show larvae and adult parasites in section in the mucosa. The filarial complement-fixation test is invariably positive and of diagnostic help in difficult cases. Barium studies may show thickening and deformities of the small bowel owing to inflammatory edema

Treatment. As so little is known about the conditions governing development of serious infections, all patients should be treated with thiabendazole, 25 mg. per kilogram twice daily for two days. Given orally, this drug is effective, with few side effects. The tablets should be chewed; they have an orange taste. Assessment of parasitologic cure requires repeated stool examinations using special techniques. The eosinophilia should fall within eight weeks. The prognosis is good in otherwise healthy subjects, but may be poor in the exceptional circumstances described above. Prophylaxis involves avoiding unsanitary conditions when infection is likely. Strongyloides of nutria and raccoons have caused transient creeping eruptions (cutaneous larva migrans) in Louisiana trappers.

Bras, G., Richards, R. C., Irvine, R. A., Milner, P. F. A., and Ragbeer, M. M. S.: Infection with *Strongyloides stercoralis* in Jamaica. Lancet, 2:1257, 1964.
Stemmerman, G. N.: Strongyloidiasis in migrants. Pathological and clinical considerations. Gastroenterology, 53:59, 1967.
Tanaka, H.: Experimental and epidemiological strongyloidiasis of Amaini Oshima Island. Jap. J. Exp. Med., 28:159, 1958.

CAPILLARIASIS

Until recently the genus Capillaria appeared to infect man so rarely that it would not have merited inclusion in a general work of this kind. The most common form, *Capillaria hepatica* (less than 20 cases reported), was recognized by finding Trichuris-like eggs encapsulated in the liver. Species of the genus had also been reported in the lungs and skin of man.

Recently, however, a new parasite of man *Capillaria philippinensis*, has been described from the northern Philippines, where more than 1000 cases and 100 deaths have been confirmed to date. Patients with intestinal capillariasis have colicky abdominal pain, chronic diarrhea, muscle wasting, and edema, which may lead to debility and death in four months. Clinical studies have shown the presence of a severe protein-losing enteropathy in these patients with malabsorption of fats and sugars.

A tiny nematode (3 to 4 mm. by 0.03 to 0.04 mm.), *C. philippinensis* is confined to the small intestine, particularly the jejunum. The eggs detected in the stool are similar to *Trichuris trichiura* (to which the Capillaria are closely related) but are smaller, are more oval, and have less prominent bipolar plugs. There is evidence that hatching may occur in the small intestine, and tissue invasion of the bowel similar to strongyloidiasis has been noted at postmortem examination. The mode of transmission of the disease is not clear but is thought to be direct from man to man, an intermediate host not being involved. It has been speculated, however, that crustaceans may act as paratenic or transport hosts.

Apart from intravenous feeding in severe cases, success in eliminating this parasite has been reported by using high doses of thiabendazole.

Detels, R., Gutman, L., Jaramillo, J., Zerrudo, E., Banzon, T., Valera, J., Murrell, K. D., Cross, J., and Dizon, J. J.: An epidemic of intestinal capillariasis in man. Amer. J. Trop. Med., 18:676, 1969.
Whalen, G. E., Rosenberg, E. B., Strickland, G. T., Gutman, R. A., Cross, J. H., Watten, R. H., Uylangco, C., Dizon, J. J.: Intestinal capillariasis, a new disease in man. Lancet, 1.13, 1969.

HOOKWORM DISEASE
(Ancylostomiasis, Miner's Anemia)

Definition. The two common hookworms of man, *Ancylostoma duodenale* and *Necator americanus*, attach themselves to the small bowel by their buccal capsules and suck blood, thereby causing chronic blood loss. Depending on their number and the iron stores of the host, a variable degree of anemia often results. A distinction is made between hookworm infection when the load is too light to produce symptoms and hookworm disease.

Pathogenic Chain. *Etiology.* The human hookworms measure about 1 cm. in length, the female being slightly longer than the male, which is recognizable by an expanded posterior end, the copulating bursa. *A. duodenale* is larger than *Necator americanus*, and the two species are differentiated most easily by the fact that *A. duodenale* has two pairs of teeth in its buccal capsule, whereas *N. americanus* has a pair of cutting plates only. The eggs of the two species are indistinguishable and are passed in the feces. In warm moist soil the larva hatches within 48 hours. The rhabditiform larva has a free-living cycle in the soil, feeding on bacteria, during which time it molts twice. The filariform larvae resulting from the second molt are the infective stage for man and can survive several months in favorable conditions. They tend to migrate up grass stems or gain any elevation up to 3 feet, and on coming into contact with the skin of man, quickly penetrate it, enter the blood stream, and are transported to the lungs. Like Strongyloides, there they leave the vascular system and emerge into the alveoli, migrate up the bronchi and trachea, and down the esophagus to reach the small intestine where maturity is attained. Eggs appear in the stool five or more weeks after invasion, and the adults live one to nine years.

Epidemiology. Over 400 million people have hookworm infections, but in the majority the worm load is small. *Ancylostoma duodenale* is the Old World hookworm, being prevalent in Europe, North Africa, and the Middle and Far East. *Necator americanus* is found more in the New World and tropical Africa. During the past 30 years both parasites have become widely distributed, and rigid geographic demarcations are not possible.

The survival of larvae is favored by a damp sandy soil, high in humus content at a temperature of 24 to 32° C. Promiscuous defecation and the absence of shoes are the chief factors responsible for infections. Such conditions occur in mines as well as on the surface of the ground. Urban people tend to have less hookworm than agricultural rural workers at locations where night soil is often used as fertilizer. Infection can be acquired by ingesting or handling contaminated vegetables. Coffee, banana, sugar cane, rice, and sweet potato fields are ideal for the growth and development of larvae. Often one locality is used as a communal latrine in the area, and people reinfect themselves by visiting these sites again and again. *The distinction between hookworm infection and hookworm disease is important.* Methods of estimating the intensity of the infection show that in endemic areas most patients have few worms and no significant anemia. Those who have hookworm anemia have more worms, and these heavy infections could be the result of repeated exposure or a failure of immunity on the part of the host. With canine hookworm, small repeated infections give almost complete immunity. Antibodies have been demonstrated in sera of infected patients.

Pathology and Pathogenesis. Inflammatory cell infiltration is seen at the site of penetration of the hookworm larvae, and in the lungs small hemorrhages occur with eosinophilic and leukocytic infiltration. An eosinophilia is present during the invasive phase. The main feature of the established disease is the active sucking of blood by the worms. They create a negative pressure in the buccal capsule and suck in a piece of mucosa which acts as both an anchorage and a source of blood. It is still not clear what hookworms abstract from the blood. Vital preparations in vitro show red cells being vigorously expelled from the posterior end. Ancylostoma sucks between 0.16 and 0.34 ml. of blood per day and Necator, 0.03 to 0.05. The development of anemia depends upon three factors: the iron content of the diet, the state of the iron reserves, and the intensity and duration of infection.

When iron intake is high, a heavy worm load is needed to produce a significant anemia. Up to 60 per cent of the iron from the hemoglobin extracted by the hookworm is reabsorbed in the intestine. At open operation small punctate hemorrhagic spots are encountered at the site of attachment. In addition to anemia, hypoalbuminemia occurs owing to a combination of blood loss and a low rate of albumin synthesis, possibly associated with anoxia affecting liver cell function. Malabsorption is said to occur in a few cases with partial villous atrophy and chronic inflammatory cell infiltration of the lamina propria.

Clinical Manifestations. The site of skin penetration by the larvae is associated with pruritus and the development of an erythematous papular eruption (ground itch) which may last several days or even longer, depending on the host's immune response. Within a week after penetration the patient may have a transient asthmatic attack, but this is not as commonly seen as in invasive ascariasis.

Established hookworm disease is associated with general symptoms of anemia, weakness, fatigue, dyspnea, palpitation, and mental and physical retardation. Pica may be noted. On examination the skin and mucus membrane are pale. Peripheral edema is due possibly to a variety of factors, namely, hypoalbuminemia, a rise of capillary venous pressure, and tissue anoxia. In severe cases there is evidence of congestive cardiac failure. The pulse is rapid with a high pulse pressure. On auscultation of the enlarged heart, a third heart sound and an ejection type of systolic murmur are commonly heard; regurgitant systolic and even diastolic murmurs may occur and disappear when the anemia is corrected. For this reason it is very unwise to diagnose a valvular lesion clinically in such anemic patients until that anemia has been corrected. The hemoglobin may be very low (2 grams per 100 ml.) and the patient still ambulant. The patient may complain of upper abdominal pain, and radiologic changes suggestive of a duodenitis have been reported.

Diagnosis and Differential Diagnosis. Stool microscopy, either by a direct smear or by a concentration technique, reveals hookworm ova. Quantitation of the egg excretion enables the physician to decide whether the patient has a significant worm load. This is done by diluting a known volume of stool and counting a sample (Stoll technique). Hookworm ova are 60 to 70μ long by 35 to 40μ wide and have a characteristic morphology with a clear shell and developing embryo inside. They must be distinguished, however, from both Trichostrongylus and *Ternidens deminutus*, both of which have larger eggs. Test tube cultivation of ova and differentiation of the resultant larvae are of value in doubtful cases. A skin test using an extract of *Necator americanus* larvae of standard nitrogen content has proved useful in screening a hookworm-infected population. Fluorescent antibody, complement-fixation, and hemagglutination tests have been developed but have little clinical application.

The anemia of hookworm disease is a classic iron deficiency anemia with a low hemoglobin, mean corpuscular hemoglobin concentration and serum iron, and a high iron-binding capacity. On the film the red cells are microcytic and hypochromic. Folic acid deficiency may sometimes be superimposed on macrocytosis. The serum albumin is low, and liver function tests may be abnormal. In the edematous patient there may be confusion with kwashiorkor, wet beriberi, or the nephrotic syndrome. The anemia has to be differentiated from other iron deficiency anemias.

Treatment. Tetrachloroethylene in a dose of 0.1 mg. per kilogram of body weight is effective (maximum of 5 ml. in a single dose). It is usually dispensed in 1-ml. gelatin capsules or in a liquid that should be kept in the refrigerator in a dark bottle. It is given in the morning on an empty stomach; all food should be withheld for six hours and any fatty foods withheld for the rest of the day.

Repeated treatments may be necessary. Vertigo, vomiting, and dizziness may follow therapy. Bephenium hydroxynaphthoate (Alcopar) is more expensive but is being increasingly used. The standard dose for an adult is 5 grams containing 2.5 grams of bephenium base; it is taken as granules in a glass of water on an empty stomach. Three daily doses may achieve total eradication. Loose stools, nausea, and vomiting have followed treatment. Both drugs will remove a large number of worms at the first dose, but to get rid of the last 5 to 10 per cent is often very difficult. In many areas total eradication may not be desirable or necessary. In general, tetrachloroethylene is said to be more effective in *Necator americanus* infections. If Ascaris are also present, Alcopar is preferred, or both Ascaris and hookworm will respond to thiabendazole. Tetrachloroethylene irritates Ascaris and may cause migration.

The anemia responds well to ferrous sulfate, 200 or 400 mg. three times daily. Occasionally the hemoglobin is so low, or there is an associated acute infection, that the patient presents in extremis owing to heart failure. Pregnancy may also precipitate acute heart failure. Intraperitoneal blood transfusion or exchange transfusions have been life-saving. The prognosis is good in most cases. It is wise to delay treating the hookworm infection until the hemoglobin is above 50 per cent after oral iron. Without treatment of the worm infection, the anemia will relapse when iron therapy is discontinued. *Prevention* involves the sanitary disposal of human excreta and the prevention of soil pollution. The wearing of shoes cuts down the opportunities for infection.

Gilles, H. M., Williams, E. J. W., and Ball, P. A. J.: Hookworm infection and anemia. Quart J. Med., 33:1, 1964.
Roche, M., and Layrisse, M.: Nature and causes of hookworm anemia. Amer. J. Trop. Med., 15:1031, 1966.
Stoll, N. R.: On endemic hookworm, where do we stand to-day? Exp. Parasit., 12:241, 1962.
Stoll, N. R.: For hookworm diagnosis is finding one egg enough? Ann. N.Y. Acad. Sci., 98:712, 1962.

CUTANEOUS LARVA MIGRANS
(Creeping Eruption)

Cutaneous larva migrans is considered at this point because its most common cause is *Ancylostoma braziliense*, although it may be produced by a variety of other helminths. It is characterized by an erythematous, serpiginous, intracutaneous track or burrow, the anterior end of which is observed to migrate at the rate of 1 to 2 cm. per day. There is often intense irritation, and secondary infection may result from scratching. This migration is due to the infective larva of *A. braziliense* (the cat and dog hookworm), which does not visceralize in man but wanders around in the skin. This migration may last for 2 to 50 weeks before the larva dies. Rarely some larvae reach the lungs, causing high eosinophilia and patchy pulmonary infiltration.

Patients are often infected by lying on beaches contaminated by dog or cat feces. The feet, legs, and hands are the most common sites, and the appearance of the lesion is usually diagnostic. It is virtually impossible to remove the larva from the skin.

Ancylostoma braziliense is found in the southern United States, Central America and tropical South America, as well as in tropical Africa and parts of the Far East, especially the Malay peninsula. There have been several reports of the worm maturing in the gut of man and eggs appearing in the feces, so there is not an absolute host specificity. Two other dog hookworms, *Uncinaria stenocephala* and *Ancylostoma caninum*, can produce similar lesions. Occasionally the ground itch of the two common human hookworms may persist and resemble creeping eruption in immune subjects.

The larva migrans track of *Strongyloides stercoralis* tends to be a short line, erythematous and rapidly moving (larva currens). Rodent Strongyloides may produce similar lesions but no mature worms. A form of myiasis with the horse bot fly maggot (Gasterophilus) can produce a larger deeper migrating form of cutaneous larva migrans.

Treatment. Thiabendazole by mouth, 25 mg. per kilogram per day for two days, is usually effective. If not, the dose can be doubled and repeated. Alternatively, the advancing end of the burrow can be treated with topical thiabendazole sprinkled on elastoplast or in a cream containing 15 per cent thiabendazole powder in a hydrosoluble base. This drug has completely superseded the other, more unsatisfactory treatments such as ethyl chloride spray and Hetrazan.

Battistini, F.: Treatment of creeping eruption with topical thiabendazole. Texas Rep. Biol Med., 27 (Supplement 2):645, 1969.
Beaver, P. C.: Larva migrans. Exp. Parasit., 5:587, 1956.
Stone, O. J.: Systemic and topical thiabendazole for creeping eruption. Texas Rep. Biol. Med., 27 (Supplement 2):659, 1969.

GNATHOSTOMIASIS

Although Gnathostoma species are more closely related to Ascaris, this group is mentioned at this point because it also presents as *creeping eruptions* or, more commonly, as *migratory swelling in the subcutaneous tissues*. More than 100 human infections with the immature stages of *Gnathostoma spinigerum* have been reported from the Far East, particularly Thailand. Normally a parasite of wild felines, dogs, and foxes, Gnathostoma infects man when he eats the larvae in undercooked fish (fermented fish is a Thai delicacy). The larva causes a migratory swelling, often in the subcutaneous tissues, associated with an intense eosinophilia. Occasionally the larva comes to the skin surface and resembles cutaneous larva migrans, but the area of involvement is larger. Sometimes the larva burrows deep into the internal tissues and may lodge in the gut wall or elsewhere and produce an abscess. Indeed, secondary infection frequently occurs. Brain involvement in fatal cases with eosinophilic meningitis has been reported. Eye involvement with iritis and orbital cellulitis is also described. If the worm does not reach the body surface, the symptoms can persist for months. Some recommend extraction of the worm, but Hetrazan has been said to be useful. There is insufficient experience with thiabendazole thus far to permit a definite statement of its value, but its trial seems reasonable.

Miyazaki, I.: On the genus Gnathostoma and human gnathostomiasis with special reference to Japan. Exp. Parasitol., 9:338, 1960.

OESOPHAGOSTOMIASIS

Oesophagostomiasis is more closely related to hookworm and Strongyloides than to Gnathostoma, but like Gnathostoma it may rarely form a tumor in the human gut wall. Again, man is not the definitive host. The infection is often carried by pet monkeys, and the clinical picture is usually one of intestinal obstruction. Bacterial infection of the tumor nodule is common. Surgical excision of the tumor shows it to contain worms of Oesophagostomum species.

Gordon, J. A., Ross, C. M. D., and Affleck, A.: Abdominal emergency due to an oesophagostome. Ann. Trop. Med. Parasit., 63:161, 1969.
Haaf, E., and Van Soest, A. H.: Oesophagostomiasis of man in North Ghana. Trop. Geogr. Med., 16:49, 1964.

ASCARIASIS

Definition. Ascariasis is infection with *Ascaris lumbricoides*, the large roundworm of man. The adults mature in the small intestine and can produce disease by intestinal obstruction or migration. The passage of larvae through the lungs may result in pneumonitis.

Etiology. Ascariasis is a large whitish nematode; the female (20 to 35 cm.) is larger than the male (15 to 30 cm.), which often has a curly tail. The vulva of the female is situated ventrally at the junction of the anterior and middle thirds of the worm. Frequent copulation is necessary to ensure the continuous production of fertile eggs. A female worm has a reproductive capacity of 26 to 27 million eggs and a daily output of 200,000. The life span of the adult worms is relatively short (12 to 24 months). They are not attached to the wall of the jejunum, but bridge themselves across the lumen and by their muscle tone maintain themselves against the fecal stream. In a largely anaerobic environment they obtain nourishment from the semidigested food of the host and possibly from epithelial cells of the intestinal mucosa. The high protein and vitamin content of the parasite suggests that they deprive the host of nutrients.

The brownish eggs with a thick shell and albuminous coat become infective ten days after being passed in the stool. Fertile and infertile eggs have a different morphology. On ingestion of infective eggs by man, the larvae hatch in the small intestine, and, penetrating its wall, are carried by the blood and lymphatic system to the lungs. It has been suggested that this migration is necessitated by the need for oxygen, which is not available in the intestine, at this stage of the life cycle. Here, like hookworm and Strongyloides, the larvae migrate up the respiratory passages to the epiglottis and down to the esophagus. A new generation of eggs appears in the feces approximately two months after the ingestion of embryonated eggs.

Epidemiology. Although cosmopolitan, this worm is most abundant in the tropics, where sanitation is poor. One in every four people in the world is infected with *Ascaris lumbricoides*. The eggs are killed by direct sunlight and temperatures above 45° C.; nevertheless, under optimal conditions they may remain viable for one year. The eggs pass unchanged through the intestine of animals with the possible exception of the pig. The pig Ascaris, *Ascaris suum*, is morphologically identical to the human Ascaris, and there is some evidence that cross infections can occur. The susceptibility to infection is greatest in childhood, reaching a peak at puberty, and transmission is by fecal contamination of food and drink. Circulating antibodies appear to play some role in host immunity.

Pathology and Clinical Manifestations. Light infections of a dozen or so worms often pass unnoticed, especially in adults. During the phase of larval migration, especially if many eggs have been ingested, respiratory symptoms may appear 4 to 16 days after infection. The pulmonary migration of larvae is associated with fever, cough, occasionally hemoptysis, and either crepitations or more rarely the signs of consolidation on auscultation of the chest. The sputum contains larvae and eosinophils, and there is a high blood eosinophilia. Sections of the lungs at this stage would show larvae in the bronchioles with patchy infiltration of alveoli with polymorphs and eosinophil leukocytes. Aberrant larvae may lodge in the liver, producing granulomatous lesions and hepatomegaly. More rarely such larvae, which fail to re-enter the circulation, are found in other abdominal organs.

When adult worms are present in the intestine, the established infection is often associated with occasional colicky abdominal pain and some abdominal distention. These adults may produce complications by mechanical effects within the gastrointestinal tract, or by wandering outside it, or more rarely by producing allergic manifestations in a sensitized host.

Heavy loads of worms may particularly be associated with intestinal obstruction, intussusception, volvulus, appendicitis, and hernial strangulation. A bolus of Ascaris may be a common cause of intestinal obstruction in childhood in an endemic area. Before undertaking bowel surgery, an Ascaris infection should always be excluded, because these worms are difficult to control once the bowel is opened, and considerable peritoneal soiling may result. Migration of adult worms may occur spontaneously or as a result of some stimulus such as fever or tetrachloroethylene. The Ascaris adults may perforate a suture line or cause a bile or pancreatic duct obstruction. Occasionally they migrate into the stomach and are vomited up, or pass down into the large bowel and out with the stool. Adult worms have been described issuing from umbilical fistulas, and even from the nose or ear. Obstruction of the bile duct is associated with cholangitis, and eggs may be deposited in the liver. *A. lumbricoides* has been said by some to be second only to *E. histolytica* in producing liver abscesses. Blockage of the pancreatic duct results in acute pancreatitis. Once the adult worm has left the bowel, it often dies, releasing foreign protein that may produce a reaction in a sensitized host. These reactions range from facial edema and giant urticaria to acute local necrosis and anaphylaxis. Laboratory personnel who work with Ascaris invariably become sensitized to the worms. Young pigs infected with Ascaris do not gain weight normally, and it is possible that heavy loads of human Ascaris may affect children similarly, as the worms will consume much food in the actively growing phase.

Diagnosis. Examination of the feces reveals the characteristic ova. Usually in view of the number of ova produced, they can be found in ordinary direct smear. Although fertilized eggs are easy to recognize, unfertilized eggs assume bizarre shapes and may be mistaken for debris. Rarely one encounters infections of immature worms or only male worms. Sometimes an infection is diagnosed in barium meal examination, as the barium can be seen in the Ascaris gut. Although many serologic tests have been developed for Ascaris, including complement-fixation, hemagglutination, and gel diffusion, they are seldom used for diagnostic purposes.

Treatment. Piperazine citrate is the drug of choice in the treatment of Ascaris infestations. The piperazine salts are simple, safe, and efficient. They act by blocking the neuromuscular junctions of the worm. The paralyzed worm can no longer bridge itself across the intestinal lumen and is carried along in the fecal stream and passed in the stool. Piperazine citrate is given in a dose of 75 mg. per kilogram to a maximal single dose of 4 grams. This will clear 75 per cent of patients of their worms, but the dose can be repeated the following day with safety. No special preparation or purgation is necessary. Neurotoxic effects from piperazine have been reported in patients with renal failure who cannot excrete the drug.

Thiabendazole in the same dose as for strongyloidiasis and Alcopar in the same dose as for hookworms are both effective in ascariasis as well. In the presence of Ascaris plus one or another of these intestinal parasites, single drug therapy may be preferred. However, neither of these drugs is as effective in ascariasis as piperazine. In multiple intestinal helminthic infections, Ascaris should always be treated first.

When examining stools for ova after therapy, it must be remembered that eggs may be passed in the stool for up to a week after the worms have been eradicated owing to the delay in the colonic circulation of feces.

The following regimen is suggested to deal with intestinal obstruction owing to Ascaris. Initially conservative treatment with nasogastric suction, intravenous fluids, and piperazine therapy should be tried for 48 hours. If no improvement follows, at laparotomy it is often possible to manipulate the bolus of worms into the large bowel through the terminal ileum. Only if this is not possible should enterotomy and worm extraction be performed.

Prevention. This consists of disposal of human excreta in sanitary privies and toilets. Children must be taught to use these facilities and avoid contamination of food with ova.

Chang, C. C., and Han C. T.: Biliary ascariasis in childhood. A clinical analysis of 788 cases. Chin. Med. J. (Peking), 85: 167, 1966.

Gelpi, A. P., and Mustafa, A.: Seasonal pneumonitis with eosinophilia: A study of larval ascariasis in Saudi Arabia. Am. J. Trop. Med., 16:646, 1967.

Lejkina, E. S.: Research in Ascaris immunity and immunodiagnosis. Bull. WHO, 32:699, 1965.

Otto, G. F., and Cort, W. W.: The distribution and epidemiology of human ascariasis in the United States. Amer. J. Hyg., 16.657, 1934.

The Control of Ascariasis. World Health Organization Technical Report, Series No. 379, 1967.

TOXOCARIASIS
(Visceral Larva Migrans)

Toxocariasis is an accidental human infection with the cat and dog Ascaris (*Toxocara cati* and *Toxocara canis*). The eggs of these species are infective two to three weeks after being passed, and if ingested by man the second stage larvae emerge. These penetrate the intestinal wall and reach the liver. The majority remain in the liver but others migrate to other organs, particularly the brain and the eye. Rarely they complete their cycle of development in man and produce adult worms in the bowel. Children are particularly susceptible because of more frequent soiling of the fingers and habits of playing with puppies, in which the incidence of infection is very high. Initially reported from the southern United States, these parasites are common in dogs and cats in many parts of the world. Although many reports have come from North America and Europe, it is likely that this syndrome also occurs in other parts of the world.

The migrating larvae produce "eosinophilic trails" and tissue inflammation in the affected organ. Usually a granuloma forms with epithelial cells, fibroblasts, lymphocytes, plasma cells, and occasional giant cells. A fibrous capsule eventually encloses the larva, which may remain alive for months. The granulomas can be seen macroscopically as small grayish-white spots. Such granulomas have been found in the lungs, eyes, brain, heart, kidney, and striated muscle.

The most common clinical form is that of a patient with a mild fever and tender hepatomegaly. Routine investigation reveals a marked eosinophilia (50 to 60 per cent), and further questioning often brings to light a history of contact with dogs. These signs and symptoms may persist for 18 months. The serum globulins may be elevated and anti-τ globulins are found. Another clinical form is as an *endophthalmitis* with a space-occupying granuloma visibly distorting the contour of the retina on funduscopy. In the past such granulomas were often mistaken for retinoblastomas, and the eye was removed. Several such series of "retinoblastomas" have been examined, and many of the tumors were found to consist of granulomas containing Toxocara larvae. Many mild infections are asymptomatic.

The syndrome of tender hepatomegaly and eosinophilia must be distinguished from invasive schistosomiasis or fascioliasis. A variety of nematodes can produce visceral larva migrans in special circumstances, among them *Ascaris lumbricoides, Necator americanus,* and *Strongyloides stercoralis.* Other nonhuman nematodes such as Gnathostoma, Capillaria, Hepaticola, and Dirofilaria may be involved in granuloma formation in the liver. Sarcoidosis and periarteritis nodosa may mimic this disease. Blind liver biopsy is seldom helpful, but where facilities exist, direct visualization of surface granulomas of the liver with a peritoneoscope may enable biopsy of a granuloma to be made. A definitive diagnosis can often be made by examination of this granuloma. A diagnosis of second-stage rhabdoid Toxocara larva can be made on a section at mid-gut level, showing a maximal width of 12 to 20 μ and lateral alae. A variety of serologic tests are available but lack specificity, as they cross-react with other helminthic infections. However, in areas where such infections are rarely encountered, a fluorescent antibody test or an indirect hemagglutination test may be helpful.

Treatment. Diethylcarbamazine (*vide infra,* Bancroftian Filariasis) has been used and does kill some larvae in the tissues of infected mice. A resolution of symptoms has followed the use of thiabendazole in one case in a dose of 25 mg. per kilogram twice daily for seven days. The prognosis is good if the source of infection is removed by treating the dog with piperazine. Care must be taken to worm pets regularly, especially puppies, if they are in contact with children.

Huntley, C. C., Costas, M. C., Williams, R. C., Lyerly, A. D., and Watson, R. G.: Anti-γ-globulin factors in visceral larva migrans. J.A.M.A., 197:552, 1966.
Kagan, I. G.: The serological diagnosis of visceral larva migrans. Clin. Pediat., 7:508, 1968.
Mok, C. H.: Visceral larva migrans: A discussion based on a review of the literature. Clin. Paediat., 7:565, 1968.
Nelson, J. D., McConnell, T. H., and Moore, D. V.: Thiabendazole therapy of visceral larva migrans: A case report. Amer. J. Trop. Med., 15:903, 1966.
Woodruff, A. W.: Toxocariasis. Brit. Med. J., 3:663, 1970.

ANISAKIASIS

Although the full life cycle is still unknown, it appears that man is occasionally infected by the ascarid *Anisakis marina,* which has its larval stages in herrings. The adult worms develop in marine mammals such as seals, dolphins, porpoises, and whales. Man is infected by eating raw or undercooked herrings, and infection has occurred where such food is considered a delicacy, namely, north eastern Europe (Denmark particularly) and Japan. The larvae appear to burrow into the wall of the stomach or small bowel to produce an eosinophilic granulomatous mass that may be mistaken for a malignancy. Perforation of the bowel wall has been reported, as has stenosis following granuloma formation. Usually the correct diagnosis is not made until the specimen is examined after surgical resection.

Van Thiel, P. H.: The final hosts of the herring worm *Anisakis marina.* Trop. Geogr. Med., 18:310, 1966.
Yokogawa, M., and Yoshimura, H.: Clinicopathologic studies on larval anisakiasis in Japan. Amer. J. Trop. Med., 16:723, 1967.

TRICHURIASIS
(Whipworm Infection, Trichocephaliasis)

In trichuriasis, the adult worms are shaped like a whip. The long anterior threadlike portion of the worm consists of a cellular esophagus buried deep into the submucosa of the colon, making it difficult to dislodge. These adults are pinkish-gray and are 30 to 50 mm. long. The male is distinguished from the female by its coiled caudal extremity. The female produces 5000 to 10,000 eggs per day. The eggs are 50 to 55 microns long, golden brown with prominent characteristic bipolar plugs. Under favorable conditions they become infective in three to five weeks, and when ingested by man the first stage larva hatches in the small intestine and spends three to ten days in the intestinal villi. Then it passes down to the large bowel where it matures in 30 to 90 days. The adult worms live for years.

Of worldwide distribution, trichuriasis is most frequently encountered in the tropics. Often in a particular endemic locality, the infestation has a patchy distribution because of dense shade, heavy rainfall, and the clay soils that hold water as well as fecal pollution, thus facilitating transmission. In the United States, whipworm infection is found in the southern Appalachians and southwestern Louisiana; it is not infrequent in Puerto Rico.

The great majority of infections are asymptomatic; only heavy loads of worms cause clinical illness. The worms are distributed throughout the colon and rectum, and heavy infections may be associated with colic and diarrhea with blood. *Trichuris trichiura* abstracts 0.005 ml. of blood per worm from the host each day. In children in precarious iron balance a load of over 800 worms may be associated with an iron deficiency anemia. Up to 5000 worms have been recovered from heavily infected children. In such infections rectal prolapse may complicate the diarrhea, and the appearance of the congested mucosa associated with the whitish bodies of the worms has been described as the "coconut cake" rectum. Early infections may be associated with a mild blood eosinophilia. Trichuris has been implicated as a predisposing factor to acute amebic dysentery by causing an initial breach of the mucosa, this suggestion being based on finding a higher incidence of Trichuris in patients with acute bowel amebiasis than is normal for the area. Trichuris is often associated with other helminthic and protozoal infections. Appendicitis and peritonitis with the presence of worms in the peritoneal cavity have been described.

Diagnosis is made by finding the eggs in the feces, either on direct smear or by concentration methods. In the rare Trichuris dysentery the eggs may appear in aggregates in the mucoid stools, together with eosinophils and Charcot-Leyden crystals. Egg counts below 10,000 per gram are unlikely to be associated with symptoms.

Treatment is not very satisfactory. Dithiazanine iodide was formerly used, but it has caused nine deaths, and has been withdrawn from the market. Treatment should be confined to heavily infected individuals presenting with symptoms and to those employed as food handlers, nurses, and so forth. Thiabendazole in a similar dose to that used in Strongyloides (25 mg. per kilogram of body weight twice daily for two days) eradicates the infection in one third of cases, and the course can be repeated after one week. Stilbazium iodine (Monopar) appears to have a slightly higher cure rate, but is still under trial. Dichlorvos, a cholinesterase inhibitor, has been shown to be very effective in adults, but further trials are needed.

Boon, W. H., and Hoh, K. K.. Severe whipworm infection in children. Singapore Med. J., 2:34, 1966.
Franz, K. H., Schneider, W. J., and Pohlman, M. H.: Clinical trials with triabendazole against intestinal nematodes infecting humans. Amer. J. Trop. Med., 14:383, 1965.
Jung, R. C., and Jelliffe, D. B.: The clinical picture and treatment of whipworm infection. W. Afr. Med. J., 1:11, 1952.
Layrisse, M., Apariedo, L., Martinez Torres, C., and Roche, M.: Blood loss due to infection with *Trichuris trichiura.* Amer. J. Trop. Med., 16:613, 1967.
Peña Chavarria, A., Swartzwelder, J. C., Villarejou, V. M., Korcher, E., and Arguedas, J.: Dichlorvos, an effective broadspectrum anthelmintic. Amer. J. Trop. Med., 18:907, 1969.

ENTEROBIASIS
(Oxyuriasis, Pinworm or Seatworm Infection)

Infestation with the pinworm, *Enterobius vermicularis,* is not limited to rural communities and the poor as with many intestinal nematodes, but occurs also in urban communities. Reportedly worldwide in distribution, it appears to be much rarer in the tropics. Children are more commonly infected than adults.

The adult female worm is 8 to 13 mm. long, and the male, which is rarely seen, 2 to 5 mm. Both live in the cecum and adjacent large and small bowel. The females migrate at night to the anal orifice, where they deposit their eggs. Within a few hours larvae develop in the eggs, which are then infectious and on ingestion hatch in the duodenum and migrate to the large bowel where they mature in 15 to 28 days. The ova can be transferred from the anal margin to the mouth by contamination of the hands, and ova lodge under the nails following

scratching of the anal margin. The eggs also become widely disseminated in the environment, notable in bedclothes and dust samples. It has been suggested that hatching of larvae on the anal margin may result in the colon's being colonized from below as a form of autoinfection. Fortunately the eggs are relatively susceptible to drying, and in a warm dry environment survive only a few days.

Usually pinworm is harmless infestation and is often asymptomatic. Pruritus ani is the chief complaint caused by the migrating female worms. Numerous other symptoms have been described, including enuresis, irritability, and insomnia, which may result from the pruritus. Less convincing reported manifestations are abdominal pain, teeth grinding, nausea, and weight loss.

Rarely the female worm may penetrate into the mucosa of the bowel, where it has been a primary cause of appendicitis. Occasionally female worms migrate into the vagina, causing an intense vulvitis. Prostatitis is a rare complication in the male, and secondary ischiorectal abscesses may follow perianal eczema. Granulomas may form around worms that enter tissues, and such granulomas have been described in the uterus, fallopian tubes, and peritoneum, presumably associated with migration of worms up the female genital tract. A rare case not reported in the literature occurred in a mentally deficient child who developed pulmonary eosinophilic granulomas owing to massive inhalation of Enterobius eggs present in the dust of the mental institution.

The best method for finding Enterobius eggs is by means of the sealing tape (Scotch tape) swab. A piece of Scotch tape 2 inches long is folded, sticky side out, over the end of a wooden tongue depressor and pressed firmly against the perianal region. The tape is then stuck to the slide, acting as a coverslip, and the specimen is scanned for the typical eggs, which are 50 to 60 μ in length, are flattened on one side, and contain a developing embryo. The patient can be given six such swabs, and he does the examination every morning for six mornings on rising and before taking a bath. All can then be examined at the laboratory. Adult worms are rarely observed in feces or on the perianal skin, or seen with the sigmoidoscope. All members of the family should be examined in view of the frequency with which whole families are infected. The eosinophil count is rarely elevated in this infection.

Treatment with piperazine citrate, 65 mg. per kilogram (maximal daily dose 2.5 grams) daily for eight days, is usually effective. Single-dose treatment is becoming more fashionable with either pyrvinium pamoate, 5 mg. per kilogram (maximum, 250 mg.), which can be repeated after two weeks, or thiabendazole, 25 mg. per kilogram twice daily for one day, repeated seven days later. Pyrvinium pamoate (Povan) turns the stool red, and may occasionally be associated with vomiting, diarrhea, and skin rashes. The methods of transmission should be explained to the patient, and care of personal hygiene (short nails, frequent baths, and clean underclothes) instituted before treatment. Follow-up tape swabs are necessary. There is a tendency for some patients to become overanxious about this infection, occasionally with the development of a "worm neurosis." They should be strongly reassured.

Cram, E. B.: Studies on oxyuriasis, xxviii. Summary and conclusions. Amer. J. Dis. Child., 65:46, 1943.

Deruiter, H., Rijpstra, A. C., and Swellengrebel, N. H.: Ectopic *Enterobius vermicularis*; variations on its pattern. Trop. Geogr. Med., 14:375, 1962.

Most, H., Gellin, G. A., Yager, R., Aron, B., Friedlander, M., and Quarfordt, S.: Enterobius (pinworm infection): A study of 951 Puerto Rican and 315 non-Puerto Rican children in New York City. Amer. J. Trop. Med., 12:65, 1963.

TISSUE NEMATODES

TRICHINOSIS*
(Trichiniasis, Trichinellosis)

Definition and Etiology. Trichinosis is a self-limited infection of the intestine (by the adult parasite) and of the striated muscle (by the larvae) produced by a small nematode, *Trichinella spiralis*. The same animal host thus acts as both the final and the intermediate host, harboring the adults temporarily and the encysted larvae for long periods. When infected meat containing larvae is ingested, these larvae are released into the upper small intestine by the action of digestive juices. They become adult in five to seven days, the males and females mate, and the fertile female begins to deposit larvae into the mucosa. These larvae pass into the circulation through the hepatic and pulmonary filters, and are carried to all parts of the body. They burrow into the muscles and encyst and complete their development in striated muscle. In other tissues such as the myocardium, brain, and eye, the larvae disintegrate and are absorbed. Among the muscles heavily parasitized are the diaphragmatic, masseteric, intercostal, laryngeal, extraocular, nuchal, pectoral, deltoid, gluteus, biceps, and gastrocnemius. A total of 1500 larvae are liberated by each female worm, usually in four to eight weeks but up to 16 weeks, after which the females die.

Larvae attain a size of 0.4 by 0.025 mm. in a cyst in the muscle by the thirty-fifth day. The capsule is complete in three months, and calcification occurs within six months to two years. Recent evidence suggests that there may be strain differences in relation to host susceptibility. The parasite is chiefly found in man, hogs, rats, bears, foxes, walruses, dogs, and cats, but any carnivorous or omnivorous animal may be infected.

Epidemiology. Generally of worldwide distribution, the parasite has not been reported from the islands of the Pacific or Australia. It occurs more frequently in the Northern Hemisphere than in the tropics. It is common in Europe and the United States. Fatal cases have recently been described from Kenya and Chile. It is rare east of the Suez Canal. In the United States there has been a marked reduction in the incidence of the infection, owing to laws requiring the cooking of garbage fed to hogs, storage of meat at low temperature, and education of the public resulting in thorough cooking of pork.

Until quite recently, trichinosis was relatively common in New York City, as pork was being obtained from garbage-fed hogs in New Jersey. However, hog-rearing in this way has substantially declined. Pigs become infected by eating infected meat and occasionally infected rats. Rats are infected in the same way. One of the main methods of transmission is in sausages, wursts, or hamburgers in which the beef is diluted (or actually contaminated in mechanical grinders) with a little pork. Infections from bear and walrus meat have been reported. The low incidence in the tropics is probably due to the fact that meat of any kind is a luxury to many people. Hindus, Jews, and Moslems eschew pork, and the Chinese cook it very well.

Pathology and Pathogenesis. Three to four days after invasion of the muscle, the fiber becomes edematous, loses its cross striations, and undergoes basophilic degeneration. The nuclei increase in number and size, and there is interstitial inflammation around the muscle with a chronic inflammatory cell infiltrate. The severity of the disease depends on the adult worm load, the age of the patient, and the degree of host resistance as well as the numbers of organs involved.

In the heart a focal interstitial myocarditis may occur. Acute nonsuppurative meningitis may be associated with larvae in the cerebrospinal fluid. Larvae may cause lesions in the choroid and retina. Catarrhal enteritis, pulmonary edema, and bronchopneumonia may occur in the early stages of the disease.

Clinical Manifestations. The cardinal features of trichinosis are fever, orbital edema, myalgia, and eosinophilia. Only a small percentage of infected patients have sufficient parasites, however, to produce such clinically recognizable disease. The clinical picture can be divided into distinct stages in a symptomatic infection. First, there is the stage of adult maturation during the first weeks after infection associated with transient gastrointestinal symptoms. From the seventh to the fourteenth day larviposition begins, and muscle penetration commences. This is usually associated with an irregular persistent fever (100 to 105° F.), urticarial rash, and occasionally respiratory symptoms in the form of cough and bronchospasm. Muscle pains become prominent and unusual, but the characteristic physical signs are bilateral orbital edema and subungual hemorrhages. A severe infection may result in death four to eight weeks after infection from toxemia, secondary pneumonia, myocardial failure, or trichinous encephalitis. Severe muscle involvement may render breathing, masticating, swallowing, or locomotion painful. An eosinophilia beginning seven days

---

*The present article is based extensively on the article on trichinosis prepared by Dr. Harold W. Brown for the twelfth edition of this book. Little new clinical information has been developed in the interval; what has appeared has been incorporated in the basic article.   P.M.

after the infection may rise to very high levels (70 per cent) and persist for months. Serum transaminases are also elevated in the invasive stage.

Diagnosis and Differential Diagnosis. Although the rising eosinophilia together with a suggestive clinical picture leads one to suspect this diagnosis, it is proved by finding the larvae in a muscle biopsy. This should be done in the fourth week of infection when a small piece of muscle is removed from the deltoid or gastrocnemius. Crushed between two microscope slides and examined under the low-power objective of the microscope, the living coiled larvae can be seen. In light infections when the direct examination is negative, the biopsy specimen can be incubated overnight in an acid-pepsin mixture and the centrifuged deposit examined for larvae.

Calcified cyst and calcified larvae represent older infections, as calcification usually takes 18 months, but the larva may live inside the calcified cyst for many years. Calcified cysts appear as tiny white spots in fresh muscle, but are too small to be detected radiologically.

A variety of serologic tests are available. The bentonite flocculation test is as sensitive as the complement-fixation test and much easier to perform. It is usually positive four weeks after infection, but may be present earlier. A change from a negative to a positive test during the illness is significant. The indirect fluorescent antibody test detects some infections at an earlier stage. Few other parasitic infections are associated with such persistent fever or generalized muscular aches and tender muscles. Polymyositis of nonparasitic etiology may present like this and be associated with eosinophilia. Periarteritis nodosa may also mimic trichinosis.

Treatment. Patients with symptomatic trichinosis should be confined to bed and given a smooth high-calorie, high-protein diet. Congestive cardiac failure should be searched for and, if present, should be treated. Mild analgesics can be given for the muscle pain. Anti-inflammatory steroids (prednisolone, 5 mg. three times daily) relieve fever, edema, and muscle pain in severe acute cases but are said not to affect the adult worms' fecundity or the number of larvae settling in the muscle. In patients with central nervous system involvement this effect of steroids is dramatic.

Thiabendazole, in a dose of 25 mg. per kilogram of body weight for five to seven days, has also produced a marked resolution of the symptoms of fever and muscle pain, but living larvae have still been recovered on muscle biopsy after much larger courses of the drug. In severe infections the use of corticosteroids and thiabendazole may be life-saving, but when the parasite load is not considerable, the prognosis is good even without treatment.

Prevention. The ultimate prevention of trichinosis is dependent on its elimination in hogs, and the incidence in these animals can be greatly reduced by heat-sterilizing garbage. Freezing meat at −32° C. for a few hours (or at 15 to 30° C. for several weeks) kills larvae, as does gamma radiation of the meat. Pigs fed on a diet containing 0.1 per cent thiabendazole fail to incubate *T. spiralis* on challenge. Routine meat inspection does not detect the infection, and serologic and skin tests on pigs have not been helpful in detecting infected animals. The chief safeguard at present is the thorough cooking of pork at 140° F. for 30 minutes for each pound of meat.

Gould, S. E.: Trichinosis. Springfield, Ill., Charles C Thomas, 1945.
Hennekeuser, M. H., Pabst, K., Poeplau, W., and Gerok, W.: Thiabendazole for the treatment of trichinosis in humans. Texas Rep. Biol. Med., 27 (Supplement 2):581, 1969.
Maynard, J. E., and Kagan, I. G.: Trichinosis (serology). Practitioner, 191:622, 1963.
Proceedings of the International Commission in Trichinellosis: No. VI. Wiad. Parazyt., 14:127, 1968.
Zimmerman, W. J., Steele, J. H., and Kagan, I. G.: The changing status of trichiniasis in the U.S. population. Public Health Rep., 83:957, 1968.

ANGIOSTRONGYLIASIS
(Eosinophilic Meningoencephalitis)

Eosinophilic meningoencephalitis, a syndrome caused by *Angiostrongylus cantonensis* (the rat lung worm), was first recognized in New Caledonia in 1950, and has since been reported from Hawaii, Tahiti, other Pacific Islands, Indonesia, and Thailand. The human disease has only been reported from the Far East and the Pacific to date, although infected rats have been found in Madagascar, Mauritius, Ceylon, and Sarawak.

The life cycle was described by workers in Australia in 1955 before the importance of the worm as a human pathogen was known. A delicate filiform nematode, 17 to 25 mm. in length, the adult lives in the lungs of rats, and the eggs are coughed up, swallowed, and pass out in the feces as first-stage larvae. Further development occurs in slugs and snails to the third-stage infective larvae. These larvae are ingested by man either while in this intermediate host or after they have been shed by it onto some other article of food, e.g., lettuce. Crabs and freshwater prawns have also been found to be infected with these metastrongyloid larvae, but probably act as paratenic hosts. The dispersal of the giant African land snail *Achatina fulica* may have assisted the spread of the infection. When infective larvae are ingested by the rat, they migrate to the brain and reach young adulthood in four weeks. They then migrate to the pulmonary arteries and after two more weeks start laying eggs. Unfortunately if man accidentally ingests these infective larvae, they migrate to the brain (as in the rat), and there produce the clinical picture of a meningoencephalitis associated with fever, signs of cerebral irritation, mental deficit, and varying degrees of loss of consciousness. Mild blood eosinophilia is present, and lumbar puncture reveals a fluid under increased pressure with increased protein and many eosinophils (from 100 to 3000 per cubic millimeter.) Occasionally patients present with a facial nerve lesion or complaints of diplopia and parasthesia. A complement fixation test using an extract of adult worms as antigen has been developed. The illness usually persists for some weeks or months and then the patient recovers spontaneously.

Young adult worms have been found in the brain and cerebrospinal fluid of man, and experimental infection of monkeys produces a similar syndrome. The pathology of the brain in fatal cases is one of focal areas of softening, the meninges and subarachnoid space being infiltrated with plasma cells, lymphocytes, eosinophils, and neutrophils. There is perivascular cuffing with chronic inflammatory cells in the brain substance. Careful sectioning of the brain is necessary to find the 0.16 to 8 mm. nematodes.

This condition must be differentiated from a variety of other parasitic infections involving the central nervous system. In Thailand cerebral gnathostomiasis and Angiostrongylus infections occur. Cerebral paragonimiasis could be an important differential diagnosis in parts of the Far East. In other situations the syndrome of eosinophilic meningitis could be produced by cysticercosis, hydatid, schistosomiasis, fascioliasis, trichinosis, and possibly strongyloidiasis. Refinements of serologic diagnostic techniques will help in this sometimes difficult clinical problem.

The author has been able to trace no references to treatment with thiabendazole, although this would seem to be the drug to try. Prevention entails education regarding dangerous foods such as raw crabs and prawns and undercooked snails, and making sure that lettuce is free of slugs and snails. Freezing of crustaceans and molluscs at $-15°$ C. for 12 hours has been found to be effective in destroying the infective larvae of *A. cantonensis*.

Alicata, J. E.: Present status of *Angiostrongylus cantonensis* infection in man and animals in the tropics. J. Trop. Med., Hyg., 72:53, 1969.

Mackerras, M. T., and Sanders, D. F.: The life history of the rat lungworm *Angiostrongylus cantonensis* (Chen) (Nematoda; Metastrongylidae). Aust. J. Zool., 3:1, 1955.

Schollhaminer, G., Aubry, P., and Rigaud, J. L.: Quelques réflexions sur la méningite à eósinophiles a Tahiti. Étude clinique et biologique de 165 observations, à propos d'un cas atypiqùe. Bull. Soc. Path. Exot., 59:341, 1966.

FILARIASIS

General Considerations

To talk of filariasis as such is to use a general term like anemia, for there are seven types of nematodes found in man belonging to the superfamily Filarioidea, as well as one member of the superfamily Dracunculoidea (the guinea worm), which is usually included in a consideration of this group. Of these Filarioidea, the embryos or microfilariae are found in the blood in five and in the subcutaneous tissues in two species. The adults are viviparous, and the blood microfilariae demonstrate a periodicity in the peripheral blood, depending on the species. They may remain ensheathed in their elongated egg shell or have no sheath. These microfilariae are distinguished on their criteria as well on as the pattern of distribution of nuclei seen in stained specimens in their tails. Giemsa stain can be used, but better results of sheath staining are obtained with Delafield's hematoxylin or Mayer's acid hemalum.

In Table 2 the species are listed and the characteristics of their microfilariae shown. The adult worms live for many years, whereas blood microfilariae have a life of three to six months. After being bitten by an infected arthropod it may take 1 year to 18 months before microfilariae are present in the peripheral blood, a long prepatent period. The controlling mechanism for periodicity has never been satisfactorily explained for many of these human species. However, Hawking's recent work suggests that at least two circadian rhythms are involved, one mechanism within the microfilariae themselves, and the other some physiological tide in the host (body temperature for certain animal species). This periodicity fits the habits of the insect vector; for instance, the Loa insect vector flies by day but most bancrofti infections are transmitted nocturnally. The geographic distribution of these species is of particular importance, because in some it is markedly restricted. For instance *Loa loa* is a filarid of Equatorial Africa, and *Mansonella ozzardi* is only found in South America.

Not all the species listed are significantly pathogenic. Few symptoms have been ascribed to *Mansonella ozzardi* infections, and the case for the pathogenicity of *A. perstans* is very shaky. Two of these filarial infections are notable in terms of their importance in man. These are the *Wuchereria-Brugia complex,* which produces bancroftian filariasis with lymphatic obstruction and elephantiasis, and *onchocerciasis,* which is a common cause of blindness in endemic areas. Multiple infections occur, in endemic areas, for instance, in parts of West Africa a patient may be seen infected with *Loa loa,* bancrofti, perstans, and onchocerciasis.

TABLE 2. COMMON FILARIOIDEA OF MAN AS DISTINGUISHED BY MICROFILARIAE CHARACTERISTICS

	Periodicity of Microfilariae	Sheathed or Unsheathed	Tail Morphology
Microfilariae in blood:			
Wuchereria bancrofti	Majority nocturnal	Sheathed	Nuclei not to tip of tail
Brugia malaya	Majority nocturnal	Sheathed	Two distinct nuclei in tail tip
Loa loa	Diurnal	Sheathed	Nuclei to tip of tail
Acanthocheilonema perstans	Nocturnally subperiodic	Not sheathed	Nuclei to tip of tail
Mansonella ozzardi	Nonperiodic	Not sheathed	Nuclei not to tip of tail
Microfilariae in subcutaneous tissues:			
Onchocerca volvulus	Nonperiodic	Not sheathed	Nuclei not to tip of tail
Acanthocheilonema streptocerca	Nonperiodic	Not sheathed	Nuclei to tip of tail, which is crooked

This final group of the most modified nematodes will be considered in the order in which they are listed in Table 2, except that the guinea worm will be considered first. Dirofilariasis and pulmonary tropical eosinophilia will then be reviewed, followed by a note on occult filariasis and the problem of eosinophilia in relation to helminthic disease.

Hawking, F.: Advances in filariasis. Trans. Roy. Soc. Trop. Med. Hyg., 59:9, 1965.
Hawking, F., Moore, P., Gammage, K., and Worms, M. J.: Periodicity of microfiliae. XII. The effect of variations in host body temperature on the cycle of *Loa loa, Monnigofilaria setariosa, Durofilaria immitis,* and other filariae. Trans. Roy. Soc. Trop. Med. Hyg., 61:674, 1967.

Dracontiasis

(Guinea Worm)

Infection with the guinea worm (*Dracunculus medinensis*) usually presents as a skin ulceration at the site of emergence of the female adult worm. Man is probably the only reservoir, although monkeys and dogs can be experimentally infected. Human infections are widespread in the tropics, occurring in local distribution in West Africa and the Nile Valley, the Middle East, India and Pakistan, the Caribbean Islands, Guiana, and Brazil. Infection occurs on ingesting infected water fleas (Cyclops) present in drinking water from shallow wells or ponds. The infective larvae in the Cyclops penetrate the intestinal walls and mature in the loose connective tissue under the skin, especially that of legs and feet. The male worm is small and dies after copulation. The female requires a year to become gravid, and then measures up to a meter long and is 2 mm. in diameter. When ready to discharge larvae, she approaches the skin surface, and a blister is produced by secretion of a toxic substance from the anterior end of the worm. The blister breaks down to form an ulcer a few centimeters across, and the anterior end of the worm protrudes into this ulcer. On contact with water the head of the worm ruptures, and the uterus periodically discharges the tightly coiled larvae infective to the water flea. Secondary infection of the ulcer with resultant cellulitis is common. Generalized allergic symptoms may occur prior to the blister formation or when surgical removal of the worm is attempted. Multiple infections are common. The lesion is usually on the lower leg, but may occur on the genitalia, buttocks, or upper limbs. In water carriers lesions have been observed on the back, suggesting that the worm is positively hydrotropic. Alternatively, the mature female may never reach the surface of the body and may be absorbed or calcify in the tissue. The radiologic appearance is pathognomonic because the worm is so large. If a gravid worm dies in situ or is broken during extraction, cellulitis and secondary infection often occur. This may give rise to contractures. Also *Clostridium tetani* may contaminate the wound and tetanus may result. Rarely the adult worm involves serous cavities, the extradural space, or joints. Guinea worm arthritis appears to be due to the presence of the adult worm or larvae in the joint. A microscopic diagnosis can be made by finding embryos in the exudate from the guinea worm ulcer after exposure to a few drops of water.

Gradually winding the worm out of the ulcer by turning it on a stick a few centimeters a day is still common practice. Surgical extraction is also practiced. Recently niridazole (Ambilhar) has been reported to be lethal to the adult worm, which can readily be withdrawn after a course of 25 mg. per kilogram of body weight for seven days. Thiabendazole is also effective. Prevention involves constructing water sources that cannot be contaminated and killing cyclops by chlorination or boiling water to be used for drinking.

Kothari, M. L., Pardnani, D. S., Lopa Mehta, and Kothari, D. L.: Niridazole in dracunculiasis: A controlled study. Trans. Roy. Soc. Trop. Med. Hyg., 63:608, 1969.
Raffier, G.: Efficacy of thiabendazole in the treatment of dracunculiasis. Texas Rep. Biol. Med., 27(Supplement 2):601, 1969.
Reddy, C. R. R. M., and Sivaramappa, M.: Guinea worm arthritis of the knee joint. Brit. Med. J., 1:155, 1968.

Bancroftian Filariasis

Etiology. Bancroftian filariasis is caused by the filarial worm *Wuchereria bancrofti*. The adult worms reside in the lymphatic system and produce recurrent lymphangitis with fibrosis and obstruction. The infection is transmitted by culicine and anopheline mosquitoes.

The threadlike adult worms are 4 to 10 cm. long and live for decades. The female worm is viviparous, producing microfilariae 130 to 320 μ long which are found in the peripheral blood; in some forms this occurs only at night, whereas during the day the microfilariae are in the lungs. If ingested by a suitable mosquito, these microfilariae develop in the thoracic muscles of the insect and are present in the mouth parts after two weeks. They enter the skin through the puncture wound when the mosquito next feeds, and finding their way to the lymphatics of the host the males and females mate and mature. More than a year after infection microfilariae appear in the peripheral blood.

Epidemiology. Man is the only definitive host of this common type of filariasis. Periodic bancroftian filariasis is found throughout tropical Africa and North Africa, as well as in the tropical coastal borders of Asia and Queensland. It is endemic in the West Indies and the northern countries of South America. In the northern Pacific bancroftian filariasis exhibits nocturnal periodicity, but in the Pacific Islands east of 160 degrees of longitude (including New Caledonia, Fiji, Samoa, The Ellis and Cook islands, Society Islands, and the Marquesas) the microfilariae are nonperiodic, being present in the peripheral blood throughout the 24-hour period. The term *W. bancrofti var. pacifica* has been applied to this strain.

Pathology. The severity of the lesions probably depends on the adult worm load and their site of development and the susceptibility of the host.

Light infections are often asymptomatic, and microfilariae are detected on incidental blood examinations. Maturing adults in the lymphatics are associated with endothelial thickening, fibrin deposition, and infiltration with eosinophils, histiocytes, and lymphocytes. Giant cells occur. Fibrotic and inflammatory changes tend to obstruct the lymphatics, and this process is exacerbated by death of the worms, which may calcify. There is reactive hyperplasia in the lymph nodes, and small granulomas are seen. An eosinophilic endophlebitis of the small veins is present in the lymph nodes. The testicles and epididymis often show similar changes with evidence of chronic inflammation. Worms may not be present at the site of inflammation. Secretions of the worm, especially after molting, are thought to be responsible for some of these changes. As lymphatic obstruction becomes more extensive, chronic edema develops in the infected areas. Recently lymphedema has been produced in laboratory animals with longstanding bancrofti infections.

Clinical Manifestations. Attacks of fever, headache, and lymphadenopathy sometimes associated with urticarial rashes are known as filarial fever and occur in the acute phase of the disease. Often, however, no history of this early phase can be obtained. Epididymitis may occur as a lone lesion. Lymphatics most affected are those of the inguinal region, upper arms, and spermatic cord. Chronic lymphadenopathy is often the only sign of infection for years. Retrograde lymphangitis may be noted. In a small proportion of infected individuals, with increasing lymphatic obstruction over the years, all degrees of chronic edema occur, affecting especially the lower limbs and scrotum. Initially the edema is pitting, but as organization of collagen occurs in the edematous subcutaneous tissues, it becomes nonpitting. Eventually the giant limbs of elephantiasis are produced. The skin over the affected part, at first smooth, later becomes scaly and is fissured at the points where the fascia is attached to the skin. Hyperkeratosis produces warts and nodules. Varicose nodes in the groin are the result of lymphatic dilatation and may lead to scrotal lymphedema. Infection may supervene in any of these lesions with formation of a chronic discharging sinus. Chronic inflammatory disease of the testicle and epididymis with or without hydrocele occurs.

Chyluria may be renal or vesical in origin, depending on the level at which the lymph varix communicates with the urinary tract. Cystoscopy and intravenous or retrograde pyelography help to establish the site of communication.

Diagnosis. In the early stages and when lymphadenopathy only is present, microfilariae are usually present in night blood films. Although the motile microfilariae are easily seen in fresh films, staining is necessary for identification. Microfilariae may be absent in the late stage; thus, only 4 per cent of patients with elephantiasis and 30 per cent of patients with hydrocele had microfilariae in one series. Concentration techniques are available for microfilariae, and they may be found in the chylous urine or hydrocele fluid.

Eosinophilia is not a constant finding. The filarial complement-fixation test and skin test, although only group specific, are useful in suggesting a filarial cause for a lymphedema. Lymphangiograms reveal the extent of the lymphatic obstruction and may be a useful preoperative measure. It is rarely justified to remove an enlarged lymph node to find the adults because this still further prejudices the lymphatic circulation. In an endemic area surgeons frequently encounter adult worms when operating on the groin.

The differential diagnosis depends on the type of clinical syndrome. Lymphadenopathy caused by other infections and neoplasms must be considered. Elephantiasis may be associated with congenital defects of the lymphatic drainage as well as tuberculous inguinal lymphadenitis. Tuberculosis, *Schistosoma haematobium*, and gonorrhea produce epididymitis, and relatively few hydroceles are filarial. Lymphatic obstruction caused by many other agents may produce lymphedema and chyluria.

Treatment. Diethylcarbamazine (Banocide, Hetrazan) is believed to kill a large proportion of adults as well as microfilariae. A dose of 3 mg. per kilogram of body weight is given, rising to a maximum of 12 mg. per kilogram over four days. This dose is then given daily for 14 days. Reactions are mild in comparison with those seen in onchocerciasis, but fever, nausea and vomiting, and skin rashes may occur as with any drug. The arsenical Mel W and the antimonial Astiban (sodium dimercaptosuccinate) kill adult filariae, but are too toxic for general use. All patients with microfilaremia should receive an adequate course of treatment.

The management of lymphedema depends on its severity. Mild degrees are best treated with elevation of the foot of the bed and an elastic stocking. Careful instructions regarding foot care should be given, as ascending streptococcal cellulitis is common in the edematous tissues and further prejudices the lymphatic circulation. Some workers believe the Streptococcus to be more important in producing lymphangitis than the worms themselves. Any foot sepsis requires early and vigorous treatment with antimicrobial drugs. Tinea infections should be eradicated. Banocide therapy is often given in elephantiasis on the grounds that it may prevent further lymphatic damage, but clinical improvement is seldom observed.

A variety of surgical operations have been devised to remove the edematous subcutaneous tissue from the leg, scrotum, and breasts. Success depends on the type of operation and the skill of the surgeon. In scrotal elephantiasis care must be taken to preserve the testicles. Hydroceles can be treated by the injection of sclerosing agents. Chyluria of bladder origin can be terminated by fulgurating the leaking bladder lymphatics. Renal chyluria is best left alone, although in the past kidneys have been wrapped in cellophane with the subsequent production of renal hypertension.

Prevention. Diethylcarbamazine, 3 mg. per kilogram per month for 12 to 18 months, has been effective in mass treatment for preventive purposes. Residual DDT or dieldrin is effective against many of the mosquito vectors, and systematic destruction of mosquito-breeding sites has also met with success. Biologic control of mosquito vectors is receiving intensive field trials, but thus far they have not resulted in methods for mass application.

Malayan Filariasis

A disease similar to bancroftian filariasis is produced by a closely related filarial worm, *Brugia malayi*. The sheathed microfilariae of this species have two distinct caudal nuclei. Transmitted by mansonoides mosquitoes, it is the only filarial infection of man in Malaya and Borneo, whereas in India, Ceylon, and tropical China it coexists with *W. bancrofti*. *Brugia malayi* is responsible for only mild lymphedema in man, usually below the knee, with enlargement of the popliteal and femoral nodes. In contrast to bancroftian filariasis, the microfilaremia rates in the Malayan form are quite high in children younger than five years. In this infection, also, there are two types of organisms, one with nocturnal periodicity, and another subperiodic form. The latter is found in many animals (primates, carnivores, and rodents) and is a true zoonosis.

Galindo, L., Von Lichtenberg, F., and Baldison, C.: Bancroftian filariasis in Puerto Rico: Infection pattern and tissue lesions. Amer. J. Trop. Med., 11:739, 1962.

Nelson, G. S.: The pathology of filarial infections. Helminth. Abst., 35:Pt. 4, 311, 1966

Schacher, J. F., and Sahyoun, P. F.: A chronological study of the histopathology of filarial disease in cats and dogs caused by *Brugia phangi* (Buckley and Edeson, 1956). Trans. Roy. Soc. Trop. Med. Hyg., 61:234, 1967.

Turner, L. H.: Studies on filariasis in Malaya: The clinical features of filariasis due to *Wuchereria malayi*. Trans. Roy. Soc. Trop. Med. Hyg., 53:154, 1959.

Wilson, T.: Filariasis in Malaya—A general review. Trans. Roy. Soc. Trop. Med. Hyg., 55:107, 1961.

Loiasis

Loa loa infection is characterized by the appearance of transient swellings mainly on the limbs; these are thought to be the site of the migrating adult worms in the subcutaneous tissue. Occasionally a worm will traverse the conjunctiva of the eye.

The male adult worm is 30 mm. long and the female 70 mm. They live for many years, and gain access to the body through the proboscis of biting flies (deer flies of the genus Chrysops). These worms appear to be in a state of continuous migration in the subcutaneous tissues of the body. It is not clearly understood how the sexes locate each other, but they meet and mate, and the female produces microfilariae that appear in the blood during the day and are infective to the insect vector.

Man is the only reservoir host, with the possible exception of monkeys. Human loiasis is restricted to Africa, mainly the West Coast. It occurs from Sierra Leone to the Cameroons and extends into the heart of Africa in the region of the Congo basin.

Clinical Manifestations. The main clinical manifestation is the repeated occurrence of hot erythematous swellings (5 to 10 cm. or more) called Calabar swellings after the endemic area of Calabar. These occur in the upper limbs particularly, are painful, and subside in a few days. They are associated with the presence of an adult worm. A similar swelling occurs around the eye when the adult worm crosses the eye beneath the conjunctivae. The patient notices the worm in his line of vision ("like a submarine, doctor") and it is worth inquiring for such a history. Calabar swellings seem to occur more frequently in the extremities. Why this is so is not known. Routine roentgenography in endemic areas often reveals calcified dead worms lying between the metacarpals. Rarely, neurologic symptoms may be associated with the infection if the Calabar swelling involves a peripheral nerve. Also the parasite has been found in the cerebrospinal fluid associated with a meningoencephalitis.

Diagnosis. The initial diagnosis is usually based on a history of Calabar swellings in a patient coming from an endemic area. Examination of the daytime blood reveals sheathed microfilariae with a characteristic distribution of caudal nuclei. In early loiasis, microfilariae may not be detected even by concentration techniques. Very high eosinophil counts are encountered at this stage (50 to 70 per cent). A positive filarial complement-fixation test is usually present. Occasionally the adult worm can be extracted as it crosses the eye. It has been suggested that another human filarid, *Acanthocheilonema perstans*, may cause Calabar swellings.

Treatment. Diethylcarbamazine (Hetrazan) kills both adults and microfilariae. One course of 12 mg. per kilogram of body weight for 14 days is all that is necessary. Reactions are rare.

Woodruff, A. W.: Loiasis. *In* Fairley, N. H., Woodruff, A. W., and Walters, J. H. (eds.): Recent Advances in Tropical Medicine. London, J. & A. Churchill, Ltd., 1961, pp. 178–194.

Mansonella Ozzardi

Mansonella ozzardi is found only in the New World, occurring in South America and certain foci in the Caribbean. The adult worms are embedded in visceral adipose tissue. Although they are usually regarded as nonpathogenic, fever, headache, lymphadenitis, and erythematous irritant skin rashes have been reported in association with their presence. Cold extremities, the result of peripheral vasoconstriction caused by a postulated filarial toxin, have been reported. The microfilariae show no particular periodicity and are about twice the size of perstans and have a different caudal morphology. *Simulium amazonicum* has been implicated as the vector, and midges of the genus Culicoides have also been suggested.

Undiano, C.: Importance and present-day concepts of the pathogenicity of Mansonella infections. Fev. Fac. Cienc. Med. Univ. Cordoba, 24:183, 1966.

Acanthocheilonema Perstans

Filakiasis caused by *Acanthocheilonema perstans* has an extensive distribution in Equatorial Africa, the Carribbean, and South America, where it sometimes overlaps with *Mansonella ozzardi*. The adult worms are found in association with the serous cavities of the body, usually behind the limiting membrane. They may be seen at postmortem examination moving behind the peritoneum or pleura. The small (100 μ) unsheathed microfilariae are found in the blood throughout the 24 hours, but there is a peak in the peripheral blood population at night. A Culicoides species, a small black midge, is responsible for transmission.

The vast majority of patients exhibiting microfilaremia have no symptoms, but there have been recent reports of clinical symptoms associated with this infection. These reports include fever, Calabar swellings, arthritis, and upper abdominal pain associated with hepatomegaly. A high eosinophilia is often present in cases with scanty embryos, and such a finding in a patient from an endemic area should prompt a careful search for these. Acute encephalomyelitis with *A. perstans* in the cerebrospinal fluid has been described. Diethylcarbamazine (Hetrazan) has little effect on the adults or on the microfilariae.

Dukes, D. C., et al.: Cerebral filariasis due to *A. perstans*. Cent. Afr. J. Med., 14:21, 1968.

Wiseman, R. A.: *Acanthocheilonema perstans:* A cause of significant eosinophilia in the tropics. Comments on its pathogenicity. Trans. Roy. Soc. Trop. Med. Hyg., 61:667, 1967.

Onchocerciasis
(River Blindness)

River blindness is a form of cutaneous filariasis caused by infection with *Onchocerca volvulus* and is characterized by skin irritation, corneal opacities, and skin nodules.

Etiology. The threadlike adult worms lie tangled together in fibrous nodules in the subcutaneous tissues or fascial planes. Microfilariae produced by the females become widely distributed in the surrounding skin. Female black flies (buffalo gnats) of the genus Simulium ingest these larvae while taking a blood meal. After development in the fly for one week, the larvae are infective for man and are deposited when the fly next bites. They take more than a year to mature, mate, and produce microfilariae. Adult worms live 7 to 15 years.

Epidemiology. Human onchocerciasis is found on the West Coast of Africa from Sierra Leone to the Congo and in the east from the Sudan to Nyasaland. It also occurs in Guatemala, Mexico, Eastern Venezuela, and Surinam. Simulium larvae and pupae are usually found in rapidly running highly oxygenated water. Small insects (3 mm. long), the flies bite low on the legs in Africa, but more around the head in Central America, which may account for the high incidence of nodules on the head in the latter locality. In East Africa *Simulium naevi* larvae and pupae evaded detection for many years until they were found on the shells of freshwater crabs.

Pathogenesis and Pathology. An initial inflammatory reaction around the adult worm is followed by a foreign body granulomatous reaction and fibrous capsule formation. The nodules are literally the graveyards of the adult worms, for these eventually die and degenerate, sometimes with secondary abscess formation. The microfilariae in the surrounding subcutaneous tissues produce a low-grade inflammatory reaction with lymphocytes, plasma cells, and eosinophils. Thickening of the epidermis and dermis owing to fibrosis eventually occurs, with destruction of elastic fibers and sometimes reduction in pigmentation.

Microfilariae migrate into the tissues of the eye to produce important inflammatory lesions which may result in blindness. Punctate keratitis is associated with death of microfilariae in the cornea, and such multiple corneal opacities may result in permanent corneal scarring. A low-grade iritis and iridocyclitis result in pupillary distortion and even occlusion. Choroidoretinitis also occurs.

Clinical Manifestations. Any patient who has a persistent irritating skin rash or visual disturbances and has been in one of the endemic areas may have onchocerciasis. More rarely, the presenting complaint takes the form of deep-seated muscular pains. The early skin lesions consist of an erythematous papular irritant rash. In heavy infections definite thickening and hyperkeratosis of the skin occurs (craw-craw or crocodile skin). Rarer late complications are depigmentation and pendulous bags in the groins containing sclerosed lymph nodes.

Nodules vary much in size from a few centimeters to as big as a tennis ball. They are frequently detected over bony prominences such as the greater trochanter, the iliac crest, the olecranons, ribs, and occiput. Often the adult worms are located deep in the fascial planes, and no nodules are palpable. To detect the small milky dots of punctate keratitis near the limbus the eyes should be examined with a strong pencil torch, the beam directed obliquely across the cornea. Signs of iritis may be present. With a slit lamp, microfilariae may be visible in the aqueous humor. Funduscopic examination may reveal the much rarer posterior segment lesion.

Diagnosis. Skin shavings are used to demonstrate microfilariae. Thin sections of the superficial skin are removed with a razor blade, mounted in saline, teased out, and examined. Many motile microfilariae emerge from these snips within an hour after they have been made. Blood contamination can be avoided if the shavings are superficial, and this is important if there is a coexistent blood microfilaremia. If there is a definite site of skin irritation, shavings should be taken from this area. In lightly infected patients multiple shavings may be necessary to detect microfilariae, and quite often they are not found. The reaction to a test dose of 50 mg. of diethylcarbamazine

(Mazzotti's test) in the form of an exacerbation of the itching rash is suggestive, as are an eosinophilia and a positive filarial complement-fixation test.

Scabies and superficial mycoses are the most common irritant skin rashes of the tropics and are important differential diagnoses. Streptocerciasis caused by infection with the rare, closely related filarid *Acanthocheilonema streptocerca* also presents as an irritating rash and requires only mention. Although an infection with no mortality, the recurrent irritation of onchocerciasis can be most distressing. Severe ocular lesions may induce total blindness, and this is the blinding filarid.

Treatment. When practicable, all nodules should be excised; this simple measure will reduce the load of adult worms. Suramin is effective in killing adult worms. The side effects and method of administration of this drug are mentioned in the article on African trypanosomiasis. A suitable course for onchocerciasis is 1 gram weekly for six weeks. As the drug is nephrotoxic, treatment should be stopped if more than 30 mg. per 100 ml. of protein appears in the urine.

Diethylcarbamazine is effective in killing microfilariae but does not kill the adult worms. In sensitized individuals, reactions occur when the microfilariae die in the tissues. Skin irritation becomes more intense, and there may be edema of the skin with fever, headache, and malaise. More serious is acute inflammation of the eye which may prejudice sight. As these reactions are dose related, it is usual to start therapy with a small dose of the drug (0.5 mg. per kilogram) and increase gradually to the doses recommended in the previous article. Eye reactions can be controlled with 1 per cent cortisone acetate eye drops and the general reactions controlled with antihistamines and, in severe cases, with systemic steroids.

Prevention. Simulium larvae and pupae are very sensitive to small concentrations of DDT in the river water (less than 1 part per million), and this has been the most effective form of control of the insect vector. Personal prophylaxis is possible to a limited extent by avoiding places where biting Simulium are numerous.

Duke, B. O. L.: Onchocerciasis. Brit. Med. J., 4:301, 1968.
Nelson, D. S.: Onchocerciasis. In Dawes, B. (ed.): Advances in Parasitology. Volume 8. New York, Academic Press, 1970, p. 173.
W.H.O. Expert Committee on Onchocerciasis. World Health Organization Technical Report Series No. 335, 1–92, 1966.
Woodruff, A. W., Choyce, D. P., Muci-Mendoza, F., Hills, M., and Pettitt, L. E.: Onchocerciasis in Guatemala, a clinical and parasitological study with comparison between the disease there and in East Africa. Trans. Roy. Soc. Trop. Med. Hyg., 60:695, 1966.

Streptocerciasis

Acanthocheilonema streptocerca is carried by midges of the genus Culicoides. It occurs in Central Africa, particularly in the Congo and neighboring countries. The adult worms are found in the region of the shoulder girdle, and the micro-

filariae produced in the skin cause a reddish brown irritant rash which may be associated with some degree of edema. Skin shavings reveal the unsheathed microfilariae with the crooked tails and the nuclei going down to the tip. Treatment with diethylcarbamazine is effective.

Duke, B. O. L.: A case of streptocerciasis in a European. Ann. Trop. Med. Parasit., 51:364, 1957.

Dirofilariasis

Several Dirofilariae have been reported to occasionally cause symptoms in man, particularly in the United States. Such infections have also been reported from the Mediterranean basin, South America, and Africa. In Louisiana and Texas a subcutaneous filarid of raccoons (*Dirofilaria tenuis*) occasionally invades man, but does not mature. It produces a painful subcutaneous nodule, consisting of an eosinophilic inflammatory reaction around the worm; this may be a granuloma or may be located in a lymph node. The diagnosis is usually made after biopsy. Mosquitoes transmit the infection.

Other species found in man include *D. conjunctivae, D. repens,* and *D. immitis.* Adult worms have been detected in the heart and great vessels and in the eye. They have also caused infarcts in the lung and "coin" lesions at the hila which may be mistaken for a bronchial carcinoma and excised before the nature is known. In sections the worm is seen in cross section in the center of an infarcted area infiltrated with eosinophils.

Beaver, P. C., and Orihel, T. C.: Human infection with filariae of animals in the United States. Amer. J. Trop. Med., 14:1010, 1965.
Beskin, C. A., Colvin, S. H., Jr., and Beaver, P. C.: Pulmonary dirofilariasis, cause of a pulmonary nodular disease. J.A.M.A., 198:665, 1966.

Pulmonary Tropical Eosinophilia
(Eosinophilic Lung, Weingarten's Syndrome)

Since the early part of this century Indian physicians have recognized a syndrome of paroxysmal cough and nocturnal bronchospasm associated with high eosinophilia, and have called it pulmonary tropical eosinophilia. Low fever, dyspnea, and malaise may be accompanying symptoms. The absolute eosinophil count is above 3000 per cubic millimeter, and may reach very high levels. Chest films may show increased reticulation, prominence of bronchovascular markings, or diffuse miliary mottling of the lung fields. In Ball's series of 1000 cases the great majority were Indian; the condition is much more common among Indians in Singapore. It is now generally accepted that this syndrome is caused by occult filarial infections. The evidence that this is so can be listed as follows: (1) Patients have a consistently high titer of filarial complement-fixing antibodies in the absence of evidence of microfilariae in the blood. (2) There is a clinical, hematologic and serologic response to therapy with the antifilarial drug diethylcarbamazine. (3) The syndrome has been produced in a volunteer by inoculation of *Brugia malayi* infective larvae and *Brugia pahangi* (a feline filaria). (4) Microfilariae have been demonstrated in lung granulomas in such cases by several groups of workers.

It is possible that eosinophilic lung results from an alteration in host immunity to the filarial parasite, giving rise to allergic phenomena manifested by persistent hypereosinophilia and pulmonary symptoms. What is not yet settled is the precise identification of the parasite. It is likely that several species of filaria of the genera Wuchereria and Brugia, some human, some animal, may be involved, depending on the locality in which the syndrome occurs. The high incidence in Indians is noteworthy and may suggest a genetic predisposition in certain racial groups. The course of diethylcarbamazide recommended is similar to that for bancroftian filariasis. Often the symptoms get temporarily worse after starting the drug, but invariably, they resolve, and a second course of the drug or the use of carbarsone as an alternative is seldom necessary.

The question of occult filariasis has recently been reviewed, and it has been pointed out that in many instances it has not been possible to identify the helminth responsible because of the difficulty of interpreting the microfilariae in tissue sections even if they are found. Quite apart from the well defined clinical entity of pulmonary tropical eosinophilia there are patients presenting with signs of reticuloendothelial activation (enlarged lymph nodes, hepatosplenomegaly) and eosinophilia for which it is difficult to find a cause.

Ball, J. D.: Tropical pulmonary eosinophilia. Trans. Roy. Soc. Trop. Med. & Hyg., 44:237, 1950.

Donohugh, D. L.: Tropical eosinophilia, an etiologic enquiry. New Eng. J. Med., 269:1357, 1963.

Danaraj, T. J., Pacheco, G., Shanmugaratnam, K., and Beaver, P. C.: The etiology and pathology of eosinophilic lung (tropical eosinophilia). Amer. J. Trop. Med., 15:183, 1966.

Islam, N.: Tropical eosinophilia. East Pakistan, Islam A. Chittagong, 1964.

Lie Kian, J., and Shandosham, A. A.: The pathology of clinical filariasis due to *Wuchereria bancrofti* and *Brugia malayi* and a discussion of occult filariasis. *In* Sandosham, A. A., and Zaman, V. (eds.): Proceedings of Seminar on Filariasis and Immunology of Parasitic Infections, and Laboratory Meeting. Kuala Lumpur, Malaysia, Rajiv Printers, 1969, p. 125.

TROPICAL PYOMYOSITIS
Philip D. Marsen

This is a condition of a large deep-seated abscess, single or multiple, occurring in any voluntary muscle. Strange lumps for diagnosis in the tropics sometimes turn out to be deep-seated abscesses. By far the most frequent organism isolated is *Staphylococcus aureus*, and in Uganda 60 per cent of such organisms are phage gpII. Histologically there are areas of focal muscle necrosis with inflammatory cell infiltration. The regional lymph nodes are rarely affected, and there may be no fever or leukocytosis in the peripheral blood. The cause is unknown. Subcutaneous helminthic infection, particularly filaria, and sickle cell disease have been suggested as predisposing conditions, but as yet there is no convincing evidence to this effect. Treatment consists of antimicrobial therapy (initially with penicillin) and surgical drainage.

Marcus, R. T., and Foster, W. D.: Observations on the clinical features, aetiology and geographical distribution of pyomyositis in East Africa. East Afr. Med. J., 45:167, 1968.

EOSINOPHILIA IN RELATION TO HELMINTHIC INFECTIONS
Philip D. Marsden

Hypereosinophilic states are considered elsewhere in this book, and conditions such as periarteritis nodosa, eosinophilic leukemia, and allergic diseases are discussed in appropriate sections. However, the author believes that a number of the cases of unexplained eosinophilia seen today in diagnostic units will in time be explained on the basis of helminthic infections, and it is worthwhile making one or two general points in relation to such infections.

As can be seen from the preceding articles, almost all helminthic infections in contrast to protozoal infections are at some time or other associated with eosinophilia. In terms of the parasites for which man is the definitive host, the eosinophilia often coincides with the invasive phase of a trematode, cestode, or nematode infection, and the diagnosis may not be apparent until several weeks or months later when the adults begin to produce progeny. For this reason obscure eosinophilia should always be kept under observation, and stool or tissue specimens reexamined. Some parasites are notorious in presenting a problem of eosinophilia for diagnosis, notably Strongyloides and Trichinella infections. After effective treatment of helminthic infections, particularly those in close contact with body tissues, there is often a pronounced rise in circulating eosinophils.

Perhaps more interesting is the clinical situation in which a patient has a significant human helminth load and yet little or no expected eosinophilia in the absence of cortisone therapy. Recent work suggesting that sensitized lymphocytes play an important role in the genesis of eosinophilia may throw some light on this problem.

Eosinophilia is a prominent feature of infections with nonhuman helminths, e.g., Angiostrongylus, and situations in which there is an abnormal host response, e.g., pulmonary tropical eosinophilia.

It appears that a small number of nonhuman helminths passing through man's tissues may engender marked eosinophilia and even hypergammaglobulinemia, e.g., toxocariasis, gnathostomiasis. To find the helminths responsible is impossible in many patients, and when found they may be very difficult to identify. Our elucidation of this clinical problem appears to rest on the elaboration of more specific and sensitive serologic tests, and the techniques of indirect hemagglutination, gel diffusion, fluorescent antibody tests, and similar procedures are useful here to detect host response to helminthic antigens. However, much difficult work will be needed to characterize these complex antigens.

Finally in a clinical consideration of this problem, common things occur commonly. A survey of a series of patients with occult eosinophilia in a large teaching hospital in New York City revealed a few cases of strongyloidiasis, but eosinophilia was most frequently one of the signs of a reaction to drug therapy.

ARTHROPODS AND LEECHES
AS AGENTS OF DISEASE
Philip D. Marsden

LEECHES
(Hirudiniasis)

Belonging to the class Hirudinea of the phylum Annelida, the leeches form an appropriate group to link the helminths to the arthropods. All blood-sucking species of medical importance live in fresh water or are terrestrial. They possess anterior and posterior suckers used for locomotion and attachment; the anterior sucker contains the mouth and cutting plates. When attachment to a host is gained, the skin is quickly perforated, and suction begins until the leech has taken several times its own weight in blood. In sucking blood, leeches secrete an anticoagulant, hirudin, the action of which continues after detachment. Leeches can survive for years without food. They can pass through boot eyelets and the fabric of loosely woven cloth to reach the skin of the host.

Both external and internal forms of hirudiniasis occur. *External hirudiniasis* is due to both land and aquatic leeches. In Southeast Asia particularly, as well as in India, tropical Australia, and parts of South America, land leeches drop in considerable numbers from jungle vegetation onto man. Large numbers may result in considerable blood loss, and even one or two may have a considerable psychologic impact. To remove these leeches, a lighted cigarette, match, or salt applied to the leech will cause it to release its jaws. The wound should be washed in antiseptic and an antibiotic cream or dressing applied; otherwise, secondary infection commonly occurs. The rarer *internal hirudiniasis* is usually due to accidental ingestion of small immature leeches in raw drinking water. They become attached to the buccal mucosa, pharynx, or larynx, and may grow there to produce signs of hemorrhage and obstruction. Manual removal of the leech with forceps may be difficult. An epinephrine nasal spray may induce it to release its hold. In the rare cases of urethral or vaginal involvement, strong salt solution has caused detachment prior to surgical removal.

Protection against aquatic and terrestrial leeches can be in the form of protective clothing or the use of repellents. Some repellents are rather soluble in water and need to be reapplied, but the use of diethyltoluamide in lanolin may overcome this problem.

Chin, T. M.: A further note on leech infestation of man. J. Parasit., 35:215, 1949.

Mann, K. H.: Leeches (Hirudinea): Their Structure, Physiology, Ecology, and Embryology. Oxford, Pergamon Press, 1962.

Salzberger, M.: Leeches as foreign bodies in the upper passages in Palestine. Laryngoscope, 38:27, 1928.

Walton, B. C., Traub, R., and Newsom, H. D.: Efficacy of clothing impregnants M-2065 and M-2066 against terrestrial leeches in North Borneo. Amer. J. Trop. Med., 5:190, 1956.

Arthropoda of Medical Importance

The phylum Arthropoda is the largest in the Animal Kingdom, containing at least three quarters of a million species. Some classes of arthropods include species of medical importance. These are the Pentasomida (tongue worms), Chilopoda (centipedes), Diplopoda (millipedes), Arachnida (scorpions, spiders, ticks), and Insecta. The latter are especially important. The major characteristic of arthropods is a segmented body that is invested with a rigid or semirigid cuticle of chitin.

PENTASTOMIDA
(Pentastomiasis, Porocephalosis, Porocephaliasis, Linguatulosis, Armilliferosis)

The class Pentastomida is considered first because its members that occasionally infect man look very much like helminths, although, in fact, they are modified arthropods with rudimentary legs and annulated but not segmented bodies.

Two families of medical interest, the Linguatulidae, and the Porocephalidae, contain the genera Linguatula (with flattened adults) and Porocephalus (with cylindrical adults).

Linguatula serrata is found in adult and nymphal stages in the nose and paranasal sinuses of carnivorous animals and as larvae and encapsulated nymphs in herbivorous animals throughout the world. Rarely, human infection with the adult occurs in the lungs. More commonly larvae and nymphs encyst in the mesenteric lymph nodes, liver, spleen, kidneys, and intestinal wall. Infection is acquired by ingesting eggs discharged in the nasal secretions of canines. This parasite is found in 4 per cent of necropsies in Chile. The syndrome of parasitic pharyngitis (halzoun) may be caused by the larvae.

The genus Porocephalus contains 20 species, of which two, *P. armillatus* and *P. moniliformis*, have been found in man in Africa and Asia, respectively. The adult is a parasite of the respiratory tract of snakes (pythons and others) and crocodiles, and the nymph is found in a wide variety of mammals. Humans acquire infection by ingesting pond or drinking water contaminated by snakes or by eating snake meat. The ingested eggs hatch in the intestine, and the larvae bore through the wall to lodge in any viscus, where they undergo nine molts in six months to a year to form infective nymphs. In man the infection usually comes to a blind end, as they have to be ingested by the definitive host. Human infection with encysted larvae or nymphs on the surface of the liver or in the intestinal mucosa, peritoneal cavity, or lung is fairly common in Africa, particularly in the Republic of the Congo. Painful inflammatory lesions may result, or the parasites may be asymptomatic and their resultant calcification give a characteristic crescentic opacity between 4 and 7 mm. in size (1.4 per cent of abdominal x-rays, in Ibadan, Nigeria, show this sign).

A recent report describes the findings of encysted nymphs in 45 per cent of autopsies on Malaysian aborigines. A range of lesions was observed from the encysted pentosomal nymph still viable with relatively little reaction, to the formation of a necrotic granulomatous reaction, with death followed by fibrosis and calcification. It is worth noting in relation to the discussion on eosinophilia (*vide supra*) that this parasite must also be considered because a blood eosinophilia can occur, especially after death of the larvae. Rarely, the parasite has caused intestinal obstruction, pneumonitis, meningitis, pericarditis, nephritis, and obstructive jaundice.

Burns Cox, C. J., Prathap, K., Clark, E., and Gillman, R.: Porocephaliasis in Western Malaysia. Trans. Roy. Soc. Trop. Med. Hyg., 63:409, 1969.

Prathap, K., Lau, K. S., and Bolton, J. M.: Pentastomiasis: A common finding at autopsy among Malaysian aborigines. Amer. J. Trop. Med., 18:20, 1969.

Schacher, J. F., Saab, S., Germanos, R., and Boustany, N.: The aeriology of halzoun in Lebanon: Recovery of *Linguatula serrata* nymphs from two patients. Trans. Roy. Soc. Trop. Med. Hyg., 63:854, 1969.

Steinbach, H. L., and Johnstone, H. G.: The roentgen diagnosis of Armillifer infection (porocephalosis) in man. Radiology, 68:234, 1957.

CHILOPODA
(Centipedes)

Flattened dorsoventrally, centipedes have a single pair of legs to each body segment. They feed on other arthropods, and the appendages of the first segment are modified as poison claws through which venom is injected into the prey. Although not fatal to man, their bite can produce intense fiery pain, and the area at the site of the bite may be inflamed. Regional lymph nodes enlarge, and rarely there are signs of meningism. Treatment consists of analgesics and the use of local anesthetics at the site of the bite. Recurrence of the local edema and arthritis has been noted. Corticosteroids have been helpful.

Haneveld, G. T.: Centipede bites. Brit. Med. J., 2:592, 1957.

DIPLOPODA
(Millipedes)

These have a rounded body contour and two pairs of legs per segment. They are vegetarian, but as a defense mechanism secrete noxious fluids from body pores when attacked. These secretions may produce a vesicular dermatitis in man.

ARACHNIDA
(Scorpions and Spiders)

SCORPIONIDA
(Scorpions, Eight Legs)

Envenomation of man or scorpiasis is common in some tropical areas. About 20,000 cases of scorpion sting occur annually in Mexico, and approximately 5 per cent are fatal, these deaths occurring mainly in small children. There are ten times more deaths from scorpion stings in Mexico than from snake bite. Scorpions are armed with a single curved caudal sting with which they inject their venom and paralyze their prey—usually other arthropods. Scorpions are nocturnal and hide beneath debris during the day.

The effects of envenomation vary with the species. Violent pain may occur at the site of the sting with radiation into the affected limbs. Chills with abundant cold sweats may be associated with severe thirst and vomiting. Venoms may have neurotoxic effects with paralysis and convulsions or cardiovascular effects with myocarditis and tachycardia, or may cause intravascular hemolysis. Death is often due to respiratory paralysis. Pancreatitis and defibrination syndromes have recently been described. Stings by scorpions with neurotoxic venom may not produce much local reaction.

Immediate treatment, as with snake bite, is aimed at delaying absorption of the venom. A tourniquet is applied to the limb and released every 20 to 30 minutes. If available, ice packs should be applied to the site and the patient kept at rest. Specific antiserum is available in some areas and should be given if signs occur in the central nervous system. Phenobarbital may control convulsions. Spraying DDT or benzene hexachloride (BHC) will cut down the scorpion population.

Bartholomew, C.: Acute scorpion pancreatitis in Trinidad. Brit. Med. J., 1:666, 1970.
McIntosh, M. E., and Watt, D. D.: Biochemical immunochemical aspects of the venom from the scorpion *Centruroides sculpturatus. In* Russell, F. E., and Sanders, P. R. (eds.): Animal Toxins. London, Pergamon Press, 1967, p. 47.
Poon-King, T.: Myocarditis from scorpion stings. Brit. Med. J., 1:374, 1963.
Sita Devi, S, et al.: Defibrination syndrome due to scorpion venom poisoning. Brit. Med. J., 1:345, 1970.
Whittlemore, F. W., Jr., Keegan, H. L., and Barowitz, J. L.: Studies of scorpion antivenoms: 1. Paraspecificity. Bull. WHO, 25:185, 1961.

SPIDERS

(Eight Legs, Abdomen Joined to Cephalothorax by a Narrow Waist)

Most spiders possess venom apparatus in the form of a pair of chelicerae terminating in sharp fangs and associated venom glands. The degree of development of this apparatus varies, and the glands contain only a small amount of venom suitable for paralyzing other arthropods. Of the 200 genera described, only eight contain species reported to be poisonous to man. Human fatalities have occurred following the bite of species of Latrodectus, Loxosceles, Phoneutria, and Atrax.

Latrodectus. It is likely that all species in this genus are poisonous to man, but the black widow (*L. mactans*) and the gray widow (*L. geometricus*) are most important. Males have much less venom than the aggressive females. These spiders are represented in most warm parts of the world and occur in the Americas from Southern Canada to Chile. They spin their webs in dark places, often outhouses. In Texas 90 per cent of spider bites occur on the buttocks and genitals because of the tendency to spin webs under lavatory seats in outside privies. The bite may pass unnoticed; two tiny red spots may be seen at the site, or a severe local reaction occurs. The neurotoxic fraction in the venom is a protein of low molecular weight which affects the cord and nerve endings. Absorption is accompanied by pain and numbness in the affected part. In 15 minutes to a few hours generalized agonizing muscular pains appear, together with symptoms of shock. The blood pressure falls, and there are marked sweating, a feeling of weakness and nausea, and labored respiration. The marked rigidity of the muscles of the abdominal wall may simulate tetanus or an acute abdomen. Paralysis and coma may be followed by cardiac or respiratory failure in severe cases.

An intravenous injection of 10 ml. of a 10 per cent solution of calcium gluconate administered slowly will relieve muscular spasm. If this fails, a muscle relaxant such as mephenesin can be given. An antivenin is available in some endemic areas where there is a demand for it. It is effective against most species of Latrodectus. The spiders are sensitive to DDT spraying.

Loxosceles. The hairy brown spiders, *L. reclusa*, of the United States and *L. laeta* of Central and South America, occur in houses among furniture. Pain occurs at the site of their bite, followed by erythema, edema, and local necrosis. A rarer cutaneovisceral form is associated with toxic nephritis and hepatitis, the venom being cytotoxic. Local pain and edema decrease after parenteral antihistamine and corticosteroids have suppressed systemic reactions.

Phoneutria. This is a genus responsible for fatalities in children in some South American countries (Chile, Brazil). The venom acts on both the central and peripheral nervous systems.

Atrax. The Australian funnel web spider also produces neurotoxic symptoms.

Editorial: Spider bites. Lancet, 2:509, 1969.
Horen, W. P.: Arachnidism in the United States. J.A.M.A., 185:839, 1963.
Levi, H. W., and Spielman, A.: The biology and control of the South American brown spider *Loxosceles laeta* (Nicolet) in a North American focus. Amer. J. Trop. Med., Hyg., 13:132, 1964.
McCrone, J. D., and Hatala, R. J.: Isolation and characterisation of a lethal component from the venom of *Latrodectus mactans. In* Russell, F. E., and Sanders, P. R. (eds.): Animal Toxins. London, Pergamon Press, 1967, p. 29.
Smith, C. W., and Micks, D. W.: Comparative study of the venom and other components of three species of Loxosceles. Amer. J. Trop. Med., 17:651, 1968.

ACARINA
(Ticks and Mites)

GENERAL CONSIDERATIONS

Families in the order Acarina (ticks and mites) are responsible for carrying some important human infections. The family Ixodoidea contains the hard ticks responsible for transmitting the rickettsia of tick typhus. The Argasidae are the soft ticks, some of which transmit tick-borne relapsing fever (*Borrelia duttoni*). The mites are also of medical importance. The family Trombiculidae contains the important genus of red mites, Trombicula, which transmit scrub typhus caused by *Rickettsia tsutsugamushi* (*orientalis*). The larvae of other similar mites cause an unpleasant, irritating skin rash (chiggers, red bugs, or harvest mites). About 24 hours after feeding, small red macules appear, and there may be hundreds if infection is severe. The diagnosis is made by finding the six-legged orange red larvae on the skin. BHC dusting powder destroys mites in their habitats and dibutyl phthalate or benzyl benzoate is quite effective for about a week if dusted over clothing. The house mouse mite Allodermanyssus transmits *Rickettsia akari* of rickettsinlpox. One other mite, however, not considered elsewhere in this book, is *Sarcoptes scabiei*, which is responsible for one of the most prevalent skin diseases in the world. Tick paralysis, a little-diagnosed entity, must also be briefly considered under this heading.

TICK PARALYSIS

Tick paralysis is a rapidly progressive flaccid paralysis, usually symmetrical, with loss of tendon and superficial reflexes. It follows tick bite and is probably caused by a neurotoxin in tick saliva. Several pathogenic chains have been suggested, including a conduction block in the somatic motor fibers, interference of the monosynaptic pathways, a depolarizing block at neuromuscular junctions, and an actual muscle lesion.

Symptoms may not come on until five to six days after attachment of the tick, when the patient becomes restless and irritable and may have numbness or tingling of the extremities, lips, throat, and face. Difficulty in walking is rapidly followed by inability to stand. Within a day or two there is paralysis of the limbs and trunk muscles, and a bulbar lesion will lead to dysphagia, slurred speech, and impaired vision. Death may result from respiratory failure or aspiration pneumonia. Pain and fever are rare, but there may be local skin change around the site of the bite, and morbilliform rashes have been reported. Providing that the paralysis is not too far advanced, rapid and complete recovery follows removal of the tick, although recovery may take more than a week. The cerebrospinal fluid is normal; bulbar and respiratory failure must be treated symptomatically, and a respirator may be life-saving. The paralysis is often confused with poliomyelitis. In polyneuritis, myelitis, syringomyelia, and spinal cord tumor, sensory loss is usually present. Sensory signs are very rare in tick paralysis. *Like leeches, ticks should not be pulled off* but should be persuaded to detach by the application of a lighted cigarette or carbon dioxide snow to their posterior end.

Children are more frequently affected than adults. In one series of 119 cases, 79 per cent, including all the fatal cases, were in children under 16; two thirds were girls. Late removal of ticks is more probable in children, particularly in girls with long hair, for in these patients 70 per cent of the ticks are attached to the head and neck. There appears to be no correlation between mortality and the proximity of tick attachment to the brain. With rapid overseas travel, this diagnostic problem may confront a physician anywhere in the world. Various tick species are responsible. *Dermacentor andersoni* and *D. variabilis* are the chief offenders in the Rocky Mountains of North America, *Ixodes holocyclus* in Australia, and *Rhipicephalus simus* in Africa. The paralysis occurs in travelers to tick-infested areas who are likely to intrude into tick habitats by camping, picnicking, fishing, or hunting.

Ransmeier, J. C.: Tick paralysis in the Eastern United States. J. Pediat., 34:299, 1949.
Tick paralysis. Brit. Med. J., 2:314, 1969

SCABIES

Scabies is the most common skin disease encountered in some parts of the world, and is usually associated with poor living conditions. It is due to infection of the skin by the mite *Sarcoptes scabiei*. Hyperinfections with crusting and pustulation are termed "Norwegian" scabies. Scabies should be considered in every patient who complains of a persistent itch, and this symptom, together with papules, vesicles, and pustules on the extremities and follicular papules on the trunk, should be regarded as being due to scabies until proved otherwise.

The female mite is acquired by sharing a bed with an infected person or by other close personal contact, and in this sense in adults it can be likened to a venereal disease. The mite burrows into cracked and folded regions of the skin, the tunnel being limited to the stratum corneum except at the anterior end. Burrowing is by means of jaws and the sharp cutting edges on the terminal joints of the first two pairs of legs. Both copulation and egg production occur in the burrow, the rarely seen male ranging over the skin in search of the female. About two eggs are produced daily for two months. The hatched six-legged larvae make their own burrows and develop into adulthood in a fortnight. About one month after the establishment of the first burrow the patient begins to itch, probably because he becomes sensitized to acarine products. The scratching limits the population of mites by depriving them of a roof over their heads and crushing them. In experimentally induced infections Mellanby found that the population reached a maximum within three months and varied from 20 to 400 egg-laying females. Examination of nearly 900 men with scabies showed a mean population of 11.3 adult females per man, and more than half the patients harbored five adult acari or fewer.

The skin eruption has two aspects: the burrows which have to be searched for, and the changes resulting from sensitization and secondary infection which are obvious. The burrow of the ovigerous female appears as a narrow, slightly raised white gray or black line. The white shiny dot sometimes seen at one end, which may be associated with a small vesicle, is the site of the mite.

The *burrows* are commonly found on the sides and webs of the fingers, the ulnar border of the hand, the volar aspect of the wrists, the points of the elbows, the axillary folds, the areolae of the nipples in women, the external genitalia in men, the buttocks, and the margins or soles of the feet.

The face and scalp are never affected in adults. Sometimes a typical burrow cannot be found. *There is a widespread rash* of follicular papules usually well marked on the abdomen, buttocks, inner sides of the thighs, and axillary folds. Scratch marks, crusted papules, and pustulation demonstrate the effects of scratching. An infected eczema sometimes develops on the fingers and wrists, nipples, or glans penis. Patients who are unable to scratch do not develop such lesions.

The *diagnosis of scabies* is probable if other members of the household are found infected. The mite can be identified by scraping a burrow along its length with the edge of a scalpel blade held at a right angle to the skin. The resultant material is mounted in 10 per cent potassium hydroxide under a coverslip, and microscopy reveals the mite. It has a body shaped like a tortoise with two pairs of legs in front and two pairs behind. The forelegs end in "suckers" and the hindlegs in long bristles. The female is about 400 μ long and coated in short bristles. Eggs or immature forms may also be present.

The typical clinical picture of scabies is subject to a number of variations. In babies the scalp may be affected, which means that the topical preparation must be carefully applied. Clean people usually have few lesions, and scabies may be overlooked in nurses for this reason. A localized eczema may be the presentation, or persistent sepsis of the skin. The amount of itch is very variable. In Norwegian scabies two million mites may be present, and the stratum corneum may be honeycombed with burrows on biopsy. Clinically, Norwegian scabies resembles exfoliative dermatitis. Often itching is absent, and this has been offered as the explanation of this hyperinfective state. However, some of these patients do itch, and other hypotheses attribute this state to topical or systemic corticosteroids or vitamin A deficiency.

The differential diagnosis includes atopic eczema, neurodermatitis, dermatitis herpetiformis, and two conditions considered later in this article, pediculosis and papular urticaria. Papular urticaria is due to the bites of various insects, often fleas or bed bugs, but may also result from bites of various mites, either cheese straw or grain mites or the Sarcoptes of dogs and cats mentioned at the end of this article.

The three essential aspects of treatment are to treat all members of the household simultaneously, to use an application that will kill the parasites, and to apply it to the whole skin area. Since the acaricides mentioned destroy all adults, larvae, and nymphs, but not the eggs, a further treatment should be given after a week. Suitable topical preparations for total body application are: (1) *benzyl benzoate, 25 per cent emulsion (60 ml. for each application)*. It is slightly irritating and may cause secondary eczematization and conjunctivitis if it is carried to the eyes. It has a rather penetrating smell, but is a very effective acaricide. (2) *gamma benzene hexachloride (Gamma BHC) as a 1 per cent cream (25 grams for each application)*. This is odorless, nonirritant, and effective against associated pediculosis as well.

A bath before the first application is desirable, and clean underclothes and sheets should be used after it. The itch may persist for some weeks after treatment, and soothing calamine lotion can be prescribed. Oral antimicrobial drugs may be necessary to combat skin infection and should be given concurrently. Most "failures" of treatment are due to unsatisfactory therapy, but it has recently been suggested that there may be benzyl benzoate-resistant Sarcoptes. As scabies is often transmitted in the course of sexual contact, the possibility of an associated veneral disease should be borne in mind. For effective treatment of scabies in a community where it occurs in high incidence, a treatment center is necessary. During World War II in Britain, scabies clinics brought the disease under control, and a scabies order gave personnel powers to enforce treatment. This species of parasite is comprised of a number of physiologic forms specific to the various vertebrate hosts; the disease in man is produced by *Sarcoptes scabiei var. hominis*. Other forms include *S. scabiei var. canis*, the cause of sarcoptic mange. This parasite and the cat mite *Notoedres cati* can cause severe papular urticaria in man although the classic burrow is not seen as these mites are specific to their normal hosts and incapable of burrowing and breeding in man.

Herridge, C. F.: Norwegian scabies (crusted scabies). Brit. Med. J., 1:239, 1963.
Lyell, A.: Diagnosis and treatment of scabies. Brit. Med. J., 1:223, 1967.
Mellanby, K.: Scabies. New York, Oxford University Press, 1943.
The scabies epidemic. Brit. Med. J., 2:193, 1967.
Thomsett, L. R.: Mite infestations of man contracted from dogs and cats. Brit. Med. J., 2:93, 1968.

INSECTA

Numerous insects are implicated in disease, and the purpose of this article is to mention those entities not covered elsewhere. We shall consider stinging insects, urticating insects, myiasis, and ectoparasitic insects in that order.

STINGING INSECTS

HYMENOPTERA
(Bees, Wasps, Hornets, Ants)

All stinging insects are included in this order, which contains 60,000 species. The stinging apparatus consists of a modified ovipositor and paired poison glands that discharge into a reservoir — the poison sac. In bees the venom apparatus is usually torn away from the body when the insect is brushed off. The average bee sting contains

0.3 mg. of venom. The venom of bees and wasps contains a number of fatty acids and saponin-like substances.

A direct action (increase in vascular permeability at the site of the sting) is associated with the presence of histamine, serotonin, and a particular kinin. In addition to the effect of these substances there is an indirect effect, depending, among other things, on the properties of histamine liberated from the damaged tissues, probably by an enzymatic mechanism. The position of the sting is of great importance. If it occurs in the buccal or pharyngeal mucosa, a serious edema of the glottis and asphyxia may result. If venom is directly inoculated into a blood vessel, rapid absorption can cause syncope and even death.

In parts of Africa and Asia some varieties of bees are especially aggressive, and a number of deaths have resulted from multiple stings. The total number of simultaneous stings necessary for a fatality is about 500. Apart from deaths owing to multiple stings, many fatalities occur in hypersensitive patients, in whom death may occur in one hour owing to anaphylaxis and laryngeal edema. The allergen occurs in all parts of the insect, and hypersensitive patients can be desensitized by injection of wasp and bee extract. In the United States more deaths were caused by stinging insects than by snakes in the period 1950–1954. In such allergic states intense pruritus after stinging is followed by severe angioneurotic edema and asthma. Severe abdominal pain and convulsion may occur.

Stings should be removed from the wound, with care taken not to express more venom into the wound by squeezing the poison sac. Acute allergic reactions should be treated with 0.5 ml. of 1:1000 epinephrine intramuscularly. This can be repeated as often as necessary, together with an intramuscular injection of an antihistamine. Hydrocortisone, 100 mg., should be injected intravenously in patients with severe laryngeal edema; tracheostomy may be life-saving. Milder reactions can be relieved by black coffee plus 30 mg. of epinephrine. Sensitized persons should carry sublingual tablets of isoproterenol and antihistamines and have epinephrine ampules available.

Barnard, J. M.: Cutaneous responses to insects. Types and mechanism of reactions. J.A.M.A., 196:259, 1966.

Beard, R. L.: Insect toxins and venoms. Ann. Rev. Entom., 8:1, 1963.

Mann, G. T., and Bates, M. R., Jr.: The pathology of insect bites: A brief review and report of eleven fatal cases. South. Med. J., 53:1399, 1960.

Shaffer, J. H.: Stinging insects: A threat to life. J.A.M.A., 177: 473, 1961.

ANTS

Although most ants possess venom apparatus, only a few are capable of injuring man. The Tucandeira ant of the Central American forests possesses a powerful sting that may result in fever for several hours. Allergic reactions to ants have been reported. The fire ant (*Solenopsis saevissima richteri*) has now established itself in the southern United States, and produces a pustular, markedly erythematous rash following multiple stinging owing to a necrotizing toxin solenamine.

Adrouny, G. A.: The fire ant's fire. Bull. Tulane Univ. Med. Fac., 25:67, 1966.

Cavill, G. W. K., and Robertson, P. L.: Ant venom, attractors and repellents. Science, 149:1337, 1966.

Middleton, E.: In combined staff clinic on poisoning by venomous animals. Amer. J. Med., 42:118, 1967.

URTICATING INSECTS

A number of moths and butterflies (Lepidoptera) and beetles (Coleoptera) possess urticating qualities and can cause irritant dermatitis and conjunctivitis.

Lepidoptera. The caterpillars of a large number of moths and some butterflies possess urticating hairs or spines singly or in clusters over the body. If such a caterpillar is handled, these penetrate the skin, and venom passes through an opening at the tip. The hairs frequently break and remain in the skin. When the caterpillar pupates, the urticating hairs are frequently present in the cocoon that surrounds the pupa, and are also carried on the wings and body of the adult insect when it emerges.

Dermatitis produced by caterpillars is very widespread. Outbreaks have occurred in Israel and Japan. In 1956, 250,000 cases of dermatitis were estimated on Honshu Island. In Texas 2130 cases of caterpillar stings were reported in 1968. The hairs can be removed by application of adhesive tape. If cellophane tape is used, the hairs can then be mounted on a slide for microscopic examination. Washing the affected area with mild antiseptic should be followed by the application of calamine. Severe urticaria may require parenteral epinephrine and antihistamines. Adult moths have been recorded as producing similar lesions.

Hellier, F. F., and Warin, R. P.: Caterpillar dermatitis. Brit. Med. J. 1:346, 1967.

Zaias, N., Ioannides, G., and Taplin, D.: Dermatitis from contact with moths (Genus Hylesia). J.A.M.A., 207:525, 1969.

COLEOPTERA
(Beetles)

Two families of beetles that contain urticating substances are the Staphylinidae (rove beetles) and the Meloidae (blister and oil beetles). Eight staphylinids of the genus Paederus cause dermatitis, especially in tropical countries. The irritant is present in the coelomic fluid, and when the beetle is crushed on the skin, erythematous blistering and pigmentary lesions occur. Pederin, a powerful vesicating toxin, comprises 1 per cent of the tiny beetle's body weight. Staphylinids are so small that they are not usually noted in the skin.

Several genera of Meloidae have urticating properties, including Mylabris, Epicanita and Lytta. *Lytta (Cantharis) vesicatoria* is familiarly known as Spanish fly. These beetles are night-flying and are frequently attracted to artificial light. The urticating substance occurs in the hemolymph, which is extruded through the integument if the insect is disturbed or escapes when the insect is crushed. Large blisters are produced if the insect contacts the human skin, and blindness may occur if the conjunctiva is affected. The pathogenesis of these lesions is explained in a way similar to that of attacks by gaseous vesicants, namely, by a blocking of enzymes of the SH groups. Like these enzymes, cantharidin inhibits glucide metabolism. *It should be noted that cantharidin has no aphrodisiac effect, and that the fatal dose is less than 60 mg.* Topical treatment of the blisters with magnesium sulfate and methyl alcohol packs has been recommended. Other tropical beetles producing vesicants are in the families Paunidae and Oedemeridae.

Two other conditions associated with beetles can be mentioned here.

Scarabiasis is the term used for the presence of adult dung beetles in the stool of man. Certain beetle larvae survive in the fecal stream, notably the meal worms (Tenebrio) ingested in contaminated cereals.

Carpet beetles can be used as an example of harmless insects which may be associated with delusions of parasitosis and the production of a type of dermatitis artifacta. However, there is at least one report of a patient who became sensitized to the varied carpet beetle (*Anthrenus verbasci*) which can be brought into the house on cut flowers.

Armstrong, R. K., and Winfield, J. L.: *Paederus fuscipes* dermatitis. An epidemic on Okinawa. Amer. J. Trop. Med. Hyg., 18:147, 1969.
Ayres, S., and Mihan, R.: Delusions of parasitosis caused by carpet beetles. J.A.M.A., 199:675, 1967.
Browne, S. G.: Cantharidin poisoning due to a blister beetle. Brit. Med. J., 2:1290, 1960.
Cormia, F. E.: Carpet beetle dermatitis. J.A.M.A., 200:799, 1967.
Giglioli, M. E. C.: Some observations on blister beetle, family Meloidae, in Gambia, West Africa. Trans. Roy. Soc. Trop. Med. Hyg., 59:657, 1965.
Halprim, K. M.: The art of self mutilation. II. Delusions of parasitosis. J.A.M.A., 198:1207, 1966.
Kerdel Vegas, F., and Gothman Yahr, M.: Paederus dermatitis. Arch Derm. (Chicago), 94:175, 1966.
Rosin, R. D.: Cantharides intoxication. Brit. Med. J., 3:33, 1967.
Scarabiasis. J. Trop. Med. Hyg., 70:49, 1967.

MYIASIS
(Maggots)

Myiasis may be defined as the infection of vertebrates with the larvae (maggots) of Diptera (flies) which feed on the tissues of the host. The maggots are usually identified by the form of their posterior spiracles, but this may be difficult to define in the early molts. Rearing the larvae to adults makes identification easier, especially with immature stages. Myiasis is a far greater problem in sheep,

cattle, and deer than in man, and there is no form of myiasis found exclusively in man. For the purposes of a textbook of medicine, it is permissible to abandon the scientific classification of the responsible species and consider the clinical type of myiasis produced. For a description of the genera of flies, a textbook of entomology should be consulted. Primary myiasis occurs in the absence of debility of the host or tissue injury; this is in contrast to secondary myiasis.

PRIMARY MYIASIS

Furuncular Myiasis

Furuncular myiasis is a good descriptive term, because the skin lesion looks like a boil but in fact contains a maggot which breathes through a hole in the tip of the lesion. When mature, the maggot drops to the ground to pupate. There are two distinct types occurring in Africa and the Americas, respectively. (1) The African Tumbu fly (*Cordylobia anthropophaga*). The eggs are sometimes laid on clothing or else the larvae actively seek the host and burrow into the skin to feed. Multiple lesions are common. The normal hosts are wild rodents. (2) The human botfly (*Dermatobia hominis*). The botfly is found in South America, Central America, and Mexico. The eggs are frequently laid on a hematophagous insect (mosquito or stable fly) by the female and thence transported to the host. The secondarily infected "boil"-like lesion also occurs in other mammals in endemic areas.

The application of vaseline to the lesion to block the spiracles often brings the suffocating larvae wriggling out backward, especially when mature. Immature larvae can be excised, but if possible it is better to let them mature and drop out.

Creeping Myiasis

Creeping myiasis is a form of larva migrans caused by flies of the genera Gastrophilus and Hypoderma. The former larvae do not mature and, being restricted to the stratum corneum, leave an obvious trail. Hypoderma penetrates more deeply and can complete its development in some instances and perforate the skin to escape.

The behavior of these two species is easily understood if their lives in their normal hosts are mentioned. *Gastrophilus*, normally a parasite of Equidae, has a period of migration as a young larva in the tongue epithelium but matures in the lumen of the intestine. *Hypoderma* is classically a parasite of bovids. *H. bovis* migrates via nerve trunks to gain the spinal canal and paravertebral muscle mass, and *H. lineatus* penetrates, migrating via the mucosa of the upper gut and gaining the same muscles via the esophagus. Both cause voluminous subcutaneous paravertebral abscesses, ruining the hide. It is not surprising, therefore that when man is the host, the larvae may wander widely and even gain the eye, causing blindness.

Ophthalmomyiasis

A painful conjunctivitis can be produced by the first-stage maggots of *Oestrus ovis* hatching from eggs laid by the female near the conjunctiva. Hypoderma maggots may penetrate the globe of the eye. Such maggots can be irrigated from the conjunctiva or mechanically removed

Other Forms of Primary Myiasis

Genitourinary myiasis owing to Fannia or Calliphora maggots has been rarely reported, the eggs being laid in the vicinity of the urethra. Maggots of these genera and the genera Sarcophaga and Musca have been found in freshly passed stools and can develop in the fecal stream. Tetrachloroethylene is effective. Intestinal myiasis is cosmopolitan and relatively common. In North America the drone fly (*Tubifera tenax*) larvae is the most frequently encountered species. The larvae of *Auchmeromyia luteola* (the Congo floor maggot) are temporary blood-sucking parasites of Africa; the larvae emerge from hiding places at night to suck blood, but after a meal retire to rest.

SECONDARY MYIASIS

Invasion of the body by maggots can occur in very debilitated individuals and in those with destructive or ulcerative lesions. Thus wounds may be infected by maggots of various fly genera, including Wohlfahrtia, Callitroga, and Chrysomyia. Similarly, myiasis of the nose, upper respiratory passages, or ear is caused by the screwworm fly maggots invading infected debilitated tissues. They should be picked out with forceps; otherwise they can penetrate the base of the skull and invade the brain.

PREVENTION

Reduction of screwworms, hobflies, and warble fly maggots in sheep and cattle reduces the chances of human infection. This can be done with various dips of insecticides. Auchmeromyia larvae can be killed by dusting houses with insecticides. Clothing should be ironed and not hung out of doors for Cordylobia to lay eggs on it. Repellents and bed nets will reduce the incidence of Dermatobia lesions. The proper control of refuse disposal will reduce the number of blue- and greenbottle flies. It is worth noting that the eradication of the screwworm fly from Curaçao by releasing sexually sterile males is one of the few instances of a successful form of biologic control.

Baumhover, A. H.: Eradication of the screwworm fly: An agent of myiasis. J.A.M.A., 196:240, 1966.

Flew, G. P., and Grundy, J. H.: Infection with *Dermatobia hominis* occurring in British Guiana. J. Royal Army Med. Corp., 113:148, 1967.

Günther, S.: Furuncular Tumbu fly myiasis of man in Gabon, Equatorial Africa. J. Trop. Med. Hyg., 70:169, 1967.

James, M. T.: The flies that cause myiasis in man. United States Department of Agriculture Misc. Publ. No. 631, 1947.

Palmer, E. D.: Entomology of the gastrointestinal tract. Milit. Med., 135:105, 1970.

Zumpt, F.: Myiasis in Man and Animals of the Old World. London, Butterworth and Company (Publishers), Ltd., 1965.

ECTOPARASITIC INSECTS
(Fleas and Lice)

Both fleas and lice are ectoparasites of man in the sense that they live outside his body on the skin but are dependent on him for food. Lice are more dependent than fleas and cannot survive long if separated from man because they need his body warmth and his tissues for their frequent feedings. Fleas are more exploratory and are capable of fantastic leaps, thus enabling them to transfer easily from host to host. Lice are flattened dorsoventrally, enabling them to hug the surface of the skin whereas fleas are laterally compressed, enabling them to slip between the upright hairs. Lice have no true metamorphosis in their life cycle, the young resembling the adults, whereas fleas have a conventional true cycle of metamorphosis with larvae and pupae.

Both ectoparasites play important roles in the transmission of human disease. Louse-borne typhus (*R. prowazeki*) and louse-borne relapsing fever (*Borrelia recurrentis*) are mainly transmitted by the body louse, and in conditions of poverty, war, and famine, great epidemics have occurred. Apart from plague, fleas also transmit endemic or murine typhus owing to *Rickettsia typhi* (*R. mooseri*).

PEDICULOSIS
(Head, Body, and Pubic Lice)

Man provides food and shelter for two genera of lice. *Pediculus humanus var. capitis* infests the head and *P. humanus var. corporis*, the body and clothing. *Phthirus pubis* (crab lice) usually lives in the pubic area, but on occasion extends its range to the axilla, chest hairs, and even the eyebrows and eyelashes. The eggs or nits are found attached to the hairs of the host, and in the case of the body louse are found on clothing. All three lice suck blood frequently and can exist only a short time away from the host. Their saliva produces an *irritant roseate papular dermatitis*. Scratching leads to secondary bacterial infection of the skin with crusting and induration, and pigmentation may be present in severe infestations (vagabond's disease). Enlargement of local lymph nodes is common, especially the posterior auricular group in severe capitis infections. *Phthirus pubis* infestation of the eyelashes leads to blepharitis. The irritant cutaneous lesions suggest the diagnosis, which is confirmed by finding the eggs or adults. The eggs can be combed out of the hair with a fine-toothed comb.

Treatment. In the treatment of head lice an ointment of 1.0 per cent hexachlorocyclohexane in vanishing cream (Kwell) should be rubbed on the scalp thoroughly. This treatment is also effective for pubic lice when the ointment is massaged into the skin of the infested area. Lice and eggs can be removed individually from the eyelashes or eliminated by the application of 0.25 per cent physostigmine ophthalmic ointment. Body lice are destroyed by sterilizing the clothing by heat, using the ointment on infested areas of the body. A 10 per cent DDT in pyrophyllite dusted onto the head, body, and clothing without undressing is highly effective. Lice in Korea and Egypt have developed resistance to DDT, and 1 per cent hexachlorocyclohexane or pyrethrum powder may be substituted for it. The secondary pyoderma should be treated with appropriate antimicrobial drugs.

Prevention. The prevention of lousiness consists primarily in personal cleanliness and the avoidance of infected persons, bedding, and clothes. *Phthirus pubis* is usually transmitted by sexual intercourse. The rise of the "hippies," with their low standards of personal hygiene and tendency to increasing sexual promiscuity, has resulted in an increase in the incidence of crab lice. Lice are quite host-specific; thus unlike fleas, the lice of domestic animals are not attracted to man.

Ackerman, A. B.: Crabs—The resurgence of *Phthirus pubis*. New Eng. J. Med., 278:950, 1968.
Buxton, P. A.: Louse: An Account of the Lice Which Infect Man, Their Medical Importance and Control. London, Edward Arnold (Publishers), Ltd., 1939.

FLEAS

Pulex irritans is primarily a human flea. The fleas of the cat and dog (Ctenocephalides) and of the rat and mouse (Xenopsylla) also frequent man. They usually migrate over the body until a tight garter or belt obstructs their passage, and there they proceed to suck blood. Individuals vary greatly in their reaction to the salivary secretion of fleas. Some are unaffected. On those who are severely irritated, raised red edematous lesions are produced (papular urticaria). Fleas are sensitive to applications of DDT.

The control of fleas requires their destruction in the home. Vacuum cleaning of rugs and removal of debris will eliminate adults as well as eggs, larvae, and pupae. Insecticide sprays such as 5 per cent DDT in oil are effective. The living quarters of dogs and cats and the animals themselves should also be treated. As DDT is rather toxic to young cats, a 4 per cent Malathion powder can be used for them. Bird fleas can also cause papular urticaria; hen runs may require treatment, and birds' nests should be removed from under eaves of affected houses.

TUNGIASIS
(Tunga Penetrans)

The common names jigger or chigoe are to be avoided because they are easily confused with chigger, the name given to trombiculid harvest mites. A highly modified flea, *Tunga penetrans*, parasitizes man, pigs, and dogs, as well as a variety of other mammals. It is common in Africa and South America. The adult female is a permanent parasite of the subcutaneous tissues of warm-blooded animals and is embedded in the skin with just the anal core having access to the exterior. The male copulates with the embedded female, and several hundred eggs are laid, after which the female dies.

The embedded females are most common on the sole of the foot and the root of the nail, where they cause pain. In debilitated people lying in infested huts many lesions may be present, all on one side of the body including the face. Secondary infection commonly results from the severe irritation. Septicemia, thrombophlebitis, tetanus, and gas gangrene may be complications. The swelling containing the ovigerous female is about the size of a pea and may be mistaken for myiasis. However, the lesion is recognized by the tip of the flea's abdomen appearing as a black dot in the center of the lesion.

Embedded females are best removed individually. After cleansing the skin with antiseptic, the opening hole of the flea pustule is enlarged with a sterile needle, and the intact insect can then be enucleated or expelled by gentle pressure. Antimicrobial therapy may be needed for secondary bacterial infection. Prophylaxis with DDT powder to the feet and socks or benzyl benzoate application is effective.

Bolam, M. R., and Burtt, E. T.: Flea infestation as a cause of papular urticaria. Brit. Med. J., 1:1130, 1956.
Jelliffe, D. B.: Tungiasis. *In* Simons, R. D. G. P. (ed.): Handbook of Tropical Dermatology. New York, American Elsevier Publishing Company, Inc., 1953, p. 895.

ARTHROPODS AS MECHANICAL CARRIERS OF DISEASE

FLIES

The common house fly and its relatives, the stable fly, greenbottle, bluebottle, blow fly, and flesh fly, breed and feed on human and animal feces and garbage. Typhoid fever, bacillary dysentery, amebiasis, and cholera may be transported on the fly's body from feces to man's food, and are found in the feces and vomitus of flies. Poliomyelitis and infectious hepatitis conceivably could also be transmitted in this way. Small flies called eye gnats may act as carriers of pathogens causing acute purulent conjunctivitis and yaws.

Control of flies by spraying breeding habitats with 10 per cent DDT in kerosene is effective. Garbage should be tightly sealed or destroyed to prevent fly access. Houses and particularly food cabinets should be rendered flyproof. Outdoor privies and septic tanks should be disinfected.

COCKROACHES
(Blattidae)

These common hospital and home insects may serve as mechanical transmitters of intestinal bacteria, virus, or Protozoa by their contact with filth and food. Cleanliness in the kitchen is essential for their control. The following are effective against roaches: Chlordane, 5 to 10 per cent dust; Chlordane, 2 per cent, and DDT, 5 per cent, in kerosene; or Malathion, 2 per cent in oil.

BEDBUGS
(Cimex)

Bedbugs are reddish brown and wingless, and have a disagreeable odor. As with fleas, the bites of bedbugs may result in papular urticaria. Because they suck human blood, they would seem to be likely disease transmitters, but all attempts to demonstrate this have failed. Although in the laboratory they can be infected with numerous human pathogens, they do not appear to transmit them in nature. In small African babies numerous bites are said to have resulted in iron deficiency anemia. A 5 per cent kerosene solution of DDT or 0.1 per cent lindane oil on infested bed frames, furniture, and wall crevices will control this insect. Infested mattresses should be discarded.

ARTHROPODS AS INTERMEDIATE HOSTS OF INFECTIOUS DISEASE

The infectious agents for which arthropods serve as vectors and the hosts in which these pathogens can develop are considered elsewhere in this book. In concluding the present section, it is worth emphasizing that for the medical man with biologic interests the field of medical entomology still holds considerable research possibilities and is worthwhile exploring. To aid in this interest some general references are given below.

Busvine, J. R.: Insects and Hygiene. London, Methuen and Company, Ltd., 1951.

Gordon, R. M., and Lavoipierre, M. M. J.: Entomology for Students of Medicine. London, Blackwell Scientific Publications, Ltd., 1962.

Herms, W. B.: Medical Entomology. 5th ed. Revised by M. T. James. New York, The Macmillan Company, 1961.

Horsfall, W. R.: Medical Entomology, Arthropods, and Human Disease. New York, The Ronald Press Company, 1962.

Leclercq, M.: Entomological Parasitology. Translated by G. Lapage. New York, Pergamon Press, Inc., 1969.

Smart, J.: A Handbook for the Identification of Insects of Medical Importance. London, The British Museum, 1965.

IMMUNE MECHANISMS
IN DISEASE

INTRODUCTION
Henry G. Kunkel

Some type of immunologic aberration has been implicated in an extremely wide and varied group of diseases. These include the allergic disorders in which the alterations involved are relatively clear, also diseases such as thyroiditis, systemic lupus erythematosus, and acquired hemolytic anemia, in which some insight concerning an immunologic mechanism has been gained, and finally such conditions as rheumatoid arthritis, ulcerative colitis, and certain types of liver disease, in which the evidence for an immunologic disorder remains very tentative. Interest has centered in particular on the challenging question of autoimmunity and its possible pathogenic role in many of these disorders. Considerable difficulty, however, has been encountered in assessing the exact significance of observed autoimmune phenomena; despite the active investigations undertaken in recent years, few conclusive answers have been obtained. Part of the problem stems from the gradual realization that the occurrence of autoantibodies is by no means a rare phenomenon limited to specific diseases. Many normal persons appear to possess such antibodies; perhaps all normal persons do. It has become increasingly clear that the "horror autotoxicus" concept with its dire implications as elaborated by Ehrlich requires considerable revision. Some autoantibodies appear to be without harmful effects, and the possibility exists, at least in certain instances, that they may be of benefit. The term "physiogenic autoantibodies" has been applied to this type and serves to distinguish them from the rarer "pathogenic autoantibodies."

Examples of widely prevalent autoantibodies that in most situations appear to be without harmful effects are immunoconglutinin or antibody to complement, the anti-γ-globulins frequently termed rheumatoid factors, and the antinuclear antibodies of many different types. All of these have been found in the sera of normal persons as well as in those with a wide variety of microbial diseases. Evidence has been obtained, however, that under certain conditions harmful effects can be produced by certain types of antinuclear and anti-γ-globulin antibodies. Characteristics such as concentration in serum, exact specificity (particularly toward antigens encountered in the serum), and physical properties such as solubility appear to govern this question.

One immunologic mechanism of tissue injury that is coming increasingly to the fore is the direct effect of antigen-antibody complexes from the circulation. This is particularly true of renal injury. Such a process appears to be involved in a number of diseases in which renal injury is manifest such as systemic lupus erythematosus and glomerulonephritis. The antigen reacting with antibody to form complexes may come from external sources such as streptococci and administered drugs, or it may come from autologous tissue breakdown products. The injury from such complexes is not limited to the kidney, a particularly sensitive target organ, but may also involve the blood vessels as a potential mechanism of vasculitis. Platelet damage represents a well documented example; complexes of drugs such as quinidine and its antibody in sensitive individuals adhere to platelets and bring about their destruction.

One way to classify the varied mechanisms of immunologic injury is according to the antigens or presumed antigens involved. Another is according to the type of antibody or other immunologic response, with particular emphasis on cellular immunity. The following subsections describe in some detail the types of antigens and the various immune responses thought to be involved in different diseases.

DIRECT SENSITIVITY TO
FOREIGN ANTIGENS

Direct sensitivity to foreign antigens, the most common type of potentially injurious immunologic reaction in man, is usually a result of antigenic stimulation by foreign protein or polysaccharide antigens. These may gain entrance to the body through parenteral, oral, respiratory, or other routes. The classic example is serum sickness, usually resulting from the administration of horse or rabbit immune serum. An Arthus reaction is initiated through the direct union of antigen and antibody in the tissue spaces. Precipitates in and around small blood vessels cause secondary damage to cells, or, when antigen is in excess, soluble complexes are formed that may deposit in certain sensitive organs in the blood vessel walls and cause local inflammatory reactions.

In most of the human allergies such as hay fever and food allergy the exact mode of sensitization to external antigens is not directly apparent. Numerous factors such as heredity, intestinal absorption, respiratory secretion, and even emotional state appear involved. In such sensitive or atopic individuals the reaction to foreign antigens is more commonly of the anaphylactic type. Here the binding of antibody to tissue cells appears to play an important role. Local anaphylaxis results from the association or passive absorption of antibodies to local sites that come in contact with antigen. Not all antibodies have this property, and the newly described class of immunoglobulins, the γE class, is primarily involved. This question will be discussed in more detail in a later section. The antigen in turn reacts with the antibody and injures these cells, which then cause the release of histamine and other pharmacologic mediators into the tissue fluid and circulation. In the skin this gives rise to the wheal and erythema at the site of antigen introduction, as in ordinary prick and scratch diagnostic tests. Hay fever and allergic asthma are local manifestations of such reactions. Extensive urticaria may also represent an expression of local cutaneous anaphylaxis.

The antigens involved in these local allergic reactions are a very diversified group. A number have been isolated and partially characterized. The major allergen of ragweed pollen has been found to be a protein of approximately 37,000 molecular weight and represents a very small portion of the extractable solids of the pollen. The biologic activity of the isolated material is very high; as little as 10^{-12} grams cause a positive intracutaneous wheal and erythema reaction in sensitive individuals. A highly active protein has also been isolated from the timothy hay pollen. Low molecular weight nonprotein allergens have also been isolated. The best example of these is chloragenic acid, which is the active material from castor beans. Just how this is effective is not clear, but the general hypothesis is that it acts as a hapten and combines with body proteins to become a complete antigen. Similar sensitivity to a wide variety of chemicals, particularly those belonging to the group of nitrogenous aromatic substances, has been observed.

The drug reactions represent an analogous type of sensitivity that may become manifest in an extremely variable manner. These are described in detail later. There is a growing awareness of the possibility that sensitivity to unknown foreign materials may play a role in a variety of diseases that at present remain obscure or have been classified as possibly autoimmune in nature. Particular insight into a variety of mechanisms of immunologic cell injury has been gained from the study of the sensitization due to drugs, particularly quinidine. In some persons thrombocytopenic purpura is the result of such sensitivity; in others it is a hemolytic anemia. It now appears that this effect is primarily the fortuitous result of the physical characteristics of the antibody produced. If the antibody is of low molecular weight it forms a type of antigen-antibody complex with quinidine that has a particular predilection for platelets; if it is of high molecular weight, complexes are formed on union with the drug that affect primarily the erythrocytes. Complement is also intimately involved in the different effects. This system illustrates the vagaries involved in the selective action against individual target organs and may be of importance in consideration of disorders of unknown origin such as idiopathic thrombocytopenic purpura and "autoimmune" hemolytic anemia.

The possibility of involvement of unknown foreign antigens, particularly haptens, is not excluded.

It has become increasingly evident that many antigens gain entrance into the body via the intestinal tract through the consumption of food. This has been demonstrated best for bovine milk proteins, and antibodies to a wide variety of these proteins have been found in the serum of many children and some adults. Clear precipitin reactions between bovine protein fractions and these human sera are readily observed. Some evidence has been obtained that "cot death" in infancy involves sensitivity to milk proteins. Usually, apparently, no ill effects result from these antibodies despite the fact that some bovine products that remain antigenic continue to gain entrance into the circulation. However, this is only one example of an antibody response to food products; many others must exist that may have important implications in, for example, certain of the intestinal disorders of unknown origin such as ulcerative colitis.

INDIRECT SENSITIVITY TO FOREIGN ANTIGENS

A very important type of reaction to nonautologous antigens is that produced by maternal-infant incompatibility. Hemolytic disease of the newborn is the outstanding example in which the mother produces antibodies that cause destruction of the erythrocytes in the fetus or newborn. The incompatibility leading to such effects may involve Rh antigens or those of the ABO system. Analogous phenomena have been described for leukocytes and platelets. Cytolytic or cytotoxic reactions occur in which complement is usually but not always necessary to effect the cellular damage. Many other antigens probably are involved in similar maternal-infant incompatibility, but the extent to which they lead to disease is not clear at present. One outstanding example that has become manifest recently is that for genetic types of γ-globulin. A high percentage of infants who lack the genetic γ-globulin character of the mother develop antibodies. These usually appear at approximately the sixth month after delivery and remain throughout the life of the individual. Antibodies to γA globulins appear to have special significance with regard to transfusion reactions. Most of these appear in individuals who lack all γA in their serum and probably arise either through maternal immunization or through the administration of blood products.

Another indirect type of reaction to foreign antigens involves antigenic cross reactions between such antigens and autologous tissues. In this situation an immune response is stimulated by a foreign antigen such as a bacterium, but since a constituent of the organism is antigenically similar to a constituent of the host the immune reaction damages the host tissue. The exact role of such a mechanism in disease remains to be determined, but the possibility exists that presumed autoimmune reactions may be initiated in certain instances by such foreign stimuli. Evidence has been obtained that material from the cell wall of hemolytic streptococci is related antigenically to human cardiac myofibers and the smooth muscle of blood vessel walls. This finding has led to the hypothesis that the cardiac damage of rheumatic fever thus results secondarily from the immune response to the streptococcal infection that preceded it.

SENSITIVITY TO AUTOLOGOUS ANTIGENS

No definitive evidence is available concerning the exact mechanism by which certain persons develop immunologic reactivity against autologous tissue antigens. In some instances it may be through the reaction to an unknown foreign organism that contains antigens, particularly polysaccharides, that cross react with similar polysaccharides in the body tissues. In other instances it may arise through tissue breakdown with release of antigens into the circulation that are ordinarily buried and not subject to the usual tolerance mechanisms. Recent studies in laboratory animals indicate that autologous proteins such as γ-globulin readily become antigenic through slight alteration of the molecule. Antibodies are produced to new determinants not ordinarily exposed but, in addition, as immunization continues, additional antibodies may be produced that involve the native configuration of the protein and will react directly.

One of the best examples of autosensitization in human disease is that found in thyroiditis. There are many features that remain poorly understood, but the evidence is overwhelming that the various degrees of lymphadenoid change in the thyroid gland, particularly in Hashimoto's disease, involve some type of immune reaction against antigens in the thyroid gland. The fact that similar lesions can be produced in laboratory animals by immunization with autologous thyroid antigens in Freund's adjuvant lends strong support to such a view. Even in laboratory animals it remains unclear whether some type of cytotoxic antibody or a cellular autoimmunity plays the dominant role in the tissue injury.

In Goodpasture's disease antibodies reactive with autologous antigens of basement membranes have been demonstrated. These react primarily with renal and pulmonary tissues and have been eluted from these diseased organs obtained at autopsy. Clear evidence of a pathogenic role of the basement membrane antibodies in the renal disease of these patients has been obtained. The antibodies eluted from the human kidneys produce glomerulonephritis in monkeys following infusion. The evidence for a role in the pulmonary disease of these patients is more indirect. It has been demonstrated that antibodies eluted from the lung fix to renal glomerular basement membrane, and antibodies eluted from the kidney fix to pulmonary membranes. The origin of these anti-bodies remains obscure. Similar antibodies also appear to be involved in a few cases of idiopathic glomerulonephritis.

In many blood diseases antibodies occur in the serum that react with autologous cells and in some instances clearly produce disease. The cold agglutinin syndrome is perhaps the clearest from the standpoint of the effect of the abnormal antibody in producing erythrocyte destruction. Anemia, jaundice, and hemoglobinuria can all be traced directly to the action of the cold agglutinin. An "idiopathic" type of the syndrome and one associated with reticulosarcoma and lymphoma offer no clues as to the mechanism by which the cold agglutinin was produced. Another type of disease that is usually of shorter duration follows viral or mycoplasmal pneumonia. Paroxysmal cold hemoglobinuria of the Donath-Landsteiner type is closely related and usually is associated with prenatal syphilis, although many nonsyphilitic cases have been reported. The much more common idiopathic, acquired hemolytic anemia of the warm antibody type presents a more obscure picture. Here the relationship of the erythrocyte damage to a variety of abnormal γ-globulins and presumed antibodies is much more tentative. Only in a minority of cases can the antibodies be shown to have a definite specificity. In these instances it is directed against an Rh antigen, usually anti-e. Again no clue is available concerning the origin of these γ-globulins that react with autologous erythrocytes.

Idiopathic thrombocytopenic purpura is another disease in which circulating antibodies react with autologous cells — in this case platelets — and cause disease through the resulting cellular injury. These antibodies have proved surprisingly difficult to detect by conventional immunologic methods, but it is now clear that they are present. The role of leukocyte auto-agglutinins as a cause of leukopenia has proved even more difficult to assess. Many of the antibodies reported by early workers have been shown to result from transfusions given to these patients, with the production of isoantibodies. However, most workers still believe that auto-agglutinins do occur and are responsible for some cases of leukopenia.

Systemic lupus erythematosus (SLE) is probably associated with a greater variety of antibodies with autospecificity than any other condition. The best known of these are the antinuclear antibodies, certain of which are responsible for the LE cell phenomenon. Special interest has centered on the DNA antibodies because of evidence for an association with disease activity. Antibodies to native double-stranded DNA as well as antibodies specific for the single-stranded form are found in the sera of these patients. Recently antibodies to double-stranded RNA have been detected. It has become evident that antibodies to a wide spectrum of polynucleotides are uniquely present in this disease. Numerous additional antibodies to protein and carbohydrate antigens extracted from the cytoplasm as well as the nucleus of human cells have been described. Some of these appear to be responsible for various secondary manifestations of the disease as, for example, hemolytic anemia. This is associated with a positive Coombs test, suggesting the occurrence of antibodies to autologous erythrocytes. Idiopathic thrombocytopenic purpura, probably involving antiplatelet antibodies, also occurs in these patients. Abnormalities involving blood coagulation have been of special interest to investigators; antibodies to specific clotting factors appear to be involved. The origin of these many antibodies as well as others not discussed remains obscure. Some of them appear to represent a marked elevation of antibodies found at low levels in normal persons, which is compatible with the concept that in SLE a general hyperreactivity of the immune system exists. The high prevalence in females and the familial trend of the disease have not as yet been fitted into the immunologic concepts. Recent work with various strains of mice, particularly the New Zealand NZB strain, has shown that manifestations of a disease with many features resembling SLE occur in a high proportion of the animals. Most striking is the renal disease and the hemolytic anemia. This experimental model shows a marked similarity to the human disease, and the unique antibodies to double-stranded DNA and RNA are present. Studies in these mice have suggested a significant role for secondary viral infections in potentiating various disease manifestations. Whether this also applies to the human disease remains to be proved. The antibodies specific for double-stranded RNA observed in the patients are difficult to explain on any basis other than that of viral origin.

The possibility has been considered that a large number of other diseases in which the cause is unknown may have as their origin some type of autoimmune mechanism. This is particularly true of rheumatoid arthritis, primarily because it is associated with uniquely high incidence and levels of an unusual group of antibodies called rheumatoid factors. These have been clearly demonstrated to be antibodies to γ-globulin and are capable of reacting with autologous γ-globulin. No evidence is available to suggest that the rheumatoid factors play a direct role in the arthritis; however, many workers think they may be indicative of an as yet undefined immunologic reaction. The fact that they are produced at least in part in the synovial tissue of the joints from local accumulation of plasma cells adds some weight to this concept. On the other hand, it has also become clear that the rheumatoid factors could develop as a response to some type of foreign organism. Antibodies to the organism following reaction with the particulate antigen or fragment thereof would form secondary anti-γ-globulins to these antigen antibody complexes. This possibility has been strengthened by the experimental production of anti-γ-globulins in rabbits following injection of coliform organisms, as well as their appearance in human sera following various types of infection. In bacterial endocarditis, for example, the rheumatoid factors disappear following elimination of the organism

with antimicrobial therapy. Similar attempts with such therapy in rheumatoid arthritis patients is without effect on the rheumatoid factors. The accumulated evidence indicates that there must be some profound immunologic stimulus present in the rheumatoid arthritis patient to sustain the rheumatoid factors at the extreme levels often observed and for the prolonged periods in which they are present. The nature of this stimulus remains unknown.

Another type of suggestive evidence that the derangement in rheumatoid arthritis might be immunologic stems from its association with various other disorders in which an immunologic basis is more apparent. This is particularly true with relation to SLE. Manifestations of this disease have been reported frequently in patients with rheumatoid arthritis, and the overlap between the two disorders has been frequently noted. In addition, serologic reactions with nuclear antigens and antinuclear antibodies detected by immunofluorescence have an impressive incidence in rheumatoid arthritis patients.

Another disorder showing profound immunologic abnormalities associated with arthritis similar to that in rheumatoid arthritis is Sjögren's syndrome. It also has been considered a possible connecting link between rheumatoid arthritis and SLE. Extreme elevation of γ-globulin similar to that found in SLE patients is observed along with many similar antinuclear and anticytoplasmic antibodies. In addition, the vast majority of these patients have rheumatoid factors, often at extreme levels. Serologically they show the findings of both rheumatoid arthritis and SLE. The lesions observed in the lacrimal, salivary, and other glands of patients with Sjögren's syndrome are highly suggestive of a local immunologic reaction. They closely resemble that observed in the thyroid gland in chronic thyroiditis, in which an immunologic alteration has been more evident.

The immunologic aspects of pernicious anemia are of considerable interest. Antibodies to intrinsic factor have been demonstrated in a large number of cases, and antibodies to the parietal cells of the gastric mucosa are frequently found. These have been revealed by a variety of classic immunologic procedures. In addition, the intrinsic factor antibody inhibits labeled B_{12} absorption in in vivo tests. Many of the antibodies appear to be autoantibodies and are found in untreated cases; others appear to represent antibodies to hog intrinsic factor as a result of therapy. A direct role in the pathogenesis of the disease has not been established, but they at least are important in certain therapeutic considerations.

The serum of patients with myasthenia gravis contains a number of unusual antibodies directed at muscle constituents. These have been demonstrated primarily by fluorescent antibody techniques, a procedure that has proved unusually hazardous when dealing with muscle sections. However, precipitating and complement-fixing antibodies have also been found. No direct role for these antibodies in the disease has been demonstrated, but they certainly raise the possibility of an immunologic mechanism. The frequent association of thymic disease with myasthenia gravis is well documented and adds further weight to a possible immune basis for this disease. One of the most important developments in immunology in recent years is the recognition of the profound role of the thymus gland in the development of immunity. It is also known that some infants born of myasthenic mothers have a transient myasthenic syndrome that could be due to placental transfer of antibody.

Antibodies with autospecificity of various types have been found in a variety of other diseases. In ulcerative colitis, antibodies to colon tissue and cellular immunity to colon cells have been described. Patients with liver disease show a wide variety of antibodies to autologous cell constituents. Antibodies reactive with mitochondria are of special interest because of their specific occurrence in primary biliary cirrhosis. They are of diagnostic value, but a pathogenic role remains to be demonstrated. Pancreas antibodies have been described in patients with pancreatitis, and adrenal antibodies in patients with Addison's disease. In all these instances the major possibility that these represent antibodies secondary to tissue breakdown in the disease has not been excluded. As stressed earlier, autoantibodies are far more common than had previously been thought, and any assessment of an injurious role in a specific disease is extremely difficult.

IMMUNE COMPLEX DISEASE

When artificially made antigen-antibody complexes are injected into laboratory animals, they are deposited in a number of organs with resultant tissue injury. By far the most sensitive organ is the kidney, and acute and chronic renal disease has been produced in a number of species by this procedure. The complexes are trapped in the glomeruli and form lumpy deposits along the glomerular basement membrane. These have distinct histologic characteristics by electron microscopy and by fluorescent antibody staining techniques. In human glomerulonephritis similar deposits are frequently observed when these same procedures are utilized. In systemic lupus erythematosus such deposits in the glomeruli are particularly striking, and a large accumulation of additional evidence for antigen-antibody complex mediated renal injury is available.

Extensive studies in a number of different laboratories have demonstrated that DNA–anti-DNA complexes represent one type involved in SLE. Antibodies to DNA aroused considerable interest when they were first described in SLE approximately 12 years ago. However, they were relegated to the position of scientific curiosities, and it has only been recently that their harmful potential has been realized. Antibodies to double-stranded DNA have special significance because double-stranded DNA antigens can appear in the circulation as a result of tissue breakdown; antigen-antibody complexes are formed with fixation of complement and deposition in the most vulnerable organ, the kidney. Elution of antibody from isolated glomeruli of diseased kidneys has proved to be a very effective technique for the detection of antibodies deposited in the kidney. DNA antibody has been found in such eluates at specific concentrations as high as 1000 times those in the serum. DNA antigen has also been demonstrated in the granular deposits observed in the glomeruli. Other, more indirect evidence such as the close clinical relationship among the appearance of DNA antibodies, serum complement depression, and exacerbations of disease has also aided in establishing the significance of the DNA system. Further studies are required to determine the relevance of the many other antibodies in the serum of these patients; some of these, if they can encounter specific antigen, may be involved as well.

Another type of renal disease in which evidence for immune complexes is rapidly accumulating is that associated with various types of drugs. Some of these may present a picture very analogous to that of serum sickness; in others, chronic drug administration may lead to a slowly progressive glomerulonephritis. The latter situation is well illustrated in the case of penicillamine. Numerous instances of nephritis have been reported following long-term administration of this material for the treatment of cystinuria, Wilson's disease, or rheumatoid arthritis. Granular deposits of γ-globulin and complement along the glomerular basement membrane are readily visualized in fluorescent antibody studies which closely resemble those produced in experimental animals by injection of complexes.

The presence of granular and "lumpy" deposits of γ-globulin and complement detected by fluorescent antibody techniques may be well visualized in renal biopsy specimens and have been found in a variety of different conditions such as malaria, bacterial endocarditis, and thyroiditis. Cases of chronic glomerulonephritis of unknown cause frequently show such a pattern. However, supporting evidence for specific antigen-antibody complexes is as yet unavailable for most of these. In post-streptococcal nephritis similar characteristics of complex-induced nephritis are present, and suggestive evidence for streptococcal antigens in the deposits has been obtained.

Eluates obtained from glomeruli isolated at autopsy from kidneys of patients who had subacute and chronic glomerulonephritis have in a number of instances shown high concentrations of γ-globulin. This appears to represent specific antibody, but its nature remains a mystery. The search is on in a number of laboratories for specific antigens that might react with such γ-globulin. Particular attention is being paid to various human viruses since recent work in laboratory animals has demonstrated complexes of virus and antibody in the kidneys of mice with chronic lymphocytic choriomeningitis infection. The task is a difficult one, however, and human tissue antigens, bacterial antigens, and even unknown drugs may be equally reasonable candidates. The possibility also seems likely that multiple antigen-antibody systems are involved in the different cases of idiopathic glomerulonephritis.

Another type of antigen-antibody complex that appears to be involved in some types of renal disease is that composed of γG globulin and anti-γG globulin. Such complexes are widely distributed in human sera and reach unusual levels in rheumatoid arthritis. Usually these are quite soluble but in some patients they precipitate out in the cold as mixed cryoglobulins. Patients with such mixed cryoglobulins show a rather ill-defined clinical syndrome, but renal lesions are common. The components of such complexes along with complement have been identified in the glomeruli of these patients.

Evidence has been obtained that injury to circulating cells, particularly platelets, may be mediated by antigen-antibody complexes. A number of drug-induced thrombocytopenias fall into this category. Particular interest is currently centered on similar mechanisms in the joint inflammation of SLE and rheumatoid arthritis. Gamma globulin complexes are well known in the latter, and high concentrations have been observed in joint fluid, in which they appear to be involved in local complement depletion. Much work remains before a direct cause-and-effect relationship can be established. Lack of an adequate experimental model similar to those available for immunologic renal injury has hampered progress in this field.

PROPERTIES OF THE ANTIBODIES INVOLVED

Five major classes of human antibodies have been characterized: γG or 7S γ-globulin, γM or 19S γ-globulin, γA globulin, γD globulin, and γE globulin. These classes differ markedly in physical and biologic properties so that some understanding of their structural characteristics is essential for an evaluation of specific antibodies in disease. Prior to the clear delineation of these antibody types considerable controversy arose concerning the antibody nature of γ-globulins with unusual properties in certain human sera. This has been especially true of the rheumatoid factors, which belong primarily in the γM or 19S class and were not considered antibodies in many quarters because of the very properties now known to be characteristic of such antibodies.

All antibodies are now known to be made up of two types of polypeptide chains, the light and heavy chains. The five classes differ markedly in the character of the heavy chains but have similar light chains. In the common γG globulin, the 7S molecule is made up of two heavy and two light chains and these are linked by disulfide bonds. In the case of the γM or 19S antibody type, a similar four-chain monomeric unit is further polymerized

into a macroglobulin consisting of five such units linked by disulfide bonds. The γA globulin is more variable and sometimes consists of a simple four-chain 7S molecule and in other instances is polymerized to various larger sizes. Less is known about the γD type, but this also appears to be a 7S protein made of two light and two heavy chains. The proteins of the γE class also consist of two light and two heavy chains. However, longer heavy chains are present, making the four-chain molecule considerably larger. These classes differ from each other in carbohydrate content, which plays an important role in solubility differences. They also differ in their ability to cross the placenta, an important property with regard to maternal-infant antibody relationships. The γM and the γA show little or no placental passage, in marked contrast to γG globulin, which in cord blood reaches similar levels to that in maternal serum. A very significant special property of γA antibodies is their occurrence as the dominant antibody in all external secretions. Saliva, tears, intestinal secretions, colostrum, and other body fluids contain primarily γA antibodies.

In addition to the four major classes of γ-globulin, various subgroups of each type have become apparent that also involve basic differences in the heavy chains. These may well prove to be of considerable importance in disease because it is apparent that they differ in such properties as skin-sensitizing activity. Current evidence indicates that each antibody, even within a particular subgroup, has its own specific primary structure and that amino acid sequence differences are at the basis of the different specificities of individual antibodies. The specific property of antibodies to combine with antigens appears to reside in the heavy chains, although the four-chain monomeric unit is essential for maximal activity. The genetic mechanism by which plasma cells gain the capacity to produce the sequence variations necessary to explain the huge number of different known antibodies remains a mystery. However, with this extreme diversity of molecules, it is not surprising to find certain γ-globulins with unusual solubility, as mentioned earlier (see article on Plasma Cell Dyscrasia).

Antibodies with autospecificity have been found that belong in each of the five main classes of γ-globulin, with the exception of γD, and γE. Most of the diverse antibodies encountered in the sera of SLE patients are of the γG type, which goes along with the usual marked elevation in the total serum γG globulin. A few, however, have been described that fall into the γM and γA class, particularly among the antinuclear antibodies. The rheumatoid factors as well as the majority of other anti-γ-globulins are primarily γM macroglobulins. Most of the cryoglobulins are macroglobulins; this is also true of the cold agglutinins. Decreased solubility in the cold is a general characteristic of the antibodies of high molecular weight. It is known that these antibodies are also very sensitive to sulfhydryl compounds such as cysteine and penicillamine, which act on the disulfide bonds responsible for their polymeric structure. Attempts have been made to utilize this effect for therapeutic purposes, particularly for the cold agglutinin disease, but with limited success thus far. The antibodies of high molecular weight usually fix complement very effectively and as a result produce severe cellular injury when cells are involved as antigens. Many such antibodies are involved in hemolytic reactions of erythrocytes. In other instances the specific properties of macroglobulin antibodies make them more benign. The γ-globulin–anti-γ-globulin complexes found in rheumatoid arthritis sera are readily soluble under most conditions, permitting them to circulate at high concentrations with surprisingly few harmful effects.

The skin-sensitizing antibodies or reagins that appear to be responsible for most of the harmful effects in the allergic diseases have many unique properties. The most striking of these is the persistence in the skin for periods of weeks after transfer to normal persons. The demonstration that these properties are characteristics of antibodies of the γE class has been a significant recent development in immunology. Quantitatively this is a very minor class, representing only approximately 0.05 per cent of the total immunoglobulins of the serum. However, it has become clear that it is specifically involved in histamine release from leukocytes and other cells. The finding of two myeloma proteins of the γE type has aided greatly in our understanding of the specific characteristics of proteins of this class. Their molecular weight is somewhat higher than γG proteins and their sedimentation rate is approximately 8S. They are rich in carbohydrate and do not fix complement. It is of particular interest that γE forming cells are concentrated in the mucosal system of the nose and respiratory tract as well as the regional lymph nodes, raising the possibility that locally formed γE may be involved in respiratory allergy. Other types of antibodies to allergens are also found in the sera of sensitive patients that do not have the unique skin-sensitizing properties and rapidly diffuse away from the site of the injection. These antibodies, which have been termed blocking antibodies, appear to be typical γG globulins, in contrast to the reagins. They also combine with antigen and may prevent a reaction with the skin-sensitizing antibody.

DELAYED TYPE OF HYPERSENSITIVITY

Another kind of allergic reaction is broadly operative that does not involve the usual varieties of circulating antibodies. The term "delayed type of hypersensitivity" arose from the delayed response of sensitive subjects to antigen; the reaction does not begin for several hours and reaches a maximum after two or three days. The term "cellular immunity" has also been used, primarily because transfer of sensitivity requires tissue cells of sensitive persons and cannot be accomplished with serum. Some investigators have postulated the involvement of antibody with a high affinity for antigen that may be present in very small amounts in the serum. Others have observed "cytophilic antibodies" with strong adsorptive capacity for cells, and these are thought to be important. However, most immunologists consider this form of immunity to be an integral property of cells of the lymphoid series without direct involvement of antibody. Two major types of delayed hypersensitivity have been most widely studied: that induced by infection, and the other, termed contact sensitivity, resulting from exposure to a variety of substances ranging from oily resins of plants to simple chemicals employed for domestic, industrial, and medical purposes. Delayed hypersensitivity to autologous antigens has been difficult to demonstrate in humans, although it can be produced in laboratory animals by immunization with autologous antigens.

Delayed-type hypersensitivity is more strikingly evident in certain specific infections such as tuberculosis, brucellosis, lymphogranuloma venereum, mumps, vaccinia, and some fungal infections. Skin tests that depend on this type of cellular immunity have been utilized in these diseases. Tuberculin reactions have been extensively studied in humans and laboratory animals as a model for the delayed type of hypersensitivity. The skin reactivity to tuberculin can be transferred to normal recipients by means of cells from lymphoid tissue, peritoneal exudate, and peripheral blood. In laboratory animals viable cells are required, but in humans the supernatant fluid of disrupted leukocytes can transfer the reactivity. Considerable interest is focused on the character of the active principle involved in the human transfer experiments, and recent studies indicate that this substance is readily dialyzable and therefore of relatively low molecular weight.

Homograft rejection results primarily from cellular immunity, which in certain respects resembles the tuberculin type. Some evidence indicates that circulating antibodies may also play a role. Recent interest has been centered on in vitro models of cellular reactivity against incompatible tissues that might be utilized for screening donors for skin and kidney grafts. It has been found that mixtures of lymphoid cells from two unrelated individuals cause cell division and uptake of labeled thymidine in tissue culture to a much greater extent than occurs when cells from identical twins are mixed. Various modifications of this technique are currently employed to gain an index of the compatibility of donor cells with those of a projected graft recipient. (For further discussion see the article on Transplantation of Kidney in Diseases of the Renal System.)

The migration of leukocytes from the end of a capillary tube has become a widely used system for assessing the delayed type of hypersensitivity. Cells from sensitive individuals are inhibited in such migration following the addition of the specific antigen to which the individual shows delayed hypersensitivity. The technique has been most widely used for the demonstration of sensitivity to various bacterial antigens. However, a sensitivity to a few autologous antigens has also been demonstrated. In pernicious anemia, for example, the cell migration studies have shown specific inhibitory effects of extracts of adrenal tissue.

Another probable manifestation of delayed-type hypersensitivity, or at least cellular immunity, is the graft versus host reaction. This has sometimes been termed "homologous disease." It is largely a disorder of laboratory animals that are able to accept foreign bone marrow or lymphoid cells because they have been irradiated or otherwise treated so that these cells are not rejected. These foreign cells then react against various antigens in the host animal, resulting in a variety of clinical manifestations. The skin lesions are most characteristic: edema, erythema, and ulceration followed by thickening, scaling, and loss of hair. Lesions of the joints and of the heart are also observed and these have aroused considerable interest because of certain similarities to those observed in some of the connective tissue disorders. Hemolytic anemia with a positive Coombs reaction has also been described. The possibility has been raised that in certain human diseases immunologically active cells react against the host in a fashion similar to that of the transferred cells in the laboratory animal experiments. The origin of such cells has been ascribed to some type of failure of tolerance mechanisms or to an alteration of host cells through somatic mutation.

Cohen, S., and Milstein, C.: Structure and biological properties of immunoglobulins. In Dixon, F. J., and Kunkel, H. G. (eds.): Advances in Immunology, Vol. 7. New York, Academic Press, 1967.

Ishizaka, K., and Ishizaka, T.: Human reaginic antibodies and immunoglobulin E. J. Allerg., 42:330, 1968.

Koffler, D., and Kunkel, H. G.: Mechanisms of renal injury in systemic lupus erythematosus. Amer. J. Med., 45:165, 1968.

Kunkel, H. G., and Tan, E. M.: Autoantibodies and disease. In Dixon, F. J., and Humphrey, J. H. (eds.): Advances in Immunology, Vol. 4. New York, Academic Press Inc., 1964.

Lerner, R. A., Glassock, R. J., and Dixon, F. J.: The role of antiglomerular basement membrane antibody in the pathogenesis of human glomerulonephritis. J. Exp. Med., 126:989, 1967.

Miescher, P. A., and Müller-Eberhard, H. J.: Textbook of Immunopathology, Vol. 1. New York, Grune & Stratton, Inc., 1968.

Roitt, I. M., Greaves, M. F., Torrigiani, G., Brostoff, J., and Playfair, J. H. L.: The cellular basis of immunological responses. Lancet, 2:367, 1969.

Samter, M., and Alexander, H. L.: Immunological Diseases. Boston, Little, Brown & Company, 1965.

IMMUNOLOGIC DEFICIENCY STATES

Fred S. Rosen

Definition. The immunologic deficiency states are a group of syndromes which may be characterized by (1) marked deficiency of immunoglobulins and impairment of antibody synthesis, (2) a severe deficit in cellular immunity, or (3) both. Frequent or recurrent infections are common to all immunologic deficiency states.

Etiology and Pathogenesis. The hypogammaglobulinemias, which constitute the first group of syndromes, are the result of diminished rates of synthesis of the gamma globulins (primary agammaglobulinemias), or of increased catabolism of gamma globulin (secondary hypogammaglobulinemia) (Table 1). The primary forms are associated with morphologic alterations of lymphoid tissue and the absence of plasma cells from lymph nodes, spleen, and bone marrow. The thymus gland is normal. Secondary hypogammaglobulinemias result from increased rates of loss of gamma globulin into the intestinal tract because of exudative enteropathy, from the skin because of exfoliative dermatitides, or in the urine as in the nephrotic syndrome.

Cellular immunity is mediated by small lymphocytes. Defects in cellular immunity result from (1) failure of maturation of lymphocytes or their precursors, (2) absence of the thymus gland which plays a vital and as yet undefined role in the maturation and functioning of lymphocytes, (3) entrapment of lymphocytes such as occurs in intestinal lymphangiectasia, or (4) neoplasia or immune destruction of lymphoid cells (Table 2).

Symptoms and Signs. The hypogammaglobulinemias are manifested clinically by recurrent, severe pyogenic infections, usually caused by pneumococci, staphylococci, streptococci, meningococci, or *Hemophilus influenzae*. These result in sinusitis, conjunctivitis, otitis media, pneumonia, furunculosis, septic arthritis, meningitis, and sepsis. Viral infections are tolerated normally. In addition to the aforementioned pyogenic infections, patients with defects in cellular immunity also sustain invasive infection by enteric pathogens, persistent moniliasis, severe viral infections, particularly with the herpes-pox group which may progress to a fatal outcome, and interstitial pneumonia caused by *Pneumocystis carinii*.

Complications. Recurrent suppuration may result in destruction or impairment of affected anatomic structures. Progressive bronchiectasis is common in the untreated agammaglobulinemias. Nonsuppurative complications include chronic arthritis and other collagen-like diseases. Lymphoreticular malignancies occur with high frequency, particularly in patients with defects in cellular immunity.

Laboratory Findings. Agammaglobulinemia can be recognized by any immunochemical method for quantitation of the immunoglobulins. Absence of antibodies may be shown by failure to detect isohemagglutinins in serum or by a positive Schick test despite immunization with diphtheria toxoid. In defects of cellular immunity, peripheral blood lymphocytes may be diminished and unresponsive to phytohemagglutinin stimulation. Prolonged survival of a skin allograft and absence of tuberculin-like delayed hypersensitivity reactions to such common antigens as monilia or streptokinase are found.

TABLE 1. HYPOGAMMAGLOBULINEMIAS

Type	Etiology or Mechanism	Globulin Levels*	Lymphoid Tissue
Primary			
1. Transient	Delayed maturation of lymphoid tissue	<400 mg. per 100 ml. γG; absent γA, γM	Follicles hypoplastic; few plasma cells
2. X-linked	Genetic	<100 mg. per 100 ml. γG; absent γA, γM	Absent plasma cells and follicles
3. Acquired	A. Lymphoma or leukemia B. Idiopathic	<500 mg. per 100 ml. γG; absent γA, γM	Absent plasma cells; follicles abiotrophic or hypertrophied
4. Dysgammaglobulinemias A. Decreased γG, γA, elevated γM	A. Genetic B. Idiopathic	>100 mg. per 100 ml. γM, <100 mg. per 100 ml. γG; absent γA	Abundant plasmacytoid cells; follicles absent or normal
B. Isolated γA deficiency	A. ?Genetic B. "Autoimmune" C. Idiopathic	Normal γG, γM; absent γA	Normal
C. Isolated γG deficiency	Idiopathic	Normal γA, γM; <500 mg. per 100 ml.	Hypoplastic follicles; few plasma cells
Secondary			
1. Nephrotic syndrome	A. Increased catabolism B. Urinary loss	γG and albumin decreased, γA, γM usually normal	Normal
2. Hypercatabolic	A. Intestinal loss B. Loss through skin	Decreased γG, γA, γM, and albumin	Normal

*Normal levels: γG 600 to 1500 mg. per 100 ml.; γA 200 to 300 mg. per 100 ml.; γM 75 to 150 mg. per 100 ml.; absent indicates <1 per cent of normal values.

TABLE 2. DEFECTS IN CELLULAR IMMUNITY

Type	Etiology	Comments
1. Thymic aplasia	Congenital	Thymus and parathyroids aplastic; immunoglobulins normal; normal function established by fetal thymic grafts
2. Thymic alymphoplasia or dysplasia	A. X-linked B. Autosomal recessive	Thymus embryonic; lymphoid tissue absent; immunoglobulins usually absent; normal function established by transplants of histocompatible bone marrow
3. Lymphangiectasia	A. Congenital B. Idiopathic	
4. Hodgkin's lymphoma	Neoplasia	
5. Immune destruction	A. Exogenous B. Idiopathic	Antilymphocyte serum used to prolong graft-survival; lymphocytotoxin may arise spontaneously
6. Wiskott-Aldrich syndrome	X-linked	Thrombocytopenia; eczema; frequent lymphoma; no antibody response to polysaccharide antigens
7. Ataxia-telangiectasia	Autosomal recessive	Absent serum γA in 80 per cent of cases; frequent lymphoma; thymus hypoplastic; onset of ataxia in second year of life; telangiectasia on exposed body surfaces appear later in first decade of life

Treatment. Acute bacterial infections require appropriate antimicrobial therapy which may have to be prolonged when structural damage such as bronchiectasis is present. Replacement therapy with human gamma globulin provides adequate prophylaxis in patients with primary agammaglobulinemias against recurrent pyogenic infections. It has been found empirically that a dose of 0.6 ml. per kilogram of a 16.5 per cent solution of gamma globulin injected intramuscularly at monthly intervals, or in divided semimonthly doses, is adequate to achieve a maintenance level of serum gamma globulin. Initially, three times this amount, or 1.8 ml. per kilogram, should be administered as a loading dose.

Good, R. A., Kelly, W. D., and Rotstein, J.: Immunologic deficiency diseases. Progr. Allergy, 6:187, 1962.
Rosen, F. S., and Janeway, C. A.: The gamma globulins. III. Antibody deficiency syndromes. New Eng. J. Med., 275:709, 769, 1966.

DEFECTS IN PHAGOCYTOSIS: CHRONIC GRANULOMATOUS DISEASE

Definition. Chronic granulomatous disease is a syndrome characterized by recurrent and progressive microabscess formation in viscera and lymphoid tissue as a result of defective intracellular bacterial killing by phagocytic cells.

Etiology and Pathogenesis. Bacteria, and possibly other microbial forms, are prepared for phagocytosis (opsonization) by interaction with antibody or antibody and complement. Phagocytic cells have a membrane receptor for γG globulin which facilitates phagocytosis. However, the opsonization of virulent pyogenic organisms involves antibody (γG or γM globulin) and the first four reacting components of complement—C1, C4, C2, and C3. Opsonized bacteria are engulfed by the cell membrane of the phagocyte so that they are ingested in a vacuole formed from a portion of the cell membrane. During the ingestion, the following metabolic events occur: (1) a net increase in lipid biosynthesis, possibly to repair the recently created breach in the cell membrane; (2) a burst of respiratory activity with increased shunting of glucose through the pentose pathway; (3) the generation of peroxide by one or more oxidases acting on reduced NAD and/or NADP; and (4) the rupture of lysosomes with discharge of their contents of hydrolytic enzymes and bactericidal cationic peptides into the phagocytic vacuoles. Phagocytic cells (both mononuclear and polymorphonuclear forms) from patients with chronic granulomatous disease fail to exhibit increased respiratory activity and generation of peroxide during phagocytosis. Their phagocytes are deficient in NADH oxidase activity. However, subsequent to ingestion, new lipid synthesis and lysosomal rupture appear to proceed normally.

Patients with this defect exhibit particular susceptibility to staphylococci and certain enteric coliform bacteria. The restricted spectrum of bacterial forms, which are associated with infection in these patients, has in common synthesis of catalase and absence of H_2O_2 production by the bacteria. Peroxide, together with a lysosomal enzyme, myeloperoxidase, and halide ion appear to peroxidize the bacterial cell wall, and may be one important mechanism for killing bacteria in phagocytic cells. Thus, adequate peroxide generation during phagocytosis is vital in the destruction of catalase-producing bacteria. Defective intracellular killing of bacteria has also been found in a single kindred whose phagocytes lack myeloperoxidase and also in children with Chediak-Higashi syndrome (see Miscellaneous Hereditary Disorders), whose phagocytic lysosomes are extraordinarily stable and fail to rupture during phagocytosis.

Signs and Symptoms. Affected children usually exhibit the initial symptoms of chronic granulomatous disease during the first year of life. Cervical adenitis, leading to chronic drainage of purulent material, is the most common first symptom. An eczematoid seborrheic rash is frequently noted. Subsequent involvement of the liver and spleen with microabscess formation results in prominent hepatosplenomegaly. Ultimate pulmonary infection can resemble miliary tuberculosis roentgenographically. Coalescence of the microabscesses leads to consolidation. Extensive pulmonary involvement or sepsis causes death within the first two decades of life.

Laboratory Findings. Total white cell counts and leukocyte morphology are normal. When leukocytes are tested for their ability to ingest and kill staphylococci or certain coliform bacteria, they are found to be grossly defective in this regard. However, intracellular killing of streptococci and pneumococci, as well as other noncatalase-producing organisms, is normal.

The metabolic defect can readily be quantitated by measuring reduction of pale yellow nitroblue tetrazolium dye to a deep purple formazan by leukocytes during phagocytosis of latex particles. Patients' phagocytes fail to reduce the dye.

The defect is transmitted, in most cases, as an X-linked recessive phenomenon. Heterozygous female carriers can be detected by intermediate degrees of dye reduction by their phagocytes. In other cases, in which the disease appears to be transmitted as an autosomal recessive phenomenon, the presumed heterozygosity in parents of affected females cannot be discerned by any test.

Treatment. There is no known therapy which specifically corrects or overcomes the defect in chronic granulomatous disease. Culture of lesions and appropriate antimicrobial therapy have prolonged the life of affected children.

Alper, C. A., Abramson, N., Johnston, R. B., Jr., Jandl, J. H., and Rosen, F. S.: Increased susceptibility to infection associated with abnormalities of complement-mediated functions and of the third component of complement. New Eng. J. Med., 282:349, 1970.

Baehner, R. L., and Nathan, D. G.: Quantitative nitroblue tetrazolium test in chronic granulomatous disease. New Eng. J. Med., 278:971, 1968.

Klebanoff, S. J., and White, L. R.: Iodinating defect in the leukocytes of a patient with chronic granulomatous disease of childhood. New Eng. J. Med., 280:460, 1969.

Lehrer, R. I., and Cline, M. J.: Leukocyte myeloperoxidase deficiency and disseminated candidiasis: The role of myeloperoxidase in resistance to Candida infection. J. Clin. Invest., 48:1478, 1969.

Quie, P. G., White, J. G., Holmes, B., and Good, R. A.: In vitro bactericidal capacity of human polymorphonuclear leukocytes: Diminished activity in chronic granulomatous disease of childhood. J. Clin. Invest., 46:668, 1967.

HAY FEVER AND ALLERGIC RHINITIS

*William B. Sherman**

Definition. *Allergic rhinitis* is a reaction of the nasal mucosa manifested by edema, sneezing, itching, and increased mucous secretion, resulting from allergy to a specific antigen. When caused by allergy to pollens, it is called *hay fever* or *pollinosis* and is characterized by seasonal recurrence during the period of pollination of the causative plants. Allergic rhinitis due to antigens other than pollens is called *nonseasonal* or *perennial allergic rhinitis*. The term *vasomotor rhinitis* is applied both to perennial allergic rhinitis and to morphologically similar chronic edema of the nasal mucosa due to nonantigenic irritants, or probably in some cases to neurogenic and psychosomatic causes.

Etiology. The allergic sensitization producing hay fever is the same "wheal and erythema" type associated with infantile eczema, atopic dermatitis, bronchial asthma, and certain forms of food allergy, so that persons manifesting one of these diseases frequently develop others of the group. Although diseases of this group tend to occur in certain families, neither the particular disease manifestation nor allergy to a specific antigen is inherited, only a tendency to become allergic to antigens to which the individual is exposed.

In general, only those plants which depend on the wind for cross-pollination and produce an abundance of buoyant, windborne pollen are important factors in the causation of hay fever. These include grasses, many families of weeds, and most of the trees of temperate climates. Plants with showy and odoriferous blossoms, including roses and goldenrod, are adapted to insect pollination, produce relatively small amounts of heavy, sticky pollen, and rarely cause hay fever. Immunodiffusion studies show most pollens to be mixtures of many distinct antigens, but the pollens of various species of each genus of trees and weeds are so similar that the use of pollen of one species of a genus in testing and treatment suffices. The pollens of all the common genera of the grasses occurring in the northern United States and southern Canada are antigenically quite similar, so that for practical purposes a mixture of the pollens of three or four of the grasses most common in a given area may be used as if a single antigen. Bermuda grass, which grows from Virginia through the South, is a different antigen.

Specific diagnosis of hay fever requires a knowledge of the flora of the patient's locality and the seasons of pollination of the plants. Throughout the greater portion of the United States and southern Canada, spring hay fever (April and May) is due to tree pollens, early summer hay fever (June and July) to grass pollens, with plantain and sorrel also important in some areas, and late hay fever (August and September) to weed pollens.

*Deceased.

The important trees vary considerably in different areas; ash, beech, birch, cedar, hickory, maple, oak, sycamore, and poplar produce an abundance of antigenic windborne pollen and may be presumed important where they grow commonly. The pollens of the pines and other conifers are relatively less antigenic and less often cause hay fever, even where abundant. The grass pollens are everywhere important, their season being prolonged through much of the year in the extreme south. In the East and Middle West ragweed is by far the most important weed pollen; it also occurs in most of the Far West, except for the north Pacific coast, but its importance in the mountain and coast areas is less than that of sage, amaranth, and Russian thistle. For detailed accounts of the windborne pollens causing hay fever in various areas of the United States and southern Canada the reader should refer to the works of Wodehouse and Samter and Durham. The tree and grass hay fever seasons in northern Europe correspond closely to those of the United States; the weed pollens are relatively much less important, ragweed not being indigenous to the area.

Prevalence. It has been estimated that 8 to 10 per cent of the population of the United States is affected by hay fever, but a large proportion of these cases are not severe enough to require medical treatment. All races appear equally susceptible, and both sexes are equally affected. In areas where ragweed is abundant, approximately 75 per cent of hay fever sufferers are affected by this pollen; in 50 per cent, it is the only significant cause. About 50 per cent are affected by grass pollens alone or in combination with other pollens. Tree hay fever is less common and usually occurs in patients also affected by grass or weed pollens.

Pathogenesis. As one of the chief functions of the nose is to warm and purify the inhaled air, a large proportion of suspended dust particles are deposited on its mucosa, which is therefore peculiarly exposed to inhaled allergens. Sensitization of the type causing hay fever consists in the development of sensitizing antibodies present in the conjunctiva, nasal mucosa, skin, and blood plasma. Contact of the allergenic pollen with the sensitized mucosa elicits an antigen-antibody reaction that is manifested by engorgement of the blood vessels, edema, increased secretion of watery mucus, and itching that gives rise to sneezing. The physiologic effects of the antigen-antibody reaction are believed to result mainly from the release of histamine, which can be demonstrated when specific antigen is added to the patient's blood in vitro. There is little evidence that the central nervous system is involved.

Although the symptoms produced by inhalation of pollen are localized to the mucosa with which it comes in contact, the sensitization is systemic. Injection of too large a quantity of antigen into a highly allergic patient in a diagnostic skin test or in treatment may elicit a *constitutional reaction* similar to experimental anaphylactic shock. It is manifested within 20 minutes or less by coughing, sneezing, asthma, urticaria, or general flushing and itching of the skin and, in severe cases, collapse. Such reactions may be serious or even fatal if not promptly treated.

Repeated injections of the antigen for the specific treatment of hay fever stimulate the formation of blocking antibody, distinct from the pre-existing sensitizing antibody and eventually cause a decrease of sensitizing antibody. This blocking antibody appears to be responsible for the increase of tolerance for injected antigen and plays some part in the clinical benefits of treatment, but the latter are more closely related to the decrease of sensitizing antibody with prolonged treatment.

Clinical Manifestations. The symptoms of hay fever characteristically recur each year at the same season with the beginning of pollination of the causative plant, the date of onset in a given locality rarely varying by more than a week or so, although the amount of pollen produced and, hence, the severity of symptoms vary considerably from year to year depending on the weather. During the season, symptoms are worse on dry, windy days and decrease during heavy rain. They usually tend to be worse in the morning. The termination of symptoms at the end of the pollen season is less abrupt than the onset, owing to the persistence of pollen in the air and, in many cases, to the complicating effects of nonseasonal allergens and superimposed respiratory infections.

The most characteristic symptom is sneezing, usually in paroxysms of several sneezes in rapid succession. The nasal mucosa is congested and there is an increased flow of watery mucoid secretion. The conjunctivae are red and itchy, and there is increased lacrimation. Itching of the soft palate and pharynx is usual, and in severe cases the ears may also itch severely. Cough, wheezing, and dyspnea are commonly present but are actually indicative of pollen asthma rather than of hay fever itself.

Diagnosis. When the pattern of seasonal recurrence has become established, the diagnosis of hay fever is easy, and the causative pollen is usually apparent to the physician acquainted with the pollen seasons of the area. During the first season, differentiation from infective rhinitis may be difficult, although the paroxysmal sneezing, the itching of the eyes and pharynx, the watery nasal discharge, the normal temperature, and the absence of sore throat and of general malaise are helpful, as is a personal or family history of allergies of the wheal and erythema type. In doubtful cases, smears of the nasal secretion may be stained with Wright's stain; an abundance of eosinophils is characteristic of allergic rhinitis.

Allergic rhinitis due to antigens other than pollens, particularly airborne molds such as Alternaria and Hormodendrum, and seasonal insects, may have a seasonal exacerbation during warm weather but lacks the precise onset and cessation characteristic of pollen allergy. Occasional cases of allergic rhinitis due to fruits or vegetables eaten at certain seasons may be confusing but can be distinguished by skin tests. The diagnosis of hay fever is established, and the

specific cause demonstrated, by skin tests with the antigen, performed with the technique and precautions outlined in the introduction to the section on Immune Mechanisms of Disease. Both the *scratch test* and the *intracutaneous test* are useful. The scratch test is simpler and involves less danger of a general constitutional reaction; the intracutaneous test is more sensitive and more useful in estimating the degree of sensitization. For the typical case of seasonal hay fever, a few tests with pollens appropriate to the season and locality suffice. If the season is prolonged, additional tests with mold spores and other inhalants may be added. (See Nonseasonal Allergic Rhinitis, *infra*.)

Reactions are read after 10 to 15 minutes. A slight but definite wheal is considered one plus; a moderate reaction (wheal 6 to 10 mm., without pseudopods), two plus; a wheal of 10 to 15 mm. (with pseudopod formation), three plus; and wheals larger than 15 mm., four plus.

The initial intracutaneous tests with pollens should be made with solutions of antigen containing no more than 10 protein nitrogen units per milliliter, and not more than six tests should be done at one time. If little or no reaction is obtained, subsequent tests may be made with solutions containing 100 units and then 1000 units per milliliter until a two or three plus reaction is elicited.

The degree of sensitivity is roughly indicated by the highest dilution producing a three plus skin reaction in the intracutaneous test: Class A, highly sensitive, 10 units per ml.; Class B, average, 100 units; and Class C, less sensitive, 1000 units. A moderate (two plus) reaction to the 1000-unit strength is evidence of sensitivity if consistent with the seasonal incidence of symptoms. Many patients with definite allergy to one pollen show slight or moderate reactions to other pollens. These indicate slight or potential allergy, but specific treatment is indicated only for those that the history shows to be important.

Prognosis. Hay fever is essentially a permanent idiosyncrasy, more troublesome than disabling and without danger to life. Variations in severity may occur spontaneously or as a result of a change of residence or habits that alters the intensity of exposure to pollen. Since hay fever is a manifestation of allergy of the wheal and erythema type, patients affected by it often develop other diseases of this type, particularly asthma. This complication eventually occurs in approximately 30 per cent of untreated patients, but the incidence is greatly reduced by specific treatment. Patients with hay fever are unusually susceptible to upper respiratory infection, and the development of sinusitis is a common complication, especially of the autumn type, which persists until the cold weather, when respiratory infections are prevalent.

Treatment. The treatment of hay fever consists of (1) avoidance of the causative pollen, (2) palliative drug therapy, (3) lessening of sensitivity by injections of the specific antigen. When treatment is started during the season of symptoms, the first two methods produce the most immediate relief, but the most satisfactory results over the long term are achieved by antigen injections started at least two months before the season and continued throughout the year.

Avoidance. When the severity of symptoms warrants it, relief may be obtained by a trip to an area known to be free of the causative pollen or by a sea voyage. Exposure to pollen may also be lessened by air conditioning, the use of suitable pollen filters in the windows, or to a lesser degree by simply remaining indoors with windows and doors closed.

Palliative Treatment. The most useful drugs are the antihistaminics, which produce satisfactory relief in a majority of cases. Tripelennamine (Pyribenzamine), 50 mg., and chlorprophenpyridamine (Chlor-Trimeton), 4 mg., are examples of the many suitable drugs of the group. They may be taken after each meal and, if necessary, every four hours at night. Phenergan (promethazine), 12.5 to 25 mg., has a more potent and lasting antihistaminic action and is useful at bedtime but is too sedative for general use during the day.

Patients with severe symptoms or with coexisting pollen asthma not relieved by the antihistaminics may be given prednisone or prednisolone, 5 mg., every six to eight hours, or corticotrophin gel, 40 units intramuscularly daily. The dose of either drug should be reduced by 25 to 50 per cent as soon as relief is obtained and is generally continued for seven to ten days at the height of the pollen season.

For relief of the conjunctival symptoms, eye drops containing cocaine hydrochloride, 0.3 per cent, epinephrine hydrochloride, 0.025 per cent, and boric acid, 3 per cent in rose water, are useful, one drop in each eye two or three times a day if necessary.

Specific Treatment. Treatment with specific pollen antigen is initiated with a series of 12 to 16 subcutaneous injections of gradually increasing doses of antigen, given at intervals of three to seven days, starting two or three months before the season. The accompanying table shows approximate doses, which must be modified according to the patient's reaction.

The injections are given on the lateral aspect of the upper arm or the thigh, with a rubber tourniquet and epinephrine, 1:1000, at hand for use in case of a constitutional reaction. The patient is kept under observation for 20 minutes after the injection.

Normally the injections produce a slight local swelling that subsides within 24 hours. If the local reaction is troublesome or lasts longer than 36 hours, the same dose is repeated after the usual interval, then increased or again repeated as indicated by the resulting reaction.

If a constitutional reaction follows the injection, a rubber tourniquet is applied promptly proximal to the site of the injection and 0.4 to 0.6 ml. of epinephrine 1:1000 is injected every ten minutes until relief is obtained. Mild constitutional

DOSAGE IN PROTEIN NITROGEN UNITS FOR TREATMENT OF HAY FEVER

Dose	Class A (Highly Sensitive)	Class B (Average Case)	Class C (Less Sensitive)
1	2	10	20
2	5	20	40
3	10	40	80
4	20	80	150
5	35	140	250
6	50	200	400
7	75	300	600
8	110	400	850
9	150	600	1200
10	200	800	1800
11	300	1000	2500
12	400	1500	3500
13	600	2000	5000
14	800	3000	6500
15	1000	4000	8000
16	1000	5000	10000

reactions may be relieved by tripelennamine (Pyribenzamine), 50 to 100 mg. orally or 25 mg. subcutaneously, but since they may rapidly become more serious, the inexperienced physician is wise to use epinephrine. When a constitutional reaction has occurred, the dosage should be dropped back two steps on the schedule and then increased more gradually. If a second constitutional reaction occurs at the same dosage, the subsequent dosage should be kept below that level.

The dose that has been reached at the beginning of the season is repeated weekly during the period of active pollination, without further increase.

Such *preseasonal treatment* produces satisfactory results in at least 75 per cent of cases and may be supplemented with drug treatment if necessary. No lasting benefit is expected, and it must be repeated each year.

Better clinical results and gradual loss of sensitivity are produced by *perennial treatment,* in which approximately the same number of injections are given throughout the year. After the end of the first season, the dose that has been reached is repeated every four weeks until the following spring. When a fresh supply of extract is obtained, the dose must be reduced 50 to 60 per cent to allow for the deterioration of the year-old antigen; it can then be gradually increased to the previous or a somewhat higher dose by giving injections every two weeks. Skin tests with the pollen antigen are repeated annually, and patients showing decreased sensitivity are subsequently treated with doses appropriate to their new classification. Continuation of such treatment for several years usually leads to a marked and persistent decrease in sensitivity.

Loveless and others have reported good results from *repository treatment* with one or two injections each year of pollen extract emulsified in mineral oil. Since the injected mineral oil is not eliminated and sometimes produces chronic local inflammations, this simplified treatment is not advised for general use.

NONSEASONAL ALLERGIC RHINITIS, VASOMOTOR RHINITIS

Allergic rhinitis due to nonseasonal antigens is essentially similar to hay fever and often affects the same persons, but if exposure to the antigen is persistent, it assumes a chronic form. Perennial allergic rhinitis may be due to inhaled antigens (inhalants) or to allergic reactions to the bacteria of the nose and paranasal sinuses, and rarely to foods or ingested drugs. Ordinary house dust which contains antigens distinct from the known substances contributing to its formation, but possibly resulting from their deterioration, is one of the most important inhalant antigens.

Vasomotor rhinitis, practically indistinguishable from chronic allergic rhinitis, may result from prolonged exposure to nonantigenic irritants, of which the most frequently encountered are vasoconstricting nose drops such as ephedrine, Privine, and Neo-Synephrine. When these drugs have been used persistently, they frequently prove to be the principal cause of prolonged rhinitis, and there is considerable improvement within a week after their discontinuation. A similar edema of the nasal mucosa can also result from psychosomatic factors, which may occasionally be the sole cause, but more often represent a contributory cause in allergic cases.

In rhinitis due to any of these causes, the nasal mucosa is swollen and presents a dull red or grayish appearance. In chronic cases there are often mucous polyps, particularly in the ethmoid region. The nasal secretion is increased in amount and is mucoid, and there is an abundance of eosinophils in the stained smear.

To evaluate the importance of extrinsic allergens, skin tests with 18 or 20 of the principal inhalants should be done as outlined in the discussion of asthma. Tests with food antigens are indicated only if the history is suggestive or if the inhalant tests give negative results. Skin tests are not satisfactory for determining the existence of bacterial allergy in the causation of vasomotor rhinitis. It may be suspected in the presence of associated chronic sinusitis, particularly hyperplastic sinusitis, and is strongly suggested by the coexistence of nasal polyps. If the patient has been using vasoconstricting nose drops persistently, their use should be discontinued before the importance of other factors is estimated. The importance of psychogenic factors in certain cases of vasomotor rhinitis, either as the principal cause or as a contributory factor in allergic patients, must be judged by the history, by the careful elimination of allergic and infective causes, and by observation over a period of time.

Treatment. Therapy is best directed to the cause. In cases due to specific inhalant antigens such as feathers or animal danders, elimination of contact is far more effective than injection treatment. Allergy to inhalants with which contact is unavoidable, such as house dust and airborne mold spores, is treated by injection of antigens in progressive dosage similar to that advised for pollen antigens. For symptomatic treatment, the antihistaminic drugs in the doses advised for hay fever are useful, but are somewhat less effective in chronic than in acute cases. Prednisone, prednisolone, and corticotrophin are highly effective in severe cases, but the relief is only temporary, and prolonged use involves risk of undesirable side effects.

Perennial allergic rhinitis, like hay fever, is not dangerous to life, but if specific treatment is neglected, it is often followed by asthma. Susceptibility to nasal and sinus infection is also greatly increased.

Blackley, C. H.: Experimental Researches on the Cause and Nature of Catarrhus Aestivus. London, 1873.

Loveless, M. H.: Repository immunization in pollen allergy. J. Immun., 79:68, 1957.

Samter, M., and Durham, O. C.: Regional Allergy of the United States, Canada, Mexico and Cuba. Springfield, Ill., Charles C Thomas, Publisher, 1955.

Wodehouse, R. P.: Hay Fever Plants. Waltham, Mass., Chronica Botanica Co., 1945.

ASTHMA

See Respiratory Diseases.

URTICARIA

William B. Sherman

Definition. Urticaria, or hives, is an eruption of the skin characterized by transitory, sharply demarcated, elevated, flat-topped wheals, usually accompanied by erythema and itching. This rash may occur without other symptoms or as one manifestation of a systemic disease.

Etiology. Urticaria may be due to a variety of different causes, the relative importance of which varies in different localities and in different types of practice.

1. Allergy to foods is probably the most frequent cause of acute urticaria, but it is relatively less important in chronic cases. Shellfish, fish, nuts, berries, and other fruits are common offenders, but almost any other food may be the cause. The urticarial reaction to food may be immediate or delayed for 12 hours or more. Skin tests are usually helpful only in the immediate reactions. In severe, acute cases, gastrointestinal and respiratory manifestations of food allergy may also be present.

2. Allergy to drugs, particularly penicillin, is a frequent cause. Urticaria due to penicillin frequently is part of a reaction resembling serum sickness, with an incubation period of a week or more and lasting another week or two, but it may persist for months without further exposure to the drug. (See articles on Drug Allergy and Serum Sickness.)

3. Biologic medications containing protein may produce urticaria either as an immediate allergic reaction or as delayed serum sickness. In addition to heterologous antiserum, insulin and allergen extracts are common offenders in the immediate type of reaction.

4. Allergy to substances touching the skin surface, such as silk, wool, and animal pelts, is occasionally a cause.

5. Infections of the teeth, tonsils, sinuses, and occasionally of other sites are among the commonest causes of chronic urticaria. Fink and Gay reported that infection was the cause in 30 per cent of 170 chronic cases.

6. Infestation by parasitic worms is an important factor in localities where they are prevalent. In susceptible persons, scabies, lice, mosquitoes, bedbugs, and other biting insects may produce typical urticaria.

7. Physical allergy to cold, light, heat, or scratching occasionally is the primary cause. More often, heat and scratching act as secondary factors in urticaria due to other causes.

8. Stress and emotional factors are major causes of chronic urticaria. Often they are contributory factors in cases primarily due to other causes, but in many cases no other cause can be established.

9. Endocrine factors, particularly menstruation, menopause, and thyroid insufficiency, are reported to play a part in some cases.

In a large proportion of chronic cases, variously estimated from 25 (Fink and Gay) to 90 per cent (Hopkins and Kesten), no cause can be clearly established.

The incidence of urticaria is higher in people with a personal or family history of allergies of the familial type, but the condition is by no means limited to this group.

Pathogenesis. The urticarial wheal consists of edema of the skin and results from dilatation of the small vessels and transudation of fluid through the walls of the capillaries in the affected area. The reaction is inhibited by adequate doses of antihistamine drugs, and similar lesions may be produced in normal skin by the intracutaneous injection of histamine or histamine liberators, suggesting that the local release of histamine is a factor in pathogenesis. There is some evidence that acetylcholine and other intermediaries may also be involved.

In urticaria due to heterologous serum, parasitic worms, or insect bites, and in the immediate urticarial reactions to foods, the release of histamine results from an antigen-antibody reaction of the immediate allergic type. Circulating antibodies are usually present, and an urticarial wheal may be produced by a skin test with the antigen. In urticaria resulting from infection, nonprotein drugs or delayed allergic reactions to foods, such an antibody mechanism is rarely demonstrable, but some allergic phenomenon is believed to be involved. The mechanism by which stress pro-

duces urticarial wheals has not been clearly established.

Clinical Manifestations. The typical lesions are multiple rounded areas, 1 to 4 cm. in diameter, with sharply defined edges, palpably raised above the surrounding skin surface. Both the wheal and the surrounding skin are erythematous, but if the skin is gently stretched, the wheal blanches and stands out clearly. The individual lesions usually fade in 6 to 24 hours, but successive crops may appear in the same or different areas. The palms, soles, and scalp are rarely affected. When the eyelids, lips, or genitalia are involved, the lesions are less sharply defined and are accompanied by subcutaneous edema, producing the picture of angioneurotic edema (see following article). Itching is usually severe, and scratching often produces new lesions of elongated form. The total duration of the attack may be a few hours, or it may persist for weeks or months.

Diagnosis. Simple urticaria should be distinguished from urticaria pigmentosa, an infiltration of the skin (and often other tissues) by mast cells, in which urticarial wheals subside to leave permanently pigmented brownish macules. Differentiation from insect bites is not always easy, since allergic persons may react to them with typical urticaria. Usually the bite shows a central puncture and, as the wheal fades, an itching papule persists for a day or more.

Treatment. Symptomatic relief of acute cases is usually afforded by injection of epinephrine 1:1000, 0.5 ml. hypodermically, repeated after 15 to 30 minutes if necessary, or ephedrine, 25 to 50 mg. by mouth. Antihistamine drugs, such as tripelennamine (Pyribenzamine), 50 to 100 mg., diphenhydramine (Benadryl), 50 to 100 mg., or chlorprophenpyridamine (Chlor-Trimeton), 8 mg., every four to six hours, are more suitable in prolonged attacks. For patients in whom psychogenic factors are evident, hydroxyzine (Atarax), which combines tranquilizing and antihistaminic actions, may be helpful. If these drugs are not effective, prednisone or prednisolone, 5 to 10 mg. every 6 to 12 hours, may be used for periods of a week or two. Calamine lotion with phenol is helpful as a local application for the relief of itching. If the onset of urticaria follows injection of penicillin, penicillinase (Neutrapen), 800,000 units, should be injected daily for two or three days, although the value of this procedure has not been established by controlled tests.

Fink, A. I., and Gay, L. N.: A critical review of 170 cases of urticaria and angioneurotic edema followed for a period of from two to ten years. Bull. Hopkins Hosp., 55:280, 1934.

Graham, D. T., and Wolf, S.: The pathogenesis of urticaria. J.A.M.A., 143:1396, 1950.

Hopkins, J. G., and Kesten, B.: Urticaria. Arch. Derm. (Chicago), 29:358, 1934.

Sheldon, J. M., Mathews, K. P., and Lovell, R. G.: The vexing urticaria problem: present concepts of etiology and management. J. Allerg., 25:525, 1954.

ANGIONEUROTIC EDEMA

William B. Sherman

Definition. Angioneurotic edema (angio-edema or giant urticaria) is characterized by transitory, localized, painless swellings of the subcutaneous tissue or submucosa of various parts of the body. It occurs in two forms: a relatively rare hereditary form due to profound hereditary defects of the enzymatic mechanisms of permeability control, and a more common sporadic or nonhereditary type, a giant form of urticaria, apparently due to the same causative factors. The dermal manifestations of the two types are similar, but the hereditary type is more often associated with visceral lesions involving the respiratory and gastrointestinal systems.

Etiology. The *hereditary form* shows a strong familial tendency; the 503 cases reviewed by Austen occurred in only 61 families. It is apparently due to lack of specific enzyme inhibitors, inherited as a mendelian dominant. Donaldson and Evans reported a lack of inhibitor of complement ($C'1$-esterase) and Landerman et al. deficiency of inhibitor for serum globulin permeability factor and/or plasma kallikrein. Present knowledge of permeability factors does not adequately explain the relationship between these two effects. Extrinsic antigens, such as those produced by infections, are of secondary importance, although mild trauma may determine the localization of individual lesions.

The *nonhereditary or sporadic type* is essentially a giant form of urticaria, often occurring with simple urticaria and due to similar causes, notably allergy to foods or drugs, infection, and emotional stress. This type is more commonly seen in, but is not limited to, people with a personal or family history of other manifestations of allergic disease.

Pathogenesis. The development of angioedema, like that of urticaria, results from dilatation of the small blood vessels and transudation of fluid through the capillaries, but the lesion of angioedema is primarily in the subcutaneous tissue. The overlying skin may or may not be affected. The vascular change is believed to result from local derangement of permeability control, possibly by release of histamine, kinins, and other permeability factors.

Clinical Manifestations. The lesion is most often single, but may be multiple. It consists of a tense, nonpitting, rounded swelling a few centimeters or more in diameter. The edema is localized, but lacks the sharply defined, raised border typical of urticaria. The overlying skin is usually normal in color and temperature, but may be slightly reddened. There is no pain, and itching is rare; the chief sensation is one of distention. The individual lesions persist for one to three days and leave no residual changes. Successive attacks may involve the same or different locations. The face, hands, feet, and genitalia are the skin areas most often affected. Involvement of the lips, tongue, and pharynx is not unusual. In the hereditary form, laryngeal edema is a frequent cause of death, but this lesion occurs less often in the sporadic type. Involvement of the gastrointestinal system is also common in the hereditary form, with abdominal pain and vomiting suggestive of an inflammatory or obstructive disease.

Diagnosis. The nature of the lesion is generally apparent from the absence of pain and heat and usually of redness. The presence of simple urticaria elsewhere on the body is also helpful. The underlying structures—for example, the teeth and sinuses in lesions of the face—should be carefully examined for evidence of infection. Edema persisting a week or more without remission is rarely angioneurotic edema. In doubtful cases, a therapeutic trial with the drugs noted below may be helpful. A distinction between the sporadic and the hereditary forms is important. Austen reports that this is best accomplished by determination of the second component of complement ($C'2$), the natural substrate of the enzyme involved.

Prognosis. In the hereditary form, frequent recurrences and visceral manifestations are expected. Death from edema of the glottis is the most frequent termination, occurring in 23 per cent of persons afflicted. In the nonhereditary form, this complication is rare, but periodic recurrences over a period of months or years are common unless an extrinsic cause is found.

Treatment. The response of large swellings to symptomatic medication is slow. Epinephrine is indicated, particularly if the tongue, pharynx, or larynx is involved. One or two doses of 0.5 ml. of the 1:1000 aqueous solution may be followed by 1.0 ml. of the 1:500 suspension in oil intramuscularly for a prolonged effect. Relatively large doses of the antihistamine drugs are required. Tripelennamine (Pyribenzamine) or diphenhydramine (Benadryl), 50 to 100 mg., may be given every four hours. In severe or resistant cases, prednisone or prednisolone, 10 to 15 mg. may be given every six hours until the lesion subsides, or corticotrophin gel, 40 to 80 units, may be injected intramuscularly.

When the pharynx or larynx is affected, vigorous treatment and close observation are essential. Preparations should be made for a prompt tracheotomy, if necessary.

In recurrent or persistent cases of the nonhereditary type, an effort should be made to determine the cause, and treatment should be directed at its elimination. Infections of the teeth, tonsils, paranasal sinuses or other organs should be treated appropriately. Food allergens suspected as causative factors on the basis of history, observation, or skin tests should be avoided. The role of physical or emotional stress should be carefully evaluated.

Austen, K. F., and Shepper, A. L.: Detection of hereditary angioneurotic edema by demonstration of a reduction in the second component of human complement. New Eng. J. Med., 272:649, 1955.

Donaldson, V. H., and Evans, R. R.: Biochemical abnormality in hereditary angioneurotic edema; absence of serum inhibitor of C′1-esterase. Amer. J. Med., 35:37, 1963.

Landerman, N. S., Webster, M. E., Becker, E. L., and Ratcliffe, H. F.: Hereditary angioneurotic edema. II. Deficiency of inhibitor for serum globulin permeability factor and/or plasma kallikrein. J. Allerg., 33:330, 1962.

SERUM SICKNESS

Fred S. Kantor

Definition. Serum sickness is a disease characterized by fever, arthralgia, skin eruptions, and edema which appears following injection of a foreign serum or serum proteins and is dependent upon an immune response of the patient to the injected serum. Hypersensitivity reactions to a variety of drugs may produce an identical illness.

Etiology. With the advent of antimicrobial therapy, the use of serum for the treatment of microbial diseases has declined markedly; the most common cause for "serum sickness" at the present time is not serum itself but exogenously administered drugs, particularly the antimicrobials. Serum therapy is still used primarily for the neutralization of bacterial toxins such as tetanus and botulinus toxins and also in the form of rabies antiserum.

The incidence and severity of the disease are clearly related to the type of serum preparation as well as to the amount administered. Of patients given prophylactic tetanus antitoxin prepared in horses, approximately 2 to 5 per cent will develop symptoms of serum sickness. The figure is considerably higher for those patients receiving equine rabies antiserum; approximately 16 per cent of these patients develop serum sickness. In general, there is an increasing incidence and severity through childhood, adolescence, and adulthood. Reactions in children are quite mild, lasting from one to four days, whereas in patients over the age of 15, the disease is more frequent and more severe.

Different methods of production of various equine antisera may have a profound effect upon the serum sickness liability of the product. Most tetanus antitoxin preparations involve a peptic digestion which does not impair antitoxic properties while hydrolyzing many of the proteins present in the serum. In contrast, antirabies antiserum is not subjected to peptic digestion because of the great loss of antibody encountered with the enzymatic treatment. The most important factor concerned with the development of serum sickness is the total amount of serum administered. Recommended doses of tetanus antitoxin and rabies antisera vary considerably from time to time; from 5 to 10 ml. of tetanus antitoxin may produce serum sickness in 5 to 10 per cent of patients, whereas 80 ml. will almost always result in illness. Age and dose relationships in serum sickness resulting from drugs are not as clear cut as with serum or serum proteins. In most cases the drug by itself is not capable of inducing the disease and must combine with a protein of the patient to form a complete antigen or immunogen. In such a situation the genetic potential of the patient of forming complete antigens and producing antibodies to them must be considered in addition to the patient's age and the dose and duration of the drug given.

Mechanism. The essential basis of serum sickness is antigen-antibody interaction. A blood level of circulating foreign protein can be measured in patients shortly after beginning serum treatment. In the early stages the administered protein is catabolized in a manner similar to that seen in the animal from which it came. This is the latent period and usually lasts from four to ten days, during which time the patient develops an immune response that is evidenced by the appearance of antibody directed against the injected protein. This antibody is not easily measured at the onset of illness because it forms soluble complexes with the circulating foreign antigen. These complexes have a varied fate depending upon their nature and the ratio of antigen to antibody in the complex. Since the antibody response is a heterogeneous one, only certain antigen-antibody complexes may be expected to lead to serum sickness. Experimental studies, in the rabbit primarily, have shown a deposition of antigen-antibody complexes beneath the endothelium of blood vessels and within the basement membrane of these vessels. Complexes shown to fix complement seem to be most important in this disease. With fixation of complement containing complexes in the wall of the blood vessels, polymorphonuclear leukocytes are attracted to the site, and appear to injure the vessel by release of potent enzymes found in their lysosomal granules. The vascular injury mediated by complement and polymorphonuclear leukocytes may lead to thrombosis and hemorrhage, typified by the petechial or ecchymotic rash attendant on serum sickness.

Another manifestation of the interaction of antigen and antibody is the release of potent vasoactive materials such as histamine, serotonin, bradykinin, and slow-reacting substance (SRSA), all of which lead to vasodilatation and leakage of protein and fluid from the vascular space into the tissues, resulting in edema. The disease varies from species to species in laboratory animals and, as most of the work has been done in the rabbit, it is pertinent to note that the renal disease, which is a frequent and important aspect of immune complex disease in the rabbit, is often nonexistent or a very mild component in the usual human patient.

Continuation of disease is dependent upon a continual supply of antigen. Removal by the reticuloendothelial system of the immune complexes is signified by a rise in serum antibody directed against the foreign proteins, and reduction of symptoms and signs of illness. Unless the foreign proteins are readministered, the disease is self-limited. During convalescence and for long periods thereafter antibodies against the foreign proteins are readily demonstrable in the patient's serum. Readministration of foreign antigen promptly leads to formation of immune complexes and clinical manifestations of disease, which continue until antigen is entirely removed from the circulation.

Clinical Manifestations. The onset of disease is often heralded by itching and discomfort, frequently at the site of serum injection. Fully developed serum sickness is a miserable disease. The unfortunate patient lies on his side in bed with a swollen, distorted face, often resulting in closure of both eyes so that he cannot see, with a skin itching all over and often covered with an urticarial or erythematous rash. He is reluctant to scratch his skin because of the pain in all his muscles and joints upon movement, and so he lies quietly in bed suffering from headache, itching, and joint pain. Especially frightening and discomforting is the appearance of neurologic manifestations which may result in weakness of an extremity or a sensory deficit, or occasionally an isolated facial palsy. Compounding the patient's difficulties may be abdominal pain, nausea, and vomiting. Upon examination a generalized lymphadenopathy may be palpated, especially prominent in the regions draining the site of injection of the serum. At that site there may be a local rash with erythema and either urticaria or tenderness, and this may provide a potent clue for the physician as to the nature of the illness. Occasionally, auscultation of the chest reveals a cardiac arrhythmia or a pericardial friction rub. The spleen is usually not palpable. A common manifestation is fever of 101 to 102° F. and, in addition to the subjective complaints of joint pain, the patient may manifest objective arthritis with swelling, redness, and accumulation of fluid in joints. The skin may show a petechial or purpuric rash in addition to the more common urticarial eruption.

Laboratory Studies. Examination of the blood may reveal a mild leukocytosis, and circulating plasma cells have been observed. The sedimentation rate is usually normal or only slightly elevated. Eosinophilia occurs, but is relatively uncommon. The urine may show slight proteinuria, a few red cells, and occasionally a few casts; but there are rarely significant evidences of renal impairment. Examination of the serum proteins of the patient reveal circulating horse γ-globulins and macroglobulins present early in the disease, and predominantly anti-horse γA globulin antibodies late in the disease and during convalescence. The development of antibodies to horse alpha-2-macroglobulin in the sera of patients recovering from serum sickness suggests that this component of the equine serum which lacks any antibody value could be deleted in manufacture without impairing the antitoxic benefits of the serum. Serum complement levels are reduced for variable periods during the disease and then return to normal.

Treatment and Prognosis. Very mild symptoms of pruritus and skin rash may be controlled by an antihistamine, such as brompheniramine, 4 mg.

given every four hours. Epinephrine and sympathomimetic amines have been recommended in the past for the treatment of the urticaria of serum sickness, and salicylates for the treatment of joint pains. However, for all but the mildest symptoms, adrenocortical steroids in the form of prednisone can be given with great safety and efficacy, and the patient need not suffer with less effective medications. As this is a self-limited disease with a natural course of one to three weeks, the usual hazards of steroid therapy are not realized before treatment is stopped. A treatment course of 40 mg. per day for four or five days may be sufficient, even for quite severe disease. Symptomatic improvement appears often within hours of the onset of steroid therapy and sometimes is remarkable within 24 hours.

Prevention. Tetanus antitoxin prepared from *human* serum is now commercially available in many parts of the world. When this is available, there is no reason to choose horse serum to obtain antitoxic benefits. When equine sera must be used in treatment, patients should be carefully questioned concerning prior exposure and for allergic symptoms to other horse products, such as horse dander or horsehair, as found in horsehair mattresses. All patients, regardless of history, should be skin tested by production of a minimal wheal (0.01 to 0.02 ml.) of a 1:10 dilution of the serum to be tested. After 15 to 20 minutes the skin site is examined for an urticarial wheal, and in its absence treatment may be instituted. If the patient is allergic and the necessity for serum treatment is great, desensitization may be attempted by repeatedly injecting small amounts of serum beginning in dilutions of 1:100 and doubling the tolerated amount about every 15 or 20 minutes until the appropriate dose is achieved. Such treatment is hazardous because of possible anaphylaxis, and the indications for it should be scrutinized carefully.

In patients who have developed serum sickness following tetanus antitoxin, active immunization should be begun during the patient's convalescence from serum sickness. It is generally advisable to immunize against tetanus all individuals who are seen by the physician in connection with unrelated allergic disease and found to be sensitive to horse dander or horse products. The immunization can be accomplished by use of tetanus toxoid. Occasionally, in the course of serum therapy an acute anaphylactic reaction occurs, consisting of sudden vascular collapse, severe pruritus of the face, hands, and feet, and is often accompanied by bronchospasm and incontinence of stool and urine. Such events must be treated promptly with epinephrine and not adrenocortical steroids. A tourniquet should be placed proximal to the injection site of the drug or serum, and 0.2 ml. of epinephrine injected into the site of injection which will slow absorption from the site. An additional 0.3 to 0.5 ml. of 1:1000 aqueous solution of epinephrine should be given subcutaneously above the tourniquet if the patient has an effective blood pressure. In the absence of adequate blood pressure, the epinephrine must be given intravenously notwithstanding the hazard of production of cardiac arrhythmia, as subcutaneous or intramuscular administration will not result in effective therapeusis because the drug will not be absorbed from the periphery.

Dixon, F. J.: Experimental serum sickness. *In* Samter, M., and Alexander, H. L. (eds.): Immunological Diseases. Boston, Little, Brown & Company, 1965, p. 161.

Kojis, F. G.: Serum sickness and anaphylaxis. Amer. J. Dis. Child., 64:93, 313, 1942.

Vaughan, J. H., Barnett, E. V., and Leadley, P. J.: Serum sickness: Evidence in man of antigen-antibody complexes and free light chains in the circulation during the acute reaction. Ann. Intern. Med., 67:596, 1967.

von Pirquet, C., and Schick, B.: Serum Sickness. Baltimore, Williams & Wilkins Company, 1951.

DRUG ALLERGY

Fred S. Kantor

The value of therapeutic agents should constantly be weighed against their potential liability. Hypersensitivity reactions must be distinguished from two other untoward effects of drugs. The first is that of intolerance, in which the usual undesirable toxic effects occur at dosages of the drug well below that expected in a normal population. An example of this type of reaction includes visual disturbances and alterations in cardiac rhythm with very small doses of digitalis. The second form of drug reaction to be distinguished from hypersensitivity is that of idiosyncrasy. Whereas intolerance is a quantitative difference, idiosyncrasy is qualitative and is based upon a biochemical alteration in the way the patient handles the drug. Such a reaction does not depend on prior exposure to the drug, is not dose dependent, and does not resemble the other pharmacologic manifestations of the drug. An example of idiosyncrasy is the hemolytic anemia produced in patients with glucose-6-phosphate dehydrogenase deficiency when treated with primaquine. Altered reactivity (von Pirquet combined these two words to produce the word "allergy") on the part of the patient always follows prior exposure, even though this may not be apparent, and its mechanism is related to the hypersensitive state as reflected by delayed hypersensitivity or antibody production.

Incidence. Any drug may produce a hypersensitivity reaction but some drugs have a much higher liability in this regard than do others. Digitalis and tetracycline have a low liability in producing allergic drug reactions, even though reports of documented cases have appeared. On the other hand, several of the antimicrobials, notably novobiocin, and certain anti-inflammatory agents, such as phenylbutazone, may have a high incidence of drug reaction. In addition to the variations produced by different drugs, equal liability is not shared by all patients for development of drug reactions to a single drug, such as penicillin.

Patients with a history of allergic disease or previous drug reactions, as well as patients with certain inflammatory diseases such as lupus erythematosus, are generally thought to be more prone to the development of new drug allergies.

Pathogenesis. Certain therapeutic agents such as insulin are complex protein molecules which are known to be immunogenic. The majority of drugs represent classes of simple chemicals which require complexing with a tissue or serum protein of the patient in order to form an antigenic or immunogenic molecule. Drugs which are highly reactive chemicals usually are the most frequent sensitizers, and conversely the more inert members of the drug armamentarium are of less allergenic potential. Sensitization by means of a simple chemical involves the formation of covalent bonds with host protein which forms a hapten-carrier conjugate. Antibodies and hypersensitivity are directed against the hapten or the hapten and a closely adjacent portion of the carrier molecule, but never to the carrier protein itself. To form a hapten-protein conjugate, the administered drug may have to undergo considerable chemical rearrangement. This may occur during the metabolism of the drug, producing an antigenic determinant which is different from the administered drug. The necessity of chemical rearrangement of the drug to form the allergenic hapten-protein complex predicts difficulty of testing in vitro for drug allergy, since the laboratory must know what the antigenic determinant is.

Drug allergy has been investigated with respect to the antigenic determinant in only a limited number of cases. One of the most recent and extensive investigations has been in the case of penicillin and a derivative, the penicilloyl determinant. This has been labeled the major determinant, and as many as three — and perhaps many more — as yet undescribed chemical rearrangements may account for minor determinants, all of which can produce sensitization in given individuals and produce allergic symptoms upon administration of the drug. It should be borne in mind that not all drug immunization implies drug allergy. A good example of this is that all patients recently treated with penicillin will have developed antibodies directed against the penicilloyl determinant.

Hypersensitive reactions have been divided into *delayed hypersensitivity* and two varieties of immediate hypersensitivity: *wheal-and-flare* and *Arthus reactivity*. Serum sickness, which was discussed in the preceding article, is an excellent example of an immediate type of hypersensitivity involving complement-fixing antibody and producing reactions to the so-called "Arthus" type.

The other type of immediate hypersensitivity, i.e., wheal-and-flare, is manifested in two major, clinically recognizable situations, urticaria and anaphylaxis. In these cases, the interaction of the drug-protein conjugate with IgE antibodies leads to release of active mediators resulting in vasodilatation and smooth muscle contraction. In this form of reaction, the hapten-protein conjugate and its respective antibody do not enter into the pathogenesis of the reaction but merely cause the release of the vasoactive material which produces the clinical effects. The last type of well recognized mechanism is that of cellular or delayed hypersensitivity. In this form of immunity, circulating antibody is not important, and the interaction of the drug-protein conjugate is with sensitized cells, causing a release of a variety of biologically active materials which lead to perivascular accumulation of mononuclear cells and the development of induration. The best example of delayed hypersensitivity induced by drugs is skin sensitization resulting from direct contact with a variety of medications. Paradoxically, antihistamines, which have been incorporated into a variety of topical preparations for treatment of itching, burning, or allergic skin conditions, are themselves skin-sensitizing, and by combining with skin proteins form potent sensitizing agents which lead to delayed hypersensitivity and the development of the typical skin lesions of contact sensitivity. A combination of reaction types is often present in typical drug allergy, but one or another of the reaction types usually predominates and treatment is most efficacious when directed against this reaction type.

Clinical Manifestations. Fever may develop immediately after administration of a drug or, more commonly, may increase in a stepwise fashion after the seventh or eighth day of administration. The fever may show a sustained or remittent course and is usually low-grade in the range of 100 to 102° F., although hectic fevers are often observed, accompanied by constitutional symptoms. In general, the patient appears less ill than would be anticipated from the height of the fever. A drug reaction may mimic the septic picture entirely, but it usually pursues a more indolent course. Cessation of fever within a day or two of discontinuing the offending drug is to be expected. In some cases of fever alone, and if the drug reaction involves other organ systems, such as the skin and the joints, it may take several days, up to a week, for the symptoms to slowly subside. Penicillin, diphenylhydantoin (Dilantin), and barbiturates are frequent causes of drug fever.

Skin Rash. Skin rash as a manifestation of drug allergy may take several forms. A maculopapular, very fine rash appearing in the softer skin of the axillary line and on the extensor surfaces of the extremities and along the trunk may be unnoticed by the patient. Usually, urticarial rashes are reported because they are accompanied by pruritus. Persistent administration of an offending drug causing maculopapular eruptions may lead to confluent erythroderma and subsequent exfoliative dermatitis. Similarly, a rash may progress to an eczematous eruption with weeping papulovesicular lesions and ill-defined patches of erythema and edema, accompanied by intense pruritus. Erythema multiforme-like eruptions may be produced by a variety of drugs and are characterized by the formation of sharply circumscribed lesions that are usually symmetrical in distribution. The individual lesions seem to spread peripherally and clear centrally to form an annular pattern with secondary and tertiary rings evolving into a "target" or "iris" lesion.

Symmetrical lesions of the lower extremities closely resembling typical erythema nodosum may also be caused by drugs, including sulfones, penicillin, and iodides. The term "fixed eruption" is used to describe an erythematous and sharply defined lesion which recurs at the same site and in the same form upon re-exposure to the same drug. Withdrawal of the drug usually leads to healing, but hyperpigmentation of the area involved may remain. Photosensitivity reactions characterized by erythema, edema, and mild scaling are sharply limited to areas exposed to light, and a clue to the examiner may be provided by the V-shaped area at the neckline, usually at the site where the collar leaves the skin exposed to light and it becomes involved. Sulfonamides and thiazide derivatives are examples known to engender photoallergic reactions.

Other Organ Systems. Drug allergy is often manifested by reactions involving the hematopoietic system. Sedormid, a once popular sedative, resulted in thrombocytopenic purpura, which was shown to depend upon the presence of drug, a serum factor demonstrated to be antibody, and the presence of platelets. Several other drugs, such as quinine and quinidine, thiouracil, and the anticonvulsant hydantoin group, have been implicated as causes of thrombocytopenic purpura. Hemolytic anemia and agranulocytosis are also common adverse reactions ascribed to drugs. Sulfonamides and thiouracil have caused both types of reaction, but aminopyrine and phenylbutazone produced mainly agranulocytosis. Care should be taken in the interpretation of allergic causality of pathologic events leading to agranulocytosis or hemolytic anemia. One of the outstanding examples of a purported allergic hemolytic anemia was that induced by the fava bean. It was later shown that the presence of an enzyme defect in the red cells of these patients resulted in their shorter life span when exposed to drug and that sensitization in the immunologic sense was not required. Aplastic anemia, involving all the formed elements of the blood, is rarely associated with drug administration; in particular it is described with chloramphenicol, gold, and the sulfonamides.

Gastrointestinal symptoms are common adverse reactions to the administration of therapeutic agents, but the mechanism of action is rarely allergic in nature. The kidney is involved in periarteritis nodosa caused by drugs. In this disease, antimicrobial drugs, notably the sulfonamides, have been frequently implicated. Interstitial nephritis has been described with the penicillinase-resistant penicillin preparation methicillin in association with hematuria, rash, and marked eosinophilia.

The lupus erythematosus syndrome has been described following ingestion of certain drugs, particularly hydralazine, procainamide, and the hydantoin derivatives. The severity of the syndrome induced by drug ingestion may vary from only a serologic manifestation, such as a positive lupus test, to the full-blown picture of fever, arthritis, polyserositis, and hematologic manifestations. Pulmonary infiltration and eosinophilia (PIE syndrome), peripheral neuritis, and hemorrhagic encephalitis have all been ascribed to allergic drug reactions, and probably represent varieties of allergic vascular injury resident in the particular organs involved. Liver damage has been attributed to treatment with heavy metals, thorazine, and sulfonamides; the evidence supporting the allergic basis of these reactions is meager. In recent times, the introduction of halothane, a potent, widely used anesthetic agent, has led to a series of symptoms, primarily involving liver dysfunction, which in some patients strongly suggest an allergic basis.

Generalized Anaphylaxis. Generalized anaphylaxis as a manifestation of drug allergy is a clinical catastrophe with which the physician must be prepared to deal promptly. The disease is usually initiated by an injected drug, although an orally administered tablet has been reported to produce a fatal reaction. Frequently the initial symptoms are generalized pruritus, particularly on the soles of the feet and the palms of the hands, and the general development of a hyperemia of the skin, particularly about the ears, so that the individual often looks as though he had acquired a recent sunburn. Angioneurotic edema may cause distortion of the face, swelling of the eyelids, and rapid loss of effective plasma volume, leading to vascular collapse and shock. The risk of developing an anaphylactic reaction, particularly to penicillin, is enhanced by the patient's having had a prior, less serious reaction, such as a maculopapular rash.

Diagnosis. Avoidance and challenge is still the best diagnostic means available to the physician, although it is often inadvisable because of the danger to the patient. Certainly in cases of anaphylactic reactions or urticarial eruptions, the challenge to the patient subsequent to the subsidence of the symptoms is not warranted and is extremely dangerous. However, in drug fever, when that condition appears alone, a fractional dose may be administered after the fever subsides to further identify the cause. Unfortunately, laboratory tests performed in vitro have been very disappointing. The basophil degranulation test, lymphocyte stimulation test, skin window technique, and others have been reported with some success from isolated laboratories, but in general they have been found to be difficult to reproduce and have not come into general usage. The necessary information concerning the intermediary metabolites of each drug and the development of specific antigenic determinants is not available for the majority of drugs which cause allergic reactions. Until this information is known, laboratory tests are not likely to be useful in this area. The leukocyte count may be high or low, and therefore not useful; eosinophilia is not a regular occurrence.

Treatment and Prophylaxis. Subsidence of allergic reactions to drugs usually occurs promptly after discontinuance of the drug, often within one or two days, but in many instances prolongation of symptoms for several days and, indeed, in some instances for several weeks and months, is well recognized. Many of our foodstuffs are contaminated with drugs: Chickens are fattened with estrogenic hormones, hogs are fed antimicrobials, and cows, when suffering from mastitis, may be treated with large doses of penicillin which appears in the milk. When strongly suspecting a drug hypersensitivity which fails to subside after cessation of the drug, inadvertent environmental drug administration should be carefully investigated. In general, treatment of the drug reaction should be directed against the altered physiology. In the reactions involving vasoactive substances, the use of a direct vasoconstrictor such as epinephrine may be lifesaving and should be used first, instead of the more glamorous, but less effective, group of adrenocortical steroids. The latter group of agents are very useful in the treatment of the Arthus type of immediate hypersensitivity as manifested by serum sickness and polyarteritis, as well as in many forms of delayed hypersensitivity. Epinephrine should be given in dosages of 0.5 to 1 ml. of 1:1000 dilution of aqueous epinephrine, given subcutaneously. Antihistaminics such as diphenhydramine (Benadryl, 50 mg.) or brompheniramine (Dimetane, 4 mg.) may be administered orally or parenterally, but the intravenous use of diphenhydramine is to be avoided because serious adverse reactions to this medication have occurred. Drug reactions are self-limited diseases, and the use of steroids in these diseases is most efficacious and generally does not impose the usual liabilities of steroid therapy. Accordingly, therapy may be instituted with full doses of 40 to 60 mg. a day, and 40 mg. a day may be given for three or four days, dropped to 20 mg. a day for an additional several days, and discontinued without a long tapering regimen.

Ackroyd, J. F.: Sedormid purpura: An immunological study of a form of drug hypersensitivity. *In* Kallos, P.: Progress in Allergy, Vol. 3. New York, Interscience Publishers, 1952, p. 531.

Chase, M. W.: Hypersensitivity to simple chemicals, Harvey Lectures, 62:169, 1966.

Demis, D. J.: Allergy and drug sensitivity of skin. Ann. Rev. Pharmacol., 9:457, 1969.

Levine, B. B.: Immunochemical mechanisms of drug allergy. Ann. Rev. Med., 17:23, 1966.

Parker, C. W.: Drug Reactions. *In* Samter, M., and Alexander, H. L. (eds.): Immunological Diseases. Boston, Little, Brown & Company, 1965, p. 663.

Shulman, N. R.: Mechanism of blood cell destruction in individuals sensitized to foreign antigens. Trans. Ass. Amer. Physicians, 76:72, 1963.

CONNECTIVE TISSUE DISEASES ("COLLAGEN DISEASES") OTHER THAN RHEUMATOID ARTHRITIS

Introduction

K. Frank Austen

The connective tissue ("collagen") diseases or systemic rheumatic diseases are a group of clinicopathologic entities considered together because of common or overlapping clinical and histologic features. The term "collagen diseases" was introduced by Klemperer for such reasons and not because of any conviction about a common etiology. Each of the major entities within this grouping has prominent nonspecific constitutional manifestations coupled with patterns of organ involvement which determine the clinical designation, i.e., rheumatoid arthritis, rheumatic fever, systemic lupus erythematosus, scleroderma, dermatomyositis, and periarteritis nodosa (polyarteritis nodosa). The common histologic features are widespread inflammatory damage to connective tissues and blood vessels, at times associated with deposition of fibrinoid material. Fibrinoid refers to an amorphous material staining deeply eosinophilic with hematoxylin and eosin, which is deposited along connective tissue fibers and within vessel walls, and most probably represents a nonspecific response of connective tissue to injury. Clinical findings which have been invoked to support a common grouping include cardinal features of more than one entity in the same patient; transitions between one entity and another within the same patient; possible familial aggregation; and serologic abnormalities which may predominate in one entity but have an appreciable incidence in others.

Progressive systemic sclerosis (scleroderma), polymyositis alone or with cutaneous manifestations (dermatomyositis), and systemic lupus erythematosus (SLE) have distinct clinicopathologic and/or serologic features. By contrast, periarteritis nodosa has neither a characteristic morphologic, biochemical, or immunochemical abnormality nor a clinical presentation that is easily distinguished from systemic necrotizing angiitis of other types, including those which may be associated with any of the other connective tissue diseases. It seems pertinent, therefore, to review historically the problem of necrotizing angiitis and to include an operational classification based almost entirely upon clinical considerations. Detailed consideration of the structure and

function of the structural proteins, collagen and elastin, ground substance, and cellular elements of connective tissue is contained in the article on Rheumatoid Arthritis, presented in the section on Diseases of Joints.

HISTORICAL REVIEW OF ANGIITIS

The term *periarteritis nodosa* was aptly introduced by Kussmaul and Maier in 1866 to designate a morbid process manifested by numerous nodules along muscular-type arteries. Infiltration of the media with polymorphonuclear leukocytes and to a lesser extent eosinophils, plasma cells, and lymphocytes, disruption of the internal elastic lamina, fibrinoid necrosis, and extension to the adventitia and intima are characteristic. Proliferation of the intima leads to partial or total occlusion, and segmental scarring of the entire wall is responsible for the visible and/or palpable aneurysms. It is characteristic of the lesions to be in all stages of evolution from acute to healed. Additional characteristic features of periarteritis nodosa are the sparing of capillaries and veins except for involvement by spread from contiguous arteries, and the absence of involvement of pulmonary arteries despite the location of nodules in the bronchial arteries.

In 1923 Ophüls reported a patient with a periarteritis nodosa-like illness with the additional features of pulmonary vessel lesions, extensive involvement of small arteries and veins, granulomatous vascular and extravascular reactions, and an intense eosinophilic infiltration of vascular and pulmonary parenchymal lesions. The granulomas often included an eosinophilic core of altered collagen and necrotic eosinophils surrounded by radially arranged macrophages, lymphocytes, plasma cells, and varying numbers of polymorphonuclear leukocytes, both neutrophilic and eosinophilic. A detailed study of similar patients in 1951 by Churg and Strauss emphasized the striking clinical feature of severe progressive asthma with peripheral eosinophilia followed by fever, and prompted these authors to term this entity *allergic angiitis and granulomatosis*. Rose and Spencer

(1957) also appreciated these unique clinico-pathologic features but preferred the term poly-arteritis with pulmonary involvement to distinguish this group from classic polyarteritis.

In 1926 von Glahn and Pappenheimer considered that the *arteritis of rheumatic fever* could be distinguished from periarteritis nodosa by the absence of arterial thrombosis (or eosinophils), involvement of small arteries, and minimal fibrinoid necrosis. In the heart, Aschoff bodies represent a key extravascular histologic finding, although the clinical manifestations are predominantly related to rheumatic carditis.

Still another type of necrotizing vascular lesion, originally believed to be limited to the cranial arteries and characterized by the presence of multinucleated giant cells, was recognized by Horton, Magath, and Brown in 1934 and established as a clinical entity by Kilbourne and Wolff in 1946. The process usually involves the innermost layer of the media with predominantly a lymphocyte infiltration, the presence of multinucleated giant cells, fragmentation of the internal elastic lamina, and associated fibrinoid necrosis. The infiltration may extend to involve the adventitia and the intima, leading to intimal thickening with subsequent thrombosis. This entity, *giant cell arteritis,* can be predominantly local—presenting as cranial, especially temporal, or aortic arch (Takayasu's) arteritis—or it may be systemic. The syndrome of polymyalgia rheumatica may be associated with a local or systemic form of giant cell arteritis with or without arterial occlusion.

Necrotizing vascular lesions associated with the administration of horse antiserum and the development of clinical serum sickness were described by Clark and Kaplan in 1937. Rich observed similar lesions (1942) which he considered to be periarteritis nodosa not only in cases of serum sickness but also in circumstances of sulfonamide hypersensitivity. However, the more recent and prevailing view proposed by Zeek in 1952 is that hypersensitivity to drugs and serum, termed *hypersensitivity angiitis,* is distinguishable from periarteritis nodosa. Hypersensitivity angiitis involves small arteries, arterioles, and venules in a process of fibrinoid necrosis, occurring in the subendothelial ground substance and extending from the intima to involve the entire vessel wall; the accompanying cellular reaction is pleomorphic with polymorphonuclear leukocyte predominance frequently including eosinophils. Hypersensitivity angiitis often involves the pulmonary system and is characterized by virtually all lesions being at a similar evolutionary stage.

An unresolved issue is whether or not allergic granulomatosis and angiitis as defined by Churg and Strauss encompasses *Wegener's granulomatosis.* This disease, described by Wegener in 1936, is characterized by necrotizing granulomatous lesions of the upper and lower respiratory tract, generalized focal necrotizing lesions of both arteries and veins, and a glomerulitis typified by fibrin thrombi, focal necrosis of tufts, and on occasion a granulomatous reaction. This complex is somewhat similar to allergic granulomatosis and angiitis, but it is noteworthy that Wegener's granulomatosis is not associated with progressive asthma and prominent peripheral eosinophilia and does not exhibit a prominence of eosinophils in the necrotizing lesions. Thus for the present it seems reasonable to list this entity separately; lethal midline granuloma may be a related condition or a local variant. (See Granulomatous Diseases of Unknown Etiology.)

The final category includes miscellaneous entities. Atrophic malignant papulosis, described by Degos in 1954, refers to a characteristic clinical triad associated with necrotizing vascular lesions of the skin, gastrointestinal tract, and brain. Erythema elevatum diutinum is manifested by a chronic erythematous-papular and often purpuric skin eruption with or without systemic signs such as arthritis; it will probably be shifted to the hypersensitivity angiitis group when more information is available. A variety of purely cutaneous vasculitis syndromes have been described, and only time will tell whether these are distinct or are merely limited manifestations of a systemic entity.

OPERATIONAL CLASSIFICATION OF NECROTIZING ANGIITIS

Necrotizing angiitis is a convenient generic term for the entire group of syndromes in which vascular lesions, arterial or venous or both, may involve all three layers of the vessel wall with fibrinoid necrosis and various cellular infiltrates (see accompanying table). The clinical manifestations are caused largely by partial or complete vascular occlusion; the lesions are segmental, and the clinical patterns depend on the size and characteristic distribution of the lesions. Zeek recognized five major syndromes in this group: peri-

NECROTIZING ANGIITIS

Periarteritis nodosa (polyarteritis nodosa)

Allergic angiitis and granulomatosis of Churg and Strauss ("polyarteritis nodosa with pulmonary involvement")

Connective tissue disease ("collagen disease"), associated with
    Rheumatoid arthritis
    Scleroderma
    Poly- and dermatomyositis
    Rheumatic fever
    Erythema nodosum

Giant cell arteritis

Hypersensitivity angiitis
    Drug reaction
    Henoch-Schönlein purpura
    Systemic lupus erythematosus
    Mixed cryglobulinemia
    Goodpasture's syndrome

Wegener's granulomatosis

Miscellaneous
    Degos' disease (malignant papulosis)
    Erythema elevatum diutinum

arteritis nodosa, allergic angiitis and granulomatosis, rheumatic fever, giant cell arteritis, and hypersensitivity angiitis. With some modification this tabulation continues to be operationally useful.

Rheumatic fever can be placed under a category broadened to include those collagen diseases in which necrotizing vascular lesions are present but are not the most prominent aspect of the entity, i.e., rheumatoid arthritis, scleroderma, dermatomyositis, polymyositis, and possibly erythema nodosum. The category of hypersensitivity angiitis is particularly diverse and contains a variety of clinical entities distinguishable on the basis of precipitating events, serologic abnormalities, and relative frequency of involvement of various organ systems – drug reactions, Henoch-Schönlein purpura, serum sickness, systemic lupus erythematosus, mixed cryoglobulinemia (IgG-IgM complexes), and Goodpasture's syndrome. Separate categories are introduced for Wegener's granulomatosis and for a miscellaneous grouping.

Such an operational classification is a justified interim measure because there are associated implications as to prognosis, treatment, and etiology. A classification based on mechanism is a further goal, and to this end a few cautionary comments about the immunopathologic approach are in order. The fibrinoid in the lesions of systemic lupus erythematosus contains protein residues of nuclear origin, acid mucopolysaccharides derived from altered ground substance, and fibrinogen (or derivatives), immunoglobulins, and complement proteins. These findings are interpreted to mean the presence of immune complexes, consisting of nuclear antigen and antibody, complement fixation, and secondary deposition of fibrinogen and alteration of ground substance. In Goodpasture's syndrome the fibrinoid necrosis of the alveolar wall and in the glomerulus is associated with deposition of complement and immunoglobulins with a specificity against basement membrane. Whereas in systemic lupus erythematosus and in Goodpasture's syndrome the specificity of the antibodies contributing to or responsible for the clinicopathologic manifestations of the disease is known, such is not the case for the other entities shown in the table. Thus, the contribution of immunologic events to their lesions is a matter of speculation. Immunoglobulins and complement have been observed in the glomerular lesions of Henoch-Schönlein purpura, in the vascular lesions of periarteritis nodosa, and in the granulomatous response of allergic angiitis and granulomatosis (often with fibrinogen), but not in Wegener's granulomatosis. Such proteins could deposit nonspecifically owing to trapping, transudation or exudation, or because of aggregation of gamma globulin. Studies should be directed toward determining the specificity of the deposited immunoglobulins. Arguments to favor specific deposition could be based on demonstration of antigen in the lesion, recognition of the antibody specificity following elution, and demonstration that the predominant L chain type or H chain subgroup in the deposit is different from the ratio observed in the circulation. Each of these criteria has been met with regard to the lesions of systemic lupus erythematosus.

Churg, J., and Strauss, L.: Allergic granulomatosis, allergic angiitis, and periarteritis nodosa. Amer. J. Path., 27:277, 1951.

Kilbourne, E. D., and Wolff, H. G.: Cranial arteritis: Critical evaluation of syndrome of "temporal arteritis," with report of a case. Ann. Intern. Med., 24:1, 1946.

Klemperer, P.: The concept of collagen disease in medicine. Amer. Rev. Resp. Dis., 83:331, 1961.

Kussmaul, A., and Maier, R.: Über eine bisher nicht beschriebene eigenthümliche Arterienerkrankung (Periarteritis nodosa), die mit Morbus Brightii und rapid fortschreitender allgemeiner Muskellähmung einhergeht. Deutsch. Arch. Klin. Med., 1:484, 1866.

Wegener, F.: Über generalisierte, septische Gefässerkrankungen. Verh. Deutsch. Ges. Path., 29:202, 1936.

Zeek, P. M.: Periarteritis nodosa: A critical review. Amer. J. Clin. Path., 22:777, 1952.

Systemic Sclerosis

(Scleroderma)

Edward D. Harris, Jr.

General Considerations. *Scleroderma* is a term used to describe a disease of the skin manifested by dermal fibrosis and fixation of the skin to underlying structures. It is complicated by atrophy, ulceration, calcinosis, and/or pain. Carlo Curzio of Naples described the cutaneous changes in 1753. It was not until the 1900's that sclerosis and dysfunction in visceral organs were recognized as part of the same process. This *systemic sclerosis* or *generalized scleroderma* can appear in two forms: a diffuse one in which progressive fibrosis of internal organs as well as of the skin of the trunk, face, and extremities occurs; and acrosclerosis in which Raynaud's phenomenon, arthralgias in finger joints, and thickening or edema with progressive immobility of skin over the hands is noted before visceral involvement. The acrosclerotic form is more common. *Localized scleroderma*, a term which includes morphea and linear scleroderma, involves the skin exclusively.

Systemic sclerosis may begin in children or in patients more than 80 years of age, but most patients develop symptoms first between the ages of 25 and 55. Women are affected two to three times more often than men. The disease is infrequent, and this makes it impossible to determine its true incidence. Mortality each year is approximately five per million in the general population. There is evidence that black women have a poorer prognosis than either black men or whites of either sex.

Pathogenesis and Pathology. *Pathogenesis.* No abnormality of collagen structure or metabolism in systemic sclerosis has been demonstrated. Studies of shrinkage temperature, determinations of tensile strength, and x-ray diffraction patterns of dermal collagen have been normal, and analyses of the amino acid composition of the collagen have revealed no significant abnormality. Collagen is stabilized in fibrous form by both intra- and intermolecular crosslinks. There is no evidence that intramolecular crosslinks in collagen from patients with systemic sclerosis are abnormal, and intermolecular crosslinks have not been examined. Although specific collagenases have been found in a number of mammalian tissues, including human skin, no defect in the collagenase system in scleroderma has yet been reported. A number of patients have been demonstrated to have more collagen per unit volume of dermis than do normal controls, and it may be that the abnormality of collagen in systemic sclerosis is quantitative, not qualitative. One unproved hypothesis is that in systemic sclerosis, abnormal types or amounts of proteinpolysaccharides are responsible for an increase in the deposition of collagen in tissues.

The clinical correlations between Raynaud's phenomenon and decreased esophageal motility, pulmonary hypertension, small bowel and colon hypotonia, and the acute and severe renal hypertension seen in systemic sclerosis have suggested to many that the primary lesion in scleroderma is neurogenic, perhaps related to neurovascular abnormalities. By this concept changes in the autonomic nervous system would lead to an excessive and poorly regulated deposition of collagen by fibroblasts. However, numerous attempts to demonstrate a specific abnormality in the synthesis or release of catecholamines in systemic sclerosis have failed, and it remains difficult to relate the finding of increased amounts of collagen in systemic sclerosis to the predominant symptom complex which suggests autonomic (or neurovascular) dysfunction. Electron microscopic studies of blood vessels in muscle have revealed an increase in mean diameter of capillaries and a characteristic laminated appearance in the basement membranes, but the significance of these findings is not known.

No support is available for the hypotheses that microbial agents or endocrine abnormalities are responsible for the development of systemic sclerosis. The immunologic abnormalities mentioned above do not constitute evidence for a cause of the disease. High titers of antinuclear factor and other serologic findings mentioned previously link systemic sclerosis to systemic lupus erythematosus (SLE). Contrary to findings in SLE, however, in which gamma globulin has been found deposited at the basement membranes in the kidney, immunohistochemical analyses of the fibrinoid vascular lesions in systemic sclerosis have not shown deposition of gamma globulin or complement.

Pathology. The result of systemic involvement in scleroderma is sclerosis. The *reticular dermis* is usually thickened. It may have a normal collagen-bundle pattern or show broad, homogeneous, acellular deposits of collagen with indistinct bundle patterns. Other findings include atrophy of the rete pegs of the epidermis, atrophy of the hair follicles and sweat glands, perivascular lymphocytic infiltration, and hyalinization of arterioles. During acute, early phases of the disease edema may be present in the dermis. Pathologic changes in the musculoskeletal system include acute and chronic inflammation in the *synovium* with no pannus formation and with more sclerosis than is found in rheumatoid synovium with an equivalent inflammatory response. Fibrin deposits are laid down around *tendons,* and in *muscles* there are a variety of abnormalities, the most common being fibrosis of the perimysium and epimysium, scattered cellular infiltrates, and atrophy and necrosis of muscle fibers similar to that seen in polymyositis.

In the internal organs mild inflammation and edema in connective tissue are followed by increased deposition of fibrous tissue in both appropriate and inappropriate loci. This leads to distortion of the architecture of the tissues affected. In the *lungs,* a relatively low-grade interstitial pneumonitis is followed by interstitial fibrosis, most marked in lower lobes. Following this, cyst formation and bronchiectasis may develop. Arteriolar thickening (concentric intimal proliferation or medial hypertrophy) is seen, particularly in those patients with clinical evidence of pulmonary hypertension. In the gastrointestinal tract, the *esophagus* is frequently involved with muscle atrophy and fibrosis. Lesions secondary to reflux of gastric contents are present in 20 per cent. Fibrosis around Brunner's glands in the submucosa of the *duodenum* occurs and can be recognized on specimens obtained by *peroral* biopsy. Involvement of the *small bowel* begins with patchy subserosal fibrosis and may progress to almost complete replacement of smooth muscle in the ileum by fibrous tissue and marked thickening of the serosa. Dilation, muscle atrophy, and fibrosis are seen in the *colon;* the fibrosis is irregular, leading to the characteristic sacculations and diverticuli. The *heart* is frequently enlarged and may be the only organ weighing more than predicted for the subject's body weight. Small patches of interstitial myocardial fibrosis are commonly found. In very severe cases as much as 60 per cent of cardiac muscle is replaced by dense, relatively acellular and avascular fibrous tissue. Endocardial or valvular thickening is unusual and rarely of hemodynamic significance. Fibrinous pericarditis is found quite often, even in the absence of uremia. *Kidneys* in scleroderma are normal in size or small and frequently have small cortical infarcts. In patients dying with uremia, intimal proliferation in the interlobular arteries, fibrinoid necrosis of small arteries and arterioles (including the glomerular tufts), and thickening of the basement membrane (the "wire-loop" lesion) may all be present. These changes are identical to those seen in kidneys from patients with malignant hypertension and occasionally may be present in the absence of renal failure or severe hypertension.

Clinical Manifestations and Diagnoses. The disease usually begins insidiously. Vague weakness, weight loss, diffuse stiffness and aching, polyarticular arthritis, diffuse edema of the hands, or Raynaud's phenomenon are the most common initial symptoms. Cutaneous involvement usually precedes visceral symptoms. If the illness progresses, it generally does so slowly, and is marked by characteristic organ system changes. Rarely, rapid progression to severe cutaneous and visceral involvement may occur in less than six months.

Cutaneous System. The patient with classic, well-developed systemic sclerosis presents with taut, thickened or edematous skin, bound tightly to subcutaneous tissues in the hands and fingers.

Feet and toes are involved less often than hands, forearms, and neck. Normal skin folds at the knuckles disappear. Atrophy and chronic, recurrent painful ulcerations at the ends of the digits and over pressure points develop, and the fingers themselves may shorten through progressive resorption of the terminal phalanges. This complication develops more often in patients with severe Raynaud's phenomenon. Joints become immobilized from tight encasement in thickened skin as well as from contractures of muscles and tendons. Telangiectasia, increased or decreased pigmentation, and subcutaneous calcification are common. Hair becomes thin, and the skin of the face appears smooth and waxy. The skin around the mouth constricts, restricting lip movement and preventing adequate dental hygiene. The normal sweating mechanism is often impaired; involved skin feels leathery and dry. The CRST syndrome (calcinosis, Raynaud's phenomenon, sclerodactyly, and telangiectasia) and the Thibierge-Weissenbach syndrome (diffuse deposition of insoluble calcium phosphates in subcutaneous tissue in the presence of acrosclerosis) are variants of the cutaneous expression of systemic sclerosis.

Musculoskeletal System. Almost half the patients with systemic sclerosis present with joint pain or develop it during the first year of their illness. Small joints are involved more often than large ones. Joint deformity and immobility in systemic sclerosis do not result from an invasive, erosive synovitis as in rheumatoid arthritis, but are the result primarily of fibrous contractures of the overlying skin and neighboring muscles. Muscle wasting is often severe in areas such as the hands, in which joint mobility is impaired by progressive tightening of the overlying skin.

Gastrointestinal Tract. Of the internal organ systems, the gastrointestinal tract is the one most often involved in systemic sclerosis. *Oral* symptoms include xerostomia and a progressive decrease in the size of the mouth. Sjögren's syndrome is seen occasionally. Symptoms referable to the *esophagus*, ranging from simple dysphagia to heartburn, nausea, and substernal fullness, are found in 45 to 60 per cent of cases. As the disease progresses patients may be unable to swallow solid foods, and if reflux esophagitis is a persistent complication, stricture may develop. Virtually all patients with Raynaud's phenomenon and generalized scleroderma have evidence of diminished esophageal peristalsis, as do many patients with Raynaud's phenomenon associated with other connective tissue diseases. Vomiting, abdominal distention, and pain or diarrhea may indicate involvement of the *small intestine*. The patient with small bowel disease in systemic sclerosis may have a fulminant and toxic course in the absence of significant skin changes. As with the esophagus, involvement of the small bowel is manifested by atony and dilation. Transit time is increased, and there may be malabsorption secondary to intraluminal stagnation with concomitant bacterial overgrowth, similar to the blind loop syndrome. Functional bowel complaints secondary

to pathologic changes in the *colon* are common, but rarely disabling.

Heart and Lungs. Dyspnea is the most common cardiorespiratory symptom in systemic sclerosis and is present in more than 50 per cent of patients. Early in this process, physical examination of the lungs may be normal. Fine, dry crackles at the bases of the lung are the first abnormality found. In some patients progression to cyanosis, repeated infections, respiratory insufficiency, and death from hypoxemia without CO_2 retention may occur when pulmonary fibrosis is marked. Those exposed in their occupation to silicate dust have a predilection to develop this form of the disease. Restriction of chest wall expansion by dermal fibrosis around the thorax rarely affects respiratory function. A few patients with severe cystic and fibrotic changes in the lungs have developed multifocal alveolar cell carcinomas.

Catheterization studies have revealed a striking lack of correlation between the extent of pulmonary fibrosis and the severity of pulmonary hypertension. Signs of elevated pulmonary vascular resistance may develop independently of parenchymal changes in the lungs and lead to cor pulmonale and congestive heart failure.

Replacement of myocardium with fibrous tissue on a primary basis (the so-called "scleroderma heart disease") is rarely the only cause for heart failure. More often, impaired cardiac function can be attributed to right ventricular failure secondary to pulmonary hypertension, or to left ventricular failure caused by systemic hypertension. Symptoms or signs of acute pericarditis during the course of scleroderma are occasionally present.

Kidneys. The development of significant albuminuria, pyuria, and casts in the urine is frequently associated with malignant hypertension resistant to therapy and uremia progressing rapidly to death. This complication may come on at any stage of the disease. It is impossible to predict which patient will develop this form of renal disease, although 5 to 20 per cent of patients with scleroderma die from this complication. A few studies suggested that acute renal failure was somehow related to treatment with corticosteroids; more data must be accumulated to evaluate this possibility.

Nervous System. Involvement of the nervous system is rare. Facial pain, questionably related to a trigeminal neuropathy, is seen in occasional patients and may be disabling.

Course Untreated. The course of the disease varies among patients. Systemic sclerosis and particularly the cutaneous manifestations may not progress and may even show signs of regression. Some patients may manifest slowly progressive acrosclerosis with painful crippling of the hands, and others will have few symptoms manifest in the extremities yet develop rapid involvement of the lungs or gastrointestinal tract, or severe hypertension and uremia. Estimates of the 50 per cent survival time after onset of the disease have ranged from two to ten years in different studies.

The most frequent causes of death are renal and cardiopulmonary involvement.

Laboratory Findings. The erythrocyte sedimentation test is elevated in most patients with systemic sclerosis, and a mild microcytic anemia may be present. Leukopenia or hemolysis is most unusual. A number of serologic abnormalities link systemic sclerosis to other connective tissue diseases. Mild hypergammaglobulinemia is present in 30 to 50 per cent of patients, and rheumatoid factor is present in 20 to 40 per cent. Using immunofluorescent techniques, antinuclear antibodies have been demonstrated in sera of 30 to 60 per cent of patients. A lesser number have antinucleolar antibodies in serum. Lupus erythematosus cells in blood are demonstrable in less than 10 per cent of patients. Recent studies have determined that serum aldolase and urinary creatine levels correlate with clinical evidence of weakness and loss of muscle mass better than histologic examination of muscle biopsy. Urinary hydroxyproline excretion, an index of collagen turnover, has been shown by Rodnan to be greater than normal in some patients, particularly in those with acute disease. However, this finding reflects nonspecific abnormality shared by other diseases of connective tissue, particularly some metabolic diseases of bone.

Roentgenography. Roentgenograms are important for the diagnosis and follow-up evaluation. The findings of soft tissue atrophy, subcutaneous calcinosis, and resorption of the tufts of the terminal phalanges without loss of apparent joint spaces between phalanges are virtually pathognomonic of systemic sclerosis when seen on hand films. The peridontal membrane is occasionally thickened. Upper gastrointestinal films reveal a dilated, atonic esophagus in about 60 per cent of patients. Occasionally a column of air in the esophagus may be seen on lateral chest roentgenograms, a finding not seen normally. Small bowel studies may demonstrate segmental atony and dilation in the duodenum and the first part of the jejunum. Linear pneumatosis (air in the wall of the gut) is occasionally seen in flat plates of the abdomen of patients with severe small bowel involvement. Barium studies of the colon reveal wide mouth, asymmetrical diverticuli in 20 to 40 per cent of patients; progression to a dilated, atonic megacolon rarely occurs. Chest roentgenograms reveal a diffuse reticular pattern with a honeycomb appearance in the lower lung fields of patients with pulmonary involvement. Serial films may document progression to a picture of dense interstitial fibrosis amid radiolucent cystic areas.

The electrocardiogram shows nonspecific abnormalities in almost 50 per cent of patients. The pattern of conduction defects with very low voltage is seen only in those uncommon patients with marked myocardial replacement by fibrous tissue.

Eighty per cent or more of patients have some abnormality demonstrable on pulmonary function tests. A restrictive defect is found in early lesions with a decreased vital capacity, decreased lung compliance, and a reduction in diffusion capacity.

As the normal architecture of the lungs is destroyed by the fibrotic changes and as abnormalities in the ventilation-perfusion ratio develop, increased venous admixture and an increased physiologic dead space are found.

Differential Diagnosis. When systemic sclerosis presents as persistent symmetrical polyarthritis involving the hands without previous skin changes, it may be impossible to differentiate it from rheumatoid arthritis or systemic lupus erythematosus, or, if the overlying skin becomes edematous or red, from dermatomyositis. In fact, "overlap" syndromes combining clinical or serologic manifestations of several of these entities are being described with increasing frequency, and one should avoid hasty classification of any clinical picture that is consistent with more than one of the connective tissue diseases.

The atrophic changes in the skin in systemic sclerosis must be differentiated from those seen in Werner's syndrome, progeria (Hutchinson-Gilford syndrome), chronic hypostatic edema or myxedema, lichen sclerosus et atrophicus, porphyria cutanea tarda, and/or scleredema. Unlike systemic sclerosis, Werner's syndrome affects the feet more severely than the hands, and has associated with it a high-pitched voice, growth abnormalities, and premature cataracts, arteriosclerosis, and diabetes. Sclerodermatous changes have been reported in skin of patients with progeria, but the dwarflike stature, characteristic facies, and premature death from coronary insufficiency set this syndrome apart. Porphyria cutanea tarda may have skin changes simulating scleroderma but can be differentiated on the basis of urinary or fecal porphyrin excretion. Scleredema (scleredema adultorum of Buschke) is a brawny edema which appears abruptly, involves skin of the neck and chest initially, and is characterized pathologically by the presence of a material resembling acid mucopolysaccharide diffusely interspersed among collagen bundles in the dermis. This is a self-limited process, perhaps related to a previous bacterial infection, and has a good prognosis. The cutaneous telangiectasia of scleroderma resembles Osler-Weber-Rendu disease (hereditary telangiectasia).

Diseases or pathologic findings associated with Raynaud's phenomenon which must be differentiated from scleroderma include occupational trauma; anatomic lesions, e.g., scalenus anticus syndrome and cervical ribs; vasomotor syndromes resulting in disuse atrophy, e.g., Sudek's atrophy or the shoulder-hand syndrome; peripheral vascular arteriosclerosis; heavy metal or ergot poisoning; and hematologic abnormalities, e.g., polycythemia vera, paroxysmal cold hemoglobinuria, and presence of cold agglutinins or cryoproteinemia.

Involvement of viscera in systemic sclerosis can mimic many other illnesses. The abnormalities in pulmonary function and roentgenographic findings seen are similar to those found in idiopathic pulmonary fibrosis (Hamman-Rich syndrome), the pulmonary fibrosis of rheumatoid arthritis, or advanced sarcoidosis. Scleroderma heart disease must be differentiated from infiltrative cardiomyopathies as well as fibrosis from diffuse coronary artery disease. The dysphagia of scleroderma is completely nonspecific, and disease of the bowel rarely can simulate sprue or any of the malabsorption syndromes, partial intestinal obstruction, or megacolon. The diagnosis of localized symmetrical scleroderma or morphea can be made only by failure to demonstrate visceral fibrosis with dysfunction by appropriate studies.

Treatment. Patients with slowly progressive systemic sclerosis can lead productive and useful lives. The most important goal in therapy is to preserve function in and prevent injury to the hands. Vocational and/or climatic change may be indicated. Hand care must be stressed, including instructions for active and passive exercises to prevent flexion contracture. Early signs of local infection in fingertips must be treated immediately before they progress to large ulcerations.

Because there is so little known about the underlying defect in scleroderma or its pathogenesis, no specific treatment is available. The one exception to this is the use of broad-spectrum antimicrobials in treatment of the malabsorption associated with bacterial overgrowth in the upper small intestine. If esophageal motility is decreased, antacid therapy is used liberally to prevent secondary esophagitis and stricture. If stricture develops, bouginage will be needed. Salicylates in pharmacologic doses may decrease clinical signs of inflammation, e.g., elevated sedimentation rates, joint pain, erythema, present in most patients at some time in the course of their disease. There is no evidence that high doses of corticosteroids effectively retard progression of systemic sclerosis; small doses (equivalent to 5 to 10 mg. of prednisone per day) may be used as a supplementary anti-inflammatory agent during the acute, edematous phases of the disease.

Based on different hypotheses of the basic lesion in scleroderma, many different therapeutic rationales have been used. Reserpine and ganglionic blocking agents have been used in patients afflicted severely with Raynaud's phenomenon; sympathectomy has been performed for the same reasons, and although early results in some patients are rewarding, the disease in most continues to progress. Potassium p-aminobenzoate, ethylenediaminetetraacetic acid, 6-aminocaproic acid infusions, and dimethyl sulfoxide applications have been employed by a few investigators, but none of these drugs has yet proved to be generally effective in treatment. D-penicillamine is being studied in patients because of its ability to inhibit formation of crosslinks in collagen. Pilot studies have not proved that alkylating agents or immunosuppressive drugs are beneficial.

D'Angelo, W. A., Fries, J. F., Masi, A. T., and Shulman, L. E.: Pathologic observations in systemic sclerosis (scleroderma). Amer. J. Med., 46:428, 1969.

Rodnan, G. P.: Progressive systemic sclerosis (diffuse scleroderma). In Samter, M., and Alexander, H. L. (eds.): Immunological Diseases. Boston, Little, Brown & Company, 1965.

Sackner, M. A.: Scleroderma. Modern Medical Monographs. New York, Grune & Stratton, Inc., 1966.

Polymyositis and Dermatomyositis

H. Richard Tyler

General Considerations. The disorder termed *polymyositis* refers to an illness in which muscle weakness is the principal clinical feature. It was first described by Wagner in 1863. Inflammatory, degenerative, and regenerative changes can be seen in the muscles. In most instances, it is not possible to establish a definite etiology, but in some cases a specific infection is the cause. When skin changes occur and are prominent, the cases are referred to as *dermatomyositis*. This subgroup was first delineated by Unverricht in 1887. The muscular lesions of dermatomyositis are identical to those seen in noninfectious polymyositis. Because of the dramatic skin lesions, dermatomyositis was more widely recognized until recently. Appreciation that muscular syndromes are more common than dermatomyositis resulted from the increased use of muscle biopsy and the clinical awareness that insidious onset and absence of muscle pain are common. If there are changes indicative of some nerve damage, the term *neuromyositis* is occasionally used. Some authors prefer the nonspecific and noncommittal term *polymyopathy* and identify as separate entities only those cases whose specific etiology is known. Others reserve the term polymyositis for cases with evidence of inflammatory changes in muscles. Until the etiology of the majority of the cases is more clearly identified, one has to accept the need to re-evaluate nomenclature periodically. All these disorders form a large spectrum which ranges from the very acute cases with myoglobinuria to the very chronic localized disorders that mimic muscular dystrophy.

No reliable figures exist as to the incidence of polymyositis. As a cause of acute or subacute muscle weakness in an adult, it is much more common than muscular dystrophy (Walton and Adams). In one teaching hospital with 400 beds, 52 cases were noted in a six-year period (Pearson;

Rose and Walton). In five counties in England with a total population of 3,294,000, 89 cases were identified over a ten-year period.

The disease can appear at any age, but the most common period is between the ages of 40 and 60. Females are affected about twice as frequently as males. In most instances, no precipitating cause is obvious, but some cases have followed a viral-like illness or the use of antimicrobial drugs. Hypersensitivity has been implicated by some because of the association with malignancy, the frequent relation to a previous infection, and the association with symptoms common to the other collagen diseases.

It has not been possible to demonstrate antimuscle antibodies in these patients. The presence of antimyosin antibody and other immune reacting proteins in some patients is nonspecific as it is also found in patients with muscular dystrophy and neuronal atrophy. It has been possible to produce a myositis in guinea pigs similar to human polymyositis by use of muscle plus Freund's adjuvant. In tissue culture preparations of rat skeletal muscle, "sensitized" lymph node cells from animals previously injected with muscle plus adjuvants destroyed the muscle cells, whereas unsensitized lymph node cells did not. The significance of these experiments for human disease remains uncertain.

Pathology. The muscle biopsy may show active inflammation with plasma cells and polymorphonuclear cells, especially around the vessels in the interstitial tissue, or individual muscle fiber necrosis with phagocytic infiltration and attempts at regeneration. The muscle tissue from the more chronic cases often shows surprisingly little change under the light microscope. This may consist of smaller muscle fibers, which vary significantly in cross-section diameter, associated with proliferation of sarcolemmal nuclei. In the polymyositis associated with Sjögren's syndrome, the muscle may be heavily infiltrated with plasma cells and lymphocytes. In the few studies utilizing the electron microscope, no changes were noted.

In the childhood form of dermatomyositis, there is intense perivascular inflammation with active arteritis and phlebitis. There is often occlusion of vessels with fibrin thrombi and infarction of muscles, nerves, and viscus (Banker and Victor). Other forms of more limited or less intense polymyositic syndromes in children have pathologic changes similar to those previously described.

The three useful laboratory tests, serum enzymes, electromyography, and muscle biopsy, are not always abnormal. Any one or even two may yield normal findings in a particular case. In one series, electromyography was abnormal in 89 per cent and muscle biopsy was confirmatory in 63 per cent. Serum enzymes are usually elevated except in some slowly progressive or stable chronic cases.

Clinical Manifestations and Diagnosis. The patient usually notes the insidious development of weakness in proximal muscles. The weakness is more common at the hips than in the shoulders. Some weakness in the flexors of the neck is almost always present. Muscle discomfort or tenderness is common but can be completely absent. When present, it is more common in the shoulders, back, and arms than in the thighs. Muscular wasting is a late sign, and when it occurs it is usually in proximal muscles such as the quadriceps. The weakness is out of proportion to the loss of muscle bulk. Reflexes are depressed in proportion to muscle weakness.

The development and the rate of progression of the weakness may show great variations from patient to patient, and even in the same patient at different stages of the illness. Weakness can progress until the patient becomes bedridden, but this is unusual. Contracture of muscles may develop quickly.

A skin rash may or may not be present. It usually takes the form of an erythema over the face, shoulders, and arms. It can mimic erythema nodosum, eczema, or exfoliating dermatitis, or can manifest itself by thickened, brawny, edematous skin. On occasion, the skin lesions appear primarily in areas exposed to sunlight. Erythematous, slightly raised lesions occur over bony prominences, i.e., elbows, knuckles, knees, and medial malleoli. These lesions often become scaly and atrophic. Hyperemia around the nail beds is not uncommon. In childhood forms a violaceous suffusion of the upper eyelids, called a "heliotrope" rash, is very diagnostic of this disorder.

Dysphagia, secondary to weakness of pharyngeal muscle and hypotonicity of the upper part of the esophagus, is frequent. About one third of the patients have arthralgias and Raynaud's phenomenon. Other visceral manifestations are rare. Many patients will have a tachycardia. Electrocardiograms may show nonspecific T wave changes. Interstitial fibrosis and pericarditis have been noted on histologic examination. A transitory pneumonitis has also been reported. Transitional cases with some features to suggest scleroderma have occasionally demonstrated severe gastrointestinal symptoms with malabsorption, severe myopathy, and only slight skin changes. If the muscle weakness comes on acutely with much muscle necrosis, myoglobinuria will occur. This can result in acute renal failure. Polymyositis may also be seen with Sjögren's syndrome.

The childhood form of dermatomyositis may be much more pernicious. It starts out with skin changes, anorexia, and fatigue. Weakness, stiffness, and pain in muscles usually follow. Low-grade fever, dysphagia, contractures, and calcinosis usually develop. A perforated viscus or mediastinitis is often the immediate cause of death.

Course Untreated. The condition can progress to severe disability and death, but most patients either improve spontaneously or proceed to a chronic phase. In earlier series, including patients primarily recognized as having dermatomyositis, mortality rates of 50 per cent were common. In one series of adult patients with polymyositis, it was noted that about two thirds were alive after ten years. About 50 per cent of these had complete recoveries, and the rest had some degree of residual disability. Many of the patients in this series had received some steroid therapy.

In a survey in which cases were accumulated from the literature, tumors were present in nearly 20 per cent, or five times the expected incidence. When polymyositis develops in an adult male, there is a greater than 50 per cent chance that a tumor will be discovered (Sheard). In another series, it was noted that when polymyositis appeared after the age of 50 a cancer was found in 71 per cent of males and 24 per cent of females. The muscular weakness may precede the detection of the tumor by two or three years despite diligent search. In this series, all nine males above 50 who were followed for three years or more had an associated neoplasm (Shy). In the male, the usual carcinoma is in the lung, stomach, intestine, or prostate; and in the female, in the ovary, uterus, or breast.

Childhood dermatomyositis appears to be a very specific subgroup of polymyositic disorders. It is severely disabling and is associated with a very high mortality.

Laboratory Findings. The sedimentation rate is usually elevated, and there may be mild leukocytosis, especially in the acute cases. A number of enzymes which arise in muscle are usually elevated in serum. Creatine phosphokinase and aldolase are the most specific, but lactic dehydrogenase and transaminase (SGOT) are usually elevated also. Serum protein changes occur in about 50 per cent of the patients. These most commonly consist of elevations of the $\alpha2$ and γ globulins. This is especially true of that form of polymyositis associated with Sjögren's disease. Rheumatoid factors are positive in 10 to 50 per cent, depending on the series. About 5 per cent will have a positive LE prep. Myoglobinuria is transient and found only with acute and severe muscular degeneration.

In patients with dysphagia, the roentgenograms often reveal pooling of barium in the vallecular and pyriform sinuses. Hypomotility of the esophagus is present in about one third of the cases. The roentgenograms frequently reveal no abnormalities except the rare deposition of subcutaneous calcification in the childhood form of the disease. Electrocardiograms often show minor abnormalities.

Electromyography is almost always abnormal in the clinically affected muscles. There is excessive irritability of muscle when the needle is initially inserted. The motor units (which are made up of many muscle fibers supplied by a single nerve) often show a loss of height, indicating a reduction in the number of functioning muscle fibers of each motor unit. Polyphasic discharges are common, indicating a loss of individual muscle fibers of the unit. Positive potentials and fibrillary potentials are seen, indicating some denervation or separation of a portion of the muscle from its afferent nerve supply. Repetitive discharges of pseudomyotonic firing are not uncommon. When the changes indicating denervation are prominent, the term "neuromyositis" has been used. The electromyogram is useful in indicating which muscles to biopsy. The site of biopsy should be selected to ensure that a proper sampling of abnormal muscle is being taken.

Differential Diagnosis. The major causes of weakness, which must be differentiated from polymyositis, are those due to muscular dystrophy and disorders of the peripheral and central nervous system. Muscular dystrophy is usually a familial disorder which is long-standing and can often be traced to childhood. The involvement of proximal muscles and neck flexor weakness would be unusual in most adult forms of muscular dystrophy. In myotonic dystrophy, the only dystrophy which often demonstrates neck flexor weakness, there is a distal weakness of muscles in the extremities. There are also cataracts and myotonia to percussion. Fascioscapulohumeral muscular dystrophy and other proximal dystrophies usually spare neck flexors. All the dystrophies are characterized by family history, significant muscle wasting, and weakness; the deep tendon reflex loss is usually early and prominent. In polymyositis, reflexes are often relatively spared until severe weakness occurs.

The weakness in peripheral neuritis tends to be distal, and careful examination usually enables one to find mild sensory loss, autonomic dysfunction, and distal areflexia. Weakness from spinal cord disease has characteristic reflex changes, such as extensor plantar responses and hyperreflexia. Occasionally, motor neuron disease (the primary muscular atrophy variant) presents as a myopathic disorder. Muscle biopsy and EMG usually distinguish between the two conditions.

Of the muscular syndromes, the metabolic myopathies most closely mimic the distribution of muscle weakness and the weakness seen with polymyositis. Chronic thyroid myopathy is characterized by its involvement of proximal muscles with significant loss of muscle bulk. The reflexes are usually quite brisk. Although there are no distinctive features, the clinical signs of thyrotoxicosis and the presence of clinical tests to support hyperthyroidism usually make it easy to distinguish this group. The most common myopathy seen today is probably the one induced by excess or chronic use of corticotrophin or steroids. It is identical to that seen with hyperadrenalism. The weakness is primarily proximal, most often involving the pelvic girdle. Early wasting of the quadriceps muscle is especially prominent. Pain and discomfort is unusual. Reflexes usually persist, and severe disabling syndromes are unusual. Muscle biopsy tends to show surprisingly little change, and then only very scattered and in single muscle fibers. These changes are usually much less than one would anticipate from the clinical status of the patients.

Since steroids are often used in the treatment of a number of clinical syndromes, it may be very difficult to establish whether progressive weakness is due to the underlying disease or the steroid treatment. Often one will have to either decrease the steroid dose sharply or increase it significantly to make such judgments. If pain is a significant problem, one must be cautious about the clinical evaluation of weakness or its disappearance with the use of high doses of steroids.

Hyperparathyroidism and hyperinsulinism have rarely been associated with syndromes of muscular weakness and must be separated from idiopathic polymyositis primarily by the associated laboratory findings.

There are a number of parasitic diseases such as trichinosis or toxoplasmosis which should be considered in acute or subacute syndromes, especially when generalized symptoms and eosinophilia are noted. These are fully discussed elsewhere in this text.

Polymyalgia rheumatica characteristically is associated with significant muscular discomfort. Changes in serum enzymes or muscle biopsy are usually not present to any significant degree. There are noticeable short term and even daily fluctuations of symptoms. Significant objective weakness is not common, although complaints of pain and fatigue and feelings of muscular weakness are often voiced by the patient. Although the findings in some are related to those seen with temporal arteritis, the findings in others are very similar to those of some patients seen with epidemic neuromyasthenia.

Treatment.   The physician's obvious goal is to eradicate the active disease process, if possible, and improve the functional capacity of the patient. In almost all cases prolonged management and long-term follow-up will be necessary. Often the chronic nature and the severe disability caused by the illness make it essential for the physician to play an active role as a counselor and friend.

Many of these patients achieve significant symptomatic improvement of muscle function when treated with corticotrophin, steroids, or salicylates. The use of immunosuppressive medication has been promising in a few cases. The disorder is rarely "cured," however, and relapses are common, especially if steroids are abruptly withdrawn. Patients may require medication for many years. The initial dose of corticotrophin or steroids should be high (60 to 80 mg. of prednisone) and tapered over months. It is useful to monitor serum enzymes during this period as they often give an early indication of the patient's likely course. Relapses are common when steroids are withdrawn in the first two years, but less frequent if treatment lasts at least three years. When steroid-treated and presteroid series of patients are compared in terms of long-range follow-up, the group receiving steroid treatment has fared better (Rose and Walton). Some of the adult forms usually do well. The childhood forms of dermatomyositis do not respond to steroids alone.

Banker, B. Q., and Victor, M.: Dermatomyositis (systemic angiopathy of childhood. Medicine, 45:261, 1966.
Pearson, C. M.: Polymyositis. *In* Milhorat, A. T. (ed.): Explanatory Concepts in Muscular Dystrophy and Related Disorders. Amsterdam, Excerpta Medica Foundation, 1967.
Rose, A. L., and Walton, J.: Polymyositis: A survey of 89 cases with particular reference to treatment and prognosis. Brain, 89:747, 1966.
Sheard, C.: Dermatomyositis. Arch. Intern. Med., 88:640, 1951.
Shy, G. M.: The late onset myopathy. World Neurol., 3:149, 1962.
Walton, J. N., and Adams, R. D.: Polymyositis. Edinburgh, Livingstone, Ltd., 1958.

Systemic Lupus Erythematosus

Peter H. Schur

General Considerations.   Systemic lupus erythematosus (SLE), a chronic disease of unknown etiology, can affect many organ systems, either individually or in a variety of combinations. The disease can be described, but not defined. The classic facial "butterfly rash" facilitates diagnosis, although the rash need not be present. The clinical course may be fulminant or indolent, but generally is characterized by periods of remissions and relapses. Patients with SLE typically develop a host of autoimmune phenomena, including anticell, anticytoplasmic, and especially antinuclear antibodies. A diagnosis of SLE has frequently been established or confirmed by the finding of these antibodies, especially the one causing the LE cell phenomenon.

Lupus, which is the Latin name for wolf, has been used since about 1230 as a term to describe cutaneous conditions which resemble the malar erythema of a wolf. Numerous publications in the nineteenth century by, among others, Bateman, Biett, Hebra, and Kaposi, described what we know now as lupus of the skin. In 1851 Cazenave first used the term "lupus érythémateux." Kaposi, in 1872, noted the systemic involvement in lupus, and in 1875 noted that the rash resembled a butterfly. Osler described the systemic complications of lupus and noted that they could occur in the absence of skin disease. The clinical recognition of SLE has changed greatly since Hargraves first described the LE cell test in 1948 and by the development of the immunofluorescent antinuclear factor test by Friou in 1957.

Incidence and Etiology.   Systemic lupus erythematosus is not a rare disorder. In a study in New York City, the prevalence rate was 2.6 per 100,000 population. The disease occurs more frequently in Negroes than in whites and is extremely rare among Asians. It occurs five to ten times more frequently among females than males and has been diagnosed in patients ranging from 2 to 97 years old. However, the majority of patients are first discovered to have SLE while in their third and fourth decades of life.

The cause of SLE remains at present undiscovered. Many factors have been shown to be associated with exacerbations of SLE. Infections or exposure to sunlight or ultraviolet radiation, viz., sunlamps, often have been followed by the prompt appearance of the facial butterfly rash or a rash on other exposed skin surfaces. Recent attention has focused more on the relation of SLE to drugs such as hydantoins, hydralazine, heterologous antiserum, gold salts, and antimicrobials, notably penicillin and sulfonamides.

In view of the heavy preponderance of the disease in females, endocrine factors have been thought to influence the development of SLE. The disease tends to remit during the last two trimesters of pregnancy and to relapse during the first trimester and again post partum. Ovulation inhibitors often cause an exacerbation of SLE.

The high incidence of SLE among females might also be considered to reflect a genetic (X chromosome) predisposition to this disease. This hypothesis is supported by observations of a higher incidence of "collagen diseases," dysgammaglobulinemia and autoimmune phenomena, among relatives of many patients with SLE than in the general population. Thus, family members of patients with SLE may be found to have SLE, rheumatoid arthritis, dermatomyositis, thyroiditis, rheumatic fever and hemolytic anemia, hyper- and agammaglobulinemia, antinuclear factors (15 per cent), rheumatoid factors, false positive Wasserman reactions, positive Coombs tests, and thyroglobulin antibodies. Supporting evidence for a genetic role in SLE comes from studies in certain strains of inbred mice. Mice of the NZB or NZW strains develop a condition with characteristics similar to human SLE, including hemolytic anemia, renal disease, and autoimmune phenomena. However, when these two strains of mice are mated, the F_1 hybrid generation, especially the females, develop the disease more frequently, at an earlier age, and with a much higher incidence of autoimmune phenomena.

Systemic lupus erythematosus is characterized particularly by autoimmune phenomena. Patients develop antibodies to many of their own cells, cell constituents, and proteins. The origin of these autoantibodies is as obscure as is the etiology of SLE. However, they do reflect a loss of tolerance to so-called self antigens. Mice of the NZB strain have been found to lose their tolerance for foreign antigens much more rapidly than do other mice. Loss of tolerance may be influenced by viral infections. In this regard, paramyxovirus-like particles have been found in biopsies from some SLE patients, and antibodies to viral RNA have been found in the sera from others. These data suggest that a viral infection, in genetically predisposed patients, may alter the delicate balance between immunity and tolerance, and may result in the development of antibodies to cell structures altered by virus; these antibodies then cross-react with the normal cell structure.

Pathogenesis and Pathology. Many of the manifestations of SLE appear to result from the deposition of antigen-antibody complexes in tissues. Although immune complexes have not been isolated from SLE patients, certain evidence is consistent with their presence. In laboratory animals, when immune complexes are formed in the circulation, serum complement levels fall and nephritis develops. In patients with SLE, especially in those with anti-DNA antibodies, a fall in complement levels is associated with the development of nephritis. In addition, some patients with serum antibodies to DNA develop fever and nephritis as the antibody disappears to be replaced by free DNA—presumably representing immune complexes in antigen excess. Using the immunofluorescent technique, immunoglobulins (especially γG), complement (including C1q, C4, C3 proteins), and antigens (DNA) have been detected in a granular and lumpy distribution along the renal glomerular basement membrane. By eluting the gamma globulin off the glomeruli, it has been possible to demonstrate that it consists of mostly antinuclear, and some anticytoplasmic, antibodies. As the immune complexes on the kidney contain complement components, they attract polymorphonuclear leukocytes, whose lysosomal enzymes are instrumental in initiating the acute inflammatory reaction.

The pathologic changes of SLE, even in organs and tissues known from clinical observation to have been involved, are often minor when examined by routine histologic methods. Fibrinoid deposition is common: it is an eosinophilic amorphous material deposited along tissue fibers and in blood vessels. Fibrin and serum proteins, including immunoglobulins, complement, and DNA, have been detected in fibrinoid, possibly representing deposits of immune complexes. Serous membranes, including pleura, pericardium, and synovia, may be edematous and contain deposits of fibrinoid. Vasculitis can involve venules, capillaries, arterioles, and occasionally arteries. Hematoxylin bodies appear to represent in vivo LE bodies analogous to the cytoplasmic inclusions in LE cells. They are rounded, hematoxylin-stained masses roughly the size of nuclei and are found in areas of inflammation.

Skin biopsies may show acute inflammation with liquefaction, degeneration of the basal layer with vacuolization of basal cells, edema of the dermis, and fibrinoid necrosis in the dermis and local blood vessels with cell infiltration; or, in chronic lesions, they may show hyperkeratosis with follicular plugging.

The spleen is the site of "onion skin lesions," which are characterized by concentric perivascular fibrosis around central and penicilliary arteries.

Libman-Sacks verrucous nonbacterial endocarditis consists of vegetations on the valves or chordae tendineae. Fibrinoid is deposited in the superficial connective tissue with infiltration of neutrophils, lymphocytes, and histiocytes. The myocardium may be involved by vasculitis.

Renal lesions are highly variable—from mild to severe. The mildest form of renal lesion consists of the deposits of immunoglobulin (mostly γG) and complement (particularly C3) in the mesangium and along the glomerular basement membrane, without any other observable histologic abnormality. The most common renal lesion is focal glomerulitis, with minimal increase of cellularity, focal thickening of the capillary basement membrane, and fibrinoid change. In glomerulonephritis, these lesions are more generalized and severe and are usually a mixture of proliferative and membranous changes, with hypercellularity of endothelial, mesangial, epithelial, and inflammatory cells, capsular inflammation leading to crescent formation, and focal thickening of the basement membrane. Some kidneys are found to have only a diffuse membranous glomerulonephritis, with few cells but considerable thickening of the basement membrane. Basement membrane thickening, when associated with fibrinoid changes, results in the so-called "wire loop" lesions. There may also be hyaline thrombi in glomeruli, focal necrosis, and, occasionally, hematoxylin bodies. Tubular degenerative changes are common.

Clinical Manifestations. The clinical recognition of SLE has changed greatly since Hargraves first described the LE cell test in 1948. Previously, a diagnosis of SLE was made primarily in young women with a butterfly rash and systemic complications, and the outcome was usually fatal. With the advent of the LE cell test, and the subsequent, even more sensitive, antinuclear factor (ANF) test, patients with much more varied symptoms and signs have had confirmed diagnoses of SLE. Most patients complain of some fatigue, arthralgia, rashes, and fever. When specific organs are involved, other symptoms may develop: pleurisy, pericarditis, edema, dyspnea and cough, Raynaud's phenomenon, bleeding, and purpura, or seizures. The disease is now considered a chronic illness with periods of remission and activity.

Musculoskeletal System. Most patients will complain of pain in their joints (arthralgia) at some time. Commonly this affects the hands, wrists, knees, ankles, and elbows. Even when pain is severe, the affected joint infrequently is swollen, erythematous, or tender (arthritis). Although slight deformities at the metacarpophalangeal and proximal interphalangeal joints may occur, major joint swelling with synovial thickening, flexion deformities with subluxations, and ulnar deviation are uncommon. X-rays rarely show the joint narrowing or cystic changes seen in rheumatoid arthritis. The appearance of deforming or destructive joint lesions suggests a diagnosis of rheumatoid arthritis or the "rupus" (rheumatoid arthritis–lupus) overlap syndrome. Muscle pain is a frequent complaint and is accompanied, occasionally, by proximal muscle atrophy. The bones are rarely affected, but an increased prevalence of aseptic necrosis of the femoral head has been noted, especially in those patients receiving corticosteroids.

Mucocutaneous Manifestations. The classic "butterfly rash" is seen in less than half the patients with SLE. There may be only a blush and swelling or a scaly erythematous maculopapular rash on both cheeks and the bridge of the nose after exposure to the sun. This may clear spontaneously, only to recur. Other skin areas, particularly those exposed to the sun, may be involved. The lesions are called "discoid" when they scale, are associated with follicular plugging, and heal with atrophy, scarring (telangiectasia), hyperpigmentation, or hypopigmentation (vitiligo). Discoid lupus, per se, is not accompanied by systemic complications. Involvement on the face often spreads to the forehead and scalp, resulting in alopecia. Patchy hair loss is frequent and usually is reversible, but discoid lupus with scarring can lead to permanent partial baldness. In these days of well-fitted hairpieces, alopecia is often undetected on cursory examination. Periungual erythema and telangiectasia, although found in only 10 per cent of patients with SLE, is said to be characteristic. Small ulcerations signifying an underlying vasculitis often develop on the fingertips and may progress to gangrene. Raynaud's phenomenon is common in both hands and feet. Painful ulcers are seen frequently on the buccal mucosa and gums. Purpura and ecchymoses usually reflect an underlying blood platelet and clotting problem, renal insufficiency, or the side effects of corticosteroids. Urticaria and angioedema may be present.

Renal Disease. Kidney involvement is seen in about half of SLE patients, and usually occurs within two years of the onset of symptoms. Acute nephritis or the nephrotic syndrome may be the presenting manifestation of SLE. The most common abnormality is a mild glomerulitis which is associated with minimal proteinuria or hematuria or both. This lesion generally responds well to therapy initially, but often recurs in mild form or as even more severe renal involvement. Acute lupus glomerulonephritis occurs less often and is associated with varying degrees of pyuria, hematuria, proteinuria, fluid retention, edema, hypertension, and azotemia. The nephrotic syndrome is associated with variable proteinuria, with fluid retention, and frequently with normal serum cholesterol levels. The finding of pyuria with fever in patients with SLE, especially in young women receiving corticosteroids, may reflect a urinary tract infection rather than lupus nephritis. This distinction is important, especially in providing therapy, and a renal biopsy in such a case may be helpful.

Most patients recover well from attacks of acute nephritis, with loss of edema and azotemia, but usually some proteinuria and decreased glomerular filtration rate (GFR) persist. Patients have recurrences, and some develop chronic glomerulonephritis with hypertension and proteinuria.

Cardiovascular Manifestations. The endocardium, myocardium, and pericardium may be involved in nearly half the patients with SLE. Although EKG changes, such as nonspecific ST, T wave changes are not uncommon, clinical myo-

TABLE 1. FREQUENCY OF CLINICAL SYMPTOMS IN SYSTEMIC LUPUS ERYTHEMATOSUS

	Per Cent
Arthritis, arthralgia	91
Fever	84
Skin	76
Butterfly rash	47
Photosensitivity	32
Alopecia	20
Raynaud's phenomenon	18
Purpura	15
Urticaria	7
Renal	54
Nephrotic syndrome	21
Gastrointestinal	55
Pulmonary	
Pleurisy	49
Effusion	29
Pneumonia	30
Cardiac	
Pericarditis	33
Murmurs	24
EKG changes	18
Adenopathy	46
Splenomegaly	10
Hepatomegaly	23
Central nervous system	30

carditis is seen less frequently. Myocarditis should be suspected when tachycardia is disproportionate to either fever or anemia. Frank cardiomegaly with congestive failure is rare. Precordial chest pain may be due to either pleurisy or pericarditis. Careful, frequent auscultation may be rewarded by hearing a pericardial friction rub. Tamponade or constrictive pericarditis is rare. Libman-Sacks or nonbacterial verrucous endocarditis usually occurs on the mitral valve and is recognized by murmurs which cannot be explained by fever or anemia; but generally this is a postmortem diagnosis. Bacterial endocarditis may develop on an already damaged valve, especially in patients receiving corticosteroids. Thrombophlebitis may be the first manifestation of SLE. Occlusion of major arteries may occur rarely. Equally rare is pulmonary hypertension.

Pulmonary Involvement. Pleuritic pain is a common complaint and often is the first clue to the diagnosis of SLE. It generally is accompanied by a friction rub and a variable amount of fluid accumulation, but the effusions are often painless. There may be pulmonary infiltrates which are quite difficult to distinguish from those due to infections. X-rays show bilateral patchy infiltrations which may shift from lobe to lobe. The involvement can progress to atelectasis, and to marked pulmonary insufficiency and cyanosis. Most pulmonary symptoms respond well to intensive corticosteroid therapy.

Neurologic and Psychologic Manifestations. Many patients have read in a dictionary or have heard that SLE is invariably a fatal illness, and this understandably leads to great anxiety. Or the patient may be told that he or she has arthritis, which leads to ungrounded fears of disabling deformities. These natural fears and anxieties of a chronic illness are complicated frequently by organic neurologic disturbances. The latter manifest themselves as behavioral disturbances, including hyperirritability, confusion, hallucinations, obsessional and paranoid reactions, and frank organic psychosis. The psychosis of SLE may easily be confused with, and in fact is difficult to differentiate from, a steroid-induced psychosis; other symptoms and signs of active SLE usually accompany the organic disease. Organic brain damage most commonly manifests itself as convulsions, which occur in at least 15 per cent of patients. Other neurologic findings, found less frequently, have included peripheral neuropathy, hemiparesis, motor aphasia, ptosis, diplopia, and nystagmus.

Cytoid bodies are fluffy white exudates in the nerve fibers of the retina. They are usually associated with some visual disturbance, are present with other signs of active SLE, and generally are reversible.

Gastrointestinal Manifestations. Anorexia, nausea, vomiting, and abdominal pain are common. The etiology is obscure, but may be due to peritonitis, enteritis, pancreatitis, or a paralytic ileus. Some patients have had repeated operations without the cause being found. Diarrhea and hematochezia have been noted. The liver is often found to be enlarged because of chronic passive congestion, but this is usually only transitory. Liver biopsy is either negative or shows fatty infiltration and/or fibrosis.

These manifestations in SLE should not be confused with *lupoid hepatitis*, which is a condition primarily of young women with progressive active hepatitis leading to chronic liver disease and failure. The serum in lupoid hepatitis contains high levels of gamma globulins, positive LE cell preparations, or positive ANF tests. It is also distinguishable from SLE by the fact that lupus nephritis does not occur, and serum complement levels remain normal or elevated.

Lymph Nodes and Spleen. Lymph nodes, characteristically, are enlarged in SLE but are not tender. The enlarged nodes have been mistaken for lymphoma. Splenomegaly, considered very common years ago, is seen now in about 15 per cent of patients.

Menses and Pregnancy. Menses are frequently irregular or heavy or both. In patients with circulating anticoagulants, bleeding may be profound. Although pregnancy carries some increased risk of miscarriage in the first trimester, most SLE patients without renal disease do well through term. It should be noted, however, that there is a considerable risk of postpartum exacerbation of the disease.

Course Untreated. It is difficult to discuss the natural history of SLE today because improved laboratory methods of diagnosis have widened greatly the clinical spectrum of SLE and because most patients are treated. Patients usually have recurrences of the same symptoms, such as arthritis, pleurisy, or nephritis; or they may develop variable symptoms and signs years apart. Remissions and relapses may be protracted or brief.

The prognosis for patients seems to improve each year, as patients with the disease are diagnosed before permanent tissue injury develops. There is no doubt, though, that the mortality rate remains higher during the first year after diagnosis. Using actuarial tables, it was shown in a study reported in 1956 that 15 per cent of patients died within three months after the diagnosis was made, and 50 per cent within four years. In 1968, 90 per cent of adults without renal disease and 80 per cent with renal disease were surviving five years. The prognosis in 1968 for children was worse, probably because the diagnosis was not considered earlier: 72 per cent without renal disease and 49 per cent with renal disease survived five years. The prognosis was poorest for those patients with diffuse proliferative glomerulonephritis.

Laboratory Findings. Hematologic. Anemia occurs in 71 per cent of the patients with SLE and is generally mild, normochromic, or normocytic. Anemia may also be due to infection, renal insufficiency, gastrointestinal bleeding, or a circulating anticoagulant. Autoagglutination of red blood cells may be observed. The Coombs test frequently is positive, but severe hemolytic anemia is uncommon. Leukopenia occurs in 57 per cent of the patients. The differential cell count is usually normal, although mononuclear cells may be more suppressed than neutrophils. Complicating infections generally result in a rise of the white blood cell count either into the normal or elevated range. Corticosteroid therapy also may result in leukocytosis. Thrombocytopenia, with or without purpura, may precede other manifestations of SLE by years or may disappear, leaving other manifestations of the disease. A circulating anticoagulant may be present in as many as 25 per cent of patients with SLE. This anticoagulant, either as antibody to factor VIII or more commonly as an inhibitor to the formation of "prothrombinase," results in prolonged clotting and prothrombin times and may be associated with mild or, rarely, severe hemorrhages.

Renal. Renal dysfunction occurs in over half the patients. Most patients have only some impairment of concentrating ability, a few red and/or white blood cells in the urine, and perhaps some proteinuria (<0.5 gram per day). Active nephritis is defined when there is either hematuria (>5 rc/hpf), pyuria (>5 wc/hpf), erythrocyte casts, increasing proteinuria, or a decreasing glomerular filtration rate. Hematuria and pyuria are rarely seen in lupus nephritis in remission.

Plasma Proteins. The erythrocyte sedimentation rate is often elevated. Serum albumin levels are low, especially in the nephrotic syndrome. Gamma globulin levels which are elevated in many patients may be low in nephrotics. Hypoalbuminemia and hypergammaglobulinemia may result in abnormal flocculation, e.g., cephalin, and turbidity, e.g., thymol, tests. Cryoglobulins, consisting of immunoglobulins and complement components, have been noted frequently, especially in patients with renal disease.

Abnormal Immunologic Reactions. Biologic false positive tests (BFP) for syphilis have been noted in 15 per cent of the patients with SLE, especially in those with circulating anticoagulants.

The BFP may be the first laboratory clue to the diagnosis of SLE and may precede symptoms by years. Rheumatoid factors have been found in 14 per cent of patients with SLE, even in the absence of clinical rheumatoid arthritis.

Most characteristic of SLE are the large number of autoantibodies which react with cells and their nuclear and cytoplasmic constituents. Historically of greatest significance is the LE cell phenomenon. The LE cell is formed in vitro as follows: some leukocytes are traumatized and release nucleoprotein (DNA-histone); the nucleoprotein reacts with a γG antibody; and the complex is phagocytized by the remaining viable leukocytes. The LE cell consists of a leukocyte with a large purplered homogeneous globulin inclusion body which compresses the nucleus against the cell membrane, leaving only a thin rim of cytoplasm. Because LE cells are not always present in patients with SLE, more sensitive tests have been developed for the detection of various antinuclear antibodies (ANA). An immunofluorescent (IF) technique, employing rodent liver or kidney as the source of nuclei, detects ANA in over 99 per cent of SLE patients. The antibodies may be of IgG, IgA, IgM, or IgD classes. Circulating DNA and other antigens may block the detection of the ANA. Employing this IF technique, different patterns of nuclear fluorescence reflect antibodies to different nuclear structures. The "homogeneous" or "diffuse" pattern reflects antibodies to nucleoprotein. The "peripheral," "rim," or "shaggy" pattern reflects primarily antibodies to DNA. The speckled pattern detects antibodies to a group of nuclear proteins, easily extractable with saline. A nucleolar pattern has also been observed, but this antigen is not well characterized.

Antibodies to some antigens, especially to DNA,

TABLE 2. LABORATORY ABNORMALITIES

	Per Cent
Hematologic:	
Anemia	71
Leukopenia	57
Thrombocytopenia	10
Hemolytic anemia	2
Circulating anticoagulant	1
Rheumatoid factor	14
Biologic false positive test for syphilis	15
Hypoalbuminemia	48
Hypergammaglobulinemia	62
LE cell test	83
Antinuclear factors	99.5
Anti-DNA antibodies	61
Hypocomplementemia	95

TABLE 3. AUTOANTIBODIES IN SLE

Antinuclear	Nucleoprotein
	DNA
	Histone
	Soluble extract ("Sm")
	Residue
Anticytoplasmic	Mitochondria
	Lysosomes
	Microsomes
	Ribosomes
	Cytoplasmic sap glycoprotein ("Ro")
Anti-RNA	Ribosomal RNA
	Double-stranded RNA (? viral)
	Single-stranded RNA
Anticell	Red cell
	White blood cell
	Platelet
Anticlotting factors	
Antithyroid	
Rheumatoid factor	
Biologic false positive test for syphilis	

have also been detected by other methods, including precipitation, diffusion in agar, complement fixation, agglutination, binding (Farr technique), and fluorescent spot test. The titers of antibodies to DNA and, to some extent, to nucleoprotein and ribosomes, tend to be higher during periods of clinical activity, especially nephritis, than during clinical remissions. Antibodies to double-stranded RNA have been noted.

Complement levels are depressed in 95 per cent of patients with SLE at some time during their illness. Markedly depressed complement levels are seen primarily in patients with active lupus nephritis. The low levels reflect in vivo activation and fixation of complement components by circulating immune complexes. Serial determination of whole complement levels (CH50) or of individual complement components (C4 and C3) may be useful in following and managing patients with SLE.

Diagnosis. The diagnosis of SLE should be suspected in those patients—especially young females—presenting combinations of butterfly rash after sun exposure, arthralgia or arthritis, unexplained fever, pleurisy, Raynaud's phenomenon, alopecia, leukopenia, anemia, renal disease, or purpura. However, SLE should also be suspected in patients with thrombocytopenia, easy bruising, diffuse adenopathy, hepatosplenomegaly, peripheral neuropathy, seizures, psychosis, endocarditis, myocarditis, pericarditis, interstitial pneumonitis, peritonitis, aseptic meningitis, or drug reactions, or in those having a false positive test for syphilis. Patients frequently are first diagnosed as having rheumatoid arthritis, rheumatic fever (especially children), glomerulonephritis, tuberculosis, scleroderma, vasculitis (including periarteritis), idiopathic thrombocytopenic purpura, lymphoma, anemia, or neutropenia. The LE cell is specific for SLE, if rheumatoid arthritis, lupoid hepatitis, or drug reactions can be excluded. Although the LE cell test is quite often negative, the antinuclear factor test is positive in 99.5 per cent of patients with SLE. The antinuclear antibodies have also been detected in 68 per cent of patients with Sjögren's syndrome, 40 per cent of patients with scleroderma—especially the speckled pattern—22 per cent of patients with juvenile rheumatoid arthritis, and 15 to 25 per cent of patients with rheumatoid arthritis—especially the homogeneous pattern. However, the antinuclear factors are present in higher titers in patients with SLE than in other disorders. Antibodies to DNA are a positive indication of SLE.

Diagnostic problems always arise in patients with the so-called overlap syndromes, that is, a mixture of signs and symptoms of SLE and other related diseases such as rheumatoid arthritis ("rupus syndrome"), Sjögren's syndrome, scleroderma, and dermatomyositis. These patients are best considered, and treated, for their primary symptoms and complaints.

Drug-induced SLE. Drugs that induce lupus can be divided into two categories: drugs that frequently induce a lupus-like syndrome in many individuals, and drugs associated with exacerba-tions of SLE. In the former group are hydrazides (hydralazine and isoniazid), anticonvulsants (Dilantin), and procainamide. A high percentage of subjects taking these drugs develop antinuclear factors—50 to 68 per cent of those taking procainamide. In one study of procainamide about 25 per cent of those with antinuclear factors developed symptoms consistent with SLE, but the symptoms generally cleared in a few weeks after discontinuation of the drug, even though positive tests persisted for months. Although few relatives of patients with the procainamide-lupus syndrome had "collagen disorders," this was not the case for the hydralazine-lupus syndrome. This suggests that certain people have a genetic predisposition to have a lupus-like reaction to certain drugs. These drug-induced lupus patients rarely have renal disease, and the disease subsides and does not recur after cessation of the drug. Other drugs, including penicillin, sulfonamides, and oral contraceptives, are associated with true exacerbations of SLE, and do not cause SLE-type symptoms or positive tests in normal persons.

Therapy and Management. The main goals of management and therapy should be prevention of exacerbations. However, when relapses occur, they should be treated aggressively so as to prevent permanent tissue injury and return the individual as soon as possible to normal daily activities. Although there is no cure, treatment can result in prolonged remissions. Certain measures are helpful in prevention of exacerbations. Antimicrobial drugs, especially penicillin and sulfonamides, should be avoided when possible. Sunlight and ultraviolet radiation should be avoided by most patients. Immunizations, blood transfusions, surgery, and nonessential drugs should be used with discretion.

In the long-term management of this illness, both patient and physician must learn to recognize those symptoms and signs that herald exacerbations. Although these symptoms may involve fever and joint pains in some patients, they may appear as alopecia, mucosal ulcers, pleurisy, or simply weight loss and fatigue in others. It is also helpful to follow certain laboratory "indicators," for many patients will have a single characteristically recurrent abnormality before frank clinical symptoms develop. This may be a high sedimentation rate or a low hematocrit, white blood cell count, platelet count, or serum complement; or it may be an abnormal urinalysis.

The acute erythematous maculopapular rash responds well to the avoidance of sunlight, local application of corticosteroid cream, and the systemic introduction of antimalarials such as hydroxychloroquin. Systemic corticosteroids are rarely warranted. The chronic lesion, or discoid lupus, responds to these same measures to a variable degree. Severe, extensive lesions have been treated with large doses of antimalarials when all else failed. However, the patient should be cautioned about the relative risks of retinal damage when taking large doses of antimalarials. Arthralgia and arthritis respond well to rest, physical therapy, splinting, salicylates, and anti-malarials. Steroids should not be needed.

Fever quite often responds to simple rest, sponge baths, and salicylates. Antimalarials may be beneficial. Persistent fever not responsive to these measures usually coincides with other signs of activity and responds to moderate doses of corti-costeroids.

Pericarditis and pleurisy respond well to rest and corticosteroids. Fluid, if present in moderate amounts, is best removed. Myocarditis should be treated with moderate doses of steroids, fluid restriction, and careful digitalization.

Hemolytic anemia and thrombocytopenia need not be treated unless symptomatic. They generally respond well to steroids. If not, immunosuppressive agents or a splenectomy may be necessary.

Involvement of the central nervous system responds poorly to treatment. Organic psychosis, in addition, may be difficult to differentiate from a steroid-induced psychosis. Because of the risk of permanent brain damage, large doses of steroids (2 mg. of prednisone per kilogram of body weight per day) are recommended until maximal improvement is achieved, at which time the dosage of steroids is gradually tapered.

Mild focal glomerulitis with minimal urinary abnormalities may respond on occasion to bed rest; however, these patients and those with acute glomerulonephritis generally require systemic corticosteroid therapy. Prednisone has been given with good results according to the following schedule depending on renal function: blood urea nitrogen (BUN) less than 30 mg. per 100 ml., 1 mg. of prednisone per kilogram of body weight per day; BUN 31 to 100 mg. per 100 ml., 2 mg. per kilo-gram; BUN over 100 mg. per 100 ml., 3 mg. per kilogram. The dose is maintained until hematuria clears and serum complement levels return to normal; this usually occurs within about three weeks. The LE cells, proteinuria, elevated sedimentation rate, and high titers of antinuclear antibodies may persist. The prednisone dosage is then tapered slowly — 10 mg. every five days. Complete blood counts, urinalyses, serum creatinine levels, and serum complement levels are checked weekly to detect relapses; relapses usually respond either to holding the dosage at that level or increasing it by 5 to 10 mg. of prednisone per day. Many patients can have the steroid dosage reduced to 5 to 10 mg. per day; some can tolerate steroids on alternate days; a few can discontinue steroids and remain asymptomatic. Continued careful monitoring and early treatment of even slight relapses may avoid more severe exacerbations.

Patients with chronic membranous glomerulonephritis and nephrotic syndrome respond less well to corticosteroids or immunosuppressives. Some, usually those with normal complement levels, may have fixed proteinuria.

Dubois, E. L. (ed.): Lupus Erythematosus. New York, McGraw-Hill Book Company, 1966.
Kunkel, H. G.: Immunological aspects of connective tissue disorders. Fed. Proc., 23:623, 1964.
Pollak, V. E., and Pirani, C. L.: Renal histologic findings in SLE. Mayo Clin. Proc., 44:630, 1969.
Rothfield, N.: Lupus erythematosus. In Fitzpatrick, T., et al. (eds.): Dermatology in General Medicine. New York, McGraw-Hill Book Company, in press.
Schur, P. H., and Sandson, J.: Immunological factors and clinical activity in lupus erythematosus. New Eng. J. Med., 278:533, 1968.

Periarteritis Nodosa

(Polyarteritis Nodosa)

K. Frank Austen

Definition. Kussmaul and Maier introduced the term periarteritis nodosa in 1866 to designate a morbid process manifested by numerous grossly visible or palpable nodules along the course of medium-sized muscular arteries. The lesions are segmental in distribution, have a predilection for the crotch of bifurcations and branchings, and involve all but the pulmonary arteries. The clinical manifestations are disparate and polymorphic, and result from partial or complete arterial occlusion, hemorrhage, and glomerulitis. In view of the necrotizing nature of the process, involving the entire arterial wall, Ferrari in 1903 suggested the alternate name of polyarteritis acuta nodosa.

The incidence, age distribution, and male-to-female ratio of periarteritis nodosa are difficult to determine because a diagnostic serologic procedure is lacking, and the spotty distribution of lesions makes biopsy uncertain. Nonetheless, the condition has been reported to occur from infancy to old age, with a peak incidence in the fifth and sixth decades of life, and the male to female ratio has been estimated at from 2 to 3:1.

Pathology. The lesions of polyarteritis involve arteries of medium and small caliber, especially at bifurcations and branchings. The segmental process involves the media, with edema, fibrinous exudation, fibrinoid necrosis, and infiltration of polymorphonuclear neutrophils and varying numbers of eosinophils, and extends to the adventitia and intima. Thrombosis and infarction or hemorrhage occur at this stage. Subsequently, the regions of fibrinoid necrosis are replaced by cellular granulation tissue, and the intima proliferates. Finally the involved segment is replaced by scar tissue with associated intimal thickening and periarterial fibrosis. These changes produce partial occlusion, thrombosis and infarction, and palpable or visible aneurysms with occasional rupture.

The glomerulitis is characterized by capillary microthrombi, focal fibrinoid necrosis, polymorphonuclear neutrophil infiltration, and capsular proliferation. With progression, the necrotizing feature of the glomerulitis is less apparent, and the process is difficult to distinguish from glomerulonephritis of other causes.

Clinical Manifestations and Diagnosis. The widespread distribution of the arterial lesions produces diverse clinical manifestations, which reflect the particular organ systems in which the arterial supply has been impaired. In addition, no study including a large number of living patients has or even can limit its patient population to those with classic periarteritis as defined by Kussmaul and Maier. The available studies are likely to include an admixture of patients with allergic angiitis and granulomatosis (see Introduction to this section). Among the early general symptoms and signs of periarteritis nodosa are tachycardia, fever, weight loss, and pain in viscera and/or the musculoskeletal system so that the differential diagnosis is of fever of unknown origin. Striking and specific presenting signs may relate to abdominal pain, acute glomerulitis, polyneuritis, or myocardial infarction. Pulmonary manifestations, especially intractable bronchial asthma, would indicate allergic angiitis and granulomatosis rather than classic polyarteritis nodosa.

Renal. Renal involvement in two forms, renal polyarteritis and a glomerulitis, may occur separately or together. Renal polyarteritis was the most common lesion in the postmortem studies of Rose and Spencer (see accompanying table), and in the comparable analysis performed at the Armed Forces Institute of Pathology by Mowrey (1954). Manifestations of the renal involvement include intermittent proteinuria and microscopic hematuria with occasional hyaline and granular casts. The glomerulitis is manifested by marked microscopic and even macroscopic hematuria, proteinuria, cellular casts, and progressive renal failure; survival of the acute phase is followed by progressive hypertension. It is no longer the prevailing view that hypertension precedes or occurs in the initial phase of periarteritis nodosa, but rather that it reflects healing renal polyarteritis, progressive glomerulitis, or both. Such renal involvement is the cause of death in about two thirds of patients with classic periarteritis nodosa and about one third of those with allergic angiitis and granulomatosis.

Gastrointestinal. Characteristic arterial lesions are commonly found in one or more abdominal viscera. The principal manifestation is pain, especially in the umbilical region or right upper quadrant; anorexia, nausea, and vomiting are less prominent. Impaired arterial supply to the bowel can produce mucosal ulceration, perforation, or infarction with melena or bloody diarrhea. Involvement of appendix, gallbladder, or pancreas can simulate cholecystitis, appendicitis, or hemorrhagic pancreatitis. Liver involvement can range from hepatomegaly with or without jaundice to the signs of extensive hepatic necrosis. Splenomegaly is uncommon.

INCIDENCE OF NECROTIZING ANGIITIS IN VARIOUS ORGANS AT NECROPSY*

	Polyarteritis Nodosa (Classic)	Allergic Angiitis and Granulomatosis ("Polyarteritis with Pulmonary Involvement")
	Per Cent	Per Cent
Lungs (pulmonary arteries)	0	47
Heart	35	60
Kidneys: Glomerulitis	30	57
Renal polyarteritis	65	60
Stomach and intestines	30	40
Liver	54	37
Pancreas	39	17
Spleen	35	43
Brain	4	3
Periadrenal connective tissue	41	40
Voluntary muscle	20	33

*Reproduced in modified form from Rose and Spencer: Quart. J. Med., 26:43, 1957. There were 54 cases in periarteritis group and 30 with the diagnosis of allergic angiitis and granulomatosis.

Central and Peripheral Nervous System. Neurologic manifestations are generally late occurrences in the course of periarteritis nodosa, and their particular presentation reflects the specific brain area compromised. Headache, convulsive seizures, papillitis, and retinal hemorrhages and exudates occur with or without localizing signs referable to the cerebrum, cerebellum, or brainstem; meningeal irritation may occur as a result of subarachnoid hemorrhage. Multineuritis multiplex, that is, involvement of several or even many individual nerves at the same or different times, is a common finding and is attributed to arteritis of the vasa nervorum. The peripheral neuropathy is usually asymmetrical with both sensory and motor distribution. The former can be extremely painful, but the latter, with attendant muscular degeneration, has on occasion been so severe as to dominate the clinical presentation.

Articular and Muscular. Arthralgia and myalgia are frequent in polyarteritis nodosa. Arthralgia is migratory, generally without swelling, and apparently due to small localized arterial lesions rather than extensive synovitis. The interpretation of those rare instances of synovitis with deformity and arterial changes of periarteritis nodosa is difficult, but it seems preferable to consider such cases as rheumatoid arthritis. Muscle pain or weakness reflects either direct involvement of the arterial supply or a peripheral neuropathy from involvement of the vasa nervorum.

Cardiac. Polyarteritis of the coronary arteries and their branches has a frequency approaching that of renal polyarteritis, and heart failure is responsible for or contributes to death in from one sixth to one half of the cases. The clinical manifestations of cardiac involvement are those of partial or complete arterial occlusion as modified by the superimposition of renal hypertension and an appreciable incidence of acute pericarditis without effusion. Whereas the combination of infarction and hypertension commonly leads to left-sided failure, an occasional patient with allergic angiitis and granulomatosis will present with predominantly right-sided decompensation.

Genitourinary. Involvement of the ovaries, testes, and epididymis is frequent, though usually asymptomatic. Mucosal ulceration in the bladder can occasionally precipitate gross hematuria with dysuria.

Cutaneous. Cutaneous involvement of some form is believed to occur in over 25 per cent of those affected with periarteritis nodosa. The acute cutaneous manifestations of periarteritis nodosa include polymorphic exanthemata—purpuric, urticarial, and multiform in character—and severe subcutaneous hemorrhage, resulting from necrotizing arteritis, with secondary gangrene. Ulcerations and a persistent livedo reticularis are associated with the more chronic stage of the disease. A most characteristic but uncommon finding is cutaneous and subcutaneous nodules; these occur at any time in the disease course. The nodules tend to group, appear in crops, are usually movable, may regress in days or persist for months, range in size from a pea to a walnut, and may cause the overlying skin to become reddened or to ulcerate.

Allergic Angiitis and Granulomatosis ("Polyarteritis with Pulmonary Involvement"). Pulmonary lesions are absent in classic polyarteritis nodosa but almost always precede the onset of polyarteritic lesions in other organs in the process termed allergic granulomatosis and angiitis by Churg and Strauss. Such patients typically present with bronchitis, bronchial asthma, or the findings of pneumonia. The asthma is intractable and associated with a marked peripheral eosinophilia. The pneumonic episodes are transient or progressive and can include hemoptysis or pleuritic pain. The appearance and superimposition of polyarteritis in other organs is followed by a rapid deterioration, respiratory involvement accounting for half the deaths.

Course Untreated. The course of periarteritis nodosa is progressive with destruction of vital organs. Intermittent acute episodes resulting from thrombosis of vital or nonvital structures are prominent. Death is most frequently attributed to renal involvement in cases of classic periarteritis nodosa and to pulmonary lesions in those cases classified as allergic angiitis with granulomatosis. Cardiac failure caused by a combination of infarction and renal hypertension is an additional frequent cause of death in both groups, and acute vascular accidents in the gastrointestinal tract or central nervous system account for much of the remaining mortality. In the retrospective postmortem study of Rose and Spencer, the five-year survival rate was about 10 per cent in classic periarteritis nodosa, and about 25 per cent in allergic angiitis and granulomatosis if onset was dated from the start of respiratory symptoms. The more recent report of the British Medical Research Council in 1960 placed the 54 months' survival rate in polyarteritis nodosa at nearly 50 per cent. Rare patients with polyarteritis limited to nonvital sites have been reported to experience an unusually long course or even a lasting remission.

Laboratory Findings. Leukocytosis, predominantly polymorphonuclear, is apparent in over 75 per cent of the cases of periarteritis nodosa or allergic angiitis and granulomatosis, eosinophilia often being marked in the latter group. The erythrocyte sedimentation rate is customarily elevated with or without some increase of the globulins. Abnormalities in the urine sediment, especially hematuria and proteinuria, reflect renal involvement. Abnormalities of the electrocardiogram and electroencephalogram are those expected on the basis of arterial occlusive disease or those secondary to the metabolic disturbances of uremia. Lesions apparent on chest roentgenograms are the rule in patients with allergic angiitis and granulomatosis. The findings range from transient or progressive infiltration to consolidation, cavitation, or scarring; upper and lower lobes are involved with equal frequency. As none of these findings is specific, antemortem diagnosis of polyarteritis depends upon biopsy. Since the arterial involvement is segmental and spotty in distribution, it is advisable to obtain tissue from a symptomatic site, and it is essential to section completely the entire specimen. A deep, open surgical biopsy including subcutaneous tissue and underlying muscle should be obtained whenever possible from a skeletal muscle exhibiting pain and tenderness. Involvement of the epididymis and testes is sufficiently common to make this a useful biopsy site, especially if palpation reveals the typical nodularity of segmental vascular lesions. There are insufficient data on needle and surgical biopsies of internal organs, such as liver or kidney, to permit assessment of their usefulness or complications.

Differential Diagnosis. The differential diagnosis of classic periarteritis nodosa includes all those conditions associated with necrotizing angiitis (see Introduction to this section). The absence of pulmonary lesions distinguishes classic periarteritis nodosa from allergic angiitis and granulomatosis. The other connective tissue diseases are recognized by their clinical characteristics even when necrotizing arteritis becomes prominent. For example, cases of rheumatoid arthritis with ulcerating cutaneous lesions and peripheral neuropathy often exhibit prominent rheumatoid nodules and a high titer of rheumatoid factor. Giant cell arteritis, in its limited form, cranial (especially temporal) or aortic arch (Takayasu's) arteritis, or in its disseminated state lacks the glomerulitis, peripheral neuropathy, and cutaneous manifestations notable in periarteritis nodosa. The drug-induced hypersensitivity angiitis group

who, for unexpla
phage-neutralizin
with the difficulty
in sarcoidosis an
may even be enha
between the two i
anism promote gr
tivity to pine poll
ents after being et
results. Autoimmu
the immunologic t
steroid therapy, bu

That unrecogn
possibly influence
high prevalence at
born immigrants t
a significantly inc
ronmental factors
occurrence or the e

PATHO

If an exogen
sis, its portal
route via the
adenopathy is
clinical manife
studies made
closed parench
ographically c
ment is preser
the liver, bor
also made at tl
granulomas, e
tiating attack
the portal of
agent in sarco
nodosum favor
numerous mic
known to evok
are all of exog

Almost any orga
flammatory process
pattern. The tissue
confluent follicles
epithelioid cells w
elongated vesicular
be present within th
and eosinophils are
Caseation is abser
necrosis are someti
cellular inclusion b
(concentrically lam
and calcium salts),
of granulomas occu
by their replaceme
scars. Epithelioid g
decade or longer af
volvement has disa

The ultrastructu
granulomatous dise
cutaneous Kveim t
microscopic observa
a complicated inter
lated organelle-rich
chondria, rough er
numerous vacuoles
well as phagocytic
synthesized substan
sis is not known.

The cellular evolu

---

may be difficult to separate on purely clinical grounds, although the history of antecedent drug administration, the frequency of pulmonary involvement, infrequency of gastrointestinal manifestations, and absence of nodules along arteries are useful points. The clinical presentation in Henoch-Schönlein purpura, mostly in children and with a relatively good prognosis, is distinctive. The combination of progressive nephritis and pulmonary hemorrhage seen in Goodpasture's syndrome is unlike polyarteritis nodosa. The findings in the immunoglobulins which accompany active systemic lupus erythematosus or mixed cryoglobulinemia are distinctive; in addition, in the presence of active renal disease both entities manifest a reduced serum complement level not observed in periarteritis nodosa.

The key morphologic differences between periarteritis nodosa and other causes of necrotizing angiitis are noted in the Introduction and include the absence of extravascular granulomas, sparing of the pulmonary arteries, failure of venous involvement except by contiguous spread, and predilection for medium-sized arteries. For allergic angiitis and granulomatosis the striking granulomatous response excludes all but Wegener's granulomatosis. The prominence of bronchial asthma, peripheral eosinophilia, and the usual absence of necrotizing lesions in the upper respiratory tract permit a tentative clinical distinction between allergic angiitis and granulomatosis (termed by some polyarteritis nodosa with pulmonary involvement) and Wegener's granulomatosis. Additional entities to be considered in the differential diagnosis are certain microbial and occlusive diseases with diverse manifestations, notably chronic meningococcemia, subacute bacterial endocarditis, trichinosis, certain rickettsial diseases, leptospirosis, and syphilis. A few vascular occlusive diseases, including Degos' disease and thrombotic thrombocytopenic purpura, must also be considered. Necrotizing papulosis of Degos, with its occlusive arterial lesions of the skin, gastrointestinal tract, and brain, is best characterized by the cutaneous manifestations. These lesions typically involve the trunk and extremities, begin as pink to gray papules, undergo central umbilication, and persist for variable periods with depressed (porcelain-like) centers covered with a removable scale and surrounded by a red elevated margin. The absence of both thrombocytopenia and intravascular hemolysis distinguishes periarteritis nodosa from thrombotic thrombocytopenic purpura. Additional points of help in the differential diagnosis of periarteritis nodosa in general are the rarity of Raynaud's phenomenon, the absence of the nephrotic syndrome, and the lack of lymphadenopathy.

Treatment. The therapy of periarteritis nodosa and allergic angiitis and granulomatosis is clearly unsatisfactory. Nonetheless, such patients can remain ambulatory and professionally active for periods of months to years after the clinical onset of the disease. The commonly employed anti-inflammatory agents such as salicylates or phenylbutazone have little or no clear effect, and thus corticosteroids have been employed most widely. Large doses, in the range of 40 to 60 mg. of prednisone per day, afford symptomatic relief and apparently do improve the one-year survival statistics. On the other hand, the study by the Medical Research Council of England did not reveal a better 54 months' survival period in a steroid-treated group as compared with a control series. Experience with antimetabolites, such as azathioprine or cyclophosphamide, is insufficient to allow a conclusion as to their efficacy.

Churg, J., and Strauss, L.: Allergic granulomatosis, allergic angiitis, and periarteritis nodosa. Amer. J. Path., 27:277, 1951.
Collagen Diseases and Hypersensitivity Panel: Report to Medical Research Council. Brit. Med. J., 1:1399, 1960.
Mowrey, F. H., and Lundberg, R. A.: The clinical manifestations of essential polyangiitis (periarteritis nodosa) with emphasis on the hepatic manifestations. Ann. Intern. Med., 40:1145, 1954.
Rose, G. A., and Spencer, H.: Polyarteritis nodosa. Quart. J. Med., 26:43, 1957.

physicians of the multifaceted character of sarcoidosis. In countries where tuberculosis is still commonly encountered, the true prevalence of sarcoidosis tends to be obscured.

It has been estimated from mass roentgenographic surveys in Denmark that for every recognized case of sarcoidosis, there are at least four cases which go undetected in the same population. Consecutive autopsy observations in Malmo, Sweden, show that the ratio of detected to undetected cases is only one in ten.

Ethnic rather than geographic factors appear to account for the differences in national prevalence rates. The highest reported prevalence rates of sarcoidosis have come from Sweden, 64 per 100,000; Eire, 33; Norway, 26; Holland, 21; and Britain, 20. There have been no nationwide roentgenographic surveys in the United States, but data from the Armed Forces and Veterans Administration hospitals have revealed that intrathoracic sarcoidosis is 10 to 20 times as prevalent among Negroes as it is in the white population, regardless of birthplace or residence in the United States. Women may be slightly more often affected than men, the highest rates occurring between 18 and 35 years, but children and persons in older age groups can also be affected. Cases have been reported among parents and children as well as in several siblings, but there is no evidence of person-to-person transmission.

CLINICAL MANIFESTATIONS AND COURSE

The manifestations of sarcoidosis vary according to the duration of the disease, the extent of involvement, and the degree of activity of the lesions. Sarcoidosis almost always begins silently and very often runs its entire course asymptomatically. The chest roentgenogram holds the key to detection, as more than 90 per cent of patients show abnormal chest film findings at some stage of the illness. In areas with well-developed medical facilities which include mass chest roentgenography, about 40 per cent of the patients finally diagnosed are first identified through this means.

SUBACUTE AND CHRONIC SARCOIDOSIS

The spectrum of clinical patterns encountered in sarcoidosis can best be appreciated through an awareness of how the disease evolves and in what chronologic order the wide variety of manifestations appear. Patients with sarcoidosis fall into two broad groups: those with *subacute* sarcoidosis, who by rough estimate have had their lesions for less than two years; and those with *chronic* disease with lesions of more than two years' duration. In published reports of large numbers of cases, the patients in the subacute stage outnumber those in the chronic stage by 3 or 4 to 1. This proportion in part reflects the high rate of spontaneous remission in sarcoidosis, especially among the growing number of patients now being detected through

routine or survey chest roentgenography in the presymptomatic stage. These asymptomatic patients usually escape the chronic stage and recover without significant residual disability.

Patients with subacute sarcoidosis tend to be younger than 30 years of age, exhibit transient lesions with few extrathoracic foci of involvement, infrequently require corticosteroid therapy, and have a good prognosis. An acute attack of erythema nodosum and polyarthritis may usher in the disease, especially among Swedish, Irish, and Puerto Rican-born women of childbearing age. These attacks are usually accompanied by fever, which may last for six weeks to three months, and are especially prevalent in the spring of the year. Recurrences are uncommon after resolution of lesions.

In contrast, patients presenting with chronic sarcoidosis are somewhat older, have persistent lesions with extensive intra- and extrathoracic organ involvement, often require corticosteroid therapy, and may become disabled by pulmonary or renal insufficiency with a fatal outcome within five years of 5 to 10 per cent.

PRESENTING SYMPTOMS

The onset of sarcoidosis is often insidious, and in about half the patients there are either no symptoms or relatively insignificant ones. Symptoms when present result from the cumulative deposits of granulomas in the various organs over a period of months or years, and the nature of the symptoms is determined by the sites of such deposits. There is a marked disparity between the patient's sense of well being and the massiveness of the hilar and paratracheal node enlargement sometimes accompanied by extensive pulmonary mottling which the chest film may disclose. In about 20 per cent of patients, respiratory symptoms are already present when the patients are seen initially. Early symptoms include cough, low-grade fever, vague substernal discomfort, and a sensation of being unable to "fill the lungs." Dyspnea and wheezing occur during the chronic stage when extensive pulmonary scarring and endobronchial involvement are present.

Less frequent modes of onset of *extrathoracic origin* include dimness of vision resulting from acute uveitis, swelling of salivary and lacrimal glands, facial palsy, and, later, superficial lymphadenopathy. Cutaneous eruptions other than erythema nodosum may first call attention to the disorder when the patient has already passed into the chronic stage. Other late symptoms include polyuria and polydipsia caused by persistent hypercalciuria, with renal damage, keratoconjunctivitis sicca, and unexplained neurologic and myocardial disorders.

Intrathoracic Sarcoidosis

Mediastinal Nodes and Lung. Despite the systemic nature of sarcoidosis, it is the intrathoracic localization which dominates in its influence on diagnosis, prognosis, and treatment of the disorder. Most systems of classification of intrathoracic sarcoidosis are based on the roentgenographic appearance of the chest which can be divided into three broad stages. The earliest stage (*stage I*) is characterized by symmetrical bilateral hilar adenopathy with or without paratracheal node enlargement and with roentgenographically clear lung fields. This pattern is the most frequent one and holds a key position in the diagnostic hierarchy. It has been speculated that all clinical sarcoidosis begins with hilar adenopathy along with roentgenographically undetectable granulomas within the lung parenchyma. Characteristically, the bronchopulmonary nodes in the right hilar area tend to stand away from the right border of the heart more than they do in lymphomatous and metastatic neoplastic nodal involvement (see accompanying figure). In the latter conditions, the shadow of the nodes tends to fuse with the right cardiac border.

In three quarters of the patients with hilar adenopathy, complete or substantial regression of nodal enlargement occurs within a one- to three-year period. In about 10 per cent of patients, hilar node enlargement may become chronic and persist for a decade or more. The remaining 15 per cent of stage I cases progress to stage II with pulmonary mottling supervening. In contrast to sarcoidosis, mediastinal adenopathy in Hodgkin's disease tends to be less symmetrical and is more often located in the anterior and superior mediastinum with a lesser tendency to enlargement of the intercalated bronchopulmonary nodes. Unilateral mediastinal lymphadenopathy is more common in primary tuberculosis and fungal infections as well as in metastatic nodal involvement in bronchogenic carcinoma. Hilar node enlargement without pulmonary mottling is not seen in either beryllium disease or pneumoconiosis. Lung function studies show few abnormalities in stage I; a slight lowering in the diffusing capacity may be demonstrated.

In almost one third of the patients, the presenting chest film shows both bilateral hilar adenopathy and pulmonary mottling (*stage II*). The mottling takes the form of localized or disseminated miliary and sometimes larger nodules in both lung fields. The nodular densities may coalesce and assume a cotton-wool appearance. Miliary nodules and confluent shadows are usually seen one year or less after sarcoidosis is detected but may appear in the second year of illness. Often the hilar node enlargement regresses and may completely disappear, leading rapidly to stage III. Miliary nodulation in sarcoidosis may mimic miliary tuberculosis, pneumoconiosis, beryllium disease, lymphangitic carcinoma, idiopathic hemosiderosis, and alveolar microlithiasis, but in most of these conditions the hilar adenopathy is not likely to be prominent. The cotton-wool, fluffy infiltrations may simulate exudative pulmonary tuberculosis, metastatic neoplasms, eosinophilic pneumonia, and Wegener's granulomatosis.

Symptoms are variable in stage II, and fever, weight loss, and easy fatigue may be present as well as symptoms referable to extrathoracic involvement. But even at this stage, the patient may remain relatively asymptomatic as is also sometimes the case with advanced silicosis or pulmonary tuberculosis. Two thirds of the patients presenting in stage II eventually show complete or substantial clearing of nodal and pulmonary lesions. The remaining third show little change for prolonged periods or progress to stage III with extensive or localized pulmonary fibrosis.

Lung function studies in stage II may show a reduced vital capacity, diminished lung compliance, an increase in both dead space ventilation and venous admixture, and a significant lowering of the diffusing capacity. On the other hand, maximal voluntary ventilation is well maintained.

About one in seven patients presents in *stage III* with a roentgenographic pattern of diffuse, sometimes confluent pulmonary mottling with fine and coarse reticulation and streaking intermixed with nodules 1 to 5 mm. in size. Enlarged hilar nodes are no longer visible. Over a two- to seven-year period, irreversible and dense fibrosis of the lung fields and of the hilar structures ensues with retraction upward of both lung roots. Lucencies of bullae appear, occasionally of giant size, and these combined with the dense fibrosis in the upper zones of both lungs may simulate closely the pattern seen in advanced pulmonary tuberculosis. In the more severely affected patients, the right ventricle gradually enlarges foreshadowing cor pulmonale and fatal respiratory insufficiency.

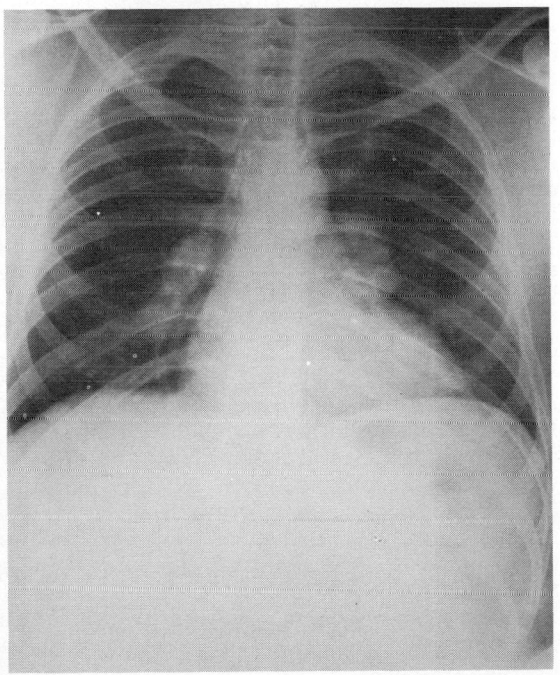

Chest x-ray of a 24-year-old Negro male who had had a normal routine film four months previously. The film now reveals bilateral hilar node enlargement, and, characteristically, the right hilar shadow is separated from the shadow of the right cardiac border.

Patients in stage III have the least favorable prognosis. They may be disabled by progressive pulmonary fibrosis, and they suffer a significant mortality, making up a major portion of the 8 per cent of patients who die within a five-year period after detection.

Cough and dyspnea are outstanding complaints, and these symptoms may be accompanied by those of chronic ocular and cutaneous involvement. Lung function studies in stage III show similar but more severe derangements than are present in stage II. In the terminal stages of pulmonary insufficiency, ventilatory impairment occasionally supervenes with alveolar hypoventilation, hypercapnia, and respiratory acidosis. The chest x-ray patterns of stage III may be easily confused with diffuse idiopathic pulmonary fibrosis, progressive systemic sclerosis, rheumatoid lung, pneumoconiosis, congestive heart failure, and advanced bullous emphysema when bulla formation is present. When both upper zones are the seat of coarse nodules and streaks and hilar node enlargement is no longer present, it becomes difficult to exclude the possibility of tuberculosis of both upper lobes. This is particularly true when small lucencies are present within dense fibrotic areas and the trachea is deviated by contraction of scar tissue within the lung.

Patients with normal chest film findings when first seen are paradoxically most often in a chronic stage of sarcoidosis and manifest ocular, cutaneous, or other extrathoracic involvement. When chest films have been made some months or years before the appearance of the extrathoracic lesions, bilateral hilar adenopathy or pulmonary mottling is commonly found to have been present and to have undergone complete resolution by the time the patient presents himself.

Endobronchial Involvement

Granulomatous involvement of the bronchial wall is common and has been demonstrated by random bronchoscopic biopsy in 40 per cent of patients in stage I and in 70 per cent of patients in stages II and III. The mucosal and submucosal granulomas do not ulcerate but may cause narrowing of segmental bronchi, causing focal and segmental atelectasis and nonspecific infections in the lung distal to the obstruction. Bronchial involvement is often clinically silent, but cough, expectoration, hemoptysis, and wheezing may be present. Multiple random bronchoscopic biopsy is a useful diagnostic measure, especially in stage III. Pleural and pericardial effusions are infrequently encountered.

Extrathoracic Involvement

Ocular Involvement. Ocular lesions are encountered in approximately 25 per cent of patients and include bilateral, acute and chronic iridocyclitis, conjunctival follicles, chorioretinitis, periphlebitis, and, as late complications, keratoconjunctivitis, secondary glaucoma, and phthisis bulbi.

Although acute uveitis associated with bilateral hilar adenopathy and erythema nodosum has a good prognosis, the outcome of chronic ocular lesions associated with skin plaques, bone cysts, and pulmonary scarring is not nearly so favorable. The triad of anterior uveitis, parotid enlargement, and facial palsy is known as Heerfordt's syndrome.

Salivary and Lacrimal Gland Involvement. Painless swelling of the parotid and submaxillary glands, sometimes accompanied by xerostomia, occurs in less than 10 per cent of patients. Enlargement of lacrimal glands may lead to the sicca syndrome. Displacement of the globe by a hugely enlarged lacrimal gland may be mistakenly attributed to a malignant retro-orbital tumor. Salivary and lacrimal gland enlargement usually regresses spontaneously without residua.

Superficial Lymphadenopathy. Discrete and painless symmetrical enlargement of cervical, supraclavicular, epitrochlear, and inguinal lymph nodes occurs in approximately 40 per cent of patients and only becomes clinically manifest a year or more after the appearance of hilar adenopathy and erythema nodosum. The granulomatous nodes do not break down to form sinuses. They are firm and discrete and, on cut section, have a granular, yellow-pink surface. Enlarged nodes tend to undergo spontaneous shrinkage but sometimes persist for months or years.

Skin. Cutaneous and subcutaneous lesions other than erythema nodosum occur in 20 to 25 per cent of patients and are of three types: maculopapular, which occur in the subacute stage; nodular; and plaquelike, including lupus pernio, in the chronic stage. The maculopapular lesions are small and are usually clustered about the alae nasi, around the lips, eyelids, forehead, and back of the neck near the hairline. The lesions are transient and regress spontaneously. Nodular and plaquelike lesions including lupus pernio are persistent and tend to recur when suppressive therapy is halted. Nodular lesions are waxy, pale, or erythematous and are distributed on the face, trunk, and extensor surfaces of the extremities. The lesions around the nose may extend into the mucosa of the nares, but the nasal mucosa may be involved even in the absence of skin lesions. In lupus pernio the tip of the nose and sometimes the ears are swollen and are dark violet in color, causing gross disfigurement. Sarcoid skin lesions rarely ulcerate or suppurate but may be crusted. Itching is not a prominent symptom. With healing, the lesions show central blanching and atrophy with circinate pigmentation at the margins. Sarcoidosis may begin with swelling of an old, healed cutaneous scar which, on biopsy, shows fresh epithelioid granulomas embedded in a fibrous matrix.

Neurologic Involvement. Neurosarcoidosis occurs in about 5 per cent of patients and affects three nervous system areas: the central nervous system, including the brain, spinal cord, and meninges; peripheral nerves; and cranial nerves. Cranial and peripheral nerve involvements usually manifest themselves in the early stage of sarcoidosis, whereas central nervous system involvement tends to appear later in the course. Facial palsy, a frequent finding, is transient, but peripheral nerve lesions last longer before improving. On the other hand central nervous system lesions fare poorly with slow recovery, which is often incomplete. Diabetes insipidus can result from hypothalamic or posterior pituitary lesions.

Musculoskeletal Involvement. *Joints.* Articular symptoms are relatively common in sarcoidosis, occurring in 10 to 20 per cent of cases. Two broad categories of joint affection are encountered. By far the most common is an acute but transient self-limiting attack of polyarthritis occurring early in the course and often associated with erythema nodosum. Chronic polyarthritis is much less common and may appear early or late in the course, recurring with acute exacerbations over a period of years, especially when the lesions of disseminated sarcoidosis remain florid. Joint deformity can sometimes occur in the chronic form, especially in uncommon instances when localized involvement of a joint results from extension of a contiguous granulomatous bone cyst. Synovial biopsy may reveal the characteristic granulomas.

Muscle Involvement. Granulomas of systemic sarcoidosis are frequently observed histologically in skeletal muscles on random biopsy, but they are not often associated with muscle symptoms or signs, and hence their frequency has been underestimated. Asymptomatic muscle involvement is found almost exclusively in the subacute stage, whereas symptomatic involvement of muscles with weakness, wasting, tenderness, and myopathic electromyographic abnormalities are rare and are only found in the chronic stage. Occasionally, patients present with acute myalgia and muscle tenderness, generally accompanying the acute polyarthritis of erythema nodosum.

Bones. Cystic lesions in the phalanges are roentgenographically visible in approximately 5 to 10 per cent of patients, the frequency depending upon the proportion of patients with chronic sarcoidosis in any given series. But unless cutaneous sarcoidosis is also present, the likelihood of detecting bone cysts in the hands or feet is small. Cystic lesions in the skull, long bones, and vertebrae have also been reported. The cysts tend to persist for years.

Liver. Hepatomegaly is encountered in 20 per cent of patients, usually in the second year of illness or later. Silent granulomas in this organ are considerably more frequent and have been found in up to 75 per cent of patients when needle aspiration biopsy is systematically practiced. Elevation of serum alkaline phosphatase and low-grade fever are common accompaniments of liver involvement. Jaundice, biliary cirrhosis, and ascites are rare. Spontaneous healing of granulomas by resorption and inconsequential scarring is the usual course.

Spleen. Moderate to giant-sized enlargement of the spleen occurs in about 20 per cent of patients mainly in the chronic stage. Anemia, leukopenia,

and reduction in blood platelets can be striking, and spontaneous bleeding can result. On occasion, the weight of the enlarged spleen may produce marked abdominal discomfort, and the capsule may rupture with mild trauma, necessitating emergency splenectomy.

Kidney. There are no accurate estimates of the frequency of granulomatous involvement of the kidneys since the tubercles produce no symptoms and infrequently impair renal function. Renal damage does result with persistent hypercalciuria, which is found in 25 per cent or more of patients, especially during the chronic stage. Urolithiasis, pyelonephritis, and nephrocalcinosis may eventually lead to renal failure and a fatal outcome. Sarcoidosis of the epididymis and testis is unusual.

Heart. Pulmonary hypertension and cor pulmonale are the usual sequelae of progressive pulmonary fibrosis in sarcoidosis. Granulomas in the myocardium have been detected in as high as 20 per cent of autopsy cases, but clinical manifestations from such involvement are an infrequent occurrence. Conduction disturbances with arrhythmias of varying severity and persistence may be observed. Sudden death in patients whose sarcoidosis is first detected on postmortem examination may be the result of cardiac standstill produced by severe granulomatous involvement of conduction pathways.

LABORATORY FINDINGS

Blood. The hemogram and bone marrow aspirates are usually normal, but leukopenia is common, even in patients with freshly appearing bilateral hilar adenopathy. Eosinophilia may occur but can often be related to concomitant intestinal parasitic infestation. The sedimentation rate is elevated, particularly in patients with lesions in three or more organ systems. Hypersplenism may cause marked reduction in all blood elements.

Chemical Studies. Hyperglobulinemia, especially of the gamma fraction, is encountered in one third to one half of the patients, especially in the chronic stage and particularly among Negro patients. Serum IgA, IgM, and IgG as well as serum complement levels are all elevated during the active phase but tend to recede with recovery. Cryoglobulins may also be demonstrated and are of unknown significance. The normal sequence of formation of IgM antibodies on initial immunization with typhoid-paratyphoid vaccine and of IgG antibodies following later booster injections is maintained in sarcoidosis. The latex fixation test may be positive in one third or more of the patients, but this finding is unrelated to arthritic manifestations.

Hypercalciuria is common, but hypercalcemia is less so, occurring in 15 to 25 per cent of patients. Increased intestinal absorption of calcium is thought to result from loss of calcium from bone stores, a disturbance which has been attributed to hypersensitivity to some vitamin D-like substance which patients with sarcoidosis (and beryllium disease) may be synthesizing. Hypercalcemia generally reaches its peak during the summer months when exposure to the sun is at its maximum. Uric acid blood levels may also be elevated without apparent renal damage, as are levels of alkaline phosphatase, notably with liver involvement. When the central nervous system is affected, the cerebrospinal fluid may show pleocytosis, increased protein, and a reduction in sugar content. Biologic false positive serologic tests for syphilis are sometimes seen.

Skin Tests. The tuberculin reaction is negative to 250 TU (second-strength PPD) in almost two thirds of the patients. Only about 10 per cent of patients respond to the conventional dose of 1 or 10 TU (first and intermediate strength PPD), the remainder being weakly sensitive and responding only to 250 TU. The level of tuberculin sensitivity shifts within a narrow range during the course of sarcoidosis, but, once lost, tuberculin sensitivity is not usually regained even after apparent recovery. Superimposed infection with *M. tuberculosis* usually causes conversion to a positive tuberculin status but not invariably so. Cutaneous anergy extends to a wide group of bacterial, viral, and fungal antigens. Patients with sarcoidosis also exhibit a decreased capacity to become sensitized to 2,4-dinitrochlorobenzene and other contact sensitizers. Allergic reactions of the immediate histamine type with wheal and flare responses are unaffected in sarcoidosis.

Kveim Test. The Kveim test consists of the intracutaneous injection of a previously validated saline suspension of human sarcoidal tissue, usually of splenic or lymph node origin. The test suspensions are very stable and possess a high level of specificity. In responsive subjects, a slowly enlarging papule 3 to 8 mm. in diameter appears at the injection site, usually reaching its largest diameter in four to six weeks when a biopsy is performed. In a positive reaction, there are characteristically discrete epithelioid cell follicles which strongly mimic morphologically, histochemically, and ultrastructurally the epithelioid cell granulomas present in the organs.

Microscopically positive Kveim reactions are observed in about three fourths of patients with active sarcoidosis, but almost half of these patients lose their capacity to respond when retested after three to five years. False positive reactions are reported in 2 to 5 per cent of nonsarcoid subjects. Kveim reactivity is partially or completely depressed by corticosteroid therapy.

The pathogenesis of the Kveim reaction is ill understood, but it is generally interpreted as an immunologic response. However, no specific antibody has yet been demonstrated nor is it known whether the active principle in the Kveim suspensions is truly an antigen. Available data suggest that the active principle is of protein nature. Supplies of standardized Kveim suspensions are not yet commercially available and remain scarce.

DIAGNOSIS

A definitive diagnosis of sarcoidosis depends upon the correlation of a characteristic constellation of systemic organ involvement with the demonstration of epithelioid cell granulomas on organ biopsy or in an excised Kveim papule. The initial clue to the diagnosis is often the chance discovery of bilateral hilar adenopathy with or without pulmonary mottling in an asymptomatic patient who has undergone routine chest roentgenography. When the finding is associated with skin anergy, erythema nodosum, acute bilateral uveitis, or swelling of salivary or lacrimal glands or a Bell's palsy, the clinical diagnosis of sarcoidosis is almost assured. Histologic corroboration by means of organ biopsy or a positive Kveim test when validated suspensions are available closes the diagnostic circle.

Biopsy Procedures. In the early subacute stage when intrathoracic localization alone may be apparent, fruitful sources of tissue biopsy include mediastinal node biopsy via mediastinoscopy, scalene fat pad biopsy, random biopsy of striated muscle especially in patients with erythema nodosum, and biopsy of old cutaneous scars showing recent swelling. Needle aspiration of the liver is of value when there is a typical clinical pattern of sarcoidosis, but in atypical cases it is less useful because granulomas are encountered in many hepatic disorders unrelated to sarcoidosis. Later in the subacute stage, it is frequently possible to perform biopsies of palpable peripheral lymph nodes or of enlarged lacrimal glands and to make random biopsies of the palatal mucosa. In the presence of pulmonary mottling, random bronchoscopic biopsy may be done, in which normal-appearing bronchial mucosa is removed from multiple carinal sites. Open lung biopsy may occasionally become necessary when other histologic confirmation is lacking or when the roentgenographic pattern of lung involvement suggests several diagnostic possibilities.

In the chronic stage, biopsy of cutaneous lesions and enlarged peripheral nodes is most useful. Biopsy of bronchial mucosa, nasal mucosa, lung, lacrimal gland, and palatal mucosa is also applicable, especially when the Kveim reaction is no longer positive. The finding of acid-fast bacilli or fungi on tissue stain and culture may confirm the presence of tuberculosis, nontuberculous mycobacterial disease, or fungal disease. If the finding of acid-fast bacilli in tissues is associated with granulomatous lesions in the uveal tracts, salivary glands, striated muscle, or phalangeal bones, coexisting sarcoidosis is highly probable; this is especially the case if the delayed type of skin sensitivity to mycobacterial and fungal antigens is depressed.

Epithelioid cell granulomas with little or no necrosis are not pathognomonic of sarcoidosis and can be evoked by a host of agents. Their exclusion in patients presenting with clinical and roentgenographic patterns not entirely typical of sarcoidosis may present formidable difficulties. But in the case of cutaneous "sarcoid reactions," leprosy, and Crohn's disease involving small bowel, large bowel, and stomach, the absence of the distinctive systemic distribution of lesions found in sarcoidosis aids in their differentiation.

The chest roentgenographic patterns of beryllium disease, tuberculosis, lymphomatous disorders, and some fungal, viral, and bacterial infections may closely approximate that of sarcoidosis, and intensive search for the known agents may be required before a correct diagnosis can be established. These difficulties are heightened when extrathoracic lesions of sarcoidosis are associated with a normal chest x-ray pattern, a finding not unusual in patients with hypercalcemia, hypersplenism, isolated cutaneous sarcoidosis, and chronic neurologic involvement.

TREATMENT

Because of the predominantly asymptomatic nature of sarcoidosis and the high rate of spontaneous remission, less than 30 per cent of patients with sarcoidosis require treatment. The three effective agents most commonly employed are corticosteroids, chloroquine, and oxyphenbutazone. Their mode of action is suppressive rather than curative.

Corticosteroid Therapy. On serial biopsies the resolution and healing of epithelioid cell deposits under the influence of corticosteroids begin within ten days and have been found to be histologically similar to spontaneous healing. But with therapy the cicatrization and hyalinization are accelerated, occurring within weeks rather than in months and years. Hastening the healing process with corticosteroid treatment results in no greater scarring than occurs spontaneously. The lack of excessive scarring is clearly demonstrated in the reversal of fresh ocular lesions under therapy. Since corticosteroids suppress new granuloma formation, treated patients with widely distributed lesions have less scarring to contend with eventually than they might when granulomatous deposits are allowed to accumulate unhindered. Corticosteroids have no effect on lesions already scarred.

Indications for Corticosteroid Treatment. The indications for prompt therapy are ocular lesions, diffuse pulmonary lesions with symptoms of alveolar-capillary block, lesions in the central nervous system (meninges, brain, and spinal cord), myocardial lesions, splenic involvement with hypersplenism, and persistent hypercalcemia and hypercalciuria with renal damage. These indications apply to about 10 per cent of the patients.

In another 20 per cent, corticosteroids are also employed but only when clinical observations over several months indicate that the disease is progressing. In this category in which delay of therapy is permissible are patients with a slowly deteriorating pulmonary status, with persisting constitutional symptoms, with disfiguring lesions of the skin, salivary glands, and superficial lymph

nodes, with lesions of nasal, pharyngeal, and bronchial mucosa, and with persistent facial palsy and prolonged joint and muscle involvement.

Treatment is generally not required for patients with enlarged hilar nodes or those with localized pulmonary involvement which is asymptomatic, particularly when fibrosis or some regression has already taken place. Other manifestations which are left untreated because of their good outlook are erythema nodosum, minor superficial lymph node enlargement, asymptomatic hepatosplenomegaly, and isolated bone cysts. Even if the patient has asymptomatic miliary seeding in both lungs, one can temporize with corticosteroid therapy, as spontaneous resolution is observed frequently. But it is prudent to employ corticosteroids early when widespread flocculent infiltrations occupy large areas of lung parenchyma even when symptoms are minimal or absent. If such patients are left untreated, a fair proportion will exhibit diffuse fibrosis and pulmonary insufficiency within three to seven years.

Dosage. The proper dose of the hormone is the amount required to suppress the manifestation being treated. In sarcoidosis, relatively moderate initial and maintenance dosages are effective. The initial daily dose of prednisone and prednisolone is 20 to 30 mg., which is followed by a gradual drop to a maintenance level of 7.5 to 15 mg. a day, or double those amounts if alternate-day therapy is followed. Methyl prednisolone, triamcinolone, dexamethasone, and betamethasone may also be used in equivalent doses with maintenance dosage being kept at half or less the initial daily dose. Salt restriction and potassium supplements are sometimes necessary.

Duration of Treatment. Treatment usually extends over a period of six to nine months, but in patients with extensive progressive lesions therapy for a year or more may be required. Patients with late-stage pulmonary fibrosis may have to receive maintenance therapy for many years. When maximal enduring benefit appears to have been achieved, the drug is gradually tapered over a two- to four-week period. The side effects on these dosage schedules are few aside from Cushingoid facies, hirsutism, and occasionally retention of fluid. The incidence of pulmonary tuberculosis complicating sarcoidosis in corticosteroid-treated patients is the same as it is among untreated patients, amounting to less than 2 per cent in both groups.

Results of Corticosteroid Therapy. Regression of granulomatous lesions occurs within a month or two in relatively fresh lesions. In chronic pulmonary lesions with fibrosis and bullous transformation, relief of cough and dyspnea may be striking in spite of little roentgenographic change in the lung fields.

Relapse. Relapse after discontinuation of corticosteroids occurs in about half the treated group but, in the main, these relapses are mild and only half of the relapsed group require retreatment. Cutaneous sarcoids respond with regularity, but long-standing lesions have a strong tendency to recur once the drug is withdrawn. Because cutaneous lesions can be extremely unsightly, many patients accept long-term low-dosage maintenance therapy at slight risk rather than bear the disfigurement.

Chloroquine. Chloroquine is especially effective in chronic cutaneous sarcoidosis. However, occasional instances of toxic retinitis, which is irreversible, and corneal opacification, which is reversible, have to a degree discouraged the use of this agent in sarcoidosis. The usual dosage is 250 mg. once or twice a day.

Oxyphenbutazone. This anti-inflammatory agent is given in oral doses of 100 mg. four times a day and is especially employed in patients with lesions of less than one year's duration which require treatment. Like corticosteroids, oxyphenbutazone represses Kveim reactivity.

PROGNOSIS

The outcome of sarcoidosis is generally favorable, more than two thirds of the patients recovering completely or with inconsequential residua of healing. In less than 10 per cent of clinically recognized patients, there is a fatal course, 5 per cent resulting from sarcoidosis and less than 5 per cent from unrelated causes. The death rate in sarcoidosis is two and one-half times the predicted rate for all causes in the general population of similar makeup. This represents a significant excess of deaths in a disease often considered to be almost entirely benign. Deaths from sarcoidosis are predominantly caused by progressive pulmonary insufficiency and cor pulmonale, a lesser proportion dying of renal insufficiency resulting from persistent hypercalcemia, central nervous system lesions, and myocardial involvement. A sudden massive hemoptysis may be the terminal event in patients whose bullous air spaces have become colonized by *Aspergillus fumigatus* with the production of a mycetoma.

In general, patients whose pulmonary lesions clear or improve within the first year of observation have an excellent prognosis. A poorer outcome can be expected in patients with chronic lesions of two or more years' duration, among those with three or more organ systems involved, as well as among those whose lesions require sustained corticosteroid therapy for their control. Patients whose lesions undergo spontaneous regression infrequently experience recurrence of disease. But in a minority of patients a smoldering course with periodic flareups can span a decade or more.

James, D. G., Carstairs, L. S., Trowell, J., and Sharma, O. P.: Treatment of sarcoidosis: Report of a controlled therapeutic trial, Lancet, 2:526, 1967.

Proceedings of the Second International Conference on Sarcoidosis. Amer. Rev. Resp. Dis., 84(Suppl):1, 1961.

Proceedings of the Third International Conference on Sarcoidosis: Acta Med. Scand., 176(Suppl 425):1, 1964.

Proceedings of the Fourth International Conference on Sarcoidosis: *In* La Sarcoidose. Paris, Masson et Cie, 1967.

Proceedings of the Fifth International Conference on Sarcoidosis. Acta Univ. Carol. [Med.] Prague, 1, 1970 (Summary of Conference, Amer. Rev. Resp. Dis., 100:888, 1969).

Scadding, J. G.: Sarcoidosis, London, Eyre and Spottiswoode, 1967.

Siltzbach, L. E.: The Kveim test in sarcoidosis. A study of 750 patients. J.A.M.A., 178:476, 1961.

Siltzbach, L. E.: Sarcoidosis—Clinical features and management, Med. Clin. N. Amer., 51:483, 1967.

Lethal Midline Granuloma

Paul B. Beeson

Lethal midline granuloma is a horrid, rare, chronic destructive disease affecting the midline structures of the face and nearly always terminating in death. The process most often affects males aged 20 to 50 and usually begins with symptoms of nasal obstruction with purulent, sometimes bloody discharge. Months or years later the skin of the nose and inner eyelid become red, then necrotic, with the formation of fistulas and with progressive loss of facial tissue. Owing to a tendency to thrombosis of blood vessels it progresses by causing necrosis of hard or soft tissues leading to destruction of the nasal septum, the hard or soft palate, the paranasal sinuses, and the orbital cavities. There is little tendency for regional lymph nodes to become enlarged, and the process does not ordinarily affect the lungs. Pain and fever are variable. Death may result from inanition, hemorrhage, or sepsis (notably when the destructive process has exposed the meninges).

A disease conforming to the aforementioned description can be caused by several specific infections, e.g., syphilis, yaws, leprosy, mucormycosis, by carcinoma arising in the nose or paranasal sinuses, and by lymphomas. Sometimes despite prolonged and intensive study including repeated biopsy, the specific causes are identified only late in the disease or at autopsy. Some writers have classified lethal midline granuloma and Wegener's granulomatosis together, but that seems wholly unwarranted. Kassel and his colleagues take the view that most cases of lethal midline granuloma are forms of neoplastic disease, some of which eventually are found to resemble accepted types of lymphoma, others a less easily recognized form which has been called "polymorphic reticulosis."

As might be expected from scattered reports of an unusual clinical disorder probably comprising more than one pathogenetic entity, recommendations as to treatment have varied. Radiation therapy to the affected regions seems the procedure most likely to palliate or arrest the process. Occasional benefits from the use of cytotoxic drugs (cyclophosphamide, methotrexate, chlorambucil) are on record. Steroid hormones do not help. Antimicrobial therapy may be called for from time to time to combat secondary infection by bacteria or fungi.

Kassel, S. H., Echevarria, R. A., and Guzzo, F. P.: Midline malignant reticulosis (so-called lethal midline granuloma). Cancer, 23:920, 1969.
Eichel, B. S., and Mabery, T. E.: The enigma of lethal midline granuloma. Laryngoscope, 78:1367, 1968.

Wegener's Granulomatosis

Paul B. Beeson

The major pathologic lesion in Wegener's granulomatosis is a granuloma which tends to affect arterial walls, leading to necrosis. The principal sites of the lesions are in the upper and lower respiratory tract, but there is also a generalized vasculitis, which may severely damage the kidney.

Persons of both sexes and all ages are affected, but the highest incidence appears to be in mid-adult life. In the "classic" picture, i.e., that which was first delineated, the initial involvement is usually in the nose and paranasal sinuses. The patient suffers for some weeks or months because of nasal stuffiness and discharge and may have undergone a series of medical and surgical treatments for "sinusitis." Later there is extension to the lower respiratory tract, with symptoms and signs caused by single or multiple lesions in the lungs. This may lead to erroneous diagnosis of neoplastic disease. Vasculitis outside the respiratory tract may provide other manifestations: fever, weight loss, and various neurologic signs caused by localized lesions in the central or peripheral nervous system. The most sinister aspect of the disease is its tendency to cause diffuse glomerulitis, with severe impairment of renal function. The urine contains excess protein, red cells, and red cell casts. Renal failure is the most common cause of death in Wegener's granulomatosis. Hypertension rarely develops despite the severity of renal disease.

Limited Forms of Wegener's Granulomatosis. Carrington and Liebow have called attention to a group of cases in which the major pathologic change is in the lungs, and in which there is little evidence of disease in the nose or paranasal sinuses, or of generalized vasculitis. They have also described a subgroup, in which the histology is suggestive of lymphoma.

Diagnosis. The diagnosis can be suspected on clinical grounds but can only be made by histologic examination of affected tissue. Routine blood studies, including eosinophil counts, are usually normal. Biopsy from the nasal structures or lung will show the characteristic granuloma with special involvement of arteries and resulting tendency to necrosis. Biopsy of the kidney may show focal necrotizing glomerulitis.

Course. The illness is generally progressive; in most of the early case reports death occurred within a year of onset. As experience has grown, and particularly with recognition of the "limited forms," it has become apparent that some patients may live several years and that in some the disease may even go into long periods of remission. Generally, however, this still must be thought of as a disease which tends to progress and to end fatally within months or a year or two.

Treatment. No treatment has been satisfactory for either amelioration or arrest of the process. Most patients are treated with antimicrobials; these may be required from time to time to deal with secondary infections, but certainly do not affect the primary disease. Many patients have had steroid therapy without notable benefit. A trial of immunosuppressive drugs seems warranted in a disease with such discouraging outlook.

Carrington, C. B., and Liebow, A. A.: Limited forms of angiitis and granulomatosis of Wegener's type. Amer. J. Med., 41: 497, 1966.
Fahey, J. L., Leonard, E., Churg, J., and Godman, G.: Wegener's granulomatosis. Amer. J. Med., 17:168, 1954.

Some Uncommon Eosinophilic Syndromes

Paul B. Beeson

GENERAL CONSIDERATIONS

Many diseases characterized by eosinophilia are dealt with in other sections of this book, for example, parasitic infestations, polyarteritis nodosa, and Hodgkin's disease. In addition there remains a group of poorly understood, uncommon syndromes in which substantial eosinophilia is a striking clinical feature. Some of these will be described in this chapter, and some bibliographic citations are appended. It must be emphasized that these conditions almost certainly comprise a heterogeneous group; doubtless with further study better understanding and more rational classification will be possible.

Despite a considerable amount of investigation there remains a vast ignorance about the role of the eosinophil. In the minds of many people it is merely a granulocyte which stains peculiarly and tends to proliferate when an allergic reaction develops. It resembles the neutrophil in morphology and has similar phagocytic ability, but differs in possessing a peroxidase not found in the neutrophil, in having a crystalline structure (the internum) within its granules, and in its behavior after administration of adrenal cortical steroid. It tends to lodge in tissues that have contact with the environment and to congregate in the neighborhood of antigen-antibody complexes and to ingest them. Although much has been written about the relationship of the eosinophil to histamine, there is no convincing evidence in man that the eosinophil makes histamine, neutralizes histamine, or is subject to a chemotaxis by histamine.

Indubitably the behavior of eosinophils is altered in some allergic states and immune processes. Their number in the circulation increases, and this is almost certainly a reflection of increased production in the marrow. Common factors of many diseases characterized by eosinophilia are constant on repeated exposure to comparatively large quantities of foreign material. Recent work has shown that increased production of eosinophils by hematopoietic tissue follows the general pattern of immune responses and that it is mediated by the lymphocyte.

EOSINOPHILIC PULMONARY SYNDROMES

The term *Löffler's syndrome* is applied to a benign illness usually lasting less than a month, characterized by transient pulmonary infiltrations, low fever, and peripheral eosinophilia. Some instances of this are associated with parasitic infestations in which circulating parasites lodge in the lungs, causing inflammatory reactions there.

More often, however, the same clinical picture is found in patients who show no sign of parasitic infestation. A somewhat similar clinical picture may develop as a manifestation of sensitivity to nitrofurantoin.

A form of illness which resembles Löffler's syndrome except for longer duration and greater severity has been designated *pulmonary infiltration with eosinophilia or P.I.E. syndrome.* This can cause marked disability because of fever, cough, and breathlessness and can persist for some years. Here again there is no clue to the etiology.

A wide variety of etiologic entities goes by the name *tropical pulmonary eosinophilia.* Doubtless many of these are either parasitic disorders or allergic responses to an inhaled antigen. This term has been used so broadly that it has little more significance than "nephritis" or "dermatitis."

Some patients exhibit pulmonary infiltration and eosinophilia during the course of bronchial asthma or polyarteritis nodosa. These entities can usually be distinguished from the aforementioned syndromes.

Liebow and Carrington have described a group of patients who had chronic pneumonia characterized by infiltration with eosinophils. They make the point that, although there is usually an increased number of eosinophils in the blood, this is not always true; but on the basis of the lung lesions they use the diagnostic term *eosinophilic pneumonia.* The consistent anatomic feature is an alveolar exudate made up of a mixture of large mononuclear cells and eosinophils. In most cases of this type the etiology cannot be determined; certainly the clinical picture can be caused, among other things, by parasites, fungi, and drugs or other chemical agents.

EOSINOPHILIC SYNDROMES AFFECTING OTHER ORGAN SYSTEMS

Eosinophilic Endomyocardial Disease (Löffler's Endocarditis). Löffler described cases in which there was a marked and prolonged eosinophilia of the blood, associated with increasing cardiac disability. Autopsy in such cases discloses cellular infiltration of the myocardium and parietal endocardium in which eosinophils are prominent. Frequently there is also an eosinophilic infiltrate in other tissues. Differentiation between Löffler's myocarditis and diffuse eosinophilic collagen disease (see below) is sometimes impossible.

Eosinophilic Meningitis. From countries bordering on the Pacific come occasional case reports of a subacute meningitis characterized by pronounced eosinophilia in the cerebrospinal fluid. It seems likely that these are due to parasitic invasion of neural tissue, but proof of such an association is usually lacking despite intensive search. One such case, however, has been shown to be due to invasion of the human central nervous system by a rat lung-worm (see Microbial Diseases).

Eosinophilic Collagen Disease. A few cases are recorded in which multisystem illness resembling the connective tissue of "collagen" diseases has been accompanied by striking eosinophilia. Clinically these have shown greater resemblance to dermatomyositis than to other diseases of connective tissue in that muscle and joint pain have been especially prominent. In most of them the myocardium has been affected, but the kidneys have been spared.

Eosinophilic Leukemia and the Hypereosinophilic Syndromes. Whether there is such an entity as *eosinophilic leukemia* continues to provoke controversy. Numerous cases have been described under that title. They have been characterized by prolonged clinical course, marked elevation of the eosinophil count in blood and bone marrow, hepatomegaly, splenomegaly, and fatal termination; at autopsy eosinophilic infiltration of various tissues has been noted. Doubt has been expressed about the designation of leukemia in some of these, principally because the eosinophils in the blood and tissues are mature forms; nevertheless some of those reported seem to satisfy conventional criteria for the diagnosis.

Hardy and Anderson believe that it is possible to depict a broad spectrum of hypereosinophilic syndromes extending from the most benign, Löffler's syndrome, to a clinically malignant form often confused with eosinophilic leukemia. This last group is characterized by manifestations of cardiac and pulmonary infiltration as well as marked enlargement of the liver and spleen, and often terminates fatally. These authors liken the spectrum of hypereosinophilic syndromes to that of *Lichtenstein's histiocytosis X* which is thought to embrace a group of clinical disorders varying greatly in manifestations as well as in severity and prognosis.

Steroid Treatment in the Eosinophilic Syndromes. In this heterogeneous group of diseases the efficacy of steroid treatment has been variable. Sometimes there has been a prompt and dramatic response, with apparent clinical cure. In others prolonged therapy has been required to suppress the hepatic and pulmonary manifestations. In a further group steroid therapy has had little or no beneficial effect.

Benvenisti, D. S., and Ultmann, J. E.: Eosinophilic leukemia. Ann. Intern. Med., 71:731, 1969.

Crofton, J. W., Livingston, J. L., Oswald, N. C., and Roberts, A. T. M.: Pulmonary eosinophilia. Thorax, 7:1, 1952.

Hailey, F. J., Glascock, H. W., Jr., and Hewitt, W. F.: Pleuropneumonic reactions to nitrofurantoin. New Eng. J. Med., 281:1087, 1969.

Hardy, W. R., and Anderson, R. E.: The hypereosinophilic syndromes. Ann. Intern. Med., 68:1220, 1968.

Klein, N. C., Hargrove, L., Sleisenger, M. H., and Jeffries, G. H.: Eosinophilic gastroenteritis. Medicine, 49:299, 1970.

Liebow, A. A., and Carrington, C. B.: The eosinophilic pneumonias. Medicine, 48:251, 1969.

Pierce, L. E., Hosseinian, A. H., and Constantine, A. B.: Disseminated eosinophilic collagen disease. Blood, 29:540, 1967.

Reeder, W. H., and Goodrich, B. E.: Pulmonary infiltration with eosinophilia (PIE syndrome). Ann. Intern. Med., 36:1217, 1952.

Rosen, L., Chappell, R., Laqueur, G. L., Wallace, G. D., and Weinstein, P. P.: Eosinophilic meningoencephalitis caused by a metastrongylid lung-worm of a rat. J.A.M.A., 179:620, 1962.

Cranial Arteritis and Polymyalgia Rheumatica

(Temporal Arteritis, Giant Cell Arteritis, Arteritis of the Aged, Anarthritic Rheumatoid Disease)

Paul B. Beeson

The two clinical syndromes of cranial arteritis and polymyalgia rheumatica are described together, because they are often associated and because of the probability that they represent different expressions of one process. The age distribution of patients is almost unique, and the diseases seem to follow similar courses. Most persons affected are more than 60 years of age; occurrence before age 50 is exceedingly rare. Although symptoms may come on quite abruptly and may cause serious incapacity for a time, the natural tendency is toward gradual improvement, with complete subsidence after a few months or at most a few years. The remarkable age incidence and self-limited course must figure prominently in any attempt to determine the nature of these disorders.

POLYMYALGIA RHEUMATICA

Polymyalgia rheumatica is a distinctive kind of muscular rheumatism in old people, more frequent in women than in men. It is characterized by pain and stiffness in the neck, shoulders, and back, and sometimes of the pelvic girdle. Tenderness and true muscle weakness are usually lacking. The stiffness may be particularly troublesome in the morning so that patients are barely able to get out of bed. There may be headache or painful areas over the cranium. Systemic manifestations aside from occasional low-grade pyrexia are not prominent. The patients have a vague sense of malaise simply described as "feeling rotten." Unfortunately these people are too often dismissed as being complaining types or with the assumption that symptoms are caused by degenerative joint disease about which little or nothing can be done.

The distinctive laboratory finding is marked elevation of the erythrocyte sedimentation rate, i.e., more than 80 mm. by the Westergren method. Mild anemia is not uncommon, and some hematologists are reporting cases of unexplained anemia in old people which, like the muscular symptoms, respond promptly to steroid therapy. Other laboratory tests are of little help. Muscle biopsy generally reveals no significant inflammatory change even when the tissue is taken from areas which seem to be the site of much pain and stiffness. Blood enzymes which sometimes become elevated in other disorders of muscle are normal in this disease. There may be slight elevation of the alpha 2 globulin. Electromyographic findings are normal. The affected muscles do not atrophy.

Because of the frequent association of polymyalgia rheumatica with cranial arteritis, and especially because cranial arteritis may cause sudden blindness, some experienced clinicians believe that biopsy of a temporal artery should be carried out in all patients with polymyalgia rheumatica. Others regard this as unnecessary because a trial of steroid therapy, which would be effective for cranial arteritis as well as for the polymyalgia, will be carried out in any event.

In the differential diagnosis rheumatoid arthritis and degenerative joint disease may present problems; however, careful questioning and examination will show that polymyalgia is a disease of muscles, not joints. Various neoplastic diseases, including multiple myeloma, have to be considered in the differential diagnosis. Similarly the collagen diseases, especially dermatomyositis, may resemble polymyalgia rheumatica.

Therapy with adrenal steroids is remarkably effective, usually bringing about prompt amelioration of symptoms. It should be begun with a moderately large dose, e.g., 40 to 60 mg. of prednisone daily for the first week, with gradual reduction over the next few weeks to a maintenance dose of 7 to 12 mg. daily for four to six months. Treatment may be required at that level for long periods; usually the disease gradually subsides in six months to four years. There are cases on record, however, in which the symptoms have persisted for as long as ten years. Usually, by occasional trials of reduced dosage and by following the sedimentation rate, the physician can determine when to terminate steroid therapy.

Davison, S., and Spiera, H.: Concepts and treatment in polymyalgia rheumatica. J. Mt. Sinai Hosp., 35:473, 1968.

Dixon, A. St. J., Beardwell, A. K., Wanka, J., and Wong, Y. T.: Polymyalgia rheumatica and temporal arteritis. Ann. Rheum. Dis., 25:203, 1966.

Fessel, M. J., and Pearson, C. M.: Polymyalgia rheumatica and blindness. New Eng. J. Med., 276:1403, 1967.

Hunder, G. G., Disney, T. F., and Ward, L. E.: Polymyalgia rheumatica. Mayo Clin. Proc., 44:849, 1969.

CRANIAL (GIANT CELL) ARTERITIS

This entity, like polymyalgia rheumatica, occurs only in people past middle age. In a substantial proportion of cases, symptoms resembling those of polymyalgia rheumatica are present weeks or months before the onset of the severe headache which characterizes cranial arteritis. In contrast with polymyalgia rheumatica there is a distinctive histologic lesion in the large and medium-sized arteries of the upper part of the body, especially the temporal vessels.

Cranial arteritis often has an abrupt onset, with severe pain usually in one temple but sometimes in the occipital area, face, jaw, or side of the neck. This may be associated with exquisite hyperesthesia so that the patient dislikes touching the scalp, combing the hair, or washing. The pain may have a throbbing character. Pain in the tongue, blanching of the tongue, and even gangrene of the tongue have been described in this disorder, doubtless ascribable to involvement of lingual arteries. Peripheral neuropathy with both sensory and motor components has also been described. When the temporal artery is affected it may be tender, thickened, and nodular. Conversely the vessel may be pulseless and impalpable. The erythrocyte sedimentation rate is elevated, and there may be a substantial fever and polymorphonuclear leukocytosis.

The most feared complication of cranial arteritis is impairment of vision, as the blood supply to the retina can be affected. This may lead to sudden onset of blindness in one or both eyes. A precise estimate of the frequency of this complication cannot be made because patients with visual symptoms receive special medical attention. The danger is real, and it is generally agreed that all patients with active cranial arteritis should receive steroid treatment for some months, especially to prevent visual loss. There is also suggestive evidence that patients with cranial arteritis are at special risk of certain other vascular accidents, including cerebral and coronary occlusion.

Although it cannot be doubted that the arteries most often affected are branches of the external carotid (accounting for the use of such names as cranial arteritis and temporal arteritis), it should be recognized that other arteries may also be the site of giant cell arteritis. Autopsy has disclosed arteritis in the aorta and even in the hepatic and renal vessels. Instances of aortic aneurysm thought to be due to giant cell arteritis are on record.

Steroid therapy should be given according to the plan outlined for polymyalgia rheumatica and should be continued until all clinical and laboratory evidence of activity has subsided.

Harrison, M. J. G., and Bevan, A. T.: Early symptoms of temporal arteritis. Lancet, 2:638, 1967.

Ross Russell, R. W.: Giant-cell arteritis. Quart. J. Med., 28:471, 1959.

Fibrosing Syndromes

(Multifocal Fibrosclerosis)

Paul B. Beeson

In rare instances the delicate fibrous areolar tissue in certain anatomic regions becomes the site of a chronic low-grade inflammatory process, leading to deposition of dense sclerotic plaques, which may obstruct or limit the movement of adjacent viscera. When the process is in the active phase, there are characteristic findings of chronic or granulomatous inflammation, featured by mononuclear cell infiltration and occasional giant cells. In the end stages the pathologic lesion is simply that of scar tissue so that by the time this process causes clinical manifestations there may be little evidence of the initial inflammatory reaction. In most cases a clue to the inciting mechanism is lacking, hence the frequent use of the term "idiopathic" in describing the various syndromes. Indubitably this pattern of response may follow different kinds of injury. For example, there is an association between therapy with methysergide and some cases of retroperitoneal fibrosis, and the suggestion has been made that fibrosing mediastinitis can occur as a sequel to infection with *Histoplasma capsulatum*. Similarities in anatomic location and pathologic picture have led some writers to suggest that mesenteric panniculitis and retroperitoneal fibrosis may be steps of the same disease process.

Although most of these syndromes have been described as separate entities depending on the clinical manifestations and the interests of the writers who have reported them, it should be emphasized that several anatomic areas may become affected in one person. For example, retroperitoneal fibrosis and sclerosing mediastinitis may be present at the same time. Even more interesting is the report by Comings and his associates, of two brothers, offspring of a consanguineous marriage, who exhibited varying combinations of retroperitoneal fibrosis, mediastinal fibrosis, sclerosing cholangitis, Riedel's thyroiditis, and pseudotumor of the orbit (familial multifocal sclerosis). This remarkable constellation of syndromes in two siblings brings up the possibility of a genetic predisposition to disease of this character, but of course does not exclude other precipitating factors, e.g., common exposure to some chemical.

Retroperitoneal Fibrosis (Peri-ureteral Fibrosis). In retroperitoneal fibrosis the fibrosing process is most commonly located over the promontory of the sacrum with extension laterally to the ureters and up as high as the level of the second or third lumbar vertebra. Less commonly the lesion develops in other extraperitoneal areas, for example, contiguous with the kidneys, duodenum, descending colon, or urinary bladder.

In some cases there has been an associated vasculitis in the skin and subcutaneous tissues, manifested by the formation of nodules, erythematous discolorations, and ulcerations. Similarly, inflammatory changes in small vessels at the sites of the sclerosis have been noted.

The occurrence of retroperitoneal fibrosis in patients taking methysergide for migraine has been reported with greater frequency than could be due to chance, and that drug must be listed as one etiologic factor. It has also been thought that continued use of amphetamine compounds may evoke this process.

The manifestations of retroperitoneal fibrosis are variable, depending on the anatomic location of the process. Pain is the most common symptom; it is vague and tends to be located in the low back and may be accompanied by symptoms referable to the gastrointestinal tract. The patient is likely to lose weight and have low-grade fever. There may be some anemia and elevation of the erythrocyte sedimentation rate. Although the ureter is the structure most often affected, symptoms referable to the urinary tract are uncommon until obstructive uropathy has led to azotemia and other clinical manifestations of renal insufficiency. The fibrosing process may surround the inferior vena cava, but signs of obstruction of that vessel are uncommon; this contrasts with mediastinal fibrosis in which the most common expression is superior caval obstruction.

Diagnosis of retroperitoneal fibrosis is difficult because of the lack of localizing manifestations. It is most often suggested by the findings at intravenous pyelography: displacement of the ureters toward the midline and evidence of obstruction usually at the level of the pelvic brim. One or both ureters may be affected. Less often a mass can be palpated in the pelvis or on the posterior abdominal wall. Once the presence of a mass has been disclosed, by roentgenography, by palpation, or at laparotomy, the main problem in differential diagnosis lies in distinguishing retroperitoneal fibrosis from retroperitoneal tumor.

Surgical treatment, if employed before there has been severe renal damage, is often highly successful. Inasmuch as the fibrosing process is seldom invasive, the constricted organ can often be freed by blunt dissection so that normal movement or flow is restored. Paramount relief of ureteral obstruction is usually achieved simply by dissecting this structure free of its fibrous encasement and bringing it out on the anterior surface of the sclerotic mass. Occasionally, however, the obstruction recurs months or years after such treatment. The claim has been made that prolonged steroid therapy may be helpful, but the evidence for this is unconvincing, and prompt surgical relief should be attempted whenever the risk is not very great. When the inferior vena cava is obstructed, surgical relief is technically difficult and risky; here it may be preferable to temporize, in the hope that development of collateral pathways may alleviate the circulatory block.

The long-term outlook is fairly good if the disease is recognized and if its obstructive consequences can be treated suitably by surgical means. Prolonged observations of some successfully treated patients indicate that the disease tends to run its course and subside so that the life expectancy may not be shortened. Most deaths have been caused by renal failure.

Mediastinal Fibrosis. Taut bundles of collagenous tissue form in the superior and anterior mediastinum with impingement on the aorta, trachea, and pericardium, but the predominant manifestations are those caused by obstruction of the superior vena cava: puffy, suffused appearance of the face and conjunctivae, nonpitting edema of the face, neck, and upper extremities, and distended veins in the neck and upper extremities. The main task in differential diagnosis is to distinguish this relatively benign condition from obstruction caused by tumor. Roentgenographic examination of the chest may reveal little or no abnormality, but angiographic studies will show the obstruction of the superior vena cava and its large tributaries. Thoracotomy may be required for histologic diagnosis.

As already mentioned some evidence suggests that histoplasmosis may be a cause of mediastinal fibrosis; therefore it should be considered, and when tests for this infection are positive a trial of appropriate chemotherapy seems justified.

Some patients with this syndrome have shown gradual improvement over months or years, presumably because of development of collateral circulation. Attempts to remove the fibrosing tissues from the large veins are technically difficult and hazardous.

Sclerosing Cholangitis. A diffuse fibrous sheath sometimes envelops the common bile duct, the hepatic ducts, and the gallbladder. The clinical manifestations are pain and tenderness in the right upper quadrant and prolonged, gradually deepening jaundice. Liver function tests reveal changes of extrahepatic biliary obstruction. This condition may progress to death, with the picture of biliary cirrhosis.

Treatment is not very satisfactory. Steroid therapy has rarely seemed to help. It is suggested that prolonged T-tube drainage of the bile ducts may ameliorate the situation until the disease regresses.

Fibrosclerosis in Other Organs. *Riedel's thyroiditis* is a rare form of fibrotic disease affecting the structures in the anterior part of the neck. This differs from Hashimoto's thyroiditis in being equally common in males and females and in the tendency of the fibrotic process to involve not only the thyroid but also its neighboring structures.

Peyronie's disease is a sclerotic induration of the corpora cavernosa of the penis. This disease has been encountered in association with sclerosing processes in other parts of the body.

Pseudotumor of the orbit causes unilateral exophthalmos and is likely to be confused with tumor. It has been seen in association with Riedel's thyroiditis, as well as in other fibrosclerosing syndromes.

Dupuytren's contracture has been thought by some to be another expression of the systemic fibrosclerosing syndromes; however, it is so often independent that the case for similar pathogenesis seems weak.

Carton, R. W., and Wong, R.: Multifocal fibrosclerosis manifested by vena caval obstructions and associated with vasculitis. Ann. Intern. Med., 70:81, 1969.

Comings, D. E., Skubi, K. B., Van Eyes, J., and Motulsky, A. G.: Familial multifocal sclerosis. Ann. Intern. Med., 66:884, 1967.

Glenn, F., and Whitsell, J. C., III: Primary sclerosing cholangitis. Surg., Gynec. Obstet., 123:1037, 1966.

Hewlett, T. H., Steer, A., and Thomas, D. E.: Progressive fibrosing mediastinitis. Ann. Thorac. Surg., 2:345, 1966.

Packham, D. A., and Yates-Bell, J. G.: The symptomatology and diagnosis of retroperitoneal fibrosis. Brit. J. Urol., 40:207, 1968.

Salmon, H. W.: Combined mediastinal and retroperitoneal fibrosis. Thorax, 23:158, 1968.

CERTAIN CUTANEOUS DISEASES WITH SIGNIFICANT SYSTEMIC MANIFESTATIONS

Introduction
Clayton E. Wheeler, Jr.

The history of medicine contains numerous examples of diseases such as lupus erythematosus and sarcoidosis that were first described on the basis of their dermatologic characteristics but were later recognized as having important manifestations elsewhere in the body. Cutaneous lesions are in fact described in connection with scores of diseases classified in other parts of this textbook. The disorders presented in this section are often treated by the specialist in dermatology, but they deserve mention in a textbook of medicine because their pathogenesis may provoke lesions in organs other than the skin and because some knowledge of them is needed by the general practitioner or the specialist in internal medicine.

Cutaneous Manifestations of Internal Malignancy
Clayton E. Wheeler, Jr.

Skin manifestations of internal malignancy are of two types: those in which there is invasion with malignant cells and those in which malignant cells cannot be identified.

Almost any internal malignant process may invade the skin. Lymphomas, melanomas, and metastases from carcinoma of the breast, kidney, prostate, lung, bronchus, stomach, colon, thymus, ovary, and testicle are the most common. Infiltration with malignant cells may produce firm to hard, nontender macules, papules, nodules, tumors, or plaques, which may be skin-colored, pink, red, violet, brown, or black. Lesions may be single or multiple, intact or ulcerated. Alopecia may appear at the infiltrated site. An erysipelas- or scleroderma-like picture may be produced by lymphatic involvement, especially in carcinoma of the breast. Colored, configurate, or ulcerated lesions are more likely to occur in lymphomas, and the skin of generalized exfoliative dermatitis may contain lymphoma cells. All areas should be examined carefully when internal malignancy is suspected; lesions of the scalp, umbilicus, and anogenital region are frequently overlooked.

Tumor cells cannot be identified in the skin in a wide variety of cutaneous manifestations of internal malignancy. In most of these there is no real understanding of pathogenesis; hormonal, immunologic, enzymatic, and toxic mechanisms have been postulated. Although patterns produced in the skin are often highly suggestive of internal malignancy, they may also be caused by benign conditions. The relationship of the skin manifestation to malignancy has been proved in many instances by subsidence of cutaneous changes upon removal of the tumor and recurrence with tumor regrowth at the original or metastatic sites. Cutaneous changes may antedate, coincide with, or follow clinical diagnosis of malignancy. A brief account of these cutaneous manifestations follows.

Pruritus may be localized, generalized, intermittent, migratory, constant, mild, or severe. It may be unassociated with detectable abnormalities of the skin except for punctate and linear excoriations or prurigo-like nodules, or it may accompany lichenoid, eczematous, or bullous eruptions. It is often recalcitrant to the usual symptomatic measures; at times it can be relieved only by successful treatment of the underlying malignant disease. It is more common with lymphomas, especially Hodgkin's disease.

Pallor of anemia or, rarely, *erythema* and *cyanosis* of polycythemia may be present. A tan to dark brown color may result from diffuse *melanosis.* This may be localized to small areas or may be generalized with accentuation of normally hyperpigmented sites. The mechanism of melanosis is obscure in most carcinomas and lymphomas; infrequently, tumors that secrete melanocyte-stimulating hormone may be found. *Altered keratinization* may result in localized or diffuse dryness and scaling that may closely resemble ichthyosis. Hyperkeratosis of the palms and soles, alopecia, and varying degrees of cutaneous atrophy may also be present. This type of acquired ichthyosis is most likely to occur with Hodgkin's disease.

Toxic erythema, urticaria, erythema nodosum, or erythema multiforme may be due to any type of internal malignant disease. Chronic forms of erythema multiforme (figurate erythemas) characterized by persistent or migratory rings, arcs, or polycyclic lesions are suggestive of internal carcinoma.

Persistent, circumscribed, or diffuse *eczematous dermatitis* may signify internal malignancy. Pruritus, excoriation, lichenification, and secondary pyoderma may be present, especially if associated with lymphomas.

Generalized exfoliative dermatitis that may be associated with alopecia, loss of nails, lymphadenopathy, defective temperature regulation, and increased peripheral blood flow is more often a manifestation of lymphoma. Skin biopsy may show cells characteristic of the lymphoma or nonspecific inflammation.

Vesicular and *bullous eruptions* that resemble dermatitis herpetiformis, bullous pemphigoid, or pemphigus may be due to internal carcinoma or, less commonly, lymphoma.

Purpura may be due to vasculitis, thrombocytopenia, hypoprothrombinemia, and hypofibrinogenemia. *Migratory, superficial thrombophlebitis,* which is often refractory to treatment with anticoagulants, may affect the extremities or trunk. It may be due to carcinoma of the lung, stomach, ovary, or pancreas. In some instances there is an associated thrombocytosis.

Cold urticaria, acral cyanosis, or *gangrene* may occur in lymphomas or myelomas in association with cryoglobulinemia and macroglobulinemia.

Alopecia mucinosa is characterized by grouped follicular papules or plaques, usually on the scalp, face, or neck. Alopecia is due to mucinous degeneration of the hair follicle. In older patients the condition may be an early manifestation of mycosis fungoides or other lymphomas.

Acanthosis nigricans, as discussed elsewhere, is often associated with adenocarcinoma arising in the abdomen or pelvis.

Dermatomyositis in patients over 40 years of age is frequently associated with an internal malignant disease, usually carcinoma. Myopathy

without dermatitis, various neuropathies, and myasthenic states may also be associated with an internal malignant condition.

Clubbing of the digits, periostitis, osteoarthropathy, and *gynecomastia* may be associated with carcinoma of the lung or other tumors.

Pachydermoperiostosis is characterized by cutaneous thickening, coarsening of facial features, cutis verticis gyrata, keratosis of the palms, excessive sweating and sebaceous gland secretion, macroglossia, clubbing, osteoarthropathy, and enlargement of the hands. The condition may be confused with acromegaly. It is usually seen in males with carcinoma of the lung.

Reduced resistance to infection is frequently present in persons with internal malignant conditions, especially lymphomas. Pyodermas are likely to be deep and severe and may result in generalized infections, at times with more than one microbial species. There is an increased incidence of herpes zoster, which tends to be accompanied by a chickenpox-like eruption. Herpes simplex infections are more extensive, deeper, and longer in duration. Progressive vaccinia may occur. Complicating tuberculosis, moniliasis, histoplasmosis, cryptococcosis, aspergillosis, mucormycosis, and cytomegalic inclusion disease tend to be progressive and fatal.

Bowen's disease is characterized by one or more circumscribed, scaly, crusted, erythematous plaques that may resemble psoriasis or eczema. Lesions may be found anywhere on the skin and may occur on mucous membranes. Intra-epidermal carcinoma is present microscopically. A high percentage of these patients eventually develop internal carcinoma, which may not appear until years after the Bowen's disease.

Paget's disease usually produces eczematoid changes of the nipple as an indication of an underlying ductal carcinoma. Extramammary Paget's disease of the perineum or elsewhere is associated with carcinoma of underlying apocrine glands.

Primary amyloidosis associated with multiple myeloma may produce macroglossia, purpura, and waxy, flesh-colored papules, nodules, or plaques on the face, trunk, or extremities.

Hormone-secreting tumors may arise from endocrine glands, and malignant tumors arising in nonendocrine tissues may secrete hormones that are identical or closely related in activity to their normally secreted counterparts. An ever-increasing list of malignant tumors, usually carcinomas but some sarcomas, is involved. The cutaneous and other manifestations of these tumors correspond to the action of the particular hormone involved. Substances with activities similar to the following hormones may be produced: corticotrophin, melanocyte-stimulating hormone (MSH), estrogen, gastrin, erythropoietin, insulin, norepinephrine, antidiuretic hormone, thyroid-stimulating hormone, chorionic gonadotrophin, parathyroid hormone, and serotonin.

Gardner's syndrome is characterized by dominant inheritance, multiple cutaneous cysts, osteomas, and polyps in the colon. Carcinoma of the colon develops in over half of these patients by the age of 40.

Cormia, F. E., and Domonkos, A. N.: Cutaneous reactions to internal malignancy. Med. Clin. N. Amer., 49:655, 1965.

Greenberg, E., Divertie, M. B., and Woolner, L. B.: A review of unusual systemic manifestations associated with carcinoma. Amer. J. Med., 36:106, 1964.

Johnson, S. A. M.: The Skin and Internal Disease. New York, McGraw-Hill Book Company, 1967, pp 58–65

Lipsett, M. B., Odell, W. D., Rosenberg, L. E., and Waldmann,

T. A.: Humoral syndromes associated with nonendocrine tumors. Ann. Intern. Med., 61:733, 1964.

Plotnick, H., and Abbrecht, M.: Alopecia mucinosa and lymphoma. Arch. Derm. (Chicago), 92:137, 1965.

Rosato, F. E., Shelley, W. B., Fitts, W. T., Jr., and Miller, L. D.: Nonmetastatic cutaneous manifestations of cancer of the colon. Amer. J. Surg., 117:277, 1969.

Skog, E.: Cutaneous manifestations associated with internal malignant tumors with particular reference to vesicular and bullous lesions. Acta. Dermatovener. (Stockholm), 44:114, 1964.

Van Dijk, E.: Ichthyosiform atrophy of the skin associated with internal malignant disease. Dermatologica (Basel), 127: 413, 1963.

Erythemas

Clayton E. Wheeler, Jr.

Disorders to be discussed under this heading are toxic erythema, erythema multiforme, and erythema nodosum. Urticaria, a close relative, is described elsewhere. Although the erythemas vary in morphology, there are features which group them into a common category. All result from reactions of small blood vessels in the skin or subcutaneous tissue. All are doubtless secondary manifestations of a wide variety of underlying disorders, although in many instances the basic condition cannot be identified. Finally, a given underlying disorder (drug reaction, for example) may cause toxic erythema, erythema multiforme, erythema nodosum, or urticaria in different individuals or simultaneous combinations of these vascular reactions in a single individual.

TOXIC ERYTHEMA

Toxic erythema is an extremely variable eruption that ranges from diffuse faint erythema to a generalized morbilliform exanthem. It is secondary to a wide variety of disorders, the most common of which are drug reactions and microbial diseases. Almost any drug may be incriminated, and infection with almost any organism may be involved. In addition, the eruption may be associated with foods and with noninfectious systemic diseases such as lymphomas, internal malignant processes, and the diseases of connective tissue. In a significant number of patients the underlying condition cannot be determined. When the causative disorder is established, the term toxic erythema is frequently discarded in favor of an etiologic diagnosis. Some examples of this are scarlet fever, infectious mononucleosis, and drug reactions.

Cutaneous manifestations result from vascular dilatation and mild inflammation in and about small blood vessels. Pathogenesis is often uncertain and probably varies with the underlying cause. Vascular changes may result from toxins, hypersensitivity reactions, or direct involvement with infectious agents.

Onset is usually abrupt with the appearance of diffuse erythema or erythematous macules. Small areas may be involved initially, but the eruption tends to become generalized and may be universal. In some instances there is a characteristic pattern of distribution and evolution—e.g., measles, scarlet fever, and erythema infectiosum—and in others there is random distribution. There is a tendency for the eruption to begin and to remain more intense at sites of minor irritation. Diffuse eruptions may be faint pink or bright red and are often scarlatiniform. Macular eruptions frequently coalesce to produce a morbilliform pattern. Erythema usually disappears with pressure on the skin, but a purpuric component may be present. Mild eruptions are transient and disappear without sequelae, whereas more severe reactions last for several days, and are followed by scaling or desquamation. The cutaneous changes may induce no symptoms or various degrees of itching, burning, or chilliness. Conjunctivitis is a common accompaniment, and the oral or genital mucous membrane may be involved.

Systemic manifestations depend primarily upon the underlying disorder. Fever is common, and chills may occur. Lymphadenopathy is frequent. Arthralgia or arthritis is occasionally present. Leukocytosis or leukopenia occurs, and the differential count may be abnormal.

The diagnosis depends upon clinical manifestations. Sometimes the eruption is so characteristic as to indicate the nature of the underlying disorder, but more often it is nonspecific. Final diagnosis of the primary condition depends upon careful history, physical examination, and laboratory study.

The primary objective of treatment is elimination of the underlying disease. Treatment of the cutaneous component is unnecessary in mild instances. In more severe cases symptomatic measures such as colloidal baths, topical calamine liniment, and oral antihistaminics may be helpful.

Dry, scaly skin may be benefited by application of a bland emollient.

ERYTHEMA MULTIFORME

Definition. Erythema multiforme is an acute inflammatory systemic disease that produces a spectrum of clinical patterns from a few inconsequential lesions on skin or mucous membrane to a severe, sometimes fatal multisystem disorder. The disorder is a symptom complex secondary to a wide variety of diseases and conditions.

Division of the disease into types such as erythema multiforme minor (Hebra) or erythema multiforme major (*Stevens-Johnson syndrome*) based on the severity or extent of the morbid process seems only to confuse the picture. The disease pattern in many instances falls between these extremes and therefore defies classification into such a scheme. Although of historical importance, synonyms such as *ectodermosis erosiva pluriorificialis, dermatostomatitis, new eruptive fever,* and *mucosal-respiratory syndrome* offer no special advantage. Descriptive titles such as erythema multiforme iris, erythema multiforme bullosum, and erythema multiforme exudativum place too much emphasis upon single morphologic features.

Etiology. There are two main theories concerning etiology: (1) The disease has a single cause, probably some infectious agent. (2) It is a symptom complex secondary to a variety of underlying disease states. In favor of the single cause theory is a close clinical resemblance to the acute exanthems. Efforts to identify specific bacterial, fungal, or viral agents have been negative or inconclusive, and there is no epidemiologic evidence that the disease is contagious. The symptom complex theory finds support in the large number of conditions with which erythema multiforme has been associated. An incomplete list of these follows: (1) microbial diseases including pneumonia, meningitis, cholera, glanders, typhus, measles, mumps, herpes simplex, vaccinia, orf, mycoplasmal pneumonia, lymphogranuloma venereum, psittacosis, and malaria; (2) drug reactions from antimicrobials, anticonvulsants, codeine, thiouracil, arsenic, barbiturates, antipyrine, belladonna, quinine, mercury, aspirin, butazolidine, chlorpropamide, and antitoxins; (3) vaccination against poliomyelitis, smallpox, or tuberculosis (BCG); (4) internal malignant conditions, including carcinoma and lymphoma; (5) deep x-ray therapy; (6) contact dermatitis, especially poison ivy; and (7) connective tissue disease.

Present consensus is that erythema multiforme is always secondary, but there remains a significant number of cases in which no underlying cause can be identified despite extensive diagnostic effort.

Incidence and Prevalence. Figures are heavily weighted in favor of the unusually severe forms of the disease, e.g., Stevens-Johnson syndrome, which are reported in preference to milder examples. If all degrees of severity are included, erythema multiforme is a common disease. Severe forms are rare in infancy, early childhood, and old age, and males are affected about twice as often as females. The disease is worldwide and there is no racial predilection.

Pathology. Nonspecific inflammatory changes secondary to vasculitis are present in skin, mucous membranes, and internal organs. The degree of inflammation correlates with clinical manifestations. The pathogenesis is incompletely understood. A symptom complex secondary to many diseases and drug reactions points to a mechanism of toxicity or hypersensitivity. The relatively common simultaneous occurrence with erythema nodosum and the frequent appearance of urticarial lesions in mild forms of erythema multiforme are further reasons to consider hypersensitivity. The appearance of the disorder a few days to three weeks after herpes simplex, vaccination for smallpox, infection with *Coccidioides immitis,* administration of penicillin, contact dermatitis from poison ivy, or deep x-ray therapy suggests that immunologic mechanisms play a role. The development of erythema multiforme after administration of antipyrine to certain persons, especially Negroes, may indicate that genetic enzymatic defects or differences are involved.

Clinical Manifestations. Perhaps half the patients experience a prodromal period of a day to two weeks, characterized by fever, malaise, cough, coryza, sore throat, chest pain, vomiting, muscular aches, and arthralgia in various combinations and severity. Following this, or in patients without prodrome, skin or mucous membrane lesions develop suddenly, together with some systemic reaction and often with evidence of visceral involvement.

Skin lesions are often the first and sometimes the only clinically detectable manifestations of the disorder. They usually develop rapidly, are distributed symmetrically and in crops. There may be few lesions, or almost the entire skin may be involved. There is a predilection for wrists, backs of the hands, ankles, tops of the feet, knees, elbows, face, palms, and soles. No area is exempt, although the scalp is affected infrequently. The polymorphous eruption usually includes red or violet macules, wheals, papules, vesicles, and bullae in various combinations. When vesicles and bullae are present they usually develop in pre-existing macules, papules, or wheals. Hemorrhage into the affected areas is common. Lesions are usually sharply demarcated from normal skin and tend to assume an annular configuration. Merging produces gyrate, serpiginous, or arciform patterns. At times central fluid-containing areas are surrounded by concentric rings of varying shades of erythema; these are the *target, iris,* or *bull's eye* forms which should bring the consideration of erythema multiforme into focus. As the disease progresses, erosions, superficial ulcerations, crusts which are often hemorrhagic, and scaling areas may occur. Paronychias and shedding of nails occur in severe cases. In mild cases healing takes place in a few days to three weeks without scarring, although hyperpigmentation or depigmentation may persist much longer. In severe cases scarring may result, and healing may take six weeks or more.

Mucous membrane involvement usually accompanies the cutaneous eruption, but in mild forms either may occur separately. One or all mucous membranes may be affected, and few or many lesions may be present. The spectrum includes macular erythema, edema, vesiculation, bleb formation, erosion, ulceration, crusting, fissuring, and bleeding. On mucous membranes vesicles and bullae rupture early, forming erosions or ulcerations. A gray or white pseudomembrane may form at the sites of previous blisters, especially in the mouth. The mouth is the most commonly involved orifice. In severe cases the lips are red, swollen, fissured, eroded, and covered with a bloody crust. The gums are swollen, eroded, and bleed easily. The tongue, buccal mucosa, pharynx, and larynx show any or all of the mucous membrane changes described above. As a result there may be pain, difficulty in eating and drinking, salivation, fetor oris, and hoarseness. Depending upon severity, the process lasts a few days to several weeks and usually heals without scarring. Lesions in the nose cause bleeding, crust formation, and obstruction. Tenesmus and bleeding may accompany anal disease. Urethral lesions, especially in the male, may cause dysuria, hematuria, pyuria, and even urinary retention in severe instances. Balanitis has led to adherence of glans to prepuce, and in females vulvovaginitis can result in formation of fibrotic bands or in partial stenosis of the vagina.

The eye is the site of attack almost as often as the mouth. The eyelids may be swollen and covered with any of the various skin lesions. Mild cases show transitory conjunctivitis. Purulent or membranous conjunctivitis is present in more severe instances. Subconjunctival hemorrhage occurs, and vesicles and bullae may appear. The cornea is usually spared except in severe cases, when it may be eroded or perforated. Iritis, iridocyclitis, and panophthalmitis have been seen. Inflammation usually subsides in a few days in mild cases but may persist for weeks. Partial or complete loss of vision may result from scarring of the cornea or panophthalmitis. Adhesions of bulbar to palpebral conjunctiva have occurred. Severe ocular damage has been less frequent since the advent of antimicrobial drugs.

Systemic manifestations may occur at any time in relation to skin or mucosal manifestations. Symptoms include fever, malaise, dehydration, muscle and joint pains, toxemia, and prostration. Respiratory manifestations include cough with or without sputum, hemoptysis, dyspnea, cyanosis, bronchitis, pneumonitis, pulmonary consolidation, and pleural effusion. Arthralgia and arthritis, often of multiple joints, have occurred frequently. Possible gastrointestinal symptoms are nausea, vomiting, dysphagia, hematemesis, abdominal pain, diarrhea, and melena. Inflammatory changes of the esophagus or colon account for most of these symptoms. Urinary tract findings have included albuminuria, hematuria, urinary retention, and anuria. Nephritis and uremia may develop, at times when skin and mucous membrane lesions are improving. Nervous system symptoms have been drowsiness, convulsion, confusion, coma, delirium, radiculitis, nystagmus, unequal pupils, and abnormal tendon reflexes. Cardiac arrhythmia, pericarditis, and electrocardiographic changes suggesting myocarditis have occurred. Regional lymphadenopathy has been common but generalized lymphadenopathy infrequent. Splenic and hepatic enlargement are rare. Endoscopic examinations have shown annular, erosive, or ulcerative pseudomembranous lesions of the esophagus, larynx, and colon.

Toxic epidermal necrolysis (scalded skin syndrome) may be a variant of erythema multiforme or a disease in its own right. It is characterized by ease of separation of top layers from underlying layers of epidermis. In adults it is often drug-induced; in children it is often due to staphylococcal infection. Erythema and tenderness are followed by the formation of large, denuded areas and flaccid bullae. The Nikolsky sign (see Pemphigus) is positive. Patients present varying degrees of toxicity and fever. Mortality rate is approximately 25 per cent. Treatment is the same as for erythema multiforme.

No laboratory test is specific for erythema multiforme. Abnormalities depend upon structures involved and degree of damage. Some degree of leukocytosis is common although the leukocyte count may be normal or decreased. Eosinophilia occurs occasionally. The platelet count is usually normal but it may be much decreased. Rarely, tourniquet tests are positive. Albuminuria, pyuria, hematuria, and casts are not uncommon. On rare occasions there may be increased cells and protein in the cerebrospinal fluid. Roentgenograms of the chest may show patchy pneumonitis or changes similar to those of mycoplasmal pneumonia. Electrocardiographic abnormalities include conduction defects and alterations suggesting myocarditis. Laboratory studies for infectious agents, tumors, and "collagen diseases" may establish the underlying cause.

Diagnosis. The diagnosis depends upon the presence of skin and mucous membrane lesions. An incomplete symptom complex without involvement of skin or mucous membrane has not been recognized. Polymorphous skin lesions that form annular and configurate patterns and bullous erosive involvement of mucous membranes usually differentiate erythema multiforme from the acute exanthems. *Pemphigus* is more protracted in course, usually exhibits less polymorphism and configuration, and skin biopsy shows acantholysis. *Pemphigoid* and *bullous dermatitis herpetiformis* are more chronic, have less mucous membrane involvement and fewer systemic symptoms, and biopsy may be helpful. *Bullous contact dermatitis* can usually be distinguished by location and configuration suggesting external factors, by lack of mucous membrane or systemic involvement, and by history and patch test. *Lymphomas* at times give rise to polymorphous skin lesions, but the clinical picture and biopsy usually suffice for differentiation. Severe forms of erythema multiforme may be confused with *septicemia* or *systemic lupus erythematosus,* but consideration of the nature of skin and mucous membrane involvement and other clinical and laboratory findings makes differential diagnosis possible.

Treatment. Underlying disease should be sought and eliminated when possible. Mild erythema multiforme requires little treatment: topical application of calamine liniment, oral antihistamines, and colloidal baths. Severe forms of the disorder require prompt active treatment of many types. Fluid and electrolyte imbalance due to improper intake, vomiting, diarrhea, and renal dysfunction must be corrected. Secondary bacterial infection, especially of the eye, in which staphylococcal infection may be prominent, must be combated with topical or systemic antimicrobials or both. High doses of corticotrophin or adrenal steroids are often helpful in severe erythema multiforme and usually need be given only for short periods of time.

Prognosis. Data concerning duration, complications, recurrences, and mortality are generally based upon studies of patients with severe forms of the disease (Stevens-Johnson syndrome). They are worthless therefore in considering erythema multiforme as a whole. Mild forms, which constitute the majority of cases, subside in a few days to two or three weeks without sequelae. Severe forms last three to six weeks or longer; sequelae include neurologic changes, corneal opacities, blindness, keratoconjunctivitis sicca, conjunctival, vaginal, or preputial synechiae, and esophageal strictures. When all forms of erythema multiforme are included, the mortality rate is low (less than 0.5 per cent). The mortality rate of severe cases has been reported as high as 10 per cent. Treatment appears to decrease the duration and severity of the disease and the mortality rate. Recurrences are likely in some forms of the disease (reports give recurrence rates as high as 25 per cent). The pattern of recurrence is variable. Some attacks are severe and some mild; some patients have only skin or mucous membrane changes, and others have most of the features of the symptom complex.

ERYTHEMA NODOSUM

Definition. Erythema nodosum is probably a hypersensitivity reaction characterized by inflammatory nodules in the dermis and subcutaneous tissue. It is regarded as secondary to a variety of underlying disorders, especially bacterial, fungal, and viral infections, and drug reactions.

Etiology. In the light of present knowledge, the cause should be regarded as hypersensitivity

vasculitis due to a multiplicity of diseases and conditions, the commonest of which are viral, bacterial, and fungal infections, and drug reactions. Among the associated disorders are tuberculosis, streptococcal pharyngitis, primary atypical pneumonia, leprosy, whooping cough, gonorrhea, lymphogranuloma venereum, measles, cat scratch disease, histoplasmosis, coccidioidomycosis, trichophytosis, chronic ulcerative colitis, syphilis, sarcoidosis, and reactions to iodides, oral contraceptives, sulfonamides, bromides, salicyclic acid, arsphenamine, phenacetin, or other drugs. In spite of extensive clinical study, an underlying disorder cannot be diagnosed in one quarter to one half of the patients. This probably reflects inability to recognize a primary condition and does not mean that erythema nodosum is a disease *sui generis.*

Incidence and Prevalence. The disorder occurs at any age but is rare in early childhood and in the elderly. After puberty it is considerably more common in women. The underlying cause varies from one geographic area to another. Thus, in New England, streptococcal pharyngitis is regarded as the commonest cause; in Scandinavia, primary tuberculous infection is frequently the underlying disorder; and in the San Joaquin Valley of California, primary infection with *Coccidioides immitis* is the most common cause.

Pathology. The pathologic picture is characteristic irrespective of the underlying cause. Inflammatory changes appear in the upper subcutaneous tissue and the dermis. Vasculitis, especially endothelial reaction in veins, is associated with infiltration with neutrophils, lymphocytes, histiocytes, and, occasionally, eosinophils. In later stages lymphocytes, epithelioid cells, and foreign body giant cells predominate.

Pathogenesis. The extensive epidemiologic and clinical studies of coccidioidomycosis carried out in California have provided useful information on the pathogenesis of one form of erythema nodosum. Typical skin lesions develop in approximately one of twenty persons during primary infection with this fungus. Lesions make their appearance ten to twenty days after the onset of the infection, at about the same time the coccidioidin skin test becomes positive. Erythema nodosum accompanied by a strongly positive skin test indicates an excellent prognosis for complete recovery from the fungal infection. This seems to link the cutaneous nodules with the delayed, or tuberculin, type of sensitivity reaction. Complement-fixing antibodies appear in the serum much later in the course of coccidioidomycosis and, therefore, seem unrelated. In tuberculosis, also, erythema nodosum appears at about the time the skin test becomes positive; in fact, skin tests with tuberculin may precipitate or aggravate the disorder.

Clinical Manifestations. Erythema nodosum is characterized by red, tender nodules which usually develop in skin and subcutaneous tissue over the shins. The anterior thighs and extensor surfaces of the forearms are not uncommonly involved, and more rarely lesions appear on the backs of the upper arms and about the head, face, and eyes. A few to several dozen lesions appear, often in crops. The lesions are usually discrete, and an individual nodule reaches 2 to 5 cm. in diameter or larger. As the lesion develops it becomes red, hot, and tender; as it involutes, the bright red color gives way to darker red and finally varying shades of green or yellow which simulate a bruise. During healing a fine cigarette-paper scale may appear on the surface. Individual lesions last a few days to two or three weeks, and usually heal without suppuration, depression, or scar formation.

Many of the symptoms associated with erythema nodosum are doubtless due to the underlying disorder or to the hypersensitivity reaction of which the cutaneous nodules are but one manifestation. There may be no systemic symptoms or varying degrees of malaise, chills, fever, sore throat, and cough. Cervical lymphadenopathy is common. Joint symptoms, present in about 75 per cent of patients, may precede, coincide with, or follow skin lesions, and they range from arthralgia to arthritis. Joint involvement has probably led to the idea that erythema nodosum is a manifestation of rheumatic fever, but follow-up studies indicate that there is only an occasional association.

Transient albuminuria and mild secondary anemia may be present. The total leukocyte count may be normal, decreased, or increased. The sedimentation rate is often elevated, and gamma globulin may be increased. Depending upon the underlying disease, skin tests with tuberculin, coccidioidin, and streptococcal antigens are positive. Chest roentgenograms have shown hilar lymphadenopathy and various types of pulmonary infiltration and pleural reaction. The electrocardiogram is usually normal.

Diagnosis. Clinical manifestations usually suffice for diagnosis. Biopsy is rarely necessary. The inflammatory lesions of adipose tissue that occur in *Weber-Christian disease* usually appear on the thighs although other areas of subcutaneous or visceral fat may be involved. These lesions tend to break down and discharge an oily liquid, and involution is usually associated with a depressed scar. *Erythema induratum* affects the calves more than pretibial regions, and the lesions are more indolent, often ulcerate, and heal with scarring. The shape of the lesion of *migratory*

thrombophlebitis often proclaims its association with a blood vessel. Nodules of *sarcoidosis, polyarteritis nodosa*, and *metastatic neoplasm* occasionally simulate erythema nodosum on the legs or other sites.

Treatment. The most important aspect of management is identification of the underlying cause. Symptomatic treatment for the erythema nodosum, such as bed rest, salicylates, or other analgesics, is usually sufficient. Corticotrophin or adrenal cortical steroids cause involution of the lesions, but these agents are indicated only in the most severe cases and should be used only when the underlying disease will not be worsened by them.

Prognosis. Erythema nodosum usually disappears in three or four weeks, but perhaps 10 per cent of the patients have continuing croplike appearance of new lesions or recurrences after free intervals.

Erythema Multiforme

Bloom, A., and Lovel, T. W. L.: Erythema multiforme with renal and myocardial injury. Proc. Roy. Soc. Med., 57:175, 1964.

Comaish, J. S., and Kerr, D. N. S.: Erythema multiforme and nephritis. Brit. Med. J., 2:84, 1961.

Lowney, E. D., Baublis, J. V., Kreye, G. M., Harrell, E. R., and McKenzie, A. R.: The scalded skin syndrome in small children. Arch. Derm. (Chicago), 95:359, 1967.

Ludlam, G. B., Bridges, J. B., and Benn, E. C.: Association of Stevens-Johnson syndrome with antibody for *Mycoplasma pneumoniae*. Lancet, 1:958, 1964.

Lyell, A., Dick, H. M., and Alexander, J.: Outbreak of toxic epidermal necrolysis associated with staphylococci. Lancet, 1:787, 1969.

Lyell, A., Gordon, A. M., Dick, H. M., and Sommerville, R. G.: The role of *Mycoplasma pneumoniae* infection in erythema multiforme. Proc. Roy. Soc. Med., 61:1330, 1968.

Shelley, W. B.: Herpes simplex virus as a cause of erythema multiforme. J.A.M.A., 201:153, 1967.

Erythema Nodosum

Browne, S. G.: Erythema nodosum in leprosy. J. Chronic Dis., 16:23, 1963.

Fine, R. M., and Meltzer, H. D.: Chronic erythema nodosum. Arch. Derm. (Chicago), 100:33, 1969.

Pinski, J. B., and Stansifer, P. D.: Erythema nodosum as the initial manifestation of leukemia. Arch. Derm. (Chicago), 89:339, 1964.

Riska, N., and Selroos, O.: Clinically diagnosed sarcoidosis in Finland in 1960. Acta Tuberc. Scand., 44:267, 1964.

Sams, W. M., Jr., and Winkelmann, R. K.: The association of erythema nodosum with ulcerative colitis. South. Med. J., 61:676, 1968.

Sellers, T. F., Jr., Price, W. N., Jr., and Newberry, W. M., Jr.: An epidemic of erythema multiforme and erythema nodosum caused by histoplasmosis. Ann. Intern. Med., 62:1244, 1965.

Weinstein, L.: Erythema nodosum. D. M., 1-30, June 1969.

Contact Dermatitis
(Dermatitis Venenata)
Clayton E. Wheeler, Jr.

Definition. Contact dermatitis is an inflammatory, frequently eczematous dermatitis that results from contact of the skin surface with a variety of substances. It is usually classified as (1) allergic contact dermatitis, (2) primary irritant dermatitis, or (3) contact photodermatitis.

ALLERGIC CONTACT DERMATITIS

Etiology. A specific sensitization process is required for the development of allergic contact dermatitis, which appears to be a form of delayed hypersensitivity.

Although almost anything that touches the skin of man may induce or elicit allergic contact dermatitis, several broad groups of substances are frequently involved. These include cosmetics, clothing, dyes, topical medicaments, industrial chemicals, plants, insecticides, detergents, cleansers, foodstuffs, costume jewelry, paints, varnishes, lacquers, rubber, and plastics.

Incidence and Prevalence. Allergic contact dermatitis, a common disorder, affects both sexes and all races. It is rare in infancy and unusual in early childhood, and the incidence declines in old age. Many occupations provide special exposure that results in contact dermatitis.

Pathology. Allergic contact dermatitis shows spongiosis (intracellular edema) and intraepithelial vesicle formation with many mononuclear cells in the vesicles. Edema and perivascular infiltrate with mononuclear cells appear in the dermis.

Pathogenesis. Four phases are recognized during sensitization: (1) In the *refractory phase* the allergen contacts the skin without initiating sensitization. This phase lasts usually a few days to a few weeks, but substances that have touched the skin for years may finally sensitize. Materials that sensitize a high percentage of contacts (strong sensitizers) tend to initiate the process rapidly; weak sensitizers may contact the skin over prolonged periods before sensitizing. Some patients may never become sensitive even after multiple exposures to strong sensitizers, some become sensitive quickly upon exposure to weak sensitizers, and some show weak reactions to strong agents or vice versa. Both sensitizer and person, as well as the degree and manner of exposure, are important in the net result. In addition, damaged skin appears to become sensitized more easily than normal skin. (2) The *period of incubation* is the time between onset of sensitization and clinical evidence of sensitivity. This interval may be as short as 5 days or as long as several weeks, but it is usually between 7 and 21 days. The refractory phase plus the period of incubation results in an interval of 10 days to several weeks between initial exposure and evidence of sensitivity. If

allergic contact dermatitis appears within 5 days after exposure, prior sensitivity existed to the agent or a close chemical relative. (3) The *reaction time* is the interval between exposure to the allergen and development of dermatitis in a sensitized person. The usual interval is 24 to 48 hours, but it may be less than 12 hours or more than 90. An important point is that there is always a latent interval between exposure and clinical evidence of dermatitis. (4) The *period of persisting sensitivity* is usually months or years and may be a lifetime.

The hypersensitivity produced is specific for the allergen involved or for close chemical relatives (cross-sensitivity). There are many examples of cross-sensitization, but only one will be given here: Primary sensitization to benzocaine may result in sensitivity to procaine, paraphenylenediamine, para-aminobenzoic acid, and the sulfonamides. The phenomenon of cross-sensitization introduces a complicating factor in diagnosis and treatment since the patient now reacts to many substances, and removal of the original allergen may not eliminate the dermatitis because of unrecognized continued exposure to chemical relatives.

Allergic contact dermatitis is usually restricted to the point of contact of the allergen with the skin. If the patient is highly sensitive or if large amounts of antigen are used, the reaction may become generalized. In addition, sites of previous dermatitis may become active when minute amounts of allergen are applied to remote areas, a reaction lacking satisfactory explanation. The entire skin is usually sensitive, but there are infrequent instances of localized sensitivity, especially to heavy metals.

Clinical Manifestations. The first symptom is usually itching, burning, or erythema; in mild cases the dermatitis may subside at this stage. With greater exposure or a higher degree of sensitivity, vesiculation and edema appear in a few hours, and these are followed by weeping and crusting. Provided that there is no further exposure, the skin becomes dry and scaly, loses its erythema, and finally heals, usually without scarring, in one to three weeks. More severe reactions may be associated with hemorrhagic vesicles, bullae, or small areas of denudation, but actual necrosis is unusual. Repeated exposures result in continuing or intermittent dermatitis that is likely to induce lichenification and hyperpigmentation or hypopigmentation. Secondary infection with staphylococci or streptococci, injudicious treatment, and excessive rubbing and scratching may complicate the picture.

Systemic symptoms are usually absent, but extensive dermatitis may result in chilliness, impaired temperature regulation, shocklike symptoms, leukocytosis, eosinophilia, and decreased serum protein.

Diagnosis. The morphologic diagnosis and specific allergen may be evident at a glance, or the nature and cause of the dermatitis may elude the best efforts. The first requirement for diagnosis is an inflammatory or eczematous dermatitis that exhibits a location and configuration compatible with an external source. Given proper morphology, the diagnosis may be established and the offending allergen identified by history of exposure and proper time relationships. In more difficult cases helpful information may be gained by removal of the patient from the suspected source, which should result in healing, and then re-exposure, which should cause recurrence. Once the list of suspected allergens is cut to a reasonable number, skin tests may be helpful in identifying the specific agent.

Two types of skin test are commonly performed. In each, nonirritating concentrations of test substances are applied to the skin. In one method, useful with liquids or semisolids, the substance is applied to a small area on two or three successive days without covering. The other method involves application of test material and covering with an adhesive, which is usually left in place 48 hours. In both tests, persistent erythema or vesiculation confined to the test site constitutes positive results. False positive results occur with irritating concentrations, sensitivity to agents having nothing to do with the dermatitis, reaction to adhesive, contamination of test substances, and over-reactive skin. False negative results occur with inappropriate concentrations, poor contact with skin, or application of the wrong chemical. The complexity of skin testing makes experienced handling mandatory, and results must be interpreted in conjunction with clinical manifestations.

Disorders to be differentiated from allergic contact dermatitis are primary irritant dermatitis, contact photodermatitis, lichen simplex chronicus, superficial fungal infection, atopic eczema, seborrheic dermatitis, and infectious eczemoid dermatitis.

Treatment. The most important part of management is elimination of exposure to the allergen. Otherwise, treatment consists of nonirritating symptomatic measures calculated to allow the skin to heal. Mild dermatitis may require no treatment. When erythema, edema, and vesiculation are present, open wet compresses of 1 per cent magnesium sulfate solution for two to three hours twice a day alternated with calamine liniment applied six to eight times a day are helpful. As the reaction subsides and the skin becomes dry, these measures are replaced by bland creams or ointments which may contain adrenal corticosteroids. Generalized eruptions may require colloidal baths. If secondary infection is present, antimicrobials may be incorporated in calamine liniment or bland ointment. Systemic antimicrobials may be utilized in the case of extensive or deep secondary infection. Antihistamines may allay itching and may provide some helpful sedative effect. Systemic adrenal steroids or corticotrophin should be used only for extensive and severe dermatitis and only if there are no contraindications to their use.

Desensitization is of little benefit (poison ivy included); indeed, institution of this procedure during active dermatitis may be harmful. Protective clothing and barrier creams are helpful in some instances.

Prognosis. Cure can be attained if the allergen is identified and removed. If this cannot be accomplished, the dermatitis is likely to persist or recur, although it may decrease in intensity with time.

Prophylaxis. Federal regulations guard against release of highly sensitizing food preservatives or colorings, drugs, clothing, cosmetics, and other items. Physicians in industry are continuously on guard against sensitizing agents, recommending the use of materials with low sensitizing capacity whenever possible, protective clothing, proper cleansing and ventilation, and other measures.

CONTACT PHOTODERMATITIS

Contact photodermatitis is an inflammatory reaction in skin from topical application of a photosensitizing compound and exposure to light. The dermatitis is localized to light-exposed sites such as the face, V of the neck, backs of the hands, forearms, and lower legs. Areas which are less involved or spared are the hairy scalp, upper eyelids, undersurface of the chin, and flexor surfaces of the arms. Two types of contact photodermatitis occur. Phototoxic dermatitis usually resembles an exaggerated sunburn and, under proper conditions, it occurs in a large percentage of the population upon first exposure. Photoallergic dermatitis is likely to be eczematous. It occurs in only a small percentage of exposed individuals, and it is a result of specific sensitization. Diagnosis of contact photodermatitis may be aided by photopatch testing. Treatment is the same as for other forms of contact dermatitis with added avoidance of exposure to light.

PRIMARY IRRITANT DERMATITIS

Primary irritant dermatitis, the most common type of contact dermatitis, is due to exposure of the skin to irritating and cytotoxic chemical and physical agents. Immunologic mechanisms are not involved; sufficient exposure will result in dermatitis in all persons. The eczematous nature of the dermatitis and its location and configuration often provide morphologic resemblance to allergic contact dermatitis. Minor differences in histopathology fail to distinguish between the two. Primary irritant dermatitis is less likely to be intermittent, it is not elicited by nonirritating materials, and the latent period between exposure and dermatitis is short or absent. Primary irritants can, of course, be sensitizers, and some patients present combinations of allergic and primary irritant dermatitis. Treatment is similar to that for allergic contact dermatitis, but it is usually easier to identify and eliminate the cause of primary irritant dermatitis. Complete avoidance of offending agents is often not necessary for cure since the skin may be able to tolerate irritants in small amounts.

Baer, R. L.: Allergic eczematous sensitization in man 1936 and 1964. J. Invest. Derm., 43:223, 1964.
Epstein, E., Rees, W. J., and Maibach, H. I.: Recent experience with routine patch test screening. Arch. Derm. (Chicago), 98:18, 1968.
Epstein, S.: The photopatch test. Ann. Allerg., 22:1, 1964.
Fisher, A. A.: Contact Dermatitis. Philadelphia, Lea and Febiger, 1967.
Ison, A. E., and Tucker, J. B.: Photosensitive dermatitis from soaps. New Eng. J. Med., 278:81, 1968.
Macher, E., and Chase, M. W.: The fate of labeled picryl chloride and dinitrochlorobenzene after sensitizing injections. J. Exp. Med., 129:81, 1969.
Macher, E., and Chase, M. W.: The influence of excision of allergenic depots on onset of delayed hypersensitivity and tolerance. J. Exp. Med., 129:103, 1969.
Odom, J. C., and O'Quinn, S. E.: Allergic contact dermatitis. A study of 100 consecutive cases. South. Med. J., 61:1378, 1968.

Behçet's Disease

Clayton E. Wheeler, Jr.

Behçet's disease is a multisystem disease of unknown cause characterized by pyodermas, mucous membrane ulcerations, joint manifestations, thrombophlebitis, and nervous system abnormalities. The disorder is more prevalent in the Middle East and usually affects young adult males. Both venous and arterial vasculitis may enter into pathogenesis. Tissue examination usually reveals nonspecific inflammation.

Behçet's disease is characterized by chronicity, with frequent recurrences at irregular intervals; these vary in duration and intensity and involve several systems in a changing pattern. Oral lesions may be the initial manifestation, and they occur in almost all cases at some time during the disease. They may resemble canker sores or may be larger and deeper. An outstanding and almost constant feature is pyoderma that includes pustules, impetigo, folliculitis, furuncles, acnelike lesions, cellulitis, and ulcers. Nodose lesions that resemble but are probably distinct from erythema nodosum may appear on the legs or elsewhere. Genital changes consist of various pyodermas, herpes-like lesions, and ulcers of the scrotum, vulva, and urethra. Epididymitis is found occasionally. A peculiar feature is the development of papules and pustules after pricking with a sterile needle or injection of sterile saline.

Eye involvement is the most frequent cause of disability; the most common lesions are iridocyclitis or uveitis with hypopyon. Chronic, recurring inflammation often leads to partial or complete loss of vision. This may begin unilaterally, but in time both eyes are affected. Other ocular changes are conjunctivitis, keratitis, retinitis, choroiditis, and optic nerve atrophy.

Most patients experience arthralgia and some develop polyarthritis. Thrombophlebitis, often migratory, is found in about one quarter of the cases. Neurologic complications are being recognized with increasing frequency; they include multiple sclerosis-like disorders, cranial nerve palsies, brainstem syndromes, meningomyelitis, meningoencephalitis, and confusional states. Pulmonary and gastrointestinal symptoms develop occasionally. Fever and malaise often accompany recurrences, and leukocytosis, elevated sedimentation rate, and serum protein abnormalities are common. Cultures from cutaneous lesions usually yield staphylococci or mixed flora.

Antimicrobials and adrenal steroids are of benefit in some cases. Immunosuppressives (cyclophosphamide, azathioprine) and fibrinolytics (phenformin, ethyloestrenol) have been suggested. Prognosis is unpredictable. Spontaneous cures occur or recurrences may continue relentlessly until blindness results. Central nervous system complications are serious and most deaths result from them.

Buckley, C. E., III, and Gills, J. P., Jr.: Cyclophosphamide therapy of Behçet's disease. J. Allerg., 43:273, 1969.
Cunliffe, W. J., and Menon, I. S.: Treatment of Behçet's syndrome with phenformin and ethyloestrenol. Lancet, 1:1239, 1969.
Enoch, B. A., Castillo-Olivares, J. L., Khoo, T. C. L., Grainger, R. G., and Henry, L.: Major vascular complications in Behçet's syndrome. Postgrad. Med. J., 44:453, 1968.
Haim, S.: Contribution of ocular symptoms in the diagnosis of Behçet's disease. Arch. Derm. (Chicago), 98:478, 1968.
Hills, E. A.: Behçet's syndrome with aortic aneurysms. Brit. Med. J. 4:152, 1967.
Oshima, Y., Shimizu, T., Yokohari, R., Matsumoto, T., Kano, K., Kagami, T., and Nagaya, H.: Clinical studies on Behçet's syndrome. Ann. Rheum. Dis., 22:36, 1963.
Wolf, S. M., Schotland, D. L., and Phillips, L. L.: Involvement of nervous system in Behçet's syndrome. Arch. Neurol. (Chicago), 12:315, 1965.

Pemphigus

Clayton E. Wheeler, Jr.

Definition. Pemphigus vulgaris is an uncommon disease characterized by bullae and erosions on the skin and mucous membranes, acantholysis, intercellular antiepithelial antibody, chemical alterations in the blood, and high mortality rate.

Etiology. The cause remains unknown despite extensive search for toxic, viral, metabolic, immunologic, and enzymatic factors.

Incidence and Prevalence. The disease affects either sex and all races; there is a higher incidence among Jews. It usually begins between the ages of 40 and 60; onset earlier in life is unusual.

Pathogenesis. Although the mechanism of bulla formation is unknown, the characteristic histologic feature of acantholysis indicates that defective intercellular attachment is involved. In acantholysis, the cells of the malpighian layer lose their prickles, become separated from each other, and lie singly or in clumps in blister fluid. On electron microscopy tonofilaments retract from their desmosomal attachments and clump in the cytoplasm of the cell. The role of recently demonstrated intercellular antiepithelial autoantibody in acantholysis is not clear.

Defective intercellular attachment accounts for the *Nikolsky sign*, characteristic of all forms of pemphigus: Firm pressure with a finger on the top of an intact blister results in extension at the edge, or application of a steady shearing force to the skin with a tongue depressor causes the top layers of the epidermis to slide over underlying cells. Epidermal separation demonstrated by this sign takes place at the site of most prominent acantholysis.

Blister fluid contains water, electrolytes, and protein. The composition resembles serum, although total protein is usually lower and albumin higher. Loss of these substances into bullae and from denuded areas explains most of the changes in the blood, which parallel the duration and severity of the disorder. Total serum protein may fall as low as 3.6 grams and there may be a correspondingly low level of albumin. Alpha$_1$ and alpha$_2$ globulins are increased. Gamma globulin and fibrinogen are usually increased. Sodium, chloride, and calcium are decreased and potassium is normal or increased. Plasma and interstitial fluid volume are increased. Anemia is common and may be due to inanition, serum loss, and infection. Anemia and increased globulin, especially fibrinogen, probably account for the increased sedimentation rate. The leukocyte count is usually elevated with an increase of immature forms. Cutaneous inflammation and infection are important causes of leukocytosis. Eosinophilia may be present.

Pathology. Characteristic changes develop in the skin and orificial mucosa. Intercellular edema in the lower malphigian layer is followed by loss of intercellular bridges, acantholysis, and cleft formation. An intra-epithelial bulla is formed just above the basal layer. Healing may result in normal-appearing epidermis or there may be hyperkeratosis, acanthosis, and papillomatosis. Simple or granulomatous inflammation is present in the dermis, and tissue eosinophilia is often prominent.

There are no specific changes in internal organs. Examination of persons dying early in the course of pemphigus may show surprisingly little. Common but variable findings are pulmonary congestion and edema, atelectasis, bronchopneumonia, hydropericardium, focal myocarditis, and brown atrophy. Myeloid hyperplasia of the bone marrow and increased numbers of normoblasts are common. Adrenal changes have included depletion of lipoid, degeneration, and inflammation followed by scar and regeneration, hemorrhage, necrosis, and vein thrombosis. Nonspecific degeneration may involve areas of brain, cord, or ganglia.

Clinical Manifestations. Flaccid or tense bullae are characteristic. These lesions often spread at the edges and show little tendency to heal, and they rupture easily. Localized involvement may be present for months or the disease may begin with a generalized eruption. Skin lesions are randomly distributed, but there is a predilection for areas of friction or pressure. Frequently affected sites are the scalp, axillae, groin, elbows, knees, back, inframammary area, umbilicus, hands, feet, nose, and eyelids. Bullae arise on normal appearing skin or at previously involved sites. Coalescence and extension often result in large denuded areas. The contents of bullae may be serous, seropurulent, or hemorrhagic, and crusting often develops. Healing takes place with little or no scarring. Secondary infection is a common complication, and hyperpigmentation, hypopigmentation, and milium formation are frequent sequelae. Itching is usually mild or absent. Denudation often causes burning or pain. The Nikolsky sign is positive over intact bullae and sometimes can be elicited over normal-appearing skin.

The oral mucosa is involved in almost all patients with pemphigus vulgaris. In half to two thirds of the cases mouth lesions precede skin lesions by weeks to a year or more. The thin-walled bullae rupture early, leaving erosions which often assume figured patterns. The gums, sides of the tongue, and buccal mucosa along the bite line are preferential sites. The lips frequently become fissured, crusted, or warty. Pain, salivation, and bleeding may make eating and drinking difficult. Bullae, erosions, and inflammation commonly involve the mucosa of the pharynx, larynx, nose, conjunctiva, genitalia, and anus.

Extensive skin and mucous membrane involvement, loss of fluid, electrolytes, and protein, inability to eat and drink, and secondary cutaneous and systemic infection contribute to weakness, weight loss, toxemia, and the severely ill appearance of these patients.

Other Types of Pemphigus. Other types are pemphigus vegetans, pemphigus foliaceus, pemphigus erythematosus, and fogo selvagem. *Pemphigus vegetans* is less severe than pemphigus vulgaris, of which it is probably a variant, and is characterized by warty, vegetating, pustular, and hyperkeratotic lesions at the axillae, groin, anogenital area, interdigital spaces, and lips. *Pemphigus foliaceus* is characterized by incompletely formed bullae, more crusting and scaling, frequent absence of mucous membrane involvement, milder but longer course, lower mortality rate, more spontaneous cures, and higher position of the bullae in the epidermis. It usually begins on the face or upper trunk and slowly becomes generalized, at which time it resembles exfoliative dermatitis. *Pemphigus erythematosus* may be an abortive form of pemphigus foliaceus or pemphigus vulgaris. Crusting and erythema about the face, mid upper back and chest produce a superficial resemblance to seborrheic dermatitis and lupus erythematosus. *Fogo selvagem* (Brazilian wildfire) resembles pemphigus foliaceus except for its endemicity in central South America and its frequent onset at an early age.

Diagnosis. The clinical diagnosis should be confirmed by biopsy and smears of skin and mucosal lesions. Multiple sampling of lesions may be necessary to show acantholysis. Intercellular antiepithelial autoantibodies can be demonstrated in skin lesions and serum by immunofluorescence. The most difficult differential diagnosis is that of *pemphigoid*, a chronic bullous disease of unknown cause in which the bullae are usually smaller, more tense, rupture less easily, and often show grouping or arise on an inflamed base. Mouth involvement is less severe and less frequent; systemic symptoms are less intense, and the mortality rate is lower. Bullae are subepidermal, acantholysis is absent, and autoantibodies are found in the basal membrane area. Bullous *erythema multiforme* shows more polymorphism and configuration, the onset is acute, fever is often high, the disease is self-limited, and acantholysis is absent. Bullous *drug eruption* follows the pattern of bullous erythema multiforme. Benign *mucous membrane pemphigoid* is characterized by chronic bullous and erosive lesions of the mucous membranes, especially of the eye, in which scarring is prominent. *Contact dermatitis* can usually be differentiated by localization and configuration of lesions, lack of systemic symptoms, infrequent mucosal involvement and self-limited course. In *familial benign chronic pemphigus*, lesions are usually limited to the neck, axillae, groin, and small areas of the trunk. Mucous membrane involvement and systemic symptoms are absent, and biopsy is usually characteristic. *Pemphigus neonatorum* is a bullous form of impetigo which can be differentiated by age, cultures, and response to appropriate antimicrobials. *Exfoliative derma-*

titis lacks bulla formation and mucosal involvement, and biopsy shows chronic dermatitis without acantholysis.

Treatment. Adrenal steroids and corticotrophin control but do not cure pemphigus vulgaris. In view of the seriousness of the disorder, there is probably no absolute contraindication to steroid therapy. The dose depends upon clinical response and varies from patient to patient. The objective is to bring the disease under control as rapidly as possible and then to decrease the dose gradually until a maintenance level is attained. On some occasions spontaneous remissions occur and maintenance medication can be stopped, but most patients require continued treatment. An initial dosage of 120 to 300 mg. per day of prednisone or its equivalent usually suffices to stop new lesions and start healing of old lesions within a week. After complete healing of skin and mucous membrane lesions the amount of drug is cautiously reduced until the maintenance level is reached; this is usually between 15 and 30 mg. per day of prednisone or its equivalent. Some patients require much higher doses than outlined above, and some succumb despite adrenal steroid therapy. Measures must be taken to combat salt and water retention, potassium depletion, osteoporosis, and peptic ulcer. Immunosuppressive agents (methotrexate, 20 to 25 mg. once a week per os, or cyclophosphamide, 100 to 200 mg. per day) may help to control the disease and make reduction in maintenance steroid dosage possible. Psychotic disturbances caused by steroid or pemphigus may require tranquilizers or sedatives. Transfusions and measures to correct abnormalities of serum protein and electrolytes are often necessary. Cutaneous and internal infection (bacteremia, bronchopneumonia, and urinary tract infection) must be combated with appropriate topical and systemic antimicrobials. Good nursing care, encouragement to eat and drink, soothing mouth washes, and a cheerful environment are important. Colloidal or potassium permanganate baths and topical use of calamine liniment may add to the patient's comfort.

Prognosis. The mortality rate of untreated pemphigus vulgaris confirmed by biopsy is greater than 90 per cent. Average duration of life after onset is fourteen months, with a range of one month to six or seven years and, rarely, longer. In addition, the uncomfortable state of the patients during much of their course adds greatly to the gloomy picture. Patients die of toxemia, cachexia, shock from protein and electrolyte abnormalities, pulmonary edema, bronchopneumonia, sepsis, or adrenal insufficiency.

Current therapy has cut the mortality rate approximately in half. This is only part of the story because control of the disease allows most patients to lead comfortable and useful lives. Complications of steroid therapy, such as perforated peptic ulcer, congestive heart failure, suicide, uncontrollable infection, and thromboembolic phenomena, must be added to the list of causes of death, but judicious management keeps these to a minimum.

Beutner, E. H., Lever, W. F., Witebsky, E., Jordan, R., and Chertock, B.: Autoantibodies in pemphigus vulgaris. J.A.M.A., 192:682, 1965.

Ebringer, A., and Mackay, I. R.: Pemphigus vulgaris successfully treated with cyclophosphamide. Ann. Intern. Med., 71:125, 1969.

Jordan, R. E., Ihrig, J. J., and Perry, H. O.: Childhood pemphigus vulgaris. Arch. Derm. (Chicago), 99:176, 1969.

Lever, W. F.: Pemphigus and Pemphigoid. Springfield, Ill., Charles C Thomas, 1965

Lever, W. F., and Goldberg, H. S.: Treatment of pemphigus vulgaris with methotrexate. Arch. Derm. (Chicago), 100:70, 1969.

Peck, S. M., Osserman, K. E., Weiner, L. B., Lefkovitz, A., and Osserman, R. S.: Studies in bullous diseases. Immunofluorescent tests. New Eng. J. Med., 279:951, 1968.

Acanthosis Nigricans

Clayton E. Wheeler, Jr.

Definition. Acanthosis nigricans is an uncommon dermatosis characterized by hyperpigmentation and epidermal hypertrophy. Two forms are recognized: (1) malignant or adult, associated with internal cancer, and (2) benign or juvenile, which may be related to developmental, endocrine, or metabolic abnormalities. This terminology is illogical, however, because the dermatosis itself is never malignant and because the adult type may be seen in children and the juvenile form in adults.

Etiology. By definition, malignant acanthosis nigricans is always associated with internal malignancy; adenocarcinoma is the predominant type of cancer, although epidermoid carcinoma and malignant lymphoma have been reported. Almost 70 per cent of the associated malignancies arise in the stomach and more than 90 per cent in the abdomen and pelvis. Sites of origin are the stomach, colon, esophagus, liver, gallbladder, pancreas, ovary, uterus, chorion, kidney, lung, bronchus, mediastinum, breast, and thyroid. Skin changes appear before clinical evidence of carcinoma in 20 per cent; the two appear simultaneously in 60 per cent; and acanthosis follows the diagnosis of malignancy in 20 per cent. Progression of the dermatosis parallels the course of the carcinoma. In a few instances acanthosis has regressed following x-ray or surgical treatment of cancer, only to recur with reactivation of the malignancy.

Benign acanthosis nigricans may be associated with a large number of developmental, metabolic, or endocrine abnormalities that seem to have little in common in the light of present knowledge. These include diabetes mellitus, pituitary tumors, adrenal hyperplasia, hypogonadism, acromegaly, gigantism, congenital total lipodystrophy, hypothyroidism, Addison's disease, Stein-Leventhal syndrome, von Recklinghausen's neurofibromatosis, arachnodactyly, achondroplasia, epilepsy, mental retardation, and degenerative disease of the cord. Familial incidence and occurrence in two and three generations suggest that hereditary factors are important. Lupoid hepatitis and administration of nicotinic acid, stilbestrol, and corticosteroids have been associated with skin lesions resembling acanthosis nigricans.

Incidence and Prevalence. The disorder is world-wide, affects all races and occurs in either sex. The peak incidence of malignant acanthosis nigricans is between the ages of 40 and 60, but it occurs at all ages. Benign acanthosis nigricans usually appears between the ages of 10 and 20, but the disorder may be present at birth, and it occurs in early childhood and middle age. Intensification and spread commonly occur at puberty if the disorder has existed previously.

Pathology. Characteristic changes are limited to the epidermis, where there are hyperkeratosis, acanthosis (increased thickness of the prickle cell layer), and papillomatosis. Melanin is increased in the basal layer. Benign and malignant forms do not differ histologically, and cancer is not found in the skin in the malignant type.

Pathogenesis. The pathogenesis of acanthosis nigricans is unknown. In the malignant type, theories include humoral or biochemical effects of the cancer, peculiarities of the host triggered by carcinoma, or a common cause for acanthosis and carcinoma. Benign acanthosis nigricans may be related to disturbances of germ plasm or endocrine function.

Clinical Manifestations. Skin changes in malignant acanthosis nigricans are bilateral and symmetrical and exhibit a predilection for flexural and intertriginous areas. The axillae, groin, genital region, and neck are the most common sites of involvement; other areas in approximate order of frequency are face, inner thighs, flexor surfaces of elbows and knees, umbilicus, perianal area, and eyelids. The palms and soles occasionally become hyperkeratotic, the backs of the fingers are sometimes involved, and in extreme and rare instances the disorder becomes generalized. Involved skin is usually dark brown or black, although light brown and yellow may be seen. The epidermis becomes thickened, and normal skin lines are exaggerated. A soft, velvety, papillomatous appearance develops, and frequently pedunculated growths or warty lesions are scattered over the area. The disorder is distinctly localized, with involved regions blending imperceptibly into normal skin. In some cases there may be loss of scalp or eyebrow hair, and dystrophy of nails may occur. The lips, mouth, tongue, epiglottis, and vagina may be affected. Involved mucous membrane becomes thickened, granular, and warty.

Benign acanthosis nigricans shows the same changes, but the degree and extent are often less, and mucous membrane involvement is unlikely. The cutaneous lesions of both forms are asymptomatic. Systemic symptoms depend upon associated internal disease.

Diagnosis. The diagnosis is based on clinical appearance, histologic findings, and associated internal disease.

Addison's disease and *hemochromatosis* cause more generalized hyperpigmentation, and involved sites lack epidermal hypertrophy, papillomatosis, and warty changes. *Arsenical hyperpigmentation* is generalized, and arsenical keratoses are small and hard and uncommonly affect flexural or intertriginous sites. *Ichthyosis hystrix* shows less predilection for flexural and intertriginous areas, there is more hyperkeratosis, and the palms and soles are more often involved. Obese persons, especially brunets, sometimes develop hyperpigmentation, acanthosis, and papillomatosis of the axillae, groin, and neck. These alterations have been called pseudoacanthosis nigricans, but they probably represent a form of benign acanthosis nigricans.

Treatment. The most important aspect of management is determination of whether internal malignancy is present. If it is, prompt treatment should be instituted. In the benign type, associated developmental or endocrine disorders may require treatment. There is no effective therapy for the dermatosis, although temporary amelioration of cutaneous changes may occur after irradiation or surgical treatment of carcinoma. Correction of endocrine abnormalities appears to have little or no influence on the skin changes.

Prognosis. The outlook for the patient with acanthosis nigricans and malignancy is gloomy. The associated carcinoma is highly malignant, and average survival after its discovery is one year. Seldom do persons live longer than two years after the skin lesions appear, and progressive skin changes are a bad omen. Few, if any, have been cured, but earlier discovery and improved methods of treatment may alter the picture. The prognosis in benign acanthosis nigricans is good and depends upon associated abnormalities and their amenability to treatment.

The dermatosis tends to progress when associated with malignancy. Skin lesions in the benign form are likely to reach a peak and remain static or regress slowly.

Brown, J., and Winkelmann, R. K.: Acanthosis nigricans: A study of 90 cases. Medicine, 47:33, 1968.
Curth, H. O., Hilberg, A. W., and Machachek, G. F.: The site and histology of the cancer associated with malignant acanthosis nigricans. Cancer, 15:364, 1962.
Hollingsworth, D. R., and Amatruda, T. T., Jr.: Acanthosis nigricans and obesity. Arch. Intern. Med. (Chicago), 124:481, 1969.
Reed, W. B., Dexter, R., Corley, C., and Fish, C.: Congenital lipodystrophic diabetes with acanthosis nigricans. Arch. Derm. (Chicago), 91:326, 1965.
Tuffanelli, D. L.: Acanthosis nigricans with lupoid hepatitis. J.A.M.A., 189:584, 1964.

Mast Cell Disease
(Mastocytosis)
Clayton E. Wheeler, Jr.

Mast cell disease will be discussed under two divisions: (1) urticaria pigmentosa of childhood and (2) systemic mastocytosis.

URTICARIA PIGMENTOSA OF CHILDHOOD

Definition. This chronic disease usually begins in early childhood and disappears partially or completely by adolescence. Characteristic skin lesions are single or multiple pigmented macules or nodules that urticate on rubbing and contain large numbers of mast cells.

Incidence. Although uncommon, the disorder is seen yearly in most dermatologic and pediatric practices. Light-skinned persons are affected most often, and it is slightly more common in males. The disorder has been reported in a parent and child in several families and in both members of monozygotic twins. More than 10 per cent of cases are present at birth; over half develop by six months; and the majority appear before puberty. Onset after puberty raises the question of systemic mastocytosis.

Etiology. The probable origin of mast cells from connective tissue cells of histiocytic type suggests that the disorder is one of the reticuloendothelioses. Urticaria pigmentosa may be a systemic disorder, but its benign course appears to separate it from systemic mastocytosis.

Pathogenesis. Human mast cells contain histamine, heparin, and possibly hyaluronic acid. The function of these cells is incompletely understood, but they may be important in connective tissue formation, repair, or maintenance. Local release of histamine on rubbing results in capillary dilatation and edema with erythema and wheal formation, whereas its absorption into the general circulation causes flushing, a shocklike state, and gastrointestinal disturbance. Pigmentation of cutaneous lesions is due to increased melanin production, which presumably results from repeated inflammatory episodes.

Pathology. The characteristic finding is accumulation of mast cells in the dermis. The number of cells determines the macular or nodular nature of the lesion. Mast cells are large and contain round or oval nuclei. The cytoplasm contains large basophilic granules that stain metachromatically and can be demonstrated by fixation with 10 per cent formalin or absolute alcohol followed by staining with Giemsa, methylene blue, or toluidine blue. Lesions that have been rubbed may show edema, eosinophilia, and degranulation of mast cells. Melanin is increased in the basal layer and dermal chromatophores.

Clinical Manifestations. One, few, or innumerable lesions may be present. Frequently they appear in crops for weeks before the final extent of the disease is reached. The trunk is the site of predilection, but the neck, face, scalp, extremities, palms, soles, and oral mucosa may be involved. Although macular eruptions predominate, nodular and plaquelike forms are common. Superimposed bullae or vesicles may occur in young children. Lesions are round, oval, or irregular and vary from a few millimeters to several centimeters. They are discrete except in extensive cases. The color varies from yellow to brown or sepia.

A significant number of patients display symptoms of histamine release into the general circulation. These include episodic bright red flushing, itching, hypotension, weakness, dizziness, headache, dermographism, nausea, vomiting, and diarrhea.

Although the extent of mast cell infiltration has been incompletely studied, the occasional finding of lymphadenopathy, splenomegaly, increased mast cells in bone marrow, and cystic or proliferative bone lesions suggests that urticaria pigmentosa is a systemic disease.

Diagnosis. The diagnosis can usually be made when pigmented lesions exhibit erythema and edema upon rubbing (*Darier's sign*). This sign is absent in some cases, especially when previous stroking has exhausted the supply of histamine. Biopsy confirms the diagnosis. Increased eosinophil content of the blood is sometimes found, and increased amounts of histamine may be present in the urine.

Pigmented nevi, nevoxanthoendothelioma, xanthoma, myoblastoma, lymphoma, insect bites, and Letterer-Siwe disease can usually be differentiated by histologic findings and the absence of Darier's sign.

Treatment. There is no effective treatment. Antihistamines may attenuate some of the symptoms. Trauma should be avoided. Solitary lesions may be excised. Once systemic mastocytosis is excluded, watchful waiting and reassurance of the parents are essential features of management.

Prognosis. Aside from cosmetic considerations and uncomfortable effects of histamine release, the disease is benign. Lesions disappear completely by adolescence in the majority of patients; in the remainder pigmented macules persist without activity.

SYSTEMIC MASTOCYTOSIS

Systemic mastocytosis, a rare, recently recognized disease, is being reported with increasing frequency. It affects both males and females and usually begins in adult life. The cause is unknown. The clinical manifestations and course may resemble those of lymphoma or leukemia, and it seems likely that the disorder should be classified with the reticuloendothelioses. (See Histiocytosis X in Hematologic and Hematopoietic Diseases.)

Skin or mucous membrane lesions may resemble childhood urticaria pigmentosa, but significant differences that indicate systemic mastocytoses are (1) onset after puberty, (2) multiple, small, confluent macules with persistent telangiectasia, (3) papules and nodules resembling leukemia cutis, (4) chronic lichenified dermatitis, (5) generalized infiltration of skin with a "scotchgrain" appearance, (6) less pigmentation, (7) less tendency to redden and urticate on stroking, (8) extensive involvement of oral, nasal, or rectal mucosa, and (9) progressive cutaneous change.

Histamine release into the general circulation is less likely than in childhood urticaria pigmentosa, yet patients may have flushing, shocklike episodes, and increased histamine in the urine. Diarrhea is often a prominent feature, and peptic ulcer occasionally develops.

Persistent or progressive cutaneous eruption may be the only evidence of the disease, although asymptomatic bone changes can be demonstrated by roentgenographic examination in many cases. These changes consist of solitary or multiple, irregular or round lytic lesions or local or general new bone formation, which causes thickening of the cortex and trabeculae and narrowing of marrow spaces. In more severe instances, lymphadenopathy, splenomegaly, and hepatomegaly are prominent early manifestations, and bone marrow aspiration shows abnormal accumulations of mast cells. The disorder may remain static at this point or may progress with weakness, weight loss, cachexia, nausea, vomiting, diarrhea, and malaise. In these patients anemia, leukopenia, thrombocytopenia, and leukemoid features develop, presumably from the proliferative effect of mast cells in bone marrow. Other blood abnormalities are eosinophilia, lymphocytosis, and monocytosis. Liver function may be impaired by mast cell invasion and associated periportal fibrosis. A malabsorption syndrome may develop. Bleeding tendencies are usually due to combinations of thrombocytopenia and prothrombin deficiency, but there may be a circulating heparin-like substance. Tissue mast cell leukemia, somewhat like other leukemias, is found on rare occasions. Abnormal numbers of mast cells are found at autopsy in almost all tissues. In mild forms, mast cells appear normal, but in severe forms, especially leukemia, anaplasia indicates malignant transformation.

Prognosis varies with the form of the disorder. Disease confined to skin and bone is compatible with long life and little morbidity, but there is always the threat of extension of the morbid process. Extensive reticuloendothelial involvement results in death in a few months to several years. Patients die from pancytopenia, infection, hemorrhage, cachexia, gastroenteritis, perforated peptic ulcer, and leukemia. Therapy is palliative and symptomatic and includes transfusions, antimicrobials, antihistamines, adrenal steroids, corticotrophin, roentgen irradiation, and nitrogen mustard.

Bank, S., and Marks, I. N.: Malabsorption in systemic mast cell disease. Gastroenterology, 45:535, 1963.
Barer, M., Peterson, L. F. A., Dahlin, D. C., Winkelmann, R. K.,
and Stewart, J. R.: Mastocytosis with osseous lesions resembling metastatic malignant lesions in bone. J. Bone Joint Surg. (Amer.), 50:142, 1968.
Burgoon, C. F., Graham, J. H., and McCaffree, D. L.: Mast cell disease. Arch. Derm. (Chicago), 98:590, 1968.
Caplan, R. M.: The natural course of urticaria pigmentosa. Arch. Derm. (Chicago), 87:146, 1963.
Clement, A. C., Fishbone, G., Levine, R. J., James, A. E., and Janower, M.: Gastrointestinal lesions in mastocytosis. Amer. J. Roentgen., 103:405, 1968.
Miller, R. C., and Shapiro, L.: Bullous urticaria pigmentosa in infancy. Arch. Derm. (Chicago), 91:595, 1965.
Sagher, F., and Even-Paz, Z.: Mastocytosis and the Mast Cell. Chicago, Year Book Publishers, Inc., 1967.
Shaw, J. M.: Genetic aspects of urticaria pigmentosa. Arch. Derm. (Chicago), 97:137, 1968.
Ultmann, J. E., Mutter, R. D., Tannenbaum, M., and Warner, R. R. P.: Clinical, cytologic and biochemical studies in systemic mast cell disease. Ann. Intern. Med., 61:326, 1964.

Lethal Cutaneous and Gastrointestinal Arteriolar Thrombosis

(Degos' Disease)

Clayton E. Wheeler, Jr.

Lethal cutaneous and gastrointestinal arteriolar thrombosis is a progressive, usually fatal, disease in which characteristic cutaneous, gastrointestinal, and central nervous system lesions result from spotty occlusive vascular disease. The cause is unknown. Most cases of this uncommon disorder occur in young adult males. Cutaneous manifestations usually precede gastrointestinal or nervous system symptoms by weeks or months, although the reverse sequence may occur. Indolent, slowly progressive, rose-colored papules 2 to 5 mm. in size appear on the trunk or proximal extremities and occasionally elsewhere. In a few days or weeks the papules develop porcelain-like central umbilication covered by white scale and surrounded by a slightly elevated violaceous telangiectatic border. In time the entire lesion becomes white, depressed, and atrophic. There are usually fewer than 100 lesions, and they appear in crops, so that several stages of development are represented at any one time.

Central nervous system symptoms may be mild, localized, evanescent, and migratory in the initial phases, but eventually they become severe, extensive, and permanent. Numbness, weakness, headache, slurred speech, aphasias, seizures, hemiparesis, paraplegia, optic atrophy, and cranial nerve palsies may be found. To date, gastrointestinal involvement has not been reported in patients with prominent central nervous system disease.

Initial gastrointestinal symptoms may be mild and vague and may be associated with asthenia and weight loss, or the onset may be abrupt with signs indicating perforation, ileus, and peritonitis. Laparotomy reveals multiple, oval, white, subserosal patches of atrophy varying from pinpoint to 2 cm. in size and irregularly distributed in stomach, ileum, jejunum, and colon. Perforation and peritonitis frequently occur, and there may be localized areas of gangrene.

The basic pathologic abnormality is an obliterative endothelial reaction affecting small arteries and arterioles and corresponding veins. Ischemic infarcts, necrobiosis, or atrophy occurs at involved sites in all layers of the skin and intestinal tract, and similar lesions are found in the central nervous system. The mouth, esophagus, rectum, anus, liver, pancreas, genitalia, bladder, kidney, lung, pleura, heart, retina, choroid, sclera, and conjunctiva have also been involved. Disease of smaller vessels, with emphasis on endothelial reaction, appears to distinguish the disorder from Buerger's disease and periarteritis nodosa.

Treatment with antimicrobials, adrenal corticosteroids, anticoagulants, and methotrexate is ineffectual. Surgical intervention in persons with gastrointestinal symptoms is of temporary or no benefit because of the multiplicity and recurrence of lesions. Patients succumb to either gastrointestinal or nervous system involvement.

Culicchia, C. F., Gol, A., and Erickson, E. E.: Diffuse central nervous system involvement in papulosis atrophicans maligna. Neurology (Minneap.), 12:503, 1962.

Howard, R. O., Klaus, S. N., Slavin, R. C., and Fenton, R.: Malignant atrophic papulosis (Degos' syndrome) Arch Ophthal. (Chicago), 79:262, 1968.

Lomholt, G., Hjorth, N., and Fischermann, K.: Lethal peritonitis from Degos' disease (malign and atrophic papulosis). Acta Chir. Scand., 134:495, 1968.

Winkelmann, R. K., Howard, F. M., Jr., Perry, H. O., and Miller, R. H.: Malignant papulosis of skin and cerebrum. Arch. Derm. (Chicago), 87:54, 1963.

Angiokeratoma Corporis Diffusum

(Fabry's Disease)

Clayton E. Wheeler, Jr.

Definition. Fabry's disease is an inherited disorder of glycolipid metabolism characterized by telangiectatic skin lesions, hypohidrosis, corneal opacities, acral pain and paresthesias, febrile episodes, gastrointestinal symptoms, renal failure, cardiovascular disease, and central nervous system disturbances.

Etiology. An X-linked, incompletely recessive error in glycolipid metabolism is manifested by a deficiency of ceramide trihexosidase with accumulation of ceramide trihexoside and other neutral glycolipids. Trihexosidase activity is essentially absent from intestinal mucosa of homozygotic males and is less than normal in heterozygotic females.

Prevalence. The disease is uncommon. Males exhibit the full-blown disorder. Females are asymptomatic carriers or develop mild forms of the disease.

Pathology. A glycolipid that is doubly refractile, periodic acid–Schiff positive, and has an affinity for Sudan black B and other histochemical properties is deposited in endothelial cells and smooth muscle of blood vessels, arrectores pilorum muscles and heart muscles. Similar deposits are found in cells of the renal glomeruli, distal convoluted tubules, loop of Henle, urinary sediment, cornea, sweat glands, central nervous system, spleen, liver, lymph nodes, and bone marrow. Skin biopsies may show glycolipid in vessels or appendages at sites distant from telangiectases. Telangiectases are dilated vessels in the upper dermis or blood-filled spaces enclosed by epidermis. Cultured skin fibroblasts accumulate ceramide trihexoside and stain metachromatically with toluidine blue.

Clinical Manifestations. Cutaneous lesions usually appear in childhood or around puberty and consist of telangiectatic spots varying in size from barely visible to several millimeters. They are bright red to blue-black, and some are covered with slight scale. They are nonpulsatile lesions that may be partially blanched in diascopy. Telangiectases tend to cluster about the umbilicus, glans penis, scrotum, buttocks, hips, and thighs; but they occur anywhere, including the oral mucosa. A few lesions are found initially, but as the disease progresses they may appear in profusion. Skin lesions may be absent. Sweating is often decreased. Hair may be scanty; many patients shave infrequently. Paresthesias of the hands and feet and episodes of very severe burning pain in the extremities, at times accompanied by fever, may be early symptoms that may be precipitated by exposure to heat or cold or by physical exertion. Attacks of nausea, diarrhea, and abdominal pain are common. A Raynaud-like phenomenon and pain in the muscles and joints may also occur. Patients may complain of dizziness, weakness, and headache. Edema may occur in the absence of renal or cardiac failure.

Dilated, tortuous venules may be found in the palpebral and bulbar conjunctiva and the retina. Corneal opacities are usually, if not always, present and lens opacities may be found. Hypertension develops in older persons, and there may be evidence of myocardial infarction, congestive failure, or cerebrovascular disease.

An early finding, which may be discovered at routine examination, is albuminuria. "Maltese cross" material may be found in the urine on polaroscopy. "Mulberry cells" containing glycolipid may be discerned in the urinary sediment. Later in the disease there are casts, hematuria, and low, fixed specific gravity, azotemia, and anemia.

Diagnosis. Cutaneous telangiectases, albuminuria, glycolipid in cells of skin and renal biopsies, glycolipid in urinary sediment (both ceramide trihexoside and ceramide dihexoside), and a positive family history are diagnostic. In addition, slit-lamp examination of the cornea shows characteristic findings, even in female carriers.

Senile angiomas (de Morgan or ruby spots) are usually brighter red, are more numerous on the upper trunk, and do not cluster together. Angiokeratomas of the scrotum (Fordyce) are common lesions of older men. Lesions of Osler-Weber-Rendu disease are brighter red, less grouped, and occur chiefly in the mouth, nose, and lips and on the fingers.

Treatment. Treatment is symptomatic.

Prognosis. The disease is slowly progressive in males, who usually die in the fourth or fifth decades of renal failure complicated by cardiovascular disease. Longevity is essentially uninfluenced by the mild form that occurs in women.

Brady, R. O., Gel, A. E., Bradley, R. M., Martensson, E., Warshaw, A. L., and Laster, L.: Enzymatic defect in Fabry's disease. New Eng. J. Med., 276:1163, 1967.

Ferrons, V. J., Hibbs, R. G., and Burda, C. D.: The heart in Fabry's disease. Amer. J. Cardiol., 24:95, 1969.

Matalon, R., Dorfman, A., Dawson, G., and Sweeley, C. C.: Glycolipid and mucopolysaccharide abnormality in fibroblasts in Fabry's disease. Science, 164:1522, 1969.

Philippart, M., Sarlieve, L., and Manacorda, A.: Urinary glycolipids in Fabry's disease. Pediatrics, 43:201, 1969.

Urbain, G., Philippart, M., and Peremans, J.: Fabry's disease with hypogammaglobulinemia and without angiokeratomas. Arch. Intern. Med. (Chicago), 124:72, 1969.

Von Gemmingen, G., Kierland, R. R., and Opitz, J. M.: Angiokeratoma corporis diffusum (Fabry's disease). Arch. Derm. (Chicago), 91:206, 1965.

Wise, D., Wallace, H. J., and Jellinek, E. H.: Angiokeratoma corporis diffusum. Quart. J. Med., 31:177, 1962.

Incontinentia Pigmenti

(Bloch-Sulzberger Syndrome)

Clayton E. Wheeler, Jr.

Incontinentia pigmenti is a congenital disorder characterized by bizarre skin lesions and defects in many structures of epidermal and mesodermal origin. The cause is unknown. Theories include anomalies of ectodermal and mesodermal development and maternal viral infection. The disorder may be inherited, since multiple cases have occurred in families, and members of two or three generations have been affected. The disease has been reported in Caucasians, Negroes, Japanese, and Chinese. Females are affected approximately ten times as often as males.

Cutaneous lesions are usually present at birth but may not appear for a few weeks or a year or two. The process is likely to be localized initially but tends to spread and become generalized. The lesions are papules, vesicles, and bullae that arise in areas of inflammation. At first there is little tendency toward a configurate pattern but, later, groups, patches, and lines are observed. Lesions often come and go in crops, and the pattern shifts from time to time. After weeks or months, the inflammatory phase either passes directly to a pigmented macular stage or blends into a warty or papillomatous stage that subsequently develops into pigmented macules. The most characteristic feature of the skin involvement is the striking and bizarre pattern assumed by pigmented macules and, to a lesser extent, by preceding warty and inflammatory lesions. Streaks, flecks, lines, whorls, patches, spidery forms, arborizations, and zebra and marble and fudge ripple patterns are found. The lines and streaks do not correspond to nerve, blood vessel, or dermatome distribution and frequently cross the midline. The macules are usually chocolate-brown, gray-brown, or slate-colored. They may persist relatively unchanged or fade gradually, leaving normal, depigmented, or atrophic areas. The hair may be thin, and a common finding is localized atrophic alopecia of the scalp. Occasionally other cutaneous defects develop such as dystrophic nails, localized atrophy, small keratotic areas, tylosis of palms and soles, and areas simulating localized scleroderma.

Other abnormalities of structures of ectodermal or mesodermal origin occur in approximately two thirds of the patients. *Dental anomalies* include delayed eruption, fewer teeth than normal, and conical crowns of the incisors, canines, and bicuspids. Both deciduous and permanent teeth are affected. Possible *eye changes* are strabismus, corneal opacities, cataracts, optic atrophy, blue scleras, retinal pigmentary abnormalities, retrobulbar glioma, and ablatio falciformis. *Nervous system involvement* includes spastic paralysis, motor disturbances, epilepsy, microcephaly, mental retardation, nystagmus, decreased hearing, and homonymous hemianopsia. Osseous change, retarded growth and development, patent ductus arteriosus, urachal cyst, supernumerary ears, absence of or supernumerary nipples, and unilateral lack of breast tissue occasionally occur in patients with incontinentia pigmenti.

In the inflammatory, vesicular phase of the disease, blood eosinophilia of 30 to 50 per cent is common, and vesicle fluid eosinophilia may reach 95 per cent. Anemia occasionally occurs at this time.

Diagnosis is difficult in the vesicular or bullous phase. Blood and tissue eosinophilia and roentgenograms of unerupted teeth in infants may be helpful. As the bizarre configuration and the warty and pigmented macular phases develop, diagnosis usually becomes easy. Bullous incontinentia pigmenti must be differentiated from dermatitis herpetiformis, congenital syphilis, epidermolysis bullosa, erythema multiforme, bullous impetigo, virus diseases, and contact dermatitis. Warty and pigmented macular phases resemble systematized epithelial nevi. Roentgenographic dental changes must be distinguished from congenital syphilis and congenital ectodermal defect.

No effective prevention or treatment is known. Adrenal steroid administration has had temporary beneficial effect on the bullous phase but has not been fully evaluated.

Morbidity and longevity depend upon the structures affected and the severity of the process.

Cutaneous involvement alone or in association with minor defects of other structures is compatible with a normal life. Involvement of the nervous system or heart may carry a serious prognosis.

Curth, H. O., and Warburton, D.: The genetics of incontinentia pigmenti. Arch. Derm. (Chicago), 92:229, 1965.
Jackson, R., and Nigam, S.: Incontinenti pigmenti: A report of three cases in one family. Pediatrics, 30:433, 1962.
Reiner, R. M., Cyrus, G., and Gurevitch, A. W.: Oral changes in incontinentia pigmenti. J. Amer. Dent. Ass., 76:795, 1968.

Hereditary Anhidrotic Ectodermal Defect

Clayton E. Wheeler, Jr.

Hereditary anhidrotic ectodermal defect is an uncommon, genetically determined developmental defect of ectodermal, entodermal, and mesodermal structures in which dysgenesis of the epidermis and its appendages is the main feature. Predominance of the disease in males is explained by the two forms of inheritance: X-linked recessive and autosomal dominant with greater manifestation in males. Defective development probably arises in the second or third month of embryonic life when epidermal appendages are being differentiated.

The *facies* is often so characteristic that unrelated persons appear to be siblings. Wide, high, scanty eyebrows, prominent frontal bones, saddle nose, thick swollen lips with radiating furrows, underdeveloped maxillas and mandibles, and pointed chin are distinctive features. The patient may be small and delicately proportioned, and the skin is likely to be thin, dry, white, and soft, producing a feminine appearance. Petechiae and purpura are occasionally seen, and the tourniquet test may be positive.

Absence of or greatly decreased numbers of sweat glands, which are often rudimentary, account for restricted sweating or none at all. Regulation of bodily temperature in a hot environment is defective because of inadequate sweating; thus, the disorder is one of the causes of fever, especially in the newborn. Lanugo, scalp, eyebrow, eyelash, axillary, and pubic hair are scant or absent. Sebaceous glands are decreased in number and activity. Nails may be normal or exhibit slow growth, ridging, or decreased thickness. Permanent and deciduous teeth may be absent or decreased in number and they are likely to be widely spaced, peg-shaped or conical, pigmented or fragile. Abnormalities of the lens include cataracts, subluxation, and absence. Mucous glands of the mouth, pharynx, larynx, trachea, and bronchi may be essentially absent. This may predispose to frequent respiratory tract infections. Chronic rhinitis contributes to the development of saddle nose. Defective lacrimal glands result in deficient tearing. Lack of sweat pores of the palmar dermal ridges and x-ray evidence of defective dentition have diagnostic value.

Less common abnormalities include primary hypogonadism, hypospadias, epispadias, absence of nipples, absence of mammary glands, satyr ears, cleft palate, mental deficiency, central nervous system defects, supernumerary fingers and toes, and micro-ophthalmia.

Histologically, the skin shows decreased epidermal and dermal thickness, absence of or rudimentary sweat glands, absence of or small pilosebaceous apparatus, and poorly developed arrectores pilorum muscles.

Treatment is entirely symptomatic and includes protection from heat, use of dentures, and plastic repair of nasal defects. Measures to improve appearance are morale builders. Longevity is usually good.

Awaad, S., and El Essawy, M. C.: Hereditary anhidrotic ectodermal dysplasia. Arch. Pediat., 77:496, 1960.
Blattner, R. J.: Hereditary ectodermal dysplasia. J. Pediat., 73:444, 1968.
Capitanio, M. A., Chen, J. T. T., Arey, J. B., and Kirkpatrick, J. A.: Congenital anhidrotic ectodermal defect. Amer. J. Roentgen., 103:168, 1968.
Frias, J. L., and Smith, D. W.: Diminished sweat pores in hypohidrotic ectodermal dysplasia. J. Pediat., 72:606, 1968.
Isaa, H.: Total anodontia with ectodermal dysplasia. Brit. Dent. J., 118:537, 1965.
Mohler, D. N.: Hereditary ectodermal dysplasia of the anhidrotic type associated with primary hypogonadism. Amer. J. Med., 27:682, 1959.
Richards, W., and Kaplan, J. M.: Anhidrotic ectodermal dysplasia. An unusual cause of pyrexia in the newborn. Amer. J. Dis. Child., 117:597, 1969.

Neurofibromatosis of von Recklinghausen

Clayton E. Wheeler, Jr.

Neurofibromatosis is a relatively common disease (one case in about 3000 births) characterized by dominant inheritance, café au lait spots, freckling, and neurofibromas of the skin and internal organs. Cause and pathogenesis are unknown.

Café au lait spots occur in more than 90 per cent of the cases. They are often present at birth, but more may appear up to adult life. In old age the number may decrease. The spots are light brown macules that vary considerably in shape and size. More than five such lesions over 1.5 cm. in size are diagnostic (small numbers occur in normal persons). Axillary or generalized freckling, when present, is a characteristic sign. Normal or increased numbers of melanocytes are present in pigmented spots and normal-appearing skin. Giant pigment granules may be found in prickle cells and melanocytes.

Neurofibromas appear at any cutaneous site including the genitalia, palms, and soles. There may be few or many, and they vary greatly in size and shape. The tumors are of two types: (1) small, dome-shaped, or nipple-like, violaceous dermal lesions that can often be pressed into the skin like small hernias, and (2) subcutaneous nodules along the courses of nerves. These may be knotted, plexiform, or pendulous and may attain great size.

The most frequent sites of internal involvement are bone, central nervous system, and pheochrome tissue. Neurofibromas in or near bone produce localized proliferative erosions or cystic lesions. Other frequent bony abnormalities are scoliosis, lordosis, kyphosis, and pseudoarthrosis. Neurofibromas may develop in almost any part of the central nervous system or in the eyes; the symptoms depend upon the size and location of the tumor. Of the cranial nerves, the acoustic and optic are most often involved. Mental deficiency is not unusual. There may be an increased number of brain tumors that are not neurofibromas. The incidence of pheochromocytoma in neurofibromatosis is probably less than 1 per cent. On the other hand, 5 to 20 per cent of patients with pheochromocytoma have neurofibromatosis. Other internal involvement includes gastrointestinal bleeding, intestinal obstruction, lung cysts, pulmonary fibrosis, and hypertension due to abnormalities of renal arteries. Sarcomatous degeneration of neurofibroma is reported in 2 to 16 per cent of cases, depending upon the series studied. Patients are often underdeveloped somatically and sexually, and fertility may be decreased.

Diagnosis is based upon café au lait spots, neurofibromas, bone roentgenograms, the histologic picture, and a positive family history. Treatment is palliative and includes surgical removal of neurofibromas that are large or interfere with function, sarcomas, pheochromocytomas, and various brain tumors. Prognosis is usually good, but it is influenced by malignancy, pheochromocytoma, and skeletal deformities.

Benedict, P. H., Szabo, G., Fitzpatrick, T. B., and Sinesi, S. J.: Melanotic macules in Albright's syndrome and in neurofibromatosis. J.A.M.A., 205:618, 1968.

Crowe, F. W.: Axillary freckling as a diagnostic aid in neurofibromatosis. Ann. Intern. Med., 61:1142, 1964.

Curtis, B. H., Fisher, R. L., Butterfield, W. L., and Saunders, F. P.: Neurofibromatosis with paraplegia. J. Bone Joint Surg. (Amer.), 51:843, 1969.

D'Agostino, A. N., Soule, E. H., and Miller, R. H.: Sarcomas of the peripheral nerves and somatic soft tissues associated with multiple neurofibromatosis (von Recklinghausen's disease). Cancer, 16:1015, 1963.

Halpern, M., and Currarino, G.: Vascular lesions causing hypertension in neurofibromatosis, New Eng. J. Med., 273:248, 1965.

Massaro, D., Katz, S., Matthews, M. J., and Higgins, G.: Von Recklinghausen's neurofibromatosis associated with cystic lung disease. Amer. J. Med., 38:233, 1965.

Ainhum
(Dactylolysis Spontanea)

Clayton E. Wheeler, Jr.

Ainhum is characterized by spontaneous amputation of the fifth toe. The disorder is rare in the United States but common in parts of Africa. It affects primarily Negroes and other dark-skinned persons, and shows a peak incidence between 30 and 40 years of age. The fifth toe is usually affected, although the fourth toe may be involved. Bilateral cases are common. Hyperkeratotic constriction develops at the undersurface of the toe at or between the plantar creases. This gradually encircles and constricts the toe until bone absorption occurs and the distal portion hangs by a thin pedicle. Inflammation or ulceration is often present. After months or years (average five years) the toe undergoes spontaneous, bloodless amputation. Neurologic and circulatory changes (plethysmographic studies are normal) are absent. Varying degrees of pain are common due to sepsis, ulceration, and possibly pressure on nerves. There are no constitutional symptoms. Pathologic findings are nonspecific and probably result from chronic inflammation. The cause is unknown, but a plausible theory is that the small toes are predisposed to spontaneous amputation following trauma, chronic infection, and inflammation. The condition may be related to poor protection and care of the feet; most of the patients have gone barefoot. Cure is accomplished by spontaneous or surgical amputation.

Browne, S. G.: True ainhum: Its distinctive and differentiating features. J. Bone Joint Surg. (Brit.) 47:52, 1965.

Cole, G. J.: Ainhum. An account of fifty-four patients with special reference to etiology and treatment. J. Bone Joint Surg. (Brit.), 47:43, 1965.

Grossman, J., and Harrison, H. D.: Ainhum (dactylolysis spontanea). New York J. Med., 68:1741, 1968.

Peterka, E. S., and Karon, I. M.: Congenital pseudoainhum of the fingers, Arch. Derm. (Chicago), 90:12, 1964.

Warts

Clayton E. Wheeler, Jr.

Warts are circumscribed benign, virus-induced epithelial growths of the skin and adjoining mucous membrane. The virus does not grow in the skin or cornea of laboratory animals or in tissues of the chick embryo, and it is doubtful if it has been grown in any type of tissue culture. Experimental inoculation of ground, filtered wart tissue into human skin results in development of warts at the sites of injection in a few weeks to a few months.

Viral particles are 45 to 75 mμ in size and roughly spherical. They tend to be closely packed in a crystalline arrangement. One virus (or closely related strains) appears to cause several different morphologic types of wart, depending upon local tissue differences and varied host reactions. The principal pathologic condition is in the epidermis, where there is varying hyperplasia of the prickle cell, granular, or horny layers, depending upon the type and location of the wart. Characteristic large, vacuolated cells without intercellular bridges appear in the upper prickle cell and granular layers. The nuclei of these cells presumably contain viral inclusions.

Warts are extremely common; their distribution is worldwide, and they affect both sexes at all ages. There is a peak incidence between 10 and 20 years. Warts are auto-inoculable, as demonstrated by kissing lesions, satellites, and new lesions along scratch lines passed through older warts. The disorder is contagious, but the source and method of infection are frequently unknown. Minor breaks in the epithelium may be important in establishing the infection.

Warts occur anywhere on the skin or mucous membrane adjacent to the skin. They may be single or multiple and are well circumscribed. Several morphologic types occur: (1) Sessile or common warts are often found on the hands, feet, arms, legs, and digits, and about the nails, face, and neck. They vary in size from a few millimeters to a centimeter or two. They are raised, gray, or brown lesions with a rough surface that exhibits black dots or red spots from thrombosed or active papillary vessels (the layman's seed wart). (2)

Filiform warts, which are a few millimeters in diameter and several millimeters long, occur chiefly about the face, neck, and scalp. (3) Plantar warts are often painful and frequently occur at pressure sites. They are usually flat and demarcated from normal skin by a hyperkeratotic ring. Shaving away the horny surface reveals thrombosed or tiny bleeding vessels, a useful point in differentiating callouses or corns. Frequently a number of lesions coalesce to produce patches called mosaic warts. (4) Flat warts are only slightly elevated and are 1 to 3 mm. in diameter. They usually occur about the face, neck, and back of the hands. (5) Moist warts (condylomata acuminata) involve anogenital skin and mucosa most frequently, although they may affect other moist sites such as the conjunctiva or between the toes. These lesions are usually pink or white and they cluster together to produce small or large cauliflower-like growths.

Treatment is empirical and must be adjusted to the number, location, and type of wart, the age and type of patient, and the experience of the physician. Conservative measures should be employed and harmful scarring, excessive local irritation and drug reactions avoided. Most sessile, filiform or flat warts can be treated with light electrodesiccation or freezing with liquid nitrogen. Weekly application of 25 per cent podophyllin in tincture of benzoin usually is adequate for moist warts. Plantar warts are especially stubborn, and several measures may be required. Daily application of 40 per cent salicylic acid plasters or flexible collodion containing 10 per cent salicylic acid and 10 per cent lactic acid may be helpful.

Spontaneous disappearance of warts occurs in 10 to 75 per cent of cases observed over 3 to 24 months. Whether spontaneous regression is related to immunologic, psychologic, or other mechanisms is not known, but it is a major consideration in the evaluation of any type of treatment, and it is likely that many therapeutic methods rely heavily upon spontaneous involution.

Goffe, A. P., Almeida, J. D., and Brown, F.: Further information on the antibody response to wart virus. Lancet, 2:607, 1966.

Massing, A. M., and Epstein, W. L.: Natural history of warts. Arch. Derm. (Chicago), 87:306, 1963.

Noyes, W. F.: Verrucae: Virus structure, localization of antigens, and comparison with Shope papilloma. Cancer Res., 28:1321, 1968.

Oroszlan, S., and Rich, M. A.: Human wart virus: In vitro cultivation. Science, 146:531, 1964.

Rowson, K. E. K., and Mahy, B. W. J.: Human papova (wart) virus. Bact. Rev., 31:110, 1967.

Thorne, N.: The treatment of warts. Brit. J. Clin. Pract., 22:313, 1968.

Weber-Christian Disease
(Relapsing Febrile Nodular Nonsuppurative Panniculitis)
Paul B. Beeson

Weber-Christian disease will be used to describe several clinical syndromes which may or may not be variants of the same disease. The feature shared by all is the occurrence of localized inflammatory lesions in adipose tissue. Histologically these show chronic inflammation with mononuclear cell infiltration; sometimes the mononuclear cells are filled with fatty material. Giant cells occur occasionally, and in more acute lesions polymorphonuclear leukocytes may be present. There is a tendency to inflammatory occlusion of small blood vessels, and necrosis is common.

The term *Weber-Christian disease* is usually applied to a clinical syndrome in which the principal involvement is in the panniculus adiposus. Women are affected more frequently than men with this form of the disease. It is characterized by development of multiple tender nodules in the subcutaneous fat, from 5 mm. to 10 cm. in diameter. The lesions are located principally on the thighs and trunk and in the breasts. They are tender, and there may be some reddening of the skin. Occasionally necrosis of the skin leads to sinus formation with discharge of an oily liquid. The course is usually indolent, crops of lesions developing from time to time over periods of months or years. When the inflammation subsides, there often remains an area of loss of subcutaneous tissue which causes dimpling of skin. Systemic manifestations are usually mild, but may include malaise, low-grade fever, leukocytosis, and eosinophilia. Enlargement of the liver and spleen are reported in some cases. The illness may grumble along for months or several years and then cease.

A more serious expression of this pathologic process has been termed *systemic Weber-Christian disease*. Here there is widespread inflammation affecting not only the panniculus adiposus but similar tissue within the abdominal and thoracic cavities. There may be parenchymatous inflammation, affecting thoracic or abdominal organs, including lungs, pericardium, pleura, bowel, spleen, kidneys, and adrenal glands. At least a dozen cases are recorded in which this form of disease has led to death.

The term *mesenteric panniculitis* has been applied to an obscure disease characterized by inflammation of the mesenteric fat. This has been encountered mainly in males, and reports of the syndrome have appeared principally in surgical journals. Symptoms include recurrent episodes of fever, abdominal pain, nausea, vomiting, and malaise. At operation the mesentery is found to be thickened, with red or yellow patches, and biopsy reveals the characteristic panniculitis, which cannot be differentiated from the lesions of Weber-Christian disease.

Several writers have suggested that these forms of inflammation in the retroperitoneal adipose tissue may represent the initial lesion in at least some cases of retroperitoneal fibrosis.

There is no specific therapy. Some writers have reported considerable relief of symptoms by use of large doses of steroids, but in other instances this has not proved helpful. Antimicrobial drugs should not be given. The use of immunosuppressive or cytotoxic agents could be considered, especially when there is evidence of systemic extension of the panniculitis.

Milner, R. D. G., and Mitchinson, M. J.: Systemic Weber-Christian disease. J. Clin. Path., 18:150, 1965.

Ogden, W. W., II, Bradburn, D. M., and Rives, J. D.: Mesenteric panniculitis. Ann. Surg., 161:864, 1965.

Disorders of Melanin Pigmentation

Aaron B. Lerner

Melanin is formed in the cytoplasm of melanocytes by oxidation of tyrosine catalyzed by tyrosinase, a copper-containing enzyme. Melanocytes are derived embryonically from the neural crest. Before the third month of fetal life the melanocytes have migrated to their resting places in the skin at the epidermal-dermal junction, in the eyes along the uveal tract, and in the central nervous system in the leptomeninges. Pigmented nevi are composed of clusters of melanocytes. Most of them form after birth. Occasionally, however, large nevi are present at birth; they represent abnormal migration of melanocytes from the neural crest.

Melanin formation is impaired by a congenital decrease of tyrosinase in albinism (see the article on albinism in the section of this textbook devoted to miscellaneous hereditary disorders) and by inhibition of tyrosinase in phenylketonuria. Severe trauma to the skin may destroy melanocytes and produce localized hypopigmentation. A common and important manifestation of hypopigmentation is vitiligo. This abnormality affects about 1 per cent of the population and is generally transmitted as a dominant trait. It has been suggested that vitiligo is caused by excessive release of a neurogenic factor, e.g., acetylcholine, that acts directly on the melanocytes to keep them in a light-colored state or to cause their disappearance from the skin. The hypopigmentation of vitiligo occurs in the exposed areas, particularly the face and dorsal aspects of the hands; on the axillae and genitalia; surrounding body orifices (mouth, eyes, nose, nipples, and rectum); at sites of pressure and trauma; about pigmented nevi; and in hair. Patients with vitiligo are usually in good general health. However, the incidence of vitiligo is increased in patients with hyperthyroidism, pernicious anemia, and adrenocortical insufficiency. In fact, vitiligo tends to occur in patients who are becoming hyperpigmented, so that there may be lightening in some areas and darkening in others. Hypopigmentation distinct from vitiligo is seen in patients with scleroderma. Patches of hypopigmentation and less frequently partial albinism are seen in patients with tuberous sclerosis.

In most clinical problems accompanied by hyperpigmentation, endocrine function is abnormal. Specific hormones induce cytoplasmic changes in the melanocytes, and tryosinase activity increases. The melanocyte-stimulating hormone, β-MSH, when released in excessive quantities by the pituitary gland, causes darkening of the skin in patients with adrenocortical insufficiency. Pituitary activity increases as a result of decreased steroid production by the adrenal cortex. However, the same kind of hyperpigmentation can occur in the presence of a pituitary tumor that releases an excess of MSH. Usually pituitary tumors first produce increased amounts of corticotrophin which stimulate the adrenals and lead to the development of Cushing's syndrome. If a pituitary tumor is not suspected and the patient undergoes bilateral adrenalectomy, the tumor will continue to grow and the skin may become very dark. Initially the tumor produces only large amounts of corticotrophin, but subsequently MSH peptides also are made. In some patients a pituitary tumor may release excess MSH but not corticotrophin, so that adrenocortical hyperplasia does not occur.

A few patients with metastatic carcinomas develop similar problems of hyperpigmentation. The carcinomas produce peptides related to or identical with corticotrophin and MSH. Some of these patients develop both Cushing's syndrome and hyperpigmentation, although others show only hyperpigmentation. Assay of some of the tumors has shown MSH and corticotrophin-like substances to be present. Hyperpigmentation also may be seen in 10 to 15 per cent of women receiving potent synthetic progesterones and estrogens for birth control. Although these substances are not as effective darkeners of melanocytes as are the MSH and MSH-like peptides, they do produce facial pigmentation or melasma.

There is evidence to support the view that MSH brings about an increase in intracellular cyclic AMP, which in turn induces tyrosinase synthesis.

Severe hyperpigmentation is seen occasionally in patients with hyperthyroidism, xanthomatous biliary cirrhosis, sprue, or hemochromatosis. However, the skin of some patients with hemochromatosis may be slate gray in color because iron pigments together with melanin may be deposited deep in the dermis. Chronic illness or ingestion of drugs such as busulfan (Myleran) or 4-amino pteroylglutamic acid (Aminopterin) also induces hyperpigmentation. It is likely that alteration of hormones other than MSH may be responsible for the pigmentary changes in these conditions.

All adults have many nevi, and most melanomas arise from nevi. Melanoma is an uncommon malignancy that accounts for about 1 per cent of cancer deaths. In a few patients with metastatic melanoma moderate amounts of tyrosine oxidation products made in the tumors are carried by the blood to the kidneys and are excreted in the urine. In air they become oxidized to melanin, giving the urine a dark color. These patients are said to have melanuria. In exceptional cases of metastatic melanoma, great quantities of tyrosine oxidation products form, reach the skin, and are converted to melanin. The patient first acquires the slate gray color of argyria and later becomes intensely brown or black.

Abe, K., Nicholson, W. E., Liddle, G. W., Island, D. P., and Orth, D. N.: Radioimmunoassay of β-MSH in human plasma and tissues. J. Clin. Invest., 46:1609, 1967.

Lerner, A. B., and McGuire, J. S.: Melanocyte-stimulating hormone and adrenocorticotrophic hormone: Their relation to pigmentation. New Eng. J. Med., 270:539, 1964.

Lerner, A. B., Snell, R. S., Chanco-Turner, M., and McGuire, J. S.: Vitiligo and sympathectomy. Arch. Derm. (Chicago), 94:269, 1966.

RESPIRATORY DISEASE

Introduction

M. Henry Williams, Jr.

In recent years, there have been dramatic changes in the field of chest medicine. New techniques, advances in therapy, and awareness of new diseases have changed and greatly increased the demands upon the knowledge and skill of both internist and pulmonary specialist.

Major advances have been made in the treatment of tuberculosis. Modern chemotherapy has led to substantial decrease of morbidity and mortality and has made it possible to treat the disease successfully on an ambulatory basis. Nevertheless, tuberculosis remains prevalent in the large cities, and it is apparent that many social and personal factors are important in its pathogenesis and in response to therapy. In treating tuberculosis the physician must concern himself with the frequently coexistent problems of alcoholism, drug addiction, and, particularly, failure of the patient to take prescribed medication regularly and for a sufficient period. Because the treatment of tuberculosis belongs rightfully within the province of the internist, because it should be treated as an infection in general hospitals instead of in sanatoriums, and because it still ranks as a major cause of undiagnosed febrile, pulmonary, or hematologic disease, the practicing physician must be thoroughly familiar with its manifestations and with the principles of therapy. This disease is discussed in detail in preceding sections of this text (see Tuberculosis).

Pneumonia also remains a common problem in medical practice, and the mortality among patients sick enough to be hospitalized is still distressingly high, despite antimicrobial therapy. Pneumococcal infection is the most common cause of pneumonia, but infections with Staphylococcus, Klebsiella, and other organisms are sufficiently frequent and the proper choice and use of antimicrobial drugs is so important that the physician must be familiar with the clinical features of the different infections (see Pneumonia).

In particular, he must be skilled in obtaining and interpreting sputum smears so as to institute appropriate therapy at the earliest possible moment and to avoid the use of unnecessary drugs.

Lung cancer and chronic obstructive pulmonary disease (COPD), each discussed in detail in a following section, have both emerged as major health problems during the past decade. Treatment is far from satisfactory for either. The physician can provide some measure of comfort to the patient with COPD, can successfully treat life-threatening episodes of ventilatory failure, and by discriminating radiographic study can select an occasional patient whose cancer can be resected.

Nevertheless, hope for cure of these diseases is bleak, and efforts must be directed at prevention, especially by combating cigarette smoking.

The interstitial pneumonias and alveolar proteinosis are some of the newly described diseases with which the physician must now be familiar, and they are discussed in the section on interstitial lung disease. Sarcoidosis, particularly as manifested by asymptomatic hilar adenopathy, has emerged as an extremely common disease, rivaling tuberculosis in prevalence in many places. Although sarcoidosis commonly involves the lung and hilar lymph nodes, it can involve any organ of the body, and it is discussed in the section on granulomatous diseases.

The organization of the following section on respiratory disease has been based partly on common anatomic features (bellows, airways, air spaces, lung parenchyma, pleura, and pulmonary circulation) and partly on common clinical features (irritants and neoplasm). Major emphasis is placed on principles of pathophysiology; diseases which have been well studied and which illustrate important principles have received special emphasis.

Evaluation and treatment of respiratory disease requires an understanding of pulmonary physiology and of the meaning and value of tests of pulmonary function. The section on pulmonary structure and function is not a complete exposition of anatomy and physiology, but it is designed to build on a framework of basic knowledge and to relate the basic material to clinical phenomena. The purpose of this article is to emphasize pulmonary physiology as it relates to clinical medicine, to refresh the reader about important physiologic principles, and to bridge the gap between the basic text and the clinical problem. In addition to understanding how the lung works, the physician should know when and why to perform various tests. Serial studies of arterial blood gas composition are essential to the appropriate management of ventilatory failure; measurement of peak expiratory flow provides useful, moment-to-moment evaluation of the patient with asthma; spirographic measurement is as much a part of the evaluation of the chest patient as an electrocardiogram is part of the evaluation of the cardiac patient; and a measurement of diffusing capacity may be the only clue to the presence or extent of diffuse interstitial pulmonary disease. Abnormalities of pulmonary function have differing degrees of therapeutic urgency. Arterial oxygen unsaturation is a potentially lethal condition which requires treatment, whereas impaired diffusion is seldom of consequence to the patient, but knowledge of its presence is vital for accurate diagnosis and prognosis.

A number of clinical problems and diagnostic techniques cut across the material presented in this section and elsewhere. Ventilatory failure is a serious complication of many types of neuromuscular disease and is discussed in the section on the nervous system as well as here under COPD. Hemoptysis is a significant clinical entity requiring appropriate diagnostic study and management (articles on tuberculosis, lung abscess, and lung cancer). The physician must be familiar with the specific physical findings in each illness, but today it is even more important to have a working familiarity with the x-ray of the chest. Every

patient with pulmonary disease should have an anteroposterior, lateral, and apical lordotic film, and the physician should know when to request oblique views, tomograms, bronchograms, and angiograms and how to evaluate localized and diffuse densities when they are present. Specialized procedures, such as needle biopsy of lung and pleura, are important tools for the chest physician, who should also be aware of the value, limitations, and risks of bronchoscopy, bronchography, mediastinoscopy, and thoracic surgery. As in all medicine, the risk and discomfort of a thoracic diagnostic procedure must be balanced carefully against the likelihood of obtaining useful and important information.

Structure and Function

GENERAL CONSIDERATIONS
M. Henry Williams, Jr.

The primary function of the lung is the exchange of respiratory gases—the elimination of carbon dioxide and the uptake of oxygen. The actual gas exchange occurs in the alveoli and is governed by the physical laws which govern the diffusion of gases. In order for gas exchange to occur and for arterial blood gas composition to be maintained at normal, the alveolar gas composition must be kept constant and normal despite the continuing extraction of oxygen and addition of carbon dioxide. This is achieved by periodic ventilation of the alveolar gas with fresh air containing 21 per cent oxygen and essentially no carbon dioxide. Closely related to this primary function is the maintenance of a normal partial pressure of oxygen and of carbon dioxide in the arterial blood. For this system to operate successfully, all the blood perfusing the tissues must come from the lung, and all the blood leaving the tissues must be pumped to the lung for repletion of oxygen and removal of carbon dioxide.

Since all the blood leaving the cells is pumped through the lungs, the pulmonary cells and capillaries are subject to assault by a variety of potentially noxious materials: blood clots, foreign proteins, and other toxins. Mechanisms must be present to deal with these insults. Likewise, the air which ventilates the alveoli may contain organic and inorganic materials which are capable of producing disease, and the lung must maintain an effective defense against these invaders. In addition, the lung itself is an organ that must remain viable and maintain itself by cellular replication and other metabolic functions. Although the following section is organized around consideration

of the primary, gas-exchanging function of the lung, mention will be made of important metabolic functions as well as of the structural characteristics of the system which are essential to its proper functioning.

In studying pulmonary function, physiologists have developed a battery of tests which have proved useful to the physician. Sometimes these tests provide direct and critical insight into pathophysiologic processes; they often shed light on the ways in which the primary function of the lung is faulty, but even more often they provide quantitative information of clinical significance even when the over-all function of the system remains adequate to maintain normal arterial blood gas composition.

VENTILATORY FUNCTION
M. Henry Williams, Jr.

LUNG VOLUMES, PLEURAL PRESSURE, AND THE RESPIRATORY CYCLE

The most obvious and easily measured aspect of pulmonary function is ventilatory function. Inspiration consists in the enlargement of the thorax by contraction of the diaphragm and intercostal muscles, each contributing to about 50 per cent of the tidal volume. By forceful contraction of inspiratory muscles, it is possible to inspire considerably more air than the tidal volume. Chest expansion is limited largely by the structural, fibrous restraints within the lung parenchyma. Measurement of the *total lung capacity* (TLC), the volume of air in the lung at the end of a maximal inspiration, provides useful clinical information. In some patients with emphysema, destruction of lung tissue and reduced resistance to lung expansion is associated with an increased TLC. Reduction of the TLC results from imperfect function of the thoracic bellows (chest deformity, pleural disease, muscle paralysis), from increased resistance of the lung to stretch (pulmonary fibrosis), or from diseases in which air-containing tissue is replaced by abnormal tissue (inflammation, neoplasia, or granulomatous disease).

Expiration is largely the result of the passive recoil of the lung which becomes greater as the lung is stretched by an inspiration. The tendency of the lung to collapse is counterbalanced by the tendency of the thoracic cage to enlarge. As the lung empties and gets smaller, its elastic recoil becomes less, whereas the outward recoil of the thorax increases. When these opposing forces become equal, expiration ends. The lung volume at which this occurs, the *functional residual capacity* (FRC), is determined by the mechanical properties of the lung and the thorax. Increased retractive force of the lung or decreased retractive force of the thorax causes reduction of the FRC, whereas reduced retractive force of the lung or increased retractive force of the thorax leads to an increase of the FRC. The inherent tendency of the lung to collapse at all volumes above residual is responsible for the negative intrapleural pressure, the magnitude of which is directly proportional to the lung volume. Normally the pleural pressure is minus 2 cm. H_2O at FRC, decreasing to minus 6 cm. H_2O at the end of an inspiration and to less than minus 20 cm. H_2O at TLC. Although the pleural pressure is always negative, the alveolar pressure is atmospheric at the end of inspiration and of expiration. During inspiration, enlargement of the thorax generates additional negative intrapleural pressure which, transmitted to the alveoli, causes air to enter the lung. The opposite occurs during expiration when the tendency of the chest to collapse makes the intrapleural pressure and the alveolar pressure less negative so that air leaves the lung.

By forceful contraction of expiratory muscles, additional air can be expelled from the lung. Forced expiration is limited by airway closure, by loss of lung recoil, or by weakness of the muscles of expiration. Generally, however, an increase of residual volume (RV), the volume of air left in the lung after maximal expiration, signifies airway obstruction. The *vital capacity* is the maximal volume of air expired from full inspiration and is one of the oldest and most useful indices of pulmonary function. It is determined by the total lung capacity and by the degree to which the lung can be emptied. The vital capacity is reduced in patients whose respiratory muscle strength is abnormal, in patients in whom the lung is rendered indistensible by fibrous tissue or by chest wall deformity, in patients whose air-containing tissue is replaced by tumor or inflammatory disease, and in patients with obstructive disease leading to complete occlusion of airways at an increased residual volume.

SPIROMETRY

The dimensions of the conducting system through which air must move in and out of the lung are so large that inspiration and expiration can be accomplished easily and quickly. In various types of obstructive pulmonary disease, the airways become so narrow as to limit the rate of air flow into and out of the lung. This impairment is easily assessed by spirometry. Obstruction to air flow is particularly obvious during expiration, both because the diameters of the airways narrow as lung volume becomes smaller and because the positive intrapleural pressure which tends to drive air from the lungs during a forced expiration also tends to collapse the conducting airways. As a result, attention is generally focused on air flow during a forced expiration. Useful indices of airway obstruction include the *timed vital capacity*, the percentage of the total which can be expired in one, two, and three seconds (normally at least 70, 85, and 95 per cent), and the volume of air expired in the first second, the *forced expiratory volume* (FEV_1), or during the middle half of expiration, the *maximal midexpiratory flow rate* (MMF: normal 2 to 4 liters per second). Patients with chronic obstructive pulmonary disease always have an MMF below 1 liter per second, and generally below 0.5 liter per second. In these patients the MMF is relatively constant and little improved by administration of a bronchodilator. In patients with bronchial asthma, the MMF may or may not be very low, and when low generally increases with therapy. The *peak expiratory flow rate* (PEFR) is a very simple and convenient method of evaluating ventilatory function, particularly when one wishes to obtain frequent serial measurements, as in asthma. Normally, the PEFR exceeds 400 liters per minute, and in asthma associated with such severe airway obstruction as to cause death from asphyxia the PEFR is less than 80 liters per minute. In general, asthmatic patients with a PEFR less than 120 liters per minute should be considered seriously ill and in need of constant medical attention.

The presence of audible rhonchi and wheezes signifies turbulent air flow, suggesting the presence of obstructive disease, and the physician can obtain a semiquantitative index of the problem by timing the duration of a forced vital capacity by listening over the larynx. By measuring intrapleural (esophageal) pressure, and simultaneously recording the air flow at the mouth, the physiologist can obtain more precise measurements of respiratory mechanics. *Lung compliance*, defined as change of volume per change of pressure, is an index of the mechanical properties of the lung, and *airway resistance*, defined as the pressure required to generate flow through the airways, is an index of the dimensions of the tracheobronchial tree. Both these measurements vary with lung volume, the lung becoming stiff (less compliant) as it is inflated and the airways becoming wider and less resistant to flow as the lung volume increases.

Although these measurements provide interesting information, a study of expiratory flow rates and vital capacity generally provides adequate clinical assessment of restrictive and obstructive disease so that the more precise measurements are seldom necessary.

MINUTE VENTILATION

Measurements of the lung volumes, expiratory flow rates, and lung mechanics provide useful information about the respiratory system. They do not, however, indicate whether or not the minute ventilation is normal. Patients with severe abnormality of lung volumes or mechanics may or may not have reduced ventilation. The effectiveness of ventilatory function must be considered in terms of the purpose of the minute ventilation, which is to add oxygen to the alveolar air and to remove carbon dioxide in accordance with the metabolic needs of the body. The ventilation is regulated to meet these metabolic needs so as to maintain a normal alveolar gas composition: a Pco_2 of 40 mm. Hg and a Po_2 of 100 mm. Hg. Increased metabolic rate, as in fever or muscular exercise, is matched by an appropriate increase of ventilation so that alveolar gas composition remains constant. Under a variety of conditions, to be discussed subsequently, ventilation may not be maintained at the appropriate level, resulting in increase of alveolar Pco_2 and a decrease of alveolar Po_2. It should be emphasized that the alveolar Pco_2 and the arterial Pco_2, which are essentially identical, actually measure the effectiveness of ventilation. Hypercapnia indicates that ventilation is reduced, and hypocapnia means that ventilation is increased in relationship to metabolic needs.

The alveolar Po_2 also reflects the level of ventilation, a high Po_2 indicating hyperventilation and a low Po_2 hypoventilation. Hyperventilation will cause the alveolar Po_2 to be elevated about as much above 100 mm. Hg as the Pco_2 is reduced below 40 mm. Hg, and in hypoventilation the Po_2 will be as much below 100 mm. Hg as the Pco_2 is above 40 mm. Hg. However, alveolar gas is often neither uniform nor measurable, and assessment of hypoventilation is best based on arterial blood measurements. Since many abnormalities can cause reduction of arterial Po_2 but not hypercapnia, adequacy of ventilation is best assessed by the arterial Pco_2.

Although the clinician may form some conclusions about ventilatory function by listening to the breath sounds generated by movement of air in and out of the lungs and by observation of the movement of the chest cage, these observations are grossly inexact, and accurate assessment of total ventilation requires a measurement of tidal volume and respiratory rate. Evaluation of the adequacy of the ventilation requires a measurement of arterial Pco_2.

ALVEOLAR AIR

Although gas exchange actually occurs across the walls of individual alveoli, the basic unit of the lung is now considered to be the acinus, the alveolar ducts and alveoli supplied by a terminal bronchiole. This unit of respiratory function is ventilated with each inspiration, and the air spaces are so small as to allow practically instantaneous diffusion of gases within the unit so that alveolar gas composition is essentially uniform throughout. Indeed, alveolar "ventilation" is largely the result of diffusion of gas molecules within the small airways and alveoli, and is not due to mass movement of air much beyond the large bronchi. Only a small portion of the lung volume within the acinus is actually turned over with each breath. The existence of a large alveolar volume, even at the end of a maximal expiration, may be considered to be a homeostatic adjustment to the fact that gas exchange across the alveolar capillaries is continuous, whereas ventilation is discontinuous—fresh air only enters the alveoli during inspiration. If the volume of the unit were not large compared to the amount of gas exchanged, the alveolar Po_2 would fall and the alveolar Pco_2 would rise from the end of one inspiration until the beginning of the next, and there would be large fluctuations of arterial blood gas composition. Thus, one may consider that the function of the lung volume is to maintain constancy of the alveolar and arterial blood gas composition throughout the respiratory cycle.

RESPIRATORY CONTROL

Respiration serves several purposes, including metabolic gas exchange, communication, and heat regulation. In addition, the respiratory system is endowed with a number of protective reflexes, some of which influence the respiratory rate and depth; others induce coughing, sneezing, and yawning. The principal integration and regulation of these several functions are achieved by respiratory neurons located in the medulla oblongata and lower pons. This "respiratory center" is, in turn, influenced by structures at higher levels of the nervous system as well as by changes in its local chemical environment. In the metabolic regulation of ventilation, priority is awarded to the maintenance of a normal Pco_2. Increased arterial Pco_2 leads to increase of the Pco_2 within tissue fluids and, hence, to a decreased pH within the chemosensitive neurons of the respiratory center. This is followed by increased respiratory activity. The resultant increase of ventilation causes decreased Pco_2 and, hence, decreased respiratory drive. This feedback control system maintains the arterial Pco_2 within narrow limits unless there is gross disturbance of the effector system (the lungs and the chest cage) or of the respiratory center itself. In addition, chemosensitive arterial receptors respond to hypercapnia, to an increased hydrogen ion concentration, and to hypoxia, the last accounting for the mild hyperventilation which exists at altitude or in subjects with hypoxemia. This is generally considered to be an emergency mechanism, and it plays little part in normal regulation of ventilation. A variety of reflex pathways also exist in lungs and other tissues which directly or indirectly affect respiration. Of these the most important clinically are afferent stimuli from pulmonary vessels stretched by pulmonary hypertension or from lungs stiffened by edema, fibrosis, or granulomatous disease.

Increased respiratory drive in excess of CO_2-determined stimulation leads to increased ventilation and hypocapnia. Decreased respiratory drive causes hypoventilation and hypercapnia and is usually the result of depressant drugs or impaired mechanical performance of the lung and chest bellows so that extra muscular effort is needed to achieve a given minute ventilation.

A clear distinction should be made between hyperventilation and dyspnea. The latter is the patient's subjective awareness of respiratory discomfort. This symptom, which is present in many diseases, may have as its physiologic basis an inappropriate shortening of respiratory muscle fibers in response to respiratory need. Respiratory need is determined by all the chemical and nervous stimuli to respiration and cannot be measured. However, one can measure the mechanical properties of the lung and ascertain that excessive muscular effort is being spent on the act of ventilation or that excessive ventilation is indeed taking place, in which case the patient might be "entitled" to dyspnea. But beyond that, the subjective nature of the symptom, attenuated and amplified by emotional factors, precludes quantitative assessment.

ABNORMALITIES IN RESPIRATORY CONTROL
Fred Plum

Neurologic or neuromuscular disorders frequently produce breathing abnormalities. Diseases of the cerebrum or upper brainstem commonly induce disturbances in the respiratory rate and rhythm which do not interfere with gas exchange. Diseases of the lower brainstem, spinal cord, nerves, or muscles can produce respiratory failure, and this is often the most serious aspect of such illnesses.

Abnormal Respiratory Rhythms in Neurologic Disease. The abnormal, irregular breathing rhythm of medullary disease is discussed below.

Patients with disease at upper pontine or low midbrain levels sometimes show *central neurogenic hyperventilation*. Such patients are usually in stupor or coma, and their metronomically regular hyperpnea must be distinguished from the other causes of hyperpnea listed in Table 1.

Cheyne-Stokes respiration is a regularly oscillating pattern of respiratory rhythm in which hyperpneic and apneic periods alternate, one full cycle requiring twice the circulation time. Usually such periodic breathing reflects bilateral neurologic damage at subcortical or diencephalic brain levels. Occasionally, particularly when the hyperpneic phase is brief and the apneic phase relatively long, periodic breathing can be a manifestation of severe lower brainstem injury at pontine levels.

Respiratory Failure in Neurologic Disease. Neurologic or muscular disease may cause either peripheral or central respiratory failure.

Peripheral respiratory failure results when the skeletal musculature of the diaphragm, chest wall, abdomen, and neck becomes so weakened that the chest bellows cannot move sufficient air to ventilate the lungs. Potential causes of peripheral respiratory failure are listed in Table 2; those that are most frequent or tend to create medical emergencies are marked with an asterisk.

The symptoms of peripheral respiratory failure depend partly upon which muscles are affected first. Patients suffering progressive paralysis of chest wall or abdomen may have few symptoms until their diaphragms are involved, at which time no respiratory reserves are left. On the other hand, patients whose diaphragms are paralyzed first may feel breathless almost immediately. Those who need to cough may become incapacitated rapidly if they lose their abdominal muscles. These considerations imply that whenever faced with the diseases listed in Table 1, the alert physician must evaluate respiratory function, using serial vital capacity measurements to estimate the qualitative functional impact of paralysis. Gross indices of respiratory function such as attention to respiratory rate, inspecting the apparent magnitude of chest expansion, and checking for dyspnea usually are unreliable. Patients with acute peripheral respiratory failure almost never become anoxemic or hypocarbic until ready to collapse, so that therapy, to be effective, must be started before cyanosis appears or abnormalities appear in blood gases.

Central respiratory failure results when the

TABLE 1. CONDITIONS CAUSING HYPERPNEA WITH STUPOR OR COMA

Respiratory Alkalosis	Metabolic Acidosis
Central neurogenic hyperventilation:	Diabetic coma
Brainstem infarcts	Uremia
Secondary brainstem compression	Ingested organic acids
Severe hypoglycemia	Methyl alcohol
Acute anoxia	Ethylene glycol
Hepatic coma	
Salicylate poisoning (adult)	
Sepsis	

Plum, F.: The effects of neurological disease on the act of breathing. In Howell, J. B. L., and Campbell, E. J. M. (eds.): Breathlessness. Oxford, Blackwell Scientific Publications, Ltd., 1966.

TABLE 2. THE NEUROLOGIC CAUSES OF RESPIRATORY FAILURE

A. Peripheral

I. Diseases of the respiratory muscles
  Progressive muscular dystrophy
  Myotonic muscular dystrophy
  Polymyositis
II. Diseases and disorders of the myoneural junction
  Myasthenia gravis*
  Botulism*
  Anticholinesterase poisons* (parathione, DFP etc.)
  Hypersensitivity to curare in patients with
    pseudomyasthenia (malignancy)
III. Peripheral neuropathies
  Guillain-Barré syndrome*
  Diphtheria
  Acute intermittent porphyria
IV. Anterior horn cell diseases
  Poliomyelitis*
  Amyotrophic lateral sclerosis
V. Lesions of the spinal conducting pathways
  High cervical trauma*
  Acute myelitis
  High spinal compression or malignancy

B. Central

I. Infections
  Encephalitic poliomyelitis
  Postexanthematous or disseminated encephalomyelitis
II. Trauma, brainstem hemorrhage, or neoplasm (rare)
  Craniovertebral abnormalities
III. Drug depression
  Barbiturates
  Opiates
  Other depressants

respiratory integrating neurons in the medulla oblongata become damaged or diseased. Common causes are listed in Table 2. Central respiratory failure produces defects in the respiratory rate and rhythm, and symptoms usually evolve through progressive stages. At first, a subtle respiratory irregularity appears, which is most pronounced during drowsiness or rest. Patients may report that it is impossible to sleep or that they must concentrate on the breathing act. By this time, the pattern of breathing may be frankly irregular. In those with drug-induced depression, the respiratory rate is slow and the volume shallow; intermittent, irregular apneic periods may occur. Respiratory sensitivity to carbon dioxide is reduced and anoxia or CO_2 retention may develop unless treatment is instituted. By this point, progressive failure and decompensation usually are rapid.

The treatment of respiratory failure is artificial respiration. There are many satisfactory respirators. Both the "iron lung" and positive-pressure types create intrapulmonary pressures that cyclically exceed external pressures on the chest. However, individual models vary widely, and the physician would do well to familiarize himself with available devices before trying to use them in emergencies. When treating respiratory failure, careful and constant attention is required to see that the airway is unobstructed. If there is any doubt, tracheotomy should be performed.

CONDUCTING AIRWAYS
M. Henry Williams, Jr.

The airways leading to the acini are tubes which branch by irregular dichotomy and provide increasing surface area at each branching. As a result, the highest resistance to flow through the conduction system occurs in the major bronchi and trachea, the smaller airways actually contributing relatively little resistance to airflow. Narrowing of the large bronchi has more effect on expiratory air flow than a similar narrowing of peripheral bronchioles, and a patient must develop widespread occlusive disease of peripheral airways before symptoms of chronic obstructive disease develop.

The airways are designed to conduct tidal volume in and out of the alveoli, and their size must represent a compromise between a large surface for conducting air with little resistance and a minimal dead space, the latter being that portion of the inspired air which remains in the airways and is not available for gas exchange. Normally about a third of each breath is so wasted. The *physiologic dead space* is measured by relating the expired to the arterial carbon dioxide tension, the difference between the two being essentially a measure of the amount of dead space air which dilutes the alveolar gas to form the expired air. Measurement of physiologic dead space is useful in determining total ventilatory requirements of a patient. The measurement also has clinical value, since an increase of physiologic dead space rarely stems from increased volume of the conducting airways but, rather, reflects ventilation of alveoli which are not perfused with blood. Air going to such units remains unaltered in composition and is wasted ventilation. The physiologic dead space is extremely variable, even in a single subject, but is closely related to the tidal volume, and the ratio of dead space to tidal volume (V_D/V_T) is essentially constant. This ratio is normally less than 0.30, and increase or decrease signifies worsening or improvement of matching of ventilation to perfusion.

Because, as mentioned above, inspired air contains a variety of inorganic and organic pollutants which may settle anywhere along the tracheobronchial tree, mechanisms must be present to remove these potential pathogens from the lungs. The bronchial mucus, secreted by goblet cells and mucous glands, serves this function. The mucus is propelled up the tracheobronchial tree by the constant beating of cilia. Any material which settles on the airways, or is brought there by alveolar macrophages, is carried up this mucous escalator to the mouth and is expectorated or swallowed. Normally, about 100 ml. of mucus is produced per day, and this amount is greatly increased in those exposed to air pollution, particularly cigarette smoke. Excessive secretion of mucus, which is accompanied by morphologic evidence of hypertrophied mucous glands, is the cardinal symptom of chronic bronchitis.

ALVEOLAR STRUCTURE AND FUNCTION
M. Henry Williams, Jr.

DIFFUSION

The actual process of gas exchange takes place in the 300 million alveoli. The alveolar wall consists of a thin epithelial lining separating the air space from the pulmonary capillary. The design of the structure provides maximum exposure of circulating blood to alveolar gas over some 80 square meters of surface area and through a minimal layer of separating tissue. This permits such rapid diffusion of gases that, in normal subjects, there is no discernible difference between the partial pressure of oxygen in the alveolar air and in the blood leaving the alveolar capillary. In patients with extensive loss or thickening of this diffusion surface, by emphysema or inflammatory disease respectively, diffusion may be imperfect, leading to measurable reduction of the end-capillary P_{O_2}. It is rare for this impairment to be so severe as to cause detectable unsaturation of arterial blood. As carbon dioxide is 20 to 30 times as "diffusible" as oxygen, hypercapnia is never a result of diffusion impairment. Although diffusion is rarely a cause of blood gas abnormality, measurement of the *diffusing capacity* of the lung is a very useful index of pulmonary structure and function. In many patients with diffuse lung disease, reduction of the diffusing capacity may be the only indication that parenchymal disease is present, and the measurement provides useful information about prognosis and the effects of therapy.

METABOLIC FUNCTION

The alveolar walls are not dry, but are lined by a complex substance, *surfactant*, which has the property of reducing surface tension, particularly at small lung volumes when the high surface tension would tend to collapse the small alveoli into larger units with correspondingly lower internal pressure. This surfactant is undoubtedly important in maintaining stability of alveolar structure and in preventing atelectasis, but the role of surfactant deficiency in human disease is uncertain. The surface-active material is apparently synthe-sized by alveolar lining cells, one of the many metabolic functions of the lung that are essential to maintenance of its functional integrity. In addition, the alveolar lining cells probably form the macrophages within the alveolar wall, an important defense against very small particles which diffuse into the alveoli from inspired air and which are potentially capable of causing disease. Finally, either in the alveoli or in the conducting airways, there are cells which possess the property of synthesizing immune globulins which are important in host defense and, possibly, in causing allergic disease.

VENTILATION-PERFUSION RELATIONSHIPS

One of the extraordinary features of pulmonary function is the correspondence between ventilation and circulation in individual lung units. Although there is considerable variation of ventilation to various parts of the lung, the upper lobes receiving less than the lower, normally there is, in general, a matching of perfusion so that the well-ventilated units receive more circulation than those that are poorly ventilated. This is very important, since ventilation of nonperfused lung would be wasted dead-space ventilation, and perfusion of nonventilated lung would, in effect, constitute a right-to-left shunt of venous blood through the lung. Imbalance of ventilation and perfusion is common in chronic pulmonary disease and, indeed, represents the major cause of arterial unsaturation (see below, e.g., hypoxemia). A number of mechanisms provide for the matching of ventilation and diffusion. It is likely that an alveolus of normal size represents the least resistance to blood flow so that alveoli which are collapsed and nonventilated because of complete obstruction, or which are overexpanded because of partial obstruction, hinder blood flow and so are correspondingly poorly perfused. In addition reduction of the oxygen tension in the alveolar air is capable of causing vasoconstriction which prevents perfusion of poorly ventilated alveoli. Likewise, reduction of the P_{CO_2} in the alveoli elicits bronchial constriction, tending to reduce the alveolar ventilation to a unit of lung which has been deprived of circulation. These mechanisms are imperfect in extreme disease but are valuable contributors to normal pulmonary function.

OXYGEN AND CARBON DIOXIDE TRANSPORT

The function of the lung is to maintain an appropriate alveolar environment with respect to oxygen and carbon dioxide and to permit the rapid diffusion of oxygen into the blood and of carbon dioxide from the venous blood into the alveoli. Maintenance of cellular function by provision of adequate oxygen supplies and carbon dioxide removal also depends upon the transport function of the blood.

Most of the carbon dioxide is carried in the form of bicarbonate (HCO_3), which is in equilibrium with carbonic acid (H_2CO_3). The concentration of the latter is determined by the concentration of CO_2 in the blood, which is, in turn, dependent upon the P_{CO_2}. These relationships are discussed in more detail in the article on acid-base balance.

Although a little oxygen is dissolved in blood (approximately 0.03 ml. per 100 ml.), most of the oxygen is bound to hemoglobin, which has the unique property of combining with large amounts of oxygen when the P_{O_2} is high and of releasing oxygen as the P_{O_2} falls. At a normal arterial P_{O_2} of 100 mm. Hg and in the absence of anemia, approximately 20 ml. of oxygen is carried in 100 ml. of blood. In the tissues, where the oxygen tension is lower, substantial quantities of oxygen are given up to the cell. Furthermore, the oxy-hemoglobin dissociation curve has the additional feature of a flat, upper portion so that there can be considerable reduction of arterial oxygen tension before appreciable hypoxemia develops.

PULMONARY CIRCULATION
M. Henry Williams, Jr.

PRESSURE FLOW AND RESISTANCE

The pulmonary circulation is unique in two important respects: the entire cardiac output passes through the lung, and the function of this circulation is to replenish the blood with oxygen rather than to deliver oxygen to metabolically active tissue. The pulmonary artery and its branches are so capacious as to offer minimal resistance to blood flow and to permit passage of blood through the large alveolar capillary network with a pressure head only one fifth of that required to pump blood to the rest of the body. Since there is no need to vary blood flow in the lung with the metabolic needs of competing tissues, the muscular arterioles which are present in the other organs of the body are not needed here. Another characteristic of the pulmonary circulation is its enormous capacity for expansion. Doubling of cardiac output by muscular exercise or of the blood flow through one lung by occlusion of the contralateral pulmonary artery is associated with relatively little increase of pulmonary artery pressure because the total cross section area of the pulmonary vascular bed expands in response to a small rise of intraluminal pressure. In acute experiments, 75 per cent of the pulmonary vascular bed must be obstructed before pulmonary hypertension develops, and the presence of severe pulmonary hypertension implies the existence of widespread vascular disease.

REGIONAL CIRCULATION

Because of the low pressure in the pulmonary artery, variation of hydrostatic pressure caused by gravity has a relatively large effect on the perfusion pressure at the apex and the base of the lung. At the top of the lung, the pressure inside the small arteries may actually be less than the atmospheric pressure on the outside, within the alveoli, so that the vessels are totally occluded and there is no blood flow. At the bottom of the lung, the hydrostatic pressure is large, and blood flow is correspondingly great. The gravitational effects on the lung volume also tend to divert more ventilation to the lower lung zones than to the upper. This is due to the fact that the pleural pressure is less negative at the bottom of the lung than at the top. As a result, at FRC the upper lobes are under greater stretch, are larger and less compliant, so that they fill less with a given inspiratory change of pleural pressure than do the less expanded and more compliant lower lobes.

A number of isotope techniques have been developed for studying regional circulation through the lung, of which the most widely used is lung scanning with I^{131}-labeled microaggregates of albumin. Aggregates of albumin are injected into the pulmonary circulation where they embolize functioning capillaries and are detected by appropriate scintillation counting. Albumin aggregates do not embolize areas of lung not perfused with blood; hence these appear as nonradioactive areas on the lung scan. Such filling defects are encountered in patients who have suffered pulmonary embolization or in patients in whom areas of the pulmonary circulation have been obstructed because of inflammation, collapse, or even over-inflation, as in bronchial asthma.

BRONCHIAL CIRCULATION

The main nutritive circulation to the lung is provided by the systemic blood brought by the bronchial arteries. As a result, total occlusion of a pulmonary artery does not necessarily lead to necrosis of pulmonary tissue, or even to x-ray changes so long as the bronchial circulation remains intact. The bronchial circulation assumes clinical importance when it becomes excessive, as in chronic suppurative lung disease (bronchiectasis) or after interruption of the pulmonary artery circulation. An expanded bronchial circulation represents a flow load on the left ventricle which pumps blood round and round through the affected pulmonary tissue, and an expanded bronchial circulation is a rare cause of left ventricular failure. Of greater importance is the fact that these systemic vessels are a potential source of serious hemoptysis. Modern techniques of angiography have made it possible to visualize the main bronchial arteries radiographically after injection of contrast material.

PULMONARY HYPERTENSION

As mentioned, significant elevation of the pulmonary artery pressure implies the presence of severe obstruction to the pulmonary circulation. This subject is considered in detail in the last article in this section (see Pulmonary Hypertension in Circulatory Disorders).

DISABILITY EVALUATION
M. Henry Williams, Jr.

PULMONARY FUNCTION TESTING

As is the case with dyspnea, disability evaluation can only be partially aided by pulmonary function testing because of the importance of subjective factors. The physician can learn whether or not an abnormality which might limit performance is present, but he cannot say that it does or will. For example, patients with apparently similar degrees of severe obstruction to airflow show marked variation in their exercise capacity.

In normal subjects, physical activity is limited largely by cardiac rather than by pulmonary performance. Even at maximal exercise, the limits of ventilation are not reached, and there is no decrease of arterial oxygen tension, implying that total pulmonary performance is perfectly adequate. Theoretically, severe obstruction of airways or severe stiffening of the lungs might make it impossible to achieve levels of adequate ventilation commensurate with the high metabolic rate induced by heavy exercise, but one rarely encounters patients in whom exercise is actually associated with worsening hypercapnia and hypoxemia. In practical terms, there is a rough correlation between the severity of obstructive airway disease and extent of disability so that a patient with a maximal midexpiratory flow rate (MMF) of 1 liter per second may be expected to be unable to do heavy work and a patient with an MMF of 0.2 liter per second can probably do no more than walk slowly on the level. Likewise, when the vital capacity is reduced to 1 liter by severe restrictive lung disease, the effort to achieve more than a slight increase of minute ventilation, such as that induced by slow walking, may become intolerable.

Disability is not synonymous with disease. Extensive involvement of the lung by metastatic disease or with granulomatous disease, as in sarcoidosis, may be associated with little impairment of pulmonary function because of preservation of large areas of normal lung. On the other hand, diffuse microscopic alteration of the alveolar capillary membrane may lead to sufficient impairment of oxygen diffusion as to result in arterial unsaturation, particularly with exercise, and to sufficient stiffening of the lung as to make breathing difficult on mild effort. It may be important for the physician to know that an inhaled pollutant, such as beryllium, has led to extensive lung disease, which may only be evident by measurement of the diffusing capacity; but this need not imply that the patient has limited ability to work. A careful assessment of the type and extent of lung disease and evaluation of whether or not the disease has led to mechanical impairment of the respiratory system and/or to blood gas abnormalities at rest or on exercise are the essential ingredients of disability evaluation.

PREOPERATIVE EVALUATION

A special type of disability evaluation is represented by the patient who is being considered for pulmonary resectional surgery. In performing this evaluation, the physician must first determine whether or not the resected tissue is functioning, since nonfunctioning tissue can be removed with relative impunity. Isotope studies of regional ventilation and perfusion now make this estimation possible. Indeed, if it is determined that an area of lung is ventilated but not perfused, resection may be of benefit in that this tissue is of no value to the patient, and its ventilation actually represents wasted effort. Likewise, a perfused but nonventilated lung contributes to hypoxemia and is of little value to the patient.

Since, as in the case of the pulmonary circulation, there is a tremendous reserve of pulmonary function available for ventilation and for gas diffusion, large amounts of pulmonary tissue may be resected from a normal individual without causing hypoxemia or even respiratory discomfort. Often, however, one must decide whether a patient with restrictive or obstructive lung disease is capable of withstanding removal of some functioning lung tissue, generally in connection with cancer surgery. One useful guide is a study of exercise tolerance. If a patient can sustain exercise requiring twice the normal resting oxygen consumption, one can anticipate that he could tolerate removal of half of his functioning lung. Calculation of the extent to which the lung to be resected is contributing to gas exchange, most easily based on studies of regional perfusion with lung scan coupled with measurements of ability to increase oxygen uptake with exercise, permits a reasonable assessment of whether or not surgery can be carried out. Other evidence of severe functional impairment may represent compelling contraindications to surgery. Most physicians feel that a patient with resting hypercapnia represents such a risk as to preclude a thoracotomy. Likewise, pulmonary hypertension, at rest or after balloon occlusion of the segment of lung to be resected, is considered a contraindication to surgery. Beyond that, although severe obstructive or restrictive diseases represent relative contraindications to surgery, assessment must be made on the basis of the patient's general health, age, and vigor and of the indications for operation.

HYPOXEMIA
M. Henry Williams, Jr.

HYPOXIA

Tissue hypoxia occurs when the supply of oxygen to the cells is inadequate to meet metabolic needs. The two general causes of hypoxia are reduction of blood flow and reduction of oxygen concentration within the blood. Reduction of blood flow may be localized, as in occlusive arterial disease, or general when the cardiac output is reduced. Arterial oxygen concentration may be diminished if there is impairment of the transport function of the blood. Impaired transport is most commonly the result of anemia, and the oxygen-carrying capacity is reduced in direct proportion to the reduction of hemoglobin concentration. Reduced transport also results from replacement of normal hemoglobin by abnormal hemoglobin such as methemoglobin or carbon monoxide hemoglobin. Heavy smokers may have as much as 10 per cent of their hemoglobin combined with carbon monoxide instead of with oxygen, and they are at a further disadvantage in that the carbon monoxide hemoglobin affects the oxygen dissociation curve of the remaining hemoglobin so that there is interference with release of oxygen to the tissues. Impaired transport also occurs when the amount of oxygen in the arterial blood is reduced because the oxygen tension is reduced. Reduced arterial oxygen tension and saturation is always, with the exception of right-to-left intracardiac shunts, the result of impaired pulmonary function.

ARTERIAL UNSATURATION

Reduced arterial oxygen saturation may, if severe, be evident clinically as cyanosis of the skin or mucous membranes. Since mild degrees of arterial unsaturation are not detectable as cyanosis and since cyanosis can result from any condition which will lead to increased amounts of reduced hemoglobin in the capillaries, such as polycythemia and reduced blood flow, accurate assessment of the arterial oxygen saturation requires its measurement. Since arterial oxygen unsaturation may be an important cause of tissue dysfunction and since it also has clinical implications concerning the type and extent of pulmonary disease present, the measurement should be carried out routinely in patients in whom hypoxemia is suspected to be present.

Hypoxemia may result from four types of impairment of pulmonary function: reduced alveolar ventilation, impaired diffusion of oxygen, right-to-left shunts, and abnormal ventilation-perfusion relationships. Two or more of these abnormalities often coexist in a given patient.

Alveolar hypoventilation is characterized by hypercapnia out of proportion to hypoxemia. Reduction of alveolar ventilation causes proportional increase of arterial P_{CO_2} and reduction of arterial P_{O_2}, but the flat portion of the oxygen dissociation curve of hemoglobin permits substantial reduction of arterial P_{O_2} before the arterial oxygen saturation falls appreciably. Thus, a patient with an arterial P_{CO_2} elevated from 40 up to 80 mm. Hg would have significant respiratory acidosis, but the concurrent reduction of the arterial P_{O_2} from 100 to about 50 mm. Hg would be associated with only mild arterial unsaturation of little clinical significance. Alveolar hypoventilation may occur after overdosage of drugs, in acute paralytic disease of muscles, or, rarely, in individuals with isolated abnormality of the respiratory center (alveolar hypoventilation syndrome), but it is associated most commonly with severe obstructive pulmonary disease, which leads to hypoxemia for other reasons.

The diffusing capacity of the lungs for oxygen is so large that even during heavy exercise the arterial oxygen tension is only slightly lower than the alveolar oxygen tension, and the diffusing capacity must be severely reduced by disease before arterial oxygen unsaturation develops. When hypoxemia is present because of impaired diffusion, as in advanced pulmonary fibrosis, it is characteristically exaggerated by exercise and is not accompanied by hypercapnia.

Right-to-left shunts produce hypoxemia in direct proportion to the magnitude of the shunt, and they are found most commonly in patients with intracardiac defects. Since the venous carbon dioxide tension is only 6 mm. higher than the arterial, even a large shunt leads to little elevation of the arterial P_{CO_2}. A 50 per cent shunt would cause the arterial P_{CO_2} to be increased by only 3 mm. Hg, whereas the oxygen saturation would be substantially reduced because of the much lower venous oxygen saturation.

Mismatching of ventilation and perfusion is the most important cause of hypoxemia. Arterial unsaturation results from the fact that well-perfused but poorly ventilated alveoli have a very low oxygen tension and the blood leaving these alveoli contains low concentrations of oxygen. Since these alveoli are relatively well perfused, they contribute large amounts of blood to the total cardiac output and, hence, cause substantial reduction of arterial oxygen saturation. Hypercapnia is also a feature of this condition, but is mitigated by the fact that alveoli which are excessively ventilated but underperfused contain correspondingly low concentrations of carbon dioxide, and the blood coming from these alveoli tends to counterbalance the CO_2-rich blood from underventilated alveoli. There is no similar compensation for oxygen because the extra ventilation does not serve to increase the oxygen saturation above the normal 98 per cent.

OXYGEN THERAPY

Most types of hypoxemia are corrected completely and easily by oxygen breathing. Inspiration of air containing a higher than normal concentration of oxygen will lead to an increase of the oxygen concentration in all the ventilated alveoli. Thus, if a patient breathes 31 per cent oxygen instead of 21 per cent oxygen, the inspired air will contain an oxygen tension which is 70 mm. Hg higher than normal, and all the ventilated alveoli will have an oxygen tension which is elevated by approximately 70 mm. Hg. This will more than suffice to raise the oxygen tension to a level capable of saturating the hemoglobin passing through these alveoli whether the hypoxemia is due to total alveolar hypoventilation, regional hypoventilation, or impaired diffusion. Hypoxemia caused by a right-to-left shunt will not be corrected fully by this treatment since the inspired oxygen fails to affect the blood passing through the shunts. Inspiration of 100 per cent oxygen will have some effect on arterial oxygen saturation because it will dissolve an extra 2 volumes per cent of oxygen in the blood which does circulate through ventilated lung. This will increase the arterial oxygen saturation 10 per cent in a patient with a normal hematocrit.

Knowledge of arterial blood gas composition during air and oxygen breathing makes possible an accurate assessment of the type of pulmonary malfunction which is causing hypoxemia, and it also provides an indication of the severity of the disease. Since high concentrations of oxygen may increase the tendency to atelectasis within the lung and adversely affect the metabolic functions of the lung, the physician should use as little additional inspired oxygen as necessary to correct hypoxemia. Measurement of the arterial oxygen saturation is the proper guide to rational oxygen therapy.

ACCLIMATIZATION

One of the extraordinary adaptations of which man is capable is the acclimatization to chronic hypoxia. Whereas acute reduction of arterial oxygen saturation to 70 per cent in a normal subject is associated with gross evidence of cerebral dysfunction and slightly lower levels of saturation will cause death, patients with chronic hypoxia, due either to chronic pulmonary disease or to prolonged residence at high altitude, are capable of normal function with an arterial oxygen saturation as low as 25 per cent. Some of this acclimatization results from polycythemia, which increases the oxygen-carrying power of the blood and from a change in the oxygen-combining character of hemoglobin, which releases oxygen more readily to the tissues. Arteriolar dilation and increased cardiac output permit a more rapid flow of blood and oxygen to the tissues. A fundamental and major adaptation undoubtedly resides in the expansion of the capillary network throughout the body. This brings the oxygen in the capillaries nearer to the cells and makes possible the diffusion of oxygen into the cells even though the partial pressure of oxygen in the capillaries is very low.

Bates, D. V., and Christie, R. V.: Respiratory Function in Disease. Philadelphia, W. B. Saunders Company, 1964.

Briscoe, W. A.: The current status of pulmonary function tests. Arch. Environ. Health, 16:531, 1968.

Comroe, J. H. Jr., Forster, R. C., DuBois, A. B., Briscoe, W. A., and Carlsen, E.: The Lung. Clinical Physiology and Pulmonary Function Tests. 2nd ed. Chicago, Year Book Publishers, 1962.

Howell, J. B. L., and Campbell, E. J. M. (eds.): Breathlessness. Philadelphia, F. A. Davis Company, 1966.

Hugh-Jones, P., and Campbell, E. T. M. (eds.): Respiratory physiology. Brit. Med. Bull., 19:1, 1963.

Liebow, A. A., and Smith, D. C. (eds.): The Lung. Baltimore, Williams & Wilkins Company, 1968.

The Diaphragm

J. B. L. Howell

The diaphragm is the most powerful muscle of inspiration and is responsible for the major part of the tidal volume in quiet breathing. Developmentally, the mesodermal partition which separates the thoracic and abdominal cavities, the septum transversum, is invaded by premuscular tissue derived principally from the fourth cervical myotome, and forms the muscular diaphragm. The motor nerve supply is bilateral and is derived from the third, fourth, and fifth cervical segments via the phrenic nerves. Sensory fibers are also derived from the lower six or seven intercostal nerves.

Congenital Defects. In the diaphragm, the posterolateral foramen of Bochdalek and less commonly the anterior foramen of Morgagni, owing to persistence of the pleuroperitoneal canal, may be the sites of herniation of abdominal viscera into the thoracic cavity. Herniation may also occur through normal foramina, especially the esophageal opening (see Hiatus Hernia in Diseases of the Digestive System).

Paralysis of the Diaphragm. Paralysis of the diaphragm may occur from interruption of its nerve supply, from muscular atrophy, or temporarily from diaphragmatic pleurisy. Unilateral diaphragmatic paralysis is usually the result of phrenic nerve interruption in the mediastinum caused by bronchial carcinoma or other tumors. Phrenic crush or section was once used therapeutically in the treatment of pulmonary tuberculosis; it may still occur inadvertently during cervical sympathectomy.

Congenital atrophy, called *eventration*, of one half of the diaphragm, is a rare and usually symptomless finding on routine roentgenography with a prevalence of about 1 in 12,000. It is more common on the left side. Its main significance is that it may be confused with the potentially more sinister phrenic paralysis. Occasionally, left-sided eventration is associated with mild dyspepsia.

Phrenic paralysis causes elevation of the affected hemidiaphragm, which shows paradoxic movement on sniffing, the basis of its fluoroscopic diagnosis. Unilateral or bilateral diaphragmatic paralysis occurs in high cervical cord injuries, motor neuron disease, paralytic poliomyelitis, infectious polyneuritis (Landry-Guillain-Barré syndrome), peripheral neuritis associated with diphtheria, tetanus, measles, typhoid, and rheumatic fever, or may occur following antitetanus serum injection into the deltoid region as part of a cervical radiculitis.

The main disturbance of pulmonary function tests in diaphragmatic paralysis is reduction in the vital capacity, especially when the patient is supine. Symptoms are orthopnea and difficulty in inspiration. Arterial oxygen saturation may be reduced, but hypoventilation does not occur.

Inflammation of the Diaphragm. Inflammation of the diaphragm and its serous surfaces may occur in viral infections, e.g., epidemic pleurodynia, or as extensions of pneumonia, pleurisy, or peritonitis. The clinical significance is that of the underlying condition, except that diaphragmatic, like thoracic wall, pleurisy may cause pain referred to the abdomen or to the shoulder, leading to diagnostic confusion.

Rupture of the Diaphragm. Rupture of the diaphragm is due to trauma, especially when associated with abdominal compression injuries. Direct trauma to the chest may also be responsible. On the right side, the liver may herniate into the thorax. The diagnosis should be suspected when roentgenographic features of paralysis of a hemidiaphragm follow thoraco-abdominal injury, especially if breathlessness is disproportionately severe.

Myotonia Dystrophica and Hemiplegia. The diaphragm may also be involved as part of generalized muscular disease in myotonia dystrophica. Unless extremely severe, spirometry, resting ventilation, and the ventilatory response to CO_2 are normal; however, sedatives readily induce respiratory depression. In hemiplegia, diaphragmatic movement is in a normal direction. Chest movements are reduced on voluntary breathing maneuvers, but not when breathing is stimulated by CO_2. This indicates that although supramedullary innervation of the respiratory muscles is bilateral, it is not symmetrically represented.

HICCUP

Hiccup is an involuntary spasm of the inspiratory muscles followed by abrupt closure of the glottis which is responsible for the characteristic sound. Normal subjects may experience hiccup, especially after eating or drinking, but it may also be a symptom of disease. It may occur in conditions which irritate vagal nerve endings in the abdomen or thorax. These include gastritis, peritonitis, pleurisy, pericarditis, and mediastinitis. It may also occur as a very troublesome symptom in uremia, when it is thought to have a central origin. When no cause is found, the psyche may be blamed, but there is no evidence to support this. In most instances, hiccup is a short-lived symptom and can sometimes be induced to stop by a variety of maneuvers such as taking a deep breath, breath holding, or drinking cold water. Rebreathing from a paper bag may sometimes help. If symptoms still persist, chlorpromazine, 25 to 50 mg. intravenously, may be successful. In the small number of cases in which hiccup has proved resistant to these simple measures, local anesthesia of one of the phrenic nerves has been successful, block of the left nerve usually being tried first.

The Chest Wall
J. B. L. Howell

SCOLIOSIS

Definition. Scoliosis means lateral curvature of the spine which may occur in the lumbar, thoracolumbar, or thoracic regions. The higher the location of the scoliosis in the vertebral column, the greater the likelihood of severe deformity and of disturbance of cardiopulmonary function (heart failure of the hunchback). Lumbar scoliosis is relatively benign. Thoracic scoliosis is associated with rotation of the spine and prominence of the posterior angles of ribs which form the hump or gibbus, and gives rise to the hunchback appear-

ance. Although commonly called kyphoscoliosis, forward angulation of the spine or kyphosis is usually not the major component of kyphoscoliosis; indeed marked lumbar or cervical lordosis is characteristic.

Etiology and Mechanism. Four types of scoliosis are recognized. The largest group is *idiopathic*, developing in childhood and adolescence during the period of bone growth. When idiopathic scoliosis occurs in infancy, boys predominate in the ratio of 6 to 4, and the curvature is usually to the left; when it occurs in adolescence, girls predominate in the ratio of 9 to 1, and the curvature is usually to the right.

Congenital scoliosis results from a variety of

developmental abnormalities, including hemivertebrae, fused vertebrae, spina bifida, and absent ribs. Other congenital abnormalities are commonly associated. *Paralytic* scoliosis resulting from poliomyelitis is especially likely to cause deformity and disability owing to the associated muscular paralyses.

Genetic abnormalities may be due to autosomal dominant conditions such as neurofibromatosis, osteogenesis imperfecta, Marfan's and Ehlers-Danlos syndromes, or autosomal recessive conditions, including Morquio's disease, Hurler's syndrome, and diatrophic dwarfism. The mechanism of the deformity is probably a combination of abnormal bone growth, usually in the vertebrae, and altered distribution of muscular forces. The importance of each factor will vary according to the type of scoliosis. The degree of deformity varies between individuals and at different ages. In one series, two thirds of the patients with thoracic idiopathic scoliosis had curvature of the spine greater than 70 degrees, and in over a fourth it was greater than 100 degrees. Scoliosis may also follow fibrotic disease of the lungs and pleura, e.g., tuberculous empyema. This is not as severe as the scoliosis that may develop in the aforementioned varieties, and cardiopulmonary disturbances are due largely to the thoracic disease.

Clinical Manifestations. Deformities with less than 70 degrees of angulation rarely cause symptoms other than those due to their psychologic effects. When more severe deformities interfere with pulmonary function the first symptom is breathlessness on exertion. With progression of the deformity or with superadded bronchitis, disturbance of pulmonary function increases, and arterial hypoxia develops; breathlessness now becomes more severe. If ventilatory failure supervenes, more severe cyanosis and signs of congestive cardiac failure develop. These findings are similar to those of chronic cor pulmonale developing in association with chronic obstructive bronchitis; however, symptoms of morning chest tightness and bronchial irritability are not present in scoliosis unless bronchial disease coexists. Abnormal physical signs are those associated with congestive cardiac failure but allowance must be made in their elicitation and interpretation for the deformity and displacement of the viscera.

Laboratory Tests. In all patients with significant deformity, total lung capacity, vital capacity, and residual volume are reduced in relation to the degree of deformity. The FEV_1/VC is essentially normal. Airway resistance in relation to lung volume is normal or slightly raised. Maximal breathing capacity is particularly reduced in paralytic scoliosis. In patients with mild deformity, Sa_{O_2} is normal. With increasing severity, Sa_{O_2} becomes reduced while Pa_{CO_2} first remains normal; but when congestive cardiac failure develops Sa_{O_2} is reduced further, Pa_{CO_2} is elevated, CO_2 sensitivity is reduced, and polycythemia may develop. Intrapulmonary gas mixing and diffusing capacity are usually not markedly abnormal. The electrocardiogram may show evidence of right ventricular hypertrophy. Interpretation of the chest film may be very difficult, owing to the distortion of the bony cage and displacement of the thoracic contents.

Mechanism of Cardiorespiratory Failure. The deformity of the bony thoracic cage reduces its capacity, it also impairs the action of the inspiratory muscles, resulting in reduced total lung capacity and its component volumes. The work of breathing is increased largely because of increased elastic resistances in the chest wall and altered mechanical advantage of the muscles. This results in more rapid shallow breathing which increases dead space ventilation and causes arterial unsaturation. Initially, over-all alveolar ventilation is maintained, but with progression of the deformity the work of breathing and arterial desaturation are further increased, and alveolar hypoventilation develops in association with impaired ventilatory response to CO_2. Hypoxemia becomes more severe, resulting in polycythemia and increased pulmonary vascular resistance. This, together with the reduction in the pulmonary vascular bed resulting from the low lung volumes, causes pulmonary hypertension and congestive cardiac failure. The end result is similar to the cardiorespiratory failure of primary alveolar hypoventilation, and of chronic obstructive bronchitis ("blue bloater" form).

Pathologic Conditions of Lungs and Heart in Scoliosis. Characteristically, the lungs are small and may appear atrophic; areas of atelectasis are common. Emphysema is not a feature. When the deformity has arisen in infancy, hypoplasia of the air spaces and vascular bed may be found. In patients dying with cardiorespiratory failure, there is usually right ventricular hypertrophy as well as other evidence of pulmonary hypertension.

Prognosis. The factors which influence the progression of minor degrees of scoliosis in childhood are poorly understood. In some it may disappear, but in others, apparently similar, rapid deformity may develop. Cardiopulmonary abnormalities are most likely with thoracic deformities, especially when due to muscular paralysis and when the deformity has occurred in infancy and early childhood rather than later in life.

Treatment. *Prophylaxis.* Prevention of progressive deformity may require the use of a Milwaukee brace (frame), which applies distraction between the pelvis and the head, and pressure on the prominent angles of the rib, or surgical intervention, although there is no general agreement on the best surgical procedure. Prevention and treatment of recurrent bronchitis (see below) is important as the pulmonary damage is additive to the effects of the deformity.

Cardiopulmonary Failure. The treatment of acute cardiopulmonary failure is similar to that occurring in chronic obstructive bronchitis (see below). It includes the treatment of bronchial infection and retained secretions with antimicrobial drugs and physiotherapy, controlled administration of oxygen, venesection for polycythemia, and diuretics. Chronic cardiopulmonary failure requires attention to bronchial toilet, diuretics, and digitalis, and repeated venesection to maintain the hematocrit below 55 per cent. Surgical correction of the deformity at this late stage is not feasible; surgery is usually restricted to the prevention of paraplegia if early signs of spinal cord damage appear. A period of assisted ventilation may be necessary for acute cardiorespiratory failure, but intubation may be difficult owing to the marked cervical lordosis. The ethical problems involved in this decision are similar to those of chronic ventilatory failure in association with chronic lung disease (see below).

ANKYLOSING SPONDYLITIS

Ankylosing spondylitis results in bony ankylosis of posterior intervertebral, costovertebral, and sacroiliac joints; there is also ossification of the spinal ligaments and the margins of the intervertebral discs. As a result, the bony thoracic cage becomes rigid and immobile, and respiratory movement becomes increasingly dependent upon diaphragmatic movement. It was once thought that respiratory illnesses were unduly common in this condition, but this has been shown not to be the case. Respiratory symptoms are not common, and pulmonary function shows few abnormalities. In the most severely affected patients, the vital capacity and maximal breathing capacity may be reduced to approximately two thirds of normal. Total lung capacity remains normal, but the residual volume and functional residual capacity are increased, suggesting that the chest is fixed in an inspiratory position. Diffusing capacity for carbon monoxide is reduced only in the most severely affected group. At autopsy, the lungs are normal.

Deformities of the Anterior Chest Wall

Three types of deformity are recognized: depression of the sternum (pectus excavatum or funnel chest), prominence of the sternum (pigeon chest), and depression of the rib cage anterolaterally in the region of the sixth rib (Harrison's sulcus). Of these deformities, only the first-named may cause any disturbance of cardiopulmonary function.

Pectus excavatum is a congenital abnormality of the anterior chest wall in which the sternum is depressed, being most marked just above the xiphisternal junction, with symmetrical or asymmetrical prominence of the ribs on either side. Occasionally, the xiphoid may project backward as a xiphoid horn. The cause of this deformity is uncertain; some believe that it is due to exces-

sive diaphragmatic traction on the lower sternum, but others believe it is secondary to displacement of the heart into the left hemithorax. Symptoms are not common and appear to be of cardiac origin. They include breathlessness on exertion, precordial pain, palpitation, and dizziness; rarely congestive cardiac failure has been reported. The electrocardiogram may show arrhythmias and changes suggestive of ischemia, but there is no supporting evidence of myocardial disease. Hemodynamic studies have rarely demonstrated restriction of ventricular filling similar to that which occurs with constrictive pericarditis. It is unlikely that disturbed pulmonary function ever plays any part in the disability. Tests are usually normal, but with very severe deformity the vital capacity and maximal breathing capacity may be reduced. Surgical correction has been reported to afford immediate symptomatic benefit, although there is a high incidence of recurrence of the deformity.

PRIMARY OR IDIOPATHIC ALVEOLAR HYPO-VENTILATION

Definition. The term primary or idiopathic alveolar hypoventilation denotes a rare clinical syndrome occurring in patients with normal pulmonary and thoracic cage mechanics in whom the primary abnormality is alveolar hypoventilation. The syndrome is characterized by symptoms of headache, drowsiness, or somnolence, exertional dyspnea, and signs of cyanosis and congestive heart failure.

Etiology. The causes of this syndrome are not known. Resistances to breathing and respiratory muscular power are essentially normal, which distinguishes it from hypoventilation occurring in chronic bronchitis, in neuromuscular disorders, in skeletal abnormalities of the thorax, e.g., kyphoscoliosis, or in extreme obesity. Associated central nervous system disorders, such as the sequelae of encephalitis, neurosyphilis, and mental retardation with or without epilepsy, have been reported in over half the patients, but no specific lesions have been found in the region of the respiratory center at autopsy. Alveolar hypoventilation has also been reported in a small proportion of patients following bulbar poliomyelitis, sometimes many years after apparent recovery, and it seems likely that in these patients central nervous system disease is responsible.

Incidence and Prevalence. Primary or idiopathic hypoventilation is a rare disease; it was first described in 1955, and since then fewer than 30 cases have been reported. The majority of patients have been between 30 and 50 years, with a preponderance of males.

Clinical Manifestations. Symptoms have usually been present for many years, but occasionally the presentation has been more acute, usually in response to a respiratory infection. The dominant symptoms include breathlessness on exertion, drowsiness, or even somnolence suggesting narcolepsy. When the symptoms are severe, the patient is cyanosed, the face being dark and suffused, sometimes with chemosis; tachycardia, raised jugular venous pressure, hepatomegaly, and peripheral edema are present. Crepitations at the bases are common. Clinical evidence of cardiac enlargement, pulmonary hypertension, right ventricular hypertrophy, and systemic venous congestion is commonly present. Periodic breathing may be prominent during sleep. Laboratory findings include raised Pa_{CO_2} (55 to 75 mm. Hg), usually with good compensation of the respiratory acidosis; there is arterial desaturation (70 to 80 per cent), mainly resulting from ventilation-perfusion abnormality, and the hematocrit is usually greater than 60 per cent. The ventilatory response to inhaled CO_2 is markedly depressed. The vital capacity may be slightly reduced, but the FEV_1/VC ratio is normal. Physiologic dead space ventilation is increased.

Diagnosis. The aforementioned findings in the absence of other disorders of the lungs and thorax are highly suggestive of idiopathic alveolar hypoventilation. This diagnosis is supported if the patient can temporarily restore the blood gas tensions to normal by a period of voluntary hyperventilation. Differential diagnosis includes other causes of congestive cardiac failure, cyanosis, polycythemia, and somnolence, the most common being chronic obstructive bronchitis ("blue bloater" form) and cyanotic congenital heart disease; the syndrome may also be confused with primary polycythemia or narcolepsy. Severe metabolic alkalosis caused by prolonged vomiting, as in anorexia nervosa or chronic pyloric stenosis, may be accompanied by severe hypoventilation. It is not certain whether the cardiorespiratory failure of extreme obesity is an essentially different disorder or not.

Pathology. No specific disease has been found in the central nervous system. In two patients substantial increase in the number and size of capillaries was found at autopsy in the floor of the fourth ventricle, reticular substance, periaqueductal region, mamillary body, and hypothalamus. There was no evidence of neuronal loss. There are usually right ventricular hypertrophy and evidence of chronic pulmonary hypertension. Thromboses of large branches of the pulmonary artery with pulmonary infarcts are common.

Pathogenesis. The primary abnormality in primary alveolar hypoventilation is impaired responsiveness of the respiratory center to carbon dioxide, leading to ventilatory failure. As a result of this reduced CO_2 sensitivity, the center is unable to increase its motor output to the inspiratory muscles by the normal amount when alveolar ventilation is reduced by increased resistances to breathing. Although the normal subject will double or treble the resting power (rate of work) of the inspiratory muscles in response to a rise in the Pco_2 of only 1 mm. Hg, these patients are unable to do so even with a rise in Pco_2 of 20 to 30 mm. Hg. Consequently, normally trivial events like acute bronchitis or increase in body weight may cause profound underbreathing, with further elevation of alveolar Pco_2 and fall in alveolar Po_2. Because of altered ventilation-perfusion relationships which accompany underbreathing, Pa_{O_2} is reduced even further until it becomes the dominant ventilatory stimulus and stabilizes ventilation at a new reduced level. Administration of oxygen is likely to be harmful by reducing or removing ventilatory drive, increasing hypercapnia, and leading to increased drowsiness or even unconsciousness. A similar response may follow small doses of sedatives or narcotics, and a number of cases have been recognized for the first time by this striking response. The hypoxemia causes polycythemia, increased pulmonary vascular resistance, and increased cardiac output, resulting in pulmonary hypertension, right ventricular hypertrophy, and systemic venous congestion. Although most patients have various degrees of ventilatory failure, some patients with this syndrome maintain alveolar ventilation at virtually normal levels, alveolar Pa_{CO_2} and Po_2 being only slightly abnormal, providing that they do not have respiratory obstruction. It is the failure to maintain adequate alveolar ventilation in the face of increased mechanical hindrance that characterizes the syndrome.

Mechanism of Impaired Sensitivity of the Respiratory Center to Carbon Dioxide. Reduced CO_2 sensitivity is not peculiar to this syndrome. It has been reported in association with a wide range of disorders, including chronic bronchitis and airway obstruction, scoliosis and kyphoscoliosis, obesity, and brainstem disorders; it also occurs as a normal event during sleep. Experimentally, reduced CO_2 sensitivity has been observed in man following vagal blockade and narcotic drugs, and has been thought to occur during partial curarization. The control of breathing is a complex process involving the integration of a variety of sensory inputs from mechanical and chemical receptors, and of motor outputs to the ventilatory apparatus. Theoretically, control may be impaired at any of a number of points, and it is possible that in different diseases interruption of normal control mechanism occurs at different sites. It is generally believed that the abnormality in primary alveolar ventilation is in the central nervous system, but its nature is unknown.

Treatment. Treatment of congestive cardiac failure usually improves the ventilatory failure as well. Oral diuretic therapy with, for example, chlorothiazide, 1 gram, or furosemide, 40 to 80 mg. daily; venesections to reduce the hematocrit to between 50 and 55 per cent; and digoxin, 0.25 mg. twice daily, will reduce pulmonary congestion and peripheral edema, with improvement in arterial Pco_2 and Po_2. Sometimes, when these measures are not successful, a short period of artificial or assisted ventilation to reduce the arterial Pco_2 and raise Po_2 may be followed by prompt diuresis. Cuirass ventilators permit ventilation to be assisted without endotracheal intubation, and in some patients regular artificial ventilation at night in a cuirass ventilator may maintain them in an improved state. Attempts to increase ventilation with acetazolamide, progesterone, aminophylline, and analeptics have not been successful. Instruction in voluntary increased breathing and electrophrenic stimulation with surface electrodes have been successful in the short term only. All other abnormalities likely to hinder breathing, e.g., bronchitis, asthma, and obesity, should be treated as effectively as possible.

Prognosis. There is insufficient information at present to estimate the prognosis with accuracy. Without effective treatment of congestive cardiac failure, the prognosis is very poor. With treatment, patients may continue in reasonable health for several years, requiring only intermittent therapy for acute pulmonary infections and venesections if polycythemia becomes severe. One patient has been reported to have maintained normal arterial P_{CO_2} for nine months after three years of continuous hypercapnia and repeated episodes of ventilatory and cardiac failure; this was attributed to voluntary increase in ventilation.

CARDIORESPIRATORY FAILURE OF EXTREME OBESITY

Cardiorespiratory failure similar to that of primary alveolar hypoventilation has been described in association with extreme obesity, the average weight being approximately 325 pounds. The similarity in appearance and behavior of these patients to the description of the fat boy, Joe, in *Pickwick Papers*, has led to this association being termed the pickwickian syndrome. The main symptoms are breathlessness on exertion and somnolence. Apart from obesity, the physical signs and physiologic abnormalities are similar to those in idiopathic alveolar hypoventilation. Periodic breathing is common during sleep. Prominent cyanosis, tachycardia, raised central venous pressure with cardiac dilatation, functional tricuspid incompetence, hepatomegaly, and peripheral edema may be observed. Investigations reveal diminished total lung capacity and its component volumes, decreased lung compliance, and increased airway resistance at functional residual capacity owing to the low lung volume. Physiologic dead space is increased. Arterial saturation is reduced to about 80 per cent; this is due partly to underbreathing but mainly to increased venous admixture. The P_{CO_2} is usually 60 to 70 mm. Hg. Ventilatory response to CO_2 is markedly reduced. Cardiac output is normal or increased; there is pulmonary hypertension usu-

ally of the order of 75 systolic and 30 diastolic in mm. Hg. There may also be systemic hypertension, which is common in obesity. With voluntary overbreathing patients can restore the blood gases to normal.

Pathogenesis. The mechanism of the cardiorespiratory failure associated with obesity is obscure. First, it has been attributed to the increased work of breathing which occurs in obesity. Two observations make this unlikely; only a minority of patients with this degree of obesity develop the syndrome, and small amounts of weight reduction of the order of 25 pounds may be associated with marked improvement. Second, this syndrome may be essentially similar to the idiopathic alveolar hypoventilation syndrome, obesity being either a fortuitous association or the result of an underlying central nervous system lesion, e.g., in the hypothalamus, which is responsible for both features. Against this are reports of the restoration of normal ventilatory control in those patients in whom weight has been restored to normal. Third, a combination of increased respiratory work resulting from obesity and low sensitivity to carbon dioxide, which occurs in a proportion of normal people, may initiate a vicious circle of events. Thus gross obesity may cause a small reduction in ventilation with increase in P_{CO_2} and arterial unsaturation; this leads in turn to further reduction in CO_2 sensitivity, further underbreathing, and more severe arterial unsaturation and the development of congestive cardiac failure. This increases respiratory work and causes further ventilatory failure. A sequence of events such as this would explain the reversibility of the condition, but at present insufficient knowledge is available concerning the range of CO_2 sensitivity in these patients when nonobese.

Treatment. Weight reduction and the measures described under idiopathic alveolar hypoventilation, i.e., diuretics, venesection, digitalis, and antimicrobial drugs, as well as attention to bronchial toilet result in marked reduction in ventilatory failure and circulatory abnormalities, and improvement in the ventilatory responsiveness to CO_2. Uncontrolled administration of oxygen is likely to cause severe underbreathing and CO_2 narcosis.

Diaphragm, Scoliosis and Ankylosing Spondylitis

Bergofsky, E. H., Turino, M., and Fishman, A. P.: Cardiorespiratory failure in kyphoscoliosis. Medicine, 38:263, 1959.

Fluck, D. C.: Chest movements in hemiplegia. Clin. Sci., 31:383, 1966.

Gillam, P. M. S., Heaf, P. J. D., Kaufman, L., and Lucas, B. G. B.: Respiration in dystrophica myotonica. Thorax, 19:112, 1964.

McCredie, M., Lovejoy, F. W. J. R., and Kaltreider, N. L.: Pulmonary function in diaphragmatic paralysis. Thorax, 17:213, 1962.

Moghissi, K.: Long-term results of surgical correction of pectus excavatum and sternal prominence. Thorax, 19:350, 1964.

Wachtel, F. W., Ravitch, M. M., and Grishman, A.: The relation of pectus excavatum to heart disease. Amer. Heart J., 52:121, 1956.

Zorab, P. A.: The lungs in ankylosing spondylitis. Quart. J. Med., 31:267, 1962.

Zorab, P. A. (ed.): Proceedings of a Symposium on Scoliosis.

National Fund for Research into Poliomyelitis and Other Crippling Diseases. London, 1965.

Idiopathic Hypoventilation Syndrome and Obesity

Burwell, C. S., Robin, E. D., Whaley, R. D., and Bickelman, A. G.: Extreme obesity associated with alveolar hypoventilation — A pickwickian syndrome. Amer. J. Med., 21:811, 1956.
Fishman, A. P., Goldring, R. M., and Turino, G. M.: General alveolar hyperventilation: A syndrome of respiratory and

cardiac failure in patients with normal lungs. Quart. J. Med., 35:261, 1966.
Oliva, P. B., Williams, M. H., and Park, S. S.: Alveolar hypoventilation syndrome. Amer. Rev. Resp. Dis., 96:805, 1967.
Rhoads, G. G., and Brody, J. S.: Idiopathic alveolar hypoventilation: Clinical spectrum. Ann. Intern. Med., 71:971, 1969.
Seriff, N.: Alveolar hypoventilation with normal lungs: Syndrome of primary or central alveolar hypoventilation. Ann. N.Y. Acad. Sci., 121:691, 1965.

Airway Obstruction

J. B. L. Howell

LOCALIZED AIRWAY OBSTRUCTION

The causes of localized airway obstruction may be grouped as endomural, intramural, and extramural. Endomural causes include bronchial secretions and aspirated foreign bodies; intramural causes include benign and malignant neoplasms, edema, and fibrous strictures; extramural causes are mainly due to enlargement of lymph nodes and other structures with airway compression. The effects of obstruction vary according to its location and whether it is complete or partial.

Laryngeal Obstruction. Laryngeal obstruction may be caused by laryngeal spasm, carcinoma, partial paralyses of the vocal cords, or collapse of the cartilaginous elements of the larynx as in rheumatoid arthritis or polychondritis.

Tracheal Obstruction. Tracheal obstruction is uncommon. Foreign bodies either impact in the larynx or descend beyond the bifurcation. Tracheal carcinoma, benign cylindroma, and amyloid tumors are rare. An increasingly common cause is tracheal stricture following tracheostomy or endotracheal intubation. It occurs at the site of the cuff or lower end of the tube and, if severe, may cause marked airway obstruction both during inspiration when it is associated with stridor and during expiration when a Starling resistor mechanism may operate (see Mechanisms of Airway Obstruction below). Surgical excision may be required.

External compression of the trachea may occur from goiter, thymic tumors, or neoplastic lymph nodes. Such pressures initially cause an irritating nonproductive cough but may progress to severe obstruction with stridor.

Localized Bronchial Obstruction. Localized bronchial obstruction does not cause interference with resting airflow unless it is severe; it is more likely to cause infection distally by interfering with mucous flow. When obstruction is nearly complete, overdistention of the distal lung tissue (obstructive emphysema) may occur; complete obstruction results in atelectasis.

ATELECTASIS

Definition. Strictly, the word atelectasis means imperfect expansion, and pathologists often use the term in this sense to describe the failure of expansion of the lungs at birth. In clinical practice, it usually implies airlessness which has developed in lung which had once been normally aerated.

Etiology and Pathogenesis. Airlessness of lung tissue may arise in two ways. First, alteration in the alveolar surfactant material by increasing alveolar surface tension may permit alveoli to deflate completely, thus expelling the air through the bronchial tree. This occurs in the lungs of premature infants and contributes to the *respiratory distress syndrome of the newborn*. Damage to alveolar surfactant is believed to occur in oxygen toxicity when multiple atelectases and sometimes massive collapse may develop. Second, when a bronchus is occluded, continued perfusion of the distal alveoli results in absorption of the air (absorption atelectasis). Bronchial occlusion may occur as a result of obstruction such as secretions, foreign body, or neoplasm in its lumen when the atelectasis is termed "absorption atelectasis." Alternatively, when the lung is permitted to relax to its minimal volume by the presence of large quantities of air or liquid in the pleural cavity, as in pneumothorax or pleural effusion, collapse of the small bronchi or bronchioles occurs. The final removal of air is again by absorption into the perfusing blood, but the atelectasis is termed "relaxation atelectasis."

Absorption of alveolar gas occurs because the total pressure of the gases in mixed venous blood is less than that in the alveoli since, in its passage through the tissues, oxygen tension falls by approximately 60 mm. Hg and is replaced by a rise in carbon dioxide tension of only 4 to 6 mm. Hg. The absorption of air takes a few hours because of its poorly soluble nitrogen content; if the subject has been breathing pure oxygen, absorption may be complete within a few minutes. Following relaxation atelectasis, the lung tissue remains undamaged, and reinflation with normal function is said to be possible after prolonged airlessness.

With obstructive atelectasis, obstruction may interfere with bronchial toilet and lead to infections, abscesses, and fibrosis.

Clinical Manifestations. Atelectasis of one or more pulmonary segments is a common complication of acute tracheobronchial infections and is diagnosed only as a result of chest roentgenograms. The atelectatic areas usually disappear with recovery from the generalized bronchitis without any specific therapy. The sudden development of atelectasis in larger segments of lung, e.g., a lobe or even a whole lung, may cause severe symptoms of dyspnea and chest pain associated with cyanosis, and, if very large, with sweating and peripheral circulatory failure. This is common in the postoperative period, especially with upper abdominal operations. A similar picture may be seen with foreign body inhalation. Over a period of a few hours, the symptoms often subside as the circulation through the atelectatic area is reduced. Lobar or segmental atelectasis resulting from bronchial neoplasm is often symptomless presumably because of its slow evolution. Segmental or lobar atelectasis may occur in patients with mild asthma, and is attributed to obstruction by secretions; however, atelectasis is an uncommon finding at autopsy in status asthmaticus. Atelectasis may also be a component of pulmonary infarction resulting from embolism. Plate atelectases have been described in drug addicts who administer their drugs intravenously.

Physical signs depend upon the size of the atelectatic area. If large enough, chest movement and tactile fremitus are diminished, the mediastinum is deviated toward the affected side, the percussion note is impaired, and breath sounds are characteristically absent. Atelectasis is confirmed by roentgenography, but unless the cause is obvious, bronchoscopy is indicated. Aspiration of occluding material may occasionally be possible through the bronchoscope.

Treatment. Treatment of atelectasis is directed at the underlying cause. For conditions requiring medical treatment, antimicrobial drugs and chest physiotherapy are given. Specific therapy of the atelectasis is seldom indicated, most conditions resolving spontaneously. When associated with bronchiectasis, the treatment is the same as for bronchiectasis. In relaxation atelectasis, removal of fluid from the pleural cavity usually causes re-expansion, often associated with transient precordial pain and violent coughing.

Lemoine, J. M.: L'atelectasie pulmonaire. Étude critique. Bronches, 17:109, 1967.

RIGHT MIDDLE LOBE SYNDROME

The right middle lobe bronchus is especially prone to involvement during primary tuberculosis because its origin is surrounded by a ring of lymph nodes draining both the middle and lower lobes of the right lung. Enlargement of these nodes readily compresses the narrow bronchus, causing atelectasis; extension of the infection into the bronchial wall leads to subsequent stricture with the eventual development of bronchiectatic changes distally. In later life, these changes may lead to recurrent infection, and the combination of recurrent pneumonic illness, hemoptysis, and right middle lobe atelectasis has been given the name of right middle lobe syndrome.

However, post-tuberculous bronchostenosis is only one of the causes of this syndrome. Other causes include chronic suppuration, foreign body, and bronchial neoplasm. Full investigation including bronchoscopy is essential; if the etiology remains uncertain, thoracotomy should be considered.

Albo, R. J., and Grimes, O. F.: The middle lobe syndrome: A clinical study. Dis. Chest, 50:509, 1966.

Brock, R. C., Cann, R. J., and Dickinson, J. R.: Tuberculous mediastinal lymphadenitis in childhood. Guy's Hosp. Rep., 87:295, 1937.

Clements, J. A., and Tierney, D. F.: Alveolar instability associated with altered surface tension. In Handbook of Physiology, Section 3: Respiration. Baltimore, Williams & Wilkins Company, 1965, p. 1565.

Graham, E. A., Burford, T. H., and Mayer, J. H.: Middle lobe syndrome. Postgrad. Med., 4:29, 1948.

Hinshaw, H. C.: Diseases of the Chest. 3rd ed. Philadelphia, W. B. Saunders Company, 1969, pp. 241 et seq.

Hutcheson, S., and Guerrant, J. L.: Atelectasis in asthma. A report of five cases and a review of the literature. Virginia Med. Monthly, 94:629, 1967.

Lindskog, G. E., and Spear, H. C.: Middle lobe syndrome. New Eng. J. Med., 253:489, 1955.

Rahn, H.: The role of N_2 gas in various biological processes with particular reference to the lung. Harvey Lectures Series, 55:173, 1959–1960.

GENERALIZED AIRWAY OBSTRUCTION: CHRONIC OBSTRUCTIVE LUNG DISEASE

GENERAL CONSIDERATIONS

The term chronic obstructive lung disease embraces a number of clinical syndromes of varying etiology and pathology, with the common feature of increased hindrance to the flow of air out of the lungs resulting from an intrapulmonary pathologic condition. In some, airflow obstruction is intermittent, and the clinical presentation is one of asthma; in others, airflow obstruction is continuous, often associated with chronic bronchitis or emphysema or both, and the clinical presentation varies depending upon the degree to which the pulmonary condition results in disturbance of pulmonary and circulatory function. In recent years, considerable advances have been made toward understanding the basic pathophysiology of airflow obstruction and of gas exchange in these various conditions; many studies have correlated the clinical features, pulmonary pathology, and disturbances of pulmonary function. It is now possible to recognize a number of different patterns of disorder within the ill-defined group called chronic nonspecific lung disease (CNSLD), which includes simple chronic bronchitis and chronic obstructive disorders associated with chronic bronchitis, emphysema, and allergic disorders of the bronchi.

Ultimately, an etiologic classification of generalized obstructive disorders of the lungs may be possible, but at present knowledge is incomplete and classification depends largely on differences in clinical presentation supplemented by what is known about their mechanism and pathology.

CHRONIC BRONCHITIS

Definition. Chronic bronchitis is characterized by increased mucous secretion by the tracheobronchial tree, resulting in cough productive of mucus present at some time of the day for at least three months of two consecutive years. It may be diagnosed on this history providing that a localized pulmonary cause such as bronchiectasis, tuberculosis, or tumor has been excluded. The definition is often interpreted less rigidly to include those with chronic or recurrent cough productive of sputum of unspecified duration. It is therefore a clinical diagnosis made solely upon the history. It has a close pathologic counterpart in an increase in the mucus-secreting glands and goblet cells of the bronchial mucosa.

Etiology and Epidemiology. The United Kingdom has the highest recorded mortality attributed to chronic bronchitis in the world. It is 4 to 5 times that of Western Europe and more than 15 times that of Scandinavia and the United States.

Factors predisposing to chronic bronchitis have been identified from epidemiologic studies carried out mainly in Europe and North America. Cigarette smoking has been shown to be the most important single factor; because of its almost overwhelming effect, the contributions of other factors have been partly obscured. Studies comparing the prevalence of chronic bronchitis in urban and rural communities, in workers in different occupations and of different social class, have shown that, in addition to cigarette smoking, air pollution, dusty occupations, poorer social and economic circumstances, and, especially, increasing age all lead to a higher prevalence of chronic bronchitis. An indication of the magnitude of these factors can be seen from recent statistics of death rates attributable to chronic bronchitis in England and Wales. The standard mortality rate (SMR) was six times greater in males living in a heavily air-polluted area of the industrial Northwest of England compared with a South coast holiday resort. It was five times greater in the lowest social class (Class V) compared with social class I. The effect of occupation is shown by an approximately tenfold increase in SMR in coal miners and laborers compared with clergymen, teachers, and doctors.

There is mounting evidence that during childhood environment is important in influencing both the frequency of lower respiratory tract infections and the ventilatory capacity. In recent epidemiologic studies in the United Kingdom, peak flow rates were found to be significantly lower in children living in areas of high air pollution and were further reduced in those with a past history of bronchitis or pneumonia. The prevalence of acute bronchitis in children is similarly increased by air pollution and also by cigarette smoking; it has been reported also to be more common among children of smokers than of nonsmokers. These influences in childhood probably play an important part in the development of chronic bronchitis and obstructive lung disease in adult life, a view which is supported by the observation that deaths attributed to this cause are higher in male immigrants from Europe to the United States of America than in native-born males. As only a proportion of individuals exposed to adverse provoking factors develop chronic bronchitis, other factors which make the individual more susceptible to their effects and which might be termed endogenous must exist, although we have little information about them in most instances.

There are two special circumstances about which more is known. First, the genetically determined abnormality of mucus production, mucoviscidosis, impairs bronchial clearance and protective mechanisms leading to recurrent or, more commonly, chronic bronchial infection. Second, and more common, bronchial allergies may themselves increase secretion of mucus by direct stimulation of the glands, or alternatively, cause increased liability to bronchial infections.

Pathology and Pathogenesis. In the majority of patients with chronic productive cough, mucous gland hyperplasia and increased numbers of goblet cells, especially in the smaller bronchioles, are present. The degree of mucous gland hyperplasia and hypertrophy may be expressed as the ratio of the thickness of the mucous glands to thickness of the bronchial wall between cartilage and epithelium (Reid index) and is normally between 0.14 and 0.36. In chronic bronchitis the ratio is increased; for example, in patients with symptoms of five years' duration or longer, the ratio was found to be from 0.41 to 0.79. In the epithelium increased numbers of goblet cells and areas of squamous metaplasia reduce the numbers of ciliated cells. Scanning electron microscope studies have revealed unsuspected marked irregularities of the bronchial surface even in the absence of gross infection. If infection is present, the bronchial wall is infiltrated with inflammatory cells and congested by dilated capillaries and lymphatics, and, if severe, small abscesses may form. Healing of these more severe infections may lead to fibrosis and deformity of the bronchial wall; bronchitis deformans, stenosans, or obliterans; or bronchiectasis. The combination of increased bronchial mucus, fewer cilia, and irregularities of the bronchial wall impairs the rate of mouthward movement of mucus, and the bronchial protective mechanisms are therefore less effective.

Normally the trachea and bronchi yield no bacteria on culture, but in chronic bronchitis a variety of organisms may be isolated, and pus cells may be seen on microscopy. The organisms include those which are normally commensals in the oropharynx and recognized pathogens such as *D. pneumoniae* and *H. influenzae.* Any factors which further impair the clearance mechanisms or other defenses against infection may lead to the development of acute purulent bronchitis. This is presumably a common mechanism of the recurrent "winter" bronchitis to which these patients are prone, although in a number of cases various respiratory viruses, especially respiratory syncytial virus and *Mycoplasma pneumoniae,* have been isolated. Many exacerbations are not associated with recognizable infecting agents. When resulting from an allergic cause, a purulent appearance of the sputum may be due not to bacterial infection with pus cells but to heavy infiltration with eosinophils.

Diagnosis. The diagnosis of chronic bronchitis is made on the history. Confirmation of the associated pathologic changes of mucous gland hyperplasia may be made by bronchial biopsy, but this is a research, not a routine, procedure. Bronchography may reveal dilated enlarged ducts of hypertrophied glands, and the bronchi themselves may be irregular, giving a "concertina" appearance.

Clinical Manifestations. The productive cough of chronic bronchitis is often not regarded as abnormal and is dismissed as a "smoker's cough." The patient expectorates mucus each morning shortly after rising and may produce only a few pieces of mucoid sputum at times during the remainder of the day. This stage is called "simple chronic bronchitis." However, two other manifestations may occur, and standard terminology has been recommended by the Chronic Bronchitis Committee of the Medical Research Council of Great Britain. First, the sputum may become purulent, either continuously or for at least a part of the day, usually in the morning; this is termed *chronic or recurrent mucopurulent bronchitis.* Second, airflow obstruction may develop, the condition becoming *chronic obstructive bronchitis,* which will be discussed in more detail later. All forms of chronic bronchitis may be subject to acute exacerbations with increased volumes of sputum with or without purulence. These acute exacerbations frequently follow a head cold, exposure to smog, or other irritants.

Treatment. Simple Chronic Bronchitis. A careful history to establish the likely role of smoking, occupational hazard, or presence of allergies must be taken. The patient must be urged to stop smoking, and realization that only a minority will succeed should not deter the attempt. Most patients are unlikely to change occupations, and the physician must not lightly advise it without also considering the social and economic circumstances of the patient. Chronic bronchitis occurring in a nonsmoker is unusual; it should raise the suspicion of an allergic cause. Mucoviscidosis is a much less common cause of chronic bronchitis. In the relatively small number of patients in whom there is suspicion of allergy, the diagnosis is strengthened by the finding of eosinophils in the sputum or blood or both; attempts to identify the allergen by history and skin testing then may be worthwhile. (Treatment of bronchial allergies is considered under Asthma.)

Mucopurulent Bronchitis. In addition to the aforementioned measures, administration of the appropriate antimicrobial drug may be successful in removing evidence of infection. Occasionally, despite administration of the whole range of antimicrobials, the infection persists. This usually implies structural damage to the bronchi, possibly with bronchiectatic areas and grossly impaired bronchial clearance. In a small number of such patients, infection is due to organisms such as *P. aeruginosa,* Proteus, and *E. coli.* (For management of the last-named group of infections see the article on Klebsiella and Other Necrotizing Pneumonias.)

In nonhospital practice, it is not necessary or feasible to obtain sputum culture during each acute exacerbation. Treatment should be started with a minimum of delay and is best achieved by self-administration at the earliest sign of infection of either tetracycline, 500 mg. four times a day, or ampicillin, 500 mg. four times a day, for seven to ten days. The patient must be instructed that, should his condition not improve within 48 hours, or deteriorate within this time, he should seek medical advice without further delay.

A variety of other antimicrobials may be used. These are usually variants of tetracycline or penicillin. Tetracycline is particularly effective in mycoplasma infections. In infections with *H. influenzae,* ampicillin, 1 gram every six hours for seven to ten days, is particularly effective when started in the acute phase, and may reduce the frequency of subsequent exacerbations. Chloramphenicol, 250 to 500 mg. four times a day, is very effective, but fear of blood dyscrasia has limited its use largely to situations in which delay in using an effective drug would be very dangerous, e.g., in association with ventilatory failure.

Long-term Antimicrobial Therapy for Mucopurulent Chronic Bronchitis. In controlled studies, long-term treatment with oxytetracyline, 2 grams daily, did not affect the frequency of acute exacerbations but reduced the duration of illness. Pneumonias were less frequent but did occur; there was no change in the frequency of isolation of *H. influenzae.* When combined with chloramphenicol, the incidence of exacerbations was reduced in patients with frequent exacerbations. Superinfection with drug-resistant bacteria was not found to be a problem. Equally good results have been obtained from prompt intermittent therapy, and most physicians consider that unless the frequency of recurrences is so great that virtually continuous therapy is being given, individual therapy of exacerbations is the method of choice.

Chronic Obstructive Bronchitis. The special additional features of management in patients with chronic obstructive bronchitis are considered later.

Prognosis. Reduction in cough and sputum may be expected if the provoking irritant can be removed, and some regression of the histologic changes has been recorded. Mortality depends largely on whether generalized obstructive changes develop in the bronchi.

Prevention. Chronic bronchitis is usually a preventable disease. Education in the dangers of cigarette smoking, control or elimination of dusty atmospheres in occupations with known hazards, and prompt effective treatment of bronchial infections in childhood are measures that would reduce chronic bronchitis to a minor disorder. Although the medical profession has a leading role to play in alerting the public to the dangers, in the last analysis it is the community as a whole which must provide the solutions. There is one exception: recognition of allergic factors and their elimination or effective treatment comprise one area in which the physician alone is responsible.

Air Pollution and Health. Summary and Report on Air Pollution and Its effects on Health by the Committee of the Royal College of Physicians of London on Smoking and Atmospheric Pollution. London, Pitman Medical and Scientific Publishing Company, Ltd., 1970.

American Thoracic Society: Statement on bacteriologic considerations in the therapy of chronic suppurative bronchitis and bronchiectasis. Amer. Rev. Resp. Dis., 82:743, 1960.

Carilli, A. D., Gohd, R. S., and Gordon, W.: A virologic study of chronic bronchitis. New Eng. J. Med., 270:123, 1964.

Holland, W. W., Bennett, A. E., and Elliot, A.: Factors influencing the onset of chronic respiratory disease. Brit. Med. J., 2.205, 1969.

Medical Research Council Report of the Committee on Etiology of Chronic Bronchitis: The definition and classification of chronic bronchitis for clinical and epidemiological purposes. Lancet, 1:775, 1965.

Reid, L.: Emphysema with chronic bronchitis. *In* Pathology of Emphysema. London, Lloyd-Luke Ltd., 1967, Chap. 12, p. 158.

Report to Medical Research Council—The value of chemoprophylaxis and chemotherapy in early chronic bronchitis. Brit. Med. J., 1:1317, 1966.

Stuart-Harris, C. H.: Chronic bronchitis. Abstracts of World Medicine, 42:649, 737, 1968.

ASTHMA

Definition. Asthma is not a disease entity but one form of clinical presentation of a variety of disorders of the bronchi in which marked changes in bronchial caliber may occur over short periods of time, either spontaneously or in response to treatment.

Because the degree of reversibility of bronchial narrowing may vary widely from complete to the barely measurable, it is not possible, nor even desirable, to define asthma in more quantitative terms. The term merely describes that end of the spectrum of reversibility of bronchial narrowing at which the changes both in the bronchi and in the clinical state of the patient are unequivocal.

Many cases are encountered in which the variability in the state of the patient is less dramatic and in which categorization as asthma is uncertain. However, the management of the individual patient does not require that this uncertainty of categorization be resolved; it is the etiology and mechanism by which the disorder is produced that must be recognized if effective therapy is not to be withheld. Most patients with this clinical entity have an allergic basis for their bronchial disorder. Nevertheless, other nonallergic mechanisms are sometimes responsible so that the presence of asthma is not in itself unequivocal evidence of the presence of an allergic disorder.

Mechanism and Etiology. In asthma, there is a continuous state of hyper-reactivity of the bronchi, during which exposure to a wide variety of bronchial irritants will precipitate an asthmatic attack.

Bronchial Hyper-reactivity. In normal subjects, inhalation of histamine or carbachol may cause small increases in airway resistance. By contrast, the bronchi of patients with asthma are highly reactive and show marked bronchoconstriction in response to these substances. This phenomenon is termed *bronchial hyper-reactivity.* In addition to these pharmacologic agents, bronchial hyper-reactivity has also been shown to occur with a variety of nonspecific irritants such as dusts and cold air. This reaction is not restricted to asthmatic patients; it may also occur in many patients with chronic bronchitis and chronic airflow obstruction. It may sometimes be seen in normal subjects, especially for short periods following an acute tracheobronchial infection. This state of hyper-reactivity may be reversible; in subjects with seasonal grass-pollen asthma, hyper-reactivity increases during the pollen season whether attacks are occurring or not. In children with perennial asthma, removal from an urban environment to the Swiss Alps has been followed by progressive reduction in the degree of hyper-reactivity. In subjects with hyper-reactivity associated with nonallergic states, e.g., chronic bronchitis, clinical observation of the effects of removal of inhaled irritants such as smoking or moving to a less polluted environment suggests that some degree of reversibility is possible.

At least two types of mechanism are involved in hyper-reactivity. The bronchoconstriction induced by cold air, for example, is blocked by atropine, indicating that a nervous reflex is involved. By contrast, the actions of histamine and SO_2 are less affected by atropine, and it is believed that an alteration in the tissues themselves is responsible.

Bronchial Irritants. A number of factors may cause hyper-reactive bronchi to constrict, and for convenience they are all termed irritants. Although the end-result of their action is similar, it is important clinically to decide whether the irritant acts by inducing an allergic reaction or by some other mechanism, because specific therapy is available only for the allergic type.

Allergic or Presumed Allergic Factors. Allergic or presumed allergic factors are involved in most cases of asthma. Immediate, Type I allergic reactions are the only ones unequivocally known to be involved. However, in studying responses to inhaled organic dusts in nonatopic patients with allergic alveolitis, Pepys observed some patients who, in addition to the characteristic inflammatory reaction in the alveoli, developed bronchospasm several hours later. This suggests that allergic reactions (Type III) involving circulating precipitating antibodies may also be involved in certain forms of clinical asthma. There is as yet no firm evidence that other types of allergic reaction are involved in asthma, although in hay fever there is evidence that delayed, Type IV, cell-mediated hypersensitivity may play a part. Common antigens involved in Type I reactions include grass pollens, tree pollens, mold spores, fungi including Aspergillus, animal dander, and house dust. In the last case, the allergen is frequently due to the presence of a mite (Dermatophagoides) of which a number of different species have been identified. In certain occupations, exposure to specific antigens may occur, e.g., bakers and millers exposed to grain dust and flour, in which again a mite has recently been claimed to be responsible. Food allergies, e.g., to eggs, shellfish, fish, and chocolate, may also cause asthma but are more likely to cause urticaria.

Physical or Chemical Irritants. Irritants such as inert dusts, sulfur dioxide and other atmospheric pollutants are often responsible for asthma; for example, so-called Tokyo-Yokohama asthma is believed to be due to the high levels of atmospheric irritants in these cities, acting on individuals with pre-existing bronchitis or asthma. Evidence has been accumulating that the active principle of certain house dusts resides in the presence of floor mites (*Dermatophagoides pteronyssimis*). A number of industrial chemicals, for example, aluminium solder flux and toluene diisocyonate (TDI), a chemical widely used in the plastics industry, may induce asthma. The mechanism is not known, and at present it is uncertain whether there is an allergic basis for these hypersensitivities or not.

Psychologic and Nervous Factors. Bronchoconstriction may occur in response to psychologic stress or as part of a conditioned reflex. This does not mean that the psyche is a primary cause of asthma, but merely that in patients with bronchi already hyper-reactive from some other cause, psychologic factors may induce an exacerbation. Presumably the hyper-reactive bronchi are showing an exaggerated response to efferent autonomic nervous activity.

Physical Exertion. Although the immediate effect of brief exercise may be to induce bronchodilatation in an asthmatic subject, many patients experience chest tightness and breathlessness if exercise is prolonged for several minutes; this may be especially noticeable after stopping the exercise. It is due to bronchoconstriction and is particularly common in children and young adults with mild asthma. The mechanism is uncertain and may be caused by different factors in different people. Hyperventilation with a lowering of P_{CO_2} or release of a circulating bronchoconstrictor substance during exercise has been suggested, but neither mechanism will explain all cases. The response is usually not blocked by the administration of atropine, but isoproterenol and cromolyn sodium have been reported to be effective. Occasionally exercise-induced attacks are the only clinical manifestation of asthma for years before spontaneous attacks begin to occur.

Infections. Respiratory infections, especially viral, are commonly associated with attacks of asthma. Whether this represents an allergic reaction to the infecting agent or is merely a nonspecific response of hyper-reactive bronchi to the infection is uncertain. There is still no firm evidence that chronic infections such as chronic sinusitis, tonsillitis, or dental sepsis are a cause of asthma in those patients in whom clear evidence of allergy is lacking (intrinsic or "infective" asthma). Lack of correlation between exacerbations of asthma and degree of activity of infection, together with failure of removal of infected foci or of long-term antimicrobial therapy to influence the course of the disease, casts doubt on the relevance of this mechanism. Skin tests to bacterial antigens are usually negative, but this may merely mean that an immediate Type I allergic reaction is not involved.

Mechanism of the Asthmatic Response to Allergens. Initial exposure to antigen in a subject with the appropriate genetic constitution results in the production of highly reactive "reaginic" antibody which attaches itself to cells, notably in the bronchi and in the skin. This antibody was until recently known to be present only by its biologic effects. Thus when the cells of the skin are brought in contact with antigen by scarification or injection intradermally, a wheal and flare reaction results. However, in 1966 the Ishizakas in the United States and Johannsen in Sweden identified the antibody in the serum of patients with allergic asthma and categorized it as IgE. Johannsen subsequently demonstrated that IgE concentration is raised in patients with asthma associated with positive skin tests, but not in patients with so-called intrinsic asthma. When the appropriate antigen combines with the cell-fixed IgE, substances (spasmogens) including histamine, slow-reacting substance of anaphylaxis (SRS-A), bradykinin, and rabbit aorta-contracting substance (RACS) are released directly or indirectly by mast cells and cause increased secretions, mucosal edema, and bronchial smooth muscle contraction which are the characteristics of an attack of asthma.

The mechanism and cause of asthma associated with negative skin tests (intrinsic asthma) are uncertain. This type is sometimes called nonallergic or infective, but it is probable that a different form of allergic process is involved. Some workers have denied any fundamental difference between intrinsic and extrinsic asthma, believing that if only the appropriate antigen were used for testing, all patients would be found to be extrinsic in origin. However, there are other features of patients in the two categories of asthma which indicate other differences between them, and these differences are listed in the accompanying table.

A clear-cut separation as suggested by this table is not always evident, but there can be little doubt that the distinction between the two types is a valid one. It does not necessarily follow that these are two diseases. It is also well recognized that some patients with extrinsic asthma in childhood may develop intrinsic asthma in middle age.

Pathology. Pathologic studies of asthma are largely related to the lungs of patients who die in status asthmaticus. The lungs are voluminous, and the smaller bronchi are largely occluded by mucous plugs. Histologically, large numbers of eosinophils are present in the bronchial walls together with varying numbers of lymphocytes and neutrophils and plasma cells. Hypertrophy of bronchial mucous glands and bronchial smooth muscle is usual; shedding of the epithelium is common.

Clinical Manifestations. Asthma occurs characteristically as episodes which may last from a few minutes to several days with a wide range of severity; between attacks the patient is well. Alternatively, the condition may be associated with chronic airflow obstruction, and some symptoms may then be present continuously though of varying severity.

Episodic Asthma. The attack may begin within minutes of exposure to antigen and may or may not be associated with symptoms of hay fever. Alternatively, it may be precipitated by exertion, irritants, emotional stress, excitement, or infection; often there is no known precipitating factor. The patient experiences a sensation of chest tightness, with coughing and wheezing, which increases in severity. Dyspnea may become severe, and expiration is usually felt to be more difficult than inspiration. If untreated, the attack may last a variable time from a few minutes to several hours, but the prompt inhalation of an aerosol of isoproterenol or similar substance may abort the attack.

Sometimes attacks happen only at night, usually waking the patient between 2 and 4 A.M. Nocturnal attacks may occur sporadically for months or years before occurring during the day.

CONTRASTING FEATURES OF EXTRINSIC AND INTRINSIC ASTHMA

	Extrinsic	Intrinsic
Age of onset	Childhood or young adulthood	Middle age
Family history of allergies	Positive	Negative
Nasal symptoms	Hay fever	Nasal polyps
Aspirin sensitivity	Not a feature	Significant association
Skin tests	Positive	Negative
IgE levels	Raised	Normal

The natural history of patients with episodic asthma is variable. Frequently asthma begins in childhood, often in association with other evidence of atopy, especially infantile or flexural eczema. It may be particularly troublesome once the child begins school, possibly because of additional emotional stress and exposure to upper respiratory tract infections. Exercise-induced asthma may prevent the child from participating in games. It is at this stage that the etiologic role of psychologic factors is liable to be overrated; instead they should be recognized as only one of several possible provoking factors. Parental anxiety is especially liable to be blamed but only leads to even greater stress if not dealt with sympathetically.

Asthma with Chronic Airflow Obstruction. In some patients, there is a gradual change in the character of the disorder. Attacks become less frequent and less severe, but the degree of recovery between them is less complete. The patient develops chronic narrowing of the bronchi with airflow obstruction, and his capacity for physical exertion is progressively reduced. This state is associated with chronic cough and sputum (chronic bronchitis), and liability to episodes of purulent bronchitis is increased.

The Attack of Asthma. In a severe attack, the patient is extremely dyspneic, orthopneic, and often cyanosed. He is agitated and may be confused. He is often most comfortable sitting forward with his arms leaning on some support, a point to remember when asking the patient to lean back on the pillows to be examined. There is indrawing of the soft tissues of the neck, and the accessory muscles are active. The chest is overinflated with diminished hepatic and cardiac dullness to percussion, and respiratory movement is reduced. The larynx is pulled downward and the lower lateral rib cage inward with inspiration. High pitched, sibilant rhonchi, often associated with coarse crepitations in some areas, occur during inspiration as well as expiration. It is important to remember that when airflow obstruction becomes extreme, rhonchi may disappear. The pulse is rapid and blood pressure is normal. Pulsus paradoxicus may be present, but, unlike the situation in pericardial tamponade, there is no associated engorgement of the cervical veins on inspiration. The sputum is usually viscid and difficult to expectorate; it may contain branched white bronchial casts and spirals of condensed mucus up to a few millimeters long, so-called Curschmann's spirals. A purulent appearance is commonly due to infection but may be due solely to the presence of large numbers of eosinophils. If the attack has been present for many hours or days without remission despite treatment, the patient has "status asthmaticus." This is often associated with signs of exhaustion and dehydration. Tachycardia is the rule, and, if greater than 130 per minute, indicates severe hypoxemia. Rarely, in patients with very prolonged severe airflow obstruction, edema of the feet and ankles may occur without other clinical evidence of heart failure.

Laboratory Tests. Vital capacity, FEV_1, and FEV_1/VC ratio are diminished. Residual volume is increased, and, if airflow obstruction is severe and prolonged, total lung capacity may also be increased. Airway resistance is markedly increased. Arterial Po_2 is reduced owing to disturbed ventilation-perfusion relationships. An FEV_1 of less than 1 liter is almost always associated with reduction in arterial Po_2, and in status asthmaticus the arterial Po_2 may reach alarmingly low levels but is usually above 50 mm. Hg. In moderate asthma, the Pco_2 is often low, indicating hyperventilation. A raised Pco_2, for example above 50 mm. Hg, is of grave significance, for it indicates that the resting ventilation is virtually the maximum of which the patient is capable and that further increase in airway resistance, or reduction in drive to breathe either through exhaustion or because of the use of sedatives or opiates, may be rapidly lethal. The arterial Po_2 may not return to normal between attacks because of persisting ventilation-perfusion disturbances which have been demonstrated using radioactive xenon studies.

The peripheral blood often shows eosinophilia. A slight polymorphonuclear leukocytosis is not uncommon. Microscopy of the sputum reveals eosinophilia and also long narrow crystals, Charcot-Leyden crystals, which are believed to be derived from eosinophils and with which they are always associated. The chest roentgenograph usually shows signs of overinflation, but occasionally patchy radiopacities may be present. These are particularly common in association with aspergillosis. Heart size is normal.

Prognosis and Prevalence. It is usual for attacks to become less frequent and severe during middle and late adolescence, and they may disappear completely. Approximately 50 per cent of children with asthma will become symptom free before adult life, and only 5 to 10 per cent continue to have severe disability, this unfortunate outcome being more likely when asthma has begun in infancy in association with eczema. This presumably reflects their greater tendency to develop hypersensitivity reactions. Often those not wholly symptom free in adulthood will experience only occasional mild attacks at infrequent intervals, but sometimes severe attacks may recur years or decades later. In adult asthmatics of the intrinsic type, followed for at least 15 years, Rackemann found that 22 per cent were symptom free, 44 per cent were improved, 33 per cent were unimproved, and 3 per cent had probably died of their asthma. Sinusitis and nasal polyps were more common in the unimproved group. There is general agreement that deaths are most common in patients with severe disabling chronic symptoms.

Asthma occurs in approximately 1 to 2 per cent of the population. There is a higher prevalence in children; various studies in the United States and the United Kingdom report asthma to be present in from 2.3 to 4.8 per cent of this age group. Asthma occurs more frequently in boys up to ten years of age, but the ratio becomes even wider during adolescence. Severe childhood asthma is much more common among boys.

Spontaneous pneumothorax and mediastinal emphysema may occur but are not common. Conjunctival hemorrhages are common after a severe attack. Emphysema of the lungs does not occur unless chronic airflow obstruction develops.

Sudden deaths in asthma have occurred more frequently in recent years. In the United Kingdom the over-all death rate from asthma increased by 42 per cent, from 2.7 to 3.8 per 100,000 between 1959 and 1964. However, in the age group 5 to 14 the increase was 330 per cent. The causes of this increase are uncertain. Corticosteroid therapy has been blamed, but there is no firm evidence to support this; in fact, use of steroids may have reduced the death rate in children. Excessive use of isoproterenol and other similar inhalant aerosols has also been blamed. Severe reactions have been recorded resulting from hypersensitivity to penicillin, aspirin, indomethacin, and radiopaque contrast media.

Differential Diagnosis. States of increased ventilation may be confused with asthma. These include severe metabolic acidosis, e.g., "renal" asthma, hyperventilation syndrome, and pulmonary embolism in which bronchospasm may also occur. Airflow obstruction with wheezing also occurs in certain patients with left ventricular failure, and inhalation of isoproterenol may give temporary relief. Paroxysmal nocturnal dyspnea caused by left ventricular failure may be confused with asthma. Large airway obstruction, e.g., laryngeal carcinoma and tracheal growths or compression from lymph nodes, may sometimes cause confusion, but inspiratory stridor should indicate the mechanism. Asthma may sometimes occur in association with other disorders of immunologic mechanisms; in association with polyarteritis nodosa, marked eosinophilia is characteristic. Carcinoid tumors are a rare cause of asthmatic attacks associated with flushing.

Management of Asthma. Obviously the most direct form of management of the patient with asthma is to terminate the exposure to responsible allergens or irritants. This may give complete relief and is most likely to be effective with occupational exposures or specific sensitivities, e.g., to animal dander. If avoidance of the allergen is not feasible, attempts may be made to *hyposensitize* the patient by injections of graded doses of the antigen at regular intervals. This produces "blocking antibodies" which interfere with the antigen-antibody reaction. This procedure, which is particularly successful for hay fever, is less successful for the relief of asthma, although sometimes dramatic success occurs with complete relief of symptoms for varying periods up to several years. Further courses of antigen injection may not be so successful. It is not possible to predict which patients will benefit, and therefore it is always worth trying in patients with continuing disability whenever other methods of treatment have failed.

Reversal of the Asthmatic Reaction. *Acute exacerbations* of asthma may be promptly relieved by inhalation of 0.1 mg. of isoproterenol, and 0.1 ml. of 1:1000 epinephrine subcutaneously or 1:100 by nebulizer. The last-named agent is least liable to induce tachycardia and, unlike isoproterenol, has been reported not to cause a further lowering of arterial Po₂. Unfortunately, the more severe the asthmatic reaction, the less is the response to these drugs, and the shorter their duration of action. It is in these circumstances that repeated doses are taken at short intervals and the danger of overdosage is present. In some individuals, a rebound bronchoconstriction occurs as the bronchodilator effect wears off.

For continuous symptoms, the most successful drugs are those which stimulate β-adrenergic receptors. Ephedrine, 15 to 30 mg., may be given twice or three times daily. This should be first given in low dosage as it may cause palpitation and tremor and, in the elderly male, urinary retention. Other effective drugs are isoproterenol 5 to 20 mg. sublingually as required, and aminophylline, 100 to 300 mg. three times a day. Aminophylline is liable to cause gastric irritation, but there are several proprietary chemical analogues which are better tolerated. Nocturnal symptoms may be relieved by suppositories of aminophylline, 360 mg. rectally on retiring at night. In persistent asthma potassium iodide, 0.6 gram three times a day after meals, is often valuable in thinning tenacious sputum.

Although the aforementioned drugs are often given in combination, they should be first administered singly and with caution to patients with heart disease, hypertension, and hyperthyroidism. Antihistamines are rarely of much value in asthma and may cause drowsiness, but because of occasional successes should be considered in special situations. In a small number of patients, aspirin may be beneficial despite the apparent paradox that in intrinsic asthma severe hypersensitivity may exist. Methysergide, the antagonist of serotonin, and the fenamates, antagonists of bradykinin, have not been found of significant value in asthma, although trials have been reported only in patients with severe chronic disease.

Suppression of Allergic Reactions. If the asthmatic response is not controlled by simple measures, suppression of the allergic reaction should be attempted. Three types of drugs may be employed: corticosteroids, corticotrophin (ACTH), and cromolyn sodium. The mode of action of *corticosteroids* in asthma is uncertain. They will not suppress the acute asthmatic response to inhaled antigen but are effective in suppressing clinical extrinsic and intrinsic asthma in most cases. It has been suggested that they reduce the inflammatory reaction and may therefore act mainly by reducing edema and mucous secretion as well as bronchial hyper-reactivity. A large number of different corticosteroid preparations are available, each with different dosage schedules. For simplicity, dosages will be described for prednisone or prednisolone; dosages of other preparations should be adjusted accordingly.

Acute Attack. For the treatment of an acute attack comparatively large doses, 30 to 60 mg. daily, may be given for a few days with safety, and after relief has been obtained reduction in dosage at a rate of 5 mg. daily is usually possible without early recurrence. The occasional use of large doses of prednisone in this way is without significant risk of side effects except in patients with peptic ulceration in whom gastrointestinal bleeding may be induced. In children, as many as 15 courses of steroids have been given in a year without any detectable side effects developing.

Continuous Symptoms. For continuous symptoms which recur during or shortly after the course of corticosteroids administered as described above, there are two alternative forms of dosage. In the one form (intermittent therapy) the treatment is given for one to three days with the lowest dose of corticosteroids which will permit them to be omitted for a similar period without return of symptoms. The aim is to minimize the dangers of side effects and adrenal suppression. In the other form (continuous therapy) a large initial dose is given to produce quick suppression, followed by a rapid reduction to an intermediate dose level, after which a slow reduction is carried out until symptoms begin to recur. Thereafter, minor adjustments of dosage are made, preferably by the patient himself if he can demonstrate his willingness and capacity to cooperate in this way.

Continuous Therapy. An initial dose of prednisolone is given sufficient to produce effective, rapid suppression of symptoms, for example, 10 mg. three times a day (range usually 20 to 60 mg. daily). In rapid reduction, when definite improvement has occurred (usually within four days) the daily dosage may be reduced by 2.5 mg. (half tablet) daily (or at longer intervals if experience indicates). In slow reduction, when the daily dosage is down to 15 mg. daily (that is, one to two weeks after start), reduction by 1 mg. once or twice weekly may be continued until either symptoms begin to recur or it has been found possible to discontinue treatment. If troublesome symptoms recur while reducing dosage, the daily dose may be increased by 3 to 5 mg., and the procedure restarted.

Intermittent Therapy. The patient will usually find a dosage below which reduction is always followed by recurrence of symptoms. Once this is accomplished, an intermittent regimen can be scheduled. Whether the intermittent or the continuous regimen is being used, superimposed acute exacerbations should be treated promptly with a large increase in dosage for a few days; then a progressive reduction may be followed as before.

Corticotrophin, natural or synthetic, may be used in place of corticosteroids for continuous symptoms. By using depot preparations, a satisfactory regimen of intermittent injections can usually be achieved. Initially, 1 mg. of depot ACTH may be given daily and reduced to once weekly. The need for reducing the dose to the minimum which will maintain adequate control is the same as for oral corticosteroids. Corticotrophin has been reported to cause less retardation of growth in children than oral corticosteroids. Suppression of pituitary secretion of ACTH may occur and abrupt cessation of therapy may lead to acute adrenocorticoid insufficiency. Allergic reactions have occurred to the natural hormone, and a case of sensitivity to the synthetic preparation has recently been reported.

Cromolyn Sodium (Disodium Cromoglycate. Cromolyn sodium is a new drug that has been reported to be effective in the prophylaxis of allergic asthma. It is administered by inhalation and is virtually ineffective orally. Unlike corticosteroids, it inhibits the asthmatic response to inhaled antigen in sensitive subjects only if given before the antigen. It also inhibits both the immediate reagin-mediated, and the late, precipitin-mediated asthmatic and febrile responses to inhalation of Aspergillus and of avian protein in sensitive subjects. However, there have been no reports to date of its use in the therapy or prophylaxis of allergic alveolitis.

The mechanism of action of cromolyn sodium is uncertain; although it does not prevent antigen and reaginic antibody from combining, it prevents the combination from disrupting mast cells and thereby releasing spasmogens. There are considerable differences in its effect in different tissues and in different species; it is effective in the lungs of human subjects and in only a limited number of animal species. It does not inhibit in vitro any of the known spasmogens such as histamine, SRSA, or bradykinin. Recent observations suggest that, in addition, it may possess alpha-adrenergic blocking properties, although the therapeutic significance of this is yet to be established.

Because of its mode of action, it is not used to treat the existing attack but to prevent further attacks. At present, the degree of improvement to be expected from cromolyn sodium cannot be predicted with confidence. Complete relief or considerable improvement is most likely in young patients with extrinsic asthma, and more than 80 per cent may be expected to show worthwhile improvement. The response of older patients with intrinsic asthma is often less satisfactory, and only approximately two thirds are likely to improve. Improvement may be reflected in a number of ways such as reduction in the number of attacks, reduced cough and sputum, reduced bronchodilator and corticosteroid requirements. It is generally accepted that these changes may sometimes occur without corresponding improvement in the results of spirometry.

In a group of patients already receiving continuous corticosteroid therapy, cromolyn sodium permitted an average reduction of steroid dosage of 40 per cent in approximately two thirds of cases; it was rarely possible to discontinue corticosteroids. The only known side effect is irritation of the throat by the dry powder.

Cromolyn sodium is prepared as a powder in capsules containing 20 mg. of drug dispersed with lactose, and is inhaled through a specially designed insufflator. For patients in whom the dry powder induces irritation of hyper-reactive bron-

chi, a preparation containing 0.1 mg. of isoproterenol is available in the United Kingdom only. The usual dose schedule is inhalation of the contents of one capsule (20 mg.) four times a day, but this may be adjusted to the minimal dose that maintains suppression of symptoms.

Immunosuppressive Therapy. Immunosuppressive therapy similar to that used in tissue or organ transplantation has been used in attempts to suppress the allergic reaction in asthma. In a small number of trials using azathioprine, chlorambucil, and methotrexate in chronic severe asthma, conflicting results have been reported, and their value has yet to be determined.

Status Asthmaticus. The majority of patients with asthma improve rapidly following admission to hospital, administration of corticosteroids, and bronchodilator therapy. Subcutaneous epinephrine should not be administered because the patient may already have taken large doses of isoproterenol before admission. Sedatives are potentially dangerous and are absolutely contraindicated if the Pco_2 is raised; with lesser degrees of severity, their cautious use may be helpful. When improvement is delayed, particular attention must be paid to humidification of the inspired air, preferably by an ultrasonic nebulizer, although occasionally this aerosol is itself a bronchial irritant. Oxygen may be administered freely since CO_2 sensitivity is not impaired. Hydration of the patient must be maintained, with intravenous fluids if necessary. Occasionally hypovolemia is present and requires more rapid rehydration.

Intravenous hydrocortisone, 100 to 200 mg., may be repeated hourly if necessary, and some workers advocate even higher dosage up to 1 gram repeated as necessary. However, gastrointestinal hemorrhage has been reported on such a regimen. If severe respiratory acidemia is present, intravenous sodium bicarbonate, 50 to 100 mEq., may be beneficial. Serial measurement of Pa_{CO_2} and Pa_{O_2} is helpful in monitoring ventilatory status and oxygen therapy.

A decision which is often difficult is that of when to use *assisted ventilation.* This is made on the basis of the over-all state of the patient, with particular attention paid to whether he is becoming exhausted, is unable to cooperate in bronchial toilet, or if the Pa_{CO_2} is rising progressively. It should not be made on any arbitrary level of Pa_{CO_2} or Pa_{O_2}. Endotracheal intubation has replaced tracheostomy in this situation; in addition to assisting ventilation, it enables bronchial toilet to be improved.

Altounyan, R. E. C.: Changes in responsiveness to histamine and atropine as a guide to diagnosis and evaluation of therapy in obstructive airway disease. *In* Proceedings of a Symposium on Disodium Cromoglycate in Allergic Airways Disease. London, Butterworth & Co., Ltd., 1970.

Altounyan, R. E. C., and Howell, J. B. L.: Treatment of asthma with disodium cromoglycate. Respiration, 26(Suppl.:131, 1969.

Curry, J. J.: The action of histamine on the respiratory tract in normal and asthmatic subjects. J. Clin. Invest., 25:785, 1946.

De Vries, K., Booij-Noord, H., Goei, J. T., Grobler, N. J., and Orie, N. G. M.: Inhalation tests. The influence of nonspecific irritants on the airways. Acta Allerg. (Kohenharn), (Suppl. 8):131, 1967.

Johansson, S. G. O.: Raised levels of a new immunoglobulin class (IgND) in asthma. Lancet, 2:951, 1967.

Jones, R. S.: Assessment of respiratory function in the asthmatic child. Brit. Med. J., 2:972, 1966.

McNeill, R. S., Nairn, J. R., Millar, J. S., and Ingram, C. G.: Exercise-induced asthma. Quart. J. Med. (N.S.), 35:55, 1966.

Rackemann, F. M., and Edward, M. C.: Asthma in children. New Eng. J. Med., 246:815, 1952.

Read, J.: The reported increase in mortality from asthma: A clinico-functional analysis. Med. J. Aust., 55:879, 1968.

Rees, H. A., Millar, J. S., and Donald, K. W.: A study of the clinical course and arterial blood gas tensions of patients in status asthmaticus. Quart. J. Med., 37:541, 1967.

Szentivanyi, A.: The beta adrenergic theory of the atopic abnormality in bronchial asthma. J. Allerg., 42:203, 1968.

Warren, W. P., and Rose, B.: Hypersensitivity bronchopulmonary aspergillosis. Dis. Chest, 55:415, 1969.

Wharton, G. W.: Mites and commercial extracts of house dust. Science, 167:1382, 1970.

Williams, M. H., Jr., and Kane, C.: Treatment of bronchial asthma with cromolyn. J.A.M.A., 209:1881, 1969.

BRONCHIECTASIS

Definition. The Greek word "ectasia" means widening; hence bronchiectasis means widening of the bronchi. There are no symptoms or signs directly related to widening of the bronchi. However, to the clinician, bronchiectasis usually means more than the anatomic lesion; it includes in addition the chronic or recurrent bronchial infection and hypersecretion of mucus which usually accompanies it.

Etiology. The causes of bronchiectasis are varied and their relative frequency has changed since the introduction of antimicrobial drugs and the control of pulmonary tuberculosis. In the pre-chemotherapy era, the most common causes of bronchiectasis were postbronchopneumonic atelectasis and pulmonary tuberculosis. Aspiration of a foreign body, pulmonary complications of surgery, pertussis, and measles were also responsible, but in approximately 25 per cent of cases no cause could be identified. Since the advent of antimicrobial drugs the incidence and the problems in management of bronchiectasis have become much less. It now occurs mainly following the pneumonias that may complicate pertussis or measles, although all the previous causes may still occasionally be responsible. Bronchiectasis secondary to infected obstructive atelectasis resulting from bronchial neoplasm is being seen more frequently. So-called congenital bronchiectasis is probably the result of infections and collapse in infancy, but bronchiectasis associated with chronic sinusitis and situs inversus (Kartagener's syndrome) is probably truly congenital. Mucoviscidosis may also result in widespread bronchiectasis, the ectatic regions sometimes tending to extend more centrally. Bronchiectasis localized to a proximal region of a segmental bronchus, with normal bronchial distribution distal to it, is sometimes seen with pulmonary aspergillosis when the bronchial wall is infiltrated and weakened by the fungus.

Pathogenesis. The caliber of intrapulmonary bronchi depends upon a balance between the inward acting forces of the connective tissues of the bronchial wall and the outward traction of surrounding lung tissue. An increase in outward traction is insufficient to cause dilatation; weakening of the wall resulting from chronic inflammation must also occur. Both these factors may occur following obstructive atelectasis with chronic infection; the atelectasis tends to increase traction and the chronic infection causes damage to the connective tissue and bronchial smooth muscle. Irregular dilatation of the bronchus and damage to the epithelial lining interfere with bronchial drainage; secretions are retained and chronic bronchial suppuration becomes established.

Pathology. Bronchiectasis usually affects segmental bronchi and may involve one or more segments, a lobe, or rarely a whole lung. It is often distributed in patches over a number of segments, and is frequently bilateral. The regions most frequently involved are the basal segments, right middle lobe, and lingula. Upper lobe bronchiectasis is usually secondary to tuberculosis.

The affected bronchus may become dilated into thick-walled sacs, *saccular bronchiectasis*, cyst-like spaces, *cystic bronchiectasis*, or may cause irregular widening over the affected length to form *fusiform* or *cylindrical bronchiectasis*. In saccular bronchiectasis approximately only four generations of bronchi, widely dilated and distorted, can be identified; the distal generations of bronchi and alveoli are usually obliterated by inflammatory tissue and fibrosis. In fusiform bronchiectasis, the distal bronchi are occluded with mucus and pus but are usually not obliterated. Extension of infection to the pleural surface causes pleurisy and adhesions to the chest wall. Histologically, some bronchi are infiltrated with lymphocytes and have lymphoid nodules in their walls; mucus-secreting glands and cells are prominent. This is likely in children with fusiform bronchiectasis of lower lobe bronchi. In saccular bronchiectasis particularly, the walls of the sacs are fibrous and contain granulation tissue in places lined with metaplastic squamous epithelium. The normal structures of the bronchial walls are destroyed. The bacterial flora is similar to that of chronic mucopurulent bronchitis. The usual commensals of the nasopharynx are present, and *H. influenzae,* pneumococci and staphylococci may also be found. Sometimes various species of spirochete and the fusiform bacilli are present and are largely responsible for the offensive fetor.

Clinical Manifestations. The clinical manifestations of bronchiectasis are dominated by the chronic infection and hypersecretion of mucus in the ectatic bronchi. *Cough* productive of copious purulent sputum, occurring especially with changes of posture, is the classic symptom. In a minority of cases, infection is minimal (dry bronchiectasis), and recurrent hemoptysis associated with episodes of infection is the major symptom.

In the heavily infected extensive case, the sputum may have a fetid odor and volumes of 400 to 500 ml. daily may be seen. After adequate drainage and control of infection this may be reduced to a few milliliters a day. Hemoptysis is common and occasionally may be profuse. Coexisting chronic sinusitis, especially of the maxillary antrum, is common, but its relationship to the bronchiectasis is uncertain. *Chest pain* usually occurs as a result of pleurisy during an infective episode, but occasionally there may be a continuous ache in the region of the bronchiectasis. Shortness of breath on exertion and edema of the ankles may occur when the bronchiectasis is complicated by chronic cor pulmonale. General symptoms caused by chronic infection include tiredness, fatigue, and, in children, stunted growth. Sometimes, bronchiectasis is entirely without symptoms and is a fortuitous finding on routine chest roentgenography or on physical examination.

The physical signs depend on the extent and degree of purulence of the bronchiectasis and on whether generalized obstructive bronchial changes have developed.

If the bronchial changes are extensive and associated with airway obstruction, the patient may be dyspneic and cyanosed. With extensive purulent bronchiectasis the fingers are clubbed. There may be flattening of the thorax and the mediastinum may be deviated to the side of the lesion. Movement is diminished, tactile fremitus is reduced, and there may be dullness to percussion. Breath sounds may be bronchial in quality over consolidated segments. Crepitations occur over affected regions and have a characteristic coarse character, well expressed by the term "leathery" crepitations; they do not clear but may be altered by coughing.

Complications. These include recurrent pneumonia, hemoptysis, lung abscess, brain abscess, empyema, pyopneumothorax and, if long standing, amyloid disease. The frequency of these has been greatly reduced with the improved management of bronchiectasis.

Disturbance of pulmonary function is more frequent in bronchiectasis than is generally realized but is due mainly to the associated generalized bronchitis. In a recent study, increased airway resistance and residual volume–total lung capacity ratio and reduced maximal breathing capacity were present in over half the patients. Physiologic dead space–tidal volume ratio and nitrogen washout, indicating alteration in the distribution of inspired gas, was abnormal in the majority. However, arterial oxygen saturation below 90 per cent and slightly raised arterial Pco_2 was seen in only 10 to 15 per cent. These disturbances of pulmonary function were rarely severe but increased in proportion to the number of segments involved. The effects of cylindrical and saccular bronchiectasis on pulmonary function tests were similar. The persistence of *H. influenzae* was correlated with a lower maximal breathing capacity, but no deterioration was observed over a period of three years in any of these patients irrespective of whether *H. influenzae*

was eliminated from the sputum by antimicrobial drugs. The rate of deterioration is related to the frequency of lower respiratory infections.

Diagnosis. The clinical diagnosis may be confirmed by roentgenography, and the chest roentgenogram is nearly always abnormal in some respect. Increased, coarse-meshed lung markings are seen in over half the patients. Evidence of lobar atelectasis occurs particularly in young patients; a honeycomb appearance is less common. Sometimes with saccular and cystic bronchiectasis, ring shadows with fluid levels are present. The diagnosis, extent, and location of the bronchiectasis is established by *bronchography* in which a radiopaque oil is introduced into the trachea and allowed to spread evenly through the tracheobronchial tree, followed by chest roentgenograms in the anteroposterior, lateral, and right anterior oblique positions. It is inadvisable to fill both sides at one examination if there is evidence of impaired pulmonary function. If a primarily endobronchial cause of the bronchiectasis is suspected, bronchoscopy must be performed. A microcytic anemia, neutrophil leukocytosis, and an elevated erythrocyte sedimentation rate, all due to chronic infection, may be present.

There is a spectrum of chronic purulent disease of the bronchi, ranging from mucopurulent bronchitis with little ectasia at one end to gross bronchiectasis at the other. In certain intermediate cases, therefore, the categorization is arbitrary.

Treatment. *Medical.* After identification of the affected segment or segments, a rational program of postural drainage can be introduced, usually twice or thrice daily. In selected cases of basal bronchiectasis, drainage throughout the night by elevation of the foot of the bed may be beneficial. After improvement has occurred, postural drainage should be continued routinely even if it is unproductive of sputum during drainage; the secretions are often moved and coughed up later. Antimicrobial drugs appropriate to the sputum culture should be administered for a limited course, but should not be administered continuously because of possible superinfection, although this rarely seems to occur. With adequate postural drainage, sputum should be reduced to small quantities daily even though it remains purulent. The drugs should be reserved for acute exacerbations when they should be administered with minimal delay. The choice of drug regimen is the same as in the treatment of chronic bronchitis and is discussed in that article and in the article on Klebsiella and Other Necrotizing Pneumonias.

Surgical. If bronchography shows localized unilateral bronchiectasis which is causing sufficient symptoms to be troublesome, usually as a socially disturbing productive cough, surgical removal of the affected segment or lobe should be considered, providing that over-all lung function is adequate. Rarely, bilateral disease may be treated in this way. Sequential resections for recurring disease will result in a greater loss of lung function than if the diseased segments had been removed at one point in time. Prognosis is poorer with left lobe bronchiectasis owing to frequent recurrence in the lingula. The best results are obtained with unilateral bronchiectasis affecting patients less than 30 years old.

Incidence and Prevalence. There is little recent information about the prevalence of bronchiectasis. It has been estimated to affect 1.3 per 1000 persons, but certainly significant clinical problems arising from this cause are becoming rare. Cylindrical bronchiectasis is reported to complicate bronchopneumonia in approximately 4 per cent of cases.

Prognosis. The prognosis has altered substantially since the introduction of antimicrobial drugs. With good control of infection, either by medical or surgical treatment, life expectancy is normal. If extensive suppuration cannot be controlled, the outlook is poor, and it has been estimated that approximately one third will die within ten years. The development of chronic airway obstruction is a serious complication and affects prognosis accordingly.

Cherniak, N. S., and Carton, R. W.: Factors associated with respiratory insufficiency in bronchiectasis. Amer. J. Med., 41:562, 1966.

Gudbjerg, C. E.: Bronchiectasis—Radiological diagnosis and prognosis after operative treatment. Acta Radiol. (Suppl. 143), 1957.

James, U., Brimblecombe, F. S. W., and Wells, J. W.: The natural history of pulmonary collapse in childhood. Quart. J. Med., 25:121, 1956.

Perry, K. M. A., and Holmes Sellers, T. (eds.): Chest Diseases. London, Butterworth, Ltd., 1968.

Prolonged antibiotic treatment of severe bronchiectasis. Clinical Trials Committee of the British Medical Research Council. Brit. Med. J., 2:255, 1957.

CHRONIC AIRWAY OBSTRUCTION

Chronic airway obstruction denotes an alteration in the mechanical properties of the lungs characterized by poorly reversible increased hindrance to expiratory airflow; it is usually but not necessarily accompanied by increased resistance to inspiration. It occurs mainly in association with primary disorders of the lungs such as chronic bronchitis, emphysema, and asthma, but rarely may complicate systemic disorders such as polyarteritis nodosa. The two main abnormalities responsible for this obstruction are, first, generalized narrowing of the bronchi and, second, destruction of the pulmonary parenchyma. An understanding of the interaction of these two factors is important in order to appreciate the significance of the abnormalities involved and the nature of the disability experienced by the patient.

MECHANISMS OF AIRWAY OBSTRUCTION

During inspiration, the inspiratory muscles lower alveolar pressure, and air flows into the alveoli at a rate which depends upon the caliber of the bronchi. During expiration, recoil of stretched elastic tissues expels air from the lungs by raising intra-alveolar pressure above mouth pressure. The rate of flow will depend upon the pressure difference and the resistance of the airways. In normal subjects, this mechanism is sufficient to meet ventilatory needs even under conditions of severe exercise. In subjects with increased resistance to airflow, elastic recoil alone may not be sufficient to achieve the ventilation required, and active expiratory muscular efforts may be made. However, the increased intrathoracic pressure which results from this expiration muscle effort introduces a new factor in expiratory airflow, a tendency to compression of the large airways. *The key to understanding this new factor is that elastic recoil of the lung is solely responsible for raising intrabronchial pressure above intrathoracic pressure.* Providing that the pressure within the bronchi is higher than intrathoracic pressure, there is no airway compression. However, when expiratory airflow is increased in subjects with raised airway resistance, the greater pressure drop along the bronchial tree may cause the pressure inside the trachea and large bronchi to fall below the surrounding intrathoracic pressure, and these structures will be compressed unless there is sufficient rigidity in their walls to resist it. Once compression occurs, no amount of further effort will increase airflow because the pressure within the bronchi cannot be increased without simultaneously increasing the surrounding pressure. In this way, compression which usually occurs in the larger segmental or main-stem bronchi forms a flow-limiting mechanism (often called a Starling resistor), and determines maximal rate of expiratory airflow. This mechanism cannot operate during inspiration; the rate of inspiratory airflow is always effort-dependent.

The maximal rate of expiratory airflow will therefore be reduced by (a) increased resistance to airflow due to structural narrowing or increased tone; (b) decreased elastic recoil of the lung parenchyma; and (c) decreased rigidity of larger airways.

Increased Airway Resistance. Increased airway resistance may be due to increased secretions; thickening of the wall of the airways caused by infiltration, edema, or glandular hypertrophy; or constriction resulting from smooth muscle contraction or fibrosis; deformity of the bronchi may also contribute. The dominant mechanism varies in different circumstances. When associated with chronic bronchitis, increased resistance of the small airways is thought to be largely the result of chronic inflammation with fibrosis, and mucous plugging and histologic changes consistent with this mechanism may be seen in some areas. The role of infection is doubtful; it has not been possible to establish a correlation between the rate of progression of airway obstruction and the frequency of infective bronchial episodes, although during acute infections airway obstruction is temporarily increased. In some areas, complete occlusion of bronchi requires that ventilation of distal areas is by collateral channels, thereby increasing airway resistance. It is possible that narrowing of chronic airways may involve increased smooth muscular tone at least in the initial stages before irreversible structural changes develop. Two observations suggest that some process additional to the results of chronic inflammation and fibrosis may be involved. First, hyper-reactivity of the bronchi is a feature of most patients with narrowing of the small airways; second, airway resistance is reduced, albeit to a small degree, following administration of isoproterenol and atropine aerosols.

Diminished Elastic Recoil. The most important cause of diminished elastic recoil is emphysema. This word is derived from the Greek word meaning "an inflation" and was introduced by Laennec to describe the overinflated and partially destroyed state of the lung "vesicles." Unfortunately, many workers later adopted this term for the clinical syndrome of breathlessness, cough, and sputum with which emphysema is often associated. This resulted in confusion because a similar clinical picture may occur without emphysema. There is now general agreement to restrict the use of the word emphysema to its original meaning as a pathologic term. The most generally accepted definition at present is that agreed on by the World Health Organization (1961): "Emphysema is a condition of the lung characterised by increase beyond the normal in the size of air spaces distal to the terminal bronchiole, with destructive changes in their walls." There is still difference of opinion whether dilatation caused by distention without destruction should be included in the definition.

Destructive changes and dilatation may be restricted to the respiratory bronchioles (centriacinar or centrilobular emphysema), or may be more extensive with destruction of the whole of the acinus (panacinar emphysema), involving both air spaces and vascular bed. These may coalesce or distend to form bullae and cysts. Changes restricted to the periphery of the acinus (paraseptal emphysema) are never extensive and are without functional significance.

Gradual stretching but not rupture of lung tissue occurs with age (senile emphysema) and with longstanding overdistention as in severe chronic airway obstruction or status asthmaticus. Rupture of connective tissue requires weakening or destruction of the connective tissue, but little is known about the factors responsible. Infection extending from the bronchi or deposition of dusts is believed to be responsible for some cases of centrilobular emphysema, but in others the appearances suggest atrophy. The causes of the extensive destructive changes of panacinar emphysema are quite unknown. The nature of the evidence that would be essential to establish causation has been presented by Wright and Kleinerman (1963). One clue to causation in those with emphysema is suggested by the finding of Laurell and Erikksen of an association with deficiency of serum antitrypsin.

If the process is extensive, panacinar emphysema may be a major factor in limiting the maximal rate of expiratory airflow by reducing elastic recoil. The reduction in recoil is not due to alteration in the properties of the elastic fibers themselves; it is due largely to the increased size of the affected air spaces, occupying a larger proportion of the thorax and allowing less room for distention of the normal parts of the lung. This is reflected in a reduction of the maximal intrathoracic pressure which may be developed at full inspiration from the normal of 20 to 30 cm. of water to as low as 3 to 5 cm. of water.

Diagnosis of Emphysema during Life. There are no clinical stigmas of emphysema, and the diagnosis cannot easily be made during life because it requires evidence of the pathologic lesion. Extensive emphysema, especially centrilobular, may be present without roentgenographic abnormality. The presence of emphysema may be inferred from the chest roentgenogram if it shows reduction in the caliber and number of the peripheral branches of the pulmonary artery, usually associated with increased transradiancy of the lung field. This is the most reliable radiologic sign. Other abnormalities such as low, flat diaphragm and increased retrosternal space, although commonly present, are actually evidence only of overinflation of the lungs.

Decreased Rigidity of the Walls of Larger Airways. A diminished rigidity of the trachea and bronchi is a common feature of chronic mucopurulent bronchitis. In itself, it is not responsible for reducing maximal expiratory airflow but predisposes toward airway compression when the other factors are present.

CLINICAL FEATURES OF CHRONIC AIRWAY OBSTRUCTION

Typically, the patient with chronic airway obstruction is a male cigarette smoker, between 50 and 60 years old, who may or may not have a long history of chronic bronchitis with recurrent winter bronchitis. His cardinal symptom is breathlessness on exertion, often with wheezing; it is worse in the morning, associated with a sensation of tightness until he has expectorated the night's accumulation of sputum. Intolerance of sudden exposure to cold air or smoky atmospheres which induce coughing, tightness, and breathlessness (bronchial irritability) is usually present when dyspnea is of sufficient severity to interfere with everyday activity. Similar symptoms may be precipitated by involvement in argument or other emotional situations. There is often orthopnea, along with shortness of breath on stooping. These features are attributable to disturbance of the bronchi and are common to nearly all patients with chronic airway obstruction. However, in some patients varying degrees of disturbance of pulmonary gas exchange may occur, leading to a wider range of clinical presentation; some patients have little evidence of disturbances of cardiopulmonary function, but others become cyanosed and edematous.

Professor Dornhorst of London caught the clinical imagination when he described the extremes of this range as "pink and puffing" and "blue and bloated." A number of studies have correlated these presentations with pulmonary pathology and pulmonary function disturbances, leading to the introduction of other descriptive terms, for example, emphysematous or bronchitic, "fighters or nonfighters," Type A or Type B. It must be emphasized that these are not two distinct diseases but the extremes of a range of presentation; some patients intermediate in type might well be called "blue puffers."

Type A, Emphysematous Type, "Pink Puffers." This patient is severely breathless on exertion. He is underweight, his appearance often suggesting hyperthyroidism. The mucous membranes are pink; there is no finger clubbing. The chest is overinflated, and the accessory muscles are prominent. Cardiac and hepatic dullness are diminished or absent, and resonance extends down to the region of the eleventh to twelfth rib posteriorly. The larynx and trachea are pulled down with each inspiration. On auscultation, breath sounds are quiet, expiration is prolonged, and forced expiration induces fine sibilant rhonchi. The forced expiratory time (the time taken to deliver the forced vital capacity) is prolonged beyond four seconds.

The apex beat is usually impalpable, but pulsation is often seen and felt in the epigastrium where the heart sounds are also heard best. The chest roentgenogram confirms the overinflated state of the chest and usually shows roentgenographic evidence of emphysema. The cardiac shadow is long and narrow.

Laboratory Findings. Total lung capacity, residual volume, and residual volume–total lung capacity ratio are increased. The vital capacity, FEV_1, and the FEV_1/VC ratio are reduced. Other indices of airflow obstruction such as peak flow rate and maximal midexpiratory flow rate are also reduced. Pa_{CO_2} is normal and Pa_{O_2} may be slightly reduced. The transfer factor (diffusing capacity) for carbon monoxide is reduced.

Many of these patients have little increase in inspiratory airway resistance, expiratory airflow obstruction being dominated by *reduced pulmonary elastic recoil*. Flow limitation may be present even during quiet breathing in severe cases, and is best seen when flow-volume curves of the lung are displayed. CO_2 sensitivity is characteristically normal or near normal, and this together with the reduction in ventilatory capacity accounts for the severe exertional dyspnea.

Pathology. Panlobular emphysema is the dominant pathologic lesion in most cases. Mucous gland hyperplasia and hypertrophy may or may not be present. The heart is usually normal.

Type B, Bronchitic Type, "Blue Bloaters." Typically, the history can be considered in three stages. First, there is a long history of chronic bronchitis with recurrent mucopurulent exacerbations. At this stage there may be no reduction of exercise capacity, although spirometry may reveal reduc-

tion in maximal ventilatory capacity. The second stage usually merges gradually with the first as the reduction in ventilatory capacity progresses to the stage at which shortness of breath on exercise becomes noticeable. Sometimes, as in Type A, this may develop relatively suddenly after an acute infective exacerbation. Usually, before shortness of breath becomes very severe, the third stage begins when the patient notices ankle edema, at first in the evenings but gradually becoming more marked and persistent.

Characteristically, the patient is well covered with a plethoric appearance. He is cyanosed at rest with warm extremities. The chest is overinflated but usually less so than in Type A. The signs of increased airway obstruction may be similar to those of Type A, but breath sounds are usually well heard and rhonchi and basal crepitations may be prominent; expiration is prolonged. The forced expiratory time is prolonged. There may be cardiac enlargement, right ventricular hypertrophy, raised jugular venous pressure, and hepatic enlargement together with edema. These signs often become more prominent during an acute exacerbation.

Laboratory Findings. Although the type B patient may have severe airway obstruction, it is not uncommon for the airway obstruction to be relatively mild (FEV_1, 1 to 1.5 liters) even though the Pco_2 is raised. Total lung capacity is usually normal, but residual volume is raised. There is arterial desaturation of varying degree, but it is not often lower than 80 per cent. Secondary polycythemia occurs with the more severe degrees of desaturation. The Pa_{CO_2} is raised, usually less than 55 mm. Hg in the early phases of the illness, but may progress to severe ventilatory failure with Pa_{CO_2} 65 to 75 mm. Hg. This is usually well compensated but with higher levels of Pco_2 may fall to below about 7.35. During acute exacerbations more severe changes may develop.

Airway resistance is increased during both inspiration and expiration. Diffusing capacity is normal. CO_2 sensitivity is depressed. This is not usually measured as a routine clinical procedure, but can readily be observed if a rebreathing method for measuring Pco_2 is used.

The chest roentgenogram shows good bronchovascular markings with thickening of bronchial walls, but characteristically there is no roentgenographic evidence of emphysema. The heart is usually enlarged. The electrocardiogram may show evidence of right ventricular hypertrophy. In acute exacerbations, Kerley B lines, indicating edema of interlobular septa, may be seen; in addition to pulmonary hypertension, cardiac catheterization may reveal raised left ventricular end-diastolic pressure, indicating left ventricular failure. A raised blood urea is common during an acute exacerbation; this is temporary and is corrected when the patient improves.

Pathology. The lungs usually show a combination of centrilobular and panacinar emphysema, but centrilobular emphysema is the more prominent. Occasionally emphysema is absent, but mucous gland hyperplasia is said to be present always. The right ventricle is usually hypertrophied, and there may be evidence of hypertensive changes in the pulmonary artery. Thrombosis of branches of the pulmonary artery is common.

Mechanism and Significance of Differences between the Type Extremes of Clinical Prototypes. The "pink puffer" may be regarded as an otherwise normal subject with severe reduction of ventilatory capacity resulting from the development of a flow-limiting mechanism. The pulmonary pathology does not lead to gross disturbance of ventilation-perfusion relationships, and arterial blood gas composition is virtually normal, at least at rest. Ventilatory control mechanisms are intact. By contrast, the "blue bloater" has, in addition to airflow obstruction, gross disturbance of ventilation-perfusion relationships and impairment of CO_2 sensitivity of the respiratory center. The ventilation-perfusion abnormality leads to a chain of abnormalities, beginning with arterial hypoxemia and followed by polycythemia, pulmonary hypertension, right ventricular hypertrophy, and systemic venous congestion with edema. The mechanism of impaired CO_2 sensitivity of the respiratory center is unknown; it leads to chronic ventilatory failure with hypercapnia and impairs the ability to maintain ventilation in the face of increased airway resistance.

DIAGNOSIS OF CHRONIC AIRWAY OBSTRUCTION

Clinical Diagnosis. Patients presenting with dyspnea on exertion may be suffering from a wide variety of disorders. *Symptoms of bronchial irritability and morning tightness strongly suggest that airway obstruction is the cause of the dyspnea.* Although rhonchi are highly suggestive, they may be absent even with severe airway obstruction. *Prolonged expiration and forced expiratory time are the only reliable signs of airway obstruction.*

Etiologic Diagnosis. In the present incomplete state of knowledge, one of the most important decisions to be made is whether the patient's condition is likely to improve with specific antiallergic therapy, i.e., corticosteroids or disodium cromoglycate or both (see Asthma above). *Two symptoms suggestive of allergy are recurring chest tightness during the day and nocturnal dyspnea, usually between 2 and 4 A.M.* A personal and family history of allergy is suggestive, but eosinophilia of the sputum and sometimes of the blood is the most important single objective finding. Patients who show good clinical response to steroids and disodium cromoglycate usually have a poor response of the FEV_1 to inhalation of atropine methonitrate compared with isoprenaline (Altounyan's test). A similar poor response to atropine is seen in patients with asthma. Alternatively, a therapeutic trial of these drugs may be given, but it is sometimes difficult to separate specific from general effects of corticosteroids.

Assessment of Severity of Airway Obstruction. Sim-

ple clinical assessment of the severity of airflow obstruction and reduction in ventilatory capacity may be obtained from the vital capacity and FEV_1, or from peak flows. More detailed measurements are seldom needed for initial clinical assessment. The following are rough correlations between FEV_1 and physical activity. If the FEV_1 is greater than 1.5 liters, the subject can usually undertake moderate exercise. With an FEV_1 between 1.0 and 1.5 liters, the subject can usually undertake light activity but is somewhat short of breath on hurrying or climbing stairs. With an FEV_1 below 1.0 liter, he is usually breathless on slight exertion, although there are wide differences according to clinical type and personality. If the degree of disability grossly exceeds the severity of the airway obstruction, other causes of shortness of breath should be sought. These include heart disease, pulmonary hypertension, anemia, thyrotoxicosis, and metabolic acidosis. An important but often overlooked cause is a psychologic disturbance. This diagnosis is supported by symptoms suggesting attacks of hyperventilation, i.e., paresthesia, dizziness, and, if severe, carpopedal spasm. The psychiatric disturbance may be one of three types: first, an hysterical reaction in patients with an hysterical premorbid personality; second, an anxiety reaction in patients with strong obsessional traits; and, third, a depressive illness.

Detection of Early Changes.   Macklem has pointed out that because of the very low resistance of small bronchioles, considerable pathologic changes may be present without causing a significant increased airway resistance. Thus, doubling the resistance or halving the number of the peripheral airways will result in only a 10 per cent increase in over-all airway resistance, because this region normally contributes only 10 per cent of the total. This raises problems in the early detection of airway disease. Measurements reflecting airway resistance are relatively insensitive, and it is now considered that abnormalities in the distribution of inspired gas (single breath N_2 test) or the demonstration of frequency dependent compliance are more likely to reveal early peripheral bronchial disease.

TREATMENT OF AIRWAY OBSTRUCTION

Despite ignorance of basic causes of chronic airway obstruction, it is nevertheless possible to reduce the effects of these disturbances by attention to detail in management.

Removal of Irritants and Treatment of Infection. Removing atmospheric irritants and stopping cigarette smoking may cause a gradual reduction in the volume of mucus and the degree of hyperreactivity of the bronchi and a moderate decrease in airway obstruction. One of the most potent irritants is bronchial infection, and this should be eradicated or minimized by appropriate antimicrobial therapy.

Bronchodilatation. Oral and aerosol bronchodilator drugs as discussed under Asthma may be helpful. However, more prolonged bronchodilatation in subjects without an allergic cause for their bronchial narrowing can be achieved with an aerosol of atropine methonitrate (0.04 mg.). Its action is slower in onset, and for this reason commercial preparations combine isoproterenol or its variants and atropine.

Bronchial Toilet and Mucolytics. Attention to humidification of inspired air and active bronchial toilet with physiotherapy may induce considerable improvement in airway obstruction. Inhalation of mucolytic drugs such as acetylcysteine may occasionally be helpful, but in allergic subjects hypersensitivity reactions have been recorded. Bromhexine (8 mg. three times a day) by disrupting the mucopolysaccharide fibers of non-infected sputum aids expectoration and in controlled studies has been shown to improve airway obstruction.

Respiratory Stimulants. Oral analeptics, e.g., amiphenazole, 100 to 200 mg. thrice daily, and prethcamide, 400 mg. three or four times daily, have been advocated for the treatment of chronic ventilatory failure. They may result in transient slight reduction in P_{CO_2}, but there is no evidence that they afford clinical benefit. Acetazolamide, 250 to 500 mg., or dichlorphenamide, 50 to 100 mg. twice a day, has been reported to improve the breathlessness of some patients with airway obstruction. These carbonic anhydrase inhibitors may cause reduction in P_{CO_2} up to 8 to 10 mm. Hg, but this fall does not correlate with subjective improvement. Paresthesia, headache, and general malaise may occur as side effects which disappear rapidly on stopping the drug.

Circulatory Management. The use of diuretics, e.g., chlorothiazide, 0.5 to 1.0 gram, furosemide, 40 to 80 mg. orally from twice weekly to daily, has greatly improved management of edematous patients. Adequate diuresis may cause considerable improvement in pulmonary gas exchange and mechanisms. Daily administration requires supplements of potassium (600 to 1200 mg. four times a day). Digoxin (0.25 mg. twice daily) is often given, but its value in this type of systemic venous congestion is disputed. It should not be given during acute respiratory failure because of the danger of inducing ventricular arrhythmias. If the hematocrit is raised above 55 to 60 per cent, repeated venesection should be used to reduce the hematocrit to about 55 per cent.

Oxygen Therapy. This has been used in two ways: first, intermittently during exercise and in the recovery phase. Portable oxygen cylinders which provide small supplements of O_2 in the inspired air are available, but self-consciousness in wearing the equipment often deters patients from using them. Second, long-term oxygen therapy has been studied in patients with the Type B, "blue bloater" form of the disease and has been shown to reduce the severity of the circulatory abnormalities.

Surgery of Emphysema. Removal of large localized emphysematous bullae or regions may reduce airway obstruction by permitting increased inflation of the remaining lung tissue and therefore increased elastic recoil. Selection of suitable patients is difficult; the best results have been obtained following removal of a single large cyst or when emphysematous changes have been in lower rather than in upper lobes. Excision or plication of multiple emphysematous bullae has sometimes been beneficial.

PROGNOSIS IN CHRONIC AIRWAY OBSTRUCTION

The prognosis in chronic airway obstruction is related to the severity of the lung disease; it is worse when airway obstruction is severe, when the diffusing capacity is markedly reduced, and when cor pulmonale is, or has been, present. It is worse at altitude than at sea level, presumably because of the greater hypoxemia. The length of history and the age of onset of symptoms are not related to mortality.

In a group of chronic bronchitics with or without airway obstruction in London, 54 per cent died within ten years; 57 per cent of these died of respiratory causes, and 8 per cent died of bronchial carcinoma. The prognosis of 200 patients with airway obstruction has been studied in more detail in a group of patients in Chicago. The severity of ventilatory impairment, resting pulse rate, and mixed venous P_{CO_2} were the most predictive of poor survival. The conclusions were that if there is no resting tachycardia, chronic hypercapnia, or severe impairment of diffusing capacity, a five-year survival may be expected in 80 per cent of cases when the FEV_1 exceeds 1.2 liters; in 60 per cent when FEV_1 is close to 1 liter; and in 40 per cent when the FEV_1 is below 0.75 liter. If the factors listed initially are present, the percentage of survival figures is reduced by 25.

The development of weight loss is of bad prognostic significance. Intensive treatment with bronchodilator aerosols or with antimicrobial drugs is without influence on the rate of deterioration of airflow obstruction.

ACUTE RESPIRATORY FAILURE

The greatest risk to the life of a patient with chronic airway obstruction is the development of an acute increase in bronchial secretions and airway obstruction which occurs in response to an acute bronchial infection or on exposure to irritant atmospheres such as smog. In patients of the "blue bloater" type, a rise in P_{CO_2} will almost certainly occur; it is unusual in the "pink puffer" patient, in whom an elevation of P_{CO_2} implies very severe airway obstruction. If P_{CO_2} rises above 50 mm. Hg or Pa_{O_2} falls below 60 mm. Hg, respiratory failure is said to be present. It is very unusual for the P_{CO_2} to exceed 80 mm. Hg because of the concomitant development of hypoxemia.

Higher values generally imply the prior administration of oxygen.

Management of this life-threatening situation requires appreciation of three things. First, the acute situation has been caused largely by increased secretions and increased airway obstruction. Second, the immediate danger is hypoxemia. Third, hypercarbia and acidemia, if present, may cause clouding or even loss of consciousness and an inability by the patient to cooperate in his therapy.

The assessment of the patient therefore requires the following two immediate decisions: Can the patient raise the secretions by coughing? And does the patient need oxygen?

Ability to Raise Secretions by Coughing. Ability of the patient to raise the secretions by coughing can only be ascertained by instructing the patient to cough; the response to this is the most useful single physical sign in this situation. If he is unable to do so unaided, skilled physiotherapy may yet be successful, especially if effective humidification can be achieved. Administration of aminophylline, 250 mg. intravenously over three to five minutes, may enable an effective cough to be produced. If the patient is too drowsy to cooperate, he may be roused sufficiently by this treatment or by the administration of nikethamide, 500 to 1000 mg. intravenously, or some equivalent analeptic. There is no place in this situation for continuous intravenous analeptics unless combined with intensive chest physiotherapy.

The expectoration of even a few pieces of sputum may result in dramatic improvement. If the patient cannot raise secretions despite all efforts, there is no alternative but bronchoscopy and tracheal suction or, preferably, endotracheal intubation with regular tracheal suction and a period of assisted ventilation. Tracheostomy should be avoided unless prolonged assisted ventilation becomes necessary.

Oxygen Need. The presence of severe hypoxemia does not *necessarily* mean that tissue damage is occurring because increased perfusion may transport sufficient oxygen to the tissues to permit aerobic metabolism to continue. It has been shown that an arterial Po_2 even below 30 mm. Hg can be adequate for tissue oxygenation *providing that a good circulation is maintained;* but usually Pa_{O_2} values below this level are associated with evidence of tissue hypoxia in the form of lactic acidosis and raised serum transaminase levels. Because of the steep slope of the hemoglobin dissociation curve for oxygen at these levels, relatively small increases in inspired oxygen will move the patient away from the brink of tissue hypoxia. The danger of administration of high concentrations of oxygen is that by correcting hypoxemia, the main source of ventilatory stimulation will be removed, thus converting a conscious, cyanosed patient capable of cooperation into a pink unconscious patient in whom secretions accumulate and in whom intubation and assisted ventilation become mandatory. With care, the cautious administration of oxygen in inspired concentrations of 24 to 28 per cent, e.g., using a Venturi device, will increase arterial oxygen tension sufficiently without seriously reducing ventilatory drives in the majority of patients. With improvement in ventilatory capacity, progressive increases in oxygen concentration will be tolerated.

The absolute indications for oxygen may be taken as, first, evidence of poor peripheral circulation, i.e., poor volume pulse, low blood pressure, poor capillary filling; and second, an arterial Po_2 below 30 mm. Hg. In practice, when arterial Po_2 levels may not be available, it is advisable to administer 24 to 28 per cent O_2, e.g., using a Venturi device, to all patients and to measure Pco_2 serially. If the Pco_2 does not rise more than a few millimeters over the next one to two hours, it may be possible to increase the concentration of oxygen further. If adequate improvement in Pa_{O_2} cannot be achieved by these means without causing a progressive rise in Pa_{CO_2}, then assisted ventilation must be considered.

Other Therapeutic Measures. While these more urgent measures are being instituted the sputum should be obtained for culture. A broad-spectrum antimicrobial drug should be started, e.g., tetracycline, 500 mg. four times a day, or ampicillin, 500 mg. four times a day orally or parenterally, unless there are clinical indications for a different drug. A diuretic, e.g., furosemide, 40 to 80 mg. intravenously, should be given if there is any evidence of pulmonary congestion or peripheral edema. Digitalis should be given with caution in the acute severely hypoxemic state because of the danger of inducing a ventricular dysrhythmia.

Prophylaxis. In view of the seriousness of acute exacerbations, advice about minimizing their occurrence should be given. The patient and his relatives should be warned of the signs of acute exacerbation and the need for attention to bronchial toilet and prompt antimicrobial therapy. A patient with previous history of respiratory failure should be admitted to hospital without delay if no rapid improvement occurs. Influenza vaccination should be administered annually.

Bates, D. V., and Christie, R. V.: Respiratory Function in Disease. Philadelphia, W. B. Saunders Company, 1964.

Burns, B. H., and Howell, J. B. L.: Disproportionately severe breathlessness in chronic bronchitis. Quart. J. Med., 38:277, 1969.

Burrows, B., and Earle, R. H.: Prediction of survival in patients with chronic airway obstruction. Amer. Rev. Resp. Dis., 99:865, 1969.

Burrows, B., Fletcher, C. M., Heard, B. E., Jones, N. L., and Wootliff, J. S.: The emphysematous and bronchial types of chronic airways obstruction. Lancet, 1:830, 1966.

Cotes, J. E.: Lung Function: Assessment and Application in Medicine. 2nd ed. Oxford and Edinburgh, Blackwell Scientific Publications, 1968.

Filley, G. F., Beckwitt, H. J., Reeves, J. T., and Mitchell, R. S.: Chronic obstructive bronchopulmonary disease. II. Oxygen transport in two clinical types. Amer. J. Med., 44:26, 1968.

Gent, M., Knowlson, P. A., and Prime, F. J.: Effect of bromhexine on ventilatory capacity in patients with a variety of chest diseases. Lancet, 2:1094, 1969.

Hogg, J. C., Macklem, P. T., and Thurlbeck, W. M.: Site and nature of airway obstruction in chronic obstructive lung disease. New Eng. J. Med., 278:1355, 1968.

Knudson, R. J., and Gaensler, E. A.: Surgery for emphysema. Ann. Thorac. Surg., 1:332, 1965.

Lane, D. J., Howell, J. B. L., and Giblin, B.: Relation between airways obstruction and CO_2 tension in chronic obstructive airways disease. Brit. Med. J., 3:707, 1968.

Nash, E. S., Briscoe, W. A., and Cournand, A.: The relationship between clinical and physiological findings in chronic obstructive disease of the lungs. Med. Thorac., 22:305, 1965.

Oswald, N. C., Medvie, V. C., and Waller, R. E.: Chronic bronchitis: A ten year follow up. Thorax, 22:279, 1967.

Sykes, M. J., McNicol, M. W., and Campbell, E. J. M.: Respiratory Failure. Oxford and Edinburgh, Blackwell Scientific Publications, 1969.

Tarkoff, M. P., Kueppers, F., and Miller, W. F.: Pulmonary emphysema and alpha$_1$-antitrypsin deficiency. Amer. J. Med., 45:220, 1968.

Uses and Dangers of Oxygen Therapy. Report of a Sub-Committee of the Standing Medical Advisory Committee. Edinburgh, Her Majesty's Stationery Office, 1969.

Woolcock, A. J., and Read, J.: Lung volumes in exacerbations of asthma. Amer. J. Med., 41:259, 1966.

Abnormal Air Spaces

Richard V. Ebert

GIANT BULLOUS EMPHYSEMA
(Vanishing Lung)

Lungs examined at autopsy frequently contain small blebs or bullae. These are most commonly found in older men. Bullae are air-containing structures resembling cysts but with a wall which is trabeculated and not lined with epithelium. The lesion is derived from the terminal air spaces of the lung, and the trabeculae represent remnants of the blood vessels and fibrous tissue of the lung. Similar lesions occurring just beneath the visceral pleura are called blebs. Occasionally these lesions may be of great size and give rise to a characteristic appearance on the roentgenogram of the chest. These giant bullae may or may not be associated with generalized emphysema of the lung.

Large solitary bullae are observed occasionally. The lesion is usually not associated with symptoms. Pulmonary function studies may reveal no abnormality. If the bulla becomes huge, it may produce dyspnea and impair pulmonary function. The term "anepithelial air cyst" has been used to describe these lesions.

More commonly, multiple large bullae are found. These may be confined to one lobe or to one lung, or they may involve both lungs. They usually occur in the upper lobes. The lesions are commonly seen in relatively young persons, being found in approximately 1 in 1000 routine roentgenograms of the chest. The patient may be asymptomatic. If the lesions are large or if there is associated generalized emphysema, the patients may complain of exertional dyspnea. Physical examination may reveal increased resonance to percussion and diminished breath sounds over the involved area. Pneumothorax is a common complication. The bullae rarely become infected or filled with fluid. In the roentgenogram of the lungs the area involved is devoid of lung markings. The wall of the lesion is extremely thin and may not be visible. This has given rise to the term *vanishing lung*. The roentgenographic appearance can be easily confused with a pneumothorax. Pulmonary function studies are variable because the lesions may be either well ventilated or poorly ventilated and because there may be generalized emphysema that is not visible on the roentgenogram. There may or may not be adequate expansion of the remaining normal lung. If the lesions are not accompanied by diffuse pulmonary emphysema, the usual findings are a relatively normal vital capacity, a considerable increase in functional residual capacity, a normal or only slightly impaired maximal breathing capacity and rate of expiratory air flow, and normal blood gases. With very large bullous lesions there may be more severe impairment of pulmonary function. Finally, some patients present the typical clinical picture of chronic obstructive lung disease, and in addition demonstrate giant bullous lesions on the roentgenogram of the lungs.

The therapy of giant bullae is surgical excision, but there seems to be little reason to remove these lesions if the patient is asymptomatic. Occasionally, repeated pneumothorax may be an indication for surgery. A difficult problem is presented by those patients who are symptomatic. The dyspnea may be related to diffuse pulmonary emphysema rather than to the bullae. In this case removal of the bullae will be of little or no benefit. In certain patients the bullae may be important in the production of symptoms. This occurs if the bullae interfere with the function of the remaining normal lung. If the bullae reach sufficient size to occupy much of the thorax, the intrathoracic pressure may not be sufficiently negative to expand the remaining lung. The normal portion of the lung may be partially atelectatic and poorly ventilated. Removal of the bullae may lead to significant improvement. Careful evaluation of the roentgenogram of the chest and of pulmonary function studies is necessary for a proper decision as to the need for surgery.

Boushy, S. F., Kohen, R., Billig, D. M., and Heiman, M. J.:
Bullous emphysema. Clinical, roentgenologic and physiologic study of 49 patients. Dis. Chest, 54:327, 1968.

Davies, G. M., Simon, G., and Reid, L.: Pre- and postoperative assessment of emphysematous bullae. Brit. J. Dis. Chest, 60:120, 1966.

LUNG CYSTS

The classification of lung cysts is somewhat confusing, since any air-containing structure in the lung can enlarge and form a cyst or cavity. There is tension on the wall of all air-containing structures in the lung because the pressure within fluctuates about atmospheric pressure, whereas the intrathoracic pressure is negative. If there is obstruction to the egress of air from a cyst or cavity, the pressure within may be considerably in excess of atmospheric pressure. The tension on the wall of a sphere such as a lung cyst is proportional to both the pressure difference across the wall and to the radius of curvature. For this reason a thin-walled cyst or cavity in the lung tends to continue to enlarge.

Thin-walled cavities may form in the lung as a result of destruction of lung substance and formation of a communication with a bronchus. Such cavities may be seen in pulmonary tuberculosis, the pulmonary mycoses, and lung abscess. These are called cavities and not cysts, but their appearance on the roentgenogram may be similar to that of lung cysts. Cystlike lesions can also form in bronchiectasis.

Belcher, J. R., and Siddons, A. H. M.: Air-containing cysts of the lung. Thorax, 9:38, 1954.

BRONCHOGENIC CYSTS

These cysts arise from the bronchi, as indicated by the name. It is thought that in most instances they are caused by a congenital defect. The cyst is lined with epithelial cells. The wall of the cyst may contain glands, smooth muscle, and cartilage.

The patient with a bronchogenic cyst may be asymptomatic. Symptoms are usually the result of secondary infection and consist of a productive cough, hemoptysis, and fever. The roentgenographic appearance is variable. The cyst may contain only air or may be filled with fluid. In the latter case the cyst may be confused with a solid tumor of the lung. The cyst may have an air-fluid level, in which case it is often mistaken for a lung abscess. The treatment of symptomatic lung cysts is surgical removal.

Congenital cysts in the lower lobe of the lung may be associated with an anomalous artery arising from the aorta near the diaphragm. This complex developmental abnormality is called *intralobar bronchopulmonary sequestration*. A knowledge of this abnormality is of some importance because the artery may be inadvertently cut during surgery, with serious hemorrhage.

HONEYCOMB LUNG

Honeycomb lung describes a pathologic state in which the lung contains many small cystic structures that are several millimeters in diameter. These cysts are derived from the bronchioles and are lined by epithelium. Fibrous tissue and smooth muscle are found about the cysts. Honeycomb lung has been described in association with eosinophilic granuloma, rheumatoid lung disease, and idiopathic interstitial pulmonary fibrosis. It occurs in association with advanced fibrosis and represents the end stage of the disease. A similar pathologic lesion may be found in association with tuberous sclerosis.

The major symptom is dyspnea. Spontaneous pneumothorax is a common complication. The roentgenogram of the lungs reveals a fine or coarse reticular appearance. Small rounded translucencies may be seen.

Heppleston, A. G.: The pathology of honeycomb lung. Thorax, 11:77, 1956.

ACQUIRED CYSTS

As mentioned above, any air-containing structure in the lung can enlarge and form a cyst or cavity. Lung abscess as a cause of such cavities is discussed immediately below. The other necrotizing lung diseases are considered in the articles on Tuberculosis, Fungal Infections, and Bacterial Pneumonia in the section on Microbial Diseases.

LUNG ABSCESS

Definition. Lung abscess is a suppurative infection of the lung resulting in destruction of lung parenchyma with the formation of a cavity containing fluid and air.

Etiology. *Aspiration of infectious material* into the lung is the most common cause of lung abscess (primary lung abscess). A history of an episode of stupor or unconsciousness is often obtained. This is most commonly the result of excessive drinking. Careful inquiry will reveal that a high proportion of persons with lung abscess are chronic alcoholics. Other causes of unconsciousness predisposing to aspiration lung abscess are convulsive seizures, anesthesia, diabetic coma, ingestion of large amounts of sedatives, and various neurologic lesions. The infected material aspirated is usually from the mouth. Most people with lung abscess will be found to have periodontal disease with accumulation of infected materials about the teeth and gums. Lung abscess is rare in an edentulous person. Aspiration of infected materials during surgery on the oral cavity or tonsils was common at one time, but is rare now because of improvements in anesthetic techniques. Aspiration is common in cancer involving the upper respiratory passages or esophagus.

As might be anticipated, the pus from a primary lung abscess contains a mixture of bacteria. Cultures performed on material aspirated from the abscess cavity prior to the use of antimicrobial drugs demonstrated gamma streptococci, diphtheroids, and a variety of anaerobic organisms.

Pneumonia caused by *Staphylococcus aureus* or *Klebsiella* may be complicated by abscess formation. Primary pneumococcal pneumonia is rarely associated with abscess formation. Treatment of patients with therapeutic agents which interfere with the normal body defenses, such as high doses of corticosteroids or the chemotherapy for cancer, predisposes to necrotizing pneumonia with abscess formation. In many hospitals lung abscesses occur almost exclusively in patients with terminal cancer.

Bronchial obstruction may lead to a lung abscess. The obstructing lesion is most commonly a bronchogenic carcinoma but may be a foreign body or an enlarged lymph node causing compression of a bronchus.

Metastatic lung abscess may result from septic emboli secondary to right-sided bacterial endocarditis or pelvic thrombophlebitis. Lung abscess may occur in association with septicemia.

Rare causes of lung abscess include amebic abscess of the lung, melioidosis, glanders, actinomycosis, and nocardiosis.

Incidence and Prevalence. The exact incidence of lung abscess has not been determined. Recent reports indicate that five to ten instances of primary lung abscess are seen each year in a large general hospital. The disease was more common prior to the introduction of antimicrobial drugs. Lung abscess occurs as a terminal event in a variety of illnesses.

Pathogenesis. The sequence of events to be described is thought to be the mechanism of formation of lung abscess in those cases in which aspiration of infected material is the initiating agent. Although this mechanism of abscess function cannot be proved in every case, there is a large body of circumstantial evidence which supports this mode of pathogenesis.

When infected material is aspirated into the tracheobronchial tree it lodges in a small bronchus in the dependent portion of the lung. As aspiration usually occurs in the supine position, the posterior segment of the upper lobe and the superior segment of the lower lobe are most commonly involved. Pneumonia develops in the surrounding tissue. The critical event is the formation of a cavity. This occurs as a result of necrosis and liquefaction of the pneumonic lung. The liquid is discharged into the bronchus draining the area, thus creating a cavity. For the lung parenchyma to be disrupted the collagen and elastic framework of the lung must be destroyed. The frequent finding of fragments of elastic tissue in the sputum is evidence of this destruction. The exact means by which liquefaction necrosis occurs is not known. It has been suggested that thrombosis of small vessels leads to ischemia of the pneumonic area. The liquefaction and destruction of the connective tissue framework of the lung must result from liberation of proteolytic enzymes.

Clinical Manifestations. Patients with primary lung abscess often give a characteristic history. The illness begins with fever, sweats, malaise, loss of appetite, and loss of weight. After a few days or weeks a productive cough develops. The amount of sputum increases until several hundred milliliters are produced daily. The patient and his associates may note a foul odor to the sputum. Some patients give a history of suddenly coughing up large amounts of foul sputum. Hemoptysis occurs in about 40 per cent of the cases. Pleuritic chest pain may occur, but is not common. In some cases the characteristic abundant foul sputum may be absent. This is most commonly seen in patients receiving antimicrobial drugs. Careful questioning of both the patient and his relatives may elicit a history of a period of unconsciousness or of excessive use of alcohol. When lung abscess complicates pneumonia caused by Staphylococcus or Klebsiella, the symptoms are those of a severe pneumonia. Abscess formation is detected on the chest roentgenogram.

The patient with lung abscess usually appears acutely ill and is febrile. Periodontal disease is often present, and infected material may be seen about the teeth and gums. Examination of the lung most commonly shows fine or medium moist rales over the involved area. Dullness and change in breath sounds may or may not be detected. Clubbing of the fingers is seen in about one fourth of the patients.

In primary lung abscess the sputum is usually copious, forms several layers on standing, and has a putrid odor. Occasionally the sputum is scanty or absent. Culture of the sputum will reveal the specific organism if the abscess is caused by Staphylococcus or Klebsiella. In lung abscess resulting from aspiration, a variety of mouth organisms are cultured. These include alpha hemolytic streptococci and neisseria. In patients receiving penicillin a variety of gram-negative organisms may be cultured. The important anaerobic organisms described earlier are not cultured by the routine methods used in most clinical laboratories.

The diagnosis of lung abscess is usually made from the roentgenogram of the lung. A cavity containing fluid surrounded by alveolar infiltrate is found. A fluid level in the cavity can usually be demonstrated and can be confirmed by roentgenograms taken in different body positions. Approximately one third of the abscesses related to aspiration are found in the posterior segment of the right upper lobe. Other common locations are the superior segments of the right and left lower lobes and the apical posterior segment of the left upper lobe. With treatment the surrounding pneumonic infiltrate may rapidly disappear and fluid may no longer be seen if good drainage is obtained. Ultimately a thin-walled cavity is left. In most cases this will eventually disappear.

Complications. Empyema with or without bronchopleural fistula may complicate lung abscess. This usually occurs in the neglected cases, and rarely is seen once antimicrobial therapy has been initiated. If therapy of lung abscess is begun weeks or months after the onset of the disease, complete healing may not occur, and a residual thick-wall cavity remains. Scarring may be associated with local bronchiectasis. Recurrent infection may occur and lead to prolonged disability. Other complications are rare. Brain abscess and amyloidosis are almost never seen with present methods of therapy.

Diagnosis. The tentative diagnosis is made from the appearance of the roentgenogram of the lungs, and particularly from the presence of a cavity with an air-fluid level. Differentiation from other diseases simulating lung abscess is made by analysis of the history, examination of the sputum, and careful study of serial roentgenograms of the chest after initiation of therapy.

The most common mistake in diagnosis is the confusion of bronchogenic carcinoma and primary lung abscess. Bronchogenic carcinoma can simulate lung abscess in two ways. A true lung abscess can develop peripheral to the obstructed bronchus, or a large tumor can undergo necrosis and cavitate. The latter event usually occurs with a squamous cell bronchogenic carcinoma but may occur with metastatic carcinoma. The diagnosis of an obstructing carcinoma can usually be made by bronchoscopy. Diagnosis of a peripheral cavitating carcinoma is difficult, and bronchoscopy is usually of no aid. The diagnosis may be suspected if the predisposing factors to an aspiration abscess are absent, if the sputum is not foul, if the location of the abscess is in the anterior portion of the lung, if the wall of the abscess is irregular, and if there is failure to respond to therapy. Examination of the sputum for neoplastic cells may establish the diagnosis in some cases.

The differentiation of lung abscess from pulmonary tuberculosis is less difficult. Tuberculosis has a more insidious onset and less systemic symptoms. The sputum is not foul. The cavity usually does not contain a fluid level. Examination of the sputum for tubercle bacilli by microscopy and culture should always be done and will establish the diagnosis. Cavitating fungal infection of the lungs, such as histoplasmosis or coccidioidomycosis, can usually be distinguished from lung abscess without difficulty.

An infected lung cyst may simulate a primary lung abscess. Differentiation may be made by a careful history and by the lack of severe systemic symptoms or foul sputum. The wall of the cavity as seen by x-ray is thin and not surrounded by an area of pneumonitis. Previous films may show an air-containing cyst. Occasionally a bullous lesion containing fluid may be seen in an area of resolving pneumonia and may be mistaken for a lung abscess.

Other lesions occasionally simulate lung abscess. At times a bland infarct of the lung will cavitate. Cystic bronchiectasis may be confused with lung abscess. There is a history of long-standing chronic cough, and the cavities are usually multiple and basal in location. Echinococcus cyst of the lung is extremely rare in the United States. Rheumatoid nodules and the lesions of Wegener's granulomatosis may cavitate, but are readily differentiated from lung abscess.

Treatment. The cornerstone of therapy in lung abscess is the administration of the appropriate antimicrobial drug in adequate dosage for a sufficiently long period. In abscesses complicating pneumonia caused by Staphylococcus or Klebsiella, the drug should be chosen on the basis of the susceptibility of the organism isolated from the sputum. In aspiration lung abscess, however, a variety of organisms are isolated. Moreover, the important anaerobic bacteria may not be cultured. Nevertheless, on an empirical basis penicillin in large doses has been found to be highly effective and is the antimicrobial drug of choice.

As a clearly definable syndrome, lung abscess is usually quite readily distinguishable from the cavitation so prominent in the pneumonias produced by klebsiellae, staphylococci, or tubercle bacilli (for treatment of these three diseases see Microbial Diseases). Selection of the proper drug therapy for lung abscess, however, is quite a different type of medical judgment than is involved in selecting drugs for microbial diseases produced by a single clearly identifiable agent. For the lung abscess the choice must be based on knowledge of the pathogenesis of the condition rather than on the identity of the microbial species isolated from the sputum. The latter, more often than not, have no etiologic significance or, at the very least, their relationship to the disease is by no means assured. Whether this syndrome of lung abscess is wholly microbial in origin and, if so, whether only a single microbial species is involved has not been established. Several lines of evidence, including the rarity of lung abscess in the edentulous person and the similarity of the flora in peridental and pulmonary abscesses, indicate that anaerobic microbes are significantly involved. Recent studies, especially those by Moon of Virginia, reveal that man has a large and diverse anaerobic flora that has previously gone unrecognized. With this new knowledge it may be possible to characterize microbial roles in lung abscess. In the meantime, as a practical matter, lung abscess can be regarded as a cavitating pneumonia caused by anaerobic microbes. Because penicillin is known to maintain its effectiveness in anaerobic environments and is demonstrably of high effectiveness in lung abscess, it represents the major drug for the treatment of this condition. Five to ten million units of crystalline penicillin daily by continuous intravenous drip may be used initially. After improvement has occurred, 600,000 units intravenously every four to six hours can be substituted. Therapy should be continued until the lesion heals or until continued improvement fails to occur. This usually requires four to six weeks. An alteration in the bacterial flora of the sputum with penicillin therapy is to be expected, but change to another antimicrobial drug should not be made unless there is clear evidence that penicillin is ineffective. Postural drainage facilitates emptying of the cavity and may be useful early in the course of therapy.

Surgery is no longer performed early in the disease. The usual indication for surgical intervention is a residual thick-walled cavity persisting after antimicrobial therapy. Thin-walled cavities or cystic lesions need not be removed and will often heal spontaneously. Residual lesions requiring surgery usually occur in patients in whom antimicrobial therapy has been delayed or was inadequate.

Abernathy, R. S.: Antibiotic therapy of lung abscess: Effectiveness of penicillin. Dis. Chest, 53:592, 1968.

Bernhard, W. F., Malcolm, J. A., and Wylie, R. H.: The carcinomatous abscess. A clinical paradox. New Eng. J. Med., 266:914, 1962.

Flavell, G.: Respiratory tract disease. Lung abscess. Brit. Med. J., 1:1032, 1966.

Perlman, L. V., Lerner, E., and D'Esopo, N.: Clinical classification and analysis of 97 cases of lung abscess. Am. Rev. Resp. Dis., 99:390, 1969.

Petty, T. L., and Mitchell, R. S.: Suppurative lung diseases. Med. Clin. N. Amer., 51:529, 1967.

UNILATERAL HYPERLUCENT LUNG

Unilateral hyperlucent lung is discovered by examination of the roentgenogram of the chest. One lung is translucent as compared with the other. The vascular markings of the hyperlucent lung are diminished, and the pulmonary artery may be inconspicuous. Fluoroscopy demonstrates a shift of the mediastinum away from the involved lung on expiration. Dilatation and irregularity of the small bronchi are visible on bronchograms. Pathologic examination of the diseased lung demonstrates an extensive bronchitis and bronchiolitis. The alveoli may be enlarged, but typical destructive emphysema is not usually found. The pulmonary artery is present. One theory of pathogenesis is that a severe pulmonary infection occurred in childhood, with consequent altered development of the lung.

The patient usually gives a history of a productive cough. Dyspnea and hemoptysis may be present. Breath sounds are often diminished over the affected lung, and rales may be heard. Abnormalities of pulmonary function are best demonstrated by bronchospirometry. The involved lung has a reduced vital capacity with evidence of air trapping; the ventilation and oxygen uptake are decreased.

Treatment consists of management of infection. Surgery is not usually performed.

Hamilton, C. R., Jr., Ballinger, W. F., II, and Cader, G.: The unilateral hyperlucent lung syndrome. Bull. Hopkins Hosp., 123:222, 1968.

Diffuse Lung Disease

Richard V. Ebert

INTERSTITIAL LUNG DISEASE

The normal alveolar wall is made up of capillaries, connective tissue, and thin alveolar epithelium. A network of delicate collagen, reticulin, and elastic fibers gives strength and support to the tissue. Coarser and more abundant connective fibers surround the alveolar ducts, bronchioles, and small bronchi. Except for the lobular septa there is surprisingly little fibrous tissue in the peripheral portions of the lung. A group of diseases is associated with cellular infiltration and increase in fibrous tissue in the walls of the alveoli. The etiology of many of these diseases is unknown. All are associated with similar roentgenographic findings in the lungs and have similar symptoms and physiologic findings.

ROENTGENOGRAPHIC, CLINICAL, AND PHYSIOLOGIC FEATURES

Roentgenographic Findings. The changes in the lungs are diffuse and consist of fine mottling and reticulation. Early in the disease the change may be subtle and can be readily overlooked. Later the shadows may be dense. Annular shadows may appear, giving a honeycomb appearance. In contrast to alveolar disease the vascular shadows persist and may be accentuated.

Clinical Manifestations. The major symptom is exertional dyspnea. This begins insidiously and in the early stages may be disregarded by the patient. The symptoms are usually progressive, and ultimately ordinary activities become limited by shortness of breath. In the advanced form of the disease dyspnea may be present at rest. Wheezing is not present, but a dry cough is common. Purulent sputum is not seen unless there is secondary bronchitis. Examination of the lungs may reveal no abnormal findings, or crackling fine rales may be observed over the lower portions of the lung. Clubbed fingers are common in diffuse interstitial pulmonary fibrosis. Cyanosis and evidence of right heart failure occur in the terminal phase of the illness.

Physiologic Features. The pulmonary function is usually altered. The changes in function differ from those in obstructive lung disease, there being no evidence of impairment of expiratory air flow. The breathing is rapid and shallow. The total pulmonary ventilation is increased both at rest and on exercise. The vital capacity and total lung capacity may be normal but are usually reduced to a variable degree. The maximal breathing capacity is normal or only slightly reduced, and the ratio of the volume of air forcibly expelled in one second to the vital capacity is normal. The diffusing capacity for carbon monoxide is reduced, and the reduction parallels the severity of the disease. In the milder forms of the disease the oxygen saturation of the hemoglobin of the arterial blood may be normal at rest and on exercise. In more severe disease the oxygen saturation is markedly decreased on exercise and may be abnormal at rest. The carbon dioxide tension of the arterial blood is normal or decreased. The basis for these changes in pulmonary function is complex. Capillaries are obliterated and alveoli destroyed by fibrosis. Other alveoli have thickened walls, and others are normal. Contrary to common opinion the alveolar capillary membrane is usually not thickened. These changes in the structure of the lung result in alterations in the mechanical properties of the lung and in gas exchange. The compliance of the lungs is reduced, resulting in an increased work of breathing. The irregular distribution of pathologic changes in the lung produces regional differences in ventilation-perfusion and ventilation-diffusion ratios, resulting in inadequate oxygenation of blood leaving certain regions of the lung (venous admixture).

CAUSES OF INTERSTITIAL LUNG DISEASE

Diffuse Interstitial Fibrosis. In 1944 Hamman and Rich described a group of patients with intense dyspnea, cyanosis, and right heart failure. The disease was rapid in its course, only a few months elapsing between the onset of symptoms and death. The lungs at autopsy showed thickening of the alveolar walls with edema and fibrin deposition, together with extensive interstitial proliferation of fibrous tissue. The term Hamman-Rich syndrome was used to describe this clinical and pathologic entity. Subsequently it was found that there was a larger group of patients with diffuse thickening and fibrosis of the alveolar walls who exhibited a more prolonged clinical course. The term idiopathic diffuse interstitial fibrosis or fibrosing alveolitis has been used to describe these patients. No specific cause has been found.

Approximately 1 to 2 per cent of patients with *rheumatoid* arthritis will have diffuse interstitial fibrosis. Most of these have a high titer of rheumatoid factor in the blood. Approximately 20 per cent of patients with diffuse interstitial fibrosis in whom there are no joint changes have an elevated titer of rheumatoid factor in their blood. Diffuse interstitial fibrosis associated with rheumatoid arthritis or with rheumatoid factor in the blood does not differ from the idiopathic type of fibrosis. A peculiar type of fibrosis involving the upper portion of the lung and associated with cyst formation has been described in ankylosing spondylitis. This differs from diffuse pulmonary fibrosis complicating rheumatoid arthritis, and is not usually associated with a positive test for rheumatoid factor.

Diffuse interstitial fibrosis is also found to occur in association with *scleroderma.* The fibrosis in scleroderma is not accompanied by a cellular reaction. The changes are usually more marked at the bases of the lungs.

Eosinophilic Granuloma. Eosinophilic granuloma of the lung may produce clinical and roentgenologic findings which are indistinguishable from those in diffuse interstitial fibrosis. Bone lesions may or may not be demonstrable. (For further description see section on Granulomatous Diseases of Unproved Etiology.)

Idiopathic Pulmonary Hemosiderosis. Idiopathic pulmonary hemosiderosis is described elsewhere. In severe cases interstitial fibrosis of the lungs develops, and the roentgenogram of the lungs may then resemble other types of diffuse fibrosis.

Chemical and Physical Irritants. Chemical and physical irritants may lead to interstitial fibrosis (see next section).

Sarcoidosis. Sarcoidosis involving the lung may lead to a diffuse interstitial involvement of the pulmonary parenchyma. Initially the lesions are granulomas, but later fibrosis may be present. The roentgenologic appearance of the lung may simulate diffuse interstitial fibrosis. The hilar lymph nodes are usually but not always enlarged. (See section on Granulomatous Diseases of Unproved Etiology.)

Tuberculosis and Fungal Disease of the Lungs. Tuberculosis and fungal diseases of the lungs may lead to a diffuse interstitial lesion with granuloma formation. Miliary tuberculosis results from hematogenous spread of the tubercle bacilli. Early in the illness the lesions may not be visible in the roentgenograms of the lungs. Later diffuse, fine miliary density is seen. Healing occurs with chemotherapy, and the patient is usually left with no functional disability. Histoplasmosis may also give a diffuse granulomatous lesion of the lung. Healing is often associated with multiple small areas of calcification of the lung.

DIAGNOSIS

The appearance of the roentgenogram of the lungs usually establishes the pulmonary lesion as interstitial in character. The differentiation of the various interstitial lesions may be difficult. Inquiry should always be made regarding exposure to various dusts. This should include a review of the various jobs held during a lifetime of work. Special emphasis should be placed on possible exposure to silica or asbestos. Physical examination may give evidence of rheumatoid arthritis or scleroderma. Enlarged lymph nodes may be discovered and on biopsy show the lesions of sarcoid. Bone x-rays may demonstrate the lesions of eosinophilic granuloma or sarcoid. Serologic studies, including tests for rheumatoid factor and complement fixation tests for histoplasmosis and blastomycosis, should be done.

In spite of careful study a group of patients remain in whom diagnosis is obscure. Most of these will fall into the category of diffuse interstitial fibrosis of unknown etiology. A much smaller group will have eosinophilic granuloma or one of the other granulomatous diseases. A firm diagnosis in these doubtful areas can be established only by lung biopsy. This need not be done in every case but should be strongly considered if there is any question of the clinical diagnosis being correct. Biopsy can be done by means of a needle or by an open surgical technique.

TREATMENT

Treatment will depend on the cause of the interstitial lesion. Idiopathic diffuse interstitial fibrosis is often treated with adrenal steroids. Results are difficult to evaluate, as no controlled clinical trials have been carried out.

The course of idiopathic pulmonary fibrosis is variable. The disease is fatal in a few months in some patients, and may continue with only slow progress for many years in others. Development of hypoxemia at rest usually means that the end of life is approaching. Cor pulmonale with right heart failure often follows and leads to death. A few patients die with alveolar cell carcinoma.

Livingstone, J. L., Lewis, J. G., Reid, L., and Jefferson, K. E.: Diffuse interstitial pulmonary fibrosis. A clinical, radiological, and pathological study based on 45 patients. Quart. J. Med., 33:71, 1964.

Marks, A.: Diffuse interstitial pulmonary fibrosis. Med. Clin. N. Amer., 51:439, 1967.

Scadding, J. G.: Chronic diffuse interstitial fibrosis of the lungs. Brit. Med. J., 1:443, 1960.

Sharp, J. T., Sweancy, S. K., and Van Lith, P.: Physiologic observations in diffuse pulmonary fibrosis and granulomatosis. Amer. Rev. Resp. Dis., 94:316, 1966.

Siltzbach, L. E.: Diffuse pulmonary granulomatosis and fibrosis: Diagnosis and treatment. Advances Cardiopulm. Dis., 4:306, 1969.

Walker, W. C., and Wright, V.: Pulmonary lesions and rheumatoid arthritis. Medicine, 47:501, 1968.

DIFFUSE ALVEOLAR DISEASES OF THE LUNG

ROENTGENOGRAPHIC, CLINICAL, AND PHYSIOLOGIC FEATURES

A variety of diseases may lead to replacement of air in the alveoli and alveolar ducts by fluid. The alveoli may be filled by edema fluid (pulmonary edema), by inflammatory exudate (pneumonia), by blood (pulmonary infarct, bleeding from bronchi and aspiration, Goodpasture's syndrome), by exudate containing a high lipid content (alveolar proteinosis, lipoid pneumonia), or by cancer tissue (alveolar cell carcinoma). The roentgenographic appearance of the lungs is similar in all of these and can usually be differentiated from the roentgenographic changes produced by interstitial lung disease. The shadows on x-ray examination form a homogeneous density with fluffy ill-defined edges. The infiltrates tend to obliterate the vascular markings and, at times, an air bronchogram may be seen. In chronic lesions a pattern related to filling of acini is seen at the edge of the lesion. This is a rosette-like lesion measuring several millimeters in diameter.

The clinical manifestations of alveolar disease will depend on the nature of the underlying lesion, the duration of the disease, and the extent of involvement. Cough and dyspnea are the two major symptoms. Fever may or may not be present. If the cough is productive, examination of the sputum grossly and with the microscope may cast light on the nature of the alveolar lesion. The sputum in pulmonary edema is thin, and white or pink in color. The sputum in pneumonia is tenacious and purulent, and may contain blood. The sputum in pulmonary hemorrhage consists of pure blood. The degree of dyspnea is related to the acuteness of the lesion and the amount of lung involved. Diffuse pulmonary edema or pneumonia will be associated with rapid, shallow, labored breathing at rest. A chronic alveolar lesion such as alveolar proteinosis may result only in exertional dyspnea.

The physiologic changes will also be dependent on the extent of the lesions and whether they are acute or chronic. The vital capacity will be reduced. The change in blood gases will depend on whether blood flows through the capillaries of the involved alveoli or not. Blood often continues to flow through areas of lung involved by acute lesions, with resultant shunting of unoxygenated blood into the pulmonary venous system. In more chronic lesions the blood flow from the pulmonary artery into the involved area is diminished or absent. The decrease in oxygen saturation of the arterial blood will be dependent on the magnitude of the shunt. If the shunt is large, hypoxia will persist while the patient is breathing high concentrations of oxygen. With massive filling of alveoli with fluid, death occurs from hypoxia in spite of oxygen administration. Hypoxia may also result from alteration in the ventilation-perfusion ratio in alveoli adjacent to the lesion. These alveoli may be poorly ventilated and well perfused, resulting in inadequate oxygenation of blood in the pulmonary capillaries. Administration of oxygen will correct this type of hypoxia. In alveolar disease the carbon dioxide tension of the arterial blood remains low or normal until massive involvement of the lung occurs.

Felsen, B.: The roentgen diagnosis of disseminated alveolar diseases. Seminars Radiol., 2:3, 1967.

Goodman, N.: Differential diagnosis of pulmonary alveolar infiltrates. Amer. Rev. Resp. Dis., 95:681, 1967.

CAUSES OF DIFFUSE ALVEOLAR DISEASE

PULMONARY EDEMA

Mechanism of Formation of Edema of the Lungs. The formation of edema in the lungs bears a certain similarity to the formation of edema in the subcutaneous tissues. In both instances the forces involved are the same, namely, the hydrostatic pressure in the capillaries, the colloid osmotic pressure of the plasma and interstitial fluid, and the interstitial fluid pressure. There are, however, major differences in the anatomy of the tissues and the hemodynamics in the two locations which lead to differences in the mechanism of formation of edema.

The anatomy of the lung is designed to permit efficient exchange of gas between the alveoli and the pulmonary capillaries. The alveolar septa are made up largely of capillaries. Between the capillaries is a very small amount of connective tissue, including ground substance, collagen, and elastin fibers. The plasma in the capillaries is separated from the air in the alveolus by a thin membrane consisting of capillary endothelium, basement membrane, and alveolar epithelial cells. Thus there is little interstitial space in the alveolar septa, and none separating the capillary from the alveolar epithelium. There is more abundant connective tissue about the bronchi and blood vessels and in the interlobular septa. The pulmonary capillary pressure is below 10 mm. Hg in normal human beings. As a result, the difference between pulmonary capillary pressure and colloid osmotic pressure of the plasma is large and creates a force tending to move fluid into the capillary. Another important force is created by the surface tension at the fluid-air interface in the alveoli. This force is related to the radius of curvature of the alveoli and the surface tension. The latter is influenced by a lipid on the surface of the alveolar wall (surfactant). The effect of this force is to make the interstitial fluid pressure negative.

Recent experimental work has elucidated the mechanism of formation of pulmonary edema. As a result of alteration in the hydrostatic forces or increase in capillary permeability to protein, fluid moves from the capillary into the interstitial space in the alveolar septum. As the interstitial fluid increases, it moves into the connective tissue about the blood vessels and bronchi and into the interlobular septa. Lymphatic flow is increased and removes some of this fluid. If the interstitial fluid continues to accumulate, fluid dissects between the capillary endothelial cells and the adjacent basement membrane, resulting in damage to the capillary wall. Finally, fluid moves through the alveolar epithelium into the alveolus. This fluid contains plasma protein and often fibrinogen and red cells.

Roentgenogram of the Lungs. The roentgenogram of the lungs mirrors the pathologic changes. During the phase of interstitial edema linear shadows may be seen (Kerley's A and B lines) which represent edema of the septa of the lungs. There may be thickening and loss of definition of the shadows of the bronchi and vessels. A perihilar haze may be seen. In some circumstances the edema may remain interstitial and not progress to intra-alveolar edema. Intra-alveolar edema results in confluent shadows of uniform density. These may be diffuse, confined to the lower portion of the lung, or seen at the hila of the lungs (butterfly pattern). Occasionally the shadows are unilateral.

Symptoms and Signs. During the period of development of interstitial edema there is intense suffocating dyspnea, and the breathing is rapid and shallow. A severe attack of paroxysmal nocturnal dyspnea resulting from left ventricular failure exemplifies the symptoms of interstitial edema. During the attack the patient is in the sitting position and breathing rapidly and in a labored manner. His face gives evidence of apprehension and is sweating. He may have difficulty in talking because of the urge to continue breathing. In spite of the intense dyspnea, examination of the lungs may fail to demonstrate rales, and the roentgenogram may not show intra-alveolar edema. If interstitial edema has been present for some time as in mitral stenosis, the patient may be free of dyspnea at rest, although exertional dyspnea is present.

With the development of intra-alveolar edema the patient continues to be severely dyspneic at rest and may cough up white or pink frothy sputum. Examination of the lungs reveals numerous moist rales. Cyanosis may be present if the edema is severe. If formation of edema fluid continues, the patient drowns in the edema fluid.

Alterations in Pulmonary Function. The rapid shallow breathing characteristic of developing pulmonary edema is believed to be the result of neurogenic stimuli arising from the parenchyma of the lungs. As a result of the abnormal stimulus to ventilation, the carbon dioxide tension of the arterial blood is decreased. With interstitial edema the oxygen saturation of the arterial blood may show little change, but with the development of alveolar edema hypoxia occurs. The oxygen tension of the arterial blood may fall to extremely low levels in severe diffuse intra-alveolar edema in spite of the administration of high concentrations of oxygen. Death results from hypoxia.

Edema of the lung leads to changes in the mechanics of ventilation. The vital capacity is decreased, and the course of pulmonary edema can be followed by repeated use of this simple bedside measurement. The total lung capacity is also reduced. This reduction is associated with a change in the elastic properties of the lung. A greater change in intrapleural pressure is required to produce a given volume change in the lung (decrease in compliance of the lung). This in turn leads to an increase in the work of breathing. With early edema there is usually no change in the resistance to air flow in the lung. Later, obstruction to flow of air may result from fluid in the bronchi. Occasionally this obstruction is severe and associated with wheezing, giving rise to the term cardiac asthma.

Causes of Pulmonary Edema. *Increase in Pulmonary Capillary Pressure.* This increase is the most common cause of pulmonary edema. The usual mechanism is failure of the left ventricle with rise in left ventricular end diastolic pressure. Hypertension, aortic valve disease, and acute myocardial infarction are common causes of acute failure of the left ventricle. Mitral stenosis leads to elevation in pulmonary capillary pressure by obstructing blood flow to the left ventricle. As a consequence the edema of the lungs is often chronic and interstitial in character. Mitral stenosis may also be associated with acute intra-alveolar edema usually precipitated by severe exertion or a sudden increase in heart rate.

The pulmonary capillary pressure may be elevated by an increase in blood volume. A general increase in blood volume is accompanied by an increase in pulmonary blood volume, which in turn leads to an elevation in pulmonary vascular pressures. Administration of large amounts of blood may precipitate pulmonary edema in a normal person. More commonly, the administration of blood or salt solution leads to pulmonary edema in an individual with previous disease of the heart or kidney. Great care must be taken in administering blood or saline to a person with a history of left ventricular failure, as small amounts of fluid may precipitate pulmonary edema. A combination of left ventricular failure and increase in blood volume may produce pulmonary edema in patients with severe chronic anemia who are receiving blood transfusions.

Pulmonary edema complicating renal disease involves fluid overload and left ventricular failure. If the patient is oliguric, as in acute tubular necrosis or acute glomerulonephritis, and receives excessive fluid orally or intravenously, the blood volume increases, and pulmonary edema may

occur. Often hypertension is present and predisposes to left ventricular failure. In chronic renal disease left ventricular failure plays an important role in the formation of pulmonary edema. Uremic pneumonia is thought to be a form of pulmonary edema occurring in patients with severe renal insufficiency.

Pulmonary edema may complicate intracranial lesions. The most common cause is marked increase in intracranial pressure secondary to head injury or spontaneous intracranial hemorrhage. It has also been described in association with brain tumors and following generalized convulsive seizures. The mechanism of production of the edema is not completely understood, but is thought to be related to reflex effects on peripheral circulation and heart with massive peripheral vasoconstriction.

High altitude pulmonary edema is a poorly understood disorder. It occurs in those recently arrived at high altitude who have engaged in vigorous exercise. The clinical picture is similar to other types of pulmonary edema. Recovery is the rule with suitable treatment and evacuation to lower altitudes.

Lowered Colloid Osmotic Pressure of Plasma. Pulmonary edema is rarely caused by diminution in the concentration of plasma proteins unless other predisposing factors are present. In the nephrotic syndrome there may be massive peripheral edema, yet the lungs remain free of fluid. In edema of the lungs produced by massive infusion of saline, the lowered plasma proteins contribute to edema formation. This is particularly true if the plasma proteins have been depleted by hemorrhage. In renal disease decrease in the concentration of plasma proteins may be one of several factors contributing to pulmonary edema.

Negative Intrapleural Pressure. Sudden reexpansion of the lung by the rapid removal of large amounts of pleural fluid may result in unilateral pulmonary edema. Edema may also result from the rapid expansion of a lung collapsed by a pneumothorax. The edema is thought to result from the application of a large negative intrapleural pressure to the lung.

Increased Capillary Permeability. Certain gases when inhaled into the lungs damage the pulmonary capillaries and increase the permeability of the capillary wall to protein. Among these gases are phosgene, chlorine, and nitrogen dioxide. The latter may result from fermentation of corn in a closed space (silo-filler's disease).

Pulmonary edema may occur as an idiosyncratic reaction to certain drugs. Self-administration of large doses of heroin has frequently been reported to cause edema of the lungs. Other drugs reported to cause increased capillary permeability with edema include hexamethonium, nitrofurantoin, busulfan, and hydrochlorothiazide. Pulmonary edema has been reported following a single blood transfusion as a result of hypersensitivity.

Pulmonary edema has been described complicating shock associated with bacteremia. In some instances this is the result of the administration of excessive volumes of fluid intravenously, but it has been described in the absence of excessive fluid administration. The exact mechanism of production of pulmonary edema is not known.

Certain pneumonias resemble pulmonary edema. Fulminating pneumonia may occur with influenza virus infection, and death may occur in 24 hours. The alveoli are filled with edema fluid, fibrin, red blood cells, and mononuclear cells. The pneumonia associated with *Pneumocystis carinii* infection is more chronic. The alveoli contain a foamy amorphous exudate.

There is considerable evidence that the administration of a high concentration of oxygen for long periods of time will cause damage to the pulmonary capillaries. It has been known for many years that damage to the lungs of animals could be produced by the prolonged administration of pure oxygen at atmospheric pressure. More recently interstitial edema and hyaline alveolar membranes have been described in patients receiving high concentration of oxygen in association with mechanical ventilation. During life there is a progressive fall in the oxygen tension of the arterial blood in spite of continuing high concentration of oxygen in the inspired air.

Treatment. The treatment of pulmonary edema consists of general measures and therapy specific for the underlying cause. Examples of specific therapy are digitalis for left ventricular failure, appropriate treatment of arrhythmias, and the use of antihypertensive drugs in heart failure precipitated by severe hypertension.

Morphine will produce dramatic relief of symptoms if administered during the interstitial phase of edema or in the early stages of alveolar edema. The pattern of breathing may return to normal, and apprehension is relieved. Morphine is of special value in attacks of pulmonary edema resulting from acute left ventricular failure. The drug is given subcutaneously in a dose of 15 mg. If rapid action is desired or shock is present, it may be given intravenously. The administration of morphine to patients with chronic obstructive lung disease under the mistaken impression that pulmonary edema is present should be avoided at all costs. Morphine should also be avoided in the late stages of pulmonary edema when respiration is depressed because of severe hypoxia.

Oxygen should be administered, as hypoxia may be present. In mild pulmonary edema an adequate concentration of oxygen in inspired air can be obtained with a nasal catheter. A high concentration of oxygen may be required in severe pulmonary edema. This may be given in association with intermittent positive pressure breathing. The increase in intra-alveolar pressure resulting from positive pressure breathing is believed to inhibit the movement of fluid into the alveoli. The use of high concentrations of oxygen for prolonged periods of time in the treatment of pulmonary edema should be avoided, as further damage to pulmonary capillaries may ensue.

Reduction in pulmonary blood volume is imperative in pulmonary edema associated with high pulmonary capillary pressure. This can be accomplished by pooling blood in the extremities or by venesection. Placing the patient in the sitting position with legs dependent will pool blood in the legs. Additional blood can be pooled by the application of venous tourniquets to the upper thighs. Venesection of 500 to 700 ml. of blood is particularly useful in those cases in which the attack of pulmonary edema has been precipitated by administration of blood or the excessive use of intravenous fluids. Diuretics have also been found valuable. Ethacrynic acid given intravenously in a dose of 50 mg. will produce a prompt massive diuresis with consequent reduction of blood volume.

Adriani, J., Zepernick, R., Harmon, W., and Hiern, B.: Iatrogenic pulmonary edema in surgical patients. Surgery, 61:183, 1967.

Ducker, T. B.: Increased intracranial pressure and pulmonary edema. Part 1: Clinical study of 11 patients. J. Neurosurg., 28:112, 1967.

Heitzman, E. R., and Ziter, F. M.: Acute interstitial pulmonary edema. Radiology, 98:291, 1966.

Roy, S. B., Guleria, J. S., Khanna, P. K., et al.: Hemodynamic studies in high altitude and pulmonary edema. Brit. Heart J., 31:52, 1969.

Staub, N. C., Nagano, H., and Pearce, M. L.: Pulmonary edema in dogs, especially the sequence of fluid accumulation in the lungs. J. Appl. Physiol., 22:227, 1967.

Steinberg, A. D., and Karliner, J. S.: The clinical spectrum of heroin pulmonary edema. Arch. Intern. Med. (Chicago), 122:122, 1968.

Teplitz, C.: The ultrastructural basis for pulmonary pathophysiology following trauma. Pathogenesis of pulmonary edema. J. Trauma, 8:700, 1968.

PULMONARY ALVEOLAR PROTEINOSIS

Pulmonary alveolar proteinosis is a recently described pathologic entity. The microscopic appearance of the lungs is typical. Large groups of alveoli are filled with a proteinaceous material containing a high concentration of phospholipid. The material gives a positive reaction with periodic acid–Schiff stain. A few large cells containing stainable lipid are present in the alveoli and along the alveolar septa. The septa themselves are remarkably normal, although changes in the alveolar capillary basement membrane have been described in studies using the electron microscope.

Symptoms consist of gradually progressive dyspnea and a productive cough. Physical examination of the lungs may be normal. The roentgenogram reveals bilateral diffuse soft densities seen most commonly at the hila or bases of the lungs. The vital capacity is reduced to a variable degree. The maximal breathing capacity is normal or slightly reduced. The oxygen saturation of the hemoglobin of the arterial blood may be normal or reduced. Complicating infection occurs. Fungal infection is common, Nocardia being the most frequent offending organism. The disease may remain stable for considerable periods of time and spontaneous improvement may occur, but it is eventually fatal in about one third of the patients.

Pulmonary alveolar proteinosis must be differentiated from diseases of the heart with pulmonary edema and from the pulmonary fibroses, pneumoconioses, sarcoidosis, and fungal infections of the lung. *Pneumocystis carinii* infection can present with a similar clinical picture and similar pathologic findings. Lung biopsy is usually necessary to clarify the diagnosis.

Various methods of treatment have been attempted. These include the use of proteolytic enzymes and instillation of a solution of heparin in saline into the trachea. Lavage of the lung appears to be the most promising. One lung is lavaged at a time using several liters of saline containing heparin. The washings contain material with a high lipid content similar to that seen in the alveoli. Clearing of the pulmonary lesions has been described following lavage.

Davidson, J. M., and Macleod, W. M.: Pulmonary alveolar proteinosis. Brit. J. Dis. Chest, 63:13, 1969.

Divertie, M. B., Brown, A. L., and Harrison, E. G., Jr.: Pulmonary alveolar proteinosis: Two cases studied by electron microscopy. Amer. J. Med., 40:351, 1966.

Ramirez-R., J., and Harlan, W. R.: Pulmonary alveolar proteinosis. Nature and origin of alveolar lipid. Amer. J. Med., 45:502, 1968.

Rosen, S. H., Castleman, B., and Liebow, A. A.: Pulmonary alveolar proteinosis. New Eng. J. Med., 258:1123, 1958.

DESQUAMATIVE INTERSTITIAL PNEUMONIA

The tissue response in desquamative interstitial pneumonia consists of proliferation and desquamation of large alveolar cells with slight thickening of the walls of the distal air spaces.

Patients with this disease complain of cough and shortness of breath, which is gradually progressive. Rales may or may not be heard on physical examination of the chest. The roentgenogram demonstrates a ground-glass appearance in the basilar portion of the lungs. Diagnosis must be made by lung biopsy. The course is chronic, the lesions persisting for months or years. Steroids are said to have a beneficial effect.

There is some question whether this entity is distinct and separate from diffuse interstitial fibrosis (fibrosing alveolitis). Cases are seen which are intermediate between the two entities with varying degrees of alveolar wall thickening and varying numbers of cells in the alveoli. There is evidence that patients with typical desquamative interstitial pneumonia may develop interstitial fibrosis after several years.

Gaensler, E. A., Goff, A. M., and Prowse, C. M.: Desquamative interstitial pneumonia. New Eng. J. Med., 274:113, 1966.

Liebow, A. A., Steer, A., and Billingsley, J. G.: Desquamative interstitial pneumonia. Amer. J. Med., 39:369, 1965.

Scadding, J. G., and Hinson, K. F.: Diffuse fibrosing alveolitis (diffuse interstitial fibrosis of the lungs). Correlation of histology at biopsy with prognosis. Thorax, 22:291, 1967.

LIPOID PNEUMONIA

Lipoid pneumonia can be exogenous or endogenous in type. In the exogenous variety mineral oil or animal fats are introduced into the lung by aspiration. A common cause is the use of nose drops with a mineral oil as a base. The oil has ready access to the larynx and trachea when applied through the nose. Another cause is the habitual use of mineral oil to regulate bowel movements. In certain persons the mineral oil is aspirated into the trachea and lungs. This is most commonly seen in the elderly in whom the protective reflexes may be dulled. Animal fats may be introduced into the lungs in chronic disease of the esophagus where regurgitation of food occurs. Achalasia of the esophagus is often associated with a chronic pneumonitis as a result of aspiration.

In pneumonia caused by mineral oil the earliest reaction is phagocytosis of the oil by alveolar macrophages. The alveolar walls become thickened, and there is an increase in fibrous tissue. Lymphocytes and globules of oil are seen in the interstitial tissue. Ultimately extreme fibrosis of the involved area of the lung occurs.

The endogenous form of lipoid pneumonia consists of a chronic inflammatory process involving a segment or lobe of the lung. The alveoli contain large mononuclear cells with a vacuolated cytoplasm. These cells are also found in the walls of the alveoli. Lymphocytic infiltration and fibrosis of the alveolar walls are present. The lipid present in the lesion is cholesterol. This type of pneumonitis not infrequently occurs secondary to an obstructed bronchus. Occasionally it is present without evident cause.

The symptoms of lipoid pneumonia are extremely variable. The patient may be virtually asymptomatic and the lesion be detected on routine roentgenogram of the chest, or productive cough and dyspnea may be present. The earliest change on the roentgenogram is the presence of an alveolar type of infiltrate. An acinar pattern may be visible at the periphery of the lesion. Later evidence of fibrosis is present, and there may be contraction of the involved area of the lung. In the exogenous form of the disease the lesions are usually seen in the basilar or posterior segments of the lung.

An important method of diagnosis is the demonstration of oil-containing macrophages in the sputum. The sputum should be collected before breakfast and after cleansing the mouth. Appropriate fat stains should be used. In some cases lung aspiration or biopsy may be necessary to establish the diagnosis.

There may be difficulty in differentiating lipoid pneumonia from bronchogenic carcinoma. The failure to demonstrate an obstructed bronchus is of great importance in diagnosis. The history of aspiration and the lack of tumor cells in the sputum or bronchial washings confirm the diagnosis of lipoid pneumonia.

There is no specific treatment except prevention of aspiration of oil or fat. If symptoms are troublesome and persistent, resection of the segment or lobe involved should be considered.

Miller, A., Bader, R. A., Bader, M. E., Teirstein, A. S., and Selikoff, J.: Mineral oil pneumonia. Ann. Intern. Med., 57:627, 1962.

Robbins, L. L., and Sniffen, R. C.: Correlation between roentgenologic and pathologic findings in chronic pneumonitis of the cholesterol type. Radiology, 53:187, 1949.

Wagner, J. C., Adler, D. I., and Fuller, D. N.: Foreign body granulomata of the lungs due to liquid paraffin. Thorax, 10:157, 1955.

Weill, H., Ferrans, V. J., Gay, R. M., and Ziskind, M. M.: Early lipoid pneumonia. Roentgenologic, anatomic and physiologic characteristics. Amer. J. Med., 36:370, 1964.

GOODPASTURE'S SYNDROME AND IDIOPATHIC PULMONARY HEMOSIDEROSIS

Goodpasture's syndrome is a rare disease characterized by repeated episodes of hemorrhage into the pulmonary alveoli associated with glomerulonephritis. The presenting symptoms are hemoptysis and dyspnea. Roentgenographic examination of the lungs demonstrates fluffy infiltrates in both lungs. An iron deficiency anemia is present, and the urine contains albumin, red blood cells, and casts. The course of the disease consists of remissions and exacerbations. Repeated episodes of hemoptysis and pulmonary infiltration occur. Progressive impairment of renal function is common, and uremia often results. The disease has a poor prognosis, and recovery is rare. There is no specific therapy. The pathology of the disease is of great interest. There is hemorrhage, and hemosiderosin-containing macrophages are in the alveoli. The alveolar septa may be thickened with an increase in collagen. A proliferative type of glomerulonephritis is found in the kidneys. An important finding is the presence of gamma globulin and complement in the basement membrane of the renal glomeruli and of the pulmonary alveoli demonstrated by immunofluorescence. Globulins eluted from lung tissue react with glomerular basement membrane. These findings suggest that antibodies against kidney and lung basement membrane are important in the pathogenesis of the disease.

The pulmonary lesions of *idiopathic pulmonary hemosiderosis* bear considerable similarities to those of Goodpasture's syndrome, but no renal lesion is present. The disease occurs most commonly in children, but may occur in young adults. The earliest symptom is hemoptysis. This is associated with transient confluent infiltrates seen on the roentgenogram of the lungs. The hemoptysis and pulmonary infiltrates come and go. Pallor develops which can be ascribed to an iron deficiency anemia. The patient ultimately develops chronic dyspnea. The chest roentgenogram now may show a reticular appearance with fine stippling. Biopsy of the lung will demonstrate hemosiderin-laden macrophages in the alveoli and an increase in interstitial fibrous tissue. Hemosiderin-containing macrophages can also be found in the sputum. Massive hemoptysis is not uncommon and may lead to death. The mortality is high, and there is no specific therapy.

Koffler, D., Sandson, J., Carr, R., and Kunkel, H.: Immunologic studies concerning the pulmonary lesions in Goodpasture's syndrome. Amer. J. Path., 54:293, 1969.

Proskey, A. J., Weatherbee, L., Easterling, R. E., et al.: Goodpasture's syndrome. A report of five cases and review of the literature. Amer. J. Med., 48:162, 1970.

Repetto, G., Lisboa, C., Emparanza, E., et al.: Idiopathic pulmonary hemosiderosis. Pediatrics, 40:24, 1967.

Soergel, K. H., and Sommers, S. C.: Idiopathic pulmonary hemosiderosis and related syndromes. Amer. J. Med., 32:499, 1962.

Weiss, E. B., Earnest, D. L., and Greally, J. F.: Goodpasture's syndrome. Case report with emphasis on pulmonary physiology. Amer. Rev. Resp. Dis., 97:444, 1968.

ALVEOLAR MICROLITHIASIS

Alveolar microlithiasis is a rare disease characterized by the presence of round calcified bodies in the alveoli. The origin and exact nature of these bodies are not known. The disease develops in young adults, and multiple cases may be seen in a family. It is most commonly discovered by examination of a routine roentgenogram of the chest. The appearance of the lungs is characteristic. Fine miliary calcific densities are distributed throughout the lung. The lesions are most prominent at the bases of the lung. The shadows may coalesce, giving a uniform density in portions of the lung. Early in the disease the patient is asymptomatic. Later dyspnea and cough are present. The course is prolonged over many years, and death occurs from pulmonary insufficiency.

Fulechon, F. J. D., Abboud, A. T., Balikian, J. P., and Nucho, C. K. N.: Pulmonary alveolar microlithiasis. Lung function in five cases. Thorax, 24:84, 1969.

Sosman, M. D., Dodd, G. D., Jones, W. D., and Pillmore, G. U.: The familial recurrence of pulmonary microlithiasis. Amer. J. Roentgen., 77:947, 1957.

Chemical and Physical Irritants

Margaret R. Becklake

Man, in taming his environment and in developing his complex industrial society, has become increasingly exposed to a wide variety of materials which may act as chemical and physical irritants to his lungs. The industrial physician is sensitized to the need for a detailed occupational history. However, in many communities, working men and women first seek medical advice from their personal physician, who may not have a high index of suspicion or an appreciation of the wide variety of inhalation hazards and the number of occupations at risk. Thus, the busy physician may fail his patient through inadequate curiosity concerning the patient's place of occupation and the nature of his work.

Today, industrial lung disease covers the reaction of the lung to a variety of physical and chemical irritants, extending beyond those conditions originally described by the term *pneumoconioses*, which refers to lung diseases consequent on the inhalation of dust. The term, in keeping with its Greek derivation, was originally applied only to inorganic (mineral) dusts, but has subsequently been extended to cover organic (vegetable) dusts as well. A large number of variants of this term have been coined to describe specific occupations at risk or specific dust diseases, and probably serve more to confuse than to clarify.

The classification of lung irritants outlined below may imply an understanding of mechanisms of lung response more precise than is justified by current knowledge. But to provide a necessary skeleton for discussion, *lung irritants* may be classified as follows:

1. Inorganic dust, producing:
   a. *Nodular pneumoconiosis:* (1) due to dust macules containing much dust and little fibrosis, e.g., coal, carbon, tin, iron; (2) due to classic silicotic nodules containing little dust and much fibrosis
   b. *Diffuse pneumoconiosis* characterized by generalized interstitial fibrosis, e.g., asbestos, aluminum (in certain circumstances), very fine and fume silica
   c. *Complicated pneumoconiosis* characterized by conglomerate fibrotic lesions, and complicating (a) and (b) above
2. Organic dust, producing:
   a. *Allergic alveolitis* in association with exposure to molds in hay, bagasse, and similar organic compounds
   b. *Byssinosis* in association with exposure to cotton, hemp, flax, and sisal
3. Chemical irritants, producing:
   a. Immediate effects primarily on large airways, e.g., sulfur dioxide, hydrochloric acid (aspirated from stomach)
   b. Delayed effects primarily on small airways and parenchyma, e.g., oxides of nitrogen
   c. Reactions suggesting sensitization, e.g., the diisocyanates
4. Radiation

INORGANIC DUSTS: DOSAGE, CLEARANCE, AND CELLULAR REACTION

The biologic effects of inorganic dusts depend on their retention in the lungs of man for long periods of time, measured usually in years, not months. It has been suggested that any mineral dust, if relatively insoluble and not immediately toxic, can produce a pneumoconiosis when inhaled in sufficient quantities. The physician is probably better advised to adopt this oversuspicious attitude to mineral dusts than to fail in recognizing old as well as new pneumoconioses.

Human lungs have been aptly called *"size-selective dust samplers."* Airborne dust, when inspired into the lung, undergoes a process of separation based on size and falling rate. Likewise, breathing patterns and minute ventilation affect penetration and deposition. About 80 per cent of larger particles (6μ and over) impact on the mucous lining of the larger airways to be removed, usually quite rapidly, by ciliary escalation; however, some particles of considerable length, e.g., asbestos fibers up to as much as 100μ in length, may penetrate as far as terminal respiratory units. Small dust particles penetrate more deeply, but only the fine particles (below 2μ) penetrate the alveolar spaces. The retention rate is high (about 60 per cent) in the 1 to 2μ size, probably even higher in those below 0.2μ, and probably minimal in the 0.2 to 0.5μ range.

Since the respiratory bronchioles and alveoli are lined with surfactant, not mucus, dust particles settling here are removed by alveolar phagocytosis; dust-laden phagocytes migrate toward the alveolar ducts and terminal bronchioles; if not extruded into the airways they may penetrate into lung interstitium and lymphatics. Furthermore, clearance mechanisms may be provoked, i.e., mucus and surfactant production, ciliary activity, and endocytosis all increase, in response to the inhalation of irritants, particularly if exposure is intermittent. Heavy doses, on the other hand, may overwhelm the removal mechanisms, and their efficiency may also be reduced by associated pollutants, either industrial or personal (tobacco smoke).

The *lung tissue response to inorganic dust* has been likened to the color spectrum to emphasize the variety in the type of response and its intensity. It is almost certainly dose related, the consequence of the integrated personal exposure less the integrated clearance over the years. It is also thought to depend on the quantity and particle size of the dust, its physicochemical and, perhaps, its antigenic properties, as well as on the presence or absence of infection, and possible synergistic or antagonistic effects of other respirable materials in the environment. Two broad patterns of response are seen, a discrete *nodular type of pneumoconiosis,* caused by relatively insoluble dusts, and a *diffuse type of pneumoconiosis,* caused by relatively soluble dusts and, occasionally, by ultrafine insoluble particles; both may progress to a *complicated pneumoconiosis,* characterized by large, irregular, fibrotic lesions.

sumption (going from rest to maximal exercise) by a factor varying from 20 in the young athlete to perhaps 10 in the middle-aged man. In its early stages pneumoconiosis may produce only very minor measurable changes in function, affecting performance at high levels of exercise only, and this may well be interpreted by the subject as the natural consequence of aging. As the condition progresses, dyspnea may be more easily related to demonstrable changes in lung function. In the following section, an attempt is made to describe the usual clinical picture caused by the different pneumoconioses in their different stages of development. *In the individual case,* however, *there is no substitute for the detailed study of pulmonary function at rest and on effort,* providing that these are interpreted in the light of industrial history, dust exposure (quality and quantity), medical history (in particular, previous and present heart and lung disease), and appropriate laboratory investigations.

DIAGNOSIS, LUNG FUNCTION, AND DISABILITY IN THE INORGANIC DUST PNEUMOCONIOSES

The *diagnosis* of these pneumoconioses depends on the characteristic changes in the chest roentgenogram, *providing that the subject in question has had a suitable history of dust exposure.* In other words, there may be no physical signs and no impairment of physical performance. In the absence of an exposure history, it may be necessary to resort to mediastinal node biopsy or to open or needle lung biopsy to establish a diagnosis. Adequate tissue samples should be sent for chemical assay and mineralogic study with x-ray diffraction as well as histopathology. The electron microprobe may ultimately allow precise characterization of mineral in very small tissue samples, or even in the single ferruginous (asbestos) body. Since most pneumoconioses develop as a consequence of occupational exposure, *precise evaluation of disability* is frequently called for, with a view to establishing compensation; hence, the many studies of pulmonary function in pneumoconiosis. It would be incorrect, however, to conclude that the interrelationship between the dyspnea and measurable disturbance of static or dynamic pulmonary function has been satisfactorily defined in pneumoconiosis, or, indeed, in lung disease in general. To date, the most acceptable theory is that dyspnea is felt when the respiratory effort (either minute volume or muscular effort) for a given task is greater than the subject habitually experiences. In health there exists a tremendous reserve of cardiopulmonary function, indicated by the capacity to increase O_2 con-

NODULAR PNEUMOCONIOSES RESULTING FROM DUST MACULES CONTAINING MUCH DUST AND LITTLE FIBROSIS
(Examples: Coal Workers' Pneumoconiosis; Siderosis in Welders and Hematite and Magnetite Miners; Stannosis in Tin Miners; Baritosis in Barium Miners; Pneumoconiosis in Chromite and China Clay Miners, and in Workers with Fuller's Earth)

Pathogenesis and Mechanisms. The dusts mentioned above are those which elicit minimal fibrotic response. They can accumulate in large amounts, usually in phagocytes which accumulate in the alveolar spaces or penetrate the interstitial pulmonary tissue to collect as discrete macules, or as sheaths of cells around the respiratory bronchioles. Although considerable amounts of dust (up to 20 grams) may be recoverable from the lungs at autopsy, only small amounts of fibrous tissue develop in these macules, usually in a radial rather than a concentric fashion. The intensity of the fibrosis, never marked, is thought to be related to quartz contamination in the dust, and variations in quartz content probably explain such regional differences as exist, for example, among the dust macule of the Welsh soft coal miner, the more fibrous macule of his counterpart in Belgium, and the *stellate "mixed dust" nodule* of the foundry worker. In addition, the radio-density of the nodules appears to be related to their iron content, endogenous iron accumulating around dust as it does around other foreign bodies. In time the respiratory bronchioles around the dust foci dilate, and a characteristic form of *focal emphysema* develops, involving primarily the respiratory bronchioles.

The pathologic changes of chronic bronchitis and more generalized emphysema (discussed else-where in Respiratory Diseases) may also be seen in lungs which are affected by these nodular pneumoconioses. To what extent these changes are attributable to dust exposure and perhaps to the presence of a simple nodular pneumoconiosis is not known. It is generally believed, however, that such changes occur more frequently and to a more disabling degree (leading to pulmonary hy-pertension and right heart failure) in certain geographic areas, e.g., the iron mines of Lorraine and the coal mines of Belgium.

Clinical Manifestations. The term "tattooing" of the chest roentgenogram has been applied to this group of *"benign" nodular pneumoconioses*, be-cause even in the presence of diffuse radiologic nodular densities symptoms and signs of chest disease are rarely present. Likewise, most tests routinely used to evaluate pulmonary function such as lung volumes, flow rates, diffusing capacity at rest, and even pulmonary mechanics, have been found to be within the normal limits in keeping with the histology of the dust macules. However, abnormalities of gas exchange (reflected in in-creased A-a O_2 differences) have been shown to exist. These changes, demonstrable at rest and exaggerated during effort, presumably reflect regional inequalities in ventilation vis-à-vis perfusion. Such changes probably do not impair function enough to cause symptoms unless there are the associated complications of chronic ob-structive lung disease.

Epidemiology and Prognosis. The prevalence rate of simple pneumoconiosis varies very much from operation to operation, even within the same industry; for example, rates range from 90 to 480 per 1000 underground workers in the coal mining industry of Great Britain, and are estimated at 68 per 1000 working Appalachian coal miners, where, however, case reporting is not yet mandatory. In small uncontrolled operations prevalence may well be higher. These differences are thought to be related to the dust exposure levels, and prevalence usually falls dramatically as dust control becomes effective, e.g., in the Dutch coal miners rates fell from 270 to 160 per 1000 working miners over a seven-year period.

Most studies indicate an *increased prevalence of chronic obstructive lung disease* (as measured by questionnaire or simple ventilatory tests or both) in coal mining communities; in some instances this appears to be determined by occupa-tion and in others by environment, e.g., when bronchitis appears to be as common among miners'

wives as among the miners themselves. Nor can the contribution of personal air pollution be ignored since miners are frequently heavy smokers. Thus attributability is a taxing and diffi-cult problem for compensation commissions, especially as it is unusual for the nodular pneu-moconioses in this group per se to produce signifi-cant disability.

It is not, however, usual for these pneumoconio-ses *to develop for the first time or to progress after exposure has ceased,* but this does occur. Likewise, the disappearance of radiologic changes following removal from exposure, though unusual, has been described, and is in keeping with animal experi-ments showing that dust nodules are not static structures but are the site of continuing phago-cytic activity. Life expectancy does not appear to be affected by the presence of these "benign" pneumoconioses, especially if exposure stops, and they are not complicated by obstructive lung dis-ease.

NODULAR INORGANIC DUST PNEUMOCONIOSES RESULTING FROM THE CLASSIC SILICOTIC NODULE CONTAINING LITTLE DUST AND MUCH FIBROSIS

(Examples: Classic Silicosis of Hard-rock Miners; Silicosis in Iron and Steelworkers and Sandblasters, in the Pottery Industry, in Industries Using Silica Flour, and in Silica Mines)

Pathogenesis and Mechanisms. If the dusts of carbon and coal represent those at the low end of the response spectrum, free crystalline silica dust represents the opposite end, with its almost unique biologic capacity to evoke a powerful fibrogenic tissue response. Reaction to silica ap-pears to start with an alteration of the lung macrophages, though by what mechanism is not fully understood; neither a mechanical nor a simple solubility theory fully explains the biologic findings. There is support for the view that damaged macrophages release altered cell mate-rial which is antigenic and which activates the reticuloendothelial system. A fibroblastic reaction follows (peribronchiolar, perivascular, or both) which leads to the accumulation of hyaline material at the site of the macrophage collections, and ultimately to the development of the *characteristic fibrous silicotic nodule* made up of layers of whorled connective tissue, like an onion. Extensive and marked fibrosis may be present in the lungs at autopsy with only relatively small amounts of dust (5 to 6 grams). Involvement of the hilar and mediastinal and sometimes abdominal lymph nodes is common, occasionally with *egg-shell calcification.* In nature, free crystalline silica occurs almost exclusively as quartz; however, other free crystalline silicas, e.g., crystobalite, tridymite, though rare in natural geologic formation, may be formed from quartz in steelmaking and in other high-heat smelting processes, and probably have a more powerful silicosis-producing action than quartz.

Clinical Manifestations. Even in nodular silicosis (in which the radiologic lesions are fibrous nodules, not dust macules, as in the "benign" pneumoconioses) there may be no clinical manifestations, and apparently no impairment in pulmonary function. The proportion of cases without signs and symptoms is probably about 20 per cent, in contrast to about 90 per cent in the "benign" pneumoconioses of equivalent radiologic category.

The first complaint in nodular silicosis is commonly shortness of breath, brought on by moderate, and then progressively less, exercise until it is present at rest. This symptom is probably due to the increased muscular work required to ventilate incompliant lungs and is aggravated by increased minute ventilation to offset impaired gas exchange. Lung volumes are reduced as the nodular disease becomes more widespread. However, in a certain number of cases, the symptoms, signs, and classic lung function pattern of chronic obstructive lung disease are present, even though the radiologic pattern is primarily that of diffuse nodular pneumoconiosis.

Epidemiology and Prognosis. Prevalence rates vary from operation to operation, depending chiefly on the efficiency of dust control. Thus in the Witwatersrand gold mining industry, rates fell from 40 per 1000 underground miners in the 1920's to less than 10 per 1000 in the 1950's, although the average period of mining service prior to diagnosis rose from 10 to 23 years over this period. However, the simple silicosis of gold miners is undoubtedly a less benign disease than the simple pneumoconiosis of coal miners, even though it does not appear to affect life expectancy. Thus, figures for Sweden indicate that, following withdrawal from exposure, x-ray changes never regress, about 40 per cent of cases progress to a higher category of simple pneumoconiosis within ten years, and a further 40 per cent to a complicated silicosis, invariably related to tuberculosis (see accompanying diagram). The prevalence of chronic obstructive lung disease does not appear to be occupationally related to classic silicosis, other than that which can be accounted for by a man's smoking habits.

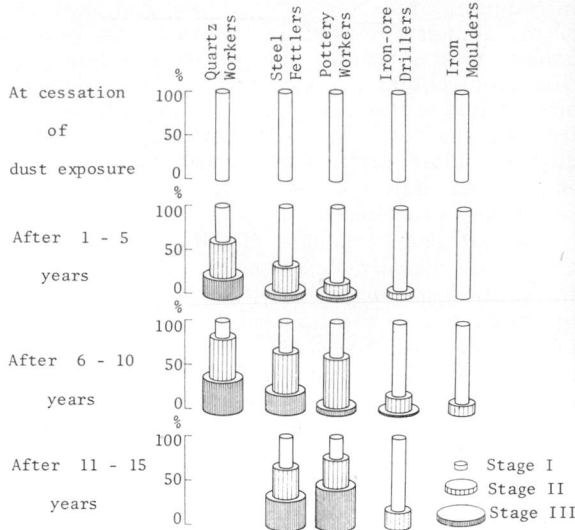

Rate of progression of different pneumoconioses following removal from dust exposure. The figures are based on five occupational groups of Swedish workers (each containing a minimum of ten cases) followed for 15 years after dust exposure ceased. (From Bruce, T., Nystrom, A., and Ahlmark, A. L.: Scand. J. Resp. Diseases, Supp. 63, 1968.)

DIFFUSE INORGANIC DUST PNEUMOCONIOSES
(Examples: Asbestosis, Aluminosis [as in Shaver's Disease]; Talcosis [in Talc Miners and Millers], Chronic Beryllium Disease of the Lung)

Pathogenesis and Mechanisms. Asbestos, the most important mineral in this group, occurs in several forms: *chrysotile* (a magnesium silicate, occurring as long, white, flexible fibers), the chief asbestos of commerce, mined primarily in Canada, Italy, Rhodesia, and South Africa, as well as the U.S.S.R.; and the *amphiboles,* iron silicates (occurring as brittle fibers such as amosite, anthophyllite, and blue crocidolite) mined in South Africa, Australia, and Finland. Exposure occurs in mining and milling, and in the manufacture of a wide variety of the commodities used by modern man, e.g., insulation in homes, brake shoes, and clutch linings of cars; components in the construction industry such as tiles, floorings, walls, and cement products such as gutters; and the spinning of resistant cloths for protective clothing, ironing boards, and oven cloths.

Inhaled fibers are thought to excite an inflammatory reaction. This causes them to be enveloped in a smooth protein film which becomes iron-impregnated, giving rise to the typical drumhead, golden-brown *asbestos bodies.* In this form, they may remain inert for long periods if not indefinitely; few penetrate the lymphoid deposits, and fewer still reach the lymph nodes and the pleura. Nevertheless, pleural reactions to exposure may be severe, e.g., *pleural plaques* and *calcification,* dense fibrous adhesive pleurisy, and malignancy in the form of *mesothelioma;* and these may occur even when there is little or no pulmonary fibrosis. It is thought that the fibrotic response in pulmonary tissue may be precipitated by disruption of asbestos bodies with release of the mineral which is thought to act as a direct stimulus to fibroblasts. The reaction frequently starts in the peribronchiolar areas and then extends widely into lung parenchyma, obliterating air spaces and replacing them with cystic spaces lined by flattened epithelium (*"honeycomb" lung*). Other mineral dusts which produce this pattern of diffuse fibrosis are talc, diatomaceous earth, and some of the very fine silicas currently used in industry, particularly if the exposure is heavy. Caplan's syndrome (see below), though more frequently recognized in coal workers, may be seen in relation to exposure to asbestos, silica, and probably most dusts.

Generalized pulmonary fibrosis may also be found in *chronic beryllium disease* of the lung, and should be regarded as a manifestation of systemic poisoning with this mineral rather than as a pneumoconiosis. The early signs are characterized by chronic interstitial pneumonitis, which is frequently granulomatous. The granulomas may vary from loose collections of histiocytes to large circumscribed granulomas, often containing giant cells with various calcific inclusion bodies, and are indistinguishable histologically from sarcoidosis. The end result is frequently fibrosis of varying severity. Diagnosis can only be made with certainty by isolation of the element beryllium in tissues or body fluids. There is often a very long period of latency. Thus, cases related to the manufacture of fluorescent light in the United States during World War II continue to be reported even today. The "epidemic" of the late 1940's, however, is almost certainly over because the use of beryllium in the fluorescent lamp industry ceased in 1949. Although its modern uses in military defense and space exploration appear to be better controlled, new cases continue to be added to the U.S. Beryllium Registry at the Massachusetts General Hospital.

Clinical Manifestations. These are no different from those of diffuse pulmonary fibrosis, whatever the underlying etiology. In some subjects *dyspnea* is the first symptom, brought on at first by considerable exertion and then by progressively less effort, until it is eventually present at rest. In other subjects, an *irritating dry cough* precedes the awareness of shortness of breath, often by many years. With the progress of the disease, the cough may become productive, and *spells of chest pain* may be associated with the coughing. When the condition is advanced, there are usually diffuse basal rales, but the lung signs may be modified by the presence of pleural thickening or calcification. Respiratory failure usually appears late in the course of the disease, as does pulmonary hypertension, right heart strain, and right heart failure. Nor is the victim of these diffuse pneumoconioses immune from the attack by general atmospheric pollutants, which may encourage the development of chronic bronchitis and bronchiectasis and increase the risk of bronchial neoplasm.

The established cause of asbestosis is associated with changes in pulmonary function characteristic of restrictive lung disease, i.e., small volumes, impaired gas exchange with reduced diffusing capacity, and hyperventilation on effort and eventually at rest. The earliest function changes, however, may be reduced vital capacity and increased exercise ventilation, tests which may eventually prove useful in the longitudinal surveillance of exposed workers. In addition, chronic obstructive lung disease may complicate the picture, particularly in workers who smoke.

In certain parts of the world, e.g., Finland, *pleural calcification* may appear as the only manifestation of exposure to asbestos, and less commonly to talc and mica. It is rarely seen under 20 years of industrial exposure, and neighborhood cases are seen with diminishing frequency as the circumferential distance of the place of residence from the industry increases.

Epidemiology and Prognosis. The *attack rate of asbestosis* varies in different industries (probably in relation to the heaviness of exposure) from 7 per cent of working miners in open mining, as in Quebec, up to over 72 per cent in men with over 20 years' exposure in the insulation and construction industries.

The epidemiology of *population exposure to asbestos* has been established from the search for asbestos bodies in lung scrapings or extruded lung fluid in routine autopsies. Positive results are reported in many parts of the world, varying from around 30 per cent in men in Cape Town (South Africa) and Miami (U.S.) to over 90 per cent when lung tissue is examined more extensively. However, it must be emphasized that the presence of *ferruginous bodies* (as experts now urge that they be called) indicates exposure, not disease. Furthermore, other types of fibers, e.g., glass, wool, cotton, talc, may constitute their core, and the lung probably uses this method to "inactivate" a large variety of inhaled particles.

There is some epidemiologic evidence to indicate that exposure to asbestos increases the *attack rate of neoplasia,* though it is not certain that all types of the mineral are equally implicated. Thus exposure, particularly in the manufacturing as opposed to the producing industries, appears to increase the attack rate (probably in a dose-related fashion) of *carcinoma of the bronchus* in smokers, suggesting a synergism between carcinogens. There may also be an increased risk of gastric neoplasia, presumably because of dust swallowing. Finally, a rare tumor, *mesothelioma of the pleura or peritoneum,* appears to occur with greater frequency in certain exposed populations. However, further studies will be needed to clarify this relationship because the latent period is frequently long (up to 40 years), creating in many instances uncertainty about the exposure history. Slight exposures, however, are suspected e.g., neighborhood exposure for a short while in childhood, and the physician should be alert to this possible hazard.

COMPLICATED PNEUMOCONIOSIS

(Progressive Massive Fibrosis of Coal Workers, Conglomerate Silicosis, Caplan's Syndrome)

Pathogenesis and Mechanisms. The inorganic dust pneumoconioses can progress to progressive massive fibrosis whether or not exposure continues. The lesions of *massive fibrosis in coal workers* consist of dust irregularly mixed with bundles of coarse, hyaline collagen fibers. Few blood vessels and air passages are seen, but the persistence of internal elastic lamellae suggests that they have been obliterated by invading fibrous tissue. Sclerosis of the vessel walls and intimal thickening at the periphery of the lesions are common. Histologic and/or bacteriologic evidence of tuberculosis is found in about half the cases, even though only a very small proportion have tubercle bacilli found in their sputum during life.

Conglomerate silicosis is the result of the matting together by fibrosis of silicotic nodules, frequently associated with caseous areas, which, however, do not always show conclusive histologic evidence of tuberculosis. Right heart strain, hypertrophy, and failure may develop subsequently, perhaps as a consequence of the pulmonary vascular bed's being reduced by the fibrosis and tissue loss associated with emphysematous changes in the adjacent lung. A reversible element in the pulmonary hypertension may also be present, related perhaps to hypoxia or hypercapnia or both.

Several mechanisms may be important in the development of complicated pneumoconiosis: the overwhelming of clearance mechanisms by lung dust; aseptic necrosis owing to interference with blood supply; infection by *M. tuberculosis* or atypical bacteria (the recovery rate of organisms during life increases as recovery efforts increase, and at autopsy has exceeded 50 per cent in several studies); significant silica contamination of the coal dust; and, finally, reaction on an immunologic basis, analogous to the lung changes in *Caplan's syndrome.* Caplan observed an association between rheumatoid arthritis and a particular radiologic picture, characterized by well-defined opacities 0.5 to 5 cm. in diameter, widely distributed and developing rather more suddenly than progressive massive fibrosis, often on a background of slight or no pneumoconio-

sis. Some lesions eventually cavitate, then shrink, perhaps with calcifications, and, in time, become incorporated into a mass radiologically indistinguishable from progressive massive fibrosis. Histologically, the rheumatoid nodule is distinguished by wide concentric bands of necrotic collagen separated by bands of dust, with a peripheral zone of active inflammation and a well-marked arteritis in the adjacent vessels. Tubercle bacilli cannot be isolated from these lesions as they can in progressive massive fibrosis. Caplan's syndrome, though first recognized and most frequently seen in coal miners, has been described in workers in foundries, asbestos, potteries, sandblasting, and boiler scaling.

Clinical Manifestations. Clinical manifestations depend on the "background" pneumoconiosis. Thus in the "benign" pneumoconioses, e.g., coal workers' pneumoconiosis, the appearance of progressive massive fibrosis usually marks the onset of symptoms and signs of lung disease. The first symptom is commonly *dyspnea* on heavy effort, and subsequently at lesser work loads until it becomes evident at rest. The changes in function initially suggest loss of functioning volume rather than a generalized restrictive lung disease. The symptom of cough does not appear to be more common in the earlier stages of complicated pneumoconiosis than in simple pneumoconiosis. *Melanoptysis* (sudden coughing up of a moderate amount of jet black fluid) is not uncommon, and frequently relates to cavitation. *Chest pain,* dull and aching, and diffusely located, is common, and there is an increasing tendency to *acute, purulent bronchitis.* Pulmonary hypertension and right heart hypertrophy, leading ultimately to *right heart failure,* is present in many instances, with the usual symptoms and signs. When infection with *M. tuberculosis* appears to be the factor which has led to the development of the complicated pneumoconiosis, it is seldom accompanied by the usual systemic symptoms, i.e., fever, weight loss, and hemoptysis.

When the chest roentgenogram suggests Caplan's syndrome (see above), serum tests for rheumatoid factor are present in 80 per cent of cases, whereas arthritis, already present in about 50 per cent of cases, will often develop subsequently in some of the others, though it may take several years.

When *complicated pneumoconiosis* develops *on a background of classic silicosis,* the symptoms, signs, and clinical presentation usually represent a progression from an already symptomatic state. The lung function pattern may suggest restrictive disease but frequently shows a pattern characteristic of obstructive disease, or there may be a mixed picture. Infection with *M. tuberculosis* is more likely to be demonstrable in conglomerate silicosis than in the progressive massive fibrosis of coal workers, and is more likely to behave and progress as in the nonsilicotic lung with constitutional symptoms. Right heart strain and failure may complicate the picture, particularly if chronic bronchitis and emphysema are present.

Epidemiology and Prognosis. Attack rates of progressive massive fibrosis in Welsh coal miners increase from 1 per cent in the lowest category of simple pneumoconiosis to 30 per cent in advanced simple pneumoconiosis, and appear to be highest in the younger men working on heavier jobs. Rheumatoid pneumoconiosis occurs in 2 to 6 per cent of United Kingdom coal miners affected by pneumoconiosis. This suggests that in any industry, prevalence rates will relate to the prevalence of pneumoconiosis in that industry (which, in turn, relates to dustiness), as well as to the prevalence of tuberculosis. It is therefore somewhat disappointing to find that vigorous antituberculosis measures in coal-mining communities have not reduced attack rates of progressive massive fibrosis as dramatically as hoped.

TREATMENT AND PREVENTION OF THE INORGANIC DUST PNEUMOCONIOSES

Treatment. There is no specific treatment for the simple nodular or diffuse inorganic dust pneumoconioses. The medical management of associated chronic obstructive lung disease and right heart failure and pulmonary heart disease is the same whether or not it coexists with pneumoconiosis (see elsewhere in this section). Progression of the condition, particularly to complicated pneumoconiosis, appears to depend as much on past as on subsequent exposure. Thus, the physician faces the difficult question of whether he should advise the individual patient to find other employment. A reasonable decision must be based on an accurate knowledge of what determines progression of simple pneumoconiosis and the attack rates of complicated pneumoconiosis in the particular operation concerned. Such knowledge is accumulating in the larger industries which can mount well-planned research operations, e.g., the coal mining industry in Great Britain, but cannot necessarily be applied to other situations, e.g., a welder in a small local plant. In general, most physicians, when faced with such a problem, permit continued employment, with the proviso that regular medical surveillance be available.

Likewise, in complicated pneumoconiosis, medical management is concerned with treatment of the complications. When active tuberculous infection can be demonstrated, appropriate chemotherapy should obviously be instituted. However, many physicians go farther and recommend a two-year course of tuberculosis chemoprophylaxis in all cases (see article on Tuberculosis). Since complicated pneumoconiosis is invariably accompanied by disability, often associated with right heart failure, most patients with complicated pneumoconiosis will have already left the industry concerned. Opinion is divided on the advisability of withdrawal from exposure if the patient is still so occupied.

Dust Control. Inorganic dust pneumoconioses cannot be treated effectively, but they can be prevented, and prevention means, essentially, dust control. Attack rate increases with exposure, and there is a dust dose–disease relationship. Thus *control should be at an epidemiologic level,* aiming at controlling the exposure of the community at risk, rather than at a personal level with the use of masks or respirators. Dust can seldom be completely eliminated from industrial operations. However, disease could be controlled if the minimal exposure which produces pneumoconiosis in a given industry were known; and throughout industrial nations, research by governments, compensation boards, and industry is being pursued along these lines. It is possible to envisage that eventually, from cumulative ongoing records of each worker's exposure to date, industries could plan their operations so that no worker would be likely to exceed the exposure known to produce disease within his working life. Such an ambitious scheme, already under way in the West German coal mining industry, is possible only in large industries able to mount extensive research programs. However, for smaller industries, it is quite valid to assert that *less dust means less disease;* definitions of low-risk levels of exposure for different dusts (threshold limit values) are annually revised by bodies such as the American Conference of Governmental Industrial Hygienists and provide general reference standards.

Tuberculosis Control. Medical attention should be directed toward reducing the attack rates of complicated pneumoconiosis and silicotuberculosis. All subjects with pneumoconiosis are at a higher risk in terms of tuberculosis than the general population; in addition the circumstances of employment may favor exposure to infection, e.g., recruitment of workers from populations in which infection with tubercle bacilli occurs relatively late in life. Case finding and control of tuberculosis should thus be of a particularly high standard in populations exposed to an inorganic dust hazard; at the very least this should include the annual chest roentgenogram.

Prophylactic Substances. Studies in laboratory animals have indicated that certain substances (ferric oxide, iron, coal, aluminum, and more recently poly-2-vinyl-pyridine-N-oxide or PVNO) inhibit the biologic effects of silica dust. Aluminum prophylaxis was introduced in the hard rock mines of Ontario in 1943, using the technique of dispensing the powder in tightly sealed change rooms; at last review (in 1961 after 15 years' use) no new cases of silicosis had occurred. However, its effectiveness can only be adequately assessed by a review of attack rates when the trial has lasted for at least 23.7 years, i.e., the mean exposure time before diagnosis up to 1943. Furthermore, it will be difficult to evaluate the contribution of improved worker hygiene. A prophylactic trial of PVNO has been started in the West German coal industry. It seems improbable, however, that prophylaxis will provide a better solution than programming the individual's exposure to less than a disease-producing dose in his lifetime.

ORGANIC DUST PNEUMOCONIOSES: EXTRINSIC ALLERGIC ALVEOLITIS
(Farmer's Lung, Bagassosis, Mushroom-worker's Lung, Maplebark-stripper's Lung, Suberosis [of Cork Workers], Sequoiosis, Malt-worker's Lung)

Pathogenesis and Mechanisms. The reaction of the lung to organic dusts appears to depend on whether an individual concerned is *atopic*. The list of organic dusts capable of producing the bronchial asthma type of reactions in atopic subjects is almost unlimited, and such subjects frequently withdraw voluntarily from an occupation involving exposure. In the *nonatopic individual,* however, these dusts may produce an allergic alveolitis, and it is this reaction which has been referred to as an organic dust pneumoconiosis. This reaction occurs providing that the dusts can penetrate the alveoli in sufficient numbers initially to sensitize (with the production of serum precipitins) and subsequently to elicit an alveolitis (probably a Type III Arthus allergic reaction). Furthermore, the heavier the dust (or antigen) exposure, the greater the attack rate among exposed nonatopic persons. Identification of the major source of allergen in *farmer's lung* (the spores of the thermophilic actinomyces, *Micropolyspora faeni,* found in moldy hay) has led to the recognition of an increasing number of diseases of similar origin; undoubtedly more will be documented in the future. The main examples currently recognized are *bagassosis,* from the spores of *Thermoactinomyces vulgaris* in moldy bagasse (sugar-cane residue used in the production of hard board, acoustic, and other thermal boards); *mushroom-worker's lung,* usually from the spores of both *T. vulgaris* and *M. faeni* in mushroom compost; and *malt-worker's lung* from the spores of *Aspergillus clavatus* and *Aspergillus fumigatus* in moldy barley and malt dust. All these spores are of the order of 6 μ or less in size, but there is evidence that spores up to 10 μ may penetrate the lung in adequate numbers to elicit alveolitis. Lung biopsy in the early stages shows a cellular

infiltration involving the alveoli and sometimes small bronchioles, with lymphocytes, plasma cells, mononuclear cells, histocytes, and multinucleated cells containing crescent-shaped basophilic inclusions. Granulomas may develop and have been attributed to a foreign body reaction resulting from the cellular removal and sequestration of large antigen-antibody complexes. These changes may resolve completely or go to fibrosis, which may also involve the organization of endobronchial exudates with bronchiolitis obliterans.

Clinical Manifestations. Symptoms usually develop within six to eight hours of exposure, commonly appearing in the evening after a day's work with moldy hay, bagasse, or some other spore source. *Fever, chills, malaise,* and generalized non-pleuritic *chest pain* are characteristic, together with a dry irritant *cough,* productive of scanty sputum, and respiratory distress. *Weight loss* is common. On clinical examination in the acute stage, rales are heard, often less widespread than anticipated, and rhonchi are not usually prominent. The chest roentgenogram, sometimes normal, characteristically shows a widespread reticular pattern and, occasionally, fine, nodular shadows, which may become confluent. Pulmonary function measurements are in keeping with the location of the disease in alveoli and small airways, i.e., gas exchange is impaired, although expiratory flow rates are usually normal. Only occasionally does an obstructive function pattern predominate.

In the absence of further exposure, clinical, radiologic, and function changes may resolve fully, only to recur with re-exposure. *A chronic form* appears to follow the superimposition of repeated acute episodes, particularly if the initial acute episode is not severe (usually because spore dose is lower) and the victim is not aware of its association with his occupation. In these individuals the chest film is more suggestive of a diffuse pulmonary fibrosis, sometimes complicated by cystic changes and associated with appropriate effects on lung function. The long-term complications include pulmonary hypertension, right heart strain, and failure.

Diagnosis and Treatment. Diagnosis during the acute attack is made on the basis of a characteristic clinical pattern, providing that there is a suitable exposure history. The chest film and lung function tests may add confirmatory evidence. A high percentage of cases have positive serologic tests (such as the demonstration of precipitins, double diffusion tests, and immunoelectrophoresis) in the acute episode, but the number diminishes with time thereafter. Taken on their own, however, positive reactions are evidence of exposure rather than evidence of disease. In subjects seen in remission, in whom serologic tests are negative, the cautious use of provocation tests involving inhaled aqueous extracts of the appropriate allergen is suggested; these result in symptoms and lung function changes several hours after the challenge. The diagnosis of the chronic case may be more difficult because of its nonspecific character, particularly if there have been no acute episodes which are clearly exposure related.

In the treatment of the acute episodes, the usual general measures are advised, together with adrenal corticosteroids which, in some cases, produce very satisfactory remissions, though it is uncertain whether they can always prevent progression to fibrosis. Avoidance of re-exposure is of prime importance to prevent repetitive episodes with progression to chronic form.

Epidemiology and Prevention. It is difficult to estimate attack rates in undefined exposed populations (as, for instance, in self-employed farmers). Furthermore, attack rates vary with spore dose, and this again will vary with the seasonal conditions predisposing to moldy hay, bagasse, or sequoia dust as the case may be. Bagassosis, once considered a rare entity, has been reported in half the workers in a Puerto Rican factory, and on another occasion in 10 per cent of employees of a West Indian sugar plant.

Prevention of extrinsic allergic alveolitis at an epidemiologic level, i.e., by removal of exposure hazards, is not easy, because the conditions favoring fungus growth and spore formation occur only intermittently. Nor is the prevention at the individual case level very practicable since masks appear to be capable only of reducing, not of wholly excluding, particles of small size such as the $1\ \mu$ spores of *M. faeni*. Furthermore, the increased resistance to breathing on exercise imposed by even the best mask limits their regular use. The only safe course is to ensure that the subject who has suffered one acute episode avoid altogether any further exposure, a drastic recommendation which may involve a farmer, for instance, in giving up his means of livelihood.

ORGANIC DUST PNEUMOCONIOSES: BYSSINOSIS

Clinical Manifestations. The diagnosis of byssinosis is made on the basis of a characteristic symptom pattern in a subject with suitable exposure to cotton, flax, or soft hemp dusts; sisal and jute dusts are probably not implicated. Symptoms are *cough, tightness in the chest,* and *breathlessness,* occurring at first occasionally on return to work after the weekend break with improvement during the working day (Grade ½), then regularly on Monday morning (Grade 1), then persisting beyond Monday (Grade 2), and finally persisting throughout the week (Grade 3), when it is indistinguishable from nonindustrial chronic obstructive lung disease. In the early stages symptoms are accompanied by parallel changes in expiratory

flow rates—$FEV_{1.0}$ and FVC. There are no specific radiologic changes. Byssinosis differs from atopic asthma in several important respects: attack rates may reach over 90 per cent of exposed populations and may first appear many years after first exposure; a family history of atopy, with hypersensitivity to inhaled histamine, is unusual; immediate skin reactions to cotton dust are infrequent. On the other hand, *Monday morning dyspnea,* like atopic asthma, is associated with reduction in forced expiratory flow rates with effects on flow volume curves which can be improved by isoproterenol inhalation. Antihistaminic drugs may also improve the flow rates in byssinosis without necessarily affording subjective relief, a finding pointing to the probable importance of small airway involvement.

Pathogenesis and Mechanisms. It is thought that some fraction of the offending dusts (probably the protein fraction) causes the nonantigenic release of histamine and perhaps other pharmacologically active substances; these reduce the caliber of large and/or small airways, the site of action perhaps being related to dust size and site of maximal deposition. Information on the nature of the long-term effects comes from the few published autopsy reports in which chronic bronchitis and emphysema were noted, together with occasional "ferruginous" bodies containing what was assumed to be cotton fibers; in addition, the lungs contain somewhat increased amounts of nonspecific dusts, probably carbonaceous. A single report of extensive fibrosis with plasma cell infiltration suggests an immunologic background for the disease, indicating the need for further study.

Epidemiology. Studies of the epidemiology of byssinosis indicate that the attack rate in the population at risk may vary very widely, from 0 per cent in some Egyptian mills and about 50 per cent in many Swedish, Dutch, and British mills, to 92 per cent in Egyptian villagers working flax in their homes. There are no recent data on how many patients with byssinosis eventually develop chronic obstructive lung disease. However, the proportion is probably not insignificant; indeed the recognition of byssinosis resulted from the observation of increased mortality and morbidity rates for cardiovascular and respiratory disease in certain Lancashire cotton workers.

Prevention. The control of byssinosis undoubtedly lies in the hands of industrial engineers, providing that risk dust levels (size and particle number) can be defined accurately. It might also be possible to remove the noxious agent from the dust, if this could be identified. Inadequate knowledge of the natural history of the disease makes it difficult for a physician to advise whether a worker should leave his employment. There seems little doubt that cigarette smoking aggravates the frequency and severity of symptoms. Regular medical surveillance of workers should be carried out, both from the point of view of identifying cases and as an index of engineering dust control.

CHEMICAL IRRITANTS PRODUCING IMMEDIATE EFFECTS PRIMARILY ON LARGE AIRWAYS
(Mists of Sulfurous Acid [H_2SO_3]; Sulfur Dioxide [SO_2], Used Widely in the Pulp and Paper Industry; Ammonia [NH_3], Used in Refrigeration Processes; Chlorine [Cl_2])

Pathogenesis and Mechanisms. The acutely irritant effects of these gases and mists can probably be attributed to their high solubility; of the physiologic gases, CO_2 is the most soluble (56.7 vols. per cent in water at 37° C. at 1 atmosphere); however, equivalent values for SO_2 (280 vols. per cent), Cl_2 (257 vols. per cent), and NH_3 (139 vols. per cent) indicate their very much greater solubility. Accidental inhalation of high concentrations results in rapid solution in the mucous membranes of the upper airways with the formation of irritant compounds, e.g., H_2SO_3 from SO_2, NH_4OH from NH_3, HCl from Cl_2. The initial irritation causing *bronchorrhea* is rapidly followed by sloughing and a *frank necrotizing bronchitis*. If exposure is prolonged or unduly heavy, the lower respiratory tract becomes exposed, with the development of an *acute chemical pulmonary edema*. Recovery may be complete. However, residual mucosal scars and submucosal thickening are not uncommon, particularly if the mucosal sloughs were deep and secondary infection prominent. Acute chemical irritation may also result from the *aspiration of vomited or regurgitated material high in HCl content,* an event more common in the frail and elderly than is generally supposed, or in relation to blunting of the gag reflex as in anesthesia, head injuries, and alcoholic or other intoxications. If the aspirate is chiefly water or saline in small amounts, absorption is quick and the consequences usually slight. Large food particles on the other hand may obstruct large or small airways.

Clinical Manifestations. When exposure to a chemical irritant is heavy, clinical manifestations are invariably immediate, the patient is alerted to his exposure, and he makes every effort to remove himself therefrom. *Conjunctivitis, irritation* and burning in the *mucosa* of the mouth and throat, *cough, laryngitis, laryngospasm,* and *difficulty in breathing* are in keeping with the usual site of damage, i.e., upper respiratory tract, and coarse *rhonchi* are a characteristic physical finding, often with profound *mucorrhea,* which may be bloodstained. More profound *dyspnea* usually implies alveolar involvement resulting from either chemical edema or aspiration of bron-

chial sloughs. These complications can frequently be suspected from chest roentgenograms and may result in profound impairment of pulmonary blood gas exchange with *severe arterial hypoxemia* and a low arterial CO_2 tension. Nausea, vomiting, and stupor may complicate the picture. If the patient survives the acute event, complete recovery is usual. However, some patients may be left with chronic bronchitis or saccular bronchiectasis or both, sometimes of considerable severity, with residual effects on pulmonary function.

Chronic irritation from long-term exposure to low doses, e.g., SO_2, as in city air pollution, Cl_2, as in chlorine plants, may perhaps be more important in terms of community health, particularly in relation to the etiology of chronic obstructive lung disease.

Treatment. *Acute chemical bronchitis* and *acute chemical pulmonary edema* are *medical emergencies.* In the acute phase, survival depends on maintaining airway patency and adequate oxygenation. To aspirate sloughs, it may be necessary to employ intubation, lavage with saline, and even bronchoscopy. Controlled oxygen administration is usually necessary, and frequently must be supplemented with positive pressure respiration, assisted in mild cases, controlled in the severe ones. Corticosteroids, thought to modify the acute inflammatory reaction at the gas-exchanging surface, should always be given in the presence of pulmonary edema and indeed are recommended by some in all cases of exposure on a prophylactic basis. Heavy initial doses should be reduced as the clinical picture improves. Infection should be controlled by the use of antimicrobial drugs.

CHEMICAL IRRITANTS PRODUCING DELAYED EFFECTS, PRIMARILY ON SMALL AIRWAYS AND LUNG PARENCHYMA
(Oxides of Nitrogen; Phosgene)

Pathogenesis and Mechanisms. Oxides of nitrogen and phosgene are considered separately because of their unusual but characteristic clinical presentation. The immediate clinical effects may be mild, but a severe, chemical pulmonary edema, often fatal, may develop after a *delay of several hours to several days.* The physiochemical processes underlying this delay are not fully understood.

If the acute event is not immediately fatal, healing by fibrosis may lead to the development of *bronchiolitis fibrosa obliterans,* usually four to eight weeks after initial exposure, often with a fatal result. Autopsy studies show widespread organization of exudates, primarily located in the terminal bronchioles; atelectasis is not seen, however, presumably because of collateral ventilation recently recognized to be extensive in man.

Clinical Manifestations. Immediate effects of exposure, which may include cough, chest irritation, and sputum, are often so mild that the victim may even fail to report to the first-aid post, only to return from hours to several days later with the symptoms, signs, and chest roentgenogram of *acute, severe, pulmonary edema.* By contrast, in the mild case of edema, symptoms may escape attention, changes on the chest film may be at the most equivocal, and the diagnosis depends on the finding of coarse rales, sometimes lasting over a short period only, with a transient hypoxemia. Clinical management has been discussed above; steroid therapy should probably be prolonged for six to eight weeks to cover the period when the subacute complication of bronchiolitis obliterans is likely to develop. This complication, probably avoidable if steroid therapy is given early, should be suspected when symptoms recur or appear at three to six weeks, and also appears to respond to steroid therapy. The residual effects, though presumably dependent on the extent of the initial damage and the vigor with which treatment is pursued, are usually slight, probably because of the location of the subacute lesions in small airways.

Epidemiology. Large scale heavy exposure to, for instance, oxides of nitrogen occurs only in relation to mass disasters, e.g., in the Cleveland clinic fire in 1929 owing to the burning of stored x-ray film, and in the Cocoanut Grove fire in Boston in 1943 owing to the burning of nitrogen-containing plastics. Many modern plastics no longer contain nitrogen. However, in most fires involving domestic buildings in which wood is used, circumstances exist in which these fumes could be evolved, and three or four cases annually are seen in most city hospitals. Other circumstances favoring the release of oxides of nitrogen are welding in closed spaces, combustion of rocket fuel, and blasting in enclosed areas. Finally, in rural communities where large silos are used for storage, exposure may occur on first entering a silo in which the ensilage was stored green (*silo-filler's disease*). Phosgene may be liberated from many chlorinated substances, such as carbon tetrachloride in fire extinguishers or chloroform in laboratory fires.

CHEMICAL IRRITANTS PRODUCING REACTIONS SUGGESTING SENSITIZATION

(Organic Isocyanates Used in Manufacturing and Applying Lacquers, Resins, Plastic Foams and Allied Material; and in Upholstery, Toys, and Insulation)

Isocyanate vapors are an irritant to the mucous membranes of the eyes, mouth, and upper respiratory tract, but the threshold limit value, a ceiling value, for toluene 2-4-diisocyanate is 0.02 ppm., probably well below the levels at which such symptoms occur. Nevertheless, after a period which seems to vary from one week to several months, these very low levels appear capable of inducing a sensitization so that if a temporary rise in concentration occurs even up to 0.2 ppm., for example, after spillage, *acute symptoms suggesting asthma* develop *in the sensitized person.* These include breathlessness, chest tightness, diffuse rhonchi, and sometimes severe mucorrhea and sputum, with a marked fall in expiratory flow rates. Symptoms subside after removal from exposure, and function may return to normal within days. However, re-exposure regularly results in recurrence, often more violent. The number of people who become sensitized varies and may be related to exposure level (estimated at 4 per cent in a well-controlled plant and 100 per cent in a poor one). Nor are the victims characteristically atopic individuals; demonstrable skin sensitivity and positive reactions to inhaled histamine are unusual. Indeed, most exposed persons show some reduction in expiratory flow rates during working hours, a change eliminated by the oral administration of an aminophylline compound. Experiments in laboratory animals suggest that isocyanates may act antigenically, but precipitating antibodies have not been looked for in exposed humans. There is some evidence that prolonged exposure may lead to chronic bronchitis. Diagnosis depends on a high level of suspicion, and treatment consists in removal from exposure.

RADIATION

Increased use of x-irradiation in the treatment of cancer of the breast and of various intrathoracic organs led to the recognition that the lungs themselves may be affected by this procedure. *Acute changes* may come on within weeks of the onset of treatment up to six months after its cessation. These include an alveolar cellular reaction followed by desquamation and in some instances by hyaline membrane formation, and there may be focal necrosis of the bronchial mucosa, small vessel thrombosis, and lymphectasia. These changes may resolve or go on to loss of lung volume, sometimes of marked degree, occurring rather suddenly, and usually ascribed to fibrosis, shrinkage, and hyalinization, particularly if there has been infection. Studies in animals suggest, however, that the loss of volume may, on occasion, be due to atrophy and that the hyalinization may be in part due to autohypersensitivity, the consequence of new cell antigens formed as a result of the ionizing radiation.

There may be no clinical manifestations of *radiation pneumonitis* even in the face of definite radiologic changes. The most common symptom is a persistent, hacking dry cough. Fever, some dyspnea, and weakness may be seen, and the symptoms of radiation esophagitis are common. On physical examination the effects of radiation on the skin of the thorax are usually evident; rales and a friction rub may be found. The chest film characteristically reveals regional or diffuse haziness. Spontaneous remission over weeks is frequent. Recommended therapy includes steroids (to lessen the chances of healing by fibrosis) and anticoagulants (to lessen the ischemic effects of small-vessel thrombosis commonly seen at autopsy), though the value of these measures has not been conclusively demonstrated (see article on Thromboembolic Diseases). When *radiation fibrosis* supervenes, clinical presentation will depend on how much functioning lung tissue is lost and on the function in the remaining lung. Respiratory failure, pulmonary hypertension, and right heart failure may all follow.

Following x-irradiation to the thorax mild radiation pneumonitis is probably common if not invariable, though symptoms occur in a small percentage of these cases only, and progression to radiation fibrosis is rare. Factors thought to affect the attack rate include total dose as well as the time over which it is given, and the technique of application. The age of the patient, the chest wall thickness, and the presence of complicating disease may also be important. Individual factors remain to be identified, however, since identical doses can be harmless to one person and cause a severe reaction in another.

Inorganic Dusts

Becklake, M. R.: Pneumoconioses. *In* Handbook of Physiology, Respiration II. Baltimore, Williams & Wilkins Company, 1965, Chapter 71, p. 1601.

Biological effects of asbestos. Ann. N.Y. Acad. Sci., 132:338, 1965.

Bruce, T.: Occupational diseases of respiratory system. Scand. J. Resp. Dis., 63(supp.):73, 1968.

Davies, C. N. (ed.): Inhaled Particles and Vapours. II. Oxford, Pergamon Press, Ltd., 1967.

Gilson, J. C.: Industrial Pulmonary Disease. *In* Schilling, R. S. F. (ed.): Modern Trends in Occupational Health. London, Butterworth & Company, Publishers, Ltd., 1960, p. 50.

Hatch, T. F., and Gross, P.: Pulmonary Deposition and Retention of Inhaled Aerosols. New York, Academic Press, Inc., 1964.

King, E. J., and Fletcher, C. M. (eds.): Industrial Pulmonary Diseases. London, J. and A. Churchill, Ltd., 1960.

Orenstein, A. J. (ed.): Proceedings of the Pneumoconiosis Conference, Johannesburg, 1959. London, J. and A. Churchill, Ltd., 1960.

Selikoff, I. J., Bader, R. A., Bader, M. E., Churg, J., and Hammond, E. C.: Asbestosis and neoplasia. Amer. J. Med., 42:487, 1967.

Stoeckle, J. D., Hardy, H. L., and Weber, A. L.: Chronic beryllium disease: Long-term follow-up of sixty cases and selective review of the literature. Amer. J. Med., 46:545, 1969.

Organic Dusts

Bouhuys, A., Heaphy, L. J., Schilling, R. S. F., and Welborn, J. W.: Byssinosis in the United States. New Eng. J. Med., 277:170, 1967.

El Batawi, M. A., Schilling, R. S. F., Valic, F., and Walford, J.: Byssinosis in the Egyptian cotton industry; Changes in ventilatory capacity during the day. Brit. J. Industr. Med., 21:13, 1964.

Hearn, C. E. D.: Bagassosis: An epidemiological, environmental and clinical Survey. Brit. J. Industr. Med., 25:267, 1968.

Hogg, J. C., Macklem, P. T., and Thurlbeck, W. M.: Site and nature of airway obstruction in chronic obstructive lung disease. New Eng. J. Med., 278:1355, 1968.

Pepys, J.: Monographs in Allergy. 4. Hypersensitivity Diseases of the Lungs due to Fungi and Organic Dusts. Basel, S. Karger, 1969.

Schilling, R. S. F.: Byssinosis in cotton and other textile workers. Lancet, 2:261, 319, 1956.

Chemical Irritants

Bates, D. V., and Christie, R. V.: Respiratory Function in Disease. Philadelphia, W. B. Saunders Company, 1964.

Connor, E. H., DuBois, A. B., and Comroe, J. H.: Acute chemical injury of the airways and lungs. Anesthesiology, 23:538, 1962.

Lancet Leading Article: Hazards of di-isocyanates. Lancet, 1:32, 1966.

Morrow, P.: Adaptations of the respiratory tract to air pollutants. Arch. Environ. Health (Chicago), 14:127, 1967.

Moskowitz, R. L., Lyons, H. A., and Cottle, H. R.: Silo-filler's disease: Clinical, physiological and pathological study of a patient. Amer. J. Med., 36:457, 1964.

Radiation

Smith, J. C.: Radiation pneumonitis: A review. Amer. Rev. Resp. Dis., 87:647, 1963.

Neoplasms of the Lung

Alvan R. Feinstein

The benign or malignant clinical consequences of pulmonary neoplasms depend on their biologic behavior, as demonstrated by the site, anatomic dissemination, and functional effects of the tumors, rather than by histologic type alone. A histologically "benign" tumor can become lethal by leading to such complications as exsanguinating hemoptysis, pneumonia, or lung abscess. Conversely, a histologically "malignant" tumor may not be fatal if it grows slowly enough to be found and removed before it disseminates. Uncommonly, a slow-growing carcinoma may be undetected during life and first found at necropsy after the patient has died of some other disease.

Anatomic Locations and Histologic Types. Tumors of the lung can arise from any part of the trachea, bronchi, bronchial tree, pulmonary parenchyma, or pleura. Although larger bronchi are the most common sites of primary lung tumors, only about 25 per cent of the tumors are central enough to be seen at bronchoscopy.

Despite occasional dissents, most pathologists believe that the tissue types of lung tumors can be usefully and consistently classified. No current scheme of histologic classification is used universally, however, and diverse discrepancies have been reported in reclassifications of the same tumor. Most current histologic classifications include such cellular types as epidermoid (or squamous), large cell anaplastic, small cell anaplastic (or "oat cell"), and alveolar cell carcinomas, as well as adenocarcinomas, adenomas, hamartomas, mesotheliomas, and a variety of other types.

Metastatic Neoplastic Disease of the Lung. The lung is a frequent site of metastasis from carcinomas originating elsewhere, particularly in the kidney, thyroid, breast, testis, or intestine. The cellular types and biologic behavior of the metastases in the lung usually depend on the characteristics of the primary tumor. When multiple lesions are found on a chest roentgenogram, an extrapulmonary tumor can be suspected; when the lesion is solitary in an asymptomatic patient, its differentiation from a primary lung tumor may be difficult and is sometimes resolved only after surgical exploration.

Primary Neoplastic Disease of the Lung. Carcinomas are the most common type of primary lung neoplasm. Among 785 primary lung tumors diagnosed consecutively in adults at a single medical center in the United States, 708 were carcinomas, 18 were bronchial adenomas, 10 were hamartomas, 8 were pleural mesotheliomas, and 3 were primary tracheal tumors. The remainder consisted of 2 teratomas, 2 fibromas, 2 lymphosarcomas, 1 fibrosarcoma, 1 sarcoma, 1 neurofibroma, and 1 Hodgkin's disease. These patterns and ratios of occurrence are similar to those reported in England and in Israel. The proportion of different cellular types in primary carcinomas will vary at any medical center according to the histologic criteria used by the pathologist. In general, squamous cell tumors are the most common, followed in frequency by anaplastic tumors and adenocarcinomas.

Bronchial adenomas, which are particularly common in women, usually have a central location and during their slow growth often produce repeated small hemoptyses or bouts of pulmonary infection that may recur for a long time before the patient seeks medical attention. Peripheral tumors are often detected before they become symptomatic, particularly in countries where diagnostic roentgenograms are readily available. A routine roentgenogram may show an unexpected circumscribed shadow that, when circular, is often called a "coin lesion." *Hamartomas* of the lung are usually peripheral and are often found by surgical exploration of such a symptomatically silent coin lesion. *Adenocarcinomas* tend to be peripherally located, whereas most other types of primary carcinoma are central. *Mesotheliomas* arise in the pleura and produce clinical manifestations related to pleural effusion or invasion of the chest wall.

Aside from these morphologic distinctions, neoplasms of the lung show no constant correlations between histologic type and clinical manifestations. Primary carcinoma, as the predominant neoplasm in this group of tumors, will be the topic of the remainder of this discussion.

PRIMARY CARCINOMA OF THE LUNG

Occurrence. The occurrence rate of cancer of the lung is difficult to estimate because the annual statistics for a particular population depend on the likelihood of a correct diagnosis being established in members of the population who have the disease. The opportunity to establish a correct diagnosis has sharply increased in recent years, with the frequent use of chest roentgenograms and with the availability of such diagnostic techniques as bronchoscopy, biopsy of affected structures, and cytologic examination of sputum and other fluids. Moreover, many tumors unidentified by these techniques are now found either during life by greater use of exploratory thoracotomy or after death through the increasing performance of necropsy. These augmented diagnostic techniques lead to the detection of many cases of lung cancer today that might have been unrecognized years ago. During the past few decades, the occurrence rates of lung cancer have risen markedly, particularly in countries where the cited diagnostic aids are available and in general use.

In addition to these distinctions, several other features of diagnostic selectivity tend to cloud the epidemiologic picture. Patients referred to medical centers for specialized modes of therapy, such as thoracic surgery, high voltage radiotherapy, and new chemotherapeutic agents, may not reflect the true distribution of lung cancer in that community or in other regions. Certain cancers formerly regarded as metastatic have been called primary in the past few decades, after pathologists recognized that nonbronchogenic lung cancers can arise peripherally and disseminate widely to other parts of the body. The opportunity for cancer to develop is enhanced by the increased life span of people who formerly might have died at a young age because of microbial diseases that today are prevented or cured by sanitation, vaccination, and the various agents of modern therapy.

For all these reasons, cancer of the lung is now diagnosed more frequently than ever before. The epidemiologic significance of the increase is difficult to evaluate, but the clinical significance of this increased occurrence rate is that lung cancer is now perhaps the most commonly recognized form of carcinoma in man.

Etiology and Prevention. No single cause for lung tumors has been identified. Most public health authorities are now convinced that cigarette smoking is a major factor, particularly for squamous cell tumors. Tobacco has had a less striking role in undifferentiated tumors, however, and has not been proposed as a cause of human adenocarcinomas and other forms of lung neoplasia. The statistical evidence associating smoking and lung cancer has been accepted generally but not unanimously, because none of the groups under investigation contained a truly random sampling of a nonvolunteer population, and the statements on death certificates were not examined for "false negative" diagnoses of cancer. Nevertheless, in each study the rates of lung cancer were higher in smokers than in nonsmokers. Although the statistical controversy is not yet settled, reduction or cessation of cigarette smoking may help prevent certain forms of lung cancer and may be beneficial in various other pulmonary or cardiac diseases.

Among the other agents variously invoked as contributory factors in causing lung cancer are atmospheric fumes and pollution (among urban dwellers), air-borne radiation (among uranium miners), proliferating scar tissue (in patients with previous pulmonary infections), and sauna bathing (in Finland). Inhalation of asbestos fibers appears to have a dose-related role in the lung cancers found in asbestos workers, and has been suspected as a cause of mesotheliomas. Genetic factors may be implicated by reports that relatives of lung cancer patients have a higher death rate from lung cancer than matched controls.

The many conflicting claims and counterclaims about the cause of lung cancer will probably not be resolved until prolonged, well-designed clinical epidemiologic studies can be conducted.

The Spectrum of Clinical Patterns

By metastasis or by many other mechanisms, a lung cancer can affect the structure or function of almost any system in the body. The functional disorders can be "direct" effects, due to the physical presence of the tumor at the involved site, or "indirect" effects, occurring without anatomic dissemination of tumor to the affected site or system.

Some of the effects are *pulmonic*, arising from the affected lung, pleura, or chest wall. Others are *extrapulmonic*, arising more remotely from involvement of the mediastinum or of regions beyond the thorax. The extrapulmonic effects can be *systemic* or *metastatic*, or both. Because these different manifestations of cancer of the lung can occur alone or in various combinations, the disease has a wide, protean spectrum with many different patterns of appearance.

Figure 1 is a Venn diagram that shows the clinical spectrum of lung cancer according to the presence or absence of any of the described pulmonic, systemic, and metastatic features. The numbers in each subset of this diagram indicate the proportionate distribution of these clinical features at the time of diagnostic detection of lung

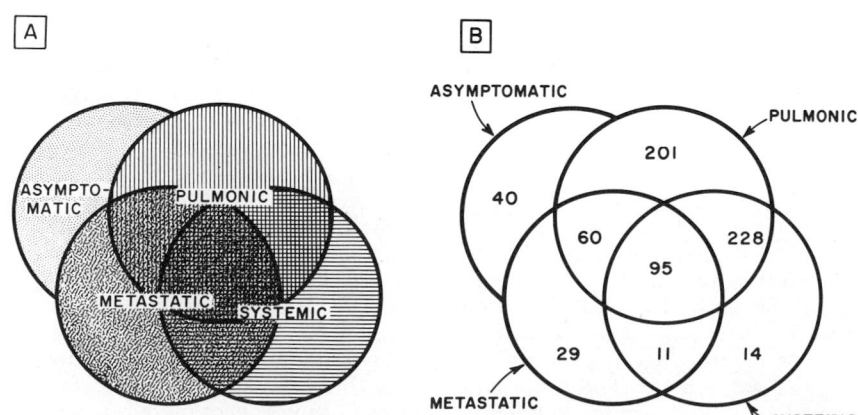

FIGURE 1. The clinical spectrum of lung cancer. The three main circles of the Venn diagram in part A are shaded to demonstrate sets of patients with pulmonic, systemic, or metastatic manifestations, as described in the text. The overlap of the circles produces seven subsets, in which these manifestations are present alone or in various combinations. An eighth subset, containing asymptomatic patients, is appended at the upper left of the diagram. Part B, for which the shading is removed, demonstrates the number of patients in each of these subsets at the time of clinical detection of lung cancer in 678 cases.

cancer in 678 consecutive patients. The most common pattern of appearance was the combination of pulmonic and systemic symptoms, which were present in 228 patients. Of the other patients in this series, 201 had pulmonic symptoms only, 95 had a combination of pulmonic, systemic, and metastatic features, 40 were asymptomatic, 29 first presented only with metastatic features, and the remaining cases were distributed as shown.

Diagnosis

As shown in Figure 1, patients with lung cancer frequently seek medical attention after development of a cough, often with hemoptysis and with an associated infection or chest pain. Anorexia and weight loss may also be present, and the chest roentgenogram almost always shows an abnormal shadow or shadows.

Although no single pattern of clinical and roentgenographic features is either characteristic or pathognomonic for diagnosis, certain manifestations are particularly suggestive. Lung cancer is suggested clinically by the combination of hemoptysis, weight loss, and clubbing in a patient who has no evidence of infection, congenital heart disease, or previous lung disease. The roentgenographic findings that most suggest lung cancer are (a) a mass arising in the hilar area; (b) an apparently pneumonic infiltrate that persists long after improvement of concomitant clinical symptoms; (c) a mass that obstructs a bronchus, usually demonstrated by tomography; and (d) a localized peripheral or coin lesion that shows no calcium in tomographic views. Nevertheless, all of these and other clinical and roentgenographic manifestations associated with lung cancer can be produced by such diseases as tuberculosis or tuberculomas, various chronic pneumonias, granulomas, and many other entities.

In diagnosis, therefore, the patient's signs and symptoms serve mainly to suggest the presence of a pulmonary lesion whose existence and extent can be shown with roentgenographic evidence, which can also be used to detect lesions in asymptomatic patients. To specify the identity of a pulmonary lesion, however, additional tests are necessary to exclude causes other than cancer, and to provide cytologic or histologic evidence of the neoplasm. Many infectious or inflammatory causes of lung lesions can be identified by appropriate examination of sputum or blood, although their demonstration does not exclude the possible coexistence of an underlying lung cancer.

Papanicolaou smears of the sputum are often positive in patients with primary carcinoma, particularly if special techniques are used to induce sputum when it is absent, and particularly when the tumor is centrally located. Peripheral cancers, however, may not communicate well with the bronchial tree or may not exfoliate enough cells to yield positive results on cytologic examination. In these circumstances, the tests of sputum may produce "false negative" results; a rare "false positive" may occur in patients who have chronic bronchial inflammation rather than cancer.

Bronchoscopy is useful both for grossly visualizing the tumor (when possible) and for obtaining bronchial specimens for histologic or cytologic examination. Most other pathologic specimens used for the diagnosis of lung cancer are obtained by biopsy of metastatic sites or from the fluid of a neoplastic pleural or pericardial effusion. A favorite location of metastasis for lung cancer is the mediastinal and supraclavicular lymph nodes. Mediastinoscopy and biopsy of the scalene nodes are often done to obtain histologic evidence when none is otherwise available, and also to exclude metastasis, although a scalene node biopsy is seldom positive for tumor unless the node is palpably enlarged.

In some instances, when no other cytologic evidence is obtainable, needle biopsy of a peripheral lung lesion may disclose the tumor. More often, however, when diagnostic tests have failed to identify the roentgenographic lesion, exploratory thoracotomy is performed. Because the risk is low, surgical thoracic exploration is now a common diagnostic procedure in these circumstances. A benign tumor, granuloma, or a metastasis from a "silent" primary site may sometimes be found, but just as often a lung cancer is discovered in a still curable state. Among patients with "operable" lung cancer, about 70 per cent do not have a specific histologic diagnosis established until thoracotomy.

Correlation of Anatomic, Functional, and Clinical Manifestations

The direct and indirect effects of lung cancer can produce a variety of anatomic, clinical, and other manifestations.

Pulmonic Manifestations. These manifestations can be bronchial, parenchymal, and parietal.

Bronchial Manifestations. Irritation of bronchial mucosa by tumor or by inflammation adjacent to the tumor may cause a change in the pattern of a chronic cough or may produce a wholly new cough. Hemoptysis of bright red blood, flecks of blood, or "rusty" sputum may be due to vascular invasion or to pneumonia developing behind the tumor. Occasionally, the tumor may occlude enough of a large bronchus to make the patient notice a respiratory wheeze.

Parenchymal Manifestations. An obstructed bronchial lumen may cause retention of secretions, predisposing to parenchymal infection; if the lumen is completely obstructed, the distal parenchyma may become atelectatic. Although roentgenographically apparent atelectasis may be asymptomatic, parenchyma that is infected or inflamed may produce all of the classic clinical, bacteriologic, and roentgenographic manifestations of a pneumonia. After conventional treatment of the pneumonia, the patient may have a conventional symptomatic and bacteriologic response, but the roentgenogram may then fail to clear because of the underlying neoplasm. In this circumstance, the "unresolved pneumonia" becomes the clue that leads to further tests and discovery of the tumor. A lung abscess can sometimes be produced at the site of such a pneumonia, although an alternative cause of lung abscess is necrosis of the interior of a large tumor.

As a parenchymal manifestation, dyspnea is the direct result of metastasis when the tumor either replaces large amounts of parenchymal tissue or, more commonly, invades the pleural surface, a subsequent effusion reducing the space available for ventilation. In many other circumstances, however, dyspnea may be indirect, occurring because (1) parenchymal inflammation extending to the pleura initiates a pleural effusion (as described in the next section), (2) the primary tumor may locally obstruct the trachea or carina, or (3) the amount of secondary parenchymal inflammation or atelectasis may be great enough to impair ventilation in a patient whose respiratory reserve had been reduced — by chronic lung disease or by poor cardiac compensation — before the tumor developed.

Parietal Manifestations. Involvement of the pleural surface can produce inspiratory chest pain, the physical findings of an effusion, or dyspnea if the effusion is massive. In one form of indirect pleural involvement due to the inflammatory extension of pneumonia developing behind the primary tumor, the pleural fluid is often pink or bloody. Another form of indirect pleural involvement, usually associated with a serous pleural effusion, occurs when the primary tumor obstructs appropriate vascular and lymphatic channels draining the pleura. In both of these indirect circumstances, the pleural fluid contains no tumor cells. In other circumstances, however, the pleura can be directly invaded via contiguous spread from a peripherally located tumor or by lymphatic metastases from a tumor in the bronchus. A neoplastic pleural effusion is seldom clinically different from one that is inflammatory or hydrostatic, but the fluid is more likely to be bloody and will usually contain cancer cells.

Although pleural involvement is the most common single cause of chest pain in lung cancer, inspiratory chest pain may also occur when a peripheral tumor extends through the pleura to the chest wall, involving muscle, bone, or both. Rib invasion may alternatively occur as a distant metastasis from a central tumor, rather than by direct extension of a peripheral tumor. Chest pain that lacks inspiratory accentuation can develop with invasion of an upper rib, sternum, or thoracic vertebra. The tumor may sometimes extend beyond the vertebra or rib to involve a thoracic nerve, with pain in the anatomic distribution of the nerve.

Extrapulmonic Manifestations. The many possible extrapulmonic manifestations of lung cancer include *systemic features,* which are often indirect, and *metastatic features,* which are due to direct spread of tumor to the affected site.

Systemic Manifestations. *General.* Anorexia may occur indirectly because of persistent infection, pain, or other discomforts of the pulmonic features just cited. With decreased food intake, the patient may then lose weight and become easily fatigued. Alternatively, however, anorexia and other digestive disturbances can be the direct result of hepatic, peritoneal, or other intra-abdominal metastases.

Hypertrophic Pulmonary Osteoarthropathy. Clubbing of the fingers and/or pain in the articular extremities of long bones can occur with either central or peripheral tumors of the lung. One or both manifestations may appear before or after other clinical evidence of the tumor, and they may sometimes be the earliest or the only clinical clues that suggest the presence of a lung cancer.

The clubbing has no physical characteristics to distinguish it from the clubbing sometimes found in congenital heart disease, chronic lung disease, and other non-neoplastic entities; and careful criteria are often needed to establish that the fingers are indeed clubbed. "Curving" of the nail bed must be distinguished from true clubbing and familial clubbing from that due to an acquired pathologic lesion.

The osteoarthropathy is actually a "periostopathy" and, when present, involves the distal third of a long bone, commonly in the leg. The proliferative periostitis makes the affected bone exquisitely tender to pressure; an associated synovitis is sometimes present and may make the subcutaneous tissues swollen and the joint painful on movement. Although the articular surface of the neighboring joint is not affected, the clinical symptoms and signs in the knees or ankles may mimic a primary arthritis, and may receive such a diagnosis until the periosteal changes are noted roentgenographically. By palpating tenderness in the bone well beyond the region of the joint, the clinician can suspect osteoarthropathy before the radiologist finds it.

The mechanisms of clubbing and of hypertrophic osteoarthropathy are unknown. A neural pathway has been suggested because vagotomy may sometimes relieve the manifestations even though the tumor remains intact. Since the manifestations are also commonly improved by direct treatment that removes or shrinks the primary tumor, the mechanism may be hormonal, due to some substance secreted by the tumor.

"Endocrine" Effects. With the availability of modern laboratory techniques, many "hormonal" effects, although not common, have been reported with almost any type of lung tumor, most often with "oat cell" cancers. So many different systems have been involved that lung cancer seems to have the occasional capacity for either acting like an auxiliary pituitary gland or for producing other nonpituitary hormonal effects.

When a patient with lung cancer has an endocrine problem resulting from a *decrease* in hormone, the cause is usually destruction of the glandular site by metastasis. An *increase* in hormone may represent one of the functional "endocrinopathies" – discussed in detail under Endocrinology – that can produce adrenal hyperfunction, inappropriate antidiuresis, hypercalcemia, or the carcinoid syndrome. The hypersecretive endocrine problems can often occur without metastasis and can sometimes be the first evidence of the tumor.

The weakness often associated with lung cancer was long regarded only as a nonspecific systemic effect until the discovery in recent years that many instances of weakness were due to *neurologic lesions*, occurring without metastasis and presumably caused by a secretory product of the tumor. The lesions can include cortical cerebellar degeneration, peripheral neuropathies, encephalomyelitis, and various myopathic syndromes.

Metastatic Manifestations. Mediastinal. Hoarseness occurs when tumor impinges on the mediastinal portion of the recurrent left laryngeal nerve. The subsequent paralysis of the left vocal cord is demonstrated at laryngoscopy (or bronchoscopy).

The superior vena cava syndrome can be produced by metastases in mediastinal nodes. Lung cancer today is the most common cause of the suffusion and brawny edema that occur in the face, neck, or upper arms as a consequence of compression or invasion of the superior vena cava.

Involvement of the esophagus by lung cancer in the mediastinum can produce the same clinical pattern of *dysphagia* noted in esophageal carcinoma.

Although *myocardial involvement* is rare in lung cancer, direct invasion of the pericardium is more common. Neoplastic cells found in a bloody pericardial effusion may sometimes be the first evidence of the cancer.

Superior Sulcus Tumors. Carcinomas arising in the apex of the lung, which are sometimes called Pancoast tumors, can invade adjacent bone or the nerve bundles that pass through the thoracic inlet. Involvement of the first or second rib can produce local pain; involvement of the brachial plexus can produce sensory or motor disturbances in the arm; and involvement of the sympathetic nerve chain can produce a Horner's syndrome on the affected side.

Extrathoracic Manifestations. Cancer of the lung can metastasize to any structure of the body. The brain has been a distant metastatic site so commonly that pulmonary examination is often performed to exclude metastasis from a lung cancer in any adult suspected of having a primary brain tumor.

Among the other diverse extrathoracic metastatic manifestations of lung cancer are pathologic fractures of bone, the development of multiple cutaneous nodules, hypoadrenalism due to metastatic replacement of the adrenal glands, diabetes mellitus due to destruction of the pancreas, gastrointestinal bleeding from metastasis to small bowel, jaundice from metastasis to periportal nodes, ascites from peritoneal invasion, and various peripheral neurologic manifestations from metastasis to vertebrae or to spinal cord.

Prognosis and Treatment

Therapeutic procedures in lung cancer begin with the diagnostic and epidemiologic effort to detect the tumor in a premetastatic state, suitable for surgical resection. The effort depends on the hope that symptomatic patients will seek medical aid promptly and that asymptomatic patients, not under medical surveillance, will be found by widespread use of routine roentgenography of the chest.

This hope of "early discovery" followed by surgical cure, which currently seems to be the most effective form of therapy, is often thwarted by diverse biologic behavior in the rate and direction of growth of the cancer. Symptomatic patients with a rapidly growing tumor may seek medical aid promptly but may already have metastases. Conversely, the initial symptoms of a slowly growing tumor may be so mild and unprovocative that a long time elapses before the patient decides to see a physician; yet the lesion may still be curable by surgical resection despite the apparently "late" treatment. Among asymptomatic patients with no previous roentgenograms, a shadow found unexpectedly in a routine film often represents a slowly growing curable tumor. If the shadow is found on the *subsequent* film of an asymptomatic patient, the increment of size in the interval between "negative" and "positive" film helps denote the rate of growth of the tumor; and for a rapid-growing tumor, even an "early" asymptomatic discovery may sometimes come too "late."

The Venn diagram of Figure 2*A* shows the same clinical spectrum depicted in Figure 1, but the eight subsets are rearranged to form five clinical stages of disease. Stage I contains the subset of patients who were detected while asymptomatic. Stages II and III are formed by dividing, into two parts, the subset of patients with pulmonic manifestations only. In Stage II the duration of symptoms was "long," i.e., six months or more, before diagnostic detection of the disease, and in Stage III, the duration was "short," i.e., less than six months. Stage IV combines the two subsets of patients in Figure 1 who had either systemic manifestations only or pulmonic and systemic manifestations – but no metastatic features. Stage V combines the four subsets of patients in Figure 1 who had metastatic manifestations, with or without systemic and with or without pulmonic features.

For the entire series of 678 patients shown in Figure 2*B*, 56 (8 per cent) were alive five years later; but a distinct prognostic gradient occurred in the five-year survival rates among the five stages, ranging from 28 per cent in Stage I progressively downward to 0.5 per cent in Stage V. The biologic explanations for these differences are that metastatic symptoms denote an unfavorable outcome regardless of rate of growth of the tumor,

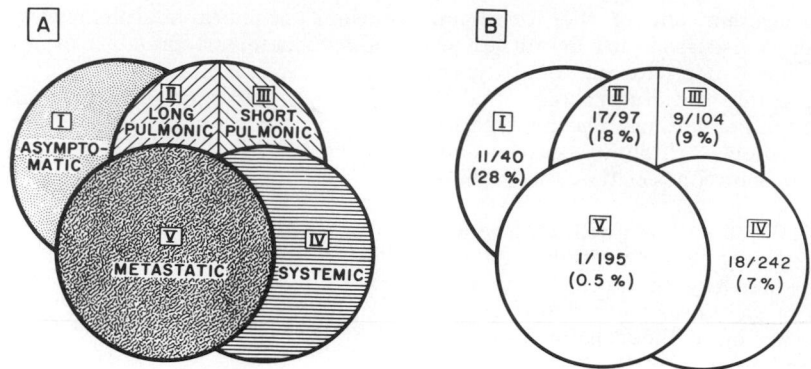

FIGURE 2. Clinical stages and prognosis in lung cancer. In part A, the Venn diagram of Figure 1A is rearranged to portray the five clinical stages described in the text, and identified here with Roman numerals. Part B shows the five-year survival rates, regardless of therapy, for patients in these five stages. The denominators indicate the number of patients initially detected in each stage, the numerators indicate the number who survived five years or more, and the percentages are the five-year survival rates. Further details are presented in the text and in the table.

and that, when metastatic symptoms are absent, patients in Stages I and II would be more likely to have slowly growing, functionally favorable tumors than those in Stages III and IV.

The appended table contains additional data showing the biologic and post-therapeutic differences of these 678 patients. Although the total operability rate was 43 per cent, surgical thoracic exploration was performed in 83 per cent of patients in Stage I and in 63 per cent of those in Stage II. For the 207 patients in whom surgical resection was possible, the over-all five-year survival rate was 27 per cent, but this rate was significantly higher (37 to 38 per cent) in the patients of Stages I and II. Even in patients whose tumors were regarded either as inoperable or as unremovable during surgical exploration, a distinct biologic prognostic gradient was present among the five clinical stages. Although only one of the 471 patients with unresectable tumor was alive five years later, 11 per cent of these patients lived more than one year, and the best one-year survival rates (20 to 25 per cent) occurred in the patients with unresectable tumors of Stages I and II.

These biologic distinctions must be borne in mind for selecting and evaluating different modes of therapy. Unless patients are analyzed according to both morphologic and clinical features, the compared populations will not be similar, and many triumphs attributed to therapy may actually be due to unrecognized aspects of the neoplasm's biologic behavior. The slow production of symptoms by slowly growing tumors is probably responsible for the better survival rates in patients of Stage II, whose tumors were discovered "late," than in Stage III patients with similar symptoms but "early" discoveries.

A morphologic prerequisite to surgical resection is location of the tumor at a resectable site, i.e., not in the trachea or carina. A functional prerequisite is the ability of the patient to tolerate both the operation itself and the subsequent reduction in functioning lung tissue. For the resection, some surgeons routinely perform pneumonectomy and radical dissection of mediastinal nodes regardless of the apparent gross extent of the tumor. Other surgeons—hoping to preserve as much normal lung tissue as possible—confine resection to the smallest amount of lung in which

PROGNOSIS AND TREATMENT IN 678 CASES OF LUNG CANCER

Clinical Stage	Clinical Characteristics	Patients Who Had Surgical Exploration	Patients Without Surgical Resection; 1-yr. Survival Rate	Patients Who Had Surgical Resection; 5-yr. Survival Rate
I	Asymptomatic	33/40 (83%)	2/10 (20%)	11/30 (37%)
II	Pulmonic symptoms only, for 6 months or more	61/97 (63%)	13/52 (25%)	17/45 (38%)
III	Pulmonic symptoms only, for less than 6 months	52/104 (50%)	11/63 (17%)	9/41 (22%)
IV	Systemic symptoms; No metastatic symptoms	118/242 (49%)	15/163 (9%)	17/79 (22%)
V	Metastatic symptoms	26/195 (12%)	12/183 (7%)	1/12 (8%)
TOTAL		290/678 (43%)	53/471 (11%)	55/207 (27%)

the tumor appears grossly contained. At operation, some surgeons may decide against resection of primary tumor if metastatic deposits are adjacent to the aorta, pericardium, or other critical mediastinal structures; other surgeons remove both the primary tumor and any deposits that do not actually invade the adjacent structures. A "palliative" resection of the primary tumor is sometimes performed despite apparent "incurability" in order to relieve hypertrophic pulmonary osteoarthropathy or lung abscess.

Irradiation may be used before or after surgery or when surgery is unfeasible. By "shrinking" a juxtacarinal lesion or mediastinal nodes, irradiation may sometimes permit subsequent surgery in a previously "inoperable" case. Radiotherapy is particularly valuable for pain due to bony metastasis and for alleviating such symptoms as osteoarthropathy, superior vena cava syndrome, and vocal cord paralysis. Malignant pleural effusions are sometimes treated by instillation of radioactive gold or other radiotherapeutic or chemotherapeutic substances.

Antineoplastic chemotherapy is usually reserved for widely disseminated tumors beyond help by either surgery or irradiation. In the panorama of available chemotherapeutic agents, the nitrogen mustard group has often had transiently good results with the superior vena cava syndrome and in cutaneous metastases. No antineoplastic agent has been consistently successful in metastatic cancer, but new agents are constantly becoming available. Although l-asparaginase has not had striking results, cyclophosphamide may prove useful.

Supportive care is needed to help the patient maintain good nutritional intake. Rhizotomy or cordotomy can be attempted for pain relief when other measures have failed, and narcotics or sedatives should be used liberally in appropriate circumstances. Such complications as infections and hormonal imbalances require appropriate treatment.

Many rapidly growing tumors produce death within six months. A patient who survives more than six months, however, is likely to have a slowly growing tumor. For such patients the best therapeutic attitude, even when metastases are present, is to regard the cancer as a chronic incurable disease for which a great deal can still be done. By maintaining an attitude of hope, by suitable attention to remediable or improvable situations, and by attention to the personal aspects of clinical care, the physician can often prolong useful life, prevent needless suffering, or permit death to come, when it must, in circumstances of tranquility and dignity.

Boucot, K. R., Cooper, D. A., Weiss, W., and Carnahan, W. J.: The natural history of lung cancer. Am. Rev. Resp. Dis., 89:519, 1964.

Brownlee, K. A.: A review of "Smoking and Health." J. Amer. Statist. Ass., 60:722-739 (Sept.), 1965.

Doll, R., and Bradford Hill, A.: Mortality in relation to smoking: Ten years' observations of British doctors. Brit. Med. J., 1:1399, 1460, 1964.

Feinstein, A. R.: Symptomatic patterns, biologic behavior and prognosis in cancer of the lung. Practical application of Boolean algebra and clinical taxonomy. Ann. Intern. Med., 61:27, 1964. See also Nature, 209:241, 1966, and New Engl. J. Med., 279:747, 1968.

Garland, L. R., Coulson, W., and Wollin, E.: The rate of growth and apparent duration of untreated primary bronchial carcinoma. Cancer, 16:694, 1963.

Kreyberg, L.: Histological lung cancer types. Acta Path. Microbiol. Scand., Suppl. 157, 1962.

LeRoux, B. T.: Bronchial Carcinoma. Edinburgh, E. & S. Livingstone, Ltd., 1968.

MacDonald, I.: The individual basis of biologic variability in cancer. Surg. Gynec. Obstet., 106:227, 1958.

Smoking and Health: Report of the Advisory Committee to the Surgeon General of the Public Health Service. U.S. Department of Health, Education, and Welfare, 1964.

Watson, W. L. (Ed.): Lung Cancer. A Study of Five Thousand Memorial Hospital Cases. St. Louis, C. V. Mosby Company, 1968.

Diseases of the Pleura

William W. Stead

Pleura is the continuous thin elastic membrane which covers the lung (visceral) and the mediastinum, diaphragm, and chest wall (parietal). A thin film of lymph lubricates the surfaces and permits them to slide smoothly during respiration. The elastic recoil of the lungs creates a negative intrapleural pressure of 4 to 6 cm. of water. Accumulation of detectable amounts of pleural transudate as in congestive heart failure is called simple hydrothorax. Inflammation of the pleura without detectable fluid is called fibrinous pleurisy. When pleurisy is accompanied by a detectable amount of exudate, it is called pleurisy with effusion. Pleurisy and pleural effusion are both signs of disease, but neither should be considered a diagnosis.

FIBRINOUS OR DRY PLEURISY

Inflammation of the pleura without grossly detectable exudate is described as dry or fibrinous pleurisy. The most common cause is bacterial pneumonia, but it may be the result of trauma of the chest wall or polyserositis accompanying systemic diseases such as disseminated lupus or rheumatic fever. Pleurodynia (due to Coxsackie B virus) and psittacosis may produce dry pleurisy, but mycoplasmal pneumonia and other forms of primary atypical pneumonia rarely involve the pleura. Pulmonary tuberculosis, pulmonary infarction, lung abscess, and bronchiectasis may also produce dry pleurisy.

The cardinal symptom of pleurisy is a stabbing pain accentuated by deep inspiration. The pain may be severe enough to produce grunting respiration or may be mild and described as a "catch" or "stitch" in the side with deep breathing or coughing. The pain is usually located in the chest wall but may be referred to the shoulder when the medial aspect of the diaphragm is involved or to the abdominal wall when the lower thoracic nerves are affected. The latter is occasionally misinterpreted as an acute intra-abdominal process.

Physical signs of pleurisy are intercostal tenderness and friction rub during respiration. The presence of pain and tenderness imply spread of the reaction to the contiguous parietal pleura because the visceral pleura contains no pain fibers.

Fibrinous pleurisy usually resolves as the inciting disease abates but may progress to pleural effusion. The great frequency of pleural adhesions observed at autopsy indicates that fibrinous pleurisy is more common than is clinically recognized. Occasionally a dry pleurisy persists for months without indication of other disease. Treatment will be considered in the discussion of Pleurisy with Effusion.

PLEURAL EFFUSION

Abnormal accumulation of fluid in the pleural space, from whatever cause, may be massive or slight. Rigler has shown that amounts less than 300 ml. can rarely be detected by a standard x-ray of the chest, and probably 500 ml. would be required for detection on physical examination. The physical signs are flatness to percussion accompanied by absence of tactile fremitus and voice and breath sounds. If massive, the mediastinum and trachea may be shifted toward the opposite side. Smaller amounts may be detected by an x-ray taken in a posteroanterior projection while the patient is lying on the affected side (lateral decubitus x-ray). This maneuver causes free fluid to shift from the diaphragm to the lateral chest wall. If the fluid lies entrapped in a pulmonary fissure, it will not shift with change in body position but may be readily detected on a film taken in the lateral projection. Occasionally even large amounts of fluid lie beneath the lung and mimic a fixed elevation of the diaphragm. The fluid nature of the density can best be demonstrated by the lateral decubitus x-ray.

PLEURAL TRANSUDATE OR SIMPLE HYDROTHORAX

Serous fluid containing little protein may accumulate in one or both pleural spaces as the result of transudation in excess of absorption in congestive heart failure, cirrhosis of the liver, edematous renal disease, benign tumor of the ovary (Meigs' syndrome), myxedema, and in conjunction with lymphedema and yellow fingernails. The protein concentration is that of edema fluid, usually less than 2.5 grams per 100 ml., although in myxedema and Meigs' syndrome and lymphedema it may exceed 3.0 grams per 100 ml. Aspiration may be indicated for diagnosis and when the fluid is sufficient to cause dyspnea. Transudates subside as the primary disease is controlled. Failure to do so suggests disease affecting the pleura itself and calls for further diagnostic studies, including a thoracentesis.

PLEURAL EXUDATE OR PLEURISY WITH EFFUSION

Regardless of whether the fluid is clear or cloudy, a protein content of 3 grams or more per 100 ml. usually indicates an extensive involvement of the pleura itself by infection, pulmonary infarction, or a neoplastic process. When the gross appearance of the fluid is distinctive, it may point rather directly to specific diseases. Thus a purulent fluid indicates an empyema usually secondary to pneumonia, but occasionally to lung abscess, tuberculosis, or an abscess in the mediastinum or subphrenic space. A bloody effusion may occur in pulmonary infarction, contusion, pleural or pulmonary malignancy, or following myocardial infarction or acute hemorrhagic pancreatitis. In company with pericarditis a bloody effusion points to carcinoma or a severe infection with Coxsackie B virus. A milky chylous fluid suggests disease or injury of the thoracic duct. A cloudy fluid with a light yellow or green metallic sheen suggests a cholesterol effusion (q.v.). Chocolate brown effusion may indicate penetration of the pleura by an amebic abscess of the liver.

The present discussion will center on cases in which the effusion is a clear yellow exudate which can be distinguished from a transudate by a protein content of 3 grams per 100 ml. or more or a specific gravity over 1.014. Perhaps it is most useful to view the finding of such clear exudate as intermediate between a simple fibrinous pleurisy and the development of a fluid having more characteristic physical properties such as purulence or bloodiness.

Diagnosis. *History and General Examination.* The history should give a clue to the type of process responsible for the involvement of the pleura, i.e., chills, fever, and purulent sputum point to pneumonia; sudden pain, breathlessness, and sweating to pulmonary infarction; chronic cough, loss of weight, and hemoptysis to malignancy of the lung; and mild illness, loss of weight, and night sweats to tuberculosis. Physical examination may contribute additional information, such as findings suggestive of pneumonia, clubbing of the fingers, or supraclavicular nodes suggestive of carcinoma. The total and differential leukocyte count may help distinguish an acute pyogenic process from other causes. If indicated by earlier findings, an elevated lactic acid dehydrogenase level in the serum may help in diagnosing pulmonary infarction; a rising antistreptolysin antibody titer suggests recent rheumatic fever; the presence of LE cells indicates lupus erythematosus; and elevated RA antibodies suggest the presence of rheumatoid arthritis.

Thoracentesis. Thoracentesis should be performed as soon as possible to obtain a specimen of the fluid which often yields the first direct evidence as to the nature of the process. Even in a very sick person enough fluid can usually be obtained for diagnostic study. When there is only a small amount of fluid, it can be obtained most easily and safely by performing the thoracentesis with the patient lying on the affected side on an examining table with the posterior thorax near the edge of the table. Fluid can then be obtained by anesthetizing the appropriate area near the posterior axillary line and inserting the needle into the chest from below. The air-filled lung floats above the fluid, thus lessening the chance of its being torn by the needle. In addition there is much less chance of syncope during the procedure ("pleural shock") than when the patient is in an upright position.

Fluid may be blood stained from trauma inflicted by the needle. If present early in the withdrawal of fluid, blood caused by trauma usually clears as withdrawal proceeds. If the lung is torn later in the course of withdrawal of fluid, the blood-staining develops near the end of the procedure. Contrary to common belief, the development of a clot in the fluid upon standing gives no indication of whether it is a transudate or exudate, since either occasionally may clot. Nor does clotting affect the validity of the protein content in distinguishing a transudate from an exudate, as the only protein removed by clotting is fibrinogen, and the bulk of the protein remains in solution. Fractionation into albumin and globulin fractions has not proved helpful thus far. If the fluid is an exudate, the white blood cell count and differential should be determined as an aid in distinguishing acute pyogenic, allergic, and chronic processes. Examination of the fluid by Papanicolaou's technique is helpful in finding malignant cells. Other tests which may be useful as indicated by the clinical picture and other findings are LDH, amylase, cholesterol, and glucose. A sample of fluid should always be submitted for culture for pyogens and tubercle bacilli.

Biopsy of the Pleura. Widespread use of biopsy of the parietal pleura has greatly increased the proportion of cases in which the cause of pleurisy can be established. It is quite a safe procedure in experienced hands, and the slight risk is well balanced by the advantage of an accurate diagnosis on which to base therapy. The accompanying illustration shows two examples of diagnostic tissue obtained with a biopsy needle.

If the pleura is thickened, a Vim-Silverman needle may be used satisfactorily. In the absence of chronic pleural thickening, however, an Abrams or Cope needle is preferable. Premedication with

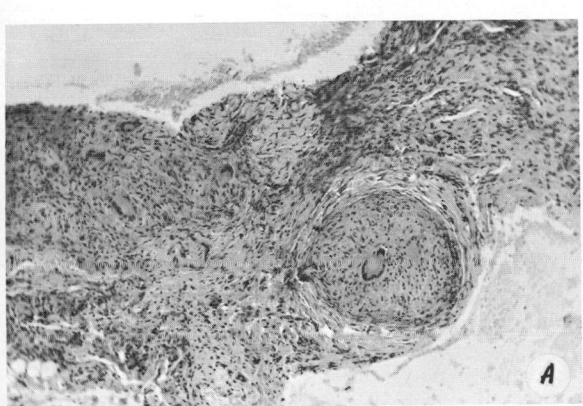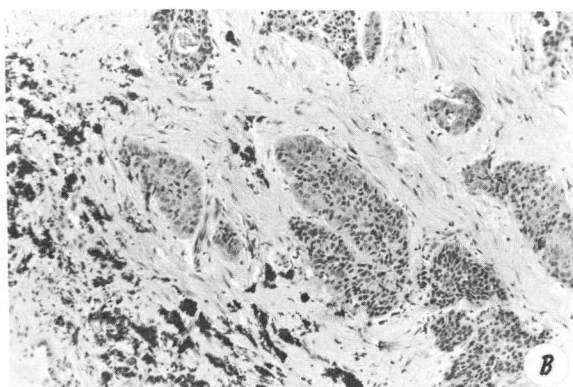

Examples of tissue obtained by needle biopsy of the pleura. *A,* Tuberculous pleuritis showing the typical picture of epithelioid-cell granuloma including several Langhans' giant cells. Tissue was obtained from a case of "idiopathic" pleural effusion in a 22-year-old woman. *B,* Squamous cell carcinoma invading the pleura, with resultant increase in fibrous stroma.

a barbiturate lessens the risk of reaction to the local anesthetic. The procedure is not unduly painful if care is taken to achieve adequate local anesthesia with procaine or lidocaine. Several fragments of pleura should be obtained to increase the chance of obtaining diagnostic material. Specimens should be submitted to the laboratory for culture and histologic sections. A second attempt may be made a few days later if the first attempt has failed to yield diagnostic material. If that fails also and the diagnosis has still not been made, an open surgical biopsy of pleura and lung should be considered.

General Treatment. The first consideration is relief of discomfort, since specific treatment must await completion of diagnostic studies. If fluid is causing respiratory embarrassment, enough should be removed by thoracentesis to relieve dyspnea. Removal of more than 600 ml. at once may precipitate pulmonary edema. If pain is severe, codeine, 15 to 30 mg., or Darvon, 65 mg., may afford relief. Occasionally meperidine, 50 to 100 mg., or morphine, 8 to 15 mg., may be required. Local heat is often comforting. Tight chest binders and adhesive taping are of little value.

More lasting relief of pain can be obtained by several means. In order of ascending complexity they are (1) calcium gluconate, 1 gram given intravenously. Why this should be effective is not clear, but it often is. Its effectiveness suggests a role of muscle spasm in the genesis of the pain; (2) Anesthetizing the painful area with ethyl chloride spray. (3) Intercostal nerve block. Premedication with pentobarbital serves both to allay apprehension and to reduce the chance of an anesthetic reaction. A small needle (No. 25 or 26) is used for skin anesthesia and then a 1½-to 2-inch No. 23 needle to inject about 2 ml. of 1 per cent solution of procaine or lidocaine between the appropriate ribs proximal to the site of pain. No attempt should be made to inject the nerves themselves, as the agents are effective if merely injected close to nerves. Care must be taken not to inject into a blood vessel and not to penetrate deeply enough to tear the lung. This can usually be avoided by probing with the needle for the outer surface of the rib and then advancing the needle 1 cm. further over the upper edge of the rib. Relief of pain from any of these procedures is often permanent in spite of the short pharmacologic effects of the agents employed.

CAUSES OF PLEURAL EXUDATES

Pneumonia. The fibrinous pleurisy surrounding acute pyogenic pneumonia may progress to form an exudate which may be clear at first and purulent later. The preceding clinical picture of pneumonia is of great aid in suggesting this type of effusion. The predominant cell is the polymorphonuclear leukocyte. In most instances vigorous specific antimicrobial therapy serves to abort the pleural infection at this early stage, but if the fluid is purulent, other measures may be indicated (see Empyema). Mycoplasmal pneumonia only rarely involves the pleura, but influenza A infection, psittacosis, and Coxsackie B viruses may do so. The rarity of mycoplasmal pleuritis should be kept in mind whenever one is tempted to ascribe a pleural exudate to "virus pneumonia."

Pulmonary Infarction. Pleural effusion may develop as part of a typical clinical picture of pulmonary infarction, or it may be the only roentgenographic abnormality observed. It may be clear initially but is commonly blood stained. It contains polymorphonuclear leukocytes, mesothelial cells, and often eosinophils. Pleural biopsy often reveals mesothelial reaction which superficially may mimic adenocarcinoma. Treatment is that of pulmonary infarction unless pain requires special attention (see above).

Myocardial Infarction. Pneumonitis and pleural exudate may develop as part of a postmyocardial infarction syndrome and be difficult to distinguish from pulmonary infarction. The treatment of pulmonary infarctions is discussed in the article on Thromboembolic Diseases.

Malignancy. Primary mesothelioma is rare but may cause a persistent pleural exudate, particularly when malignant. Although always bloody eventually, the fluid may be clear at an early stage. Mesothelioma is much more frequent in persons with a remote past history of exposure to asbestos dust, and the finding of plaques of calcium in the pleura may be very helpful in suggesting this possibility. Diagnosis can usually be made by cytologic examination of the exudate or by pleural biopsy, but open biopsy may be necessary.

Involvement of the pleura by metastatic malignancy is a common cause of bloody pleural exudate. The most common tumor is a bronchogenic carcinoma, but more remote tumors may involve the pleura also, e.g., breast, pancreas, stomach, uterus, or prostate. Cytology and pleural biopsy often help in diagnosis. Hodgkin's disease and lymphoblastoma may involve the pleura and evoke an exudate.

Treatment of Malignant Effusion. Treatment is largely palliative and is directed at reducing the rate of formation of fluid which produces dyspnea and lowers body protein stores. This appears to be accomplished at times by the removal of as much fluid as possible with a small catheter, followed by the instillation of antineoplastic or other compounds. The agents that have been employed include atabrine, chloroquine, chlorambucil, thio-tepa, radioactive gold, and powdered talc instillation. Prednisone may also be given because it may reduce the inflammatory reaction. A transient febrile reaction is frequent. Some have advocated pleurectomy to achieve pleural symphysis as a means of controlling formation of fluid from pleural malignancy, but most believe this to be more radical than warranted.

TUBERCULOUS PLEURAL EFFUSION

("Undiagnosed" or "Idiopathic" Pleurisy with Effusion)

When no cause can be found for pleurisy with a lymphocytic effusion, it is often called *idiopathic*. However, experience has taught that such effusions are *most commonly due to tuberculosis* in the early postprimary stage.

Etiology and Pathogenesis. Tuberculous pleurisy is secondary to tuberculosis near the surface of the lung. Simple inflammation of overlying pleura produces a fibrinous pleurisy. When there is a detectable effusion, it is the result of a reaction of the pleura when a small superficial tuberculous lesion of the lung erodes the pleura and actually extrudes a small amount of caseous material into the pleural space. The eroding lesion is usually so small that it escapes roentgenographic detection and does not permit air to escape with the caseous material. When a large lesion ruptures it may give rise to a bronchopleural fistula and tuberculous empyema.

The role of hypersensitivity in tuberculous pleurisy was demonstrated by Paterson in 1917. Upon injection of tubercle bacilli into the pleural space of previously uninfected guinea pigs, the organisms multiplied rapidly, little fluid formed, and the animals died promptly of disseminated tuberculosis. By contrast, when tuberculin-reactive guinea pigs were so treated, multiplication of organisms was much delayed, and a significant pleural effusion was formed. Jacobeus observed tuberculous lesions beneath the pleura, and Stead and associates showed that tuberculous effusion was the result of extrusion of material through the pleura.

Pathology. The pleural reaction is a granulomatous inflammation of both visceral and parietal surfaces which may lead to considerable fibrosis as it heals. Stead and associates showed that, although the granulomatous thickening of the pleura is widespread, there is usually one point at which the pleural reaction is inseparable from a fibrocaseous lesion of the lung which has eroded through the visceral pleura.

Clinical Manifestations. Tuberculous pleural effusion may develop at any stage of tuberculous infection. It is most common in the early postprimary stage in young adults but may be seen in older persons in whom chronic tuberculosis is the result of late recrudescence of infection decades after the primary infection. In younger persons the parenchymal lesions usually have too little radiodensity to be seen by x-ray, but in older persons chronic pulmonary tuberculosis is often apparent.

The first symptom is usually pain accentuated by deep breathing. If massive, the effusion produces dyspnea, but usually not otherwise. Systemic symptoms suggestive of tuberculosis may be present, but are inconstant because early postprimary tuberculosis often produces little illness. Rarely the onset may occur with a chill, but more often there is a low-grade fever in the evening or sweating during the night.

It is important to realize that clearing of a pleural effusion, either spontaneously or in association with drug therapy, offers little evidence against tuberculosis because primary tuberculosis tends to subside initially and to enter a dormant phase. It may be months or years before chronic tuberculosis makes its appearance in lung, bones, or kidney if the infection is not properly treated early in its course.

Diagnosis. A positive tuberculin skin test using 5 test units of PPD (intermediate strength) is usually present. Occasionally second-strength PPD may be required to elicit a reaction in persons who are clinically ill. Now that only about 5 per cent of young adults react to intermediate PPD owing to an infection acquired in childhood, the finding of a reaction to this dose in a young adult who has a pleural exudate is often enough to warrant a presumptive diagnosis of early postprimary tuberculosis as the cause of the pleurisy.

Direct evidence of the tuberculous nature of the process may be difficult to obtain. Thoracentesis and examinations of the fluid are of paramount importance in identifying the lymphocytic and exudative nature of the fluid, but do not always yield positive evidence of the cause of the effusion. Tubercle bacilli are by no means invariably isolated on culture. Biopsy of the parietal pleura usually reveals typical epithelioid granulomas (see illustration), but often fails to reveal bacilli on microscopy. Culture of the pleural biopsy should be made, but is positive with any frequency only if a liquid culture medium is used which enables growth of bacilli present in small numbers. An open biopsy of the pleura and lung almost always provides proof of the diagnosis. However, in many instances experienced clinicians accept the diagnosis of tuberculosis in a case of "idiopathic" pleurisy with effusion simply on grounds of probability and institute appropriate antituberculous chemotherapy. Culture of sputum or gastric washings yields tubercle bacilli in about one third of cases proved or presumed to be of tuberculous origin. This fact is consistent with a parenchymal focus of tuberculosis as the cause of the pleurisy.

Treatment. Whether the diagnosis of tuberculous pleurisy is confirmed or presumed on clinical grounds, the patient should be given an adequate course of antituberculous chemotherapy. Two effective drugs, including isoniazid, should be employed for the first several months and then isoniazid should be continued for no less than one year. Bed rest is of importance only in the acute phase and rarely need last more than two to three weeks. For details of treatment, see the section on Tuberculosis.

It was once the practice to attempt to drain as much of the exudate from the chest as possible to prevent the development of a restricting fibrothorax. With the very effective antituberculous chemotherapy now available, this is no longer necessary. Therapy for several weeks with corticosteroids in addition to the antimicrobial therapy is advocated by some to hasten subsidence of the granulomatous pleuritis and resorption of fluid. The prompt response of the tuberculous process to effective chemotherapy, however, makes it difficult to prove the benefit of steroid therapy. There appears to be no necessity for instillation of hydrocortisone into the pleural space.

Prognosis. Without specific antituberculous therapy, the likelihood of developing chronic tuberculosis of the lung, bone, or kidney by a group with effusion was found by Roper and Waring to be 67 per cent within a five-year period, regardless of whether the diagnosis was confirmed bacteriologically or was merely presumed on clinical grounds. With intensive initial and adequately prolonged antituberculous therapy, the prognosis is excellent, and recovery is almost always complete and lasting. Shorter courses of therapy may be marred by the late appearance of chronic tuberculosis in a significant number of cases.

Berlin, S. O.: Exudative tuberculous pleurisy. Acta Tuberc. Scand., Suppl. 40, pp. 1-134, 1957.

Falk, A., and Stead, W. W.: Antimicrobial therapy in the treatment of primary tuberculous pleurisy with effusion: Its effect upon the incidence of subsequent tuberculous relapse. Amer. Rev. Tuberc., 74:897, 1956.

Paterson, R. C.: The pleural reaction to inoculation with tubercle bacilli in vaccinated and normal guinea pigs. Amer. Rev. Tuberc., 1:353, 1917.

Roper, W. H., and Waring, J. J.: Primary serofibrinous pleural effusion in military personnel. Amer. Rev. Tuberc., 71:616, 1955.

Stead, W. W., Eichenholz, A., and Stauss, H. K.: Operative and pathologic findings in twenty-four patients with syndrome of idiopathic pleurisy with effusion, presumably tuberculous. Amer. Rev. Tuberc., 71:473, 1955.

LESS COMMON CAUSES OF PLEURAL EXUDATES

Diseases of Connective Tissue ("Collagen Diseases"). A polymorphonuclear exudate may be a manifestation of pleural involvement in systemic lupus erythematosus, acute rheumatic fever, scleroderma, dermatomyositis, polyarteritis nodosa, and rheumatoid arthritis. In the last the fluid is characterized by virtual absence of glucose and may contain a very high concentration of cholesterol (up to a gram or more per 100 ml.) which may be in solution or crystalline.

Viral Infections. Pleural involvement is not a feature of mycoplasmal pneumonia. When this diagnosis is invoked to explain a pleural effusion in a young adult, there is a strong possibility that postprimary tuberculosis is being overlooked. Pleural involvement may occur in infectious mononucleosis, influenza A infection, and psittacosis,

but such a diagnosis should not be accepted without clear-cut changes in the titers of appropriate serologic tests.

Epidemic pleurodynia resulting from Coxsackie B5 virus may give rise to an exudative pleurisy which may be bloody and is often accompanied by a similar pericarditis. It can be recognized with confidence only when it occurs as part of an epidemic which appears in late summer or autumn. The illness usually begins as a coryza with a sore throat which subsides but returns with the onset of severe pleuritis pain (devil's grip) which may be costal in location or referred to the shoulder and abdomen. Diagnosis is made by isolation of Coxsackie virus from the stool or by changing serum titers of complement-fixing antibodies. There is no specific treatment, but the disease is usually self-limited.

Systemic Fungal Infections. Although it is rare, the pleura may be invaded from parenchymal lesions in coccidioidomycosis, histoplasmosis, actinomycosis, blastomycosis, or cryptococcosis. Infection with less pathogenic fungi may occur in patients receiving steroids and various immunosuppressive drugs. Diagnosis is made by culture of fluid and sputum.

Subdiaphragmatic Abscess. A "sympathetic" exudate may form in the pleural space when there is a subdiaphragmatic abscess caused by rupture of a hollow viscus. If caused by a ruptured duodenal ulcer, the fluid may contain enough amylase to suggest hemorrhagic pancreatitis as its cause. An air-fluid level beneath the diaphragm is strong evidence of a ruptured viscus. The fluid is a polymorphonuclear exudate.

Pancreatitis. Acute hemorrhagic pancreatitis or ruptured pseudocyst may produce an exudate in the left pleural space secondary to peritoneal involvement. It is commonly bloody but may be clear early in its course. It is characterized by a predominance of polymorphonuclear leukocytes and an elevated amylase (often well above 1000 units).

Splenic Hematoma. A bloody effusion at the left lung base following a fall on the left thorax and accompanied by anemia suggests the possibility of a splenic injury with an enlarging hematoma. Unless the condition is recognized and the spleen removed, it may rupture fatally one to three weeks following the injury.

Meigs' Syndrome. In addition to producing a pleural transudate, as mentioned earlier, fibroma and other ovarian tumors may give rise to a peritoneal and pleural exudate (usually on the right side). The route by which the fluid reaches the pleural space is not clear, but it appears to be by lymphatics or defects in the diaphragm, which are not rare. Removal of the ovarian tumor usually causes the exudate to subside promptly.

Amebiasis. A chocolate-colored purulent exudate in the right thorax suggests the presence of amebic pleuritis secondary to amebic abscess of the liver. Diagnostic studies should include complement fixation titer for amebiasis and search for *E. histolytica* in the fluid and stool.

Eosinophilic Pleural Effusion. Eosinophilia in a pleural exudate has no specific significance. It may be seen in exudates accompanying Loeffler's eosinophilic pneumonia, pneumothorax, pulmonary contusion or infarction, Hodgkin's disease, echinococcal infection, histoplasmosis, allergies to various drugs, and occasionally in connective tissue diseases but rarely in tuberculosis. Pleural biopsy should be performed for diagnosis.

Drug Allergies. Pleurisy may arise from allergic reaction to various drugs. The resulting fluid may be characterized by eosinophilia.

Cholesterol Effusion. Pleural fluid of golden or light green color and iridescent sheen suggests a high concentration of cholesterol (as high as 1000 mg. per 100 ml. or more), which may even be in crystalline form. The cause may be a metabolic disorder, rheumatoid arthritis, or a late stage of a very chronic tuberculous pleurisy.

Chylous Effusion. Injury to the thoracic duct by trauma or invasion of a malignant tumor or lymphoma may produce a milky pleural fluid resulting from accumulation of chyle in the thorax. It is more common on the right side. Characteristic findings include fat droplets seen with Sudan III stain, elevated lipid content, and a normal or mildly elevated cholesterol. Treatment must be directed at the cause of the damage to the thoracic duct, but pleural symphysis may be necessary to control the loss of chyle which makes adequate nutrition difficult to maintain.

EMPYEMA THORACIS

Empyema thoracis is the presence of pus in the pleural space. The most common cause is a contiguous pneumonia or lung abscess, but it may result from infection of the mediastinum (ruptured esophagus) or a subdiaphragmatic abscess. It may result from necrosis of a pyogenic or tuberculous lesion which erodes both the pleura and a branch of the bronchial tree. This dire event gives rise to a bronchopleural fistula and produces a pyopneumothorax. The presence of gross infection in the pleural space is the one instance in which specific therapy for the pleural involvement is urgently indicated. Treatment must include closed drainage of the pus in addition to appropriate specific antimicrobial therapy for the infectious process. Tuberculous empyema usually contains a preponderance of lymphocytes; others, a predominance of polymorphonuclear leukocytes. Treatment of pyogenic empyema is discussed elsewhere (see Pneumonia).

FIBROSIS OF THE PLEURA

Most inflammatory reactions of the pleura heal by fibrosis. If localized, pleurisy is followed by local fibrous adhesion of the visceral and parietal surfaces. If generalized the lung may be encased in a layer of fibrous tissue thick enough to impair pulmonary function. Occasionally this leads to obvious retraction of a hemithorax. Pleural fibrosis can mimic pleural fluid on both physical and roentgenographic examination to such an extent that they can be differentiated only by inability to obtain fluid by a careful thoracentesis. The principal means of combating pleural fibrosis is prompt and adequate therapy of pleurisy early in its course. Surgical removal of a thick fibrous pleura usually does not improve pulmonary function significantly.

Emerson, P. A.: Yellow nails, lymphoedema and pleural effusions. Thorax, 21:247, 1966.

Ferguson, G. C.: Cholesterol pleural effusion in rheumatoid lung disease. Thorax, 21:577, 1966.

Leininger, B. J., Barker, W. L., and Langston, H. T.: A simplified method for management of malignant pleural effusion. J. Thorac. Cardiov. Surg., 58:758, 1969.

Lemming, R.: Meigs' syndrome and pathogenesis of pleurisy and polyserositis. Acta Med. Scand., 168:197, 1960.

Sulavik, S., and Katz, S.: Pleural Effusion. Springfield, Ill., Charles C Thomas, 1963.

PNEUMOTHORAX

Definition. The pleural "space" normally contains no air and only a few milliliters of lubricating fluid. When air enters the space, the lung collapses in proportion to the amount of air present. It may be so little as to escape detection or so massive as to threaten life (tension pneumothorax). Prompt recognition of the latter is of utmost importance if life is to be saved.

Pulmonary rupture may be spontaneous or traumatic. Spontaneous pneumothorax is usually the result of rupture of a superficial emphysematous bulla and may occur in apparently healthy persons or in association with chronic pulmonary disease. It is usually unilateral but may become bilateral if air reaches the mediastinum and ruptures into both pleural spaces. Traumatic pneumothorax may be caused by a penetrating wound, pleural or lung biopsy, fractured rib, excessive respiratory pressure, faulty tracheostomy, or difficulty in inserting a subclavian needle or catheter.

Clinical Manifestations. Spontaneous pneumothorax is usually of abrupt onset and accompanied by dyspnea and pleuritic pain of the chest wall or shoulder. A history of unusual exertion is uncommon and the onset may even occur during sleep. Dyspnea varies with the amount of air and pre-existing diffuse pulmonary disease (emphysema or fibrosis). The pain is limited to the affected side and is frequently aggravated by deep inspiration. It may be referred to the upper abdomen or shoulder but does not radiate into the arm. A nonproductive cough is occasionally noted. About 10 per cent of patients report no symptoms. The condition is fairly common among healthy persons of college age, with a preponderance of 5:1 in the male. In persons over the age of 40 it is usually seen as a complication of other pulmonary diseases, particularly emphysema, diffuse pulmonary fibrosis, sarcoidosis, histiocytosis X, berylliosis, and scleroderma. During infancy it most often accompanies staphylococcal pneumonia. It is rare in active tuberculosis, except when a large tuberculous lesion ruptures and produces a bronchopleural fistula and empyema.

Occasionally a small amount of bleeding occurs from the site of rupture and may be detected as fluid on the roentgenogram. Rarely, bleeding may be massive. A small amount of exudate may be formed which is characterized by eosinophilia. Whenever an air-fluid level is observed on x-ray, a thoracentesis should be performed without delay to determine whether it is due to hemopneumothorax or pyopneumothorax. A ball-valve mechanism may develop at the site of rupture and pump air into the pleural space under pressure, giving rise to a tension pneumothorax which is life-threatening and must be relieved promptly (see Treatment). Extravasated air may dissect into the mediastinum (pneumomediastinum) and from there to subcutaneous tissues of the neck and chest wall (subcutaneous emphysema). These may be detected by hearing a crunching sound synchronous with systole (Hamman's sign) and by feeling subcutaneous crepitation.

Chronic pneumothorax may result if the lung continues to leak. In one series 10 per cent of the cases became chronic. When this occurs a layer of fibrin is gradually deposited on the visceral pleura which interferes with both re-expansion and function of the lung. An abnormally high intrapleural pressure then develops, causing a chronic hydrothorax which recurs to the same extent whenever the fluid is removed.

Diagnosis. Physical findings of pneumothorax are rarely dramatic and must be carefully searched for. The affected side is slightly hyper-resonant, and both breath and transmitted sounds are distant and indistinct. Occasionally the trachea may be shifted to the contralateral side in the suprasternal notch and the apex impulse of the heart displaced. A crunching systolic sound over the heart is common and indicates the presence of air in the mediastinum.

The diagnosis must be made roentgenograph-

ically. When the lung is filled with air in inspiration, there is little contrast between the lung and the air surrounding it. A film exposed in expiration affords considerably greater contrast and makes diagnosis easier.

Treatment. Most cases of small pneumothorax require no specific treatment for the first attack. The patient should be confined to quarters for a few days and avoid strenuous activity for several weeks. Air is resorbed over a period of 10 to 20 days by an interesting physiologic "pump" mechanism: partial pressure of oxygen falls within a few hours from about 140 mm. to about 30 mm. Hg; this difference is only partially compensated by a rise in P_{CO_2} from near zero to about 45 mm. Hg, thus creating a P_{N_2} well above that of the blood. This causes nitrogen to be absorbed which increases the P_{O_2} enough so that more oxygen is absorbed or metabolized. This process continues until all gas has been absorbed.

If the degree of collapse is large (50 per cent or more), most experienced clinicians prefer to insert a plastic or soft rubber catheter to aspirate the air from the chest.

Tension pneumothorax should be suspected when respiratory distress is great and x-ray reveals a great collapse of the lung. The pressure is often great enough to push out the plunger of a wet glass syringe when a needle is inserted into the chest. The pressure may be measured with a manometer similar to that used for determination of central venous pressure. If positive pressure is identified, it is imperative to insert a catheter for suction or underwater drainage without delay.

Recurrent or Chronic Pneumothorax. Thirty per cent of patients with spontaneous pneumothorax experience a recurrence on either the same or the contralateral side and occasionally bilaterally. At the time of a second episode and in case of chronic pneumothorax, steps should be taken to create a symphysis of the parietal and visceral pleura. Various nonsurgical methods have been used but are not very reliable. These include injection of various irritating solutions into the pleural space (sucrose, silver nitrate, and aerosolized powdered talc). The most reliable method appears to be to rub the pleural surfaces with dry gauze to create widespread inflammatory pleuritis. Then the two surfaces can be made to adhere by keeping the lung expanded for a few days by continuous intrapleural suction. Some surgeons prefer to remove the parietal pleura surgically to achieve the same result.

Beumer, H. M.: A ten-year review of spontaneous pneumothorax in an Armed Forces hospital. Amer. Rev. Resp. Dis., 90: 261, 1964.

Dickie, H. A.: Spontaneous mediastinal emphysema and spontaneous pneumothorax. A report of 20 cases. Ann. Intern. Med., 28:618, 1948.

Macklin, M. T., and Macklin, C. C.: Malignant interstitial emphysema of the lungs and mediastinum. Medicine, 23:281, 1944.

Ruckley, C. V., and McCormack, R. J. M.: The management of spontaneous pneumothorax. Thorax, 21:139, 1966.

Circulatory Disorders

PULMONARY HYPERTENSION
*John R. Hickam**

The normal upper limit of pulmonary arterial pressure in resting man is usually accepted as 25/12 mm. Hg, with a mean pressure of 15 mm. Hg. Many disorders of the cardiovascular and respiratory systems cause acute or chronic elevations of this pressure, sometimes to levels above the aortic pressure. Chronic pulmonary hypertension causes hypertrophy and eventual failure of the right ventricle. Although the disorders which produce pulmonary hypertension are many, the recognized mechanisms by which they have this effect are relatively few. In particular instances these factors may operate singly or in combinations. Our growing understanding of these mechanisms has greatly simplified the diagnosis, management, and prognostic evaluation of individual patients with pulmonary hypertension and consequent right ventricular hypertrophy and failure. For this reason, the subject will be introduced by an account of some general pathogenetic and pathologic features of pulmonary hypertension. Details pertinent to various disease states will be further discussed under the appropriate sections.

THE NORMAL PULMONARY CIRCULATION

The normal pulmonary circulation has been described in full elsewhere, and only pertinent aspects are presented here.

Structure. The media of pulmonary arteries down to an external diameter of 1000 to 500 μ consists of elastic connective tissue. In the fetus, the elastic lamina of the large pulmonary arteries are long, parallel, and dense, like those of the aorta. During the first two years after birth they become progressively more fragmented, irregular, and sparse to achieve the adult pattern. Below this size and down to a diameter of 100 to 70 μ are the muscular pulmonary arteries, thought to be the principal site of active changes in pulmonary vascular resistance. The media of these vessels is composed of smooth muscle, with both an internal and external elastic lamina. Relative to systemic arteries of this size, the media is thin and the lumen wide. In smaller vessels, the arterioles, the smooth muscle coat disappears and the vessel wall becomes attenuated to a thin layer of collagen fibers, a single elastic lamina, and a lining of endothelial cells. The capillaries, which branch at large angles from the arterioles, are wide but flattened in the alveolar septa. The arteries are distributed with the bronchial tree, but the

venules and veins lie separately in the connective tissue septa of the pulmonary parenchyma. Venules resemble arterioles. Veins greater than 80 μ in diameter acquire a smooth muscle coat, but they contain more elastic and fibrous tissue and less muscle than the arteries. The pulmonary veins have a single internal elastic lamina. Near the heart, a layer of cardiac muscle extends into the major pulmonary veins. The pulmonary arteries and veins are accompanied by lymphatics. Bronchial arteries supply the bronchial tree to the level of the terminal bronchiole, below which parenchymal nutrition is maintained by the pulmonary circulation. In the terminal areas of the bronchial circulation there is free anastomosis between pulmonary and bronchial veins.

Hemodynamics. Normally, the pulmonary vessels contain 500 to 600 ml. of blood, about 90 ml. of which is in the pulmonary capillaries and approximately two thirds of the entire amount in the veins. The system has a relatively low compliance and tolerates moderate changes in volume with only small pressure changes; however, a 100 ml. increase in volume will cause a twofold increase in pulmonary vascular pressures. This *relatively* low compliance is more pronounced on the venous side, which thus serves a reservoir function for the left ventricle.

The pulmonary arterial pressure is normally low, and the vessels are compliant and only weakly reactive. In consequence, the distribution of flow is much affected by gravity and various intrathoracic forces. Pulmonary arterial pressure is determined by the rate of blood flow, the resistance to flow through the vessels, and the opposing left atrial pressure on the venous side. Resistance is often calculated as an index of the state of the small vessels. It is defined as

$$\text{Pulmonary vascular resistance} =$$

$$\frac{\text{mean pulmonary artery pressure} - \text{mean left atrial pressure}}{\text{cardiac output}}$$

The requisite measurements are made during cardiac catheterization with left atrial pressure determined either directly or as wedge pressure. Resistance is expressed as "units" in mm. Hg/liter/min. or as dyne sec. cm.$^{-5}$, representative normal values being about 1.5 and 120, respectively. Narrowing of the pulmonary vascular bed by vasoconstriction or disease elevates the resistance, and dilatation decreases it. However, the interpretation of resistance changes must be made with caution, especially when pulmonary artery pressures are low, since resistance can be altered by factors not intrinsic to the vessels themselves.

In normal man at rest the pulmonary vessels are not all open. In the erect position the upper lung receives little or no pulmonary flow because the arterial pressure, reduced by gravity, is less than the intra-alveolar pressure, and the capillaries are closed. Below this is a second zone where effective

*Deceased.

arterial pressure is greater and forces blood through the capillaries, but alveolar pressure is still higher than venous pressure. Here the distal capillaries are partially collapsed and act as a sluice or Starling resistor. In the third, or lowest, zone venous pressure is higher than alveolar pressure, the capillaries are open, and the major site of resistance is in the small muscular arteries. Still further down the lung all intraluminal pressures are progressively increased by gravity, the thin-walled vessels are more and more distended, and resistance is progressively decreased. Lowering arterial and venous pressures will reduce the over-all size of the perfused vascular bed and increase resistance, and raising these pressures will have the opposite effect, without any changes in vascular tone. Overexpanding the lungs raises vascular resistance at the alveolar-capillary level. Increased expiratory resistance can have the same effect. Atelectasis collapses small pulmonary vessels. When the right ventricular output is increased, as by exercise, small increases in pulmonary arterial and venous pressure readily open vascular channels, and calculated resistance falls. For this reason the pulmonary arterial pressure rises only slightly during exercise until the cardiac output is about three times the resting value. Thereafter, the vascular bed is filled, and pressure begins to rise more or less in proportion to output. At high cardiac outputs the lung is fairly evenly perfused, and the capillary surface available for gas diffusion is considerably greater than in the resting condition.

Although the adult human pulmonary circulation is largely controlled by passive response to extravascular factors, it also exhibits vasomotor reactions to certain stimuli, and some of these reactions are clearly important to local regulation of flow. The pulmonary vessels are supplied with vasomotor nerves by way of the autonomic system, and both constrictor and dilator responses have been shown to be mediated by these nerves in animals. In man, the role of the nervous system in control of the pulmonary vessels is not yet well understood. Alveolar hypoxia constricts the muscular pulmonary arteries and possibly the small veins as well. This raises vascular resistance and shunts blood away from locally hypoxic regions. When hypoxia is generalized, the over-all pulmonary vascular resistance and arterial pressure may be increased by as much as 50 per cent. The mechanism of hypoxic vasoconstriction is apparently dependent on a decrease in the potassium ion content of the muscle cells of the pulmonary vessels. Oxygen diffuses readily from the alveoli into the walls of the muscular arteries, and a drop in the alveolar oxygen tension causes a drop in oxygen tension of the vessel wall. The effect on the vessel can thus be direct and local. It has also been shown in animals, and in man under special circumstances, that raising the hydrogen ion concentration of the blood will produce pulmonary vasoconstriction.

The pulmonary vessels respond to a number of other vasoactive substances, both naturally occurring and synthetic. Since there is much variation in response from one species to another, results in laboratory animals need not apply to man. The problems of interpreting measurements of pulmonary vascular resistance have allowed only very limited conclusions to be drawn from observations on normal man, but much additional information is available from studies on patients with increased resistance.

Pulmonary vascular resistance can be decreased in the normal subject by infusion of bradykinin. When the resistance is abnormally increased, it can often be lowered some 20 to 30 per cent by the infusion of acetylcholine into the pulmonary artery at a rate of about 1 mg. per minute, by the inhalation of oxygen, by the intravenous administration of isoproterenol, by aminophylline, and occasionally by the infusion of tolazoline into the pulmonary artery. When the vascular resistance is lowered, as by acetylcholine, in patients with lung disease, there is often a fall in systemic arterial oxygen saturation, presumably because of increased flow through poorly ventilated lung regions previously shut off by hypoxic vasoconstriction.

Pulmonary vascular resistance can be increased in man by phenylephrine, angiotensin, and, incidentally, by bretylium tosylate. The effects of epinephrine and norepinephrine are unsettled. Serotonin elevates resistance in some animals, but not in man, at least in tolerable doses.

PATHOGENESIS OF PULMONARY HYPERTENSION

Severe pulmonary hypertension is caused primarily by *high pulmonary vascular resistance,* which in turn may develop in the course of disorders that affect the respiratory system, the pulmonary vasculature, or the heart. Such disorders elevate pulmonary vascular resistance through a number of different pathogenetic mechanisms. These mechanisms and their interactions are not yet completely understood, and some which appear to be distinct may operate through a common path. Others almost certainly remain to be discovered. Presently recognized mechanisms are:

1. Obstruction of the pulmonary vessels as by blood clot, primary disease of the vessel wall, external pressure, or distortion.

2. Loss of part of the vascular bed in the course of destructive lung disease or surgery.

3. Vasoconstriction in response to alveolar hypoxia, and to increased blood hydrogen ion concentration.

4. Vasoconstriction in response to elevation of pulmonary venous pressure and perhaps arterial pressure as well.

5. The development of occlusive vascular changes in high flow states, as ventricular septal defect.

6. The development of secondary structural changes in the arteries of patients who already have chronic pulmonary hypertension, with conse-

quent further increase in resistance. If the original cause of hypertension can be corrected, these vascular changes may gradually regress, or they may be irreversible.

The mechanisms which increase pulmonary vascular resistance are further discussed under various specific disorders. In most cases, increased resistance appears to depend on both structural changes and increased constrictor tone of the blood vessels. The constrictor tone can be demonstrated by drop in resistance on administering vasodilators such as acetylcholine or oxygen.

Additional mechanisms have been postulated but not established as yet. Apart from changes in the vascular system, resistance may be elevated by increasing blood viscosity, as with polycythemia.

With a high vascular resistance the *pulmonary arterial pressure* varies roughly in proportion to the rate of blood flow, since there are no "reserve" vascular channels to open as the pressure rises. Factors which commonly increase flow and consequently raise pressure are exercise, inotropic drugs, fever, hypoxia, the development of arterial bronchopulmonary anastomoses, and left-to-right shunts in congenital heart disease. Venous hypertension can make a significant passive contribution to pulmonary arterial hypertension, as elevation of the left atrial pressure raises pressure through the the entire system.

Pathology. In chronic pulmonary hypertension the elastic arteries show dilatation, intimal thickening and atheromatosis, medial thickening, and in severe cases degenerative changes in the media. When hypertension is present from birth, as in congenital heart disease, the medial elastic laminae retain the fetal pattern.

The muscular arteries have increased thickness of the media which may partly result from being in a constricted state but also appears to represent true hypertrophy of the smooth muscle coat. Longitudinally oriented muscle bundles also appear, and these are not normally present. A smooth muscle coat may be found in vessels as small as 30 μ well into the arteriolar size. The intima shows proliferation, at first cellular, then more fibrous or fibroelastic. This proliferation may go so far as to occlude the vessel. Intimal thickening also affects the arterioles.

With severe disease, as in primary pulmonary hypertension or progressive hypertension in congenital heart disease, additional changes occur. The elastic arteries can show degenerative alterations, such as metachromasia and medial necrosis. In the muscular arteries, so-called dilatation lesions develop. One example is the plexiform lesion in which a muscular artery, which at first shows medial hypertrophy and fibrosis, intimal thickening, and a narrow lumen, further in its course undergoes aneurysmal dilatation embraced by a plexus of narrow channels separated by connective tissue strands. The vessels beyond have thin, atrophic walls. Such lesions may develop from thromboses, but their origin is not certain.

In advanced pulmonary hypertension, dilated atrophic vessels, presumably distal to sites of high resistance, may be very numerous. In occasional patients fibrinoid necrosis of the media occurs, sometimes with a surrounding inflammatory response. There may be associated thrombosis of the vessel. In many cases of progressive pulmonary hypertension, arterial and venous thrombosis contribute to increasing vascular obstruction. With high flow states as in atrial septal defect, intimal fibrosis, sometimes marked, may affect both large and small pulmonary arteries and veins.

When venous hypertension evokes a substantial increase in vascular resistance, the muscular arteries show medial thickening and intimal fibrosis; but more advanced changes are not usual. The veins also demonstrate medial hypertrophy, and they may acquire an external elastic lamina, thus simulating the arterial structure. Venous intimal fibrosis often develops. In mitral stenosis, which is much the most common cause of longstanding venous hypertension, these vascular changes are most pronounced in the lower lobes. The capillaries are distended, and small hemorrhages occur, with the ultimate accumulation of hemosiderin-containing macrophages in alveoli and septal walls. Apparently in response to these cell aggregates and to recurrent edema, pulmonary interstitial fibrosis commonly develops. Lymphatic vessels around arteries and veins can be markedly distended. In the connective tissue septa of the lung, distention of lymphatic vessels and septal edema sometimes produce transient horizontal lines (Kerley's lines) visible in x-rays at the lung base. The bronchial veins acquire numerous anastomoses with pulmonary veins and become distended and sometimes telangiectatic. Rupture of bronchial telangiectases can produce brisk hemoptysis.

When pulmonary arterial hypertension is associated with chronic hypoxia, as in high altitude dwellers and some patients with obesity or chest deformity, constriction and medial hypertrophy of muscular arteries is a common lesion. In chronic obstructive lung disease medial hypertrophy of these vessels is often less pronounced, even though the right ventricular wall may be distinctly hypertrophied. Episodic arterial constriction nevertheless seems likely from the transient hypertension during bouts of respiratory insufficiency and the acute fall in resistance in response to pulmonary vasodilators. The more characteristic anatomic lesion is intimal fibrosis, which is most common in small muscular arteries near the respiratory bronchioles, possibly as a reaction to repeated bronchial inflammation. The capillaries are stretched around distended air spaces, and special studies have demonstrated considerable loss of the capillary network in emphysema, suggesting that significant flow resistance may occur at the capillary level.

Diffuse interstitial fibrosis, including that caused by scleroderma, dermatomyositis, x-radiation fibrosis, sarcoidosis, and the idiopathic varieties, may produce pulmonary hypertension by destroying the vascular bed. The alveolar walls are thickened by fibrous tissue which compresses and finally obliterates the capillary network. Secondary changes of medial hypertrophy, intimal fibrosis, and thrombosis affect the muscular arteries. Tuberculosis obliterates vessels but usually does not, by itself, cause clinically significant pulmonary hypertension. Massive and diffuse pneumoconiotic fibrosis, of which silicosis is an excellent example, can easily obliterate enough of the vascular bed to cause severe pulmonary hypertension.

Thromboembolism is discussed elsewhere. In some parts of the world pulmonary schistosomiasis is a frequent cause of severe pulmonary hypertension. Ova lodge in the pulmonary arteries and initiate a granulomatous arteritis which ultimately closes the vessels. Very occasionally, pulmonary hypertension is caused by the diffuse spread of neoplastic tissue through the blood or lymphatic vessels of the lung.

In bronchiectasis, large anastomoses may occur between bronchial and pulmonary arteries in the affected area, with a resultant left-to-right shunt. This rarely causes clinically significant pressure overload on the right heart or volume overload on the left, but rupture of these dilated arteries in the wall of a bronchiectatic sac can cause severe hemoptysis.

Serial lung biopsies after the inciting cause of pulmonary hypertension has been surgically corrected in congenital or rheumatic heart disease have demonstrated marked regression of muscular medial hypertrophy and intimal fibrosis. The dilatation lesions of advanced disease do not regress.

With chronic pulmonary hypertension right ventricular hypertrophy develops. This is probably most reliably measured at autopsy by the weight of the right ventricular free wall, which normally is less than 75 grams. The ratio of left ventricular weight, including the septum, to that of the right ventricular wall is normally between 2 and 3.5. In severe right ventricular hypertrophy secondary to lung disease, a slight increase in septal weight may occur. The weight of the left ventricular free wall is usually normal, but may be increased without apparent cause.

General Clinical Assessment. Pulmonary hypertension may result from (1) disorders producing chronic generalized pulmonary venous hypertension, (2) high altitude hypoxia and hypoventilation of extrapulmonary origin, (3) chronic obstructive bronchopulmonary disease, (4) restrictive lung disease, and (5) pulmonary vascular disease including thromboembolism, primary pulmonary hypertension, and congenital heart disease, with or without increased pulmonary blood flow. Before describing these categories some general observations are in order on the clinical detection of pulmonary hypertension and evaluation of its cause.

The existence of pulmonary hypertension may be very easy to suspect because of the obvious presence of cardiac or pulmonary disease which might cause it. It may be overlooked, however, when heart or lung disorders are not obvious or not considered appropriate in kind or degree to cause pulmonary hypertension. Such disorders include chronic embolic disease of the pulmonary circulation, primary pulmonary hypertension, alveolar hypoxia and hypercapnia of extrapulmonary origin, or diffuse interstitial fibrosis which is not apparent on chest films.

Undue exertional dyspnea is the most characteristic symptom of pulmonary hypertension. In severe hypertension, angina, exertional syncope, and extreme fatigability are common. The classic physical signs of pulmonary arterial hypertension are described in Primary Pulmonary Hypertension. Abnormalities which can limit ventilation such as kyphoscoliosis, extensive thoracoplasty, obesity, and neuromuscular disease should raise the possibility of pulmonary hypertension. Marked restriction of respiratory excursion, intercostal retraction, and a shower of fine crackling rales during vigorous inspiratory effort may uncover diffuse interstitial fibrosis.

Roentgenograms are helpful but not diagnostic. There is no well-established contour pattern of right ventricular enlargement. The right ventricular outflow tract and main pulmonary artery may produce an abnormal convexity of the left heart border below the aortic arch in the posteroanterior film and may fill in the retrosternal space in the lateral or right oblique views. With pulmonary arterial hypertension the central arteries are distended and the peripheral lung fields are relatively avascular. This pattern is modified by associated disorders. With venous hypertension the lung fields may be congested, showing enlarged veins, local areas of edema, and Kerley's short horizontal lines at the lung base. With high flow states there is generalized increase in vascularity. With obstructive lung disease the heart is relatively narrow and vertical, the central vessels large, and the peripheral fields avascular. In serial films increasing pulmonary artery pressure is often manifested by increasing size of the central arteries and transverse heart diameter, and falling pressure by the opposite changes. Pulmonary arteriography demonstrates central dilatation and peripheral pruning of the pulmonary arteries. It can be especially helpful in the detection of thromboembolic disease by showing irregularities in the lumen of the large arteries and abrupt occlusion of some vessels, rather than a symmetrical distribution of contrast material. Regional reduction or loss of blood flow can also occur with lung tumors and other causes of bronchial obstruction. Localized regions of diminished perfusion can be demonstrated by scintillation scan after the intravenous injection of macroaggregated human albumin tagged with a suitable gamma emitter, such as I^{131}.

The *electrocardiogram* often, but not always, shows changes indicating right heart hypertrophy in patients with chronic pulmonary hypertension.

The pattern may be modified, especially in patients with obstructive lung disease by shifts in heart position and changes in the degree of electrical insulation offered by the lung.

With right atrial hypertrophy, and with a vertical heart position, the mean P vector in the frontal plane is deviated rightward. This can produce a P wave which is abnormally tall (over 2.5 mm.) in II, III, and aVF. The wave is not abnormally wide, like a "p mitrale," since the right atrium begins depolarization before the left, and any prolongation of its depolarization because of hypertrophy rarely extends beyond the time of left atrial depolarization. This "P pulmonale" is especially characteristic of right heart enlargement in obstructive lung disease.

Right ventricular hypertrophy caused by substantial chronic pulmonary hypertension characteristically produces right axis deviation, dominant R or R' in V1, inverted T waves in the right chest leads, and a deep S wave in V5 and V6. With chronic obstructive lung disease the QRS pattern is influenced by a tendency toward vertical position and clockwise rotation of the heart. There is right axis deviation. Most commonly the precordial leads show an rS pattern which may change to an Rs unusually far over on the left chest, or may be maintained through V6. The right precordial T waves are usually upright, but may be inverted during cardiopulmonary insufficiency. Less commonly the precordial leads show the characteristic pattern of right ventricular hypertrophy, with a dominant R1, inverted right precordial T waves, and prominent SV5 and SV6. Occasionally, there may be partial or complete right bundle branch block.

Arrhythmias are not uncommon in patients with pulmonary hypertension. They include atrial and ventricular extrasystoles, supraventricular tachycardia, sometimes with atrioventricular block, atrial flutter, and atrial fibrillation.

When pulmonary hypertension is suspected or known to be present, *pulmonary function tests* may provide useful information about the nature and severity of the underlying disorder. In respiratory system disorders, simple spirometry and measurement of arterial blood gases will help identify and estimate the extent of hypoventilatory, obstructive, and restrictive disease. Obstructive disease is identified by primary impairment in rate of air movement out of the lung (for example, FEV_1/VC less than 80 per cent, and restrictive disease by impairment of excursion of the lung (reduced VC). Patients with chronic hypoventilation from extrapulmonary causes characteristically show a decreased arterial blood Po_2 and increased Pco_2, but this may be somewhat variable during the excitement of an arterial puncture. An elevated plasma bicarbonate and, less reliably, polycythemia are sometimes more stable indicators of chronic change in ventilatory function. Pulmonary hypertension in obstructive disease classically appears in episodes of respiratory impairment, when pulmonary vasoconstriction is induced by alveolar hypoxia and hypercapnia. The systemic arterial blood, with much reduced Po_2 and increased Pco_2, reflects these alveolar gas changes, and arterial blood gas measurements are essential for optimal detection and management of these episodes. Restrictive lung disease causes pulmonary hypertension by obliteration of small vessels. Oxygen uptake is impaired by ventilation-perfusion imbalance, including virtual shunts, and to some extent by diffusion defects. Accordingly, arterial Po_2 is reduced, and the attendant hyperventilation in lung regions which can still effectively unload CO_2 usually reduces arterial Pco_2 as well.

Occasionally a patient with pulmonary hypertension resulting from widespread obliteration of the capillary network through interstitial fibrosis, scleroderma, or other cause may have a chest film which shows no lung disease, and spirometric or blood gas measurements in a normal or equivocal range. In such cases, measurement of the diffusing capacity for carbon monoxide (DL_{CO}) may pinpoint the abnormality by the finding of much reduced values, such as 30 to 50 per cent of normal.

Thromboembolic disease tends not to reduce DL_{CO} greatly because the capillaries are still intact and may have some circulation through bronchopulmonary anastomoses. DL_{CO} measurements by standard methods reflect the presence of capillaries containing blood but are not sensitive to the rate of blood flow through the capillaries. Thromboembolic disease, however, does have the effect of substantially shutting off blood flow from some portions of the lung and increasing flow elsewhere. The presence of many alveoli which still have ventilation but little exchange of oxygen and carbon dioxide with blood produces a measurable increase in the volume of "dead space" or wasted ventilation, and in the Pco_2 difference between arterial blood and alveolar gas. Measurements of dead space ventilation and arterial-alveolar Pco_2 gradients therefore have some value in thromboembolic and other occlusive vascular disease, but the sensitivity of these tests is diminished by the tendency of the lung to reduce ventilation by bronchoconstriction in regions with poor blood flow.

When infiltrative or vascular obstructive disease of the lung is known or suspected to be present as the cause of pulmonary hypertension, lung biopsy can provide very valuable information as to the nature of the process and the possible utility of steroid, anticoagulant, or other therapy. Vascular lesions of the lung may be somewhat irregularly distributed, and this must be taken into account in the interpretation.

Cardiac catheterization, by which pulmonary arterial and pulmonary venous or wedge pressures can be measured, the pulmonary blood flow estimated, and shunts detected, yields the most definitive functional information about the pulmonary circulation. The pressure and resistance values characteristic of various disorders are described under the appropriate disease categories.

LEFT ATRIAL AND PULMONARY VENOUS HYPERTENSION

Chronic high-grade elevation of the pulmonary venous pressure is commonly caused by mitral stenosis, to a lesser extent by mitral insufficiency and chronic left ventricular failure, and much more rarely by a variety of uncommon disorders, including left atrial tumors, mediastinal tumors compressing the pulmonary veins, cor triatriatum, and diffuse pulmonary veno-occlusive disease of unknown cause. The clinical features of pulmonary venous hypertension have been studied most extensively in patients with mitral stenosis, and the subsequent discussion is based on this group.

In *mitral stenosis* left atrial pressures of 20 to 30 mm. Hg are not uncommon at rest, and during exercise pressure may rise by 50 per cent or more. This pressure is transmitted through the entire pulmonary vascular system and is, in itself, a cause of significant pulmonary arterial hypertension. A substantial minority of patients with resting left atrial pressures above 20 mm. Hg also develop a large increase in pulmonary vascular resistance. In Wood's large series, about 30 per cent of patients coming to surgery for mitral stenosis had a resistance exceeding 6 units (normal 1.5) and 12 per cent had a resistance above 10 units, which approximates the normal systemic vascular resistance. Present evidence suggests that resistance increase depends not only on the level of left atrial pressure but also on individual susceptibility.

The cause of increased resistance is not clear, but it appears to depend in part on active vasoconstriction, apparently of the muscular pulmonary arteries, possibly in response to high intraluminal pressure. Resistance can be lowered acutely but only partially by acetylcholine and other pulmonary vasodilators. In these patients, pulmonary vascular resistance is often abruptly increased when the left atrial pressure is sharply raised by exercise. Secondary structural changes in the pulmonary vessels, as described above, must play a considerable part, and in some instances fibrotic changes in the alveolar walls may reduce the capillary bed. As noted before, vessels in the dependent segments of lung are much more narrowed than those in the upper portions. Correspondingly, special studies have shown that the normal distribution of pulmonary blood flow is reversed in patients with advanced mitral stenosis, so that the upper lung is much more richly perfused than the base. In isolated lung preparations perfused under high venous pressure, a similar flow distribution develops, associated with the appearance of thick cuffs of edema around pulmonary arteries and veins of 100 μ and larger diameter in the lower lung. It has been postulated that perivascular edema may reduce the elastic distending support which these vessels receive from the surrounding lung parenchyma, allowing their partial closure.

Whatever the relative roles of active vasocon-

striction, structural changes in the vessels and alveolar walls, and perivascular edema, the pulmonary vascular resistance sometimes falls dramatically after surgical relief of left atrial hypertension. Even high-grade resistance may fall by 50 per cent in 48 hours after surgery and be halved again in eight to ten days. Usually there is a more gradual fall over a period of months to values which are substantially reduced or normal. The surgical mortality of mitral valve repair or replacement is considerably increased in patients with high-grade pulmonary vascular resistance, but the end result of a successful operation can be most satisfactory.

A few cases of *diffuse pulmonary veno-occlusive disease* of unknown etiology have been reported, predominantly in women. The small and medium-sized veins are narrowed and occluded by fibrous tissue and thrombosis without inflammatory change in the vein wall. The changes in pulmonary arteries and lung parenchyma resemble those in severe mitral stenosis with increased pulmonary vascular resistance. The clinical picture is much like that of primary pulmonary arterial hypertension except for the occasional appearance of orthopnea and rather modest x-ray evidence of congestion in the form of Kerley's lines and mottling in the lower lung fields. The course has been relentless, with survival ranging from a few weeks to five years after the onset of symptoms.

HIGH ALTITUDE HYPOXIA

The occurrence of mild to moderate pulmonary hypertension in dwellers at high altitude is well established. School children living in Colorado at about 10,000 feet were found to have a mean pulmonary artery pressure averaging 25 mm. Hg, rising to 54 mm. Hg on exercise, and in individual cases going much higher. Similar results have been obtained in Peruvian Indians, who exhibit slightly higher pressures at more extreme altitudes. Breathing oxygen produces a relatively small immediate fall in pulmonary arterial pressure and pulmonary vascular resistance, but after residence at low altitudes for one or two years pressures are generally normal. Right ventricular hypertrophy and medial hypertrophy of the muscular pulmonary arteries have been found in high altitude dwellers, and progressive rightward deviation of the frontal QRS vector has been observed in populations living at progressively higher altitudes up to nearly 15,000 feet. There is striking individual variation in the propensity to high altitude pulmonary hypertension.

CHRONIC OBSTRUCTIVE PULMONARY DISEASE

This entity, which has been defined elsewhere, often leads to pulmonary hypertension, right ventricular hypertrophy, and right heart failure. It accounts for the majority of patients with "cor pulmonale," defined by the World Health Organization as "hypertrophy of the right ventricle resulting from diseases affecting the function and/or the structure of the lung, except when these pulmonary alterations are the result of diseases that primarily affect the left side of the heart or of congenital heart disease." Cor pulmonale has been estimated to account for 5 to 10 per cent of organic heart disease. Perhaps a quarter of patients with chronic obstructive pulmonary disease ultimately show clinical evidence of cor pulmonale.

Pathologic Physiology. Hypertrophy and failure of the right heart in chronic obstructive lung disease are caused by pulmonary hypertension, possibly abetted by the deleterious effects of hypoxia. Structural changes which reduce and distort the pulmonary vascular bed in obstructive disease have been previously described. Between bouts of respiratory insufficiency these patients do not usually have pulmonary hypertension at rest, but with exercise the pressure tends to rise steeply as the cardiac output increases, reflecting loss of the normal ability to distend and recruit additional channels. With respiratory insufficiency, alveolar hypoxia and hypercapnia develop in most of the perfused regions of the lung. Hypoxia and acidosis have individually been shown to produce pulmonary vasoconstriction and to have mutually reinforcing effects in this regard. In patients with obstructive lung disease, progressive acidosis makes the pulmonary artery pressure more and more sensitive to hypoxia, but progressive hypoxia makes the pressure more and more sensitive to acidosis. Respiratory insufficiency, commonly caused by respiratory infection, thus precipitates pulmonary hypertension. During right heart failure, pressures of the order of 70/35 with a mean of 50 mm. Hg are commonly found but they subside markedly over a few days or weeks as respiratory insufficiency and congestive failure respond to treatment.

When hypoxia is relieved by giving oxygen during failure, there is an immediate, but small, drop in pulmonary artery pressure. With continuing therapy the resting pressure during air breathing gradually subsides, and the administration of oxygen continues to produce small pressure drops. This gradual fall in pressure over days or weeks is not closely correlated with the relief of acidosis. Once an increase in pulmonary vascular resistance has been well established, it declines relatively slowly even when hypoxia and acidosis are quickly relieved.

During right heart failure in obstructive lung disease the cardiac output is usually normal or only moderately decreased, although it does not rise much on exercise. The blood volume is considerably increased, and it appears that these patients are more prone to retain salt and water than patients with most other causes of cardiac insufficiency. Patients with obstructive lung disease who have never been edematous have been shown to have subnormal renal plasma flow and glomerular filtration rate.

Despite the occasional finding of left ventricular hypertrophy in patients dying of obstructive lung disease, the pulmonary wedge pressure is characteristically not elevated during bouts of failure, and measurements of left ventricular function have shown little or no abnormality, even during failure.

Clinical Manifestations. Many patients with chronic obstructive lung disease never have heart failure. Those with predominant bronchitis who readily become hypoxic and hypercapnic may have repeated bouts of failure. Those with predominant emphysema are slower to fail but often do poorly once they have failed.

A typical patient is a middle-aged or elderly male with a long history of chronic cough and progressive dyspnea, both acutely worse in recent days. There may have been an obvious respiratory infection, but even without this history low grade fever and purulent sputum are frequently present. The patient is acutely ill, dyspneic, cyanotic, and confused. Congestive failure is often evident from distended neck veins, ankle edema, and tenderness of the liver. The diaphragms are low, breath sounds are distant, crepitant rales are heard, particularly at the lung bases, and scattered expiratory wheezes may be present. The heart rate is usually well over 100 per minute, and the rhythm is generally regular. The apex impulse is not palpable to the left of the sternum, and the heart size cannot be estimated by percussion. Auscultation is difficult because of interfering respiratory sounds, except in the subxiphoid region, where a diastolic gallop may be heard. In some patients failure may develop much more insidiously, with gradually increasing dyspnea, and there may be difficulty in recognizing the presence of failure.

The plasma bicarbonate content is almost always elevated, and the hematocrit may be elevated. Oxygen saturation of arterial blood is usually below 80 per cent and the P_{CO_2} above 60 mm. Hg.

Chest x-rays do not usually show convincing right heart enlargement, but increase in heart size and in the width of the major pulmonary arteries is evident by comparison with prefailure films.

The electrocardiogram has been previously described (General Clinical Assessment).

Diagnosis. The diagnosis is usually made easily from the features described above. In some cases in which failure is evident there may be uncertainty whether obstructive lung disease is the cause. If it is, blood gas changes will be marked, and pleural fluid, Cheyne-Stokes breathing, and a palpable apex impulse are unlikely. In subtle cases, failure may be diagnosed only in retrospect after diuresis and decrease in heart size. In early stages, diminishing pulmonary function and increases of plasma bicarbonate, hematocrit, body weight, and roentgenographic heart size are suggestive.

Treatment. In chronic obstructive lung disease with pulmonary insufficiency and heart failure, relief of hypoxia and improvement of alveolar ventilation are basic in treatment. The management of this problem is described elsewhere. Otherwise, conventional therapy for congestive failure is employed, consisting of bed rest, sodium restriction (500 mg. per day), digitalis (intoxication is common), and chlorothiazide, 500 mg. twice a day or equivalent. Other diuretics may be required.

When hypoxia and hypercapnia are relieved by successful treatment of ventilatory insufficiency in patients with heart failure caused by obstructive pulmonary disease, the pulmonary arterial pressure fails, diuresis occurs, and the patient returns substantially to his prefailure state in the course of a few weeks. Recurrence of failure within a few months or years is very common, but may be long delayed by proper maintenance therapy.

HYPOVENTILATION OF EXTRAPULMONARY ORIGIN

Disorders of the ventilatory apparatus which result in chronic alveolar hypoventilation can cause pulmonary hypertension and right heart failure. Among such disorders are *structural abnormalities of the chest* such as kyphoscoliosis, extreme obesity, constrictive pleuritis, and thoracoplasty; and *neuromuscular disease* such as poliomyelitis, muscular dystrophy, and "respiratory center" dysfunction.

Pathologic Physiology. It is by no means clear why persons who have managed well for years despite limited mobility of the thoracic cage ultimately decompensate and develop ventilatory insufficiency. Progressive reduction in thoracic compliance, loss of muscular strength with age and sedentary life, gradual accommodation of the respiratory center to abnormal proprioceptive and chemical stimuli, and respiratory tract infection have all been suggested as playing a part. With onset of alveolar hypoventilation, hypoxia, and hypercapnia, pulmonary hypertension develops, and right heart failure follows, much as in the ventilatory insufficiency of obstructive lung disease.

Clinical Manifestations. As a group, these patients yield with relatively little struggle to advancing ventilatory insufficiency. Dyspnea is not a prominent complaint. Weakness, somnolence, confusion, and headache are more characteristic. These symptoms and the appearance of plethora, polycythemia, and elevated plasma bicarbonate in a patient with thoracic cage dysfunction should alert the physician to the possibility of ventilatory insufficiency. The diagnosis is confirmed by arterial blood gas measurements. The rare patient with "primary" hypoventilation, perhaps due to a central nervous system lesion, presents a similar picture, but without a visible reason for ventilatory insufficiency.

The signs of right heart failure are most obvious in obese patients with ventilatory insufficiency, are often less pronounced in persons with kypho-scoliosis or old thoracoplasty, and are frequently overshadowed by central nervous system manifestations of hypoxia and hypercapnia in persons with neuromuscular dysfunction.

The essential features of the x-ray and electrocardiogram have been described (General Clinical Assessment).

Treatment. The principles of treatment are the same as in obstructive pulmonary disease. Once compensation has been regained, weight reduction is mandatory for the obese patient, to avoid a recurrence. Physical therapy and breathing exercises to maintain muscular vigor and mobility of the thoracic cage may be very helpful for other persons with impaired mobility of the chest cage.

Prognosis. Once failure has occurred, recurrence is common within a year or two. Occasionally patients will remain compensated and active for prolonged periods.

RESTRICTIVE LUNG DISEASE

Extensive fibrotic and granulomatous disorders of the lung frequently cause pulmonary hypertension, primarily by destruction of more than two thirds of the vascular bed. Included in this category are silicosis and other pneumoconioses with massive fibrosis, radiation fibrosis, scleroderma, dermatomyositis, diffuse interstitial fibrosis of unknown cause, sarcoidosis, berylliosis, and eosinophilic granuloma.

For most of its course the clinical picture is dominated by the underlying lung disease, which produces dyspnea, fatigability, cyanosis, and often digital clubbing. Ventilation-perfusion imbalance, impaired oxygen diffusion, and frank intrapulmonary shunts progressively decrease arterial blood oxygen tension and saturation, with worsening on exercise. These patients hyperventilate enough in lung regions which still exchange gas to maintain normal or reduced arterial blood carbon dioxide tensions.

When pulmonary hypertension develops, the cardiovascular signs resemble those described under Primary Pulmonary Hypertension, and the roentgenographic and electrocardiographic manifestations of pulmonary hypertension and right ventricular hypertrophy appear (General Clinical Assessment).

In most cases pulmonary hypertension and failure are unyielding, but when steroid therapy favorably affects the pulmonary disease they can be forestalled.

VASCULAR DISEASE

Congenital Heart Disease

This subject is discussed fully elsewhere, but a résumé of some aspects pertinent to pulmonary hypertension is presented here.

Pathologic Physiology. When a large defect connects the left and right cardiac chambers or great vessels downstream from the tricuspid valve, pulmonary hypertension is often present, and the pulmonary vascular resistance is high. Examples are ventricular septal defect, patent ductus arteriosus, aorticopulmonary septal defect, and persistent truncus arteriosus. As the high fetal pulmonary resistance begins to regress in postnatal life, large left-to right shunts may cause failure. Usually, pulmonary flow is limited by incomplete regression or early re-establishment of the increased pulmonary resistance at the expense of causing pulmonary hypertension. With many defects resistance is normal or low. It is often elevated but stable with large defects. In a minority of patients with large defects, pulmonary resistance and pressure increase progressively, and the shunt finally begins to reverse. This course is nearly always determined in early life. Only 12 per cent of a large series of patients with ventricular septal defect showed a rise in pulmonary arterial pressure on prolonged follow-up. There was no progression if the initial systolic pressure was under 50 mm. Hg.

Whether re-establishment of high resistance depends on high pulmonary flow, high intravascular pressure, or elevation of left atrial pressure during systolic closure of the mitral valve against a high pulmonary flow is debated. After defect repair, residual elevations in resistance gradually decline, and medial and intimal thickening of the arteries regresses. When resistance is very high and dilatation lesions of the pulmonary arteries are present, resistance is fixed and defect closure has a forbidding mortality.

The common large shunts upstream from the tricuspid valve have a different history. The major examples are atrial septal defect and partial anomalous pulmonary venous drainage. With large defects there is a large left-to-right shunt and a large pulmonary blood flow. The pulmonary arteries are dilated and thin walled, and the pulmonary vascular resistance is low. In a minority of patients, estimated at 9 to 13 per cent in some series and less in others, the pulmonary vascular resistance begins to rise in later life, usually between 20 and 40 years of age. The primary cause of increased resistance appears at first to be intimal fibrosis in the arterioles. Subsequently, medial hypertrophy, dilatation lesions, and other degenerative changes, including thrombosis, affect larger arteries. As these changes progress, pulmonary hypertension becomes severe, the right ventricle hypertrophies, the shunt reverses, and failure ultimately develops. Closure of the defect at this stage has a poor prognosis. A somewhat more common unfavorable course for patients with atrial septal defect in adult life is the development of atrial fibrillation and failure with only slight or moderate pulmonary hypertension.

PULMONARY EMBOLISM

This subject is discussed under Pulmonary Embolism and Infarction.

PRIMARY PULMONARY HYPERTENSION

Primary pulmonary hypertension is a progressive disease, predominantly affecting young parous women, in which severe pulmonary hypertension results from increased arterial resistance of unknown cause. The differentiation between this disorder and repeated embolization of small arteries is difficult.

Incidence. Primary pulmonary hypertension occurred in 0.17 per cent of 10,000 cases of heart disease seen in Wood's clinic. In 93 collected case reports the age range was 1 to 68 years, most patients being from 20 to 40. Females exceeded males in a ratio of 3:1. A number of instances of familial pulmonary hypertension have been reported. In one family, inheritance appeared to be by way of a Mendelian dominant gene with variable penetrance.

Pathologic Physiology. The pathologic findings have been described. Pulmonary arterial pressure may exceed systemic arterial pressure at rest. It is usually found to be 65 to 90 mm. Hg, systolic. The pulmonary vascular resistance is high, averaging about eight times normal. The wedge pressure is not elevated. The cardiac output is reduced. A variable drop in pulmonary vascular resistance occurs on infusing dilator drugs such as acetylcholine, isoproterenol, or tolazoline into the pulmonary artery, indicating a labile resistance component. This lability is more pronounced in young persons and apparently in early cases. The arterial blood oxygen saturation may be normal or slightly reduced, and it often falls a little on exercise. Central cyanosis does not occur, however, except when a patent foramen ovale and elevated right ventricular diastolic pressure permit right-to-left shunting. The arterial blood Pco_2 is usually reduced by hyperventilation.

Clinical Manifestations. Primary pulmonary hypertension provides a clinical model of severe progressive pulmonary hypertension in the absence of other disorders of the heart and lungs.

Most of the *symptoms* are brought on by exertion. The most common symptoms are easy fatigability and severe exertional dyspnea. Exertional syncope and angina occur with significant frequency. Occasionally, there are small hemoptyses, ascribed to pulmonary infarcts.

Distinctive *physical findings* are usually present. Because of low cardiac output, peripheral cyanosis, cold extremities, and a small pulse are often noted. The cardiac rhythm is at first normal, but paroxysmal or fixed atrial flutter or fibrillation may appear later. The jugular venous pulse characteristically exhibits a giant "a" wave of atrial contraction which may later disappear with right heart failure or be obscured by tricuspid insufficiency. Coincident with the "a" wave, a prehepatic or precordial pulsation may be felt. In most cases a systolic right ventricular heave can be seen or felt along the left sternal border. The closing shock of the pulmonic valve is easily felt.

A right atrial gallop is heard as a dull, low-frequency sound, usually loudest at the lower left sternal border, although occasionally well transmitted to the apex region when this is occupied by the right ventricle. Tricuspid regurgitation is frequent, and a pansystolic murmur of this origin is usually heard at the lower left sternal border, though it also may be heard well at the right sternal border or the xiphoid region. When the right ventricle extends to the cardiac apex, this murmur may be heard well to the left. It may be musical or harsh, varies greatly in intensity from one patient to the next, and may be associated with a palpable thrill. The murmur is increased during inspiration. A pulmonic ejection sound is common. This is best heard in the second and third left intercostal spaces, and characteristically has a sharp, high-pitched clicking quality. The loud closure sound of the pulmonic valve is the most characteristic of all auscultatory sounds of pulmonary hypertension. It is best heard at or near the pulmonic area but may be widely transmitted. The second heart sound, as a whole, tends to be quite closely split, with accentuation of the second or pulmonic component when this can be distinguished. When right ventricular failure occurs, the split may be widened. The Graham Steell murmur of pulmonic incompetence can be heard in a sizable minority of these patients. It is heard best in the second and third intercostal space and is prolonged and high pitched. Occasionally it is accompanied by a thrill. A pulmonic ejection murmur is not characteristic. With failure, a diastolic ventricular gallop often appears. Of all the physical signs, the right ventricular heave and loud pulmonic closure point most convincingly toward right ventricular hypertrophy and pulmonary hypertension.

The chest film and the electrocardiogram have been described (General Clinical Assessment).

Diagnosis. The diagnosis of pulmonary hypertension can usually be made with a high degree of certainty from the clinical picture outlined above. To make the diagnosis with absolute certainty it is necessary to measure pressures in the lesser circulation by cardiac catheterization. This procedure is also most helpful in deciding among the various causative possibilities when conventional clinical data are inadequate. The diagnosis of primary pulmonary hypertension must be made by exclusion of other etiologic possibilities. This may require extensive investigation, and it should be remembered that these patients have a propensity to die suddenly in the course of procedures which are usually well tolerated, such as cardiac catheterization, angiography, and open lung biopsy.

The most important alternative diagnosis to consider is recurrent pulmonary embolism because of the therapeutic implications. Other possibilities which can be differentiated by special studies include high-grade mitral stenosis with greatly reduced output and loss of the characteristic murmur, severe hypertension in congenital heart disease with modification or loss of the usual physical signs, and diffuse interstitial fibrosis not evident on x-ray. Pulmonary veno-occlusive disease has a course much like that of primary pulmonary hypertension and is difficult to distinguish during life.

Treatment. Treatment has been most unsatisfactory. Anticoagulant therapy is often used against the possibility of undetected thromboembolic disease and in the hope of retarding thrombosis in the pulmonary arterial tree. A few efforts have been made to relax pulmonary vasoconstriction in early cases by prolonged administration of acetylcholine or other dilators through an inlying pulmonary catheter. Conventional treatment for congestive heart failure should be used.

Prognosis. The outlook is extremely poor. The average duration of life from the onset of symptoms is three years. Persons with familial pulmonary hypertension sometimes have a much more prolonged course.

OTHER CONDITIONS

Other disorders which affect the pulmonary vasculature and may cause hypertension are bilharziasis, polyarteritis nodosa and other arteritis, malignant embolism, and multiple thrombosis in sickle cell anemia.

Bergofsky, E. H.: Cor pulmonale in the syndrome of alveolar hypoventilation. Progr. Cardiov. Dis., 9:414, 1967.

Oakley, C. M., and Goodwin, J. F.: The current status of pulmonary embolism and pulmonary vascular disease in relation to pulmonary hypertension. Progr. Cardiov. Dis., 9: 495, 1967.

Wagenvoort, C. A., Heath, D., and Edwards, J. E.: The Pathology of the Pulmonary Vasculature. Springfield, Ill., Charles C Thomas, 1964.

Williams, J. F., Jr., Childress, R. H., Boyd, D. L., Higgs, L. M., and Behnke, R. H.: Left ventricular function in patients with chronic obstructive lung disease. J. Clin. Invest., 47: 1143, 1968.

Williams, M. H., Jr., Adler, J. J., and Colp, C.: Pulmonary function studies as an aid in the differential diagnosis of pulmonary hypertension. Amer. J. Med., 47:378, 1969.

Wood, P.: Diseases of the Heart and Circulation. 3rd ed. Philadelphia, J. B. Lippincott Company, 1968.

DISEASES OF THE CARDIOVASCULAR SYSTEM

Heart Failure

Alfred P. Fishman

The heart is subject to a wide array of congenital, metabolic, inflammatory, and degenerative disorders, not only of its muscular walls, its linings, and its valves, but also of its nutrient vessels. Some of its diseases, such as coronary atherosclerosis, progress so slowly and insidiously as to become evident only when the disorder is far advanced. Others, such as myocardial infarction, the major complication of coronary atherosclerosis, are often dramatic in onset and catastrophic in course.

When signs and symptoms of heart disease do appear, they are of two different kinds: those referable to the heart itself, such as pain and palpitation, and others that are extracardiac and originate in congested circulatory beds and hypoperfused organs. Considered out of context, each extracardiac manifestation may be disappointingly nonspecific. For example, breathlessness is a common symptom that is shared by disorders of the heart, the lungs, and the brain. Nonetheless, when breathlessness develops in a patient with left heart disease, in association with other evidence of congested and edematous lungs, and grows worse when the patient lies flat, there is little question that the patient is suffering from left heart failure.

The following parts of this section will deal with individual cardiac disorders. The present part will be concerned with heart failure, a final common pathway for many of the diverse etiologies and pathogenic mechanisms that will be discussed subsequently.

PATHOPHYSIOLOGY OF HEART FAILURE

PATHOGENIC INTERPLAY

The heart consists basically of two primary muscular pumps (ventricles), two less muscular, booster pumps (atria), and their directional valves. The performance of each ventricle as a muscle and the competence of its valves determine its effectiveness as a pump. The two ventricles empty in unison, simultaneously dispatching venous blood to the lungs for arterialization and arterialized blood to the rest of the body for metabolic purposes. In order to fulfill these functions, heart muscle has to generate tension and shorten.

Since Starling's observations on the isolated heart about 50 years ago, it has been common knowledge that the heart possesses a considerable degree of intrinsic control and that much of this capacity is a function of the properties of its myocardium. Less appreciated has been the fact that for fulfilling its obligations with respect to the changing metabolic needs of daily life, the normal heart depends more on elaborate extrinsic neurohumoral controls than on the intrinsic properties of its muscle.

Heart Failure. In principle, the heart has failed to fulfill its function as a pump when it can no longer deliver an adequate supply of oxygenated blood to the tissues for their individual metabolic needs, both at rest and during usual levels of exercise. In practice, this concept has little practical application, because metabolic needs are more easily established in the experimental laboratory than at the bedside, and proper therapeutic measures depend on a clear definition of which part of the pumping mechanism is at fault, i.e., muscle, valves, or pericardium.

Definitions. Here, the designation "heart failure" will be used as a synonym for *myocardial* failure. This definition excludes valvular defects, such as mitral insufficiency, unless they strain the left ventricle enough to bring about myocardial failure. Not only does this restricted usage have practical value with respect to treatment, but it also makes it possible to relate pathogenesis to biochemical and molecular alterations in heart muscle.

The definition has several other implications. For example, it excludes states of peripheral circulatory collapse, such as that which follows severe hemorrhage, in which cardiac output is low because of an inadequate venous return rather than poor myocardial performance. It also draws a sharp distinction between a "congested state," such as may be produced by overtransfusion, in which the heart performs splendidly despite the overfilled circulation, and "congestive heart failure," in which the same degree of pulmonary and systemic venous congestion indicates that both ventricles have failed.

Finally, by restricting "heart failure" to myocardial failure, the definition automatically excludes electrophysiologic failure (cardiac arrest or ventricular fibrillation) as well as mechanical occlusion of the circulation, e.g., ball-valve thrombus of the mitral valve, embolus to the main pulmonary artery.

Load versus Myocardial Capacity. Clinical heart failure is usually chronic, the end stage of a sustained disproportion between hemodynamic load and the capacity of the heart muscle to handle the load; the load may be in the form of venous return (preload), resistance to ejection (afterload), or both. Rarely, as in acute mitral insufficiency that follows rupture of a papillary muscle, or after the sudden appearance of an abnormal communication between cardiac chambers in the course of myocardial infarction, does myocardial failure run an accelerated course. Both chronic and acute heart failure evoke compensatory adjustments, such as increased peripheral resistance, redistribution of blood flow, and heightened erythropoietic activity. But the adaptive mechanisms may be quite different in type, degree, intensity, and even in direction. For example, acute left atrial distention stimulates water diuresis, whereas chronic left atrial distention is associated with salt and water retention. These differences, particularly in reflex and humoral effects on remote organs such as the kidney, may be misleading when chronic heart failure in man is compared with experimental heart failure in animals, since the latter is generally acute in onset, fulminating in course, and abrupt in termination.

Left ventricular failure is much more common than right ventricular failure simply because of the prevalence of coronary atherosclerosis, systemic arterial hypertension, and rheumatic heart disease which affect the left side of the heart. However, in time, as left ventricular failure persists, the right ventricle will also fail because of the pulmonary hypertension that the incompetent left ventricle generates. Indeed, left ventricular failure is the most common cause of right ventricular failure, the combination being responsible for the clinical picture of "congestive heart failure."

Conceivably, an imbalance between load and capacity may arise in two ways: (1) an inordinate load, such as systemic hypertension, or (2) a damaged myocardium, in which ventricular performance is impaired by infection, coronary atherosclerosis, or pharmacologic agents. In most instances, heart failure is the consequence of a combination of the two, the proportion of each depending on the etiology of the heart disease.

Different loads are managed differently by the myocardium. Thus, overloading by high flow, e.g., arteriovenous shunt, aortic and mitral insufficiency, and anemia, generally evokes a gradual response in the form of dilatation and hypertrophy of the ventricle. On the other hand, in response to a sustained high resistance to emptying, as in aortic stenosis, or to a high blood pressure, as in systemic arterial hypertension, hypertrophy occurs well in advance of dilatation. Only after a long period of hypertrophy does the heart dilate

appreciably. Indeed, if the load continues, dilatation may progress to the point of rendering the mitral valve incompetent, thereby adding to the load; thereafter, the heart and its regulatory mechanisms deteriorate rapidly. Compared with these effects of overloading, a primary myocardiopathy generally elicits an extraordinary dilatation and hypertrophy. Although the different ways in which the myocardium responds to injury and overloading suggest that it has alternative biochemical and physiologic adaptations, the nature of these adjustments is entirely unclear.

Compensatory Mechanisms. The overloaded heart resorts to many of the same mechanisms that operate automatically in daily life to adjust cardiac output to the changing levels of activity. These include (1) The Frank-Starling (length-tension) relationship, (2) enhanced inotropic activity, and (3) tachycardia. A supplementary adaptive mechanism is hypertrophy.

The *Frank-Starling law of the heart* relates the end-diastolic volume of the ventricle to the energy that is liberated during the following systole. In effect, as in the case of skeletal muscle, it relates the initial length of the myocardial fibers to the tension that they develop. For the heart, end-diastolic pressure is usually used as a rough estimate of initial length, and stroke output or work is substituted for tension. This relationship is exploited by the ventricle to sustain a normal or near-normal stroke output by increasing its end-diastolic volume. The relationship is illustrated in Figure 1 by a family of curves. The position of each curve indicates the contractility of the heart. For example, enhanced contractility, as after sympathetic nervous stimulation, moves the normal curve toward one in which more stroke work is done at lower filling pressures. As contractility becomes progressively impaired and the heart continues to dilate, the relationship shifts to a lower curve instead of slipping, as originally pictured, over the hump of a single curve on to a descending limb. In the normal heart, the Frank-Starling mechanism serves principally to match the stroke outputs of the two ventricles. But in heart failure, or in heart that has been deprived

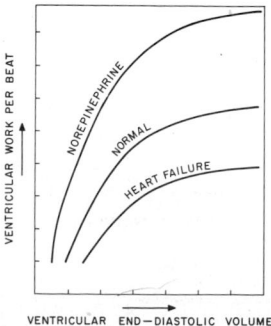

FIGURE 1. Hypothetical Frank-Starling relationships for different states of myocardial contractility. (Modified from Sarnoff, S. J., and Mitchell, J. H.: The control of the function of the heart. *In* Hamilton, W. F., and Dow, P.: Handbook of Physiology. Washington, D. C., American Physiological Society, 1962, p. 506.

of its extrinsic neurohumoral controls, it assumes much greater significance as an adaptive mechanism.

Enhanced inotropic activity is the dominant compensatory mechanism for the normal heart. In contrast to the Frank-Starling mechanism, an increase in the force and velocity of contraction occurs without a corresponding increase in the end-diastolic ventricular volume. The increase in myocardial contractility is accomplished by adrenergic nervous and humoral factors which, under normal conditions, tend to obscure the Frank-Starling mechanism. In heart failure, the adrenergic mechanism is impaired, denying to the heart the support that it requires for enhanced performance during stress such as exercise. Thus, the myocardium is poor in norepinephrine, the intrinsic adrenergic transmitter, and lacks ability to replenish this store. Because of this poverty, it has only a blunted inotropic and chronotropic response to stimulation of the cardiac adrenergic nerves. Therefore, it has to rely on blood-borne norepinephrine, released by the adrenals, for its sympathetic nervous support rather than on its own intrinsic supply. Further depletion of the heart of its catecholamines, as by guanethidine, aggravates the heart failure. In many respects, the performance of the human heart that has failed resembles that of both the "denervated" heart and the isolated heart-lung preparation that Starling used.

Tachycardia in normal subjects has little effect on the cardiac output as long as the heart rate is not excessive. Thus, up to heart rates of approximately 100 per minute, reciprocal changes in heart rate and stroke volume operate to keep cardiac output virtually unchanged. However, in heart failure, the cardiac output is rate-dependent because the stroke output is relatively fixed.

Hypertrophy differs from the other compensatory mechanisms in that it takes time to develop. During hypertrophy, both muscle mass and capillary vessels increase proportionately to sustain the over-all contractile performance of the heart despite the increased load. But within hypertrophy is contained the seed of heart failure. Thus, even though the hypertrophied heart does succeed in sustaining over-all contractile performance at normal levels, abnormalities in details of contraction appear during hypertrophy, quite similar to those of the heart that has failed. For example, both the rate at which the myocardium develops tension during contraction and the rate of contraction are abnormally low in hypertrophy. Consequently, once hypertrophy has begun, the myocardium has also started on the road to failure.

Why the hypertrophied heart begins to fail is still a mystery. The traditional notion that implicated myocardial hypoxia which developed as the enlarging muscle mass outgrew its capillary blood supply is not supported by anatomic evidence. Nor is there convincing anatomic reason to believe that the calibers of the large coronary arteries become inadequate as the muscle mass and capillary circulation enlarge. Even less tenable is the

proposition that disproportionate hypertrophy of the outflow tract impedes ventricular emptying. More intriguing but still to be proved is the idea that each hypertrophied myocardial fiber is slightly less adequate than the normal fiber. According to this notion, hypertrophy entails the addition of inadequate functional units; when the total sum of inadequacies exceeds the advantages of hypertrophy, the heart starts its decline to failure. Although each of these hypotheses has its proponents, the ultrastructural and biochemical bases for hypertrophy still remain to be settled.

Dilatation. Progressive dilatation marks the transition between ventricular hypertrophy and failure. For a long while, dilatation may serve as a compensatory mechanism, increasing the contractile force of the heart by way of the Frank-Starling relationship. But dilatation gradually becomes inadequate to maintain the stroke output.

Several different mechanisms seem to be involved in the ultimate inability of the dilated heart to maintain its output. (1) Slippage and rearrangement of sarcomeres during progressive dilatation; as a result, they neither produce a coordinated contraction nor are properly stretched to enhance contractility as the heart dilates further. (2) High wall tension in accord with the law of Laplace (Fig. 2); as the volume of the ventricle increases, its wall tension for a given pressure in the ventricular cavity during contraction is greater than normal. (3) Protracted maintenance of high wall tension during contraction; in contrast to the normal heart, in which the wall tension decreases in the course of systole, wall tension remains high in the dilated heart. (4) High energy requirements coupled with an inefficient conversion of chemical to mechanical energy; despite the decrease in stroke output, the dilated heart does more internal work and has a higher myocardial oxygen consumption than does the normal heart. Because of these limitations, chronic enlargement is an inefficient and ill-fated mechanism for achieving sustained improvement in cardiac performance.

Overshoot of Compensatory Mechanisms. Be-

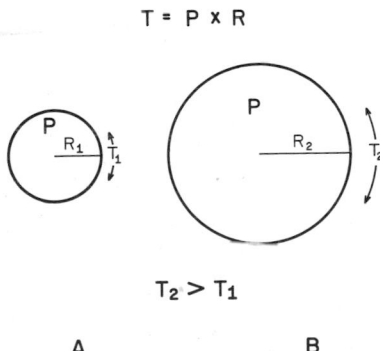

$$T = P \times R$$

$$T_2 > T_1$$

A   B

FIGURE 2. An illustration of the law of Laplace ($T = P \times R$). *A,* The tension in the wall of a hollow cylinder (T_1) is directly proportional to the product of the tube's radius (R_1) and the pressure (P) that the wall is supporting. *B,* Dilatation of the cylinder (R_2) at the same pressure (P) is associated with an increase in its wall tension (T_2).

yond a certain point, "compensatory" mechanisms not only become inadequate but may even do harm. A familiar example is the episode of heart failure that has been precipitated by an excessively rapid heart rate; this tachycardia fails to sustain the cardiac output because of the abbreviated ventricular filling time while taxing the myocardium by imposing inordinate requirements for energy.

The Kidneys in Heart Failure. In normal subjects, the fluid compartments of the body are held remarkably constant as the result of an automatic interplay among *intake* (governed by thirst and appetite), *transcellular exchanges* of fluid and electrolytes (governed by passive and active mechanisms), and *excretion* (regulated mainly by the kidneys). In heart failure, this automatic balance tends to be upset mainly because of inordinate retention of salt and water by the kidneys. The result is an isosmotic expansion of the extracellular fluid in which the circulating blood volume shares. It is conceivable that early in heart failure the conservation of salt and water may serve a useful purpose by expanding the blood volume either to sustain venous return to the failing heart or to relieve the arterial baroreceptors from undue stimulation as the cardiac output fails. But this teleologic explanation no longer applies when the myocardium can no longer respond to increased filling pressures and volumes, and the retention of salt and water only aggravates congestion and edema.

Several features characterize the kidneys in heart failure: the glomerular filtration rate is either low or normal; the renal blood flow is consistently decreased; the filtration fraction is regularly increased. But the fundamental renal defect in heart failure is disproportionate reabsorption of sodium for the level of the filtration rate. This avidity of the tubules for sodium is part of an over-all sodium-retaining syndrome, as the concentrations of sodium are low in the sweat and saliva as well as in the urine. Also, natriuretic agents, such as thiazides, mercurials, or spironolactone, which are particularly active on the distal tubule, can completely relieve the edema of heart failure even though they exert no direct effect on the heart.

Several different mechanisms seem to be involved in the inordinate reabsorption of sodium by the renal tubule: a heightened secretion of aldosterone; a decrease in glomerular filtration; intrarenal hemodynamic changes, signified by the high filtration fraction and the redistribution of blood flow within the kidney; and "third factor," the sum of all influences on conservation of sodium by the kidney except for aldosterone and the filtration rate.

The Signal from Heart to Kidney. The myocardium, per se, is not the unique source of the signal to the kidney since the sodium-retaining response also occurs in patients with valvular heart disease in whom the myocardium is normal. Instead, the signal seems to stem from a distortion or stretch of strategically disposed stretch receptors. Whether these receptors are located in the atria, kidneys, or arterial tree, or in all three sites, is not settled. But it is clear that expansion of the extracellular fluid volume, which prompts the elimination of sodium by the kidney when the heart is normal, fails to do so when the heart has failed.

How the heart notifies the kidney that it is failing is unclear. The connecting links may be nervous, humoral, hemodynamic, or a combination of all three. Moreover, these links need not be the same in different types of heart failure. But it does seem likely that no matter what the nature of the connections, the final common pathway for sodium retention in heart failure is the renin-angiotensin-aldosterone system.

The Endocrines in Heart Failure. Once heart failure is complicated by edema, heightened mineralocorticoid activity appears in the blood. Although not entirely conclusive, mainly because of the complicated analytic techniques and the few patients that have been studied, several different lines of evidence have assigned a major role to the renin-angiotensin-aldosterone system in the pathogenesis of edema during heart failure. Paramount among these are the heightened renin-angiotensin activity and the high concentrations of aldosterone in the plasma of many patients in heart failure, as well as the reversal of these changes during sodium depletion. The response of this system to sodium depletion in heart failure is opposite to the normal response. In contrast to the renin-angiotensin-aldosterone system, enhanced activity of the antidiuretic hormone is not essential for the formation of edema in heart failure.

PERFORMANCE OF THE FAILING HEART

Traditionally, the performance of the failing heart has been considered in terms of the heart as a pump and as a component of the circulation. For this purpose, hemodynamic principles and techniques have been applied. More recently, principles and techniques of muscle mechanics and energetics, originally developed for skeletal muscle, have been extended to heart muscle.

The Heart as a Pump: Hemodynamics of Heart Failure. If the heart muscle is badly damaged, it is usually quite easy to demonstrate on clinical, fluoroscopic, and even angiographic grounds that it is contracting poorly. Graphic evidence may also be gained at the bedside where combinations of noninvasive methods, such as the simultaneous registration of the electrocardiogram, phonocardiogram, and carotid arterial pulse, may be useful in showing that in a poorly contracting heart the pre-ejection phase of systole is prolonged at the expense of the ejection phase. On the other hand, lesser degrees of reduced contractility remain difficult to detect and to express in quantitative terms.

For a long while after the introduction of cardiac catheterization in man, the quantitative appraisal of cardiac performance focused on the Frank-Starling (length-tension) mechanism. By changing the load on the heart, ventricular performance was assessed in terms of the relationship between stroke output or stroke work and end-diastolic volume; as a practical expedient, end-diastolic pressure was substituted for end-diastolic volume. From these observations, certain useful generalizations about heart failure in man were established: (1) In the ventricle that has failed, the end-diastolic pressure is abnormally high at rest (usually more than 10 mm. Hg), the degree of emptying is abnormally low, i.e., less than two thirds of the expanded end-diastolic volume, the mean rate of ejection is slower than normal, and peak-systole is often delayed. (2) Even though the cardiac output may be normal at rest in heart failure, the increments in cardiac output during graded exercise are disproportionately low with respect to the increments in oxygen consumption. (3) In heart failure, the arteriovenous difference for oxygen is abnormally wide due, almost entirely, to the low oxygen content of venous blood returning to the heart rather than to impaired arterialization in the lungs. (4) The administration of digitalis to the patient in heart failure increases the cardiac output (and external work) even though the end-diastolic pressure (and volume) decreases. (5) After recovery, the cardiac output, at any level of activity, is higher than during heart failure.

Taken separately, and unless decidedly abnormal, some of these indices of heart failure may be difficult to interpret in terms of myocardial performance. For example, although end-diastolic pressure has proved to be a reliable qualitative guide to directional changes in end-diastolic volume, it is unreliable as a quantitative measure because of the changes that different kinds and degrees of heart disease impose on the distensibility characteristics of the ventricle (see below); the end-diastolic volume, in turn, is strongly influenced not only by the contractile behavior of the heart but also by extracardiac factors which determine venous return. Nonetheless, despite such reservations and difficulties in varying cardiac load without eliciting a variety of reflex cardiac adjustments, the Frank-Starling relationship has proved to be a useful approach to the performance of the failing heart in man, particularly when the response of the same heart is compared before and after treatment.

Relaxation and Distensibility of the Failing Heart. Although most studies of ventricular performance during heart failure have centered around the contraction phase, the course of the relaxation phase (diastole) influences the pattern of the subsequent cardiac contraction. The filling of the ventricle during diastole depends not only on the time available but also on the pattern of relaxation. Relaxation consists of two components: an active one, which promotes relaxation by way of intrinsic mechanisms; and a passive one, arising from extension of the fibers by the inflowing blood. Incomplete relaxation would be expected not only to increase the filling pressure of the heart but also to dissipate energy. In the normal heart, the active and passive components appear to work synergistically to minimize losses in chemical energy. But in heart failure the viscous and elastic properties of the heart muscle seem to change so that there is a diminished resistance to filling (decreased "impedance") and an increased extent of ventricular expansion on filling (increased "compliance"). Thus, not only the velocity and duration of relaxation but also changes in the physical properties of the muscle seem involved in heart failure.

The Heart as a Muscle: Myocardial Contractility. The sine qua non of heart failure is reduced myocardial contractility. Although conventional pressure-flow measurements provide information about ventricular performance, particularly during exercise, they do not separate contractility, per se, from the mechanical loading conditions which alter it. Thus, a change in either the preload (the length of the ventricular fibers at end-diastole) or the afterload (the force developed in the ventricular muscle during systole) can modify ventricular performance considerably without affecting contractility. Also, since hemodynamic measurements do not take heart size into account, it is not possible to compare contractility in hearts of different sizes.

As a result of these ambiguities, more specific indices of myocardial contractility have been sought. Among these have been the *total* tension developed during systole, the level of systolic pressure achieved by the ventricle, the stroke output, and the work done by the heart. However, none has provided an accurate guide to impaired contractility. Much more promising as measures of contractility are the *rates* at which ventricular pressure and tension increase during systole, and the velocity of contraction.

Rates of Increase in Ventricular Pressure and Tension during Contraction. The rate at which ventricular pressure increases during contraction (dp/dt) has been shown in animals and in isolated papillary muscles to be a sensitive index of myocardial contractility as long as loading conditions (end-diastolic fiber length and developed tension) remain unchanged. In practice, dp/dt can be determined as the first derivative of the ventricular pressure. At present its application in man is handicapped by the need for extraordinarily high fidelity recording systems and by the difficulty in reproducing loading conditions. Although it holds considerable promise for comparisons of contractile performance in a single patient before and after intervention, it has little prospect for comparing different hearts. Attempts to obtain a related kind of information using an end-catheter velocity gauge to determine the rate at which blood is ejected into the aorta are promising but are still in their infancy.

As in the case of pressure, the rate of development of wall tension is also decidedly abnormal.

Moreover, in contrast to the normal heart in which wall tension decreases during systole, in heart failure wall tension remains high throughout systole so that both the velocity and degree of shortening are abnormal.

Velocity of Contraction. The use of the velocity of contraction as a measure of contractility involves the force-velocity relationship originally developed by A. V. Hill for skeletal muscle (Fig. 3). According to this relationship, the velocity of shortening in skeletal muscle is inversely related to the magnitude of the tension that the muscle develops, i.e., the greater the load that the muscle is obliged to lift during contraction, the slower its speed of shortening. Applying this relationship to the myocardium, the position of the force-velocity curve would be affected both by a change in end-diastolic fiber length (initial stretch or preload) and by a change in inherent inotropic activity. But the effects would be different. Thus, a change in the degree of initial stretch of the heart muscle, and presumably in the number of active sites at which the chemical reactions of contraction can occur, would modify the total force that the muscle develops; in Figure 3, this change would shift the horizontal, but not the vertical, intercept. In contrast, a change in inotropic activity (Fig. 3) by cardiotonic agents, on the one hand, or myocardial failure, on the other, would be expected not only to affect the horizontal intercept (total force) but also to displace the force-velocity curve with respect to the vertical axis (rate of force-generating processes). Indeed, the observations on skeletal muscle even suggested that an ideal measure of contractility might be obtained by extrapolating the force-velocity relationships to the vertical axis (V_{max}), as shown in Fig. 3, thereby determining the maximal velocity of shortening that would exist at zero load. Unfortunately, V_{max} for heart muscle has proved to be better in theory than in practice. Indeed, it

is now clear that much more reliable information about contractility can be obtained by actually determining force-velocity values at *small* loads than by attempting the uncertain extrapolation to zero load.

It should be stressed that the assessment of force-velocity relations in the human heart is still in its infancy. At present, the assessment is a technical feat which involves a combination of cineangiography, high fidelity recording of ventricular pressures, and an assumed geometric model of the ventricular cavity as a basis for relating wall stress to the velocity and extent of shortening. But these practical limitations should not obscure the conceptual values of the new approaches to contractility. Moreover, even though direct determinations of force-velocity relationships have yet to be made on the human heart in failure, there is little reason to doubt that in the human heart, as in the isolated papillary muscle, myocardial failure will prove to be associated with a decrease in both the force and velocity of myocardial contraction.

Energetics. The heart does work and expends energy in developing contractile tension within its walls during systole. The contraction of the heart depends on the conversion of the chemical energy of oxidizable substrates into the mechanical energy of muscular contraction. ATP participates in this process as the principal store of energy released by oxidation; its breakdown by myosin ATPase is the principal way by which chemical energy is transformed into mechanical energy. ATP resynthesis in the myocardium is accomplished chiefly through oxidative phosphorylation. The rate of ATP breakdown and the quantity of energy used by the myocardium depends chiefly on the tension that is developed in the myocardial fibers rather than on the degree of shortening or the work done; this developed tension causes the ventricular walls to contract and the blood to be ejected. The energy which the contracting ventricle confers on the blood that it ejects is the external work of the ventricle.

The energy cost per beat is closely related to the blood pressure and heart rate, and, to a lesser extent, to the cardiac output. From a biochemical point of view, the muscle of a ventricle has failed when its generation of free energy, or its utilization of that energy in the process of contraction, is insufficient for the circulatory load which it has to handle.

About 1950, studies were begun to determine whether specific biochemical abnormalities could be implicated in the contractile defects of myocardial failure. Of particular concern was the question of energetics. Although this question is still not entirely resolved, certain aspects do seem clear for the usual types (low cardiac output) of heart failure: (1) no consistent abnormalities have been found in the production or conservation of energy at a time when myocardial contractility is definitely impaired; (2) although myocardial energy stores are often slightly depressed in heart failure, there is no evidence that this

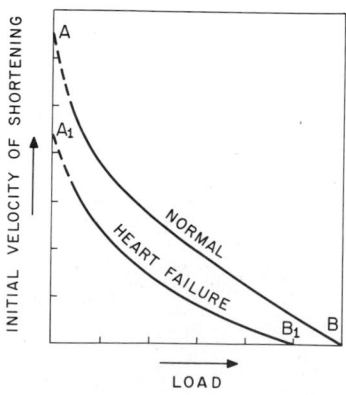

FIGURE 3. Hypothetical representation of force-velocity changes in heart failure. Under controlled conditions, the position of the force-velocity curve is determined by the contractile state of the myocardium. The force-velocity relationship would be expected to shift during heart failure, theoretically decreasing both the maximal velocity of shortening (A to A_1) and the maximal developed tension (B to B_1). (Modified from Braunwald, E., Ross, J., Jr., and Sonnenblick, E. H.: Mechanisms of Contraction of the Normal and Failing Heart. Boston, Little, Brown & Company, 1968.)

depression is causally related; (3) specific abnormalities have not been identified in either the calcium or potassium content of the failing heart; (4) no consistent defects have been found in either the structure or physicochemical properties of the contractile proteins, actin or myosin; and (5) the major biochemical defect in the usual types of heart failure seems to be a defective conversion of chemical energy to mechanical work, i.e., although the failing myocardium seems to channel the available chemical energy properly into the contractile mechanism and even though it converts chemical energy into mechanical work at a normal efficiency, for some reason the rate at which this conversion proceeds is considerably reduced. Many abnormalities could explain the ineffective use of energy by the heart muscle once it has failed—such as overstretched myofibrils before the start of systole, diminished ATPase activity, or discoordinated interactions among the ultrastructural components of the contractile machinery—but the problem remains unsettled.

Certain types of heart failure, such as those associated with high cardiac output, do seem to have particular defects in myocardial energetics, e.g., decrease in oxidative phosphorylation and in energy stores. However, these defects are apparently related to the fundamental disease, e.g., anemia, beriberi, or thyrotoxicosis and are not the common denominators of impaired contractility.

The Heart as a Component of the Circulation. As a ventricle fails, signs of venous congestion or of inadequate organ perfusion may predominate. On this basis, clinicians have long distinguished between "backward" and "forward" failure. Although this distinction may have clinical value, it makes little physiologic sense because, in a closed circuit, the inability of the heart to match its output to the level of metabolic activity and the pooling of blood on the venous inflow side must go hand in hand, even though the evidences of one or the other may predominate.

In either circuit, the origin of venous hypertension during heart failure may be traced to inadequate ventricular emptying: as the volume (and pressure) increases at the end of systole, atrial emptying is impeded, and atrial pressure increases. Several other elements contribute to the venous hypertension: (1) heightened venomotor tone, (2) expansion of the blood volume as a consequence of sodium retention by the kidney, and on occasion (3) regurgitation of blood from ventricle to atrium as the atrioventricular valve becomes incompetent either from ventricular dilatation or from improper closure during an arrhythmia.

It has been pointed out above that a decrease in cardiac output is a hallmark of most types of heart failure. Accompanying the decrease in cardiac output are a variety of neurohumoral adjustments. Most prominent are peripheral vasoconstriction and readjustment of blood flow among the various tissues and organs so that kidneys, liver, and skin are underperfused for the sake of maintaining flow to the brain and heart. These changes account for the characteristic oliguria and clammy skin of heart failure. A similar rearrangement occurs in diving mammals during submersion and in normal man during exercise; in patients with heart failure, exercise exaggerates this pattern. Part of the circulatory changes seem attributable to increase in the adrenal secretion of constrictor substances; much more is due to heightened autonomic nervous activity.

"Low Output" Failure versus "High Output" Failure. A regular feature of "hyperkinetic" circulatory states is high cardiac output. Consequently, it has become expedient, with the advent of cardiac catheterization, to classify myocardial failure according to the level of the cardiac output. This practice has served at least two purposes: (1) it has separated, on clinical and physiologic grounds, a type of myocardial failure in which the circulation remains vigorous and the extremities remain warm despite venous congestion, edema, and a lower cardiac output than existed prior to the heart failure; and (2) it has emphasized that the state of the circulation during myocardial failure is, in large degree, a consequence of the size of the circulating blood volume and the level of the cardiac output that existed prior to heart failure.

The separation into "high" and "low" output failure is concerned with the consequences, rather than the causes, of myocardial failure. But it is also a hemodynamic frame of reference to which the anatomist and the biochemist can relate the myocardial origins of heart failure. For example, "high output" failure probably has different biochemical bases from "low output" failure. Moreover, not all types of "low output" or "high output" failure are apt to have the same biochemical bases. For example, it is unlikely that the "high output" failure of a peripheral arteriovenous fistula has the same anatomic or biochemical beginnings and evolution as the "high output" failure of severe anemia or malnutrition.

Heart Failure versus Congested State. It has been noted earlier that congestion of both venous circulations, without myocardial failure, may be induced by rapid infusions; it may also occur in the course of "hyperkinetic" circulatory states as diverse as severe anemia and peripheral arteriovenous fistula. Similar but less dramatic venous congestion may also complicate Paget's disease or beriberi. In all these situations venous hypertension may arise from a combination of an expanded circulating blood volume and heightened venomotor tone, rather than failure of heart muscle.

Any of these "hyperkinetic" congestive states may, in time, cause the heart muscle to fail from overwork. But the onset of myocardial failure may be difficult to detect on clinical grounds, since the hyperkinetic circulation persists and the congestion may be only slightly increased during myocardial failure. At this time, cardiac catheterization may suggest myocardial failure by demonstrating an inadequate increase in cardiac output during exercise and a considerable increase in cardiac output after digitalis. Fortunately, this distinction between "congested state" and "congestive heart failure" is of greater theoretical than practical importance since therapeutic measures, such as the administration of diuretics and the replacement of particular nutrients, e.g., thiamine in beriberi, are effective in both situations. However, digitalis would be expected to improve myocardial performance much more in myocardial failure than in an overfilled circulation in which the heart is already performing well.

MANIFESTATIONS OF HEART FAILURE

Depending on which ventricle has failed and on the nature and severity of the initiating mechanisms, the signs and symptoms of heart failure may have different origins: from the heart, congested and edematous lungs, prolonged circulation time, systemic venous congestion, hypoperfused and congested organs, or from the accumulation of edema fluid in the tissues and body cavities.

The Heart. The heart generally calls little attention to itself in heart failure. Pain is rare unless a complication, such as myocardial infarction, coexists; palpitation is also uncommon unless an arrhythmia has been initiated by overdigitalization, usually in combination with electrolyte disorders produced by the overzealous administration of potent diuretic agents.

Gallop Rhythm. In a middle-aged or elderly patient with heart disease, the appearance of a third heart sound during diastole indicates serious heart disease, often heart failure; systolic triple rhythms do not have the same serious import. Three kinds of gallop rhythm occur in heart failure: (1) *Ventricular or "S-3" gallop* occurs in the dilated heart during the stage of rapid ventricular filling, i.e., in protodiastole, presumably originating in the vibrations of the ventricular walls as the rapidly inflowing blood is abruptly arrested; although its timing is the same as that of the normal third heart sound in most normal young children and in many young adults, in the older patient it is generally a reliable sign of ventricular failure. (2) *Atrial or "S-4" gallop* is attributed to the forceful presystolic distention of the ventricle by atrial contraction; it usually accompanies hypertrophy of a ventricle which causes reduced compliance and increased resistance to filling. (3) *Summation gallop* is a triple rhythm which occurs during tachycardia because of the coincidence of the atrial and ventricular gallops; in general, it has the same meaning as diastolic gallop rhythms in general, but it is considered to be benign if it disappears when the heart is slowed, as by carotid compression.

Pulsus Alternans. The regular alternation of one strong beat and one weak beat, either over the heart or at the pulse, is designated pulsus alternans. It is a serious sign of heart failure, commonly found in patients with systemic hypertension, coronary atherosclerosis, aortic stenosis, and idiopathic myocardiopathy. It is not to be confused with an arrhythmia which takes the form of a bigeminy, and only rarely is it associated with electrical alternans. Instead, it is entirely a mechanical phenomenon, generally attributed to alternating initial fiber lengths and contractility.

Congested, Edematous Lungs. As the lungs progress from congestion to edema, they produce characteristic signs and symptoms.

Dyspnea. Like pain or anxiety, dyspnea is a subjective phenomenon. The subject becomes conscious of his breathing, and he verbalizes this awareness as "breathlessness." The sensation may appear either at rest or during mild exertion; a similar awareness, often complicated by an element of distress, occurs in normal subjects after severe exertion, such as a desperate dash for the bus. Awareness rather than discomfort is usually the hallmark of dyspnea. Indeed, the subject who is preoccupied or distracted may manifest tachypnea (increased rate of breathing) or hyperpnea (increased depth of breathing) without complaining of dyspnea.

A wide variety of clinical disorders of the heart, lungs, acid-base balance, musculoskeletal system and nervous system, and many different pathogenic sequences may lead to dyspnea. In left heart failure, dyspnea is a characteristic consequence of pulmonary congestion, edema, and stiff lungs. Failure of the right ventricle, which frequently occurs after prolonged left ventricular failure, may, by decreasing pulmonary congestion, relieve the dyspnea.

In left ventricular failure, as the volume of blood and extravascular fluid in the lungs increases at the expense of the air volume, the vital capacity decreases. Also, as the lungs grow stiffer (less compliant) from a combination of pulmonary edema and congestion, the work and energy cost of breathing increase. A new breathing pattern of rapid shallow breathing is automatically adopted for the sake of minimizing the work and energy spent in breathing. Thereafter, the patient may either continue to be dyspneic, or he may verge on dyspnea, only becoming breathless if the fluid volume of the lungs increases acutely, as during anxiety of exertion, or when a complication occurs, such as pulmonary embolus, hydrothorax, or pneumonia.

There is no clearer idea about the genesis of dyspnea in left heart failure than in other states. Most theories center around the increased work and energy cost of breathing: some emphasize the inordinate total amount of work, energy, or force; others favor length-tension "inappropriateness," i.e., the disproportion between the inordinate amount of energy that is spent and the ventilation that is produced. But how much fatigue of the respiratory muscles contributes is unsettled. Nor is it clear how the diverse stimuli – ranging from abnormal gas tensions to Hering-Breuer reflex and musculoskeletal receptors – interrelate to generate the sensation. Particularly frustrating is the fact that nerve receptors, which can elicit dyspnea when stimulated, have yet to be identified.

Orthopnea. Dyspnea that appears when the subject lies down is called orthopnea. When the patient with left heart failure is flat, the increased venous return that is delivered to the lungs by the competent right ventricle cannot be handled by the left ventricle; pulmonary congestion and edema ensue. The patient becomes breathless. Since the excess fluid may be in the interstitial space and not in the alveoli, rales may not be present. Of the same clinical significance as orthopnea is the appearance of a distressing cough when the patient lies flat, presumably originating in edematous tracheobronchial walls. In contrast to patients with dyspnea from left ventricular failure, patients with dyspnea from intrinsic pulmonary disease or musculoskeletal disease generally do not experience orthopnea.

Paroxysmal Nocturnal Dyspnea. The patient with the congested lungs of left heart failure is a candidate for paroxysmal nocturnal dyspnea, particularly if he suffers from orthopnea. During sleep, he slides from the sitting position, thereby mobilizing toward the lungs the fluid and blood that have accumulated during the day in the lower part of the body. As fluid accumulates in the lungs, he suddenly wakes to find himself desperately short of breath. He struggles to get up, gasping and afraid that he is going to suffocate. Not only acute pulmonary edema but also anxiety contributes to the picture: the patient is pale and in a cold sweat as he struggles for air; tachycardia is a regular feature; gallop rhythm is common. Improvement generally begins before the physician arrives since the upright position has freed the apices of the lungs of fluid; reassurance remarkably accelerates the recovery. But although this frightening episode may subside quickly and spontaneously, it has heralded the presence of severe left heart failure.

Cardiac Asthma. If the bronchi share in the acute pulmonary edema, the clinical picture may be indistinguishable from asthma. Indeed, the acute onset of asthma in a middle-aged or elderly individual who has no history or manifestations of allergy should suggest the possibility of left heart failure. An underlying bronchitis predisposes to this occurrence. Rales may be absent, depending on the localization of the pulmonary edema, i.e., an interstitial space or alveoli. The precipitating mechanism is the same as that for paroxysmal nocturnal dyspnea, i.e., acute pulmonary engorgement resulting from an imbalance between the right and left ventricles.

Cough. Cough and expectoration are frequent complaints in patients with cardiac failure. The cough is produced by reflexes from the congested lungs and bronchi. Rarely, except in mitral valvular disease, does enlargement of the left

atrium produce cough by pressure on the bronchi. The cough produced by pulmonary congestion may be severe enough to interfere with sleep; frequently a paroxysm of coughing will trigger an acute attack of nocturnal dyspnea.

Hemoptysis. Rusty sputum, laden with "heart failure cells" (alveolar macrophages containing hemosiderin), occurs frequently in severe left heart failure. Frankly bloody sputum is generally a sign of pulmonary infarction. In severe pulmonary edema caused by left ventricular failure, the frothy fluid that pours from the bronchial tree is often pink, i.e., blood-tinged, owing to the escape of red cells into the alveoli from the congested minute vessels of the lungs.

Prolonged Circulation Time. The circulation time depends on the cardiac output and the volume of blood interposed between the sites of sampling and detection. In failure of either ventricle, the time for detectable concentrations of a test substance to pass from the site of intravenous injection to the site of detection is prolonged. For example, in left heart failure, the arm-to-tongue (Decholin) time is prolonged well beyond the normal limits of 10 to 15 seconds, presumably because of delays in traversing the pulmonary circulation and dilated left heart, and by excessive dilution of the tracer by the expanded thoracic blood volume; the arm-to-breath (ether) time, as well as the arm-to-tongue time, is prolonged in right heart failure because of delayed (beyond four to eight seconds) transit from the arm vein to the lungs. By considering the central venous pressure and the circulation times together, it is often possible to verify at the bedside which ventricle has failed. For example, in isolated left heart failure, central venous pressure and ether time will be normal whereas Decholin time will be prolonged. Although serial measurements of the circulation time have also been used to follow the course of patients in heart failure, the information obtained is generally not worth the effort.

Periodic Breathing (Cheyne-Stokes Respiration). In many patients with congestive heart failure the usually regular sequence of respiratory movements is replaced by alternate periods of hyperventilation and apnea. This waxing and waning of the level of ventilation is accompanied by cyclic changes in arterial O_2 and CO_2 tensions.

Normally arterial blood gas tensions are maintained within circumscribed limits by compensatory changes in ventilation which diminish any deviation of arterial O_2 and CO_2 tensions from their usual levels. This self-adjusting behavior is characteristic of control systems in which the controller is informed of the effects of its actions by negative feedback. Cheyne-Stokes breathing seems to be a result of unstable behavior on the part of the negative feedback system which is supposed to control the level of ventilation and arterial blood gas tensions. Because of this instability, ventilation either undershoots or exceeds its proper level, and arterial blood gases oscillate instead of remaining at their normal level.

Two important mechanisms may produce such

an instability in the control of breathing: (1) a heightened sensitivity of the respiratory controller in the brain to changes in arterial CO_2 tension; this mechanism plays an important role in producing Cheyne-Stokes breathing in certain patients with strokes, in normal individuals at altitude, and in a few patients with heart failure, particularly those with concomitant cerebrovascular disease; and (2) a delay in feedback, as by a prolonged circulation time, so that cerebral arterial blood fails to notify the respiratory controller promptly about the changes in the gaseous composition of the blood that the controller has effected in the lungs by changing the level of ventilation; in general, the longer the circulation time, either experimentally or in human heart failure, the longer the cycles of hyperventilation and apnea.

No matter how the Cheyne-Stokes breathing is produced, the *arterial* O_2 tension reaches its peak, and the *arterial* CO_2 tension its nadir, during apnea; the opposite changes occur during hyperventilation. On the other hand, the *alveolar* O_2 tension reaches its peak, and the *alveolar* CO_2 tension its nadir during hyperpnea. Thus, the cyclic changes in arterial blood gases seem to *cause* the swings in ventilation, whereas the swings in alveolar gas tensions (and of the pulmonary venous gas tensions) are the *effects* of the changes in ventilation. The gas tensions in the systemic (cerebral) arterial blood and pulmonary venous blood are out of phase because of the time required for blood to pass from the pulmonary veins to the systemic arteries.

The periodic changes in the level of ventilation seen in Cheyne-Stokes breathing are often accompanied by cyclic neurologic and cardiovascular changes. During apnea the patient with Cheyne-Stokes breathing is often dizzy or stuporous, cerebral blood flow decreases, and the electroencephalogram is characterized by low frequency waves. During hyperventilation the patient may be excited, cerebral blood flow increases, and the electroencephalogram consists mainly of high frequency waves. Cyclic changes in pupillary diameter may occur in synchrony with the changes in ventilation. In some patients, fluctuations in blood pressure and heart rate also accompany the periodic swings in ventilation; the changes in heart rate appear to be caused by variations in levels of vagal activity since they can be abolished by the administration of atropine. Atrioventricular conduction time may also vary and is usually longest at the end of apnea. These changes in conduction time may be sufficient to trigger cardiac arrhythmias in certain patients with Cheyne-Stokes breathing. The phase of hyperpnea in Cheyne-Stokes breathing may also precipitate attacks of cardiac asthma by increasing pulmonary blood volume.

Not all periodic breathing is Cheyne-Stokes respiration. In patients with blunted ventilatory response to CO_2 because of depressed medullary function, a periodic pattern of ventilation may appear characterized by irregular bursts of respiratory activity. This type of breathing seems to be produced by failing respiratory neurons and not by instability in the operation of the respiratory control system.

Systemic Venous Congestion. A characteristic feature of ventricular failure is hypertension in the venous circuit that feeds the ventricle that has failed. Quite evident is the systemic venous hypertension that accompanies right ventricular failure: as the right atrial pressure climbs to more than 10 to 15 cm. of water, the distended systemic veins act like manometric extensions of the atrium, accurately reflecting its high pressures. Much more indirect is the evidence for pulmonary venous hypertension since systemic venous pressures, including those in the central veins, remain normal even though left atrial and pulmonary venous pressures mount to high levels. Indeed, for evidence of pulmonary venous hypertension, symptoms (dyspnea and orthopnea) rather than signs (tachypnea, rales) become the main criteria for recognition. Only after left heart failure and pulmonary venous hypertension have led to enough changes in the pulmonary circulation to produce pulmonary arterial hypertension and right heart failure, will the systemic venous pressures follow, to any appreciable extent, left heart pressures.

Several different influences contribute to the genesis of systemic venous hypertension: (1) the inability of the ventricle that has failed to cope with the venous return; this topic has been considered earlier in this section; (2) the quantity of blood that returns to the heart; this depends not only on the size of the circulating blood volume but also on its distribution; and (3) heightened venomotor tone; this is part of an over-all increase in sympathetic neurohumoral activity that affects the entire circulatory tree.

The total blood volume is regularly increased in heart failure but often not to the same extent as the extracellular fluid volume. Thus, in moderate heart failure, the plasma volume may increase by only 10 to 30 per cent even though peripheral edema is present, and the increase in extracellular fluid volume is much more marked. This disparity emphasizes the complicated relationship between the circulating and extravascular fluid volumes in heart failure, an interplay which is exaggerated by the various therapeutic measures which promote diuresis and reduce the blood volume.

Heightened systemic venous pressure is largely responsible for the characteristic hepatomegaly, splenomegaly, and peripheral edema of right heart failure. Less apparent are the congestion and edema of the gastrointestinal tract.

Hypoperfused and Congested Organs. Changes in the performance of certain tissues and organs provide many of the striking features of heart failure.

Skin. A blue discoloration of the skin and mucus is designated as cyanosis. It is rarely striking in uncomplicated heart failure except in severe forms of right heart failure. It is due to an abnormal concentration of reduced hemoglobin (more than 5 grams per 100 ml. of blood). In large part, its intensity varies with the amount of reduced hemoglobin that is visible through the skin, but a variety of modifying influences make the visual impression of the degree of cyanosis an unreliable index of the degree of arterial oxygenation. Since the skin over the nailbeds, lips, tip of nose, ears, and cheeks is quite thin, cyanosis is usually most intense in these areas. Because of anatomic arrangement, the blood in the subpapillary venous plexus (rather than in the superficial capillary loops) is the major determinant of the cyanotic hue. In right heart failure, engorgement of these vessels with poorly oxygenated red cells accounts for the cyanosis; in left heart failure, cyanosis is usually due to a complication, e.g., pneumonia, and not to the heart failure.

In any instance of cyanosis, the amount of reduced hemoglobin may be high for two reasons: (1) delivery to the tissues of a large volume of blood that has escaped oxygenation in the lungs, either owing to lung disease or to venoarterial shunts ("central cyanosis"), or (2) a considerable extraction of oxygen by underperfused tissues. It is the latter that obtains in virtually all cases of left heart failure since arterial oxygen saturation is consistently higher than 90 to 92 per cent and perfusion of the skin is poor; CO_2 retention is also absent. The poor perfusion accounts for the pale, ashen cyanosis of heart failure and contrasts with the ruddy cyanosis of secondary polycythemia.

In the elderly confused patient who is seen for the first time, the distinction between "central cyanosis" and "peripheral cyanosis" may be critical. If the arterial blood sample indicates no appreciable hypoxemia or hypercapnia, the conventional program of cardiotonic agents, sedation, and oxygen may effect quick relief; but if there is arterial hypoxemia and hypercapnia (from lung disease or depressed ventilation), the same program may be lethal by inducing CO_2 narcosis.

Liver. Hepatomegaly and mild abdominal discomfort are common in right heart failure. As the volume of blood in the liver increases, and the liver blood flow decreases, oxygen tensions in the vicinity of the central veins become very low, leading to atrophy and necrosis of hepatic cells in their vicinity; the venous and hepatic sinusoidal hypertension lead to hepatic edema, most marked around the central veins. Elsewhere in the liver, lobule fat accumulates. If the capsule stretches gradually, there is generally more discomfort than pain.

Hepatic function generally remains good despite the hepatomegaly, although mild elevations in the serum bilirubin level and abnormal tests of hepatic cell function (SGOT) are not uncommon. Moderate splenomegaly is a common concomitant of a swollen liver. The enlarged spleen is firm and nontender.

When right heart failure is severe enough to be associated with functional tricuspid insufficiency, the liver pulsates with each heart beat. Manual pressure over the congested liver causes the cervical neck veins to distend abruptly (hepatojugular reflux) since the displaced blood cannot be adequately handled by the incompetent right heart.

Acute swelling of the liver is apt to occur during rapidly developing right heart failure. The liver is enlarged and tender from the sudden stretching of the liver capsule. The pain in the right upper quadrant is usually a constant ache; occasionally, it is colicky. Such pain is quite common in right heart failure and may be severe enough to suggest an acute abdomen or a pulmonary infarction.

As the result of repeated bouts of right heart failure extensive fibrosis of the liver may occur (cardiac cirrhosis). This is most common when very high hepatic venous pressures have been present for many months. Often it is difficult to decide whether cardiac cirrhosis is a separate entity or an unrecognized Laennec or postnecrotic cirrhosis.

Many patients with heart failure develop hyperbilirubinemia, but few develop enough bilirubin in their serum to become jaundiced. When jaundice does occur, hepatic and pulmonary congestion have been severe and long-standing; often there has been a recent pulmonary infarction. The hyperbilirubinemia is usually due to a combination of quick and slow-reacting bilirubin, and presumably is a consequence of anoxia of hepatic cells produced by inadequate hepatic perfusion and hepatic venous hypertension.

In severe and sustained biventricular heart failure, associated with severe reduction in cardiac output and marked systemic venous hypertension, profound *hypoglycemia* may occur. This is presumably the result of an inadequate store of glycogen in the liver and the increased breakdown of glucose to lactic acid because of anoxia.

Gastrointestinal Tract. Anorexia, nausea, and vomiting are common in congestive failure, and may originate in a number of ways: reflex, central, local, or due to the effects of drugs, such as digitalis or potassium. Congestion of the abdominal viscera may cause nausea and vomiting. Central stimulation of reflex pathways may produce vomiting. When systemic venous congestion is severe, congestion and edema of the bowel wall may produce a protein-losing enteropathy.

Brain. Symptoms of cerebral dysfunction are common in heart failure, although they do not usually become marked until the patient has reached the end-stages of heart failure, i.e., when dyspnea is continuously present. At that time, cardiac output has presumably decreased to a degree sufficient to impair the metabolism of the brain. As the heart failure intensifies and cerebral blood flow decreases further, irritability, restlessness, and difficulty in fixing attention develop. Preterminally, stupor and coma may occur. It may well be that the changes in cerebral metabolism caused by heart failure have a more complicated mechanism than the reduction of the blood supply to the brain, as there are widespread disorders in intermediary metabolism produced by the decreased blood supply to the liver, endocrine glands, gastrointestinal tract, and other organs of the body. If, for any reason, heart failure is complicated by hypoxemia, e.g., from independent lung disease, cerebral symptoms are more likely to occur and to be severe.

Kidney. Oliguria occurs in both left and right heart failure but is much more striking in the latter. As the heart improves, urinary output increases. The urine is poor in sodium but has a high specific gravity (1.020 to 1.030). Proteinuria is common but not severe. A variety of casts accompany the proteinuria. Renal function, as determined by clearance techniques, is only slightly depressed except in severe right heart failure of long standing. Azotemia is common and generally moderate except when there is independent renal disease, e.g., arteriosclerosis, and after vigorous diuresis.

Edema. In heart failure, excess fluid accumulates in the tissues because of an upset in the normal balance between capillary filtering and reabsorptive forces in favor of the outflow of fluid. For edema to remain or accumulate, not only must capillary pressures be sufficiently high to force fluid into the tissues, but salt and water retention by the kidney is essential to replace the fluid that has left the circulation. According to the low protein content of edema fluid, neither increased capillary permeability nor lymphatic obstruction plays any appreciable role in cardiac edema.

What initiates the retention of sodium and fluid that leads to edema is unclear. The circulating plasma volume shares in the expansion of extracellular fluid; the retained salt and water are localized in areas where capillary pressure is high and tissue pressure is low. During the day, because of the upright position, the excess fluid tends to accumulate in the lower parts of the body; in the recumbent position, redistribution occurs as capillary pressures become more uniform. If pulmonary venous pressure is high because of left ventricular failure, the excess fluid may be sequestered in the lungs.

Subcutaneous Edema. Dependent edema, manifested as swelling of the feet or ankles, which gradually develops during the day and subsides by the morning, is a characteristic feature of right heart failure. Its formation is invariably associated with signs of systemic venous congestion, such as distended neck veins and hepatomegaly; but, after diuresis, subcutaneous edema may disappear much more slowly than does the other evidence of systemic venous hypertension. Subcutaneous edema may be the first obvious sign of abnormal fluid retention in right heart failure. More often it is preceded by an appreciable gain in weight, i.e., up to 10 to 20 pounds. If unchecked, fluid accumulation may increase until the stage of persistent pitting edema of the lower limbs. Such edematous legs are liable to complications: low-grade cellulitis is not uncommon and, on occasion, edema becomes so massive that the skin

ruptures and drains fluid. During this sequence of increasing dependent edema, evidences of systemic venous congestion become more striking, and fluid tends to accumulate in body cavities.

Hydrothorax. The accumulation of excess fluid in the pleural cavities is designated hydrothorax. Although the association of pleural effusion and heart failure has been recognized for years, the mechanisms responsible for the accumulation of abnormal quantities of fluid in the thoracic cavities are still unclear. Indeed, it is not even entirely settled whether fluid is more apt to accumulate in one hemithorax (the right) than in the other during heart failure.

In general, fluid movement in the pleural space, as in the lungs and subcutaneous tissues, is in accord with Starling's law of transcapillary exchange. Some have interpreted the high concentration of protein in the pleural fluid (2 to 3 grams per 100 ml., approximately ten times as much as in peripheral edema fluid) as a sign of high capillary permeability. Unfortunately this premise is unreliable since the high concentration could just as well be due to a heightened reabsorption of water from the pleural space. Nonetheless, the high protein in the pleural fluid enhances the effect of high capillary pressures by negating the osmotic pressure of plasma proteins.

Actually there are different sets of capillaries at the pleural surfaces. In the parietal pleura, the capillaries are systemic; in the visceral pleura, they are both systemic and pulmonary. Consequently, fluid can move into the pleural space from either circulation when capillary pressures are sufficiently high and can be reabsorbed into the circulation when capillary pressures are sufficiently low. In addition, fluid may be removed by the pleural lymphatics. In reality, the situation is even more complicated with respect to fluid accumulation in the pleural space because of uncertainties not only about the values for pleural capillary pressure in either of the circuits, but also for the corresponding interstitial pressures. Despite these uncertainties, it is clear that hydrothorax is more common in combined heart failure (right and left) than in failure of either ventricle per se. This is reasonable since in combined heart failure both capillary beds in the pleura are at high pressure; moreover, since systemic venous pressure is high, lymphatic drainage from the lungs is also likely to be impeded.

Ascites. Appreciable quantities of free fluid accumulate in the abdominal cavity after hepatic venous engorgement as a consequence of hepatic capillary hypertension. This ascites is a late manifestation of right heart failure, often occurring in conjunction with severe peripheral edema and hydrothorax. It is a consequence of sustained right heart failure or of any other mechanism for producing systemic venous hypertension between the liver and the right ventricle, such as constructive pericarditis or tricuspid valvular disease; it does not occur when the inferior vena cava is ligated below the liver. Like pleural fluid, ascitic fluid is rich in protein (2 to 3 grams per 100 ml.), and its formation is promoted by a hypoproteinemia, e.g., by protein-losing enteropathy. Without salt and water retention, ascites cannot either form or progress.

Pericardial Effusion. In severe and persistent heart failure, appreciable quantities of fluid may accumulate in the pericardial sac. However, the amount is insufficient to cause tamponade.

Anasarca. This is a severe manifestation of right heart failure in which edema is massive and generalized, affecting all parts of the body including the abdominal wall, thorax, genitalia, and arms. Only rarely, if the patient sleeps flat, is the face involved.

Other Manifestations. In severe congestive heart failure, the accumulation of edema may obscure the gradual loss of tissue mass. Often this tissue wasting is associated with *weakness.* In extreme instances, extreme *cachexia* may develop. At this late stage, the patient is usually suffering from anorexia, gastrointestinal upsets, anemia, and electrolyte upsets. Part of the picture undoubtedly stems from organ hypoperfusion and congestion. But often a large contribution has been made by overvigorous use of diuretics and digitalis.

Anxiety. It is not surprising that patients with organic heart disease become anxious. Indeed, anxiety is a regular feature by the time the heart fails. But not always is it an easy matter to distinguish between cardiac complaints as manifestations of anxiety or of the cardiac disorder. Part of the difficulty stems from the nonspecific nature of complaints, such as breathlessness, especially if the patient does have organic heart disease. The difficulty is compounded if the patient misinterprets or exaggerates his symptoms unconsciously. For example, the severely anxious patient may hyperventilate to the point of alkalosis, producing the characteristic lightheadedness, cold hands, and tingling fingers of hypocapnia, reduced cerebral blood flow, and peripheral vasoconstriction, thereby reinforcing his view of the organic nature of his breathlessness. Palpitation is also commonly misinterpreted by the patient suffering from anxiety as a tell-tale sign of organic heart disease.

The standard approach for the physician is the separate assessment of the organic versus the psychosomatic aspects of the heart disease. Particularly helpful in this regard are excessive or inconsistent complaints for the extent of the cardiac disease. Not infrequently, hemodynamic measurements may be required to settle the role of organic heart disease in producing the clinical symptoms.

"Cardiogenic Shock." This is an ambiguous clinical term for a state of severe left heart failure associated with massive infarction of the left ventricle. Severe peripheral circulatory failure is combined with severe pulmonary congestion because of the inability of the left ventricle to handle the blood returned to it by the right ventricle. The syndrome will be considered in the article on Shock and Circulatory Failure.

CLINICAL MANAGEMENT OF HEART FAILURE

The aim of treatment in heart failure is to arrest and reverse the pathogenic sequence that led to the clinical signs and symptoms, to increase the cardiac output, and to mobilize excess fluid from the lungs and periphery. Early in the course of heart failure, the response to treatment is usually dramatic. But successive bouts of heart failure are apt to become more refractory to treatment, not only because of progressive deterioration of the myocardium, but also because of untoward effects of the therapeutic agents, particularly when they are administered for protracted periods in large doses.

Increased Cardiac Output. In most forms of chronic heart failure, the cardiac output can be made to increase by decreasing the cardiac load, by improving myocardial contractility, or by a combination of the two. In the elderly patient with a very slow heart rate, especially following myocardial infarction, acceleration of the heart by right ventricular pacing often improves the cardiac output in heart failure that may otherwise be refractory to conventional therapy. Recently, techniques for artificially augmenting the performance of the infarcted heart by means of mechanical devices ("circulatory assist") have been tried. Although the initial trials have been disappointing, the future outlook of these devices seems promising.

Decreasing the Work of the Heart. The overburdened heart may be carrying an extra pressure or volume load. The extra pressure load commonly originates in arterial vasoconstriction; the excess volume of blood to be handled by the heart may stem from diverse causes, ranging from the physiologic expansion of the blood volume in late pregnancy to the pathologic overload of severe anemia, beriberi, arteriovenous fistula, or congenital left-to-right shunt.

All therapeutic programs designed to decrease the cardiac load begin with *rest.* In the normal subject, the amount of blood that the heart is called upon to eject is matched, in some mysterious way, to the level of metabolic activity, automatically rising and falling with the oxygen consumption. By decreasing the metabolic requirements via restricting activity, the work required of the heart is decreased.

Rest has to be both physical and mental; it may be required for days to weeks and be succeeded by a new life pattern of lessened activity. The anxious patient who is confined to bed may not only maintain a level of metabolic activity comparable to that of mild exercise but also add to it peripheral arterial constriction. Often reassurance, in conjunction with sedatives or tranquilizers (such as chloral hydrate, 0.5 to 1.0 gram, or phenobarbital, 15 to 30 mg., or diazepam, 2 to 10 mg., taken orally, three times per day and at bedtime), will suffice for relaxation, particularly as the patient improves. Except for acute pulmonary edema, narcotics are rarely needed in heart failure. Excessive sedation, to the point of immobilizing the patient, enhances the risk of venous thrombosis and embolism, particularly in the elderly.

By having the patient in left heart failure assume a sitting or semisitting position, either in bed or in a chair, tachypnea and dyspnea usually decrease spontaneously as fluid drains from the apices of the lungs, so that the patient does less work in breathing; often he falls asleep as he is relieved of the distress of labored breathing. Oxygen by nasal catheter (4 to 6 liters per minute) also seems to relieve dyspnea, more often as a consequence of reassurance than of its role in relieving hypoxemia. Prevention of constipation and of urinary retention also contribute to the mental rest of the patient.

A major restriction to the use of sedatives, tranquilizers, or narcotics in heart failure is CO_2 retention. The hypercapnic state is identified by abnormally high values either for carbon dioxide (> approximately 45 mm. Hg in arterial blood) or for the concentration of bicarbonate in serum (> approximately 28 mEq. per liter). Carbon dioxide retention is almost a regular feature of the heart failure that complicates certain types of cor pulmonale, e.g., right heart failure in patients with chronic obstructive disease of the airways. Not only does CO_2 retention occur in right heart failure, but it has also been encountered recently as part of the metabolic alkalosis that follows the massive diuresis produced by potent diuretic agents, such as furosemide, in the treatment of left heart failure. Whatever the cause, CO_2 retention is associated with depression of sensitivity of the respiratory center to CO_2 and heightened dependence on the hypoxic stimulus to breathing. Consequently, in CO_2 retention either further depression of the respiratory center by sedatives or complete relief of the hypoxia by high concentrations of inspired oxygen (> approximately 40 per cent O_2 in N_2) may depress ventilation to dangerously low levels.

It is remarkable how often the proper use of rest as the initial step in treatment will promote a vigorous diuresis, slow the heart rate, and relieve dyspnea, thereby allowing a more leisurely use of other cardiotonic agents, such as digitalis and diuretics. On the other hand, if metabolic demands remain high, as during undetected thyrotoxicosis, the heart failure may prove refractory to the conventional cardiotonic program until the thyroid overactivity is curtailed.

Improving Myocardial Contractility. Since impaired contractility is at the root of heart failure, success in any cardiotonic program depends on readjusting the balance between myocardial capability and load. Some agents improve contractility by a direct (inotropic) effect; others, such as diuretics, by lessening the load.

Digitalis. The time-tested agent for improving myocardial contractility in heart failure is digitalis. Although the full picture of how digitalis exerts its inotropic effect on the heart is still obscure, certain features are becoming distinguishable. Thus, the effect seems to begin with a direct inhibition of sodium plus potassium activated adenosine triphosphatase ($[Na^+ + K^+]$ ATPase) in the membranes of heart muscle; it seems to end in an increased concentration of calcium ions at the sites of interaction between the thick and thin filaments of the sarcomere during each contraction. Linking these two steps is an increased concentration of intracellular Na^+ ions, a consequence of the inhibition of the membrane ATPase, and a mechanism for freeing Ca^{++} ions to act at the force-generating sites. Accompanying the inhibition of membrane ATPase and the increase in intracellular Na^+ ions is cellular depletion of K^+ ions. This intracellular hypokalemia, especially when the concentration of potassium in serum is low, predisposes to arrhythmias by promoting the emergence of ectopic foci and re-entrant mechanisms.

The unique property of digitalis as an inotropic agent stems from its ability to improve myocardial contractility in heart failure without simultaneously eliciting antagonistic effects, such as peripheral vasoconstriction or tachycardia. After digitalis has been given in effective doses and myocardial contractility has increased, the heart shrinks in size, and cardiac output increases even though the end-diastolic volume and pressure decrease; in the veins leading to the failing ventricle the blood pressure decreases, and evidences of venous congestion and of organ hypoperfusion disappear. Peripheral vascular resistance decreases. This decrease in peripheral resistance in heart failure is the result of a complicated interplay by which the heightened sympathetic tone of heart failure decreases reflexly as the performance of the heart improves, overwhelming the direct constricting effect of digitalis on arterioles and veins. In the reordering of the circulation that occurs after digitalis has relieved congestive heart failure, blood which had been sequestered in the splanchnic venous bed is redirected to the systemic veins by appropriate adjustments in vascular tone, thereby helping to sustain the improved cardiac output.

Digitalis improves the contractility of the failing myocardium regardless of the type of heart failure, the rate, or the rhythm. Once heart failure is recognized, even if only by the more subtle signs of pulsus alternans, gallop rhythm, or mild dyspnea, digitalis should be given. The fact that rest, salt restriction, and diuretics have eliminated the signs and symptoms should not obscure the fact that digitalis will be needed as soon as activity is resumed. In some instances, such as inflammatory disease of the myocardium or severe hypoxia in cor pulmonale, digitalis may be discontinued once the initiating mechanism has been abolished.

The problem with using digitalis for its inotropic effect is its other pharmacologic actions. Some of these are turned to advantage in treating heart failure. For example, if rapid atrial fibrillation is present during heart failure, the slowing of atrioventricular conduction by digitalis—a "side effect" as far as contractility is concerned—decreases the number of atrial impulses reaching the ventricle. Indeed, in heart failure associated with atrial fibrillation, slowing of the ventricular rate is a useful guide to digitalis dosage. On the other hand, during sinus rhythm or tachycardia, the heart rate is often a poor guide to the therapeutic effect of digitalis on contractility, particularly if a complication such as pulmonary embolism is sustaining the rapid rate.

Many practical lessons have been learned about the clinical use of digitalis since Withering urged, in 1785, that digitalis leaf be continued "until it either acts on the kidneys, the stomach, the pulse or the bowels: let it be stopped upon the first appearance of any one of these effects." By substituting digitalis glycosides for digitalis leaf, pure substances of constant and uniform potency were obtained. Although none of these proved to have any intrinsic advantage over another with respect to beneficial effect on myocardial contractility, there are considerable differences in their speeds of action, time course of effectiveness, and rates of dissipation and elimination. Also, despite Withering's admonition, rarely is it necessary to produce minor toxicity in order to be sure of the full inotropic effect of digitalis, since half-therapeutic doses have been shown to produce considerable improvement in contractility, and the therapeutic dose has often proved to be only 50 to 60 per cent of the toxic dose.

In starting a therapeutic program with digitalis, it is important to know whether digitalis, in any form, has been taken during the preceding week or two. Usually, unless renal failure is present, two weeks is allowed for digitalis to be entirely eliminated. If digitalis is administered intravenously to a patient who has recently received the drug, ventricular tachycardia or fibrillation may ensue.

Clinical manifestations and the electrocardiogram are the key guides to dosage. As the circulation improves, signs and symptoms of heart failure abate: diuresis occurs; dyspnea and orthopnea lessen; distended neck veins become less turgid; the heart rate tends to slow unless a hypermetabolic state, such as fever or hyperthyroidism, or myocarditis or pulmonary embolism is present; during exercise, the heart rate does not increase as much as it did before failure. As indicated above, the most dramatic ventricular slowing occurs during atrial fibrillation, increasing the pulse deficit.

By changes in the ST segments and T waves, the electrocardiogram only indicates that appreciable quantities of digitalis are on board; changes in contour provide no guide to either toxic or therapeutic levels. For this, serum levels of the glycosides are now being determined. On the other hand, particularly if the heart rate fails to slow during digitalization, the electrocardiogram may show an arrhythmia from digitalis toxicity, e.g., paroxysmal atrial tachycardia with block or ventricular tachycardia.

The particular digitalis preparation that is used depends on the clinical circumstance. Most physicians rely on one or two oral and intravenous preparations: one for short and one for prolonged action; another for emergency use. Among the oral preparations, digoxin and digitoxin are currently the most popular; of the intravenous preparations, ouabain and lanatoside C (Cedilanid) are most widely used.

Digitalization may be accomplished rapidly or slowly. Small doses have a cumulative effect, and even "maintenance" doses tend to accumulate in the body; therefore it is possible to digitalize over a period of weeks, using small ("maintenance") doses. At the other extreme, it is possible to digitalize rapidly, i.e., within a matter of minutes, using an intravenous preparation. Large intravenous doses, e.g., 2 to 3 mg. of digoxin in four hours, may produce toxicity even in patients who have not previously had digitalis. Rarely is intravenous digitalis required in heart failure, even if acute pulmonary edema exists, unless paroxysmal atrial fibrillation with a rapid ventricular rate has produced a life-threatening situation.

The *extracardiac toxic effects* of digitalis are anorexia, aversion to food, nausea, vomiting, diarrhea, mental confusion, and disturbances in vision. They generally precede cardiotoxicity and are more likely to occur with one preparation, e.g., digitalis leaf, than another, e.g., digoxin. Cardiotoxicity may take the form of a wide variety of abnormalities in impulse generation and conduction, ranging from ventricular premature beats to ventricular tachycardias, atrial fibrillation, and various degrees of heart block. Atrial flutter is rare.

The toxic effects of digitalis on the heart are probably independent of the effects on contractility. Their occurrence is strongly influenced by the electrolyte pattern in the serum and, presumably, in the heart muscle. Serious derangements in these patterns are produced by certain diuretic agents (see below) and occur in uremia. Most familiar are hypokalemia, which potentiates the toxic effects of digitalis, and hyperkalemia, which nullifies them. The role of other electrolyte disturbances is not as clear, but violent upsets undoubtedly affect the toxic manifestations of digitalis.

The cardinal rule that applies when disturbances in rhythm and conduction suggest that overdigitalization has occurred, is not only to stop the digitalis but also to discontinue those diuretic measures which promote hypokalemia. If renal function is adequate, potassium salts (4 to 6 grams of potassium chloride per day) may be administered orally; care should be exerted to administer a palatable form of potassium. For urgent correction of ectopic beats or tachycardia resulting from digitalis overdosage, potassium salts may be administered intravenously. The usual preparation is 40 mEq. of potassium in a 500-ml. solution of 5 per cent glucose in water; this is administered slowly, i.e., at a rate of 40 mEq. per hour. Venous irritation at the site of infusion may be troublesome. The electrocardiogram is monitored throughout, both for arrhythmias and for peaking of T-waves. Hypotension may limit the amount of potassium that can be safely given by vein. Lidocaine (1 to 2 mg. per kilogram in one to two minutes by intravenous injection or as a continuous infusion) has been used to control premature ventricular beats and ventricular tachycardia resulting from digitalis. It has the advantage over procaine amide of not causing hypotension.

Other measures are less reliable or necessary than the administration of potassium salts. Propranolol, 2 to 5 mg., and diphenylhydantoin sodium, administered intravenously at a rate of 5 to 10 mg. per kilogram during 5 to 15 minutes, have their advocates. Quinidine and chelating agents have also been used on occasion. Electroconversion by DC shock, which is remarkably effective for many arrhythmias, may produce serious paroxysmal ventricular arrhythmias in overdigitalized patients.

The oral preparations are illustrated by digoxin and digitoxin in Table 1. These may be used not only orally, but also intramuscularly (if digitalis cannot be tolerated by mouth) and intravenously. In practice, digitoxin is rarely administered intravenously since it is long-acting. Intramuscular administration of either agent is rarely used (because of uncertain absorption and local irritation) unless medication by mouth is not tolerated.

Digoxin is the most widely used oral preparation of digitalis. As may be seen in Table 1, an oral dose of 1 mg. usually produces a digitalis effect in one to two hours and peak effect in six to eight hours; additional doses of 0.25 to 0.5 mg. every eight hours are commonly used to complete digitalization. The subsequent maintenance dose is usually 0.25 to 0.5 mg. per day. This schedule can be modified considerably, and digitalization

for as long as one week may be used on the basis that approximately 2.5 mg. is the total amount required for 24 to 36 hours and that 0.25 mg. per day is eliminated. The rapid elimination of digoxin makes it useful in case of toxicity but also provides wider swings in level than does digitoxin.

Digitoxin is used by many as the long-acting drug of choice. It is completely absorbed after oral administration so that oral and intravenous dosages are identical. It is quite similar to digitalis leaf with respect to onset and peak of action and to the rate of dissipation and elimination, but is about 1000 times as powerful (0.1 mg. of digitoxin equals 0.1 gram of digitalis leaf). Its slow dissipation and elimination afford the prospect of less variation in levels from hour to hour than digoxin. But the drug accumulates insidiously so that maintenance doses which suffice at the onset (0.1 to 0.2 mg. per day) often prove to be toxic in time.

Not shown in the table is gitalin, a glycoside mixture obtained from *Digitalis purpurea*. Its rate of elimination or dissipation (three to four days) is equal to, or a little slower than, digoxin but more rapid than digitoxin. It has the same pharmacologic and toxic effects as the other glycosides; the original proposition that it has an unusual effectiveness and favorable toxic-to-therapeutic ratio has not been proved. The average digitalizing dose by mouth or intravenous injection ranges between 3.0 and 10.5 mg., with a maintenance dose of 0.25 to 0.5 mg. per day.

Intravenous preparations (Table 2) are, as a rule, reserved for life-threatening situations since digitalization by the oral route is usually sufficiently rapid. The possible indications include acute heart failure during an episode of atrial fibrillation with rapid ventricular rate, massive life-threatening pulmonary edema as part of acute left ventricular failure, and heart failure or a serious arrhythmia during operation. In general, the larger the dose the greater the incidence of serious ventricular arrhythmias.

Ouabain is the traditional digitalis preparation for intravenous use. It is a pure crystalline substance which is unsuitable for oral use because of poor absorption from the gastrointestinal tract.

TABLE 1.   ORAL DIGITALIS PREPARATIONS

	Digoxin	Digitoxin
Source	*Digitalis lanata*	*Digitalis purpurea; Digitalis lanata*
Tablets available, mg.	0.25	0.05, 0.1
Initial dose, mg.*	1.0	0.75
Total digitalizing dose (24–36 hrs.), mg.†	2.5 (1.5–3.75)	1.5 (1.2–2.0)
Maintenance dose, mg.†	0.25 (0.25–0.75)	0.1 (0.05–0.2)
Absorption from gastrointestinal tract, percentage administered‡	60–80	90–100
Onset of activity, hrs.‡	1–2	0.5
Peak effect, hrs.‡	6–8	8–12
Duration of effect, days‡	1–3	4–7
Period of elimination, days‡	3–6	14–12

*Presupposes no digitalis during previous two weeks.
†Average values and ranges. These are rough estimates: toxicity has been observed with doses much smaller than the lowest extremity of the range; conversely, full digitalization may not occur with the highest dosages.
‡Approximate values.

TABLE 2. INTRAVENOUS DIGITALIS PREPARATIONS

	Ouabain	Cedilanid D	Digoxin
Source	*Strophanthus gratus*	*Digitalis lanata**	*Digitalis lanata**
Dosages available, mg.†	0.25, 0.5	0.4, 0.8	0.5
Initial dose, mg.	0.25	0.8	0.5
Subsequent intravenous dosages	0.1 mg. per 0.5 hr.	0.2–0.4 mg. per 2–6 hrs.	0.25 mg. per hr.
Maximum intravenous dose/24 hrs., mg.	1	1.6	1.5
Onset of activity, min.‡	3–10	10–30	10–30
Peak effect, hrs.‡	0.5–1	1–2	2–3
Duration of effect, days‡	1–3	0.5–1.5	2–3
Period of elimination, days‡	0.5–3	3–6	3–6

*Digitalis glycosides should not be given intravenously if patient has received digitalis during previous two weeks.
†In ampules (sterile solutions) for intravenous or intramuscular injection.
‡Approximate values.

Its latency period is exceedingly brief (less than five minutes); its rapid elimination disqualifies it for maintenance of digitalization. The initial intravenous dose is 0.3 mg. (slowly); an additional 0.15 or 0.3 mg. may be given again after 24 hours.

Deslanoside (Cedilanid D), which is related to digoxin, is gradually replacing ouabain. Because it has a shorter latent period and is more rapidly eliminated than digoxin, it is less satisfactory for oral use and for maintenance of digitalization. It is administered intravenously; hardly ever is it given intramuscularly. After intravenous injection, a digitalizing effect appears in 10 to 30 minutes, reaching peak effect in 1 to 2 hours, regressing in 24 hours. For rapid intravenous digitalization, the full 1.6 mg. may be given at once, or, preferably, 0.8 mg. may be followed by another 0.8 mg., either in four hours or in divided doses, at two- to four-hour intervals for two or three additional doses. Maintenance of digitalization is preferably done by oral digoxin or digitoxin. But if desirable, 0.4 mg. may be given intravenously or intramuscularly at 8- to 12-hour intervals.

Digoxin is preferred by some for intravenous as well as for oral use. After an initial intravenous dose of approximately 0.5 (or 0.75) mg., additional doses are usually given by mouth. If desirable, an additional few doses of 0.25 (or 0.5) mg. may be administered intravenously before switching to the oral medication. The suggested total dosage given intravenously in 24 hours is less than the corresponding oral dosage.

Acetylstrophanthidin is a partial synthetic which, because of its exceedingly rapid onset of action and dissipation, has been advocated more as a diagnostic test for under- and overdigitalization than as a therapeutic agent for heart failure. In practice, repeated injections of the substance (0.25 mg. in 5 ml. of glucose in water) are made until toxic or therapeutic effects are observed. Unfortunately, it is potentially dangerous, and other tests, such as short-acting cholinesterase inhibitors (Tensilon) are replacing it. At present, the most useful indices of under- and overdigitalization remain the clinical signs and the electrocardiogram; although immunoassay techniques are currently being applied to determine concentrations of digitalis glycosides in serum as a guide to digitalization, these procedures are still in the developmental stage.

Sympathomimetic Amines. Although fashions in diuretics have changed considerably over the years, no inotropic agent has as yet been found as a successor to digitalis. Replacements have been sought among the sympathomimetic amines which also stimulate the myocardium but differently from digitalis. The qualifications that have been sought include effectiveness after oral administration, improved contractility in conjunction with peripheral vasodilatation, increased renal excretion of sodium, and a greater increase in coronary blood flow than in myocardial oxygen consumption. Three catecholamines have been singled out for close scrutiny because of their ability to stimulate the heart and to decrease peripheral resistance: epinephrine, isoproterenol, and dopamine. Unfortunately, none of these is on a clinical par with digitalis: all three provoke tachycardia; epinephrine decreases the elimination of sodium by the kidney, whereas isoproterenol usually has no effect on sodium excretion; dopamine has to be given intravenously, acts briefly, and causes undesirable increments in systemic arterial pressure.

Glucagon, a polypeptide hormone produced chiefly by the α cells of the pancreas, has recently attracted considerable attention as a possible adjunctive measure in the treatment of the patient in refractory heart failure who can tolerate no more digitalis. Like the catecholamines, glucagon presumably exerts its cardiotonic effects by activating adenyl cyclase. It has been given by continuous intravenous infusion (2 to 4 mg. per hour for 10 to 13 days) and by injections of large single doses (10 to 25 mg.). In these doses, the major side effect was nausea; abnormalities in blood sugar levels were uncommon. Unfortunately, enthusiasm for this agent has begun to wane, because of recent evidence that the effects of glucagon on myocardial contractility are far less consistent in chronic heart failure than in the normal heart.

Cardiac Assistance Devices. In some clinics, attempts have been made to provide a temporary respite for the heart in acute refractory failure, using devices which share the load for hours to days while the heart recuperates. The most popular methods are (1) venoarterial bypass, which assists the heart by diverting blood from the heart and returning it by a pump to the arterial tree, and (2) counterpulsation, which is synchronized with the heart beat to modify aortic pressure by rhythmically changing either the blood volume in the aorta, using an external pump, or the capac-

TABLE 3. USEFUL DIURETICS AND

Type of Diuretic	Example	Relevant Chemical Structure	Major Site of Renal Action	Preferred Route of Administration	Onset of Action	Duration of Diuretic Effect
Chloruretic sulfonamide	Chlorothiazide (Diuril)	Benzothiadiazine derivative	Distal tubule	Oral	Within 1 hour	12–24 hrs.
Mercurials	Meralluride (Mercuhydrin)	Theophylline plus organic mercurial	Distal tubule	IM	1–2 hrs.	12–24 hrs.
Potassium-sparing	Triamterene (Dyrenium)	Pteridine derivative	Distal tubule	Oral	1–2 hrs.	16–24 hrs.
Ethacrynic acid	Ethacrynic acid (Edecrin)	Ketone derivative of aryloxyacetic acid	Ascending limb of Henle's loop	Oral*	1 hour	6–8 hrs.
Carbonic anhydrase inhibitors	Acetazolamide (Diamox)	Sulfanilamide derivative	Proximal tubule (Na–H exchange)	Oral	1 hour	5–8 hrs.

*For acute pulmonary edema, 20 to 50 mg. is administered intravenously; its diuretic action starts almost immediately. Furosemide, a nonthiazide sulfonamide with a benzosulfamyl group, has practically the same effect in the same dosage.

†Higher dose is for severe heart failure.

‡Ethacrynic acid and furosemide may become more popular for milder cases of heart failure when more is learned about how to use these powerful agents.

¶Hazardous in renal insufficiency.

§Hypokalemia may precipitate digitalis intoxication.

ity of the aorta, using an intra-aortic balloon. All methods aim to reduce the external work of the heart, the developed tension, and the myocardial oxygen consumption while improving coronary perfusion. As yet, technical problems have restricted the use of these devices in man to desperate circumstances and for as brief a period as possible.

Mobilization of Excess Fluid. For edema to form, excessive amounts of sodium and water must be retained by the kidneys. Restriction of sodium intake, not only as the chloride but in other forms, such as sodium-containing medications, should always start a program designed to get rid of edema. Reduction of water intake is usually unnecessary except in severe heart failure, in which hyponatremia and water intoxication are apt to occur. In mild heart failure, salt intake is generally restricted to less than 3 grams per day; in severe congestive heart failure, an intake of less than 0.5 gram per day is often needed to promote diuresis and to reduce the blood volume and the venous pressure. The total burden of excess fluid may be gauged by daily weighing, before breakfast and after urinating. Although the advent of potent diuretics has liberalized dietary controls, the side effects of diuretic therapy make it preferable to control body sodium by intake rather than to rely heavily on the kidney. The combination of severe sodium restriction plus potent sodium-losing diuretics may, particularly if renal disease is present, lead to weakness, oliguria, and azotemia.

Diuretic Therapy. Digitalis and salt restriction may not suffice to eliminate edema. Diuretics do this, not by influencing cardiac contractility, but by promoting the loss of water and electrolytes by the kidney. The most important diuretics act by depressing the renal tubular absorption of water and electrolytes; some of the ancillary diuretics also affect the filtration rate. Large losses of edema fluid (more than 1 to 2 kg. per day) are upsetting to electrolyte balance and may cause muscle cramps, weakness, gastrointestinal upset, and digitalis toxicity.

Three types of "first-line" diuretics are in common use: chloruretic sulfonamides (benzothiadiazine derivatives), mercurials, and furosemide or ethacrynic acid. The "second-line" diuretics include aldosterone inhibitors, xanthines, and carbonic anhydrase inhibitors. The effects of diuretic agents may usually be potentiated by proper combinations (Table 3) since they act by different mechanisms, and often at different sites.

The *chloruretic sulfonamides* are the agents of choice for mild to moderate cardiac edema. They exert their major effect by blocking absorption of sodium and chloride; to a much lesser extent they also inhibit carbonic anhydrase. The prototypes of this group are *chlorothiazide* and *hydrochlorothiazide*, both of which are extraordinarily

SOME OF THEIR CHARACTERISTICS

Usual Dosage Per Day	Suggested Pattern of Therapy	Major Electrolyte Changes in Urine	Major Electrolyte Changes in Blood	Typical Toxic Effects	Remarks
500–2000 mg.†	Few days on; few days off	Increased excretion of Na, Cl, K	None (small doses) to hypochloremic alkalosis; hypokalemia§	Nausea, vomiting; skin rashes; hyperuricemia; hyperglycemia	May need potassium supplements or potassium-sparing diuretic¶
2–6 ml.†	To start treatment or as adjunct	Increased excretion of Na, Cl; variable K	Hypochloremic alkalosis	Mercury intoxication; sudden death (after IV injection); occasional agranulocytosis; minor systemic effects	Inactivated by hypochloremic alkalosis; hazardous in oliguria¶
100–300 mg.	For one month or so, in conjunction with more potent diuretics	Decreased excretion of K and H; slight increase in Na, Cl, HCO_3	Hyperkalemia	Generally nontoxic; GI upset; gynecomastia; rare agranulocytosis	Synergistic with thiazides and ethacrynic acid,¶ avoid potassium supplements
40–300 mg.†	Refractory edema‡	Increased excretion of Na, Cl, HCO_3, K, H	Hyponatremia, hypochloremia, hypokalemia§	ECF depletion; hypotension; azotemia; contraction alkalosis; GI upsets; hyperuricemia; agranulocytosis; diabetogenic	Causes renal (cortical) vasodilatation; effective in renal insufficiency
250–500 mg.	When blood bicarbonate is high or before (not during) mercurial injections	Increased excretion of Na, K, HCO_3; decrease in H	Hyperchloremic acidosis; hypokalemia§	Generally nontoxic; mild GI and mental upsets; occasional sulfonamide idiosyncrasy	Not very potent; loses effectiveness with continued administration¶

effective by mouth. Although there are now many derivatives of chlorothiazide, they do not differ appreciably in mode of action or in potency when optimal doses are given; but they do differ with respect to duration of effect. In mild heart failure, effective doses (500 mg. per day of chlorothiazide) increase the output of sodium, chloride, and, to a lesser extent, potassium without appreciable change in urinary pH or in the rate of bicarbonate excretion. In severe cases, in which higher doses (2000 mg. per day) are used, the carbonic anhydrase inhibitory effect becomes manifest so that bicarbonate excretion increases and the urine becomes alkaline; potassium excretion is also increased. The urine produced by chlorothiazide diuresis is richer in sodium chloride than that produced by mercurials, suggesting that chlorothiazide acts on a more distal part of the tubule. With large or continuing doses, potassium serum levels may fall below 2 to 3 mEq. per liter since supplementation by diet is often inadequate; full doses of potassium salts are then needed to avoid hypopotassemia. Potassium salts, particularly the chloride, cause gastrointestinal discomfort. The need for potassium supplementation can be lessened either by using smaller doses of thiazides or by adopting an intermittent dosage schedule, e.g., three days on and four days off, or by combining treatment with an aldosterone inhibitor. Complications of the thiazide deriva-

tives include nausea, vomiting, mild skin rashes, hyperuricemia (rarely clinical gout) and hyperglycemia (or exacerbation of diabetes). Less common are the more serious complications, such as exfoliative dermatitis, thrombocytopenia, agranulocytosis, jaundice, pancreatitis, and glomerulonephritis. As with other agents that cause potassium loss, digitalis intoxication may be a complication of excess kaliuresis.

Mercurial diuretics are the traditional auxiliary agents in heart failure. Many of these are combinations of an organic mercurial and theophylline. Compounds are available for intravenous or intramuscular (meralluride), subcutaneous (sodium mercaptomerin), and oral (chlormerodrin) use; the intramuscular route is most often used. When given intravenously for severe heart failure, meralluride has to be administered slowly (in 100 ml. of 5 per cent glucose in about one-half hour) because of potential cardiac toxicity. After intramuscular injection, absorption is usually complete in one hour; up to 90 per cent may be recovered in the urine in 24 hours. When first used, daily administration elicits sustained diuresis and natriuresis. In time, especially with intensive treatment, refractoriness results from one or two causes: (1) the development of a hypochloremic alkalosis (with fairly normal sodium levels) from which responsiveness may be restored by ammonium chloride, or (2) the development of a *low-salt syndrome*, in which sodium as well as chloride levels in serum are severely depressed; occasionally when this state does not respond to fluid restriction, the cautious infusion of hypertonic saline (3 to 5 per cent) may prove helpful but runs the risk of precipitating a bout of pulmonary edema.

Ethacrynic acid and *furosemide* are the most potent of the diuretic agents. Although they differ chemically, they are quite similar in their physiologic effects. They are particularly useful when other diuretics have failed or for the emergency treatment (intravenous) of acute pulmonary edema. Both interfere with sodium reabsorption in the ascending limb of the loop of Henle, but large doses seem also to affect proximal tubular reabsorption. Like the thiazides, they produce diuresis, natriuresis, and kaliuresis, and interfere with the diluting mechanisms; unlike the thiazides, they also induce hydrogen depletion and interfere with the concentrating mechanisms. Problems in their use arise almost exclusively from the perturbations in electrolyte concentrations which they induce, particularly in continued doses.

Among the "second-line" diuretics, probably the most useful are the *aldosterone inhibitors*. Spironolactone, a typical aldosterone inhibitor, blocks both the sodium-retaining and the potassium-losing effects of aldosterone (endogenous or exogenous). Oral doses of 50 to 600 mg. per day are well tolerated for months, virtually free of toxic effects. Unfortunately, this agent is quite expensive. Its unique value is in promoting natriuresis and diuresis without causing increased excretion of potassium. Its absorption is often poor, and there may be a latent period of a few days unless it is used in conjunction with other diuretic agents. Because of its potassium-sparing effect and its unusual mode of action, spironolactone may be a valuable diuretic agent in complicated or prolonged heart failure either to potentiate the effects of a "first-line" diuretic or to avoid the consequences of potassium depletion. Hyperkalemia is a serious threat if potassium salts are given orally in conjunction with aldosterone inhibitors.

Another potassium-sparing diuretic is *triamterene*. In contrast to spironolactone, it is nonsteroidal, and it is potassium-sparing even after adrenalectomy. In full dosage (200 mg. per day) it is a mild diuretic and natriuretic agent; it acts mainly on the distal tubule. Its chief value is in retarding the loss of potassium during protracted administration of thiazides. It may cause mild hyperchloremic acidosis. Amiloride (MK 870) is like triamterene and may even prove to be more effective. But it is still too new for full appraisal.

Aminophylline, a xanthine derivative, has little use in severe heart failure; in mild heart failure it may be useful (as a suppository) for its bronchodilating as well as diuretic effects, and as a spacer between doses of more potent diuretics.

Acetazolamide, a carbonic anhydrase inhibitor, is a mild diuretic which promotes excretion of sodium, potassium, and bicarbonate; the excretion of titratable acid and ammonia decreases. It acts by suppressing the sodium-hydrogen exchange mechanism in the kidney, leading to the preferential excretion of potassium as hydrogen formation is decreased. It loses its effectiveness in a few days and is only useful for interrupted treatment. Like ammonium chloride, it is valuable to prepare for a mercurial diuresis because of the hyperchloremic acidosis produced. When given *simultaneously* with thiazides, it potentiates the excretion of sodium and potassium. Severe acidosis (as from renal failure) is a contraindication to its use.

Osmotic diuretics, such as *mannitol*, block the reabsorption of sodium and water at the proximal tubule, and increase renal blood flow. Mannitol may be useful in managing refractory cardiac edema, especially in conjunction with distal tubular blocking agents, such as mercurials, thiazides, ethacrynic acid, or furosemide, but it may produce cardiocirculatory overload owing to the volume expansion if diuresis is delayed.

When intensive or long-continued diuretic therapy is required, a combination of diuretics, such as those in Table 3, may prove to be less upsetting to the water and electrolyte balance than increasing the dosage of any particular one. For example, the diuretic effects of ethacrynic acid may be safely augmented by adding chlorothiazide and a potassium-sparing drug. Indeed, a carbonic anhydrase inhibitor may be used to complete the diuretic picture since it acts differently from the others, i.e., by interfering with proximal tubular reabsorption of sodium bicarbonate, thereby delivering more sodium bicarbonate to the loop of Henle where the ethacrynic acid acts.

Refractory Heart Failure. Ultimately, if the myocardium continues to deteriorate, an end-stage of refractory or intractable heart failure is bound to ensue. But in many instances "refractory" has proved to be a relative term. Not infrequently, heart failure merely becomes unresponsive simply because of a combination of inadequate attention to details of treatment, such as the low sodium diet and digitalis dosage, and severe upset in water and electrolyte balance that has been produced by the overzealous administration of potent diuretics. Bizarre water and electrolyte disturbances may take the form of "contraction alkalosis," hyponatremia and hypo-osmolarity of the extracellular fluid, and abnormal partition of potassium between cells and circulating fluids. Restoration of water and electrolyte balance is quite difficult in such instances since the withholding of water may cause intense thirst, and the administration of hypertonic saline may precipitate pulmonary edema. In some instances peritoneal dialysis has been used in the attempt to restore a near-normal electrolyte pattern in the serum.

Elimination of excessively rapid, slow, or irregular heart rates may convert refractory heart failure to one that is manageable. For example, reversion of atrial fibrillation to a normal sinus rhythm may make the heart failure more amenable to conventional treatment. Conversely, acceleration of a slow heart rate, such as may occur in complete heart block, may make it possible to treat heart failure successfully.

One eternal hope in treating refractory heart failure is to uncover an obscure but treatable basis for the disproportion between myocardial capacity and load. The list of candidates is long. impaired myocardial performance from rheumatic fever, myxedema, or beriberi; constrictive pericarditis; hypermetabolic states produced by hidden infection or hyperthyroidism; inordinate cardiac loads produced by pheochromocytoma, arteriovenous fistula, valvular heart disease, or coarctation of the aorta; arrhythmias, which cause excessively rapid rates on the one hand and severe bradycardia on the other; and multiple pulmonary emboli. All of these are potentially treatable and have been responsible for supposedly "refractory" heart failure.

The prognosis in refractory heart failure is grim unless the contractile performance of the heart can be improved. Glucagon may prove to be a useful supplement to digitalis. In addition, attention is currently being paid to mechanical devices that can assist the overburdened heart as well as to procedures for "electroaugmentation," by which a positive inotropic effect is produced by electrical stimulation of the heart instead of by drugs.

Acute Pulmonary Edema. This is a distressing and potentially life-threatening situation generally arising from an acute inability of the failing left heart to handle the blood that the competent right ventricle is delivering to it. As a result, pulmonary venous pressure increases abruptly to high levels, alveoli are flooded and gas exchange begins to suffer, particularly as fluid begins to overflow the alveoli into the distal ramifications of the bronchial tree. Depending on the distribution of fluid within the lungs, i.e., interstitium, alveoli, and airways, the blood gases may or may not be abnormal. Thus, if edema is confined to the pulmonary interstitial space, the stiff lungs, and the resulting increase in respiratory frequency, would be expected to cause respiratory alkalosis. On the other hand, respiratory acidosis would not be unexpected should fluid mount into the airways and cause bronchiolar and bronchial obstruction.

Acute pulmonary edema occurs most often as a complication of left ventricular failure resulting from ischemic heart disease, hypertension, or aortic valvular disease. It also occurs frequently in young people with tight mitral stenosis. Even in normal subjects, it may be produced by excessive administration of fluid intravenously. It is not uncommon after raised intracranial pressure and head injury. It complicates pulmonary embolism. It has been observed sporadically after strenuous exertion of visitors to high altitudes. In cardiac patients, it is particularly apt to occur during acute arrhythmias, acute myocardial infarction, physical or mental exertion, discontinuation of a cardiotonic program, fluid overload, use of cardiodepressant drugs, e.g., propranolol, or sodium retention (dietary indiscretions or steroids).

The onset of acute pulmonary edema may be with a cough with wheezing or with breathlessness and a sense of oppression in the chest. Physical signs are tachypnea and rales, heard at first in the dependent parts of the lungs, then extending progressively upward as the attack worsens; rales are a late sign, marking the presence of free fluid in the airways rather than in the interstitial space and alveoli. In severe attacks, pallor, sweating, cyanosis, and frothy sputum are present.

Ambulant patients with mitral stenosis sometimes suffer mild bouts of pulmonary edema after sudden exertion. Cough, increased dyspnea, and sometimes frothy or pinkish sputum, with transient moist or asthmatic rales, are frequent findings. A short rest usually relieves the attack.

Hypertensive patients may develop a severe form of pulmonary edema, characterized by intense anxiety, cough, and pressure in the chest, followed by orthopnea, labored and hyperpneic dyspnea, and sometimes cardiac asthma. Cyanosis, moist or asthmatic rales, pallor, sweating, and further increase in pulse and blood pressure are evident on examination.

In acute pulmonary edema resulting from acute left ventricular failure, meperidine, 50 mg., or morphine, 10 to 15 mg., may be administered intravenously for restlessness or dyspnea. Morphine is the traditional agent but distressing side effects, such as nausea, vomiting, and urinary retention, have detracted from its popularity. For ease in breathing, the patient regularly assumes an upright position, thereby shifting fluid to the lung bases. Diuresis should be instituted promptly to reduce the circulating (and extravascular fluid) volume, using a rapid-acting diuretic which is administered intravenously (ethacrynic acid or furosemide). Prompt and dramatic relief may be accomplished by reducing venous return to the right heart; this may be done by either one or two small phlebotomies (250 ml. of blood), by rotating tourniquets (releasing one at a time for five minutes every half hour), or by intermittent positive pressure breathing which raises pleural pressure, thereby impeding venous return. Even though arterial oxygenation may be near normal, high concentrations of humidified oxygen, 50 to 100 per cent, are frequently used empirically to relieve dyspnea, restlessness, and confusion. Severe hypotension is a contraindication to phlebotomy and to artificial respiration.

In the approach outlined above, the emphasis has been on decreasing the volume load that returns to the left heart. Rarely is specific treatment needed for the high blood pressure that apprehension and anxiety effect during almost any episode of acute pulmonary edema, because this type of hypertension is generally transient, almost invariably subsiding as the pulmonary edema clears. On the other hand, if the condition has been precipitated by a paroxysm of systemic arterial hypertension, small doses of ganglionic blocking agents may be needed to lower the arterial blood pressure and bring the attack under control.

Digitalis (digoxin or lanatoside C, 1.0 mg.) may be administered intravenously if the patient has had none during the preceding two weeks, but the urgency for intravenous administration has decreased considerably since the advent of the potent, rapid-acting diuretics. On the other hand, there may be more urgency for digitalis if a paroxysmal bout of arrhythmia, such as atrial fibrillation, which usually responds to digitalis, is responsible for the episode of pulmonary edema. Alternatively, if the situation seems to have reached a critical stage because of a ventricular or supraventricular ectopic tachycardia, it may be necessary to use DC electroshock to interrupt the arrhythmia.

Face to face with a patient in pulmonary edema, the physician often feels compelled to apply a battery of strenuous measures in rapid succession or simultaneously. Especially for patients in poor condition, this treatment may be worse than the disorder, which is usually self-limited once the upright position has been assumed, mental rest accomplished, and a potent diuretic administered. As soon as the crisis is over, a more conventional cardiotonic program is begun and a search made for the etiology of the left heart failure as well as for the mechanism that precipitated the episode.

The role of left heart failure in producing high-altitude pulmonary edema is not clear. In any event, prompt recovery usually follows bed rest, descent to lower altitude, and the administration of oxygen.

Braunwald, E., Ross, J., Jr., and Sonnenblick, E. H.: Mechanisms of Contraction of the Normal and Failing Heart. Boston, Little, Brown & Company, 1968.

Brugan, E., Kozonis, M. C., and Overy, D. C.: Glucagon therapy in heart failure. Lancet, 1:482, 1969.
Genest, J., Granger, P., DeChamplain, J., and Boucher, R.: Endocrine factors in congestive heart failure. Amer. J. Cardiol., 22:35, 1968.
Kirkendall, W. M., and Stein, J. H.: Clinical pharmacology of furosemide and ethacrynic acid. Amer. J. Cardiol., 22:162, 1968.
Koch-Weser, J.: Mechanism of digitalis action on the heart. New Eng. J. Med., 277:416, 1967.
Linzbach, A. J.: Heart failure from the point of view of quantitative anatomy. Amer. J. Cardiol., 5:370, 1960.
Longobardo, G. S., Cherniack, N. S., and Fishman, A. P.: Cheyne-Stokes breathing produced by a model of the human respiratory system. J. Appl. Physiol., 21:1839, 1966.
Marshall, R. J., and Shepherd, J. T.: Cardiac Function in Health and Disease. Philadelphia, W. B. Saunders Company, 1968.
Mason, D. T., Spann, J. F., and Zelis, R.: New developments in the understanding of the actions of the digitalis glycosides. Prog. Cardiov. Dis., 11:443, 1969.
Meerson, F. Z.: The myocardium in hyperfunction, hypertrophy and heart failure. Cir. Res., 25 (Supp. II):1, 1969.
Sarnoff, S. J., and Mitchell, J. H.: The control of the function of the heart. In Hamilton, W. F., and Dow, P. (eds.): Handbooks of Physiology. Washington, D.C., American Physiological Society, 1962, p. 506.
Suah, P. M., Gramiak, R., Kramer, D. H., and Yu, P. N.: Determinants of atrial (S4) and ventricular (S3) gallop sounds in primary myocardial disease. New Eng. J. Med., 277:753, 1968.
Wildenthal, K., Mullins, C. B., Harris, M. D., and Mitchell, J. H.: Left ventricular end-diastolic distensibility after norepinephrine and propranolol. Amer. J. Physiol., 217:812, 1969.

Shock and Circulatory Collapse

Alfred P. Fishman

No single unifying concept or definition of shock will satisfy all concerned. On the other hand, each clinic that treats shock is inevitably forced to develop its own operational definition, tacit or expressed, simply as a practical basis for treatment. The present section describes the approach used in our clinic, in which one unambiguous type of shock, i.e., hemorrhagic shock, is taken as the standard, and other related syndromes are considered, implicitly or explicitly, as deviations from this norm.

Definition. The designation "shock" is reserved in our clinic for a state of circulatory insufficiency in which the clinical picture is dominated by manifestations of organ hypoperfusion and of heightened sympathetic activity; invariably the cardiac output is low and is associated with generalized peripheral vasoconstriction. Usually, this syndrome of vasoconstricted shock is initiated by an insufficient return of blood to the heart. Less often, other etiologic agents and mechanisms, such as those listed in the table, may produce the same picture. Even though each initiating mechanism imposes its own imprint on the syndrome, the common denominator is the decrease in the discharge of blood by the left ventricle into the systemic circulation, selective organ hypoperfusion, and reflex neurohumoral adjustments.

According to this definition, shock, like chronic heart failure, which was considered previously, is one type of circulatory failure. Indeed, included in the table are types of shock in which the heart is at fault as the initiating mechanism. However, in contrast to *chronic* heart failure, in which neurohumoral adjustments are gradual because the myocardium fails slowly, circulatory inadequacy in shock is acute in onset and fulminating in course, thereby eliciting a more rapid, intense, and, occasionally, different series of compensatory mechanisms.

Clinical Syndrome. Not only in shock after hemorrhage but also after the other causes listed in the table, the patient appears to have been drained of blood; he is exceedingly pale and the skin is cool and moist. He seems to have been smitten by a blow which has sapped him of strength and will. Early, he may be restless and agitated; later, he is likely to be apathetic and somewhat confused. His sensorium is blunted. Breathing is rapid and shallow. Although he complains of thirst, he cannot tolerate more than sips of water because of nausea. His urinary output is low. The pulse is rapid but thready. The arterial blood pressure, particularly the systolic, tends to be low and the pulse pressure narrow.

This stereotype is only characteristic of late

CAUSES OF SHOCK

Pathogenesis	Initiating Mechanism
1. *Decrease in Venous Return*	
A. Decrease in blood volume	Hemorrhage; trauma; burns
a. Loss of blood or plasma	Vomiting; diarrhea; intestinal obstruction; diabetic acidosis;
b. Depletion of extracellular fluid	Addisonian crisis; heat exhaustion
B. Decrease in effective blood volume	Gram-negative bacteremia; peritonitis
2. *Impaired Cardiac Filling*	
A. Obstruction to venous return	Pericardial tamponade; tension pneumothorax
B. Inadequate diastolic filling times	Severe tachycardias
3. *Impaired Cardiac Pumping*	
A. Myocardial injury	Myocardial infarction ("cardiogenic shock"); myocarditis
B. Acute valvular insufficiency or cardiac defects	Ruptured valve cusp or chorda; perforated ventricular septum
4. *Mechanical Obstruction*	Massive pulmonary embolus; severe valvular stenosis; ball-valve thrombus of mitral valve; atrial myxoma

shock. Indeed, early in the evolution of shock, some of these features are generally absent. For example, during bleeding, the arterial blood pressure may remain at normal levels a long while if the bleeding is slow and the patient is sheltered and undisturbed. Conversely, it may plummet to hypotensive levels if hemorrhage is brisk and profuse; or if the stage of hypovolemia persists or is protracted; or if additional insult, in the form of pain or forced activity, is imposed; or if environmental stress, such as undue heat, upsets the unstable vascular adjustments.

Because of the different initiating mechanisms, as well as the modifying influences described above, there is no single clinical hallmark of shock, such as arterial hypotension or tachycardia, except in the late stage. Instead, particularly with respect to treatment, shock is best regarded as a syndrome of organ hypoperfusion and heightened sympathetic activity, which is particularly apt to follow certain initiating mechanisms and which has a poor prognosis unless the initiating mechanisms are arrested and adequate therapeutic measures are promptly instituted.

Initiating Mechanisms. The etiologic bases for shock are conventionally sorted into groups, such as those shown in the table. The circulatory inadequacy may result from (1) an acute reduction in venous return to the heart as the blood volume decreases or as a portion of it is withheld in peripheral and splanchnic veins, (2) inadequate cardiac filling, (3) total inadequacy of the heart as a pump for the circulation, or (4) almost complete obstruction to the egress of blood from the heart. Although the etiologic bases are listed separately in the table, some may overlap. For example, some instances of cardiogenic shock are associated with hypovolemia.

Decrease in Venous Return. Hemorrhage, trauma to skeletal muscles, and burns produce shock by depleting the blood volume. In a healthy young man, at least 1 liter of blood must be withdrawn quickly in order to elicit manifestations of shock; prompt return of the blood relieves the signs

and symptoms. Trauma to skeletal muscles causes shock because of bleeding into the muscles. After hemorrhage or trauma, hemodilution results; after burns, there is hemoconcentration because of preferential loss of plasma. Despite these differences, the distinction between shock caused by loss of blood and of plasma is not critical since prompt restoration of the blood volume restores the circulation to normal in either case. After burns or extensive trauma to muscle, the effects of depleted blood volume are complicated by the products of local infection and dead tissue.

The blood volume may be depleted by ways other than direct loss from the blood stream. The same end-result may be produced by vomiting, diarrhea, intestinal obstruction, diabetic acidosis, and Addison's disease, all of which cause severe loss of water and electrolytes.

Endotoxin shock is a complication of bacteremia caused by gram-negative enteric organisms. In addition to the direct effects of the toxins, the lipopolysaccharide complex that is released from the bacteria seems to promote the release of a variety of humoral substances, including histamine and catecholamines. The complicated nature of this type of shock is illustrated by the demonstration at autopsy of some of the features of the generalized Shwartzman reaction, i.e., intravascular coagulation, deposition of fibrin in glomeruli, and bilateral renal cortical necrosis. Evidences of hypoperfusion of organs and tissues, such as lactic acidosis and oliguria, are generally striking, and the tendency to intravascular conglutination of formed elements is marked. This condition is discussed in the article on Coliform Bacterial Infections.

Impaired Cardiac Filling. Shock may develop in patients with pericardial tamponade from causes as varied as stab wounds of the heart, perforation of the heart by a cardiac catheter, or after myocardial infarction. The same effect may be produced by excessively rapid heart rates which sharply curtail diastolic filling or by an acute tension pneumothorax which impedes systemic venous return. Characteristically, the systemic venous pressure is high, and the normal respiratory fluctuations in arterial pressure are greatly exaggerated (pulsus paradoxus).

Impaired Cardiac Pumping. Acutely impaired cardiac pumping may produce a state of shock in a patient with massive infarction of the left ventricle (*"cardiogenic shock"*); the normal right ventricle pumps blood into the lungs in quantities which the left ventricle cannot handle. Characteristically, this type of shock – which coexists with acute left heart failure – is complicated by congestion and edema of the lungs; the edema is first interstitial but, as the patient survives and other compensatory mechanisms for enlarging the blood volume become operative, signs of alveolar edema (rales) appear. If this state persists, the sequence of pulmonary venous and capillary hypertension may lead to pulmonary arterial hypertension, right heart failure, and systemic venous hypertension.

Myocardial infarction may also be complicated by acute mitral insufficiency or a perforated ventricular septum. These may be catastrophic in onset with shock as part of the syndrome. Acute bacterial endocarditis, causing a perforation of the aortic valve or rupture of a chorda, can also produce a state of shock.

Mechanical Obstruction. Shock may be produced by a massive pulmonary embolus or by a ball-valve thrombus or an atrial myxoma which impedes flow through the mitral valve. A similar result may occur from obstruction of the peripheral pulmonary circulation by neoplastic tissue or by pulmonary emboli. The situation in multiple pulmonary emboli is complicated not only by reflex stimuli that arise from the occluded areas but also by the effects of cellular contents that are released from infarcted areas in the lung.

Pathogenic Sequence. Continuing efforts over the years to relate the diverse initiating mechanisms to a common pathogenic sequence have been singularly unsuccessful. Outstanding among the discarded theories is the concept that the usual forms of shock stem from paralysis of the systemic arterioles so that the peripheral circulation acts like a limp bag, withholding blood from the heart. It will be shown later that this is a mechanism for vasodilated hypotension rather than for conventional forms of shock.

Among the concepts currently in vogue, three are attracting particular attention: (1) reticuloendothelial failure to cope with the normal quantities of endotoxin which enter the blood stream from the intestine, (2) local liberation of histamine in the vicinity of precapillary sphincters causing capillary stagnation in certain vascular beds, and (3) disseminated intravascular coagulation.

General Physiologic Features. Accompanying the decrease in cardiac output is an increase in sympathetic nervous activity, manifested not only by tachycardia but also by generalized vasoconstriction, affecting arteries, arterioles, veins, and venules. This increase in vasomotor activity is not uniform, varying not only from organ to organ, but also within organs and even from segment to segment along the course of the vascular tree. One result of this nonuniformity is the curtailment of the blood supply to the skin and kidneys in favor of the blood supply to the brain, heart, and liver, a pattern reminiscent of that observed in diving mammals. At first, the selective vasoconstriction is manifested by the pale, cold skin and oliguria; later the cerebration is affected, and the function of the liver and heart becomes impaired. In such a vasoconstricted patient, even a slight fall in systolic blood pressure signals not only a decrease in cardiac output but also the generalized redistribution of blood flow under the influence of the sympathetic nervous system.

As the result of the diminished cardiac output and the sympathetic hyperactivity, blood flow through the minute vessels of the vasoconstricted organs becomes sluggish, and the formed elements of the blood tend to clump. In turn, the abnormal capillary circulation causes cells to become hypoxic and damaged, releasing lactic acid and enzymes, such as lactic dehydrogenase and glutamic oxaloacetic transaminase, into the blood. Unless shock is promptly ameliorated, the ischemic organs are candidates for irreparable injury.

The Heart. Depending on the initiating mechanism (table) and the duration and severity of the shock, the heart is involved to different degrees. Thus, in the most common types of shock, which are simply due to an acute decrease in venous return, the heart is rarely affected seriously, except if hypoperfusion is prolonged. At the other extreme is sudden injury to the heart as in myocardial infarction, or disruption of a valve in the course of an endocarditis, or a severe uncontrollable tachycardia, each of which may cause shock. Although exhaustion of the myocardium in a patient with severe refractory heart failure or mitral valvular disease may mimic most of the clinical features of shock, the collapse of the circulation in these chronic disorders is simply the consequence of progressive deterioration of the heart, culminating in an exceedingly low cardiac output and exhaustion of compensatory mechanisms, rather than of an *acute* circulatory derangement.

The Lungs. Early in shock, unless the airway or chest is abnormal, the lungs generally pose no clinical problem. At this time, alveolar ventilation is usually high, and even though there is some evidence of ventilation-perfusion imbalance, arterial hypoxemia and hypocapnia are slight and generally insignificant. Indeed, it is even doubtful that the abnormal gas exchange is an intrinsic feature of cardiogenic shock since dogs in experimental cardiogenic shock, which receive no opiates, sedatives, or high-oxygen–inspired mixtures and are not immobilized, do not show this abnormality in gas exchange.

As shock continues and grows worse, pulmonary performance deteriorates. Arterial hypoxemia then becomes more marked, principally because of continued blood flow through atelectatic or fluid-filled lung. This situation may be aggravated to an irreversible stage by narcotics and sedatives which depress alveolar ventilation, by inspissated bronchial secretions which block ventilation in perfused parts of the lungs, by oxygen toxicity which damages the alveolar-capillary membrane, and by overtransfusion which causes pulmonary edema. The final stage of pulmonary insufficiency is one of total disruption in external and alveolar-capillary gas exchange, producing the "shock lung."

The shock lung is characterized by a combination of pulmonary congestion, edema, atelectasis, hyaline membrane, hemorrhage, and thrombi; pneumonia is also often present. It is not clear whether shock lung is a distinct entity. Suspicion is currently rife that prolonged oxygen therapy, using very high concentrations of oxygen, may contribute to the development of this complication. Indeed, shock lung that occurs after prolonged systemic hypotension may prove to be an example of a nondescript reaction of the lungs to a wide variety of insults, including hypoperfusion and oxygen poisoning.

The Liver. Blood flow through the liver increases early in shock, but decreases later. Portal venous pressure increases throughout as hepatic vascular resistance increases, leading to the sequestration of blood in the splanchnic venous bed. As the blood flow through the liver decreases and is rearranged, the effectiveness of the liver in detoxification and in performing its metabolic activities decreases; organic acids accumulate in the blood in conjunction with hyperglycemia and hyperkalemia.

The Kidneys. Oliguria and anuria are common, particularly if systemic arterial hypotension is marked; pre-renal azotemia may be marked. As the circulation is restored and blood pressure increases, urinary output improves and the azotemia disappears. But if severe hypotension and renal vasoconstriction have persisted for hours, particularly in patients who have abnormal pigments from hemolysis or muscle trauma in the blood, irreversible injury to the kidneys may occur from tubular necrosis.

Hemodynamic Correlates. Because of the diverse causes, it is not surprising that there are few strict hemodynamic correlates for the clinical picture. Indeed, one outstanding feature of vasoconstricted shock is the excessive physical and mental incapacity for the degree of hemodynamic derangement.

Cardiac Output. A low cardiac output is a regular occurrence in shock. Somewhat puzzling is the fact that, for the same decrease in cardiac output, the patient in chronic left ventricular failure is almost invariably better off than is the patient in shock. Two reasons may account for this discrepancy: (1) the difference in onset and course of circulatory insufficiency; the longer duration of chronic heart failure must influence the extent and degree to which compensatory mechanisms, such as salt and water retention by the kidney and the engagement of the autonomic nervous system, are involved; and (2) differences in organ perfusion and congestion in the two conditions; for example, in left heart failure,

in which the pulmonary circulation is engorged, left atrial and pulmonary venous stretch receptors—which reflexly affect the behavior of remote organs such as the kidneys—must be differently stimulated than in those types of shock in which pulmonary blood volume is severely depleted.

Arterial Blood Pressure. It has been noted above that heavy reliance on an appreciable drop in systemic arterial blood pressure as a prerequisite for the diagnosis of early shock is ill advised. Thus, a decrease in systolic blood pressure to levels of 70 or 80 mm. Hg is more of a sign of advanced shock and of failing compensatory mechanisms than of early shock. Indeed, early in shock, when anxiety and pain may stimulate the release of large quantities of catecholamines into the circulation, arterial blood pressure may be high rather than low. But this hypertensive phase is fleeting and apt to be followed by a calamitous drop in blood pressure unless provision has been made to support the circulation if the blood pressure should begin to fall below normotensive levels.

When shock is severe and peripheral vasoconstriction is intense, the sphygmomanometer may give artificially low values in shock because of the low cardiac output and the narrow pulse pressure. Consequently, many clinics use arterial cannulation to follow the course of the blood pressure during shock. The cannula affords the additional advantage of providing blood samples for the determination of arterial oxygen tension and pH.

Peripheral Vascular Resistance. Calculations of peripheral vascular resistance, expressed as the ratio of drop in blood pressure across the systemic circulation to the cardiac output, are commonly made in patients with shock and are presumably used as a basis for treatment. In the types of shock described above, in which sympathetic nervous activity is high, the ratio is generally increased, but to different degrees, e.g., often more in endotoxin shock than in cardiogenic or hemorrhagic shock. But there is still no convincing proof that this calculation is any more informative with respect to treatment than is the clinical appearance of the patient, the warmth of his skin, the level of the blood pressure, the rate and fullness of his pulse, and his urine output. Moreover, because of the nonuniform effects of heightened sympathetic activity, such calculations often tend to obscure the complicated and heterogeneous involvement of the different systemic vascular beds in the different types of shock.

Irreversible Shock. This concept is a relic from experiments in animals involving volume replacement in hemorrhagic shock. It is currently still being used to indicate a state of shock that has become refractory despite all therapeutic efforts. The term has no clinical meaning and can only be applied retrospectively after the patient has died. By the time of death, not only the initiating mechanism but also disorders of the hypoperfused lungs, heart, liver, kidneys, gastrointestinal tract, adrenals, and even pancreas may be contributing to the fatal outcome.

OTHER HYPOTENSIVE STATES

Vasodilated Hypotension. Some refer to this syndrome as vasodilated "shock" because of unwarranted preoccupation with arterial hypotension as a manifestation of shock. But the clinical picture is entirely different in appearance and in prognosis from those states of circulatory insufficiency described heretofore, in which sympathetic venous activity and systemic vasomotor tone are regularly high and in which systemic arterial hypotension represents failure in sympathetic vasomotor adjustments. Vasodilated hypotension is a much rarer form of circulatory collapse which originates from intense peripheral vasodilatation. Because the resistance vessels of the arterial circulation dilate, the arterial blood pressure decreases; the cardiac output is normal or nearly normal; the renal blood flow and the urine volume remain within the normal range. There are no evidences of organ hypoperfusion: for example, the concentration of lactic acid in the blood is not increased; acidosis is not present. A clear example of this hypotensive syndrome follows paralysis of the peripheral vasomotor nerves, as by anesthetics or drugs, or severe abdominal trauma; related, but more complicated is the vasodilated shock that may complicate bacteremias with *gram-positive* organisms or serious infections, such as lobar pneumonia or malaria. Anaphylaxis also causes a state of vasodilated hypotension but, in this instance, arteriolar vasodilatation is complicated by leakage of vessels, hemoconcentration, and the release of neurohumoral substances, such as histamine.

Syncope. Syncope is a form of circulatory inadequacy in which consciousness is transiently lost because of a decrease in cerebral blood flow. Arterial hypotension is a regular feature. For comparable levels of arterial hypotension, syncope is distinguished from shock by its sudden onset, its brief duration, and its immediate response to the initiating mechanism. Syncope may originate in the heart, e.g., an episode of ventricular arrest or fibrillation; in the great vessels, e.g., aortic stenosis; or, most often, in collapse of the peripheral circulation. (See article on Syncope.) The most familiar example of syncope is the *common faint.*

The common *faint,* or *vasovagal syncope,* stems from a sudden and precipitous fall in peripheral resistance, probably involving both arterioles and veins, and unaccompanied by the increase in cardiac output that usually follows peripheral vasodilatation. The subject becomes pale, breaks out in a cold sweat, and complains of nausea. The arterial pressure falls precipitously, and the pulse usually slows. The cardiac output shows only a slight decrease or no decrease below the precollapse level. It is often seen in anxious subjects *after* they are convinced that they will come to no harm, in blood donors after only small quantities of blood have been let, or in subjects with indwelling arterial needles who develop a persistent gnawing dull pain at the puncture site as the local anesthetic wears off. If the subject is seated or upright, the combination of hypotension and bradycardia causes the cerebral blood flow to fall precipitously, leading to syncope. Vasovagal syncope usually clears promptly when the subject lies or falls down; rarely is atropine needed.

TREATMENT OF SHOCK

Critical elements in the successful treatment of shock are early recognition and prompt attention to the initiating mechanism. For example, anaphylactic shock requires the immediate administration of epinephrine intravenously; pericardial tamponade often has to be relieved without delay if the circulation is to be restored; overwhelming infections may require the intravenous administration of antimicrobial drugs, and often of corticosteroids, as soon as an intravenous cannula can be placed. On the other hand, a surgical procedure designed to remove the initiating mechanism, e.g., a perforated appendix, may have to be delayed until blood pressure is restored, even if it means going to the operating room with the intravenous infusion in place.

General Measures. Attention to certain simple measures helps to arrest shock and to restore the adequacy of the circulation. Among the general measures are (1) placing the patient in a supine position, with legs slightly elevated, to improve cerebral blood flow; (2) relief of pain and restlessness, using morphine (15 mg.) or meperidine (100 mg.) administered intravenously, as nausea and a slowed circulation preclude the use of the more conventional routes; (3) withholding food, even though sips of water are allowed for thirst, because of the danger of vomiting and aspiration; and (4) ensuring adequate respiration and gas exchange and administering oxygen, as simply as possible, e.g., by nasal catheter, if more than slight degrees of arterial hypoxemia exist.

Almost reflex on the part of the physician once the diagnosis of shock is made is the introduction of a venous cannula for the administration of fluids and medications. But if the general measures and the intravenous fluid do not effect immediate improvement, steps are taken in rapid succession for more intensive treatment. Blood is withdrawn for typing and cross-matching. A catheter is advanced into a large vein near the right atrium for monitoring central venous pressure, for administration of fluids, and for blood sampling. If the patient is oliguric or anuric, a urinary catheter is placed for reliable determinations of urine flow. A cannula may also be inserted into a peripheral artery not only for serial determinations of blood pressure but also to provide blood samples for Po_2 and pH.

Once these general measures—volume replacement and provisions for monitoring—have been instituted, a decision has to be reached concerning priorities: continued transfusions to replenish the decreased circulating blood volume; use of autonomic agents to change the calibers of systemic blood vessels; cardiotonic agents, such as digitalis, to improve cardiac performance.

Replenishment of the Circulating Blood Volume. In all types of shock associated with hypovolemia, intravenous administration of fluids is the first line of treatment. If blood has been lost, it should be replaced. While waiting for the appropriate cross-matching and typing, some other kind of fluid must be given. Crystalloid solutions, such as isotonic saline or glucose, have traditionally been used for this emergency, but their effects are fleeting because of the rapidity with which they leave the circulation. Preferable are substances which remain longer in the circulation. Most popular at present is a dextran of low viscosity and molecular weight (about 40,000) which not only is an excellent expander of the plasma volume but is also inexpensive and readily available. Except in states of hypofibrinogenemia and bleeding dyscrasias, it is remarkably free of side effects. It is usually administered intravenously as a 6 per cent solution, either in physiologic saline or glucose solution. Five hundred milliliters generally expands the blood volume by an average of approximately 1200 to 1800 ml.; the effect is over in a few hours because of its loss via the kidneys unless an additional slow infusion is administered. If oliguria persists during the infusion, there is danger of overexpansion of the plasma volume and of precipitating pulmonary edema. Colloidal solutions of albumin (25 grams in 100 ml. of 0.9 per cent saline) are as effective but much less available. Albumin is preferable to plasma because it does not entail the risk of hepatitis.

The desirable end-point in the administration of fluids is the reestablishment of an adequate circulating volume and a near-normal distribution of blood flow among organs and tissues without severely upsetting the electrolyte balance. If treatment is prolonged, different sequences and combinations of fluids are generally needed, depending on whether the problem is to maintain electrolyte balance, to provide energy, or to combat acidosis. Assuming the judicious selection of fluids, the key clinical guides for the administration of adequate amounts of fluid intravenously are clearing of the sensorium, improved circulation to the skin, restoration of the arterial blood pressure, slowing of the heart rate, and increase in urine flow. Unfortunately, consecutive determinations of blood volume have proved to have little practical value as guides to fluid replacement because of the changing nature of most kinds of shock and the inevitable delays that are involved between the times of sampling, the analysis, and the final reporting.

Arterial blood pressure continues to be an important index for fluid replacement when shock has progressed to the stage of hypotension. But as a single index, the arterial blood pressure has often proved to be unreliable not only because of the complicated baroregulatory mechanisms that sustain it, but also because overzealous attempts to restore arterial blood pressure to normal

levels by the administration of fluids have precipitated pulmonary edema. Recently, the central venous pressure has gained ascendancy as the simplest way to avoid overtransfusion.

The determination of *central venous pressure* involves the measurement of blood pressure in a large intrathoracic vein. Normally, this value is of the order of 2 to +5 cm. of water. Unfortunately, like the arterial blood pressure, the value may be difficult to interpret since central venous pressure is a function not only of blood volume but also of venous tone, of the competence and distensibility of the right ventricle, and of intrathoracic pressure. Often in shock central venous pressure is high because of the recent administration of vasopressor agents which increase venous tone. In practice, the central venous pressure is used as follows: Fluids are administered intravenously in an attempt to increase the arterial blood pressure and the urine output without driving the central venous pressure to abnormally high levels (to more than 10 to 15 cm. of water); should the central venous pressure start mounting excessively, particularly if it does so abruptly, the right ventricle is assumed to have failed. However, because the monitoring of central venous pressure provides no measure of left ventricular performance, pulmonary edema may occur as the left ventricle fails from overtransfusion even though the right ventricle continues to perform well and the central venous pressure remains normal. Indeed, when the competency of the left heart is in question, the pulmonary arterial diastolic pressure, as an approximate index of left ventricular end-diastolic pressure, is a more meaningful guide for the intravenous administration of fluids than is the central venous pressure.

Autonomic Agents. A wide variety of sympathomimetic amines are currently in vogue for the treatment of shock. Exerting their effects on α or β receptors, their actions are either excitatory, inhibitory, or a combination of the two. α-excitatory drugs, such as methoxamine (Vasoxyl) cause vasoconstriction; β-excitatory drugs, such as isoproterenol (Isuprel), relax vascular smooth muscle while exerting positive inotropic, chronotropic, and dromotropic effects on the myocardium. Norepinephrine (levarterenol) exerts both α and β effects and is particularly useful in producing vasoconstriction in conjunction with inotropic and chronotropic effects on the myocardium. Metaraminol can serve the same purpose if the stores of catecholamines in myocardium and vascular smooth muscle are not depleted; it has the advantage of avoiding serious injury and necrosis at the site of infusion should the agent inadvertently escape into the tissues.

Strong and divergent opinions are rampant concerning the proper place of autonomic agents in the treatment of shock. Some investigators do not use vasoconstrictors at all for the conventional forms of shock, relying entirely on transfusions and vasodilators; others use them gingerly, discontinuing them promptly if blood pressure and urine output do not increase in response to small doses. Another group can see no role for vasodilators except to relieve "harmful vasoconstriction" to which excessive use of vasoconstrictors has generally contributed. For these divergent views, few convincing conclusions can be reached because the patients and the protocols are not comparable. But they do serve as reminders that there still is no single treatment for shock and that indiscriminate use of these vasoactive substances may convert manageable to refractory shock.

Despite these divergent views and incomplete data, most clinics have adopted rules of thumb, such as the following, for the use of autonomic agents in treating the usual types of shock in which sympathetic activity is high: (1) Vasoconstrictive and inotropic agents, such as norepinephrine, are most likely to be effective if the blood volume is not substantially below normal. (2) Since increasing the level of arterial blood pressure by vasoconstrictors generally increases flow to the brain and heart at the expense of flow to other organs, such as the kidneys, the use of any one of these agents should be as brief and in as small a dose as possible. (3) Acidosis, a regular concomitant of severe shock, lessens the effectiveness of certain vasoconstrictive agents, tempting the physician to administer larger doses, thereby increasing the likelihood of undesirable side effects. (4) Once volume expansion has been carried to its tolerable limit and vasoconstriction is at a maximum, either spontaneously or because of vasoconstrictors, judicious use of vasodilators may help to undo "harmful vasoconstriction." (5) Prolonged and severe oliguria that has resisted both volume expansion and the administration of vasoconstrictors during shock may respond to renal vasodilators, such as furosemide, thereby helping to prevent serious renal injury. (6) Massive doses of adrenal cortical steroids, such as hydrocortisone, may be useful in states of bacteremic shock and merit trial in other instances of refractory shock; they have an unequivocal role in *preventing* shock in those patients on maintenance doses of steroids for systemic illness, e.g., rheumatoid arthritis, who are about to be subjected to the stress of anesthesia or surgery.

Oxygen Therapy. It has been noted above that patients in shock are candidates for a wide variety of pulmonary disorders, including atelectasis, pneumonia, and pulmonary edema; the prospects of these grave complications increase as shock persists. Early in shock, the abnormalities in pulmonary performance are generally mild and are manifested by low values for arterial oxygen tension which rarely require more serious attention than the administration of oxygen by nasal catheter. But if shock is severe and protracted, pulmonary performance becomes more disordered, culminating in pulmonary insufficiency which may persist even after the circulation is restored. At that time, some patients may even require assisted ventilation because of ineffective alveolar ventilation (mounting arterial Pco_2) and labored breathing. Unfortunately, the use of positive-pressure respirators to improve gas exchange entails the risk of aggravating shock because of impeding venous return. Assisted circulation in shock should be undertaken only by experts.

Cardiotonic Agents. Even though the normal myocardium may suffer somewhat in early shock from being hypoperfused, rarely is it sufficiently compromised to require the support of digitalis. More justifiable is the administration of digitalis in protracted shock if the heart has previously been damaged by disease or by aging. Even then, extraordinary care is required in digitalization because of the potentiating effects of acidosis, hypoxia, and electrolyte disturbances in severe shock on the production of ventricular arrhythmias and conduction disturbances by digitalis. Glucagon is currently being tested for its inotropic effects in such cases of severe and sustained shock.

Although inotropic effects are rarely the principal concern in treating early shock, some of the agents do improve contractility even though they are administered for other purposes. For example, catecholamines, such as levarterenol, combine an inotropic effect on the heart with peripheral arterial vasoconstriction. Dopamine also enhances myocardial contractility, but its major attraction at the moment is its role in producing renal vasodilatation. Isoproterenol has staunch advocates among those who attempt to elicit an inotropic effect on the heart while relieving "harmful vasoconstriction." Unfortunately, isoproterenol may not only fail to increase the blood pressure because of its opposing effects on heart and systemic circulation, but may complicate the situation further by its tendency to produce arrhythmias.

Intravascular Coagulation. Defects in coagulation are common in shock, but bleeding is uncommon. Despite the tendency to intravascular aggregation and clotting disorders, none of these seem to require anticoagulant therapy. Improvement in the circulation suffices to correct these deficiencies.

Concluding Comment. Because the mortality from severe shock remains high, new forms of treatment continue to be sought. Some recent attempts, such as hyperbaric oxygenation, have already been abandoned. Others, such as hypothermia plus antihistamines, are currently under investigation. Mechanical assistance is being tried as a last resort for some patients who are in cardiogenic shock. But both the old and the new therapeutic measures remain deeply rooted in empiricism, emphasizing the pressing need to sort out the various types of shock and to enlarge the number of reliable physiologic and biochemical bases for treating each type and stage individually.

TREATMENT OF VASODILATED HYPOTENSION

As in the treatment outlined above for shock in which vasoconstriction predominates, the treatment of hypotension from peripheral vasodilatation begins with attention to the arrest of initiating mechanisms and the removal of influences which tend to perpetuate or aggravate the hypotension. In general, despite the same sense of urgency in starting treatment, the intensity of the therapeutic effort is tempered by the awareness that prognosis is better in vasodilated hypotension because there is less threat of irreparable damage from organ hypoperfusion. Using central venous pressure as a guide, treatment of vasodilated hypotension, like that of hemorrhagic shock, begins with volume expansion, on the assumption that the *effective*, rather than the *actual*, circulating blood volume has been reduced by the vasodilatation. But should volume expansion fail to restore the circulation promptly, vasoconstrictors, such as levarterenol or metaraminol, seem more warranted than in conventional types of shock in which vasoconstriction may already be quite intense.

Hardaway, R. M., III: Clinical Management of Shock. Springfield, Ill., Charles C Thomas, 1968.

Jacobson, E. D.: A physiologic approach to shock. New Eng. J. Med., 278:834, 1968.

Lluch, S., Moguilevsky, H. C., Pietra, G., Shaffer, A. B., Hirsch, L. J., and Fishman, A. P.: A reproducible model of cardiogenic shock in the dog. Circulation, 39:205, 1969.

Loeb, H. S., Pietras, R. J., Tobin, J. R., Jr., and Gunnar, R. M.: Hypovolemia in shock due to acute myocardial infarction. Circulation, 40:653, 1969.

Mills, L. C., and Moyer, J. H. (eds.): Shock and Hypotension, New York, Grune and Stratton, Inc., 1967.

Weil, M. H.: Diagnosis and Treatment of Shock. Baltimore, Williams & Wilkins Company, 1967.

Congenital Heart Disease

Howard B. Burchell

INTRODUCTION

Definition. Persons born with a cardiac anomaly or defect are classed as having congenital heart disease. The range of significance of anomalies is tremendous, and varieties are practically infinite.

Incidence. In no other category of heart disease is the incidence so well known and predictable as that of congenital cardiac disease. Of infants born at or near term, nearly 1 per cent have a cardiac defect; but a more practical value is the 0.5 per cent obtained when one excludes stillborns and infants with multiple defects who do not survive the first month. Thus, in the United States among about 4,250,000 live births a year, there should be about 25,000 new cases of clinical congenital cardiac disease. Although careful screening in the nurseries will identify most cases among the newborn, many will be manifest only after some years. The stethoscope remains the main instrument in case finding, and roentgenographic surveys of the chest are a trailing second.

Pathogenesis. The causes of congenital cardiac anomalies may be classed as follows: genetic forces, fetal injury, and dynamic forces. It has been stated in the past that congenital heart disease is not inherited; for the pragmatist, this statement was satisfying and adequate, because the incidence of afflicted offspring of parents with congenital cardiac lesions appeared not to be statistically increased. However, a sibling of one child with congenital cardiac disease has more than twice the normal chance of having a heart defect. The aggregation of defects in family groups gives the strong clinical impression of a trend to stereotypy, and occasional examples of amazingly exact replicas of unusual cardiac defects in siblings are seen, supporting the view that there is a maintained identity of a genetic template. Although identical (monozygous) twins occasionally may demonstrate the same cardiac anomaly, the likelihood of heart disease in the twin of an afflicted child is but little increased. Concordance in defects in twins may be expected in approximately a quarter of instances. Although various syndromes characterized by chromosome aberration, for example, Down's syndrome, are prone to include congenital cardiac anomalies, isolated heart defects are usually associated with a normal chromosome pattern.

From the experimental production of cardiac defects in animals by various agents, which may be called teratogenic, and from the now accepted role of rubella in the first trimester of pregnancy, repeatedly evidenced by recent epidemics, as a cause of cardiac malformation, fetal injury as the main cause of congenital heart disease has had a proper vogue. The "rubella syndrome" is classically characterized by cataracts, deafness, pulmonary arterial stenosis, and a patent ductus arteriosus. Multiple disorders, including severe purpura, may be manifest and in the infant may shed virus for many months.

The contribution of the experimentalists is not to be deprecated, but whether fetal injury is the outstanding cause of congenital heart disease is yet to be established. The relationship of asplenia and multiple spleens, wherein specific but complex syndromes are recognized, to congenital cardiac defects is of unique interest. The recently developed efficacious rubella vaccine should be administered under the pediatrician's guidance, to young girls—never to the pregnant woman.

The tragic deformities of infants related to thalidomide intake by the mother during pregnancy re-emphasize the potential dangers of environmental factors in fetal development, the timing of the agent's presence being more important than the dose. The prominent deformity has been associated with the limbs (in its most severe form, a phocomelia), but cardiac defects also occur.

If one visualizes from memory the beating of the embryonic heart of the chick, perhaps one may better capture the concept of an inseparable relationship of function and form. Even as structure may determine hemodynamics, so may hemodynamics mold structure. Thus, the final malformation, as the anatomist views it, is the result of a dynamic, ever-changing and ever-compensating growth process that is also attempting to obey the background morphogenic energy that forces a pattern to the great vessels, the myocardium, and the whole organ.

Certainly one must have a multifactorial etiologic concept of congenital heart disease. In certain instances the possibility of chance alone determines vascular anomalies, as in the development of anomalous pulmonary veins with a vascular plexus many possibilities for the eventual arrangement of vessels exist.

The spontaneous closure of the ductus arteriosus in normal infants is a fascinating phenomenon, and the forces in operation still have mysterious aspects. Lack of closure in infants may be regarded as equally mysterious in most instances in which this defect is isolated. The closure and the failure of the ductus to close in the immediate postnatal period have been clearly demonstrated in lambs to be related to the local oxygen tension. That infants born at high altitudes have a higher incidence of patent ductus and that patent ductus has been a frequent sequel to fetal rubella are established facts.

In the pathogenesis of congenital defects one must also consider the inherited disorders wherein the heart may be initially or subsequently affected, as in Marfan's syndrome (dilatation of great vessels, aortic dissection, mitral incompetence), gargoylism, glycogen-storage disease, and Friedreich's ataxia (myocardial deterioration).

Classification. Since myriad forms of cardiac anomalies are encountered, any attempted complete classification inevitably becomes involved and unwieldy, particularly when used as a platform for clinical diagnoses. There are three approaches to classification, namely, that of the hemodynamic pattern, that of the structural abnormality, and that of the clinical picture; thus, in essence, there are the physiologic, anatomic, and clinical approaches. As one shapes an orderly categorization of defects, one blends these disciplinary approaches, with emphasis on the hemodynamic state.

In decades past, the simple classification of cyanotic or noncyanotic was accepted, and the physician may still properly so categorize his patients. However, he will encounter the problem of how to classify the patients with right-to-left shunts and mild hypoxemia who are not cyanosed. The clinician will also wish to categorize the status of pulmonary blood flow, deciding whether the lungs may be plethoric or oligemic, to which goal roentgenograms of the chest are of limited aid, particularly in infants.

For each anatomic defect that is chosen to be designated the primary one, there will generally be a subclassification dependent upon the associated defects; for example, tricuspid atresia is classified according to whether there is associated pulmonary stenosis or not and whether the great vessels are transposed or not.

Relative Incidence of Various Congenital Cardiac Defects. The frequency of one lesion relative to others plays a role in diagnosis, and in rough approximations the relative percentages of various defects in pediatric practice are ventricular septal defect 20 per cent, tetralogy 12 per cent, ductus arteriosus 12 per cent, atrial septal defect 10 per cent, pulmonary stenosis (isolated) 10 per cent, coarctation 6 per cent, transposition of great arteries 4 per cent, aortic stenosis 4 per cent, A-V cushion defects 3 per cent, tricuspid atresia 3 per cent, and miscellaneous 16 per cent.

A Suggested Classification

I. No intercommunication between right and left sides of heart
   A. Somatic asymmetry — dextrocardia, dextroposition, levocardia
   B. Obstruction to ventricular outflow
      1. Pulmonary stenosis ("pure," "isolated")
         a. Valvular
         b. Subvalvular, supravalvular, multiple branch stenoses
      2. Aortic stenosis
         a. Valvular
         b. Subvalvular
         c. Supravalvular
   C. No obstruction to ventricular outflow
      1. Valvular malformations
         a. Mitral incompetence
         b. Tricuspid disease — Ebstein's malformation
         c. Isolated pulmonary incompetence
      2. Coronary anomalies
      3. Myocardial
         a. Endocardial sclerosis
         b. Cardiomyopathies
II. Intercommunication between right and left sides of heart. Level of atria, ventricles, or great vessels
   A. With pulmonary stenosis
   B. Without pulmonary stenosis
   C. With pulmonary hypertension (obstructive vascular states)
III. Anomalies of great vessels
   A. Transposition
      1. Complete
      2. Physiologically "corrected," ventricular inversion
   B. Truncus
   C. Coarctation
      1. Preductal
      2. Postductal
IV. Anomalies of veins
   A. Pulmonary veins — partial, complete anomalous drainage with and without venous outflow obstruction
   B. Systemic veins, coronary sinus
V. Miscellaneous syndromes

Physiologic Studies, Adaptive Mechanisms, Clinical Effects. Often those infants with very serious congenital cardiac disease are retarded in growth and development. The most pitiable appearing infants, whose weight may not exceed a normal birth weight for months, are those who have practically no mechanism for the transfer of oxygen from the lungs to the body. Among these are many with transposition of the great vessels and the rarer forms of multiple and complex defects.

The degree of unsaturation of the arterial blood

compatible with life is astonishing; one occasionally sees children who are conscious and capable of some activity who have saturations of arterial blood at a level of (30) per cent. Such infants also are subject to severe metabolic acidosis. A gross erythrocytic response may require some months to develop and may not reach massive proportions for years.

The stimulus for hematopoiesis has not been identified but is assumed to be a hormonal factor that produces a generalized response of the marrow. In a situation in which there is differential cyanosis, the saturation of arterial blood to one area of bone marrow being normal and that to another area being quite low (ductus with reversed flow), the bone-marrow activity is equal in the two areas.

It has been hypothesized that an adaptive hypometabolic state is present in the severely hypoxemic child, but proof of such a hypothesis is hard to come by, for there is no good measure of the mass of metabolically active tissue in cachectic, underdeveloped children and of what the basal normal uptake of oxygen should be. Confusion regarding the metabolic rate is increased by some data purporting to show a hypermetabolic state.

Clinical cyanosis and hypoxemia are not synonymous; as a most elastic generality, cyanosis is not readily apparent until the saturation of arterial blood is less than (80) per cent. Coincidentally, this level of oxygen saturation with its attendant oxygen tension appears to be that below which the hematopoietic stimulus becomes increasingly evident, though one cannot determine any exact threshold values. The difficulties of clinically recognizing cyanosis and attributing it to a central venous admixture of a right-to-left shunt and resultant hypoxemia do not necessarily become easier with long-continued practice; indeed, one becomes more aware of the difficulty. For this reason a simple classification of congenital heart disease into cyanotic and noncyanotic has lost exact meaning. The student, from his knowledge of the basic sciences, will equate the absolute concentrations of reduced hemoglobin with the degree of cyanosis and will readily appreciate the role of polycythemia and of a relatively stagnant peripheral subcutaneous venous (venule) pool in abetting the cyanotic appearance.

On introduction to studies of cyanosis, one would be unlikely to appreciate the large amount of systemic venous blood that needs to be shunted into the arterial circuit, bypassing the lungs, to produce blueness; in patients who are obviously cyanotic, one finds right-to-left shunts of 40 to 80 per cent. The actual figure denoting percentage shunt is significant, but cardiac output in its widest sense gains significance. This concept may be illustrated by constructing a graph (Fig. 1) of isoshunt lines which show the large venous admixture that could be present without significant cyanosis if the systemic venous saturation were high. If the right-to-left shunt, in terms of percentage, and the oxygen uptake by the tissues remained constant and the cardiac output were increased, the arterial oxygen saturation would rise consequent to a rise of systemic venous saturation (narrowing of the arteriovenous difference); or, assuming constancy of the right-to-left shunt and little or no increase in cardiac output but increase of peripheral oxygen uptake, as in exercise, and increase of arteriovenous oxygen difference, the shunted systemic venous blood would be of darker hue, and cyanosis would deepen.

Patients who have congenital heart disease with cyanosis (hypoxemia) vary greatly in their ability to exercise, but as a group they do not have a normal increment in cardiac output (regardless of its distribution to the systemic and pulmonary circuits); thus, arteriovenous oxygen difference abnormally increases and cyanosis is deeper. Increased cyanosis with exercise in patients with

FIGURE 1. A graph of isoshunt lines illustrating that the same percentage shunt may be associated with a wide range of arterial oxygen saturations. At the same shunt value in percentage, an increase in venous oxygen saturation will cause a rise in the arterial oxygen saturation. With an increased cardiac output into both the aorta and the pulmonary artery, the arterial saturation rises concomitantly with the venous saturation.

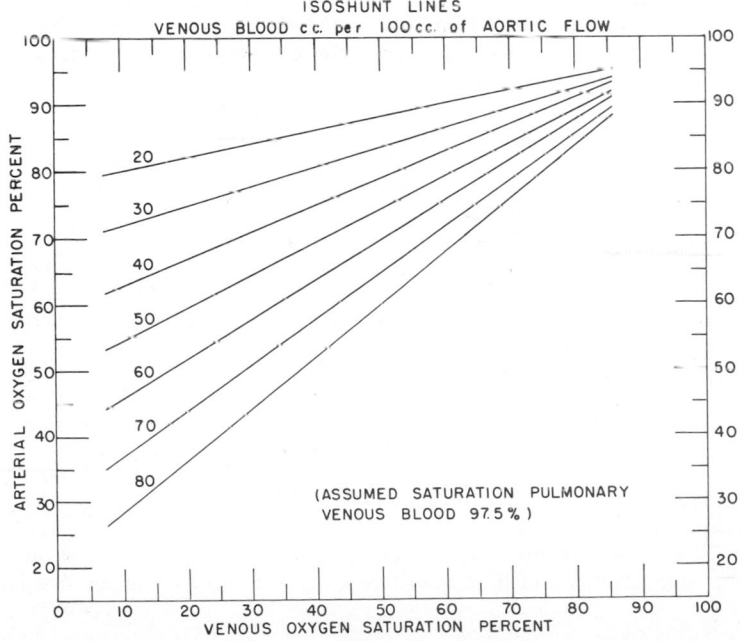

ISOSHUNT LINES
VENOUS BLOOD c.c. per 100 c.c. of AORTIC FLOW

(ASSUMED SATURATION PULMONARY VENOUS BLOOD 97.5%)

ARTERIAL OXYGEN SATURATION PERCENT

VENOUS OXYGEN SATURATION PERCENT

pulmonary stenosis is related not only to decrease in saturation of the systemic venous blood but also, frequently, to some increase in percentage shunt, which in some patients becomes critical when exercise leads to syncopal reactions.

In situations in which there is what might be called "common ejectile ventricular force," as in patients with a large ventricular septal defect or a single ventricle, the distribution of the ejected blood depends upon the relative resistances in the systemic and pulmonary circuits. If there is an organic fixed obstruction to pulmonary inflow (pulmonary valvular stenosis), pulmonary flow depends primarily on systemic resistance. If systemic resistance is lowered during exercise, there is an increased diversion of the stroke volume of the heart into the aorta. In a severe hypotensive episode, systemic recirculation dominates the picture, little blood reaching the lungs, and cyanosis becomes so deep that a child may be a bluish-black color. In systemic hypertension, the arterial oxygen saturation may rise because of the higher pressure gradient across the pulmonary stenotic orifice and the higher pulmonary flow. Systemic hypertension, however, is not encountered as a natural adaptive mechanism in pulmonary stenosis with ventricular septal defect. Undoubtedly, the moderate increase of blood pressure with age plays a role in the mild absolute increase of pulmonary blood flow in patients with tetralogy, and transient hypertension might contribute to the recovery from syncope. Even in severely cyanotic children with evidence of cerebrovascular insufficiency or evidence of renal dysfunction with gross albuminuria and erythrocyturia without azotemia, hypertension is rarely encountered.

Occasionally the muscular infundibulum of the right ventricle may play a dynamic role in reducing pulmonary flow—for instance, under sympatheticoamine stimulation, for example, with isoproterenol infusion and with the reversal of the effect by propranolol. Probably multiple factors may operate nefariously in decreasing pulmonary flow with exercise—a catecholamine effect on the infundibular myocardium, a drop in pH, and marked venous oxygen desaturation with resultant increase in the pulmonary vascular resistance, and a decrease in systemic resistance relative to the resistance into the pulmonary circuit.

Hypoxemia acts as a stimulus to cardiac output, without a specifically determined threshold, but it is operative at about 80 per cent arterial saturation; in an occasional patient there is an apparent response to this stimulus, and even if the apportionment of the blood to the lungs and the periphery remains constant, the increased cardiac output may be a factor holding the arterial saturation above critical levels. The shape of the O_2 dissociation curve will favor O_2 delivery when acidosis is present. The degree of the polycythemic response, particularly in adults, is frequently in excess of its usefulness, values of twice normal for hemoglobin and hematocrit readings between 70 and 80 per cent being *common*. The increased oxygen transport related to mild polycythemia is helpful, but polycythemia that gives hematocrit readings in excess of 70 per cent, with high blood viscosity, seems detrimental to the efficiency of the circulation.

Young children with cyanotic heart disease, specifically tetralogy of Fallot, characteristically squat. This phenomenon has long intrigued students of congenital heart disease. The child learns the maneuver himself. As normal youngsters may be seen to squat occasionally when tired, one can assume that the fatigued cyanotic child quickly acquires the habit. In such a position, the cyanotic child will have a rise in arterial (and systemic venous) saturation. It cannot be claimed that there is a clear understanding of the mechanism of acquired comfort the child experiences; multiple factors are probably operative.

Left-to-Right Shunts and Pulmonary Arterial Pressure. In a population of persons with left-to-right shunts of the same order of magnitude, pulmonary hypertension is most common in those with ventricular septal defect, uncommon in those with patent ductus, and least common in those with atrial septal defect. Likewise, the incidence of development of progressive pulmonary vascular obstruction is so distributed. That a high pulmonary flow per se cannot be the cause of an outstanding pulmonary vascular change is evidenced by the rarity of such change in atrial septal defect. In the large ventricular septal defect and patent ductus, however, the left ventricular pulse is propagated into the pulmonary vascular bed. It is not known what factors are responsible for the varied pulmonary vascular susceptibility to pathologic changes in patients with large ventricular septal defects.

The factors determining the direction and magnitude of the left-to-right shunt in patients with a ventricular septal defect or a patent ductus are the size and resistance to flow at the defect, the vigor of the ventricular contractions, and the ratio of the total resistances in the pulmonary and systemic circuits. In large atrial septal defect, there is no resistance to flow across the defect, and the pressures into the two atria are so nearly equal that usual methods of measurement do not reveal the gradient. If one accepts the filling pressures into the ventricles as equivalent, the respective distributions into them must be related to their compliance or distensibility. The compliance of the left ventricle being less, a larger flow will occur toward the more compliant right ventricle. (This is an acknowledged oversimplification of the hemodynamic determinants.)

When the right ventricle is hypertrophied or physiologically overdistended, its compliance decreases, its ready filling is impeded, and the shunt decreases. On the other side, with hypertrophy of the left ventricle, perhaps in association with a coincidental aortic stenosis, the left-to-right shunt increases. In practice, a left-sided lesion favoring a left-to-right transatrial flow is mitral stenosis, a combination of defects, known as _Lutembacher's syndrome,_ that is relatively rare.

Because diastolic pressures in the two ventricles in a patient with a large atrial septal defect tend to equalize, any rise in venous pressure will be present in both ventricles in late diastole. If venous pressure were used as a yardstick of myocardial failure, the conclusion would be reached that both ventricles had failed, perhaps the left being mainly at fault. The phenomenon of failure in a patient who has an atrial septal defect with a maintained large left-to-right shunt is complex, as exemplified by the fact that some patients have not only a large pulmonary flow but also a high normal systemic flow. The situation regarding distribution of blood volume is unique, for the blood cannot be selectively apportioned to the greater or the lesser circulation, and increases will distend the total system, excluding the state of each ventricle operating independently regarding the filling pressure.

A patient who has an atrial septal defect with a large left-to-right shunt may also have a small right-to-left leak, originating from inferior vena caval inflow. This may be exaggerated by such maneuvers as exercising and raising the legs or the Valsalva maneuver and may be evidenced in recordings by transient slight decreases in arterial oxygen saturation.

With exercise, patients who have a large left-to-right shunt increase their total cardiac output, with systemic flow usually increasing much more than pulmonary flow; thus the _percentage_ of the blood shunted decreases. In patients with high pulmonary vascular resistance the direction of the shunt may be reversed, and in a rare case the ratio of pulmonary to systemic resistance may be reversed. With the breathing of mixtures rich in oxygen, the left-to-right shunt characteristically increases; with breathing a subnormal oxygen mixture, the left-to-right shunt decreases. The extent of these changes is not predictable but is more prominent and more readily quantitated in the presence of moderately or severely elevated pulmonary pressures. With acetylcholine infusions many patients show some decrease in pulmonary vascular resistance, that is, increased flow at a slightly lower pressure, and an occasional patient shows a dramatic decrease.

Pulmonary Hypertension. The pathogenesis of progressive pulmonary hypertension in patients with congenital cardiac defects, particularly as it relates to the vasomotor activity of the pulmonary vasculature and the mechanisms of resistance and morphologic change, remains one of the great challenges in the field. It will be readily appreciated that in the case of a single ventricle with free egress of blood to the aorta and pulmonary artery, the systolic pressures in these two vessels will be equivalent. A similar state will be present with a large ventricular septal defect and with a free communication between the aorta and the pulmonary artery. In the former instance the

diameter of the defect must be in excess of 1 cm. for equivalent pressures to pertain; to correct for patient's age, the critical size appears to be 1 sq. cm. in area per square meter of body surface. Some reservation must be held in regard to the significance of any simple measurement in the dead or nonbeating heart, for there is good evidence that there may be a narrowing of some defects with systole.

When a common pressure source for the two great vessels is present, respective flows into them will be related to the respective resistances in the lungs and systemic circuit. As the vital factor driving the heart in regard to its output is related to the oxygen transport to peripheral tissues, the systemic (tissue) blood flow (Q_s) in the compensated state is normal, and the shunting of blood through a ventricular septal defect and creating a volume overloading of the left ventricle (and some volume and pressure overloading of the right ventricle), depends on the pulmonary resistance. In essence, the work load placed on the left ventricle in large left-to-right shunts with a ventricular septal defect or a patent ductus is roughly akin to that placed on the whole heart from the leak across a systemic arteriovenous fistula, wherein the effective systemic (tissue) flow is normal in the absence of heart failure, though the aortic flow (cardiac output) is grossly increased. In both instances an increase in blood volume is part of the adaptive process.

The critical aspects of the hemodynamic state in patients with huge ventricular septal defects (and the other dynamically similar defects) hinge thus on pulmonary vascular resistance. If this is inadequate, the left ventricle cannot maintain adequate systemic flow despite a tremendous output, and the concomitant flooding of the lungs may add to a lethal situation. On the other hand, if pulmonary resistance is or becomes high, pulmonary blood flow is choked off and, with pulmonary resistance greater than systemic resistance ($R_p > R_s$), the direction of the shunt reverses ($Q_p < Q_s$) or systemic flow exceeds pulmonary flow ($Q_s > Q_p$). While a large pulmonary flow contributes to pulmonary hypertension (hyperkinetic hypertension), in all cases in which pulmonary and aortic pressures approach equality the pulmonary arteriolar resistance is elevated. The status of the pulmonary vasculature frequently is the focus of any hemodynamic appraisal of patients with ventricular septal defect, and on its proper evaluation largely rest the predicted risks of surgical closure of a defect and the over-all benefit to be anticipated if the patient survives.

Considerable controversy pertains to the circulatory adjustments made in the neonatal phase and over the years by babies with large ventricular septal defects. More specifically, the main questions are: How large a defect in the ventricular septum may close spontaneously? Do all infants with ventricular septal defect have a period of lowered vascular resistance and large pulmonary flow, or do some have a maintained high resistance and never have plethoric lungs and an enlarged, overactive heart? Is there eventually a progressive relentless pulmonary vascular disease in all persons with an initially *very* large left-to-right shunt? To what degree can one discriminate between a normal morphologic adaptation and a true disease process in vessels?

The following generalizations will hold if one keeps the whole profile of the population with ventricular septal defect in view. A large number, possibly 30 per cent, of the ventricular septal defects present at birth spontaneously close. Although a drop in pulmonary vascular resistance is probable in all infants with large ventricular septal defects in the neonatal period, it will vary markedly in degree and duration, and clinically one will have a rough, early separation into two categories: those with quiet and those with overactive hearts (and absence or presence of pulmonary plethora). Over the years, many patients do not change their basic hemodynamic profile, but others develop pulmonary vascular obstruction and eventual reversal of their shunt. In infancy, maintenance of life may depend on the development of a mild to moderate increase in pulmonary vascular resistance. When obstructive pulmonary vascular changes are evident after a year of age, it cannot be expected that reversal to normal will occur.

In the categorization of patients, pulmonary pressure per se may have little discriminating value; it is necessary to know pressure and flow, and their nonlinear relationship is the conventional factor, resistance $(R = \dfrac{Pr}{Q})$, to which the main contributory element is vessel caliber. The resistance is, in part, fixed (organic), in part, dynamic (vasomotor). To generalize, there is a sizable dynamic aspect to the resistance in *some* cases of pulmonary hypertension related to a ventricular septal defect (or ductus), as evidenced by decreases, in such cases, in the calculated values on breathing mixtures high in oxygen content, on infusion of acetylcholine or tolazoline (Priscoline), and after operation with the defect repaired and pulmonary flow reduced. In occasional instances reduction of left atrial pressure may have had an important dynamic role in the postoperative reduction of total pulmonary resistance. The drop in pulmonary arterial pressure may be much greater than the decrement in left atrial pressure; the explanation for this may be in the abolishment of a veno-arterial constrictive mechanism in the lung, that is, a rise in venule pressure resulting in a localized constriction in the arteriole of the area. Such changes must be studied together with change in blood volume and changes in the basic ventricular work curves.

In patients with equivalent systolic pressures in the two ventricles, there often is lower minimal diastolic (and higher pulse) pressure in the pulmonary artery than in the aorta. The slope of the diastolic pressure is steeper, but this is more related to the compliance characteristics of the system than to the rate of (diastolic) flow. Rarely, pulmonary valvular incompetence may play a role in this finding.

Heart Failure in Infancy. The occurrence of heart failure in infancy has special connotations, particularly in regard to the possibility of curative surgical treatment. Specific defects have their characteristic time of appearance and the problem of neonatal heart failure deserves to be called a subspecialty by itself. Two general categories may be defined: that in which flow is obstructed, and that in which flow is excessive. As examples, in the former category are (1) patients with coarctation of the aorta, (2) patients with severe pulmonary stenosis with an intact ventricular septum, and (3) patients with obstructed anomalous pulmonary veins. In the second category, with plethoric lungs, is the patient with either a large ventricular septal defect or a patent ductus arteriosus. More complicated forms of cardiac defects may also give the picture of heart failure, with increased venous pressure and an enlarged heart and prominent liver.

Heart failure in the infant does not present the edematous picture seen in the adult. More characteristic are pallor, restlessness ("fretting"), inability to nurse, lack of ease in breathing, perspiration, and growth failure.

Diagnostic Techniques. *Clinical Examination. History.* The intelligent parent will give most useful information pertaining to diagnosis, in particular, information on maternal illnesses during the pregnancy, the rate of growth and development, feeding patterns, occurrence of respiratory infections, time that murmur was first detected, syncopal or cyanotic spells, squatting, time of appearance of increased cyanosis, breathing distress, and fatigability. Such a history is essential, although only rarely will it give a clue to the exact anatomic diagnosis.

The time of appearance of symptoms may give a clue to the diagnosis, for example, transposition of the great arteries with poor mixing between the two circulations, creating an emergency procedure within the first few days of life.

Physical Examination. Thoroughness in physical examination, with an orderly approach and attention to detail, will give high rewards in patients with congenital heart disease. Often, however, the exact diagnosis will depend on data obtained from cardiac catheterization and angiocardiography.

There are so many specific features to be recognized as present or absent that one might wish to have a "check list" akin to that used by a pilot in a modern aircraft before take-off and landing. The use of electronic computers as a diagnostic aid further emphasizes the necessity for collecting specific items and assigning each a certain value without emotional content; there would be no argument that this is how a cerebral computer should also work.

Each variety of cardiac defect in infancy must be emphasized as having possibly unique features, but the principles of examination are the same. In general, physical signs tend to have less diagnostic specificity in infants than in older children; this is particularly true of murmurs.

On inspection, the facies, general development, state of nutrition, presence, and distribution of cyanosis, deformities of the thorax, nature of the breathing effort, and character of the jugular pulse should all be quickly noted.

On palpation, the activity of the heart, the location and force of the apex beat, the presence of thrills, and the nature of the femoral pulse are tallied.

With auscultation, the cardiologist is traditionally at his best. In the majority of cases, the mass of evidence supporting his clinical diagnosis will be based on what he hears, and what he hears will be related to what he listens for. The loudness of a murmur may well dominate the auscultatory experience in the novice, but soon the trainee will be properly noting the duration of the murmur, its frequency and intensity profile, its position in the cardiac cycle, the effect of respiration, its intensity distribution on the chest wall, and its relation to other events such as a thrill. In addition, the quality and intensity of the first and second sounds, and particularly the degree of splitting of the second sound, will be noted (Fig. 2).

Roentgenograms. Roentgenographic examination of the chest may be properly regarded as part of the bedside diagnostic procedure. Although he ought not to express preference for such practice, the diagnostician might properly study the roentgenogram before examining a child. The first assessments from the roentgenogram are those of cardiac size and pulmonary flow; the extremes are readily recognized, but not always the mild changes. In infants particularly, estimation of pulmonary flow is fraught with difficulty. The examiner notes the relationship of the size of the proximal arteries to the size of the peripheral arteries and is sensitive to the possibility that pulmonary venous congestion might be misinterpreted as increased flow. The size of the main pulmonary artery, the presence of the aortic knob, and the size and shape of the silhouette are noted. In most cases of congenital heart disease, the clinician demurs in identifying enlargement of specific chambers; only occasionally may dogmatism be warranted. In some syndromes, as exemplified by coarctation, various forms of anomalous pulmonary venous drainage, isolated pulmonary valvular stenosis, and, occasionally, transposed great vessels, the roentgenographic appearance may be practically diagnostic.

Electrocardiographic Diagnosis. The approaches to electrocardiographic interpretation in patients with congenital heart disease differ

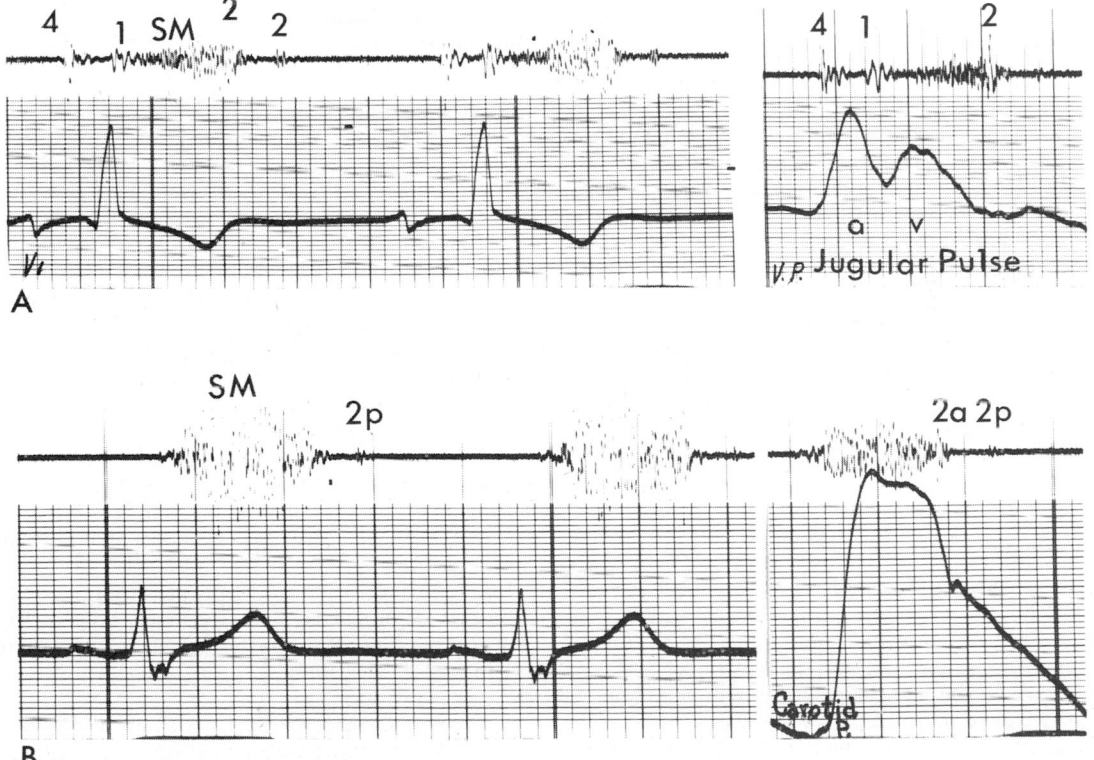

FIGURE 2. Types of murmur in pulmonary stenosis. *A,* Severe pulmonary stenosis (right ventricular systolic pressure, 150 mm. of mercury) showing a presystolic (atriogenic) murmur (atrial systolic pressure exceeded simultaneous pulmonary pressure), a giant A wave in the jugular pulse, a prolonged systolic murmur overlapping the aortic second sound, and a delayed, muted second pulmonary sound. The characteristic electrocardiogram of right ventricular hypertrophy ("pressure overloading") is present in the right precordial lead. *B,* Man, age 31 years. Moderate infundibular pulmonary stenosis (right ventricular pressures 85/3–25/3 and ventricular septal defect with small left-to-right shunt (15 per cent), demonstrating the holosystolic murmur and wide splitting of the second sound (the pulmonary component was not audible). The degree of splitting (0.12 second) would suggest the presence of infundibular stenosis per se if a ventricular septal defect were known to be present.

from those of routine practice in adults. In adults, one generally assumes that aberrations of the tracings result from disease processes in a heart likely to have had at one time a relatively normal structure. With congenital defects, one may be confronted with unusual positions of the heart within the thorax, complete absence of a functioning chamber, peculiarities of structure such as transposition or inversion of chambers of the heart, and distortions of the anatomic patterns of specialized conducting tissue, as well as changes resulting from selective hypertrophy and enlargement of parts of the heart.

Electrocardiographic interpretations are not necessarily more difficult in patients with congenital heart disease, but one must have a larger frame of reference. The normal evolution of the electrocardiogram of the healthy infant must be known. In congenital cardiac problems wherein all chambers are present, one may encounter the purest expressions of hemodynamic effects: what has been called "overloading patterns." Some specific congenital diagnoses suggested by the electrocardiogram are empirical rather than rational deductions. Exaggerations in voltage of P waves from right atrial excitation are particularly striking in some cases of tricuspid atresia and pulmonary stenosis. The P vector may sometimes be the main clue to the relationship of the atria in patients with isolated dextrocardia or levocardia. Magnitude of the QRS voltages and the spatial orientation of the mean QRS have important connotations, and the registration or calculation of the vectorcardiogram in the frontal, sagittal, and horizontal planes is now commonplace practice. Advantages are possessed by both scalar electrocardiography and vectorcardiography, but some lead with a time base is necessary for the evaluation of the PR and QT intervals. Although the precordial leads generally best reflect the anatomic position of the greatest myocardial mass and, hence, in the presence of two ventricles, the relative hypertrophy of these two chambers, the axis deviation as derived from the standard leads (mean QRS in the frontal plane) often gives important diagnostic information.

The diagnosis of right ventricular hypertrophy rests basically on right axis deviation and high-voltage R waves in the right precordial leads; that of left ventricular hypertrophy, on a trend to left axis deviation, either actual or relative for the age group, and high-voltage R waves in the left precordial leads. This oversimplified analysis requires amplification and refinement for accurate interpretations: for instance, the use of the ratio of R and S in the precordial leads and the time of the intrinsicoid deflections when it can be assessed. To illustrate, an rS complex from the precordial "2" position (S more than 2 mv.) and a prominent Q (more than 0.2 mv.) from the precordial "6" position with moderate R voltage may reflect left ventricular hypertrophy as clearly as tracings having high potentials from the left precordium.

The concept of "strain" or of "overloading" has added to the understanding of the relationships of physiologic events and the electrocardiogram, and the terms "systolic overloading" and "diastolic overloading" (or preferably, "pressure overloading" and "volume overloading") have had some popularity. The discriminatory diagnostic value of such patterns is established. Exceptions to the expected pattern, however, are not infrequent, and the terms are losing popularity.

In essence, volume overloading tends to cause increased QRS duration and prominent T vectors in the same direction as the QRS vectors, whereas pressure overloading tends to give a simpler high-voltage QRS with a discordant T vector in the opposite sextant. The so-called partial form of right bundle-branch block (an rSR in right precordial leads) is particularly characteristic of volume overloading of the right ventricle. In the presence of severe pulmonary stenosis and intact ventricular septum, a very simple pattern—a narrow QRS vectorial loop pointed to the right, upward and forward (an axis of about +220° in the frontal plane) and the T wave the reverse in space—is characteristic. Thus, one may have an S_1, S_2, S_3 in the standard leads, an R and a negative T in V_1, and an S and a positive T in V_6.

In interpreting tracings, the normal right ventricular hypertrophy of the newborn may be re-emphasized. A small but useful item is the direction of the T wave in right precordial leads, normally upright at birth and normally inverting in a few weeks. If it remains positive with a prominent R wave, one has a reliable clue to persistent right ventricular hypertension, probably equivalent to systemic pressure.

Some cardiac malformations characterized by helpful, sometimes practically diagnostic electrocardiograms are tricuspid atresia, Ebstein's malformation of the tricuspid valve, atrial and ventricular septal defects originating from defects of the embryonic atrioventricular valvular cushions ("ostium primum defect" of the atrial septum, "atrioventricular canal"), and in some cases "corrected transposition" of the great vessels and anomalous origin of the left coronary artery.

The electrocardiogram is usually normal in children with such conditions as coarctation of the aorta, small patent ductus, small ventricular septal defect, and mild to moderate aortic or pulmonary stenosis. Even severe aortic stenosis in children may be associated with a normal electrocardiogram.

Intracardiac electrocardiograms obtained at the time of catheterization of the heart help to indicate the position of the catheter and to give limited aid in the diagnosis of Ebstein's malformation of the tricuspid valve.

Cardiac Catheterization. Although the techniques of cardiac catheterization and angiocardiography will be discussed separately, they are inseparably wedded in the modern diagnostic laboratory. In their beginnings, cardiac catheterization gave basic and diagnostic data particularly in regard to pulmonary pressure and left-to-right shunts, and angiocardiography, in regard to right-sided malformations and right-to-left shunts.

With refinements in both techniques, particularly in indicator-dilution methods in cardiac catheterization and selective ejection sites in angiocardiography, they are increasingly mutually complementary.

The basic information that may be obtained from catheterization of the right side of the heart is gained from the fluoroscopic course of the catheter, the pressure recorded from it, and the saturation of the blood or the concentration of an indicator substance withdrawn through it. Some findings are then obvious, such as (1) the high right ventricular pressure of pulmonary stenosis or (2) a high saturation of the blood with oxygen ("arterialization"), as would occur at the atrial level in atrial septal defect, at the ventricular level in ventricular septal defect, and at pulmonary-artery level in patent ductus arteriosus, when such lesions are in their common form with increased pulmonary flow. If there is a right-to-left shunt at any level and an indicator is introduced at the level of the shunt in the right side of the heart or at any place proximal (upstream) to it, part of the indicator will pass directly to the aorta and may be recorded from an artery by a proper sensing device. As an example, in patent ductus with reversed shunt, injection of dye into the pulmonary artery or sites upstream from it will result in early appearance of dye in the femoral artery, but little or none in the right radial artery, for the shunt is distal to the origin of the innominate. In the presence of left-to-right shunting, an indicator injected into the right side of the heart recirculates in part in the pulmonary vessels, so that the dilution curve is characterized by a diminished maximal concentration and a prolonged disappearance slope. Although such records are diagnostic for large left-to-right shunts, the method is relatively insensitive, not detecting shunts of less than 20 per cent with certainty, and it has no localizing value.

The number of variations of the method, including various types of indicator, is legion. The same principles pertain to the modifications (Fig. 3). It is apparent that, if an indicator is injected into the pulmonary circuit and is sampled from the right side of the heart at the site of a left-to-right shunt (or downstream from it), the shunt would be detected from the early appearance of the indicator. This scheme is the basis of the demonstration of left-to-right shunts by sampling from the right side of the heart. If a person takes a breath of a foreign gas, such as methyl iodide tagged with radioiodine or Freon,* the blood returned from the lungs is labeled, and if a catheter is sampling in the right side of the heart, a left-to-right shunt may be identified by early appearance of the indicator. A high degree of accuracy in the quantitation and localization of a left-to-right shunt may be obtained also by a double-catheter technique in which the distal catheter is used for injection of indicator, the proximal one for sampling.

The success of the double-catheter technique utilizing a dye material depended on the discovery of a dye that could be sensed independently of the relative amounts of oxyhemoglobin and reduced hemoglobin. A green dye (indocyanine green) has attained considerable popularity as an indicator. As an example, if the dye is injected into a distal pulmonary artery in the presence of a left-to-right shunt at the level of the great vessels, early-appearing dye will be recorded from the second catheter when it is in the main pulmonary artery, but not when it is in the right ventricle or the right atrium. If the left-to-right shunt is at the ventricular level, early-appearing dye will be present in the right ventricle (and pulmonary artery) but not at the atrial level. Proper allowances in interpretation must be made for the possibility of incompetent valves, but this can be defined in addition by the injection of indicator at a site that normally is immediately "downstream" to the valve and sampling immediately "upstream" to it.

Indicator-dilution techniques have other uses in diagnostic catheterization procedures. Examples are (1) the identification of the great vessel in which the catheter tip lies, (2) determination of the flow patterns from various areas, as in anomalous venous connections, or (3) the proving of two outlets from the right ventricle. Such techniques allow great versatility in cardiac catheterization procedures. Recording apparatus that displays the data without significant delay is required.

In some catheterization procedures, only a few specific measurements are needed to make the clinical diagnosis complete. In other cases in which the diagnosis is much in doubt, there should be an orderly progression in the catheterization procedure, the direction of each step being determined by the cumulative information that has been obtained prior to the newly projected step. With multiple sampling sites, experience, and good planning, a precise differential diagnosis may be made: for example, the differentiation of (1) a patent ductus and an aorticopulmonary "window" or (2) anomalous pulmonary veins and atrial septal defect and their combination.

Ordinarily one expects the catheter to enter all available chambers from the right atrium, and hence a defect may be directly demonstrated. When it is not possible to enter the pulmonary artery, an abnormal position of its origin is suggested, that is, transposition. The catheter may enter many unusual places as well as the usual, and the operator will be rewarded by his knowledge of possible anomalies, such as a persistent left superior vena cava, an azygos system replacing the inferior vena cava, the internal mammary vein, and anomalously connecting pulmonary veins.

The recording of sounds and murmurs from within the cardiac chambers and great vessels by a sensitive transducer at the end of a catheter sound (a phonocatheter) has elucidated the site of production of murmurs and has demonstrated diagnostic potentialities. The complexities of

---

*Freon is the trade name of DuPont fluorinated hydrocarbons.

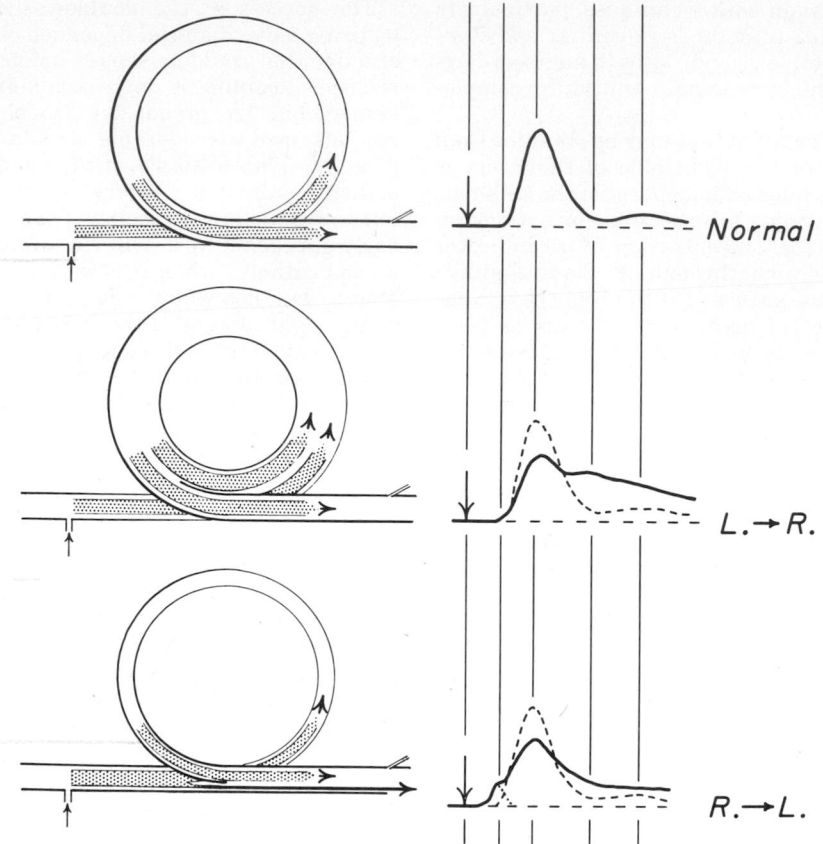

FIGURE 3. Diagrams to illustrate the circulation and indicator-dilution curves in the normal, in left-to-right shunting, and in right-to-left shunting. In the normal, the dye travels through the loop (representing the lungs) and has dispersion related to minor differences in length of the pathway and in mixing; at the sampling site, there is a normal rise and fall in concentration of the indicator, followed by a small recirculation peak. In the left-to-right shunt, the indicator recirculates in the lungs, a smaller quantity reaching the periphery initially and giving a smaller major deflection, and the disappearance slope is prolonged, being related to a maintained release of indicator from the pulmonary circuit and also obscuring the secondary systemic recirculation peak. In the right-to-left shunt the defect allows, and pressure relationships cause, some of the indicator to bypass the lungs and appear early at the systemic sampling site. The second concentration peak represents the indicator passing through the normal route and arriving at the normal time. From the relative areas of the reconstructed two curves or their initial portions, the right-to-left shunt may be quantitated; the amount represented in this illustration is small.

In the left-to-right shunt, it may be visualized that if an indicator is placed in the pulmonary circuit, either by inhalation or by means of a catheter in the pulmonary artery, proximal sampling will sense the indicator prematurely if, because of a defect, some of the material is allowed to enter the right side of the heart instead of all of it passing through the normal circuit of the left side of the heart to the aorta.

In young children with rapid transit times and a large right-to-left shunt, the peripheral dye curve from a central injection might mimic in contour that of a left-to-right shunt. In the former case, the appearance time is short, and the slow decline of the slope is related to multiple time courses of the blood entering the lungs—for example, from the bronchial arteries.

A fourth diagram might illustrate complete separation of the two circuits as in transposition of the great vessels, wherein, however, a minimal calculable amount of blood needs to reach the lungs and an equivalent amount needs to return to the systemic circuit to maintain volume balance, oxygenation of the tissues, and life. An indicator injected into the pulmonary circuit is delayed in reaching a sampling site in the systemic artery, and the resulting concentration is of low magnitude and very prolonged in duration.

recording have apparently gainsaid any widespread application to routine diagnostic work.

Angiocardiography. Angiocardiographic methods have long been of established value in diagnosis of congenital cardiac defects, and refinements have allowed diagnosis of minute anatomic details. Angiocardiography is indispensable for assessment of defects in young infants, as exemplified by various forms of single ventricle, pulmonary atresia, and transposed great vessels. Venous angiocardiography, the injection of contrast media by a needle in a peripheral vein, has been replaced by selective angiocardiography, that is, the injection of media by catheter placed in the desired cardiac chamber.

Selective angiocardiography contributes most when supervised by an expert, when the catheter is placed properly, when an adequate amount of material is injected rapidly, and when a rapid sequence of roentgenograms is made in two planes. The need for proper roentgenologic techniques of exposure and development of films is self-evident. These requirements and the ultimate interpretation of the shadows establish cardiac roentgenology as a true subspecialty in roentgenology.

Cineangiography, the rapid photographing of the passage of dye through the heart or parts thereof and subsequent cinematic projection of the photographs, has been possible through the utilization of image-amplifier screens. Review of such films gives one an understanding of the hemodynamics and patterns of blood flow not otherwise available. In general, large angiocardiographic roentgenograms display anatomic details that cannot be appreciated from most cineprojections or enlargements. Occasionally one can clearly see in cineangiographic projections small shunts not revealed by the more widely spaced angiocardiographic exposures. However, such revelations may not be as important diagnostically as demonstration of fine details of structure—for example, whether a ventricular chamber has the internal form of a right or a left ventricle. Theoretically, the methods should have nearly equal value, and the rewards that accrue from either are in large part related to the skill and experience of the user.

The application of special techniques is not justified on the sole grounds of obtaining a diagnosis, but rather it must depend upon the objective of determining definitive therapy. However, because of advances in surgical methods, most young people with congenital cardiac disease are candidates for operation, and early exact diagnoses are mandatory.

Initial enthusiasm for angiocardiographic methods in patients with large right-to-left shunts was tempered by the occurrence of occasional deaths, apparently due to the entrance of a large bolus of medium into the cerebral or coronary circulation or both. With greater experience such complications have virtually disappeared, but the laboratory personnel must be attuned to, and capable of, handling cardiac arrest. Perforation of the heart by a catheter, in infants particularly, is a recognized hazard.

NONCYANOTIC DEFECTS

DEXTROCARDIA

Dextrocardia has been classified as true or false. True dextrocardia indicates that there is a derangement of the cardiac chambers, false dextrocardia that there is a displacement of the heart to the right. *Dextroposition* of the heart is preferred to "false dextrocardia"; the condition is seen in malformations of the thorax and lungs. True dextrocardia may occur as part of the picture of complete situs inversus, which has an incidence of approximately 0.01 per cent in the general population, and in which structurally and functionally the heart is frequently normal, or as isolated dextrocardia, in which complex intracardiac defects are to be expected. The incidence of significant congenital cardiac defects in persons born with situs inversus is not established, but a reasonable approximation is 10 per cent. One form of isolated dextrocardia associated with a functionally normal heart is properly called *dextrotorsion*, as there is a simple dextrorotation of the heart, the left ventricle becoming anterior. One condition stereotyped sufficiently to earn the appellation of a syndrome is that of an anomalous right pulmonary vein connecting to the inferior vena cava, partial agenesis of the right lung and displacement of the heart into the right side of the chest. This is sometimes referred to as the "scimitar syndrome," the coiners of the term likening the shadow of the vein to the curve of a scimitar.

In simple dextrocardia with a mirror rearrangement of the chambers, the electrocardiogram is diagnostic, with lead I "upside down," although the electrocardiographer may be able to say only, "Either dextrocardia or a technical mistake of reversing the right and left arm leads in the normal subject."

The normal position of the organs is designated by the term "solitus," the mirror position, by "inverted." When partial inversion of the organs is present, there is the helpful clinical rule that the liver, right (venous) atrium, and inferior vena cava will be on one side, and the stomach, thoracic aorta, and left atrium will be on the other. With multiple spleens there is an unusual development with the organs on both sides resembling the normal left-sided ones.

In complicated cases, including isolated levocardia with otherwise situs inversus as well as isolated dextrocardia, angiocardiographic studies give the best answers as to the abnormality present, those studies being done in conjunction with cardiac catheterization. Catheterization alone may reveal the general hemodynamic derangement, but from catheterization data the prediction of the anatomic derangement is fraught with difficulty or is impossible.

MALFORMATIONS OF THE AORTA

Coarctation of the aorta and various anomalies of the aortic arches are discussed elsewhere. The varied symptom complexes, particularly in infants, in whom treatment may be urgently needed, require continued emphasis. Coarctation may be associated with a patent ductus, which causes a different clinical picture related to its position, that is, proximal or distal to the stricture. The terms "preductal" and "postductal" are in common use, and in the latter it is evident that a right-to-left shunt will continue after birth. The subclavian vessels may arise below the coarctation, leading to reverse flow in the vertebrals. Coarctation may be associated with various types of "vascular ring" and cause symptoms suggesting heart disease by tracheal or bronchial obstruction.

ANOMALOUS CORONARY CIRCULATION

The architecture of the coronary arteries in the normal person varies but little from the basic pattern of two arteries, the left having an early bifurcation into the anterior descending and circumflex branches. A single coronary artery is rare, and is not directly associated with symptoms. When the great vessels are transposed and the ventricles are inverted (corrected transposition), there is also inversion of the coronary architecture, the vessels arising from the posterior aspect of the aorta and the right coronary having the pattern of the usual left coronary.

The anomaly of main importance to the clinician is that in which a coronary artery arises from the pulmonary artery, and any clinical trouble relates, as a rule, to an anomalous *left* coronary. A variety of syndromes result from this. In the infant the combination of episodic distress interpreted as angina, cardiac enlargement, and electrocardiographic evidence of anterior myocardial ischemia or infarction is characteristic, but such a complete or classic syndrome is rare. More often there is the appearance of heart failure with left ventricular enlargement simulating the course of a myocardiopathy or endocardial sclerosis. In a very rare patient with cardiac enlargement, mitral incompetence dominates the clinical picture.

The untoward functional consequences of the origin of a coronary artery from the pulmonary artery are related not to desaturation of the venous blood in the anomalous vessel but rather to the inadequate perfusing pressure. Evidence is now adequate to support an earlier hypothesis that in many cases there is actual retrograde flow in the anomalous vessel and that hemodynamically a coronary arteriovenous fistula is simulated.

The diagnosis may be suspected, but it is often difficult to prove, and both aortography and pulmonary angiography may be indicated if the diagnosis is necessary as a prerequisite to surgical treatment. Although simple ligation of the anomalous vessel at its origin has a rational basis, it is expected that surgical transplantation of the anomalous orifice to the aorta will be practiced with greater frequency.

CORONARY ARTERIOVENOUS FISTULA

Coronary arteriovenous fistula, involving as a rule the right coronary artery and coronary sinus, may be suspected from the presence of a continuous bruit. It may be demonstrated best by aortography. Hemodynamically related malformations with a similar clinical picture are those with a communication between a coronary artery and the right ventricular chamber (aortocameral fistula) or with a vessel draining into the atrium or a pulmonary artery.

ANOMALIES OF THE CORONARY SINUS

There are no clinical syndromes associated with anomalies of venous drainage of the heart. The coronary sinus may be the site of connection with anomalous pulmonary veins. There is, however,

the rare, interesting situation in which the orifice of the coronary sinus is sealed and there is either drainage into the left atrium by way of an "unroofed" portion of the coronary sinus or, very rarely, drainage by retrograde flow into a small persistent left superior vena cava. It will be appreciated that when a large left superior vena cava is present the coronary sinus is huge. In cases of persistent left superior cava the P-wave vectors may be oriented superiorly and anteriorly in a biphasic display, and this has led to the conjecture that the pacemaker may be in the left atrium near the opening of the coronary sinus.

PURE PULMONARY STENOSIS

Pulmonary stenosis with an intact ventricular septum is an essentially noncyanotic condition. In its severe forms associated with some increase of right atrial pressure, if there is an interatrial communication such as a foramen ovale, there is a right-to-left shunt at the atrial level. Pulmonary stenosis is an important cause of heart failure in the first weeks of life or may give rise to difficulty only in late adult life. The valvular deformity varies; sometimes there is a dome-shaped structure, the movements of which have been beautifully demonstrated by angiocardiographic studies. The aperture of these valves is usually central and varies in size; in many cases there is associated subvalvular stenosis. The relative incidence of the valvular and infundibular forms of stenosis and the extent to which the infundibular form may be hypertrophic, consequent to the valvular obstruction, are still points of argument. Pure infundibular stenosis with a normal valve is uncommon; however, in patients with it, the pressure tracings recorded during the withdrawal of a catheter from the pulmonary artery to the right ventricle are diagnostic, showing a low-pressure infundibular zone.

Diagnosis. Mild forms of pulmonary stenosis may readily be overlooked clinically (for example, pressure gradients of 20 to 30 mm. of mercury across the valve), because the only finding may be a systolic murmur. When pulmonary stenosis is severe, the striking findings allow one to predict the anatomy with considerable accuracy. The more severe the stenosis, the more prominent is the A wave in the jugular pulse, the louder and longer is the murmur, the greater is the split of the second sound (pulmonary valve closure, however, may be muted), the more evident usually is the post-stenotic dilatation of the pulmonary artery, and the more clearly portrayed in the electrocardiogram is the right ventricular hypertrophy. Cardiac catheterization readily confirms the diagnosis, though the risk of this procedure may be slightly increased for patients with severe stenosis and with transatrial shunt. Presumably, this risk is related to a syncopal reaction in which the blood may circulate practically entirely in the systemic system alone until hypoxic death occurs. The severity of the obstruction may occasionally be

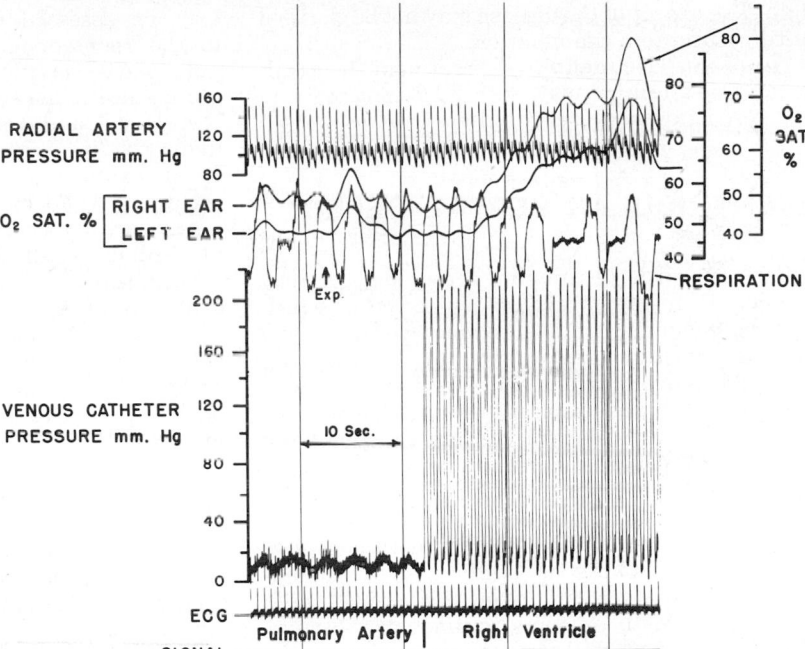

FIGURE 4. Reproduction of a portion of a record taken during catheterization of a 22-year-old man with severe pulmonary stenosis and patent foramen ovale. The very high right ventricular pressure (210 mm. of mercury) and the low saturation of the arterial blood (ear oximeter readings) when the catheter was through the pulmonary valve are to be noted. When the catheter was pulled from the pulmonary artery to the right ventricle, a dramatic rise in arterial saturation followed within a few seconds.

demonstrated by significant blockage of the pulmonary orifice by the cardiac catheter, and an increased venous-arterial shunt may be recorded (Fig. 4). In the presence of valvular stenosis, one may or may not be able to show an associated infundibular narrowing by records of pressure across the area. However, one can diagnose with assurance infundibular stenosis and absence of valvular narrowing if such is the condition present. Right ventricular angiocardiography portrays the anatomic condition with remarkable exactitude, including the syndrome of hypertrophied, anomalous-appearing muscle bands in the outflow tract. In infants angiocardiography is mandatory for diagnosis.

Treatment. The treatment of severe pulmonary stenosis is surgical. In moderate stenosis a gradient of 70 mm. of mercury across the pulmonary outflow area has been the usual criterion for operation, such a figure being modified according to the patient's age, his cardiac output, the circulatory response to exercise, the size of the pulmonary artery, and the electrocardiographic evidence of hypertrophy of the right ventricle. The surgeon should have an operative plan that incorporates a method to relieve infundibular as well as valvular stenosis, unless the former has been excluded by good angiocardiographic studies.

AORTIC STENOSIS

The varieties of aortic stenosis are discussed in another chapter. As in coarctation, the obstruction to left ventricular outflow may be critical in infants, and prompt evaluation of the site and nature of the obstruction may be urgent. Each variety of stenosis has unique multidisciplinary interest, for example, the relationship in some cases of supravalvular aortic stenosis to hypercalcemia, mental deficiency, and characteristic facies (widely spaced eyes and thick lips) as outstanding features. Aortic stenosis in children presents often a trying therapeutic problem, as frequently the valvular deformity does not lend itself to successful surgical repair.

ENDOCARDIAL SCLEROSIS
(Fibroelastosis)

Endocardial sclerosis may be either apparently primary or secondary to long-standing ventricular enlargement. The former may present in the form of either a small ventricle or a large ventricle, usually the latter, and rarely there may be a varying degree of associated involvement of the aortic or mitral valve. Its cause is unknown, although antibody studies had implicated the mumps virus as a possibility. Its importance lies in its responsibility for prolonged intractable cardiac disability. Death occurs from heart failure, sometimes in infancy but oftener in late childhood.

Diagnosis. The diagnosis is suspected from cardiac enlargement and the suggestion of left ventricular hypertrophy (often with ST depressions of the ischemic type) in the electrocardiograms; frequently there is no murmur. The differential diagnosis should consider chronic pericardial effusion, primary cardiomyopathy, and anomalous origin of a coronary artery from the pulmonary artery. Although the clinical picture is often adequate for the tentative diagnosis, cardiac catheterization and angiocardiographic studies are often justified to obtain supportive data. The extent of the disease may not be clarified until postmortem examination.

Treatment. No definitive treatment is available. Heart failure may respond temporarily to salt restriction and use of digitalis.

VENTRICULAR SEPTAL DEFECT

Patients with ventricular septal defects may present a variety of syndromes, three of which may be exemplary: (1) no symptoms but a loud systolic murmur (*bruit de Roger*) as the only sign; (2) an overactive heart, a loud systolic murmur and often a soft apical diastolic (mitral-flow) murmur, biventricular enlargement, and plethoric lungs; and (3) a quiet heart, perhaps no murmur, a very loud pulmonary component of the second sound, evidence of right ventricular hypertrophy in the electrocardiogram, and the roentgenologic picture of a choking off of the peripheral pulmonary vasculature. All gradations between these types exist. With advanced pulmonary vascular obstruction, cyanosis becomes obvious in the picture called "Eisenmenger's syndrome," a term that is properly losing favor because of lack of specific criteria for its use. The evidence has accumulated to indicate that many defects of the ventricular septum may close spontaneously during infancy. Another postnatal development in the heart with a ventricular septal defect is that of infundibular hypertrophy with right ventricular outflow obstruction, a left-to-right shunt being replaced by a right-to-left shunt.

The physician should remember that a ventricular septal defect may communicate with the right atrium and may be complicated by moderate pulmonary stenosis (but still a left-to-right shunt), by the association of inverted ventricles and transposed great vessels, by an atrial septal defect, by a patent ductus, or by the origin of both great vessels from the right ventricle. He should also be aware of the possibility of associated rare acquired defects such as aortic incompetence and mitral incompetence. The syndrome of aortic incompetence with a ventricular septal defect is well recognized, and it is usually the aortic regurgitation that dominates the clinical picture.

Diagnosis. The diagnosis of the usual forms of ventricular septal defect may be made with considerable accuracy by clinical findings, allowing disposition, including surgical scheduling, to be made without special complicated procedures. The characteristic murmur is holosystolic, reaching its greatest intensity in early systole; it is located in the midsternal area and may be heard well toward the base. When the murmur is heard well at the apex, the suggestion may be ventured that the defect is in the apical muscular portion of the septum or, if it is prominent to the right of the sternum, that the defect communicates with the right atrium, but such predictions are not reliable. In problem cases associated with severe pulmonary hypertension, the hemodynamic state

may be assessed with confidence by attention to the roentgenogram of the chest and to the pulmonary vascular pattern, the electrocardiogram since it may reflect right or left ventricular "overload," and the arterial oxygen saturation under conditions of rest and exercise as measured by an oximeter on the ear. With a premium on accuracy, when risk and success of intracardiac repair are of concern, intensive investigations by cardiac catheterization are deemed advisable.

Treatment. The therapy for ventricular septal defect associated with a significant left-to-right shunt, for example, 40 per cent or more of left ventricular output, is surgical. At present, surgical treatment for small defects, with small shunts and normal pressure in the pulmonary artery, is not indicated. Controversy persists in respect to the incidence of progressive pulmonary vascular obstruction. Whether to attempt surgical treatment in patients with pulmonary hypertension and severely reduced pulmonary flow ($Q_p/Q_s < 1.5$) is one of the most difficult decisions in the field of congenital heart disease. When pulmonary vascular resistance is equal to or greater than systemic resistance, surgical measures are contraindicated, with rare exceptions in very young children who have had evidence of pulmonary plethora in the recent past. With infants whose lives were in jeopardy by reason of large shunts, surgical constriction, or banding, of the pulmonary artery has been a lifesaving procedure, but medical management followed by complete repair is in general preferable.

VENTRICULAR SEPTAL DEFECT AND AORTIC INCOMPETENCE

Aortic valvular incompetence is occasionally the outstanding hemodynamic problem in a patient with a ventricular septal defect. This is an acquired defect, but it may appear early in childhood. It is attributed to prolapse of the aortic leaflets inadequately supported in the region above the ventricular defect. The ventricular defect is often of only moderate size, and the right anterior aortic cusp is most often the seriously prolapsed one. The combination of lesions often includes a mild infundibular stenosis of the right ventricular outflow tract.

Clinical Manifestations. Aortic regurgitation dominates the clinical picture, and the ventricular septal defect is suspected when there is a history of a murmur heard early in life. The vascularity of the lungs is increased to a degree consistent with the left-to-right shunt. Diagnosis is substantiated by cardiac catheterization, and usually aortography is indicated.

Treatment. Surgical therapy is advised when the hemodynamic load is severe. The long-term results of the aortic valvuloplasties have been, in general, disappointing. For the severe problems often a prosthetic valve or a homograft will be needed.

RUPTURE OF AN AORTIC-SINUS ANEURYSM

Rupture of an aneurysm at the base of one of the aortic sinuses is of unusual interest because of the characteristic clinical picture, the neatness of the physiologic-pathologic correlations, and the availability of surgical cure.

It is almost invariably the posterior or right anterior aortic sinus from which the aneurysm originates. Rupture from the posterior sinus takes place into the right atrium; from the right anterior, into either the infundibular area of the right ventricle or the right atrium. The site of "arterialization" in the right side of the heart will indicate the probable site of origin of the aneurysm.

Clinical Manifestations. Some patients give the story of a sudden, occasionally dramatic, change in their exercise tolerance, and a loud continuous bruit is present over the midsternal area. The pulse is collapsing in type, and the left ventricle gives a strong forcible apex beat. Thus, in the clinical picture there is the suggestion of both aortic regurgitation and patent ductus. The heart shows progressive enlargement, and the lung fields typically show moderate increase in vascularity. The electrocardiogram may be slow to change, but eventually shows the pattern of left ventricular hypertrophy. If it is known that there has been a systolic murmur since infancy, the diagnosis of an associated ventricular septal defect may be made, and this also indicates the location of the aneurysm to be at the base of the right anterior aortic cusp.

Treatment. Surgical treatment is now recommended, and the results are excellent.

ABNORMAL ORIENTATION OF THE GREAT VESSELS WITH VENTRICULAR SEPTAL DEFECT

Three variations of the great vessels with a ventricular septal defect are sufficiently recurring in practice to deserve special mention: (1) "corrected transposition" (levotransposition of the aorta with inverted ventricles), (2) both great vessels arising from the right ventricle, and (3) partial transposition with a biventricular origin of the pulmonary artery (Taussig-Bing complex), that is, double outlet with the ventricular septal defect high in the septum, above the crista, under the pulmonary valve. Pulmonary vascular obstruction may be associated with all three, and this factor largely determines the direction of the shunt. All three variations have special interest for both the anatomist and the surgeon who would like either to avoid or to attempt repair.

The complex of "corrected transposition" (Fig. 5) with inverted ventricles (the right atrioventricular valve and ventricle simulating the usual left, and vice versa) may exist without a ventricular septal defect, but is more usual with such a defect and a left-to-right shunt. The syndrome may be further characterized by left-sided atrioventricular-valve regurgitation and by partial or complete heart block.

The complex of the double outlet of the great vessels from the right ventricle may masquerade clinically as a usual type of ventricular defect when the defect is low in the septum below the crista supraventricularis, or, when pulmonary stenosis is present, as tetralogy of Fallot.

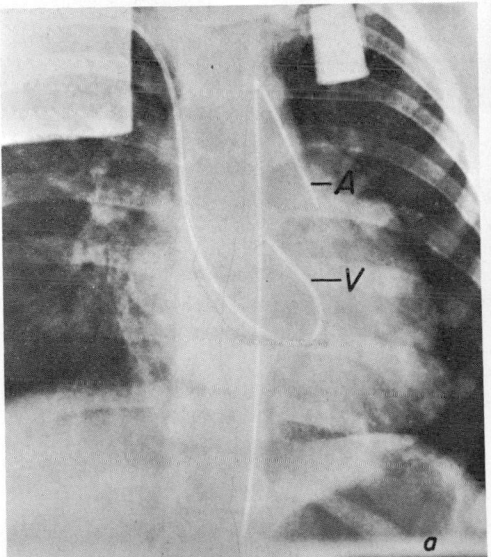
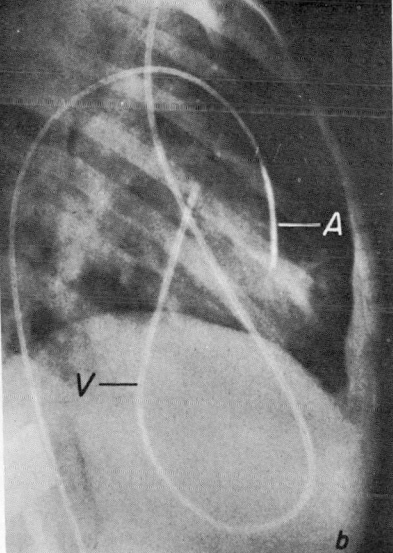

FIGURE 5. Presence of transposition of great vessels confirmed by positions of catheter in a two-year-old boy with ventricular septal defect. Catheters introduced into the heart by vein *(V)* and artery *(A)*, the ends of the catheter in each instance being just above the semilunar valves. The anatomic picture may be best portrayed by selective angiographic studies.

The *Taussig-Bing complex* is an exceedingly rare condition in which the pulmonary artery overrides the ventricular septal defect. The great vessels appear partially transposed and a conus structure exists at the outlet of both the right and left ventricles. It is characterized roentgenographically by a large pulmonary artery. As there is recirculation through the pulmonary circuit, the saturation in the pulmonary artery characteristically exceeds that in the aorta.

In all three syndromes, selective angiocardiography in combination with cardiac catheterization is the proper method of investigation. Attention is paid not only to the (anterior and sinistral or dextral) position of the aorta and the (medial and posterior) position of the pulmonary artery, as in "corrected transposition," but also to the abnormal (same level and plane) relationships of the pulmonary and aortic semilunar valves.

ATRIAL SEPTAL DEFECTS

There are three common forms of atrial septal defect. The most common one is in the region of the original ostium II of the atrial septum or at the site of the fossa ovalis. The second is in the lower part of the atrial septum in the region of ostium I and is associated with various degrees of deformity of the tricuspid and mitral valves. The third is a cephalad-located defect under the entrance of the superior vena cava into the right atrium. There is an assorted terminology. The first is called "usual type" or "secundum type"; the second, "ostium primum type," "atrioventricular-cushion malformation type" or "common atrioventricular-canal (AV commune) type"; and third, "superior vena cava syndrome" or "sinus venosus type." The last type is associated with anomalously connected pulmonary veins. There are additional forms such as multiple fenestrations and a caudally located communication through the coronary sinus when this has communicated with the left atrium as well as the right.

Diagnosis. The diagnosis of atrial septal defect in adults is usually readily made on the basis of the forceful lift of the right ventricle, a pulmonary systolic (ejection) murmur, frequently a faint early diastolic murmur, and a prominently split second sound that changes little, if at all, during the respiratory cycle. On physical examination, one cannot identify the various types or clearly distinguish them from anomalous pulmonary veins, although one may suspect an atrioventricular-cushion deformity when there is a loud holosystolic murmur inside the apex, heard well toward the sternum, suggesting mitral incompetence. When anomalously connected pulmonary veins from one lung are present and the atrial septum is intact, the second sound has, on inspiration, a normal increase in split and thus suggests the diagnosis; however, a normal splitting is also present in some cases of atrial septal defect.

The electrocardiograms of patients with atrial

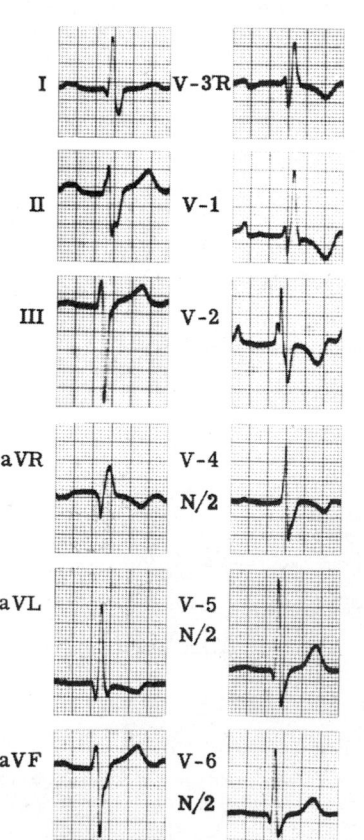

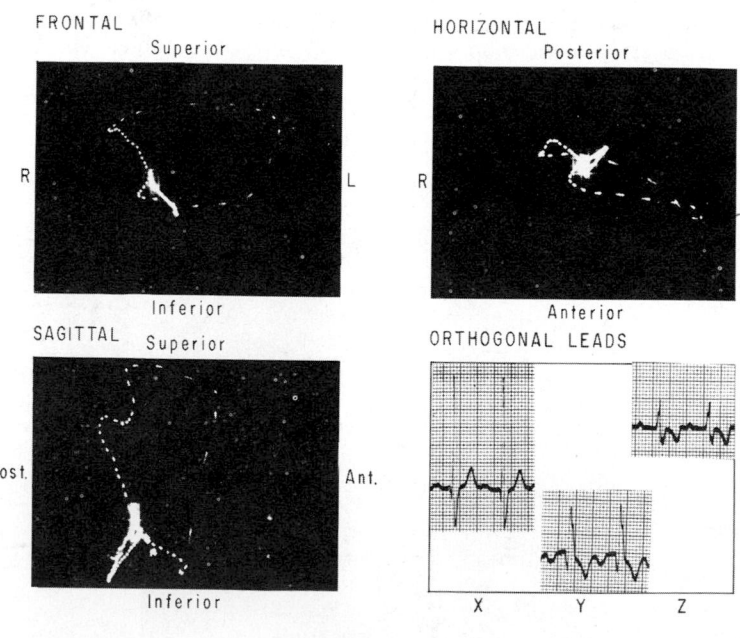

FIGURE 6. Electrocardiograms on a 4½-year-old patient with a surgically proved atrioventricular-cushion defect. The interventricular communication was small, the mitral incompetence severe. At the time of operation the right ventricular pressure was 50, the left 100 mm. of mercury.

defect characteristically show evidence of right ventricular volume overloading characterized particularly by an rSR complex in the right precordial leads, but they may be normal. Tracings may be diagnostically discriminatory in that the low atrial defect of the atrioventricular-cushion type characteristically shows left axis deviation, and such records may be relied upon with confidence as support for such a diagnosis (Fig. 6). The routine roentgenogram of the thorax reveals in the usual case, large vascular shadows extending out toward the periphery of the lung, enlargement of the right ventricle and sometimes the right atrium, and prominence of the main pulmonary artery. Years ago, emphasis was placed on the excessive pulmonary artery pulsations (hilar dance) observed on fluoroscopy, but this may not be of diagnostic value in patients with moderate shunts.

In patients with the clinical diagnosis of atrial septal defect, confirmation of the diagnosis is sought by right-heart catheterization and is usually substantiated. The technique utilizing two catheters and indicator-dilution studies will give a very accurate value for the shunt, but the general hemodynamic profile is usually satisfactorily established by a single catheter.

The differentiation of various types of AV cushion defects may be difficult even with angiocardiography. The deformity of the ventricular septum, the size of an associated interventricular communication, and the details of the valvular distortions are difficult to assess.

Despite the ease with which an atrial septal defect should be diagnosed, it may be readily mistaken for rheumatic valvular disease in middle-aged and elderly adults.

Treatment. The treatment of atrial septal defects is surgical except when they are associated with advanced pulmonary vascular disease. In the uncomplicated case, the risk is very low. When surgery is delayed and symptoms are severe, the over-all results are palliative rather than approaching curative value. In all probability, with adequate casefinding in childhood, the disease as such will become rare in adult cardiologic practice. Patients with heart failure, tricuspid incompetence, and mild arterial unsaturation may be accepted for surgical treatment despite a high risk if pulmonary flow exceeds systemic flow. In patients who have had repair of the ostium primum type of defect, it is expected that a mitral defect will persist, but the over-all results have been satisfactory. When the AV cushion defect is "complete," with a single atrioventricular valve and a serious defect in the ventricular septum, surgical treatment has had an almost forbidding risk, but new techniques give promise of both acceptable surgical risk and postoperative results.

ANOMALOUS PULMONARY VEINS

Pulmonary veins may be anomalously connected to the superior vena cava, left innominate vein, inferior vena cava, and coronary sinus. When the atrial septum is intact, the anomalously drained lung functions normally as an organ, yet it does not function normally in relation to the body as a whole. For example, life could not continue with an anomalously draining lung if the normally draining lung were excised (or massively collapsed). Clinically, nonobstructing anomalous pulmonary veins present a picture akin to that of atrial septal defects, and the two conditions are frequently associated.

When a vein from the right lung drains into the inferior vena cava, there are often associated various degrees of agenesis of the right lung and dextroposition of the heart. Part of the right lung may also be supplied from a systemic artery. The anomalous vein frequently may appear quite distinct in routine roentgenograms or may be more dramatically displayed in tomograms. The curvature of the vein coursing downward in the right lower lung field has suggested the term "scimitar syndrome."

In total anomalous venous connection, all the oxygenated blood from the lungs mixes with the systemic venous blood, and for maintenance of systemic blood flow an atrial defect is necessarily present. The ratio of pulmonary to systemic blood flow can be reasonably predicted by knowledge of the arterial oxygen saturation alone; in general, if the arterial saturation is more than 80 per cent, the pulmonary flow will be at least twice the systemic flow. When the pulmonary veins enter the superior vena cava, the saturation of blood in the pulmonary artery often slightly exceeds that in the aorta, because of preferential flow from the superior vena cava into the right ventricle and from the inferior vena cava into the left atrium and ventricle.

Two basic forms of total anomalous pulmonary venous drainage are of outstanding clinical importance: one is associated with obstruction and is observed in infants with a common vein either entering the abdomen to join a systemic vein such as the ductus venosus or ascending through the mediastinum to the left innominate vein; the other occurs when there is no venous obstruction and a free interatrial communication exists. In the former, early heart failure, sometimes with venous distention, is outstanding, and although it is undoubtedly present, pulmonary congestion may not be as prominent a part of the clinical or roentgenographic picture as might be expected.

A familiar form of total anomalous drainage in the child or adult is that in which a common pulmonary venous chamber communicates with a (dilated) superior vena cava, producing a roentgenographic shadow in the superior mediastinum. This shadow has been given the roentgenologic designation "figure-of-eight" or "snow man." Despite the complete admixture of systemic and pulmonary venous blood, patients with this syndrome are frequently not overtly cyanosed, which correlates with the fact that, with high pulmonary flows, the arterial oxygen saturation may be held as high as 90 per cent and may not, even with exercise, drop below 80 per cent.

In the absence of advanced pulmonary vascular

disease, the treatment is surgical. Good results are to be expected. The surgical treatment of infants with an obstructive type of anomalous pulmonary vein drainage has been associated with a high risk.

COR TRIATRIATUM

Cor triatriatum is a condition in which a common pulmonary venous chamber exists as part of the left atrium, being separated from the part overlying the mitral orifice by a diaphragm-like septum that has a small obstructive aperture. The condition is thus clinically akin to mitral stenosis and may be suspected if findings of mitral stenosis are present in early childhood or when there is no history of rheumatic fever. Because of the possibility of potential surgical cure, a specialist may hope but will be unlikely to encounter and diagnose such a condition more than a few times in his lifetime.

PATENT DUCTUS

Patent ductus arteriosus has a venerated position in cardiologic lore, as it was the first congenital defect that was readily diagnosed clinically with confidence and the first to be completely corrected by surgical means.

Diagnosis. In uncomplicated patent ductus there is a leak from the aorta to the pulmonary artery analogous to that of arteriovenous fistula, and a continuous bruit with a late systolic accentuation is characteristic. In infancy a systolic murmur alone may be present. In the unusual patient who has an associated severe pulmonary vascular obstruction, there may be either a systolic or a diastolic murmur—or, indeed, no murmur at all. In the latter condition an idiopathic pulmonary hypertension is clinically simulated. A large patent ductus may result in heart failure in early infancy, and its differentiation from ventricular septal defect is not always easy. The simple procedure of evaluating the femoral pulse, which usually has a collapsing character in patent ductus, frequently has a differentiating value, and the same features may be reflected also in a hyperdynamic aortic pulse on fluoroscopic examination. Patent ductus and a ventricular septal defect are occasionally associated, and, although in older children the sites of two murmurs may be identified, this is not true for infants. It should be remembered that patent ductus may be associated with coarctation and that the ductus may be above, at, or below the coarctation. When the last type is complete, the descending aorta is a direct continuation of the ductus, and equivalent high pressures and equal desaturation of the blood are present in the pulmonary artery and the femoral arteries.

Even as in ventricular septal defect, pulmonary vascular obstruction may occur with patent ductus and may be manifest as either of two varieties: the one, having been present in a relatively stable form for years; the other, having been recently acquired after the long existence of a large left-to-right shunt. The first is associated with a small heart, the second with a large heart. In either case, reversal of flow through the ductus may occur, and differential cyanosis may be recognizable, the feet (and to a lesser extent the left hand) being cyanotic, the right hand not. In the adult the routine roentgenogram may show unusual prominence of the aortic knob and a small fleck of calcification in the area of the ductus.

The differential diagnosis of patent ductus focuses usually on the causes of a continuous bruit heard over the anterior part of the thorax. These causes include an aorticopulmonary defect above the semilunar valves, ruptured aortic-sinus aneurysm, ventricular septal defect with aortic incompetence, focal constriction of a pulmonary artery branch, coronary arteriovenous aneurysm, and, rarely, truncus arteriosus.

The diagnosis of patent ductus can usually be made clinically, but the lesion lends itself readily to demonstration by several methods—cardiac catheterization with or without indicator-dilution curves, cineangiography, angiocardiography, or aortography.

Treatment. The treatment of patent ductus associated with a left-to-right shunt is surgical; indeed, there is no better example of surgical cure of heart disease. When the shunt and heart are large, operation should not be delayed. When they are small, operation may be deferred to a convenient time. Technically and psychologically the preadolescent period may be ideal.

DEFECTS CHARACTERIZED BY CYANOSIS

TRANSPOSITION OF THE GREAT VESSELS

Diagnosis. Transposition of the great vessels is characterized by severe and early cyanosis and progressive cardiac enlargement. The diagnosis implies recirculation in both the systemic and pulmonary circuits. It is amazing how life may continue in some patients with complete transposition of the great vessels and with minimal intercommunications between the right and left sides of the heart. In patients having patent ductus, one may rarely see differential cyanosis, the deeper hue, when present, being in the upper part of the body (the opposite of that in reversing ductus). The site of the cyanosis is related to the fact that ductus flow from the pulmonary artery (arising from the left ventricle) carries oxygenated blood to the descending aorta (the aorta arising from the right ventricle).

The clinical patterns observed largely depend on the presence or absence of a ventricular septal defect and/or pulmonary stenosis. Pulmonary vascular disease in the former situation may develop very early in infancy.

The cardiac silhouette in transposition varies considerably. Characteristically the heart is large and globular, the superior vascular shadow narrow, and the pulmonary vascular shadows normal or increased. The electrocardiographic findings are not sufficiently consistent to help, but indirectly they may help exclude diagnoses of other cyanotic conditions. In practically all cases, angiocardiographic studies are necessary for clear appraisal of the defect.

Treatment. Surgical treatment is not standardized nor to be considered established, but an increasing number of hemodynamic cures are being reported from intra-atrial reconstructions in which pulmonary venous drainage was directed into the right ventricle and the flow from the superior and inferior venae cavae into the left ventricle. The outstanding recent advance has been the introduction of balloon septostomy (Rashkind), whereby desperately ill infants may be markedly improved, allowing survival and later other surgical procedures. The factors limiting surgical success are the difficulties in closing a ventricular septal defect, if present, sometimes advanced pulmonary obstructive vascular change, rarely tricuspid valve incompetence, and occasionally some postoperative obstruction to venous inflow.

SINGLE VENTRICLE

Often when a single ventricle exists it may not be the primary anomaly, but rather the sequel to other abnormalities. The genetic force operates to mold right and left ventricular structure, but is thwarted by atretic valvular areas or the dynamic force of blood flow. The single ventricle is advantageously considered clinically as a single pump, although the anatomic realities are a challenge to the embryologist. Sometimes an arbitrary decision may have to be made between the tremendous ventricular septal defect that is virtually a "functional single ventricle" and a single ventricle. Cyanosis is usually present in patients with a single ventricle, not because of the ventricular anomaly but because of the frequent association of either pulmonary stenosis or pulmonary vascular disease. From determinations of the oxygen saturations alone one could readily err in the diagnosis of single ventricle, as saturation in the pulmonary artery may be either considerably lower or higher than in the aorta, related to inadequate mixing in the ventricle and streaming of blood into the two often transposed great arteries.

In the approach to the problem of the single ventricle, one may initially group together pul-

monary, tricuspid, mitral, and aortic atresias, or combinations thereof, as there is one basic ventricular pump. The anatomic arrangements, however, for maintenance of quasi-adequate circulation are multiple; for example, in aortic atresia, the ductus becomes the functional aortic channel, the tiny proximal aorta supplies the coronary arteries, and the left ventricle is a diminutive relic. In pulmonary atresia, which functionally may be regarded at the extreme end of the range of "tetralogy," the pulmonary circulation is attained by bronchial arteries; the right ventricle, in free access to the aorta, usually develops, however, and, despite dynamic unity of the ventricular chambers, there is usually ventricular septal development. In the therapeutic approach to cyanotic patients, the important question, and the one to which angiocardiographic studies will give definitive answers, is often whether a patent right ventricular outflow tract exists or whether two ventricles are present.

TETRALOGY OF FALLOT

An adage of the past stated that if one saw a cyanotic child (not infant) one could diagnose tetralogy of Fallot without an examination and be right 90 per cent of the time. This percentage reflected undue optimism and was inadequate for precise specialty practice in any case. This citation does serve the purpose of emphasizing the frequency of the defects that are termed "tetralogy" but that are recognized now not only to have a wide anatomic variation but also to present a varied physiologic picture. The historic clinical picture of a child cannot be accurately reconstructed from postmortem examination of the heart alone. Although cyanosis is traditional and characteristic, it may be mild, and persons with pulmonary stenosis and ventricular septal defect may indeed have a left-to-right shunt at the ventricular level. An occasional infant with tetralogy may be well nourished and have a normal rosy color when first seen, yet have the history of severe cyanotic episodes with unconsciousness.

Morphology. The term "tetralogy of Fallot" has had such traditional international use that it will probably not be readily discarded, despite invalidity of a true tetrad or Fallot's proprietary right to an eponym. Classically, the four abnormalities were pulmonary stenosis, ventricular septal defect, dextroposition of the aorta, and right ventricular hypertrophy. The latter two conditions are entirely secondary to the first two abnormalities.

Clinical Manifestations. The typical clinical picture of tetralogy is that of cyanosis, a short systolic murmur of the stenotic "ejection" type, right ventricular hypertrophy as indicated by the roentgenogram and the electrocardiogram, and oligemic lungs as evidenced by the roentgenogram. The roentgenogram may also reveal a suggestion of a small main pulmonary artery. The intensity and duration of the murmur vary inversely with the severity of the stenosis, the reverse of the relationship when the ventricular septum is intact. The second sound is single and loud over a large area of the precordium. When the second sound is particularly intense to the left of the upper sternum, however, one should suspect the possibility of an anteriorly placed (levotransposed) aorta.

The general development of the child and the degree of cyanosis and polycythemia will reflect the degree of the inadequacy of the pulmonary blood flow, which may be further quantitatively revealed by the level of the arterial oxygen saturation (as may be measured by an ear oximeter) at rest and during exercise.

In the typical patient, the diagnosis may be confidently made without cardiac catheterization or angiography, but angiography will be required in most infants and in many other patients in whom the murmur is faint or otherwise atypical or when the cardiac silhouette lacks a shadow of the main pulmonary artery or is otherwise unusual.

Treatment. Some cases constitute emergency situations with early shunts from the aorta to a pulmonary artery indicated. In a few patients with cyanotic spells, propranolol has been of value. Complete surgical reconstruction has been satisfactory at acceptable operative mortality (less than 5 per cent in some centers) in children over four years of age, and in adults, but in small infants in dire need of help there still remains a place for anastomotic operations diverting some aortic flow into the pulmonary arteries. The very long-term results of complete reconstruction are yet to be evaluated, but it is expected that the successes achieved so far will not be significantly altered by the passage of time. Some pulmonary incompetence, often difficult to recognize clinically and frequently the necessary byproduct of complete relief of the stenosis, may constitute a handicap in some patients over many years. A rare patient with the ventricular septal defect closed and residual pulmonary stenosis may develop severe tricuspid regurgitation.

TRICUSPID ATRESIA

The condition of tricuspid atresia (Fig. 7) deserves special mention because of its relative frequency among the less common defects, its clinical simulation of a tetralogy when it is associated with pulmonary stenosis, its commonly characteristic electrocardiographic appearance (Fig. 8), and its ease of diagnosis by cardiac catheterization and angiocardiography. A classification of types of tricuspid atresia that has been generally used is dependent on the presence or absence of (1) transposition of the great vessels and (2) pulmonary stenosis. The size of the ventric-

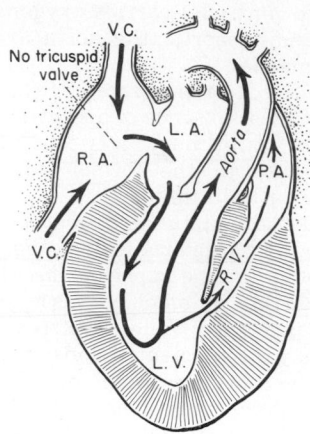

FIGURE 7. Flow diagram for one type of tricuspid atresia, illustrating complete admixture of systemic and pulmonary venous blood and a stenotic channel representative of a ventricular septal defect and the right ventricle as a pathway for pulmonary flow. Vessels are not transposed. (Reproduced by permission from Dry, T. J., Edwards, J. E., Parker, R. L., Burchell, H. B., Rogers, H. M., and Bulbulian, A. H.: Congenital Anomalies of the Heart and Great Vessels: Clinicopathologic Study of 132 Cases. Part I and Part II. Postgrad. Med., 4:231–263, 1948; 4:327–360, 1948.)

ular septal defect is of obvious importance in the control of pulmonary flow when the great vessels are normally related.

Treatment. If the pulmonary artery is unobstructed (and pulmonary hypertension is present), no surgical therapy is possible. If pulmonary stenosis is present and disability is severe, a systemic-pulmonary artery anastomosis of the Blalock type is of benefit. In certain clinics, diversion of superior vena caval blood to the distal end of the right pulmonary artery by an end-to-end anastomosis is the favored surgical treatment.

LOCALIZED CONSTRICTION OF PULMONARY ARTERIES

This anomaly, if associated with a ventricular septal defect, may give a clinical picture like that of tetralogy, but characteristically a continuous bruit is present. The condition lends itself to diagnostic angiocardiographic studies. The anomaly is rare, may be a sequel to rubella, and surgical correction may still be regarded as formidable.

TRUNCUS ARTERIOSUS

When a single large arterial trunk arises from the heart, it arises from the right ventricle and there is necessarily a ventricular septal defect. The latter defect is usually, but not necessarily, of adequate size to conduct the oxygenated blood from the left side of the heart. If the deformity

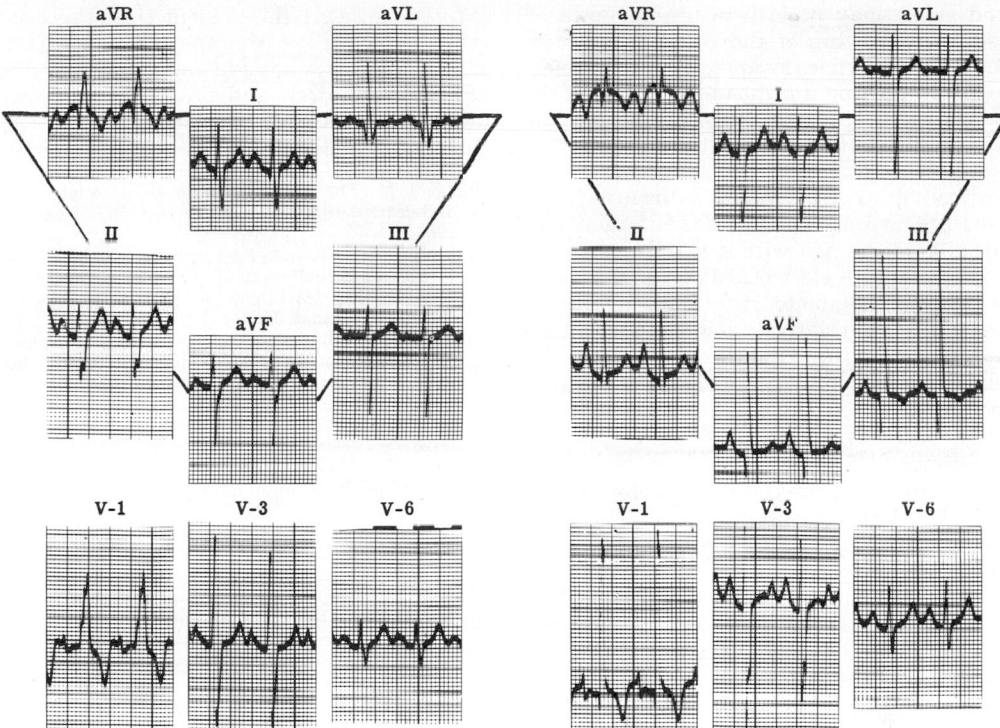

FIGURE 8. Electrocardiogram characteristic of tricuspid atresia (left) compared with that of mitral atresia (right). Pulmonary stenosis was associated in each instance. Although the precordial leads have certain similarities, the standard leads (axis deviation) are very dissimilar.

involves only the proximal part of the trunk, a short main pulmonary artery and its two branches are identifiable, or various combinations of the pulmonary arteries may arise as single branches. In a rare form the pulmonary arteries, as such, may be absent, and the blood supply to the lungs is through enlarged bronchial arteries. The aortic arch is frequently on the right.

A useful classification exists dependent upon the origin of the pulmonary arteries. A functionally similar situation exists in the presence of a completely atretic main pulmonary artery, the pulmonary arteries being supplied through a large ductus. The embryologic background and detailed anatomy are quite dissimilar, and the term "pseudotruncus" is commonly used for the latter condition.

Diagnosis. The presence, diagnosis, and degree of arterial unsaturation depend on the pulmonary blood flow (and there is a functional analogy to other conditions wherein there is opportunity for a nearly complete admixture of systemic and pulmonary venous blood). The diagnosis is difficult to make clinically, but may be suspected if there is a crescendo-decrescendo systolic murmur fitting a ventricular septal defect, a continuous bruit over the upper sternal area, and a narrow vascular shadow in the posteroanterior roentgenographic view. The second sound is loud and single but often with resonating frequencies, producing a "split" sound. The continuous bruit is rather uncommon in pseudotruncus and quite rare in the true form. The electrocardiogram shows dominant right ven-

tricular forces, but the terminal vectors sometimes do not swing as far into the area of right axis deviation, and occasionally a simple clue may be thus a diminutive R in aVR.

Pertinent here is the general axiom of the need of special studies when the clinical diagnosis is not clear and amenability of the lesion to surgical treatment has not been decided. Selective right-heart angiocardiograms and frequently, in a particularly difficult situation, a retrograde aortogram will clarify the anatomic details.

It may be appreciated that a defect between the root of the aorta and the root of the pulmonary artery is in essence related to a truncus, but hemodynamically it is more like a huge patent ductus arteriosus.

Treatment. When the main pulmonary arteries and high pulmonary flow are present, recent surgical advances allow definitive operations in some patients, a homograft being placed between the right ventricle and the pulmonary arteries and the ventricular septal defect being closed.

EBSTEIN'S ANOMALY

Ebstein's anomaly of the tricuspid valve consists of a downwardly displaced and variously distorted tricuspid valve, which results in inadequate function of the right ventricle. The degree of distortion of the valve and the right ventricle varies greatly; characteristically the functional right atrium is huge, and there may be either incompetence of the valve or narrowing of the channel between the atrium and ventricle. Frequently the foramen ovale is open, allowing a right-to-left shunt; if so, the cyanosis increases with the years because of inadequate right ventricular function.

Diagnosis. The diagnosis is supported by a loud third sound, a short systolic murmur in the low sternal area, right-sided cardiac enlargement, relatively oligemic lungs with a small main pulmonary artery, and an electrocardiogram that may simulate that of complete right bundle-branch block but is often of relatively low voltage. Intracardiac electrocardiograms may be practically diagnostic, showing the usual type of right ventricular cavity potentials from the low functional atrial area. Some patients exhibit a Wolff-Parkinson-White syndrome. Of some interest is the occurrence of Ebstein's malformation in the physiologic left ventricle when corrected transposition (inverted ventricles) is present. Angiocardiographic and catheterization procedures will substantiate the diagnosis (it is about the only cyanotic cardiac defect without elevation of right ventricular pressure), but the exact detailed anatomy of the tricuspid valve is not accurately revealed.

Treatment. At the present time there is no established curative therapy, though anastomosis of the superior vena cava and the distal pulmonary artery in children and prosthetic-valve implacement in adults have had limited success.

Brown, J. W.: Congenital Heart Disease. 2nd ed. London, Staples Press, 1950.

Campbell, M.: The mode of inheritance in isolated laevocardia and dextrocardia and situs inversus. Brit. Heart J., 25:803, 1963.

Edwards, J. E., Dry, T. J., Parker, R. L., Burchell, H. B., Wood, E. H., and Bulbulian, A. H.: An Atlas of Congenital Anomalies of the Heart and Great Vessels. Springfield, Ill., Charles C Thomas, 1954.

Ivemark, B. I.: Implications of agenesis of the spleen on the pathogenesis of cono-truncus anomalies in childhood. Acta Paediat., 44(suppl. 104):1–101 (Nov.) 1955.

Keith, J. D., Rowe, R. D., and Vlad, P.: Heart Disease in Infancy and Childhood. 2nd ed. New York, The Macmillan Company, 1967.

Kjellberg, S. R., Mannheimer, E., Rudhe, U., and Jonsson, B.: Diagnosis of Congenital Heart Disease: A Clinical and Technical Study by the Cardiologic Team of the Pediatric Clinic, Karolinska Sjukhuset, Stockholm. 2nd ed. Chicago, Year Book Publishers, 1959.

Nadas, A. S.: Pediatric Cardiology. 2nd ed. Philadelphia, W. B. Saunders Company, 1963.

Taussig, H. B.: Congenital Malformations of the Heart. 1st ed. New York, The Commonwealth Fund, 1947.

Watson, H. (ed.): Pediatric Cardiology. St. Louis, C. V. Mosby Company, 1968.

Chronic Valvular Heart Disease

Eugene Braunwald

MITRAL STENOSIS

Etiology. Mitral stenosis is, with very rare exceptions, rheumatic in origin, the scarring of the valve leaflets leading to their retraction as active rheumatic endocarditis heals. The mitral commissures fuse, the chordae tendineae shorten, the valvular tissue becomes rigid and calcified, and these changes in turn lead to narrowing of the mitral orifice. Pure or predominant mitral stenosis occurs in approximately 40 per cent of all patients with rheumatic heart disease and is the most common chronic valvular abnormality following rheumatic fever. Two thirds of all patients with mitral stenosis are females.

Clinical Manifestations. A history of one or more attacks of acute rheumatic fever can be elicited from approximately two thirds of adult patients with predominant or pure mitral stenosis. When the degree of valvular obstruction is trivial, the murmur and many of the other physical signs of mitral stenosis can be present in the absence of symptoms of diminished cardiovascular reserve. In the presence of more significant mitral obstruction, blood can flow from the left atrium to the left ventricle only if propelled by an abnormally elevated left atrioventricular pressure gradient. The elevated left atrial pressure in turn raises the pulmonary venous and capillary pressures, resulting in exertional dyspnea, which is an important early symptom in mitral stenosis. In many patients the first bouts of dyspnea are precipitated by situations associated with increased rate of blood flow across the mitral orifice, which results in further elevation of the left atrial pressure. Extreme exertion, excitement, fever, paroxysmal tachycardia, sexual intercourse, pregnancy, anemia, and thyrotoxicosis may precipitate elevations of pulmonary capillary pressure and lead to dyspnea in patients whose mitral orifices are large enough to accommodate a normal blood flow with only trivial elevations of left atrial pressure. As mitral stenosis progresses, the events that precipitate dyspnea become less extreme, and the patient becomes limited in his daily activities. Since the majority of symptomatic patients are in their third and fourth decades, when family and professional responsibilities are maximal, the obstruction to left atrial emptying interferes significantly with vocational or homemaking activities. As stenosis progresses, the redistribution of blood from the dependent portions of the body to the lungs, which occurs when the patient assumes the recumbent position, leads to orthopnea and paroxysmal nocturnal dyspnea. Acute pulmonary edema occurs when there is a sudden increase in flow rate across a seriously narrowed mitral orifice, and rarely this complication may be fatal.

Hemoptysis results from rupture of pulmonary

bronchial venous connections and occurs most frequently in patients who have elevated left atrial pressures without markedly elevated pulmonary vascular resistances; this complication is almost never fatal. True hemoptysis must be distinguished from the bloody sputum that occurs in the presence of pulmonary edema, recurrent bronchitis, and pulmonary infarction, all of which occur with increased frequency in the presence of mitral stenosis.

When the pulmonary vascular resistance rises in patients with mitral stenosis, symptoms secondary to pulmonary congestion tend to become ameliorated, and the episodes of acute pulmonary edema and hemoptysis diminish in frequency and severity. Elevation of pulmonary vascular resistance further increases right ventricular systolic pressure, ultimately leading to symptoms of right ventricular failure. Fatigue, weakness, abdominal discomfort due to hepatic congestion, and ankle swelling are prominent features of this stage of the disease. If tricuspid stenosis or regurgitation develops in a patient with mitral stenosis, sudden surges of blood into the pulmonary vascular bed are reduced and the frequency of episodes of acute pulmonary congestion also diminishes.

As the left atrium enlarges, it often becomes the site of origin of premature contractions, of atrial tachycardia, or of paroxysms of atrial flutter and fibrillation. The rapid ventricular rate associated with untreated atrial fibrillation reduces the time available for flow across the mitral valve and therefore is frequently responsible for acute exacerbation of dyspnea. The development of permanent atrial fibrillation often marks a turning point in the patient's course and is generally associated with acceleration of the rate at which symptoms progress.

Thrombi may form in the left atria of patients with mitral stenosis, particularly in the enlarged atrial appendages. When these thrombi are dislodged they embolize to the systemic vessels, most commonly the kidneys, spleen, extremities, and brain. This complication occurs much more frequently in patients with atrial fibrillation, in older patients, and in those with a reduced cardiac output. However, it is not more frequent in patients with extremely severe than in those with only moderate degrees of obstruction, and systemic embolization is occasionally the presenting complaint in otherwise asymptomatic patients with mild mitral stenosis. At operation, thrombi are not found more frequently in the left atria of patients with a past history of embolization than in those without this complication, indicating that it is usually the freshly formed clots that embolize. Rarely, a large pedunculated thrombus or a free-floating clot may suddenly obstruct the stenotic mitral orifice. Such "ball-valve" thrombi produce syncope, angina, and changing auscultatory signs with alterations in position. Left atrial thrombi may be detected by means of angiocardiography, particularly when the contrast medium is injected into the left atrium or by scintillation scanning

after administration of I^{131} antibodies to human fibrinogen.

The elevated blood volume and cardiac output associated with pregnancy frequently intensify the symptoms of mitral stenosis. In patients not seriously limited prior to conception, a successful outcome may be expected if medical treatment is intensified during pregnancy. In patients with severe stenosis in whom pulmonary congestive symptoms progress during early pregnancy in spite of conservative management, mitral valvulotomy may be performed, preferably during the first trimester. Following delivery, most patients recover the clinical status that existed prior to pregnancy, although the condition of some women continues to deteriorate. The increased physical activities resulting from the augmented family responsibilities also tend to increase the mother's symptoms.

Recurrent pulmonary infarctions are an important cause of morbidity and mortality late in the course of mitral stenosis, occurring most frequently in patients with right ventricular failure and markedly elevated pulmonary vascular resistance. Pulmonary infections, i.e., bronchitis, bronchopneumonia, and lobar pneumonia, commonly complicate untreated mitral stenosis and are probably related to pulmonary venous hypertension. Essential hypertension is rare in mitral stenosis, and angina pectoris is not a prominent symptom. When the latter occurs, however, it is usually due to cardiac ischemia related to a severely depressed cardiac output, previous coronary embolism, or associated coronary artery disease. Cholelithiasis and chronic cholecystitis tend to occur with greater frequency in patients with mitral stenosis. Bacterial endocarditis is relatively uncommon in pure mitral stenosis, particularly in patients with atrial fibrillation in whom the mitral valve is calcified.

Peripheral and facial cyanosis occurs commonly in patients with extremely severe mitral stenosis. Typically, there is a malar flush and the facies appears pinched and blue. Inspection of the jugular venous pulse reveals prominent a waves due to vigorous right atrial systole in patients with sinus rhythm who have severe associated pulmonary hypertension or tricuspid stenosis. When atrial fibrillation is present, the jugular pulse reveals only a single expansion during systole (c-v wave). The systemic arterial pressure is usually normal or slightly low. Examination of the heart generally reveals a tap along the left sternal border, signifying an enlarged right ventricle, and pulmonary hypertension. In patients with associated pulmonary hypertension the impact of pulmonary valve closure can usually be felt in the second and third left intercostal spaces just to the left of the sternum; the left ventricle is not palpable in severe, pure mitral stenosis. A diastolic thrill may frequently be felt at the cardiac apex, particularly if the patient is turned into the left lateral recumbent position; however, the absence of a thrill does not indicate that mitral stenosis is either absent or mild. The apex cardiogram, i.e., a recording of the movement of the cardiac apex, reveals a slow rate of left ventricular filling during early diastole; when a rapid left ventricular filling phase is present, either the mitral stenosis is very mild or there is associated mitral or aortic regurgitation.

Since the mitral valve cannot close until the left ventricular pressure reaches the level of the elevated left atrial pressure, the first heart sound is often slightly delayed, and it is usually loud and snapping. The pulmonary (second) component of the second heart sound is also often accentuated, and in patients with severe pulmonary hypertension the two components of the second heart sound may be closely split. A pulmonary systolic ejection click may be heard in patients with severe pulmonary hypertension and extensive dilatation of the pulmonary artery. The opening snap of the mitral valve is heard best in expiration at, or just medial to, the cardiac apex, but may also be easily audible at the left sternal edge or at the base of the heart. This sound generally follows the sound of aortic valve closure by 0.06 to 0.12 second, and occurs after the pulmonic valve closure sound. Since the opening snap of the mitral valve occurs at the instant at which the left ventricular pressure falls below the left atrial pressure, the time interval between aortic closure and the opening snap will tend to be shorter the higher the left atrial pressure and the more severe the mitral stenosis. When the time interval between the electrocardiographic Q wave and the beginning of the first heart sound exceeds the time interval between aortic valve closure and the opening snap by 0.02 second or more, the mitral obstruction is generally moderate or severe.

The opening snap usually ushers in a low-pitched, rumbling, diastolic murmur, heard best at the apex with the patient in the left lateral recumbent position and often accentuated by mild exercise just before auscultation. In general, the more severe the mitral stenosis, the longer the duration of the diastolic rumbling murmur. In patients with sinus rhythm the murmur may reappear or may become reaccentuated during atrial systole, as atrial contraction re-elevates the rate of blood flow across the narrowed orifice. Soft, short (grade I or II/VI) systolic murmurs are commonly heard at the apex or along the left sternal border in patients with mitral stenosis and do not necessarily signify the presence of mitral regurgitation. However, the longer and louder the apical systolic murmur, the greater the likelihood of serious mitral regurgitation. When severe pulmonary hypertension is present, a loud pansystolic murmur produced by functional tricuspid regurgitation may be audible along the left sternal border. This murmur is often accentuated by inspiration, diminishes during forced expiration or during performance of the Valsalva maneuver, may disappear as compensation is restored, and should not be confused with the apical pansystolic murmur of mitral regurgitation. This distinction is of particular clinical importance since surgical management may be quite different, depending

upon whether mitral stenosis is complicated by regurgitation of the tricuspid or mitral valves.

The presence of a presystolic murmur and an accentuated first heart sound may be taken as evidence against the presence of serious associated mitral regurgitation. On the other hand, when the first sound and/or the opening snap is soft or absent in a patient with mitral valve disease, it is likely that significant mitral regurgitation and/or serious calcification of the deformed mitral valve leaflets is present. A third heart sound heard at the apex generally signifies that the degree of associated mitral regurgitation is more than trivial. This sound is generally duller, lower pitched, and occurs later than the opening snap. Occasionally, in patients with pure mitral stenosis, severe pulmonary hypertension, and right ventricular failure, a third heart sound may originate from the right ventricle and may be audible along the left sternal border. In patients with severe pulmonary hypertension the enlarged right ventricle may rotate the heart, and the enlarged right ventricle may form the cardiac apex, giving the examiner the erroneous impression of left ventricular enlargement. Under these circumstances the rumbling diastolic murmur and the other auscultatory features of mitral stenosis become less prominent or may even disappear. When severe congestive heart failure exists in a patient with calcific mitral stenosis, none of the auscultatory findings typical of severe mitral stenosis may be detectable, but these may become apparent as compensation is restored. The presence of associated tricuspid stenosis also tends to obscure many of the physical signs of mitral stenosis. The *Graham Steell murmur* of pulmonary regurgitation, a high-pitched, diastolic, decrescendo blowing murmur along the left sternal border, results from dilatation of the pulmonary valve ring and occurs in patients with mitral valve disease and serious pulmonary hypertension. This murmur may be indistinguishable from the more common murmur produced by mild aortic regurgitation.

Hepatomegaly, ankle edema, ascites, and the physical finding of pleural effusion, particularly in the right pleural cavity, may occur in patients with mitral stenosis and right ventricular failure.

Electrocardiogram. In mitral stenosis and sinus rhythm the P wave suggests left atrial enlargement; it is notched and broad in lead II and is diphasic, with a prominent negative component in lead V_1. It may become tall and more peaked in lead II and upright in V_1 when severe pulmonary hypertension or tricuspid stenosis complicates mitral stenosis and right atrial enlargement occurs. When atrial fibrillation is present in patients with mitral valve disease, the base line shows coarser undulations than when this arrhythmia occurs as a consequence of coronary artery disease. The QRS complex may be normal even with critical mitral stenosis. However, with severe pulmonary hypertension, right axis deviation and electrocardiographic signs of right ventricular hypertrophy are often present. Electrocardiographic evidence of left ventricular hypertrophy in patients with mitral stenosis generally indicates that an additional lesion that places a burden on the left ventricle, such as mitral regurgitation, aortic valve disease, or hypertension, is present.

Roentgenographic Features. In patients with mild or moderate mitral stenosis the cardiac silhouette is not grossly enlarged. The earliest changes are straightening of the left border, prominence of the main pulmonary arteries and backward displacement of the esophagus by an enlarged left atrium; the aortic knob is usually small. Dilatation of the upper lobe pulmonary veins may be observed roentgenographically even in mild mitral stenosis. In severe mitral stenosis, all chambers and vessels behind the narrowed valve are prominent, including the pulmonary veins and arteries, right ventricle, right atrium, and superior vena cava. The degree of dilatation of the main pulmonary arteries, in general, reflects the pressure in these vessels. Kerley B lines are fine, dense, opaque, horizontal lines that are most prominent in the lower and mid lung fields and that result from distention of interlobular septa and lymphatics with edema. These lines usually signify a resting mean left atrial pressure of at least 20 mm. of mercury. As the pulmonary arterial pressure rises, the smaller pulmonary arteries become attenuated, at first in the lower and then in the mid lung fields. Deposits of hemosiderin occur in the lungs of patients who have had multiple hemoptyses; the hemosiderin-containing macrophages fill the air spaces, and if the deposits become large enough may result in a fine, diffuse nodulation most prominent in the lower lung fields. Ossified nodules are also more common in the lower lung fields and are produced by true lamellar bone, which tends to develop in areas of recurrent interstitial pulmonary edema.

Hemodynamics. In normal adults the mitral valve area is approximately 4 square centimeters. Few if any symptoms are present until the orifice has been reduced to less than 2 square centimeters. When the mitral valve opening is reduced to 1 square centimeter, a left atrial pressure of approximately 25 mm. of mercury is required to maintain a normal cardiac output. A diastolic atrioventricular pressure gradient is the hemodynamic hallmark of mitral stenosis; this gradient is largest in early diastole. However, in sinus rhythm, the gradient rises again during atrial contraction. Since blood flow across stenotic heart valves is turbulent, the transvalvular pressure gradient is not a simple linear function of the flow, but rather is directly proportional to the square of the flow rate. Thus, a doubling of blood flow across a stenotic mitral valve is associated with approximately a quadrupling of the pressure gradient. Accurate determination of the severity of valvular stenosis by measurement of the transvalvular pressure gradient alone is therefore not possible, since the gradient is influenced importantly by the flow as well as the size of the orifice. From these considerations it is clear that in order to assess the severity of obstruction it is necessary to measure the transvalvular flow rate and pressure gradient, simultaneously if possible. When valvular regurgitation exists, the flow rate across the valve is the sum of the effective cardiac output and of the regurgitant flow. Since most clinical techniques for measuring blood flow record only the effective cardiac output, the valvular flow rate may be seriously underestimated, and the severity of the stenotic lesion may therefore be falsely exaggerated if allowance is not made for associated regurgitation. In addition, since alterations in heart rate modify the fraction of the cardiac cycle during which blood flows across cardiac valves, changes in rate alter the velocity of transvalvular blood flow at any given level of cardiac output; an increase in heart rate shortens diastole more than systole and diminishes the time available for flow across the mitral valve. Therefore, at any given level of minute cardiac output tachycardia augments the gradient across the mitral valve, but tends to reduce the transaortic pressure gradient.

The left ventricular diastolic pressure is normal in pure mitral stenosis; when this pressure is elevated, mitral regurgitation, aortic valve disease, rheumatic myocarditis, systemic hypertension, coronary artery disease, or cardiomyopathy is possibly responsible. In pure mitral stenosis the left atrial and pulmonary artery wedge pressure pulses usually show elevation of the mean pressure and gradual y descents, the latter resulting from the obstruction to left atrial emptying; prominent atrial contraction waves are usually present in patients with sinus rhythm. In patients with mild to moderate mitral stenosis without elevation of the pulmonary vascular resistance, the pulmonary arterial pressure may be normal at rest and may rise only with exercise. However, when mitral stenosis is severe and whenever the pulmonary vascular resistance is significantly increased, the pulmonary arterial pressure is elevated with the patient at rest, in extreme cases exceeding even the systemic arterial pressure. The right ventricular end-diastolic and mean right atrial pressures are frequently elevated in patients whose pulmonary arterial systolic pressure exceeds 60 mm. of mercury.

Cardiac output varies considerably in patients with mitral stenosis. Thus, the hemodynamic response to a given degree of mitral obstruction may be characterized in some patients by a normal cardiac output and an elevated left atrioventricular pressure gradient, or at the opposite end of the hemodynamic spectrum, by a greatly reduced cardiac output and small pressure gradient. In some patients with moderately severe mitral stenosis, the cardiac output is normal at rest and rises normally during exertion, and, under these circumstances, the elevated atrioventricular pressure gradient is responsible for symptoms of pulmonary congestion. In other patients the cardiac output is normal at rest, but rises subnormally during exertion. In patients with severe stenosis, particularly those in whom the pulmonary vascular resistance is elevated, the cardiac output is subnormal at rest and may remain constant or even decline during exercise.

The clinical and hemodynamic picture of mitral stenosis is dictated largely by the level of the pulmonary vascular resistance. Pulmonary hypertension results from (1) the passive backward transmission of the elevated left atrial pressure, (2) arteriolar constriction that can be relieved by the infusion of acetylcholine and that presumably is triggered by left atrial and pulmonary venous hypertension, and (3) organic obliterative changes in the pulmonary vascular bed. On histologic examination, the major pulmonary arteries show arteriosclerotic changes, and there is thickening of the media and intima associated with luminal narrowing in all segments of the pulmonary vascular bed; the lower lobes are the sites of predilection for these changes. The resultant elevation of pulmonary vascular resistance may be considered a complication of mitral stenosis, and, if it continues, will result in right heart failure as well as in tricuspid and pulmonary incompetence. However, these changes in the pulmonary vascular bed may also be considered to exert a protective effect on the patient with mitral stenosis. The elevated precapillary resistance reduces the likelihood of pulmonary congestive symptoms by tending to restrain blood from surging into the pulmonary capillary bed and damming up behind the stenotic mitral valve. It is particularly important to identify patients with mitral stenosis who have a significantly elevated pulmonary vascular resistance, since surgical relief of the obstruction is usually followed by regression of the changes in the pulmonary vascular bed and striking clinical improvement.

Parenchymal Pulmonary Changes. In addition to the changes in the pulmonary vascular bed, extensive fibrosis of the alveolar walls and thickening of pulmonary capillary walls occur commonly in mitral stenosis. The vital capacity, total lung capacity, maximal breathing capacity, and oxygen uptake per unit of ventilation tend to be reduced, and the latter fails to rise normally during exertion in patients with severe stenosis. In advanced cases there is uneven distribution of ventilation and later of blood flow, resulting in physiologic right-to-left shunting and enlargement of the physiologic dead space. Normally, with the patient in the erect position, blood flow is much greater at the lung bases than at the apices; this difference is abolished in mitral stenosis. In other patients, the diffusing capacity during exertion may be lowered as a result of structural changes in diffusing surface and reduction of pulmonary capillary blood volume. The reduction of pulmonary compliance that occurs generally correlates directly with the severity of the dyspnea and inversely with the left atrial pressure. In some patients airway resistance is abnormally increased.

All these changes are due in part to increased transudation of fluid from the pulmonary capillaries into the lungs as a consequence of the elevated pulmonary capillary pressure. A combination of the above-mentioned alterations in pulmonary function, particularly the diminution of pulmonary compliance, contributes to the increase of respiratory work and plays an important role in the genesis of dyspnea in mitral stenosis. However, the thickening of the alveolar and capillary walls tends to impede the transudation of fluid into the alveoli and the development of pulmonary edema at times when the pulmonary capillary pressure exceeds the plasma oncotic pressure.

Differential Diagnosis. A number of cardiac and noncardiac conditions may be confused with mitral stenosis. Significant *mitral regurgitation* may be associated with a prominent diastolic murmur at the apex, but there is often clear-cut evidence of left ventricular enlargement on physical examination, roentgenography, and electrocardiography. In addition, a pansystolic murmur of grade III/VI intensity or louder, as well as a third heart sound at the apex, should arouse the suspicion of significant associated regurgitation. Similarly, the apical mid-diastolic murmur associated with *aortic regurgitation (Austin Flint murmur)* may be mistaken for mitral stenosis. However, the absence of an audible opening snap or of presystolic accentuation in a patient with aortic regurgitation and sinus rhythm would tend to exclude mitral stenosis. The presence of *tricuspid stenosis*, a valvular lesion that rarely occurs in the absence of mitral valve disease, may mask many of the clinical features of mitral stenosis.

Exertional dyspnea and *recurrent pulmonary infections* may be falsely ascribed to pulmonary emphysema in patients with both chronic lung disease and mitral stenosis. Careful auscultation, however, will generally reveal the characteristic opening snap and rumbling diastolic murmur of mitral stenosis. Similarly, the hemoptysis that occurs in many otherwise asymptomatic patients with mitral stenosis may be improperly attributed to bronchiectasis or tuberculosis. Actually, the latter condition is uncommon in patients with significant mitral obstruction.

Primary pulmonary hypertension results in a number of the clinical and laboratory features of mitral stenosis. It is seen most frequently in young women. However, the opening snap and diastolic rumbling murmur are absent, there is no left atrial enlargement on the electrocardiogram or roentgenogram, and the pulmonary artery wedge and left atrial pressures are normal in primary pulmonary hypertension. *Cor triatriatum* is an unusual congenital malformation that consists of a fibrous ring within the left atrium. It results in elevation of the pulmonary venous, capillary, and arterial pressures. This lesion can be recognized most readily by means of left atrial angiography.

A left *atrial myxoma* may obstruct left atrial emptying, resulting in dyspnea, a diastolic murmur, and hemodynamic changes that resemble those of mitral stenosis. However, patients with left atrial myxoma often demonstrate findings suggestive of a systemic disease, with weight loss, fever, anemia, systemic emboli, elevated erythrocyte sedimentation rate, and increases in the serum gamma globulin concentration. Usually an opening snap is not audible, there is no clinical evidence of associated aortic valve disease, and the auscultatory findings frequently change with body position. The diagnosis can be established by demonstrating a lobulated filling defect in the left atrium by angiocardiography.

The Role of Specialized Techniques. Right and left heart catheterization can now be performed with a very low mortality, and although these techniques need not necessarily be applied in the majority of patients with mitral stenosis, they are of considerable value in patients who present particular problems. Left heart catheterization is probably of greatest importance in deciding whether valvulotomy is necessary in patients in whom it is difficult to estimate the severity of obstruction by clinical means alone. Similarly, when this procedure is combined with left ventricular angiocardiography, it is particularly valuable in the detection and estimation of associated mitral regurgitation and in the detection and estimation of coexisting lesions such as aortic stenosis and regurgitation. Left atrial thrombi may be detected by angiocardiography, particularly when the contrast medium is injected directly into the left atrium. Left heart catheterization is also helpful in the detection of conditions that impair left ventricular function and would thereby contraindicate or reduce the effectiveness of mitral valvulotomy. Detailed physiologic investigations are indicated for most patients who have undergone previous mitral valve operations and who have redeveloped serious symptoms; in such patients clinical assessment is particularly difficult, and the hemodynamic studies allow intelligent planning of the operative procedure and aid in estimating the risk.

Treatment. In the asymptomatic adolescent with mitral valve disease, penicillin prophylaxis of β-hemolytic streptococcal infections and vocational counseling are particularly important; the choice of a physically strenuous occupation should be avoided so that premature retirement will not be necessary should symptoms develop later. In symptomatic patients considerable improvement can be expected with restriction of sodium intake and maintenance doses of oral diuretics. Digitalis glycosides are necessary for slowing the ventricular rate of patients with atrial fibrillation and for reducing the manifestations of right heart failure in the advanced stages of the disease. Particular attention must be directed to detecting and treating anemia and infections. Hemoptysis is treated by measures designed to diminish pulmonary venous pressure, including bed rest, the sitting position, salt restriction, and diuresis. Anticoagulants are indicated for patients who have suffered systemic and/or pulmonary embolization.

If atrial fibrillation is of relatively recent origin in a patient whose mitral stenosis is not severe enough to warrant surgical treatment, reversion to sinus rhythm, either by means of electrical countershock or quinidine, is indicated. Conversion to sinus rhythm is rarely helpful in patients with severe mitral stenosis, particularly those in whom the left atrium is particularly enlarged or in whom atrial fibrillation has been present for more than a year, since it is frequently impossible to maintain sinus rhythm, and reversion back to atrial fibrillation is common. However, after successful surgical treatment of the mitral valve lesion, conversion of atrial fibrillation is usually indicated, since sinus rhythm can then often be maintained with quinidine.

Surgical treatment is indicated for the symptomatic patient with pure mitral stenosis whose effective orifice is less than approximately 1.5 square centimeters. Unless recurrent systemic embolization has occurred, valvulotomy is not indicated for patients who are truly asymptomatic, regardless of hemodynamic findings. In uncomplicated cases, the surgical mortality should be less than 3 per cent, and a comparison of the natural history of patients with serious symptoms treated by valvulotomy with those who did not receive the benefits of surgical therapy has shown considerable improvement following the operation. However, there is no evidence that surgical treatment improves the prognosis of patients with slight or no functional impairment. When there is little symptomatic improvement following valvulotomy, it is likely that the procedure was ineffective or induced regurgitation, or that another valvular or myocardial lesion was present. The recurrence of symptoms several years after an excellent clinical and hemodynamic result may be due to restenosis of the mitral valve, but myocardial failure or mitral regurgitation is occasionally responsible. Since some degree of scar formation, contraction, and refusion of commissures occurs postoperatively in almost all patients, symptoms of mitral stenosis tend to recur most rapidly in patients in whom the valvulotomy was least adequate.

There is no unanimity among surgeons concerning the most effective and safest operative techniques. A closed operation is often preferable for patients with pure mitral stenosis who have not been operated upon before, who have no detectable valvular or perivalvular calcification on fluoroscopic examination, and in whom there is no suspicion of left atrial thrombosis. Transventricular instrumental dilatation of the mitral valve usually results in more effective relief of stenosis than transatrial finger fracture, and the importance of loosening any existing subvalvular fusion of papillary muscles and chordae tendineae is now generally appreciated. In a number of patients with uncomplicated mitral stenosis, closed valvulotomy may be ineffective or may result in severe regurgitation. For these reasons, the ready availability of an extracorporeal system is helpful. Patients with extremely severe obstruction, significant associated mitral regurgitation, valvular calcification, left atrial thrombi, or a mitral valve distorted by previous operative manipulation are usually managed most effectively under direct vision, utilizing open-heart techniques. Total prosthetic replacement of the valve may have to be carried out in those patients who were severely symptomatic preoperatively and in whom the surgeon does not find it possible to improve valve function significantly, even under direct vision. Since the operative mortality and the postoperative morbidity and mortality of prosthetic replacement of the mitral valve are substantially higher than those of valvulotomy, patients in whom preoperative evaluation suggests the possibility that prosthetic replacement may be required should be operated upon only if they are severely limited and symptomatic on ordinary activity.

MITRAL REGURGITATION

Etiology. In contrast to mitral stenosis, pure or predominant rheumatic mitral regurgitation occurs more frequently in males. In most patients, mitral regurgitation is caused by chronic rheumatic heart disease; the rheumatic process produces rigidity, deformity, and retraction of the valve cusps, as well as fusion, shortening, and contraction of the chordae tendineae. Mitral regurgitation may also occur as a congenital anomaly, most commonly as a consequence of a defect of the endocardial cushions; it may occur with rupture of the papillary muscles following myocardial infarction or fibrosis, as well as rupture of chordae tendineae or valvular perforation consequent to bacterial endocarditis. Mitral regurgitation resulting from papillary muscle dysfunction is due to a change in the normal spatial relationship between various elements of the mitral valve apparatus. Closure of the valve may be prevented by inadequate restraint which allows a portion of the leaflet to evert into the atrium. Prolapse of an elongated posterior leaflet may be associated with myxomatous degeneration of the mitral valve. This so-called "floppy valve" has been attributed to Marfan's syndrome, but similar changes also occur in osteogenesis imperfecta. Functional mitral regurgitation may occur with marked left ventricular dilatation of any cause, and idiopathic hypertrophic subaortic stenosis may distort the mitral valve so as to render it regurgitant. Massive calcification of the mitral anulus, which occurs most commonly in elderly women and is of unknown cause, can also be responsible for significant mitral regurgitation. Congenitally short or long chordae, abnormal valvular insertion of chordae, and papillary muscle involvement in endocardial sclerosis and cardiomyopathy are other causes of mitral regurgitation.

Mitral regurgitation of any cause tends to be a gradually progressive disorder, since enlargement of the left atrium places tension on the posterior mitral leaflet, which is pulled away from the mitral orifice, thereby aggravating the valvular dysfunction. Similarly, the dilatation of the left ventricle increases the regurgitation, which in turn further enlarges the left atrium and ventricle.

Clinical Manifestations. It must be appreciated that only a small fraction of all patients with rheumatic mitral regurgitation ever experience cardiac difficulty. An uncomfortable awareness of the heart beat may be the first complaint and is usually followed by fatigue, exertional dyspnea, orthopnea, and nocturnal dyspnea. Since fluctuations of the mean pulmonary capillary pressure are less in mitral regurgitation than in mitral stenosis, symptoms of pulmonary congestion tend to be less episodic; indeed, acute paroxysmal pulmonary edema is rare. Similarly, hemoptysis and systemic embolism occur far less frequently in mitral regurgitation than in stenosis. On the other hand, fatigability, weakness, and exhaustion are more prominent symptoms and occur most frequently in patients with marked reduction of cardiac output. Right heart failure, characterized by painful hepatic congestion, ankle swelling, distended neck veins, ascites, and evidence of tricuspid regurgitation, is observed commonly in patients with associated pulmonary vascular disease.

Severe symptomatic mitral regurgitation may exist for many years and may lead to generalized wasting and debilitation. Although the blood pressure is usually normal, the arterial pulse is often characterized by a sharp upstroke. The jugular venous pulse shows abnormally prominent *a* waves in patients with sinus rhythm and severe pulmonary hypertension. A systolic thrill is usually palpable at the cardiac apex. The left ventricle is hyperdynamic, and may extend to the midaxillary line. The apex cardiogram reveals a prominent rapid filling wave during early diastole. When the left atrium is markedly enlarged, it may extend anteriorly, and its expansion may be palpable during ventricular systole. The combination of retraction of the left ventricle and expansion of the left atrium during systole may produce a characteristic rocking motion of the chest with each cardiac cycle. A right ventricular tap and the shock of pulmonary valve closure may be felt in patients with severe pulmonary hypertension.

The first heart sound at the apex is generally absent, soft, or buried in the systolic heart murmur; conversely, an accentuated mitral closure sound is useful in excluding severe regurgitation. The splitting of the second heart sound is usually normal, although in patients with severe regurgitation aortic valve closure may occur early, resulting in wide splitting of the second heart sound. An opening snap indicates associated mitral stenosis but does not exclude predominant regurgitation. A low-pitched, third heart sound, occurring 0.12 to 0.17 of a second after the aortic valve closure sound at the completion of the rapid filling phase of the left ventricle, is believed to be caused by the sudden tensing of the papillary muscles, chordae tendineae, and valve leaflets, and is an important auscultatory feature of severe mitral regurgitation. The absence of a third heart sound suggests that if mitral regurgitation exists it is not severe. The third heart sound ushers in a rumbling, mid-diastolic murmur, which is usually shorter in duration than the murmur that follows the opening snap of the mitral valve in patients with mitral stenosis. A fourth heart sound is present in patients with acute severe mitral regurgitation, as occurs in rupture of chordae tendineae. A presystolic murmur is not ordinarily heard in patients with pure regurgitation and sinus rhythm, but is produced by significant mitral stenosis.

A systolic murmur, Grade III/VI intensity or louder, is the most characteristic auscultatory finding in patients with severe mitral regurgitation. It usually lasts throughout systole but occasionally is confined to early or late systole. It may be crescendo-decrescendo in configuration, and there is a rough correlation between the intensity and duration of the murmur and the magnitude of the regurgitant flow. The systolic murmur usually radiates into the axilla, but in a minority of patients, particularly those with ruptured chordae tendineae or primary involvement of the posterior mitral leaflets the regurgitant jet strikes the left atrial wall adjacent to the aortic root, and the systolic murmur is referred to the base of the heart and therefore may be confused with the murmur of aortic stenosis. However, the systolic murmur of aortic stenosis usually ends just before aortic valve closure, whereas that of mitral regurgitation ends with, or immediately after, the aortic closure sound. In patients with ruptured chordae tendineae the systolic murmur may have a cooing or "seagull" quality. (Mitral regurgitation owing to prolapse of the posterior mitral leaflet is often associated with a midsystolic ejection click followed by a late systolic murmur.)

Electrocardiogram. The electrocardiographic signs of ventricular hypertrophy are variable; in many patients, there is no clear-cut electrocardiographic evidence of enlargement of either ventricle. In severe regurgitation the signs of left ventricular hypertrophy are usually present, although in many patients associated right ventricular hypertrophy is apparent. Electrocardiographic signs of pure right ventricular hypertrophy occur in patients with severe pulmonary hypertension and, although unusual in patients with pure mitral regurgitation, they do not exclude this diagnosis. In patients with sinus rhythm the electrocardiogram characteristically shows evidence of left atrial enlargement, but right atrial hypertrophy may be present when pulmonary hypertension is severe. Evidence suggestive of posteroinferior ischemia may occur in patients with prolapse of the posterior leaflet. Prolonged, severe mitral regurgitation with marked left atrial enlargement usually results in atrial fibrillation.

Roentgenographic Features. The left ventricle and left atrium are the dominant chambers, and the latter may be enlarged to aneurysmal proportions. Although both mitral stenosis and regurgitation tend to increase left atrial size, the presence of marked left atrial enlargement usually indicates that regurgitation is the predominant

lesion and that it has existed for years. On fluoroscopic examination the left ventricle is hyperdynamic and the left atrium exhibits vigorous systolic expansions. Calcification of the mitral leaflets occurs commonly in patients with combined severe regurgitation and stenosis, but is uncommon in patients with pure regurgitation in whom the calcium may be confined to the mitral anulus.

Hemodynamics. The initial compensation to acutely induced mitral regurgitation consists of more complete systolic emptying of the left ventricle. However, a progressive increase in left ventricular end-diastolic volume occurs as the severity of the regurgitation increases and the function of the left ventricle deteriorates. The atrial contraction wave in the left atrial pressure pulse (*a* wave) is not as prominent as it is in mitral stenosis, but the *v* wave is often much taller, since it is inscribed during ventricular systole, when blood regurgitates from the left ventricle into the left atrium. Following the opening of the mitral valve, there is a particularly rapid *y* descent as the distended left atrium suddenly empties. The left ventricular end-diastolic pressure is either near the upper limits of normal or somewhat elevated. The effective cardiac output at rest may be well maintained for many years in spite of the presence of severe regurgitation, but it is usually depressed in seriously symptomatic patients. Although a left atrioventricular pressure gradient persisting throughout diastole indicates the presence of significant associated mitral stenosis, a brief, early diastolic gradient may occur in patients with pure regurgitation as a result of the torrential flow of blood across a normal-sized mitral orifice.

The diagnosis of mitral regurgitation can be established by means of indicator-dilution curves, the prompt appearance of indicator in left atrial blood following its injection into the left ventricle signifying the presence of mitral regurgitation. When the indicator is sampled from a peripheral artery, the curve characteristically ascends rapidly, but exhibits a gradual descending limb as indicator is washed back and forth between the left ventricle and left atrium. The regurgitant volume can be measured by determining the total left ventricular stroke volume angiocardiographically, while simultaneously measuring the effective forward stroke volume by the Fick method. The results of such studies suggest that the regurgitant volume may be of the same magnitude as the effective forward stroke volume or may even exceed it in patients with severe regurgitation. Qualitative, but clinically useful, estimates of the severity of regurgitation may be made by cineangiographic observation of the degree of left atrial opacification following the injection of contrast material into the left ventricle.

Patients with severe mitral regurgitation may be divided into several subgroups, depending on the compliance, i.e., the pressure-volume relationship, of the left atrium and pulmonary venous bed, which appears to be capable of modifying profoundly the clinical and hemodynamic picture.

Three major groups of patients with severe mitral regurgitation have been identified: (1) *Normal or reduced compliance.* In this group there is little enlargement of the left atrium but considerable elevation of the mean left atrial pressure, and particularly of the v wave. In many patients in this group severe mitral regurgitation developed acutely, as in those in whom it followed rupture of chordae tendineae or a tear of a mitral leaflet. Marked elevation of pulmonary vascular resistance frequently occurs in this group, and therefore right heart failure is a common clinical manifestation. Sinus rhythm is usually present, as is a fourth heart sound. (2) *Moderate increase in compliance.* By far the most common group consists of patients whose clinical and hemodynamic features are midway between those in the other two groups; moderate enlargement of the left atrium and significant elevation of the left atrial pressure are present. (3) *Marked increase in compliance.* At the other end of the spectrum from group 1 is a group of patients with severe chronic mitral regurgitation, massive enlargement of the left atrium, and normal or minimally elevated left atrial pressure. The pulmonary artery pressure and pulmonary vascular resistance are also normal or only slightly elevated. Clinically, these patients are usually disabled with fatigue and exhaustion because of a low cardiac output, but the symptoms of pulmonary congestion are less prominent. The mitral regurgitation is long-standing, and atrial fibrillation is almost invariably present. It is believed that long-standing mitral regurgitation may, in some instances, alter the physical properties of the left atrial wall and thereby displace the atrial pressure-volume curve, allowing a normal pressure to exist in a greatly enlarged left atrium.

Treatment. The medical management of mitral regurgitation is to restrict those physical activities that regularly produce extreme fatigue and dyspnea, to reduce sodium intake, and to enhance sodium excretion with the appropriate diuretics. Digitalis glycosides play a more important role in the treatment of mitral regurgitation than of mitral stenosis, since these drugs augment the output of the overburdened left ventricle. However, the same considerations apply to the reversion of atrial fibrillation to sinus rhythm, as in patients with mitral stenosis. In the late stages of the disease anticoagulants and leg binders are used to diminish the likelihood of developing peripheral venous thrombi and pulmonary emboli.

Although nonrheumatic mitral regurgitation can sometimes be treated by direct surgical repair of the defective valve, or by narrowing the widened anulus, effective surgical treatment of rheumatic mitral regurgitation generally requires total valvular replacement with a suitable prosthesis. The mortality rate of the latter procedure usually ranges from 10 to 20 per cent, depending on the level of compensation and the patient's general condition, as well as the experience and skill of the operative team. Although most patients who survive operation appear to be greatly improved, some degree of myocardial dysfunction may persist. The development of thrombi around the prosthesis, which may block the valvular orifice or result in systemic embolization, remains a serious hazard in the early as well as the late postoperative periods. The use of anticoagulants and newer prostheses which reduce the risk of thrombosis may minimize this complication.

In the selection of patients for surgical treatment, the chronic, often slowly progressive nature of the disease must be balanced against the immediate risks and long-term uncertainties attendant upon valve replacement. At the present time, patients with hemodynamically severe mitral regurgitation who are asymptomatic or who are limited only during severe exertion should not be considered as candidates for surgical treatment, since they may live for many years with relatively little deterioration. However, surgical treatment should be considered for patients so disabled that they are no longer able to work or perform normal household activities. The risks of valve replacement rise sharply when the disease advances so that the patient is symptomatic at rest, has developed congestive heart failure refractory to medical therapy, or has associated severe tricuspid regurgitation. However, operative treatment may be indicated even at these advanced stages of the disease, since conservative management has little to offer and the clinical and hemodynamic improvement following surgical treatment is occasionally dramatic. It is likely that both the immediate and long-term results of surgical treatment will improve considerably in the future, and the physician will be able to recommend operative treatment for selected patients with mitral regurgitation even before they become disabled.

When surgical treatment is contemplated, detailed hemodynamic investigations and selective left ventricular angiocardiography are generally indicated. These studies are helpful in confirming the presence of severe regurgitation, and aid in the identification of patients with primary myocardial disease and relatively mild functional mitral regurgitation who usually do not benefit from operation. Hemodynamic studies are also helpful in detecting and assessing the severity of associated valve lesions that may have to be dealt with at the time of operation or that might limit the patient's ultimate improvement if left untreated.

AORTIC STENOSIS

Etiology. Aortic stenosis may be congenital or secondary to rheumatic inflammation of the aortic valve or to calcification of the aortic cusps of unknown cause. The congenitally affected valves may be stenotic from birth and gradually become calcified during the first three decades of life and progressively more stenotic. Alternatively, the valve may be congenitally bicuspid, without serious narrowing of the aortic orifice during childhood, its abnormal architecture apparently makes the leaflets susceptible to a variety of hemodynamic stresses that ultimately lead to valvular calcification, increased rigidity, and narrowing of the aortic orifice. Rheumatic endocarditis of the aortic leaflets produces commissural fusion, most commonly between the two coronary cusps, resulting in a bicuspid valve, the leaflets of which are also susceptible to local trauma, ultimately leading to calcification and further narrowing. By the time the obstruction to left ventricular outflow causes serious disability and the valve is examined, either at operation or at autopsy, it is usually a rigid calcified mass, and even careful examination does not permit differentiation between rheumatic or congenital origin. The latter is more likely in males with isolated aortic stenosis, whereas rheumatic cause is favored by a history of active rheumatic fever, by clinical, hemodynamic or pathologic evidence of involvement of the mitral and tricuspid valves, and by associated severe aortic regurgitation. Idiopathic calcific stenosis in the elderly is rarely associated with fusion of the valve cusps, and although this process may give rise to many of the characteristic physical signs of aortic stenosis, the valvular obstruction is usually relatively mild.

In some patients with calcific aortic stenosis the calcium extends inferiorly from the left ventricular aspect of the aortic valve onto the anterior leaflet of the mitral valve. It may also invade the ventricular septum and rarely may be responsible for complete heart block. Occasionally, a calcific spur from the aortic aspect of the valve may obstruct a coronary ostium. Post-stenotic dilatation of the aorta occurs in the majority of patients with hemodynamically significant aortic stenosis.

Aortic stenosis occurs in about one fourth of all patients with chronic valvular heart disease, and pure or predominant aortic stenosis is approximately twice as frequent as pure or predominant aortic regurgitation. Approximately 80 per cent of adult patients with symptomatic valvular aortic stenosis are male.

Clinical Manifestations. Aortic stenosis rarely becomes of hemodynamic or clinical importance until the valve orifice has narrowed to approximately 25 per cent of normal. Even then the left ventricle is usually capable of compensating for the increased burden for many years by becoming hypertrophied, and decompensation develops only when the thickened left ventricle is no longer capable of sustaining the extra work. Thus, in contrast to mitral stenosis, which results in symptoms as soon as the obstruction becomes critical because the chamber just proximal to the narrowed valve provides little compensation, severe aortic stenosis may exist for many years without producing clinical disability.

Most patients with pure or predominant aortic stenosis do not become symptomatic until the fourth or fifth decade. *Exertional dyspnea, angina pectoris,* and *syncope* are the three cardinal symp-

toms. Dyspnea results from elevation of the left ventricular end-diastolic pressure, which in turn increases the mean left atrial and pulmonary capillary pressures. Angina pectoris usually develops somewhat later and resembles the pain of myocardial ischemia that occurs in patients with coronary artery disease. Severe angina pectoris in patients with aortic stenosis does not necessarily signify coexisting coronary artery disease; more commonly it is a consequence of the imbalance between myocardial oxygen requirements and oxygen availability; the oxygen needs of the hypertrophied left ventricle are elevated, while coronary flow is impeded by the resistance to coronary inflow produced by the elevated intramyocardial tension. Exertional syncope may result from a decline in arterial pressure caused by vasodilation in the exercising muscles in the face of a fixed cardiac output, or from a sudden fall in cardiac output and arterial pressure produced by an arrhythmia. If prolonged, the syncopal episode may be accompanied by convulsions and loss of sphincteric control. Many patients experience frequent episodes of dizziness or presyncope ("graying out") and learn to avoid frank unconsciousness by immediately discontinuing physical activity.

Since the resting cardiac output is well maintained until a late stage of the disease, marked fatigability, debilitation, peripheral cyanosis, and other clinical manifestations of a low cardiac output are usually not prominent until this stage is reached. Symptoms of left ventricular failure, with marked orthopnea, paroxysmal nocturnal dyspnea, and pulmonary edema also occur in the advanced stages of the disease. Preterminally there may be right ventricular failure with systemic venous hypertension, hepatomegaly, atrial fibrillation, and tricuspid regurgitation. Occasionally, aortic stenosis causes sudden death, although rarely in patients who previously were totally asymptomatic. In contrast to mitral stenosis, systemic embolization is uncommon in aortic stenosis, but when it does occur it usually results from the dislodgement of small calcific fragments from the diseased valve.

The general appearance, development, and nourishment of the patient with pure aortic stenosis are normal except in the terminal stages of the disease. The systemic arterial pressure is usually within normal limits. In the late stages, however, the systolic pressure often declines, and the pulse pressure narrows. Severe systemic hypertension is extremely unusual in patients with critical aortic stenosis, and a basal systolic arterial pressure exceeding 200 mm. of mercury practically excludes critical stenosis. On palpation, the peripheral arterial pulses characteristically rise slowly, with a delayed peak. Indirect recordings of the carotid pulse exhibit a gradually ascending limb, often with a prominent anacrotic notch or shoulder on the upstroke, as well as a delayed peak, with coarse systolic vibrations. A palpable double systolic wave, the so-called pulsus bisferiens, excludes pure or predominant aortic stenosis, and signifies the presence of dominant or pure aortic regurgitation or of idiopathic hypertrophic subaortic stenosis. In the late stages of the disease, when the stroke volume and the pulse pressure are reduced, the pulse amplitude is so small that the anacrotic nature of the pulse and the delay in its upstroke may become more difficult to appreciate. The jugular venous pulse may be normal, although in many patients the *a* wave is accentuated because of the diminished distensibility of the right ventricular cavity caused by the bulging, hypertrophied, interventricular septum and/or the presence of pulmonary hypertension. A prominent jugular venous *v* wave, signifying tricuspid regurgitation, is extremely rare in aortic stenosis and is observed only in the latest stages of the disease.

A precordial bulge suggests that cardiomegaly was present during early childhood and thus favors a congenital origin. On palpation, the apex beat is usually accentuated and displaced inferiorly and laterally, reflecting the presence of left ventricular hypertrophy. A double apical impulse may be appreciated, particularly with the patient in the left lateral recumbent position; the first outward expansion occurs during atrial systole and reflects the important contribution made by atrial contraction to ventricular filling, whereas the second outward expansion commences during early systole and is well sustained during most of ejection. The right ventricle is rarely prominent on palpation, except when pulmonary hypertension develops in the late stages of the disease. A systolic thrill is usually easily palpable at the base of the heart, in the jugular notch, and along the carotid arteries, but occasionally it may be felt only if the patient leans forward and expires forcibly. In patients who do not have severe pulmonary emphysema, a particularly thick chest wall, thoracic deformity, or a markedly depressed stroke volume, the absence of a systolic thrill signifies that the aortic stenosis is relatively mild.

On auscultation the rhythm is generally regular, and the presence of atrial fibrillation should alert the examiner to the possibility of associated mitral valve disease. An early systolic ejection sound, actually the opening snap of the aortic valve, is frequently audible in children and adolescents with noncalcific valvular aortic stenosis. When the valve becomes calcified and rigid, this sound usually disappears. Similarly, the sound of aortic valve closure can be identified most frequently in patients with aortic stenosis who have pliable valves; calcification tends to diminish the intensity of this sound as well. As aortic stenosis increases in severity, left ventricular systole may become prolonged, so that the aortic valve closure sound no longer precedes the pulmonic valve closure sound, and the two components may become synchronous, or aortic valve closure may even follow pulmonic valve closure. The latter condition, paradoxical splitting of the second heart sound, may be recognized by auscultation, or phonocardiographically by the finding that the time intervals between the two components do not widen but actually narrow during inspiration. Paradoxical splitting of the second sound in the absence of left bundle branch block usually excludes mild obstruction to left ventricular outflow, although the converse is not true in that the second sound behaves normally during respiration in some patients with severe aortic stenosis. A fourth heart sound, i.e., an atrial gallop, is audible at the apex in many patients with severe aortic stenosis. It reflects the presence of considerable left ventricular hypertrophy and an elevated left ventricular end-diastolic pressure. A third heart sound, i.e., a ventricular gallop, generally occurs in adult patients with aortic stenosis when the left ventricle dilates and fails.

The systolic murmur in aortic stenosis is characteristically ejection in quality; it commences not simultaneously with, but shortly after, the first heart sound, increases in intensity to reach a peak toward the middle of the ejection period, and diminishes progressively thereafter to end just before aortic valve closure. The murmur is usually low-pitched, rough and rasping, and is loudest at the base of the heart, usually in the second intercostal space just to the right of the sternum. It is transmitted upward to the jugular notch, along the carotid arteries, and may occasionally be heard as far distant as the brachial artery. In patients with trivial degrees of obstruction the murmur may be relatively soft and brief and confined to the middle of systole. However, in almost all patients with significant aortic stenosis, the murmur is loud, at least grade III/VI, and its intensity and duration are not particularly helpful in distinguishing moderate from severe stenosis. However, when left ventricular failure supervenes and the stroke volume declines, the murmur may again diminish in intensity. In some patients the murmur is transmitted downward and to the apex, and may be confused with the systolic murmur of mitral regurgitation. However, in the latter condition the murmur is usually holosystolic, but it is diamond-shaped and of the ejection type in aortic stenosis.

Electrocardiogram. The electrocardiogram reveals evidence of left ventricular hypertrophy in most patients with severe aortic stenosis. In advanced cases, in addition to the voltage criteria for left ventricular hypertrophy, there are ST segment depressions and T wave inversions in standard lead I, aVL and left precordial leads. However, there is no close correlation between the electrocardiogram and the hemodynamic severity of obstruction. The electrocardiographic signs of an old myocardial infarction do not necessarily exclude severe aortic stenosis, but suggest that symptoms of myocardial ischemia or left heart failure may be related to coronary artery disease as well as to obstruction to left ventricular outflow. The presence of left bundle branch block or intraventricular conduction defects with QRS prolongation suggest diffuse fibrotic involvement of the myocardium. Atrial fibrillation or electrocardiographic signs of left atrial enlargement are rarely seen in patients with pure aortic stenosis; their presence should suggest the possibility of associated mitral valve disease.

Roentgenographic Features. Because the development of concentric left ventricular hypertrophy is the initial response to obstruction to left ventricular outflow, the chest roentgenogram may show no or little over-all cardiac enlargement for many years. Considerable hypertrophy without dilatation may produce some rounding of the cardiac apex in the frontal projection and slight backward displacement in the lateral view; significant aortic stenosis is often associated with post-stenotic dilatation of the ascending aorta. Aortic calcification is usually readily apparent on fluoroscopic examination with an image intensifier or on films obtained by means of body section laminagraphy. As the disease progresses and the left ventricle dilates, there is progressively more evidence of left ventricular enlargement. In the late stages of the disease there may also be roentgenologic signs of pulmonary congestion, as well as enlargement of the left atrium, pulmonary artery, and right side of the heart.

Hemodynamics. The primary hemodynamic abnormality in valvular aortic stenosis is the pressure gradient between the left ventricle and aorta during the systolic ejection period. There is now considerable evidence that a large pressure gradient may exist for years without producing any symptoms. As stenosis progresses in severity, the left ventricular systolic pressure continues to rise, but rarely exceeds 300 mm. of mercury. As with mitral stenosis, in order to estimate the severity of obstruction, it is necessary to measure both the transvalvular pressure gradient and blood flow, preferably simultaneously. A peak systolic pressure gradient exceeding 50 mm. of mercury in the face of a normal cardiac output or an effective aortic orifice less than 0.7 square centimeter per square meter of body surface area is generally considered to represent critical obstruction to left ventricular outflow. The left ventricular pressure pulse exhibits a rounded summit as the contraction of this chamber becomes progressively more isometric, and pulsus alternans in the left ventricle is frequent in patients with severe stenosis. The elevated left ventricular end-diastolic pressure observed in most patients with severe aortic stenosis does not necessarily signify the presence of left ventricular failure, but may instead reflect diminished compliance of the hypertrophied left ventricular wall.

A large *a* wave in the left atrial pressure pulse is usually present in patients with severe aortic stenosis, because of unusually forceful atrial contraction, diminished ventricular compliance, or a combination of these factors. Atrial contraction tends to raise left ventricular end-diastolic pressure without producing a concomitant elevation of mean left atrial pressure. This "booster pump" function of the left atrium prevents the pulmonary venous and capillary pressures from rising to levels that would produce pulmonary congestion, while at the same time maintaining

left ventricular end-diastolic pressure at the elevated level necessary for effective left ventricular contraction. Loss of an appropriately timed, vigorous atrial contraction, as occurs in atrial fibrillation or atrioventricular dissociation, occasionally results in a rapid aggravation of symptoms or in cardiovascular collapse, even when the ventricular response is not particularly rapid.

The cardiac output and stroke volume at rest are within normal limits, but are usually fixed and show little elevation during exercise in most patients with critical aortic stenosis. Late in the disease the cardiac output and stroke volume may decline, and the mean left atrial, pulmonary artery wedge, pulmonary arterial, and right ventricular systolic pressures usually become elevated while the left ventricular-aortic pressure gradient falls. A prominent *a* wave in the right atrial pressure pulse is also commonly found. Hemodynamic evidence of mitral regurgitation, with a tall left atrial *v* wave and sharp *y* descent, may occur in the later stages of the disease in association with marked left ventricular dilatation.

Angiocardiographic studies with left ventricular injection of contrast material are helpful in defining the size of the left ventricular cavity, the thickness of the wall, the motion of the left ventricular wall, the site of obstruction, and the degree of deformity and mobility of the aortic valve cusps, as well as the diameter of the ascending aorta. In patients with critical narrowing, a jet of contrast substance passing through the aortic orifice is readily visualized, but left ventricular angiography is not as useful as left heart catheterization in determining the severity of obstruction. When contrast substance is injected into the ascending aorta, the aortic valve cusps can also be outlined, and any associated aortic regurgitation can be detected and its severity evaluated.

Left heart catheterization and angiographic studies are indicated for most patients suspected of having severe aortic stenosis, and should be performed before a final decision concerning operative treatment is made. These investigations are particularly indicated for (1) young, asymptomatic patients with noncalcific aortic stenosis in order to define the severity of their aortic obstruction, since operation may be indicated if aortic stenosis is critical; (2) patients in whom it is suspected that the obstruction to left ventricular outflow is not at the aortic valve, but rather that it is either sub- or supravalvular; (3) patients with clinical signs of aortic stenosis and symptoms of myocardial ischemia in whom associated coronary artery disease is suspected; it is important to determine whether aortic stenosis and/or coronary atherosclerosis is responsible for the symptoms in this group of patients, and coronary arteriography may have to be done in addition to left heart catheterization; and (4) patients with multivalvular disease in whom the role played by each valvular deformity must be defined before operative treatment is planned.

A significant number of patients with rheumatic

aortic stenosis have associated mitral valve disease. Aortic stenosis intensifies the severity of mitral regurgitation by increasing the pressure driving blood from the left ventricle to the left atrium. The dilatation of the left ventricle, which occurs late in the course in some patients with aortic stenosis, further intensifies the magnitude of the mitral regurgitant flow. When aortic stenosis and mitral stenosis coexist, the mitral obstruction masks many of the clinical findings of aortic stenosis. The reduction of cardiac output induced by mitral stenosis lowers the pressure gradient across the aortic valve, diminishes the frequency of anginal and syncopal episodes, and retards the development of aortic calcification and severe left ventricular hypertrophy. On the other hand, symptoms considered more characteristic of mitral stenosis, such as pulmonary congestion, hemoptysis, and atrial fibrillation, occur more frequently in patients with the combined stenotic lesions than in those with isolated aortic stenosis. Careful physical, electrocardiographic, and roentgenologic examinations in patients with aortic and mitral stenosis generally reveal more evidence of left ventricular enlargement than in patients with pure mitral stenosis, and left heart catheterization is helpful in defining the relative importance of each valvular abnormality.

Treatment. Strenuous physical activity should be restricted in cases of severe aortic stenosis with evidence of left ventricular hypertrophy, even in the asymptomatic stage. Nitroglycerin is helpful in relieving angina pectoris, and digitalis glycosides, salt restriction, and diuretics are indicated in the treatment of congestive heart failure. The most critical decision in the management of aortic stenosis concerns the advisability of surgical treatment. The indications for and results of operation, as well as the techniques, differ considerably depending on the patient's age and the nature of the valvular deformity.

In children and adolescents with noncalcific, congenital aortic stenosis considerable improvement of the hemodynamic state can be expected from simple commissural incision under direct vision. When carried out by an experienced surgeon, this procedure can be expected to enlarge the size of the valvular orifice significantly without increasing the magnitude of aortic regurgitation. The mortality rate is less than 5 per cent. Accordingly, this operation is recommended not only for symptomatic patients but also for asymptomatic children and adolescents with hemodynamic evidence of severe obstruction to left ventricular outflow, with a peak systolic pressure gradient exceeding 50 mm. of mercury when the cardiac output is normal, or a calculated effective orifice less than 0.7 centimeter per square meter of body surface area. From the technical point of view it is well to consider that the smaller the patient's aorta, the more difficult the surgical procedure; for this reason, operation is generally deferred until the patient's weight exceeds 15 to 17 kg. The procedure is always performed during total cardiopulmonary bypass. The ascending aorta is occluded, and the aorta is opened just above the aortic valve. The coronary arteries are perfused with oxygenated blood, and the fused commissures divided. Although the operation can be expected to result in complete or almost complete relief of obstruction in most patients, the valves cannot be rendered entirely normal anatomically, and it is possible that they will later become deformed, calcified, and stenotic again.

The surgical problems presented by the adult patient with calcific aortic stenosis are more serious. The difference between the results of simple commissurotomy in children and in adults is largely attributable to the seriousness of the deformity and the calcification of the valve that is almost invariably present in adults with severe aortic stenosis, regardless of the underlying cause. In most adults with calcific aortic stenosis satisfactory valve function cannot be restored, even by deliberate sculpturing procedures carried out under direct vision, and prosthetic replacement of the aortic valve is necessary. In addition, since patients with calcific aortic stenosis are usually elderly, particular attention must be directed to the levels of hepatic, renal, and pulmonary function before valve replacement is recommended.

Aortic valve replacement is associated with a higher immediate mortality than is aortic commissurotomy in childhood—10 to 20 per cent in most centers—and the long-term results and complications associated with the use of presently available prostheses still have not been defined completely. Accordingly, a more conservative approach to operative treatment is warranted for the adult with calcific aortic stenosis than for the child with noncalcific stenosis. However, it is now clear that the outlook for survival is limited for patients whose symptoms are believed to result primarily from aortic stenosis and who have hemodynamic evidence of severe obstruction, as defined above. If possible, operation should be performed before the development of frank left ventricular failure, as the operative risk in such patients is extremely high, and evidence of myocardial disease may persist even if the operation is technically successful. Nonetheless, in view of the very poor prognosis of such patients when treated medically, there is usually little choice but to advise surgical treatment.

In patients in whom severe aortic stenosis and coronary artery disease coexist, successful relief of stenosis may result in striking clinical improvement, presumably because of the diminution of the pressure load on the left ventricle and the resultant decrease in myocardial oxygen requirements. However, replacement of the aortic valve can relieve only one aspect of the problem, and the presence of associated coronary artery disease certainly raises the risk of operation and diminishes the likelihood of complete symptomatic recovery.

The management of asymptomatic patients with severe calcific aortic stenosis continues to pose a difficult problem. In most instances it seems prudent to postpone operation since the prognosis is not necessarily poor in such patients, and they may survive for years before disability develops. However, it is likely that as the results of total prosthetic replacement of the aortic valve improve, many of these patients will become candidates for operation before their disease reaches the symptomatic stage.

OTHER FORMS OF OBSTRUCTION TO LEFT VENTRICULAR OUTFLOW

Although valvular aortic stenosis is the most common form of obstruction to left ventricular outflow, three other lesions may be responsible for this physiologic abnormality.

Idiopathic Hypertrophic Subaortic Stenosis

Idiopathic hypertrophic subaortic stenosis is characterized by severe hypertrophy of the left ventricle, involving in particular the interventricular septum and the left ventricular outflow tract. During systole the hypertrophied muscle in the outflow tract may constrict this region sufficiently to obstruct left ventricular ejection, and in some hearts the hypertrophied septum bulges into and encroaches on the right ventricular outflow tract as well. Most patients with hypertrophic subaortic stenosis are males, and in about one third of the cases the disease occurs in more than one member of a family. The most common symptoms are dyspnea, angina, dizziness, syncope and left ventricular failure. On physical examination the arterial pulse is usually sharp, a fourth heart sound is regularly audible, and a systolic murmur of the ejection type is heard most easily along the left sternal border or at the apex, rather than at the aortic area or along the carotid vessels.

The electrocardiogram reflects the presence of left ventricular hypertrophy, and in some patients there are abnormally deep and broad Q waves, which result from gross septal hypertrophy rather than from myocardial infarction. On roentgenologic examination left ventricular enlargement is usually present, although aortic valvular calcification or dilatation of the ascending aorta is generally not apparent. The indirect carotid pulse tracing rises rapidly and exhibits a double peak during systole. The obstruction can be localized to the left ventricular outflow tract by demonstration of a pressure gradient between the left ventricular cavity and the subvalvular area at left heart catheterization. In addition to obstruction to ventricular outflow, hypertrophic subaortic stenosis is characterized by an abnormally reduced ventricular compliance, an important consequence of which is interference with left ventricular filling.

The variability of the hemodynamic findings from moment to moment is an important feature of this condition. Obstruction is intensified after an extrasystole and leads to a characteristic reduction of the post-extrasystolic arterial pulse pressure. Since the obstruction to left ventricular outflow results from systolic contraction of the hypertrophied muscle in the walls of the left ventricular outflow tract, the size of the left ventricular cavity during systole, the force of left ventricular contraction, and the transmural pressure that distends the outflow tract during systole are the principal determinants of the severity of obstruction. Reduction in ventricular volume produced by the Valsalva maneuver, isoproterenol, nitroglycerin, digitalis glycosides, and muscular exercise tends to intensify the obstruction. Conversely, administration of phenylephrine, expansion of the blood volume, and general anesthesia increase ventricular volume and tend to diminish the severity of obstruction.

The natural history of idiopathic hypertrophic subaortic stenosis is extremely variable. Sudden death occurs in a small number of patients, including some who were previously asymptomatic or who had only mild left ventricular outflow tract obstruction. In general, however, the disease progresses only slowly. Seriously ill patients should be treated either with beta-adrenergic receptor blocking agents or surgical incision of the hypertrophied outflow tract.

Discrete Congenital Subvalvular Aortic Stenosis

Discrete congenital subvalvular aortic stenosis is produced by either a membranous diaphragm or a fibrous ridge just below the aortic valve. The clinical features are similar to those in valvular congenital aortic stenosis except that the systolic ejection sound is rarely heard and the diastolic murmur of aortic regurgitation is somewhat more common. Also, no valvular calcification is evident roentgenographically, even in adults. The differentiation between valvular and discrete subvalvular aortic stenosis can be made with certainty only by demonstrating a pressure gradient at the time a catheter is withdrawn across the left ventricular outflow tract or by actually visualizing the obstruction by means of left ventricular angiocardiography. Bacterial endocarditis involving the aortic valve is not uncommon. The operative indications are similar to those in congenital valvular aortic stenosis, and surgical treatment, which consists of excising the membrane or fibrous ridge, is usually effective.

Supravalvular Aortic Stenosis

Supravalvular aortic stenosis is an uncommon congenital anomaly produced by narrowing of the ascending aorta or by a fibrous diaphragm with a small opening just above the aortic valve. The malformation may be associated with diffuse tubular hypoplasia of the ascending aorta, and with multiple peripheral stenoses of branches of the pulmonary arteries. Frequently it occurs in families. In the nonfamilial cases it may be associated with mental retardation and a peculiar facies; the latter finding may be related to infantile hypercalcemia. The clinical findings in supravalvular aortic stenosis are similar to those observed in patients with valvular aortic stenosis except that the aortic closure sound is frequently accentuated and the transmission of the murmur along the carotid vessels may be unusually prominent. Generally there is no systolic ejection sound nor any post-stenotic dilation of the aorta, and there may be inequality of the arterial pressures in the upper extremities. The definitive diagnosis of supravalvular aortic stenosis is established by demonstrating a pressure gradient just above the aortic valve by retrograde aortic catheterization and a constriction in this region by aortography. Patients with severe obstruction and severe left ventricular hypertrophy should receive surgical treatment, which consists of enlarging the opening in the fibrous diaphragm or excising the affected portion of the aorta and replacing it with a graft.

AORTIC REGURGITATION

Etiology. The disease is rheumatic in origin in approximately 80 per cent of instances. Rheumatic fever causes thickening, deformation, and shortening of the individual aortic valve cusps, changes that prevent their proper closure during diastole. Less commonly, bacterial endocarditis may attack a valve previously affected by rheumatic disease, a congenitally deformed valve, or a normal aortic valve, and may perforate or erode one or more leaflets. Patients with discrete membranous subaortic stenosis may develop thickening of the aortic valve leaflets, which in turn leads to mild or moderate degrees of aortic regurgitation and makes these valves particularly susceptible to bacterial endocarditis. Aortic valvular regurgitation may also occur in patients with congenital bicuspid aortic valves. Prolapse of an aortic cusp resulting in progressive aortic regurgitation occurs in approximately 15 per cent of patients with ventricular septal defect. Although traumatic rupture of the aortic valve is an uncommon cause of aortic regurgitation, it is still the most frequent serious lesion observed in patients surviving nonpenetrating cardiac injuries. Congenital fenestrations of the aortic valve occasionally produce mild or moderate degrees of aortic regurgitation. In patients with aortic regurgitation due to primary valvular disease, dilatation of the aortic ring may occur secondarily and may intensify the regurgitation.

Aortic regurgitation may also be due entirely to severe aortic dilatation without primary involvement of the valve leaflets; in these patients widening of the aortic anulus and separation of the aortic leaflets are responsible for the aortic regurgitation. Syphilis and ankylosing rheumatoid spondylitis may be associated with cellular in-

filtration and scarring of the media of the thoracic aorta, changes that often lead to aortic dilatation, aneurysm formation, and severe regurgitation. In syphilis of the aorta the involvement of the intima may also narrow the coronary ostia, which in turn may be responsible for coronary insufficiency. Cystic medionecrosis of the ascending aorta—which is frequently but not always associated with Marfan's syndrome—idiopathic dilatation of the aorta, and severe hypertension may also widen the aortic anulus and lead to progressive aortic regurgitation. Occasionally, retrograde dissection of the aorta to the aortic anulus produces aortic regurgitation.

The association of aortic stenosis of hemodynamic significance occurs only in patients with aortic regurgitation who have rheumatic or congenital disease and, for all practical purposes, the presence of hemodynamically significant aortic stenosis, not merely a systolic murmur, excludes all of the rarer forms of aortic regurgitation. Approximately 75 per cent of patients with pure or predominant regurgitation are males; however, females predominate among patients with aortic regurgitation who have associated mitral valve disease.

Clinical Manifestations. The average time interval between the first episode of acute rheumatic fever and the development of significant aortic regurgitation is approximately seven years, and this period is followed by an asymptomatic interval of approximately ten years, during which the severity of the aortic regurgitation may continue to increase. In patients with cardiovascular syphilis the latent period between the primary infection and the development of hemodynamically significant aortic regurgitation averages 15 years, and these patients usually remain asymptomatic for about another seven years. Once symptoms of left heart failure develop, the prognosis is usually worse in patients in whom the aortic regurgitation is due to syphilis than in those with rheumatic disease.

A careful history is often helpful in determining the cause of aortic regurgitation. A family history may frequently be elicited from patients with Marfan's syndrome, and a history of heart murmur heard early in life may be obtained from patients with congenital aortic regurgitation. Patients with aortic regurgitation of obscure cause should also be questioned in detail about prior chest trauma. A history compatible with subacute bacterial endocarditis may sometimes be elicited from patients with rheumatic or congenital involvement of the aortic valve; the infection often precipitates or seriously aggravates pre-existing symptoms.

As already indicated, severe aortic regurgitation may exist for many years without producing symptoms. The first complaint is often an uncomfortable awareness of the heart beat, especially on lying down. Sinus tachycardia occurring during exertion or with emotion or premature systoles may produce particularly uncomfortable palpitations, as well as pounding in the head. These complaints may persist for many years before the development of exertional dyspnea, usually the first symptom of diminished cardiac reserve. This is usually followed by angina pectoris, orthopnea, paroxysmal nocturnal dyspnea, excessive diaphoresis, and, very late in the disease, by dyspnea at rest.

Angina occurs frequently in younger patients with severe aortic regurgitation, and it is not necessary to invoke the presence of coronary artery disease to explain its origin. Myocardial ischemia occurs in patients with aortic regurgitation because both left ventricular dilatation and the increased left ventricular systolic pressure characteristic of this disease tend to elevate the systolic tension developed by the myocardium and thereby increase myocardial oxygen requirements. However, the major portion of coronary blood flow occurs during diastole, when aortic, i.e., coronary, perfusion pressure is lower than normal. The clinical features of angina pectoris in patients with aortic regurgitation may differ from those commonly observed in patients with coronary artery disease or predominant aortic stenosis. Thus, anginal pain may develop at rest as well as during exertion in patients with aortic regurgitation. Nocturnal angina is a particularly troublesome symptom and is frequently accompanied by profuse sweating. The anginal episodes may be prolonged, associated with profound diaphoresis, and often do not respond satisfactorily to sublingual nitroglycerin. Late in the course of the disease symptoms of systemic fluid accumulation, including painful congestive hepatomegaly, ankle edema, and ascites, may develop. Patients with severe aortic regurgitation do not tolerate high fevers, infections, or cardiac arrhythmias, and may die in pulmonary edema as a result of one of these complications.

The general examination should be directed toward the detection of causes predisposing to aortic regurgitation, such as Marfan's syndrome, rheumatoid spondylitis, syphilis, essential hypertension, and ventricular septal defect. As one approaches the patient with free aortic regurgitation, the jarring of the entire body and the bobbing motion of the head with each systole can be appreciated; the large stroke volume may even rock the bed in which the patient is lying. The abrupt distention and collapse of the larger arteries are easily visible in patients with severe regurgitation. On palpation there is a rapidly rising "water-hammer" pulse, which collapses suddenly as arterial pressure falls rapidly during late systole and diastole (Corrigan pulse). Capillary pulsation (Quincke pulse), an alternate paling and flushing of the skin at the root of the nail while pressure is applied to the tip of the nail, may also be observed. A booming, "pistol-shot" sound can be heard over the femoral arteries, and a to-and-fro murmur (Duroziez's sign) is audible if the femoral artery is lightly compressed with a stethoscope.

The arterial pulse pressure is widened; the systolic pressure is elevated, sometimes to as high as 200 mm. of mercury, and the diastolic arterial pressure is depressed. The measurement of arterial diastolic pressure with a sphygmomanometer may be complicated by the fact that systolic sounds are frequently heard with the cuff completely deflated. However, the level of cuff pressure at the time of muffling of the Korotkoff sounds generally corresponds reasonably well with the true arterial diastolic pressure. The severity of aortic regurgitation does not always correlate directly with the arterial pulse pressure; in many instances severe regurgitation exists in patients with arterial pressures in the range of 140/60 mm. of mercury. As the disease progresses and the left ventricular end-diastolic pressure and peripheral vascular resistance rise, the arterial diastolic pressure may rise to levels higher than those that existed at earlier stages of the disease.

The apex beat is displaced laterally and inferiorly. In patients with free regurgitation the left ventricle is particularly hyperdynamic. The systolic expansion and subsequent retraction of the apex contrast sharply with the sustained systolic thrust observed in patients with severe aortic stenosis. A diastolic thrill is frequently felt along the left sternal border in patients with severe regurgitation, and a prominent systolic thrill may be palpable in the jugular notch and transmitted upward along the carotid arteries. This thrill and the accompanying systolic murmur are due to the markedly increased blood flow across the aortic orifice; they do not necessarily indicate that aortic stenosis is present. Palpation or indirect recording of the carotid arterial pulse reveals it to be bisferiens, i.e., with two systolic waves separated by a trough, in many patients with pure aortic regurgitation or with combined stenosis and regurgitation.

In the presence of severe aortic regurgitation the sound of aortic valve closure is usually diminished or absent, and the indirectly recorded carotid arterial pulse does not usually show a clear-cut incisura. A third heart sound is common, and occasionally a fourth heart sound may also be heard. A loud systolic ejection sound is common and presumably results from the sudden dilatation of the aorta by a greatly increased stroke volume. At least three distinct heart murmurs can usually be distinguished in patients with severe regurgitation. The murmur of aortic regurgitation is a high-pitched, blowing, decrescendo diastolic murmur usually heard best at Erb's point in the third intercostal space to the left of the sternum. In patients with mild regurgitation this murmur is brief, usually lasting less than one third of diastole. However, as the severity of regurgitation increases, the murmur generally becomes louder and longer, and in patients with free aortic regurgitation it is usually holodiastolic. When the murmur is soft, it can be heard best with the diaphragm of the stethoscope and with the patient sitting up, leaning forward, and holding the breath in forced expiration. As this murmur increases in intensity it tends to radiate widely, particularly down the lower sternal edge. In patients in whom the regurgitation is caused by primary valvular disease, the diastolic murmur is usually louder along the left than along the right sternal border. However, when the decrescendo diastolic murmur is heard best along the right sternal border, it suggests that the aortic regurgitation is caused by dilatation or an aneurysm of the aortic root.

The murmur of aortic regurgitation may be difficult to distinguish from that of pulmonic regurgitation in patients with multivalvular rheumatic heart disease. However, on a purely statistical basis, a diastolic blowing murmur along the left sternal border is much more commonly caused by aortic than by pulmonic regurgitation, even in a patient with mitral valve disease. Unless it is trivial in magnitude, aortic regurgitation can also be recognized by peripheral signs, such as a widened pulse pressure or a collapsing pulse. On the other hand, the Graham Steell murmur of pulmonary regurgitation is usually accompanied by clinical evidence of severe pulmonary hypertension, including a loud and palpable pulmonary component of the second heart sound, and it is usually not well heard in the second interspace at the left sternal margin. In addition, on phonocardiograms the murmur of aortic regurgitation begins with the aortic second sound and therefore commences somewhat before the murmur of pulmonary regurgitation.

A systolic ejection murmur is generally heard best at the base of the heart and is transmitted to the jugular notch and along the carotid vessels. This murmur may be as loud as grade V/VI without reflecting organic obstruction; it is often higher pitched and less rasping in quality than in patients with predominant aortic stenosis.

The third murmur frequently heard in patients with aortic regurgitation is the Austin Flint murmur, soft, low-pitched, and rumbling. It is probably produced by the aortic regurgitant stream displacing the anterior leaflet of the mitral valve and producing functional mitral stenosis. However, this displacement of the mitral valve does not appear to be associated with significant obstruction to left ventricular filling. This murmur may also be produced by late diastolic mitral regurgitation. In patients with rheumatic aortic regurgitation it may be difficult to distinguish the Austin Flint murmur from the rumbling diastolic murmur of mitral stenosis. Both are loudest at the apex, but the murmur of mitral stenosis is usually accompanied by a loud first heart sound and follows the opening snap of the mitral valve, whereas the Austin Flint murmur is usually associated with a soft first sound and follows a ventricular diastolic gallop. The Austin Flint murmur is usually shorter in duration than the murmur of mitral stenosis, and in patients with sinus rhythm the latter more frequently exhibits presystolic accentuation. The presence of atrial fibrillation or electrocardiographic evidence of left atrial enlargement favors organic mitral stenosis. A blowing holosystolic murmur at the apex, which is transmitted to the axilla, may also

be heard in patients with marked left ventricular dilatation and functional mitral regurgitation.

Electrocardiogram. In patients with mild aortic regurgitation there may be no electrocardiographic abnormalities, but as the severity of aortic regurgitation increases so do the electrocardiographic signs of left ventricular hypertrophy. In addition to the abnormally tall R waves over the left precordium and the deep S waves over the right precordium, patients with severe aortic regurgitation frequently exhibit ST segment depressions and T wave inversions in leads 1, aVL, V_5 and V_6. Electrocardiographic signs of previous myocardial infarction generally indicate associated coronary artery disease. Left axis deviation in the frontal plane and/or QRS prolongation denote diffuse myocardial disease, generally associated with patchy fibrosis, signs usually associated with a poor prognosis.

Roentgenographic Features. Although mild aortic regurgitation is not accompanied by roentgenographic changes, moderate or severe degrees of regurgitation are always associated with varying degrees of left ventricular enlargement. The apex is displaced downward and to the left on the frontal projection, and frequently the cardiac shadow appears to extend below the left diaphragm. Left ventricular enlargement can also be appreciated in the left anterior oblique and lateral projections, in which the left ventricle is displaced posteriorly and encroaches on the spine. In patients in whom primary valvular disease is responsible for the aortic regurgitation, the ascending aorta and aortic knob may be moderately dilated and extend further to the right than the right atrial shadow in the frontal view. On fluoroscopic examination the aorta and left ventricle pulsate vigorously in opposite directions during systole. When aortic regurgitation is caused by primary disease of the aortic wall, there may be aneurysmal dilatation of the aorta roentgenographically, and the aorta may fill the retrosternal space in the lateral view.

Hemodynamics. The total stroke volume expelled by the left ventricle is increased in aortic regurgitation, since it consists of the sum of the effective forward stroke volume and the volume of blood that regurgitates back into the left ventricle. In contrast to mitral regurgitation, in which a fraction of the left ventricular stroke volume is delivered into the low-pressure left atrium, in aortic regurgitation the entire left ventricular stroke volume is ejected into the aorta, a higher pressure chamber. An increase of the left ventricular end-diastolic volume constitutes the major hemodynamic compensation to aortic regurgitation, and the total stroke volume is augmented through the operation of the Frank-Starling mechanism. Recent measurements of aortic regurgitant flow by means of angiocardiographic techniques, as well as with electromagnetic flowmeter probes placed on the aorta during operation, have revealed that in patients with free aortic regurgitation the volume of regurgitant flow may be of the same order of magnitude as the effective forward stroke volume. Dilatation of the left ventricle allows this chamber to expel a larger stroke volume without requiring increase in the relative shortening of each myofibril. On the other hand, through the operation of Laplace's law, left ventricular dilatation increases the left ventricular systolic tension required to develop a given level of systolic pressure. As left ventricular function deteriorates, the end-diastolic volume increases without further elevation of the aortic regurgitant volume. Considerable thickening of the left ventricular wall also occurs with chronic aortic regurgitation, and at autopsy the hearts of these patients may be among the largest encountered, occasionally exceeding 1000 grams in weight.

The reduction of aortic diastolic pressure in aortic regurgitation shortens the left ventricular isometric contraction period, which is helpful in allowing a longer left ventricular ejection period. The reverse pressure gradient from aorta to left ventricle, which is responsible for the aortic regurgitant flow, falls progressively during diastole, accounting for the decrescendo nature of the diastolic murmur. Equilibration between aortic and left ventricular pressures may occur toward the end of diastole, particularly when the heart rate is slow, and the left ventricular end-diastolic pressure may be elevated, occasionally to extreme levels (> 40 mm. of mercury). Rarely, the left ventricular pressure exceeds the left atrial pressure toward the end of diastole, and this reversed pressure gradient closes the mitral valve prematurely, or in patients with mitral disease produces diastolic mitral reflux.

In patients with free aortic regurgitation the effective forward cardiac output is usually normal or slightly reduced at rest, but fails to rise normally during exertion. In the most advanced cases there may be considerable elevation of the left atrial, pulmonary artery wedge, pulmonary arterial and right ventricular pressures, and the cardiac output at rest declines. A rough estimate of the severity of aortic regurgitation is generally provided by the recording of aortic and left ventricular pressures. In addition, indicator dilution techniques with left ventricular injection and arterial sampling are helpful since they show an unusually prolonged descending limb. A qualitative index of the severity of aortic regurgitation may also be obtained by determining the intensity of left ventricular opacification and the size of the left ventricle during thoracic cineaortography. This technique also allows the detection of associated mitral regurgitation. The volume of aortic regurgitant flow, like that of mitral regurgitant flow, may be determined by quantitative angiocardiography.

Treatment.   The left ventricular failure of aortic regurgitation at first usually responds to treatment with digitalis glycosides, salt restriction, and diuretics. Digitalis may also be indicated for patients with severe regurgitation and dilated left ventricles without symptoms of frank left ventricular failure, as it may retard the development of the latter complication. Cardiac arrhythmias and infections are poorly tolerated by patients with free aortic regurgitation and must be treated particularly promptly and vigorously. Although nitroglycerin and long-acting nitrites are not as helpful in relieving anginal pain as in patients with coronary artery disease or aortic stenosis, they are worth a trial. Patients with syphilitic aortitis should receive a full course of penicillin therapy.

As in patients with aortic stenosis, the most critical decision in therapy concerns the advisability and proper timing of surgical treatment. Total replacement of the aortic valve with a suitable prosthesis is generally necessary in patients with rheumatic aortic regurgitation and in many patients with other forms of regurgitation. Rarely, when a leaflet has been perforated during an episode of bacterial endocarditis or torn from its attachments to the aortic anulus, surgical repair may be possible. When aortic regurgitation is due to aneurysmal dilatation of the anulus and ascending aorta, rather than to primary valvular involvement, it may be possible to reduce the regurgitation by narrowing the anulus or by excising a portion of the aorta without operating directly upon the aortic valve itself. More frequently, however, regurgitation can be eliminated only by replacing the aortic valve, excising the aneurysm responsible for the regurgitation and replacing the latter with a graft. This formidable procedure carries with it a higher risk than aortic valve replacement alone, since the diseased, dilated aortic wall, particularly in the presence of cystic medionecrosis, does not hold sutures well. As in patients with aortic stenosis, the risks of aortic valve replacement are largely dependent on the stage of the disease. Surgical treatment should be considered only for patients who have free aortic regurgitation and who are symptomatic on ordinary activity in spite of maximal medical therapy. It is likely, however, that further reductions of operative mortality and increased confidence in the long-term effects of valvular prostheses will make it possible to recommend operative treatment to asymptomatic or minimally symptomatic patients with severe regurgitation and cardiomegaly.

TRICUSPID STENOSIS

Tricuspid stenosis is a relatively uncommon valvular lesion and is generally rheumatic in origin; unusual causes are carcinoid heart disease, fibroelastosis, and endomyocardial fibrosis. Rheumatic tricuspid stenosis does not usually occur as an isolated lesion or in patients with pure mitral regurgitation, but most commonly is observed in association with mitral stenosis, and sometimes with combined mitral and aortic stenosis. Hemodynamically significant tricuspid stenosis occurs in 5 to 10 per cent of patients with severe mitral valve disease, and is seen predominantly in females. In most patients the valvular deformity does not result in pure stenosis but in a combination of stenosis and regurgitation.

Since mitral stenosis generally precedes the development of tricuspid stenosis, many patients initially have symptoms of pulmonary congestion. However, the presence of tricuspid stenosis prevents the abrupt increases in pulmonary blood volume that are characteristic of mitral stenosis and that are responsible for the occurrence of paroxysmal dyspnea. Thus, an amelioration of the symptoms of pulmonary congestion in a patient with mitral stenosis should lead to the suspicion that tricuspid stenosis may be developing. Characteristically, patients with hemodynamically significant tricuspid stenosis complain of relatively little dyspnea for the degree of hepatomegaly, ascites, and edema they present. In some patients tricuspid stenosis may be suspected for the first time when symptoms of right ventricular failure persist after an adequate mitral valvulotomy.

Severe tricuspid stenosis is associated with marked hepatic congestion, often resulting in cirrhosis, jaundice, malnutrition, severe edema, and ascites. The jugular veins are usually distended, and in patients with sinus rhythm there may be giant *a* waves that reach the angle of the jaw in the sitting position. The *v* waves are less conspicuous, and since the presence of tricuspid obstruction impedes right atrial emptying during diastole, there is a slow, gentle, almost imperceptible *y* descent. In patients with sinus rhythm there may be prominent presystolic pulsations of the enlarged liver.

The right ventricle and the shock of pulmonary valve closure are usually not readily felt. Indeed, a giant *a* wave in the jugular venous pulse without palpatory evidence of pulmonary hypertension or right ventricular enlargement should always suggest the possibility of tricuspid stenosis. An opening snap of the tricuspid valve may be heard or recorded phonocardiographically approximately 0.06 second after pulmonary valve closure occasionally. The diastolic rumbling murmur of tricuspid stenosis has many of the qualities of the mitral diastolic murmur, and since tricuspid stenosis almost always occurs in the presence of mitral stenosis, the less common valvular lesion may be missed unless the examiner considers the possibility of its presence. However, the tricuspid murmur is generally heard best along the left sternal margin and over the xiphoid process. It is augmented during inspiration, when negative intrathoracic pressure increases the velocity of blood flow across the tricuspid orifice, and it is reduced during expiration and particularly during the Valsalva maneuver, when tricuspid blood flow is reduced. As the stethoscope is inched laterally, the diastolic murmur may diminish in intensity or disappear, only to intensify or reappear as the

mitral murmur at the apex. In patients with sinus rhythm the presystolic component is often louder at the tricuspid than at the mitral area. Since right atrial contraction precedes left atrial contraction, the tricuspid presystolic murmur commences before the mitral and it often is of the crescendo-decrescendo type.

Electrocardiographically, the most striking features are tall, peaked P waves in lead II, as well as prominent upright P waves in V_1; the P waves may actually be taller than the QRS complexes in V_1. The absence of electrocardiographic evidence of right ventricular hypertrophy in a patient with right heart failure who is believed to have mitral stenosis should suggest the possibility of associated tricuspid valve disease. Chest roentgenograms in patients with combined tricuspid and mitral stenosis show particular prominence of the right atrium and superior vena cava without much enlargement of the pulmonary artery and less evidence of pulmonary vascular congestion than occurs in patients with pure mitral valve disease.

A diastolic pressure gradient between the right atrium and right ventricle is the hemodynamic hallmark of tricuspid stenosis. This gradient can be recorded most conveniently by means of a double lumen cardiac catheter, with the distal lumen in the right ventricle and the proximal lumen in the right atrium. The pressure gradient is augmented during inspiration and reduced during expiration. A mean diastolic pressure gradient exceeding 5 mm. of mercury is usually sufficient to elevate the mean right atrial pressure to levels that result in systemic venous congestion and, unless sodium intake has been restricted or diuretics have been given, is associated with ascites and edema. In patients with sinus rhythm the right atrial *a* wave may be extremely tall and may even approach the level of the right ventricular systolic pressure; the latter, as well as the pulmonary artery and pulmonary artery wedge pressures, usually show little elevation. Hemodynamically significant tricuspid stenosis is usually associated with a depressed resting cardiac output that fails to rise during exercise. The low cardiac output is responsible for the normal or only slightly elevated left atrial, pulmonary arterial, and right ventricular systolic pressures in the presence of mitral stenosis.

Since patients with tricuspid stenosis generally exhibit marked systemic venous congestion, intensive salt restriction, digitalization, and diuretic therapy are required during the preoperative period. Such a prolonged preparatory period may diminish the hepatic congestion and thereby improve hepatic function sufficiently so that the risks of operation are diminished. In patients with mild tricuspid stenosis with effective orifices exceeding 2 square centimeters, surgical treatment of the tricuspid valve is not ordinarily indicated at the time of mitral valve surgery. On the other hand, definitive surgical treatment of the tricuspid stenosis should be carried out, preferably at the time of mitral valvulotomy, in patients with moderate or severe tricuspid stenosis, with mean diastolic pressure gradients exceeding 5 mm. of mercury and tricuspid orifices less than 1.7 square centimeters. Tricuspid stenosis is almost invariably accompanied by significant tricuspid regurgitation, and simple finger fracture valvulotomy often does not produce significant hemodynamic improvement, but may merely substitute severe regurgitation for stenosis. Open operations utilizing cardiopulmonary bypass may permit improvement of tricuspid valve function, but most frequently prosthetic replacement of the tricuspid valve is required.

TRICUSPID REGURGITATION

Most commonly, tricuspid regurgitation is functional and is secondary to marked dilatation of the right ventricle and the tricuspid valve ring. Functional tricuspid regurgitation may complicate right ventricular failure of any cause and is commonly seen in the late stages of heart failure due to rheumatic or congenital heart disease with severe pulmonary hypertension, as well as coronary artery disease or hypertension. Rheumatic fever may also produce organic tricuspid regurgitation, which is associated with tricuspid stenosis in some instances. Less commonly, tricuspid regurgitation is produced by congenital heart disease, and occurs with defects of the atrioventricular canal as well as with Ebstein's malformation of the tricuspid valve. Carcinoid heart disease, endomyocardial fibrosis, bacterial endocarditis, and trauma may also produce tricuspid regurgitation.

The symptoms of tricuspid regurgitation result primarily from systemic venous congestion and reduction of the cardiac output. When functional tricuspid regurgitation develops, the pre-existing clinical manifestations of right failure are usually intensified. On physical examination, peripheral cyanosis resulting from reduced systemic blood flow may be present, and the neck veins are generally distended with prominent v waves. Severe hepatomegaly, ascites, pleural effusions, edema, systolic pulsations of the liver, and a positive hepatojugular reflux are common. The right ventricle is usually hyperactive, with a prominent right ventricular pulsation along the left parasternal region. A blowing holosystolic murmur is heard best along the left sternal margin; this murmur is generally intensified during inspiration and reduced during expiration or the Valsalva maneuver. A fourth sound (pre-systolic gallop) may be audible if tricuspid regurgitation develops acutely. However, atrial fibrillation is usually present in patients with significant tricuspid regurgitation, and the absence of a properly coordinated atrial contraction may intensify the regurgitation.

There are no electrocardiographic features characteristic of tricuspid regurgitation, but on roentgenographic examination both the right ventricle and right atrium are enlarged, and the latter chamber expands during systole. The cardiac output is often greatly reduced, and the right atrial pressure pulse may exhibit no x descent during early systole, but a prominent c-v wave with a rapid y descent. The mean right atrial and the right ventricular end-diastolic pressures are often elevated.

Treatment of the underlying cause of heart failure usually reduces the severity of functional tricuspid regurgitation. In patients with mitral valve disease and tricuspid regurgitation due to massive right ventricular enlargement, surgical correction of the mitral valvular abnormality frequently relieves the tricuspid regurgitation as the pulmonary vascular changes regress and the right ventricular pressure falls. However, when tricuspid regurgitation is severe and due to rheumatic involvement, then either tricuspid valve replacement or narrowing of the tricuspid anulus by means of an anuloplasty may be necessary.

Braunwald, E.: Mitral regurgitation: Physiological, clinical and surgical considerations. New Eng. J. Med., 281:425, 1969.

Braunwald, E., Lambrew, C. T., Rockoff, S. D., Ross, J., Jr., and Morrow, A. G.: Idiopathic hypertrophic subaortic stenosis: I. A description of the disease based upon an analysis of 64 patients. Circulation, 30(Suppl. 4):3 1964.

Morrow, A. G., Roberts, W. C., Ross, J. Jr., Fisher, R. D., Behrendt, D. M., Mason, D. T., and Braunwald, E.: Obstruction to left ventricular outflow. Current concepts of management and operative treatment. Ann. Intern. Med., 69:1255, 1968.

Perloff, J. K., and Harvey, W. P.: Clinical recognition of tricuspid stenosis. Circulation, 22:346, 1960.

Segal, J., Harvey, W. P., and Hufnagel, C.: A clinical study of one hundred patients with severe aortic insufficiency. Amer. J. Med., 21:200, 1956.

Symposium on Mitral Insufficiency. Progr. Cardiov. Dis., 5:119, 1962.

Werko, L.: The dynamics and consequences of stenosis or insufficiency of the cardiac valves. In Hamilton, W. F., and Dow, P. (eds.): Handbook of Physiology, Circulation, Vol. I. Washington, D.C., American Physiological Society, 1962, p. 645.

Wood, P.: An appreciation of mitral stenosis. Parts I and II. Brit. Med. J., 1:1051 and 1113, 1954.

Wood, P.: Aortic stenosis. Amer. J. Cardiol., 1:553, 1958.

Ischemic Heart Disease

Thomas Killip

ANGINA PECTORIS

Definition. Angina pectoris is a clinical syndrome caused by inadequate oxygenation of the heart, characteristically precipitated by exertion relieved by rest or sublingual nitroglycerin.

Historical. Although there were several earlier reports, the condition since known as angina pectoris was masterfully described by William Heberden in 1772 in a paper entitled "Some Account of a Disorder of the Breast." The word angina refers to the sensation of strangling and anxiety which accompanies an attack. Heberden pointed out that the condition is common; that the seizure occurs while walking, especially uphill or after a meal; that the uneasiness vanishes with standing still; that prior to an attack the subjects appear perfectly well; that the pain is in the sternal area but may go to the left arm; that males past 50 are the most common victims; and that sudden death may terminate an attack.

Clinical Manifestations. *Pain.* The discomfort of angina may vary from mild to most intense. It may persist as a vague ache, and although the patient is aware of the sensation, he may continue his activities. On the other hand, once started, angina may rapidly build up to the point of intolerance, forcing the victim to stop and seek immediate relief. The pain of angina is usually not as severe as the intense precordial crushing sensation associated with acute myocardial infarction. It is usually described as pressing, boring, or gripping. The patient may feel as though a weight is on his chest. The chest feels tight, and there is often a sensation of heavy breathing. It may be difficult at times to determine whether the patient is complaining of angina, dyspnea, or both. Many sufferers, in describing angina, will make a fist as they grope for words to describe the discomfort. This gesture is a helpful clue.

The pain of angina characteristically is a deep, visceral sensation—dull, aching, or heavy. Sharp, fleeting sensations are not typical of angina. Patients who complain of lightning pains in the anterior chest usually have some other process. Although the patient may feel that his chest is tight or squeezed so that his breath is restricted, the pain is not exaggerated by inspiratory movements. It is not searing, knifelike, or hot.

Angina may be attributed to indigestion. In some patients the sensation felt in the epigastrium is described as burning. It may be accompanied by considerable abdominal distress, including bloating and belching. The need to belch during an attack is common, and this may even relieve the attack. Intermingling of gastric and cardiac symptoms does not ease the diagnostic task of the physician.

Some patients do not refer to the discomfort of angina as pain; rather they describe it as an ache or a vague awareness of discomfort. The reaction to angina is highly variable. Those with mild discomfort may ignore the sensation and carry on normal activities, whereas in other patients there may be an acute fear of death. Often a strong element of denial makes obtaining an accurate history of the frequency, nature, and intensity of angina very difficult. Patients with more severe forms may markedly limit activity to avoid triggering another attack. Activity may be so restricted that few attacks occur. A careful history should enable the physician to recognize the true intensity of the condition.

The discomfort of angina is characteristically substernal. It is not felt on the surface of the chest, but may be located beneath the upper, middle, or lower portions of the sternum. Most commonly it is described in the midsternal region. The pain may also be felt beneath the precordium. It is important to emphasize that angina is seldom felt in the region of the cardiac apex. The pain may radiate widely. Typically the sensation is felt in the left arm and shoulder. It may radiate from the substernal region as intensity increases, or it may be felt predominantly in the arm, with minimal or no chest component. Usually the discomfort radiates down the medial side of the arm and may go to the fingers. Occasionally the pain may radiate down the right arm or both arms. A relationship between the localization of cardiac ischemia and the pattern of pain radiation has not been established. The pain may radiate to the back, neck, or jaw, or discomfort may be localized in the intrascapular area. Occasionally, it is felt in the upper or lower abdomen. In all the areas of remote pain, the sensation retains the deep and aching character of visceral pain.

Precipitating Factors. Angina is characteristically episodic and triggered by *physical activity.* A patient may be able to predict discomfort by a specific act, for example, climbing a flight of stairs, but in other patients the effort of exertion is variable. Walking may be tolerated, but climbing a small hill may precipitate an attack. Angina is frequently induced by a *heavy meal,* especially if followed by exertion. Some patients are forced to change their habits and eat several small meals to avoid discomfort. *Cold weather* is especially prone to produce angina. Sometimes the first contact with cold air on leaving a warm room is sufficient, even though the patient is standing still. Many patients are able to walk indoors and perform labor, although they cannot do the same outdoors without discomfort.

Emotion is a well-known trigger for angina. An argument, a tense encounter, an anxiety-producing situation, or sexual excitement may induce pain. Angina may occur when the patient is resting quietly, seemingly without stimulation (angina decubitus). It is thought to imply more severe

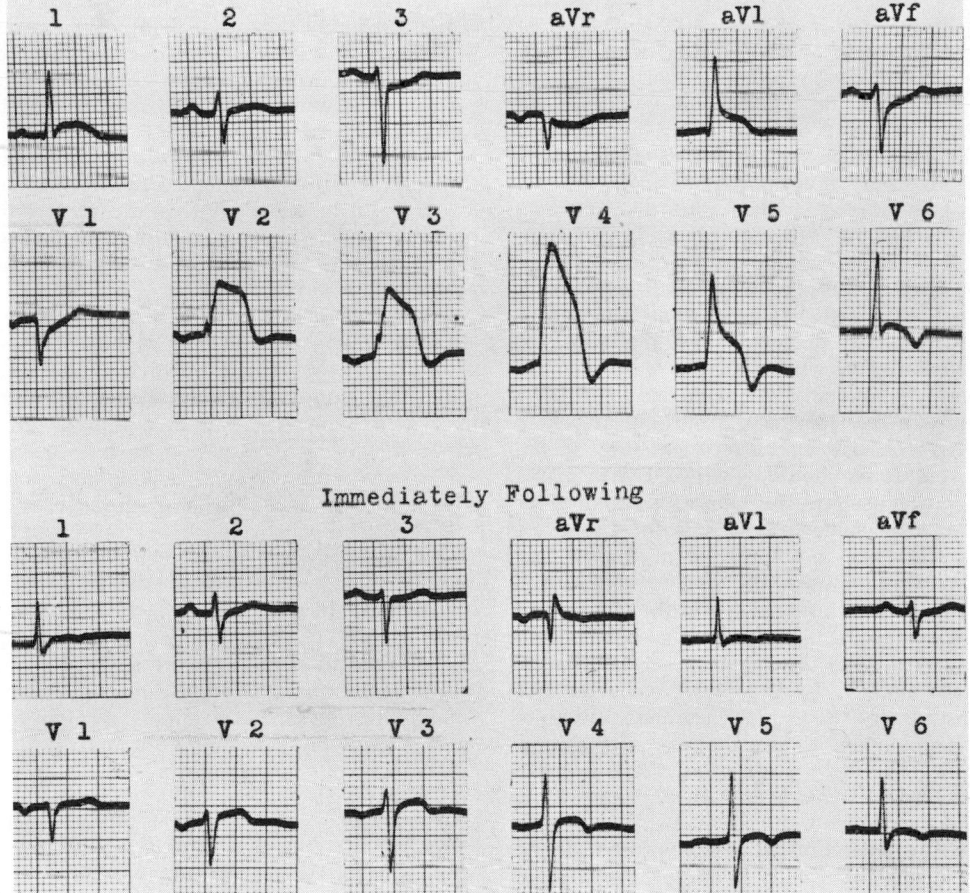

FIGURE 1. Electrocardiogram recorded in a 57-year-old man during an episode of angina pectoris. *Top:* During the attack. *Bottom:* After pain had spontaneously subsided. The electrocardiogram shows extensive abnormality of the ST segments and T waves. During angina the ST segments are elevated in several leads, especially V₂-V₅. The electrical location of these changes suggests epicardial ischemia of the area of myocardium supplied by the anterior descending coronary artery. As the angina improved, the electrocardiogram reverted to the pattern recorded at rest in this patient. The tracing obtained following angina is abnormal.

disease and to have a worse prognosis than other forms. Most instances of angina decubitus are probably triggered by emotion.

Nocturnal angina may be troublesome. In this form the patient has awakened from an apparently sound sleep with angina. It is important to differentiate this condition from nocturnal dyspnea secondary to left ventricular failure, which usually responds to digitalis. Recent investigations have correlated changes in the electroencephalogram and rapid eye movement with intermittent periods of dreaming. It has been shown that nocturnal angina is frequently preceded by a dream in which the subject is emotionally stimulated or is exercising. The dreams are often accompanied by striking increases in respiration, heart rate, and blood pressure. In one reported example the subject dreamed he was riding a bicycle up hill, and awoke with angina.

Although most individuals will stop exertion with the onset of angina, some will carry on and "walk through" the pain. Studies have revealed three patterns of response if exertion continues with angina. In some patients the angina eventually subsides, and physical activity can continue without discomfort. In others the pain persists, is of only moderate intensity, does not progress, and the patient is able to tolerate the level of discomfort. He continues his activity. In a third group, however, the pain becomes progressively intense and forces the subject to obtain relief by rest or medication. Most patients fall into the last category.

Duration and Relief. Anginal pain usually persists no more than three to five minutes. The duration is somewhat variable, depending on the stimulus triggering the attack. When the pain is related to exertion, such as walking, it characteristically subsides, becoming progressively less severe, if the sufferer promptly stops and rests. Most patients with angina have pain only a few times a week. Since hurrying may precipitate angina, many victims learn to saunter and stop frequently to rest.

Spontaneous angina decubitus or angina increased during emotional tension may be especially severe in intensity and duration. Such episodes tend to persist for 10 to 15 minutes or longer and to be of agonizing intensity. The blood pressure may rise to an extraordinary degree, with development of striking diastolic hypertension during these attacks.

Some patients with clear-cut angina complain of long periods of chest discomfort lasting an hour or more. The sensation tends to be low grade, almost at the threshold of awareness. The patient equates the sensation with angina, describing it as an ache or an annoyance, but carries on his normal activities. Exertion or emotion may precipitate a full-blown attack. It seems likely that the complaint reflects a mild, chronic myocardial ischemia. It may or may not be relieved by nitroglycerin.

Usually the characteristics of angina are reasonably constant for the individual patient. The type of stimulus, whether emotional or physical, and the intensity, frequency, radiation, and duration of the pain are fairly regular from one attack to another. Any change in pattern causing an increase in symptoms should be viewed with grave suspicion. Increase in frequency, intensity, or duration or any lowering of the threshold for triggering the pain may presage an impending coronary syndrome. Both the physician and the patient should be aware of the significance of an increase in symptoms. This subject is discussed in more detail later.

Causes of Pain. Many theories have been proposed in an attempt to explain the mechanism of cardiac pain. Although painful spasm of the coronary arteries has been postulated, there is little evidence to support this thesis. Spasm may occasionally be recognized during the filming of a coronary arteriogram, but it is most often induced by the catheter tip. Even when not mechanical in origin, the spasm apparently occurs without causing symptoms.

The pain of angina is most likely directly related to metabolic changes caused by ischemia. Electrocardiographic abnormalities may precede awareness of pain or may occur in absence of pain, suggesting that an accumulation of active substances to some threshold necessary to cause pain is occurring. Such substances might be H$^+$, K$^+$, and possibly components of the kallikrein system. There are two networks of sensory nerve fibers in the heart: a perivascular network encircling the coronary arteries, and fibers running beside the vessels and terminating between muscle bundles. Presumably the latter are stimulated by the ischemic process.

The pain of angina pectoris and that of myocardial infarction are similar in quality. The pain of infarction tends to be more intense, and may persist for several hours. Prolonged pain implies continued ischemia, not infarction. Once death of myocardium has occurred, pain is no longer present. One explanation for the occasional sudden improvement in previously stable angina is infarction of the chronically ischemic area.

Ischemic cardiac pain and the pain of intermittent claudication presumably have a similar mechanism. Both are described as deep, visceral sensations. Both occur with increased muscular work, and are relieved by rest. Both are usually secondary to obstructive vascular disease.

The nerve pathways from the myocardium travel through the superficial and deep cardiac plexus and the thoracic cardiac nerves to the first four or five thoracic ganglia. They enter the spinal cord via the white rami of corresponding thoracic segments. Cord segments D1 to D5 also receive pain fibers from the precordium, the medial portion of the anterior surface of the arm, and the forearm. Convergence within a common anatomic pathway of nerve impulses doubtless accounts for the characteristic radiation of the pain of angina pectoris.

Physical Findings. Between attacks, patients who suffer from angina may or may not have signs of organic heart disease. During an angina episode the patient usually becomes apprehensive. He may begin to sweat. Often he will press hard on the sternum with his hands. If he has had previous experience with the medication, he is anxious to take a nitroglycerin tablet as quickly as possible.

During the attack the heart rate usually rises. The blood pressure is frequently elevated, occasionally to alarming levels. Heart sounds may become more distant. The apical impulse may be more diffuse. Careful inspection and palpation of the precordium may reveal a localized systolic bulging or a paradoxic movement. This finding is thought to represent the effects of segmental myocardial ischemia producing a localized area of noncontracting myocardium. The second sound may become paradoxically split during angina so that the components close during inspiration and widen during expiration. This reversal of the normal splitting is thought to reflect a more prolonged left ventricular ejection time during the ischemic episode, as normally the aortic valve closes before the pulmonic valve.

In some patients a systolic murmur may appear in the region of the cardiac apex during angina. Characteristically the murmur begins in mid or late systole after the first sound. It is rather shrill and not exceptionally loud. This murmur is ascribed to papillary muscle dysfunction secondary to localized ischemia. If the papillary muscles are involved in the ischemic process, they become incapable of holding against left ventricular pressure during systole. During the latter half of systole, the mitral valve is forced open, and regurgitation occurs. The condition is often self-limited, for the murmur may not be detected when the patient is free of pain.

Careful observation and examination of the patient during an attack of chest pain may be extremely rewarding. Detection of abnormal cardiac findings and the disappearance of the findings with the subsidence of the complaints may help considerably in establishing the diagnosis.

Electrocardiogram. It must be emphasized that the resting electrocardiogram may be entirely within normal limits in the patient who has clear-cut and indisputable angina pectoris. Too many physicians still harbor the erroneous belief that if the electrocardiogram is normal, the patient cannot have angina. The electrocardiogram is more likely to be normal when the syndrome first begins.

Perhaps 20 to 30 per cent of patients first experiencing angina have a normal electrocardiogram on initial examination. The electrocardiogram is almost always abnormal when angina has persisted for a year or more.

Chronic Changes. The presence of chronic electrocardiographic abnormality does not establish a diagnosis of angina. These changes may indicate the presence of organic heart disease. The chronic abnormalities that may be present include evidence of left ventricular hypertrophy, ST segment and T wave change, bundle branch block, or pathologic Q waves suggesting old myocardial infarction. Abnormalities of the ST segments or T waves in the electrocardiogram are frequently nonspecific, and one must avoid overinterpretation. It is important to know whether the patient is receiving digitalis, which will reduce T wave amplitude and produce an ST segment depression in most leads. In the normal person the effects of digitalis may be difficult to detect in the electrocardiogram, and consist largely of some decrease in amplitude of the T wave and a very slight ST segment depression. In the patient with organic heart disease, on the other hand, digitalization may produce more striking changes. T waves may become inverted, and ST segments markedly depressed. A pattern of "left ventricular strain" may appear when prior to digitalis the electrocardiogram was essentially normal.

Scarring, owing to small infarcts, may cause abnormalities of the T waves and ST segments. A characteristic "ischemic" sign is said to be a flat ST segment depression from the end of the QRS complex to the onset of the T waves. Since there are many variations of ST segment depression and the changes are usually nonspecific, it is seldom possible to utilize the electrocardiogram obtained in the absence of pain to confirm the diagnosis of angina pectoris.

Significant Q waves suggesting old myocardial infarction are helpful in confirming a diagnosis of coronary artery disease. Bundle branch block patterns may be difficult to evaluate. Right bundle branch block is perhaps a more benign lesion, in terms of diagnostic implications and prognosis, than is left bundle branch block. Blockage of the right bundle causes a delay of terminal QRS forces, and hence does not interfere with the recognition of abnormal Q waves of myocardial infarction. It is generally held that left bundle branch block implies disease of the left ventricle, either fibrosis or coronary artery disease. The abnormality in blockade of the left bundle is a prolongation of the initial QRS vector and a change in direction. Hence the pattern of old or recent infarction may be obscured in the presence of left bundle branch block by the absence of expected Q waves.

Acute Changes. An acute, self-limited, and reversible abnormality of the electrocardiogram may be recorded during an attack of angina. One experienced cardiologist has reported that the electrocardiogram is abnormal during angina in approximately 80 per cent of cases; my view is that the electrocardiogram is abnormal in virtually all patients with angina, providing that sufficient observations with appropriate leads are obtained. The recording of an electrocardiogram continuously during an attack of chest pain may be of inestimable value in establishing the diagnosis of angina pectoris. During angina there are dramatic changes, the so-called "ischemic" pattern, in the repolarization waves of the electrocardiogram, the ST segment and the T waves. Sometimes QRS changes may appear also. The R wave may increase or decrease in height, and Q waves may appear temporarily. Intraventricular conduction disturbances or bundle branch block occasionally develop. Usually the most striking electrocardiographic change during an acute attack of angina is in the ST segments and T waves. The T waves may flatten and invert. If already inverted, they may become upright. "Ischemic" ST segments consisting of depression of 0.1 mV. or more may appear. At times the depression is truly striking, reaching 0.4 mV. or more. In some patients the ST segments become markedly elevated in leads with upright R waves. The changes resemble those seen in the so-called "hyperacute" stage of myocardial infarction, but promptly subside after the pain is relieved. If infarction were present, the electrocardiographic abnormality would gradually evolve rather than rapidly return to the control tracing. It has been said that the form of angina with ST segment elevation represents a special syndrome or angina variant, but this seems unlikely. More probably, the presence of ST segment elevation represents dominant ischemia in the subepicardial layer, whereas the more typical ST segment depression is an expression of subendocardial circulatory and metabolic change.

Exercise Tolerance Tests. An extensive literature has accumulated attesting to the value of the electrocardiogram obtained during exercise as an aid in the diagnosis of coronary artery disease and in the evaluation of the patient with chest pain. Despite the widespread use of these tests, much of the support for their value has been of a testimonial nature, and until recently correlation of the electrocardiographic interpretation with anatomic or metabolic abnormality of the heart has been limited. The introduction of the techniques of coronary arteriography and sampling of blood from the coronary sinus during stress has lent a measure of objectivity to the electrocardiographic diagnosis of myocardial ischemia.

In the patient with coronary artery disease, an episode of myocardial ischemia induced during exercise is usually associated with the development of significant electrocardiographic abnormalities during or after the exercise. It is not necessary to induce angina to precipitate the electrocardiographic change. The electrocardiographic patterns observed are similar to those described earlier as occurring during an episode of angina pectoris.

The hallmark of an abnormal "ischemic" elec-

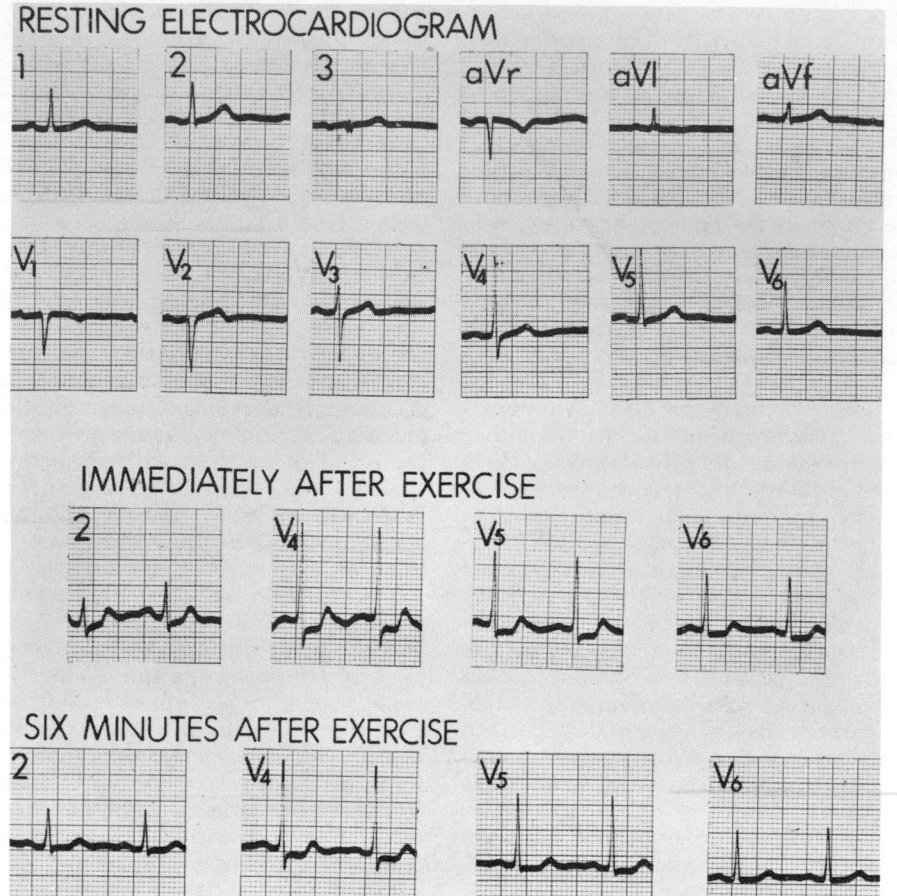

FIGURE 2. An abnormal electrocardiogram response to exercise in a 49-year-old man. The exercise tolerance test was performed by having the patient complete 40 trips over and back on a specially constructed 2-step. The electrocardiogram obtained at rest is normal. During exercise, heart rate rose from 75 to 105 beats per minute. The patient did not have angina during the test. Immediately after exercise, the ST segments in the leads recorded are depressed more than 1.5 mV. Six minutes after exercise, ST segment depression is less. These changes constitute an abnormal electrocardiographic response to exercise.

trocardiographic response to exercise is ST segment depression or the development of an ST segment vector essentially opposite in direction to the mean QRS vector. Although many criteria have been proposed, most authorities would agree that ST segment depression of 0.5 to 1.0 mV. is of borderline significance, but that depression of greater than 1.0 mV. is definitely abnormal. It has been shown recently that in many patients the electrocardiographic abnormalities induced by exercise, endocardial pacing, or infusion of isoproterenol are accompanied by metabolic evidence of anaerobic metabolism with excess lactate in the coronary sinus, thus indicating that reversible ischemia has developed.

It is important to bear in mind two essential points. First, demonstration that a patient has an abnormal electrocardiographic response to exercise does not prove that his chest complaint is angina unless the symptom recurred during exercise and was associated with characteristic electrocardiographic change. Second, a diagnosis of ischemic heart disease owing to coronary artery abnormality as a result of a positive exercise test is inferential. Many conditions may be associated with a positive exercise tolerance test, e.g., digitalis administration, valvular heart disease, myocardiopathy, and diseases of the small coronary arteries. A syndrome, discussed in greater detail below, has been described which occurs mostly in young women, and is characterized by an angina-like pain, abnormal electrocardiographic exercise tolerance test, and a normal coronary arteriogram. In some patients excessive hyperventilation during exercise is associated with changes in the cardiogram, especially T wave inversion. The abnormality is apparently related to increased blood pH and decreased plasma potassium. It may be prevented by breathing 5 per cent carbon dioxide during the test and by administration of potassium salts intravenously.

The results of an exercise tolerance test must be interpreted with caution. The implications of a diagnosis of ischemic coronary artery disease are so important that there must be continued awareness of the possibility of a false positive result. The incidence of false positive or false negative tests is not established. This is due in part to lack of precise anatomic, electrocardiographic, and physiologic correlations and in part to lack of standardization of the exercise tolerance tests themselves. It appears that the patient with typical angina will have an abnormal electrocardiogram during exercise if the stress is sufficiently vigorous. Data from coronary arteriography suggest that patients with angina will have significant obstruction of at least one major coronary artery, confirming Blumgart's observations on autopsy specimens more than 30 years ago.

The purpose of an exercise test is to increase muscular work, heart rate, and oxygen consumption to the point that ischemia of the myocardium, as reflected in the electrocardiogram, will be induced. Two types of exercise are currently employed, the *two-step test* and *exercise on the treadmill*. Proponents of the two-step test have prescribed the height and width of the steps and specified the number of trips according to age and weight of the patient. In the treadmill test the instrument is adjusted for speed and grade to increase muscular work. Recent reports indicate that exercise tests performed on the treadmill may have a reliability greater than 90 per cent if the exercise is sufficient to increase heart rate to 80 to 90 per cent of predicted maximum for the individual patient. Tables are available relating predicted maximal heart rate during exercise to sex and age.

Although the exercise tolerance test is a potentially dangerous maneuver in a patient with severe ischemic heart disease, relatively few serious accidents have been reported. The test is contraindicated when the resting cardiogram is unstable or suggests acute ischemia or infarction. Patients with crescendo angina or frequent, severe attacks of pain, or those in whom a diagnosis of myocardial infarction is suspected should not be exercised.

Pathogenesis. According to current understanding, angina pectoris develops when cardiac work, and hence myocardial oxygen need, is greater than the ability of the coronary arterial system to supply oxygen, per unit time. Angina can be precipitated by an increase in cardiac work and hence oxygen need, or, conversely, angina may occur following a decrease in the oxygen supply secondary to obstruction of coronary flow or a reduction of arterial oxygen content. Angina most commonly results when cardiac work and hence myocardial oxygen need exceed the available oxygen supply because coronary blood flow to certain regions is restricted. Obstruction of coronary flow owing to coronary atherosclerosis is the most common anatomic finding in the presence of angina. Other conditions which greatly increase cardiac work, such as aortic stenosis, hypertrophic subaortic stenosis, and aortic regurgitation, may be associated with angina despite anatomically normal coronary arteries. Although spasm of the arteries has frequently been invoked as a cause of angina, there is no substantial body of evidence to support this concept.

Oxygenated arterial blood is supplied by the two main coronary arteries. Coronary blood flow occurs mainly during diastole because the systolic contraction of the ventricles so increases the resistance in the coronary tree that nutrient flow is largely blocked. An adequate coronary blood flow is therefore dependent on adequate diastolic pressure. When the aortic diastolic pressure drops abruptly, as in aortic regurgitation, coronary blood flow may be severely diminished.

The oxygen content of blood obtained in the coronary sinus is the lowest occurring in any vein draining a major organ. Usually the coronary sinus blood oxygen content, saturation, or Po_2 varies but little despite marked variations in cardiac work. Increase in myocardial oxygen consumption is met not by increased extraction from arterial blood but by increased coronary blood flow. Coronary vascular resistance is rather precisely adjusted, by mechanisms that are incompletely understood, to regulate blood flow in relation to oxygen need. Thus when cardiac work and oxygen utilization increase, coronary vascular resistance falls, permitting an increase in coronary

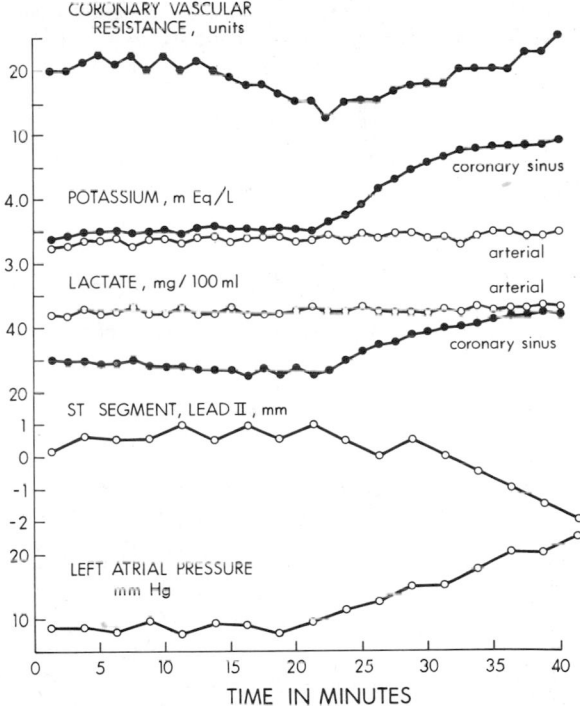

FIGURE 3. Physiologic and metabolic changes in experimental myocardial ischemia. A cannula is inserted into the left coronary artery, and myocardial blood flow is measured. Serial blood samples are obtained from an artery and the coronary sinus. The electrocardiogram and ventricular pressures are recorded continuously. Nutrient flow through the left coronary artery is progressively reduced in this experiment in a dog, and a series of sequential changes occur. Coronary vascular resistance declines and reaches a minimum at 20 minutes. When coronary resistance reaches a low point, the following changes occur: onset of potassium efflux into the coronary sinus; change of myocardial metabolism from lactate utilization to lactate production; appearance of ST segment depression in the electrocardiogram; and development of progressive rise in left ventricular filling (left atrial) pressure. Thus in this experiment, myocardial ischemia develops when reduction of coronary vascular resistance can no longer compensate for deficient coronary blood flow. With the onset of ischemia there are progressive changes in myocardial cell membranes and metabolism, in the electrocardiogram, and in the function of the left ventricle. (After Case.)

blood flow and oxygen delivery. Conversely, when oxygen demand falls, coronary vascular resistance rises, and coronary blood flow and oxygen delivery decline. Implicit in this mechanism is the maintenance of relatively constant coronary sinus oxygen levels, because changes in extraction of oxygen from arterial blood are relatively minor.

Changes in arterial P_{O_2}, as influenced by hypoxia or abnormal ventilation, may lessen myocardial oxygenation. It has been suggested, but not firmly established, that increased affinity of hemoglobin for oxygen, which would increase the oxyhemoglobin saturation or content for a given P_{O_2}, may precipitate myocardial ischemia. A number of hemoglobin variants with abnormal affinity for oxygen are now known, but their relation to ischemic heart disease has not been clarified.

Carbon monoxide may be important in myocardial ischemia. It has an affinity for hemoglobin some 200 times that of oxygen, and displaces oxygen from the hemoglobin molecule; thus a given level of carbon monoxyhemoglobin reduces the blood oxygen content that can be reached even with inspiration of 100 per cent oxygen. Carbon monoxyhemoglobin levels in people who smoke cigarettes may reach 6 to 10 per cent or even higher. Thus, it has been suggested that CO plays an important role in the increased risk of cigarette smokers for myocardial infarction and sudden death.

Under normal conditions, myocardial metabolism is entirely aerobic, there being little capacity to maintain normal function anaerobically. A wide variety of substrates are utilized as fuels, depending on their availability. These include free fatty acids, glucose, ketones, lactate, and pyruvate. Under ischemic or anaerobic conditions, glycolysis is activated through the Embden-Meyerhof cycle to derive high energy phosphate. In these circumstances pyruvate becomes the hydrogen acceptor, substituting for oxygen, and lactate is produced.

Clinically the most useful metabolic index of myocardial ischemia is demonstration of myocardial lactate production via coronary sinus sampling during angina or myocardial stress. Myocardial stress may be induced by pacing the heart at a rapid rate or by intravenous infusion of isoproterenol, which increases both heart rate and myocardial contractility, thus increasing oxygen need. Production of lactate with myocardial stress generally indicates a 90 per cent or greater occlusion of a major coronary artery.

It is difficult to obtain precise metabolic data during an episode of myocardial ischemia or angina in man. Certain animal experiments are pertinent, however. When coronary blood flow is gradually reduced, but cardiac work is kept constant, a sequence of events may be identified. Myocardial extraction of oxygen is near maximal initially, so that coronary sinus P_{O_2} falls but little. Coronary vascular resistance declines progressively to reach a low plateau. Further reduction in blood flow and hence oxygen delivery is followed by metabolic and physiologic evidence of ischemia. The myocardium switches from lactate extraction to lactate production. Coronary sinus blood pH falls. Potassium loss from the myocardium is detected. Electrocardiographic abnormalities appear, and the ST segments are depressed. Ventricular performance begins to deteriorate, and left ventricular filling pressure and left atrial pressure rise.

In man, during spontaneous angina pectoris or ischemia induced by exercise, pacing, or isoproterenol, metabolic and functional changes can be detected similar to those described in animals. Lactate is produced. Potassium efflux occurs. The electrocardiogram becomes abnormal, and frequently left ventricular diastolic pressure rises. These changes are reversed during recovery. Application of the technique of cardiac catheterization combined with metabolic studies is especially useful for evaluating puzzling, angina-like syndromes and in determining the late effects of surgical procedures designed to improve nutritional coronary flow.

The major determinants of myocardial oxygen consumption are heart rate, systolic tension or pressure, and contractility. In the occasional patient whose angina is made worse by digitalis, increased myocardial oxygen demand secondary to the effect of digitalis on the contractile mechanism has been postulated. Any mechanism by which heart rate, ventricular systolic pressure, or contractility is increased may induce angina. Studies during exercise or cardiac pacing have shown that some patients with angina will predictably develop metabolic or electrocardiographic signs of ischemia or pain when cardiac work reaches a given value for the individual patient. Thus, the level of cardiac work required to induce angina may be reproducible under laboratory conditions.

Studies during spontaneous angina have shown that the subjective awareness of pain is usually preceded by an increase in heart rate and a rise in blood pressure. In some patients electrocardiographic changes appear one to three minutes before the pain, suggesting a buildup of metabolic substances prior to stimulation of pain receptors. Blood pressure usually continues to rise as the ischemic attack progresses. If the angina is not relieved by medication, the blood pressure, both systolic and diastolic, may rise to alarming levels. I have observed levels as high as 200/150 in a patient who was normotensive between attacks. The rise in systemic blood pressure and increase in heart rate during angina represent a potentially disastrous feedback system: the higher the blood pressure and the faster the heart rate, the greater the unmet myocardial oxygen need. In patients who become severely hypertensive during angina, prompt treatment with vasodilators such as nitroglycerin or amyl nitrite is mandatory. Narcotics such as morphine will frequently relieve the pain, but not lower the pressure significantly. Careful evaluation of the patient with prolonged, excruciating angina will often reveal paroxysmal hypertension, presumably in response to the pain. Adequate treatment of the pressor response will ease the angina in most instances.

The cause of the rise of blood pressure in angina is not established. It does not appear to be related to adrenal cortical function.

The mechanism by which exposure to cold induces angina has been elucidated by recent studies. During such exposure arterial pressure and peripheral vascular resistance reflexly rise. Cardiac work may be suddenly and sharply increased, thus inducing an ischemic attack. The exposed skin of the face is an important cold receptor triggering the reflex. This susceptibility of the face to cold may be an atavistic expression of the diving reflex found in aquatic mammals and birds. The wearing of a face mask in cold weather may reduce the frequency of angina.

Pathology. Coronary artery disease with atherosclerosis of major vessels is the most common cause of angina pectoris. Pathologic studies in patients who die almost invariably reveal extensive atherosclerosis. Blumgart showed many years ago in postmortem perfusion studies that the patient with angina had occlusion of at least one major coronary artery. Coronary arteriography has demonstrated that angina is almost invariably associated with a significant obstruction of a major coronary artery, greater than 90 per cent. At autopsy, the myocardium frequently also shows small scars and areas of fibrosis. This observation suggests that patients with angina may have multiple small and clinically silent myocardial infarcts. Angina is more common in males than in females, and the incidence increases with age. Children in their teens or young adults with familial hypercholesterolemia (Type II lipoprotein disorder) may have angina secondary to precocious coronary atherosclerosis. The abnormal lipoprotein patterns observed in patients with carbohydrate intolerance and mild and severe forms of diabetes mellitus also predispose to atherosclerosis and angina. Diabetes may also be complicated by pathologic change in the small (less than 1 mm.) coronary arteries.

Any condition which obstructs coronary flow or increases cardiac work may be associated with angina. *Syphilitic aortitis* is often complicated by angina, because the inflammatory process may lead to constriction of the coronary ostia. Patients with hemodynamically significant *aortic stenosis* are especially susceptible to angina. Indeed, the onset of angina is an important symptom implying poor prognosis. Its presence should suggest careful evaluation of the hemodynamic severity of the obstructive lesion, and surgical intervention should be considered. Three factors contribute to the association between angina and aortic stenosis. First, the obstructive lesion markedly increases cardiac work because of increased left ventricular systolic pressure, especially during exercise. Second, excrescences from the degenerative process of calcific aortic stenosis may obstruct the coronary ostia. Third, patients with aortic stenosis tend to be males in the sixth or seventh decade, and concomitant coronary artery disease is not uncommon.

Occasionally nonsyphilitic *aortic regurgitation* is complicated by angina. Although flow work, high cardiac output, is less costly in terms of oxygen requirement than pressure work, systolic pressure in severe aortic regurgitation is quite high. The ventricle is enlarged because of the very large stroke volume, and wall tension is increased. Diastolic pressure is correspondingly low. Coronary blood flow which occurs predominantly in diastole is reduced, and ischemic attacks may occur.

Angina is a complication of *hypertrophic subaortic stenosis*. The myocardium in this condition may be massively hypertrophied. Angina appears to be related to the markedly increased pressure—work and left ventricular wall tension—associated with this condition, because usually the coronary arteries are large and patent.

Angina is said to complicate advanced *mitral stenosis*. It is frequently difficult to separate anamnestically a sensation of chest tightness owing to acute dyspnea from that of angina. In my experience, patients with mitral stenosis and angina have had concomitant coronary artery disease. It is possible that angina may reflect right ventricular ischemia in some patients with advanced pulmonary vascular change secondary to mitral stenosis.

Angina may be associated with *severe right ventricular hypertension* in congenital heart disease such as severe pulmonic stenosis, primary pulmonary hypertension, or tetralogy of Fallot. The so-called hypercyanotic angina or pain of pulmonary arterial hypertension is most likely right ventricular angina. There is no convincing evidence that distention of the pulmonary arteries is painful.

Anemia, hyperthyroidism, and *hypothyroidism* may be complicated by angina. In most instances there is severe pre-existing coronary atherosclerosis. The patient with myxedema may present a special problem. Restoration of a euthyroid state with thyroid medication may precipitate severe angina. There is a significant risk of acute myocardial infarction or sudden death if excessive doses of thyroid are used. Most authorities recommend a prolonged treatment period with small increments of thyroid.

Angina and Normal Coronary Arteries. Since the advent of coronary arteriography, a syndrome of angina pectoris with anatomically normal coronary arteries has been recognized. This variant amounts to 5 to 10 per cent of patients referred for arteriography. The condition occurs predominantly in young women. In some cases the history suggests classic angina. In others the story is less clear, and the physician may be uncertain about the true diagnosis. Attacks may be precipitated by exercise or emotion, but often occur spontaneously. Since current techniques for coronary arteriography can visualize vessels no smaller than 1 mm., it has been postulated that the syndrome reflects small vessel disease. Pathologic evidence is not available to support this thesis. It is possible that occasionally obstruction of the coronary arteries is overlooked through failure to obtain high quality films or multiple views. Injection of dye following administration of nitroglycerin may be necessary to ensure that no local obstruction exists in the coronary tree. Many patients are heavy smokers, and coronary spasm has been proposed but not proved as a cause. Raynaud's phenomenon is but rarely found in association with this syndrome. Increased affinity of hemoglobin for oxygen or local metabolic abnormality has also been postulated, but confirmation is lacking.

Diagnosis. Angina pectoris is a clinical diagnosis, largely dependent on the history. In some cases the diagnosis may be established by direct observations during an attack. In the vast majority of patients, however, the diagnosis is evident to the experienced physician from the history alone, and confirmatory tests are not needed.

The electrocardiogram may be utilized to confirm the diagnosis. In doubtful cases the recording of typical electrocardiographic "ischemic" changes, as described earlier, during an attack of pain will often be diagnostic. However, use of exercise tolerance tests with electrocardiographic recording to confirm the presence or absence of angina is frequently unsatisfactory. As usually performed in the doctor's office, occurrence of pain, the patient's complaint, is uncommon. The tests are poorly standardized and the amount of physical work may vary. False negative and false positive tests are frequent. A positive test, in the absence of pain, does not confirm the presence of angina. It does suggest, however, the presence of ischemic or coronary artery disease.

In atypical cases the response to nitroglycerin may be utilized as a critical diagnostic test. Angina pectoris is characteristically relieved in from 90 seconds to 3 minutes after sublingual administration of nitroglycerin. Failure of the patient's complaint to be relieved promptly by nitroglycerin should cast suspicion on the diagnosis of angina. Many patients have a poor sense of timing, and cannot accurately describe the duration of an attack or the quickness of relief following medication. It is important to emphasize to the patient the necessity for accurate information before drawing the conclusion that nitroglycerin is not useful and therefore that the diagnosis is in doubt.

Coronary Arteriography. Demonstration of coronary artery obstruction may be made by coronary arteriography. The technique most widely used involves selective cannulation with a specially shaped catheter that is passed to the aortic root from the brachial or femoral artery. Use of the brachial artery usually requires a cut-down and incision of the vessel. Following repair of the vessel, loss of the brachial pulse may occur in up to 30 per cent of cases. Utilization of larger vessels such as the femoral artery permits a percutaneous technique, as described by Seldinger, in which the vessel is punctured with a needle and a guide wire inserted. The needle is then withdrawn and a catheter advanced over the guidewire to the desired location. The wire is then withdrawn, and the catheter is flushed with heparinized saline or other fluid.

The coronary arteriogram is obtained when radiopaque dye is injected into the coronary ostia. Usually the pictures are recorded on 35-mm. cine film exposed at 60 frames per second. Several injections are filmed in various oblique views so that all vessels may be visualized in multiple projections. In doubtful cases arteriograms are obtained before and after administration of nitroglycerin. The vasodilation following nitroglycerin may reveal areas of obstruction not previously recognized.

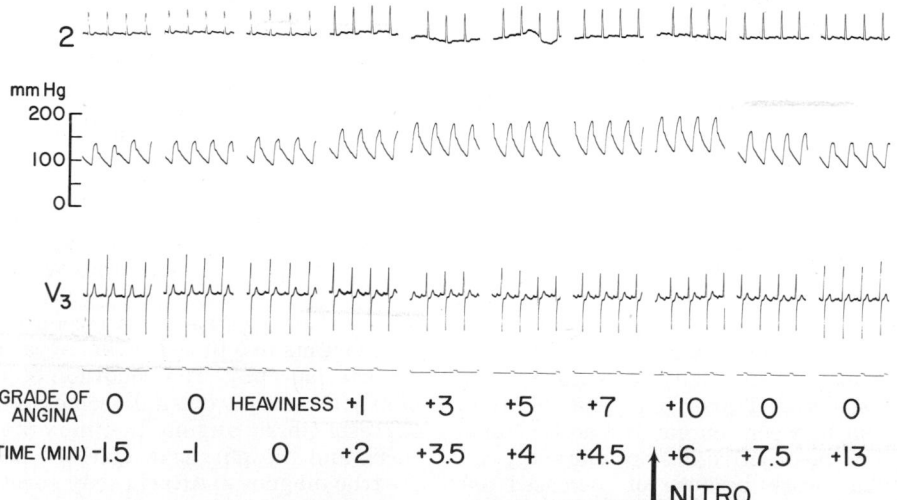

FIGURE 4. Physiologic changes during spontaneous angina pectoris in a 53-year-old man. The patient was able to grade the intensity of angina on a scale of 0, "no discomfort," to 10, "worst pain ever." Figure shows from top, lead 2 of electrocardiogram, brachial arterial pressure recorded directly; lead V_3 of electrocardiogram, 1 second time marker, grade of angina, and time in minutes. Arterial pressure before onset of angina is 135/90 mm. Hg and heart rate is 60 beats per minute. One minute before onset of sensation of heaviness in chest, heart rate and arterial pressure have increased moderately, and slight ST segment depression has appeared, best seen in V_4. During the next five minutes intensity of angina progressively increases, electrocardiographic changes are more marked, blood pressure and heart rate increase. When angina is most severe, arterial pressure has risen to 210/135 mm. Hg. Following sublingual administration of nitroglycerin, angina is relieved within 90 seconds. Arterial pressure falls coincident with improvement of symptoms.

Coronary atherosclerosis is recognized by narrowing, beading, or occlusion of the arteries. Vessels as small as 1.0 mm. may be demonstrated with good technique. Collateral vessels may be seen bridging obstructed areas or providing retrograde filling of a proximally obstructed artery.

A complete examination usually includes injection of dye into the left ventricle to obtain a left ventriculogram, and measurement of left ventricular end-diastolic pressure. Although the latter is influenced by many factors, including the stiffness of the ventricle, elevated levels suggesting compromised ventricular performance are frequently observed in patients with severe coronary artery disease. Myocardial contractility and size may be evaluated in a general way by scrutiny of the ventriculogram. The ratio of the volume of blood ejected during systole to the volume remaining at end-systole may be calculated. Normally, approximately 50 per cent of the end-diastolic volume is ejected with each beat. Smaller fractions suggest myocardial disability and increased residual volume. Areas of abnormal contractility owing to an old scar or infarction may be observed. Ventricular aneurysms may be outlined by appropriate studies.

Specific indications for coronary arteriography include the following: (1) To determine whether coronary artery disease is present. This may be necessary for evaluation of signs or symptoms. For example: an airline pilot develops T wave abnormalities not previously present on routine electrocardiogram. Unless significant coronary artery disease is ruled out by arteriogram he will be permanently grounded. (2) To determine the location and extent of disease in patients being considered for coronary artery surgery and revascularization procedures. (3) To evaluate the possibility of coronary artery fistulas, aneurysm, or anomaly as a guide to planning specific surgical therapy.

Coronary angiograms are frequently performed to evaluate the cause of atypical chest pain. As mentioned earlier, the procedure cannot establish the presence of angina; nevertheless, in some patients with incapacitating chest pain the finding of a normal coronary arteriogram can provide helpful reassurance. Attention can then be directed to symptomatic management and search for other causes of pain.

Complications of the procedure include precipitation of angina, dissection of a coronary artery, acute myocardial infarction, and asystole or ventricular fibrillation. Asystole usually responds to a blow on the chest. Atropine in a dose of 1.0 mg. intravenously is a useful preventive in susceptible subjects. Immediate DC precordial shock usually reverts ventricular fibrillation. To be successful, the shock must be applied within a few seconds of the onset of fibrillation. *Mortality* from coronary arteriography is approximately 0.1 to 0.5 per cent in skilled hands. *Morbidity* is largely related to complications of the arterial puncture or cut-down.

A diagnosis of ischemic heart disease may be confirmed by demonstration of lactate production into the coronary sinus during myocardial stress induced by isoproterenol infusion or endocardial pacing. Catheterization of the coronary sinus is utilized in some centers as part of the evaluation prior to coronary artery surgery. Successful relief of ischemia should be accompanied by postoperative evidence of reversal of anaerobic lactate production previously produced by stress.

Differential Diagnosis. Many conditions cause pain in the chest, but few, if any, truly mimic angina pectoris. The syndrome of angina is so characteristic in the majority of patients that errors in diagnosis are usually the result of careless history taking or failure by the physician to listen to what the patient is actually saying. In obtaining an accurate history it is best first to allow the patient to describe his problem in his own way, and then to amplify the story by a series of questions.

Diseases of the gallbladder and gastrointestinal tract, chest wall disorders, abnormalities of the cervicodorsal spine, and pulmonary conditions may cause discomfort in the chest. Costochondral separation may be a source of confusion, but is readily diagnosed by demonstration of exquisite point tenderness at one or more costochondral junctions on the anterior chest. Evaluation of the role of peptic ulcer disease, gallbladder abnormality, or hiatus hernia may be troublesome. Many patients with angina suffer from one or more of these conditions. It may be difficult to recognize that the patient actually has two or more complaints. Clinical experience supports the view that disease of the upper gastrointestinal tract may exacerbate angina. In some cases removal of a diseased gallbladder reduces the incidence of angina. In many patients symptoms of hiatus hernia trigger angina, especially at night; treatment with antacids and elevation of the head of the bed may improve the angina. Electrocardiographic changes have been reported during gallbladder attacks or symptomatic hiatus hernia. Usually these are nonspecific ST segment or T wave changes. They probably reflect the presence of coronary artery disease and represent an abnormal response to fever or tachycardia. Reflex changes have also been postulated as causative.

Complications. Heberden recognized that *sudden death* may occur in angina pectoris. Presumably the mechanism is ventricular fibrillation triggered by ventricular premature beats occurring in the vulnerable period of the ischemic heart. Heart block may also develop, especially in patients with certain pre-existing conduction disturbances, such as left axis deviation combined with right bundle branch block. The incidence of sudden death with angina is quoted as approximately 10 per cent, but it may actually be higher.

Most patients with angina pectoris eventually develop acute *myocardial infarction.* Our own studies suggest that the infarction is usually preceded by an intensification of symptoms and the development of progressive or crescendo angina. Any increase in frequency, duration, intensity, or lowering of the threshold for onset of pain should be viewed with grave suspicion. Such patients should be put to bed in a neutral environment and sedated; visitors should be restricted, and hypertension or heart failure treated appropriately. The aim of therapy is to forestall an impending myocardial infarction.

Treatment. An effective plan of treatment must be based on a thorough understanding of the severity and intensity of the patient's complaint. The physician should carefully explore the circumstances in which angina occurs, as well as its relation to physical exertion, emotional outbursts, and other causative factors. Often, minor adjustments in the patient's activity will reduce the frequency of attacks. Angina often occurs repeatedly during the same activity. Avoidance of that specific activity or administration of nitroglycerin before onset will usually reduce symptoms. Should an attack occur, most patients will stop, rest, and administer a nitroglycerin tablet. Some will ignore the discomfort and continue their exertion. Progressive increase in intensity of pain usually forces the subject to stop. Occasionally the pain will improve despite continued activity. Although the development of angina usually indicates significant obstruction of one or more vessels by coronary atherosclerosis, it is important to emphasize the generally good prognosis in patients with stable angina. The patient should be encouraged to report any change in the pattern of angina promptly to his physician.

The association of angina and a moderately severe *depression* is not uncommon. Angina may remind the patient that he is growing older, and that his activity is becoming restricted. Physician and patient should take an optimistic and realistic point of view. With appropriate therapy and some adjustment of the daily living pattern, activity may be nearly normal. Angina may persist for many years. During this time the patient may continue to work and to enjoy recreation and normal family relationships. There may be considerable anxiety, especially on the part of the spouse, about *sexual activity*. The patient may reasonably be encouraged to engage in those activities as long as they do not precipitate disturbing symptoms.

Before treatment for angina is advised, possible contributing conditions should be carefully evaluated. There is no doubt about the striking relationship between *smoking* and increased risk of sudden death or myocardial infarction with coronary artery disease. Patients with coronary artery disease and angina pectoris should be encouraged in the strongest possible terms to cease smoking. The evidence for an adverse effect of smoking on the natural history of coronary artery disease is overwhelming. Epidemiologic data indicate that, following cessation of smoking, the risk of myocardial infarction or sudden death declines to that of a nonsmoker in a few weeks.

Many patients who develop angina are *overweight*. Reduction of body mass to more normal values may be associated with clinical improvement. It is frequently useful to treat even mild

diastolic hypertension, levels of 90 to 100 mm. Hg, with an agent such as hydrochlorothiazide, 50 mg. daily. In older patients systolic pressure is usually increased because of increased vascular stiffness. Although this systolic hypertension may increase left ventricular work, treatment of systolic blood pressure elevation of itself is not usually recommended.

In an occasional patient, angina is a manifestation of left ventricular failure. Treatment of the *heart failure* may produce dramatic improvement of the angina. The onset of exertional dyspnea prior to the perception of pain is a clue suggesting the possibility that angina is precipitated by left ventricular failure. Rarely digitalis intensifies angina, and the drug must be discontinued. Rapid paroxysmal *arrhythmia* may precipitate angina even in the absence of coronary artery disease. Usually, however, angina in the presence of arrhythmia in the older patient indicates coronary atherosclerosis. Treatment aimed at prevention of the arrhythmia may forestall chest pain. Angina may be complicated by arrhythmia, especially ventricular premature beats. Their presence may increase the risk of sudden death and should be treated promptly.

Drug Therapy. *Immediate Treatment. Nitroglycerin (glyceryl trinitrate* sublingual tablets) in doses of 0.15 to 0.60 mg. sublingually is the single most effective agent for treatment of the acute episode in most cases. With the exception of amyl nitrite, no other agent can approach it in general usefulness. Onset of action begins in one and one half to three minutes. Relief is usually dramatic and immediate. Occasionally the patient will take a second dose a few minutes after the first for complete effect. A large number of tablets may be ingested daily with few side effects. A fullness or pounding in the head is common, but most patients tolerate this well. An occasional patient will refuse to continue the medication because of intolerable headache. Fortunately such occurrences are rare. Because the drug is an effective peripheral vasodilator, the individual should first test its effectiveness while sitting or lying to avoid the possibility of syncope. It has been said that nitroglycerin loses its potency during storage and that some patients may become tolerant of the drug through prolonged usage. Although these possibilities should be kept in mind, they do not appear to be troublesome in practice.

Nitroglycerin is a potent smooth muscle vasodilator. Following administration, a decline in coronary vascular resistance and an increase in coronary blood flow can be demonstrated in laboratory animals and normal man. In the past it was thought that the drug relieved angina by its direct action on the coronary vascular tree. Recent studies have shown, however, that sublingual administration of the drug has little primary influence on coronary vascular resistance or coronary blood flow in patients with advanced coronary artery disease. This is not surprising when one considers the intimal and medial distortion characteristic of atherosclerosis. Injection of nitroglycerin directly into coronary ostia in diseased vessels causes a fleeting increase in coronary flow as revealed by disappearance curves of radioactive krypton or xenon. It is unlikely that the effectiveness of nitroglycerin in angina can be ascribed to a direct action on the heart. Following sublingual nitroglycerin there is a fall in systemic blood pressure and a decrease in calculated systemic vascular resistance. The great veins dilate, causing pooling of venous return, and cardiac output declines. The net result of these systemic effects is a marked decrease in cardiac work. Since angina results from an imbalance between oxygen demand and oxygen delivery, any mechanism that restores a more favorable relationship by either increasing delivery (coronary blood flow) or reducing demand (cardiac work) should theoretically be therapeutic. Current evidence strongly suggests that nitroglycerin is dramatically effective because it rapidly reduces cardiac work, thus reversing myocardial ischemia in patients with abnormalities of the coronary arteries.

Amyl nitrite is an extremely potent vasodilator that was first described in the treatment of angina more than 100 years ago. The drug is extremely volatile; it is contained in small, 0.3 ml. ampules which are crushed, and the vapor is briefly inhaled. It has a strong, clinging odor, and is best used in a room with good ventilation. Because of its extreme potency, the drug should be applied only when the patient is lying down. The ampule is crushed and wafted under the nose two or three times. A deep breath or two is generally all that is needed to obtain an effect. If the drug is administered by a second person, caution is advised to avoid his inhaling too much drug.

Amyl nitrite causes a profound peripheral arterial vasodilation. Blood pressure will fall precipitously with adequate dosage. In contrast to nitroglycerin, it has relatively little effect on the great veins, and venous pooling is not marked. For this reason cardiac output increases considerably following inhalation of the drug. Because of these effects on peripheral resistance and flow, amyl nitrite has been utilized to evaluate certain heart murmurs, such as those associated with aortic stenosis or mitral regurgitation, and to reveal the characteristic pressure pulse in hypertrophic myocardial disease. Following amyl nitrite, the murmur of aortic stenosis is accentuated because of the increased cardiac output, whereas the murmur of mitral regurgitation declines in intensity because of the marked drop in peripheral resistance.

The use of amyl nitrite is currently unfashionable. It is, however, extremely effective in the occasional patient with severe, persistent angina and concomitant hypertension with high levels of diastolic pressure. The hypertension may be secondary to the angina and represent an exaggerated pressor response to pain. In the author's experience, amyl nitrite is extremely effective in this situation, relieving the hypertension and pain most impressively. In some patients with angina complicated by hypertension, amyl nitrite is the only consistently effective form of therapy.

Drugs Given to Lessen the Frequency of Attacks. Long-acting nitrites are said to provide relief of angina throughout the day by virtue of sustained blood levels of active substances. These include erythrityl tetranitrate (10 to 30 mg.), pentaerythritol tetranitrate (10 to 20 mg.), and isosorbide dinitrate (5 to 30 mg.) taken three or four times daily. Although large amounts of these drugs are dispensed and many physicians and patients are satisfied with their usefulness, objective evidence of significant clinical effect is lacking. Evaluation of the treatment of angina is difficult because the response to therapy is often highly subjective and depends on the patient's assessment of his own symptoms. A skillful physician with positive transference from the patient may be extremely effective in managing angina, but aside from the acute effects of nitroglycerin and amyl nitrite, the role of other agents such as long-acting nitrites is difficult to measure. Carefully executed double blind studies have failed to provide convincing data on the efficacy of the long-acting agents.

Sedation is a useful adjunct to therapy in many instances. Neither phenobarbital nor any of the many available tranquilizers have specific cardiac action in small dosage, but may reduce anxiety and fearfulness. Alcohol in moderation may be helpful for some patients. In patients with a major component of depression, the antidepressant agents such as Tofranil, Elavil, and Ritalin may be useful.

Propranolol, a beta adrenergic blocking agent, is effective in selected patients for reducing the frequency and severity of angina. In the opinion of some experienced workers, the introduction of propranolol in the treatment of angina represents the most significant advance in medical management since the advent of nitroglycerin. Stimulation of the sympathetic nerves to the heart or infusion of isoproterenol intravenously increases cardiac rate and augments contractility, or the strength and velocity of the cardiac contraction. These functions are specifically blocked by propranolol.

Recent clinical experience attests to the efficacy of propranolol in the treatment of angina. At least 50 per cent of patients offered a therapeutic trial of the drug are significantly improved. Dosage ranges from 80 to 300 mg. or more daily in three or four divided doses. In treating patients with propranolol it is best to begin with a low dose, 40 to 80 mg. daily, and continuously increase the dosage, if the drug is well tolerated, in an attempt to achieve the desired therapeutic effect.

Propranolol reduces heart rate and decreases myocardial contractility. Studies in man have shown that administration of the drug is associated with a fall in cardiac output and a reduction in maximal dp/dt. Left ventricular end-diastolic pressure may rise. The normal response to exercise is blunted so that the anticipated increase in heart rate and cardiac output is limited. During exertion left ventricular end-diastolic pressure in patients maintained on propranolol may increase sharply, suggesting severe impairment of function. In addition to slowing the rate, propranolol has a quinidine-like effect on the transmembrane action potential, and is thus an antiarrhythmic. Propranolol may induce heart block and should be used cautiously in patients with known atrioventricular conduction disturbance. The drug is contraindicated in patients with advanced forms of heart block, such as a greatly prolonged PR interval, intermittent atrioventricular block with dropped beats, or complete heart block.

The mechanism of action of propranolol in the treatment of angina appears to be related to its direct myocardial action, reducing cardiac stroke work by decreasing myocardial contractility. The drug also reduces resting and exercise heart rate, thus contributing to a decline in cardiac work per minute. Myocardial oxygen need is largely controlled by systolic pressure, contractility, and heart rate. Since propranolol reduces all three, oxygen demand is lower following administration of the drug. The drug does not increase coronary blood flow or oxygen delivery; indeed, these parameters may actually decline.

In general, large doses of propranolol are required for successful treatment of angina. If effective doses are well tolerated, the number of nitroglycerin tablets ingested daily declines. Patients note fewer angina episodes and remark that those that do occur are less intense. The majority of patients develop *heart failure* on high doses of the drug, and it is best to administer digitalis and even mild diuretics such as hydrochlorothiazide, 25 to 50 mg. daily, with appropriate potassium replacement before beginning propranolol. In some patients severe bradycardia or the development of heart block necessitates the withdrawal of treatment. Propranolol is an extremely potent agent and it must be used with caution under close medical supervision. Postural hypotension and exaggeration of bronchospasm in patients with asthma are occasionally troublesome side effects.

Surgical Treatment.   Many surgical procedures have been advocated to provide additional coronary blood supply or relieve obstructed vessels. Talcum powder has been dusted in the pericardial space in the hope of stimulating anastomotic vessels between pericardium and epicardium. Evidence of improved myocardial nutrient flow following this operation is not convincing, and the procedure has been generally abandoned.

The implantation of an internal mammary artery into a myocardial tunnel (*Vineberg procedure*) with various modifications has been extremely popular among surgeons during the past decade. In selected cases mortality is approximately 5 per cent. The artery must be implanted in viable and presumably ischemic tissue. Implantation in an area of low coronary flow, as in a scar, is useless. If the implanted area is ischemic, a network of fine anastomotic vessels gradually develops between the implanted artery and the coronary vessels. Full development takes several months, and clinical improvement is not usually noted until at least two or three months postoperatively. About three fourths of the implanted arteries remain patent, as demonstrated by postoperative angiography. Skeptical physicians have questioned the value of the Vineberg procedure. Does the implantation really provide nutrient flow? Angiography six or more months after operation with injection of contrast agent into the root of the artery implanted in the myocardial tunnel frequently reveals dye running into the heart, causing a myocardial blush, and then draining into the coronary sinus. Metabolic studies have also shown reversal of myocardial lactate production at rest or during myocardial stress in some patients following the procedure. It is likely, therefore, that increased nutrient flow can result from the Vineberg procedure. Difficulties in evaluating the results of surgical therapy relate to the selection of patients and the variable nature of angina. An acute myocardial infarction may occur as a complication of surgery, and this event may explain the immediate benefit observed in some patients.

It is now technically feasible to anastomose small vessels to the coronary arteries either directly or by utilizing vein grafts. If arteriography shows proximal obstruction of one or more coronary arteries and the patient is symptomatic, such operations may be indicated. Postoperative angiograms have frequently been impressive and have shown that the anastomoses function and provide increased blood flow to large areas of the coronary vasculature. In contrast to the Vineberg procedure, the direct anastomoses are effective immediately. In patients with extensive coronary artery disease the heart is frequently enlarged, contractility is poor, end-diastolic pressures are high, and the ejection fraction (stroke volume/end-diastolic volume) is low. It has been claimed that these abnormalities are improved when coronary blood flow is augmented by direct anastomotic procedures. Such an observation would have great significance in the treatment of coronary artery disease, but the claim requires further substantiation.

Indications for surgical revascularization of the heart focus predominantly on the relief of angina. Surgery may be considered in the patient with frequent episodes of angina which seriously hinder normal activity and are unresponsive to medical therapy. The decision regarding surgery should be made by consultation between physician and surgeon. The patient's interests are best served when he is evaluated first by a physician who works closely with a cardiac-surgical group and who has a continuing experience in the pre- and postoperative management of patients undergoing cardiovascular surgery.

Although unremitting angina is the prime indication for surgery, it has been suggested that patients with premature coronary artery disease or myocardial infarction should also be considered. There is solid evidence accumulating that angina is improved or relieved in some patients following revascularization procedures. It will be many years before their influence on long-term mortality can be evaluated. Furthermore, long-term treatment with propranolol may improve prognosis. One study suggested that the long-term influence on mortality from either a Vineberg procedure or propranolol therapy was essentially the same. The results of any new surgical therapy must be compared with the effect of more conservative medical management, because angina pectoris is a capricious disorder which waxes and wanes according to a variety of influences, including extent of disease, occurrence of myocardial infarction, emotional state, weather, medications, and attitude of the physician.

Another form of surgical therapy that has attracted considerable interest is stimulation of the sinus nerve with an implanted battery-powered device. Sinus nerve stimulation reduces cardiac work by slowing heart rate and reducing arterial pressure secondary to vasodilation. The patient may voluntarily turn on the stimulator when he develops an angina attack. This technique is both clever and intriguing. Initial results with its use show considerable promise.

Prognosis. In some patients angina may gradually improve and even disappear. Most patients with angina carry on their daily activity with relatively little discomfort for many years. By avoiding trigger situations and taking nitroglycerin prophylactically prior to stressful situations, they may have relatively few severe attacks. Angina persisting for more than 10 years is not uncommon, and many patients survive 20 years or more.

Any worsening of angina should be viewed with grave suspicion. Intensification of symptoms may represent new coronary occlusion or loss of collateral blood supply. Progressive or crescendo angina may herald the onset of acute myocardial infarction—the so-called *impending coronary syndrome*. Hospitalization with sedation, strict bed rest, possibly anticoagulation, and treatment of increased blood pressure, if present, may be called for in an attempt to prevent overt myocardial infarction. Many experienced observers have postulated that sudden improvement in angina implies a small infarction in the ischemic area, an infarction too small to be detected clinically by electrocardiogram or blood enzyme change. This idea is supported by the high incidence of small left ventricular scars found at autopsy in patients with a history of angina.

The prognosis is actually best in patients with coronary artery disease, despite the hazards of sudden death or acute myocardial infarction. Angina complicating valvular or congenital heart disease usually implies a far advanced process, and has a poor prognosis.

ACUTE MYOCARDIAL INFARCTION

Definition. Acute myocardial infarction is a clinical syndrome resulting from deficient coronary arterial flow to an area of myocardium with eventual cellular death and necrosis. It is characterized by severe and prolonged precordial pain, similar to, but more intense than, that of angina pectoris, and signs of myocardial damage, including acute electrocardiographic changes and a rise in activity of certain serum enzymes.

Etiology and Pathology. Although it is attractive to view acute myocardial infarction as the direct result of a sudden obstruction of a major coronary artery, current pathologic studies indicate that this is not always the case. Infarction without occlusion and occlusion without infarction may be observed pathologically. Occlusion, when present, is found in large extramyocardial coronary arteries, usually within 1 to 2 cm. of their origin. An occlusion may result from an acute thrombosis, subintimal hemorrhage, or rupture of an atheromatous plaque which may initiate clot formation.

The development of coronary artery thrombi apparently depends on the time and mechanism of death. Clots in the coronary arteries have been observed in approximately 25 per cent of patients who die suddenly. Patients who survive myocardial infarction for several hours or days and then die from heart failure or cardiogenic shock manifest a high incidence of coronary thrombi; an incidence of up to 60 or 70 per cent has been reported. In many instances, however, the thrombosis appears to be younger than the associated infarction, suggesting that the myocardial damage caused the clot. In an extensive international study on death from myocardial infarction, it was found that 25 per cent of the patients had no recognized coronary occlusion in large vessels, had less coronary artery disease than expected, and had died within a few hours of the onset of the acute attack.

Significant coronary artery disease can usually be demonstrated in the vessel directly supplying the area of infarction. Extensive collateral development may make correlation of precise myocardial and vascular relationships difficult. In the presence of collaterals, an acute arterial occlusion may not produce ischemia or infarction. If an area is dependent on collateral flow, on the other hand, a remote occlusion or a change in the balance of vascular resistance may produce an infarction considerably removed from the source of difficulty.

The possibility that evanescent platelet agglutination may precipitate myocardial infarction has recently attracted considerable interest. Platelets have been shown to adhere to collagen and basement membrane, and these structures may be exposed in injured vessels. When injured, platelets release adenosine diphosphate which accelerates the agglutination of platelets to form an adherent or obstructing clump. Platelets release many other active factors which adhere to the vessel wall. It has been shown experimentally that the injection of adenosine diphosphate causes platelet aggregation within the coronary arteries. The peripheral platelet count falls. Although platelet thrombi can be observed on microscopic sections shortly after injection of the adenosine diphosphate, the clumps are no longer apparent after ten minutes. Acute myocardial infarction can be recognized pathologically in two hours, yet by this time the coronary arteries are no longer obstructed. The theory that platelets may play a role in the development of acute myocardial infarction or angina pectoris remains an intriguing but as yet an unproved possibility.

A myocardial infarct is termed *transmural* when it extends from endocardium to epicardium and *nontransmural* when the necrosis does not reach the inner or outer surface. A *subendocardial* infarct involves the endocardial and subendocardial layers. In general, transmural infarcts tend to be larger than nontransmural infarcts and are associated with more severe complications of ventricular dysfunction. Subendocardial infarcts may also be quite extensive, and are associated with occlusive disease of all three of the major coronary arteries. Since the subendocardial layer is subjected to the greatest amount of wall tension, subendocardial infarcts may result from prolonged hypotension or shock owing to noncardiac causes, and may complicate hemorrhage, anesthesia, or extensive surgical procedures.

Acute myocardial infarction is predominantly a disease of the left ventricle and the inner ventricular septum. Occasionally the infarct extends into the right ventricle, and the atria may also be involved. The extent and location of the infarct depends upon the causative factors, the extent of coronary artery disease, the presence of collateral blood supply, and whether previous infarctions have occurred. Any condition which tends to increase cardiac work, and hence oxygen need, will tend to enlarge the infarction. Thus hypertension, tachycardia, cardiac enlargement with consequent increased wall tension, or acute change in contractility may aggravate the extent of infarction. Decrease in coronary blood flow or coronary perfusion pressure, as with hypotension or shock, will have similar effects.

Other Causes. *Coronary embolization* may complicate bacterial endocarditis or left atrial thrombosis, resulting in acute infarction or sudden death. Embolization of calcified excrescences may occur in *aortic stenosis*. Myocardial infarction without coronary obstruction may complicate aortic stenosis if coronary perfusion pressure drops, with syncope or hypotension, although ventricular systolic work is maintained at a high level because of the fixed obstruction. Acute myocardial infarction secondary to *arteritis* has been described in periarteritis nodosa and acute hypersensitivity syndromes. In Marfan's syndrome, *cystic necrosis* of the media may involve the coronary arteries as well as the aorta. In acute aortic dissection, the separation may extend to the base of the aorta and include a major coronary artery. Electrocardiographic changes suggesting subendocardial ischemia or necrosis may be observed following prolonged *surgical procedures,* often with extensive blood loss and replacement, or secondary to hypotension or shock from a variety of causes.

Clinical Manifestations. The outstanding characteristic of acute myocardial infarction is severe, prolonged pain. The pain is usually qualitatively similar to that of angina, but is more intense and persists much longer. It is usually present for at least half an hour, but may last for many hours. Nitroglycerin affords no relief, or only temporarily abates the attack. The pain is usually relieved by administration of opiates, although repeated doses may be required.

The pain is described as pressing or crushing, like a deep ache inside the chest. Often patients will press on the sternum or state that it feels as though there were a great weight on the chest, such as a rock or someone sitting on it. The pain is a deep visceral discomfort, and usually it is not described as sharp or lancelike. The radiation of pain is similar to that of angina: it may be felt in the right or left arm but usually the left, in the elbow and down to the fingers, in the jaw, in the back, or in the upper epigastric area. Although the symptoms have never occurred before, many patients will state that they are having a heart attack. Intense fear of impending death or doom is common. If pulmonary edema and cardiogenic shock are early complications, the pain may be obscured.

Although the typical patient with acute infarction presents with severe pain, the range of response is wide. The pain may be brief and not severe. Occasionally, an electrocardiogram will reveal evidence of acute or recent infarction without a history of pain. Patients who have associated gastrointestinal disease, such as peptic ulcer, hiatus hernia, or gallbladder disorders, may have difficulty separating the pain of infarction from that of the other conditions. In patients with preexisting angina pectoris, infarction may be heralded by a more intense episode of pain, unrelieved by nitroglycerin or rest. Should the infarction precipitate acute pulmonary edema, the pain becomes a minor complaint. Acute arrhythmia, especially heart block or ventricular tachycardia, may be the presenting sign. Atrioventricular dissociation is relatively common in diaphragmatic-inferior infarctions, and the first symptom may be weakness or syncope owing to marked bradycardia. Patients with severe coronary artery disease may develop myocardial infarction with any prolonged circulatory disorder such as heart failure, hypertension, or arrhythmia. Sometimes it is difficult to be certain which came first, the circulatory disorder or the acute infarction.

In patients who survive to be hospitalized for acute infarction, *prodromata* are common. In one study, two thirds treated in a coronary care unit had prodromal symptoms, usually chest pain, prior to the acute infarction. Prodromata are most common in patients with angina pectoris, and are usually manifested by progressive or crescendo angina. The pain is more easily triggered, lasts longer, and is more intense than usual. Any change in the pattern of previously stable angina pectoris should be viewed as possibly a forewarning of impending acute infarction.

Physical Findings. The patient with acute infarction is usually restless, apprehensive, and in severe pain. His color may be poor, the face ashen, and the nailbeds cyanotic. Sweating is frequent, and the skin is cool. Examination of the lungs may reveal essentially normal findings. Alternatively there may be signs suggesting early heart failure or acute pulmonary edema. The heart sounds are often distant and muffled. Paradoxical splitting of the second sound may appear. Usually a fourth heart sound and sometimes a third are present. Auscultation may reveal a soft murmur, suggesting mitral regurgitation. The pulse may be thready and the blood pressure reduced. A careful examination provides the physician with an evaluation of myocardial performance, but it can neither establish nor deny the possibility of a diagnosis of acute infarction.

Laboratory Findings. Routine laboratory examinations reveal abnormalities compatible with necrosis of tissue. The temperature is usually elevated for the first three to five days after acute infarction. The rise is usually modest, to 100° or 101° F., but occasionally the temperature becomes quite high, up to 104° F. In an occasional patient continued high fever, apparently caused by myocardial necrosis, threatens survival, and extraordinary measures to reduce the temperature, including cooling baths and cold blankets, may be necessary.

Leukocytosis occurs regularly, but usually persists no longer than five days to a week. White counts of 12,000 to 15,000 cells per cubic millimeter with a shift to the left are usual. Counts above this level should be viewed with suspicion and possible complications assiduously sought.

Serial analysis of activity in blood of a variety of enzymes normally found intracellularly is of great value in establishing the diagnosis of acute myocardial infarction. It has been shown experimentally that infarction of as little as 1 gram of myocardium will result in a detectable serum enzyme rise. If the enzyme activity is not elevated in a patient suspected of having acute infarction, it is assumed that no infarction occurred or that the tissue damage was so small that it could not be detectable by current techniques. Proper interpretation of serum enzyme patterns requires measurement of enzyme activity for several days after the presumed acute infarction.

Glutamic oxaloacetic transaminase (GOT) is an enzyme present in high concentration in myocardium, skeletal muscle, liver, brain, and kidney. Normal serum activity is 20 to 40 Frank-Karmen units, or 30 to 60 international units. Following myocardial infarction, serum activity rises, reach-

ing a peak in 48 hours, and gradually falling to normal by five days. Providing that liver necrosis has not also occurred, the peak levels correlate in a rough way with the extent of myocardial damage. Levels of over 300 Frank-Karmen units are usually associated with extensive infarction complicated by heart failure or shock. Serum GOT activity increases also in a wide variety of disorders associated with hepatic necrosis, including central necrosis of the liver, heart failure, hypotension, or shock. Narcotics such as morphine and, to a lesser extent, meperidine may be associated with a rise in serum activity, presumably secondary to spasm of the sphincter of Oddi.

Lactic dehydrogenase (LDH) is found in a variety of tissues, and elevations of serum activity are usually not specific for a diagnosis of myocardial infarction. Of the five isoenzymes of LDH, fraction 1 (termed fraction 5 in the European nomenclature) is normally found in serum in small concentration, and increase of this fraction in blood strongly suggests recent myocardial necrosis. Serum *creatine phosphokinase* activity, an enzyme occurring in high concentration in heart and skeletal muscle, rises rapidly, reaching peak levels approximately 24 hours after acute myocardial infarction. Serum activity returns to normal within 72 hours.

Electrocardiogram. The electrocardiogram is extremely useful in evaluating the patient with a tentative diagnosis of acute myocardial infarction, providing that the tracing is interpreted with full knowledge of the wide variety of nonspecific factors which may induce abnormality. The hallmark of *acute transmural infarction* is the appearance of Q waves of sufficient amplitude and duration to be termed significant. The electrocardiogram is usually diagnostic when obtained during the pain. It has been said that changes may not occur for two to five days after infarction in some patients, but this seems unlikely. Late appearance of ECG abnormality usually indicates that an impending infarction syndrome finally culminated in infarction and death of cardiac tissue. During the early stage of infarction the ST segments are markedly elevated in those leads depicting the area of infarction with reciprocal ST segment depression elsewhere. As the infarct evolves electrically the ST segments become depressed and the T waves inverted. Varying degrees of abnormality persist, although in some patients recognition of healed transmural infarction from the ECG may be difficult.

In *nontransmural* and *subendocardial infarction,* abnormalities in the ECG are primarily in the ST segments and T waves. The ST segments may be elevated, but are usually depressed in leads reflecting the area of infarction, and the T waves are usually inverted. Interpretation of the ECG may be difficult because of the nonspecific nature of the ST segment and T wave change. Serial tracings over several days may be helpful, especially if the abnormalities progressively improve toward the preinfarction pattern.

Diaphragmatic or inferior infarctions are reflected in leads 2, 3, and aVf. Anterior-septal infarctions influence leads V_2 to V_4, whereas anterior-lateral infarctions involve leads V_3 to V_6. Strictly posterior infarctions are recognized by changes in V_1 and V_2. Subendocardial damage usually results in development of an ST and T vector opposite in direction to the mean QRS vector. Left bundle branch block frequently obscures the recognition of acute infarction because of the abnormal initial QRS vector, but right bundle branch block does not.

Diagnosis. The diagnosis of acute transmural myocardial infarction is straightforward when the patient presents with severe, crushing precordial pain lasting 30 minutes or more, and the electrocardiogram reveals characteristic Q waves and ST segment elevation of the "hyperacute" stage. Myocardial infarction, however, has a wide range of clinical manifestations, and recognition of the acute episode may be difficult.

Diagnosis is based on a clinical triad: (1) prolonged cardiac pain, more severe and longer lasting than angina, (2) abnormal electrocardiograms with a progressive evolution of pattern, and (3) rise and fall in serum enzyme activity. At least two of these should be present to support the diagnosis. In some patients pain either does not occur or is not recognized as representing a serious illness. Denial is an important component of the initial response to the symptoms of acute infarction in many patients, making interpretation of the history difficult. As with angina, the pain may be ascribed to indigestion or other gastrointestinal complaint. When acute infarction is a complication of a surgical procedure, anesthesia, trauma, or other disease such as gastrointestinal hemorrhage, hypertension, or shock, pain may be absent. The diagnosis is then suspected from changes in the electrocardiogram, and may be corroborated by serial analysis of blood enzyme activity.

In acute transmural infarction the electrocardiogram is usually diagnostic when obtained during or after the pain. Interpretation of the electrocardiogram in nontransmural or subendocardial infarction may be difficult. Frequently the tracing was previously abnormal, and changes in the ST segments or T waves may not be marked. The electrocardiogram may be surprisingly unrevealing in some patients with one or more previous infarctions and extensive atherosclerosis of the three major coronary vessels. Probably the widespread yet discrete abnormalities cancel each other out on the surface electrocardiogram. In an occasional patient a clinical diagnosis of acute infarction seems certain, but the electrocardiogram remains unchanged.

Serial assay of blood enzyme activity is most useful when the clinical story is not helpful or is imprecise. Acute abnormality of the electrocardiogram followed by resolution toward normal coupled with a characteristic rise and fall of enzyme activity will usually be diagnostic. There are many situations in which it is not possible to prove or disprove the diagnosis of acute infarction,

yet the wise clinician chooses to treat the patient as though infarction had occurred.

Differential Diagnosis. The most frequent problem is determining whether the patient has had a prolonged attack of angina or an infarction. Electrocardiographic abnormalities develop during angina, but the changes revert to the previous pattern when the pain subsides. Fever and leukocytosis are not present. The serum enzymes do not rise following angina pectoris. Persistent electrocardiographic abnormality after a severe pain of angina suggests that subendocardial or nontransmural infarction has developed, especially if accompanied by changes in serum enzyme activity. Although great reliance is often placed on assay of serum enzymes, it seems likely that small, discrete infarctions may occur without a detectable rise in enzyme activity.

A diagnosis of impending infarction is made when episodes of cardiac pain are prolonged and progressive or crescendo in nature. During the pain, which is usually exceptionally severe, the patient may become fearful and apprehensive and break into a sweat. Blood pressure may climb to exceptionally high levels. The attack may be accompanied by acute electrocardiographic changes, either marked depression or elevation of the ST segments and inversion of the T waves. QRS amplitude may fall, or occasionally increase. Following the attack the electrocardiogram returns to the pre-pain form, and serum enzyme activity remains normal. The preinfarction syndrome is a manifestation of a dynamic change in coronary circulation—either a progressive diminution in the caliber of some vessels or a marked increase in cardiac work and, hence, oxygen need. Some patients respond to bed rest, sedation, a quiet environment, and anticoagulation, and the condition subsides. In other patients acute infarction eventually occurs, and the attacks of pain cease.

Acute pericarditis may be mistaken for acute myocardial infarction. The pain of pericarditis is often made worse by deep inspiration. Relief is obtained by sitting up and leaning forward. The hallmark of pericarditis is a precordial friction rub which characteristically has three components: presystolic, early diastolic, and systolic. Faint rubs with only one or two components are often missed or mistaken for soft murmurs. The electrocardiogram in acute pericarditis shows moderate ST segment elevation initially with upright T waves. Later the ST segment may be slightly depressed and the T waves become inverted. Q waves do not occur in pericarditis.

Pulmonary embolus may cause chest pain and electrocardiographic changes, but the pleuritic pain is seldom suggestive of myocardial infarction. The electrocardiogram in pulmonary embolus may reveal an S1, S2, S3 pattern, complete or incomplete right bundle branch block (usually evanescent), or clockwise rotation of the precordial pattern suggesting right ventricular overload.

Other conditions which may be confused with myocardial infarction include *ruptured aortic* aneurysm, acute aortic dissection, acute pneumo-thorax, gallbladder disease, pneumonia, and acute arrhythmia. Errors in diagnoses can frequently be ascribed to inadequacies of the history and physical examination or overinterpretation of nonspecific changes in the electrocardiogram.

Complications. **Sudden Death** Sudden, unexpected fatality occurs in as many as 30 per cent of patients with acute myocardial infarction. The incidence is not related to the severity of the infarction and is most likely to develop in the first four to six hours after clinical onset, the frequency decreasing exponentially thereafter. Observations from monitoring units suggest that the mechanism is probably ventricular fibrillation in most cases, although acute heart block may be the initial arrhythmia in some.

Sudden death outside the hospital may be the first manifestation of coronary artery disease. When death occurs within one hour in the setting of apparent previous good health, pathologic examination will reveal evidence of advanced coronary artery disease in the majority of cases. Almost one third have had a previous infarction, and more than half have a history of ischemic heart disease. In ambulatory and asymptomatic patients in middle age the incidence of sudden death is increased some seven to ten times if premature ventricular beats are recorded on routine electrocardiography. The high incidence of sudden death in the first few hours after onset of attack is the major reason for strong emphasis on early recognition and treatment of acute myocardial infarction.

Arrhythmia. More than 90 per cent of patients hospitalized with acute infarction have arrhythmia, especially during the first 72 hours. Some dysrhythmias are trivial, some are potentially life-threatening, and some have such immediate consequences that their mere recognition should impel prompt, vigorous therapy. Abnormal rhythms may affect cardiac performance by adversely influencing ventricular rate, altering the sequence of atrial and ventricular contraction, or initiating depolarization from an abnormal focus. Of greatest importance clinically is the adequacy of the ventricular rate. In general if the ventricular rate is reasonable (60 to 110 beats per minute) and well tolerated, treatment of an abnormal rhythm may not be especially urgent. On the other hand, if the ventricular rate is either too fast or too slow, prompt correction of the situation is usually indicated. Patients with myocardial damage often have fixed stroke volumes so that minute volume, or cardiac output, is dependent upon heart rate. If the heart rate is too slow, as in sinus bradycardia or heart block, cardiac output may fall.

A sinus rate greater than 110 beats per minute is often an ominous sign. *Sinus tachycardia* may reflect a low stroke volume or impending shock. If evidence of heart failure is present, the rate may slow following cautious administration of digitalis. *Sinus bradycardia* occurs in 10 to 15 per cent of patients with acute infarction. Presumably it is a reflection of sinus node dysfunction secondary to alteration of blood supply, although reflex "vagotonia" has been postulated. Bradycardia is usually an early complication and lasts but a few hours.

Arrhythmia of atrial or nodal (junctional) origin may reflect atrial infarction, the development of heart failure, hypokalemia, digitalis excess, or a combination of factors. Atrial premature beats are often the forerunner of sustained *atrial dysrhythmia*. Atrial tachycardia is uncommon in myocardial infarction. *Atrial fibrillation or flutter* occurs in about 10 per cent of patients and has a marked tendency to spontaneous reversion followed by relapse within minutes.

Prolongations of the PR time (*first degree block*) and Wenckebach phenomenon (*second degree block*) are due to disorders of conduction in the region of the A-V node. They are frequent complications of inferior-diaphragmatic infarctions (electrocardiographic changes in leads 2, 3 aVf) and reflect disturbance of blood supply to the AV node from the posterior surface of the heart. This form of block is almost always temporary, and improves after a few hours or a day or two. In inferior-diaphragmatic infarctions the normal sinus and the AV nodal pacemaker may discharge at approximately the same rate. The dominant pacemaker oscillates between the two nodes, depending on their respective rates. The QRS complex is normal in form, and the ventricular rate is usually above 55. This arrhythmia is not a form of heart block, because the normal conduction pathways will be utilized whenever a sinus node impulse arrives in the region of the AV node after ventricular repolarization. Specific treatment is not required.

Complete heart block is a dangerous and potentially lethal complication of acute myocardial infarction. The mortality is approximately 50 per cent. In the form known as Mobitz type II, AV block develops suddenly without previous prolongation of the PR interval or dropped beats. Direct recordings of the electrogram from the bundle of His indicate that this conduction disturbance is almost always caused by bilateral bundle branch block. It seldom occurs without prior conduction abnormality, such as right or left bundle branch block or marked left axis deviation. When complete heart block complicates acute infarction, the ventricular response is usually slow, and the QRS complexes are wide and bizarre. About half the patients with pre-existing bundle branch block develop acute heart block as a complication of myocardial infarction. The incidence is especially high with the QV_1-RBBB pattern. Some authorities advocate the placement of a temporary pacemaker-electrode in the right ventricle in all patients with pre-existing bundle branch block because of the danger of developing bilateral bundle branch block.

Ventricular premature beats are common in acute myocardial infarction, occurring in about 75 per cent of monitored patients. Premature beats are important because they may initiate ventricular tachycardia or ventricular fibrillation if sufficiently premature to strike the vulnerable period of the diastolic repolarization phase of the cardiac cycle. The vulnerable period occurs during the latter portion of the relative refractory period, and coincides with the ascending limb of the T wave. The more closely coupled a ventricular premature beat is to the preceding normal beat, the more likely it is to initiate tachycardia or fibrillation.

Ventricular tachycardia, defined as three or more consecutive ventricular beats, and *ventricular fibrillation* occur in about 10 per cent of patients hospitalized with acute infarction. When the rate in ventricular tachycardia is slow, the arrhythmia is usually well tolerated. With fast rates, however, the circulation rapidly deteriorates, requiring immediate emergency treatment. Ventricular tachycardia may progress to ventricular fibrillation. Fibrillation is usually heralded by preceding ventricular premature beats or tachycardia. In some instances, termed primary fibrillation, the arrhythmia develops suddenly without warning ectopic beats. Primary fibrillation is probably an important factor in sudden death, as its incidence is greatest in the first 12 hours after infarction.

Heart failure, pulmonary edema, and shock are common complications of acute myocardial infarction. About two thirds of patients surviving to reach the hospital will develop some form of *heart failure.* Mortality varies directly with the clinical severity of heart failure, averaging about 5 per cent in the absence of failure, 15 per cent when failure is moderate, 35 per cent with pulmonary edema, and 80 to 90 per cent in cardiogenic shock. Direct measurements in patients with transmural infarction have revealed that left ventricular end-diastolic pressures may be considerably elevated, reaching 25 mm. Hg or more (normal is less than 10 mm. Hg). Mean left ventricular filling pressure is proportionately increased, suggesting that marked dysfunction of the left ventricle is relatively common. Despite the evidence of high pulmonary venous pressure, however, clinical signs of heart failure are not always evident.

Cardiogenic Shock. This develops in about 10 per cent of hospitalized patients. The condition is characterized by low blood pressure and signs of inadequate peripheral circulation, including cold skin, mental confusion, peripheral cyanosis, decreased urine flow, and tachycardia. Patients with shock tend to be in the older age group, but shock may occur at any age. Previous clinical history of infarction, hypertension, diabetes, or other complications is not helpful in predicting shock. Shock may develop at any time up to several days after the onset of infarction. In the hospitalized patient it is often precipitated by a clinical episode suggesting extension or reinfarction. Survival is uncommon. Autopsy usually reveals extensive old and recent infarction, the damaged area exceeding 50 per cent of the left ventricular myocardium.

Embolism. Both systemic and pulmonary emboli may complicate acute myocardial infarction. The combination of liberal use of anticoagulants and less restrictive bed rest with attention to movement of the extremities has reduced the frequency of these hazards. The current incidence of clinically recognizable episodes is probably less than 3 per cent. Pulmonary emboli from the right heart tend to be small and nonfatal, whereas those from the deep veins may be massive and may cause sudden death. Systemic emboli have their source in the mural thrombi which form on the endocardium of the infarcted left ventricle.

Cardiac Rupture. Rupture of the heart occurs in about 5 per cent of fatal cases. It is the only complication of acute infarction that is more common in women than in men. Rupture develops in transmural infarction usually within the first ten days. Death is caused by acute hemopericardium and tamponade. The condition is characterized clinically by sudden loss of blood pressure without arrhythmia. Sinus tachycardia often persists for several minutes, although the patient is unresponsive. Occasionally the rupture is sealed by the pericardium, and survival for several months is possible.

Rupture of the intraventricular septum is heralded by the appearance of a loud systolic murmur with a thrill along the left sternal border. The dynamic effects depend on the size of the tear and volume of left to right shunt. Successful surgical repair of acquired ventricular septal defect has been accomplished, but is usually not attempted for several weeks after the acute event.

Insufficiency of the Mitral Valve. Mitral regurgitation is a common complication of acute infarction, usually caused by dysfunction of the papillary muscles, secondary to the ischemic process. Heikkila reported that 30 per cent of patients with acute infarction develop murmurs of mitral insufficiency detected by repeated, daily auscultation. The murmur is usually soft and blowing, is heard at the apex, and may be holosystolic or confined to the latter half of systole. Rupture of the papillary muscle may precipitate acute and intractable pulmonary edema. The murmur is loud and holosystolic. Differentiation from rupture of the ventricular septum may not be easy. In the patient with refractory heart failure, emergency replacement with an artificial mitral valve may be indicated.

Weakening of the Ventricular Wall. Aneurysm of the left ventricle results from scarring and thinning of the ventricular wall following transmural infarction. When large, the aneurysm bulges outward during systole and this paradoxical movement may be appreciated by careful palpation of the precordium. Large aneurysms are usually lined with clot, and systemic embolus is a hazard. Aneurysm of the left ventricle may be recognized on a chest film when the bulge is especially prominent. Cineangiography with injection of contrast medium into the left ventricle has revealed that localized disorder of ventricular contraction is common following myocardial infarction. Small aneurysms that were not suspected clinically are frequently observed in the angiogram. When the area of disordered contraction is large, the ventricle is usually dilated and the ejection fraction (stroke volume/end-diastolic volume) is reduced. Removal of the dyskinetic muscle has been attempted surgically in the hope of increasing the ejection fraction and improving ventricular performance.

Postinfarction Syndrome. A postinfarction syndrome has been described occurring a week or more after acute infarction and characterized by pericarditis with pleuritis and pleural effusions. This condition is similar to the postpericardiectomy syndrome observed occasionally after cardiac surgery. It responds dramatically to moderate doses of corticosteroids.

Treatment. The aims of treatment are (1) to make the patient comfortable, (2) to reduce the demands on the heart by maintaining the patient at rest during the healing phase, (3) to prevent complications, or (4) to treat them. No techniques are currently available which are known to influence the rate of healing or scar formation.

Prehospital Management. Fatal arrhythmia or heart block is now recognized as such a hazard in the immediate postinfarct period that serious consideration should be given to the administration of an antiarrhythmic drug if there is evidence of bradycardia, heart block, or ventricular ectopic beats when the patient is first observed. In the acute situation, treatment with a potent drug may be necessary despite lack of exact electrocardiographic diagnosis. When the heart rate is slow, administration of atropine, 0.5 mg. to 1.0 mg. intravenously, is useful. The dose may be repeated after five minutes if the response is inadequate. Frequent ventricular ectopic beats usually respond to 50 to 100 mg. of lidocaine given intravenously. The dose may be repeated in three to five minutes. The administration of either drug without precise electrocardiographic control is not without hazard, and in the acute situation the physician must judge what is in the best interest of the patient. When possible the physician should attempt to stabilize the cardiac rhythm and transport the patient to a hospital with adequate monitoring and resuscitative facilities.

Hospitalization. Generally, complications cannot be managed well in the home, and when proper facilities are available it is advantageous to admit the patient to a Coronary Care Unit. The Coronary Care Unit contains devices for constant monitoring of heart rate and rhythm and is staffed by highly trained nurses readily available 24 hours a day. In the Coronary Care Unit are concentrated facilities and personnel which previously were scattered about the hospital. Constant monitoring enables recognition and treatment of life-threatening arrhythmias and prevention of serious complications. Despite the wide variety of electronic monitoring instruments available, the only body function which has been shown to be useful to monitor routinely and continuously is the rate and rhythm of the heart as revealed by the electrocardiogram. Since the physician is only intermittently in attendance, nurses and other personnel are trained to interpret electrocardiograms and initiate therapy for abnormal rhythm.

Symptomatic Care. *Environment.* The patient should be put to bed in a quiet, calm area. Rest and relaxation should be encouraged. Most patients prefer a single room, although this may not be possible in all situations. Light should be subdued and noise kept to a minimum. Usually visitors are sharply restricted during the first few days of illness. Radio, newspapers, and television are reduced to a minimum. A clock and a calendar provide the patient with considerable security and prevent a sense of isolation from the outside world.

Pain and Apprehension. Morphine sulfate, 8 to 15 mg. parenterally, is usually effective for pain or restlessness. In severe cases it may be necessary to repeat the drug in smaller dosages every three to four hours. Morphine depresses respiration, reduces myocardial contractility, and is a potent vasodilator. Hypotension, which can usually be overcome by elevation of the lower extremities, or bradycardia, responsive to atropine, may develop. Meperidine, 50 to 100 mg., is also useful, although not as effective as morphine. The patient who is confused and restless may be suffering from cerebral dysfunction or delirium owing to heart failure or shock. It is well, therefore, to be cautious in administering narcotics, especially in repeated doses.

Mood changes with apprehension are common. A well-trained sympathetic nursing staff under the direction of an understanding physician to interpret and explain the illness and treatment is essential. Specific treatment with barbiturates, such as phenobarbital, 32 to 64 mg., or chlordiazepoxide (Librium), 10 mg. three or four times a day, may be helpful.

Bowel Function. Maintenance of reasonably normal bowel function and the avoidance of straining at stools are important aspects of treatment. An effective therapy is milk of magnesia, 30 ml. twice daily. Dioctyl sodium sulfosuccinate (Colace), 100 mg. twice daily, may be added if necessary. This program usually produces a satisfactory stool in mid-morning. Milk of magnesia combined with cascara tends to cause bloating, cramps, and excessive flatus, as does Colace when used alone.

Bed Rest. Time-honored treatment calls for strict bed rest for two to three weeks. This is probably excessively confining for most patients. It is well to maintain strict bed rest for the first three or four days. If no serious complications develop, the patient may then be allowed modified bed rest with some activity, sitting in a chair. Use of a bedside commode is much appreciated by the patient. In an uncomplicated infarction, after ten days to two weeks of chair rest, progressive ambulation may begin to prepare the patient for discharge three to four weeks after the acute attack. At home activity is gradually increased, and the patient may anticipate returning to work in two to three months.

Bladder. Urinary retention resulting from bladder neck obstruction is not uncommon in older patients during prolonged bed rest. If urinary retention is suspected, the physician should not hesitate to insert an indwelling catheter with aseptic technique. After the cardiac problem has improved, definitive therapy may be undertaken if necessary.

Diet. Acutely ill patients usually have little appetite, although modest amounts of tastily prepared food may be appreciated. Usually the patient is offered a soft diet, moderately reduced in calories, 1500 to 1800, and in sodium, 2 to 3 grams (87 to 130 mEq.) as soon as he wishes to eat. A number of adequate salt substitutes are available. Salt intake and the variety of food may be liberalized after the first week if no evidence of heart failure has been detected. For the overweight patient, the close supervision of the convalescent period may offer an opportunity for weight reduction.

Oxygen. Debate over the usefulness of oxygen continues to rage. Administration of oxygen may (1) increase arterial Po_2 in patients with pulmonary congestion or shock, and (2) increase oxygen tension in the ischemic myocardium bordering the infarcted zone, thus (hopefully) reducing the size of infarction. High concentrations of oxygen approaching 100 per cent are seldom indicated except in the presence of acute pulmonary edema or cardiogenic shock. Unfortunately most patients do not tolerate a tight-fitting mask well, and such masks are difficult to apply effectively. The loose-fitting Venturi mask is comfortable and efficient. Models are available which deliver 28, 35, or 40 per cent oxygen. An oxygen tent is an inefficient and expensive way to deliver therapy. With careful nursing techniques and flow rates of 12 to 15 liters per minute, the concentration of oxygen in the inspired area may reach 40 to 50 per cent, but it is usually much lower. The tent may be useful in providing a cool, moist atmosphere but has the distinct disadvantage of preventing easy access to the patient. Other methods for delivering oxygen should be utilized wherever possible. A nasal cannula can provide 35 to 40 per cent oxygen at flow rates of 6 to 8 liters per minute with relatively little discomfort. Despite the uncertainty about the importance of oxygen therapy, it seems reasonable to provide an atmosphere of increased oxygen to most patients during the first few days, utilizing either the Venturi mask or nasal cannula.

Anticoagulation. The usefulness of anticoagulants and the importance of thromboembolic phenomena on the morbidity and mortality of myocardial infarction remain moot. Many of the earlier studies of anticoagulation were faulty in design, and their conclusions are not currently applicable. At the present time, with emphasis on the treatment of heart failure, early ambulation, reduced sedation, and limb movement in bed, it is apparent that the morbidity is low and the mortality essentially nil from thromboembolism complicating myocardial infarction. It is questionable whether anticoagulants influence the formation of mural thrombosis. There is no evidence to suggest that anticoagulants influence the course of the infarction itself. Although most patients hospitalized with acute myocardial infarction in the United States today probably receive anticoagulant therapy, the decision to use anticoagulants is largely elective. Their use should be based on the patient's past history, the quality of the supporting laboratory, and the experience of the physician with anticoagulant drugs. Recent phlebitis or embolism favors treatment. History of ulcer, bleeding tendency, or hemorrhage would argue against anticoagulation. The most commonly utilized agents are coumadin derivatives. Heparin is indicated only occasionally when thrombosis or embolism appears as a life-threatening complication.

Arrhythmia. *Sinus Bradycardia.* Reduction of the heart rate below 55 owing to failure of the normal sinus mechanism may be accompanied by evidence of low cardiac output, development of heart failure, or hypotension. Intravenous atropine, 0.5 to 1.0 mg., is usually effective. Occasionally 2.0 mg. may be required. Atropine is not practical for long-term maintenance. Repeated use of the drug is limited by occasional central nervous system effects, urinary retention, and the rare precipitation of acute glaucoma. Overdosage may cause unpleasant tachycardia. Slowing of the sinus rate is usually temporary, and responds to the treatment outlined. Occasionally the condition persists, and temporary pacing with an electrode inserted into the right atrium or right ventricle is required.

Atrial Arrhythmia. Frequent atrial premature complexes are often the harbinger of atrial fibrillation or flutter, and they usually respond to digitalis. If atrial flutter and fibrillation are well tolerated, without hypotension or heart failure, they are best treated with digitalis. If complications develop or the patient is not tolerating the arrhythmia well, DC precordial shock should be utilized. Supraventricular arrhythmias are frequently recurrent, but after the acute illness subsides, spontaneous reversion is the rule.

Atrial-Ventricular Block. An important guide to therapy of heart block is the ventricular rate. In atrioventricular dissociation with an AV nodal rhythm, the QRS configuration is usually normal, and the heart rate is well maintained. Thus treatment may be expectant. However, when there is intermittant atrial capture of the ventricle with dropped beats (second-degree heart block) or complete AV block with a slow idioventricular rate characterized by wide QRS complexes (third-degree heart block), therapy is usually required. An intravenous infusion of isoproterenol may be immediately effective. Isoproterenol, 0.4 to 1.0 mg., is dissolved in 500 ml. of 5 per cent glucose in water and carefully administered intravenously by a slow drip. The rate of infusion and the concentration of the drug should be adjusted according to the ventricular response. Isoproterenol may induce both atrial and ventricular arrhythmia, and its use requires constant, close medical supervision.

In most forms of heart block with slow ventricular rate, transvenous pacemaking with an electrode catheter in the right ventricle is the most effective form of therapy. The electrode should be activated by a battery powered demand-type pacemaker. Heart block in acute myocardial infarction is almost always self-limited. Established heart block following recovery from infarction is rare. Thus, if a satisfactory ventricular rate can be maintained for a few days, conduction will almost invariably resume through normal pathways, and the pacemaker catheter can then be withdrawn.

Sudden complete heart block, Mobitz Type II, is usually due to bilateral bundle branch block. Recent studies have shown that more than 50 per cent of patients with right or left bundle branch block prior to acute infarction develop bilateral bundle branch block during the acute illness. The mortality in sudden acute complete heart block is high, averaging more than 50 per cent. In view of the risk, it seems appropriate to recommend "prophylactic" insertion of a temporary electrode catheter into the right ventricle in all patients with acute myocardial infarction and pre-existing bundle branch block.

Ventricular Premature Beats; Unsustained Ventricular Tachycardia. The appearance of more than three ventricular premature beats per minute or bursts of ventricular contractions requires urgent treatment. They may be the forerunners of cardiac arrest, and prompt, aggressive treatment may forestall a catastrophe. The most effective and rapidly acting agent currently available is lidocaine hydrochloride intravenously in doses of 50 to 100 mg. by rapid injection (bolus). The dose may be repeated in three to five minutes to achieve the desired result—obliteration of extrasystoles. When the ectopic beats have disappeared following bolus injection, a constant intravenous drip of lidocaine may be administered and the drip rate adjusted to maintain an infusion rate of 1.0 to 5.0 mg. per minute. The infusion rate may be gradually reduced after several hours if there is no recurrence, and may be discontinued in 24 to 36 hours. Recurrence of extrasystoles may require extra immediate doses of lidocaine followed by an increase in the infusion rate.

Lidocaine is a local anesthetic and may cause sensations of body numbness or tingling or twitching of the face muscles. Large doses often cause drowsiness. Convulsions may occasionally occur with excessive dosage, especially in the presence of cerebral anoxia.

If lidocaine is not effective, procaine amide, 0.5 gram intramuscularly every 4 to 6 hours, or quinidine sulfate, 0.2 to 0.4 gram every 2 to 4 hours, may be useful in suppressing ectopic beats. Diphenylhydantoin, 100 to 200 mg. every 4 to 8 hours, is also occasionally effective. In refractory situations it may be useful to overdrive the ventricle with a pacemaker and maintain a rate considerably in excess of the basic sinus rate. Overdriving shortens electrical diastole and suppresses the tendency for ectopic beats to develop. This technique has proved extremely useful in a limited number of desperate clinical situations.

Ventricular Tachycardia and Ventricular Fibrillation. These two arrhythmias are considered together, as ventricular tachycardia often precedes and degenerates into ventricular fibrillation. If blood pressure is maintained without circulatory collapse in the presence of ventricular tachycardia, 100 mg. of lidocaine may be administered rapidly intravenously. If there is no effect within three to five minutes, DC precordial shock is applied. If blood pressure is not maintained and the patient develops clinical cardiac arrest, immediate treatment with precordial shock is mandatory.

Ventricular Fibrillation. The proper therapy of this arrhythmia is immediate defibrillation. If the defibrillator is available, time is wasted attempting to ventilate the patient or attempting closed-chest cardiac massage. In older patients there are approximately 60 seconds in which to administer an effective shock and revert ventricular fibrillation to normal rhythm before the development of serious metabolic disturbance or brain damage. In the well-run coronary care unit, defibrillation for unexpected cardiac arrest can frequently be applied by the trained nurse within 30 seconds of onset.

Asystole. Sudden, unexpected asystole is uncommon in acute infarction. Most often it is the culmination of a gradual decline in cardiac function in severe heart failure or shock. A series of thumps on the chest or closed chest cardiac massage may restore cardiac action. If an electrode catheter is in place or can be rapidly inserted, artificial pacemaking may be effective.

Pulmonary Edema. The initial manifestation of acute infarction may be the sudden development of pulmonary edema, a complication especially likely to appear during the first few hours of illness. The aims of therapy are to improve cardiac function, reduce airway resistance and the work of breathing, and increase arterial oxygen tension. If the blood pressure is well maintained, the patient is propped into a sitting position. Morphine sulfate, 8 to 15 mg. parenterally, is effective. Oxygen is administered, preferably by mask, in high concentration. If the patient can tolerate a tightly fitting mask, oxygen under positive pressure or with positive pressure on exhalation is useful, because the increased intrathoracic pressure impedes venous return and lowers ventricular filling pressures. Blood pressure should be carefully followed because positive pressure inhalation is contraindicated in hypotension or shock. Rotating tourniquets are extremely useful because they impound a significant portion of the circulating blood volume in the extremities. Tourniquets should be applied to three limbs tightly enough to inhibit venous return yet permit transmission of the arterial pulse, and should be rotated every 20 minutes.

The usefulness of digitalis and diuretics in the treatment of acute pulmonary edema is debated. Digitalis is usually not necessary in the immediate treatment unless the condition has been precipitated by acute supraventricular arrhythmia, especially rapid atrial fibrillation or flutter. The drug is usually indicated for long-term management, and may be necessary in refractory cases. Furosemide, 40 to 80 mg., and ethacrynic acid, 50 to 100 mg., are potent diuretic agents which will initiate diuresis within 15 minutes of intravenous administration. Both are frequently utilized in patients with pulmonary edema and probably are effective in acutely reducing plasma volume, thereby lowering venous filling pressure. Other measures include phlebotomy of 300 to 500 ml. of blood or more, administration of aminophyllin as a suppository (0.5 gram) or intravenously in a slow infusion in a dosage of 250 to 500 mg. Mercurial diuretics, meralluride (Mercuhydrin) and mercaptomerin (Thiomerin), in 2-ml. doses intramuscularly, are also utilized.

Heart Failure. Congestive heart failure is fairly common in acute myocardial infarction, occurring in approximately two thirds of hospitalized patients. Early signs of pulmonary congestion may be treated with diuretics or reduction of salt intake. Opinions vary whether digitalis should be utilized liberally or conservatively in acute myocardial infarction. There is strong experimental and clinical evidence to support the view that the infarcted heart is sensitive to the toxic effects of digitalis. On the other hand, the response to digitalis in the patient with clear clinical and hemodynamic evidence of heart failure is frequently gratifying. Digitalis should not be withheld when clearly indicated. Because of the increased hazard of arrhythmia, it is reasonable to give somewhat smaller doses of digitalis to patients with acute infarction and to observe blood potassium levels closely. Additional drug can always be given in cases of need. It is impossible to remove an overdosage.

Many different digitalis preparations are available, but it is best to avoid administration of more than one agent to a single patient, as judgment about the level of digitalization becomes exceedingly difficult. *Digoxin* is a useful preparation. It is rapidly absorbed and excreted; hence dosage depends upon frequency and route of administration. In patients who are acutely ill the author prefers intravenous administration, as there is certainty about the time and amount given. A reasonable schedule is 0.5 mg. initially intravenously, followed by 0.25 mg. every two to four hours for three doses. The total dose is less than optimal, but this schedule will usually avoid any problem of digitalis intoxication. For oral dosage 0.5 mg. is given every four to six hours for three doses, and a maintenance schedule of 0.25 to 0.5 mg. is given daily thereafter. *Ouabain,* available only in an intravenous preparation, has been advocated in

the treatment of heart failure complicating acute myocardial infarction by some authorities. This drug has the same physiologic half-life as digoxin, and a convenient dosage schedule is as follows: 0.4 mg. intravenously as an initial dose, followed by 0.1 to 0.2 mg. every two hours for two or three additional doses. This drug will usually have a detectable effect within 20 minutes, with a peak action at about two hours.

Hypotension. In many patients the blood pressure falls, yet they remain alert and warm, have an adequate urine output, and are not in shock. Generally such hypotension should be managed expectantly, and a treatable cause searched for. The fall in blood pressure may be caused by drugs, particularly sedatives, or narcotics such as morphine. If hypotension is due to peripheral venous pooling, elevation of the lower extremities is an effective countermeasure. Occasionally the fall in blood pressure is a reflection of reduced blood volume, and central venous pressure is low. This form of hypotension has been observed in patients previously treated for acute pulmonary edema who then become hypotensive following brisk diuresis. The most common precipitating factor is use of the new and potent diuretic agents such as ethacrynic acid or furosemide.

Thus, when central blood pressure falls, venous pressure of less than 80 mm. of saline suggests the possibility of hypovolemia. Infusion of 100-ml. increments of half-normal saline or low molecular weight dextran with careful monitoring of the venous pressure is initiated. If blood pressure increases with little or no change in venous pressure, hypovolemia is indeed present. Some patients may receive 2 or 3 liters of fluid before venous pressure increases. However, if venous pressure rises promptly as the fluid is infused, it is unlikely that hypovolemia is a contributing factor to the hypotension.

Cardiogenic Shock. The patient in shock has a systolic blood pressure less than 90 mm. Hg, is usually restless, has reduced mental awareness, cyanosis, oliguria (less than 20 ml. per hour) or even anuria, and cool, moist extremities. Hemodynamic studies reveal that cardiac output and stroke volume are markedly reduced in cardiogenic shock, averaging one third of normal or less. Peripheral resistance is variable but is usually moderately increased. Myocardial oxygenation is inadequate, and the heart produces lactate. Progressive metabolic acidosis is a hallmark of shock, and arterial pH should be measured frequently. Mortality in shock is approximately 90 per cent. Autopsy almost invariably reveals massive myocardial infarction with extensive coronary artery disease.

Treatable causes such as cardiac tamponade, hypovolemia, or serious arrhythmia should be sought and vigorously managed. Tamponade may be suspected when hypotension or shock is accompanied by marked distention of the neck veins or very high venous pressure. To evaluate the possibility of hypovolemia central venous pressure should be measured, and, if low, the response to volume replacement, as described above, carefully evaluated.

Treatment of cardiogenic shock is unsatisfactory. Infusion of isoproterenol will increase cardiac output, but blood pressure does not increase. Mean arterial pressure and, hence, coronary artery perfusion pressure fall. Since isoproterenol increases myocardial oxygen demand and induces lactate production in the ischemic heart, its overall effect in cardiogenic shock may be deleterious. Norepinephrine increases peripheral vascular resistance and improves myocardial contractility. Despite extensive use and many eloquent testimonials, convincing evidence that infusion of norepinephrine improves mortality in cardiogenic shock is lacking. Administration of so-called alpha blocking agents such as phenoxybenzamine or phentolamine or of large doses of adrenal corticosteroids has been advocated. Although these agents are apparently effective in certain types of experimental shock, there is no evidence supporting their effectiveness in cardiogenic shock secondary to acute myocardial infarction. Because of the inadequacy of current treatment, a number of techniques for temporarily supporting the circulation have been prepared, including cardiopulmonary bypass, external counterpulsation, and insertion of an intra-aortic counterpulsating balloon. If these measures are to be successful, they must be applied early in the hope that a significant portion of the extensive myocardial damage is reversible so that adequate cardiac function can be restored.

Prognosis. Mortality is greatest during the first few hours, before most patients reach a hospital. The risk declines rapidly from onset of the acute attack. Studies from both Belfast and Edinburgh have revealed essentially the same findings: 50 per cent of the deaths from acute myocardial infarction occur within the first 2 hours and 15 minutes after the onset of the illness. Approximately three fourths of all deaths occur within the first 24 hours. The majority of the early deaths are sudden, owing to electrical instability of the heart, and are not necessarily related to the size of the infarct or the development of heart failure.

Reliable data for total mortality outside and inside the hospital in acute myocardial infarction are difficult to obtain. Mortality rates in excess of 60 per cent have been reported. Oliver observed that 42 per cent of all patients under 70 died during the first four weeks. At the end of six months the total mortality was 49 per cent. The greatest risk was incurred by women from 60 to 69 in whom the mortality was 52 per cent at four weeks and rose to 59 per cent after six months.

The patient who is admitted to a hospital has already survived a considerable risk. Prior to the development of the Coronary Care Unit, mortality of the hospitalized patient probably averaged about 35 per cent, varying somewhat in different communities and in different types of hospitals. In the well-run Coronary Care Unit, mortality currently averages 12 to 18 per cent in patients in whom myocardial infarction is diagnosed utilizing strict criteria.

Prognosis after recovery depends upon many factors, including age, history of previous infarctions, presence of diabetes, presence of heart failure, mental attitude, type of employment, and employment policies. Patients who have survived ventricular fibrillation and successful resuscitation have an excellent prognosis in the absence of heart failure. Persistent heart failure and frequent ventricular ectopic beats warrant a guarded prognosis. If cardiac function is well maintained six weeks after acute infarction, most patients are able to return to previous employment and a full range of normal activity.

Case, R. B., Nasser, M. G., and Crampton, R. S.: Biochemical aspects of early myocardial ischemia. Amer. J. Cardiol., 24:766, 1969.

Epstein, S. E., et al.: Treatment of angina pectoris by electrical stimulation of the carotid-sinus nerves. New Eng. J. Med., 280:971, 1969.

Fulton, M., Julian, D. G., and Oliver, M. F.: Sudden death and myocardial infarction. Circulation, 50(Suppl. IV):182, 1969.

Heikkila, J.: Mitral incompetence as a complication of acute myocardial infarction. Acta Med. Scand. (Suppl. No. 475, pp. 1-139), 1967.

International Anticoagulant Review Group: Collaborative analysis of long-term anticoagulant administration after acute myocardial infarction. Lancet, 1:203, 1970. Leading Article: Long-term anticoagulants after acute myocardial infarction. Ibid., 1:226, 1970.

James, T. N.: Anatomy of the coronary arteries in health and disease. Circulation, 32:1020, 1965.

Kagan, A., Livisic, A. M., Sternby, N., and Vihert, A. M.: Coronary-artery thrombosis and the acute attack of coronary heart-disease. Lancet, 2:1199, 1968.

Killip, T., and Kimball, J. T.: A survey of the coronary care unit: Concept and results. Progr. Cardiov. Dis., 11:45, 1968.

Kimball, J. T., and Killip, T.: Aggressive treatment of arrhythmias in acute myocardial infarction: Procedures and results. Progr. Cardiov. Dis., 10:483, 1968.

Likoff, W., Segal, B. L., and Kasparian, H.: Paradox of normal selective coronary arteriograms in patients considered to have unmistakable coronary heart disease. New Eng. J. Med., 276:1063, 1967.

Most, A. S., Kemp, H. G., and Gorlin, R.: Postexercise electrocardiography in patients with arteriographically documented coronary artery disease. Ann. Intern. Med., 71: 1043, 1969.

Mustard, J. F., and Packham, M. A.: Platelet function and acute myocardial infarction. Circulation, 50(Suppl. IV, 20), 1969.

Parker, J. O., West, R. O., Case, R. B., and Chiong, M. A.: Temporal relationships of myocardial lactate metabolism, left ventricular function, and S-T segment depression during angina precipitated by exercise. Circulation, 60:97, 1969.

Scheidt, S., Ascheim, R., and Killip, T.: Shock after acute myocardial infarction: A clinical and hemodynamic profile. Amer. J. Cardiol., Vol. 26, December 1970.

Solomon, H. A., Edwards, A. L., and Killip, T.: Prodromata in acute myocardial infarction. Circulation, 60:463, 1969.

Weinblatt, E., Frank, C., Shapiro, S., and Sager, R.: Prognostic factors in angina pectoris—A prospective study. J. Chron. Dis., 21:231, 1968.

Weinblatt, E., Shapiro, S., Frank, C., and Sager, R.: Prognosis of men after first myocardial infarction: Mortality and first recurrences in relation to selected parameters. Amer. J. Public Health, 58:1329, 1968.

Thromboembolic Diseases
(Thrombophlebitis, Phlebothrombosis, Pulmonary Embolism, and Infarction)

Sol Sherry

Thrombosis is the formation from the constituents of the blood of a solid mass or plug in the heart or blood vessels. The thrombus which forms may be dislodged in whole or in part to another vascular site; when this occurs the thrombus or its fragment is referred to as an embolus. Collectively the states associated with such thrombi or emboli are referred to as the thromboembolic diseases or disorders.

Alterations in blood flow, damage to the vessel wall, and changes in the coagulability of the blood have been stressed as the major factors responsible for thrombus formation in vivo. In the arterial system, a vascular lesion is generally accepted as the most frequent primary cause of an acute thrombotic event. Thrombi originate in the immediate proximity of a lesion in the arterial wall and are composed primarily of a large white head containing platelets and some fibrin; a variable amount of fresh clot then extends from this white head. It is postulated that platelets adhere to the exposed collagen fibers at the site of vascular injury, e.g., fissured or ulcerated atheromatous plaque, and this adherence, when followed by platelet aggregation, initiates the arterial thrombotic event.

The pathogenesis of venous thrombosis is less well understood except when there is direct injury or infection of the vein wall which leads to a thrombus much like that in an artery. However, in most instances, thrombus formation takes place in the absence of a demonstrable vascular lesion since the venous intima, unlike the arterial intima, is much less exposed to injury from pressure, turbulence, or atherosclerosis. Furthermore, in contrast to the arterial thrombus, the venous thrombus is composed primarily of a red gel-like mass similar to a test tube blood clot; a white platelet head is either inconspicuous or absent. Thus, although platelet sticking and aggregation may or may not initiate venous thrombosis, the event appears to be dominated by activation of the clotting mechanism. Stasis, a common predisposing factor to venous thrombotic disease, probably accounts for this by serving to sustain the action of activated components of the clotting mechanism, as in the animal model developed by Wessler. In the latter, immediately following the systemic injection of early activated components of the clotting mechanism (either in partially purified form or as serum), isolation of a venous segment by ligatures or clamps, so as to effect stasis, results in the rapid formation of a thrombus in situ; thrombosis is not seen in the freely flowing circulation and is markedly delayed in the isolated venous segment of control animals.

Considering the frequency of thromboemboli in all sites of the circulatory system (heart, arteries, and veins), the thromboembolic diseases, when viewed as an entity, are the leading cause of serious illness and death in the Western world and are likely to grow in importance as longevity increases. Unfortunately and in contrast to cancer, thrombosis is considered only as a finding associated with disease in many organs rather than as a disease which affects many organs. Accordingly, the thromboembolic disorders involving the heart, systemic arteries, and selected veins, e.g., hepatic, portal, renal, are considered elsewhere throughout this text, and the present chapter is concerned primarily with peripheral venous thrombotic disease and its major complication, pulmonary artery embolism.

THROMBOPHLEBITIS AND PHLEBOTHROMBOSIS

The presence of a thrombus in a vein is referred to clinically as thrombophlebitis or phlebothrombosis. In the peripheral vessels, such thrombi usually begin in the valve pockets and then extend either up along the vein wall or into the flowing circulation, or they may completely obstruct the entire vascular lumen. Adherence to the vein wall incites an inflammatory reaction with local symptoms, and because of the associated phlebitis the process is referred to as thrombophlebitis. When the thrombus is poorly adherent and extends primarily into the free-flowing circulation, the local symptoms of phlebitis may be minimal or absent, and the process may be referred to as phlebothrombosis. Since the two thrombotic states are, for the most part, identical and subject to the same complications, little virtue attaches to such a clinical differentiation; hereafter only the term thrombophlebitis will be used.

Etiology, Pathogenesis, and Prevalence. Multiple causes probably exist for the initiation of venous thrombosis. Injury to the vessel wall by mechanical trauma, infection, chemical irritants, or the process of thromboangiitis obliterans is responsible for some cases, particularly of the superficial variety. Stasis, with slowing of blood flow and venous distention, appears to be a major predisposing factor in many others. Peripheral venous thrombi frequently complicate the use of constricting garments. Such clinical conditions or states as the hyperviscosity syndromes, including polycythemia vera, severe obesity, varicose veins, the postoperative state, trauma (particularly when extensive or involving fractures of the pelvis or femur), pregnancy and parturition, acute myocardial infarction, heart failure, hemiplegia, debility, and cachexia may be precipitating factors. Protracted periods of cramped sitting, e.g., in travel or watching television, or in fact any state involving prolonged periods of partial or complete immobilization, because of the loss of the normal pumping action of the leg muscles, is subject to an increased incidence of venous thrombosis.

Alterations in blood components have received much attention, but such a "hypercoagulable state," i.e., one predisposing to thrombus formation, has defied simple description. Rather it is recognized that many disorders of the blood may be associated with venous thrombosis. These include thrombocythemia as well as certain thrombocytopathies, particularly those involving increased platelet aggregation and reactivity, dysfibrinogenemias, accelerated thromboplastin generation, constitutionally elevated levels of plasma factors V and VIII, heightened antifibrinolytic activity, and decreased antithrombin activity.

Finally a variety of other clinical conditions are associated with an increased incidence of thrombophlebitis, but the responsible factors have not been adequately elucidated. These include ulcerative colitis, malignancies of all types (possibly more so of the pancreas), homocystinuria, and the prolonged administration of large doses of estrogens or estrogen-containing oral contraceptive agents. When thrombosis occurs without evidence of a known predisposing factor or associated clinical condition, the disease is called idiopathic thrombophlebitis.

Thrombosis in the veins occurs most commonly in the peripheral vessels and is most frequently observed in the deep and superficial veins of the lower extremities. The thrombus extends proximally into larger vessels, frequently progressing to involve the common femoral and iliac vein. More rarely the inferior vena cava is also affected. Next in frequency are thrombi in the pelvic venous network, the right cardiac chambers, and the veins of the upper extremities. However, thrombi may occur in any vein (retinal, cerebral, renal, hepatic, portal, mesenteric) and contribute significantly to disease of the organ system involved.

Current data on the incidence and frequency of peripheral venous thrombi are inadequate, for many of these are inapparent clinically. Leg vein dissections are not routinely done in postmortem examinations, and certain problems preclude the routine use of phlebography. Their incidence must be large indeed, as attested to by the observations in one series in which thrombi were found in the deep veins in more than half of 351 consecutive autopsies on middle-aged patients confined to bed. Furthermore, considering that probably no more than 15 to 20 per cent of venous thrombi embolize, the incidence of venous thrombosis must be several-fold greater than the high frequency noted for pulmonary embolism.

Clinical Manifestations and Diagnosis. Thrombophlebitis occurs suddenly or gradually. Superficial thrombophlebitis is not difficult to diagnose since the thrombosed vessel can usually be felt beneath the skin as a tender cord, and the lesion may be accompanied by a surrounding area of localized inflammation. With the more extensive use of the venous route both for therapy and drug abuse, the incidence of this form of thrombophlebitis has increased sharply. Though usually benign, a significant number of patients may become infected, e.g., following the use of contaminated equipment or when intravenous catheters have been left in situ for periods greater than 48 hours, and this may lead to a serious septic state.

Deep vein thrombophlebitis is much more difficult to diagnose since it may or may not be accompanied by local (pain and tenderness) and systemic (fever) symptoms. In the absence of local findings, the diagnosis should be suspected when there is an unexplained increase in the circumference of the limb, and the presence of a positive *Homans' sign* (pain in the calf and/or popliteal space on dorsiflexion of the foot). The sphygmomanometer cuff pain test of Lowenberg also may prove useful. A blood pressure cuff around the involved part of the extremity is slowly inflated to 200 mm. Hg and then deflated. During inflation, discomfort is normally experienced at or above 160 mm. Hg. In venous obstructive disease, discomfort is evident at a lower level (60 to 150 mm. Hg). The test may often be positive when other symptoms and signs are absent, but it is not sufficiently specific to be considered diagnostic. Other useful diagnostic techniques include the use of ultrasound and phlebography. Though the latter is the most specific, it has limitations: The sural vessels are not well visualized, the radiologic interpretation and clinical findings have not correlated too well, and the procedure may predispose to further thrombosis or embolization.

Unless the patient has local complaints, the signs of venous thrombosis are often overlooked until the occurrence of pulmonary embolism calls attention to the limbs. Therefore, special attention should be paid to the possibility of venous thrombi in all patients who are predisposed, and frequent observations should be made in older patients immobilized for any period of time.

Local tenderness in the calf and pain on forced dorsiflexion of the foot should suggest involvement of the deeper branches of the popliteal vein. Edema and mottled cyanosis will be present when the superficial femoral vein is affected; these findings are absent when adequate collateral channels exist. When the disease extends to involve the common femoral and iliac veins, there is the rapid appearance of edema and cyanosis of the leg, often with a diminished pulsation of the femoral artery. A particularly serious form is called *phlegmasia cerulea dolens* in which cyanosis and swelling of the extremity are associated with a disappearance of the arterial pulses; the leg becomes cold; gangrene appears imminent and may follow. This form is associated with massive venous occlusion involving the deep, superficial, and intercommunicating veins so that there is almost total outflow obstruction; the rapid rise in tissue pressure compromises the arterial inflow and produces the picture of combined arterial and venous occlusive disease.

Damage to the venous valves resulting from an extensive episode or repeated attacks of deep vein thrombophlebitis may cause venous stasis and insufficiency; this leads to chronic edema, fibrosis, pigmentation, and trophic ulceration in the limb. The eventual deformity in this *postphlebitic syndrome* may be extreme and disabling. However, the most frequent and serious complication of thrombophlebitis is pulmonary embolism, a subject discussed later in this chapter.

Prophylaxis. Stasis should be eliminated whenever possible, particularly in the older patient. This includes the use of frequent leg exercises during periods of immobilization or illness or following surgery, trauma, or fracture; avoidance of long periods of cramped sitting and of constricting garments about the abdomen and lower extremities; and the wearing of elastic or supportive hose in the presence of varicose veins. Early mobilization following illness, surgery, or trauma is to be encouraged. Although the value of wearing elastic hose during periods of immobilization has not been substantiated, such supports should prove useful, particularly for the unaffected limb in cases of established thrombophlebitis. *Iatrogenic* thrombophlebitis can be minimized by avoiding the prolonged use of intravenous catheters or administration of solutions which are hypertonic or chemically irritating.

Prophylactic therapy with anticoagulants is to be considered in high risk groups, i.e., those most likely to develop venous thrombi and pulmonary embolism. Included in this category are patients over the age of 50 who will be bedridden or immobilized for extended periods of time as a result of extensive fractures, particularly of the femur, or other forms of trauma, debilitating disease, or operation. The pharmacologic basis for the use of anticoagulation in the prevention of venous thrombotic disease is sound, and its effectiveness in reducing thromboembolic complications following fractured hips or extensive trauma and during the postoperative state has been established in several series of observations. When indicated, anticoagulant therapy should be instituted immediately and can be carried out solely with oral agents (coumarin or indandione compounds), for though these agents take several days to induce a hypocoagulable state, the danger period for thrombosis usually begins somewhat later. Anticoagulation should be continued until full mobilization is completed, since the risk of thrombosis remains as long as stasis exists. Such anticoagulation is not a contraindication to surgery or other procedures. Surgery can be performed without much danger shortly after the institution of anticoagulants, since hemostasis is not impaired for several days; later, in the more chronically anticoagulated

patient, surgery can be undertaken following reduction of the level of anticoagulation with careful attention to wound hemostasis. Nevertheless, despite its proved value, physicians have been reluctant to use such prophylactic anticoagulant therapy except in cases of recurrent thrombophlebitis or pulmonary embolism; cited are the hazard of bleeding and the difficulties in maintaining adequate anticoagulation in older patients. Since these problems would be circumvented by the use of such antiplatelet aggregates as aspirin and dipyridamole, the efficacy of the latter agents in preventing venous thrombotic disease is under evaluation at present.

Treatment. *General Measures.* Acute superficial thrombophlebitis is most often a self-limited disease, unless infected, and usually responds promptly to analgesics, bed rest, warm moist packs, and elevation of the affected limb. Antimicrobial drugs are not indicated except in the management of septic phlebitis, in which the choice of agent depends on the organism responsible for the infection.

Acute deep vein thrombophlebitis must be managed more aggressively because of the tendency of these thrombi to extend, embolize, and produce serious venous obstruction and damage (not infrequently sufficient to result in a postphlebitic syndrome). In addition to the local measures described above, the objectives of treatment are to prevent further disease and, if indicated, to remove the obstructing thrombus.

Anticoagulants. Currently the principal therapeutic agents for the prevention of further extension and embolization are the anticoagulants, and with their use alone most cases can be managed successfully and without complication. In the absence of contraindications (bleeding diathesis, hemorrhagic lesion, malignant hypertension, known allergy to heparin) anticoagulation should be instituted immediately with heparin, for it is the most effective of the agents available and induces an immediate antithrombotic state.

Heparin can be administered intravenously or by the intramuscular and subcutaneous routes. Based on control of antithrombotic effects, the intravenous route is most often recommended, particularly for the first several days of therapy. Even with the intravenous route, dosages and regimens vary. A suggested procedure is to use a total of 60,000 I. U. the first day either by continuous intravenous infusion or by intermittent injections every four hours through an indwelling plastic catheter inserted into a superficial forearm vein. If the infusion technique is used, therapy should be instituted with an initial loading dose of 75 I. U. per pound of body weight. Beginning on the second day, dosage control is regulated by measurements of the Lee-White clotting time; for continuous infusions the clotting time is maintained between 30 and 45 minutes; for intermittent injections, the clotting time should be at the same level within one hour before the next dose. After several days it is usually more convenient to use intermittent intravenous injections, and once the dose requirement has been established, the clotting time may be checked once daily at an appropriate time to exclude a possible increase or decrease in the anticoagulant effect of the drug and to allow for variations in heparin requirement during the course of therapy. Not infrequently, patients in whom thrombosis is occurring require more heparin in the first 24 to 48 hours of treatment than is required several days after the institution of therapy. Heparin therapy is recommended for periods of seven to ten days before relying solely on oral anticoagulation with coumarin drugs; this will ensure the most potent antithrombotic state and allow the underlying thrombus to become firmly fixed to the vessel wall.

Heparin therapy carries a significant risk of bleeding; in one series it was as high as 50 per cent in women over the age of 60. When significant bleeding occurs, the heparin in the circulation can be immediately neutralized with protamine sulfate; the latter reacts with heparin stoichiometrically and on a milligram per milligram basis. Protamine is administered slowly intravenously after dilution in physiologic saline in an amount equivalent to half the last dose of heparin but not in excess of 100 mg.

Oral anticoagulation with coumarin compounds should be instituted several days before the discontinuation of heparin therapy. It should be continued for six weeks to six months, unless the phlebitis is associated with immobilization, in which case the drug should be continued until full physical activity is resumed. If thrombi recur when anticoagulants are discontinued, anticoagulants should be resumed, and long-term therapy may be necessary. Patients with known recurrent episodes of phlebitis often require prophylactic anticoagulant therapy extending over years.

The action of coumarin compounds is indirect, i.e., the induction of a hypocoagulable state, in contrast to the direct action of heparin as a thrombin inhibitor. Thus the aim of therapy is to reduce the level of the prothrombin complex factors (factors II, VII, IX, and X) to approximately 20 per cent of normal and sustain it there. This is achieved by regulating dosage so as to prolong the one-stage prothrombin time test to one and a half to two times the control time, equivalent to 17 to 23 per cent prothrombin activity by the Quick test or 7 per cent activity by the thrombotest.

There is little difference in the onset of effect or smoothness of control among the various coumarin derivatives, and vitamin K_1 is equally effective in counteracting their action. With most of the coumarins, in the doses commonly employed, maximal effects usually are seen after 24 to 48 hours. A suggested regimen is to give warfarin, 0.75 mg. per kilogram (for elderly and debilitated patients) to 1.0 mg. per kilogram but not to exceed 50 mg., in one dose on the first day; none is given on the second day; dosage thereafter is dictated by the prothrombin time. Maintenance doses vary from 2 to 15 mg. daily but are usually in the range of 5 to 10 mg. A variety of other drugs affect the responsiveness to these prothrombinopenic agents, and this should be taken into consideration in planning therapy. Bleeding is a significant hazard with oral anticoagulation, occurring in 3 per cent or more of patients on therapy; vitamin K_1 in doses of 5 to 10 mg. is usually corrective. In patients receiving heparin and coumarin agents simultaneously, prothrombin times should be carried out on blood taken just before the next heparin dose and preferably when the clotting time has returned to normal or near-normal levels.

Low molecular weight dextran infusions, based on their ability to improve flow rates by expanding plasma volume and possibly to inhibit platelet adherence and aggregation, have been recommended by some as a useful adjunct in the management of acute thrombophlebitis; the value of such therapy remains to be proved, and at present there is little justification to have it *replace* anticoagulant therapy. Also there is considerable current interest in the use of defibrinating agents which completely "defuse" the clotting mechanism and produce the most potent antithrombotic state yet achieved in man. The most promising agent in this respect is a highly purified fraction (Arvin) obtained from the venom of the Malayan pit viper. Therapy with this agent is under investigation at present; it remains to be established whether it will have advantages over heparin.

Surgical Therapy. Surgical procedures may be helpful in the management of some cases of thrombophlebitis; proximal interruption of venous flow can be employed to prevent embolization, and thrombectomy to relieve obstruction. The surgical procedures of choice to protect adequately against pulmonary embolization from the lower extremities and pelvis are inferior vena caval ligation and plication; either of the latter two procedures has its adherents, but plication obviates the difficulty of sudden acute fluid sequestration with hypovolemia and impaired venous return, an event which may be tolerated poorly by people with underlying heart disease. Since these procedures carry a significant incidence of distressing sequelae, both immediate and late, and do not permanently protect (large collaterals develop in several months and may provide a new route for embolization), they are not given consideration except in the presence of pulmonary embolism, or when the latter has been known to occur in the past and there is a contraindication to the use of anticoagulant therapy.

Thrombectomy, including the use of Fogarty and similar types of catheters, has been employed successfully in the management of phlegmasia cerulea dolens. However, since this procedure is often followed by venous rethrombosis as well as complicating the subsequent use of anticoagulation, it is currently indicated only for those cases in which acute fluid sequestration and high tissue tension sufficiently jeopardize the arterial circulation as to threaten the survival of the limb.

Thrombolytic Therapy. Clot-dissolving agents

ultimately should prove useful as adjuncts in the management of deep vein thrombophlebitis, for they provide the only medical means for directly affecting a thrombus already formed. The most useful agents for thrombolytic therapy are streptokinase and urokinase, activators of the naturally occurring human fibrinolytic enzyme system. *Streptokinase* is a secretory product of the hemolytic Streptococcus and can be produced readily in large quantities and relatively inexpensively for therapeutic purposes. Its major disadvantage is its antigenicity; this poses problems in dosage and, more important, in retreatment should thrombosis recur. *Urokinase,* a normal constituent of human urine, is nonantigenic and simpler to use therapeutically, but is more expensive. Both agents are given intravenously: for thrombophlebitis, a suggested procedure for streptokinase is to give 250,000 units as a loading dose over a 20- to 30-minute period, followed by a sustaining infusion of 100,000 units per hour for 48 to 72 hours; with urokinase, 2000 units per pound of body weight is given as a loading dose, followed by a sustaining infusion of the same amount per hour for 48 hours. Heparin therapy is instituted at the termination of the fibrinolytic therapy so as to prevent rethrombosis. Though both agents when used in appropriate dosage are capable of lysing large thrombi in the deep leg veins, the therapeutic efficacy of the treatment is still under evaluation, and neither agent is as yet commercially available in the United States. The only available preparation, human fibrinolysin, is in reality a mixture of streptokinase and human plasmin. At the dosages recommended by the manufacturer, the fibrinolytic activity induced in the patient is extremely variable, and currently little enthusiasm exists for using this material for thrombolytic purposes.

Follow-up Therapy. When the systemic symptoms and signs of thrombophlebitis have subsided and the involved limb is pain-free and nontender, the patient can begin ambulation with the leg supported by elastic stockings unless such activity is followed by a return of symptoms. Following ambulation, the patient should be advised to elevate the extremity above heart level for several half-hour periods a day. Elastic stockings should be worn until measurement of the extremity reveals no accumulation of edema fluid. Early and persistent therapy is important to prevent the development of the postphlebitic syndrome. Once the brawny swelling and induration of the postphlebitic limb have occurred, they may be relieved somewhat by long periods of elevation, elastic compressions, vigorous massage, special exercises, and mechanical devices, providing that there has been no recent recurrence of phlebitis. Gross deformities, ulcerations, and persistent or repeated infections ultimately may require one or more surgical procedures.

PULMONARY EMBOLISM AND INFARCTION

Definition. Pulmonary embolism is the impaction in the pulmonary vascular bed of previously detached thrombus or foreign matter. Its major complication, pulmonary infarction, is the necrosis of lung parenchyma resulting from interference with blood supply. Since pulmonary embolism is the more common event, is not invariably accompanied by infarction, and has distinguishing features of its own, this section will be devoted primarily to pulmonary embolism; however, discussion of pulmonary infarction will be included as indicated.

Etiology. Pulmonary embolism is a complication, not a primary disease; therefore its etiology is considered in terms of the nature and source of the offending embolus. Almost all pulmonary emboli originate as thrombi; on occasion nonthrombotic materials such as amniotic fluid, fat, air, bone marrow, or tumor may embolize to the lung. Fat embolism is considered below.

Peripheral venous thrombi in the lower extremities are the most common source for pulmonary emboli, accounting for 80 per cent. Another important source for pulmonary embolization (10 per cent) is thrombi in the pelvic veins and prostatic plexus. Prostatic vein thrombosis may be seen with malignant disease of the prostate but more frequently accompanies prostatic surgery. In the female, thrombosis in the pelvic veins may follow parturition or surgery; a particularly severe form, with frequent and protracted embolization, may complicate septic abortions. The other 10 per cent of pulmonary emboli usually arise from the right heart and are seen in association with cardiac failure, atrial fibrillation, myocardial infarction, the primary myocardiopathies, and bacterial endocarditis (involving the tricuspid or pulmonic valves). Thrombi in the right heart frequently embolize and account for approximately 25 per cent of pulmonary emboli among cardiac patients.

The factors controlling the detachment of the whole or part of a venous thrombus into the general circulation are even less well understood than thrombus formation itself; frequently such thrombi will break away without apparent cause. It was formerly believed that embolization occurred more frequently with phlebothrombosis, but evidence to support this concept is lacking, and symptomatic thrombophlebitis is frequently complicated by embolization as well. Of more importance are factors that acutely change pressure relationships in veins or suddenly increase venous blood flow; these include straining at stool, exertion, and ambulation following long periods of immobilization.

Once a thrombus is released into the venous circulation, it usually proceeds rapidly through the great veins and right heart into the pulmonary arteries, except under those circumstances in which the embolus is shunted, through a patent foramen ovale or other defect, into the left heart and systemic circulation (*paradoxical embolization*). However, even the latter tends to occur most frequently after a bout of pulmonary embolism, for the associated pulmonary hypertension predisposes to paradoxical embolization.

Incidence and Prevalence. Pulmonary embolism with or without infarction is a common disorder and a most important cause of morbidity and mortality. It is frequently misdiagnosed. If not second to all forms of pneumonia combined, it is the most common pulmonary lesion seen in hospitalized patients today; 30 per cent of pulmonary emboli occur in cardiac patients, another 30 per cent occur among medical noncardiac cases (particularly among the aged), and most of the remainder occur postoperatively. The over-all incidence of pulmonary embolism in general autopsy series ranges from 5 to 14 per cent, but the incidence is considerably higher (25 per cent) in custodial institutions involving older aged patients, and highest (30 to 45 per cent) among cardiac patients; noteworthy is a series that cites evidence for old or recent pulmonary emboli in 64 per cent of a group of consecutive autopsies at a large general hospital.

Massive pulmonary embolus, i.e., involving the main pulmonary artery or its primary branches so as to occlude acutely the major portion of the circulation through the lungs, though less frequent than embolism of smaller vessels, is an important cause of sudden death (5 per cent) and occurs in about 3 per cent of general autopsy series but with antemortem diagnosis of only one in eight.

Embolism to small-sized arteries and capillaries or sublobar vessels, is observed approximately three to five times more frequently in autopsy series than is massive embolism, but, since the former is commonly not fatal and often is recurrent, the actual incidence of acute episodes is relatively much greater. Furthermore, in contrast to massive embolism, the presence of medium-sized emboli at autopsy can be considered only as incidental in two thirds of the cases; in the other third, the clinical features are such as to suggest some relation to the fatal termination. Pulmonary infarction complicates embolism of medium-sized arteries in less than 25 per cent of cases. In cardiac patients, the incidence of infarction following such embolism is considerably increased; in one autopsy series, more than 90 per cent of the lungs of cardiac patients with emboli were found to have areas of infarction.

Embolism to small-sized arteries and capillaries probably occurs with great frequency, but the incidence is difficult to assess. As an isolated and focal lesion, such embolization has little clinical significance, for it is not large enough to produce a macroinfarction, and in routine autopsies the lesion is likely to be overlooked unless there are associated thrombi in the larger vessels. However, multiple small emboli scattered throughout the lungs are frequently observed in association with thrombotic occlusions of larger vessels; under these circumstances they contribute significantly to the impairment of pulmonary circulation and associated morbidity. Miliary small vessel occlusion is also the major cause of morbidity when nonthrombotic emboli, such as fat, amniotic fluid, air, or nitrogen, are involved.

Pathology. Pulmonary emboli may be single or multiple and vary in size from microscopic particles to large saddle emboli that completely occlude the pulmonary artery and its major branches. In addition, a large impacting embolus may immediately break up and not only obstruct a major vessel but further embolize into one or more smaller branches in both lung fields.

With occlusion of the main pulmonary artery or of both its primary branches, there is acute mechanical obstruction to pulmonary blood flow; the pulmonary artery is distended by the presence of both clot and blood, the right ventricle is acutely dilated, the peripheral veins are engorged, and the liver is congested. Acute infarction rarely occurs; either the lung parenchyma is fairly normal or there are moderate atelectasis and edema. The low incidence of acute infarction is probably attributable to the rapidity with which death occurs (75 per cent of these patients die within two hours); other factors ultimately may be invoked to account for this phenomenon. Occasionally a pleural effusion is found, and in 40 per cent of the cases there is evidence of previous embolization and infarction.

Emboli small enough to pass beyond the pulmonary artery and its major branches tend to impact the arteries of the lower lobes, more often on the right than on the left. Embolism to the other lobes is much less frequent; combined, they account for only 25 per cent of the cases. The more frequent involvement of the lower lobes is believed to be due to the fact that these areas lie in the more direct stream of the pulmonary arteries; this is particularly true when thrombi are coming from the lower extremities or pelvis.

When infarction occurs, it spreads to involve a pleural surface, either peripheral or interlobar. The infarcted area is airless and hemorrhagic; the hemorrhage is both interstitial and alveolar. Because of the associated pleuritis, hypoventilation, and pre-existing disease, there may be surrounding atelectasis and edema as well. Although occlusion of the larger medium vessels, e.g., interlobar arteries, tends to be associated with infarcts of larger size, the relation between size of vessel occlusion and infarction is a poor one; other factors appear to be more critical in determining the presence and size of the infarct. By roentgenography, infarcts are poorly visualized on the first day. Thereafter, they usually appear as wedge-shaped or, less commonly, as rounded shadows. When they occur near the bases, considerable diaphragmatic elevation and restriction of motion may be observed. In 30 to 40 per cent of cases, infarcts are associated with a variable amount of pleural effusion that may be serous, serosanguineous, or frankly hemorrhagic; usually the specific gravity is in the range of 1.014 to 1.017, and there is a mild to moderate pleocytosis.

Some infarcts clear rapidly (two to three days) on roentgenographic examination and have been referred to as "incomplete" infarcts; however, it is not certain that this clearing represents true resolution of an infarct or reventilation of a surrounding atelectatic and congested area. "Complete" infarcts clear slowly over a two- to three-week period, ending as an area of linear fibrosis.

Mechanisms of Disease. Emboli lodging in the pulmonary arterial tree acutely reduce the circulation distal to the site of obstruction. Potentially, the effects are threefold: (1) Less blood proceeds through the pulmonary circuit to the left heart and systemic circulation, (2) there is a damming back of blood behind the mechanical obstruction, and (3) hemorrhagic necrosis of the ischemic area may occur.

Except for the occurrence of infarction, which must be considered as a localized or focal disorder, the average person is believed capable of tolerating considerable obstruction of the pulmonary arterial bed without serious consequences to the vascular dynamics; in animals, a 60 to 70 per cent obstruction is usually well tolerated. Nevertheless, exceptions occur, both in the congested lung, where less extensive occlusions may elevate pulmonary arterial pressure or significantly reduce pulmonary venous outflow, and where pulmonary circulation has been previously impaired by disease or prior embolization.

With massive occlusion of the main pulmonary artery or both primary branches, the effects are acute and primarily mechanical: rapidly rising pulmonary artery pressure, failure of the right ventricle, cyanosis, venous engorgement, and hepatic congestion. The consequences of impaired pulmonary venous return are sharp reduction in left ventricular filling, diminished cardiac output, reduced coronary and cerebral blood flow, hypoxia, dyspnea, pallor, tachycardia, and hypotension, usually progressing quickly to shock and death. Sudden dyspnea and retrosternal pain frequently are the most prominent initial complaints; the dyspnea is believed to be due to anoxia, apprehension, and stimulation of Hering-Breuer and other reflexes; the angina is usually attributed to acute coronary insufficiency, but direct stimulation of sensory nerves in the wall of a rapidly distending pulmonary artery may also play a significant role.

The effects of embolization to medium-sized vessels depend on the number, size, and distribution of the emboli and the prior state of the lung and circulation. Several patterns may be observed. (1) There may be no observable effects; a transient episode of dyspnea may be the only clue to its occurrence. (2) The picture may be predominantly one of pulmonary infarction with hemoptysis, pleuritic chest pain, friction rub, and abnormal roentgenographic shadows. Often, however, some elements of this pattern may be absent, notably the hemoptysis or the evidence of pleural involvement. (3) There may be an acute picture similar to but frequently not as severe as that seen with massive embolization, in which pattern the primary difficulty is one of extensive and sudden compromise of the pulmonary arterial circulation by multiple emboli or recurrent embolization; it may or may not be complicated by infarction. (4) There may be a chronic and insidiously developing syndrome of cor pulmonale from progressive pulmonary hypertension that has evolved slowly following repeated episodes of embolization with or without infarction. This is often superimposed and obscured by the presence of other underlying chronic disease.

Controversy exists relative to the factors that acutely compromise the pulmonary circulation when emboli impact in medium-sized or smaller vessels. Some hold that vasoconstriction (pulmonary and perhaps coronary), mediated either through reflexes emanating from occluded arterioles or by the local release of serotonin or other vasoactive substances, plays an important role. It seems probable, however, that the effects of most pulmonary emboli on the circulation of the lungs are primarily mechanical; when a major segment of the circulation is organically occluded, pulmonary hypertension and decreased venous outflow result. The suggestion has been made, and experimental studies have been cited to support the concept, that idiopathic pulmonary hypertension and pulmonary arteriosclerosis may result from repeated small pulmonary emboli.

The mechanism of pulmonary infarction is poorly understood. It does not result from ligation of pulmonary vessels and is unusual after embolization in animals with normal lungs; however, it does occur with great frequency in the congested, infected, or hypoventilated lung. Currently the best working hypothesis is that, when medium-sized embolization occurs, enhancement of the circulation through the bronchial artery collaterals and bronchopulmonary vascular anastomoses distal to the embolus ordinarily serves to sustain the lung. However, in the presence of congestion or other conditions that predispose to local intrapulmonic circulatory stasis, augmentation of the collateral circulation is delayed or its benefits voided, and infarction occurs.

Hemorrhagic necrosis of the lung tissue and the overlying pleural inflammation that incites are responsible for the characteristic clinical features of pulmonary infarction; the former accounts for the hemoptysis, cough, and fever, the latter for the pleural friction rub and pain. Since both lung tissue and the visceral pleura are devoid of sensory nerves, infarcts that do not extend to the outer surface of the lung to involve the parietal pleura do not cause pleural pain. When pain is present, it usually occurs over the ribs in the axillary region, but occasionally it may appear in the abdomen along the costal margin, or, when there is involvement of the parietal diaphragmatic pleura, in the shoulder or neck. The mechanism of the pain has usually been attributed to friction over an inflamed pleura, but an alternative explanation that may better explain its features (accentuation only on inspiration) is tension exerted during inspiration on those sensitized nerve ends of the pleura that are attached to the intercostal muscles.

Clinical Manifestations. The manifestations of pulmonary embolism include sudden dyspnea; precordial or substernal oppressive pain, occasionally with radiation to shoulders and neck; evidences of right-sided cardiac dilatation and failure; tachycardia; restlessness; anxiety; syncope, occasionally with convulsions; and hypotension.

With massive embolism, death may be sudden or may occur over a period of several hours. In the latter instance, shock with vascular collapse becomes prominent. In some 15 per cent of the cases, death may be delayed from one to several days but, when blood pressure spontaneously returns to normal, recovery is likely. The physical signs noted include pulsation in the second left interspace, accentuation of P_2, a pseudo- or pleuropericardial friction rub, systolic or diastolic murmurs in the second left interspace, an interscapular bruit, gallop rhythm, increased cardiac dullness to the right, distended neck veins, increased venous pressure with an hepatojugular reflex, and enlarged liver. Dislodgment of a large obstructing embolus may be associated with the dramatic transient appearance of a "red arterial wave" suddenly passing over a pallid cyanotic face.

Serial electrocardiographic observation reveals transient changes in most patients. These include arrhythmias, the development of an S_1Q_3 pattern, deep S waves in the standard leads, S-T segment depression in leads I and II, T wave inversion in leads II and III, right axis deviation, clockwise rotation of the heart, right bundle branch block, peak P waves in leads II, III, and AVF, and inverted T waves with S-T segment deviations in the right precordial leads. These changes result from the acute strain and dilation of the chambers of the right side of the heart and from myocardial ischemia. The presence of Q waves in leads II and III and AVF with inverted T waves may be interpreted erroneously as evidence of an acute myocardial infarction. Roentgenographically, pulmonary embolism may result in the appearance of a large pulmonary arterial shadow that is dilated and terminates abruptly; in some cases the ischemia may produce an increased radiolucency of portions of the lung field.

When embolization involves the medium-sized or smaller vessels, the clinical manifestations may vary from a transient episode of dyspnea or the sudden or insidious worsening of an underlying pulmonary or cardiac disease to the full-blown picture described above; however, when pulmonary infarction occurs, its manifestations may also be superimposed.

The manifestations of pulmonary infarction are usually less dramatic. They vary in intensity from silent lesions to those characterized by pleuritic chest pain, hemoptysis, cough, moderate dyspnea, fever, tachycardia, pleural friction rub, areas of dullness or flatness on percussion, diminished breath sounds, occasionally with tubular breathing, and rales. The leukocyte count is usually elevated, the sedimentation rate is accelerated and, subsequently, the serum bilirubin and serum lactic dehydrogenase levels rise. Roentgenographic examination may show typical wedge-shaped shadows; on occasions the lesions are rounded or indistinguishable from pneumonic infiltrates. At other times, a pleural effusion may be the only clue to an underlying infarct. The average patient with pulmonary infarction runs a moderately febrile course for a few days, which is followed by clearing of roentgenographic and physical signs in one to three weeks.

Diagnosis. Despite the introduction of such excellent diagnostic aids as pulmonary isotopic photoscanning and selective pulmonary angiography, the diagnosis of pulmonary embolism with or without infarction is accurately made in no more than 50 per cent of cases when compared to autopsy findings. Frequently the diagnosis is overlooked, because the disorder appears in the guise of congestive heart failure or pneumonia rather than as a distinctive syndrome; furthermore, the cardinal features do not occur with any great regularity. *In half of the patients subsequently proved to have recurrent infarction, no evidence of phlebitis, pleural pain, pleural friction rub, or hemoptysis is present, and in any one episode the incidence of each of these features is less than 20 per cent.* Thus in the absence of classic features, the diagnosis must be made on the basis of a high index of suspicion followed by confirmatory laboratory findings.

Pulmonary embolism with or without infarction should be suspected in all cases of chest pain of unknown cause, atypical pleural effusion, or bronchopneumonia. The possibility of this complication should also be considered most carefully in any critically ill patient with congestive heart failure, for the incidence among these patients approaches 50 per cent and is much higher among those who exhibit unexplained fever or the triad of tachycardia, digitalis toxicity, or edema unresponsive to diuretic therapy.

Actually, the presence of one or more of the following symptoms, signs, or laboratory findings should raise the possibility of pulmonary embolism for consideration: sudden or increased dyspnea, tachypnea, or cough; substernal or pleuritic chest pain; hemoptysis; phlebitis; acute right-sided failure or sudden worsening of congestive heart failure; shock; pulmonary consolidation; pleural friction rub; roentgenographic evidence of pulmonary infiltration, elevated diaphragm, or pleural effusion; electrocardiographic changes consistent with acute right-heart strain or dilatation; pulmonary function studies indicating an increased ventilatory dead space, i.e., a reduction in the mean alveolar carbon dioxide tension in the presence of a normal or nearly normal arterial carbon dioxide tension; or unexplained fever, leukocytosis, elevated erythrocyte sedimentation rate, serum bilirubin, and lactic dehydrogenase.

Confirmation of the diagnosis often can be achieved through the use of either selective pulmonary angiography or pulmonary isotopic photoscanning with radioactively labeled macro-aggregated human serum albumin; on occasion, both techniques will be necessary. Since selective *pulmonary angiography* provides for direct visualization of the vascular tree, it is the more definitive of the two procedures, and is the choice for establishing the diagnosis of pulmonary embolism. However, there are limitations to its usefulness. It is an expensive procedure and requires a skilled team; catheterization of the pulmonary artery is associated with some morbidity; the technique does not distinguish between new and old emboli; the smallest vessels are not visualized adequately; and there may be errors in interpretation unless the emboli are actually visualized.

Pulmonary isotopic photoscanning has the advantages of convenience and lack of significant morbidity, and allows for repeated observation in following the course of the patient. However, unlike pulmonary arteriography, photoscanning does not visualize the pulmonary arterial tree; rather, it is a measure of pulmonary capillary perfusion, and defects in perfusion may be misinterpreted as to cause, especially in the presence of any underlying pulmonary lesion, e.g., infiltrates, blebs, cysts, emphysema, or alterations in perfusion as a result of previous or associated disease. The technique is most useful for demonstrating the perfusion defect of a pulmonary embolism when the chest roentgenogram is normal; it may also be diagnostic by revealing multiple perfusion defects (indicative of multiple pulmonary embolism) when only an isolated infiltrate or lesion is present roentgenographically. Resolution of the perfusion defect following embolism occurs progressively (50 per cent in two weeks), and this too may be useful diagnostically.

Acute pulmonary embolism may be most readily confused with acute myocardial infarction, pulmonary edema, an acute asthmatic attack, atelectasis, pericarditis, spontaneous pneumothorax, ball-valve thrombus in the left atrium, dissecting aneurysm, and pulmonary artery thrombosis. The latter occurs rarely as a primary form of obscure cause or as a complication of a partially obstructing embolus, invading tumor, narrowed vascular lumen, or atherosclerotic plaque.

The differential diagnosis of pulmonary infarction includes pneumonia, pleurisy, other forms of pleural effusion, neoplasm, acute upper abdominal conditions, and the various causes of pulmonary hemorrhage.

To distinguish between an infarct and pneumonia may be difficult, yet this question arises frequently. Findings that are frequently helpful in pointing to the diagnosis of infarct are a history or the presence of one of the preconditions of infarct, e.g., recent surgery, trauma, or cardiac disease; an extremely rapid appearance of roentgenographic abnormalities from the time of the first respiratory symptom; illness that seems disproportionately mild in relation to the extent of the pulmonary involvement, or leukocytosis; and relative lack of cough or lack of preceding respiratory disease.

A spontaneous form of pulmonary infarction occurs in sickle cell disease, in the mixed sickle cell hemoglobinopathies, or in persons with sickle cell trait who are exposed to high altitude.

Treatment. General Measures. Supportive treatment for the usual acute embolism should include bed rest, an analgesic or narcotic (morphine or preferably meperidine hydrochloride [Demerol]) for pain and apprehension, and oxygen as indicated. The administration of antimicrobial drugs to prevent bacterial disease of the lungs is not indicated unless a septic infarct is suspected. All sudden effort should be avoided, especially straining at stool. Stool softeners and colonic lavages may prove useful. Pleural effusions may require aspiration, particularly if dyspnea is progressive. Digitalization is indicated if cardiac failure appears or worsens, but usually results in little benefit.

In the more severe cases, continuous oxygen therapy should be employed, and positive pressure oxygen may prove particularly useful when pulmonary edema is present. Cardiac arrhythmias, which occur in 10 per cent of cases, should be treated appropriately. If shock occurs, fluids and vasopressors should be given. Intravenous fluids should be monitored by central venous pressure measurements but maintained below 150 mm. saline to prevent pulmonary edema. For hypotension, norepinephrine in high concentration, 4 to 8 mg. per 100 ml., can be given intravenously slowly to sustain the systolic blood pressure at about 100 mm. Hg (preferably at 120 mm. Hg in previously hypertensive patients). Methoxamine (Vasoxyl) in 10 to 15 mg. doses, metaraminol (Aramine), 2 to 10 mg., and mephentermine (Wyamine), 15 to 35 mg., are also effective when given intramuscularly. Aminophylline, 250 to 500 mg. (by suppository, intramuscular, or slow intravenous administration) may prove useful, particularly when dyspnea is prominent or pulmonary edema is present. Venesection may be dangerous, however, because of impaired left ventricular filling. The value of pulmonary vasodilators, e.g., papaverine, and bronchodilators, e.g., atropine, are still highly controversial.

Anticoagulants. In the absence of contraindications, heparin therapy should be instituted immediately in all patients with pulmonary embolism to lessen the danger of a recurrent and frequently fatal embolic accident (when heparin allergy is present, anticoagulation should be instituted immediately with coumarin compounds). Hemoptysis from pulmonary infarction is not a contraindication to anticoagulant therapy. The regimen for heparin therapy and subsequent oral coumarin anticoagulation is as described under the treatment of thrombophlebitis. Coumarin therapy is continued for at least six weeks unless there is a chronic disease, e.g., cardiac failure, that predisposes to repeated venous thrombus formation; under these circumstances anticoagulant therapy should be continued for prolonged periods.

Thrombolytic agents undoubtedly will find a place in the management of acute pulmonary embolism, both to relieve the pulmonary arterial obstruction and to lyse the original source of embolization. At present the specific indications and best regimen of therapy have not been defined, though such a regimen is likely to be shown to be most beneficial in the management of patients with extensive or massive pulmonary embolization. Arvin, the defibrinating agent, is also likely to be of benefit in the management of acute pulmonary embolism, but its advantage over heparin remains to be established.

Surgical Therapy. Inferior vena caval ligation or plication should be reserved for those patients in whom anticoagulants are contraindiated or whose disease for one reason or another cannot be successfully managed with this form of therapy. Since these procedures carry a significant incidence of sequelae, they are not indicated unless there has been massive embolism or there is evidence of recurrent embolization (a minor recurrence is observed in about 10 per cent of patients during the first few days of heparin therapy, and should not be considered as a failure of anticoagulant therapy unless the episode is significant clinically or continues to recur); however, in the presence of septic emboli to the lungs from foci of infection in the pelvic veins, e.g., following septic abortion, caval interruption should be performed immediately.

Surgical embolectomy may be life-saving in critically ill patients. However, this procedure requires cardiac bypass, and because of the condition of the patients, the mortality in patients treated with surgical embolectomy is still very high. At present, the indication for embolectomy is limited to those patients with angiographic evidence of massive embolism and with a sustained peripheral hypotension despite the use of appropriate supportive measures. Pulmonary embolectomy may also be considered for those patients who have survived a massive embolism but in whom pulmonary hypertension resulting from the presence of the embolus is leading to the development of cor pulmonale.

Prognosis. The prognosis of pulmonary embolism is difficult to establish because the clinical diagnosis is frequently obscure. The mortality from an acute episode, excluding those who die immediately or in the first few hours, is of the order of 10 per cent, but the likelihood of death is increased with succeeding embolic attacks. The greatest hope for the management of this problem lies in its prevention.

Unfortunately, such measures as the use of elastic stockings or bandages, leg exercises for immobilized patients, and early ambulation postoperatively have not greatly affected the high incidence of pulmonary embolism; nevertheless, the intelligent use of such measures is to be encouraged. In addition, serious consideration should be given to the use of anticoagulants for all patients predisposed to thrombus formation. When used carefully, anticoagulants have significantly reduced the incidence of pulmonary embolism following fracture of the femur and in cases of congestive heart failure. This form of therapy should not be undertaken lightly, because the hazards, in any specific case, may outweigh the benefits to be derived.

Debakey, M. E.: Collective review: A critical evaluation of the problem of thromboembolism. Int. Abstr. Surg., 98:1, 1954.

Fletcher, A. P., and Sherry, S.: Thrombolytic agents. Annual Rev. Pharmacol., 6:89, 1966.

Gillenwater, J. Y., Breslow, I. H., and Lisker, S.: Phlegmasia cerulea dolens. Circulation, 25:39, 1962.

Gorham, L. W.: A study of pulmonary embolism. Arch. Intern. Med. (Chicago), 108:8, 189, 418, 1961.

McLachlin, A. D., McLachlin, J. A., Jory, T. A., and Rawling, E. G.: Venous stasis in the lower extremities. Ann. Surg., 152:678, 1960.

Sasahara, A. A., and Stein, M. M.: Pulmonary Embolic Disease—Symposium. New York, Grune and Stratton, Inc., 1965.

Sautter, R. D.: Massive pulmonary thromboembolism. Experience with 12 pulmonary embolectomies. J.A.M.A., 194:336, 1965.

Sevitt, S.: Venous thrombosis and pulmonary embolism. Their prevention by oral anticoagulants. Amer. J. Med., 33:703, 1962.

Sherry, S., Genton, E., Brinkhous, K. M., and Stengle, J. M. (eds.): Thrombosis. Washington, D. C., National Academy of Sciences, 1969. (Excellent reference source for all aspects of thrombosis and thromboembolic diseases.)

Spencer, F. C., Quattlebaum, G. K., Quattlebaum, G. K., Jr., Sharp, E. H., and Jude, J. R.: Plication of the inferior vena cava for pulmonary embolism: A report of 20 cases. Ann. Surg., 155:827, 1962.

Thomas, D. P.: Treatment of pulmonary embolic disease. New Eng. J. Med., 273:885, 1965.

Wessler, S., and Gaston, L. W.: Pharmacologic and clinical aspects of heparin therapy. Anaesthesiology, 27:475, 1966.

FAT EMBOLISM

This is a form of embolization involving fat globules that may follow extensive crushing injuries to soft tissues and long bones or, less commonly, following closed chest cardiac massage or extensive surgery on bone or fatty tissue. Under these circumstances, liquid fat from ruptured fat cells is forced into the circulation; myriads of fat globules are then formed as a result of surface tension, and diffusely embolize the small pulmonary capillaries. The acute obstruction of the pulmonary circulation results in severe hypoxia, cyanosis, dyspnea, and tachypnea. In addition, many of the fat emboli escape through pulmonary arteriovenous shunts or are forced from the pulmonary capillaries into the systemic circulation, where they occlude and damage peripheral capillaries; these effects may be observed readily in the brain, skin, and kidneys.

In the brain, the fat emboli have a predilection for obstructing and injuring small vessels of the white matter; such cerebral lesions in conjunction with hypoxia produce restlessness, delirium, and transient neurologic changes (twitchings and convulsions). In the skin, petechiae are common and have been described as more brownish than usual, a phenomenon possibly related to the presence of fat in the hemorrhage. The renal glomerular lesions are focal and unassociated with significant renal functional impairment, but fat globules escape into the urine and can be identified for diagnostic purposes.

Diagnosis. The clinical picture is usually characteristic but is variable in severity; about 10 to 20 per cent of clinically recognized cases are fatal. The patient suddenly develops dyspnea, tachypnea, and cyanosis on the first or second day following injury; restlessness and anxiety rapidly follow and may progress to delirium and coma. On the second to third day, petechiae appear over the upper trunk and may be observed in the conjunctivae and retina. Although most patients recover, dis-

orientation, with periods of lucidity, may persist for up to two weeks. The development of coma is a poor diagnostic sign. The diagnosis may be established early in the course of the disease by the finding of fat globules in the sputum or on the surface of the urine; heating of the urine surface may produce the crackling sound of burning fat.

Treatment. No specific therapy is available. Oxygen is the single most beneficial agent and may be particularly useful when given under positive pressure. Other supportive measures are used as indicated. Heparin, because of its lipemia-clearing effect, has been recommended, and hypothermia may prove useful when coma supervenes.

Jackson, C. T., and Greendyke, R. M.: Pulmonary and cerebral fat embolism after closed chest cardiac massage. Surg. Gynec. Obstet., 120:25, 1965.

Love, J., and Stryker, W. S.: Fat embolism: A problem of increasing importance to the orthopedist and the internist. Ann. Intern. Med., 46:342, 1957.

Sevitt, S.: Fat Embolism. London, Butterworth & Co. Ltd., 1962.

Arterial Hypertension

W. S. Peart

Definition. A statement that a given arterial pressure is above normal requires a knowledge of the range of normality. For a true definition of a raised arterial pressure, such as is used in epidemiologic studies, a rise above the mean of a population studied under standard conditions is usually used. It is easy to say that an arterial pressure of 120 systolic, 80 diastolic in mm. of mercury is normal from the age of 15 years on and that an arterial pressure of 250 systolic, 150 diastolic in mm. of mercury is abnormal at any age. The intermediate ranges are decided somewhat arbitrarily. In clinical practice this is of little help. It is wise when there is some doubt not to state either that hypertension exists or that it does not exist, but to substitute observation over a period of time to make sure that casual arterial pressure readings are consistently on the higher side of what is usually encountered in a completely normal subject. Again, it must be realized that single readings taken with a sphygmomanometer under varying circumstances may not reflect the usual arterial pressure in a given person. Measurements taken with automatic apparatus over 24-hour periods have shown considerable lability of pressure in many persons. This does not mean that high casual pressures may not be harmful, but in an individual case it must not be readily assumed that they are, since in these days of intensive therapy and investigation a great deal depends on this decision.

There are thus the two approaches: epidemiologic, which may have to depend upon isolated single readings of large populations that give information only about the range of casual read-

ings, and the clinical approach, in which other factors have to be taken into account. It seems quite clear that most manifestations of disease in patients with raised arterial pressure are the consequences of, or are made worse by, the presence of raised pressure. This applies, for example, to the incidence of atheroma and other vascular disease. There is no doubt either that the higher the arterial pressure, whether systolic or diastolic, the higher the morbidity and mortality, and there is a distinct quantitative relation between these factors in many population studies. The fact that some patients withstand high arterial pressures without showing very many significant changes in their vascular systems compared with other patients with lower pressures and more serious vascular diseases does not invalidate this thesis. One individual's blood vessels may be of better quality than another's.

Some patients have mainly a rise in systolic arterial pressure. This particularly applies to the elderly, in whom such figures as 200 systolic, 90 diastolic in mm. of mercury are not uncommon. It is likely that this mainly systolic hypertension represents increasing rigidity of the aorta and main vessels with less effect on the arterioles. There are all gradations from rise of the diastolic pressure with a relatively small rise in the systolic pressure to rise in the systolic pressure with a relatively smaller rise in the diastolic pressure. Too much has been made of the greater importance of diastolic hypertension in morbidity. It is highly likely that rise in the mean pressure is of greatest importance whatever way it is produced.

Measurement of Arterial Pressure. The ordinary sphygmomanometric method of measuring has been shown to be subject to considerable error. This has emerged in epidemiologic studies of distribution of arterial pressure and must be taken into account clinically, particularly in following the results of treatment. Quite apart from the influence of arm circumference, so that those with fat upper arms have higher recorded pressures than those with thin arms for the same true direct intra-arterial measurements, observer error creeps in. Many observers show conspicuous digit preference in measuring the arterial pressure, and this can make 10 mm. of mercury difference in one reading.

Causes of Hypertension. In most cases of hypertension (high arterial pressure) it is impossible at the present time to establish a cause. These cases, probably about two thirds of all those seen, are called "essential" or "idiopathic" hypertension. Fortunately, inroads are continually being made into this majority as greater knowledge accrues about disorders known to cause raised arterial pressure. These may be classified as follows:

I. Nonrenal causes
  A. Adrenal cortical overactivity
    1. Cushing's syndrome: Overproduction of hydrocortisone and corticosterone
    2. Conn's syndrome: Overproduction of aldosterone
    3. Pseudohermaphroditism: Overproduction of androgenic steroids
    4. Deoxycorticosterone production due to enzyme defect
  B. Adrenal medullary overactivity
    1. Pheochromocytoma: Overproduction of epinephrine, norepinephrine, and occasionally other amines such as hydroxytyramine
  C. Pregnancy
    Although pregnancy exacerbates the effects of underlying renal disease, the arterial pressure may be raised without any obvious renal disease as part of the "toxemia of pregnancy" syndrome.
  D. Coarctation of the aorta
    Although the coarctation has to take place above the level of the renal arteries for hypertension to exist, no conclusive evidence of renal involvement has yet been provided.
  E. Miscellaneous
    1. Ovarian tumors of varying histologic type: Overproduction of various steroid hormones similar to those in Cushing's syndrome is sometimes seen.
    2. Porphyria during acute attacks
    3. Lead poisoning during acute phase
    4. Raised intracranial pressure, more usually of acute onset, as with subarachnoid hemorrhage
    5. Administration of monoamine oxidase inhibitors followed by cheese ingestion
    6. Licorice usually used for peptic ulcer treatment
II. Renal causes
  Practically all renal diseases known have been associated with hypertension. Important examples are:
  A. Acute and chronic glomerulonephritis
  B. Pyelonephritis
  C. Diabetic kidney
  D. Polyarteritis nodosa
  The probable link is interference with blood supply to the kidney, best exemplified by renal artery stenosis due to atheroma, extrinsic bands, or fibromuscular disease.

Incidence and Prevalence. In a given population group there is no comprehensive information about the distribution of causes. Attempts have been made to define this in selected groups of the population. It has been found, for example, by population study in both Wales and Jamaica, that there is a similar incidence of symptomless bacilluria in some subjects with hypertension, but whether cause or effect is uncertain. It is not known how many patients have atheromatous renal artery stenosis or fibromuscular hyperplasia of the renal arteries, or even chronic glomerulonephritis. To completely exclude a renal cause of hypertension requires considerable investigation in depth, including pyelography, arteriography, and renal biopsy, and even with such aids the presence of occult pyelonephritis as a scattered disease of the kidney may be missed. It still seems likely, however, that the bulk of cases picked up in epidemiologic surveys will have no known cause at present with the most intensive of our investigations. The prevalence varies widely in different parts of the world and among various races. For example, Negroes in Georgia have a very high incidence of hypertension, as do coastal dwellers in northern Japan. In the former case, no cause can be attributed, although environmental factors are incriminated theoretically; in the latter, high ingestion of salt has been indicted. In some areas hypertension is very uncommon, for example, in the Gilbert Islands.

Epidemiology. Much effort has been devoted to the epidemiology. Most of the studies depend upon casual arterial pressures taken under reasonably standard conditions, and the results show certain definite features. In general, arterial pressure in urban communities rises with age. This tendency is less marked in some communities, for example, in the Gilbert Islands. This applies to both the systolic and diastolic pressures in both males and females, although the rise in females is greater from the age of 30 to 40 years. This difference in the female has been noted in widely separated populations in different parts of the world. There is a quantitative likeness in the arterial pressure of blood relatives. Despite the common occurrence of hypertension in certain families, over all there is no evidence of a common dominant genetic inheritance but rather of multiple factors. Environment as well as genetic inheritance has a common role in families. For example, the husbands of multiparous women in a study in South Wales had a lower than average arterial pressure, as did their wives. Unexpected correlations of this sort emerge in epidemiologic studies. Another is the higher incidence of hypertension among the relatives of subjects with hypertension and pyelonephritis. Nevertheless, identical twins may develop severe hypertension at about the same age even though they have spent their lives apart.

Pathology. Certain changes are common to all forms of hypertension and may properly be regarded as due solely to the level of arterial pressure. Other changes are peculiar to each cause of high arterial pressure, and they will be considered separately. In nearly all diseases associated with hypertension, the malignant phase may follow, so that a complicated picture due to the presence of the disease and the effects of malignant hypertension may be seen. Despite occasional suggestions to the contrary, the best evidence points to the malignant phase (necrotizing or accelerated phase) of hypertension as being mainly related to the absolute height of the mean pressure or the rate of rise of the mean pressure. Efforts to segregate malignant hypertension as a peculiar disease in its own right have been unrewarding, and the fact that some patients have all the evidence of malignant hypertension at mean pressures lower than other patients who have been withstanding higher pressures for many years does not disprove this general thesis. In any study of a large number of patients, those with malignant hypertension have a higher arterial pressure than those without. The manifestations of malignant hypertension in pathologic terms are acute vascular changes with fibrinoid necrosis in arterioles. The brunt of the damage is borne by vessels in the kidney, pancreas, mesentery, adrenal, and retina. It is rarely seen in voluntary muscle, and no cause can be suggested for this type of distribution. Since the kidney is always involved in all forms of hypertension, it is often difficult to be sure of the difference between primary change causing the hypertension and secondary damage because of the hypertension. It is reasonably certain that there is a primary disease in the kidney when the changes are most clearly seen in the glomeruli, as in glomerulonephritis, disseminated lupus erythematosus, amyloidosis, and diabetes. The glomerular changes with interference of blood flow lead to tubular atrophy, and in those cases in which the blood pressure is elevated, the most common changes are initially hypertrophy of the muscular wall of the afferent arteriole; next, hyalinization; and finally, in the malignant phase, intimal hyperplasia of the onion skin variety, which occurs also in slightly larger arteries, as well as the definitive fibrinoid arteriolar necrosis. In the larger arteries within the kidney, from the interlobar to the arcuates, hypertension causes intimal thickening, replication of the internal elastic lamina, and fibrosis with atheromatous deposits, sometimes in a very uniform manner but often as a nodular process. It is thought that this change, when it occurs in the apparently normal kidney, may be responsible for perpetuation of hypertension when the opposite abnormal kidney, the seat of pyelonephritis or involved by renal artery stenosis, is removed. The signs of ischemic change are best seen when the main renal artery is stenosed. The kidney volume shrinks; the glomeruli are crowded but generally appear normal; the juxtaglomerular apparatus in the afferent arteriole, the cells surrounding, and the macula densa of the distal convoluted tubule hypertrophy, sometimes grossly, and become hypergranulated, whereas the tubules between the glomeruli are atrophic and the interstitium may be expanded or fibrotic. The opposite kidney may show all the signs of hypertensive change previously described. The effects of acute narrowing of the arteriolar

lumen on the performance of the relevant organs are seen, so that, in the case of the kidney, diminution of function with proteinuria, microscopic hematuria, and even frank hematuria occur. In the retina, exudation and hemorrhage due to small infarcts, and papilledema associated with a raised intracranial pressure, which is of uncertain origin, are the main features. When this process occurs in the brain, various disturbances result, according to the part of the brain affected; fits and unconsciousness are not rare and are given the clumsy name of hypertensive encephalopathy. Arteriolar spasms may underlie some of these attacks as opposed to cerebral edema, previously implicated, and full recovery may occur. Because the impact may be apparently greater in some organs than in others, it is possible to find fibrinoid necroses in renal biopsies without any characteristic change in the retina. The converse is perhaps less common. In most cases this disorder runs its course, if untreated, to death within two years of diagnosis. The features it shares with all other hypertensive manifestations are those due to the increased load put upon the heart and the blood vessels in different territories. A main finding is the increased incidence of atheroma, both experimentally and pathologically. The increased pressure leads to hypertrophy of the left ventricle and a tendency to angina pectoris and myocardial infarction. The increased load on the left heart leads to raised pulmonary venous pressure, pulmonary edema, raised pulmonary artery pressure, and congestive cardiac failure. The increased pressure in the vessels to the brain leads to a high incidence of strokes due to cerebral hemorrhage, thrombosis, and subarachnoid hemorrhage. The site of these is probably the arterial microaneurysms originally described by Charcot. Vascular damage in the kidney leads to renal failure. It must be emphasized again that all these manifestations may be linked quantitatively with the level of arterial pressure. There is no doubt that in such conditions of acute onset as acute glomerulonephritis and eclampsia, the manifestations of malignant hypertension, particularly in the retina, may appear at lower pressures and may seem more florid in the presence of renal failure. The latter, however, is not essential to the appearances. It is likely that the rate of rise of pressure at least in part governs the severity of the signs.

The Mechanisms of Hypertension.   *Circulatory Pattern.*   The major factors controlling the arterial pressure are the cardiac output and the total peripheral resistance. If the cardiac output rises, the arterial pressure will rise unless there is a corresponding drop in the peripheral resistance. Most peripheral resistance occurs in the arterioles and is governed by contraction of their muscular walls. A given level of arterial pressure depends on the interplay between these two major factors and, in order to describe the pattern of the circulation, it is necessary to be able to say what the peripheral resistance is and in which part of the body the major changes are occurring. Although it has been claimed that changes in cardiac output are responsible for rises in pressure and may even ultimately lead to persistent high arterial pressure, the evidence for this is weak. In most cases of high arterial pressure, either experimental or in man, the one uniform feature is a raised peripheral resistance. The cardiac output in most cases of established hypertension in man is within normal limits. Theoretically, it might be thought that to know the particular pattern of peripheral resistance could give important clues to the cause of high arterial pressure. In only one form of high arterial pressure is there a very distinctive pattern, and this is pheochromocytoma. Epinephrine and norepinephrine, the amines most commonly released by these tumors, are particularly potent as vasoconstrictors in the skin. Measurements of skin blood flow show very low levels in such patients, unlike other causes of high arterial pressure. Removal of the tumor is followed by a rise in skin flow. If there were a wide variety of different agents raising the arterial pressure by increasing the peripheral resistance in various territories, certain characteristic patterns might emerge. However, in either renal hypertension or hypertension of unknown origin, the pattern is strikingly the same, so that the distribution of resistance is much the same from patient to patient. Admittedly, simultaneous measurements of flow in different parts of the body have not been done. Certain organs show the increased resistance most, the kidney and splanchnic area in particular. The general impression is, however, of a widely distributed increase of peripheral resistance in every tissue and organ of the body except the voluntary muscles.

Increased Cardiac Output. There are a few situations in which increased cardiac output seems to play an important role in raising the arterial pressure: renal failure, toxemia of pregnancy, and acute glomerulonephritis. Most studies have been made of patients with renal failure; these patients are particularly susceptible to fluid load, and the arterial pressure may rise abruptly when the patients are overloaded with water.

Cause of Rise in the Peripheral Resistance. This is unknown in all cases of hypertension except those associated with pheochromocytoma. Hypertension itself causes changes in peripheral resistance in the sense that at a high arterial pressure the vessels contract, whereas lowering the arterial pressure causes decreased contraction. This is presumably a direct effect of pressure on the smooth muscle of the arteriolar wall, as was first shown by Folkow and his colleagues (1958). At one extreme, Borst (1963) has claimed that the sequence may be retention of salt and water, rise in the cardiac output, rise in arterial pressure, secondary contraction of peripheral arterioles leading to further rise in arterial pressure. Others believe that there is a primary cause for a rise in peripheral resistance, leading inevitably to a rise in arterial pressure. There are no firm data to support either view convincingly. There is no evidence of overactivity of the sympathetic nervous system either on the heart or on the peripheral resistance. The following major fields require deeper discussion.

Hypertension Associated with Retention of Water and Salt, with or without the Action of Adrenocortical Steroids. The best example, mentioned before, is of the patient with renal failure who tolerates fluid load badly and who is incapable of adjusting cardiac output and peripheral resistance so as to maintain his arterial pressure at normal levels. Removing body fluid by dialysis and lowering the salt intake will readily control this high arterial pressure in most instances. Even here another renal factor is revealed by the further lowering of arterial pressure brought about in this type of patient by total nephrectomy prior to renal transplantation. It was in animals that the condition of "renoprival hypertension" was described, but from closer studies made recently it seems that the hypertension that develops without kidneys is most likely to be due to increased sensitivity to salt and water overload with a rise in cardiac output. One of the experimental links of hypertension with salt and water metabolism is the observation that salt feeding in the rat leads to hypertension and also to renal damage, particularly if deoxycorticosterone (DOCA) is administered subcutaneously. Dahl and his colleagues have shown that there are salt-sensitive and salt-insensitive strains of rats, so that the possibility exists of a genetic factor acting in conjunction with an environmental one to produce high arterial pressure. The high incidence of hypertension and cerebral hemorrhage in northern Japan may be related since there is a high salt intake in that area, but the exact mechanism is uncertain. In Cushing's syndrome with excess secretion of cortisol from hyperplastic adrenals, hypertension may be very severe and is associated with sodium and water retention as well as increased potassium excretion. The condition may be cured by removal of the suprarenals.

Renal Hypertension. That the kidney is directly and primarily responsible for some cases of raised arterial pressure is shown by the successful cure of hypertension by unilateral nephrectomy when one of the two kidneys is diseased. Among the many renal diseases known to be associated with curable hypertension, pyelonephritis, tuberculosis, carcinoma, and, perhaps most important, obstruction to the main renal artery by atheroma or fibromuscular hyperplasia need to be mentioned. The link seems to be interference with blood supply to the kidney. Similar arguments can be applied to bilateral disease. It is not yet clear how the kidney raises the arterial pressure in any of these conditions, including the experimental application of a clip to the renal artery, first successfully accomplished by Goldblatt and his colleagues (1934).

Following are some of the major ways in which the kidney may be associated with elevation of the arterial pressure.

Failure to Excrete or Destroy an Extrarenal Pressor Substance. This has been partly touched on in the discussion of renoprival hypertension, in which the emphasis was on extracellular fluid volume sensitivity, but certain experimental observations suggest that some metabolic function of the kidney might be important apart from its effect on extracellular fluid volume. The hypotensive effect of introducing a normal kidney into the circulation of an animal with hypertension due to a renal clip and the way in which a kidney with normal blood supply yet deprived of excretory function by a ureteric tie prevents the rise in pressure due to a clip on the opposite renal artery point to this suggestion. The ready reversal of renal stenosis hypertension both in man and in animals by removal of the obstruction, even with hypertension of long duration, argues against a very potent extrarenal pressor system.

Failure to Produce a Vasodilator. The hypothesis that the kidney has its main effect on the arterial pressure by providing a vasodilator to keep the arterial pressure down and that hypertension may be due to a failure of vasodilator production has received much recent study. Various extracts, particularly of the medulla of the kidney, have appeared to lower the arterial pressure on injection into animals. Some of these substances seem certainly to be prostaglandins. Before these findings can be assumed to have any physiologic or pathologic meaning, it will be necessary to demonstrate the release of such substances into the circulation.

Increased Response of a Normal Pressor Mechanism. An obvious candidate for this role is the sympathetic nervous system and its higher neural centers. If the kidney produced some substance that increased the over-all activity of the sympathetic system, this might be reflected in high arterial pressure. There is no substantial evidence in favor of this view and much strong evidence against. Studies of norepinephrine metabolism have not indicated serious overproduction. Investigations of the normal or pathologic state of activity of the sympathetic nervous system suffer, however, from a lack of sufficiently precise techniques in the whole animal or man.

Another way in which an increased response in the body could occur would be for the arterioles to respond more markedly than usual to a normal stimulus. For example, if the degree of contraction produced by a given dose of norepinephrine were markedly increased, then a state of high arterial pressure might follow. In hypertension, renal or otherwise, most of the evidence points to decreased response in pathologic situations to substances like norepinephrine and angiotensin rather than to increased response, so at present this view lacks substantial support.

Decreased Response of Baroreceptors. The view has been proposed that the fault in hypertension may lie in the baroreceptors and that by an alteration in their response the arterial pressure is allowed to rise to a higher level. There is no direct evidence to support this hypothesis, but it is clear that the baroreceptor mechanism in the carotid sinus is easily modified and seems to respond only to change or rate of change in pressure, so the depressor mechanism rapidly becomes reset at higher levels of arterial pressure and operates again only when the arterial pressure is even further elevated. There is need for much greater knowledge of baroreceptors, both central and peripheral in man, and merely to consider the carotid sinus is inadequate.

Stimulation of an Extrarenal Pressor System. The relation between the kidney and the adrenal is of the greatest importance in this respect. The discovery by Conn of hypertensive patients with tumors in the suprarenal secreting aldosterone in large amounts soon led to the finding that many patients with severe hypertension had an increased production of aldosterone. Experimental work in animals has clearly linked the kidney with the adrenal, and the demonstration that angiotensin stimulates aldosterone production has completed this foundation. It seems clear that the renin-angiotensin system is often a prime stimulator of aldosterone production but that apart from the cases of Conn's tumor, in which hypertension may be cured by removal of the tumor, the role of aldosterone in most cases of hypertension is purely additional to whatever is the primary cause. In relation to the mechanism of hypertension produced by excess aldosterone, it is noteworthy that the high pressure can be lowered by spironolactone, which blocks the action of aldosterone on sodium-potassium exchange not only in the renal tubule but also across other membranes and presumably the arterial wall. This important relation between the renin-angiotensin system and aldosterone has much wider implications than hypertension. From study of subjects under different conditions using a very sensitive assay for renin (Brown and colleagues [1963–1966]), it has been possible to show that renin levels in the plasma are increased in association with sodium deprivation and lowered plasma sodium as in Addison's disease, in association with ascites due to cirrhosis of the liver, and in normal pregnancy. The renin plasma level can be reduced by sodium loading, by retransfusion of blood after bleeding and by the effects of aldosterone as in Conn's syndrome. In the presence of a renal artery stenosis, either experimental or pathologic, the plasma renin level may be high or normal. From other experimental work it is clear that a renal artery clip or obstruction leads to increased amounts of renin in the plasma. The measurement by a radioimmunoassay of the small amounts of angiotensin in the normal circulation (about 5 picograms per ml. venous plasma) led to a more precise definition of the end product of the renin-angiotensin system, but no serious discrepancy between measures of renin activity and angiotensin level has emerged. In experimental renal clip hypertension, although the level rises initially for a day or two, it drops down to normal quickly even as the arterial pressure continues to rise. In human hypertension resulting from renal artery stenosis, even when the level of angiotensin is raised, it very rarely rises above a level equivalent to the infusion of 0.25 μg. per minute into a normal subject, and this is only just enough to elevate the pressure slightly. It is more difficult to understand the precise relationship between the renin-angiotensin-aldosterone system when the group of patients with low plasma renin activity and angiotensin level and either a normal or low plasma aldosterone level are considered. Some of these patients initially thought to have distinct tumors of the suprarenal cortex are found at operation to have bilateral hyperplasia so that the possibility of a response of both the renin-angiotensin system and the suprarenal cortex to some other undescribed factor in hypertension must be considered. Consideration must be given to a possible tertiary hyperaldosteronism in which primary renal disease could lead to stimulation of the adrenal cortex to produce aldosterone followed by the development of an autonomous tumor, the activity of which leads to a suppression of the renin-angiotensin system. The one certain statement is that there is no clear relation between a given level of plasma renin or angiotensin and the arterial pressure.

Production of a Vasoconstrictor. Since the discovery of renin as the enzyme in the kidney that acts on its substrate in the plasma to produce angiotensin, which was originally found to raise the arterial pressure by directly contracting arterial smooth muscle, it seemed clear that this was the mechanism of renal hypertension including that due to renal clip. Direct measurement of angiotensin has never shown amounts sufficient in any form of experimental or human hypertension to equal that needed to raise the arterial pressure on intravenous infusion. This led to a search for increased sensitivity to normally sub-pressor doses or to an indirect action by the nervous system centrally or peripherally, but so far there is no convincing evidence. It has certainly been possible to develop renal hypertension in animals immunized against angiotensin so that they are unable to respond to renin or angiotensin given intravenously, so the case for other factors seems even stronger. Further, despite the direct action of angiotensin on the kidney to cause sodium retention in man, independent of the effect on aldosterone secretion, there is no evidence that brings this action clearly into the field of hypertension.

Clinical Manifestations. The symptoms and signs are usually secondary to effects on blood vessels in the various organs and tissues or to the increased load borne by the heart.

Cerebral. *Headache* is common, and the early morning occipital headache with stiffness of the neck, sometimes awakening the patient from sleep, commonly associated with vomiting attended by relief, is almost diagnostic of hypertension. Many patients only have headache on Saturday or Sunday mornings when they sleep later. The mechanism of this typical headache is uncertain. It is not closely related to the level of arterial pressure, and many patients with severe hypertension never experience it. It is most likely to be related to changes in cerebrospinal fluid pressure,

as in patients with cerebral tumors. Various other forms of headache are associated, and even migraine of classic type may develop. *Giddiness* short of true vertigo is a common complaint. Although disturbances in the balancing mechanisms are suggested by this, no direct evidence can be offered. *Personality changes* are not uncommon with the severe forms of hypertension and are presumably secondary to vascular damage. Some of these can be reversed by lowering the arterial pressure effectively; for example, ill-defined symptoms of anxiety may disappear. With extreme vascular disease, of course, *fits*, including jacksonian epilepsy, *minor strokes*, and *cerebral deterioration*, all occur. The experimental demonstration that the blood vessels in the brain may contract vigorously in response to high arterial pressure must obviously be related to these manifestations collected under the term *hypertensive encephalopathy*, quite apart from any more permanent vascular change induced by hypertension.

Thoracic. *Angina pectoris* is common and that it is linked to the high pressure and not necessarily to pure narrowing of coronary arteries is demonstrated by its alleviation on lowering the arterial pressure by drugs. An early symptom is *shortness of breath* on effort. This presumably is due to a change in the physical properties of the lung, leading to the sensation of dyspnea. This is often ascribed to left ventricular failure but perhaps more accurately should be attributed to a rise in left atrial pressure and consequently in pulmonary venous pressure. This process may occur acutely at night when the patient has been recumbent and asleep for, usually, about two hours. The typical attack of *cardiac asthma* ensues in which the patient has to sit up, gasping for breath. He dangles his legs over the edge of the bed and may get up and sit by an open window until his breathing is restored to normal. In extreme cases, frank pulmonary edema occurs and may be recognized by the coughing up of pink, frothy sputum. Listening over the chest reveals crackling sounds of all degrees from fine to coarse, depending on the degree of edema, and even wheezing noises may be produced, leading occasionally to confusion with so-called bronchial asthma. Acute lowering of the pressure by drugs alleviates these attacks dramatically. A surprising and unexplained feature is the fact that when the patient resumes his slumbers, he is very rarely reawakened by a second attack.

Because of the increased tendency to vascular disease, *myocardial infarction* may be superimposed on angina or may occur without warning. This may in some patients lead to a permanent cure of the hypertension, presumably because of reduced cardiac output. After a period in which there has been shortness of breath on effort and cardiac asthma, right-sided heart failure may follow, with improvement in the shortness of breath and cardiac asthma but with the other consequences of congestive cardiac failure. Some patients who have had few or no previous symptoms present for the first time in *congestive cardiac failure*. No convincing explanation has been offered for this, but perhaps the response of the pulmonary vasculature in some patients is different, so that the symptoms of left heart failure are minimized until the load on the right heart produces its own failure.

Vascular. The peripheral arteries may be observed to be either occluded in part or conspicuously tortuous. In this respect, a curly right carotid is common, as are tortuous brachial and radial arteries. The heart may show obvious hypertrophy of the left ventricle with an apex outside the midclavicular line, forcefully lifting the ribs above it. Auscultation of the heart typically reveals a presystolic triple rhythm heard usually best between the apex and the sternum. This disappears with successful treatment of the hypertension. The second sound in the right second space is loud and may have a distinctly twangy quality. Otherwise, in the absence of secondary cardiac disease, the sounds are unremarkable.

A rare observation is the presence of *pulsus alternans*, occasionally appreciated by variation in the strength of alternate beats at the wrist. Pulsus alternans may be observed more easily on taking the arterial pressure with a sphygmomanometer; the apparent rate of the pulse doubles as the pressure is slowly decreased. This again may be abolished by lowering the arterial pressure. The presence of failure of all types may be readily recognized from the rales in the lungs or the raised venous pressure, edema, hepatic enlargement, and congestive failure.

Bleeding from unexpected sites occurs in the higher ranges of arterial pressure. Nosebleeds, in the absence of uremia, and hemospermia are not rare.

In addition to the vascular disease already mentioned, involvement of the blood vessels to the legs is perhaps most commonly indicated by the complaint of *intermittent claudication*. This feature may, in fact, be made worse when the arterial pressure is lowered since the usual cause is a block in the arteries somewhere between the external iliac and the popliteal.

A rare cause of *absent or delayed femoral pulses* is coarctation of the aorta. Although this is often diagnosed in childhood, it may present in young adults. It is fairly easily recognized clinically by the pulse changes. The collateral vessels are clearly seen and felt around the posterior scapular margin and the intercostal spaces, particularly on the back. In the other main vessels, the most striking occurrence is dissecting aneurysm through the media, which is practically always associated with hypertension in the older age group. Aneurysmal dilatation of other vessels and the rupture of berry aneurysms within the skull indicate other types of strain imposed on the vascular system.

Ocular. Patients commonly present with *vascular manifestations in the eye*, and bilateral or unilateral blurring of vision or scotoma is common. In the malignant phase, the changes include papilledema, in which characteristically the swelling is in the retina around the disc and encroaches on the edge, eventually involving the whole; a small circumscribed so-called "hard" exudate, often arranged like grains of salt, between the disc and the macula; the "cotton-wool" exudate commonly associated with acute rise of arterial pressure as in acute glomerulonephritis and eclampsia, but especially florid in uremia; the typical macular fan or star figure of white lines of exudate between the nerve fibers leading from the macula; and hemorrhages, both linear and round. Papilledema is occasionally unilateral without hemorrhages or exudates, and, conversely, hemorrhages and exudates of all varieties may occur without papilledema; yet all are associated with this accelerated phase. Less severe changes are tortuosity in the arteries and nipping of the veins so that they are distended distally from crossings. Actual white sheathing of the arteries from the disc may be seen as well as variations in caliber. Spontaneous variations in caliber have been reported in severe hypertension, but this must be an extremely rare observation. One of the most common retinal changes is segmental venous thrombosis, usually starting in the vessels on the temporal side of the retina and clearly occurring at a point of arteriovenous crossing. Central venous obstruction is another similar manifestation. Less common are central retinal arterial obstruction and, perhaps surprisingly, segmental arterial obstruction.

Renal. The symptom due purely to hypertension and not related to the underlying renal disorder is increased *nocturnal frequency*. This may be an early manifestation of hypertension, usually occurring when the diastolic pressure is 120 in mm. of mercury or more, and it may be alleviated by lowering the arterial pressure by any means. In severe hypertension of recent onset, diuresis may be extreme and associated with increased water, sodium, and potassium loss, leading to thirst, weakness, and cramps. Long-standing hypertension with vascular damage to the kidneys leads to all the secondary consequences of renal failure and ultimately to uremia.

Special Investigations. *Urine.* The presence of protein in the urine is a most important sign in hypertension. It may indicate the presence of the malignant phase, congestive cardiac failure, or a primary renal disease causing hypertension. When proteinuria is associated with glycosuria and ketones, a diabetic kidney, as in the Kimmelstiel-Wilson syndrome, may be present. Alternatively, glycosuria with very little proteinuria may raise the suspicion of a pheochromocytoma with associated hyperglycemia. Examining the centrifuged deposit may reveal the red cells and red cell casts typical of acute glomerulonephritis, polyarteritis nodosa, or the malignant phase of hypertension. Pus cells and motile bacteria characterize urinary infection and point to pyelonephritis. Greater precision is given to the diagnosis of chronic pyelonephritis with sterile urine by quantitative demonstration of the increased rate of cellular excretion, particularly when further stimulated by intravenous injections of prednisolone.

If proteinuria persists, it may be impossible to decide the underlying renal disease without percutaneous renal biopsy and light or electron microscopy. The presence of chronic glomerulonephritis, lupus erythematosus, and other renal diseases causing hypertension may readily be shown by this procedure. It is of much less help in the absence of proteinuria.

One other striking feature of the urine in hypertension is persistent alkalinity in the presence of potassium deficiency, which is most important because it points to hyperaldosteronism. The presence of an inappropriately high potassium excretion for the level of plasma potassium is further evidence of hyperaldosteronism. Estimation of the catecholamine content of the urine, including the free amines epinephrine and norepinephrine, together with measurements of their metabolic products, vanillylmandelic acid and the metanephrines, adds precision to the diagnosis of pheochromocytoma. A simple test of renal function is failure to raise the specific gravity above 1.010 or the osmolality above 500 mOsm. per liter after overnight water deprivation.

Blood. The level of blood urea gives only a rough indication of renal performance since it is much influenced by dietary protein, and a better estimation, particularly in following the results of treatment, is that of creatinine clearance, which is still probably the most reliable and easily repeated of the tests of renal function. Electrolyte patterns have become of very great importance and are essential to the investigation of any case of hypertension. A low potassium and high bicarbonate point to hyperaldosteronism, and if associated with a higher than normal sodium level they are strongly suggestive. The most common cause, however, of low plasma potassium and raised bicarbonate is previous administration of a thiazide or similar diuretic. With a suspicion of hyperaldosteronism, either primary or secondary, the use of radioactive isotopes to measure total exchangeable sodium which is high and potassium which is low, is often helpful. It is still difficult to measure plasma levels of aldosterone, and this is also true of measurements of aldosterone secretory rate from measurements on the urine. Although circulating levels of epinephrine and norepinephrine can be measured fluorometrically, it is a difficult technique, and the diagnosis of pheochromocytoma is best made upon urinary excretion of catechol derivatives. Plasma renin activity and angiotensin levels will be considered later.

Feces. The sodium and potassium content in the stools reflects the function of the colonic wall which is under the influence of mineralocorticoids like aldosterone. Alteration in the sodium-to-potassium ratio can indicate hyperaldosteronism.

Chest Roentgenogram. In the roentgenogram of the chest, signs purely related to the hypertension and not to its cause are increased size of the heart, particularly the left ventricle, and increased vascularity of the lung fields due to pulmonary venous congestion, often with edema. The heart may not appear obviously enlarged according to ordinary roentgenologic criteria, even though enlargement is clinically obvious by the thrust of the left ventricle. Special signs occur in coarctation of the aorta, in which the notching of the lower margin of the rib by the collateral intercostal arteries is diagnostic.

Electrocardiogram. Even with well marked hypertension, the electrocardiogram may show no definite changes but probably the most reliable evidence of left ventricular hypertrophy is high voltage in the precordial leads. Left axis deviation is common, and depression of the ST segments and T wave inversion over the lateral chest leads are usually present in a well established case of severe hypertension. This is often termed "left ventricular strain pattern," but it is uncertain whether this is on an ischemic basis, particularly as it may merge with the changes of ischemia resulting from coronary artery disease.

Intravenous Pyelography. Using this technique it is possible to pick out those patients with a nonfunctioning kidney and those in whom the clubbed calices and the irregular outline of the scarred kidney point to pyelonephritis. Dilatation of the pelvicaliceal system points to the need to look for obstruction in the urinary tract since, particularly when associated with infection, this type of obstruction from the urethra upward can be a cause of hypertension. Naturally stone or calcification in the kidney can be seen and may be relevant to the hypertension. It is worth examining the pelvic films carefully for evidence of iliac arterial calcification. On pyelography the delayed appearance on one side of a small volume system in rapid sequence films taken at one-minute intervals up to five minutes, together with increased contrast of dye in the later films up to twenty or thirty minutes, is typical of renal artery obstruction, especially when associated with a smaller kidney. Retrograde ureteric pyelography is only used when obstruction is either apparent or suspected and calyceal anatomy is indistinct. The use of high dose intravenous pyelography has reduced the frequency and need for retrograde examination. The size and shape of the kidney may be better appreciated by the use of tomography, which, when combined with presacral air insufflation will not only give better indication of these factors, but may also show tumors in the suprarenal or renal areas.

Arteriography. In the search for renal causes of hypertension, arteriography is used only when surgical intervention is intended should an appropriate renal disorder be discovered. The clearest pictures are given by selective catheterization of each renal artery. Small scars or poor cortical filling can be seen by this technique as well as major blocks in the main renal arteries. Pheochromocytomas can be demonstrated, using aortography as long as epinephrine-blocking drugs are given.

Venography. Catheterization of the renal vein is performed mainly selectively to enter the left adrenal vein and to show the anatomy of the suprarenal gland by retrograde dye injection. In some cases it is possible to enter one adrenal vein on the right from the cava. This technique has also been used for collecting blood from the renal vein for assay of renin and the adrenal vein for assay of corticosteroids.

Renography. Most information is gained by comparing the curves of radioactivity obtained from the two kidneys simultaneously after the administration of I^{125}-hippuran. This gives quantitative information about individual renal function which is extremely useful in relation to vascular and parenchymal disease as well as obstructions in the urinary tract. Combined with scanning techniques, either instantaneous using a gamma camera, or slowly using a scintillation scanner, information about both function and morphology can be gained.

Divided Renal Function Studies. Divided renal function tests, in which the urine is collected through separate ureteric catheters and the composition is compared, are the ultimate tests of renal function, despite their technical difficulties and the rapid improvement in renography. For example, in stenosis of the main renal artery, water reabsorption increases markedly, leading to increased concentration but reduced clearance of such filtered substances as creatinine, inulin, and para-aminohippuric acid (PAH). The sodium concentration in contrast drops markedly. In parenchymal disease, as for example pyelonephritis, the water reabsorption is reduced and the concentration, as well as the clearance, of inulin, creatinine, and PAH drops, and the sodium concentration may be higher or no different than on the normal side. As a preliminary to surgery of the kidneys, such tests are essential.

Essential (Idiopathic) Hypertension. Hypertension for which no recognizable cause can be found is called essential or idiopathic. It should be emphasized that even if a known cause appears to exist—for example, renal disease—an etiologic relationship has not been established conclusively. Frequently the removal of an apparently diseased kidney is not followed by a fall in arterial pressure. (In some cases, secondary damage in the vascular system or opposite kidney may account for this.)

A great deal of controversy has gone on over the role of inheritance in hypertension. The most reasonable position on the basis of data now available seems to be that many factors, predominantly environmental but also inherited, lead to similar arterial pressures in members of certain families. In some families there is perhaps a stronger inherited tendency than in others; for example, twins have been described who developed malignant hypertension at about the same age while in different environments. The tendency to develop high arterial pressure certainly seems to be present at an early age and long before high arterial pressure itself is present. This is shown by the effects of pregnancy. In some women a high arterial pressure may occur for which no cause can be discovered; the arterial pressure may drop after pregnancy and may rise again later in life. They usually come from families with a history of high arterial pressure.

No consistent factor in hypertension of unknown origin has yet emerged that tells us anything about mechanism apart from these few clues.

Prognosis and Treatment. The outlook for a patient with high arterial pressure may in general be quantitatively related to the level of arterial pressure. The higher the pressure, the lower the survival rate over any given period. This has been shown repeatedly in population studies. In an attempt to differentiate the outlook for various patients with hypertension, the terms *benign* and *malignant hypertension* have been used; the latter is also called the *accelerated* or *necrotizing phase* to describe both the rapidity of the course and the fibrinoid arteriolar necroses that define the histologic condition. The term "benign" should be abandoned because it is a poor description for a condition that leads to death by stroke, myocardial infarct, and renal failure. It is easier from the epidemiologic viewpoint in describing large populations to give a quantitative prognosis, but in the individual patient seen for the first time the wise clinician takes account of all the variable factors discussed previously that may influence a particular value measured on the sphygmomanometer. This analysis, of course, influences his decision about whether the patient needs treatment or not.

There is no doubt in malignant hypertension that, unless the arterial pressure is successfully lowered, the patient will be dead usually within two years. It has been shown many times that it is possible to prolong life well over ten years by successful medical or surgical treatment of this phase of hypertension. Now that controlled trials of treatment in less severe grades of hypertension have been carried out, it is clear that improvement in outlook is conferred by successful treatment. In these cases, the prognosis depends on many factors, such as the presence of obvious vascular disease in major organs and the level of arterial pressure in relation to age. Although malignant hypertension may arise abruptly in a patient with previously normal pressure, it commonly supervenes after many years of moderately severe hypertension and seems clearly related to a rise over some months. Adequate treatment keeps this sort of patient out of this dangerous situation. The treatment depends in part on whether a potentially curable cause has been found. The curable causes of hypertension include pheochromocytoma, Cushing's syndrome, Conn's syndrome, unilateral renal disease, and, occasionally, bilateral renal disease due to surgically correctable renal artery stenosis. By "cure" in these cases is meant that the arterial pressure is returned to a completely normal level after operation.

Philosophy of Investigation and Treatment. *The first decision* a physician has to make is whether the arterial pressure as measured is too high for the individual, considering both the circumstances of the measurement and any of the other factors that can influence a single arterial pressure reading. *Time is on the side of the physician,* and repeated measurements under similar conditions, weeks or months apart, are often necessary to determine this point in the absence of any obvious signs of the effects of hypertension. It is also good to take the pressure three times in succession at one visit since it is striking in many patients that the second and third pressures are lower when the stimulus of the initial cuff tightening has worn off. Measurements made over 24 hours by portable apparatus have shown how variable a pressure may be and how it may only be elevated when being measured by the physician. The next decision to be made after deciding that the arterial pressure is too high is given by the answer to the question, *"Am I seeking a cure or merely alleviation?"* Clearly in a young person with severe hypertension and no evidence of vascular disease, a cure is always sought. In a patient of 65 years with evidence of vascular disease of considerable degree, the answer may well be alleviation. In the first place this means that all the investigations that are currently available will be used to obtain a diagnosis, whereas in the second, one will be content with a few investigations useful in the management but concentrating on treatment by drugs. This is a good rule for other conditions than hypertension. The next important therapeutic rule is to make sure that the *symptoms complained of are caused by hypertension* and that the treatment by drugs is not going to cause more trouble than the underlying condition. Too many elderly patients in their seventies with pressures of 190 systolic, 90 diastolic in mm. of mercury are treated with potent hypotensive drugs for symptoms of giddiness due to positional changes or for headaches as a manifestation of anxiety or depression that have nothing to do with hypertension, and are made much worse. Age needs no additional therapeutic hazards.

With severe hypertension it is unusual to be able to control the pressure by one major drug alone. A diuretic is needed in at least two thirds of the cases.

There is no particular "best" drug for the treatment of high arterial pressure. One of the mysteries of high arterial pressure is the way in which some patients respond well to one drug, some to another, without any other obvious difference between the patients. It is best to become accustomed to the actions and side effects of a small variety of drugs and to use them on all the patients who need treatment, exploiting each one to the full or to the limit of side effects before adding the adjunct or shifting to a new major drug. In the higher range of drug dose in which side effects accrue, multiple therapy is to be encouraged and not sneered at. Some patients do better, for example, on alpha-methyldopa plus guanethidine plus chlorothiazide than on either of the main drugs alone.

Curable Hypertension. Out of this group, two are of immediate interest because of the problems posed.

Renal Artery Stenosis. Once clearly diagnosed, prediction as to success of either nephrectomy or reconstructive arterial surgery depends upon other factors. It is best to be under 40 years with fibromuscular hyperplasia of one renal artery on the left side and a high peripheral plasma renin activity or angiotensin level with a higher concentration of renin in venous blood from the affected kidney than from the other side, and with a PAH clearance on the normal side that is well above 200 ml. per minute. This enables the surgeon to bring down the splenic artery distal to the stenosis with the knowledge that if the blood flow can be restored satisfactorily, the arterial pressure will be lowered and not maintained, for example, by disease in the opposite kidney. The plasma renin activity is useful in conjunction with clear evidence of ischemia determined by pyelography, renography, and divided renal function studies. By contrast, it is bad to be over 40 years with an atheromatous block and other evidence of atheromatous vascular disease elsewhere as, for example, in the coronary arteries, and an absence of the criteria noted above.

Conn's Syndrome. Although initially primary hyperaldosteronism associated with a single tumor of the suprarenal cortex was believed to be easily identified by the presence of hypokalemia, moderate hypertension, raised plasma aldosterone or aldosterone secretion, and a suppressed plasma renin activity, it has now become clear that there are patients with all these criteria who have bilateral hyperplasia of the suprarenal cortex and whose hypertension is not cured by adrenalectomy. In general, however, a plasma renin activity which fails to rise in the upright posture with stimulation by low sodium diet or injections of a potent diuretic, is associated with an adenoma and curable hypertension if the aldosterone plasma level is elevated.

Medical Treatment. From the results in large series of patients medically treated for hypertension, there is no doubt that morbidity and mortality are both reduced so long as the arterial pressure has been consistently lowered. Symptoms and signs both improve, as shown, for example, by the early relief of angina and the diminution in cardiac size roentgenographically. The occurrence of a cerebrovascular stroke in hypertension is an indication for lowering the pressure in order to lessen the risk of further stroke. Similarly, the presence of renal damage with hypertension is usually an indication for lowering the pressure to minimize further deterioration. The creatinine clearance may drop for a short time on lowering the arterial pressure but usually rises again, often to higher levels than at the outset if successful treatment is maintained. This temporary drop must not be used as an argument for lessening the vigor of treatment.

The *drugs used in treatment* have known major actions as well as a number of others that are not altogether well defined. It is fair to say that very few of the drugs in current or in past use have had their action of lowering the arterial pressure completely explained. Various types of drugs are used, as follows:

Ganglion Blockers. The best example of these is hexamethonium. The basic chemical structure of this drug has been altered in various ways to produce substances of more desirable properties that are capable of predictable absorption by mouth and predictable duration of action. Acting on parasympathetic and sympathetic ganglia, these agents produce a widespread blockade, leading to changes in peripheral resistance and in venous tone, so that part of their action, seen best with the patient in the standing position, is due to venous pooling and diminished cardiac output. Most of these drugs will lower the arterial pressure in many patients, particularly in the standing or sitting position. The major undesirable side effects are dryness of the mouth, paralysis of ocular accommodation, constipation, and impotence.

Pempidine tartrate may be used in a dose of 5 mg. three times a day, which may be increased by 5 mg. on each dose. This is probably the best of this type of drug for oral use. It should not be used in patients with distinct uremia (blood urea nitrogen over 50 mg. per 100 ml.), since paralytic ileus is a real risk. This drug, because of its quick onset of action and relatively short duration, is best given three times daily. The paralysis of ocular accommodation may be overcome by the use of pilocarpine hydrochloride 0.5 per cent eye drops. There is now very little place for this type of drug except as an adjunct in a very severe and resistant hypertensive patient.

Sympathetic Blockers. These have largely replaced the ganglion blockers, and either deplete or interfere with catecholamine metabolism at nerve endings or centrally. A prototype is *guanethidine*, which is concentrated in the postganglionic sympathetic fibers and interferes with the release of norepinephrine from the nerve endings. It also clearly has central effects, shown by the sleepiness and depression produced in some patients. Like the ganglion blockers, these agents produce a fall in pressure, mainly with the patient in the standing position, and, because of the sympathetic blockade, a distinct slowing in heart rate is seen. The major side effects are tiredness, peculiar muscular achings, giddiness and postural hypotension on exercise due to failure of vasoconstriction, diarrhea, and occasional impotence.

Guanethidine sulfate in a starting dose of 10 to 25 mg. daily is recommended. The full effects of the drug take a few days to become apparent, so that increases of dose should not be made more frequently than about every four or five days. Since it has a prolonged action, it need only be given once daily.

Bethanidine is like guanethidine in its actions but is quicker in onset and shorter in duration of action and has the merit of not causing diarrhea. The initial dose is 10 mg. three times daily.

Debrisoquine sulfate has few central effects psychologically, does not cause diarrhea, and has a prolonged action. The starting dose is 10 mg. twice daily.

Reserpine (various extracts of *Rauwolfia serpentina*), depletes nerve endings and organ stores of norepinephrine and epinephrine. It can be useful as long as a dose of 0.5 mg. daily is not exceeded; beyond this amount, its major side effect of depression, even to suicide, becomes common. It is best used in a dose of 0.25 mg. daily in conjunction with a thiazide diuretic, and even then the physician must remember that depression may slowly occur after several apparently trouble-free months; this can be reversed by removing the drug.

Alpha-methyldopa, among its other actions, serves as a competitive substrate for dopa decarboxylase on the route of production of norepinephrine via dopamine. It has marked central effects with tiredness and depression. Patients commonly seem to escape from its effects after some months of treatment. The starting dose is 250 mg. either twice or three times daily, with a warning to the patients that they will feel extremely sleepy for the first few days, but that this usually wears off. The dose may be increased slowly as with guanethidine; because of its sedative action, it is well to begin by increasing the night dose. Occasional cases of jaundice and hemolytic anemia have been reported.

Propranolol hydrochloride is different from the above-named group in that it is mainly a beta blocker and acts not only on blood vessels, but also on the heart. It perhaps lowers the supine pressure relatively more than the other group of drugs and, apart from its beneficial effect in angina pectoris, it may provoke cardiac failure in those patients with a poor myocardium. The starting dose is 20 mg. three times daily. *RENIN INHIB*

Pargyline hydrochloride is a monoamine oxidase inhibitor, has a marked central effect, and is often useful in the depressed patient with hypertension. Like all other drugs of this type, it is dangerous if the patient is not warned about taking cheese, yeast and beef extracts, and heavy red wine, all of which may provoke severe hypertension and cerebral hemorrhage. Nevertheless some patients do well.

Adjuvant Drugs. Various drugs are used mainly as adjuvants to these main lines of treatment. They include hydralazine hydrochloride (starting dose 20 mg. three times daily), whose mode of action is obscure, and phenoxybenzamine hydrochloride (starting dose 10 mg. three times daily), which antagonizes the action of norepinephrine or epinephrine on the vessel wall but is surprisingly ineffective by itself.

Diuretics. In any case of severe hypertension, one of the previously described drugs is usually used in conjunction with a diuretic. The addition of a diuretic increases the hypotensive action and may make possible the use of a smaller dose of the major drug. The most commonly used are the thiazide derivatives and there is nothing to choose between any of them. For example, chlorothiazide, 0.5 gram daily, is an adequate adjuvant. Because of the potassium loss induced by the thiazide, it is usually necessary to give potassium chloride (1 gram twice daily), or alternatively — and better — the thiazide may be omitted for two days per week, e.g., Saturday and Sunday. The initial mode of action is probably by sodium depletion and reduction in plasma volume, but action still continues when the plasma volume and sodium have been repleted, probably by diminished peripheral resistance. Combined tablets of thiazide and potassium chloride should not be given, as small gut ulceration and stricture occur. The thiazides may also occasionally precipitate diabetes mellitus, and more commonly gout. Although it was initially thought that only mild cases of hypertension would respond to a thiazide, experience has shown that quite severe cases may often respond to a thiazide alone; and if there is no particular urgency, then it is worth using, for example, 25 mg. of hydrochlorothiazide twice daily, with a slow release tablet of potassium chloride (1.2 grams twice daily). The full effect may take three to six weeks to be demonstrated but is undoubted.

Spironolactone. Although this can also be used as an adjuvant, it has a place of its own quite apart from its use in lowering the arterial pressure of patients with definite Conn's syndrome. In a dose of 25 mg. twice daily, it can be introduced and the dose increased. It must be taken after meals since otherwise it may cause nausea; it is contraindicated in the presence of peptic ulcer which it may cause to bleed. In some males it causes gynecomastia; in fewer females, interference with the menstrual cycle occurs, presumably because of its estrogenic effects. In the presence of renal failure, it should be used cautiously because of the elevation of plasma potassium it causes. Given together with a thiazide, it can provide a smooth, well controlled, and symptomless control of hypertension. Suitable treatment is hydrochlorothiazide, 25 mg., spironolactone, 25 mg., each twice daily, or a combination tablet of spironolactone, 25 mg., and hydroflumethiazide, 25 mg., twice daily. Unless there is urgency, this is the best initial approach to the treatment of even severe hypertension.

Treatment of Acute Pulmonary Edema and Hypertensive Encephalopathy. Two situations in hypertension demand emergency treatment in which it is essential to bring the arterial pressure down as rapidly as possible. The first is pulmonary edema due to left ventricular failure, and the second is the state of fits and unconsciousness called hypertensive encephalopathy. In the first, if the patient is overloaded with fluid as in acute glomerulonephritis, the best form of treatment is to reduce the extracellular fluid volume, either by bleeding or by dialysis, although when renal function is not seriously impaired, the intravenous injection of fursemide, 40 mg., provides a rapid

diuresis. If there is no obvious fluid overload, the dyspnea may be relieved by use of pentolinium tartrate in a dose starting at 1.5 mg. intramuscularly and increasing until the pressure is brought down. The patient should, if possible, be sitting up for this procedure. Good results have been obtained with other drugs such as reserpine (5 mg. intramuscularly), alpha-methyldopa as an intravenous injection (50 mg. per ml., total 250 mg.), guanethidine sulfate as an intramuscular injection (25 mg.), and sodium nitroprusside by continuous intravenous infusion (25 to 400 μg. per minute); in a particular patient it may be necessary to try various of these in sequence. Relief of symptoms can be dramatic. It is dangerous to use guanethidine sulfate intravenously since the release of norepinephrine raises the arterial pressure even higher. Diazoxide (300 mg. intravenously) given as a rapid injection which produces flushing, nausea, and often vomiting, nevertheless can occasionally produce a dramatic fall in arterial pressure which may last 12 to 24 hours before a further injection is needed. Its mode of action is quite unknown and, if given over a long period, it may cause pancreatitis. It is at its best in fulminating hypertension.

Typical Drug Dosages. Pempidine, 5 to 20 mg. three times daily; guanethidine, 10 to 100 mg. daily; bethanidine, 10 to 30 mg. three times daily; debrisoquine, 10 to 40 mg. twice daily; reserpine, 0.25 to 0.5 mg. daily; alpha-methyldopa, 250 mg. twice daily to 750 mg. three times daily; propanolol, 10 to 80 mg. three times daily; pargyline, 10 to 25 mg. twice daily. To each of these drugs in moderate to severe hypertension, hydrochlorothiazide, 25 mg., or equivalent thiazide is added on five of seven days.

Combined therapy in severe resistant hypertension: e.g., alpha-methyldopa, 250 mg. three times daily, guanethidine, 25 mg. daily, and hydrochlorothiazide, 25 mg. on five of seven days. Hydrochlorothiazide, 25 mg. daily to 25 mg. twice daily, with potassium chloride or equivalent, 1 gram twice daily. Spironolactone, 25 mg. twice daily to 50 mg. three times daily, always after meals.

Combined therapy: spironolactone, 25 mg. twice daily with hydrochlorothiazide, 25 mg. twice daily.

Conclusion. Finally, the main aim of treatment is that the patient should live a more comfortable life than before treatment. The patient with diarrhea, impotence, tiredness, and a normal arterial pressure is not a therapeutic triumph. To treat hypertensive subjects requires patience, perseverance, optimism, and a belief that the drugs can be manipulated in most cases to lower the arterial pressure while keeping the patient comfortable.

Britton, K. E., and Brown, N. J. G.: The clinical use of C.A.B.B.S. renography. Brit. J. Radiol., 41:570, 1968.
Conn, J. W.: Aldosteronism and hypertension: Primary aldosteronism versus hypertensive disease with secondary aldosteronism. Arch. Intern. Med. (Chicago), 107:813, 1961.

Dahl, L. K., Heine, M., and Tassinari, L.: Effects of chronic excess salt ingestion. Role of genetic factors in both DOCA-salt and renal hypertension. J. Exp. Med., 118:605, 1963.

Gross, F. (ed.): Antihypertensive Therapy, Principles and Practice. Proceedings of the Symposium held in Siena, Italy, June 28 to July 3, 1965, sponsored by CIBA. Berlin and Heidelberg, Springer-Verlag, 1966.

Leishmann, A. W. D.: Merits of reducing high blood pressure. Lancet, 1:1284, 1963.

Page, I. H., and Bumpus, F. M.: Angiotensin. Physiol. Rev., 41:331, 1961.

Page, I. H., and McCubbin, J. W. (eds.): Renal Hypertension. Chicago, Year Book Medical Publishers, Inc., 1968.

Peart, W. S.: Hypertension and the kidney. In Black, D. A. K. (ed.): Renal Disease. 2nd. ed. Oxford, Blackwell Scientific Publications, 1967, p. 638.

Peart, W. S.: The renin-angiotensin system. Pharmacol. Rev., 17:143, 1965.

Pickering, G. W.: High Blood Pressure. 2nd ed. London, J. & A. Churchill, Ltd., 1968.

Pickering, G. W.: The Nature of Essential Hypertension. London, J. & A. Churchill, Ltd., 1961.

Quinn, E. L., and Kass, E. H.: Biology of Pyelonephritis. Henry Ford Hospital International Symposium. Boston, Little, Brown & Company, 1960.

Stamey, T. A., and Good, P. H.: Diagnostic tools in the evaluation of renal vascular disease. In Brest, A. N., and Moyer, J. H. (eds.): Hypertension: Recent Advances—The Second Hahnemann Symposium on Hypertensive Disease. Philadelphia, Lea & Febiger, 1961, p. 189.

Symposium: Primary hyperaldosteronism. Arch. Intern. Med. (Chicago), 123:113, 1969.

Cardiac Arrhythmias

PHYSIOLOGIC PRINCIPLES
Stanley A. Briller

NORMAL MECHANISMS

Spread of Activation. The sequence of activation of the heart is directly related to electrical events at a cellular level (Fig. 1). Pertinent information has been gathered by the use of a microelectrode, an ultrafine glass capillary tube filled with a conducting fluid. If a microelectrode is thrust into a cell in the region of the sinoatrial node during earliest diastole, a voltage difference of about 60 millivolts is measured between the microelectrode and a second electrode placed elsewhere. This voltage appears as soon as the cell

membrane is penetrated; the polarity is such that the inside of the cell is negative. During diastole, the voltage difference or "resting potential" steadily declines (diastolic depolarization). Upon reaching a critical value of about 40 millivolts, the resting potential is suddenly further reduced, and the inside of the cell becomes briefly positive to the extent of about 10 millivolts. This rapid change in voltage (depolarization) is followed by further, slower voltage changes (repolarization), which culminate in the restoration of the resting potential. The voltage changes of depolarization and repolarization are known collectively as the monophasic action potential.

The pacemaker property of sino-atrial tissue is dependent upon diastolic depolarization. Atrial cells surrounding the sino-atrial node generate monophasic action potentials fairly similar to

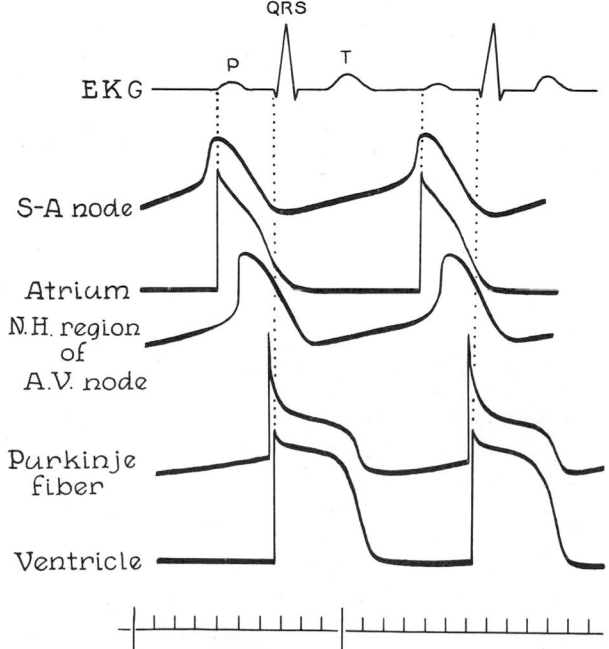

FIGURE 1. The relationship between the electrocardiogram and the intracellular electrical events in five tissues of the heart during two beats of a normal sinus rhythm. The pacemaker (S-A node) and potential pacemaker regions (N-H region of the A-V node and Purkinje fiber) are tissues that fail to maintain a constant voltage during diastole (diastolic depolarization). The rate of diastolic depolarization is greatest in the S-A node and least in Purkinje fibers. The dotted lines indicate that the electrocardiogram detects electrical activity originating in the atria and ventricles. Depolarization of the S-A node, A-V node, and Purkinje fibers is not discernible in the electrocardiogram. The electrocardiogram is approximately 1/100 the amplitude of the intracellular voltages, although all electrical events are shown at roughly equal size for clarity. (Adapted from Hoffman, B. F., and Cranefield, P. F.: Electrophysiology of the Heart. New York, McGraw-Hill Book Co. 1960.)

those generated by the node. However, the resting potential of atrial cells is constant. The depolarization spike of sino-atrial tissue abruptly reduces the constant resting potential of the adjacent atrial cells, and they in turn become depolarized. Depolarization of the remaining atrial tissues in dogs has recently been shown to be highly complex, very likely modulated by preferential spread over interatrial and internodal tracks which exhibit diastolic depolarization. The rich quadrupole (nondipole) content of the P wave of surface electrocardiograms of human subjects with and without heart disease is consistent with the above observation in dogs. Over-all spread of excitation in the atria takes about 0.1 second or, stated otherwise, occurs with a *mean* velocity of approximately 0.3 M/sec.

Although cells in the distal (N-H) region of the atrioventricular node adjacent to the bundle of His exhibit diastolic depolarization similar to that of the sino-atrial node, the rate of depolarization is slower. Consequently N-H atrioventricular nodal cells will not have reached excitation threshold prior to the activation of atrial and adjacent proximal (N) atrioventricular nodal cells. Elevation to threshold level of the end-diastolic voltage of all atrioventricular nodal cells is accomplished by a further spread of the chain reaction from the atrial cells. In this way the rhythm of the atrioventricular node is set by the sino-atrial node, provided the discharge rate of the latter exceeds that of the former. Successive depolarization from cell to cell in the atrioventricular node is very slow (0.05 M/sec.) compared with the spread of excitation in the other portions of the heart.

Fully polarized, resting cells at the origin of the bundle of His are depolarized by active cells at the distal end of the atrioventricular node. Spread of excitation through the large cells (Purkinje fibers) of the bundle of His, the bundle branches, and the terminal arborization beneath the ventricular endocardium is fairly rapid (2.0 M/sec.) Studies with the microelectrode have revealed cells with a fixed resting potential as well as others within this tissue in which very slow diastolic repolarization is present. Ventric-

ular cells are stimulated by the action potential spikes of terminal arborization fibers. Spread of excitation through ventricular tissue proceeds at about half the rate of spread through the Purkinje fibers. The resting potential of ventricular cells is constant and similar to that of atrial tissue.

The Ionic Basis of Resting and Action Potentials. The presence of intracellular nondiffusible anion (protein) accounts in large part for the intracellular:extracellular ratios of the relatively diffusible potassium (approximately 20:1) and chloride (approximately 1:20) ions. It is generally accepted that these transmembrane ion ratios in turn produce a difference in electrical voltage across the membrane that agrees in sign and magnitude with the negative intracellular resting potential. Sodium ion, which permeates the resting cell membrane less easily than either chloride or potassium, is both driven into the interior of the cell by the greater concentration of extracellular sodium and attracted to the intracellular space by the negative charge within the cell. Continuous extrusion of sodium against these forces is necessary if a constant intracellular concentration of this ion is to be maintained. Energy for this process is believed to arise from metabolic intracellular synthesis of an as yet unidentified substance that combines with and carries sodium across the membrane: the "sodium pump." It is likely, but unproved, that those tissues (sino-atrial nodal, N-H atrioventricular nodal, and some Purkinje cells) that exhibit the phenomenon of diastolic depolarization gradually lose their initial diastolic permeability to potassium ion. Since the resting potential is related to a differential concentration of diffusible potassium ions across cell membranes, decreasing potassium permeability would then account for the diastolic decline in resting potential.

Depolarization (phase 0) (Fig. 2) is accompanied by a sudden increase in cellular membrane permeability to sodium accompanied by presumed inactivation of the sodium pump mechanism. The intracellular:extracellular sodium ratio (almost the reverse of the potassium ratio) in the presence of free movement of this

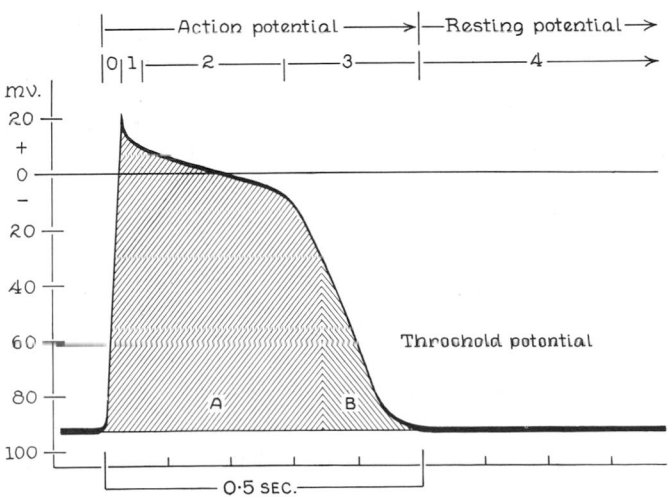

FIGURE 2. The time course of electrical events during one beat of a ventricular muscle cell is subdivided into the four phases of the action potential (0, 1, 2, 3) and the resting potential (4). Initially an electrical impulse from adjacent active tissue raises the resting potential from a level of about −90 millivolts to about −62 millivolts (threshold potential). The potential spontaneously continues to rise rapidly past 0 to a level of approximately +20 millivolts (depolarization or phase 0 of the action potential). Phases 1, 2, and 3 of the action potential are arbitrary subdivisions of the repolarization process that culminate in phase 4 or the resting potential. The absolute refractory period (A) includes phases 0, 1, 2, and the first portion of phase 3, whereas the latter portion of phase 3 is synonymous with the relative refractory period (B). (Modified from Brooks et al.: Excitability of the Heart. New York, Grune and Stratton, 1955, Chapter V.)

ion across the membrane has two effects: (1) The interior of the cell briefly becomes positive in voltage, and (2) a small number of sodium ions enter the cell. Repolarization begins with a decline in membrane permeability to sodium and a fall of the transmembrane voltage to a near zero value (phase 1). The voltage remains at zero (phase 2) for the greater portion of the action potential. During the latter half of phase 2, membrane permeability to potassium rises, the intracellular voltage rapidly becomes negative again (phase 3), and a few potassium ions leave the cell. Immediately the resting potential (phase 4) is restored, the sodium pump is reactivated, and the sodium ions that entered during depolarization are extruded. This process is coupled with the return to the cell interior of potassium lost during the latter portions of repolarization. These ionic adjustments coincide in time with the relative refractory period and, possibly, the U wave.

The Mechanism of Control of Heart Rate. Sino-atrial tissue responds to epinephrine by increasing the rate at which the resting potential declines. Consequently, the threshold potential is reached more quickly, increasing the rate of spontaneous discharge. Acetylcholine or vagal stimulation has the opposite effect: the slope of diastolic depolarization becomes more gradual, and a reduction in heart rate is the consequence. In general, neither sympathetic nor parasympathetic mediators influence the shape of the action potentials of cardiac tissues. The resting potential of atrial and ventricular tissue is unaffected by these neurohumoral mediators.

Relationship between Cellular Events and Surface EKG. The short-circuiting effect of extracardiac body tissues greatly attenuates the magnitude of electrical currents that originate within the various portions of the heart and flow to the body surface. Small units of the heart such as the sino-atrial node, the atrioventricular node, and the Purkinje system contribute such diminutive electrical currents that no evidence of their activity can be identified in body surface leads. An intracardiac electrode, strategically placed near the coronary sinus, is required to demonstrate activity of structures such as the His bundle in man. On the other hand, activity of the atrial and ventricular masses is signified by the P and QRST deflections, respectively, in conventional body surface leads.

A complex relationship exists between cellular electrical activity and the resultant surface electrocardiogram. Although additional factors such as the velocity, direction, and magnitude of cellular depolarization and repolarization participate in this relationship, the rate of change of voltage (first derivative) during the various phases of the intracellular action potential is a good approximation of the wave form of the body surface electrocardiogram. Since the diastolic resting potential (phase 4) of both atrial and ventricular tissues is constant, its rate of change is zero, and no voltage is present on electrocardiographic leads during electrical diastole. The sequential depolarizations (phase 0) of atrial and ventricular cells consist of rapid intracellular voltage changes and give rise to the appreciable P and QRS deflections. During phase 2 of the repolarization process in these tissues, the fairly invariant nature of the intracellular voltages is reflected in surface leads by isoelectric P-R and S-T intervals. Transit of the excitatory process through the atrioventricular node and proximal portions of the Purkinje fibers begins during the inscription of the P wave and ends during the QRS complex. The fairly rapid voltage changes present during phase 3 of the repolarization of ventricular cells give rise to the T wave. Phase 3 of the repolarization of atrial cells occurs during the inscription of the QRS deflections, and the atrial T wave (P_T wave) is ordinarily obscured by the much larger ventricular complex.

ABNORMAL MECHANISMS

Escape. Transient suppression of sino-atrial impulse formation by vagal or other influences may allow lower rhythmic centers to originate one or more heart beats. Since the only areas below the sino-atrial node that exhibit diastolic depolarization are scattered pacemaker cells throughout the atria, the N-H portion of the atrioventricular node, the bundle of His, and the Purkinje fibers, one or the other of these may discharge (escape) during a long diastolic interval. If the escape beat originates in pacemaker tissue proximal to the Purkinje system, spread to the ventricles is guided by the normal or near normal Purkinje route, and the QRS complex resulting may have little morphologic change from the preceding normal complex. The excitatory process may spread retrogradely from any such focus to capture the atria, producing a deformed or inverted P wave that may precede, be superimposed upon, or follow the QRS complex. Occasionally retrograde conduction of an atrioventricular nodal escape beat to the atria will be blocked. In this case the atrioventricular nodal escape focus will not activate the atria, and, if a P wave is present, it originates in a higher focus.

If an element of the more distal Purkinje system is the nidus of the escape beat, conduction through the ventricles is abnormal. Under these circumstances the resulting ventricular escape beat appears as a bizarre QRS that is usually unassociated with a retrograde P wave.

Ectopic Beats and Rhythms. The pacemaker function of the sino-atrial node may be pre-empted by any element of cardiac tissue (an ectopic focus) beyond the sino-atrial node. Most frequently, a single beat or premature systole is the result. On the other hand, a rapid succession of such beats constitutes an ectopic tachycardia.

The mechanism of *re-entry* probably underlies many ectopic rhythms. The proponents of this theory surmise that areas of depressed function within the heart may have prolonged refractory periods. An impulse approaching such an area would be diverted to adjacent excitable regions. If the excitatory path through normal tissue is sufficiently circuitous, the impulse will again reach the depressed area (by now excitable) late in electrical systole. Upon traversing it, the excitatory process is free to re-enter normal regions and thereby to restimulate the chamber or entire heart. Repetition of the foregoing cycle is possible and would generate an ectopic tachycardia. The close coupling between the preceding normal beat and a premature systole or the onset of an ectopic tachycardia is a consequence of the re-entry mechanism.

Location of a single re-entry mechanism within the ventricle would account for ventricular tachycardia, ventricular flutter, and ventricular premature systoles. The presence of a similar mechanism within the atria, usually termed the circus theory, may account for atrial flutter. The most frequent common denominator in flutter is the electrocardiographic presence of continuous electrical activity from either the atrial or ventricular locus of the re-entrant mechanism. Fragmentation of a single re-entrant path into multiple smaller cycles is believed to account for fibrillation of either the atria or ventricles.

The theory of re-entry has been strengthened by the demonstration in many subhuman mammals of two pathways in the atrioventricular node that conduct an impulse at different velocities. It was demonstrated that a very early premature atrial impulse might be propagated over the slower path to the ventricles, only to return to the atria over the faster atrioventricular nodal path. On several occasions, this re-entrant cycle was self-perpetuating, resulting in a supraventricular tachycardia. A similar mechanism could reasonably explain the generation of atrial or nodal tachycardias and atrial or nodal premature systoles. Since the re-entry cycle is contained within the atrioventricular node which is electrocardiographically silent, the continuous electrical activity present in such arrhythmias as atrial flutter and ventricular tachycardia is not seen. As the re-entrant cycle passes each end of the atrioventricular node, the atria and the ventricles are successively stimulated. The result is a rapid, but discrete, repetition of P, QRS, and T.

Rare ectopic ventricular beats that occur approximately midway between two normal beats (interpolated ventricular extrasystoles) as well as the phenomenon of parasystole are examples of ectopic rhythms that are apparently not the consequence of re-entry. These arrhythmias are attributed to a focus of cells that is suddenly endowed with an augmented rate of diastolic depolarization or impulse formation. Local metabolic abnormalities are usually cited as the underlying cause, but the precise cellular mechanism is unknown. The persistence of the ectopic ventricular focus in interpolated extrasystoles and in parasystole, despite the otherwise orderly sequence of ventricular contractions of sino-atrial origin, is

attributed to *entrance block*: a halo of refractory cells about the ectopic center that prevents its discharge by nonectopic impulses.

Interference and Block. Once depolarized, normal cardiac tissue is incapable of being restimulated for the greater portion of the duration of the action potential. This interval of nonresponsiveness (the absolute refractory period) is followed by gradually increasing excitability (relative refractory period) when greater than usual stimulus intensity is required to elicit a response (Fig. 2). Shortly after repolarization, normal responsiveness is regained. Although the duration of the refractory period is reduced when the cardiac rate is increased, there is a minimum beyond which further shortening does not occur. Of all portions of the heart, atrioventricular nodal tissue manifests the least reduction in duration of the refractory period with increasing heart rate. Inability of the atrioventricular node of the adult to conduct to the ventricles more than 200 to 250 atrial impulses per minute is a normal consequence (*interference*) of the minimal atrioventricular nodal refractory period. The beating of the ventricles at a fraction of the atrial rate in atrial flutter is a simple instance of this principle. A more complex situation occurs when two pacemakers compete for control of the heart (a *dissociated* rhythm), and interference prevents reexcitation of each pacemaker's dominion by the other. If, for example, the atria are depolarized by the sino-atrial node during the period of retrograde spread of activation from a low atrioventricular nodal center, the latter pacemaker will fail to invade the atria but will depolarize the ventricles alone. Impulses originating in the atrioventricular node and the sino-atrial node meet high in the atrioventricular node, where interference occurs and terminates further excitation in either direction. In other circumstances the meeting place of impulses from two pacemakers may be located within the ventricular or, uncommonly, atrial myocardium. When an ectopic beat invades a portion of a chamber otherwise depolarized by an impulse of sino-atrial or atrioventricular nodal origin, the resultant systole is known as a *fusion* beat.

In contrast to interference, a normal protective mechanism of cardiac tissue, heart *block* is a manifestation of abnormal function. The precise physiologic mechanism underlying heart block is speculative. If fibrosis, congenital malformation, or inadvertent surgical interruption is implicated, it may be assumed that inexcitable tissue through which transmission cannot occur is responsible. On the other hand, localized edema, anoxia, electrolyte disorders, neurohumoral factors, or drug effects may produce block by prolonging the refractory period, raising the excitability threshold, increasing the resting potential or, conceivably, by diminishing the action potential spike of junctional tissue. These latter, potentially reversible pathophysiologic mechanisms, are naturally to be suspected when the observed block is of an evanescent or transient nature. Block in impulse transmission may occur at any level between the sino-atrial node and the ventricular muscle. If the impulse is delayed in transit, but eventually reaches its destination, block is described as partial or incomplete. Under such circumstances, the rhythm of the heart is undisturbed and the presence of incomplete block ordinarily depends upon the electrocardiographic demonstration of a prolonged P-R or QRS interval.

When the conduction defect results in total interruption of a portion of the conduction system, the block is categorized as complete. Complete bundle branch block that involves one but not both of the bundle branches is the only instance of complete block of a section of the conduction mechanism in which the basic rhythm is undisturbed. If complete block occurs at the level of either the atrioventricular node or the sino-atrial node, perpetuation of the heart beat is dependent upon the emergence of a pacemaker below the level of the block (escape). In the case of complete A-V block, only distal elements of the conduction system (the common bundle, the bundle branches, and their subendocardial arborizations) are capable of pacemaker function. Their inherent rate of diastolic repolarization is slow and so is their rate of impulse formation. If the cells assuming pacemaker function lie in the common bundle, the resultant so-called idioventricular rhythm is manifest electrocardiographically by a succession of normal-appearing QRS complexes at a rate ranging from 50 per minute downward. If the idioventricular focus is located in a more distal element of the Purkinje system, the resultant QRS complexes will be wide and bizarre. Sino-atrial impulse formation with subsequent spread through the atria and the formation of normal P waves is uninhibited by the presence of complete A-V block. The repetition rate of such P waves is usually faster and always unrelated to the idioventricular rate. In sino-atrial block the heart beat is usually maintained by an atrioventricular nodal pacemaker whose rate of impulse formation is usually higher than that of the more distal idioventricular foci. The resulting QRS complex is only minimally deformed, if at all, since the conduction system is uninvolved. However, atrial activation can occur only by retrograde impulse transmission from the A-V nodal focus.

Briller, S. A., and Conn, H. C.: The Myocardial Cell. Structure, Function and Modification by Cardiac Drugs. Philadelphia, University of Pennsylvania Press, 1966.

Langer, G. A.: Ion fluxes in cardiac excitation and contraction and their relation to myocardial contractility. Physiol. Rev., 48:708, 1968.

Manning, G. W., and Ahuja, S. P.: Electrical Activity of the Heart. Springfield, Ill., Charles C Thomas, 1969.

Moore, E. N.: Microelectrode studies on retrograde concealment of multiple premature ventricular responses. Circ. Res., 20:88, 1967.

Spach, M. S., King, T. D., Barr, R. C., Boaz, D. E., Morrow, M. A., and Herman-Giddens, S.: The electrical potential distribution surrounding the atria during depolarization and repolarization in the dog. Circ. Res., 24:857, 1969.

CLINICAL PRINCIPLES
Calvin F. Kay

DISORDERS OF IMPULSE FORMATION

DISORDERS ARISING IN THE SINUS NODE

Sinus Tachycardia. Sinus rhythm with a rate over 100 is usually not a disorder but a physiologic response to exertion, to fever, or to emotional or physical stress. The magnitude of this response is usually greater in the young, in the ill, and in women. It is not uncommon to observe rates of 110 to 120 in routine examinations of emotionally labile but otherwise healthy adults. Under severe physiologic stress, as in shock, the pulse rate may rise to as high as 160. Sinus tachycardia is a feature of hyperthyroidism and may indicate persisting carditis in rheumatic fever. Differential diagnosis from atrial flutter or from paroxysmal atrial tachycardia may occasionally be difficult. Sinus tachycardia differs from these in that the heart rate changes gradually rather than abruptly or not at all, either spontaneously or as induced by exertion, rest, or measures that augment vagal tone. Sinus tachycardia may cause palpitation, but it usually disturbs heart function very little. It is of clinical significance principally as an index of an emotional or physical state toward which therapy, if necessary, is directed.

Sinus Bradycardia. Sinus rhythm with a rate below 60 is not uncommon in resting normal males. It is observed in patients with excessive vagal stimulation under the influence of emotion, nausea, anoxia, vagotonic drugs (neostigmine, morphine, and digitalis), or when it is deliberately induced by gagging, eyeball compression, or carotid sinus massage. Bradycardia is also caused by drugs that cause catechol depletion or blockade, e.g., reserpine, propranolol, and it is commonly present in hypothyroidism and in severe jaundice. It is usually transient and of little consequence, but it may cause weakness, faintness, or, rarely, syncope if the subject is standing. Bradycardia sometimes develops in acute myocardial infarction, in pulmonary embolism, or in shock. It then predisposes to major, even lethal, ventricular arrhythmias. *Atrial arrest* lasting for a period of several seconds may occur as an extension of progressive bradycardia or it may abruptly interrupt a normal rate in severely damaged hearts, in the presence of digitalis toxicity, or as one of the mediating mechanisms of carotid sinus syncope. Ordinarily an escape mechanism from a lower center will intervene before serious functional impairment occurs. Treatment is usually unnecessary, but atropine sulfate, 0.5 to 1.0 mg., may be given orally, subcutaneously, or intravenously depending upon the urgency of the situation. A

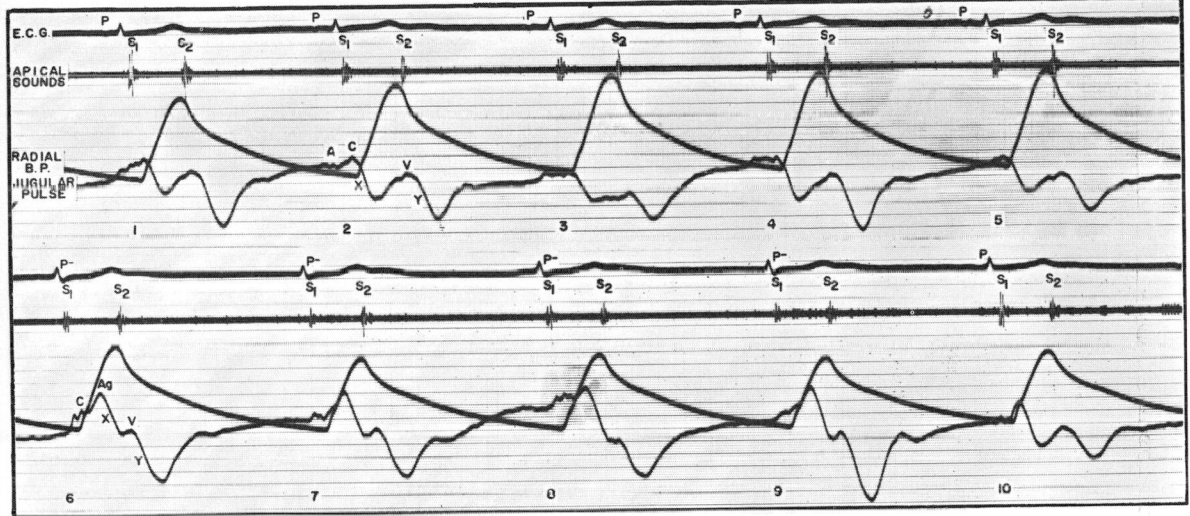

FIGURE 1. Wandering pacemaker—continuous lead II. The focus wanders from S-A to A-V node. P-R 0.16 in beats 2, 3, 4, and 5; 0.13 in 1; and 0.06 in beat 10. Retrograde, inverted P waves are barely visible at end of QRS in beats 6, 7, 8, and 9. First heart sounds (S_1) are loud in beats 1 and 10 with short P-R intervals, faint in nodal beats 6 and 9, and of intermediate intensity in the other (P-R 0.16) beats. In beats 1 to 5, with normal P-R, the radial pulse wave amplitude is greater and the second sounds (S_2) are louder than in beats 6 to 10. Atrial activity is indicated in the jugular pulse by small presystolic undulations (A) in beats 1 to 5. These are absent in beats 6 to 10. Instead, a giant A wave (A_G) is present between the first and second sounds. With each of these beats the patient experienced a thrusting sensation, and the venous pulsation was easily visible. In beat 10, A_G is relatively early, relating to earlier atrial contraction than in beats 6 to 9. The C waves, venous reflections of ventricular ejection, follow S_1 in all beats. The X descent, venous collapse during downward displacement of the A-V valves during systole, is exaggerated in beats 6 to 10 in which blood had been regurgitated into the neck. It is followed by the V wave of atrial filling in late systole and then by the Y descent of atrial emptying into the ventricles.

pacemaker may occasionally be required. Atrial arrest may be sufficiently protracted to cause syncope.

Sinus Arrhythmia. A variable rate of impulse discharge from the sinus node is of two types. In the more common respiratory type, the heart rate increases with inspiration and slows with expiration in response to reflex stimulation. This form is normally present in infants and children, and may be exaggerated during active rheumatic carditis. It may also be seen in adults with acute myocardial infarction or after the administration of morphine. It diminishes or disappears with acceleration of the heart rate. A second type of sinus arrhythmia is observed during Cheyne-Stokes respirations. The pulse rate increases and then slows again during the apneic phase. Sinus arrhythmia is not a cause of symptoms or disability and requires no treatment.

Wandering Pacemaker. A slight change in the rate from beat to beat in association with a varying contour of the P wave and variations of the PR interval is common in the aged. The focus wanders from the sinus node to and from atrial or sinoatrial nodal tissues (see Nodal Rhythm and Fig. 1).

DISORDERS ARISING IN THE ATRIA

Atrial Premature Beats. Atrial premature beats arise from an atrial ectopic focus. They are common in elderly persons and occasionally are present in healthy young persons. They are frequent in those with serious heart disease of any type, especially in those disorders, e.g., mitral stenosis or hyperthyroidism, that usually lead to the subsequent development of more serious atrial disorders (fibrillation, flutter, or paroxysmal supraventricular tachycardia). Digitalis occasionally induces them. This arrhythmia is usually asymptomatic and causes no significant cardiac functional disability. In the electrocardiogram (Figs. 2 and 3), the premature P wave configuration is usually similar to the normal; sometimes it is considerably altered. Identification of the P wave may be difficult if it is concealed within the preceding T wave. The P-R interval may be shorter

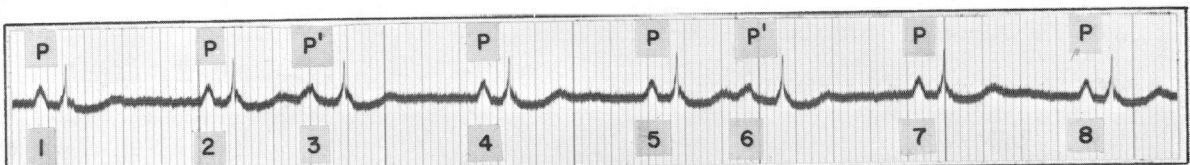

FIGURE 2. Atrial premature beats. P-P interval of sinus beats 0.88 second. P' of beats 3 and 6 are premature and deformed with P-P' intervals of 0.55 and 0.50 respectively. P-R of premature beats 0.19, compared with P-R of 0.14 of sinus beats; P'-P intervals slightly longer than P-P intervals. The $R_2 - R_4$ interval is 1.46, and the $R_5 - R_7$ interval is 1.44, considerably less than twice the normal R-R interval ($2 \times 0.88 = 1.76$): no compensatory pause. Aberrant conduction is not present in this example.

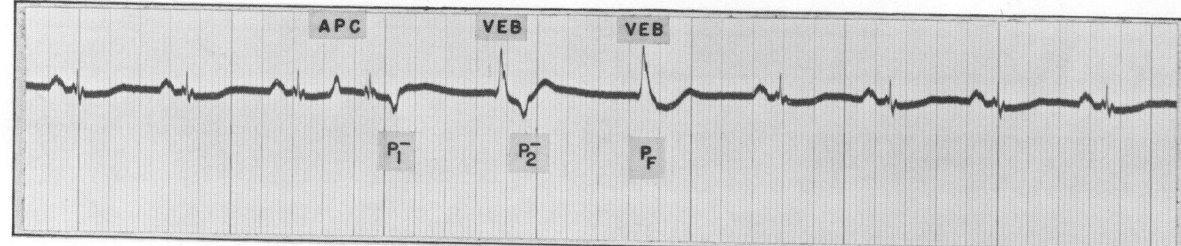

FIGURE 3. Sinus rhythm, rate 83, P-R 0.15, interrupted by atrial premature contraction with deformed P wave, P-R 0.21, followed by retrograde, inverted P wave (P_1), R-P 0.16. Sino-atrial activity is depressed because of three discharges in a short interval, allowing time for an independent ventricular focus to initiate a beat (ventricular escape beat) which, in turn, induces retrograde activation of the atria as indicated by another retrograde P wave (P_2). Sino-atrial discharge occurs during or following this atrial activation rather than preceding it, as is normal. Hence, the P-P interval is longer than the normal P-P interval, and the following P wave is obscured in the second ventricular escape beat, but interferes with a repeat of the retrograde activation of the atria. Normal sinus activation is then resumed. The beats labeled VEB may arise from a nodal focus, with aberrant conduction to the ventricles.

or longer than in the normal beats, but it is always more than 0.12 second. If the premature P wave falls early in diastole, the P-R interval may be much longer than in the normal beats, or the beat may not reach the ventricle at all: a blocked atrial premature beat. The QRS complex may be slightly or considerably altered (aberrant atrioventricular conduction). The interval from the normal beat to the premature beat is shorter than the normal beat-to-beat interval. The interval from the premature QRS to the following normal QRS may be a little longer than the normal beat-to-beat interval for two reasons. Time is required for transmission of the ectopic impulse from its origin in the atrium to reach and discharge the sinus node, and the sinus node is transiently depressed as a result of premature excitation. The sum of these two intervals (from the QRS before to the QRS after the atrial premature beat) is appreciably less than two normal intervals; the *compensatory pause* is incomplete or absent. This is of some help in differentiation of atrial from nodal or ventricular premature beats. It is not a reliable guide because, rarely, the sinus node may not be discharged by the atrial premature beat. In this case, the compensatory pause is complete; the interval from the beat before to the beat after the premature beat equals two normal intervals. Conversely, an incomplete compensatory pause results if nodal or, very rarely, ventricular ectopic stimuli discharge the sinus node. Except as a warning of a possible impending major atrial arrhythmia, atrial premature beats are of little consequence and require no treatment.

Atrial Paroxysmal Tachycardia. This is clinically indistinguishable from *nodal paroxysmal tachycardia*; in fact, differentiation may not be possible even in the electrocardiogram. The term *supraventricular paroxysmal tachycardia* is used to designate either variety. In this arrhythmia the atrial musculature contracts with small, rapid (160 to 220), regular motions that are not very effective dynamically. The ventricles usually contract in a 1:1 ratio with the atrial contractions. It is much less common than atrial fibrillation and somewhat more common than atrial flutter.

In most patients who have paroxysmal supra-

ventricular tachycardia, evidence of other heart disease is lacking. Attacks may recur sporadically from early childhood to late adult life. Some people may experience only a few attacks in a lifetime; in others a hundred or more paroxysms may occur each year. Often a series of attacks occurs over a period of a few days or weeks, followed by a protracted interval of freedom before the disorder reasserts itself. Emotional or physical stress clearly precipitates attacks in some persons. Others relate their seizures to allergy, minor infections, menses, coffee, tobacco, or fatigue; in many, no predisposing factor can be identified, but *thyrotoxicosis* should always be considered.

Isolated attacks of paroxysmal supraventricular tachycardia may complicate acute or chronic heart disease of almost any type. It may also be a manifestation of digitalis intoxication, especially when accompanied by partial AV block. A special form is associated with accessory AV conduction.

Supraventricular paroxysmal tachycardia is symptomatically characterized by a sudden sensation of pounding or fluttering in the chest or throat, persisting for a few minutes to several hours, rarely for days. Faintness, weakness, or breathlessness is commonly associated with a paroxysm, especially in those with structural cardiac disease. Syncope may occur. Most patients are less certain of the cessation of the attack than of its onset. Polyuria may occur when attacks have lasted for an hour or more. Diagnosis can usually be made from the patient's description. The abruptness of onset and regularity of the palpitation are, to him, impressive features.

In the electrocardiogram (Fig. 4), the first beat of a paroxysm is premature, with or without a P wave to guide in identification of the site of genesis. It is followed by QRS complexes regularly spaced at a rate of 150 to 220 beats per minute in adults. The end of the paroxysm is often followed by a brief period of asystole and then by normal sinus beats, by varying intervals of nodal rhythm, or by short runs of atrial premature beats before resumption of sinus rhythm. RST and T depression is common during the paroxysm, and T wave inversions may persist for hours or days after protracted attacks. During an attack the QRS patterns are usually the same as they were before it,

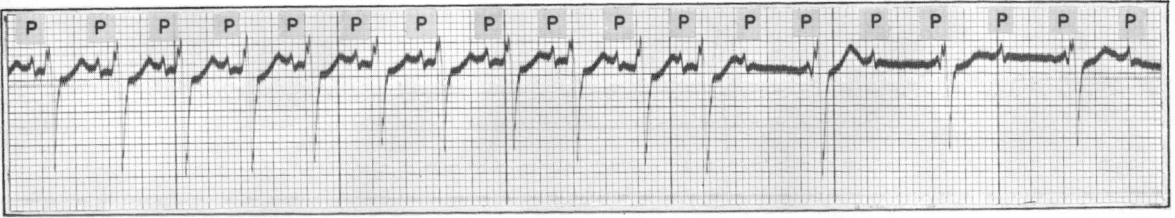

FIGURE 4. Supraventricular paroxysmal tachycardia. Deformed P waves at rate of 152/minute. Ventricular response is 1:1 with P-R interval of 0.10, changing abruptly to 2:1 with P-R reduced to 0.05.

but they may be prolonged and bizarre in configuration, especially when the heart is seriously diseased. The clinical and electrocardiographic differentiation from ventricular paroxysmal tachycardia may, then, be difficult. Supraventricular paroxysmal tachycardia also clinically resembles paroxysmal atrial flutter, in which the rate is usually somewhat slower and the attack more protracted. Differentiation is usually apparent in the electrocardiogram, and the response to vagotonic procedures is quite different.

At times, the ventricular response is not regular, and *clinical* differentiation from atrial fibrillation may be impossible. Careful inspection of the electrocardiogram (Fig. 5) will reveal regularly spaced P waves at a rate of 150 to 200, with irregular ventricular response. Further inspection will usually reveal some measure of consistency in the rhythm of sequences of ventricular beats; a regular trigeminy or quadrigeminy may be present, and in these a progressively prolonged P-R interval is followed by a dropped beat at the end of each sequence (*Wenckebach phenomenon*). Irregular

ventricular response is fairly common when supraventricular paroxysmal tachycardia occurs in patients with seriously diseased hearts, but digitalis toxicity should be immediately suspected by the examiner, especially if the P wave rate is less than 160. It may be a serious error to confuse paroxysmal atrial tachycardia with block with atrial fibrillation because, if the arrhythmia has resulted from digitalis toxicity, further administration of the drug is hazardous.

Treatment. A recurrent attack of supraventricular tachycardia in a person with an otherwise normal heart rarely requires vigorous measures. The danger is small, and spontaneous termination can be expected before serious functional embarrassment develops. Patients with recurrent attacks usually develop an effective treatment plan including self-induced *vagal stimulation* by straining, gagging, or self-manipulation of the right carotid sinus and *rest* with or without drug assistance (secobarbital 0.1 or 0.2 gram). A single 0.2 gram tablet of quinidine sulfate is possibly useful, but two or three tablets in

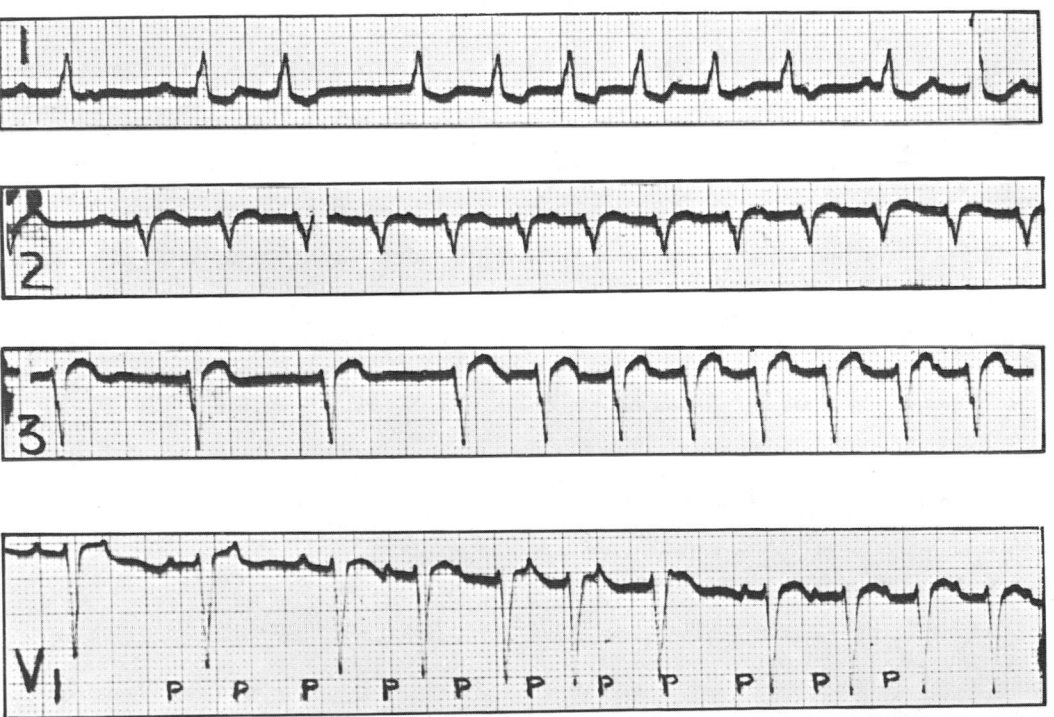

FIGURE 5. Paroxysmal atrial tachycardia with block. Easily mistaken clinically and in limb leads for atrial fibrillation. Lead V₁ shows regular P waves at rate 145/minute. Successive prolongation of P-R intervals followed by nonconducted beat (Wenckebach phenomenon). Overdigitalized patient; normal rhythm was restored with potassium.

a single dose are more likely to exert a favorable effect. If these measures are ineffective, additional quinidine may be given under medical supervision; or other measures, usually reserved for more hazardous cases, may be necessary.

If the rate is unusually rapid, if the attack is unusually persistent, or, most especially, if serious cardiac disease coexists, paroxysmal atrial tachycardia may be an alarming disorder. The management of such an attack requires a more vigorous program and continuous medical attention with electrocardiographic monitoring. Immediate attention should be directed to massive abdominal distention, tension pneumothorax or hydrothorax, or severe hyperpyrexia, if these exist. Eyeball compression has been recommended, but the danger of retinal detachment is appreciable. Gagging or straining may be effective. Carotid sinus massage is the most effective of the vagal stimulating maneuvers, but it may induce a cerebral vascular accident in elderly patients. If carotid pulsation can be felt on *both* sides of the neck, carotid sinus massage for 10 to 15 seconds, first on the right side, then on the left side, may be tried. (*Never massage both sides at once!*) Morphine sulfate, 10 mg. subcutaneously or 5 mg. intravenously, is given promptly if the patient is in severe distress. It allays apprehension and is a vagal stimulant. Narcotics must be avoided for those with frequently recurrent attacks.

Hypotension is common in serious attacks. Methoxamine, 10 to 20 mg. intramuscularly or 5 to 10 mg. intravenously, averts shock, and, through restoration of coronary circulation and reflex vagal effect, may terminate the arrhythmia. Phenylephrine, 5 mg. subcutaneously; metaraminol, 5 mg. intramuscularly; or levarterenol 4 to 8 mg. in 500 ml. as an intravenous drip, are alternatives. If there is reason to suspect digitalis toxicity, special measures may be indicated (see Ventricular Paroxysmal Tachycardia). If the patient is not already digitalized, digoxin, 2.0 mg. orally or 1.0 mg. intramuscularly, may be given when distress is not severe, or, if it is, 0.5 mg. of digoxin or lanatoside C may be given intravenously, repeated every 15 minutes, to a total of three doses (3×0.5 mg.) if necessary. Since each of these measures stimulates vagal activity, vagotonic maneuvers, originally ineffective, may be tried again from time to time. If all these measures fail, quinidine sulfate should be used. To an adult of average size, 0.4 gram orally, repeated every two to three hours to a total of four doses, may be given. Nausea, occasional vomiting, or mild diarrhea is not necessarily a sign of serious toxicity, but aggravated blood pressure depression or shock, gross widening of the QRS complexes, or the appearance of ventricular arrhythmias precludes further medication. Sometimes urticaria, chills and fever, purpura, or other manifestations of idiosyncrasy appear with the first or subsequent doses of quinidine and contraindicate its further use. Quinidine in doses greater than those described above is attended by a rising hazard of major drug toxicity. Cardioversion is then a safer and more effective method (*vide infra*).

Except in digitalis toxicity, it is indicated early, in place of vigorous drug therapy, in those with associated serious heart disease.

Prophylaxis. For those with brief attacks at long intervals, instruction in measures to be taken with each attack is sufficient. In the prevention of recurrent attacks, the possibility of hyperthyroidism should always be considered and treated, if present. Quinidine sulfate, 0.8 to 1.6 grams in four to six divided doses throughout the day and night, or its equivalent in more sustained action quinidine preparations, is highly effective in some patients and of some help in most. Digitalization should be tried if quinidine is ineffective, although it is infrequently helpful in preventing attacks, and it does not influence the rate of the heart when an attack occurs. Occasionally it is impressively effective. Propranolol, 40 to 200 mg. in four or five divided doses, is often highly effective. Excessive bradycardia, postural hypotension, and other side effects are sufficiently frequent to place it behind quinidine and digitalis in order of trial for prophylaxis, and in larger doses it may induce congestive failure. Procaine amide, 250 mg. four times daily, is an alternative, but over protracted periods the development of lupus-like reaction is an infrequent but distressing complication. Other rarely used alternatives are chloroquine, 250 mg. twice daily, or reserpine, 0.25 to 0.5 mg. daily. I[131] therapy of euthyroid subjects has been largely abandoned. Phenobarbital or meprobamate may be helpful in patients whose attacks are associated with emotional outbursts.

Atrial Fibrillation. In this condition, the atrial myocardium is in continuous, incoordinate, vermicular motion that is dynamically functionless. It is the most common of the major arrhythmias. It may occur in the absence of heart disease as a paroxysmal disorder after thoracic surgery, following pulmonary embolization, in the presence of severe infections or high fever, or in the elderly, but it is most common in persons with intrinsic heart disease. In general, the more severe the functional impairment, the more likely it is that atrial fibrillation will occur. In mitral valve disease, either stenosis or insufficiency, it is almost always present when congestive failure has developed, and it frequently appears before functional impairment is great. Fibrillation sometimes is permanent from the moment it first appears. More commonly, transient periods of fibrillation become progressively more frequent and protracted, eventuating in the chronic permanent state.

The development of atrial fibrillation reduces resting cardiac output and reserve output capacity by abolishing the atrial contribution to ventricular filling and, of greater importance, by increasing ventricular rate to beyond the level of optimal dynamic efficiency. Some beats may transmit a feeble or imperceptible pulse wave to the periphery, resulting in a *pulse deficit* when beats recorded at the wrist are compared with the audible beats at the apex. This is especially evident when the ventricular rate is rapid.

In everyday practice, a completely irregular

rhythm is most often due to atrial fibrillation. The ventricular response in untreated patients with fibrillation is usually between 90 and 160. It may be as high as 200, especially in paroxysmal fibrillation without intrinsic heart disease or in thyrotoxicosis. It may be as low as 50 in older persons with arteriosclerotic heart disease or after digitalis medication. The ventricular rate depends upon the physiologic characteristics, especially the refractory period, of the conductive tissues below the atrial level. Whatever the rate, the rhythm is always completely irregular unless a dissociated rhythm is present, with the ventricle under the control of an ectopic focus in the lower portions of the AV node or in the ventricle. Irregularity may occasionally be difficult to ascertain by radial palpation, especially when the pulse is very slow. On auscultation, heart sounds are irregular in both rhythm and intensity. The presystolic murmur of mitral stenosis never coexists with atrial fibrillation. Atrial fibrillation is clinically important not only because of its influence upon cardiac function, but because clots frequently form within the atria, especially in the left atrium when the mitral valve is diseased. Peripheral and pulmonary embolization are serious hazards.

In the electrocardiogram (Fig. 6), P waves are replaced by fibrillation waves, usually best seen in lead V_1. These are continuous undulations varying in amplitude and configuration, having a frequency in the range of 300 to 600 beats per minute.

Treatment. With few exceptions, the immediate therapeutic indication is to give a digitalis preparation to reduce ventricular rate by direct and vagal influences upon the refractory period of the atrioventricular conduction tissues. The dose and route of administration are governed by exigencies of the situation. When the rate is excessively rapid and serious intrinsic heart disease exists, when congestive failure is acutely developing, or when shock or pulmonary edema is present, a rapidly acting preparation administered intravenously is indicated. Digoxin, 0.5 mg. intravenously, will usually be sufficiently helpful within 30 minutes that further therapy may be given orally. If necessary, a second and third injection of 0.25 mg. may be given at 15-minute intervals. In the great majority of instances, oral administration is selected because it is safer.

Many oral digitalis preparations are available. Digitalis leaf, 1.2 to 1.5 grams to an adult in a single dose or, preferably, in divided doses over a 24-hour period, will usually establish an effective level of digitalization with little hazard of toxicity (unless the patient has already received digitalis or is hypokalemic). As an alternative, digitoxin, 1.2 to 1.5 mg. in the first 24 hours, or digoxin, 2.0 to 2.5 mg. in the first 24 hours, is equally effective. All digitalis preparations have approximately the same margin of safety between efficacy and toxicity. They differ principally in the rate at which they influence the heart and the duration of biologic effects (see Fig. 7).

The ventricular rate usually serves as a useful guide to the adequacy of digitalis therapy in atrial fibrillation. Insufficient medication may be associated with adequate slowing at rest but a sharp rise with exertion. This indicates a predominantly vagal effect, and further benefits are likely to attend a higher dosage. When the ventricular rate is already slow in an untreated patient, but congestive failure is present, inotropic benefits of digitalis will almost always precede any hazardous further reduction in ventricular rate, but the drug should be given with greater caution than usual, and the effects should be followed closely. Digitalis cardiotoxicity in a patient with atrial fibrillation may manifest itself in excessive slowing of the ventricular rate; complete AV block may be induced, or coupled or erratic ventricular premature beats may appear. If the rate becomes more regular and rapid as digitalis is given in larger doses, nodal paroxysmal tachycardia or ventricular tachycardia may have developed. These are cardinal warnings of impending disaster — ventricular fibrillation. They demand instant cessation of digitalis medication and, usually, potassium administration. In chronic atrial fibrillation, maintenance digitalis is usually continued indefinitely. The dose is variable in different patients, but 0.15 mg. of digitoxin, 0.375 mg. of digoxin, or 0.15 gram of digitalis leaf is the average daily dose. In those who have had an embolic complication, long-term anticoagulant therapy is usually recommended.

When atrial fibrillation has been present for only a short time, quinidine sulfate may be used in an attempt to convert it to normal sinus rhythm. In determining whether to attempt conversion, one should be governed by the principle that *unless* conversion occurs the patient may be temporarily worse because of the myocardial depressant action of the drug. Hence, quinidine is usually given after digitalis therapy. It should never be continued once it is apparent that conversion of the fibrillation is not going to occur.

Quinidine sulfate is also of value in the attempted conversion of a patient who has been in fibrillation for months or years, but in whom a

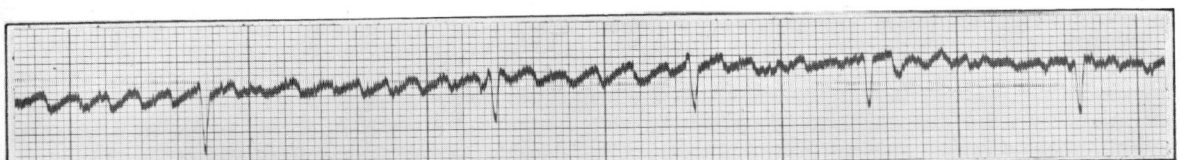

FIGURE 6. Atrial fibrillation. In first portion of record, atrial activity has a semblance of order at approximate rate of 350/minute (flutter-fibrillation). In latter portion it is completely irregular. Ventricular beats are erratic in timing, average about 50/minute. A slow ventricular rate is often present in elderly persons or after digitalis therapy. Otherwise, ventricular rate is usually much more rapid than in this illustration.

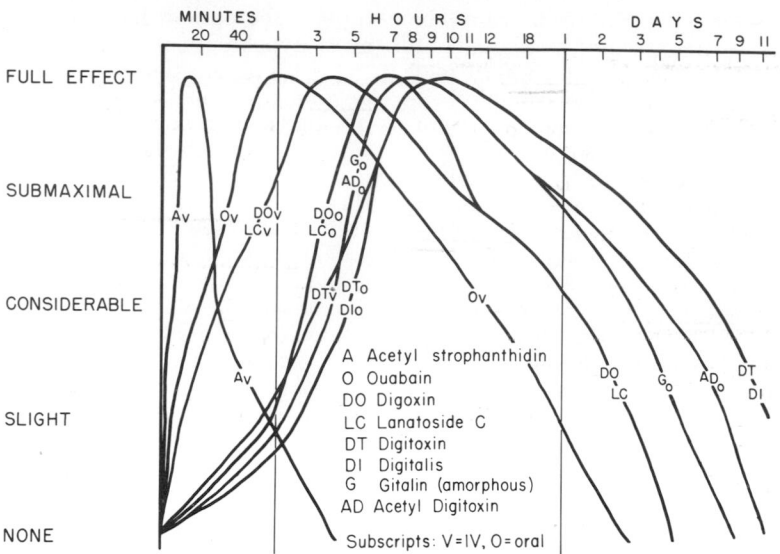

FIGURE 7. The accumulation and decline of biologic effects of single doses of cardioactive glycosides in man. (Adapted from Circulation, 12:123, 1955.)

toxic or mechanical factor contributing to the induction and perpetuation of the arrhythmia has been abolished. This particularly applies to those who have had successful mitral valve surgery or relief of chronic thyrotoxicosis. During quinidine therapy, digitalis may be continued, but ordinarily at a slightly reduced maintenance dose. Not uncommonly, atrial fibrillation changes to flutter during quinidine therapy. This does not contraindicate further trial at higher dosage, but, when flutter develops, successful conversion is unlikely to occur. In some instances, atrial fibrillation that fails to respond to quinidine in the usual therapeutic dose range might be reverted to normal sinus rhythm if therapy were administered with sufficient vigor. However, quinidine in large doses carries a high immediate risk. Quinidine sulfate in doses of 0.2 gram every four hours for 48 hours is sometimes effective, and it is attended with relatively little hazard in an adult. A course of the drug in a dose of 0.4 gram every three hours for four doses, starting early in the morning, is preferable for hospitalized patients under observation. Much larger doses have been effectively used in the past, but it is safer and more effective to induce conversion electrically (vide infra) than to give quinidine in doses appreciably larger than 1.6 grams within a nine-hour period.

Conversion of atrial fibrillation, especially if it has been present for a long time, is attended by some risk that an atrial embolus will be dislodged. A period of several weeks of anticoagulant therapy before attempting conversion may reduce this risk.

Prophylaxis. In those who have had recurrent paroxysms of atrial fibrillation, and in those in whom reversion to normal sinus rhythm has been effected, quinidine is used to prevent recurrence of the arrhythmia. It is not always effective. The usual dosage is 0.2 gram of quinidine sulfate four to eight times daily, or an equivalent dosage of a long-acting preparation. Propranolol, 40 to 200

mg. daily in divided doses, is sometimes useful as an adjuvant to quinidine but must be used cautiously in patients with borderline congestive failure. It is rarely of value alone. The control of hyperthyroidism, if present, is essential. Therapeutic thyroid depression may rarely be indicated in euthyroid subjects to eliminate recurrent paroxysms of fibrillation or to reduce the ventricular rate in those with chronic fibrillation who respond inadequately to digitalis.

Atrial Flutter. This arrhythmia is much less common than atrial fibrillation. A sequence of electrical and mechanical atrial events repeats itself in the atrium at an exactly regular rate that may range from 220 to 360 times per minute and is usually between 270 and 320. At any one time, some fibers are in systole and others are in diastole; hence the dynamic effectiveness of the atrial contraction is small. In experimental preparations, atrial flutter can be produced either as a cyclic reentry around a ring of tissue or as a repetitive outgoing wave from a single ectopic focus. Whether the circus hypothesis or the unitary focus hypothesis or both are applicable to man is controversial, but this arrhythmia clearly differs in several important respects from atrial paroxysmal tachycardia.

Atrial flutter is closely related to atrial fibrillation. Many patients will shift back and forth between the two from moment to moment or day to day, and change from one to the other is frequently induced by drugs: flutter to fibrillation with digitalis and the reverse with quinidine. Impure flutter and flutter fibrillation are terms employed to describe an in-between state in which atrial activity is not quite regular in rate or in electrocardiographic configuration, and in which the ventricular response is erratic in relation to the atrial beats (Fig. 6). Flutter, like fibrillation, is more often a protracted than a transient paroxysmal disorder and is much more often associated with serious intrinsic heart disease than with otherwise normal hearts. A 1:1 ratio of atrial to ventricular beats is rare. The ventricular rate is then 250 or more, and circulatory collapse may be expected. When the ratio is 2:1, as is most common, some degree of cardiac functional impairment usually is present, and the symptoms and clinical findings may be indistinguishable from those of paroxysmal supraventricular tachycardia. At higher ratios (4:1 or 6:1, but very rarely 3:1), the ventricular rate is sufficiently slow that symptoms may be slight or absent. A perfectly regular pulse of 140 to 160 is usually due to flutter. Rarely is it possible to identify atrial flutter waves in the cervical venous pulse. The most reliable guide in clinical differentiation from paroxysmal supraventricular tachycardia or sinus tachycardia is the response to carotid sinus massage. If, for the duration of the manipulation, the ventricular rate slows abruptly to one half or two thirds of the former rate, signifying a change from 2:1 to 4:1 or 3:1 respectively, the diagnosis of flutter is very probable. Even a change from regular to irregular rhythm at a slower rate, resulting from transient and erratic changes in AV ratio, is strongly suggestive. Characteristically the original ratio and rate return promptly when massage is discontinued.

In the electrocardiogram (Fig. 8), the flutter waves are classically seen as a saw-tooth pattern in leads 2 and 3, with ventricular complexes falling regularly and in a fixed position on every second or fourth (rarely third) flutter wave. When the ratio is 2:1, flutter waves may be difficult to distinguish from T waves. Carotid sinus massage often causes a transient change in ratio and clarifies the nature of the arrhythmia.

Treatment. Either digitalis or quinidine or both are used in the treatment of atrial flutter. Electrical conversion is less often successful than in atrial fibrillation, but should be tried when drugs are ineffective. Digitalis, in addition to its inotropic effect, is usually of value in one or more of several ways. It may slow the ventricular rate by converting a 2:1 to a 4:1 or 3:1 block by its effect upon AV conduction. This change is usually transient and unstable even though digitalis is continued. Rarely, conversion to normal rhythm occurs directly. Much more often, the flutter is converted to atrial fibrillation with an irregular but slower ventricular rate than before. This may require unusually large doses of a digitalis preparation, bordering on toxic levels. In patients with serious heart disease, especially if flutter or fibrillation has been present for a long time, further improvement cannot be expected. When the duration of the arrhythmia has been brief or when the cardiac status has been modified favorably by surgery or by relief of thyrotoxicosis, reversion to normal rhythm may occur during the digitalis therapy or when it is abruptly discontinued. If, instead, atrial flutter returns, as it often does, quinidine should be tried. It is advisable to continue digitalis at a modest dosage level during quinidine therapy.

The therapy of atrial flutter with quinidine provides an unusual opportunity in clinical pharmacology. The therapeutic program is essentially the same as in the elective reversion of atrial fibrillation. With quinidine, the flutter rate slows progressively as successive doses are given. According to the "circus theory" of flutter, this is caused by a progressive slowing of conductivity in the "ring." It is hoped, however, that prolongation of the refractory period will predominate over conduction slowing in order that the most advanced point on the cyclic wave will fall upon refractory tissue, terminating the flutter. Usually this is accomplished before the atrial rate has slowed by more than 30 per cent, e.g., 300 to 210, or not at all. Quinidine sometimes changes the ratio from 2:1 to 4:1 by an imbalance of reciprocal vagal and direct effects upon AV conduction, but this tendency to increase the ratio is usually counteracted by the longer periods between stimuli arriving at the AV tissue as the atrial flutter rate slows. There is some hazard that 2:1 will convert to 1:1 at a dangerously high ventricular rate, especially in young persons or in those who are not receiving concomitant digitalis. Widening of the QRS complex forewarns of dangerous quinidine toxicity, which may result in ventricular tachycardia, flutter, fibrillation, or arrest.

It is recommended that electrical conversion be employed in preference to either quinidine or digitalis if very large doses are required. If conversion succeeds, long-term quinidine therapy is usually required.

DISORDERS ARISING IN THE AV NODE

Nodal Premature Beats. Less frequent than atrial premature beats, nodal premature beats occur under similar circumstances. The ectopic focus in the AV node activates the ventricles and usually the atria also. If the retrograde activation of the atria discharges the SA node, the compensatory pause is absent or incomplete. As with a premature beat of any type, the ventricular stroke output is small relative to a normal beat. In the electrocardiogram (Fig. 1), the nodal origin of the

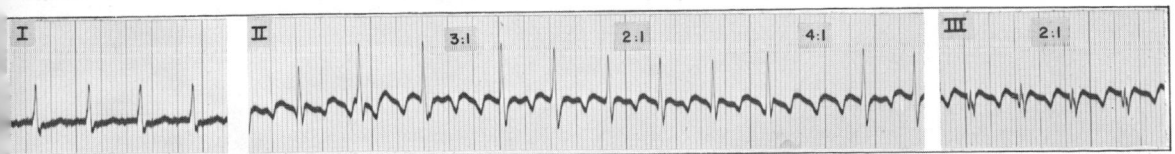

FIGURE 8. Atrial flutter. Continuous atrial activity, with regular rhythm at rate 290/minute, best seen in leads II and III. Regular 2:1 ventricular response in most of tracing. In lead II, varying A-V block with 3:1 and 4:1 intervals, induced by left carotid sinus stimulation during lead II recording.

beat is identified by the P wave. The timing of the P wave with respect to the QRS relates to the relative conduction velocities downward to the ventricles vs. upward to the atria. The P wave may precede the QRS by 0.11 second or less; it may be concealed within the QRS or may follow it. If a P wave precedes the QRS, it may be deflected in the normal direction, but it is deformed in configuration. As it more closely approaches the QRS or falls behind it, the direction of the deflection reverses from the normal. An upright P wave in AVR is almost always nodal in origin. When the nodal beat is conducted only to the ventricles, a normal P wave of sinus origin may be present at its normal time; in this instance after the nodal premature QRS. If so, it may not be conducted to the ventricles because of interference at the AV node. The QRS of a nodal beat is more likely to be deformed (aberrant conduction) than that of an atrial premature beat. Isolated nodal premature beats cause insignificant dynamic disturbance and require no therapy.

Nodal Escape Beats.   These occur when the sinus rate slows excessively. They are *post*mature rather than premature but otherwise resemble nodal premature beats. They provide the most common safety mechanism to sustain the heartbeat when the sinus mechanism fails to do so.

Nodal Rhythm.   When the ventricles are under the control of an atrioventricular nodal focus, the rhythm is said to be nodal (Figs. 1 and 9). It usually occurs as an escape mechanism in any circumstance in which the sinus node is depressed. In other instances, it is present because the rate of spontaneous discharge in the nodal focus rises above that of the sinus node. It is not uncommon in patients with normal hearts, especially in the elderly, or under emotional stress, during anesthesia, or when vagotonic drugs have been given. It also occurs in acute myocardial infarction, particularly if shock is present, after excessive digitalis medication, and in acute rheumatic fever. Nodal rhythm is almost always a transient, unstable mechanism, with variation of the site of the focus in the AV node from beat to beat and wandering of the pacemaker to and from the sinus node in an ever-changing pattern. When the nodal focus activates the atria as well as the ventricles, as it

usually does, variations in the P wave configuration, in the direction of deflection, and in timing in relation to the QRS complex occur as in nodal premature beats. Less often, the atria remain under the control of the sinus focus beating at a slightly slower or faster rate than the nodal focus. A succession of P waves of normal and unchanging configuration progressively approach the QRS, become lost within it, and then appear after it. These P waves are not conducted to the ventricles because the nodal stimulus has discharged the conduction pathways. This is a form of *AV dissociation* because of *interference* and it should not be confused with AV block, although the two may coincide. As the P waves fall progressively behind the nodal-induced QRS, the conducting pathways to the ventricles are no longer refractory, and the sinus beat is conducted for one or several beats; this is *ventricular capture*, and the first such beat of a series is premature. The faster nodal focus subsequently resumes control of the ventricles, and the cycle is repeated.

Nodal rhythm is characterized by some interesting symptoms and physical findings (Fig. 1). Many patients are aware of a forceful thrust or "turning over" in the chest or in the root of the neck with each nodal beat, but not with the sinus beats. With continuing nodal rhythm, the patient may be conscious of each heartbeat, an annoyance that may be the principal complaint. On examination, the nodal, symptomatic beats are associated with forceful venous distention (*a giant "a" wave*) in the neck, faint first heart sound, and small pulse volume. These phenomena occur when atrial contraction coincides with ventricular systole. Since atrial blood cannot be ejected into the contracted ventricles, it is regurgitated into the veins. If the atrial contraction immediately precedes that of the ventricles, the first heart sound may be louder than in the sinus beats. Nodal rhythm is usually of little physiologic or pathologic significance and requires no therapy.

Nodal Paroxysmal Tachycardia.   This disorder, often indistinguishable from atrial paroxysmal tachycardia, has already been discussed under the latter heading. A special form occurs as an unusual but important manifestation of digitalis toxicity. When, in patients with atrial fibrillation,

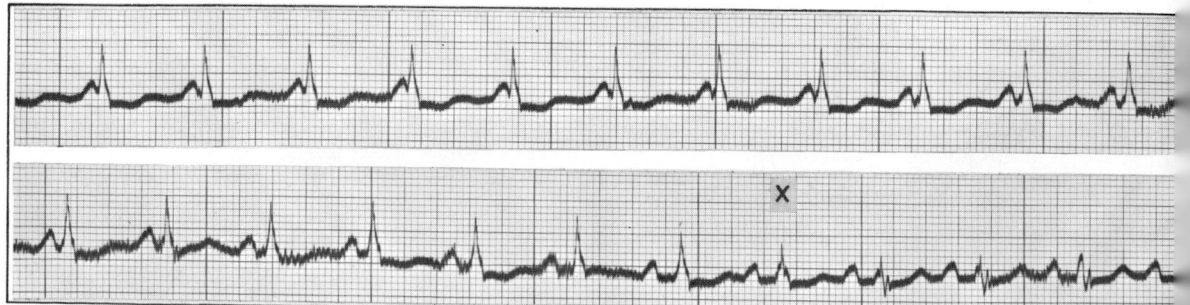

FIGURE 9.   Nodal rhythm. The sinus node, activating the atria, is slightly faster than the nodal focus activating the ventricles in the first portion of this continuous lead II. P waves, concealed within the QRS complexes, progressively precede them. The atria do not activate the ventricles because of interference. At X, the P-R interval reaches 0.19 second. Thereafter, the ventricular rate is slightly faster and the QRS follows each P wave at a fixed interval (ventricular capture). Aberrant activation of the ventricles, present during the period of nodal rhythm, disappears as sinus rhythm begins.

the rhythm becomes regular and progressively rapid as digitalis administration is augmented or as potassium depletion develops, potentially serious digitalis toxicity should be suspected.

DISORDERS ARISING IN THE VENTRICLES

Ventricular Premature Beats. These constitute the most common disorder of rhythm. It occurs as a benign disturbance in persons with otherwise normal hearts, increasing in frequency as age advances. Such beats are first noted in some subjects in early adult life and recur thereafter, especially during periods of stress or fatigue. They are common in healthy persons during anesthesia and are occasionally induced by epinephrine, ephedrine, or amphetamine medication. Not all ventricular premature beats are benign; they are frequently a manifestation of damaged, anoxic, or toxic heart muscle. They are especially associated with ischemic heart disease, and may occur during and shortly after acute infarction, during anginal seizures, and in patients with areas of old myocardial scarring. Serious heart disease of any type is likely to be associated with ventricular premature beats, especially if heart failure exists or is impending. Digitalis toxicity should always be considered as a possibility when this arrhythmia is present.

Whether the arrhythmia is benign or is the product of myocardial distress, ventricular premature beats are most commonly isolated, single beats interspersed between relatively long sequences of normal beats. Clinical significance increases as the premature beats become more frequent. Coupled beating or bigeminy may be caused by other arrhythmias, but is usually the result of a ventricular premature beat following each normal beat. It should immediately suggest digitalis toxicity. Runs of two or more ventricular premature beats, whether regularly recurrent or an erratic phenomenon, multifocal beats, or beats that fall during the so-called "vulnerable period" shortly after the peak of the T wave, warn of impending ventricular paroxysmal tachycardia or fibrillation.

The stroke output of a premature beat is small, resulting at times in a radial pulse deficit. The output of the post premature beat, which comes after a compensatory pause, is usually greater than normal. As a result, cardiac output is relatively little reduced unless the premature beats are very frequent or occur in runs. Many patients are conscious of the cardiac arrhythmia, especially while lying quietly in bed. It is generally stated that the forceful, post-premature beat is the one felt, but this is incorrect. The sensation coincides with the premature beat in the majority of instances. The symptom is then evidently induced by atrial regurgitation into the veins as in some nodal premature beats. The first heart sound may be relatively louder or softer, depending on the position of the AV valves at the moment of systole. The second sound is almost always faint, and may be absent if systolic ejection does not occur.

In the electrocardiogram (Fig. 10), ventricular premature beats are characterized by prematurity (differentiating them from ventricular escape beats), by the absence of preceding P waves and by bizarre configuration of the QRS with a duration of 0.12 second or more. They must be differentiated from supraventricular premature beats with aberrant conduction. Usually the premature beats are similar to each other if not identical. Discharge from multiple ectopic foci results in gross differences in QRS configuration from beat to beat and suggests a serious cardiac disorder. *Fixed coupling* (a constant interval between the normal and the premature beat) suggests digitalis toxicity. Fixed coupling and fixed QRS shape suggest a re-entry mechanism. In a parasystolic mechanism, the interval between the ectopic beats is always the multiple of the discharge rate of the parasystolic focus, which is usually at a much slower rate than the supraventricular focus, and fails to discharge the ventricles when its activation falls within the refractory period of the ventricle. Sometimes the ventricular premature beat is transmitted backward through the AV node to stimulate the atria and produce a retrograde P wave. Even when this occurs, the sinoatrial focus is rarely disturbed. If the sinus rate is slow, an interpolated ventricular premature beat may fall between two normal beats.

Treatment. Ventricular premature beats per se rarely call for treatment. In healthy persons

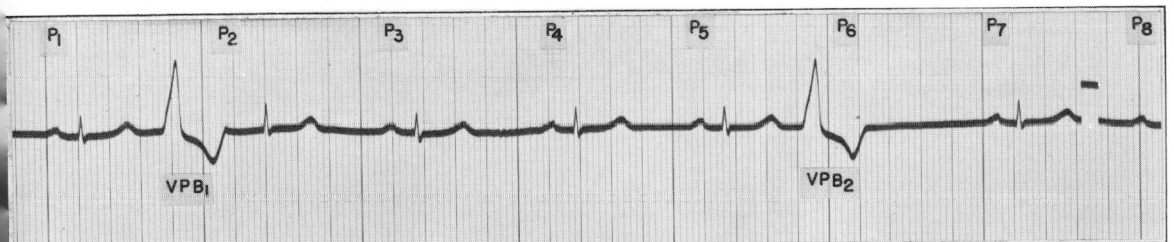

FIGURE 10. Sinus rhythm with slight sinus arrhythmia (P_3-P_4 equals 1.04 seconds, P_7-P_8 equals 0.96 second). Ventricular premature beats. VPB_1 is interpolated; hence there is not a compensatory pause, although R of the postpremature beat is slightly delayed because the P-R interval is prolonged, resulting from retrograde invasion of the A-V node (concealed conduction). VPB_2 is of the common type. P_6 is blocked because of interference, and the compensatory pause is complete (P_2-P_4 equals 1.98 seconds, P_5-P_7 equals 1.92 seconds). Sinus arrhythmia accounts for the slight discrepancy. The coupling is not fixed. Examination of full tracing shows that this is not parasystole.

disturbed by awareness of the beats, reassurance is helpful; in some instances it may be advisable to give quinidine (0.2 gram three to four times daily), reserpine (0.25 mg. daily), or sedation. When there is reason to suspect digitalis toxicity, appropriate measures must be taken. This arrhythmia is not a contraindication to the use of digitalis; on the contrary, premature beats may disappear from a failing heart after digitalization. If ventricular premature beats are caused by intrinsic disease, treatment is primarily directed toward the disorder. When ventricular premature beats become numerous during an acute cardiovascular illness, or if at any time they are multifocal, in runs of two or more, or if the premature beat is superimposed upon the T wave of the preceding beat, this constitutes warning of threatened paroxysmal tachycardia, flutter, or fibrillation. Atropine, quinidine, procaine amide, or lidocaine should be administered appropriately (see Myocardial Infarction), or potassium or phenylhydantoin if digitalis toxicity is probable.

Ventricular Paroxysmal Tachycardia. A run of ventricular premature beats that continues for six beats or more is called ventricular paroxysmal tachycardia. In this clinically important disorder, the ectopic ventricular pacemaker drives the heart in successful competition with a coexistent supraventricular pacemaker (dissociation) or, when AV block exists, at a rate greatly in excess of that of the usual ventricular focus. In apparently normal persons, in rare instances, this arrhythmia may develop during or after operative procedures, electroshock therapy, or serious infections, otherwise it develops almost exclusively in patients with obvious serious heart disease. The majority of these have old or recent myocardial infarction; about half are, or have been, in congestive failure; and in an appreciable number of these, digitalis toxicity is a contributing or precipitating factor. In a few instances, this arrhythmia is a toxic manifestation of quinidine, procaine amide, or chloroquine therapy.

Attacks are usually preceded by ventricular premature beats, first individually, then in short runs. Paroxysms may last only a few seconds, returning again and again, or may last for minutes, hours, or days. The death rate in ventricular tachycardia is relatively high, from abrupt ventricular fibrillation or arrest, or from progressive shock or congestive failure. Occasionally, embolism is a lethal complication.

During most attacks the ventricular rate is between 140 and 175, but ranges from 110 to 250

are observed. Ventricular tachycardia differs from other types of rapid heart action in several respects. Slight beat-to-beat variations (0.01 to 0.03 second) are usually present, and the average rate may change by 10 beats per minute or more in attacks that persist for several hours, or in different attacks in the same individual. Carotid sinus massage has no effect.

In the electrocardiogram (Figs. 11 and 12), this arrhythmia is characterized by QRS complexes of over 0.12 duration, often with slight variation in beat-to-beat contour as well as in rate. A considerable change in QRS configuration may develop if the attack persists. *Electrical alternans* (slight alternate change in contour) may be seen, especially when the rate is relatively rapid. Direction reversal in alternate complexes carries an especially unfavorable prognosis and particularly suggests digitalis toxicity. The QRS complexes often, but not always, resemble isolated ventricular premature beats recorded before or after the paroxysm. The atrial activity may be difficult to identify, but sometimes P waves at a slower rate may be discovered. These are obvious in esophageal leads using a Brody electrode or in intra-atrial leads, now in use in some intensive care units. If so, the diagnosis is established. Rarely, the atria are activated by retrograde impulses, with a 1:1 atrial response or with progressive prolongations of the R-P interval and periodic dropping of P waves (*retrograde Wenckebach phenomenon*).

Treatment. Ventricular tachycardia is one of the most dangerous of the arrhythmias. Constant professional surveillance is demanded First consideration should be given to the pos-

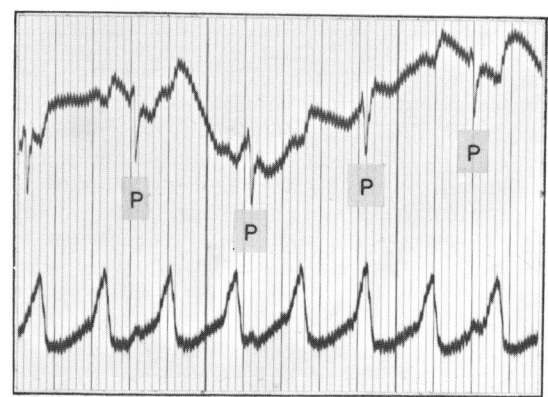

FIGURE 11. Ventricular paroxysmal tachycardia. Esophageal lead (above) records regular P waves. In lead I, below, the QRS complexes are wide and deformed; rate 178 with slight irregularity. P waves can be identified in this lead.

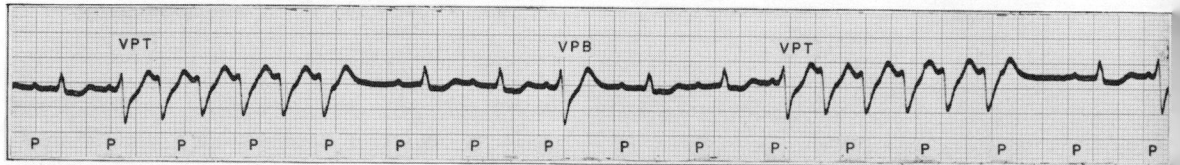

FIGURE 12. Ventricular paroxysmal tachycardia. During two paroxysms, each of six beats, there is complete A-V dissociation with undisturbed atrial activation from sinus focus at rate 104. P waves are obscured (visible in last complex of each paroxysm?). Ventricular rate 188, rhythm slightly irregular. Single ventricular premature beat resembles first beat of paroxysms. Ventricular tachycardia became persistent shortly after this recording. It disappeared immediately with intravenous phenylephrine.

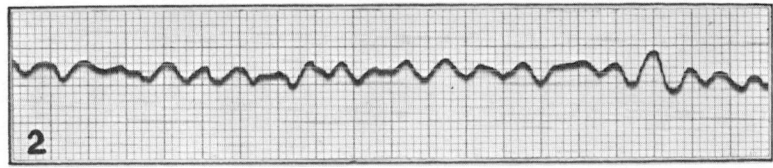

FIGURE 13. Ventricular fibrillation. Completely erratic electrical activity of ventricle. No atrial activity can be identified in this example.

sibility that digitalis has been a precipitating factor. If this is a reasonable possibility, a serum potassium determination should be made, and pending the report and unless hyperkalemia is suspected, KCl, 3 grams in 500 ml. of 5 per cent glucose, is given intravenously at 4 to 6 ml. per minute. This is continued until the arrhythmia has been controlled, the potassium serum level is normal, or 9 grams has been given, to be then followed with oral administration. Diphenyl-hydantoin, 100 mg. intravenously every three minutes for four doses, or propranolol, 1 to 3 mg. intravenously over a period of 10 minutes, is highly effective in digitalis-induced tachycardias.

In ventricular tachycardia *not* the result of digitalis toxicity, therapy depends upon the clinical situation. Bursts of tachycardia unattended by circulatory distress may be treated with oral quinidine, 400 to 600 mg. followed by 200 mg. ever two to three hours, or by procaine amide orally, 750 mg. followed by 250 mg. every three hours, or intravenously, 50 mg. per minute to 300 mg., then 50 mg. every four minutes to a maximum of 1000 mg. When the tachycardia is more persistent and the clinical setting is more ominous, lidocaine is the drug or choice, 50 to 100 mg. as a bolus intravenously followed by 1 to 4 mg. per minute as an intravenous drip. Excessive dosage results in restlessness, and occasionally in convulsions. Isoproterenol, 2 mg. in 500 ml. 5 per cent dextrose, administered intravenously at about 1 ml. per minute may be used for circulatory support during any of the above measures.

Electrical conversion has largely superseded drug therapy in the management of sustained ventricular paroxysmal tachycardia except that which is due to digitalis toxicity. It is sufficiently superior that considerable effort is justified to bring the patient to the equipment or vice versa.

When ventricular tachycardia complicates pre-existing AV block, relief with antiarrhythmic agents occasionally results in ventricular arrest. If possible, a pacemaker should be available in the event that this development should occur. Rarely, pacemakers are used to capture the rhythm, preventing a return to ventricular tachycardia. This is especially likely when the atrial rate is slow.

Ventricular Flutter. This is a form of paroxysmal ventricular tachycardia in which the heart rate is usually about 200 per minute. The electrocardiograph records a continuous undulation approximating a sine wave. Ventricular flutter is rarely a stable state and frequently precedes either ventricular arrest or fibrillation. During ventricular flutter, some useful cardiac function continues, but cardiac output is grossly deficient and attended

by faintness, shock, syncope, or rapidly developing pulmonary congestion.

Ventricular Fibrillation. This is a state of electrical and mechanical chaos of the heart: the "bag of worms" to direct palpation, devoid of any dynamic function. It is a terminal state in many kinds of death, and is the most common mechanism of death after electrical shock. When it occurs, with or without the forewarning of ventricular premature beats, tachycardia, or flutter, the circulation stops. It is not possible to differentiate this disorder from ventricular standstill except with the electrocardiograph (Fig. 13). Spontaneous recovery has occurred in a few instances. Drugs are useless once fibrillation exists. Closed chest resuscitation and electrical defibrillation are necessary for recovery (*vide infra*).

DISORDERS OF IMPULSE PROPAGATION

DISORDERS ARISING IN THE SINUS NODE

Sinoatrial Block. Impulses are generated in the sinus node, but one or more of the impulses fail to excite the adjacent atrium. This rare arrhythmia may occur sporadically or regularly, with the drop of every second, third, or fourth beat. Occasionally two or more successive sinus impulses are blocked, resulting in transient faintness. This disorder develops under circumstances that are essentially the same as in atrial arrest, but it should especially suggest a digitalis effect. It can be differentiated from atrial arrest by the fact that the PP interval bracketing the dropped beat or beats is usually a nearly exact multiple of the usual PP interval. A nonconducted atrial premature beat with the P wave obscured in the T wave may be confused with sinoatrial block, but the PP interval is less than twice the normal interval. Treatment, if necessary, is like that for atrial arrest.

DISORDERS ARISING IN THE AV NODE

Atrioventricular Block. Impulses arising in or above the AV node are delayed or obstructed in passage to the ventricles. The conduction impairment may be in the lower portions of the AV node, in the bundle of His, or in both bundle branches. It may result from permanent structural damage or transient inflammation, or from physiologic disturbances induced by drugs, anoxia, or intense vagal stimulation. Often two or more of these factors are concurrent. The majority of patients have arteriosclerotic heart disease with recent or old myocardial infarctions or myocardial fibrosis and degeneration. In young persons, rheumatic fever is frequently responsible. Digitalis may be implicated alone or in combination with other factors. A list of the conditions associated with AV block includes anoxia, hyperkalemia, fibrocalcific aortic stenosis, congenital septal defects, bacterial endocarditis, trichinosis, diphtheria, gummatous syphilis, and various drugs, especially quinidine, procaine amide, and cholinergic preparations. Atrioventricular block is one of the mechanisms by which carotid sinus syncope is mediated. Although this disorder is generally attributed to hypersensitivity of the carotid sinus and resulting excessive vagal discharge, it is probable that hypersusceptibility of the diseased myocardial conducting tissues to vagal stimulation is largely responsible.

In all instances of atrial fibrillation, and in most instances of flutter, not all supraventricular impulses are conducted to the ventricles. This fortunate circumstance is a product of normal physiologic functioning of the AV node and is not a manifestation of block. When the idioventricular focus is rapid as in ventricular paroxysmal tachycardia, atrial impulses may not be transmitted to the ventricles because of interference, resulting in atrioventricular dissociation; this also must be differentiated from block. Atrioventricular block, partial or complete, may be present in association with supraventricular arrhythmias of any type.

Atrioventricular block is classified according to the severity of the conduction defect. In *first-degree block*, all supraventricular beats are conducted to the ventricles, but with excessive delay at the AV node. Accordingly, the PR interval lengthens beyond the normal maximum of 0.20 second. Since neither pulse rate nor rhythm is disturbed, first-degree block is difficult to identify clinically, but two physical findings may suggest its presence. The first heart sound may become fainter. Also, because atrial contraction falls earlier in the diastolic phase, its dynamic effect may augment passive ventricular filling, and this may amplify or initiate gallop sounds, which are called *summation gallop* sounds.

In *second-degree block*, some or many of the supraventricular impulses fail to reach the ventricles. Beats may be dropped regularly or irregularly, and as the block increases, two or more successive beats are not transmitted (Fig. 14). As the ventricular rate slows, escape beats appear, and with increasing block, these become the dominant mechanism with only an occasional transmitted beat to disturb the rhythm of an otherwise complete block. Instability is the rule rather than the exception in second-degree block. A change to first-degree block or to complete heart block may occur in a short space of time with changes in atrial rate, in vagal tone, or in degree of anoxia. When ventricular beats are dropped, the PR interval after the dropped beat is usually relatively short, then progressively prolonged in subsequent beats until another beat is dropped. This stepwise sequence is known as the *Wenckebach phenomenon*. Second-degree block may sometimes be identified by observation of atrial waves in the neck veins, or by beat-to-beat changes in heart sound intensity or in gallop sounds.

In some instances one or more P waves are not followed by a ventricular response without significant variation of PR interval in the conducted beats (Mobitz block). This block is lower in the conduction system and has a more hazardous prognosis than Wenckebach block. Not infrequently two of the three conduction conduits to the ventricles have ceased to function, as for example when right bundle branch block is associated with left axis deviation resulting from block of the anterior division of the left bundle branch, a frequent precursor of Mobitz or bilateral bundle branch block.

With further conduction impairment, *third-degree* or complete heart block occurs. Survival demands an escape mechanism: an *idioventricular* focus below the block. It may be in the lower-most portion of the AV bundle or in the bundle of His, in which case (unless bundle branch block is also present) the QRS complexes will resemble those of conducted beats. If it is below the bifurcation, as is more common, the QRS will be bizarre in configuration as in ventricular premature beats. The ventricular beat is usually at a rate of 28 to 42, but may be 20 or less or as fast as 60 to 70. The beat-to-beat interval often varies slightly, but, over a period of time, considerable changes of rate occur. In rare instances, the rate rises appreciably with exertion or emotion, and it almost always rises temporarily in those who have been given isoproterenol (Fig. 15).

Complete heart block should always be suspected when the ventricular rate is below 50. Atrial venous waves beating independently of the ventricular contractions may sometimes be seen.

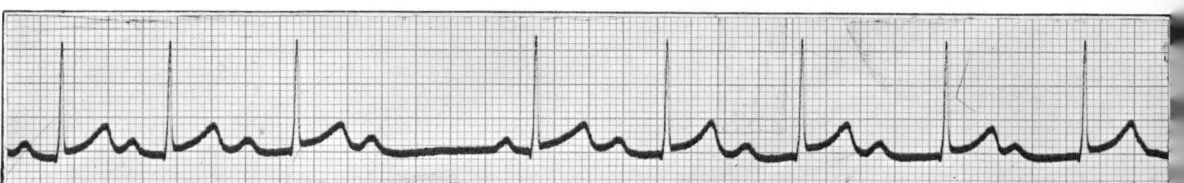

FIGURE 14. Second degree A-V block with Wenckebach phenomenon. Sinus arrhythmia. P-R interval 0.24 in beat 1, 0.26 in beat 2, 0.34 in beat 3. The P wave in beat 4 is not conducted to the ventricles. A short P-R (0.20) resumes in beat 5 and becomes progressively longer in succeeding beats.

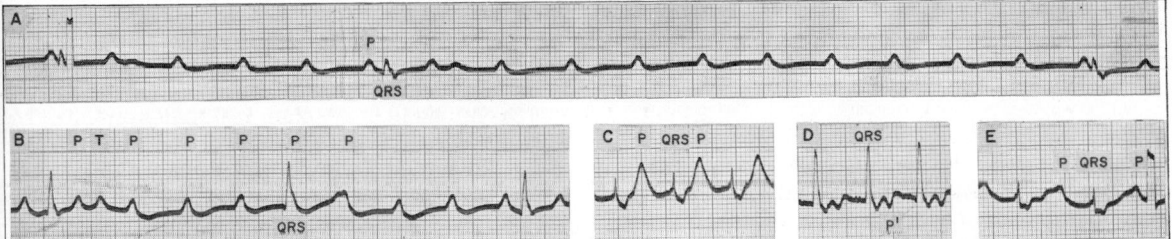

FIGURE 15. A-V block with syncope. Treatment with intravenous isoproterenol. *A*, Complete A-V block. Atrial rate 110. Ventricular rate average 14, rhythm irregular. Broad (0.13 second), bizarre QRS bear no temporal relation to P waves. *B*, Isoproterenol 5 mg./L, i.v. at 1 ml./min. for 10 minutes. Complete A-V block. Atrial rate 132. Ventricular rate 30, regular rhythm. QRS narrower, completely dissociated temporally from P waves. Ectopic focus in lower A-V node or common bundle. *C*, After 20 minutes at 1 ml./ minute. First degree A-V block. Atrial rate 120. P waves obscured in T waves. PR about 0.30. Right bundle branch block. Infusion slowed to 0.5 ml./minute. *D*, Five minutes later. Nodal rhythm with tachycardia (rate 140). Retrograde P waves with R-P interval of 0.11. QRS resembles B. Infusion stopped. *E*, Thirty minutes later. First degree A-V block. Rate 98. PR 0.28. QRS as in *C*.

Intermittently, when atrial and ventricular contraction coincide, regurgitated atrial blood causes a giant venous wave. When the atrial contraction immediately precedes that of the ventricle, the ensuing heart sound is unusually loud (cannon sound). This is usually attributed to a favorable positioning of the AV valves for maximal sound generation in closure. The arterial pulse wave of such a beat is larger than that of other beats. Conversely, first heart sounds are faint and pulse waves are weak when atrial contraction long precedes ventricular contraction. A widened pulse pressure may be expected, as in any bradycardia. Cardiac size is increased not only because of the intrinsic heart disease but also as a direct result of the protracted diastole with augmented ventricular filling. The cardiac output is usually reduced when complete AV block is present. To a considerable extent the reduction may be attributed to the usually associated heart disease. At rates below 40, cardiac output is always low, and the hypodynamic influence of the bradycardia per se is progressive as the rate falls.

Severe bradycardia, with a rate under 35, is almost always symptomatic. Weakness, faintness, dyspnea, and congestive failure are commonly present. The hazards of complete AV block relate not only to the direct physiologic effects of the bradycardia, but to the pronounced predilection of these patients to have changes in ventricular mechanism (severe bradycardia or arrest or ventricular tachycardia, flutter, or fibrillation) that result in syncope or sudden death.

Treatment. Factors in therapy include type and severity of underlying heart disease, degree of block, functional incapacity resulting from the bradycardia per se, and occurrence of syncopal seizures. Extracardiac factors, e.g., anoxia or vagotonic drugs, should be eliminated if possible. When the block is due to an acute inflammatory disorder, as in acute rheumatic fever, steroids are indicated. Atropine (0.5 to 1.0 mg. subcutaneously) should usually be tried. Ephedrine (30 to 60 mg. orally every four to six hours) may be of some benefit, but when used in effective doses it usually causes disturbing psychic stimulation and may predispose to ventricular fibrillation. Epinephrine (3 to 5 ml. of 1:1000 solution subcutane-

ously) is more effective, but also more hazardous. Of the sympathomimetic drugs, isoproterenol is the safest and most effective. Unless the dosage is excessive, it may be given with little danger that it will induce ventricular tachycardia or fibrillation. In fact, these hazards are definitely reduced by the drug in patients with complete heart block. Isoproterenol has relatively little effect upon the peripheral circulation. Its cardiac effects are multiple. Contractile force is increased and atrioventricular conductivity is enhanced. If complete heart block persists after the drug has been given, the higher idioventricular pacemakers are selectively excited. This may result in the establishment of a new focus with a faster rate and a reduced proclivity for arrest, tachycardia, or fibrillation. Sublingual isoproterenol, 10 to 15 mg., usually exerts effects upon heart rate and force of contraction in 10 to 20 minutes. The obvious evidences persist for 30 to 90 minutes, but even after the rate has returned to the premedication level, effects upon AV conductivity and upon the ventricular level of the pacemaker, and inhibition of chaotic rhythms may continue for three to five hours. Sustained-action oral tablets have been introduced. In emergencies, isoproterenol may be given intravenously (about 1 to 2 ml. per minute of a solution of 5 mg. in 500 ml. of glucose is usually sufficient to sustain an adequate ventricular rate) for short periods or for several days. Alternatively, it may be given intramuscularly in doses of 0.1 to 0.5 mg. Sodium lactate in molar or half-molar solution may be a useful emergency measure for severe bradycardia or arrest, especially if hyperkalemia is responsible. Doses of 10 to 15 ml. per minute up to 100 ml. may be given. Larger doses may be given over a period of several hours.

Although syncopal seizures caused by second or third degree heart block may occasionally be averted completely by maintenance of a rigid schedule of medication, especially of isoproterenol, a pacemaker (*vide infra*) is usually indicated in chronic disease states, and occasionally in acute problems.

Digitalis is not, of course, given as therapy for AV block, but neither is it necessarily contraindicated. In AV block of any degree, digitalis may be given if congestive failure is present unless evidence indicates that the block has been caused by digitalis. If so, the drug is discontinued and potassium therapy is instituted as described previously.

SHORT P-R INTERVAL WITH WIDENED QRS COMPLEXES
(Anomalous, Accessory or Accelerated AV Conduction; Pre-excitation; Wolff-Parkinson-White Syndrome)

The term Wolff-Parkinson-White syndrome is appropriate especially when recurrent paroxysmal tachycardia is associated with the electrocardiographic abnormality. A congenital defect in AV conduction is probably present in all cases, and a familial incidence has been observed. The electro-

cardiographic pattern occurs in approximately 0.1 to 0.4 per cent of the tracings recorded, depending upon the rigidity of the diagnostic criteria and the selection of cases. The syndrome is more common in males than in females and may be present at any age.

This disorder is important because 25 to 50 per cent of those who have the electrocardiographic pattern also have recurrent paroxysmal tachycardia. In addition, the pattern may obscure electrocardiographic evidences of other disease states or, if not recognized, may lead to erroneous diagnosis of infarction, bundle branch block, or nodal rhythm. It should be suspected in all persons who have recurrent paroxysmal tachycardia and indeed is found in 5 to 10 per cent of patients with that disorder. Otherwise, it has no distinguishing clinical features and the diagnosis

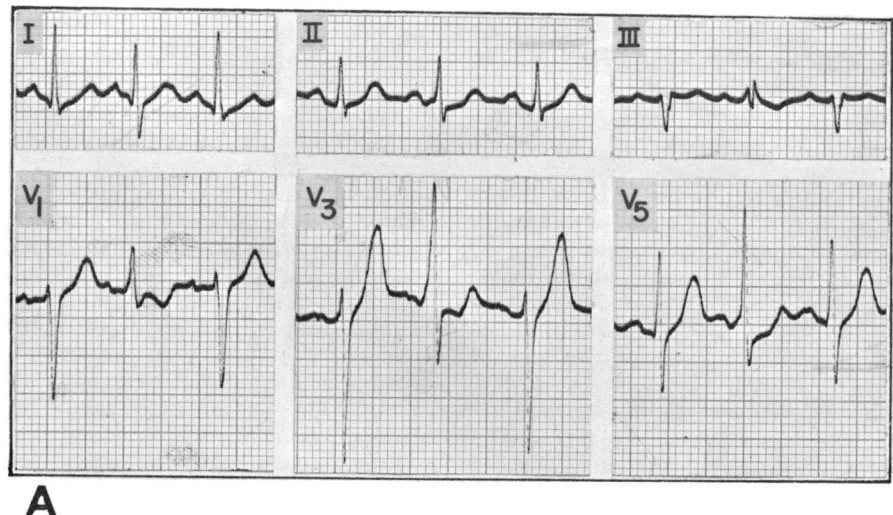

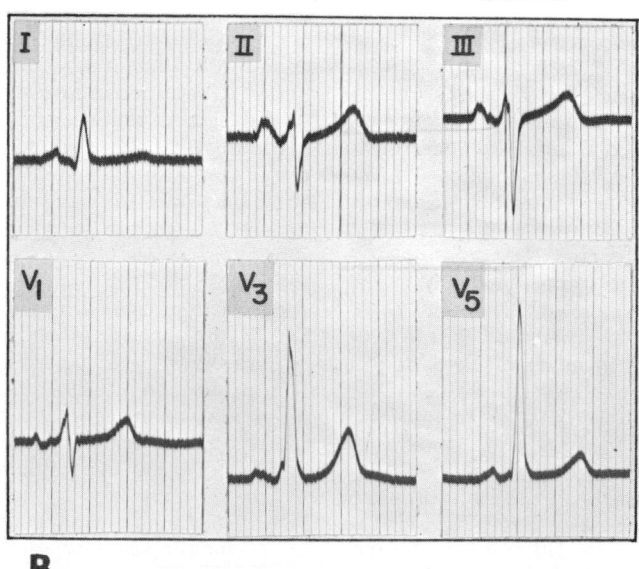

FIGURE 16.   Accessory (anomalous, accelerated) A-V conduction.

A, Healthy male, age 31. The middle beat of each record is abnormal with short (0.09) P-R interval and relatively broad (0.11) and deformed QRS complexes. Slurred R upstroke (delta waves) in II and chest leads. RST and T abnormalities in abnormal beats. Regular alternation of normal and abnormal beats in this tracing. At other times all beats normal or all abnormal.

B, Male, age 42, healthy except for many attacks of paroxysmal tachycardia. P-R 0.12 is not as short as is commonly observed in this disorder. Deformed QRS complexes with delta waves. *Wolff-Parkinson-White syndrome.*

is entirely based upon the electrocardiogram (Fig. 16). The classic features are P waves of normal configuration; P-R interval of 0.10 second or less; widening and deformity of the early portions of the QRS complexes with resulting delta waves especially in those leads that are predominantly monophasic; normal or slightly shortened total PQRS duration; T wave deformity approximately parallel in degree to the QRS deformity. In some persons these electrocardiographic abnormalities are present only intermittently, sometimes coming and going from beat to beat, or alternately present or absent for long periods of time. In the majority of instances, an electrocardiographic defect is constantly present, with or without some variation in the degree of abnormality. Quinidine, atropine, amyl nitrate, sympathomimetic amines, and exercise have some tendency to normalize, and digitalis and carotid sinus stimulation some tendency to accentuate, the electrocardiographic pattern, but these effects are highly inconstant.

During attacks of paroxysmal tachycardia, the widening of QRS usually disappears, and neither the electrocardiographic pattern nor the clinical features can be distinguished from supraventricular tachycardia of the ordinary variety. Rarely the QRS remains broad during attacks, which are particularly likely to be protracted, and differentiation from ventricular paroxysmal tachycardia may be difficult. Other arrhythmias, especially atrial fibrillation, are more common among persons with the pre-excitation pattern than in the normal population; rarely, sudden death may occur.

This disorder results from a dual pathway of the transmission of impulses from atrium to ventricle. In addition to the normal pathway via the AV node and bundle, an accessory pathway exists, either remote from the AV bundle or contained within it. Transmission in the accessory pathway is not subject to the normal physiologic delay of the AV node. As a result, a portion of the ventricle is prematurely activated. It is assumed that, when paroxysmal tachycardia occurs, the impulse descends via the normal pathway to the ventricles and re-enters the atrium via the accessory pathway, establishing a self-perpetuating circus. Both the electrocardiographic abnormality and the paroxysmal tachycardia have been simulated in animals by providing an accessory AV pathway and appropriate electronic circuitry. The occasional appearance of an electrocardiographic abnormality of this type during cardiac catheterization or induction of anesthesia has not been satisfactorily explained; perhaps a latent anomaly is activated.

Treatment and prophylactic measures relate entirely to the paroxysmal tachycardia. It is managed in the same way as the ordinary variety, except that quinidine is somewhat more likely to help, and digitalis less likely to do so. In a very few instances, the anomalous path has been sectioned surgically.

DISORDERS ARISING IN THE VENTRICLES

Bundle Branch Block. The downward progress of the wave of excitation is obstructed in either the right or the left branch of the AV bundle. In either case, the normal sequence of ventricular activation is disturbed. Anatomically, the right bundle branch is a discrete group of conducting fibers parallel and proximate to each other for an appreciable length. On the left, the bundle divides into an anterior and a posterior division. Block of various combinations of one or the other division, with or without right bundle branch block, can now be recognized by electrocardiography. Complete left bundle branch block requires a much more widely distributed lesion than on the right. Right bundle branch block is sometimes a congenital lesion, and it is occasionally a random discovery in the routine electrocardiographic examination of an apparently healthy adult. When acquired, coronary occlusive disease, especially of the right coronary artery, is the most common cause. Left bundle branch block is almost invariably acquired; it is also most common in association with arteriosclerotic heart disease. Neither right nor left bundle branch block has an important influence upon cardiac

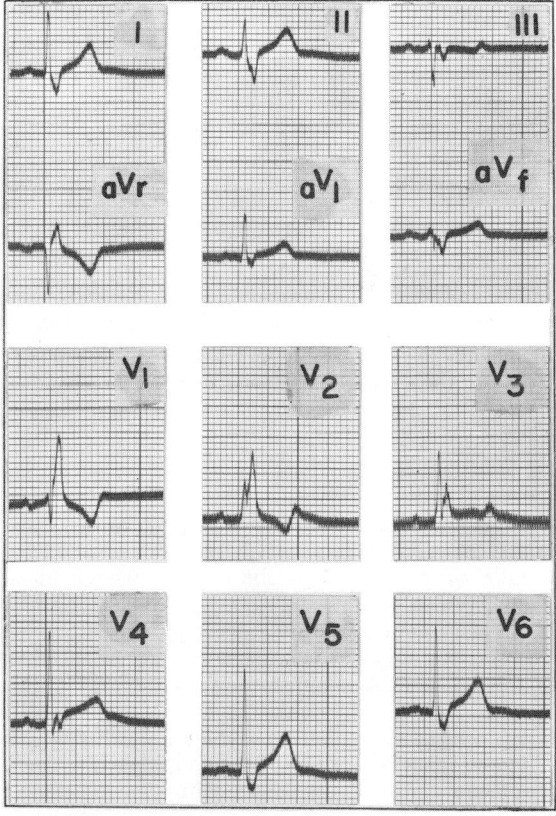

FIGURE 17. Right bundle branch block. Increase in QRS duration to 0.12 second or more. Deformity of the late portions of the QRS in all leads with a tall, broad R' in V₁ and broad S wave in V₆. T waves normal or nearly so in all leads except V₁-V₃.

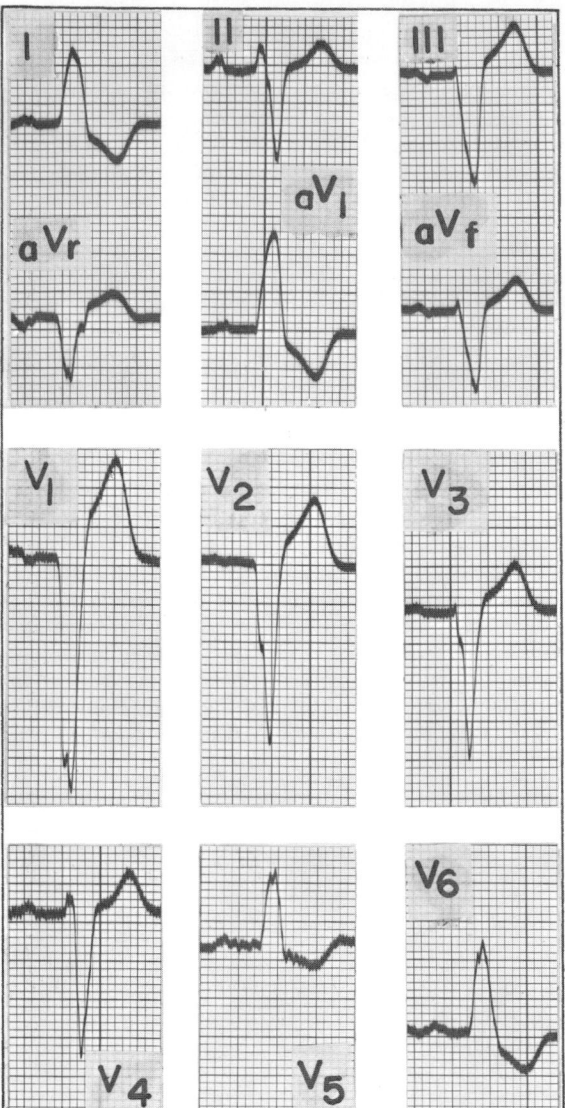

FIGURE 18. Left bundle branch block. QRS duration 0.12 second or more. Deformity of all portions of all QRS complexes with a slowly rising, broad R in V_6 and deep Q (with or without a small R) in V_1. RST elevated and T waves abnormally large in direction opposite to principal QRS deflection.

CLOSED CHEST RESUSCITATION; ELECTRICAL DEFIBRILLATION AND CONVERSION; PACEMAKERS

These are now standard tools in the management of many major acute and chronic arrhythmia problems. A circulation sufficient to sustain life for periods of as long as an hour may be induced by rhythmic manual compression of the sternum, while respiration is sustained by mouth-to-mouth breathing. Ventricular fibrillation, if responsible for the circulatory arrest, may be terminated by one or more electrical shocks administered through electrodes placed upon the chest, with current delivered from a defibrillator. The appropriate equipment is now available in almost all hospitals, usually in conjunction with the apparatus used for conversion of other arrhythmias to normal sinus rhythm. The use of this apparatus, usually called a *cardioverter*, is especially indicated as an emergency measure in the treatment of patients in shock or with pulmonary edema, or when these are impending, with rapid ventricular rates resulting from ventricular tachycardia or supraventricular tachycardia that does not respond promptly to appropriate medications. It is not to be used in sinus tachycardia. In arrhythmias (other than ventricular fibrillation) caused by digitalis toxicity, cardioversion should be used only in the most pressing emergencies, when potassium and other measures have failed, since a lethal ventricular fibrillation, unresponsive to further shock, may be induced. If used for digitalis toxicity, the apparatus should be set for low output (50 watt-seconds).

The apparatus energizes large electrodes placed on the front and back of the chest delivering 100 to 400 watt-seconds in a single brief discharge to the lightly anesthetized patient. The discharge is triggered to occur during the early part of ventricular depolarization, to avoid the induction of ventricular fibrillation. It is discharged manually when ventricular fibrillation is already present, since no appropriate ventricular signal is present to trigger the discharge. Defibrillation and cardioversion have largely displaced intensive drug therapy for the conversion of hazardous arrhythmias, but concomitant drug therapy is almost always necessary to sustain the conversion.

Cardioversion is commonly used as an elective measure for the conversion of atrial fibrillation to normal sinus rhythm. Occasionally, it is employed in atrial flutter or protracted supraventricular paroxysmal tachycardia. Quinidine is given in a dose of 0.6 gram shortly before the procedure and is continued in a dose of 0.2 gram every four hours for 24 hours; this is followed by long-term suppressive therapy. Digitalis should be canceled

function, although functional impairment is commonly a part of the disease responsible for the bundle branch block. Right bundle branch block is entirely an electrocardiographic diagnosis since it is not manifested clinically. Left bundle branch block commonly causes reduplication of the first heart sound and paradoxical splitting (in expiration) of the second sound. The two types of bundle branch block have distinctive electrocardiographic patterns (Figs. 17 and 18). The prognosis and treatment are those of the underlying heart disease.

for 24 hours before the procedure, and attempted conversion should be postponed if digitalis toxicity is suggested. About 90 per cent of patients will be successfully converted, but only about 50 per cent can be maintained in sinus rhythm on long-term quinidine therapy. The percentage of sustained success is appreciably higher in patients with good heart function, in those with small hearts, in those in whom the arrhythmia has been present for a few months or less, and in those in whom the basis for the arrhythmia has been ameliorated (postoperative mitral stenosis) or removed (thyrotoxicosis). The percentage is lower in those with major functional impairment, large hearts, protracted arrhythmias, rheumatic lesions other than pure mitral stenosis, ischemic heart disease, or cardiomyopathies. Embolism may occur in rare instances (less than 5 per cent), often some hours after the conversion, usually as a transient benign event, but sometimes extremely serious. In those with a past history of embolism, especially if repeated, anticoagulants should be given for two months before conversion is attempted. Ventricular fibrillation may occur as an immediate complication; if so, fibrillation, unresponsive to further shock, may be induced.

Pacemakers are now widely employed in the prevention of syncopal seizures associated with circulatory arrest, usually in those with intermittent or sustained atrioventricular block. A catheter with electrodes at the tip is inserted into the right ventricle via the jugular vein, and the leads are coupled to an external pacer. This form of pacer is especially useful in acute problems, as in myocardial infarction with heart block, but it has been used for months or years in many patients. Local irritation or infection, embolism despite anticoagulants, and ventricular perforation are among the complications. When such a pacer fails, the batteries may be exhausted, the lead wires may be broken, or the catheter tip may have become dislodged into the atrium or pulmonary artery. Commonly, electrode-tissue resistance rises in time and the current must be increased, or, if the rate is set too slow, paroxysms of ventricular premature beats are seen. Implanted pacemakers are now generally used when the indication is other than temporary. Several varieties are available. Infection is less likely, and the patient is not encumbered with apparatus, but when function becomes defective, repair is more difficult. A fine catheter that may be floated into the heart via the veins is now in use for emergency pacing in intensive care units.

Various types of electronic circuitry are used to drive the heart. For the most part, fixed rate pacemakers are used for permanent complete heart block. Demand pacemakers fire at any time that the ventricle has not been activated spontaneously at a sufficient rate. They are used when block or bradycardia is intermittent.

Biggers, J. T., Jr., Schmidt, D. H., and Kutt, H.: Relationship between plasma level of diphenylhydantoin sodium and its cardiac antiarrhythmic effects. Circulation, 38:363, 1968.

Brody, D. A., Harris, T. R., and Romans, W. E.: A simple method for obtaining esophageal electrocardiograms of good quality. Amer. Heart J., 50:923, 1955.

Epstein, S. E., and Braunwald, E.: Beta adrenergic receptor blocking drugs. New Eng. J. Med., 275:1106, 1966.

Furman, S., Escher, D. J. W., and Solomon, N.: Experience with myocardial and transvenous pacemakers. Amer. J. Cardiol., 23:66, 1969.

Gianelly, R., Griffin, J. R., and Harrison, D. C.: Propranolol in the treatment and prevention of cardiac arrhythmias. Ann. Intern. Med., 66:667, 1967.

Jelliffe, R. W.: An improved method of digoxin therapy. Ann. Intern. Med., 69:703, 1968.

Kay, C. F.: The clinical use of digitalis preparations. Circulation, 12:116, 291, 1955.

Lasser, R. P., Haft, J. I., and Friedberg, C. K.: Relationship of right bundle branch block and marked left axis deviation (with left parietal or peri-infarction block) to complete heart block and syncope. Circulation, 37:429, 1968.

Lau, S. H., Damato, A. N., Berkowitz, W. D., and Patton, R. D.: A study of atrioventricular conduction in atrial fibrillation and flutter in man using His bundle recordings. Circulation, 40:71, 1969.

Lown, B., Kosowsky, B. D., and Klein, M. D.: Pathogenesis, prevention, and treatment of arrhythmias in myocardial infarction. Circulation, 40 (Supp. IV):261, 1969.

Rosenbaum, M. B., Elizari, M. V., and Lazzari, J. O.: Intraventricular trifascicular blocks. Amer. Heart J., 78:450, 1969.

Schamroth, L.: Principles governing 2:1 AV block with interference dissociation. British Heart J., 31:980, 1969.

Pericarditis*

James V. Warren

Pericardial disease may occur as an isolated process or as a subordinate and clinically unsuspected manifestation of disease elsewhere in the body. Acute pericarditis is an inflammatory process involving the pericardium, at times accompanied by an outpouring of fluid into the pericardial sac. This fluid may be serous, exudative, bloody, or purulent, depending upon the cause. This is *pericardial effusion,* which also may result from noninflammatory disturbances of fluid balance or hemorrhage. If it occurs with rapidity or in great amounts, impairment of the circulation may result, and *pericardial tamponade* is said to exist. Chronic fibrotic disease of the pericardium, causing impairment of heart function, is called *constrictive pericarditis.*

*The assistance of Drs. James J. Leonard and Arnold M. Weissler in preparation of this article is gratefully acknowledged.

ACUTE PERICARDITIS

Etiology. Pericarditis has many causes such as bacterial infection, viral infection, chemical changes, or poorly understood diseases such as systemic lupus erythematosus. The more common of these are enumerated in the accompanying table.

Pathologic Physiology. The basic lesion is an acute inflammatory process involving the pericardium. The visceral pericardium and part of the parietal pericardium are not supplied with pain nerve fibers, but the diaphragmatic and the lower parietal pericardium are so supplied. This would appear to account for the variable nature of the pain noted in pericarditis and for its occasional absence. There may be inflammatory involvement of contiguous structures, particularly pleura and lung. The myocardium is frequently involved, which probably accounts for the electrocardiographic changes in pericarditis and, in part, for cardiac enlargement. Unless pericarditis is associated with appreciable myocardial disease, an arrhythmia, or pericardial tamponade, there is no circulatory impairment.

Clinical Manifestations. Pericardial disease may be present without symptoms. *Pain*, the most frequent symptom, is variable in expression. If present, it is usually precordial rather than substernal, and may vary greatly in intensity. At times it is relatively superficial, but on other occasions is deep, simulating that seen in myocardial infarction. It is frequently varied by respiration and is often relieved by leaning forward or turning, and worsened by recumbency. At times it may have the radiation characteristic of pain accompanying myocardial ischemia, that is, to the left arm, neck, or shoulder. Often it is worsened by coughing. Because of proximity to the esophagus, there may be pain on swallowing. With large effusions there may be a heavy or "dragging" sensation in the lower thoracic region. *Dyspnea* is common, but frequently difficult to explain. In some instances it seems related to associated pleuritic involvement. General symptoms of *fever, chills, fatigue,* and the noxious *effects of systemic infection* are present in many instances, depending on the nature of the underlying disorder.

Physical Examination. The most striking physical sign of pericarditis is the pericardial friction

CAUSES OF ACUTE PERICARDITIS

1. Acute nonspecific pericarditis
2. Pericarditis due to living agents
   a. Tuberculous
   b. Purulent
   c. Protozoal
   d. Mycotic
   e. Viral
3. Connective tissue disorders and allergic diseases
4. Chemical and metabolic disturbances
5. Neoplastic processes
6. Myocardial infarction and heart disease
7. Trauma

rub. This auscultatory finding, often described as sounding like the creaking of bending leather, is superficial and "close to the ear." It varies considerably with position and respiration and may come and go as the patient is observed, over a period of hours. It is best heard with the diaphragm of the stethoscope tightly applied to the thorax. When fully developed it has at least three components that give it a "to-and-fro" character: the first, presystolic related to atrial contraction, the second caused by ventricular systole, and the third in early diastole associated with rapid ventricular filling. When it is incompletely developed, and when there is variability with respiration, one should suspect a so-called pleuropericardial rub. The true pericardial rub remains present with transient cessation of respiratory activity. Usually the heart sounds in pericarditis are of good quality, but at times, in the presence of an effusion, they are muffled and distant. Especially in the presence of effusion or constriction there may be a loud early diastolic extra heart sound, sometimes called a pericardial knock. This sound appears to be a variant of the normal third heart sound or the so-called ventricular gallop sound. When pericardial effusion or appreciable myocardial involvement is present, there may be signs of increased heart size. In acute pericarditis unaccompanied by pericardial tamponade, neither venous pressure elevation nor paradoxical pulse is present.

Diagnosis. The "to-and-fro" friction rub is the most characteristic clinical finding indicating presence of pericarditis. It should be differentiated from a pleuropericardial rub, the so-called xiphosternal crunch, the sound of mediastinal emphysema (Hamman's sign), and certain types of relatively high-pitched murmurs. If the friction rub is not present, a sudden increase in heart size may be the key to diagnosis. Without either of these findings, and in the absence of tamponade or constriction, the diagnosis may be exceedingly difficult.

Laboratory Studies. Laboratory studies may indicate the systemic reactions to inflammation or the presence of an underlying disease process. The leukocyte count is often elevated. The serum enzymes are not elevated unless there is appreciable myocardial involvement. The *electrocardiogram* frequently yields useful information. Early, the characteristic pattern is concordant upward displacement of the RST junction and the S-T segment without T wave inversion. The vector of this injury current is directed toward the apex. Later, irregular abnormalities of the T wave appear with inversion indicating delayed repolarization. The T vector now tends to point away from the apex. These findings occur only when pericarditis is active, and often are detected only by serial tracings. When the above sequence of electrocardiographic alterations appears, it can usually be differentiated from the changes caused by myocardial infarction or digitalis administration, but if not fully developed this differentiation may be difficult.

Roentgenographic studies usually demonstrate a normal cardiac silhouette, but may show evidence of increase in heart size if there is myocardial involvement or effusion. This at times is demonstrated only if serial roentgenograms have been obtained. Pericardial fluid in amounts of more than 200 to 300 ml. causes roentgenographic changes; there is a tendency for the lower part of the cardiac silhouette to bulge outward and form a pear-shaped or "water-bottle"-shaped heart. There may be diminished cardiac pulsations along the lateral margin of the heart silhouette, but this may occur in other causes of cardiac enlargement. Other diagnostic procedures are available if fluid is present; these will be described later under Pericardial Effusion.

Course. The course of pericarditis depends upon the underlying disease. In myocardial infarction it may be transient, mild, and asymptomatic, whereas other conditions such as tuberculous pericarditis may be severe and lead to death. So-called acute benign pericarditis is particularly likely to relapse. Some forms of pericarditis, such as tuberculous and staphylococcal, may become chronic and lead to pericardial constriction of the heart.

Therapy. Therapy depends upon the nature of the underlying disease. In many instances appropriate general therapy is adequate for management of pericarditis. So-called acute benign pericarditis, despite some reports of improvement with antimicrobials, appears best treated by simple supportive means. Specific infectious agents should be treated with appropriate medications. At times, but to a decreasing degree, open surgical drainage of the pericardium may be necessary in the management of purulent pericarditis.

INDIVIDUAL FORMS OF PERICARDITIS

Rheumatic Pericarditis. Pericarditis is a serious manifestation of rheumatic fever, and usually indicates the presence of underlying heart disease. It is reported to occur in 3 to 13 per cent of patients with rheumatic fever. Associated with it are the more serious manifestations of rheumatic fever. It may or may not be accompanied by pericardial effusion.

Uremic Pericarditis. Pericarditis occurs in probably more than half of the patients with chronic renal failure and in somewhat fewer of those with acute renal insufficiency. Its pathogenesis is not clearly understood. The pericarditis is often asymptomatic and is not regularly accompanied by effusion; however, pain, bleeding into the pericardial sac, and pericardial effusion have been reported. Pericardial tamponade may occur. In general, pericarditis has been considered an ominous sign, but survival for months is not uncommon, and may be even longer with hemodialysis. It may be present and disappear in patients with reversible renal insufficiency. It is considered by some as a signal indicating the need for dialysis. The fluid balance and blood volume changes associated with dialysis introduce special problems in maintaining an adequate circulation in these patients.

Purulent Pericarditis. Purulent pericarditis is caused by a variety of bacteriologic agents, particularly staphylococci, pneumococci, and hemolytic streptococci. There is usually severe systemic reaction to the infectious process, and signs of pericarditis are well developed. There may be moderate amounts of purulent fluid, but it is usually not excessive. Appropriate antimicrobial therapy has reduced mortality to between 25 and 50 per cent. Surgical drainage is required much less frequently than in the past, predominantly in those patients whose infecting organism is insensitive to antimicrobial agents.

Tuberculous Pericarditis. The patient may or may not have clinical evidence of tuberculosis elsewhere. Presumably, the pericardial lesion results from a direct infection of the pericardium. At times there may be a rapid outpouring of fluid with minimal evidence of active infection of the pericardium itself. On the other hand, the infection may advance relentlessly and lead to relatively early constrictive pericarditis. The symptoms are often vague and insidious in onset. Pain may be absent or mild, rarely severe. At times it is related to the appearance of effusion. Diagnosis is established by aspirating the pericardial effusion and demonstrating the organisms either by culture or guinea pig inoculation. Although this was formerly a highly fatal illness, modern chemotherapeutic methods of treating tuberculosis have reduced the mortality to as low as 10 per cent.

Acute Nonspecific Pericarditis. This illness, which has been described under many names, is a form of acute pericarditis prone to recur, and of unknown cause. There is evidence that in some patients it is caused by viral infection. The patients are usually healthy persons who are stricken rapidly by pain associated with variable degrees of systemic reactions to infection. Frequently there is a history of an upper respiratory infection during the preceding two weeks. In a majority appreciable effusion does not occur, but it may occur and uncommonly may lead to pericardial tamponade. Rarely, if ever, does it lead to constrictive pericarditis. In the acute phase, the leukocyte count is elevated to 15,000 to 20,000, and classic electrocardiographic changes of pericarditis are usually present. Most authorities believe that antimicrobial and other specific methods of therapy are not of value.

Traumatic Pericarditis. Trauma to the pericardium through actual penetration of the chest wall or through nonpenetrating blows to the chest wall may result in pericardial irritation, the development of a friction rub, and at times bleeding into the pericardial sac. This may, on occasion, lead to pericardial tamponade. Following direct injury and particularly after surgical procedures on the heart, a syndrome apparently related to the development of hypersensitivity may result in pericarditis, friction rub, and pericardial effusion. There is usually a delay in onset of two or more weeks following injury. The clinical picture is similar to that of "acute nonspecific pericarditis." This has been found in some instances to be effectively treated by the use of steroid hormones.

Pericarditis with Myocardial Infarction. In the first few days following myocardial infarction, transient pericarditis is common. Clinically this is usually detected only by hearing a friction rub, and pain is rare. Uncommonly, pericardial effusion may occur, and in patients receiving anticoagulant therapy, a form of hemorrhagic pericarditis with bleeding into the pericardial cavity has been described. This may lead to tamponade and death. Fortunately, it is a most infrequent complication of anticoagulant therapy, but is serious when it occurs. During the months following myocardial infarction, various syndromes have been described characterized predominantly by recurrent bouts of precordial pain, apparently not due to myocardial ischemia and thought by some to be related to hypersensitivity reactions. This *postmyocardial infarction syndrome* may be confusing to the physician, and only on careful study can it be differentiated from extension or new myocardial infarction or other forms of pericarditis.

Pericarditis Associated with Neoplastic Disease. Various neoplastic diseases may involve the pericardium and cause pericarditis that is clinically significant. Carcinoma of the lung or breast and the lymphomas are perhaps the most frequent offenders. There may be direct gross implants in the pericardial sac, and resultant from these may be massive effusion or hemorrhage. Primary tumors of the pericardium also occur, but are rare. They also may give rise to bloody pericardial effusion. These neoplastic causes of pericardial effusion are often characterized by a persistent tendency to recur. If the diagnosis cannot be made by other means, the pathologic examination of the pericardial fluid may reveal the presence of tumor cells. In some instances, the instillation of tumor-depressing agents into the pericardial cavity has been recommended.

accumulates rapidly or there is inadequate stretch of the pericardium, pericardial tamponade occurs.

A pericardial effusion may be suspected on physical examination by enlargement of the area of cardiac dullness. Roentgenographically, the presence of pericardial effusion may be suggested by a tendency for the lower part of the cardiac silhouette to bulge outward and form a so-called "water-bottle" heart or by diminished cardiac pulsations along the lateral margins. However, these roentgenographic signs are not usually helpful in differentiating the enlarged cardiac silhouette of effusion from that due to cardiac enlargement. Often of diagnostic help is the finding that the lung fields are strikingly clear in pericardial effusion, in contrast to pulmonary congestion usually associated with the large and failing heart. Aside from the simple means previously noted, cardiac catheterization, angiocardiography, intravenous injection of carbon dioxide, techniques involving the use of ultrasound or the scanning of the precordium following the intravenous injection of radioisotopes have been utilized to demonstrate the normal-sized cavitary chambers when effusion is causing the enlarged cardiac silhouette.

If effusion is suspected, a pericardial paracentesis may be undertaken to demonstrate fluid and to sample it for diagnostic examination. The xiphoid or apical approaches, with the patient in the sitting position if possible, are usually preferable. Electrocardiographic monitoring appears to increase the safety factor in this potentially hazardous procedure. By such techniques the needle functions as an exploring unipolar electrode. When it touches the myocardium, gross injury currents are detectable in the specific lead. Although in emergency situations it may be done at the bedside, it is preferably carried out in a laboratory with radiologic and resuscitative support. At times, it is useful following pericardial paracentesis to instill air into the pericardial sac, or preferably carbon dioxide, so that roentgenograms can demonstrate the degree of thickening of the pericardial sac. This provides some index of the nature and chronicity of the disease process.

PERICARDIAL EFFUSION

Under the circumstances of acute pericarditis or in those states accompanied by generalized edema formation, such as cardiac failure and liver disease, there may be an outpouring of fluid into the pericardial cavity. In myxedema particularly, at times there is an accumulation of fluid in the pericardial space with massive pericardial effusion. This may produce a large increase in the cardiac silhouette detectable either by physical examination or roentgenogram. Often there is associated cardiomegaly. If the fluid accumulation is slow and the pericardium stretches, no impairment of the circulation occurs. If the fluid

CHRONIC PERICARDIAL EFFUSION

Although in most instances pericardial effusion appears suddenly and then subsides, there are a number of situations in which effusion persists over a period of time, even as long as ten years. It may be asymptomatic and discovered only by chance examination or roentgenography. The enlarged cardiac silhouette in the absence of symptoms may be the only diagnostic clue. Special studies such as angiography or other procedures noted earlier may be necessary to distinguish between cardiomegaly and pericardial effusion. Such chronic effusion often complicates underlying heart disease, may be related to pericardial neoplasm, or may be associated with a generalized disease process such as lupus erythematosus, scleroderma, or myxedema. At times, no specific cause can be identified. The electrocardiogram does not usually have the classic pattern of acute pericarditis, but there may be low voltage or other nonspecific alterations. The pericardial fluid is usually clear and straw-colored, but may have a high protein content approaching that of blood plasma. In some instances, the fluid may become blood-stained or frankly hemorrhagic. This may occur after repeated tapping. In patients with so-called *cholesterol pericarditis*, a special form of chronic pericardial effusion may occur. The fluid is often described as resembling gold paint, and it contains a large number of cholesterol crystals. This form is particularly common in myxedema, but may be seen in other forms of chronic effusion. Repeated pericardial paracenteses may not be effective in controlling the disorder. If this is the case, surgical therapy with either pericardial fenestration or pericardiectomy may be required.

PERICARDIAL TAMPONADE

Pericardial tamponade results when pericardial fluid accumulates rapidly or in amounts sufficient to produce enough increased intrapericardial pressure to impair cardiac filling and cause circulatory embarrassment. In this category should be included penetrating wounds of the heart such as stab wounds or those inflicted during bone marrow biopsy of the sternum, and bleeding into the pericardial sac caused by anticoagulant therapy.

Mild pericardial tamponade produces diagnostic signs with few or no symptoms. In more severe form, serious circulatory impairment occurs, and the clinical picture of shock with low arterial pressure, rapid pulse, and cold, clammy extremities develops. In contrast to other forms of shock, that complicating pericardial tamponade is accompanied by increased venous pressure so that the neck veins may be noticeably distended. At times a visible increase in venous pressure may occur on inspiration (Kussmaul's sign). There is frequently a *pulsus paradoxus* with waxing and waning of the arterial pressure on respiration, although the heart rate remains regular. Inspiration normally produces a slight fall in arterial pressure not exceeding 6 to 8 mm. of mercury. With a paradoxical pulse the change may be striking so that the pulse may actually disappear during the inspiratory phase. Small degrees of paradoxical pulse may best be determined by means of a blood pressure apparatus, listening as one keeps the cuff inflated near systolic pressure. It should be remembered that a paradoxical pulse may be found in other disorders, such as airway obstruction in bronchial asthma and in some cases of congestive heart failure or shock. In the latter instances, the finding is usually not prominent. The combination of pulsus paradoxus, high venous pressure, and normal heart size is practically diagnostic of pericardial disease.

The mechanism producing pulsus paradoxus has been the subject of debate for many years. It has been thought by some that the distended or fibrotic pericardium fails to transmit the normal respiratory variations in intrathoracic pressure to the interior of the heart, thus creating accentuation of the normal respiratory variations in ventricular output and blood pressure. More recent evidence indicates that when tamponade or pericardial constriction exists, inspiratory right ventricular filling is enhanced. Because of the limited space available for blood within the pericardial sac, there is less space available for left ventricular filling, and therefore left ventricular output is diminished, causing a transient fall in arterial pressure. In other words, there appears to be a competition for the available space within the now limited pericardial cavity. Changes in ventricular distensibility as a result of movement of the diaphragm have been suggested as an additional factor. Final resolution of the problem is not yet available. Nevertheless, it remains a valuable physical sign. Coupled with inspiratory congestion of the neck vein, it is a strong indicator of pericardial disease.

The diagnosis of pericardial tamponade calls for rapid removal of the fluid from the pericardium as described under Pericardial Effusion. In uncomplicated situations, the removal of a relatively small amount of fluid will result in immediate benefit. Further treatment of the disorder depends on the nature of the underlying disease. In uremic patients, changes in blood volume may occur in the course of dialysis which may endanger a patient with tamponade. Adequate filling pressure must be maintained to overcome the elevated intrapericardial pressure. In patients with penetrating wounds of the pericardium and heart, surgical therapy may be required if pericardiocentesis does not produce permanent improvement. Rarely, if fluid removal is impossible, intravenous fluids raising venous pressure or drugs causing venous constriction such as metaraminol (Aramine) are useful until more definitive therapy can be undertaken.

CHRONIC CONSTRICTIVE PERICARDITIS

Constrictive pericarditis is a chronic disorder of the pericardium characterized by interference with the heart's action and congestive circulatory failure.

Etiology. In the past, tuberculosis has been considered as the most frequent etiologic factor, although today studies appear to indicate that idiopathic forms are increasing in number. Specific agents, such as the Staphylococcus and other pyogenic organisms, histoplasmosis, neoplastic involvement, and tissue reactions to hemorrhage are among the other causes of constrictive pericarditis. It is of particular note that rheumatic fever and acute nonspecific pericarditis are considered to be causative only under the most unusual circumstances.

Pathologic Physiology. The constrictive process involving the pericardium interferes with diastolic filling of both the left and the right ventricles. It undoubtedly also interferes with their emptying. At times there has been evidence indicating that the obstruction results from involvement of a specific part of the heart or great vessels, but this is probably not common. It was originally thought that the process primarily affected the right side of the heart, but this has not been borne out by more recent studies. Although clinical evidence of pulmonary congestion is not common, pulmonary pressures have been found to be elevated. Pulmonary edema and paroxysmal nocturnal dyspnea are rare. Undoubtedly in all patients there is an element of myocardial involvement. At times this may be considerable, and it is important in determining the outcome of surgical procedures.

Clinical Manifestations. The symptoms often appear insidiously. It is predominantly a disease of adults; children are much less frequently affected. As in heart failure of any cause, respiratory symptoms and manifestations resulting from accumulation of edema are present. The accumulation of edema may become severe, particularly in the abdomen (ascites) and legs. At times a picture mimicking that of cirrhosis of the liver or the nephrotic syndrome is present. Respiratory symptoms are usually not striking; paroxysmal nocturnal dyspnea and pulmonary edema are rare. Although pain may be present in the active and early part of the disease as in other forms of pericarditis, it occurs only rarely otherwise. Cardiac arrhythmias, particularly atrial fibrillation, are occasionally present.

Physical Examination. The patient shows evidence of fluid retention. There is frequently venous distention and elevation of venous pressure. The heart may be only minimally enlarged or normal in size; only rarely is it grossly enlarged. The rate is usually increased and there may be atrial fibrillation. On auscultation, the heart sounds are usually not remarkable except for a striking early diastolic sound that occurs somewhat earlier and is much sharper than the conventional ventricular (protodiastolic) gallop rhythm. This is at times referred to as a pericardial knock. The arterial pressure is sometimes slightly reduced and the pulse pressure lessened, and there is frequently a pulsus paradoxus. Although there may be pleural effusion, signs of pulmonary congestion are usually minimal. There is often hepatomegaly.

Electrocardiogram. In most instances the total voltage of the QRS complexes is diminished and the T waves are frequently flattened or inverted. Atrial fibrillation is common. Otherwise no specific electrocardiographic changes are present. On roentgenographic examination, the silhouette of the heart is usually within normal limits or only moderately enlarged. The pulsations of the heart may be diminished dramatically. The superior vena cava is said to be prominent. In approximately half the patients with constrictive pericarditis, there is calcification of the pericardium. At times, this may be difficult to observe on the conventional anterior-posterior roentgenogram so that other views must be obtained. Careful fluoroscopy may be useful. Calcification of the pericardium, however, does not necessarily indicate the presence of constrictive pericarditis.

Laboratory findings reveal that the serum protein levels are often reduced, particularly the albumin fraction. Albuminuria may be present, but is usually not excessive. The venous pressure is frequently elevated, often dramatically, and the circulation time may be moderately prolonged. Studies by cardiac catheterization indicate normal arterial oxygen saturation. The cardiac output at rest is usually below conventional normal values and responds little to exercise, or in fact actually may decrease. The stroke volume is diminished and the cardiac output would be very low, except for the presence of tachycardia. Pressures in all chambers of the heart are usually elevated. Pressure tracings obtained from the right heart have been described as showing an M- or W-shaped contour with an early diastolic dip in pressure rising to a high plateau in presystole. Apparently this is caused by rapid filling of the ventricle early in diastole and its abrupt cessation caused by the cardiac constriction. Although such tracings were originally considered to be pathognomonic of constrictive pericarditis, they have also been described in various forms of diffuse myocardial disease with serious heart failure.

Differential Diagnosis. Constrictive pericarditis may present a clinical picture simulated by certain other forms of heart disease and also by noncardiac disease. Of the former, diffuse myocardial disease or advanced arteriosclerotic heart disease at times may present a similar clinical picture. In general, the increase in heart size is greater in these disorders than in constrictive pericarditis, and there is a greater prominence of symptoms related to the pulmonary circulation, such as paroxysmal nocturnal dyspnea. Complete studies often may be required for differentiation, and at times it is difficult even with these. Cirrhosis of the liver and the nephrotic syndrome may present a picture similar to that of constrictive pericarditis. In these clinical situations, however, the venous pressure is usually not elevated, and in the nephrotic syndrome there is usually more profuse albuminuria.

Treatment. The disease should be prevented if possible. For this reason there is increased interest in early therapy, both medical and surgical, particularly for those patients with acute pericardial disease known to be of a type predisposing to constrictive pericarditis. This is true especially of tuberculous pericarditis, in which chemotherapeutic agents have diminished the need for surgical treatment, either early or late.

If the clinical picture of fully developed constriction is present, surgery offers hope of benefit in about 60 per cent of patients. The mortality rate immediately following operation, formerly as high as 25 to 30 per cent, recently has dropped to levels of 10 to 15 per cent in most clinics. If there is a large element of myocardial degeneration, this may dispose toward less satisfactory surgical results.

When surgery cannot be attempted, or if it has been done and results have not been satisfactory, the patient with constrictive pericarditis must be managed medically. The value of digitalis has been debated, but there is enough evidence of myocardial involvement in most instances to warrant a trial of this medication. Diuretic therapy, as in ordinary congestive heart failure, may be used, and at times is extremely efficacious. Following the use of diuretic agents, the venous pressure often falls and edema is lessened.

Alfrey, A. C., Goss, J. E., Ogden, D. A., Vogel, J. H. K., and Holmes, J. H.: Uremic hemopericardium. Amer. J. Med., 45:391, 1968.

Bailey, G. L., Hampers, C. L., Hager, E. B., and Merrill, J. P.: Uremic pericarditis. Clinical features and management. Circulation, 38:582, 1968.

Beaudry, C., Nakamoto, S., and Kolff, W. J.: Uremic pericarditis and cardiac tamponade in chronic renal failure. Ann. Intern. Med., 64:990, 1966.

Bedford, D. E.: Chronic effusive pericarditis. Brit. Heart J., 26: 499, 1964.

Bishop, L. H., Jr., Estes, E. H., Jr., and McIntosh, H. D.: The electrocardiogram as a safeguard in pericardiocentesis. J.A.M.A., 162:264, 1956.

Dorhorst, A. C., Howard, P., and Leathart, G. L.: Pulsus paradoxus. Lancet, 1:746, 1952.

Evans, E.: Symposium on pericarditis. Amer. J. Cardiol., 7:1, 1961.

Feigenbaum, H., Waldhausen, J. A., and Hyde, L. P.: Ultrasound diagnosis of pericardial effusion. J.A.M.A., 191:711, 1965.

Golinko, R. J., Kaplan, N., and Rudolph, A. M.: The mechanism of pulsus paradoxus during acute pericardial tamponade. J. Clin. Invest., 42:249, 1963.

McGuire, J., Kotte, J. H., and Helm, R. A.: Acute pericarditis. Circulation, 9:425, 1954.

McKusick, V. A., and Harvey, A. McG.: Diseases of the pericardium. In Dock, W., and Snapper, I. (eds.): Advances in Internal Medicine. Chicago, Year Book Publishers, 1955, p. 157.

Disease of the Myocardium

Wallace Brigden

General Considerations. Many diseases of the heart which lead to failure of the pump and the circulation are initiated by mechanical faults concerned with valve defects, deprivation of fuel supplies, or increased cardiac work. However, the myocardium, though showing remarkable reserves, is eventually secondarily affected, and its failure often finally determines the course of events. This section is concerned with those rather less common conditions which are primarily localized in the myocardium leading to defective muscle function and its final failure.

These primary myocardial diseases are probably much more common than is generally recognized. Their true incidence is unknown because serious investigation into these disorders has developed only in the last two or three decades. Furthermore, diagnostic errors are common not only because physical signs are often inconspicuous, but also because symptoms and signs may suggest one of the more well known disorders which affect the heart of man. The incidence of primary myocardial diseases is greatly affected by socioeconomic and geographical factors, and it happens that primary myocardial diseases are most common in underprivileged parts of the world such as central Africa where sophisticated medical care with modern diagnostic methods is thinly spread.

Innumerable terms have been used for these disorders, but most are unsatisfactory and must remain so until the etiologic processes are fully understood. Primary myocardial disease indicates a process often of obscure etiology and is localized in the myocardium; cardiomyopathy indicates a somewhat wider range and includes processes which, although dominantly affecting the myocardium, may be of a generalized nature. Myocarditis, in keeping with usage of the suffix, should be restricted to disorders of an infectious or inflammatory nature. Myocardosis is an unsatisfactory term sometimes used to embrace all the noninflammatory processes. Classification is as unsatisfactory as terminology and for similar reasons. However, it is apparent that the myocardium may be damaged by any of the known disease processes which affect man; thus genetic, infective, metabolic, nutritional, and immunologic disorders may be found among the causes of cardiomyopathy. It would be rational, in such a classification, to include muscle disease resulting from vascular disorders, but habit and the magnitude of the problem have naturally led to isolation and separate consideration of coronary disease. However, there are rare cases of diffuse small vessel coronary occlusion which result in diffuse myocardial fibrosis causing clinical features which resemble other forms of cardiomyopathy. The following features concern primary myocardial disease in general.

Clinical Manifestations. The primary myocardial diseases present in diverse ways and clinical features, depending on the site, extent, and nature of the myocardial disorder and consequent disturbance of hemodynamics. Almost any of the symptoms and signs of heart disease (and any combination thereof) which arise in the whole field of heart disease may occur in the cardiomyopathies.

Dyspnea is the most common symptom. All

forms are met, but since most myopathies dominantly affect the left ventricle, orthopnea and nocturnal asthma are common. *Syncope* is especially likely to occur in those forms of myocardial disease which cause heart block and paroxysmal arrhythmia; it may also result from effort when there is outflow tract obstruction (see Hypertrophic Cardiomyopathy) as in other obstructive disorders of the cardiovascular system. *Cardiac pain* is not common, but when it occurs an erroneous diagnosis of coronary disease is often made. True angina is a feature of idiopathic hypertrophic subaortic stenosis (see below). Myocarditis, possibly when associated with pericarditis, may cause prolonged cardiac pain. Hepatic pain arising and increasing during effort may superficially resemble angina pectoris. *Palpitation* from frequent extrasystoles or other arrhythmia is common, especially in the familial forms, in alcoholic cardiomyopathy, and in myocarditis. Occasionally a primary muscle disorder may masquerade as an innocent paroxysmal tachycardia in the early stages of the disease process.

Physical examination and cardiovascular investigation may show any one of a number of dynamic disturbances which depend on the site and nature of the pathology. These may be classified in various ways. A division into congestive, constrictive, and hypertrophic (including obstructive) types, depending on the dominant hemodynamic derangement, has been suggested. From increasing experience with these conditions, it is clear that although there are such clear-cut hemodynamic disorders, there is also much overlap. However, the hypertrophic obstructive type is sufficiently discrete to be considered a separate and possibly single disease entity (see below).

Chronic hypokinetic heart failure (congestive type) occurs in many forms of primary myocardial disease, but is probably most common in post-inflammatory cardiomyopathy, active myocarditis, and familial cardiomegaly. The heart is very large and relatively "quiet" on fluoroscopy, and lung fields are often clear owing to right ventricular failure. All signs point to a chronic low cardiac output. At *necropsy* the heart weight is usually well above average, but the ventricular wall may appear thinner than normal because of the great dilatation. Macroscopic appearances of the muscle vary from normality to patchy fibrosis, and even large areas of damage may be found. Mural thrombi in varying stages of organization are common.

"Constrictive" forms of cardiomyopathy are not uncommon and cause confusion with constrictive pericarditis. This disorder is produced by restriction of ventricular filling because of diminished compliance of thick abnormal muscle or because of obstruction at the atrioventricular valves by masses of ventricular myocardium, or by massive endocardial thrombi and fibrosis (see Endomyocardial Fibrosis). However, in many cases of cardiomyopathy the resemblance to constrictive pericarditis is relatively superficial. The venous pressure is high, an early diastolic sound is usual, and the right ventricular pressure curve shows a sharp early diastolic dip coincident with the *y* descent and a late diastolic plateau of the J.V.P. The *x* descent of the venous pulse (or R.A. pressure pulse) is usually shallow in primary myocardial disease in contrast to constrictive pericarditis. Furthermore, the electrocardiogram in constrictive cardiomyopathy usually shows a very abnormal QRS-T, whereas in constrictive pericarditis the QRS tends to remain near normal. However, the greatest diagnostic difficulty arises in some forms of endomyocardial fibrosis when the bulk of the muscle mass may be relatively normal, resulting in a nearly normal QRS complex. Calcification of the pericardium is absent, but difficulty may arise when there is myocardial or endomyocardial calcification. Cardiac amyloidosis and the African form of endomyocardial fibrosis often cause features of the constrictive syndrome.

HYPERTROPHIC CARDIOMYOPATHY

A group of patients have primary myocardial disease which is essentially of a hypertrophic nature. This hypertrophy may be of such magnitude that it causes dynamic derangement of an *obstructive nature* which may embarrass inflow to, or outflow from, either ventricle. The clinical features, laboratory findings, and pathologic changes are sufficiently uniform to justify consideration of this condition as a single disease entity variously known as *asymmetrical hypertrophy, idiopathic hypertrophic subaortic stenosis,* and *hypertrophic obstructive cardiomyopathy.* The cause is unknown, but in at least 30 per cent of patients there is a strongly positive family history of the same disease.

Pathology. Necropsy shows great ventricular hypertrophy which is often asymmetrical, and the ventricular cavity tends to be obliterated. The heart weight is always above normal and often greatly so. Diffuse fibrosis may be apparent, but large areas of fibrosis are not usually seen. The microscopic picture is of a bizarre arrangement of large muscle fibers separated by connective tissue. Fibrosis is common in the center of the muscle bundles. Using histochemical methods and electron microscopy, Pearse found widespread dystrophy of grossly hypertrophic muscle fibers accompanied by glycogen storage and mitochondriosis. There is also abnormal shortness of myofibers, proliferation of connective tissue with functional hyperplasia of arterioles and capillaries, and a proliferation of sympathetic nerve fibers (sympathosis) with consequent noradrenosis. At the electron microscopic level there is a close resemblance of cardiomyopathic fibers to normal atrial fibers; thus there is a possibility that developmental abnormality lies behind the syndrome. However, the proliferation of the sympathetic nerves may indicate a primary role of the autonomic nervous system.

Etiology. It is clear that many patients with hypertrophic obstructive cardiomyopathy have familial cardiomyopathy (see below); however, in many cases there is no evidence of a familial disorder. A real division into familial and non-familial groups is supported by a different sex incidence which appears to be equal in the familial form, whereas males predominate in the non-familial forms. Furthermore, sudden death is much more common in the familial disease. It is possible that obstructive features may develop in any condition causing extreme ventricular hypertrophy associated with long survival. Thus it appears to be most common in congenital cardiomyopathy. Its rare appearance in such conditions as hypertensive heart disease and aortic valve disease is possibly due to the limited "natural history" imposed by other factors such as coronary disease.

Clinical Manifestations. The clinical features of obstructive cardiomyopathy depend on the site and severity of the obstruction, which is most commonly in the outflow of the left heart. Individuals of any age may be affected; although most commonly recognized in early adult life, the condition has been recognized in infants and in elderly subjects in whom diagnosis may be particularly difficult. The outstanding complaints in order of frequency are dyspnea, fatigue, cardiac pain, faintness, and syncope on effort; nocturnal dyspnea and palpitation are not uncommon.

A group of signs characterizes idiopathic hypertrophic subaortic stenosis: a fast rising pulse of bisferiens quality, a prominent fourth sound, a systolic murmur which may occur in early or late systole but never fills it, and sometimes an atrial systolic murmur. In contrast to valve stenosis an ejection click is absent. In some a palpable atrial pulse may be recognized in the precordium. In others a double precordial pulse may be due to two distinct phases of systole. The murmur and bisferiens pulse may be accentuated by the use of amyl nitrite. In many patients there is clear evidence of mitral incompetence, which may be due to distortion of the anterior mitral valve leaflet coupled with high ventricular pressure. Although the foregoing applies to the distinctive syndrome, it must be emphasized that there are many marginal cases and others in which a mixed picture of obstruction in the right ventricle overlaps with the subaortic obstructive syndrome.

The *electrocardiogram* shows clear evidence of left ventricular hypertrophy in most cases. P waves showing right and left atrial hypertrophy are common. In anterior chest leads deep S waves and sometimes Q waves are the result of great septal hypertrophy, and varying degrees of T wave abnormality are found in the left chest leads. Wolff-Parkinson-White syndrome has been reported in several patients. *Roentgenography* usually shows some cardiac enlargement and a rather globular silhouette. A bulge on the left border is common.

Diagnosis may be confirmed by *left heart catheterization* and *angiographic* examination. Studies of the left heart pressure pulses show that the degree of obstruction depends on the many factors which govern myocardial action and the resistance to systolic ejection. It is not surprising therefore that there is great variation in pressure gradients under changing circulatory conditions from day to day, and even from beat to beat. The aortic pressure pulse shows an early rapid rise followed by a dip and a second rise. Simultaneous left ventricular cavity and aortic pressure curves show that an increasing gradient develops during systole. Gradients across the right ventricular outflow tract are not uncommon. The *left ventricular angiocardiogram* shows the abnormal thickness of the wall in anterior and lateral projections. The cavity is narrowed, becoming slitlike in systolic films, and it is encroached upon by masses of hypertrophic muscle. Diminished relaxation of the ventricle in diastole may also be appreciated.

Obstruction to *right ventricular filling* from a very thick septum may be associated with idiopathic hypertrophic subaortic stenosis or may appear in almost pure form, resembling tricuspid stenosis. The clinical features of this condition are not uncommon in the African type of endomyocardial fibrosis in which the right ventricular cavity may be almost obliterated by massive mural thrombus. Obstruction to left ventricular filling by hypertrophic muscle, "rigid" muscle, or endomyocardial thrombi may produce clinical features resembling mitral stenosis. However, this is rare.

Pharmacodynamics. The effect of vasoactive drugs on this condition is of considerable interest. Digitalis glycosides cause an increase of the obstruction which may be due to their inotropic effect on the myocardium in the area of the obstruction. Exercise has a similar influence. Likewise isoproterenol with its powerful inotropic action causes an increase of obstruction; furthermore, in some patients isoproterenol provokes significant pressure gradients in the ventricle where there was no obstruction at rest. Nitroglycerin and amyl nitrite increase the obstruction, suggesting that these drugs may be contraindicated in obstructive myopathy. This effect may be due to lowered peripheral resistance and increased cardiac output. Beta-adrenergic blocking agents, e.g., propranolol, diminish the obstruction, and the increase of systolic gradient caused by exercise is reduced by beta-adrenergic blockade. However, these drugs have little effect on patients at rest.

Patients with idiopathic hypertrophic subaortic stenosis may be divided into five groups on the basis of their hemodynamic findings and responsiveness to drugs (Braunwald): (1) those who have intraventricular pressure gradients under all conditions; (2) those who have obstruction in the basal state, but in whom the gradient may be abolished by methoxamine and phenylephrine or angiotensin; (3) those with intermittent obstruction in the basal state; (4) those who do not have evidence of obstruction in the basal state but in whom obstruction develops with one of the provocative tests (isoproterenol, nitroglycerin, exercise, the Valsalva maneuver, or premature contractions); and (5) those with evidence of left ventricular hypertrophy who are relatives of patients in the first group but who do not develop obstruction under any circumstances.

Natural History. Many patients are apparently asymptomatic for many years. Even those with severe symptoms may undergo a period of remission, and symptoms may remain unchanged over a long period. Prognosis is difficult, but it appears to be less serious than might be anticipated from the severity of symptoms and signs. Sudden death is most likely to occur in the familial form and may occur in asymptomatic patients as well as in incapacitated ones.

Treatment. There is no effective treatment, but long-term medication with propranolol is under investigation. Restriction of physical activity should be advised as this may provoke arrhythmia, and it is known that the pressure gradient is increased by effort. A prolonged rest with sodium restriction or thiazide diuretics may help those with dyspnea or other evidence of heart failure. Digitalis is not advisable. Beta-adrenergic blocking drugs should be beneficial, but long-term results of treatment with these drugs are not available. *Surgical treatment* is indicated for patients with serious progressive symptoms from obstruction. Operative relief by resection of obstructing muscle or myotomy can be consistently accomplished even in severely ill patients, and survivors show striking symptomatic and hemodynamic improvement. Complete heart block is sometimes a complication of the operation, and postoperative left bundle branch block is usual though not invariable, and is not essential for a good result.

FAMILIAL CARDIOMYOPATHY

Some forms of primary myocardial disease are perhaps best regarded as congenital cardiomyopathy. These include so-called *idiopathic familial cardiomegaly, obstructive cardiomyopathy* (idiopathic hypertrophic subaortic stenosis), some forms of *endocardial fibroelastosis*, and certain hereditary neuromuscular disorders which also involve the myocardium.

Familial cardiomyopathy may be a single disease entity which presents in a variety of ways, including hypertrophic obstructive disorder (see above), congestive cardiac failure, and dysrhythmia. In some cases there is evidence of inheritance as a mendelian dominant, and transmission appears most commonly through the female parent, possibly because males die at a younger age; but there is no evidence of sex linkage. Birth order is not important, as most pedigrees suggest an erratic distribution in the family. It has been suggested that this may be the same disease as the cardiomyopathy associated with familial muscular dystrophies and ataxias, but the history of families with primary cardiomyopathies does not generally reveal other members with neuropathy. However, cardiomyopathy may be apparent before the development of neurologic features in Friedreich's ataxia and in myotonia, and a few families affected by neuropathy have been reported with only one member with cardiomyopathy alone. It has also been suggested that familial heart disease is a result of intrauterine myocarditis from an infection such as toxoplasmosis, but the evidence for this is poor. Organisms have not been found in the myocardium in familial cardiomegaly, although inflammatory reactions have been reported, and, on a priori grounds, it is unlikely that latent infection could persist through many generations, or be transmitted through the male as it is in some affected families.

At necropsy the heart is often very large, and heart weights tend to be greater in this condition than those found in other cardiomyopathies. Histologic examination shows giant fibers with vacuolation and varying amounts of fibrous tissue. Electron microscopy and histochemistry show interesting and possibly specific features at least in the variety presenting as subaortic obstructive myopathy.

The symptoms of familial cardiomyopathy include palpitation from arrhythmia, giddy attacks and syncope, either from arrhythmia or following effort in obstructive cardiomyopathy, and dyspnea from varying degrees of heart failure. The age at onset of symptoms is variable, but it is usually between 5 and 30 years. Pregnancy may precipitate heart failure in the last trimester or early in the puerperium, thus leading to an erroneous diagnosis of "puerperal cardiomyopathy." Sudden death in previously asymptomatic individuals is not uncommon and has been recorded in most writings on the subject. Various arrhythmias have been described in this condition, including atrial fibrillation, atrial flutter, multiple ventricular extrasystoles, and heart block.

As in other cardiomyopathies the electrocardiogram is not specific but gross conduction defects, left ventricular preponderance, and widespread Q waves are common. Radiology provides no special evidence in diagnosis, but some degree of cardiomegaly is usual, the left ventricle being most commonly affected. The left atrium is selectively enlarged when mitral valve regurgitation is a feature as in some cases. Angiography may show the characteristic appearance of left ventricular outflow tract obstruction in a minority; in others there is ventricular dilatation.

There is no specific treatment for familial cardiomyopathy. Arrhythmias are usually difficult to control. However, the poor prognosis of patients in heart failure may be considerably improved by prolonged rest, a low salt regimen, thiazide diuretics, and indefinite restriction of physical activity. Considerable reduction in heart size may be achieved by these means. Surgical treatment may be indicated when there is dominant left ventricular outflow obstruction (see Hypertrophic Cardiomyopathy).

INFLAMMATORY OR INFECTIVE CARDIOMYOPATHY
(Myocarditis)

The term "myocarditis" should be restricted to inflammatory disease of the myocardium. Clinicians have been reluctant to diagnose myocarditis, but there is no doubt that the myocardium may be damaged in many different infections of viral, rickettsial, bacterial, protozoal, and even metazoal origin. Myocarditis is mainly incidental in the course of a generalized infection and remains relatively unimportant. However, it may dominate the clinical picture and determine the outcome of the disease, and sometimes it appears to be "isolated" with no evidence of generalized infection. Fatal heart failure 'and sudden death may result from severe myocarditis, but most attacks are probably subclinical or mild and are easily overlooked by the unwary. The long-term effects of such infection may lead to myocardial damage and fibrosis, but such sequelae are difficult to investigate and prove. It is probable that idiopathic myocardial hypertrophy, diffuse myocardial fibrosis, subendocardial fibrosis, and idiopathic cardiomyopathy are in some instances the residue of previously unrecognized acute or subacute myocarditis. Such sequelae may follow any type of myocardial inflammation.

Fiedler's myocarditis is not a specific disease, and the eponym should be dropped. The lesions found in the heart muscle in hypersensitivity diseases, serum sickness, diseases of connective tissue, hypokalemia, and many other states without evidence of an infectious inflammatory nature are not classified here as myocarditis.

Clinical Manifestations. Clinical manifestations include almost the whole range of symptoms and signs found in heart disease. They clearly depend on the nature of the infection, the severity and site of the myocardial damage, the resistance of the host, the capacity of the damaged myocardium to recover, and other associated factors such as anemia, nutritional status, and the presence or absence of pre-existing cardiovascular disease.

In acute cases substernal discomfort and even pain (possibly due to accompanying pericarditis) are common. Dyspnea will depend on the degree of damage to left ventricular function. The most frequent physical signs of myocarditis are tachycardia, dysrhythmia, gallop rhythm, and evidence of developing congestive cardiac failure. The electrocardiogram provides good evidence of myocardial damage; it may show evidence of myocarditis before enlargement of the heart is seen on x-ray or before physical signs of abnormality appear.

Viral Myocarditis. Poliomyelitis, measles, mumps, viral pneumonias, encephalitis, infectious hepatitis, psittacosis, choriomeningitis, influenza A, rabies, varicella, and infectious mononucleosis may be complicated by myocarditis, but proof of direct viral invasion is almost invariably lacking. However, during the past decade there have been many reports of *Coxsackie Group B* myocarditis in infants and children, and as in suckling mice, it was thought that the virus was especially cardiotropic at this age. Coxsackie myocarditis does not produce a specific histologic picture, but interstitial edema, infiltration with mononuclear cells, and areas of myocardial necrosis are usual. The criteria for the diagnosis of a Coxsackie myocarditis, apart from the evidence of myocardial disease, are the isolation of the virus from blood, feces, or throat swabbings, and the demonstration of a rising titer of neutralizing antibodies against the virus recovered from a patient. Pericarditis is the most common manifestation of Coxsackie carditis in adults.

Myocarditis is a common feature in *poliomyelitis* and its prevalence probably varies in different epidemics. Histologic examination may show capillary dilatation and perivascular infiltration with lymphocytes and polymorphonuclear leukocytes, and in some cases the myocardial fibers are necrotic. The lesions are similar to those found in influenza A infection and are probably produced by the direct invasion of the poliomyelitis virus which has been recovered from human heart muscle by transfer to monkeys. Some myocardial damage may be due to the anoxia which occurs in most cases prior to death.

Although many filterable viruses — possibly all of those which cause disease in man — may cause myocarditis, it is probable that other factors which impair myocardial metabolism make the myocardium susceptible to infection. Pre-existing disease, anoxia, digitalis, steroids, alcohol, and electrolyte disturbances are possible determinants. Indeed, it has been shown in laboratory animals that those procedures which reduce the supply of oxygen to the heart result in a high incidence of myocardial lesions in laboratory animals infected with Virus III. Furthermore it is possible that in some viral diseases the mechanism of heart damage may concern biochemical disturbances, lesions of the central nervous system, or autoimmune reactions rather than direct viral invasion.

Bacterial Myocarditis. Bacterial myocarditis rarely if ever occurs in isolation. The incidence of pyogenic myocarditis has fallen with the use of antimicrobials for all bacterial infections. Myocarditis associated with bacterial endocarditis remains an important component of the disease — indeed, late-developing heart failure after cure of the infection is in some cases due to myocardial damage rather than to increased valve disease.

The most important effect of specific bacterial

...ction is by an indirect action of which rheu-...atic carditis and diphtheritic myocarditis are the well known common examples. Streptococcal fever may cause a myocarditis (other than rheumatic); diffuse parenchymatous and focal interstitial reactions have been observed. Although clinical evidence may suggest that recovery is complete, it is possible that healing may result in fibrosis which, with hypertrophy, appears as a chronic cardiomyopathy many years later.

Diphtheritic Myocarditis. Diphtheritic myocarditis, though now uncommon, remains the most serious sequel of diphtheritic infection, and is responsible for more than half of the deaths from diphtheria. Myocardial cells are primarily damaged, but an interstitial reaction occurs which may be a nonspecific response to muscle death. The clinical picture varies in intensity, and in severe cases the development of hypokinetic failure or severe hypotension carries a bad prognosis. The electrocardiogram shows various abnormalities. Conduction defects are especially common, and complete heart block may lead to Adams-Stokes syndrome.

Toxoplasma Myocarditis. Toxoplasmosis may involve the heart in both its congenital and acquired forms. The organism has been observed in heart muscle in the acquired generalized form and, although myocarditis is usually part of the generalized illness, it may be the presenting and dominant feature of the disease. There are several well documented fatal cases of toxoplasmic myocarditis, the diagnosis being proved by finding the organism on histologic examination or by inoculation of heart muscle into a mouse. It has been suggested that some cases of familial cardiomyopathy are due to toxoplasmosis; pregnancy may reactivate toxoplasmosis in the mother, resulting in fetal infection. It is thus clear that in cases of subacute myocarditis, familial cardiomegaly, or isolated chronic cardiomyopathy, the possibility of toxoplasmosis should be considered although proof is generally unobtainable.

Trichinosis. It is known that the heart muscle may be infected in trichinosis. The parasite may be seen in heart muscle, but this is unusual even in cases in which there has been evidence of myocarditis in life. Trichinosis may be mistaken for rheumatic fever because of arthralgia, fever, epistaxis, and electrocardiographic abnormalities; ventricular ectopic beats are common. These signs of myocarditis may disappear with the administration of corticotrophin or cortisone, which probably suppresses the inflammation following invasion by the larvae which later became encysted.

Trypanosomiasis. The myocardium may be damaged in both the acute generalized and chronic forms of infection with *Trypanosoma cruzi* (Chagas' disease). Interstitial myocarditis and even extensive necrosis of muscle may be found in the acute form. Chagas' disease should be regarded as an essentially cardiotropic infection by the trypanosome. The acute form occurs mainly in infants and children, and the heart is affected in most cases. In chronic cases, arrhythmias and conduction defects are especially common. Sometimes chronic lesions of the heart are associated with megaesophagus, and men between 20 and 50 are more often affected than women. As in other forms of myocarditis it is probable that the healing process is associated with fibrosis and hypertrophy of undamaged muscle, although even in chronic cases some degree of inflammatory reaction persists.

Treatment. The management of acute myocarditis concerns the causal disease process (if known) and the heart disease per se. The former is dealt with in the appropriate section of this book. From the cardiac point of view absolute rest is indicated for any form of active myocarditis, and rest should be continued until clinical and laboratory evidence indicates that active myocarditis has subsided. Heart failure demands treatment by routine methods as soon as the most minimal evidence appears. A slight elevation of venous pressure, the presence of a gallop sound, or venous congestion on x-ray is an indication for the use of a thiazide diuretic, and a maintenance dose of digitalis should be given providing that there is no electrocardiographic sign of developing heart block. A light diet with sodium restriction is an obvious requirement. Adrenal corticosteroids have a favorable effect in myocarditis associated with rheumatic fever and other hypersensitivity forms of myocarditis, but indications for their use in isolated myocarditis and the infectious forms mentioned above are not clear. However, because occasional favorable effects have been observed, a trial is indicated when activity of the myocarditis is not subsiding with rest or when a life-threatening deterioration develops.

NUTRITIONAL CARDIOMYOPATHY

The association of myocardial disease and malnutrition has been recognized for a long time. Several distinct but overlapping syndromes have been described, and it is probable that multiple factors are involved in most cases. Mixed vitamin deficiencies, repeated infection and infestation, disturbed immunologic mechanisms, anemias, hypoproteinemia, hypomagnesemia, and hypokalemia are some known factors, and no doubt there are many unknowns which may cause disturbed myocardial function. Thus exact pathogenesis remains obscure in most cases.

In Africa two distinct syndromes of nutritional heart disease have been recognized. A *form of hypokinetic heart failure occurs in the Bantu,* which is reversible when an adequate mixed diet is given, although in the most seriously affected patients deterioration continues in spite of treatment. At necropsy there is hepatic cirrhosis and patchy fibrosis in the heart without hydropic change. A second form occurs in *kwashiorkor* which is due to protein deficiency in the growing child after weaning, and, as in other severe nutritional disorders, recovery occurs when the condition is treated early enough.

Beriberi causes the most well known form of nutritional cardiomyopathy, but this disease is relatively rare among the more affluent peoples of the world. Beriberi heart disease, although occurring in alcoholics, is perhaps the least common form of myocardial disease associated with alcohol. It has been known for a long time that not all patients with beriberi have a hyperkinetic circulatory state; indeed some investigations have shown that chronic myocardial disease with hypokinetic heart failure is more common. Some confusion arises here from the use of the term "beriberi," which should be restricted to patients with a hyperkinetic circulatory state and with a clear response to thiamin.

Potassium deficiency may cause cardiomyopathy. Myocardial damage and patchy necrosis result in some animals from feeding potassium deficient diets. Similar abnormalities have been found in man; after chronic potassium deficiency extensive myocardial fibrosis has been found in the absence of coronary disease. A low potassium level should be corrected completely if permanent myocardial injury is to be avoided.

Alcoholic Cardiomyopathy. Perusal of case histories presented in the many papers on noncoronary myocardial disease reveals a frequent mention of alcohol, sometimes ignored by the authors. A causal relation has, however, long been recognized, with varying degrees of conviction, by many writers. It is now clear that there is an association in some patients between a long-standing high consumption of alcohol and the development of cardiomyopathy.

Adult males are most commonly affected, and three clinical syndromes which depend on the dominant derangement of circulatory function at any one time have been recognized. *Cardiac beriberi* (thiamin-responsive disease) is the least frequent and least serious disorder, occurring especially in very heavy beer drinkers (not averse to spirits as well) who have an additional adverse nutritional status for economic, psychiatric, or gastrointestinal reasons. Therapeutic response to vitamin B_1 and withdrawal of alcohol is effective, but relapse occurs on resumption of previous habits. A chronic myocardial fault may be indicated by persistent abnormality in the electrocardiogram. *Arrhythmia*—especially atrial fibrillation—with or without varying degrees of heart failure is probably the most common mode of presentation in alcoholic cardiomyopathy. The ventricular rate tends to be fast, and multifocal ventricular ectopies are common. Fast heart rates, frequent ventricular extrasystoles, cardiomegaly, and abnormal QRS-T complexes in the electrocardiogram distinguish the condition from so-called idiopathic atrial fibrillation. Treatment with digitalis, diuretics, and conversion of the rhythm meets with varying degrees of success. Reasonable health may be maintained if total abstinence is observed, especially when the development of an arrhythmia with accompanying palpitation draws attention to alcoholic heart disease before irreversible damage has been done.

A few patients present with *hypokinetic heart failure*, cardiomegaly, and electrocardiographic evidence of severe myocardial disease. Response to treatment is poor, and an episodic downhill course is usual.

The electrocardiogram in alcoholic cardiomyopathy shows a wide range of abnormality as in other forms of myocardial disease. A normal or nearly normal electrocardiogram strongly supports a diagnosis of beriberi heart disease. There is a fairly close correlation between the degree of cardiographic abnormality and the severity of the myocardial disease as judged by heart size and response to treatment. Mild polycythemia, which is probably a response to low-grade chronic cardiac insufficiency, and low serum cholesterol levels, probably the result of dietary replacement by ethanol, are common findings. Differential diagnosis may be difficult. "Silent" coronary occlusion, "fallen" hypertension, and thyrotoxicosis (because of tremor, atrial fibrillation, tachycardia, and low cholesterol) are common errors.

Necropsy shows moderate left ventricular hypertrophy and small areas of macroscopic fibrosis. Microscopically there are scattered small areas of muscle degeneration, showing fibrosis or recent necrosis with a slight cellular reaction. The histochemical findings show an accumulation of neutral lipid in the myocardial fibers and varying degrees of mitochondrial damage. These findings are nonspecific and indicate a process of chronic myocardial degeneration, the end result of which is cell death and healing by fibrosis. There is some evidence that electron microscopy may show more specific features.

It is clear that there is some causal relationship between a high consumption of alcohol and myocardial disease, but the pathogenesis of the lesion and the nature of individual susceptibility remain obscure. The following theories merit consideration: (1) That alcohol acts as a direct myocardial toxin; however, there is little evidence for this and it would not explain great variation in individual and organ susceptibility. (2) That alcohol exhausts thiamin and resources, but few patients are helped by thiamin therapy, and the clinical features are unlike those of thiamin depletion. (3) That alcohol causes hypomagnesemia and thence hypokalemia; certainly histologic appearances are similar to those produced by hypokalemia, which may be associated with magnesium depletion known to occur in some alcoholics. (4) That alcoholic injury to the myocardium provides conditions for viral invasion. (5) That myocardial necrosis caused by alcohol in one way or another initiates an autoimmune process which is self-perpetuating; however, none of the usual clinical features of hypersensitivity are found.

Treatment. Total abstinence is indicated. A

first attack of heart failure should respond well to routine measures, but relapse is inevitable unless rest is prolonged and alcohol avoided altogether. When there is atrial fibrillation an attempt at conversion by DC countershock after treatment of heart failure, and under anticoagulant therapy, should be made. Excellent recovery even in patients with long-standing heart failure and cardiomegaly has been achieved by prolonged bed rest under sanatorium conditions.

CARDIAC AMYLOIDOSIS

Cardiac amyloidosis usually appears in primary amyloid; it also occurs in some 15 per cent of patients with myelomatosis, and accounts for between 5 and 7 per cent of all forms of isolated noncoronary myocardial disease in adults. The sexes are equally affected. Small amounts of amyloid may be found in perhaps 2 per cent of elderly hearts (in patients over age 60), but cardiac amyloidosis of sufficient severity to cause death from heart failure is a relatively rare disease; however, some 56 per cent of patients with primary amyloidosis die of heart failure.

Pathology. At necropsy the heart weight is usually moderately increased. Any structure in the heart may be the site of amyloid deposition, and the amount may vary from an occasional small nodule or vascular cuff to almost total replacement of the myocardial mass. The pericardium is frequently affected, and small nodules may be seen on its surface. Occasionally both layers are diffusely thickened and gray. Histologic examination may show perivascular amyloid in the small vessels of the epicardial fat. In patients who have died from heart failure, the greatest amount of amyloid is found in the myocardium, both atria and ventricles being frequently affected. The muscle is curiously stiff, and presumably this diminished compliance of the ventricular mass is the main factor in creating the hemodynamic features of restricted ventricular filling which closely resemble those of constrictive pericarditis. Histologically the muscle cells appear surrounded by rings of amyloid apparently deposited on the cell surface or in the perivascular reticulum of the interstitium. In most severely affected hearts the muscle fibers appear atrophic, necrotic, completely replaced by amyloid, or actually transformed into amyloid substance. Hypertrophic fibers, presumably responsible for the increased heart weight, may be seen in less damaged areas. The valves are occasionally affected.

Clinical Manifestations. Most patients with cardiac amyloidosis are over 50 years old, and the sex distribution is about equal. The majority present with insidious heart failure, though occasionally palpitation or syncope resulting from arrhythmia may be the first symptom. Cardiac pain may occur, and when it is associated with the finding of abnormal Q waves in the cardiogram, an erroneous diagnosis of coronary disease may be made. Effort dyspnea is the most common symptom, but it may be conspicuously absent in patients with the "constrictive" syndrome, which occurs when both sides of the heart are equally affected. Paroxysmal nocturnal dyspnea develops when disease mainly affects the left side of the heart. Uneven deposition of amyloid within the heart may affect the clinical features. Thus deposition in papillary muscle and the mitral valve may cause left atrial enlargement and even a mitral diastolic murmur, although murmurs are absent in most cases. Arrhythmia including atrial fibrillation, nodal and ventricular extrasystoles, and various degrees of heart block are not uncommon. Deposition of amyloid in the lung parenchyma and small vessels may increase dyspnea from heart failure, and possibly cause obstructive pulmonary hypertension.

Diagnosis is helped by finding evidence of amyloid in other organs. Macroglossia and infiltration of the base of the tongue may cause difficulty in speaking and swallowing. Cutaneous manifestations are important from the diagnostic point of view and include purpura, papules, and localized nodular deposits. The central nervous system is usually unaffected, but a few patients have presented with minor degrees of peripheral neuropathy. Hoarseness may be due to amyloid infiltration of the larynx, and biopsy of vocal cord nodule has led to correct antemortem diagnosis. Although clinical evidence of renal disease is uncommon in patients with dominant cardiac amyloidosis, the kidneys are affected in about one third of cases at necropsy. Diarrhea, meteorism, and gastrointestinal bleeding may result from gastrointestinal amyloid, but this is rare in primary cardiac amyloid.

The electrocardiogram is always abnormal in clinically significant cardiac amyloid. The findings, though not specific, are perhaps more suggestive of the nature of the underlying disease than in most other forms of cardiomyopathy. P waves are often small, and the P-R interval may be prolonged. The most characteristic abnormalities are low voltage of the QRS-T complex, especially in the frontal plane leads, and abnormal Q waves indicating extensive myocardial disease. Both forms of bundle branch block have been reported, and T waves are almost invariably flat or inverted. Cardiac catheterization may show great elevation of both right and left atrial pressures as in other forms of severe myocardial failure. Restricted ventricular filling (probably owing to diminished compliance of ventricular myocardium) and diminished contractility result in low arterial pulse pressures and a low cardiac output. As a reasonably accurate assessment of hemodynamic status can be made at the bedside, there seems little indication for cardiac catheterization, for the findings are not specific. Confirmation of diagnosis is best obtained by biopsy of some accessible part that appears to be affected, but even a "positive" specimen may be misinterpreted or missed because of the variable tinctorial character of amyloid. The Congo red test is positive in less than 50 per cent of the patients in whom it has been performed. Hypoproteinemia and hyperglobulinemia (moderate increase in alpha-2 and gamma-fractions) support a diagnosis of amyloid, but as serum protein studies are abnormal in only 15 per cent of cases they do not provide much help in diagnosis.

The outlook for patients with clinical cardiac amyloidosis is uniformly bad. Progressive heart failure usually leads to death in less than two years. Rest, digitalis, and diuretics may improve heart failure temporarily, but the response is mostly unsatisfactory. Various treatments have been suggested, including large doses of liver, ascorbic acid, corticotrophin, and cortisone, but none has been clearly effective.

OTHER CARDIOMYOPATHIES

Endomyocardial Fibrosis.   Minor degrees of endocardial fibrosis are common in myocardial disease but this should not be confused with an obscure cardiopathy which occurs commonly in tropical Africa and sporadically elsewhere. It is characterized by extensive endocardial and subendocardial fibrosis. The disease appears to be a specific entity, but its etiology remains unknown. Indirect evidence suggests that it is of an infectious nature, the organism or its vector being responsible for the geographical distribution of the disease (Parry). Malnutrition is not likely to be a factor, for this disease occurs in well-fed Africans, and it has been seen in well-nourished expatriates from Africa residing in the United Kingdom.

At necropsy the cavities of either or both ventricles are partially obliterated by dense fibrous tissue which may be organized into a dense white thick lining. Fibrous tissue may bind papillary muscles and chordae to the posterior wall of the ventricle, producing gross mitral reflux.

The clinical manifestations are varied and depend on which ventricle is most severely affected. Insidious heart failure of a "constrictive" type results from uniform biventricular disease. Dominant left ventricular disease may present with symptoms of left ventricular failure with or without severe mitral reflux. A few patients develop severe reactive pulmonary hypertension which dominates the clinical picture. Pure right ventricular disease is not uncommon, and its features have been described by Abrahams (1962). Ascites and hepatomegaly without peripheral edema are usual, the jugular venous pressure is very high, and roentgenography shows an aneurysmal right atrium.

There is no specific treatment. Routine treatment of heart failure may delay the inevitable deterioration which occurs in this extraordinary disease.

Löffler's Fibroplastic Endocarditis.   See article on Hypereosinophilic Syndromes.

Sarcoidosis.   See article on Sarcoidosis.

Peripartum Cardiomyopathy (Puerperal Myocarditis).   Peripartum cardiomyopathy is probably not a single disease entity. It describes a condition of heart failure arising in the last trimester of pregnancy or the puerperium and is due to idiopathic myocardial disease. It is unrelated to toxemia of pregnancy but may be difficult to differentiate from "silent" pulmonary thromboembolism; however, the heart failure tends to be mainly of left ventricular origin. It is probable that the late stages of pregnancy and/or the metabolic effects of involution in the puerperium in some unknown way have an adverse effect on hitherto asymptomatic myocardial disease. Clinical recovery is usual, but the electrocardiogram usually reveals the continuation of myocardial disease. Furthermore, subsequent pregnancies are likely to be followed by heart failure. No specific treatment is known.

Myocardial Disease and Neurologic Disorders. Friedreich first recorded that the heart was affected in the congenital neurologic disorder named after him. This finding has been amply confirmed since; indeed, some have considered that the disease is as much an affection of the heart as of the nervous system. The left ventricular myocardium is the site of degenerating fibers, interstitial fibrosis, and hypertrophy. The electrocardiogram may be abnormal in infancy before neurologic features appear. Furthermore, the author of this article has seen cardiomyopathy without neurologic manifestations in a man whose several adult siblings suffered from ataxia. Arrhythmias and congestive cardiac failure are the usual outcome.

Myocardial disease also occurs in association with the *myotonic dystrophies*. Cardiac manifestations may arise at any time in the natural history of the disease, and arrhythmia is the most common presenting feature.

TUMORS OF THE HEART

Primary tumors of the heart are rare but important, as the majority may be cured by surgery. *Myxomas* are the most common; they are benign in the oncologic sense, but malignant insofar as they cause death by obstruction or embolism. *Rhabdomyoma, fibroma,* and *lipoma* are other very rare benign tumors. Malignant *sarcomas* are also rare and may arise from any part of the heart or pericardium.

Myxomas are of special interest not only because they are the most common and can be cured, but also because of their clinical features, which mimic other diseases and pose difficult problems in diagnosis. They may occur at any age. Myxomas

...se from atrial endocardium, most commonly in the left heart, and produce features resulting from obstruction, a generalized systemic disturbance, or peripheral embolism. Obstruction at the atrioventricular valves may cause signs resembling mitral or tricuspid stenosis, but because these tumors may move, the symptoms and signs characteristically vary from time to time. Acute transient obstruction may be caused by a change in posture, leading to syncope, and there may be a periodic change in venous congestion of the lung. Occasionally the mitral valve cusps may be kept open in systole, leading to an erroneous diagnosis of valvar mitral reflux. Systemic symptoms probably due to an abnormal immunologic response to the tumor may sometimes dominate the clinical picture. They comprise vague aches and pains, low-grade fever, a raised sedimentation rate, and abnormal serum proteins. When present these features may lead to an erroneous diagnosis of bacterial endocarditis or collagen disease. Sudden embolism of a major artery may be the presenting feature, and diagnosis has been made on histologic examination of emboli removed at emergency surgery. Diagnosis depends on the physician's having a high index of suspicion followed by selective angiography when an atrial filling defect is confirmatory.

These tumors should be removed under cardiopulmonary bypass. Successful surgery is followed by rapid resolution of the mechanical and immunologic features.

Metastatic tumors in the heart are much more common than primary ones. Various necropsy series in malignant disease place the incidence between 10 and 20 per cent. Bronchial cancer accounts for one third; breast and esophageal neoplasms are other common sources. Pericarditis with effusion is the usual mode of presentation; indeed, this occasionally provides the first evidence of a bronchial carcinoma.

Abrahams, D. G.: Endocardial fibrosis of the right ventricle. Quart. J. Med., 31:1, 1962.
Boyer, S. H., Chisholm, A. W., and McKusick, V. A.: Cardiac aspects of Friedreich's ataxia. Circulation, 25:493, 1962.
Braunwald, E., Brockenbrough, E. L., and Morrow, A. G.: Hypertrophic subaortic stenosis. Circulation, 26:161, 1962.
Braunwald, E., Lambrew, C., Morrow, A., Pierce, G., Rockoff, S. D., and Ross, J.: Idiopathic hypertrophic subaortic stenosis. Circulation (Supps.), 1964.
Brigden, W.: Cardiac amyloidosis. Progr. Cardiov. Dis., 7:142, 1964.
Brigden, W., and Robinson, J.: Alcoholic heart disease. Brit. Med. J., 2:1283, 1964.
Burch, G. E., and DePasquale, N.: Viral Myocarditis. Cardiomyopathies. Ciba Foundation Symposium, 1964, p. 376.
Goodwin, J. F.: Diagnosis of left atrial myxoma. Lancet, 1:464, 1963.
Goodwin, J. F.: Cardiac function in primary myocardial disorders. Brit. Med. J., 1:1527, 1964.
Gore, I., and Saphir, O.: Myocarditis. Amer. Heart J., 34:827, 1947.
Hudson, R. E. B.: Tumors of the heart. *In* Cardiovascular Pathology. London, Edward Arnold, Ltd., 1965, Vol. 2, p. 1563.
Mattingly, T. W.: Clinical features and diagnosis of primary myocardial disease. Mod. Conc. Cardiov. Dis., 30:677, 683, 1961.
Meadows, W. R.: Idiopathic heart failure in the last trimester of pregnancy and the puerperium. Circulation, 15:903, 1955.
Parry, E. H. O.: Endomyocardial Fibrosis. Cardiomyopathies. Ciba Foundation Symposium, 1964, p. 322.
Pearse, A. G. E.: Histochemistry and Electronmicroscopy of Obstructive Cardiomyopathies. Ciba Foundation Symposium, 1964.
Webster, R. H.: Cardiac complications of infectious mononucleosis. Amer. J. Med. Sci., 234:62, 1957.
Whitefield, A. G. W.: Familial cardiomyopathy. Quart. J. Med., 30:119, 1961.
Whitehead, R.: Isolated myocarditis. Brit. Heart J., 27:220, 1965.

Bacterial Endocarditis

Paul B. Beeson

Definition. A disease caused by dissemination of an infective agent from a focus on the lining of the heart or a large blood vessel; characterized by bacteremia, fever, splenomegaly, embolic manifestations, and usually a heart murmur; nearly always fatal unless treated appropriately.

Problems of Terminology. The designation *endocarditis* is not perfect, because the site of infection is most often on a valve leaflet, and it may even be located outside the heart, for example, at the site of aortic coarctation or arteriovenous fistula. In such cases the term *endarteritis* is more suitable. The word *bacterial* is also unsatisfactory, since the same clinical disease is caused not only by bacteria but also by fungi, rickettsiae, or spirillar organisms. The adjective formerly employed, *infective*, therefore seems more nearly correct. The disease is usually described in two forms: "*subacute*" and "*acute*," although some writers have preferred to substitute the term "*chronic*" for "subacute." Classification into acute and subacute forms involves difficulties, because there are many borderline cases with features of both; nevertheless the general separation is useful. Therefore the special characteristics of acute and subacute forms of the disease will be referred to frequently in the pages to follow.

Etiology. The *subacute or chronic form* is usually associated with infection by micro-organisms having comparatively little capacity to act as primary invaders in other tissues. The related group of nonhemolytic streptococci normally found in the mouth, which will be grouped here under the term *Streptococcus viridans*, accounts for approximately 50 per cent of bacteremic cases. Enterococcus (or *Streptococcus faecalis*) and coagulase-negative staphylococci are each responsible for 5 to 10 per cent of cases. Micro-aerophilic and anaerobic streptococci are also encountered from time to time. The remainder includes literally dozens of other micro-organisms, most of which are rarely if ever associated with other forms of clinical illness. Also, the disease has been caused by organisms resembling *Spirillum minus*, the rickettsia of Q fever and several fungi.

The *acute form* of bacterial endocarditis is usually caused by organisms capable of primary invasion of other tissues, such as *Staphylococcus aureus*, pneumococcus, and gonococcus. The incidence of staphylococcal infections is presently increasing, whereas pneumococcal and gonococcal endocarditis have become comparatively rare.

Recent reports on bacterial endocarditis, which do not differentiate between acute and subacute clinical forms, list *Staphylococcus aureus* as the responsible agent in 10 to 20 per cent of bacteremic cases. The proportion of cases caused by the *Streptococcus viridans* group appears to be diminishing.

Pathogenesis. Bacteremia. *Subacute* bacterial endocarditis develops as a chance event in a transient bacteremia. Bacteria from mucous surfaces probably commonly gain access to the blood stream, as has been demonstrated following dental treatments and even vigorous cleansing of the teeth. Urethral instrumentation and parturition have also been shown to cause escape of bacteria into the blood stream. In most instances such a bacteremia is harmless, but when a suitable nidus exists on the lining of the cardiovascular system the micro-organisms may be able to settle and multiply.

The Original Nidus. It has commonly been suggested that the initial nidus for bacterial growth is in a tiny platelet thrombus on a roughened surface, and that the vegetation develops in response to some stimulus provided by bacterial growth. Angrist proposes, instead, that there may be a much larger pre-existing structure—so-called *nonbacterial thrombotic endocarditis*. Grossly visible masses of platelets and fibrin are often encountered at autopsy in about the same sites as the vegetations of bacterial endocarditis. Angrist suggests that in the pathogenesis of subacute bacterial endocarditis an area of the heart subjected to injury and stress may develop a vegetation of nonbacterial thrombotic endocarditis, and this in turn may be colonized during an episode of bacteremia, resulting in the development of the lesion of bacterial endocarditis.

Sites of Predilection. As a rule, bacterial endocarditis develops on a cardiac valve leaflet; frequently more than one valve may be involved. The valves on the left side are affected much more often than those on the right, approximately as follows: mitral 85 per cent, aortic 55 per cent, tricuspid 15 per cent, and pulmonic 1 per cent. Infection is *confined* to the right side of the heart in less than 5 per cent of cases.

Subacute bacterial endocarditis usually occurs on valves already damaged by another disease, especially rheumatic fever (about 70 per cent) and congenital defects (about 10 per cent). Other kinds of valve injury, such as those due to arterio-

sclerosis, syphilis, or cardiac surgery, are also associated. It is noteworthy that the process is almost never engrafted on the roughened surface of a sclerotic artery or on a mural thrombus.

Acute bacterial endocarditis, i.e., that caused by an inherently virulent organism, is also more frequently encountered on the left side than on the right, although the proportion of right-sided cases is somewhat greater than with the subacute form.

The curious tendency of subacute bacterial endocarditis to develop in some areas and to spare others has excited much speculation. Vegetations usually develop at the site of a regurgitant stream. Rodbard points out that the dynamics of flow in such areas would provide little or no lateral perfusing pressure, a situation in which platelets and fibrin could collect and offer shelter to circulating bacteria. Eventually a typical lesion of bacterial endocarditis would then develop. The combination of factors identified by Rodbard are: (1) a high pressure source (left ventricle, aorta), (2) a narrow orifice (insufficient valve, ductus arteriosus), and (3) a low pressure chamber beyond the orifice (atrium, ventricle during diastole and pulmonary vein). This fits with the frequent development of endocarditis on the mitral and aortic valves, small ventricular septal defects, coarctation of the aorta, ductus arteriosus or arteriovenous fistula; and with the rarity of endocarditis on the roughened aorta or in association with atrial septal defect or a large ventricular septal defect. Also in line with this concept is the tendency of subacute bacterial endocarditis to occur in patients with comparatively mild heart disease without failure and without atrial fibrillation. In the presence of the latter complications, decreased pressure gradients and flow rates would perhaps be less likely to favor the initiation of a lesion.

The factors listed by Rodbard might affect nutrition of the wall and fluid dynamics at the sites of predilection in such a way as to lead to development of the nonbacterial lesions emphasized by Angrist. The concepts of Rodbard and Angrist are thus compatible, and they comprise the most acceptable explanations currently available for development of this unique infection.

Course of an Established Infection. After infection has been established, on a heart valve or other intravascular focus, steady and continuous bacteremia usually ensues. Investigations in such patients, whereby samples of blood were withdrawn simultaneously from different parts of the circulatory system, have shown that the apparent constancy of the bacteremia results from an equilibrium between steady replenishment of the blood with fresh organisms and their efficient removal from blood passing through areas of reticuloendothelial activity. A notable characteristic of this constant bacteremia is absence of metastatic foci of infection. Most of the organisms are filtered from the blood and quickly destroyed in reticuloendothelial tissue, and those that may lodge elsewhere do not seem capable of establishing infection.

he distinguishing feature of subacute bacterial endocarditis is its chronicity and durability. This lesion, caused by micro-organisms often incapable of persisting in or infecting any other tissue, becomes responsible for a progressive disease, nearly always fatal unless treated with antimicrobial drugs. The host usually responds with formation of antibodies specific for the infecting organism and with a vigorous outpouring of polymorphonuclear leukocytes; but these, though capable of preventing development of metastatic infection in other parts of the body, are not able to destroy the micro-organisms in the vegetations. One obvious explanation is the meager inflammatory response exhibited there. Capillaries do not extend into all areas of the vegetation; consequently, comparatively few phagocytic cells can reach the nests of bacteria. It appears therefore that bacteria can colonize superficial portions of the vegetations, safe from phagocytosis, yet capable of drifting out into the circulating blood at a comparatively even rate. Their presence in the vegetation doubtless provides a stimulus to further deposit of fibrin and platelets. The lesion may at the same time cause gradual erosion of the underlying structures, leading to destruction or perforation of the valve leaflet and worsening of a pre-existing insufficiency.

Pathology. Mechanisms of the formation of the primary lesion—*the vegetation*—have already been discussed. Other characteristics of the disease may be attributed either to the bacteremia or to embolization of fragments of vegetation. Enlargement of the *spleen* with follicular hyperplasia is doubtless an example of the acute splenic tumor that develops in response to continued bacteremia or to antigen administration. The spleen may also be the site of infarction by emboli from the vegetations. The *kidney* may be infarcted grossly or may show evidence of multiple small emboli ("flea-bitten kidney"); there may also be lesions resembling glomerulonephritis, and this is the process which can cause renal failure. It is doubted that embolic injury is ever sufficiently widespread to be responsible for renal insufficiency. Other sites of major embolization include the *brain* and *mesentery*. Myocardial infarction due to emboli in the coronary vessels is an occasional event; more commonly the heart shows focal myocarditis, which is probably caused by multiple small emboli. Lesions called *mycotic aneurysms* may develop in the walls of large or medium-sized arteries, usually at sites of bifurcations. They are thought to begin as embolic lesions in vasa vasorum. They are particularly hazardous within the cranial cavity, where rupture may produce manifestations of subarachnoid or intracerebral hemorrhage. Rupture elsewhere may cause severe localized pain and swelling.

Acute bacterial endocarditis often develops as a metastatic focus of infection, secondary to established infection elsewhere, e.g., septic thrombophlebitis, furuncle, pyelonephritis, pneumonia, or osteomyelitis. In such cases a previously healthy heart valve may be invaded by circulating bacteria, and rapid destruction of tissue at this site may follow. The endocarditis often seems to develop in the course of a severe sepsis and to be unrecognized until a murmur is noted or cardiac decompensation develops.

In acute bacterial endocarditis the causative organisms are capable of producing abscesses in other tissues, such as brain, kidney, spleen, or lung, with the usual manifestations of these processes. A characteristic local extension of the infection is the so-called *valve-ring abscess* that develops at the base of a vegetation, spreading into the subjacent myocardium. It appears to have grave significance, possibly playing a part in the too frequent failure of antibacterial therapy of acute bacterial endocarditis.

Manifestations of Subacute Bacterial Endocarditis. In fully half of all cases the disease begins insidiously, without an identifiable predisposing factor. Many of the other patients give a history of a respiratory infection at about the time the cardiac infection seems to have begun, but this may represent only the coincidental occurrence of a common ailment or erroneous interpretation of early nonspecific symptoms. In 5 to 10 per cent of cases there is a history of dental extraction or other manipulation within two or three weeks of the onset. In an even smaller proportion of cases the illness has been preceded by urologic instrumentation or by parturition. Opinions differ regarding the role of dental sepsis, but probably gingival or peridental infection can add to the hazard. Certainly *Streptococcus viridans* endocarditis is very rare in edentulous persons.

The *onset* in most cases is subtle, with malaise and low-grade fever—patients usually think they have "the flu." Occasionally there is a more dramatic beginning with high fever or with an embolic accident. *Elevation of body temperature,* although present in nearly every case, is variable in extent, sometimes not more than 1° F.; in other cases there may be hectic variations accompanied by chilliness and sweating. In addition to malaise, other accompaniments of fever such as fatigue, weight loss, and anorexia may be noted.

Heart murmur is present in the great majority of cases. Percentages as high as 98 or 99 have been reported, but this is somewhat misleading. There may of course be no cardiac murmur if the vegetations are outside the heart, as in coarctation or infected arteriovenous fistula. Occasionally even when the infection is on a valve leaflet there may be no murmur early in the illness, but a bruit may become audible later in the course. This seems especially common in middle-aged men with aortic valve endocarditis. Right-sided endocarditis too is notorious for frequent absence of heart murmur. Acute bacterial endocarditis may develop on a previously normal valve, but the destructive nature of this disease may quickly erode part of a valve, resulting in the sudden appearance of a loud murmur. Changing murmurs are often said to be characteristic of subacute bacterial endocarditis; actually the day-to-day changes are more likely to be caused by changes in cardiac output secondary to fluctuations of temperature and heart rate than to changes due to sloughing of a vegetation or perforation of a leaflet. Infected patent ductus arteriosus may, however, be characterized by significant changes in character of the murmur from time to time. *Pericardial friction rubs* are notably rare in this disease. *Splenomegaly* is demonstrable in about 80 per cent of cases, but the organ seldom becomes greatly enlarged. The spleen may be tender after infarction or in acute endocarditis when it harbors an abscess. *Clubbing of the fingers* (and toes) develops in at least half the long-standing cases, but nowadays, with early recognition and effective therapy, this physical sign may not have time to develop.

Findings in the *skin and mucous membranes* may be characteristic and helpful in diagnosis, especially late in the course. Petechiae appear on any part of the body, although some clinicians have the impression that they are especially likely to be found over the clavicles and about the ankles. These are small, red or purple macular lesions that do not blanch on pressure. Because of difficulty in distinguishing them from cherry angiomas, it is often helpful to mark questionable lesions and to inspect them again after a day or two, an interval in which petechiae should fade. Petechiae in the conjunctiva or oral mucosa are especially easy to recognize and are not likely to be confused with any other lesion. Sometimes they have white centers. Hemorrhages in the nail beds usually have a linear distribution near the distal end; hence, the name *"splinter hemorrhages."* These can be helpful diagnostic signs, but it must be emphasized that *they are by no means pathognomonic of bacterial endocarditis*, since they often occur in patients with other chronic diseases of the heart and lungs, apparently being caused by dissemination of tiny thrombi, and they can frequently be found in people who do hard manual work. *Osler's nodes* are acute, painful, barely palpable nodular lesions in the pulps of the fingers and toes. There may be reddening of the overlying skin. *Pallor* due to anemia is present when the disease has existed for a few weeks or longer. Older descriptions of the disease mention a *café-au-lait color of the skin*. This is not a prominent feature today; it may have been related to long-standing untreated infection associated with renal decompensation. In acute bacterial endocarditis, especially when the causative organism is the Staphylococcus, there may be painless red-blue dermal lesions on the palms or soles, a few millimeters in diameter, which are called *Janeway lesions*. Another lesion characteristic of acute endocarditis, found by ophthalmoscopic examination, is called the *Roth spot*: usually located near the optic disc, it is an oval, pale area surrounded, especially on the dependent side, by hemorrhage.

Neurologic manifestations are common, and may constitute the chief complaint. Cerebral embolism (see below) may simulate cerebrovascular disease. Less commonly there may be the picture of encephalopathy, meningitis, or convulsions. Peripheral neuropathy develops occasionally.

The *blood picture* is not distinctive in bacterial endocarditis. Mild normochromic anemia, without reticulocytosis, develops in cases untreated for more than a few weeks. The leukocyte count is usually in the high normal range or moderately elevated because of increase in granulocytes. *Abnormal histiocytes* may be found in the peripheral blood in this disease, especially when the specimen examined is the first drop of blood obtained by puncture of an ear lobe. The characteristic cells are bizarre in appearance and may contain erythrocytes or other leukocytes. Their demonstration has occasionally been helpful when the diagnosis of bacterial endocarditis has been under consideration.

Dramatic clinical events may accompany the occurrence of *large emboli* in arteries throughout the body at any time in the course. *Cerebral embolism* may lead to hemiparesis or other focal neurologic signs. *Coronary embolism* may cause myocardial infarction. *Splenic infarction* is manifested by tenderness and sometimes by pain on respiration. In rare instances this is complicated by local abscess formation, curable only by splenectomy. In contrast to splenic infarction, *renal infarction* unless massive is usually asymptomatic but may reveal itself by sudden appearance of hematuria. Embolism of the *mesenteric arteries* can lead to severe abdominal pain, ileus, distention, and melena. Occlusion of a superficial artery may cause *gangrene* of a digit, the tip of the nose, or the ear.

Heart failure is a frequent and important complication that merits discussion under manifestations of bacterial endocarditis. The mechanism of failure may be either impairment of valvular efficiency or injury to the myocardium. The former may result from perforation of a valve cusp or leaflet or from rupture of a papillary muscle or chorda tendinea. It is especially likely when the aortic valve is affected; here there may be sudden intensification or alteration in character of the regurgitant murmur, accompanied within hours or days by evidence of worsening cardiac status. The myocardium may be injured by multiple small emboli or by larger ones affecting whole areas of the coronary circulation. In any event the development of signs of heart failure during the acute or convalescent stage of bacterial endocarditis has grave prognostic significance. These patients may be cured of their infection only to die of heart failure within a few weeks or months.

Rheumatic manifestations — pains in muscles and joints — are fairly common in bacterial endocarditis. Occasionally there are swelling and heat in one or more joints that may be difficult to differentiate from an exacerbation of rheumatic fever; indeed the conditions can probably coexist.

Mild or moderate *proteinuria* may occur, and microscopic *hematuria* is a frequent and helpful ostic finding. In untreated cases death may ...lt from *renal failure*; this is rare now except when the true nature of the underlying disease is unrecognized. As already mentioned, the serious form of kidney damage is that which resembles glomerulonephritis morphologically. Interestingly the evidences of renal decompensation may disappear after successful antimicrobial therapy.

Age and Sex Incidence. The disease is comparatively uncommon before puberty, but may be encountered at any later period of life. It is by no means a rarity in advanced age, when, however, recognition may be especially difficult. The incidence is higher in males, especially in older age brackets.

Special Situations. *Following Labor or Urologic Treatment.* In contrast to the infections that occur subsequent to dental procedures, those related to urogenital tract manipulation are more likely to be caused by the enterococcus or by enteric bacteria. This point is to be borne in mind when prescribing prophylactic medication to patients with valvular defects.

Infected Arteriovenous Fistula. Perhaps 20 such cases have been reported. The infecting organism in most of them has been *Streptococcus viridans.* In about a third of the reported cases bacterial endocarditis has later developed on the aortic valve. Presumably here the fistula, by causing circulatory strain, has rendered the valve liable to infection. This seems analogous to the observations of Lillehei in animals with surgically induced arteriovenous fistulas, in which there is increased susceptibility to bacterial endocarditis.

Following Cardiac Surgery. The incidence of bacterial endocarditis as a sequel to cardiac surgery seems to vary widely, as judged by reports from different clinics. With mitral valvotomy the risk is slight, but aortic valve surgery, implanting of prostheses, and employment of extracorporeal circulation are attended by a substantial hazard of infection, at times as high as 5 to 7 per cent of cases. The differential diagnosis may be difficult, other possibilities including postcardiotomy syndrome, drug fever, active rheumatic fever, and sepsis. In the reported cases there has been a low incidence of characteristic signs such as splenomegaly, petechiae, and major emboli. The Staphylococcus, coagulase positive or negative, is by far the commonest infecting organism, but Candida, hemolytic Streptococcus, Pseudomonas, and other enteric bacilli may also be responsible. The prognosis is especially grave in postcardiotomy infections; very few cures have been achieved.

Endocarditis in the Aged. The death rate from endocarditis in elderly patients is high. The diagnosis may be made later or not at all in these people, because systolic heart murmurs and cerebral vascular accidents are likely to be attributed to arteriosclerotic processes, and temperature elevations may be ascribed to respiratory or urinary tract infection.

Heroin Addicts. Acute bacterial endocarditis is one of the hazards of heroin addiction. These people inject the drug intravenously, usually without sterile technique. There appears to be an increased likelihood of tricuspid valve endocarditis under these circumstances, so that the principal clinical manifestations may be pulmonary, resulting from septic embolization, and heart murmur may not be detected. The clinical impression is likely to be pneumonia with septicemia. *Streptococcus viridans* is not likely to be the etiologic agent here; the most common is *Staphylococcus aureus,* and other possibilities include esterococcus, Candida, and various gram-negative bacilli.

Right-Sided Endocarditis. A considerable proportion of the reported cases has been in young children. The etiologic agent is most often a primarily pathogenic organism, such as Staphylococcus, pneumococcus or enterococcus. Contrary to some statements, blood culture is positive about as often as in left-sided endocarditis. Heart murmur may not be present or may develop late, since the causative organisms can invade normal valves. Petechiae and splenomegaly are less frequently observed. An additional clinical feature is evidence of pulmonary embolization and infection. Metastatic infections often develop in other organs, especially the kidney, brain, and lungs. Peripheral arterial embolism is rare.

Characteristics of Certain Etiologic Agents. Certain etiologic agents may induce somewhat different syndromes from the "textbook picture" of subacute bacterial endocarditis. Reference has already been made to the distinguishing features of acute bacterial endocarditis caused by inherently pathogenic micro-organisms: attack on previously healthy valves, fulminant course, absence of murmurs, metastatic infections, Janeway and Roth spots.

Pneumococcal Endocarditis. The likelihood of an associated endocarditis should always be considered in a case of pneumococcal meningitis. Austrian estimates that the two forms of infection are combined in a quarter to a third of patients with pneumococcal meningitis. Rupture of the aortic valve cusp is especially likely to occur in such cases; this is almost invariably followed by intractable heart failure.

Enterococcal Endocarditis. Middle-aged or elderly men with urologic disease or women in the child-bearing period are the usual victims of enterococcal infection; hence, there is little question that the urogenital tract is an important portal of entry. The clinical features resemble those of *Streptococcus viridans*, except for greater tendency to metastatic suppurative foci, including splenic abscess.

Gonococcal Endocarditis. Two distinctive features have been reported. About half the patients show an unusual kind of fever: a double rise and fall during each 24-hour period. This has not been characteristic of any other form of endocarditis, and an explanation is lacking. The second noteworthy feature is evidence of hepatic dysfunction. The liver is conspicuously spared in most kinds of endocarditis, but jaundice is relatively common when gonococcus is the infecting organism.

Fungal Endocarditis. The clinical features in the several dozen cases of fungal endocarditis that have been reported are similar to those of bacterial endocarditis. In some the valvular involvement has been only one aspect of an overwhelming septicemic process, but in the majority the endocarditis has been the central lesion. Quite a few cases have now been reported following cardiac surgery. Most fungal infections are caused by Candida or Histoplasma, but a few instances of infection with Aspergillus, Blastomyces, Coccidioides, Cryptococcus, and Mucor have been reported. One notable characteristic is embolic occlusion of large arteries; this may be related to the bulkiness of vegetations induced by fungi.

Diagnosis. The possibility of bacterial endocarditis must always be kept in mind because it is a curable disease, but it is fatal if unrecognized. In the absence of another clear-cut cause of the illness, the concurrence of fever and heart murmur imposes on the physician an obligation to consider the likelihood of bacterial endocarditis — *and to draw blood cultures.* Waiting for the appearance of such "cardinal" manifestations as clubbing of the fingers, splenic enlargement, anemia, changing murmurs, and petechiae is inexcusable.

Firm diagnosis can be achieved only by demonstration of bacteremia, which is possible in about 80 per cent of cases. As already discussed, bacteremia, if present at all, is usually a fairly steady, continuous process. Cultures are no more likely to be positive at a particular time of day or when the patient's body temperature is high or low. The best practice, therefore, is to draw four to six samples of blood for culture during the first day or two. If the patient had been receiving antimicrobial therapy, it is desirable to terminate that and to wait two or three days until the drug has been eliminated before obtaining the cultures. Blood from the antecubital vein is as likely to yield positive cultures as arterial blood. No advantage is gained by culturing bone marrow. If an organism with unusual growth requirements is suspected, special culture media may have to be employed.

Diagnosis is considerably more difficult in abacteremic cases, which comprise about 20 per cent of the total. It is impossible to discern why, in this proportion of cases, bacteria rarely, if ever, gain access to the blood stream, in contrast to the more common state of affairs when they are demonstrable almost continuously. Doubtless some agents cannot be demonstrated by the usual blood culture techniques; for example, cases caused by the rickettsia of Q fever will be identified only by testing specifically for serologic evidence of this infection. At any rate, the clinician must recognize the existence of this type of case and must weigh the indications for proceeding with a "blind" trial of antimicrobial therapy, as described later under Treatment.

Certain laboratory findings may provide some support for the diagnosis. *Rheumatoid factor* has been demonstrated in about half the patients

tested. The positive reaction in this disease is only transiently present and tends to disappear within a few weeks after the infection has been brought under control. *Cryoglobulins* can also be demonstrated occasionally. *Serum complement* level may be very low in patients who show evidence of nephritis during the course of bacterial endocarditis, perhaps because of the same mechanism that is responsible for the low complement level in acute glomerulonephritis or lupus nephritis. Elevation of the *gamma globulin* fraction of the blood is common, though not of much specific help in diagnosis, since so many diseases that cause prolonged fever are also likely to be accompanied by this abnormality.

Differential Diagnosis. Bacterial endocarditis is one of the most familiar causes of prolonged fever of obscure origin. When bacteremia can be demonstrated the diagnosis is relatively easy; the abacteremic cases present the main difficulty. A treatise on the differential diagnosis of this disease could be of great length. Here it is possible only to mention some of the most common diseases with which bacterial endocarditis can be confused.

Systemic lupus erythematosus may present many of the findings of bacterial endocarditis, e.g., fever, heart murmur, anemia, hematuria, arthralgia, and petechiae. A positive test for LE factor and negative blood cultures are the usual criteria for differentiation. Therapeutic trials of antimicrobial drugs and of steroids may give some assistance in diagnosis.

It may be extremely difficult to distinguish between *acute rheumatic fever* and bacterial endocarditis. Erythema marginatum, pericarditis, and severe disabling arthritis are findings that would point toward acute rheumatic fever. Changing titers of antibody to beta hemolytic streptococcal antigens would also favor that disease.

Sickle cell disease can cause fever, anemia, heart murmur, arthralgia, and abnormal kidney function. Demonstration of sickling or of abnormal hemoglobin should identify this disorder.

Atrial myxoma can mimic bacterial endocarditis. There may be fever, arthralgia, changing heart murmurs, petechiae, splinter hemorrhages, and embolic manifestations. Several patients with this rare disease have been treated for bacterial endocarditis — a fatal clinical error in view of possible surgical cure.

Nonbacterial thrombic endocarditis. As discussed earlier, it is possible that bacterial endocarditis begins with bacterial invasion of a preexisting lesion composed of masses of fibrin and platelets. Such lesions are common findings at autopsy of people who have suffered long wasting illnesses. It is now well established that this process can cause symptoms by embolization in the arterial circulation of sterile pieces of vegetation. The most common reported sites of large infarcts are spleen, kidney, and brain. Thus these patients may have heart murmur, fever, and embolic manifestations.

Drug reactions resulting in fever and anemia

commonly suggest the possible presence of bacterial endocarditis. Discontinuing medications and careful clinical observation will resolve the issue.

Other well-known causes of obscure febrile illness such as *miliary tuberculosis* and *lymphoma* or *other neoplasms* may cause confusion if the patient happens to have a heart murmur.

The differential diagnosis in *acute bacterial endocarditis* includes various serious acute infectious diseases such as pneumonia, meningitis, pyelonephritis, and biliary tract infection.

Treatment. Bacterial endocarditis stands out among infectious diseases as one in which cure depends on use of drugs capable of killing bacteria in the tissues, unaided by phagocytosis or other defense mechanisms. Ample clinical experience has demonstrated that those antimicrobial agents that generally have only a bacteriostatic effect, such as sulfonamides, tetracyclines, and chloramphenicol, are seldom capable of curing bacterial endocarditis. Although their use is often followed by clinical improvement and negative blood cultures, the disease relapses shortly after treatment is terminated. The penicillins are by far the most valuable agents in treatment, and streptomycin sometimes helps, as an adjunct to penicillin. Occasionally, especially in gram-negative bacillary infections, cure is achieved by use of drugs such as neomycin, colistin, or polymyxin, and in a few cases of fungus infection amphotericin B and 5-fluorocytosine have been effective. But the central role of the penicillins in saving lives of patients with bacterial endocarditis can hardly be overemphasized. When the infecting organism is resistant to this family of drugs, or when the patient is so allergic to them that one dares not give them, the chance of achieving cure is lessened.

A second requirement for successful drug therapy is prolonged administration. Unlike most infections, in which an antibacterial effect sufficient to tip the balance in favor of host defenses will suffice, the cure of bacterial endocarditis seems to depend on the drug alone. Therefore, opportunity must be provided for every microorganism in the vegetation to enter a phase of growth in which it is susceptible to killing by the drug. Perhaps also some time is required for erosion of the surface of the vegetation, exposing the nests of bacteria that lie embedded there. A few cures have been reported in cases treated for only ten days, and many cases have been successfully treated in fourteen-day courses. On the other hand, there is ample experience to demonstrate that treatment should extend for many weeks in certain kinds of cases, as will be described subsequently.

Before effective chemotherapy was available, a few cases of endarteritis in arteriovenous fistulas or in patent ductus arteriosus were successfully treated purely by surgical obliteration of the fistulous connection. Nowadays it seems preferable to eradicate, or at least control, the infection by drugs before attempting surgical intervention.

The question of combining antimicrobial therapy with anticoagulant or fibrinolytic agents to inhibit further deposition of fibrin and platelets on the vegetations has often been raised. There is, however, little or no evidence to show that this is beneficial; on the other hand, anticoagulant therapy has been associated with fatal hemorrhagic complications, usually intracranial. Therefore this form of treatment seems contraindicated.

Certain considerations should influence the decision on how soon to begin therapy, once the diagnosis seems probable and blood cultures are in process. Because excessive delay in instituting treatment undoubtedly permits further damage to heart valves and opportunity for serious embolic accidents, there is a tendency to initiate antimicrobial therapy immediately. Indeed, when the manifestations are those of fulminating infection, with the probability that the causative microorganism is a true pathogen, or when the aortic valve is affected, it is advisable to proceed at once with therapy, using the best guess as to appropriate drug and dose, making changes later when laboratory results are available. On the other hand, waiting until the diagnosis has been confirmed by blood culture, so that an appropriate plan of chemotherapy can be based on secure knowledge of the etiology, also has advantages. When the clinical manifestations are mild, and the probability of *Streptococcus viridans* infection can be assumed, there is little danger in waiting until the diagnosis can be confirmed by blood culture, and sensitivity tests can provide information on the best drug to use and the proper dosage.

When bacteremia has been demonstrated, the organism should be kept viable in the laboratory until conclusion of treatment, because further tests to confirm or improve the efficacy of the treatment regimen may be desired.

Even when penicillin appears to be the drug of choice, the quantity to be given daily may have to be varied considerably. When the etiologic agent is *Streptococcus viridans*, sensitive to 0.1 unit per milliliter or less, therapy consisting of 2 million units of penicillin G daily, given parenterally at six-hour intervals, is sufficient. For strains less sensitive to penicillin, e.g., 0.1 to 1.0 unit per milliliter, considerably larger doses of penicillin, up to 20 million units per day, may be required, and it is common practice to add probenecid (Benemid), 0.5 gram four times a day, to retard penicillin loss via the kidneys. In cases of enterococcus infection, one is dealing with an organism generally exhibiting some degree of resistance to penicillin. Here the requirement is for large daily doses of penicillin and the use of streptomycin in combination. The amount of penicillin required may be 20 million to 100 million units daily, together with 1.0 gram of streptomycin per day, in four doses. Quantities of penicillin of this magnitude must be given by continuous intravenous infusion because of the severe local inflammatory response to intramuscular injection of large quantities.

When the causative organism is a penicillinase-producing organism, especially *Staphylococcus aureus*, cure may be effected by use of a semi-synthetic penicillin such as methicillin or oxacillin. These drugs are given in doses of 4 to 18 grams daily intramuscularly or intravenously.

It is generally believed that penicillin should be administered parenterally in this disease, although some good results have been obtained by giving the drug orally. This practice may gain favor in the future because of availability of semi-synthetic forms of penicillin that resist gastric acid and are well absorbed. It would seem essential to ascertain that suitable levels in body fluids are being attained with this method of administration by testing the antibacterial activity of the patient's serum from time to time during the course of therapy.

Occasionally the patient is so allergic to penicillins that administration would threaten his life. Attempts may be made to suppress the allergic manifestations by steroid therapy, but this can lead to most serious difficulty. Here it seems preferable to employ cephaloridine, in doses of 4 to 12 grams per day, since most patients allergic to penicillin seem to tolerate cephaloridine without evidence of a cross-reaction to it.

When the causative organism is resistant to the penicillins, certain other bactericidal drugs may be employed, such as vancomycin (2 to 4 grams per day, intravenously) or bacitracin (25,000 units intramuscularly, four times a day). In gram-negative bacterial endocarditis, the drugs mentioned so far may be ineffective, but cure may yet be accomplished by use of neomycin or kanamycin (0.25 to 0.5 gram intramuscularly, four times a day) or polymyxin sulfate or colimycin sulfate (40 to 75 mg. intramuscularly four times each day). These are all capable of serious toxic side effects on the auditory apparatus or on the kidney and must be used with care, but their use even to the point of serious renal or otic toxicity is justified when no other agent will control the infection.

In rare instances resistant cases of bacterial endocarditis have been handled successfully by use of combinations of bacteriostatic and bactericidal drugs, e.g. tetracycline, chloramphenicol, and streptomycin. Laboratory guidance regarding combinations of three or more drugs is difficult to obtain and is somewhat uncertain because of the fluctuating concentrations that exist in the patient's tissues.

One of the most reliable guides to proper therapy is to test the blood serum of the patient against his own infecting organism during the course of the treatment. Successive dilutions of serum in broth are tested against small inocula (less than 10,000 organisms). These can then be subcultured after 24 hours' incubation, so that information regarding both bactericidal and bacteriostatic activity can be obtained. For probability of favorable clinical result, bactericidal action of the patient's serum in a dilution of 1 to 8 or greater is desired.

Treatment of abacteremic cases is especially difficult, because there is no laboratory guide available for selection of drugs and dosages. In view of the probability of gram-positive infection, a reasonable program of treatment is the following: Begin with 10 million units of penicillin and 1 gram of streptomycin daily. If the patient's condition improves and his temperature level falls during the next 72 hours, continue with this program. If there is no evidence of clinical effect in three days, raise the dose of penicillin to 100 million units daily, and continue treatment for three days. If there is still no sign of benefit, discontinue penicillin G and streptomycin and try methicillin or oxacillin, 12 grams daily for three days. If this does not appear to be effective, change to vancomycin, 4 grams daily, by continuous intravenous drip, for another three days. If the causative agent is a gram-positive organism, one of the foregoing plans of treatment should have been effective. With the possibility of gram-negative bacterial infection under consideration, one could then try the effect of neomycin or kanamycin, 0.5 gram four times daily by intramuscular injection. The chemotherapy of the various mycotic infections is discussed in the articles devoted to them. If none of these plans of treatment shows an effect, the infection is probably one for which there is at present no satisfactory treatment.

Regarding *duration of treatment,* it is permissible to stop in two or three weeks in cases in which all signs are favorable: short duration of illness, sensitive organism, and prompt improvement after beginning therapy. On the other hand, in abacteremic cases, in those in which the disease has already existed many weeks or months (presumably with large masses of vegetations), and in those in which the infecting organism is relatively resistant, it is wiser to continue treatment for six to ten weeks.

At the conclusion of a planned course of antimicrobial therapy, if the patient appears to have responded well, the temperature should be normal, the spleen should have diminished in size, and the patient should be relatively free of complaints. After therapy has been discontinued, the patient should be carefully observed for evidence of persisting infection. Several blood cultures should be obtained during the first week, others at two weeks and six weeks. If there has been no return of symptoms by the end of six weeks, and if blood cultures have remained negative, it is safe to assume that cure has been accomplished. Second attacks of bacterial endocarditis are by no means unknown, whereas relapse of the original infection after a free interval of six weeks would be most unlikely. Prophylactic chemotherapy to prevent development of a second infection is not recommended, but prophylaxis at the time of dental or urologic procedures is indicated for patients cured of bacterial endocarditis just as it is for anyone with chronic valvular or congenital heart disease.

Surgical Measures. Even before the advent of modern chemotherapy, a few cures of this disease were achieved by excising an infected arteriovenous fistula or patent ductus arteriosus. Infections superimposed on surgically implanted prosthetic devices are exceedingly difficult to eradicate by chemotherapy; at times, therefore, it may be necessary to replace a plastic valve or remove suture material in order to control infection.

When patients develop severe aortic insufficiency as a result of bacterial endocarditis, it may be necessary to attempt to construct a better aortic valve after the infection has been eradicated.

Prophylaxis of Bacterial Endocarditis. Chemotherapy. In view of the indubitable role of dental and urologic manipulations in pathogenesis of some cases of bacterial endocarditis it is considered proper practice to "protect" people with valvular or congenital heart disease by a short course of chemotherapy at the time of the procedure. Some authorities recommend that the therapy begin one day before the procedure and be continued for two or three days; others begin therapy the morning of the operation and continue for two days. For dental procedures, in which infection with *Streptococcus viridans* is most likely, penicillin is the agent usually given. The recommended dosage is 400,000 units of penicillin V, one hour before the procedure, repeating this dose at six-hour intervals for two days thereafter. For urologic instrumentation, in which enterococcus or a gram-negative bacillus is more likely to gain entry to the blood stream, tetracycline, 250 mg. four times a day, may be preferable. There is no question that these programs of treatment diminish the frequency with which bacteremia can be demonstrated following the procedure, but their effectiveness in preventing bacterial endocarditis is difficult to prove, because the numerical risk is not great in any event—estimated at about one chance of infection per 500 tooth extractions in patients with chronic valvular heart disease. In any case, prophylactic treatment of persons known to be at risk is so well established that considerable blame may fall on the physician who neglects to carry it out.

Dental Care. Infection by *Streptococcus viridans* is rarely encountered in edentulous patients. For this reason it is recommended that patients with valvular defects have special attention devoted to their teeth and that indications for extraction be interpreted liberally.

Prognosis. Most reports of series of cases of bacterial endocarditis treated with modern chemotherapy indicate that the infection can be eradicated in 60 to 70 per cent of cases; a few have claimed success in as high as 80 per cent of cases. It must be emphasized, however, that eradication of infection is not the whole story, because a significant proportion of patients in whom infection is eradicated have nevertheless suffered permanent cardiac damage, and these may succumb to

heart failure within a few months. Furthermore, occasional patients have permanent disability caused by the occurrence of cerebral embolism during the course of the disease. As an over-all figure, it may be said that somewhat less than 50 per cent of patients will be well and free of cardiac failure five years after treatment, but this figure is remarkably good when viewed in the light of the almost certain fatal outcome without chemotherapy.

Factors that indicate a poor outlook are: (1) *Insusceptibility of the causative organism* to penicillin and other bactericidal drugs. Results are likely to be less favorable in infections due to staphylococci, gram-negative bacteria, enterococci, or fungi. (2) *Heart failure*, appearing during treatment. This is likely to resist supportive therapy and may lead to death within a few weeks or months. (3) *Aortic valve involvement.* The likelihood of serious valvular damage and intractable failure seems much greater when the aortic valve is one of those infected. (4) *Old age.* Patients who develop bacterial endocarditis after the age of 60 only occasionally make a good recovery. (5) *Abacteremic disease.* In most series the survival rate for abacteremic cases is about half that for bacteremic cases. Several reasons may be offered. Diagnosis is likely to be delayed and treatment begun later. Without laboratory aid in studying the sensitivity of the infecting organism the treatment must be by guesswork, guided by clinical response, which may mean further delay before an effective program is hit upon. Other factors may render chemotherapy less effective in those cases in which the bacterial colonies do not lie close enough to the circulating blood to give bacteremia. (6) *Infection of a prosthetic device.* Chemotherapy usually fails to eradicate infection on the surface of a prosthesis. (7) *Delay in institution of therapy.* Failure to think of the possibility of this diagnosis may lead to loss of precious days or weeks. The common practice of prescribing a broad-spectrum antimicrobial such as tetracycline or chloramphenicol for any patient with fever may lead to long delays in recognition and institution of proper treatment.

Angrist, A. A.: Pathogenesis of bacterial endocarditis. J.A.M.A., 183:249, 1963.

Cherubin, C. E., Baden, M., Kavaler, F., Lerner, S., and Cline, W.: Infective endocarditis in narcotic addicts. Ann. Intern. Med., 69:1091, 1968.

Jones, H. R., Jr., Siekert, R. G., and Geraci, J. E.: Neurologic manifestations of bacterial endocarditis. Ann. Intern. Med., 71:21, 1969.

Kerr, A., Jr.: Subacute Bacterial Endocarditis. Springfield, Illinois, Charles C Thomas, 1955.

Lerner, P. I., and Weinstein, L.: Infective endocarditis in the antibiotic era. New Eng. J. Med., 274:199; 323; 388, 1966.

Rodbard, S.: Blood velocity and endocarditis. Circulation, 27:18, 1963.

Diseases of the Aorta

J. Willis Hurst

ELONGATION AND KINKING OF THE AORTA

Medial sclerosis (*Mönckeberg's sclerosis*) is one of the most common disease processes affecting the larger arteries. In this condition the media shows varying degrees of loss of muscular and elastic tissue along with calcification.

The cause of medial sclerosis is not known, but it begins in middle life and increases with advancing age. The abnormality of the media causes the vessels to elongate and is responsible for the firm and tortuous nature of the temporal, brachial, and radial arteries observed in some middle-aged and most elderly people. This process in itself does not lead to occlusion or rupture of a vessel. The disease may be associated with atheromatous changes in the media, which, of course, may lead to more serious complications.

The decrease in elastic and muscular elements of the media plus calcification of the area causes systolic hypertension that requires no therapy. The aorta, as well as the visible peripheral arteries, becomes long and tortuous. The abnormality and the medial calcification may be detected on a roentgenogram of the chest. The elongated aorta may simulate an aneurysm. The esophagus tends to follow the course of the aorta because it is bound intimately to it. Accordingly, when the aorta takes an unusual course because of the effects of medial sclerosis, the barium-filled esophagus will be seen to do the same when viewed under the fluoroscope or on the roentgenogram of the chest. The unusual path taken by the esophagus in such cases may simulate posterior displacement of the structure by the heart.

The aortic arch may elongate until it becomes kinked or folded downward in the region of the ligamentum arteriosum. The condition is called *"pseudocoarctation."* There may be mild obstruction in rare cases. (See Figure 1A and B.) This abnormality can resemble mediastinal tumor. An aortogram may occasionally be needed for its identification.

Robbins, S. L.: Pathology. Philadelphia, W. B. Saunders Company, 1967, pp. 578 ff.

ANEURYSM OF THE AORTA

Definition. An aneurysm is a localized or diffuse enlargement of an artery. When one or all of the layers of the aorta make up the sac of the aneurysm, it is called a *true aneurysm*. When the aorta is injured by trauma or infection, a pulsating hematoma may develop due to destruction of the wall of the vessel; perivascular clot and connective tissue make up the wall of the enlargement—in this case, a *false aneurysm*. A *saccular aneurysm* has a pouchlike appearance and appears to be a sac attached to the side of the aorta. A *fusiform aneurysm* is spindle-shaped and involves the entire circumference of the aorta.

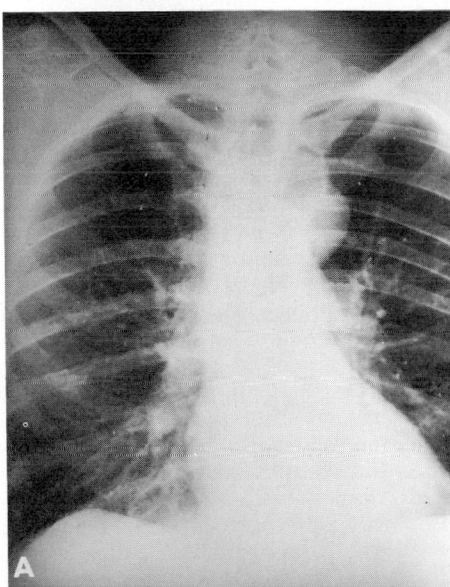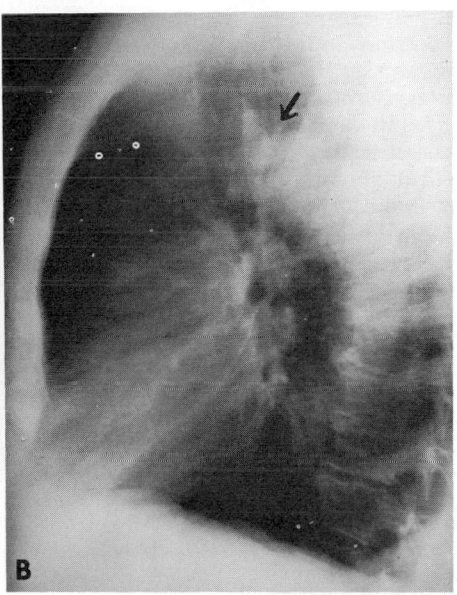

FIGURE 1. Posteroanterior *(A)* and lateral *(B)* roentgenograms of the chest showing an "elongated" aorta with pseudocoarctation.

Etiology. Aneurysms of the aorta may be due to arteriosclerosis, syphilis, medial cystic necrosis, trauma, infection (mycotic aneurysm), and congenital vascular disease. The discussion dealing with arteriosclerotic and syphilitic aneurysms of the aorta will make up the major portion of this section. Dissecting aneurysm, traumatic aneurysm, mycotic aneurysm, and aneurysms of the sinuses of Valsalva will be discussed separately.

Pathogenesis. Although the pathologic processes associated with production of aortic aneurysm are varied, certain factors are common to all. The media of the normal aorta must remain intact in order for the aorta to withstand the systolic blood pressure. When the media is damaged, there is progressive dilatation at the weakened area and an aneurysm gradually develops. Once an aneurysm develops it tends to gradually increase in size, being restrained only by blood clots and scar tissue; hence there is the likelihood that the aneurysm may finally rupture.

Incidence. The incidence of aneurysms at autopsy is approximately 2 per cent. The majority of aortic aneurysms are found in patients between 40 and 70 years of age, and the incidence is higher in men than in women. Syphilitic aneurysms of the arch of the aorta are still found, but are fortunately decreasing in frequency. Today most aneurysms of the aorta seen in the United States are due to arteriosclerosis, regardless of location, even those of the ascending aorta.

Clinical Manifestations. The signs and symptoms depend upon the size and location of the aneurysm. Venous distention and edema of the face, neck, and shoulders may develop when an aneurysm compresses the superior vena cava. Impingement on the trachea and bronchi may produce cough and dyspnea, and compression of the esophagus can produce dysphagia. An aneurysm may impair the function of the recurrent laryngeal nerve and cause hoarseness. A syphilitic aneurysm of the first portion of the aorta may erode the sternum (Fig. 2). Severe pain may occur when a syphilitic aneurysm of the arch and early descending aorta erodes the vertebra and ribs. Death may be the result of hemorrhage into the trachea, bronchi, pleural space, or pericardium. An arteriosclerotic aneurysm of the abdominal aorta may cause no symptoms until rupture occurs. The patient or his physician may discover the aneurysm because of a pulsating mass in the abdomen. The aneurysm may cause pain in the upper portion of the abdomen, the lower portion of the back, the groin, and occasionally in the testicles. The mechanism of such pain may be associated with rupture, sudden enlargement or a small leak into the retroperitoneal space. The pulsating mass, usually felt without difficulty, may extend from above the umbilicus into the pelvis. The mass may be nontender and movable, but tends to become tender and fixed when there has been recent symptomatic enlargement.

A thoracic aortic aneurysm can usually be identified on posteroanterior and oblique roent-

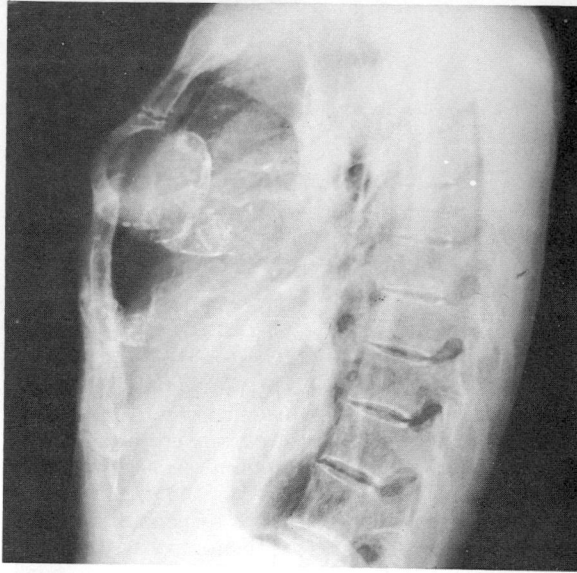

FIGURE 2. Lateral roentgenogram of the chest showing the erosion of the sternum by a syphilitic aortic aneurysm.

genograms of the chest. The pulsation of the mass can be studied during fluoroscopic examination. Pulsations may be absent, however, because thrombosis in the aneurysm may prevent movement. Since some solid tumors located adjacent to the heart appear to pulsate, it is occasionally necessary to resort to aortography in order to differentiate an aortic aneurysm from a tumor. An abdominal aneurysm can often be identified in the ordinary roentgenogram of the abdomen (particularly in the lateral view) because calcification of the aortic wall is frequently present. Aortography may be needed to establish the diagnosis in some cases.

Prognosis. Aortic aneurysm is a serious disease with poor prognosis. According to Estes, one third of patients with arteriosclerotic aneurysm of the abdominal aorta die within a year after the diagnosis is made. Three fourths of the patients die within five years after diagnosis, usually from rupture. Kampmeier's study of aneurysms of the thoracic aorta indicated that the average duration of life, after the onset of symptoms, was six to eight months, and De Bakey found that over 90 per cent of patients with aneurysms of the thoracic aorta died within five years.

Treatment. There is no medical treatment for aortic aneurysms. The discovery of an aortic aneurysm forces one to consider resection of the lesion and replacement by a plastic graft. When an aneurysm of the abdominal aorta is found and the patient has no other recognizable disease, surgical resection is usually possible; the operative mortality is about 7 per cent. When the patient is older than average, say in the eighth decade of life, or when there is clear evidence of heart, cerebrovascular, renal, or other serious disease, the operative mortality may be 25 per cent or more. It is obvious also that, if such a patient survives the operation, his life expectancy will be less than that of a normal person because of the underlying disease. Generally speaking, then, all aneurysms of the abdominal aorta should be surgically resected, regardless of symptoms or size. Resection should not be attempted for asymptomatic lesions if the patient has associated disease that will shorten his life anyway or will greatly increase the operative risk. If the aneurysm has actually ruptured or if symptoms suggest that rupture may be imminent, operation should be attempted regardless of associated disease, even through the operative risk is high.

Surgical treatment of aneurysms of the thoracic aorta carries a higher operative mortality rate than that for aneurysm of the abdominal aorta. Even in expert hands the operative mortality is about 30 per cent. A saccular aneurysm can at times be resected at its neck and the wall of the aorta repaired. Fusiform aneurysms are more difficult to resect. The mortality varies with the location of the aneurysm. Although it is possible to resect an aneurysm of the entire aortic arch, the death rate from the procedure is very high. Techniques have been developed that prevent cardiac strain and provide blood to the heart, brain, spinal cord, and kidneys, while the aorta is occluded, using extracorporeal circulation, temporary bypass shunts, and hypothermia. The prognosis of thoracic aneurysm is so grave that one is forced to consider resection of the lesion despite the high operative mortality. Accordingly, if resection seems technically possible and no serious associated disease precludes the procedure, an attempt should be made.

Blakemore, A. H., and Voorhees, A. B., Jr.: Aneurysm of the aorta: A review of 365 cases. Angiology, 5:209, 1954.
Cranley, J. J., Herrmann, L. G., and Preuninger, R. M.: Natural history of aneurysms of the aorta. Arch. Surg., (Chicago), 69:185, 1954.
Estes, J. E., Jr.: Abdominal aortic aneurysm: A study of 102 cases. Circulation, 2:258, 1950.
Joyce, J. W., Fairbairn, J. F., II, Kincaid, O. W., and Juergens, J. L.: Aneurysms of the thoracic aorta. Circulation, 29:176, 1964.
Lord, J. W., Jr., and Imperato, A. M.: The abdominal aortic aneurysm. Its importance to the internist. J.A.M.A., 176:93, 1961.

DISSECTING ANEURYSM

Definition. Dissecting aneurysm of the aorta is really a dissecting hematoma. Blood enters the wall of the aorta and splits the media of the vessel.

Etiology and Pathology. Medial cystic necrosis is usually considered to be the abnormality responsible for dissecting aneurysm. Actually the problem is complex because dissecting aneurysm may occur when medial cystic necrosis is absent or slight, or, on the other hand, medial cystic necrosis may be found without dissection. The cause of medial cystic necrosis is not known. It is considered by some to be a nonspecific change in the aorta in response to hemodynamic stresses. The disease process is usually most severe in the ascending aorta and decreases progressively to-

ward the distal aorta, but may be extensive throughout the aorta and major vessels.

Dissecting aneurysm and rupture of the aorta can be produced experimentally by feeding growing rats *Lathyrus odoratus* (sweet pea) meal, which contains B-aminopropionitrile. The rats develop skeletal abnormalities and medial degeneration of the aorta.

Dissecting aneurysm is common in *Marfan's syndrome*. This condition is characterized by severe medial cystic necrosis, which, like the remainder of the syndrome, is genetically determined. In fact, some persons with dissecting aneurysm may appear normal, yet are found in a family group whose other members have typical Marfan's syndrome. In addition, the incidence of dissecting aneurysm seems to be increased in patients with skeletal deformities, e.g., scoliosis, pigeon breast, and funnel depression of the thorax.

The relation of *hypertension* to dissecting aneurysm is not clear. Although hypertension is frequently associated with dissecting aneurysm, it is notable that the younger the patients in a series, the larger is the proportion without hypertension. Some believe that hypertension, by increasing hemodynamic stresses on the aorta, accelerates the development of medial cystic necrosis.

Dissecting aneurysm may occur during *pregnancy*; many case reports are available emphasizing this point. Patients with *coarctation of the aorta* may die of dissecting aneurysm. Dissecting aneurysm has also been reported to be associated with *aortic stenosis* and with *myxedema*.

Atheromatous disease of the aorta is not the direct cause of medial cystic necrosis, although the two diseases may occur together. Occasionally bleeding into the media of the aorta may originate at the edge of an atheromatous ulcer. Syphilis is not the cause of medial cystic necrosis, and the syphilitic process does not prevent dissection in situations in which both diseases occur together. Other lesions, such as an aortic abscess, may initiate dissection of the aorta.

De Bakey classified dissecting aneurysm into three types. Type I begins as a transverse tear in the intima of the ascending aorta and extends distally for a variable distance. Type II is said to be present when the dissection is confined to the ascending aorta. Type III is used to signify the condition when the process begins distal to the arch vessels. When the dissection proceeds distal to the intimal tear it may also involve the branches of the aorta and may re-enter the lumen of the aorta some distance from the origin. (This can produce a double barreled aorta.) Occasionally an intimal tear is absent; this has led to speculation that an intramural hematoma developed because the vasa vasorum ruptured as a result of medial cystic necrosis. Some have extended the reasoning to state that the intimal tear itself occurred because the medial supported it so poorly. Braunstein's study refutes this idea and supports the concept that dilatation and hypertension promote the intimal tear by increasing the tension on the intima of the aorta.

Incidence. Dissecting aneurysm of the aorta is far less common but far more serious than myocardial infarction. Men are affected twice as often as women except in the advanced age groups. The peak incidence is in the fourth to seventh decades. Type I dissection is more common than Type III dissection, and Type II is comparatively rare.

Clinical Manifestations. The clinical features and prognosis associated with dissecting aneurysm are determined by the anatomic derangement which characterizes the three types of the condition. Dissecting aneurysm is frequently mistaken for and treated as myocardial infarction. It can be misdiagnosed as pulmonary embolism. In view of the fact that the arteries supplying blood to the brain and cord, the abdominal viscera, and the extremities branch off the aorta, it must be borne in mind that dissecting aneurysm can mimic cerebral vascular accident, acute abdominal crises, or peripheral vascular occlusions. The following points are useful in differential diagnosis:

Pain. Although the majority of patients with dissecting aneurysm of the aorta have chest pain, it is now clear that some do not. Painless dissection occurs especially with Marfan's disease. It must be remembered that a severe neurologic deficit, caused by the dissection, may prevent the patient from giving a history of pain. The patient usually experiences severe anterior chest pain, however, and it is for this reason that the condition is frequently misdiagnosed as myocardial infarction. Dissecting aneurysm should be considered under the following circumstances: when the chest pain is excruciating and when considerable morphine is needed for relief; when the pain is maximal at the onset rather than gradually increasing, as it frequently does with myocardial infarction; when the pain radiates to the back or predominates in the back; when the pain is widespread and radiates to the abdomen, legs, head, and neck; and when the pain shifts to a lower level in the body as the dissection extends.

Pain may be the only manifestation of the condition in patients with Type III dissection, whereas patients with Types I and II are likely to have pain plus other physical abnormalities.

Level of Blood Pressure. Although the patient may have the appearance of being in shock, with anxiety, pallor, sweating, tachypnea, and tachycardia, the blood pressure is elevated in most patients with dissecting aneurysms. This occurs because many patients have hypertension prior to the catastrophic event and there may be an increase in blood pressure during dissection as a result of severe pain. In addition, the heart may function well in such circumstances, unlike myocardial infarction, in which a portion of the myocardium is destroyed. Marked elevation of systemic blood pressure is more common in patients with Type III dissection as compared with those with Type I dissection. Frank shock levels of blood

pressure are seldom observed in patients with Type III dissection but may be seen in 20 per cent of patients with Type I dissection.

Arterial Pulsations. The carotid, brachial, radial, and femoral arteries must be palpated repeatedly for change in pulsation. Absence or inequality of pulsations is an important clue and indicates arterial occlusion. The degree of pulsation may vary from hour to hour because of arterial spasm. When signs and symptoms of peripheral arterial occlusion occur within a few hours after chest pain, dissecting aneurysm should be considered rather than myocardial infarction, since an embolic episode due to infarction is delayed until several days after the onset of chest pain. Alteration of the pulsation of the various arteries is more common in patients with Type I dissection than in those with Type III dissection.

Aortic Regurgitation. The murmur of aortic regurgitation may be heard in about one third of patients with dissection of the aorta. It is more common in patients with Type I dissection. Aortic regurgitation occurs because the integrity of the aortic ring is altered and because the support of the aortic valve cusps may be destroyed. On rare occasions a peculiar fluttering sound can be heard in diastole, probably caused by a piece of the intima vibrating in the blood stream during diastole. Chest pain followed by the development of aortic regurgitation should suggest dissecting aneurysm.

Pulsation of the Sternoclavicular Joint. Pulsation of the right or left sternoclavicular joint may be noted in dissecting aneurysm. This unusual pulsation can also be produced by other types of aortic aneurysms. A rare cause of right sternoclavicular pulsation is an anomalous right aortic arch.

Neurologic Abnormalities. Neurologic abnormalities are common and result from decreased blood flow to the brain and cord associated with shock or obstruction of the arteries by the dissecting hematoma. Neurological complications are more often associated with Type I dissection. Coma, hemiplegia, confusion, and visual disturbances may occur. Weakness and even paralysis of the lower extremities may be caused by ischemia of the spinal cord or ischemia of the legs. The weakness may be associated with pain, paresthesia, and sensory and reflex changes in the extremities. Severe chest pain accompanied by severe weakness of the lower extremities should always suggest the possibility of a dissecting aneurysm.

Abdominal Findings. When abdominal symptoms predominate in a patient with dissecting aneurysm, laparotomy may be performed because of the diagnosis of "acute abdomen." At operation, the bowel, gallbladder, or other organs are found to be ischemic or blood is found leaking into the abdominal cavity.

When the renal arteries are involved, hematuria and suppression of urine flow may result.

Cardiovascular Findings. A pericardial friction rub may be noted. Such a finding does not invariably mean that the aorta has dissected into the pericardial space since a rub may occur when the beads of blood surrounding the injured vasa vasorum of the ascending aorta leak into the pericardial space. (The pericardium encloses a small part of the aorta.) Neck veins may be distended because of superior vena caval obstruction or because of bleeding into the pericardial space with subsequent cardiac tamponade. The latter is almost always followed by death. The precordial thrust may be large and sustained because of left ventricular hypertrophy due to previously existing hypertension. Aortic regurgitation has already been mentioned. The electrocardiogram may show left ventricular hypertrophy, nonspecific S-T and T changes, rhythm disturbances, and pericarditis. Dissection of the coronary arteries may occur, and this usually leads to death.

Roentgenographic Findings. Enlargement of the aortic shadow is the most common roentgenographic sign of dissecting aneurysm (Fig. 3). Unfortunately the roentgenogram must be made with the patient recumbent because of his critical state. Bedside techniques for roentgenography of the chest produce considerable distortion of the heart and great vessels, thereby making accurate interpretation of a wide upper mediastinum difficult. Progressive enlargement of the aorta over a period of days or weeks may be noted. Occasionally the width of the aortic wall may be identified if intimal calcification is present, thereby marking the internal limit of the aortic wall. When a hematoma is present, the wall thickness is greater than the normal 2 to 3 mm. In many instances angiocardiography may be needed to determine the presence and extent of dissection (Fig. 4). This procedure should not be done routinely, but in selected cases venous angiography and angioaortography are indicated, especially if surgical intervention is contemplated. Modern aortographic techniques have assisted in clarifying the

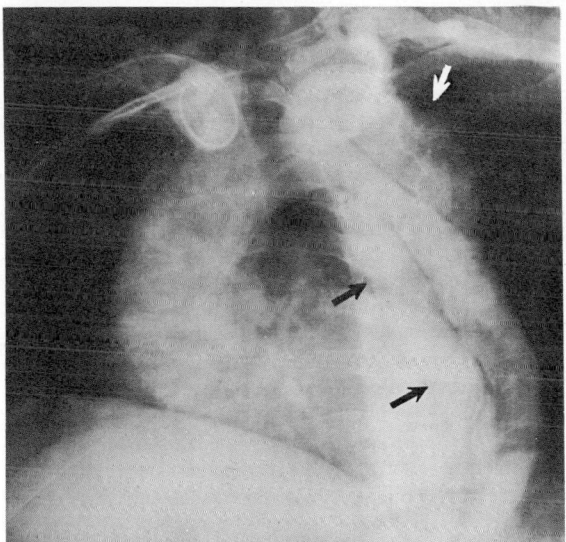

FIGURE 4. Aortogram showing a "double lumen" aorta secondary to dissecting aneurysm.

clinical spectrum of this condition. The identification of Type III dissection has improved considerably since the development of aortography.

Laboratory Findings. Leukocytosis may develop in a few hours and may reach 25,000 cells per cubic millimeter. Anemia may develop, and hyperbilirubinemia may occur occasionally. Urinalysis may show erythrocytes, albumin, casts, and gross hematuria because of renal artery occlusion.

Prognosis. Dissection of the aorta is a serious disease and is usually fatal within hours or days. The natural history of dissecting is poorly understood and this fact makes it difficult to assess therapeutic intervention. In one report (Lindsay and Hurst) of 62 patients, the initial and long-term survival was far better in patients in whom the ascending aorta was spared by the disease process. No patients in this series in whom the ascending aorta (Type I) was involved survived more than 3 weeks, whereas 8 of 19 patients whose disease began distal to the arch of the aorta (Type III) were known to survive 6 to 69 months.

Death is usually due to hemopericardium and cardiac tamponade, hemothorax, hemomediastinum, retroperitoneal hemorrhage, myocardial infarction, shock, neurologic abnormalities, congestive heart failure, renal failure, and rarely gangrene of the bowel.

Treatment. The treatment of patients with dissecting aneurysm is unsatisfactory. Pain must be relieved with opiates, blood should be replaced when needed, and oxygen may be administered. Anticoagulants are absolutely contraindicated. Wheat, Palmer, et al. have pioneered in the use of drugs to reduce the arterial blood pressure and pulsatile forces in patients with dissecting aneurysm. Trimethapan, guanethidine, α-methyldopa, and parenteral reserpine may be used to lower the systolic blood pressure to 100 to 120 mm. of mercury as quickly as possible. It may not be

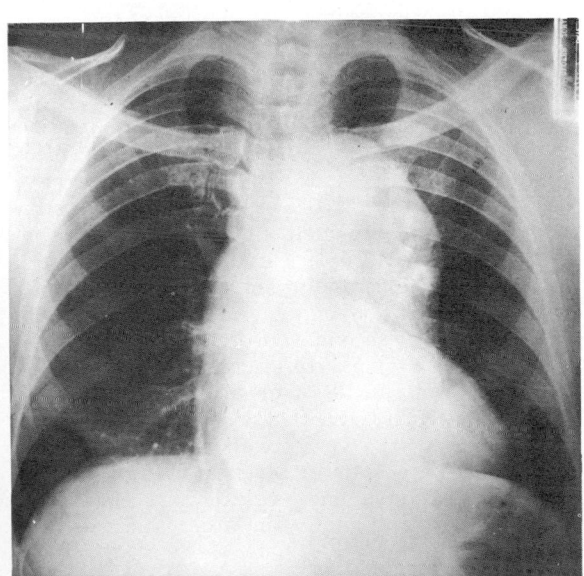

FIGURE 3. Roentgenogram of chest showing a wide aorta due to a dissecting aneurysm.

possible to use such therapy when the blood pressure is already low, when ventricular arrhythmias are present, or when oliguria is present. The exact place of this form of therapy has not been established, but it seems likely that it alters the acute course of dissection in a favorable way.

Operation is not indicated during the acute stages of disease because the risk is prohibitive, although it is occasionally attempted during the acute stage of the disease if a limb appears to be dying from lack of blood supply or if there appears to be a slow leak from the aorta. After several days, when the dissection is presumed to be no longer progressing, operation may be considered. On rare occasions the dissection may be well localized, and excision with aneurysmorrhaphy may be possible. A re-entry passage may be created into the true lumen of the descending aorta, and the false lumen can be obliterated by suture. When possible, it seems wise to use some form of excisional therapy and aortic replacement with the use of left atriofemoral bypass perfusion, external bypass graft, or hypothermia. Aortic regurgitation has occasionally been corrected by means of a Starr-Edwards ball-valve prosthesis. The operative mortality experienced by the De-Bakey team is about 25 per cent. Follow-up observations for more than five years reveal that many vascular problems have occurred in the group of survivors.

The treatment of dissecting aneurysm is now being studied in many medical centers. The trend in therapy seems toward a combination of drug therapy and surgical therapy. Unfortunately the treatment remains unsatisfactory.

Braunstein, H.: Pathogenesis of dissecting aneurysm. Circulation, 28:1071, 1963.
De Bakey, M. E., Henley, W. S., Cooley, D. A., Morris, G. C., Crawford, E. S., and Beall, A. C.: Surgical management of dissecting aneurysms of the aorta. J. Thorac. Cardiov. Surg., 49:130, 1965.
Hirst, A. E., Johns, V. J., Jr., and Kime, S. W., Jr.: Dissecting aneurysm of the aorta. A review of 505 cases. Medicine, 37:217, 1958.
Lindsay, J., Jr.: The therapy of dissecting aneurysm of the aorta. Mod. Conc. Cardiov. Dis., 38:13, 1969.
Lindsay, J., Jr., and Hurst, J. W.: Clinical features and prognosis in dissecting aneurysm of the aorta: A reappraisal. Circulation, 35:880, 1967.
Lindsay, J., Jr., and Hurst, J. W.: Drug therapy of dissecting aortic aneurysms: Some reservations. Circulation, 37:216, 1968.
Shuford, W. H., Sybers, R. G., Weens, H. S., Lindsay, J., Jr., and Hurst, J. W.: Aortographic findings in dissecting aneurysm of the aorta. Amer. J. Cardiol., 24:111, 1969.
Wheat, M. W., Jr., Palmer, R. F., Bartley, T. D., and Seelman, R. C.: Treatment of dissecting aneurysms of the aorta without surgery. J. Thorac. Cardiov. Surg., 50:364, 1965.

TRAUMATIC ANEURYSM

Injury of the aorta may be caused by penetrating wounds or by blunt trauma. Damage to the thoracic aorta may be produced by injuries that do not produce rib fractures. The most common cause of such injuries is automobile accidents.

Ruptures and tears with subsequent aneurysm formation are usually found at points where the aorta is relatively fixed in position—just distal to the origin of the left subclavian artery at the site of the ligamentum arteriosum, and in the ascending aorta just beyond the aortic valve. When a severe accelerative or decelerative force is sustained, the remainder of the aorta moves more freely than the fixed points, producing an injury to the vessel. An injury to the aorta that tears all layers of the aorta causes death, but when the tear involves only the intima it may cause only a hematoma in the media or, on rare occasion, a dissecting aneurysm.

A tear in the aorta may cause mediastinal hemorrhage, which may be diagnosed by the mediastinal widening in chest roentgenograms. Repeat roentgenograms of the chest should be made in such cases in order to detect the appearance of aortic aneurysm, which may become visible in a few weeks. The aneurysm may be noted first on a routine chest film made years after the injury.

Resection is usually indicated for traumatic aneurysms of the aorta. Since this type of aneurysm is not necessarily related to other diseases, the general vascular status in patients is frequently good. Accordingly, the operative risk for the resection of traumatic aneurysms is less than it is for other kinds of aneurysms.

De Bakey, M. E., and Crawford, S. E.: Surgical considerations of acquired diseases of the aorta and major peripheral arteries. I. Aortic aneurysms. Mod. Conc. Cardiov. Dis., 28:557, 1959.
Goyette, E. M., Blake, H. A., Forsee, J. H., and Swan, H.: Traumatic aortic aneurysms. Circulation, 10:824, 1954.

MYCOTIC ANEURYSM

Mycotic aneurysm of the aorta may be associated with bacterial endocarditis, septicemia, or the extension of a neighboring abscess into the aortic wall. Microscopic examination of the vessel wall shows inflammatory cells and destruction of tissue. The offending organisms include streptococci, staphylococci, and salmonellae.

Mycotic aneurysm or suppurative arteritis due to salmonellae is being recognized more frequently than before. Sower and Whelan have reported that three types of vascular lesions may be produced by salmonellae: (1) a diffuse suppurative arteritis with rupture and the development of a saccular or false aneurysm; (2) a focal arteritis with the formation of a mycotic aneurysm and rupture; or (3) a secondary infection superimposed upon a pre-existing arteriosclerotic aneurysm. A normal vessel can be involved when an infected embolus becomes lodged on its wall, or organisms gain access to the vessel wall through the vasa vasorum. The vessels involved in many of the reported cases have had pre-existing lesions, including dissecting aneurysm, atherosclerosis, and syphilis.

Once a mycotic aneurysm of the aorta has developed, surgical resection offers the only possibility of cure.

Allen, E. V., Barker, N. W., and Hines, E. A.: Peripheral Vascular Diseases. 3rd ed. Philadelphia, W. B. Saunders Company, 1962.

Sower, N. D., and Wholan, T. J.: Suppurative arteritis due to salmonella. Surgery, 52:851, 1962.

ANEURYSMS OF THE SINUSES OF VALSALVA

An aneurysm of one of the sinuses of Valsalva may be due to syphilitic aortitis, bacterial endocarditis, medial cystic necrosis, or a congenital defect. The lesion is described in the section on Congenital Heart Disease.

SYPHILIS OF THE AORTA

Syphilis is described elsewhere in this textbook. The discussion here is confined to its effect on the aorta (and the heart).

Pathology. Although syphilitic myocarditis, gummas of the myocardium, and syphilitic involvement of the coronary arteries are known to occur rarely, it is safe to assume that the aorta is always involved in cardiovascular syphilis. Syphilitic aortitis begins with perivascular inflammation of the vasa vasorum in the adventitia. Treponemas subsequently invade the media via the lymphatics, producing medial inflammation and destruction. The ensuing fibrous proliferation results in intimal wrinkling and the characteristic "tree bark" appearance. It seems likely that many of the lesions of the aorta just described are secondary to changes that have occurred in the vasa vasorum that result in a diminished blood supply to the aorta itself. As a rule, the pathologic process is limited to the thoracic portion of the aorta. Gummatous lesions of the aorta may occur but they are not common.

Clinical Manifestations. Uncomplicated syphilitic aortitis is difficult to diagnose during life. There are no reliable clinical signs that allow one to make a diagnosis. The majority of patients who have had inadequate treatment of syphilis during its early stages show syphilitic aortitis at autopsy. Diagnosis of uncomplicated aortitis is not based on signs and symptoms.

Syphilitic aortitis may lead to *dilatation of the aorta*. This almost always occurs in the ascending portion, and no symptoms are produced by it. There are no clearly diagnostic physical findings. It has long been said that the second heart sound is accentuated and has a tambour-like quality when there is syphilitic aortitis. Dilatation of the aorta secondary to systemic hypertension or atherosclerosis can also be associated with a loud second heart sound. Since these diseases are far more common than dilatation of the aorta due to syphilis, the sign is not of diagnostic value. Dilatation of the ascending aorta may produce a nonspecific systolic murmur in the aortic area. Visible and palpable pulsations in the upper parasternal region may be noted. When there is moderate dilatation or aneurysmal formation of the ascending aorta, pulsation of the right or left sternoclavicular joints may be detected (see Fig. 2). When the ascending aorta is dilated, the upper parasternal dullness may be wider than normal.

Dilatation of the ascending aorta may be detected at fluoroscopic examination of the heart and aorta and on roentgenograms of the chest utilizing the oblique positions. Unfortunately, it is not easy to state when the aorta has attained definitely abnormal size. The width of the root of the aorta can be studied far more adequately by angiocardiography. This is not always needed but it may occasionally be justified. The surest sign of syphilitic aortitis is calcification of the early portion of the ascending aorta (Fig. 5). About one fifth of the cases of syphilitic aortitis have the sign. The calcification is actually due to the atherosclerosis of the aorta. Ordinarily calcification of the intima of the aorta due to atherosclerosis is seen roentgenographically in the aortic knob. The atherosclerotic process seems to increase in the root and ascending portion of the aorta where the syphilitic process is most severe.

Aortic regurgitation, the most frequent complication of syphilitic aortitis, is mainly due to the dilatation of the aortic ring. The syphilitic process also extends into the base of the valve leaflet. The result is separation of the valve commissures and deformity of the cusps. This deformity, plus the dilated aortic ring, produces insufficiency. Aortic stenosis never develops as a result of syphilis.

Aortic regurgitation due to syphilis usually appears between the ages of 35 and 50. It is seen earlier in Negroes. Men have the condition far

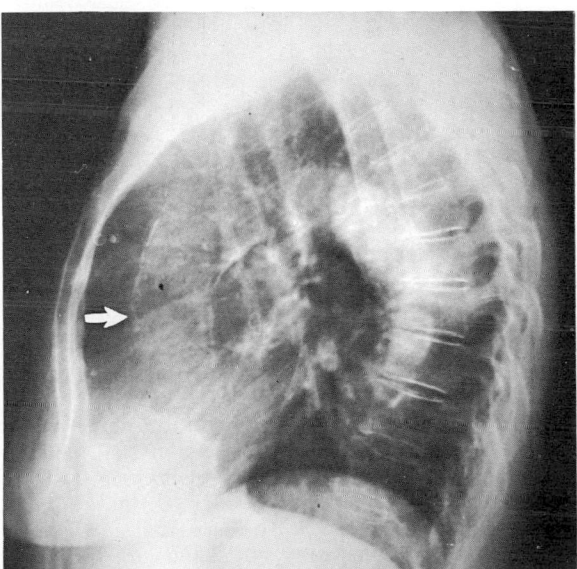

FIGURE 5. Lateral roentgenogram of chest showing calcification of the early portion of the aorta. This type of calcification is characteristic of atherosclerosis superimposed on syphilitic aortitis.

more often than women. It occurs in about half of all cases of cardiovascular syphilis.

The signs and symptoms of aortic regurgitation due to syphilis depend upon the degree and duration of the abnormality. Symptoms and signs of heart failure are likely to ensue within three to four years after aortic regurgitation is discovered. Heart failure may develop gradually or may be heralded by acute pulmonary edema. Therapy may be beneficial for a time and a few patients survive more than a decade after heart failure has developed, but the majority do not live more than a few years. Sudden and unexpected death may occur in patients with severe aortic regurgitation.

Syphilitic aortitis may cause *narrowing of the ostia of the major arterial branches* of the thoracic aorta. There may be diminished pulsation of the carotid arteries, and the blood pressure and pulsations of the upper extremities may be altered. (See discussion of Aortic Arch Syndrome.) Narrowing of the coronary ostia, when mild, causes no symptoms. Angina pectoris in patients with syphilitic aortitis is usually due to a combination of factors, including narrowed coronary ostia, the hemodynamic effects of aortic regurgitation, the increased demand of associated left ventricular hypertrophy, congestive heart failure, and associated coronary atherosclerosis. Angina pectoris in this clinical setting may be more severe and less responsive to nitroglycerin than usual. Myocardial infarction is an uncommon autopsy finding in patients with cardiovascular syphilis, but prolonged chest pain and sudden death are not rare. It is not wise to make a diagnosis of isolated coronary ostial disease due to syphilis with no other evidence of syphilitic aortitis. Coronary atherosclerosis is so common that it is likely to be the cause of angina pectoris in such cases.

Rimsa, A., and Griffith, G. C.: Trends in cardiovascular syphilis. Ann. Intern. Med., 46:915, 1957.

THROMBOSIS OF THE TERMINAL AORTA

Thrombosis of the terminal aorta may occur suddenly or may develop gradually, usually on atheromatous lesions. Most often it occurs in males between the ages of 40 and 65, although it has occurred at a younger age.

Sudden thrombosis of the terminal aorta may simulate embolic obstruction when the aortic lumen has been almost normal in size prior to the formation of the clot. If sudden thrombosis is superimposed on a partially obstructed aorta, the signs and symptoms may be less severe because collateral circulation has had time to develop prior to the acute thrombosis. Pain and weakness of the lower extremities may occur after sudden thrombosis of the aorta. The pain may radiate to the lower back and inguinal regions. The arterial pulses below the obstructed area are absent. The legs may be pale, mottled, cyanotic, or white, and signs of shock may be present. It may be impossible to differentiate a saddle embolus to the aortic bifurcation from sudden thrombosis of the terminal aorta. When a heart lesion is present that could be the source of an embolus, the diagnostic scale tips in that direction.

When thrombosis of the aorta occurs with normal aortic lumen, the outlook is poor. The treatment is similar to that of saddle embolus. When thrombosis of the aorta occurs in a partially occluded aorta with a better collateral circulation, the outlook may be somewhat less grave. Surgical resection and grafting of the occluded portion of the aorta is usually indicated as an emergency procedure.

Gradual thrombosis of the terminal portion of the aorta has been called the *Leriche syndrome.* This condition differs from sudden occlusion of the aorta and is far more common. The patient feels distress produced by walking and relieved by rest. The discomfort develops in the thighs, hip region, or buttocks and represents intermittent claudication at a high level. The arterial pulses are absent or decreased in the lower extremities. Feeble pulsations are sometimes found when collateral circulation has developed to a moderate degree. Bruits may be heard over the abdominal aorta and over the iliac and femoral arteries. Atrophy of leg muscles may develop in time. Many patients with the Leriche syndrome have good nutrition to the skin of the extremities because of the adequate collateral circulation that develops when the vascular obstruction is high. In fact, the good prognosis with regard to limb survival should be emphasized. Some patients do have coldness, pallor, cyanosis, trophic changes of the legs, and, rarely, gangrene of the feet, but it is likely that the smaller peripheral vessels are also diseased when these signs of arterial insufficiency are present. Many cases of Leriche syndrome are misdiagnosed as osteoarthritis of the lumbosacral spine or hip, ruptured intervertebral disc, or bursitis of the hip. The majority of these patients die as a result of cerebral or coronary atherosclerosis. Rarely, the renal arteries may become occluded by cephalad extension of the aortic thrombus.

Aortography is not usually needed to make the diagnosis of thrombosis of the aorta. It is useful, however, in determining the site and extent of the obstruction, estimating the collateral circulation, and determining the amount of disease in the distal vessels. The modern contrast media and newer techniques have made aortography much safer than formerly.

The usual conservative therapy for chronic occlusive peripheral vascular disease is indicated. Surgical treatment is indicated when the intermittent claudication is severe enough and disabling enough to justify the mortality and morbidity risk of such treatment. Recognizable cerebral, coronary, and other serious diseases are usually contraindications to operation. Three operative procedures are utilized; thromboendarterectomy, excision with graft replacement, and bypass graft. The operative risk reported by De Bakey is only about 2.5 per cent, and relief of symptoms and restoration of pulses were obtained in 96 per cent of cases. Operation on the aorta of course does nothing to prevent the complications of cerebral and coronary atherosclerosis in these patients.

De Bakey, M. D., and Crawford, S. E.: Surgical considerations of acquired diseases of the aorta and major peripheral arteries. III: Atherosclerotic occlusive vascular disease, Mod. Conc. Cardiov. Dis., 29:571, 1960.

Juergens, J. L., Barker, N. W., and Hines, E. A.: Arteriosclerosis obliterans: Review of 520 cases with special reference to pathogenic and prognostic factors. Circulation, 21:188, 1960.

Leriche, R., and Morel, A.: The syndrome of thrombotic obliteration of the aortic bifurcation. Ann. Surg., 127:193, 1948.

Massarelli, J. J., Jr., and Estes, J. E.: Atherosclerotic occlusion of the abdominal aorta and iliac arteries. A study of 105 patients. Ann. Intern. Med., 47:1125, 1957.

EMBOLISM AT THE BIFURCATION OF THE AORTA

An embolus lodging at the bifurcation of the aorta is called a *saddle embolus*. Perhaps no more than 5 per cent of all systemic arterial emboli lodge at this point, but when one does, a true emergency is created.

Large emboli almost always originate in the heart. In patients with rheumatic heart disease who have mitral valve disease and a dilated left atrium, left atrial clots may be the source of emboli. Emboli are more often associated with mitral stenosis than with mitral regurgitation. They occur with higher frequency when there is atrial fibrillation rather than normal sinus rhythm. The presence of heart failure does not seem to increase the frequency of emboli from this source. Occasionally an embolus seems to be related to a change in cardiac rhythm from atrial fibrillation to normal sinus rhythm. An embolus may follow mitral valve surgery. A large, friable, left ventricular thrombus may develop secondary to myocardial infarction, and it may break off and be swept by the blood to the bifurcation of the aorta, where it lodges. This has occurred with decreasing frequency since anticoagulants have been used in the treatment of myocardial infarction. Emboli can occur from such a source a week or several weeks after the myocardial infarction. The presence of heart failure increases the possibility of left ventricular thrombosis and peripheral emboli in such cases. The emboli related to bacterial endocarditis are usually too small to cause a saddle embolus. Rarely an embolus may arise from the systemic veins and pass through an atrial septal defect into the systemic arteries. Thrombi in aortic aneurysms or on ulcerated atherosclerotic lesions of the aorta may be the source of emboli.

Although a rather large clot is required to produce a saddle embolus, the clot need not be as large as the aorta itself. Edema of the aortic wall and intense arterial spasm of the involved collateral vessels occur very quickly after an embolus. These factors, along with secondary thrombosis, can convert a partial block into a complete one.

Clinical Manifestations. Pain in the legs usually develops suddenly, but may come on gradually. Abdominal or sacral pain may occasionally predominate. Paresthesia, anesthesia, and muscular weakness of the lower extremities may follow the pain or may develop without pain. The clinician must be alert when a patient with reason for peripheral arterial embolus complains that his leg has "gone to sleep." The skin of the lower extremities may be cold, pale, mottled, or cyanotic. Pulsations of the femoral, popliteal, posterior tibial, and dorsalis pedis vessels are usually not felt. Saddle embolus of the aorta must be differentiated from thrombosis of the terminal aorta and thrombophlebitis with associated severe arterial spasm.

It should be emphasized that more distal peripheral emboli may proceed or follow the embolus to the bifurcation of the aorta.

Patients with saddle block embolus frequently die or lose a limb unless embolectomy can be performed promptly. Even with surgical intervention the mortality is high, especially when the embolus occurs subsequent to myocardial infarction. The technique described by Cranley et al., using an "embolectomy catheter" with a balloon, has been employed with moderate success. Heparin should be administered as soon as the diagnosis of arterial embolism is made. Heparin and drugs useful for long-term anticoagulation should be used postoperatively. At times, cardiac valve abnormalities should be corrected surgically when they are thought to be responsible for the intracardiac thrombi.

Cranley, J. J., Krause, R. J., Strasser, E. S., Hafner, C. D., and Fogarty, T. S.: Peripheral arterial embolism: Changing concepts. Surgery, 55:57, 1964.

Crave, C.: Embolism to the bifurcation of the aorta. New Eng. J. Med., 258:359, 1958.

Deterling, R. A.: Acute arterial occlusion. Surg. Clin. N. Amer., 46:587, 1966.

Whitman, E. J., and McGoon, D. C.: Surgical management of aorto-iliac occlusive vascular disease. J.A.M.A., 179:923, 1962.

THE AORTIC ARCH SYNDROME

The term "aortic arch syndrome" is given to a group of disorders leading to occlusion of the vessels arising from the arch of the aorta. (The term "pulseless disease" is often used synonymously with the term "aortic arch syndrome.") The disease may be due to nonspecific arteritis (*Takayasu's disease*). It may be due to the obstructive lesions found in arteries associated with *supravalvular aortic stenosis*. Years ago *syphilitic arteritis* was a common cause of the obstructive lesions of the vessels arising from the aortic arch. Today the majority of patients seen in the United States with pulseless disease are in the middle and older age groups, and the pathologic lesion causing the occlusive disease of the arteries is almost invariably *atherosclerosis.* The signs and symptoms associated with obliterative disease of the vessels arising from the arch of the aorta are predictable when one considers the blood supply of the brain, eyes, face, and arms.

The rare disease known as *Takayasu's disease* has been observed as early as age 11 and as late as age 64. The diagnosis is usually made during the third decade of life. For unexplained reasons, most patients with the syndrome are females. Reports from many countries prove that the condition is not confined to Japan, as it was once thought to be. The clinical features include vertigo, syncope, convulsions, aphasia, headache, transient cerebral ischemia resulting in hemiplegia or hemiparesis, absence of palpable carotid arteries on one or both sides, transient episodes of blindness, amblyopia, rapidly developing cataracts, retinal atrophy or pigmentation, photophobia, optic atrophy, atrophy of the iris, sluggish blood flow in the retinal vessels, decreased intraocular arterial pressure, muscular atrophy of the face, thin pigmented skin of the face, ulcerated nose and palate, claudication of muscles of mastication, decreased or absent audible blood pressure in the arms and increased blood pressure in the lower extremities (hence the term "reversed coarctation"), absence of subclavian, brachial and radial pulses, claudication of upper extremities, palpable collateral arteries in the neck and intercostal spaces, rib notching, and continuous murmurs in the neck and upper chest. Calcification of the intima of the ascending aorta, aortic regurgitation, angina pectoris, and myocardial infarction may occur. This multitude of symptoms and signs can be kept in mind if one remembers that they are associated with ischemia of the brain, eyes, face, and upper extremities. Leukocytosis and elevated sedimentation rate are common.

Histologically the lesions are characterized by an arteritis of all layers of the involved vessels with giant cell infiltration and obliteration of the lumen. The pathologic process is usually limited to the innominate, subclavian, and carotid arteries as well as the coronary ostia. It has also been observed to involve the thoracic and abdominal aorta and the mesenteric arteries.

Patients with this syndrome usually die of cerebral ischemia or heart disease. No figures are available to indicate the average length of life after onset of the disease. After the onset of symptoms, patients have lived from one and one-half to fourteen years. Long-term anticoagulant treat-

ment has been recommended in an effort to prevent arterial thrombosis. Surgical treatment, including endarterectomy, local resection, and vessel grafts, may be applicable in suitable cases.

Cheitlin, M. D., and Carter, P. G.: Takayashu's disease. Unusual manifestations. Arch. Intern. Med. (Chicago), 116: 283, 1965.
Judge, R. D., Currier, R. D., Gracie, W. A., and Figley, M. M.: Takayasu's arteritis and the aortic arch syndrome. Amer. J. Med., 32:379, 1962.
Kalmansohn, R. B., and Kalmansohn, R. W.: Thrombotic obliteration of the branches of the aortic arch. Circulation, 15: 237, 1957.
Shimizu, K., and Sano, K.: Pulseless disease. J. Neuropath. Clin. Neurol., 1:37, 1951.
Vinijchaikul, K.: Primary arteritis of the aorta and its main branches (Takayasu's arteriopathy): A clinicopathologic study of eight cases. Medicine, 43:15, 1967.

RHEUMATOID AORTITIS

Aortitis may be recognized in a small percentage of patients with rheumatoid arthritis. A rheumatoid etiology for aortic regurgitation is especially likely when there is rheumatoid spondylitis, uveitis, or psoriasis. Some observers believe that this type of aortitis is specifically seen when there is ankylosing spondylitis and that it does not occur in rheumatoid arthritis without spinal involvement. When the murmur of aortic regurgitation develops during an exacerbation of rheumatoid arthritis, particularly in the presence of uveitis, it is considered to be diagnostic of rheumatoid aortitis and aortic valve disease. Aortic regurgitation due to rheumatoid aortitis and aortic valve disease is differentiated from syphilitic heart disease when the serologic tests for syphilis are negative and when the murmur occurs at an early age in a patient with rheumatoid arthritis.

Although the clinical features of rheumatoid aortitis and aortic valve disease are similar to the findings in rheumatic heart disease, the pathologic findings are more distinctive. The cusps of the aortic valve do not fuse at the commissures as they do in rheumatic aortic valve disease. Plaquelike lesions of the aortic intima near the valve commissures found in rheumatoid aortitis have not been observed in rheumatic fever. The lesions in the aorta usually do not extend beyond the ascending portion of the vessel. The entire clinical and pathologic picture forces one to support the idea that rheumatoid aortitis is a specific complication of rheumatoid arthritis.

When surgical treatment for aortic regurgitation is deemed necessary in patients with rheumatoid spondylitis, the newest surgical techniques, including the placement of a Starr-Edwards prosthetic valve, can be utilized.

Clarke, W. S., Kulka, J. P., and Bauer, W.: Rheumatoid aortitis with aortic regurgitation; An unusual manifestation of rheumatoid arthritis (including spondylitis). Amer. J. Med., 22:580, 1957.
Graham, D. C., and Smythe, H. S.: The carditis and aortitis of ankylosing spondylitis. Bull. Rheum. Dis., 9:171, 1958.

OTHER CAUSES OF AORTITIS

Aortitis may develop in association with a variety of conditions. These include scleroderma and Hodgkin's disease.

Giant cell arteritis may involve the aorta and produce the aortic arch syndrome, aneurysm of the ascending aorta, aortic regurgitation, and dissecting aneurysm. This condition is being recognized with increasing frequency.

Behçet's syndrome, consisting of mouth and genital ulcerations, blindness, central nervous system involvement, thrombophlebitis, and arterial involvement, may be associated with aortic aneurysms.

Austin, W. G., and Blennerhassett, J. B.: Giant cell aortitis causing an aneurysm of the ascending aorta and aortic regurgitation. New Eng. J. Med., 272:80, 1965.

Fraumeni, J. F., Jr., Herweg, J. C., and Kissane, J. M.: Panaortitis complicating Hodgkin's disease. Ann. Intern. Med., 67:1242, 1967.

Hills, E. A.: Behçet's syndrome with aortic aneurysms. Brit. Med. J., 4:152, 1967.

Hunder, G. G., Ward, L. E., and Burbank, M. K.: Giant-cell arteritis producing an aortic arch syndrome. Ann. Intern. Med., 66:578, 1967.

Roth, L. M., and Kissane, J. M.: Panaortitis and aortic valvulitis in progressive systemic sclerosis (scleroderma). Amer. J. Clin. Path., 41:287, 1964.

CONGENITAL ANOMALIES OF THE AORTA

A right aortic arch may occur as an isolated and asymptomatic abnormality. It may produce pulsation of the right sternoclavicular joint and is usually identified on the chest roentgenogram. The anomaly may be associated with other cardiovascular defects. For example, 25 per cent of patients with tetralogy of Fallot and truncus arteriosus and 5 per cent of patients with tricuspid atresia have the aortic arch on the right side.

The right subclavian artery may arise from the descending aorta (*aberrant right subclavian artery*). The anomaly may be unassociated with other abnormalities, but an association with tetralogy of Fallot has been reported. The vessel passes posterior to the esophagus and for this reason is usually identified by observing an indention of the barium-filled esophagus during fluoroscopy. This anomaly is occasionally associated with a large aneurysmal diverticulum of the aorta (*Kommerell's diverticulum*). An aberrant right subclavian artery is found in approximately 1 per cent of routine barium studies of the esophagus. It is almost always asymptomatic but has been claimed to cause dysphagia on rare occasions. Aneurysmal dilatation and rupture of an aberrant subclavian artery have been reported.

A number of vascular anomalies of the aortic arch may contrive to encircle the esophagus and trachea and produce a *vascular ring*. Although many varieties of rings are possible, the two common types are *double aortic arch* and *right aortic arch with retroesophageal segment with a left-sided ligamentum arteriosum*. Vascular rings may produce noisy respiration, brassy cough, recurrent pulmonary infections, and dysphagia during early life. Infants may be more comfortable with the neck hyperextended. The vascular abnormality may be suspected in a routine roentgenogram of the chest if the air column of the trachea is constricted at the proper location. More often the condition is identified by fluoroscopic examination of the barium-filled esophagus. More exact delineation of the vessels can be accomplished by aortography (Fig. 6). When obstructive lesions are severe, surgical correction is indicated.

Atresia of the aortic arch may be the cause of heart failure during the first few days of life. In fact, heart failure at this age is a clue to the diagnosis. Death usually occurs in a few days to weeks. On rare occasions pulmonary arteriolar disease protects the lungs and prolongs survival time. The atretic area is usually located between the left common carotid artery and the ductus arteriosus. Arterial unsaturation is found in the lower extremities.

Supravalvular aortic stenosis may be misdiagnosed as ordinary valvular aortic stenosis. This less common condition occasionally occurs as a familial trait and is characterized by unusual facies, occasional mental retardation, a pressure difference in the two arms (lower in left arm), obstructive lesions of the vessels arising from the aortic arch (including obstruction of the coronary arteries), associated pulmonary stenosis, multiple pulmonary artery stenoses, and hypercalcemia, in addition to the murmur of aortic

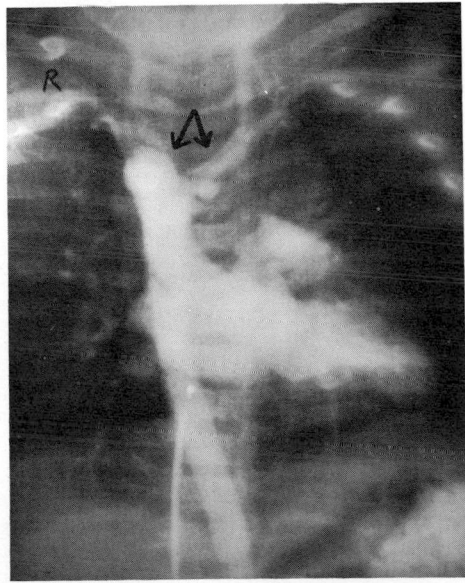

FIGURE 6.   Angiocardiogram showing double aortic arch.

obstruction. Surgical correction of this condition is not entirely satisfactory since multiple abnormalities may be present.

COARCTATION OF THE AORTA

The constriction of the aorta that characterizes coarctation of the aorta is usually located just distal to the left subclavian artery near the site of the ligamentum arteriosum. This abnormality is more common in males than in females, but is seen with increased frequency in females with ovarian agenesis (*Turner's syndrome*). The patient with coarctation of the aorta is usually asymptomatic. The condition is suspected because of a heart murmur and hypertension in the upper extremities. The muscular development of the upper extremities may be prominent compared with that of the legs. It is extremely rare for intermittent claudication of the legs to be noted. Collateral vessels on the back may be detected in the adolescent child.

Not all patients with coarctation of the aorta have hypertension, but the majority have slight to moderate elevation of the systolic and diastolic pressure. The hypertension is probably due to altered renal hemodynamics rather than to mechanical obstruction. Normally the blood pressure recorded in the legs is higher than the blood pressure in the arms. This is, of course, largely artifactual because the thigh, where the pressure is usually recorded in the leg, is larger than the upper arm. When there is coarctation of the aorta, the blood pressure reading in the arms is higher than that in the legs. Occasionally the arterial pulse and blood pressure in the left arm may be absent or lower than that of the right arm if the left subclavian arises from the constricted area or from the aorta below the coarctation. There may be relative hypotension in the right arm, either because of a stenotic origin of the subclavian or innominate artery or because of an aberrant right subclavian artery. Normally the pulsation of the femoral artery is strong and is easily felt, and arises at the groin at about the time the radial pulse is felt. When coarctation of the aorta is present the femoral artery pulsation is weak and when felt may be noted to occur after the radial artery pulsation. Coarctation of the aorta may be simulated by thrombosis of the terminal aorta in middle-aged adults. Careful palpation of the abdominal aorta may help differentiate these two conditions.

The patient with isolated coarctation of the aorta usually has a systolic murmur along the left upper sternal border, aortic area, and neck. A systolic ejection click may be heard at the cardiac apex. The systolic murmur may be heard quite well on the left back between the spine and scapula. Continuous murmurs may be heard over collateral vessels. Aortic regurgitation may be present because of dilatation of the aorta. A bicuspid aortic valve occurs in about 25 per cent

of patients with coarctation and may give rise to the murmurs of aortic stenosis and regurgitation.

The heart size may be normal, but the apex impulse may be characteristic of left ventricular hypertrophy.

Retinal hemorrhages and exudates are uncommon and the urinalysis values are normal. When advanced abnormalities are found in the retina and when the urinalysis reveals albumin and red cell casts, primary renal disease should be suspected in addition to coarctation of the aorta.

The routine chest roentgenogram may show the dilated left subclavian artery high on the left mediastinal border. There may be left ventricular prominence. Notching of the lower border of the ribs, secondary to dilatation and tortuosity of the intercostal arteries, may be seen after age six (Fig. 7). The barium-filled esophagus may show the E sign. It is produced by the dilated aorta above the coarctation, the coarctation area and the dilatation below the stenotic area.

The electrocardiogram may be entirely normal. Young children with no other abnormalities may have some residual right ventricular hypertrophy. The electrocardiogram of older patients may show increased QRS voltage with a normal mean QRS axis. When severe left ventricular hypertrophy is found, an associated lesion, such as aortic stenosis, should be considered.

Complications of Coarctation. Life may be threatened by congestive heart failure during the first year of life, usually between one week and three months of age. Many of these infants have associated defects such as aortic stenosis, patent ductus arteriosus, ventricular septal defect, transposition of the great vessels, and endocardial fibroelastosis. Congestive failure seldom occurs between the ages of one and thirty. Congestive failure may also occur in older patients, but it is

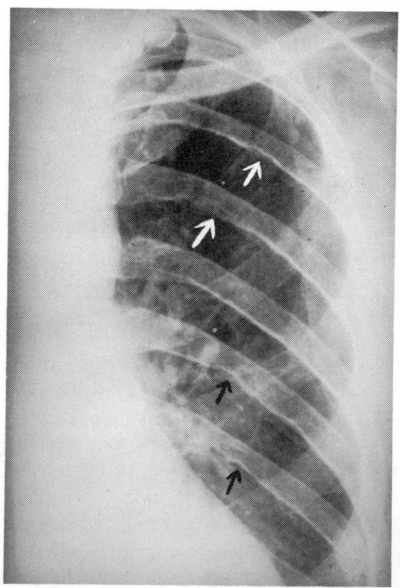

FIGURE 7. Roentgenogram of the chest showing rib notching associated with coarctation of the aorta.

wise to search for additional factors that might be responsible for the failure. Hypertensive encephalopathy has been noted. Rupture of a berry aneurysm in the brain is the cause of death in about 10 per cent of patients. Rupture of the ascending aorta with dissection into the pericardial space is found in 20 per cent of autopsy cases. Rupture may occur in late pregnancy and after trauma. Bacterial endocarditis may occur at the site of coarctation or on an associated abnormality such as a bicuspid aortic valve.

Diagnosis. Congestive heart failure in the young infant requires that a search be made for coarctation of the aorta. Hypertension is usually the first clue to the diagnosis, and it is necessary to record the blood pressure in all the extremities of patients with an elevation of arm pressure. Even when the blood pressure is normal, it is wise to carefully evaluate the femoral arterial pulsation and to record the pressure in the four extremities. Occasionally the cardiac murmur is the first clue to the diagnosis. To the embarrassment of the physician, the radiologist may suggest the diagnosis after finding rib notching on the roentgenogram of the chest. Cardiac catheterization is rarely indicated but may be necessary to exclude associated abnormalities. Aortography may be used to delineate the exact area of aortic constriction.

Treatment. Congestive heart failure during infancy due to coarctation of the aorta is a serious condition. Medical therapy should be vigorous.

If the patient does not improve satisfactorily, diagnostic studies are indicated, and surgery may be necessary. The optimal time for surgical correction of the asymptomatic patient is between the ages of eight and twenty years. The majority of patients should have the procedure.

The blood pressure in the upper extremities may remain elevated for several weeks after the obstruction in the aorta has been removed. On rare occasions, necrotizing arteritis of the bowel may occur between the fifth and tenth postoperative days. This may be associated with necrosis of the bowel, progressive hypertension, abdominal pain, and leukocytosis. Antihypertensive therapy is indicated for this condition.

Advice regarding prophylaxis against bacterial endocarditis must not be neglected. It is often necessary to continue the protection after surgical correction of the coarctation because of the commonly associated aortic valve abnormality.

Blake, H. A., and Manion, W. C.: Thoracic arterial arch anomalies. Circulation, 26:251, 1962.

Griffith, G. C., Oblath, R. W., and Jones, J. C.: Unusual manifestations of coarctation of the aorta. Circulation, 12:1080, 1955.

Harris, J. S., Sealy, W. C., Young, W. G., Jr., and Callaway, H. A., Jr.: Treatment of paradoxical hypertension and necrotizing arteriolitis following resection of coarctation of the aorta. Amer. J. Dis. Child., 94:423, 1957.

Hurst, J. W., and Logue, R. B.: The Heart. 2nd ed. New York, McGraw-Hill Book Company, 1970.

Stewart, J. R., Kincaid, O. W., and Edwards, J. E.: An Atlas of Vascular Rings and Related Malformation of the Aortic Arch System. Springfield, Ill., Charles C Thomas, 1964.

Diseases of the Peripheral Vessels

Jay D. Coffman

PERIPHERAL VASCULAR DISEASES DUE TO ORGANIC ARTERIAL OBSTRUCTION

ARTERIOSCLEROSIS OBLITERANS

Definition. Arteriosclerosis obliterans is caused by arteriosclerotic narrowing or obstruction of large and small arteries supplying the extremities; symptoms and signs are produced by ischemia.

Etiology. The etiology of arteriosclerosis is discussed in the section on obesity.

Incidence. Arteriosclerosis obliterans is the leading cause of obstructive arterial disease of the extremities after age 30. The lower extremities are involved most commonly; the superficial femoral artery is affected by stenosis or obstruction in approximately 90 per cent of patients. The

aorto-iliac and popliteal areas are the next most common sites. The greatest incidence of superficial femoral and more distal arterial disease occurs in the seventh decade, but aorto-iliac disease has its peak a decade earlier. The disease is more common in males than in females, especially before the menopause (about 9:1). Patients with diabetes mellitus develop arteriosclerosis obliterans more frequently and at an earlier age than nondiabetics. Diabetics have the same incidence of femoro-popliteal disease but a greater frequency of vessel involvement below the knee than nondiabetics. In patients with isolated aorto-iliac disease, high plasma cholesterol and total lipids are frequent findings, but diabetes mellitus is not.

Pathology. It should be emphasized that the stenotic or occlusive process is usually segmental, for surgical therapy depends on this characteristic; however, the intima also displays widespread arteriosclerotic changes proximal and distal to the segmental lesion. Although the occlusive or stenotic lesions causing symptoms are usually proximal to the knee, the incidence of lower leg arterial occlusions is high (45 per cent in some surveys) and rises steeply with increasing age. Of the small vessels in the calf, the posterior tibial artery is most often affected. A specific lesion of arteriolar and capillary endothelial proliferation has been described in diabetes by some investigators but has not been found by others. In patients with diabetes the development of indolent ulcers in the presence of adequate pulses may be due to diabetic neuropathy and not to small vessel disease.

Pathophysiology. Symptoms and signs are produced by inadequate oxygenation of the tissues distal to the arterial lesion, secondary to the decrease in blood flow or pressure at rest or during exercise. Large and medium-sized arteries must have a decrease in cross-sectional area of 70 to 90 per cent before a decrease in blood flow or pressure occurs at rest; during exercise a 60 per cent decrease may suffice. The critical stenosis diameter which decreases flow or pressure is dependent on the velocity of flow and therefore the peripheral resistance; the length of the stenotic segment has a lesser effect. Factors affecting peripheral resistance are discussed below. In patients who develop ischemic symptoms only during exercise, the calf blood flow may be normal at rest; however, during exercise the blood flow may stop or be abnormally slow. The decreased blood pressure in the artery distal to the obstructing lesion allows the force of the contracting muscle during exercise to partially or completely obstruct arterial flow. Also, if full vasodilatation (reactive hyperemia) is produced in an involved limb, the total blood flow is usually much less than in the normal limb.

Although all the vessels of a system contribute to its total resistance, the arterioles and precapillary sphincters are of greatest importance. Peripheral resistance is regulated reflexly by the sympathetic nervous system and locally by the formation of vasodilator metabolites. Activity of the sympathetic nervous system usually causes cutaneous vasoconstriction, thereby increasing peripheral resistance. This normal activity, i.e., reflex vasoconstriction when exposed to cold, can be harmful to an ischemic extremity. Removal of vasoconstrictor activity in an extremity results in vasodilatation. Blood vessels in skeletal muscle also are affected by sympathetic activity but only to a very limited extent during exercise when vasodilator metabolites are active.

Blood supply to the limb distal to an obstructing or stenotic arterial lesion is via collateral blood vessels. Most of these collaterals are present in the normal limb but unused until an obstruction occurs; they appear almost immediately following an acute arterial occlusion. Little is known concerning the reactivity of the collateral vessels in man; in animals, vasodilating or constricting stimuli or agents have little effect on them. Blood flow can be increased through collateral vessels by raising the systemic blood pressure.

Clinical Manifestations. The most common symptom of arteriosclerosis obliterans is *intermittent claudication* (intermittent limping). The patient experiences cramping pain, tightness, numbness, or severe fatigue in the muscle group being exercised. The amount of exercise producing the pain is relatively constant in each patient, and the pain is relieved promptly by rest. In a few patients, pain may disappear on further walking, perhaps because of an unconscious slowing of gait. Intermittent claudication is most frequent in the calf muscles because femoral artery disease is so common. However, even in more proximal lesions (aorto-iliac disease) the calf is the most common site of claudication because these muscles do the most work in walking. Low back, buttock, thigh, and foot claudication may also occur; the site of the symptoms localizes the obstructing lesion proximally.

Rest pain is the other important symptom of obstructive arterial disease. Rest pain is a grave sign indicating that the blood supply is not sufficient even for the small nutritional requirements of the skin. It may be localized to one or more toes but often has a stocking distribution. The latter distribution means that ischemic neuritis is not usually the cause of rest pain. Rest pain is worse at night and is relieved somewhat by dependency and by cooling.

Other symptoms of arteriosclerosis obliterans include coldness, numbness, paresthesias, and color changes in the involved extremity.

Examination of the patient with intermittent claudication reveals diminished or absent pulses below the site of obstruction. Although the dorsalis pedis pulse may be absent congenitally in more than 10 per cent of people, the posterior tibial pulse is absent in only 2 per cent, and both pulses in approximately 0.5 per cent. If pulses are palpable in the presence of an obstructive lesion, exercise will make the pulses disappear; this is often a valuable diagnostic test. If pulses cannot be detected with the fingertips, an oscillometer is often useful. The oscillometer gives a qualitative measure of the pulse beneath a blood pressure cuff. It will reveal pulsations in the presence of edema and obesity when vessels are too deep to be palpated, and sometimes when vasospasm rather than complete obstruction is present. Marked differences in oscillometric readings between two limbs at symmetrical positions or between different levels on the same limb are important. The second important part of the examination is to listen with the stethoscope over the aorta and peripheral arteries. The presence of a systolic or continuous bruit indicates a proximal obstructive or stenotic lesion; a continuous bruit denotes a very low diastolic pressure distal to the obstruction and therefore an inadequate collateral blood flow.

Examination may also reveal signs of ischemia. Distal to an arterial obstruction, the limb is often cool when compared with the proximal part of the same extremity or the symmetrical part of the opposite extremity. Skin temperature may vary widely in health, and even profound coldness, if present in all extremities, particularly in a cool environment, may be physiologic. Severe coldness that persists in a warm environment usually is abnormal, and, if unilateral, definitely abnormal. A warm extremity with normal color but absent pulses means collateral blood flow is adequate. The involved extremity may also show color changes: pallor, owing to a markedly decreased blood flow; cyanosis, caused by a diminution in blood flow not sufficient to cause blanching of the skin; rubor, a persistent red or reddish-blue discoloration of a cold extremity secondary to persistent dilatation of the cutaneous capillaries and venules owing to injury from anoxemia. Trophic changes may develop; the subcutaneous tissue becomes puffy and thickened; the skin becomes dry, atrophic, shiny, and tightly drawn with an absence of hair; and the toenails become hard, brittle, thickened, ridged, and deformed. Indolent ulceration and gangrene indicate severe local ischemia. Ischemic ulcers on the toes, and sometimes over the anterior and lateral lower calf, are usually quite painful and sensitive.

Isolated aorto-iliac disease (Leriche's syndrome) produces a characteristic picture. Intermittent claudication of the low back, buttock, thighs, or calves may be present. Global atrophy of the limbs and pallor of the legs and feet are frequent findings. Other trophic changes are usually absent; if present, concomitant femoro-popliteal disease is often found. Hypertension may be present in the upper extremities; impotence has been emphasized as a symptom but is not frequent. All pulses are usually absent in the legs, but weak femorals may be felt if the collateral circulation is well developed or if the occlusive process is only partial. A systolic murmur is often heard over both femoral arteries and lower abdomen.

Diagnosis. By careful palpation of pulses and auscultation for bruits, the diagnosis and site of obstruction or stenosis are easily determined in most patients. The presence of coldness, discoloration, and trophic changes indicates the degree of ischemia. A triad of tests can be used to evaluate the degree of ischemia and collateral circulation. With the patient supine, the involved limb is raised to a 45 degree angle. Normally the plantar surface remains pink; pallor indicates a deficient blood supply. If pallor occurs only after ankle exercise, the circulation is not as compromised. Then the patient sits up quickly, allowing the extremities to assume a dependent position, and flushing and filling of the veins of the feet are timed. Flushing should occur immediately; veins should fill in about 10 seconds. Flushing and venous filling times of greater than 20 and 30 seconds, respectively, denote a severely ischemic limb with inadequate collateral circulation. These tests should be performed in a warm room to rule out vasospasm; varicosities invalidate the venous filling time.

The presence or absence of calcification by x-ray of the extremities is usually meaningless. *Arteriography* may be necessary if the diagnosis is in doubt. It is always performed if surgery is being considered to reveal the exact location and extent of the obstructive lesion and the collateral circulation. In doubtful cases, an exercise test may be performed while blood flow is measured by the disappearance of a radioisotope (I^{131}, Xe^{133}) from the involved muscle. During exercise the disappearance rate either stops or is abnormally slow in claudicators compared with that in normal subjects. The postexercise disappearance rates are also usually abnormal in obstructive arterial disease. Postexercise or postischemic flow can also be measured with a plethysmograph, but there is some overlap of values between claudicators and normal persons. A variety of equipment has been used to demonstrate the small, rounded pulse with a slow upstroke and downstroke and absent dicrotic notch, or to show the decrease in systolic pressure below an obstructing or stenotic lesion. These tests can be valuable, but it is important that the "normal ranges" are first established for the particular combination of methods or procedures used.

Intermittent claudication may occur in *severe anemia* and in *McArdle's syndrome*; both are easily distinguished from arteriosclerosis obliterans by the presence of normal pulses. The pain of *arthritis* may radiate to the thighs or calves, but is present at rest and not usually worse with exercise. *Arterial embolism* pain does not develop as insidiously as arteriosclerotic ischemic symptoms. In occasional patients with *lumbar disc, spinal canal or cauda equina disease,* pain may occur only with exercise; also vasospasm may be intense so that distal pulses cannot be felt. Usually neurologic signs are present or appear with exercise. Even large vessel pulsations may disappear in patients taking *vasoconstrictive drugs* (see Ergotism and Methysergide); patients should be carefully questioned concerning the use of these drugs.

Ischemic ulcers resulting from arteriosclerosis obliterans must be differentiated from ulcers that occur in patients with hypertension (*Hines' ulcers*). In hypertensive ischemic ulcers, pulses in the leg and foot are normal, and signs of ischemia are absent elsewhere in the extremity. The hypertensive ulcer is most commonly located on the lateral aspect of the leg or ankle, but arteriosclerotic ulcers usually are on the toes. Hypertensive ulcers are more common in females and are extremely painful. They begin as a purplish plaque which develops into a hemorrhagic bleb; the bleb then ulcerates, leaving a lesion with purplish red margins.

Prognosis. Often intermittent claudication is the first symptom of generalized arteriosclerotic vascular disease, and most patients die eventually from myocardial infarctions or cerebral vascular accidents. Seventy to 90 per cent of patients with femoral artery disease remain stable in their symptoms or improve over a nine-year follow-up period. If diabetes mellitus is present, the prognosis is grave, for progression of the disease almost always occurs. The prognosis after surgical revascularization appears good in large vessel (aortic or femoral artery) disease.

Treatment. If the patient has only intermittent claudication with a normal appearing limb, he should be treated conservatively. He will be able to walk farther without pain if he slows his gait and loses excess weight. Tobacco should never be used in any form, for it causes cutaneous vaso-constriction via the sympathetic nervous system. The patient is advised to exercise frequently to the development of pain but to rest until the pain totally disappears. It is hoped that exercise will stimulate further growth of collateral blood vessels, but proof is lacking for this point. Patients should protect their limbs from cold or trauma; careful attention to keep the skin scrupulously clean, dry, and soft is important. Even minor infections such as the dermatophytoses may produce problems. Toenail trimming should be done regularly and with care.

If the claudication is found to be progressively worse over a 6-month to 2-year observation period, if it interferes seriously with the patient's daily activity, if even minor ischemic symptoms such as numbness or paresthesias are present, or if diabetes mellitus exists, surgery should be considered. Since the lesion is often localized and segmental, restoration of circulation beyond segmental stenotic or obstructive areas by thrombo-endarterectomy or graft bypass is the treatment of choice. Currently autogenous saphenous vein grafts are used most frequently because the incidence of thrombosis is less than with grafts made of synthetic materials. Often patch grafts are used on one portion of the vessel. Thrombo-endarterectomy is performed when there is minimal medial and adventitial involvement of the artery by the sclerotic process. Bypass grafts are favored over excision and graft replacement since collateral circulation is not destroyed with the bypass method. Before a grafting procedure can be performed, arteriography must be done to determine that there are patent vessels below the obstruction ("good runoff"). However, connection of a graft to an "isolated" popliteal segment (no calf vessels patent) may produce good results with healing of trophic lesions. Vein grafts have been connected to the posterior tibial artery in the lower calf in attempts to save ischemic, even gangrenous, feet. In patients with aorto-iliac disease who cannot undergo major surgery, subcutaneous axillo-femoral or, if one femoral is patent, femoro-femoral grafts have been an evidently successful innovation. In patients with more than one obstructing lesion in the vessels supplying an extremity, correction of the most proximal obstruction often produces relief of symptoms. The success of a surgical attack on involved vessels is proportional to the size of the vessel involved; aorto-iliac operations have a 90 per cent or better success rate; femoro-popliteal, 70 to 80 per cent; and posterior tibial artery, 50 per cent.

If surgery cannot be performed because of poor runoff or other serious disease, and rest pain or gangrene is present, rest in bed is essential. The affected extremity should be kept 20 to 30 degrees below the horizontal, for the dependent position increases blood flow and occasionally is the only position the patient can tolerate. If edema is pres-

ent, the extremity should be kept horizontal but never elevated. External local warmth, if used at all, is best applied by means of a thermoregulated cradle kept at a temperature below 38° C. (100.4° F.). Direct application of external heat should never be used because ischemic tissue blisters and burns at much lower temperatures than normal tissue. Rest pain may require the use of aspirin, phenobarbital, propoxyphene (Darvon), or even narcotics. The injection of alcohol or the crushing of peripheral nerves produces anesthesia that persists for two to six months, after which the operation may, if necessary, be repeated. Ulcers caused by ischemia are treated the same as rest pain; warm saline soaks should be used to keep the ulcer open, moist, and clean. Enzymatic debridement is not advised because of possible local allergic reactions. If infection is present, the appropriate systemic and local antimicrobial drug should be used as determined by culture and sensitivity tests.

Preganglionic lumbar sympathectomy may be performed to increase skin blood flow when ulcers, rest pain, or small areas of gangrene are present. Before surgery, it must be demonstrated that the sympathetic nervous system is intact in the extremity, especially in diabetics in whom peripheral neuropathy sometimes produces an autosympathectomy. To assess sympathetic activity in an extremity, plethysmographic foot blood flow, toe pulse, or skin temperature may be measured before and after a procedure to remove sympathetic activity. Methods used to remove sympathetic activity are (1) a warm environment, (2) local anesthesia of sympathetic ganglia, (3) local anesthesia of appropriate mixed nerves, (4) spinal anesthesia, or (5) autonomic blocking agents. An increase in the parameter being measured after one of these procedures indicates that a sympathectomy may be beneficial. Sweating of the involved extremity is also an indication of sympathetic activity. Although superficial ulcers often heal after the operation, sympathectomy alone rarely improves intermittent claudication.

Arteriosclerotic gangrene often necessitates amputation of the limb. In the presence of gangrene with ascending infection (advancing lymphangitis, fever, and leukocytosis), antimicrobial chemotherapy is indicated. Prompt amputation must be considered because the efficacy of the antimicrobial agents may be limited by the ischemia of the affected tissues and by local necrosis. The level of amputation is determined by palpable pulses and the presence of warm viable tissue of good color. The percentage of patients who become ambulatory after amputation is much higher with below-the-knee than above-the-knee operations.

Vasodilator drugs and agents are widely advertised but have little, if any, place in the treatment of arteriosclerosis obliterans. They are consistently ineffective in relieving intermittent claudication but may increase muscle or skin blood flow at rest in some patients. The efficacy of drugs with prolonged vasodilator action depends upon the degree to which structural disease has rendered the peripheral arteries rigid and incapable of dilatation; it has yet to be shown that they are active on the collateral vessels. Vasodilator drugs often lower systemic blood pressure so that flow to the ischemic limb may be decreased; even intra-arterial administration has been shown to decrease foot flow in some patients. Before use in patients with severe peripheral ischemia, a parameter of blood flow should be measured before and after drug administration to be sure no harmful effect will result.

Agents that act directly on blood vessels to relax them include ethyl alcohol (0.5 ml. per kilogram of body weight three times a day), papaverine (0.03 to 0.06 gram three times a day) and nicotinic acid preparations (50 mg. three times a day). Tolazoline (Priscoline, 25 mg. three times a day) is a sympatholytic and adrenolytic agent intended specifically to reduce adrenergic cutaneous vasoconstriction. Agents chemically similar to epinephrine, possessing its vasodilator effect in muscle, are nylidrin (Arlidin, 6 to 12 mg. three times a day) and isoxsuprine (Vasodilan, 10 to 20 mg. three times a day).

Long-term anticoagulation has also been recommended for treatment of arteriosclerosis obliterans, but conflicting results have been reported. The use of fibrinolytic therapy has not been adequately evaluated but, in view of the pathology of the disease, should not be effective.

Coffman, J. D.: Peripheral collateral blood flow and vascular reactivity in the dog. J. Clin. Invest., 45:923, 1966.

Coffman, J. D., and Mannick, J. A.: An objective test to demonstrate the circulatory abnormality in intermittent claudication. Circulation, 33:177, 1966.

Cooke, T. D. V., and Lehmann, P. O.: Intermittent claudication of neurogenic origin. Canad. J. Surg., 11:151, 1968.

Friedman, S. A., Holling, H. E., and Roberts, B.: Etiologic factors in aorto-iliac and femoro-popliteal vascular disease. New Eng J. Med., 271:1382, 1964.

Kouchoukos, N. T., Levy, J. F., Balfour, J F., and Butcher, H. R.: Operative therapy for femoral-popliteal arterial occlusive disease. Circulation, 35 (Suppl. 1), 174, 1967.

Mannick, J. A., and Nabseth, D. C.: Axillofemoral bypass graft. New Eng. J. Med., 278:461, 1968.

Schadt, D. C., Hines, E. A., Jr., Juergens, J. L., and Barker, N. W.: Chronic atherosclerotic occlusion of the femoral artery. J.A.M.A., 175:937, 1961.

Wilkins, R. W., and Coffman, J. D.: Tests of peripheral vascular efficiency. Practitioner, 188:346, 1962.

THROMBOANGIITIS OBLITERANS

(Buerger's Disease)

Definition. Thromboangiitis obliterans is an obliterative vascular disease or syndrome, probably inflammatory in type, affecting chiefly the peripheral arteries and veins. Identified first as endarteritis obliterans (von Winiwarter, 1879), it was described more fully and given its present name by Buerger (1908).

Incidence. All races are subject to thromboangiitis obliterans, but the greatest incidence is in the Ashkenazim Jews, of whom 20 in 100,000

develop the disease compared with 7 or 8 per 100,000 in the general population. The disease is also common in the Orient. The incidence of the disease in the United States has decreased markedly in the last two decades. Men are affected far more frequently than women, in a ratio of about 75 to 1 Thromboangiitis obliterans has been observed at all ages but occurs more frequently between 20 and 45.

Etiology. Although many agents, toxic and infectious, have been suggested, no etiology has received general acceptance. Cigarettes are used moderately or excessively by many, but not all, patients with thromboangiitis obliterans and have been thoroughly investigated as a causative agent, since smoking aggravates the disease. An increased skin sensitivity to tobacco has been reported by some investigators but not found by others. Recent research has been directed at a thrombotic etiology; the thromboplastin generation test has been reported abnormal, and higher levels of heparin precipitable fraction of fibrinogen in plasma have been found in patients with thromboangiitis obliterans than in normal persons or patients with arteriosclerosis obliterans. A rise in adhesive platelet counts has also been described in the disease and apparently correlates with tobacco smoking.

Considerable skepticism has been expressed that this disease is an entity different from arteriosclerosis occurring in young people. Evidence has been presented that its clinical and pathologic pictures are specific; however, it may be a syndrome with more than one cause.

Pathology. The lesions are segmental in that diseased sections of arteries or veins are separated by normal areas. In the acute stage cellular proliferation of the intima is accompanied by the formation of red thrombi in small and medium-sized vessels. Polymorphonuclear leukocytes, lymphocytes, and giant cells infiltrate all coats of the artery and extend into the thrombus. The formation of sterile microabscesses within the thrombi is a specific finding in this disease. Additional segments of artery or vein are involved acutely at intervals from days to years; hence, a single long artery may exhibit many stages, ranging from the acute picture to dense scar formation. Late stages cannot be distinguished pathologically from arteriosclerosis obliterans.

Pathophysiology. The disease is characterized by alternating periods of activity and quiescence. Depending upon the time relation between the developing occlusion and compensation by collateral circulation, the onset and course vary from insidious to fulminant. Usually occlusion gradually outstrips the developing collateral circulation, and definite peripheral ischemia brings the patient under medical care within one to four years after the first mild symptoms appear. The disease often has an initially more active course of six to twelve years, and then advances much less rapidly; at this stage it is very difficult to differentiate from arteriosclerosis obliterans.

Clinical Manifestations. The typical patient

with thromboangiitis obliterans is a young male who smokes cigarettes, presents symptoms of peripheral vascular ischemia, and may have a history of thrombophlebitis. The lower extremities are affected most commonly, and the most frequent presenting complaint is persistent coldness of the limbs. The upper extremities are involved in more than 70 per cent of patients (sometimes without symptoms), the digital arteries being affected more frequently than the ulnar or radial. Raynaud's phenomenon, hyperhidrosis, and ulcers of the digits are common. In comparison with other vascular diseases, the pain is often excruciating. Migratory thrombophlebitis may precede or accompany arterial involvement and occurs in approximately 40 per cent of patients. Tender, red, elevated areas about 1 cm. in diameter appear suddenly in the skin near the valves of small, superficial veins and gradually disappear during two to three weeks, to be followed after irregular intervals by new lesions. Other symptoms and signs (intermittent claudication, rest pain, ulcers, gangrene) are the same as in arteriosclerosis obliterans except that femoral artery disease is less frequent and aorto-iliac, rare. Thromboses of the mesenteric, coronary, cerebral, and renal arteries have been described but are uncommon. Myocardial infarction is frequent in patients with thromboangiitis obliterans but has not been shown to be secondary to the disease process.

Diagnosis. The diagnosis may be suspected when a young male presents with peripheral vascular insufficiency and thrombophlebitis, but it can be definitely proved only by biopsy of an active lesion. The age group, sex, thrombophlebitis, frequent involvement of upper extremities, Raynaud's phenomenon, and normal blood cholesterol and glucose tolerance test help differentiate the disease from arteriosclerosis obliterans. Arteriography can be helpful in demonstrating normality of vessels between lesions, absence of atheroma, a characteristic tree root configuration of the collateral vessels around the point of abrupt occlusion, and asymptomatic involvement of the upper extremities. Since Raynaud's disease is rare in men, affects the upper extremities more severely, and does not obliterate arterial pulsation at the wrist or ankle, it should not be confused with Raynaud's phenomenon in thromboangiitis obliterans. Migratory thrombophlebitis without symptoms or signs of arterial involvement cannot be diagnosed as thromboangiitis obliterans unless histologic proof is obtained.

Prognosis. The prognosis for life is good, but amputation of extremities is common, especially in the fulminant form. In the late stages, the prognosis and course are similar to arteriosclerosis obliterans.

Treatment. The treatment is the same as that outlined for arteriosclerosis obliterans, but it is imperative that tobacco never be used in any form. Nicotine produces transient vasoconstriction and probably favors extension of the disease. Bilateral preganglionic sympathectomy has been advocated for established, gradually advancing thrombo-angiitis obliterans, especially if vasospasm is prominent. This major operation is not indicated in mild cases responding well to medical treatment or in advanced cases with massive gangrene. Opinion is still divided concerning the usefulness of sympathectomy in this disease. In thromboangiitis obliterans resistance to infection is fairly high and collateral circulation usually good, so that minor amputations may be performed more safely than in arteriosclerotic gangrene.

Barker, N. W.: Diagnosis and treatment of thromboangiitis obliterans (Buerger's disease). Minnesota Med., 39:303, 1956.

Brown, G. E., et al.: Thrombo-angiitis Obliterans. Philadelphia, W. B. Saunders Company, 1928.

Craven, J. L., and Cotton, R. C.: Haematological differences between thromboangiitis obliterans and atherosclerosis. Brit. J. Surg., 54:862, 1967.

DeCamp, P. T., Carrera, A. E., and Ochsner, A., Jr.: The hypercoagulable state. Surgery, 63:173, 1968.

Goodman, R. M., Elian, B., Mozes, M., and Deutsch, V.: Buerger's Disease in Israel. Amer. J. Med., 39:601, 1965.

McKusick, V. A., Harris, W. S., Ottesen, O. E., Goodman, R. M., Shelley, W. M., and Bloodwell, R. D.: Buerger's disease: A distinct clinical and pathologic entity. J.A.M.A., 181:5, 1962.

Wessler, S., Ming, S. C., Gurewich, V., and Freiman, D. G.: A critical evaluation of thromboangiitis obliterans. New Eng. J. Med., 262:1149, 1960.

ARTERIAL EMBOLISM

Definition. Fragments of centrally located thrombi or atheromatous material may embolize and occlude large or small peripheral blood vessels.

Etiology. Emboli usually originate from mural or valvular thrombi in the left side of the heart (atrium or ventricle), less commonly from an atheromatous ulcer in the aorta or a more peripheral artery, and from thrombi in aneurysms. Paradoxical emboli originate from the right side of the heart and pass through a patent foramen ovale. Most emboli occur in association with atrial fibrillation, myocardial infarction, mitral valve disease, chronic congestive heart failure, or endocarditis. With the advent of surgical replacement of heart valves, prostheses have become a common source of emboli.

Pathophysiology. Emboli lodge at bifurcations of arteries and at narrowed arteriosclerotic areas. The most common site is at the junction of the femoral artery with the profunda femoris; emboli at the origin of the iliac arteries from the aorta (*saddle emboli*) are also frequent. The embolus stops blood flow through the artery and is followed within a few hours by secondary progressive arterial thrombosis below and sometimes above the point of obstruction. Secondary vasospasm has been assumed to be an important factor causing ischemia of the affected extremity, but convincing experimental evidence has not been presented to support this theory. The amount of muscle and skin ischemia that occurs depends on the degree of collateral circulation development.

Pathology. Emboli from the heart or aneurysms show the same pathology as the parent thrombi.

Emboli lodged in arteries usually organize by the ingrowth of connective tissue, and later recanalization may occur. However, fragmentation of the embolus before organization is not uncommon with fragments lodging in more distal vessels. Emboli that originate from friable, ulcerated atheromatous lesions either produce large vessel obstruction by amorphous debris or arteriolar and capillary blockage by a variable combination of cholesterol crystals and lipoid material. The cholesterol crystals incite an inflammatory response which leads to fibrosis and complete vessel obstruction.

Clinical Manifestations. In approximately half of patients, there is the sudden onset of severe pain in the extremity distal to the site of embolization. The other cases have an insidious beginning over one to several hours; numbness and paresthesias may precede the pain. Pain is present in 80 per cent of patients and may become excruciating within one or two hours, particularly if the patient exercises the limb. Paresthesias occur in about 60 per cent of cases, and 20 per cent develop muscular weakness or actual paralysis. When large arteries are involved, fainting, nausea, vomiting, and abdominal pain may precede a shocklike state.

Examination of the involved extremity reveals pallor and coldness, sharply demarcated distal to the site of embolization, viz. at the inguinal ligaments or sometimes as high as the umbilicus in saddle embolus, at the lower third of the thigh in femoral artery embolus, and at midcalf in popliteal artery embolus. Arterial pulses are absent below the embolus by palpation or oscillometry. In the arms, because of the easy palpability of the brachial artery, the site of embolus lodgment can be determined by the disappearance of the pulse. Occasionally there is tenderness directly over the embolus in an artery. The extremity may also show collapsed veins, decreased to absent reflexes and sensation, and weakness and paralysis. Later the initial pallor changes to a blotchy cyanosis. If collateral circulation is good, the extremity soon shows signs of improvement in color and temperature, but muscle tenderness and pitting edema may develop. If the collateral circulation is inadequate, massive gangrene follows with bleb formation, spotty vermilion discoloration of the skin, and mummification.

Large emboli from thrombi or amorphous atherosclerotic debris show the above picture. Smaller emboli may produce only local digital cyanosis with or without pain. Atheromatous microemboli (cholesterol crystals and lipoid material) may produce sudden leg pain, tender muscles, cool legs with pulses, petechiae, livedo reticularis, and plaquelike reddened elevations of the skin. Pedal pulses may disappear later in this syndrome. The spontaneous appearance of painful dusky discoloration of a toe or toes in the presence of pulses should suggest atheromatous microembolism.

Diagnosis. The diagnosis of embolization is not difficult in the patient with the acute onset of a painful, ischemic extremity who demonstrates a source for embolus formation. Acute arterial thrombosis can be distinguished from an embolus only by the presence or absence of underlying etiologies; absent or decreased arterial pulsations in the opposite limb support a diagnosis of acute thrombosis. Patients with acute iliofemoral thrombophlebitis sometimes have no palpable pulses in the affected extremity and may show signs resembling those of arterial embolus. Detection of a feeble pulse by oscillometry, distended veins, and massive edema of the extremity helps rule out embolus. In patients with symptoms and signs of embolization or microembolization and normal pulses, angiography must be performed to look for ulcerative atherosclerotic lesions or aneurysms in the proximal large vessels. Microembolization is often confused with polymyositis or polyarteritis nodosa; muscle biopsy may be necessary to demonstrate the cholesterol crystals.

Prognosis. The prognosis in acute arterial embolization depends on several factors, including size of vessel affected, age of patient, collateral blood supply, and speed of treatment. The larger the artery involved, the worse the prognosis without treatment. Gangrene is much more common after the age of 60 years, probably because of concomitant arteriosclerotic involvement of the blood vessels and collaterals. The development of collateral circulation is very important, for sufficient collaterals may save a limb without treatment. The presence of patent companion vessels, i.e., around the elbow, gives a favorable outlook. The earlier an embolus can be removed surgically, the better the prognosis for survival of the severely ischemic limb.

With any method of treatment, the mortality in most studies is usually greater than 20 per cent, due to the underlying disease and recurrent embolization to vital areas. The incidence of embolus recurrence is very high. Following either medical or surgical treatment, limb incapacity from muscle fibrosis with tendon shortening or intermittent claudication is common.

Treatment. Although embolectomy should restore the normal physiology and is strongly recommended in the surgical literature, conservative medical management often gives as good end results. The exception is emboli at the aortic bifurcation, when surgery is the optimal treatment. When the patient is first seen, treatment should be instituted to improve blood flow to the extremity, and a vascular surgeon should be immediately called in consultation. Anticoagulation with heparin should be started at once to prevent thrombus formation below and above the embolus, and further embolization (long-term anticoagulation is usually indicated to prevent recurrent emboli). The limb should be positioned in 15 degree dependency and adequate analgesics given to relieve the pain. The affected limb should be kept comfortably warm, as in a thermoregulated (30 to 34° C., 86 to 93.2° F.) cradle, and the body and uninvolved extremities warmed in an effort to produce reflex vasodilatation in the involved limb. Every precaution should be taken to prevent burning during heat application; ischemic limbs burn at much lower temperatures than normal limbs. Lumbar sympathetic block by paravertebral injection of procaine or xylocaine has been recommended to relieve vasoconstrictor tone and vasospasm if present; if used it should be performed before anticoagulation. Vasodilator drugs have also been recommended. The intra-arterial route may be successful in increasing blood flow to the limb, but there is a danger of decreasing flow to the ischemic limb if the blood pressure is lowered by systemically administered vasodilator agents. Other therapy not adequately evaluated at present includes the use of fibrinolysins and dextran.

If conservative medical therapy is not effective in greatly improving the extremity in two to four hours and the underlying condition of the patient will allow surgery, embolectomy is indicated. Early diagnosis is essential as the greatest success with embolectomy is within eight to ten hours of the incident. In recent years, embolectomy has been performed longer than 48 hours after the acute insult with some success, although less than with earlier operations. Muscle tenderness and edema often occur after embolectomy and may be mistakenly diagnosed as thrombophlebitis. In cases presenting with gangrene, amputation is usually necessary. In atheromatous embolization or emboli from aneurysmal thrombi, surgical attack on the proximal lesion may be successful in preventing further emboli.

Baird, R. J., and Lajos, T. Z.: Emboli to the arm. Ann. Surg., 160:905, 1964.
Darling, R. C., Austen, W. G., and Linton, R. R.: Arterial embolism. Surg., Gynec. Obstet., 124:106, 1967.
Eliot, R. S., Kanjuh, V. I., and Edwards, J. E.: Atheromatous embolism. Circulation, 30:611, 1964.
Haygood, T. A., Fessel, W. J., and Strange, D. A.: Atheromatous microembolism simulating polymyositis. J.A.M.A., 203:423, 1968.
Jacobs, A. L.: Arterial embolism in the limbs. Edinburgh, E. and S. Livingstone, Ltd., 1959.
Silverblatt, C. W., Wasserman, F., and Wolcott, M. W.: Pulmonary artery embolism and paradoxical embolization. Arch. Intern. Med. (Chicago), 107:105, 1961.
Szekely, P.: Systemic embolism and anticoagulant prophylaxis in rheumatic heart disease. Brit. Med. J., 1:1209, 1964.
Wessler, S., Sheps, S. G., Gilbert, M., and Sheps, M. C.: Studies in peripheral arterial occlusive disease. III. Acute arterial occlusion. Circulation, 17:512, 1958.

PERIPHERAL ARTERITIS AND GANGRENE IN SYSTEMIC INFECTIONS

Symptoms and signs of peripheral vascular disease, mild or severe, appear occasionally as complications in bacterial, viral, rickettsial, and fungal infections. Bacterial arteritis and abscess of the wall of an artery are uncommon complications of bacterial endocarditis and septicemias and may lead to hemorrhagic lesions or aneurysm formation. The rickettsial diseases, especially typhus and Rocky Mountain spotted fever, may cause endothelial proliferation of the arterioles, capillaries, and venules followed by degeneration

and necrosis of the media; thrombosis of larger arteries may occur rarely. In infectious arteritis with direct vascular involvement, signs of subacute or acute arrest of peripheral blood flow occur with necrosis of skin and sometimes massive gangrene. However, peripheral ischemia may be transitory and, in large part, vasospastic.

Tuberculosis of the peripheral arteries is rare, but occasionally metastatic infection or embolism produces panarteritis or endarteritis with fully developed tubercles in thrombosed vessels. Direct involvement by extension from adjacent tuberculous lesions, although common in centrally located vessels, is rare in the extremities.

Syphilis may diminish peripheral circulation by producing periarteritis, obliterative intimal hyperplasia, or panarteritis, but the media is much less affected than in the large arteries. True gummas have been found in the vessels of gangrenous limbs. Peripheral vascular complications of syphilis are more common in men than in women. Peripheral ischemia, vasospastic or organic, appears insidiously or suddenly, but gangrene is rare. Active antisyphilitic therapy usually arrests the acute progress of the disease and relieves vasospasm, but organic occlusion remains.

Collins, R. N., and Nadel, M. S.: Gangrene due to the hemolytic Streptococcus—a rare but treatable disease. New Eng. J. Med., 272:578, 1965.
Derick, C. L., and Hass, G. M.: Diffuse arteritis of syphilitic origin. Amer. J. Path., 11:291, 1935.
Learmouth, G. E.: Gangrene of the lower extremities complicating scarlet fever. Canad. Med. Ass. J., 15:69, 1925.
Slaughter, W. H.: Symmetrical gangrene of malarial origin. J.A.M.A., 86:1607, 1926.

SHIN SPLINTS AND ANTERIOR TIBIAL COMPARTMENT SYNDROMES

The anterior tibial compartment is a closed space in which the muscles and blood vessels are surrounded by nonexpanding fascia and bone. Swelling of the tissues in this compartment can cause mild to severe complications.

Shin splints is a frequently encountered syndrome of pain and discomfort in the lower anterior part of the leg following repetitive, unusual exertion. The syndrome is presumably a result of ischemia from an abnormally high tissue pressure compressing the blood vessels. It often occurs in athletes or dancers early in the season. The pain in the front of the legs occurs during or after exercise and is only slowly relieved by rest. Tenderness is most frequent at periosteal attachments of the muscles to the tibia or interosseous membrane. Mild swelling and a slight rise in local skin temperature may be present. When the pain is reproduced by repeated dorsiflexion of the foot against resistance, the anterior tibial muscles become very hard and bulge prominently; a pulsation may become visible over the front of the legs. Arterial pulses are normal. Treatment consists of rest of the muscles, supportive strapping, and a program of graduated exercise.

The *acute anterior tibial compartment syndrome* is a rare condition caused by the rapid onset of ischemic necrosis of muscles in the anterior tibial space. Swelling of the muscles compresses muscles, nerves, and blood vessels. The cause is unknown, but there is usually a history of excessive exertion. A dull, aching pain which becomes progressively severe is the major symptom; it is unrelieved by rest and sometimes by analgesics. Extreme tenderness is present over the entire anterior tibial compartment, and the fascia rapidly becomes tense and boardlike. The skin becomes glossy, erythematous, and edematous as muscle necrosis occurs; a slight fever and leukocytosis may be present. Loss of dorsiflexion of the great toe and foot then occurs, and sensation may be lost between the first and second toes (deep peroneal nerve compression). The dorsalis pedis pulse may be present or absent. Treatment must be immediate and involves surgical decompression of the anterior tibial compartment by fasciotomy. If treatment is delayed, complete necrosis of the muscles occurs with a resultant permanent footdrop.

A *chronic anterior tibial compartment syndrome* also has been described with pain similar to intermittent claudication in the front of the lower leg on severe exertion but not with ordinary walking. The discomfort disappears with rest. Tenderness is present over the entire compartment when the pain occurs; arterial pulses are normal. The syndrome is thought to be due to an abnormally small compartment. Treatment is usually unnecessary, but a fasciotomy will relieve the symptoms.

French, E. B., and Price, W. H.: Anterior tibial pain. Brit. Med. J., 2:1290, 1962.
Leach, R. E., Zohn, D. A., and Stryker, W. S.: Anterior tibial compartment syndrome. Arch. Surg. (Chicago), 88:187, 1964.
Slocum, D. B.: The shin splint syndrome. Amer. J. Surg., 114: 875, 1967.

PERIPHERAL VASCULAR DISEASE DUE TO ABNORMAL VASOCONSTRICTION OR VASODILATATION

RAYNAUD'S PHENOMENON AND DISEASE

Definition. Raynaud's phenomenon is a syndrome characterized by paroxysmal, bilateral ischemia of the digits induced by cold or emotional stimuli and relieved by heat.

Etiology. Raynaud's phenomenon may be secondary to an underlying disease or anatomic abnormality, but the most common cause is *Raynaud's disease*, which is of unknown etiology. It is less common before puberty and after age 40 but may occur at any age. Women are affected more frequently than men (5:1). Raynaud concluded from his early studies (1862, 1874) that excessive sympathetic activity was responsible for the attacks, but Lewis found that the digital vessels were abnormally reactive to local cold. Catecholamines have been implicated as important; norepinephrine and epinephrine have been found elevated in wrist venous blood of patients. The amine oxidase content of digital arteries may be decreased. About a dozen cases of Raynaud's phenomenon associated with pulmonary hypertension have been reported, suggesting that a neurohumoral mechanism may be operative in causing both syndromes. Recently an increased viscosity of the blood associated with a raised plasma fibrinogen concentration and increased red blood cell aggregation has been reported in Raynaud's disease. This could lead to sludging and slowing of blood flow, especially in the acral parts and more so when exposed to cold. Since ischemic attacks can still be induced after sympathectomy, it may be concluded that there is a local fault in the blood vessels or in the blood in Raynaud's disease which is aggravated by the normal degree of reflex sympathetic nervous activity.

Raynaud's phenomenon may occur in occlusive arterial disease (thromboangiitis obliterans, arteriosclerosis obliterans, arterial emboli), collagen disease (especially scleroderma), following trauma (pneumatic hammer disease, injuries to pianists or typists, after gangrene from any cause), drug intoxication (ergot, methysergide), blood dyscrasias (cryopathies, cold hemagglutinins), and neurogenic lesions (thoracic outlet compression syndromes, poliomyelitis, syringomyelia, causalgia). In Raynaud's phenomenon from secondary causes, the syndrome is caused usually by irritation of the sympathetic nerves, pathologic alterations in the small blood vessels, or sludging and agglutination of red blood cells.

Pathologic Physiology. The paroxysmal ischemia of the digits is due to constriction of the digital and palmar or plantar arteries; initial pallor indicates that vasoconstriction involves the small cutaneous vessels. Later the digital capillaries and venules become dilated, and the slowed blood flow allows the hemoglobin to release more of its oxygen, producing cyanotic, cold digits. When the vasoconstriction is relieved, blood flow increases greatly (reactive hyperemia), imparting a red color to the previously ischemic digits.

Pathology. In the early stages of the disease, the blood vessels are histologically normal. Later, in progressive cases, the intima is thickened and the muscular coats of the arteries are hypertrophied. Eventually thrombosis of small arteries may occur and focal gangrene of the digital tips may form, although elsewhere the arteries are still histologically normal or show only slight hypertrophy.

Clinical Manifestations. In typical Raynaud's

phenomenon, the fingers of both hands blanch on exposure to cold and then may turn cyanotic; sometimes only cyanosis occurs. During recovery, a bright red color (reactive hyperemia) replaces the cyanosis. During the ischemic phase, the digits are cold, numb, and covered with perspiration. In the reactive hyperemia phase, throbbing pain, tingling, swelling, and a rise in skin temperature are found. The digits are affected to different levels in each patient (sometimes extending to the wrist), but the terminal phalanges are always most severely involved. Initially, attacks may be unilateral and involve only one or two digits, but they soon become bilateral and can be induced by emotional upsets as well as by cold exposure.

In Raynaud's disease, the onset is usually gradual with attacks only in the winter. Attacks may be rare, or they may occur several times a day; they may last a few minutes in mild cases to two hours or more in severe cases. They end spontaneously or can be terminated by immersing the hands in warm water. Between episodes, the digits are normal or, in severe cases, mildly cyanotic.

The hands alone are affected in half the cases, hands and feet in the remainder; nose, cheeks, ears, and chin are affected much more rarely. The course of the disease varies; after onset it may persist indefinitely in mild form, improve spontaneously, or become more severe. In the small number of cases that are progressive, the attacks become more frequent, persist during the summer, and last longer; finally, mild cyanosis may be present constantly. Hand blood flow in patients without trophic changes is usually in the normal range in a warm environment but is decreased in patients with nutritional lesions of the fingers.

Trophic changes appear in progressive cases, usually one to four years after onset. The fingers become thin and tapering and their skin smooth, shiny, less mobile, and eventually tightly stretched (sclerodactyly). The nails grow slowly and are ridged or curved. Recurrent infections, blisters, and small areas of local cutaneous gangrene appear on the fingertips, but gangrene of a whole digit is rare. The gangrenous areas are extremely painful and, on healing, leave tiny depressed scars.

Diagnosis. Criteria which should be present in patients with Raynaud's phenomenon in order to diagnose Raynaud's disease include (1) absence of any disease or anatomic abnormality to which paroxysmal digital ischemia might be secondary; (2) digital pallor or cyanosis occurring in intermittent attacks, induced by cold or emotion and followed by recovery with reactive hyperemia; (3) symmetrical or bilateral involvement of digits; and (4) gangrene, if present, usually limited to small areas of skin. Previously, presence of symptoms for two years with no evidence of an underlying cause had been considered a fifth diagnostic point; however, Raynaud's phenomenon may precede the diagnosis of scleroderma by 12 years. It is probably unsafe to diagnose the idiopathic disease in the presence of an elevated sedimentation rate or minor symptoms or signs suggestive of an underlying disease (arthralgias, telangi-

ectasis). Raynaud's phenomenon is diagnosed by discovering an underlying disease or condition known to cause attacks.

Raynaud's disease and phenomenon are distinguished from acrocyanosis by the intermittency of attacks. The cyanotic, cold, and edematous limb affected by poliomyelitis or other diseases causing paralysis is also persistent in nature. The cause of sudden "bilateral gangrene of the digits" (Lewis), which appears rarely in children or young adults without previous attacks of discoloration and without cold exposure, is unknown. The fingers, toes, nose, and ears become permanently cyanotic, and within a few days gangrene develops in the distal phalanges of one or more fingers, often symmetrically and bilaterally. The gangrene is extensive and is due to sudden thrombotic occlusion of the final end branches of the digital arteries. The relationship of this syndrome to Raynaud's disease is uncertain, although typical cyclic color changes may appear during the healing stage.

Prognosis. Mild cases of Raynaud's disease improve slowly or remain stationary for years, and the attacks, being few and avoidable, are merely an inconvenience. In a large series of cases, the disease caused no deaths and very little disability; amputations of terminal phalanges were necessary in only 0.4 per cent, and the phenomenon improved or disappeared in 46 per cent. The progressive form, with recurring infection and local gangrene, becomes increasingly painful and disabling, usually despite treatment, but only rarely results in the loss of more than the distal phalanges. The prognosis for secondary Raynaud's phenomenon depends on the underlying cause. Generalized scleroderma and rheumatoid arthritis, which are frequently associated with Raynaud's phenomenon, may produce extreme deformity and disability.

Treatment. Mild cases of Raynaud's disease with infrequent attacks limited to cold exposure, and without trophic changes or gangrene, may be relieved by reassurance, sedatives or tranquilizers, and protection from cold exposure. Smoking has been shown to produce cutaneous vasoconstriction, and the use of tobacco should, therefore, be avoided. Rauwolfia products in continued small oral doses (reserpine, 0.25 to 0.5 mg. daily) will often decrease the severity and frequency of attacks. If necessary, a vasodilator drug (tolazoline long-acting tablets, 80 mg. every 12 hours) can be added to the therapeutic regimen. The addition of thyroid substances and androgens has been recommended but helps little, if any. Antiserotonin treatment has not been evaluated adequately as yet.

Vasoconstrictor tone due to sympathetic nervous system activity is an important factor in bringing on and maintaining attacks of digital ischemia, whether or not the local arteries are abnormally reactive to cold. Removal of vasoconstrictor impulses by regional sympathectomy may be of benefit for the progressive type of Raynaud's disease with indolent ulcers or local gangrene. The success of the sympathectomy depends upon the extent to which the normal capacity for vasodilatation is preserved, as shown by the vasodilator response to body warming or sympathetic ganglion nerve block with lidocaine. In early Raynaud's disease of the lower extremities, lumbar sympathetic ganglionectomy gives complete relief of symptoms. For the upper extremity, preganglionic cervicodorsal sympathectomy is the operation of choice but usually is of only temporary (six months to two years) benefit.

The treatment of Raynaud's phenomenon secondary to an underlying disease or anatomic abnormality is directed at the secondary causes. Sympathectomy is of little or no benefit in scleroderma or arthritis but may be helpful in Raynaud's phenomenon secondary to pneumatic hammer disease or causalgia (reflex sympathetic dystrophy).

Baddeley, R. M.: The place of upper dorsal sympathectomy in the treatment of primary Raynaud's disease. Brit. J. Surg., 52:426, 1965.

Farmer, R. G., Gifford, R. W., Jr., and Hines, E. A., Jr.: Raynaud's disease with sclerodactylia: a followup study of seventy-one patients. Circulation, 22:13, 1961.

Gifford, R. W., Jr., and Hines, E. A., Jr.: Raynaud's disease among women and girls. Circulation, 16:1012, 1957.

Guntheroth, W. G., Morgan, B. C., Harbinson, J. A., and Mullins, G. L.: Raynaud's disease in children. Circulation, 36:724, 1967.

Kontos, H. A., and Wasserman, A. J.: Effect of reserpine in Raynaud's phenomenon. Circulation, 34:259, 1969.

Lewis, T., and Pickering, G. W.: Observations upon maladies in which the blood supply to digits ceases intermittently or permanently, and upon bilateral gangrene of digits; observations relevant to so-called "Raynaud's disease." Clin. Sci., 1:327, 1934.

Pringle, R., Walder, D. N., and Weaver, J. P. A.: Blood viscosity and Raynaud's disease. Lancet, 1:1086, 1965.

Winters, W. L., Jr., Joseph, R. R., and Learner, N.: "Primary" pulmonary hypertension and Raynaud's phenomenon. Arch. Intern. Med. (Chicago), 114:821, 1964.

ACROCYANOSIS

Acrocyanosis (Croq, 1896; chronic acro-asphyxia, Cassirer, 1900) is a symmetrical cyanosis of the hands and, less commonly, the feet with few or no symptoms and no complications.

Etiology and Pathology. It is primarily a vasospastic disturbance of the smaller arterioles of the skin of unknown cause, but is probably due to local cold sensitivity. When compared with normal digits, acrocyanotic digits have a heightened arteriolar tone at average room temperature. Secondary dilatation of the capillaries and the subpapillary venous plexus occurs, and the slower blood flow allows the hemoglobin to release a greater part of its oxygen content, accounting for the blue color. Acrocyanosis occurs without special age or sex incidence, and may be associated with various endocrine disorders or asthenias as well as with certain anxiety states. No specific pathology has been described.

Clinical Manifestations. Patients usually present with an unevenly blue and red discoloration of the skin which may extend from the digits to the wrists and ankles but is most intense distally. The digits are also persistently cold and sweat

profusely. Puffiness of the digits and mild hypesthesia may be present, but other trophic changes are rare. The cyanosis is intensified by cold or emotional upsets and is relieved by warmth.

Diagnosis. Acrocyanosis can be distinguished from Raynaud's disease by the persistent nature of the discoloration. The presence of normal arterial pulses rules out obstructive arterial disease. Since the discoloration is limited to the hands and feet and disappears when the extremities are warmed, it should not be confused with various types of generalized cyanosis.

Treatment. Except for reassurance, treatment is usually unnecessary. Possible endocrine abnormalities should be investigated. To prevent reflex sympathetic vasoconstriction, general body protection from cold, as well as local measures, help to decrease the intensity of the discoloration. For cosmetic reasons, vasodilator drugs (tolazoline long-acting tablets, 80 mg. every 12 hours, or nicotinyl alcohol, 50 mg. every 6 hours) may be used. Sympathectomy is helpful but seldom warranted.

Elliot, A. H., Evans, R. D., and Stone, C. S.: Acrocyanosis: A study of the circulatory fault. Amer. Heart J., 11:431, 1936.

Larsson, Y.: The vasoconstrictor tone of the cutaneous arterioles in acro-asphyxia, hypertension, and in the cold pressor test. Acta Med. Scand., (Supp. 206), 130:146, 1948.

Lewis, T., and Landis, E. M.: Observations upon the vascular mechanism in acrocyanosis. Heart, 15:229, 1930.

Lottenbach, K.: Vascular response to cold in acrocyanosis. Helv. Med. Acta, 33:437, 1966.

ERGOTISM AND METHYSERGIDE TOXICITY

Definition. Intense vasoconstriction of small and large blood vessels, producing symptoms and signs of peripheral vascular ischemia, may result from the ingestion of ergot or methysergide.

Etiology. Ergotism results from the use of ergot-containing drugs or the ingestion of bread made from rye or wheat infected with the ergot fungus (*Claviceps purpurea*). It formerly occurred in epidemic form, but is now seen only sporadically (due to the fungus), or after the repeated administration of ergotamine (Gynergen, Cafergot) for migraine or pruritus or of ergot in abortion. Methysergide is a synthetic serotonin antagonist useful in the treatment of migraine headaches. Approximately 7 per cent of patients develop peripheral vascular symptoms or signs with methysergide ingestion, usually following large doses, although as little as 1 mg. has caused symptoms in some patients.

Pathophysiology and Pathology. Both drugs induce large and small blood vessel vasoconstriction. Ergot induces vasoconstriction by a direct action on vascular smooth muscle and can lead to secondary intimal hyperplasia and thrombosis. Gangrene may result if thrombosis occurs. The pathology of methysergide toxicity is unknown as is the mode of action, but it does potentiate the effect of catecholamines on blood vessels.

Clinical Manifestations. *Acute ergotism* produces diarrhea, colic, and vomiting followed by headache, vertigo, paresthesias, convulsive seizures, and occasionally gangrene of the digits, nose, and ears. It is rarely seen with the drug ingestion. In *chronic intoxications*, intermittent claudication, muscle pains, numbness, coldness and pallor of the digits, and even Raynaud's phenomenon may occur. Examination reveals only cool, pale digits or mottling of the skin with normal or decreased arterial pulsations; however, complete absence of medium- and large-vessel pulsations in the extremities may occur. Gangrene may develop in the severe cases. A similar picture of peripheral vascular ischemia may follow methysergide ingestion. Abdominal angina and angina pectoris have also been caused by these drugs. Methysergide has been implicated as an etiologic agent in periureteral or retroperitoneal fibrosis which can extrinsically obstruct arteries and veins.

Diagnosis. The diagnosis is made from the history of drug ingestion associated with symptoms and signs of peripheral ischemia. Arteriography characteristically shows diffuse or segmental narrowing of large arteries and often very constricted distal vessels with collateral vessels present. Arteriosclerosis obliterans, Raynaud's disease, and acrocyanosis are differentiated from ergotism and methysergide toxicity by the history of drug ingestion and by arteriography.

Prognosis. The prognosis is excellent if gangrene has not appeared before treatment and if drug administration is stopped.

Treatment. Treatment involves anticoagulation to prevent thromboses and the use of vasodilators, e.g., tolazoline, 25 mg., intra-arterial or intravenous, to counteract the vasoconstriction. Body warming is recommended to produce reflex vasodilatation in the involved extremities, but is often unsuccessful as is vasodilator drug therapy. With avoidance of the offending drug, the vasoconstriction usually subsides in one to three days. Sympathetic nerve block or sympathectomy may be necessary in pregangrenous or gangrenous cases.

Cranley, J. J., Krause, R. J., Strasser, E. S., and Hafner, C. D.: Impending gangrene of four extremities secondary to ergotism. New Eng. J. Med., 269:727, 1963.

Graham, J. R.: Methysergide for prevention of headache. New Eng. J. Med., 270:67, 1964.

Haynes, C. D., and Davis, M. E., Jr.: Ergotism: Report of case with localized arteriographic changes in femoral vessel. Angiology, 19:199, 1968.

Rackley, C. E., Mengel, C. E., Pomerantz, M., and McIntosh, H. D.: Vascular complications with use of methysergide. Arch. Intern. Med. (Chicago), 117:265, 1966.

ERYTHROMELALGIA
(Erythermalgia)

Definition. Erythromelalgia (Mitchell, 1872) is a rare syndrome of paroxysmal, bilateral vasodilatation of the feet and, less often, the hands, associated with burning pain, increased skin temperature, and redness of the skin.

Etiology and Pathology. The cause is unknown. It has occurred as an hereditary affliction. Increased blood flow is usually present, but symptoms may occur in a limb in which the arteries are occluded by a blood pressure cuff. Therefore it is thought that there is a hypersensitivity of the skin to heat or tension. No uniform pathologic condition has been found but data are scarce. The syndrome occurs without special age or sex incidence.

Clinical Manifestations. The patient with erythromelalgia complains of attacks of bilateral burning pain, superficial or deep, involving circumscribed areas on the soles or palms, the entire foot or hand, or even the whole extremity. The attacks follow stimuli that normally induce only physiologic peripheral vasodilatation or engorgement such as local heat, a warm environment, exercise, standing, or simple dependency of the extremity. The onset is gradual, and symptoms may remain mild for years or may become so severe and continuous that total disability results. Examination during an attack (which may be produced by exposure to a 32 to 36° C. environment) usually reveals that the affected skin is hot and red and often sweats profusely; arterial pulsations are normal. Trophic changes, gangrene, and ulceration do not occur, but swelling may be present.

The syndrome may be either idiopathic or secondary to polycythemia vera or hypertension. The condition may precede the polycythemia by as long as 12 years. Secondary erythromelalgia occurs more commonly in an older age group, is more often unilateral, and produces pain of lesser intensity than idiopathic erythromelalgia.

Diagnosis. Arteriosclerosis obliterans may produce localized and often unilateral burning pain and redness but, unlike erythromelalgia, is not associated with normal pulses or a rise in skin temperature. Neuritis, infectious ganglionitis, and poisoning by thallium, lead, or arsenic may produce painful peripheral hyperemia. Chronic inflammatory states produce in the skin a "susceptible state" with diminished capillary and arteriolar tone. Burning pain (erythralgia, Lewis) is then induced by mild grades of heat, cold, friction, and congestion that leave normal skin unaffected. A temporary reactive vasodilatation of the cutaneous vessels also normally occurs after prolonged exposure to cold in response to a histamine-like substance liberated by local tissue damage (Lewis). This is easily distinguished from erythromelalgia by the history.

Treatment. Attacks can be avoided or aborted by rest, elevation of the extremity, and cold applications. Aspirin (0.6 gram orally) quickly relieves pain in some cases, and the remarkable response is of diagnostic value. Vasoconstrictor agents such as ephedrine (25 mg. orally) may be useful; methysergide (1 to 4 mg. orally) has also produced relief. Even vasodilator agents (isoproterenol, nitroglycerin) have been reported to be helpful. Contrast baths, using heat below the threshold for pain, often afford considerable but temporary relief. Severe attacks require liberal doses of sedatives, and the therapy is generally unsatisfactory. Occasionally section or alcohol injection of peripheral nerve is required; sympathectomy has been successful in the treatment of three cases.

Prognosis. The prognosis in idiopathic erythromelalgia is guarded since the severe pain may become disabling. Prognosis of secondary cases depends on the underlying disease; treatment of polycythemia often relieves the symptoms.

Babb, R. R., Alarcon-Segovia, D., and Fairbairn, J. F., II: Erythermalgia. Review of 51 cases. Circulation, 29;136, 1964.
Catchpole, B. N.: Erythromelalgia. Lancet, 1:909, 1964.
Cross, E. G.: The familial occurrence of erythromelalgia and nephritis. Canad. M.A.J., 87:1, 1962.
Lewis, T.: Clinical observations and experiments relating to burning pain in extremities and to so-called "erythromelalgia" in particular. Clin. Sci., 1:175, 1933.
Telford, E. D., and Simmons, H. T.: Erythromelalgia. Brit. Med. J., 2:782, 1940.

PERIPHERAL VASCULAR DISEASES DUE TO EXPOSURE TO COLD

Exposure to cold induces vasoconstriction by a direct action on blood vessels and also by reflex sympathetic nervous system activity. Cold application to the forehead or to one extremity stimulates vasoconstriction in all extremities. The decreased blood flow and local anoxia may lead to tissue damage, depending on the degree and duration of exposure and the susceptibility of the patient.

Even brief exposure to nonfreezing cold is followed in sensitive persons by an exaggerated and prolonged type of reactive vasodilatation, low-grade edema, and tingling pain. Similar exposure in more susceptible patients produces pronounced edema of the angioneurotic or urticarial type on exposed areas; even mucous membranes may be involved on ingesting cold substances. A systemic reaction with increased pulse rate, decreased blood pressure, flushing of the face, and even syncope may accompany the edema. Following swimming in cool water, this reaction has proved fatal in some instances. A histamine-like substance has been shown to be released and is measurable in the urine in about 50 per cent of patients. Diagnosis is made by exposure of a hand or arm to 12 to 14° C. (53 to 57° F.) water; edema will develop during or after exposure. Antihistamines may be of use in the treatment of cold sensitivity, but protection of the patient from cold exposure is most important.

IMMERSION FOOT
(Trench Foot)

Definition. Immersion foot is due to prolonged exposure of the extremities to water; syndromes characterized by only painful, swollen feet or hands to the more serious manifestations of muscle necrosis, ulceration, and gangrene may result.

Etiology. Although prolonged exposure (greater than 48 hours) to dampness or water is the important factor in the production of immersion foot, immobility and dependency of the lower extremities, constricting garments, chilling of the body, trauma, exhaustion, or dehydration, and, in some instances, semistarvation with deficient intake of protein and vitamins are often contributing causes. Two types, cold water and warm water (tropical) immersion foot, exist and present different clinical pictures. The combination of wetness plus cold (not necessarily freezing) temperatures produces the most serious condition.

Pathophysiology. The factors causing cold water immersion foot tend to decrease blood flow to the extremities. Vasoconstriction is caused by direct and reflex cold stimulation; actual cellular damage and the ensuing hyperemia are important in producing the clinical and pathologic picture. Persistent local anoxia leads to tissue necrosis and injures the capillary walls. Capillary filtration increases remarkably, and plasma and protein pass freely into the interstitial tissue, producing a tense edema. The resultant increased viscosity of the blood leads to stasis and occlusion of small vessels. The local anoxia may also produce Wallerian degeneration of the nerves in the affected area.

Warm water immersion foot is thought to be caused by waterlogging and swelling of the stratum corneum together with abrasion from footwear. *Pseudomonas aeruginosa* can usually be cultured from the affected areas and may contribute by digesting human callus with its proteolytic enzymes.

Pathology. The early pathologic picture of the cold type has not been studied. In late stages, a nonspecific picture of vascular occlusion, desquamation of skin, deep fibrosis, and superficial gangrene is seen. The nerves may be embedded in contracting fibrous tissue, and fibrosis of the media of arterioles and venules is present. The pathologic features of the warm water type have not been investigated.

Incidence. Cold water immersion foot was common in most wars and is seen in training camps where appropriate conditions exist. Non-Caucasians are thought to be more susceptible to the disease, perhaps on the basis of acclimatization.

Warm water immersion foot has recently been described as a common entity in the Vietnam war but was also seen, though not fully recognized, in the Pacific in World War II.

Clinical Manifestations. At the time of rescue from sea, or when first seen in trench warfare, cold water immersion foot often presents as pulseless, cold, red feet with a sock distribution of hypesthesia or anesthesia. The condition may develop insidiously with only numbness, paresthesias, and slight swelling as long as the tissues are supported by boots or shoes. As soon as the support is removed, edema, tingling, itching, and severe pain occur. The skin later becomes mottled yellow, blue, or black. This is called the prehyperemic stage and lasts a few hours to a few days. A hyperemic stage follows, characterized by red, hot, dry feet, burning paresthesias, and intense pains, shooting or stabbing in nature. Pulses are now bounding. Edema increases with formation of blisters, which may weep serous fluid and then slowly heal. In severe cases, muscle weakness and wasting, ulcerations, and gangrenous patches develop. Gangrene is often superficial, and the necrotic skin sometimes sheds in large pieces leaving healthy skin beneath. Even in the absence of gangrene, extensive exfoliation is common. This stage lasts one to ten weeks, depending on the grade of initial injury.

The recovery stage (posthyperemic) blends indistinguishably with the hyperemic stage; there is a return of vascular tone with restoration of normal skin color and temperature. Recovery may be complete in mild cases within two to five weeks, but severe cases often require three to twelve months. A few patients show late sequelae such as sensitivity to cold with Raynaud's phenomenon; general or marginal hyperhidrosis; paresthesias that are increased by warmth, dependency, or exertion; rigid toes caused by fibrosis of muscles; contracted joints in the feet and toes; or painful, indolent ulcers of the digits or their stumps.

Warm water immersion foot presents with painful and extremely tender feet, especially over pressure areas. Wrinkled, white, convoluted plantar surfaces and even maceration are seen on examination. Symptoms and signs subside within a week, usually leaving no residua.

Prophylaxis. Drying of the feet overnight is the best method to prevent immersion foot. Avoidance of constricting clothing, prolonged dependency, or immobility; frequent rest periods; and several changes of clothes and boots will also help. If these conditions are impractical, application of silicone grease once a day will reduce the incidence of the affliction.

Treatment. In the prehyperemic stage bed rest and body warming are important. It is probably best to keep the extremities at heart level until pulses are present. Vasodilator drugs have been recommended, but their value is unknown. Treatment of the hyperemic stage consists of complete bed rest, cooling of the hyperemic tissues to control pain and edema, keeping the body warm, elevation of the extremities above heart level, and cor-

rection of dietary deficiencies. If cleansing is necessary, light washing with dilute hexachlorophene solution may be used. Infected tissue and epidermophytosis should be treated with appropriate agents. For cooling, it may be sufficient to expose the extremities to room air, but sometimes electric fans with water sprays or ice bags are needed. With cooling, pain is usually relieved in a few hours, but in some instances, it is necessary to discover an optimal temperature since too low a temperature may again produce pain. Analgesics must be used. Tobacco smoking is prohibited. The patient is ready to walk when edema does not occur on dependency.

Sympathectomy has not been helpful in the hyperemic stage but appears to improve late sequelae such as chronic painful ulcers, persistent vasospasm, and hyperhidrosis.

The treatment of warm water immersion foot involves bed rest with extremity elevation until edema and pain entirely disappear. Other measures are usually unnecessary; the symptoms and signs disappear in one to seven days.

Clayton, A. J. W.: Twenty-one cases of immersion foot. Med. Ser. J. Canada, 23:857, 1967.
Lange, K., Weiner, D., and Boyd, L. J.: The functional pathology of experimental immersion foot. Amer. Heart J., 35:238, 1948.
Montgomery, H.: Experimental immersion foot; review of physiopathology. Physiol. Rev., 34:127, 1954.
Taplin, D., and Zaias, N.: Tropical immersion foot syndrome. Milit. Med., 131:814, 1966.
White, J. C.: Vascular and neurologic lesions in survivors of shipwreck. I. Immersion foot syndrome following exposure to cold. II. Painful swollen feet secondary to prolonged dehydration and malnutrition. New Eng. J. Med., 228:211, 1943.

CHILBLAIN AND PERNIO

Chilblain and pernio (*erythrocyanosis*) occur commonly in patients, especially females, with a history of cool limbs in summer as well as winter. The etiologic and pathogenic factors are unknown, but the disease is seen only in cold, damp climates. However, it is much more frequent in England than in areas of the United States with comparable climates.

Acute chilblain occurs on the dorsum of the digits, hands, or feet as localized, warm, red, intensely pruritic swelling that may disappear spontaneously in a few days. Pernio is probably the same disease but involves the lower parts of the legs, especially in women who, because of their mode of dress, do not adequately protect their legs from cold weather. Rarely, indolent lesions, dull red or violaceous, proceed to painful bleb formation. The blebs contain blood-stained serous fluid and often lead to ulcer formation.

In some patients exposed repeatedly to cold, recurrent and chronic lesions, often appearing in crops, may develop. The lesions are erythematous and ulcerative and may leave residual scarring, fibrosis, and atrophy of the skin and subcutaneous tissues. The disease is more active during the cooler months and subsides in warm weather. Bilateral and symmetrical parts of the extremities are involved. This state is called chronic chilblain or pernio (erythrocyanosis frigida crurum).

Treatment is nonspecific. Corticosteroid creams may be used for itching and inflammation, antimicrobials for sepsis. Reserpine (0.25 mg. orally daily) has been reported to ameliorate the disease.

Eskell, J.: Reserpine in the treatment of chilblains. Practitioner, 189:792, 1962.

Lewis, T.: Observations on some normal and injurious effects of cold upon the skin and underlying tissues. II. Chilblains and allied conditions. Brit. Med. J., 2:837, 1941.

McGovern, T., Wright, I. S., and Kruger, E.: Pernio: A vascular disease. Amer. Heart J., 22:583, 1941.

Thomas, E. W. P.: Chapping and chilblains. Practitioner, 193:755, 1964.

FROSTBITE

Definition. Frostbite is due to freezing of tissues which may result in damage to skin, muscle, blood vessels, and nerves.

Etiology. Superficial freezing of tissues evidently begins when the temperature of deeper tissues reaches about 10° C. (50° F.). During the Korean War, most cases of frostbite occurred at −6.5° C. (20° F.) or below, following 7 to 18 hours' exposure. High winds, dampness, and general chilling of the body make frostbite more likely at above freezing temperatures. Predisposing factors include any type of peripheral vascular insufficiency, improper clothing, exhaustion, and previous cold injury. Lack of acclimatization and geographic origin have also been implicated; the black race is more susceptible to frostbite. Most frostbite is of the slow freezing type, but a rapid frostbite (occurring in a few minutes) takes place at high altitudes with extremely low temperatures and has a predilection for the extremities rather than the face and ears.

Pathophysiology. Whether actual tissue freezing or decreased blood flow from vasoconstriction is most important in producing cell injury is unknown. Damage is probably due to a combination of direct freezing with the formation of extracellular ice crystals, inducing dehydration of cells, and to intense vasoconstriction. The vasoconstriction is due to direct cold exposure of the tissues but may also involve reflex vasoconstriction from chilling of other body areas. The reduced blood flow leads to capillary stasis and arteriolar and capillary thromboses. Capillary permeability is increased and results in edema formation.

Pathology. The pathologic findings vary with the stage of the disease and the depth of tissue affected. In early stages, low-grade vasculitis and inflammation in all tissues is seen. Later the skin is atrophied and may be keratinized, muscle is necrosed and shows waxy degeneration, arterioles and capillaries are thrombosed, and nerves demonstrate fibroblastic proliferation and neurolysis.

Clinical Manifestations. The first indication of frostbite is often a sharp, pricking sensation that draws attention to a yellowish-white, numb area

of hardened skin. However, cold itself produces numbness and anesthesia that may allow freezing of tissue without warning. When the freezing is superficial, thawing leads to local reddening and wheal and flare formation. When freezing involves deep tissues, subcutaneous edema occurs with thawing, followed by formation of vesicles and bullae. A hyperemic, reddish zone may be apparent between frozen and normal tissue. As the edema subsides in a day or two, necrosis and gangrene may become evident. However, it may take two to three months before final demarcation between viable and dead tissue can be ascertained. In the healing phase, a black eschar usually covers the area.

The traditional classification of frostbite has been from first to fourth degree depending on the depth of tissue injury. Since the true extent of tissue damage cannot be judged on initial examination, a simpler classification of superficial and deep frostbite is more practical. The prognosis depends on the depth of freezing, as superficial cases usually have no sequelae, although deep freezing may finally end in amputation.

Prophylaxis. Frostbite is preventable and occurs rarely among those who have been instructed how to protect themselves. Prophylactic measures include observance of each other for signs of frostbite; wearing adequate, loose fitting, dry clothing and mittens; exposure for only brief periods when exercise is not possible; and avoidance of smoking before and during exposure. Feet and socks should be kept dry.

Treatment. Superficial frostbite can be treated immediately by rewarming; affected areas on the face and ears can be warmed with the hands, hands can be placed in the axillae, or frostbitten parts can be warmed on the exposed torso of a partner. Frostbitten areas should not be rubbed with snow or exercised.

Treatment of deep frostbite should be delayed until adequate facilities for rewarming are available. Therapy should always be very conservative since the depth of tissue damage is difficult to ascertain, sometimes for months. It is best to rewarm the tissues as rapidly as possible in 40 to 44° C. water (104 to 111° F.). Massage, exposure to too high temperatures, and reactive hyperemia should be avoided because they tend to increase pain and edema. Analgesics usually are needed during rewarming. After rewarming, which usually requires about 20 minutes, the frostbitten area is exposed to room air (21 to 26° C., 70 to 78° F.). Although pressure dressings may be used, the open method with sterile surroundings is usually preferred. Vesicles, bullae, and eschars are left untouched. Antimicrobial drugs are indicated if infection is present. Tobacco smoking should be prohibited. Regional sympathectomy has been reported as beneficial, both clinically and experimentally, if performed at an optimal time of 24 to 48 hours after frostbite occurs. Sympathectomy may conserve tissue and lead to earlier demarcation, cessation of pain, and healing of tissue.

Vasodilator drugs (alcohol, papaverine, isox-suprine, nicotinic acid) have been recommended but have been shown of value only in animal experiments. Low molecular weight dextran and anticoagulants have received both favorable and unfavorable reports.

Eventual recovery is usually surprisingly good, the black eschar peeling off to leave normal tissue beneath. Sensitivity to cold, paresthesias, and a predilection to repeated frostbite often persist. In severe frostbite, fibrosis of tissue may lead to disability, and gangrenous extremities may require amputation.

Golding, M. R., Martinez, A., DeJong, P., Mendosa, M., Fries, C. C., Sawyer, P. N., Hennigar, G. R., and Wesolowski, S. A.: The role of sympathectomy in frostbite, with review of 68 cases. Surgery, 57:774, 1965.

Lapp, N. L., and Juergens, J. L.: Frostbite, Mayo Clin. Proc., 40:932, 1965.

Meryman, H. T.: Tissue freezing and local cold injury. Physiol. Rev., 37:233, 1957.

Washburn, B.: Frostbite. What it is, how to prevent it, emergency treatment. New Eng. J. Med., 266:974, 1962.

PERIPHERAL VASCULAR DISEASES DUE TO ABNORMAL COMMUNICATIONS BETWEEN ARTERIES AND VEINS

ARTERIOVENOUS FISTULA

Definition. Arteriovenous fistulas are abnormal communications, single or multiple, between arteries and veins by which arterial blood enters the veins directly without transversing a capillary network.

Etiology. Acquired arteriovenous fistulas, usually single and saccular, may develop after a bullet or stab wound involving an artery and a contiguous vein. Fistulas of the iliac vessels may occur following surgery for intervertebral disc disease. Congenital fistulas are present from birth and are usually multiple; they result from defects in differentiation of the common embryologic anlage into artery and vein. There is no special sex incidence, and any part of the body may be involved.

Pathophysiology. Arterial blood, following the path of least resistance, flows directly into the vein, bypassing the corresponding capillary bed. The arterial pressure is transmitted to the venous side of the fistula; the distal vein pressure is increased, but the proximal vein pressure may actually be negative. The elevated venous pressure leads to the development of varicose veins and venous stasis changes in the limb. Increased blood flow makes the tissues near the fistula abnormally warm, and diminished flow distal to the fistula may produce peripheral coldness and trophic changes. Large fistulas impose a burden on the heart; the cardiac output must be increased above normal by an amount proportional to the size of the fistula in order to maintain the general circulation. Total blood volume may be increased. The low peripheral resistance of the involved area tends to decrease diastolic and increase systolic and pulse pressure systemically. Large fistulas may lead to cardiac decompensation.

Pathology. In the region of the fistula, the intima and media of the involved veins become thickened, and newly developed elastic fibers appear. The arteries show a thinning of their walls with loss of elastic tissue and muscular fibers in the media.

Clinical Manifestations. Patients complain of aching pain, edema, varicosities, or hypertrophied extremities. Occasionally, cardiac symptoms such as palpitation, substernal pain, and dyspnea on exertion are present. Examination reveals tortuous, dilated superficial veins in the extremity, and venous pulsation can be felt unless the fistula is small and deeply placed. In congenital fistulas, the skin temperature is usually elevated locally but decreased distal to the fistulas, although in acquired lesions, the temperature of the digits may be greater than in the opposite normal limb. A bruit and thrill are common over acquired fistulas; the bruit lasts throughout systole and diastole and has a coarse machinery-like quality. The tissues near the fistula may be tender, edematous, and either red or slightly cyanotic. The circumference of the extremity is increased by edema or true hypertrophy, but bony structures are hypertrophied only if the fistula was present before epiphyseal closure. Stasis pigmentation and chronic indurative cellulitis with or without indolent ulceration may be present distal to the fistula. In contrast to the postphlebitic limb in which ulcers form around the medial malleolus, the ulceration of fistulas may affect the distal parts of the foot. Rarefaction of bone in the extremity may also occur. Temporary compression of the artery supplying a large fistula diminishes the heart rate (*Branham's sign*) and may be a helpful diagnostic sign.

Diagnosis. If the diagnosis cannot be made from the clinical manifestations, other examinations may be helpful. The oxygen saturation of blood removed from fistula veins will be found to be greater than that of blood removed from corresponding veins in the opposite extremity. Arteriography will reveal the lesion, its location, and the number and size of communications. Edema of one or both extremities following surgery for intervertebral disc disease should suggest the possibility of a fistula. Thrombophlebitis and the postphlebitic extremity can be distinguished from fistulas by the oxygen studies and arteriography.

Prognosis. The prognosis of acquired and single congenital fistulas is good following surgical repair. In acquired iliac vessel fistulas, congestive heart failure develops in two thirds of patients, and immediate repair is important. Without surgical repair, which is often not possible in multiple fistulas, the outlook is for a chronically swollen limb with varicosities, stasis pigmentation, and ulceration. Bacterial infection of acquired fistulas occurs but is rare.

Treatment. Single fistulas can be repaired surgically by re-establishing the continuity of the involved artery and vein walls by a variety of procedures (arteriorrhaphy, end to-end suture, grafting). Ligation of the involved artery and vein leads to a high incidence of arterial and venous insufficiency of the extremity and should be avoided if possible. If the arterial supply depends upon a large anomalous artery, ligation of this vessel, followed by sclerosing injections of the dilated veins, may be effective. Multiple fistulas are much less amenable to surgery. Ulcers, edema, and pain may be relieved by wearing elastic bandages or stockings; pressure on the veins encourages blood flow to follow the arterial pathway. Amputation is required for large inoperable fistulas producing cardiac decompensation or gross deformity.

Binak, K., Regan, T. J., Christensen, R. C., and Hellems, H. K.: Arteriovenous fistula: Hemodynamic effects of occlusion and exercise. Amer. Heart J., 60:495, 1960.

Lawton, R. L., Tidrick, R. T., and Brintnall, E. S.: A clinicopathologic study of multiple congenital arteriovenous fistulae of the lower extremities. Angiology, 8:161, 1957.

Nickerson, J. L., Elkin, D. C., and Warren, J. V.: The effect of temporary occlusion of arteriovenous fistulas on heart rate, stroke volume, and cardiac output. J. Clin. Invest., 30:215, 1951.

Spittell, J. A., Jr., Palumbo, P. J., Love, J. G., and Ellis, F. H., Jr.: Arteriovenous fistula complicating lumbar disk surgery. New Eng. J. Med., 268:1162, 1963.

Wakim, K. G., and Janes, J. M.: Influence of arteriovenous fistula on the distal circulation in the involved extremity. Arch. Phys. Med., 39:431, 1958.

GLOMANGIOMA OR GLOMUS TUMOR

Definition. Glomangioma or glomus tumor designates painful enlargement of a glomus body.

Pathology. The pathology consists of hypertrophy of the glomus body which contains an arteriovenous anastomosis with its associated smooth muscle coat, nonmyelinated nerve fibers, and connective tissue. Histologically, the lesion is encapsulated, occasionally diffuse but never invasive, and contains numerous epithelioid cells with no inflammatory cells.

Clinical Manifestations. Glomus tumors are extremely tender but inconspicuous subcutaneous nodules which develop slowly during adult life. Pain may be present before the nodule becomes visible. They are found in various parts of the upper and lower extremities, but most frequently (30 per cent) beneath the fingernail. The diameter of the tumor is usually only a few millimeters. The nodule has a flat or slightly raised surface

with reddish-blue to purplish discoloration. Excruciating burning or shooting pain, both local and referred up the extremity, occurs spontaneously or is produced by the slightest pressure. Heat, cold, and even contact with clothing may become intolerable so that protection is required continuously day and night. The tumor may pulsate slightly, and skin temperature may be elevated locally. In glomus tumors beneath nails, a small excavation of the phalanx from erosion by the tumor can often be seen by roentgenography.

Treatment. Surgical excision leads to complete and immediate relief without recurrence.

Bailey, O. T.: The cutaneous glomus and its tumors—glomangiomas. Amer. J. Path., 11:915, 1935.

Horton, C., Maquire, C., Georgiade, N., and Pickrell, K.: Glomus tumors: An analysis of 25 cases. Arch. Surg. (Chicago), 71:712, 1955.

Stabins, S. J., Thornton, J. J., and Scott, W. J. M.: Changes in the vasomotor reaction associated with glomus tumors. J. Clin. Invest., 16·685, 1937.

DISEASES OF THE PERIPHERAL VEINS

THROMBOPHLEBITIS

This subject is discussed elsewhere.

VARICOSE VEINS AND THE POSTPHLEBITIC SYNDROME

Definition. Varicose veins are distended, tortuous veins with incompetent valves. The postphlebitic syndrome denotes the chronically swollen extremity with trophic changes secondary to chronic venous stasis; despite the name, a previous history of thrombophlebitis is often not obtainable.

Etiology. Varicose veins are caused either by congenitally defective valves or by a condition that deforms valves or obstructs venous outflow over long periods of time. Varicosities resulting from congenital defects are most common and may develop early in life. Since increased forearm vein distensibility has been demonstrated in patients with lower extremity varicosities, a generalized abnormality of the veins has been suggested as the predisposing factor. Thrombophlebitis leads to deformation or destruction of venous valves and venous obstruction, and is the second most frequent etiologic factor. Pregnancy, ascites, abdominal tumor, excessive weight or height, or prolonged weight bearing may lead to increased venous pressure in the legs, distention of veins, and finally incompetency of valves.

Incidence. Varicose veins are very common, appearing in approximately 40 per cent of women; the incidence is less in men. The saphenous veins in the lower extremities are most frequently affected.

Clinical Manifestations. The dilated, tortuous, sacculated varices are easily visible. Some patients with extensive superficial varicosities have no other symptoms or signs, but others have aching pain on easy fatigability of the calf muscles and edema after weight bearing. The edema usually disappears with bed rest overnight. When the communicating or deep veins are incompetent, symptoms and signs are more common. Chronic venous insufficiency is manifested by edema, which may later become fibrosed to produce a brawny induration. Extravasation of blood locally may cause a brownish pigmentation; an itchy, eczematoid rash may appear in the area. Finally the skin may ulcerate, producing an indolent, nonpainful lesion, usually above the medial malleolus near a palpable, incompetent communicating vein. This picture of chronic swelling and stasis dermatitis is called the postphlebitic syndrome. Arterial pulses are normal. When the deep venous system is blocked, pain similar to intermittent claudication may rarely occur.

Diagnosis. The diagnosis can be made from the clinical picture. Retrograde flow of blood past incompetent valves can be demonstrated by the Trendelenburg test and its variations. The leg of the recumbent patient is elevated to empty the veins, and then a tourniquet is applied to occlude the superficial veins. The patient quickly assumes a standing position, the tourniquet is released, and the veins will become distended immediately if back flow is present. If two tourniquets are applied and left in place when the patient stands, filling of the saphenous veins between the tourniquets indicates an incompetent communicating vein. Application of the tourniquets to different levels on the limb can delineate exactly the sites of vein pathology. Venography may be used in doubtful cases or to be certain the deep venous system is patent. In a patient with varicosities and edema, other causes of edema, e.g., cardiovascular and renal disease, should be investigated.

Prognosis. The prognosis for simple superficial varicose veins is good with treatment. Once the postphlebitic syndrome has developed, progressive disability usually can be expected despite treatment.

Treatment. Uncomplicated varicose veins respond well to support with elastic stockings or bandages to prevent progression. Panty girdles should never be worn. When edema or other mild complications are present, frequent periods of elevation of the extremity above heart level, high ligation with stripping of the saphenous veins, and injection of sclerosing solutions may also be necessary. Venous stasis ulcers are treated with sponge rubber pressure dressings or gelatin boots; local or systemic antimicrobials are indicated if infection is present. Sometimes the entire fibrosed area must be removed and a skin graft applied to heal an indolent ulcer.

Bauer, G.: Pathophysiology and treatment of the lower leg stasis syndrome. Angiology, 1:1, 1950.

Fegan, W. G., Fitzgerald, D. E., and Beesley, W. H.: A modern approach to the injection treatment of varicose veins and its applications in pregnant patients. Amer. Heart J., 68:757, 1964.
Mullarky, R. E.: The Anatomy of Varicose Veins. Springfield, Illinois, Charles C Thomas, 1965.
Wood, J. E.: The Veins. Boston, Little, Brown & Company, 1965.
Zsotér, T., and Cronin, R. F. P.: Venous distensibility in patients with varicose veins. Canad. M.A.J., 94:1293, 1966.

DISEASES OF THE PERIPHERAL LYMPHATIC VESSELS

Lymph is formed by the transudation of plasma through capillary walls into tissue spaces. The plasma that is not reabsorbed into the venular end of the capillaries is collected by a rich intercellular network of tiny lymphatic vessels. These vessels become larger as they convey lymph to the regional lymph nodes; then the lymph travels through trunk lymphatics to the thoracic duct and finally to the left internal jugular vein. In the extremities, there are superficial and deep lymphatic systems which probably are joined by communicating vessels. The flow of lymph depends on intrinsic, rhythmic contractions of the lymph vessels, muscular contraction, respiratory movements, and, to a certain extent, gravity.

LYMPHEDEMA

Definition. Lymphedema is a form of chronic unilateral or bilateral edema of the extremities caused by the accumulation of lymph secondary to abnormalities or blockage of the lymph vessels or pathologic conditions of the lymph nodes.

Etiology. Primary lymphedema may be a hereditary disease or may occur sporadically. Various classifications exist according to whether the lymphedema is present at birth (*congenital*), appears at or near puberty (*praecox*), occurs after age 35 (*tarda*), or is familial and congenital (*Milroy's disease*). The mode of inheritance is probably dominant but has not been thoroughly investigated. An increased incidence occurs in ovarian dysgenesis syndromes. Primary lymphedema affects females predominantly (about 8:1); the onset of the disease occurs before age 40 in more than 90 per cent of cases.

Secondary lymphedema is most commonly caused by inflammation and follows recurrent lymphangitis (see below). In tropical and subtropical regions, filariasis often leads to lymphedema. Neoplasms are the second most common cause either by invasion or compression of lymph vessels or nodes. Surgical removal of lymph nodes and the fibrosis following irradiation may also cause lymphedema. Secondary cases have no special sex incidence and are uncommon before age 40.

Pathology. Examination of primary lymphedematous limbs by lymphangiography has revealed aplasia, hypoplasia, or hyperplasia (varicosities) of the lymphatic vessels. The lymph nodes may also be aplastic or hypoplastic, producing an obstructive type of lymphedema. No specific pathologic picture has been correlated with the current classification system, but the few cases of Milroy's disease examined have revealed aplasia (or absence) of the lymphatic vessels. There is some indication that lymphedema may be part of a generalized defect in lymphatic vessels. Patients with lymphedema have been reported to have chylous pleural effusions, chylous ascites, and even intestinal lymphangiectasis. A syndrome of yellow nails, recurrent pleural effusion, and lymphedema occurs and is believed to be secondary to lymphatic abnormalities in each area. In secondary lymphedema, innumerable small, irregular lymphatics are usually seen beside normal or tortuous, sometimes varicose, vessels.

Clinical Manifestations. Primary lymphedema is usually gradual in onset and asymptomatic; the distal portion of the extremity or whole extremity, or even a portion of the trunk, may increase in size. The edema is soft and pitting at first and disappears with treatment but later becomes firm and nonpitting, and cannot be relieved completely by treatment. At this stage, the skin becomes thickened and resists wrinkling; hair follicles are prominent. The lower extremities are involved most often; about half the patients develop bilateral swelling. The edematous tissue is especially susceptible to episodes of lymphangitis and cellulitis, which add to the deformity.

Secondary lymphedema is seldom bilateral. Lymphedema of the inflammatory type follows recurrent episodes of lymphangitis. Each attack leaves more residual edema after the inflammation subsides. The skin finally becomes thick, coarse, folded, and hard so that the eventual deformity may be extreme (elephantiasis). Secondary lymphedema resulting from neoplasm and other noninflammatory causes produces painless swelling of an extremity. Painless swelling of an extremity in an elderly male must be considered secondary to carcinoma of the prostate until proved otherwise.

Diagnosis. Painless chronic swelling of an extremity suggests the diagnosis of lymphedema. Differentiation from venous insufficiency may be made by the lack of prominent veins, stasis dermatitis, and ulceration; lymphangiography and venography may be necessary. Mixed lymphangiomatous and hemangiomatous malformations that cause enlarged limbs can be diagnosed by the obvious tumor mass. In lipodystrophy, lymphangiography is necessary to delineate the normal lymphatics displaced by the lipomatous masses.

Prognosis. Primary lymphedema usually progresses inexorably to a chronically swollen limb or limbs despite treatment. However, the lymphedema associated with gonadal dysgenesis may disappear spontaneously in months to years. Secondary lymphedema caused by infection may be controlled with adequate treatment. The prognosis is that of the underlying disease in other causes.

Treatment. In primary lymphedema, the most important aim of therapy is to keep the involved extremities free of edema in order to prevent fibrosis and recurrent infection. Frequent elevation of the extremity (including sleeping with the extremity above heart level), elastic support applying graded pressure from the foot proximally when ambulatory, low sodium diet, and diuretics are usually necessary. Local infection and obvious lesions, such as epidermophytosis, should be eradicated. Conflicting results have been reported with the use of corticosteroid treatment. Surgical attack in advanced cases with fibrosis and resistant edema (Kondoleon operation and its modifications) has produced some relief but is usually disappointing.

Dilley, J. J., Kierland, R. R., Randall, R. V., and Shick, R. M.: Primary lymphedema associated with yellow nails and pleural effusions. J.A.M.A., 204:670, 1968.

Gough, M. H.: Primary lymphedema: Clinical and lymphangiographic studies. Brit. J. Surg., 53:918, 1966.

Hall, J. G.: The flow of lymph. New Eng. J. Med., 281:720, 1969.

Homans, J.: The treatment of elephantiasis of the legs. New Eng. J. Med., 215:1099, 1936.

Kinmouth, J. B., and Taylor, G. W.: The lymphatic circulation in lymphedema. Ann. Surg., 139:129, 1954.

Schirger, A., Harrison, E. G., Jr., and James, J. M.: Idiopathic lymphedema: Review of 131 cases. J.A.M.A., 182:14, 1962.

Smith, R. D., Spittell, J. A., Jr., and Schirger, A.: Secondary lymphedema of the leg: Its characteristics and diagnostic implications. J.A.M.A., 185:80, 1963.

LYMPHANGITIS

Definition. Lymphangitis is an acute or chronic inflammation, usually pyogenic, of the lymphatic vessels.

Etiology. In the majority of cases of lymphangitis the hemolytic Streptococcus is the infecting agent; second most common is the coagulase-positive Staphylococcus. The bacteria enter the skin via areas of local trauma, trichophytosis, or arterial ischemic or venous stasis ulcers, although a portal of entry cannot always be discovered. Infection then spreads by the lymphatic vessels to the local lymph nodes; an accompanying diffuse cellulitis of the extremity is often present. An immune response to previously present bacteria or their products has been postulated as a cause of lymphangitis when an organism cannot be isolated, but proof of this is lacking.

Pathology. Acute, subacute, or chronic inflammation is found in the subcutaneous tissues and regional lymph nodes.

Clinical Manifestations. Attacks of lymphangitis may be ushered in by malaise, headache, nausea, vomiting, and shaking chills followed by fever. Fever may reach as high as 105° F. Systemic symptoms, however, may not be present. Red streaks appear in the affected extremity, originating at the portal of entry and following the pathway of lymphatic vessels. Regional lymph nodes are usually enlarged and tender. There may be a surrounding area of cellulitis with tenderness and red discoloration in the lower part of the extremity, which is usually swollen with a soft, pitting edema.

Diagnosis. The clinical picture is usually typical and allows the diagnosis to be made easily. A leukocytosis is often present. The inciting organism should be sought by culturing the portal of entry if obvious or by needle puncture of the subcutaneous tissues. A difficult diagnosis to rule out is acute thrombophlebitis, especially when a diffuse cellulitis is present, for symptoms and signs are similar; it is often wise to administer therapy for both diseases simultaneously.

Prognosis. For an initial attack in a limb without underlying disease, the prognosis with treatment is excellent. However, some patients have recurrent attacks, often mild, which can lead to the development of lymphedema. In recurrent cases, the limb may remain somewhat larger after each attack.

Treatment. Systemic antimicrobial drugs should be administered as indicated by culture (and sensitivity studies if necessary). If no organism is cultured, penicillin should be given because the Streptococcus is so commonly the etiologic agent. Drainage of any focus of origin is also extremely important. Adjunctive measures include rest, elevation of the extremity above heart level, and warm wet dressings. Possible fungal infections in the feet and causes of secondary lymphedema should be sought. When attacks subside, elastic support should be worn on the extremity for three months to prevent residual swelling. In recurrent cases, either with or without underlying lymphedema, prophylactic long-term antimicrobial therapy should be instituted. Lymphangitis is especially dangerous in the ischemic tissues of patients with obstructive arterial disease; only under these unfavorable conditions is prompt amputation sometimes required.

Babb, R. R., Spittell, J. A., Jr., Martin, W. J., and Schirger, A.: Prophylaxis of recurrent lymphangitis complicating lymphedema. J.A.M.A., 195:871, 1966.

Edwards, E. A.: Recurrent febrile episodes and lymphedema. J.A.M.A., 184:858, 1963.

DISEASES OF THE KIDNEYS

Investigation of Renal Function

D. N. S. Kerr

The common effects of disease on the function of the renal parenchyma are increased excretion of protein, alteration in the formed elements in the urine, reduction in renal blood flow and glomerular filtration rate, impairment of tubular reabsorption and secretion, and alteration in the secretion rates of erythropoietin and renin. Accurate study of these functions is an essential part of renal research, but most of the precise methods are too demanding or tedious for routine clinical use and are employed only at specialist units and for particular purposes. Plasma renin and angiotensin assay are employed almost exclusively in the investigation of hypertension. Assay of erythropoietin is still too imprecise and difficult to be of use outside research laboratories. Individual tubular functions other than concentrating power are tested in the investigation of renal tubular acidosis, other inherited and acquired tubular disorders, and renal calculous disease, and the appropriate tests are described in articles dealing with these subjects.

The study of proteinuria and urine microscopy are important in differential diagnosis. Measurement of glomerular filtration rate has little value in diagnosis, except in distinguishing early renal disease from physiologic states such as postural proteinuria, but is important in following the progress of disease and the response to treatment. Renal blood flow would be of some value diagnostically were it not so difficult to measure. Concentrating ability has been used more as a test for early renal damage than as one of specific tubular function, but in the latter role it has a limited value in differential diagnosis.

Proteinuria. The urine of normal adults contains about 40 to 100 mg. of protein per 24 hours during sedentary activity. The very low concentrations in normal urine are difficult to measure accurately, and the mean figure quoted varies quite widely. Conventionally the upper limit of normal is taken as 150 mg. per 24 hours in the ambulant subject and 0.03 mg. per minute during short collection periods in recumbency. The most sensitive screening test for urinary protein is the formation of a white cloud on heating filtered urine saturated with sodium sulfate and acidified with a few drops of 3 per cent acetic acid; this detects about 5 to 10 mg. per 100 ml. as a faint trace. A definite positive with any clinical test therefore indicates a protein concentration higher than the normal should achieve under resting conditions, and "proteinuria" has been accepted as the term to describe excessive proteinuria.

All such screening tests have a considerable observer error. The formation of a cloud with 25 per cent salicylsulfonic acid and the appearance of a green color on paper impregnated with bromophenol blue and a buffer (Albustix, Labstix) are much simpler than the heat test, and this compensates for their slightly lower sensitivity. All three tests give a very crude guide to the concentration of protein, the +, ++, +++, and ++++ corresponding roughly to 30, 100, 300, and 1000 mg. per 100 ml. in the case of bromophenol blue. However, the middle part of the range has poor reproducibility, and a more accurate test is necessary even for general medical use. A turbidimetric method using salicylsulfonic acid can be performed in the ward laboratory and a biuret method in the automated laboratory; both are sufficiently accurate (about ± 10 per cent) for clinical work.

Normal urinary protein contains at least 30 components, the largest of which is a mucoprotein with a molecular weight of about 7 million, called *Tamm-Horsfall protein*, which originates in the cells lining the renal tubules from the loop of Henle downward. Precipitation of this protein in the distal tubule forms the basis of renal casts. Other components include most of the plasma proteins of small molecular weight, with albumin the most prominent, and several proteins derived from the prostate and seminal vesicles. The normal glomerulus has been shown to have a high selectivity, i.e., to filter predominantly small colloid molecules, by studies with graded dextrans.

Increased protein excretion occurs with heavy exertion, fever, heart failure, and operative trauma without any known changes in renal structure or permanent change in renal function. Proteinuria from these sources is usually under 500 mg. per 24 hours and rarely over 1 gram per 24 hours; its major component is albumin and its presumed origin, the glomerular filtrate. Proteinuria is detected in about 5 per cent of children and adolescents at school medical examinations; the majority of the "positives" prove to have benign exercise or postural proteinuria. Nearly all adolescents and about 50 per cent of young adults can produce proteinuria by adapting a lordotic position, e.g., bent backward over a chair. The proteinuria may be quite heavy, but has no pathologic significance. A smaller proportion (about 5 per cent of adolescents and a few younger children and young adults develop proteinuria simply from standing erect. During prolonged standing the proteinuria may become quite heavy—up to 14 mg. per minute has been recorded—but over 24 hours the loss is usually less than 2 grams and virtually never results in the nephrotic syndrome. This *orthostatic proteinuria* in an adolescent or young adult with no other sign of renal disease is nearly always benign, and often disappears around the age of 20. It is, however, important to confirm on several occasions that proteinuria completely disappears on recumbency, as postural accentuation of slight proteinuria is common in early renal disease. At least three early morning samples, taken on first rising, the patient having emptied his bladder the last thing before retiring, should be protein-free to heat testing. A faint trace of protein is sometimes found in morning urine from contamination with urine left in the urinary dead space the previous night. In this case it is necessary to collect successive hourly samples with the patient recumbent, and to confirm that proteinuria disappears completely within an hour or two. Lordotic and orthostatic proteinuria are generally attributed to temporary obstruction of the renal venous outflow, but their origin within the kidney is uncertain. The proteinuria is unselective (*vide infra*), but glomerular permeability is normally selective as judged by the dextran test, suggesting that some of the larger proteins originate below the glomerulus, possibly from renal lymph. On the other hand, changes in the glomerular epithelial foot processes, similar to those in childhood nephrosis, have been shown to appear on standing, and to disappear on lying down, in a few patients with orthostatic proteinuria.

Persistent proteinuria is always pathologic.

Even if there is no other evidence of renal disease, biopsy usually reveals glomerular or vascular disease. Pathologic proteinurias can be subdivided by concentrating urine (when necessary) and examining it electrophoretically and by immunologic methods. A characteristic pattern, with only a small proportion of albumin, large components of alpha$_1$, alpha$_2$, and beta$_1$ globulins, and an abnormally high proportion of beta$_2$ microglobulin, is found in patients with active pyelonephritis, congenital tubular disorders, hypokalemic nephropathy, and some types of transplant rejection; it is referred to as "tubular proteinuria" and rarely exceeds 1 gram per 24 hours. In some forms of myelomatosis, the light chains of the abnormal immunoglobulins, being small enough to pass through the glomerular filter easily, appear in the urine as *"Bence Jones proteinuria."* All other patterns of proteinuria are attributed to increased permeability of the glomerular filter. The normal glomerulus allows macromolecules to enter the filtrate at a rate proportional to the logarithm of their molecular size (Fig. 1). This relationship still holds approximately when the glomerulus becomes excessively leaky, but the slope of the graph varies according to the disease. In nephrotic syndrome with minimal change (childhood nephrosis) it remains steep, so that only the smaller plasma proteins such as albumin appear in the urine in detectable quantities (Fig. 2). In several diffuse diseases of the glomeruli, including membranous glomerulonephropathy and amyloidosis, the graph is less steep, and very large molecules such as alpha$_2$ macroglobulin can be detected in the urine. Proliferative glomerulonephritis occupies an intermediate position, but yields rather variable results. This is probably due to the patchy nature of the lesion; tests of selectivity based on proteins in plasma and urine exaggerate the loss of selectivity in this condition, probably because protein

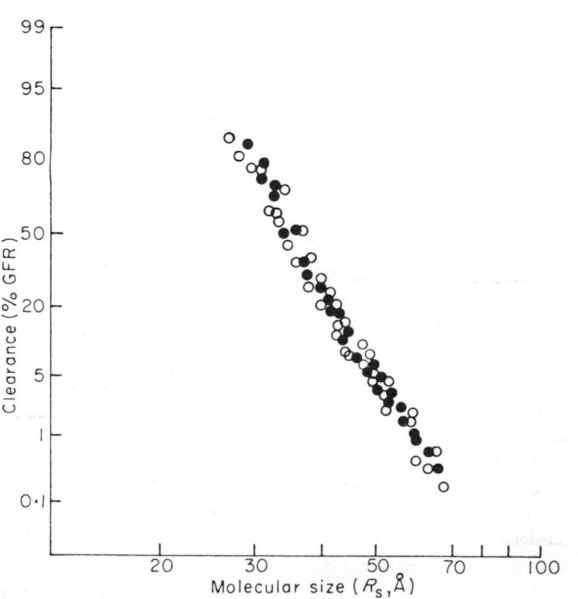

FIGURE 1. Relationship between the molecular size and the glomerular clearance of large polymers (○ = allyl-Dextran; ● = polyvinylpyrrolidone) in normal rabbits. (From Hardwicke, J., et al.: Clin. Sci., 34: 509, 1968.)

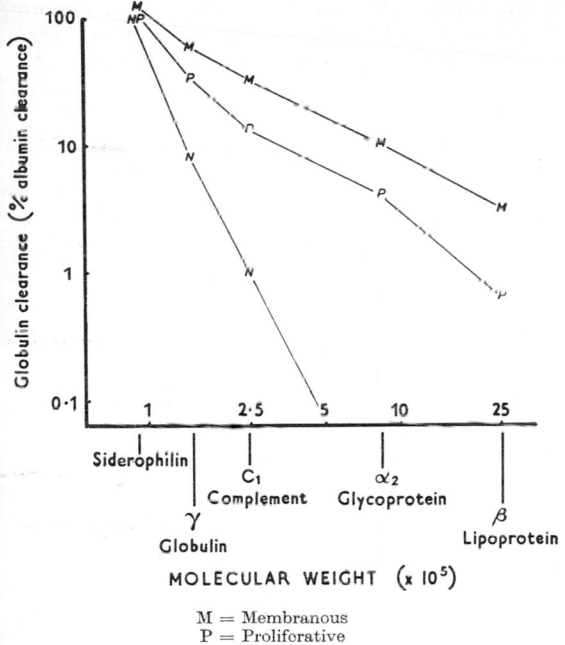

M = Membranous
P = Proliferative
N = 'Minimal'

FIGURE 2. Relationship between molecular weight and relative clearance of plasma proteins in the three main types of nephrotic syndrome (M = membranous, P = proliferative, N = 'minimal'). (From Blainey, J. D., et al.: Quart J. Med., 34:235, 1959.)

is reabsorbed in the tubules of the least affected nephrons. A simplified test for selectivity of proteinuria in which transferrin and IgG or alpha$_2$ macroglobulin are measured in serum and urine with the aid of immunoplates is now a standard laboratory test much simpler than electrophoresis of concentrated urine. Its main value is in the nephrotic syndrome of childhood in which selective proteinuria makes a response to corticosteroids so likely that renal biopsy may often be avoided.

Urine Microscopy. Urine should be collected in midstream with the same precautions as for culture at a time when the urine is likely to be concentrated. It should be handled by a constant technique, e.g., by centrifuging 10 ml. at top speed in a bench centrifuge and resuspending the sediment in the last 0.5 ml. of urine. It should be examined with a good quality, well-maintained microscope equipped with a variable illuminator and preferably a polarizer. A thick drop should be examined under low power for casts and crystals, and a thin film in a hemocytometer under high power for red cells, white cells, bacteria, and the exact identification of casts.

Red cells are normally excreted at a rate of about 150 to 300,000 per 24 hours, with an approximate upper limit of 1 million per 24 hours or 1000 per minute in short collections. Only an occasional red cell should be seen on qualitative microscopy as described above. White cells are excreted at an average of about 70,000 per hour in both sexes, but this applies only to urine entirely free from contamination in the female. If there has been

much contamination with vaginal secretion, as indicated by large numbers of squamous epithelial cells, leukocyturia cannot be interpreted unless it is extremely heavy. The upper limit of normal leukocyte excretion is 200,000 per hour, which yields one or two leukocytes per high-power field in qualitative microscopy of a concentrated urine. Leukocytes are difficult to distinguish from nonsquamous epithelial cells from the renal tubules, and the two are usually counted together. The increase in leukocyte excretion following pyrogen injection or prednisolone has been proposed as a test for chronic pyelonephritis, but it is so difficult to obtain non-catheter-timed urine samples from females free from vaginal contamination that it is seldom employed in practice. Qualitative examination for leukocytes is nonetheless of great importance in the detection of urinary infection, renal tuberculosis, and analgesic nephropathy.

Hyaline casts consist of precipitated Tamm-Horsfall protein only; they have a refractive index close to that of urine and are easily missed if the illumination is too high. Up to 10,000 per 24 hours are excreted by normal subjects, but at this rate only a very occasional one is seen even on the thick drop under low power. Numerous hyaline casts are seen in nearly all renal diseases associated with glomerular proteinuria; hyaline casts with few or none of the other varieties described below are seen in benign essential hypertension and nephrotic syndrome with minimal change. Hyaline casts are mainly of roughly constant diameter corresponding to the lumen of the distal convoluted tubule, but short thick casts, formed in the collecting duct, are seen in chronic renal failure and recovering tubular necrosis or glomerulonephritis. Misshapen, long, and branching casts are formed in the late stages of chronic renal diseases, particularly chronic nephritis, reflecting the distorted shape of some nephrons.

Granular casts are speckled or barred, sometimes to the point of appearing almost black in low illumination. It was thought until recently that they represented degenerate cellular casts, but it has now been shown that the granules are plasma proteins, mainly immunoglobulins. Granular casts may appear in normal urine after severe exercise or during orthostatic proteinuria. In the resting afebrile subject they almost invariably indicate renal pathology, but do not point to any particular disease.

Red blood cell casts, which have a faint orange tinge, much harder to detect than most descriptions suggest, indicate glomerular bleeding, and are found in acute glomerulonephritis, polyarteritis, and malignant hypertension. Leukocyte casts are usually indicative of pyelonephritis. Epithelial cell casts, with numerous free epithelial cells, are said to suggest tubular necrosis; but they are also found in glomerulonephritis, which is often the important differential diagnosis. Fatty casts, staining red with Sudan III and showing "Maltese crosses" in polarized light, accompany heavy proteinuria and are probably due to the leakage of lipoproteins through the glomerular filter. Oval fat bodies—degenerate tubular cells—and free fat globules have the same significance.

The recognition of casts is a very important step in establishing the existence of renal disease; they are particularly helpful in the investigation of proteinuria and hematuria, indicating a probable renal origin for the latter. However, their role in distinguishing between renal diseases has probably been exaggerated, and the prognostic significance attributed to them in the past is unfounded; heavy cast excretion, including renal failure casts, can continue for years without appreciable decline in renal function, and there are in any case better ways of determining the prognosis.

Glomerular Filtration Rate. If a substance is filtered at the glomerulus in proportion to plasma water and is not reabsorbed or secreted by the tubule, it can be used to estimate glomerular filtration rate (GFR) because the excretion rate is then determined only by the plasma level and the GFR.

$$\text{GFR (clearance rate of marker substance)} = \frac{\text{excretion rate}}{\text{plasma level}}$$

The one universally accepted marker substance is inulin, a mixture of fructose polymers with an average molecular weight of about 5200, but it has the disadvantages of being a variable mixture, of having a low solubility, and of hydrolyzing to fructose during the boiling necessary to dissolve it. The analytic methods for inulin are also difficult. Polyfructosan, with a narrow range of molecular weight and better solubility, is probably superior but less familiar. Any exogenous substance used for measurement of GFR must be infused at a constant rate for long enough to allow complete stabilization of the blood level, and then continued until several urine samples can be obtained of sufficient volume to minimize bladder-emptying errors. Consequently accurate measurement of GFR with inulin, without bladder catheterization, takes four to six hours, and is unsuitable for routine clinical use.

Several substances more easily measured than inulin, which are also not protein bound, freely filtered, and little affected by tubular secretion or reabsorption, are available, including [131]iodine-labeled inulin or diacetrizoate and ^{51}Cr-labeled EDTA. As all these substances, like inulin, have a very low rate of extrarenal excretion, they can be used to measure GFR approximately by a single injection technique. After an initial delay for equilibration in its volume of distribution, the plasma level of the marker substance falls exponentially, and the slope of the line is a measure of GFR. This technique gives a reproducibility of about ± 5 per cent using multiple plasma samples, and a little poorer result using an external counter to avoid blood sampling. The method is now provided by many hospital physics departments on a routine basis, and is sufficient for clinical purposes,

as the GFR is in any case subject to a diurnal variation of about ± 10 per cent, reaching its peak in the afternoon and its trough during the night; it is also readily disturbed by exercise or emotional disturbance.

The most popular rough estimate of GFR is the endogenous creatinine clearance, using a 24-hour collection and a single plasma sample. Timing of the plasma sample is not critical, as plasma creatinine varies little during the day if renal function is stable, and it can even be drawn soon after the end of the collection period in outpatients. The automated technique used in most hospital laboratories, based on the Jaffe reaction, measures creatinine plus some of the creatinine-like chromogen, but its reliability is better than that of the manual methods measuring true creatinine.

Creatinine clearance has poor reproducibility and high interlaboratory variation in surveys of laboratory accuracy, particularly when the result is close to normal. When the plasma creatinine is less than 1 mg. per 100 ml., the error of the plasma estimation alone is about ± 10 per cent. Reliance should never be placed on a single estimation. Two or three consecutive collections should be employed and the results averaged to compensate for bladder-emptying errors. Creatinine clearance considerably, and unpredictably, overestimates GFR in nephrotic syndrome, after renal transplantation, and in terminal renal failure, probably because of tubular secretion of creatinine. It is most useful in the range of GFR 10 to 50 ml./per minute.

Urea clearance in the normal subject and in the early stages of chronic renal disease is dependent on urine flow as well as GFR. The relationship is complex; below about 0.35 ml./per minute urea clearance is proportional to urine volume. From 0.35 to about 2 ml. per minute it increases in proportion to the square root of urine flow rate. Above 2 ml./per minute it increases only very slowly with urine flow. The maximal urea clearance, i.e., clearance measured at a flow rate of 2 ml./per minute or above) is about 60 to 70 per cent of GFR. Maximal urea clearance was once the most popular test of glomerular function, and it is still occasionally employed. The results are hopelessly unreliable unless a constant diuresis can be induced by giving fluid at half-hourly intervals and unless at least three urine samples can be collected at a flow rate over 2 ml. per minute. This minimizes errors resulting from the washout of urinary dead space. Plasma samples must be drawn in each collection period because plasma urea falls during the test. This test should not be employed in late renal failure because of the risk of water intoxication. As renal failure advances, urea clearance becomes less dependent on urine flow and approaches the GFR. At a GFR below 5 ml. per minute it is about 90 per cent of GFR. At the same time fluctuations in plasma urea throughout the 24 hours, expressed as a percentage of the mean, diminish so that urea clearance can be estimated on 24-hour urine samples. Some laboratories automatically measure urea and creatinine on the same samples, and provide an average of urea and creatinine clearance, as an approximation to GFR, in renal failure.

The most widely used indices of excretory function are the plasma urea and creatinine. The clinician translates them subconsciously into estimates of GFR, as in Table 1. It is a very crude estimation. Several studies of ambulant patients have shown that there is a wide scatter of plasma urea and creatinine at all levels of GFR and that plasma urea levels within the normal range can be encountered with a GFR down to about a third of normal. Both plasma urea and creatinine usually fall below the predicted level in late renal failure when extrarenal removal of urea and tubular secretion of creatinine become important. Plasma urea is influenced not only by GFR and protein intake but also by net catabolism and anabolism of body protein and by variations in fluid intake until late in renal failure; a stable plasma urea is only achieved after about a fortnight of constant intake in the metabolic ward. Changes in plasma urea do not necessarily indicate changes in excretory function. On the other hand, creatinine production is proportional to muscle mass and is largely uninfluenced by dietary protein intake. Changes in plasma creatinine therefore reflect changes in GFR, providing that there is no major alteration in muscle mass caused by starvation, refeeding, or intercurrent illness. It is the more useful measurement for following the progress of renal failure between accurate estimations of GFR.

Plasma urea and creatinine are more helpful in establishing renal impairment than in excluding it. A plasma urea above 60 mg. per 100 ml. or a creatinine above 2.0 mg. per 100 ml. almost certainly indicates depression of GFR (temporary or permanent), but a plasma urea and creatinine within the normal range do not exclude it.

The more important use of plasma urea and creatinine is as measures of the retention of metabolic end products in renal failure; in this role they are complementary. Urea represents those compounds produced in proportion to protein intake; creatinine, those which are influenced only by cell turnover. Many other important compounds have characteristics between the two. During peritoneal and hemodialysis urea is removed faster than almost any other compound, and gives an unduly optimistic picture of the over-all retention of end products; creatinine is removed much more slowly. The clinician who asks for a plasma urea needs a plasma creatinine as well, and he should base his treatment on the worse result of the two.

Renal Blood Flow. Renal blood flow can be estimated by dye dilution methods or by the elution curve of radiokrypton if the renal artery and vein are catheterized. These techniques are sometimes employed clinically after renal transplant when fine catheters can be left in the donor organ at operation and kept in situ during the first few weeks. A fall in renal blood flow is probably the first detectable sign of rejection of a homograft. In other situations renal plasma flow is usually measured as the clearance rate of para-amino hippurate (PAH) on the assumption that PAH is both filtered at the glomerulus and secreted by the tubules so that it is cleared almost completely from the plasma in a single passage through the kidney. PAH is easy to measure accurately, and it equilibrates in the body more rapidly than inulin so the performance of PAH clearance is relatively simple. In the normal subject the removal of PAH from blood traversing the kidney is about 92 per cent, which is near enough to the theoretic 100 per cent to make the test useful; it has been employed to show that renal blood flow varies more widely than GFR with exercise and emotion but has about the same and parallel diurnal variation. In renal disease the extraction ratio of PAH may be well below 92 per cent so PAH clearance cannot be equated with renal plasma flow unless the extraction ratio can be measured simultaneously with the aid of a renal vein catheter—seldom a justifiable clinical procedure.

Glomerular filtration rate and renal blood flow are both related to body size, and surface area has been found to correlate with them most closely in the adult. They are therefore corrected to a standard surface area of 1.73 square meters before comparison with the normal range. This correction is of course unnecessary when they are used serially to follow the progress of disease. In infants under one year the GFR and renal blood flow are low in relationship to surface area, but this is probably a reflection of the high surface area of the infant rather than a reduced renal reserve. On other criteria, e.g., using body volume as a standard, the GFR reaches adult proportions at about one month. Both GFR and renal blood flow rise in pregnancy, reaching a peak at about 36 weeks, so it is essential to compare results in pregnancy with the normal range for the same stage of gestation.

TABLE 1. PREDICTED RELATIONSHIP BETWEEN GFR, PLASMA CREATININE AND PLASMA UREA IN PATIENTS WITH STABLE LEAN BODY MASS

GFR (ml./min.)	Plasma Creatinine (mg./100 ml.)		Plasma Urea (mg./100 ml.)	
	Male	Female	40 Gram Protein Diet	80 Gram Protein Diet
120	1.0	0.75	16	32
60	2.0	1.5	29	58
30	4.0	3.0	53	106
15	8.0	6.0	91	182
5	24.0	18.0	238	576

Assumptions used in these predictions: (1) Creatinine clearance is equal to GFR. (2) Average 24 hour urea clearance rises from 50 per cent GFR at 120 ml. per min. to 80 per cent GFR at 5 ml. per min. (3) Average creatinine excretion in male is 1800 mg. per 24 hours—a little below most published figures for normal populations. (4) Female creatinine excretion is about 75 per cent that of male. (5) No extrarenal removal of urea or creatinine.

Urinary Concentrating Power. The ability to concentrate urine is impaired as the population of nephrons declines with disease, and it is seldom worthwhile testing concentrating power at a GFR less than 20 ml. per minute. It is impaired disproportionately by any disease affecting the loop of Henle or the collecting duct. The concentration test has often been described as a sensitive index of early renal damage, but the reproducibility is so low and the normal range so wide that it cannot be more than a crude index. To obtain maximal concentration reliably, it is necessary to deprive the patient of fluid for more than 24 hours, which makes the test inapplicable to outpatients and dangerous to those in renal failure. If the urine reaches an osmolality over 700 mOsm. per liter after 16 hours of fluid deprivation, i.e., in a morning specimen, dry meals taken since previous lunch time, or if this level is found in a spot early morning sample, it is probable that the concentrating mechanism is normal. Pitressin tannate in oil, 5 units intramuscularly, produces urine concentration three to five hours later which is close to that after water deprivation in patients with defective concentration. The pitressin test gives results about 100 mOsm. per liter lower than water deprivation in the normal person. Tradi-

tionally urine SG has been used as the criterion of urinary concentration, but as it bears an inconstant relationship to osmolality (which is the best measure of the work of concentration), particularly in the presence of proteinuria, glycosuria, and some exogenous substances such as contrast media, it should now be abandoned in favor of osmolality, which can be measured more accurately on a much smaller sample and, with modern instruments, almost as quickly. An osmolality of 700 corresponds roughly to an SG of 1.020.

Hamburger, J., Richet, G., Crosnier, J., Funck-Brentano, J. L., Antoine, B., Ducrot, H., Mery, J. P., de Montera, H., and Royer, P. (Translator, Walsh, A.): Nephrology. Philadelphia, W. B. Saunders Company, 1968, Chapter 5.

James, J. A.: Renal Disease in Childhood. St. Louis, C. V. Mosby Company, 1968, Chapter 5.

Kerr, D. N. S.: Renal function tests. *In* Innes Williams, D. (ed.): Paediatric Urology. London, Butterworth and Co. (Publishers), Ltd., 1968, pp. 73, 548.

Peterson, P. A., Evrin, P. E., and Berggard, I.: Differentiation of glomerular, tubular and normal proteinuria: Determinations of urinary excretion of β_2-microglobulin, albumin and total protein. J. Clin. Invest., 48:1189, 1969.

Relman, A. S., and Levinsky, N. G.: Clinical examination of renal function. *In* Strauss, M. B., and Welt, L. G. (eds.): Diseases of the Kidney. London, J. & A. Churchill, Ltd., 1963, Chapter 3.

Wesson, L. G., Jr.: Physiology of the Human Kidney. New York, Grune and Stratton, Inc., 1969, Chapters 6, 7, 14, and 23.

Chronic Renal Failure
D. N. S. Kerr

ETIOLOGY

Permanent renal damage arises from many causes, and every clinician has his own classification based on etiology or some other criterion. In Table 2 the major causes are arranged in a manner intended to aid differential diagnosis. Those in the last group should usually be recognized from other features of the primary disease. Many in the second and third groups will also be identified by involvement of the bladder or other systems. Diseases in the first group usually present with features of renal disease alone. These divisions are, of course, incomplete. Some diseases in Group 1 may have extrarenal manifestations—e.g., epididymitis with renal tuberculosis, back pain with retroperitoneal fibrosis—whereas some in Group 4, e.g., gout, diabetes, atheroma, subacute bacterial endocarditis, occasionally have renal failure as their presenting feature. Nonetheless, if a good history and examination have failed to reveal a systemic cause for chronic renal failure, the likely possibilities are in Groups 1 and 3.

The incidence of diseases causing renal failure is dependent on the age of the patient. In early infancy congenital cystic disease of the infantile type, hypoplasia, and urinary obstruction by valves in the posterior urethra (in males) are im-

portant causes. In later childhood, chronic pyelonephritis, usually associated with vesicoureteral reflux and other congenital anomalies, becomes the most important cause; but medullary cystic disease, oxalosis, cystinosis, congenital nephritis, chronic proliferative glomerulonephritis, and hemolytic uremic syndrome (in the postacute stage) are responsible for a significant number of cases. Between the ages of 15 and 50, chronic proliferative glomerulonephritis, chronic pyelonephritis, and essential hypertension together provide about three quarters of all cases. Analgesic nephropathy is a major cause in Australia, Scandinavia, and Switzerland, and is of greater importance in Great Britain and the United States than is generally recognized. Polycystic disease of the adult type assumes increasing importance in those older than 40, and is responsible for 10 to 15 per cent of all cases of chronic renal failure in adult life in Great Britain. In old age chronic pyelonephritis again emerges as a major cause in both sexes; prostatic enlargement leading to urinary obstruction and infection is the most common precipitant in men.

The problem that has been most hotly disputed is the relative contributions of pyelonephritis and glomerulonephritis in older children and young and middle-aged adults. Both diseases may pre-

TABLE 2. A CLINICAL CLASSIFICATION OF THE CAUSES OF CHRONIC RENAL FAILURE

Local Causes:
  Diseases in which the kidneys are predominantly involved and in which the presenting features are usually those of renal disease
    Proliferative glomerulonephritis
    Membranous glomerulonephropathy
    Chronic pyelonephritis
    Tuberculous pyelonephritis
    Renal calculi
    Congenital nephritis
    Polycystic disease
    Medullary cystic disease
    Renal hypoplasia
    Renal tubular acidosis
    Balkan nephropathy
    Upper urinary tract obstruction
      Hydronephrosis
      Retroperitoneal fibrosis
      Neoplasm

Lower Urinary Tract Obstruction:
  Presenting features often those of bladder dysfunction, but may present in renal failure
    Prostatic enlargement
      Adenoma
      Neoplasm
    Urethral stricture
    Urethral valves
    Bladder neck obstruction
    Neurogenic bladder

Systemic Diseases and Intoxications:
  (a) In which renal failure is not infrequently a presenting feature
    Malignant essential hypertension
    Polyarteritis nodosa
    Disseminated lupus erythematosus
    Primary and secondary amyloidosis
    Analgesic overconsumption
    Potassium deficiency
    Hypercalcemia
    Cystinosis
    Oxalosis
    Consumption coagulopathies
      Hemolytic uremic syndrome
      Thrombotic thrombocytopenic purpura
      Postpartum renal failure
    Lead or cadmium poisoning
  (b) In which renal failure is usually a late feature or overshadowed by other manifestations
    Benign essential hypertension
    Atheroma
    Systemic emboli
      Subacute bacterial endocarditis
      Rheumatic heart disease
    Gout
    Diabetes
    Heart failure
    Cirrhosis

sent at a late stage when pyelography is unrewarding and renal biopsy or autopsy merely reveals small scarred ("end stage") kidneys. In Great Britain in the late 1950's deaths from "nephritis and nephrosis" heavily outnumbered those from "infection of the kidney," according to death certificates. Ten years later the proportions were reversed, but the total deaths under both headings were virtually unchanged. More accurate diagnosis during life and an increasing use of autopsy no doubt contributed to the change, but the main cause was probably an alteration in certification habits as the medical profession became more aware of chronic pyelonephritis. Several other sources of information, more accurate than death certification, suggest that glomerulonephritis is still the most common cause of chronic renal failure between the ages of 15 and 50. Recipients of transplants—in whom accurate diagnosis is usually facilitated by bilateral nephrectomy—and candidates for regular dialysis suffer from glomerulonephritis more than twice as often as they do from pyelonephritis.

There is also some difficulty in separating the roles of chronic glomerulonephritis and essential hypertension. Rapidly progressive malignant hypertension in young adults causes afferent arteriolar necrosis and the rapid onset of renal failure with kidneys of normal size which are not easily confused with those of nephritis. However, more slowly progressive, severe hypertension causes medial and intimal thickening of interlobular arteries and hyaline degeneration of afferent arterioles which lead to diffuse scarring of the kidney. In its late stages this "hypertensive nephrosclerosis" is difficult to distinguish from chronic glomerulonephritis with secondary hypertension.

The effects of hypertension also merge into those of atheroma, which frequently complicates it but which also occurs in normotensive subjects. Atheroma of the renal arteries may lead to superimposed renal hypertension, atheroembolism, or thrombosis with renal infarction, any of which will hasten the decline in renal function.

The kidney is involved histologically in almost all patients with gout, and renal failure has been quoted as the cause of death in 18 to 30 per cent. This is probably an overstatement based on selected hospital series. The renal failure usually occurs late in the course of gout, progresses slowly, and may be retarded by treatment with allopurinol. Consequently gout provides few of the candidates for regular dialysis and transplantation—only 0.3 per cent in European centers in the 1960's.

THE INVESTIGATION OF CHRONIC RENAL DISEASE

Investigation has three objectives: recognition of the primary disease, assessment of the degree of renal failure, and detection of any aggravating factors.

Recognition of the Primary Disease. When chronic renal disease is detected at an early stage, the accurate identification of the causative disease is obviously required, but many patients still see their doctors for the first time when renal failure is well advanced and most of the damage to the kidneys is irreparable. Full investigation at this stage is often uncomfortable, expensive, and unrewarding and sometimes hazardous. Renal biopsy is difficult when the kidneys are small and fibrotic, and its dangers are increased by hypertension and advanced uremia. Retrograde pyelography may introduce infection to a damaged kidney. The ability to distinguish, for instance, between the end stages of chronic pyelonephritis and chronic glomerulonephritis confers no therapeutic benefit, and strenuous efforts in this direction will only be justified when we have specific therapy for the late stages of one of these diseases. Nonetheless, considerable information can usually be obtained without discomfort to the patient, and several reversible causes of renal failure must always be sought with care. Correction of urinary obstruction and removal of calculi will sometimes result in improvement even in advanced renal failure. Withdrawal of analgesics from a patient with analgesic nephropathy will halt the decline in renal function and occasionally reverse it. Retroperitoneal fibrosis often improves spontaneously or with steroid therapy if methysergide is withdrawn; it is also amenable to surgery. Lupus nephritis often responds to corticosteroids and other immunosuppressive drugs.

The history should include a lifelong survey of previous renal complaints, occupation, and drug consumption. Specific inquiry should be made about symptoms suggestive of urinary infection and the intake of analgesics, other phenacetin-containing compounds, and methysergide, because these are often overlooked by the patient. The family history should include specific inquiry about renal disease, hypertension and its sequelae, gout, collagenoses, preeclampsia, and deafness. The facets of physical examination and general medical investigation that may be important comprise most of the physician's repertoire.

Investigations that are virtually always required include urinary pH and osmolality on an early morning sample, microscopy, and midstream culture, qualitative test for glycosuria and quantitative test for proteinuria, plasma or serum urea, electrolytes, creatinine, urate, calcium, phosphorus, alkaline phosphatase, total protein, electrophoresis and cholesterol, and straight roentgenography of the renal tract. Chest roentgenogram, electrocardiogram, serum magnesium and creatinine clearance are also included in the initial screening but not for the sake of differential diagnosis. If the renal size is not obvious from the straight roentgenogram, it is often revealed by tomography. High-dose or infusion pyelography will usually provide acceptable pictures down to a glomerular filtration rate (GFR) of about 7 ml. per minute and will help to detect hydronephrosis, polycystic disease, and other conditions not calling for fine calyceal detail, down to a GFR of 2 to 3 ml. per minute.

Proteinuria exceeding 3 grams per 24 hours is unusual in chronic pyelonephritis, analgesic nephropathy, benign hypertension, urinary obstruction, calculous disease, and renal tubular acidosis; it is usual or common in chronic glomerulonephritis, membranous glomerulonephropathy, amyloidosis, diabetic nephropathy, polyarteritis, disseminated lupus, and malignant hypertension. Proteinuria may diminish in the latter group of diseases as renal failure advances, but this does not always happen—very heavy proteinuria can be encountered with a GFR below 5 ml. per minute. Mild hypoproteinemia accompanies fluid overload in many forms of renal disease, but more severe hypoproteinemia (below 5 grams per 100 ml.), particularly if associated with a nephrotic electrophoretic pattern and hypercholesterolemia, strongly suggests that heavy proteinuria was present in the recent past even if no longer demonstrable. It takes weeks, and sometimes months, for the electrophoretic pattern to return to normal after the patient maintained by dialysis has become anuric.

Numerous cellular casts in the urinary deposit suggest some form of glomerulonephritis, including the collagenoses, or malignant hypertension. They are seldom encountered in chronic pyelonephritis or analgesic nephropathy, in both of which an increased output of white cells is often the only abnormality of microscopy. Hyaline casts predominate in membranous glomerulonephropathy and hypertensive nephrosclerosis without malignant hypertension.

Hyperchloremic acidosis suggests chronic pyelonephritis, analgesic nephropathy, renal tubular acidosis, or polycystic disease; it is also found after urinary diversion into the bowel. Hypercalcemia is occasionally found in secondary hyperparathyroidism, but it should always raise the question of whether the hypercalcemia is the cause of the renal failure and not vice versa. Paper or cellulose acetate electrophoresis and search for Bence Jones protein in the urine will detect most examples of renal failure caused by myelomatosis, but other techniques such as immunoelectrophoresis are required to demonstrate the monoclonal gammapathies that underlie most instances of "primary" renal amyloid—one of the diseases that most frequently eludes detection until renal biopsy is performed.

Very large kidneys are typical of obstruction or polycystic disease, though in some instances polycystic kidneys are impalpable and are first detected at autopsy or bilateral nephrectomy. Renal failure with kidneys of normal size should always alert the clinician to the possibility of acute rather than chronic renal failure, though several forms of chronic renal disease—amyloidosis, rapidly progressive nephritis, membranous glomerulonephropathy—may reach the end stage without much contraction of the kidney. Small symmetrical kidneys with preservation of the calyceal pattern are found in many chronic renal diseases, notably chronic glomerulonephritis. Chronic pyelonephritis is confirmed by asymmetrical and irregular scarring with clubbing and outdrawing of the calyces; pyelography is the most useful test in diagnosing this disease. Typical findings in analgesic nephropathy are small kidneys with scalloped outlines—sometimes misinterpreted as fetal lobulation—and clubbed calyces corresponding to the sloughed papillae; however, the pyelogram may remain normal even in late renal failure; rare but diagnostic signs are encirclement of a separated papilla by contrast medium ("ring sign") and calcification of papillae.

Urinary infection is still present in about half the patients with chronic pyelonephritis currently seen in chronic renal failure; it is also a common accompaniment of calculous disease, analgesic nephropathy, and lower urinary tract obstruction. It is often said that superimposed pyelonephritis is common in all forms of chronic renal disease, but this is an opinion based on one interpretation of histology. In practice positive cultures are seldom obtained from patients with chronic glomerulonephritis or malignant hypertension who have not undergone instrumentation of the urinary tract. Nonetheless it is sound practice to screen all patients with chronic renal failure for urinary infection; three midstream urines should be cultured at intervals of at least a week when the patient is receiving no antimicrobial drugs. If these cultures are all negative, it is extremely unlikely that he harbors persistent renal infection. However if he is known to have had infection in the past and has recently received an antimicrobial such as a penicillin which acts on cell walls, special media should be used to detect bacterial L-forms.

Assessment of the Degree of Renal Failure. The most important parameter is the glomerular filtration rate. It is most accurately measured by timed urine collection during constant infusion of inulin or of some substitute which is more easily measured, is not protein-bound, and is handled like inulin, e.g., ^{131}I-labeled inulin or diacetrizoate, ^{51}Cr-labeled EDTA. However, this involves urethral catheterization or collection over several hours and is of no practical use outside research laboratories. A single-dose modification, using one of the labeled markers and surface counting, estimates the GFR with an error of about ± 5 per cent, and is provided as an outpatient service in some general hospitals. Most clinicians must rely on endogenous creatinine clearance, using a 24-hour collection and a single plasma sample. Timing of the plasma sample is not critical, as plasma creatinine varies little during the day if renal function is stable, and it can even be drawn after the end of the collection period in outpatients. The automated technique used in most hospital laboratories measures creatinine plus some of the creatinine-like chromogen, but its reproducibility is better than that of the manual methods measuring true creatinine.

Creatinine clearance is one of the estimations with the poorest reproducibility and highest interlaboratory variation in surveys of laboratory accuracy, particularly when the result is close to normal. Reliance should never be placed on a single estimation; two or three consecutive collections should be employed and the results averaged to compensate for bladder-emptying errors. Creatinine clearance overestimates GFR considerably and unpredictably in nephrotic syndrome, after renal transplantation, and in terminal renal failure, probably because the tubules secrete creatinine. It is most useful in the range of GFR 10 to 50 ml. per minute.

Urea clearance in the early stages of chronic renal disease, as in the normal, is dependent on urine flow, and maximal urea clearance is about 60 to 70 per cent of GFR. As renal failure advances, urea clearance becomes less dependent on urine flow and approaches the GFR. At a GFR below 5 ml. per minute it is about 90 per cent of GFR and can be measured on 24-hour samples. Some laboratories automatically measure urea and creatinine on the same samples and provide an average of urea and creatinine clearance, as an approximation to GFR, in renal failure.

The most widely used indices of excretory function are the plasma urea and creatinine. The clinician translates them subconsciously into estimates of GFR, as discussed in the preceding article. It is a very crude estimation. Several studies of ambulant patients have shown a wide scatter of plasma urea and creatinine at all levels of GFR and that plasma urea levels within the normal range can be encountered with a GFR down to about a third of normal. Both plasma urea and creatinine usually fall below the predicted level in late renal failure when extrarenal removal of urea and tubular secretion of creatinine become important. Plasma urea is influenced not only by GFR and protein intake, but also by net catabolism and anabolism of body protein and by variations in fluid intake until late in renal failure; a stable plasma urea is only achieved after about a fortnight of constant intake. Changes in plasma urea do not necessarily indicate changes in excretory function. On the other hand, creatinine production is proportional to muscle mass and is largely uninfluenced by dietary protein intake. Changes in plasma creatinine therefore reflect changes in GFR, providing that there is no major alteration in muscle mass caused by starvation, refeeding, or intercurrent illness. It is the more useful measurement for following the progress of renal failure between accurate estimations of GFR.

Plasma urea and creatinine are more helpful in establishing renal impairment than in excluding it. A plasma urea above 60 mg. per 100 ml. or a creatinine above 2.0 mg. per 100 ml. almost certainly indicate depression of GFR (temporary or permanent), but a plasma urea and creatinine within the normal range do not exclude it.

The more important use of plasma urea and creatinine is as measures of the retention of metabolic end products in renal failure; in this role they are complementary. Urea represents those compounds produced in proportion to protein intake; creatinine, those which are influenced only by cell turnover. Many other important compounds have characteristics between the two. During peritoneal and hemodialysis urea is removed faster than almost any other compound, and gives an unduly optimistic picture of the over-all retention of end products; creatinine is removed much more slowly. The clinician should ask for both plasma urea and plasma creatinine, and should base his treatment on the worse result of the two.

Detection of Aggravating Factors. Glomerular filtration rate may be depressed by hypovolemia from renal sodium loss, vomiting and diarrhea, systemic infections, surgery, trauma, hemorrhage, urinary infection, sudden reduction of long-standing hypertension, rapid rise in blood pressure, and administration of nephrotoxic drugs. The production rate of urea and other metabolic end products may be increased by excessive protein intake, tissue wasting from starvation, infection, trauma and surgery, resorption of hematoma, bleeding into the gut, and administration of corticosteroids or tetracyclines.

These aggravating factors should be sought and corrected in every patient seen for the first time in chronic renal failure, and no subsequent deterioration should be blamed on the primary disease until they have been excluded as contributory factors. When doubt exists, the patient should be kept alive for several weeks, if necessary by peritoneal dialysis or hemodialysis, to provide time for investigation and for his recovery from complications.

THE PATHOPHYSIOLOGY OF CHRONIC RENAL FAILURE

Chronically diseased kidneys often support life in comfort until about 90 per cent of their glomerular filtration has been lost, and they maintain some sort of life until 97 to 99 per cent has gone. This statement applies to most of the conditions listed in Table 2 and is the justification for considering them together. It implies that even in the late stages of disease the kidneys retain some ability to respond to the demands of the body by varying the output of water and important solutes. The most popular explanation for this response of the diseased kidney to physiologic stimuli is the "intact nephron hypothesis."

According to this theory the deformed nephrons seen in histologic preparations and nephron dissections are largely nonfunctional; excretory function is maintained by a remnant of surviving nephrons in which both glomerulus and tubule have escaped irreparable damage. In these nephrons the glomerulus produces an increased volume of glomerular filtrate. Hypertrophy of the tubule enables it to handle this extra filtrate within limits, but the additional solute load causes an osmotic diuresis which has the same effects as a saline or urea diuresis in the normal subject. Urine is produced at a nearly constant rate throughout the 24 hours, at an osmolality which is eventually fixed around 300 mOsm. per kilogram (specific gravity, SG, about 1.010)—a state referred to as isosthenuria. This condition becomes established only when the GFR is reduced to about a quarter of normal. It results in nocturia, one of the most common symptoms of early renal failure (but one which often fails to alert the patient to his condition; the accompanying polyuria leads to thirst, and the nocturia is blamed on an increased consumption of fluid in the evenings).

There is substantial evidence in support of the intact nephron hypothesis, and the events outlined in the last paragraph probably underlie most of the adaptations to chronic renal failure. However, there are important exceptions. The grotesquely deformed nephrons of polycystic disease retain some excretory function, and the same may apply to other renal diseases. Those conditions in which medullary damage is a prominent feature—particularly chronic pyelonephritis, analgesic nephropathy, and medullary cystic disease—are often characterized by severe polyuria with hypotonic urine, suggesting that many functioning nephrons have lost their concentrating mechanism, and there is other evidence of impaired distal tubular function in these patients. At the other end of the scale are diseases such as rapidly progressive nephritis, in which glomerular damage is widespread and roughly uniform in time, which do not pass through an isosthenuric phase, so that patients enter the terminal stage of renal failure without ever having experienced nocturia.

Water. Polyuria commonly accompanies isosthenuria. It reaches a peak while the GFR is declining through the range 25 to 5 ml. per minute, then gives way to oliguria in the preterminal phase of chronic renal failure, except in a minority of patients with predominant medullary damage who remain polyuric to the end. Thirst is a constant accompaniment of polyuria, and if the patient has free access to water he will usually maintain his water balance with reasonable accuracy. The once popular practice of "pushing fluids" to reduce the plasma urea is unnecessary and potentially dangerous. Thirst is sometimes excessive, because dryness of the mouth is common in late renal failure. This symptom is occasionally due to overbreathing from acidosis, but is usually the result of an unexplained reduction in salivary flow.

Large water loads are excreted more slowly than in the normal subject; hyponatremia follows their ingestion for several hours; convulsions are occasionally precipitated. Conversely, obligatory water loss through the kidneys is increased, and patients are therefore sensitive to water deprivation, caused by drowsiness or vomiting.

Sodium. The excretion of most solutes, like that of water, can only be varied over a restricted range in renal failure. The patient remains in reasonable health if his intake is adjusted to the ability of his kidneys to excrete, but he faces trouble if it is close to one of the extremes tolerated by normal persons. A normal individual can adapt equally well to a sodium intake of a few milliequivalents (mEq.) a day and to one of several hundred mEq. per day. He adjusts his sodium excretion to match his intake by altering the secretion rate of aldosterone and "third factor," which is probably an unidentified natriuretic hormone. His extracellular volume and GFR are virtually the same on the high and low intakes. A patient with chronic renal failure placed on a very low sodium diet, e.g., the traditional 22 mEq. per day, is often unable to reduce his sodium output by hormonal control alone because of the osmotic diuresis in his surviving nephrons. He goes into negative sodium balance and excretes a corresponding volume of water, his extracellular fluid volume, plasma volume, and GFR all fall. This reduces the osmotic load per nephron and permits more avid sodium retention. Sodium balance is re-established at the price of some decline in glomerular filtration rate.

If the patient is now placed on a high-sodium intake, he passes into positive sodium balance, retaining water in proportion, expanding his extracellular fluid volume, and raising his GFR. This increases the osmotic load per nephron until sodium output again equals intake. This new equilibrium is achieved at the price of an expanded extracellular fluid volume, which may be detectable as peripheral or pulmonary edema and which is often interpreted by the clinician as heart failure. Quite often, however, several liters of tissue fluid are accommodated without overt edema; the overloaded subcutaneous tissue conceals the wasting of muscle and fat characteristic of chronic renal failure, giving the patient a false appearance of adequate nutrition, which is rapidly corrected when his surplus fluid is removed at the start of regular dialysis.

A fortunate minority of patients remain normotensive even when grossly edematous. The majority develop hypertension when their extracellular fluid (ECF) volume is overexpanded. When the hypertension is of recent origin, it can usually be controlled by removing the surplus ECF and preventing its reaccumulation by dietary restriction. This is the treatment employed when the patient becomes dependent on regular hemodialysis. Control of hypertension is usually followed by the disappearance of any remaining excretory function which is unimportant at this juncture. At an earlier stage in renal failure the same control of blood pressure can be achieved with diuretics and low sodium diet, but at the cost of some reduction in GFR. There is therefore no ideal sodium intake for an individual in chronic renal failure; he must often choose between being normovolemic and normotensive with a low GFR, or edematous and hypertensive with a higher GFR. The choice must be guided by his future prospects. If he is a candidate for regular dialysis or transplantation, he would be far better off starting dialysis a few months early with a normal blood pressure than persisting with conservative treatment and enduring the effects of hypertension.

As GFR declines to a few milliliters per minute, the proportion of filtered sodium excreted in the urine must rise if sodium balance is to be maintained. The normal subject excretes only about 1 per cent of his filtered sodium, but in terminal renal failure some patients lose about 30 per cent of the filtered sodium in their urine—about the same as a normal subject under maximal osmotic diuresis. However, a substantial proportion are unable to approach this theoretic maximum, and they can be maintained in sodium balance only by severe dietary restriction or high-dose diuretic therapy. Their hypertension is accordingly difficult to control, and regular hemodialysis may be required for control of blood pressure before being required on other grounds. Low sodium dieting in this group can be inadvertently vitiated by the use of medicines; indigestion mixtures and antidiarrheal preparations, e.g., magnesium trisilicate mixture NF and kaolin and morphine mixture NF, are the main offenders, providing 20 to 40 mEq. of sodium per day at standard dosage.

At the other extreme a minority of patients excrete a high proportion of their filtered sodium even in early renal failure, and are liable to become sodium depleted if they fail to keep up a high dietary intake. The condition is sometimes referred to as "salt-losing nephritis," but it is not a separate pathologic entity. Most of these patients suffer from chronic pyelonephritis; a few suffer from analgesic nephropathy, medullary cystic disease, or adult polycystic disease. They are often pigmented, and may be thought to have Addison's disease. A helpful point in differentiation is the almost invariable presence of hyperchloremic acidosis in those with renal disease. Most of these patients are normotensive and tolerate dietary supplements (usually as sodium bicarbonate or citrate, with a liberal use of sodium chloride as condiment) without trouble. A few live on a knife edge between sodium depletion and hypertension, and require particularly careful control.

Potassium. Hypokalemia is found in a minority of patients with early renal failure. It is usually caused by diuretic therapy, diarrhea, vomiting, or purgation, but is sometimes due to spontaneous potassium loss in the urine. In a very few patients potassium loss is sufficient to cause severe hypokalemia and muscular paralysis. The condition has been called "potassium-losing nephritis," but is not a separate disease; it is an unusual manifestation of chronic pyelonephritis, renal tubular acidosis, ureterosigmoid anastomosis, and very occasionally other renal diseases. Excessive sodium and calcium loss in the urine sometimes coexist. When the potassium leak is an isolated defect, differentiation from Conn's syndrome can be difficult; a hyperchloremic acidosis strongly suggests a renal cause and a complete response to spironolactone an aldosteronoma, but diagnosis has sometimes awaited adrenal exploration.

During most of the course of renal failure most patients maintain normal plasma potassium, and their potassium excretion varies with their intake. As renal failure advances, potassium excretion may exceed the filtered potassium, presumably as a result of increased exchange for sodium in the distal tubule aided by the osmotic diuresis. However, the maximal capacity to excrete potassium is impaired even in early renal failure. An oral or intravenous dose causes an excessive rise in plasma potassium, which is corrected only over an extended period. Dangerous hyperkalemia may therefore follow endogenous release of potassium following hemolysis, trauma, or infection, or its administration medicinally or in stored blood. Deaths have resulted from the use of potassium citrate in chronic urinary infection (in which it is of doubtful value), and care must be exercised in prescribing potassium supplements and spironolactone during diurectic therapy.

Hyperkalemia is common in terminal renal failure; at this stage even dietary ingestion of excess potassium as fruit, fried potatoes, meat, and meat products can be hazardous. Occasional patients complain of muscle weakness or paresthesias when the plasma potassium reaches dangerous levels (over 7 mEq. per liter), but the majority are unaware of the condition until cardiac arrest occurs. The only warning signs are those detected by electrocardiography—flattened P wave, widened QRS complex, and peaked T wave.

In patients with a potassium leak, hypokalemia usually reflects severe depletion of total body potassium, but in other situations in renal failure the plasma level is not a reliable guide to body stores. Plasma potassium rises in acidosis and falls rapidly when this is corrected with sodium bicarbonate, without appreciable change in body potassium. Some hyperkalemic patients in terminal renal failure or on regular dialysis have diminished total body potassium, but this may be a reflection of reduced muscle mass rather than cellular potassium deficiency and is not to be regarded as an indication for potassium therapy.

Magnesium. Mild asymptomatic hypomagnesemia is not uncommon in early renal failure. It is due to an increased fecal loss which is accentuated by high calcium diet, because calcium and magnesium compete for the same absorptive mechanism. Hypomagnesemia of more than slight degree is usually due to diuretic therapy.

For most of the course of renal failure serum magnesium is usually normal, but hypermagnesemia appears with increasing frequency when the GFR falls below 30 ml. per minute, and is the rule in terminal renal failure. Serum magnesium rises in the presence of acidosis or tissue trauma; very high levels (over 3.5 mEq. per liter) are nearly always due to administration of magnesium salts as antacids, purgatives, or enemas (magnesium is well absorbed from the colon). Little is known about total body magnesium in chronic renal failure, but severe magnesium depletion has been reported in the presence of hypermagnesemia.

Spontaneous hypermagnesemia impairs nerve conduction time but probably plays no part in the development of neuropathy and may even protect against it; it is probably not responsible for any of the symptoms of renal failure. The very high levels (3.5 to over 8 mEq. per liter) that have followed magnesium medication or the use of hard water for hemodialysis have produced drowsiness, light coma, muscle weakness, and skin irritation.

Hydrogen Ion. Nonrespiratory acidosis virtually always develops during the progression of chronic renal failure, though it can be reversed temporarily by vomiting. In patients without predominant medullary damage it becomes pronounced only after the GFR falls below about 20 ml. per minute. A renal bicarbonate leak can be demonstrated in some patients with chronic renal failure when their plasma bicarbonate level is restored to normal with sodium bicarbonate. It is sufficiently severe to play a major role in the initial fall in plasma bicarbonate and, if confined to a minority of nephrons, it could be important even in later renal failure. However, the proportion of patients displaying a bicarbonate leak is uncertain, and the orthodox view is that it plays no part in the acidosis of late renal failure when bicarbonate is undetectable in the urine.

As renal acidosis progresses, urine becomes more acid, eventually reaching a pH of about 5—close to the minimum achieved by normal subjects after acid loading. This does not imply normal urinary acidification, as the patient achieves this urine pH at a much lower plasma bicarbonate level than normal. Moreover he excretes a considerably smaller quantity of hydrogen ion at any given urinary pH than normal. This is mainly due to a defect in ammonia production shown by a lower excretion of ammonium. Titratable acidity is normal or slightly reduced for the urine pH, because the main buffers (monohydrogen phosphate and creatinine) are excreted in nearly normal amount until late in renal failure.

It is now possible to calculate with fair accuracy the hydrogen ion produced by a stated diet. It is derived mainly from the oxidation of sulfur-containing amino acids to sulfuric acid, the hydrolysis of phosphate esters to phosphoric acid, the metabolism of purines to uric acid, and the production of intermediary acids during carbohydrate metabolism. Balance studies show that patients in renal failure excrete only about three quarters of their acid production, retaining 10 to 20 mEq. of hydrogen ion per day. In spite of this, their plasma bicarbonate level changes very slowly; the extra acid is believed to be neutralized by calcium carbonate in bone. This probably accounts in part for the negative calcium balance in renal failure, and may be a factor in the genesis of renal bone disease.

Respiratory compensation for the acidosis occurs in a predictable manner if there is no lung disease, the uremic subject behaving in the same manner as a normal subject ingesting ammonium chloride. Pa_{CO_2} falls by about 1.2 mm. Hg for every 1 mEq. per liter fall in plasma bicarbonate. This does not completely correct the blood pH, which falls in a roughly linear relationship to the plasma bicarbonate, reaching the lower limit of normal (7.35) when the plasma bicarbonate is about 15 mEq. per liter. In terminal renal failure the plasma bicarbonate falls below 10 mEq. per liter, and there is deep sighing (Kussmaul) respiration which produces a low Pa_{CO_2}, but blood pH is well below the normal range. Any interference with respiratory compensation by chest infection, pulmonary edema, heavy sedation, or coma leads to a rapid increase in the acidosis, and the plasma bicarbonate then ceases to be a reliable guide to the severity of the condition.

Rapid correction of extracellular acidosis by fast hemodialysis or infusion of sodium bicarbonate is followed by a respiratory alkalosis which persists for up to 24 hours. Bicarbonate diffuses slowly into the CSF, which therefore remains acid and continues to stimulate the respiratory centers on the anterior surface of the medulla, inappropriately lowering the Pa_{CO_2}.

In the genetic form of renal tubular acidosis urinary pH remains high (above 5.5, usually over 6.0) in the presence of an acidosis. A similar, but less severe, defect in urinary acidification is found in chronic pyelonephritis and particularly in analgesic nephropathy; in both conditions the urinary pH remains higher than in other renal diseases at the same level of GFR. In these three diseases the fall in plasma bicarbonate is often accompanied by a rise in plasma chloride which may exceed 110 mEq. per liter. Presumably when there is a reduced bicarbonate concentration in glomerular filtrate some other anion must be reabsorbed with sodium; in early renal failure the readily available anion is chloride. Hyperchloremic acidosis therefore indicates impairment of hydrogen ion excretion greater than would be expected from loss of nephrons alone. It is also found in some patients with distal tubular lesions owing to polycystic disease, amyloidosis, systemic lupus, and ischemic damage or rejection in renal homografts. It is found after urinary diversion into the bowel, partly from the associated pyelonephritis, and partly from the action of bowel mucosa on retained urine. When acidosis develops later in renal failure, plasma chloride is usually normal or depressed, the anion concentration in plasma being made up by retained sulfate and phosphate.

Calcium and Phosphate. Renal calcium excretion falls early in renal failure before there is any change in the serum calcium level. This has been attributed to the rise in plasma parathyroid hormone level which begins early in the course of renal failure, as parathormone depresses calcium excretion. However, recent work suggests that it is simply a reflection of the decline in GFR and that the fraction of filtered calcium appearing in the urine actually rises in renal failure. As urinary calcium falls, there is a parallel decrease in intestinal absorption and rise in fecal calcium. In late renal failure urinary calcium falls below 100 mg. per day, but this is more than offset by the increased fecal excretion, and negative calcium balance is usual. Positive balance can be restored by the administration of vitamin D in large doses (1 to 7.5 mg. per 24 hours). Negative calcium

balance often persists during regular hemodialysis in spite of the absence of significant urinary loss; it is corrected by successful transplantation if steroid therapy is not excessive.

Serum calcium declines in late renal failure, often reaching 6 mg. and occasionally 4 mg. per 100 ml. The proportion of total serum calcium which is ionized and complexed is increased so that ultrafilterable calcium remains close to normal until serum calcium is depressed below about 8 mg. per 100 ml. Even in the presence of very low serum calcium, which must be accompanied by a fall in ionized calcium, tetany is unusual in renal failure. It may be precipitated by the infusion or ingestion of sodium bicarbonate or lactate to correct acidosis, and may then be accompanied by grand mal seizures. However, the common forms of muscle cramp, muscle twitching, and convulsion seen in terminal uremia are probably not related to the serum calcium, and are seldom alleviated by calcium infusion.

Hypercalciuria accompanying the hypercalcemia of parathyroid adenoma, sarcoidosis, and hypervitaminosis D disappears when renal failure develops, but the hypercalciuria of renal tubular acidosis, medullary cystic disease, and other tubular disorders may persist in the presence of renal failure. A high urinary calcium is also found in a minority of patients with medullary damage, usually in association with a sodium leak.

Plasma phosphate remains in the normal range until the GFR has fallen to about 30 ml. per minute. This is the result of a normal urinary phosphate excretion in the face of a falling GFR, probably owing to the elevated plasma parathormone level, which in late renal failure reaches about ten times the normal level. The rise in plasma phosphate which occurs in late renal failure bears no constant relationship to the simultaneous changes in serum calcium. Patients on regular hemodialysis maintain nearly stable serum calcium in the face of wide fluctuations in plasma phosphate, and those receiving vitamin D may experience a simultaneous rise in plasma phosphate and serum calcium.

Bone disease can be detected histologically in the majority of patients dying of chronic renal failure, although it is a major cause of symptoms in less than 5 per cent of those treated conservatively if one omits the small minority with renal calcium or phosphate leaks. Rickets or osteomalacia sufficiently severe to cause bone pain, bending, and pseudofractures is usually found in patients with chronic pyelonephritis, obstructive uropathy, analgesic nephropathy, and polycystic disease. These are characterized by severe acidosis and by slowly progressive, and therefore prolonged, renal failure. Opinion is sharply divided on which of these characteristics is important for the genesis of osteomalacia. Even in those patients without clinical or radiologic bone disease, autopsy usually reveals some increase in the proportion of uncalcified osteoid.

Secondary hyperparathyroidism, shown by

proliferation of both osteoclasts and osteoblasts, scalloping, and bone marrow fibrosis, is almost invariably found at autopsy, and its severity correlates well with the size and activity of the parathyroids and with the level of plasma parathormone. Severe changes are associated with the radiologic signs of hyperparathyroidism, of which subperiosteal erosions on the phalanges and arterial calcification are the most constant, but bone symptoms are unusual.

Quantitative histology shows an increased total mass of bone, and even the area of calcified bone is normal or increased—an observation difficult to reconcile with the negative calcium balance of chronic renal failure. Bone mineral is redistributed in the skeleton with local patches of osteosclerosis, particularly at the upper and lower margins of the vertebra, giving rise to the radiologic appearance of "rugger jersey spine." Striking generalized osteosclerosis is occasionally seen after prolonged vitamin D therapy.

During regular hemodialysis, hyperparathyroidism slowly diminishes and its radiologic stigmata disappear; osteomalacia does not always heal. The total mass of bone diminishes, and a severe progressive osteoporosis with bone pain and pathologic fractures develops after two or three years of dialysis in some parts of the world; its peculiar geographical distribution is unexplained.

There is no constant pattern of blood biochemistry associated with these varieties of renal bone disease. Serum calcium and plasma phosphorous are on average lower in those patients with rickets and osteomalacia than in those with severe hyperparathyroidism, but there is a wide scatter in both groups and considerable overlap. Serum alkaline phosphatase is usually elevated in both conditions, but is often normal in the osteoporosis of dialyzed patients.

Following successful transplantation, parathyroid overactivity may persist for months despite the return of normal renal function. This has been quoted as evidence for the autonomy of the parathyroid glands in renal failure. An alternative explanation is that very large parathyroids have a high obligatory output of hormone which declines only when the glands return to normal size over many months; surgeons who have left the parathyroids in situ after transplantation have usually found that the hypercalcemia disappeared spontaneously within about a year.

Patients with secondary hyperparathyroidism often suffer from generalized *pruritus*, which has been attributed to calcium phosphate deposition in the skin in the presence of a high serum calcium x phosphate product. Aluminium hydroxide has been administered by mouth to prevent phosphate absorption, lower plasma phosphate, and reduce the calcium × phosphate product; metastatic calcification in subcutaneous tissue, cornea, and conjunctiva is partially reversed, but itching is seldom relieved. Dramatic relief has followed parathyroidectomy within a few hours, suggesting some more direct connection between high circulating parathormone level and skin irritation.

Plasma vitamin D–like activity is low in renal failure, but its restoration to normal with conventional dietary supplements does not heal osteomalacia or restore positive calcium balance. Uremic serum inhibits the calcification of cartilage in vitro, suggesting that it contains some antagonist to the action of vitamin D. Recently vitamin D has been shown to be rapidly degraded to inactive metabolites in renal failure, but whether this increased breakdown is sufficient to account for the enormous doses of the vitamin that are sometimes required to heal renal bone disease is uncertain.

Trace Elements. Regular hemodialysis has permitted study of the role of trace elements in the manifestations of renal failure. Many trace elements are present in tap water, and they may accumulate in anuric patients exposed to large volumes of dialysis fluid made from raw water. Fatal copper poisoning has resulted from solution of copper pipes by acid dialysis fluid, and zinc uptake has resulted from the use of zinc oxide plaster on coils. However, no important accumulation of the elements so far investigated—including copper, zinc, manganese, arsenic, and selenium—has been demonstrated in undialyzed patients. During renal failure plasma fluoride may rise to two or three times the range for normal subjects in areas where tap water is fluoridated, and it rises to about 100 times the control value after some years of regular dialysis in these areas. An association with renal bone disease in dialyzed patients has been suggested, but the evidence is not conclusive.

Sulfate. Sulfate is produced from the metabolism of sulfur-containing amino acids and is therefore in approximate proportion to protein ingestion. The plasma sulfate level rises as GFR declines, roughly parallel with plasma urea. Sulfate retention is not the direct cause of any known symptom of renal failure, but the excessive secretion of sulfate into the gut may be one factor that limits calcium absorption.

Urea and Ammonia. Urea diffuses into all body secretions. If the plasma level is very high, it occasionally crystallizes out of sweat, leaving "urea frost" on the skin. The breakdown of urea to ammonia in a dry and crusted mouth is probably the cause of the unpleasant taste and "uremic odor" of terminal renal failure.

In normal subjects about 20 per cent of the daily production of urea is secreted into the gut and broken down by bacteria to ammonia and carbon dioxide. The ammonia is reabsorbed and resynthesized into urea in the liver. In chronic renal failure the proportion of urea production removed extrarenally may rise as high as 80 per cent; most of this is probably broken down and resynthesized to urea, as in the normal person. However, ammonia can be used as a substrate for the synthesis of amino acids, and a patient in renal failure who has an adequate supply of essential amino acids, but an over-all protein deficiency, will utilize a considerable proportion of the ammonia released in his gut for protein synthesis; this observation is the basis of the Giordano-Giovannetti dietary regimen. Even in terminal renal failure the large supply of ammonia from the gut does not elevate the blood ammonia level of peripheral blood, which is usually subnormal. However, simultaneous hepatic and renal failure cause a rapid rise in blood ammonia and the early onset of coma.

"Sterilization" of the bowel with antimicrobial drugs does not prevent the utilization of urea for protein synthesis, suggesting that the urea production cycle can be made to "back pedal" under appropriate circumstances, but the proposition is difficult to prove, as some bowel bacteria survive any antimicrobial onslaught.

Urea was long regarded as nontoxic, but the Giovannetti diet, which reduces plasma urea without much change in other plasma constituents, relieves nausea, vomiting, and diarrhea, and raises the hemoglobin level. Ammonia released by bacteria from urea in the gastrointestinal tract has been blamed for vomiting, hematemesis, and uremic ulceration of the gut, but there are alternative explanations for these symptoms and signs.

Uric Acid. A rise in plasma urate level begins very early in chronic renal disease, but it is so slight that the level only becomes consistently abnormal when the GFR falls to about 15 ml. per minute. This stability of the plasma urate in the face of a normal production rate and a declining GFR is the result of increased distal tubular secretion of urate and increased uricolysis in the gut. In late renal failure there is a further increase in fractional urate clearance so that plasma urate rises less steeply than plasma urea or creatinine. Levels at least as high as those in gout are often encountered in terminal renal failure, but secondary gout is rare except in lead nephropathy and analgesic nephropathy, or during regular dialysis. Urate crystals are often found in the kidneys of patients with secondary hyperuricemia, and may accelerate the decline in renal function.

Plasma urate correlates much better than plasma urea with the onset of uremic pericarditis, but urate crystals are not found in the inflamed pericardium, and pericarditis is a rare complication of primary gout.

Carbohydrate. More than 50 per cent of patients in late renal failure have glucose intolerance as severe as in mild diabetes but with a normal fasting blood dextrose and often without glycosuria. It is not a cause of symptoms unless a large dose of glucose is administered during intravenous therapy, peritoneal dialysis, or hemodialysis, when severe hyperglycemia can be provoked. Fructose, galactose, and sorbitol tolerance are normal, showing that there is no defect in hepatic glycogenesis. Plasma insulin levels are appropriate to blood sugars, or nearly so, and there is

a reduced response to injected insulin, implying peripheral antagonism to insulin action. Plasma growth hormone levels are usually normal, and potassium deficiency is only occasionally implicated. Glucose tolerance returns to normal after one or two weeks of adequate dialysis, suggesting the presence of a dialyzable insulin antagonist.

Lipids. Total plasma lipids are raised in late renal failure, mainly owing to a rise in triglycerides; phospholipids and cholesterol are normal or slightly elevated. There is a consistent rise in pre-β lipoproteins. More striking elevation in plasma lipids is found in those who remain nephrotic in renal failure. Hyperlipidemia may act synergistically with hypertension to produce a high incidence of atheroma in older patients with renal failure.

Other Compounds Implicated in Uremia. "Uremia" comprises those symptoms and signs of renal failure which are not explained by water and electrolyte imbalance or hypertension. Most of these features correlate only approximately with the plasma levels of urea, creatinine, uric acid, and other substances that have been thoroughly investigated. Current contenders for the role of "uremic toxins" include guanidines, amines, and phenolic acids. They are difficult to measure accurately, and it is uncertain whether they correlate with symptoms any more closely than urea, but some of them, e.g., methylamine and methylguanidine, produce convulsions, coma, vomiting, and other uremic symptoms in laboratory animals at concentrations found in uremic plasma.

Many of the symptoms of renal failure are mimicked by the side effects of drugs that accumulate when GFR is depressed. The claim that "the best thing you can do for a uremic is to stop all his drugs" has a germ of truth.

CLINICAL FEATURES OF RENAL FAILURE AND THEIR TREATMENT

PLAN OF MANAGEMENT IN IRREVERSIBLE RENAL FAILURE

Patients younger than about 55 without extensive vascular disease and with no systemic disease which threatens life, should receive conservative management on a moderately restricted (40-gram protein) diet until the first incapacitating symptoms of uremia begin to appear or until working time is lost—usually when the GFR is around 5 ml. per minute. Regular hemodialysis should then be instituted until a well-matched cadaver transplant is available. If this plan is followed, these patients sacrifice a few months of independence in increasing discomfort, but escape most of the clinical features listed below and should require therapy only for hypertension and, in some cases, bone disease. The following description applies mainly to those patients for whom definitive treatment is not available.

Skin. Pruritus is common and often distressing. It is particularly associated with secondary hyperparathyroidism, but occurs in the absence of radiologic bone disease; it is sometimes caused by sensitivity to *Candida albicans*. The skin is often dry, flaky, and affected by erythematous and maculopapular rashes which become excoriated with scratching. Pigmentation, which is common in slowly progressive renal failure, is due to melanin, not to urochromes. The sallow complexion of the uremic becomes a healthy tan when he is tranfused.

Itching occasionally responds to oral aluminium hydroxide gel. Phenothiazine antipruritics are not very effective, and their cumulation in renal failure causes mental blunting and parkinsonism; oculogyric crises are sometimes misinterpreted as uremic fits. Hydrocortisone cream is useful in areas of skin rash.

Gastrointestinal Tract. Dry mouth, metallic taste, and uremic odor can be helped a little by chewing gum. Anorexia is a common early symptom, progressing to nausea and vomiting. Vomiting is sometimes effortless and unexpected, but in the terminal stage continuous dry retching becomes a distressing feature. The disorder responds to the Giovannetti diet, providing that an anorexic patient can be persuaded to eat it. Preliminary treatment with peritoneal dialysis and intravenous feeding may be required until appetite returns. Antiemetics are of little value in restoring appetite, but they do have a role in controlling the retching of terminal uremics for whom no better treatment is available. Metoclopramide, 10 mg., or prochlorperazine, 25 mg., three times a day may be tried orally, but can be given intramuscularly in the same dosage if necessary. Thiethylperazine, 10 mg., can be given as a suppository. In the last resort, stupor caused by large doses of chlorpromazine is preferable to continuous retching.

Diarrhea is often described as a feature of chronic renal failure, but it is seldom encountered before the very last stages of the illness unless produced by antihypertensives, antimicrobial drugs, or the high vegetable content of some Giovannetti diets. Constipation is a much more common complaint.

There is probably an increased incidence of hematemesis and melena in uremic patients even before they are subjected to intermittent anticoagulation for hemodialysis. Autopsy used to reveal ulceration of nasopharynx, mouth, stomach, or bowel in about a quarter of all uremics, but these features are now uncommon.

Nutrition and Growth. Anorexia and vomiting cause inadequate caloric intake, leading to wasting of fat and muscle. Dry, straggly, and depigmented hair is common in malnourished uremics. Gain of weight and improvement in hair texture occur during adequate hemodialysis and, to a lesser extent, during successful Giovannetti dieting.

Children with a GFR below about 20 per cent of normal have impairment of growth and are often below the third percentile for height. Bone age is retarded, and a late growth spurt may occur during adequate dialysis or after transplantation. Loss of height is often accentuated by bone bending owing to renal rickets.

Endocrine Function. The onset of puberty is delayed by several years in children with renal insufficiency. In adults, libido and potency decline in the last few months of the illness in males. Libido is depressed, ovulation suppressed, and amenorrhea common in females. However, contraception is advisable, because pregnancy can occur late in renal failure, and is associated with decline in renal function, increased hypertension, slow fetal growth, and high fetal mortality. As a general guide, pregnancy is hazardous and unlikely to produce a live child if the plasma urea is consistently raised on a normal diet and hypertension is present in the first trimester. It is usually uneventful for mother and child if the renal disease is static or slowly progressive, and the plasma urea and the blood pressure are normal at the start of pregnancy. Immunologic tests for pregnancy often give false positives in the presence of proteinuria.

Hypertension. Hypertension develops at some stage in more than 80 per cent of patients with chronic renal failure. It is associated with sodium and water retention; plasma renin is usually normal except in malignant hypertension. The complications are similar to those of any type of hypertension, but a malignant phase and resistance to drug therapy are more common in renal failure. After the primary disease, hypertension is the most important determinant of survival; it leads to a vicious spiral of declining renal function, further sodium retention, and rising blood pressure. The aim of treatment should be the restoration of normal blood pressure in all postures. This demands persistence and close supervision—weekly outpatient visits for many months in resistant cases.

Methyldopa is a common first choice, in a starting dose of 250 mg. twice daily increased every few days. Side effects appear at a lower dose in renal failure than in essential hypertension as it is partly dependent on renal excretion, and depression and drowsiness are common if the dose exceeds 2 grams per day. Many patients are uncontrolled by this dose and require one of the sympathetic blockers—bethanidine, debrisoquine, or guanethidine—all in an initial dose of 10 mg. daily and with increments every few days. These drugs all produce incapacitating postural and exercise hypotension if supine blood pressure is restored to normal. It is a salutary experience to check blood pressure of the patient supine, standing, and after exercise at each examination.

Propranolol reduces blood pressure without postural change and may become a first line drug with longer experience. The initial dose is 10 mg. three times a day, and it can be increased to 320 mg. per day or more. Heart failure or bronchial asthma is occasionally precipitated; bradycardia below 50 per minute calls for a reduction in dose.

Thiazide diuretics lose their diuretic—and probably their antihypertensive—action below a GFR of about 15 ml. per minute. Fursemide and ethacrynic acid in high doses still produce a diuresis down to a GFR of about 3 ml. per minute; ethacrynic acid occasionally causes deafness in renal failure. Fursemide is given in an initial dose of 40 to 80 mg. daily and is increased until adequate diuresis is obtained. In terminal renal failure a daily dose of 1 to 2 gm. may be required. No antihypertensive effect is exerted without a diuresis. Hypokalemia can occur even in renal failure, and potassium supplements may be required; regular estimation of plasma potassium is essential.

Edema. Edema may be due to hypertensive heart failure, impaired sodium and water excretion, or nephrotic syndrome. The last should be recognized by the heavy proteinuria, the electrophoretic pattern, and the hyperlipidemia, as it may call for high protein feeding except in late renal failure. Heart failure and salt and water retention are difficult to distinguish, but the treatment is the same—sodium and water restriction plus diuretics if necessary. Cardiac glycosides confer little benefit if rhythm is normal, and are dangerous when plasma potassium is varying, particularly during dialysis which removes potassium faster than the glycosides. If they are employed, the dose should be reduced by about a third to compensate for the loss of renal excretion, but they are best avoided except in atrial fibrillation.

Pulmonary edema is a common complication of renal failure with hypertension; it is characterized by attacks of nocturnal dyspnea, basal crepitations, and "bat's wing" perihilar shadows on chest roentgenograms. After repeated attacks the lung becomes infiltrated with macrophages and the fibrous septa thickened, a condition sometimes called *"uremic lung"* in this situation, but it is essentially the same as the *"hexamethonium lung"* of inadequately treated essential hypertension. Vital capacity, forced expiratory volume, and diffusing capacity are all reduced, particularly the last. Acute pulmonary edema responds rapidly to fluid removal by diuretics, peritoneal dialysis, or hemodialysis. The oral administration of 150 ml. of 70 per cent sorbitol to produce an osmotic diarrhea is equally effective but undignified.

Pericarditis. Pericarditis was once the harbinger of death. It occurred in about half the patients dying of chronic renal failure, and they seldom survived its onset by more than two months. It is now a sign that dialysis has been delayed or ineffective and calls for urgent treatment.

The onset is usually signaled by pain, which is often felt on the left side of the chest on inspiration for the first few hours, but may be central from the start. Pain is frequently severe, mimicking myocardial infarction, but it may appear after the friction rub and disappear long before it. The friction rub is usually loud, generalized, and palpable, and it may persist when the pericardial cavity contains half a liter of fluid and fatal tamponade is imminent. Tamponade was rare until the 1960's, but is now a major cause of death in the early weeks of regular hemodialysis. The important signs are falling blood pressure and pulse pressure, paradoxic fall in blood pressure with inspiration, cold, poorly perfused extremities, and raised jugular venous pressure. Paradoxic movement of the neck veins is a late and inconstant sign. On chest roentgenogram the typical globular shape of the heart may be seen in first attacks, but recurrent pericarditis produces a dense fibrous parietal pericardium which alters little in shape when fluid accumulates. The effusion can be confirmed by superimposing a radioalbumin scan on the chest film or passing a cardiac catheter into the right atrium to demonstrate that the edge of the cardiac shadow is beyond the atrial wall. The fluid should be removed by paracentesis, repeatedly if necessary, and intensive dialysis should be instituted. Hemorrhagic effusion is the rule in uremia and it occurs before heparinization for dialysis. The hematocrit of the aspirated effusion is usually about half that of circulating blood.

In the acute stage there is a fibrinous exudate over the visceral pericardium. After several attacks, sometimes after a single attack, an adherent pericardium thickens and within a few months to a few years produces constrictive pericarditis, usually without calcification, which must be treated surgically. The whole affected pericardium should be stripped off the heart.

Other Cardiovascular Effects. Deposits of calcium phosphate are found in the heart in severe hyperparathyroidism, and calcium oxalate and urates are deposited after some months of inadequate regular hemodialysis. Sudden cardiac arrest or arrhythmias result from deposition in the conducting tissue.

A uremic myocarditis, not due to crystal formation, hypertension, or atheroma, and causing a clinical picture similar to constrictive pericarditis, has been described by several authors, but its existence is not universally accepted.

Anemia. Anemia is so nearly universal in chronic renal failure that a uremic patient with a normal hemoglobin must be presumed to have acute renal failure until proved otherwise. Red cells are normochromic or have a slightly reduced MCHC, about 30 to 31. The major cause is a reduction in plasma erythropoietin level which results in relative hypoplasia of the marrow. The red cell precursors in the marrow are normal or slightly increased, the reticulocyte count, when corrected for red cell count, is one to four times normal, and radioiron transit time through the marrow is normal or reduced; but in each case the level of activity is well below that which occurs in anemia of the same degree from other causes.

Uncommon exceptions to this rule are a few patients with urinary obstruction, renal artery stenosis, and polycystic disease who overproduce erythropoietin and maintain a normal or even increased hemoglobin in early renal failure. Polycystics as a group have significantly higher hemoglobins than other patients with renal failure throughout the course of the illness and into their experience of regular hemodialysis.

Mild degrees of folate deficiency can be demonstrated by leukocyte lobe counts and marrow morphology in a minority of patients in late renal failure, but response to folic acid is slight. Deficiency of folic acid and pyridoxine, which are dialyzable, and deficiency of iron become important after the start of regular hemodialysis.

Uremia may be responsible for some of the marrow hypoplasia. Improvement in erthropoiesis occurs during regular hemodialysis, but may be partly explained by the appearance of erythropoietin of nonrenal origin. Bilateral nephrectomy causes a temporary fall in hemoglobin, but a stable hematocrit can eventually be maintained.

A more important effect of uremia is the occurrence of mild hemolysis. Red cell life is shortened to about half normal when the blood urea exceeds 200 mg. per 100 ml. Burr cells, helmet cells, and other misshapen red cells appear in the blood film as uremia increases. An improvement in red cell survival and hemoglobin level occurs when plasma urea is lowered by the Giovannetti diet. Much more striking hemolysis and deformation of red cells occur in malignant hypertension and in association with several diseases that cause renal failure, such as thrombotic thrombocytopenic purpura.

Anemia becomes a major cause of symptoms in uremia only when the hemoglobin falls below about 7 grams per 100 ml. It is then responsible for dyspnea, may precipitate angina and claudication, and produces ejection systolic murmurs, raised cardiac output, and elevated venous pressure.

Two groups of drugs are said to raise the hemoglobin level in chronic renal failure by a modest 1 to 3 grams per 100 ml., but in neither case has the claim been established by controlled trial. Salts of cobalt probably act by inducing tissue anoxia, and have therefore been condemned as illogical and dangerous, though more on theoretic grounds than on published evidence of toxicity. Androgens and related anabolic steroids increase the hemoglobin level of normal women in small doses and normal men in larger doses. In very high dosage they sometimes initiate a remission from hypoplastic anemia. They act on the marrow directly, as well as through an increased output of renal erythropoietic factor. Success has been claimed in the anemia of renal failure in patients of both sexes, with and without kidneys and before and after regular hemodialysis, but their current widespread use is based on rather flimsy evidence of efficacy. Little harm can result from the use of testosterone proprionate, 150 mg. intramuscularly per week, in men, and it may incidentally help to restore flagging libido. In females nonicterogenic steroid of low androgenicity, such as nandrolone decanoate, 25 mg. intramuscularly per three weeks, seldom causes troublesome side effects, and its anabolic effect at least is well established. Patients should be warned to report

hair growth and skin thickening, which are reversible, because the voice change which follows them may be permanent.

Transfusion was the mainstay of treatment until recently. Packed red cells are given in small volume (200 to 500 ml.) with particular caution if the patient is hypertensive. The fear that a rise in hematocrit might imperil renal function by reducing renal plasma flow has been dispelled in clinical trial; renal function declines only if heart failure is precipitated by overtransfusion. However, the benefit is short lived; donor cells have the same shortened life span as the patient's own red cells, and erythropoiesis is depressed by even a small transfusion. Transfusion once begun must therefore be continued on a regular basis every one to three weeks. Until 1967 blood was transfused at a rate of 2 to 4 pints per month after the start of regular hemodialysis, but the practice fell into disrepute as it caused the development of cytotoxic leukocyte antibodies which endanger subsequent renal transplant, and it may have contributed to the numerous outbreaks of hepatitis on renal units. A hemoglobin level compatible with reasonable activity can be maintained without transfusion during regular hemodialysis if blood losses are kept to a minimum; after successful transplantation the hemoglobin rises to, or even above, normal. Symptomatic anemia in a patient destined for regular dialysis or transplantation is therefore an indication for expediting definitive treatment. Patients who are precluded from these forms of treatment may require regular transfusion, but they should be segregated as far as possible and their sera checked regularly for hepatitis-associated antigen.

Bleeding Tendency. A hemorrhagic tendency is common in late renal failure. Epistaxis, menorrhagia, gastrointestinal hemorrhage, and excessive bleeding or bruising after trauma are common manifestations; purpura is unusual. Whole blood clotting time and prothrombin time are usually normal, although deficiencies of factors V and VII are occasionally described. The total platelet count is normal or slightly reduced, and the life span of platelets is normal; but defects of platelet function can usually be detected and are thought to be the major cause of uremic bleeding. The proportion of sticky platelets is reduced, platelet aggregation with ADP impaired, the prothrombin consumption test abnormal, and platelet factor III availability decreased. The bleeding time is often prolonged but a modification of the Ivy test, using multiple punctures and measurement of blood loss, may be required to demonstrate it. The platelet defect is roughly proportional to plasma urea, is corrected when plasma urea is reduced by dialysis or low protein diet, and can be reproduced in normal persons by feeding urea, but it is not produced by addition of urea to blood in vitro.

Plasma fibrinogen level is usually raised in renal failure, the mean elevation being about 30 per cent. Plasma fibrinolytic activity is depressed, as indicated by a prolonged euglobulin lysis time, but fibrin degradation products can often be demonstrated in plasma, suggesting excessive intravascular deposition and removal of fibrin. As the kidney is a major source of plasminogen activator, it is tempting to attribute the reduced blood fibrinolytic activity in renal failure to the loss of renal mass, but this is probably not the true explanation, because regular hemodialysis restores the fibrinolytic activity to normal, even after bilateral nephrectomy. Plasma fibrinogen also returns to normal during regular dialysis.

Troublesome bleeding in uremia is best controlled by peritoneal dialysis or hemodialysis with reduced, or regional, heparinization. Infusion of inhibitors of fibrinolysis, such as aminocaproic acid (EACA) in an initial dose of 100 mg. per kilogram of body weight over four hours, is helpful if local measures and dialysis fail to control bleeding externally or into the gut. It should be used only in dire emergency for bleeding into the urinary tract or internal cavities because of the risk of producing indissoluble clot.

Infection. Susceptibility to bacterial infection is characteristic of uremia; it is the main cause of death in acute renal failure and a major source of morbidity in chronic renal failure. The neutrophil count is normal and rises normally in response to infection, but the ability of the cells to ingest and kill bacteria is impaired. Total serum immunoglobulins are normal, unless reduced by the primary disease or by heavy proteinuria, and the anamnestic response to antigens such as tetanus toxoid is normal, but the appearance of antibodies to new antigens is delayed and their titer low, at least in laboratory animals. The Mantoux and similar tests show impairment of delayed hypersensitivity which is not corrected by regular hemodialysis. The circulating lymphocyte count is reduced. The prolonged tolerance of homografts in uremia is further evidence of altered cellular immunity.

Two common and important problems in renal failure are colonization of the nose and other carrier sites by staphylococci, leading to recurrent infection of the operation wounds and arteriovenous shunts, and infection with *Candida albicans.* Both are encouraged by repeated exposure to antimicrobials and the hospital environment, and may reflect this rather than a specific vulnerability of the uremic patient. On the tongue and buccal mucosa, Candida forms painful white plaques which may make eating almost impossible and which are the usual cause of "uremic ulceration of the mouth." It spreads to the esophagus, causing dysphagia and a moth-eaten appearance on barium swallow. In the gut it causes diarrhea, and may produce generalized allergic rashes as well as pruritus ani. In the vagina it causes discharge and pruritus vulvae.

Strenuous efforts should be made to identify the causative organisms before starting antimicrobial therapy and to follow the change in the bacterial flora during treatment. In seriously ill patients it is worthwhile swabbing the usual carrier sites and wounds and culturing sputum, blood, urine, and stool every few days in an effort to keep one jump ahead of the bacteria. Pathogens found in the nose on Monday are likely culprits in a pneumonia or wound infection developing on Friday; their antimicrobial sensitivities can guide therapy during the first 48 hours while the new invaders are being identified.

If the causative organism can be identified, narrow-spectrum antimicrobials should be employed when there is a choice. If broad-spectrum therapy is needed, and in all seriously ill uremics receiving antimicrobials, antifungal agents, e.g., nystatin suspension 500 mg. four times a day should be given orally to prevent Candida superinfection, and particular care should be taken with mouth toilet. Established Candida infection of mouth and esophagus should be treated with amphotericin lozenges (10 mg.) sucked continuously, at a rate of 10 to 20 per day. If response is slow, the lesions should be painted with gentian violet solution, 1 per cent three times a day.

The loading dose of antimicrobials is unchanged in renal failure, but the size or spacing of maintenance doses must be adjusted to renal function (Table 3). When the drug is wholly dependent on excretion by glomerular filtration, the blood level produced by a standard regimen will vary up and down with the alterations in GFR that commonly occur in the course of infections in renal failure. If the drug has a low margin of safety, e.g., all ototoxic antimicrobials, the dose should be adjusted daily on the basis of blood antimicrobial measurements; these can now be performed in most hospital laboratories, and the results are

TABLE 3. MAINTENANCE DOSE OF ANTIMICROBIALS IN RENAL FAILURE

Group 1. Major extrarenal pathways of elimination. Normal dose schedule can be used.

Methicillin	Novobiocin
Cloxacillin	Fusidic acid
Ampicillin	Chloramphenicol
Erythromycin	Sulfadimidine

Group 2. Minor adjustment in dosage is needed. Doses should be spaced more widely than normal, but not more than 24 hours apart. Exact timing is not critical as there is some extrarenal excretion and/or the drugs are not toxic at moderately elevated blood levels.

Penicillin G	Carbenicillin
Cephalothin	Trimethoprim-sulfamethoxazole
Cephaloridine	Nalidixic acid
Lincomycin	Isoniazid
Clindamycin	

Group 3. Major adjustment is required—doses 24 hours or more apart in severe renal failure.

Tetracycline	Gentamicin*	Cycloserine
Oxytetracycline	Vancomycin*	Para-amino-
Methacycline	Polymyxin B*	salicylate
Streptomycin*	Colistin*	
Kanamycin*	Amphotericin B*	

Group 4. Avoid altogether.

Chlortetracycline
Nitrofurantoin

*Daily estimation of blood level is highly desirable to avoid risk of ototoxicity or nephrotoxicity.

available within 24 hours, provided that only one or two drugs are used at a time.

Peripheral Neuropathy. Nerve conduction slows with uremia, falling to about half normal in the legs in terminal renal failure; the arms are less affected. The abnormality is gradually reduced during regular hemodialysis and corrected by successful transplant. Hypesthesia of the feet and diminished ankle jerks can often be detected in the most severely affected patients, but they seldom cause spontaneous complaint, and severe neuropathy was rare until the advent of regular hemodialysis. The first symptom is usually numbness of the toes and feet, sometimes accompanied by unpleasant tingling and burning. Ascending anesthesia, areflexia, and muscle weakness may progress rapidly over a few days or weeks to quadriplegia. The condition may deteriorate during the first few weeks of regular hemodialysis, even if it is adequate, but the most disabling permanent neuropathies have occurred during inadequate hemodialysis. Sural nerve biopsy shows axonal degeneration and segmental demyelination.

The incidence of fulminant uremic neuropathy varies between geographic centers. This is partly explained by local fashions in drug therapy; nitrofurantoin is an important cause of neuropathy in the uremic, and the onset of symptoms demands a careful review of drug therapy.

The only effective treatment is intensive hemodialysis — 30 to 40 hours per week on the Kiil dialyzer or its equivalent. Multivitamin supplements, including thiamin, pyridoxine, and hydroxycobalamin, are usually given to protect against any deficiency caused by anorexia, diet, or dialysis, but they have no therapeutic effect. All but the most advanced cases of neuropathy remit completely within a few months of successful transplant.

The tingling and numbness of neuropathy must be distinguished from the similar symptoms produced by hypocalcemia, which are usually precipitated by feeding sodium bicarbonate, and from Raynaud's phenomenon. The latter is common in renal failure, particularly in patients whose hypertension has been controlled by sodium and water removal.

Myopathy. A proximal myopathy accompanies renal osteomalacia and may be severe enough to produce a waddling gait and prevent stair-climbing. Wasting is slight and tendon reflexes paradoxically brisk. This rare syndrome becomes more common after the start of regular hemodialysis in those centers where bone disease is a major problem.

Cramps. Muscle cramps in the calves, thighs, and flexors of the toes are common in early renal failure, particularly at night. They may also occur in the upper limbs and during the day when they are precipitated by stretching, awkward posture, or repetitive exercise such as knitting. They accompany sodium depletion or dehydration through the artificial kidney, and are then relieved by infusion of saline, but they also occur commonly in the absence of any specific electrolyte abnormality. Nocturnal cramps are alleviated by a nightly dose of quinine sulfate, 300 mg. orally.

Other Nervous and Muscular Symptoms. Muscle twitching affects single muscles or groups in late renal failure. It wakes the patient as he dozes off, and, when severe, interferes with activities such as writing or holding a cup. Flapping tremor, which is demonstrated by dorsiflexing the wrist of an outstretched arm, is due to a similar sudden involuntary relaxation of muscle groups. A common complaint, probably of central origin, is restlessness of the limbs, particularly the legs. The limbs or the whole body must be moved to relieve an uncomfortable feeling which the patient finds it hard to describe. The symptom is at its worst during the first hour after lying down to sleep. It may be accompanied by a feeling as of insects crawling under the skin — a sensation so unpleasant that it may be described as a pain. This dysesthesia and restless limbs may be precursors of a state of extreme hyperexcitability and muscular overactivity, seen at its worst in patients undertreated by peritoneal or hemodialysis, which is rapidly fatal unless treated by intensive dialysis. As a symptomatic measure, diazepam, 5 to 10 mg. intravenously, is effective and may be repeated every four hours.

Persistent hiccup is common in terminal renal failure, and it occasionally affects a patient at an earlier stage, exhausting him over the course of a few days. There is no really effective treatment short of very heavy sedation, but chlorpromazine, 25 mg. orally three times a day, will sometimes abort an attack.

Insomnia is common and, although sometimes due to restless limbs or pruritus, it often persists beyond the first hour in bed when these are at their worst. It is accompanied by lethargy during the day and may represent reversal of normal sleep rhythm. Recourse to nocturnal sedatives is often necessary; barbiturates, nitrazepam, and methaqualone are currently most popular and about equally effective. They are given in full dosage, and all but the longest-acting barbiturates are well tolerated without troublesome hangover in spite of the fact that they all depend partly on renal excretion.

Tiredness is almost universal in uremia, although the level at which it occurs is variable; some patients are active in business with a blood urea over 200 or even 300 mg. per 100 ml. Its causes include sleep disturbance, anemia, hypertensive heart failure, muscle weakness, and drug side effects, but there is probably a specific effect of uremia that is noticeably relieved by the first one or two hemodialyses.

Increased mental fatigability may begin early in renal failure and is succeeded by loss of concentration, reduced performance at mental arithmetic and other demanding skills, impaired memory, and in terminal renal failure by drowsiness, disorientation, stupor, and coma. Episodes of toxic psychosis with confusion, hallucinations, delusions, and intervals of insight are particularly associated with infections and pericarditis in late renal failure. Major electroencephalographic changes accompany these severe mental symptoms; spike potentials occur sporadically in bursts, and slow waves come to dominate the recording, the mean frequency falling as low as 2 or 3 per second. Toxic *psychosis* and *confusion* respond to intensive peritoneal or hemodialysis, but some caution must be exercised during initial treatment. A "disequilibrium syndrome" of headache, vomiting, confusion, coma, and convulsions with further deterioration of the EEG occurs when patients with severe uremia are treated by rapid dialysis. It was a common and sometimes fatal problem in the days when hemodialysis was instituted at a blood urea of 400 mg. per 100 ml. with large membrane area machines. It has almost disappeared from those centers at which dialysis is performed early and at a reasonable pace, and is there encountered almost exclusively in the treatment of already confused patients with chronic renal failure. It is attributed to cerebral edema caused by the removal of osmotically active substances—urea and in some cases sodium and chloride—from the extracellular compartment. It can be prevented by using a slow method of dialysis, e.g., peritoneal dialysis, for the first 24 to 48 hours and by inducing a compensatory hyperglycemia. This is achieved by using dialysis fluid with an increased dextrose content and monitoring blood sugar every few hours. The main dangers of the syndrome are convulsions and inhalation of vomitus; anticonvulsants should be given prophylactically and the stomach kept empty with the aid of a gastric tube.

Convulsions. Convulsions can be precipitated in terminal renal failure by a variety of alterations in plasma composition, of which water intoxication is the most common. Intravenous therapy should be planned to correct abnormalities slowly. However, the most important precipitant is severe hypertension, which is responsible for about two thirds of all uremic fits and for nearly all such episodes in early renal failure. Acute hypotension initiates some fits, particularly in the course of hemodialysis. In terminal renal failure convulsions may occur without any obvious precipitant. They are usually of grand mal type, occasionally jacksonian. They often recur in rapid succession, and carry a formidable mortality from asystole or ventricular fibrillation. They are a dire medical emergency and must be controlled rapidly, by anesthetizing the patient and maintaining him on a respirator if necessary. Usually they can be managed less drastically with intravenous diazepam, 10 mg., or sodium amylobarbitone, 125 to 250 mg., repeated every hour or two initially. If fits recur, sedation should be heavy enough to allow the insertion of an intratracheal tube, as it is vital to prevent anoxia; the stomach should be aspirated hourly. Intravenous sodium phenytoin, 200 mg., should be given at the start and may be repeated two or three times in the first 24 hours. Maintenance therapy with phenobarbitone, 60 to 120 mg. daily, and sodium phenytoin, 50 to 100 mg. three times a day, should be

continued until definitive treatment for uremia has begun. Phenobarbitone accumulates in renal failure, and its blood level should be checked if the patient develops depression, drowsiness, or mental blunting; phenytoin has other pathways of excretion. Severe hypertension should also be corrected as an emergency. A useful regimen is hydralazine, 20 to 40 mg. intramuscularly hourly until the blood pressure is controlled, if an initial test dose of 10 mg. is well tolerated. Methyldopate hydrochloride, 250 to 1000 mg. every 6 hours by infusion, acts more slowly, reducing blood pressure over 6 to 12 hours.

The brain of a patient dying in uremia shows areas of nerve cell depopulation in addition to the acute neuronal damage, scattered petechiae, and edema attributable to uremia or convulsions. Some permanent decline in cerebral function probably occurs if the patient survives, and one survey suggested an average drop of 10 to 15 per cent in IQ in a group treated by regular hemodialysis. However, the most striking examples of failing intelligence and impoverished personality are seen in hypertensive patients; these probably reflect vascular damage in the brain rather than the effects of uremia.

Ocular Manifestations. The most important changes in the eye are those of *hypertensive retinopathy*. In spite of many references to "albuminuric retinopathy" there are no features that distinguish these changes from those of hypertension in the patient with normal renal function. Visual acuity is usually impaired in the presence of papilledema, and scotomas corresponding to large hemorrhages may be noticed by the patient. Control of hypertension is followed in sequence by the clearing of hemorrhages, resolution of papilledema, and disappearance of exudates, the macular star often persisting for some months after blood pressure is normal. Vision usually returns to nearly normal, but some patients are left with optic atrophy and permanent loss of acuity.

Retinal detachment, usually of globular shape in the lower half of the eye, occurs in patients with severe hypertensive retinopathy, renal failure, and fluid overload; hypertension is probably the most important precipitant, but the condition often resolves spontaneously even if the blood pressure is poorly controlled. It is due to serous effusion below the retina. Resolution is usually complete if hypertension and fluid overload are treated rapidly by dialysis.

"Red eyes" in renal failure are caused by conjunctival vasodilatation with calcium deposition as plaques on the conjunctiva and as a thin line just inside the limbus ("band keratopathy"). It is caused by a high calcium × phosphate product, and is a hazard of vitamin D therapy for bone disease and the treatment of hyperkalemia with calcium phase resins. Calcium can be detected by slit-lamp examination before the onset of symptoms, and this is a useful screening test for metastatic calcification during these forms of treatment. If the condition is allowed to progress, smarting and watering of the eye develop. This can sometimes be reversed by oral aluminium hydroxide to control plasma phosphate, and it is corrected by parathyroidectomy or successful transplant.

Low Protein Diet. Protein restriction was introduced because animal experiments suggested that it could retard the progress of renal disease. The hope that this applied to man has long been abandoned, and diet is now used solely as a symptomatic measure. It is important that the treatment should be more tolerable than the disease and that it should improve the patient as well as his biochemical data. A common fault is the prescription of diet before it is really needed. The only symptoms consistently relieved are anorexia, nausea, and vomiting, though improvement in mental symptoms, muscle twitching, and pruritus are described often enough to suggest that they are genuine.

With 40 grams of predominantly first-class protein per day a diet can be constructed with a calorie content sufficient for light work which is reasonably attractive to patients with some culinary skill and an adventurous palate. Extra calories for heavy workers can be provided in electrolyte-free carbohydrate supplements such as Hycal or Caloreen which are less sweet than natural carbohydrates and can be disguised in other food.

The diet is much less attractive when simultaneous restriction of sodium, potassium, or water becomes necessary. It is expensive, involves a change from traditional food, and is unacceptable to other members of the family. It is rarely consumed conscientiously unless supported by detailed initial training and prolonged follow-up with dietary counseling by medical staff as well as dietitians. Poorly instructed patients, fobbed off with a diet sheet, merely consume a calorie-deficient, truncated version of their normal diet.

A 40-gram protein diet should be started when symptoms first develop on free diet—a variable point in the course of renal failure, but on average at a GFR of about 10 ml. per minute. When these symptoms recur on the 40-gram diet, it has been usual to reduce the protein intake further to 30 or 20 grams per day, but this results in negative nitrogen balance, and the patient wastes away. One reason is the near impossibility of providing adequate calories in 20-gram mixed protein, sodium-restricted diet, because most standard calorie sources such as cereals have a considerable content of second-class protein. However, a diet containing only 18 grams of protein will maintain nitrogen balance after an initial period of nitrogen loss, reduce plasma urea, and relieve many uremic symptoms, if at least two thirds of the protein is first class, providing a high proportion of essential amino acids. This is achieved in the *Giordano* or *Giovannetti diet* by using cereals, from which most of the protein has been removed as calorie sources, and egg with a little milk or meat to provide the protein. This high egg content makes the diet nauseating to some, and acidosis is increased by the metabolism of phospholipids in

yolk. Bread and spaghetti made from protein-free flour are stodgy and flavorless. Many modifications have been devised to suit local tastes. Egg white can be baked into the bread to improve its texture. Potatoes have a better amino acid mixture than cereals and can be used without protein extraction, but their potassium content must be reduced by preboiling. With ingenuity the diet can be made just tolerable to most patients with GFR down to 3 ml. per minute, but even its conscientious use adds only a few months to the average life span of the patient in renal failure. If facilities for dialysis and transplantation are available, this short respite does not justify the effort involved.

General Reviews

Hamburger, J., Richet, G., Crosnier, J., Funck-Brentano, J. L., Antoine, B., Ducrot, H., Mery, J. P., de Montera, H., and Royer, P. (translator, Walsh, A.): Nephrology. Philadelphia, W. B. Saunders Company 1968, Chapter 7.

Proceedings of the Fourth International Congress of Nephrology (1970). Copenhagen, Munksgaard (In press).

Rosenheim, M. L., and Rosi, E. J.: Chronic renal failure. *In* Black, D. A. K. (ed.): Renal Disease. Oxford, Blackwell, Scientific Publications, Ltd., 1967.

Seldin, D. W., Carter, N. W., and Rector, F. C., Jr.: Consequences of renal failure and their management. *In* Strauss, M. B., and Welt, L. G. (ed.) Diseases of the Kidney, London, J. & A. Churchill, Ltd., 1963, Chapter 5.

Pathophysiology and Clinical Features

Adamson, J. W., Eschbach, J., and Finch, C. A.: The kidney and erythropoiesis. Amer. J. Med., 44:725, 1968.

Berlyne, G. M., Mallick, M. P., and Gaan, D.: Dietary treatment of chronic renal failure. *In* Wrong, O. (ed.): Fourth Symposium on Advanced Medicine, London, Sir Isaac Pitman & Sons, Ltd., 1968.

Bricker, N. S.: On the meaning of the intact nephron hypothesis. Amer. J. Med., 46:1, 1969.

Coburn, J. W., Popovtzer, M. M., Massry, S. G., and Kleeman, C. R.: The physicochemical state and renal handling of divalent ions in chronic renal failure. Arch Intern. Med., 124:302, 1969.

Eknoyan, G., Wacksman, S. J., Glueck, H. I., and Will, J. J.: Platelet function in renal failure. New Eng. J. Med., 280: 677, 1969.

Epstein, F. H.: Calcium and the kidney. Amer. J. Med., 45:700, 1968.

McPhaul, J. J.: Hyperuricaemia and urate excretion in chronic renal disease. Metabolism, 17:430, 1968.

Stanbury, S. W.: Bone disease in uremia. Amer. J. Med., 44:714, 1968.

Steele, T. H., and Rieselbach, R. E.: The contribution of residual nephrons within the chronically diseased kidney to urate homeostasis in man. Amer. J. Med., 43:868, 1967.

Tyler, R. H.: Neurologic disorders in renal failure. Amer. J. Med., 44:734, 1968.

van Ypersele de Strihou, C., and Frans, A.: The pattern of respiratory compensation in chronic uraemic acidosis. Nephron, 7:37, 1970.

Wesson, L. G.: Physiology of the Human Kidney. New York, Grume and Stratton, Inc., 1969.

Wilkinson, R., Scott, D. F., Uldall, P. R., Kerr, D. N. S., and Swinney, J.: Plasma renin and exchangeable sodium in the hypertension of chronic renal failure: The effect of bilateral nephrectomy. Quart J. Med. 39:377, 1970.)

Treatment

Berlyne, G. M.: Nutrition in Renal Disease. Edinburgh, Livingstone, 1968.

Lewis, E. J., and MacGill, J. W. (eds.): Conference on the Nutritional Aspects of Uremia. Amer. J. Clin. Nutr., 21:346, 1968.

Schwartz, W. B., and Kassirer, J. P.: Medical management of chronic renal failure. Amer. J. Med., 44:786, 1968.

Acute Renal Failure

Neal S. Bricker

Definition. Acute renal failure is a clinical syndrome characterized by a sudden decrease in glomerular filtration rate, often to values of less than 1 to 2 ml. per minute. Acute renal failure is usually associated with oliguria (urine volumes of less than 400 ml. per day), and is always associated with biochemical consequences of the reduction in glomerular filtration rate such as a rise in blood urea nitrogen (BUN) and serum creatinine concentrations. The occurrence of other abnormalities in body fluids such as metabolic acidosis and hyperkalemia will depend upon the duration and severity of the renal failure, the nature and severity of any underlying injury or disease process, and the intensity of treatment.

Acute renal failure so defined encompasses many different forms of disease with widely varying pathogeneses, natural histories, and prognostic implications. For example, a sudden decrease in glomerular filtration rate may occur in association with profound reduction in effective extracellular fluid volume or fall in blood pressure, and may be readily reversible by volume expansion or blood pressure elevation. More commonly acute renal failure is due to intrinsic disease of the renal parenchyma; but some forms are ultimately (albeit not immediately) reversible, and others are not. Finally, this syndrome may occur in consequence of urinary tract obstruction or occlusion of the renal arteries or veins.

Because of the diversity of etiologic and pathogenic events which can culminate in acute renal failure, because recognition of the immediately reversible forms of the syndrome, can lead to prompt restitution of normal renal function while failure of recognition may lead to persistence of uremia and permanent nephron destruction, because the syndrome so frequently is superimposed upon major injuries or serious systemic disease, and because a substantial percentage of patients will survive their disease if therapy is dedicated and skillful, this group of abnormalities stands among the most challenging problems in clinical medicine.

The discussion in this article will deal principally with one form of acute renal failure, *acute tubular necrosis.* Other types of the syndrome will be considered, but primarily as they relate to the differential diagnosis of acute tubular necrosis.

Acute tubular necrosis is defined as a special form of acute renal failure caused by an intrinsic abnormality of the renal parenchyma that is potentially reversible after an interval ranging from several days to several weeks. It may follow exposure to a nephrotoxic drug, or a primary extrarenal injury or disease, or occasionally may appear without an obvious predisposing abnormality. Most characteristically there is a period of oliguria, followed by gradually increasing rates of urine flow, culminating in a period of polyuria. Recovery of renal function toward the pre-illness level then occurs in patients who survive.

Causes of Acute Renal Failure. Acute Tubular Necrosis. *Nephrotoxic Drugs or Chemicals.* Acute tubular necrosis may follow exposure to a host of different chemical agents, some when administered in therapeutic doses. Sulfonamides and many of the commonly used antimicrobial drugs, including kanamycin, colistin, cephaloridine, amphotericin, bacitracin, neomycin, vancomycin, gentamicin, and polymixin have been incriminated as the causal agents in the induction of acute tubular necrosis. This necrosis has occurred following exposure to organic iodonated x-ray contrast media. It may also follow either accidental or intentional exposure to a variety of nephrotoxic agents. Included among these are organic solvents (especially carbon tetrachloride and tetrachloroethylene); ethylene and diethylene glycol; inorganic mercurials and other heavy metals, including bismuth, uranium, lead and, rarely, organic mercurials; methyl alcohol; and massive doses of salicylates and paraldehyde. This subject is dealt with in greater detail in the article on Toxic Nephropathy.

Systemic Injury or Illness. Acute tubular necrosis may follow severe trauma such as crushing injuries or major operative procedures, especially when blood loss and/or hypotension occur. It may also follow severe febrile illnesses, gram-negative septicemia, major losses of extracellular fluid volume, or major translocations of this volume, into gut, soft tissues, and skin (in burns). Acute tubular necrosis may develop in the course of complicated pregnancies, particularly when hemorrhage or hypotension occurs. It may follow an incompatible blood transfusion and, occasionally, intravascular hemolysis resulting from other mechanisms. In most of the foregoing entities, one or more of the following events frequently occurs: (1) profound depletion of actual or effective extracellular fluid volume, (2) hypotension, (3) hemoglobinuria, or myoglobinuria.

Acute Tubular Necrosis Occurring de Novo. In some patients, the disease occurs without known exposure to any nephrotoxic agent and in the absence of a detectable fall in blood pressure, obvious change in circulatory dynamics, loss or translocation of extracellular fluid volume, intravascular hemolysis, or myoglobinuria. Indeed, it may in some instances occur without any apparent predisposing illness or injury and in an apparently healthy individual.

Other Parenchymal Diseases. *Bilateral Renal Cortical Necrosis.* Cortical necrosis may be diffuse or patchy. In the former instance, acute renal failure is severe, and may be characterized by total anuria. In patchy cortical necrosis, the occurrence and severity of the renal failure will depend upon the extent of cortical destruction. Return of enough renal function to support life is unusual in patients with diffuse bilateral cortical necrosis; it is not infrequent in patients with patchy cortical necrosis.

Glomerulitis. Severe acute renal failure may be seen occasionally in poststreptococcal acute glomerulonephritis, particularly in the adult. Acute renal failure may also be seen in the acute glomerulitides associated with systemic lupus erythematosus, hypersensitivity angiitis, rapidly progressive glomerulonephritis, Henoch-Schönlein purpura, Goodpasture's syndrome, and malignant nephrosclerosis. It may also be seen in accelerated scleroderma in which the predominant site of involvement is in the small arterioles of the kidney.

Papillary Necrosis. Renal papillary necrosis appears classically in patients with diabetes mellitus, in urinary tract obstruction (especially when accompanied by severe pyelonephritis), and in patients who have ingested excessive quantities of analgesic agents, including phenacetin. The severity of the renal failure, as well as the potential for ultimate recovery, will depend upon the number of renal papillae that escape destruction.

End-Stage Chronic Renal Disease. Acute renal failure may occur under two circumstances in patients with chronic progressive renal disease: (1) when the nephron population diminishes below a critical level and oliguria supervenes; and (2) when an acute complicating process (such as extracellular fluid volume depletion, acute glomerulitis, or urinary tract obstruction) results in a sudden but potentially reversible decrement in renal function from the previous steady-state level.

Miscellaneous Forms of Parenchymal Involvement. Severe *hypercalcemia* may be associated with the rapid onset of acute renal failure. In most instances the rising BUN is accompanied by polyuria rather than oliguria; but occasionally, particularly with extremely high levels of serum calcium, urine volumes may fall to the oliguric range. *Hyperuricemia* can lead to acute renal failure when the plasma levels increase very rapidly and to high levels. The renal failure presumably is due to intrarenal obstruction caused by deposition of uric acid precipitates in collecting ducts and the renal papillae. The renal failure may occur during the course of *multiple myeloma.* In some instances this is the result of severe (but reversible) hypercalcemia; the disease may also follow a period of fluid deprivation, usually for purposes of performing intravenous pyelography, in patients with Bence Jones proteinuria. The renal failure is presumed to be due to the inspissation of proteinaceous materials in the tubular lumina. Whether the x-ray contrast media per se play a role in this form of the disease is not clear. Another cause which is being seen with increasing fre-

quency is *homograft rejection* in transplanted kidneys. Treatment of the rejection often results in reversal of the acute renal failure.

Occlusion of the Renal Arteries or Veins. Acute interruption of the blood supply to the kidneys may occur following embolization, in situ thrombosis, or dissection of the aorta. For renal failure to occur, virtually the entire nephron population of both kidneys must be deprived of blood supply and, with the exception of aortic surgery, when "sludge" may flow into both renal arteries during or following release of aortic clamping, arterial occlusion is an unusual cause of the renal failure. Bilateral renal vein thrombosis also is an unusual cause of the disease, for the involvement must be bilateral (if there are two kidneys), and the luminal occlusion must be complete or virtually complete.

Hemodynamic Alterations (Prerenal Azotemia). Prerenal azotemia is a reversible abnormality characterized by a functional reduction in glomerular filtration rate per nephron. The latter may be secondary to a decrease in mean arterial blood pressure and/or to intrarenal vascular adjustments initiated by marked depletion of effective extracellular fluid volume. This loss may be extracorporeal, or it may represent a sequestration of fluid in areas of the body such as the intestinal (following major surgical procedures), skin bullae (in burns), etc. If prerenal azotemia is not recognized and treated, it may lead to the development of acute tubular necrosis.

Hepatorenal Syndrome. Acute renal failure may occur in the course of severe hepatic or biliary tract disease, or following biliary tract surgery. In some instances it is due to acute tubular necrosis; but it may also be due to the hepatorenal syndrome, an abnormality that typically is irreversible. The etiology and pathogenesis of the syndrome are unknown, and there are no characteristic pathologic changes in the kidneys. From a pathophysiologic point of view, the hepatorenal syndrome resembles prerenal azotemia rather than acute tubular necrosis (the differences will be discussed under Pathologic Physiology); thus the implication exists that the renal failure is of hemodynamic origin.

Urinary Tract Obstruction. For obstruction of the urinary tract to produce acute renal failure, the obstructing process must interfere with the flow of urine from the vast majority of nephrons. Thus if the obstructing lesion is above the uretero-vesical junction, it must be bilateral if both kidneys are functioning.

Pathogenesis of Acute Tubular Necrosis. Several theories have been proposed for the pathogenesis of acute tubular necrosis. Each has its proponents, and there are at least some supporting experimental data in animals. But for each, contradictory evidence has also accrued; and for none is there universal acceptance.

The most prominently considered theories are the following: (1) *Obstruction of tubular lumina* secondary to inspissated debris; the debris may be composed of hemoglobin or myoglobin, or of sloughed epithelial cells and protein. (2) *A profound reduction in glomerular filtration rate per nephron,* with or without tubular obstruction. The decrease in glomerular filtration rate would be sufficiently severe to eliminate the great majority of nephrons from the urine-forming group, and would presumably affect the cortical nephrons preferentially. (3) *"Back-leak" of tubular fluid into the renal interstitium through areas of discontinuity in the tubular walls.* The accumulation of tubular fluid in the interstitium would result in obstruction of contiguous nephrons. Back-leak could occur with or without nephron obstruction and with or without a decrease in glomerular filtration rate per nephron.

Essential to each of the hypotheses is damage to the tubular epithelial cells. The proponents of tubular obstruction believe that the damaged cells contribute to the luminal occlusion. Proponents of the reduced glomerular filtration rate thesis view the damage as impairing sodium reabsorption in proximal tubules. An increase in volume or sodium concentration of tubular fluid reaching the macula densa would follow. The sensors in the macula densa, in turn, would initiate the release of renin from the juxtaglomerular granules, and the renin would lead to high local concentrations of angiotensin. The angiotensin finally would produce vasoconstriction of the afferent arteriole and a decrease in glomerular filtration rate. In the "back-leak" hypothesis, damage to the epithelial cells and basement membranes would account for the discontinuity of the tubular walls, and thus the cycling of tubular fluid from nephron lumina into interstitial spaces.

In at least some forms of experimental acute tubular necrosis, there is little evidence of widespread cast formation, of diffuse tubular dilatation, or of increase in intratubular pressure in individual surface nephrons. Thus distal tubular obstruction is not a universal phenomenon. Moreover, direct measurement of glomerular filtration rate in single nephrons indicates that a primary or at least causal reduction in the filtration rate is not universal. Finally in some models, inulin injected directly into proximal tubules has been recovered essentially completely in the urine, thus indicating that back-leak is not universal. The ambiguity, in all probability, relates to the fact that many different techniques have been used to produce acute tubular necrosis in the animal; and there may be differences in pathogenesis among these entities. Hence, it is conceivable that tubular obstruction, reduction in single nephron glomerular filtration rate, and even back-leak may contribute either alone or in combination to the pathogenesis of the acute renal failure in the laboratory animal. But acute tubular necrosis in man also arises in a wide spectrum of circumstances and following a multiplicity of different insults; and it is equally conceivable that there is more than one pathogenic pathway leading to the development of the human disease.

Pathology. On gross examination, kidneys with acute tubular necrosis appear enlarged and swollen. On cut section they exhibit a pale cortex and a dark congested medulla. Microscopically the changes are largely confined to the tubules, and neither the glomeruli nor the vessels show consistent abnormalities. The changes in the tubular epithelia tend to be scattered and nonuniform, and in some cases no abnormalities can be seen on light microscopy. Usually, however, the proximal tubular epithelia tend to appear flattened, and mitotic figures may be seen. Frank necrosis may be observed in the proximal tubule, particularly after exposure to a nephrotoxic agent. The distal tubules appear dilated, and the epithelia are low and basophilic with dense staining nuclei and occasional mitotic figures. Casts of varying types may appear within the distal segments of the nephrons. Tubular basement membranes may be disrupted in scattered areas in nonnephrotoxic acute tubular necrosis, but this change is unusual when the necrosis is secondary to a nephrotoxic drug. Within several days of the onset of necrosis, round cell infiltration and edema of the interstitial spaces occur in most cases. The edema may become quite pronounced in overhydrated patients.

Electron microscopic examination has revealed structural alterations in the mitochondria of tubular epithelial cells, loss of the microvilli in the proximal tubular epithelia, and loss of endoplasmic reticulum; there may also be disruption of continuity of the tubular basement membrane.

Pathologic Physiology of Acute Tubular Necrosis. With normal renal function, less than 1 per cent of the water filtered at the glomeruli is ordinarily excreted in the urine, and only about 0.5 per cent of the filtered sodium is excreted on an average salt intake. In a typical patient with oliguric acute tubular necrosis, from 10 to 20 per cent of the filtered water and from 5 to 10 per cent of the filtered sodium are excreted. Considering the marked decrease in glomerular filtration rate, these increased *fractional* excretion rates are appropriate in direction, however, the changes are much less marked than in patients with chronic renal failure. For example, a patient with chronic uremia and a filtration rate of 1 ml. per minute may excrete as much as 50 per cent of the filtered water and 50 per cent or more of the filtered sodium. The consequences of these excretory patterns are as follows: At a glomerular filtration rate of 1 ml. per minute, the patient with acute tubular necrosis typically will excrete less than 300 ml. of urine and less than 20 mEq. of sodium per day, whereas the patient with chronic renal disease may excrete approximately a liter of urine and as much as 100 mEq. of sodium per day.

Two questions about the patterns of salt and water excretion in acute tubular necrosis thus emerge: (1) Are the increments in fractional salt and water excretion regulatory in nature or are they fortuitous consequences of intrinsic damage to the tubular epithelial cells? (2) Why are the responses not greater? Does it take time to build up natriuretic forces in a patient with uremia; or do the functioning nephrons in acute tubular necrosis fail to respond to these forces? To date the answer to these questions is not available. However, the fact that patients with acute tubular necrosis do spontaneously excrete a moderately high percentage of filtered water and filtered sodium (regardless of the mechanism) provides a clear explanation for "nonoliguric" tubular necrosis and for certain of the characteristics of the diuretic phase of the disease.

In most patients with the disease, the glomerular filtration rate (as estimated by endogenous creatinine clearance) drops to values of 1 ml. per minute or less. Such patients are oliguric. However, in some patients the drop in the filtration rate is not as severe, and values may stabilize at a level of 3 to 5 ml. per minute. Urea synthesis will still far exceed urea excretion, and the BUN will rise progressively. Creatinine and phosphate concentrations also will rise, and acidosis and hyperkalemia may develop. The patient thus may develop all the symptoms and signs of acute uremia. However, if 20 per cent of the filtered water is excreted at a glomerular filtration rate of 4 ml. per minute, urine flow will be almost 1200 ml. per day, and this urine may contain 60 or more mEq. of sodium. Hence there will exist a seeming paradox wherein the patient will present with stigmas of mounting uremia but with urine volumes that are not reduced, i.e., nonoliguric acute tubular necrosis.

A similar physiologic basis exists for the continued rise of the BUN during the first few days of the diuretic phase of tubular necrosis. If 20 per cent of the filtered water is excreted, urine volumes may exceed 1.5 to 2 liters per day before the glomerular filtration rate becomes high enough to allow for the filtration (and thus the excretion) of an amount of urea equal to that produced. The more catabolic the patient is, the higher must be the filtration rate (and the rate of urine flow) before the BUN will start to decline.

As the GFR increases progressively during the recovery phase of acute tubular necrosis, urine volumes may rise to very high levels. Two factors appear to have a profound influence on the magnitude of the diuresis. The first is the degree to which urea and other endogenous solutes accumulate in the blood during the oliguric phase; the second is the degree of expansion of the extracellular fluid volume. If urea is allowed to accumulate in body fluids rather than being removed by repeated dialysis, the retained solute will be excreted as the filtration rate rises toward normal. And because the urine remains isosmotic in acute tubular necrosis, every 300 mOsm. of extra solute excreted will obligate the excretion of approximately a liter of water. If the BUN concentration is lowered by 20 mg. per. 100 ml. in a 24-hour period, approximately 18 grams of urea

(equal to 300 mOsm.) will be excreted in a 70-kg. man, and this will increase the 24-hour urine volume by about 1 liter.

The second factor that may influence the magnitude of the diuresis is the degree of expansion of extracellular fluid volume. If effective extracellular fluid volume is supernormal, natriuretic forces will be mobilized, and as the diuretic phase proceeds, the nephrons will respond to these forces and excrete an increasing fraction of filtered sodium and water. This phenomenon can lead to a fluid vicious cycle wherein urine volume increases in consequence of fluid volume expansion, and the rate of fluid administration in turn is increased to keep up with the rising urine volumes.

Clinical Manifestations. When there is an inciting event, the onset of acute renal failure follows the insult by an interval varying from hours to as long as two days. The oliguric phase may last from a few hours to three or more weeks, and in some instances it appears not to occur at all. The diuretic phase lasts from a few days to a week or longer. The recovery phase is characterized by progressive rise in glomerular filtration rate and restoration of renal responsiveness to the volume needs of the organism. With recovery, renal function is restored toward the pre-tubular necrosis level, but in most patients some permanent nephron loss probably occurs.

The presenting picture is usually that of an oliguric patient with a rising concentration of blood urea and creatinine. If the oliguria has been present for some period of time and has not been recognized, or if an effort was made to restore normal renal function by overzealous fluid administration, salt and water retention, occasionally of massive proportions, may be present. Hyperkalemia may also be present when the patient is first seen. In untreated patients, the symptoms and signs of uremia may develop rapidly, and if there is an underlying injury or illness, the total constellation of clinical abnormalities will reflect the primary disease plus the superimposed manifestations of advancing uremia. Uremic manifestations tend to be particularly severe in patients with acute renal failure; for in contrast to the patient with chronic progressive renal disease who gradually adapts to the chemical abnormalities, the patient with acute renal failure is thrust from a normal to a uremic environment virtually overnight. Patients with acute tubular necrosis thus tend to be more symptomatic than patients with chronic renal disease with a comparable degree of uremia.

Uremia in acute tubular necrosis may affect many organ systems. *Gastrointestinal manifestations* include anorexia, nausea, and vomiting; if water must be restricted, thirst may become a disturbing symptom. *Central nervous system manifestations* include asterixis, subtle to overt changes in mentation (including organic psychosis), convulsions, and coma. *Cardiovascular changes* include an increase in cardiac output presumably resulting from anemia and acidosis, an increase in blood pressure in some patients, acute left ventricular failure in patients who are markedly hypervolemic, and pericarditis. Electrocardiographic changes are principally those of hyperkalemia, and may include the successive development of tall peaked tent-shaped T waves, prolongation of the P-R interval, prolongation of the QRS interval, disappearance of P waves, and ultimately disintegration of the electrocardiographic pattern with a so-called sine wave appearance. For any given level of elevation of plasma potassium concentration, the cardiotoxic effects tend to be greater when either severe acidosis or hyponatremia is also present.

Therapy will exercise a profound influence on the clinical course of acute tubular necrosis. If dialysis is performed early and at frequent intervals, the patient may progress through the entire course of his illness with few symptoms or signs attributable to the renal failure and without the burden of severe dietary restrictions. If the patient is treated with optimal conservative therapy, but without dialysis, he will develop progressive manifestations of uremia, and moreover will be required to restrict markedly his fluid intake and protein intake. He also may require special treatment for preventing a dangerous rise in plasma potassium concentration. The diuretic phase will be more exaggerated. *In all instances the clinical course is influenced greatly by the nature and severity of any underlying illness or injury*. Patients with acute tubular necrosis need no longer die of uremia, but many continue to die of the underlying abnormality that precipitated the renal failure.

During the recovery phase patients not infrequently exhibit reactive mental depression. They also may require a longer period of recuperation, particularly if catabolism has been severe. Finally, at the end of the diuretic phase, body weight may be substantially less than the clinical estimate of dry weight. This reflects the fact that lean body mass often decreases far more than is suspected during the course of the illness, and the decrease is masked by unrecognized extracellular fluid volume expansion.

Treatment. The treatment of the renal failure in acute tubular necrosis is best accomplished by early and frequent dialysis. Either peritoneal or hemodialysis may be employed. If hemodialysis is preferred or is required because peritoneal dialysis is contraindicated, an arteriovenous shunt may be placed in an extremity at the beginning of the illness to facilitate dialysis on a daily or every-other-day basis. When frequent dialysis is employed, only modest salt and water restriction is needed, and a moderate amount of protein, e.g., 40 to 60 grams per day, may be allowed in the diet. However, when dialysis is not used on a frequent basis, the amount of water, sodium, and potassium must be regulated carefully so as to minimize chemical and volumetric abnormalities of body fluids.

The standard principles of management in a patient who is not dialyzed repeatedly include fluid restriction sufficient to effect the loss of approximately half a pound of body weight per day. In general this amounts to the administration of 400 to 500 ml. of fluid plus the amount lost in the urine and gastrointestinal tract. Excessive fluid administration carries the risk of inducing congestive heart failure and pulmonary edema. If the patient is able to take food by mouth, a diet providing approximately 2000 calories which is potassium and protein-free and essentially sodium-free is recommended; there are some observers, however, who favor the inclusion in the diet of a small amount of protein (ca. 20 grams per day), containing the minimal daily requirements of essential amino acids. If parenteral alimentation is necessary, it is the general practice to infuse dextrose (at least 100 grams per day) and vitamins; but the caloric requirements may also be partially fulfilled by intravenous fat emulsions. When glucose is administered, it must usually be given as a hyperosmotic solution because of the requirement for fluid restriction. Precautions are required to prevent venous thrombosis and infection of the venous catheter.

Particular attention may be necessary to prevent the development of progressive hyperkalemia. The administration of a potassium-binding resin either by mouth or by enema two to four times daily will generally serve to prevent serious elevations of plasma potassium concentrations.[*] If marked hyperkalemia is present when the patient is first seen, intravenous glucose and insulin, sodium bicarbonate, or calcium chloride all will protect temporarily against the cardiotoxic effects of potassium. But potassium exchange resins and/or dialysis should be initiated promptly to prevent the recurrence of hyperkalemia. Metabolic acidosis can generally be corrected and controlled by dialysis. If dialysis is not available, or the acidosis progresses despite dialysis, the administration of $NaHCO_3$ in carefully regulated amounts is indicated to keep the plasma bicarbonate concentration above 15 mEq. per liter. Hyponatremia can best be controlled by preventing progressive water retention and can best be corrected by dialysis. *Hyponatremia should not be treated by the administration of hypertonic saline.* Anemia will develop routinely in the course of acute tubular necrosis, and ordinarily no effort should be made to maintain the hematocrit in excess of 20 volumes per 100 ml. If blood transfusion does become necessary because of a pro-

---

[*]The resin generally used in the United States is a sodium cycle resin (Kayexalate), and in a standard dose of 15 to 60 grams per day over 30 mEq. of Na may be released into the gastrointestinal tract. To obviate sodium retention, part or all of the resin may be given as a calcium cycle resin if the latter is available.

gressive fall in hematocrit or cardiovascular complications, packed red blood cells using fresh blood should be employed. In treating hemorrhage, fresh whole blood may be preferable. Hyperphosphatemia may occasionally become very pronounced, and may be attended by the development of hypocalcemia. The latter ordinarily does not produce manifestations of tetany; but if ionized calcium concentrations become reduced inordinately, as may occur if the patient becomes alkalotic from the infusion of bicarbonate in excessive amount or from vomiting, tetany and even seizures may develop. Hyperphosphatemia is best controlled by protein restriction and/or frequent dialysis, but the administration of phosphate binding gels, e.g., aluminum hydroxide gel, 30 to 60 ml. every six hours by mouth may be of great value.

All drugs from antimicrobials to digitalis glycosides must be administered with full knowledge of their route of degradation and excretion. Drugs which are neither detoxified, metabolized, nor excreted by the kidney may be given in full dosage. But these are the exception rather than the rule. Most drugs, including many antimicrobials, will have to be given in reduced amounts and at prolonged intervals. It is tragic indeed to have a patient recover from acute tubular necrosis only to have a permanent vestibular or auditory defect owing to streptomycin or kanamycin toxicity. Digoxin is the recommended digitalis glycoside. A digitalizing dose of 2 to 3 mg. and a maintenance dose of 0.25 mg. every other day will provide a therapeutic effect without toxicity in most adult patients with acute tubular necrosis.

If the renal failure is treated satisfactorily, the outcome will depend almost entirely upon the natural history of any underlying illness or injury. Thus the intensity of treatment of a surgical wound, an area of necrotic tissue, or a burn should not be diminished because of the existence of acute tubular necrosis; quite the contrary: any delay in appropriate treatment may compromise the survival of the patient. Removal of necrotic tissue is, if anything, more urgent in the patient with acute renal failure than in the patient with normal renal function; and surgical procedures, even major ones, are not contraindicated if they are considered to have life-saving importance. Finally, although prophylactic antimicrobial drugs are contraindicated, infection must be treated promptly with the correct drugs but with prorated dosages. And in the same context, careful attention must be given to avoiding the introduction of secondary infection. Thus, after the first day of the disease, the use of a bladder catheter solely to monitor urine volumes is not justified, and intravenous catheters should be treated aseptically and never left in the same vein for more than three days.

Differential Diagnosis. The fact that the patient with acute tubular necrosis characteristically excretes a relatively large percentage of filtered salt and water may be very helpful in differentiating the disease from the oliguric states associated with volume depletion, acute glomerulitis, and the hepatorenal syndrome.

As indicated previously, a normal person with normal salt and water intake will excrete less than 1 per cent of his filtered sodium and water. If extracellular fluid volume depletion occurs, the appropriate response is to *decrease* fractional salt and water excretion. If volume losses are profound, the glomerular filtration rate may fall markedly, in which case the patient will present not only with oliguria but with a rising level of BUN and creatinine. Thus he will fulfill the criteria for acute renal failure. But in contrast to the patient with acute tubular necrosis, the patient with volume depletion will typically excrete less than 5 per cent of his filtered water, and may have a sodium-free urine. A similar picture evolves early in the course of a severe glomerulitis and in the hepatorenal syndrome.

The urine/plasma (U/P) creatinine ratio is a readily available test for estimating the fraction of filtered water excreted. The accompanying table compares the U/P ratios with the fractional rate of water excretion. A U/P ratio of 10 indicates that approximately 10 per cent of the filtered water is excreted. A U/P ratio of 5 is equivalent to the excretion of 20 per cent of the filtered water, and a ratio of 2 signifies the excretion of 50 per cent of the filtered water. In acute tubular necrosis, creatinine U/P ratios typically range between 5 and 10, and rarely exceed 20. In extracellular fluid volume depletion, acute glomerulitides, and the hepatorenal syndrome, creatinine U/P ratios typically exceed 10, and often are well above 20. The urinary sodium concentration (U_{Na}) in acute tubular necrosis typically exceeds 20 mEq. per liter, and in most patients ranges from 40 to 90 mEq. per liter. In volume depletion, acute glomerulitis, and hepatorenal syndrome, U_{Na} is usually less than 20 mEq. per liter, and often is less than 10 mEq. per liter. Calculation of the fraction of filtered sodium excreted may also be very helpful. This value is equal to the U/P ratio for sodium divided by the U/P ratio for creatinine and expressed as a percentage. In acute tubular necrosis 5 per cent or more of the filtered sodium

THE RELATIONSHIP BETWEEN CREATININE URINE/PLASMA (U/P) RATIOS AND THE PERCENTAGE OF FILTERED WATER EXCRETED

Creatinine U/P ratio	Per Cent Filtered H_2O Excreted
100	1
50	2
20	5
10	10
5	20
2	50

is typically excreted; in volume depletion, acute glomerulitis, and the hepatorenal syndrome, less than 5 per cent and often less than 2 per cent of the filtered sodium is excreted. In chronic end-stage renal disease, the values will depend upon the glomerular filtration rate and the salt intake; but at a rate of 2 ml per minute and with an average salt and water intake, about 30 per cent of the filtered salt and water are excreted.

The creatinine U/P ratio, U_{Na}, and the U/P Na U/P creatinine ratio are thus of help in the differential diagnosis of acute renal failure. But there are substantial gray zones where the patterns overlap, and these biochemical values must in all instances be viewed in light of the historical and clinical findings. There are also sources of error in utilizing the biochemical values. One of these is that acute renal failure secondary to volume depletion may progress to acute tubular necrosis; and if the urine examined was produced prior to the advent of acute tubular necrosis, it will be low in sodium and have a high creatinine U/P ratio. Another source of error exists in a patient with true tubular necrosis in whom there is a profound stimulus to sodium retention. For example, in tubular necrosis associated with burns, the translocation of extracellular fluid into the affected areas results in a striking decrease in effective fluid volume. The patient thus may present with oliguria, a glomerular filtration rate below 1 ml. per minute, a creatinine U/P ratio of less than 10, but virtually no sodium in the urine. A low U_{Na} has also been observed in acute tubular necrosis following bypass cardiac surgery and mercury poisoning.

Error in using the creatinine U/P ratio and U_{Na} also may occur in patients with glomerulitis, after the occurrence of compensation but before the filtration rate rises appreciably. After enough salt and water have been retained to expand extracellular fluid volume appreciably, natriuretic forces may be mobilized and fractional reabsorption of sodium (and water) in the urine-forming nephrons may be markedly depressed. Thus creatinine U/P ratios may fall below the 10 to 20 range and U_{Na} may be high when acute renal failure is superimposed on underlying chronic renal disease, e.g., from volume depletion or acute glomerulitis; the creatinine U/P ratio may remain low, and the U_{Na} high.

Other Aids in Differential Diagnosis. *Urine Volume.* Total anuria is very rare in acute tubular necrosis unless it is due to the ingestion of bichloride of mercury. Total anuria is seen in severe acute glomerulitis, bilateral cortical necrosis, and urinary tract obstruction. If there is a history of an abrupt change in urine volume from very low to high levels in a short period of time, obstruction is strongly suggested.

Urinary Sediment. Red blood cell casts are unusual in acute tubular necrosis (but they occur) and are the rule in glomerulitides (but they may be absent). Qualitative measurements of protein in urine in the disease rarely exceed 1 to 2+, whereas they often are 3 to 4+ in glomerulitides.

Urine Osmolality. The osmolality of the urine is the same as that of the plasma in patients with tubular necrosis. In patients with severe volume depletion, glomerulitides, and hepatorenal syndrome, the urine may occasionally be hyperosmotic to the plasma. *Consequently isosmotic urine is not of value in differential diagnosis, although hyperosmotic urine favors volume depletion, acute glomerulitis, and the hepatorenal syndrome, and virtually excludes acute tubular necrosis.*

Response to Mannitol or Volume Expansion. A limited increase in urine volume may occur in the disease following both mannitol administration and volume expansion. However, unless the increase is progressive and is attended by a substantial rise in glomerular filtration rate, continuous administration of either mannitol or a synthetic extracellular fluid solution is contraindicated in patients with acute renal failure of unknown variety. The differential diagnostic implications of a small increase in urine volume and sodium excretion following the administration of potent diuretics such as furosemide are not yet clear; but large increments in urine volume point away from the diagnosis of acute tubular necrosis.

Prognosis. In uncomplicated cases of acute tubular necrosis, in which there is no serious underlying disease and treatment is optimal, survival rates in excess of 80 per cent are common. On the other hand, when there is a serious underlying disease or injury, the death rate exceeds 50 per cent, and in severely traumatized patients may exceed 70 per cent. Judging from the experience in the Vietnam war, as contrasted with the Korean war, the speedy evacuation of wounded and rapid treatment of blood loss and shock will substantially reduce the incidence of acute tubular necrosis; but unfortunately once it does develop, the mortality rate among wounded patients requiring hemodialysis remains at about 70 per cent.

Prevention. The likelihood of occurrence of acute tubular necrosis following a given insult is influenced by the composite physiologic adversities. Thus the better the supportive therapy, the lower should be the incidence of the disease. The war experience just cited supports this view.

The role of mannitol in preventing acute tubular necrosis is uncertain. Some observers have favored the view that administration of mannitol to an oliguric patient will confer a substantial degree of protection by eliminating the contribution of luminal obstruction to the disease. However, at the very least, obstruction is not a universal factor in its pathogenesis; moreover, it can be induced in the experimental animal with myoglobinuria despite the presence of high rates of urine flow per nephron. Mannitol also may increase renal blood flow, and conceivably some protective effect could derive from this. But it seems most reasonable to confine the use of mannitol chiefly to patients in whom there is an increase in the creatinine U/P ratio and a decrease in urinary sodium concentration, but no evidence of hypervolemia. (Furosemide may be used in the latter group.) The mannitol should be administered only for a limited period of time and in an amount not to exceed 25 to 50 grams; if no substantial rise in glomerular filtration rate and/or urine flow occurs, its use should not be continued.

In patients with extracellular fluid volume depletion and oliguria, volume repletion should be effected as expeditiously as possible. When hypotension exists, this also should be corrected as rapidly as possible. The use of sodium bicarbonate intravenously in patients with intravascular hemolysis is of dubious value.

The early recognition of urinary tract obstruction is not only of importance for the prompt reversal of acute renal failure, but for the prevention of progressive nephron destruction. When obstruction is suspected in a patient with acute renal failure, either bladder catheterization or unilateral retrograde pyelogram should be performed without delay.

Biber, T. U. L., Mylle, M., Baines, A. D., Gottschalk, C. W., Oliver, J. R., and MacDowell, M. C.: A study by micropuncture and microdissection of acute renal damage in rats. Amer. J. Med., 44:664, 1968.

Heptinstall, R. H.: Acute renal failure. In Pathology of the Kidney. Boston, Little, Brown and Company, 1966, p.645.

Merrill, J. P.: Acute renal failure. In Strauss, M. B., and Welt, L. G. (eds.): Diseases of the Kidney. Boston, Little, Brown and Company, 1970.

Muehrcke, R. C.: Acute Renal Failure: Diagnosis and Management. St. Louis, C. V. Mosby Company, 1969.

Treatment of Irreversible Renal Failure by Dialysis and Transplantation

Priscilla Kincaid-Smith

The clinical application of cadaver transplantation to the treatment of renal failure has been one of the most revolutionary therapeutic developments in the past decade. Experience has shown that renal allografts from cadavers may function for years, and these results have been particularly rewarding because renal failure is a major cause of death in young people whose other organs are healthy. The parallel development of the artificial kidney has been a very important contributing factor to the success of renal transplantation. Prospective recipients can be kept alive for months or years by hemodialysis while awaiting a suitable transplant from a cadaver. In spite of some conflict in the past about the relative merits of dialysis and transplantation, these techniques are now combined in the treatment of chronic renal failure. All suitable patients should be accepted for treatment, and this can only be achieved in a program whose primary aim is to treat patients by renal transplantation, although dialysis plays an important part in maintaining patients who are waiting for a suitable transplant. In addition there will be a small number of patients in whom transplantation is contraindicated for medical or immunologic reasons, the latter group perhaps after failure of one or more transplants. For such patients dialysis may be used as a permanent method of treatment.

This approach has been shown in Australia to permit the acceptance of nearly all patients presenting for treatment of terminal renal failure.

THE PROBLEM OF IRREVERSIBLE RENAL FAILURE IN THE COMMUNITY

The enormous cumulative costs of treating a large number of patients by maintenance dialysis and the high initial costs of transplantation have led to a critical assessment of the number of patients likely to present with end-stage renal failure and the costs of and facilities required for their treatment.

It is estimated that 20 to 40 people per million of the population below the age of 60 will present each year with irreversibile renal failure. In the over-60 age group degenerative vascular disease and other factors make it unlikely that either dialysis or transplantation will be successful.

Even a figure of 20 to 40 per million of the population means that each year in the United States between 4000 and 8000 people may present for treatment. Although the initial costs of providing facilities for the treatment of these patients would amount to many millions of dollars, it is not the initial cost but the cumulative maintenance costs that prohibit the use of dialysis as a definitive method of treatment for all patients with renal failure. Maintenance costs of $40,000,000 to $80,000,000 each year for the first 4000 to 8000 patients added to the costs of a new patient load of 4000 to 8000 patients each year soon run into billions of dollars. Both doctors and governments question the wisdom of making such huge amounts available to maintain a relatively small number of patients in a state of chronic renal failure, which is all that dialysis achieves. Restoration of normal renal function by a successful renal allograft is therefore a more worthwhile goal.

These factors led the Gottschalk committee to recommend that a program attempting to deal with the problem of chronic renal failure in the community must be strongly oriented toward renal transplantation to avoid the enormous cumulative costs of maintenance dialysis.

In the United Kingdom an ambitious program to treat patients by maintenance dialysis was established in 1965. Here, in spite of a fully nationalized health service and strong financial backing, between May 1966 and May 1969 less than 10 per cent of the number of people estimated to require treatment for end-stage renal failure were accepted for dialysis. One hundred and thirty patients a year have been started on dialysis compared with estimated numbers of 1000 to 2000 requiring treatment each year. The enormous requirements in terms of buildings, equipment, and trained staff probably caused the program in the United Kingdom to fall so far short of its goal. Considerable expansion of transplantation facilities is now being planned to deal more effectively with the large number of patients presenting for treatment.

One can contrast the centrally planned and heavily subsidized program in the United Kingdom with the situation in Australia. Here there is no compulsory health insurance scheme, and payment for medical treatment is the individual responsibility of the patient. No separate government funds have yet been made available for the treatment of chronic renal failure in Australia, but active transplantation programs have been developed with minimal financial support in teaching hospitals in major cities. Early experience at the Royal Melbourne Hospital suggested that with very slender dialysis facilities cadaver transplantation permitted the treatment of all patients presenting with chronic renal failure. This has now been confirmed by experience throughout Australia and New Zealand. Approximately 200 renal allografts from cadavers are now done each year in Australia and New Zealand, and thus already between two thirds and three fourths of the estimated numbers of patients requiring treatment are being treated; in fact all medically suitable patients are being accepted at major centers.

Dialysis facilities are still very small because these cannot be expanded without strong financial backing. In spite of this the problems of renal failure in the community have been very largely solved.

A registry of cadaver grafts done in Australia and New Zealand over the past two years shows that, when cadaver transplantation is regarded as the treatment of choice for chronic renal failure, much better results can be achieved than the over-all results throughout the world. Thus the latest figures from the Boston Registry show a 29 per cent two-year survival for 1084 cadaver grafts between 1964 and 1969, whereas over the same period Australasian registry figures show a 55 per cent two-year survival for 345 cadaver grafts. Patient survival is of course much better than this because many patients have received more than one graft or are alive on dialysis awaiting a second transplant.

When cadaver transplantation is used as the main method for the treatment of chronic renal failure, the rapid turnover allows the small numbers of patients unsuitable for this method of treatment to be trained for home dialysis by gradual expansion of home training facilities.

PREVENTION OF RENAL FAILURE

A program which aims to treat renal failure in the community must include adequate provisions for prevention. Renal failure can be prevented by both the application of modern methods of treatment to renal disease and improvement of present methods of treatment through research. All major renal units should include facilities for research and for adequate diagnosis and treatment of renal disease at all stages. Even by applying present methods of treatment the numbers requiring dialysis and transplantation may decrease substantially. Detection and treatment of asymptomatic bacteriuria and hypertension are very likely to reduce the numbers presenting with chronic renal failure. Glomerulonephritis is the most common cause of renal failure in patients presenting for dialysis and transplantation, and although treatment of this condition has usually proved ineffective, promising results with newer forms of treatment including anticoagulants, are likely to diminish the numbers presenting each year with irreversible renal failure.

Analgesic nephropathy is a totally preventable disease which has led many patients to transplantation in some programs in Australia. This disease, which results from prolonged high doses of proprietary analgesic drugs, would disappear completely if such preparations were only available on a doctor's prescription.

SELECTION OF PATIENTS

One of the most distressing aspects of treatment of terminal renal failure has been the publicity given to the selection of patients for the very limited number of places available in a dialysis program.

All patients who have terminal renal failure and are considered medically suitable, as well as sufficiently cooperative and intelligent to carry out the instructions, should be accepted for treatment. Practical experience has shown that this can be done if the program is clearly orientated toward transplantation as the primary form of treatment.

It is critically important, if all suitable patients are to be accepted, that the numbers must not be exaggerated by accepting patients before they really require treatment. It has been stated recently that dialysis must be started early before the patient develops terminal renal failure. Clearly treatment must be instituted when any serious consequences such as peripheral neuropathy are developing on conservative management. It is unethical, however, to accept a patient for dialysis before this is necessary unless one is able to accept all patients presenting. The course of some forms of chronic renal disease is unpredictable and it should not be forgotten that the best that dialysis and transplantation can offer at present is a 50 per cent chance of living for five years.

Certain diseases, notably polycystic renal disease and analgesic nephropathy, may show considerable fluctuations in renal function over many years. Patients with renal failure resulting from analgesic nephropathy may even recover to normal blood urea levels and show radiologic hypertrophy continuing for years after apparent terminal chronic renal failure. Simple measures such as the administration of sufficient salt to patients with chronic renal failure tend to be forgotten in the wave of enthusiasm for the dramatic and expensive methods of treatment.

RENAL TRANSPLANTATION

Transplantation was the first method of treatment shown to be capable of prolonging life in patients with terminal renal failure. The famous Boston series of isografts established the undoubted value of transplantation in identical twins. In spite of the surprising success of some of Hume's cadaver transplants in 1955, many years passed before transplantation became accepted as an effective means of treatment in chronic renal failure. Early deaths were mainly due to immunosuppressive methods, including total body irradiation; the beginning of real clinical success of renal transplantation dates from the introduction of the drug azathioprine in 1963. This is the major immunosuppressive drug used in renal transplantation.

As far as treatment of renal failure in the community is concerned, only cadaveric transplantation can offer treatment to everyone, although the better results obtained with related living donors have persuaded some units to concentrate on this method of treatment. There is no doubt that a well matched transplant from a related living donor offers a much better chance of rapid return to a normal way of life than a cadaver transplant. Nevertheless, living donors will only provide a very small number of the kidneys needed. Cadaveric transplantation should, therefore, be the aim in all patients accepted for treatment of irreversible renal failure unless there is a definite contraindication to transplantation.

Histocompatibility Testing. The HL—A system of leukocyte antigens is thought to represent the major histocompatibility locus in man. Its relevance to renal transplantation has been reviewed by Walford. It appears that the HL—A locus comprises two or three subloci, each being multiallelic. However, there are still a number of undetected alleles at each of these subloci, and this adds to the difficulty of matching donors and recipients for renal transplants.

Despite gaps in our present knowledge of the HL—A system, matching by leukocyte typing of living related donors and recipients can be very precise. The reason for this is that the definition of a number of leukocyte antigens through the members of a family allows the transmission of the two chromosomes carrying the HL—A locus in each parent to be traced in the children. Thus siblings can be identified who share the same chromosomes carrying the HL—A locus (HL—A identical siblings), who differ at one chromosome, and who differ at both chromosomes. Generally each child will share only one chromosome with each parent. If this genotyping information can be obtained, then it is irrelevant that all alleles at the HL—A locus cannot be detected. Transplants performed between HL—A identical siblings are usually trouble-free, many requiring no steroid therapy post-transplant.

A much more difficult situation exists when the donor and recipient are unrelated, for here few assumptions can be made about the presently undetected alleles. The chances of an unrelated donor and recipient being truly identical at the HL—A locus are poor, perhaps of the order of 1 in 500. Nevertheless early reports suggest some correlation between the outcome of unrelated grafts and matching by leukocyte typing, suggesting that most badly matched grafts have a poor course, although many reasonably well-matched grafts also do badly. This is understandable when it is remembered that the whole HL—A system cannot yet be identified.

At present leukocyte typing is an essential and accurate method of selecting histocompatible, living related donors and recipients. In cadaver transplantation it seems reasonable to anticipate that as definition of the HL—A system becomes more precise, matching will significantly improve results. Because of the complexity of the leukocyte antigenic systems, however, it will be necessary to have regional or even national pools of donors and recipients to ensure good matches for the majority of patients awaiting cadaver transplants.

Finally, an essential part of this serologic matching system is a cross match between the recipient's serum and a potential donor's white cells. If a positive cross match is found as a result of prior sensitization of the recipient by transfusions, pregnancy, or a previous renal graft, then transplantation is definitely contraindicated, as hyperacute rejection of the transplant will usually result.

Supply of Donors. If all the kidneys were available from road-accident victims, the number of donors would far exceed the patients with chronic renal failure awaiting transplant. This would provide an ideal situation whereby a well matched cadaver transplant could be provided without the need for a large recipient pool which is so costly to maintain on dialysis.

Pathologic Features of Rejection. Although intense cellular infiltration is a prominent feature in the unmodified rejection reaction seen in animals, this is not a prominent feature in patients in whom rejection is modified by treatment with steroids and azathioprine. The major lesions seen in renal allografts in man are in the vessels and may involve all blood vessels from the main artery vein to the glomerular capillaries and intertubular sinusoids.

Polymorphonuclear leukocytes may accumulate within the blood vessels of the allograft within minutes in so-called "hyperacute" rejection in which very florid thrombotic vascular lesions develop within days of grafting. Such patients often have preformed antibody in their serum prior to transplantation. The vascular lesions of hyperacute rejection are the same as those occurring in acute and chronic rejection. The differences between the three are differences of degree and rate of progress, but the essential pathogenesis as seen in percutaneous biopsy specimens is similar. Platelet and fibrin thrombi may be demonstrated within vessels of all sizes in the acute stages, and the glomerular and vascular lesions seen months or years after transplantation represent the residual lesions following organization of these thrombi. This process of organization may result in lesions which resemble atheroma in the main renal artery, intimal proliferation, and narrowing of branch arteries and occlusion or narrowing of glomerular capillaries by subendothelial material which persists after fibrin thrombi disappear.

The rejection process is most active during the first three months; subsequently severe acute lesions are rare. However they may occur in episodes as long as three and one half years after transplantation. Preliminary evidence suggests that antithrombotic and anticoagulant drugs may modify and reduce the vascular lesions of rejection.

Clinical Course in Patients with Renal Allografts. The grafted kidney from a living donor usually functions at once, and many cadaver kidneys also function immediately if the blood pressure and oxygenation of the donor have been well maintained prior to death and the warm ischemic time is short. Acute tubular necrosis may cause oliguric renal failure for a few days or even weeks in cadaver grafts.

Once the kidney is functioning, the most sensitive index of rejection is deterioration in renal function. The renal blood flow falls a day or two before other parameters alter; a fall in urine volume and sodium content, rise in the serum urea and creatinine, and fall in the glomerular filtration rate may be accompanied by proteinuria, rise in the urine lymphocyte count, and pyrexia. Needle biopsy may be valuable in confirming the diagnosis, particularly during the stage of oliguric renal failure. Transplants from well matched living related donors do not usually reject, but patients who have received cadaver grafts usually have one more clinical episodes of rejection.

The clinical course in a patient with a renal allograft is almost entirely governed by the severity of the rejection process. The postoperative management varies in different centers, but if no complications arise, the patient is fit to be discharged from hospital a week or ten days after operation, although some consider that patients should be kept in a low pathogen area for a period of about six weeks. Frequent clinical assessment and tests of renal function are advisable in the first six to twelve weeks, particularly in cadaver allografts because rejection is likely to occur and is more easily reversed if treated promptly.

If rejection does not occur or is adequately controlled, the patient is usually fit to return to a normal active life six weeks to two months after operation. Thereafter weekly attendances at the hospital are usually necessary for three months, and monthly visits are advisable even a year or more after transplantation. If rejection episodes are frequent, removal of the graft may be necessary to avoid death from the complications of high doses of steroids or immunosuppressive drugs. The decision about the time to remove a graft is difficult and requires experience and careful consideration of the clinical and histologic state of the graft. Several rejection episodes in the early months may be compatible in a few patients with prolonged satisfactory graft function.

Treatment. Treatment regimens vary. In related living donor grafts and in well matched cadaver grafts, the dosage of both azathioprine and steroids and the rate of reduction of steroids will be different from those in poorly matched cadaver grafts.

The introduction of antilymphocyte globulin has reduced the doses of azathioprine and steroids given in the early weeks after transplantation in some units.

Azathioprine. This drug is usually given in a dose of 3 mg. per kilogram per day in the early stages. The dose must be reduced to 1.5 mg. per kilogram per day if oliguric renal failure is present. Reduction in dosage is also necessary if leukopenia or thrombocytopenia occur. The drug is continued indefinitely, although in some centers the dose is greatly reduced. Cessation of azathioprine even when it is being given in a very small dose may precipitate acute rejection years after transplantation. Within 24 hours of stopping azathioprine percutaneous biopsy may show lymphocytes within the vessels of the graft. Azathioprine dosage is usually kept constant at the time of rejection.

Steroids. Most centers now use a high initial dose of steroids. Prednisone, 100 mg. daily or an equivalent dose, is given in the first few days after grafting and then reduced; the rate of reduction varies considerably. Less steroids are necessary in related living donor transplants, and the dose can be more rapidly reduced if rejection episodes do not occur. In a cadaver graft program most patients who survive a year would be taking 10 mg. of prednisone daily, and doses of this order do not cause troublesome complications of steroid therapy.

Rejection episodes are usually treated by increasing the dose of prednisone to 100 to 300 mg. for one day and then rapidly reducing it to a level just above the dose at which rejection occurred. Intravenous preparations are sometimes used in the treatment of rejection. Actinomycin C, 200 to 400 μg., and local irradiation in a dose of 150 r have also been widely used at the time of rejection episodes.

Antilymphocyte Globulin. An antiserum to human lymphocytes may be prepared by repeated injections of lymphocytes from spleen, thymus, or thoracic duct into horses or other animals. Thoracic duct lymph is said to be one of the most satisfactory sources of lymphocytes for this purpose. The antiserum can then be purified, and antilymphocyte globulin prepared for injection into patients. Clinical trials which have not yet been satisfactorily controlled suggest that antilymphocyte globulin reduces the requirements of azathioprine and steroids and improves graft function. However, results in man have been disappointing by comparison with the outstanding results reported in some laboratory animals. Large injections of antilymphocyte globulin in mice given at the same time as small doses of antigen have produced lasting tolerance to grafted tissue.

Among the immediate clinical disadvantages of antilymphocyte globulin are the great pain and local reaction that accompany intramuscular injection and the thrombosis that follows intravenous injection. However, the major problem in its use is the lack of an in vitro assay to measure its immunosuppressive activity. Thus there is no guarantee that a standard immunization of a horse with human lymphocytes will result in an immunosuppressive antilymphocyte globulin.

Complications. Many complications are directly attributable to steroid therapy or immunosuppressive drugs.

Ureteric Fistula. The most common postoperative surgical complication is a ureteric fistula. This is serious because of the inevitable accompanying infection. It may heal spontaneously over a period of six weeks, but in our experience may be more satisfactorily managed by early surgical intervention before local infection supervenes.

Hypertension. Many patients who have received a renal transplant have temporary or persistent hypertension after operation. Severe hypertension may be associated with high renin levels and may be due to ischemic lesions distal to vessels narrowed by rejection changes. Renal artery stenosis caused by the intimal changes of rejection in the main renal artery has been common in our experience.

Urinary Infection. This is one of the most frequent complications of renal transplantation. The incidence varies with the surgical method and the use of catheter in the postoperative period. The use of neomycin, 0.5 per cent in the bladder at the time of operation and before withdrawal of the catheter may diminish the incidence. Prevention or eradication of infection early in the course of a graft is important because, once it becomes established, chronic bacteriuria is liable to persist for years. The site of infection in these cases can be shown to be renal, and the infection may cause recurrent episodes of septicemia in grafted patients who are particularly susceptible to this complication because of their steroid-azathioprine treatment.

Other Infections. Pathogenic bacteria are more likely to cause serious infection, including septicemia, in transplant patients. Organisms not normally pathogenic may also cause serious infections, particularly in patients who require prolonged high doses of steroids. Among the fungi and yeasts, *Candida albicans*, *Nocardia*, and cryptococcus have been prominent. They may cause widespread infection and abscess formation. *Listeria monocytogenes* may cause serious infection, including fatal meningitis. Virus infections may also be serious in patients with transplants, and such minor infections as herpes simplex may cause serious spreading, destructive lesions, and death of the patient. At autopsy cytomegalovirus and *Pneumocystis carinii* can usually be demonstrated in the organs. There is some doubt about the clinical significance of their presence, although it has been suggested that these organisms may cause "transplant lung."

Transplant Lung. Transplant lung is an entity that usually occurs within the first few months of transplantation in patients who have had frequent episodes of rejection. Breathlessness is the main symptom, and on examination there may be crepitations and impaired percussion or there may be no abnormal physical signs. Diffuse or nodular opacities are found in the lungs on roentgenography. Respiratory function studies show a serious diffusion defect, resulting in poor oxygen exchange, and death may occur in a few days. Various forms of antimicrobial and antifungal treatment have been used without great benefit. Our own studies suggest that a vascular lesion in the lungs similar to that in the kidneys may be the underlying process in the syndrome of transplant lung.

Aseptic Necrosis of Bone. This lesion usually affects the hip joint and may be bilateral. It occurs in patients who have had prolonged high doses of steroids, but seems to be a more frequent complication of steroid therapy in transplant patients than in others, such as patients with disseminated lupus who require long-term steroids. This may be related to the renal osteodystrophy which precedes transplantation in many patients.

Other Steroid Complications. Any of the well recognized complications of steroid therapy such as peptic ulceration, diabetes, and cataract may develop in patients who have received transplants.

Prognosis in Patients Who Have Received Renal Allografts. The ultimate fate of renal allografts cannot yet be assessed. Only a few patients with cadaveric renal allografts have survived for five years because the operation has been done on a large scale only recently. The survival curves seem to flatten out after two years, and renal function remains steady or may even improve. It is possible that five-year and even ten-year survival figures may be similar to two-year survival figures, which have already been quoted, although histologic changes in many of the kidneys after one to two years suggest that the life expectancy of these kidneys may be measured in one to five years.

Rehabilitation. In the case of a successful transplant full rehabilitation is usually achieved within two to three months of operation. A few patients will die, but those in whom repeated treatment for rejection is necessary may never be fully rehabilitated; in such cases it would be better to remove the allograft and attempt to obtain better results with a subsequent transplant.

MAINTENANCE DIALYSIS

The artificial kidney was first developed for the temporary treatment of patients with reversible acute renal failure. Its use in this way was suggested as early as 1913 by Abel, Rowntree, and Turner. Advances in methods of dialysis, and particularly in arteriovenous shunts which permit repeated dialysis, have made it possible to keep people alive in this way for years after kidney function has ceased.

Although a successful transplant is the more acceptable permanent form of treatment, the chances of survival in the first two years are better on dialysis in an experienced unit than with a cadaver graft. In spite of this the enormous costs of dialysis and the inability to expand facilities rapidly have convinced even the most enthusiastic protagonists that dialysis alone cannot succeed as a method of dealing with the problem of renal failure in the community.

It is now envisaged that maintenance dialysis will fulfill two main functions. For most patients dialysis will be used until a suitable matched cadaver kidney becomes available. In a small minority of patients in whom transplantation is contraindicated for medical or immunologic reasons, it will be used as a permanent form of treatment. Because permanent center dialysis is not a practical proposition, such patients should be trained for home dialysis.

METHODS OF DIALYSIS

Peritoneal Dialysis. In peritoneal dialysis the dialyzing fluid is introduced into the peritoneal cavity, and the peritoneum acts as the semipermeable membrane across which dialysis occurs. In repeated peritoneal dialysis infection is a serious complication leading to the formation of adhesions that prevent effective dialysis.

Automatic cycling machines and a closed sterile system for the whole period of dialysis have made it possible to avoid infection and use peritoneal dialysis over long periods of time. However, results are unlikely to be as good as those of hemodialysis.

Hemodialysis. Repeated hemodialysis depends upon flow of the patient's blood at 150 to 300 ml. per minute through a dialyzer.

The Scribner shunt first made repeated dialysis possible. At present either an external shunt of this type or repeated needle punctures of the large vessels that form around an arteriovenous fistula are used to connect the patient to the dialyzer.

Two dialysis systems are in common use: the coil type and the flat plate type. The most commonly used coil dialyzer is the Kolff twin coil, which consists of two coils of cellulose tubing wound around a central core and is supported by a fine fiberglass or criss-cross polypropylene screen. The coil is inserted into a canister, and dialysis fluid is pumped up through the coil. The blood circulates through the cellulose coils and because of the resistance in the coil a blood pump is essential to maintain adequate blood flow.

The Kiil dialyzer consists of three polypropylene boards with two sheets of cuprophane membrane between each board. The blood compartment lies between the cuprophane sheets. The dialysis fluid compartment is between the grooved surface of the polypropylene boards and the cuprophane sheets. As this provides a low resistance system of dialysis, a flow of 150 to 200 ml. can be maintained by blood pressure alone; thus a blood pump is not usually necessary.

With either type of instrument it is usual to dialyze patients for a minimum of 14 hours twice a week or 8 to 10 hours three times a week.

A number of other forms of dialyzer are available or are being developed. One of the most promising new developments is the hollow fiber kidney which uses multiple hollow tubes of deacetylated cellulose triacetate 200 to 230μ in diameter. Ten thousand fibers 18 cm. long are used. The blood flows through the fibers, and the dialysis fluid flows in the opposite direction around the fibers.

Ultrafiltration, or removal of fluid from the blood because of a pressure gradient between the blood and dialysis fluid, is obligatory with the coil type of dialyzer because of the high perfusion pressure. With the Kiil system a pressure gradient is achieved by lowering the pressure in the dialysis fluid compartment by a simple siphon mechanism.

Dialysis Fluid. The composition of dialysis fluid is fairly standard, although different centers vary the concentration, particularly those of sodium potassium and calcium. The usual concentrations are as follows: sodium 134.0 mEq. per liter; potassium, 2.6 mEq. per liter; calcium, 2.5 mEq. per liter; magnesium, 1.5 mEq. per liter; chloride, 104.0 mEq. per liter; sodium acetate, 36.6 mEq. per liter, and anhydrous dextrose, U. S. P. 2.0 grams per liter.

A potassium-free bath may be used under certain circumstances, and some centers prefer a bath calcium concentration of 3 mEq. per liter, which achieves a positive dialysis calcium balance. Sodium concentrations are also varied in relation to blood pressure control.

Dialysate Supply Systems. Central fluid supply for eight or ten dialyzers has been widely used in the past, and is still useful for center dialysis in patients awaiting transplants.

Recent development has been mainly related to home dialysis units. Dialysate supply systems satisfactory for use in the home must be fully monitored for safety, and units are usually compact proportioning pump units which mix tap water and fluid concentrate in the correct proportions for delivery to the dialyzer. They include safety monitors for conductivity which will detect change in dialysate concentration, temperature, and blood leaks, and can thus be used without supervision in the home.

PROBLEMS ASSOCIATED WITH MAINTENANCE DIALYSIS

Cost. The major barrier to effective use of dialysis for the treatment of chronic renal failure is the cost.

Diet. The main dietary requirements for maintenance dialysis are restriction of protein, sodium, potassium, and water. Of these, restriction of sodium and water are the most troublesome to the patient. Sodium is usually restricted to 500 mg. per day. This requires salt-free bread, butter, and milk as well as no salt added to any foods. Potassium is restricted to 2.5 grams per day; departure from this restriction may cause a lethal rise in the serum potassium between dialyses.

Shunt Problems. Even in the most experienced centers *clotting* in Teflon-Silastic shunts has been a serious problem. Average shunt survival times have varied from four to nine months, but have been as short as 25 days in some units. Considerable restriction of physical activities have been necessary to protect the shunt, and patients are taught to regard this as their lifeline. The procedure of declotting a shunt may be associated with serious permanent and at times fatal neurologic complications due to retrograde embolization of the cerebral vessels. Shunt *infections* are also common

and potentially serious. They often lead to thrombosis and occasionally cause septicemia.

The frequency of shunt infections and clotting have led to the increasing use of internal arteriovenous fistulas for maintenance hemodialysis in the home as well as in hospital. These permit a more normal active life with participation in physical activities previously prohibited, as well as removal of anxiety about the shunt and reduction of the incidence of infection. The disadvantage of this method is that a blood pump must be used to achieve a blood flow of 200 ml. per minute through needles inserted into the anastomotic arteriovenous channels.

Hepatitis. Hepatitis is perhaps the greatest single threat to the use of maintenance dialysis. Few units which have functioned for more than two or three years have avoided outbreaks of hepatitis among patients and staff. In a single outbreak 50 per cent or more of the patients may contract the disease, and deaths among members of staff have been a feature. Both infectious hepatitis and serum hepatitis have been suspected in different outbreaks. The high occurrence rate of hepatitis on dialysis units is probably related to frequent contact with blood as well as the repeated contact between the same group of patients and staff over very long periods of time. Risks from contaminated equipment can be avoided by using separate Kiil plates for each patient. The staff should wear gloves and gowns and should not eat or smoke in the dialysis area. Patients' bed clothes and excreta should be dealt with in such a way as to eliminate the risk of spread of infection.

The prophylactic use of immunoglobulin probably protects the staff against infectious hepatitis, although there is some doubt about its value in serum hepatitis. Routine screening tests for Australia antigen are being used at present in our unit, and this has led to the detection of hepatitis in two patients before the serum transaminase or serum bilirubin showed any abnormality. Early transfer of such patients to separate isolation facilities may reduce the spread of infection within the unit.

It was hoped that home dialysis would put an end to the problem of hepatitis in patients on maintenance dialysis. However, a recent outbreak of hepatitis in a large home dialysis service in the United Kingdom has affected many patients. Thus it appears that they too run this risk.

PROBLEMS THAT APPLY PARTICULARLY TO HOME DIALYSIS

The difficulties of home dialysis may have been underrated; there are certain factors which may limit its widespread use.

High Capital Cost. The initial capital cost for home dialysis is far greater than that for center dialysis. Each patient must have his own dialyzing unit, and this should be fully automatic and must be fully monitored. The cost of such units is still about $5000. In addition, alterations to the home will cost $500 to $1000.

Apart from the cost of the equipment, certain socioeconomic standards must be met for home dialysis to be a practical proposition, and this automatically limits the number of suitable patients in most communities.

Suitability of Patients for Home Dialysis. The patient must be psychologically stable and sufficiently intelligent and cooperative to become fully independent in all aspects of dialysis; thus children and adolescents are unsuitable. A cooperative spouse or other close relative is another essential requirement. Because it is difficult to persuade patients on hospital dialysis to accept the extra work and responsibility of dialysis in the home, a program aimed at home dialysis from the start, in which the patient participates fully in dialysis techniques in hospital in the training period, is essential.

Influence of Home Dialysis on the Family. Dialysis in the home has a profound impact on the family. Major psychological problems associated with a home dialysis program have been reported in the spouse and other members of the family in as many as 25 per cent of relatives in one series.

DIALYSIS PROBLEMS RELATED TO RENAL FAILURE

The reported pre- and postdialysis serum creatinine levels vary in different units. Acceptable figures in experienced units may be as high as 14 to 16 mg. per 100 ml. before dialysis and 4 to 6 mg. per 100 ml. after dialysis. This serves as a reminder that patients on maintenance dialysis have the biochemical features of persistent moderate-to-severe renal failure. In view of the constant elevation of blood urea and serum creatinine, it is not surprising that problems associated with renal failure may arise.

Anemia. This major problem of maintenance dialysis can be treated by repeated transfusion, but transfusions increase the risk of hepatitis and of hemosiderosis. They also increase the likelihood of rejection of subsequent kidney grafts because of the formation of leukocyte antibodies which react with histocompatibility antigens.

For these reasons and also because of cost, blood transfusions are now given only for acute blood loss or major symptoms attributable to anemia. The packed cell volume is usually below 20 if patients are not transfused, but it may rise gradually after some months at this level. The anemia is due to increased destruction and decreased production of red cells, and although serum iron and folate levels may be low, no response is seen when iron and folic acid supplements are given.

Renal Osteodystrophy and Metastatic Calcification. This complication of chronic uremia has been prominent in most maintenance dialysis programs. Progressive decalcification of bone and increasing metastatic calcification together with other typical radiologic features of renal osteodystrophy may occur in about half the patients on maintenance hemodialysis. Although most authors have reported that these abnormalities could not be controlled by dialysis, some claim improvement with adequate dialysis. The level of calcium in the dialysis fluid may be important in determining the onset and severity of renal osteodystrophy. It has been claimed that lesions will heal when a positive dialysis calcium balance is achieved by raising the dialysis fluid calcium from 2.5 mEq. per liter to 3.0 mEq. per liter. The plasma phosphate level should be controlled by administration of aluminum hydroxide so that the calcium phosphate product does not exceed 75. A combination of these measures together with longer and more frequent dialysis seems to have led to the disappearance of serious metastatic calcification in patients on dialysis.

Recurrent arthritis associated with progressive periarticular calcification is now rarely seen, probably because of more adequate dialysis and control of the calcium phosphate product by aluminum hydroxide administration.

Frank osteomalacia may develop if the plasma phosphate level is allowed to fall too low either spontaneously or following aluminum hydroxide.

Peripheral Neuropathy. This complication of chronic uremia was prominent in early reports of patients on maintenance dialysis. It is now clear that symptomatic peripheral neuropathy is related to inadequate dialysis and does not develop with current dialysis methods.

Nerve conduction times are abnormal in far more patients than those presenting with symptoms of peripheral neuropathy. These do not invariably improve on dialysis although they may do so.

CONTROL OF THE BLOOD PRESSURE ON DIALYSIS

In view of the great fluctuations in response to hypotensive drugs in the pre- and postdialysis periods, a reduction of sodium and water intake provides a more satisfactory method of controlling the blood pressure in patients on dialysis.

It is usual to reduce the patient's weight in the early weeks of dialysis by reduction in the salt and water intake and increased removal of water during dialysis by ultrafiltration. When the blood pressure is normal in the predialysis period, an attempt is made to maintain the weight at this level. This is sometimes called the optimal dry weight. In a small number of patients the blood pressure remains difficult to control, and in such patients bilateral nephrectomy may have a dramatic effect. After operation the blood pressure is lower and permits a more generous salt and water intake between dialyses. Patients with blood pressure resistant to control by salt and water depletion alone may show very high renin activity in the serum.

PSYCHOLOGICAL PROBLEMS ASSOCIATED WITH MAINTENANCE DIALYSIS

Like other patients with fatal illnesses patients on dialysis commonly develop reactive depression which, if it becomes excessive, may lead to frank psychosis. Severe anxiety depression and suicidal reactions are commonly described, and may seriously interfere with successful institution of dialysis.

After starting on dialysis, anxieties and problems are often related to the arteriovenous shunt on which so much depends.

Some psychological problems are undoubtedly related to the financial stress of maintenance dialysis. Private individuals can rarely afford this form of treatment, and there are only a few countries in which the total costs are provided by the state. Even if the actual costs are met, the earning capacity of any particular dialysis patient is likely to be reduced even when full rehabilitation is possible.

REHABILITATION

Most people who have been on dialysis for a period of a few months are able to return to full employment. Anemia and external shunts exclude them from certain forms of occupation, particularly those that are physically demanding.

CONCLUDING REMARKS

By far the most attractive way of dealing with the problem of chronic renal failure in the community is by prevention. Rapid advances in all aspects of nephrology make it likely that the number of patients presenting for treatment of irreversible renal failure will be considerably reduced by applying known methods of treatment of renal disease. Improved methods of treatment are likely to result from research in the renal field.

An aggressive and active approach to the treatment of early renal failure will considerably reduce the need for dialysis and transplantation within a particular hospital.

The importance of prevention in dealing with the problem of renal failure in the community cannot be overemphasized, and any provision for the treatment of end-stage renal disease would be shortsighted if it did not also provide for research into new methods of treatment and proper application of present methods of treatment of renal disease.

Treatment of terminal renal failure presents a serious public health problem because of the very high costs of treatment for each patient and the fact that both dialysis and transplantation carry with them a high mortality and morbidity risk. Indeed, the results of conservative treatment may be better in some forms of renal disease than the application of the dramatic and expensive methods of dialysis and transplantation. This is particularly true in conditions that may gradually improve, such as analgesic nephropathy.

Experience has shown that only a program whose primary aim is the provision of a suitably matched cadaver allograft for every patient can adequately meet the needs of the community in relation to irreversible renal failure. Maintenance dialysis has an important part to play in keeping prospective recipients alive until a suitable donor is found. It will also be required as a definitive form of treatment for a small number of patients unsuitable for transplantation for immunologic or medical reasons, but because of the reduced costs of home dialysis such patients should be trained for treatment in the home.

Burton, B. J.: Kidney Disease. Program Analysis. A Report to the Surgeon General. U. S. Public Health Service Publication. No. 1754, 1967.

Curtis, J. R., Eastwood, J. B., Smith, E. K. M., Storey, J. M., Vermont, P. J., de Wardener, H. E., Wing, A. J., and Wolfson, E. M.: Maintenance hemodialysis. Quart. J. Med. (N. S.), 38:49, 1969.

Gottschalk, C. W.: Report of the Committee on Chronic Kidney Disease to the U. S. Bureau of the Budget, 1967.

Kincaid-Smith, P.: Modification of the vascular lesions of rejection in cadaveric renal allografts by dipyridamole and anticoagulants. Lancet, 2:266, 1969.

Moorhead, J. E., Baillod, R. A., and Hopewell, J. P.: Home Dialysis. Proceedings, Fourth International Congress of Nephrology (in press).

Porter, K. A.: Tissue and organ transplantation. J. Clin. Path., 20 (Suppl.), 1967.

Rapaport, F. T., and Dausset, J.: Human Transplantation. New York and London, Grune & Stratton, Inc., 1968.

Walford, R. L.: The isoantigenic systems of human leucocytes. Series Haematologica, 2:1, 1969.

Glomerular Disease
O. M. Wrong

INTRODUCTION

Diseases which affect mainly glomeruli display such important features in common that they can usefully be considered together and contrasted with diseases commencing in other parts of the kidney. Numerically glomerular disease accounts for approximately half of the patients with severe renal disease seen in most communities, and over two thirds of the patients accepted for renal replacement by units undertaking intermittent hemodialysis or renal transplantation.

Each glomerulus consists of a complex branching system of capillaries, and, thus, even though these capillaries are highly specialized, glomerular disease can be regarded as a form of capillary disease. In many forms of glomerular disease small blood vessels in other parts of the body are also diseased, but because the glomerular circulation is particularly vulnerable to pathologic insult the effects of renal damage often dominate the clinical picture. Many glomerular diseases, particularly the inflammations, are the result of an antigen-antibody reaction; others are degenerative or infiltrative, e.g., diabetic renal disease, amyloid, Fabry's disease.

Most forms of glomerular disease are macroscopically diffuse, affecting equally the cortex of both kidneys, and one part of the cortex as severely as another. Consequently the small amount of material which can be removed by percutaneous renal biopsy usually yields a histologic picture which is representative of the kidneys as a whole, and this investigation has been valuable in both diagnosis and study of the natural history of glomerular disease. Histologically glomerular lesions may be either *diffuse,* involving all parts of all glomeruli, or *focal,* affecting only some glomeruli or glomerular segments, and these topographic distinctions are of help in categorizing glomerular disease further.

Proteinuria. Increased loss of protein in the urine, in excess of the 30 to 130 mg. per day excreted normally, is almost an invariable accompaniment of glomerular disease; it is a direct result of increased glomerular permeability to plasma proteins caused by the disease process. The amount of protein lost in the urine is often much greater than in other forms of renal disease. In practice it is found that losses of more than 3 grams per day are not seen except in glomerular disease, and this finding therefore has great diagnostic value. The main urinary protein is always albumin, but variable amounts of the other plasma proteins are also lost, depending on the type of glomerular disease. When urinary protein losses of more than 5 grams a day persist, hepatic synthesis may not be able to increase sufficiently to maintain the serum albumin, and hypoalbuminemic edema may result. The triad of proteinuria, hypoalbuminemia, and edema is known as *nephrotic syndrome,* and is discussed in detail later.

Hypertension. Hypertension may complicate any form of renal disease, but is particularly common and severe in glomerular disease, although even here it is not invariable. It is now known that renal hypertension has at least two causes: (1) increased secretion of renin by the juxtaglomerular apparatus (JGA), and (2) increased extracellular fluid and blood volume caused by diminished renal ability to excrete salt and water, e.g., the "renoprival" hypertension that follows bilateral nephrectomy. Both factors play a part in the hypertension of glomerular disease, but their relative contributions differ from case to case. The JGA may be directly involved, or rendered ischemic, by the primary disease, and hypertension may be caused by resultant hypersecretion of renin. When glomerular disease has led to renal failure, a renoprival type of hypertension may develop simply from failure to excrete salt and water. The development of severe hypertension in glomerular disease is an ominous sign, as it leads to further damage from the effects of hypertension on the renal circulation. Prompt control of hypertension is therefore of vital importance in the care of such patients.

Sodium Loss. Patients with glomerular disease only rarely show a renal sodium-losing tendency. Experiments involving dietary sodium deprivation have shown that patients with glomerular disease are often unable to reduce urinary losses of sodium as efficiently as normal subjects, but their obligatory losses are usually well below the amount supplied by a normal diet, and it is exceptional for a sodium supplement to be required. The clinical demonstration of renal sodium-wasting in a patient with renal disease is therefore evidence against glomerular disease, and particularly suggests pyelonephritis or obstructive renal disease.

In clinical practice use of the aforementioned principles will usually distinguish glomerular disease from other forms of renal disease. However, it is frequently difficult to distinguish between different forms of glomerular disease, even with the assistance of all modern diagnostic laboratory aids. To some extent this is the result of artificial distinctions between so-called disease entities, which may represent merely groups of commonly associated clinical features, rather than the results of distinct etiologic processes. But the problem is also due to the very limited way in which glomeruli can respond to different pathologic insults, which means that the same histologic and clinical picture may result from several different pathologic processes.

GLOMERULONEPHRITIS

Definition. Although the term "glomerulonephritis" has been loosely applied to almost all types of glomerular disease, its use is usually confined to those forms characterized by an inflammatory reaction, with leukocytic infiltration and cellular proliferation of the glomeruli, and exudation of erythrocytes, leukocytes, and plasma protein into Bowman's space. In chronic forms of glomerulonephritis the inflammatory element is less apparent, and cellular proliferation, glomerular adhesions, and scarring are the most conspicuous histologic features; these changes are thought to represent a less acute and more prolonged form of the same type of glomerular disease.

Etiology. Repeated attempts to isolate microorganisms from the lesions of glomerulonephritis have failed, and the disease is not considered to be a direct result of bacterial invasion of the kidneys. It is more difficult to exclude the role of viruses, but at present there is no good evidence that any form of human glomerulonephritis is caused by the presence of viruses in the glomeruli.

The detailed pathogenesis of glomerulonephritis is still obscure, but there is considerable evidence that an antigen-antibody reaction plays a part in initiating the glomerular lesions in most forms of glomerulonephritis. The evidence can be summarized as (1) demonstration of complexes of antigen-antibody and complement either on or within the glomerular basement membrane in many forms of glomerulonephritis; (2) marked lowering of serum β_1C globulin (the third factor of complement) in many cases of active nephritis; and (3) experimental production of glomerular lesions resembling human glomerulonephritis either by injections of anti-kidney antibodies prepared from other species or of nonspecific antigen or antigen-antibody complexes.

There is still disagreement on the exact form of immune injury to the glomeruli in the different forms of glomerular disease, and the evidence will be discussed under the appropriate titles. It is generally agreed that the presence of products of an antigen-antibody reaction, whether or not the reaction primarily involves glomerular antigen, initiates an inflammatory response with cellular proliferation, leukocytic infiltration, and phagocytosis. In addition thromboplastic material is liberated within the glomerular capillaries, leading to the formation of fibrin and platelet clots in the capillary lumen with further impairment of glomerular function. Erythrocytes circulating through damaged glomerular capillaries may themselves be damaged, with resultant intravascular hemolysis and the appearance of fragmented and distorted red cells in the peripheral blood film. These changes have been described as *microangiopathic hemolytic anemia,* or more dramatically as the "Waring Blendor syndrome." Marked hemolytic anemia and thrombocytopenia are usually indications that the underlying vascular disease has involved tissues in addition to the kidney, as in the Moschcowitz and hemolytic-uremic syndromes.

Logical therapeutic attempts to interrupt the aforementioned sequence have included cytotoxic drugs (such as the nitrogen mustards, cyclophosphamide, and azathioprine) to reduce antibody formation, steroids or other anti-inflammatory agents to reduce the effect of immune injury on the kidney, and anticoagulants to lessen the secondary intravascular coagulation. Such rational forms of therapy have in general proved disappointing; the occasional success is mentioned when appropriate.

Brain, M. C., Dacie, J. V., and Hourihane, D. O.: Microangiopathic haemolytic anaemia: The possible role of vascular lesions in pathogenesis. Brit. J. Haemat., 8:358, 1962.

Dixon, F. J.: The pathogenesis of nephritis. Amer. J. Med., 44: 493, 1968.

Heptinstall, R. H.: Pathology of the Kidney. Boston, Little, Brown and Company, 1966.

ACUTE POST-STREPTOCOCCAL GLOMERULONEPHRITIS

This is the best documented and most understood form of glomerulonephritis. Although its course is complex and variable, it does demonstrate almost all the possible features of glomerular disease, and therefore has served in the past as the usual starting point and reference in discussing glomerulonephritis. To some extent this emphasis has been unfortunate in that it has tended to delay recognition of the many forms of glomerulonephritis which are unrelated to the Streptococcus, and which are now becoming relatively more important because of the falling incidence of streptococcal infection. However, post-streptococcal nephritis is still common enough to deserve emphasis in its own right. Hence this article is deliberately detailed, whereas the articles on other forms of glomerulonephritis are brief and stress particularly how they differ from the post-streptococcal variety.

Etiology. In 1836 Richard Bright recognized that acute glomerulonephritis usually followed an infection, particularly scarlet fever. Since then scarlet fever has become much less common, and the incidence of post-scarlatina nephritis has likewise fallen. It is now recognized that acute nephritis can follow streptococcal infection in any part of the body, although the pharynx is the usual site, and is unrelated to the production of erythrotoxin by the organism. Only certain strains of Streptococcus are "nephritogenic" (capable of initiating nephritis); all the offending organisms are group A β-hemolytic streptococci, and the majority are of type 12. Other less common nephritogenic strains are types 1, 4, 25, 41, and 49 (Red Lake strain); the last has been incriminated in outbreaks of streptococcal pyoderma causing nephritis.

Symptoms of acute glomerulonephritis do not usually develop until 7 to 20 days after the streptococcal infection, by which time the patient appears to have recovered from the local infection. Transitory mild proteinuria and microscopic hematuria are common during the initial streptococcal infection, particularly in persons who subsequently develop clinical nephritis, but it is not clear whether these are the first manifestations of nephritis or merely represent the urinary changes common in any severe infection. The long delay, before full manifestations of the disease appear, does suggest that the renal disease is not a direct result of streptococcal toxins, but depends on a reaction on the part of the host which takes some days to develop. The marked reduction in serum $\beta_1 C$ globulin and the more recent finding that the glomerular lesions contain complexes of gamma globulin (particularly IgG) and complement both suggest that the disease is a result of an antigen–antibody reaction. There are two differing views on the nature of this reaction; the first is that, because of an antigenic similarity between the Streptococcus and glomerular basement membrane, antibody formed as a consequence of the streptococcal infection reacts against the glomerulus, much as an anti-kidney serum causes nephritis when injected into an animal. The second view, at present marginally favored, is that nephritis is a form of immune-complex disease, which results from the formation in the plasma of complexes of streptococcal antigen, human antibody, and complement; these complexes are deposited in the glomeruli where they cause an inflammatory response. There is experimental evidence to support both views, but much work remains to be done before the story is complete.

Incidence. Acute post-streptococcal nephritis occurs in all parts of the world. Males are affected about twice as frequently as females. No age is exempt, but the disease is particularly common in children and adolescents, perhaps because of the increased risk of acquiring a streptococcal infection from exposure at school. In temperate climates the disease is most common in the winter months, when streptococcal infections are at their peak. The relationship of acute nephritis to certain streptococcal strains explains some epidemiologic features of the disease, such as its tendency to cause small epidemics in homes or schools, as well as the variations in incidence in persons known to have had streptococcal infections—from nil with a non-nephritogenic strain to as high as 40 per cent with a strain known to be highly nephritogenic. By contrast the incidence of rheumatic fever in those with streptococcal infections who have not previously had the disease is fairly constant at 2 to 3 per cent.

Pathology. Acute nephritis is rarely fatal, and most knowledge of its pathology comes from material obtained by biopsy. The occasional necropsy has shown symmetrical renal enlargement and pallor of the cortex. Histologically the glomeruli are nearly all similarly affected, with enlargement of the whole glomerulus and marked increase in the number of nucleated cells, consisting mainly of endothelial and mesangial cells and mononuclear leukocytes, although polymorphonuclears are prominent early in the course of the disease. The glomerular lobules are swollen and relatively bloodless, with reduced capillary lumina and scanty erythrocytes and occasional necrotic and thrombosed capillary loops. Electron microscopy shows the presence of humps of what appear to be antigen–antibody complement complexes adhering to the outside of the capillary basement membrane, but in general the basement membrane does not show marked change.

Even within the first two or three weeks of a clinical attack of post-streptococcal nephritis, renal biopsy may show proliferation of the cells lining Bowman's capsule, with adhesions and early crescent formation. However, this change is more characteristic of the subacute and chronic forms of the disease described below, and is not conspicuous in biopsies from patients who subsequently appear to make a complete recovery. The more usual course is for all histologic features to resolve slowly; one of the last features to remain is slight hypercellularity, most marked in the vicinity of the glomerular stalk or mesangium, in which it may be detectable several months after apparently complete clinical recovery.

Clinical Manifestations. Most patients have a fairly clear history of preceding streptococcal infection. Usually the infection is a pharyngitis which has been sufficiently severe to keep the patient away from school or work, but occasionally the infection lies elsewhere—for example, an otitis media, a leg ulcer, or a surgical wound. Sometimes the infection can only be demonstrated by a positive bacteriologic culture, or presumed from the finding of a raised anti-streptolysin O titer.

The patient has usually recovered from the initial infection when manifestations of nephritis appear, some 7 to 20 days after onset of the original infection. The most common presenting symptom is edema, noted particularly in the face on first arising. Hematuria is also a common first symptom; usually the urine has a smoky brown color, but occasionally it is frankly blood-stained. Less commonly the patient complains of reduced urine output, or of bilateral dull loin pain, which is probably caused by stretching of the renal capsules.

It is important to note that the edema present at the onset of the disease is invariably caused by fluid retention, which itself is the result of reduced renal excretion of salt and water. In an adult of average size the presence of generalized edema implies a weight gain of at least 5 kg. At this stage patients have not lost enough protein in the urine to develop hypoalbuminemic edema (nephrotic syndrome), although this complication may develop later; nor is there any good evidence for the earlier views that the edema of acute nephritis is caused either by increased capillary permeability or by heart failure.

Vague malaise, nausea, and headache are common in acute nephritis, but fever is unusual, and patients do not usually feel really ill, although they are often distressed by the appearance of edema. In mild cases the patient may be quite asymptomatic; the disease may be picked up only by examining the urine of a person known to have had a recent streptococcal infection.

Physical examination usually shows generalized edema and mild hypertension of the order of 140 to 160 systolic, 90 to 110 diastolic. Very occasionally hypertension is severe, with retinal hemorrhages and exudates, papilledema, or hypertensive encephalopathy. Fluid retention, if marked, may lead to the signs of congestive cardiac failure, with cardiac enlargement and triple rhythm, venous engorgement, hepatic distention, and gross pulmonary and systemic edema.

Urine output is usually reduced, although the reduction is often not noticed by the patient. Complete suppression of urine is rare, and indicates a very severe attack of nephritis; this complication may develop within a few days of the onset, or urine output may gradually fall to nothing over several weeks. As might be expected, fluid retention is particularly severe in such cases, and unless rigid restriction of sodium and water has been instituted early, edema and hypertension are particularly marked. Unless renal function returns rapidly, the symptoms of renal failure eventually appear, with nausea and vomiting, twitching and pruritus, acidotic respirations, and progressive anemia.

Urine. Urinary concentration is usually in the range of 350 to 600 mOsm. per kilogram (corresponding to a specific gravity of 1.014 to 1.020 when correction is made for protein content), but appears more concentrated because of the presence of red cells. Moderate quantities of protein are present, and occasionally mild renal glycosuria occurs. The urinary deposit contains large numbers of red cells and leukocytes, particularly the former, and a smaller number of renal tubular cells. Casts, particularly the granular variety, are also present; erythrocyte and hemoglobin casts indicate bleeding into the tubules, and are particularly suggestive of acute glomerulonephritis.

Laboratory Tests. Mild renal failure, with blood urea (not BUN) concentrations of 40 to 150 mg. per 100 ml., is very common in the initial stage of the disease. Conventional tests of glomerular function show the expected reduction in clearance values. In the rare case of severe renal failure the biochemical sequelae are similar to those of renal failure from other causes except that

hyperkalemia seems particularly common, probably because these patients are usually previously fit and active young people who rapidly lose muscle mass during their illness.

A nephritogenic strain of Streptococcus can be cultured from the pharynx of many patients, except those treated with effective antimicrobial drugs, even when all clinical evidence of local infection has disappeared. Occasionally cultures taken from the throats of other members of the family will reveal the presence of a nephritogenic Streptococcus when this can no longer be cultured from the patient's own throat.

The serum anti-streptolysin O titer is usually raised, indicating recent streptococcal infection, but the titer may fall rapidly to normal and so pass unnoticed, or it may not rise at all if the streptococcal infection is rapidly aborted by use of antimicrobials. Unfortunately, as has been pointed out by Rammelkamp, not all nephritogenic strains of streptococci produce streptolysin O (nor do they invariably cause β-hemolysis in culture), and so detection of the preceding streptococcal infection by this means may be difficult. The serum titer of type specific antibody to streptococcal M antigen is more difficult to measure, but remains raised for considerably longer after a streptococcal infection (often for years), and has the added advantage of indicating whether an infection was caused by a strain known to be nephritogenic. A marked drop in serum complement is characteristic of acute post-streptococcal nephritis, but this finding is not absolutely diagnostic as it may occur in other forms of nephritis, e.g., systemic lupus erythematosus and the nephritis of bacterial endocarditis, and few laboratories can provide the measurement as a routine.

The erythrocyte sedimentation rate is moderately raised. The hemoglobin concentration is usually slightly reduced (to 11 to 12 grams per 100 ml.) as a result of dilution. In addition a mild hemolytic anemia of microangiopathic type is seen in a few patients. In those who develop renal failure a normocytic normochromic type of anemia, owing to reduced erythropoiesis, appears after a few weeks.

Course and Prognosis. A diuresis usually starts 7 to 14 days after the onset of symptoms, and over the space of a few days the patient loses edema and hypertension. Renal clearances and the blood urea concentration return to normal, but microscopic hematuria and proteinuria persist longer, and may not disappear for weeks or months. During this period clinical relapses may occur, particularly at the time of nonspecific respiratory infections.

Occasionally urinary losses of protein during the first few weeks are sufficiently large to cause hypoalbuminemic edema, which first reveals itself when renal excretory function improves and the expected diuresis does not materialize. Although the development of nephrotic syndrome is of grave import if it first appears after several months, its rapid appearance at this early stage of the disease does not necessarily carry a bad prognosis, and patients with this syndrome may recover completely within the next few weeks.

It is difficult to ascertain what proportion of patients recover completely, for hospital series are weighted by the more severe cases. Most estimates state that 90 to 95 per cent of children and about 60 per cent of adults eventually make a full clinical recovery. But it is difficult to recognize when an individual patient has recovered, for microscopic hematuria and mild proteinuria, often postural, may disappear after as long as two years, and renal biopsy has sometimes shown mild but definite mesangial cellular proliferation in the glomeruli even when proteinuria has ceased. Indeed, it may be incorrect ever to talk about *complete* recovery, for even when *clinical* recovery has occurred months or years earlier, renal biopsy may show an occasional hyalinized glomerulus or glomerular segment clearly incapable of further recovery, although the rest of the renal biopsy has returned to normal.

In the early years of this century, post-streptococcal nephritis in the acute stage caused death in about 5 per cent of patients. Death was usually due to pulmonary edema, the complications of hypertension, or intercurrent infection. Nowadays these complications can usually be prevented, and most fatalities are the result of acute renal failure with anuria or severe oliguria. Even these patients can be kept alive by peritoneal dialysis or hemodialysis, and some patients so treated, particularly children, experience a return of renal function after days or weeks. If renal recovery does not ensue, or is inadequate to maintain life, and renal biopsy shows irrecoverable glomerular damage, patients may be treated by intermittent hemodialysis. Renal transplantation has also been used, but at the present time most centers are avoiding this form of treatment, as there is evidence that the transplanted kidney may develop acute glomerulonephritis.

The most distressing cases of glomerulonephritis are those in which the patients survive the acute illness but do not recover completely, and enter a phase of subacute or chronic glomerulonephritis, in which the glomerular lesions progress inexorably, with increasing cellular proliferation, crescent formation, scarring and eventual glomerular hyalinization. This process may take a few weeks or last many years, and for long periods there may be no apparent progression in the disease. In a few patients the disease appears to become completely inactive after months or years, leaving the patient with some degree of renal failure or hypertension. However, the usual course is one of slow deterioration. During this period sudden transient exacerbations of hematuria and decreased renal function may occur, usually in association with nonspecific systemic infections.

Unfavorable features which suggest that satisfactory recovery will not take place are (1) delayed or absent diuresis, (2) persistent renal failure, (3) persistent hypertension, (4) prolonged or increasing proteinuria, often leading to the nephrotic syndrome, and (5) severe changes in the renal biopsy, particularly obliteration of Bowman's space by epithelial crescents and disappearance of glomerular capillaries.

Patients who recover from acute glomerulonephritis are not immune to second attacks, but these are uncommon because of the development of type-specific antibodies which protect against infection by the original strain of Streptococcus and exert an effect for many years. Most apparent second attacks of acute post-streptococcal glomerulonephritis are in reality exacerbations of a long-standing chronic glomerulonephritis.

Diagnosis. The condition most easily confused with acute post-streptococcal nephritis is exacerbation of a subacute or chronic glomerulonephritis, with transitory hematuria and further reduction in renal function. Such exacerbations may be precipitated by many different infections, even those caused by viruses, but are particularly common after streptococcal infection; and in the absence of previous evidence of renal disease this situation closely resembles an initial attack of post-streptococcal nephritis. Features suggestive of chronic nephritis are the absence of an interval between infection and renal symptoms, and the presence of renal failure, severe hypertension, or hypoalbuminemia early in the attack. Subsequent complete disappearance of all features of renal disease suggests a post-streptococcal nephritis.

The transient proteinuria and microscopic hematuria that accompany many severe systemic infections may also be mistaken for post-streptococcal nephritis, but these signs occur at the height of the infection, and are not usually associated with other features of renal disease.

It may be difficult to distinguish acute post-streptococcal nephritis from other forms of acute glomerulonephritis, such as Henoch-Schönlein nephritis (which may also be precipitated by a streptococcal infection) systemic lupus erythematosus, the microscopic form of polyarteritis nodosa, recurrent focal nephritis with hematuria, and the nephritis of bacterial endocarditis. Here the physician will be guided by features suggesting systemic involvement and by evidence of recent streptococcal infection. Renal biopsy may also help by showing a glomerular lesion more focal than that of post-streptococcal nephritis.

Less often, acute post-streptococcal nephritis may be confused with primary malignant hypertension, with various forms of hemolytic anemia with hemoglobinuria, or with acute tubular necrosis, particularly when the latter is precipitated by a systemic infection. A more serious error is to overlook some surgical cause of hematuria, such as renal calculus or acute pyelonephritis. An intravenous pyelogram may be required to exclude such possibilities.

Treatment. It has not been convincingly shown that any form of treatment alters the course of the glomerular lesion, but individual manifestations and complications frequently require treatment.

Infection. In the acute stage penicillin is usually given either by mouth or injection to eradicate any remaining streptococcal infection; this treatment has much to commend it, but there is no evidence that it alters the subsequent evolution of the glomerular disease. Penicillin should also be used prophylactically to treat close contacts, particularly members of the family who may have contracted streptococcal infection from the patient, unless this possibility is excluded by bacteriologic tests. Oral penicillin V (phenoxymethyl penicillin, 250 mg. twice a day) is often recommended after attacks of acute nephritis to reduce subsequent respiratory infections which might cause exacerbations of nephritis; if used it is best continued through the next winter season when streptococcal infections are rife.

Edema. Fluid retention during the oliguric phase of the disease should be prevented by careful attention to body weight. Salt and fluids should be restricted if edema is present or a weight gain of more than 2 to 3 kg. occurs. In these circumstances oral fluids should be limited to no more than 500 ml. per day, plus a volume equal to the urine output of the previous day, and dietary sodium should be reduced as far as possible, preferably to 20 mEq. per day. If severe edema is already present, or develops despite these measures, a diuresis may occasionally be obtained by oral diuretics, particularly furosemide in doses of 40 to 500 mg. twice a day. Digitalis is ineffective in this situation, despite the presence of many classic features of congestive cardiac failure, because the circulatory troubles are due to excess of extracellular fluid, and not to a primary cardiac cause. In the rare case in which fluid overload threatens life, and diuresis cannot be obtained by drugs, the excess fluid should be removed by dialysis.

Uremia. There is no convincing evidence that dietary protein influences the course of the glomerular lesion, but early in the disease it is wise to restrict protein intake moderately (40 to 70 grams per day) until it is clear that the patient is not likely to develop renal failure. Patients who do develop severe renal failure should be treated by more drastic protein restriction, with or without some form of dialysis, as described in the article on renal failure.

Hypertension. If fluid retention is carefully controlled, there is usually no need to treat hypertension specifically. But the patient with severe fluid overload may require treatment for hypertensive encephalopathy with convulsions, or retinopathy with failing vision; in these emergencies parenteral hydralazine, reserpine, or diazoxide are the drugs of choice.

Other Drugs. Steroids, anticoagulants, and cytotoxic drugs, either alone or in various combinations, have been used in the acute stage of the disease, particularly in patients with severe renal failure, but there is no good evidence that they alter the outcome.

Rest. In the acute stage of the disease bed rest is advisable. The patient does not usually wish to be active, and the recumbent position facilitates diuresis. Once macroscopic hematuria, edema, and hypertension have disappeared and the blood urea has returned to normal, the value of rest is uncertain. Many authorities recommend that bed rest continue as long as proteinuria is diminishing, but there is no evidence that this alters the course of the disease, and it may be impractical or economically disastrous for the patient whose proteinuria persists for months.

Continued Observation. Because of the difficulty in deciding when a patient has recovered from the disease, it is valuable to follow all patients until at least a year after the last clinical evidence of nephritis. Frequent determination of blood pressure, urinary protein and deposit, and blood urea concentration are the most useful indications of disease activity. The purpose of this follow-up is to observe any exacerbation of the disease, so that renal failure, nephrotic syndrome, or hypertension can be immediately recognized and treated. Acute urinary infections, which are common in such patients, can also be recognized and treated.

Bright, R.: *In* Osman, A. A. (ed.): Original Papers of Richard Bright on Renal Disease. London, Oxford University Press, 1937.

Dodge, W. F., Spargo, B. H., Bass, J. A., and Travis, L. B.: The relationship between the clinical and pathologic features of poststreptococcal glomerulonephritis. A study of the early natural history. Medicine, 47:227, 1968.

Jennings, R. B., and Earle, D. P.: Post-streptococcal glomerulonephritis: Histopathologic and clinical studies of the acute, subsiding acute and early chronic latent phases. J. Clin. Invest., 40:1525, 1961.

Kassirer, J. P., and Schwartz, W. B.: Acute glomerulonephritis. New Eng. J. Med., 265:686, 736, 1961.

McCluskey, R. T., and Baldwin, D. S.: Natural history of acute glomerulonephritis. Amer. J. Med., 35:213, 1963.

Rammelkamp, C. H.: Etiology of glomerulonephritis. *In* Black, D. A. K. (ed.): Renal Disease. 2nd ed. Oxford, Blackwell Scientific Publications, 1967, p. 209.

OTHER FORMS OF ACUTE DIFFUSE GLOMERULONEPHRITIS

Frequently patients with acute glomerulonephritis show no evidence of a preceding streptococcal infection, even though in almost every other way their disease is typical of post-streptococcal nephritis. It is impossible to be sure that any patient has *not* had a streptococcal infection, and probably many of these patients have had an infection which cannot be detected in retrospect. However, it is now recognized that an acute glomerulonephritis may follow infections caused by microorganisms other than streptococci. It seems likely, from a consideration of the probable pathogenesis, that human glomerulonephritis may, like the experimental model, be precipitated by exposure to a variety of foreign proteins, which need not be exclusively of infective origin.

When pneumococcal pneumonia was a common disease, before the advent of antimicrobial drugs, it was frequently reported to be a cause of acute glomerulonephritis. The disease was similar to the post-streptococcal variety, except that the latent interval was shorter and fluid retention and hypertension were less apparent. In most instances the possibility of a complicating streptococcal infection was not adequately excluded, and there must be considerable doubt as to the existence of such an entity.

Acute glomerulonephritis has also been reported after typhoid fever and diphtheria, and after many virus infections—such as mumps, measles, chickenpox, infective hepatitis, mononucleosis, and infections with echovirus and adenovirus. Although in many instances a complicating streptococcal infection has not been excluded, the number of these reports is so great that it is difficult to accept that they all represent cases of post-streptococcal nephritis. In several recent cases a renal biopsy has been obtained, or the patient has come to necropsy, and morphologic glomerular changes very similar to those of post-streptococcal nephritis have been found.

The concept of an acute diffuse glomerulonephritis which results from non-streptococcal infections has thus been established, but it should be emphasized that nephritis is much rarer after these infections than it is after infections with nephritogenic strains of group A streptococci.

The natural history of glomerulonephritis caused by other than streptococcal infections is not fully known. The disease appears to behave like post-streptococcal nephritis in that the majority of patients recover completely, but a few are left with a continuing process with progressive impairment of renal function, which may be complicated by nephrotic syndrome or severe hypertension.

Leading article. Renal damage in chicken pox. Brit. Med. J., 3:264, 1968.
Seegal, D.: Acute glomerulonephritis following pneumococcic lobar pneumonia. Arch. Intern. Med. (Chicago), 56:912, 1935.

GLOMERULONEPHRITIS IN INFECTIVE ENDOCARDITIS

(Focal Embolic Nephritis)

The acute or subacute glomerulonephritis that complicates viridans endocarditis has often been regarded simply as a form of acute glomerulonephritis caused by streptococcal infection. This view is misleading for several reasons: (1) This strain of Streptococcus does not cause glomerulonephritis when it infects other parts of the body; (2) it is being increasingly realized, perhaps because of longer survival, that patients with other forms of infective endocarditis, e.g., pneumococcus, Staphylococcus, and *H. influenzae*, also develop glomerulonephritis; and (3) the glomerulonephritis of infective endocarditis is a mixture of a focal

and a diffuse glomerulonephritis, and can thus be distinguished histologically from post-streptococcal nephritis. A common alternative hypothesis, that the disease is caused by bacterial embolization to the glomeruli, would explain the focal glomerular lesions, but not the fact that bacteria cannot be demonstrated in the glomeruli or the diffuse glomerulonephritis. A more plausible explanation, in view of present evidence of the role of the immune process in glomerulonephritis, is that the renal lesions are caused by circulating antigen-antibody complexes initiated by bacterial antigen arising from the infected heart valves, and that embolization to some extent determines the distribution of these complexes among the glomeruli.

Patients with infective endocarditis do not usually show evidence of glomerulonephritis until they have had infection for several weeks, and the condition is therefore most common in patients with *Streptococcus viridans* endocarditis, and is not usually seen with infections which prove to be rapidly fatal. The condition presents with hematuria and proteinuria, and less frequently with impairment of renal function, which is often first mistakenly attributed to severe cardiac failure and resulting reduced renal perfusion. Hypoalbuminemic edema and hypertension have not been features of most reports. Severe renal failure is seldom seen except in patients in the terminal stage of a prolonged endocarditis.

In most cases the diagnosis presents no difficulty because the symptoms and signs of the underlying endocarditis are prominent. Rarely this is not so, and the disease may be confused with diffuse forms of vasculitis, such as polyarteritis or systemic lupus, because of fever and evidence of a systemic disease, necrotic and hemorrhagic skin lesions, or renal biopsy finding of a mixed focal and generalized glomerulonephritis. In such patients the true diagnosis may only be revealed by repeated blood culture, by the finding of splenomegaly, or by evidence of a cardiac lesion.

Successful treatment of the underlying valvular infection leads to healing of the glomerular lesions, with disappearance of the urinary findings and slow improvement in renal function when this is impaired.

RENAL INVOLVEMENT IN CONNECTIVE TISSUE DISEASES

Many generalized diseases of connective tissue may affect the kidney, where they cause glomerular lesions which may be very difficult to distinguish, either on clinical or histologic grounds, from other forms of glomerulonephritis.

Systemic Lupus Erythematosus. Here are found glomerular lesions which show pronounced focal distribution. The most common lesions are localized areas of cellular proliferation with underlying fibrinoid necrosis of part of a glomerular lobule, patchy thickening of the glomerular basement membrane ("wire loop" lesions), intracapillary hyaline thrombi, epithelial crescents, and glomerular scarring. Such lesions are not specific for lupus erythematosus, but their appearance in a patient with the serologic and systemic manifestations of the disease is sufficient to establish the diagnosis. (Hematoxylin bodies, although specific for the disease, frequently cannot be demonstrated in the glomerular lesions.) The diagnosis can be very difficult if extrarenal manifestations of the disease are unconvincing and the histologic picture is unusually diffuse, resembling post-streptococcal nephritis or idiopathic membranous glomerular disease.

Renal involvement may present clinically as a symptomless proteinuria which remains unchanged for months or years, with nephrotic syndrome, or with a severe progressive acute glomerulonephritis. Once renal failure has developed, the progress of the disease is usually one of steady deterioration, leading to death in renal failure within a few months. Treatment is unsatisfactory; steroids or cytotoxic drugs have often been used, and seem to help a few patients, particularly those in an active phase of their disease, but in most patients the progress of the disease is not altered, or is influenced only by very high doses that cause serious side effects.

Polyarteritis. Small arteries of the kidney may be affected, leading to macroscopic infarcts of the renal substance, or there may be the microscopic form described by Davson, Ball, and Platt, in which glomerular arterioles and capillaries are involved, leading to a glomerulonephritis which closely resembles acute post-streptococcal nephritis, but usually shows a more focal pattern.

The clinical presentation is protean and depends on what other tissues of the body are involved, as well as on the size of the affected arteries. Pulmonary involvement is common, usually presenting with hemoptysis; roentgenography shows fleeting areas of pulmonary infiltration or, more rarely, nodular lesions which may cavitate. Skin lesions are common and very helpful in diagnosis; most characteristic are small (2 to 4 mm.) tender cyanosed areas, representing infarcts, in the pulp of the fingers or toes. Fever and leukocytosis occur, out of proportion to the severity of any complicating infection. Occasionally the systemic manifestations are so mild that the true nature of the disease is not suspected until renal biopsy, in a patient with unexplained renal disease, shows characteristic glomerular or vascular lesions.

The renal presentation may be that of repeated renal infarction with local pain and hematuria, of chronic glomerulonephritis with proteinuria and steady reduction in renal function, or of severe oliguric acute nephritis. Renal hypertension is common.

Usually the course is progressive deterioration, particularly in those with the microscopic form of the disease. Large doses of steroids appear to halt the progress of the disease in a small proportion of cases, and steroid-induced remissions of several years' standing have been recorded. Rarely the disease appears to become stationary spontaneously, or there may even be temporary periods of improved renal function.

Wegener's Granulomatosis. This entity is discussed in the section on Granulomatous Diseases of Unproved Etiology. The renal lesions may contain small granulomas in relation to blood vessels and glomeruli; otherwise, the renal disease cannot be distinguished from classic polyarteritis. The course is usually rapidly progressive renal failure, uninfluenced by treatment, leading to death in uremia, usually within a few months of the first renal manifestations.

Anaphylactoid Purpura (Henoch-Schönlein Syndrome). In anaphylactoid purpura hematuria may be caused by bleeding from the mucosal surface of the ureters, bladder, or urethra. Occasionally, however, anaphylactoid purpura causes a true glomerulonephritis, which clinically resembles a post-streptococcal acute glomerulonephritis. This resemblance is enhanced if the disease follows a streptococcal infection, as is often the case. However, serum complement is not diminished, and renal biopsy shows a focal rather than a diffuse glomerulonephritis. It is generally believed, although the evidence is not convincing, that complete renal recovery is less common than after a post-streptococcal nephritis; but it must be remembered that recurrent attacks of anaphylactoid purpura are common, and the possibility of permanent renal damage may be greater for that reason. The course of the disease in patients whose glomerulonephritis does not resolve completely is very like that of other forms of chronic glomerulonephritis, except that nephrotic syndrome appears to be less common.

Goodpasture's Syndrome (Lung Purpura and Nephritis). Goodpasture's syndrome is a form of acute progressive glomerulonephritis accompanied by massive capillary hemorrhage into the lungs. The eponym "Goodpasture" is unfortunate, although firmly entrenched by usage, for there is considerable doubt whether the patients described by him suffered from the condition that now bears his name.

The primary cause of the condition is still unknown, but there is evidence that the glomerulonephritis is caused by circulating antibodies directed against the glomerular basement membrane, perhaps the only spontaneous form of human glomerulonephritis (other than rejection of a transplanted kidney) for which this is true. The association between pulmonary and glomerular lesions appears to be the result of an immunologic similarity between the capillary basement membranes at these two sites.

Histologically the renal lesion is an acute progressive glomerulonephritis, which may initially be focal, but rapidly becomes generalized. The lungs show massive confluent alveolar hemorrhage, identical with that seen in the rare condition *idiopathic pulmonary hemosiderosis;* the pulmonary capillaries show patchy basement membrane changes, but it is usually difficult to see changes gross enough to account for the amount of blood in the alveoli. In some otherwise typical patients an arteritis of pulmonary arterioles can be demonstrated; by convention this is regarded as microscopic polyarteritis, but the borderline between the two conditions is not precise.

No age is exempt, but the disease is most common in the second and third decade. Males are affected three or four times as often as females. The first symptom is usually recurrent hemoptysis, and only after days or weeks do manifestations of nephritis occur, most often hematuria. The pulmonary hemorrhage is often very severe, with symptoms and signs of acute blood loss; after repeated episodes an iron deficiency anemia may appear, owing to loss and sequestration of large amounts of iron in the lungs as hemosiderin. Occasionally the first manifestations are those of subacute glomerulonephritis, and only after several weeks does pulmonary hemorrhage indicate the presence of a generalized disease.

In most cases the renal lesion progresses rapidly to total glomerular destruction, often passing through a nephrotic phase, and leading to death in uremia within a few weeks or months of the onset of symptoms. Death may also result from pulmonary hemorrhage, either because of asphyxia or from acute blood loss. Treatment is usually without influence on the course of the disease, but there have been occasional reports of long remissions after treatment with steroids.

Hemolytic-Uremic Syndrome. This affects infants and young children, and is characterized by thrombocytopenia, microangiopathic hemolytic anemia, and acute progressive renal failure. Histologically the renal lesion is a proliferative glomerulonephritis, less frequently a patchy cortical necrosis.

The hematologic manifestations appear to be secondary to an underlying vasculitis, which may be generalized or confined to the glomeruli. Minor degrees of the same blood changes are common in all forms of acute glomerulonephritis or diffuse small vessel vasculitis, and for this reason many authorities do not accept the hemolytic-uremic syndrome as a separate disease entity, but regard it as a syndrome with many causes, including acute post-streptococcal nephritis and polyarteritis. However, because the condition has sometimes occurred in small local outbreaks, and is much more common in some communities, e.g., Argentina and Chile, than in others, it has been suggested by some that there might be an infective basis.

The condition often starts with evidence of an acute gastroenteritis, with bloody diarrhea, but whether this is infective or due to vascular lesions in the bowel is uncertain. Fever, upper respiratory symptoms, cutaneous purpura, and neurologic features (especially convulsions and coma) are common. It is difficult to ascertain in an individual case whether the diffuse organ involvement is caused by underlying vasculitis or by local hemorrhage resulting from the thrombocytopenia, which is often profound.

Renal involvement is shown by hematuria and the rapid development of oliguric renal failure, without clinical remissions. Milder cases occur, but most patients who develop renal failure die in uremia; the few recoveries that have been reported have often followed treatment with steroids or heparin.

Moschcowitz's Syndrome (Thrombotic Thrombocytopenic Purpura, TTP). This rare disease, also discussed elsewhere, first described by Moschcowitz in 1925, has close similarities to hemolytic-uremic syndrome, and may be regarded as a variant of the same theme.

The characteristic morphologic lesion is occlusion of the small arterioles and capillaries of many organs by conglutinations of platelets and fibrin. In the kidney the most conspicuous feature is eosinophilic thrombi in the capillaries of the glomerular tuft, with some degree of focal glomerular proliferation. The disseminated vascular lesions appear to be the result of primary disease of the vessels themselves. Generalized intravascular coagulation leads to thrombocytopenia and hypofibrinogenemia, accompanied by profound hemolytic anemia of microangiopathic type.

The disease runs an acute or a chronic relapsing course; it can affect any age, but is most common in young adults. Clinically it is characterized by anemia, cutaneous purpura, rapidly progressive renal failure, and neurologic features such as convulsions and hemiplegia. Formerly it was thought to have a uniformly fatal course, but steroids may have a beneficial effect, and use of heparin in the acute stages of the disease has sometimes been followed by prolonged remission.

The distinction between hemolytic-uremic syndrome and Moschcowitz's syndrome is probably artificial. However, as currently defined, hemolytic-uremic syndrome affects younger patients, and morphologically shows fewer and less severe lesions in organs other than the kidneys. Both conditions have a very poor prognosis, but a chronic relapsing course is common in Moschcowitz's syndrome, whereas patients with hemolytic-uremic syndrome who do recover usually have no further attacks of glomerulonephritis.

The Kidney in Systemic Sclerosis (Scleroderma). Although systemic sclerosis may affect the kidney, it is unusual among connective tissue diseases in that it does not cause glomerulonephritis. Instead there is a slowly progressive obliteration of renal arteries of interlobular size or smaller, and of the renal arterioles, morphologically identical to the vascular involvement of other organs. Histologically the vascular changes closely resemble those of malignant hypertension and radiation nephritis. The usual clinical manifestations, if indeed there are any, include mild proteinuria, slowly progressive renal failure, and renal hypertension, which may be severe. Treatment of hypertension may be required, but otherwise there is no treatment for the renal lesion.

Allen, D. M., Diamond, L. K., and Howell, D. A.: Anaphylactoid purpura in children (Schönlein-Henoch syndrome): Review with a follow-up of the renal complications. Amer. J. Dis. Child., 99:833, 1960.

Benoit, F. L., Rulon, D. B., Theil, G. B., Doolan, P. D., and Watten, R. H.: Goodpasture's syndrome: A clinicopathologic entity. Amer. J. Med., 37:424, 1964.

Clarkson, A., Lawrence, J., Meadows, R., and Seymour, A.: The haemolytic uraemic syndrome in adults. Quart. J. Med., 39:227, 1970.

Davson, J., Ball, R., and Platt, R. P.: The kidney in periarteritis nodosa. Quart. J. Med., 17:175, 1948.

Lock, S. P., and Dormandy, K. M.: Red-cell fragmentation syndrome: A condition of multiple aetiology? Lancet, 1:1020, 1961.

McLean, M. M., Jones, C. H., and Sutherland, D. A.: Haemolytic-uraemic syndrome. Arch. Dis. Child., 41:46, 1966.

Moschcowitz, E.: An acute febrile pleiochromic anemia with hyaline thrombosis of the terminal arterioles and capillaries: An undescribed disease. Arch. Intern. Med. (Chicago), 36:89, 1925.

Pollak, V. E., Pirani, C. L., and Schwartz, F. D.: The natural history of the renal manifestations of systemic lupus erythematosus. J. Lab. Clin. Med., 63:537, 1963.

Roberts, F. B., Slater, R. J., and Laski, B.: The prognosis of Henoch-Schönlein nephritis. Canad. Med. Ass. J., 87:49, 1962.

Rodnan, G. P., Schreiner, G. E., and Black, R. L.: Renal involvement in progressive systemic sclerosis (generalized scleroderma. Amer. J. Med., 23:445, 1957.

Rose, G. A., and Spencer, H.: Polyarteritis nodosa. Quart. J. Med., 26:43, 1957.

Rothfield, N. F., McCluskey, R. T., and Baldwin, D. S.: Renal disease in systemic lupus erythematosus. New Eng. J. Med., 269:537, 1963.

Shumway, C. N., and Terplan, K. L.: Hemolytic anemia, thrombocytopenia and renal disease in childhood: The hemolytic-uremic syndrome. Pediat. Clin. N. Amer., 11:577, 1964.

FOCAL GLOMERULONEPHRITIS WITH RECURRENT HEMATURIA
(Essential or Benign Hematuria)

The term *focal nephritis* has often been used in the European literature to designate a form of renal disease characterized by repeated attacks of profuse hematuria after systemic infection, which attacks leave little residual renal damage. The renal lesion is a focal glomerular inflammation, but the disease otherwise has little in common with other forms of focal glomerulonephritis, such as polyarteritis or the renal lesions of bacterial endocarditis. The etiology is completely obscure.

Clinical Manifestations. The disease is most common in the second and third decades of life, and affects males much more frequently than females. The characteristic feature is recurrent attacks of hematuria, which usually start about the age of puberty and continue at the rate of several a year for as many as 20 or 30 years. Attacks may occur without an obvious precipitating cause, but most often follow a febrile illness or, less frequently, some strenuous unaccustomed exertion. Unlike post-streptococcal nephritis, hematuria may develop within a few hours of the

evidence of systemic infection, and is seldom delayed more than two days. There is no constant relationship to group A streptococci or to any particular form of infection, and often the manifestations of the precipitating illness (usually an evanescent pyrexia and myalgia) are so slight that this cannot be diagnosed with certainty.

Even during the attack of hematuria it is unusual for hypertension, renal failure, or edema to develop, though the urinary deposit is characteristic of an acute glomerulonephritis. Renal biopsy discloses focal areas of glomerular proliferation, usually affecting only a segment of a glomerulus here and there.

Prognosis. At first the urine clears completely after each attack, but in older patients mild proteinuria and microscopic hematuria often persist between attacks. The disorder is usually regarded as benign, because renal failure and hypertension do not commonly develop. However occasionally patients do develop these complications, or more rarely the nephrotic syndrome, and in such patients renal biopsy shows that the glomerular lesions, although still focal, have caused very severe glomerular destruction.

Management. The history of the condition is so distinctive that a diagnosis can usually be made with confidence from this alone. However, it is often valuable to demonstrate the characteristic histology by renal biopsy, either in order to reassure the patient that he has a form of renal disease that does not usually shorten life, or to put an end to the repeated urologic investigations which these patients have often endured.

Patients with focal nephritis should be advised to avoid infections or any activities which they know are liable to precipitate an attack. Penicillin prophylaxis, to reduce bacterial respiratory infections, is often tried, but the results have been disappointing. The usual benign course of the condition does not justify routine use of steroids, nor is there any evidence that they influence the disease.

Bodian, M., Block, J. A., Kobayashi, N., Lake, B. D., and Shuler, S. E.: Recurrent haematuria in childhood. Quart. J. Med., 34:359, 1965.

Ross, J. A.: Recurrent focal nephritis. Quart. J. Med., 29:391, 1960.

HEREDITARY NEPHRITIS
(Alport's Syndrome)

Definition. Hereditary nephritis is a form of hereditary renal disease, characterized histologically by glomerulonephritis and interstitial nephritis, and frequently associated with nerve deafness.

Genetic Aspects and Incidence. The disease is inherited as an autosomal dominant. Males and females are approximately equally affected, but the disease usually takes a more serious form in men. Patients with renal disease frequently have nerve deafness, and some members of the family may have deafness with normal renal function. Ophthalmologic defects, such as cataracts and lenticonus, occur less frequently.

About 100 cases have been reported, but it is very difficult to make the diagnosis in sporadic cases, or in families without deafness, and the true incidence is probably many times greater.

Etiology and Pathology. The nature of the underlying defect in the kidney is unknown. Histologically the renal lesion may be a chronic proliferative glomerulonephritis, often with segmental glomerular lesions; in other patients the glomeruli may appear normal but there is an extensive interstitial nephritis which resembles pyelonephritis or analgesic nephropathy. Most writers have remarked on an abundance of fat-laden foam cells in the interstitium, but these are common in other forms of renal disease, and their presence cannot be regarded as diagnostic.

Clinical Manifestations. The first symptom of the disease is usually hematuria, often noticed in childhood, and frequently preceded by some systemic infection. Proteinuria is usually present, but seldom severe enough to cause the nephrotic syndrome. Occasionally frank attacks of pyelonephritis occur, with positive urine cultures. The usual course of the renal disease is slow deterioration in renal function, often with hypertension, leading eventually to death in uremia in the third to fifth decade. Nerve deafness can develop at any age; initially it affects high tones predominantly, and may be unsuspected until revealed by audiometry.

Diagnosis. The diagnosis is often difficult because no single known feature of the disease is absolutely diagnostic. The most helpful features are nerve deafness in the patient or immediate relatives and familial renal disease. However, to be convincing, a family history should include more than one generation, for the presence of glomerulonephritis in several sibs might be the result of simultaneous infection with a nephritogenic Streptococcus during earlier childhood. Sporadic cases may be confused with other forms of chronic glomerulonephritis, with the syndrome of focal nephritis and recurrent hematuria described above, or with familial renal tubular defects which are occasionally associated with nerve deafness.

Treatment. No treatment is known to alter the progress of the renal disease, but patients may require treatment for urinary infections, for renal hypertension, or for symptomatic renal failure. Renal replacement, by intermittent hemodialysis or renal transplant, is well worth considering in the terminal stages.

Alport, A. C.: Hereditary familial congenital haemorrhagic nephritis. Brit. Med. J., 1:504, 1927.
Perkoff, G. T.: Familial aspects of diffuse renal diseases. Ann. Rev. Med., 15:115, 1964.

CHRONIC GLOMERULONEPHRITIS

Definition. Chronic glomerulonephritis is a chronic inflammatory condition affecting the renal glomeruli which can result from many different disease processes. Histologically the lesion is a proliferative glomerulitis leading to fibrosis and finally to complete obliteration. The course is progressive, with eventual renal failure.

Etiology. Chronic glomerulonephritis has often been described, as in earlier editions of this book, as if it were usually the sequel of a post-streptococcal glomerulonephritis. Undoubtedly this sequence does occur, but only a minority of cases are likely to have this origin, for nowadays the proportion of cases in which there is a history of an acute nephritic episode is no greater than 15 to 20 per cent; even fewer have a history suggestive of streptococcal infection.

The nature of the diseases giving rise to most cases of chronic glomerulonephritis is obscure. An uncertain number are sporadic instances of hereditary nephritis. Others are cases of vascular disease such as polyarteritis or anaphylactoid purpura, in which the extrarenal manifestations are less conspicuous than usual; this suspicion arises particularly when the glomerular histology shows focal characteristics. Others may be examples of membranous nephropathy (see below), a condition which is not strictly a glomerulonephritis, as it does not show evidence of glomerular inflammation, but which in its late stages can show a histologic picture like the late stages of a chronic glomerular inflammation. In some parts of the tropics a chronic proliferative glomerulonephritis may result from long-standing infection with quartan malaria; renal involvement usually presents as a nephrotic syndrome in childhood. However, in temperate zones most patients with chronic glomerulonephritis elude precise diagnosis, and within this group there may be several different disease entities not as yet defined.

Even when one considers cases of glomerulonephritis which can be assigned to one or another diagnostic category, there is at present little evidence why some patients, particularly those with post-streptococcal glomerulonephritis, recover completely from their disease, whereas others who are initially similar show continued progression of their disease, which thus becomes "chronic glomerulonephritis." There is some evidence, particularly from studies of serum complement and immunofluorescence of renal biopsy material, that progression is due to continuing immune injury. The suggestion has been made that the initial episode of glomerular damage so alters some glomerular constituents that they themselves become antigenic, and so perpetuate the process. However, this lacks adequate confirmation and fails to explain the extreme variations in clinical course in patients who initially seem similarly affected.

Incidence. In America and Europe chronic glomerulonephritis can affect any age, but is most common in the third to sixth decade. Men and women are equally affected. It is difficult to obtain figures for its absolute incidence, but an idea of its relative prevalence can be gained from its frequency in relation to other forms of renal disease; in most series it accounts for slightly less than half of the deaths from renal failure, and two thirds or more of the patients treated by maintenance hemodialysis or renal transplantation.

Pathology. The essential lesion is chronic glomerular inflammation, with cellular proliferation and leukocytic infiltration. Both changes occur in various forms of acute recoverable glomerulonephritis, but in the chronic form they are accompanied by progressive destructive changes, including necrosis of glomerular segments, fibrosis, adhesions between the capillary loops of the glomerular tufts, and obliteration of Bowman's space by glomerular adhesions and epithelial crescents (Fig. 1). Eventually many glomeruli are destroyed entirely, to be replaced by structureless hyaline material. Renal shrinkage, particularly of the cortex, proceeds at the same time, largely owing to ischemic atrophy and fibrosis of the tubules which comprise the main part of the renal bulk. In long-standing cases shrinkage and distortion of the normal architecture may be so extreme that it is difficult to distinguish the disease from the final stages of chronic pyelonephritis or hypertensive renal disease; this difficulty is compounded by the fact that both of these are common complications of chronic glomerulonephritis.

Differentiation has often been made between a subacute glomerulonephritis, in which histologic changes are more exudative, necrosing, and proliferative, and the clinical course is rapidly progressive, leading to total destruction of renal excreting function within a few months; and a more chronic form of glomerulonephritis, with more extensive glomerular fibrosis, which takes as many as 20 or 30 years to run the same course. However, the term "rapidly progressive" is more satisfactory, because the expression "subacute glomerulonephritis" has been reserved by some European workers for the nephrotic phase of the disease. Even so, it must be stressed that every degree of clinical chronicity is seen. In general it is not possible to predict the length of survival, or the likelihood of development of nephrotic syndrome or hypertension, from the appearances shown by renal biopsy. A possible exception to this generalization is the appearance known as "chronic lobular glomerulonephritis" (Fig. 2), in which interglomerular proliferation is marked but epithelial crescents are inconspicuous; this appearance seems to be a particularly common sequel of post-streptococcal nephritis, and is often associated with the nephrotic syndrome.

Clinical Manifestations. The most common forms of clinical presentation are symptomless proteinuria, nephrotic syndrome, renal hypertension, and azotemic renal failure. Patients may pass through each of these phases in turn, usually in the sequence listed. Although the course is almost invariably progressive, the rate of deterioration may be so slow that survival is prolonged for 30

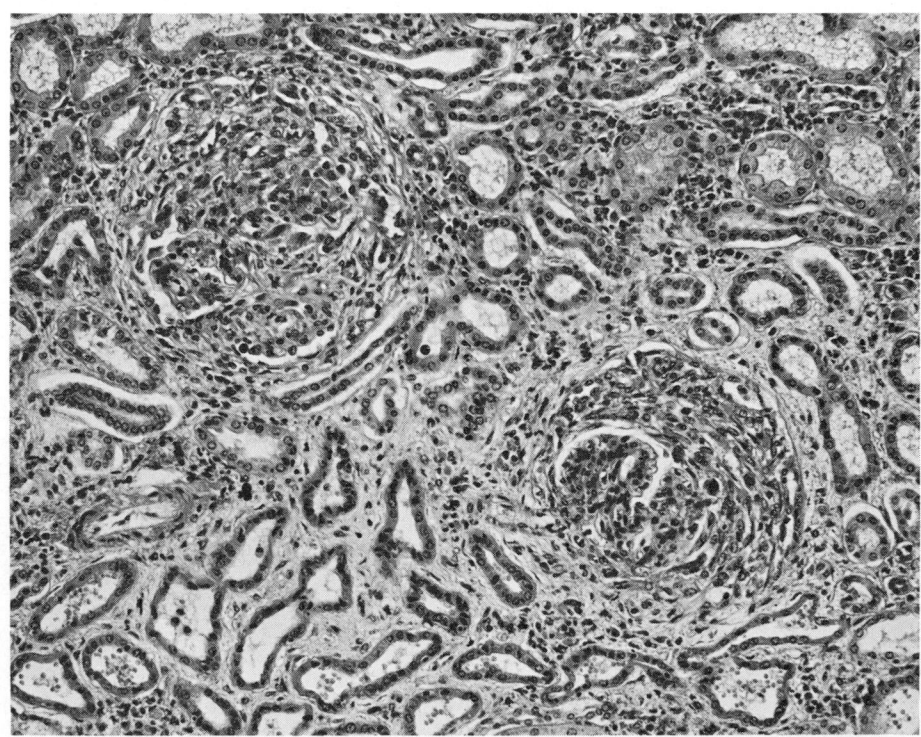

FIGURE 1. Abundant crescent formation in a 13-year-old girl with rapidly progressive glomerulonephritis. No good history of streptococcal infection was obtained. (H and E, × 150.) (From Heptinstall, R. H.: Pathology of the Kidney. Boston, Little, Brown and Company, 1966.)

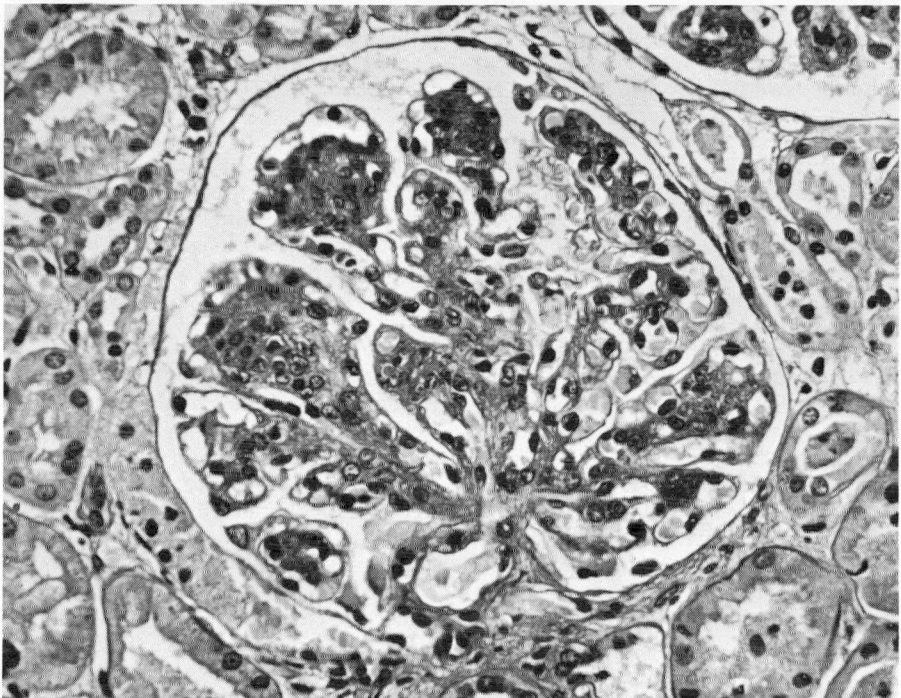

FIGURE 2. Lobular form of glomerulonephritis. (H and E, × 400.) (From Heptinstall, R. H.: Pathology of the Kidney. Boston, Little, Brown and Company, 1966.)

years or more. However, the development of accelerated hypertension at any time in the course of the illness is associated with rapid deterioration in renal function.

Proteinuria is invariable; cylindruria and microscopic hematuria are usually present. Urinary protein losses of over 3 grams a day are common; some of these patients develop all the features of the nephrotic syndrome, but in others the rate of albumin synthesis is sufficient to prevent the development of edema. Occasionally proteinuria may be very slight or intermittent; in such cases it is usually more marked after exertion or when the patient is up and about. This situation is easily confused with benign postural proteinuria.

Patients with long-standing glomerulonephritis are particularly prone, because of their long survival, to the complications of chronic renal failure, such as secondary gout, hyperparathyroidism, and soft tissue calcification (discussed in the article on Chronic Renal Failure).

Management. No known treatment will definitely alter the course of the underlying renal disease. Steroids and cytotoxic drugs have been tried and in rare cases have appeared beneficial, although the possibility of spontaneous partial remission cannot be excluded. If these forms of treatment are used at all, they should be restricted to patients with the more rapidly progressive and more cellular glomerular lesions, for in patients with the more chronic forms of glomerulonephritis it is difficult to see how the fibrotic or hyalinized glomeruli could be altered by treatment, and the natural course of the disease is so long that pro-

longed treatment would carry an unacceptable risk of drug toxicity.

The main complications of chronic glomerulonephritis—the nephrotic syndrome, renal hypertension, and renal failure—may all require special treatment, and this is discussed under the appropriate titles. Treatment of hypertension is particularly important, as the development of accelerated hypertension leads to a rapid further deterioration in renal function which is usually permanent. Mild degrees of hypertension, e.g., 150 systolic, 100 diastolic, are permissible, but a diastolic pressure consistently 120 mm. Hg or more must be treated. In patients with renal failure hypertension may be partly or entirely due to sodium retention, and a low sodium regimen or diuretics, such as furosemide, may be required.

Relman, A. S.: Clinical aspects of chronic glomerulonephritis. *In* Strauss, M. B., and Welt, L. G. (eds.): Diseases of the Kidney. Boston, Little, Brown and Company, 1963, p. 320.

MINIMAL CHANGE GLOMERULAR DISEASE
(Lipoid Nephrosis)

Definition. This is a glomerular disorder causing heavy proteinuria, characterized by absence of obvious histologic glomerular changes on light microscopy.

The term "lipoid nephrosis" was introduced by Munk in 1913, and refers to the presence of fat bodies in the urine and fatty change in the tubular cells. These changes are now known to be the result of a glomerular protein leak, but with the light microscope it is not usually possible to see glomerular abnormalities, and it was not until the advent of the electron microscope that glomerular changes were shown to be present invariably. Hamburger's suggestion that the term "minimal change" should be used to describe the glomerular lesions has been widely followed.

Etiology, Incidence, and Pathology. The etiology is unknown. There is no convincing evidence that the disease is the result of immune injury to the kidney, despite the fact that it occasionally follows exposure to foreign protein and responds dramatically to steroid treatment.

The disease is most common in infancy and childhood, a fact largely responsible for the good prognosis of nephrotic syndrome in childhood. The peak incidence is between three and four years, but no age is exempt. Males are affected more often than females, in a ratio of 3:2.

Light microscopy usually shows no glomerular abnormalities, but there may be occasional small areas of glomerular proliferation or adhesions to Bowman's capsule. The tubules usually show protein casts and doubly refractile lipid vacuoles in the cells of the proximal tubule; edema of the interstitium is often present and may cause considerable renal enlargement. The electron microscope invariably shows changes in the glomeruli, consisting of swelling and coalescence ("smudging") of the foot processes of the epithelial cells on the outer side of the basement membrane. The basement membrane itself usually has a normal appearance, but sometimes contains small vacuoles or shows irregular thickening.

Until recently the view was widely held that this form of renal disease represented an early form of a glomerulonephritis which would eventually show destructive glomerular changes. This view is no longer tenable; serial renal biopsies have shown that the glomerular lesions do not usually progress; indeed, they disappear after a spontaneous or steroid-induced clinical remission. Although a few patients who do not remit have subsequently shown generalized thickening of the basement membrane and have eventually developed renal failure, these are in the minority, and it has been argued that they can be recognized at the time of their initial renal biopsy by demonstration of definite basement membrane abnormalities on electron microscopy and a lack of selectivity in their glomerular protein leak (see below).

Despite the absence of gross changes in the basement membrane on light microscopy, it is likely that the protein leak is the result of change in the basement membrane itself. The change in the foot processes is probably indicative of the presence of protein within Bowman's space, for an identical appearance can be produced in animals by intravenous injection of proteins that cross the glomerular filter. This histologic appearance is also a feature of other forms of glomerular disease with heavy proteinuria, and is in no way specific for minimal change glomerular disease, although here it is the only constant glomerular finding.

The permeability characteristics of the glomerulus in this disease have been well worked out (Squire, Blainey, Hardwicke, and Soothill). The urinary protein consists almost entirely of the plasma proteins of lower molecular weight, particularly albumin (molecular weight, 68,000) and transferrin (90,000), whereas plasma proteins of larger size, such as β-lipoprotein (molecular weight, up to 2,500,000) are almost completely absent. The same pattern of glomerular permeability can be demonstrated after intravenous injection of dextrans of different molecular sizes, when only the smaller molecules are found in the urine. The glomerular protein leak is thus highly selective, whereas in almost all other forms of glomerular disease the leak is nonselective or poorly selective in that plasma proteins of every molecular size are found in the urine.

Clinical Manifestations. The most common first symptom is edema, which develops insidiously and often reaches mammoth proportions. Examination at this stage reveals all the characteristics of the nephrotic syndrome — heavy proteinuria (more than 5 grams per day), hypoalbuminemia, and usually hypercholesterolemia. The urine sediment contains hyaline, granular and fatty casts, and occasional red cells; gross microscopic hematuria and red cell casts are not found. Hypertension is unusual. The blood urea and serum creatinine are usually normal; however, azotemia is not uncommon in the early stages of the disease, and a transitory oliguric renal failure rarely develops — perhaps the result of tubular damage caused by proteinuria or obstruction of tubules by protein casts.

The disease has a remarkable tendency to remit. This may take place spontaneously, may follow systemic infections such as measles, or may result from treatment with steroids or cytotoxic drugs. Remissions are usually complete, with disappearance of all signs of the disease, but partial remissions with continuing mild proteinuria are common. Relapses are unfortunately frequent, and may exactly replicate the initial attack of the disease. Repeated relapses may occur over a period of many years (over 20 years in one case personally known to the author) without deterioration in renal excreting function or the appearance of destructive changes in the glomeruli.

Treatment. The chief hazard of the disease lies in the complications of edema, particularly infection, which have been greatly reduced by modern diuretics and antimicrobial drugs. Before the advent of penicillin, pneumococcal peritonitis was a common cause of death, but this is now very rare. Treatment of edema is discussed in connection with the nephrotic syndrome. Two other hazards of the disease require mention. Hypogammaglobulinemia, owing partly to reduced synthesis and partly to urinary losses of gamma globulin, itself carries a risk of infection; hypercholesterolemia, as in other forms of nephrotic syndrome, may eventually lead to early atheroma and a predisposition to arterial thrombosis.

The disease is one of the very few forms of glomerular disease in which the underlying glomerular fault can be remedied by treatment. When given steroids or corticotrophin (ACTH), most patients rapidly lose their proteinuria and all other signs of the disease. Serial renal biopsies have shown that the glomerular foot processes simultaneously return to normal. It is not known how adrenal steroids exert this remarkable effect, and the dose of steroids required varies from case to case, usually being in the range of 20 to 60 mg. of prednisolone, or equivalent, daily. Relapses often follow withdrawal of steroids, even when the dose has been reduced very gradually. A minority of patients do not appear to respond to steroids; as mentioned above, some authorities believe that such patients are the ones who show patchy areas of basement membrane thickening at the onset of their disease. These nonresponding cases sometimes show a good response to cytotoxic drugs, among which cyclophosphamide currently appears to be the best available. This treatment may also have value in the case of patients who respond to steroids but develop severe side effects and who persistently relapse when attempts are made to withdraw steroids.

Treatment with steroids should not be lightly undertaken. It must be realized that this is the only form of nephrotic syndrome which shows a satisfactory response at all frequently, and that this treatment has definite dangers. The diagnosis should not rest on clinical manifestations alone, but should be based on the appearances of renal biopsy and on the finding of a highly selective proteinuria. In children, in whom high doses of steroids are less dangerous, and in whom most cases of nephrotic syndrome are caused by this process, it is justifiable to commence steroids without the evidence of renal biopsy or protein clearances, provided that treatment is gradually withdrawn if no effect is seen within three weeks. Conversely in a few elderly patients, even those who have been shown by renal biopsy to have the disease, the risks of long-continued steroids, particularly gastric ulcer, may be greater than the risks of nephrotic syndrome, provided that edema can be satisfactorily controlled.

Once a decision is made to employ steroid treatment it is wise to begin with a high dose, e.g., 60 to 80 mg. of prednisolone per day in an adult, or 40 to 60 mg. in a child. This dose should be maintained for about three weeks and then reduced to a maintenance dose of one half to two thirds the original dose if a satisfactory response (disappearance or marked lessening of proteinuria) occurs; if not, the treatment should be gradually withdrawn. Maintenance treatment should be continued for about three months; then periodic attempts can be made to reduce dosage further or stop altogether;

if clinical relapse occurs, it will be necessary to increase the dose temporarily. Troublesome side effects of steroids are common, particularly retarded growth in children, but there is some evidence that they can be prevented or lessened by giving steroids on alternate days, without a loss of therapeutic effect; alternatively steroids can be replaced by cyclophosphamide. It is unwise to regard complete abolition of proteinuria as the sole aim of treatment, for in some cases this requires an unacceptably high dose of steroids, whereas a much smaller dose will sufficiently lessen proteinuria to return the plasma albumin to normal and so remove the risk of edema.

Black, D. A. K., Rose, G., and Brewer, D. B.: Controlled trial of prednisone in adult patients with the nephrotic syndrome. Brit. Med. J., 3:421, 1970.

Connolly, M. E., Wrong, O. M., and Jones, N. F.: Reversible renal failure in idiopathic nephrotic syndrome with minimal glomerular changes. Lancet, 1:665, 1968.

Farquhar, M.: Ultrastructure of the nephron disclosed by electron microscopy: A review of normal and pathologic glomerular ultrastructure. In Metcoff, J. (ed.): Proceedings, 10th Annual Conference on the Nephrotic Syndrome. New York, National Kidney Disease Foundation, 1959, p. 2.

Hamburger, J.: In Wolstenholme, G. E. W., and Cameron, M. P. (eds.): Renal Biopsy. London, J. & A. Churchill, Ltd., 1961, p. 139.

Hardwicke, J., and Soothill, J. F.: Proteinuria. In Black, D. A. K. (ed.): Renal Disease. 2nd ed. Oxford, Blackwell Scientific Publications, Ltd., 1967, p. 252.

Moncrieff, M. W., White, R. H. R., Ogg, C. S., and Cameron, J. S.: Cyclophosphamide therapy in the nephrotic syndrome in childhood. Brit. Med. J., 1:666, 1969.

Squire, J. R., Blainey, J. D., and Hardwicke, J.: The nephrotic syndrome. Brit. Med. Bull., 13:43, 1957.

(See also references following next article.)

IDIOPATHIC MEMBRANOUS GLOMERULAR DISEASE
(Membranous Nephrosis)

Definition. This is a glomerular disease of unknown etiology, characterized by thickening of the capillary basement membrane, without cellular infiltration.

The condition is often called membranous "glomerulonephritis," but this term is inappropriate inasmuch as there is usually no evidence of glomerular inflammation.

Etiology, Incidence, and Pathology. Although the etiology is obscure, the finding of gamma globulin on the thickening basement membrane has led to the suggestion that this is a form of immune glomerular injury.

The disease affects all ages, but is most common in adults; males are affected more often than females, particularly in middle age and later life.

Histologically the disease can be recognized with the light microscope by the presence of a more or less uniform thickening of the capillary basement membrane of every glomerulus. This thickening is often obvious in sections stained with hematoxylin and eosin (Fig. 3), but is particularly

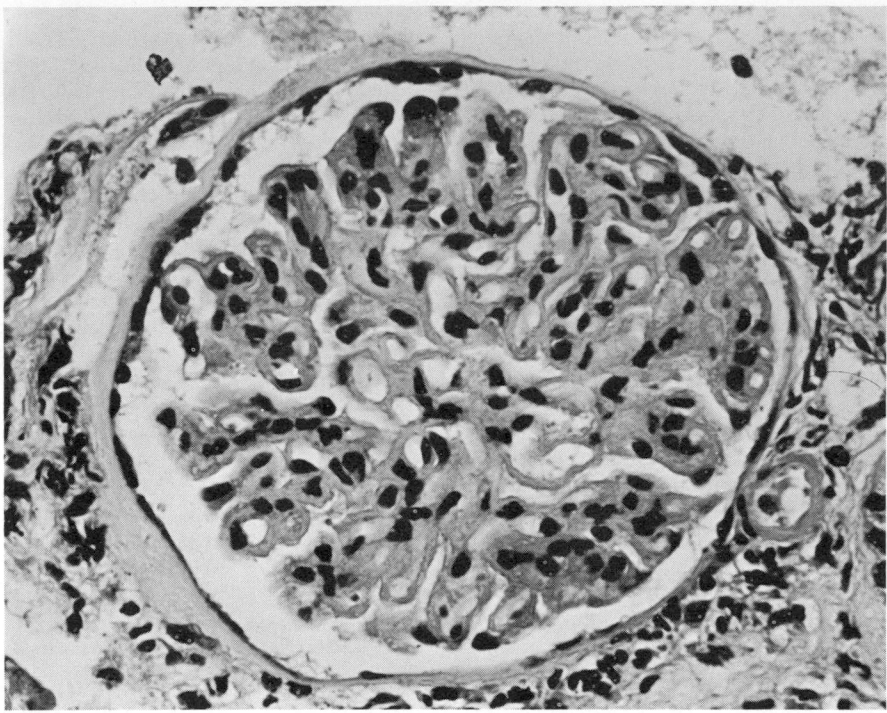

FIGURE 3. Renal biopsy from patient with idiopathic membranous disease and nephrotic syndrome. Widespread capillary basement membrane thickening but no nuclear increase. (H and E, × 500.) (From Heptinstall, R. H.: Pathology of the Kidney. Boston, Little, Brown and Company, 1966.)

apparent in thin sections (less than 2 μ) stained with periodic acid–methenamine–silver. The thickening may be so marked that the capillary lumen is reduced in caliber or obliterated, but there is no increase in glomerular cellularity. Under the electron microscope the glomerular capillaries show an irregular accumulation of electron-dense material between the lamina densa of the basement membrane and the fused foot processes of the epithelial cells. Secondary tubular changes, with interstitial edema and fibrosis, are common as in other forms of glomerular disease.

The membranous form of glomerular disease is generally believed to be distinct from other forms, not merely a stage in the evolution of another process. This view is supported by serial renal biopsies, which have shown a worsening in the glomerular alterations with time, but no real change in nature. However, renal biopsies from patients with nephrotic syndrome sometimes show a mixed picture of membranous and proliferative change. These are usually considered to be variants of the proliferative glomerulonephritis of chronic glomerulonephritis, but they do point up the unsatisfactory state of our present morphologic classification of glomerular disease.

Clinical Manifestations. Membranous glomerular disease usually presents with nephrotic syndrome, less often with asymptomatic proteinuria, renal hypertension, or chronic renal failure. All features of the nephrotic syndrome may be found, but the condition may be distinguished from minimal change glomerular disease by the higher average age of patients, the frequent presence of hypertension and renal failure, the nonselective nature of the proteinuria, and the rarity of clinical remission. Microscopic hematuria is slightly more common than in minimal change glomerular disease, but hypercholesterolemia is less frequent.

The disease runs a slowly progressive course; usually many years elapse before renal failure is a serious problem. Very occasionally a fulminant course is followed, oliguric renal failure developing within a few months of onset. No treatment is known to alter the course. Remissions do not occur, although there are a few reports that proteinuria has temporarily disappeared without any change in renal histology.

Blainey, J. D., Brewer, D. B., Hardwicke, J., and Soothill, J. F.: The nephrotic syndrome: Diagnosis by renal biopsy and biochemical and immunological analyses related to the response to steroid therapy. Quart. J. Med., 29:235, 1960.

Pollak, V. E., Rosen, S., and Pirani, C. L.: Natural history of lipoid nephrosis and of membranous glomerulonephritis. Ann. Intern. Med., 69:1171, 1968.

RENAL VEIN THROMBOSIS

Increased renal venous pressure can give rise to heavy proteinuria alone or to all the manifestations of the nephrotic syndrome. This association has occasionally been reported in constrictive pericarditis, congestive cardiac failure, or thrombosis of the inferior vena cava, but it is much more often the result of thrombosis of the renal veins.

There are four main varieties of renal vein thrombosis:

1. *Thrombosis of the inferior vena cava with secondary involvement of the renal veins.* Usually patients have a history of deep venous thromboses of the legs, or repeated pulmonary emboli. The full clinical picture of inferior vena caval obstruction, with conspicuous superficial anastomotic veins, takes time to develop, and is not always apparent.

2. *Obstruction of the renal veins or inferior vena cava by external pressure or neoplasm.* Renal carcinoma, which often grows along the lumen of the renal veins, is one of the common causes in this category.

3. *Renal vein thrombosis secondary to primary renal disease.* This is the most common type of renal vein thrombosis. The main predisposing factor to thrombosis is probably reduced renal blood flow. Thrombosis starts in the renal vein radicles, and only later extends into the main renal veins, whence parts of the thrombus may break away and cause pulmonary emboli. Renal amyloidosis is by far the most common form of underlying renal disease, but various forms of renal vasculitis are also common, and indeed any severe form of renal disease may be complicated by venous thrombosis.

4. *Primary renal vein thrombosis* may complicate acute gastroenteritis, particularly in infants, perhaps as a result of increased blood viscosity caused by saline depletion. In other instances thrombosis develops without obvious predisposing cause.

Pathology. When renal vein thrombosis is sudden and complete, as in the primary variety in children, the result is a hemorrhagic infarction of the kidney. More often thrombosis is slowly progressive, allowing time for an anastomotic circulation to develop. The kidneys enlarge as a result of interstitial edema. The glomeruli show surprisingly little histologic change, and in some cases are virtually normal or merely enlarged. However, there is usually a mild diffuse thickening of the capillary basement membranes, which resembles idiopathic membranous disease, even under the electron microscope, except that the thickening tends to be less marked. There is often considerable tubular atrophy and interstitial cellular infiltration. None of these histologic changes is specific, and the findings on renal biopsy are not usually diagnostic except on the rare occasion when the biopsy includes a thrombosed vein.

Clinical Manifestations. Local pain and swelling may result from edema of the kidney with stretching of the renal capsule. Other clinical features depend very much on the cause of the thrombosis, but two developments are usual — nephrotic syndrome and renal failure. In patients who already have these features because of primary renal disease there is sudden deterioration which often enables the diagnosis to be suspected. In patients without primary renal disease the picture is very similar to the insidious onset of nephrotic syndrome owing to idiopathic membranous disease, and no doubt many patients are incorrectly so diagnosed; features which should arouse suspicion are severity of the nephrotic syndrome (protein losses of 40 to 80 grams a day may occur), presence of local pain, coincident development of renal failure early in the course, pulmonary emboli, caval thrombosis, and the presence of marked interstitial edema and cellular infiltration in the renal biopsy.

Radiology may make a significant contribution to diagnosis. Venography of the inferior vena cava may show obstruction to this vein, thrombi protruding into the cava from the orifices of the renal veins, or reduced streaming of blood from the renal veins; when combined with the Valsalva maneuver, in which caval blood usually refluxes into the renal veins, phlebography may reveal obstruction of the main renal veins or filling of an anastomotic venous circulation. Aortography and direct injection of contrast medium into the renal substance or anastomotic veins have also been helpful, but at present there is no general agreement on their place in diagnosis. The technique of Gillot and Stuhl, in which contrast medium is injected into the inferior vena cava, which is blocked both above and below by inflated balloons, has given good results and deserves further trial.

Prognosis. In those with underlying renal disease the outlook is grave, and even with all modern resources these patients usually die in a few days or weeks; however, they are suitable for a renal replacement program unless their underlying renal disease or general state prevents this.

In those without prior renal disease the prognosis is less serious, although renal failure, gross nephrotic syndrome, and the risk of pulmonary embolization are all dangerous hazards. Fortunately renal function usually improves eventually, either because of recanalization or the opening up of anastomoses, but further attacks of renal vein thrombosis may occur. Renal hypertension is not usually a problem, but there is a risk of secondary pyelonephritis. In patients who survive, the features of nephrotic syndrome gradually relent, although they may take years to disappear.

Treatment. Nephrectomy is often recommended in acute renal vein thrombosis of childhood when the disease is unilateral; the value of operation is controversial, but its proponents claim that removal of the infarcted organ may prevent local infection or hypertension, and may reduce the spread of thrombosis. In adults nephrectomy has not been popular, although it is reasonable to believe that it would cure the nephrotic syndrome in the rare cases of unilateral renal vein thrombosis. The main aspects of treatment are anticoagulation, which needs to be continued for very long periods, treatment of the complicating nephrotic syndrome and renal failure, and, when necessary, the use of some form of dialysis in the hope that renal function will improve.

Gillot, C., and Stuhl, L.: La phlébographie rénale occlusive: documents pathologique obtenus en sériographie. Presse Méd., 74:1041, 1966.

Harrison, C. V., Milne, M. D., and Steiner, R. E.: Clinical aspects of renal vein thrombosis. Quart. J. Med., 25:285, 1956.

Rosenmann, E., Pollak, V. E., and Pirani, C. L.: Renal vein thrombosis in the adult: A clinical and pathological study based on renal biopsies. Medicine, 42:269, 1968.

HYPERTENSIVE NEPHROPATHY

The term *nephrosclerosis*, introduced by Fahr in 1919, is often employed when referring to the renal damage caused by hypertension. The term is misleading and should be abandoned, for it implies that the kidney is hardened, which is usually not the case, and it does not include any reference to the increased blood pressure that is the cause of the renal damage.

ACCELERATED HYPERTENSION
(Malignant Hypertension)

Accelerated hypertension is defined clinically by the association of hypertension and papilledema, and pathologically by fibrinoid necrosis of afferent glomerular arterioles and endarteritis fibrosa ("onion-skin" thickening) of the interlobular arteries of the kidney. The latter changes cause renal ischemia, and hence renal failure, and are responsible for over 80 per cent of the mortality of accelerated hypertension. Although papilledema and the histologic criteria of accelerated hypertension usually go hand in hand, they do not invariably do so; in rapidly progressive hypertension it is quite common to see patients with the renal vascular changes who have retinal hemorrhages and exudates but no papilledema.

Hypertensive adults do not usually enter the accelerated phase unless their diastolic blood pressure is persistently 120 mm. Hg or more; young children occasionally develop the condition with blood pressures in the range 100 to 120 diastolic.

Clinical Manifestations. Accelerated hypertension from any cause, including primary renal disease, causes renal damage; the only exception is hypertension caused by stenosis of a renal artery in which the blood vessels distal to the stenosis are protected from the effects of hypertension.

In patients with pre-existing renal disease there is usually rapid deterioration in renal function, which is apt to be confused with the natural course of the underlying disease. In patients with nonrenal causes of hypertension, the first sign of renal damage is proteinuria, accompanied by microscopic hematuria and cylindruria. Occasionally there is gross hematuria ("renal apoplexy"). Proteinuria may be heavy enough to cause nephrotic syndrome, but usually renal failure develops too rapidly for this sequence to occur. Nonrenal manifestations, such as visual impairment owing to retinal changes, the transient neurologic features known as hypertensive encephalopathy, and congestive cardiac failure, develop side by side with the renal complications. Often the peripheral blood film shows a microangiopathic picture, but hemolytic anemia is usually not a clinical problem.

Unless hypertension is treated, renal failure usually develops within weeks or months. Occasionally the final event is oliguric renal failure, which may come on so suddenly as to suggest acute glomerulonephritis or acute tubular necrosis.

Prognosis. More than 90 per cent of untreated patients die within two years, the majority from renal failure. The use of antihypertensive drugs has radically altered the prognosis, and now many patients live ten years or more, depending on when treatment is started and how successfully hypertension is controlled. In hypertension caused by underlying renal disease the prognosis obviously depends largely on the course run by that disease.

If treatment of hypertension is commenced after renal failure is manifest, it is common to see a further deterioration before renal failure stabilizes. However, prolonged treatment is sometimes followed by slow recovery of renal function, probably because of hypertrophy of surviving nephrons and the resolution of the changes in vessels not completely obstructed by the disease.

Treatment. The treatment of hypertension with drugs is described elsewhere, and the general principles enunciated there apply to patients with accelerated hypertension and renal damage. It is often thought that such patients, with a diseased renal circulation, need an especially high renal perfusion pressure to maintain renal blood flow. This view is incorrect, and disregards the fact that the vascular damage is the direct result of a high perfusion pressure and the experimental findings in animals that the vascular changes regress when the blood pressure is reduced. Obviously it is wise to avoid hypotension when lowering the blood pressure, but control of the diastolic pressure at 90 to 110 mm. Hg achieves the purpose of reducing blood pressure below the critical level, with little risk of hypotensive episodes which might further reduce renal function. Methyldopa, guanethidine, and bethanidine are at present the drugs of choice, and are preferable to the ganglion-blocking drugs which may give rise to sudden hypotension. Diuretics and dietary salt restriction are also important aspects of treatment, because saline retention caused by renal failure contributes to the hypertension.

BENIGN HYPERTENSION

Whether hypertension in its so-called "benign" phase causes clinical renal disease is a moot point. Degrees of hypertension less than those defined as "accelerated" (by the criteria just described) can cause marked thickening of the intima and media of the arteries in the kidney. Study of patients with benign essential hypertension has shown that a few have reduced measurements of renal function, particularly renal plasma flow. Histologically kidneys from such patients may show complete hyalinization of some glomeruli, whereas others show segmental atrophy, fibrosis, and thickening of the basement membrane, changes thought to be caused by ischemia. These features resemble those found in the kidneys of nonhypertensive elderly subjects, possibly the changes are caused more by age than by high blood pressure.

Although mild degrees of renal impairment may result from benign hypertension alone, it is most unusual for symptomatic renal failure to be due to this cause, and the diagnosis can only be accepted when all other possible causes of renal failure have been excluded.

Fishberg, A. M.: Hypertension and Nephritis. 5th ed. Philadelphia, Lea & Febiger, 1954.

Kincaid-Smith, P., McMichael, J., and Murphy, E. A.: The clinical course and pathology of hypertension with papilloedema (malignant hypertension). Quart. J. Med , 27:117, 1958.

Mroczek, W. J., Davidov, M., Gavrilovich, L., and Finnerty, F. A.: The value of aggressive therapy in the hypertensive patient with azotemia. Circulation, 40:893, 1969.

Pickering, G. W.: High Blood Pressure. 2nd ed. London, J. & A. Churchill, Ltd., 1968.

Wilson, C., and Byrom, F. B.: Renal changes in malignant hypertension; experimental evidence. Lancet, 1:136, 1939.

RENAL CHANGES IN OTHER SYSTEMIC DISEASES

DIABETES MELLITUS

Although the renal complications of diabetes mellitus include papillary necrosis and pyelonephritis, the most serious and relentlessly progressive lesion is *intercapillary glomerulosclerosis* (Kimmelstiel-Wilson lesion) in which nodular deposits of eosinophilic material arise within the lobules of the glomerular tuft, and are associated with diffuse mesangial thickening, thickening of the basement membrane, and gradual obliteration of the glomerular capillaries. Histologically the lesion has similarities with glomerular amyloid or idiopathic membranous thickening.

The glomerular lesions may be present in the prediabetic state, but it is unusual for them to give rise to clinical features until after development of overt diabetes, and they are first seen most commonly in patients who have been known to have diabetes for at least 10 to 15 years. Although the pathogenesis of the lesions is not clear, it seems likely that they are part of a generalized small vessel change which is also responsible for diabetic retinopathy and neuropathy. These three complications of diabetes usually develop at about the same time, and careful clinical examination of a patient with diabetic glomerulosclerosis usually shows evidence of the other complications. There is no good evidence that careful control of diabetes influences the development of the glomerular lesion.

Patients with known diabetes usually have their urine tested frequently, and the first sign of glomerulosclerosis is therefore apt to be proteinuria, which may persist unchanged for years, Sooner or later the proteinuria increases and gives rise to the nephrotic syndrome. From then on the course is more rapidly progressive, with steady deterioration in renal function, leading within months to renal failure, often accompanied by severe hypertension. No treatment is known to alter the course of the renal disease. Patients with end-stage uremia may be kept alive by intermittent hemodialysis, but are not usually considered suitable for renal transplantation because of the difficulty experienced in controlling diabetes in patients given large doses of steroids.

Gellman, D. D., Pirani, C. L., Soothill, J. F., Muehrcke, R. C., and Kark, R. M.: Diabetic nephropathy: A clinical and pathological study based on renal biopsies. Medicine, 38:321, 1959.

Kimmelstiel, P., and Wilson, C.: Intercapillary lesions in glomeruli of kidney. Amer, J. Path., 12:83, 1936.

AMYLOIDOSIS

Although systemic amyloidosis exists in several different forms that tend to affect different groups of organs, all forms of amyloid are liable to attack the kidney, and renal failure is the most common cause of death from amyloidosis.

In the early stages renal amyloid gives rise to considerable renal enlargement, but later the kidneys shrink to normal or subnormal size. The glomeruli and small arteries are the usual sites of deposition; tubules are affected less often. Glomerular involvement resembles histologically that of idiopathic membranous disease, except that the lesions are more nodular and often appear to be on the capillary side of the basement membrane. Renal amyloid usually stains well with Congo red, methyl violet, or thioflavin T; occasionally it does not take up these dyes and then can only be recognized with certainty by the electron microscope, which shows a characteristic fibrillary structure with a periodicity of 80 to 100 Å.

The first sign of renal amyloid is usually proteinuria, which may persist unchanged for years, but occasionally disappears temporarily. More severe renal involvement causes nephrotic syndrome or renal failure. It was formerly believed that renal amyloidosis does not cause hypertension; this view is incorrect, although hypertension may be less common than in other forms of glomerular disease. Renal vein thrombosis is a very serious complication of amyloidosis, and should be suspected whenever a patient suddenly develops oliguric renal failure or marked worsening of nephrotic syndrome.

Although it is widely believed that cure or surgical removal of sepsis leads to regression of secondary amyloid, this is certainly a rare event as far as the kidney is concerned, and usually amyloid persists or accumulates further despite removal of the cause. Certainly it is not justifiable to submit patients to heroic surgery, which would not otherwise be warranted, simply because of the existence of amyloid. Treatment of nephrotic and renal failure caused by amyloid follows conventional lines. The value of prophylactic anticoagulants in preventing renal vein thrombosis is uncertain.

Very occasionally patients show a sodium-losing tendency and require a small salt supplement. This feature, so unusual in glomerular disease generally, may here be the result of deposition of amyloid in the adrenal cortex or distal renal tubules. Rarely other tubular syndromes, including nephrogenic diabetes insipidus and renal tubular acidosis, have been encountered in renal amyloidosis with unusually severe tubular involvement.

Patients with severe uremia from amyloidosis are eligible for intermittent hemodialysis, but they are usually unsuitable for renal transplantation because of the danger that the steroids and cytotoxic drugs given to suppress transplant rejection will lead to a flare-up of the original sepsis.

NEPHROTIC SYNDROME

Definition. In the first half of this century the term *nephrosis*, introduced by Müller in 1905, was widely used in at least two quite different senses: (1) as a descriptive histopathologic term for renal diseases without an inflammatory component, and (2) to describe the clinical picture caused by heavy urinary protein losses. Much confusion was caused by this double usage, and as a result the word has been largely abandoned. By general agreement the term *nephrotic syndrome* has been adopted for the second of these meanings, and refers to the *clinical association* of *heavy proteinuria, hypoalbuminemia,* and *generalized edema,* irrespective of the underlying pathology, it being further understood that the serum albumin is low as a result of urinary albumin loss and the edema is due to hypoalbuminemia. In general these criteria are not fulfilled unless at least 5 grams of protein a day are lost in the urine at some time in the course of the disease, and the serum albumin (determined electrophoretically) is less than 3 grams per 100 ml.

The aforementioned definition does not include reference to renal excreting failure, to hypertension, or to hypercholesterolemia. At various times attempts have been made to include one or another of these features as obligating items, particularly

hypercholesterolemia. However, the advantages of simplicity are lost if the definition includes features not closely linked causally, such as hypertension and renal failure, or of which the mechanisms are uncertain, such as hypercholesterolemia.

Etiology. The nephrotic syndrome has many causes. The accompanying table, drawn mainly from Kark et al. and Schreiner with some more recent additions, shows those that have been fully substantiated. The list includes almost all recognized forms of glomerular disease, and *only* forms of glomerular disease, for urinary protein losses in other forms of renal disease are not gross enough to give rise to hypoalbuminemia. (It has sometimes been claimed that pyelonephritis can give rise to nephrotic syndrome, but the patients referred to have probably had glomerular disease complicated by pyelonephritis.) The most important items in the table have already been separately described; in some of the others, such as nephrotic syndrome caused by penicillamine or secondary syphilis, the glomerular morphology

CAUSES OF NEPHROTIC SYNDROME

Inflammatory forms of renal disease
　Acute post-streptococcal glomerulonephritis
　Other forms of acute glomerulonephritis
　Glomerulonephritis in infective endocarditis
　Glomerulonephritis in connective tissue diseases
　　Systemic lupus erythematosus
　　Polyarteritis
　　Anaphylactoid purpura
　　Goodpasture's syndrome
　　Hemolytic-uremic syndrome
　　Moschcowitz's syndrome
　Focal glomerulonephritis with recurrent hematuria
　Familial nephritis
　Chronic (proliferative) glomerulonephritis
　Glomerulonephritis in quartan malaria

Glomerular disease in other systemic diseases
　Secondary syphilis
　Accelerated hypertension
　Diabetic glomerulosclerosis
　Amyloidosis

Other idiopathic types of glomerular disease
　Minimal change glomerular disease
　Idiopathic membranous glomerular disease

Mechanical causes
　Renal vein thrombosis
　Constrictive pericarditis
　Obstruction to inferior vena cava

Toxins
　Mercury, inorganic or organic
　Gold
　Trimethadione (Tridione) and paramethadione
　　(Paradione)
　Penicillamine
　Allergy to pollen, insect bites, snake bites, or plant
　　toxins
　Serum sickness

Miscellaneous
　Toxemia of pregnancy
　Renal transplant

has not been fully established. There is some overlap between parts of the table; thus the nephrotic syndrome caused by various foreign proteins is due to a proliferative glomerulonephritis, and that seen in renal transplants may be either a proliferative or a membranous picture.

Many of the causes listed give rise to transient nephrotic syndrome which in itself is neither a diagnostic nor a therapeutic problem. Persistent nephrotic syndrome, on the other hand, is a major diagnostic and therapeutic problem to all who deal with renal disease. In Europe and North America about 75 per cent of cases are caused by three idiopathic types of glomerular disease—minimal change disease, membranous disease, and chronic glomerulonephritis with predominantly proliferative lesions. The frequency of these three types varies between centers, partly because of variations in classification of cases with mixed membranous and proliferative change, but in most centers minimal change disease causes the majority of cases in children, and one fifth to one third of adult cases. Proliferative glomerulonephritis is slightly more common than membranous disease except in elderly men. Lawrence et al. carefully studied the glomerular histology of patients with proliferative glomerulonephritis causing nephrotic syndrome and found that only 25 per cent of them showed histologic features suggestive of post-streptococcal disease. The main causes of the disease in the remaining 25 per cent of nephrotics who do not have idiopathic glomerular disease are diabetic glomerulosclerosis, amyloidosis, various forms of focal glomerulonephritis (including lupus and anaphylactoid purpura), and renal vein thrombosis.

Clinical Manifestations. Generalized edema, often accompanied by ascites and pleural effusions, is the *sine qua non* of the nephrotic syndrome. The edema is primarily due to the reduced plasma oncotic pressure caused by hypoalbuminemia; but numerous other factors, such as salt intake and mineralocorticoid activity, play parts in its development, and because of these there is no predictable relationship between the amount of edema and the level of the serum albumin. In children gross edema of the face may develop early in the course of the disease, but in adults the legs are usually most affected. In severe cases the weight of the body may be increased by 50 per cent simply from accumulation of edema fluid.

Hypertension is present in some patients, but its presence depends on the type of glomerular disease. The low plasma volume which results from a very low serum albumin may occasionally cause severe vascular collapse with hypotension. Protein malnutrition caused by the high urinary losses may lead to muscle wasting (often obscured by the generalized edema) or growth retardation in children. Increased opacity (whiteness) of the fingernails is found in some patients, and occasionally it is possible to estimate how long they have had nephrotic syndrome by the position of the discolored area.

Urine is often scanty while edema is accumulating, and contains more than 5 grams of protein a day. The features of the urinary deposit and degree of renal impairment depend on the underlying glomerular pathology, but transient renal failure may occur from hypovolemia or tubular damage without implying a destructive glomerular disease. Children with nephrotic syndrome sometimes develop evidence of multiple renal tubular defects, with renal glycosuria, aminoaciduria, and potassium-losing tendency.

The serum albumin is invariably reduced below 3.0 grams per 100 ml. The usual value is between 1.0 and 3.0 grams per 100 ml., but occasionally concentrations as low as 0.5 grams per 100 ml. are seen; in such cases signs of hypovolemia (particularly postural hypotension) are common, and the edema is often resistant to treatment. The plasma proteins other than albumin may be normal, but electrophoresis often shows a decrease in alpha and gamma globulins, and an increase in alpha$_2$ and beta$_1$ globulins which is mainly due to increases in alpha-glycoprotein and beta-lipoprotein. The concentrations of the relatively small molecular weight transferrin and ceruloplasmin are reduced, whereas fibrinogen concentrations are increased.

The other characteristic chemical change in the blood is hyperlipemia. This involves not only cholesterol, which for technical reasons is the only blood lipid measured in most laboratories, but all the major lipid components of plasma, including triglycerides and phosphatides. Plasma cholesterol may rise to 1500 mg. per 100 ml., but the level of this and the other lipids varies considerably, even in patients with the same type of nephrotic syndrome. Little prognostic or diagnostic value can be attached to the determination except that an abnormal value appears to be less common in lupus erythematosus than in other forms of nephrotic syndrome. The mechanism of the hyperlipemia is obscure, but seems intimately linked to the low albumin concentration.

Differential Diagnosis. Two complex investigations, *renal biopsy* and *differential protein clearances*, have proved of great value in establishing the morphologic diagnosis in individual cases. Nephrotic syndrome is now one of the main indications for renal biopsy. The diseases that cause the syndrome are nearly always diffuse, so that needle biopsy yields a representative picture. The procedure is not usually technically difficult unless the kidneys are small, which is unusual. Frequently it is possible to base treatment and prognosis on the histologic findings. This matter is discussed under the various disease headings, and will not be further elaborated here.

The diagnostic value of differential protein clearances was largely established by Squire and his colleagues (for references, see under minimal change glomerular disease). The principle is that the abnormal glomerulus in nephrotic syndrome permits the passage of increased amounts of protein, and that the selective pattern of this permeability varies in different diseases. Some glomerular diseases permit only the smaller proteins, e.g., albumin and transferrin, to escape into the urine, whereas in others all the plasma proteins are found. A crude idea of glomerular permeability can be obtained by electrophoresis of urinary protein; a highly selective proteinuria is seen to consist almost entirely of albumin with small peaks of alpha₁ and gamma globulin, whereas a poorly selective proteinuria shows an electrophoretic pattern similar to that of normal plasma. However, electrophoresis is an unsatisfactory method for the study of glomerular selectivity, for the electrical change and molecular weight of proteins are not closely related, and more satisfactory results can be obtained by measurement of individual proteins. A useful indication of selectivity, suggested by Cameron and Blandford, is the ratio of the clearance of gamma G globulin to that of transferrin; in highly selective proteinurias values below 0.2 are obtained. The major cause of a highly selective proteinuria is minimal change glomerular disease, which carries a good prognosis and usually responds well to steroids. The forms of nephrotic syndrome likely to be confused with this disease, which have a much worse prognosis and do not respond to steroids, i.e., membranous change and chronic glomerulonephritis, show poor selectivity in their pattern of protein excretion. There appear to be only two exceptions to the general rule that a highly selective proteinuria indicates a good prognosis, and both are uncommon—congenital nephrotic syndrome, a rare and invariably fatal disease, and occasional cases of renal amyloidosis.

Treatment. Treatment of the common diseases causing nephrotic syndrome has already been discussed under specific diseases. The treatment of many other causes of nephrotic syndrome listed in the table is obvious; for example, the nephrotic syndrome caused by mercury, trimethadione, and penicillamine usually improves rapidly when exposure to these substances ceases. It remains to say something of the treatment of nephrotic syndrome itself.

Although the cause of the edema is the low serum albumin resulting from the glomerular leak, there is no practical way of increasing plasma albumin while urinary protein losses persist. High protein diets have been advocated for years; occasionally they cause a marginal increase in plasma albumin, but usually their most obvious effect is to increase urinary protein losses. Moreover, protein is the most costly item of the diet, and many patients are unable to take a high protein diet because of its expense. Intravenous protein, given as salt-poor human albumin, is occasionally of value in the treatment of hospital patients with circulatory collapse caused by hypovolemia, or to initiate diuresis in a patient with refractory edema, but it produces a transitory effect and is impractical for chronic treatment.

The main factors in treatment of edema are dietary sodium restriction and diuretics. Sodium restriction should not be pushed to extremes; diets containing 20 to 50 mEq. a day contain enough salt to keep the food palatable, and will not lead to the reappearance of edema in most patients who are simultaneously given diuretics. Water restriction is not required except for patients with renal failure who may accumulate water in excess of salt. The diuretic regimen required varies from patient to patient; in general the oral diuretics are best, and it is wise to start treatment with a relatively gentle drug, such as a thiazide, and only use the more powerful diuretics, e.g., furosemide and ethacrynic acid, if initial treatment fails to produce diuresis. If diuretics are given more than three times a week, potassium deficiency usually develops unless the patient also takes a potassium supplement or spironolactone, but in renal failure potassium depletion is less of a problem, and both these forms of treatment may precipitate hyperkalemia. Modern diuretics are now so efficient that there is no longer a place for local fluid removal by paracentesis abdominis or Southey's tubes, though occasionally benefit may be obtained by aspiration of pleural effusions if these do not disappear rapidly.

When following the progress of edema, body weight rather than fluid balance is the most helpful guide. However, it must be remembered that treatment of edema is palliative only, and mild edema of the lower extremities carries little risk to life. Treatment of edema should not be pushed to the point at which the patient suffers severe postural hypotension or is unable to tolerate the prescribed diet, and it may be good judgment to allow mild edema to persist, particularly when the serum albumin is below 1.0 gram per 100 ml.

Nephrotic syndrome is usually a chronic disease, and it is wise therefore to encourage patients to follow their normal activities as far as possible. Frequently the physician will be asked by young female patients about the possible risks of pregnancy. The dangers depend largely on the underlying renal disease and the risk that because of this the pregnancy will be complicated by hypertension and placental insufficiency. Hypoalbuminemic edema does not per se contraindicate pregnancy (although edema frequently gets temporarily worse during pregnancy), and many women with nephrotic syndrome, particularly that resulting from minimal change glomerular disease, have had completely normal pregnancies.

Cameron, J. S., and Blandford, G.: The simple assessment of selectivity in heavy proteinuria. Lancet, 2:242, 1966.
Kark, R. M., Pirani, C. L., Pollak, V. E., Muehrcke, R. C., and Blainey, J. D.: The nephrotic syndrome in adults: A common disorder with many causes. Ann. Intern. Med., 49:751, 1958.
Lawrence, J. R., Pollak, V. E., Pirani, C. L., and Kark, R. M.: Histological and clinical evidence of post-streptococcal glomerulonephritis in patients with the nephrotic syndrome. Medicine, 42:1, 1963.
Shreiner, G. E.: The nephrotic syndrome. *In* Strauss, M. B., and Welt, L. G. (eds.): Diseases of the Kidney. London, J. & A. Churchill, Ltd., 1963.

BENIGN POSTURAL PROTEINURIA
(Orthostatic Proteinuria)

Definition. Benign postural proteinuria is a functional anomaly in which the kidney is normal morphologically, the urine contains protein when the patient is erect or in the lordotic position, but the proteinuria disappears in recumbency.

Benign postural proteinuria (often called *orthostatic*, although few physicians know what is meant by *orthostasis*) was believed to be a common condition in the years before renal biopsy was a standard investigation. The diagnosis was usually made in young military recruits, of whom a small proportion (2 to 3 per cent) were found by routine urine testing to have proteinuria, which disappeared in urines passed after a period of recumbency. Proteinuria could often be reproduced by placing the patient in a lordotic position while still recumbent. Many theories were advanced to explain the association of proteinuria with posture. The relationship of this form of proteinuria to that which occurs during fever or after excretion by normal subjects is unknown.

It is generally recognized that proteinuria resulting from organic renal disease is often more marked in the upright position, and may almost disappear during recumbency. The explanation for this phenomenon is obscure. Many patients with so-called benign postural proteinuria have been found on careful investigation to have organic renal disease, most often some form of chronic glomerular disease or a chronic pyelonephritis. The numbers of patients diagnosed to have benign postural proteinuria appear to have decreased in recent years, and it may be that the increased sophistication of renal investigations, particularly renal biopsy, is responsible for less frequent diagnosis. A recent report that postural proteinuria may disappear during treatment with steroids suggests that it is sometimes due to a mild form of minimal change glomerular disease. Because of this possibility it is impossible to acquit any subject with postural proteinuria of organic renal disease unless a renal biopsy has been examined by both the light and electron microscopes.

No large recent survey of patients with postural proteinuria, using renal biopsy and electron microscopy, has been reported, but studies of small groups of patients have shown that morphologic changes, often minor, in the kidney are very common. Until a large-scale investigation with several years of follow-up has been reported, it would be wise to keep an open mind on the existence of the syndrome, and to investigate patients who have the criteria of the condition just as carefully as those with persistent proteinuria.

Robinson, R. R.: Idiopathic proteinuria. Ann. Intern. Med., 71:1019, 1969.

Toxemia of Pregnancy
Thomas F. Ferris

Toxemia of pregnancy is a disease occurring in late pregnancy characterized by hypertension, edema, and proteinuria. Historically, convulsions have been the hallmark of toxemia, and the disease has been divided into eclampsia (Greek, eclampsis: a sudden flash) and preeclampsia, based upon whether a convulsion has occurred. Although the presence of convulsions is usually indicative of severe disease, separating toxemia on this basis does not imply different etiologies, and may have no more validity than separating other hypertensive processes associated with convulsions, e.g., acute glomerulonephritis and malignant hypertension.

Incidence. The disease occurs in 5 to 10 per cent of pregnancies, but the reported incidence depends upon criteria used to make the diagnosis and on the population studied. Hypertension alone has been reported to occur during the first pregnancy in 25 per cent of women in Great Britain. There is a bimodal frequency of the disease with peak incidences in young primiparous women and in multiparous women over 35. Toxemia is more common with pre-existing renal disease, hypertension, and diabetes, with twin pregnancies, and in Negroes.

Clinical Manifestations. The usual sequence of manifestations is edema and hypertension followed by proteinuria; occasionally proteinuria precedes hypertension. Because normal pregnancy is characterized by a reduction in blood pressure, particularly in the second trimester, blood pressures higher than 130 systolic and 80 diastolic should be considered abnormal during pregnancy. Diastolic hypertension is more striking than systolic with toxemia, and systolic blood pressures greater than 180 to 200 mm. Hg usually indicate that preceding hypertensive disease existed. Toxemia typically begins after the thirty-second week of pregnancy, but may occur as early as the twenty-fourth week, particularly in women with pre-existing renal disease or hypertension. It can occur during the first trimester with a hydatidiform mole. Excessive weight gain during pregnancy predisposes to its development, probably through mechanisms similar to those associating obesity with essential hypertension; but sudden weight gain is caused by edema. The edema is similar to that seen in acute glomerulonephritis, with a prominent distribution in the periorbital region, hands, and ankles. Headache, visual disturbances, or midepigastric pain are frequently present. On funduscopic examination segmental arteriolar narrowing and a wet glistening retina ("retinal sheen") are often seen. The presence of increased light reflex and tortuosity of the arterioles points to hypertensive disease having preceded the toxemia. Retinal hemorrhages or exudates are rare. The spinal reflexes may be hyperactive, and are important parameters to follow in assessing the degree of central nervous system excitability. Proteinuria ranges from trace amounts to levels seen in the nephrotic syndrome, 5 to 10 grams per 24 hours. Microscopic examination of the urine may reveal a few red blood cells, but significant hematuria or pyuria is more consistent with the presence of a primary renal disease. Although reduction in glomerular filtration rate occurs with toxemia, azotemia is seldom prominent because of the increase in glomerular filtration rate accompanying pregnancy. The low blood urea nitrogen (9 ± 2 mg. per 100 ml.) and creatinine (0.75 ± 0.2 mg. per 100 ml.) in late pregnancy are indicative of this increase, and even with a 50 to 75 per cent fall in glomerular filtration rate, the blood urea nitrogen and creatinine can remain within the normal range. A disproportionate reduction in urate clearance occurs in toxemia so that hyperuricemia usually precedes the development of azotemia.

Pathogenesis.   The cause of toxemia is unknown. Nonspecific changes have been described in the liver, brain, heart, and adrenals, and renal biopsies have demonstrated consistent findings. The glomeruli are swollen, and the glomerular lumen is occluded by cytoplasmic swelling of the endothelial cells. Electron microscopy may reveal focal basement membrane thickening, but this finding is inconstant and not prominent. These glomerular changes are distinctive for toxemia and are not seen in other hypertensive diseases.

The mechanism of the hypertension is unclear. Salt retention, caused by the reduction in glomerular filtration rate, might exacerbate the hypertension but alone would not cause it. The recent finding of renin in human uterus is of interest because there is a large amount of clinical evidence to suggest uterine ischemia as a factor in the pathogenesis of toxemia. If renin is involved, the sequence of events resulting in hypertension has not been elucidated. Plasma renin falls with the onset of toxemia, but since this accompanies salt retention, extracellular fluid expansion, and increased sensitivity to angiotensin, the effect of a specific level of plasma renin on blood pressure is difficult to evaluate. Any explanation of the pathogenesis of toxemia must account not only for hypertension but also for the renal pathology and central nervous system excitability which are disproportionate to the magnitude of the hypertension.

Treatment.   Control of weight gain during pregnancy and the use of diuretics when edema appears reduce the incidence of complete expressions of the disease. With the onset of toxemia, bed rest, salt restriction, diuretics, and sedation constitute the initial therapy. If hypertension becomes severe or does not abate with the aforementioned measures, antihypertensive drugs should be instituted. For immediate control of the blood pressure intravenous hydralazine (Apresoline), 25 to 40 mg. in 500 ml. dextrose and water, diazoxide, 300 mg., and methyldopa (Aldomet), 500 mg., have been efficacious. Magnesium sulfate has been widely used in toxemia, because it has both a depressant effect upon the central nervous system and a mild antihypertensive action. Barbiturates are useful in controlling central nervous system hyperexcitability, and should be used if convulsions appear imminent. The definitive therapy is termination of the pregnancy, and, providing that the fetus is viable, this should be accomplished as soon as the patient's condition is stable. When fetal size makes viability of concern, control of the disease with antihypertensive drugs and diuretics may allow for further fetal development. If proteinuria or azotemia persists despite therapy, delivery should be accomplished; there is little evidence that fetal growth occurs in the face of persistent toxemia. Eclampsia is sufficient reason for inducing delivery, because convulsions significantly increase maternal and fetal mortality.

Prognosis.   Maternal death with toxemia is now rare. Blood pressure usually returns to normal within two weeks after delivery, although the proteinuria may persist longer. However, women who develop toxemia have a higher incidence of hypertension in later life, and the role toxemia plays in its development has been a subject of concern and controversy. The unresolved question is whether toxemia causes subsequent hypertension or simply occurs more frequently in women with latent hypertension. In women having toxemia with a multiparous pregnancy, two findings favor an underlying hypertensive diathesis as a factor in the toxemia. First, the incidence of late hypertension is greater following multiparous than primiparous toxemia; indeed, in white women with eclampsia, a higher incidence of late hypertension can be demonstrated only following a multiparous toxemia. Second, the recurrence of toxemia with subsequent pregnancies is over 50 per cent following multiparous toxemia, but only 25 per cent in women developing toxemia with the first pregnancy.

An interesting finding in women having toxemia is that hypertension follows preeclampsia more often than eclampsia. This has been interpreted by some to indicate that the fulminant nature of eclampsia has prevented the toxemia from being of sufficient duration to produce permanent renal damage, the cause of ultimate hypertension. An equally plausible explanation is that preeclampsia occurs more frequently in those women destined to develop essential hypertension.

Eastman, N. J. (ed.): Williams' Textbook of Obstetrics. 13th ed. New York, Appleton-Century-Crofts, 1966.

Pollak, V. E., and Nettles, J. B.: The kidney in toxemia of pregnancy: A clinical and pathological study based on renal biopsies. Medicine, 39:469, 1960.

Pyelonephritis

Paul B. Beeson

DEFINITION

The term pyelonephritis refers to immediate and residual effects of bacterial infection in the kidney. The clinical manifestations are generally conceived of as existing in two forms: *acute pyelonephritis,* and active pyogenic infection, usually accompanied by local and systemic symptoms of infection; and *chronic pyelonephritis,* wherein the principal manifestations are caused by the injury sustained in preceding active infections. Actually, considerable uncertainty exists regarding the relationship between acute and chronic pyelonephritis. For example, many patients known to have had multiple attacks of acute pyelonephritis show no indication of progression to chronic pyelonephritis even after intervals of many years. Furthermore, comparatively few patients with chronic pyelonephritis give a history of acute infection of the urinary tract. The possibility exists, therefore, that some cases of the disease we are now calling "chronic pyelonephritis" result from something other than bacterial infection of the kidney. Reasons for this uncertainty include inadequacy of diagnostic procedures for diagnosis of chronic pyelonephritis and erroneous interpretation of bacteriologic findings.

Thus, after acknowledging that important questions remain unanswered in respect to pathogenesis and differential diagnosis, not only between acute and chronic pyelonephritis, but also between chronic pyelonephritis and other chronic renal diseases, we shall nevertheless proceed to outline the concepts of these entities commonly held at present.

ACUTE PYELONEPHRITIS

Etiology. More than 95 per cent of cases of acute pyelonephritis are caused by gram-negative enteric bacilli. The role of these organisms in urinary tract infections, including pyelonephritis, is discussed elsewhere in this book. A minor proportion of cases of acute pyelonephritis is caused by gram-positive cocci, enterococcus, and Staphylococcus. From the standpoint of the pathologic lesion and the general clinical picture, these infections resemble the gram-negative bacillary infections, and we may consider them here as a group.

Factors in Pathogenesis. Perhaps half of all cases of acute pyelonephritis begin in healthy people without discernible precipitating factors. Among the remainder certain obvious associations with other conditions can be discussed. Following are the most important predisposing factors: (1)

Obstruction. Any impediment of urine flow renders the kidney far more susceptible to acute bacterial infection. Acute pyelonephritis occurs 12 to 20 times more frequently in persons with obstructive lesions than in those without obstruction. (2) *Age and sex.* A comparatively high incidence of acute pyelonephritis during the first 18 months of life is generally attributed to the frequency of lower urinary tract infection in this age group, perhaps caused by fecal soiling of the urethral meatus. Female infants are affected somewhat more frequently than males. Acute pyelonephritis is perhaps ten times as common in women of childbearing age, i.e., 18 to 40 years, as in males at this age. Factors here may be trauma to the urethra during sexual intercourse and the physiologic loss of tone in the ureters during pregnancy, usually in the latter half. (3) *Instrumentation of the urinary tract.* There can be no question that, despite every precaution, bacteria are liable to be carried into the bladder urine (from which they may ascend to the kidneys) during catheterization, cystoscopy, or other instrumentation of the lower urinary tract. (4) *Autonomic disturbances of bladder function.* Persons with various kinds of neuropathy, e.g., spinal paraplegia, poliomyelitis, tabes dorsalis, frequently develop urinary tract infection and pyelonephritis. In all probability the sequence here is: inability to void → catheterization → infection of the bladder urine → infection of the kidney. Immobilization of the patient occasioned by such lesions may contribute, because of demineralization of bone and formation of urinary calculi with consequent obstruction of urine flow. (5) *Vesicoureteral reflux.* Improved techniques of roentgenographic study have disclosed the occurrence of reflux from the bladder into the ureters during micturition in a substantial proportion of patients with recurrent acute pyelonephritis. This defect would provide a means for transporting bacteria to the kidney, and would also serve to impair the mechanism by which the bladder rids itself of bacteria. (6) *Sickle cell trait.* Acute pyelonephritis occurs more frequently in persons with the sickle cell trait than in comparable persons lacking the trait. Inasmuch as the sickling phenomenon has been shown to take place more readily in hypertonic media, a possible explanation for increased susceptibility to infection in these patients may be sickling and thrombus formation in blood vessels of the renal medulla. (7) *Diabetes mellitus.* It is usually stated that acute pyelonephritis is somewhat more common in patients with diabetes mellitus, but there are no reliable data to substantiate this. Undoubtedly a very severe form of acute pyelonephritis, renal medullary necrosis, is much more common in the diabetic, as described more fully at the end of this article.

Pathology. Knowledge of the pathologic process is meager because uncomplicated acute pyelonephritis does not lead to death. Nevertheless, on the basis of occasional chance opportunities and experiments in animals, it is possible to describe the probable form of the lesion with reasonable assurance. One or both kidneys may be affected. The lining of the renal pelvis and calyces is diffusely inflamed. Infection of the renal substance is usually confined to one or more wedge-shaped areas, the apices being in the medulla. In this zone of acute inflammation there are micro-abscesses, some of which may bulge under the capsule of the kidney, but they almost never rupture into the perinephric area. Collections of polymorphonuclear leukocytes can be seen in and around the lumina of the tubules throughout their length. The glomeruli are usually spared structurally, but may become functionless because the tubular part of the nephron is destroyed. The infectious process tends to remain confined within the originally involved segment of renal tissue and to subside gradually over a period of one to three weeks. As healing takes place, the area contracts, polymorphonuclear leukocytes are replaced by mononuclear cells, and scar tissue is deposited. Eventually a linear scar involving a streak of medulla and corresponding cortical tissue is all that remains. Remnants of glomeruli and tubules filled with a colloid-like material lie in this fibrous matrix.

A considerable amount of work has been done on the pathogenesis of pyelonephritis in laboratory animals. The kidney can be infected either by the intravenous route or by introducing bacteria into the urinary tract; the lesion is the same regardless of the route of inoculation. In order to infect the kidney by way of the blood stream it is necessary to inject large numbers of bacteria, probably because only a minute proportion of the inoculum is trapped by the kidney. As a general rule, coliform bacteria, although the most common cause of human pyelonephritis, are incapable of infecting a normal kidney, although pathogenic strains of Staphylococcus, enterococcus, occasional strains of Proteus, and rare strains of coliform organisms will do so. In the presence of an obstructive lesion, however, the susceptibility of the kidney to infection by all these bacteria, including the coliforms, is greatly increased. Obstruction has been produced by introducing artificial calculi into the bladder, by partial or complete ureteral ligation, or by mechanical injury of the kidney. Even small injuries of the medulla caused by needle puncture lead to obstruction of a few collecting tubules and localized susceptibility to infection. Experiments of this kind have demonstrated that bacterial multiplication begins in the medulla and then spreads into the corresponding area of cortex. It is thought, therefore, that infection spreads in retrograde manner from the obstructed collecting tubules in the medulla throughout the nephron. Characteristic wedge-shaped areas of acute pyelonephritis involving both medulla and cortex are also produced when small numbers of bacteria, e.g., 10 to 100 living organisms, are inoculated into the medulla. By contrast, as many as 100,000 coliform bacteria must be inoculated into the cortex in order to establish even local infection. A conspicuous feature of the areas of acute pyelonephritis produced in laboratory animals is lack of tendency for infection to invade neighboring, unobstructed areas of renal parenchyma. The process remains confined to the area of intrarenal hydronephrosis, eventually "burns out," and shrinks to a scar, leaving adjacent kidney unaffected. This seems compatible with acute pyelonephritis in man, wherein there is usually no measurable evidence of even temporary impairment of renal function despite evidence that both kidneys are acutely infected. It is reasonable to presume, therefore, that the disease in man is one of patchy renal involvement, leaving large segments of tissue unaffected. Evidence obtained in animals indicates that the medullary zone is the critical one from the standpoint of pathogenesis of acute bacterial infection. Factors that may be responsible include the following: (1) *Ammonia formation.* Evidence has been obtained that high local concentration of ammonia, as may be present when the body is dealing with an acid load, may be sufficient to inactivate complement, thus rendering ineffective a major defense mechanism against bacterial infection. (2) *Hypertonicity.* The unusual osmolarity in this area of the body may be sufficient to affect the activity of complement and phagocytes, as well as to permit survival of bacterial protoplasts. (3) *Differences in the blood supply.* The blood flow to the medulla is far less than that to the cortex.

Clinical Manifestations. The clinical picture may be characteristic: sudden rise of body temperature to 102° to 105° F., shaking chills, aching pain in one or both costovertebral areas or flanks, and symptoms of bladder inflammation. Physical examination reveals tenderness in the region of one or both kidneys; at times a tender kidney may be detected by palpation. Laboratory tests show polymorphonuclear leukocytosis, and the urine is laden with leukocytes. Stain of the sediment reveals numerous bacteria, usually gram-negative bacilli, and culture confirms this. In a small proportion of cases blood culture is also positive. There are no signs of impaired renal function of of acute hypertension as is sometimes seen in acute glomerulonephritis.

In the absence of an obstructive lesion of the urinary tract, such as stone or tumor, this illness is self-limited, rarely lasting more than a week or ten days.

The clinical picture just described is easy to recognize and is seldom confused with anything else. Yet there must also be subclinical forms, because typical evidence of previous attacks of acute pyelonephritis is encountered at autopsy in patients lacking a history of symptoms of urinary tract infection. Possibly the size of the area of renal tissue involved in an episode is the determining factor. In addition to the "classic" clinical picture and the subclinical form, acute pyelonephritis at times presents with symptoms that do not point to the urinary tract. Dysuria may be lacking, and there may be no fever. There may only be backache, without demonstrable tenderness in the kidney region. Some patients have pain in either the upper or the lower abdomen, together with symptoms of disturbed gastrointestinal function. Others complain only of general fatigue. Mild anemia may be caused by repeated episodes of acute pyelonephritis. The urine can be free of pus cells or bacteria for brief periods. Repeated urinalyses on succeeding days should, however, always reveal presence of pus cells and bacteria.

Acute urinary tract infection, complicated by pyelonephritis, frequently arises in debilitated patients in hospitals and nursing homes who have been subjected to urethral instrumentation, especially the indwelling catheter. In such people the infection may take a fulminating course, with bacteremia and shock, and can in fact be the terminal event of prolonged illness. Gram-negative sepsis and bacteremic shock are described in another article.

Diagnosis. In the absence of more obvious symptoms and physical findings, the diagnosis of active urinary tract infection can be made when pus cells and bacteria are demonstrated in the urine. It is often difficult, indeed impossible, to differentiate between infection confined to the lower urinary tract and that which involves the renal substance, i.e., pyelonephritis. Presence or absence of fever is one of the most helpful guides in this situation. It is a reasonable clinical practice to infer that the infection involves renal substance when the patient has fever. On the other hand, absence of fever should not exclude the possibility of renal involvement. Demonstration of an obstructive lesion in a patient with urinary tract infection makes the diagnosis of pyelonephritis highly probable. There are no characteristic roentgenographic signs of acute pyelonephritis. Needle biopsy of the kidney is unlikely to disclose the process because of its patchy distribution; furthermore, it could conceivably be harmful in this situation.

Treatment. Treatment of acute pyelonephritis is discussed elsewhere in this book as part of the problem of bacterial infections of the urinary tract.

CHRONIC PYELONEPHRITIS

As mentioned in the opening paragraph of this article, the term "chronic pyelonephritis" is employed to indicate the renal disease resulting from cicatricial effects of pre-existing bacterial infection, as well as the progressive disease resulting from persisting and recurring bacterial infection. The concept that this represents one of the most common and most important kinds of chronic renal disease has gained general acceptance only relatively recently, i.e., since about 1940. Before that time the term "chronic pyelonephritis" was scarely mentioned in classifications of chronic renal disease. Doubtless many pathologic processes now

being called "chronic pyelonephritis" were formerly designated "nephrosclerosis," "chronic interstitial nephritis," etc. There is reason to believe that current opinion may have gone too far and that the name "chronic pyelonephritis" is being given to some forms of renal disease not caused by bacterial infection, since pathologists frequently make this diagnosis solely on the basis of a pattern of morphologic change regardless of evidence of present or previous infection. Yet we know that many kinds of renal injury can lead to changes similar to those caused by infection, examples being injury by chemical agents, obstructive uropathy, electrolyte abnormalities, vascular disease, and inflammation due to immune mechanisms. Furthermore, even when bacterial infection is present, it may be a secondary process, engrafted on a kidney injured in some other way. Obviously, pathologists currently differ in readiness to diagnose chronic pyelonephritis, as indicated by reported incidences at autopsy ranging from as high as 10 to 15 per cent to as low as 2.5 to 3 per cent.

Pathology. The most distinctive feature of chronic pyelonephritis is its patchy distribution throughout the kidney. The external surface may reveal U-shaped scars, and the cut section shows linear streaks of scarring extending from the medulla out into cortical tissue. Microscopic examination shows, in addition to areas of scarring between tubules and around glomeruli, patches of mononuclear cell infiltration. Glomeruli may be crowded together, and tubules may be filled with a colloid-like material resembling that in the thyroid gland.

A common accompaniment of the scarring process just described is *admixture of areas of acute pyelonephritis*; indeed, this may account for the progressive nature of chronic pyelonephritis and for continued outpouring of pus and bacteria in the urine. The scarring of a previous area of acute infection may in turn lead to development of an adjacent area of intrarenal hydronephrosis which then becomes a susceptible focus for fresh infection, thus tending to perpetuate a cycle: infection → scarring → infection.

Clinical Manifestations. Generally there are no symptoms of infection in chronic pyelonephritis. Less than half the patients have a history of preceding bouts of urinary tract infection. Usually manifestations of chronic renal insufficiency come on insidiously in persons who have previously been well. The patient may notice fatigue, headache, poor appetite and some weight loss. Polyuria and excessive thirst are fairly common. The period of renal insufficiency may be unusually long. Many persons have lived in relative comfort for years despite moderate anemia and azotemia. Edema and other manifestations of the nephrotic syndrome are rarely, if ever, seen in chronic pyelonephritis.

Some patients with chronic pyelonephritis show considerable enlargement of the spleen, and this may be associated with anemia greater than is usually found in chronic renal disease.

Symptoms of an obstructive lesion may be present, e.g., difficulty in voiding, passage of stones or blood. There may or may not be evidence of _bacterial infection_ in the urinary tract; if infection is present, the evidence resembles that of acute urinary tract infection, the coliform bacteria accounting for the majority of cases. On examination of urine sediment the finding of _leukocyte casts_ is strongly suggestive of the presence of pyelonephritis, and is regarded by many as the most distinctive finding in this disease. When supravital stains are applied to the urine sediment, large pale-staining polymorphonuclear leukocytes containing granules that show active brownian motion are sometimes found in considerable number. These, called _"glitter cells,"_ seem to be polymorphonuclear leukocytes altered by the low osmolarity of the urine. They can be found in other renal disease and in lower urinary tract infection, and are not by themselves diagnostic of pyelonephritis. A special test for chronic pyelonephritis is based on acute changes in urine cellular content following intravenous injection of bacterial endotoxin or prednisolone. Within the first two to four hours there may be a several-fold increase in the number of leukocytes and renal tubular epithelial cells in the urine of patients with chronic pyelonephritis, whereas in other kinds of chronic renal disease there is usually little or no change in cellular excretion. The response, although not absolutely specific for pyelonephritis, may be of diagnostic value when considered in conjunction with other studies.

Proteinuria is not prominent in pyelonephritis; output of more than 3 grams per day should suggest some other kind of renal disease. _Intravenous pyelography_ can be a helpful diagnostic procedure, especially in young patients. It may reveal evidence of obstructive uropathy; patchy renal scarring is suggested by asymmetry and deformity of the renal pelvic shadows; and one or both kidneys may appear smaller than normal. Needle _biopsy_ of the kidney may reveal pathologic changes already described, but its value is limited because the extent of these changes is difficult to estimate, and the small sample obtained may miss areas showing characteristic lesions.

Renal Function. The severe injury of acute pyelonephritis is likely to cause permanent destruction of a group of nephrons. Thus, the end result of a series of acute lesions is loss of some nephron units, leaving intact and hypertrophied nephrons to carry out renal work. Clearance studies may therefore show reduction in mass of functional tissue. Eventually destruction reaches the point where reserve is inadequate, and manifestations of insufficiency make their appearance. An effect on tubular function may become evident first—i.e., impaired capacity to secrete concentrated urine—but elevation in the blood nonprotein nitrogen level follows soon after. In addition, some students of renal disease believe that at times specific tubular functions are affected predominantly, giving rise to such syndromes as sodium-losing or potassium-losing nephritis, to hyperchloremic acidosis, or to nephrogenic diabetes insipidus.

Relation between Chronic Pyelonephritis and Hypertension. There is no unanimity of opinion regarding the role of chronic pyelonephritis in the etiology of hypertension. In general, it may be said that about 15 per cent of patients with hypertension also have significant changes in renal architecture consistent with chronic pyelonephritis. Cures of hypertension by nephrectomy for unilateral renal disease have been obtained in patients with undoubted chronic pyelonephritis. Some pathologists have claimed that malignant hypertension is almost always associated with chronic pyelonephritis. On the other hand, it must be emphasized that many patients succumb to severe renal insufficiency due to chronic pyelonephritis without developing hypertension at any time. We must recognize too that primary vascular disease may lead to scarring of the kidney that resembles the lesions remaining after infection has subsided; furthermore, the scarring due to vascular disease could lead to increased susceptibility to infection. Hence, it seems highly likely that, in some patients who have hypertension and bacterial infection of the kidney, the latter exists only as a secondary phenomenon.

Course. Chronic pyelonephritis is usually an insidious process compatible with many years of life. Obvious pathologic changes may be found in persons who have exhibited no evidence of impaired function. Even when decompensation appears, it usually progresses slowly so that an affected person may be able to maintain his activity despite considerable azotemia for months or even years. Death may result from uremia or from intercurrent infection. In chronic pyelonephritis associated with hypertension, coronary or cerebral vascular disease may be the cause of death.

Treatment. If bacterial infection is present, it should be treated vigorously, as outlined elsewhere for urinary tract infections. Improvement in well-being and renal function may sometimes follow eradication of smoldering infection even in the absence of fever or pyuria. _As with any form of urinary tract infection, efforts should be made to find and relieve an obstructive lesion._ Improved renal function is often observed following relief of obstruction as, for example, in prostatic disease. Treatment of the manifestations of renal insufficiency is outlined elsewhere.

RENAL MEDULLARY NECROSIS
(Renal Papillary Necrosis, Necrotizing Papillitis)

Renal medullary necrosis is a severe complication of pyelonephritis—ischemic necrosis of the renal papilla and adjacent portions of the renal medulla. The lesion is most often, though not invariably, associated with severe acute and chronic pyelonephritis. It is especially common in patients with diabetes and pyelonephritis, about half the reported cases having involved such persons. Obstruction of the urinary tract is also regarded as a predisposing factor, but this may relate only to the aggravating effect of obstruction on infection in the kidney. European clinicians report fairly frequent occurrence of renal medullary necrosis in women who have habitually ingested large quantities of analgesic medicines containing phenacetin for headache. These patients also usually have infection of the urinary tract. The relative roles of infection and phenacetin in the pathogenesis of the lesion cannot be specified with certainty.

Although infection appears to be the most important factor in the pathogenesis of this lesion, there can be little doubt that the peculiarities of blood supply of the medulla must also be factors. This could help to explain the frequent occurrence of the lesion in patients with diabetes and generalized vascular disease, as well as the role of obstruction, which must impair the blood supply of this area.

The zone of necrosis may occur throughout the pyramid from the extreme tip as far proximally as the corticomedullary junction. Eventually this usually sloughs, so that chunks of necrotic tissue often migrate down through the urinary passages.

The clinical manifestations of renal medullary necrosis are intensification of symptoms of preexisting pyelonephritis. There may be pain in the lumbar region, colicky pain along the ureteral radiation, and hematuria. Fever may be high. Manifestations of gram-negative bacteremia may supervene. This lesion should be considered always in elderly patients with diabetes who show rapid deterioration in clinical status with signs of active pyelonephritis and increasing renal decompensation.

The diagnosis can sometimes be made by finding pieces of renal medullary tissue in the urine sediment. Pyelography may also be of assistance: in addition to the scarring and asymmetry of chronic pyelonephritis, cavities and sinuses in the region of the papillae may be demonstrated.

Therapy is not notably effective, but should be directed toward control of infection, and whatever measures can be employed to improve the status of patients who have diabetes mellitus or who are habitual abusers of analgesic medicines.

Beeson, P. B.: Urinary tract infection and pyelonephritis. *In* Black, D. A. K. (ed.): Renal Disease. 2nd ed. Oxford, Blackwell Scientific Publications, 1967.

Bengtsson, U.: A comparative study of chronic non-obstructive pyelonephritis and renal papillary necrosis. Acta Med. Scandinav., Suppl. 388, 1962.

Gilman, A.: Analgesic nephrotoxicity. A pharmacological analysis. Amer. J. Med., 36:163, 1964.

Heptinstall, R. H.: The limitations of the pathological diagnosis of chronic pyelonephritis. *In* Black, D. A. K. (ed.): Renal Disease. 2nd ed. Oxford, Blackwell Scientific Publications, 1967.

Hodson, C. J.: Natural history of chronic pyelonephritic scarring. Brit. Med. J., 2:191, 1965.

Kass, E. H. (ed.): Progress in Pyelonephritis. Philadelphia, F. A. Davis Company, 1965.

Kincaid-Smith, P., and Bullen, M.: Bacteriuria in pregnancy. Lancet, 1:395, 1965.

Kleeman, C. R., Hewitt, W. L., and Guze, L. B.: Pyelonephritis. Medicine, 39:3, 1960.

Pawlowski, J. M., Bloxdorf, J. W., and Kimmelstiel, P.: Chronic pyelonephritis. A morphologic and bacteriologic study. New Eng. J. Med., 268:965, 1963.

Other Specific Renal Diseases

William B. Schwartz

THE NEPHROPATHY OF POTASSIUM DEPLETION

Potassium depletion often produces characteristic structural and functional disturbances in the kidney. The changes occur regardless of the cause of the depletion; primary aldosteronism, Cushing's syndrome, renal tubular disorders such as Fanconi's syndrome, and gastrointestinal losses from diarrhea or vomiting can all produce a deficit great enough to induce renal injury. It is not certain how long potassium deficiency must be present before renal abnormalities can occur. Occasionally, renal disease has been recognized in a patient who has been depleted for only several weeks, but in most instances depletion has been present for months or years.

The characteristic histologic changes in the kidney consist of multiple vacuoles in the tubular epithelium, usually most numerous in the proximal convolutions. These vacuoles (which do not contain fat or glycogen) are virtually pathognomonic of the disease. In most patients, however, the tubular abnormalities are less specific and are limited to mild degenerative changes or to diffuse foamy swelling. The glomeruli and blood vessels are usually not involved. Occasionally, despite striking functional abnormalities, the histologic appearance of the kidney is entirely normal.

The most frequent and striking functional abnormality is an inability to concentrate the urine even after prolonged restriction of water or after the administration of vasopressin. Diluting ability, on the other hand, is usually well preserved. The exact nature of the defect in concentrating power in man is not known, but it would appear from studies in animals that inability to establish a normal degree of medullary hypertonicity and reduced permeability of the collecting ducts to water are both important factors.

Many patients have no urinary symptoms, but in some, nocturia, polyuria, and polydipsia are prominent complaints. Occasionally these symptoms are of sufficient severity to suggest the diagnosis of diabetes insipidus. The polyuria and related symptoms probably result from impaired concentrating ability, although it has also been proposed that excessive fluid intake induced by a primary abnormality of the thirst mechanism may contribute.

Examination of the urine may reveal slight proteinuria and cylindruria, but often no abnormalities are found. Tubular excretion of phenol-sulfonphthalein and para-aminohippurate is often reduced. Blood urea nitrogen and creatinine concentrations are ordinarily within normal limits or only slightly elevated, but frank azotemia may be induced by complications such as sodium depletion, hypotension, or pyelonephritis. Renal potassium wasting is *not* a feature of the disease; its presence indicates that an underlying disorder of adrenal or renal origin is responsible for the potassium depletion.

Pyelonephritis is said to occur with unusual frequency in patients with the nephropathy of potassium depletion, but, in view of the relative frequency with which pyelonephritis complicates virtually all types of renal disease, it is difficult to attach any special significance to this observation.

In some instances, urinary abnormalities, slight azotemia, and inability to concentrate the urine lead to an erroneous diagnosis of irreversible renal disease such as chronic glomerulonephritis. In other instances, kidney injury resulting from potassium depletion may complicate pre-existing renal disease and contribute to the development of serious renal failure.

Correction of the potassium deficiency is usually followed within several months by improvement or correction of renal functional abnormalities. Serial renal biopsies indicate that in most instances the structural abnormalities can be completely reversed within a few months to a year.

Hollander, W., Jr., and Blythe, W. B.: Nephropathy of potasssium depletion. *In* Strauss, M. B., and Welt, L. G. (eds.): Diseases of the Kidney. Boston, Little, Brown and Company, 1971.
Schwartz, W. B., and Relman, A. S.: Effects of electrolyte disorders on renal structure and function. New Eng. J. Med., 276:383, 452, 1967.

THE NEPHROPATHY OF HYPERCALCEMIA

Hypercalcemic nephropathy is characterized in its early stages by tubular injury and polyuria, and in its late stages by progressive renal insufficiency. The changes in structure and function of the kidney are similar, regardless of the metabolic disturbance responsible for elevation of serum calcium concentration. The usual causes of hypercalcemic nephropathy are *hyperparathyroidism, sarcoidosis, vitamin D intoxication, excessive ingestion of milk and alkali (milk-alkali syndrome, Burnett syndrome), multiple myeloma, malignant disease,* and, less frequently, *immobilization* (particularly in *Paget's disease*) and *hyperthyroidism.*

The characteristic pathologic changes are in the collecting ducts and in the distal convoluted tubules, the epithelium in both areas showing degenerative changes and often necrosis and calcification. Calcified casts, which form in sites adjacent to tubular injury, lead to obstruction of nephrons with resultant dilatation of proximal segments. In long-standing hypercalcemia, calcification of the interstitium and occasionally of the glomeruli and vessels leads to progressive scarring and loss of renal mass. At this stage hypertension often develops, and the resultant nephrosclerotic changes may come to dominate the histologic picture.

Clinical findings vary with the duration and severity of the hypercalcemia. Moderate elevations of serum calcium concentration produce a clinical picture characterized initially by evidence of tubular dysfunction. Injury to the distal nephron impairs the countercurrent mechanism for concentrating the urine, and leads to polyuria and polydipsia. Tubular secretory capacity is affected, as evidenced by the impairment of phenolsulfonphthalein excretion. Azotemia develops only after a prolonged period and is a consequence of obstruction of nephrons rather than of primary glomerular injury. The urine frequently contains a small quantity of protein as well as casts, erythrocytes, and leukocytes. Roentgenographic examination of the abdomen may demonstrate *nephrocalcinosis,* which is usually seen chiefly in the area of the renal pyramids. Patients with hypercalcemia are likely to have hypercalciuria and therefore to develop *renal calculi,* often complicated by pyelonephritis. It is worth emphasizing that, when an elevated serum calcium concentration is found in a patient with renal insufficiency, it should be assumed, at least initially, that the calcium disorder is primary since renal failure with secondary hyperparathyroidism rarely produces hypercalcemia. Hypercalcemia occurs with significant frequency, however, in patients with chronic renal failure who undergo successful renal transplantation; in these patients persistence of the parathyroid hyperplasia characteristic of secondary hyperparathyroidism may lead to a state of *autonomous hyperparathyroidism (tertiary hyperparathyroidism)* and to elevations in serum calcium concentration sufficient to threaten the integrity of a transplanted kidney.

Hypercalcemic nephropathy is best treated by correcting the underlying metabolic disorder. Removal of a parathyroid adenoma, control of hyperthyroidism, discontinuance of excessive milk and alkali intake, or ambulation of the patient with Paget's disease usually leads to prompt reduction of the serum calcium concentration to normal. Reduction in serum calcium concentration following withdrawal of excessive vitamin D is generally slower, but can be hastened by administration of corticosteroids. Steroids may also be effective in the hypercalcemia of a sarcoidosis, metastatic bone disease, and multiple myeloma.

Severe hypercalcemia (15 to 20 mg. per 100 ml.) presents a special therapeutic problem because it may produce rapidly progressive renal failure, oliguria, confusion, lethargy, and coma. This syndrome of so-called *hypercalcemic crisis* is seen most frequently in association with hyperparathyroidism and with malignant disease. It usually proves fatal within a short time unless a prompt reduction in serum calcium concentration is effected. As an initial approach to accomplishing such a reduction it is current practice to administer 2 to 3 liters of normal saline intravenously over a period of six to nine hours; such treatment is often accompanied or immediately followed by a significant fall in serum calcium concentration that takes the patient out of danger. This effect is mediated, at least in part, by a diuresis of sodium which increases the renal excretion of calcium. If hypercalcemia does not respond adequately to saline infusion, it can usually be quickly controlled by the intravenous administration of inorganic phosphate. Phosphate salts are thought to act by both increasing calcium deposition in bone and by diminishing bone resorption. The usual program of treatment consists of the infusion of 500 ml. of a buffered 0.1 molar phosphate solution (1.5 grams of phosphorus) over eight or nine hours. The chief risk attendant on such treatment is that of producing severe hypocalcemia; but, with the regimen described above, such an occurrence is uncommon unless renal failure and a diminished ability to excrete phosphate lead to marked hyperphosphatemia. In the patient with renal insufficiency the period of infusion should generally be extended to 24 hours; serum calcium concentration should be measured several times during this interval.

Phosphate therapy may also be of use for the prolonged management of mild or moderate hypercalcemia that cannot be controlled by therapy directed toward the underlying disease state. For example, in certain patients with malignancies the daily oral administration of 1 to 3 grams of phosphorous (as sodium phosphate) may provide the only effective means of holding calcium concentration at or near normal levels. Whether or not such treatment entails the risk of producing clinically significant soft-tissue calcification has not as yet been clearly determined.

The prognosis in hypercalcemic nephropathy depends on the severity and chronicity of the renal disease. Renal failure of recent onset induced by acute hypercalcemia is often completely reversible. However, renal insufficiency that has developed gradually in association with chronic hypercalcemia is often little affected by restoration of a normal serum calcium concentration; when improvement occurs, it is likely to be slow, sometimes taking many months. The prognosis is particularly poor if severe hypertension and nephrosclerosis are present. Nevertheless, in every instance of hypercalcemia a vigorous effort should be made to restore the serum concentration to normal in the hope of preserving remaining renal function or of at least slowing the advance of renal insufficiency.

Epstein, F. H.: Calcium and the kidney. Amer. J. Med., 45:700, 1968.
Goldsmith, R. S., and Ingbar, S. H.: Inorganic phosphate treatment of hypercalcemia of diverse etiologies. New Eng. J. Med., 274:1, 1966.
Massry, S. G., Mueller, E., Silverman, A. G., and Kleeman, C. R.: Inorganic phosphate treatment of hypercalcemia. Arch. Intern. Med. (Chicago), 121:307, 1968.
Schwartz, W. B., and Relman, A. S.: Effects of electrolyte disorders on renal structure and function. New Eng. J. Med., 276:383, 452, 1967.

RENAL TUBULAR ACIDOSIS

Renal tubular acidosis (RTA) is an uncommon disorder in which there is a tubular defect either in urinary acidification or in bicarbonate reabsorption. Hyperchloremic acidosis and hypokalemia are characteristic features, and both osteomalacia and nephrocalcinosis are often present. In the early stages of the disease neither blood urea nitrogen nor creatinine concentration is increased appreciably.

Renal tubular acidosis occurs in primary and secondary forms. The *primary* or *classic* type is of unknown origin and can be seen either as a transient disturbance during the first 12 to 18 months of life or as a permanent disorder that begins most commonly in adolescence or early adulthood. The adult form occurs more commonly in females than in males (2 to 1), and in some cases appears to be hereditary. In primary RTA, acidosis usually results from an inability of the distal tubule to establish a normally steep concentration gradient for hydrogen, the urine pH rarely falling below a value of 6.0 even in the face of severe acidosis.

The *secondary* form of RTA may occur in a variety of clinical settings. It may be seen as a complication of the ingestion of *paraldehyde*, *outdated tetracycline*, or *amphotericin B*, in diverse *hypergammaglobulinemic states*, and in certain inherited disorders such as *Wilson's disease*. It also occurs in a number of other circumstances, such as after *renal transplantation* and in association with *hypercalcemia*. In most instances of secondary RTA, acidosis results from an impaired proximal reabsorption of bicarbonate that increases delivery of alkali to the distal tubule and thus overwhelms the normal acidifying mechanism. The inherent capacity of the distal tubule to acidify the urine is preserved, however; if plasma bicarbonate concentration (and thus filtered load of bicarbonate) is reduced sufficiently to allow complete reabsorption of bicarbonate, urine pH falls to a level of less than 5.5. The ability to acidify the urine in response to metabolic acidosis (induced by an NH_4Cl load) serves to differentiate the proximal (bicarbonate-wasting) from the distal (gradient) form of the disease.

Experience with the long-term course of most secondary states of renal tubular acidosis is as yet quite limited, and for this reason the following discussion of clinical manifestations is based chiefly on studies of the primary form of the disease.

Osteomalacia. Hypophosphatemia and a high rate of phosphate excretion, i.e., increased phosphate clearance, are typical features of the primary form of renal tubular acidosis, and are often accompanied by roentgenologic evidence of rickets or osteomalacia. The clinical and roentgenologic manifestations are thus similar to those encountered with vitamin D deficiency or with resistance to vitamin D. In addition to the disturbance in phosphate metabolism, an important contributory factor to the development of osteomalacia appears to be the metabolic acidosis. In some patients osteomalacia produces bone pain, and this may be the presenting problem; in others the initial clinical difficulty is a disturbance in gait resulting from abnormal skeletal growth.

Hypercalciuria and Renal Calculi. Hypercalciuria is an almost constant feature of renal tubular acidosis, and frequently leads to the formation of renal calculi. A low urinary citrate excretion is also thought by some investigators to contribute to the tendency to form stones. Symptoms of renal colic are frequent and may be the first manifestations of the underlying tubular disease. Complications of renal calculi, such as obstruction or pyelonephritis, are encountered commonly and are often responsible for both secondary renal damage and hypertension. Diffuse calcification of the renal medulla (*nephrocalcinosis*) is a characteristic though not consistent roentgenologic finding and at times is an important clue to diagnosis.

Hypokalemia and Muscle Weakness. A low serum potassium concentration accompanied by continued excretion of large quantities of potassium is a frequent abnormality. In "distal" RTA the loss of potassium results in part from an impaired ability of the distal tubule to secrete hydrogen at sites of sodium-cation exchange. As a result a larger than normal fraction of sodium reabsorption takes place by exchange with potassium. Secondary hyperaldosteronism resulting from renal sodium loss and slight hypovolemia also promotes excessive potassium secretion. In "proximal" RTA, potassium wasting presumably results from flooding of distal exchange sites with sodium bicarbonate and consequent acceleration of sodium reabsorption and potassium secretion.

As a result of potassium deficiency patients often suffer from chronic weakness and fatigue. In instances of severe potassium depletion, frank paralysis with quadriplegia may occur. Such episodes of paralysis often appear intermittently and may simulate the syndrome of familial periodic paralysis. Long-standing potassium deficiency is also prone to produce *hypokalemic nephropathy*.

Treatment. The treatment of renal tubular acidosis consists of the administration of alkalinizing salts, such as sodium bicarbonate or sodium citrate, in quantities sufficient to restore plasma bicarbonate concentration to normal or nearly normal levels. In "proximal" RTA, in which there may be a gross defect in bicarbonate reabsorption, large quantities of alkali (as much as 5 to 7 mEq. per kilogram of body weight per day) are sometimes required in order to achieve this goal. Supplementary potassium may be needed in order to correct hypokalemia. If severe bone disease is present, it may also be necessary to administer large doses of vitamin D; but if such therapy must be employed, careful observations of serum calcium concentration must be carried out because of the risk of hypercalcemia. In some instances hypercalcemia will develop before the therapeutic goal of restoring serum phosphorous concentration to normal is achieved.

Course. Slowly progressive renal failure, occurring over a period of many years, is characteristic of sustained renal tubular acidosis and is usually accounted for by complications such as obstruction or infection. It should be noted, parenthetically, that renal tubular acidosis may also occur as part of a more complex syndrome of tubular defects such as Fanconi's syndrome. This disorder is discussed in detail in the section on Miscellaneous Hereditary Disorders.

Milne, M. D.: Renal tubular dysfunction. *In* Strauss, M. B., and Welt, L. G. (eds.): Diseases of the Kidney. Boston, Little, Brown and Company, 1971.

Morris, R. C.: Renal tubular acidosis; mechanisms, classification and implications. New Eng. J. Med., 281:1405, 1969.

Soriano, J. R., Biochis, H., Stark, H., and Edelmann, C. M., Jr.: Proximal renal tubular acidosis: A defect in bicarbonate reabsorption with normal urinary acidification. Pediat. Res., 1:81, 1967.

THE NEPHROPATHY OF ACUTE HYPERURICEMIA

Acute uric acid nephropathy occurs as the result of a sudden, marked elevation of serum uric acid concentration in patients undergoing intensive treatment for leukemia or lymphoma. This disorder, though relatively infrequent, is a serious complication that can lead to progressive renal failure, anuria, and death. It can occur with any form of therapy, such as cortisone, radiation, or nitrogen mustard, that abruptly reduces the number of circulating white cells or diminishes the mass of splenic and lymphoid tissue. The increase in the size of the uric acid pool results primarily from the metabolism of nucleic acid released during the process of cellular destruction. With massive cellular destruction, uric acid concentration occasionally reaches a level as high as 50 to 75 mg. per 100 ml.

Severe hyperuricemia is most likely to occur in patients with pre-existing hyperuricemia or in whom there is already some impairment of renal function that restricts the ability to excrete an abnormally large uric acid load. The untoward effects on kidney function result either from obstruction of ureters and pelvis by masses of uric acid or from intrarenal precipitation of uric acid within the collecting ducts and the distal tubules. Deposition in the proximal tubules ordinarily does not occur. The observed pattern of deposition can readily be understood if it is appreciated that at a pH above 7.0 uric acid (pK 5.5) is present almost entirely as the highly soluble urate anion, whereas at a pH of 5 to 6 a large fraction is present as the un-ionized and poorly soluble uric acid. Thus it is only in the distal tubule and collecting duct, in which marked acidification of the filtrate takes place, that conversion of urates to uric acid creates a condition favorable to uric acid precipitation. Abstraction of water by the distal nephron and the resulting increase in uric acid concentration in the urine are undoubtedly additional factors favoring precipitation in the tubules and the pelvo-ureteral system.

The single most important consideration in uric acid nephropathy is *prophylaxis*. Until the last several years the most effective means of preventing renal injury was through the administration of alkalinizing agents in quantities sufficient to keep the urine pH above 7, the excess uric acid in both tubules and urinary tract thus being maintained in a soluble state. To achieve this goal sodium bicarbonate has to be administered at frequent intervals during the day and a carbonic anhydrase inhibitor (such as Diamox) at bedtime. Allopurinol, a potent inhibitor of xanthine oxidase, has provided an even more reliable and physiologic approach to prophylaxis. Allopurinol, by blocking the conversion of hypoxanthine and xanthine to uric acid, prevents a rise in serum uric acid concentration (and in uric acid load delivered to the kidney), even in the face of extensive destruction of neoplastic tissue. When used in doses of 200 to 800 mg. per day it virtually eliminates the hazard of acute uric acid nephropathy. Allopurinol has proved to have few, if any, significant side effects.

When a patient presents with the problem of uric acid nephropathy and azotemia, cystoscopy and retrograde examination should be carried out in order to make certain that extrarenal obstruction is not present. If uric acid deposits are found to be blocking the pelvis and ureters, irrigation may serve to relieve the obstruction, but in some instances a pyelostomy will be necessary. In those instances in which obstruction is intrarenal rather than extrarenal, one should attempt to reduce uric acid concentrations and to alkalinize the urine in the same fashion as described above in the consideration of prophylaxis.

In some instances, osmotic diuresis with mannitol is said to be helpful in initiating urine flow in the oliguric patient. If such efforts are ineffective, and if anuria or severe azotemia persists, some form of dialysis should be used for the purpose of removing uric acid and dealing with the clinical and chemical manifestations of the uremic state. Despite all these measures, there is a high mortality rate among patients who develop severe hyperuricemic nephropathy, and, as mentioned earlier, prevention of renal damage should always be the primary concern.

DeConti, R. C., and Calabresi, P.: Use of allopurinol for prevention and control of hyperuricemia in patients with neoplastic disease. New Eng. J. Med., 274:481, 1966.
Frei, E., III, Bentzel, C. J., Rieselbach, R., and Block, J. B.: Renal complications of neoplastic disease. J. Chron. Dis., 16:757, 1963.
Muggia, F. M., Ball, T. J., and Ultmann, J. E.: Allopurinol in the treatment of neoplastic disease complicated by hyperuricemia. Arch. Intern. Med. 120:12, 1967.

BALKAN NEPHRITIS

During recent years a chronic and progressive nephritis of unknown cause has been noted in a large percentage of the population living in certain areas of Yugoslavia, Bulgaria, and Rumania. The disease occurs only in small villages located in valleys along river bottom land, and is not seen in neighboring cities or in adjacent foothills or mountains. Approximately one third of the population in the endemic areas has been found to have some evidence of renal disease, such as proteinuria, and between 5 and 10 per cent have been found to have significant azotemia. Several members of the same family are often affected by the disease. Proteinuria occurs in adolescents and in young adults, but azotemia is rarely encountered in patients under the age of 30 to 40 years.

The cause is unknown, and epidemiologic studies to date have not been fruitful. The renal lesion is apparently not the consequence of a previous streptococcal infection, of urinary tract infection, or of the excessive use of analgesics such as phenacetin. It is not related to exposure to toxic agents such as cadmium or lead, or to other factors such as the water supply, nutrition, alcohol intake, or economic status. A curious feature is that people who move out of the affected area do not subsequently develop the disease, whereas those who move into the area frequently develop renal disease, usually in a period of about ten years. Further studies on various environmental factors are obviously required and are, in fact, in progress.

The kidneys in the patient with the advanced form of the disease are characteristically small, their weight averaging 40 to 60 grams. The most severe atrophy is noted at the outer portion of the cortex, the deeper portions of cortex being more or less spared. From both biopsy and postmortem examination it appears that the primary lesion involves the interstitium and the tubules rather than the glomeruli. Interstitial fibrosis is prominent and there is a minimal infiltration of round cells. Many tubules are atrophied, and the remaining tubules are often hyperplastic and show mitotic figures. The glomeruli are relatively uninvolved and appear to degenerate only late in the course of the disease, apparently as a consequence of the interstitial lesion.

The clinical picture in Balkan nephritis is characterized by an insidious onset, usually without a history of edema or hematuria. The urine is found to contain small quantities of protein, usually not exceeding 1 gram per day; and the sediment is scanty, containing only a few leukocytes and erythrocytes and an occasional cast. It is noteworthy that blood pressure is usually normal, though in a small percentage of cases hypertension has been noted. Diminished concentrating ability occurs early, a finding consistent with the histologic observation that tubular damage is a prominent feature of the disease. Hyperchloremic acidosis gives further evidence that injury to tubules is out of proportion to glomerular injury. Renal failure, once present, generally progresses slowly, usually over a five- to ten-year period, to a fatal termination. There is no specific treatment. The most pressing problem remains that of determining the cause.

Griggs, R. C., and Hall, P. W.: Investigations of chronic endemic nephropathy in Yugoslavia. *In* Metcoff, J. (ed.): Renal Metabolism and Epidemiology of Some Renal Diseases. York, Pennsylvania, The Maple Press Company, 1964, p. 312.
Hall, P. W., Dammin, G. J., Griggs, R. C., Fajgelj, A., Zimonjic, B., and Gaon, J.: Investigation of chronic endemic nephropathy in Yugoslavia. II. Renal pathology. Amer. J. Med., 39:210, 1965.
Wolstenholme, G. E. W., and Knight, J. (eds.): The Balkan Nephropathy. Boston, Little, Brown and Company, 1967.

Obstructive Nephropathy

George E. Schreiner

Functional and anatomic damage to the renal parenchyma may occur whenever urine flow proceeds against functional or anatomic resistance. Obstruction may be acute, intermittent, or chronic. Back pressure is generated from (1) hydrostatic (filtration) pressure working against the outflow resistance, the proximal intraluminal pressure rising to approach capillary filtration pressure, and (2) the hydraulic pressure of bladder contraction when the ureterovesical "valve" is incompetent. The patient then voids "backward" into his kidneys.

Etiology. Obstruction may exist anywhere in the urinary conduit from the kidney to the tip of the urethra. Calyces may be obstructed by space-occupying tumors or cysts. The kidney may be involved in congenital generalized fibromatosis. Vessels, fibrous bands, and extensive masses may impinge on the pelvis or close the ureteropelvic junction. A pathologic condition occurs in the presence of obstruction anywhere from kidney to urethra. Peristaltic propulsion from pelvis to bladder is accomplished by a well innervated muscle system which exhibits an electrical and contractile phase analogous to the myocardium. The rhythm and the force of contraction may be affected by infection, pregnancy, drugs, and a variety of pathologic states. The causes of increased resistance to urine flow include (1) inadequate lumen, e.g., bladder neck contracture, stenosis, ureteral stricture, atresia; (2) intrinsic blockade, e.g., calculus, clots, crystals, exudates; (3) extrinsic compression, e.g., aberrant vessels, fibrous bands, tumors, cysts, endometriosis, prostatic hyperplasia, median bar; (4) anomalies of form, e.g., angulation, ptosis, diverticula; (5) disease of the wall, e.g., ureteritis, periureteral fibrosis, malakoplakia; and (6) functional inadequacy, e.g., atony, neuropathy, drugs, infection, pregnancy, surgery. Increased resistance to bladder emptying induces work hypertrophy. Trabeculation signifies hypertrophy of detrusor muscle bundles. They separate and the mucosa evaginates. Saccules develop, the bladder wall thickens, and diverticula may form. Alternatively (or eventually with decompensation) hypertrophy may yield to dilatation, bladder enlargement, increased capacity, incomplete emptying (residual), and atony (bladder decompensation or "congenital failure"). A most intricate neural mechanism controls bladder function. The oblique angulation of the intramural portion of the ureters may straighten or lose its normal ability to occlude during micturition. Vesicoureteral reflux on one or both sides may be shown by micturition cystograms and may be inferred from the physiologic consequences of backflow or the anatomic development of hydroureter, redundancy, lengthening and angulation, and lastly, hydronephrosis. Bell found a 3.8 per cent incidence of hydronephrosis in 32,360 autopsies.

Principles of Pathophysiology. In anatomic obstruction, dilatation is cephalad or proximal to the site of the lesion. In drug-induced, neurologic, or functional states, dilatation is uniform in the involved segment, but may extend upward. The bladder, as the expansible lake in the stream system, must dilate massively to involve healthy ureters. Disuse atrophy is more theoretic than real. Transplant patients have recovered bladder function quickly after years of nonuse while being maintained on hemodialysis. In high ureteral obstruction, the pelvis is the only reservoir distal to the nephron. Capacity to dilate is greater if the pelvis is anatomically extrarenal (a congenital variant), and sacs holding several liters have been found at autopsy.

Physiologic Consequences of Obstruction. Mild partial urinary tract obstruction producing slow dilatation may exist without functional impairment. Some skepticism, however, is warranted on the interpretation of renal clearances measured in the presence of increased dead space and irregular emptying. Urine flow should be augmented to a brisk diuresis, and collection periods should be lengthened. Pelvic pressures above 30 to 50 mm. of mercury may reduce function and produce pain if the elevation is acute. Conversely, intraureteral pressures up to 150 to 190 mm. of mercury do not always produce colic.

Endogenous creatinine and urea clearances are often reduced, and widely different values may be obtained in successive clearance periods, highlighting the difficulties in collection. Such differences are a diagnostic clue to the presence of obstruction. An elevated serum urea–creatinine ratio is seen in lower tract obstruction, i.e., > 10:1, often 15 to 50:1. Using 15-minute fractions in the PSP test may reveal a rising or flattened curve instead of the normal major excretion in the first 15 minutes. Maximal concentrating ability is often impaired. In unilateral obstruction discrete function tests may be necessary to bring out dysfunction, the evidence of which may be cancelled by bladder-mixing of two disparate urines. The I^{131} hypinate renogram washout curve may be useful in unilateral obstruction, as are the radioactive mercury scan, measurements of relative renal size, and the appearance time of the two-, three-, and five-minute nephrogram.

Moderate obstruction may reduce the relationship between filtration rate and renal blood flow (low $\frac{C_{in}}{C_{pah}}$). The reduced $\frac{C_{in}}{C_{pah}}$ is more striking since ascending pyelonephritis of moderate severity (prevalent in obstructive nephropathy) characteristically produces elevation in $\frac{C_{in}}{C_{pah}}$. Renal hyperemia relative to tubular function is also found in obstruction (high $\frac{C_{pah}}{Tm_{pah}}$ ratio). In acute unilateral experimental obstruction involving elevation of intraureteral pressure to 60 to 80 cm. of water, sodium concentration is lower and osmolality higher than the control side. The obstructed kidney thus excretes a smaller fraction of its filtered sodium and water. The sodium difference is exaggerated by volume expansion with saline, although the hyperosmolality is minimized. Thus the functional results closely simulate those produced by constriction of one renal artery. In chronic obstruction, the filtration rate declines, but so do sodium concentration and osmolality. Urinary acidification may be impaired with suboptimal urinary pH in acidotic states. The obstructed kidney thus excretes a larger fraction of filtered sodium and water. Persistent complete obstruction for seven days in dogs produces permanent damage to nephrons. No change in Tm glucose occurs until ureteral pressure reaches 30 per cent of mean blood pressure. Therefore, significant depression occurs. Obstruction increases DNA synthesis and cell division as compared to the control kidney.

Upon removal of obstruction these physiologic variations rapidly revert toward normal, provided secondary renal trauma is not irreversible. The contralateral kidney may exhibit transient reactive hyperemia subsiding during continued recovery of the drained kidney.

In patients with long-standing obstruction (bladder neck or ureter) of sufficient degree to produce an anuric obstruction, e.g., periureteral fibrosis, prostatic hypertrophy, obstruction of catheter, etc., release may be followed by a polyuric, hyposthenuric phase lasting several days to several months. This has all the features of an osmotic diuresis, viz., minimum U/P ratios of inulin below 8, excretion of more than 60 per cent of filtered urea ($\frac{C_{urea}}{C_{in}}$ exceeds the augmentation limit of a water diuresis), osmolar clearance greater than 5 per cent of filtered water, and large daily electrolyte excretion capable of producing depletion syndromes. Most of the solute is salt. Hyponatremia may result. Experimental hydronephrosis leads to erythrocytosis associated with elevated erythropoietin levels in 60 per cent of rabbits. Human polycythemia caused by hydronephrosis has been relieved by nephrectomy. The acidification defect reverses with a lower maximal pH of the urine.

Thus incomplete acute and chronic obstruction produces a decreasing filtration rate, progressing to anuria when obstruction is complete. The effects on sodium, water, and hydrogen ion excretion are variable, and differ in the acute, chronic, and postrelease states.

Clinical Manifestations. Unfortunately, the kidneys may be silently mutilated by obstruction. Excessive diagnostic zeal is justified by the tragic consequences of missing a treatable obstructive nephropathy. Infection is the calling card of obstruction. Any part of the clinical spectrum of transient cystitis or pyelonephritis in children and recurrent pyelonephritis in adults should be an invitation to investigate. Most frequent presenting signs and symptoms in order are fever, pain in the flank, abdomen, or suprapubic area, positive features in the micturition history, gastrointestinal complaints, abnormalities noted at birth, abdominal or palpable mass, polydipsia, irritability, respiratory distress, convulsions, and anemia. Pain patterns may mimic those produced by any abdominal pelvic organ, and patients with urinary obstruction have had operative intervention on the appendix, small intestine, colon, liver, stomach, spleen, uterus, and fallopian tubes. Micturition abnormalities and changes in the urinary sediment are the most frequently overlooked features of obstructive nephropathy. They include slow onset of voiding, infrequent voiding, incontinence, urinary frequency, enuresis, urgency, straining, dysuria, nocturia, and suprapubic pain on voiding. Micturition history must be painstaking and specific. Gastrointestinal complaints include failure to thrive, nausea and vomiting, diarrhea, failure to gain weight on good dietary intake, and interruption of normal growth pattern. Pain may be referred to the pelvis, back, hips, thighs, or rectum.

Urinary Sediment. Urinary findings include hematuria, pyuria, bacteriuria, and, in the case of bladder neck infections, the sloughing of small clumps of pavement epithelial cells or round cells from the bladder neck. These may show granules with streaming or brownian movement. Ghosts of tubules or fragments of papillae may be recovered from strained urine in the presence of papillary necrosis. Telltale crystals may be found in obstruction owing to cystine, urate, or calcium oxalate stones.

Roentgenographic Findings. These include increased size and dilatation of pelvis, broadening of the base of major calyces progressing to sacculation, flattening or clubbing of the minor calyces progressing to obliteration, progressive shortening of the papillae, change in the insertion angle of the ureter progressing to elongation, dilatation, angulation, and redundancy. An anatomically extrarenal pelvis may dilate to huge capacity, and an intrarenal pelvis may produce greater parenchymal damage with less volume expansion. Ureteropelvic, vesicoureteral obstructions and stenosis produce areas of narrowing with proximal dilatation. A change in the normal peristaltic pattern of the ureter may be the first sign of obstruction. A completely dye-filled ureter should not be considered normal. The upright cystoureterogram is the best technique to demonstrate increased bladder size and vesicoureteral reflux. Cinefluorography during micturition with dye in the bladder may demonstrate early functional defects. In one study of 100 selective arteriograms, 42 had filling defects produced by vascular compression. In complete obstruction dye will be diluted in the dilated calyces and nonvisualization reported. Delayed films up to 12 hours may be helpful. A good nephrogram will help to distinguish obstructive uropathy from vascular causes of anuria. The isotope renogram will show a flat and delayed washout segment on the obstructed side. Cystoscopy may be valuable for lateralization (urine coming from one orifice). Inserting a catheter beyond an obstruction is not an act to be taken lightly, because it may introduce infection into a stagnant area.

Differential Diagnosis. While investigating micturition abnormalities, the physician must be mindful of the major disease processes affecting micturition. They include spinal cord injury, multiple sclerosis, diabetic neuropathy, tabes dorsalis, poliomyelitis, herpes zoster, degenerative neurologic diseases, congenital lesions of the spinal cord, trauma, and a variety of psychiatric causes.

Many popular drugs affect micturition, produce bladder atony, and may mimic obstructive nephropathy. Included are the anticholinergic agents, the ganglionic blocking drugs, reserpine, hydralazine and other anti-hypertensives, adrenergic drugs such as ephedrine and dextroamphetamine, antihistamines, isoniazid, and potent diuretics acting indirectly via sudden bladder distention. Some contraceptive pills may induce changes which mimic the ureteral dilatation of early pregnancy.

Special Forms. *Retroperitoneal Fibrosis.* The condition is presently regarded as an exaggerated fibrocytic response to varied stimuli (notably infection and neoplasm) involving retroperitoneal structures, particularly the ureter, and at times the aorta, inferior vena cava, and contiguous structures. The colon and bile ducts have also been affected, and an associated vasculitis has been reported. This condition may be the same disorder that, in the thoracic cavity, is called idiopathic mediastinal fibrosis. The condition predominates in middle-aged white men presenting with back pain or chronic and progressive abdominal pain. This may be colicky or in the flank, and is often associated with nausea, vomiting, and weight loss and malaise. Forty per cent become anuric. Physical examination is unrevealing. Anemia is a constant feature along with varying azotemia, unilateral or bilateral. Hydronephrosis or ureteral obstruction may be identified on retrograde pyelography. Bacterial clumps and microabscesses may be found embedded in the fibrous tissue. The prognosis is good with correct treatment, which includes prolonged antimicrobial therapy and relief of obstruction by ureterolysis, pyeloplasty, and plastic reconstruction of damaged segments of ureter or pelvis. Diabetes insipidus-like syndrome and hypertension have been ascribed to the disease.

Methysergide Fibrosis. Graham in 1963 encountered two patients who developed periureteral fibrosis while being treated with methysergide (Sansert), an ergot preparation for migraine headaches. Since then this diagnosis has been established in a considerable number of other patients. One additional patient took ergot preparations other than methysergide. The symptoms were as described above. The patients ingested 4 to 28 mg. per day of methysergide for periods of one to five years. Some speculations on the mechanism include rebound from the antiinflammatory and antiserotonin effects of methysergide, a disturbance of tryptophan metabolism, and the effects of prolonged edema or vasoconstriction. Withdrawal of the drug may result in regression of the fibrosis, or plastic surgery may be required.

Lower Urinary Tract Obstruction in Children. About half the children found to have lower urinary tract obstruction are unaware of urinary tract disease at the time the diagnosis is made by an alert physician or in the course of routine diagnostic work-up. Among the anatomic causes are (1) muscular hypertrophy of the bladder neck or absence of the plexiform dilator fibers (*Marion's disease*); this produces obstruction just beyond the internal sphincter that may be relaxed by spinal anesthesia and is analogous to pylorospasm; (2) persistent posterior valves arising from deficient integration of wolffian ducts into the wall of the urethra, abnormal location of the original orifices of wolffian ducts in the cloaca, or abnormal course in their terminal ends; (3) diaphragm at the bulbomembranous junction (mucosal fold, "iris" deformity, mucosal stricture with or without fibrosis), generally recognizable only by skillful cystoscopy; (4) polyp or inflammatory hypertrophy of the verumontanum, usually producing the picture of intermittent obstruction; (5) cysts of the bladder neck; (6) diverticulum of the urethra; and (7) meatal stenosis.

Prognosis and Treatment. The fundamentals of treatment include decompression and hydration of the patient. The choice of method depends upon the obstructive site and may include dilatation, indwelling catheter, suprapubic cystotomy, ureterostomy, pyelostomy, and nephrostomy. Vigorous and prolonged treatment of the associated infection is indicated. Electrolyte depletion syndromes should be prevented or corrected, and the correct anatomic diagnosis defined. The uremic syndrome may require treatment by dialysis preceding surgical intervention. When the patient is in the best possible metabolic condition, definitive removal of the obstruction should be attempted.

Plastic Procedures Intended to Reduce Dead Space. New and still experimental developments in urologic plastic surgery have transformed this area from one of dreary outlook to one of exciting challenge. They include focal steroid suppression of fibroblast proliferation, wedge resections of the bladder neck, tunneling and implantation of ureters, vesical and ureteroplasty, pyeloplasty, and bridging of gaps by transplants and regeneration. It is imperative that corrective measures be taken before irreplaceable loss of nephrons.

When azotemia is not reversible by decompression or relief of obstruction, management is identical with that of any other cause of chronic renal failure. Advantage may be taken of the salt-losing tendency to sustain an osmotic diuresis by salt administration. Chronic smoldering infection requires long-term antimicrobial therapy. Children with a tolerable degree of renal failure may become worse during the pubertal growth spurt when small damaged kidneys cannot sustain enlarging bodies. We have experimentally closed epiphyses with estrogen-androgen therapy to prevent growth in such a situation. We are also studying the potential for long-term regeneration after correction of reflux.

Baum, S., and Gillenwater, J. Y.: Renal artery impressions on the renal pelvis. J. Urol., 95:139, 1966.

Benitez, L., and Shaka, J. A.: Cell proliferation in experimental hydronephrosis and compensatory renal hyperplasia. Amer. J. Path., 44:961, 1964.

Bricker, N. S., Klahr, S., Lubowitz, H., and Rieselbach, R. E.: Renal function in chronic renal disease. Medicine (Balt.), 44:263, 1965.

Bricker, N. S., Schwayri, E. I., Reardan, J. B., Kellogg, D., Merrill, J. P., and Holmes, J. H.: An abnormality in renal function resulting from urinary tract obstruction. Amer. J. Med., 23:554, 1957.

Edvall, C. A.: Influence of ureteral obstruction (hydronephrosis) on renal function in man. J. Appl. Physiol., 14:855, 1959.

Graham, J. R., Suby, H. I., LeCompte, P. R., and Sadowsky, N. L.: Fibrotic disorders associated with methysergide therapy for headache. New Eng. J. Med., 274:359, 1966.

Jaworski, Z. F., and Wolan, C. T.: Hydronephrosis and polycythemia: A case of erythrocytosis relieved by decompression of unilateral hydronephrosis and cured by nephrectomy. Amer. J. Med., 34:523, 1963.

Kerr, W. S., Jr.: Effect of complete ureteral obstruction for one week on kidney function. J. Appl. Physiol., 6:762, 1953.

Knowlan, D., Corrado, M., Schreiner, G. E., and Baker, R.: Periureteral fibrosis, with a diabetes-insipidus-like syndrome occurring with progressive partial obstruction of a ureter unilaterally. Amer. J. Med., 28:22, 1960.

Kuru, M.: Nervous control of micturition. Physiol. Rev., 45:425, 1965.

McGovern, J. H.: The presenting manifestations of obstructive urinary anomalies in children. Pediatrics. 27:3, 1961.

Suki, W., Eknoyan, G., Rector, R. C., Jr., and Seldin, D. W.: Patterns of nephron perfusion in acute and chronic hydronephrosis. J. Clin. Invest., 45:122, 1966.

Teng, P., Warden, M. J., and Cohn, W. L.: Congenital generalized fibromatosis (renal and skeletal) with complete spontaneous regression. J. Pediat., 62:748, 1963.

Witte, M. H., Short, F. A., and Hollander, W., Jr.: Massive polyuria and natriuresis following relief of urinary tract obstruction. Amer. J. Med., 37:320, 1964.

Toxic Nephropathy

George E. Schreiner

Toxic nephropathy is a functional or structural change in the kidney caused by a chemical or biologic product. By extension, the concept is often applied to the renal effects of physiologic substances circulating in abnormal concentrations. This situation obtains in hypercalcemic, hyperuricemic, hypokalemic, and hypomagnesemic nephropathies, which are considered in detail in another article. The classification of toxic nephropathy is contained in Table 1, and a partial list of nephrotoxins is shown in Table 2.

The peculiar susceptibility of the kidney to an enormous range of drugs and biologically active materials stems from its huge blood supply relative to weight, its large endothelial vascular surface, its high oxygen consumption and glucose production, the fact that excreted compounds are concentrated along the luminal surface of the nephron, and the fact that many drugs occupy, at least transiently, an intracellular position if they are involved in secretory or reabsorptive transport processes. It is possible that some reabsorbed drugs may be concentrated along with sodium in the hypertonic interstitial tissues of the papillae.

Toxic nephropathy accounts for an appreciable fraction of all reported series of acute renal failure. In the past 15 years at Georgetown Hospital it represents 20 per cent of the total experience with acute renal failure. The most frequently encountered nephrotoxins in the series were carbon tetra-

TABLE 1. CLASSIFICATION OF TOXIC NEPHROPATHY

Class 1. Drugs, chemicals, or their metabolites with a reasonably *direct* effect, producing an identifiable morphologic or persisting functional change in the nephron. Model: bichloride of mercury.

Class 2. Compounds producing sensitivity disease identifiable as the *nephrotic* or *nephritic* syndrome in which the initial step may be subtle alteration in the renal cell or alteration of a protein, producing an immune reaction. Model: aminonucleoside nephrosis and nephroallergens producing the nephrotic syndrome.

Class 3. Compounds producing sensitivity reactions of the angiitis or vasculitis type involving the kidney as a vascular organ. Model: sulfa sensitivity.

Class 4. Compounds that may produce *chronic nephrotoxicity,* when the mechanism extends over a period of months or years and the evidence remains largely epidemiologic or circumstantial. Model: lead nephropathy.

Class 5. Compounds that aggravate pre-existing renal disease or predispose to secondary renal disease such as pyelonephritis. Model: diuretics and cathartics predisposing to pyelonephritis via potassium deficiency.

chloride, mercury, sulfonamide drugs, radiographic contrast media, analgesics, ethylene glycol, and antimicrobials.

Toxic nephropathy may also account for a significant segment of so-called geographic renal diseases. The World Health Organization has cited some 25,000 cases of an interstitial nephritis that has been reported by various investigators as Yugoslavian, Bulgarian, and Balkan nephritis. This disease has a distribution conforming to specific altitudes and river valleys. Pathologically it resembles a toxic nephropathy, but the specific agent has not been identified. As more sophisticated renal diagnostic techniques are correlated with renal biopsy and histochemistry, it is likely that the number of recognized nephrotoxins will increase during the next decade—both chemicals now in existence and substances still to be produced through the remarkable ingenuity and industry of the organic chemists.

TABLE 2. A PARTIAL LIST OF NEPHROTOXINS

Metals: Mercury (organic and inorganic), bismuth, uranium, cadmium, lead, gold, arsine and arsenic, iron, silver, antimony, copper, and thallium

Organic solvents: Carbon tetrachloride, tetrachlorethylene, methyl cellosolve, methanol, and miscellaneous solvents

Glycols: Ethylene glycol, ethylene glycol dinitrite, propylene glycol, ethylene dichloride, and diethylene glycol

Physical agents: Radiation, heat stroke, and electroshock

Diagnostic agents: Contrast agents in high concentration (pyelography and aortography) and bunamiodyl

Therapeutic agents: Antimicrobials: Sulfonamides, penicillin, streptomycin, kanamycin, vancomycin, bacitracin, polymyxin and colistin, neomycin, tetracycline, and amphotericin. *Analgesics:* Salicylates, para-aminosalicylate (PAS), ? phenacetin, phenylbutazone, zoxazolamine, pheninedione, puromycin, tridione, paradione

Osmotic agents: Sucrose, mannitol

Insecticides: Biphenyl, chlorinated hydrocarbons

Miscellaneous chemicals: Carbon monoxide, snake venom, mushroom poison, spider venom, nephroallergens, cresol, beryllium, hemolysins, aniline, and other methemoglobin formers

Abnormal concentration of physiologic substances: Hypercalcemia, hyperuricemia, hypokalemia, hypomagnesemia, etc.

SPECIFIC NEPHROTOXINS

MERCURY AND OTHER HEAVY METALS

Mercury. Mercury in various forms acts as a nephrotoxin. Acutely it produces tubular necrosis with renal failure. In organic form or with prolonged exposure it may produce the nephrotic syndrome or chronic renal damage. Frequently encountered mercuric compounds are chloride, iodide, oxide, cyanide, and salicylate. Mercurous compounds include the chloride (calomel), iodide, and oxide salts. Organic mercuric compounds associated with nephrotoxicity include merbromin (Mercurochrome) and the mercurial diuretics.

Epidemiology. Inorganic mercury poisoning usually occurs by accident, in suicide attempts, or following its use as an abortive agent. Poisoning has occurred in a wide variety of industries, including the manufacture of paint, alloys, and scientific instruments. Agricultural exposures are due to disinfectants and pesticides. Medical poisoning stems from mercurial diuretics, ammoniated mercury ointments, and absorption from the skin of widespread dermatoses, such as psoriasis. Inhalation toxicity may occur. The urinary excretion of inorganic mercury normally ranges from 0.1 to 1 μg. per liter. Patients with chronic industrial exposure often excrete amounts in excess of 300 μg. per liter. Psoriatic patients have had mercuriuria demonstrated from 500 to 1000 μg. per liter.

Clinical Manifestations. Mercury produces a lingering, bitter, metallic taste that may be followed by a sensation of constriction in the throat, suffocation, substernal burning, esophagitis, gastritis, abdominal pain, nausea, and vomiting. Ulcerations occur on the palate or lips; diarrhea may be blood-tinged. Circulatory collapse is signaled be feeble pulse, peripheral vasoconstriction, syncope, and shock with oliguria and anuria. It is important to obtain urine before oliguria sets in. The urine usually shows albumin, epithelial cell casts, erythrocytes, glycosuria, aminoaciduria, and increased mercury content, particularly in the precipitable fractions. Leukocytosis is the rule.

Pathology. Mercurial vapor, dust, or liquid dissolves locally on moist surfaces of the mucous membranes. Mercuric salts are well absorbed by the gastrointestinal tract and vagina and ammoniated mercury by the intact skin. Absorbed mercury is bound quickly to circulating protein, and appears in blood, kidney, liver, heart, brain, and some endocrine organs. Inorganic salts are excreted largely by the colon, kidneys, salivary glands, biliary system, and skin, and organic materials predominantly by the kidney. The most striking pathologic changes occur in the form of granular or vacuolar degeneration of the proximal tubules. Mitotic figures and basophilic cytoplasm may be seen in the early phases of healing. Early calcification of the site of necrosis may occur. In severe cases all segments of the tubule may be involved, and patchy tubulorrhexis may occur. Extrarenal autopsy findings include induration of surface membranes in pharynx, esophagus, and stomach, erosive gastritis, softening of the muscular coat of the intestine, severe colitis, congestion of liver and spleen, degeneration of myocardium, and focal hemorrhages in the cerebral cortex. It appears that mercury initiates cellular destruction by combining with the sulfhydryl groups of protein in the mitochrondrial membrane, leading to the disintegration of mitochondria and necrosis of nuclei and subsequent loss in enzyme activity.

Fourteen cases of acute renal failure caused by mercury have been studied at Georgetown Hospital. The dose expressed as inorganic mercury ranged from 0.4 to 10 grams. Oliguria occurred within the first 48 hours, and persisted for an average of 15 days (range 7 to 22). Tissue necrosis was a catabolic factor, and the BUN increased an average of 31 mg. per 100 ml. per day during the first week. Thirteen patients required hemodialysis, and three died. None of the patients died who underwent hemodialysis within 48 hours after the ingestion of mercury and the administration of BAL. Six cases of nephrotic syndrome secondary to mercury have been observed.

Treatment. Prevention is exceptionally important. The use of mercuric salts for douching and surgical irrigation should be discouraged. Bottles should be labeled as poison and should be secured in a safe place. Acute ingestion is a medical emergency. Emesis usually occurs, but if not, the stomach should be emptied with a large lavage tube, and rinsed with egg white or concentrated albumin or medicinal charcoal. A useful lavage solution combines one pint of skim milk, 50 grams of glucose, 20 grams of sodium bicarbonate, and 3 eggs beaten into a mixture. One gram of medicinal charcoal can combine with 850 mg. of mercuric chloride. After absorption, BAL (2,3-dimercapropanol) acts as an effective antidote since it appears to compete with biologically important sulfhydryl groups. Injections of 2.5 to 3 mg. of BAL per kilogram of body weight should be given every four hours up to six injections, depending on the severity of poisoning. BAL may produce transient nausea, vomiting, diarrhea, burning stomatitis and excessive lacrimation. It is a mild hypoglycemic agent. In severe poisoning large doses of BAL are given immediately, and dialysis is carried out shortly thereafter to remove the mercury-BAL complex; the patient is then re-treated with BAL. Exchange transfusion may also be of value. Patients who remain oliguric should be given the same conservative management as other patients with acute renal failure (see Acute Renal Failure).

Treatment of patients with nephrotic syndrome caused by mercury calls for immediate removal of the agent, administration of adrenocortical steroids, and a regimen similar to that recommended for other patients with the nephrotic syndrome. These patients may be subject to repeated renal damage by mercurial diuretics. Hypersensitivity reactions to mercurial diuretics have included generalized pruritus, urticaria, asthma, exfoliative dermatitis, and sudden death. Cystine, penicillamine, BAL, or other sources of sulfhydryl compounds may be used to augment the treatment of mercury sensitivity and especially ventricular fibrillation, which is the cause of sudden death.

Acrodynia (pink disease) occurs in children throughout the world, and is characterized by irritability, emaciation, stomatitis, and erythema of acral parts. The children have fever, leukocytosis, albuminuria, and mercuriuria from mercury used in teething powder or diaper rinses.

Bismuth. Bismuth toxicity arises chiefly from industrial poisons, antisyphilitic therapy, and soluble bismuth compounds such as the subcarbonate and the mixed thioglycolates. Bismuth may produce either acute renal failure or nephrotic syndrome. Sore mouth, diarrhea, peripheral neuritis, stomatitis, obstructive jaundice, and pigmentation of the gum margins may occur, together with evidence of acute renal failure with hyposthenuria, cylindruria, and the desquamation of renal tubular epithelial cells.

Uranium. Uranium causes proximal tubular necrosis in a distribution similar to that of mercury. Uranium nitrate may produce a central lobular lesion in the glomeruli. Uranium has been implicated in some cases of geographic nephritis.

Cadmium. Cadmium is widely used in the metal plating and industrial chemical industries. Interstitial nephritis may follow chronic exposure, and acute poisoning produces proteinuria and proximal renal damage. The most significant feature of cadmium nephrotoxicity is a peculiar proteinuria, ranging from 70 to 2600 mg. per 24 hours. There is a low molecular weight protein (20,000 to 30,000) that precipitates with nitric acid but not with boiling, and migrates as an alpha globulin. Cadmium proteinuria is clinically significant and is best treated by removing the patient from the toxic environment. Cadmium is soluble in acid; acid foods and beverages placed in cadmium-plated containers such as ice cube trays may be a source of poisoning.

Lead. Lead nephrotoxicity has been implicated in severe renal disease produced from the drinking of whiskey made in stills improvised from automobile and truck radiators. In Queensland, Australia, the eating of paint or drinking of rain water from porches painted with lead paint has been found to result in a high incidence of chronic nephritis associated with increased skeletal lead content and increased lead in the urine. Unexposed subjects may excrete about 0.08 mg. per liter of lead, and asymptomatic exposed subjects may excrete up to 0.15 mg. per liter. Patients with lead poisoning may excrete from 0.15 to 0.30 mg. per liter. Lead nephropathy is a predominantly tubular syndrome with renal glycosuria, aminoaciduria, albuminuria, casts, and increased excretion of lead, delta-amino-levulinic acid, co-proporphyrin, urobilinogen, urobilin, and bile pigments. Roentgenograms show typically the increased density at the ends of the shafts of the long bones. Ziehl-Neelsen acid-fast, intranuclear inclusion bodies may be seen on renal biopsy. Treatment of lead nephropathy lies in immediate removal of the subject from the source of exposure. Attempts may be made to increase excretion by such agents as sodium citrate, dimercaprol, and disodium calcium ethylenediamine tetraacetate.

Gold. Gold salts are used in rheumatoid arthritis in the form of gold sodium thiosulfate, sodium aurothiomalate, aurothioglucose, and aurothioglycanide. Cutaneous manifestations of hypersensitivity include urticaria, purpura, itching, maculopapular to exfoliative dermatitis, and polyneuritis. Bone marrow depression may be encountered. Nephrotoxicity is usually heralded by proteinuria and microscopic hematuria. The nephrotic syndrome may supervene. Brun et al. studied the localization of gold in renal biopsies of patients receiving gold therapy. Deposits of the metal were found in the proximal tubules shortly after injection. Subsequently (one to four years) they were localized in the distal tubules. In the interstitial tissues gold was stored in macrophages, and could be demonstrated up to 28 years after the last injection. At Georgetown Hospital four patients with the nephrotic syndrome following gold therapy have been observed. Three subsequently developed laboratory features of systemic lupus erythematosus.

Arsine. Arsine intoxication produces shock, hemoglobinuria, and acute tubular necrosis, which has been successfully treated by hemodialysis.

Arsenic. Arsenic may produce a toxic nephritis leading to oliguria and uremia, aggravated by the dehydration from associated diarrhea. The urine contains albumin, casts, erythrocytes, and leukocytes. Arsenic may be recovered in the dialysate of such patients treated with hemodialysis.

Silver. Silver may produce renal tubular degeneration, with sparing of the glomeruli, interstitial deposits of silver, and interstitial edema. It has been reported in persons who regularly handle photographic developers.

Iron. Acute tubular necrosis has been reported with a mortality rate of 50 per cent in children who accidentally ingest large doses of ferrous sulfate. It is presumably related to the mucosal damage in the gastrointestinal tract, metabolic acidosis, hepatic damage, and shock. Chronic renal failure, interstitial fibrosis, and iron deposition may be seen in hemochromatosis and severe transfusion hemosiderosis. In rabbits saccharated iron oxide produces a nephrotoxic lesion.

Antimony. As used therapeutically for leishmaniasis, antimony can lead to transient oliguric renal failure.

Copper. Copper sulfate ingestion can produce vomiting, dehydration, hypotension, sulfhemoglobinemia, and acute renal failure. Tubular degeneration and necrosis are seen, particularly in the ascending loop and distal convolution.

Thallium. Thallium is used in rat poisons, depilatories, and denaturing agents for alcohol. It causes albuminuria, tachycardia, colic, and a neurologic syndrome.

SOLVENTS

Carbon tetrachloride is used as a cleaning agent, grease solvent and vermifuge, and in fire extinguishers. It is heavier than air. Nephrotoxicity may occur after either inhalation or ingestion. It is aggravated by the simultaneous ingestion of alcohol, even in small amounts. The initial symptoms are irritation at the exposure site, followed by headache, mental confusion, coma, and convulsions. Narcosis, encephalomyelitis, cerebellar degeneration, and optic and peripheral neuritis may occur. Gastrointestinal symptoms are prominent, particularly when the substance has been ingested, and include nausea, vomiting, and abdominal pain. The delayed manifestations are toxic hepatitis with jaundice, tender hepatomegaly with hepatic failure, and a toxic nephropathy with anuric acute tubular necrosis. Renal involvement may be insidious and delayed for as long as a week after exposure. The urine is typical of acute renal failure, with proteinuria, cylindruria, pyuria, hematuria, and desquamation of renal tubular epithelial cells. Bleeding manifestations, particularly scleral and periorbital hemorrhages, epistaxis, and hypoprothrombinemia may be seen. In the Georgetown Hospital experience, the most frequent signs and symptoms encountered were oliguria, nausea and vomiting, hepatomegaly, and abdominal pain. Half or less than half of the patients had bleeding, fever, hypertension, jaundice, rash, edema, ascites, and renal tenderness. Patients were azotemic, but the creatinine/BUN ratio averaged 16 per cent, considerably higher than the 11 per cent ratio in the entire group of acute renal failure. This may reflect some impairment of hepatic urea synthesis. The patients were usually hyperuricemic, hyponatremic, hypokalemic, hypochloremic, hypophosphatemic, and acidotic. Serum glutamic oxaloacetic transaminase was elevated. Hyperbilirubinemia, hyperglycemia, abnormal thymol turbidity, cephalin flocculation tests, and alkaline phosphatase levels were usual.

Treatment consists of removing the patient from the area of exposure and providing adequate ventilation, gastric lavage, and catharsis. The use of unsaturated oils by mouth has been suggested but not clinically proved to be helpful. People chronically exposed to carbon tetrachloride should be warned about the synergism with alcohol. After hepatic or renal failure has ensued, standard therapy for these complications should be employed. Hemorrhagic phenomena require the judicious use of blood transfusions.

GLYCOLS

Ethylene glycol is commonly encountered in antifreeze solutions. Part of the compound is rapidly converted to oxalic acid, which may be deposited in the kidneys and other organs such as the moninges. In the kidney there is destruction of epithelial cells with preservation of the basement membrane, focal regeneration, and tubules filled with masses of calcium oxalate crystals that are birefringent on polarized light. Nephrons are dilated above the crystalline obstruction. Focal mononuclear cell infiltrates and interstitial edema are also seen.

The clinical events may be divided into three stages: During the first 12 hours central nervous system effects resemble those of ethanol intoxication. In severe poisoning this may include stupor, coma, convulsions, and death. During the second 12 hours the manifestations are predominantly cardiopulmonary, with tachypnea, cyanosis, pulmonary edema, and death in cardiac failure. After the first day the problem is mainly renal injury, with slight pain, tenderness over the kidneys, proteinuria, oliguria, and anuria; death may result from uremia.

Ethylene glycol poisoning is a medical emergency, and should be treated with immediate hemodialysis aimed at removal of the circulating alcohol to diminish the substrate for conversion to glycolic and oxalic acid. Gastric lavage and parenteral solutions of sodium bicarbonate may also be used. After anuria has supervened, the treatment is the same as for acute renal failure in general.

PHYSICAL AGENTS

Radiation nephritis is encountered clinically following radiation of tumors in or near the kidneys. The kidney is said to be the most radiosensitive of all major organs. The major syndromes include acute and chronic nephritis and benign and malignant hypertension. Clinically, radiation nephritis is characterized by proteinuria, hypertension, anemia, cardiomegaly, congestive heart failure, encephalopathy, and chronic uremia. In *acute* cases the mortality rate is about 50 per cent; survivors generally begin to improve within six months from the onset. In *chronic* radiation exposure the nephritis may be manifested only by proteinuria, anemia, hyposthenuria, and slowly progressive decline of renal function. These symptoms may occur as a continuum from the acute disease or may be discovered later in patients who have never presented with an acute syndrome.

Histologic study reveals marked thickening of the renal capsule, hyaline obliteration of the glomeruli, focal necrosis of the fibrinoid or hemorrhagic type, proliferation of Bowman's capsule, pericapsular fibrosis, tubular degeneration and atrophy, diffuse interstitial fibrosis, and fibrinoid necrosis of arterioles. There is a remarkable tendency to development of malignant hypertension and necrotizing arteriolitis.

The treatment is not essentially different from that for acute and chronic nephritis from other causes; the hypertension should be treated vigorously with antihypertensive drugs. When radiation nephritis is unilateral, the resulting hypertension may be benefited by nephrectomy.

Heat stroke may be encountered in hyperthermal industrial environments or military situations in the desert, and acute renal failure may be the dominant manifestation. Lack of acclimatization may be a primary factor in pathogenesis. Hemolysis, shock, hemoconcentration, volume depletion, and hypernatremia have been prominent clinical features. Acute renal failure ensues in up to 10 per cent of the patients who survive heat stroke.

DIAGNOSTIC AGENTS

Contrast media: Iodide is an essential component of all absorbable contrast media. A significant percentage of persons manifest iodine hypersensitivity in the form of urticaria, skin rashes, glottal edema, and occasionally anaphylactoid reactions with shock and acute tubular necrosis. Excluding hypersensitivity, organic iodides are, nevertheless, nephrotoxic. The highest incidence seems to be associated with an oral contrast medium, bunamiodyl (Orabilex), and with other double doses of dehydration techniques that have been used for attempted visualization of diseased gallbladders. Toxicity is also associated with abdominal aortography, especially when high concentrations of contrast material are used by direct rapid injection.

The numerous mechanisms suggested to explain the nephrotoxicity of contrast media have included renal vasoconstriction, erythrocyte agglutination and crenation from hyperosmolar injections, and loss of the dispersing effect of albumin, coagulation defect, and high concentration of the material in the tubular cell of a patient who has impaired hepatic excretion. Experimentally it has been shown that stasis with obstruction to urinary flow potentiates the toxicity.

Pathologic changes follow the particular route of pathogenesis: vasculitis in some cases of iodine hypersensitivity, proteinuria, and glomerular damage from vasoconstriction and capillary thrombi, and acute tubular necrosis from shock or direct toxicity to the tubular cell. Recent reports suggest a specific reaction between the myeloma kidney and contrast material. Some may be due to dehydration incurred in preparation for pyelography. McAfee surveyed 13,207 abdominal aortograms and uncovered 12 fatal and 27 serious nonfatal instances of nephrotoxicity. Crawford noted reduced renal function in 50 per cent of patients receiving more than 40 ml. of Urokon above the renal artery.

Intravenous pyelography, using less concentrated material, appears to produce fewer complications in even the presence of renal insufficiency. Retrograde pyelography carries the risk of infection from instrumentation and edema of the ureters, producing obstruction, and has been associated with papillary necrosis.

Cholecystography: It has been estimated that more than 100 cases of acute renal failure have been caused by bunamiodyl. The major pathologic finding is tubular necrosis, accompanied by deposition of birefringent green-brown crystals at the base of the tubular epithelial cell that are anisotropic with polarized light. Bunamiodyl is more completely absorbed from the intestine than other cholecystographic media and is, therefore, delivered in higher concentrations to the kidney, particularly in the presence of liver disease and an abnormal gallbladder. Wennberg recently demonstrated depression of glomerular filtration rate due to bunamiodyl. Renal failure has also occurred in patients with underlying renal disease subjected to dehydration and specialized techniques of rapid intravenous or double-dose cholecystography.

THERAPEUTIC AGENTS
(Antimicrobial Drugs)

In the presence of infectious disease and its circulatory consequences, recognition of nephrotoxicity from antimicrobial agents may be difficult. Dehydration, hypotension, vomiting, and allergic reactions may lead to renal failure that is not, properly speaking, direct nephrotoxicity. However, a number of antimicrobials do appear to produce direct renal damage.

Sulfonamide compounds may precipitate in the nephron or calyces, and may be excreted in high concentrations into a urine with a low pH. This can produce sulfonamide concretions, obstructive uropathy, and parenchymal damage from crystals. Occasionally direct tubular necrosis, interstitial nephritis, or necrotizing angiitis may also occur. Other lesions have been reported from acetazolamide.

Streptomycin may produce necrosis of the proximal tubular epithelium, cylindruria, and albuminuria. Since the excretion of streptomycin is predominantly renal, underlying kidney disease may be associated with higher and more toxic blood levels.

Kanamycin has been associated with proteinuria and microscopic hematuria in 10 and 20 per cent of the patients, respectively, at dosage levels of 25 to 50 mg. per kilogram per day. Oliguria may develop, and tubular necrosis seems to be aggravated by prior therapy with streptomycin or viomycin.

Bacitracin produces renal tubular necrosis. *Polymyxins* A, B, C, D, and E have nephrotic properties of varying severity. Only polymyxin B has received extensive clinical use. It may produce albuminuria, casts, epithelial cells in the urine, decrease in concentrating ability, and tubular degeneration. Polymyxin B accumulates if renal function is impaired or if the dose exceeds 3 mg. per kilogram per day. Nephrotoxicity is dose-related.

Colymycin (colistin) is chemically similar to polymyxin and has a similar nephrotoxicity.

Neomycin is not normally well absorbed from the gastrointestinal tract. It produces foamy vacuolization of the epithelial lining of the proximal convoluted tubules, and progressive renal failure has been reported following intraperitoneal administration.

Tetracycline accentuates azotemia by its catabolic effect in increasing nitrogen turnover. Deteriorated tetracycline, used after its expiration date, has produced a largely reversible Fanconi type of syndrome consisting of reduced renal function, polyuria, polydypsia, glycosuria, aminoaciduria, hyperphosphaturia, hypercalciuria, hypophosphatemia, hypokalemia, hyperuricemia, and severe metabolic acidosis with debilitating lethargy. Instances have also been demonstrated of heavy Bence Jones proteinuria, transient hyperglycemia, and a macular papular rash. The characteristic lesion is tubular degeneration with desquamation of epithelial cells, granular cytoplasm, vacuolization, hemosiderosis, evidence of reparative epithelial cell regeneration and pale staining nuclei. Among the degradation products believed to account for the syndrome, two have been biochemically identified as epianhydrotetracycline and anhydrotetracycline. Clinical manifestations may appear in three or four days following ingestion of as little as 10 to 12 capsules.

Amphotericin B is dangerous chiefly because of renal damage. Cylindruria is the first manifestation, and may be accompanied by hematuria, pyuria, and proteinuria. The glomerular filtration rate and renal blood flow may decline by half or more. Maximal concentrating capacity decreases; serum urea and creatinine increase. Therapy may have to be terminated. Examination of kidney tissue shows necrosis and degeneration of proximal and distal tubules with flattened epithelium, regenerative foci, and calcification prominent in casts and interstitial tissue. Thickening of the glomerular basement has been noted in some patients.

ANALGESIC ABUSE
(Phenacetin Nephropathy)

Mixed analgesic preparations are among the most frequently used drugs in medical therapy and self-medication. In 1953 Spuhler and Zollinger noted an increase in interstitial nephritis and a

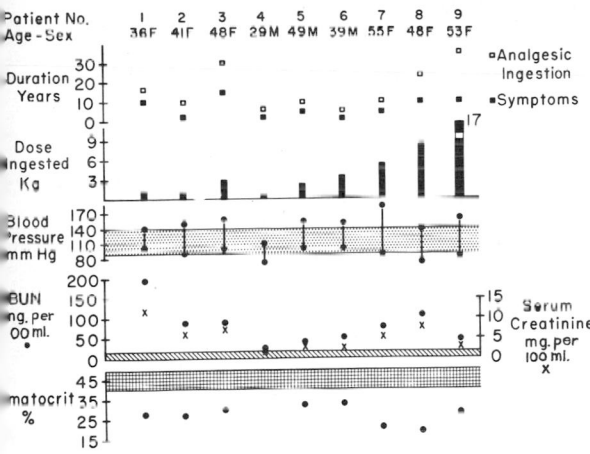

NEPHROPATHY OF ANALGESIC ABUSE

anuria has been reported following exposure to *chlordane*.

Aye, R. C.: Renal papillary necrosis. Diabetes, 3:124, 1954.

Becker, C. G., Becker, E. L., Maher, J. F., and Schreiner, G. E.: Nephrotic syndrome after contact with mercury. A report of five cases, three after the use of ammoniated mercury ointment. Arch. Intern. Med. (Chicago), 110:178, 1962.

Brun, C., Olsen, S., Raaschou, F., and Sorensen, A. W. S.: The localization of gold in the human kidney following chrysotherapy. A biopsy study. Nephron, 1:265, 1964.

Crawford, E. S., Beall, A. C., Moyer, J. H., and De Bakey, M. E.: Complications of aortography. Surg. Gynec. Obstet., 104:129, 1957.

Doolan, P. D., Walsh, W. P., Kyle, L. H., and Wishinsky, H.: Acetylsalicylic acid intoxication: Proposed method of treatment. J.A.M.A., 146:105, 1951.

Freeman, R. B., Maher, J. F., Schreiner, G. E., and Mostofi, F. K.: Renal tubular necrosis due to nephrotoxicity of organic mercurial diuretics. Ann. Intern. Med., 57:34, 1962.

Frimpter, G. W., Timpanelli, A. E., Eisenmenger, W. J., Stein, H. S., and Ehrlich, L. I.: Reversible "Fanconi syndrome" caused by degraded tetracycline. J.A.M.A., 184:111, 1963.

Goodman, L., and Gilman, A.: The Pharmacological Basis of Therapeutics. 3rd ed. New York, The Macmillan Company, 1965.

Lauler, D. P., Schreiner, G. E., and David, A.: Renal medullary necrosis. Amer. J. Med., 29:132, 1960.

Longcope, W. T., and Leutscher, J. A.: The treatment of acute mercury bichloride poisoning with BAL (2,3 dimercaptopropanol). Med. Clin. N. Amer., 34:469, 1950.

Luessenhop, A. J., Gallimore, J. C., Sweet, W. H., Struxness, E. G., and Robinson, J.: The toxicity in man of hexavalent uranium following intravenous administration. Amer. J. Roentgen., 79:83, 1958.

Maher, J. F., and Schreiner, G. E.: Cause of death in acute renal failure. Arch. Intern. Med. (Chicago), 110:493, 1962.

Maher, J. F., and Schreiner, G. E.: The clinical dialysis of poisons. Trans. Amer. Soc. Artif. Intern. Organs, 9:390, 1963.

McAfee, J. G.: A survey of complications of abdominal aortography. Radiology, 68:825, 1957.

Pendergrass, E. P., Hodes, P. J., Tondreau, R. L., Powell, C. C., and Burdick, E. D.: Further consideration of deaths and unfavorable sequelae following the administration of contrast media in urography in the United States. Amer. J. Roentgen., 74:262, 1955.

Rich, A. R.: The role of hypersensitivity in periarteritis nodosa as indicated by 7 cases developing during serum sickness and sulfonamide therapy. Bull. Hopkins Hosp., 71:123, 1942.

Schreiner, G. E.: Dialysis of poisons and drugs: Annual review. Trans. Amer. Soc. Artif. Intern. Organs, 16:544, 1970.

Schreiner, G. E.: The nephrotoxicity of analgesic abuse. Ann. Intern. Med., 57:1047, 1962.

Schreiner, G. E., and Maher, J. F.: Toxic nephropathy. Amer. J. Med., 38:409, 1965.

Schreiner, G. E., Maher, J. F., Marc-Aurele, J., Knowlan, D., and Alvo, M.: Ethylene glycol—two indications for hemodialysis. Trans. Amer. Soc. Artif. Intern. Organs, 5:81, 1959.

Schwartz, W. B., Hurwit, A., and Ettinger, A.: Intravenous urography in the patient with renal insufficiency. New Eng. J. Med., 269:277, 1963.

Setter, J. G., Maher, J. F., and Schreiner, G. E.: Acute renal failure following cholecystography. J.A.M.A., 184:102, 1963.

Spuhler, O., and Zollinger, H. U.: Die chronischinterstitielle Nephritis. Z. Klin. Med., 151:1, 1953.

Strauss, M. B., and Welt, L. G.: Diseases of the Kidney. 2nd ed. Boston, Little, Brown & Company, 1971.

Wennberg, J. E., Okun, R., Hinman, E. J., Northcutt, R. C., Greip, R. J., and Walker, W. G.: Renal toxicity of oral cholecystographic media. J.A.M.A., 186:461, 1963.

Yow, E. M., Moyer, J. H., and Smith, C. P.: Toxicity of polymyxin B. II. Human studies with particular reference to evaluation of renal function. Arch. Intern. Med. (Chicago), 92:248, 1953.

high incidence of medullary necrosis in patients who had abused analgesic therapy. Many such patients have now been reported from Switzerland, the Scandinavian countries, Australia, New Zealand, South Africa, Canada, and the United States. At Georgetown Hospital, nine patients with this entity have been studied, and some of the findings are summarized in the accompanying figure.

Satisfactory understanding of the pathogenesis of analgesic nephropathy is lacking. Anti-inflammatory effects, salicylates as uncoupling agents, hypokalemia, manufacturing contaminants (acetic-4-chloranilid), methemoglobinemia and sulfhemoglobinemia, sensitivity reactions, and predisposition have all been suggested as playing a role in the disease. Direct toxicity has not been demonstrated in animals except when excessive amounts of phenacetin have been used; similar levels of aspirin ingestion are fatal. In general, clinical cases have occurred in which the cumulative ingestion calculated as phenacetin is in excess of 1 kg. Continuing investigation may add more epidemiologic and circumstantial evidence for an association between chronic interstitial nephritis, renal papillary necrosis, and/or a unique susceptibility to pyelonephritis of patients who chronically ingest analgesic mixtures.

INSECTICIDES

Biphenyl is a citrus fungicide that produces polyuria and focal tubular dilatation resembling small cysts. Chronic exposure to *DDT* may produce fatty degeneration of the tubular epithelium, and

Renal Calculi

William C. Thomas, Jr.

Renal calculi are concretions consisting of crystals and a matrix of organic matter. Crystals usually make up the greater portion of the mass of a calculus, but calculi occurring as a consequence of urinary tract infections are occasionally composed largely of matrix material. Renal calculi are to be distinguished from calcific deposits *within* the renal parenchyma. Such deposits occurring at sites of previous inflammation or degenerative change are designated by the term "nephrocalcinosis." Elsewhere in the text are specific presentations of a number of disorders often complicated by nephrolithiasis; this article is largely limited to a discussion of broadly applicable principles in the cause and management of renal calculi.

Etiology. *General Factors.* Our knowledge of the cause of various types of calculi is incomplete, but from available evidence it appears that a combination of factors rather than any single event is most often responsible for calculus formation. The likelihood and type of calculus disease is modified by geographic factors, sex, race, and probably diet. In the United States the incidence is greatest in the Southeast, but there are other areas of the country where the incidence is also high. South Africa, portions of India, and Southeast Asia are additional regions where calculus disease frequently occurs. In the Southeastern United States "hard water" has been thought by some to be the important factor favoring calculus formation, but such a correlation fails to explain why calculi are infrequent in other "hard water" regions of the world. In India and Southeast Asia protein-poor, predominantly cereal diets have been considered, largely from epidemiologic surveys, to promote development of calculi, and efforts are now being made to test this thesis. Although these and other suggested explanations to account for the regional incidence of calculi may have some validity, none have the necessary investigative support to warrant acceptance.

Recurrent calculi composed of calcium oxalate and phosphate crystals are relatively uncommon in women and rare in Negroes of either sex. The disproportionate occurrence of such calculi in Caucasian males is unexplained, but holds true even in the high incidence areas of the Southeastern United States and South Africa. Women, however, are more susceptible than men to urinary tract infections. Thus, women with magnesium-ammonium-phosphate or calcium phosphate stones that develop as a complication of infection with urea-splitting organisms outnumber similarly affected men. Certain disorders predisposing to calculus formation, especially hyperparathyroidism, overcome the protective influence of sex or race, and this provides a diagnostic lead when searching for the cause of calculi in Caucasian women or Negroes.

Structure and Composition of Calculi. Examination of sectioned calculi usually reveals a distinct lamellar and sometimes radically striated organization. In most stones there is a small identifiable "nucleus" around which the bulk of the calculus appears to have developed. In calcium oxalate stones, the most common variety, this nucleus often consists of calcium phosphate, frequently in hydroxyapatite form. There is evidence that such nuclei may originate within the substance of renal pyramids or beneath the papillary epithelium. It has been suggested that many calculi may be formed by apposition of crystals and matrix onto the tiny nuclei which have been extruded into the renal pelvis. Whether the organic matrix present in all calculi can be formed from the proteinaceous material and cellular debris present in most urine, or whether it depends on the presence of specific products secreted by cells lining the urinary tract, has not been determined.

Although all calculi must initially be small and the matrix essential, it is the dense aggregation of crystals into a hard mass which accounts for the medical significance of renal stones, i.e., except for the previously mentioned largely matrix calculi occurring in some severely infected patients. The crystalline components of calculi are formed from the less soluble crystalloids predominant in the urine at the time the stone was developing. Crystallization may be promoted in several ways: increased excretion of crystalloids to a degree exceeding solubility limits, as in cystinuric patients or those with oxalosis; alteration of urinary pH in subjects who form urine persistently more acid than normal, and are thus susceptible to development of uric acid stones; or conversely, the production of excess ammonia and resulting increased urinary pH caused by infection with urea-splitting organisms, favoring crystallization of magnesium-ammonium-phosphate and calcium phosphate complexes. A variable degree of hypercalciuria is present in most patients with calcareous calculi, but often the increase in urinary calcium is slight. In addition to increased concentration of crystalloids or alteration of urinary pH, reduction in those urinary constituents which normally account for the supersaturated state of urine may also promote crystal formation. This type of change is now thought to be possibly more important in the genesis of calculi, particularly in those with calcareous stones, than is altered calcium excretion.

Composition of Urine. Normally, urine contains in solution a number of ions, e.g., calcium, magnesium, phosphate, oxalate, urate, at concentrations exceeding those achievable in water. The solubility of these ions is enhanced by the presence of urea. Organic acids, especially citrate, which form soluble chelates with calcium or magnesium, contribute to the solubility of these elements in urine, but the potential of organic acids to chelate metal ions is markedly decreased when the urine is acid.

In recent years specific inhibitors to the crystallization of calcium salts have been detected in urine and in serum. These biologic "water conditioners" may be important in determining susceptibility to calculus formation. One of them, inorganic pyrophosphate, has been studied in considerable detail. It is a product of intermediary metabolism and exists in serum at concentrations of 75 to 160 μg. per 100 ml. Urinary excretion of pyrophosphate by subjects receiving dairy-product-free diets ranges from 4 to 10 mg. per day, and, within limits, the amount in urine varies directly with orthophosphate excretion. Although urinary pyrophosphate may be a protective constituent, the amount excreted is the same in calculous and normal subjects, and is insufficient to account for the solution stability of urine.

More potent inhibitors of crystal formation than inorganic pyrophosphate have now been identified in urine. Very small amounts of these prevent crystallization of calcium salts from highly supersaturated solutions. They are water-soluble acidic compounds of low molecular weight, but of undefined composition. Although possibly of major importance, there are presently only a limited number of observations indicating a decreased urinary excretion of these "biologic water conditioners" by patients with idiopathic hypercalciuria and calcareous calculi. From several types of observations, however, comes evidence that calcium-containing crystals form more readily from urine of patients with calcareous calculi than from urine of normal subjects. Whether the difference is due to altered excretion of inhibitor compounds or to other unrecognized stabilizing constituents remains to be determined. Although it is tempting to assign to various inhibitors of crystallization a role in determining susceptibility to calculus formation, additional data are required to establish the concept.

Diagnosis. *History.* The history is important in evaluating patients with calculi. Infection as an etiologic or complicating factor is suggested by a history of fever preceding the initial episode of renal colic. Also, in postpartum women with calculi it is important to ascertain whether urinary tract infection occurred during pregnancy. Is there a family history of calculi? Genetic disorders such as renal tubular acidosis and cystinuria are expected in kindred, but idiopathic calcareous calculi may also occur in families. Chronic diarrheal states are accompanied by increased incidence of calculi. A number of medications have been causally related to renal stone formation, and patients should be questioned about chronic use of medicines, particularly acetazolamide, absorbable alkalis, trisilicates, and allopurinol. The type of water used and unusual dietary habits are additional items of relevant information.

Symptoms. Many patients with renal calculi are asymptomatic. Inflammation or infection resulting from calculi may lead to symptoms, but passage of a calculus into the ureter with resulting renal colic is the classic manifestation of calculus disease. Passage of small, gravel-like concretions with relatively little pain is not uncommon, particularly with uric acid lithiasis and sometimes in patients with calcium oxalate stones. Gross hematuria, especially in the absence of accompanying renal colic and a demonstrable ureteral calculus, should be regarded with suspicion as possibly indicative of infection or a coexistent neoplasm. Microscopic hematuria, however, is quite regularly present in patients with calculi. The malingerer, feigning renal colic in order to obtain narcotics, may demonstrate considerable ingenuity in developing a symptom complex.

Laboratory Findings. Careful examination of fresh urine provides immediate, valuable information. For example, an acid urine and urate crystals may be present in those with uric acid calculi, or a high urine pH (7.0 or higher) may signify infection or a renal tubular disorder. The presence of bacteria in fresh uncentrifuged urine usually indicates significant infection. As mentioned, microscopic hematuria is usual, and there may be few to many white blood cells. The pH of each freshly voided specimen of the patient's urine should be determined for 24 hours. The paper-strip method is adequate for this purpose. If the pH is consistently high and infection is present (values between 8.5 and 9.0 always indicate infection), the pH determinations should be repeated after eradication of the infection. In normal persons receiving a regular diet, urine pH will be less than 6.0 at some time during the 24 hours. If this degree of acidity is not achieved, the presence of renal tubular acidosis is likely, and should be confirmed by definitive tests. A persistently acid urine occurs in some patients with uric acid calculi.

A qualitative test for cystine should be performed in every patient with calculi, using freshly voided urine for the analysis. This disorder is much more common than is recognized.

Urine culture should also be obtained. The persistent occurrence of staphylococci in urine cultures should not be discounted as unimportant to stone formation, for some staphylococci are capable of splitting urea.

Urinary calcium should be determined in patients with radiopaque stones; this is conveniently done by having the patient abstain from dairy products (milk, cheese, and ice cream) for one to two days and then, while continuing the diet restriction, collecting urine for one or two 24-hour periods. The calcium ingested with such a regimen will usually be less than 300 mg. per day, and the amount excreted by normal subjects will be less than 170 mg. per 24 hours. Urinary calcium is increased in most patients with calcareous calculi, but will be normal in patients whose primary problem is infection. The urinary phosphorus reflects dietary phosphorus, and is a useless measure unless the amount ingested is accurately known.

In patients with calcareous calculi, serum analyses are required chiefly to establish the presence or absence of hypercalcemic states, particularly hyperparathyroidism or renal tubular acidosis. With the patient in a postabsorptive state, determinations of carbon dioxide, chloride, uric acid, phosphorus, and calcium are sufficient. Abnormal values should be rechecked. The serum concentrations of carbon dioxide and chloride may be normal in patients with mild renal tubular acidosis. Phosphorus concentrations in the sera of patients with idiopathic calcium oxalate or phosphate calculi are often slightly less than those of normal subjects.

When the calculus is available, both its central and peripheral portions should be subjected to chemical or crystallographic (by x-ray diffraction) analysis. Much information as to cause and treatment may be gained from this.

Radiologic Findings. It is often best to delay contrast urography until completion of blood and urine analyses, but a plain film of the abdomen or renal tomography in a patient properly prepared with laxatives is often informative. Roentgenographic visualization of the urinary tract should not be delayed if an infected patient is suspected of having ureteral obstruction. Uric acid and the rare xanthine calculi are radiolucent and may be large or small. Large or staghorn-shaped radiopaque calculi are usually the result of infection and are composed of magnesium-ammonium-phosphate or calcium phosphate, but cystine stones may achieve a similar size and configuration. Detectable laminations are not uncommon in large calculi resulting from infection. Calcium oxalate calculi are usually small (2 to 5 mm. in diameter), dense, and frequently multiple. Such calculi in children may indicate the presence of oxalosis. When large (diameter greater than 10 mm.) extremely dense stones are present in children or adults, hyperoxaluria should be suspected. The coexistence of nephrocalcinosis and renal calculi is not uncommon as a sequel of infection, but may also indicate the presence of renal tubular acidosis, hyperparathyroidism, sarcoidosis, and rarely oxalosis.

Stones are often of mixed composition, particularly when infection has supervened; for example, at the core of a large calculus there may be either a radiolucent area composed of urates or a radiologically dense oxalate stone. The rare calculus consisting largely of matrix material may be barely visible radiologically.

Finally, roentgenographic visualization of the urinary tract may reveal anatomic abnormalities conducive to calculus formation, presumably because of localized stagnation of urine.

Treatment. **General.** Avoidance of dehydration is important in calculus disease of all types, but especially so in patients with cystinuria, those with a susceptibility to uric acid concretions, and those with urinary tract infections. To maintain continuously dilute urine usually requires a daily intake of approximately 4 quarts of liquids, which should be distributed *throughout the 24 hours.* Although dairy products are frequently omitted during test procedures, there are no data to suggest that continued avoidance is beneficial in reducing the incidence or growth of calcareous calculi.

Every effort should be made to eradicate infection promptly. In paraplegic patients in whom high incidence of calculi correlates with urinary tract infections, dramatic reduction in stone development has been achieved by prompt and effective treatment of incipient infections. The size of ureteral calculi that can be passed spontaneously is surprising. Therefore it is often wise to delay instrumental intervention until it is certain that the calculus will not be extruded.

Specific. Details regarding the rationale for treatment of patients with cystinuria, renal tubular acidosis, and uric acid calculi are recorded in other parts of this text. Suffice it to say here that if treatment with absorbable alkali is to be instituted, the amount required varies, depending on renal function, but for adults with normal glomerular filtration rates it is usually from 100 to 250 mEq. of cation per day irrespective of the salt used. Cystinurics to be treated in this manner require the larger amounts because of the need to maintain urinary pH in the range of 8.0. Dosage with alkali should be spaced equally throughout the 24 hours to ensure continuous control of urinary pH.

Patients with single or very infrequent calcareous calculi that are passed without undue difficulty should be advised to drink copious amounts of liquid, but usually need not be considered candidates for continuous treatment. Several, largely empiric, modes of therapy are currently being evaluated in those patients with recurrent calcareous calculi. Orthophosphate salts have been extensively used, and administration of 6 to 9 grams in three or four divided doses has almost uniformly prevented formation of additional calculi. Sodium or potassium phosphate or a neutral mixture of these salts may be used. Diarrhea is the only adverse symptom, and is corrected by reducing the dose to a tolerated amount. Phosphate administration is followed by increased excretion of inorganic pyrophosphate and possibly other inhibitors of crystal formation, and usually a modest reduction in urinary calcium. Whether these changes are sufficient to account for the cessation of calculus formation is unknown.

Hydrochlorothiazide administration decreases urinary calcium and increases excretion of magnesium. In a limited experience this compound apparently prevents formation of calcareous calculi, but its use requires close supervision, and possible complications are numerous. Magnesium oxide has been advocated on the basis that increased urinary magnesium promotes oxalate solubility, but experience with this mode of therapy is too limited to assess its merit.

Patients with calculi caused by infection are the most difficult to manage. None of the regimens mentioned has had the desired effectiveness. The infection should be treated, but it is rarely possible to prevent recurrence. Treatment directed to reducing the urinary phosphorus to several hundred milligrams per day has been used by a number of investigators. This program requires that the patient avoid dairy products, and, to further decrease phosphate absorption, ingest 30 ml. of aluminum carbonate gel after each meal and at bedtime. When infection cannot be eradicated by anti-microbial drugs, and especially when calculi are larger, their surgical removal is advisable.

Hodgkinson, A., and Nordin, B. E. C. (eds.): Renal Stone Research Symposium. London, J. & A. Churchill Ltd., 1969.

Kolb, F. O. (ed.): Symposium on treatment of kidney stones. Mod. Treatm., 4:461, 1967.

Maurice, P. F., and Henneman, P. H.: Medical aspects of renal stones. Medicine, 40:315, 1961.

Shorr, E., and Carter, A. C.: Aluminum gels in the management of renal phosphatic calculi. J.A.M.A., 144:1549, 1950.

Smith, L. H., Jr. (ed.): Symposium on stones. Amer. J. Med., 45:649, 1968.

Cysts of the Kidney

George E. Schreiner

POLYCYSTIC DISEASE

Polycystic disease is the most prevalent renal cystic disease (Table 1). It is inherited as a dominant, non-sex-linked disease emerging at two prominent age peaks, in infancy and in adult life. Progressive dilatation of renal tubules leads to obstruction, infection, rupture of cysts, bleeding, or chronic renal failure. There may be associated anomalies, such as cysts in the liver or other organs or berry aneurysm of the cerebral vessels. Sporadic cases are found without familial history and scattered through childhood. More often the adult disease emerges after the next generation has already been "planted." The infantile type may be autosomal recessive, but the adult disease is a hereditary dominant. Penetrance is high and rises with increasing age. Clinical surveys in large families usually reveal that half or more of the members are afflicted. In advanced age penetrance is almost total.

Embryology. Older theories no longer accepted for the pathogenesis of polycystic disease include fetal papillitis with secondary fibrosis and obstruction, cyst formation as a neoplastic process, congenital syphilis, and fetal interstitial nephritis. Popular theories include (1) "nonunion" of ureteric bud and tubules, (2) noncanalization owing to lack of "organizer," and (3) persistence of primitive nephrons that fail to atrophy. A microdissection study subclassified four types: (a) hyperplasia of interstitial portion of collecting tubules, (b) inhibition of ampullary activity, (c) multiple developmental anomalies, and (d) urethral obstruction. Infantile cysts may be totally isolated; adult cysts near the capsule are large, glomerular, and do not connect. In deeper cortex they have entering and exiting tubules. In the medulla the cysts involve collecting ducts and may be related to a calyx.

Physiology. Analyses of cyst fluid have shown concentrations of Na$^-$ from 3 to 150 mEq. per liter, K of 4.6 to 58 mEq. per liter, H ion from 13 to 9800 nanoEq. per liter, and creatinine 11 to 87 mg. per 100 ml. Inulin and PAH may enter polycysts, and water may be removed. Cyst-plasma ratios of creatinine are often above 1.0 in deep cysts. Amino acids may concentrate and add 50 to 100 mOsm. per kilogram of water to the osmotic concentration of cyst fluid. Protein, red cells, bacteria, and cellular debris may be found.

Incidence. Since early diagnosis is difficult, the clinical incidence varies with the vigor of the diagnostic pursuit. Widespread application of the renal scan enhances the diagnostic yield. Polycystic disease is still often a surprise diagnosis at autopsy. Some representative incidence figures are summarized in Table 2.

Pathology. The kidneys are enlarged and often asymmetrical. They have a nodular surface produced by projecting cysts that may be filled with watery, serous, hemorrhagic, pustular or viscid fluid, or clear urine. Cut surface reveals the entire parenchyma honeycombed by cysts protruding from various levels. About one fifth of polycystic patients have intracranial aneurysm and 4 per cent of patients with clinical aneurysms have polycystic disease. Cysts may coexist in liver, spleen, lungs, and pancreas, but are rarely clinically significant. Mild renal cysts may occur in hepatic cystic disease and may be clinically subordinate. Histologically, cysts of various caliber, location, and content may be demonstrated. The

TABLE 1. SIMPLE CLASSIFICATION OF CYSTIC DISEASE

A. Polycystic disease
    Infantile
    Adult
B. Multicystic disease
C. Multilocular cysts
D. Simple cysts
E. Medullary cystic disease
F. Medullary sponge kidney
G. Dysplasia
H. Miscellaneous cysts of renal origin
I. Miscellaneous cysts of nonrenal origin

TABLE 2. SOME REPRESENTATIVE INCIDENCE FIGURES

Year	Place	No. Polycystic Cases	Ratio to Autopsies
1897	Kiel	16	1:636
1928	Leningrad	192	1:261
1933	Mayo	9	1:1019
1934	New York	14	1:428
1935	Gottingen	38	1:222
1949	Great Britain	16	1:375
1950	Minnesota	70	1:779
1954	Copenhagen	143	1:773
1955	Mayo	35	1:323
1965	Georgetown	——	1:165

Total = 533 + Avg. = 1:498

internal lining may be flattened or cuboidal and rarely may have papillary projections or glomerular tufts. Recently, it has been shown that interruptions of the elastic laminae of small renal arteries, ruptured arteries, and microaneurysms can be demonstrated in the renal parenchyma. It is not clear whether vessel rupture is cause or effect. Degenerative changes from pressure, calculi and secondary infection may be seen. Many cases of renal carcinoma have been reported in polycystic kidneys. Renal biopsy studies are needed in polycystic families since little is known of the natural history of cysts in the presymptomatic decades.

Diagnosis. The *infantile type* is usually diagnosed by palpation of bilateral renal masses, roentgenographic findings, or presentation with uremia. Nausea, vomiting, dehydration, and abdominal distention are the most prevalent. We have one such patient six years old. The small cyst variety is the most difficult to diagnose. The *adult type* may be totally asymptomatic for several decades, with a chance finding on roentgenographic examination or even at autopsy. With progressive enlargement, presenting symptoms include lumbar or abdominal pain (28 per cent), palpable mass (20 per cent), hypertension (17 per cent), bladder symptoms of frequency, urgency, and dysuria (17 per cent), painless hematuria (17 per cent), and painful hematuria (10 per cent). Other patients may present with any of the manifestations of renal failure. On examination, hypertension and palpable enlarged kidneys are present in about three quarters of the patients at the time of diagnosis. Kidneys growing to a size of 6 kg. or more produce weakness, a dragging sensation, increasing abdominal girth, and the displacement of other organs.

Complications. Many patients with polycystic disease present or die with complications such as vascular accidents from ruptured aneurysms or hypertensive disease, secondary pyelonephritis, infected cysts, perinephric abscess, gross hematuria, calcification of cyst wall and formation of urinary calculi, and associated renal carcinoma. Both erythrocytosis and polycythemia have been noted. Dalgaard found calculus and/or colic in 18 per cent of 350 patients. Rarely dystocia has been reported owing to distended abdomen of the fetus from infantile cystic disease. We have seen subdiaphragmatic abscess from ruptured infected cysts and obstructive uropathy from enlarging cysts in the lower pole obstructing the ureteropelvic junction and reversible by surgical decompression of the offending cyst. A family history of polycystic kidneys can readily be obtained in the majority of cases by taking a detailed history and surveying causes of death in siblings. Spurious histories are commonly encountered in families with a pathetic desire to hide the trait. General problems we have encountered include psychologic "block" to family surveys, the problem of marriage and pregnancy, questions of elective surgery and procedures, economic problems generating from inability to get life, health, hospital, or disability insurance or to meet medical requirements of a job, and the emotional impact of watching other members of the family die from a known affliction of the observer.

Laboratory Findings. These include albuminuria, hematuria, pyuria, passage of epithelial cells, and all of the progressive laboratory findings associated with renal failure. Hyperchloremic acidosis may be seen. A salt-losing tendency with dehydration, increasing azotemia, and hyponatremia is much more frequent than in other renal diseases.

Roentgenography. Important roentgenographic findings include enlarged or displaced kidneys with varying densities, loculation, or calcification, elongated pelves, crescentic deformities of calyces (wine-glass sign), hydronephrosis and other obstructive phenomena, and "unfolding" of the calyceal system. The small cyst, infantile type, is best diagnosed by observation of nephrographic phenomena persisting up to 72 hours. This parenchymal opacification results from concentration of iodine in tubular cells and excretion into the lumina of dilated tubules. Less than 10 per cent of polycystic disease is unilateral. Recently nephrotomography has been found useful in differentiating neoplasm from cyst, and the renal scan may give a characteristic appearance of "holes," as seen in the accompanying figure.

Prognosis. The *infantile type* is rapidly fatal from uremia or complications. The adult type may be latent and rarely may not interfere with longevity. Progressive cystic disease proceeds to hypertension, uremia, vascular accidents, infections, and death, with the peak mortality in the latter half of the fifth decade. Prognosis can be improved by continuous medical care and treatment of infection and acute obstruction, management of chronic uremia, and avoidance of—or special care during—pregnancy. Polycystic patients often do not tolerate strict salt restriction. The age of diagnosis and the subsequent life expectancy are related. Under 50, one third of males are alive 12½ years later. Over 50, only 14 per cent are alive 2½ years later.

Treatment. The treatment is medical. Marsupialization, bivalving with unroofing, puncture and aspiration, and unilateral nephrectomy have all been tried and have failed. Decompression or heminephrectomy is justified only when extrarenal obstruction is demonstrated. Treatment for infection is as outlined in the article on urinary tract infections. Treatment of acute renal failure and chronic renal failure is detailed elsewhere. Bed rest is indicated for hematuria and transfusions for symptomatic anemia of blood loss. In patients suffering recurrent pain from enlarging cysts, we have had some success with the use of acetazolamide, 500 mg. daily, as a single dose, or with combinations of acetazolamide and a thiazide diuretic. Management of hypertension and edema may be helpful. Sympathetic understanding of the psychological problem is important. The diagnosis of polycystic kidneys carries with it the responsibility to conduct a family survey and advise the patient and family members concerning the basic diagnosis and management of possible complications.

Hemodialysis has been successfully used for transient exacerbations of renal failure caused by infection, obstruction, dehydration, hyponatremia or hypotension. It may occasionally result in prolonged improvement even in apparently moribund patients. Recent history of a good urinary volume forms a reasonable guide in selection of patients for dialysis. Polycystic patients often make good transplant candidates because the graft does not acquire the disease of the recipient. Erythrocytosis may follow the relief of azotemia and may be reversed by removal of a cystic kidney.

Bialestock, D.: The morphogenesis of renal cysts in the stillborn. A study of microdissection technique. J. Path. Bact., 71:51, 1956.

Bricker, N. S., and Patton, J. F.: Cystic disease of the kidneys. A study of dynamics and chemical composition of cyst fluid. Amer. J. Med., 18:207, 1955.

Brown, R. A. P.: Polycystic diseases of the kidneys and intracranial aneurysms, etiology and inter-relationship of these conditions: Review of recent literature and report of seven cases in which both conditions co-existed. Glasgow Med. J., 32:335, 1951.

Dalgaard, O. Z.: Polycystic disease of the kidneys. In Strauss, M. B., and Welt, L. G. (eds.): Diseases of the Kidney. Boston, Little, Brown and Company, 1963. p. 907.

Gardner, K. D., Jr.: Composition of fluid in twelve cysts of a polycystic kidney. New Eng. J. Med., 281:985, 1969.

Smith, C. H., and Graham, J. B.: Congenital medullary cysts of the kidneys with severe refractory anemia. Amer. J. Dis. Child., 69:369, 1945.

Strauss, M. B.: Clinical and pathological aspects of cystic disease of the renal medulla: An analysis of 18 cases. Ann. Intern. Med., 57:373, 1962.

Strauss, M. B.: Cystic disease of the renal medulla. In Strauss, M. B., and Welt, L. G. (eds.): Diseases of the Kidney. Boston, Little, Brown and Company, 1963, p. 938.

OTHER CYSTS

Serous or *solitary* cysts are thin sacs with flattened epithelium frequent in the lower pole and rarely communicating with a nephron. Congenital in origin, they may grow to 12 liters, produce backache, dragging sensation, palpable mass, obstruction, or urographic abnormality. They may contain blood and calcification. Solutes generally approximate those of plasma water. *Multilocular* cysts have septa or a honeycombed interior. When large they may resemble polycystic disease and may account for some older reports of unilateral poly cysts. *Lymphatic* cysts are found near the hilus and are associated with veins and vascular atresias. They begin 1 to 2 cm. in diameter in the newborn but may enlarge. *Diverticula* of pelvis and calyces are associated with infection and obstruction, and they may appear as *cystic dilatations* of the parenchyma. They are suspected by their location. *Perirenal* cysts may follow traumatic extravasation or may be neoplastic. The latter originate in aberrant mesodermal tissue (wolffian or müllerian ducts, lymph channels), are varied in form, are usually unilateral, and are on the left side in females. *Renal hematomas* may liquefy and cavitate. *Angiomas* may produce profuse bleeding over long periods. *Mesenteric* cysts form below the kidney and simulate tumor or cause obstruction. *Dermoid* cysts contain all germ layers and may contain hair, bones, teeth, and other tissues. Infectious erosion of the renal parenchyma or disso-

Isotope scan of a kidney; the cystic areas are indicated by areas of diminished or absent radioactivity.

lution of infected infarcts in *pyelonephritis* may produce cystlike areas, filled with fluid or pus. *Renal tuberculosis* may produce *caseocavernous abscesses* or ulcerations of the pelvis. Retention cysts of chronic glomerulonephritis are rarely of clinical importance. *Echinococcus cysts* occur from infestation by the larval stage of the dog tapeworm. This is prevalent in certain sheep-raising countries. The manifestations include tumor, pain, dysuria, hematuria, eosinophilia, and excretion of ova, hooklets, and scolices in the urine. A complement-fixation test may be positive. *Toxoplasma* may produce microscopic pseudocysts in the kidney. *Renal aneurysm* may produce flank pain, hematuria, hypertension, and urographic filling defects. Renal cysts are associated with angiomatous tumors of the cerebellum in *Lindau's disease* and of the retina in *von Hippel–Lindau disease.*

Treatment of most cysts depends on type, location, and manifestation. Known serous and pustular cysts may be aspirated by needle. More often, because of the threat of malignancy, most cysts require surgical exploration and removal. Normal parenchyma should be preserved whenever possible. Erythrocytosis may be reversed by cyst removal, but cysts rarely contain granular cells or significant erythropoietin. They probably stimulate erythropoietin production in nearby tissue. Advances in renal plastic surgery now permit more frequent choices between partial and total nephrectomy. The latter should be avoided in benign conditions.

Isaac, F., Schoen, I., and Walker, P.: An unusual case of Lindau's disease: Cystic disease of the kidneys and pancreas with renal and cerebral tumors. Amer. J. Roentgen., 75:912, 1956.

More, T.: Unilateral cystic kidneys. Brit. J. Urol., 29:3, 1957.

Parkkulainen, K. V., Hjelt, L. V., and Sirola, K.: Congenital multicystic dysplasia of the kidney: Report of nineteen cases with discussion on the etiology, nomenclature, and classification of the cystic dysplasias of the kidney. Acta Chir. Scand., Suppl. 244, 1959.

Vertel, R. M., Morse, B. S., and Prince, J. E.: Remission of erythrocytosis after drainage of a solitary renal cyst. Arch. Intern. Med. (Chicago), 120:54, 1967.

UREMIC MEDULLARY CYSTIC DISEASE

Uremic medullary cystic disease and the familial juvenile nephronophthisis described by Fanconi et al. now appear to be facets of the same disease with minor variations. There is definite hereditary predisposition exhibiting in various pedigrees as a recessive, a dominant, or an incomplete recessive affecting young children, older children, young adults, and a few rare survivors in the fifth and sixth decades. The disease presents an insidious onset with pallor, polyuria, anemia, or failure to thrive and grow. The normochromic anemia is refractory. The urine is deceptively benign, although modest proteinuria is frequent in older patients. Salt wasting is almost the rule. Hypertension is rare. The patients progress inexorably, but at varying rates, into uremia, with any or all of its features. Prominent are hyponatremia, hypochloremia, hypocalcemia, hyperphosphatemia, hyperphosphatasemia, metabolic acidosis, retarded growth, bone age, demineralization, and other features of osteodystrophy, parathyroid and adrenal hyperplasia, and myelofibrosis. All tubular defects are distal with impaired concentrating ability, poor response to ADH, impaired acidification, impaired ammonium excretion, salt wasting, and a tendency to hyperkalemia. Infection is rare except after instrumentation. Notably absent are phosphaturia, glycosuria, aminoaciduria, or any disorder of proximal tubular function.

Pathologically, the kidneys are contracted (45 to 100 grams), granular, and lobulated. There are glomerulosclerosis, periglomerular fibrosis, diffuse, severe interstitial fibrosis, tubular atrophy and dilatation, colloid casts, localized lymphangiectasia, and cysts widespread in medulla, but often randomly distributed elsewhere. Mongeau and Worthen reviewed 103 cases. Postmortem studies in 50 revealed macroscopic cysts in 32 and microscopic cysts in 18. Cut sections from patients with nephronophthisis and medullary cystic disease are indistinguishable. Overemphasis on macroscopic cysts and their anatomic distribution has confused the issue. Goldman et al. have traced 50 members of a family through five generations and found a dominant pattern. Eighteen of 25 persons in the first three generations had either overt renal failure or transmission to offspring. In other families it has been recessive. In some cases there is no family involvement. The cause and progression resemble human toxic nephropathy from a variety of agents, including heavy metals, and the lesions resemble early diphenylamine intoxication in rats. The disease could be an inborn error of metabolism that permits accumulation of a toxic substance, affecting distal tubular development in fetal life or early infancy.

Treatment consists in genetic counseling, management of abnormal physiology such as the salt depletion, treating the full range of defects seen in the nephrotic syndrome, especially osteodystrophy and anemia, and ultimately resorting to the definitive therapy of terminal renal failure—dialysis or transplantation. Patients with renal transplants in place for more than two years have not acquired the defect, indicating that medullary cystic disease is purely renal in origin.

Fanconi, G., Hanhard, E., Albertini, A., von Uhlinger, E., Dolivo, G., and Prader, A.: Die familiare juvenile Nephronophthise (die idiopathische Schrumpfniere). Helv. Paediat. Acta, 6:1, 1951.

Goldman, S. H., Walter, S. R., Merigan, T. C., Jr., Gardner, K. D., Jr., and Bull, J. M. C.: Hereditary occurrence of cystic disease of the renal medulla. New Eng. J. Med., 274:984, 1966.

Herman, R. C., Good, R. A., and Vernier, R. L.: Medullary cystic disease in two siblings. Amer. J. Med., 43:335, 1967.

Levin, N. W., Rosenberg, B., Zwi, S., and Reid, F. P.: Medullary cystic disease of the kidney, with some observations on ammonium excretion. Amer. J. Med., 30:807, 1961.

Mongeau, J. G., and Worthen, H. G.: Nephronophthisis and medullary cystic disease. Amer. J. Med., 43:345, 1967.

Strauss, M. B.: Clinical and pathological aspects of cystic disease of the renal medulla. Ann. Intern. Med., 57:373, 1962.

Strauss, M. B., and Sommers, S. C.: Medullary cystic disease and familial juvenile nephronophthisis. New Eng. J. Med., 277: 000, 1967.

SPONGE KIDNEY

(Nonuremic Medullary Cystic Disease)

Sponge kidney, first recognized in 1939, has now been recognized in several hundred patients. It is a congenital anomaly which can be manifested by pain, colic, calculi, recurrent infection, or hematuria; but more often it is asymptomatic and discovered as an incidental finding on roentgenography, biopsy, or autopsy. Branching, radial ducts and cysts are found ramifying from calyces along the pyramids. They may fill on intravenous pyelography, and may *not* fill on retrograde pyelography. Flow is slow, and contrast material hangs behind. They may be uni- or bilateral, segmental, or focal. The roentgenographic appearance has been likened to a sponge, grapes, flowers, and twigs. The cysts are filled with fluid, cellular debris, and concretions. Calcium apatite, carbonate,

oxalate, and triple phosphate have been found. Nephrocalcinosis may occur. Hypercalciuria, pyelonephritis, and hypertension may supervene. Distal tubular defects have been noted, but so uncommonly that they may be related to the complications rather than the disease. Similar cysts have been noted in congenital hepatic fibrosis. Reported cases in Ehlers-Danlos syndrome, hemihypertrophy, and congenital pyloric stenosis may be special forms of sponge kidney. The roentgenographic pattern has been seen in two generations of one family and in two siblings, but is generally nonfamilial. The prognosis is related to infection, obstruction, and calculous disease. The asymptomatic form is benign and usually without any counterpart functional disorder. Instrumentation should be avoided.

Abeshouse, B. S., and Abeshouse, G. A.: Sponge kidney: A review of the literature and a report of five cases. J. Urol., 84:252, 1960.

Copping, G. A.: Medullary sponge kidney: Its occurrence in a father and daughter. Canad. Med. Ass. J., 96:608, 1967.

Lagergren, C., and Lindvall, N.: Medullary sponge kidney and polycystic diseases of the kidney: Distinct entities. Amer. J. Roentgen., 88:153, 1962.

MacDougall, J. A., and Prout, W. G.: Medullary sponge kidney: Clinical appraisal and report of twelve cases. Brit. J. Surg., 55:130, 1968.

Morris, R. C., Yamauchi, H., Palubinskas, A. J., and Howenstine, J.: Medullary sponge kidney. Amer. J. Med., 38:883, 1965.

Tumors of the Kidney

George E. Schreiner

Neoplasia of the genitourinary tract accounts for about one fifth of adult tumors and about one quarter of childhood tumors. Renal masses are considered malignant until proved otherwise. Our ignorance of the mechanisms of renal neoplasia parallels our general lack of knowledge of the pathogenesis of unrestrained cell growth. A classification of renal tumors is given in the accompanying table.

Unending subclassifications of tumors and morphologic grading have generally proved to be a sterile pathologic exercise. Older designations, such as hypernephroma, adenocarcinoma, alveolar carcinoma, and embryonic carcinoma have been dropped in favor of "renal carcinoma" or tumors of epithelial cell origin. Multiple sections often reveal more than one histologic type.

Pathology. Tubular epithelium gives rise to adenocarcinoma. The epithelial lining of the pelvicalyceal system yields transitional cell carcinomas, and immature parenchymal tissue is the source of Wilms' tumor. Carcinoma accounts for 80 per cent of renal malignancy. Cell types are *clear* and *granular*. Anatomic staging is as follows: IA—intracapsular tumor; IB—intrarenal but extracapsular (invasion through tumor capsule); II—

perinephric microscopic; III—perinephric gross; and IV—distant metastases. Renal carcinoma has a male preponderance, with a peak incidence at 45 to 60 years of age. Extension into the renal veins or through the renal capsule offers a bad prognosis (vein invaded—30 per cent five-year survival, versus 60 per cent when the vein is not invaded). Degeneration and calcification are a good prognostic feature. Renal carcinoma may spontaneously regress. A metastatic lesion may regress after removal of primary site, or may occur as late as 20 years after primary removal. Spread is by direct invasion or by vascular and lymphatic channels. Venous occlusion may result from spread of the tumor up the inferior vena cava. Favorite metastatic sites are lungs, liver, bones, and brain. They may be solitary.

Embryonal nephroma (Wilms' tumor) may occur in the fetus or rarely in later life. Seventy-five per cent appear before the age of five; about two thirds occur before two years of age. Eight per cent are bilateral. More than 50 confusing names have been applied to this tumor. It grows rapidly, may approach the weight of the rest of the body, and metastasizes most frequently through the veins to the lungs or through the lymphatics to

CLASSIFICATION OF RENAL TUMORS

1. Neoplasms of renal parenchyma
   A. Benign tumors
      Fibroma
      Adenoma
      Papillary cystadenoma
      Endometriosis

   B. Epithelial neoplasms
      Renal carcinoma
      Embryonal nephroma (Wilms' tumor, nephroblastoma)

   C. Mesothelial neoplasms
      Sarcoma
      Neurogenic tumors
         Neuroblastoma
         Schwannoma
         Sympathicoblastoma

2. Neoplasms of the pelvis and calyces
   Papilloma
   Papillary carcinoma
   Squamous cell carcinoma
   Hemangioma

3. Tumors of the renal capsule
   Fibroma
   Fibrolipoma
   Malignant sarcoma
   Angiosarcoma
   Chondroma

4. Perirenal tumors and cysts

5. Tumors metastatic to the kidney

the periaortic nodes. Widespread metastases in many organs may be seen.

Clinical Manifestations. Since early renal tumors are asymptomatic, diagnoses are achieved by way of accidental or routine diagnostic studies. The classic triad of hematuria, mass, and pain must now be considered a later finding. Fever, leukocytosis, evidence of metastases, abdominal and flank pain, albuminuria, anorexia, weight loss, nausea, and vomiting are the most common symptoms. Even so, in less than half the children with Wilms' tumor is diagnosis achieved within one month of onset of symptoms. Demonstration of hematuria varies with the skill and persistence brought to the urinalysis. Erythrocytes in urine should never be considered a normal finding; suspicion of tumor should become greater during a systemic exclusion of other causes of hematuria. Because of venous extension and vascular spread, examination of patients with nephroma should be cautious, and treatment should be instituted as early as possible. Hypertension has been reported with widely varying incidence in embryonal nephroma; it may not revert on tumor removal. Presumably the tumor produces pressors directly or indirectly via ischemia. Nephroma may simulate or coexist with infantile polycystic disease.

In adult renal cell carcinoma the most prominent manifestations, in order, are hematuria, weight loss, lassitude, flank pain, fever, and abdominal pain. A firm spherical mass may be demonstrable by palpation, or roentgenographic studies may reveal it. Distant metastases may be observed before local signs appear. Notable are "cotton ball" metastases to the lung, osteolytic lesions in the long bones (femur, humerus), and involvement of lymph nodes, liver, adrenals, and contralateral kidney. No organ is exempt; unusual cases have been diagnosed by finding lesions in such places as the eye and vagina. Pelvic angiography and pulmonary fluoroscopy with an image intensifier have revealed asymptomatic metastases unrecognizable by other means.

Unusual Features. Renal carcinoma may present curious features and it has been called the "internist's tumor." These features include large tumor without distortion of the calyceal system, leukemoid reaction with leukocytes ranging up to 100,000 per cubic millimeter, polycythemia, eczematoid dermatitis, hypertension, hypercalcemia, peripheral nephropathy, plasmacytosis, and amyloid disease. Renal carcinoma has emerged as a major consideration in fevers of unknown origin. It may mimic a prolonged septic disease, or it may form an arteriovenous fistula to produce congestive heart failure. Both adult carcinoma and Wilms' tumor have been associated with erythemia and polycythemia. Elevated blood and tumor levels of erythropoietin have been reported. Renal carcinoma has been diagnosed in several patients considered to have polycythemia vera, and we have seen secondary polycythemia including granulocytosis and thrombocytosis in a patient with a small renal carcinoma not demonstrable roentgenologically.

Transitional cell tumors of the renal pelvis have been reported in patients with analgesic abuse and papillary necrosis.

Laboratory Findings. In addition to anemia or polycythemia, renal carcinoma characteristically brings about an unusually high sedimentation rate (up to 150 mm. per hour). On electrophoresis, serum albumin is reduced, and alpha$_2$ globulin is elevated. A special form of tumor, the clear-cell PAS-positive renal carcinoma, has been associated with evidence of increased glucoprotein synthesis and abnormal serum glucoproteins.

Roentgenographic findings include irregularity of renal margin, multiple calcifications, deformity of infundibulum or calyces, and displacement of the kidney by outward growth. Renal tomography, renal arteriography, and renal scan are all recent techniques contributing to earlier diagnosis. Perinephric insufflation has also been used.

Prognosis and Treatment. Embryonal nephroma was once 90 per cent fatal. The combination of early diagnosis, restriction of palpation, preoperative irradiation, prompt nephrectomy, and postoperative irradiation has dramatically reduced mortality, so that half or more of the patients can survive. Actinomycin D has also been used postoperatively. Earlier diagnosis and prompt nephrectomy have also bettered the former 20 per cent survival in renal carcinoma, but the outlook is still grave. Statistics are confused by the delayed appearance of metastases. Renal carcinoma may stimulate fibrosis such as that seen in periureteral fibrosis. The resulting obstruction can falsely simulate metastases or contralateral spread. The physician who diagnoses or suspects a space-occupying lesion has an urgent obligation to achieve definitive diagnosis and surgery when indicated. There is no infallible way to distinguish clinically between a solitary cyst and a potential malignant disease. Papillary tumors of the renal pelvis yield positive exfoliative cytology in the urine.

Anonymous: Analgesic abuse and tumours of the renal pelvis. Lancet, 2:1233, 1969.

Bottiger, L. E.: Studies in renal carcinoma. I. Clinical and pathologic anatomical aspects. II. Biochemical investigations. Acta Med. Scand., 167:443, 1960.

Clarke, B. J., and Goade, W. J., Jr.: Fever and anemia in renal cancer. New Eng. J. Med., 254:107, 1956.

Foot, N. D., Humphreys, G. A., and Whitmore, W. F.: Renal tumors: Pathology and prognosis in 295 cases. J. Urol., 66.190, 1951.

Johnson, S. H., III, and Marshal, M., Jr.: Primary kidney tumors of childhood. J. Urol., 74:707, 1955.

Rubin, P.: Cancer of the urogenital tract: Kidney: Localized renal adenocarcinoma. J.A.M.A., 204:219, 1968.

Miscellaneous Renal Disorders

George E. Schreiner

INFARCTION

Definition. Infarction is the ischemic death of tissue. Total ischemia of the cortical area is better termed *renal cortical necrosis* (*cf.* Acute Renal Failure). Bland infarction without reaction is the same as *focal cortical necrosis* and may be seen in trauma, preeclampsia, infectious shock, and in most of the causes of cortical necrosis. The term *renal infarct* is usually applied to the segmental type. These are usually due to *arterial* obstruction such as *embolism* (mural thrombi, cholesterol plaque material, endocarditis), *thrombosis, trauma,* surgical injury, intrarenal *narrowing* (scleroderma, malignant nephrosclerosis), stasis (shock, diabetic acidosis), and sickle cell disease, or to *venous* thrombosis as seen in neoplastic states (hypernephroma, lymphoma), dehydration (infantile diarrhea), septicemia, and hypercoagulable states. In one study of 205 human infarctions, about 77 per cent accompanied a cardiac lesion. The early red lesion evolves rapidly into a central and peripheral dead zone and a marginal area which is presumably the source of the pressor materials that produce the often-accompanying hypertension.

Diagnosis. The diagnosis is suggested by history, flank pain, renal tenderness, transient hematuria and albuminuria, and a space-occupying lesion or change of size or nonfunctioning kidney on pyelography. Total renal infarction with recovery is followed by calcification of the necrotic tissue and hypertrophy of the contralateral kidney. Infarction may produce acute or accelerated hypertension, and should be suspected when that is coupled with history of trauma to the kidney or renal surgery. The hypertension usually peaks at two to three weeks after a single infarction, and may subside as the ischemic tissue progresses to scar formation. Renal infarcts presenting as space-occupying lesions have to be distinguished from cysts and tumors. Nephrograms with "black" areas, scintigrams with "cold" areas, or anomaly in the distribution of dye in the segmental arteriogram may be an aid to diagnosis. Identification of small renal infarcts as embolic phenomena may be the clue that leads to a primary diagnosis, e.g., asymptomatic myocardial infarction.

Heparin perfusion during selective arteriography may have therapeutic benefit.

Treatment. Embolectomy or endarterectomy should be considered as emergency treatment when the blood supply to one kidney is threatened. Aortic repair may be indicated when dissection involves the renal artery. Vascular prostheses with a side arm have also been used to bypass an irreparably damaged renal artery involved in the Leriche syndrome. Anticoagulant therapy may be indicated for a central source of embolization. When diagnostic studies indicate unilateral renal infarct as a cause for accelerated hypertension, surgical intervention may be indicated if the hypertension does not spontaneously ameliorate within two months.

Baum, S.: Renal ischemic lesions. Radiol. Clin. N. Amer., 5:543, 1967.

Halpern, M.: Acute renal artery embolus: A concept of diagnosis and treatment. J. Urol., 98:552, 1967.

Howard, J. E., Berthrong, M., Gould, D. M., and Yendt, E. R.: Hypertension resulting from unilateral renal vascular disease and its relief by nephrectomy. Bull. Hopkins Hosp., 94:51, 1954.

Hoxie, H. J., and Coggin, C. B.: Renal infarction: Statistical study of 205 cases and detailed report of an unusual case. Arch. Intern. Med. (Chicago), 65:587, 1940.

Lauler, D. P., and Schreiner, G. E.: Bilateral renal cortical necrosis. Amer. J. Med., 24:519, 1958.

Thurlbeck, W. M., and Castleman, B.: Atheromatous emboli to the kidneys after aortic surgery. New Eng. J. Med., 275:442, 1957.

CHYLURIA

Chyluria is lymph in the urine. The entity has been known since Hippocrates. Biochemically the urine contains a colloidal suspension of fat in molecular form, albumin, lecithin, cholesterin, fibrinogen, and soaps producing a milky or creamy appearance resembling lactescent serum. The major component is usually triglycerides. The proteinuria may be sufficient to produce the *nephrotic syndrome.*

Parasitic (tropical) chyluria is caused by *Filaria sanguinis-hominis* (*W. bancrofti*). *Nonparasitic chyluria* is due to a rupture of a lymphatic into the collecting system resulting from observation of lymphatics anywhere between the intestines and the thoracic duct. Specific causes include tumors, fibrosis, pregnancy, and trauma. Pyelonephritis may be associated.

Milky urine, intermittent (postural) or constant, is the major sign. It may be mistaken for pyuria. Milky urine is stable, containing 2 to 4 per cent fat, and does not exhibit fat droplets on microscopy. Retrograde pyelography may demonstrate pyelolymphatic backflow. Oral fats labeled with Sudan 3 or isotopic I^{131} will appear in the urine. Ether will extract both chyle and the label.

Major items to be differentiated are lipiduria and pyuria. *Lipiduria* has fat droplets that rise to the top on centrifugation. It may be associated with fractures, eclampsia, diabetes, phosphorus, arsenic, and carbon monoxide poisoning.

Primary treatment is identification and removal of the obstruction. A low fat diet reduces chyluria.

Caserta, S. J.: Description of chyluria: Report of a case. New Eng. J. Med., 255:1239, 1956.
Tuller, M. A., Feuer, M. M., Schapira, H. E., and Ho, Peh-Ping.: Recumbent chyluria: Demonstration of unilateral renal-lymphatic communication. Amer. J. Med., 33:951, 1962.
Yamauchi, S.: Chyluria: Clinical laboratory and statistical study of 45 personal cases observed in Hawaii. J. Urol., 54:318, 1945.

PNEUMATURIA

Pneumaturia is the passage of gas bubbles in the urine.

In noninfected patients, pneumaturia is usually due to a vesicovaginal or vesicoenteric fistula. Vegetable fibers and fecal contamination may be found in the urine. Such fistulas may be congenital in infants, may result from gross infections or neoplasms, or may follow radical pelvic surgery. Bubbles may also be caused by gas-forming bacteria proliferating in urine. *E. coli, A. aerogenes,* or yeast may be involved. The gas is carbon dioxide. Pneumaturia, although rare, is most frequent in elderly diabetic women.

Bubbling or frothing urine is noted by the patient at the end of micturition or by physician and nurse in the last drainage by catheterization. A gas shadow may be seen in the bladder on roentgenographic study.

Treatment consists of reassuring the patient; finding and repairing the fistula, if present; or treating a specific infection and eliminating glycosuria.

NEPHROPTOSIS

Definition. Nephroptosis is excessive mobility of the kidney. It is to be distinguished from *ectopia,* which is congenital or acquired permanent abnormal placement of the kidney, and *malrotation,* or pivoting of the kidney on its vertical axis, the pelvis and ureter deviating from the normal position. When observing the percutaneous biopsy needle during normal respiratory excursions, most physicians are amazed by the normal mobility of the kidney, which has a fascial attachment to the diaphragm. It is, therefore, difficult to say how much mobility is "excessive." On palpation the fingers should not be able to slide above the upper pole. On urography the ureteropelvic junction should not descend on standing more than one to one and a half vertebral spaces.

Nephroptosis occurs in about one fifth of adult women and much less frequently in men. There is a right-sided predominance. It is more common in thin, hyperkinetic people.

Pathogenesis. The kidney is held within its normal excursion by its vascular supply (pedicle), its fascia (Gerota) anchored to the diaphragmatic attachments, peritoneal adhesions, intra-abdominal pressure and support of other organs, and its form-fit to the lumbar gutter. Nephroptotic kidneys usually have diminished renal fat and poorly developed fascia. A long, thin torso, shallow lumbar gutter, generalized visceroptosis, faulty posture, atrophy of abdominal muscles, and multiple pregnancies may all be contributing causes.

Clinical Manifestations. Nephroptosis is largely asymptomatic, but has been too often made the organic focus for neurotic or hypochondriacal personality. Other than a vague dropping or dragging sensation, specific symptom complexes come from torsion, kinking, ureteral obstruction, infection, and stretching of the vascular pedicle. Recently, orthostatic hypertension and postural hyperaldosteronism (via angiotensin) have been identified with nephroptosis, accounting for 7 of 47 operated patients in one series of renal hypertension. Fibromuscular hyperplasia may accompany the condition. The arteriogram, renin excretion, and aldosterone secretion may be abnormal *only* in the upright position. *"Dietl's crisis"* is an acute prostrating ureteral colic coming on shortly after assuming the upright posture or after postural fatigue, e.g., in a waitress. The severe pain can be accompanied by nausea, vomiting, hypotension, oliguria, swelling, and tenderness of the kidney. It is relieved by a short period in the Trendelenburg position, followed by horizontal resting, at which time the urine may increase in volume and may contain albumin and erythrocytes. It is thought by some that, in the absence of nephroptosis, Dietl's crisis may occur owing to spasm of the renal pelvis characterized by decreased intrapelvic volume and increased frequency and intensity of peristalsis, analogous to spastic colon.

Diagnosis. Diagnosis is usually made by relating symptoms to posture or occupation and relief by assumption of the horizontal position. Physical examination is performed with the patient in the supine and standing positions, the weight on the leg opposite the side being palpated. Intravenous pyelography in the conventional supine position followed by a view of the upright position is a valuable adjunct. Urinalysis may reveal hematuria and albuminuria from vascular distention of pyuria and bacteria from secondary infection.

Treatment. Reassurance and explanation are the major components of treatment. Weight-gain regimens and exercises to strengthen the abdominal wall may be helpful. Short rest periods in the horizontal position and sensible shoes may work wonders for women whose jobs cause standing fatigue. Often a change of occupation or prolonged rest may be necessary to establish the postural relationship. Patients with recurrent pyelonephritis related to postural fatigue accompanied by ureteral kinking may occasionally benefit from nephropexy. When fibromuscular hyperplasia is present, nephropexy should be combined with arterial repair. The uncomplicated nephroptotic kidney should not be subjected to surgery or used as a psychosomatic crutch.

Derrick, J. R., and Hanna, E.: Abnormal renal mobility and hypertension. Amer. J. Surg., 106:673, 1963.
Ginn, H. E., Jr., and Parry, W. L.: Postural hypertension and edema caused by excessive mobility of the kidneys. Southern Med. J., 57:735, 1964.

ANOMALIES OF THE GENITOURINARY TRACT

Because of the complex embryologic development of the various specialized structures in the genitourinary tract, developmental mishaps are more common than in any other organ system and affect more than 10 per cent of all humans. Anomalies of the kidney include deviation in number, size, structure, form, and location. In addition, anomalies of the pelvis, ureter, bladder, and urethra may lead to obstruction or infection secondarily involving the kidney.

Kidney. *Bilateral renal agenesis,* often associated with malformations of the ear, is incompatible with life. Toxic or environmental factors would be most damaging at the fourth week of pregnancy. *Unilateral agenesis (solitary kidney),* which has an incidence of about 0.16 per cent, results from failure of the renal bud, the nephrogenic blastema, or the vascular supply. Arrested development of the wolffian duct results in associated nondevelopment of the rest of the urinary tract on the involved side. No ureteral orifice or ridge is revealed on cystoscopy. Solitary kidney may give rise to anuria when it becomes involved in acute parenchymal disease. As a cardinal principle, the presence of two kidneys should be established before doing any instrumentation or surgical procedure. *Supernumerary kidney,* completely separated and free, is extremely rare. *Fused supernumerary kidney* has an incidence of about 0.025 per cent. *Renal aplasia* may consist of unorganized parenchyma surrounded by fat, and may produce hypertension. *Renal hypoplasia* is generally unilateral and medial in position. In the adult this must be distinguished from renal atrophy secondary to pyelonephritis. Hypoplastic kidneys frequently become infected, demonstrate constant albuminuria, are symmetrically reduced in size, and show small nephrons on biopsy together with atrophic blood vessels. *Renal hypertrophy* may exist congenitally contralateral to a hypoplastic kidney or may be acquired. Functional hypertrophy regularly occurs in transplanted kidneys. *Fetal lobulation* is normal in infants, but persists in about 5 per cent of adults. Fusion of the two kidneys, which is found in about 0.2 per cent of people, may occur at the lower poles, at the lower or upper pole tips (*horseshoe kidney*), at both poles (*doughnut kidney*), throughout (*cake kidney*), or at the contralateral upper and lower poles (*sigmoid kidney*). The common variety, the lower-pole horseshoe kidney, lies close to the spine, with anterior rotation of the pelves. The vascular supply is almost always anomalous. Surgical separation is sometimes feasible for intractable infection or stone. *Congenital ectopia* (incidence 1 per cent) usually results in a pelvic location for the kidney and has been mistaken for tumor. The position of congenital ectopia is defined by the length of the ureter and vascular supply. In acquired ectopia the ureter and blood vessels were originally of normal length, but upon loss of fascial support the vascular pedicle lengthened and the ureter became redundant. *Malrotation* is frequent in ectopic kidneys. In *crossed ectopia,* the kidney crosses the midline, and lies adjacent to or fused with its mate.

Renal Pelvis. The normal renal pelvis is flask-shaped, with upper, middle, and lower major calyces branching into minor calyces. Increase in number of major calyces up to six has been observed. "*Double kidney*" is really double pelvis, and results from the reduplication of the ureteral bud. It is found in about 4 per cent of urograms. The duplication has varying degrees of completion, and may or may not be accompanied by double ureter. "*Spider pelvis*" is a congenitally long, thin pelvis simulating compression. *Congenital hydronephrosis* may result from a variety of conditions present in fetal life. *Extrarenal pelvis* should be considered a normal variant from *intrarenal pelvis.* It becomes important, however, in the pathophysiology of obstructive uropathy.

Blood Vessels. Anomalies of the blood vessels are receiving increased attention because of their possible role in unilateral renal disease with hypertension. They are being discovered with increasing frequency since the advent of the radiohippuran and other radioiodide renograms and increased use of transaortic or retrograde aortography and renal angiography. *Arterial anomalies* include *congenital atresia, tortuosity,* and *aberrant vessels*. Minor anomalies are present in about 25 per cent of people. Renal arteries and veins may derive from the pedicle, aorta, vena cava, adrenals, pancreas, and liver. Anomalous vessels usually involve either pole, and upon crossing the upper portion of the ureter or the ureteropelvic junction may produce obstruction. *Renal artery aneurysm* and intrarenal *arteriovenous fistula* are rare but do occur.

Ureter. Ureteral malformations include agenesis, duplication, triplication, ectopia, ureterocele, herniation, postcaval ureter, aplasia, congenital stricture, congenital valves or folds, hydroureter, diverticula, torsion, kinks, and involvement with aberrant vessels.

Bladder. Malformations of the bladder include agenesis, hypoplasia, reduplication, diverticula, hypertrophy, urachal cysts and fistulas, trigonal folds, and cloaca formation. Vesical neck anomalies are discussed in the article on obstructive nephropathy.

Related Congenital Anomalies. Congenital cysts are discussed under Cysts of the Kidney. Malformed ears, particularly asymmetrical, are associated with some genitourinary anomalies.

Congenital deficiency of the abdominal musculature is regularly associated with genitourinary problems. Renal anomalies have been described in the Marfan syndrome. Nerve deafness is associated with hereditary nephritis.

Diagnosis. The diagnosis of congenital renal and urinary anomalies is usually made during the course of investigation for other anomalies, as an incidental urographic finding, or when symptoms develop because of infection or obstruction. Most malformed and malrotated kidneys have defects in drainage and are liable to ascending pyelonephritis. Anomalous structures can be mistaken for cysts or tumors and may become significant factors in the course of pregnancy or of surgical procedures on nearby structures. The longest recorded survival in renal agenesis is 39 days.

Benjamin, J. A., and Tobin, C. E.: Abnormalities of kidneys, ureters and perinephric fascia: Anatomic and clinical study. J. Urol., 65:715, 1951.

Campbell, M. F.: Principles of Urology. Philadelphia, W. B. Saunders Company, 1957, Chapter 6.

Loughridge, L. W.: Renal abnormalities in the Marfan syndrome. Quart. J. Med., 28:531, 1959.

Ravitch, M. M., and Wilder, R. J.: Pediatrics (non-cardiac anomalies). Ann. Rev. Med., 10:343, 1959.

Smith, E. C., and Orkin, L. A.: Clinical and statistical study of 471 congenital anomalies of kidneys and ureter. J. Urol., 53:11, 1945.

DISEASES OF THE DIGESTIVE SYSTEM

Introduction

Marvin H. Sleisenger

The thirteenth edition of this textbook includes a number of new and exciting advances in clinical gastroenterology. These developments, which directly affect diagnosis and care of patients with gastrointestinal disease, have resulted from the continued growth and interest in clinical research and relevant investigation in the basic sciences. In the articles which follow, new information about motor disturbances, disease, and disorders of secretion, absorption, the hepatobiliary system, the small bowel, the colon, and neoplasia of the gut will be presented. A brief summary of some of these advances appears to be in order.

Tracings of esophageal motility, along with pH recordings, now clearly indicate that gastroesophageal reflux may occur with or without the presence of a hiatus hernia, accounting for the oft-noted lack of correlation between heartburn and hiatus hernia. Esophageal tracings in patients with alcoholism and diabetic neuropathy have revealed disordered motility in both conditions and some impairment of the gastroesophageal sphincter in the latter, perhaps accounting in part for the esophagitis in these patients.

The chemical similarity between gastrin and cholecystokinin has stimulated investigation which revealed that the two hormones share all actions, but differ in potency for a given action. Gastrin and cholecystokinin exhibit competitive interaction suggesting common receptor sites.

The advent of immunoassay for gastrin has greatly stimulated continuing investigation of the physiology of this hormone as well as its possible role in the pathogenesis of duodenal ulcer. To date the evidence is against hypergastrinemia as a cause of peptic ulcer. Gastrin levels are elevated in the well-known Zollinger-Ellison syndrome, pernicious anemia, and atrophic gastritis.

Once again work is going forward on characterizing intestinal inhibition of gastric acid secretion. Whether or not intestinal hormones are important in the pathogenesis of duodenal ulcer has not been determined at this point; however, it remains a fruitful area for investigation. Secretin is now completely characterized chemically; its use in medicine is still largely confined, however, to testing pancreatic secretion. Important work is now in progress on the interrelationships of gastrin, glucagon, secretin, and cholecystokinin-pancreozymin in hepatobiliary and pancreatic secretion.

Treatment of peptic ulcer is still frustrating, despite increasing acceptance of the thesis that diet (except for interdiction of alcohol, caffeine-containing compounds, and, perhaps, smoking) is unimportant in therapy; frequent feedings are still an accepted part of ulcer management, as are the use of effective antacids and sedatives or tranquilizers. Vagotomy (particularly selective) with pyloroplasty seems to be gaining widespread acceptance as the operation of choice for peptic ulcer, if technically feasible, but it is yet too early to tell whether this will prove to be the best operation. We must watch carefully for the incidence of recurrent ulcer following these procedures and compare the disadvantage of this long-term complication with other well-known symptoms that follow partial gastrectomy and vagotomy.

The now classic work of Davenport on "back diffusion" of gastric acid appears to offer an exciting lead in the understanding of the pathogenesis of gastric ulcer. Extensions of his work on factors affecting the mucosal barrier indicate that lowering it may, in some instances of drug ingestion (salicylates, phenylbutazone), result in gastric ulcer from an accelerated rate of "back diffusion" of acid. Also, gastric ulcer patients appear to reflux bile more commonly than normal subjects, and bile acids have likewise been shown to impair the gastric mucosal barrier.

Since the last edition of this book, advances in our knowledge of the role of the gut in various immunologic mechanisms has accelerated with localization of secretion of IgA plus "transfer piece" to gut mucosal cells. Absence or marked diminution of IgA is frequently associated with diarrhea and in some cases with malabsorption. Whether some breakdown of the normal immunologic processes is involved in ulcerative (and granulomatous) colitis is not yet known; current work on the cytotoxicity of lymphocytes in these diseases suggests that a cell-mediated, delayed type of hypersensitivity may be operative, but conclusive evidence is not yet at hand. Granulomatous disease of the colon is apparently more common than had previously been suspected; however, its separation from ulcerative colitis purely on the basis of differences in pathology is not yet wholly satisfying. Further, "mixes" of the two types of inflammatory disease are not uncommonly noted. When discrete etiologies are unveiled we may discover that our distinctions today are relatively artificial.

The types of "allergic gastroenteritides," including eosinophilic gastroenteritis, have been better defined. Allergic gastroenteropathy of childhood and eosinophilic gastroenteritis of youth and adulthood may be related, although the relationship of this gut reaction to various offending substances that are ingested (milk, meat, and cereals) is not so firm in the latter as in the former condition.

Absorption and malabsorption continue to be areas of intense clinical interest and investigation. The micellar theory for fat solubilization has been confirmed by further studies of bile acid metabolism, showing that diminution of the bile salt pool (resulting chiefly from distal small bowel resection) or decreased critical concentration of conjugated bile acids in the jejunum (resulting chiefly from overgrowth of anaerobic organisms or acid pH) is associated with decreased micellar lipid following ingestion of triglyceride. Much yet remains to be understood concerning the interrelationships of small bowel resection, plasma bile acids, and hepatic function. Unabsorbed bile acids in patients with distal small bowel resection cause what has been described as "choleretic enteropathy"; this condition is due to inhibition of absorption of water and electrolytes in the colon. Therapeutically, medium chain triglycerides (MCT) seem to be gaining a wide acceptance in the therapy of the diseases of malabsorption, particularly in individuals having massive resection of the small intestine, but also as an adjunct to more definitive therapy of other diseases of malabsorption such as pancreatic insufficiency or adult celiac disease.

Much has been learned about the pathogenesis of cholelithiasis from work on the physical chemistry of bile and the solubilization of cholesterol in bile. Epidemiologic studies of the prevalence of gallstones in the American Indian population has also contributed valuable information. There appears to be little doubt that precipitation of cholesterol in bile is important, but whether the bile is unable to hold cholesterol in solution when it leaves the hepatic cell or whether hepatic secretion of bile "supersaturated" with cholesterol is the cause is not yet settled, although the latter possibility is the more likely. Also, some mystery shrouds the origin of the nidus for cholesterol

stone formation; is it bilirubinate, glycoprotein, or bacterial breakdown substances? The recent studies of the Indian population have taught us that the "fat, fair, forty, and fertile" individual may not be a universal prototype for this disease, because young, nulliparous Indian women eating a diet similar to Caucasians have an extremely high incidence of gallstones.

The discovery of the so-called "Australia antigen" has perhaps been the most exciting advance in the field of liver disease for the past two decades, and has opened up a new horizon for research directed toward isolation of the virus. Presently, testing for the Australia antigen has been of help in diagnosis of serum hepatitis (long-incubation virus) and in screening of blood donors. Conventional immunologic testing for the antigen is about to give way to sensitive radioimmunoassay techniques which promise to increase the yield of positive diagnosis in the early stages of infectious hepatitis (short-incubation virus). If, in fact, the Australia antigen is a part of the virus, its isolation from the serum may be the first step in successfully culturing the organism.

The efficacy of prophylactic portacaval shunt for complications of portal hypertension is excellent; however, it has not increased the survival rate of those who have had the procedure. Detection of the source and nature of the lesion causing upper gastrointestinal bleeding has been greatly facilitated by the advent of flexible endoscopes with camera attachments. In selected instances angiography may also be of great benefit in localizing the site of hemorrhage.

Little progress has been made in the field of gut cancer except that studies of cell replication in colon polyps already indicate an abnormal pattern. Although the debate still rages, most authorities are willing to avoid surgery in patients with isolated adenomatous polyps of the colon with stalks. The Japanese seem to be doing well in their mass screening programs for gastric cancer, with a five-year survival rate approaching 90 per cent after surgery in asymptomatic individuals. On this side of the world we have abandoned large-scale screening for gastric cancer, perhaps because the disease appears to be steadily diminishing in incidence.

Disorders of Motility

Thomas P. Almy

GENERAL CONSIDERATIONS

Most gastrointestinal symptoms have as their immediate cause some disturbance of the motility of the gut, and the most common intestinal disorders in clinical practice are those in which

disturbed motility is unassociated with a recognizable morphologic or biochemical lesion, i.e., they are "functional" disorders. Much less commonly, the most impressive physiologic and clinical effects of a morphologically definable disease process are disturbances of gut motility, the understanding of which represents the key to effective therapy. These two kinds of disorder are considered together in this section.

Rhythmic contractility is an intrinsic property of the intestinal wall. In the absence of extrinsic nerves or humoral influences, peristalsis is maintained by local reflexes for which the afferents arise in the mucosa, and the efferents include the myenteric ganglia. Extrinsic neural and humoral mechanisms serve to regulate and adapt the intrinsic motility of the gut to the needs of the total organism. A purposeful alternation of propulsive and nonpropulsive patterns of activity, adapted to civilized habits of eating, working, sleeping, and defecating, is referred to as normal intestinal function. The most common and clinically important disorders of intestinal motility occur during periods of stress in persons with normally innervated intestines, when the aforementioned patterns are long sustained as bodily accompaniments of emotional tension.

By contrast certain disorders, such as achalasia, congenital megacolon, and the esophageal disorder in diabetic neuropathy, are based upon permanent defects in integrative mechanisms. The high pressures generated at the sites of colonic and esophageal diverticula appear to result from patterns of disordered motility, the neural basis of which is as yet unclear.

Our knowledge of these disorders has been extended rapidly in recent years through the improvement of methods for the observation and recording of intestinal motility in intact man. The comparison of electromanometric recordings of intraluminal pressure with cineradiographic images of the barium-filled intestine has contributed much to our understanding of mechanisms, and at times has directly aided the diagnosis. The true diagnostic limitations of these methods, however, have not been fully defined.

DISORDERS OF SWALLOWING

Normal deglutition is accomplished by peristaltic movements, triggered by reflexes arising from voluntary contractions of the muscles of the buccal and pharyngeal cavities. The elevation of the tongue and larynx thrusts the food bolus against the posterior wall, raises the pressure in the pharynx, and seals off the aditus of the larynx. A fall in the pressure follows immediately (see Fig. 1) in both the superior (cricopharyngeal) and inferior (vestibular) esophageal sphincters, and a gradient of pressure is established favorable to propulsion of the bolus. The wave of high pressure generated in the pharynx then sweeps progressively downward to the stomach. The reflex pathways subserving this mechanism lie in the fifth, seventh, ninth, tenth, and eleventh cranial nerves, and the effectors include both skeletal muscle (tongue, pharynx, larynx, upper one third of the esophagus) and smooth muscle (lower two thirds of the esophagus). In the latter region the efferent pathway is autonomic and

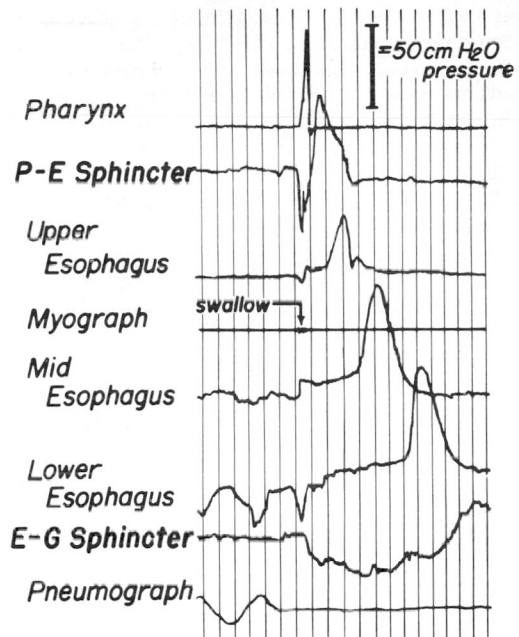

FIGURE 1. A composite of electromanometric recordings showing simultaneous pressure changes throughout pharynx and esophagus during a single swallow. Read from left to right; interval between vertical lines = 1 second. P-E Sphincter = pharyngoesophageal sphincter. E-G Sphincter = esophagogastric sphincter or lower esophageal sphincter. (Adapted from Code, C. F.: An Atlas of Esophageal Motility in Health and Disease. Springfield, Illinois, Charles C Thomas, 1958.)

cholinergic, the postganglionic neurons lying in the esophageal wall (Auerbach's plexus).

Difficult swallowing, or *dysphagia*, may result from a defect or disorder in any part of the mechanism outlined above or from mechanical obstruction to the bolus propelled by this mechanism. In other patients a complaint of dysphagia will be found to relate entirely to difficulty in initiating the voluntary act of swallowing or to defects in the reflex coordination of oropharyngeal movements. When dysphagia is due to motor dysfunction, difficulty is experienced with both liquids and solids, whereas, in the presence of a mechanical obstruction or stenosis, the strong peristaltic movements above the lesion serve to propel through it any particle smaller than the stenotic lumen. Thus the patient with an obstructing carcinoma may experience the sudden onset of dysphagia on swallowing a bolus of meat or toast, and, as the lumen progressively narrows, may have to limit his diet to semiliquid and ultimately liquid foods.

Pain on swallowing, if mild, is likely to be incorporated in the experience of dysphagia. Its location often accurately reflects the level of the esophagus principally affected. At times esophageal pain is more severe, outlasts the normal duration of the deglutition, or is dissociated from it in time. Its location is usually substernal, beneath the xiphoid process, and in the episternal notch. It may radiate to the anterior neck and lower jaw, the dorsal spine, the sides of the chest, the shoulders and arms, and the epigastrium. Rarely it may originate in one of these sites. Its quality is most often either crushing or burning. The latter sensation, commonly called *heartburn*, characteristically radiates upward to the neck, and results from inflammation of the mucosa of the lower esophagus usually brought about by reflux of gastric juice.

Esophageal *regurgitation* is a common manifestation of obstructive disorders, and is to be distinguished from vomiting by the absence of nausea, the tendency to occur during or immediately after meals, the lack of digestion of regurgitated food, and the absence of bile or of a sour or bitter taste.

DISORDERS OF THE UPPER (PHARYNGOESOPHAGEAL) SEGMENT

The "lump in the throat" is a familiar transitory sensation accompanying fear or acute anxiety. Related is the "globus hystericus," in which a person suffering emotional conflict is incapable of initiating the voluntary movements of deglutition.

In any *disease of the brain stem,* the *cranial nerves,* or the *muscles* of this segment, the coordinated contraction of the pharyngeal musculature and relaxation of the pharyngoesophageal sphincter may fail to develop, with resultant gagging, coughing, and regurgitation of fluids through the nose. The specific cause is usually made obvious by associated symptoms and signs, and may be pseudobulbar palsy, bulbar poliomyelitis, myasthenia gravis, dermatomyositis, ocular myopathy, myotonic dystrophy, or sarcoidosis. The prognosis and treatment are those of the underlying disease.

SIDEROPENIC DYSPHAGIA
(Plummer-Vinson Syndrome, Paterson-Brown-Kelly Syndrome)

Sideropenic dysphagia is a disorder characterized by dysphagia referable to the upper segment, atrophy of the mucous membranes of mouth and pharynx, koilonychia, hypochromic microcytic anemia, hypoferremia, gastric achlorhydria, and stenoses or webs of the upper esophageal mucosa demonstrable by roentgenography or by endoscopy. It occurs mainly in women subsisting on low intakes of iron and vitamins, chiefly those of the B complex. The prognosis is excellent in most cases, but these patients should be observed for later development of carcinoma of the pharynx or esophagus, to which they are unusually susceptible. It is effectively treated with a good general diet, at first soft or semiliquid in consistency, with oral or parenteral iron in the amounts used for iron-deficiency anemia and vitamin supplements. Occasionally the stenotic lesions require bouginage.

DISORDERS OF THE LOWER (ESOPHAGOGASTRIC) SEGMENT

The motility of the lower esophagus may be altered by diffuse disease of the muscular wall or by disturbances of intrinsic neural mechanisms. In systemic lupus erythematosus and other connective tissue diseases, disordered swallowing is strikingly associated with *Raynaud's phenomenon.* It is commonly seen in *scleroderma* (progressive systemic sclerosis), where it may antedate the appearance of cutaneous changes. In an advanced case the esophagogram reveals dilatation and absent peristalsis, a patulous vestibule allowing free regurgitation of barium from the stomach. In milder instances, and often in the absence of dysphagia, the patient with scleroderma will show defects in peristalsis only while swallowing barium in the recumbent position or when recorded electromanometrically (Fig. 2A). Esophagoscopy may reveal peptic esophagitis, to which acute or chronic blood loss may be due. The therapy is that for regurgitant esophagitis and other aspects of scleroderma (q.v.).

Healthy persons may fail to generate a primary peristaltic wave, and instead exhibit incoordinate contraction of the lower esophagus after 1 to 10 per cent of swallows. These phenomena may occur after the majority of swallows in elderly persons (presbyesophagus) and in a number of disorders of the nervous system, including multiple sclerosis, amyotrophic lateral sclerosis, parkinsonism, pseudobulbar palsy, and both diabetic and alcoholic neuropathy. In many of these diseases, the esophagogastric sphincter may fail to relax. These defects of neuromuscular activity are seen in exaggerated form in three disorders apparently localized to the esophagus—diffuse spasm, hypertensive esophagogastric sphincter, and aperistalsis—which appear together or sequentially in the same patient with significant frequency, and hence may be pathogenically related.

DIFFUSE ESOPHAGEAL SPASM
(Corkscrew Esophagus, "Curling")

Particularly in some elderly persons, deglutition may evoke strong, uncoordinated, nonpropulsive contractions of the body of the esophagus (Fig. 2B). Although in most instances this condition is asymptomatic, it may induce dysphagia or substernal pain, at times simulating angina pectoris. On barium swallow, the esophageal lumen appears in the form of an irregular series of concentric narrowings, or a spiral coil (curling, Fig. 3). In some cases the esophagus is abnormally sensitive to methacholine (see Aperistalsis).

This disorder is usually chronic and nonprogressive. Rarely, it is followed by typical aperistalsis. When required, pain can be prevented or relieved by an anticholinergic agent, e.g., propantheline, 15 to 30 mg. three times daily, or

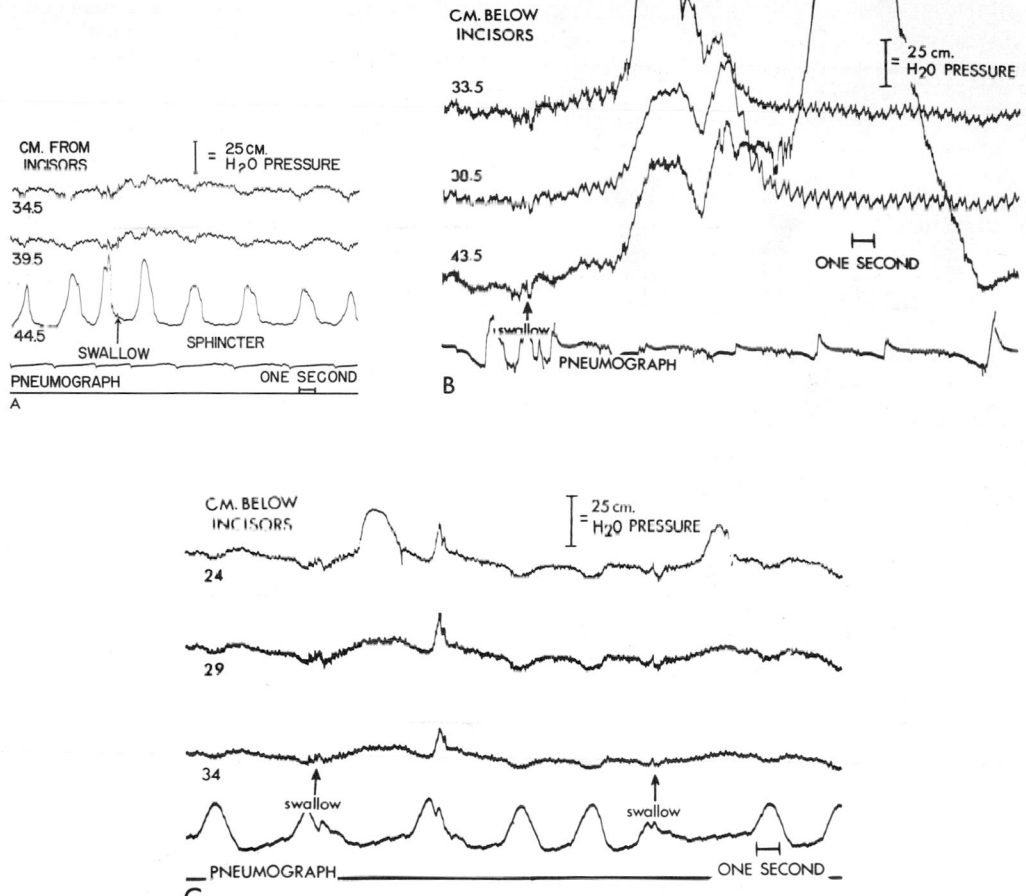

FIGURE 2. Electromanometric recordings from lower esophagus and lower esophageal sphincter. *A, Scleroderma.* Note absence of peristalsis; fluctuations in sphincter pressure coincide with inspiration. *B, Diffuse esophageal spasm.* Note extremely large, sustained or repetitive contractions beginning simultaneously at three levels. *C, Aperistalsis* (achalasia). Note absence of peristalsis; pressure in the sphincter (here at 34 cm.) does not fall on swallowing. (Reproduced from Kelley, M. L., Jr., by permission.)

isopropamide, 5 to 10 mg. twice daily orally. Severe cases may require a long esophagomyotomy for relief of symptoms.

HYPERTENSIVE ESOPHAGOGASTRIC SPHINCTER

In rare instances the resting pressure in the esophagogastric sphincter has been shown to exceed by far the normal upper limit of 40 cm. of water. At times of spontaneous or induced emotional conflict, both roentgenographic and manometric studies indicate the occurrence of varying degrees of "spasm" of this sphincter, unassociated with disturbed peristalsis in the body of the esophagus, yet often giving rise to a sensation of obstruction at the xiphoid level. Long persistence of this phenomenon and more severe pain and dysphagia are seen when it is associated with diffuse spasm or hiatus hernia. Treatment is based largely on psychophysiologic principles (see Irritable Colon) if other lesions have been excluded.

APERISTALSIS
(Achalasia of the Esophagus, Cardiospasm, Megaesophagus)

Definition. Aperistalsis is a chronic disorder of motility that leads to obstruction at the level of the esophagogastric sphincter. The commonly accepted name, *cardiospasm,* is actually inappropriate, as the "cardiac" sphincter (or vestibule) is not contracted with excessive force, but only fails to relax (achalasia) in the act of swallowing. Moreover, it is clear that the disturbance of motility also involves the lower two thirds of the body of the esophagus, in which the normal progressive wave of contraction fails to develop on swallowing. Thus the most inclusive and satisfactory concept, including the absence of both moving waves of contraction and receptive relaxation, is that of *aperistalsis* of the esophagus.

Prevalence, Epidemiology, and Etiology. Although one of the more common causes of esophageal obstruction, aperistalsis is a relatively rare disease in medical practice in the United States, where no regional, ethnic, or familial predisposition has

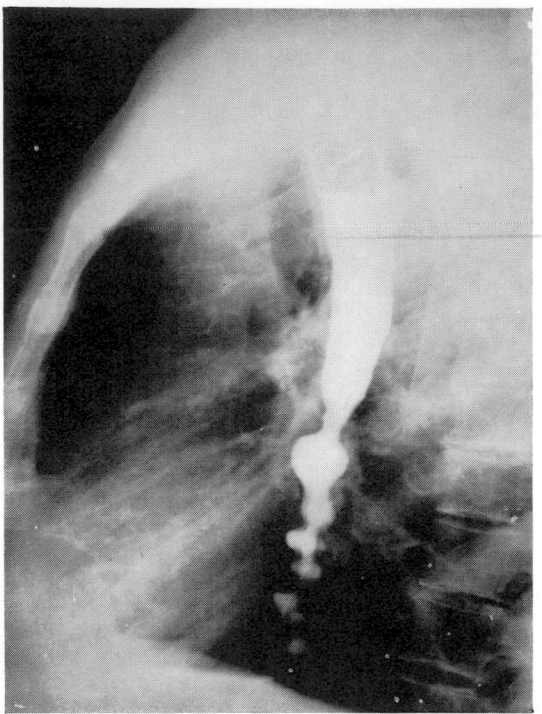

FIGURE 3. Diffuse esophageal spasm.

been recognized. It develops usually in the third to sixth decades, and is rare in children. No environmental factors of etiologic importance are known.

In Latin America, however, an identical disorder occurs endemically among the poor, chiefly in rural districts, in whom an association with Chagas' disease is suggested by epidemiologic and serologic evidence. In such patients the esophageal disorder is often associated with disturbances elsewhere, such as megaureter or megacolon (see Chagas' Disease).

Pathology and Pathologic Physiology. The fundamental lesion in aperistalsis is degeneration of the ganglion cells of the myenteric (Auerbach's) plexus or of the vagal motor nuclei. This varies greatly in degree, at times amounting to complete atrophy and at times being undetectable by ordinary histologic criteria, and appears to be proportional to the duration and severity of the motility disturbance.

Even in those cases without evident structural damage to the ganglia, physiologic abnormalities are demonstrable at any time. In manometric studies the total motor activity in the resting state varies widely; but, consistently on swallowing, a moving peristaltic wave fails to develop in the body, and the vestibule fails to relax normally (Fig. 2C). Whereas the motility of the normally innervated esophagus is altered by methacholine only when given in subcutaneous doses of 25 mg. or more, injection of only 5 to 10 mg. in a patient with aperistalsis is sufficient to induce a strong, sustained, incoordinated, often painful contraction of the body of the esophagus. In accordance with "Cannon's law," stating that a tissue deprived of its autonomic nerve supply is excessively sensitive to the chemical transmitter of the nerve impulse, this is held to be pharmacologic evidence of partial or complete aganglionosis.

With failure of relaxation of the vestibule on swallowing, food and liquid accumulate in the esophagus until, in the vertical position, the hydrostatic pressure exceeds the resistance of the sphincter, and the contents passes bit by bit into the stomach. The esophagus may be greatly dilated and elongated (Fig. 4), but, if the level of total motor activity is high, may long remain of normal caliber. The wall of the esophagus often becomes greatly thickened, although just above the vestibule conspicuous thinning or a pseudodiverticulum may appear. With severe retention, the mucosa and submucosa are often inflamed. Rarely, carcinoma of the lower esophagus appears to be a complication of long-standing megaesophagus. Because patients often lie down before the esophagus empties itself, acute and chronic aspiration pneumonia is a moderately common complication.

Clinical Manifestations. The leading symptom, *dysphagia*, is usually insidious in onset; but in many instances it may begin suddenly and may be intermittent or of variable severity, despite the persistence of the morphologic and physiologic changes in the esophagus. From the beginning, some difficulty will be experienced in swallowing liquids as well as solids. Nevertheless, the patient often learns that he can obtain relief by drinking a liquid after a meal, presumably because the added fluid raises the hydrostatic pressure in the lower esophagus sufficiently to

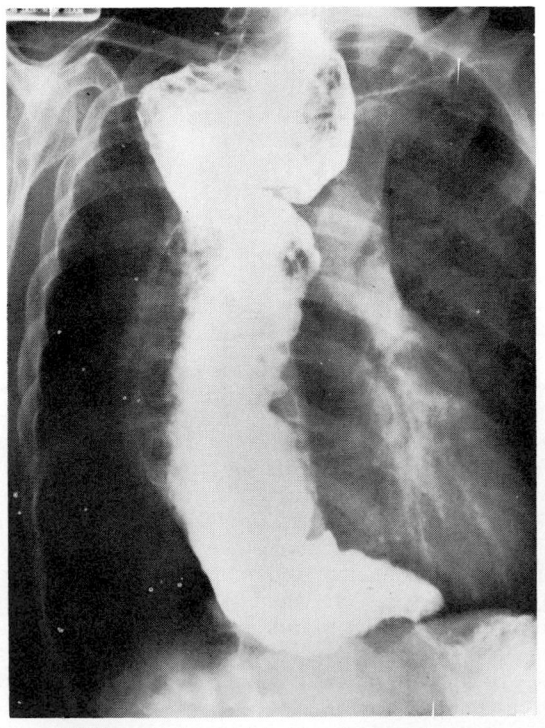

FIGURE 4. Aperistalsis. Far advanced changes.

open the sphincter. Substernal *pain* after eating, lasting a few minutes, occurs variably in some patients, apparently because of spasm of the body of the esophagus.

In the more severe and chronic cases, there may be striking *loss of weight* or symptoms of *pneumonia* or lung abscess resulting from aspiration of esophageal contents.

Diagnosis. The symptom of dysphagia should lead promptly to the observation of a barium swallow; in a typical case of advanced aperistalsis the dilated, elongated, tortuous body of the esophagus, together with an elongated, firmly contracted vestibule, permits easy recognition. Sometimes the disease is suspected because the esophagus produces the shadow of a large paramediastinal mass on plain film of the chest. When the esophagus is less strikingly enlarged, fluoroscopic study in the horizontal position will still reveal defects in the primary peristaltic wave, and "spot" films of the terminal esophagus will show the point of narrowing as a symmetrically tapered cone. Esophagoscopy confirms this and, because the vestibule usually dilates to allow passage of the instrument into the stomach, permits exclusion of an organic stricture. Manometric studies of swallowing and of the response to methacholine (see above) may be of great diagnostic value. In some cases of minimal dilatation of the esophagus, it is impossible to make a clear distinction between aperistalsis and diffuse esophageal spasm on the clinical and manometric findings.

By these means, aperistalsis can and must be differentiated from *carcinoma* of the fundus of the stomach or terminal esophagus. In such instances, during endoscopy direct biopsy of the lesion or (better) cytologic study of aspirated contents may reveal neoplastic cells. In *scleroderma* of the esophagus comparable defects in peristalsis are seen in the body of the esophagus, but the esophagogastric sphincter is most often patent and there is no abnormal sensitivity to methacholine. In *regurgitant esophagitis* the manometric findings are not typical of aperistalsis, and evidence of regurgitation, of mucosal inflammation, of stricture, or of hiatal hernia is usually obtained by fluoroscopic study, by esophagoscopy, and by measuring the pH of the lower esophageal contents.

Treatment and Prognosis. Initial conservative management is recommended because many patients are able to eat adequately and with minimal distress when freed from stress and emotional tension. The only medication frequently useful is a mild sedative. Anticholinergic drugs, such as atropine sulfate, 0.5 to 1.0 mg., or propantheline, 15 to 30 mg., can prevent or relieve painful spasms of the body of the esophagus, but do not relax the esophagogastric sphincter. Amyl nitrite inhalation (or glyceryl trinitrite, 0.4 mg. sublingually) relaxes the sphincter, but only transiently.

The damage done to the innervation of the esophagus in this disease is, nevertheless, irreversible, and truly effective therapy requires that this be compensated by lasting damage to the esophagogastric sphincter, permitting drainage of the esophagus by gravity. Forcible stretching or rupture of the muscle fibers is accomplished by bougies and other dilators passed and positioned in the sphincter under fluoroscopic control. Although use of the pneumatic, hydrostatic, or mechanical (Starck) dilators is attended by pain and a small risk of esophageal perforation, lasting relief of dysphagia is obtained in 60 to 80 per cent of patients after one or two treatments. These procedures are recommended for any case of aperistalsis in which severe dilatation and significant retention are regularly present and in which accurate placement of the dilator is technically feasible.

When adequate dilatation has not been possible or its results have been unsatisfactory, surgical division of the sphincter often becomes necessary. Yet the more radical and successful the destruction of the sphincter, the more likely is the postoperative occurrence of regurgitant esophagitis (discussed later) here worsened by the ineffective clearing of regurgitated material because of defective peristalsis. The most satisfactory compromise appears to be the Heller procedure, in which the muscle of the vestibule is sectioned longitudinally and the mucosa left intact. About 80 per cent of the patients may be expected to remain free from dysphagia, to gain weight, and to escape the symptoms of esophagitis.

Whether the sphincter has been damaged by dilatation or by surgery, measures should be instituted to prevent regurgitant esophagitis. The patient should not lie down for one to two hours after eating, straining and chronic coughing should be controlled, and tight corsets should be discarded.

Ellis, F. H., Jr., and Olsen, A. M.: Achalasia of the Esophagus. Philadelphia, W. B. Saunders Company, 1969.
Gillies, M., et al.: Diffuse esophageal spasm. Brit. Med. J., 1: 527, 1967.
Ingelfinger, F. J.: Esophageal motility. Physiol. Rev., 38:533, 1958.
Kramer, P.: Progress in gastroenterology: The esophagus. Gastroenterology, 54:1171, 1968.
Leading Article: Esophageal dysfunction in diabetes. Brit. Med. J., 2:466, 1969.

DIAPHRAGMATIC HERNIA, HIATAL HERNIA, AND REFLUX ESOPHAGITIS
(Regurgitant Esophagitis, Peptic Esophagitis)

Definition. Gaps in the diaphragm resulting from congenital defects, relaxation of supporting tissues, or trauma may permit the stomach, colon, or other abdominal organs to herniate into the chest. *Traumatic hernia* may result in acute chest pain, dyspnea, hiccup, vomiting, and shock, usually in association with other internal injuries; on the other hand, large herniations may result but remain asymptomatic, later to be discovered on routine roentgenographic examinations. *Non-*

traumatic hernia may be present at birth or delayed until adult life and may involve (1) the pleuroperitoneal hiatus (foramen of Bochdalek), (2) the gap (usually posterior) left by congenital absence of a portion of the diaphragm, and (3) an anterior substernal opening (foramen of Morgagni). By far the most common and clinically important, however, is (4) *herniation through the esophageal hiatus*, a slitlike opening, bounded by muscle bundles from the right crus of the diaphragm, in which the vestibule of the esophagus is normally located, bound in turn to the inferior surface of the diaphragm by the phrenoesophageal ligament. The clinical manifestations of esophageal hiatal hernia are due in large part to one of its complications, reflux esophagitis. Therefore, although the latter has other causes, these conditions are here described together.

Prevalence and Pathology. The true prevalence of hiatal hernia is not known. Because it is essentially a dynamic process, estimates based on autopsies are too low. In roentgenographic surveys it is extremely common, especially in older women. Peptic esophagitis is the most common benign cause of dysphagia and persistent esophageal pain. In about 75 per cent of instances the hernia is of the *sliding* type, in which the esophagogastric junction lies inside the thorax at the apex of the herniated mass. In these a "short esophagus" exists—the result rather than the cause of the herniation; congenital primary short esophagus is exceedingly rare. In 25 per cent the hernia is *rolling* or *paraesophageal*, in which the apex of the herniated mass is some portion of the greater curvature of the stomach, which has rolled upward, medially and anterior to the vestibule, which may remain in its normal position or may be displaced above the diaphragm. (The latter hernia is often called the *mixed* type.) With the sliding and mixed types, mucosal inflammation may be found in the terminal 1 to 5 cm. of the esophagus. Early lesions show only edema and vascular engorgement, but with advancing disease mucosal erosions, hemorrhage, cellular infiltration, and fibrosis appear. In the end, an elongated, smoothly tapered stricture may be found.

Etiology and Pathogenesis. To open the esophagogastric junction is normally easy from above and difficult from below. The main mechanisms preventing reflux from the stomach include (1) the esophagogastric sphincter, maintained at a resting pressure which is greater than those of the adjacent esophagus and stomach, and which increases adaptively with increasing pressure or acid secretion in the stomach; (2) the muscular sling from the right crus of the diaphragm, which assists in occluding the esophagus in the Valsalva maneuver and during coughing; and (3) the intra-abdominal segment of the esophagus, which allows intra-abdominal pressure to be exerted directly on the terminal esophagus and assist its closure. When as the result of pregnancy, obesity, ascites, or repeated or prolonged eructation, coughing, or vomiting the sphincter is held or raised repeatedly above its usual position in the hiatus, the intra-abdominal segment of the esophagus disappears, and the force of the muscular sling is added to the intragastric rather than the sphincteric pressure; some of the adaptive increases in sphincteric pressure are then lost, and reflux occurs with or without a visible sliding hiatus hernia. The pressures generated within the hernia and the probability of severe reflux esophagitis appear to be the greater, the *smaller* the hernia. Once inflammation occurs in the terminal esophagus, sustained contraction of its musculature raises the local pressure and reflexly diminishes the pressure within the (more distal) sphincter, thus accentuating the reflux.

Reflux esophagitis also occurs in other settings: (1) in prolonged use of intragastric tubes, especially postoperatively; (2) following operative disturbance of the diaphragmatic crura or the esophagogastric sphincter; (3) in scleroderma, in which the sphincter is immobilized by inflammation; and (4) in chalasia of infants, in which innervation of the sphincter is retarded. It can occur in the absence of hydrochloric acid or, indeed, of the stomach; it is likely that bile salts have a primary injurious effect.

Hemorrhage in cases of hiatal hernia is believed to arise either from the inflamed esophagus or from the hernial sac itself. Usually it is due to multiple erosions, but often when severe it can be traced to a discrete ulcer in the engorged mucosa of the herniated stomach.

Clinical Manifestations. The majority of hiatal hernias are virtually or wholly asymptomatic, and the most common problem for the physician is to judge whether this condition is in fact responsible for the complaints of the patient. There is no relation between the severity of symptoms and the size of the hernia unless, as some suggest, pain is *inversely* related to size.

In the absence of complications, *pain* usually is described as a dull, early postprandial, retrosternal fullness, disappearing spontaneously after a few minutes to one hour; it is often associated with belching or hiccup. It is often worse on lying down or on exertion after heavy meals; sometimes it radiates to the back, the jaws, the shoulders and down the inner aspects of the arms, closely simulating angina pectoris. Particularly with large hernias, and with displacement of thoracic structures, there may be dyspnea, palpitation, or cough.

The earliest manifestation of esophageal reflux is usually *heartburn*. It is worse after heavy meals, on lying down, and on bending forward, as in tying a shoe; conversely, it is often improved by sitting or standing upright, by draughts of any liquid and by ingestion of an effective antacid. With development of true esophagitis the pain becomes more severe, lasts longer, and is worsened by irritating food and drink of all kinds. Still later, dysphagia appears, worse for solid foods, and as it progresses the development of a severe stricture may be indicated by some amelioration of the heartburn.

Hemorrhage may take the form of acute hematemesis and melena or chronic blood loss. In the latter instance, the stools are usually not discolored and are only intermittently positive for occult blood, and the presenting manifestation may be a sideropenic anemia of unknown cause. Neither in acute nor in chronic hemorrhage should hiatal hernia be accepted as the cause until a search has been made for other potential sources.

Diagnosis. The positive diagnosis of hiatal hernia rests usually upon roentgenographic findings or upon such findings considered together with clinical manifestations. With large hernias, the recognition above the diaphragm of a portion of the stomach, marked by its coarse rugae (Fig. 5), is usually simple. Diagnosis of the smaller sliding hernias depends upon precise location of the esophagogastric junction and the demonstration of reflux by fluoroscopy and cineradiography, and is aided by tilting the head downward and by the Valsalva maneuver. Rarely, the displacement of the vestibular sphincter upward into the chest may be recognized at esophagoscopy or by manometric techniques.

In the presence of a hiatal hernia or other predisposing cause, the existence of *reflux esophagitis* should be suspected when there is recurrent or persistent heartburn or otherwise unexplained, usually mild, upper gastrointestinal bleeding. Esophagoscopy may reveal mucosal inflammation, confirmed by punch or suction biopsy, but negative findings do not exclude the diagnosis. Such esophagitis may rarely be due to *syphilis* or *tuberculosis*, or, more commonly, to *candidiasis*, particularly in children or debilitated adults with concomitant thrush (see Candidiasis in Mycoses). The regurgitation of gastric juice can be confirmed by aspiration of lower esophageal contents and measurement of its pH, with the patient supine. It may be helpful to infuse into the lower esophagus 0.1N HCl at the rate of 10 ml. per minute for 30 to 60 minutes or until pain is experienced. Reproduction of the pain by this means strongly supports the diagnosis of reflux esophagitis.

Strictures of the lower esophagus resulting from chronic peptic esophagitis must be differentiated from those due to lye or other corrosive poisons, to prolonged intubation, to foreign bodies, or to congenital stenosis or atresia, as well as from carcinoma or aperistalsis (achalasia).

As it is capable of causing substernal pain radiating to the shoulders and arms, hiatal hernia may enter importantly into the differential diagnosis of angina pectoris, myocardial infarction, dissecting hematoma of the aorta, gallbladder disease, pancreatitis, and the "splenic flexure syndrome." Patients frequently exhibit two or more of these disorders simultaneously; management therefore requires thorough clinical and laboratory study and judgment based upon careful and repeated inquiry into the setting in which the attacks occur.

Treatment. In the conservative treatment of hiatal hernia, control of symptoms is attempted through avoidance of overdistention with food, control of gastric acidity, and reduction of intraabdominal pressure. The patient receives daily six feedings of bland food, with interval use of nonabsorbable antacid, as recommended elsewhere for peptic ulcer. The last feeding should be given at least two hours before bedtime. Anticholinergic drugs should *not* be used, because

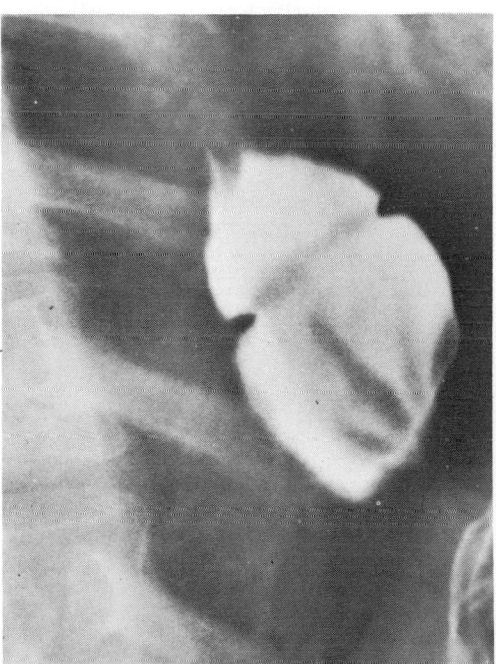
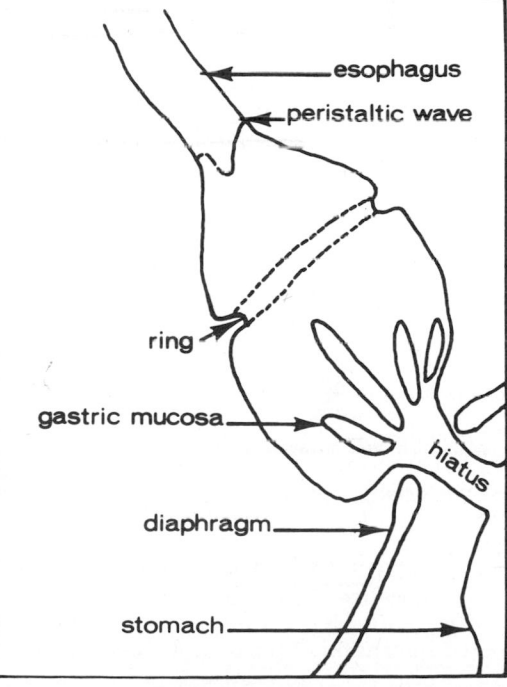

FIGURE 5.   Roentgenogram of a small sliding hiatal hernia, with an associated Schatzki ring (contraction ring).

they delay the emptying of both the esophagus and the stomach and thus favor both regurgitation and esophageal retention. Any patient who is overweight should be helped to reduce his weight, and measures should be taken to control chronic coughing or to eliminate bending forward, as in scrubbing floors or weeding gardens. Tight clothing, such as corsets, should be discarded. The head of the bed should be elevated about 10 inches on blocks or stout chairs.

The vast majority of symptomatic cases of hiatal hernia and early reflux esophagitis will be relieved by careful adherence to the aforementioned regimen. Frequent recurrence of substernal pain, heartburn, or dysphagia under these conditions is a clear indication for more radical measures. These are directed at repair of the hernia, reduction of gastric acidity, and the relief of lower esophageal obstruction.

In most instances, surgical reduction of the hernia and reconstruction of the hiatus, performed through either the abdomen or the posterior thorax, is the treatment of choice. If an early esophageal stricture exists it may be necessary preoperatively to pass metal bougies of gradually increasing diameter over a previously swallowed string as a guide. In patients with complicating diseases creating a high operative risk, control of gastric acidity by radiation therapy over the fundus of the stomach has yielded some good results. Because the sacrifice of the esophagogastric sphincter is an invitation to postoperative recurrence of esophagitis, surgical resection of the strictured zone is regarded as a measure of last resort. In recent years the interposition of a loop of jejunum or descending colon between the resected esophagus and the fundus of the stomach has seemed to prevent or delay this complication, but the precise value of this procedure has not yet been determined.

The results of surgical repair are usually excellent in rolling hernias, but only about 80 per cent successful in controlling symptoms of the sliding hernia. With painstaking reconstruction of an intra-abdominal segment of esophagus, however, recurrence rates as low as 7 per cent have been reported.

ESOPHAGEAL DIVERTICULA

Most diverticula of the esophagus occur at one of three locations, and at each of these the lesion has distinctive features.

The hypopharyngeal (or Zenker's) diverticulum is an evagination of the mucosa and submucosa directed posteriorly between the lower margin of the inferior constrictor muscle of the pharynx and the upper border of the cricopharyngeus muscle. It is considered a *pulsion* diverticulum, resulting from sharply localized increase in pressure at this point when swallowing occurs without perfectly coordinated relaxation of the pharyngoesophageal

sphincter. It is usually seen in men over 50 years of age, and enlarges progressively downward to the left of the cervical spine, eventually displacing and compressing the upper esophagus. Symptoms include dysphagia for both liquids and solids; regurgitation with aspiration of food and coughing, chiefly at night; and ultimately loss of weight. The sac may sometimes be felt as a mass in the left side of the neck, but is usually first identified on a lateral roentgenogram of the barium-filled pharynx and upper esophagus. Small diverticula usually require no treatment; when dysphagia and weight loss have been severe, the patient should be repleted by tube feeding and the diverticulum surgically resected in one stage, with myotomy of the pharyngoesophageal sphincter.

The *midesophageal* diverticulum is usually located at the level of the bifurcation of the trachea, and extends anteriorly and laterally from the esophagus. All layers of the esophageal wall are included, and the orifice is wide. Its formation is attributed to the contraction of adherent inflammatory tissue (usually tuberculous lymph nodes), or to the persistence in adult life of an incomplete tracheoesophageal fistula. It usually causes no symptoms, and is recognized by its roentgenographic appearance.

The *epiphrenic* diverticulum, rarest of the three, is located a few centimeters above the vestibule and is thought to result from the high pressures of incoordinate contractions in achalasia, diffuse esophageal spasm, or reflux esophagitis. The symptoms and indicated management are usually pertinent to these associated conditions.

LOWER ESOPHAGEAL RING

In many elderly patients, roentgenographic study of the lower esophagus reveals a symmetrical, annular, shelflike constriction a few centimeters above the diaphragm (Fig. 5). The diameter of the ring may be as small as 5 to 10 mm.; yet its detection requires careful fluoroscopy or cineradiography, with the esophagus well distended with barium. It usually lies below the esophagogastric sphincter, at the junction of esophageal and gastric mucosa; it is often associated with hiatus hernia.

In some such patients, attacks of severe lower substernal pain occur acutely on swallowing large and poorly chewed boluses that become lodged in the ring. Relief is afforded in some cases by bouginage and in others by actual cutting of the ring.

Cross, F. S.: Esophageal diverticula: Related neuromuscular problems. Ann. Otol., 77:914, 1968.
Fleischner, F. G.: Hiatal hernia complex. J.A.M.A., 162:183, 1956.
Johnson, H. D.: The fluid mechanics of the control of reflux. Lancet, 2:1267, 1966.
Schatzki, R., and Gary, J. E.: The lower esophageal ring. Amer. J. Roentgen., 75:246, 1956.
Wilkins, E. W., Jr., and Skinner, D. B.: Medical progress: Surgery of the esophagus. New Eng. J. Med., 278:824, 887, 1968.

DISORDERS OF GASTRO-DUODENAL MOTILITY

The motility of the stomach and the duodenum may logically be considered together, as these two organs have the common purpose of mixing the food with digestive juices and as the interaction of these two segments is considerable.

On the ingestion of food, initially a small amount is propelled through the stomach into the duodenum, after which the pylorus appears to close and the body of the stomach to dilate progressively as the remainder of the meal enters from the esophagus. Following a period of nonpropulsive churning movements, a series of peristaltic waves appears, beginning at or slightly above the antrum and carrying through the pylorus to the second portion of the duodenum. Under normal conditions the stomach is emptied in this manner, after which peristalsis ceases.

Gastric emptying is known to be retarded by the instillation into the duodenum of acid solutions, hypertonic solutions of sugar or sodium chloride, or fat. It is accelerated by administration of alkali. Thus, a form of servomechanism exists, regulating the rate of gastric emptying and relating that process to the need for dilution and digestion of ingested food.

"GASTRIC" SYMPTOMS AND SYNDROMES

Disturbances in this motor pattern have been correlated with a number of important digestive symptoms. Vigorous gastric peristalsis in the absence of food has, of course, long been associated with normal *hunger*. The sensation of *nausea*, on the other hand, clearly is accompanied by cessation of gastric phasic contractions and by simultaneous sustained contraction, or spasm, of the descending portion of the duodenum. Probably, *anorexia* is associated with similar changes of lesser degree. It is of interest, nevertheless, that both hunger and nausea can occur in gastrectomized persons, and corresponding behavior may be observed in eviscerated animals. Hence the gastroduodenal motor patterns are probably only peripheral manifestations of a disturbance arising in the brain.

Vomiting. Whether or not preceded by nausea, the mechanism of vomiting involves close coordination of visceral and somatic movements. The gastric fundus and corpus are flaccid, the antrum and the proximal duodenum strongly contracted, and the esophageal vestibule (cardia) relaxed. The pharyngoesophageal sphincter is likewise relaxed, the glottis closed, and the larynx and soft palate elevated. At the moment of emesis the diaphragm forcibly descends and the abdominal wall contracts, squeezing the flaccid stomach and causing ejection of its contents. All of this activity is triggered by the vomiting center in the floor of the fourth ventricle on chemical, humoral, reflex neural, or psychic stimulation. Persistent vomiting is most readily treated by drugs that depress this center or the vestibular apparatus, or both. The most effective short-term medication is a phenothiazine such as prochlorperazine, 5 to 10 mg. (or promethazine, 10 to 20 mg.) three times a day. For more prolonged use meclizine, 25 to 50 mg. daily (or cyclizine, 50 mg. daily), is safer and may be effective.

The Mallory-Weiss Syndrome. This signifies the hematemesis or melena that follows typically upon many hours or days of severe vomiting and retching, and that is traceable to one or several slitlike lacerations of the mucosa, longitudinally placed at or slightly below the esophagogastric junction. These lacerations may extend to or even through the muscularis, with rupture of blood vessels mainly in the submucosa. They are attributed to incoordination of the act of emesis, resulting from fatigue of the vomiting center and consequent forcible distention of the cardiac portion of the stomach while the vestibule remains contracted. Although usually recognized only at autopsy, the characteristic history of hematemesis following prolonged vomiting, usually after alcoholic indulgence, may often lead to the detection of these lesions by emergency esophagoscopy. Supportive medical treatment is indicated unless the threat of exsanguination makes emergency surgery mandatory.

Aerophagia. Aerophagia, or the swallowing of air, is well nigh universal at meal times, though differing widely in degree. Its symptomatic results include belching, epigastric pain or fullness related to distention of the stomach, pain in the right lower quadrant, or in the right or left upper quadrant associated with distention of various parts of the colon, and the passage of flatus by rectum. All these symptoms, or any one of them, may be signified by the term *flatulence* or "gas." As aerophagia is for the most part a compulsive habit and a manifestation of emotional tension, it should be treated as such. The patient's consciousness of the habit can be increased by having him hold a tongue blade between his teeth, thus making swallowing much more difficult.

Acute Gastric Dilatation and Volvulus. Aerophagia may lead to serious overdistention of the stomach under two conditions: (1) during complete or partial *paralytic ileus* (*vide infra*), following surgery, trauma, or acute medical conditions, when *acute gastric dilatation* may occur; and (2) in *torsion* or *volvulus* of the stomach, in which the most dependent portion of the greater curvature rotates forward, upward, and to the left, bringing both the cardia and the pylorus below the level of contained liquid and preventing the escape of air. Under both conditions the rise in intragastric pressure may lead to increased gastric secretion and congestion of the gastric wall. The upper abdomen on examination is distended and tympanitic; a plain roentgenogram of the abdomen reveals the greatly enlarged gastric air bubble, which in volvulus characteristically presents a broad, smooth upward convexity beneath the left diaphragm.

Milder degrees of distention may give rise only to a feeling of pressure and pain in the epigastrium and left hypochondrium, relieved at times on change of position leading to escape of the gas by belching or, after traversing the intestines, on passage of flatus. In such cases decompression by stomach tube and constant suction of gastric contents should give prompt relief. Prevention of recurrences may demand effective treatment of aerophagia (*vide supra*).

In some instances of severe distention or torsion, a large volume of potassium-rich fluid is lost to the gastric lumen from the extracellular space, and the gastric circulation is impaired to the point of necrosis of the gastric wall, with resulting muscular weakness, severe shock, and death if the process is unchecked. In such cases, rapid parenteral repletion of extracellular water and electrolytes, followed by operative intervention, may be lifesaving.

PYLORIC STENOSIS

Definition. Pyloric stenosis, broadly defined, is any obstruction of the pyloric canal. What is commonly called pylorospasm is actually only the failure of relaxation of the sphincter in the absence or diminution of antral propulsive waves. True spasm of the pylorus, especially in adults, is usually associated with nearby duodenal or gastric ulcer or severe gastritis, and is to be differentiated from infiltration of the wall with inflammatory cells, fibrous tissue, or malignant cells.

Congenital hypertrophic pyloric stenosis is an obstructive narrowing due to thickening of the pyloric muscle, possibly resulting from immaturity of enzymatic mechanisms in its intrinsic ganglion cells. It occurs in up to 3 per 1000 live births (four times more frequently in male than in female infants, and apparently as the expression of a single dominant gene. Never found before the fifth day of life, it is influenced also by multiple environmental factors affecting early infant feeding.

Clinical Manifestations. Typically, an infant between the ages of ten days and three months develops projectile vomiting, constipation, dehydration, and rapid loss of weight. Curiously, the appetite is well preserved, and feeding may be resumed immediately after vomiting. The vomitus may contain blood but no bile. Inspection after a feeding may reveal visible peristaltic waves passing from left to right across the upper abdomen. In many instances a firm tumor mass, 1 to 2 cm. in diameter, is felt a few centimeters below the costal margin at the external margin of the right rectus muscle. Roentgenograms after a barium meal indicate gastric dilatation and a symmetrically narrowed, elongated pylorus.

In those patients not treated surgically (*vide infra*), attacks of nausea and vomiting occur at intervals for many years, sometimes throughout life. Rarely, such attacks begin in adult life and lead to the discovery of an identical hypertrophy of pyloric muscle.

Treatment. Initially an infant with this disorder is continued on breast milk or a formula yielding soft curds, supplemented with thick cereals. It may be necessary to make up deficits of water and electrolytes parenterally. Traditionally, atropine sulfate (0.06 mg.) is given before each feeding, but the value of anticholinergics is not clearly documented. Phenobarbital (8 mg.) may be combined to good effect with each dose of atropine. In most instances, as soon as dehydration has been corrected and acid-base balance restored, a Rammstedt operation (pyloromyotomy) should be performed. This requires a longitudinal incision that severs all the circular muscle fibers of the pylorus, leaving the mucosa intact. Although the mortality rate of this procedure is from 1 to 5 per cent, permanent cure is the rule.

In older children and adults, initial treatment of presumed pyloric stenosis should be the same as for peptic ulcer with obstruction (*vide infra*). Anticholinergics should not be used. During this interval the possible diagnosis of gastric cancer is studied by cytologic and gastroscopic means, and that of pyloric or duodenal ulcer by repeated roentgenographic examination. Unless the obstruction disappears completely within four to six weeks, it should be relieved surgically by pylorotomy or gastrojejunostomy.

MEGADUODENUM

The term *megaduodenum* is applied to gross dilatation of the duodenum from its upper end to the middle of the transverse portion. No point of true stenosis is to be found. The muscularis is hypertrophic, but the myenteric ganglion cells are damaged or absent. Although physiologic studies are so far lacking, the pathogenic mechanism is considered to be aperistalsis, comparable to the disorder in congenital megacolon, with which it is sometimes associated. A similar phenomenon has been observed in certain cases of South American trypanosomiasis (Chagas' disease), in which megacolon and megaesophagus may also be present.

This form of obstruction of the lower duodenum is to be differentiated from stenosis due to malignant disease at the same site and from "superior mesenteric ileus," in which the transverse duodenum appears to be compressed between the lumbar vertebrae and the superior mesenteric artery near its origin from the aorta. Treatment is by duodenojejunostomy.

Barnett, W. O., and Wall, L.: Megaduodenum resulting from absence of the parasympathetic ganglion cells of Auerbach's plexus. Ann. Surg., 141:527, 1955.

Carter, C. O.: The inheritance of congenital pyloric stenosis. Brit. Med. Bull., 17:251, 1961.

Jones, F. A., and Gummer, J. W. P.: Clinical Gastroenterology. Oxford, Blackwell Publications, Ltd., 1960, pp. 102-117.

Swenson, O.: Pediatric Surgery. 2nd ed. New York, Appleton-Century-Crofts, 1962, pp. 262-270.

DISORDERS OF INTESTINAL MOTILITY

Among the significant disorders of intestinal motility, some are adaptive mechanisms of general occurrence among persons under stress. Paralytic ileus and the irritable colon are both here interpreted in this light. These interrelated disorders are presented in the following pages, together with mechanical obstruction of the intestine, so often important in differential diagnosis.

Other disorders are thought to be due to excessive stimulation by humoral agents. These are the metastatic carcinoid syndrome and the diarrhea seen in patients with medullary carcinoma of the thyroid. Still others are known to be related to defects in the efferent cholinergic nerves regulating intestinal motility (megacolon), or thought to result from defects in the afferent limb of intestinal reflex arcs (diabetic pseudotabes; tabes dorsalis).

NORMAL COLONIC FUNCTION

The human colon has two main functions: (1) the absorption of water and crystalloids, and (2) the formation of a reservoir to permit the orderly and convenient evacuation of feces. The fluid mass it receives from the ileum is subjected over long periods to slow phasic contractions, kneading or accordion-like movements, which facilitate absorption. During this time the colon is sacculated or haustrated in outline. At long intervals, usually following the ingestion of food, this pattern of motility is replaced by one of mass peristalsis, in which haustra disappear, the proximal portions contract and the distal ones relax, and the entire colon undergoes shortening. In this manner feces are advanced rapidly.

The rectum is usually empty until part of the contents of the sigmoid is forced into it by mass peristalsis. This distends the rectal walls, produces discomfort in the sacral area, and initiates the defecation reflex by which the contraction of skeletal muscles of the abdominal wall and the coordinate relaxation of the anal sphincter assist in the emptying of the terminal colon. Voluntary inhibition of the reflex can be achieved by vigorous contraction of the external sphincter and a thoracic pattern of breathing. With time the walls of the rectum become adapted to the fecal mass; their tension decreases, and the stimulus to defecation subsides until renewed by further additions to the rectal contents.

DIARRHEA

Definition. Diarrhea signifies the passage of excessively liquid or excessively frequent stools. Never a complete diagnosis in itself, its recognition demands careful study to determine its cause. Its duration and course vary widely, depending upon the natural history of the underlying disease.

Etiology. The many causes for diarrhea may be briefly outlined as follows:

I. *Functional disorders,* including adaptive colitis, allergy to ingested food and drugs, defective gastric or pancreatic digestion, defective absorption, vitamin deficiencies, and abuse of cathartics.

II. *Generalized disorder or disease affecting the intestine,* including uremia, Graves' disease, Addison's disease, cardiac decompensation, portal hypertension, neurologic disease, and poisoning with heavy metals.

III. *Intrinsic disease of the intestine,* due to (1) specific viral, bacterial, fungal, protozoan, or metazoan parasites; (2) alterations in intestinal flora, antimicrobial therapy, fistula, blind loops, or small intestinal stasis; (3) nonspecific inflammatory disease such as regional enteritis or ulcerative colitis; or (4) benign or malignant tumors and other causes of partial intestinal obstruction.

Differential Diagnosis. The formidable task of identifying the one or the several causes of diarrhea in a given case can be facilitated by efforts to estimate, in succession, the *location* and the *nature* of the disease process. The location is suggested by the character of the stools and the zone of reference of pain. If each stool is *large* in volume, it may be presumed that the distal colon is reacting as it would to an enema and is itself not diseased, and therefore that the chief site of the disorder is in the proximal colon or small intestine. In such instances, any accompanying pain is usually referred to the periumbilical area or the right lower quadrant. On the contrary, if some stools, though attended by notable urgency, are of *small* size, the conclusion is justified that the distal colon does not tolerate accumulation of a normal amount of feces, and therefore that it is diseased. In such instances, the stool is more likely to contain visible mucus or flecks of blood, and pain is felt in the lower abdomen or the sacral region. The *nature* of the disease process is estimated from its manner of onset and course over time; history of exposure to toxic, infectious, and allergenic agents; the extent of debility; and the personality and life situation of the patient. The diagnostic study of the patient usually includes sigmoidoscopy, gross and microscopic examination of the stools and cultures for pathogenic bacteria, and barium enema, in the order named. Other useful laboratory tests are mentioned elsewhere in the sections on specific diseases.

Treatment. It is frequently necessary to mitigate the diarrhea or its consequences before the recognition of the true cause permits specific therapy. In most acute infectious diarrheas, the disease is brief, and the diarrhea serves a useful purpose in ridding the body, at least subtotally, of the offending agent. Hence, the first indication is to replace the losses of fluid and electrolytes, usually with infusions of physiologic saline and 5 per cent glucose, guided by measurements of urinary output and plasma volume. Replacement of potassium and further adjustments of acid-base balance are guided by serial determinations of serum sodium, potassium, chloride, and bicarbonates. If oral fluids are tolerated, warm weak tea, broth, and, ultimately, thin cooked cereals are given in sufficient quantity to maintain a urinary output in excess of 1500 ml. per day. Cold liquids and concentrated sweets are poorly tolerated.

Lying flat in bed, with constant use of heating pad or hot water bottle, is usually helpful. Most of the conventional binding agents, such as bismuth, pectins, and kaolin, are of a low order of effectiveness. Aluminum hydroxide gel in large doses (20 to 40 ml. four times a day) is often useful. Codeine sulfate, 0.03 to 0.06 gram, or morphine sulfate, 0.008 to 0.015 gram, may be given every three to four hours during acute diarrhea, but will produce severe distention and cramps in most instances. The synthetic opiate, diphenoxylate hydrochloride, carries apparently less risk of addiction and is often effective in doses of 5 to 10 mg. three times daily before meals and at bedtime. Camphorated tincture of opium (paregoric) is used in doses of 4 ml. after each bowel movement until diarrhea is controlled. In prescribing any of these agents, the physician assumes the responsibility for eventually freeing the patient from dependence upon them.

Steinberg, H., and Almy, T. P.: The choice of an anti-diarrheal agent. *In* Modell, W. (ed.): Drugs of Choice 1964-65. St. Louis, C. V. Mosby Company, 1964, pp. 359-364.

CONSTIPATION

(With Emphasis on Habitual Constipation or Rectal Constipation)

Definition. Constipation ordinarily signifies the passage of excessively dry stools or the evacuation of the bowels less often than every other day. By many patients, however, the same term is used to refer to a sense of incomplete emptying of the rectum or to the small size of their stools.

Pathogenesis. Inadequate propulsion of feces may result from mechanical obstruction (as in carcinoma of the sigmoid colon), from diminished contractions of the proximal intestine, e.g., paralytic ileus, or from failure of the distal colon to relax, e.g., irritable colon and congenital megacolon. In most instances, however, constipation results chiefly from failure of the defecation reflex (habitual constipation, rectal constipation, or dyschezia).

Early in childhood, despite great variations in the intensity of "toilet training," the habits of defecation become subject to complex patterns of conditioned reflex behavior. Their disruption in adult life is usually associated with major changes in the pattern of living, e.g., travel or going away

to school, with intercurrent illness, with emotional tension, or with willful neglect. The mechanical efficiency of defecation may be impaired by the use of high toilet seats, of bedpans, or other departures from the primitive squatting position. Weakness of the muscles of the back or of the abdominal wall due to neurologic disorders or to multiple pregnancies is occasionally an important factor. Failure of relaxation of the anal sphincter may be due to neighboring painful lesions such as anal ulcers or thrombosed hemorrhoids. These are, however, more often a result of the constipation than a cause.

Prolonged retention in the rectum (or rarely in the sigmoid colon) results in excessive dehydration or *impaction* of feces. This may lead to cramping lower abdominal pain and to paradoxical diarrhea, as watery brown stools are passed around the hardened mass. Many patients with constipation complain also of anorexia, bloating, belching, passage of flatus, headache, malaise, weakness, or faintness. Such symptoms are related in part to the attendant disturbances of intestinal motility and in part to the anxiety aroused by the constipation itself.

Diagnosis. In any constipated patient who has not recently been given an enema or a laxative, the finding of more than a few grams of feces on digital examination of the rectum indicates that habitual constipation is present. (Conversely, the usual finding in irritable colon or in megacolon is an empty rectum.) The search for localized anal and rectal lesions should be made carefully with both anoscope and sigmoidoscope. In most instances a barium enema, and in some an upper gastrointestinal roentgenographic series, is indicated to exclude intrinsic intestinal disease. Careful thought should be given to the possible etiologic importance of constipating medications such as opiates, anticholinergics, ganglionic blocking agents, and nonabsorbable antacids. Search should be made for systemic diseases such as myxedema, hyperparathyroidism, lead poisoning, scleroderma, and mental depression, of which constipation may rarely be the presenting symptom.

Management. The goal of treatment is an empty rectum, or the maximal possible restoration of normal habits of defecation, with minimal disturbance of normal intestinal motility. In bedridden patients, or in others whose daily habits are greatly disrupted, this must be postponed, and an effort is made to avoid fecal impaction by tapwater enemas or mild laxatives at one- or two-day intervals. Any painful anal lesion such as an ulcer or thrombosed hemorrhoid should be treated at once with sitz baths, local anesthesia by ointments or suppositories, and nightly mineral oil. Fecal impactions should be digitally broken, softened by a retention enema of cottonseed oil (150 ml.) or dioctyl sodium sulfosuccinate (5 ml. of a 1 per cent solution diluted to 90 ml. in water), and evacuated by enemas of tapwater or soapsuds.

The cooperation of the patient is enlisted through explanation of the mechanisms of his constipation and of the goal of therapy. He must be persuaded that a daily bowel movement is desirable but not necessary. A large breakfast is prescribed, to contain fruit, cereal, toast or rolls, preserves, and coffee or milk; no other dietary regulation is needed. He is required to sit on the toilet daily within the hour after breakfast, remaining ten minutes, and to distract his attention by a newspaper, magazine, or other device. All previous cathartics or enemas are forbidden; in their place a rounded teaspoon of a hydrophilic colloid (psyllium or agar) is taken with 400 ml. of water at bedtime and again on arising. Mineral oil, 15 to 45 ml. at bedtime only, may be substituted.

The patient is warned that one to four weeks are required for the achievement of desired results and that his bodily discomfort may in the meantime increase. When relief of this distress is needed, at intervals of two or three days, an enema of tapwater or of prepared hypertonic solutions (Travad, Clyserol, Sigmol) is taken after the morning toilet visit. As normal habits are restored, the enemas and mild laxatives are cancelled; they may be recommended for future prophylactic use when the patient's habits of living are again disturbed.

Miner, R. W. (ed.): The colon: Its normal and abnormal physiology and therapeutics. Ann. N.Y. Acad. Sci., 58:293, 1954.
Steinberg, H., and Almy, T. P.: The choice of a cathartic. In Modell, W. (ed.): Drugs of Choice 1964-65. St. Louis, C. V. Mosby Company, 1964, pp. 350-359.

IRRITABLE COLON

(Mucous Colitis, Spastic Colon, Unstable Colon, Adaptive Colitis)

Definition. Irritable colon signifies a variety of disturbances of colonic function that accompany emotional tension and participate in the general bodily adaptation to nonspecific stress.

This disorder is considered to account for more than 50 per cent of all gastrointestinal illnesses, and ranks with the common cold as one of the leading causes of recurrent minor disability.

Symptoms and Their Mechanisms. *Abdominal pain* of some degree occurs in most patients. It is usually located in the hypogastrium or left lower quadrant; it is commonly felt in the other quadrants of the abdomen but very rarely in the periumbilical region. In some instances severe pain is felt far laterally over the left costal margin and radiates to the precordium, the left shoulder, and the inner aspect of the left arm (the *splenic flexure syndrome*). In most instances, the pain of irritable colon is relieved by the passage of feces or gas. Hence, it is believed to be due to distention or spasmodic contractions of the colon at various points (explaining its variable location). *Constipation* is probably related to heightened nonpropulsive activity (spasm), chiefly in the sigmoid colon, and *gaseous distention* of the proximal colon and *passage of flatus* are commonly associated. *Diarrhea* of varying severity may occur, together with urgency and tenesmus, usually in the morning before and after breakfast. Commonly the *stools are small*, whatever their consistency (hence the term "irritable colon"); they often contain visible *mucus*, or mucus alone may be evacuated with no fecal residues. Diarrhea and myxorrhea appear to represent the motor and secretory response of the colon to exaggerated cholinergic stimulation.

Extracolonic symptoms, often encountered in these patients, emphasize the generalized character of the body's adaptive response. Thus *anorexia, nausea, belching,* and *occasionally vomiting* indicate a concurrent disturbance of gastroduodenal motility. The syndrome of *neurocirculatory asthenia*, including palpitation, shortness of breath, precordial discomfort, and fatigue on mild exertion, is often present. *Headache* is common, and sweating, flushing, faintness, sighing respirations, and hyperventilation may be noted.

Natural History and Pathogenesis. This disorder may begin at any age, but usually in early adult life or in adolescence. Its course is extremely variable, but in most instances individual episodes of illness can be measured in terms of days, weeks, or months. In some persons a single symptom consistently predominates, but in most constipation and diarrhea appear alternately, and pain occurs irregularly. There is rarely any significant dehydration or loss of weight.

The onset and recurrences of irritable colon usually coincide with periods of life stress and emotional conflict, and the symptoms often disappear spontaneously when these influences abate. Relevant disturbances of colonic function have been observed in the laboratory when emotional conflicts have been induced in patients through stressful interviews (Fig. 6) and have appeared as normal bodily manifestations of emotion, not unlike blushing and weeping. The emotional state accompanying constipation has been described as one of assertive independence, defensiveness, or self-confident resistance to a noxious situation. The attitudes commonly observed with diarrhea are those of dependence, helplessness, and self-reproach. These impressions have been consistent in both clinical and laboratory studies. The pathways by which these reactions are mediated probably include the central and peripheral portions of the autonomic nervous system, as comparable disturbances have been produced transiently by administration of methacholine or neostigmine. Presumably other neurohumoral factors, such as serotonin, are involved.

Diagnosis. The diagnosis of irritable colon must be based upon (1) the recognition of characteristic symptoms, (2) the exclusion of other disease processes suggested by the symptoms, and (3) repeated and conscientious testing of the hypothesis that the symptoms are related to life stress and emotional tension. On examination of the patient one commonly finds a palpable, tender sigmoid colon, enlarged areas of tympany over

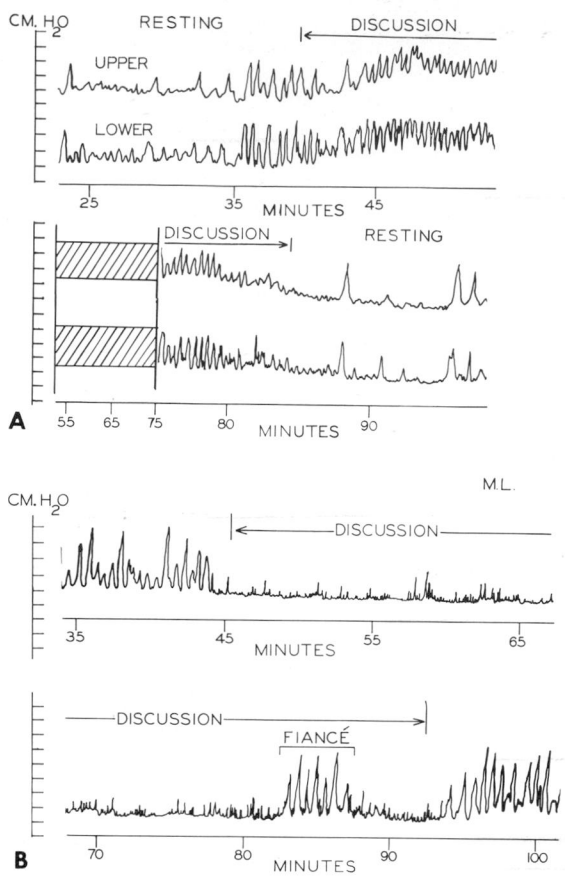

FIGURE 6. A, Heightened nonpropulsive contractions of sigmoid colon during stress interview in subject with spastic constipation. (Tandem balloons.) B, Reduced phasic activity of sigmoid colon during stress interview in a subject with functional diarrhea. (Single balloon.)

the proximal colon, and proctoscopic signs of mucosal engorgement, spasm, and excessive mucous secretion; yet none of these findings is specific for the disease or is a significant departure from the normal. The condition cannot be diagnosed, but may be suggested, by roentgenographic examination of the colon.

The syndrome of irritable colon may be mimicked very closely by abuse of cathartics; by specific infections of the colon such as amebiasis, shigellosis, or lymphogranuloma venereum; by allergy to ingested food or drugs; and by intolerance of specific disaccharides, particularly lactose. The differentiation from early ulcerative colitis or from carcinoma of the colon can usually be made by proctoscopy and barium enema. Differentiation from diverticular disease may be more difficult, as the symptoms and motor disturbances of the colon in this disease closely resemble those of irritable colon, and the two conditions may coexist or be interrelated (see Diverticula of the Intestines).

Broadly, irritable colon must be differentiated from all the various causes of abdominal pain, constipation, and diarrhea. Of particular note, the pain of gallbladder disease may be simulated by

gaseous distention of the hepatic flexure, the pain and tenderness of acute or chronic appendicitis by distention of the cecum, and the migration of pain to the precordium in the "splenic flexure syndrome" may simulate angina pectoris or myocardial infarction.

Because of the ubiquity of stress and emotional tension, symptoms of irritable colon may be superimposed upon those of other and more serious diseases, or may reflect the anxiety occasioned by them. Careful consideration of the significance of each process is required, lest a carcinoma go undetected or the removal of a symptomless gallbladder prove useless in the relief of unrelated abdominal distress.

The establishment of a diagnosis of irritable colon on positive grounds depends upon a profound understanding of the social history and personality of the patient. As the process of acquiring this understanding is of both diagnostic and therapeutic value, it is described under the heading of Management.

Management. The recognition of irritable colon as a bodily reaction to stress calls for treatment directed to the patient as a whole rather than to his colon. As in the relief of blushing or weeping, both the environment and the attitudes of the patient must be considered.

At the first visit, the patient is called upon for a brief autobiography, including his relations with parents, marital partner, employers, and others. He is asked to compare his own personality with that of a sibling or a good friend. His speech and expression are observed for evidences of emotion, and topics of special meaning for him are thus usually easily recognized. The several visits required for adequate laboratory investigation and early symptomatic management provide opportunities for further discussion of these topics. Careful note is made of the dates of important events, so that a "life chart" may be constructed, correlating these with the course of bowel symptoms.

After several visits, such a procedure permits the reasonably certain acceptance or rejection of the diagnosis of irritable colon on the positive grounds of coincidence with life stress and correlation with emotional tension. A decision should then be made as to the prognosis and needs for future therapy. Those patients whose episodes of illness appear but little related in time to easily recognizable stress situations and who have made a uniformly inadequate adjustment to major personal problems may be considered the "more neurotic" group. They should be referred to a psychiatrist for consultation, if feasible. The further efforts of the physician are best limited to reassurance regarding the benign character of the illness, manipulation of important environmental factors, explanations to responsible relatives, sympathetic listening, and the conscientious use of placebos.

On the other hand, the "less neurotic" patient who has made a satisfactory adjustment to most life situations, whose bowel symptoms are intermittent and closely related in time to specific difficulties, e.g., new job or military service, can profit by relatively brief and simple psychotherapy in the hands of the general physician. This begins with *reassurance* as to the absence of serious disease and usually a simple explanation of his illness as an expression of emotional tension. He is urged to ventilate his feelings to the physician or members of his family or friends, or to sublimate them through more active and vigorous pursuit of sports, games, or hobbies. He is encouraged to make his own changes in ways of living as a result of the insight acquired.

Concurrently, symptomatic management may be required. The most common problem is habitual *constipation*, which should be treated as outlined. With *diarrhea* the usual binding agents are ineffective. The most rational therapy is an anticholinergic drug in sufficient dosage to dry the mouth, i.e., propantheline, 15 to 30 mg., or tridihexethide, 25 to 50 mg. This should not be given continuously but in anticipation of the hours of more severe diarrhea, usually in the early morning or just prior to social or business engagements. In some cases diphenoxylate hydrochloride, 5 mg. three times daily before meals and at bedtime, is indicated and is more effective. In view of the chronic and benign nature of the illness, even temporary use of opiates is rarely desirable. Severe abdominal *pain* is best relieved by a hot water bottle or a warm tapwater enema.

Sedatives, tranquilizers, and other measures may be required to deal with extreme degrees of anxiety and insomnia. Their use should be guided by the principles set forth in the article on The Psychoneuroses, and they should not be routinely prescribed for patients with irritable colon. The most convenient "placebo" is tincture of belladonna in doses of 10 to 15 drops in water three times daily before meals.

Prognosis. The "more neurotic" patients, as defined above, may be expected to have symptoms of varying severity, mitigated only temporarily by the solicitude of the physician or favorable life situations. The "less neurotic" should have symptoms at long intervals, reduced in frequency and severity, but rarely abolished, by a high degree of insight and alteration of their environment.

Almy, T. P.: Experimental studies on the irritable colon. Amer. J. Med., 10:60, 1951.
Chaudhary, N. A., and Truelove, S. C.: The irritable colon syndrome. Quart. J. Med. (N.S.), 31:307, 1962.

INTESTINAL OBSTRUCTION
(Ileus)

Definition. Intestinal obstruction is broadly defined as any impairment, arrest, or reversal of the normal anad flow of intestinal contents. This concept thus includes obstruction due to mechanical factors and that due to failure of peristalsis for reasons of deficient neural stimulation (paralytic ileus) or vascular insufficiency.

Etiology. The majority of severe cases are due to *mechanical factors* that locally occlude the intestinal lumen. The most common of these are extramural, constricting the entire circumference of the gut, and include *hernias* (especially inguinal and femoral), peritoneal *adhesions* due to previous operations or local inflammatory disease, and *volvulus* (usually of the sigmoid or ileocecal regions). *Mural thickening* due to disease or congenital defect of the intestinal wall may narrow or obliterate its lumen—examples are benign and malignant tumors; inflammatory strictures due to diverticulitis, regional enteritis, or previous operative anastomoses; and congenital atresia or imperforate anus. Least common are *intramural* factors, including fecal impactions, meconium, foreign bodies, intussusception, gallstones, and large worms.

Another large group of cases is due to general or regional *failure of peristalsis (adynamic ileus)*. In minor form, this may occur in many severe, acute diseases, such as pneumonia and myocardial infarction. It is an impressive feature of many painful conditions in the thoracolumbar area, such as renal and biliary colic, retroperitoneal hematoma, or spinal injuries, but is most severe in the presence of peritonitis. In these conditions it is held to be the result of excessive adrenergic neural influence on the gut, and motility has often been restored by lumbar sympathetic blockade. An initially identical picture may result from *ischemia* of the bowel wall due to *vascular insufficiency*. The term *spastic ileus* is sometimes used to describe a failure of peristalsis orad to a zone of known spasm, which is usually in the distal colon. Such local spasm is probably present in most cases of adynamic ileus and may be considered an acute and extreme form of irritable colon.

In many cases more than one of these mechanisms play a part, and the operation of a secondary factor may convert a case of mild or partial obstruction into a complete and most serious one. Thus, postoperative adynamic ileus may lead to volvulus and subsequent ischemia of the twisted loop. The possible combination of mechanical and physiologic factors calls for periodic reconsideration of the diagnosis in individual cases.

Pathogenesis. Whatever the etiologic mechanism, the immediate effect of ileus is to interrupt the normal pathways of intestinal propulsion and absorption of liquid and gas. *Even in the absence of oral intake* 7 to 10 liters of water and contained solutes enter the upper gastrointestinal tract each day, most of which is to be absorbed at lower levels. In intestinal obstruction, this cycle is interrupted. Even if vomiting does not occur, this liquid is withdrawn from the body fluid compartments to lie in the intestinal lumen. The result is dehydration, loss from extracellular fluid of sodium and chloride ions, alkalosis, and shift of potassium ion from intracellular to extracellular fluid to compensate for loss of potassium into the gut. Hypovolemia and hypokalemia may lead to acute renal insufficiency, even in the absence of arterial hypotension. Hypokalemia itself further inhibits peristalsis.

Stasis within the gut leads to multiplication of its bacteria, absorption of indoles and other of their metabolic products, and accumulation of gas produced by bacterial action, diffusion from the blood, and air swallowing. The resultant distention of the gut leads to dangerous increases in intraluminal pressure, especially in closed-loop obstructions due to hernia or volvulus, or in complete occlusion of the colon, in which the contents are trapped proximally by the ileocecal valve. With rise in pressure there is at first venous stasis in the mucosa, with resultant hypoxia and transudation of fluid into the lumen. Ultimately the terminal mesenteric arterial branches are compressed, and the wall of the gut becomes necrotic. Early in the course of necrosis the selectivity of the intestinal membrane is lost, and plasma proteins and blood ultimately exude into the lumen, whereas bacteria and their toxins pass across the gut wall to peritoneum and blood even in the absence of gross free perforation.

Clinical Manifestations. The cardinal manifestations of acute intestinal obstruction are *abdominal pain, vomiting, constipation*, and *distention*. Variations in the character and sequence of these symptoms may be valuable in establishing the primary location and mechanism of the disorder. In general, obstructions high in the intestine produce more severe and rapidly progressive symptoms. The presence of strangulation is indicated by continuous pain, rapid dehydration, prostration, and hypotension.

Pain, referable most often to the periumbilical area, is usually the first symptom of acute mechanical obstruction. It is characteristically intermittent, lasting a few seconds to a few minutes, and corresponds to the strong peristaltic contractions above the obstruction. Thus, the cramps are more frequent and intense with higher obstructions, are least severe with colonic lesions, and tend to abate as distention increases and peristalsis weakens. Paroxysmal pain is not a feature of adynamic ileus.

Vomiting occurs early in small intestinal obstruction, but may be much delayed or absent following occlusion of the colon. After ingested food has been raised, the vomitus appears bilestained or gray and opalescent. Brownish discoloration and fecal odor may later appear, even with a small intestinal obstruction, because of the proliferation of intestinal bacteria.

Constipation is a certain feature in all cases, but its appearance may be delayed by the evacuation of intestinal contents below the obstruction. Especially in cases of colonic occlusion, blood or blood and mucus may appear in the stool.

Examination of the patient with ileus *in its early stages* does *not* support the impression of severe illness, and the findings are usually *confined to the abdomen. Distention* of the abdomen may or may not be present on the initial examination; it is usually generalized, but is less noticeable with high jejunal ileus, and may be localized or inapparent with a colonic lesion.

Auscultation of the abdomen is of prime importance. Early in the course, audible borborygmi are prominent in mechanical obstruction, but are absent in adynamic ileus. Paralleling the intestinal cramps in timing, intensity, and frequency, they occur in higher pitch and at shorter intervals when the obstruction is high in the intestine. As with the pain, their progressive subsidence coincides with loss of peristalsis and the appearance of distention. Bowel sounds should not be considered absent except after continuous auscultation for three minutes or more. At times the peristaltic waves are visible through a thin abdominal wall.

With the development of strangulation, additional physical signs appear. Persistent direct and rebound *tenderness* and *rigidity* of the abdomen signal the development of peritonitis. *Dehydration* may become clinically evident, and *shock* will manifest itself by an anxious facies, elevated pulse rate, cold clammy extremities, and ultimate fall in blood pressure. Fever is a late and unimpressive feature.

Laboratory Findings. Early in the course, the fluid shifts are manifested by diminished urinary output, fall in serum chloride and potassium, and rise in plasma bicarbonate and pH and in the blood urea nitrogen. As these abnormalities worsen, the hematocrit may rise, and urinary specific gravity and osmolality may become fixed. With strangulation the peripheral leukocyte count rises, far out of proportion to the body temperature.

Early and repeated *roentgenographic examination* of the abdomen is essential. Films taken of the patient in the prone position aid in localization of the obstruction in the small or large intestine, as gaseous distention of portions of the colon usually appear only in the latter case. The degree of accumulation of fluid and gas can be estimated from films taken in the lateral or upright position, which reveal characteristic fluid levels in distended loops. These features are presented in both mechanical and adynamic ileus, but the volume of gas is often much less when the primary mechanism is vascular occlusion. Cautious performance of a barium enema, without preparatory cleansing of the bowel, is often indicated in localizing a point of colonic obstruction, but barium or other contrast media should rarely be given by mouth.

Treatment. The effective management of cases of intestinal obstruction calls for frequent re-evaluation of the status of the patient by clinical and laboratory methods and modification of the therapeutic plan to deal with the changing conditions thus discerned. The cardinal principles of therapy are *replacement* of metabolic losses, *decompression* of the intestine, and *removal of the cause* of obstruction.

Intake of fluid and food by mouth is suspended, and an infusion of equal parts of 0.9 per cent sodium chloride and 5 per cent dextrose in water is begun. As soon as the adequacy of renal function can be estimated or the serum potassium level has been reported, potassium chloride should be added to the infusion and delivered at a rate not exceeding 40 mEq. of potassium per hour. An electrocardiogram should be taken before therapy; repeated observation of the T waves and ST segments can serve, along with repeated determinations of serum potassium and chloride, to gauge the effectiveness of replacement. Once hypokalemia has been corrected, any residual alkalosis may be treated with additional chloride in the form of parenteral solution of ammonium chloride or lysine monohydrochloride. In the presence of strangulation, hypotension, and rising hematocrit, the blood and plasma volumes should be estimated, and infusions of human albumin, plasma, or whole blood should be given in sufficient amounts to restore normal values. If parenteral alimentation is continued longer than 24 to 48 hours, infusion of protein hydrolysates is indicated to compensate for nitrogen catabolism.

In adynamic ileus, *morphine* sulfate, given subcutaneously in doses of 10 to 15 mg. at three- to six-hour intervals, may be helpful in restoring intestinal tone. When strangulation is suspected, antimicrobial drugs are used in the manner recommended for cases of vascular occlusion.

Decompression of the intestine is accompanied by intubation with a long, balloon-tipped tube (Miller-Abbott or Cantor type), advancement of the tube under observation by repeated roentgenographic examination until it lies as close as possible to the site of obstruction, and constant suction. Such a procedure will greatly diminish the symptoms of the patient, but will not benefit his fluid and electrolyte depletion, and may render less clear the signs of strangulation. For this reason, intubated patients must be carefully observed and, if local tenderness and leukocytosis are not diminished after 24 to 36 hours, the probability of strangulation is so great that surgical intervention is required.

Removal of the cause of ileus requires *operation* in most cases of complete mechanical obstruction and in many cases of severe adynamic ileus. It must be postponed in all instances until dehydration, electrolyte loss, and shock have been overcome; but, in the face of evident strangulation or closed loop obstruction of the colon, it must be accomplished as rapidly as possible. Just before operation, intensive antimicrobial therapy should be started; penicillin, 1 to 2 million units, and streptomycin, 1 gram, should be given in divided doses daily, or ampicillin, 0.5 to 1.0 gram every six hours. The surgical procedure depends upon the findings at laparotomy and the judgment of the surgeon, particularly as to the viability of the bowel.

Some cases of volvulus tend to right themselves on conservative management, permitting later surgery at a time of election, and rare cases of ileocolic intussusception in childhood are relieved by the intracolonic pressure exerted by a barium enema.

Prognosis. The outlook for recovery from intestinal obstruction depends chiefly upon the presence or absence of strangulation and its consequent toxemia, and the presence or absence of renal insufficiency resulting from excessive loss of fluid and electrolytes. These are in turn influenced by the type, location, and degree of obstruction, the existence of related primary disease (such as peritonitis leading to paralytic ileus), and the extent of delay in initiation of effective therapy. For persons recovering from ileus, the outlook for recurrence depends upon the underlying causes; with most patients with mechanical obstruction who recover without emergency operation, the probability of recurrence is so great as to dictate interval elective surgery.

Cantor, M. O.: Intestinal Obstructions. Baltimore, Williams & Wilkins Company, 1957.
Ochsner, A., and Granger, A.: The roentgen diagnosis of ileus. Ann. Surg., 92:947, 1930.
Wangensteen, O. H.: Intestinal Obstruction. Springfield, Ill., Charles C Thomas, 1942.

THE CARCINOID SYNDROME
(The Malignant Carcinoid Syndrome, the Metastatic Carcinoid Syndrome, Carcinoidosis)

The carcinoid syndrome connotes the occurrence of cutaneous flushing, diarrhea, wheezing, and valvular heart disease in association with carcinoid tumors (argentaffinomas), usually those which have metastasized to the liver. These tumors, though described as early as 1808 by Merling, were generally regarded until the past 30 years as benign and symptomless. Since then their malignant potentiality has been clearly recognized, and their capacity to secrete serotonin (5-hydroxytryptamine, 5-HT) and other bioactive amines has been established. In 1954, Thorson, Waldenström, and their associates published the classic clinical description of the syndrome, and in 1955, Sjoerdsma, Weissbach, and Udenfriend announced the first practical diagnostic test, based on the metabolism of serotonin. Since then, although its pathogenic importance relative to other substances produced by the tumor has become less certain, knowledge has accumulated regarding its role in normal intestinal function and in certain disturbances of motility and absorption unrelated to neoplastic disease.

Biochemistry and Physiology. About 90 per cent of the serotonin of the body is found in argentaffin (Kultschitzky) cells, where it is believed to be formed locally from the enzymatic hydroxylation and decarboxylation of tryptophan. Its formation from 5-hydroxytryptophan can, however, also be demonstrated in liver, lung, brain, and kidney, as well as in carcinoid tumors. It is metabolized in the presence of monoamine oxidase to 5-hydroxyindoleacetic acid (5-HIAA), which is excreted in the urine. It is present in bound (inactive) form in platelets and in many tissues; it is found in high concentration in bananas, plantains, tomatoes, and pineapples. Experimental studies, both in vivo and in vitro, indicate that it sensitizes intestinal mucosal stretch receptors by which the peristaltic reflex is activated, and augments gastric acid secretion. It appears to contract smooth muscle; to constrict arteries and veins, but dilate capillaries; and to increase intravascular volume, but decrease the rate of blood flow. Its active metabolism in basal areas of the brain gives it a presumptive role in the regulation of behavior.

Reflecting these postulated regulatory functions, increased excretion of 5-HIAA has been shown in malabsorption, in some instances of diverticulosis of the colon and of intestinal spasm, in experimental intestinal obstruction, and in allergic asthma. High levels of blood 5-HT and reduced urinary 5-HIAA have been found in some patients with motor disorders of the gut classified with "irritable colon"; and a role of 5-HT in the postgastrectomy "dumping" syndrome has been suggested.

Pathology and Pathogenesis. Carcinoid tumors are firm, yellow, usually spherical or ovate, and arise chiefly in the argentaffin cells of the intestinal tract, most often in the appendix, the terminal ileum, or a Meckel diverticulum. The malignant carcinoid usually arises in the ileum, and produces metastases, often massive, in the liver. As serotonin produced in the ileal tumor is oxidized in the liver, secretion by the metastases into the hepatic vein is the usual source of the high levels (up to 0.5 to 3.0 μg. per milliliter) in the circulating blood. Significant exceptions are the carcinoids of the bronchus, ovary, or testis, the secretions of which bypass the liver. Serotonin secreted by the liver tumor is partly inactivated in the lung by monoamine oxidase; endocardial fibrosis and valvular stenosis are observed in 50 per cent of late cases, but chiefly on the right side of the heart. Some tumors (of stomach, pancreas, and bronchus) secrete 5-hydroxytryptophan rather than serotonin. The typical cutaneous flush is thought to result from the action of epinephrine in releasing from the liver tumors both 5-HT and kallikrein, which then lead to the production of bradykinin and the release of histamine from normal tissue stores.

Clinical Manifestations. The most distinctive feature is an episodic *cutaneous flush*, at first dark red and later violaceous, spreading from the face and neck to the chest and extremities, usually several minutes to hours in duration. Associated are feelings of palpitation, giddiness, blurred vision, fullness in the face, and labile blood pressure. Commonly there are simultaneous *midabdominal pain*, watery *diarrhea, wheezing*, and urgency of urination. Such episodes are often precipitated by emotion, physical exertion, eating, or ingestion of alcohol. They may be followed by a persistent telangiectasia in the flush area, and by periorbital edema. Additional findings may include marked enlargement of the liver, enlarged heart, signs of tricuspid or pulmonic stenosis,

marked inanition, and a pellagra-like hyperpigmentation and keratosis of the skin.

Diagnosis. In the presence of characteristic symptoms, markedly elevated urinary excretion of 5-HIAA is diagnostic. The 24-hour output is 50 to 1000 mg. in the carcinoid syndrome, as compared with 2 to 10 mg. in normal persons and 10 to 30 mg. in nontropical sprue. When more than 40 mg. is excreted, development of a purple color with a nitrosonaphthol reagent affords a screening test. False positives may be seen in patients given reserpine or in those eating bananas or pineapples, and mephenesin and phenothiazine drugs interfere with the reaction. Elevated levels of serotonin itself in blood or urine may also be found.

Prognosis. The course is variable, both in the frequency of attacks and the duration of life. Survival for 10 to 20 years with known metastases is recorded. Death comes from heart failure, hepatic decompensation, inanition, or intercurrent infection.

Treatment. Medical treatment includes a diet high in calories and animal protein, supplemented with niacin and other vitamins, and restoration of fluid and electrolyte deficits. Phentolamine, dibenzyline, and prednisone may alleviate the cutaneous flushing, and chlorpromazine and cyproheptadine may reduce diarrhea. Alphamethyldopa is useful in some cases. Surgical resection of both primary and secondary tumor masses, even in the presence of large metastases, is justified by the palliation thus afforded through reduction of serotonin production, and by the prolonged survival of some patients with slowgrowing tumors. (For a full discussion of carcinoid syndrome see Diseases of Endocrine System.)

Leading Article: Humoral basis of carcinoid flush. Lancet, 2:1013, 1966.

Roberts, W. C., and Sjoerdsma, A.: The cardiac disease associated with the carcinoid syndrome (carcinoid heart disease). Amer. J. Med., 36:5, 1964.

Sjoerdsma, A., and Melmon, K.: The carcinoid spectrum. Gastroenterology, 47:104, 1964.

Sjoerdsma, A., Weissbach, H., and Udenfriend, S.: Simple test for diagnosis of metastatic carcinoid (argentaffinoma). J.A.M.A., 159:397, 1955.

Sokoloff, B.: Carcinoid and Serotonin. In Rentchnick, P., (ed.): Recent Results in Cancer Research. Vol. 15. New York, Springer-Verlag, 1968.

Thorson, A.: Studies on carcinoid disease. Acta Med. Scand. Supp. 334, 1958.

CONGENITAL MEGACOLON
(Idiopathic Megacolon; Hirschsprung's Disease)

Definition. The term *megacolon* is often loosely used to describe any unusually dilated, elongated, or redundant colon recognized by barium enema or at laparotomy. Such an appearance may or may not be associated with sluggish motility, and the size of the colon probably has no etiologic importance in constipation. *Congenital megacolon*, or *Hirschsprung's disease*, is a specific disorder of intestinal motility, usually observed in infants, and resulting in severe constipation.

Etiology and Pathology. Congenital megacolon occurs once in 2000 births, more commonly in male children, and with significantly increased frequency in sibs. The basic lesion is a congenital absence of myenteric ganglion cells in a distal segment of the colon, with neighboring autonomic nerve fibers increased in number or size. The aganglionic segment may be located just inside the anal margin or may extend upward a variable distance into the rectum and sigmoid, or less often as high as the distal ileum. Because its muscle is persistently contracted, it presents a functional obstruction to the passage of feces. This narrow, usually empty segment connects by a short conical portion with a greatly dilated, more proximal segment. The dilated segment has normal myenteric ganglia, hypertrophic muscular coats, and normal propulsive activity; it is usually filled with putty-like feces. On the subcutaneous injection of methacholine, the phasic motility of the dilated portion often diminishes, as does that of the distal colon in many normal persons. The narrow segment, because of its disturbed innervation, fails to relax. Megaloureter and megalobladder may be associated abnormalities.

Wherever *Chagas' disease* (South American trypanosomiasis) is prevalent, this disorder is often found as a late complication, due to destruction of the ganglia by the tissue reaction to the parasite.

Clinical Manifestations. Many patients will have had an episode of intestinal obstruction in the first few days of life. After a remission of several weeks or months there is the gradual return of severe and continuous constipation, sometimes with occasional vomiting. Weeks or months may pass without a bowel movement. The abdomen progressively enlarges, the costal margin flares, and colonic peristalsis may be plainly visible. Nutrition is poor and growth may be retarded. A mild anemia is common.

Diagnosis. A plain roentgenogram of the abdomen may reveal the fecal retention as a large ovoid mass mottled by small irregular gas shadows. The narrow segment can be demonstrated on barium enema in the lateral or oblique headdown position. Pressure studies of the anal canal reveal a failure of the normal relaxation of the internal sphincter on distention of the rectum. Final diagnosis presently requires demonstration of absent ganglia on open biopsy of the wall of the narrowed rectum, performed *per anum* under general anesthesia.

Treatment and Prognosis. A large majority of cases of obstinate constipation in infants are of functional origin, and will respond to toilet training as recommended in the article on habitual constipation. In most instances it is advisable to reserve roentgenographic studies for those infants not greatly benefited or relieved by such a regimen.

In a small minority of cases of true megacolon with a very short aganglionic segment near the anus, the colon can be successfully emptied by the daily use of laxatives (magnesia magma, cascara, or senna) and enemas of physiologic saline or soap suds. Rarely, such a patient grows to early adulthood in a fair state of health, but with continuous dependence on these measures.

All the remainder of the cases require surgical relief. The procedure of choice is the resection of the aganglionic segment, with end-to-end anastomosis of the normally innervated upper colon to the stump of the rectum just inside the anus (Swenson's "pull-through" procedure). Histologic study of the segment removed is necessary to ensure that the anastomosis has been made to normally innervated bowel. If this condition is satisfied, the results are lasting and almost uniformly excellent.

Davidson, M., et al.: The pathologic physiology of congenital megacolon. Gastroenterology, 29:803, 1955.

Passarge, E.: The genetics of Hirschsprung's disease. New Eng. J. Med. 276:138, 1967.

Schnaufer, L., et al.: Differential sphincteric studies in the diagnosis of anorectal disorders of childhood. J. Pediat. Surg., 2:538, 1967.

Swenson, O.: Congenital megacolon. Pediat. Clin. N. Amer., 14:187, 1967.

Swenson, O.: Pediatric Surgery. 2nd ed. New York, Appleton-Century-Crofts, 1962, pp. 388-449.

DIABETIC DIARRHEA

Definition. Persistent or episodic watery diarrhea in patients with diabetes represents a now well-defined functional disorder best referred to as diabetic diarrhea. It occurs infrequently, even among diabetics; its importance lies in the social disability imposed by the symptoms and in the availability of striking benefits from therapy.

Etiology and Pathogenesis. This disorder is most frequent among those whose diabetes has been poorly controlled by therapy and is complicated by neuropathy, particularly by other signs of visceral neuropathy, i.e., impotence, urinary incontinence, defects of sweating, pupillary abnormalities, gastric atony, and orthostatic hypotension. Degenerative changes in autonomic ganglia and in dorsal nerve roots have been occasionally observed at postmortem examination. The clinically evident disturbances in motility of the bowel are believed to be associated with defective innervation, which may be confined to afferent pathways. The recent accidental observation of dramatic improvement in some cases with the use of antimicrobial therapy (*vide infra*) has provoked the thought that some substance produced by the normal intestinal flora is directly responsible for the diarrhea.

Clinical Manifestations. The diarrhea in this disorder usually occurs in the form of severe and explosive attacks lasting one to a few days each, and separated by periods of either normal bowel function or constipation of variable severity. Less often, diarrhea is continuous. Movements characteristically are associated with great urgency, often waking the patient from sleep, and the penalty for sound sleep is often fecal incontinence. The stools are voluminous, watery, brown, and foul;

they only rarely contain gross blood. The attacks are associated with little pain, and usually do not lead to serious dehydration or shock.

Physical examination reveals little except collateral evidence of peripheral or autonomic neuropathy (*vide supra*) or of the ocular or vascular complications of diabetes. Gastrointestinal roentgenograms may show atony and delayed emptying of the stomach; the small intestine appears normal in pattern, but passage time may be greatly accelerated or delayed. Chemical examination of the stools may or may not reveal an excess of fat, and the pancreatic juice is normal in volume and enzyme content.

The diagnosis should be suspected whenever explosive watery diarrhea recurs or persists, especially with nocturnal attacks of fecal incontinence. The probability is increased by the finding of neuropathy. The diabetes is not always clinically apparent or previously recognized.

Treatment. Control of the diabetes (maintenance of normal weight through adequate diet and insulin, freedom from ketosis, minimal glycosuria and hyperglycemia) is sufficient to eliminate or substantially diminish the symptoms in about half the cases. Standard medicaments for symptomatic control of diarrhea, including anticholinergics and opiates, are generally ineffective. Recently the tetracyclines have been shown to terminate attacks in a few cases within an hour of the ingestion of a single dose, e.g., chlortetracycline, 250 mg. When diarrhea occurs frequently or continuously, the same dose may be given once daily or even once weekly (see article on Malabsorption).

Prognosis. Even without therapy, this disorder is not progressive in severity, but attacks may be expected to recur with variable frequency over many years or even decades. Severe electrolyte disturbances or dietary deficiencies seldom result. Health and survival are usually limited instead by the other complications of diabetes.

Malins, J. M., and French, J. M.: Diabetic diarrhea. Quart. J. Med. (N. S.), 26:467, 1957.

Rundles, R. W.: Diabetic neuropathy. Medicine, 24:111, 1945.

Whalen, G. E., et al.: Diabetic diarrhea. Gastroenterology, 56:1021, 1969.

MESENTERIC VASCULAR INSUFFICIENCY

Definition. A variety of acute and chronic intestinal disorders result from narrowing or obstruction of the mesenteric vessels. Most familiar is acute infarction of the bowel due to *mesenteric thrombosis* or *embolism*. Less extensive infarcts may be confined to the mucosa and result in *ischemic enteritis* or *colitis*. In recent years the syndrome of *chronic mesenteric arterial insufficiency* has been increasingly recognized and has received the descriptive terms *abdominal angina, midgut ischemia,* and *intestinal claudication.* Inasmuch as this syndrome of insufficiency

may sometimes precede the appearance of an intestinal infarct, it is useful to consider these topics together.

Etiology. Mesenteric vascular disease occurs at all ages and in both sexes, but it is most common and severe in old men. The most common direct causes are, in order of frequency, venous thrombosis, arterial thrombosis, and arterial embolism. Venous thrombosis usually is a complication of abdominal and pelvic infections; not uncommonly, it complicates malignant disease or cirrhosis with portal obstruction. Arterial thrombosis or embolism is seen in advanced atherosclerosis, endocarditis, thromboangiitis obliterans, and polyarteritis. Vascular occlusion is an important complication of mechanical obstruction of the intestine and, less often, of polycythemia vera or the use of oral contraceptive agents. Rarely, it is the result of rupture of or trauma to the mesenteric vessels.

Pathophysiology and Pathology. The mesenteric circulation is rich in collateral channels and may contain a large share of the total body blood volume; local blood volume and flow are extremely labile, however, and may be sharply reduced by vasoconstriction. At low rates of flow the mucosa becomes especially hypoxic, in the face of its high metabolic requirements, because of the collapse of small vessels, increased viscosity, and a countercurrent exchange of oxygen from arteriole to venule.

As a consequence, half the cases of infarction of the bowel are due to *nonocclusive ischemia,* in which the aforementioned processes are set in motion by shock, hypoxia, and congestive heart failure. On the other hand, given time for development of collaterals, major occlusions of the mesenteric vessels are found frequently at autopsy without evidence of present or previous intestinal infarction. Because of the relative paucity of available collaterals, occlusion of the superior mesenteric vessels has the most serious import.

In the slow evolution of intestinal infarction, two stages are recognized. In the first, only the more vulnerable mucosa is involved, necrosis and ulceration leading to mural inflammation, intraluminal hemorrhage, transudation of fluid and electrolytes into the lumen, and spasm of the hypoxic muscle layers. Necrosis may be limited to small patches on the antimesenteric border; the process may heal spontaneously with fibrosis and stricture. In the second, necrosis extends through the entire wall, with paralysis of muscle layers, dilation of the bowel, and serosanguineous fluid in the peritoneum. Shock results from both reduction in blood volume and absorption of bacterial toxins.

In patients with chronic arterial insufficiency the usual findings are atheroma and thrombosis limited to the first few centimeters below the points of origin of these trunks from the aorta. This fact not only explains the effective collateral flow but offers the surgeon an opportunity to restore the circulation. The moderate hypoxia of the intestinal mucosa leads to malabsorption of fat and other nutrients and, by still unknown mechanisms, to disturbances of motility.

Clinical Manifestations. In both the chronic and the acute forms of vascular insufficiency, the symptoms are much more impressive than the physical findings.

The syndrome of chronic or intermittent ischemia includes abdominal pain, weight loss, and diarrhea. The pain is usually periumbilical in location, may be constant, but always is worse in the period from 15 minutes to 3 hours after eating, and in proportion to the size of the preceding meal (intestinal angina). It usually becomes progressively more severe, and the periods of remission between meals gradually disappear. The patient fears food, reduces his intake, and loses weight; nausea and vomiting may also occur. There are changes in bowel habit, more often diarrhea than constipation, and grossly fatty stools are sometimes seen. Physical examination usually reveals only evidence of weight loss and of occlusive arterial disease of the extremities, brain, or heart, but a localized abdominal bruit may also be found. The stools may yield positive tests for occult blood or for excessive fat by chemical analysis. Roentgenograms of the gastrointestinal tract are usually negative, but selective abdominal angiography (especially in lateral projections) may reveal proximal stenoses of the superior mesenteric artery and the other arterial trunks.

The symptoms of mesenteric vascular occlusion may have either an insidious or a dramatically sudden onset. Early in the course, there is severe and generalized abdominal pain and vomiting. The pain is unremitting and almost always is the first symptom. There may be diarrhea, melena, or hematemesis. On examination the abdomen is slightly or moderately distended, and tympany is notably absent. There is variable tenderness and little rigidity; the bowel sounds are hyperactive early, but later disappear. The temperature is at first normal and only later elevated, but the blood leukocyte count is soon elevated to 15,000 to 25,000 per cubic millimeter. Films of the abdomen show very little gas in the bowel but often a "ground-glass" appearance indicative of peritoneal fluid. On aspiration this fluid is found to be serosanguineous. Over the course of a few hours, unless promptly treated, the condition of the patient rapidly worsens; dehydration and shock appear, at first detectable by a rising hematocrit, diminished blood volume, and decreased urinary output.

Segmental or mucosal infarcts of the small intestine may be manifested by periumbilical pain, melena, and vomiting. In the more common event of ischemic colitis, the main features are cramps in the lower abdomen, diarrhea, and grossly bloody stools. On barium enema, the affected segments of colon reveal ulceration and luminal narrowing caused by irregular edema and hemorrhage in the mucosa and submucosa ("thumbprinting").

These lesions and the associated symptoms often resolve in weeks or months, leaving behind asymmetrical strictures sometimes as little as 2 cm. in length.

Diagnosis. Mesenteric arterial insufficiency should be suspected in elderly persons who have evidence of occlusive vascular disease elsewhere and who have characteristic pain, weight loss, and diarrhea but normal gastrointestinal roentgenograms. This condition must be differentiated from gastric ulcer, pancreatitis, other causes of malabsorption, and obstructive lesions such as regional enteritis. Definitive diagnosis may require visceral angiography, exploratory laparotomy, or both. Acute vascular occlusion must be thought of in the differential diagnosis of all acute abdominal emergencies, especially intestinal obstruction, acute pancreatitis, or perforation of a viscus. When characteristic symptoms and signs occur in an elderly man with predisposing vascular disease, small gas shadows on an abdominal roentgenogram, serosanguineous peritoneal fluid, and a rising hematocrit, the diagnosis can be made with considerable confidence. Ischemic colitis and segmental infarction with fibrosis of the small bowel must be differentiated from granulomatous colitis and regional enteritis, respectively. In the former instance, the characteristic localization of the lesion in the sigmoid or in the splenic flexure (where the superior and inferior mesenteric circulations meet) may favor its recognition.

Treatment. Acute vascular occlusion most urgently requires operative intervention, and rapid preoperative restoration of blood volume and fluid and electrolyte losses is essential. The principles and procedures are identical with the preoperative management of intestinal obstruction with strangulation (vide supra). In nonobstructive infarction, the microcirculation may be improved by infusion of low-molecular-weight dextran preparations. Additional measures to be used in the treatment of shock associated with absorption of bacterial toxins include parenteral administration of antimicrobials (penicillin, 2 million units, and streptomycin, 2.0 grams; or ampicillin, 2.0 to 4.0 grams, in divided doses each day) and adrenal corticosteroids (hydrocortisone, 200 to 300 mg. intravenously, then prednisolone, 25 mg. every six hours, or other steroids in equivalent doses).

Surgery in fully developed infarction usually consists of resection of the bowel with immediate or later anastomosis, particularly with venous occlusion. In very early occlusion of a large arterial trunk, embolectomy or even thromboendarterectomy is occasionally feasible. In chronic arterial insufficiency, the stenotic portions of major vessels may be bypassed by a Dacron or a venous graft.

Prognosis. Prognosis in acute vascular occlusion is usually grave; the early mortality is from 60 to 90 per cent. The extensive bowel resections needed to save life often leave in their wake crippling diarrhea and steatorrhea (the "short bowel syndrome"). The lesions of segmental occlusion often undergo virtually complete spontaneous healing.

Conner, L. A.: A discussion of the role of arterial thrombosis in the visceral diseases of middle life based upon analogies drawn from coronary thrombosis. Trans. Ass. Amer. Physicians, 47:67, 1932.

Harkins, H. N.: Mesenteric vascular occlusion of arterial and of venous origin; Report of 9 cases. Arch. Path., 22:637, 1936.

Leading Article: Patterns of intestinal ischemia. Lancet, 2:1222, 1964.

Marston, A., et. al.: Ischemic colitis. Gut, 7:1, 1966.

Mikkelsen, W. P., and Zaro, J. A., Jr.: Intestinal angina. New Eng. J. Med., 260:912, 1959.

Price, W. E., et. al.: Mesenteric vascular diseases (editorial). Gastroenterology, 57:599, 1969.

GASTROINTESTINAL ALLERGY AND FOOD INTOLERANCE
(Food Idiosyncrasy)

Introduction. The gastrointestinal mucosa is rich in lymphocytes and plasma cells and is exposed to a myriad of potential antigens in food, in drugs and other chemicals, and in micro-organisms, resulting in a great variety of antigen-antibody reactions. In addition, it apparently has the capacity to form and react with autoantibodies, as has been postulated in atrophic gastritis. Any and all clinical phenomena resulting from antigen-antibody reactions in the intestinal wall are connoted by the term *gastrointestinal allergy*, and these may include some aspects or some cases of established disease entities of uncertain or variable etiology, e.g., ulcerative colitis. The term *food allergy*, on the other hand, includes all manifestations of hypersensitive reactions to ingested foods, many of which, e.g., urticaria, are in tissues other than the intestine. *Food intolerance* or *food idiosyncrasy* connotes a variety of gastrointestinal disorders attributed in whole or in part to non-allergic mechanisms incited by specific foods or properties of foods.

Pathogenesis and Symptoms. The mucosa is slightly permeable throughout life to whole proteins, but markedly so in the neonatal period, when sensitization of its lymphatic tissue is most likely to occur. Probably as a result of this, many asymptomatic persons have circulating serum precipitins to proteins of cow's milk, hen's eggs, and other foods. Sensitization to chemicals and drugs may occur at any age and may be occult, as when milk from penicillin-treated cows is ingested. In a minority of those sensitized, later exposure to an antigen may give rise to reactions in the gut mucosa characterized pathologically by edema, vascular engorgement, ecchymoses, erosions, excessive mucous secretion, and often spasmodic muscular contractions. The resulting symptoms vary in nature and in time of onset with the segment of gut affected, but commonly include abdominal pain, nausea and vomiting, diarrhea, and mucoid stools. Urticarial eruptions and wheezing may be associated; and in severe cases hematemesis, melena, purpura, arthralgias and prostration may occur (see article on Vascular Hemostatic Mechanisms). In such acute cases recovery is usually prompt and complete, but in others of more insidious onset the course of symptoms is prolonged and highly variable.

Management. The presumptive diagnosis of intestinal allergy often can be made from a careful history, establishing a consistent temporal relationship between exposure to antigen and onset of symptoms. This impression, the more convincing if a single foodstuff is involved, can be confirmed prospectively by a food diary and notation of the time of symptoms, and then can be tested by elimination and reintroduction of the suspected allergen. The latter is best accomplished without the patient's knowledge, by stomach tube or by admixture with barium given for gastrointestinal roentgenograms, permitting (with suitable controls) observation of the motor effects of contact with the allergen. The gastric or colonic mucosa may be directly viewed by endoscopy following exposure to suspected antigens and to control materials. These methods can give valid information if practiced with great care. Skin tests, levels of serum antibodies, and changes in circulating leukocytes are of little value. According to present evidence, the levels of antibodies in the stool or in intestinal secretions (coproantibodies) more closely reflect antigen-antibody reactions in the gut mucosa, and may be diagnostically useful.

Once an offending antigen is recognized, its removal should constitute effective treatment, provided all sources of the antigen can be identified. Food additives, insecticides, and bread molds are examples of sources often difficult to eliminate. In some conditions, e.g., hypersensitivity to milk protein in ulcerative colitis, reaction to the exogenous antigen may constitute but one of many pathogenic factors in the disease, and the results of total exclusion are of doubtful value.

Differential Diagnosis. The symptoms of gastrointestinal allergy are nonspecific and may be mimicked by a wide range of gastrointestinal disorders, most commonly food poisoning and the irritable colon.

Many other reactions to ingestion of food are based on either nonallergic or questionably allergic mechanisms. The inconsistency in the clinical responses to exposure to the postulated food stimulus is based both on variations in the other influences on intestinal function and on the need for a threshold amount of the offending substance to evoke a clinically evident reaction. Some food idiosyncrasies are clearly *spurious* in that they are not, on repeated careful testing, consistently enough evoked by the suspected food. Intolerance of *roughage* is truly rare, and of probable significance only with marked stenosis of the esophagus, the large bowel, an abdominal stoma, or the anus. It should be remembered that food residues constitute only one third to one half of the bulk of the stool. Often certain foods are poorly tolerated because of previous *conditioning*, having been eaten under conditions of anxiety, depression, or disgust. In other instances, *motor disturbances* are brought about by physiologic mechanisms, such as the delayed emptying of the stomach (and feeling of fullness) after a fatty meal, and the osmotically induced distress of the postgastrectomy "dumping" syndrome (see article on Peptic Ulcer).

Most clearly recognized nonallergic mechanisms of intolerance are related to defects of *digestion and absorption.* Gastric achylia may be manifested by a distaste for meat, and pancreatic achylia by steatorrhea on ingestion of fat. Intolerance of wheat, rye, and barley appears to be due to deficiency of a peptidase in the jejunal mucosa (*gluten enteropathy*—see Diseases of Malabsorption), and intolerance of milk seems most often due to *deficiency of intestinal lactase* or, in some infants *sensitivity to cow's milk proteins,* with resulting steatorrhea and severe electrolyte depletion. In the latter instance it is still not clear whether the intolerance is due to hypersensitivity or to defects in peptidase activity. Aside from lactase deficiency, bloating of the abdomen commonly attends the ingestion of beans and other legumes, apparently because of *bacterial fermentation of their nonabsorbable carbohydrates,* such as raffinose. Bloating that follows the eating of onions and cabbage appears to be due to their content of flavone compounds which directly inhibit intestinal motility. Considering the many unknowns in the chemistry of foods, many other nonallergic mechanisms must await discovery.

Fries, J. H.: Gastrointestinal Allergy. *In* Prigal, S. J. (ed.): Fundamentals of Modern Allergy. Blakiston Division, McGraw-Hill Book Co., 1960, pp. 405-411.

Ingelfinger, F. J., Lowell, F. C., and Franklin, W.: Medical progress—Gastrointestinal allergy New Eng. J. Med., 241:303; 337, 1949

Levitt, M. D., and Ingelfinger, F. J.: Hydrogen and methane production in man. Ann. N. Y. Acad. Sci., 150:75, 1968.

Pollard, H. M., and Stuart, G. J.: Experimental reproduction of gastric allergy in human beings with controlled observations on the mucosa. J. Allerg., 13:467, 1942.

Taylor, K. B., and Truelove, S. C.: Immunological reactions in gastrointestinal disease: A Review. Gut, 3:277, 1962.

DIVERTICULA OF THE INTESTINES

These outpouchings of the intestinal wall are, with the exception of Meckel's diverticulum, acquired herniations of the mucosa and submucosa through the muscular layers, which come to lie within the serosa or the retroperitoneal tissues. Because their formation is attributed in part to excessive intraluminal pressure, they are properly considered among the disorders of intestinal motility. Some of their complications are, however, discussed elsewhere (see articles on Inflammatory Diseases of the Intestine and Diseases of Malabsorption).

Diverticula of the small bowel are relatively uncommon, and their frequency decreases from the pylorus to the ileocecal junction. Diverticula of the duodenum have been reported, however, in 2 to 22 per cent of unselected cases at autopsy. In most instances they are found on the lesser curvature of the duodenum and the mesenteric border of the jejunum, at the sites of defects in the muscular wall through which major blood vessels (or the common bile duct) penetrate. In the duodenum they more often number but one or a few, whereas in the jejunum they are commonly multiple. Heterotopic gastric or pancreatic tissue is sometimes recognized in their walls. They are usually found in middle-aged or elderly subjects as an unexpected and clinically silent abnormality on barium roentgenographic studies. In a minority of patients with duodenal diverticula, abdominal pain, nausea, vomiting, and weight loss may occur without other explanation. In a few, hemorrhage, obstructive jaundice, perforation, and peritonitis may be seen. The same complications may rarely be observed in jejunal diverticula, wherein bowel obstruction is sometimes due to inflammatory stricture or muscular thickening. Of particular interest is the association of a form of malabsorption syndrome (a variant of the "blind loop syndrome") with jejunal diverticula, in which stasis of intestinal contents has permitted massive bacterial overgrowth. In the absence of complications, no treatment is required; in severely symptomatic cases, surgical resection is warranted.

Meckel's diverticulum is a common developmental anomaly of the ileum, found in 0.3 to 2.0 per cent of the population, and represents the persistence of the stalk of the fetal yolk sac. It may remain attached to the umbilicus by a fibrous cord or (very rarely) by a patent sinus, and is almost always found 2 to 3 feet above the ileocecal junction on the antimesenteric border. Its wall includes all the layers of the intestine, including the muscularis; its mucosa often contains islands of heterotopic gastric, pancreatic, or colonic glands. Though the majority of these pouches are clinically silent, symptoms may arise in a number of ways: (1) intestinal obstruction, with periumbilical cramps and vomiting, may be caused by intussusception or by volvulus around the fibrous attachment to the umbilicus; (2) impaction of intestinal content may lead to inflammation and ischemic necrosis, both pathologic and clinical features closely resembling those of acute appendicitis; and (3) peptic ulceration may result from the secretion of heterotopic gastric glands, including parietal cells, with resulting pain and often perforation or severe hemorrhage in the form of brick red or mahogany stools. In 60 per cent of instances these symptoms occur before the age of ten; hence this anomaly figures importantly in the differential diagnosis of abdominal pain, the acute abdomen, intestinal obstruction, intestinal bleeding, and peritonitis in childhood.

DIVERTICULAR DISEASE OF THE COLON
(Diverticulosis)

The presence of multiple herniations of the mucosa and submucosa of the colon through the circular muscle layer is commonly referred to as *diverticulosis.* This condition, recognizable during life only at laparotomy or on barium roentgenographic studies, probably affects 20 per cent of the American population over the age of 40 years. Although the majority of those harboring diverticula suffer no ill effects, about 20 per cent have significant symptoms and up to 1 per cent may develop inflammatory complications (*diverticulitis*) of serious import. The entire spectrum of disorders associated with these pouches is connoted by the term *diverticular disease of the colon*.

Prevalence. Both diverticulosis and diverticulitis vary greatly in prevalence in different countries. In North America and northern Europe, the frequency is extremely high, as indicated above; it is approximately 40 times more common than in certain native, nonwhite populations in developing tropical countries. The condition is exceedingly rare below the age of 35, and its prevalence rises steeply as age advances.

Morbid Anatomy and Pathogenesis. A typical diverticulum is a small pouch, the fundus of which measures 3 to 25 mm. in diameter, lying beneath the serosa and connected by a narrow neck with the lumen of the colon. It passes through the muscularis at the points of penetration of blood vessels from serosa to submucosa; hence diverticula commonly form in four parallel rows between the mesenteric and the antimesenteric taeniae. In some instances they appear uniformly distributed from cecum to sigmoid, in others virtually confined to the sigmoid and descending colon. Rarely, one or a few diverticula are found in the right colon alone; significantly the rectum, having an intact longitudinal muscle layer, is never involved. In typical cases the wall of the distal colon is thrown into many thick, arcuate or concertina-like folds, each consisting of a double layer of thickened circular muscle (myochosis); the taeniae are conspicuously shortened. The diverticula appear at the apices of the small intervening haustra.

Their protrusion is attributed to the high intraluminal pressure observed in the affected segments of bowel. Further, the folding of the wall converts the colon into a series of isolated chambers in which high pressures can be confined. In some instances, high pressure and myochosis have been apparently well developed before any significant formation of diverticula, and it is believed that the motility disturbance is the primary change, continuation of which brings about not only herniation of mucosa but also the impaction, vascular congestion, minor necrosis, and perforation which lead to diverticulitis and pericolonic abscess.

Etiology. The cause of the colonic hypermotility is unknown. Because such a change is believed to occur transiently but often in some patients with the "irritable colon," it has been suggested that diverticular disease may be a sequela of that disorder. There appears to be a motor incoordination of the affected segments of bowel, but the neural basis for this has not been recognized by morphologic or physiologic means. The great international variations in prevalence are compatible with the hypothesis that diets high in content of vegetable fiber retard development of diverticula; this is confirmed by dietary experiments on diverticulosis in aged laboratory rats.

Clinical Features. Most commonly, patients experience one or several attacks of griping *pain* in the left lower quadrant or the hypogastrium, lasting one to ten days, with exacerbation after eating. The sigmoid colon in such instances may be felt as a distinct, firm, tender mass. Unless true diverticulitis has developed, rebound tenderness, abdominal rigidity, fever, and leukocytosis are absent. In the intervals between attacks, moderate to severe constipation and a sense of abdominal fullness, relieved by passage of flatus, are commonly reported. Brief episodes of moderate or profuse *rectal bleeding* are not infrequently observed in patients with diverticular disease in the absence of inflammation. These usually cease spontaneously.

The *diagnosis* of diverticular disease depends chiefly upon the barium enema, although the pockets are readily shown following barium by mouth. The deeply folded wall of the distal colon itself gives rise to the "saw-tooth" pattern of the barium outline, and hence this does not constitute evidence for diverticulitis. In view of the high prevalence of diverticula in aged persons, caution must be exercised in attributing rectal bleeding to this source, lest a carcinoma or other more dangerous lesion go undetected.

The *treatment* of early symptomatic diverticular disease is essentially that of the irritable colon with mild constipation. Empirically, a diet high in fruit and vegetable fiber is recommended, together with additional bulk in the form of hydrophilic colloids, such as agar and psyllium seed preparations; but this regimen has not been validated by controlled studies. Relief of pain, if not obtained with warmth to the abdomen, may require use of meperidine. Opiates are contraindicated because they dangerously elevate intracolonic pressures. Antimicrobial drugs should be reserved for clearcut cases of diverticulitis.

Almy, T. P.: Diverticular disease of the colon: The new look. Gastroenterology, 49:109, 1965.
Arfwidsson, S.: Pathogenesis of multiple diverticula of the sigmoid colon in diverticular disease. Acta Chir. Scand., Suppl. 342, 1964.
Fleischner, F. G., and Ming, S.: Revised concepts on diverticular disease of the colon. Radiology, 84:599, 1965.
Morson, B. C.: The muscle abnormality in diverticular disease of the sigmoid colon. Brit. J. Radiol., 36:385, 1963.
Painter, N. S., and Truelove, S. C.: The intraluminal pressure patterns in diverticulosis of the colon. Gut, 5:201, 1964.

Acid-Peptic Disease

Joseph B. Kirsner

PEPTIC ULCER

Definition. Peptic ulcer is a sharply circum scribed loss of tissue, involving the mucosa, submucosa, and muscular layer, occurring in areas of the digestive tract exposed to acid-pepsin gastric juice: the lower portion of the esophagus, the stomach, the first portion of the duodenum, the small intestine adjoining a patent gastroenterostomy, and a Meckel's diverticulum containing functioning gastric glands.

History. Knowledge of gastric ulcer apparently dates to antiquity, and Hippocrates was probably aware of it; but all the accounts were vague until the report of Matthew Baillie in 1793. Cruveilhier in 1829 described the lesion in detail, and Brinton published a comprehensive account in 1857, based upon more than 7000 autopsies. Duodenal ulcer was apparently described in the early part of the nineteenth century, when Benjamin Trotters reported two perforations. John Abercrombie in 1828 and Budd in 1855 noted the occurrence of the pain of duodenal ulcer after meals. Classic reports relating to peptic ulcer include the observations on gastric physiology by Beaumont in 1833 and Walter B. Cannon's description in 1898 of the stomach as observed roentgenologically.

Pathology. Most peptic ulcers occur along the lesser curvature of the stomach and in the first 3 or 4 cm. of the duodenum, the duodenal "bulb." Acute and chronic ulcers differ chiefly in the amount of granulation tissue and fibroplasia. Acute erosions extend only to the muscularis mucosae, and superficial ulcers to the upper portion of the submucosa. They are often multiple, oval, or round, and vary in diameter from several millimeters to 1 or 2 cm. Subacute ulcers involve the mucosa, submucosa, and, occasionally, the muscularis propria. They vary in diameter from 5 to 25 mm. or more; the margins are sharply defined, with overhanging edges. Edema and engorgement are less pronounced than in acute ulcer.

Chronic gastric ulcer usually is single, but may be multiple. The crater is oval or elliptical, with overhanging edges. The diameter varies from several millimeters to several centimeters, and the depth from 10 to 20 mm. or more. The adjacent mucosa may be normal, inflamed, or atrophic. Microscopically, chronic gastric ulcer is a U-shaped defect, extending through mucosa and submucosa to a varying depth in the muscularis propria, and occasionally penetrating the serosal layer to the pancreas or liver. The ulcer base typically comprises four zones: on the surface, a grayish exudate of leukocytes, overlying a zone of fibrinoid necrosis, superimposed upon a layer of granulation tissue, blending with an underlying cicatricial zone. The muscular layer is interrupted completely by the ulceration and by fibrous tissue. Activity and healing coexist in the same lesion. In acute ulcers the blood vessels are normal; in

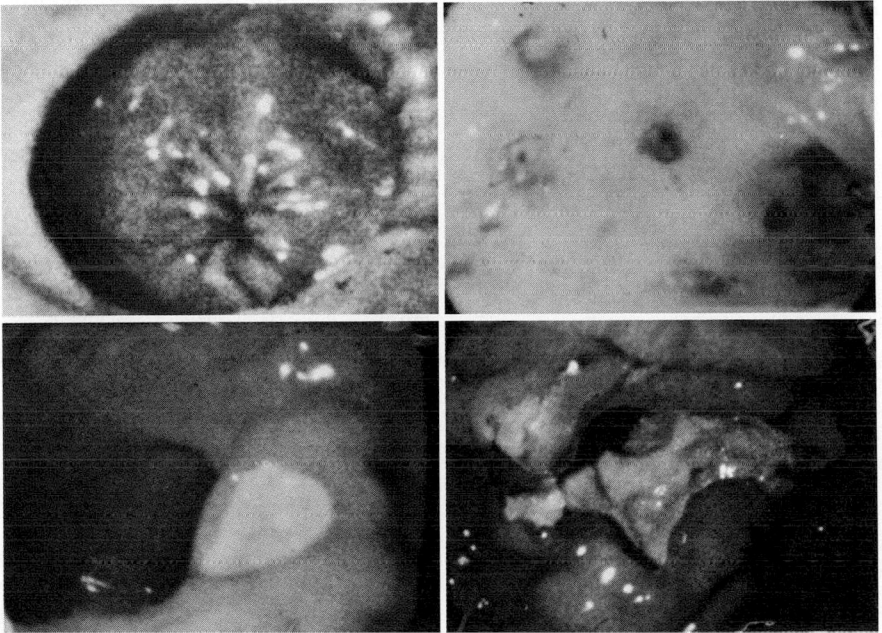

Top left, Normal gastric mucosa (antrum).

Top right, Erosions with active bleeding (antrum).

Bottom left, Benign ulcer, typically round in shape, at the gastric angulus, with a clean whitish base, sharp margin, and surrounding edema.

Bottom right, A deep, large ulcer with an irregular margin in the greater curvature of the upper portion of body of stomach. The upper and lower edges of the ulcer appeared to be eroded into the adjacent mucosa. Irregular thickening of the mucosa and discoloration are visible at the upper edge of anterior aspect in association with bleeding. These findings are compatible with a neoplastic ulcer. (Histologic diagnosis: Reticulum cell sarcoma).

subacute and chronic lesions, the vascular changes may include partially organized thrombi, arteritis, and periarteritis, and subintimal proliferation of connective tissue. There may be inflammation and degeneration of nerve fibers and disappearance of ganglion cells.

Healing of peptic ulcer occurs from below upward, with the growth of granulation tissue and young fibroblasts. In small superficial lesions, healing is complete; the glands regenerate and the muscularis mucosae is re-formed by ingrowth from the periphery. In the healing of large, acute ulcers, the glands are fewer and shorter, and the newly formed mucosa may be thinner than normal. In chronic ulcers, healing is slower; new glands are not formed; and the destroyed muscle, after cicatricial approximation of the severed ends, is replaced by fibrous and elastic tissue.

Incidence and Epidemiology. Peptic ulcer is a disorder of man. Erosions and superficial ulcerations occur spontaneously in many animals, but chronic ulcers are rare. Peptic ulcer is a common disease. The generally accepted incidence, based upon roentgenologic and autopsy surveys, is 10 to 12 per cent. The digestive tract of man everywhere is responsive to an enormous variety of "ulcerogenic" influences, and peptic ulcer is found in all parts of the world. Its occurrence is not correlated consistently with climate or food, or with economic or social class. Geographic and cultural differences exist but fit no particular pattern.

Age Distribution. Peptic ulcer occurs at all ages, but symptoms usually develop between the ages of 20 and 40; the highest incidence is between 45 and 55 years of age. In the newborn, acute ulcerations often are associated with intracranial lesions, sepsis, and burns; there is little tendency to healing, and hemorrhage and perforation are frequent. Peptic ulcer is not uncommon among children; duodenal ulcers predominate. Peptic ulcer, especially gastric ulcer, is frequent among the aged. The craters often are large, and hemorrhage and perforation are common.

Sex Differences. Until puberty, the sex distribution of peptic ulcer is the same; the incidence then increases in both sexes, but much more so in males. After artificial or spontaneous menopause, the incidence of peptic ulcer in women rises. Among adults, males predominate in a proportion of 4:1 for gastric ulcer and 10:1 for duodenal ulcer. The apparent predisposing factors in children with peptic ulcer are the same as those in adults.

ETIOLOGY

The cause of peptic ulcer remains obscure, although much is known of its development and course. Physiologically, peptic ulcer results from the inability of localized areas of the gastroduodenal mucosa to withstand the digestive action of acid-pepsin gastric content. Clinically, chronic peptic ulcer develops only in areas of the digestive tract exposed to acid gastric juice and only in persons secreting hydrochloric acid. Acute, super-

ficial ulcers may develop in an atrophic mucosa apparently not secreting acid, but they do not progress to chronic ulceration. Anacidity developing spontaneously or after gastric irradiation always induces complete healing of peptic ulcer without recurrence for the duration of the achlorhydria.

PATHOGENESIS
Gastric Secretion

The principal constituents of gastric secretion are hydrochloric acid; mucus; the proteolytic enzymes urease, carbonic anhydrase, lysozyme, and lipase; miscellaneous enzymes, including lactic dehydrogenase, B-glucuronidase, glutamic oxaloacetic transaminase, and phosphohexose isomerase; also intrinsic factor; blood group substances; the anions chloride, phosphate, and sulfate; and the cations sodium, calcium, and magnesium; and proteins, including secretion from the surface mucous cells, cytoplasm of desquamated cells, and a transudate of interstitial fluid. The parietal cells transmit their secretion into the lumen through delicate canaliculi, lying between the chief cells, extensions of a system of minute canals within the cell protoplasm. Under optimal conditions, the parietal cells secrete an iso-osmotic or slightly hyperosmotic solution of hydrochloric acid, with an acid concentration approximately between 160 and 170 mEq. per liter. The lower concentrations observed clinically reflect dilution and neutralization by the alkaline component, rediffusion of hydrogen ions into cells in contact with the secretion, and buffering and neutralization by saliva, food, and alkaline intestinal content.

Gastric acid secretion involves a complex interplay of neurogenic, humoral, chemical, and mechanical mechanisms. The energy for the process of acid secretion is probably derived from the oxidation of glucose in the mucosal cells, supplemented by aerobic glycolysis, generating high energy phosphate bonds. Increased secretion of hydrochloric acid, as induced by betazole (Histalog) or gastrin, is associated with a rise, and decreased secretion, as after truncal vagotomy, with a fall in gastric blood flow; extreme reduction in gastric blood flow can inhibit gastric secretion almost completely. Optimal blood concentrations of ions, such as calcium, and probably of hormones, such as adrenocortical steroids, are necessary to normal function of the gastric glands, as for other secretory functions.

Stimulation. The secretion of hydrochloric acid is physiologically a composite of three closely related phases: neurogenic, gastric, and intestinal. The *neurogenic* phase is initiated by stimuli such as the sight, smell, or taste of food acting upon receptors in the cerebral cortex, followed by stimulation of the vagal nucleus, the vagus nerves providing the efferent pathway to the stomach. The vagus nerves play a dominant role in the stimulation of gastric secretion. The basal or continuous secretion of gastric juice in normal man and animals is caused almost entirely by tonic impulses in the vagus nerves. The hormonal mechanism for the stimulation of gastric secretion is almost completely quiescent when there is no food in the stomach or duodenum. The taking of food causes an immediate and profound stimulation of gastric secretion. Impulses in the vagus nerves are aroused reflexly by the sight, odor, and taste of palatable food. These impulses release acetylcholine at the endings of the vagus fibers in the stomach wall, and the transmission of the nervous impulse to the acid and pepsin-producing cells is probably via this humoral agent. If the gastric content in contact with the antral mucosa is not acid in reaction, the vagus impulses also cause a small release of gastrin into the circulation, sufficient to potentiate the stimulating effect of the vagus impulses on the parietal and chief cells. The suggestion that both gastrin and vagus impulses release histamine and that histamine serves as a final common pathway for both of these types of stimulation seems improbable. Gastric juice secreted in response to vagus stimulation is rich in pepsin; that secreted in response to histamine stimulation is poor in pepsin; and that secreted in response to gastrin is intermediary in composition. If the final agent for all three is assumed to be histamine, these differences in the composition of the gastric secretion should not occur.

The *gastric* phase is mediated by the hormone gastrin, secreted by the antrum, in response to (1) distention by food or fluid, (2) vagal stimulation, and (3) contact of the digestive products of protein with the mucosa of the antrum. The release of gastrin in response to feeding is probably attributable to both vagal and local mechanisms. The vagal impulses act directly by stimulation of the gastrin-secreting cells and indirectly by increasing motility of the antrum. The more potent local mechanism is activated by contact of food with receptor cells in the antral mucosa. These cells relay the stimulus to the gastrin cells by reflex arcs which extend into the submucosa and possibly involve Meissner's plexus.

Gastrin, derived from hog antrum, has been characterized as two peptides identical in their amino acid composition and sequence (gastrins I and II). Each preparation is many times more potent than histamine in stimulating gastric acid secretion, when administered subcutaneously in low concentrations. Synthetic pentagastrin in doses of 6 μg. per kilogram of body weight subcutaneously elicits approximately the same volume and output of hydrochloric acid as 40 μg. of histamine or 2 mg. of betazole (Histalog) per kilogram of body weight subcutaneously, and with fewer side effects. Intriguing biologic interrelationships, including immunologic cross-reactivity, have been described for gastrin, pancreozymin-cholecystokinin, and caerulein. Gastrin also increases pancreatic secretion, especially enzyme output, bile flow, and gastric and intestinal motility. When given in high concentrations, gastrin

inhibits acid secretion and increases the output of pepsin.

The *intestinal* phase contributes only 5 or 10 per cent to the total stimulation of gastric secretion in man. It is initiated by the entrance of partly acidified or neutralized food into the small intestine, activating a humoral mechanism, with release of either a hormone resembling gastrin or a stimulant produced by the digestion of food. The target of these secretory stimuli is the parietal cell; varying numbers of these cells respond at a given time, depending upon the physiologic state of the stomach and upon the strength of the stimulus. The total number of responding parietal cells represents the parietal cell mass; and a correlation probably exists between the number of parietal cells and the hydrochloric acid produced in response to maximal doses of histamine, betazole (Histalog), or gastrin.

Inhibition. Gastric secretion may be inhibited under certain emotional conditions, apparently via inhibitory fibers in the vagus and splanchnic nerves and by reflex mechanisms, perhaps involving vasoconstriction. The production of hydrochloric acid is also controlled by at least two autoregulatory mechanisms. The intragastric accumulation of acid to a pH of 1.5 or lower, and, to a lesser degree, within the pH range 1.5 to 3.0, inhibits further release of gastrin by local action upon the antral mucosa, possibly via an inhibitory hormone, or by direct interference with the formation or release of gastrin. Fat in the upper small intestine, in the presence of bile salts and pancreatic lipase, elicits the release of an inhibitory hormone formerly known as *enterogastrone*, but now thought to be secretin. The passage of acid gastric contents into the duodenum causes an inhibition of gastric secretion, mediated at least in part hormonally. Experimentally, pancreatic secretin, heparin, and cholecystokinin inhibit food-stimulated secretion in Heidenhain pouches. Extirpation of the duodenum in whole or in part increases gastric secretion. Experimental operations such as the Exalto and Mann-Williamson procedures, which prevent the acid gastric content from entering the duodenum, cause an increase in gastric secretion through removal of the normal restraint on gastric secretion exerted by the duodenum. The experimental ulcers produced by these operations are in part due to this hypersecretion. Inadequacy of the "duodenal brake" on gastric secretion perhaps is involved in the hypersecretion of gastric juice in patients with peptic ulcer. Clinical procedures such as gastroenterostomy with closure of the pylorus deviate the gastric acid from the duodenum, and this is probably responsible for the poor results of this operation. The superiority of the Billroth I over the Billroth II operation is probably ascribable chiefly to better preservation of the duodenal inhibition of gastric secretion.

Pure acid gastric juice can digest all living tissues, including the stomach, but the gastroduodenal mucosa ordinarily is not exposed to pure gastric juice. The acid is diluted, buffered, and neutralized by swallowed saliva, food and liquid, gastric mucus, and regurgitated intestinal content. The mucus-secreting cells and the overlying layer of mucus provide added chemical and mechanical protection.

In man, gastric secretion is more or less continuous, but the production of hydrochloric acid is not necessarily continuous. The volume of gastric juice secreted daily under fasting conditions in the average normal adult ranges from 1000 to 1500 ml., with an acid concentration of approximately 40 mEq. per liter, but with considerable variation among individuals and in the same person at different times. In duodenal ulcer, the 24-hour volume often exceeds 2000 ml., with an average acid concentration of approximately 40 to 80 mEq. per liter; however, the output of acid may be three to twenty times normal. The volume of secretion in patients with gastric ulcer is similar to that of normal persons, but the concentration of acid usually is lower. The output of acid is lowest in patients with gastric carcinoma. On the average, acid gastric secretion in duodenal ulcer is twofold greater than normal both in the basal state and following maximal stimulation. However, there is substantial overlap in the range of individual values between groups of patients with duodenal ulcer, other gastrointestinal disease groups, and normal persons. The pH in the duodenal bulb is significantly more acid in patients with duodenal ulcer (2.9) than in normal persons (4.5). Hypersecretion in duodenal ulcer is also abnormal in that it persists in the absence of the usual stimuli for gastric secretion, i.e., between meals and during the night. It continues during the healed as well as the active phases of peptic ulcer.

HYDROCHLORIC ACID SECRETION
(AVERAGE VALUES)

	Basal (mEq./hr.)	Maximal Histamine (mEq./hr.)	Nocturnal (mEq./12 hr.)
Normal	2	20	18
Gastric ulcer	4	20	8
Duodenal ulcer	8	35	60
Zollinger-Ellison	30	45	120

Four and possibly five distinct *pepsinogens* and *pepsins* have been identified by chromatography and electrophoresis in the gastric content of man. Vagally mediated influences are the major stimuli for the sustained secretion of pepsin; the output of pepsin also may be increased by gastrin and by large doses of histamine. The output of pepsin is normal in gastric ulcer, but is increased in duodenal ulcer because of the increased volume of secretion. Hydrochloric acid alone is capable of injuring tissue cells; pepsin greatly increases this capacity. Gastric proteolysis is maximal at pH 2.5, but activity persists at several pH ranges. The role of pepsins in the production of peptic ulcer requires further investigation.

Cause of Hypersecretion. The hypersecretion in duodenal ulcer remains incompletely understood.

The basal or continuous secretion of gastric juice in patients with duodenal ulcer is probably of vagal origin since it is abolished when all or nearly all of the vagus fibers to the stomach are divided. Failure to divide all the vagus fibers may result in persistence of hypersecretion and failure of peptic ulcer to heal, suggesting that some intermediary mechanism, possibly Meissner's plexus, exists between the efferent vagus fibers and the parietal cells so that even a small vagus branch can activate the entire glandular apparatus. Anatomically, the hypersecretion of duodenal ulcer is correlated with an increased number of parietal cells. The total number of parietal cells has been estimated as 0.65 billion for gastric ulcer, 0.92 billion for the average normal stomach, and 1.72 billion for duodenal ulcer.

Psychogenic and Neurogenic Influences

In Great Britain and the United States, duodenal ulcer is more frequent among people whose occupations involve administrative and professional responsibility and competitive effort, endeavors which readily generate nervous tension; however, ulcers occur among persons in all occupations. Emotional disturbances are common in patients with peptic ulcer, and the recurrences and complications are often associated in time with periods of sustained anxiety, frustration, or other psychogenic difficulties. These relationships are more apparent in duodenal than in gastric ulcer, and among those with recurrent or complicated lesions than in patients with easily controlled ulcers. The psychogenic difficulties are presumed to predispose to peptic ulceration by increasing gastric secretion via the vagal mechanism and, sometimes, by decreasing tissue resistance. The tensions, strains, and competitive efforts of modern life apparently increase the tonus of the vagus nerves involving both motor and secretory fibers. The long-continued vagal stimulation of the gastric glands produces hyperplasia and hypertrophy with resultant increase in the parietal cell mass. Experimentally, fear in monkeys and dogs and conscious anxiety in man may be accompanied by increased gastric secretion, engorgement, and friability of the gastric mucosa. The importance of the vagal pathway is indicated by the decrease in acid production and in secretory responsiveness to psychologic stress after truncal vagotomy. On the other hand, psychogenic tension does not always cause gastric hyperfunction. Acidity may increase during emotional tension, but the effect disappears upon removal of the stimulus, whereas the hypersecretion of duodenal ulcer continues despite prolonged psychotherapy.

Tissue Resistance

The normal resistance of the stomach and duodenum to acid and other traumatic influences involves at least five components: (1) the integrity of the mucosal cells, (2) the rapid, continuous regeneration of epithelium, (3) the mucous barrier, (4) the abundant vascular supply, and (5) the permeability of the gastroduodenal mucous membrane. Unidentified protective factors within the gastroduodenal wall and secretory inhibitors in the gastric content probably contribute to this defense. Prolonged exposure to large amounts of hydrochloric acid and pepsin may decrease cellular resistance, but localization of the ulcer then remains unexplained. The *absence* of chronic gastric ulcer in patients with *pernicious anemia* and severe *gastric atrophy* indicates that atrophy alone is insufficient for chronic ulceration; hydrochloric acid and pepsin are also required. Indeed, the atrophic mucosa retains considerable potential for regeneration, as indicated by the healing of most gastric ulcers.

The gastric mucous barrier consists of three integrated units: (1) the layer of viscous mucus covering the mucosa, (2) the underlying tall columnar cells, and (3) the low cuboidal and columnar cells lining the crypts of the gastric glands. Gastric mucus, a complex mixture of mucopolysaccharides and mucoproteins, is secreted continuously, and its capacity to absorb pepsin, to neutralize and buffer acid, and to physically resist digestive activity is an important defense. An abnormality in secretion of mucus has not been demonstrated in human peptic ulcer but has been implicated in experimental ulceration induced with steroids, indomethacin, and other drugs in dogs. There is no evidence of decreased mucosal cell regeneration in peptic ulcer. The hypothesis implicating an increased concentration of acetylcholine in the gastroduodenal mucosa, with degranulation of mast cells and the release of vasoactive substances, including histamine and heparin, increasing local capillary and mucosal permeability, is unproved. Reflux of bile into the stomach after the taking of food has been implicated in the local tissue injury, especially in the development of gastric ulcer. The reflux of bile has been ascribed to reduced antral pressure, increased intraduodenal pressure, uncoordinated antral-duodenal motility, or to a combination thereof; but as yet supporting evidence is indecisive.

The stomach and duodenum are abundantly supplied by freely anastomosing blood vessels; but the submucous vascular plexus and the arteriovenous anastomoses, under autonomic nervous control, are capable of rapidly diverting blood from the mucosa, theoretically creating areas of ischemia. However, while attractive theoretically as a factor in decreased tissue resistance, focal ischemia of the stomach or duodenum has not been demonstrated in patients with peptic ulcer. The evidence for a vascular component in the pathogenesis of peptic ulcer in man is inconclusive. The association of peptic ulcer and atherosclerotic cardiovascular disease represents selected coincidence rather than causal relationship. Present statistical analyses indicate a negative correlation between peptic ulcer and cardiovascular disorders, and vascular disease directly involving the stomach is exceedingly rare. The microcirculatory changes in experimental gastric ulceration are nonspecific and are those to be expected in vessels anywhere exposed to trauma and chronic inflammation. When gastric juice is buffered to an alkaline pH, vascular changes do not develop after the administration of histamine in susceptible animals. Ulcers can be induced experimentally by vasoactive drugs but also by vasoconstrictor compounds. Ligation of 90 per cent of the nutrient arteries to the stomach does not lead to chronic ulceration. Local failure of the circulation may contribute to lowered tissue resistance to ulceration, but as yet has not been demonstrated as a significant antecedent event. Furthermore, the tendency of peptic ulcer to enlarge, bleed, and perforate indicates a penetrating process, originating in the mucosa and extending through the gastric wall, a course of events incompatible with vascular infarction.

The acute, multiple ulcerations of the upper digestive tract complicating *central nervous system lesions,* including *intracranial hemorrhage, burns, overwhelming infection, myocardial infarction, surgery,* and *shock* have been attributed to several mechanisms mediated through the posterior hypothalamus. Cholinergic and adrenergic neurohormonal agents are liberated, causing vasospasm and tissue anoxia, and thus increasing the susceptibility to acid-pepsin digestion. Hypersecretion, ascribable to parasympathetic stimulation, also may be noted. Corticotrophin is released from the anterior pituitary and stimulates the adrenal cortex to release steroids, with possible harmful effects upon the mucosa of the upper digestive tract.

Gastritis, Gastric Mucosal Atrophy, and Peptic Ulcer

All types of *chronic gastritis* are demonstrable gastroscopically and by gastric biopsy in association with peptic ulcer. Atrophy is more frequent in gastric than in duodenal ulcer, whereas a hyperplastic hypertrophic mucosa is more common in duodenal than in gastric ulcer.

Gastric atrophy is characterized by progressive secretory failure involving hydrochloric acid, pepsin, and, finally, intrinsic factor. Atrophy of the gastric mucosa is invariably present in *pernicious anemia* and *gastric polyposis*, and frequently in patients with *tropical sprue, pellagra,* and *iron deficiency anemia.* Gastric atrophy not only leads to pernicious anemia, but may also predispose to carcinoma. Duodenal ulcer is not associated with complete atrophy of the gastric mucosa.

Small amounts of IgG, IgM, and IgA are found in the normal gastric mucosa but are increased, especially IgA, in atrophic gastritis, as a corollary of the increased number of immunoglobulin-producing plasma cells. The number of IgA-containing cells may be decreased in pernicious anemia, perhaps predisposing to the gastric mucosal damage. Antibodies to incompletely defined cytoplasmic constituents of parietal cells are found in the serum of a large proportion of patients with pernicious anemia, less frequently in patients with chronic gastritis, and rarely in persons with an unequivocally normal gastric mucosa. The antibodies are 7S gamma globulins and comprise both IgA and IgG. So-called blocking or binding antibodies or both, to intrinsic factor are found in the serum of patients with adult pernicious anemia and malabsorption of vitamin B_{12}. They are generally not demonstrable in atrophic gastritis without vitamin B_{12} malabsorption, in postgastrectomy gastritis, and in normal persons. The immunologic differences between secretory IgA-binding antibody to intrinsic factor in the gastric juice of a patient with pernicious anemia and the autologous serum IgG antibodies to intrinsic factor suggest that these antibodies are products of different immunologic systems. The occasional improvement in the gastric mucosa following the administration of adrenal corticosteroids, with increased secretion of intrinsic factor and improved absorption of vitamin B_{12}, further supports an immunologic mechanism in the development of the gastric lesion. The immunoglobulin deficiency noted in very occasional patients with early or overt pernicious anemia, with an absence of antibodies to parietal cells or to intrinsic factor, suggests a delayed type of cellular immune mechanism.

Hypertrophic gastritis is characterized by hypertrophy of the gastric mucosa involving all glandular elements, parietal, chief, and mucous cells. There may be increased secretion of gastric hydrochloric acid, pepsin, and mucoprotein, or decreased outputs of acid and pepsin. The condition may be demonstrable roentgenographically and by gastroscopy as a pronounced enlargement of the gastric folds. Hypertrophic, "hypersecretory" gastritis occurs alone, as well as in association with duodenal ulcer and with the *Zollinger-Ellison syndrome*. The cause is unknown, but presumably involves factors stimulating gastric mucosal growth and function.

Menetrier's disease is characterized by giant hypertrophy of the gastric mucosa. The gastric folds are enlarged up to 1 cm. in width and 3 to 4 cm. in height, and may resemble the cerebral convolutions. The histologic features include hyperplasia of the surface epithelium, with elongation of foveolar pits; normal or decreased numbers of parietal cells; increased numbers of mucous cells; infiltration with polymorphonuclear leukocytes, lymphocytes, and eosinophils; and edema and thickening of the submucosa and muscularis mucosae. Symptoms include *epigastric distress, anorexia, nausea,* and *weight loss.* A striking feature is the excessive loss of protein, mostly albumin, into the gastric secretion, resulting in chronic *hypoproteinemia,* with *edema* and *ascites* (see article on Malabsorption). Roentgenographic and gastroscopic examinations demonstrate enlarged, tortuous mucosal folds. The cause is unknown. Treatment includes supportive measures, including the replacement of albumin.

Endocrine Relationships

There is no causal relationship between the ordinary peptic ulcer and primary endocrine disorders. However, certain endocrine (humoral) abnormalities may be associated with refractory peptic ulcer and extreme gastric hypersecretion.

The *Zollinger-Ellison syndrome* is characterized by single or multiple non-beta islet cell adenomas of the pancreas; enormous outputs of hydrochloric acid and pepsin; single or multiple ulcers in the esophagus, second, third, and fourth portions of the duodenum, and in the jejunum and ileum, in addition to the stomach and duodenal bulb; and refractoriness to medical or surgical treatment, other than total gastric resection. The parietal cell mass has been estimated as sixfold greater than normal and threefold larger than in patients with the usual duodenal ulcer. Gastric rugae and mucosal folds in the small intestine often are enlarged. Although the syndrome is relatively uncommon, it is not rare, more than 700 cases having been recorded to the present time. The disorder is more common in men, the ratio being six males to four females. It occurs in all age groups, but especially during the third to fifth decades.

Ulcer pain is present in approximately 95 per cent of patients. Symptoms exceed one year in duration in more than 80 per cent and range from five to ten years in duration in 30 per cent. Atypically located and multiple peptic ulcers (esophagus, distal duodenum, and jejunum) strongly suggest the disorder. However, three fourths of the ulcers in the Zollinger-Ellison syndrome are not atypically located and are not multiple. Jejunal and gastric ulcers develop in most patients treated by partial gastric resection. They often are multiple, usually are penetrating, and frequently perforate. Although early case reports emphasized the severe, occasionally dramatic complications of atypically located peptic ulceration, the symptoms are often indistinguishable from those of ordinary peptic ulcer, until operation removes the anatomic integrity of the stomach and duodenum and disrupts normal homeostatic mechanisms controlling acid gastric secretion. The course then usually, although not invariably, becomes more complicated, with severe ulcer pain, complicated by bleeding and perforation, the entire sequence occasionally developing very rapidly after limited ulcer surgery.

Diarrhea occurs in approximately one third of patients and may not be associated with peptic ulcer. The picture includes a profuse watery diarrhea without steatorrhea, causing symptomatic and often fatal hypokalemia and dehydration; secretion of hydrochloric acid is low or absent. Hypokalemic metabolic acidosis and dehydration occur frequently in this group, and hypokalemic nephropathy may be an initial manifestation of the syndrome. Steatorrhea is not uncommon in those patients with peptic ulcer disease and is attributable to multiple factors; acid inactivation of pancreatic lipase and precipitation of bile salts, both causing defective micelle information. Direct injury to the intestinal mucosa by the excessive hydrochloric acid and "acid injury" to the vitamin B_{12}-intrinsic factor complex have also been implicated.

Occasionally, there is no adenoma in the pancreas, but an increased number of islets and a higher proportion of non-beta to beta cells. Approximately 60 per cent of the tumors are malignant. The adenomas have a low grade of malignancy; but, like carcinoids, they may metastasize to the liver. They occur anywhere in the pancreas, but especially in the body and tail. Aberrant adenomas may be found in the hilus of the spleen, in the gastric wall, and along the lesser curvature of the second portion of the duodenum.

The most characteristic laboratory finding is the enormous "basal" secretion of hydrochloric acid, exceeding 200 ml. or 20 mEq. of hydrochloric acid per hour, with a comparatively small increment (less than 60 per cent) following maximal stimulation by histamine, Histalog, or pentagastrin. The volume of the 12-hour nocturnal gastric secretion averages 2000 ml., with recorded volumes up to 5 and 10 liters. Low gastric acidity, however, has been observed in approximately 5 per cent of patients, and the basal versus stimulated outputs of hydrochloric acid may bear the usual relationship, though the quantities of acid are large.

The gastric hypersecretion is humoral in origin, gastrin having been extracted from the pancreatic adenoma and from metastases in the liver, duodenum, or lymph nodes and identified immunochemically with the amino acid constituents of human gastrin types I and II. The carboxyl–terminal tetrapeptide amide, Try-Met-Asp-Phe-NH_2, is the biologically active component of gastrin, producing the full spectrum of actions of gastrin, but is, on a molar basis, only about one fifth as potent. Antibodies to gastrin have been produced by immunization with the C-terminal tetrapeptide amide of gastrin conjugated to carrier protein macromolecules. These antibodies react equivalently on a molar basis with the C-terminal tetrapeptide amide, the gastrin-like pentapeptide amide, and with a variety of intact gastrin molecules. Utilizing fluoresceinated antibodies to human gastrin I, it has been possible to localize gastrin within mucosal cells of the antrum of man and the hog. Immunofluorescence is restricted to numerous conspicuous cytoplasmic granules in differentiated interspersed mucosal cells present along the course of pyloric antral glands. The gastrin-producing cell in the antrum has not been identified conclusively; but interest has focused upon the D (delta) cell (the third type of cell in the pancreas, the other cells designated as alpha and beta). Electron microscopy reveals characteristic granules 150 to 250 μ in size, intermediate in electron density between the granules of the alpha and beta cells. Histochemically, similar "G" cells also have been noted in the antral pyloric area of the stomach. The staining properties of granules stored in G cells suggest the presence of an acid protein with many side chain carboxyl groups, in accord with the chemical properties of gastrin. The identity or possible interrelationship of the D and G cells and their role in the production of gastrin remain to be determined.

Although not available generally at present, diagnostic bioassay techniques of serum, gastric juice, and urine have been developed, based upon the capacity of the test biologic fluid to stimulate gastric acid secretion in animal preparations (rat, dog). The radioimmunoassay for serum gastrin provides a more sensitive and more accurate diagnostic method. With this technique, fasting serum from patients with the Zollinger-Ellison syndrome contains gastrin levels tenfold or higher than normal. Normal fasting levels of gastrin by this technique range from 10 to 300 picograms per milliliter, with a mean of 100 picograms. Similar levels apparently are found in "ordinary" peptic ulcer. In both normal persons and in patients with peptic ulcer, gastrin levels increase with age. The range in patients with the Zollinger-Ellison syndrome is 800 to 165,000 picograms. Serum levels of gastrin in three patients with histologically verified Zollinger-Ellison syndrome were 3550, 7880, and 21,000 picograms, respectively. Since some Zollinger-Ellison tumors apparently secrete intermittently, repeated analyses may be required for diagnosis. Serum gastrin levels also appear to relate directly to the plasma calcium concentration, decreasing with hypocalcemia after parathyroidectomy and increasing with infusions of calcium but not of parathormone. The humoral abnormality in the Zollinger-Ellison syndrome is not limited to the overproduction of gastrin. Blood and urine levels of various biologically active amines also may be elevated. Definite diagnosis may be established at abdominal operation by examination of the pancreas with biopsy, exploration of the duodenum for aberrant tumors, and biopsy of abdominal lymph nodes.

The Zollinger-Ellison ulcer and its complications are not controlled by the usual antacid and antisecretory therapy, by gastric irradiation, or by surgery, including vagotomy with pyloroplasty, gastroenterostomy or antrum resection, or subtotal gastrectomy. Local excision of the tumor may be considered with an adenoma in the pancreas or wall of the duodenum, when there are no evident lymph node or distant metastases. However, removal of a tumor nodule alone is usually fruitless since diffuse hyperplasia of the non-beta cells occurs in 10 per cent, the tumors are multiple in one third of cases, and metastases are present in the remaining cases. The treatment of choice at present, therefore, is complete removal of the stomach. Total gastrectomy should be performed despite the presence of multiple metastases because these tumors are often not fatal, and, in fact, may regress. Further, patients with the Zollinger-Ellison syndrome often maintain good nutrition after total gastrectomy, in contrast to individuals with gastric cancer undergoing the same operation. Active immunization with the gastrin tetrapeptide may induce resistance in rats to the acid-secretory effects of exogenous gastrin. This technique and the possible development of specific gastrin antagonists eventually may provide an effective medical approach to the gastrin-mediated hypersecretion of hydrochloric acid by patients with the Zollinger-Ellison syndrome.

Polyendocrine adenomatosis (Wermer's syndrome) is a familial disorder characterized by the presence of multiple tumors or hyperplasia of several endocrine glands. The parathyroid glands are most frequently involved, followed by the pancreatic islets, pituitary, adrenals, and thyroid glands. Bronchial and intestinal carcinoid tumors, pheochromocytomas, and lipomas are included in the syndrome. The adenomas may or may not be hormonally active in one or more glands and in any combination. Peptic ulcer is present in more than 50 per cent of cases; the sexes are affected equally; and the disease has been described in all age groups after the first decade, with the peak occurrence in the third and fourth decades. Multiple endocrine adenomatosis appears to have a genetic basis attributable to the action of an autosomal dominant gene of high penetrance. Approximately one half of the ulcers are multiple and in atypical locations. The most common presenting feature of the syndrome is peptic ulcer and its complications. Symptoms of hypoglycemia are next in frequency. *Acromegaly, pituitary dwarfism, hypogonadism, Cushing's syndrome, hyperaldosteronism,* and *hyperthyroidism* may occur alone and in any combination. Perforation, obstruction, and hemorrhage are common. Diarrhea and steatorrhea occur in 10 per cent of patients in association with ulcer. Although gastrin has been extracted from the pancreatic adenomas, all attempts to isolate gastrin or a gastric secretogogue from adenomas of other endocrine glands have failed. The peptic ulcer associated with polyendocrine adenomatosis seems identical in all respects to that of the Zollinger-Ellison syndrome. On the basis of present information, therefore, it perhaps is justifiable to regard some cases of the Zollinger-Ellison syndrome as the "gastrin-secreting, pancreatic islet-cell tumor component" of polyendocrine adenomatosis. Treatment of each endocrine abnormality follows the usual measures; management of the ulcer in polyendocrine adenomatosis is the same as for the Zollinger-Ellison syndrome. (See section on Diseases of the Endocrine System.) The incidence of duodenal ulcer is reportedly increased in patients with parathyroid adenomas and hyperparathyroidism, without pancreatic adenomas, especially among men; however, other studies do not substantiate this finding. Acute ulcers may develop during adrenocortical insufficiency, but they heal rapidly when function is restored. Peptic ulcers are not more frequent in patients with adenocortical hyperfunction, such as Cushing's syndrome.

Genetic Considerations

The striking incidence of peptic ulcer in some families, the frequency of ulcers among living sibs of ulcer patients, and the occasional ulcers in homozygous twins indicate genetic influences. The male predominance and the occurrence of peptic ulcer in only 10 to 15 per cent of the population also suggest an individual predisposition. Patients with duodenal ulcer appear to have increased taste sensitivity to 6-n-propylthiouracil, a bitter-tasting phenylthiourea. This observation, also suggesting a genetic aberration, is of interest in relation to the distribution of blood groups in patients with peptic ulcer.

Blood Groups

People with blood group O appear to develop duodenal ulcer more often than persons of groups A, B, and AB, a trend documented in many countries and among various races and nationalities. Blood group substances A and B are group-specific, but blood group substance H is not group-specific and can be found in the saliva of all secretors, regardless of their ABO blood group distribution. Persons capable of secreting A, B, and H substances in saliva, approximately 75 per cent of the population, are called *secretors;* and those without A, B, and H, 25 per cent, are called *nonsecretors.* Nonsecretors usually produce more of another blood group substance, *Lewis,* than do secretors, and the total content of blood group substances in the saliva is not decreased. Blood group and secretor status are inherited separately. Nonsecretors apparently are more liable to duodenal ulcer than secretors, independent of blood group status. The incidence of duodenal ulcer is significantly higher in those with blood group O who are "nonsecretors" than in persons with blood group O who are "secretors;" this relationship is more pronounced with stomal ulcer. The nature of this curious susceptibility is unknown. The ABO and secretor genes are not associated with an increased tendency to gastric hypersecretion.

Association of Peptic Ulcer with Other Diseases

Peptic ulcer occurs in association with practically all diseases except those characterized by complete anacidity, particularly *pernicious anemia.* Active gastric or duodenal ulcer may coexist with *gastric carcinoma.* The incidence of peptic ulcer is probably not excessive in cirrhosis of the liver, but increases after the establishment of *portacaval shunts.* The gastric hypersecretion is attributed to failure of the bypassed liver to inactivate histamine or a similar stimulant, possibly blood ammonia or an amino acid combination produced in the small intestine, especially after protein meals. The hypersecretion is not lowered by vagotomy or antrum resection jejunectomy, iliectomy, or colectomy, or by altering the intestinal flora with neomycin, but it can be decreased by fasting.

Chronic peptic ulcer is frequent in patients with *chronic pulmonary disease,* including obstructive emphysema and tuberculosis associated with CO_2 retention, and in patients with ischemic heart disease. The ulcers are principally duodenal, and complications, including hemorrhage and perforation, are common. They occur often without past history of ulcer disease, and develop rapidly. Peptic ulcer occurs in at least 20 per cent of patients with *rheumatoid arthritis.* The incidence of severe *atherosclerosis* and *coronary occlusion* appears to be increased in some surveys of patients with peptic ulcer, but the incidence of mild atherosclerosis and coronary artery disease appears similar to that in the general population. There are no unique anthropometric features in peptic ulcer; persons with all types of body build are affected.

Drug-Induced Peptic Ulcer

Peptic ulcer, with hemorrhage or perforation, may develop during the use of numerous therapeutic agents. The exact incidence and the etiologic relationships are difficult to determine because of differences in groups studied, concomitant or previous medication, emotional influences, and other factors. The mechanism of drug-induced peptic ulceration includes stimulation of gastric acidity and decreased mucosal resistance, possibly involving angiospasm. The initial and major effect of adrenergic blocking agents and reserpine is to increase gastric secretion; an accompanying vasospasm may contribute by diminishing tissue resistance. *Phenylbutazone* (Butazolidin), *cinchophen, colchicine, salicylates, indomethacin* (Indocin), and *tolbutamide* lower resistance by producing a hemorrhagic, erosive gastritis and duodenitis. The ulcerogenic mechanism for caffeine includes both the acid and tissue effects.

Acetylsalicylic acid is the most common cause of drug-induced injury to the gastroduodenal mucosa in man. The acute gastric mucosal injury is prevented by administering the acetylsalicylic acid with an alkaline solution, suggesting the un-ionized acid, rather than its sodium salt, as the irritant. The presence of hydrochloric acid is therefore important in the development of aspirin-induced gastric lesions. Acetylsalicylic acid damages the mucosal barrier as it is absorbed, apparently by disrupting the lipid-protein layer on the surface of the cells and breaking the tight junction between cells. The mucosa becomes abnormally permeable to water-soluble compounds and ions. The liberation of histamine and other products of cell injury increases the permeability of the gastric mucosa and the vulnerability of the capillaries. Hydrogen ions diffuse back through the more permeable gastric mucosa, and large amounts of interstitial fluid, sodium and potassium ions, and plasma proteins enter the gastric lumen. The back diffusion of acid injures capillaries and venules, causing bleeding; it may account in part also for the apparent gastric hyposecretion in gastric ulcer and in drug-induced

peptic ulceration. Experimental evidence suggests that the injurious effects of acetylsalicylic acid and other organic acids are also attributable in part to a decrease in the mucus content of the stomach. The drug-induced ulcer may be a new lesion or reactivation of a previous ulcer.

The frequency of peptic ulcer during the use of corticotrophin and adrenal corticosteroids is not known precisely. It ranges up to 30 per cent, increasing with large doses and prolonged administration. The ulcers are frequently gastric in location and occur on the greater as often as on the lesser curvature of the stomach. Experimentally, corticotrophin and adrenal corticoids may increase the gastric secretory response. Clinically, gastric secretion may increase, but not consistently, and the output of acid is often normal. Decreased resistance of the gastroduodenal mucosa is apparently more important in the development of steroid and aspirin-induced ulcerations and probably of other drug-induced ulcers, perhaps related in part to an alteration in the gastric mucous barrier. "Steroid ulcers" are more frequent in patients with rheumatoid arthritis and lupus erythematosus, and are uncommon in patients with bronchial asthma, pemphigus, or ulcerative colitis receiving comparable amounts of steroid for long periods. There is no apparent correlation with the type, dosage, or duration of steroid therapy. Symptoms may be typical or atypical, and the initial manifestation may be bleeding or perforation. The ulcer may heal rapidly during antacid therapy, although steroids are continued.

CLINICAL, LABORATORY, AND ROENTGENOGRAPHIC MANIFESTATIONS OF PEPTIC ULCER: DIAGNOSIS

Symptoms

The patient with a peptic ulcer characteristically complains of an aching, burning, cramplike or gnawing sensation, or a sense of fullness or pressure in the epigastrium or upper abdomen, often associated with an unpleasant sense of hunger. The pain may be mild or severe. Characteristically, it is steady rather than intermittent, continuing for a half hour to several hours unless relieved by food or antacid. It occurs in definite relationship to eating. Pain during or soon after a meal may suggest *esophageal ulcer;* pain 30 to 60 minutes later, a *gastric ulcer;* and distress two or three hours later, a *duodenal ulcer;* but, except perhaps for esophageal ulcer, the time sequences are not sufficiently precise to localize the lesion. Ulcer pain is typically absent in the morning before breakfast, unless it has recurred during the night or gastric secretion is enormous. Pain during the night occurs one to four hours after retiring, usually between midnight and 3 A.M., unless the patient has eaten late or in some other way has disturbed the usual routine. It is more likely to reappear if present earlier in the evening and controlled by an antacid; once relieved, the noctural distress ordinarily does not recur. Nocturnal pain denotes a sensitive ulcer and gastric hypersecretion; although it accompanies obstructing or penetrating ulcers, it is not pathognomonic of these complications.

Cause of Ulcer Pain. The pain of peptic ulcer is caused by the hydrochloric acid in the gastric content. The acid induces a chemical inflammation, lowering the pain threshold of the nerve endings in the margins and base of the ulcer. Vascular engorgement, with and without acute inflammation, further decreases the threshold for pain. In uncomplicated ulcer, the pain is a true visceral sensation, arising at the lesion and transmitted to the central nervous system by the splanchnic nerves. The pain mechanism remains intact after complete vagotomy, but is abolished by interruption of the splanchnic nerves. Abnormal motility, hyperperistalsis, or increased intragastric pressure is not the cause of ulcer distress, as indicated by the absence of pain in obstruction of the pylorus or duodenum, with powerful peristaltic waves distending the stomach. However, peristalsis or spasm of muscle fibers may increase the distress.

The disappearance of pain during anticholinergic medication is not ascribable to vagal inhibition or decreased gastrointestinal motility, but to delayed gastric emptying and failure of hydrochloric acid to reach the ulcer. The absence of pain in some instances and the occurrence of hemorrhage or perforation without antecedent pain are difficult to explain except on the basis of an individually high pain threshold and very rapid development of the ulcer. Peptic ulcer may penetrate rapidly with little or no pain. Further, blood may protect the crater against the action of acid.

Location of Pain. The site of peptic ulcer cannot be predicted accurately by the location of the pain. Ulcer distress is usually localized in the epigastrium, in an area 3 or 4 cm. in diameter. The pain in gastric ulcer is often situated to the left of the midline or in the left upper quadrant. In *duodenal ulcer*, it is ordinarily to the right of the midline, halfway between the umbilicus and xiphoid or slightly above the umbilicus; occasionally, it is referred toward the left upper quadrant or the right lower quadrant. Ulcers located high on the *lesser curvature of the stomach* may cause distress in the anterior chest. Gastric ulcers accompanying esophageal hiatal hernia may produce pain below the xiphoid, with substernal radiation. The pain of *esophageal ulcer* is also noted in the substernal or subxiphoid area. In *postbulbar ulcer*, the pain may be in the right upper quadrant, penetrating to the back; and relief from antacids is less prompt. The distress of *jejunal ulcer* may be in the left mid-abdomen, left lower quadrant, or hypogastrium. Infrequently, ulcer pain occurs only in the back, at the level of the eighth to tenth dorsal vertebrae; this localization may accompany chronic penetration, but is not pathognomonic of it.

Chronicity and Periodicity. In addition to rhythmicity and response to measures neutralizing gastric acidity, ulcer distress is characterized by chronicity and periodicity. The duration of symptoms may be only several days or weeks or may extend for 20 or 30 years and longer; the usual history averages between 5 and 8 years. Periodicity is the tendency for gastric and duodenal ulcer to reappear daily for several weeks, subside for months or years, and then recur. The periods of distress may last only several days or weeks, but may often continue for several months. In some patients, exacerbations may be confined to the spring and autumn, but they occur at all times of the year. The periodicity of peptic ulcer is not correlated with the level of gastric secretion. Its occurrence in all parts of the world, with varying peak incidences, excludes climatic factors. With the passage of time, the episodes of ulcer pain often increase in frequency, severity, and duration. Periodicity tends to disappear with obstructing or penetrating ulcers. However, progression is not inevitable, for in many patients recurrences become less frequent and less severe; eventually, the ulcer may heal completely.

Atypical Manifestations. The typical ulcer history usually is so characteristic as to be diagnostic. Atypical symptoms are ascribable to an incomplete history, to individual variations in pain threshold, and occasionally to complications. Nausea and vomiting, with little or no pain, may follow the same relationship to food-taking as typical ulcer distress; nausea alone, however, is an infrequent manifestation of active ulcer. Vomiting also occurs in the absence of obstruction when ulcer pain is severe, perhaps because of a reflex neuromuscular disturbance. It may also be noted when the ulcer is in the *pyloric canal*. At this site, the clinical picture is otherwise very similar to that of duodenal ulcer. With acutely inflamed ulcers, the relief from food or antacid may be transitory. Ulcer pain may occur in isolated episodes, radiating to the right upper quadrant or back and may be accompanied by vomiting, as in biliary colic. The anorexia and weight loss of elderly patients may suggest malignant disease. Symptoms in the young child often lack relationship to eating and periodicity; the abdominal pain may be periumbilical or generalized; refusal to eat and vomiting are common manifestations. The symptoms of peptic ulcer in older children are more typical. In *Meckel's* diverticulum containing acid-secreting gastric glands, peptic ulcer develops in the area exposed to the hydrochloric acid. The clinical manifestations are usually those of hemorrhage, obstruction, or perforation.

Physical Examination

The physical examination usually does not contribute significantly to the diagnosis of peptic ulcer. Localized tenderness in the epigastrium or upper abdomen may be demonstrated over the site of an active ulcer. In severe obstruction of the pylorus or duodenum, the distended stomach, containing fluid and air, is readily visible and palpated, and peristaltic waves may be apparent.

Inflammation surrounding a penetrated ulcer may produce a tender mass in the upper abdomen.

Gastric Analysis

Gastric secretion can be determined in test meals with alcohol, caffeine, and other stimulants, and by measurement of the output during the 12-hour nocturnal period. A two- to three-hour analysis in the morning, after an overnight fast, may incorporate the "basal" gastric content (one hour) and the secretion stimulated by histamine phosphate, its analogue, betazole hydrochloride or pentagastrin. The preferred gastric analysis currently is a morning "basal" one-hour test after an overnight fast, comprising four 15-minute samples, followed by pentagastrin, 6 μg. per kilogram of body weight, subcutaneously, with collections in 15-minute periods for a second hour. This procedure effectively measures gastric secretory capacity, with minimal or no side effects.

In the "maximal" histamine test for determining secretory capacity and complete achlorhydria, 0.04 mg. of histamine acid phosphate per kilogram of body weight is administered subcutaneously, and juice is collected for an additional hour in 15-minute fractions (see table). The systemic effects of histamine are counteracted by the prior (20 minutes) intramuscular injection of an anti-histaminic compound. Betazole hydrochloride may be administered in a dosage roughly equivalent to maximal histamine—1.5 mg. per kilogram of body weight. The diagnosis of true achlorhydria rests upon the absence of a secretory response to such stimulation. Proper technique obviates spurious "achlorhydrias." Measurements on each 15-minute collection include volume (milliliters), concentration of H ions (estimated electrometrically as pH), and concentration of acid determined by titration with NaOH to pH 7.0 to 7.4, utilizing phenol red as the indicator.*

The acid secretory response in gastric ulcer is the same as in normal persons. The clinical usefulness of the test relates to the diagnosis of duodenal ulcer. Basal acid outputs exceeding 15 mEq. per hour and maximal outputs exceeding 40 mEq. per hour favor the diagnosis of duodenal ulcer. Recurrent ulceration after gastric resection or vagotomy is almost always associated with high acid values, e.g., 20 mEq. per hour. Enormous outputs of acid in the basal secretion (i.e., greater than ten times normal) suggest the Zollinger-Ellison syndrome. The complete absence of hydrochloric acid in the gastric content after maximal stimulation excludes the diagnosis of benign peptic ulcer.

In the exceptional situation wherein intubation is not feasible, the presence or absence of hydrochloric acid, but not its quantity, is demonstrable by the oral administration of an ion exchange resin, combined with a basic blue dye, azure A, together with 50 mg. of Histalog and subsequent

*Values for acid secretion—basal and after stimulation—are given in the table.

examination of the urine. In the presence of acid, hydrogen ions displace base from the resin; the base is absorbed and excreted in the urine, where its presence is indicated by the development of a blue color. However, 5 to 10 per cent of negative results are false.

Other Laboratory Data

On occasion occult blood may be demonstrable in the feces in active peptic ulcer. In such instances, serial examinations provide a useful index of the effectiveness of treatment, the occult blood disappearing with healing of the ulcer. Exfoliative cytologic study usually reveals normal cells, but abnormally large cells may be observed during the healing of gastric ulcer. Iron deficiency anemia is demonstrable after occult or massive bleeding. The various chemical constituents of the blood, and hepatic, pancreatic, and adrenal functions are normal in uncomplicated peptic ulcer.

Roentgenographic Examination

Roentgenographic examination of the upper digestive tract is the most important objective method for the diagnosis of peptic ulcer. The value of the procedure depends upon the skill and interest of the examiner, and, in part, upon the clinical acumen of the physician; errors are common, both in failing to recognize an existing ulcer and in diagnosing spurious changes as ulcer. Diagnostic difficulties are presented by erosions and superficial ulcerations too shallow to retain barium, an irritable or posteriorly directed duodenal bulb, and ulcers at the lower end of the esophagus, in the second portion of the duodenum or in the jejunum. The roentgenographic diagnosis of duodenal ulcer should not be based upon the finding of an irritable bulb. Normal roentgenographic findings should not overbalance a typical ulcer history; under such circumstances, the examination should be repeated. The decisive roentgenographic criteria of peptic ulcer are crater and deformity; indirect manifestations such as gastric retention and localized tenderness may be suggestive, but they are not diagnostic.

The ulcer crater is more frequently demonstrable in the stomach than in the duodenum and jejunum (Figs. 1 to 3). The crater of a gastric ulcer is visualized, *en face*, as a dense, well-defined persistent collection of barium, varying from 1 mm. to 1 cm. or more in diameter, encircled by a translucent halo or collar of edematous tissue. In profile, the ulcer crater projects for a varying distance beyond the natural outline of the stomach. During healing, the crater decreases and disappears, leaving no trace or only an accentuation or convergence of rugae at its site (Fig. 4). The crater of duodenal ulcer similarly appears as a sharply circumscribed collection of barium, spherical or linear in shape; thin mucosal folds often radiate to the site. The crater is usually located within the first two or three centimeters of the bulb, more often toward the lesser curvature,

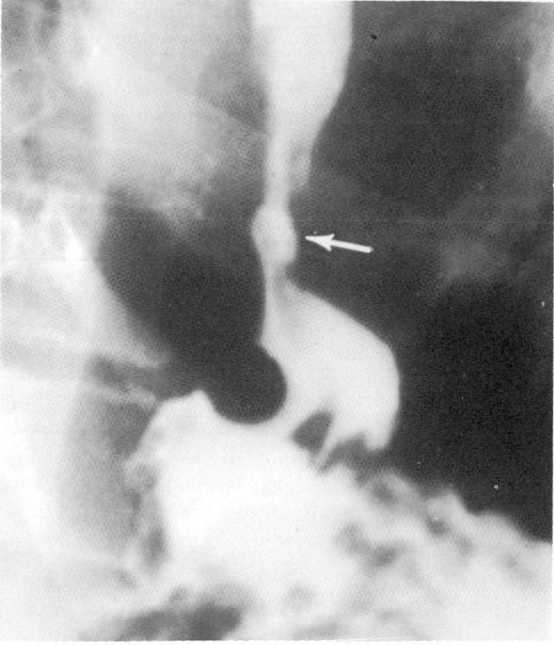

FIGURE 1. B. H., a 44-year-old housewife with intermittent dysphagia for four years and burning midepigastric pain, recurring after meals and during the night, for eight months. Esophagoscopy revealed chronic esophagitis with stricture; biopsies did not demonstrate neoplasia. The roentgenogram demonstrates an ulcer crater in the esophagus. Antacid therapy facilitated healing, and the dysphagia subsided.

and at or immediately proximal to the deformity; occasionally, it is at the apex or immediately distal. Craters may be so large as to simulate the duodenal bulb. Craters infrequently are present on both the anterior and posterior walls, the so-called "kissing ulcers." In healing, the crater diminishes more rapidly in depth than in width. Roentgenographic evidence of the disappearance of a crater precedes complete healing by weeks or months.

Since the diameter of the normal bulb, 2 to 4 cm., is much less than that of the stomach, deformity is produced more readily by spasm, by edema of mucosal folds, and by cicatricial contrac-

tion. The deformity consists of contraction of the lesser or greater curvature of the bulb, or both, at its base, midportion, or apex, narrowing the lumen at that point and producing the typical cloverleaf deformity. Distortion of the bulb may accentuate the lateral recesses of its base, creating pouchlike formations or *pseudodiverticula;* occasionally, barium in a lateral recess simulates an ulcer crater. Diagnostic difficulty may be caused by an incompletely filled or physiologically contracted bulb or by air trapped at the apex of the duodenal bulb where the duodenum angles sharply as it becomes retroperitoneal. Extensive deformity of the distal end of the stomach may handicap identification of the anatomic relationships between the antrum and duodenal bulb. In *pyloric canal ulcer*, the pyloric canal, instead of bisecting the base of the duodenal bulb, may occupy an eccentric position, often in line with the lesser curvature border.

Giant duodenal ulcers are so large as to stimulate the duodenal bulb, thereby escaping detection temporarily. They are not rare; the symptoms are the same as with ordinary ulcer craters, although pain may be severe. Postbulbar ulcers, because of their location, may be difficult to diagnose. Pain may be referred through to the right side of the back, and may be intractable. These ulcers may penetrate into the biliary tract. Hemorrhage is common.

Roentgenographically, the differential diagnosis of gastric ulcer primarily involves the differentiation of benign and malignant lesions. The demonstration of a crater and/or deformity of the duodenal bulb is pathognomonic of duodenal ulcer. Diseases of the gallbladder, bile ducts, pancreas, or duodenum rarely produce deformities resembling duodenal ulcer.

Other Diagnostic Methods

Esophagoscopy supplements roentgenography in the visualization of esophageal ulcers. *Gastroscopy* confirms the roentgenographic diagnosis of gastric ulcer, and in some instances may demon-

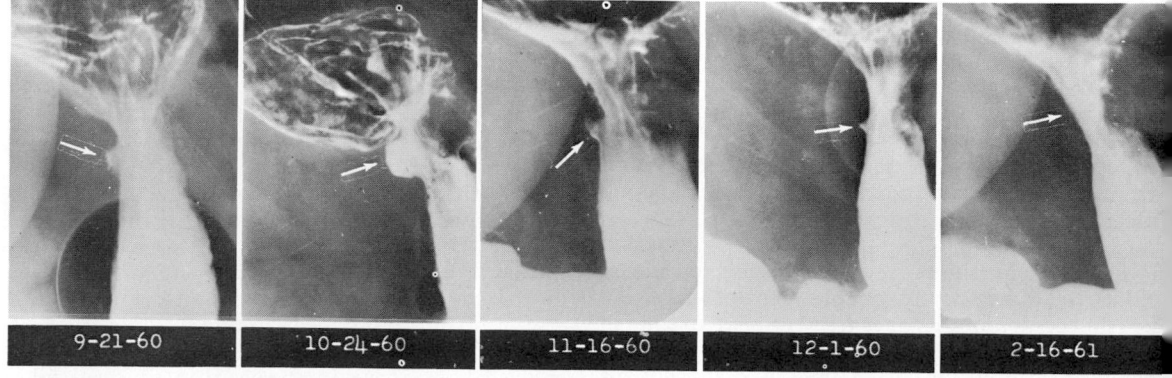

| 9-21-60 | 10-24-60 | 11-16-60 | 12-1-60 | 2-16-61 |

FIGURE 2. R. K., a 74-year-old woman with substernal burning for several years and postprandial and nocturnal epigastric pain for five months. Roentgenographic examination demonstrated an ulcer crater on the lesser curvature of the stomach near the cardia. Antacids relieved symptoms temporarily, with partial healing and then enlargement of the ulcer crater. More complete control of gastric acidity relieved symptoms completely, with gradual but total healing of the ulcer.

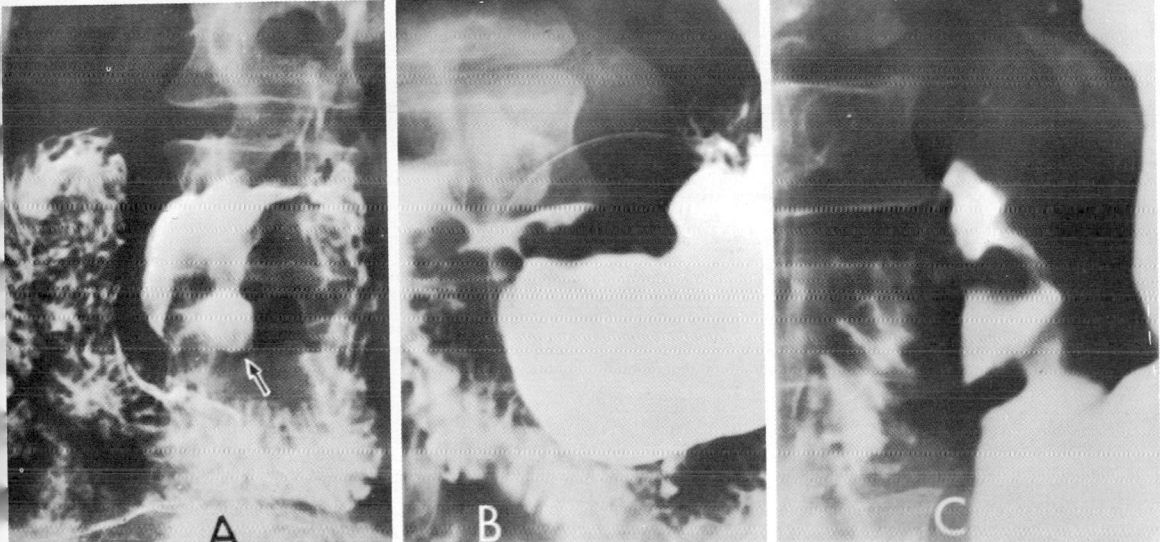

FIGURE 3. A, Large ulcer crater in the duodenal bulb of a man with rheumatoid arthritis treated with salicylates and Butazolidin. B, Deformity of the duodenal bulb with stenosis in a 40-year-old man with recurrent ulcer symptoms for 17 years. Abdominal vagotomy and posterior gastroenterostomy were performed subsequently. C, Pronounced deformity of the duodenal bulb in a 54-year-old male with a 20-year history of ulcer symptoms, responding to antacid therapy.

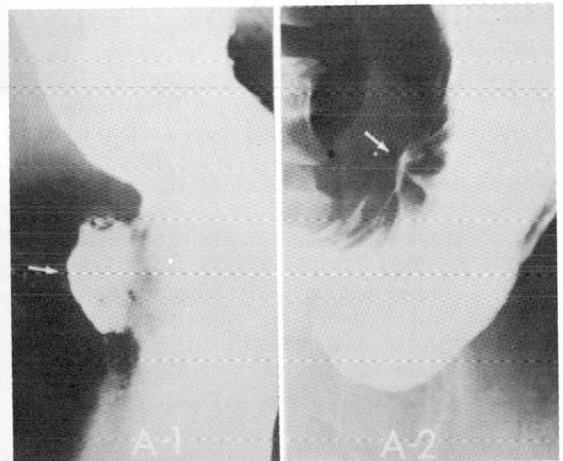

FIGURE 4. M. N., a 38-year-old housewife with intermittent pain in the left upper quadrant, radiating into the chest, occurring after meals. Studies were compatible with a benign ulcer, and the response to antacid therapy was excellent. The roentgenograms demonstrate a large ulcer crater on the lesser curvature of the stomach (A-1) and subsequent healing with mucosal folds radiating to the site of the ulcer (A-2).

strate ulcers not observed on the roentgenograms. Gastroscopy is of no value in the diagnosis of duodenal ulcer, but may demonstrate jejunal and stomal ulcers. The newly developed fiber optic duodenoscope facilitates direct visualization of duodenal ulcers and other lesions in the duodenum, but this instrument is not generally available at present.

Differential Diagnosis

The typical ulcer history presents no diagnostic difficulty. In the absence of characteristic symptoms, peptic ulcer may require differentiation from various illness. *Functional disturbances of the gastrointestinal tract* may produce ulcer-like distress with a sensation of burning or heartburn, relieved temporarily by alkalis (see article on Disorders of Motility). The discomfort lacks the relationship to food-taking, occurs typically in the morning before breakfast, tends to persist throughout the day, decreasing toward evening, and appears during the night. The differentiation is facilitated by a careful history, including the chronologic account of a "typical day." *Gastritis* may cause symptoms resembling those of peptic ulcer; the diagnosis depends upon gastroscopy. The heartburn associated with gastroesophageal reflux with or without *hiatal hernia* and with *esophagitis* is substernal in location. It lacks the ulcer-like relationship to meals, occurring during the intake of food, and may be associated with dysphagia. Often it is induced or aggravated by change in position, particularly recumbency and bending over. The occurrence of peptic ulcer in 10 per cent of patients with hiatal hernia may necessitate consideration of both diagnoses. The distress of an *ulcerating gastric carcinoma*, in the presence of hydrochloric acid, may duplicate the pain of peptic ulcer; the roentgenographic, gastroscopic, and exfoliative cytologic findings establish the diagnosis. *Benign gastric tumors, diverticulum, syphilis*, and *tuberculosis* of the stomach rarely require consideration in the differential diagnosis. *Neoplasms of the duodenum or jejunum* may cause gastric retention and pain in the upper abdomen after eating relieved by vomiting. The symptomatology suggests intestinal obstruction, and roentgenographic studies are likely to demonstrate the lesion. The pain of *bilary colic* is occasionally in the epigastrium, but its episodic, cramplike nature, with onset after a heavy meal, lack of relief from antacids, and need for opiates are distinguishing features. The pain of chronic *relapsing pancreatitis* is usually more severe, located in the left epigastrium and back, and may be accompanied by fever and mild jaundice. Diagnostic difficulty arises when an ulcer penetrates the pancreas, causing pancreatitis. The serum amylase is elevated, but not to as high levels as in primary pancreatitis. *Carcinoma of the pancreas* may be associated with ulcer-like symptoms and may produce a constant deformity of the duodenal bulb; the other manifestations of pancreatic neoplasm facilitate the diagnosis (see Pancreatic Diseases). *Insufficiency of the coronary arteries* may present as "indigestion" after meals, but without the ulcer type of sequence; the relationship to activity and the electrocardiographic findings facilitate the diagnosis. Chest pain from any *disease of the lungs* or *pleura* may radiate across the epigastrium, and epigastric discomfort may occur during *cardiac failure* as a result of distention of the hepatic capsule by the congested liver; the clinical manifestations are almost always so evident as not to pose serious diagnostic problems.

SPECIAL CHARACTERISTICS OF GASTRIC ULCER

Gastric ulcers are one tenth as common as duodenal ulcers. They occur concomitantly with duodenal ulcer in approximately 20 per cent of patients, although in some areas, as in Jamaica, this incidence is higher. The age range is higher, and more women are affected than by duodenal ulcer. Gastric ulcers may be single or multiple, large or small, acute or chronic. They occur anywhere in the stomach, but especially on the lesser curvature, proximal to the angulus, and in the area distal to the border zone formed by the junction of fundic and pyloric gland tissues. According to Dragstedt, gastric ulcer, is usually caused by hypersecretion of gastric juice of humoral origin induced by stasis of food in the stomach in contact with the gastric antrum. This stasis may result from pyloric stenosis from an accompanying duodenal ulcer or from defective gastric tonus and motility. Patients with gastric ulcer and an accompanying duodenal ulcer display the nervous hypersecretion characteristic of duodenal ulcer. Patients with gastric ulcer without organic obstruction at the pylorus usually display subnormal basal gastric secretion and a poorly emptying stomach. Many patients with gastric ulcer secrete little hydrochloric acid in the basal secretion, suggesting that the nervous phase of gastric secretion is reduced. Hypersecretion and stasis suggest decreased activity of both secretory and motor fibers of the vagi. Gastric stasis in gastric ulcer patients may not be revealed by the usual liquid barium meal but becomes evident only when the patient eats a large meal. The gradually increasing acidity of the gastric content 8 to 12 hours after eating testifies to the continuing stimulation of secretion of gastric juice by gastrin.

Gastric ulcer resembles duodenal ulcer in its clinical manifestations, course, complications, and response to medical treatment, but differs in that the secretion of hydrochloric acid is normal or less than normal (see table). Nevertheless, the digestive capacity of the gastric content apparently exceeds the resistance of the susceptible mucosa, since sustained neutralization or elimination of acid results in complete healing. The increased incidence of benign gastric ulcer among women in Australia has been related to the increased consumption of large quantities of aspirin-containing preparations, usually aspirin, phenacetin, and caffeine for tension headaches. No such correlation has been observed for men with gastric ulcer or for males or females with duodenal ulcer.

DIFFERENTIAL DIAGNOSIS OF GASTRIC ULCER AND CARCINOMA

Most gastric ulcers are *benign,* and diagnostic errors are more often made by classifying benign craters as malignant and proceeding with operation than the reverse. Diagnostic difficulty occurs chiefly because of inadequate study; accuracy exceeds 95 per cent when all methods are applied expertly. Clinically, the history, physical examination, and symptomatic response to treatment of both diseases may be identical. Occult blood disappears during therapy, both in healing benign ulcer and in healing peptic ulceration of carcinoma; but *persistent occult blood* during medical treatment suggests malignant ulceration. Gastric secretion may be normal, low or high in both benign and malignant ulceration, although it tends to be subnormal in both conditions. The unequivocal absence of hydrochloric acid, despite maximal stimulation with histamine, Histalog (*vide supra*), or pentagastrin strongly suggests carcinoma. Gastric cancer is characterized generally by reduced acid secretion, by elevation of certain enzymes, e.g., beta glucuronidase, and by an increased concentration of lactic acid.

Roentgenographically, benign and malignant ulcers occur at any site. A smooth, sharply defined, collar-button or conical crater, projecting from the lesser curvature beyond the natural outline of the stomach, almost invariably denotes a benign ulcer. The size of the crater is of no diagnostic value. Other roentgenographic features of a benign ulcer are a sharp line or narrow band of translucency about the orifice of the crater, representing the undermined mucosal edge; and a smooth ulcer floor and an intact mucosal pattern, with folds radiating to the crater. An irregular crater, with rolled margins, suggests carcinoma. Other roentgenographic manifestations of a malignant ulcer are a flat, saucer-like crater with base broader than apex, located within the confines of the gastric outline; rigidity or nodularity of the adjacent mucosa; and absence of peristalsis in the ulcer area. A decrease in the size of the crater does not necessarily indicate a benign ulcer, for peptic ulceration in carcinoma may also heal temporarily during therapy. However, complete roentgenographic and gastroscopic restitution of a carcinomatus ulcer to normal is rare.

Gastroscopy with the newer fibroptic gastroscopes is a relatively easy and useful procedure for confirming the roentgenographic diagnosis of gastric ulcer and detecting lesions of the stomach not demonstrable roentgenographically. Intragastric photography with the gastrocamera, incorporated in the fibergastroscope, increases the accuracy of diagnosis. The typical benign gastric ulcer is easy to recognize for the following features: round or oval shape, well defined edges, whitish yellow base, and mucosal folds radiating directly to the ulcer crater. The adjacent mucosa is usually normal, but may manifest erythema and edema. Atypical *benign gastric ulceration* may demonstrate multiple ulcerations, irregular shape (sometimes linear), poorly defined edges in the healing stage, dark red base after hemorrhage, nodules at the edges or in the base of the ulcer center owing to granulation tissue, and bleeding occasionally from the base or, rarely, from the margins. The *malignant ulcer* is characterized by an irregular shape, poorly defined edges, grossly nodular margins or base, frequent hemorrhage from the margins or base, irregular erythema and discoloration of the surrounding mucosa, occasional elevated margins, and irregularly disrupted converging folds.

The role of *exfoliative cytology* in the differential of benign and malignant gastric ulcers is mainly the positive identification of malignant lesions. The stomach-washing method, utilizing isotonic saline solution or chymotrypsin, has provided a useful diagnostic supplement to roentgenography and endoscopy. Direct vision cytology, whereby the lesion is brushed or lavaged under direct visualization during endoscopy, facilated by the newer Japanese fiberscopes, has yielded a diagnostic accuracy exceeding 95 per cent.

The therapeutic test, demonstrating the decrease and disappearance of gastric ulcer during medical management, is justified when the total evidence suggests a benign ulcer and when the patient can be observed carefully, preferably in the hospital. Significant healing should occur within four to six weeks. However, debilitated patients, persons in the older age group, and, occasionally, those with steroid ulcers of the antrum may require two or more months. Even large ulcers in younger people in good general health may heal completely only after several months of treatment. The objective is complete and permanent healing, as demonstrated by roentgenographic examination and gastroscopy, fortified by normal gastric cytology. Re-examination subsequently is indicated at intervals of perhaps 3, 6, and 12 months, and longer, to document the permanency of healing.

PEPTIC ULCER OF THE ESOPHAGUS

Peptic ulcer of the esophagus is caused by the same factors as are involved in gastric and duodenal ulcers. Sliding hiatal hernia with reflux, cardioesophageal reflux without hernia, reflux after surgical procedures, and prolonged intubation predispose to its development. The ulcer, caused by acid-peptic juice, but occasionally by bile after total gastrectomy, is usually single and most often is located in the lower third of the esophagus. The principal symptom is pain beneath the lower part of the sternum or high in the epigastrium, often occurring during eating and drinking, and intensified in the recumbent position. *Dysphagia* may result from accompanying spasm or from the subsequent development of a stricture. The major complications are obstruction, *perforation* into the mediastinum or upper abdomen, and *hemorrhage*. Treatment is the same as for duodenal ulcer. In addition, the patient is advised to avoid the recumbent position after eating and to elevate the head of the bed during sleep. Operation may be necessary for the complications. (See Disorders of Motility.)

MEDICAL TREATMENT OF PEPTIC ULCER

General Observations. The objectives of the medical treatment of peptic ulcer are relief of symptoms, complete healing of the ulcer, and the prevention of complications and recurrences. The results are influenced by the cooperation of the patient, by the knowledge and interest of the physician in maintaining effective therapy (including an adequate patient-physician relationship), by the age, physical and emotional status of the patient, and by the presence or absence of complications.

Physiologically, medical management seeks to protect the gastroduodenal mucosa from the digestive action of hydrochloric acid and pepsin. This goal might be achieved by increasing tissue resistance, but no method is currently available for directly improving the tissue defense in peptic ulcer. Maintenance of general health, avoidance of gastrointestinal irritants in diet, drink, and drugs, and relief from emotional difficulties may be indirectly helpful. Permanent elimination of hydrochloric acid would abolish peptic ulcer, regardless of other possible etiologic factors, but no procedure except total gastrectomy consistently produces permanent anacidity. Effective therapy requires continuously complete relief of pain; distress, though mild, signifies an inadequate program.

The relatively high incidence of "spontaneous" remission of peptic ulcer complicates the evaluation of individual components of the therapeutic program. Gonadotrophins, progestational agents and extracts of placenta, utilized because of the lower incidence of peptic ulcer and its complications in women, have proved useless. Beneficial results have been reported with estrogens, but confirmation is lacking. The hazards of feminization of the male patient and vascular problems ascribed to estrogen therapy would be disadvantages. Gastric freezing has been abandoned as treatment for peptic ulcer.

Rest and Sedation. Since sustained emotional stress may increase the secretion of hydrochloric acid and the susceptibility of the gastroduodenal mucosa to ulceration, rest and relief of tension are important. The needs vary with the individual; for some, a vacation from work may be desirable; for others, rest in bed is indicated. Many patients can be managed effectively at home, provided there are no serious domestic problems. Hospitalization is indicated for patients with severe distress and with recurrent or complicated ulcers. *Sedatives* (including phenobarbital, 0.015 to 0.3 gram four times daily) do not influence gastric secretion, but promote relaxation and sleep. Ataractic drugs (including prochlorperazine [Compazine], 5 mg., methaminodiazepoxide [Librium], 5 to 10 mg., and meprobamate, 400 mg., three or four times daily) may also be prescribed. The emotional difficulties of the ulcer patient are approached by identification of the disturbing factors and by intelligent efforts at their control. The support provided by the understanding physician can be invaluable. Psychotherapy may be useful in ulcer patients with serious emotional problems; alone, it is not adequate treatment for an active peptic ulcer; it does not lower gastric acid secretion. Since recurrences are also associated with physical fatigue, excessive physical activity should be avoided.

Diet. Although gastric ulcer is occasionally associated with malnutrition, the usual peptic ulcer is not caused by abnormal protein metabolism or nutritional deficiency, and no rationale exists for special foods or dietary combinations. There is no conclusive evidence that coarse or highly seasoned foods retard healing or that a soft diet enhances healing. However, some foods apparently increase the discomfort of individual patients, and, therefore, as a practical approach, are best avoided.

Most foods are capable of neutralizing and buffering gastric acidity. *Frequent feedings,* given at intervals of two or three hours, are chiefly for this purpose. The selection of palatable foods, an intake adequate to maintain normal nutrition, regular eating habits, and physical and emotional relaxation at the time of eating are important considerations. Food supplements may be added if a gain in weight is desirable; a low-calorie program, avoiding milk and cream and other high-calorie foods, is indicated for the obese patient. Dietary restriction during the interval of remission from active peptic ulcer does not necessarily prevent or reduce the likelihood of recurrence.

Antacids. Peptic ulcers heal despite the presence of hydrochloric acid, but healing is facilitated and recurrences are diminished when the acidity is decreased or neutralized. Control of gastric secretion is both worthwhile and possible in the treatment of *active* peptic ulcer. The purpose of antacids is constant neutralization of the acid gastric juice and decreased acidity of the duodenal content. The *ideal antacid* is characterized by effective, prolonged neutralization when administered orally in acceptable amounts, no constipating or cathartic action, no interference with digestive or absorptive processes, palatability, and no systemic effects such as alkalosis. Theoretically, ideal neutralization is maintenance of the pH of the gastric content between 4.0 and 5.0 or higher; at this hydrogen ion concentration, acid and peptic activity are practically absent. Neutralizing efficiency in patients with peptic ulcer is limited by the excessive secretion, rate of gastric emptying, solubility of the antacid preparation, and the rate of reaction.

None of the available antacids is ideal. In general, large amounts of antacid are required for effective neutralization of gastric acidity; a "standard" dose does not exist, and the actual requirements are preferably individually determined. Partial and temporary reductions in gastric acidity are useless in the sustained treatment of peptic ulcer. The most potent preparation is probably calcium carbonate, in quantities of 2 or 4 grams hourly during the day and evening. The neutralizing effect is enhanced by the administration of atropine, anticholinergic drugs, or fats, prolonging the emptying of the stomach. The principal disadvantage of calcium carbonate is constipation, especially among older patients. Acid rebound has been described after the administration of calcium carbonate, 4 or 8 grams, apparently mediated by the action of calcium ions within the gastrointestinal tract and potentiated by food. Magnesium carbonate and magnesium oxide are potent antacids, but because of their laxative effects they are prescribed to counteract the constipating ulcer regimen. Aluminum hydroxide, phosphate or carbonate, in quantities of 16 to 30 ml. hourly, also partially neutralizes acidity. The magnesium and aluminum preparations, although less potent than calcium carbonate, have the advantages of greater palatability, easier regulation of bowel function, and absence of biochemical disturbances (*vide infra*). The antacid effect of sodium bicarbonate is pronounced but transient, although gastric pepsin is denatured at the pH 8.0 occasionally achieved with bicarbonate. Antacids in tablets are inferior to powders because of less complete interaction with hydrochloric acid, but in large amounts may be helpful as adjunctive medication.

Antacids do not influence the secretory mechanism; hence, constant neutralization requires continuous administration. The "routine" administration of antacids, unmonitored by frequent checks on the adequacy of acid neutralization, does not constitute effective antacid therapy. Therapy must be sustained, since the healing time of peptic ulcer is prolonged, and ulcers recur. After the initial hourly schedule, antacids are prescribed most effectively between meals, approximately at 10 and 11 A.M., 2 and 4 P.M., 8 P.M. and bedtime, to provide with the meals, a practical but effective schedule of continuous neutralization. The excessive nocturnal gastric secretion in duodenal ulcer also requires antacids during the night especially to relieve ulcer pain completely.

Intragastric Drip. Acidity may also be lowered

by the administration of milk and cream and alkali or food supplements through an intragastric tube for the 12-hour night period or continuously for several days. The antacid effects result from neutralization locally and decrease in the neurogenic phase of secretion. Two to three thousand milliliters of milk or milk and cream, with antacids and food supplements, may be given within 24 hours. The procedure is indicated very occasionally for patients with hypersecretion and severe pain or with massive hemorrhage. The disadvantages of the intragastric drip are possible intrabronchial aspiration of fluid, esophageal inflammation or ulceration, and the hazard of immobilizing older patients. The intragastric drip is contraindicated in the presence of pyloric obstruction.

Complications of Antacid Therapy. Constipation with *fecal impaction* is the most common complication of antacid therapy. Frequent digital examinations of the rectum and the liberal use of laxative antacids are necessary to regulate bowel function.

The term *alkalosis* refers to a biochemical disturbance characterized by an increase in the serum pH. In the alkalosis produced by the ingestion of large amounts of sodium bicarbonate, the serum sodium is increased and the chloride decrease is minimal. The alkalosis caused by persistent vomiting or gastric aspiration is characterized by hyponatremia, hypokalemia, and elevations of the serum pH and carbon dioxide content. Other features are dehydration, increased blood urea nitrogen, and temporary decrease in renal function. The *milk-alkali syndrome,* complicating the excessive intake of milk and soluble alkali, is characterized by hypercalcemia without hypercalciuria or hypophosphaturia, normal or slightly elevated serum alkaline phosphatase, renal insufficiency with azotemia, milk alkalosis, conjunctivitis, and calcinosis, manifested usually as band keratitis. The symptoms include *distaste for food, nausea, vomiting, headache,* and *weakness.* This complication may occur after the ingestion of milk alone or after calcium carbonate. Differentiation from hyperparathyroidism may be difficult (see Hyperparathyroidism). The disorder subsides rapidly after discontinuance of milk and alkali and the intravenous administration of isotonic sodium chloride.

Nonabsorbable antacids containing magnesium and aluminum hydroxide limit the gastrointestinal absorption of phosphorus; fecal excretion of phosphorus is thus increased. The chemical disturbance is associated with hypercalcemia, hypophosphatemia, increased loss of skeletal calcium and phosphorus, and increased intestinal absorption of calcium. Symptoms include malaise, weakness, and anorexia. The use of magnesium containing antacids in patients with defective renal function may be complicated by the retention of magnesium. The clinical manifestations include hypotension, nausea, vomiting, coma, and slow, shallow respiration; if not recognized in time, the episode may terminate in death.

Lactose and galactose in milk facilitate the intestinal absorption of calcium and theoretically, increase the tendency to nephrolithiasis. Renal and ureteral calculi may be noted during antacid therapy, but, except in individuals drinking excessive amounts of milk and alkali, are not more frequent than in control populations.

Gastric Antisecretory Drugs. *Anticholinergic drugs* interfere with the transmission of nerve impulses mediated by acetylcholine at the neuroeffector junctions of postganglionic nerves. They suppress vagal and antral mechanisms of gastric secretion and may decrease the responsiveness of the parietal cells to peripheral stimuli. Gastrointestinal motility is depressed more readily, but this effect is not essential to the healing of peptic ulcer. The use of anticholinergic drugs in peptic ulcer is based upon the concept of a vagal mechanism in the hypersecretion of duodenal ulcer. The ideal gastric antisecretory agent has not been developed that will selectively and safely decrease gastric secretion for long periods after oral administration, with minimal or no side effects and without development of tolerance. Average doses of tincture (10 drops, four times daily) or powdered extract of belladonna (0.75 mg., four times daily) do not suppress gastric secretion. Atropine sulfate (0.5 mg. three or four times daily by mouth) is partially inhibitory when administered orally, and is more effective when injected intramuscularly; the anticholinergic effects are both central and peripheral. Synthetic atropine substitutes are less potent. Many gastric antisecretory compounds with generally similar therapeutic effects are available; representative compounds include poldine methysulfate (Nacton), 4 mg., methscopolamine bromide (Pamine), 10 to 15 mg., propantheline bromide (Pro-Banthine), 75 to 90 mg., glycopyrrolate (Robanul), 4 mg., and hexocyclium methylsulfate (Tral), 100 mg., in divided doses daily. These agents are more potent when administered intramuscularly than orally; but parenteral therapy, except for occasional hospitalized patients, is impractical. Since it is more effective against basal than against food-stimulated secretion, the medication is prescribed 30 to 60 minutes before meals. Amounts two and three times larger than average are administered at bedtime in an effort to inhibit the nocturnal gastric secretion. The dosage is adapted to the individual patient, and may be regulated by measuring the effect upon basal gastric secretion or by utilizing dryness of the mouth as an index of sufficient intake. Since the action of anticholinergic drugs is limited to the period of administration, they are prescribed continuously during the treatment of an *active* peptic ulcer.

No single anticholinergic drug excels. The compounds usually inhibiting gastric secretion also produce systemic manifestations of parasympathetic inhibition. The symptoms include *dryness of the mouth, blurring of vision, constipation, atony of the bladder* and slowing of the urinary stream (especially in older men), *intestinal atony* (especially in patients with nutritional and electrolyte depletion), *headache, drowsiness, tachycardia, choking sensation,* and *mental confusion.* The side effects tend to decrease with continued medication. Present anticholinergic drugs do not produce a "medical vagotomy," although some preparations are superior to belladonna and atropine, at least for some patients. However, their long-term value in preventing the recurrences and complications of peptic ulcer and in reducing the need for surgery remains in doubt.

The use of anticholinergic drugs alone in the management of peptic ulcer is not recommended. They are contraindicated in the presence of reduced gastric motility or *pyloric obstruction achalasia, incipient glaucoma, prostatic hypertrophy,* and *atony of the urinary bladder.*

Attempts to lower the digestive capacity of the gastric content by decreasing the concentrations of pepsins, in the absence of any change in pH, have been ineffective in man. Favorable results have been reported in the healing of gastric ulcer with a synthetic sulfated amylopectin polysaccharide, but further study of this antipepsin preparation is necessary.

Gastric Irradiation. Roentgen irradiation of the stomach may be utilized as an adjunct to medical therapy in selected cases to decrease or eliminate the secretion of hydrochloric acid. Approximately 1650 r, total depth dose, are directed in ten divided treatments to the fundus and body of the stomach, over anterior and posterior portals, 13 cm. square, outlined fluoroscopically to conform to the fundus and body of the stomach, using 250 KvP, HvL 3.0 cm. Cu, FSD 50 cm. The inhibitory action of irradiation upon gastric secretion depends upon destruction of the parietal cells. The antisecretory effect becomes evident within one to six weeks after irradiation. Complete achlorhydria develops in 10 per cent of patients, continuing from several weeks to six to twelve months, occasionally for periods of five years or longer. In approximately 40 per cent of patients, acid secretion decreases by more than 50 per cent and for long periods. The secretory decrease, though variable and unpredictable, often suffices to benefit the clinical course; recurrences and complications are diminished, and the need for surgery is reduced. Achlorhydria is followed by complete healing of peptic ulcer without recurrence so long as the anacidity persists. A single course of gastric irradiation may be considered for persons above the age of 45 with peptic ulcers that recur despite careful medical management, but without the complications of bleeding or stenosis, as well as for patients unfit for surgery because of serious medical problems, such as congestive heart failure or obstructive pulmonary disease. Damage to the left kidney has been noted after gastric irradiation for peptic ulcer utilizing larger amounts of radiation. This complication has not been observed, in our experience, after a single course of 1650 rads.

Treatment of Gastric Ulcer. The medical management of gastric ulcer is approximately the same as for duodenal ulcer. The immediate results of comprehensive medical treatment are favorable in approximately 90 per cent of patients; however, the long-term results are satisfactory in perhaps 50 to 60 per cent.

The tendency of gastric ulcer to recur is the principal reason for operation. Other indications for surgery are recurrent or uncontrollable *hemorrhage, delayed gastric emptying* accompanying pyloric stenosis or antral narrowing, and *perforation.* Operation is also indicated when an associated hiatal hernia does not respond to medical management and when malignant disease cannot be excluded. Ulcers on the greater curvature should probably be evaluated as ulcers elsewhere in the stomach. For ulcers located high in the fundus or near the cardia four-quadrant biopsy can be performed to establish the diagnosis of benign ulcer, followed by a limited wedge resection. Contraindications to resection for benign ulcer are extreme old age, poor surgical risk because of concurrent illness, and the likelihood of healing upon discontinuance of ulcerogenic drugs. Partial gastric resection is effective in preventing recurrent ulcer in almost all cases; however, this result does not justify the routine resection of benign gastric ulcer, since 15 to 20 per cent of patients will suffer symptoms attributable to partial gastrectomy (see below). Vagotomy and gastroenterostomy or pyloroplasty also has been recommended in the surgical treatment of benign gastric ulcer.

Special Problems in the Management of Peptic Ulcer

Tobacco, Alcohol and Ulcerogenic Drugs. The excessive use of tobacco may contribute to the chronicity or recurrence of peptic ulcer, perhaps because of an effect upon the gastroduodenal mucosa. The habit, therefore, should be discontinued by patients with recurrent peptic ulcer. Alcohol tends to increase the secretion of acid and to irritate the mucosa, and should be avoided. Excessive amounts of coffee, because of its caffeine content, also may irritate the mucosa, stimulate gastric acidity, and reactivate peptic ulcer. Ulcerogenic drugs, especially *salicylates, steroids, indomethacin,* and *phenylbutazone* (Butazolidin), are to be avoided, if possible, by patients with known peptic ulcer, or should be administered in conjunction with antacids.

Prevention of Recurrences

Recurrences are frequent with almost any treatment that does not adequately neutralize or eliminate hydrochloric acid secretion. The precipitating factors recognized and emphasized most often are *physical fatigue, anxiety, frustration* and other forms of *nervous tension, insomnia, excessive smoking, dietary indiscretions, irritating drugs,* and *intercurrent illness.* The tendency to recurrences may be diminished and their severity decreased by a program including (1) thorough treatment of the active ulcer and careful supervision of the patient subsequently; (2) avoidance of alcohol, tobacco, excessive coffee, and irritating drugs and foods; (3) sufficient rest and sleep; (4) resolution of emotional problems, if possible; and (5) proper management of respiratory and other intercurrent illnesses.

COMPLICATIONS OF PEPTIC ULCER

Stenosis

Stenosis is the most frequent complication of peptic ulcer. The lumen frequently is narrowed in the presence of juxtapyloric and duodenal ulcers, but not sufficiently to delay gastric emptying and produce symptoms. Obstruction occurs when the narrowing interferes with the normal passage of food into the small intestine. The usual causes are inflammatory edema surrounding an active ulcer, with and without spasm; cicatricial narrowing at the pylorus or in the duodenal bulb; ulceration, inflammation, and narrowing of the gastric antrum; and shortening of the lesser curvature of the stomach, with upward retraction of the antrum and distortion of the pylorus, as a result of chronic gastric ulcer. In the duodenum, constriction of the lumen to a width of only 1 or 2 mm. usually results in gastric dilatation and hyperperistalsis. *Vomiting*, rather than pain, is the principal symptom, the emesis consisting of sour-smelling, undigested food eaten one or two days earlier. Other symptoms are *distention* after eating, *decreased appetite* and *loss of weight*, and the *pain of an active ulcer*. The physical examination demonstrates a *distended stomach* with *visible peristalsis* and the *succussion splash* produced by fluid and air. Gastric retention also may be demonstrated by the prolonged retention of food or barium in test meals. Nightly gastric aspirates, i.e., at bedtime, four hours after the last meal, exceed 300 ml., in contrast to the normal 60 to 120 ml.; and morning aspirates, after an overnight fast, exceed 100 ml., in contrast to the usual 20 or 30 ml. The laboratory findings may include *alkalosis* (elevated serum pH, elevated carbon dioxide-combining power), *hypochloremia*, *hyponatremia*, and *hypokalemia* caused by loss of electrolytes from the stomach. The *blood urea nitrogen* is often *elevated* because of dehydration and temporarily impaired renal function.

Obstruction caused by inflammatory edema around an active ulcer and by spasm decreases during effective medical management, including an initial period of continuous gastric suction for 36 to 48 hours and replacement of electrolytes and fluids intravenously. Then a program of small liquid feedings with intermittent gastric aspiration is initiated. In the absence of significant cicatricial narrowing, gastric emptying returns to normal. The volume of nightly aspirate, within seven days or less, decreases to 90 to 120 ml. Anticholinergic drugs are contraindicated because they prolong gastric emptying. Ulcer of the pyloric canal, because of its strategic location,

often produces obstruction and gastric retention. Medical management is effective, but surgery is required frequently because of cicatricial narrowing. Occasionally, after a long period without recurrence, the lumen in a stenosing duodenal ulcer may widen substantially. *Operation* is indicated under the following conditions: persistent vomiting and weight loss, continued large gastric aspirates nightly exceeding 300 ml., and the roentgenographic demonstration of a large stomach, with narrowing of the pyloric or duodenal lumen to 3 mm. or less. For persistent obstruction associated with pyloric channel ulcer, the operative approach may include vagotomy and antral resection or selective vagotomy in the good-risk patient; and vagotomy and gastroenterostomy or, possibly, the Jaboulay type of pyloroplasty for the poor-risk patient.

Hemorrhage

General Observations. *Bleeding* occurs in at least 25 per cent of patients with peptic ulcer, and some patients tend to bleed recurrently. Melena from acute peptic ulceration is not uncommon during infancy. Bleeding is caused by penetration into an artery, vein, or capillary, or by vascular granulation tissue at the base of an ulcer. The ulcers are usually on the posterior wall; the anterior surfaces of the stomach and duodenum contain no major vessels, and the vessels are smaller than on the posterior wall. Hemorrhage is more common and tends to be more severe in gastric, postbulbar, and stomal ulcers than in duodenal ulcer, and in persons over the age of 50, though serious bleeding occurs in younger patients. The onset of hemorrhage may be associated chronologically with nervous tension, dietary indiscretions, excessive smoking, physical exertion, and the use of irritating drugs, especially acetylsalicylic acid, and alcoholic drinks; often no precipitating cause is apparent.

Clinical Manifestations. *Hematemesis* occurs frequently in bleeding gastric ulcer and occasionally in bleeding duodenal ulcer. The associated symptoms depend upon the severity of the blood loss. In mild or moderate bleeding, the only indications may be *hematemesis, melena*, or both, and a mild episode of *weakness* and *sweating*; approximately 100 ml. of blood is required to produce a tarry stool. Severe hemorrhage is indicated by hematemesis and persistent melena, and, if peristalsis is rapid, red blood appears in the feces. The clinical manifestations of hypotension are noted: *sudden weakness, faintness, perspiration, dizziness, headache, thirst, dyspnea, syncope*, and *collapse*. The patient is *pale* and *restless;* the blood pressure may fall precipitously, and the pulse rate may rise when the patient sits up. Usually, the vasomotor system regains its tone rapidly, and vascular dynamics are readjusted. In massive bleeding, however, the hypotension, tachycardia, and collapse may continue, as a result of peripheral vasodilatation, until the blood volume is restored by the transfusion of plasma and blood. After hemorrhage, blood volume is restored by tissue fluids; but complete hemodilution does not occur for some time.

Clinical assessment of the severity of bleeding initially is not simple. A pronounced vasovagal reaction may suggest greater blood loss than has occurred. Homeostatic adjustments of blood pressure and pulse may create a deceptively favorable clinical impression. The initial hemoglobin, hematocrit, and erythrocyte count does not invariably indicate persistent bleeding. Despite these limitations, the magnitude of the hemorrhage and its course can be determined by careful observation of the patient, frequent measurements of the hematocrit, hemoglobin, and red blood cell levels, inspection of the stools for subsidence of the melena, and, subsequently, chemical testing of the feces for the disappearance of occult blood.

Diagnostic Approach. Peptic ulcer is the most common source of bleeding from the upper gastrointestinal tract. Other causes include *esophageal varices,* ulceration associated with *hiatal hernia, lacerations* at the cardioesophageal area, *erosive gastritis,* *gastric polyps* and *submucosal benign tumors,* *carcinoma* and *lymphoma* of the stomach, and, infrequently, involvement of the upper digestive tract by hereditary *hemorrhagic telangiectasia, leukemia,* *polycythemia rubra vera,* and *Hodgkin's disease.* The diagnostic approach to hemorrhage from the upper digestive tract varies with individual patients. Sufficient quantities of blood are administered to correct shock and to prepare the patient for diagnostic studies.

The patient should be promptly intubated in order to ascertain the presence and probable site of the bleeding in the esophagus, stomach, or duodenum, and to help assess the rapidity of bleeding. This, however, is especially indicated when *esophageal varices,* *erosive gastritis,* or *gastric ulcer* are strongly suspected. The preferred sequence of tests, after gastric lavage with ice water, saline, or Ringer's solution, is roentgenographic examination of the esophagus, stomach, and duodenum, followed by esophagoscopy and fiberoptic gastroscopy. However, endoscopy is the initial procedure of choice in many institutions.

The "string" test may help to localize the bleeding site. The procedure consists of swallowing a soft cotton tape with transverse and longitudinal radiopaque markings and a mercury-weighted tip. Ideally, the tip is passed into the upper small intestine, and followed by a plain film of the abdomen. At this time, 20 ml. of fluorescein is injected intravenously; the string is removed four minutes later and is inspected under a Wood's lamp. Segments of fluorescence are correlated with the roentgenogram, thus indicating the approximate area of active bleeding.

Percutaneous selective abdominal angiography utilizing the celiac and mesenteric arteries with subselective catheterization of the gastric artery and other vessels, is a relatively safe, readily applied and, at times, useful procedure. Animal studies suggest that bleeding in the range of 0.5 to 6.0 ml. per minute can be detected radiologically by the extravasation of contrast material into the bowel lumen.

Treatment. Since most of the causes of hemorrhage other than peptic ulcer also involve acid pepsin digestion of gastroduodenal mucosa as a primary contributory factor, and effective initial approach is the same treatment as for peptic ulcer. Medical management is indicated for mild and moderate bleeding and initially in most instances of massive hemorrhage. Treatment requires the early and continuing cooperation of internist and surgeon, meticulous nursing care, and frequent measurement of blood pressure and pulse. Absolute rest is essential. Management should include elevation of the foot of the bed, appropriate *sedation* with phenobarbital, *frequent feedings,* and hourly administration of *antacids* day and night. Anticholinergic drugs are not administered during acute or massive hemorrhage, to avoid the interference of drug-induced tachycardia, with the usefulness of the pulse rate as a clinical guide, and to obviate the possible difficulties of intestinal atony, fecal impaction, and urinary retention. In the presence of vomiting, food and fluids are withheld temporarily; nasogastric suction is maintained continuously, and isotonic saline or distilled water, with 5 per cent glucose, is administered intravenously in quantities sufficient to maintain an adequate output of urine. Transfusions of whole blood are indicated when the systolic blood pressure falls to 100 mm. of mercury or less, the pulse rate exceeds 100, the hematocrit decreases to 30 or less, or when there is continued massive bleeding. When 2000 or 2500 ml. of blood is inadequate to replace the loss of blood, the hemorrhage probably is arterial in origin and requires surgical intervention. Replacement of blood is invaluable, but it must be undertaken judiciously because of the hazards of transfusion reactions, serum hepatitis, Rh isoimmunization, and the danger of overloading the cardiovascular system in patients with decreased cardiac reserve. Packed red blood cells may be necessary for the patient with cardiac disease. Continuous gastric aspiration may be beneficial in severe hemorrhage from known gastric or duodenal ulcer. Cessation of bleeding is indicated by return of the pulse rate and blood pressure to normal, increase in the hematocrit and red blood cell count toward normal, and disappearance of gross and occult blood from the feces.

Hemorrhage from peptic ulcer as well as from gastritis occasionally may be controlled by *gastric hypothermia,* using continuous lavage with ice water. This method is safer and easier to employ than a balloon through which chilled ethyl alcohol is circulated.

Surgical Management of Bleeding. The decision for operation is usually undertaken during the first 48 to 72 hours because of the increased hazard of death, vascular complications and/or electrolyte disturbances during prolonged bleeding, and multiple transfusions. A longer period of observation is justifiable when the general condition of the patient remains satisfactory. Most ulcer hemorrhages respond to medical management, and the initial bleeding episode does not necessarily require surgical intervention. *Operation* is indicated under the following circumstances: (1) severe hemorrhage during medical treatment, with persistent hypotension and tachycardia, (2) recurrent bleeding, (3) stomal or jejunal ulcer with hemorrhage, and (4) associated obstruction or perforation. Surgical treatment should be adapted to the individual problem, utilizing the procedure with minimal risk and providing maximal opportunity for the control of bleeding. The operations include partial gastric resection, excision of the ulcer, if possible, and ligation of the bleeding vessel; and truncal vagotomy and pyloroplasty for bleeding duodenal ulcer in poor-risk patients. However, severe bleeding may recur after vagotomy and pyloroplasty, especially in large, calloused ulcer craters and in deep, penetrating duodenal ulcers that have eroded the gastroduodenal artery itself or one of its major branches. Apparently, only direct ligation of the bleeding vessel or a bypass operation in normal tissue prevents repeated hemorrhage in this circumstance. Another procedure combines vagotomy, antral resection, and excision of the ulcer when technically feasible. Early, near-total gastric resection may be the only effective surgical approach to the control of massive hemorrhage from multiple-stress erosions and ulcerations in some patients with uncontrollable diffuse mucosal bleeding.

Mortality. The mortality from hemorrhage in peptic ulcer is correlated with the severity of the blood loss and with the effectiveness of medical treatment and of surgical intervention. The mortality is as high with the initial hemorrhage as with recurrent episodes of bleeding. It is less than 1 per cent in patients younger than 50, and may range from 5 to 15 per cent in patients older than 50 because of decreased ability of the cardiovascular system to withstand severe loss of blood and because of concurrent serious disease. Death results from loss of 40 per cent of the total blood volume and uncorrected shock because of the inadequate transfusion of whole blood, from cardiac failure or coronary insufficiency, from pulmonary infection or the aspiration of blood into the lungs, from renal failure because of prolonged shock, and from complications of emergency surgery.

Perforation

Acute perforation is the most serious complication of peptic ulcer and the most frequent cause of death. Approximately 1 to 2 per cent of all ulcers perforate; perforations recur in 1 or 2 per cent of cases. Pyloroduodenal perforations exceed gastric perforations in a proportion of 20:1 for men and 5:1 for women. Perforation occurs at all ages, but especially in the older age groups; it occurs 50 times more frequently in males than in females. The ulcers are usually on the anterior wall of the stomach or duodenum, unsupported by contiguous structures. Ulcers on the posterior wall tend to penetrate rather than perforate, and their ex-

tension is limited by adjacent solid organs. The ulcers usually are chronic, but acute lesions are common. A preceding history of ulcer distress is elicited in 75 per cent of patients. Perforations are more frequent during the day than at night, and occur most often toward the end of the afternoon or after a meal. The onset may follow a period of intense nervous strain, vomiting, coughing, straining at defecation, a blow to the abdomen, or other vigorous activity. Ulcers perforate at all times of the year, but less often during the summer and perhaps more frequently during the winter.

Clinical Manifestations. The abrupt escape of irritating gastric and intestinal contents initially produces a chemical peritonitis. The *symptoms* begin dramatically, with sudden, overwhelming, and agonizing pain in the epigastrium, extending rapidly throughout the abdomen. The patient is prostrated, pale or ashen gray, and anxious; he lies almost motionless, and struggles for breath in short, panting respirations. The abdominal muscles are held rigid; the knees are flexed and the hands are held over the abdomen to prevent even the slightest movement. Initially, the blood pressure is normal, and the pulse rate is increased only slightly; the temperature is normal or subnormal. Nausea and vomiting may occur, especially if the perforation has followed a meal. The pain may be referred to one or both shoulders because of irritation of the diaphragm, innervated by the phrenic nerves. Perforation of a gastric ulcer may cause pain referred into the thorax anteriorly and to the interscapular area posteriorly. Gravitation of the escaping gastroduodenal contents to the right paracolic gutter produces pain in the right lower abdominal quadrant.

Physical examination demonstrates a tender, rigid, boardlike abdomen. Peristaltic sounds are decreased or inaudible as a result of paralytic ileus. The usual liver dullness is absent because of interposition of free intraperitoneal air between the liver and the chest or abdominal wall; this finding is unreliable in patients with distention of the colon or with pulmonary emphysema. Rectal examination elicits tenderness in the cul-de-sac.

After several hours, the pain decreases, the body becomes warm, and the skin may regain its usual color. The patient feels better, but the abdominal rigidity and tenderness persist. Within 6 to 12 hours, the chemical irritation of the parietal peritoneum is followed by a bacterial peritonitis. The abdominal pain is less intense, though movement is painful. Distention appears, but the abdominal muscles remain rigid. The pulse increases in rate and decreases in strength. The temperature rises, respirations become more rapid and shallow, and the malaise and toxicity of generalized peritonitis ensue. During the next 12 to 24 hours, the clinical condition deteriorates. The distention increases, and the extreme abdominal rigidity disappears, presumably because of paralysis of the abdominal muscles. The temperature, pulse, and respiration remain elevated, though the temperature ominously may fall below normal. If the condition is untreated, death follows in two to five days.

Roentgenographic examination of the abdomen demonstrates free air beneath one or both diaphragms or within the peritoneal cavity in 60 per cent of cases. The leukocyte count rises to 10,000 or 15,000 per cubic millimeter or higher. The serum amylase may increase moderately from absorption of fluid containing pancreatic enzymes through the peritoneal lymphatics. The rise in serum amylase is not as high as in pancreatitis, i.e., < 300 units per milliliter, but the interpretation may be complicated by the coexistence of an acute pancreatitis.

Occasionally, the perforation is small and is closed rapidly by adherence to adjacent structures. The escape of gastroduodenal content is relatively slight, and the peritonitis is localized to the upper abdomen or right upper quadrant. The sudden severe pain is replaced within 6 to 12 hours by a dull discomfort, and may disappear completely within 24 hours. The tenderness and muscle rigidity are localized to the upper abdomen. The condition of the patient remains satisfactory, and recovery occurs within several weeks. Rarely, rupture of the protecting fibrinous adhesions causes a generalized peritonitis. A *subphrenic abscess* may become apparent four to ten days after perforation and is denoted clinically by a sharp rise in temperature and in pulse rate, subsequently following a septic pattern, pain one one side of the upper abdomen, chest and in one shoulder, hiccup, and cough from irritation of the diaphragm, pleura, and adjacent lung. The diaphragm is elevated and immobilized. Roentgenographic examination may demonstrate a pleural effusion obliterating the outline of the diaphragm and gas beneath the diaphragm. The leukocyte count is elevated to 15,000 or 20,000 per cubic millimeter, with a predominance of polymorphonuclear cells.

Massive hemorrhage may accompany an acute perforation in 10 per cent of cases. The chief causes of death from perforated peptic ulcer, in addition to peritonitis, are pulmonary infection and abdominal abscesses. The mortality rate, though less than in earlier years, approximates 10 to 15 per cent.

Chronic perforation is not unusual, especially in gastric ulcer. The base of the ulcer is formed by the capsule of the liver, pancreas, transverse mesocolon, colon, gastrohepatic omentum, or abdominal wall. Involvement of the head of the pancreas causes pain at the level of the umbilicus, radiating to the right and through to the back; penetration into the body of the pancreas produces pain low in the epigastrium, radiating bilaterally and to the back; perforation into the tail of the pancreas causes pain in the left side of the epigastrium and around or through to the left subscapular region. Ulcer symptoms may be unchanged as a result of chronic perforation. Frequently, however, the characteristic rhythmicity and periodicity of the distress disappear, and relief from food or alkali is less complete.

Differential Diagnosis of Perforation. The clinical features of acute perforation are usually pathognomonic. In individual cases, various conditions may require consideration. In *acute cholecystitis* the pain is usually in the right upper quadrant, the temperature is elevated, signs of peritoneal irritation are limited to the right upper quadrant, and the gallbladder may be palpable. Perforation of the *gallbladder* resembles ulcer perforation closely, but the pain and tenderness are in the right hypochondrium. The perforation usually occurs after apparent subsidence of an acute cholecystitis. An antecedent history of ulcer distress or biliary colic may be helpful. *Acute pancreatitis* may cause pain as severe as or more intense than that of perforated ulcer. The prostration and collapse may be more pronounced, and a peculiar slate-blue color may be apparent in the lips, ears, and fingernails. Abdominal rigidity is less pronounced and is usually not boardlike. Movement of the patient does not precipitate spasm and boardlike rigidity of the abdomen, as in perforated ulcer. Roentgenographic examination of the abdomen does not demonstrate free air in the peritoneal cavity. A past history of cholelithiasis may provide a clue. The most significant laboratory finding is an increase in the serum amylase. The serum lipase and bilirubin, blood sugar, and urinary diastase may also be elevated, as well as SGOT, SGPT, LDH, and alkaline phosphatase. (See Diseases of the Pancreas.) In *acute appendicitis* the onset of pain is less sudden; the pain usually shifts from the epigastrium to the right lower quadrant. Abdominal rigidity is less intense and localized, and prostration is minimal. Acute perforation of an ulcer is rare during adequate therapy, whereas acute appendicitis is not infrequent because of calcium concretions in the appendix. Acute *intestinal obstruction* produces colicky pain with vomiting of alkaline, light brown intestinal contents. Abdominal rigidity may develop in the presence of volvulus or strangulation, but is rarely boardlike. Tenderness is maximal in the lower abdomen. Roentgenographic examination reveals the absence of pneumoperitoneum and the presence of dilated intestinal loops. The scar of a previous abdominal operation may provide a useful clue. Diverticulitis of the colon causes pain in the left lower quadrant, with constipation or diarrhea and slight fever; there is little or no abdominal rigidity. *Renal colic*, in addition to the typical location and distribution of pain, does not produce boardlike rigidity of the abdomen. *Myocardial infarction* ordinarily produces pain or pressure in the precordium and sternum, radiating to the neck and down the arms, and the abdomen is not rigid. Occasionally, however, the distress of myocardial infarction may be upper abdominal, and the patient may have nausea or vomiting, or both. *Pneumonia* is usually heralded by fever, and the respiratory rate is increased. The accompanying upper abdominal pain may be associated with muscle rigidity, but both are mild; the pulmonic physical findings facilitate the diagnosis. *Diaphragmatic pleurisy* occasionally produces abdominal and shoulder pain, with tenderness in the upper abdomen in relation to respiration; the fever and cough direct attention to the problem. *Spontaneous pneumothorax* causes sudden severe pain, maximal above the diaphragm; there is no abdominal tenderness, and rigidity, if present, is slight and temporary. *Mesenteric thrombosis* is usually preceded by a history of cardiovascular disease; the pain is colicky, intermittent, and not as severe; however, the pattern is quite variable. Abdominal rigidity is less, and abdominal distention occurs promptly, in contrast to perforation. The intense pain of *dissecting aneurysm* of the aorta is commonly substernal and progresses downward with the dissection; abdominal rigidity is minimal or absent; cardiovascular shock and the manifestations produced by involvement with other organs indicate the correct diagnosis.

In ruptured *ectopic pregnancy* the pain and tenderness are in the lower abdomen and hypogastrium, and the rigidity is less pronounced; the evidence for pregnancy and the rarity of ulcer perforation in women facilitate the diagnosis. In the gastric crises of *tabes dorsalis*, abdominal rigidity is absent; Argyll Robertson pupils are present; the patient moves about; the general condition is not critical. Pneumoperitoneum is absent, and the leukocyte count is normal.

Treatment of Perforation. Acute perforation is the most urgent indication for surgery. Treatment is usually limited to simple closure of the perforation, utilizing a piece of omentum, and thorough cleansing of the peritoneal cavity by meticulous aspiration of the peritoneal gutters and pelvic and subphrenic spaces. The pronounced loss of fluid through the perforation, by vomiting, and from the irritated peritoneum causes significant depletion of extracellular fluid and electrolytes, especially potassium, and necessitates appropriate replacement. Gastric resection may be feasible in selected younger patients in good general health with a long history of ulcer recurrences, previous hemorrhage, perforation, or obstruction. It is also indicated when perforation is further complicated by hemorrhage, and in some patients with perforated gastric ulcer. Vagotomy and antral resection may be added to simple plication of the perforation in the good-risk patient; vagotomy and pyloroplasty may be considered in the poor-risk elderly patient.

The nonoperative approach is based upon the observation that early perforations seal rapidly if the stomach is kept empty by aspiration. It includes prompt and continuous gastric aspiration, along with administration of appropriate fluid, electrolytes, and antimicrobial drugs.

This program may infrequently be indicated for patients with localized abdominal findings who seek medical attention 24 hours or more after the perforation, and for persons who are operative risks because of concurrent serious disease. Operation is usually necessary later in such cases.

Stress *erosions* and *ulcerations* complicate other serious illnesses, including massive infection, burns, intracranial disease, traumatic injury, and myocardial infarction. They usually present as massive hemorrhage, unresponsive to medical measures. Gastric acid secretion is not excessive, and their pathogenesis has been ascribed to a defect in the ordinarily protective mucus or to some other breakdown of tissue resistance. The surgical approach includes truncal vagotomy, pyloroplasty, and attempted suture of a discrete bleeding ulcer. However, since later stress ulceration is often multiple, subtotal gastric resection is usually preferred.

Jejunal Ulcer

Jejunal (anastomotic, marginal) ulcer is a complication of the surgical treatment of peptic ulcer, developing under circumstances of ineffective control of gastric secretion and exposure of the vulnerable jejunal mucosa to the acid-pepsin gastric content. Jejunal ulcers are most frequent in the efferent loop, approximately 1 cm. beyond the anastomosis. The onset usually occurs soon after the original operation, but it may be years later. Jejunal ulcers may also develop in the absence of surgery in patients with the Zollinger-Ellison syndrome. They predominate in males 10:1.

The development of pain, resembling the original ulcer distress, after gastroenterostomy or gastric resection is highly suggestive. However, the pain tends to be poorly localized; it may be in the left lower quadrant or in the lower abdomen; it is often more severe than previously and less responsive to treatment. In perforated jejunal ulcer, it may extend to the left groin, testes, left flank, and back. The characteristic relationship to the intake of food may disappear, and nocturnal distress is frequent. Nausea and vomiting may be present if there is an associated malfunction or obstruction of the stoma. Loss of weight is common but not pronounced, unless a jejunocolic fistula develops.

The crater of a jejunal ulcer, although not always demonstrable, appears roentgenographically as a circumscribed dense collection of barium, 5 to 25 mm. in diameter. Another roentgenographic finding is spastic, inflammatory, or cicatricial narrowing of the previously normal stoma. At gastroscopy jejunal ulceration appears as a sharply defined lesion with a narrow margin of erythema and a white or yellow-white base.

Jejunal ulcer is less responsive to medical treatment than either gastric or duodenal ulcer. Penetration of the lesion results in acute, subacute, and chronic perforation. Occult bleeding is common, is often painless and is usually manifested as melena; occasionally the hemorrhage is massive. Obstruction of the gastroenterostomy stoma results from the inflammation of active ulceration, cicatrix, adhesions, and (less commonly) volvulus or herniation of a jejunal loop. Surgery is preferred in most cases: transabdominal vagotomy with or without gastric resection or excision of the ulcer and a more extensive gastric resection.

Other Complications

Gastrojejunocolic Fistula. A gastrojejunocolic fistula results from penetration of an ulcer at the anastomosis between the stomach and the efferent jejunal loop into the adjacent transverse colon. This complication is uncommon, and is demonstrable in perhaps 10 per cent of anastomotic ulcers requiring operation. It is more likely after retrocolic gastroenterostomy for duodenal ulcer; 98 per cent of the patients are men. The clinical manifestations include the pain or discomfort produced by a stomal ulcer, and, in 80 per cent of cases, diarrhea, with as many as 30 bowel movements daily. If the fistula is small and is plugged intermittently with food or mucosal folds, diarrhea may be mild or intermittent. Regurgitation of colonic material into the stomach produces fecal belching and vomiting in the absence of intestinal obstruction. Bypass of the absorptive surface of the small bowel and the diarrhea rapidly cause severe loss of weight and electrolyte and water depletion. Laboratory studies may demonstrate *anemia, hypoproteinemia, hyponatremia,* and *hypokalemia* (see Malabsorption). Gastrojejunocolic fistula is better diagnosed by barium enema examination than by barium meal. After correction of electrolyte and fluid imbalance surgery must be performed. Severe, recurrent marginal ulceration, particularly after high subtotal gastrectomy, suggests Zollinger-Ellison syndrome. Gastric secretion, despite previous surgery, is normal or even supernormal.

Obstructive Jaundice. Rarely, duodenal ulcer causes obstructive jaundice by ulceration into the common bile duct. Inflammatory obstruction of the distal end of the common duct, especially in postbulbar ulcer, may also be noted. The ulcer may penetrate into the gastrohepatic ligament, obstructing the more proximal portion of the common bile duct.

SURGICAL TREATMENT OF PEPTIC ULCER

General Observations. The most important indications for surgery in peptic ulcer are *perforation, uncontrollable or recurrent hemorrhage, persistent obstruction, unresponsive or recurrent ulcers* despite thorough medical treatment, *jejunal ulcer,* or *gastric ulcer* that either does not heal despite thorough medical treatment or in which carcinoma cannot be excluded completely. Approximately 15 per cent of patients with duodenal ulcer and 40 per cent of patients with gastric ulcer will, by these criteria, come to surgery. The requirements of an effective operation are safety, with low morbidity and minimal mortality rate, elimination of recurrences, maintenance of nutrition, and restoration of the patient to a healthy, useful life. Since no operation increases the resistance of the gastrointestinal mucosa, the value of operative treatment is largely determined by the decrease in acid-secreting potential. An important consideration in choice of operation is preservation of the normal homeostatic mechanisms, including the hormones elaborated by the duodenal mucosa, for controlling gastric secretion. The outcome is poorest when operation is undertaken prematurely after inadequate medical management for relief of pain in emotionally unstable persons and in those with extreme gastric hypersecretion, as in the Zollinger-Ellison syndrome.

Many ulcers are apparently refractory because of poor cooperation by the patient or ineffective therapy by the physician; they *do* respond to adequate treatment. Intractability properly means ulcers not responding to careful medical management in the hospital. It is more common in men than in women, in gastric and postbulbar ulcers, in deeply penetrating or chronically perforated ulcers, and in the Zollinger-Ellison syndrome (*vide supra*).

Gastroenterostomy. Posterior gastroenterostomy relieves obstruction at the pylorus or duodenum. It promotes healing by diverting acid from the ulcer and by facilitating neutralization through reflux of alkaline intestinal secretion. The gastric secretory potential is unchanged. The excessive production of hydrochloric acid in duodenal ulcer predisposes to a high incidence of jejunal ulcer. Gastroenterostomy, therefore, is not acceptable for duodenal ulcer, although it may be indicated for a very small number of older, poor-risk patients with pyloric stenosis and low acid output. Anastomosis near the pylorus avoids stasis and stimulation of the gastrin mechanism in the antrum.

Gastric Resection. Subtotal gastric resection usually involves removal of 70 to 80 per cent of the stomach, including the antrum. Operative mortality is 1 to 5 per cent, depending upon the skill of the surgeon and the adequacy of postoperative care. The anastomosis is often stomach to jejunum (Billroth II), permitting a more adequate gastric resection and providing greater protection to the ulcer area by diverting the acid. Anastomosis of the stomach to the duodenum (Billroth I) is performed in an effort to decrease the incidence of "dumping" and malabsorption associated with Billroth II (*vide infra*). Gastric secretion is lowered because of the decreased parietal cell mass and removal of the antrum; vagotomy may also be done to eliminate the neurogenic phase of secretion. Subtotal gastrectomy is the procedure of choice for gastric ulcer.

Gastric resection does not consistently eliminate hydrochloric acid. Stomal or jejunal ulcers occur in 3 per cent of operations for gastric ulcer and in 5 to 10 per cent for duodenal ulcer. Peritonitis from a leak at the duodenal anastomosis, pancreatitis, cardiac or pulmonary complications, and associated serious diseases such as cirrhosis of the liver, pulmonary emphysema, or myocardial insufficiency are important causes of death. Additional early problems after gastric resection include *gastrojejunocolic fistula, obstruction of the afferent loop, and internal herniation.* The incidence and severity of postprandial complaints such as epigastric fullness, bilious vomiting, and the dumping syndrome after surgery for duodenal ulcer are apparently little affected by the type of operation, but are related to loss of the functional integrity of the pylorus.

The *afferent loop syndrome* is associated with chronic partial obstruction of the afferent loop, after the Billroth II antecolic type of gastric resection. Following the ingestion of food, the secretion of bile and pancreatic juice causes distention and lengthening of the afferent loop and, occasionally, kinking. Duodenal distention results in pain and nausea. As pressure in the afferent loop increases, the contents are finally expelled forcibly through the anastomosis into the gastric remnant, resulting in vomiting with relief of symptoms. The corrective operative procedure of choice is conversion of the Billroth II to the Billroth I anastomosis.

The late-developing problems of subtotal resection include undernutrition, with deficiency of vitamin B^{12} in 1 to 5 per cent of patients; deficiency of folic acid in approximately 10 per cent; disordered calcium metabolism with demineralization and rarefaction of bowel resulting from decreased oral intake and reduced absorption of calcium and vitamin D; increased intestinal leakage of albumin, especially after the Polya-Finsterer type of resection; decreased absorption of iron and iron deficiency anemia; the uncovering of latent gluten enteropathy; mild to moderate steatorrhea; higher than expected incidence of pulmonary tuberculosis; and, in emotionally labile patients, addiction to alcohol or drugs. (Malabsorption following gastrectomy will be discussed in the article on Malabsorption.) The evidence for an increased incidence of cholelithiasis after partial gastric resection is inconclusive.

Vagotomy. Complete truncal vagotomy reduces the excessive gastric secretion of duodenal ulcer to normal by eliminating the neurogenic phase, diminishes the production of gastrin, and decreases the responsiveness of the parietal cells to humoral and peripheral stimuli. This procedure is indicated in the surgical management of jejunal ulcer. For duodenal ulcer, vagotomy is combined with a pyloroplasty or gastroenterostomy. Pyloroplasty, by preserving normal anatomic integrity of the gastroduodenal area, maintains normal homeostatic mechanisms controlling gastric secretion. In pyloric channel ulcer the pylorus often is so inflamed, scarred, and distorted as to prevent the usual pyloroplasty. The preferred procedure, in addition to vagotomy, is a posterior gastroenterostomy or a Jaboulay type of pyloroplasty. The combination of vagotomy and pyloroplasty is an effective operation for children with peptic ulcer requiring surgery, permitting normal growth and development. For a deeply penetrating duodenal ulcer on the posterior wall, truncal vagotomy has been combined with a pyloroplasty of the Jaboulay type or a gastroduodenostomy.

The incidence of malabsorption and dumping is considerably lower than after gastric resection. The mortality rate is less than 1 per cent. The incidence of recurrent ulcer after operation for duo-

denal ulcer ranges from 5 to 10 per cent, presumably because of incomplete vagotomy and persistence of the antral phase of secretion. Poor results for various reasons occur in an additional 5 to 10 per cent of patients. Vagotomy and pyloroplasty also have been recommended in the surgical management of gastric ulcer in patients who previously had had a duodenal ulcer.

The principal problems after vagotomy are an unexplained diarrhea (troublesome in approximately 5 per cent of patients), gastric retention, and continued stimulation of the gastrin mechanism as the result of an inadequate drainage procedure. Stasis and dilation of the gallbladder resulting in an increased incidence of gallstones have been attributed to cutting of the hepatic branch of the anterior vagus nerve, but this observation requires confirmation. Esophageal complications may include perforation, hemorrhage, or devascularization at operation. Temporary dysphagia may result from vagotomy. The gastric ulcers developing very occasionally after vagotomy and a drainage procedure have been attributed, in part at least, to hypomotility of the stomach with hyperfunction of the antrum, and to reflux of small gut contents which causes gastritis.

Selective gastric vagotomy seeks to obviate the alleged adverse effects of complete truncal vagotomy on the biliary tract, pancreas, and intestines, and to preserve the mechanism of inhibition of the antral and intestinal phases of gastric secretion. The procedure involves anterior gastric denervation, sparing the hepatic branch; posterior gastric denervation, sparing the celiac branch; and suprahiatal palpation for proximal gastric branches from the right and left vagal trunks. According to some observers, preservation of normal gastrointestinal motility obviates a drainage operation. Selective vagotomy is more difficult technically than the usual vagotomy procedure. Furthermore, as yet there is no conclusive evidence of specific advantages, such as decreased incidence of postvagotomy diarrhea, biliary dysfunction, or the dumping syndrome. Both operations effectively control peptic ulcer in 85 to 90 per cent of patients.

Antral Resection and Vagotomy. Vagotomy and antral resection eliminate the neurogenic and antral phases of gastric secretion. The morbidity, mortality and ulcer recurrence rates are thus far comparatively low. Gastrointestinal motor activity is more normal than after conventional resection, and nutrition is better maintained. The disadvantages are a somewhat higher mortality rate than for vagotomy and pyloroplasty; also a higher incidence of the dumping syndrome and lower incidence of achlorhydria. A recent study has indicated excellent or good results in approximately 75, 79, and 80 per cent in groups of patients with duodenal ulcer undergoing vagotomy and gastroenterostomy, vagotomy and antrectomy, and partial gastrectomy, respectively. Nevertheless, although there is as yet no single ideal operation for all circumstances, vagotomy and pyloroplasty or vagotomy and gastroenterostomy have emerged as the preferred operations for duodenal ulcer and

for selected gastric ulcers. The therapeutic benefits tend to diminish, and the physiologic and
metabolic consequences tend to increase, however,
with the passage of time after virtually all operative procedures.

Dumping Syndrome

The dumping syndrome is a sequence of events
caused by excessively rapid gastric emptying,
particularly following gastric resection, but also
following vagotomy and antrum resection, gastroenterostomy, or pyloroplasty, initiated by the
passage of large volumes of material from the
stomach into the proximal jejunum. Infrequently,
it occurs in the absence of gastric surgery. Food
and fluid are evacuated rapidly into the small intestine, distending the bowel. The hyperosmolar
intestinal content initiates the movement of extracellular fluid from the plasma to the lumen to
achieve isotonicity, decreasing the circulating
blood volume and inducing compensatory vasoconstriction. Although release of serotonin and
vasoactive peptides such as bradykinin have been
implicated in the vasomotor symptoms of dumping
syndrome, substantiated supporting evidence is
lacking.

The *early manifestations* (5 to 30 minutes after
eating) that result from these events include
fullness, nausea, vasomotor phenomena such as
warmth, sweating, pallor, palpitation, headache,
vertigo, diarrhea, desire to lie down, and, rarely,
syncope. The blood pressure and pulse tend to
rise, although the blood pressure may fall during
a severe attack.

The *late manifestations* result from the rapid
rise of blood glucose, which elicits an over-release
of insulin, causing *hypoglycemia* that may be
noted two to three hours after a meal, at which
time weakness, tremulousness, anxiety, sweating,
and change in personality characterize the clinical
picture.

Dumping may be precipitated by any food, but
notably by those rich in glucose and disaccharides,
particularly when taken with fluids. Emotional
tension also seems important in attacks. The intake of food is decreased in an effort to control
the dumping, leading to loss of weight. The incidence of the dumping syndrome may approximate
50 per cent soon after operation, but symptoms
subside in most patients within 6 to 12 months.
Dumping is more frequent after surgery for duodenal ulcer, in women and among emotionally
labile patients. In 5 to 15 per cent, the syndrome
persists in varying degrees and presents a difficult
although manageable problem.

Medical therapy includes a diet high in protein
and fat and low in carbohydrates. Multiple feedings may be necessary to attain an adequate intake of calories. Other measures include limitation or exclusion of liquids during and immediately
after meals, eating in the recumbent or semire-
cumbent position to delay gastric emptying and
to decrease jejunal distention, sedatives and anti-
spasmodics to lengthen gastrointestinal transit
time, and possibly the use of serotonin antagonists
to diminish the vasomotor effects of serotonin.
Conversion of a Billroth II to Billroth I anastomosis or jejunal transposition has been reported
to correct severe dumping symptoms in occasional
patients. Interposition of a short antiperistaltic
segment of jejunum between stomach and duodenum also has been attempted. The operative
readjustment of an excessively large pyloroplasty
may be helpful occasionally.

GENERAL PROGNOSIS

The immediate results of comprehensive medical treatment for peptic ulcer disease are excellent;
the long-term results are less impressive. Recurrences and chronicity are common with any type
of therapy, medical or surgical, that does not
abolish the secretion of hydrochloric acid completely. However, the outlook for patients with
peptic ulcer is generally favorable. Recurrences
are not inevitable, and the disease is often not
progressive. The majority of patients will respond
to intelligent medical treatment. Improved surgical techniques, apparently more physiologic and
less extensive than in the past, are available for
those patients with the complications of peptic
ulcer. Peptic ulcer remains an enigmatic disorder,
but it is not incurable.

Davenport, H. W.: Physiology of the Digestive Tract. Chicago,
    Year Book Publishers, Inc., 1961.
Dragstedt, L. R.: The cause of peptic ulcer. J.A.M.A., 169:203,
    1959.
Gregory, R. A., and Tracy, H. J.: The constitution and properties
    of two gastrins extracted from hog antral mucosa. I. The
    isolation of two gastrins from hog antral mucosa. II. The
    properties of two gastrins isolated from hog antral mucosa.
    Gut, 5:103, 107, 1964.
Kirsner, J. B.: Peptic ulcer: A review of recent literature. Gastro-
    enterology, 44:664, 1963; 46:706, 1964; 49:70, 1965.
Kirsner, J. B., and Palmer, W. L.: The problem of peptic ulcer.
    Amer. J. Med., 13:615, 1952.
Palmer, W. L.: Causality in peptic ulcer. Arch. Intern. Med.
    (Chicago), 106:786, 1960.
Proceedings of the World Congress of Gastroenterology. Volumes
    I and II. Baltimore, Williams & Wilkins Company, 1958.
Zollinger, R. M., and Ellison, E. H.: Primary peptic ulceration of
    the jejunum associated with islet cell tumors of the pancreas.
    Ann. Surg., 142:709, 1955.

Diseases of Malabsorption

Marvin H. Sleisenger

The malabsorption syndrome is a constellation of symptoms and signs that are the result of abnormal fecal excretion of fat (steatorrhea) and of varying degrees of malabsorption of fat-soluble vitamins as well as carbohydrate, protein, minerals, other vitamins, and water.

MECHANISM OF NORMAL ABSORPTION

In view of the wide range of absorption defects that can be involved, each instance of the malabsorption syndrome must be analyzed against the background of the processes of *normal* absorption. Accordingly, a brief review of the processes of normal absorption is presented at this time.

During absorption, the end products of digestion must leave the intestinal lumen, traverse the mucosal cells, enter the terminal branches of the vascular and lymphatic vessels, and thus gain entrance into the general circulation. Three mechanisms, acting separately or together, are important in this process: *active transport, facilitated transport*, and *passive diffusion*. Each of these is presumed to take place in relationship to a hypothetical cell membrane.

Passive diffusion requires no energy, and is the passage of a molecule across a membrane barrier according to chemical concentration and electrical gradients. *Facilitated transport* is like passive diffusion, in that it requires no expenditure of energy, but a carrier mechanism permits a degree of effective transport exceeding that predictable on the basis of passive diffusion alone. *Active transport* requires metabolic work with expenditure of energy that results in a net movement of substances against a chemical or electrical difference. An important mechanism of active transport systems is the "carrier," which makes possible penetration of the cell membrane.

Fat Absorption. The stomach plays an important role in fat digestion. It reduces the size of particles and, by slowly emptying its acid chyme into the duodenum, ensures not only a normal rate of absorption, but also an adequate stimulation for the flow of bile and pancreatic juice. Some evidence exists for a gastric lipase which splits medium and short-chain triglycerides. Finally, *gastric acid* may also be important in maintaining sterility of the upper small bowel. Heavy growth of bacterial flora in this segment interferes with fat and vitamin B_{12} absorption (*vide infra*).

Fat absorption in the jejunum depends upon many factors, principally "digestion" or breakdown. The key to normal digestion is hydrolysis of neutral fat (triglyceride) into di- and monoglycerides and thence to its component fatty acids and glycerol. For this action, *pancreatic lipase* is primarily required; this enzyme is activated at the alkaline pH of the upper jejunum. Bile, by its emulsifying action, also facilitates hydrolysis.

Conjugated bile salts form a polymolecular aggregate with fatty acids and monoglycerides in the lumen of the small intestine. This complex is called a *micelle*; by virtue of its amphipathic nature, hydrophilic substances such as cholesterol and the fatty acids of lecithin are contained inside, whereas hydrophilic groups such as the polar end of fatty acids and monoglycerides are on its surface.

Micelle formation may be impaired in several ways: *inadequate hydrolysis* of triglyceride to monoglyceride and fatty acids (as in pancreatic insufficiency); *poor mixing* of pancreatic lipase and triglyceride (following subtotal gastrectomy); or *deficiency of conjugated bile salts* (as in bacterial overgrowth, cholestatic liver disease, biliary tract obstruction, or following resection of distal ileum). Micellar lipid crosses the membrane, but the conjugated bile salts pass into the lower small intestine, where they are actively absorbed, and return to the liver for re-excretion into bile. The total bile salt pool, 4.0 grams, is thus in large part sustained.

The major site for fat absorption is the upper jejunum. For normal function, at least 90 cm. of this segment must be free of bacterial overgrowth and must contain normal villi and patent lymphatics. Triglycerides (neutral fat) after emulsification with fatty acids and bile salts *may* be absorbed unhydrolyzed, but apparently only in small quantity. Indeed, 80 to 90 per cent of neutral fat is either partly or completely hydrolyzed.

Although exact figures are not available, a considerable amount of fat may be absorbed in the absence of bile, indicating that the process is not entirely dependent upon micelles. The question of ileal absorption of fat has not been resolved.

The rate of absorption of both free fatty acids and glycerides is determined mainly by both chain length and degree of saturation of the fatty acids involved. The mechanism for penetration of the lipid cell membrane is unknown, but does not appear to require energy; the exact nonenzymatic, physicochemical process is unknown.

Conjugated bile salts also help to activate intracellular enzymes, which are required for resynthesis of triglyceride, a necessary step in chylomicron formation; although unconjugated bile salts at high concentrations may appear to inhibit uptake of lipid as well as resynthesis of triglyceride intracellularly, decreased concentration of conjugated bile salts is responsible for diminished uptake and reesterification. In the mucosal cells, fatty acids may be esterified or incorporated into phospholipids. Short-chain fatty acids (fewer than 10 carbon atoms) pass into the portal venous system without esterification. Long-chain fatty acids (more than 16 carbon atoms) are esterified and pass into the intestinal lymphatics. Recently, medium-chain triglycerides (MCT), with fatty acids of length C-8 to C-12, have been shown to be partially hydrolyzed in the absence of bile salts and pancreatic lipase. Thus, this lipid is more readily prepared for absorption than the long-chain triglycerides. Unsplit MCT also appears to be taken up by cells to some extent, and is hydrolyzed by mucosal lipase, releasing fatty acids. Further, short-chain fatty acids pass directly into the portal venous system. This independence of mucosal re-esterification and of the lymphatics is thought to be advantageous in patients with intestinal mucosal disease. Obviously, MCT may be extremely useful in the therapy of patients with malabsorption syndrome, and its indications and usefulness will be discussed under Treatment (*vide infra*, Table 6).

Absorption of *cholesterol* appears to depend upon its separation from protein and release from fatty acid esters through hydrolysis by pancreatic esterase. The intestine also synthesizes cholesterol as well as very low density lipoproteins. Dietary vitamin A, largely in ester form, undergoes hydrolysis in the intestinal lumen to the free alcohol. The absorption of both cholesterol and vitamin A alcohol requires bile salts. Indeed it now seems likely that absorption of cholesterol and all fat-soluble vitamins is more dependent upon micelle formation than are the hydrolytic products of neutral fat.

Protein and Amino Acid Absorption. Gastric pepsin may partially hydrolyze dietary protein; however, complete hydrolysis is due to the action of pancreatic proteolytic enzymes such as *trypsin*, *chymotrypsin*, and *carboxy-peptidase*. No evidence exists that peptides pass the membrane barrier of the intestinal mucosal cell under *normal* conditions. If small peptides gained access to the cell, it is almost certain that they would be rapidly split into their component amino acids. However, peptides are probably absorbed in very early infancy. Moreover, a recent study indicates that hydroxyproline peptides are absorbed after the ingestion of gelatin.

With regard to amino acid absorption, it seems that the majority of L-amino acids are transported actively and more rapidly than the D isomers, which diffuse across the membrane; the rate of uptake of the L-isomers is regulated by a saturable carrier system in the apical membrane of the absorbing cells. Eighty to 90 per cent of "liberated" amino acids are absorbed in the jejunum in man and the balance in the lower small intestine. The rate of movement into the mucosa depends greatly upon the configuration and chain length of the "R substituent" of the α carbon. Thus, mono-amino monocarboxylic amino acids are absorbed more rapidly than those with di-amino (lysine) or di-carboxylic (glutamine) groups. Some modification of the α amino group or abolition of the free carboxyl group affects active transport. An important factor influencing absorption of these substances is the mutual inhibition of constituent L-amino acids when fed as mixtures. The action of L-methionine is notable in this regard. Amino acid transfer requires sodium ions in the medium, and is oxygen dependent.

Amino acids may be synthesized into peptides in the mucosal cells; most of them pass quickly into the blood, however, and enter the general "metabolic pool." The liver is the principal organ for their metabolism.

Carbohydrate Absorption. Starch is broken down in the duodenum into nonabsorbable disaccharides, maltose and isomaltose, and some glucose. Maltose and other dietary disaccharides, sucrose and lactose, are split further by maltase, sucrase, and lactase, respectively, into their component monosaccharides, glucose-glucose, glucose-fructose and glucose-galactose. These enzymes are located in the brush border (microvillus) of the absorbing cell. The rate of absorption of hexoses in descending order is galactose, glucose, fructose. Glucose and galactose are actively transported, and fructose diffuses passively; however, its absorption may be "facilitated" by a poorly understood mechanism, and some of it is converted to glucose within the cell. Others (xylose, mannose, sorbose) apparently are not actively transported; however, it is questionable whether they pass into the gut wall in a strictly passive fashion, since these water-soluble substances must penetrate the fatty envelope of the cell. Recent evidence derived from study of the movement of pentose and other sugars into various cell preparations indicates that a true passive transfer is not likely.

The exact mechanism of carbohydrate transport has not been elucidated. It is clear, however, that phosphorylation plays no role. Active transport of glucose depends somewhat upon presence of a free OH in the second position. Although it is possible that a chemical reaction is necessary for active transport, this phenomenon has not been demonstrated for any sugar. The concentration and movement of various ions, particularly sodium, appear to be vital to glucose absorption. Indeed, the hypothesis that the transfer of glucose into and out of the cell is dependent upon the movement of sodium—the so-called "sodium pump mechanism"—is currently accepted as valid, the "carrier system" for sugar requiring a primary interaction with Na^+ at the villous membrane.

Vitamin B_{12} Absorption. Vitamin B_{12} absorption is dependent upon the presence of "intrinsic factor" (IF), a constituent of gastric juice. Vitamin B_{12} in complex with this substance adheres to the gut wall, preferentially the ileum, and then in some unknown manner, after several hours, becomes "unbound" and passes into the blood. Whether or not the uptake by mucosal cells is energy-dependent is not settled. It is fairly certain, however, that calcium ion is required for the uptake of vitamin B_{12}-IF complex by the mucosa. Alterations in bacterial flora, such as obtain in the "blind loop syndrome" (*vide infra*) or after subtotal gastrectomy and gastrojejunostomy (Billroth II), lead to decreased absorption of B_{12} that, in most instances, can be reversed by the administration of broad-spectrum antimicrobial drugs. In some manner these bacteria bind the B_{12} or the complex or somehow destroy the complex (see Table 3).

Folic Acid Absorption. Dietary folic acid is in the form of conjugated folate, linked to glutamate residues. Normal absorption depends, therefore, upon enzymatic deconjugation in the mucosa. As with hexoses, lipid, calcium, iron, water-soluble vitamins, fat-soluble vitamins, and amino acids, folic acid is absorbed in the proximal small gut.

Water and Sodium Absorption. The bulk of water and electrolyte absorption takes place in the small intestine. The rate of water absorption in the small gut is five to ten times that in the stomach. Sodium absorption, likewise, occurs rapidly in the upper small bowel. Water absorption is a passive phenomenon proximally, which is linked to, and dependent upon, active absorption of dissolved solutes, sodium and, particularly, glucose, moving with them to maintain isotonicity of intraluminal contents. Sodium transport in the ileum is an active process. The small intestine usually absorbs over 7 liters of water and about 700 mEq. of sodium per day. Potassium movement seems to be passive, diffusing from the lumen proximally and into the lumen distally.

The amount of water and sodium absorbed represents the difference between influx from lumen to blood and efflux in the reverse direction. This net flux is diminished by hypertonicity of the intraluminal solution and is increased by hypotonicity. Changes in concentration of sodium in the lumen depend on relative rates of exchange of both sodium and water between blood and lumen.

During diarrhea, sodium concentration increases with increasing stool volume, and beyond 3 liters approaches values close to that of plasma. Conversely, potassium concentration progressively decreases.

Calcium and Iron Absorption. Observation of everted gut sacs shows that calcium is absorbed actively. This transport is facilitated by *parathyroid hormone* and by *vitamin D*, and is inhibited by deprivation of this vitamin. Anaerobiosis is also inhibitory. In vivo calcium absorption depends also upon pH and concentration of phosphates and fatty acids, as well as upon vitamin D. Vitamin D absorption is necessary for calcium absorption since it stimulates synthesis of a calcium-binding protein which is a key substance in the active transport of the cation. Also, vitamin D (specifically, 25 OH cholecalciferol, its active form), stimulates Na^+ dependent ATP-ase to release calcium from its binder in the cell.

Like calcium, *iron* has been shown to be absorbed *actively* and is dependent upon oxidative metabolism. The duodenum is the principal site for uptake of both calcium and iron. Iron absorption is diminished in chronic infection and by prior administration of large amounts of iron, and apparently is increased in pregnancy and iron deficiency. Iron from hemoglobin is an important source of this substance in the human. After ingestion hemoglobin is split in the upper gut; heme is readily absorbed, from which iron is split within the cell and passes thence into the circulation where it is bound by iron-binding protein. Some iron is released from heme intraluminally and is taken up directly by the cells. In human subjects, absorption of iron depends

upon its release from dietary compounds to which it is originally bound. Administration of ascorbic acid appears to facilitate absorption, both by chelation of iron and by promoting reduction of the ferric to the ferrous form. Diminished iron absorption is associated with achlorhydria, since an acid pH is needed to solubilize ferric iron for chelation with ascorbic acid and other substances, in which form it is absorbed. Ferrous iron may be chelated at an alkaline pH. Over-all, iron absorption is regulated by the state of repletion, content of iron in absorbing cells, and factors affecting erythropoiesis. Influence of gastric and pancreatic juice proteins which bind iron is still uncertain.

CAUSES OF THE MALABSORPTION SYNDROME

The principal diseases and disorders that may give rise to the malabsorption syndrome are listed in Table 1. These conditions are discussed in detail in a subsequent portion of this article and are presented only in brief outline at this point. They can be divided conveniently into seven categories as follows:

1. Defective Intraluminal Hydrolysis. Conditions that lead to failure of normal breakdown of fat as well as of other substances include *gastrectomy, cirrhosis, biliary tract obstruction,* and *pancreatic insufficiency.* In the case of *gastrectomy,* the magnitude of the resulting steatorrhea is roughly proportional to the amount of organ excised. A 15 to 20 per cent loss of ingested fat is common in about three quarters of those with subtotal gastrectomy, and a 30 per cent or more loss is usual after total gastrectomy.

Chronic liver disease, particularly *biliary cirrhosis,* and chronic *obstruction* of the *biliary tree* (common bile duct stone, carcinoma of the bile ducts, etc.) cause impaired fat digestion principally through insufficiency of bile and, perhaps in some instances, alteration of its composition. Resection of terminal ileum by reducing resorption of bile salts and the bile salt pool may lead to serious decrease of the intraluminal concentration of bile salts in the jejunum and thus to decreased micellar lipid. Gastric hypersecretion, by inactivation of lipase, also reduces micellar lipid.

Pancreatic insufficiency results in loss of as much as 80 per cent of fat in the stool. Failure to produce lipase and/or obstruction of flow into the upper duodenum are the causes. In patients with subtotal or total gastrectomy and gastrojejunostomy, adequate stimulation of flow of both pancreatic secretion and bile is probably diminished (see Diseases of the Hepatic System).

2. Primary Mucosal Cell Abnormality. This group includes celiac disease (adult and childhood), deficiency of disaccharidases, and a-beta-lipoproteinemia. In a-beta-lipoproteinemia the mucosa is unable to form chylomicrons (inability to synthesize lipoproteins) necessary for entrance of lipid into lacteals. Also included are primary glucose-galactose malabsorption and disorders of impaired transport of dibasic amino acids, cystine, and neutral amino acids (cystinuria and Hartnup disease).

3, 4. Inadequate Absorptive Surface and Abnormalities of the Small Intestine. Jejunal exclusion, gastroileostomy, massive resection of the small intestine, and large enteroenteric fistulas form this group.

5. Lymphatic Obstruction. Failure to absorb normally in lymphoma, Whipple's disease, and tuberculosis (tabes mesenterica) and, to some extent, in granulomatous enteritis as well as lymphangiectasia is secondary to stasis of the lymphatic system of the small bowel.

6. Altered Bacterial Flora and Parasitic Infections. Such alteration is noted in the blind loops, multiple jejunal diverticula, multiple strictures, small fistulas, intestinal scleroderma, tropical sprue, Whipple's disease, strongyloidiasis, *Giardia lamblia,* and during therapy with certain antimicrobial drugs.

7. Miscellaneous. This group includes carcinoid syndrome, diabetes mellitus, hypoparathyroidism, hypothyroidism, islet

TABLE 1. CAUSES OF THE MALABSORPTION
SYNDROME

1. Defective Intraluminal Hydrolysis:
　Stomach resection
　Pancreatic insufficiency
　Gastric hypersecretion of acid
　　Non B islet cell tumor of pancreas
　　Massive small bowel resection
　Exclusion or deficiency of conjugated bile salts
　　Biliary obstruction
　　Biliary cirrhosis
　　Ileal resection

2. Primary Mucosal Cell Abnormality:
　Celiac disease
　A-beta-lipoproteinemia
　Disaccharidase deficiency
　Monosaccharide malabsorption
　Cystinuria and Hartnup disease
　Absence of B_{12}–IF receptor

3. Inadequate Absorptive Surface:
　Massive small gut resection
　Ileal resection or by-pass
　Jejunal by-pass:
　　Jejunocolic fistula (large)
　　Surgical gastroileostomy

4. Abnormalities of the Intestinal Wall:
　Ileojejunitis, granulomatous and nongranulomatous
　Infectious enteritis
　Amyloidosis
　Drug effects
　Radiation injury
　Eosinophilic enteritis
　Mastocytosis

5. Lymphatic Obstruction and Stasis:
　Lymphoma
　Tuberculosis (tabes mesenterica)
　Lymphangiectasia

6. Bacterial Overgrowth and Parasitic Infections:
　Blind loops
　Multiple jejunal diverticula
　Multiple strictures
　Enteroenteric or enterocolic fistulas
　Scleroderma
　Whipple's disease
　Tropical sprue
　Giardia lamblia
　Strongyloidiasis

7. Miscellaneous:
　Carcinoid syndrome
　Diabetic neuropathy
　Hypoparathyroidism
　Hypothyroidism
　Hypogammaglobulinemia
　Mesenteric artery insufficiency
　Vasculitis (systemic lupus erythematosus, Degos' disease)

cell tumor of the pancreas, hypogammaglobulinemia, mesenteric artery insufficiency, and vasculitis (systemic lupus erythematosus, Degos' disease). The mechanisms for impaired absorption in this group differ and in general are not well understood.

CLINICAL MANIFESTATIONS

The signs and symptoms of the malabsorption syndrome include weight loss, anorexia, abdominal distention, borborygmi, muscle wasting, and passage of abnormal stools that are characteristically light yellow to gray, greasy, and soft. In many instances frequent movements are noted, but occasionally there is only one stool per day. In addition, edema, ascites, skeletal disorders, peripheral and circumoral paresthesias, tetany, and, rarely, convulsions may be observed.

The clinical features that result from deficiencies of fat-soluble vitamins include *hyperkeratosis follicularis* (vitamin A); *bleeding*, particularly *ecchymoses* and *hematuria* (vitamin K); and *bone pain* or *fractures* (vitamin D) (Table 2). Deficiencies of the vitamin B complex are manifested by *glossitis, cheilosis, muscle tenderness, peripheral neuritis*, and *dermatitis* (Table 2). The symptoms of the malabsorption syndrome may be intermittent or low-grade, so that medical attention is not sought for a very long time—more than 35 years in some instances of adult celiac disease. The secondary manifestations of malabsorption may often overshadow the intestinal complaints. For example, about 20 per cent of patients with *adult celiac disease* will seek aid for bleeding or for skeletal pain or fractures. In many patients, *weakness, fatigue, dyspnea*, or *dizziness*, all due to anemia, may be the presenting symptoms. *Borborygmi* and *abdominal distention*, which increase during the day and are often not relieved by defecation, are among the most common complaints. An extreme degree of such distress is frequently noted in patients with *scleroderma* of the small intestine.

About 25 per cent of patients with *adult celiac disease* have abdominal pain, usually cramping. Variable degrees of pain accompany other diseases of malabsorption as well. Thus, the patient with granulomatous *ileojejunitis* may note periumbilical or right lower quadrant pain, most often following meals; those with *chronic pancreatitis* usually suffer recurrent deep epigastric pain that radiates to the mid-back; in patients with *lymphoma* of the small intestine and mesentery, the pain may be cramping (obstruction) or steady and intense (local invasion or spread).

Patients with malabsorption owing to *ischemia* of the small gut often also have periumbilical or midabdominal cramping pains 20 to 30 minutes after meals and often other evidence of either widespread arteriosclerosis, or have chronic atrial fibrillation. Those with hypo- or agammaglobulinemia may have other historic evidences of immunoglobulin deficiency (repeated infections; symptoms suggesting autoimmunity or even malignancy). *Eosinophilic gastroenteritis* is often highlighted by a specific "food allergy" or by a history of skin, nasopharyngeal, bronchial, or other allergy. Virulent peptic ulcer disease (Zollinger-Ellison syndrome) will highlight the history of malabsorption caused by *gastric hypersecretion*. Diarrhea associated with carbohydrate will be noted from childhood in those with *disaccharidase deficiency* or *monosaccharide malabsorption*. Surgical scars and associated histories will highlight cases of *massive resection, gastrectomy,* and *blind loop*.

Physical examination usually reveals *low blood pressure* and evidences of malnutrition and multiple vitamin deficiencies: *pallor, diffuse* brownish

TABLE 2. CORRELATION OF LABORATORY DATA WITH ABSORPTIVE DEFECTS AND SIGNS AND SYMPTOMS OF THE MALABSORPTION SYNDROME

Clinical Features	Laboratory Evidence	Pathophysiology
Muscle wasting; small stature; edema	↓ Serum albumin	*Impaired protein metabolism* ↓ Absorption ↓ Intake ↑ Enteric loss ? Impaired synthesis
Skeletal deformity; pain; fractures	Skeletal demineralization roentgenographically	
Weight loss; pale, bulky stools	↑ Fecal fat ↓ Serum cholesterol, carotene	*Impaired absorption and excess loss of:* Fat Fat-soluble vitamins and calcium:
Paresthesias; tetany; + Chvostek and Trousseau signs	↓ Serum Ca^{++}; ↓ or nor. PO$_4$; ↑ Alkaline phosphatase. Osteomalacia roentgenographically (Milkman's fractures)	Vitamin D and calcium
Bleeding; ecchymoses, hematuria, etc.	↑ Prothrombin time	Vitamin K
Hyperkeratosis follicularis	↓ Oral vitamin A tolerance	Vitamin A
A N E M I A — G L O S S I T I S — Paresthesias; Neuropathy	Macrocytic anemia; megaloblastosis; ↓ serum B$_{12}$ and ↓ absorption B$_{12}$ (CO^{60}B$_{12}$)	Vitamin B$_{12}$
	Macrocytic anemia; megaloblastosis; ↓ serum folic acid; ↑ formimino-glutamic acid (Figlu) in urine after histidine load	Folic acid
Koilonychia	Microcytosis, hypochromia; ↓ serum iron and ↓ saturation iron binding protein; ↓ iron in marrow	Iron
Weakness; paresthesias; tetany	↓ Serum magnesium	Magnesium
Dehydration; nocturia	↓ Plasma volume	Water
Muscle cramps, weakness	↓ Serum Na$^+$	Sodium
Muscle flaccidity, weakness; ↓ tendon reflexes; arrhythmias	↓ Serum K$^+$; EKG abnormalities	Potassium
Cheilosis; neuritis; dermatitis; glossitis, muscle weakness	↑ Urinary tryptophan metabolites (B$_6$); n-methylnicotinamide (B$_2$); ↓ red cell transketolase (B$_1$)	Vitamin B complex
Abdominal distention; flatulence; diarrhea	Low to flat oral glucose tolerance curve; ↓ absorption d-xylose; ↓ oral lactose tolerance; ↓ or absent rise of blood glucose after oral sucrose; ↓ or absent rise of blood reducing substances after oral galactose	*Impaired hydrolysis of disaccharides, particularly lactose and sucrose, or ↓ absorption of mono-saccharides*

pigmentation of the skin but not of the mucous membranes, *hyperkeratosis, petechiae* or *ecchymoses, muscle wasting, edema, abdominal distention, skeletal deformity* (particularly kyphosis), *positive Chvostek* and/or *Trousseau signs, glossitis, cheilosis, impaired vibration sense, deep muscle pain,* and *clubbing* of the fingers. In addition, signs of various underlying diseases may be noted: an abdominal mass (*lymphoma, regional enteritis*); fixation or severe limitation of joint movement and thickened skin (*scleroderma*); facial flush and hepatomegaly (*carcinoid syndrome*); puffed facies, bradycardia, hair loss (*hypothyroidism*); arthritis or skin rashes (*hypogammaglobulinemia*); nasopharyngeal congestion, skin rash, wheezing (*eosinophilic gastroenteritis*); butterfly rash, splenomegaly, etc. (*SLE*); neurologic impairments (*a-beta-lipoproteinemia*); diminished or absent peripheral arterial pulsations, cataracts, and absent or diminished deep tendon reflexes or

other evidences of diabetic neuropathy (*diabetes mellitus*); lymphadenopathy, arthritis, and signs of pulmonary disease (*Whipple's disease*).

The malabsorption syndrome may be fatal, owing to the nature of the underlying disease (*lymphoma, pancreatic carcinoma, progressive scleroderma,* or *granulomatous enteritis*) or to the complications of malabsorption, which include superimposed infection, hypokalemia, or progressive inanition.

THE PHYSIOLOGIC MECHANISMS OF THE CLINICAL MANIFESTATIONS

In Table 2 may be seen the correlation between various absorptive defects and vitamin deficiencies, the clinical signs and symptoms, and the abnormalities of the routine laboratory tests in the malabsorption syndrome. Rarely does a patient manifest all of the findings listed in Table 2, but many patients will exhibit most of them.

Impaired Protein Metabolism: Loss of Weight, Edema. Protein metabolism, reflected by decreased muscle mass and lowered serum protein levels, is impaired for several reasons. *Synthesis* is below normal owing to defective protein absorption. *Catabolism* or breakdown is accelerated because of inadequate intake and absorption of carbohydrate. Decreased serum albumin may result also from abnormal loss of protein into the lumen of the gut, so-called *protein-losing enteropathy.* Such loss is usually associated with diseases that cause malabsorption by lymphatic obstruction or in which there is an inflammatory mucosal lesion, although it has also been reported in adult celiac disease (*vide infra*). *Hypogammaglobulinemia,* both congenital and acquired, has also been associated with steatorrhea, but the defective fat absorption cannot be related directly to low plasma globulins. In some instances, *impaired hepatic function* contributes to lowered serum protein levels.

The emaciation and weakness may be extreme (Fig. 1). The finding of hypotension and diffuse pigmentation makes the picture closely resemble severe *adrenal cortical insufficiency. Hypokalemia* as well as partial atrophy may underlie muscle weakness.

Clinical Manifestations Resulting from Steatorrhea. Excess loss of fat in the stool deprives the body of substantial calories and contributes greatly to weight loss and malnutrition. Perhaps the irritative effect of unabsorbed long-chain (C18) fatty acids which are hydroxylated contributes to the diarrhea with its severe losses of water, electrolytes, and other nutrients. In addition, binding of calcium by fatty acids contributes to hypocalcemia. Flatulence and abdominal distention may be related to both diminished fat absorption and excessive carbohydrate fermentation. Failure to absorb fat-soluble vitamins A, D, and K also results in a variety of serious symptoms as recorded in Table 2.

Vitamin D Deficiency: Hypocalcemia and Skeletal Disease in Malabsorption Syndrome; Hypomagnesemia. Low serum calcium results from failure of normal absorption owing both to vitamin D deficiency and to chelation of calcium by unab-

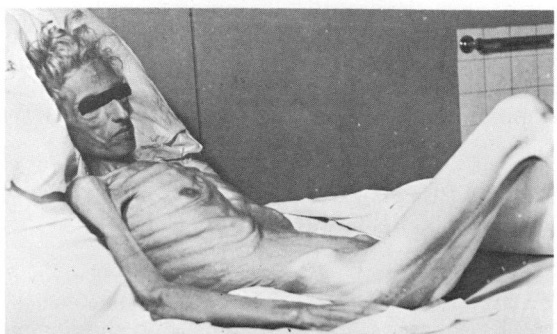

FIGURE 1. Extreme wasting in a patient with adult celiac disease (nontropical sprue).

sorbed fatty acids. Symptoms caused by depression of unbound or "ultrafilterable" calcium of the blood range from *paresthesias* of extremities and circumoral area to *carpopedal* and *laryngeal spasms* and *muscle cramps.* When levels are extremely low, the patient may even convulse. Clinically, hypocalcemia may be demonstrated by *Chvostek* or *Trousseau signs.* Obviously, the defect in calcium absorption involves more than deficiency of vitamin D, since the return of serum calcium to normal in patients with adult celiac disease who are on a gluten-free diet is more rapid than may be attributed to the action of this vitamin.

Low levels of serum calcium stimulate parathyroid activity. Increased secretion of parathormone raises the level of blood calcium both by direct effect upon bone and by a renal mechanism. These processes lead to demineralization—*osteomalacia.* Osteomalacia principally affects the spine, rib cage, and long bones, with or without fractures (Milkman's fractures), and may cause extreme pain and disability.

In patients with poor protein nutrition, in part caused by malabsorption or protein-losing enteropathy (*vide infra*), particularly postmenopausal women and elderly men, the demineralization process is aggravated by *osteoporosis* or failure to deposit bone matrix.

Hypomagnesemia may also be noted in the malabsorption syndrome, causing symptoms that are identical with those of hypocalcemia. Differentiation is accomplished by the finding of lowered serum magnesium and by disappearance of symptoms only after administration of magnesium chloride or sulfate. Hypomagnesemia also may dramatically reduce the responsiveness of the parathyroids to hypocalcemia. Indeed, correction of magnesium deficiency is essential to restoration of normal calcium by action of the parathyroid glands.

Vitamin K Deficiency: Bleeding Diathesis in Malabsorption Syndrome. As noted, *bleeding,* particularly subcutaneous, nasal, urinary, vaginal, and, occasionally, gastrointestinal, is not uncommon in the malabsorption syndrome and may be the principal symptom. Defects in coagulation are seen as a result of deficiency of plasma prothrombin owing to impaired absorption of fat-soluble vitamin K.

Vitamin A Deficiency. In the malabsorption syndrome *hyperkeratosis follicularis* may be noted, but nyctalopia is very rare.

Manifestations of Abnormal Carbohydrate Absorption. The abnormal carbohydrate absorption results in diminished glycogen stores in liver and muscle. Also, intraluminal fermentation of sugars contributes greatly to *abdominal distention* and *flatulence.* Failure to hydrolyze disaccharides, particularly lactose (*disaccharidase deficiency*), results in watery diarrhea as well as these local abdominal complaints (*vide infra*).

Anemia. Deficiency of vitamin B_{12} or folic acid may cause a macrocytic anemia with megaloblastic bone marrow changes, whereas iron deficiency will cause a microcytic hypochromic anemia. With deficiency of vitamin B_{12}, folic acid, and iron, anemia with mixed features will be present. The former type is seen in tropical sprue, following resection of a large segment of the terminal ileum, and in conditions in which there is bacterial overgrowth in the upper small intestine—"blind loops," jejunal diverticulosis, enteroenteric or enterocolic fistulas, and multiple small bowel strictures. In contrast to pernicious anemia, in these conditions simultaneous feeding of intrinsic factor does not improve vitamin B_{12} absorption. In those cases due to bacterial overgrowth as well as in tropical sprue, normal absorption of B_{12} may be restored by oral administration of a broad-spectrum antimicrobial drug—chloramphenicol, tetracycline, or ampicillin (1.0 gram daily) for 10 to 14 days (Table 3). Indeed, a brisk reticulocytosis may be noted in three to four days. Impaired absorption of vitamin B_{12} and megaloblastosis may also be noted occasionally in patients with *adult celiac disease*.

Folic Acid Deficiency. Folic acid deficiency may also underlie *megaloblastosis* and *anemia*. As there is often an associated deficiency of B_{12}, diagnosis may be established only by the finding of low blood folic acid levels (< 40 mcg.) after an oral load, or of increased urinary formimino glutamic acid (Figlu) after feeding histidine, or of a reticulocytic response to administration of minimal daily effective dosage (0.05 to 0.5 mg. parenterally).

Glossitis and Peripheral Neuropathy. *Glossitis* and *peripheral neuropathy* can in part be attributed to deficiency of vitamin B_{12}. Since combined system disease may be induced or exacerbated by administration of folic acid, normal vitamin B_{12} absorption must be established before institution of folic acid *alone* for megaloblastic anemia.

Iron Absorption. Iron absorption may be subnormal except when the malabsorption syndrome is due to uncomplicated pancreatic insufficiency. Most often the iron deficiency is caused by poor absorption owing either to mucosal disease or to inability to release inorganic iron from organic compounds. However, occult blood loss may contribute to the anemia. Iron deficiency anemia is very common in adult celiac disease and may be noted also in the later stages of tropical sprue. When associated with deficiencies of folic acid and vitamin B_{12}, iron deficiency may not become apparent until these substances are repleted. Incorporation of iron into young marrow red blood cells requires both folic acid and vitamin B_{12}.

Dehydration, Muscle Cramps and Weakness. Common in the malabsorption syndrome are *dehydration, weakness,* and *hypotension*. Large amounts of water and electrolytes are lost if diarrhea is severe or if stools are very loose or bulky. Absorption of water in adult celiac disease is slower than normal, and diuresis after a water load is delayed. Thus, patients with steatorrhea often have nocturia. *Hyponatremia* not due to renal loss responds readily to administration of sodium, and symptoms of "low salt"—weakness, lethargy, nausea, cramps —rapidly disappear. *Hypokalemia,* if severe, causes muscle flaccidity and cardiac arrhythmias.

Vitamin B Complex Deficiency: Dermatitis, Neuritis, and Cheilosis. Although *glossitis, neuritis* (peripheral neuropathy), and *dermatitis* in the malabsorption syndrome have been attributed to deficiency of B vitamins, proof of impaired absorption of these substances—vitamins B_1, B_2 and B_6—is not at hand. Perhaps deficiency results from metabolic action of abnormal bacterial flora that ordinarily do not inhabit the small bowel. However, conclusive demonstration of this mechanism also is lacking, particularly in *adult celiac disease*. Moreover, administration of vitamin B complex ($B_{1, 2, 6, 12}$) does not always cure the glossitis, which may be partially due to iron deficiency. Laboratory tests for deficiencies of components of the vitamin B complex are listed in Table 2.

DIAGNOSIS

The clues to diagnosis of the malabsorption syndrome are the history, symptoms, signs, and laboratory abnormalities listed in Tables 2 and 4 that relate to malabsorption of fat and other substances, particularly fat soluble vitamins, proteins, iron, and vitamin B_{12}. Thus the patient will complain of rather bulky, light-colored stools, often with increased frequency (but not necessarily so), abdominal distention, and variable weight

TABLE 3. DIAGNOSTIC VALUE OF Co^{60}-VITAMIN B_{12} ABSORPTION STUDIES

	Megaloblastic Anemia Associated with:				
	Pernicious Anemia and Total Gastrectomy	Adult Celiac Disease	Blind Loop Syndrome	Primary Malabsorption of Vitamin B_{12}	Tropical Sprue
	. . . Absorption . . .				
Vitamin B_{12}	Low	Low-normal	Low	Low	Low
Vitamin B_{12} + Intrinsic factor	Normal	Low No change	No change	No change	No change
Vitamin B_{12} after antimicrobial therapy	Low	No change	Normal	No change	Normal or low
Vitamin B_{12} after gluten-free diet		Normal	Low	No change	No change

loss, and will also show laboratory evidence of impaired absorption. Worthy of special mention are the patients who complain principally of bleeding tendency or of some skeletal disability, chiefly pain. Other features commonly seen in many diseases of this syndrome include *hypotension, abdominal distention, diffuse brownish pigmentation,* and *clubbing of the fingers and toes.*

It is not usually difficult to establish solely by clinical examination that the malabsorption syndrome is present. Much more precise information as to *which* absorption defects are present is necessary, however, if the physician is to treat the illness successfully. In large measure, this essential information can be obtained only by the proper use of a number of laboratory procedures.

Laboratory Diagnosis

The pathophysiologic basis for the abnormal findings of the laboratory tests has been described and is presented in Table 2. The particular uses of the individual tests in arriving at a diagnosis are considered in Table 4.

Measurement of Stool Fat: Serum Carotene. Because the most important feature in diagnosis of the malabsorption syndrome is steatorrhea, accurate measurement of fecal fat is extremely important. The only reliable method is the chemical analysis of a 72-hour stool collection, the patient ingesting 90 to 100 grams of fat per day. Normal excretion in these circumstances is 5.0 grams or less per 24 hours (Table 4).

In recent years much experience with the use of I[131] triolein in measuring fat absorption has accumulated. However, after the feeding of this substance, I[131] activity in neither the blood nor the stool quantitatively reflects the amount of fat absorbed, since about 15 per cent of patients with chemically determined steatorrhea will have normal stool radioactivity, and 28 per cent will have a normal peak of blood radioactivity. Conversely, 10 to 20 per cent of persons with normal stool fat content will have abnormal stool activity. Moreover, I[131] triolein does not yield quantitative information about *dietary* fat absorption.

Depressed levels of *serum carotene* will usually be found in patients with steatorrhea. This test is useful in "screening" those in whom the malabsorption syndrome is suspected. Recently, reports of malabsorption syndrome resulting from adult celiac disease with impaired absorption of iron or calcium without steatorrhea have appeared.

Pancreatic Function. A very important part of differential diagnosis is the evaluation of pancreatic function by measurement of volume and bicarbonate concentration of duodenal aspirates and enzyme activity of serum (amylase, lipase) after appropriate stimulation (see Diseases of the

TABLE 4. LABORATORY TESTS COMMONLY EMPLOYED TO STUDY ABSORPTION

	Normal Values	Malabsorption Syndrome
Serum:		
Albumin	4.0 to 5.2 grams/100 ml.	Diminished
Carotene	0.06 to 0.4 mg./100 ml.	Diminished
Calcium	9.0 to 10.5 mg./100 ml.	Diminished
Cholesterol	150 to 250 mg./100 ml.	Diminished
Potassium	3.5 to 4.7 mEq./L	Diminished
Magnesium	1.7 to 2.0 mEq./L	Diminished
Plasma:		
Prothrombin time	Control value	Elevated
Tolerance tests:		
d-Xylose (25 grams orally)	Urinary excretion of 4.5 grams or greater per 5 hours	Diminished (normal in pancreatic insufficiency)
Glucose (100 grams orally)	35 mg. rise over fasting plasma level	"Flat curve" in celiac disease and diseases of intestinal wall and in monosaccharide malabsorption
Vitamin A (0.22 gram/kg. of oily vitamin A which contains 60,000 units/gram)	A rise of at least 50 May units at 3 to 8 hours	"Flat curve"
Lactose (50 to 100 grams orally)	Rise in blood glucose of 20 mg./100 ml.	Low to flat curve in primary lactase deficiency; celiac disease; diseases of the intestinal wall
Galactose (1.75 grams/kg. orally)	Rise in blood reducing substance of 20 to 40 per cent of fasting level	Low to flat
Sucrose (100 grams orally)	Rise in blood glucose of 20 mg./100 ml.	Low to flat
Stool Fat:		
Chemical determination (on 100 grams fat daily)	5 grams/24 hours	Increased
I[131] Triolein (3-day collection)	0 to 4%	Increased
I[131] Oleic acid (3-day collection)	0 to 4%	Increased
Miscellaneous:		
5-Hydroxyindolacetic acid (urinary excretion)	1.7 to 8.0 mg./24 hours	9 to 20 mg. in adult celiac disease; 30 to 600 mg. in metastatic carcinoid syndrome
Indole-3-acetic acid (urinary excretion)	Less than 18 mg./24 hours	Elevated
Indican (urinary excretion)	Less than 100 mg./24 hours	Elevated

Pancreas). Subnormal response strongly indicates pancreatic insufficiency or pancreatic ductal obstruction, although normal values do not exclude these possibilities.

Roentgenographic Changes. Diagnosis of the malabsorption syndrome may be facilitated by recognition of nonspecific changes in the roentgenograms of the small bowel (Fig. 2). This "malabsorption pattern" includes dilatation of loops of small intestine, "flocculation" and "scattering" of barium, coarsening of valvulae conniventes, and rather oddly shaped collections called "moulage" (waxy casts).

The factors underlying these changes are not completely understood. Some disturbance of motility or the effect of overproduction of mucus, both perhaps caused by the collection in the gut of irritating substances such as fatty acids or substances derived from bacterial action, may be responsible. In many instances these changes cannot be correlated with the histologic picture of the small intestine, and are not present when "nonflocculating" barium is used. Differential diagnosis of various malabsorption states by roentgenographic examination of the small bowel is most difficult unless a characteristic finding for an underlying disease (tumor, stricture, or blind loop, etc.) is evident (Fig. 3).

Three aspects of malabsorption particularly helpful in differential diagnosis of the malabsorption syndrome merit special mention. These are: d-*xylose absorption;* measurement of tryptophan metabolites in the urine, *5-hydroxyindolacetic acid (50 HIAA), indole-3-acetic acid (I3AA or IAA),* and *indican;* and *histologic study,* by both dissecting and light microscopy and, very recently, by electron microscopy, of *jejunal mucosa* obtained by transoral suction biopsy.

Recently, indirect assay of small intestinal *lactase* has been carried out by oral administration of *lactose* followed by serial measurement of plasma glucose levels (*vide infra*: Disaccharidase Deficiency).

d-Xylose Absorption (Table 4). During recent years absorption of d-xylose has been measured in the study of a wide variety of intestinal disorders. Following absorption of this substance, its metabolism is not as rapid as that of glucose, and its renal excretion does not depend upon a threshold. Therefore, as a measure of carbohydrate absorption, it is more reliable than the oral glucose tolerance test. Also, about 20 per cent of normal subjects will have a flat or low glucose tolerance "curve," probably owing to delay in gastric emptying. Measurement of excretion of xylose in the urine is simple and reliable. The normal urinary excretion is at least 4.5 grams in five hours (Table 4).

Although the fate of a considerable proportion of the 25.0 gram oral load is unknown, it is clear that lowest excretion in five hours (<3.0 grams) is noted in untreated *adult celiac disease* and *tropical sprue* and separates patients with these disorders from those with pancreatic insufficiency and from

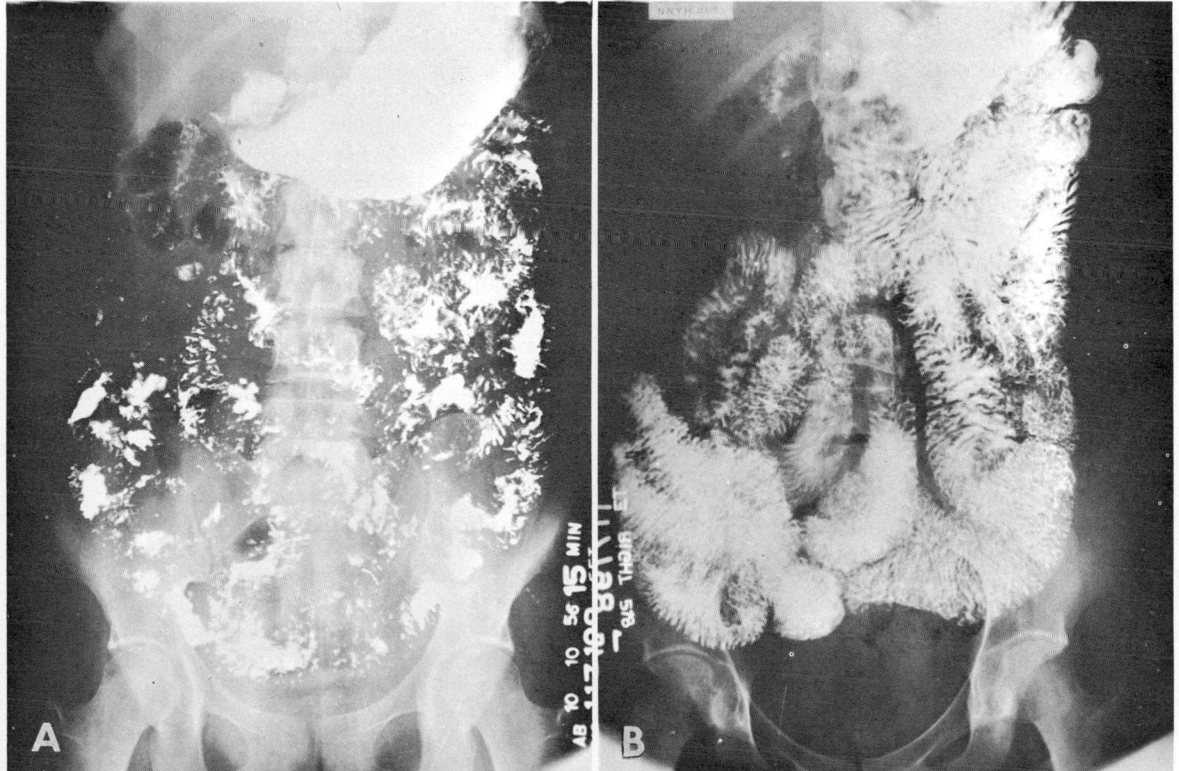

FIGURE 2. Small bowel roentgenographic series in patient (M.S.) with adult celiac disease. *A,* Before treatment. *B,* Six weeks after elimination of gluten from the diet. Note that the severely disordered pattern has improved.

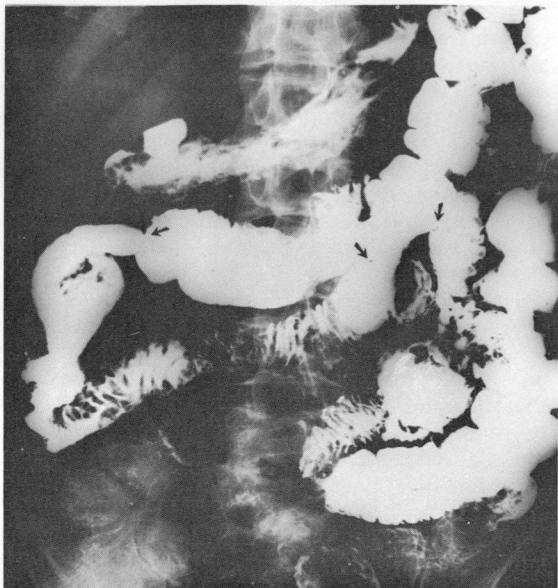

FIGURE 3. Small bowel series showing postoperative terminal ileum (arrow on left) and ileo transverse colostomy stoma (between arrows on right). Note the blind loop.

normal subjects. It has occasionally been found abnormal in *pancreatic carcinoma* with metastatic involvement of the small intestine, *scleroderma, Whipple's disease, acute staphylococcal enteritis,* extensive granulomatous and nongranulomatous enteritis, following massive resection of the small intestine, and in a number of other diseases of the small bowel.

In many patients with these as well as other diseases of malabsorption, however, excretion will be normal or only slightly depressed despite steatorrhea. In contrast to tropical sprue and *adult celiac disease,* it rarely is lower than 3.0 grams. When the excretion in any of these conditions is in this range, however, it is highly likely that the patient also has significant steatorrhea. Normal *d*-xylose absorption is strong evidence against the diagnosis of *adult celiac disease.* An abnormal result casts strong doubt upon the diagnosis of *pancreatic insufficiency.* The test is also valuable in gauging the effect of therapy when pretreatment values have been low. For proper evaluation of results, renal function must be normal. In such instances determination of blood levels may be helpful. Also, 25 per cent of healthy persons more than 65 years old will have diminished absorption of xylose.

Tryptophan Metabolites. The measurement of various urinary metabolites of L-tryptophan, particularly indole-3-acetic acid (I3AA), indican, and 5-hydroxyindolacetic acid (50HIAA), has been valuable in the study of the pathogenesis and diagnosis of malabsorptive states. Elevated urinary levels of indole-3-acetic acid (I3AA) are found in virtually all malabsorptive states, and the degree of elevation does not help in differential diagnosis. Return toward normal values may follow administration of broad-spectrum antimicrobials over a one- to two-week period. In adult celiac disease, adherence to a gluten-free diet will also result in return to normal excretion of this metabolite. Urinary *indican* is likely to be elevated in many diseases associated with the malabsorption syndrome, but is always elevated in those in which bacterial overgrowth is present (>100 mg./per 24 hours). Recent studies indicate that this test is a reliable guide in treatment of bacterial overgrowth because levels consistently fall toward normal when appropriate antimicrobial therapy is given.

The normal range of 5-hydroxyindolacetic acid is up to about 8.0 mg. per 24 hours. In adult celiac disease, however, the urinary level is elevated — 9.0 to 15.0 mg. — reflecting perhaps an increased amount of circulating 5-hydroxytryptamine or serotonin. Treatment with a gluten-free diet restores normal excretion of this substance. Except for the metastatic carcinoid syndrome, in which levels are greatly elevated (300 to 500 mg. per 24 hours), or Whipple's disease, in which an elevated level (15 mg. per 24 hours) has been reported in several instances, excretion of this substance is usually normal in the various disorders which may cause the malabsorption syndrome.

The significance of these findings is not clear, but they indicate abnormal metabolism of tryptophan. Most likely this is related in some way to stasis and bacterial overgrowth, but also, as shown by appropriate loading tests with tryptophan, to a deficiency in vitamin B_6, which is necessary for its normal metabolism. The role of indoleacetic acid in the pathophysiology of the malabsorption is not known, but there is evidence that it may have a suppressant effect upon the bone marrow.

Jejunal Histology. Histologic study of jejunal mucosa obtained by suction biopsy technique has further aided differential diagnosis of the malabsorption syndrome. The procedure is easily performed with one of several available tubes (Rubin tube, Crosby capsule, Shiner tube). Prothrombin time, as well as coagulation in general, must be normal. Characteristic findings have been associated with the *celiac syndrome* in both children and adults and in *tropical sprue, Whipple's disease, amyloidosis,* and *eosinophilic gastroenteritis.* In some instances alterations may be noted in diffuse *ileojejunitis,* in *lymphoma,* following *gastrectomy,* in *hypogammaglobulinemia* with steatorrhea, in patients with "*protein-losing enteropathy*" who have dilated lacteals, and in individuals with *radiation enteritis* or severe *drug reactions.* Fat-laden epithelial cells are found in a-beta-lipoproteinemia.

A section of normal jejunal mucosa from a specimen obtained by suction biopsy is shown in Figures 4 and 5. The villi are long, delicate, and frondlike; the lining columnar epithelium is regular with basal orientation of nuclei. The crypts are normal, and cellular infiltration of the lamina propria is minimal. Proper interpretation of jejunal histology, it must be emphasized, depends upon correct (perpendicular) sectioning of the specimen, which, in turn, requires correct mounting before fixing.

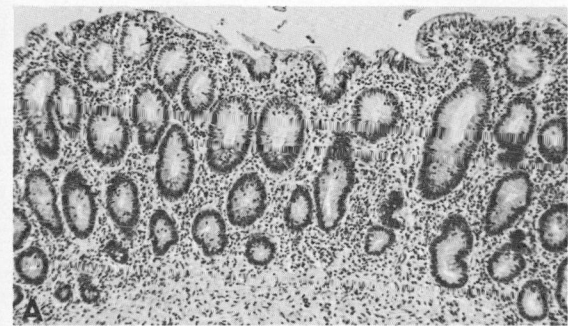
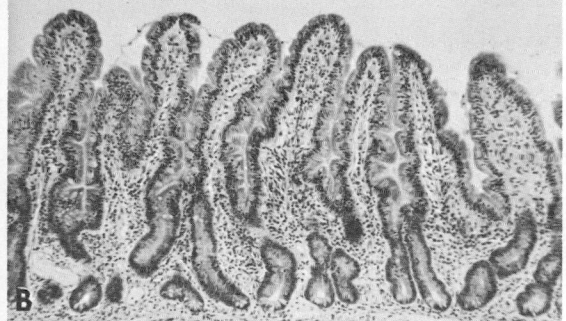

FIGURE 4. Jejunal mucosa of patient (F. G.) with adult celiac disease. *A*, Before treatment (60 ×). *B*, Twenty-eight months after elimination of gluten from the diet. Note the regeneration of the villi and the return toward normal of the columnar epithelium (60 ×).

The jejunal histology in *adult celiac syndrome and tropical sprue* is strikingly abnormal. In evaluation of small bowel biopsies from such patients, particular attention must be directed to configuration of the villi, morphology of the epithelial cells with their brush border, and the degree of the chronic inflammatory cell infiltration. The severity of changes may be graded from mild to moderate to severe. In the *severe* group (total villous atrophy) the changes consist of complete flattening of the mucosal surface without detectable villi or, at best, only very short and broad villi. Generally, there is a dense infiltration of chronic inflammatory cells and disorganization of the epithelial cells with a sparse brush border (Figs. 4 and 5). In the *mild* group (partial villous atrophy), the villi are formed but still are shorter and broader than normal. In some areas the villi approach normal in all respects. The epithelial cells with brush border generally may be nearly normal, and the cellular infiltration is mild. In the *moderate* subdivision (subtotal villous atrophy), changes ranging between those of the mild and severe groups are noted (Fig. 5).

The degree of infiltration of the lamina propria and of alteration of the epithelial cells is proportional to the extent of villous atrophy. The brush border frequently appears intact in the crypts, although it is disorganized and sparse near the midportion and tip of the villus. Although the severity of the lesion varies considerably among patients, the variation within a limited region of the proximal jejunum in a single patient is minimal; however, definite differences between samples from more distant locations in the same patient have been noted. Total villous atrophy, although characteristic of celiac disease, is not specific. Occasionally, it may be noted in *tropical sprue,* in *lymphoma,* or in *Whipple's disease,* and it has recently been reported in *diffuse nongranulomatous ileojejunitis* (often "ulcerative"), as well as in patients with *congenital hypogammaglobulinemia.* Some of the last-named will respond to a gluten-free diet and thus have adult celiac disease as well; the same coincidence may be noted in patients with diabetes mellitus (not caused by pancreatic insufficiency) and steatorrhea.

Moderate changes of this nature have also been noted in the jejunal mucosa of patients following gastrectomy, and with diffuse ileojejunitis. The number of patients with such alterations is small, and the possibility of associated adult celiac disease has not been clearly eliminated.

In *Whipple's disease* the diagnosis may be made by the demonstration of macrophages laden with periodic acid–Schiff staining material in lymph nodes or in the lamina propria of the intestinal wall. In addition, moderate villous atrophy may be noted (Fig. 6). Recent electromicroscopic studies during the active phase of the disease have revealed membranous structures, which may represent an infectious agent outside the macrophages. Deposits of *amyloid* have been found in the submucosa of the jejunum in patients with amyloidosis, particularly within the walls of arterioles.

In the past few years examination of fresh biopsy specimens under the dissecting microscope has yielded information about a number of diseases of the small intestine associated with malabsorption. The normal patterns of *finger-like villi* and *leaflike villi* are seen in Figure 5. The former are jejunal, and the latter are also normally present in the duodenum and upper jejunum. Epithelial convolutions usually indicate disease and, on histologic examination, correspond to *partial villous atrophy.* A most extreme change is noted with total villous atrophy, with *"mosaics"* or *"brain patterns"* as the picture under the dissecting microscope. Examples of this classification are presented in Figure 5.

DIFFERENTIAL FEATURES AND TREATMENT OF INDIVIDUAL FORMS OF THE MALABSORPTION SYNDROME

Because the presenting clinical picture includes a wide range of symptoms—bulky stools, flatulence, distention, anorexia, weight loss, weakness, glossitis, paresthesias, bleeding, bone pain, etc.—a careful history is of extreme importance in differential diagnosis. Particular attention must be paid to bowel habits in childhood, family history, previous illnesses and surgical operations, and dietary habits (including consumption of alcohol). A history of symptoms commonly associated with diseases that might underlie the malabsorption must be sought. Valuable clues may also be derived from a careful physical ex-

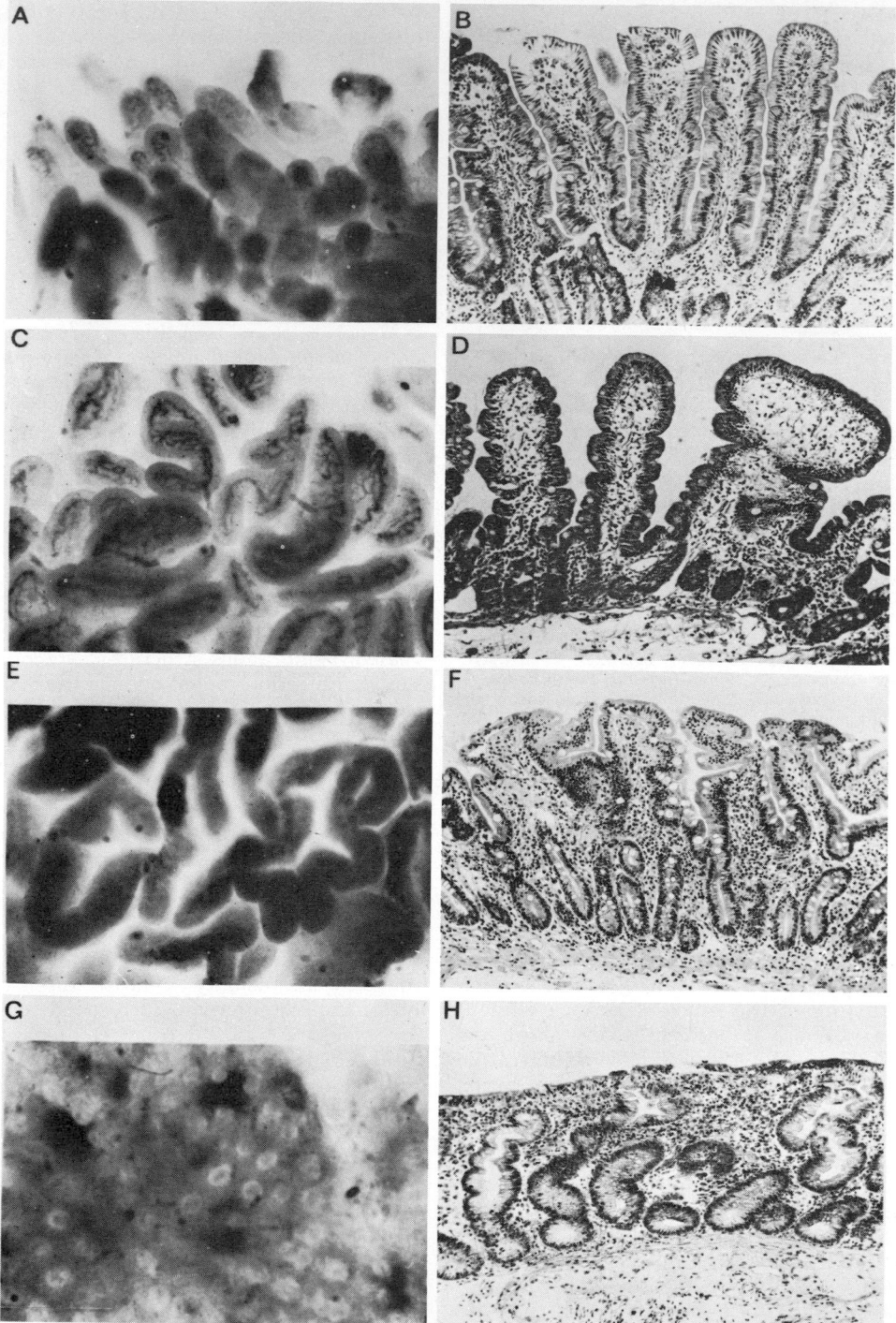

FIGURE 5. Comparison of dissecting microscopy and light microscopy of jejunal biopsy specimens. *A*, Finger-like villi vs. *B*, normal villous pattern. *C*, Leaflike villi vs. *D*, normal villous pattern. *E*, Convolutions vs. *F*, partial villous atrophy. *G*, "Mosaics" vs. *H*, total villous atrophy. *E* through *H* are specimens from patients with adult celiac disease.

amination. In this way, a diagnosis of tropical sprue or adult celiac disease, Whipple's disease, hypothyroidism, scleroderma, lymphoma, etc., may be facilitated.

The malabsorption syndrome must be differentiated from a wide variety of conditions characterized by a bleeding diathesis, by skeletal pain with or without fracture, by evidence of vitamin B

deficiency and extreme malnutrition, or by chronic diarrhea. Diagnosis of the malabsorption syndrome as a cause for these symptoms and signs must first, however, be based upon demonstration of abnormal fat absorption.

As the patient with the malabsorption syndrome may have extreme weight loss, weakness, hypotension, and diffuse pigmentation, differen-

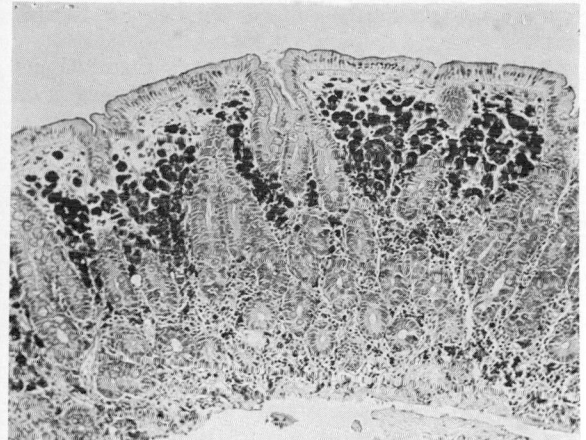

FIGURE 6. Jejunal biopsy from a patient with Whipple's disease. Periodic acid–Schiff stain. Note macrophages laden with stained material in the lamina propria.

tiation from *Addison's disease* must be made. Abnormalities of serum calcium, carotene, plasma prothrombin, etc., and impaired absorption of fat and xylose indicate the presence of the malabsorption syndrome (Table 4). Addison's disease may be excluded by the responsiveness of the adrenal gland to an intravenous infusion of corticotrophin.

The principal distinctive features of the individual forms of the malabsorption syndrome are discussed according to the seven categories mentioned previously in connection with the various causes of the syndrome.

As there are numerous conditions that can produce the malabsorption syndrome, its treatment must be individualized. In contrast to the often gratifying response to dietotherapy shown by patients with adult celiac disease, or to broad-spectrum antimicrobials and folic acid and vitamin B_{12} by patients with tropical sprue, successful management of malabsorption resulting from various other diseases or alterations of the gastrointestinal tract is often difficult. Dosage schedules for agents used in the treatment of malabsorption syndrome are listed in Table 5.

Category I: Defective Intraluminal Hydrolysis (Following Subtotal or Total Gastric Resection; Insufficient or Altered Bile; Pancreatic Insufficiency)

Steatorrhea and malabsorption after subtotal gastrectomy and gastrojejunostomy (Billroth II) or total gastrectomy are attributable to (1) loss of reservoir function with rapid ejection and dispersion of food through the small intestine, thereby hindering proper mixing with digestive ferments; (2) bypass of the duodenum after a Billroth II procedure, which diminishes stimulus to bile flow and pancreatic secretion; or (3) stasis with bacterial contamination of the afferent loop of a Billroth II gastrojejunostomy. Deficiency of vitamin B_{12} will inevitably follow total gastrec-

TABLE 5. REPRESENTATIVE DOSAGES FOR AGENTS USED IN MANAGEMENT OF PATIENTS WITH THE MALABSORPTION SYNDROME

1. CALCIUM
   Oral: Calcium gluconate (91 mg. Ca^{++}/gram), 1 to 5 grams three times daily
   Intravenous: Calcium gluconate injection, U.S.P, 10 per cent solution (9.1 mg. Ca^{++}/ml.), 10 to 30 ml. administered slowly intravenously depending upon response
2. MAGNESIUM
   Oral: Magnesium sulfate (8 mEq./gram), 1.0 to 6.0 grams daily in divided dosage
   Intravenous: Magnesium sulfate, 0.5 per cent solution, up to 1000 ml. at a rate not faster than 1.0 mEq./minute
3. IRON
   Oral: Ferrous gluconate, 0.6 gram three times daily
   Intramuscular: (Imferon). Must be calculated according to severity of anemia. Detailed instructions accompany preparation.
4. FAT-SOLUBLE VITAMINS
   a. VITAMIN A
      Oleovitamin A capsules, U.S.P. (25,000 units per capsule), 100,000 to 200,000 units daily in severe deficiencies; maintenance, 25,000 to 50,000 units daily.
   b. VITAMIN D
      Synthetic oleovitamin D, U.S.P. (10,000 U.S.P. units vitamin D/gram), 30,000 units daily; increase dosage as necessary to raise serum calcium to normal. Dosage varies considerably depending on response as determined by level of serum calcium and urinary calcium.
   c. COMBINATION A AND D VITAMINS
      Concentrated oleovitamins A and D, U.S.P. (50,000 to 65,000 U.S.P. A units and 10,000 to 13,000 U.S.P. D units/gram) may be used rather than separate preparations.
   d. VITAMIN K
      Oral: Menadione, U.S.P., 4 to 12 mg. daily. Vitamin K_1 tablets (Mephyton), 5 to 10 mg. daily.
      Intravenous: (Bleeding episodes – acute situations.) Vitamin K_1 (Mephyton), 50 mg. ampoule. Administer 50 mg. slowly over 10-minute period. Repeat in 8 to 12 hours if prothrombin time has not returned to normal.
5. FOLIC ACID, U.S.P. (5 mg. tablets)
   Dose: Initial, 10 to 20 mg. daily
   Maintenance, 5 to 10 mg. daily
6. VITAMIN B_{12} INJECTION, U.S.P. (15 mcg./ml.)
   Dose: Initial, 30 to 60 mcg. daily for 2 to 3 weeks
   Maintenance, 30 to 100 mcg. monthly
   If combined system disease is present, a more intensive program is indicated.
7. VITAMIN B COMPLEX
   Any multivitamin preparation that contains daily requirements (thiamine 1.6 mg., riboflavin 1.8 mg. and niacin 20 mg.). Use 2 or 3 tablets daily. Intramuscular preparations are available for severe deficiencies.
8. PANCREATIC SUPPLEMENTS, ORAL
   Recently these agents have been shown to be more effective when given at 6 to 12 regular intervals during the day rather than at meal times.
   a. *Pancreatin,* U.S.P. (0.3 gram tablet), 6 to 18 grams daily.
   b. *Viokase* (0.3 gram tablet), 4 to 12 grams daily in divided doses at meals or hourly per day.
   c. *Cotazym* (0.3 gram capsule), 4.0 to 12.0 grams daily, divided doses at meals or hourly per day.
9. BROAD-SPECTRUM ANTIMICROBIALS
   Oral: Chloramphenicol, tetracycline, or oxytetracycline (0.25 gram), 1.0 gram per day in divided doses for 10 to 14 days; ampicillin (0.25 gram), 2.0 to 4.0 grams per day in divided doses; kanamycin (0.5 gram), 2.0 to 4.0 grams per day in divided doses; sulfisoxazole (0.5 gram), 1.0 to 2.0 grams daily in divided doses. Repeated courses often necessary or administration for 3 to 4 days each week indefinitely.
10. HUMAN ALBUMIN, SALT POOR (0.25 gram/ml.)
    Intravenous administration of 50 to 100 grams each day for 3 to 7 days to elevate a severely depressed serum albumin level

TABLE 5. REPRESENTATIVE DOSAGES FOR AGENTS USED IN MANAGEMENT OF PATIENTS WITH THE MALABSORPTION SYNDROME *(Continued)*

11. GLOBULIN, IMMUNE SERUM (0.165 gram/ml.)
    Intramuscular injection of 0.05 ml./kg. each 3 to 4 weeks in patients with hypogammaglobulinemia and recurrent infection
12. CORTICOTROPHIN AND ADRENOCORTICOSTEROIDS
    a. Corticotrophin, 30 to 40 units intravenously each day, 10 to 21 days or longer for severely ill patients.
    b. Prednisolone or prednisone, 30 to 60 mg. orally each day as needed; 5.0 to 15.0 mg. maintenance dose.
13. MEDIUM CHAIN TRIGLYCERIDES (MCT)
    a. "Home or Hospital Mix" (MCT: 45 per cent calories; caseinate, 15 per cent; dextrose, 40 per cent). Ingredients homogenized with H_2O to one liter (MCT: 75 ml.; caseinate, 60 grams; dextrose, 160 grams). Keep at 20 C. for one year. Defrost day's formula each morning; give three ounces at meals; gradually increase between-meal feedings to six ounces.
    b. Portagen (MCT: 45.0 grams fat/quart; 30 cal./oz.; 10 per cent carbohydrate). Formula mix. Prepare according to instructions. Give 16 oz. every day.
14. ANTIDIARRHEAL AGENTS
    Oral: Diphenoxylate hydrochloride (2.5 mg.), 5.0 mg. twice or three times daily. Deodorized tincture opium, 10 drops twice to three times per day. Propantheline (15.0 mg.), 30 mg. twice or three times daily.
15. CHOLESTYRAMINE, ORAL RESIN
    4.0-gram dose, three to six times daily, before feedings.
16. DRUGS FOR PARASITES
    Oral: Thiabendazole (25 mg./kg./day). Duration of therapy depends on disease. *Strongyloidiasis,* three to four days. *Capillariasis philippensis,* 30 days.
    Oral: Quinacrine (100 mg.) 300.0 mg. in divided doses daily for seven days for *Giardia lamblia.*

tomy, the lag period being determined by the liver store of the vitamin.

Exclusion or Deficiency of Conjugated Bile Salts. Insufficient concentration of conjugated bile salt in the upper intestine, caused by severe liver disease or prolonged extrahepatic biliary tract obstruction, diminished bile salt pool, or significant reduction of conjugated bile salts resulting from bacterial overgrowth (*vide infra*), diminishes hydrolysis of neutral lipid and results in steatorrhea. The pathophysiologic mechanism is subnormal concentration (<1.5 mmoles per liter) of conjugated bile salts necessary for micelle formation. Distal iliectomy, by disrupting the enterohepatic circulation of conjugated bile salts, also causes steatorrhea, the degree proportional to the length of the resected segments (about 8 to 15 grams per 24 hours for distal 100 cm.) Decreased conjugated bile salt pool is also notable in primary or secondary biliary cirrhosis; that the steatorrhea in these cases is due to liver disease is supported by disappearance of malabsorption with improvement of liver function. It is surprising, however, that the steatorrhea of complete obstruction is moderate—indicating other mechanisms for absorption in addition to proximal uptake of micellar lipid. As yet no satisfactory preparation of conjugated bile salts is available for therapy in patients with obstruction or advanced biliary cirrhosis. Malabsorption of fat in postnecrotic (macronodular) or portal (micronodular) cirrhosis is usually mild unless chronic

pancreatitis (usually caused by alcohol) is also present.

Pancreatic Insufficiency. Pancreatic insufficiency associated with chronic relapsing pancreatitis or with carcinoma of the pancreas is due to extensive parenchymal destruction and/or obstruction of the major ductal system. In chronic pancreatitis, with malabsorption (see Diseases of the Pancreas), the patient frequently is diabetic, the gland is noted to be calcified on flat film of the abdomen, and frequently, but not always, there is a history of recurrent attacks of inflammation. Occasionally the dominant symptoms of *carcinoma of the pancreas* are those of malabsorption rather than pain, anorexia, or jaundice. Other types of pancreatic disease are also associated with the malabsorption syndrome, e.g., *mucoviscidosis* and non-insulin-secreting β *islet cell tumor* of the pancreas. *Mucoviscidosis* is most often clinically apparent in early childhood; increasingly, however, the diagnosis is being made in adults. Islet cell tumor is discussed under Category VII.

Whatever the cause of pancreatic insufficiency, failure of lipolysis results in moderate to severe steatorrhea, depending to some degree on the amount of gland remaining. Patients with this disease rarely show evidence of deficiency of either vitamin B_{12} or fat-soluble vitamins. In contrast to adult celiac disease, d-xylose absorption is normal in pancreatic insufficiency except in the unusual instance of carcinoma of the pancreas that has invaded the small intestine. Although stool examination of I^{131} after oral I^{131} triolein may be high, oleic acid is absorbed normally. This difference may be of value in the diagnosis of pancreatic disease as a cause of steatorrhea and malabsorption. As noted earlier, the diagnosis of pancreatic insufficiency is facilitated by analysis of duodenal fluid after stimulation of the pancreas. When lipolysis is markedly depressed, hydroxy fatty acids are not produced, distinguishing pancreatic steatorrhea from steatorrhea of bacterial overgrowth and other nonpancreatogenous forms of malabsorption.

Acidic pH. Since pancreatic lipase is inactivated at an acid pH, conditions characterized by excessive gastric acid secretion, such as non-β islet cell tumor of the pancreas (Zollinger-Ellison syndrome) or massive small bowel resection, are associated with significant steatorrhea. As noted, defective lipolysis causes deficient formation of micelles.

TREATMENT OF DEFECTIVE INTRALUMINAL HYDROLYSIS

Gastrectomy. Fat absorption is usually normal following the Billroth I gastric resection. Steatorrhea after the Billroth II procedure is common, and after total gastrectomy it is universal, although the severity of the clinical problem after these procedures is not directly proportional to the degree of fat loss. After a Billroth II, steatorrhea results both from insufficient stimulus for secretion of bile and pancreatic juice and from inadequate mixing of food with bile owing to the bypass of the duodenum and/or the rapidity with which food reaches the small intestine. In addition, overgrowth of bacteria in the afferent loop may play an important role (*vide infra*). Jejunal interposition after total gastrectomy, however, requires no afferent loop and thus permits food to make direct contact with the upper duodenum, but food and digestive juices still do not mix normally.

Administration of ox bile extract (8 to 16 grams daily, in divided doses before and after meals) is not helpful, probably because of its high content of unconjugated salts. As yet no preparation of pure conjugated bile salts is available for treatment. Pancreatic extracts may be tried in selected cases, although when given alone they have not produced consistent improvement. However, when pancreatic extract is combined with broad-spectrum antimicrobials (chloramphenicol, ampicillin, or tetracycline, 1.0 gram per day in divided dosage) in the treatment of patients following Billroth II operations, fat absorption may be significantly improved. These results clearly indicate that, in some patients at least, bacterial contamination – probably originating in the afferent loop – plays an important etiologic role in the malabsorption syndrome that follows this procedure.

Patients who have undergone Billroth II procedures should receive a high-caloric diet rich in protein, with frequent feedings containing as much fat as can be tolerated, in order to maintain good nutrition. After a total gastrectomy, 30 to 100 mcg. of vitamin B_{12} intramuscularly must be given monthly. Calcium, iron, and the fat-soluble vitamins may be added to this regimen as needed or when diarrhea or steatorrhea is so severe that deficient absorption of these substances may be anticipated (Table 5).

Pancreatic Insufficiency. Replacement of digestive enzymes and insulin is important in the treatment of patients with pancreatic insufficiency. Among the available sources of enzymes are a commercial pancreatic extract, pancreatin, U.S.P., a preparation containing whole raw pancreas, Viokase, and one containing hog pancreas extract, Cotazym. Doses of these preparations are listed in Table 5; occasionally it may be necessary to increase the recommended amounts. Replacement therapy may be more effective when it is given in divided doses at regular intervals six times daily or even hourly during the day than when it is limited to meal times. There is some indication that giving bicarbonate with pancreatic extracts may improve fat absorption, but this evidence is scanty.

Exclusion or Deficiency of Conjugated Bile Salts. Cases in which insufficient bile reaches the intestine pose a difficult problem in treatment. If possible, fistulas or chronic obstruction of the biliary tree should be corrected surgically. The keystone of medical management is a balanced diet without restriction of fat. It is important to provide calcium and fat-soluble vitamins A, K, and D in adequate amounts (Table 5). The demineralization of bone in patients with prolonged biliary obstruction results from osteoporosis and osteomalacia. Adequate supplements of vitamin D and calcium not only may prevent further osteomalacia but also may increase calcium deposition. The administration of a high protein diet and anabolic hormones, i.e., norethandrolone (Nilevar) or testosterone, and of estrogens intermittently, may help to correct the osteoporosis. Because inactivity contributes to the skeletal demineralization, maximal ambulation must be encouraged. (At the moment a satisfactory preparation of conjugated bile salt is not available for replacement therapy. Currently, commercial ox bile preparations often cause diarrhea and do not provide adequate conjugated bile salts in doses that do not produce this undesirable side effect.)

Medium Chain Triglycerides (MCT) (Table 5). Feeding preparations of MCT appear to be valuable in a number of diseases that cause malabsorption, including those associated with defective intraluminal hydrolysis of fat. MCT is significantly cleaved and solubilized despite diminished concentrations of lipase and conjugated bile salts. Further, it is absorbed unhydrolyzed to a greater degree than long-chain (dietary) triglycerides. Additional advantages include mucosal cell hydrolysis of MCT which gains access to the interior of the cell. Along with those fatty acids which have entered from the lumen, split fatty acids pass directly into the portal system. Thus, reesterification and chylomicron formation are not necessary, and disappearance into the circulation is not dependent upon patent lymphatics.

MCT has been used in patients with defective intraluminal hydrolysis and is most effective in those with pancreatic insufficiency (who are also being given supplement of pancreatic enzymes (*vide supra*) and in patients with deficiency of conjugated bile salts (particularly biliary tract obstruction or bile fistulas).

Indication for MCT is strongest in situations in which no specific therapy for malabsorption is available, such as after massive small bowel resection (short gut syndrome), lymphatic obstruction, and biliary atresia. It is a useful adjunct in malabsorption for which specific therapy is available (celiac disease, bacterial overgrowth, Whipple's disease, parasitism, and tropical sprue – all of which will be discussed in detail later in this article).

Category II: Primary Mucosal Cell Abnormality

Celiac Disease. An important cause of chronic malabsorption syndrome in the continental United States is adult celiac disease (gluten enteropathy or nontropical sprue). In some way, dietary gluten is related to this disease. It seems quite likely that the intestinal mucosa of these patients is incapable of hydrolyzing a peptide or group of peptides contained in this substance, probably because of a deficiency or absence of necessary peptidases. In some unknown manner, perhaps these peptides facilitate the mucosal damage that is associated with malabsorption.

As high as 25 per cent of patients in this group may have a history of childhood diarrhea or steatorrhea suggestive of celiac disease or have a family history of this disorder. Commonly, the symptoms of celiac syndrome disappear in later childhood and in adolescence, despite continued malabsorption. Although the clinical remission is sometimes permanent, the classic features of adult sprue may appear during the third to sixth decades. The patients then present an extreme degree of malabsorption with foul-smelling diarrheal stools, skeletal disorders, bleeding phenomena, and symptoms of hypocalcemia. There are no pathognomonic physical signs in this disease. There may be all degrees of malnutrition, as evidenced by muscle wasting and edema (Figs. 1 and 7). Hypotension and abdominal bloating are very common. Occasionally, there is clubbing of the fingers and pigmentation similar to that of Addison's disease.

Roentgenography of the small bowel gives findings that are characteristic but not specific. Frequently the only change is an altered pattern with segmentation and flocculation of the barium meal and some coarsening of the jejunal folds. More severe impairment is manifested by dilatation of small bowel segments and clumping of the barium meal, with a waxy cast appearance of bowel segments (the "moulage" sign) (Fig. 2). As mentioned previously, the routine laboratory studies used in establishing the presence of the malabsorption syndrome are not specific. The glucose tolerance test, however, may be of help in differentiating this condition from pancreatic diseases.

The newer, more specific techniques in diagnosis of adult celiac disease—measurement of d-xylose absorption, determination of urinary indoles and study of jejunal histology—have been discussed.

As has been noted, vitamin B_{12} absorption studies may be useful in the differential diagnosis of the malabsorption syndrome (Table 3). The defective vitamin B_{12} absorption that exists in a few cases of adult celiac disease is not corrected by intrinsic factor or broad-spectrum antimicrobial drugs, but may revert to normal after institution of the gluten-free diet.

Finally, mention should be made of a diagnostic trial of dietotherapy with these patients. That the vast majority of adult celiac disease patients will respond favorably to an adequate gluten-free diet has been well established, but there is still some question as to how often other disorders will improve with this treatment. At present, it seems safe to say that no condition other than celiac disease will respond so dramatically or so completely to this therapy. Although clinical remission within two months of institution of this therapy is the rule, nevertheless some patients may require 6 to 12 months or even longer. Occasionally patients with adult celiac disease fail to respond completely to gluten elimination because they have pancreatic

insufficiency as well. The basis for the latter condition is unknown.

Disaccharidase Deficiency and Monosaccharide Malabsorption. Certain individuals, particularly children, are unable to split disaccharides because of a lack of invertase and isomaltase or lactase. Since the intestine is unable to absorb disaccharides completely, these sugars remain in the lumen. Bacterial fermentation products cause diarrhea with stools of high lactic acid content. Steatorrhea is mild; clinical symptoms may be reversed by elimination of disaccharides from the diet. The lactase deficit is by far the most common. It appears to be much more common in Negroes, and more common in Orientals than in Caucasians. The possible effect of dietary deficiency of lactose in this situation is not clear. Adults may be affected as well as children. Indeed, recent studies indicate that a number of persons diagnosed as having "irritable colon syndrome" (see Disorders of Motility) are deficient in jejunal lactase and that removal of milk and other lactose-containing products from the diet may relieve their diarrhea. These patients complain of loose stools, abdominal distention, borborygmi, etc. Weight loss is unusual, and appetite remains good. Steatorrhea, if present, is mild. Diagnosis of lactase deficiency may be made by the measurement of blood glucose after the oral administration of lactose (Table 4). A rise of less than 20 mg. per 100 ml. is abnormal, and if the patient's blood glucose rises normally after he ingests a mixture of glucose-galactose of equal amount, lactase deficiency is extremely likely. Diagnosis may be confirmed only by the finding of low lactase activity in a jejunal biopsy specimen. Occasionally, these patients have lactosuria after administration of 50 grams of lactose during the lactose tolerance test. Omission of foods with lactose from the diet may dramatically relieve the diarrhea in some of these patients.

Depression of lactase activity is also secondary to certain diseases affecting the jejunum, particularly adult celiac disease, but has been found in nonspecific, nonbacterial jejunitis, a-beta-lipoproteinemia, infectious diarrhea of childhood, bacterial overgrowth, Giardia lamblia infection, and granulomatous (regional) enteritis. Deficiency of sucrase is rare; it is associated with deficiency of isomaltase. Recent studies indicate that it is an homozygotic deficiency affecting perhaps as many as two in 1000 individuals in the population. Symptoms include watery diarrhea and borborygmi, usually from infancy, and are caused by ingestion of sucrose and sucrose-containing foods.

Diagnosis of sucrase deficiency may be made by failure of blood glucose to rise at least 20 mg. per 100 ml. after ingestion of 100 grams of sucrose. Treatment may be either elimination or marked reduction of cane sugar and starch products. Administration of Bimyconase, 1.3 grams with meals, or sucrase tablets has been reported to help. Congenital glucose-galactose malabsorption is present from birth and is exacerbated by all sugars broken down to these hexoses. Diagnosis is made by failure of these children to absorb either of these substances. Treatment consists of feeding fructose or fructose precursor-containing foods such as tuberous sunflower. Rare defects of amino acid transport include Hartnup disease and cystinuria, details of which are presented in the section on Diseases of Metabolism.

A-beta-lipoproteinemia (Acanthocytosis). A-beta-lipoproteinemia is a disease characterized by a morphologic defect of erythrocytes, "spiny red cells," low to absent serum beta-lipoproteins, very low serum cholesterol and, in some instances, mild steatorrhea, ataxia, nystagmus, motor incoordination, and retinitis pigmentosa. The cause of the disease is unknown, but it is related to an inability of the mucosal cells to invest lipid with a protein envelope necessary for entry to the lacteals. The severity varies—milder cases have no steatorrhea or neurologic defects. Substitution of MCT for ordinary dietary triglycerides has led to weight gain in some patients since the component fatty acids enter the portal, not the lacteal, system.

Vitamin B$_{12}$ Malabsorption. Very rarely, primary malabsorption of the vitamin B$_{12}$–IF complex is noted, perhaps owing to absence of a specific but unidentified "receptor" in the ileal mucosa. These patients have been shown to have adequate IF, normal ileal histology, calcium concentration, and alkaline pH. Treatment is monthly injections of vitamin B$_{12}$ intramuscularly (Table 5).

TREATMENT OF ADULT CELIAC DISEASE

The basis for the use of the gluten-free diet in adult celiac disease lay in observations of its beneficial effect in children with celiac syndrome. Laboratory as well as clinical data strongly indicated that these patients cannot tolerate cereals with high gluten content. This substance contains a peptide or group of peptides that are noxious to the intestinal mucosa. Thus, when wheat, rye, oats, and barley were eliminated from the diet of children who had the celiac syndrome, diarrhea and steatorrhea ceased, appetite improved, and rapid weight gain ensued. Cereal starch was conclusively shown to be not related causally to the symptoms. The similarity of the clinical features of adult and childhood celiac disease naturally led to an application of this diet to the treatment of the adult disease.

The gluten-free diet excludes all cereal grains except rice and corn. To follow this diet, all labels must be carefully scrutinized to eliminate completely products that contain wheat, rye, barley, and oats. As substitutes for the usual grains, rice, corn, and soy flours may be used. Recently, a wheat starch flour (Cellu Products Company) has become available. Beer and ale must be avoided, as they contain cereal residues; however, whiskies can be used because the offending agent is not contained in the distillate. All other foods are permitted, including fats. In general, the diet should be well balanced and high in protein. The

complete diet is available in standard nutrition texts.

A substantial majority of the patients with adult celiac disease have responded to this diet, showing symptomatic improvement within a few days or a week, although a rare patient may require as long as 2 to 12 months. The following is a representative case:

M.S., a 23-year-old housewife (Fig. 7) was admitted to The New York Hospital-Cornell Medical Center in 1956 for treatment of frequent foul, yellowish stools associated with abdominal distention, rapid weight loss, and profound weakness. From the age of 15 months to two and a half years she had been followed at The New York Hospital with a diagnosis of celiac disease. Dietary and supportive therapy was employed, and she gradually improved over this period. She remained poorly developed, but asymptomatic. At 15 years of age, recurrent urticaria appeared, and skin testing revealed allergies to rye, barley, oats, chocolate, and spinach. The symptoms subsided, and she did well until the age of 22 when, during the third trimester of her first pregnancy, she noted increasing fatigability. Two months after delivery she had the sudden onset of explosive diarrhea, with six or seven daily stools that were light in color, foul-smelling, and floated on water. No blood was noted. The symptoms waxed and waned over the course of the next few months. Six months after delivery she noted bilateral ankle swelling, bloated abdomen, and progressive weight loss of 6.9 kg.

Physical examination revealed a pale, frail women who appeared chronically ill. The blood pressure was 90/40 mm. of mercury. She had 3+ pitting edema of the lower legs, a "pot belly" abdomen with no palpable organs or masses, and a positive Chvostek sign. Her appearance at this time is shown in Figure 7A, in which emaciation, breast atrophy, muscle wasting, and edema are particularly notable. All parameters reflecting absorption were highly abnormal. Small bowel roentgenographic study demonstrated dilatation of segments, coarsening of valvulas, and "moulage." After evaluation of her physical and biochemical status, she was placed on a gluten-free diet and was observed for three weeks, after which laboratory studies demonstrated improvement in all parameters.

After six weeks of treatment, carotene, cholesterol, prothrombin, calcium and albumin returned to normal, and she gained 7.0 kg., despite the loss of 5.6 kg. with mercurial diuretics. She had no diarrhea, felt entirely normal and was without abdominal distention, wasting, or edema (Fig. 7B). She continued to be well for two and half years on her diet. About two years after treatment began, healthy twins were uneventfully delivered.

The vast majority of patients with this disease treated with the gluten-free diet as the sole form of therapy have achieved clinical remission. The weight gain has been striking; nine of these patients have voluntarily restricted their caloric intake. The fact that a complete clinical remission with return to normal of pertinent blood parameters can be obtained in the majority of cases is significant, since previous treatment programs were usually only incompletely effective. Follow-up biopsies have demonstrated improvement of the mucosal histology in patients who adhered strictly to their diet. Such histologic change in one patient is shown in Figure 4B. Repeated biopsies in a few other patients, however, reveal little or no improvement. Absorption of d-xylose returns to normal as does urinary excretion of 5-hydroxyindolacetic acid within a few weeks of elimination of gluten. Steatorrhea diminishes remarkably in all instances, but fat absorption returns completely to normal only in those patients who carefully eliminate all gluten. Failure to obtain regeneration of villi and return to nor-

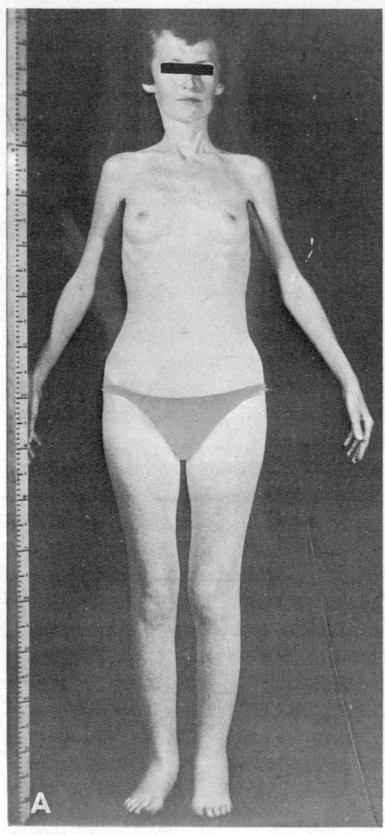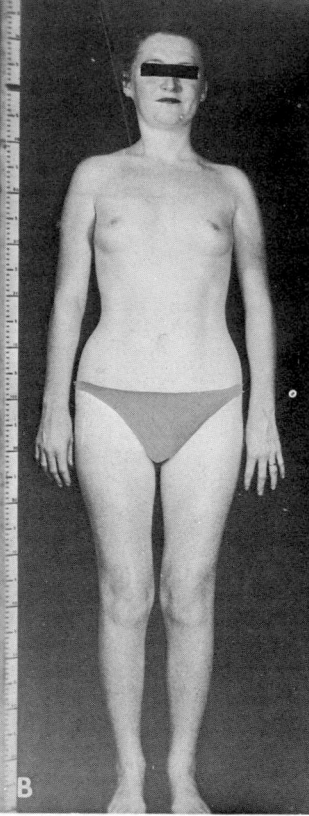

FIGURE 7. Appearance of patient (M. S.) with adult celiac disease. *A*, Before treatment. Note wasting and edema. *B*, Six weeks after elimination of gluten from the diet.

mal of fat absorption may be due either to irreversibility of the lesion or to failure of the patient to adhere strictly to the diet.

Corticosteroids have been shown to produce significant improvement in adult celiac disease without entirely correcting the steatorrhea or biochemical abnormalities. These agents should be used for long-term therapy only in cases refractory to the gluten-free diet, for impaired protein metabolism and osteoporosis are troublesome features in this chronic condition.

Occasionally, a patient with adult celiac disease is critically ill, with severe diarrhea, wasting and anorexia, and serious protein and electrolyte depletion. There may also be bleeding, tetany, and edema. This situation demands a rigorous therapeutic regimen, employing intravenous vitamin K and calcium as well as infusions of salt-poor albumin (Table 5). It is in this clinical situation that corticosteroids may be life-saving by greatly stimulating the appetite and perhaps by increasing absorption. Initially, corticotrophin, 30 units, should be given intravenously over an eight-hour period daily. After 10 to 14 days, either prednisolone or prednisone, 60 mg. a day, may be substituted. Simultaneously, a gluten-free diet should be offered, and, as the patient's condition improves, drug therapy should be discontinued by gradual reduction in dosage over three to four weeks. It would presently seem that these patients should remain on such dietotherapy permanently.

An additional helpful measure for the acutely ill patient is the limitation or elimination of lactase-containing foods, since low levels of jejunal mucosal lactase are reported during this stage of the disease.

SPECIAL CONSIDERATIONS AND COMPLICATIONS

Lymphoma and Carcinoma. The incidence of primary small bowel lymphoma and carcinoma in patients with adult celiac disease is high, about 13 per cent in a large collected series, with lymphoma contributing 10 per cent. Abdominal pain, weight loss, bleeding, obstruction, and perforation are the cardinal clinical features of this fatal complication. It is believed that lymphoma is more common in those not treated with a gluten-free diet. Perhaps relapse in those who have responded, associated with suggestive symptoms, should alert one to the possibility.

Small Bowel Ulceration. Nonmalignant ulcers of the jejunum and ileum may complicate celiac disease, and are manifested by exacerbation of severe diarrhea, abdominal pain, fever, and severe hypoproteinemia secondary to protein-losing enteropathy (*vide infra*). Perforation, bleeding, or obstruction are late manifestations.

Neurologic Complications. A syndrome similar to subacute combined degeneration of the spinal cord is noted early in celiac disease despite remission with a gluten-free diet and no vitamin B_{12} deficiency.

Celiac Disease and the Skin. *Dermatitis herpetiformis* may be associated with patchy villous atrophy of the duodenum and upper jejunum; this abnormality does not extend beyond the proximal foot or so of the small gut, perhaps explaining why malabsorption in these patients is mild or even absent. Response to a gluten-free diet is poor, and instillation of gluten into the gut causes no inflammatory response as it does in gluten enteropathy. Subtotal and complete villous atrophy have also been noted in *rosacea, atopic dermatitis,* and *psoriasis,* associated with varying degrees of steatorrhea and occasionally a dramatic response to a gluten-free diet.

Category III: Inadequate Surface

Most absorption takes place in the duodenum and first 90 cm. of the jejunum. Clinical studies of patients who have had extensive resection of the small intestine indicate that survival is now reasonably certain with 90 to 120 cm. of remaining normal small bowel, and is possible with shorter segments provided caloric intake is adequate. This length of jejunum is sufficient for normal carbohydrate absorption and, in some instances, for maintenance of positive nitrogen balance. The postoperative course is influenced by the site of resection—jejunum or ileum. Thus, vitamin B$_{12}$ absorption will be subnormal if a large length of ileum has been removed; conversely, sacrifice of a corresponding amount of jejunum will more seriously impair absorption of fat, calcium, and folic acid.

The three common causes for extensive resection of large segments of the small intestine are (1) *recurrent regional enteritis,* (2) *mesenteric vascular disease,* particularly thrombosis of the superior mesenteric artery, and (3) *malignant processes* involving the blood supply of the small bowel.

Treatment for Massive Resection and Jejunal Bypass. When possible, gastrojejunocolic or jejunocolic fistulas, or inadvertent gastroileostomies, which "sidetrack" large segments of small intestine, should be corrected surgically.

The patient who has had an extensive resection of the small intestine or jejunal bypass which cannot be corrected, requires medical care. For periods of up to 12 months postoperatively, the remaining segment of intestine will show progressive improvement in absorptive capacity, associated with elongation and dilatation. It is important to remember that, since the amount of fat absorbed is proportional to the amount presented to the absorbing surface, the maximal intake of fat that does not cause symptoms is desirable. Regardless of which segment or its part— ileum or jejunum—remains, the diet should be high in protein, and frequent feeding (six times daily) should be recommended. Vitamins A, D, and K and the B-complex vitamins as well as calcium may be given orally, except in those instances in which adequate replacement is possible only by the parenteral route (Table 5). In general, a high protein intake will adequately maintain the serum albumin; however, occasionally, infusions of salt-poor albumin must be given.

Supplementation of the diet by MCT (*vide supra;* Table 5) has been of distinct benefit to patients with massive small bowel resection, diminishing diarrhea and helping to stabilize weight by improving fat absorption; however, it must be noted that weight gain attributable principally to MCT in these patients is slight. Drugs that decrease intestinal motility, such as diphenoxylate hydrochloride (5.0 mg. twice or three times daily), anticholinergics (propantheline, 15 to 30 mg. twice to three times daily), and/or small doses of tincture of opium (10 drops twice to three times daily) may help reduce diarrhea (Table 5).

Distal Ileal Resection or Bypass. As noted, ileal resection is often required for granulomatous disease or vascular insufficiency (as part of massive small gut resection). Recently operations have been devised to bypass the ileum so that obese patients may lose weight by the malabsorption syndrome so created.

After resection of the distal ileum, the principal site of Vitamin B$_{12}$ absorption, this vitamin should be replaced parenterally, as in pernicious anemia. If the megaloblastic anemia that appears in this condition does not respond entirely to vitamin B$_{12}$, folic acid should be added to the regimen. Iron deficiency anemia, which is frequent after massive resection, should be treated by oral administration of an iron salt, but may respond only to an intramuscular preparation (Imferon) (Table 5).

Since distal ileal resection interrupts the enterohepatic circulation of bile salts, these substances come into contact with the colonic mucosa and inhibit water and electrolyte absorption, particularly in the ascending segment, resulting in three to six loose to soft movements daily. If less than 100 cm. has been resected, steatorrhea is mild to moderate (20.0 grams fecal fat daily) and treatment with cholestyramine, a bile salt binding resin, is indicated and will often ameliorate the diarrhea. Of course, in patients with more than 100 cm. resected, steatorrhea will be reduced by feeding MCT in place of dietary lipid (Table 5).

Adrenal corticosteroids have been used for patients with extensive resections, but present evidence that these steroids actually improve absorption is not conclusive. These agents may be helpful if other measures fail, but the clinician must be constantly alert to the complications of long-term therapy, i.e. *osteoporosis, intestinal ulcerations,* and *recurrent infections.* The beneficial effect may be due to stimulation of the appetite and an improved sense of well-being.

Studies of the effect of potent pancreatic extracts and/or antimicrobials (broad-spectrum) are not available.

Category IV: Abnormalities of the Small Intestine

Diffuse diseases that severely affect the mucosa of the small intestine inevitably result in deficient absorption. These diseases include *granulomatous enteritis,* *diffuse nongranulomatous ileojejunitis,* and *acute infectious enteritis,* *amyloidosis,* *radiation injury* *eosinophilic gastroenteritis,* and *drug effects.*

Diffuse Nongranulomatous Ileojejunitis. Steatorrhea and malabsorption may result not only from the complications of the granulomatous form of this disease (*strictures,* *fistulas,* or *massive resections*) (see article on Regional Enteritis), but also from nongranulomatous involvement of a large segment of the small intestine, particularly the jejunum. Frequently, the mucosa is also ulcerated.

The onset of this latter illness is abrupt, and signs and symptoms of malabsorption may predominate. A daily remittent *fever* (102° to 105° F.), *abdominal cramping pain,* usually periumbilical, and frequent *watery stools* are common complaints. *Splenomegaly,* occurring in 20 per cent of these patients with fever, may suggest an initial diagnosis of "abdominal lymphoma." Usually, diffuse inflammatory changes are noted in roentgenograms of the small bowel. Stenotic segments and fistulas are not usually seen. The small bowel pattern may be indistinguishable from that of a wide variety of conditions associated with the malabsorption syndrome. One laboratory finding of help in the differential diagnosis is elevation of the leukocyte count, often with a substantial increase in the percentage of nonsegmented polymorphonuclear cells. Diagnosis may also be facilitated by a previous misdiagnosis of appendicits. Often, however, diagnosis is made either by the response to treatment or by surgical exploration. (See article on Regional Enteritis.)

Treatment of Diffuse Nongranulomatous Ileojejunitis. In diffuse ileojejunitis, corticosteroids may have a dramatic effect upon the clinical symptoms, including those that are due to malabsorption. Steatorrhea will diminish or cease; serum calcium, carotene, and plasma prothrombin concentration will return to normal. Serum albumin, often severely depressed to levels of 1.0 to 2.0 grams per 100 ml. by "weeping" of serum protein into a large segment of inflamed gut, so-called protein-losing enteropathy (*vide infra*), likewise rises as the inflammation subsides. These improvements, as indicated by laboratory tests, accompany the disappearance of fever as well as the increase in appetite, weight, and strength. Although such a therapeutic result is most salutary, it may not, unfortunately, be permanent. Recurrence is frequent, with progress of the disease in localized areas.

The consensus is that such patients, often acutely ill with fever and diarrhea, respond best to intravenous corticotrophin, 40 units daily, given over an eight-hour period for 10 to 14 days. The oral corticosteroid preparations are used following corticotrophin in the more serious cases and may be the principal therapeutic agents throughout the course of the less severe cases. The initial dose range in either instance is 40 to 60 mg. of prednisone or prednisolone daily. The dose is gradually tapered over a week or longer to a maintenance level of 10 to 30 mg. daily. The day-to-day clinical response best regulates the dose of drug at this stage of treatment. Broad-spectrum antimicrobials are not useful except in the presence of septic complications. Unfortunately, the long-range outlook for permanent remission of this disease, is not good.

Eosinophilic Gastroenteritis. Increasingly, patients are seen with malabsorption, varying degrees of gastrointestinal bleeding, and protein-losing enteropathy (PLE), whose small gut is infiltrated by eosinophils, is edematous, but shows no vasculitis. The involvement in many instances is principally mucosal. In some cases, in which the stomach is also involved, the deeper layers of the gut, including serosa, are infiltrated. The symptoms—cramping pain, diarrhea, weight loss, nausea, fever, and a degree of malabsorption—are related to the location and extent of the disease in the small bowel. If the stomach is also involved, epigastric pain, vomiting, and bleeding are common. Frequently, the patients have allergies, particularly hay fever and asthma, and many have urticaria as well as diarrhea after eating certain foods (milk, egg, cereal, meat). Marked eosinophilia is a constant finding—15 per cent. The disease tends to be chronic with recurrent symptoms. Roentgenographic examination often reveals a nonspecific "malabsorption pattern" with coarsened folds of jejunum. Occasionally, narrowed segments may be seen. Hypoproteinemia caused by PLE may be severe and may be associated with marked edema and ascites. Iron deficiency anemia resulting from occult gastrointestinal bleeding is common in children. Disease of the stomach, particularly antral, may cause hematemesis.

Treatment of Eosinophilic Gastroenteritis. Effective therapy consists of withdrawal of offending foods, particularly milk for children. In more ill patients, prednisone, 20 to 40 mg. daily orally with gradual tapering to a low maintenance dose, will bring remission of major symptoms and decrease of eosinophilia. With remission, edema and infiltrate of the jejunal mucosa also disappear in cases with no involvement of deeper layers. In patients with brisk bleeding from the stomach, surgery may have to be performed. Laparotomy, for severe pain or bleeding resulting from transmural small bowel disease, reveals thickened loops of jejunum, involved antrum, and enlarged mesenteric nodes. Biopsy differentiates this disease from granulomatous enteritis and tuberculosis. In the majority of patients the clinical picture, typical history, eosinophilia, obvious allergies, and response to treatment are sufficient to exclude acute diffuse nongranulomatous ileojejunitis, lymphoma, and celiac disease. Transoral jejunal biopsy will also be helpful.

Amyloidosis. Either the primary or the secondary form of the disorder may affect the gastrointestinal tract and cause malabsorption. Diffuse crampy pain and ileus are the most frequent abdominal symptoms. In the primary form of the disease, *cardiac failure, macroglossia,* and *renal disease* may be noted, but the Congo red test is negative. Roentgenographically, amyloidosis is characterized by dilated loops of bowel, occasionally with thickening of the jejuno ileum and slow passage of the barium meal through the intestines. The diagnosis is made by tissue study. Gingival or tongue biopsies are frequently positive in primary amyloidosis, particularly when the disease is associated with myelomatosis; liver biopsy, although hazardous, may also establish the diagnosis. Biopsy of the liver or bowel at laparotomy, however, may be necessary in some instances. Recently, diagnosis has been made from specimens of jejunal mucosa obtained by transoral suction biopsy.

In secondary amyloidosis, the presence of a chronic inflammatory illness and hepatosplenomegaly suggest the diagnosis. Congo red tests may show greater than 90 per cent retention of the injected material by the tissues.

Injury Secondary to Radiation and Drugs. A few patients who receive high dosage x-ray therapy to the abdomen will develop a malabsorption syndrome on the basis of radiation injury to the bowel. It is difficult to assess how much of the defect in absorption is attributable to arterial damage, mucosal inflammation or atrophy. Since the reaction to injury is slow, symptoms do not appear for weeks to months after exposure. Fibrosis and stricture are occasional sequelae of severe reaction, causing obstruction, usually chronic. Jejunal biopsy may reveal patchy villous atrophy. Mucosal atrophy and malabsorption have also been documented following administration of drugs: specifically, antimicrobials, folic acid antagonists, alcohol, and some anticonvulsant drugs. Large doses (10.0 to 12.0 grams daily) of *neomycin* lead to malabsorption of fat, protein, xylose, glucose, vitamin B$_{12}$, and iron. The mechanism is not clear, but may be a combination of effects including mild structural changes of the villi, precipitation of bile salts, possible inhibition of lipase, diminution of intestinal lactase, and inhibition of bile acid absorption. Kanamycin, tetracycline, polymyxin, and bacitracin may also rarely produce mild malabsorption.

Treatment of Amyloidosis and Radiation Injury. Management of diseases affecting the intestinal wall and mesenteric lymphatic system is often supportive only, usually limited to replacement therapy. Such treatment, which is limited to the regulation of the diet with the addition of supplements to correct specific deficiencies, is all that can be offered patients with primary amyloidosis, carcinomatosis, and radiation injury. No specific beneficial effect is to be expected from corticosteroids.

Acute Infectious Enteritis. A number of such infections may cause transient but severe malabsorption. Patients with this condition will have severe steatorrhea and may have diminished xylose absorption. The serum calcium as well as the plasma prothrombin concentration may be depressed. Serum proteins may fall rapidly, largely owing to abnormal rate of loss into the inflamed gut. With recovery, absorption returns to normal.

Treatment of Infectious Enteritis. As noted, patients with acute infectious diarrhea due to staphylococci, Salmonella, Shigella, or viruses may rapidly develop severe malabsorption and hypoproteinemia. These patients may recover without specific antimicrobial therapy provided that fluids and electrolytes have been rapidly and adequately replaced. Nevertheless, antimicrobials should be administered as soon as a bacteriologic diagnosis is made, or sooner if suspicion of *B. dysenteriae* infection is high or if staphylococcal infection is suggested by history or by fecal smear. Such infection is apt to attack patients who have had abdominal surgery, particularly those also given broad-spectrum antimicrobials. Differentiation of staphylococcal enteritis from that caused by Salmonella or Shigella is extremely important because most such staphylococcal infections are penicillin-resistant and require discriminating and intensive antimicrobial therapy (see Staphylococcal Disease). Salmonella infections are best treated with chloramphenicol, whereas the tetracyclines are indicated in disease caused by Shigella. (Diagnosis and treatment of cholera is discussed in the section on Microbial Diseases).

Category V: Lymphatic Obstruction

Lymphoma. The malabsorption syndrome secondary to lymphoma of the small bowel and mesentery may be clinically and roentgenographically identical to the classic picture of adult celiac disease. Several features, however, suggest the correct diagnosis. In contrast to adult celiac disease, which predominates in females, 80 per cent of small bowel lymphomas with malabsorption occur in males. The symptoms of this disease are likely to be of much shorter duration and to include *crampy abdominal pain* and *fever. Lymphadenopathy* and *hepatosplenomegaly* do *not* appear until late in the course. Although intraluminal small bowel masses may be present in some cases, the roentgenographic study of the intestine generally does not reveal them. Unexpectedly, the usual therapeutic measures, such as diet, fat-soluble vitamins and vitamin B$_{12}$, may lead to a temporary clinical and laboratory remission. The incidence of malabsorption syndrome caused by small bowel lymphoma is difficult to ascertain. It appears that about 5 per cent of patients with adult celiac disease will develop lymphoma.

The diagnosis is usually established by laparotomy necessitated by some complication of the underlying disease, such as *bleeding, perforation,* or *obstruction.* In some patients, the diagnosis may be made from jejunal tissue obtained by peroral biopsy instruments. The average duration of this illness after onset of symptoms is 13 months, despite resection and roentgen therapy.

Treatment. Treatment of lymphoma of the small bowel and mesentery includes local resections as well as radiotherapy, and possibly therapy with chlorambucil and steroids or nitrogen mustard when the disease is disseminated. Despite this program, the course is frequently progressive, the average duration of life after onset of symptoms being about one year. In these patients, continuous supportive therapy (high caloric diet, iron, vitamins, calcium, etc., as needed) is frequently helpful and may result in successful maintenance of the patient's activity over a period of months. Indeed, these patients have also improved when given low-fat diets with vitamin and mineral supplementation.

Primary intestinal lymphoma, with malabsorption, may be a chronic condition in certain parts of the world, particularly in the Middle East in young Arabs and Sephardic Jews. The clinical picture strongly resembles adult celiac disease in terms of chronicity and jejunal villous atrophy; however, most of these patients do not respond to elimination of gluten, and peroral biopsies will show evidence of lymphoma in the majority. In contrast to primary lymphoma of the small bowel with malabsorption in North America and Europe, which carries a prognosis of death one to two years after onset of symptoms (despite surgery, radiation, and chemotherapy), the young Middle Easterners may live with their disease for as long as ten years.

Tuberculosis. Tuberculosis may result in a malabsorption syndrome through involvement of the mesenteric lymph nodes, although in some cases there may be associated disease of the intestinal wall. It is extremely rare in the United States, and it occurs almost always in persons with a history of severe pulmonary or cervical lymph node tuberculosis.

Fever, palpable abdominal masses, a positive tuberculin skin test, evidence of old or recent disease on chest roentgenography, and *calcification of mesenteric and pelvic lymph nodes* on flat film all suggest the diagnosis, which may be confirmed by *culture of sputum or gastric juice.* Occasionally, stool culture may be useful, but only if the other secretions are demonstrably free of tubercle bacilli. Roentgenographic studies—both barium enema and small bowel series—are particularly helpful when there is also deformity of the ileocecal segment resulting from hyperplastic lesions. Rarely, there may be diffuse small bowel abnormalities, such as coarsening of the folds, stricture formation, and edema, which suggest ileojejunitis. At times, exploratory laparotomy with node or bowel biopsy is necessary for diagnosis (see article on Extrapulmonary Tuberculosis).

Treatment. Tuberculous involvement of the mesenteric lymph nodes should be treated by chemotherapy, as outlined in the article on Extrapulmonary Tuberculosis. A high caloric diet should be employed with calcium and vitamins as indicated. When there is an associated hyperplastic ileocecal tuberculosis with partial obstruction, appropriate local resection may be necessary.

Other Diseases. In addition to the diseases just discussed, several other conditions may rarely cause the malabsorption syndrome by lymphatic blockade. These include certain *parasitic diseases, the reticuloendothelioses, metastatic tumor* to the mesenteric nodes, and *neoplastic invasion of the main lymphatic channels* in the retroperitoneal tissues.

Category VI: Bacterial Overgrowth—"Blind Loop" Syndrome and Infection

For many years, steatorrhea and anemia have been clinically and experimentally associated with alterations in the anatomy of the small intestine, particularly "blind loops," multiple strictures, small fistulas that do not create a large "bypass" of the small intestine, and multiple jejunal diverticula.

The common denominator in all conditions is bacterial overgrowth, which results either from stasis in a segment of small bowel or from contamination of small bowel by large bowel content. Concentration of anaerobic coliform organisms greater than 10^3 to 10^4 per milliliter, or presence of certain anaerobes, particularly bacteroides, clostridia, and lactobacilli, is responsible for impairment of intraluminal hydrolysis of lipid. Bacterial overgrowth may rarely play a role also in the malabsorption in diabetes mellitus with neuropathy (unclear), tropical sprue, and after subtotal gastrectomy and Billroth II gastrojejunostomy.

"Blind Loop." A loop of intestine is "blind" either when it is disconnected from the main stream (rare) or when intestinal contents may gain access to it but not ready egress from it. Examples would be a partly defunctionalized terminal ileal loop that has been partially excluded by either side-to-side or end-to-side ileo-transverse colostomy. Stasis and overgrowth of bacteria take place with subsequent invasion of the upper small intestine.

The mechanism of the malabsorption of vitamin B_{12} and fat in "blind loop syndrome" has recently been elucidated. Vitamin B_{12} is utilized by multiplying organisms. Fat absorption is impaired by bacterial deconjugation of bile salts. The decline in concentration of conjugated bile salts below a critical level (<1.5 mmoles per liter) impairs micelle formation, reducing uptake of lipid by the mucosa. Concentration of free bile acids is increased intraluminally; their absorption from the proximal small gut by passive diffusion is rapid, and their serum levels are elevated. Observations on patients with bacterial overgrowth (subtotal gastrectomy, intestinal strictures, enterocolic fistulas) indicate that less than 20 per cent of intraluminal fat is in a micellar phase 45 minutes after ingestion of a lipid meal (normal: >50 per cent). Since hydrolysis of fat is not impaired, steatorrhea is principally the result of impaired micelle formation.

The jejunal villi are normal in *scleroderma* and after *subtotal gastrectomy,* as they are in the majority of patients with either *enteroenteric fistulas or strictures* or true "blind loops" (unless these are due to inflammatory disease that also involves the upper jejunum). Occasionally some mononuclear infiltration of the lamina propria is noted in all these conditions, but the villous structure is intact.

Multiple Strictures and Jejunal Diverticula. Strictures result either from diffuse *granulomatous ileojejunitis* or, less commonly, from *x-radiation* therapy. Most multiple jejunal diverticula are probably acquired. Stasis of intestinal content in these pockets of bowel leads to bacterial overgrowth.

Fistulas. Fistulas may complicate gastric or intestinal neoplasm or granulomatous enteritis, involving stomach, small gut, and colon (gastroenterocolic), small gut and colon (enterocolic), or loops of small gut (enteroenteric). As already noted, malabsorption may result from exclusion of significant lengths of absorbing surface from the main stream by large fistulas (gastroileostomy).

The diagnosis is greatly aided by a history of previous chronic enteric disease or of surgical procedure. Roentgenographic examination will often establish the diagnosis by the demonstration of one of these diseases or alterations. Frequently, however, the cause may not be demonstrated.

The megaloblastic anemia commonly associated with the "blind loop" syndrome will, unlike pernicious anemia, respond to the administration of broad-spectrum antimicrobial drugs. After 10 to 14 days of such therapy (tetracycline or chloramphenicol, 1.0 gram daily in divided dose), absorption of vitamin B_{12} is usually, but not always, restored to normal (Table 3). In contrast to those with pernicious anemia, these patients usually secrete hydrochloric acid.

Tropical Sprue. Tropical sprue can be differentiated from adult celiac disease. The disease occurs primarily in persons residing in certain areas of the Far East, India, and the Caribbean. Both nutritional deficiencies and bacterial contamination of the small gut appear to play causative roles; the response to therapy solely with broadspectrum antimicrobial drugs, however, suggests, but does not prove, that the latter factor is important. Also histologic changes suggestive of tropical sprue may be noted in individuals newly arrived in the tropics; such changes may often be associated with an acute enteritis and a variable degree of malabsorption. Although the remarkable clinical improvement that follows folic acid therapy strongly suggests a vitamin deficiency, tropical sprue is not seen in some areas of the world where the population has a marginal or even inadequate diet; conversely, it has been noted in people with adequately "balanced" diets.

Clinically, three phases of the disease have been described. *In the initial phase* the patient complains only of fatigue, asthenia, and bulky stools. After weeks to months, *the second phase* of malnutrition is noted. Weight loss is prominent. Glossitis, stomatitis, cheilosis, and hyperkeratosis are observed in varying degrees. Moderate prothrom-

bin depletion is present but is rarely associated with bleeding. Manifestations of impaired calcium absorption are not clinically apparent in patients with tropical sprue, in contrast to those with adult celiac disease. Iron deficiency anemia follows depletion of iron stores. Hypoalbuminemia with edema may be a late manifestation of this disease. All laboratory criteria of impaired absorption are present (Table 4). *The third stage* is characterized by anemia and megaloblastosis and the symptoms of full-blown severe malabsorption described earlier in the chapter, although diarrhea may not be prominent. However, the clinical spectrum is wide—steatorrhea may be minimal, glossitis absent, and megaloblastosis inconstant. This inconsistent picture may indicate various etiologies.

Laboratory investigation reveals characteristic findings (Table 4). Small bowel roentgenographic findings and histologic changes of the jejunum are the same as those in adult celiac disease except that total *villous atrophy* is not as commonly encountered in tropical sprue. In many tropical areas, however, asymptomatic individuals often have histologic abnormalities suggestive of tropical sprue, making tissue diagnosis very difficult. Other routine laboratory studies, including d-xylose absorption, are also comparable in the two diseases. The gluten-free diet is ineffective, but the administration of broad-spectrum antimicrobial drugs (tetracycline, 1.0 gram, four times daily), folic acid, or vitamin B_{12} induces remission. Removal from an endemic area may also induce remission (see Treatment).

Therapy for Tropical Sprue. The therapy for this disease is very effective. The similarity of tropical sprue to pernicious anemia, particularly in its hematologic aspects, prompted the use of liver extract, folic acid, and vitamin B_{12}, and remissions have also been noted with antimicrobial drugs, a low-fat, high-protein diet, and migration to a temperate climate. Administration of a broad-spectrum antimicrobial (tetracycline, 1.0 gram daily by mouth) along with 10 mg. of folic acid daily is the best treatment and frequently brings remission with disappearance of diarrhea and glossitis, and gain in appetite and weight. However, response may be slow in some patients, and normal absorption and jejunal histology may not be noted for six months or longer. Parenteral vitamin B_{12} should be given for two months (Table 5). For those not responding completely within six months of treatment with antimicrobials and folic acid, therapy should be continued for as long as absorption continues to improve.

When remission has been achieved, 5.0 mg. of folic acid daily is the maintenance therapy. In the presence of achlorhydria, addition of vitamin B_{12} to the regimen should be considered unless absorption of Co^{60} B_{12} is normal (Table 5). If absorption of vitamin B_{12} remains subnormal after remission, monthly injections should be given.

Whipple's Disease. In Whipple's disease or lipophagic intestinal granulomatosis (intestinal "lipodystrophy"), there is a heavy infiltration of the intestinal wall and lymphatics by macrophages filled with glycoprotein. It is a generalized disease with steatorrhea as its principal feature, and it occurs predominantly in males in the fourth to seventh decades.

Although it may be difficult to differentiate this entity from lymphoma, tuberculosis, and other causes of lymphatic obstruction, there are several suggestive manifestations. These include *arthritis*, *polyserositis*, and *postprandial pain*. Indeed, arthritis is frequently the initial complaint. When gastrointestinal symptoms occur, the disease usually progresses rapidly. Physical findings that suggest this disorder include *lymphadenopathy*, found in 40 per cent of the patients, and the various manifestations of polyserositis. *Fever* may be noted in about one third of the cases. Indefinite plastic or doughy abdominal masses have been described in approximately one quarter of the patients. The most consistent findings in the routine laboratory studies are *anemia* and an increased sedimentation rate; *eosinophilia* is occasionally present. The roengenographic findings in the small bowel are nonspecific, usually showing a "spruelike pattern."

The diagnosis of Whipple's disease can be verified either by peripheral lymph node biopsy or, when this is normal, by biopsy of a mesenteric lymph node at laparotomy. Diagnosis may be established by identification of macrophages containing periodic acid–Schiff-positive material in jejunal biopsy specimens obtained perorally (Fig. 6). Electron microscopic studies have revealed bacilliform bodies in and near these macrophages that may be infectious agents. Recent studies suggest that a tetracycline-susceptible pleomorphic organism is involved. Infiltration of the lamina propria also causes enlargement of villi and thickening of the submucosa.

Treatment of Whipple's Disease. Antimicrobial drugs by mouth are effective in treating Whipple's disease. Indeed, present information indicates that continuous treatment with broad-spectrum antimicrobials — tetracycline, chloramphenicol, or ampicillin — always brings about remission. The dosage of tetracycline or chloramphenicol is 1.0 gram daily. The duration of therapy with antimicrobials is determined by the clinical response. Present data indicate that such treatment should be maintained indefinitely; otherwise, symptoms may return. Histologic as well as clinical improvement is noted after a period of weeks to months, with loss of diarrhea, reappearance of appetite, and tremendous gain of weight. The PAS-positive material slowly disappears from the mucosa, and the bacilliform bodies are no longer visible on electron microscopy. When remission has been sustained for nine months to one year, antimicrobial agents may be given intermittently, i.e., every other day or for three consecutive days each week (Table 5).

The symptoms of Whipple's disease may respond to corticosteroid therapy, as do those of other diseases characterized by arthritis and polyserositis, but the over-all result of such treatment is not satisfactory. Present evidence strongly indicates that only 40 per cent of patients achieve remission of the disease for two to six months while receiving corticotrophin or corticosteroids, and, in the majority, the disease relapses on cessation of such therapy. Many patients, particularly those whose illness is in a terminal phase, do not respond at all. The desperately ill patient should be given both corticotrophin intravenously, 40 units daily, *and* parenteral antimicrobial agents until the condition permits withdrawal of the former agent.

Scleroderma. Although a disturbance of esophageal motor function is the most common gastrointestinal manifestation of scleroderma, severe involvement of the small bowel may cause malabsorption. Atrophy of the smooth muscle of the gut, submucosal fibrosis, and damage to the myenteric plexuses severely impair or abolish peristalsis. The resulting intermittent ileus may simulate closely the picture of complete intestinal obstruction. Severe involvement of the small intestine is usually associated with esophageal involvement, thickening of the skin, or other evidence of disseminated sclerosis, e.g., soft tissue calcification, telangiectasia, pulmonary diffusion defect, so that diagnosis is not difficult. Mucosal changes of the jejunum resembling those of adult celiac disease have not been reported.

Recent studies indicate that bacterial overgrowth is the principal factor in the steatorrhea and malabsorption of patients with scleroderma involving the small intestine. As with the esophagus (see Diseases of Motility), small bowel smooth muscle is atrophic and is replaced with fibrous tissue. Motility is severely impaired; stasis and bacterial overgrowth result. Culture of small bowel content of such patients yields a heavy growth of coliform organisms and, usually, anaerobes. Some patients with diabetic neuropathy and malabsorption have responded to broad-spectrum antimicrobial drugs, indicating bacterial overgrowth as the cause; however, well-documented data of abnormal jejunal flora are scanty.

Treatment of Bacterial Overgrowth ("Blind Loop" Syndrome). Absorption of vitamin B_{12}, and occasionally of fat, is impaired with intestinal strictures, fistulas, blind loops, and multiple jejunal diverticula. The surgical correction of the strictures, fistulas, or blind loops may effect a permanent cure and is, therefore, the therapy of choice. An illustrative example follows:

Mrs. H. D., a 53-year-old housewife, had diarrhea with passage of frequent pale yellow stools and cramping periumbilical pain for 13 years. The diagnosis of terminal ileitis was made ten years before at laparotomy. Four years before admission, she developed persistent edema, and three weeks before hospitalization had ascites. She had lost 55 pounds during her illness. On examination she was emaciated, weak, diffusely pigmented, and had ascites and edema. The spleen was felt 2 cm. below the costal margin. Pertinent laboratory studies revealed anemia, lowered serum protein and calcium, and steatorrhea. Roentgenograms of the small intestine showed diffuse enteritis with areas of dilatation. Laparotomy revealed multiple areas of stricture with proximal dilatation. A large segment of jejunoileum was resected. Recovery was rapid. Repeat studies of fat absorption and measurement of serum proteins, calcium, etc., three months later showed a return toward normal values.

In some patients with malabsorption syndrome associated with either subtotal (Billroth II) or total gastrectomy, or scleroderma, long-term antimicrobial therapy should be undertaken. Tetracycline, oxytetracycline, 1.0 gram a day, or ampicillin, 2.0 to 4.0 grams a day, should be given for 10 to 14 days, and intermittently every other day or three days each week thereafter (Table 5). Chloramphenicol, also in a daily dosage of 1.0 gram, may be used in situations in which the risks of drug toxicity seem outweighed by the potential dangers of the disease. Many of these patients, similar to those with bacterial overgrowth from other disorders, require continuous treatment. Rotation of antimicrobial drugs may be necessary since organisms tend to become refractory after a period of weeks to months. Aspiration of jejunal contents for cultures and periodic drug susceptibility determinations are necessary for therapeutic guidance. If organisms are not susceptible to the more usually employed drugs, courses of kanamycin (2.0 to 4.0 grams daily orally) and sulfisoxazole (2.0 grams daily, orally), may be given. All these drugs should be used in a rotational scheme. Occasionally some patients with recurrent regional enteritis and strictures or fistulas, in whom the surgical approach is not feasible, will have to be managed in a similar fashion.

In addition to the assessment of clinical response, efficiency of antimicrobial therapy may be judged by the fall in urinary *indican* to normal or nearly normal levels.

Giardia lamblia Infection; Other Parasites. Patients with *Giardia lamblia* infection of the small bowel may suffer from malabsorption, particularly individuals with subtotal gastrectomy; hypogammaglobulinemia associated with so-called "nodular lymphoid hyperplasia"; tropical sprue; or severe malnutrition, particularly children. Thus, the role played by the parasite is not completely clear despite demonstration of its invasion of the mucosa and a report of some improvement in absorption after treatment with quinacrine (0.1 gram three times daily for one week).

Although malabsorption has been reported with *hookworm disease,* a causal relationship is unlikely in view of the strong possibility that it coexists in these instances with tropical sprue, as judged by biopsy changes in jejunal mucosa.

Malabsorption associated with *Strongyloides stercoralis* infection may be improved by therapy for this infection (thiabendazole, 0.5 gram twice daily for three to four days).

Category VII: Miscellaneous

Steatorrhea with Hypogammaglobulinemia. Patients with congenital or acquired hypogammaglobulinemia may have steatorrhea, but the precise incidence is not known. Although the number of cases so documented is small, it is steadily growing. Evidence at hand indicates that most (if not all) of these patients have a severe deficiency of IgA; the majority show very low IgG levels, and IgM may be normal or low. The intestinal histology most commonly reveals villous atrophy identical with celiac disease; occasionally it shows so-called "nodular lymphoid hyperplasia," noted to be associated also with *Giardia lamblia* infection and a rare granulomatous lesion. Occasionally, a perfectly normal jejunal architecture is found, but a marked reduction of plasma cells and a reduced number of lymphocytes are noted in the lamina propria. Other abnormalities include splenomegaly and gastric atrophy.

Of those with villous atrophy about 50 per cent will have a good to excellent response to the gluten-free diet. Antimicrobial drugs and injections of gamma globulin appear to be ineffective except in a rare patient with nodular lymphoma hyperplasia. Of interest, patients with celiac disease have normal or elevated serum IgA and normal IgG levels and have a normal distribution of immunoglobins in the plasma cells and lymphocytes of the lamina propria. Patients with so-called congenital hypergammaglobulinemia — without nodular hyperplasia — also have a high incidence of associated "autoimmune" abnormalities such as arthritis and hemolytic anemia.

Metastatic Malignant Carcinoid Syndrome. The presenting symptoms of this disease may be those of malabsorption. Steatorrhea may be caused by an increased production of 5-hydroxytryptamine (serotonin), which markedly increases gastrointestinal motility and thus impairs absorption. Other, less likely explanations for diarrhea and steatorrhea in this disease include lymphatic obstruction of the mesentery of the small bowel by tumor and niacin deficiency. Treatment is that used for carcinoid syndrome in general. Methysergide (8.0 to 12.0 mg. per day, orally) and cyproheptadine (80 mg. per day in divided doses) have been reported to decrease diarrhea in this disease. Small doses of tincture of opium, however, seem most effective for the diarrhea. Parachlorphenylalanine, which inhibits hydroxylation of tryptophan to 5-HTP, has been effective in controlling diarrhea; however, side effects may preclude its general use. (See the Carcinoid Syndrome in the section on Diseases of the Endocrine System.)

Hypoparathyroidism. The association of steatorrhea and deficient parathyroid function has been recently documented. Symptoms of malabsorption may be the earliest manifestation of deficient parathyroid function. With parathormone replacement therapy and (later) vitamin D_2, diarrhea decreases, steatorrhea disappears, serum carotene and albumin levels rise, vitamin B_{12} absorption increases, and the roentgenographic appearance of the small bowel becomes normal. Diagnosis of hypoparathyroidism as a basis for malabsorption may be established by changes in urinary phosphate excretion after intravenous infusions of parathormone or calcium (see section on Diseases of the Endocrine System).

Parathormone facilitates calcium absorption by the intestinal tract. The effect of hypocalcemia per se upon intestinal absorption is not known.

Treatment. Administration of vitamin D and calcium will alleviate malabsorption as well as other manifestations of disease (see Parathyroid).

Diabetes Mellitus. Patients with long-standing diabetes mellitus may have severe diarrhea (see Disorders of Motility). Some of those with diarrhea will also have steatorrhea and malabsorption, and these patients are usually not well controlled by dietotherapy or insulin, or both. A high percentage also have some evidence of neuropathy. Likewise, the intestinal difficulty may be due to involvement of the autonomic innervation of the small bowel, since such patients often also have orthostatic hypotension, inability to perspire, and impotence. Possibly changes in the microbial flora or mesenteric vascular insufficiency may also contribute to the malabsorptive state. Response to broad-spectrum antimicrobials supports the former hypothesis; however, careful bacteriologic studies of intestinal contents in a group of patients with diabetic neuropathy and diarrhea revealed that bacterial overgrowth is an uncommon cause for the steatorrhea of diabetic neuropathy. Although exocrine function is usually normal in diabetes, some patients have pancreatic insufficiency for which replacement therapy should also be given (Table 5) (see Diseases of the Pancreas). Adrenal corticosteroids have been reported to benefit patients with this syndrome, but no satisfactory chemical documentation of such response has been presented. A disadvantage of such therapy would be the increased requirement for insulin. An increased incidence of *adult celiac disease* has also been reported in diabetics (*vide supra*).

Islet Tumors of the Pancreas. A malabsorption syndrome has been associated with non-beta islet cell tumors of the pancreas. The syndrome may also include one or all of the following: gastric hypersecretion, severe recurrent peptic ulceration, hyperkalemia, and high incidence of malignancy of the tumor. The reasons for diarrhea and steatorrhea are not known, particularly in those few who have not had gastric hypersecretion; however, in the majority with these tumors who have steatorrhea and highly acid gastric juice, inactivation of pancreatic secretions is mainly responsible since lipolysis has been repeatedly shown to be inhibited by the acid pH of the jejunum. Minimal alteration of jejunal mucosa has also been noted, but is not likely to be an important factor despite some evidence that the jejunal mucosa in this disease takes up lipid slightly subnormally.

Mesenteric Artery Insufficiency. In recent years a number of clinical reports have emphasized the association of malabsorption with mesenteric vascular insufficiency involving primarily the superior mesenteric artery or one of its branches. Such patients are commonly in the older age group

and have evidence of obliterative arterial vascular disease affecting other organs or chronic atrial fibrillation with embolization to the mesenteric arterial tree. Periumbilical pain is often felt 30 minutes to one hour after meals and gradually subsides. As the vascular problem increases, the patient may begin to have soft, light-colored stools and progressive weight loss. Small bowel roentgenograms show an abnormal picture with thickened, blunted folds, areas of narrowing, and even rigid-appearing loops. Occasionally, a "stack of coins" pattern (seen also in small bowel intramural hematomas) in the jejunum may be noted. The mechanism for the malabsorption is obscure, but must somehow relate to impaired nutrition of the mucosa.

This malabsorption syndrome may occasionally be corrected surgically, since evacuation of a clot or resection of the vessel with or without grafting may be associated with improvement of the patients' condition; if this approach is not feasible, a trial of anticoagulant therapy might be considered.

Indeed, an occasional acutely ill patient with abdominal distention, bleeding, ileus, hypertension, who is unable to withstand surgery and is treated conservatively with nasogastric intubation, intravenous fluids, antimicrobial drugs (ampicillin, 2.0 grams four times daily, or penicillin, 1,000,000 units four times daily, along with streptomycin, 1.0 gram intramuscularly every day), and, in the instance of embolization, with anticoagulants, may survive. Malabsorption may then follow the disappearance of the symptoms and signs of the severe ischemic attack. Even following evacuation of clots (emboli) or endarterectomy with or without insertion of a graft, absorption may be subnormal, and a variable length of small intestine may be noted to be narrowed, resembling in some respects granulomatous enteritis.

Vasculitis. The blood supply to the small intestine is occasionally severely compromised in patients with so-called collagen vascular disease, particularly periarteritis nodosa and systemic lupus erythematosus (SLE). Although malabsorption syndrome has been reported in these diseases, the documentation is unclear; Degos' disease, characterized by necrotic skin lesions and vasculitis of the small gut, may also cause malabsorption, although the far more serious and common clinical manifestation is infarction of the gut. A necrotizing type of arteriolitis leading to ulceration and perforation of the small gut is a serious form of vascular complication of the collagen vascular diseases.

MALABSORPTION SYNDROME AND ENTERIC LOSS OF PROTEIN

Hypoalbuminemia without liver disease, inadequate protein intake, or albuminuria may be due to excessive loss of serum protein into the intestine. This loss has been noted in patients with mucosal ulceration of the stomach, small bowel, or colon; with mucosal disease without ulceration; or in lymphatic obstruction (Table 6). Intestinal lymphatic dilatation without obvious cause (lymphangiectasia, Fig. 8) is associated with abnormal enteric protein loss in some patients whose illness was previously termed "hypercatabolic hypoproteinemia." Many of these patients, regardless of the cause for plasma protein leakage, have some degree of malabsorption.

Edema or ascites, or both, secondary to hypoalbuminemia may overshadow enteric symptoms and, indeed, underlie presenting symptoms in patients with so-called *protein-losing enteropathy*. Most of these patients have specific diseases of the intestine. Thus, the syndrome has been reported with gastric diseases such as *giant hypertrophic rugae* (Menetrier's disease), *giant gastric ulcer, gastric cancer*, and *eosinophilic granuloma of the stomach*. A variety of inflammatory diseases of the small and large intestines are also associated with this syndrome: *granulomatous enteritis* and *enterocolitis, ulcerative colitis, granuloma* of the small bowel associated with *congenital or acquired hypogammaglobulinemia, celiac disease, tropical sprue, lymphoma* of the small intestine and *Whipple's disease*, and, as noted, *lymphangiectasia*.

Allergy to milk protein and, in rare cases, to cereals or even meat may underlie protein-losing enteropathy by affecting the small intestine. Biopsy is normal or shows mild infiltration of the lamina propria with eosinophils; the disorder usually begins in childhood; it is characterized

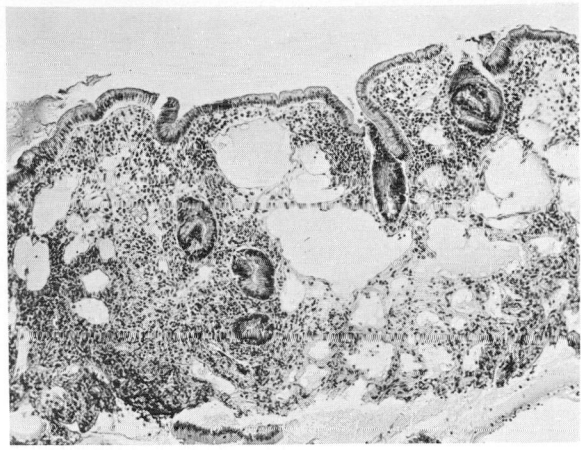

FIGURE 8. Jejunal biopsy demonstrating dilated lacteals of lymphangiectasia associated with protein-losing enteropathy.

by hypoproteinemia and edema; an iron deficiency anemia is common, as is diarrhea; eosinophilia is a permanent feature. This condition may well be a milder form of *eosinophilic gastroenteritis* in which both protein-losing enteropathy and malabsorption may be more serious (*vide supra*). Both conditions may be classified as *allergic gastroenteropathy* (Table 6). Recently, infestation with a roundworm, *Capillariasis philippensis*, has been described in the Philippines and it causes diarrhea, protein-losing enteropathy, and malabsorption, and proves fatal in two to four months.

Clinical Picture. As noted, the clinical picture may be dominated by signs and symptoms of hypoproteinemia. In most instances, the patient complains of some abdominal symptoms related to the underlying disease.

Diagnosis. The diagnosis of protein-losing enteropathy should be suspected in any patient with low serum albumin who has normal liver function and does not have an abnormal amount of protein in the urine. The abnormal loss may be confirmed by abnormal fecal excretion of Cr^{51} after intravenous injection of Cr^{51} albumin or by a rapid decay curve after intravenous Cr^{51} chloride.

Treatment of Protein-Losing Enteropathy (Table 6). Since therapy may be very successful, accurate diagnosis is extremely important. Resection of localized granuloma or ulcers of the stomach and bowel, or of localized giant gastric rugae, may lead to complete cessation of enteric protein loss. Patients with adult celiac disease and those with allergic gastroenteropathy who are sensitive to milk protein or other substances will respond to elimination of gluten or milk or other offending agents from the diet. Patients with intestinal lymphangiectasia respond to reduction of dietary fat to very low levels—5 grams or less—or to administration of MCT in place of dietary fat. These regimens will usually reverse the abnormal protein loss in this disease, and may lessen it in any disease that obstructs lymphatics. Protein loss resulting from *acute, nongranulomatous ileojejunitis*, as well as *granulomatous enteritis* and

TABLE 6. CLASSIFICATION AND THERAPY OF DISEASES ASSOCIATED WITH ENTERIC LOSS OF PLASMA PROTEIN

Disease	Therapy
A. Mucosal Ulceration:	
Gastric carcinoma	
Gastric lymphoma	Surgical resection
Multiple gastric ulcers	
Colon cancer	
Granulomatous enteritis	
Diffuse nongranulomatous ileojejunitis	Corticosteroids
B. Mucosal Disease Without Ulceration:	
Rugal hypertrophy (Menetrier's, etc.)	Resection, if local
Celiac disease	Gluten elimination
Tropical sprue	Antimicrobials; folic acid
Whipple's disease	Antimicrobials
Allergic gastroenteropathy	Elimination diet; steroids
Bacterial or parasitic enteritis	Antimicrobial drugs
Gastrocolic fistula	Resection
C. Lymphatic Abnormalities:	
Capillariasis philippensis	Thiabendazole
Primary lymphangiectasia	Low-fat diet or MCT
Lymph-enteric fistula	Resection
Lymphoma	Chemotherapy
Constrictive pericarditis	Pericardiectomy
Tricuspid valvular disease	Rx of heart failure

ulcerative colitis, may disappear during therapy with corticosteroids, or, in the case of oral enteritides, with spontaneous recovery from the infection. *Acute bacterial enteritis* caused by Shigella or Salmonella, *Whipple's disease, enteric tuberculosis,* and instances of excessive protein loss associated with bacterial overgrowth in the small intestine (*"blind loop syndrome"*), all may respond to appropriate antimicrobial therapy. *Capillariasis philippensis* is said to respond to thiabendazole, 25 mg. per kilogram per day for 30 days (see Helminthic Diseases). A similar effect has likewise been reported in enteric lymphoma after x-radiation and treatment with chlorambucil (Table 6).

Protein-losing enteropathy may be associated with *chronic constrictive pericarditis,* presumably due to mediastinal lymphatic obstruction. Pericardiolysis or parietal pericardiectomy will alleviate or even completely reverse this enteric loss. Also, effective treatment of severe *right heart failure* may alleviate protein-losing enteropathy.

PROGNOSIS

The outlook for the patient with malabsorption syndrome depends upon both the nature of the underlying disease and the institution of appropriate therapy. (Proper treatment, of course, implies correct diagnosis.)

Specific therapy for patients with adult celiac disease (gluten-free diet) and effective agents for tropical sprue are available. Intelligent replacement therapy for those with deficient digestion (gastrectomy, hepatobiliary disease, pancreatic insufficiency, massive resection of the small intestine, or iliectomy often alleviates the major symptoms.

Whipple's disease now appears entirely manageable, and perhaps even reversible, with use of broad-spectrum antimicrobial agents and adrenal steroids. The malabsorption of diffuse ileojejunitis, involving large segments of the small intestine, may be completely abolished by administration of adrenal steroids or corticotrophin. Likewise, isoniazid and streptomycin are similarly effective in tuberculosis enteritis. Elimination of an offender

in the diet and corticosteroids are an effective combination against eosinophilic gastroenteritis.

The correction of conditions in which intestinal microbes play an important role ("blind loop syndrome") may be accomplished by appropriate surgery, such as resection of fistulas or strictures, or by administration of broad-spectrum antimicrobial drugs. In either case, a normal or nearly normal state of health may be achieved.

The prognosis for patients with malabsorption associated with endocrine disorders is good. The patient with diabetes mellitus who has neuropathy and bacterial overgrowth may be helped by the intermittent administration of antimicrobial drugs. Parathormone, vitamin D, and calcium will restore absorption toward normal in cases of hypoparathyroidism. Resection of a non-insulin-secreting, non-beta-cell tumor of the pancreatic islets will diminish diarrhea and steatorrhea.

Because of the nature of the underlying disease, the outlook is bleak for a number of patients with malabsorption syndrome. These are the patients with advancing biliary cirrhosis; complicated relapsing pancreatitis; extensive granulomatous enteritis associated with recurrent fistulas, strictures, and mutilative surgery; progressive scleroderma of the intestine; lymphoma of the small bowel and mesenteric lymph nodes; and progressive occlusive disease of the superior mesenteric artery. Therapy for protein-losing enteropathy is remarkably good if the correct diagnosis is made (Table 6).

On the whole, the prognosis for the malabsorption syndrome is optimistic provided that the specific abnormality is identified and appropriate corrective measures are instituted.

Benson, G., Kowlessar, O. D., and Sleisenger, M. H.: Adult celiac disease with emphasis upon response to the gluten-free diet. Medicine, 43:1, 1964.

Handbook of Physiology. Section 6: Alimentary Canal. Vol. II. Absorption. American Physiological Society, 1967.

Jeffries, G. H., Weser, E., and Sleisenger, M. H.: Malabsorption. Gastroenterology, 56:777, 1969.

Krone, C. L., Theodor, E., Sleisenger, M. H., and Jeffries, G. H.: Studies on the pathogenesis of malabsorption: Lipid hydrolysis and micelle formation in the intestinal lumen. Medicine, 47:89, 1968.

Sleisenger, M. H.: Malabsorption syndrome. New Eng. J. Med., 281:1111, 1969.

Diseases of the Pancreas
O. Dhodanand Kowlessar

ACUTE PANCREATITIS

GENERAL CONSIDERATIONS

During the past 15 years, rapid progress has been made in the understanding of basic pancreatic physiology and biochemistry. These advances have come from studies that have elucidated the

factors controlling the secretion of pancreatic juice, the ultrastructure of the human pancreas by the use of the electron microscope, the sites of synthesis and discharge of pancreatic enzymes by the use of labeled amino acids and radioautography, the precise electrolyte and enzyme contents of pancreatic juice, and the chromatographic and electrophoretic purification of potent pancreatic hormones. The information thus obtained, supplemented by contributions of clinicians, radiologists, and surgeons, has resulted in a better understanding of the pathogenesis of pancreatic inflammation, edema, and hemorrhage. It has further resulted in more exact and reliable diagnostic tests of pancreatic disease and, through utilization of therapeutic measures directed against specific etiologic mechanisms, in more rational and efficacious treatment. A brief review of pancreatic function will be helpful in understanding the etiology and pathogenesis of acute pancreatitis.

PANCREATIC PHYSIOLOGY, BIOCHEMISTRY, AND ANATOMY

Pancreatic juice, as it appears in the duodenum, is a clear, colorless fluid, of low viscosity and alkaline pH (8.3). It is made up mainly of water, electrolytes, and a protein moiety of enzymes. The main ions are Na^+, K^+, HCO_3^-, and, in lesser concentrations, Cl^-, Ca^{++}, Zn^{++}, $HPO_4^=$, and $SO_4^=$. Secretion of pancreatic juice in man is probably continuous with an increased flow during digestion regulated by the hormones secretin and pancreozymin, as well as by neurogenic and vascular factors. The total daily volume of pancreatic juice has been estimated to be between 1500 and 3000 ml. Secretin is responsible for the water and bicarbonate secretion of the pancreas, and pancreozymin stimulates the outpouring of pancreatic enzymes. Thus, the augmentation of pancreatic secretion during digestion is the result of stimuli arising within the duodenum and acting by way of hormone and nerve mechanisms. Hydrochloric acid, by stimulating the release of secretin, produces a secretion low in enzyme activity but high in bicarbonate. The carbohydrates, although unable to induce secretin production in the resting gland, augment moderately the enzyme output of the actively secreting pancreas. On the other hand, protein and fats, as well as their intermediate products of digestion and metabolism, are powerful stimuli for enzyme secretion (pancreozymin-vagal type of secretion) but affect only minimally the production of bicarbonate. The nerve mechanism, which includes the vagus, the sympathetic nervous system, and the local duodenopancreatic reflexes, is of great significance in the regulation of pancreatic enzyme secretion during digestion.

Electrolytes are secreted by the human pancreas in a solution that is isotonic with the blood plasma. The concentrations of the cations Na^+, K^+, and Ca^{++} approximate the diffusible ionic content of the blood plasma. The Cl^- content varies inversely with the concentration of HCO_3^-, the latter increasing as the rate of secretion increases. The secretion of bicarbonate by the intralobular duct cells appears to be under the catalytic influence of carbonic anhydrase, which controls the formation of bicarbonate ion within the cell according to the following equation: $H_2O + CO_2 \rightleftharpoons H_2CO_3 \rightleftharpoons H^+ + HCO_3^-$. The main function of this balanced electrolyte pancreatic juice, apparently, is to adjust the duodenal contents to an optimal alkaline pH for the action of the pancreatic enzymes: amylase, lipase, trypsin, chymotrypsin, carboxypeptidases, leucine amino peptidase, deoxyribonuclease 1, ribonuclease 1, elastase, collagenase, and lecithinase. Trypsin and chymotrypsin are secreted in combination with specific inhibitors. The activation of these enzymes is accomplished by the enzymatic action of free trypsin and by the action of the intestinal peptidase enterokinase. These enzymes break down proteins to polypeptides, which are further broken down by specific peptidases to absorbable amino acids. Amylase, secreted in active form, is responsible for the digestion of starch, glycogen, and other carbohydrates to the disaccharide form for further splitting by intracellular intestinal enzymes. Lipase, aided by bile salts, acts on neutral fats and phospholipids, liberating glycerol and fatty acids. The nucleoproteins are broken down by deoxyribonuclease 1 and ribonuclease 1.

Both morphologic data obtained by the electron microscope and turnover studies employing labeled amino acids suggest that the pancreatic enzymes are rapidly synthesized in the microsomal fraction of the pancreas and accumulate in the zymogen granules for discharge into the pancreatic ducts for transport and function. This transfer of enzymes from the aqueous phase of the intracellular fluid across the lipoid membrane to the lumen of the duct appears to be aided by the "carrier" effect of the phosphatids, phosphoinositide, phosphatidic acid, and phosphatidyl ethanolamine.

ETIOLOGY OF ACUTE PANCREATITIS

A number of factors have been proposed for the etiology of pancreatitis. The three most important etiologic categories are gallstones, alcohol, and "idiopathic" processes, accounting for 90 to 95 per cent of all cases of acute pancreatitis; miscellaneous factors are implicated in the remaining 5 to 10 per cent of patients. The multiplicity of mechanisms for production of this disease demonstrates that this gland is capable of responding to stress of many different types with a unitary reaction of varying degree.

Biliary Tract Disease. Biliary tract disease is responsible for 10 to 95 per cent of large series of pancreatitis. This wide range is related to the incidence of alcoholism in a given patient population.

The importance of a mechanical factor in the pathogenesis of pancreatitis was stressed in the early writing of Opie, who postulated his "common channel theory" from the observation of acute pancreatitis in a patient with a small stone impacted in the ampulla of Vater. In such situations it is believed that the retrograde passage or reflux of bile into the pancreatic duct initiates the pathologic process. It seems, however, that spasm of the sphincter of Oddi coupled with pancreatic duct obstruction is the most likely initiating cause.

That bile reflux or pressure changes in the biliary tree do not cause pancreatitis has been shown by (1) absence of pathologic and chemical evidence of the presence of bile in the pancreatic duct system of patients with pancreatitis; (2) evidence that the secretory pressure is higher in the pancreatic duct than in the biliary tract; and (3) the fact that pancreatitis occurs in patients in whom the pancreatic duct and common duct enter separately, so that biliary reflux via a "common channel" is impossible.

Alcohol. Alcoholism is responsible for 8 to 75 per cent of cases, depending upon whether the patient population is derived from a private hospital (lower figure) or from tax-supported institutions (higher figure). The mechanisms whereby ethyl alcohol induces pancreatitis are not known. It is likely that following a large alcohol intake the pancreas would be stimulated through the acid-secretin mechanism to secrete a large volume of juice into a duct obstructed by alcohol-induced papillary edema and sphincter spasm. Although the mechanical hypothesis appears to be cogent, it is possible that an excess of ethyl radicals may competitively affect the metabolism of methyl groups in a chain of biochemical events analogous to the antagonism that follows administration of ethionine to laboratory animals, and is associated with severe pancreatic necrosis. Methyl alcohol can also cause pancreatitis.

Idiopathic Factors. Idiopathic factors consistently account for 20 to 50 per cent of large series and thus represent the third most common category; the precise etiology is unknown.

Miscellaneous Causes. A miscellaneous group of etiologic factors make up about 10 per cent of other causes of pancreatitis. Among these are (1) *Metabolic-nutritional disturbances,* including primary hyperlipoproteinemia (Types I, IV and V), diabetic ketoacidosis, malnutrition (kwashiorkor), uremia, pregnancy, and *hypercalcemic states* (hyperparathyroidism, multiple myeloma, and sarcoidosis), which bring about excessive activation of trypsinogen by calcium ion, or by precipitation of calcium in an alkaline milieu in the ducts leading to obstruction. An increased incidence of parathyroid carcinoma causing hyperparathyroidism has been observed in those cases associated with severe pancreatitis. Of note also are the cases of severe pancreatitis occurring within the first 24 hours after the removal of a parathyroid adenoma. *Hereditary pancreatitis* appears to be transmitted as a non-sex-linked mendelian dominant trait. The attacks begin, in most cases, in childhood or early adult life, the average age of onset being 12 years. At present, men and women have been affected with about equal frequency. Cholelithiasis and alcoholism are infrequent concomitants. Pancreatic calcifications most often appear as discrete calculi in the larger pancreatic ducts. Aminoaciduria has been observed in approximately 50 per cent of a small group of persons (with or without pancreatitis) so far studied in affected kindreds. The aminoaciduria of persons in hereditary pancreatitis kindreds resembles the "incomplete

recessive" form of cystinuria, with abnormally large excretion of lysine and cystine, and, less often and to a lesser degree, of arginine. Studies of endogenous renal clearances of amino acids in some patients reveal that excessive excretion of lysine resulted principally from impaired renal tubular reabsorption of this amino acid. Carcinoma of the pancreas was a cause of death in a few members of kindreds with this entity. (2) *Infection* secondary to the reflux of infected material into the pancreatic duct, or from such systemic infections as mumps, scarlet fever, typhoid fever, viral hepatitis, and infectious mononucleosis. (3) *Trauma:* steering-wheel injuries, postoperative pancreatitis (following surgery in the area of the pancreas, as well as distant areas from the pancreas, e.g., transurethral resection), and electric shock. (4) *Vascular and autoimmune mechanisms:* hypertension, polyarteritis nodosa and systemic lupus erythematosus. (5) *Drugs:* glucocorticoids, chlorothiazide, isoniazid, salicylates, sulfamethizole, indomethacin, and immunosuppressive drugs (6-mercaptopurine and azathioprine).

PATHOGENESIS

Pancreatitis is a chemical autolytic process, the pathogenesis of which is well documented from postmortem, operative, and experimental studies. The underlying mechanism in the production of pancreatic inflammation is the escape of activated enzymes into the interstitial tissues, and the earliest responses to this chemical irritation are edema and vascular engorgement of the pancreas. Apparently the interstitial fluid within the pancreas contains potent enzyme inhibitors, because many cases of pancreatitis without active necrosis are seen at laparotomy. Furthermore, the protease inhibitors appear to be more effective than those for lipase, as judged by the frequent finding of fat necrosis in and about the pancreas, without concomitant hemorrhage and tissue destruction.

Edema may occur anywhere in the gland, but is apt to be more severe in the head. The region affected becomes pale and indurated, with progressive engorgement of the blood vessels. In most instances, the inflammatory edema subsides spontaneously but, in a small percentage of cases, there is progression to hemorrhage, necrosis, and suppuration, or the inflammation becomes chronic. Progression of pancreatic edema to hemorrhagic necrosis is in part the result of enlargement of the pancreas within its capsule, which obstructs the pancreatic duct further and aggravates the vascular engorgement until ischemia supervenes. As elsewhere, ischemia superimposed on an inflammatory process results in infarction and hemorrhage. Activated pancreatic enzymes may bring about erosion of major blood vessels, with hemorrhage into the pancreas, the retroperitoneal tissues, and even the colon. Collections of blood, digested tissue, and pancreatic secretions may burrow along the tissue spaces into the gastrohepatic ligament and retroperitoneally into the lesser sac and flank, giving rise to the classic ascitic exudate of acute pancreatitis described as "beef broth," and to visible hemorrhagic areas in the costovertebral angle (Grey-Turner's sign). The peritoneal effusion and peritoneal irritation during the early stages of acute pancreatitis are greatest in the lesser sac and at the base of the transverse mesocolon. This localized chemical peritonitis often results in a segmental paralytic ileus of the first jejunal loop, which has been described as a diagnostic sign, the "sentinel loop" of acute pancreatitis.

Thus, the local pathology of pancreatitis at the inception is the result of edema, hemorrhage, and the onslaught of biochemical agents, i.e., the pancreatic enzymes. As the disease progresses without resolution, superimposed infection, especially by the colon-aerogenes group of intestinal bacteria, produces suppuration, and results in pancreatic abscesses, as well as purulent collections in the various abdominal fossae, the lesser sac, the cul-de-sac, and the left subphrenic space.

Resolution may occur with fibrosis and calcification. The edema and other inflammatory changes subside during the first week of illness. Areas of necrosis are autolyzed and replaced by fibrous tissue. Cellular proliferation attempts to restore normal glandular architecture. By the end of the second week histologic repair may have proceeded to such a degree that the pancreas may appear normal. On the other hand, resolution is delayed in the more severe forms, with persistence of residual fibrosis, calcification, and acinar dysfunction.

DIAGNOSIS

Clinical Manifestations. *Pain* and *shock* are the outstanding symptoms of acute hemorrhagic pancreatitis; *pain* and *metabolic disturbances* dominate the clinical picture of acute edematous pancreatitis and chronic relapsing pancreatitis. However, all three — pain, shock, and metabolic disturbances — may be absent, as in painless pancreatitis.

The *pain* in acute pancreatitis results from distention of the pancreatic capsule, retroperitoneal extravasations, chemical peritonitis, and obstruction or spasm in the pancreatic ducts, extrahepatic biliary tract, and duodenum. Characteristically, the attack is sudden, and the pain is usually severe, constant, and widespread. It is frequently more intense when the patient is lying supine than when he is sitting or lying on the side with his spine flexed. Though usually originating in the epigastrium, the pain also may be experienced in other parts of the abdomen, and may radiate to the back, substernal area, and flanks. Physical examination discloses an acutely ill patient complaining of abdominal pain, with *fever* and *tachycardia.* The blood pressure may be slightly elevated in those in whom circulatory collapse has not supervened. *Cyanosis, cold* and *clammy skin, rapid* and *feeble pulse,* and *subnormal temperature*

are present in the more severe attacks. The *abdomen* may be distended early as a result of paralytic ileus and the accumulation of peritoneal fluid. Peristalsis may be diminished or inaudible. *Tenderness* is invariably present in the epigastrium, and is associated with a moderate degree of muscular rigidity; it may be elicited elsewhere in the abdomen, depending on the sites of seepage of the pancreatic juice. Occasionally, a *mass* in the upper abdomen — an inflammatory pseudocyst — may be palpable. The systemic effects in acute pancreatitis are presumed to result from the absorption of activated pancreatic enzymes and the products of pancreatic digestion into the blood.

Shock is the outstanding systemic phenomenon in *severe acute pancreatitis,* and may be so profound that death ensues within a few hours. The shock results from a combination of the following physiologic events: (1) presumed increase in serum proteolytic activity; (2) the release of the activated enzyme kallikrein, which in turn is responsible for the formation of kinins, whose main actions are stimulation of smooth muscle, dilatation of blood vessels, and lowering of blood pressure; (3) contraction of the blood volume, as great as 30 per cent, secondary to exudation of blood and plasma into the peritoneal cavity and possible protein leak; and (4) hyperlipasemia, which may then be related to hyperlipemia, fat necrosis of the subcutaneous tissue and the bone marrow. Additional factors are (5) acute coronary insufficiency resulting from thrombosis and electrolyte disturbances (in turn, the lowered blood volume and shock contribute to the myocardial problem), and (6) pulmonary embolus.

In many cases, other metabolic disturbances can be uncovered. Serum calcium, potassium, and sodium are lowered. The depression of calcium is due partly to fixation by fatty acids in areas of fat necrosis, and possibly to increased levels of circulating glucagon. Levels of calcium below 7 mg. per 100 ml. are usually accompanied by tetany.

Disturbances of islet cell function are associated with *hyperglycemia, glycosuria,* and impaired glucose tolerance in about 50 per cent of the cases. These changes, although transient in the acute cases, may, with repeated attacks, progress to true "pancreatic" diabetes. *Coma* may be the presenting symptom of severe hemorrhagic pancreatitis; when associated with the commonly elevated blood sugar in acute pancreatitis, diabetic coma may be erroneously diagnosed.

Jaundice is seen in about 25 per cent of patients with acute pancreatitis, resulting primarily from obstruction of the terminal common duct as it traverses an edematous pancreas; in some patients, exacerbation of associated biliary tract disease may also be partly responsible. Intrahepatic cholestasis secondary to alcoholic liver disease may also contribute to the icterus.

Hyperlipemia with grossly opalescent serum has been observed in patients with pancreatitis caused by alcoholism; the mechanism of its production is not understood. Some authors have reported disseminated fat necrosis in the marrow and subcutaneous tissues. Acute and chronic bone lesions secondary to medullary necrosis have been described. *Pulmonary atelectasis, pneumonia,* and *pleural effusion,* particularly left-sided, are noted frequently. Significantly, pancreatic enzyme concentrations are higher in the pleural effusion than in simultaneously obtained serum. These enzymes are thought to reach the pleural fluid from the ascitic exudate by passage through the transdiaphragmatic lymphatic channels. Occasionally, respiratory symptoms may overshadow the abdominal complaints.

The vascular phenomena in acute pancreatitis include peripheral *venous thromboses* and *thrombophlebitis.*

Laboratory Diagnosis. Serum Enzymes. A diagnosis of acute pancreatitis may be made when an elevated *serum amylase,* usually greater than 300 Somogyi units, is found in a patient with acute, severe pain in the upper abdomen, tenderness, vomiting, fever, tachycardia, and leukocytosis. The serum amylase becomes elevated early in the course of the disease, usually within the first 24 to 48 hours. In most cases, values range from 300 to 800 but levels as high as 12,000 units have been reported. Apparently no constant relationship exists, however, between the severity of the disease and the height of the serum amylase values. Milder episodes may have considerable elevations. Conversely, in attacks with early fatality, the amylase values (as well as other enzyme levels) may be greatly decreased because of destruction of the pancreas or the formation of a large pseudocyst into which most or all of the pancreatic juice drains and from which enzymes do not pass into the circulation. The serum *lipase* usually rises later, reaching its peak in 72 or 96 hours; values greater than 2.0 ml. of N/100 NaOH are significant. Elevations of the levels of *glutamic oxaloacetic acid transaminase, alkaline phosphatase,* and *leucine aminopeptidase* are usually secondary to obstruction of the common bile duct or associated liver disease.

A variety of diseases, intra-abdominal and extra-abdominal, may be accompanied by elevation of the serum enzymes, frequently posing a difficult diagnostic problem. Hyperamylasemia is encountered in *perforation of peptic ulcer, small bowel obstruction, salivary duct occlusion, parotitis,* and *uremia,* and after administration of opiates, notably codeine and morphine. Elevations of serum lipase have been reported in patients with *carcinoma of the pancreas; obstructive jaundice due to stone, tumors, and cirrhosis of the liver; viral hepatitis; intestinal obstruction;* and *peritonitis.* It should be pointed out, however, that in these instances the serum enzyme elevations are not as high as in acute pancreatitis.

Urinary Amylase Levels. Elevation of urinary amylase concentration has been used to diagnose acute pancreatitis, in the absence of renal failure. Levels of urinary amylase higher than 4000 units per 24 hours or 300 units per hour are usually seen in patients with acute attacks of pancreatitis.

Furthermore, these levels can remain elevated from seven to ten days after the serum amylase levels have returned to normal.

In view of recent reports of patients with hyperamylasemia secondary to a serum amylase of unusually high molecular weight, it appears that both serum and urinary amylase should be determined. In patients with high molecular weight serum amylase, the urinary amylase is normal.

Other Laboratory Data. Ancillary laboratory findings must be considered in making the diagnosis. The *leukocyte count* often ranges from 10,000 to 30,000 per cubic millimeter, with an increase in immature granulocytes. In mild cases, the leukocyte count may be normal. The hematocrit and erythrocyte count are usually not significantly lowered, except when there is hemorrhage into the peritoneal cavity. Elevation of *blood urea nitrogen* is not uncommon in the more severe cases, especially when shock and oliguria are present. *Glycosuria* appears in about 11 per cent of patients with acute pancreatitis, and disappears with resolution of the process. Transient *hyperglycemia* may be found more frequently than glycosuria. The development of glycosuria and hyperglycemia in patients with acute pancreatitis has not been adequately explained.

A slight depression of serum *calcium* occurs in most patients between the third and fifteenth days of the disease, the lowest level occurring about the sixth day. Serum calcium below 7.0 mg. per 100 ml. portends a poor although not invariably fatal prognosis. Diminished serum albumin lowers the total serum calcium, so that hypoalbuminemia should be evaluated in the assessment of serum calcium and in replacement therapy. An unexpectedly normal serum calcium level in severe pancreatitis may be the first indication of hyperparathyroidism. *Hypokalemia* may be observed, and is most likely related to alkalosis, intravenous administration of saline solution, and loss of gastric juice because of continuous nasogastric suction. In severe cases, in which there is considerable tissue destruction, *shock* with oliguria causes hyperkalemia.

Electrocardiography. The electrocardiograms of some patients with acute pancreatitis may show depression of S-T segments in the limb leads and precordial leads as well as changes in the Q-T intervals. These changes may be due to the electrolyte imbalance or may be related to the shock in the more severe cases.

Roentgenographic Findings. Although in no way pathognomonic of acute pancreatitis, certain roentgenographic abnormalities are encountered with sufficient frequency to suggest the diagnosis. A survey film of the abdomen may reveal a localized paralytic ileus of jejunum ("sentinel loop"), usually in the left mid-portion of the abdomen, or calcification in the region of the pancreas (see accompanying figure) or the "colon cut-off" sign. The latter consists of an isolated gaseous distention of the ascending colon and hepatic flexure due to partial obstruction caused by spread of the in-

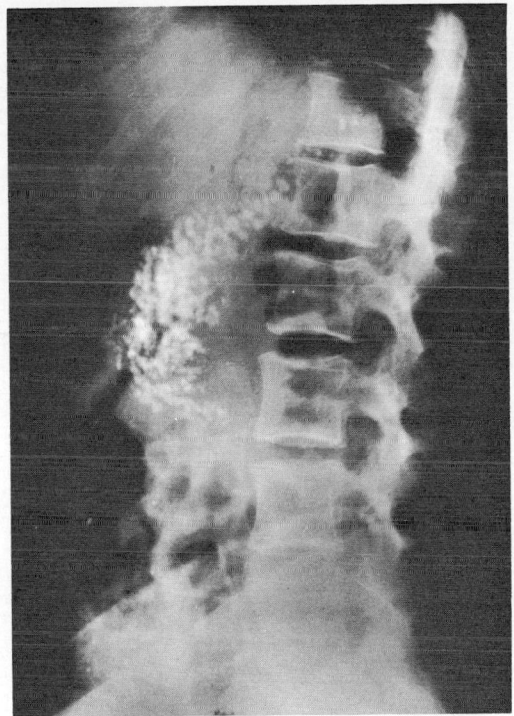

Left oblique roentgenogram of abdomen demonstrating pancreatic calcification.

flammatory process from the head of the pancreas. Barium swallow may demonstrate displacement of the stomach, enlargement of the duodenal loop, or collection and stasis of barium in the dependent parts of the duodenum caused by an enlarged head of the pancreas or an inflammatory pseudocyst. Also there may be an enlarged edematous ampulla of Vater and irritability of the stomach and duodenum. In most instances the biliary tree may be adequately visualized by intravenous cholangiography, excluding bile duct obstruction as the precipitating event. Nonvisualization of the gallbladder after either oral or intravenous administration of dye, however, is a common finding during the acute episode, but does not necessarily indicate a disease of the gallbladder. Accordingly, the roentgenographic studies should be repeated several weeks after the attack has subsided, at which time, if the gallbladder is diseased stones in the biliary tree and/or nonfilling of the gallbladder will be observed. The chest roentgenogram may show pleural effusion of linear focal atelectasis at the lung bases.

Other Diagnostic Procedures. Diagnostic tap of the peritoneum, performed under local anesthesia, in the left lower quadrant of the abdomen may reveal turbid yellow fluid in edematous pancreatitis or reddish-brown fluid in the hemorrhagic type. The peritoneal fluid amylase is considerably higher than serum amylase tested at the same time, and may remain elevated for two or three days after the serum amylase has fallen to normal levels. The determination of serum methemalbumin has been proposed as a diagnostic test for pancreatitis. However, recent evidence suggests

that elevated levels have occurred in other acute abdominal emergencies, which invalidates the test as a positive diagnostic criterion for pancreatitis.

Differential Diagnosis. The diagnosis of acute pancreatitis should be established as rapidly as clinical and laboratory facilities permit. However, the diagnosis is made difficult by the large number of abdominal catastrophes that may in many ways simulate this condition.

Perforated peptic ulcer, more than any other abdominal condition, may resemble acute pancreatitis. Usually a preceding history compatible with ulcer can be elicited, although occasionally perforation may be its first indication. Unlike pancreatitis, however, *boardlike rigidity of the abdomen* is the outstanding finding. A flat plate of the abdomen may show free air, usually under the right diaphragm. Hyperamylasemia, resulting from the escape of duodenal contents into the peritoneum or involvement of the pancreas in the process, may accompany perforation, but usually the values are not as high as in acute pancreatitis. (See Acid-Peptic Disease.)

Biliary colic may resemble acute pancreatitis by virtue of pressure changes in the biliary tree and associated inflammation of the gallbladder. Pain, tenderness, and rigidity are frequently localized in the right upper quadrant of the abdomen. *Acute cholangitis*, caused by stones in the common bile duct, is associated usually with chills, fever, and jaundice. An elevated serum amylase is seen in about 20 per cent of cases of common duct stone, and differentiation may have to await the course of the disease.

The pain of *acute cholecystitis* is usually in the right upper quadrant and may radiate to the right scapula. Tenderness and guarding are present in the right upper quadrant. A striking feature is that, despite the pain, these patients do not usually look very ill, in contrast to the patients with acute pancreatitis.

Acute *small bowel obstruction* may be a diagnostic problem in view of occasional associated hyperamylasemia. The history of vomiting and the cramplike periumbilical pain with abdominal distention and visible peristalsis are helpful. In *mechanical ileus*, auscultation will reveal high-pitched notes, succussion splashes, and peristaltic rushes. Acute appendicitis involving a retrocecal appendix in close contact with the gallbladder may require differentiation. The amylase is usually normal in this condition.

Mesenteric thrombosis may present as intestinal obstruction with a less acute onset. This may be associated with *bloody diarrhea*, which is rare in pancreatitis. Shock is more acute, and diffuse tenderness and rigidity are more common. A flat plate of the abdomen may show a large, dilated, fluid-filled loop of bowel, the site of infarction.

Dissecting aneurysm usually presents with severe pain, shock, absent pulsations in the femoral vessels, and lowered blood pressure in the legs. A pulsating mass may be felt.

Nephrolithiasis on the left side may simulate

acute pancreatitis. Hematuria and a flat plate of the abdomen revealing a stone will help in the differentiation.

Acute coronary occlusion may be present with left upper quadrant or epigastric pain, nausea, and vomiting. Electrocardiographic changes and elevation of the serum glutamic oxaloacetic transaminase occur in pancreatitis, but Q waves are not ordinarily present in pancreatitis. Also, the lack of elevation of serum enzymes of pancreatic origin will help exclude acute pancreatitis.

Acute intermittent porphyria is usually associated with a history of vomiting at intervals, severe and frequent episodes of abdominal pain, and chronic constipation. The demonstration of porphobilinogen in the urine by the Watson-Schwartz test is helpful in establishing the diagnosis.

Acute systemic lupus erythematosus and *periarteritis nodosa* may present with an abdominal picture requiring differentiation from pancreatitis. The situation is further confused by the fact that pancreatitis may be a complication of these diseases. The history, coupled with other common findings in these diseases, will help in the differential diagnosis.

TREATMENT

Acute pancreatitis varies greatly in the degree of its severity. The milder attacks are presumably due to edema of the pancreas, and in this situation therapy is directed primarily to the relief of pain. In the more severe form with hemorrhage and necrosis, and their concomitant physiologic and biochemical disturbances discussed previously, treatment may conveniently be divided into several distinct phases.

Control of Pain. The pain is usually severe, and should be treated promptly with adequate doses of analgesics. Meperidine (Demerol), with its minimal effect on the tone of the sphincter of Oddi, is probably the drug of choice and should be given parenterally in doses of 75 to 100 mg. every four to six hours to assure prompt and adequate relief. Morphine and codeine should be avoided because of their spasmogenic effects. Sympathetic nerve blocks and continuous or fractional epidural anesthesia can be used to supplement the effects of meperidine in patients whose pain is persistent.

Treatment of Shock. Circulatory collapse is often the most immediate and major problem of the severe form of pancreatitis. Whole blood is probably the most effective treatment, and, in view of the diminution of blood volume to approximately 70 per cent in severe cases, should be given promptly. Large volumes of fluid are often required; constant monitoring of central venous pressure as well as careful measurement of fluid intake and urinary output are necessary. Albumin and plasma are adequate temporary substitutes. Low-molecular-weight dextran may be highly effective and should be tried.

Inhibition of Pancreatic Secretory Activity. An important principle in the management of acute pancreatitis is the "splinting of the injured pancreas" by suppression of pancreatic secretion. Achievement of this goal is accomplished by cessation of oral intake of food, continuous nasogastric suction to minimize release of secretin through stimulation by gastric acid, and administration of drugs to inhibit pancreatic secretion. Included among these drugs are such enzyme inhibitors as acetazolamide (Diamox), which interferes with the formation of pancreatic juice at a cellular level, and atropine or a synthetic anticholinergic drug, Propantheline (Pro-Banthine) bromide, 30 mg., or methantheline (Banthine) bromide, 50 mg., given parenterally every six to eight hours, may be beneficial because of their pharmacologic effects, which include suppression of gastric acidity, relaxation of the sphincter, and partial inhibition of pancreatic enzyme production. However, in the presence of *paralytic ileus*, these drugs may be harmful and should be avoided.

Prevention of Infection. In severe cases and in those associated with biliary tract disease, broad-spectrum antimicrobial drugs should be given as prophylactic agents against the potential septic complications of pancreatic necrosis—abscess and peritonitis. Penicillin G, 600,000 units twice daily, and streptomycin, 0.5 gram twice daily, or the tetracycline drugs, 250 mg. every six hours parenterally, are efficacious agents against the usual intestinal organisms found in the peritonitis of pancreatitis, as well as in the biliary tract. Recently cephalothin (Keflin) in doses of 6 to 10 grams intramuscularly has been reported to be extremely effective against the commonly encountered organisms in severe pancreatitis with the exception of Pseudomonas.

Fluids and Electrolytes. The continued gastric suction and the abstinence from any oral intake make it necessary to replace body fluids and electrolytes carefully. The amount of normal saline with supplemental potassium chloride to be administered may vary between 3 and 6 liters daily and should be estimated by considering the insensible loss, the amount of sweating, the elevation of temperature, the volume of gastric suction, and the anticipated urinary output. Glucose must be administered cautiously, for it may aggravate a diabetic state that has been precipitated by acute pancreatitis. When hyperglycemia and glycosuria are marked and diabetic acidosis is imminent, small doses of insulin must be given.

Hypocalcemia is fairly frequent, and calcium gluconate solution may be given intravenously as needed. *Hypokalemia* is combated by cautious intravenous administration of potassium chloride. Blood potassium determinations and electrocardiograms should be done frequently to avoid potassium toxicity.

Miscellaneous Measures. Abdominal distention and ileus are usually adequately managed by gastric suction, but occasionally it may be necessary to insert a long intestinal tube to deflate the small intestine. The adynamic nature of this ileus makes the passage of such a tube rather difficult.

Many drugs have been used in the treatment of acute pancreatitis, but, since the disease is self-limiting in most instances, it is difficult to assess their efficacy. In recent years, the use of corticotrophin and cortisone has been advocated in acute fulminant pancreatitis, particularly when an abdominal exploration has been performed without previous knowledge of the existence of the disease. However, evidence has accumulated that steroids, when used in other diseases, have brought about lesions similar to those seen in pancreatitis. Thus, caution should be exercised, and these drugs should be reserved for those patients in whom shock has developed that is unresponsive to the usual measures.

Peritoneal dialysis should be attempted in those patients whose clinical symptoms fail to improve after a period of conservative th...

creatitis who develop the chronic relapsing form of the disease. Suffice it to say that continued alcoholism or neglected biliary tract disease is often associated with recurrent attacks. Another important determining factor is the degree of ductal obstruction that is the residue of the initial bout of inflammation. Correction or control of an underlying cause, e.g., an endocrine disturbance such as hyperparathyroidism, or the withdrawal of a potentially noxious drug may help to prevent further attacks.

Bank, S., Barbezat, G. O., Marks, I. N., and Silber, W.: Methemalbuminemia in acute abdominal emergencies. Brit. Med. J., 1:86, 1968.
Bolooki, H., and Gliedman, M. L.: Peritoneal dialysis in treatment of acute pancreatitis. Surgery, 64:466, 1968.
Dreiling, D. A., Janowitz, H. D., and Perrier, C. V.: Pancreatic ... y Disease: A Physiologic Approach. New York, ... Row Publishers, Inc., 1964.
...nbill, E. E., and Ulrich, J. A.: Hereditary pan...scription of a fifth kindred and summary of ...res. Amer. J. Med., 33:358, 1962.
...apport, M., and Cooperband, S. R.: The renal ...amylase in renal insufficiency acute pancreati...amylasemia. Ann. Intern. Med., 71:919, 1969.
..., Keynes, W. M., and Cope, O.: Further experi...ncreatitis as a diagnostic clue to hyperpara...New Eng. J. Med., 266:265, 1962.
...te pancreatitis. Amer. J. Med., 21:246, 1956.

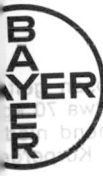
...NG PANCREATITIS AND ...NIC PANCREATITIS

...creatitis is the end result of recur...of acute inflammation. The paren...gland, subjected to cycles of fat ne...and calcification, is gradually and ...placed by fibrotic tissue with dis...acinar and islet tissue. During the ...of *relapsing pancreatitis*, the func...of the gland and its capacity for ...sis and recovery are so great that ...ncies are only transiently demon...the acute attacks. As the disease ...iently more severe in the region of ...gland, and the islets of Langerhans ...ed in the body and tail, disturbed ...etabolism appears relatively late. ...osited in the obstructed main duct ...r ducts as well as in areas of fat ...parenchyma. In the later stages, ...destruction of the parenchyma and ...he biochemical abnormalities of ...ydrate metabolism (*diabetes*), in...n of stool fat (*steatorrhea*), and ...tion of stool nitrogen (*azotorrhea*)

Etiology. The etiologic factors involved are the same as those of acute pancreatitis, including frequent association with disease of the biliary tract (approximately 50 per cent of the cases) and chronic alcoholism. Recently, because of the recurrent nature of the disease, the possibility of an autoimmune mechanism or a hypersensitive state has been suggested. Indeed, the serum of patients

PROGNOSIS

Recovery is universal for patients with acute edematous pancreatitis; however, the fatality rate among those with hemorrhagic or necrotic disease is high, approximating 50 per cent. It is difficult to state the percentage of patients with acute pan-with pancreatitis contains one or more precipitating antibodies that react with homologous pancreatic homogenate. The inability to create experimental pancreatitis by the injection of antiserum, coupled with the incomplete understanding of the mechanism of antibody formation, makes these observations only of experimental interest at this time.

Clinical Manifestations. Chronic pancreatitis begins most often in the third or fourth decade of life, but may begin in early childhood or old age. It is more common in men than in women and, unlike gallbladder disease, has no predilection for obese persons.

The clinical syndrome is readily divided into two stages. In the earlier stage the outstanding feature is recurrent attacks of severe abdominal pain (relapsing pancreatitis); the later stage is characterized by metabolic disturbances, e.g., diabetes, steatorrhea, and azotorrhea with concomitant weight loss (chronic pancreatitis). Pseudocyst formation and pancreatic calcification are also common complications.

The abdominal pain in both stages is the same as that described in the article on acute pancreatitis, and it may persist for days to weeks. Between attacks the patient may be asymptomatic except for occasional complaints of fullness, abdominal distention, and dull epigastric ache. As the disease progresses, the intervals between attacks become shorter, and the pain may eventually be continuous, requiring constant therapy with narcotics, which in some cases may lead to addiction. Nausea, vomiting, chills, jaundice, and tachycardia may be associated with these painful episodes.

Physical examination of the abdomen during an acute exacerbation may reveal the signs of acute pancreatitis. In addition, an epigastric mass may be found, representing either an inflamed pseudocyst of the pancreas or an enlarged fatty liver. With repeated attacks, the parenchymal disturbances become irreversible, and cause steatorrhea and diabetes mellitus. Loss of weight, despite a good appetite and a satisfactory caloric intake, results from faulty digestion and absorption of fat. The stools become bulky, frothy, glistening, and foul-smelling, and they may increase in frequency (see Diseases of Malabsorption). Sometimes, diabetes and/or steatorrhea first attracts attention to the existence of a destructive inflammatory process in the pancreas.

Course and Diagnosis. *Dysfunction of Acinar Cells.* The degree of disruption of acinar cells as reflected by serum levels of amylase and lipase depends on the stage of the disease. During an acute attack, levels of serum amylase and lipase are increased (vide supra). These enzyme values tend to rise early and return to normal after the acute attack. Elevations may persist when the attacks occur in rapid succession, when activity is prolonged, or in the presence of pancreatic ductal obstruction by stone. With repeated attacks, more and more of the gland is destroyed; thus, late in the disease,

even though active pancreatitis is present, serum levels of amylase and lipase do not rise. At this stage, abnormal fat excretion, usually greater than 7 grams of fat, and nitrogen excretion, greater than 2.5 grams of nitrogen daily, will be found.

Deficient secretion of pancreatic juice is consistently encountered in chronic pancreatitis. The characteristic changes in pancreatic juice are subnormal volume and bicarbonate concentration after the intravenous injection of one clinical unit of secretin per kilogram of body weight. The normal volume response is 2 ml. or more per kilogram in 80 minutes, and the maximal bicarbonate concentration should reach 90 mEq. per liter in any 20-minute specimen. Volume response as well as enzyme concentrations may be normal in the face of diminished bicarbonate except when the disease is advanced. It has not been established whether this dissociation indicates a differentiation of function between the acinar and intralobular cells or a differential loss of function of the secretory cells.

Disturbance of Function of Islet Cells. In the early stages of relapsing pancreatitis, acute attacks may demonstrate temporary islet cell dysfunction, characterized by glycosuria, hyperglycemia, and even abnormal glucose tolerance curves. However, with advanced disease, there is further destruction of islet tissue, and frank *diabetes mellitus* is encountered.

Roentgenographic demonstration of calcification in the region of the pancreas furnishes additional evidence of chronic pancreatitis (see figure in article on Acute Pancreatitis). Other roentgenographic findings, such as widening duodenal loop and displacement of the stomach, discussed under Acute Pancreatitis, are more likely to be encountered with repeated attacks and progression of the disease.

In the *differential diagnosis* of the acute painful episodes of chronic relapsing pancreatitis, the same causes of abdominal pain that were discussed in the article on acute pancreatitis must be considered. In the later stage, when steatorrhea and malabsorption are present, adult celiac disease, carcinoma of the pancreas, Whipple's disease, etc., should be excluded (see Diseases of Malabsorption). *Primary atrophy of the pancreas* should be excluded. This is a disease of unknown cause, appearing in both sexes after the fifth decade. The fully developed clinical picture of pancreatic atrophy is that of a deficiency syndrome characterized by steatorrhea, weight loss, normal or increased appetite, occasionally edema, anasarca, and diabetes mellitus. Abdominal pain, pancreatic calcification, and increase of serum enzymes are absent. By the time the disease is recognized clinically, the pancreas has undergone nearly complete atrophy. This observation underscores the great reserve capacity of this gland. The predominant chronic symptom, steatorrhea, usually begins insidiously and is generally mild. Edema and anasarca are frequently the initial signs in this disease. When there is an associated decrease of islet cells, diabetes mellitus of varying degrees develops. Exploratory laparotomy may be necessary for exact diagnosis.

Pathologically, this entity is characterized by almost complete disappearance of the acinar cells and, to a lesser extent, of the islets of Langerhans. Fatty replacement of the atrophic tissue may be an accompanying finding.

Painless Pancreatitis. Although clinically the hallmark of chronic pancreatitis is recurrent bouts of severe upper abdominal pain lasting for days or weeks and followed by epigastric tenderness for even longer periods, this disease may be painless. The diagnosis is to be suspected when one encounters a patient who, without having experienced abdominal pain, has the sequelae of chronic pancreatitis, i.e., pancreatic calcification, diabetes mellitus, and steatorrhea. All of these may coexist, or they may occur in various combinations. Infrequently, at operation, painless jaundice may be found to have resulted from obstruction of the common bile duct by a chronically inflamed pancreas. Recent evidence suggests that acute or subacute edematous forms of pancreatitis may occur without abdominal pain. In one review of 25 cases of chronic pancreatitis at necropsy in a 35-year period, the pathologist was unable to discover any clinical record that abdominal pain had occurred in 15 patients (60 per cent). Such observations suggest that acute edematous pancreatitis may occur more frequently than is suspected and that it may undergo complete resolution without recognition by either physician or patient.

Treatment. Palliation of acute symptoms and efforts to terminate the acute exacerbation have been discussed in the article on Acute Pancreatitis. Management comprises bed rest, limiting the oral intake of fluids, nasogastric suction, adequate sedation and narcotics, and appropriate fluids, electrolytes, and parenteral antimicrobial therapy.

Nonsurgical Treatment. Medical means for preventing attacks of chronic relapsing pancreatitis and halting the progression of the disease are few and of limited value. Adherence to a bland, low-fat diet, avoidance of overeating, abstinence from alcohol, and the use of anticholinergics (propantheline bromide [Pro-Banthine], 15 mg., or methantheline bromide [Banthine], 50 mg., given one half hour before meals and at bedtime) are the principal measures. Management of pancreatic insufficiency secondary to progressive pancreatic destruction requires control of diabetes and of excessive losses of fat and nitrogen, with their associated abdominal distention, cramps, borborygmi, increased flatus, passage of large, malodorous and frequent stools, and loss of weight. The dietary intake of fat is usually restricted to 70 grams a day, and 120 grams of protein and up to 450 grams of carbohydrate are offered to compensate for the calories lost by restriction of fat intake.

Potent pancreatic extracts (Pancreatin, Viokase, or Cotazym) should be given, 1 tablet every hour during the waking hours, or 3 tablets spaced at the beginning, middle, and end of each meal, plus 1 tablet with "snacks." In patients with high basal acid output, it may be helpful to give 30 ml. of an antacid before each meal, or 0.5 gram of sodium bicarbonate when a program of 1 tablet every hour is used. Sodium bicarbonate therapy should be avoided in older patients. With a greater degree of effective digestion, the insulin requirement may be increased. Multivitamin capsules will provide adequate vitamin supplements when the patient is malnourished and the intake of food is restricted. Supplementary calcium and vitamin D may have to be given (see Diseases of Malabsorption). Replacement of dietary triglyceride with medium-chain triglyceride (MCT) is reported to have had great success in patients with pancreatic insufficiency. Although MCT can be given in appetizing form, its use is not very convenient. It may be important in the management of some patients, especially in the hospital, when early weight gain is a desirable goal.

Surgical Treatment. The large number of surgical procedures employed in the treatment of pancreatitis reflects the continued efforts, too often unsuccessful, to relieve pain and to prevent progression of the disease. Temporary relief is the usual result of such surgical procedures. The major exception may be the removal of a diseased gallbladder or stones in the common duct that have caused recurrent attacks of pancreatitis. Unfortunately, in some of these instances, difficulty continues owing to obstruction of the ductal system by damage from previous acute attacks. On the other hand, if the patient has pancreatitis associated with alcoholism, such procedures are futile and inadvisable.

Attempts have been made to reduce the pressures in the common and pancreatic ducts in the presence of a "common channel" by prolonged external drainage of the common bile duct by means of a T-tube. Theoretically, at least, internal drainage such as side-to-side anastomosis between the common bile duct and duodenum or roux-Y type of anastomosis between the gallbladder and jejunum is superior. Cutting the sphincter of Oddi to relieve spasm and obstruction has also been advocated. Results of these operations have been satisfactory in only about half the patients in whom the pancreas has not already been ravaged by the disease and in those with pancreatitis secondary to biliary tract disease.

Operations directly on the pancreas include removal of pancreatic calculi (followed by T-tube drainage) to relieve pancreatic ductal obstruction or internal drainage of pancreatic pseudocysts, and partial or complete pancreatic resections. Removal of large obstructing stones in the main pancreatic ducts has been followed by good results in a limited number of cases. Surgical drainage of pancreatic pseudocysts has been relatively successful. Internal drainage of such cysts is preferable to external drainage because of the difficulties and unpleasantness of prolonged drainage of material rich in enzymes. Ninety-five per cent resection of the pancreas leaving a thin rim of pancreas, with suturing of the main pancreatic duct close to the duodenal surface, appears to be effective. Bilateral thoracolumbar sympathectomy in selected cases for relief of pain is sometimes helpful, but the relief lasts for only two or three years.

It is clear that several variables complicate appraisal of the results of surgical therapy. Such variables include the number of spontaneous remissions, the presence or absence of disease of the biliary tract, the effect of previous operations, continued alcohol ingestion, the stage of destruction and the activity of the disease in the pancreas, and the presence or absence of diabetes, calcification, pseudocysts, or external pancreatic insufficiency. Even though the results of different surgical procedures vary, there is no choice but to ask the surgeon to carry out a procedure that seems suited to the individual case.

Prognosis. Replacement therapy has made the outlook good for those patients with chronic pancreatitis and pancreatic insufficiency whose attacks have ceased or become infrequent. Recurrent attacks will usually not be prevented simply by diet and antacid medication. The best hope lies in the surgical removal of a stone in the common bile duct or pancreatic duct, in the cutting of a stenotic sphincter of Oddi, or in the establishment of normal drainage in some way. In all other instances, especially if the patient partakes of alcohol, the prognosis for health and comfort is guarded.

Gross, J. B., and Comfort, M. W.: Chronic pancreatitis. Amer. J. Med., 21:596, 1956.
Littman, A., and Hanscom, D. H.: Current concepts: Pancreatic extracts. New Eng. J. Med., 281:201, 1969.
White, T. T.: Pancreatitis. Baltimore, Williams & Wilkins Company, 1966.

CARCINOMA OF THE PANCREAS

The diagnosis of malignant tumors of the pancreas and the periampullary region is a challenging and perplexing problem. The protean manifestations of this disease and retroperitoneal location of the gland make early diagnosis difficult. Serum enzyme determinations and combined secretin and cytologic tests may be helpful adjuncts to the clinical history, physical examination, and roentgenographic studies. Fortunately, carcinoma of the pancreas is not a common disease, being encountered in 0.3 to 0.9 per cent of autopsies, and comprising 1.76 to 4 per cent of all types of carcinoma.

Pancreatic carcinoma is predominantly a disease of males, with a sex ratio of 2 or 3 to 1. The peak incidence occurs in the sixth and seventh decades. The tumors are nearly all adenocarcinomas, arising mostly from ductal epithelium. The head of the pancreas is involved in more than 60 per cent; about 20 per cent are diffuse, and the remainder arise in the body and tail. Extension of the tumor is direct by invasion of the remaining gland or duodenum and by adherence to adjacent structures. Extension via the perineural lymphatics and those accompanying the pancreaticoduodenal vessels is the rule. Metastases are most frequent to the regional lymph nodes and to the liver. Other sites of metastases, in their order of frequency, are lungs, intestines, adrenals, bone, and other organs.

Clinical Manifestations. **Symptoms.** Despite the still widely held opinion that carcinoma of the pancreas and ampulla of Vater is painless, *pain* is the most frequent first symptom. The pain is not diagnostic in any sense but is of three general types: (1) colicky, and frequently located in the right upper quadrant of the abdomen; (2) steady, dull, and midepigastric, radiating through to the low back; and (3) paroxysmal, near the umbilicus but felt over a wide area of the back, in the anterior chest, and over the abdomen. Other characteristic features of the pain are its severity, steady progression, exacerbation at night, and its nonrelationship to normal events of the digestive cycle. The next most significant symptom is *jaundice,* which occurs in about 65 to 80 per cent of cases of carcinoma of the head of the pancreas, and is the symptom which causes most patients to seek therapy. It is almost always persistent and steadily progressive, and can become extremely deep, with accompanying pruritus. *Weight loss* occurs invariably and is usually extreme, frequently averaging more than 5 pounds per month. Gastrointestinal symptoms such as *anorexia, nausea,* and *vomiting,* although not specific for carcinoma of the pancreas, are very common complaints. An aversion for or complete rejection of food, rather than true anorexia, is considered distinctive of cancer of the pancreas. A feeling of *gastric fullness* and *flatulence* is common. Diarrhea, which may or may not be associated with steatorrhea, has been observed in 15 per cent of cases. *Constipation* is more common and may be related to the anorexia. *Bleeding* into the gastrointestinal tract, manifested by occult blood in the stool, is noted in about 50 per cent of cases, and is especially significant in lesions involving the stomach or duodenum and in carcinoma of the ampulla. *Thrombophlebitis* or *phlebothrombosis,* especially of the migrating type and resistant to anticoagulants, may be the first symptom in patients with carcinoma of the body and tail of the pancreas. Emotional disturbances, especially depression and anxiety, are said to be unusually common with carcinoma of the pancreas, especially of the body and tail. Abnormal glucose tolerance or even frank *diabetes* is more common in carcinoma of the pancreas than in the general population.

Physical Findings. Abnormal findings that may be noted on physical examination are evidence of weight loss, an enlarged, frequently hard liver, a distended gallbladder, jaundice, tenderness or resistance in the upper part of the abdomen, and a mass in the region of the pancreas. The gallbladder is visibly or palpably enlarged in about

50 per cent of patients with jaundice caused by carcinoma in contrast to that in patients with jaundice and chronic pancreatitis. Ascites and peripheral edema occur in about 20 per cent of cases. Splenomegaly may occur secondary to compression or thrombosis of the splenic vein. Recently, a systolic bruit in the left upper quadrant has been described in patients with carcinoma of the body of the pancreas.

Diagnosis. *Roentgenographic Findings.* Roentgenographic studies of the upper gastrointestinal tract may reveal a number of abnormalities owing to the tumor, such as changes in the mucosal pattern and rigidity of the duodenal wall, widening of the duodenal loop, "padding" of the gastric antrum, and disturbed motor activity of the small bowel. Occasionally, evidence of invasion of the duodenal wall—the "inverted 3" sign of Frostberg—will be noted. In the presence of obstructive jaundice, percutaneous transhepatic cholangiography will aid in the diagnosis of carcinoma of the head of the pancreas. These roentgenographic findings invariably are manifestations of progressive neoplastic change in the pancreas and surrounding structures.

Serum Enzymes. Determinations of a number of serum enzymes may be helpful in establishing the diagnosis of carcinoma of the pancreas. Early obstruction of the pancreatic duct will occasionally elevate the serum lipase and amylase. It is clear, however, that if the block has been prolonged, with resultant destruction of the acinar cells of the pancreas or replacement of the gland with tumor, these levels may be low. Unfortunately, significant change in either direction is infrequent. *Serum trypsin* or *exopeptidase,* or both, have been found to be elevated in carcinoma of the pancreas; however, these tests cannot differentiate carcinoma of the pancreas from acute or chronic pancreatitis.

Leucine aminopeptidase, nonspecific alkaline phosphatase, and *5-nucleotidase* are elevated in carcinoma of the pancreas when there is an element of obstruction of the common bile duct or metastasis to the liver.

Pancreatic Drainage. Analysis of duodenal secretion after injection of *secretin* or *secretin followed by pancreozymin* is potentially of great diagnostic value. Precise localization of an obstructive lesion is possible. If both biliary and pancreatic secretions are absent, the obstruction must be in the head of the pancreas or in the ampulla of Vater. If the pancreatic and biliary flows are normal in volume, the lesion is not obstructive. If pancreatic secretions are ample despite absence of bile, the lesion must be in the extrahepatic biliary system, or duodenal obstruction is being bypassed by an anomalous pancreatic duct. With partial obstruction of the pancreatic duct the quantity of bicarbonate and enzymes in the pancreatic secretion decreases, but the relative concentrations remain the same. Cytologic examination for malignant cells after secretin enhances the chance of positive diagnosis. The accompanying table presents a summary of the findings in carcinoma of the pancreas, chronic pancreatitis, and diseases of the biliary tract and liver after secretin stimulation. A significant rise in serum amylase or lipase, or both, after injection of secretin and pancreozymin strongly indicates pancreatic obstruction.

Radioactive Photoscanning. Radioactive photoscanning of the pancreas utilizing ^{75}Se selenomethionine has shown a decreased photoscan concentration in the area of tumors of the pancreas, as well as in pseudocysts. Uptake by the liver, however, reduces the accuracy of the procedure. Utilization of ^{198}Au with ^{75}Se selenomethionine and an isotope subtraction technique may improve the accuracy of this method.

SIGNIFICANCE OF THE SECRETIN TEST

	Total Volume Flow	Maximum HCO$_3^-$ Concentration	Total Enzyme Secretion	Biliary Pigment Response
Normal	2 ml. or more/kg. body weight/80 min.	90 mEq./L. in any 20-minute specimen	Normal	Normal
Pancreatic carcinoma				
Head	Greatly diminished	Normal to diminished	Normal to diminished	—
Body	Moderately diminished	Normal	Normal	—
Tail	Normal	Normal	Normal	—
With obstruction	Diminished	Normal to diminished	Normal to diminished	Obstructive (no bile)
Chronic pancreatitis				
Moderate	Normal	Diminished	Diminished to normal	Normal
Severe	Diminished	Diminished	Diminished	Normal
Biliary tract				
Common duct stone, stricture, or neoplasm	Normal	Normal	Normal	Obstructive (no bile)
Intrahepatic				
Hepatitis, cholangitis, and cancer	Normal	Normal	Normal	Normal (nonobstructive)
Cirrhosis and hemochromatosis	High	Normal	Normal	Normal

Pancreatic Angiography. Pancreatic angiography, especially subselective angiography of vessels close to, or directly into, the pancreatic vessels, appears to help in establishing the diagnosis of carcinoma of the pancreas. Findings indicative of pancreatic disease are often subtle and include circumferential arterial stenosis, arterial occlusion, or arterial displacement—especially when combined with venous compression or occlusion in the same region. Tumor vessels are rarely seen.

Hypotonic Duodenography. Hypotonic Duodenography is a detailed roentgenographic demonstration of the paralyzed, distended duodenal loop. Spiculation (fine, sharply pointed serration along the inner aspect of the duodenal loop), flattening of folds, and nodular indentations along the inner aspect of the duodenal loop are the most reliable findings suggestive of pancreaticoduodenal cancer.

Glucose Tolerance. As 13 to 25 per cent of patients with carcinoma of the pancreas develop diabetes, measurement of glucose tolerance is mandatory in the study of any patient suspected of having a pancreatic tumor. Although the islet cells are located predominantly in the body and tail of the pancreas, diabetes associated with carcinoma of the head of the gland is due to obstruction of the main duct, which causes atrophy and fibrosis of the body and tail. Similarly, steatorrhea may occur in approximately 10 per cent of the cases as judged by abnormal chemical fat excretion.

Carcinoma of the pancreas can usually be diagnosed either grossly or by biopsy at operation, although such biopsy of the pancreas frequently reveals only inflammation. This finding is usually due to the fact that pancreatic carcinoma is surrounded by inflammatory tissue.

Treatment and Prognosis. The natural course of disease, whether it is primarily in the head or in the body and tail of the pancreas, is one of swift progression to death after onset of symptoms, regardless of whether metastases or contiguous extensions are present, and is uninfluenced by any surgical procedure except radical extirpation in very rarely suitable cases. Resection of tumors of the head of the pancreas should be attempted, for one may really be dealing with a carcinoma of the ampulla of Vater, and in such cases the prognosis following surgery is more satisfactory. Palliative surgery for relief of jaundice and pruritus can be accomplished by choledochoduodenostomy. However, life is not prolonged by this procedure, the average duration being seven months following operation. Carcinoma of the body and tail is almost never resectable, and five-year cures are extremely rare.

Clifton, E. E.: Carcinoma of the pancreas. Amer. J. Med., 21:760, 1956.

Dreiling, D. A., Nieburgs, H. E., and Janowitz, H. D.: The combined secretin and cytology test in the diagnosis of pancreatic and biliary tract cancer. Med. Clin. N. Amer., 44:801, 1960.

Eaton, S. B., Fleischli, D. J., Pollard, J. J., Nebesar, R. A., and Potsaid, M. S.: Comparison of current radiologic approaches to the diagnosis of pancreatic disease. New Eng. J. Med., 279: 389, 1968.

Gullick, H. D.: Carcinoma of the pancreas: A review and critical study of 100 cases. Medicine, 38:47, 1959.

CYSTIC FIBROSIS OF THE PANCREAS
(Mucoviscidosis)

Cystic fibrosis of the pancreas is a generalized, inheritable disease of unknown cause, associated with dysfunction of all exocrine glands, including those that are mucus-producing. Although characteristically a disease of early childhood, cystic fibrosis is now recognized with increasing frequency in adolescents and adults. The increased longevity has been attributed to earlier diagnosis, to increased use of antimicrobial drugs and other measures that control pulmonary infection, so frequently the cause of death, and to the effectiveness of potent pancreatic extracts and medium-chain triglycerides.

Etiology. The basic defect in cystic fibrosis is still unknown, and speculation as to its nature has followed various channels. Deficiency in function of the autonomic nervous system; abnormal physicochemical characteristics of mucous secretions in many areas of the body, resulting in the obstruction of single mucus-producing cells or the excretory passages of organs; a striking elevation in the concentration of sodium, chloride, and potassium in sweat and to a lesser extent in saliva; increases in organic and enzymatic constituents; and calcium and phosphorus levels in submaxillary saliva have all been proposed to explain the generalized dysfunction of exocrine glands.

Whatever the nature of the basic defect in cystic fibrosis, it appears to be genetically transmitted as an autosomal recessive trait.

Evidence is accumulating that homozygotes show the full disease picture and that heterozygotes, who probably make up the majority of adult patients seen in medical practice, exhibit either no detectable change or only partial manifestation of the disease.

Incidence. The incidence of patients with the fully manifested disease (homozygotes) is estimated as 1 per 2000 live births, and that of heterozygotes as 2 to 5 per cent of the population. It affects equally all groups of the Caucasian race, is rare in Negroes, and very rare in Orientals.

Pathophysiology. The pancreas of patients with cystic fibrosis is characterized pathologically by obstruction of the large and small pancreatic ducts with amorphous eosinophilic concretions, followed by dilatation of the acini, degeneration of the parenchyma, and fibrosis. The islets of Langerhans remain intact. In view of these changes, it is not surprising to find deficiency or absence of pancreatic enzymes, especially trypsin, lipase, and amylase, resulting in *steatorrhea* and *azotorrhea*. Carbohydrates are better utilized. *Diabetes* *mellitus* occurs in this disease, but ketosis is rare. The majority of these patients can tolerate protein better than fats, making a positive nitrogen balance possible with increased protein intake.

Generalized bronchial obstruction with secondary infection is a cardinal manifestation of the pulmonary involvement. The process leads to acute and chronic bronchitis, peribronchitis, patchy atelectasis, bronchiolectasis and bronchiectasis, poor alveolar aeration, hypoxia, hypercarbia, pulmonary hypertension, and cor pulmonale. The ventilatory dysfunction is characterized by a rise in residual lung volume, a decrease in ventilatory flow rates and vital capacity, an increase in airway resistance, and uneven gas distribution throughout the lung. In spite of their unusual susceptibility to respiratory infections, these patients are capable of developing good levels of circulating antibodies to many pathogenic bacteria to which they are exposed, and have adequate immunoglobulin responses to infections. Discovery of the constant presence of hemolytic *Staphylococcus aureus* and, more recently, of *Pseudomonas aeruginosa* in their sputum and nasopharynx suggests a metabolic basis for the striking association of these organs and cystic fibrosis.

Sweat and Salivary Electrolytes. The eccrine sweat defect is characteristic of cystic fibrosis in the pediatric age group, and is rarely seen in other pediatric disease except adrenal cortical insufficiency. A striking increase in the levels of sodium, chloride, and to a lesser extent potassium is present in virtually all homozygote patients with cystic fibrosis. In contrast, most other sweat solutes, as well as the rate of sweating and the response of the sweat gland to various stimuli, appear to be normal or nearly normal. A similar but less striking elevation of sodium and chloride has been found in the saliva of patients with cystic fibrosis *(vide infra)*. Serum electrolyte concentrations in these patients are normal when the patients are clinically well. If severe pulmonary disease is present, especially in the early phases of an attack of widespread bronchial obstruction, the patient may have an uncompensated respiratory acidosis, a low pH, and elevated carbon dioxide combining power, but normal serum chloride, sodium, and potassium levels. In the heat casualties, because of the massive outpouring of electrolytes in the sweat in a few hours, the concentrations of serum electrolytes decrease, with the exception of potassium.

Biochemistry of Secretions. The duodenal contents of most patients with cystic fibrosis contain a glycoprotein that is easily and irreversibly denatured by a 1:1 mixture of benzene and ethanol, and is rendered insoluble in water. Detailed chemical analyses of the glycoproteins of urinary macromolecules, salivary fractions, rectal mucus, and Tamm-Horsfall urinary glycoproteins fail to reveal significant quantitative differences from normal values. However, it appears that there is an interaction between calcium and glycoproteins in submaxillary saliva. The precipitation of such an insoluble calcium-glycoprotein complex may lead to many of the pathologic changes seen in cystic fibrosis.

Recent Observations. Recent observations which may have some bearing on the disease include the following: (1) The isolation of a heat-labile, nondialyzable factor which precipitates out with the euglobulin fraction from the serum of patients with cystic fibrosis and which disorganizes the ciliary rhythm in explants of respiratory epithelium. This factor was also detected in parents of children with cystic fibrosis, but in a lower concentration. It was present in only 1 of 25 control sera, the expected incidence of heterozygotes in the population. (2) Easily recognizable cytoplasmic intravesicular metachromasia, found in skin-fibroblast cultures derived from children affected with cystic fibrosis of the pancreas. A similar cytoplasmic metachromasia was seen in 13 of the 14 parents, obligatory heterozygotes.

Clinical Manifestations. *Chronic pulmonary disease* is characterized by chronic cough, wheezing, thick, tenacious sputum, and repeated respiratory tract infections, which are the hallmarks of the disease in both children and adults. With irreversible damage to the bronchi, the pulmonary disease becomes progressive and leads to the distressing picture of pulmonary insufficiency and eventually death through such complications as *lobar atelectasis, lung abscesses, cor pulmonale, pulmonary hypertension,* mediastinal and subcutaneous *emphysema, pneumothorax, hemoptysis,* and *asphyxia.* The chest is usually hyperresonant, with depressed diaphragm and increased anteroposterior diameter. Clubbing of the fingers may be present (see articles in Respiratory Diseases). *Pancreatic insufficiency,* characterized by abdominal distention, large, bulky, foul-smelling stools, diarrhea, and abdominal cramps, can occur either alone or in combination with respiratory disease. Malnutrition may be severe despite an exorbitant appetite and an apparently adequate caloric intake. This may lead to shortened stature and delayed puberty if the disease is first discovered during adolescence.

Meconium ileus, cirrhosis of the liver (multilobular biliary cirrhosis with concretions) with subsequent portal hypertension, rectal prolapse, and collapse secondary to heat exhaustion are frequent in children but are rarely noted in the past history or clinical picture in the adult. Fecal masses that may be so persistent and tenacious as to produce acute mechanical intestinal obstruction occur frequently in older children and adults (meconium ileus equivalent).

Chronic involvement of the paranasal sinuses is a regular finding and with progressive pneumatization leads to a nasal voice, postnasal drip, and formation of polyps that often require surgical removal. Enlargement of submaxillary salivary glands, pulmonary hypertrophic osteoarthropathy, and ocular lesions (dilatation of the arteries and veins of the fundus with hemorrhage and papilledema) have been reported.

Diagnosis. The diagnosis of cystic fibrosis

should be based on four criteria: (1) increase in electrolyte concentration in the sweat, (2) absence of pancreatic enzymes on assay of aspirated duodenal contents, (3) chronic lung disease, and (4) family history of the disorder. It is important to realize that, in view of the genetic nature of this disease, one or more of these criteria may be absent in the individual patient; usually two criteria are sufficient to establish the diagnosis.

An accurate *quantitative sweat test* performed by stimulation of the sweat glands by iontophoresis of a cholinergic substance (0.2 per cent pilocarpine nitrate) is mandatory. Analyses of chlorides and sodium in sweat thus obtained will reveal mean values of 30 to 40 mEq. per liter and 60 mEq. per liter, respectively, in normal children; in children with fibrocystic disease the means will be 105 to 125 mEq. per liter for chlorides and 120 mEq. per liter for sodium. Values for sweat chloride greater than 60 mEq. per liter and for sodium greater than 80 mEq. per liter are considered diagnostic for children with cystic fibrosis. Even though sweat tests have been used in the diagnosis of cystic fibrosis in adults, they are thought to be of limited value in this group. However, persistent elevated levels of sodium and chloride in the sweat of an adult or of an adolescent after strict salt deprivation constitute valid criteria for the diagnosis of cystic fibrosis of the pancreas. The clinical picture and duodenal aspiration appear to be more specific in the diagnosis of adult cystic fibrosis. A thick, viscid secretion with profound deficiency of amylase, lipase, and trypsin is obtained on duodenal drainage. Chest roentgenograms reveal generalized obstructive *emphysema* and *bilateral bronchopneumonia*. A family history of cystic fibrosis is of great diagnostic aid.

In patients with no lung involvement, but with symptoms and signs of *malabsorption,* the diagnosis of cystic fibrosis must be differentiated from that of *celiac disease,* with which it is most often confused, and from other causes of malabsorption. In celiac disease, a jejunal biopsy will show virtual absence of villi, the *d*-xylose absorption test will be abnormal, urinary excretion of 5-hydroxyindolacetic acid will be elevated, and a clinical and biochemical response to a gluten-gliadin-free diet will be obtained (see Malabsorption).

Rectal biopsies in some patients with cystic fibrosis have shown widely dilated crypts packed with mucus, which can appear lamellated. The *jejunal biopsy* usually shows normal villi and epithelial cells, with some increase in inflammatory cells of the lamina propria. However, the crypts may show the same lamellated mucus observed in the rectal biopsies.

Treatment. Therapy of the chronic lung disease with various antimicrobials deserves major emphasis, as pulmonary involvement dominates the clinical picture and determines the fate of the patient. During acute infections and when it is judged necessary to initiate therapy before definite sputum culture and drug-susceptibility results are known, the daily use of sodium cloxacillin, 500 mg. every six hours orally or parenterally should be started, because the major organisms cultured are penicillinase-producing staphylococci. Another antimicrobial effective against such organisms is parenteral sodium methicillin, 1 gram every four hours. Gentamicin, 3 mg. per kilogram per day in three equally divided doses, appears to be effective against Pseudomonas infection. Oral tetracycline, 500 mg. four times daily, can be used for mixed infections and for patients with moderate chronic disease. There is some doubt whether chemoprophylaxis is effective. It appears that it is better to treat each episode of acute infection separately.

Pulmonary physiotherapy in the form of postural drainage of each lobe three to four times daily often provides effective drainage of the involved lobe. In recent years, continuous nocturnal mist nebulization in a tent, with an appropriate small droplet nebulizer with a solution of 10 per cent propylene glycol, has been recommended. Agents such as deoxyribonuclease and N-acetyl cysteine have been recommended for daily nebulizations with the hope of diminishing the viscosity of pulmonary secretions.

Pulmonary surgery is rarely indicated, because the pulmonary disease is usually bilateral and generalized.

The malabsorption seen in these patients can be offset by a large intake of food with moderate restriction of fat intake and addition of pancreatic extracts to the diet. Concentrated pancreatic extract (Viokase or Cotazym) given hourly during the waking hours is satisfactory therapy (see Malabsorption). Medium-chain triglyceride preparations (MCT) may aid in further decreasing steatorrhea and thereby help growth, development, and weight gain.

Massive salt depletion in hot weather may represent an acute emergency requiring intravenous infusions of isotonic sodium chloride solution to reconstitute an adequate extracellular fluid volume and to avoid cardiovascular collapse. Meconium ileus and portal hypertension resulting from cirrhosis of the liver require surgical treatment.

Prognosis. The prognosis in this disease is improving as early diagnosis and treatment become more effective. The pulmonary involvement usually determines the fate of the patient. Approximately 50 per cent of affected children die before the age of 10 years, more than 80 per cent before the age of 20 years, and the majority before 30 years of age.

Meconium ileus produces symptoms of intestinal obstruction shortly after birth and, unless surgically corrected, proves fatal. However, patients who survive the operation have essentially the same outlook as those without this complication.

Uncontrollable *gastrointestinal bleeding,* secondary to portal hypertension, and massive *salt de-*

pletion in hot weather are additional hazards. In the older age group, *sinusitis* with its complications (notably polyps) has been a serious problem. Although pancreatic insufficiency is clearly present, digestive symptoms are minimal, and patients are able to tolerate an unrestricted diet. Growth is characteristically retarded in most young children but eventually proceeds normally, and these patients usually reach low normal height. Sexual maturation proceeds normally, but with slight delay. A small number of women with this disease have given birth to healthy children, although reproductive failure seems to be uniform among the affected adult males.

Danes, B. S., and Bearn, A. G.: Cystic fibrosis of the pancreas: A study in cell culture. J. Exp. Med., 129:775, 1969.

di Sant'Agnese, P. A., and Talamo, R. C.: Medical progress: Pathogenesis and physiopathology of cystic fibrosis of the pancreas. New Eng. J. Med., 277.1207, 1344, 1399, 1967

Shwachman, H., Kulczycki, L. L., and Khaw, K. T.: Studies in cystic fibrosis: A report on sixty-five patients over 17 years of age. Pediatrics, 36:689, 1965.

Spock, A., Heick, H. M. C., Criss, H., and Logan, W. S.: Abnormal serum factor in patients with cystic fibrosis of the pancreas. Pediat. Res., 1:173, 1967

Inflammatory Diseases of Intestine

Louis Zetzel

REGIONAL ENTERITIS

Definition. In 1932 Crohn, Ginzberg, and Oppenheimer described the clinical and pathologic findings of an inflammatory stenosing lesion in the terminal ileum. Subsequent reports have enlarged the anatomic distribution of these features to include the stomach, the entire small intestine, and, most recently, the colon. Regional enteritis is characterized clinically by recurrent episodes of crampy abdominal pain, usually periumbilical or in the right lower quadrant, accompanied by diarrhea and, frequently, by fever, anorexia, and weight loss. Gross rectal bleeding is rare. Complications include malnutrition, anemia, perianal abscesses, and internal as well as perirectal fistulas. Its protean manifestations make it a serious diagnostic possibility even when the clinical symptoms referable to disease of the small intestine are minimal or absent. The chronicity of regional enteritis and its high recurrence rate, morbidity, and frequent invalidism, with the number of hospitalizations averaging four per patient, give it an importance beyond its incidence.

Incidence and Prevalence. Before 1932, many cases now recognized as regional enteritis were diagnosed as hyperplastic tuberculosis, mesenteric adenitis, or appendicitis. The incidence or average annual rate of first hospitalization per 100,000 white population is 1.35 in Baltimore, 0.95 in the Oxford area of England, and 0.25 in Norway. On the basis of the Baltimore figures, some of the discrepancies among these areas may be due to the varying percentage of Jews in the respective populations, as the incidence of regional enteritis among this group was approximately nine times that found in non-Jews. The Oxford study showed the prevalence of this disease to be 12 times its incidence. If this same ratio is projected to Baltimore and the United States as a whole, the prevalence of regional enteritis among whites is 16 per 100,000. The frequency is approximately equal among the sexes. The geographic and ethnic distribution is widespread, although the incidence and the relative proportion of active versus chronic cases vary in different countries. Thus the incidence among blacks in the United States is low, and in Japan where regional enteritis is infrequent the acute type is much more prevalent than the classic chronic form of the disease. The average age-adjusted death rate for regional enteritis in the United States is 0.08 per 100,000 of the population, or approximately one fifth that for ulcerative colitis.

Etiology and Pathogenesis. The importance of a genetic factor is suggested not only by the high incidence of familial occurrence but by its frequent association with ulcerative colitis in the same family and their relatives. An apparent increase in these families of members with eczema and hay fever has been offered as further evidence for their genetic basis. The absence of a suitable laboratory model in which the disease occurs spontaneously or in response to experimental transmission has hampered the search for its cause.

Efforts to implicate tuberculosis, abdominal injury, a defect in blood supply, or foreign bodies as responsible for the granulomatous disease have been unsuccessful. The clinical picture strongly suggests an inflammatory process, but no bacterium, virus, or protozoan has been isolated in a primary role. As with ulcerative colitis, Shigella has been incriminated. At most, such a causal relationship could account for only a very small percentage of the total number of patients with regional enteritis.

In the past, this condition was most frequently confused with hyperplastic ileocecal tuberculosis. Pathologic distinction may be made on the basis of discrete, noncaseating tubercles in regional enteritis as well as failure to isolate the tubercle bacilli.

The concepts as to its pathogenesis are as

varied as those pertaining to its etiology. Granulomatous lymphatic endothelial obstruction of the mesenteric lymphatics and submucosal lymphoid hyperplasia have been suggested as the primary important features of the disease. These differences in the pathologic picture have been considered by some to be a reflection of the multiplicity of causes responsible for regional enteritis, which may then be expressed either as a diffuse nonspecific inflammation or as focal granulomas originating in lymphoid follicles or Peyer's patches of the bowel.

The possible relationship of lymphatic blockage to the striking increase in the thickness of intestine, mesentery, and lymph nodes has been confirmed experimentally by the serial injection of crystalline silica into the mesenteric and serosal lymphatics of dogs after an initial intravenous injection of E. coli.

Although the granulomatous lesions of regional enteritis resemble sarcoidosis, the distribution is different. Generalized sarcoidosis rarely involves the gastrointestinal tract and is not associated with rectal fistulas. Regional enteritis is confined to the intestine and mesenteric lymph nodes, and rarely invades the liver.

Relief of symptoms with the elimination of certain foods, especially milk, and exacerbation during the "pollen season" in some patients suggest an allergic basis for the disease. However, the blood and tissue eosinophilia seen in patients with obvious extrinsic allergens are seldom found in regional enteritis. The hypothesis that an immunologic disturbance with an antigen-antibody reaction involving cellular constituents of the gut causes the disease is attractive but has not been established.

That the repeated impact of emotional stress may give rise to dysfunction of the small intestine is suggested by the clinical observation that recurrent symptoms are, at times, chronologically related to disturbing psychologic events. Regardless of the emphasis placed on the etiologic role of these psychologic factors, effective treatment, whether surgical or medical, must encompass the emotional as well as the physical needs of the patient.

Until the problems of etiology and pathogenesis are settled, the relationship between regional enteritis and ulcerative colitis will remain controversial. At either end of the spectrum are clearcut clinical and pathologic characteristics that distinguish the two diseases. However, the ileocecal valve is no longer a rigid barrier separating the two, for ulcerative colitis may invade the ileum, and regional enteritis the colon.

Pathology. The pathologic area is usually grossly apparent. However, at times, only histologic examination will reveal inflammatory changes in a bowel which superficially appears normal. The most prominent gross feature of the disease, especially when seen at operation and most frequently in the terminal foot of ileum, is the granular, reddish-purple, edematous thickening of the bowel wall with distended loops proximal

to any area whose lumen is markedly narrowed. The mesenteric fat surrounds the serosal surface of the diseased bowel in the direction of its antimesenteric border.

The loops of intestine may be adherent and covered by exudate, or communicate by fistulous channels with each other or with contiguous structures, such as colon, rectum, vagina, or urinary bladder. There is a sharp demarcation grossly between pathologic and normal bowel, although this distinction cannot always be confirmed microscopically. The mucosal surface is red and swollen, with irregularly shaped ulcerations, usually on the mesenteric side. Occasionally, these ulcerations burrow deeply beyond the submucosa and into the mesentery, causing abscess or fistula formation.

The histologic picture is complex, not only because the material usually available for study is derived from patients with long-standing disease, but also because of the combined effects of inflammation, ulceration, tissue destruction, and repair which obscure or obliterate the initial lesion. The thickness of the bowel wall consists of the marked hypertrophy and edema of the submucosa.

The most striking microscopic features consist of dilated and tortuous lymph vessels and granulomatous structures resembling noncaseating tubercles (Fig. 1). These granulomas are made up predominantly of epithelioid cells, lymphocytes, and occasional giant cells, and are found primarily in the intestinal submucosa as well as in the mesenteric nodes. In addition, granulomas with giant cells of the foreign body type often contain residues from previous abdominal surgery such as lipids or talc. With the development of inflammation, these granulomas often lose their circumscribed borders and merge with the surrounding tissue reaction.

None of these features is specific for regional enteritis and, to a certain extent, may be found in other conditions. However, the frequency with which they are associated in regional enteritis suggests a characteristic, if not specific, pathologic picture.

Clinical Manifestations. Acute ileitis is seen in about 5 per cent of cases of regional enteritis,

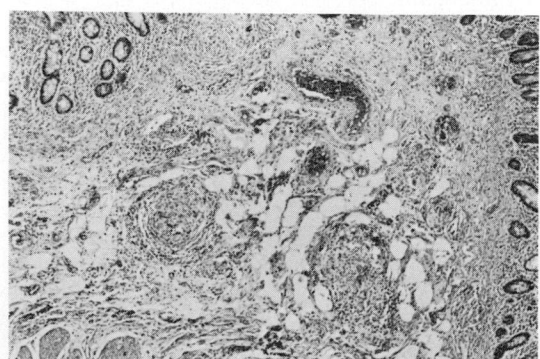

FIGURE 1. Regional enteritis. Submucosa of ileum, showing noncaseating granulomas with multinucleated giant cells. Hematoxylin and eosin stain, × 150.

except in Japan, where the value approaches 70 per cent. This disparity is in part attributable to the lack of uniform criteria for the selection of cases in this category. The infrequency with which acute ileitis is followed by the chronic form of the disease (0 to 20 per cent), its preponderance in children, the rarity of fistulas even after appendectomy, the increased incidence of free perforation, and the usual absence of granulomas in the histologic picture all suggest that "acute" ileitis as presently defined includes disease entities unrelated to chronic regional enteritis. Within this heading may be included such different entities as viral enteritis, mesenteric adenitis, eosinophilic enteritis, or acute reversible vascular impairment of the mesenteric circulation.

The syndrome of acute right lower quadrant pain and tenderness with low-grade fever, leukocytosis, and occasional vomiting is strongly suggestive of acute appendicitis, and the correct diagnosis is usually made only at operation. The tendency to spontaneous regression is sufficiently great that no surgical treatment beyond exploration, with the possible exception of appendectomy, is indicated in such a situation.

In those presenting with a picture other than acute ileitis, there are several clinical variants. Most common is the ulcerative type, in which increase in bowel movements develops abruptly or insidiously, with intermittent episodes or continuous progression of loose stools, but rarely with gross blood or pus. Tenesmus is uncommon unless the rectal region is involved in the granulomatous process, or the disease has become complicated by perianal or perirectal abscesses and fistulas. Fever, malaise, anorexia, and weight loss are variable, episodic, or continuous. When there is diffuse involvement of the ileum and jejunum, severe malnutrition with anemia, peripheral edema, and cachexia are combined to produce a serious depletion of blood, fluid, vitamins, electrolytes, and proteins.

Obstruction is the predominant clinical feature, when the lumen is uncroached upon by edema, fibrosis, adhesions, abscesses secondary to walled-off perforations, or by the matting together and kinking of bowel loops. The resulting pain is diffuse and cramplike or more prominent over one segment of the bowel, usually in the right lower quadrant. A tender mass caused by abscess or inflamed thickened loops of bowel is often felt.

The initial manifestations of the disease may result from its complications. These include acute intestinal obstruction resulting from stenosis; a variety of symptoms resulting from multiple fistulas involving the perianal region, abdominal wall, genitourinary tract, or loops of intestine; and symptoms caused by an abscess. Fever of unknown origin may be the only complaint, and the associated arthralgia, clubbing of the fingers, anemia, and weight loss will suggest only a chronic disease, unless one is suspicious enough to look for regional enteritis in the absence of diarrhea and abdominal pain.

The clinical picture of regional enteritis is in part a reflection of the linear extent of the involvement. The depth of penetration of the pathologic process determines the degree of both the narrowing of the lumen and the matting together of loops of bowel, as well as the development of abscesses and fistulas.

Enteritis of the jejunum when it occurs is usually part of universal ileojejunitis. As in the ileum, narrowing, ulceration, and fistula formation may take place. If the enteritis is sufficiently diffuse or if a substantial segment of jejunum is involved, malabsorption may result. As a consequence, there are severe constitutional effects such as anemia, prothrombin deficiency, tetany, and, in children, retardation of skeletal growth and of sexual maturation (see Diseases of Malabsorption).

In at least 10 per cent of patients, regional enteritis may involve the right colon, segmental portions of the rest of the large bowel, or, rarely, the entire colon, though usually sparing the rectum (see Ulcerative Colitis). The clinical picture resulting from disease involving both sides of the ileocecal valve is compounded of features common to both and is, on the whole, more severe than either alone. Secondary manifestations of arthritis and iritis are especially frequent in this combined group.

The clinical features of granulomatous involvement of the stomach and duodenum are mainly those of obstruction, and include fullness and vomiting caused by gastric retention, anemia, and hypoproteinemia.

Arthralgia, arthritis, iritis, erythema nodosum, and pyoderma gangrenosum complicate regional enteritis less commonly than ulcerative colitis.

Diagnosis. The diagnosis of regional enteritis should be considered in any patient presenting with the features of acute appendicitis, especially if there is an antecedent history of intermittent abdominal pain and/or diarrhea. The diagnosis should also be thought of in a patient with unexplained fever or anemia, malnutrition, migratory arthritis, or arthralgia. Anal, perianal, and perirectal abscesses and fistulas are often the presenting complaint and may precede the development of diarrhea by many months. As fistulas or abscesses occur in at least 30 per cent of patients with regional enteritis or granulomatous colitis, their presence should suggest the possibility of inflammatory disease of the small or large intestine.

Although suggestive, none of these features is pathognomonic. Roentgenographic examination and surgical exploration remain the two most reliable methods of establishing the diagnosis.

Roentgenographic Features. In approximately 5 per cent of patients there is no roentgenographic evidence of the disease. The earliest discernible changes are those of a flattening and thickening of the valvulae conniventes. In this early phase of enteritis, the prominent irritability, spasm, and edema, usually of the terminal ileum, give the appearance of a rigid contour to the diseased segment. Referred to as the string sign of Kantor, this change is a manifestation of activity, potentially reversible, and should not be confused with the fixed rigidity of the fibrosed wall in the stenotic phase. The initial irregularity in width soon gives way to a hoselike, narrowed tube as progressive scarring destroys the normal mucous membrane (Fig. 2). The bowel gradually loses its flexibility, and the matted coils cannot be separated. The barium mixture in the lumen of the diseased bowel remains fluid and homogeneous instead of segmented, as in the malabsorption syndrome. With progressive constriction, the proximal portion of the bowel dilates, and may resemble a loop of large intestine. In spite of its abnormal appearance, compounded of distention and secondary inflammatory changes, this segment of proximal bowel is capable of resuming its normal function when relieved of its distal obstruction. Fistulas are often obscured by the overlapping loops of bowel.

The bowel disease is usually demonstrable in the terminal loops of ileum during the course of a barium enema. Upper gastrointestinal examination, however, is necessary to outline the full extent of the disease proximal to the terminal ileum. Characteristically, once the roentgenographic appearance has become definitely established, linear extension of the granulomatous process seldom occurs unless the patient is subjected to surgery. Subsequent changes are in the form of progressive stenosis, abscess, and fistula formation.

Differential Diagnosis. The manifestations of fever, abdominal pain, and leukocytosis may simulate acute appendicitis, right-sided diverticulitis, or mesenteric adenitis. Although diarrhea and the infrequency of antecedent nausea and vomiting favor the diagnosis of acute ileitis, they are not sufficient to exclude acute appendicitis without laparotomy. The more generalized symptoms of fever, weakness, and anemia require consideration of disorders of many systems, so that only a high index of suspicion will lead to a study of the small bowel. Steatorrhea, anemia, and malnutrition suggest the malabsorption syndrome, and therefore differentiation must be made from adult celiac disease and other conditions in which absorption is impaired (see Diseases of Malabsorption). This situation is most likely to arise with chronic regional enteritis, especially diffuse ileojejunitis, or following multiple resections. However, fever, a localized abdominal mass and tenderness, a narrowed terminal ileum, and the presence of perirectal abscesses and fistulas should establish the diagnosis of enteritis. The characteristic mucosal biopsy changes of celiac disease should differentiate it from regional enteritis.

Carcinoma of the right colon is often associated with low-grade fever, anemia, weight loss, and an abdominal mass. However, roentgenographic examination will usually reveal the neoplasm of the right colon and a normal small bowel.

When the clinical features include diarrhea, abdominal tenderness, and a palpable mass, hyperplastic tuberculosis and carcinoid must be considered. Hyperplastic tuberculosis is rarely seen in areas where milk is pasteurized. Other forms of intestinal tuberculosis are usually associated with similar disease in the lungs. Carcinoid involving the ileocecal region may produce the symptoms and signs of regional enteritis. The facial flushing, the increased urinary levels of 5-hydroxyindoleacetic acid, and the enlarged nodular liver establish this diagnosis.

Fever, leukocytosis, diarrhea, abdominal pain, and tenderness in the lower right quadrant may be associated with right-sided diverticulitis. In the absence of perirectal abscesses or fistulas, it may be difficult to differentiate this disease from regional enteritis except by roentgenologic examination.

When the differential diagnosis rests between ulcerative colitis and regional enteritis of the small intestine or ileocolitis, the decision may be difficult. If the sigmoidoscopic and roentgenologic examinations reveal involvement of the distal colon and rectum or of the entire colon, ulcerative colitis is the likely diagnosis; on the other hand, if disease is noted only in the small intestine or in association with segments of the colon, particularly the right side, regional enteritis of the small intestine and colon (granulomatous ileocolitis) should be the presumptive diagnosis. Biopsy of the diseased rectum may provide the answer.

"Backwash" ileitis, which is seen in at least 20 per cent of patients with universal ulcerative colitis, is not to be confused with regional enteritis clinically, roentgenographically, or histologically. It is not a harbinger of progressive small bowel disease, but represents a direct extension of colitis through the ileocecal valve. The pathologic changes, seldom extending more than 20 cm., are those of mucosal inflammation, edema, and even ulceration. This is in contrast to the more extensive boggy thickness and stenosis of the bowel wall in regional enteritis.

Circumferential and obstructing ulcers of the

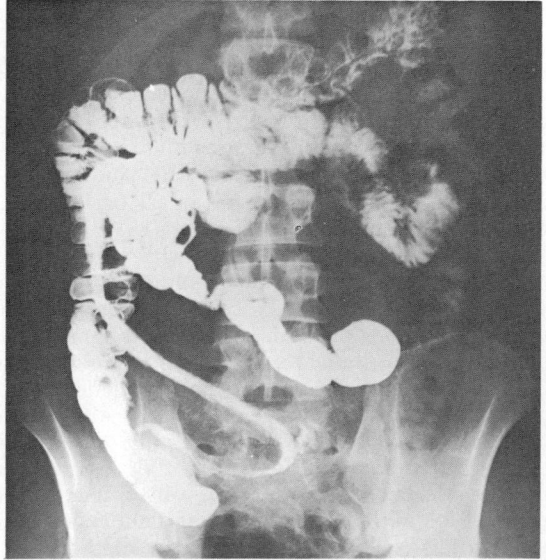

FIGURE 2. Involvement of terminal ileum in regional enteritis. Note narrowing of lumen with hoselike configuration of ileal contours.

small intestine have developed in some patients taking enteric-coated potassium salts, usually in association with chlorothiazides. This entity should be considered in patients with congestive heart failure or hypertension who complain of symptoms suggesting the obstructive phase of regional enteritis. These preparations, however, are also prescribed in the treatment of obesity and edema of pregnancy as well as that noted premenstrually. Fever, malaise, and anorexia, though common in granulomatous disease, are seldom noted with these ulcers. Roentgenographically, the string sign of bowel involvement is absent, and the narrowing is limited to a short segment in the area of the ulcer which is usually solitary. Perianal fistulas and abscesses have not been reported. The treatment of choice is surgery.

In the past few years we have begun to separate the idiopathic inflammatory entities of the intestinal tract such as regional enteritis and ulcerative colitis from those whose roentgenographic and gross appearance is compounded of bowel infarction and infection arising from bacterial or viral flora. How well the nutritional requirements of the bowel are met is directly related to its functional integrity. The role played by the impairment of this blood flow, or ischemia, in the pathogenesis of so-called nonspecific enteritis and colitis has seldom been considered, even though it has been recognized for some time that arterial insufficiency within a segment of the bowel can by itself produce the picture of mucosal ulceration and subsequent fibrosis. Ischemia of the small intestine of gradual onset may result in chronic, vague symptoms of abdominal discomfort, especially after meals, often referred to as abdominal or mesenteric angina. Roentgenographic studies of such patients may be entirely negative. When the interruption of the superior mesenteric circulation is sudden, the pathologic changes reflect the totality of the occlusion and the degree of available blood flow from the collateral circulation. The effectiveness of this compensatory mechanism will determine the irreversibility or reparative nature of the process. Thus, these changes may vary from the extremes of necrosis to ulceration of the more sensitive mucosa with complete healing or intermediate stages of submucosal hemorrhage and pseudotumor, perforation or fibrotic stenosis, and intestinal obstruction. The roentgenographic features will thus depend on the course of the disease and will include the filling defects of localized hemorrhage and edema, diffuse thickening of mucosal folds, temporary areas of narrowing resulting from spasm and irritability, focal or widespread ileus, free air in the peritoneal cavity as the result of perforation, or prominent narrowing with proximal dilatation. All these changes may resemble those seen in regional enteritis and its complications.

Impairment of the *superior mesenteric circulation* caused by emboli is seen in patients with mural thrombi resulting from myocardial infarction or in mitral stenosis with atrial fibrillation. Atherosclerosis with cardiovascular disease in the aged or in diabetics usually produces a more gradual occlusion owing to progressive thrombosis of these vessels. Thus the age of the patient and the associated pathologic findings may help distinguish the abdominal findings from regional enteritis.

More unusual causes of ischemia are *polyarteritis, diffuse lupus erythematosus,* and Schönlein-Henoch purpura. The intestinal ulceration that follows in the latter case is completely reversible.

Blunt trauma to the abdomen has been followed by infarction and stenosis of the bowel. There are several case reports of regional enteritis that was first noted after a severe blow to the abdomen; in such cases the pathogenesis may be that of segmental ischemia on the basis of intramural hematoma. The injudicious use of vasospastic drugs of the ergot family may also give rise to intimal damage and occlusion of the smaller arteries, followed by intestinal ischemia and diarrhea.

Infarction of the bowel preceded by abdominal pain and diarrhea may occur with patent mesenteric vasculature. Severe ischemia of the gut may result from the diminished cardiac output, as in myocardial infarction with hypertension or in the presence of severe congestive failure with compensatory intestinal vasoconstriction. The ileus and distention may further compromise an already diminished blood flow to the bowel.

Bleeding into the peritoneal cavity and the development of intramural hematoma are infrequent complications of anticoagulant therapy, especially with bishydroxycoumarin. The clinical course is that of varying degrees of intestinal obstruction owing either to the ileus resulting from peritoneal hemorrhage with ischemia of the bowel as a consequence of the distention, or to encroachment on the lumen by the submucosal hematoma. In contrast to other hemorrhagic disorders such as hemophilia, in which the internal bleeding usually follows abdominal trauma, that seen with the hypoprothrombinemia of anticoagulant therapy is spontaneous. The pain and distention may suggest the obstructive phase of regional enteritis, but the history of anticoagulant therapy, the acuteness of the complaints, and the predominance of jejunal involvement as the site for the hematoma and proximal distention strongly favor the latter.

Mild villous atrophy and cellular infiltration into the lamina propria in the absence of sprue have been reported in the jejunum of inhabitants of the tropics. The nonspecific nature of these findings and their reversal in American troops upon their return to a temperate climate are an indication of the bowel's limited capacity of reacting to the trauma of intestinal infection, parasitism, the use of drugs such as chloroquine, and inadequate nutrition. The history of exposure to a tropical environment, the predilection for involvement of the jejunum, and the subsequent disappearance of clinical and pathologic evidence of any abnormality should eliminate consideration of regional enteritis.

Chronic ulcerative jejunitis is a rare nongranulomatous disease occasionally associated with similar involvement of the ileum. In spite of the spotty villous atrophy, the associated ulceration in the jejunum and the failure to respond favorably to a gluten-free diet are against sprue–celiac disease. Clinically the diarrhea, malabsorption, and severe protein loss may suggest regional enteritis, but the predominance of jejunal involvement, the absence of fistulas or of obstructive phenomena, clinically or radiologically, should exclude this possibility. On pathologic examination no granulomas are found.

Eosinophilic (allergic) *gastroenteritis* is a disease of unknown etiology, though the blood (> 15 per cent) and tissue eosinophilia in patients with other stigmata of allergic disease suggest hypersensitivity. The stomach is the most constant site of involvement for the disease and, more rarely, the large bowel, peritoneum, and urinary bladder may share in the same pathologic features. This multiplicity of organ involvement is a distinctive and important factor in the differential diagnosis of regional enteritis, with which the radiologic appearance of the bowel may be confused. The lesion in the antrum and distal portion of the stomach may resemble an infiltrating carcinoma, although the pliability of the wall suggests a benign process. The small bowel may be diffusely or segmentally involved, and the patient may suffer from malabsorption and protein-losing enteropathy (see Diseases of Malabsorption). It is a self-limited disease which responds favorably with complete reversal in the milder form to normal after elimination of certain foods (particularly meat, cereals, and milk) or corticosteroid therapy. It is not to be confused with eosinophilic granuloma, in which blood eosinophilia is uncommon, and involvement of the skin, bones, and lungs is frequent.

Less than 100 cases of *eosinophilic granuloma* (see Histiocytosis X [Reticuloendotheliosis]) involving the digestive tract have been recorded in the past 25 years. The gross appearance of the lesions in the small intestine and the clinical picture of abdominal cramping suggestive of intestinal obstruction simulate regional enteritis. The macroscopic pathologic findings consist of localized projections, single or multiple, resembling intussuscepting polyps. The more diffuse type thickens the bowel wall and narrows the lumen for varying lengths. Microscopically, in addition to the edematous connective tissue stroma with increased capillaries and lymphatics, there is characteristically a massive infiltration of eosinophils, usually limited to the submucosa. Only a minority of patients have an allergic history or a corresponding blood eosinophilia. This disease may be suspected if there are lesions of bone as well as of the skin, lymph nodes, and lungs. However, the diagnosis is seldom established preoperatively because the presenting complaints are usually those of intestinal obstruction, for which surgery is promptly performed.

Hypogammaglobulinemia is an immunologic disorder in which there is depression of all serum immune globulins, especially IgA and IgG. It is characterized clinically by recurrent upper respiratory infections, fever, and occasionally infestation with *Giardia lamblia*; its possible confusion with regional enteritis is suggested by nodular lymphoid hyperplasia, diarrhea, and malabsorption (see Diseases of Malabsorption). The nodules are 1 to 3 mm. in diameter and consist of lymphoid follicles with large germinal centers uniformly distributed throughout the small intestine and occasionally the right colon. The histology of the bowel is otherwise normal. Isolated cases, however, have been recorded in hypoglobulinemia of a nonspecific granulomatous disease of the small bowel with clinical and radiologic features similar to regional enteritis. The immune globulin deficiency is somehow responsible for the appearance of giardiasis. These symptoms may improve on antimicrobial therapy, i.e., quinacrine for giardiasis, and in some instances may respond dramatically to the monthly infusion of plasma rather than commercial preparations of gamma globulin in which IgA is usually lacking. The immune globulin abnormalities will establish the correct diagnosis except in instances of protein-losing enteropathy in which the plasma immunoglobulins are depressed (see Diseases of Malabsorption).

Evolution of the Disease. Mention has already been made of the tendency of acute ileitis to undergo complete resolution, both clinically and roentgenographically. Patients in whom the disease progresses to the chronic phase resemble the majority of those who first come to medical attention because of a complication. By the time the diagnosis is confirmed, either clinically, roentgenographically, or surgically, the disease is firmly established. Subsequently, the course may progressively deteriorate and be associated with malnutrition, avitaminosis, and one or more of the systemic or local complications of the disease.

Another clinical variant is seen in the patient whose remission is of such length as to create the false impression of a cure of the disease. More often, the intervals between attacks become progressively shorter in duration and eventually give way to a stage of continuous activity. The chronic disease rarely resolves clinically or roentgenographically.

Progression of the disease may result in inanition and invalidism. Its mortality, when one considers the high morbidity, is curiously low, unless the patient has been subjected to surgery and succumbs to the complications of the procedure. The postoperative exacerbations often necessitate further resection, leading to a degree of malnutrition at times incompatible with life.

Complications. Complications are so frequent that they should be considered an integral part of the disease. Their appearance is often sudden and dramatic and may necessitate urgent surgery, not only for relief of the immediate problem, but also for resection of affected bowel. Anal and rectal inflammatory lesions may be the only clinical evidence of the disease, antedating the more common abdominal symptoms by many months. Radical local therapy, undertaken without due regard for the basic underlying disease, often leads to poor healing and anal incontinence. Such unfortunate results are likely when the patient has anemia, hypoproteinemia, and malnutrition. When the patient has little or no diarrhea, however, and the serum protein and hemoglobin values are normal, these complications may be safely treated surgically even in an active phase of enteritis.

The complications that stem directly from the bowel include intestinal obstruction, hemorrhage, perforation, cutaneous fistulas in the scars of a previous abdominal operation, enteroenteric or enterocolic fistulas, and perianal as well as perirectal abscesses and fistulas. Of these, partial intestinal obstruction is the most common and is the reason for surgical intervention in more than 75 per cent of all patients requiring operation. Edema and spasm may close an already narrowed lumen. In addition, potassium loss, by promoting atony, contributes to the picture of obstruction. When obstruction is due to fibrotic stenosis, resection is less likely to be followed by recurrent activity than when it is performed during the active phase of edema and ulceration.

Perforation usually results in a localized abscess or a fistulous tract between adjoining loops of small intestine or between ileum and colon, urinary bladder, or vagina, but it seldom causes frank peritonitis except in acute ileitis. Internal fistulas are found in 20 per cent of patients coming to operation and external fistulas in less than 10 per cent.

Massive hemorrhage is rare in contrast to its frequency in ulcerative colitis. However, occult blood in the stools is common, and is a contributing factor to the usual hypochromic anemia.

Because of the proximity of the genitourinary tract, the disease may extend to the urinary bladder, causing urinary frequency, dysuria, and, occasionally, pyuria and pneumaturia. It may also form a retroperitoneal abscess with compression of the ureter, leading to hydronephrosis and hydroureter.

Renal stones composed of uric acid and calcium have been reported in approximately 10 per cent of patients with granulomatous disease of the bowel, including those with ileocolitis. Possible mechanisms in their development are ureteral obstruction, urinary tract infection from an inflammatory mass, excretion of an acid urine, and increased calcium mobilization from prolonged bed rest, as well as relative oliguria caused by dehydration resulting in turn from persistent diarrhea.

Weight loss, anemia, and nutritional disturbances frequently complicate chronic enteritis, despite limitation of the disease to the terminal ileum. These abnormalities may be accentuated when the jejunum is also involved. The responsible mechanisms are (1) diminished caloric intake because of abdominal pain and diarrhea; (2) increased catabolism secondary to a chronic inflammatory, febrile state; (3) loss of electrolytes and essential nutrients caused by the rapid intestinal transit time, and loss of protein-rich exudate and transudate from the bowel wall into the lumen, and (4) serious diminution of the absorptive capacity of the small intestine, as in widespread ileojejunitis or even in severe localized enteritis.

Consequences of specific deficiencies such as ascites (hypoproteinemia), bleeding (malabsorption of vitamin K), and tetany (resulting from loss of calcium and vitamin D) may complicate the clinical course. Intestinal absorption and nutrition may improve with the removal of even a large segment of diseased bowel if the remaining portion (100 cm.) is structurally and functionally normal (see Diseases of Malabsorption).

Defects in vitamin B_{12} and fat absorption may be prominent as a result of the disease in the terminal ileum or after its resection. This abnormality may seriously interfere with bile salt reabsorption. The cathartic effect of these salts is an additional mechanism contributing to the diarrhea resulting from the inflammatory process in the gut or that noted after bowel resection with loss of the ileocecal valve. Further sequelae of this interference with the normal enterohepatic circulation of bile salts will result in an ever-diminishing pool of these salts available for their role in lipid absorption in the duodenum and upper jejunum. If this is not adequately compensated for by oral replacement of bile salts, not only steatorrhea but also malabsorption of fat-soluble vitamins will result. Although the bile salts that are deconjugated by colon bacteria are absorbed by the colon, they nevertheless reduce colonic absorption of water with resultant serious loss of potassium and magnesium.

If less than 100 cm. of ileum has been resected and the fecal fat is less than 20 grams, the diarrhea, but not the steatorrhea, may be improved by the use of cholestyramine, a bile salt sequestering resin, in a dosage of 4 grams three to four times daily. Its bulk and taste have made it intolerable for some. Recently, lignin, a nonabsorbable, fibrous polymer found in vegetable matter and in high-roughage foods, has been used in a dosage of 1 to 2 grams after each meal to absorb bile acids and thus diminish this form of diarrhea.

Lactase deficiency is a frequently acquired complication in regional enteritis whose contribution to the resulting diarrhea can be obviated by the removal of milk and milk products from the diet.

Involvement of other organs in regional enteritis is not as common as in ulcerative colitis. Some degree of histologic abnormality may be found in most livers, resulting from serum hepatitis, hepatotoxic drug therapy, portal sepsis, or malnutrition. These abnormalities include fatty infiltration, focal necrosis, pericholangitis, cirrhosis, and rarely granulomas. In the pancreas, periductal and interlobular fibrosis as well as gross nodular enlargement have been noted. The kidneys at necropsy may show glomerulitis with endothelial proliferation. In all these organs, the degree of histologic involvement is not associated with any significant clinical evidence of functional impairment, in spite of occasional abnormalities in laboratory tests. The incidence of *cholecystopathy* is definitely increased. The pathogenesis of this association is not clear, although the pericholangitis and the decrease in the bile acid pool are possibilities.

Amyloidosis with regional enteritis is rare and may not be correlated with the duration of the disease, its extent, the presence of fistulas, or gross suppuration. When it is diagnosed, resection of the involved bowel, if feasible, is indicated, because the amyloidosis may lead to renal failure.

The development of carcinoma in segments of diseased bowel is extremely rare, and the few cases that have been reported may represent coincidence.

Recent detailed history-taking and roentgenographic studies have raised the incidence of arthritic manifestations in regional enteritis. Active polyarthritis affecting primarily the proximal interphalangeal joints of the hands and knees is seen in 5 per cent of patients, and a past history of arthritis in twice as many. This form is usually mild, migratory, recurrent, and not deforming. Although resembling rheumatoid arthritis, the latex fixation test is negative. Ankylosing spondylitis is found in 6 per cent of patients, and in an additional 12 per cent there is roentgenographic evidence of significant sacroiliitis.

In children, disturbances in skeletal growth and gonadal function reflect the general nutritional deficiencies, although their incidence is not as high as in ulcerative colitis.

Treatment. *Nonsurgical.* The treatment of regional enteritis in the absence of complications is symptomatic and empiric. It is directed at relieving abdominal pain, maintaining nutrition, controlling diarrhea, correcting deficiencies in electrolytes, vitamins, proteins, and hemoglobin, and treating infection. No plan of medical management is uniformly successful in effecting a cure, in obtaining prolonged remissions, or in preventing serious complications. In spite of this gloomy estimate, conservative management is sufficiently effective to warrant its choice as an initial approach, especially since the recurrence rate after surgery is high. In addition, the inflammation of the acute stage remits frequently enough to avoid resection. Medical therapy is also indicated in the care of patients with diffuse ileojejunitis, with recurrent disease after surgery, and with chronic enteritis without complications.

General Measures. To meet optimal nutritional needs, it is often necessary to overcome anorexia, abdominal discomfort initiated by ingestion of food, and the debilitating effects of diarrhea. To this end it is important to avoid the unpalatability of a rigidly imposed, highly restrictive diet, unless the patient has demonstrated a specific food intolerance. To enlist his compliance in a high-caloric, high-protein diet, with adequate fat to encourage the appetite, will require in-

genuity and cooperation from the cook, as well as flexibility and understanding on the part of the physician. The temporary use of sedation and narcotics, with due regard for the danger of addiction may be resorted to in order to allay the diarrhea and thus break up the sequential relation between food, abdominal pain, and rectal urgency with tenesmus (see Ulcerative Colitis).

Antimicrobial Therapy. Except in the treatment of the purulent complications, the general use of antimicrobial drugs has proved disappointing, and at times the development of a pseudomembranous enterocolitis during such therapy has complicated the picture. The nonabsorbable sulfonamides such as succinylsulfathiazole and phthalylsulfathiazole, in doses of 2.0 to 3.0 grams every six hours, are usually well tolerated, and occasionally diminish the fever and diarrhea. More recently there has been a tendency to substitute salicylazosulfapyridine in doses of 1.0 to 2.0 grams every six hours. The use of this preparation and its indications and toxic effects are referred to in detail under Ulcerative Colitis. In general, it has not proved as effective in the treatment of regional enteritis as in ulcerative colitis.

Intermittent obstruction owing in part to edema may respond to nasogastric suction, steroids, and antimicrobials (if necessary), the patient's fluid and electrolyte needs being maintained parenterally.

Blood transfusions are indicated as replacement therapy in the rare instances of massive hemorrhage; more often they are given for the chronic anemia that results from infection, malnutrition and continuous blood loss in the stool. Because of the irritating effects of oral iron preparations on the bowel, resulting in more diarrhea, a parenteral preparation such as dextran iron complex (Imferon) is occasionally preferable to correct the iron deficiency anemia.

Steroid Therapy. The theoretical principle underlying the rationale for the use of corticosteroids and corticotrophin in regional enteritis the complications associated with their administration, and the pre- and postoperative management of patients who have received the hormones previously are discussed under Ulcerative Colitis The improvement in mood and appetite consequent to their use has encouraged patients about the possibility of over-all improvement, and has permitted physicians to gain time for the employment of other constructive measures. These agents have empirically improved the clinical course in patients with extensive involvement of the bowel, as in ileojejunitis and ileocolitis, or with repeated recurrences after successive small bowel resections. The corticosteroids are not curative, however, and relapses have occurred frequently, after an unpredictable interval, when they were omitted or the dosage was reduced Either peptic ulcer or perforation of the bowel may complicate their administration, but less frequently than in ulcerative colitis; moreover, the occurrence of these complications cannot always be attributed with certainty to the steroids. There is no clear evidence that they have exerted any strikingly favorable influence in mitigating or avoiding the complications of hemorrhage, perforation, fistula formation, or stenosis.

Immunosuppressive Agents: Nitrogen Mustard and Azothioprine. See under Ulcerative Colitis.

Radiation Therapy. Roentgen ray therapy has been advocated for patients refractory to conservative management or for those in whom extensive involvement or successive recurrences after surgery preclude further resection. The results have not been encouraging. Bleeding and increased bowel stenosis have prevented a more general acceptance of this form of therapy.

Surgical Treatment. The obvious indications for surgery in the treatment of regional enteritis are obstruction, internal and external fistulas, perforation, hemorrhage, and intra-abdominal masses. The original dictum of 1932, that "the proper approach to a complete cure is by surgical resection of the small intestine and of the ileocecal valve with its contiguous cecum," has been radically modified. Recurrence of the active disease in more than 50 per cent of patients after surgery soon led to a realization that the diagnosis of regional enteritis need not immediately or even inevitably require operation, and that even radical resection of all the obviously involved bowel may not be curative. The mounting recurrence rate after surgery following longer periods of observation should not, however, dictate a policy in which surgery is limited only to the complications of abscess and obstruction. Many patients whose clinical course is deteriorating in spite of a comprehensive medical program may be cured or improved by judicious surgical intervention. The remaining 50 per cent of patients without recurrence after surgery remain well, in spite of occasional diarrhea resulting from the markedly shortened gut, from excision or exclusion of the ileocecal valve, or as a result of bile salt catharsis. In this regard, it should be noted that roentgenologic signs of recurrence do not always indicate clinical activity.

The likelihood of surgical cure is greater in patients whose disease is first recognized when they are past the age of 50, when there is no antecedent severe steatorrhea, or if only two feet or less of the small bowel must be resected. Approximately 60 per cent of all recurrences will appear within two years and 85 per cent within five years of the initial operation. Some patients may have recurrences as long as 20 years after surgery, but in the intervening period they have been clinically well or improved to the point of leading normal lives. The recurrence is usually in the terminal ileal portion of the ileocecal anastomosis. The presence of unrecognized "skip" areas of diseased bowel may contribute to the failure of surgical treatment. What is often considered a recurrence may represent only an exacerbation in a persistent focus.

If an operation is deemed necessary because of the patient's refractoriness to medical management, it is preferable to intervene at a time when the active inflammatory process has subsided. The advantages of waiting for this optimal period, however, must be weighed against the risk that delay may lead to the development of other complications that add to the hazards of surgery. As in many other conditions for which specific therapy is unavailable, the timing of an operation is difficult, especially because the result is unpredictable. Although such intervention may avert serious complications, premature resection may be followed by rapidly spreading recurrences.

Two approaches to the surgical treatment of the intrinsic bowel disease are available. The first is radical excision of the diseased segment followed by enteroenterostomy or ileocolostomy. The other type of surgery, exclusion of the involved bowel with ileocolostomy, is reserved for patients whose general condition or local lesions make a more radical procedure undesirable. In this operation, normal proximal ileum is transected and anastomosed to the colon.

Those who favor exclusion of the diseased segment and a sidetracking ileocolostomy, followed by resection at a later date only if the former procedure proves inadequate, report a lower morbidity and equally good results. Surgery undertaken for the relief of obstructive symptoms in granulomatous involvement of the stomach and duodenum usually consists of a simple sidetracking procedure, anastomosing uninvolved jejunum to normal stomach.

Prognosis. Not more than 10 per cent of patients are cured of regional enteritis either by spontaneous remission or in response to medical management. This figure is undoubtedly subject to downward revision with the passage of time and the recognition that some of those designated as cured are merely enjoying a prolonged remission. Approximately the same number will die from causes directly related to the disease and its management. By utilizing a program compounded at times of all the components outlined above, an additional 10 per cent of patients may be maintained at a satisfactory level of adjustment compatible with social and economic usefulness, in spite of roentgenologic and clinical evidence of disease. The remaining 70 per cent of patients will require some form of surgery, averaging three major procedures per patient, with a surgical case mortality of 5 per cent.

The results of surgical treatment leave much to be desired in comparison with the surgical achievements in other diseases. However, a general assessment of the efficacy of surgery must be viewed from the perspective of the relatively recent arrival of regional enteritis on the medical scene and of our need to rely principally on empiric measures because of our lack of knowledge of its cause.

Crohn, B. B., Ginzberg, L., and Oppenheimer, G. D.: Regional ileitis: A pathologic and clinical entity. J.A.M.A., 99:1323, 1932.

Law, D. H.: Regional enteritis. Gastroenterology, 56:1086, 1969.

Rappaport, H., Burgoyne, F. H., and Smetana, H. F.: The pathology of regional enteritis. Milit. Surg., 109:463, 1951.

Shapiro, R.: Regional ileitis: A summary of the literature. Amer. J. Med. Sci., 198:269, 1939.

Van Patter, W. N., et al.: Regional enteritis. Gastroenterology, 26:347, 1954.

ULCERATIVE COLITIS

Definition. Idiopathic, nonspecific ulcerative colitis is an inflammatory disease involving primarily the mucosa and submucosa of the colon. A more accurate term, though one not commonly used, is idiopathic proctocolitis, which describes the almost constant involvement of the rectum and indicates that the ulcerative component, although frequent, is not an inevitable feature of the basic inflammation. The disease is peculiar to man, does not appear in epidemic form, is not contagious, and relapses frequently. In spite of long periods of remission, the likelihood of recurrence is ever present.

Incidence and Distribution. The incidence or average annual first hospitalization rates per 100,000 for the white population in Copenhagen, Oxford, Baltimore, and Norway are 7.3, 6.5, 3.5, and 2.0, respectively. In the Oxford series, the prevalence or total number of patients with ulcerative colitis on a given day was 12 times its incidence. Projecting this relationship onto the Baltimore figures, the prevalence of ulcerative colitis among the white population there would be 42 per 100,000. There is some evidence that the incidence among officers is higher than that among enlisted men in the United States Army, in those in a higher socioeconomic group, and in those with a higher I.Q.

The peak incidence is in the third decade; however, it frequently affects children and, occasionally, adults in the sixth, seventh, and even eighth decades. The disease is slightly more prevalent in females, and some studies report a familial incidence ranging from 1 to 17 per cent. Its true frequency, although not as high as that of peptic ulcer, carcinoma of the stomach, or irritable colon, is undoubtedly obscured by its insidious onset and low-grade activity. In the absence of a sigmoidoscopic examination, the diagnosis is often overlooked.

Ulcerative colitis is worldwide in distribution. In some series the incidence among Jews is three to four times that in the general hospital population. The disease is seen rarely among Negroes and less frequently in the Southern United States.

Etiology and Pathogenesis. In 1875 Wilks and Moxon made a distinction between specific epidemic dysentery and all other inflammatory disease of the colon of unknown etiology. From time to time various entities of specific etiology and pathogenesis have been separated from what undoubtedly still remains a heterogeneous reservoir or wastebasket. The profusion of etiologic concepts advocated for this disease and the contradictory clinical and experimental efforts to confirm them are in large measure due to the tendency to look upon all cases of ulcerative colitis as a homogeneous monolithic group, with a single causal factor and therapeutic approach.

The development of ulcerative colitis as an aftermath of bacillary dysentery suggests a bacterial origin. However, the infrequency of ulcerative colitis in more than one member of a family, the absence of consistent bacteriologic confirmation, and the failure of therapeutic agents generally effective against Shigella suggest that these organisms are responsible for only a small fraction of cases. Other organisms for which specific etiologic significance has been claimed are a diplostreptococcus, *Bacterium necrophorum*, and various fungi and viruses. Their presence in increased amount in the stool may be more properly attributable to the growth-favoring medium of blood and pus in the bowel rather than to a primary role. However, they may contribute to the mucosal damage as secondary invaders or by acting synergistically with other nonbacterial agents that have not yet been successfully cultured.

The dramatic remission that occasionally follows the omission of certain foods, especially milk, has emphasized the etiologic role of certain allergens. The frequent failure of a specific food-allergy regimen is explained on the basis of severe irreversible structural changes in the bowel complicated by secondary infection.

Immunologic considerations in the cause or perpetuation of ulcerative colitis were stimulated by the finding of colon antibodies in the serum of some patients with this disease. The cross-reactivity of these antibodies with *E. coli* in the gastrointestinal tract has suggested a mechanism whereby under certain circumstances these antigenic micro-organisms provoke the production of specific antibodies directed to the immunologically related epithelial cell. In addition, lymphocytes of a patient with ulcerative colitis (and granulomatous enteritis) have been shown to be cytotoxic for colon epithelial cells, suggesting a delayed type of hypersensitivity. This concept rests upon the hypothesis of an underlying host vulnerability which is genetically or environmentally determined.

Exacerbations of ulcerative colitis after minor attacks of infectious enteritis may result from antigenic proteins derived from cellular debris or nonpathogenic bacteria invading a damaged intestinal wall. The conjunction of ulcerative colitis with manifestations of hypersensitivity states, such as purpura, erythema nodosum, uveitis and arthritis, drug reactions, elevation of serum alpha and gamma globulins, and favorable response to corticotrophin and corticosteroid therapy, lends support to this hypothesis. For the present, colon antibodies may play one of three roles in ulcerative colitis: they may cause the disease, serve to perpetuate it, or merely result from tissue damage whatever the mechanism.

Recent observations have pointed to the presence of a specific vulnerability of the bowel in ulcerative colitis. Stroking the rectal mucosa with a cotton probe produces a sharply demarcated wheal and subsequent hemorrhage from the rupture of its superficial vessels. The similarity of this reaction to the third stage of the "triple response" to injury in skin suggests that the trauma has produced a release of histamine-like substances resulting in increased capillary permeability. The edema of ulcerative colitis may thus be interpreted as a local tissue hypersensitivity reaction, perhaps mediated by the mast cells, increased numbers of which have been reported within the bowel wall in this condition. Mast cells are rich sources of histamine and contain a heparin-like substance. The release of these chemicals may cause congestion, edema, and muscular spasm and, ultimately, ulceration of the bowel wall.

The roentgenologic appearance of "mass peristalsis" has been reproduced in normal persons by the injection of methacholine or acetylcholine, particularly in patients subjected to disturbing and emotionally charged interviews. It has therefore been postulated that the continued readiness of the bowel in ulcerative colitis for defecation may be the result of increased cholinergic stimulation induced by emotional stress or other agents capable of promoting such overactivity.

The relationship between psychologic trauma and ulcerative colitis is based on observations that stressful life situations may be reflected in disturbances of the motor, secretory, and vascular responses of the colon. The psychologic makeup of these patients, although not peculiar to them, is expressed during the active phase of the disease by hopelessness and helplessness at the loss of a key figure in their milieu by death, rejection, or removal. More graphically, such a person has been described as dependent, immature, and hypersensitive to criticism, with difficulty in assuming responsibility and maintaining appropriate interpersonal relationships. The discrepancy between the patient's superficial appearance and innermost feelings is particularly striking. Timidity, submissiveness, and passivity often conceal a smoldering hostility, aggressiveness, and resentment. This psychosomatic hypothesis is predicated upon a specific biologic vulnerability to emotional trauma. Protective homeostatic mechanisms break down, and structural bowel changes develop.

Both components of this etiologic concept i.e., the specific psychologic profile and the patient's vulnerability to emotional trauma, have been contested. Several prospective studies have failed to confirm any increased incidence of psychologic abnormality or of psychic conflict immediately preceding the onset of the disease. There is more agreement, however, that emotional stress plays an important part in recurrences and, thus, in determining the clinical course.

Pathology. The availability of biopsy material obtained in the course of endoscopic examination has made it possible to study early changes. The earliest lesion is an inflammatory infiltration with abscess formation at the base of the crypts of Lieberkühn. Coalescence of these distended and ruptured crypts tends to separate the overlying mucosa from its blood supply, leading to ulceration and even denudation of the mucosal surface. Attempts at healing often result in the production of an abnormally thin, atrophic epithelium. Residual islands of epithelial cells with granulation tissue, or elongated mucosal tags surrounded by a sea of ulceration, are frequently seen on sigmoidoscopy or roentgenography.

The inflammatory involvement is diffuse and superficial, usually limited to the mucosa and submucosa. When the necrosis extends through the muscularis, perforation results. All phases of inflammation and attempted repair may be seen during any one attack—erosions, capillary engorgement, edema, ulceration, necrosis, and fibrosis. Continuing fibrosis leads to a distorted and shortened colon and, occasionally, to progressive stenosis of the bowel and obstruction.

The fulminating phase of ulcerative colitis is considered by some to have a different primary histologic lesion. Here the wider and deeper ulceration is attributed to a diffuse, necrotizing vasculitis with thrombosis of arteries, veins, and capillaries.

Grossly, the anatomic extent of nonspecific inflammatory colitis comprises two main groups. In the larger of these, 60 per cent, the rectum is initially involved. In about 5 per cent of all patients, the disease is confined to this area. Though frequently referred to as ulcerative proctitis, the pathology is the same as in those with more extensive involvement. In another subdivision of this first group, comprising roughly 20 per cent of all patients, the disease process spreads progressively from the rectum to involve most of the sigmoid and descending colon. In the remaining patients with rectal involvement, 35 per cent of all ulcerative colitis, the disease affects the entire colon. In approximately 20 per cent of those with universal disease, the terminal ileum for a distance of about 8 to 12 inches shows varying degrees of inflammatory changes, referred to often as "backwash" ileitis.

The pathology of the second group, 40 per cent of all patients, is heterogeneous. Its common denominator is involvement of the right colon or some segment other than the rectosigmoid. Included in this group are patients with right-sided colitis, with or without coincidental involvement of the adjoining ileum, as well as those with single or multiple segmental areas of disease. It is within this group that the question is raised whether the colonic lesion is in fact ulcerative colitis rather than a variant of regional enteritis (see Differential Diagnosis, *infra*).

Clinical Manifestations. In approximately half the patients, the initial symptoms of malaise, vague abdominal discomfort, or slight change in frequency and consistency of stools are so mild that there may be difficulty in dating the onset of this illness. The clinical picture then usually becomes more concrete, and includes cramping, lower abdominal pain or rectal bleeding, soon followed by frequent, loose discharges consisting mainly of blood, pus, and mucus with scanty fecal particles. The urge to defecate is great, and tenesmus may be severe, especially if the rectum is involved. The clinical course may remain stationary at this relatively mild level or become gradually and progressively more severe.

In about one third of the patients, the onset is abrupt, with fever, bloody diarrhea, anorexia, and weight loss that become progressively worse. Although abdominal tenderness may be found in any quadrant, it is most common over the left colon. The rectum and ampulla are usually found to be spastic, often containing blood but little fecal material. Even in the absence of local complications, the rectal examination is often difficult and painful. The clinical picture is characterized by fluctuation of its signs or symptoms. Constipation rather than diarrhea may be present, especially if only the rectum is diseased or if there is an obstructing stricture in the colon. With disease limited to the descending colon, the scout film of the abdomen may show fecal stasis in the right colon, indicating a normal capacity to absorb fluid.

Acute Fulminating Colitis and Toxic Megacolon. In the remaining 10 to 15 per cent of patients, the colitis begins explosively and the patient's condition deteriorates rapidly as a consequence of universal involvement of the colon, with necrosis of the mucosa, thrombosis of the submucosal vessels, and often perforation. The severity of the constitutional reaction, with early severe diarrhea, bleeding, high fever, apathy, restlessness, extreme dehydration, diffuse abdominal tenderness, and progressive distention, reflects profound physiologic and metabolic derangements. Potassium and sodium are rapidly depleted because of inadequate intake and excessive loss in the stool; acidosis is common, further complicating the shock of acute blood loss. The diffuseness of its source and associated deficiency of vitamins C and K protract the bleeding. Dehydration causes the hematocrit to be normal or high, and thus disguises the degree of blood loss. Increased cardiac output, fever, and tachycardia are associated with peripheral vasodilation and the picture of "warm handed" shock. Because of the dehydration and peripheral vasodilation, the normal homeostatic mechanisms are unable to help replete blood volume by transfer of fluid from the extravascular to the intravascular space.

The severity and diffuseness of the inflammation and the resulting necrosis may produce extreme dilatation of the colon, so-called "toxic dilatation" of the colon, in 2 to 5 per cent of all patients with ulcerative colitis. A subserosal radiolucent line of the transverse segment may be readily demonstrable in a scout film of the abdomen in toxic dilatation. Visualization of the diseased colon by barium enema is thus not only unnecessary but dangerous, since it may be followed by increasing dilatation and even perforation. Bowel distention with a diameter at least 9.0 cm. in the scout film of the abdomen is attributable to the severe necrosis and disintegration of all layers

of the colon, especially of the muscular coat (Fig. 3). Associated factors are hypokalemia and, possibly, the destruction of the ganglion cells of the myenteric plexus. Distention may not always be apparent on physical examination, but suspicion warrants frequent scout films of the abdomen; in patients with dilatation they should be obtained daily. The injudicious and continuous use of anticholinergic preparations and/or narcotics may materially contribute to the onset of dilatation of the bowel as well as further aggravate it. In this circumstance, decrease in the number of bowel movements should not be misinterpreted as a favorable sign. The dilated and disintegrating bowel facilitates the transfer of bacteria into the portal circulation. The resulting liver disturbances of pericholangitis and fatty degeneration may add to the profound metabolic derangement of toxic dilatation.

Diagnosis. The diagnosis of ulcerative colitis involves consideration of this disease not only in patients with signs and symptoms referable to the bowel, such as abdominal discomfort and diarrhea, but also with obscure fever, anemia, weight loss, or evidence of unexplained hepatic disease.

The sigmoidoscopic examination is the single most important means for establishing the diagnosis. The earliest recognizable abnormality is a thickening and shortening of the normally sharp edges of the rectal valves. Edema and hyperemia of the mucosa are noted early, and are soon followed by fragility of the bowel wall, so that the slightest trauma may produce copious bleeding. Subsequently petechial hemorrhages and minute ulcerations progress and coalesce into deeper and wider denuded surfaces; these lesions are responsible for the frequent hemorrhagic rectal dis-

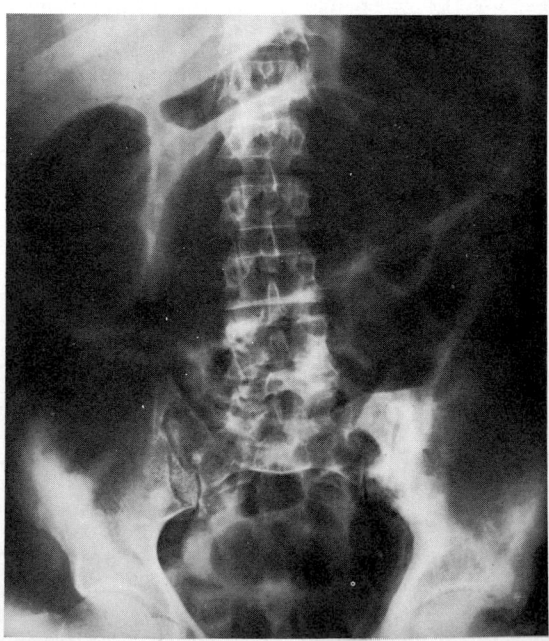

FIGURE 3. Dilatation of the transverse colon in fulminating ulcerative colitis.

charges. As the disease advances, one may encounter narrowing of the lumen or multiple excrescences of pseudopolyps that represent islands of regenerating mucosa in the midst of ulcerations (Figs. 4 and 5). When complete healing takes place in ulcerative colitis, slight granularity may be the only residual sign. The sigmoidoscopic examination is an accurate index of the activity of the disease. Rarely, however, there may be histologic evidence of pathologic lesions not recognizable grossly.

Examination by barium enema is the best means for detection of disease in the proximal bowel. In addition, it reveals the extent and depth of the bowel involvement and of complications such as stricture, polyps, or carcinoma beyond the reach of the sigmoidoscope.

The earliest roentgenographic changes of spasm and irritability may be indistinguishable from those seen in patients with the irritable bowel syndrome (see Diseases and Disorders of Motility). However, with the appearance of mucosal edema, the normal haustral markings become flattened, to be replaced by the fuzzy, serrated, irregular outline of the tiny, barium-filled ulcerations. As the bowel becomes more severely diseased, attempts at repair are reflected in a progressive fibrosis that produces a narrow, shortened, rigid, hoselike colon, offering as little resistance to retrograde flooding with the barium enema as it does to the caudad rush of the fecal stream.

The diagnosis of ulcerative colitis is strongly supported by these different clinical and roentgenographic features, but it cannot be considered firmly established until other conditions that closely resemble it have been excluded.

Differential Diagnosis. At either end of the spectrum of diseases whose chief manifestation is diarrhea are *carcinoma* of the colon and *irritable colon.* Within these two extremes of prognostic seriousness are the specific *bacterial dysenteries,*

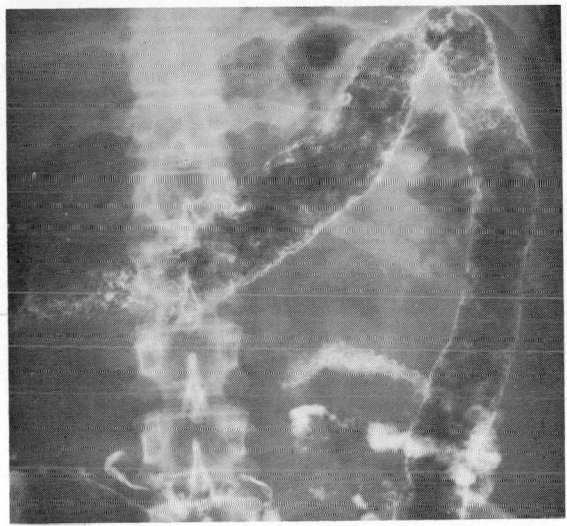

FIGURE 5. Evacuation film of colon of same patient as in Figure 4.

diverticulitis, granulomatous enterocolitis, ischemic colitis, pseudomembranous colitis, adult celiac disease, tropical sprue, and the *malabsorption syndrome,* all of which must be considered in the differential diagnosis.

The picture of *carcinoma* of the colon unassociated with ulcerative colitis usually does not suggest an inflammatory process. On occasion, it may be difficult to distinguish the obstruction of stricture caused by ulcerative or granulomatous colitis from an infiltrating scirrhous carcinoma. In this instance, study of exfoliated cells according to the methods of Papanicolaou may be helpful, but surgical exploration is often necessary.

Ubiquitous, *specific infectious enteritis* with signs and symptoms commonly observed in acute nonspecific ulcerative colitis must be considered in the differential diagnosis. The epidemic nature of the disease and the clinical setting of poor community sanitation and faulty personal hygiene suggest the diagnosis. Stool cultures, warm-stage examinations of rectal swabbings, rectal biopsy, and other appropriate microbiologic studies may identify those patients with *shigellosis, salmonellosis, amebiasis,* and *viral enteritis,* as well as *infections* caused by staphylococci, enteropathogenic *E. coli,* and *Clostridium welchii* (see Microbial Diseases). In infections caused by Shigella, *E. coli,* and Salmonella, the severe hyperemia and ulceration of the mucosal surface may be indistinguishable from ulcerative colitis. However, in all instances, the prime consideration is the correction of fluid and electrolyte deficits, though identification of the causative agent is most important for its epidemiologic value and for guidance in specific chemotherapy. Acute proctitis may be noted following broad-spectrum antimicrobial therapy (for any reason), or with gonococcal infection of the rectum.

Intestinal tuberculosis is usually associated with pulmonary disease, and has a predilection for the right colon, particularly the cecum; the regional lymph nodes show central caseation and, together

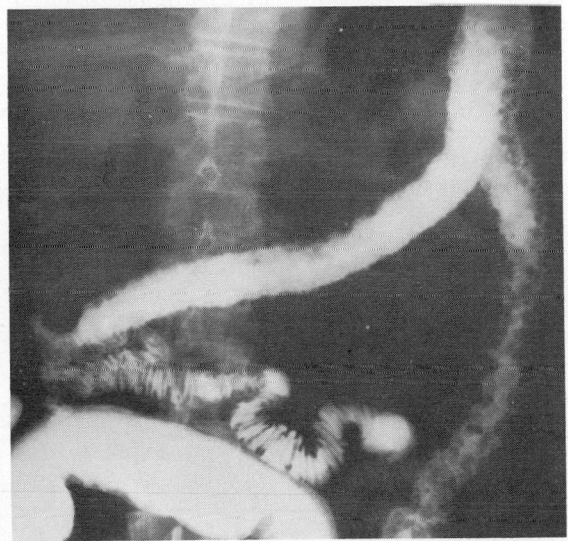

FIGURE 4. Diffuse ulcerative colitis with pseudopolyposis.

with sections of the bowel wall, may harbor tubercle bacilli. Positive Frei and complement-fixation tests, buboes, and a funnel-shaped rectal stricture favor the diagnosis of *lymphogranuloma venereum* (see Lymphogranuloma Venereum in section on Microbial Diseases).

Signs and symptoms of *acute diverticulitis* may resemble those of active ulcerative colitis. However, sigmoidoscopic examination in diverticulitis shows a normal mucosal pattern without evidence of ulceration or granularity, and the barium enema should reveal the area of involvement to lie above the rectum, usually in the sigmoid, and to be associated with diverticula (*vide infra*).

Regional enteritis limited to the small intestine may closely resemble ulcerative colitis clinically, and a barium enema or small bowel series is required to make the distinction (*vide supra*).

Ischemia of the Colon (see below). Recent contributions to the pathophysiology of intestinal vasculature have clearly defined the clinical picture of bowel disease resulting from impairment of mesenteric circulation. Many of these patients with ischemia of the colon have in the past undoubtedly been diagnosed as having ulcerative colitis or granulomatous colitis. Indeed, epidemiologic studies purporting to show a bimodal curve for age distribution in this disease may have been influenced by the inclusion of patients with ischemia of the inferior mesenteric artery. The effect of an impaired blood supply to the colon will be determined not only by the degree and rate of occlusion in this vessel but also by the state of collateral flow through other major mesenteric vessels. Occlusion of these vessels is by atherosclerosis, by emboli from the mural thrombi of myocardial infarcts or from the left atrium in atrial fibrillation, or as a complication of aortic reconstructive surgery. At times, no striking abnormality of the mesenteric vessels is apparent, and the pathophysiologic mechanism is diminished perfusion as in hypotension resulting from acute blood loss, overwhelming sepsis, or myocardial infarction, crucially reducing a marginal mesenteric blood supply. The bacterial flora of the colon contributes importantly to the ensuing inflammatory reaction, necrosis of tissue, and peritonitis.

The clinical picture of ischemic colitis will range from a transient episode so mild that it is recalled only after a barium enema reveals abnormal configuration to a catastrophic picture of severe abdominal distress, with bloody diarrhea, shock, and death owing to extensive infarction of the bowel with massive necrosis, gangrene, and peritonitis. Roentgenographically, polypoid changes caused by submucosal hemorrhage or mucosal irregularity as a consequence of ulceration and edema may be noted, perhaps to be followed by narrowing with stricture and sacculation resulting from fibrosis.

The splenic flexure and sigmoid are most frequently affected, though, occasionally, more proximal areas and, rarely, the rectum may be involved. Thus, a number of features cause ischemic disease of the colon to be mistaken for ulcerative colitis, or particularly granulomatous colitis. Onset in the older age group, acuteness, and the clinical history of cardiovascular disease should strongly suggest the former. In some doubtful cases, selective angiography should be done to confirm the diagnosis; in others, immediate exploration should be carried out with resection, if possible. Unfortunately, many of these patients succumb to shock and infection with anaerobes, particularly *C. welchii.* For those who do not have necrosis and peritonitis, response to conservative management with fluids, nasogastric suction, and antimicrobial drugs is generally favorable. Repeat barium examination later may show a stricture as the only residual sign of healing. In contrast to granulomatous colitis, the narrowing of the lumen is concentric, and skip lesions are rare in ischemic colitis.

Pseudomembranous enterocolitis is characterized clinically by the acute onset of abdominal pain and distention, nausea and vomiting, severe intractable diarrhea, and dehydration with circulatory collapse and shock. The picture may suggest the acute fulminating phase of ulcerative colitis with toxic megacolon. This inflammatory state may be considered a complication of adrenocorticosteroids or of antimicrobial therapy (or both), or of hypotension, during abdominal surgery; it may also be due to staphylococcal bowel infection or to ischemia of the intestinal tract. Pseudomembranous enterocolitis, however, has been observed in the absence of all the aforementioned factors, e.g., in the region proximal to an obstructing carcinoma of the colon or in patients with cardiac failure and uremia.

The gross pathologic picture consists of irregularly placed plaques diffusely spread over the mucosal surface and initially separated by normal-appearing bowel. Microscopically, the fecal exudate consists of mucus, epithelium, fibrin, and leukocytes, which coalesce with necrotic tissue to form a false membrane that may be passed rectally or seen on sigmoidoscopy. Smears and stain of the discharge may reveal clumps of staphylococci. The appearance of the characteristic membrane, the association with some striking clinical event or serious systemic disease, and the absence of epithelial bridging and pseudopolyps should help to distinguish these cases from ulcerative colitis.

Treatment consists of combating shock by replacing blood, fluid, protein, and electrolytes. Erythromycin, 1.0 to 2.0 grams daily, or methicillin should be given if staphylococci are present in the rectal discharge. Shock in such cases may be due to the effect of exotoxins.

Stercoraceous Ulceration of the Colon. This disorder is attributed to pressure exerted on a progressively more attenuated bowel from impacted fecal masses. Constipation is the most frequent symptom, but the occasional patient with diarrhea and rectal bleeding may suggest ulcerative colitis, especially in the elderly malnourished person. These ulcers are most frequently found in the rectosigmoid, but have been observed in all parts of the colon and even in the absence of any primary area of obstruction proximal to the impaction. Microscopically, the ischemic necrosis produced by the fecaliths affects the mucosa first. The important characteristic that differentiates these ulcerations from nonspecific ulcerative colitis is the abnormal bowel function, usually constipation, in weakened, bedridden, dehydrated patients whose sensorium is often obtunded and who may be found to be habitual users of constipating antacids such as aluminum hydroxide or calcium carbonate. Rectal and sigmoidoscopic examination may reveal inspissated fecal masses responsible for a constant urge to defecate.

Postradiation Colitis. Postradiation colitis may appear within one month to several years after exposure. Sigmoidoscopic examination reveals edema, spasm, hyperemia, and friability, often indistinguishable from acute proctitis or ulcerative colitis. The radiologic appearance varies from spasm and edema of the earlier pathologic changes to smooth scarring and narrowing of the lumen which, however, seldom completely obstructs. The history of exposure is the significant point in the differential diagnosis, although the latent period after radiation may be long.

Irritable or Spastic Colon. Irritable colon is often referred to as spastic colitis; this latter term erroneously implies an inflammatory disease of the bowel, and carries with it in the minds of the lay public the connotation of a more serious condition and prognosis. The fundamental problem appears to be psychologic rather than colonic. The symptoms are those of alternating constipation and diarrhea with tenderness to palpation over the descending colon. There is no fever, weight loss, anemia, or malnutrition, and there is no blood in the stools. The radiologic examination is either negative or shows spasm or irritability as the barium passes through the left colon, with frequent smoothing and slight narrowing of its outline (see Disorders of Motility).

Clinical Course. In about 10 per cent of patients with ulcerative colitis, or 5 per cent of all patients with idiopathic inflammatory disease of the colon, the disease is initially limited to the rectum. The pathology is the same as in ulcerative colitis. No more than one tenth of these patients with proctitis suffer proximal progression, and the clinical course is generally mild even in these patients. The most consistent complaint is rectal bleeding; diarrhea is mild or, occasionally, the patient is constipated. Even bleeding may be so mild that its cause is overlooked, and the patient is subjected unnecessarily to hemorrhoidectomy. The proctoscopic appearance may show complete healing, although recurrence with bleeding is not unusual. Systemic complications are rare. Topical steroid enemas or suppositories are most effective (see below).

When first seen, patients with ulcerative colitis may be placed in one of three categories: those with low-grade activity and minimal evidence of the disease, those with moderately severe colitis, and those with a rapidly progressive course which

may be fatal unless it responds dramatically to corticosteroid therapy or colectomy is performed.

The clinical course and pathologic progression in the first two groups of patients are unpredictable. The disease may remain mild throughout and the structural abnormalities noted on sigmoidoscopy and biopsy may disappear. More frequently, the disease becomes established in a chronic form, with remissions and relapses of varied length and severity. The course of the disease and the tendency to recurrent exacerbations are related, at least temporally, to upper respiratory or enteric infections, dietary indiscretions, surgical procedures, menses, pregnancy, and emotional trauma.

The highest mortality occurs during the first two years and is usually associated with bowel perforation and peritonitis. Fatal complications that are less frequent are massive hemorrhage, sepsis, electrolyte disturbances (particularly potassium loss), and thromboembolism, involving especially the brain and lungs. Although therapy to correct the harmful effects of infection and malnutrition has often resulted in a dramatic resolution of the acute attack, it is still too early to know whether the use of corticosteroids and sulfonamides, such as salicylazosulfapyridine, has permanently altered, rather than only temporarily influenced, the course of the disease (see below).

Complications of Ulcerative Colitis. Local. The complications of ulcerative colitis are frequent. When its associated clinical features are mild or even absent, the complications may be the presenting complaint and the first clue to the underlying disease. These include thrombosed hemorrhoids, perianal and perirectal abscesses and fistulas (much more common in the granulomatous form of the disease), perforation of the colon with peritonitis, pericolic abscesses, hemorrhage, toxic dilatation of the colon, and obstruction caused by stricture and carcinoma.

All these complications may require surgical treatment, in most cases definitive and extensive, such as colectomy and ileostomy.

Carcinoma. The over-all incidence of carcinoma in all age groups, without regard to the duration of the disease, is roughly 4 per cent. In children with the onset of colitis before the age of 16, this figure rises to 6 per cent. In patients who have had colitis for more than ten years and in whom the diagnosis is based on surgical or postmortem specimens, the incidence in some series has been reported as high as 20 per cent. The five-year survival rate for all patients with carcinoma in ulcerative colitis, with or without surgery, varies from 0 to 30 per cent in contrast to a figure of 60 per cent for those who have had resection for carcinoma of the colon and rectum in the general population. The striking characteristics of carcinoma in association with ulcerative colitis are its tendency to multicentricity, the youth of the patients involved, its appearance frequently during periods of quiescence, and the relatively poor prognosis. The risk of this complication is greatest in those with onset of the colitis before age 20, with universal distribution of the disease, and in patients who have lived with it for more than 10 years. In those with total involvement of the colon, the carcinoma is more evenly distributed than in patients without colitis, although the rectosigmoid remains in both groups the most common site. When the colitis is limited to the left colon, and especially in the case of ulcerative proctitis, the incidence of carcinoma is rare. The lag in correctly diagnosing carcinoma when it complicates ulcerative colitis may be shortened by routine cytologic studies of colonic washings. The use of periodic rectal biopsies, especially in those who have had colitis for more than ten years, has been advanced as a means of determining more precisely the cancer-prone patients; that is, "precancerous" changes of the mucosa may be noted, of the same variety that have been found in patients with invasive cancer and long-standing ulcerative colitis. In spite of theoretical objections to the validity of these epithelial changes, if prospective studies confirm their prognostic value, such a procedure will be a more reasonable approach than the routine prophylactic colectomy advocated by some for all patients who have had colitis more than 10 years, regardless of clinical status.

General Complications. *Catabolic Changes.* Iron deficiency anemia, electrolyte disturbances, and hypoproteinemia result primarily from bleeding, diarrhea, anorexia, and increased metabolism caused by inflammation and fever. The effects of hypopotassemia such as ileus, anorexia, muscle weakness, apathy, cardiac irregularities, and renal impairment may be irreversible unless promptly corrected (see Potassium Metabolism). Blood calcium may be reduced, with the clinical manifestations of tetany. Calcium and, especially, uric acid stones may be noted in patients with dehydration and chronic loss of Na^+, K^+, Cl^-, and Mg^+, which normally increase the solubility of calcium salts in the urine. Hypoproteinemia is accentuated by the abnormal loss of protein-rich exudate through the necrotic mucous membrane and, in some patients, by impaired liver function. Small intestinal absorption may also be abnormal in patients with lactase deficiency or sensitivity to milk proteins.

Renal and Pancreatic Changes. The kidneys often show glomerular endothelial proliferation, but obstruction to the capillary blood flow is found only in severe cases. Interstitial *pancreatitis* with moderate fibrosis may also be found; however, there is no evidence that these pathologic findings are of clinical significance.

Liver Disease. Fatty infiltration of the liver is common and is attributed to malnutrition and infection. These changes may be transitory and reversible, varying with the clinical status of the colitis. Of more serious import is pericholangitis, characterized by intermittent jaundice, hepatomegaly, pruritis, and an elevated alkaline phosphatase. The pathogenesis of this complication, which may lead to biliary cirrhosis, is possibly owing to portal bacteremia. The relationship between ulcerative colitis and primary sclerosing cholangitis involving primarily the larger bile ducts has recently been emphasized (see Biliary Tract Disease).

Joint Manifestations. Symptoms referable to joints may be found in 10 to 20 per cent of patients with ulcerative colitis. The frequency of ulcerative colitis in patients with spondylitis, approximately 18 per 1000, is more than 40 times that noted in the general population. Conversely, the frequency of ankylosing spondylitis in patients with ulcerative colitis is about 6 per cent, or more than 100 times the expected incidence. The severity of the arthritis of the spine and sacroiliac joints does not always parallel the clinical course of the colitis, and in most of these patients colectomy does not influence its progression; the symptoms and signs of irreversible disease continue postoperatively. Arthralgia affecting the peripheral joints or low back region, but without any clinical or roentgenographic signs of soft tissue swelling or bone damage, is a common complaint. In patients with this disorder joint symptoms correlate well with the activity of the colitis. Virtually all patients are relieved of their pain with subsidence of the disease or after colectomy.

In the remaining group are those patients with "toxic" arthritis, whose attacks of pain and swelling are limited to the large joints, appearing simultaneously with episodes of colitis. The latex fixation test is negative, indicating absence of so-called "rheumatoid factor." Improvement in the colitis, whether by medical or surgical means, is associated with complete remission of the arthritis. Thus, one might consider this type of arthritis, if severe, a reason for colectomy.

Other Complications. The complications of osteoporosis, uveitis, erythema nodosum, pyoderma gangrenosum, vascular thrombosis, and amyloidosis are less common than arthritis but, nevertheless, are noted in 1 to 5 per cent of patients. Retarded sexual development, amenorrhea, and infantilism represent serious problems in management of adolescents with this disease and their importance often overshadows all other symptoms. Normal development often will not proceed unless colectomy is performed.

Granulomatous Colitis and Enterocolitis. In the past ten years the concept of granulomatous colitis as an entity with distinctive clinical, pathologic, and roentgenographic features has been generally accepted. Soon after Crohn, Ginzberg, and Oppenheimer had described regional enteritis limited to the terminal ileum, there were sporadic case reports of a similar involvement in the colon which was variously referred to as right-sided colitis, regional migratory ulcerative colitis, segmental ulcerative colitis, and regional colitis.

Only some of the characteristic features of granulomatous colitis and those which serve to distinguish these cases from ulcerative colitis will be described here. Gross bleeding per rectum is unusual. In common with regional enteritis of the small intestine, fistulas are present in approximately 50 per cent of patients, mostly in the perirectal region, and may antedate obvious disease in the colon by months or years. The rectum is grossly spared in 30 to 50 per cent. Carcinoma has not been reported in as large a number of patients as with ulcerative colitis, although some of this disparity may be the result of earlier and more frequent colonic resection, owing to a higher incidence of complications and less effective responsiveness to medical treatment.

Radiologically, the presence of classic regional enteritis in the small intestine favors the same diagnosis for the accompanying inflammatory process in the colon. The colonic distribution is typically segmental, right-sided, and sparing the rectum, with multiple areas involved and intervening normal bowel. The asymmetric lumen, with transverse and longitudinal fissures, cobblestone mucosa, fistulas, and sinus tracts, contrasts with the findings in ulcerative colitis both on barium enema and at operation. Multiple, penetrating, transverse fissures in granulomatous colitis associated with diverticula may coalesce into a large paracolic fistulous tract for a distance of more than 8 cm. parallel to the bowel contour. Until recently, this feature had been considered characteristic of the single perforation with abscess formation of diverticulitis.

The pathologic picture is the same as in granulomatous disease of the small intestine, with noncaseating granulomas in 30 to 50 per cent and transmural involvement with edema, fibrosis, and thickening of the bowel wall, mesentery, and lymph nodes. Of 100 patients with granulomatous disease of the intestine, 50 will have disease limited to the small intestine, and 40, combined ileocolitis; in 10 the colon alone will be involved. In comparison with ulcerative colitis, more recent reports have raised its relative incidence from 10 to more than 50 per cent. In spite of sharper pathologic criteria, however, there remains a group comprising 15 to 25 per cent of all cases hitherto considered to be idiopathic ulcerative colitis, but which cannot be clearly classified, because it has pathologic and radiologic features of both.

Lacking knowledge of the cause of ulcerative colitis and granulomatous colitis, some look upon these distinctions as reflections of a difference in the host reaction to the same injury. For the present, however, it is advisable to think of them as separate diseases from the clinical point of view.

Other Special Clinical Features of Granulomatous Colitis. Since this disease may be segmental, the complaints may be unusual when an isolated area is involved, unless it narrows the lumen, causing symptoms of *obstruction*, or perforates into other loops of gut, producing the picture of *enterocolic fistula* (see Malabsorption).

In many cases, the patient complaining only of right lower quadrant pain, weight loss, and "looseness of stools" will have a well-defined *lower abdominal mass* on examination, representing matted loops of bowel with fistulas and, in some instances, abscess formation.

Patients with granulomatous colitis or enterocolitis also have the associated abnormalities of ulcerative colitis, i.e., arthritis (including spine and sacroiliac joints), uveitis, phlebitis, erythema nodosum, and pyoderma gangrenosum (see below). Some think these abnormalities are noted with greater frequency in the granulomatous form of the disease.

Occasionally, a patient with this disease will present a fever of unknown origin ("FUO") and because of arthralgia, tachycardia, elevated sedimentation rate, and perhaps erythema nodosum will be thought to have rheumatic fever. When diagnostic evidence for this latter disease or other specific diseases that cause fever is not obtained, roentgenographic investigation for chronic inflammatory bowel disease is indicated, even in the absence of a history of diarrhea or abdominal pain.

Treatment of Ulcerative and Granulomatous Colitis. Medical. The treatment of ulcerative and granulomatous colitis is based on measures designed to give symptomatic relief, correct nutritional deficiencies, restore blood volume and hemoglobin concentration, and control complications of the disease. At the outset, it is most important for the physician to establish a satisfactory relationship with the patient, who is often apprehensive, depressed, and emotionally immature. The degree of success in treatment will also depend upon the physician's judicious and discriminating use of antimicrobial agents, transfusions, adrenal corticosteroids, and psychotherapy.

A selective diet, with restriction only of very cold liquids or any food or drink that is known to stimulate excessive evacuation, promotes not only optimal caloric intake but maximal cooperation of the patient. There is no evidence that a low-residue diet is helpful except in the presence of luminal narrowing caused by a stricture. A diet with a high roughage content in addition to a stool softener, such as dioctyl sodium sulfosuccinate, may actually be necessary in the treatment of paradoxic constipation when the inflammatory process is limited to the left colon and the rest of the bowel retains its normal capacity to absorb water and produce a formed stool. Restriction of the diet to fluids or interdiction of any oral feeding may, however, be necessary for the treatment of severe and persistent abdominal discomfort and severe diarrhea with tenesmus.

Symptomatic Therapy. Diet, bed rest, sedation, and anticholinergic preparations are often necessary, and are usually sufficient to relieve the abdominal cramps or control the severe diarrhea. Tincture of belladonna is often used for its effect on excessive bowel motility and cramping pain, unless there is evidence of a dilated colon. It is usually started in a dosage of 15 drops before meals and at bedtime, with daily increments of 1 to 3 drops until the proper therapeutic effect has been obtained or undesirable reactions occur, such as tachycardia, disturbances in visual accommodation on bladder evacuation, or abdominal distention. Narcotic drugs, such as tincture of opium, 6 to 8 drops, paregoric, 4 to 8 ml., or codeine, 15 to 30 mg., every four hours, often help allay apprehension as well. Although toxic dilatation of the colon is uncommon in granulomatous colitis, these drugs must be given cautiously (vide supra).

Blood transfusions may be necessary as a temporary measure in combating the serious effects of exsanguinating hemorrhage or in the management of anemia resulting from progressive blood loss and malnutrition. Oral iron preparations are generally ineffective during activity of the disease, especially in the presence of bleeding, and may even aggravate the diarrhea. When the bleeding has ceased and the inflammation and infection have subsided, repletion of iron is necessary; if oral iron is not tolerated, parenteral preparations such as dextran iron complex (Imferon) are preferable (see Malabsorption).

Antimicrobial Therapy. Dramatic results have occasionally been observed with the use of various antimicrobials such as penicillin, 300,000 to 600,000 units twice daily intramuscularly, streptomycin, 0.5 gram twice daily intramuscularly, or tetracycline, 0.25 gram every six hours orally. Except in the treatment of the secondary bacterial invaders associated with purulent complications, such as bowel perforation, perirectal abscesses, or fistulas, the response to these agents has been inconstant and at times has been complicated by a severe staphylococcal enterocolitis. Among the sulfonamide preparations, the poorly absorbed drugs such as succinylsulfathiazole and phthalylsulfathiazole, 2 grams every four hours, are usually well tolerated, even over a long period, and occasionally improve the patient's condition.

An absorbable azo compound of sulfapyridine and salicylic acid (salicylazosulfapyridine) is the most consistently effective preparation in this group. Its metabolites are concentrated in gut tissue, but the reason for its favorable effect on the disease is not known. However, the usual initial daily dose of 4 to 8 grams (1.0 to 2.0 grams four times a day) is associated with headache, nausea, vomiting, fever, or rash in 15 to 20 per cent of patients. More serious complications such as jaundice, leukopenia, and hemolytic anemia are seen less frequently. In those who are able to tolerate it, the response to salicylazosulfapyridine may be comparable to that in patients treated with corticotrophin and corticosteroids. Although the toxic effects of the corticosteroids are more serious, the disturbances associated with salicylazosulfapyridine are more frequent. There is some evidence that maintenance therapy with 2 grams per day of this sulfa preparation is more effective than corticosteroids. In dealing with the moderately ill patient, it may be advisable to start with salicylazosulfapyridine and change to steroid therapy if the former is poorly tolerated or proves ineffective.

Corticotrophin (ACTH) and Adrenocorticosteroids. The rationale for the use of corticosteroids in ulcerative and granulomatous colitis rests on several observations and theoretical considerations. These diseases are often associated with conditions such as arthritis, iritis, and erythema nodosum, common manifestations of hypersensitivity states, for which corticosteroids have been successfully employed. Their influence on the tissue response to inflammation might reduce the severity of the toxic reaction and the degree of the local fibroblastic proliferation. Moreover, the generally favorable effect of these drugs on the patient's appetite and in producing a sense of well-being are helpful to the malnourished, anorectic, depressed patient.

Corticotrophin and corticosteroids are indicated in the management of the acute fulminating phase, in patients who have failed to improve with other measures, and as an adjunct in preparing precariously ill patients for surgery. The results of treatment are most favorable when these drugs are given early in the course of the disease and when the acute manifestations are associated with only superficial involvement of the bowel. Their success in treatment of acute exacerbations of chronic ulcerative and granulomatous colitis is less striking.

The nature of the remission may be only symptomatic and limited to an improvement in mood, fever, and diarrhea. The degree of involvement of the mucosa may be unchanged, and rectal biopsy months after remission may continue to show inflammation. A successful clinical response will usually be apparent within the first week. If a favorable effect has not been obtained by the third week, continued administration of steroids is not only futile, but may mask continuing progression of the bowel disease and even perforation. In addition, prolonged use of high doses of steroids increases the incidence of intraperitoneal infection postoperatively in those who require colectomy.

The superiority of ACTH over hydrocortisone and cortisone and their synthetic analogues, such as prednisone and prednisolone, is suggested not only by the higher percentage of favorable results with ACTH but also by its ability to improve the condition of patients previously unresponsive to other preparations. Thus, ACTH appears to be the most effective form of steroid therapy and, therefore, is indicated for the more seriously ill patients.

A satisfactory regimen for those patients consists of the daily intravenous administration of 40 to 80 units in a slow drip of 500 ml. of glucose and water throughout an eight-hour period, supplemented by 20 to 40 mEq. of potassium. Salt is restricted to 1.0 gram daily during treatment with ACTH as well as with higher doses of prednisone. With the beginning of a remission, usually within five to seven days, the corticotrophin may then be given intramuscularly in the long-acting gel form, usually 40 to 60 units every 12 hours. With continuous improvement, this dosage is gradually decreased so that after another week oral prednisone may be substituted, in an initial daily dose equal to the last previous dosage of corticotrophin, usually 40 to 60 mg. Decrements of 5 mg. every two to three days are advisable if the clinical course progresses favorably. In reaching the daily maintenance level of 10 to 20 mg. of prednisone, salt intake may be liberalized. The goal in therapy is to arrive at a maintenance dosage compatible with a satisfactory clinical remission, and yet small enough to avoid undesirable and harmful cumulative side effects.

In an effort to reduce the incidence of side effects from corticosteroid therapy, an intermittent schedule of drug therapy has been employed, i.e., a double daily dose is given every other day at breakfast. Such a program has been used in the management of asthma and rheumatoid arthritis without any apparent loss in effectiveness of therapy. There is sufficient merit in this proposal to warrant its use after the acute symptoms have been alleviated by the continous daily dosage schedule for several weeks. In practice, however, it has not always been possible to effect such a transfer and maintain a favorable state of remission in the treatment of ulcerative or granulomatous colitis.

In the less seriously ill patients the initial dosage of corticosteroids is 200 to 300 mg. for cortisone and 40 to 60 mg. for prednisone daily. Since these doses of cortisone will lead to significant sodium retention, salt should be restricted.

When the disease is predominantly rectal or there is much tenesmus, local instillation of hydrocortisone suppositories (10 mg.) two or three times daily may be helpful. When the drug is thus introduced, there is very little, if any, absorption, and hence no adverse constitutional reactions are noted. When the disease has involved the colon beyond the rectum and rectosigmoid, effective use has been made of a plastic disposable enema unit, which permits rapid self-administration rectally of 100 mg. of hydrocortisone hemisuccinate or 20 mg. of prednisolone-21-phosphate in 100 ml. of saline. (The use of 5 per cent glucose as the diluent is to be avoided because of its irritating effect.) With this procedure the enema contents may pass beyond the hepatic flexure. This treatment, given nightly until the clinical condition warrants reduction in frequency to alternate nights, has been most effective in the treatment of left-sided colitis, in part, perhaps, because 5 to 20 per cent of the steroid is absorbed and may have a systemic effect. Although some suppression of the adrenal gland by the absorbed steroid has been noted, the main effect is local. Maintenance therapy consists of instillations twice weekly for indefinite periods. In the case of universal colitis, the combination of steroid enemas and oral steroids will often produce a favorable remission with a smaller than usual dose of the systemic preparation.

The potential disadvantages of steroid therapy should be distinguished from the complications of the disease. When hypertension, hyperglycemia, acne, hirsutism, and fluid retention appear, they may properly be considered complications of the treatment, because they are not features of ulcerative colitis. Electrolyte disturbances, especially hypokalemia and hypocalcemia, are serious consequences of severe and progressive ulcerative and granulomatous colitis, which may be aggra-

vated by ACTH or corticosteroid therapy. Hypocalcemia and osteoporosis may be accelerated so that long bones and vertebrae may fracture on minimal trauma. The most common and important ocular complication of systemic corticosteroid therapy is bilateral posterior subcapsular cataracts. These may be seen in adults when more than 10 mg. of prednisone has been administered daily for more than one year; a proportionately smaller dose over a shorter treatment span may produce this complication in children. Slit-lamp examination may be necessary to detect the early lesions because visual disturbances appear late. Thus, eye examinations should be performed at least twice annually in all patients on continuous steroid therapy. Another serious complication is tuberculosis. Accordingly, all patients with evidence of previous infection should be treated with isoniazid, 300 mg. daily. Patients on steroid treatment for more than six months should be put on the same prophylactic program. Chest films should be obtained twice yearly.

Less common complications of use of systemic corticosteroids are retinopathy with hypertension, exophthalmos, ptosis, chemosis of lids, and extraocular myopathy with ocular palsy. Papilledema associated with nausea, vomiting, and headache as manifestations of increased intracranial pressure (pseudotumor cerebri) may also rarely be noted. Prepsychotic behavior or even frank psychosis, although infrequent, is a serious and disturbing complication. Acute adrenal insufficiency may result from decreasing the dose of these preparations too rapidly, as well as from severe infection in patients who had been on steroid therapy during the preceding 18 months. Under such circumstances, hydrocortisone should be given parenterally in doses of 100 to 200 mg. daily for the first 48 hours, with gradually decreasing dosages over the subsequent five to seven days as the general condition improves.

That steroids increase the likelihood of perforation of the colon in ulcerative colitis is a subject of dispute, because this catastrophe is part of the natural history of the disease. However the risk of this complication should not prevent their use. In the treatment of acute fulminating colitis with toxic dilatation, however, steroid therapy should be discontinued if it has been ineffective after five days. The frequency of reactivation of a preexisting peptic ulcer or of its de novo appearance cannot be precisely stated, but, in comparison with the incidence of steroid ulcers in rheumatoid arthritis, it is rare; these drugs, therefore, should be given when indicated for ulcerative colitis, despite a history of peptic ulcer disease. Frequent feedings and antacid medication as in the management of peptic ulcer is recommended for all patients on steroid therapy, especially for patients with histories of peptic ulcer (see Peptic Ulcer). One should avoid those antacids whose magnesium content may aggravate the diarrhea. Steroid therapy should be terminated (not abruptly) if an ulcer bleeds or perforates.

Adrenocorticosteroids and ACTH are the most

important and effective compounds available in the medical management of ulcerative colitis. Although capable of initiating a clinical and, at times, anatomic remission, their effectiveness is unpredictable. The high relapse rate following their omission, in some series as high as 80 per cent, emphasizes the suppressive rather than the curative nature of this response. Recurrences may result from premature withdrawal of the steroids, especially if symptomatic improvement alone is the goal in therapy rather than healing of the bowel. Long-term therapy may prevent invalidism in patients with chronically active colitis or in those with increasingly frequent recurrences. In comparing the steroid with the presteroid era, one must not overlook the influence of other therapeutic advances, including earlier diagnosis, more effective antimicrobial agents, better understanding of nutrition, and appropriate parenteral replacement of blood, protein, fluids, and electrolytes.

The steroid era has been associated with a decrease in mortality and morbidity. Although the total number of serious complications has decreased—attributable in whole or in part to hormonal therapy—osteoporosis, thrombophlebitis, nephrolithiasis, psychic disturbances, and massive upper gastrointestinal bleeding have increased. The total number of surgical procedures is not less, but more operations are undertaken under elective rather than emergency conditions, permitting more definitive and safer surgery in one stage.

Immunosuppressive drugs such as nitrogen mustard and azothioprine have been employed in the treatment of patients who have not responded to current methods of medical treatment. Their use is fraught with serious complications, especially those of bone marrow suppression and uncontrollable infection; because of the delay in effecting a response they are not applicable in the management of acute fulminating cases. For the present, these preparations are not advisable for routine use, and should be limited to institutions whose personnel are experienced in their administration and where the necessary supervision can be employed.

Psychotherapy. The physician must be aware of the patient's psychological problems as well as his physical requirements. An important aspect of therapy is to foster a strong physician-patient relationship based upon a willingness to accept responsibility for the needs of the patient with sympathy and understanding. An abrupt alteration of the intense involvement with his physician may cause the patient to feel hopeless and may hasten his downward course. This is especially pertinent during the acute fulminating phase of the illness, when intensive psychotherapy is contraindicated. Formal psychotherapy should be undertaken only by a psychiatrist who is experienced in the management of these patients and is aware of the vulnerability of their psychic and physical structure. His greatest usefulness will be during a relatively quiescent period when the patient may be physically and psychologically better prepared to deal with his conflicts. The care of children often requires manipulation of the home situation in order to provide a more favorable environment.

When patients are hospitalized, the personnel should be alerted to the difficulty in management posed by infantile regressive attitudes, often expressed by hostility and lack of cooperation. Because of the patient's dependency and his fear of rejection, the temporary absence of key medical personnel or a change in rotation among staff physicians may result in a serious setback, unless such events are properly anticipated.

Surgical Treatment. The course of ulcerative colitis is variable, and the response to medical management in the individual instance is unpredictable. However, either because of spontaneous remissions or therapy, more than 75 per cent of patients with ulcerative colitis do not require surgical intervention. In the remaining patients, limited surgical treatment may be indicated for local complications, such as thrombosed hemorrhoids and perianal or perirectal abscesses. Occasionally these local problems are the presenting complaint, and the more serious underlying colitis is not recognized. Rectal surgery undertaken without knowledge or consideration of the primary bowel disease may lead to a more rapid progression of the colitis, as well as to poor healing of the incised area, with consequent anal incontinence.

A better understanding of the significance of electrolyte disturbances and blood loss, improved surgical techniques, and the availability of more satisfactory ileostomy appliances have successfully challenged the medical attitude of the past, which considered colectomy and ileostomy as the last resort for a desperately ill patient.

The most common indication for extensive surgery is intractability or the failure of medical treatment to prevent chronic invalidism. Before subjecting a patient to colectomy, one must be satisfied that the proper treatment has been pursued and that sufficient patience and skill have been employed to ensure his cooperation.

The recognition of carcinoma of the colon as a complication of ulcerative colitis should lead to immediate surgery. The correlation between the incidence of carcinoma and the duration of colitis has led some to advocate prophylactic colectomy for all patients who have had ulcerative colitis for more than ten years. However, the risk of this complication is not so great nor the morbidity or mortality of ileostomy and colectomy so small as to warrant the adoption of such an extreme measure. This is particularly true if the patient is well and the course of the disease does not otherwise warrant such radical treatment. However, it must be pointed out that carcinoma often supervenes during long periods of quiescence of the disease.

The persistence of perirectal infection despite repeated local therapeutic efforts is another indication for colectomy and ileostomy. An obstructing stricture in chronic ulcerative colitis may be indistinguishable from carcinoma, particularly in the right colon. Strictures of the sigmoid and rectum are most often benign and represent hypertrophy of the muscularis rather than fibrosis. If the lesion is proximal or if doubt exists about its pathologic nature, the treatment of choice is colectomy, and the correct diagnosis may be established in such cases only after microscopic examination.

Colectomy and ileostomy are often lifesaving measures in the treatment of massive hemorrhage or perforation and for patients with toxic dilatation who do not respond to medical measures. There is general agreement that the definitive surgery for ulcerative colitis should combine colectomy with ileostomy in one or several stages. Controversy is now centered on whether the diseased rectal stump should be preserved so that an ileorectal anastomosis can be performed. Because it might be the seat of continuing inflammation and of future carcinoma, most surgeons agree that the rectum should be removed with the colon or at some time after subtotal colectomy and ileostomy, as atrophy and distortion of the rectal stump because of disuse or inflammation make it difficult to perform sigmoidoscopy and correctly interpret its findings. In contrast to surgery for cancer, permanent sexual dysfunction rarely follows removal of the rectum for colitis.

Several British surgeons, however, perform total colectomy with the removal of the rectal stump only in relatively few patients. Adequate follow-up studies are not available to permit any firm conclusion about this approach, although many reports indicate continued activity of the disease following ileoproctostomy. Thus, ileoproctostomy or ileosigmoidostomy should probably be performed only when the rectum is grossly and histologically normal.

If the patient has been on steroids during the preceding 18 months, hydrocortisone is administered parenterally in a dosage of 100 to 200 mg. daily for two days before the operation, during the day of the procedure, and for two to three days postoperatively. It is then gradually decreased over seven to ten days, during which time it may be given orally. Pulse and blood pressure, urinary output, serum sodium, and urea nitrogen are carefully observed during this period in order to detect adrenal insufficiency (see Adrenals).

The patient's acceptance of ileostomy will be proportionately influenced by the degree of discomfort and debility previously suffered. Pre- and postoperative visits by patients who have adjusted to ileostomy may help considerably. Indeed, many ileostomy patients are now organized into groups and have made themselves available for such services.

Despite its effectiveness, surgical treatment of ulcerative colitis has disadvantages that restrict its use to well-defined indications. Not all patients will accept the handicaps of the ileostomy, troublesome odors, skin irritation, and, at times, leakage around poorly functioning appliances. The complications of a malfunctioning ileostomy— bowel prolapse, retraction, stenosis, obstruction,

and electrolyte disturbances — are serious sequelae of the postoperative period that may lead to recurrent difficulty and further surgery. Varying degrees of salt and water depletion may be precipitated by episodes of gastroenteritis or excessive sweating. This mechanism should be suspected in an ileostomy patient complaining of headache, nausea, muscle cramps with oliguria, hypotension, or convulsions. To a young, unmarried patient, the psychologic handicap of an ileostomy may represent an insuperable burden, and the fear of pregnancy may be the cause of severe anxiety to a young married couple.

Acute Fulminating Colitis and Toxic Megacolon. Despite improvements in medical management and surgical techniques, acute fulminating ulcerative colitis remains the most formidable variant of the disease. The treatment must be immediate and vigorous in order to restore the fluid, electrolyte, and blood losses. The administration of more than 5 liters of fluid within the first 24 hours may be necessary for severe dehydration. Massive blood transfusions are often imperative, in spite of the theoretical objection of increasing the cardiac work load in a patient who has adapted to a relatively contracted vascular bed. Scout films of the abdomen often show evidence of marked bowel distention and perforation which is not clinically apparent. In the absence of perforation, medical measures should be instituted, but should not be continued beyond four to five days if there is not marked improvement in the fever, tachycardia, abdominal tenderness, and dilatation of the colon.

Pericolic infection resulting from small, walled-off perforations and toxemia are best combated with penicillin in a dosage of 3.0 to 6.0 million units parenterally, daily. Corticotrophin or corticosteroids are given because of their value as anti-inflammatory agents. The use of these preparations, particularly 40 to 80 units of corticotrophin in an intravenous drip of 500 ml. of 5 per cent glucose in water, supplemented by 20 to 40 mEq. of potassium daily, has decreased the risk of surgical intervention. The danger of steroids masking perforation or aggravating intra-abdominal sepsis must always be borne in mind. Oral feeding should be omitted and nasogastric suction instituted. Some authorities favor use of a long tube intubation for decompression, i.e., a tube that is passed to the terminal ileum. Surgery should be undertaken if the patient does not improve in four to five days, if free perforation occurs, or if there is evidence of abscess by abdominal palpation or rectal examination. In any event, subtotal colectomy and ileostomy should not be performed until fluid, electrolyte, particularly potassium, and blood losses have been corrected and appropriate antimicrobial therapy instituted.

Granulomatous Colitis. Distinguishing ulcerative colitis from granulomatous colitis is of more than academic interest. Like regional enteritis, granulomatous colitis, particularly ileocolitis, tends to recur postoperatively, particularly at enterocolic anastomoses. Occasionally, the stoma and prestomal ileum are the sites of new disease.

In any event, recurrences are prone to appear soon after surgery—weeks to months. Some observers, however, limit this high recurrence rate to anastomotic operations and claim the same satisfactory result ultimately for colectomy and ileostomy in this disease as in ulcerative colitis. Although the medical management of granulomatous colitis is essentially similar to that of regional enteritis of the small intestine or of ulcerative colitis, more than 70 per cent of those with granulomatous colitis will eventually require surgery. Broadly, the indications are the same as for ulcerative colitis. If the disease is segmental and the rectum is spared, the optimal procedure is a localized resection with colocolostomy or, more commonly, anastomosis of ileum to normal colon, ileotransversecolostomy for right-sided disease, or ileosigmoidostomy for more extensive disease. If the nature and severity of the recurrence make an ileostomy and colectomy necessary (in approximately 50 per cent of cases), it should be undertaken with the same prospects for ultimate cure of the disease as in the case of ulcerative colitis. The subsequent development of ileostomy dysfunction, noted more frequently than after colectomy for ulcerative colitis, and often resulting from recurrent granulomatous disease at, and proximal to, the stoma, can usually be satisfactorily managed with an ileostomy revision, with little likelihood that this will be followed by a progressively more proximal ileitis.

Colitis and Pregnancy. The course of ulcerative colitis in pregnancy is unpredictable, and the behavior in a previous pregnancy is not a satisfactory guide to the future. Pregnancy during an active rather than a quiescent stage is likely to aggravate colitis.

Ulcerative colitis that becomes manifest during pregnancy, particularly during the first trimester or in the immediate postpartum period, may be unusually severe. Severe colitis during the first trimester raises the question of a therapeutic abortion. The possibility of a spontaneous remission as the pregnancy advances must be weighed against the risk of progressive deterioration and of a transabdominal approach for termination in the second or third trimester. The patient's attitude toward her pregnancy may influence the clinical course. The psychologic significance of her pregnancy, as well as the more tangible physical aspects of the colitis, will require careful medical supervision in which a sympathetic understanding and reassuring support are important ingredients. The colitis does not adversely affect the pregnancy per se, and the prospect of a full-term delivery of a normal child is the same as for the population at large, in spite of antecedent therapy with sulfonamides and steroids.

Prognosis. The prognosis of ulcerative colitis cannot always be accurately gauged because of the variability of its natural course and the difficulty in assessing the effects of various forms of therapy. Moreover, except in the presence of carcinoma, stricture, perforation, or toxic dilatation, neither the roentgenologic appearance of the colon nor the sigmoidoscopic picture is a reliable criterion of the patient's condition or of the prognosis. Even a seriously damaged bowel may permit a normal existence.

The degree of severity of the initial attack seems related to the ultimate course. In one series, 70 per cent of those who were seriously ill when first seen became worse, whereas 65 per cent of those with mild colitis at the onset improved. The extent of colonic involvement, which is usually determined within the first year of the initial attack in most patients, also appears to influence the prognosis. Thus, the patient whose entire colon is affected at this time is more likely to have chronic disease with its complications. Patients whose colitis is confined to the distal colon by the end of the first year may suffer extension of the disease in depth, and the course thereafter depends on the severity of this process. In general, however, these patients fare better than those with universal involvement. When the colitis has been present for more than two years, no method of management has proved uniformly successful in preventing recurrences. The relapse rate is high, and only 20 per cent of patients have remained free of recurrences at the end of five years, no matter what form of therapy has been given.

In the group (10 per cent) whose disease starts before the age of 20, the prognosis is distinctly poor, judging by their subsequent clinical course and need for surgical intervention. In one series, half of the patients in this age group eventually required surgical treatment. The problem was further complicated by impairment of normal growth and an increased incidence of malignant disease.

In 10 per cent of all patients, the disease begins after the age of 50. This figure has in the past, undoubtedly, included patients with ischemic colitis. In general, half of these older patients respond favorably to conservative measures without relapse during a two-year period of observation after therapy is begun. The other half usually require surgical treatment for the initial attack or because of recurrent episodes and progressive deterioration. Frequently, the condition is incorrectly diagnosed as carcinoma or diverticulitis.

Recent experience demonstrates clearly the reduction of morbidity and mortality of total colectomy through improved pre- and postoperative management. A definite statement, however, about the long-term results of this treatment cannot be made because of insufficient follow-up data. Results of surgery as currently performed cannot be compared with those of a previous era since, in addition to improved technique and more widespread use of colectomy rather than ileostomy alone, operation is now undertaken on patients who either have not been ill for a long period or who are in vastly better condition for surgery.

The striking improvement in surgical results has weakened the position of those who persist in medical management beyond any reasonable prospect of success. The hope of obtaining a clinical and structural remission leading to the control of this disease without resorting to colectomy is a worthwhile goal, but it must not lead to endless delay beyond the point at which the chance for a successful result from operation is compromised. On the other hand, the wave of surgical enthusiasm must not sweep patients too soon into permanent ileostomy.

Banks, B. M., Korelitz, B. I., and Zetzel, L.: The course of non-specific ulcerative colitis: Review of 20 years' experience and late results. Gastroenterology, 32:983, 1957.

Engel, G. L.: Biologic and psychologic features of ulcerative colitis. Gastroenterology, 40:313, 1961.

Janowitz, H. D., Lindner, A. E., and Marshak, R.: Granulomatous colitis, Crohn's disease of the colon. J.A.M.A., 191:825, 1965.

Lennard-Jones, J. E., Lockhart-Mummery, H. E., and Morson, B. C.: Clinical and pathological differentiation of Crohn's disease and proctocolitis. Gastroenterology, 54:1162, 1968.

Marston, A.: Mesenteric arterial disease: The present position. Gut, 8:203, 1967.

Truelove, S. C., and Edwards, F. C.: The course and prognosis of ulcerative colitis. Gut, 4:299, 1963.

Wilks, S., and Moxon, W.: Lectures on Pathological Anatomy. 2nd ed. London, J. & A. Churchill, Ltd. 1875.

Zetzel, L.: Granulomatous (ileo)colitis. New Eng. J. Med., 282:600. 1970.

APPENDICITIS

Definition. Acute inflammation of the vermiform appendix is the most common surgical lesion within the abdomen. It occurs at all ages, though more frequently and typically in young adults between 20 and 30. There are approximately 200,000 cases of acute appendicitis recognized annually in the United States, with an over-all mortality of 1 per cent. Occasional appendectomies and, more frequently, drainage of appendiceal abscesses had been performed before the latter part of the nineteenth century, but the modern era of the proper surgical approach to this disease dates from the classic work of Fitz. In 1886, he established the importance of inflammation of the appendix in what had previously been considered perityphilitis and emphasized the need to operate and remove the appendix early, rather than wait for it to perforate and then to drain the complicating abscess.

Etiology and Pathogenesis. The appendix is an offshoot of the cecum, with whose lumen it shares the fecal contents of the colon. The appendix literally "hangs onto" the cecum. Its location within the peritoneal cavity is thus usually in the right lower quadrant, but it may also be found low in the pelvis, in the right upper quadrant when there is malrotation, or even in the left lower quadrant in the case of situs inversus. The small-caliber appendiceal lumen ends blindly, but in the absence of obstruction or inflammation its fecal contents are readily evacuated back into the cecum. The mechanical effects of an obstructing fecalith leading to stasis and inflammation raise the intraluminal pressure beyond the point where the terminal appendiceal artery can remain patent. The circulation is thus compromised, and, unless the obstruction is relieved, necrosis, perforation, and peritonitis develop progressively. The peritonitis may remain local with the forma-

tion of abscesses in the region of the appendix, in the pelvis, and in or around the liver. If the walling off process is inadequate, a more generalized peritonitis ensues. The appendix may also become inflamed from contiguous sources of infection in the ileocecal segment or from more distant foci via the lymphatics or blood stream. The rate of progression and the virulence of the spread will be affected by the age and general health of the patient, the duration of the disease before recognition, and the virulence of the infecting organism. Laxatives may hasten rupture.

Clinical Manifestations. The typical, classic constellation of signs and symptoms of appendicitis is found only in slightly more than 50 per cent of patients. In those able to express themselves clearly, *pain, nausea with vomiting*, and *tenderness* in the right lower quadrant are the chief abdominal manifestations. At first vague and diffuse, the ache becomes more severe in the midepigastrium or periumbilical region before localizing in the right lower quadrant. With a retrocecal appendix, lying alongside the right ureter or near the urinary bladder, pain in the anterior abdomen may be absent but referred to the thigh or right testicle, or may be felt as burning and frequency of urination.

The initial steady pain is due to serosal stretching by edema and to the inflammatory involvement of the lymphatics at the root of the mesentery. The progression of the inflammation beyond the lumen to the adjoining parietal peritoneum is responsible for pain in the right lower quadrant. Further development of necrosis and gangrene to the point of perforation may result in a short period of relief as the pressure within the distended appendix is suddenly released. With the ensuing localized or generalized peritonitis, the severe pain returns and persists until surgical drainage is effected.

Vague *anorexia* or *nausea and vomiting* usually follow the onset of abdominal pain. *Tenderness* on abdominal pressure is the most reliable and constant sign as to the location of the inflamed appendix. *Rebound tenderness* elicited by suddenly releasing manual pressure firmly applied to the abdomen will be maximally felt over the area of appendicitis before rupture and generalized peritonitis have developed. Muscle spasm may be minimal or absent if the perforated appendix is protected by adhesions, is retrocecal, or is separated from the outer abdominal wall by other organs. When the appendix is lying low in the pelvis, next to the rectal wall, tenderness on the right side on rectal examination may be the only objective sign of acute appendicitis.

Fever in acute appendicitis is usually low-grade unless the appendix has perforated. High spiking fever with chills is suggestive of a complicating pylephlebitis.

Moderate *leukocytosis* with a shift in the differential count to immature granulocytes is the rule in uncomplicated appendicitis. Levels above 15,000 suggest the presence of perforation with peritonitis or abscess. A normal white blood cell count, however, which is often found in elderly patients with acute appendicitis, does not exclude this diagnosis.

Perforation and Abscess Formation. Progression of appendicitis to perforation with peritonitis and/or abscess occurs in 1 of 6 patients and is the most important factor in determining mortality. The diagnosis of perforation is suggested by abdominal pain that persists more than 48 hours, temperature above 103° F., leukocytosis over 15,000 per cubic millimeter, a palpable abdominal mass, and physical signs of peritonitis. The development of an abscess following perforation of the appendix is often overlooked, though it occurs in approximately 5 per cent of cases and carries a mortality rate of more than 10 per cent. The signs and symptoms are usually and initially those of a perforated appendicitis in which abdominal pain may have receded, and there are, in addition to pronounced fever, leukocytosis and diarrhea, and a *palpable mass* on abdominal or rectal examination. Occasionally an abscess may first be suspected only weeks or months after an attack of acute appendicitis in which the correct diagnosis had not been established. The presence of an abdominal or pelvic mass detected by tenderness and induration on rectal examination in a patient with persistent or recurrent fever should suggest the diagnosis. The abscess may rupture spontaneously into the rectum or may require drainage.

Peritonitis. The development of a spreading, generalized peritonitis is the most serious complication of acute appendicitis. It is the major cause of death in this disease, more likely to occur in children, the elderly, and in patients with appendicitis who are given laxatives or enemas in the treatment of abdominal pain.

Differential Diagnosis. The varied clinical picture in patients with acute appendicitis makes the diagnosis one to be considered in all conditions with signs and symptoms referable to the abdominal cavity, especially in the right lower quadrant or pelvis. Reliance solely upon the classic picture for diagnosis will be responsible for delay in treatment with its increased morbidity and mortality.

Some of the conditions to be considered in the differential diagnosis, such as twisted *ovarian cyst, cholelithiasis*, and *perforated abdominal viscus*, require surgical therapy. An operation undertaken with the mistaken diagnosis of suspected appendicitis in these instances will thus usually not be harmful.

In *gastroenteritis*, nausea and vomiting precede the abdominal pain, diarrhea is common, and others in the family or community are similarly affected. Spasm of the abdominal wall musculature is lacking. Tenderness, when present, is diffuse. The patient usually has malaise, weakness, and generalized muscle aching.

Lead poisoning of the alimentary form is characteristically associated with colicky pain, at times in the right lower quadrant, and may suggest the pain of appendicitis. The periodic nature of the attacks, their severity, the absence of spasm of the abdominal musculature and of rebound tenderness between episodes of pain, the presence of anemia and of the pathognomonic leadline in the gum margin of poorly cared-for teeth, the unrelenting constipation, and history of exposure to lead should establish the correct diagnosis. (See Heavy Metals in Diseases Due to Chemical Agents.)

Mesenteric adenitis in children under 15 is much more common than acute appendicitis, but in spite of the statistical differences such as less spasm, tenderness, and leukocytosis in the former, this diagnosis may be suspected but often cannot be made accurately except at operation.

Renal or ureteral calculi may produce referred pain in the right lower quadrant, but tenderness in the right flank and the absence of significant fever and leukocytosis will usually direct attention to the genitourinary tract. Hematuria may result from irritation of the contiguous right ureter by an inflamed appendix, but there will seldom be more than 5 to 10 red blood cells per high-power field.

A *ruptured Graafian follicle* may closely simulate acute appendicitis in young females. However, fever and leukocytosis are uncommon, the resulting pain is less localized, and occurs, as its synonym Mittelschmerz suggests, in the middle of the interval between menses. In *ectopic tubal pregnancy*, pain usually develops with catastrophic suddenness, is more generalized, and is associated with rapidly progressive lowering of blood volume and shock. The severity of these clinical signs when added to the abdominal findings in a pregnant woman makes operation imperative. A *twisted ovarian cyst* produces tenderness on movement of the cervix on vaginal examination. The local physical findings are more severe and out of proportion to the relative mildness of the patient's general appearance. *Acute salpingitis* may resemble the pelvic peritonitis of a perforated appendicitis. In spite of dysuria, purulent vaginal discharge, and cervical as well as vault tenderness on pelvic examination, all suggestive of salpingitis, the suspicion of acute appendicitis may be sufficient to warrant operation.

It is well to operate if appendicitis is suspected, since the risk of overlooking this diagnosis is greater than that of laparotomy in patients with gastroenteritis, mesenteric adenitis, diverticulitis, ruptured Graafian follicle, acute salpingitis, lead poisoning, and renal colic.

In patients with *retrocecal appendicitis*, the abdominal pain and tenderness may be sufficiently high in the right upper quadrant to be confused with *acute cholecystitis.* Conversely, acute cholecystitis in patients with ptotic gallbladders may produce pain in the right lower quadrant. The history of fatty food intolerance, the occasional development of jaundice and other signs of extrahepatic biliary tract obstruction will favor cholecystitis. (See Diseases of the Gallbladder and Bile Ducts.) However, in the earlier stages of cholecystitis, it may be less hazardous to explore surgically if the diagnosis of appendicitis is in question. The same rule holds for *regional enteritis,* in which right lower quadrant tenderness, fever, and leukocytosis so suggestive of acute appendicitis, warrant operation. In fact, acute appendicitis is the most common preoperative diagnosis in acute regional enteritis.

Acute diverticulitis may give rise to pain, tenderness, and a mass in the right lower quadrant in the unusual circumstance in which the ruptured diverticulum and resulting peridiverticulitis involve the ascending colon or cecum. Diverticulitis of the sigmoid colon is much more common and may simulate acute appendicitis if the excessively mobile loop of the descending colon comes to rest in the right side of the abdomen. Though recurrent episodes of such attacks associated with diarrhea suggest diverticulitis, the localization in the right side is too much like appendicitis to forego operation (*vide infra*).

Laparotomy is dangerous and must be avoided in a number of diseases with features suggesting appendicitis: pneumonia, myocardial infarction, nephritis, and porphyria.

Right lower lobe pneumonia with diaphragmatic pleural involvement may present with abdominal pain. The absence of spasm and rebound tenderness, the severity of the leukocytosis early in the course of the disease, the presence of pain in the upper abdomen, the increased respiratory rate, cough, and positive chest roentgenographic findings should direct attention to the chest rather than the abdomen. This is one of the few situations in the differential diagnosis of acute appendicitis in which surgery is both unnecessary and harmful.

In *acute myocardial infarction* the diaphragm may be sufficiently implicated to produce abdominal pain. However, the pain is high in the abdomen, the patient is dyspneic, cyanotic, and may be in shock. The ECG should confirm the diagnosis of an acute coronary thrombosis with infarction and prevent the serious mistake of abdominal exploration.

In *acute glomerular nephritis,* nausea, vomiting, and abdominal tenderness may suggest generalized peritonitis due to a perforated acute appendicitis. However, the abnormal urinary findings and blood analyses should establish the correct diagnosis.

Severe colicky pain localized to the right lower quadrant may occasionally be seen in patients with *porphyria.* The absence of muscle spasm and of rebound tenderness and the demonstration of urinary porphobilinogen by means of the Ehrlich aldehyde test favor the diagnosis of porphyria.

Treatment. The treatment of acute appendicitis, as pointed out by Fitz in 1886, is removal of the appendix, preferably within the first 24 or 48 hours of the onset of abdominal pain. With such an approach the mortality rate should be less than one half of 1 per cent. Delay beyond this point often leads to gangrene, rupture, and peritonitis. The morbidity and mortality in appendicitis are almost entirely attributable to these

complications. Surgery undertaken in this late period may permit no more than drainage of an abscess, with removal of the appendix postponed for two or three months.

There has been a plea in some quarters for the conservative, nonsurgical treatment of a perforated appendix and abscess with antimicrobial drugs. In these circumstances, a trial of nonoperative therapy is favored, using antimicrobials and supportive measures for several days; surgery is undertaken if the inflammatory process is not resolved within this period. Such an approach is not generally accepted and is not recommended unless the perforation is late, the localization is definite, and there is no evidence of spreading peritonitis.

Chronic Appendicitis. Recurrent episodes of right lower quadrant pain have been widely attributed to chronic appendicitis. Appendectomies performed in such cases seldom reveal any evidence of local inflammation. It is highly questionable whether chronic appendicitis is to be considered an established clinical entity. The pathologic condition responsible for recurrent abdominal pain is often functional rather than organic. In these circumstances, appendectomy is not only unnecessary; it also frequently aggravates the underlying problem, with recurrence of the original symptoms. The presence of an abdominal scar and a history of surgical intervention may make subsequent diagnosis and management an increasingly complex problem. Operation-prone neurotic patients may attribute their repeated abdominal attacks to the scar and adhesions acquired in an operation undertaken for "chronic appendicitis."

Appendicitis in the Elderly. The classic picture of acute appendicitis is often missing in patients over 60. The history is either inadequate or misleading because of the age or medication and the absence of a reliable confirmatory historian. The physical examination is often confusing because of associated disease that obscures the underlying inflammation and because of the atypical nature of the usual protective mechanisms. Both leukocytosis and fever may be minimal. Because of delay in seeking medical advice and the frequent self-administration of laxatives, many patients are first seen after perforation has already taken place. The relatively poor diagnostic accuracy of 70 per cent and the high incidence of complications, greater than 40 per cent, are factors most responsible for a mortality of 10 to 15 per cent in this age group, in contrast to 1 per cent for the over-all population.

Cope, Z.: The Early Diagnosis of the Acute Abdomen. 11th ed. London, Oxford University Press, 1957, pp. 45-74.

Editorial: Appendicitis. J.A.M.A., 180:154, 1962.

Farmer, R. G., and Turnbull, R. B., Jr.: "Missed" appendicitis: A continuing diagnostic challenge. Cleveland Clin. Quart., 32:125, 1965.

Fitz, R. H.: Perforating inflammation of the vermiform appendix. Amer. J. Med. Sci., 92:321, 1886.

Williams, J. S., and Hale, H. W. Jr.: Acute appendicitis in the elderly. Ann. Surg., 162:208, 1965.

DIVERTICULA OF THE INTESTINES

A *diverticulum* (Latin, "turning aside") is a protruding pouch made up of all the coats of the bowel (true diverticulum) or a herniation of the mucosa through the muscular fibers of the bowel wall (false diverticulum). The distinction is seldom clear-cut. "False" diverticula are especially frequent in the colon and are most often acquired.

Duodenal Diverticula. These are usually found on the concave side of the second portion of the duodenum, just distal to the ampulla of Vater. These diverticula probably result from increased intraluminal pressure at the point where the bile and pancreatic ducts and blood vessels enter. Diverticula in the first portion of the duodenum or in the second portion proximal to the ampulla are related either to peptic ulcers or to traction from adhesions arising from cholecystitis or pancreatitis. Their over-all incidence is approximately 2 per cent, and they are rarely seen before the fourth and fifth decades. They are seldom clinically significant, unless they obstruct or bleed from heterotopic pancreatic or gastric tissue. When symptomatic, treatment is essentially that for peptic ulcer. Surgery is undertaken only when these methods are unsuccessful or in the presence of obstruction or hemorrhage. Their usual location in close proximity to the ampulla of Vater makes such a surgical procedure hazardous.

Meckel's Diverticulum. This vestige of the proximal end of the omphalomesenteric duct is usually found on the antimesenteric border of the ileum, within 75 to 100 cm. of the ileocecal valve. It is more common in males and is generally asymptomatic. It may remain attached to the umbilicus by a fibrous cord and thus serve as a source of small intestinal volvulus and obstruction. Aberrant gastric or pancreatic tissue within the diverticulum may ulcerate and give rise to abdominal pain or hemorrhage, especially in children and young adults.

The cause and location of these complaints are often unsuspected on the basis of the usual gastrointestinal investigation, as the diverticulum is seldom visualized on roentgenographic examination with a barium meal. Acute inflammation of the diverticulum, its most common complication, simulates acute appendicitis and is almost always first recognized at laparotomy. Excision is the treatment for symptomatic Meckel's diverticulum.

Jejunal Diverticula. Generally considered of no clinical significance in the past, massive diverticulosis of the small intestine—usually of the jejunum—may be associated with malabsorption, especially of vitamin B_{12} and fats, resulting in macrocytic anemia and steatorrhea, respectively. (See Diseases of Malabsorption.) Rarely, the diverticula bleed or perforate. The presence of air and fluid in multiple jejunal diverticula in an erect film of the abdomen may simulate the characteristic picture of small intestinal obstruction.

Diverticula of the Large Intestine. A diverticulum of the colon is a herniation of the mucosa through the bowel wall where mesenteric vessels pass through the circular muscle coat at the edge of longitudinal taenia. It has been estimated that 5 to 10 per cent of persons over 40 will develop such diverticula, although recent postmortem examinations have raised their incidence to over 40 per cent in individuals more than 50 years old. Diverticular disease is thus the most common pathologic process in the colon.

The mechanism for the formation of diverticula is still unexplained in spite of their frequency and the increasing attention paid to them since Grasser in 1899 emphasized their importance and De Quervain in 1913 first demonstrated them roentgenographically. Weakness of the colonic wall and increased intraluminal pressure seem to be the most plausible prerequisites. The exaggerated response of the bowel with diverticula to morphine and neostigmine, with the increased intraluminal pressure limited to the involved segment, suggests that spasm and incoordination of muscular contractions are responsible for the increased bowel tonus.

Frequently, diverticula may bleed severely in the apparent absence of inflammation.

Diverticulitis. *Incidence and Pathogenesis.* Approximately 20 per cent of patients with diverticula will develop diverticulitis. Acute diverticulitis is rarely limited to the mucosa. Much more frequently, the sequence of events is a micro- or macroperforation of a diverticulum, due to increased intracolonic pressure, into or beyond the colon wall, followed by periverticular inflammation, *pericolitis, abscess, fistula, or peritonitis* (Fig. 6). If the perforation remains localized, it often responds to conservative management. Recurrent episodes of acute diverticulitis probably represent fresh rupture of a diverticulum.

Diagnosis. The diagnosis is suggested by left lower quadrant pain, occasionally with loose bowel movements, fever, leukocytosis, and tenderness along the course of the left colon. A mass may be felt, and the patient may even be obstructed. Gross bleeding is unusual. Roentgenographic

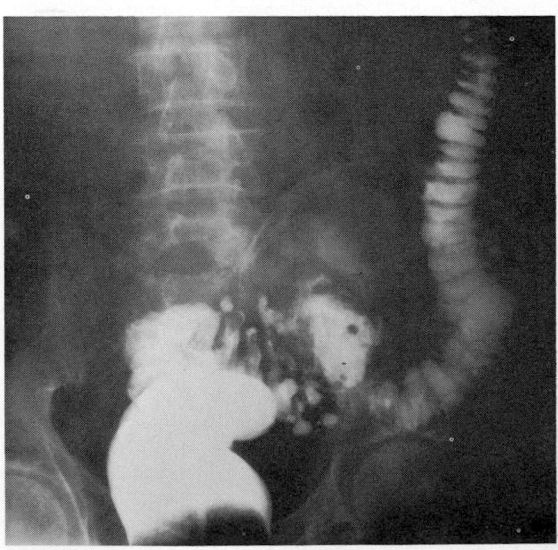

FIGURE 6. Diverticulitis of sigmoid colon with perforation.

findings consist of extravasation of barium from one or more diverticula and a unilateral shallow filling defect in the wall of the colon, associated with a soft tissue mass outside it, consistent with paracolonic inflammation. In some instances, the lumen of the colon communicates with a contiguous abscess or other segments of the bowel. *Fistulous tracts* to the urinary bladder are common and are reflected clinically in the passage of gas and feces in the urine. When the inflammatory process is circumferential, the concentric narrowing may lead to varying degrees of obstruction, and the roentgenographic picture at times may be indistinguishable from that of malignant disease of the colon.

Differential Diagnosis. Symptoms of left-sided crampy abdominal pain that, in the absence of fever and leukocytosis, suggest the diagnosis of *irritable colon*, have been erroneously attributed to diverticulitis because a barium examination of the colon revealed irregular contractions and sawtooth configuration of the sigmoid outline. Histologic examination of many such colons, however, has shown neither diverticula nor inflammation. The pain and roentgenographic configuration are rather due to bowel hypermotility and spasm, with the contracting circular musculature thrown into irregular and inconstant folds closely bunched together.

Carcinoma of the colon is the most important possibility to be considered in the differential diagnosis. Sigmoidoscopy in diverticulitis is negative except for spasm and irritability. Roentgenologic examination of the colon may be safely performed if the clysma is introduced cautiously and without undue pressure. The abrupt change in contour of the bowel and the disruption of the normal mucosal pattern caused by carcinoma are in contrast to the gradually tapering appearance of the longer segment of abnormal colon in diverticulitis. In spite of all these diagnostic measures and the varying picture presented classically by the two diseases, the correct diagnosis may not be established except after surgical exploration and histologic examination, especially since the two conditions may coexist.

Acute appendicitis, especially left-sided and in elderly patients, *pelvic inflammatory disease*, *ulcerative colitis*, and granulomatous colitis (see Granulomatous Colitis) are the other important conditions to be considered in the differential diagnosis.

Treatment. In the uncomplicated cases with fever, leukocytosis, pain, and abdominal tenderness, therapy with ampicillin, 2 to 4 grams parenterally daily, is indicated. Fluid and electrolyte needs should be maintained parenterally, and meperidine rather than morphine should be given for severe pain to avoid increasing intraluminal pressure. If the acute process subsides without any residual sequelae, the patient should be placed on a regimen designed to obviate constipation and colonic spasm. This includes adequate fluid intake, bowel habit training, a high-residue diet, and hydrophilic laxatives such as psyllium (Metamucil), in dosage of one rounded teaspoonful in a glass of water before meals one to three times daily, to increase the lumen of the colon and diminish the higher pressure in the short contracted segments of sigmoid. Removal of the sigmoid colon may be advisable for recurrent episodes of acute diverticulitis. Complications such as massive *hemorrhage*, *obstruction*, *peritonitis*, *abscess*, and *fistula*, especially into the urinary bladder, will require immediate surgery, with resection of the involved segment. The condition of the patient and the findings at operation will influence the decision whether this is to be done as a one-stage procedure or only after a diverting colostomy.

Almy, T. P.: Diverticular disease of the colon — The new look. Gastroenterology, 49:109, 1965.

Fleischner, F. G., and Ming, S.: Revised concepts on diverticular disease of the colon. Radiology, 84:599, 1965.

Painter, N. S., and Truelove, S. C.: The intraluminal pressure patterns in diverticulosis of the colon. Gut, 5:201, 1964.

Welch, C. E.: Diverticulitis of the colon. Amer. J. Gastroent., 29:374, 1958.

Williams, I.: Diverticular disease of the colon. A 1968 view. Gut, 9:498, 1968.

Diseases of the Peritoneum
William V. McDermott, Jr.

THE PERITONEUM — ANATOMIC AND PHYSIOLOGIC CONSIDERATIONS

The peritoneum by definition is the serous membrane that lines the abdominal cavity and that, by the numerous folds into which it evolves through the course of the development of the fetus, covers the surfaces of the abdominal viscera. To give some concept of the total extent of the peritoneum, its surface is roughly equivalent to the total cutaneous area of the body; each of these surfaces comprises about 2500 square inches. The peritoneum itself is of mesodermal origin and is composed of a layer of flat, serrated cells beneath which lie a layer of connective tissue and the blood vessels and lymphatics that must be considered as a functional part of the peritoneum. The peritoneal cavity that is enclosed by the various enfoldings of the peritoneum is a space that is completely closed in the male but communicates in the female with the external environment through the female reproductive system.

Physiologically the primary functions of the peritoneum consist of (1) its powers of absorption and exudation or transudation, which, under normal conditions, are so balanced that there is very little free peritoneal fluid; and (2) the specific property of the peritoneum that characteristically forms adhesions in the presence of an inflammatory process; this is a protective mechanism effecting the localization of a source of infection within the peritoneal cavity that otherwise might give rise to an overwhelming spreading peritonitis. Any of the constituents of the blood pass freely across the peritoneal barrier and, therefore, peritoneal dialysis has been used both in renal failure for removal of nitrogenous products and electrolytes and also in hepatic failure for clearance of dialyzable substances such as ammonia, which can contribute to the metabolic disorders accompanying failure of hepatocellular function.

The intraperitoneal pressure is hydrostatic, and in man measures approximately 8.0 cm. of water in both the upper and lower abdomen. Breathing causes a fluctuation of 2.0 to 4.0 cm. The above measurements are those in the supine position. In the erect position, the lower abdominal intraperitoneal pressure increases to as much as 20.0 cm. of water, although the upper abdominal pressure remains at the same level as in the supine position. Coughing, vomiting, and straining may elevate the intraperitoneal pressure to levels as high as 150 cm. of water. The intraperitoneal pressure rises in a variety of clinical conditions as, for example, in intestinal obstruction. This increase in pressure produces part of the generalized pathophysiologic changes of peritonitis, obstruction, etc., and results in (1) increased thoracic respiratory activity; (2) upward displacement of the diaphragms; (3) venous stasis within the abdomen; (4) a fall in arterial pressure contributing to the other mechanisms of shock that affect the arterial pressure; (5) electrocardiographic changes, particularly noticeable in a notching of the QRS complex; and (6) a reduction in renal flow by as much as 50 per cent and in renal oxygen consumption by almost the same degree.

PERITONITIS

Peritonitis is by definition an inflammatory process of the peritoneal cavity that may be primary or secondary and may appear in an acute or chronic form. In the acute form, from whatever cause, the motor activity of the intestinal tract is decreased, and the intestinal tract becomes distended with gas and fluid. About 70 per cent of the gas is derived from swallowed air, 20 per cent by diffusion from the blood, and 10 per cent from bacterial metabolism. Fluid accumulates as the result of obstruction to free passage of the 7 or 8 liters that are normally excreted daily into the gastrointestinal tract and absorbed from the distal small bowel and colon during the normal functioning of the intestines. Peritonitis is usually of bacterial origin, but frequently one finds an aseptic peritonitis when the inflammatory process is due to blood, urine, bile, or pancreatic juice extravasated into the abdominal cavity.

Diagnosis. The clinical picture of spreading peritonitis is one of increasing diffuse abdominal pain, distention, nausea and vomiting, inability to pass feces or flatus, fever, hypotension, tachycardia, thirst, and oliguria. On physical examination, the patient appears acutely ill and febrile with a hot dry skin and variable abdominal distention. The abdomen is usually acutely tender and tympanitic, often with "rebound." Early in the course, peristalsis is audible, but as the disease progresses, it disappears. In hours the pulse becomes weak and more rapid, and blood pressure falls. Leukocytosis of more than 20,000 cells per cubic millimeter is characteristic, and the cells visualized on Gram stain are almost entirely of the polymorphonuclear leukocyte series with many band forms. Roentgenographic examination (supine, upright, and decubitus) of the abdomen shows dilated large and small bowel with edema of the bowel wall, as evidenced by the distance between adjacent loops of gas-filled small intestine. Abdominal tap with a fine needle is valuable in determining the nature of the exudate, including whether it is chemical or bacterial in origin, and in providing material for microscopy, culture, and drug-susceptibility tests.

The special types of peritonitis will be taken up individually, and the general systemic and metabolic effects of the disease will be considered where they are most applicable under the general discussion on secondary peritonitis.

SECONDARY PERITONITIS

This term applies to the disease to which we ordinarily refer when using the general term "peritonitis." It may be due to the effects of bacteria entering the peritoneal cavity from a perforation in the gastrointestinal tract or from an external penetrating or perforating wound. It may be caused by organisms invading the peritoneum through the reproductive system. Or it may be secondary to severe chemical irritation from the release of the proteolytic enzymes of the pancreas, the digestive juices of the upper gastrointestinal tract, or bile released by perforation of, or trauma to, the biliary system.

The most common causes of bacterial secondary peritonitis are appendicitis, diverticulitis, and gangrenous obstruction of the small bowel from adhesive bands, incarcerated hernia, volvulus, etc.; any lesion resulting in the escape of intestinal micro-organisms may, of course, be the source, including perforating carcinoma, foreign body, ulcerative colitis, and a long list of esoteric diagnoses.

Because of the remarkable resistance of the peritoneal cavity, any sudden insult to the peritoneum tends to become localized, and the disease process itself is self-limiting unless continuous contamination occurs; in this case the process presents a potentially lethal hazard. Before the era of antimicrobial therapy, any continuing intraperitoneal suppuration carried a very high mortality, and even today, with the variety of chemotherapeutic agents available for treatment, it is still attended by significant morbidity and mortality. It is obvious from this initial brief description that the most effective way to treat peritonitis is to remove as soon as possible the source of the bacterial or chemical contamination that has initiated the inflammatory process. If peritonitis is well established, however, and the potentially lethal sequelae have been set in motion, one must base any treatment on a careful evaluation of the effects of peritonitis on various organ systems.

Systemic Effects of Peritonitis. *Circulatory.* Spreading peritonitis invariably places an increased demand on the circulatory system, primarily because of an exudative response that may result in dangerous decreases in the effective circulating blood volume. Fluid lost into the peritoneal cavity under these circumstances is composed of plasma in approximately 50 per cent of its volume. The total fluid, electrolyte, and plasma loss is not accounted for entirely by this exudative response into the peritoneal cavity, but is exaggerated by the accompanying adynamic ileus with increasing fluid losses into the lumen of the gastrointestinal tract. The decreased organ perfusion secondary to this plasma loss and consequent hypovolemia may be exaggerated if the source of the peritonitis is bacterial because endotoxin depresses the circulatory compensation.

Respiratory. In the presence of severe peritonitis, respiratory demands are increased. With increasing ileus and elevation of the diaphragms, ventilatory capacity and respiratory exchange may be interfered with, thus exaggerating the relative oxygen lack.

Fluid and Electrolyte Shifts. In addition to plasma loss, there is a tremendous escape of water and electrolytes into an expanded serous space formed by the peritoneal cavity itself and into the distended lumen of the intestinal tract. One of the important results is a large loss of potassium (which may be masked by hemoconcentration, making EKG's necessary), with a shift of sodium into the intracellular compartment.

Endocrine Response. There is usually an increase in adrenal activity with elevated glucocorticoids and aldosterone, further aggravating potassium loss and sodium retention. Catecholamines may be elevated as a response to decreased volume and, although this response may be effective for a time in maintaining blood pressure, the resulting peripheral vasoconstriction with increased peripheral resistance results in decreased organ perfusion most significantly affecting renal function and cardiac action.

The greatly increased energy expenditure secondary to fever and to the increased caloric requirements caused by the massive inflammatory response also has a debilitating effect.

Treatment. From this simplified description of the metabolic and clinical response to peritonitis, it is obvious that therapy depends primarily on early removal of the source of peritoneal contamination, restoration of plasma volume, replacement of fluid and electrolyte losses as indicated, maintenance of adequate pulmonary function, support of cardiac output, and the use of appropriate antimicrobial drugs to combat the effects of invasive sepsis and the potentially lethal and depressing action of bacterial endotoxin.

Reference should be made to an extremely lethal type of intestinal obstruction that is associated with established peritonitis. Despite the presence of intraperitoneal infection, it is of vital importance to restore intestinal function by lysis of obstructing bands.

The attractive hypothesis that adrenal corticosteroids might prevent the formation of adhesions following operation or other factors initiating this type of peritoneal response has not been borne out by experimental studies. Indeed, steroids often mask the clinical manifestations of the peritoneal response, a particular problem in patients with ulcerative colitis under steroid therapy, in whom lethal perforations of the large bowel may pass unrecognized until the patient is in a terminal state. The use of hyaluronidase, an enzyme with the property of hydrolyzing hyaluronic acid (one of the polysaccharides composing intracellular granular substance), prevents the formation of adhesions and their re-formation after division. It has been used with encouraging results in the peritoneal cavity of man following lysis of obstructing adhesions.

PRIMARY PERITONITIS

This term is usually applied to bacterial infection of the peritoneal cavity by streptococci or pneumococci, which is almost invariably seen in childhood between the ages of two and ten with a maximal age incidence at five. For reasons that are not clear, primary peritonitis is much more common in female children. This may be due to the existence of a portal of entry through the female reproductive tract, since it may occur without any obvious focus elsewhere in the body. In the past, the mortality was high; but with modern chemotherapy the prognosis is excellent if diagnosis can be established early and specific treatment instituted.

GONOCOCCAL PERITONITIS

Gonococcal peritonitis is not a form of primary peritonitis in the strict sense of the word, since it is ordinarily an extension from a primary focus in the female reproductive tract. The signs of inflammation are usually limited to the pelvis, but there may be findings consistent with a mild generalized peritonitis. Occasionally, the patient has right upper quadrant pain and tenderness caused by the "violin string adhesions" above the liver that are thought to be pathognomonic of previous invasion of the peritoneal cavity by gonococci.

TUBERCULOUS PERITONITIS

Tuberculosis occurs in the abdomen as (1) intestinal tuberculosis; (2) tuberculous mesenteric adenitis, formerly a common disease of childhood; or (3) tuberculous peritonitis resulting from (a) miliary tuberculosis, (b) rupture of a caseous mesenteric node, or (c) direct infection from the bowel or fallopian tubes. Four forms have been described but are not clearly demarcated; various combinations may occur in the same patient. These four types have been described as (1) the *ascitic variety*, which is characterized by a peritoneal exudate and numerous tubercles (encysted forms occur, the latter sometimes being mistaken for a mesenteric cyst or abdominal tumor); (2) an *adhesive form*, in which the bowel loops are usually matted together by tuberculous granulation tissue and later by adhesions; (3) *acute tuberculous peritonitis*, characterized by multiple tubercles and a diffuse plastic exudate in which both spleen and lymph nodes are usually concomitantly enlarged; and (4) a *caseous form*, in which there may be multiple individual tumor-shaped masses and sausage-shaped infiltrations of the omentum and mesentery; in this form, redness around the umbilicus may herald the development of a spontaneous fistula. Tuberculous peritonitis is still an important clinical entity and, if the diagnosis is established early, it is responsive to appropriate therapy. (See articles on tuberculosis.)

SUBPHRENIC ABSCESS

By anatomic definition there are six potential subphrenic spaces in which infection may localize. Two of these lie beneath the left diaphragm and four beneath the right diaphragm; of these six spaces, four are actually intraperitoneal and two are retro- and extraperitoneal. On the left side, the anterior intraperitoneal subphrenic space consists of a broad area lying to the left of the falciform ligament below the diaphragm, and the boundaries consist of the left lobe of the liver, the transverse colon and splenic flexure, and the spleen; surgical drainage may be achieved either by the anterior subcostal approach or by a posterior or posterolateral approach through the bed of the twelfth rib. The left retroperitoneal subphrenic space is defined as the area below the diaphragm and above the left kidney to which approach must be made posteriorly.

The right subphrenic area is more complicated anatomically because of the liver with its various attachments and peritoneal reflections. The right anterior subphrenic space between the liver and the diaphragm is bounded posteriorly by the right triangular ligament and medially by the falciform ligament. Access to this area for surgical drainage may be accomplished through the right anterior subcostal area, which also permits exploration and drainage of the right subhepatic space. A broad area lying between the liver and diaphragm has been referred to as the right posterior intraperitoneal space, to which access must be gained through a posterior or posterolateral approach and removal of the twelfth rib. The last of these right subphrenic spaces is extraperitoneal and consists of the area where the reflections of the peritoneum leave the posterior aspects of the right lobe of the liver denuded of peritoneum; infection may localize in this area by extension up the right gutter and form an abscess cavity lying directly posteriorly beneath the bed of the eleventh and twelfth ribs.

The diagnosis should be suspected in any patient with a *persistent or recurrent fever* following a disease or operative procedure that permitted access of environmental or gastrointestinal micro-organisms to the peritoneal cavity. Signs and symptoms depend on the subphrenic space involved, and may include localized subcostal *tenderness* anteriorly or posteriorly, pleural effusion (usually right), *elevation* of the *diaphragm*, fever, *leukocytosis*, and *shaking chills* with bacteremia. Localization by roentgenography is most valuable, as an immobile diaphragm with fluid above is highly suspicious and, as the process develops, an *air-fluid level* may be demonstrated in one of the subphrenic spaces.

Subphrenic abscess is now a rare condition. It represents a complication of various diseases associated with perforations of the gastrointestinal tract that are usually treated early. Because of its increasing rarity it has also become a dangerous complication because it may so often pass unrecognized by attending physicians and, in actual fact, may be masked by the administration of antimicrobial drugs until potentially lethal complications ensue, such as perforation of the abscess through the diaphragm into the pleural space or lung.

DISEASES OF THE OMENTUM

One might reasonably consider the omentum in any discussion of the peritoneum as a whole. No appreciable detrimental effect has ever been observed from removal of the omentum while the organism is existing in a normal state, but in the presence of intraperitoneal infection there is no doubt that the omentum exerts a very specific protective function. It does this by migrating toward a foreign body or an area of inflammation, thus assisting in the mechanism of walling off a pathologic process originating within the abdominal cavity. Torsion and infarction are the main disorders of the omentum. Torsion of a portion of the omentum may occur either spontaneously or secondary to a fixed adhesive point, and may result in devascularization of a part of this structure. The aseptic necrosis thus produced is not a lethal process but may mimic the acute abdomen, and preoperative diagnosis is difficult. Spontaneous idiopathic infarction of the omentum is difficult to diagnose because the signs and symptoms are the same as in any acute intra-abdominal process such as *appendicitis, perforated ulcer, pancreatitis, or mesenteric thrombosis.* No etiologic factors have been recognized in association with idiopathic infarction of the omentum. Although infarction or torsion of the omentum is rarely diagnosed preoperatively, the signs and symptoms of an acute abdominal crisis not accompanied by nausea and vomiting might suggest this particular diagnosis. Since spontaneous infarction usually appears in the right free border of the omentum, it will characteristically mimic the picture of acute appendicitis more than any other intraperitoneal inflammatory process.

SPECIAL PROBLEMS

PNEUMATOSIS CYSTOIDES INTESTINALIS

This term has been commonly used to designate a condition in which multiple gas-filled blebs accumulate in the endothelial-lined spaces in the intestinal wall beneath the serosal surface of the bowel. Most authors believe that the gas is originally present within lymphatic channels, which then become sealed off and cystic as the areas coalesce. The source of the gas has not been explained satisfactorily, although the mechanical theory is plausible in some instances, particularly when the cysts are associated with gastric, duodenal, or intestinal ulcerations. In instances without apparent defects in the mucosa, the cysts may result from *E. coli* infection. A specific deficiency has been suggested by experimental studies in which the disease has been reproduced in hogs fed on diets of polished rice. Regardless of speculation on etiology, most cases of pneumatosis are associated with specific ulcerations of the intestinal mucosa, particularly peptic ulcer with pyloric stenosis. The symptoms are usually due to the associated disease rather than to the condition itself.

Specific physical findings secondary to the pneumatosis do not exist, and the diagnosis is made in most cases by characteristic roentgenographic findings or at laparotomy. Occasionally, these distended subserosal cysts may rupture, resulting in spontaneous pneumoperitoneum.

PNEUMOPERITONEUM

Ordinarily, pneumoperitoneum results from a free perforation in the gastrointestinal tract, and is most commonly associated with a perforated peptic ulcer, although rupture of a diverticulum of the colon may also present with a large amount of free air in the peritoneal cavity. Spontaneous asymptomatic pneumoperitoneum is rare because ordinarily peritonitis results also from the leakage of gastric or intestinal contents. Occasionally, however, a small leak from a peptic ulcer may seal off promptly, and roentgenographic studies may surprisingly demonstrate pneumoperitoneum without symptoms; another possible cause of asymptomatic spontaneous pneumoperitoneum is the rupture of one of the gas cysts of pneumatosis cystoides. Pneumoperitoneum, of course, occurs secondary to any laparotomy, and will persist for ten days to three weeks following the operative procedure.

HEMOPERITONEUM

This term refers to the presence of blood in the peritoneal cavity. It may occur from multiple sources and is usually secondary to penetrating or nonpenetrating trauma. Probably the most common clinical condition is traumatic rupture of the spleen in which characteristically the trauma may be minor and the rupture delayed. Nontraumatic hemoperitoneum is most commonly associated with the rupture of a tubal pregnancy, which occurs ordinarily within the first six weeks of the ectopic gestation.

The initial escape of free blood into the peritoneal cavity is associated with signs and symptoms of peritoneal inflammation, although if the hemorrhage ceases, these symptoms subside promptly and no residual symptoms persist. Reabsorption occurs steadily over a period of several weeks; it is interesting that red cells as such may be absorbed directly from the peritoneal cavity.

CHYLOUS "PERITONITIS"

This term refers to the accumulation of chyle in the peritoneal cavity. The condition is sometimes associated with chylothorax. Since varying conditions may be associated with a cloudy or milky-appearing peritoneal fluid, microscopic or chemical examination is necessary to establish the diagnosis of chylous peritonitis. Chyle contains fat globules, which can be seen by the use of proper staining methods, and, on chemical examination, the fat content is high.

The etiologic factors associated with the appearance of chyle in the peritoneal cavity can be classified as (1) *trauma*, either penetrating or nonpenetrating or secondary to an operative procedure that damages a main duct in the lymphatic system within the abdomen; (2) *intestinal obstruction,* which under certain conditions may result in distention and ultimate rupture of a major lymphatic channel; (3) *congenital lymphangiectasia*; or (4) *malignant disease* or *tuberculous infection* that involves the thoracic duct, cisterna chyli, or a major lymphatic tributary.

If the accumulation of chyle is rapid and massive and requires repeated aspiration, nutritional depletion will be progressive because of the loss of fat and protein. Ordinarily, however, either the accumulation of chyle will subside spontaneously, or at exploration a suture repair of the site of the leak can be carried out successfully.

Since chyle is initially irritating to the peritoneal cavity, the sudden accumulation is accompanied by the triad of abdominal pain, signs of peritoneal irritation, and leukocytosis. Surgical exploration is frequently performed, although if untreated, the acute symptoms will usually subside within a matter of hours, leaving the patient with a distended, nontender, fluid-filled abdomen.

Newer roentgenographic techniques of lymphangiography may serve to clarify in the future the exact diagnosis and the location of chylous obstruction and leaks. With better definition of the source of the chyle leak, the condition should be remediable in most cases. In instances in which continued accumulation occurs and location of the source is not possible, a venous peritoneal anastomosis using the saphenous vein has been described. This will, of course, return the chylous fluid directly into the venous circulation, provided that the valves in the saphenous vein segment are competent.

PSEUDOMYXOMA PERITONEI

This condition is characterized by the prolific growth of mucin-containing cystic masses throughout the peritoneal cavity. The usual source of these implants is either a pseudomucinous cystic tumor of the ovary or a mucocele in the appendix that becomes implanted in the peritoneal cavity either at the time of surgery or through spontaneous rupture. When this unfortunate event occurs, these mucinous masses spread inexorably throughout the peritoneal cavity, and, although the patient may live many years with the disease and repeated surgical intervention may provide excellent palliation for long periods of time, the condition ultimately is lethal. Technically, most of the cases have been categorized as benign because of the great difficulty in finding any cells

microscopically that could be classified as malignant; but from a clinical point of view, this condition represents a low-grade malignant process.

Colloid carcinoma arising from the stomach or colon with peritoneal implants may resemble the picture of pseudomyxoma at laparotomy. The course of this type of highly malignant tumor is one of rapid cachexia and early death. The differentiation can be made by the appearance of many highly malignant cells in the peritoneal implants.

CARCINOMATOSIS PERITONEI

Many types of malignant metastatic disease, particularly those arising from the gastrointestinal tract, pancreas, and ovaries, may present with multiple peritoneal and omental implants. Invariably this type of metastatic malignancy is associated with progressive ascites with a high specific gravity and high protein content, often with large numbers of red blood cells or even gross blood. The diagnosis can be established by demonstrating malignant cells in the fluid by cytologic techniques. The clinical progress of the disease can be altered by instillations of a radioactive colloid such as isotopic gold. This is particularly true in certain types of metastatic ovarian carcinomatosis in which, with proper management, life may be measured in terms of years rather than weeks.

Peritoneoscopy. The procedure consists of making a small skin incision under local anesthesia and then introducing a peritoneoscope, which, combined with an induced pneumoperitoneum, may permit diagnostic observation of much of the abdominal contents. In skilled hands, this may be a useful tool, but the inherent limitations of the procedure have restricted its use. Under the general heading of peritoneoscopy one should also refer to the procedure of culdoscopy, inspection of the pelvic viscera by means of a small opening posterior to the uterus through the pouch of Douglas; it may be a means for preventing laparotomies for obscure or puzzling gynecologic problems.

Neoplastic Diseases of the Alimentary Tract

Malcolm L. Peterson

GENERAL CONSIDERATIONS

In the United States cancer is the second major cause of death; one third of these cancers arise in the digestive organs, mostly in the large intestine. Discussion of a clinical problem of such magnitude

is here focused on the more common neoplasms of the gut, most of which are epithelial in origin.

A few comments pertinent to the general problem of alimentary tract neoplasia provide orientation to current knowledge and areas of research that promise improved understanding of the diagnosis and treatment.

Despite epidemiologic clues that show impressive geographic differences in the incidence of various gastrointestinal malignancies, and thereby suggest environmental causes or genetic determinants of neoplasia, none of the cancers of the gut has been shown to be caused by any of the factors proposed as possible etiologic agents, e.g., ingested carcinogens (food additives, radioactive elements, or trace metals), viruses, or high temperature of foods. The striking decline in death rate from gastric carcinoma has not led to the identification of any factor that causes this neoplasm. Familial patterns in the incidence of neoplasms are not apparent for the common gastrointestinal neoplasms except carcinoma of the stomach.

The usual clinical manifestations of cancer of the alimentary tract are pain, bleeding, and obstruction, regardless of the site. Since such information is not sufficient to establish the nature of the lesion or to identify the portion of the gut that is affected, roentgenographic, endoscopic, and cytologic methods of detection and diagnosis are required. These are still being refined and evaluated to increase diagnostic proficiency and thus improve therapeutic results. Only rarely are chemical or enzymatic measurements of use in the diagnosis of gastrointestinal tumors. There are no changes in absorptive or digestive functions that are currently recognized as attributable to neoplasms per se, and most observed biochemical abnormalities are nonspecific. Search for specific serologic or chemical tests indicative of gastrointestinal malignancy has had only limited success as yet.

Surgery is the most effective means of treating gastrointestinal cancer, but most results are disappointing because metastases often occur before the primary neoplasm manifests itself. Improved therapeutic results can sometimes be achieved with preoperative radiation or postoperative chemotherapy. In only limited instances is radiotherapy itself the best treatment. Regional perfusion with antimetabolites or alkylating agents may improve operative success, but this therapeutic approach is still experimental.

NEOPLASMS OF THE ESOPHAGUS

CARCINOMA OF THE ESOPHAGUS

Etiology. No agent has been shown to cause esophageal carcinoma, but several predisposing or associated lesions have been suggested. There is an apparent correlation between sideropenic dysphagia (Plummer-Vinson or Patterson-Kelly syndrome) and carcinoma of the esophagus. The syndrome of iron deficiency anemia and dysphagia is encountered among women from the northern part of Sweden, many of whom subsequently develop carcinoma of the oropharynx or esophagus. The pathologic changes of sideropenic dysphagia are mucosal atrophy and formation of a web that bridges the lumen in the proximal esophagus. This is the same site in which these women develop carcinoma, thus suggesting the "precancerous" quality of this lesion.

No association between carcinoma of the esophagus and any other acquired lesion has been proved, although an increased incidence of the neoplasm in patients with cardiospasm, lye strictures, or congenital strictures has been suggested. In members of two large families with *tylosis*, a heritable disorder of the skin transmitted as a mendelian dominant, an extraordinary frequency of esophageal carcinoma has been observed. This has not been noted in other families with tylosis so that the significance of association is unclear.

Incidence and Prevalence. Carcinoma of the esophagus is the cause of almost 2 per cent of all cancer deaths in the United States and in the United Kingdom. The incidence is greater in some areas of the world, notably China and Japan. The mortality rate among white Americans has remained constant through the last three decades. Carcinoma of the esophagus has been reported to be more frequent in lower socioeconomic groups. Among nonwhite Americans there is a steadily rising mortality rate, owing partly to an increased longevity and to better case-finding techniques.

Over three fourths of patients with carcinoma of the esophagus are older than 50 years, although patients in their 20's have been reported to have the neoplasm. The disease is twice as common in men as in women.

Pathology. Carcinomas are particularly frequent in three sites in the esophagus: at the level of the arch of the aorta, just above the esophagogastric junction, and in the hypopharyngeal segment. About 50 per cent of the tumors are in the middle third, 30 per cent in the distal third, and the remainder in the upper third. The tumors that occur in the postcricoid area are much more common in women. This may have some bearing on the relationship to sideropenic dysphagia.

The tumors arise from the squamous epithelium and develop into lesions that range from firm, fibrotic, and intramural to friable, proliferative, and intraluminal. Regardless of whether it is primarily invasive or papillary, the neoplasm reduces the flexibility of the wall and in this manner produces the initial symptoms.

Carcinoma of the esophagus usually extends by local invasion and lymphatic spread. The tumor cells spread up and down the wall, but distal carcinomas usually extend into the gastric wall by lymphatic spread. The outward growth of the neoplasm can affect adjacent structures. Tumors in the upper third extend into the trachea. From the middle third the growth is usually into the bronchi, lungs, and major vessels and nerves. The diaphragm, vertebral bodies, pericardium, and heart can be involved by extension from a tumor in the lower third.

Lymph nodes throughout the mediastinum, as well as those of the left gastric and celiac groups, can be involved. Hematogenous dissemination of metastases is less common, but when it occurs, the organs usually affected are liver, lungs, bones, and kidneys.

Clinical Manifestations. The course of the disease correlates with the development of the tumor. While the lesion is restricted to the mucosa or is not yet hemicircumferential, there are usually no symptoms. When the malignancy involves over half of the circumference, the patient begins to experience *dysphagia*. The esophagus is so distensible that uninvolved portions of the wall can be sufficiently expanded by a bolus to permit its passage; however, when the growth has restricted distention or impaired motility, obstruction results. Gradual progression of dysphagia, initially for solids, but later for everything that is eaten, is the most common presenting story, but it is not always so straightforward. Occasionally the patient will experience very *sudden obstruction* to a bolus of food that he could have easily swallowed the day before. Such a history must alert the physician to the likelihood of esophageal carcinoma, and demands a full diagnostic investigation.

In addition to difficult deglutition, patients may experience an unusual retrosternal sensation, commonly referred to the area of the xiphoid and epigastrium, which is dull or burning and often constant, not always associated with swallowing. Such sensations have been produced by esophageal spasm (emotionally induced) or by distention of the esophagus with balloons. Other symptoms resulting from chronic obstruction include *accumulation of secretions* (usually noted on arising), *bad breath* or *bad taste*, and *constant thirst*. As the lesion grows, dysphagia worsens, and the patient chooses a softer diet. The obstruction of the lumen can result in regurgitation of undigested solid food particles and of liquids that may spill into the trachea. Thus, eating becomes an uncomfortable affair associated with severe bouts of *coughing*. All these mechanical problems result in reduced caloric intake. The ensuing *weight loss* can be accelerated by the hypercatabolic effect of *fever*, which often develops as a result of bronchopulmonary inflammation. Pain is not remarkable during the early stages. If it develops later, it is located in the back or the lower sternum. *Anemia* frequently develops in the later stage (although blood loss is not a prominent feature), and this exaggerates the patient's debility.

Metastatic spread of the tumor causes impairment of function of the organs involved. The most common symptom resulting from metastases is unremitting *hiccup* due to involvement of phrenic nerve or diaphragm. Other late complications include extension to the trachea or bronchi, producing a cough; esophageal perforation, producing mediastinitis, empyema, or tracheoesophageal or bronchoesophageal fistula (Fig. 1);

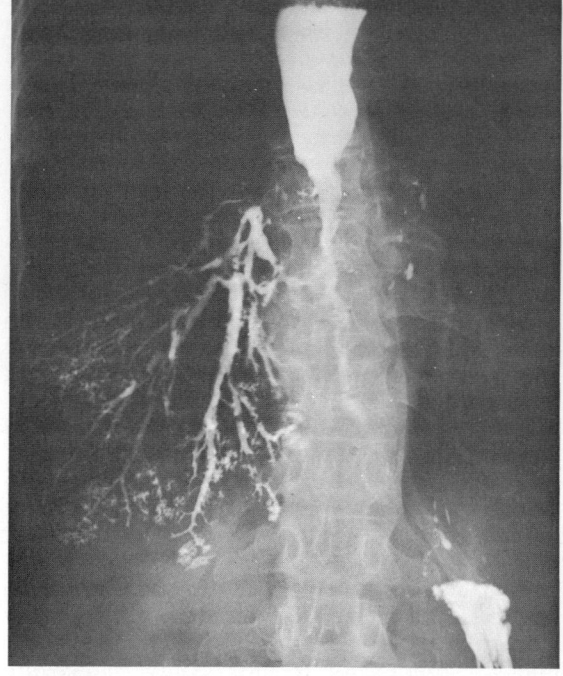

FIGURE 1. Carcinoma of the esophagus. A bronchoesophageal fistula has resulted from the extension of this tumor into the right bronchus. Note the overhanging irregular margins of the narrowing in the esophagus and slight proximal dilatation.

and extension into the major vessels, producing hemorrhage. Occasionally, recurrent laryngeal nerve involvement causes hoarseness. Depending on the sites of distant metastases, patients may also complain of jaundice, abdominal discomfort, cyanosis, and dyspnea.

Physical signs other than weight loss are lacking until progression of the tumor produces secondary states of anemia or inflammation.

Diagnosis. Investigation of the esophagus depends chiefly on roentgenologic techniques. The barium swallow must be done under fluoroscopic observation to look for filling defects or delay of the bolus and to ensure optimal positioning for roentgenograms. The usual appearance of a carcinoma is a constant filling defect with ragged margins (Fig. 1). The column of barium tapers toward the lesion and there is only slight proximal dilatation. Increased peristaltic activity is commonly noted. The regularity of the mucosal folds is destroyed by the tumor.

After the contrast study is done, it may be necessary to perform esophagoscopy. By this means, direct inspection and biopsy of the mucosal lesion can be carried out. Cells washed from the esophagoscope or obtained by appropriate washing of the esophagus should be examined by cytologic methods for evidence of malignant disease.

Differential Diagnosis. There are few diseases that can be confused with carcinoma of the esophagus. The major one is *benign stricture* secondary to peptic esophagitis. This lesion can be associated with a short history of dysphagia and with a roentgenographic appearance similar to that of a malignant neoplasm, although most tumors show evidence of a mass and erosion and destruction of the mucosa. Esophagoscopy, biopsy, and cytologic study should make the distinction possible.

Cardiospasm is a cause of dysphagia in middle age, but the history is usually of an intermittent difficulty in swallowing fluids and solids. Often the blockade diminishes to allow passage of swallowed material in contrast to the persistent obstruction caused by a neoplasm. Dysphagia resulting from cardiospasm gradually increases in severity, and in the advanced stages such obstruction may lead to regurgitation of undigested food and copious amounts of ropy mucus. The slow progress of cardiospasm usually results in dilatation of the esophagus to produce a characteristic appearance of mega-esophagus above the "beaked" stricture in the zone of the gastroesophageal junction. The esophagoscopic appearance of this stricture is that of a purse string without mucosal disruption. Studies of esophageal motility permit conclusive differentiation between cardiospasm and tumor, although one must be aware that the two conditions are known to coexist. (See Disorders of Motility.)

A *leiomyoma* of the esophagus is distinguishable from a carcinoma on the basis of their respective roentgenographic characteristics. (See Other Neoplasms of the Esophagus, *infra*.) The benign lesion, being intramural, usually produces no mucosal destruction, but has a smooth contour with a round shoulder. Malignant growths have a rough surface and produce an irregularly tapering margin of the filling defect. It is important to recall that food impacted above a stricture or other benign narrowing can give a roentgenographic appearance not unlike that of a carcinoma.

It is often difficult to decide on the basis of roentgenographic or esophagoscopic appearances whether a tumor in the distal esophagus is primary in that organ or has invaded from a carcinoma that is primary in the stomach. The distinction is often impossible without histologic evidence. Undoubtedly some of the so-called adenocarcinomas of the esophagus are tumors that arise from rests of gastric tissue in the distal esophagus. This confusion has created some difficulty in assessing therapy and the natural history of esophageal cancer.

Treatment and Prognosis. Treatment of carcinoma of the esophagus is primarily surgical. Recent experience with high voltage x-radiation promises that some improvement in the very poor therapeutic results can be achieved with preoperative radiation or even with x-ray alone, especially in proximal cancers. Patients who are free of evidence of distant metastases are considered operable. Depending on the site of the tumor, the mortality rate for esophagectomy is from 15 to 20 per cent. Staged operations for carcinoma of the middle third of the esophagus in debilitated patients have lowered the surgical mortality. Lesions in the proximal third are more difficult to resect, and have a higher operative mortality.

Even if the patient is apparently a candidate for esophagectomy, the procedure is essentially palliative because undetectable local extension has usually occurred when the patient first experiences symptoms. It is for this reason that total esophagectomy has been recommended despite an apparent lack of intramural extension. Untreated patients usually die within a year. Although the five-year survival after operation is very low (less than 5 per cent), surgery offers the patient the best hope for extended life and comfort.

When the patient is adjudged "incurable" at surgery, a palliative procedure should be performed to afford him comfort in eating and freedom from pain. For these purposes an esophagojejunostomy to bypass the lesion can be done; partial esophagectomy or esophagogastrectomy is sometimes performed.

OTHER NEOPLASMS OF THE ESOPHAGUS

Leiomyoma. Leiomyomas are the most common benign neoplasms of the esophagus. These may be more common than clinical experience indicates, since tumors less than 1 to 2 cm. in diameter often fail to produce symptoms, and are detected only as incidental findings at autopsy. The tumors arise from the muscularis and, as intramural growths, impinge on the lumen without producing any damage to the overlying mucosa until they grow large. The major symptom caused by these tumors is *dysphagia;* rarely, there may be *bleeding.* Roentgenographically a leiomyoma has a round shoulder with a smooth surface, and esophagoscopy reveals nothing but flattening of the mucosa over the tumor. Although it has been repeatedly suggested that leiomyomas undergo malignant change, there is no clinical or pathologic evidence that this is true of tumors of this type that arise in the esophagus. The treatment of esophageal leiomyomas is surgical; simple enucleation from the wall is sufficient, and resection is usually unnecessary.

NEOPLASMS OF THE STOMACH

CARCINOMA OF THE STOMACH

Etiology. *Hereditary Influences.* Despite many epidemiologic and experimental investigations, no causative agent for carcinoma of the stomach is known. Several genetic influences and a few so-called precancerous factors have been noted, but their relationship to tumor formation is unknown. An increased familial incidence of carcinoma of the stomach is well established. Studies of the incidence of gastric carcinoma in twins have shown that the frequency of this neoplasm in both members of the pair is greater in monozygotic than in dizygotic twins. Aird has demonstrated that another genetic correlation is the greater than expected frequency of blood type A among patients with carcinoma of the stomach. In the control population the frequency of group A type was 39.8 per cent, whereas in the population with gastric cancer it was 44.8 per cent. Blood group O was correspondingly lower. The probability of this having been merely chance observation was less than one in ten thousand, and such unexpected distributions have now been seen in similar studies elsewhere. Obviously having blood type A is not the *sine qua non* of the disease, but it is of interest in consideration of etiologic factors. The only other group of cancer patients in which there is such an anomalous distribution of blood type is that with tumors of the salivary glands.

Adenomatous Polyps. Aside from these hereditary influences on the incidence of gastric carcinoma, several lesions of the gastric mucosa, viz. *adenoma, atrophic gastritis,* and *peptic ulcer,* have been thought to be premalignant. Malignant change in adenomatous gastric polyps is unlikely; many gastric polyps have been observed over long periods of time in which no transformation has been found. Benign polyps are not often found in stomachs that have been removed for carcinoma, whereas almost 40 per cent of patients with a gastric adenoma have more than one. Nevertheless, there is indisputable evidence of malignant cells in parts of polyps that otherwise appear benign. Malignant polyps in the stomach are probably carcinomatous from the onset rather than transformations from adenomas to adenocarcinomas.

Atrophic Gastritis. In atrophic gastritis the histologic changes (mucosal atrophy and intestinal metaplasia) occur in those same areas in which carcinoma commonly develops; in stomachs that have been removed for carcinoma, atrophic gastritis is frequently seen in the mucosa that is not involved in the malignant process. However, this is seen with the same frequency in stomachs of patients of the same age and sex who do not have carcinoma. Diminished hydrochloric acid production is also a feature common to atrophic gastritis, carcinoma of the stomach, and advancing age. Thus, it is difficult to ascribe the role of "premalignant" to atrophic gastritis only. Among patients with *pernicious anemia* there is an increased incidence of gastric carcinoma, but the connection here is difficult to isolate because patients with pernicious anemia also have an increased frequency of group A blood type, atrophic gastritis, achlorhydria, and a higher than normal incidence of gastric adenomas. In any event, patients with pernicious anemia must be considered prime candidates for development of gastric cancer. At present the interrelationship between the occurrence of gastric carcinoma and the presence of pernicious anemia, achlorhydria, atrophic mucosal changes, and adenomas is con-

fusing, even more so if the blood group aspect is also considered. This is a problem that needs more study before a causal relationship can be assigned.

Peptic Ulcer. Peptic ulcers of the gastric mucosa have been thought capable of undergoing malignant change. There are well substantiated examples of histologic evidence of malignant cells in the margins of otherwise typical benign gastric ulcers. The problem is not decided, however, for differing explanations of the finding have been offered, and no satisfactory proof for any of them has emerged. Unquestionable histologic evidence of malignant cells in mucosal ulcers is offered as evidence that the ulcers become malignant, but opponents of this view argue that the majority of these are the result of devitalization of mucosa by an invading tumor and that the ulcer is the secondary event rather than the initiating one. It is argued also that the few patients with peptic ulceration and malignant growth are only that portion of the population with peptic ulcer who develop gastric carcinoma.

Environmental Factors. Epidemiologic studies that have detected differences in the incidence of gastric carcinoma have been designed to determine whether unique environmental factors are causative. Thus far the search has been unrewarding. Alcohol, smoked fish, formation of carcinogens such as benzpyrene in barbecued meats or heated fats, and deficiency of dietary magnesium have been implicated, but there is no direct evidence that indicts any of these.

Incidence and Prevalence. In the United States, cancer of the stomach is one of the leading causes of death. An inexplicable decrease in the mortality in the United States over the last 30 years has brought the age-adjusted death rate down by about 5 per 100,000 population in each successive decade to the present total rate of 9 per 100,000 population. This unquestionably reflects a true decline in incidence, although improved therapeutic success may be partly responsible. No such change in incidence is apparent in most other nations. Extraordinary mortality rates from gastric cancer are reported from Japan, Iceland, and Austria. Although such mortality figures must be considered perspective—for other factors affect these statistics—there are remarkable regional differences in the incidence of gastric carcinoma, even within countries. In Wales the mortality rate is three times greater than it is in southeast England.

Carcinoma of the stomach is twice as prevalent among men as among women, and this ratio is maintained regardless of the over-all incidence in the various populations. The neoplasm has been found in all age groups, but most commonly in patients 50 to 69 years of age.

In several countries it has been observed that the incidence of gastric cancer is greater in lower socioeconomic groups than in the higher ones.

Pathology. Carcinoma develops in all areas of the stomach; the sites of predilection are antrum, lesser curvature, cardia, and fundus, in descending order of frequency. Occasionally multiple tumors may be found. Morphologically the tumors can differ, most being circumscribed, exophytic, fungating growths containing ulcerations (Fig. 2), whereas some are widespread and invasive in the wall of the stomach to produce the "leather bottle" appearance of linitis plastica (Greek, meaning linen net, so-called because of the network arrangement of submucosal connective tissues interspersed with malignant cells). An even more uncommon type is the superficial spreading carcinoma, which is restricted to the mucosa, muscularis mucosae, and submucosa, and gives a finely nodular appearance to the mucosal surface. Histologically there are wide variations in tumors from well differentiated types to wildly anaplastic ones.

Carcinoma of the stomach generally spreads by direct invasion to adjacent organs and by lymphatics to the lymph nodes. Thus the liver, pancreas, or transverse colon is often incorporated into the tumor mass. The tumor grows intramurally and often crosses the esophagogastric junction to invade the lower esophagus. Such submucosal growth can extend for surprising distances and can restrict the distensibility of the esophagus. Direct extension across the pylorus from prepyloric lesions does occur (despite Rokitansky's dictum to the contrary), but it is uncommon.

Lymphatic metastasis occurs early, judging by the extent of lymph node involvement in most resected stomachs. The particular local nodes involved depend on the site of the tumor, but from the local nodes the spread is commonly to the nodes in the preaortic area, porta hepatis, and mediastinum. Distant lymphatic metastases sometimes develop in the left supraclavicular lymph nodes (Virchow's node), reputedly on the basis of thoracic duct involvement.

In addition to contiguous spread through the surrounding tissues, gastric carcinoma cells frequently seed the peritoneal cavity. Such peritoneal implants have been found in one third of autopsies on patients with this neoplasm. Such a metastasis can give rise to a Krukenberg tumor, i.e., a secondary ovarian tumor of mucus-containing signet-ring cells.

Hematogenous spread of gastric cancer results most commonly in metastatic growth in liver, lungs, and bone. Often pulmonary metastases are diffuse, giving a picture of miliary dissemination.

Clinical Manifestations. Symptoms. Unfortunately, the early phase of growth of the tumor is not associated with symptoms. By the time symptoms occur to an intensity that makes the patient seek medical advice, the tumor is usually found to have extended to tissues outside the stomach. The insidious nature of the disease is emphasized by the fact that, even after operation has disclosed extensive inoperable tumor, some patients experience no symptoms for months afterward. Apparently symptoms do not occur until *ulceration*, *obstruction*, *necrosis*, or *immobility* has been produced by the tumor.

The most frequently observed presenting complaints of patients with gastric cancer are *weight loss*, *pain* or *indigestion*, *weakness*, *anorexia*, and *vomiting*. Weight loss has been found to be the most common complaint among collected histories of patients with carcinoma. Weight loss often seems inordinately great, but is usually 10 to 15 pounds when the patient is first seen. Inadequate caloric intake usually results from combinations of anorexia, pain, vomiting, and dysphagia.

The abdominal *pain* is poorly localized and very insidious in its onset. It is usually not referred to as "pain" by the patients, but as an awareness of "pressure," "fullness," "ache," or "bloating." Most patients have difficulty describing the sensation and may call it "indigestion," "dyspepsia," or "gas." At first the patient is hardly aware that he is experiencing transient episodes of mild upper abdominal discomfort until suddenly he recognizes that his sensation has been recurrent. To about 20 per cent of patients it is similar to episodes of dyspepsia that they have had off and on for as long as they can recall. The sensation, or pain, is most commonly epigastric in location, although often it is noted to be in the right upper quadrant; less frequently it is retrosternal or in the left upper quadrant. It is apparent that pain can arise from an ulcer in the tumor itself or by invasion involving a pain-sensitive structure, e.g., pancreatic invasion is often accompanied by pain radiating through to the back. About half the patients note pain immediately after eating, but the others observe no relationship of the sensation to ingestion of food or drink. Often this discomfort can be relieved by an ulcer regimen. Such misdiagnosis or symptomatic treatment, either self-directed or by advice of a physician, may be a delaying factor that prevents effective treatment.

Anorexia is a remarkably common feature of the

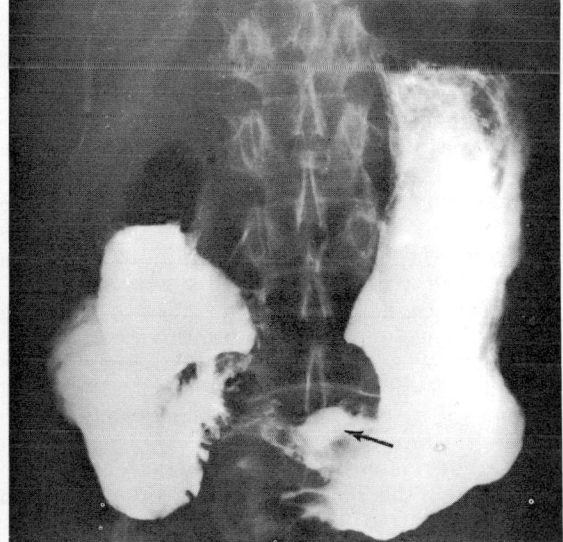

FIGURE 2. Carcinoma of the stomach. The tumor has involved the entire antrum and produced a characteristic filling defect and mucosal destruction. An ulcer within the mass is indicated by the arrow.

histories even in the absence of other complaints that would discourage eating. The patient may note that his appetite is normal until he takes one or two bites of food, and then he feels satiated or even uncomfortably full. Linitis plastica often causes severe limitation of the quantity that the patient can eat. Taking a careful history is of great importance in regard to these points. By appropriate questions one can often bring out that the patient has unconsciously altered his dietary habits, that his clothes have become loose-fitting, or that he becomes fatigued unusually easily. Weakness resulting from a deficient nutritional state is probably compounded by anemia, which is present in two thirds of the patients.

When vomiting is a feature of the history, it may indicate that the tumor involves the prepyloric area, and is causing intermittent obstruction. Hematemesis is rarely a complaint, but if it is, it is found most commonly to be associated with lesions in the cardiac area. Indeed, bleeding is rarely profuse, and relatively few patients (about 15 per cent) complain of melena despite the frequency of anemia.

Other presenting complaints have been recorded for patients with gastric carcinoma: onset of eructations (occasionally malodorous), unpleasant breath, singultus, diarrhea, awareness of an abdominal mass, or even constipation as a reflection of diminished food intake. Many of the chief complaints are manifestations of anemia: dizziness, fainting, dyspnea, pallor, and burning of the tongue.

The foregoing are mostly initial symptoms and do not necessarily carry prognostic significance; other complaints, which may not preclude successful treatment, are usually present only after other organs have been involved. These symptoms include dysphagia caused by esophageal involvement, awareness of an increased abdominal girth resulting from ascites, jaundice caused by metastases to the liver or lymph nodes in the porta hepatis, and bone pain resulting from pathologic fracture at a metastatic site. Rarely the patient may present with only a brief history of acute abdominal pain caused by gastric perforation. In one study 10 per cent of patients with perforation of the stomach were found to have carcinoma as the underlying cause.

Physical Examination. The physical examination is usually normal. The impression of chronic illness is surprisingly infrequent in most initial examinations. Palpation of the abdomen discloses a mass in less than half the patients. When a mass is palpable, it often indicates extragastric extension, although some pyloric tumors can be felt near the umbilicus. Fundal tumors are usually not palpable behind the rib cage, but tumors in the body can sometimes be felt in the epigastrium. Tenderness is usually not elicited unless a mass is present. Pallor, cheilosis, and other signs of anemia are not ordinarily seen despite the usually low hemoglobin measurements.

Hepatomegaly is relatively common, but does not always indicate metastases. On rare occasions metastatic extension is detectable by discovery of nodules on rectal ("Blumer's shelf") or pelvic examination, or by actually seeing a tumor nodule in the umbilicus. Other evidence of advanced disease is discovery of left supraclavicular lymph node enlargement.

Diagnosis. A history of vague epigastric complaints, anorexia, and weight loss usually directs the attention of the physician to the upper gastrointestinal tract as the site of disease, even though ultimately the patient may be shown to have a benign ulcer of the stomach, cholelithiasis, pancreatic neoplasm, or even angina pectoris.

Laboratory Studies. With carcinoma of the stomach in mind, the clinician must proceed to laboratory studies until an explanation for the complaints is found, and the suspicion of gastric cancer is either abolished or confirmed. Examination of the blood will disclose a hypochromic, microcytic anemia in two thirds of patients. Often the degree of anemia seems far out of proportion to demonstrable blood loss; in some patients an aspect of hemolysis has been demonstrated. Testing the stool for occult blood discloses bleeding in 45 per cent of the patients, but only 10 to 15 per cent will give a history of melena.

Roentgenologic Findings. Barium study of the upper gastrointestinal tract is essential for the evaluation of a patient suspected of having gastric cancer. Satisfactory examination requires that the patient be in the fasting state so that there are no interfering gastric contents. Fluoroscopic examination is essential because so many valuable features of the examination are not detectable in roentgenograms alone, e.g., any hold-up or splitting of the stream of barium at the cardia, impairment of peristaltic motion and immobility of the gastric wall. Fluoroscopy is necessary also to ensure optimal positioning for filming of suspicious areas. The mucosal pattern must be thoroughly studied and the fundus fully visualized. This can be done by using the air bubble for a double-contrast study. Since patient cooperation is so important for optimal examination, it is very helpful if the purpose and nature of the study be explained to the patient by the physician who recommends it.

Thorough roentgenographic and fluoroscopic examination permits the detection of tumors as filling defects (Fig. 2), areas of rigidity, ulceration, or mucosal irregularity and distortion. Most lesions can be detected on the basis of such an examination, and the diagnostic accuracy approaches 95 per cent if re-examinations are done to study questionable findings. Most lesions which are missed by barium studies have been found to lie in the fundus or cardia. A cascade stomach (the fundus is festooned to form a sacculation from which the barium cascades into the body) makes evaluation of this area particularly difficult.

In general, malignant neoplasms of the stomach appear as fixed filling defects with evidence of mural rigidity and deformity. An ulcer may be seen in the mass (Fig. 2), or it may simply appear as a crater in the mucosa. Malignant processes usually cause destruction of the mucosal pattern and irregularity of the rugae. Careful "spot-films" with abdominal pressure can often show characteristic semitranslucent halos of tumor tissue around the ulcer. Despite a highly accurate evaluation of the nature of most gastric ulcers, there are always some lesions that cannot be identified absolutely on roentgenologic grounds. Periodic roentgenologic examination of the stomach along with a study of gastric cytology (*vide infra*) is recommended for patients over 45 with pernicious anemia, in view of the high incidence of stomach cancer in this disease.

Gastroscopy. Gastroscopy is a useful adjunct to the barium examination. Visualization of gastric lesions by optical or photographic means has been greatly facilitated by use of fiberoptics instruments combined with miniaturized cameras. In experienced hands these techniques can extend the capability of detecting gastric tumors by confirming, differentiating, or even adding to the roentgenographic findings. Color photographs taken with stepwise rotation and withdrawal of the gastrocamera according to a protocol designed for maximal attention to the area in question give a permanent record of a lesion (Fig. 3). A photographic record of lesions has advantages for serial evaluation and for viewing by others than the endoscopist. Despite the technical improvements which afford better and more complete visualization with less discomfort for the patient, these methods still do not achieve complete accuracy.

Cytology. Gastric biopsy under gastroscopic control is being developed into a suitable technique, but blind aspiration biopsy is useless. Thus, the most satisfactory means of diagnostic histologic examination is the cytologic study of gastric washings. Cancer cells exfoliate more readily than normal cells, and the recognition of malignant cells in the aspirate is excellent evidence for the presence of a tumor. Several negative examinations support an opinion of absence of malignant disease, but do not exclude the possibility that a tumor is present. Unfortunately the technique is not universally applicable because a competent cytologist must be available if the results are to be confidently interpreted. In the large medical centers where meticulous technique of gastric lavage and reliable cytologic examination are available, accurate diagnoses are made in 95 per cent of patients with carcinoma of the stomach, and false positive interpretations (after repeated studies) occur only rarely. Use of this technique in conjunction with roentgenologic, gastrocamera, and endoscopic studies affords the greatest possibility of accurate diagnosis.

Observation that exfoliated malignant cells fluoresce under ultraviolet light after the patient has ingested tetracycline has led to the proposal

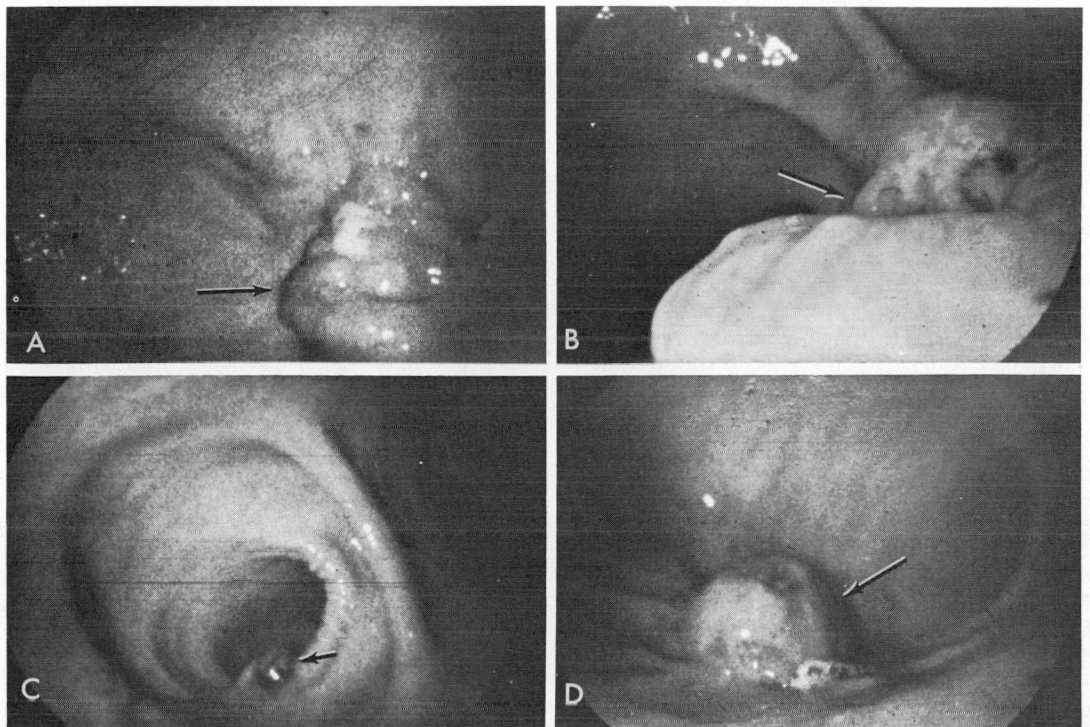

FIGURE 3. Four gastric lesions photographed with the gastrocamera (reproduced from 5 mm. color transparencies). *A*, Adenocarcinoma (arrow) seen on the posterior aspect of the stomach near the incisura angularis. *B*, Benign gastric ulcer (arrow) from a tangential view showing the incisura angularis with the antral region to the left and fundus to the right. The edematous rolled margins of the ulcer surround the typical necrotic center; there is no evidence of neoplasia. *C*, This adenomatous polyp (arrow) in the gastric antrum had bled persistently, causing the patient to become severely anemic. The 5 to 6 mm. lesion was seen in only one of several carefully performed upper GI series. Its size, shape, and smooth contours are consistent with the subsequently proved diagnosis of adenoma. *D*, Leiomyoma (arrow) on the posterior wall of the body of the stomach lying above the incisura angularis. Note the obviously submucosal character of this lesion and its typical umbilication by an apical ulcer.

of this technique for the diagnosis of gastric cancer. Unfortunately, even the most careful technique gives a large number of falsely positive and negative examinations so that this procedure falls short of the accuracy of examinations of exfoliated cells stained by the Papanicolaou method.

Other Diagnostic Procedures. Aside from the observation of the anatomic evidence of carcinoma of the stomach, there are several other diagnostic tools for further evaluation of the patient. Intubation alone can be of value because the presence of altered blood or of more than a few flecks of fresh blood in the aspirate is abnormal and may indicate presence of malignant disease. Following removal of the overnight secretions, lavage for exfoliative cytology or an augmented histamine test can be performed. (See Acid-Peptic Disease.) The augmented *histamine test* is of use when it is properly executed, offering one strong point of differentiation: an ulcer that is found in the presence of true achlorhydria is almost surely a malignant ulcer. There is a positive correlation between hypochlorhydria and gastric cancer, but the significance of this finding in the consideration of an individual patient is very small because many patients with benign peptic ulcers have hypochlorhydria.

The discovery of increased amounts of β-glucuronidase in gastric juice from patients with gastric cancer suggests that not only may this measurement be a means of detecting carcinoma of the stomach, but it can assist in the differentiation of a benign or malignant ulcer. Gastric juice of pH greater than 3.0 can be tested rapidly for β-glucuronidase; levels over 1000 Fishman units are abnormal, and indicate that gastric cancer is probably present.

Differential Diagnosis. The range of possible causes of nonspecific upper gastrointestinal symptoms is narrowed by roentgenographic studies of the gut. As soon as the physician considers gastric ulcer or neoplasm as the cause for a patient's complaints, he must proceed with a barium examination of the stomach. Too often, however, he postpones the investigation of the patient's complaint and temporizes with symptomatic treatment. If a satisfactory roentgenologic study demonstrates no gastric abnormality and evidence points to another organ as the locus of disease, the physician can justifiably redirect his attention. If a duodenal ulcer is seen, the likelihood of gastric cancer is extremely small. Similarly, gallbladder, pancreatic, esophageal, and cardiac pathology are evaluated. On the other hand, if the history warrants further consideration of the diagnosis of carcinoma of the stomach or if there are any unexplained roentgenographic findings, more extensive examination is demanded.

The diagnosis most likely to be confused with carcinoma is peptic ulcer of the stomach. By history the two diseases are similar, and roentgenologically the distinction can be very difficult. Inflammatory reaction in a peptic ulcer can produce a raised everted rim that resembles neoplastic tissue with a deep conical ulcer and distorted mucosa. A malignant process can invade the wall without much mucosal disturbance, and may show merely a small ulcer crater. Knowing that such mimicry occurs, the physician must immediately pursue further studies to determine whether the ulcer is benign or malignant. If gastroscopy, gastrocamera, gastric analysis, and cytologic studies do not resolve the question, he must consider laparotomy. However, at this point it is often useful to try to decide the nature of such a lesion by placing the patient on an intensive ulcer regimen, in the hospital if necessary, with the purpose of observing whether the symptoms improve and the roentgenologic, gastrocamera, or endoscopic appearance of the ulcer improves during four to six weeks of such a program. If the ulcer does not heal, the patient should then have a laparotomy. Operation should be done before the anticipated end of the trial if the expected improvement does not occur or if weight loss or gastrointestinal bleeding continues while treatment is in progress. A frequent criticism of this trial of therapy is that ulceration of tumors may show healing under these circumstances, but this occurs very rarely. If there is any question about the patient's intention to cooperate in such a program, it is better to recommend immediate surgery. (See Acid-Peptic Disease.)

Because of the silent growth period of carcinoma of the stomach, cancer detection surveys based on mass roentgenologic studies have been conducted. As it is manifestly impossible to have enough personnel and equipment to do upper gastrointestinal series on all the population, it has been proposed to limit the survey to persons most likely to have gastric cancer. The selections have been based on age, sex, and family history, but the most meaningful selection has been based on the presence of achlorhydria. By this means, the detection of unsuspected carcinoma of the stomach can be brought from 0.04 per cent in a random population of men and women more than 50 years of age up to 1.0 per cent in the selected population. Such public health measures are still exploratory, but the early experience has been promising enough to warrant further investigation. Against such surveys are the problems of limited money and personnel, the hazards of radiation, and the inaccuracies of the roentgenologic examination. Perhaps by the training of more medical personnel, the use of image intensifiers to reduce the radiation exposure, substitution of the fibroscope-gastrocamera technique, and the education of the public to an awareness of public health needs, surveys of this kind may become practicable on a wide scale.

Treatment and Prognosis. Carcinoma of the stomach can be treated surgically. Indeed, this is the only therapy that can favorably influence the outcome of the disease, but opinion regarding the best operative procedure is not uniform. In patients deemed operable, total resection of the stomach has recently been favored. Commonly in this procedure the spleen, tail of the pancreas, and all attendant lymph nodes are removed. The proponents of total gastrectomy argue that their operative mortality is not much more than that for subtotal resection, but that the chances of survival are much higher. In this operation the usual reconstruction is an interposed loop of jejunum or an esophagojejunostomy with Roux-en-Y. Following recovery from the operation, the patient can eat satisfactorily, gains back most of his weight, and does not develop nutritional deficiencies if vitamin B_{12} and iron are given.

Many other surgeons do partial gastric resection, taking out the tumor and at least a 4-centimeter margin of apparently healthy tissue. They argue that the more extensive procedure does little to alter the prognosis because tumor "recurrences" are distant metastases that were probably present but undetected at operation and do not arise from unresected tumor tissue in the stomach. Surgeons favoring this view usually do a modified Billroth II procedure for distal tumors and either a proximal-subtotal or a total gastrectomy for proximal ones. Perhaps the necessity for more extensive resection for high-lying tumors may explain the greater mortality rate for these lesions.

At the time of laparotomy, metastatic spread may preclude curative resection, but palliative gastroenterostomy, with or without resection of the tumor, should be performed in many cases in order to give the patients the most comfort possible.

Treatment of gastric carcinoma by x-ray has not been successful, but investigations are under way to determine whether brief preoperative radiation may improve surgical results as it has in other tumors. Chemotherapy by means of postoperative regional perfusion with antitumor compounds has not yet had sufficient study to determine whether it will afford adjunctive means for more effective treatment.

Regardless of the operative procedure, the physician is obligated to ensure that the patient is in optimal preoperative condition. Preoperative care includes specific attention to the depleted red cell mass and blood volume. The albumin pool is commonly reduced (perhaps in part because of direct intragastric loss of albumin as a result of the tumor), but this may be masked by the reduction of the blood volume so that appropriate blood, electrolyte, and fluid replacement must be carried out.

The results of surgical treatment are frustratingly poor. *The most favorable data* show that the five-year survival rate of those patients undergoing "curative" surgery, even excluding immediate postoperative deaths, is 30 per cent. The five-year survival rate of all patients with carcinoma of the stomach, whether operated on or not, is 5 to 10 per cent. Analyses of the diagnostic and therapeutic experience in this disease have shown that the most important factor influencing prognosis is the growth behavior of the neoplasm. When the lesion is confined to the stomach, the five-year survival is 35 per cent, but when metastases have occurred, this falls to 7 per cent. Do these figures reflect the efficacy of surgery or differences in growth behavior of the tumors?

Because the controllable factors, i.e., the present diagnostic and operative techniques, seem to be near the limit of improvement, there is an obvious need for improved cancer detection and more fundamental knowledge about tumor growth if the survival rate for patients with carcinoma of the stomach is to be improved.

OTHER NEOPLASMS OF THE STOMACH

Although carcinoma comprises about 90 per cent of neoplasms removed from the stomach, it is important to recognize that other histologic types are encountered. Many of these are not distinguished from carcinoma on the basis of historic, roentgenographic, or gastroscopic findings, and the diagnosis is made either at operation or in the pathology laboratory. The tissue diagnosis is very important because the prognostic and therapeutic implications are so different from those of carcinoma.

ADENOMA

Adenomas of the stomach comprise about 5 per cent of restricted gastric neoplasms. In the general population over 50 years of age the incidence of adenoma is less than 0.1 per cent, but in patients with achlorhydria it is about 2 per cent, and in patients with pernicious anemia it is about 5 per cent. The tumors have been seen in patients of all ages, but the peak incidence occurs between the ages of 60 and 70. The tumors are found more commonly in men than in women.

The tumors may be multiple. Most are in the antrum and body. Macroscopically the adenoma appears polypoid, usually pedunculated, and is clearly demarcated from the surrounding mucosa, which may be atrophic. Microscopically the tumor consists of proliferated epithelium that is in an ordered acinar arrangement. The stalk is a connective tissue strand, into which the submucosa sometimes is invaginated.

The complaints most commonly encountered among patients with gastric polyps are epigastric distress, nausea, vomiting, and bleeding. Often adenomas are discovered incidentally in patients without gastric symptoms. Frequently the patients have a hypochromic, microcytic anemia and blood in the feces. More than 80 per cent of patients with gastric polyps have hypochlorhydria.

The *diagnosis* of gastric adenoma is generally made by roentgenologic examination, and the lesions appear as circular filling defects. If the stalk is long enough, the tumor can be displaced on manipulation of the stomach during fluoroscopy to give the impression of a foreign body. Gastroscopic and gastrocamera examinations are particularly useful in the evaluation of polypoid lesions. Many of the small ones are initially detected by gastroscopy (see Fig. 3C). The benign adenoma is a berry-like growth above the surface of the mucosa.

The treatment of gastric adenomas hinges on accurate diagnosis of polypoid lesions. Exclusion of other possible benign lesions, e.g., aberrant pancreas, foreign body, leiomyoma, or inflammatory fibroid polyp, is usually possible by appropriate roentgenologic and endoscopic techniques leaving the differential diagnosis between adenoma and carcinoma. Spherical, nonulcerated polyps (especially when they are pedunculated) less than 2 cm. in diameter in patients with negative cytologic examinations can be considered benign adenomas, and surgery is not indicated unless bleeding is a problem. Even though smooth polyps greater than 2 cm. in diameter may be adenomas, operation is indicated in this instance because experience has shown that tumors of this size are often malignant. Most available evidence supports the concept that adenomas do not become carcinomas; excision of adenomas to prevent cancer is not indicated.

LEIOMYOMA

The incidence of leiomyoma in the stomach is much greater than is appreciated. In meticulous postmortem examinations the incidence is about 15 per cent, but in terms of clinical experience this type is very unusual, comprising less than 1 per cent of excised tumors. Leiomyomas occur in patients of all ages but most frequently in those 40 to 60 years old. They occur with equal frequency in men and in women. The tumors arise from the muscularis and grow submucosally, usually projecting into the gastric lumen. They are 2 to 10 cm. in their greatest dimension, but they can become huge, weighing as much as 6 kg. Two thirds of the tumors occur in the body and antrum. Macroscopically the tumor is seen to be an intramural ovoid mass over which the mucosa has been stretched. It is ulcerated or umbilicated and scarred in 60 per cent of cases. Malignant change is thought not to occur.

Of the symptoms that suggest gastric neoplasm, *bleeding* is the most common complaint among patients with leiomyomas. Generally the bleeding is gradual and sufficient to produce an iron deficiency anemia, but it may begin dramatically. Patients may also complain of *dyspepsia, epigastric pain,* and *anorexia.*

The *diagnosis* is usually first suggested on barium study, for these tumors have a characteristic smooth contour with a mucosal ulceration overlying the apex of the mass. On gastroscopy the tumor appears pale pink or slate-gray, the mucosa over the surface is smoothed out, and rugae are seen mounting the sides of the tumor. The central ulcer is visible (see Fig. 3D).

These tumors should be excised when they are discovered because it is not possible to exclude the possibility that they are malignant and because they can cause massive bleeding as well as distressing symptoms. Local excision should be performed unless the tumor is so large that partial gastrectomy is necessary.

LEIOMYOSARCOMA

Malignant smooth muscle tumors are very unusual, comprising less than 1 per cent of gastric tumors. Nothing in the history distinguishes these tumors from any of the neoplasms of the stomach except that some patients with such tumors are aware of an abdominal mass. Bleeding is common, as with leiomyomas. Ulceration is frequently seen in the summit of the tumor, which tends to be lobular. Metastatic spread is intra-abdominal in most instances. The growth behavior is slow in comparison with carcinoma, but there are no roentgenographic or gastroscopic distinctions. At operation a wide resection is recommended even though metastases are recognizable. Patients who have been operated upon have a 40 per cent five-year survival rate.

LYMPHOMA

Lymphomas of all histologic types comprise 3 to 5 per cent of malignant gastric neoplasms. The most common histologic types are the *reticulum cell sarcoma* and *small round-cell lymphocytoma,* but gastric involvement also occurs in *Hodgkin's disease, lymphatic leukemia, giant follicular lymphoma,* and *plasmacytoma.* Patients with lymphoma most commonly complain of dyspepsia, anorexia, and epigastric pain; they have anemia, bleeding, and cachexia less frequently than patients with carcinoma. Most of the patients are between ages 40 and 60. There is no difference in incidence among men and women. The roentgenographic and gastroscopic characteristics are not distinctive enough from carcinoma to permit unequivocal preoperative diagnosis; in the diffuse form the stomach may appear to be a "leather bottle." Large rugae should alert one to the possibility of lymphomatous infiltration. The mucosa may become superficially ulcerated.

The usual *management* of the neoplasm, regardless of histologic type, is resection of the tumor followed by radiation. Perhaps this sequence has been the procedure because the diagnosis is so often established operatively, following which radiation is advocated because of the radiosensitivity of lymphoid tissue. Some patients have been treated with radiation alone, and the results appear to be as satisfactory as surgical results. The five-year survival rate of patients with lymphoma of the stomach treated by surgery and radiation is 50 per cent.

NEOPLASMS OF THE SMALL INTESTINE

MALIGNANT NEOPLASMS

Many histologic types of malignant lesion in the small intestine are reported, but *carcinoma* is the most frequent. *Carcinoid* tumors are the next most numerous.

Etiology. It is impressive that, although the stomach and colon are so commonly the site of malignant processes, the mucosa of the small intestine is rarely subject to neoplastic change. No etiologic basis for carcinoma of the small intestine is known. Certainly inflammation is not a causative factor since the first portion of the duodenum, the locus of most peptic ulcers, is that portion of the gut least likely to undergo malignant change. Furthermore, regional enteritis is not associated with an increased incidence of neoplasia, in contradistinction to ulcerative colitis, which is. Patients with celiac disease appear to develop lymphoma of the small bowel with greater than expected frequency, but no pathogenic link has been found.

Incidence. Cancer of the small bowel comprises less than 1 per cent of all malignant neoplasms of the alimentary tract. It occurs in younger persons than is the case with other gastrointestinal carcinomas, and men are affected twice as frequently as women.

Pathology. The second portion of the duodenum is the site most commonly involved, although the ileum, with its greater amount of lymphoid tissue, is where most of the lymphomas occur. Epithelial tumors grow into the lumen or have a constricting growth that compromises the lumen. Spread is confined to the liver and local lymph nodes; extra-abdominal metastases are rare. Lymphomas invade the walls of the gut to produce a semirigid tube and serosal adhesions.

Clinical Manifestations. Tumors of the small bowel usually cause the patients to complain of upper abdominal pain, vomiting, and weight loss. These symptoms are due to obstruction and therefore are progressive as the growth enlarges. Tumors in the duodenum produce symptoms of pyloric obstruction, and if the ampulla of Vater or the common duct becomes obstructed, the patient may first complain of pruritus, chills and fever, or jaundice. Carcinomas of the duodenum bleed more frequently than tumors of the jejunum and ileum; evidence of anemia is seen in more than half of the patients with small bowel neoplasms. Examination of the abdomen does not commonly disclose a mass, although in lymphomatous diseases infiltrated loops of bowel frequently are palpable. Abdominal distention and tenderness are commonly seen. Patients with lymphomatous infiltration of the small bowel may develop malabsorption (see Diseases of Malabsorption) and may even present with a history of weight loss, weakness, and bulky stools suggestive of idiopathic steatorrhea. Frequently these patients have fever and a moderate to severe anemia.

Diagnosis. Examination of the small intestine by barium contrast is the most satisfactory technique for preoperatively establishing the diagnosis, but its limitations are such that in only 60 per cent of all patients can the tumor be demonstrated. However, much depends on the site of the tumor; almost 90 per cent of lesions in the second portion of the duodenum are demonstrable. Roentgenographic examination is accomplished by the serial "follow-through" technique or by small bowel "enema" via a duodenal tube. The tumors usually appear as filling defects, with a constriction of the lumen and a fixed dilated proximal loop. Lymphomas generally produce a very distorted mucosal pattern in the terminal ileum, where the differentiation from regional ileitis is very difficult.

Duodenal drainage and examination of the sediment for malignant cells by cytologic technique has been rewarding in establishing the diagnosis of proximal lesions, but this method has only limited applicability. Exploratory laparotomy has proved to be the most effective means of establishing the diagnosis.

Treatment and Prognosis. Malignant lesions of the small bowel are resected whenever possible. If the tumor cannot be removed, a bypass procedure should be done to relieve or prevent obstruction. Lesions in the duodenum are more formidable because of the frequent necessity of partial pancreatectomy and partial gastrectomy to achieve removal. The five-year survival rate after resection is affected by the type of tumor growth. For example, obstruction produced early in the development of the tumor leads to early detection and better surgical results. The five-year survival rate approaches 20 per cent in a few series, but in general the figure is less than 5 per cent. Evaluation of the efficacy of radiotherapy in addition to surgical treatment of patients having lymphoma of the small intestine cannot be made from experience thus far obtained. The five-year survival rate of patients with intestinal lymphoma is about 15 per cent.

BENIGN NEOPLASMS

In clinical experience benign neoplasms of the small bowel are less than 0.1 per cent of alimentary tract neoplasms, although autopsy records show that this low incidence merely reflects the asymptomatic quality of these tumors. As elsewhere in the gut, the most common types of benign neoplasms are adenoma and leiomyoma; usually such tumors are solitary. Hemangiomas are also encountered; they may be multiple and may be associated with vascular tumors in other organ systems.

Benign neoplasms cause *symptoms* similar to those of malignant lesions in the small bowel:

bleeding, abdominal pain, and vomiting. Patients complain of borborygmi and eructation early in the course, but later they have all the symptoms of obstruction. Perforation is uncommon. Physical signs are unremarkable unless there is obstruction. Obstruction is not due to constriction of the lumen by the tumor mass, as with malignant neoplasms, but to intussusception resulting from peristaltic propulsion of the polypoid tumor and the consequent invagination of the segment to which it is attached. Blood is frequently detected in the stools and anemia is present, but the bleeding is usually not noted by the patient.

The *treatment* is removal of the tumor that is responsible for bleeding or obstruction. Prophylactic resection of adenomas is not done because there is no evidence that they undergo malignant transformation. This is also true in the Peutz-Jeghers syndrome.

PEUTZ-JEGHERS SYNDROME

In 1921 Peutz described a clinical entity in which he listed adenomatosis of the small bowel as one of the chief features. The syndrome consists of familial gastrointestinal polyposis with distinctive mucocutaneous pigmentation. Jeghers' publications of further observations of such patients have recently stimulated the awareness of clinicians, and now more than 100 cases have been reported.

The syndrome is heritable and appears with the frequency of a non-sex-linked dominant. The genetic mechanism for pigmentation occurring with polyposis is not clear, but it is most likely a single gene. Patients of different national and racial origins have been found with the syndrome.

Polyposis is most frequently found in the ileum, to a lesser extent in the jejunum, and still less frequently in the colon and stomach. (Peutz first used the term visceral polyposis because he also noted pharyngeal and bladder polyps; however, these are very infrequent in recent cases.) On histologic section these polyps are hamartomas. They are multiple and grow in crops, i.e., they are not detectable for years after resection has been performed, and then they apparently recur in a spurt of growth. At first it was believed that these polyps became malignant, but this impression has not been substantiated by subsequent experience.

The mucocutaneous pigmentation is most noticeable on the lips and buccal mucosa, but it also appears in the skin on the fingers, palms, toes, forearms, and umbilical area. The spots in the skin may fade after puberty, but those in the mucosa are permanent.

The *clinical manifestations* of the syndrome, aside from the skin findings, which can be concealed by use of cosmetics, are *recurrent bouts of abdominal pain, borborygmi,* and *anemia.* The polyps accentuate peristaltic activity, and this leads to *intussusception.* The patient experiences transient, midabdominal, postprandial, "green apple" colic, and he finds that through contortions

of his body or vigorous abdominal manipulation he can relieve the pain. In reported observations of such therapeutic massage it has been obvious that what is accomplished is reduction of the intussusception. *Borborygmi* are remarkably loud and frequent and therefore a source of embarrassment to the patient.

The only physical sign attributable to the polyposis is the mass that is palpable at the time intussusception occurs, but this is brief. Occasionally clubbed fingers have been noted in these patients. *Anemia,* very common in patients with this syndrome, is attributable to occult gastrointestinal bleeding.

It is not surprising that the evanescent symptoms and signs and bizarre contortions have caused many of these patients to be labeled psychoneurotic. The syndrome should be considered whenever one sees a polyp in the rectum or stomach. Similarly, the discovery of pigmented spots in the buccal mucosa should lead to careful roentgenographic evaluation for polyps.

A major part of *management* of the patient with Peutz-Jeghers syndrome is providing him with an understanding of his disease. Obviously if there is bleeding or sustained intussusception (gangrene resulting from irreducible intussusception is very rarely encountered in these patients), the offending polyp must be removed. Since there is no evidence of malignancy in these polyps and they have been shown to appear in the nonresected areas, a prophylactic excision is not justifiable. This is in contrast to the situation in familial polyposis coli (see article under that heading, *infra*). Usually with the Peutz-Jeghers syndrome, the symptomatic treatment for the abdominal pain is something the patient discovers for himself.

NEOPLASMS OF THE LARGE INTESTINE

CARCINOMA OF THE LARGE INTESTINE

Etiology. No agent that causes carcinoma of the large intestine has been found. The incidence of carcinoma of the large bowel among relatives of patients with this disease is the same as it is in the general population. The only genetic influence on the incidence of this neoplasm is among patients with *familial polyposis coli* (*vide infra*), in whom the lesion is truly premalignant. In this case the question arises whether the heritable trait is a predisposition to develop benign polyps that undergo transformation into carcinoma or is a predisposition to develop adenoma *and* carcinoma.

The fact that carcinoma of the large intestine occurs with any frequency only in man has led to consideration of dietary factors in the etiology of intestinal tumors, but there is no evidence that any of the substances thus far suspected, e.g., food additives, aromatic amines, etc., can be implicated.

Aside from the well established association of carcinoma and familial polyposis coli, two other lesions that have been labeled "premalignant" are *ulcerative colitis* and *adenoma* of the large bowel. There is no doubt of the association between ulcerative colitis and the subsequent development of carcinoma. The time lag between the diagnosis of colitis and the appearance of malignancy is eight to thirty-five years, but clinical experience suggests that most neoplasms develop in those patients who have severe, unremitting colitis. There are some unusual features about these malignancies: they are often multicentric, are highly anaplastic, and appear as fibrous thickening rather than as fungating growths. They do not develop in the pseudopolyps, but arise in islands of epithelium buried deep in the submucosa during the repeated episodes of mucosal denudation and healing.

Increasing evidence militates against the older view that adenomas of the colon have a premalignant quality.

Incidence and Prevalence. Most patients with carcinoma of the large bowel are between 50 and 70 years of age, but the neoplasm has been reported in children. The incidence of carcinoma of the large intestine is equal in men and women; however, this fact conceals two interesting inequalities—that cancer of the rectum is more frequent among men and that cancer of the colon is more frequent among women. The age ranges are similar for the two sexes.

Carcinoma of the bowel is second only to carcinoma of the lung as the leading cause of cancer deaths in the United States. There are known to be wide variations in the incidence of this disease in different parts of the world. In Chile, where age-adjusted death rates from carcinoma of the stomach are among the world's highest, the age-adjusted death rates from cancer of the large intestine are lower than in all other major countries, being about one tenth of that in the United States.

Pathology. Carcinomas develop in certain parts of the large intestine more frequently than in others. About 60 per cent of the neoplasms develop in the rectum, 20 per cent in the sigmoid, 6 per cent in the cecum, and the remainder in other portions of the colon. In about 3 per cent of surgical specimens, multiple foci of carcinoma have been found, but the tumors have not usually been very far from each other.

Neoplasms in the large intestine differ greatly in their growth behavior. Macroscopically they are polypoid, ulcerating, annular, scirrhous, or colloid in type. The polypoid tumor is cauliflower-like and is the most common type found in the right colon. The scirrhous and annular lesions are the most common types found in the left colon. Rectal tumors are usually ulcerating or annular, but the polypoid type is fairly common. Of course,

a tumor in any part of the bowel can be one or a combination of these types, but to some extent the predilection for certain tumors to develop in certain regions accounts for the differences in symptoms according to tumor location. Thus, a polypoid lesion filling the lumen of the right colon does not prevent the passage of the semifluid contents, as do annular or infiltrating lesions of the left colon, which compromise the distensibility and diameter of the lumen of this segment, in which the feces are much less fluid. Obstruction produces proximal distention, and the colon, loaded with feces, undergoes a phase of dilatation and hyperperistalsis leading to hypertrophy of the muscularis. Ileal dilatation of this type may occur with lesions in the right colon. Mucosal damage develops when the fecal matter remains impacted; "stercoral ulcers" may be noted proximal to the obstruction. Perforation can occur in the ulcerated tumor or through such a stercoral ulcer.

Histologically these tumors show a spectrum from differentiated to anaplastic forms. In general, the papilliferous growth shows better differentiation than the ulcerating or invasive growths, and tumors in the colon tend to be more highly differentiated than rectal neoplasms. Classifications of degree of malignancy based on differentiation and extent of invasion have been found to correlate with the prognosis.

The spread of tumors from the large bowel occurs by four means: direct extension, lymphatic and hematogenous spread, and implantation. Any adjacent structure may be involved by the direct extension of the tumor. The reproductive organs, bladder, and ureters may be thus involved so that exenteration becomes necessary. Frequently tumor spread across serosal surfaces is only partly responsible for adherence of involved bowel to other organs; inflammation also contributes to this complication. Tumors in the transverse colon may spread to the stomach, giving rise to symptoms that are the same as those of primary gastric disease. Fistula tracts and abscesses result from the intervisceral spread of tumor. Rectovesical fistulas with pneumaturia, gastrocolic fistulas with vomiting of fecal matter, and enterocolic fistulas with diarrhea are some of the complications of such extension.

Spread of the tumor also occurs after the cells enter the submucosa and grow into the lymphatic vessels. The local paracolic lymph nodes contain metastatic growths that subsequently reach the preaortic nodes via the chain of lymph nodes along the blood supply of the affected region. Skipping of local nodes rarely, if ever, can be demonstrated. Lymphatic spread is found to have occurred in 30 per cent of colonic lesions and in 50 per cent of rectal lesions that are removed. Lymphatic metastases are more common in women than in men.

Hematogenous spread of tumor cells from neoplasms of the large intestine is found in almost half of the postmortem examinations of patients who die from carcinoma of the large intestine. The fact that the cells directly enter the blood stream is clearly shown by the frequent histologic findings of plugs of tumor cells in veins near the tumor. Malignant cells can be recovered from the peripheral circulation. The liver is the most common site of blood-borne metastatic growths, but they occur in the lungs, kidneys, bones, and adrenals also. Cerebral metastases are found in 1 per cent of the patients autopsied.

Seeding of the peritoneal cavity with metastatic cells produces multiple plaques throughout, but this is not a common metastatic route. In such instances the tumor is so far advanced that operation is of little benefit. The growth of nodules in a healed incision in the skin or other tissues damaged at time of resection does occur, although it may be possible to avert this by use of appropriate wound drapes while tumor tissue is being manipulated and by the use of cytotoxic peritoneal lavages.

Clinical Manifestations. Patients with carcinoma of the large bowel have changes in bowel habits, blood and mucus per rectum, weight loss, abdominal pain, vomiting, weakness, and tenesmus. Although these are typical symptoms, the histories differ according to the location of the tumor.

Patients with *carcinoma of the rectum* characteristically complain of rectal bleeding, change in bowel habits, weight loss, tenesmus, and mucus in the stool. *Bleeding per rectum* is the most common problem for which these patients are admitted to the hospital. The bleeding may be only slight, and may appear as blood on the stool or paper or in the water in the bowel. *The most characteristic symptom of rectal carcinoma, elicited in 80 per cent of the histories, is a change in bowel habit within recent months.* Although constipation is reported, the more common complaint is diarrhea. As soon as the patient stands up he feels an urge to defecate, but he passes only mucus, flatus, and sometimes blood. Feeling that the rectum is still not evacuated, the patient shortly has another call to stool and repeats the performance. This type of episode recurs throughout the morning, each time only a small amount of feces being passed. Later in the day the patient may have a more normal bowel movement, sometimes with tenesmus, but commonly there is a history of frequent use of laxatives despite the "diarrhea." Passage of mucus or "slime" is described by about 20 per cent of the patients. This is very rarely mentioned by patients with carcinoma elsewhere in the large bowel. Loss of weight and lassitude occur, but not as commonly as in more proximal lesions.

Carcinoma of the sigmoid colon produces a remarkably different complex of symptoms, although the major ones, viz., changes in bowel habit, rectal bleeding, and pain, are indistinguishable from those of carcinoma of the rectum. The most common complaint of patients with lesions in this area is also changed bowel habit, but constipation is more frequent than diarrhea, and the history is usually of only a few days' or weeks' duration. *Bleeding* per rectum is mentioned by only a third of these patients. The distinctive feature is *abdominal pain.* This is present in over half the patients and is described as a dull ache or colicky pain in the lower abdomen. Recollection of the fact that annular stenosing tumors are the type that commonly occur in the sigmoid will explain the less frequent bleeding and the more frequent obstructive aspects, viz., constipation and pain. *Acute obstruction,* often without premonitory symptoms, is found in about 25 per cent of patients who have carcinoma of the sigmoid. In view of the frequency of obstructive phenomena, it is not surprising that perforation, peritonitis, and abscess formation are more common when the carcinoma is in the sigmoid. Some patients complain of urinary tract symptoms, usually a manifestation of bladder involvement.

Carcinoma of the left transverse or descending colon produces another pattern of symptoms. The most common feature of these lesions is *abdominal pain,* complained of by 70 per cent of patients. The pain is on the left side and is unrelated to meals. A history of *changed bowel habit* can be elicited from 60 per cent of patients; most frequently it is constipation. Rectal bleeding is noted in about 10 per cent of these patients. About 20 per cent of them present with findings of *complete obstruction.*

Carcinomas in the cecum, ascending colon, and right transverse colon are notoriously silent lesions. The blood loss, which is almost invariably present, is so gradual that it is unnoticed, and frequently such patients are severely anemic by the time they are first seen. The symptom most commonly experienced by patients with lesions in the right colon is *abdominal pain* on that side. It is described as a steady deep ache, but episodes of severe colicky pain associated with vomiting occur in one third of patients. Often the patients note that eating a meal provokes this pain, and so, with the abdominal ache, borborygmi, and nausea, the patients classify their symptoms as indigestion. This relationship to meals frequently results in *anorexia* or a reluctance to eat. Weight loss is noted by about half of the patients with carcinoma of the right colon, but this is not commonly the chief complaint. Lassitude, weakness, dizziness, and breathlessness are symptoms that 20 per cent of patients develop. These systemic symptoms caused by *anemia* are often the most prominent feature in the history. Indeed the patient may go to his doctor because of angina pectoris or even congestive heart failure secondary to the anemia. About 10 per cent of patients complain of having noted an abdominal mass.

Late complications of carcinoma of the large bowel are usually manifestations of the spread of tumor to other viscera. Thus, derangement of hepatic function, with or without hepatomegaly, is found in patients with liver metastases. Metastases to the adrenal glands are found in moribund patients with hypotension and electrolyte imbalance. Flatus and fecal material per urethra or per vagina follow fistula formation, and fistulas can develop in the abdominal wall from a paracolic abscess.

In summary, changed bowel habits, bleeding from the rectum, abdominal pain, weight loss, anorexia, and vomiting are symptoms that occur in patients with carcinoma of the large intestine, but mechanical features of the tumors and of bowel function produce a *different complex* of these symptoms depending on the location of the tumor. In general, the more proximal the tumor, the more predominant are pain, vomiting, and systemic symptoms; the more distal the tumor, the more predominant are alteration of bowel habit and bleeding.

Physical Examination. Physical examination is very helpful in establishing a diagnosis of carcinoma of the large intestine *because the neoplasm is palpable or visible in more than three fourths of the patients.* Palpation of the abdomen will reveal an abdominal mass in 65 per cent of patients with lesions of the right colon, in which tumors tend to be large polypoid structures that have been growing silently for some time. Of the tumors in the left colon less than 25 per cent are palpable on the initial examination, partly because the left colon is less accessible for palpation but also because these tumors tend to produce symptoms before they are very large.

The fact that one third of all carcinomas of the large bowel occur within reach of the finger on rectal examination emphasizes the importance of this simple procedure and the inexcusability of not doing it. As Hamilton Bailey has observed, "He who does not put his finger in it, puts his foot it it." On digital palpation a rectal carcinoma has two characteristic features—induration and elevation. The tumor may be an indurated disc or a protuberant ulcerated growth; assessment of the location and extension of the malignancy must be made at the rectal examination. In women a pelvic examination frequently permits a more complete evaluation of the lesion and its spread.

In addition to the 35 per cent of large intestinal cancers detectable by rectal examination, another 30 per cent are visible through the sigmoidoscope. *Sigmoidoscopic examination of the colon should be considered as much a part of a physical examination as are ophthalmoscopic or stethoscopic examinations.* The use of a sigmoidoscope is no more the restricted privilege of a gastroenterologist or a surgeon than the use of a tongue blade is that of an otolaryngologist. The procedure need not be time-consuming or involved. Most successful examinations of the distal 25 centimeters of the gut can be done without the necessity of preparative enemas, but in the remainder of instances a simple proprietary enema or suppository can be administered at the time of the office visit. Most tumors are easily recognized through the sigmoidoscope, for they are raised from the normal mucosa and are a deeper red, often violaceous. Within the indurated margin an ulcer with a gray-green base is often seen. The tumor bleeds easily from swabbing or the pressure of the end of the sigmoidoscope. It is possible to get some idea of the extent of local spread by gentle pressure on the tumor with the instrument. A freely movable

mass is, of course, a promising sign. Biopsy at the time of sigmoidoscopy should be done.

Diagnosis. Obviously a strong clinical impression or a firm diagnosis of neoplasm of the large intestine is possible by history and physical examination in more than 90 per cent of patients. Barium enema with air contrast will confirm the diagnosis. The tumor is seen as a filling defect (Fig. 4) or a stricture in the barium enema. The air contrast permits evaluation of the mucosal pattern of such irregularities and the detection of intraluminal tumors as small as a few millimeters that otherwise would not be seen in the opaque column. Visualization of the colon by the double-contrast technique is a mandatory part of the evaluation of a patient who has bleeding from the rectum. The barium study must be done even in patients who are found to have a lesion, benign or malignant, by sigmoidoscopic examination because knowledge of the presence or absence of other colonic neoplasms is essential for the proper surgical approach. Multicentric carcinomas occur in 3 per cent of patients; hemorrhoids or polyps in the distal intestine can be present when malignant lesions exist higher in the colon. The one circumstance in which a barium study should not be done is when there is perforation. In patients who have evidence of obstruction the study may be limited to outlining the distal portion of the lesion, for introduction of barium beyond the stenosis may result in subsequent difficulty of return of the suspension. If large bowel obstruc-

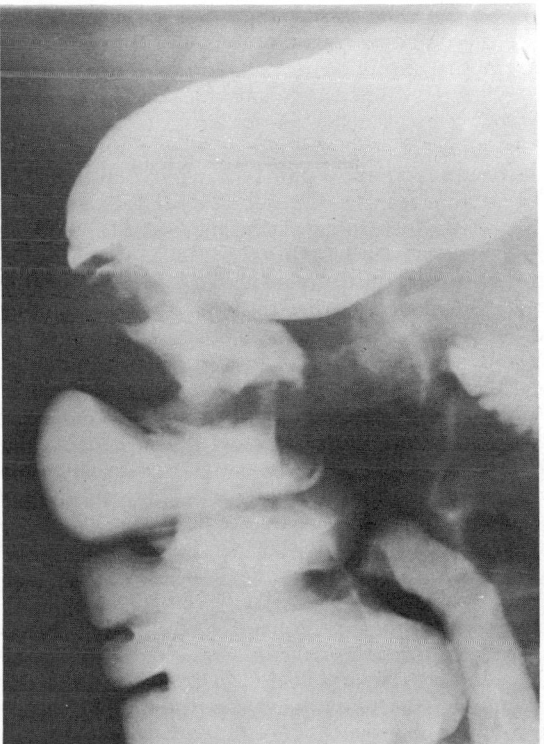

FIGURE 4. Carcinoma of the colon. This annular lesion in the ascending colon has produced a typical appearance of mucosal destruction and overhanging margins.

tion is present, barium should not be given by mouth.

In addition to visualization of the colon by means of roentgenographic examination, a histologic diagnosis should be made whenever possible by biopsy of the lesion through the sigmoidoscope. Not only is this a means of establishing the type of neoplasm that is present, but the degree of differentiation of a carcinoma may influence the surgeon in his choice of the operative procedure to be used. With regard to biopsy of a polypoid lesion, the entire tumor should be removed rather than "nibbling off" part of the head.

Experience with the use of exfoliative cytologic methods for diagnosis of malignancy in a polyp has proved that the technique is accurate, but it has found only limited use at present because it rarely extends the diagnostic range already attained with sigmoidoscopy, roentgenographic examination, and biopsy.

Differential Diagnosis. The differential diagnosis to be considered in the evaluation of a patient who has symptoms, signs, or roentgenographic findings suggestive of carcinoma of the large intestine includes other neoplasms and some inflammatory lesions. On digital, sigmoidoscopic, or roentgenologic examination a *villous adenoma* may be mistaken for carcinoma. Multiple biopsies will enable one to show the character of the tumor and search for any malignant foci. Very rare colonic neoplasms that clinically and roentgenographically can resemble carcinoma are *leiomyoma, leiomyosarcoma, lipoma, lymphosarcoma, mucocele of the appendix,* and *hemangioma.*

Carcinoma versus Diverticulitis. Inflammatory disease may produce a history that suggests carcinoma; many of the complications are similar, e.g., fistulas, abscess, or obstruction. The inflammatory process most frequently confused with carcinoma is *diverticulitis.* This can produce bleeding, abdominal pain, change in bowel habits, obstruction, perforation, abscess, fistula, and any other manifestations of carcinoma, although the history is commonly longer and the complaints are more intermittent in patients with diverticulitis. Physical examination does not permit an unequivocal choice between these diagnoses, although the findings of fever, extreme abdominal tenderness, and paralytic ileus favor diverticulitis. Roentgenographic findings can be similar because the inflammation produces a mass, constriction of the lumen, and mucosal distortion. The associated finding of diverticulosis of the colon is not helpful because 30 per cent of patients with carcinoma are found to have diverticula as well. There are no absolute distinctions, and sometimes laparotomy is necessary. The only consolation in this dilemma is that a person with a palpable mass or a filling defect resulting from severe diverticulitis requires laparotomy as much as a patient with carcinoma. Even at operation the nature of the lesion may not be apparent, and sometimes the pathologist must give the final answer.

Other Inflammatory Processes. Other inflammatory processes may be considered when evaluating a patient with symptoms of carcinoma of the colon, but usually appropriate diagnostic aids permit one to make the distinction. *Ulcerative colitis* can be distinguished by its sigmoidoscopic characteristics and more widespread involvement of the colon. *Regional enteritis* of the large bowel, which is notorious for causing perforation and fistulas, will sometimes produce a clinical picture similar to that of carcinoma. If there is any doubt, a biopsy of a lesion in the mucosa will show the giant cell reaction that is typical of this disease. Other inflammatory processes that have been confused with carcinoma are *appendiceal abscess* and *intestinal tuberculosis.*

One must be aware of the possibility of *endometriosis* of the colon producing symptoms and roentgenographic findings suggestive of carcinoma of the colon.

Treatment and Prognosis. The only treatment for carcinoma of the large intestine is surgical. The operation required depends on the site of the lesion, its extension, and the general status of the patient, but the general principle is to preserve as much function and continuity as possible. A curative procedure for carcinoma of the cecum or right colon requires a right hemicolectomy with ligation of the branches of the superior mesenteric artery and removal of all associated nodes. A curative resection of lesions in the left colon involves removal of that region of the left colon that is affected and the appropriate branches of the inferior mesenteric artery. A wider resection, left hemicolectomy with ligation of the inferior mesenteric artery, is advocated to ensure complete removal. For carcinoma of the distal sigmoid or upper rectum it is possible to save the anal sphincter and achieve anastomosis; for lower lesions the rectum must be removed and a colostomy is necessary.

The number of patients found to have "resectable" tumors varies with the economic status of the community (a measure of the availability of medical care), but, in general, 75 per cent of right-sided and 50 per cent of left-sided tumors are considered removable. In addition, operations for palliation should be performed in some of those patients known to have inoperable tumors. Such procedures generally follow the same lines as the curative ones, except that less extensive resection is performed.

Current studies using regional perfusion with chemotherapeutic agents during the immediate postoperative period may improve the survival rates of patients with malignant disease of the colon. The prognosis is a function of the growth characteristics of the tumor and the stage at which operation intervenes. Over-all, the five-year survival rates of patients with carcinoma of the large intestine is about 30 per cent. More than 90 per cent of patients who survive operation and are found to have *noninvasive lesions* live five years or more without evidence of recurrence. Unfortunately, these constitute a small fraction of patients with the disease, but better diagnostic facilities and improved operative techniques promise to improve the results of treatment. One of the most important influences on therapy is sterilization of the bowel prior to operation. The decrease in operative mortality brought about by the use of minimally absorbed antimicrobial drugs has altered the assessment of "operability" of patients with carcinoma of the large bowel.

ADENOMA OF THE LARGE INTESTINE

Definition. An adenoma of the large intestine, in contrast to pseudopolyps of ulcerative colitis, polypoid carcinomas, juvenile (retention) polyps, and villous adenomas, is a rounded mass of branching glandular tubules lined by mature mucus-secreting goblet cells. Villous adenoma and the polyps found in patients with familial polyposis are exceptional variants of the adenoma and are discussed separately.

Etiology. No causative agent for these tumors has been shown. There is no evidence for a familial propensity to develop solitary adenomas, and no epidemiologic data exist that implicate any environmental factors in their origin.

Incidence. Autopsy studies reveal that 4 to 10 per cent of people have adenomas in the colon. Even in autopsies of people less than 21 years of age, the incidence is 3 per cent. In clinical experience the incidence of adenoma is almost this high, being from 2 to 8 per cent of the population studied. Incidences as high as 19 per cent have been found in older populations by means of cancer-detection surveys. Adenomas are more common in men than in women in a ratio of 3 to 2.

Pathology. Adenomas can occur anywhere in the large intestine, but 80 per cent are found in the rectum and sigmoid. They are usually pedunculated, and the stalk may be as long as 40 mm. The bulbous tip may be as large as 40 mm. in diameter, but the average diameter is 12 mm. They are smooth or lobulated, soft, round structures with a color only slightly deeper than that of the normal mucosa. Microscopically they are closely packed tubules of adenomatous epithelium with very little stroma. The stalk usually is a thin strand of connective tissue covered with a single layer of normal epithelial cells.

Relationship to Carcinoma. Recent evidence has dispelled belief in a premalignant nature of adenomas of the colon. Carcinomatous conversion from benign polyps had been thought to occur, but discordance in sites of development of carcinomas and adenomas, equal incidence of adenomas in cancer and control populations, and clarification of the histologic basis for diagnosis of malignant polypoid lesions have been found by many pathologists to outweigh any data in support of the older concept.

Clinical Manifestations. *Bleeding* from the rectum is the most common complaint among patients who are subsequently found to have adenomas. Otherwise there are no characteristic symptoms. Vague abdominal pain and changes in bowel habit are sometimes noted in the history, but control populations, similar in age and sex to patients with adenomas, have the same frequency of these complaints.

Diagnosis. The diagnosis of an intestinal adenoma is usually made by sigmoidoscopic examination or barium enema during the evaluation of a patient with symptoms suggestive of carcinoma of the colon. Almost 75 per cent of these tumors are visible at sigmoidoscopy, and most of the others are detected by double-contrast roentgenographic examination, in which they appear as filling defects in the opaque column of barium and as small "berries" on the mucosa in the air-contrast film. Pedunculated, smooth, spherical polyps less than 10 mm. in diameter and not producing puckering of the adjacent gut wall can be interpreted roentgenographically as adenomas. Sessile, lobulated, and asymmetrical filling defects are less assuredly benign. Fecal material can produce a misleading appearance so that another examination may be necessary to verify the presence of the tumor. The differential diagnosis lies among different histologic types of polypoid neoplasms, chiefly carcinoma, carcinoid, leiomyoma, and lymphoma.

Treatment. If a polyp is bleeding, is causing intussusception, or is otherwise responsible for the patient's disability, it obviously must be removed. The dilemma lies in deciding whether to remove a polyp on the grounds that it is perhaps malignant. Since the roentgenologic and endoscopic appearance of polypoid lesions does not always permit differentiation between those that are malignant and those that are benign, the surest treatment would be to remove all polyps of the colon. This presents no problem when lesions are within the range of the sigmoidoscope; in such instances the adenomas are removed with a snare or cutting forceps through the sigmoidoscope. For those lesions beyond the sigmoidoscope the recommendation for removal must be tempered by a consideration of the necessity for major abdominal surgery. Experience has shown that the polyps that contain malignant cells are those greater than 10 mm. in diameter. Consequently it is recommended that lesions smaller than this should be observed regularly, and if there is evidence of growth, mucosal destruction, or puckering of the subjacent colonic wall, the tumors should then be removed. The mode of excision is determined by the type of polyp; sessile polyps usually should be removed by local resection and pedunculated ones by colostomy and polypectomy.

The removal of an adenoma is curative. Subsequent appearance of other tumors is regarded as *de novo* neoplasia and unrelated to the previous adenoma.

FAMILIAL POLYPOSIS COLI

Intestinal polyposis was first noted to be hereditary by Cripps in 1882. In 1925 Lockhart-Mummary described the high incidence of carcinoma among these patients. Since that time careful studies of these patients and their families have elucidated most of the features of the natural history of the disease.

More than one hundred families of patients known to have polyposis coli have been studied. The genetic pattern among these families shows that the gene behaves as a simple mendelian dominant. At birth the patient is normal and no polyps are demonstrable, but at puberty, or shortly after, polyps begin to appear. In association with the polyposis many of the patients have multiple exostoses, dermal inclusion cysts, and connective tissue tumors. The development of cancer in these patients is such that the average age of death among the untreated affected members of the families is 25 years below that of the general population with intestinal cancer. Indeed, the most recent experience suggests that these affected persons will all develop carcinoma of the colon if they are untreated and do not die of an intervening illness.

The polyps that appear in the colon are simple adenomas, but they are innumerable and are found from cecum to rectum. The polyps vary greatly in size. After they develop, the patient usually has diarrhea and bleeding from the rectum. In association with these symptoms the patient loses weight and becomes anemic.

The diagnosis of this disease is established through sigmoidoscopic and barium enema recognition of the multiple polyps. These diagnostic studies should be performed in all relatives of patients with polyposis coli in order to establish the diagnosis and to give appropriate treatment before malignant disease develops in those who are affected.

The treatment of patients with familial polyposis coli consists of removal of the colon. Relatives of patients with polyposis must be closely observed so that colectomy can be done as early as possible on those who carry the defect. Unfortunately, this is not easily accomplished because the patients are not readily convinced of the necessity of having an ileostomy rather than a few symptoms that are only relatively bothersome. Because of the resistance to optimal treatment, many patients have been treated by ileoproctostomy. In these patients the rectal remnant is examined every three months and polypectomy is done as necessary, but this is not effective prophylactic treatment because carcinoma frequently develops in such rectal remnants.

VILLOUS ADENOMA
(Papillary Adenoma)

A villous adenoma is commonly regarded as a benign variant of the solitary adenoma, but this is open to argument, for 75 per cent of these tumors show carcinoma or atypical cellular foci, and they can recur. An implantation tumor in the operative wound has been observed subsequent to a colotomy for removal of a villous adenoma that was histologically benign. It is probably incorrect to call a villous adenoma a *precursor* of carcinoma, for it

is evident from these points that their behavior is actually that of a malignant process. This is the case even though the "adenoma" may have benign characteristics on examination under the microscope. The villous adenoma is probably a unique pathologic entity and not just a variant of the adenoma. Villous adenomas constitute about 5 per cent of all "polyps" encountered clinically, and are found with equal frequency among men and women. The average age of patients with villous adenomas is 63 years.

Macroscopically the tumors are large, sessile, granular, or shaggy soft growths, most of which are found in the rectum and sigmoid. Occasionally they are circumferential, but usually they are knobby protuberances on one wall. Microscopically the frondlike surface is seen to consist of projections of loose vascular stroma covered by a single layer of epithelial cells that are taller and more deeply staining than the normal cells and contain less mucin.

The clinical manifestations of these tumors are *mucous diarrhea* and *rectal bleeding*. In about 10 per cent of patients the tumor causes prolapse of the rectum, which further increases the discharge of mucus. This often produces a state that the patient terms "diarrhea" but that really consists of simply evacuating large amounts of clear mucus. Occasionally the mucus discharged is rich in potassium, and the patients become severely *hypokalemic*, even to the point of prostration.

The diagnosis is established by discovery of the tumor on rectal or sigmoidoscopic examination, but the exact histologic diagnosis requires multiple biopsies of the tumor, properly oriented for sectioning and microscopic study, to determine whether there is evidence of carcinoma. Barium enemas are helpful in finding villous adenomas if they are more proximal, but roentgenographically they are often interpreted as being carcinomas despite characteristic differences.

Treatment of villous adenoma requires adequate local excision. This may be possible simply via the anus or by a sleeve resection of a portion of the colon, but it may entail an abdominoperineal procedure including removal of the distal rectum. The deciding factors are the location of the tumor, its size, and the extent of invasion. The prognosis is good in that 66 per cent of all patients survive for five years after such surgical attack. Simply cauterizing or snipping out the tumor is of no use because it regrows.

Ackerman, L. V.: Surgical Pathology. 3rd ed. St. Louis, C. V. Mosby Company, 1964.

Castleman, B., and Krickstein, H.: Do adenomatous polyps of the colon become malignant? New Eng. J. Med., 267:469, 1962.

Dormandy, T. L.: Gastrointestinal polyposis with mucocutaneous pigmentation (Peutz-Jeghers syndrome). New Eng. J. Med., 256:1093; 1141; 1186, 1957.

Ehrlich, A. M., Stalder, G., Geller, W., and Sherlock, P.: Gastrointestinal manifestation of malignant lymphoma. Gastroenterology, 54:1115, 1968.

Sherlock, P., Ehrlich, A. N., Pavon, E., and Paglia, M. A.: Treatment of gastrointestinal cancer: Current status and research progress. Gastroenterology, 53:630, 1967.

DISEASES OF THE HEPATIC SYSTEM

Diseases of the Liver

Graham H. Jeffries

PATHOGENIC MECHANISMS OF HEPATIC DISEASE

An understanding of the pathophysiology of liver disease provides the basis for a rational clinical approach to the patient. The articles that follow will review selective aspects of the biochemical and regulatory functions of the liver, the pathophysiology of clinical manifestations of liver disease, and the differential diagnosis and treatment of diseases of the liver.

JAUNDICE

Jaundice or *icterus* refers to a yellow discoloration of the skin or sclerae by bilirubin. It is best seen in daylight, and may not be detected under artificial illumination. The depth of jaundice depends on the concentration of bilirubin in the plasma, on factors that control capillary permeability and the diffusion of bilirubin from plasma to tissue lymph, and on the binding of bilirubin by the tissue. Bilirubin enters the tissue fluid by diffusion of albumin-bilirubin complexes through the capillary endothelium; pigment will thus appear more rapidly at sites of inflammation and more slowly in areas of edema. There is a preferential binding of bilirubin by elastic fibers in tissue.

Jaundice is usually apparent in the sclerae and skin when the serum concentration exceeds 2 to 3 mg. per 100 ml. Mucous membranes, colored by capillary blood, usually appear icteric only when serum bilirubin levels are considerably elevated. In patients with long-standing jaundice of the obstructive type, the skin may assume a greenish hue that is due in part to melanin pigmentation. The cerebrospinal fluid usually remains colorless in the jaundiced patient unless there is associated meningitis with an increased permeability of the blood-cerebrospinal fluid barrier or raised cerebrospinal fluid protein concentrations.

BILIRUBIN METABOLISM

Bilirubin is a yellow tetrapyrrol pigment derived from hemoglobin and excreted in bile.

Senescent red cells that have survived in the circulation for approximately 120 days are taken up by macrophages in the reticuloendothelial system (R-E system), and their hemoglobin is degraded rapidly to bilirubin. The intermediates in the reactions that separate iron and protein (globin) from the molecule and open the tetrapyrrol ring at the α-methene bridge have not been defined. In studies on the incorporation of N^{15}-labeled glycine into the fecal pigment *stercobilin* (urobilin) that is derived from bilirubin, a small fraction (10 to 20 per cent) of labeled bile pigment was excreted within a few days of isotope administration. This "early-labeled" bile pigment may be derived in part from hemoglobin metabolized in the bone marrow but not incorporated into peripheral red cells, and in part from the metabolism of hepatic cytochromes.

Bilirubin released from the R-E cells is transported in plasma tightly bound to albumin (1 molecule of albumin binds up to 2 molecules of bilirubin). The subsequent excretion of bilirubin depends on its transfer from the plasma to the liver cell, its conjugation to diglucuronide, and its secretion into the bile canaliculus. The mechanism of bilirubin transfer from the plasma to the liver cell is not known, but must depend on binding by membrane or intracellular receptor substances that are able to displace bilirubin from the albumin-bilirubin complex. In the liver cell, bilirubin is concentrated and esterified to bilirubin diglucuronide. Conjugation with glucuronic acid is catalyzed by a microsomal enzyme, *glucuronyl transferase*, in the presence of uridine diphosphoglucuronic acid, and converts nonpolar, lipid-soluble, unconjugated bilirubin to a polar, water-soluble compound, which is excreted in bile.

The secretion of conjugated bilirubin from the liver cell across the membrane lining the bile canaliculi is normally the rate-limiting step in bilirubin excretion. *Conjugation of the pigment is a prerequisite for its secretion into the bile.* In the absence of bilirubin glucuronyl transferase (Crigler-Najjar syndrome, *vide infra*), the bile is colorless, and bile pigment is excreted by unidentified metabolic pathways.

Bacterial enzymes in the distal small intestine and colon convert conjugated bilirubin to colorless urobilinogens, which are excreted predominantly in the feces but are partly reabsorbed in the ileum and colon. Reabsorbed urobilinogen is either cleared by the liver and re-excreted in bile or excreted in the urine.

PATHOPHYSIOLOGY OF JAUNDICE

Hyperbilirubinemia with jaundice may be due to one or several mechanisms that include excessive pigment production, reduced hepatic uptake or conjugation of bilirubin, or decreased excretion of the conjugated pigment.

Excessive Bilirubin Production. *Hemolysis,* an excessive rate of red blood cell destruction, is the most common mechanism of excessive bilirubin production. In the normal subject, the low serum bilirubin concentration predominantly in the unconjugated fraction reflects the efficient hepatic clearance of the pigment. Hepatic bilirubin excretion may increase to maximal levels when pigment production is increased by hemolysis, but the serum concentration of bilirubin (predominantly unconjugated) rarely exceeds 3 to 5 mg. per 100 ml. unless hepatic excretion is impaired by reduced blood flow, impaired hepatocellular function, or ductal obstruction.

In some patients with unconjugated hyperbilirubinemia, bile pigment may be excreted in excess of the amount derived from peripheral red cell destruction. This is typical of thalassemia and pernicious anemia, but is sometimes unassociated with hemolytic disease. *Ineffective erythropoiesis* may account for excessive bilirubin production and jaundice in these patients. Although the "early-labeled" pigment excreted in bile is partly derived from the metabolism of heme enzymes (cytochromes) in the liver, there is currently no evidence that jaundice may result from increased hepatic metabolism of cytochromes.

Reduced Hepatic Uptake of Bilirubin. A defect in the transfer of plasma bilirubin to the liver cell may explain the unconjugated hyperbilirubinemia in *Gilbert's syndrome (vide infra),* following recovery from acute *viral hepatitis,* in congestive heart failure and following portacaval shunt surgery. Certain drugs may also competitively interfere with bilirubin uptake (iodopanoic acid, novobiocin).

Reduced Hepatic Conjugation of Bilirubin. Bilirubin conjugation with glucuronic acid is essential for normal bilirubin excretion. A deficiency or inhibition of glucuronyl transferase activity causes unconjugated hyperbilirubinemia. *Neonatal jaundice* is commonly due to immaturity of the hepatic excretory system, particularly in premature infants. In the *Crigler-Najjar syndrome (vide infra),* glucuronyl transferase activity is congenitally absent, the serum concentration of unconjugated bilirubin reaches high levels, and brain damage due to deposition of pigment in the basal ganglia (kernicterus) is usual. Rare patients have survived to adulthood.

Inhibition of glucuronyl transferase activity by a steroid excreted in maternal milk is an unusual cause for neonatal jaundice (*vide infra*).

Reduced Excretion of Conjugated Bilirubin. The excretion of conjugated bilirubin into the bile canaliculus appears to be an active transport process, but bilirubin excretion is markedly influenced by the volume of bile flow controlled by excretion of conjugated bile salts. In the *Dubin-Johnson* and *Rotor syndromes* there is a congenital defect in hepatic excretion of conjugated bilirubin and other organic anions including sulfobromophthalein (BSP); the normal excretion of conjugated bile salts in these patients suggests a separate transport pathway. Impaired excretion may result from hepatocellular injury as in *virus hepatitis,* or may be due to *drugs* that interfere with cell metabolism or increase the permeability of the biliary tree (methyl testosterone, estrogens), compete for excretion in bile, or damage bile ductules (chlorpromazine). Inflammatory, granulomatous, or neoplastic *infiltration* of the liver and extrahepatic *bile duct obstruction* by gallstone, stricture, or carcinoma commonly interfere with bile excretion.

Patients with jaundice may be subdivided clinically into two groups in which the serum bilirubin is either predominantly unconjugated or conjugated. *Unconjugated hyperbilirubinemia* is due to excessive production, reduced uptake, or reduced conjugation of pigment, whereas *conjugated hyperbilirubinemia* may result from hepatocellular or biliary tract disease. The terms *hemolytic jaundice, hepatocellular jaundice,* and *obstructive jaundice* of intra- and extrahepatic types (*intra-* and *extrahepatic cholestasis*) are often used to describe these types of jaundice. *Cholestasis* refers to reduced bile flow and reduced excretion of bile constituents; pathologically, there is usually evidence of bile stasis with bile plugs in the canaliculi. Several of the mechanisms discussed in the previous sections may be responsible for jaundice in a particular patient. As an example, in acute viral hepatitis mild hemolysis may increase bilirubin production; parenchymal cell damage may impair uptake, conjugation, and excretion of pigment; and intrahepatic cholestasis resulting from disruption of bile canaliculi or inflammation may reduce bile excretion.

FECAL AND URINARY EXCRETION OF BILE PIGMENTS

Unconjugated bilirubin, tightly bound to albumin and relatively nonpolar, cannot be dialyzed from plasma and does not pass the glomerular filter; jaundice with unconjugated hyperbilirubinemia is thus *acholuric.* Bilirubin diglucuronide, less avidly bound to plasma albumin, is partly dialyzable from plasma, and is excreted in the urine by glomerular filtration.

The quantity of bile pigment excreted as urobilinogens in feces and urine is a reflection of the amount of bilirubin in the bile, the bacterial conversion of bilirubin to urobilinogens, and the capacity of the liver to excrete urobilinogen absorbed from the intestine. *Fecal urobilinogen* is increased by excessive bilirubin production, and is reduced when hepatobiliary disease impairs bilirubin excretion or when bacterial conversion of bilirubin to urobilinogens is inhibited by antimicrobial therapy. *Urinary urobilinogen* is increased when greater amounts of urobilinogen are absorbed from the intestine or when parenchymal liver disease impairs the hepatic excretion of this pigment. Reduced urinary levels suggest cholestasis or impaired renal function.

CHANGES IN THE LIVER

Liver enlargement is usually an indication of disease. A normal liver displaced by a depressed diaphragm or a Riedel lobe must be considered in the differential diagnosis. An increase in liver size may reflect changes in liver cells (infiltration with fat or glycogen, or an increase in the smooth endoplasmic reticulum) cholestasis (intrahepatic or extrahepatic) venous congestion, inflammation (hepatitis) or abscess formation, cellular infiltration (macrophages in Gaucher's disease, granuloma in sarcoidosis, hematopoietic cells in extramedullary hematopoiesis, tumor cells in primary or secondary neoplasms), or fibrosis with regeneration (cirrhosis in the alcoholic). A *small liver* is characteristic of acute and subacute hepatic necrosis and idiopathic cirrhosis. The *consistency* of the liver may indicate the nature of the underlying disease. Infiltration and fibrosis cause induration; palpable *nodules* may be neoplasm, cysts, abscesses, or regeneration nodules. *Tenderness* may be due to acute enlargement or inflammation, and may be elicited by direct palpation or by percussion over the right lower ribs. Expansile *pulsation* of the congested liver results from tricuspid regurgitation. Vascular *bruits* over the liver may be due to arteriovenous fistulas, vascular tumors, or pressure on the aorta by an enlarged liver. *Friction rubs* are usually associated with neoplastic infiltration of the liver capsule and peritoneum, but may be due to peritonitis.

PORTAL HYPERTENSION

The pressure in the portal vein normally varies from 5 to 15 cm. of saline above the right atrial pressure. The causes of increased portal venous pressure (*portal hypertension*) are as follows:

1. *Increased central venous pressure* as in constrictive pericarditis and congestive heart failure.

2. *Postsinusoidal obstruction of the hepatic veins.* Major hepatic veins may be occluded by thrombus or tumor (Budd-Chiari syndrome). Centrolobular fibrosis (without cirrhosis) may obstruct the central veins (veno-occlusive disease, sclerosing hyaline necrosis in the alcoholic). Blood flow through smaller hepatic vein tributaries may be impaired by the distorted hepatic architecture and regeneration nodules in *cirrhosis;* intrahepatic arteriovenous shunting may also contribute to the elevation of portal pressure. These lesions that interfere with the flow of blood from the liver cause *sinusoidal hypertension* as

well as portal hypertension, and are commonly associated with ascites (*vide infra*).

3. *Presinusoidal obstruction of the portal vessels.* The obstructing lesions may be *intrahepatic,* involving the distal branches of the portal vein as in *schistosomiasis* and *congenital hepatic fibrosis,* or may be *extrahepatic* with thrombosis of the portal vein.

4. *Increased splanchnic blood flow.* This may be associated with *arteriovenous fistulas* in the splanchnic bed (either congenital or acquired from rupture of splenic or hepatic artery aneurysm), or may be related to *massive splenomegaly.* Although increased portal blood flow without mechanical obstruction to the portal system might cause portal hypertension, most patients with *idiopathic portal hypertension,* i.e., without cirrhosis or portal obstruction, exhibit sclerosis and narrowing of the intrahepatic portal bed. *Tropical splenomegaly* is the most common form of idiopathic portal hypertension.

MANIFESTATIONS

The manifestations of portal hypertension are *splenomegaly,* the development of a *collateral circulation,* and *ascites.*

Splenomegaly. Splenic enlargement is commonly due to venous congestion, but may also result from lymphoid hyperplasia and cellular infiltration. The spleen is not always palpable in patients with portal hypertension, and, conversely, an enlarged spleen does not necessarily imply that a patient with liver disease has portal hypertension.

Portal-Systemic Collateral Vessels. Collateral veins draining from the portal to the systemic venous system develop in response to an *increased pressure gradient* at sites of anastomosis between portal and systemic veins—in the esophagus and lower rectum, in the falciform ligament, in the retroperitoneal space, and in adhesions between the visceral and parietal peritoneum.

Esophageal collateral vessels between the left gastric and azygos veins develop as tortuous, dilated, thin-walled submucosal veins that may extend from the fundus of the stomach to the midesophagus (*esophageal* and *gastric varices*). Collateral vessels between the inferior mesenteric and internal iliac veins may form *hemorrhoids.* Collaterals from the left branch of the portal vein through patent umbilical or paraumbilical veins in the falciform ligament to the anterior abdominal wall may form a *caput medusae*—dilated, tortuous veins radiating from the umbilicus with centrifugal blood flow to epigastric, lateral thoracic, and saphenous vessels. A *venous hum* may be audible at the umbilicus (Cruveilhier-Baumgarten syndrome). These subcutaneous collaterals are most prominent when the patient is erect, and their origin from the portal system may be proved by showing that the glucose content of variceal blood exceeds that of peripheral venous blood during glucose absorption.

Acute upper gastrointestinal *bleeding from esophageal varices* is the major complication of portal hypertension (*vide infra*).

Ascites. Ascites is an accumulation of lymph in the peritoneal cavity. Hepatic and intestinal lymph normally drains through the thoracic duct into the left subclavian vein. Ascitic fluid accumulates when hepatic, and intestinal lymph is formed in amounts that exceed the capacity of the thoracic duct to drain lymph from the abdomen. Two factors, *portal hypertension* and a *lowered plasma colloidal osmotic pressure,* contribute to the increased transudation of fluid from hepatic sinusoids and splanchnic capillaries in patients with liver disease. A third factor, *increased plasma aldosterone* concentration, augments sodium and water retention by promoting distal renal tubular reabsorption of sodium.

Portal hypertension due to hepatic venous outflow tract obstruction (hepatic vein occlusion or cirrhosis), with *increased hepatic sinusoidal pressure,* is the major factor that determines the *selective* accumulation of fluid in the peritoneal cavity of patients with liver disease. Large volumes of hepatic lymph drain from congested sinusoids through dilated hilar lymphatic vessels to the thoracic duct, or may leak from lymphatic vessels in the capsule and hilum of the liver into the peritoneal cavity. Ascites in patients with liver disease is not a stagnant pool. There is a rapid exchange of water and electrolytes between plasma and ascites across the visceral peritoneum, and an increased volume of lymph drains through the thoracic duct from the abdominal viscera and peritoneal cavity.

Portal hypertension without sinusoidal hypertension rarely causes ascites unless acute bleeding from esophageal varices precipitates hypoalbuminemia and stimulates aldosterone secretion. (See Hepatic Schistosomiasis, *infra*.)

Hypoalbuminemia with a lowered plasma colloidal osmotic pressure increases fluid transudation from hepatic sinusoids and splanchnic capillaries, and thus augments lymph flow from these congested vascular beds. Hypoalbuminemic patients without portal hypertension, however, develop ascites only as a manifestation of fluid accumulation in dependent parts as in the nephrotic syndrome.

In cirrhotic patients with ascites there are increased urinary excretion and plasma concentration of *aldosterone,* owing in part to an *increased adrenal secretion* of aldosterone and in part to *reduced hepatic metabolism* of the hormone. Although it has been shown that inferior vena caval obstruction proximal to the hepatic veins in the dog stimulates aldosterone secretion, the exact mechanism of *secondary hyperaldosteronism* in patients with cirrhosis and portal hypertension has not been defined. A relative pooling of blood in the splanchnic bed with reduced renal blood flow may be the primary stimulus for the release of *renin* from the juxtaglomerular cells in the kidney and the subsequent secretion of salt-retaining

hormone. Aldosterone secretion will be further augmented by hemorrhage, infection, and the administration of diuretic agents to these patients.

Ascites is sometimes precipitated by *peritonitis* (especially *tuberculous*) or *tumor* invasion of the peritoneal cavity. These complications must be considered in the differential diagnosis (*vide infra*).

The clinical manifestations of ascites are increasing *abdominal distention* with *weight gain* and an associated *decrease in urine output.* Distention of the abdominal wall may cause pain over the lower ribs at the insertion of the abdominal muscles, and may promote the formation of umbilical and inguinal hernias. On physical examination there may be *shifting dullness,* a *fluid wave,* and *elevation of the diaphragms.* Ascitic fluid may leak through the diaphragm to create a *pleural effusion;* this is more often seen on the right than on the left. The urinary excretion of sodium is considerably decreased and may be less than 1 mEq. in 24 hours, whereas urinary potassium excretion is increased.

NEUROPSYCHIATRIC ABNORMALITIES ASSOCIATED WITH LIVER DISEASE

The neuropsychiatric manifestations of acute alcohol intoxication, prolonged excessive use of alcohol, alcohol withdrawal, vitamin deficiency in alcoholics, and head injury are often encountered in patients with cirrhosis. These are considered in the article on addiction. *Wilson's disease* is important in the differential diagnosis of patients with juvenile cirrhosis. The neurologic changes that result from copper deposition in the central nervous system are discussed under Inborn Errors of Metabolism.

HEPATIC COMA AND PRECOMA
(Hepatic Encephalopathy, Portal-Systemic Encephalopathy)

Patients with acute or chronic liver disease may develop a *metabolic encephalopathy* characterized by a variable disturbance of consciousness, psychiatric changes, a flapping tremor with hyperreflexia and increased muscle tone, hyperventilation with respiratory alkalosis, and a typical fetor.

Pathogenesis. Hepatic coma is associated with either severe impairment of liver function or with shunting of portal venous blood through collateral vessels into the peripheral circulation. Of the several factors that may contribute to this metabolic encephalopathy, changes in *ammonium metabolism* have been studied most extensively. An increase in blood ammonium concentration parallels the severity of neuropsychiatric changes in cirrhotic patients with *chronic* encephalopathy following portacaval anastomosis. This increase in blood ammonium concentration due to enteric absorption of ammonia formed by bacterial deamination of amino acids or urea hydrolysis may be the major biochemical change that precipitates dysfunction of the central nervous system. In patients with *acute* hepatic coma, however, disturbances of ammonium metabolism may be of lesser importance, and blood ammonium levels may be normal.

The central nervous system of the patient with liver disease may be more susceptible to a variety of metabolic insults. Thus, *hypoxia*, *electrolyte* and *acid-base imbalance*, *infection*, and *depressant drugs* may each contribute to metabolic encephalopathy in these patients. Although there may be changes in the serum concentration of electrolytes, elevation of blood ammonium concentration, and/or altered blood pH in patients with hepatic coma, these changes do not necessarily parallel electrolyte and pH changes and ammonium concentrations in the central nervous system. These changes *within the brain* are of primary importance in precipitating encephalopathy; alkalosis, which favors the diffusion of ammonia across the blood-brain barrier, increases ammonia toxicity. A biochemical explanation for the changes in brain metabolism in hepatic encephalopathy has not been established.

Clinical Features. The neuropsychiatric changes in hepatic encephalopathy are nonspecific. One of the more characteristic features of the metabolic encephalopathy associated with liver disease is its *rapid fluctuation. Disturbances of consciousness* may range from mild lethargy to deep coma. *Personality changes,* with depression or euphoria, irritability, anxiety, and paranoid features, together with a loss of concern for person or property, are evident. Intellectual function is variably impaired with *memory loss, inability to concentrate,* and a loss of the capacity for abstract thought. Speech may be slow and slurred, with a loss of modulation, and writing deteriorates; there may be dysphasia, perseveration, and apraxia. The common neurologic changes are a "flapping" tremor of the outstretched hands, asterixis, an increase in muscle tone, hyper-reflexia with clonus—often with flexor plantar responses—and ataxia. Hyperventilation causes respiratory alkalosis. The electroencephalogram shows the nonspecific changes of metabolic encephalopathy; high amplitude delta waves (2 to 3 per second) may replace normal alpha waves.

The *clinical course* of hepatic encephalopathy varies with its pathogenesis. In patients with *fulminant hepatitis* there is a rapid progression; mania and convulsions may precede the development of decerebrate rigidity and terminal deep coma. In patients with cirrhosis, encephalopathy may be acute or chronic and of varying severity. Chronic encephalopathy usually improves with therapy (*vide infra*), but may progress to permanent neuropsychiatric syndromes (paraplegia, dementia) over a period of years.

CLINICAL MANIFESTATIONS RESULTING FROM IMPAIRED HEPATIC DETOXIFICATION

The liver cell is the major site of detoxification of many drugs and exogenous substances and of endogenous substances, including hormones. In general, by processes of oxidation, reduction, hydrolysis, or conjugation, mediated by enzymes in the smooth endoplasmic reticulum, relatively lipid-soluble substances are converted to water-soluble compounds that may be excreted in bile or urine.

When hepatic detoxification is impaired in patients with liver disease, the pharmacologic action of some drugs may be augmented and prolonged as higher blood levels are maintained for longer periods of time than in normal subjects.

Many of the endocrine changes seen in patients with liver disease result from altered hepatic metabolism of hormones (*vide infra*).

ENDOCRINE CHANGES

The liver has a dual role in the metabolism of hormones. Several plasma proteins, alpha globulins, which bind hormones in the plasma, e.g., *thyroxin-binding protein, transcortin,* are synthesized by the liver; hormone activity may be influenced by protein binding in the plasma. Thyroxin and adrenal and gonadal steroid hormones are conjugated in the liver and partly excreted in bile. Conjugation forms polar, water-soluble molecules that have an enterohepatic circulation and are finally excreted in the urine.

Endocrine abnormalities in patients with liver disease may be due to malnutrition or chronic illness, to specific lesions of the endocrine glands (iron infiltration in hemochromatosis), or to altered hepatic metabolism, conjugation, and excretion of hormones by the diseased liver. Disturbances of gonadal function are particularly common. In males, there may be *hypogonadism,* with small testes, reduced libido and impotence, *gynecomastia,* and delayed development or regression of secondary sex characteristics. These changes may result from a reduced secretion of pituitary gonadotrophin or altered androgen metabolism. In females there may be delayed menarche, oligomenorrhea, or amenorrhea with subnormal breast development. Normal cyclic hormonal activity is disturbed, and cessation of ovulation leads to sterility.

Cutaneous *striae,* acne, and *hirsutism* with truncal obesity and moon facies may suggest *Cushing's syndrome.* Although plasma cortisol levels may be slightly elevated in these patients, the urinary excretion of hydroxy- and ketosteroids is either normal or subnormal.

The appearance of some alcoholic patients with cirrhosis may suggest *hyperthyroidism.* There may be a tremor, peripheral vasodilatation with sweating, tachycardia, and a slight stare. Although the basal metabolic rate and the uptake and conversion of radioiodine by the thyroid may be increased (particularly if there is iodine deficiency), the serum protein-bound iodine concentration is normal.

NUTRITIONAL AND METABOLIC ABNORMALITIES IN LIVER DISEASE

Weight loss may be due to malabsorption, reduced caloric intake in patients with anorexia, or increased tissue catabolism in acutely ill febrile patients. The chronic alcoholic, deriving a major fraction of his calories from alcohol, consumes a diet that may be deficient in protein, folic acid, ascorbic acid, B vitamins, and minerals. Although body weight may be maintained by alcohol and carbohydrate, *muscle wasting* with progressive weakness is usual. *Hypokalemia,* magnesium deficiency, or alcoholic *myopathy* may accentuate muscle weakness in some patients.

Carbohydrate Metabolism. The liver has a central role in regulating blood sugar levels. During carbohydrate absorption, the monosaccharides glucose, fructose, and galactose are taken up from portal venous blood by liver cells, phosphorylated in the presence of specific hexokinases, and converted to glycogen or metabolized through pyruvate and Krebs' cycle intermediates. During periods of fasting, or with secretion of epinephrine and glucagon, glycogenolysis or gluconeogenesis maintains or increases blood sugar levels.

Symptomatic *hypoglycemia* may occur in liver disease when hepatic glycogenolysis and gluconeogenesis are impaired. When liver glycogen stores are depleted by fasting, the ingestion of alcohol, which inhibits gluconeogenesis, may precipitate hypoglycemia (*alcoholic hypoglycemia*). Lowered blood sugar levels also result from massive hepatic necrosis (fulminant hepatitis) or a deficiency of enzymes necessary for glycogenolysis (glycogen storage diseases).

Diabetes mellitus in patients with cirrhosis is often due to associated pancreatic disease (chronic alcoholic pancreatitis, or hemochromatosis), but may be coincidental. Nondiabetic cirrhotic patients often have an abnormal glucose tolerance curve owing to a reduced rate of glucose uptake and release from the diseased liver. Normal fasting blood sugar levels, with prolonged hyperglycemia and late hypoglycemia following a glucose load, are characteristic.

Triglyceride Metabolism. Postprandially, dietary triglyceride enters the circulation as a lipid emulsion (chyle) from the thoracic duct (fatty acids of chain length > C10), or passes directly as fatty acid into the portal venous blood (fatty acids of chain length < C10). During periods of fasting, free fatty acid (FFA) is mobilized from peripheral fat depots and circulates as an albumin-

FFA complex. Plasma FFA or triglyceride entering the liver cell is stored as triglyceride droplets, incorporated into plasma lipoproteins and thus transported to peripheral depots or catabolized to ketone bodies for peripheral utilization.

Triglyceride accumulates in the liver whenever there is excessive peripheral mobilization of fat or when liver cell injury prevents the normal metabolism of triglyceride. A fatty liver is commonly found in obese subjects, in diabetics, in normal subjects during starvation, and in alcoholics. The disturbances in tryglyceride metabolism caused by acute and chronic alcohol ingestion are discussed in a later section.

Cholesterol and Bile Acids. Cholesterol synthesized in the liver is either incorporated into plasma lipoproteins, excreted directly into bile, or converted to primary bile acids.

Plasma lipoproteins, containing varying amounts of cholesterol (both free and esterified), phospholipid, triglyceride, and specific proteins, are synthesized by the liver and intestinal epithelium. Cholestasis causes an increase in plasma cholesterol concentration; this is associated with an increase in high density lipoprotein with a high content of cholesterol and phospholipid. This does not cause a lipemic serum. Liver failure with impaired hepatic synthesis depresses serum concentrations of lipoprotein and cholesterol.

Cholesterol is excreted in bile as a micellar solution with conjugated bile salt and phospholipid. Changes in the concentration of these compounds may lead to the formation of gallstones (see Diseases of the Gallbladder and Bile Ducts).

The primary bile acids (cholic and chenodeoxycholic acids) are synthesized from cholesterol and are secreted in bile as their glycine and taurine conjugates (bile salts). These conjugated bile salts undergo an enterohepatic circulation with active reabsorption from the distal small intestine. Between 20 and 30 grams of conjugated bile salts are thus excreted in bile and reabsorbed daily; the daily fecal loss of bile acids (approximately 1 gram) is balanced by resynthesis from cholesterol.

The conjugated bile salts have important functions that depend on their detergent properties. In the bile they permit the formation of soluble micelles containing cholesterol; in the intestinal lumen they activate pancreatic lipase and form mixed micelles with monoglyceride and long-chain fatty acids, thus facilitating the absorption of fat and fat-soluble vitamins.

Liver disease may be complicated by *malabsorption* when biliary secretion of conjugated bile salts is insufficient to promote the formation of lipid micelles in the jejunum. The duration of malabsorption in patients with acute liver disease may be too short to cause deficiency states other than *hypoprothrombinemia* owing to malabsorption of vitamin K. In patients with chronic cholestasis (primary and secondary biliary cirrhosis, *vide infra*) steatorrhea may cause diarrhea and weight loss, while malabsorption of fat-soluble vitamins A, D, and K may lead to night blindness, bone demineralization, and hypoprothrombinemia. Severe cholestasis with bile duct hyperplasia has been produced in laboratory animals by feeding monohydroxy bile acid (lithocholic acid); this may be due to precipitation of relatively insoluble bile salt in the biliary tree. There is a possibility that human intrahepatic cholestasis may be related to the excretion of monohydroxy bile salts (formed primarily in the diseased liver, or secondarily by bacterial dehydroxylation of dihydroxy acid in the intestine), but this has not been established.

Protein Metabolism. The liver cell contains enzyme systems that permit the synthesis of nonessential amino acids, synthesis of cellular and plasma proteins from amino acids, catabolism of plasma protein and amino acids, and conversion of ammonia to urea.

Amino acids derived from digested dietary proteins are absorbed in the upper small intestine, enter the portal venous blood, and are almost completely cleared by the liver to be catabolized or utilized in protein synthesis. During periods of fasting, amino acids are converted to pyruvate and phosphorylated hexose intermediates, which support gluconeogenesis and provide a source of glucose for brain metabolism.

Perfusion studies have shown that the liver is responsible for the synthesis of plasma proteins with the exception of the immunoglobulins and antihemophiliac globulin (AHG). It is also probable that the liver is a major site of plasma protein catabolism. The factors that control the synthesis and catabolism of the plasma proteins and thus maintain their constant physiologic levels are not known. These proteins maintain the colloidal osmotic pressure of plasma, play a vital role in the transport of many substances (including iron, vitamin B_{12}, hormones, hemoglobin, bilirubin, and nonesterified fatty acids) and maintain normal blood clotting mechanisms. Hepatic synthesis of plasma proteins may be impaired by hepatocellular failure. A reduced rate of plasma protein catabolism may partly compensate for reduced synthesis, which leads to *hypoproteinemia*. Severe *bleeding* may complicate a deficiency of blood-clotting factors. Excessive urinary excretion and elevated plasma levels of amino acids is a manifestation of severe hepatocellular failure, particularly fulminant hepatitis. Although urea is synthesized by the liver, low blood urea levels are more often the result of dilution with fluid infused intravenously than of hepatocellular failure.

HEMATOLOGIC ABNORMALITIES

Anemia in patients with liver disease may be due to *blood loss* or *excessive destruction* and/or *reduced formation* of red cells. Changes in red cell morphology may reflect specific deficiency (iron or folic acid) or may result from changes in the lipid composition of the red cell membrane. Red blood cells from patients with cholestasis have an increased surface area related to the reversible accumulation of cholesterol from the plasma; these cells have a lowered osmotic fragility, and appear as target-cells on stained smears. Severe hemolysis in the alcoholic with liver disease may be associated with the appearance of poikilocytes (burr-cells) on peripheral smears.

Bleeding from the nose, upper gastrointestinal tract (esophageal varices, erosive gastritis, or peptic ulcer), or rectum (hemorrhoids) may precipitate acute anemia or chronic iron deficiency anemia. In the absence of blood loss, iron deficiency is uncommon in patients with liver disease; an increase in total body iron with hemosiderosis is more usual, particularly in alcoholic patients with pancreatic disease. The pathogenesis of this secondary hemosiderosis is not known.

Hemolysis is the most common cause of chronic anemia in patients with liver disease. Chronic, low-grade hemolysis in patients with splenomegaly is due to sequestration of red blood cells in the cortex of the congested spleen. Red cell production may fail to compensate for this increased destruction, particularly during periods of hepatic decompensation, so that the patient may exhibit a normochromic and sometimes macrocytic anemia with a normal reticulocyte count, reduced serum levels of haptoglobin, an increased serum level of unconjugated bilirubin, and a bone marrow showing cellular hyperplasia. Severe hemolytic anemia may be associated with hyperlipemia in alcoholic hepatitis (*vide infra*) (*Zieve's syndrome*), but a causal relationship between the hyperlipemia and hemolysis has not been established. Acute viral hepatitis may precipitate hemolysis in patients with *glucose-6-phosphate dehydrogenase (G-6-PD) deficiency;* particularly high serum concentrations of bilirubin usually result.

A *deficiency of folic acid* may lead to a severe macrocytic anemia with *megaloblastic* bone marrow in alcoholic patients with liver disease. An inadequate vitamin intake, together with alcohol inhibition of folic acid utilization, contributes to the anemia. Treatment with a normal diet containing folic acid or with folic acid supplements corrects this deficiency. Rarely, a normochromic, normocytic anemia may be due to *pyridoxine deficiency*.

Although *thrombocytopenia* (platelet counts < 200,000 per cubic millimeter) and *granulocytopenia* (WBC counts 4000 per cubic millimeter) may be associated with anemia in patients with liver disease and congestive splenomegaly, these abnormalities are rarely complicated by serious bleeding or infection. Severe thrombocytopenia and fatal aplastic anemia have been reported as complications of acute viral hepatitis.

CARDIOVASCULAR CHANGES

Hepatocellular failure is often associated with an *increase* in *cardiac output* manifested by tachycardia, a precordial ejection systolic murmur, and peripheral vasodilatation. The cause for these circulatory changes is not known.

Hypovolemic shock may be a terminal complication of chronic liver disease with ascites, precipitated by massive upper gastrointestinal bleeding, by infection (especially gram-negative septicemia), or by paracentesis. A lowered circulating blood volume owing to bleeding or sudden redistribution of fluid from the plasma compartment to ascitic fluid after paracentesis reduces splanchnic and peripheral blood flow. Impairment of renal function causes progressive uremia; reduced hepatic blood flow may further impair liver function; and changes in cell membrane permeability in anoxic tissues alter electrolyte distribution between extra- and intracellular fluid to precipitate hyperkalemia, hyponatremia, and metabolic acidosis.

Some patients with cirrhosis may exhibit central *cyanosis* with arterial oxygen unsaturation. In patients with portal hypertension, this may be due to portopulmonary venous shunts that bypass the pulmonary capillaries, or may result from pulmonary arteriovenous shunts or reduced aeration of basal lung segments in patients with tense ascites.

CHANGES IN RENAL FUNCTION

There are many causes for impairment of renal function in patients with liver disease. Many agents may cause acute cellular injury in both liver and kidneys; these include *hepatotoxins* (carbon tetrachloride, *Amanita phalloides*), *infectious agents* (leptospirosis, infectious hepatitis virus; *vide infra*), and *hypoxia* (shock). *Metabolic diseases* may damage both organs; in Wilson's disease the deposition of copper in the tissues is associated with cirrhosis and impaired tubular reabsorptive function with glycosuria, aminoaciduria, and hypouricemia.

In patients with cirrhosis and ascites several factors may modify or impair renal function. There may be a physiologic response to secondary hyperaldosteronism with sodium retention and potassium excretion, reversed by aldosterone-blocking drugs (*vide infra*). Abnormal excretion of a water load owing to antidiuretic hormone activity, reduced renal blood flow, or an unexplained decrease in free water clearance by the kidney may lead to dilutional hyponatremia with water intoxication. Impaired renal function with azotemia in cirrhotic patients with ascites is sometimes explained by chronic pyelonephritis, but there is often no renal lesion on postmortem examination; a reduced renal blood flow caused by a decrease in the peripheral blood volume may be the most common cause for impaired renal function in these patients.

In view of the known diversity of the many processes that may impair both hepatic and renal function, it is misleading and inappropriate to use the term "hepato-renal syndrome."

CUTANEOUS MANIFESTATIONS OF LIVER DISEASE

Pruritus. Patients with obstructive jaundice (both intrahepatic and extrahepatic cholestasis) may suffer from generalized itching. This is probably caused by retained *bile acids.* The intensity of pruritus parallels the serum concentration of bile acids, and the oral administration of the resin cholestyramine lowers serum bile acid levels and relieves itching by binding bile salts in the intestine and preventing their reabsorption. *Itching is not related to the intensity of jaundice;* anicteric patients may itch because of retained bile salts, whereas deeply jaundiced patients may be free of pruritus when cholesterol and bile acid synthesis is impaired by hepatocellular failure.

Pigmentation. An increase in *melanin pigmentation* of the skin is typical in chronic obstructive jaundice (biliary cirrhosis) and in hemochromatosis. The pathogenesis is not known.

Spider Angiomas (Vascular Spiders). These cutaneous lesions, found in areas drained by the superior vena cava, have a central pulsating arteriole from which small vessels radiate over an area 1 to 10 mm. in diameter. Multiple lesions may appear and disappear during the course of both acute and chronic liver disease, but are most numerous when liver disease is chronic and progressive. Small arterial spiders are also seen in normal subjects, and often appear during pregnancy. Their pathogenesis is not known.

Palmar Erythema. Cutaneous erythema, maximal over the thenar and hypothenar eminences and the pulp of the fingers and less often seen on the soles of the feet, is due to local vasodilatation with increased blood flow. The cardiac output is usually increased in patients with prominent palmar erythema.

Other changes in the hands include *Dupuytren's contractures* in patients with cirrhosis associated with alcohol ingestion, *clubbing* of the nails in patients with biliary cirrhosis, and white, opaque nails with loss of lunules in hypoalbuminemic patients.

Xanthomas. Prolonged obstructive jaundice with elevation of serum lipoprotein may be associated with deposits of lipid, predominantly cholesterol, in macrophages in the dermis or subcutaneous tissue. Flat lesions (*xanthelasma*) are common on the eyelids, on the neck, and in the palm creases, as yellow, slightly raised, soft deposits. Tuberous lesions, more common over areas exposed to pressure, are firm, nodular, and slightly yellow. These lesions may appear when serum cholesterol levels exceed 450 mg. per 100 ml. for several months, and may disappear when serum cholesterol levels fall below that value.

NONSPECIFIC SYMPTOMS IN PATIENTS WITH LIVER DISEASE

Many symptoms in patients with liver disease are also common manifestations of nonhepatic disorders. It is often impossible to determine whether these symptoms are primarily due to liver disease or whether they result from extra-hepatic effects of the primary noxious agent. The prodromal symptoms of acute viral hepatitis— malaise, weakness, unusual fatigability, anorexia, fever, myalgia, and headache—are good examples. Although these symptoms are nonspecific, they are often helpful in differential diagnosis.

Fever. Fever is common in patients with acute liver disease and is usually due to tissue necrosis, infection, or drug hypersensitivity. In patients with acute metabolic encephalopathy, fever may be due to dysfunction of central thermoregulatory mechanisms. This usually occurs in fulminant hepatitis and in the alcoholic with a severe withdrawal reaction (delirium tremens).

Abdominal Pain. Abdominal pain may be localized to the right upper quadrant and may result from inflammation or stretching of the pain-sensitive capsule of the liver. Epigastric or mid-abdominal pain may be due to associated peptic ulcer disease, acute gastritis, or pancreatitis. Stretching of the abdominal wall by tense ascites may cause pain over the lower costal margin.

DIAGNOSTIC PROCEDURES

TESTS OF LIVER FUNCTION

Many biochemical tests have been used to estimate liver function. In interpreting tests of liver function one must remember that no test is diagnostic of specific liver lesion, that many tests may be normal in the presence of liver disease, and that factors other than liver disease may cause abnormal tests.

Serum Bilirubin. Spectrophotometric measurement of the amount of diazo-pigment formed by the van den Bergh reaction after one minute in the absence of alcohol gives an estimate of the direct-reacting serum bilirubin concentration; this is approximately equal to the serum concentration of conjugated bilirubin, which is diazotized in the absence of alcohol. When alcohol is added in the van den Bergh reaction, unconjugated bilirubin is able to react with the diazo reagent, and the total concentration of bilirubin (direct plus indirect reacting) in the serum is estimated. Normal serum contains less than 0.2 mg. of direct-reacting pigment and less than 0.8 mg. of indirect-reacting pigment per 100 ml. Measurements of serum bilirubin (direct-reacting and total) are helpful in separating diseases associated with unconjugated bilirubinemia from those causing predominantly conjugated hyperbilirubinemia, but are of no value in differentiating jaundice resulting from hepatocellular disease from extra-hepatic cholestasis. Serial determinations of serum bilirubin concentration provide a more accurate measure of the impairment of bilirubin excretion during the course of liver disease than can be gained by a clinical assessment of the degree of jaundice.

Tests for *bilirubin in the urine* are helpful in differentiating jaundice caused by unconjugated hyperbilirubinemia; only conjugated bilirubin is excreted in the urine. Bilirubin may be excreted in the urine when the elevation of serum bilirubin is insufficient to cause jaundice.

Urinary and Fecal Urobilinogen. Urinary excretion of urobilinogen increases when the amount of urobilinogen absorbed from the intestine is increased by excessive pigment production or when hepatic excretion of urobilinogen is impaired by liver disease. Normally, urobilinogen can be detected in urine diluted to 1 in 16. *An increase in urinary urobilinogen excretion in the absence of increased fecal excretion of pigment is a very sensitive indicator of liver disease.* A quantitative measurement of the 24-hour fecal excretion of urobilinogen is of diagnostic value in hemolytic states and in patients with biliary tract disease. An increased fecal excretion of urobilinogen confirms that there is excessive bilirubin production, and a total absence of urobilinogen in the stool indicates complete biliary tract obstruction owing to atresia or neoplasm.

Sulfobromophthalein Sodium (Bromsulphthalein, BSP) Clearance. The measurement of the hepatic clearance of this organic, anionic dye is the most sensitive test of liver function. Injected BSP, bound by plasma proteins (albumin and alpha globulin), is cleared by the liver and excreted in bile. BSP excretion by the liver depends on the selective uptake and concentration of dye in the liver cell and the rate-limiting active transport of both unconjugated and glutathione-conjugated BSP into the bile canaliculi. BSP clearance varies with bile salt excretion, and can be increased experimentally by intravenous infusion of bile salt which augments excretion by increasing canalicular bile flow.

In the standard liver function test, the amount of BSP retained in the plasma is measured 30 or 45 minutes after an intravenous injection of the dye (5 mg. per kilogram of body weight). The normal subject excretes more than 90 and 96 per cent of the injected BSP in 30 and 45 minutes, respectively. A reduced plasma clearance of BSP (increased retention of dye in the plasma) may result from changes in hepatic blood flow as in congestive heart failure or portal vein thrombosis, from reduced ability of liver cells to concentrate or excrete the dye as in hepatocellular injury and metabolic abnormalities, or from obstruction to bile flow in intrahepatic and extrahepatic cholestasis. Thus, abnormal BSP excretion does not indicate a specific hepatic lesion. The dye should be injected with care, as leakage outside the vein causes severe pain and tissue necrosis.

Although the standard BSP test is a sensitive measure of liver function, the maximal capacity of the liver to excrete the dye is not measured. The maximal capacity of the liver to concentrate and to excrete BSP may be estimated by measuring plasma clearance when infusions of the dye are given. Either of these maxima may be reduced when all other tests of liver function remain normal. In some patients with liver disease, the maximal excretion rate of the dye may be reduced when hepatic storage is normal or increased.

Albumin. Normal levels of plasma albumin are maintained by an equilibrium between hepatic synthesis and degradation or loss. When synthesis is reduced in liver disease, the serum albumin concentration and the total body albumin pool decrease until a new equilibrium is established between synthesis and degradation. In view of the slow rate of albumin degradation (the half-time of plasma albumin degradation varies between 12 and 18 days), the serum concentration of albumin does not immediately reflect rapid changes in liver function, but decreases slowly when synthesis is impaired.

Globulins. Changes in the concentration of the serum globulins can be assessed by salt fractionation or by electrophoresis of serum. *Alpha and beta globulin* concentrations increase in patients with infection or obstructive jaundice and decrease when hepatocellular failure impairs their synthesis. The serum concentration of the *immunoglobulins* increases when antibody production is stimulated by exogenous or tissue antigen. Although immunoglobulin synthesis is not a function of the liver, measurements of serum gamma globulin concentrations may be helpful in diagnosis. Extreme hypergammaglobulinemia may be found in patients with postnecrotic and biliary cirrhosis. This may be associated with positive serologic tests (antinuclear, L-E).

The serum *flocculation tests* are nonspecific tests in which the plasma proteins are precipitated or flocculated by a variety of agents. Positive tests depend on relative changes in the concentration of several plasma proteins and are not specific for liver disease.

Blood-Clotting Factors. Many of the factors active in blood clotting are synthesized by the liver: prothrombin, factors V, VII, IX, and X, and fibrinogen. A lowered plasma concentration of these proteins, measured by blood-clotting tests (see Coagulation Defects in Diseases of Blood), may be due to *malabsorption of vitamin K,* which is required for the synthesis of prothrombin and factors VII, IX, and X, or may reflect *impaired* hepatic protein *synthesis*. In view of the very short half-life (two to four days) of several of the blood-clot-

ting factors, changes in the one-stage prothrombin time provide a sensitive index of sudden changes in liver function in patients with acute liver disease. An abnormal test after vitamin K has been given parenterally to correct for deficiency resulting from malabsorption indicates severe hepatic damage.

Cholesterol. Changes in serum cholesterol concentrations reflect changes in serum lipoprotein. In cholestasis, when cholesterol and bile acid excretion is impaired but cholesterol synthesis is normal, serum lipoprotein and cholesterol concentrations increase. When hepatic lipoprotein synthesis is impaired by hepatocellular disease, serum cholesterol concentrations fall.

Serum Enzymes. Increases in serum enzyme activity in patients with liver disease result from the release of intracellular enzymes from damaged liver cells (transaminases and dehydrogenases) or from an increased synthesis and/or reduced secretion of enzymes that are normally present in bile (alkaline phosphatase, 5-nucleotidase, and leucine aminopeptidase). Liver cell necrosis is associated with considerable elevation of the transaminases and dehydrogenases, whereas cholestasis leads to elevations of alkaline phosphatase, 5-nucleotidase, and leucine aminopeptidase activities.

NEEDLE BIOPSY OF THE LIVER

Percutaneous needle biopsy of the liver by an intercostal approach under local anesthesia is a simple, safe bedside procedure that provides a tissue diagnosis of liver disease without subjecting the patient to the greater risk of general anesthesia and laparotomy with open surgical biopsy.

Indications. Needle biopsy of the liver is of proved value in the following situations:

1. In the differential diagnosis of jaundice, hepatic enlargement, and splenomegaly.

2. In the differential diagnosis of unexplained fever. A liver biopsy may suggest or establish the diagnosis of *miliary tuberculosis,* sarcoidosis, brucellosis, or neoplasm.

3. To assess the degree of hepatic fibrosis in chronic hepatitis and cirrhosis, to evaluate the course of hepatitis and acute liver disease, and to estimate hepatic stores of iron in hemochromatosis.

Contraindications. Liver biopsy is contraindicated in the following circumstances:

1. In patients who are uncooperative or who cannot control movements of the diaphragm, e.g., with severe recurrent cough.

2. In patients with bleeding disorders, with clotting defects (prothrombin time elevations greater than two to three seconds over control), or with vascular tumors in the liver.

3. In patients with severe cardiopulmonary disease that would be a contraindication to surgery should a biopsy complication ensue.

4. In patients with prolonged jaundice, probably extrahepatic in origin.

Complications. Needle biopsy of the liver is usually painless, but is occasionally followed by right pleuritic chest pain referred to the shoulder; a transient pleural friction rub may be audible at the site of biopsy. Serious complications include *hemorrhage* from the biopsy site and leakage of bile from dilated intrahepatic bile ducts or gallbladder, with *bile peritonitis*; this is usually a complication of extrahepatic obstruction. The incidence of these major complications should be less than 0.1 per cent.

PROCEDURES USED TO DIAGNOSE BILIARY TRACT DISEASE

Oral cholecystography and *intravenous cholangiography* are discussed in the articles on Diseases of the Gallbladder and Bile Ducts.

A *percutaneous transhepatic cholangiogram,* in which dye is directly injected into dilated intrahepatic bile ducts, may be helpful in establishing a diagnosis of biliary tract disease (either intrahepatic or extrahepatic) in patients with obstructive jaundice. In view of the risks of bile peritonitis, this should be done as an elective preoperative procedure.

The value of *duodenal drainage* and the *secretin test* in the diagnosis of biliary tract and pancreatic diseases is also discussed under Diseases of the Gallbladder and Bile Ducts.

DIAGNOSTIC PROCEDURES IN PORTAL HYPERTENSION

Esophageal varices may be demonstrated roentgenographically by a *barium swallow,* although *esophagoscopy* is a more accurate method for their identification.

Portal venous pressure may be measured indirectly by *splenic pulp manometry,* as the pressure in the splenic sinusoids reflects portal venous pressure. Splenic pressure is measured either with a saline manometer or with a strain gauge through a needle inserted into the spleen between the lower ribs. This procedure is often combined with a *percutaneous intrasplenic portal venogram,* in which radiopaque dye injected into the spleen permits visualization of the portal venous system and collateral vessels; it is important to visualize the portal venous system in patients with portal hypertension prior to portacaval shunt surgery, because a patent portal vein is necessary for this operation. The portal circulation may also be visualized roentgenographically by *selective celiac arteriography,* or by injection of contrast material into the *catheterized umbilical vein. Hepatic vein catheterization* via the subclavian vein and right atrium with measurement of the *wedged hepatic vein pressure* provides an indirect measure of the hepatic sinusoidal pressure, i.e., the pressure in the vascular bed proximal to the site of the wedged catheter. This value is elevated when there is postsinusoidal portal hypertension as in cirrhosis of the liver and is normal when portal hypertension is due to a presinusoidal portal obstruction as in schistosomiasis.

Liver Scanning. When compounds that are concentrated in the liver (either by parenchymal or Kupffer cells) are labeled with gamma-emitting isotopes and injected intravenously, their uptake by the liver can be assessed by surface scanning. ^{131}I-labeled rose bengal, ^{198}Au colloidal gold, and ^{99}technetium have been used. Space-occupying lesions (cysts, abscesses, or tumors) appear as filling defects. In patients with cirrhosis, hepatic uptake is decreased and irregular and splenic uptake may be increased.

THE HEPATIC DISEASES

METABOLIC DISORDERS

Inborn errors of metabolism may cause chronic liver disease. In some of these conditions specific enzyme defects have been demonstrated (glycogen storage diseases, galactosemia), whereas in others the underlying metabolic abnormality has not yet been defined (idiopathic hemochromatosis, Wilson's disease, Gaucher's disease). These diseases are considered in detail under Inborn Errors of Metabolism.

Disorders of Bilirubin Metabolism. Knowledge of several metabolic disorders has contributed greatly to an understanding of bilirubin metabolism and excretion.

Unconjugated Hyperbilirubinemia. Acholuric jaundice with unconjugated hyperbilirubinemia in the absence of other signs of anemia or liver disease may be due to one of the following conditions:

1. *Compensated hemolysis* in which increased red cell production masks excessive red cell destruction. This abnormality may be suggested by lowered serum haptoglobin concentrations and increased fecal urobilinogen and reticulocyte counts, but can be confirmed only by direct measurement of red cell survival using tagged erythrocytes.

2. *Excessive bilirubin production without hemolysis* ("shunt hyperbilirubinemia"). This is a rare condition in which abnormal catabolism of hemoglobin in red cell precursors in the bone marrow results in excessive pigment production (early-labeled bilirubin) and increased fecal urobilinogen excretion; peripheral red cell survival is normal.

3. *Idiopathic unconjugated hyperbilirubinemia (Gilbert's syndrome).* Mild unconjugated hyperbilirubinemia (usually <3 mg. per 100 ml.), without hemolysis or excessive bilirubin production

is commonly recognized in healthy young subjects. Jaundice may be intermittent with exacerbations during intercurrent illness. The absence of physical abnormalities, normal liver function tests, and normal liver histology exclude a diagnosis of viral hepatitis. This syndrome appears to have an autosomal dominant inheritance; unconjugated hyperbilirubinemia was detected in 16.1 per cent of parents and 27.5 per cent of siblings of patients with this disorder.

A defect in hepatic uptake of unconjugated bilirubin is the most likely explanation for the hyperbilirubinemia. Definition of this abnormality requires a better understanding of bilirubin uptake and storage in the liver.

4. *Parenchymal liver disease* may be associated with unconjugated hyperbilirubinemia. This has been recognized in patients during recovery from viral hepatitis. Other abnormal tests of liver function (positive flocculation tests, mildly abnormal BSP), and histologic changes on liver biopsy suggest hepatitis in these patients. Unconjugated hyperbilirubinemia in patients with congestive heart failure, or following portacaval shunt surgery for portal hypertension, reflects reduced hepatic blood flow and bilirubin clearance.

5. *Impaired bilirubin conjugation.* A defect in bilirubin conjugation is usually manifest during the neonatal period, and may be due to immaturity of the liver, inhibition of glucuronyl transferase, or deficiency of this enzyme.

a. *The immature liver* of the premature infant exhibits a reduced level of glucuronyl transferase activity. It has not been established, however, that this is the primary cause for physiologic jaundice; there may be other defects in the excretory mechanism.

b. *Prolonged neonatal jaundice in breast-fed infants* may be due to inhibition of glucuronyl transferase activity by an abnormal steroid (pregnane-3α,20β-diol) excreted in the mother's milk. Jaundice is maximal during the second to third week, and subsides rapidly if breast feeding is discontinued, or over a four to eight week period with continued breast feeding.

Transient neonatal hyperbilirubinemia, described in successive infants of several mothers, has been related to the presence of an inhibitor of glucuronyl transferase in the maternal plasma during pregnancy. Several of these infants developed kernicterus.

c. *The Crigler-Najjar syndrome* (congenital, nonhemolytic, unconjugated hyperbilirubinemia with glucuronyl transferase deficiency). This syndrome, characterized by severe jaundice, usually from birth, is transmitted in some patients as an autosomal recessive defect, and in others as an autosomal dominant. Patients with the autosomal recessive defect are deeply jaundiced (mean bilirubin levels 25 to 31 mg. per 100 ml.) and develop kernicterus. Their bile is colorless, and phenobarbital administration does not lower the serum level of unconjugated bilirubin. The autosomal dominant defect may cause less severe hyperbilirubinemia so that some patients survive to

adulthood without kernicterus. When phenobarbital is given to these patients, the serum bilirubin concentration falls dramatically; this effect may be due to induction of glucuronyl transferase activity.

The homozygous *Gunn rat,* deficient in glucuronyl transferase, provides a laboratory model of the Crigler-Najjar syndrome.

Kernicterus (Bilirubin Encephalopathy). This neurologic complication of unconjugated hyperbilirubinemia usually develops in the jaundiced infant during the first week of life with the appearance of spasticity, leading to head retraction, opisthotonos, muscle twitching, or convulsions. The infant may die during the neonatal period, whereas survivors exhibit mental retardation and spastic paraplegia with athetosis. Unconjugated bilirubin, bound to plasma albumin, does not diffuse into the central nervous system. Diffusible, free bilirubin is present in serum when the total bilirubin concentration exceeds the albumin-binding capacity, or when bilirubin is dissociated from the albumin-bilirubin complex by drugs (sulfonamides and salicylates), or under conditions of metabolic acidosis. The biochemical mechanism for bilirubin encephalopathy has not been defined.

Preventive therapy depends on the early recognition and treatment of conditions that may cause severe unconjugated hyperbilirubinemia in the newborn, e.g., Rh incompatibility). Exchange transfusion may be necessary to lower serum bilirubin levels; drugs which reduce albumin binding of bilirubin should be avoided, and metabolic acidosis should be treated vigorously. The administration of phenobarbital and exposure to sunlight or intense blue light (440 mμ wavelength) have been suggested as means of decreasing bilirubin levels by increasing excretion or degradation.

The Dubin-Johnson Syndrome. This is a familial metabolic disorder caused by impaired transport of certain organic anions into the bile. Jaundice is associated with an increased serum level of conjugated bilirubin and bilirubinuria. Jaundice is usually intermittent, and exacerbations are often associated with mild right upper quadrant abdominal pain. There is no hepatic enlargement. The excretion of oral cholecystographic agents is impaired so that the normal biliary system often cannot be visualized. Although BSP is concentrated and conjugated normally in the liver cell, biliary excretion of the dye is impaired, and large amounts of conjugated BSP passing back into the plasma may elevate the two-hour plasma BSP level above the 45-minute value. Patients with the Dubin-Johnson syndrome do not suffer from pruritus; there is no evidence for abnormal biliary secretion of the conjugated bile salts. In contrast to the retention of conjugated bilirubin and BSP, serum alkaline phosphatase levels are usually normal.

The diagnosis of the Dubin-Johnson syndrome is established by needle biopsy of the liver. Macroscopically the fresh liver tissue is black, and microscopically there are deposits of melanin-like pigment in the parenchymal cells, particularly in the centrilobular areas. The Kupffer cells do not contain pigment, the bile canaliculi are normal, and the liver is free of fibrosis or inflammatory infiltrate. Recent studies on mutant Corriedale sheep with a similar defect in organic anion transport and liver pigmentation suggest that the pigment may be an oxidation product of metanephrine glucuronide, an epinephrine metabolite normally excreted in bile but poorly excreted by these animals and by patients with the Dubin-Johnson syndrome. The hepatic pigment accumulates with increasing age in both conditions. The *Rotor syndrome* is a variant of the Dubin-Johnson syndrome, differing only in the absence of hepatic pigment.

The more important considerations in managing patients with this disorder of bilirubin metabolism are the reassurance that the abnormality is benign and leads to no disability or reduction in life expectancy and the avoidance of unnecessary biliary tract surgery.

DISEASES ASSOCIATED WITH ACUTE HEPATIC INJURY

Acute liver injury may result from a variety of noxious agents—physical, chemical, viral, and bacterial. There may be necrosis of liver cells, interference with normal cellular function, or changes in the formation of bile. The acute injury may be followed by rapid clinical, biochemical, and histologic recovery, may lead to early death, or may result in chronic progressive liver disease.

ACUTE VIRAL HEPATITIS

Acute viral hepatitis is a common acute inflammatory disease of the liver caused by two strains of hepatotropic virus: virus or viruses A of acute infectious hepatitis (IH), and virus or viruses B of serum hepatitis (SH). The diagnosis of viral hepatitis is a presumptive one based on epidemiologic, clinical, biochemical, and histologic evidence that may be typical but never pathognomonic. Major advances in our knowledge of the pathogenesis of viral hepatitis and its sequelae and improved methods of prevention, diagnosis, and treatment await the isolation of the hepatitis viruses and the preparation of specific vaccines and antisera.

Etiology. Much of the information relating to the viral origin of both IH and SH has been based on indirect evidence derived from studies of epidemic hepatitis and from human transmission experiments. Both IH and SH are caused by filterable agents relatively resistant to heat and chemical disinfectants. Epidemiologic and clinical evidence suggests several differences in the biologic properties of these viruses. In IH, virus is transmitted by both parenteral and oral routes, sometimes as an endemic infection, at other times in epidemic outbreaks. The incubation period is short (two to six weeks), and the infective agent appears in both blood and feces during the prodromal and early icteric phases of illness. Infection confers immunity against further attacks of IH, but does not protect against SH. Serum hepatitis was considered to be transmitted only by parenteral inoculation of infected blood or blood products with a long incubation period of six weeks to six months. Transmission of disease following transfusion of blood from healthy donors indicated a prolonged carrier state.

A recent study by Krugman et al. clearly defined two epidemiologically and clinically distinct types of hepatitis. One had a short incubation period and caused a brief illness; the other had a long incubation period and caused a more protracted illness. Each conferred homologous but not cross immunity, and *each was transmitted by both parenteral and oral routes.* This study provides strong objective evidence that SH may be transmitted by nonparenteral routes. *Just as it is no longer valid to assume that all patients with post-transfusion hepatitis are infected with SH virus, so also it is now uncertain that patients who develop hepatitis without parenteral exposure are suffering from IH virus infection.*

Recently, a virus-like antigen has been identified in the serum of patients with hepatitis. This antigen reacts in immunodiffusion and complement-fixation tests with an antibody in the serum of patients who have received multiple transfusions, e.g., in hemophilia. The antigen was initially called *Australia antigen* because it was first observed in the serum of an Australian aborigine, or *serum hepatitis* (SH) antigen from its association with post-transfusion hepatitis; the name *hepatitis-related antigen* seems more appropriate until it has been better characterized. Hepatitis-related antigen appears in the blood during the incubation period and early clinical course of post-transfusion hepatitis, and usually disappears with clinical recovery. It has been detected in the serum of many adult patients with hepatitis (with or without a history of parenteral exposure) and in children with hepatitis of long incubation period, whereas childhood hepatitis of short incubation and point-source outbreaks of epidemic hepatitis are not associated with the antigen. Of other patients with liver disease, only those with chronic aggressive hepatitis have a significant frequency of hepatitis-related antigen in their sera.

Epidemiology. *Infectious Hepatitis.* Transmission of the IH virus is usually by the fecal-oral route, although infusion of infected blood obtained from viremic donors may cause sporadic infection. The occurrence of both sporadic and epidemic hepatitis depends on the distribution of infected material and the susceptibility of the exposed population. Thus, poor sanitation, overcrowding, and exposure of a nonimmune population will contribute to an epidemic situation. Explosive epidemics have been described following fecal contamination of drinking water and milk, and the concentration of virus by shellfish in polluted sea water has been a recent cause of several epidemics in the eastern United States. The common epidemics in institutions that house small children — orphanages, schools and homes for the mentally retarded — reflect the exposure of a nonimmune population to many cases of anicteric or pre-icteric IH.

Serum Hepatitis. Transmission of SH (long incubation period) by the parenteral route is well documented. This is a hazard of blood transfusion, particularly when many of the donors are drug addicts. Pooled plasma, fibrinogen, and vaccines contaminated with human serum, e.g., yellow fever vaccine during World War II, are likely to be contaminated with virus. The hazard of using inadequately sterilized syringes, hypodermic needles, dental and surgical instruments, tattoo needles, and razors is well recognized. Inoculation of as little as 0.0004 ml. of infected blood may transmit SH. Professional laboratory workers (particularly those who work in chronic dialysis units) are subject to occupational exposure, and heroin addicts who share infected needles constitute a major fraction of the patients with icteric hepatitis.

Post-transfusion hepatitis is a major public health problem. It has been estimated that the carrier rate among healthy donors who give no history of liver disease and who have no clinical or biochemical signs of hepatitis is approximately 1 per cent. This carrier rate is higher in an addict population. Hepatitis-related antigen has been detected in the serum of many of these carriers, but the current tests for antigen do not identify all carriers. There is currently little information relating to the factors that determine immunologic tolerance to the SH virus.

The circumstances that permit transmission of SH virus by nonparenteral exposure have not been clarified. Studies on the distribution of hepatitis-related antigen in various body fluids may provide information on this point.

Pathology and Pathogenesis. Infectious and serum hepatitis cause identical histopathologic lesions in the liver. Recent biopsy studies have shown that tissue lesions in infectious hepatitis are not confined to the liver, but are also present in the mucosa of the upper gastrointestinal tract and in the kidney. The sites of early virus multiplication and the mode of virus spread during the incubation period have not been defined. Viremia during the incubation period of IH and SH may result from the replication of virus in liver cells and subsequent release by cell lysis, or may be due to the local multiplication and release of virus from cells in the gastrointestinal tract. Similarly, the early appearance of virus in the stools of patients with infectious hepatitis may result from their presence in bile or in the intestinal mucosa.

The hepatic lesion in viral hepatitis is characterized by parenchymal cell degeneration and necrosis, proliferation of Kupffer's cells, inflammatory cell infiltration, and cell regeneration. Parenchymal cells throughout the lobule, and particularly in centrilobular areas, undergo rapid necrosis so that the cell cords are disrupted. Degenerating liver cells either show ballooning of their cytoplasm or hyalinize to form acidophilic bodies that may exhibit pyknotic nuclei. Cell necrosis is closely followed by cell regeneration; this may be recognized by the appearance of cells in mitotis and by large cells with multiple hyperchromatic nuclei. An increased number of macrophages containing a yellow, acid-fast pigment (lipofuscin) accumulate at sites of cell necrosis. Numerous lymphocytes, plasma cells, and polymorphonuclear cells, both neutrophil and eosinophil, also accumulate focally at sites of cell necrosis in the lobules and in the portal areas.

Although necrosis disrupts the normal cell cords, the reticulum framework surrounding the hepatic sinusoids is preserved, and cell regeneration restores normal lobules. During the recovery phase an increased number of fibroblasts with collagen may appear in the portal areas, together with proliferating bile ductules; these changes, together with the inflammatory cell infiltrate, disappear with full recovery.

Intrahepatic cholestasis — dilated bile canaliculi containing bile plugs — particularly in centrilobular areas, is often seen in viral hepatitis. This may be due to a disruption of bile canaliculi by parenchymal cell necrosis, or it may result from a change in the composition of bile due to cell injury.

Rarely, viral hepatitis may cause more extensive necrosis of parenchymal cells in areas that extend between lobules; collapse of the normal reticulum framework of the lobule disrupts the normal structure. This has been termed *subacute or acute hepatic necrosis*, according to the extent of the lesion and clinical manifestations. Patients with *acute* (massive) *hepatic necrosis* usually die before parenchymal cells can regenerate. The term *acute yellow atrophy* refers to the shrunken, bile-stained liver in which zones of collapsed reticulum and sinusoids lie between islands of degenerating cells. *Subacute (submassive) hepatic necrosis* may cause death during the acute illness or may lead to *posthepatitic cirrhosis*. With survival, cell regeneration does not restore normal lobular architecture but leads to the formation of large regeneration nodules; zones of collapsed reticulum undergo collagenization to form bands of fibrous tissue that contain inflammatory cells and regenerating bile ductules.

Extrahepatic lesions in infectious hepatitis appear in the gastrointestinal mucosa and the kidney. The mucosae are edematous and infiltrated with mononuclear cells; renal biopsies reveal interstitial edema without inflammation.

Clinical Manifestations. Acute viral hepatitis (IH or SH) is commonly a mild disease without jaundice, particularly in infants and children — *anicteric hepatitis*. Icteric hepatitis is usually benign but is occasionally complicated by *acute or subacute hepatic necrosis*; these complications may have a fatal outcome, or may lead to the development of cirrhosis. The factors that influence the severity of viral hepatitis include the age of the patient—hepatitis in the young is usually mild, whereas acute and subacute hepatic necrosis more often complicates hepatitis in the elderly; immunologic factors—injections of gamma globulin protect against infectious hepatitis; and associated conditions that include pregnancy, diabetes, abdominal surgery, and severe illness.

Anicteric Hepatitis. The symptoms of anicteric hepatitis are similar to those of many other viral infections; the onset of disease may resemble the prodromal (pre-icteric) period of icteric hepatitis. The diagnosis is suspected only in epidemic situations, in patients exposed to known infection, or in those who develop tender enlargement of the liver. A diagnosis is confirmed by liver function tests and liver biopsy. There is often slight hyperbilirubinemia with an increase in urinary urobilinogen and bilirubin and BSP retention. The serum enzyme changes are most helpful in diagnosis; serum transaminase and dehydrogenase levels are elevated, and serum alkaline phosphatase and 5-nucleotidase may be slightly increased. On liver biopsy, the hepatic lesion is indistinguishable from that of icteric hepatitis except for the absence of bile stasis.

Typical Acute Viral Hepatitis: Symptoms and Signs. *The Pre-icteric Phase.* The pre-icteric phase of nonspecific constitutional and gastrointestinal symptoms varies in duration from a few days to several weeks, is usually abrupt in onset in patients with IH but vague in those with SH, and may mimic other viral infections of the respiratory or gastrointestinal tract. *Fever* is usually most pronounced at the onset, and may be accompanied by a shaking chill; it is unusual, however, for shaking chills to be recurrent, although fever may persist until the early icteric phase. *Anorexia, weakness, headache,* and *myalgia* are common symptoms; there may be a striking loss of taste for cigarettes. Right upper quadrant pain with local tenderness and muscle spasm may simulate an acute abdominal emergency. Joint pains and urticarial or erythematous maculopapular rashes are sometimes seen. During this pre-icteric phase, the liver may become enlarged and tender, and the urine may become discolored with bilirubin.

The Icteric Phase. Gastrointestinal symptoms—anorexia, nausea, and vomiting with right upper abdominal discomfort—usually increase during the early period of increasing jaundice, the liver becomes more enlarged and tender, and the spleen may be palpable. Fever usually subsides a few days after the onset of jaundice. Within a few days of hospitalization and bed rest, nausea subsides, and the appetite improves in most patients. Typically, the patient is maximally jaundiced within two weeks, and thereafter clinical jaundice and serum bilirubin levels gradually return to normal within six weeks. Hepatic enlargement may subside with symptomatic improvement, but often persists during the icteric period. The maximal changes in urinary and fecal bilirubin excretion coincide with maximal serum bilirubin levels.

The Convalescent Phase. The convalescent phase leading to complete recovery and resumption of normal activity may last for several weeks or months. During this period variable tiredness and malaise with mild hepatic tenderness may persist. These symptoms may be quite troublesome to the patient. They are often precipitated by unaccustomed activity and may be accompanied by mild elevation of serum transaminase levels and minimal BSP retention.

Laboratory Features. The hemoglobin and hematocrit are usually normal early in the illness, but mild hemolysis and repeated venipuncture for laboratory tests may cause anemia later in the course of the acute disease. A normal or reduced white cell count, with atypical mononuclear cells (virocytes) on smear, is usual during the pre-icteric and early icteric periods. The erythrocyte sedimentation rate is slightly increased.

The urine contains an increased amount of both urobilinogen and bilirubin in the early icteric period; bilirubinemia increases with increasing jaundice, whereas urinary urobilinogen excretion decreases to minimal levels when jaundice is maximal. Minimal proteinuria with microscopic hematuria, pyuria, and granular casts during the early icteric period may reflect the renal abnormalities that have been demonstrated on renal biopsy.

During the icteric period both direct- and indirect-reacting bilirubin are almost equally elevated in the serum, but during the convalescent period indirect bilirubinemia may persist (see Gilbert's syndrome). Serum transaminase (glutamic-oxaloacetic or glutamic-pyruvic) levels, maximally elevated in the late prodromal or early icteric periods, may exceed 500 to 1000 i.u. These increased enzyme levels may be sustained during the icteric period but usually fall toward normal during the icteric period. Serum elevations of alkaline phosphatase, 5-nucleotidase, and leucine aminopeptidase are usually minimal and return to normal during the late icteric period. The typical changes in plasma proteins include a slight decrease in albumin and a late increase in gamma globulin, and the flocculation tests may be abnormal late in the prodromal period and return to normal during convalescence. BSP retention decreases to normal levels during the convalescent period.

Diagnosis. During the prodromal period, symptoms may suggest some other viral infection—*influenza* or *gastroenteritis.* Abdominal pain may mimic *acute cholecystitis, pneumonia,* or *acute appendicitis.* In the icteric patient, other causes for jaundice must be considered; *drug-induced or toxic hepatitis* is usually indicated by a history of drug exposure, but cannot be clearly differentiated by the pre-icteric symptoms from viral hepatitis. Choledocholithiasis with obstruction is suggested by a history of calculous disease, biliary colic, predominant cholestasis with pruritus, high alkaline phosphatase levels with only slight increases in transaminase, and signs of bacterial infection—shaking chills and polymorphonuclear leukocytosis. *Infectious mononucleosis* with hepatic involvement is distinguished by lymphadenopathy, pharyngitis, and a positive *heterophil* test. *Leptospirosis* is usually accompanied by headache and photophobia, signs of meningeal irritation with abnormal cerebrospinal fluid, persisting fever, leukocytosis, and proteinuria or renal insufficiency. It is important to exclude an exacerbation of chronic liver disease with jaundice; *acute alcoholic hepatitis* or *chronic aggressive hepatitis* may present with jaundice (*vide infra*).

HEPATITIS WITH PREDOMINANT CHOLESTASIS
(Cholestatic Hepatitis, Cholangiolitic Hepatitis)

Intrahepatic cholestasis, manifested by dilated bile canaliculi containing bile plugs and by elevation of serum alkaline phosphatase, is present in varying degree in most patients with icteric viral hepatitis. Occasionally, intrahepatic cholestasis may be the predominant manifestation of viral hepatitis with minimal evidence of liver cell necrosis.

Jaundice with pruritus, dark urine with bilirubinuria, pale stools with decreased fecal urobilinogen excretion, hepatic enlargement without impressive tenderness, and elevations of serum alkaline phosphatase, 5-nucleotidase, and leucine aminopeptidase with minimal increases in serum transaminase are characteristic of this illness. It is difficult to differentiate viral hepatitis with predominant cholestasis from drug-induced intrahepatic cholestasis or extrahepatic obstruction.

If viral hepatitis is considered to be a likely diagnosis in patients with obstructive jaundice, surgical exploration of the extrahepatic biliary system should be deferred, and a needle biopsy of the liver should be performed. If there are morphologic changes suggestive of viral hepatitis, continued medical therapy is indicated; however, a typical hepatitis lesion is not always present. If during the period of medical therapy the patient develops evidence of pancreatitis, biliary tract infection with fever, chills, and leukocytosis, or if there is no decrease in the serum bilirubin level after three weeks, an exploratory laparotomy is indicated to exclude extrahepatic biliary tract obstruction or to relieve it. A transhepatic percutaneous cholangiogram performed prior to operation is often helpful in defining a biliary tract lesion.

FULMINANT HEPATITIS
(Massive Hepatic Necrosis)

Fulminant hepatitis with acute massive hepatic necrosis is usually fatal within two weeks of the onset of illness. The pre-icteric period is usually short, with severe symptoms, particularly abdominal pain, vomiting, and high fever. The clinical features indicative of severe hepatitis leading to massive necrosis with a fulminant course are (1) high fever, severe abdominal pain, and vomiting that persist several days after the initiation of bed rest; (2) a sudden decrease in the size of the liver; (3) mental changes that include drowsiness, irritability, insomnia, and confusion, or more obvious hepatic encephalopathy; and (4) marked prolongation of the prothrombin time with or without bleeding (uncorrected by parenteral vitamin K).

Patients with fulminant hepatitis may become deeply jaundiced or may die during the early icteric period; the serum bilirubin concentration does not always reflect the severity of the illness. The serum elevation of transaminase is of no prognostic significance; values often decrease during the period of rapid clinical deterioration. Diffuse mucosal hemorrhage, ascites, and coma are terminal manifestations.

SUBACUTE HEPATIC NECROSIS
(Submassive Hepatic Necrosis)

The clinical features that suggest this complication of acute viral hepatitis include those listed under fulminant hepatitis: fever, abdominal pain, and vomiting prolonged after the first week of jaundice, or recurring during the icteric period; symptoms and signs of hepatic encephalopathy; a sudden decrease in liver size; and marked prolongation of the prothrombin time with mucosal bleeding. Whenever the serum bilirubin levels continue to rise after two weeks of jaundice or persist at peak levels, or when ascites, severe hypoproteinemia, or marked hyperglobulinemia with splenomegaly complicates acute hepatitis, this diagnosis should be considered.

Subacute hepatic necrosis with acute hepatocellular failure may have a fatal outcome within 2 to 12 weeks of the onset of icteric hepatitis. Death is usually preceded by deepening jaundice, ascites, diffuse mucosal bleeding, and hepatic coma. Some patients may exhibit progressive clinical and functional deterioration and may die from liver failure or a complication of cirrhosis many months later, whereas other patients may enter an asymptomatic period of compensated cirrhosis with almost normal liver function and develop complications of cirrhosis many years later.

CHRONIC PERSISTING HEPATITIS (PROLONGED HEPATITIS) AND RECURRENT HEPATITIS

Some patients with otherwise typical acute viral hepatitis may remain icteric with hepatic enlargement and abnormalities of liver function for several months. Others may exhibit exacerbations of symptoms (anorexia, fatigue, and hepatic tenderness) and worsening of liver function (elevation of bilirubin and serum transaminases with increased BSP retention) after a period of recovery from typical hepatitis. Liver biopsy reveals normal lobular architecture, inflammatory infiltration of the portal areas without invasion of the parenchyma by fibrous tissue, and focal necrosis of parenchymal cells typical of acute hepatitis. This histologic picture differentiates this benign form of prolonged hepatitis from *chronic aggressive hepatitis (vide infra)*.

CHRONIC AGGRESSIVE HEPATITIS
(Active Chronic Hepatitis)

This condition is characterized pathologically by a normal lobular architecture in which fibrous septa extend from enlarged portal tracts into the parenchyma, disrupting the liver cell plates adjacent to the portal zones and separating off rosettes of parenchymal cells. Piecemeal necrosis of liver cells adjacent to the expanding portal zones, infiltration of the portal areas with mononuclear and plasma cells, and reactive proliferation of bile ducts are present in varying degree according to the "activity" of the lesion. Progressive destruction of the lobular architecture and the subsequent formation of regeneration nodules lead to the development of cirrhosis (see Idiopathic Cirrhosis).

Chronic aggressive hepatitis has been documented by liver biopsy in patients with anicteric liver disease and in those whose initial illness was typical of acute viral hepatitis. In different patients, and in individual patients at different times, varying "activity" of the diffuse hepatic lesion may be reflected by varying symptoms (anorexia, nausea, malaise), signs of liver disease (hepatic enlargement with tenderness, splenomegaly, jaundice, spider angiomas), and varying degrees of abnormality of liver function (bilirubinemia, increased SGOT, hypergammaglobulinemia). Extreme hyperglobulinemia in some patients (particularly young women) may be associated with positive serologic tests (L. E., antinuclear, Wasserman, rheumatoid factor).

Whether chronic aggressive hepatitis is the result of persisting viral infection or whether immunologic injury to the liver determines this progressive lesion has not been established.

MANAGEMENT OF ACUTE VIRAL HEPATITIS

Patients with acute viral hepatitis should be admitted to hospital during the early icteric phase, unless it is possible to give optimal medical and nursing care in the home. During the early symptomatic period frequent careful clinical observation and assessment of liver function are necessary for early recognition and treatment of massive or subacute hepatic necrosis. Liver function tests should be performed several times each week, and a daily estimation of the prothrombin time after parenteral vitamin K_1 (10 mg. intramuscularly) is valuable in detecting a sudden deterioration in liver function. A daily measurement of caloric intake is also helpful in assessing the patient's progress.

A liver biopsy should be performed if the diagnosis is not firmly established on the basis of clinical and biochemical findings, or if an atypical course suggests subacute hepatic necrosis.

Rest. The value of rest in acute viral hepatitis is suggested by the remission and exacerbation of symptoms that follow bed rest and physical activity, respectively. Nevertheless, the only controlled study on the effect of rest and activity in infectious hepatitis indicated that enforced rest was of no value in therapy and that activity did not cause complications, lengthen the course of the disease, or lead to chronic residual abnormalities. This controlled study was carried out on military personnel who were young and fit and who, irrespective of therapy, suffered no mortality or long-term sequelae that could be attributed to the viral hepatitis. In a civilian population of varied age, with other disease states complicating viral hepatitis infection, there are significant morbidity and mortality from subacute and massive hepatic necrosis. *Complete bed rest during the acute phase of viral hepatitis may protect some of these patients from these complications.* Until there is further information relating to a civilian population, it is recommended that all icteric patients rest in bed during the early symptomatic period when it may be difficult to assess the severity of illness, and that limited activity during the icteric period be permitted only for young, otherwise healthy patients. Elderly patients and patients with complicating disease should be ambulated when the serum bilirubin has fallen below 2 mg. per 100 ml. It is important that ambulation to normal physical activity should be gradual for patients who have been confined to bed for long periods.

Diet. During the preicteric and early icteric periods, a poor appetite and nausea or vomiting may limit food intake. The patient should be served and encouraged to eat those foods that appeal to him. For some patients, it is possible to increase the caloric content of the breakfast when they have difficulty in eating other meals. If a total intake of 2000 calories daily is not maintained, intravenous glucose supplements should be given.

Corticosteroids. Although glucocorticoids effect a dramatic remission of symptoms and biochemical improvement in patients with viral hepatitis, it has not been established by controlled studies that these agents shorten the course of the acute disease or reduce the complications. Thus, in mild, uncomplicated hepatitis there is no indication for their use. Corticosteroids are recommended, however, for acutely ill patients whose symptoms are severe and persist for several days in spite of bed rest. A daily dose of 30 to 60 mg. of prednisolone, or equivalent doses of other steroids, maintained for a week and tapered slowly over a period of several weeks is suggested.

Sedatives. Sedatives and other drugs should be

used with caution in patients with viral hepatitis. Smaller doses may be necessary to achieve a therapeutic effect. In acutely ill patients their side effects may complicate the clinical assessment of the patient.

Surgery. All surgical procedures should be deferred to the postconvalescent period if possible. There is evidence that abdominal surgery under general anesthesia increases the risk of subacute or massive hepatic necrosis.

MANAGEMENT OF FULMINANT HEPATITIS

Although heroic measures have been used to treat patients with fulminant hepatitis in hepatic coma, there is no clear evidence that these measures have decreased the mortality of this condition.

Patients with manifestations of impending hepatic coma should receive intravenous infusions of glucose (10 per cent by central venous catheter), albumin (50 grams daily), electrolytes, and vitamins. A corticosteroid drug is usually given in high doses intravenously, e.g. prednisolone, 100 mg. daily. The patient in coma demands intensive nursing care to prevent the potentially fatal complications of the comatose state (see Management of Acute Depressive Drug Poisoning); measures which maintain an effective airway and prevent aspiration may provide greatest benefit in reducing mortality. The agitated hyperactive patient should not be heavily sedated; this will only deepen his coma (see Metabolic Brain Disease). Bleeding may be controlled by infusions of fresh frozen plasma. Exchange transfusion, cross perfusion with primate or normal human subject, and perfusion of blood through an isolated pig liver are measures that may have prolonged the lives of individual patients. Although these measures may improve the patient's central nervous system function, they may not promote regeneration of his liver.

MANAGEMENT OF CHRONIC PERSISTING AND CHRONIC AGGRESSIVE HEPATITIS

These patients with prolonged illness and the threat of chronic disability require strong emotional support and reassurance. A liver biopsy may be particularly helpful in providing information on the patient's prognosis; evidence of chronic persisting hepatitis suggests that the long-term outcome will be favorable.

Physical activity should be limited only by the patient's symptoms; strenuous activity, however, should usually be avoided.

Corticosteroids (prednisolone 10 to 30 mg.) may reduce symptoms and improve liver function (decrease in bilirubin, gamma globulin, and SGOT, and increase in BSP clearance), but a retrospectively controlled study suggests that this therapy does not modify the development of cirrhosis. If relatively high doses are required, side effects may outweigh the benefit.

Immunosuppressive agents, such as azathioprine

(Imuran), 1 to 2 mg. per kilogram daily, have been used with apparent success in treating some patients with chronic aggressive hepatitis. The therapeutic value of this agent should be assessed by a controlled clinical study.

PROPHYLAXIS OF HEPATITIS

A single dose of pooled gamma globulin (0.02 to 0.04 ml. of 16 per cent solution per kilogram of body weight, intramuscularly) protects against, or modifies, infectious hepatitis in exposed subjects. Susceptible persons probably develop anicteric rather than icteric hepatitis. Susceptible travelers to zones of known poor sanitation should receive a larger dose, 0.06 to 0.12 ml. per kilogram, to give protection for five to six months.

There is conflicting evidence relating to the value of gamma globulin prophylaxis against serum hepatitis; limited protection against post-transfusion hepatitis may be conferred by large doses of pooled gamma globulin. This is currently the subject of a prospective controlled study.

The risk of post-transfusion hepatitis may be reduced by more careful selection of blood donors and by avoiding the use of pooled fresh plasma and fibrinogen.

PROGNOSIS

Patients with acute viral hepatitis, anicteric or icteric, usually recover completely. The frequency of fulminant hepatitis among icteric hospitalized patients is less than 1 per cent. Fulminant hepatitis is usually fatal. The frequency of chronic aggressive hepatitis as a sequel to anicteric hepatitis is not known. The frequency of subacute hepatic necrosis and aggressive hepatitis among patients with icteric hepatitis varies from less than 1 per cent in young patients to 10 per cent in the elderly; the rate at which these lesions progress to decompensated cirrhosis varies from a few months to many years.

HEPATITIS DUE TO OTHER VIRUSES

The viruses of yellow fever, rubella, cytomegalic inclusion disease, and herpes simplex may cause hepatitis. Yellow fever is discussed elsewhere in this volume. Infection with *rubella, cytomegalic inclusion virus,* and *herpes simplex* may cause *neonatal hepatitis* with jaundice and hepatosplenomegaly. Rubella and cytomegalic inclusion viruses are transmitted transplacentally, whereas herpes virus infects the infant during delivery. Hepatitis resulting from these viral agents may be part of a generalized disease. Although there may be complete recovery, with normal liver function and structure, these infections may be important but previously unrecognized causes for juvenile cirrhosis.

Many viral illnesses may be accompanied by minor, nonspecific changes in liver function (positive flocculation tests and slight transaminase elevation). There may be hyperplasia of Kupffer's cells and infiltration with mononuclear cells in portal areas—nonspecific reactive hepatitis.

INFECTIOUS MONONUCLEOSIS

Infectious mononucleosis of unknown cause is discussed elsewhere (see Infectious Mononucleosis under Diseases of the Blood). Jaundice is unusual, although hepatic enlargement with mild tenderness is often seen. The disturbances of liver function are those associated with hepatic infiltration: an elevation of the serum alkaline phosphatase, 5-nucleotidase and leucine aminopeptidase, and BSP retention. Serum transaminase levels may be slightly elevated. Histologically, there is mononuclear infiltration predominantly in the portal areas with minimal evidence of cell necrosis.

No case of chronic liver disease has been proved to result from an attack of infectious mononucleosis.

LIVER DISEASE ASSOCIATED WITH BACTERIAL INFECTIONS

In bacterial infection, liver disease may result from the effect of bacterial toxins on cell metabolism, changes in liver blood flow caused by endotoxin, shock or fever, localization and multiplication of bacteria in the liver, or the effect of antimicrobial agents.

Severe infections, particularly intraperitoneal, may cause obstructive jaundice with conjugated bilirubinemia, increased alkaline phosphatase, and minimal elevation of serum transaminase. In the absence of demonstrable lesions of the extrahepatic biliary system and normal operative cholangiograms, the jaundice in these patients results from intrahepatic cholestasis resulting from unknown toxic factors.

Gram-negative septicemia with shock may cause acute hypoxic necrosis of the liver with jaundice as a terminal manifestation. The liver may be enlarged and tender. Serum transaminase levels are elevated in typhoid fever during the bacteremic phase. Focal necrosis of parenchymal cells with acute and chronic inflammatory cell infiltration is seen on liver biopsy. In leptospirosis, jaundice is usually disproportionally greater than other evidence of liver involvement; the associated renal disease may impair urinary excretion of conjugated bilirubin.

ACUTE LIVER ABSCESSES AND SUPPURATIVE CHOLANGITIS

Amebic abscesses are discussed elsewhere in this volume.

Pyogenic liver abscesses are usually associated with intra-abdominal sepsis—appendicitis with suppurative pyophlebitis, acute cholecystitis, or suppurative cholangitis, but may result from septicemia complicating distant foci of infection (gram-positive cocci).

The clinical course is usually hectic, with high spiking fever, chills, prostration, right upper quadrant pain with tender hepatomegaly and jaundice. A polymorphonuclear leukocytosis, positive blood culture, and elevations of serum alkaline phosphatase and transaminase are significant laboratory abnormalities.

The patient with liver abscesses should be treated with antimicrobial drugs and by incision and drainage. When the causal organism has not been identified, broad-spectrum antimicrobial drugs should be used.

PARASITIC DISEASE OF THE LIVER

Parasites that commonly invade the liver include amebae (E. histolytica and malarial parasites), schistosomes (S. mansoni), flukes (Clonorchis sinensis, Fasciola hepatica) and tapeworms (Echinococcus granulosus). These diseases are discussed under Microbial Diseases.

Hepatic Schistosomiasis. Hepatic involvement results from portal seeding with ova that lodge in the portal areas and stimulate an inflammatory reaction with fibrosis. In the later stage of hepatic parasitism, portal fibrosis interferes with hepatic blood flow and causes a presinusoidal portal hypertension, splenomegaly, and a collateral portal-systemic circulation. Bleeding from esophageal varices is a major complication. Liver function is usually good, so that patients may tolerate recurrent bleeding very well, and do not usually develop ascites unless bleeding or malnutrition lowers serum albumin concentrations. In view of the good liver function, portacaval shunt surgery for bleeding esophageal varices is usually well tolerated; shunt surgery may be complicated, however, by chronic portal-systemic encephalopathy.

The diagnosis of hepatic schistosomiasis is established by demonstrating ova on liver biopsy; examination of "squash" preparations in glycerol is more helpful than routine histologic examination. The presence of ova in the stools or rectal biopsy of a patient with portal hypertension and splenomegaly suggests this diagnosis (see article on Schistosomiasis).

TOXIC AND DRUG-INDUCED LIVER DISEASE

A *hepatotoxin* is defined as an agent that causes liver injury in both man and animals in a predictable manner. Liver injury is dose-related and usually manifest after a relatively short latent period. Hepatotoxins may cause liver cell necrosis or biochemical changes without necrosis; these changes may be manifest by impaired formation of bile, disturbances of lipid metabolism with fat accumulation, or altered enzyme activity. Some hepatotoxins may exert their effect indirectly by interfering with hepatic blood flow (senecio alkaloids in veno-occlusive disease).

With elimination of industrial hazards, exposure to hepatotoxins is now usually accidental or suicidal. Hepatotoxic agents are not often used pharmacologically unless the therapeutic dose is considerably less than the toxic dose, or unless therapy despite toxic side effects may still benefit the patient. The chlorinated hydrocarbon anesthetic agents, chloroform and halothane (Fluothane), are relatively nontoxic in anesthetic doses, but may exert a toxic effect if hypoxia or other unknown factors increase the susceptibility of the patient. Immunosuppressive agents and certain agents used in the chemotherapy of cancer and of tuberculosis may be hepatotoxic. Poisoning by several hepatotoxic agents—carbon tetrachloride, yellow phosphorus, and *Amanita phalloides*—is discussed under Diseases Due to Chemical Agents. The effects of alcohol (ethanol) on the liver are discussed under Chronic Liver Disease.

Carbon Tetrachloride Liver Injury. The clinical features of carbon tetrachloride liver injury are similar to those of acute viral hepatitis, but with a shorter symptomatic pre-icteric period and with more rapid recovery, unless massive necrosis causes early death or renal tubular necrosis leads to irreversible or fatal renal failure.

The symptoms that follow inhalation or ingestion of the agent are predominantly gastrointestinal, with *anorexia,* *nausea* and *vomiting,* and right upper quadrant *pain* with *tender hepatomegaly* preceding the onset of jaundice. In many patients there may be hepatic enlargement with acute elevation of serum transaminase levels without jaundice. Acute renal failure is often a more prominent manifestation of poisoning.

Pathologically, there is centrilobular necrosis without inflammation during the period of maximal liver injury, followed rapidly by regeneration of parenchymal cells and hyperplasia of Kupffer's cells. Complete restoration of structure and function follows recovery from a single exposure. There is some evidence, however, that repeated exposure may sometimes lead to cirrhosis of the liver.

Hepatotoxicity of Anesthetic Agents. Liver injury has been attributed to *chloroform* and to the recently developed volatile, nonexplosive halogenated hydrocarbon, *halothane.* Many other possible etiologic factors must be excluded before one may attribute postoperative liver necrosis to an anesthetic agent; these include hypoxia and hypercapnia, hypotension, postoperative sepsis, biliary tract disease, coincidental viral hepatitis with subacute hepatic necrosis precipitated by surgery, and reactions to other drugs. In spite of a very extensive clinical experience with halothane, hepatic necrosis is rare. It has been estimated that only seven fatal cases of massive hepatic necrosis were associated with the first five million anesthetic administrations; this frequency is no greater than with other anesthetic agents. This low frequency of hepatic necrosis following halothane anesthesia suggests that hypersensitivity may be the basis of hepatotoxic reactions. This has been well documented in one patient who developed recurrent acute hepatitis each time he was exposed to subanesthetic doses of halothane. Fever commonly precedes the overt manifestations of liver disease. Any patient who develops unexplained fever or evidence of acute liver disease following anesthesia with a fluorinated hydrocarbon should not be re-exposed to that agent. In the cases that have been documented clinically, biochemically and histologically, the changes are similar to those that result from severe viral hepatitis.

Sex Hormones and the Liver. Methyl testosterone and C-17 alkyl substituted steroids (norethandronone) may cause intrahepatic cholestasis with conjugated hyperbilirubinemia, reduced clearance of BSP (with normal hepatic uptake and conjugation), and increased serum alkaline phosphatase and 5-nucleotidase activity. This effect is dose related in man, causes no permanent liver damage or acute parenchymal cell necrosis, and is reversible. This type of cholestasis may be due to a change in the permeability of the biliary tree to bile salts.

During the third trimester of normal pregnancy there may be increases in serum cholesterol, alkaline phosphatase, and 5-nucleotidase with reduced clearance of BSP. Occasionally, impaired hepatic excretory function may cause jaundice that recurs in subsequent pregnancies—*recurrent jaundice of pregnancy.* Recent studies have shown that natural estrogens reduce hepatic BSP clearance. It is probable that the physiologic changes in liver function during the third trimester of pregnancy are due to hormone effects on the liver. These observations are of particular interest in view of the recent reports that hormones given to suppress ovulation may occasionally cause hepatic dysfunction.

Drug Hypersensitivity. Liver injury following drug therapy is more often due to a *hypersensitivity reaction* than to a hepatotoxic effect. In contrast to hepatotoxic reactions, the hypersensitivity reaction is quite unpredictable unless a previous reaction has been recorded, is not dose related, follows a variable latent period after drug exposure, cannot be reproduced in experimental animals, and may be associated with other manifestations of hypersensitivity (skin rash, fever, eosinophilia).

Drug hypersensitivity reactions involving the liver may be minor local manifestations of a generalized reaction, e.g., minor changes in liver function in patients with exfoliative dermatitis, or may be the predominant manifestation of the reaction. The common hepatic lesions are *intrahepatic cholestasis* and *parenchymal cell necrosis*. The former is illustrated by reactions to *chlorpromazine*, the latter by reactions to *iproniazid*.

Chlorpromazine Jaundice. Approximately 1 per cent of patients treated with this phenothiazine develop a hypersensitivity reaction with intrahepatic cholestasis and jaundice. A greater number of patients develop changes in excretory function without jaundice. Early symptoms, beginning acutely usually within one to four weeks of initial drug exposure, or within a few days of repeated challenge, include *nausea*, *vomiting*, and *epigastric pain* often associated with *fever*, *lymphadenopathy*, *skin eruptions*, and *arthralgias*. The liver becomes enlarged and variably tender. Jaundice is obstructive in type with severe pruritus, dark urine, and pale stools, and tests of liver function reflect predominant *cholestasis* with conjugated hyperbilirubinemia and increased serum alkaline phosphatase, 5-nucleotidase, and cholesterol levels. The serum transaminase levels may be elevated in the range of 100 to 200 i.u. The white blood count may be normal or slightly elevated, with peripheral eosinophilia.

On liver biopsy, intrahepatic cholestasis, with bile plugs in dilated bile canaliculi and bile staining of parenchymal cells, and variable periportal infiltration with mononuclear and eosinophil cells are the prominent findings. There may be minimal centrilobular necrosis of liver cells.

Jaundice usually subsides within a few days or weeks of onset, with complete recovery, but occasionally chronic intrahepatic cholestasis may develop in spite of cessation of drug therapy. The clinical features in these patients may be similar to those in primary biliary cirrhosis, but periportal fibrosis is less severe, and eventual recovery without cirrhosis is usual.

Treatment. There is no specific therapy. The offending agent should be discontinued and avoided thereafter. Cholestyramine, 2 grams every four hours orally, may relieve pruritus by lowering serum bile acid levels. Vitamin K should be given parenterally if malabsorption causes an increase in prothrombin time. Corticosteroids are of little benefit either in relieving jaundice or in reducing pruritus.

Iproniazid Hepatitis. Iproniazid, a monamine oxidase inhibitor related chemically to isoniazid, may cause acute hepatitis that is indistinguishable clinically, biochemically, and pathologically from viral hepatitis. It has been suggested, therefore, that the drug may be stimulating a latent viral infection. The clinical course, however, is more complicated than that of acute viral hepatitis; there is a high mortality from fulminant liver disease with massive necrosis, and subacute hepatic necrosis more often leads to cirrhosis. Iproniazid is seldom used today. However, a similar form of hepatitis is produced by ethionamide and by the nicotinamide derivative, pyrazinamide, which are used in special circumstances in the treatment of tuberculosis.

Hypersensitivity drug reactions with liver disease usually follow the clinical and pathologic patterns illustrated by chlorpromazine and iproniazid, and are usually constant for a given drug. Occasionally, however, there may be features of both necrosis and cholestasis.

FATTY LIVER

Fat accumulation in the liver (fatty liver) may be a physiologic response to an increase in lipid mobilization from peripheral fat, e.g., during early starvation, or may result from several disturbances of lipid transport and metabolism in a variety of disease states. Excessive lipid in parenchymal cells may arise from one or more of three sources: (1) the diet, (2) peripheral fat depots, and (3) hepatic synthesis. Lipid from any of these sources may accumulate when the supply is increased, or when a decrease in hepatic oxidation of fatty acids or reduced lipoprotein synthesis and release diminishes the clearance of lipid from the liver.

In *starvation*, free fatty acids are mobilized from adipose tissue, and are in part esterified in the liver to triglyceride. This physiologic response is probably the mechanism for the fatty infiltration of the liver observed in many patients following acute and chronic illnesses. In *protein malnutrition (kwashiorkor)*, extreme fatty liver may be related in part to fat mobilization from depots (free fatty acid concentrations in serum are elevated), and in part to impaired lipoprotein synthesis. In *obese patients*, an excessive accumulation of fat in the liver may be a reflection of the general increase in the triglyceride stores. *Diabetic ketoacidosis*, with excessive mobilization of depot fat, is usually accompanied by liver enlargement caused by fat. In each of these conditions the major clinical manifestation of fatty liver is hepatic enlargement; tenderness usually accompanies acute enlargement. BSP retention may be the only abnormality of liver function.

In several conditions fatty liver may be associated with severe derangement of liver function. This is particularly the case when fat accumulation is due to toxic injury causing decreased fatty acid oxidation or impaired lipoprotein synthesis. In *carbon tetrachloride* or *phosphorus* poisoning, fat accumulation is one manifestation of toxic liver injury. Large intravenous doses of *tetracycline* (usually > 1 gram daily), particularly in pregnant women, have caused liver failure and death; a fine fatty vacuolization of the liver cells is the major pathologic change in the liver. In two syndromes, fatty liver is accompanied by severe encephalopathy with high mortality; the clinical picture may be that of fulminant hepatitis. *Fatty liver of pregnancy* usually presents with vomiting, abdominal pain, and jaundice during the last month of pregnancy; bleeding, premature labor, renal failure, and coma with convulsions rapidly lead to death. The serum bilirubin and alkaline phosphatase elevations suggest severe cholestasis; disturbances of the clotting mechanism reflect impaired synthesis of the clotting factors. In *Reye's syndrome,* acute encephalopathy (acute nonsuppurative encephalitis) with delirium, spasticity and decerebrate posturing, and coma is accompanied by acute liver enlargement resulting from fatty infiltration; jaundice is unusual, probably because of the rapidly fatal outcome. Extremely high serum levels of transaminase and prolonged prothrombin time indicate severe liver injury. The pathogenesis of this syndrome and the relationship between liver and brain injury are unknown; the suggestion that this syndrome may complicate viral infection has not been supported by virologic studies.

The most common form of toxic liver injury leading to fatty infiltration of the liver is that due to *alcohol (ethanol) ingestion (vide infra).*

Treatment of the underlying cause of fatty liver, e.g., correction of protein malnutrition, or withdrawal from alcohol, is usually effective in lowering the fat content of the liver. In patients with acute severe liver injury associated with encephalopathy, measures used in the management of patients with fulminant hepatitis have been applied with questionable success (see treatment of fulminant hepatitis).

THE LIVER IN ACUTE HEART FAILURE AND SHOCK

Hypoxia secondary to reduced liver blood flow may cause centrilobular parenchymal cell necrosis. This often complicates *acute congestive heart failure* or *hypotension* due to any cause. The liver may be enlarged and tender if the central venous pressure is raised. The predominant clinical manifestations are those of the underlying cardiovascular disease, which determines both therapy and prognosis. The biochemical changes in acute heart failure include slight hyperbilirubinemia with slight elevation of transaminases and alkaline phosphatase and BSP retention. In shock, the serum transaminase levels are sometimes markedly elevated but return quickly to normal levels with restoration of normal blood flow and parenchymal cell regeneration. Deep jaundice may be a terminal event in patients with prolonged shock.

HEPATIC VEIN OCCLUSION
(Budd-Chiari Syndrome)

Occlusion of the hepatic veins is a rare condition usually caused by *tumor infiltration* (hepatoma, metastatic tumor) or *thrombosis* of the vessels. This may be a local lesion, or may extend from the inferior vena cava. *Polycythemia vera* is one of the more common causes of thrombosis of these veins. The major clinical manifestations of this condition are *hepatic enlargement,* with *pain* and *tenderness,* and *ascites.* In the acute form, hepatic vein occlusion is characterized pathologically by centrilobular congestion and necrosis of the adjacent parenchyma. A needle biopsy of the liver should establish the diagnosis when hepatic congestion resulting from an increase in central venous pressure has been excluded. The obstruction may be subacute or chronic when ascites and portal hypertension are the major clinical problems. *Hepatic venography* by direct injection of contrast material into a hepatic catheter is the most valuable technique for establishing the diagnosis.

Patients with chronic hepatic vein occlusion usually respond to a diuretic program (see treatment of ascites). Polycythemia vera should also be treated vigorously (see Hematologic and Hematopoietic Diseases).

CHRONIC LIVER DISEASE

CIRRHOSIS OF THE LIVER

Definition. The cirrhotic liver is one in which there is a loss of normal lobular architecture, with nodular regeneration of parenchymal cells separated by fibrous septa.

Classification. There is no satisfactory classification of cirrhosis. A *pathologic* classification may not relate to etiology and to clinical events, and may be complicated by the presence of a varying pathologic structure in many diseased livers. An *etiologic* classification is limited by the fact that a cause cannot be defined in many patients. For want of a better scheme, however, an etiologic classification is used and is as follows:

1. Cirrhosis in the alcoholic.
2. Posthepatitic and idiopathic cirrhosis.
3. Metabolic cirrhosis (hemochromatosis and Wilson's disease).
4. Biliary cirrhosis (primary and secondary).
5. Schistosomal fibrosis.
6. Cardiac cirrhosis.

CIRRHOSIS IN THE ALCOHOLIC

Pathogenesis and Epidemiology. The incidence of cirrhosis in the United States parallels the consumption of alcohol. Little is known, however, of the factors that determine individual susceptibility to cirrhosis; these would explain why many persons with a chronic heavy intake of alcohol do not develop liver disease; both genetic and dietary factors may be of importance. Some insight into the problem of liver disease in the alcoholic has been gained from experimental studies on the effect of alcohol (ethanol) on liver metabolism.

The Effects of Alcohol (Ethanol) on the Liver. Both in man and in laboratory animals, alcohol ingestion is associated with two prominent morphologic changes: the accumulation of fat (triglyceride) in parenchymal cells and degeneration of cell organelles (visible as *alcoholic hyaline-eosinophilic cytoplasmic inclusions* in man). These changes may result from a direct *hepatotoxic effect of alcohol* rather than a deficiency of dietary factors; they are seen when alcohol is substituted for carbohydrate in an adequate diet.

In the alcoholic it has been shown that a major fraction of the liver fat is derived from dietary triglyceride. Increased hepatic synthesis of fatty acids and a decrease in the hepatic oxidation of fatty acids (dietary or endogenous) lead to fatty liver.

The relation between the acute and subacute effects of alcohol on the liver and the late development of cirrhosis has not been defined; it is inferred that continual necrosis of cells damaged by alcohol leads progressively to the formation of fibrous septa separating regeneration nodules.

Pathology. The liver in *acute alcoholic hepatitis* is enlarged and firm, and on microscopic examination the parenchymal cells are distended with droplets of fat, and may contain eosinophilic cytoplasmic inclusions (alcoholic hyaline). There is variable inflammatory cell infiltration in portal areas and throughout the parenchyma, and bile stasis occurs in jaundiced patients.

Cirrhosis in the alcoholic is usually of the *Laennec type,* with small uniform regeneration nodules separated by fibrous bands containing mononuclear cells and proliferating bile ductules. The pathologic changes of acute alcoholic hepatitis—inflammation, cell degeneration, and infiltration with fat—are often seen in the cirrhotic liver. Occasionally the liver is of the *macronodular type,* with coarse, irregular regeneration nodules and broad intervening bands of fibrous tissue.

Clinical Manifestations. **Acute Alcoholic Hepatitis.** A patient with acute alcoholic hepatitis may seek medical help because of *abdominal pain* caused by acute hepatic enlargement, gastritis, or pancreatitis; *vomiting,* with or without *hematemesis,* caused by gastritis, ulcer, or sometimes esophageal varices; *jaundice; abdominal swelling* with ascites; or because of symptoms caused by head injury, alcohol withdrawal, or thiamin deficiency.

On admission to hospital, the patient is usually *febrile* and *dehydrated* and has an alcoholic fetor. An *enlarged, firm, tender liver,* abdominal distention with *ascites* and *jaundice,* with prominent *spider angiomas* and *palmar erythema,* are typically present. The early hospital course is often complicated by *delirium tremens.* Intense jaundice with *pruritus* in febrile patients may simulate extrahepatic biliary tract obstruction.

Liver function tests reveal conjugated hyperbilirubinemia, elevated serum transaminase levels (50 to 300 units), variable increases in alkaline phosphatase activity, and depression of serum albumin concentrations. The serum cholesterol concentration may be increased, normal, or depressed. *Hypokalemia* often results from increased

urinary excretion of potassium. *Hyperuricemia* resulting from depressed urinary excretion of uric acid parallels lactic acidosis. Anemia may be due to bleeding or *hemolysis;* acute severe hemolysis is sometimes associated with *hyperlipemia* (Zieve's syndrome).

Cirrhosis. *Cirrhosis* in the alcoholic may present insidiously with anorexia, fatigue, and weakness, and a gradual onset of jaundice and ascites, or may present acutely with one or several major complications: acute upper gastrointestinal *bleeding,* sudden onset of *ascites,* liver failure with *jaundice* or *coma,* or symptoms of hepatic *carcinoma.* When the cirrhotic patient shows manifestations of acute alcoholic hepatitis, the term *florid cirrhosis* is often used. In the absence of these complications the only stigmata of cirrhosis may be a firm, enlarged, nontender liver with or without splenomegaly, and the cutaneous manifestations of chronic liver disease.

In *compensated cirrhosis* the only abnormalities of liver function may be mild BSP retention and an increased urinary excretion of urobilinogen. With progressive decompensation, serum protein concentrations fall, and hyperbilirubinemia and BSP retention increase. Serum enzyme levels are usually only slightly elevated.

Differential Diagnosis. In the differential diagnosis of acute alcoholic hepatitis other causes for acute jaundice must be considered, i.e. *viral hepatitis, extrahepatic obstruction,* and *drug reactions.* Infection should be considered in the febrile patient, although fever may be due to cell necrosis. In the compensated cirrhotic, an enlarged, firm liver may be suggestive of infiltrative disease. A needle biopsy of the liver usually resolves these differential diagnostic problems.

When cirrhosis is complicated by bleeding, ascites, or coma, other causes for these complications must be excluded. In cirrhotic patients, acute upper gastrointestinal *bleeding* may come from esophageal varices; but acute gastric erosions, peptic ulcer, and neoplasm must also be considered. Esophagoscopy, gastroscopy, and roentgenologic evaluation of the esophagus, stomach, and duodenum are necessary to establish the site of bleeding (see management of upper gastrointestinal bleeding under Peptic Ulcer). Although *ascites* is usually due to portal hypertension with hypoalbuminemia, *constrictive pericarditis,* *bacterial peritonitis* (especially *tuberculous*), and *intra-abdominal neoplasm* must also be considered. Measurement of the venous pressure and a diagnostic paracentesis with analysis for protein, enzymes, bacteria, and cells are of value in differential diagnosis. In tuberculous peritonitis the protein concentration of ascitic fluid may exceed 2.5 grams per 100 ml., and the ascitic fluid white cell count usually exceeds 250 per cubic millimeter, with lymphocytes predominant. Malignant effusions are often hemorrhagic, with a protein content greater than 2.5 grams per 100 ml. and elevated lactic dehydrogenase activity; malignant cells may be found on cytologic examination.

Treatment. The most important step in the management of the alcoholic with cirrhosis is to eliminate his intake of alcohol. With continued alcoholism no medical or surgical measures will significantly prolong his life.

Patients with acute alcoholic hepatitis should be treated with bed rest, alcohol withdrawal, and a diet containing adequate protein, vitamins, minerals, and calories. Intravenous infusions of 5 per cent glucose, with potassium, magnesium, and vitamin supplements, may be needed by the febrile, dehydrated patient. Oral supplements of ferrous sulfate (0.3 gram three times a day) or folic acid (50 mg. daily) should be given to correct anemia caused by iron or folic acid deficiency. Salt intake should be restricted to 1 to 3 grams per 24 hours in patients with ascites. On this regimen clinical and biochemical improvement is usual within two to three weeks, and is accompanied by a spontaneous diuresis and disappearance of ascites. If there is no clinical improvement during this period, or if acute hepatocellular failure is severe at the time of admission, glucocorticoid therapy (prednisolone, 20 to 40 mg. daily) may be helpful in stimulating the appetite, potentiating diuresis, and improving liver function.

Portal Hypertension with Upper Gastrointestinal Bleeding. In the early management of bleeding, treatment is directed toward restoring blood volume and controlling the bleeding at the same time that diagnostic efforts are made to determine the site of bleeding. The alcoholic patient may bleed from *acute gastric erosions, peptic ulcer,* or *esophageal varices;* appropriate therapy depends on the site of bleeding. The several measures that may be used to control bleeding in cirrhotic patients include gastric lavage with ice water, local gastric hypothermia using an esophagogastric balloon, intravenous infusions of Pitressin, esophageal tamponade with an inflated balloon, or direct surgical procedures. *Lavage* with ice water is unlikely to control esophageal bleeding, but may be effective when bleeding is from gastric erosions. Gastric *hypothermia* using an intraluminal esophagogastric balloon cooled to 5° C. may control variceal bleeding but is contraindicated when the site of bleeding has not been defined. Infusions of *Pitressin* (20 units intravenously in 10 minutes) constrict the splanchnic arterioles, reduce splanchnic blood flow, and lower portal venous pressure. Bleeding from varices may thus be temporarily controlled. *Esophageal tamponade* (with a Sengstaken esophageal tube) may be the only nonoperative procedure that will control massive bleeding from esophageal varices. The disadvantage of this procedure is the many complications that result from tamponade; asphyxia resulting from upward displacement of the balloon, aspiration, and esophageal erosion by pressure necrosis.

Several surgical procedures have been recommended to control bleeding from esophageal varices. These include direct ligation of varices, transection of the esophagus with division of varices, esophagogastric resection, splenectomy,

and splenorenal or portacaval anastomosis. Each procedure carries a high risk in the poor-risk patient with hepatic decompensation. The surgical procedure of choice is a *portacaval anastomosis,* which controls bleeding by lowering portal pressure; with the subsequent disappearance of esophageal varices, recurrent bleeding is unusual.

A portacaval anastomosis is recommended for the good-risk patient with documented bleeding from esophageal varices, unless bleeding has been precipitated by acute alcoholic hepatitis. In the latter instance, portal pressure may return to normal, and varices may disappear upon recovery from acute hepatic decompensation and resolution of hepatic inflammation and fatty infiltration. When esophageal bleeding complicates hepatocellular failure, surgery is contraindicated even when medical therapy is ineffective in controlling hemorrhage. There is no evidence that a prophylactic portacaval shunt is of value in prolonging the life of a patient with portal hypertension and esophageal varices that have not bled.

Ascites. When ascites complicates acute alcoholic hepatitis, therapy aimed at improving liver function usually leads to a spontaneous diuresis as the portal pressure falls toward normal and serum albumin levels rise. Sodium intake should be restricted to 1 to 3 grams daily, but diuretics should be used with caution.

When ascites is of longer duration and is associated with sustained portal hypertension and hypoalbuminemia, diuretic agents together with a restricted intake of sodium may be necessary to control sodium and water retention. The sole use of diuretic agents that act principally on the proximal tubule (mercurials and chlorothiazides) is contraindicated. These agents do not counteract the effect of aldosterone on the distal tubule; not only are they ineffective diuretics in cirrhotic patients with secondary hyperaldosteronism, but they also augment potassium loss and may precipitate *hypokalemic alkalosis* with hepatic coma in spite of oral potassium supplements.

To promote an *effective* and *safe* diuresis, an *aldosterone blocking agent* should be given in combination with one of the above diuretic agents. Spironolactone (50 to 200 mg. daily) with hydrochlorothiazide (50 to 100 mg. daily) is recommended. Oral potassium supplements (KCl in cherry syrup, 1 gram three times a day) may be necessary during the initial two to four days of combined drug therapy to prevent hypokalemia. The complications of diuretic therapy include the following: (1) *Hyperkalemia* often results from the use of aldosterone-blocking drugs in patients with impaired renal function. (2) *Hyponatremia* may be associated with an abnormal distribution of sodium between the intracellular and extracellular fluid pools in patients with an increased total body sodium, with disproportionate water retention, or with sodium depletion after prolonged diuresis. (3) *Azotemia* may be due to contraction of the extracellular fluid pool or a decrease in renal blood flow with hypovolemia. (4)

Hepatic encephalopathy may follow rapid diuresis or disturbances of pH and electrolyte balance. These complications will be reduced if serum electrolyte concentrations and urinary electrolyte excretion are measured frequently during therapy. Diuretics should be discontinued when neuropsychiatric symptoms complicate rapid diuresis or electrolyte imbalance, and no attempt should be made to mobilize all ascitic fluid by prolonged therapy that increases the risk of complication without benefit to the patient. When long-term diuretic therapy is necessary to control ascites, diuretics should be given intermittently rather than continuously.

When ascites is associated with severe hypoalbuminemia, intravenous infusions of salt-poor albumin (50 to 100 grams daily) may potentiate a diuresis, but pulmonary edema caused by an expanded plasma volume must be avoided.

Paracentesis with removal of less than 1000 ml. of ascitic fluid should be performed for diagnostic purposes, but is now rarely indicated for therapy of ascites except when impaired renal function prevents safe or effective diuretic therapy. Ascitic fluid should then be removed slowly through a small plastic catheter, and salt-poor human albumin (50 to 200 grams) should be infused intravenously over a period of 12 to 24 hours to prevent hypovolemia and shock that may result from a shift of fluid from the intravascular compartment into the peritoneal cavity.

Hepatic Coma. When a cirrhotic patient develops hepatic encephalopathy it is important to identify the precipitating cause. It may be due to gastrointestinal bleeding; fluid and electrolyte imbalances and pH disturbances, particularly during diuretic therapy; the administration of depressant drugs, both analgesic and sedative; intercurrent infection with fever; or increased dietary intake of protein. In the treatment of hepatic coma, gastrointestinal bleeding, and infection must be controlled, depressant drugs withheld and disturbances of fluid, electrolyte, and acid-base balance corrected. In all patients, measures that lower blood ammonium concentration by reducing enteric bacterial breakdown of amino acids and urea should be instituted. These measures include dietary *protein restriction* (complete in the comatose patient, or partial—20 to 40 grams—in patients with mild encephalopathy), *cathartics* (magnesium citrate, 240 ml. twice daily), *enemas* to clear the intestine of its nitrogenous content, and *neomycin* (4 to 6 grams daily by mouth or by nasogastric tube) to reduce the bacterial flora.

Patients with chronic hepatic encephalopathy, who usually have extensive portal-systemic shunts, may be helped by long-term restriction of protein intake to 40 grams and the administration of neomycin, 2 to 3 grams daily. Lactulose, a pentose sugar that is not absorbed but is metabolized by intestinal bacteria to organic acids, is effective in lowering the blood ammonia levels of patients with chronic encephalopathy; the un-

absorbed sugar produces an osmotic diarrhea, and ammonia is retained in the fecal content at the acid pH.

A surgical approach to the management of the patient with chronic hepatic encephalopathy is excision or exclusion of the colon; the complications of surgery in chronically ill patients usually balance the potential benefit of removing a bacteria-laden gut.

In treating the alcoholic patient with cirrhosis, efforts should be directed toward the control of his addiction, upon which depends the ultimate success of all medical and surgical measures.

POSTHEPATITIC AND IDIOPATHIC CIRRHOSIS (POSTNECROTIC CIRRHOSIS)

Pathogenesis. It has been shown by serial liver biopsy studies that acute viral hepatitis (both icteric and anicteric) or toxic hepatitis complicated by subacute hepatic necrosis leads to a macronodular cirrhosis. In many nonalcoholic patients there is no history to suggest previous viral or toxic hepatitis; i.e., the cirrhosis is idiopathic. Idiopathic cirrhosis is sometimes associated with chronic ulcerative colitis; it has been suggested but not proved that chronic pericholangitis resulting from portal bacteremia may cause cirrhosis in these patients.

The association of hypergammaglobulinemia, positive antinuclear reactions, positive L-E cell phenomena, and other positive serologic reactions with idiopathic cirrhosis has led to a theory that cirrhosis may be caused by immunologic destruction of parenchymal cells; this has not been proved. An increased formation of immunoglobulins with hyperglobulinemia may be stimulated by antigens released from necrotic cells, and may have no primary etiologic significance.

Pathology. The liver in posthepatitic or idiopathic cirrhosis is typically shrunken, with irregular large regeneration nodules and broad zones of fibrous tissue. Pathologically, this is referred to as *macronodular (postnecrotic) cirrhosis*. During the phase of *progressive cirrhosis* following subacute hepatic necrosis or chronic aggressive hepatitis, there may be microscopic evidence of cell degeneration and regeneration, and mononuclear infiltration (both lymphocytes and plasma cells) is prominent in the zones of fibrosis. Intrahepatic cholestasis with bile plugs in dilated bile canaliculi varies with the degree of jaundice, and bile duct proliferation is usual.

Clinical Manifestations. The progressive cirrhosis following subacute hepatic necrosis and chronic aggressive hepatitis is often associated with malaise, weakness, anorexia, and jaundice. The patient often has a low-grade fever, and multiple spider angiomas may be seen. The liver is sometimes enlarged and tender, but is more typically shrunken and associated with increased percussion resonance over the right lower costal margin; the spleen may be slightly or massively enlarged.

Ascites or peripheral edema may complicate portal hypertension or hypoalbuminemia, and increased bruising may be due to hypoprothrombinemia. Manifestations of disturbed endocrine function—acne, striae, gynecomastia, and amenorrhea—are particularly common in juvenile patients with active cirrhosis. Hypergammaglobulinemia parallels the degree of lymphocytic and plasma cell infiltration in the liver, and may be accompanied by serologic abnormalities. The term lupoid hepatitis has been used in referring to those patients with L-E cell phenomena, but there are no other clinical features to separate this group of patients from others with active idiopathic cirrhosis. Chronic intrahepatic cholestasis with jaundice, hypercholesterolemia, and high alkaline phosphatase levels sometimes mimics primary biliary cirrhosis. It is not unusual for the biochemical evidence of hepatocellular failure to exceed the clinical evidence of this condition.

The only clinical manifestations of compensated idiopathic cirrhosis may be the cutaneous stigmata of chronic liver disease and splenic enlargement. In these patients, ascites, hepatic coma, and bleeding from esophageal varices may be late complications.

Treatment. During the period of progressive cirrhosis, limited physical activity and corticosteroids (prednisolone, 10 to 30 mg. daily) may reduce symptoms, improve liver function with lowering of serum bilirubin, transaminase, and gamma globulin levels, and decrease hepatic infiltration with mononuclear cells. There is no evidence, however, that corticosteroid therapy prevents progression of the cirrhotic lesion. The apparent beneficial effects of corticosteroid therapy in these patients must be weighed against the risk of steroid side effects—iatrogenic Cushing's syndrome, bone demineralization, and increased susceptibility to infection. Corticosteroids are of no benefit for patients with compensated idiopathic cirrhosis.

BILIARY CIRRHOSIS

Primary biliary cirrhosis (chronic nonsuppurative destructive cholangitis) is a disease of unknown etiology. Chronic intrahepatic cholestasis is associated with progressive periportal fibrosis and chronic inflammation. Cirrhosis with nodular regeneration is a late pathologic finding. Although hypersensitivity reactions to drugs sometimes cause prolonged intrahepatic cholestasis, there is no evidence that acute intrahepatic cholestasis leads to primary biliary cirrhosis. It has been suggested that the primary lesion may be an injury to small bile ducts; these are often absent in liver biopsy specimens taken early in the course of the disease, but regenerate in the cirrhotic liver. Patients with primary biliary cirrhosis may exhibit hypergammaglobulinemia with circulating antibodies reactive against cells that contain many mitochondria, but the significance of immunologic phenomena has not been established.

In secondary biliary cirrhosis, bile duct obstruction with or without infection causes periportal inflammation with progressive fibrosis, parenchymal cell destruction, and nodular regeneration.

Clinical Features. Primary biliary cirrhosis is most often diagnosed in women aged 40 to 60. The earliest symptom may be generalized pruritus. Jaundice with dark urine and pale stools and cutaneous xanthomas appear later with increasing intrahepatic cholestasis. At the time of onset of symptoms, the liver is usually firm and enlarged, and the spleen is palpable. Liver function tests at this time reflect cholestasis with good hepatocellular function; alkaline phosphatase, 5-nucleotidase, and cholesterol levels may be markedly elevated, whereas serum albumin levels remain normal. During the period of maximal cholestasis the manifestations of malabsorption may become evident: weight loss, diarrhea with pale bulky stools, bleeding resulting from hypoprothrombinemia, and collapse of vertebrae and pathologic fractures with bone demineralization caused by malabsorption of vitamin D and calcium. Xanthomas usually appear when the serum cholesterol level exceeds 450 mg. per 100 ml. Acute upper gastrointestinal bleeding is more often from a duodenal ulcer than from esophageal varices; a reduced flow of alkaline bile with normal gastric acid secretion may contribute to peptic ulcer.

The terminal stage of biliary cirrhosis is one of hepatocellular failure with rising serum bilirubin levels, a decrease in serum albumin and cholesterol with disappearance of xanthomas, and the onset of ascites.

Differential Diagnosis. The diagnosis of primary biliary cirrhosis must always be confirmed by exploratory laparotomy, with liver biopsy and operative cholangiography. Stenosing cholangitis, extrahepatic bile duct obstruction resulting from stone or stricture, and carcinoma involving the major extrahepatic or intrahepatic bile ducts should be excluded. The presence of antimitochondrial antibody is of diagnostic importance—patients with extrahepatic biliary obstruction do not exhibit this antibody.

Treatment. Supplements of fat-soluble vitamins should be given to prevent or correct deficiency caused by malabsorption. Vitamin K_1, 5 to 10 mg., and vitamins A and D, 10,000 units, should be given by mouth daily together with calcium lactate or gluconate, 6 to 12 grams. Pruritus may be relieved by methyl testosterone or norethandrolone, 10 mg. twice or three times daily, but these agents increase the jaundice. The bile acid sequestrant resin, cholestyramine, 8 to 12 grams daily in divided doses, is effective in relieving pruritus, lowering serum cholesterol levels, and reducing xanthomas when cholestasis is incomplete. Patients with duodenal ulcer or with complications of cirrhosis should be treated appropriately as outlined in other sections.

Prognosis. The average life expectancy in primary biliary cirrhosis from the time of onset of symptoms is approximately five years. With supportive therapy the patient will be more comfortable and will suffer fewer complications during this period.

CARDIAC CIRRHOSIS

Chronic congestive heart failure with valvular heart disease and tricuspid incompetence or constrictive pericarditis may cause progressive fibrosis extending peripherally from centrilobular to portal areas. Regeneration nodules are not prominent. Fat may accumulate in hypoxic cells.

The liver is usually firm, with tenderness and an increase in size during more severe episodes of heart failure. Hepatic pulsation may be detected with tricuspid insufficiency. The changes in liver function are those of acute hepatic congestion, but hypoalbuminemia may be more severe when there is excessive enteric leakage of plasma protein. (See Diseases of Malabsorption.) Although chronic congestive heart failure may raise the portal venous pressure, a portal-systemic collateral circulation, e.g., esophageal varices, does not develop in the absence of an increased pressure gradient between these systems.

CONGENITAL HEPATIC FIBROSIS

Congenital hepatic fibrosis is a variant of polycystic disease. Broad bands of fibrous tissue containing bile ducts surround the liver lobules and obstruct portal blood flow. Splenomegaly, portal hypertension, and bleeding from esophageal varices are the usual presenting manifestations in childhood or adolescence. With normal liver function these children usually tolerate recurrent bleeding and portacaval shunt surgery better than patients with cirrhosis. In adults, *polycystic disease of the liver* may cause massive liver enlargement without interfering with liver function. The complications include hemorrhage into a cyst with abdominal pain and bleeding from esophageal varices.

INFILTRATIVE DISEASE OF THE LIVER

HEPATIC GRANULOMAS

Hepatic granulomas are most commonly due to *sarcoidosis and tuberculosis,* but also occur in beryllium poisoning, brucellosis, and fungal and parasitic infections.

In sarcoidosis there are noncaseating granulomas, with mononuclear, epithelioid, and giant cells, and variable fibrosis. In patients with pulmonary tuberculosis or miliary tuberculosis, hepatic granulomas are particularly common. Small lesions may exhibit no caseation, and no organisms may be demonstrated; but larger lesions may have a central area of caseation.

Granulomatous disease of the liver may be associated with enlargement of the liver and BSP retention with elevation of alkaline phosphatase and 5-nucleotidase without jaundice. A needle biopsy of the liver should be performed to establish the diagnosis of granulomatous disease. This is particularly helpful in the diagnosis of miliary tuberculosis in an ill, febrile patient without typical radiologic changes in the chest.

SECONDARY CARCINOMA OF THE LIVER

Primary carcinomas of the lung, gastrointestinal tract, and breast are the most common neoplasms that metastasize to the liver. Abdominal swelling or pain and jaundice are the presenting symptoms, but the liver is usually massively enlarged with multiple nodules before jaundice develops. The earlier biochemical manifestations of hepatic metastases are BSP retention and elevations of serum alkaline phosphatase and 5-nucleotidase. Needle biopsy of the liver is helpful in providing a tissue diagnosis of secondary carcinoma, and may save the patient from the discomfort of an exploratory laparotomy. External radioisotopic scanning of the liver after the intravenous injection of a gamma-emitting radioisotope that is concentrated in the liver may be helpful in localizing large metastases that appear as "cold" areas in the surface scan.

SARCOMAS OF THE LIVER

Hepatic infiltration with lymphoma, lymphosarcoma, or Hodgkin's disease is usually a manifestation of disseminated disease. Firm liver enlargement and biochemical evidence of intrahepatic cholestasis are typical manifestations. Jaundice is more often the result of hepatic infiltration than invasion of the extrahepatic bile ducts by tumor; jaundice caused by intrahepatic cholestasis may develop, however, in the absence of liver infiltration.

PRIMARY CARCINOMAS OF THE LIVER (HEPATOMA)

Hepatic carcinoma usually complicates cirrhosis of the liver; it has a higher incidence in postnecrotic cirrhosis and hemochromatosis than in Laennec's cirrhosis. This lesion should be suspected whenever a cirrhotic patient exhibits unexplained clinical deterioration with enlarging liver, right upper quadrant pain, or sudden onset of ascites. A vascular bruit may be heard over these tumors. Hypoglycemia is sometimes a prominent clinical manifestation. Changes in liver function include a rising alkaline phosphatase and elevated lactic dehydrogenase. Hepatomas localized to one lobe of the liver have been excised successfully on several occasions, but usually cirrhosis and invasion of hepatic veins or local spread prevent surgical therapy.

Hepatoma can be produced with a high degree of regularity in several species of laboratory animals by injection of minute doses of the microtoxin known as *aflatoxin*. This substance is produced by Aspergillus growing on peanut (groundnut) meal that has been stored in appropriately hot, humid conditions. The incidence of hepatoma in man has long been known to show a marked geographic variation, and there is a correlation between the localities where hepatoma is the most frequently occurring carcinoma and the particular complex of circumstances that favors the production of aflatoxin. Recently Siperstein has shown that in the human liver containing a hepatoma there is unregulated cholesterol synthesis due to breakdown of a normal feedback control mechanism. He has further shown that in an animal model in which hepatoma is produced in high incidence at some time after a single injection of aflatoxin (trout), there is suppression of the normal hepatic feedback control mechanism within five days of injection of this extremely potent toxin. Obviously, it cannot be stated as yet that hepatoma in man is caused by aflatoxin, but this possibility that hepatoma is thus environmentally induced is being actively pursued in epidemiologic, clinical, and laboratory studies.

ALPHA, FETOPROTEIN

General

Scheuer, P. J.: Liver Biopsy Interpretation. London. Balliere, Tindall and Cassell, Ltd., 1968.

Schiff, L.: Diseases of the Liver. 3rd ed. Philadelphia, J. B. Lippincott Company, 1969.

Sherlock, S.: Diseases of the Liver. 4th ed. Oxford, Blackwell Scientific Publications, 1968.

Manifestations of Liver Disease

Bergström, S.: Metabolism of bile acids. Fed. Proc., 21:28, 1962.

Hoffman, A. F., and Small, D. M.: Detergent properties of bile salts: Correlation with physiological function. Ann. Rev. Med., 18:333, 1967.

Javitt, N.: Bile salt regulation of hepatic excretory function. Gastroenterology, 56:622, 1969.

Kowlessar, O. D., Haeffner, L. J., Riley, E. M., and Sleisenger, M. H.: Comparative study of serum leucine aminopeptidase, 5-nucleotidase and nonspecific alkaline phosphatase in diseases affecting the pancreas, hepatobiliary tree and bone. Amer. J. Med., 31:231, 1961.

Leevy, C. M.: Evaluation of Liver Function in Clinical Practice. Indianapolis, Eli Lilly and Company, 1965.

Lester, R., and Troxler, R. F.: Recent advances in bile pigment metabolism. Gastroenterology, 56:143, 1969.

Sherlock, S.: Jaundice. Brit. Med. J., 1:1359. 1962.

Acute Liver Disease

Chalmers, T. C., Eckhardt, R. D., Reynolds, W. E., Cigarroa, J. G., Jr., Deane. N., Reifenstein, R. W., Smith, C. W., and Davidson, C. S.: The treatment of acute infectious hepatitis. Controlled studies of the effect of diet, rest and physical reconditioning on the acute course of the disease and on the incidence of relapses and residual abnormalities. J. Clin. Invest., 34:1136, 1955.

Clain, D., Freston, J., Kreel, L., and Sherlock, S.: Clinical diagnosis of the Budd-Chiari syndrome. Amer. J. Med., 43:544, 1967.

Conrad, M. E., Schwartz, F. D., and Young, A. A.: Infectious hepatitis — a generalized disease. A study of renal, gastrointestinal and hematologic abnormalities. Amer. J. Med., 37:789, 1964.

Gocke, D. J., and Kavey, N. B.: Hepatitis antigen: Correlation with disease and infectivity of blood-donors. Lancet, 1:1055, 1969.

Klatskin, G.: Toxic and drug-induced hepatitis. In Schiff, L. (ed.): Diseases of the Liver. 3rd ed. Philadelphia, J. B. Lippincott Company, 1969, p. 498.

Krugman, S., Giles, J. P., and Hammond, J.: Infectious hepatitis: Evidence for two distinctive clinical. epidemiological and immunological types of infection. J.A.M.A., 200:365, 1967.

Netzger D. M., and Chalmers, T. C.: The treatment of acute infectious hepatitis. Ten-year follow-up study of the effects of diet and rest. Amer. J. Med., 35:299, 1963.

Prince, A. M., Hargrove, R. L., Szmuness, W., Cherubin, C. E., Fontana, V. J., and Jeffries, G. H.: Immunologic distinction between serum and infectious hepatitis. New Eng. J. Med., 282:987, 1970.

Senior, J. R.: Post-transfusion hepatitis. Gastroenterology, 49:315, 1965.

Trey, C., Lipworth, L., Chalmers, T. C., Davidson, C. S., Gottlieb, L. S., Popper, H., and Saunders, S. J.: Fulminant hepatic failure. Presumable contribution of Halothane. New Eng. J. Med., 279:798, 1968.

Chronic Liver Disease

Chalmers, T. C.: Pathogenesis and treatment of hepatic failure. New Eng. J. Med., 263:23:77, 1960.

Conn, H. O., and Lindenmuth, W. W.: Prophylactic portacaval anastomosis in cirrhotic patients wih esophageal varices. New Eng. J. Med., 279:725, 1968.

Garceau, A. J., Chalmers, T. C., and the Boston Inter-Hospital Liver Group: The natural history of cirrhosis. New Eng. J. Med., 268:469, 1963; 271:1173, 1964.

Grace, N. D., Muench, H., and Chalmers, T. C.: Present status of shunts for portal hypertension in cirrhosis. Gastroenterology, 50:684, 1966.

Klatskin, G.: Subacute hepatic necrosis and postnecrotic cirrhosis due to anicteric infections with hepatitis virus. Amer. J. Med., 25:333, 1958.

Lieber, C. S.: Metabolic derangement induced by alcohol. Ann. Rev. Med. 18:35, 1967.

Lieber, C. S., Jones, D. P., and DeCarli, L. M.: Effects of prolonged ethanol intake: Production of fatty liver despite adequate diets. J. Clin. Invest., 44:1009, 1965.

Losowski, M. S., Jones, D. P., Lieber, C. S., and Davidson, C. S.: Local factors in ascites formation during sodium retention in cirrhosis. New Eng. J. Med., 268:651, 1963.

Reynolds, T. B., Geller, H. M., Kuzma, O. T., and Redeker, A. G.: Spontaneous decrease in portal pressure with clinical improvement in cirrhosis. New Eng. J. Med., 263:734, 1960.

Schenker, S., McCandless, D. W., Brophy, E., and Lewis, M. S.: Studies on the intracerebral toxicity of ammonia. J. Clin. Invest., 46:838, 1967.

Shaldon, S., McLaren, J. R., and Sherlock, S.: Resistant ascites treated by combined diuretic therapy. Lancet, 1:609, 1960.

Sherlock, S.: Hepatic coma. Gastroenterology, 41:1, 1961.

Sherlock, S.: Primary biliary cirrhosis. Gastroenterology, 37:574, 1959.

Turner, M. D., Sherlock, S., and Steiner, R. E.: Splenic venography and intrasplenic pressure measurement in the clinical investigation of the portal venous system. Amer. J. Med., 23:846, 1957.

Van Itallie, T. B., Hashim, S. A., Crampton, R. S., and Tennent, D. M.: The treatment of pruritus and hypercholesterolemia of primary biliary cirrhosis with cholestyramine. New Eng. J. Med., 265:469, 1961.

Walker, J. G., Doniach, D., Roitt, I. M., and Sherlock, S.: Serological tests in diagnosis of primary biliary cirrhosis. Lancet, 1:827, 1965.

Wilcox, R. G., and Isselbacher, K. J.: Chronic liver disease in young people. Amer. J. Med., 30:185, 1961.

Diseases of the Gallbladder and Bile Ducts

Marvin H. Sleisenger

GENERAL CONSIDERATIONS

Inflammation, infection, and carcinoma are the major categories of disease of the gallbladder and biliary tract. Ninety per cent of patients with these disorders have cholelithiasis. The principal symptoms are *pain, jaundice,* and *fever*. Pain is by far the most common of the three symptoms.

Biliary Tract Pain. Characteristically, biliary tract pain is severe, intensifies rapidly, and is usually steady for a period of hours, although it may be intermittent (colic). It is due to increased tension of smooth muscle of the gallbladder and/or the common bile duct, associated with spasm or obstruction. Colic may occur when there are stones in the gallbladder or biliary tract or when the gallbladder is inflamed, with or without stones. The afferent nerve supply from the gallbladder and extrahepatic bile ducts is through the right and left splanchnic nerves to the posterior roots of T7 through T10; the more severe the pain, the greater is the area referred to by the patient. For example, the pain may begin in the epigastrium and, as it increases in severity, may be felt by the patient to be extending along the costal margin into the back and up beneath the right scapula and shoulder, and then to the substernal area and sometimes to the left precordial region, left costal margin, and left shoulder. The pain may be continuous or intermittent (biliary colic).

Because of overlap in the segmental distribution of nerves to the upper abdominal organs, the stomach and lower esophagus, the duodenum, and the pancreas, disease of these organs may cause pain that simulates the pattern of gallbladder or biliary tract disease.

As the calculi formed from bile are so important in the common diseases of the gallbladder and bile ducts, a consideration of the physiology of bile secretion is essential to an understanding of stone formation and the diseases of the biliary tract.

FORMATION OF BILE

Bile is a neutral or slightly alkaline fluid that is continuously secreted by the hepatic parenchymal cells into the bile canaliculi. Bile is concentrated and stored in the gallbladder. Intermittent gallbladder emptying in response to circulating cholecystokinin (pancreozymin), is coordinated with the discharge of concentrated bile and pancreatic juice into the duodenal lumen. The cholecystokinin causes an increase in the tone of the gallbladder, increasing its intraluminal pressure from 300 mm. of water to nearly 375 mm., and returning the bile to the common duct. At the same time that the gallbladder contracts, the sphincter of Oddi relaxes so that the bile flows through the ampulla of Vater into the duodenum without an increase in pressure within the common bile duct. Certain foods such as fats, egg yolk, and those high in cholesterol act as a strong stimulus for the gallbladder to empty.

The constituents of bile may be divided into those substances that are present in concentrations similar to plasma filtrate: sodium, potassium, and chloride; substances that are present in concentrations lower than in plasma: plasma proteins, glucose, phospholipids, cholesterol, and phosphate; and substances that are present in higher concentrations: bile salts (glyco- and taurocholates), conjugated bilirubin, steroid hormones, pressor amines, and enzymes (alkaline phosphatase). Exogenous substances of clinical importance are also excreted in bile: sulfobromophthalein, the radiopaque contrast media used in roentgenographic visualization of the gallbladder and bile ducts, and several antimicrobial drugs. During the process whereby the gallbladder concentrates bile salts tenfold, water containing sodium, chloride, and bicarbonate is transported through its wall back into the circulation.

The secretion of bile constituents is an energy-requiring process that may involve active transfer and concentration in the liver cell, chemical alteration (conjugation of bilirubin and steroids), and active secretion through the microvilli of the parenchymal cell membrane lining the bile canaliculus.

Bile salts (sodium glyco- and taurocholates), synthesized by the liver cell from cholesterol and secreted in concentrations of 1 to 2 per cent, have an important function not only in activating pancreatic lipase and facilitating the digestion of triglyceride fat, but also in stimulating the metabolism of intestinal mucosal cells. In biliary tract obstruction the retention of bile salts results in a decrease in the conversion of cholesterol to bile acids with increased levels of serum cholesterol, malabsorption of fat and fat-soluble vitamins owing to impaired digestion and absorption, and generalized pruritus owing to an increase in the tissue bile acid concentration.

Bile cholesterol, synthesized by the hepatic parenchymal cell, is retained in solution by complexes with bile salts and lecithin, known as *micelles*. Factors that may alter the relative concentration of cholesterol, phospholipid, and bile salts, and, presumably, the ratio of conjugated to unconjugated bile salts, play an important role in the formation of gallstones. The bilirubin content of bile (bilirubin glucuronide and sulfate) is related to hemoglobin catabolism in the presence of normal liver function.

Mechanism of Roentgenographic Visualization. (See also Choledocholithiasis, *infra.*) The diagnosis of cholelithiasis and of acute and chronic cholecystitis depends mainly upon roentgenography. Orally administered organic iodides (iodopanoic acid, Telepaque) are absorbed in the small intestine and excreted in the bile in concentrations too dilute to give roentgenographic visualization of the ductal system. Concentration of the dye in the gallbladder, however, permits the subsequent visualization of that organ and, with the emptying of the gallbladder, the common bile duct may be defined. Factors that would cause nonvisualization of the gallbladder include: (1) failure to absorb the orally administered dye; (2) failure of dye excretion in the bile (parenchymal cell dysfunction or bile duct obstruction); (3) failure of the dye to enter the gallbladder (cystic duct obstruction); and (4) impaired concentration of the dye by the gallbladder (chronic cholecystitis). Gallbladder disease may be diagnosed definitely if the organ is not opacified by dye, providing that an adequate dose is absorbed and the liver is able to excrete the dye. In some patients the diagnosis of suspected biliary tract disease may be strengthened by a flat film of the abdomen that demonstrates calcified calculi.

In the absence of the gallbladder or when partial obstruction of the common bile duct is suspected, the ductal system may be visualized after the intravenous injection of another organic iodide. This technique depends on the excretion of a dye, sodium iodopamide (Biligrafin, Cholegrafin), at a concentration that permits roentgenographic visualization of the bile ducts without further concentration of the dye in the gallbladder. On the other hand, the delayed visualization of the gallbladder during intravenous cholangiography does not necessarily signify a normal gallbladder, but only that the cystic duct is patent. Visualization by either method is unlikely if serum bilirubin is greater than 3.0 mg. per 100 ml.

GALLSTONES (CHOLELITHIASIS)

Types and Incidence. Primary consideration of gallstones is indicated because cholelithiasis is strongly linked with both inflammatory and malignant disease of the gallbladder and biliary tract. Often the liver and pancreas are secondarily involved (see Diseases of the Liver and Diseases of the Pancreas).

Gallstones are concretions that form anywhere in the biliary tract, although it is believed that most of them form in the gallbladder. They vary greatly in content, size, and shape. The prevalence of gallstones is estimated to be from 10 to 20 per cent among the adult white population of the United States, based on autopsy studies. Prospective surveys, however, indicate a prevalence of only 6 per cent in females aged 30 to 62, with peak incidence of 9 per cent for the age group 50 to 62; for males (30 to 62), the prevalence is 1.3 per cent;

peak incidence is 5 per cent in the age group 50 to 60.

The incidence of gallstones in American Indians (Navajo, Pima) is, however, considerably higher, with a prevalence of 38 per cent in women aged 30 to 62, and over 50 per cent in those over age 40. In males aged 30 to 62 the prevalence is 6 per cent. Also, the incidence of gallstones in the third decade is significantly higher in Indians than in whites.

Very rarely, stones may be composed entirely of *cholesterol.* These stones tend to occur singly and to be rounded, are of yellow-white color, and reveal a crystalline structure on cross section. They are usually fairly large. *Bilirubin-calcium* stones are black and assume various shapes, being irregular, faceted, or rounded. They vary greatly in size from sandlike particles to calculi 1 cm. or more in diameter. They are of a homogeneous structure, either crystalline, e.g., the cholesterol stones, or laminated, e.g., the mixed calculi. They constitute about 3 per cent of all gallstones. The most common form of calculus is the so-called *mixed type,* which represents essentially a cholesterol stone to which layers composed of bilirubin, calcium, cellular debris, and glycoprotein have been added. Over 96 per cent of all stones are of this type. They also vary greatly in size, shape, and consistency. They are usually laminated and have a central nucleus that is soft with superimposed concentric layers of various amounts of cholesterol, bilirubin, and calcium. Each concretion is considered to have a nidus, usually either glycoprotein, bilirubinate, or, more rarely, cellular debris. The roentgenographic appearance of stones depends on their calcium content; pure cholesterol stones are radiolucent, whereas bilirubin-calcium and mixed stones may be radiopaque (Fig. 1); however, only 20 to 30 per cent of all calculi are sufficiently calcified to be apparent on plain films of the abdomen.

Stones may be found in the biliary tract in patients of any age. They are rare in infants and infrequent in children and adolescents. Rarely, in whites they are found in young adult males and in females who have not been pregnant. They are more common in multiparous white women than in the nulliparous ones, and occur with gradual and increasing frequency in each decade after 40. However, parity does not affect the incidence in Indian women, nor, apparently, does their diet or obesity.

In infants and young children, gallstones are so rare that they are seldom considered in differential diagnosis. Their presence has been reported, however, in the newborn at autopsy. Before the age of puberty their occurrence is usually associated with hemolytic disease. In the female, cholelithiasis is one of the most frequent diseases associated with gestation among white women in North America. This association accounts for the predominance of calculi in the female (F:M::4:1). Between the ages of 35 and 55 years the incidence of gallstones in men and nulliparous women is

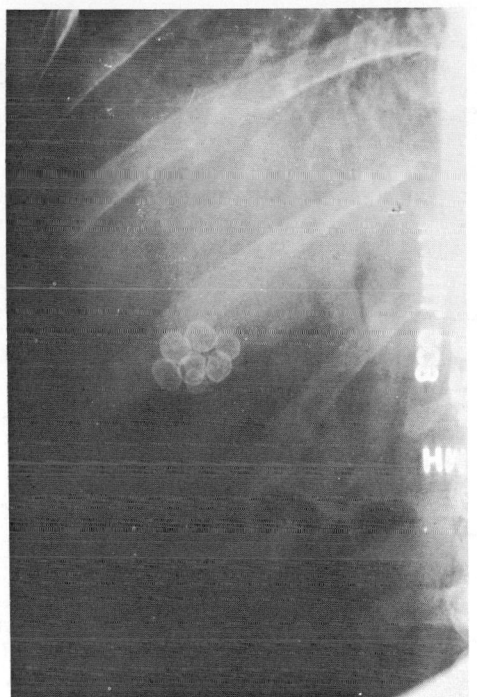

FIGURE 1. Multiple gallstones visualized on roentgenogram. Calculi consist briefly of cholesterol with peripheral deposition of calcium.

equal, and is considerably higher than the incidence in the younger age group.

Etiology and Pathogenesis. *Mechanism of Gallstone Formation.* Although the gallbladder is the usual site of gallstone formation, stones may be deposited in the intra- or extrahepatic bile ducts in the presence of infection and/or stasis.

The mechanism whereby stones are formed in the gallbladder and biliary ductal system is not completely understood, although much study has been devoted to this problem. Many isolated and easily comprehended facts have been revealed, and many more associated and complex fragments of information difficult to interpret have been brought forth by numerous investigators. Despite these intensive studies, however, there is no single theory that provides an adequate explanation for all gallstone formation. The precipitation of the bile constituents, particularly cholesterol, results from physicochemical disturbance of the *micelle* that keeps them in solution.

Cholesterol Metabolism. Recent evidence indicates that the liver secretes bile that is supersaturated with cholesterol in patients with cholelithiasis. Cholesterol crystals precipitate in gallbladder bile. Particulate matter—glycoproteins and bilirubinate—may then become the nidus for aggregation of these crystals and stone formation. Cholesterol stones, although composed mainly of cholesterol crystals about a nidus, thus are almost always mixed stones, containing bilirubin, calcium, glycoprotein, and debris, possibly bacterial in origin. The pathogenesis is due to an imbalance in the mixture of cholesterol and bile salts plus lecithin, in which there is relatively too much cholesterol to remain in micellar solution. This excess of cholesterol has been found in all studies of bile in patients with these mixed stones and even in a few instances before stones have been detected. This abnormality is noted in white and Indian populations.

The formation of these stones is also influenced by the presence of glycoproteins, perhaps in excess or in abnormal form which may serve as the nidus for cholesterol crystals, as may bilirubinate. In addition, glycoprotein interlaces the matrix of these mixed stones.

The relative excess of cholesterol may result, as noted, from hepatic dysfunction, perhaps due to a basic abnormality of the canalicular membrane which normally is dissolved by bile salts, releasing cholesterol and lecithin. If the cholesterol thus released is relatively greater in amount than lecithin, its solubilization by the micelle may be reduced. Of interest, serum concentration of cholesterol in these individuals is normal.

Serum cholesterol is elevated in *myxedema,* the *nephrotic syndrome, familial hypercholesterolemia,* and *primary biliary cirrhosis,* conditions that are *not* associated with an increased incidence of gallstones. However, diabetes mellitus has an increased incidence of cholelithiasis. Although no definite relationship has been established between diet and gallstones, racial differences in the incidence of gallstones may reflect the effect of different dietary habits on cholesterol metabolism. Thus, in most Asian people, the serum cholesterol levels are usually low and gallstones are uncommon, whereas in overweight North Americans, both hypercholesterolemia and gallstones are fairly common. However, diet does not appear to influence the incidence of cholelithiasis in the North American Indian, in whom it is extremely high despite food that is little different from that of whites who, as noted, have a significantly lower incidence. Obesity does not predispose to cholelithiasis in either race. Also, serum cholesterol levels in American Indians with gallstones are not elevated.

Bilirubin Metabolism. It is now held that the pathogenesis for formation of bilirubin stones is the splitting of bilirubin salts by glucuronidases in bile (probably of bacterial origin). Studies in patients with these stones universally show *E. coli,* whereas these organisms are not found in those with mixed stones. In conditions associated with increased red cell destruction and increased bilirubin excretion in the bile for long periods, the incidence of these stones appears to be increased.

Infection and Stasis. More than 70 years ago, Naunyn was convinced that ascending infection in the biliary tract, when there was stasis, led to stone formation. Bacteria can be isolated from gallbladders containing stones removed at operation in more than 50 per cent of the patients and from 20 per cent of stones. Streptococci, *Escherichia coli,* and various salmonellae, including *S. typhosa,* are found most frequently, but a wide variety of organisms may be encountered including staphylococci and actinomyces. These bacteria increase the ratio of free to conjugated bile salts in the *micelle* and thus lead to the precipitation of cholesterol; however, it is likely that the bacterial growth in gallbladder bile is a consequence of the disease except, as noted, in patients who form bilirubin stones (see above). Regardless, when bacteria populate bile, they further contribute to stone formation by deconjugation of bile salts, free bile salts being resorbed in the upper gut and gallbladder. Their return to the liver leads perhaps to increased release of cholesterol from canalicular membranes. Bacteria also break down lecithin to lysolecithin which does not solubilize cholesterol as well as its precursor. Further, bacteria hydrolyze conjugated bilirubin, and the liberated free bilirubin may be a nidus for stone formation by precipitated cholesterol crystals.

The role of stasis of bile alone in calculi formation has not been determined. Stones tend to form when bile stagnates, as in *pregnant women*, those with organic *obstruction* to *bile flow*, and in those who are confined to bed or are otherwise immobilized for long periods. Impaired emptying of the gallbladder increases concentration of bile. In this respect, it must be emphasized that our understanding of the pathogenesis of cholelithiasis is still imperfect. Is an enlarged gallbladder in a pregnant woman necessarily a "static" one? The organ normally is static, emptying only with stimuli following meals. The problem of stone formation appears to be more related to factors that regulate the composition of bile. Apparently, there is time enough for precipitation under normal circumstances.

THE RELATIONSHIP BETWEEN GALLSTONES AND BILIARY TRACT DISEASE

Gallstones are associated with most disorders of the biliary tract. Thus, in the consideration of biliary tract disorders, one may more concisely present a comprehensive picture of the subject by first following the natural course of gallstones and noting specifically the instances in which calculi are not involved or are relatively unimportant. Briefly stated, we may begin with stone formation in the gallbladder—the usual site of origin of most gallstones. It is true that some gallstones fail to give rise to clinical illness. It is also true that *cholecystitis*, either acute or chronic, may occur without calculus formation, but such instances are relatively few. In the usual patient, stones appear in the ductal system and produce symptoms at varying periods after their formation. A stone lodged in the cystic duct is most often the immediate cause of acute cholecystitis. Recurrent inflammation progressively impairs gallbladder function. Choledocholithiasis also increases appreciably each decade after stones have appeared in the gallbladder.

Long-standing disease of the gallbladder leads to changes in the ductal system and the liver. It is

believed that *calculi* obstruction, and *infection* in the gallbladder produce an inflammatory process that extends throughout the ductal system to involve the liver cells, probably by way of the lymphatics. This has been labeled *cholangitis* (see Choledocholithiasis), and may vary in degree from minimal involvement, evidenced only by edema microscopically, to gross suppuration. Some scarring results from each episode of inflammation and, therefore, over the years there is a cumulative injury to the liver that may eventually result in full-blown biliary cirrhosis. The exact roles and significance of the presence of *calculi, infection,* and *stasis* or *obstruction* are difficult to establish because cholangitis may also rarely be the result of blood-borne infection from the portal or systemic circulation.

Finally, malignant disease—*carcinoma* of the biliary tract—may follow in the wake of gallstone formation. The incidence of stones associated with carcinoma ranges from 50 to 90 per cent in reported series of patients with carcinoma of the gallbladder.

Natural History of Cholelithiasis. A great debate rages concerning the morbidity and mortality of untreated cholelithiasis. Accurate statistics are not at hand. Those who see the complications of the disease believe it to be high; those who ponder the high incidence of "silent stones" in the older age groups (discovered by cholecystography or at autopsy) feel that it is low. Studies which report the fate of persons with asymptomatic cholelithiasis indicate that, within 10 years of diagnosis, complications will be noticed in about 30 per cent.

ACUTE CHOLECYSTITIS

Etiology. *Acute cholecystitis* is most often the initial manifestation of cholelithiasis with or without prior impairment of gallbladder function. Occasionally (5 to 10 per cent of cases) it may develop in the absence of stones. In contrast to *chronic cholecystitis*, the acute phase presents the dramatic clinical manifestations of an acute inflammatory process, usually due to cystic duct obstruction by stone. Although the acute attack usually subsides, it can progress, and may result in *perforation* with *abscess* formation and local or generalized *peritonitis*. In addition to involvement of the gallbladder, there is almost always extension of the infection to the biliary ductal system, *cholangitis*, of varying degree. Repeated attacks, particularly when associated with jaundice, may injure the liver.

Bacterial infection, derived from the liver, the blood stream, and the lymphatic channels may rarely cause acute cholecystitis in some patients without calculi. In some cases it is possible that regurgitation of pancreatic juice is responsible, or the reaction produced by bile-salt concentration within the gallbladder. *Arteritis* and *arteriolitis* associated with terminal hypertensive cardiovascular disease or with *periarteritis nodosum* and causing mucosal ischemia may precipitate acute cholelithiasis. Any severe _systemic infection_ may be accompanied by acute cholecystitis. In years past, a history of _typhoid fever_ was frequently obtained in acute cholecystitis. In an elderly patient, an attack of acute cholecystitis may be precipitated by gallbladder _carcinoma_ obstructing the cystic duct.

Pathology. The gallbladder in the early hours of an attack is hyperemic and edematous, and its wall rapidly thickens. The cystic duct may be occluded so that no bile enters it and none is emptied through it into the common duct. Thus, the gallbladder may be distended with bile, inflammatory exudate, or pus. The microscopic changes in the mucosa and underlying fibromuscular layers range from mild acute inflammation with edema and cellular infiltration to necrosis and perforation of the gallbladder wall. In the beginning, the bile in the gallbladder is normal in appearance and consistency. It may become diluted with thin mucoid material or even blood. Early in an initial acute attack the contents of the gallbladder may be sterile, but with repeated attacks bacteria are usually present in the gallbladder lumen, in the acutely inflamed wall, and in the regional lymph nodes.

Following the subsidence of an initial attack, the mucosal surface heals, and the wall becomes scarred. Depending on the amount of tissue destroyed by the infection, the function of the gallbladder may be impaired. The impairment may be so slight that it is of no particular importance, or it may be so severe that the gallbladder is no longer capable of receiving or concentrating bile. If obstruction of the cystic duct remains when the acute inflammation subsides, the gallbladder may become distended with clear mucoid fluid—_hydrops of the gallbladder._ The initial attack of acute cholecystitis may be but the beginning of a long series of events in biliary tract disease. Recurrent attacks of acute inflammation in the presence of stone and infection lead to progressive scarring of the gallbladder with loss of function, and the residual debris from the infection at its height may provide a nidus for further gallstone formation.

So-called "cholesterolosis" of the gallbladder—deposits of cholesterol crystals in the mucosa—characterizes a high percentage of organs that contain stones.

Clinical Manifestations and Diagnosis. The manifestations of acute cholecystitis are in proportion to its severity and, in the absence of stones, the onset is less sudden than in acute cholecystitis resulting from obstructive calculi. With mild inflammation the patient may have only some "indigestion," moderate pain and _tenderness_ in the _right upper quadrant,_ accentuated by deep inspiration and occasionally, _fever._ With more severe inflammation, pain and _tenderness_ increase, and _muscle spasm_ is elicited. _Rebound tenderness_ in the right upper abdomen is noted in the more serious cases of _suppurative cholecystitis_ with peritoneal inflammation. The spread of pain,

tenderness, and rebound tenderness over the abdomen generally indicates either that _perforation_ has occurred or that there is an associated _pancreatitis_ (see Pancreatitis). The gallbladder is at times palpable in acute cholecystitis. As a rule, it is rather vague and difficult to outline, principally because of tenderness and muscle spasm. At times, however, the gallbladder is felt more distinctly as a tender sausage-like mass extending down below the right rib margin, slightly lateral to the midclavicular line. It is more often palpated in patients suffering their first attack of cholecystitis in whom there had not been prior thickening of the gallbladder wall. Occasionally, the symptoms are limited to the midepigastrium and take the form of a sudden severe sensation of localized distention.

Prostration often results from acute suppurative cholecystitis. The _temperature_ is commonly _elevated_ to 102° to 105° F. _Nausea_ and _vomiting_ are frequently observed. _Abdominal distention_ with decreased or absent bowel sounds is common. _Jaundice_ may be present, and usually indicates a calculous obstruction of the hepatic or common bile duct. Jaundice without calculous obstruction may result either from inflammatory edema of the extrahepatic bile ducts or from the direct extension of inflammation into the liver. The urine commonly contains increased amounts of urobilinogen, which usually disappear within 24 to 48 hours after the infection subsides. As a rule the attack of cholecystitis is relatively short, from a few hours to a few days. In some instances, however, _empyema_ of the gallbladder may produce persistent pain and _tenderness_ for weeks. A somewhat vague _tender mass_ representing the subacutely inflamed gallbladder may be felt for an equal period of time, eventually becoming smaller and less tender, until finally it is no longer palpable. During the state of acute inflammation, the leukocyte count is elevated (12,000 to 40,000; usually about 15,000 per cubic millimeter), with a _neutrophilic leukocytosis_ and an increase in band forms.

Fever of unknown origin may occasionally be due to subacute or chronic cholecystitis in patients with neither the symptoms and physical findings of acute cholecystitis nor those of common duct obstruction with cholangitis. In these patients, often elderly or otherwise debilitated, the gallbladder is chronically inflamed and possibly hydropic. In some instances it is thickened and shrunken with evidence of prior perforation. Rarely, abscess—subhepatic or subdiaphragmatic—which was the consequence of a prior attack of cholecystitis may be responsible for the fever.

Diagnosis is substantiated by failure of the gallbladder to visualize after either oral or intravenous cholecystography because of obstruction of the cystic duct or inability of the organ to concentrate the dye. In many cases, calculi may be seen on plain abdominal film (Fig. 1) or may be outlined by a faint concentration of dye (Figs. 3 and 4). The examinations are made during the acute attack or as it subsides. If the patient is jaundiced, the gallbladder almost certainly will not visualize.

Differential Diagnosis. If the common duct is partially obstructed, the *serum transaminases, SGOT* and *SGPT*, may be moderately elevated (200 to 500 units); however, the levels are not usually as high as in *acute viral hepatitis.* (See Diseases of the Liver.) Rarely, the values transiently (for 24 to 48 hours) exceed 1000 units. The location and character of the pain and the history of previous attacks of gallstone colic or jaundice are helpful in distinguishing cholecystitis from *peptic ulcer.* After perforation, the symptoms and findings may be identical. The presence of free gas in the peritoneal cavity, as determined by roentgenogram, however, is more likely to indicate perforation of the gastrointestinal tract than of the gallbladder. *Acute appendicitis,* particularly in persons with a high-lying cecum may offer difficulty. The history of onset of diffuse abdominal pain with subsequent localization in the right lower quadrant, rarely higher, usually serves to distinguish appendicitis. Right-sided *pyelonephritis* at times simulates cholecystitis with respect to pain. The maximal tenderness, however, is usually in the loin, and this fact, plus the urinary symptoms and findings, makes differentiation possible. A diagnosis of *acute pancreatitis* may be confirmed by measurement of amylase levels of serum or peritoneal fluid. It must be remembered however, that common bile duct obstruction often is associated with inflammation of the pancreas (see Diseases of the Pancreas). Even a normal gallbladder may not opacify on oral or intravenous cholecystography during an attack of acute pancreatitis and for several weeks after its subsidence. It will also not visualize if the patient has gastric obstruction or ileus. In all patients with right upper abdominal pain, a chest roentgenogram and an electrocardiogram should be taken to exclude a *right lower lobe pneumonia* or acute *myocardial infarction.* It is well to keep in mind with regard to *myocardial infarction* that distention of the common bile duct may cause T-wave changes in the electrocardiograms. Indeed, biliary tract infection and obstruction may precipitate myocardial infarction. In both biliary tract inflammation and myocardial infarction, the SGOT may be elevated. SGPT, however, is not elevated in myocardial disease if the patient is not in congestive failure. Occasionally, cholecystitis causes cardiac arrhythmias. The most important distinguishing features are the clinical course over a 48- to 72-hour period, including the pattern of serial electrocardiograms.

Rarely, patients with *acute hepatitis,* viral or toxic, may have severe right upper quadrant and epigastric pain as the major symptom, associated with exquisite tenderness and even rigidity, with rebound on palpation. However, the white blood count is not elevated in viral hepatitis, and abnormal lymphocytes may be noted on blood smear. Serum SGOT and SGPT in this situation are markedly elevated, SGOT usually being greater than 1000 units. (See Diseases of the Liver.)

Patients with *acute cardiac decompensation* may complain of severe epigastric pain owing to acute hepatic distention and may also show mild to marked icterus. In patients not previously studied, and especially in those about whose diagnosis doubt exists, appropriate roentgenography of the biliary tract must be performed, particularly after the jaundice has subsided.

Diagnosis of suspected acute cholecystitis may be confirmed with certainty by roentgenography of the biliary tree. The findings have been described under Clinical Manifestations and Diagnosis.

Treatment. There is general agreement that the preferred treatment of biliary tract disease is surgical. There is, however, considerable controversy as to when surgery should be undertaken in patients with acute cholecystitis. Some prefer to encourage the subsidence of the attack by placing the patient at bed rest, allowing nothing by mouth, and maintaining gastric decompression with an indwelling tube while supporting the patient with parenteral fluids, antimicrobial therapy, sedatives, and analgesics to relieve pain and discomfort. Following recovery and at some time thereafter, cholecystectomy is recommended. In sharp contrast, others recommend early surgical treatment of acute cholecystitis unless there is some contraindication. *Cholecystectomy* is the recommended procedure, particularly when there is no medical contraindication.

Cholecystostomy, a lesser procedure, may be indicated following perforation of the gallbladder, in the presence of severe jaundice caused by common obstruction, or when the general condition of the patient is so grave that a prolonged operative procedure is contraindicated. Cholecystostomy under such circumstances is a compromise procedure, but it may be life-saving by tiding the patient over a critical period. Definitive surgery, that is, cholecystectomy, should be done a few months later. Drainage of the common bile duct (choledochotomy), in addition to cholecystectomy or cholecystostomy, is indicated in acute cholecystitis when stones are present in the common duct. The diagnosis of *common duct stone* may be difficult in the patients with acute cholecystitis, but must be suspected in the patients who are jaundiced or who have had previous attacks of jaundice.

If conservative treatment is initially elected, it is usually desirable to wait several weeks after subsidence of acute symptoms before surgery is undertaken.

An acute attack may be controlled by withholding food or fluids by mouth, decompression of the stomach with an indwelling nasogastric tube, and providing fluids parenterally. Conservative measures during the acute stage also include relief of pain by injection of meperidine, 0.05 to 0.1 gram, subcutaneously every four to six hours as necessary. As a general rule, it is inadvisable to use morphine and its congeners because of possible spastic effect upon the sphincter of Oddi. Nitroglycerin, 0.65 mg. dissolved under the tongue, will often aid in controlling pain, and may be of value in relaxing the smooth muscle of the cystic duct. Nasogastric suction may be necessary for abdominal distention and vomiting. Infusions of 5 or 10 per cent glucose in saline, containing potassium, must then be administered intravenously. With subsidence of symptoms, clear liquids such as skimmed milk, thin broths, and light fruit juices may be taken, followed by small amounts of cooked cereals, tapioca, cooked fruits, and vegetables. If the attack does not subside in 24 to 48 hours, especially if high fever appears or persists after hydration, broad-spectrum antimicrobials, such as ampicillin or chloramphenicol, 1.0 to 2.0 grams, should be given parenterally in divided doses daily. Oxytetracycline should not be given intravenously in this dosage because of possible injury to the liver. Failure to respond to this program in the following 24 to 48 hours and/or the persistence or appearance of signs of severe infection or perforation indicate that the attack has become complicated and that surgical treatment will be necessary.

The "Silent Stone" Problem. The question arises as to what to advise a patient with asymptomatic cholelithiasis or with a nonfunctioning gallbladder, for in 97 per cent of such cases stones are present. It is a difficult question, and one for which no all-encompassing answer may be given. Since, as noted, about 30 per cent of patients with asymptomatic cholelithiasis will develop complications such as acute cholecystitis requiring surgery, obstruction, jaundice, or pancreatitis, it appears wise to recommend cholecystectomy for all such patients under 50. For those between 50 and 60 the problem is especially knotty, because the morbidity and mortality of elective surgery are higher, and the question is further complicated by the increasing possibility that these patients will eventually die of other causes. It appears wise, on balance, to recommend cholecystectomy for those in good health who have multiple small stones. In anyone who shows evidence of disease in the cardiac, arterial, renal, or pulmonary systems, or who may have some liver disease, operation should not be carried out. In the over-60 group, operation is not recommended. Clearly, the life expectancy in this group, despite possible complications of their disease, appears greater if elective surgery is not performed.

Complications. There are many complications of acute cholecystitis in which both gallstones and associated infection play a joint role. Among the complications are *pancreatitis* (both acute and chronic) (see Diseases of the Pancreas), *peritonitis* caused by perforation of the gallbladder, internal *biliary fistula, cholangitis* and *liver abscesses, pylephlebitis,* and, rarely, *thrombosis of the hepatic vein* and *endocarditis.*

Internal *biliary fistulas* may open into the duodenum, colon, or, rarely, the stomach. They may also extend into the peritoneal or pleural cavity or externally through the abdominal wall. By far the most frequent formation of a fistula is by *perforation of the gallbladder,* with discharge of

a stone into the lumen of an adherent viscus, usually the duodenum or jejunum. If the stone is too large to pass through the small intestine, it becomes lodged in the area where the lumen is smallest and produces a typical *acute intestinal obstruction.* Because the lumen of the ileum is the narrowest, it is a frequent site for obstruction (Fig. 2). Stones perforating into the stomach may be vomited, and those into the large bowel are passed in the feces.

The more common site for perforation is into the first or second part of the duodenum, leaving a residual fistula behind. If the stone obstructs the small bowel in its terminal portion, a triad of findings is to be observed *distended small bowel; a gallstone in the small intestine,* usually in the terminal ileum; and *air in the biliary tract.* If one keeps this triad in mind when seeing patients with intestinal obstruction, particularly in the older age group, the diagnosis may be readily made. Since it is rare for a stone that is large enough to produce intestinal obstruction to pass from the common duct through the ampulla of Vater, it should be assumed that a cholecystointestinal fistula exists.

Prognosis. Acute cholecystitis constitutes a problem of varying importance and urgency, depending on whether it occurs as an early phase of biliary tract disease, in a young woman who has recently had a baby, for example, as an episode in the later stages of chronic biliary tract disease, as with men and women in the older age group; or as a complication of a terminal systemic disease or following some operative procedure unrelated to the biliary tract. Acute cholecystitis in the young, recently pregnant woman, as well as in patients under 50, is not a serious disease; however, the prospect of future attack with

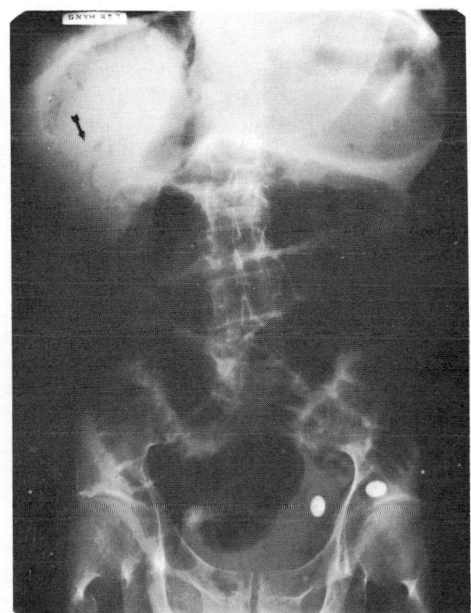

FIGURE 2. Cholecystoduodenal fistula. Plain roentgenogram reveals small bowel obstruction; laminated gallstone in right lower quadrant and air in intrahepatic ductal system.

serious complication is sufficiently great to warrant cholecystectomy either during or after an attack. The prognosis for *perforation* with *peritonitis* or for *empyema* of the gallbladder is good in this age group, providing that surgical drainage is rapidly achieved and broad-spectrum antimicrobials and fluids with electrolytes are given. The prognosis is correspondingly guarded in those over 50 and in patients with associated serious illnesses. Most of these patients have a long history of biliary tract disease. The older the patient and the longer the duration of biliary tract disease, the more common are the complications of acute cholecystitis.

By and large, the older the patient, the more difficult it is to estimate the exact nature of the process by physical examination, temperature elevation, or leukocyte count and thereby determine whether the wall of the gallbladder is gangrenous or whether perforation is impending. Furthermore, the incidence of common duct stone is greater in the older group. These patients are also more prone to develop postoperative complications, which contribute to a higher mortality rate.

CHOLELITHIASIS AND CHRONIC CHOLECYSTITIS

Definition. *Cholelithiasis* may express itself clinically in a variety of pictures, depending to some degree upon the behavior of the stones. As noted, *obstruction of the cystic duct* may lead to a dramatic attack of acute gallbladder inflammation, and repeated episodes of mild degree may be noted; in turn, *obstruction of the common duct* or of the ileum by stone leads to distinct clinical pictures. Finally cholelithiasis is associated in some with *carcinoma of the gallbladder*. We shall next consider the most common disability that may result from cholelithiasis, *chronic cholecystitis*. This is characterized by evidence of a chronic inflammatory process on gross or microscopic examination. Stones are present in a high percentage of the patients, and gallbladder function, as demonstrated by cholecystography, is usually impaired, but not always.

Pathology. The term "chronic cholecystitis" includes a wide extent of pathologic change, ranging from a stage of chronic inflammation attended with minimal changes to one in which the gallbladder wall has been reduced to dense scar tissue contracted over calculi; the gallbladder is without function, and *choledocholithiasis* and *liver damage* may be associated. The gallbladder with minimal microscopic involvement usually produces few other manifestations of disease, but occasionally such a gallbladder gives rise to severe disability. Between the two extremes there are a number of varieties and combinations of pathologic changes.

Clinical Manifestations. Unequivocal *chronic cholecystitis* is associated with discrete attacks of epigastric or right upper quadrant pain, either steady or colicky, with tenderness to palpation and lasting for hours. *Fever, dark urine,* and/or *icterus* may accompany the episode, indicating common duct obstruction caused by edema and/or a calculus. Gradually, gallbladder function is lost.

Although the attacks may not be so clear-cut, *recurrent pain,* often with *nausea* and *vomiting,* and right upper quadrant *tenderness* with episodes related to large meals strongly suggest the diagnosis.

Attribution of symptoms of "indigestion," such as postprandial "fullness," or belching, and intolerance for fat and other foods to a chronic inflammatory state of the gallbladder is much more difficult. Usually, the "attacks" in such patients are without fever, icterus, or right upper quadrant tenderness. The gallbladder often (but not always) is opacified on cholecystography, if only faintly; calculi, however, may be demonstrable. If they are present, the patient must be considered to have chronic cholecystitis, especially if the gallbladder does not fill with dye.

Obviously, a spectrum of chronic recurrent symptoms is associated with *cholelithiasis*. These symptoms do not always correlate well with either the degree of pathologic change in the wall of the gallbladder or with the number and type of gallstones. Although cholelithiasis may be found in some persons with postprandial symptoms, one cannot assume that it necessarily underlies such complaints. Perhaps those so afflicted are suffering from disturbed upper gastrointestinal motility with delayed gastric emptying — perhaps with some element of esophagitis. (See Diseases of Motility.)

The only *physical sign* that may indicate chronic cholecystitis is right subcostal tenderness in the gallbladder area. The organ is rarely palpable.

Diagnosis. As stated previously, roentgenography of the gallbladder and biliary tract is the principal means of diagnosis of cholecystitis. Calculi may be apparent on a flat film of the abdomen (Fig. 1) or by cholecystography with iodopanoic acid (Fig. 3), or even by intravenous cholangiography *(vide infra;* Fig. 4). Often the diseased gallbladder is not visualized after ingestion or injection of dye, indicating either cystic duct obstruction or advanced disease with impairment of its ability to concentrate (Fig. 5). Occasionally the gallbladder will opacify, obscuring small stones, which, however, become visible in the erect or decubitus position. With careful and proper evaluation, *chronic cholecystitis* and *cholelithiasis* may be accurately diagnosed in more than 95 per cent of the patients. Chronic cholecystitis without cholelithiasis may be more difficult to diagnose.

Differential Diagnosis. In view of the lack of specificity of the symptoms suggesting chronic cholecystitis, the patient's history, the findings on physical examination, and the laboratory data must be carefully evaluated. Roentgenographic examinations, such as a gastrointestinal series, barium enema, and an intravenous pyelogram, are necessary to exclude conditions that may give rise to similar symptoms and that indeed may coexist with gallbladder disease. The demonstration of gallbladder disease by cholecystography does not exclude the possibility of other conditions as the cause of symptoms referred to the epigastrium. The more common of these are *gastritis, irritable colon, peptic ulcer, diaphragmatic hernia, pancreatitis, renal disease,* and *lesions of the colon (diverticulitis* and *carcinoma).* Gallstones and

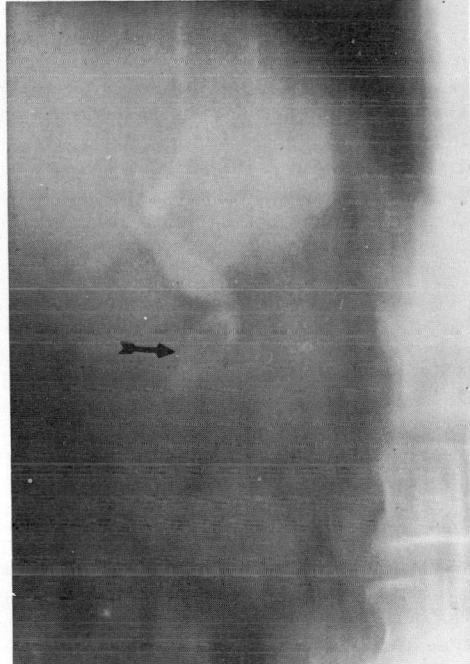

FIGURE 5. Intravenous cholangiogram. Gallbladder not visualized. Common duct is enlarged with calculus proximal to choledochal-duodenal junction.

coronary insufficiency may coexist, and cholecystectomy may reduce symptoms caused by coronary disease.

Treatment. The treatment of chronic cholecystitis with cholelithiasis is surgical; cholecystectomy is the procedure of choice. Long experience has demonstrated that, if stones are removed from a gallbladder and the organ remains, stones are likely to form again within a period of months.

When, for one reason or another, surgical treatment is not to be undertaken, there are several measures that may diminish and in part control the symptoms temporarily. These include diet and fluid intake. Foods of high lipid content, fats, eggs, and chocolate should be taken in small amounts, or not at all. Fried foods, pork products, and rich dressings may precipitate attacks or symptoms. Symptoms in a patient with biliary calculi may follow a large meal of almost any type of food. Thus, a regimen of small feedings of simple foods offers protection.

Patients who complain only of "dyspeptic" symptoms often have normal cholecystograms. These persons often have "fullness," nausea, anorexia, diffuse epigastric heaviness, etc., based on motility disturbances of the upper gastrointestinal tract (often, too, they have irritable colon). (See Disorders of Motility.) Those in whom a cholecystogram has revealed nothing more than reduced gallbladder function, i.e., faint opacification and impaired emptying, are difficult clinical problems. At operation some may be demonstrated to have calculi with gross and microscopic changes within the gallbladder wall. Some of these are relieved of their symptoms after cholecystectomy. Others, suffering essentially from motor disturbances,

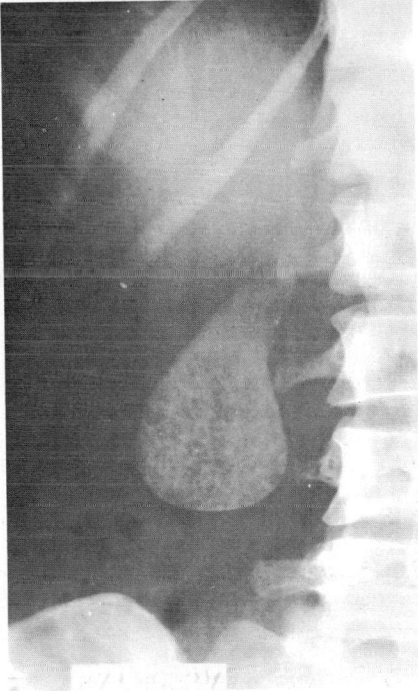

FIGURE 3. Oral cholecystogram showing enlarged gallbladder containing many calculi and a poorly functioning gallbladder.

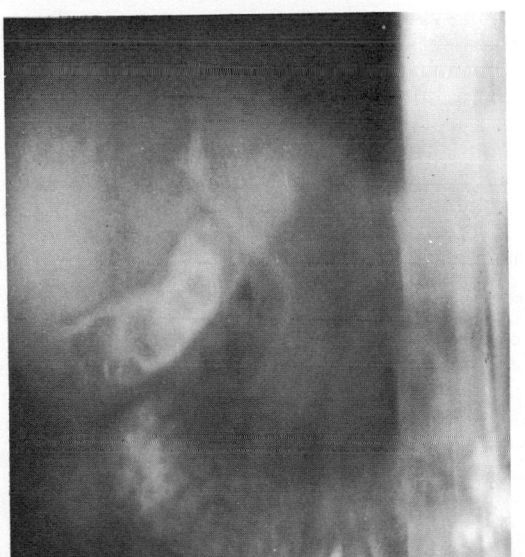

FIGURE 4. Intravenous cholecystogram and cholangiogram. Gallbladder contains large calculi; common duct is well visualized without calculi.

appear at operation to have a normal extrahepatic biliary system. For these, the results following cholecystectomy are usually unsatisfactory. Unless biliary tract disease can be unequivocally established, these patients are best treated by medical management. (See Disorders of Motility.)

Cholesterolosis and Pseudopolyps. Occasionally, upper abdominal distress may be associated with deposits of lipid, mainly cholesterol, in the epithelial cells and in the macrophages in the mucosa of a gallbladder that does not contain calculi. Although the distress is more likely to be low-grade and chronic, akin to some examples of chronic cholecystitis associated with calculi, occasionally episodes of acute cholecystitis may be experienced. In most instances, however, the condition is asymptomatic. Nevertheless, numerous deposits of lipid may be found scattered on the mucosa. The cholecystogram in this instance may reveal numerous very tiny radiolucent areas. The gallbladder functions well, however, and fills with dye and empties normally. Indeed, it has often been noted that the dye is "hyperconcentrated."

Occasionally, the mucosa surrounding the lipid deposits may become inflamed and, in this instance, the mucosa of the gallbladder looks like a "ripe strawberry." Rarely, the collections of lipids in the macrophages of the mucosal folds may appear as lucent defects in the cholecystogram. "Pseudopolyps" may result from enlargement of the Rokitansky-Aschoff sinuses associated with mucosal injury. These structures invaginate the submucosa. This type of pseudopolyposis, referred to as adenomyomatosis, is not associated with cholesterol deposits on the mucosa (Fig. 6). When the gallbladder contracts, dye may empty into these sinuses, giving a speckled appearance. Regardless of the origin of the pseudopolyps, they have no relationship to malignant disease of the gallbladder.

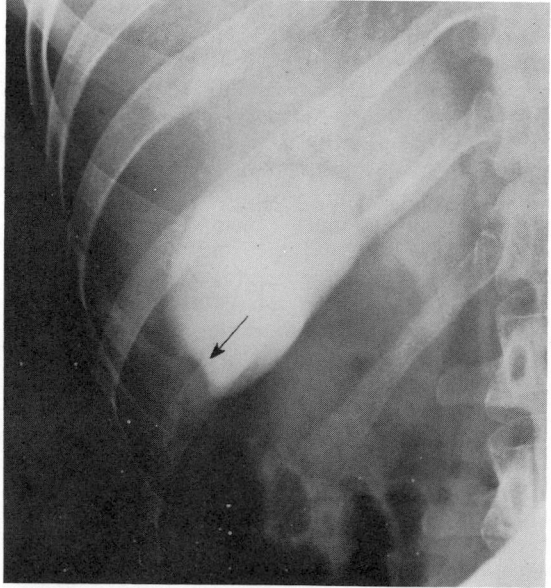

FIGURE 6. Cholecystogram. "Pseudopolyp" or adenomyoma of the gallbladder. Not related to adenoma or carcinoma.

CHOLEDOCHOLITHIASIS

Incidence and Pathogenesis. Stones in the common duct should be looked upon as a sequel or complication of calculi in the gallbladder. Although their actual incidence cannot be predicted with certainty, it is well established that it increases with both the duration of gallstones and the age of the patient. Calculi may form anywhere within the intrahepatic biliary ductal system and pass into the common duct. Once present in the common duct, they may pass into the duodenum through the ampulla of Vater or remain and increase in size and number.

Pathology. The pathologic effects of common duct stone result from both ductal obstruction and infection. The wall of the bile ducts proximal to the site of obstruction becomes thickened and the ducts dilated. With complete ductal obstruction the flow of bile ceases, and reabsorption of the pigment contained within the bile ducts may result in a pale bile (white bile) within the dilated ductal system. Bile pigment, bile salts, cholesterol, and enzymes normally excreted in the bile increase in concentration in the serum. Ductal obstruction of short duration without infection may cause no significant damage to hepatic parenchymal cells, normal bile flow being rapidly established following relief of obstruction. With obstruction of longer duration, particularly in the presence of infection within the biliary system, acute and chronic inflammation around the portal areas in the liver with necrosis of liver cells and progressive fibrosis ultimately leads to *secondary biliary cirrhosis*. (See Diseases of the Liver.)

Clinical Manifestations. The symptoms of choledocholithiasis include biliary colic, jaundice, and fever with chills. *Biliary colic* resulting from dilatation and muscular contraction of the bile duct over an impacted stone, is visceral in character with mid-dorsal segmental distribution. Attacks of pain are usually abrupt in onset, often commencing several hours after a heavy meal. The pain is colicky with a periodicity of up to 30 minutes and a total duration that rarely exceeds a few hours. The pain varies in intensity and may be accompanied by nausea, vomiting, and sweating. The patient is usually extremely restless, and may writhe, roll, double up, press his fists into his abdomen, shout, or cry because of acute distress.

Jaundice and dark urine usually become manifest within 24 hours of the onset of common duct obstruction. The development of jaundice depends, however, on the duration and completeness of ductal obstruction. The urine usually contains bilirubin within a few hours of the attack of pain, and the stools may become pale. With intermittent obstruction, jaundice, dark urine, and pale stools occur only transiently, whereas with *complete, unremitting obstruction*, jaundice, bilirubinemia, and pale stools persist, and urobilinogen disappears from the urine.

Choledocholithiasis may cause persistent jaundice without fever or infection.

Occasionally, stones are present in the common bile duct without jaundice. The patients may have fever, at times chills, intermittent pain, or combinations of these symptoms.

Fever and leukocytosis signify the presence of infection. Enteric organisms associated with stone in the bile ducts may cause no systemic manifestations until ductal obstruction ensues. At that time the release of organisms or endotoxin into the circulation causes a high paroxysmal fever with shaking chills and leukocytosis (Fig. 7). With intermittent obstruction, fever and leukocytosis may also be intermittent, as described by Charcot. When obstruction is unremitting, a continuous fever and leukocytosis will indicate infection and will vary in degree with the severity of infection. (See Acute Suppurative Cholangitis, *infra*.)

An enlarged gallbladder is unusual in patients with calculous common bile duct obstruction. Courvoisier (1890), in autopsy studies, found that the gallbladder was distended in only 20 per cent of patients with calculous obstructive jaundice, whereas it was distended in 90 per cent of the patients with neoplastic obstruction. The fibrosis resulting from previous cholecystitis limits distention of the gallbladder in patients with calculous disease.

Physical examination usually reveals tenderness in the right upper quadrant of the abdomen, with the reflex spasm of the abdominal muscles.

Diagnostic Tests. *Intravenous Cholangiography* (Figs. 4 and 5). The use of sodium iodopamide (Biligrafin or Cholegrafin) administered intravenously may permit the roentgenographic visualization of the common and hepatic bile ducts and the demonstration of calculi in patients with incomplete obstruction without jaundice. Visualization of the terminal common duct can be improved by tomography. Dilatation of the common bile duct may be demonstrated following cholecystectomy, and may erroneously suggest the presence of common duct stone. Thus, dilatation of the common duct to greater than 15 mm. is required for the diagnosis of common duct obstruction. As already noted, the ducts will not opacify if serum bilirubin is greater than 3.0 mg. per 100 ml. or if the liver is diseased, or both. Dilatation of the cystic duct stump also may be seen with this technique.

Percutaneous Transhepatic Cholangiography. During the past few years, the diagnosis of biliary tract obstruction by stone, stricture, or tumor has been facilitated by the ability to outline its passages with radiopaque dye that is injected through a needle previously inserted intercostally into the parenchyma of the liver. The values of the procedure are the accurate localization of the obstruction, if one exists, and, occasionally, the demonstration of a normal biliary tract, which effectively excludes an extrahepatic obstructive process. Usually, the biliary tract will not be visualized unless it is dilated and under increased pressure. Thus, bile may leak into the peritoneal cavity as a result of this procedure and, for this reason as well as because bleeding may result from the procedure, laparotomy is usually performed immediately following it.

Biliary Drainage. The nature of the obstructing lesion may possibly be defined by duodenal drainage. Presence of cholesterol crystals, in the absence of jaundice, indicates cholelithiasis. Bilirubinate crystals may indicate either stasis or stones. This test is now reserved for those who are sensitive to the organic dyes given orally or intravenously to diagnose biliary tract disease.

Serum Enzymes and Tests of Liver Function. Choledocholithiasis is commonly accompanied by an elevation of the *serum alkaline phosphatase*. This enzyme elevation may be transient in the presence of transient obstruction, and its degree is no indication of the nature or site of the obstructing lesion. Parallel elevations of the serum enzymes, *5-nucleotidase* and *leucine-aminopeptidase*, result from ductal obstruction. These enzymes may be significantly elevated even when serum bilirubin is only slightly abnormal. However, levels of these enzymes do not clearly differentiate extrahepatic obstructive jaundice from intrahepatic cholestasis. (See Diseases of the Liver.)

In patients with cholangitis accompanying common duct obstruction, there may be extreme elevation, often transient, of the serum *transaminases* (SGOT and SGPT) in the range of 200 to 500 units and occasionally as high as 1000 units.

Differential Diagnosis. *Biliary colic* is usually recognized without difficulty. *Renal and intestinal colic* rarely cause confusion. The pain of renal colic commences in the loin or flank and radiates downward, especially to the inner surface of the thigh, or to the genitalia; dysuria and hematuria are often present. The pain of intestinal colic is usually a more generalized crampy pain, often somewhat more severe below the level of the umbilicus. If it is due to intestinal obstruction, there is increasing emesis, distention of the abdomen, and the auscultatory finding of high-pitched or musical borborygmi in association with the colicky pain. The colic of *acute porphyria* may closely simulate gallstone colic; the

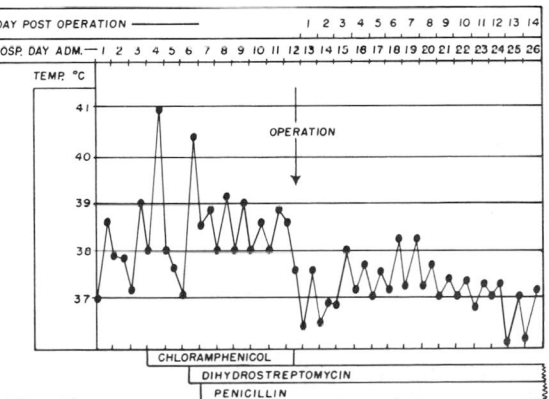

FIGURE 7. Acute suppurative cholangitis in association with common duct obstruction secondary to stone. The septic course of the patient was not interrupted by antimicrobial drugs. Dramatic response to T-tube decompression of common duct and choledocholithotomy on the twelfth day following admission is shown.

presence of dark urine owing to porphyrin (or of urine that becomes dark on exposure to light) is of decisive importance. The Ehrlich aldehyde test for porphobilinogen will help to distinguish between the two conditions. (See Porphyria in section on Miscellaneous Hereditary Disorders.)

The pain of acute *coronary thrombosis* may be confused with that caused by gallstones. In some cases coronary thrombosis causes abdominal distress, which may be limited to the right upper quadrant or epigastrium. The electrocardiogram is of aid in such instances. The presence of a pericardial friction rub is distinctive. Slight jaundice may follow an attack of coronary thrombosis, but this occurrence is less common than with biliary calculus, and it usually does not appear until several days after the attack, when it is often, but not always, associated with pulmonary infarct. Although serum SGOT may be elevated in both myocardial infarction and choledocholithiasis with cholangitis, it is rare for the former to have levels higher than 100 to 150 units except in very severe cases; also SGPT elevation will be noted in the latter, not in the former, condition. Jaundice resulting from calculous obstruction of the common bile duct must be differentiated from extrahepatic bile duct obstruction resulting from other causes (usually carcinoma of the head of the pancreas or carcinoma of the bile duct) and from intrahepatic cholestasis.

The differentiation of intrahepatic cholestasis caused by hepatitis, viral or toxic, or fatty infiltration of the liver from extrahepatic obstructive jaundice constitutes the most difficult diagnostic problem in patients with disease of the liver and bile ducts. (See Diseases of the Liver.) Tests of liver function, including serum enzymes, serum levels of conjugated and unconjugated bilirubin, cholesterol, and BSP excretion, may not be helpful in this differential diagnosis. Liver biopsy may show histologic changes that differentiate intrahepatic from extrahepatic cholestasis. (See Diseases of the Liver.)

Rarely, *acute viral hepatitis* may be associated not only with severe right upper quadrant pain but also with exquisite tenderness, rigidity, and even rebound tenderness. The differential diagnosis may be difficult (*vide infra*). Likewise, *acute congestion of the liver,* associated with cardiac decompensation, may cause intense right upper quadrant pain and even jaundice. In this instance, however, the temperature is normal, and the white count is only slightly elevated, if at all. The patient has other obvious evidence of cardiac decompensation, of which the enlarged tender liver may be only one feature (*vide supra*).

The palpation of a smooth, nontender gallbladder, in association with complete biliary obstruction, would indicate the possibility of carcinoma of the pancreas, common bile duct, or ampulla of Vater. Complete biliary obstruction, evidenced by the finding of less than 5 mg. of fecal urobilinogen per day over a four-day period, with less than 0.3 mg. of urobilinogen in the 24-hour urine, is much more frequently associated with these malignant conditions than with choledocholithiasis. Also, occult blood in the stool is often found with these diseases. Malignant obstruction of the common bile duct, pancreas, and ampulla rarely has the fever characteristic of choledocholithiasis and suppurative cholangitis (*vide infra*).

Treatment. Treatment for the acute attack is the same as for acute cholecystitis (*vide supra*). If cholangitis intervenes, broad-spectrum antimicrobials must be given (*vide infra*). In either case, the earliest possible surgical removal of the stones is strongly recommended. Preoperative correction of possible vitamin K deficiency is most important. If the liver is not diseased, the elevated prothrombin time will rapidly return to normal after intramuscular injection of 5 to 10 mg. of vitamin K. Occasionally, following common duct exploration, a postoperative cholangiogram reveals a residual stone. This stone should be removed, unless there is a contraindication to further surgery.

Complications. *Acute cholangitis* frequently accompanies ductal obstruction by stone. Suppurative cholangitis and focal hepatic abscesses may result from the presence of pathogenic organisms, and may threaten the life of the patient. Chronic obstruction with infection may lead to *secondary biliary cirrhosis.* (See Diseases of the Liver.)

Acute, recurrent, and *chronic pancreatitis* is often related to calculous biliary tract disease. (See Diseases of the Pancreas.)

ACUTE OBSTRUCTIVE SUPPURATIVE CHOLANGITIS

Etiology and Incidence. *Acute suppurative cholangitis* results from the invasion of the biliary tree by a pathogenic organism, usually a gram-negative bacillus of enteric origin, in the presence of ductal obstruction. The obstruction is most often caused by a stone within the common bile duct or biliary radicles, but may be secondary to stricture, and rarely is due to carcinoma of the bile ducts or to a lesion arising in the pancreas or duodenum.

Pathology. The bile ducts, both intrahepatic and extrahepatic, are dilated above the site of obstruction, which is usually in the common bile duct. There is inflammatory thickening of the wall of these ducts. The liver is enlarged, and in fatal cases there may be multiple abscess cavities in the hepatic parenchyma. Microscopic examination of a liver biopsy specimen reveals *pericholangitis* with acute and chronic inflammatory cells (neutrophils, lymphocytes, and plasma cells) within and adjacent to the portal spaces. Occasionally polymorphonuclear leukocytes may be visualized within small bile ducts. Necrosis of parenchymal cells may occur in relation both to the portal areas with formation of microabscesses and to the areas of extravasated bile (bile lakes).

The term "cholangitis lenta" signifies a rare

hematogenous form of suppurative cholangitis in the absence of biliary obstruction. Secondary endocarditis may occur. Seeding of the blood stream probably occurs in most patients, but bacteremia is not always demonstrable by blood culture.

Clinical Manifestations. The manifestations of acute suppurative cholangitis are those of biliary tract obstruction – obstructive jaundice with or without biliary colic – accompanied by infection. When complete obstruction to bile flow occurs within the common duct or within one or more of the major intrahepatic ducts in the presence of pathogenic enteric bacteria, an overwhelming, catastrophic syndrome may develop. It is characterized by the acute onset of *severe right upper quadrant pain* that is unremitting. *Chills, fever,* and *progressive obstructive jaundice* follow (Fig. 7). The liver enlarges and becomes exquisitely tender. The patient becomes extremely toxic. Vasomotor collapse and coma precede death. Fever is usually of the paroxysmal type accompanied by shaking chills. There is a severe leukocytosis ranging up to 30,000 or more with a shift to the left. Blood culture is usually positive. Although the primary lesion may be ductal obstruction, there is early evidence of parenchymal cell dysfunction and necrosis – hepatic tenderness, increased urinary urobilinogen, and a profound elevation of the serum SGOT and SGPT.

Diagnosis. Suppurative cholangitis is to be suspected in any patient presenting with *jaundice, chills, fever,* an *enlarged tender liver,* and *leukocytosis,* especially if that patient has had previous evidence of biliary tract disease. *Suppurative pylephlebitis, amebic abscess,* and *liver abscesses* resulting from pyogenic organisms must be considered in the differential diagnosis.

Treatment. Temporary spontaneous improvement may occur in patients in whom obstruction is partially relieved by movement of calculi within the common duct, but it is infrequent and unpredictable. *Surgery should be considered mandatory as an emergency procedure* unless there is sudden subsidence of symptoms. The primary objective of surgical treatment is to establish and maintain drainage of the obstructed bile duct system. Although it is desirable to remove the cause of obstruction, the critical condition of the patient demands the minimal operative procedure. Definitive surgery can be done later.

General supportive measures both pre- and postoperatively include fluid and electrolyte replacement, vasopressor drugs to maintain the blood pressure, and antimicrobial therapy. Plasma or whole blood should be administered if the patient has a gram-negative septicemia and depressed central venous pressure. Blood cultures are essential to establish the identity and drug susceptibility of the organism. Antimicrobials effective against gram-negative organisms should be administered intravenously; e.g., ampicillin or chloramphenicol, 2.0 to 4.0 grams daily in divided doses. Penicillin, 2 to 4 million units, and streptomycin, 1.0 gram, in divided doses intramuscularly daily may also be given if the organism is sensitive. However, the infection will not be controlled if the ductal system remains obstructed. When the bile flow has been established by surgical drainage of the common bile duct, the full effectiveness of the antimicrobial therapy can then be attained.

Stenosing Cholangitis. Rarely, the common bile duct and even hepatic ducts stenose, leading to intermittent or chronic obstruction. The cause of this entity is unknown, but it appears most frequently in patients with chronic inflammatory bowel disease. (See articles on Regional Enteritis and Ulcerative Colitis.) However, episodes of clinical cholangitis, with fever, leukocytosis, pain, and tenderness, are rare. Fibrosis of the wall of the duct may reduce the diameter of the lumen to 1.0 mm. The gallbladder rarely contains calculi, and is usually normal. Diagnosis is made by the demonstration of a markedly narrow common duct by cholangiography, either preoperatively or at abdominal exploration. Complications include intrahepatic obstruction during acute episodes with damage to parenchymal cells; chronic obstruction may lead to biliary cirrhosis.

The *treatment* consists of choledochostomy with T-tube drainage for a period of weeks or months. As a result of this procedure, the lumen may gradually enlarge, and lasting relief may be obtained after the tube is removed. Rarely cholecystenterostomy may be necessary in some patients. Some reports state that prolonged administration of low doses of prednisone, 15 to 20 mg. per day, are associated with gradual disappearance of jaundice, but no data on its effect on the caliber of the common duct are recorded.

CONGENITAL ANOMALIES OF THE BILE DUCTS

CONGENITAL ATRESIA

At a certain stage in embryonal development, the bile ducts are represented by solid cords of epithelial cells. Failure of canalization, *atresia,* occurs at some site in the biliary tree in approximately one of every 20,000 births. In approximately 16 per cent of cases, atresia involves the distal segment of the common bile duct. Following birth, unremitting jaundice develops with cessation of the maternal clearance of bilirubin from the fetal circulation. The liver becomes large, and the stools remain acholic. The differential diagnosis includes *physiologic jaundice, erythroblastosis fetalis,* and *neonatal hepatitis.*

Early surgical exploration should always be done in the hope that a communication can be established between the hepatic bile ducts or gallbladder and the intestinal lumen in order to prevent irreversible damage to the liver. Approximately one third of patients who are explored may be amenable to corrective anastomotic surgery. Even when effective drainage is accomplished, however, the prognosis may be limited by irreversible liver damage or by secondary stricture formation at the anastomotic site, with ascending infection of the biliary tree.

CONGENITAL CYSTIC DILATATION OF THE COMMON BILE DUCT

Congenital cystic dilatation of the common bile duct is rare, occurring once in every 500,000 births (over 200 cases have been reported). The cause is not known. The symptoms are those of common bile duct obstruction and cholangitis usually becoming evident in childhood, and a cystic mass of variable size may be palpable in the epigastrium. Surgical treatment consists of creating an anastomosis between the cyst and small intestine. Cholangitis, stone formation, recurrent obstruction, and carcinoma are reported complications.

CARCINOMA OF THE GALLBLADDER

Etiology and Incidence. Carcinoma of the gallbladder, the most common neoplasm of the biliary system, occurs more often in women than in men (3:1), with a peak incidence during the sixth and seventh decades. The association of carcinoma with gallstones (up to 90 per cent) suggests that chronic irritation caused by stone and associated infection may be an important factor in the initiation of carcinoma. Furthermore, the structural similarity between bile acids and the experimental carcinogen, methyl cholanthrene, suggests that bile acid derivatives may have a carcinogenic effect in man.

Pathology. Both adenocarcinomas and squamous cell carcinomas occur in the gallbladder. Infiltrating adenocarcinoma, the most common lesion, is rapidly invasive. Papillary adenocarcinomas may produce slowly growing tumor masses with late dissemination. Scirrhous and mucous adenocarcinomas and squamous cell carcinomas, which occur infrequently, are invasive tumors. Tumor spread may occur either by local invasion of adjacent tissue or by lymphatic drainage into the porta hepatis.

The site of origin of the tumor in the gallbladder may determine the spread of the tumor and the clinical manifestations that result. Fundal tumors frequently extend through the wall of the gallbladder and invade the adjacent liver and peritoneum. A firm mass may be palpable in the region of the gallbladder. Infiltration of the cystic, hepatic, or common bile ducts may occur with carcinomas originating in the body or neck of the gallbladder. Cystic duct obstruction may result in distention of the gallbladder with mucus or blood, and may precipitate an attack of acute cholecystitis. Involvement of the hepatic or common bile duct with obstructive jaundice is a late manifestation of tumor spread.

Relationship to Polyps. Although carcinoma of the gallbladder may arise in an adenomatous polyp (true polyp) of the mucosa, this relationship remains unsubstantiated, principally because of the extreme rarity of such lesions of the mucosa. The appearance of a polypoid defect (Fig. 6) on the cholecystogram is much more likely to represent either adenomyomatosis (pseudopolyp), often associated with dilated mucosal sinuses elsewhere in the gallbladder, or, very rarely, a large cholesterol deposit. Cholecystectomy is not indicated in such patients unless symptoms strongly indicate an associated cholecystitis, which is difficult to establish since calculi are usually absent and the gallbladder fills and empties normally.

Clinical Manifestations. The early symptoms and signs of carcinoma of the gallbladder are indistinguishable from those of nonmalignant disease of the gallbladder, and may be due to the associated cholelithiasis, to neoplastic obstruction of the cystic duct with secondary cholecystitis, or to local tumor invasion. Resectable lesions, confined to the gallbladder, may be discovered unexpectedly during operations for cholelithiasis or acute cholecystitis. The late symptoms and signs — weakness, anorexia, weight loss, abdominal pain, jaundice, a palpable mass, and liver enlargement — usually occur when there has been local or distant spread of the neoplasm.

Treatment. The treatment is surgical. In those instances in which the tumor has not become disseminated, radical cholecystectomy, including resection of the adjacent liver or lobectomy, is indicated, in view of the frequency of local spread into the liver. The prognosis of patients with gallbladder carcinoma has been discouraging. At the time of operation, about 60 per cent of patients have distant metastases, and of those with resectable lesions, less than half survive for more than a year.

CARCINOMA OF THE EXTRAHEPATIC BILE DUCTS

Carcinoma of the extrahepatic bile ducts may arise from the mucosa of the hepatic duct, the cystic duct, the common bile duct, or the ampulla of Vater. Often the primary site of the tumor is obscured by extension of the tumor. Primary tumors of the pancreas or duodenum may also be confused with those arising from the ampulla of Vater. Extrahepatic bile duct carcinoma is less common than gallbladder carcinoma; it occurs with equal frequency in both sexes, and the incidence of associated gallstones is lower than that with gallbladder carcinoma (incidence in reported series varies between 21 and 55 per cent).

Infiltrating and papillary adenocarcinomas are the most common neoplasms in this group. The infiltrating tumors predominate in the common bile duct, whereas papillary adenocarcinomas are more frequent in the region of the ampulla of Vater. Tumor spread may occur along the wall of the bile ducts by direct invasion of surrounding structures or by lymphatics. *Obstructive jaundice*, almost always painless, is the most common presenting manifestation, the occlusion of the bile duct usually being progressive and complete. Carcinomas of the ampulla, however, may produce incomplete or intermittent obstruction to bile flow. Papillary lesions at the ampulla may ulcerate, with intermittent relief of ductal obstruction or with erosion of blood vessels; thus, *melena, guaiac-positive stools,* and *anemia* are not infrequent manifestations. Rarely, neoplastic obstruction of the bile ducts is complicated by infection, with symptoms and signs of ascending cholangitis.

Diagnosis. A diagnosis of bile duct or ampullary carcinoma may be indicated preoperatively by clinical findings and the results of roentgenographic and pancreatic secretory studies. Complete bile duct obstruction in a patient with a palpable, distended, smooth, nontender gallbladder is evidence of a neoplastic process in the bile duct, at the ampulla of Vater, or in the head of the pancreas. Subnormal pancreatic secretion of fluid and bicarbonate following secretin stimulation is evidence of a lesion obstructing both pancreatic and common bile ducts, whereas normal pancreatic secretion localizes an obstructing lesion in the bile duct alone. (See Diseases of the Pancreas.) An *upper gastrointestinal series* — particularly with appropriate air insufflation after administration of an anticholinergic drug (hypotonic duodenography) — may show duodenal deformity indicative of a neoplasm of the head of the pancreas or a tumor mass in the region of the ampulla of Vater. Anemia with evidence of gastrointestinal bleeding may be noted in this malignant condition, but it favors an ampullary lesion. Carcinoma of the pancreas, by infiltrating the antrum of the stomach or the duodenum, also causes bleeding into the gastrointestinal tract.

Preoperative percutaneous *transhepatic cholangiography* with direct injection of contrast material into dilated intrahepatic bile ducts is a new and valuable procedure in determining the site of neoplastic obstruction before surgical exploration.

Treatment and Prognosis. Most tumors are not resectable at the time of surgical exploration; early dissemination occurs in the porta hepatis, with involvement of contiguous vascular structures. Palliative surgery has been directed toward relief of the bile duct obstruction and the relief of pain. With carcinoma of the ampulla of Vater, pancreatoduodenectomy or a more extensive radical resection is indicated in all patients in whom excision of the gross tumors seems initially possible. Although the immediate postoperative mortality and morbidity are high, this procedure offers hope of complete excision of the neoplasm. *Carcinoma of the ampulla* has a far better prognosis than that of either the gallbladder or bile ducts. Patients with carcinoma of the ampulla without spread who are treated by radical pancreatoduodenectomy have had a much longer survival period than have those with carcinoma of the gallbladder or bile ducts, many surviving more than five years without evidence of recurrence. Palliative procedures (cholecystojejunostomy) may relieve bile duct obstruction but do not prolong the life of the patient.

Bouchier, I. A. D., and Freston, J. W.: The aeteology of gallstones. Lancet, 1:340, 1968.

Comess, L. J., Bennett, P. H., and Burch, T. A.: Clinical gallbladder disease in Pima Indians. New Eng. J. Med., 277:894, 1967.

Rains, A. J. G.: Gallstone disease. Brit. Med. J., 1:295, 1968.

Small, D. M.: Current concepts of gallstones. New Eng. J. Med., 279:588, 1968.

Small, D. M., and Rapo, S.: Source of abnormal bile in patients with cholesterol gallstones. New Eng. J. Med., 283:53, 1970.

Wenckert, A., and Robertson, B.: The natural course of gallstone disease. Gastroenterology, 50:376, 1966.

DISEASES OF NUTRITION

NUTRIENT REQUIREMENTS
Nevin S. Scrimshaw

GENERAL CONSIDERATIONS

The nutrient intakes recommended by most national and international organizations are defined as the amounts sufficient for the physiologic needs of virtually all healthy persons in a population. Conceptually, they are intended to cover the mean plus two standard deviations, although the data for actually calculating a standard deviation are rarely available. It is important for the physician to recognize that existing recommended dietary allowances for nutrients do not cover the additional needs that arise from microbial disease, trauma, advanced malignancies, disorders of the gastrointestinal tract, or metabolic diseases and abnormalities. Moreover, the intake recommended for any one nutrient presupposes that the requirements for energy and for all other nutrients are fully met.

Persons receiving less than the recommended allowance are not necessarily malnourished; it depends on their individual requirements, on the margin of safety inherent in the recommendation, and on whether other deficiencies are more limiting. On the other hand, persons consuming the recommended allowance are not necessarily adequately nourished. The presence of disease may interfere with absorption, increase utilization, or accelerate loss of an essential nutrient. This should be taken into account in prescribing diets for persons with acute or chronic disease. Moreover, imbalance among nutrients can render inadequate an intake which would otherwise be ample.

The 1968 Recommended Dietary Allowances of the Food and Nutrition Board (FNB) of the National Academy of Sciences are given in Table 1. They differ from those of the United Kingdom and FAO/WHO in their higher recommendations for calcium and ascorbic acid and slightly lower recommendations for calories. They include for the first time quantitative recommendations for vitamin E activity, folacin, pyridoxine, iodine, and magnesium. They are similar to the FAO/WHO recommendations for protein, thiamin, riboflavin, and niacin, although somewhat lower for calories and higher for vitamin A and calcium.

The following nutrients have been established as necessary dietary constituents for man under physiologic or pathologic conditions, or both.

NECESSARY NUTRIENTS

Calories. The body requires a source of energy to maintain the normal processes of life and to meet the demands of activity and growth. Calorie requirements depend mainly on body size, basal metabolic rate, activity, age, sex, and environmental temperature. Clinical diseases associated with calorie deficiency are marasmus in children and cachexia in adults (see below: Kwashiorkor, Marasmus, and Intermediate Forms of Protein-Calorie Malnutrition; and Undernutrition, Starvation, and Hunger Edema). A 70-kg. male requires approximately 70 calories per hour under basal conditions and up to 600 calories per hour for very heavy muscular work, so that activity levels largely determine gain or loss of weight on a given diet. Carbohydrate and protein furnish about 4 calories per gram, alcohol about 7, and fat about 9. The report of the FAO Expert Committee on Calorie Requirements provides more detailed information.

Protein. Food proteins are split during digestion into their constituent amino acids. These in turn are utilized in the synthesis of new protein for tissue growth and maintenance. Proteins in the diet vary in their usefulness, depending on the extent to which they contain those eight essential amino acids that cannot be synthesized within the body in the proportions needed for making new tissue. When protein is severely deficient relative to calories, kwashiorkor develops (see below: Kwashiorkor, Marasmus, and Intermediate Forms of Protein-Calorie Malnutrition).

Protein requirements have two components: sufficient amounts and proportions of the essential amino acids, and adequate additional nitrogen from any utilizable source. The latter comes from both the dietarily dispensable amino acids and those essential amino acids present in excess of requirements. If the diet does not supply adequate calories, dietary protein will be utilized to meet energy needs at the expense of fulfilling requirements for protein. Protein requirements are greatly increased by microbial disease, trauma, and most other pathologic states.

Protein requirements are expressed in terms of reference protein which, in theory, is 100 per cent absorbed and utilized. Since only egg and human milk approach this ideal, recommended dietary allowances for protein must be expressed in terms of the quality of the protein of the actual diet. In industrialized countries it can be assumed that the protein of the ordinary mixed diet is about 70 per cent utilized, but for cereal-based diets in most developing countries a figure of 60 per cent or less is more appropriate. Proteins of animal origin are

TABLE 1. FOOD AND NUTRITION BOARD, NATIONAL ACADEMY OF SCIENCES—NATIONAL RESEARCH COUNCIL RECOMMENDED DAILY DIETARY ALLOWANCES,*Revised 1968†

Designed for the maintenance of good nutrition of practically all healthy people in the U.S.A.

	Age‡ (years) From Up to	Weight (kg.)	Weight (lbs.)	Height (cm.)	Height (in.)	kcal.	Protein (gm.)	Vitamin A Activity (I.U.)	Vitamin D (I.U.)	Vitamin E Activity (I.U.)	Ascorbic Acid (mg.)	Folacin§ (mg.)	Niacin (mg. equiv.)¶	Riboflavin (mg.)	Thiamin (mg.)	Vitamin B_6 (mg.)	Vitamin B_{12} (µg.)	Calcium (g.)	Phosphorus (g.)	Iodine (µg.)	Iron (mg.)	Magnesium (mg.)
Infants	0–1/6	4	9	55	22	kg × 120	kg × 2.2**	1500	400	5	35	0.05	5	0.4	0.2	0.2	1.0	0.4	0.2	25	6	40
	1/6–1/2	7	15	63	25	kg × 110	kg × 2.0**	1500	400	5	35	0.05	7	0.5	0.4	0.3	1.5	0.5	0.4	40	10	60
	1/2–1	9	20	72	28	kg × 100	kg × 1.8**	1500	400	5	35	0.1	8	0.6	0.5	0.4	2.0	0.6	0.5	45	15	70
Children	1–2	12	26	81	32	1100	25	2000	400	10	40	0.1	8	0.6	0.6	0.5	2.0	0.7	0.7	55	15	100
	2–3	14	31	91	36	1250	25	2000	400	10	40	0.2	8	0.7	0.6	0.6	2.5	0.8	0.8	60	15	150
	3–4	16	35	100	39	1400	30	2500	400	10	40	0.2	9	0.8	0.7	0.7	3	0.8	0.8	70	10	200
	4–6	19	42	110	43	1600	30	2500	400	10	40	0.2	11	0.9	0.8	0.9	4	0.8	0.8	80	10	200
	6–8	23	51	121	48	2000	35	3500	400	15	40	0.2	13	1.1	1.0	1.0	4	0.9	0.9	100	10	250
	8–10	28	62	131	52	2200	40	3500	400	15	40	0.3	15	1.2	1.1	1.2	5	1.0	1.0	110	10	250
Males	10–12	35	77	140	55	2500	45	4500	400	20	40	0.4	17	1.3	1.3	1.4	5	1.2	1.2	125	10	300
	12–14	43	95	151	59	2700	50	5000	400	20	45	0.4	18	1.4	1.4	1.6	5	1.4	1.4	135	18	350
	14–18	59	130	170	67	3000	60	5000	400	25	55	0.4	20	1.5	1.5	1.8	5	1.4	1.4	150	18	400
	18–22	67	147	175	69	2800	60	5000	400	30	60	0.4	18	1.6	1.4	2.0	5	0.8	0.8	140	10	400
	22–35	70	154	175	69	2800	65	5000	–	30	60	0.4	18	1.7	1.4	2.0	5	0.8	0.8	140	10	350
	35–55	70	154	173	68	2600	65	5000	–	30	60	0.4	17	1.7	1.3	2.0	5	0.8	0.8	125	10	350
	55–75+	70	154	171	67	2400	65	5000	–	30	60	0.4	14	1.7	1.2	2.0	6	0.8	0.8	110	10	350
Females	10–12	35	77	142	56	2250	50	4500	400	20	40	0.4	15	1.3	1.1	1.4	5	1.2	1.2	110	18	300
	12–14	44	97	154	61	2300	50	5000	400	20	45	0.4	15	1.4	1.2	1.6	5	1.3	1.3	115	18	350
	14–16	52	114	157	62	2400	55	5000	400	25	50	0.4	16	1.4	1.2	1.8	5	1.3	1.3	120	18	350
	16–18	54	119	160	63	2300	55	5000	400	25	50	0.4	15	1.5	1.2	2.0	5	1.3	1.3	115	18	350
	18–22	58	128	163	64	2000	55	5000	400	25	55	0.4	13	1.5	1.0	2.0	5	0.8	0.8	100	18	350
	22–35	58	128	163	64	2000	55	5000	–	25	55	0.4	13	1.5	1.0	2.0	5	0.8	0.8	90	18	300
	35–55	58	128	160	63	1850	55	5000	–	25	55	0.4	13	1.5	1.0	2.0	5	0.8	0.8	90	18	300
	55–75+	58	128	157	62	1700	55	5000	–	25	55	0.4	13	1.5	1.0	2.0	6	0.8	0.8	80	10	300
Pregnancy						+200	65	6000	400	30	60	0.8	15	1.8	+0.1	2.5	8	+0.4	+0.4	125	18	450
Lactation						+1000	75	8000	400	30	60	0.5	20	2.0	+0.5	2.5	8	+0.5	+0.5	150	18	450

*The allowance levels are intended to cover individual variations among most normal persons as they live in the United States under usual environmental stresses. The recommended allowances can be attained with a variety of common foods, providing other nutrients for which human requirements have been less well defined. See text for more detailed discussion of allowances and of nutrients not tabulated.

†Reprinted from Recommended Dietary Allowances. 7th Ed. Washington, D.C., National Academy of Sciences, Publication 1694, 1968.

‡Entries on lines for age range 22–35 years represent the reference man and woman at age 22. All other entries represent allowances for the midpoint of the specified age range. The recommended allowances refer to dietary sources as determined by *Lactobacillus casei* assay. Pure forms of folacin may be effective in doses less than one quarter of the RDA.

§The folacin allowances refer to dietary sources as determined by *Lactobacillus casei* assay.

¶Niacin equivalents include dietary sources of the vitamin itself plus 1 mg equivalent for each 60 mg. of dietary tryptophan.

**Assumes protein equivalent to human milk. For proteins not 100 per cent utilized factors should be increased proportionately.

generally the best utilized, followed by those from legumes, oilseeds, and rice. Most other cereal proteins are of relatively poor quality.

Carbohydrates and Fats. Carbohydrates supply dietary energy and are necessary constituents of a balanced and palatable diet. There is no fixed requirement for carbohydrates, however, since they can be completely replaced as energy sources in the diet by protein and fats. Fats supply more than twice the energy of carbohydrate and protein per gram, and thus contribute a concentrated source of calories as well as palatability in the diet. The actual requirement for fat, however, is limited to a minute quantity of linoleic, linolenic, or arachidonic acid—all polyunsaturated fatty acids. Deficiency of these in young children leads to defective growth and scaly skin.

Fat-soluble Vitamins

Vitamin A. Vitamin A (retinol) is essential for integrity of mucosal surfaces and is required in the form of its aldehyde for vision, particularly in dim light. Avitaminosis A results in skin and eye lesions and reduced resistance to infection (see below: Hypovitaminosis A), and hypervitaminosis A is equally serious (see below: Hypervitaminosis A).

Vitamin A is found preformed in animal tissue, and the beta-carotene of green and yellow vegetables is converted in the body to vitamin A with an efficiency of about 50 per cent. There are several other forms of carotene which have some activity but are still less efficiently utilized. One international unit (I.U.) is equivalent to 0.3 μg. of retinol, or 6 μg. of beta-carotene.

Vitamin D. Vitamin D is essential at all ages for maintenance of calcium homeostasis and skeletal integrity. The diseases associated with vitamin D deficiency are rickets in children and osteomalacia in adults (see The Osteomalacias in the section on Diseases of Bone). Vitamin D can be acquired by ingestion of vitamin D_2 (ergocalciferol) or D_3 (cholecalciferol) and by exposure to certain ultraviolet wavelengths of light which convert 7-dehydro-cholesterol in the skin to vitamin D_3. Vitamin D deficiency can occur only when the amount supplied by both sources is inadequate.

One I.U. of vitamin D is 0.025 μg. of pure vitamin D_3. Excessive amounts of vitamin D (of the order of 1000 to 3000 I.U. per kilogram per day) are potentially dangerous and may lead to hypercalcemia and attendant complications.

Most foods of animal origin have some vitamin D activity, and 1 quart of vitamin D–fortified milk supplies the daily requirement.

Vitamin E. The earliest evidence of vitamin E deficiency differs with the species, but eventually the hematopoietic, muscular, vascular, and central nervous systems are affected. The normal resistance of red blood cells to rupture by oxidizing agents is also markedly reduced in vitamin E deficiency. One I.U. of vitamin E is 1 mg. of synthetic *dl*-alpha-tocopherol acetate. Recommendations are based on the formula, I.U. = 1.25 × body weight in kg.$^{0.75}$

Abundant vitamin E is supplied by salad oils, shortening, margarine, fruits and vegetables, and whole-grain products. However, high intakes of polyunsaturated fatty acids may increase requirements sufficiently to induce a deficiency of this vitamin.

Vitamin K. The K family of vitamins occurs throughout nature and is required in microgram amounts by man and certain animals to maintain prothrombin and other clotting factors. The average diet apparently contains adequate amounts of vitamin K, and additional amounts are supplied by the gastrointestinal flora. Thus, few malnourished human beings have presented findings indicating inadequate dietary vitamin K. Because of the lack of reliable information, a daily allowance for this vitamin has not been established. A group of older adults experimentally depleted of vitamin K were found to require slightly more than 0.03 mg. per kilogram of body weight intravenously to obtain normal blood clotting.

Water-soluble Vitamins

Ascorbic Acid (Vitamin C). Ascorbic acid has many biochemical functions in the body and is essential for normal wound healing and resistance to infection. Man, higher apes, and the guinea pig lack the metabolic pathway to synthesize adequate amounts of ascorbic acid, and in these species a lack of sufficient dietary ascorbic acid leads to scurvy. The minimal daily intake of ascorbic acid to prevent scurvy in the adult is about 10 mg., but this does not allow tissue saturation. Despite many extravagant claims, efforts to demonstrate beneficial effects from large doses of ascorbic acid have been unsuccessful. The United Kingdom recommendation is 30 mg. per day for adults, half the amount suggested by the FNB for an adult male. Ascorbic acid is furnished by fruits, particularly citrus fruits as well as by most fresh vegetables. (For more information on ascorbic acid deficiency, see below: Scurvy).

Biotin. Biotin is essential for the activity of many enzyme systems in bacteria, animals, and, presumably, man. Biotin deficiency does not occur naturally in man because the vitamin is so widely distributed in all common foods. Experimental biotin deficiency in man, induced by feeding the metabolic antagonist avidin found in egg white, results in the development of serious clinical and pathologic changes. These include scaly dermatitis, pallor, extreme lassitude, anorexia, muscle pains, insomnia, precordial pain, and slight anemia.

Although the minimal daily requirement for biotin has not been established, diets providing a daily intake of 150 to 300 μg. of biotin are considered adequate.

CO_2 FIXATION !

Choline. Choline serves as a source of labile methyl groups in the body, and in addition is a constituent of several compounds necessary for nerve function and lipid metabolism. Choline is generally considered to be an essential nutrient in the diet, although human choline deficiency has not been demonstrated. The average mixed diet consumed by persons in industrialized countries has been estimated to contain 500 to 900 mg. per day of choline, mostly from egg yolk, vegetables, and milk. Beef liver contains about 0.6 per cent choline.

Folacin. Folacin coenzymes function in the transfer of single carbon units in a number of intracellular metabolic processes, particularly in the synthesis of purine and pyrimidine ribotides and deoxyribotides and in amino acid interconversions. A folacin deficiency may arise from inadequate dietary intake, impaired absorption, excessive demands by tissues of the body, and metabolic derangements. Megaloblastic anemias resulting from folacin deficiency have been recognized with increasing frequency (see Megaloblastic Anemias in the section on Hematologic and Hematopoietic Diseases). Although the minimal amount of folacin required by the normal adult may be as low as 0.05 mg. per day, the intake of food folacins required to provide this amount would depend on the highly variable amount destroyed by cooking. During pregnancy the requirement may be increased to as much as 0.5 mg. per day. Folic acid (phenylmonoglutamic acid) and folacin (tetrahydropteroyl glutamic acid) occur in a wide variety of foods of animal and vegetable origin, particularly in glandular meats, yeasts, and green leafy vegetables.

Niacin. The term "niacin" is generic for both nicotinic acid and nicotinamide. Nicotinamide functions in the body as a component of two important coenzymes that are primarily concerned with glycolysis, tissue respiration, and fat synthesis. Tryptophan is a precursor of niacin in man, and the efficiency of conversion is such that an average of 60 mg. of dietary tryptophan is equivalent to 1 mg. of niacin. An inadequate intake of both niacin and tryptophan results in the development of pellagra (see below: Pellagra). Good dietary sources of niacin are liver, other meats, fish, whole-grain cereals and enriched breads, dried peas, nuts, and peanut butter.

Pantothenic Acid. Pantothenic acid is of biologic importance because of its incorporation into CoA, on which acylation and acetylation and other interactions depend. Pantothenic acid deficiency induced in human volunteers by feeding the metabolic antagonist, omega-methylpantothenic acid, together with a deficient diet, resulted in serious clinical signs and symptoms within a few months. An important feature of the syndrome produced by pantothenic acid deficiency was reduced antibody formation. Neuropathy associated with low serum pantothenic acid has been observed in alcoholic patients habitually consuming extremely poor diets. A daily intake of 5 to 10 mg. is probably adequate for children and adults.

Ordinary cooking does not cause excessive losses of pantothenic acid, and the vitamin is so widely distributed in plant and animal tissues that deficiency does not occur spontaneously in human populations.

Food sources include organ meats, egg yolk, peanuts, plants of the cabbage family, and whole grains. Other meats, vegetables, milk, and fruits also contain moderate amounts of pantothenic acid. The usual diets of industrialized countries furnish 15 mg. of pantothenic acid daily.

Riboflavin. Riboflavin functions as a coenzyme or active prosthetic group of flavoproteins concerned with the oxidative processes. The requirement for riboflavin is related to body size, metabolic rate, and rate of growth. Deficiency of riboflavin produces lesions in mucous membranes, most easily seen in the tongue, lips, and cornea (see Ariboflavinosis).

The FNB expresses riboflavin requirements for adults as 0.07 mg. per kilogram to the 0.75 power to prevent tissue saturation, and FAO/WHO uses 0.55 mg. per 1000 calories to arrive at its similar recommendations.

Riboflavin is soluble in water. It is widely distributed in all leafy vegetables, in the flesh of animals and fish, and in milk, but may be destroyed when food is exposed to sunlight or cooked.

Thiamin. Thiamin functions in the carbohydrate metabolism as a coenzyme in the decarboxylation of alpha-keto acids and in the utilization of pentose in the hexose monophosphate shunt. Thiamin deficiency leads to beriberi, still seen among populations subsisting primarily on rice; but in the industrialized countries, signs of thiamin deficiency are limited almost entirely to chronic alcoholics (see Beriberi).

Thiamin is widely distributed in foods and readily available. It is soluble in water, sensitive to oxidation, and destroyed rapidly by heat in neutral or alkaline solutions. Roasting and stewing of meat may reduce the thiamin content by 30 to 50 per cent, and vegetables may lose 25 to 40 per cent in cooking.

It has been generally assumed that thiamin need is related to caloric intake, particularly to those calories derived from carbohydrate. Although dietary fat does "spare" thiamin to some extent, the reduction in requirement appears to be small. Satisfactory thiamin nutriture under normal conditions will be maintained by 0.5 mg. per 1000 calories. Because it is possible that older persons use thiamin less efficiently, it is deemed advisable to recommend that a thiamin intake of 1 mg. per day be maintained by older adults, even when they are consuming less than 2000 calories daily.

Vitamin B_6. Vitamin B_6 in the form pyridoxal phosphate or pyridoxamine phosphate has been shown to function in carbohydrate, fat, and protein metabolism. Vitamin B_6 is a collective term for a group of naturally occurring pyridines that are metabolically and functionally interrelated; namely, pyridoxine, pyridoxal, and pyridoxamine.

The vitamin appears to be part of the molecular configuration of glycogen phosphorylase. Pyridoxine deficiency has occurred in children fed a proprietary formula in which the B_6 content was largely destroyed as a result of changes in the sterilization process. Symptoms were restlessness and irritability, and some developed convulsions. Pyridoxine deficiency may be responsible for anemia in adults.

To provide a reasonable margin of safety and allow for daily intakes of 100 grams or more of protein, the FNB recommendation is 2 mg. per day for adults. Most diets provide 1 to 2 mg. per day, which is sufficient for most people. Good dietary sources are liver, other meats, whole-grain cereals, soybeans, peanuts, corn, and many vegetables.

Vitamin B_{12}. Vitamin B_{12} is essential for the normal functioning of all cells, but particularly those of the bone marrow, nervous system, and gastrointestinal tract, because it facilitates reduction reactions and participates in the transfer of methyl groups. Its chief importance seems to be in nucleic and folic acid metabolism. Deficiency of vitamin B_{12} results in the development of megaloblastic anemia and signs of degeneration of the long tracts of the spinal cord. Sore tongue, paresthesias, and amenorrhea may also be present. (See Vitamin B_{12} Deficiency in the article on Nutritional Disorders of the Central Nervous System).

Cyanocobalamin is the principal one of several compounds with vitamin B_{12} activity. As little as 1.0 μg. daily will cure most cases of megaloblastic anemia resulting from deficiency of this vitamin, but will not replenish liver stores. In a dose of 0.5 μg. more than 70 per cent is absorbed, but as the dosage of vitamin B_{12} increases, absorption gradually decreases to 30 per cent in a dose of 5 μg. If absorption is normal, a dietary intake of 5 μg. per day of vitamin B_{12} is recommended to ensure the replacement of normal losses. Average diets appear to meet these requirements in both the industrialized and developing countries. Vitamin B_{12} occurs predominantly in foods of animal origin, with very little present in vegetables. Nevertheless, except in vegetarians, deficiency states are likely to arise only as a result of superimposed infections, malabsorption, or lack of intrinsic factor (pernicious anemia).

Mineral Elements

Calcium. Calcium is a major mineral constituent of the body and makes up about 1.5 to 2.0 per cent of the body weight of the mature human, more than 99 per cent of it in bones and teeth. Active processes of bone formation and resorption constantly exchange calcium with body fluids. The small proportion of calcium distributed in body fluids and tissues contributes importantly to other functions, such as blood coagulation, neuromuscular irritability, muscle contractility, and myocardial function. An FAO/WHO Expert Committee in 1961 recommended a practical allowance ranging from 400 to 500 mg. per day to meet the needs of normal adults, a lower figure than that of the FNB given in Table 1.

Calcium is incompletely absorbed, and phytate, oxalate, and fatty acids of the diet form nonionized or poorly soluble calcium complexes, further interfering with intestinal absorption. Calcium requirements are increased during periods of growth, and in pregnancy and lactation, but intestinal absorption is more efficient as need increases.

Good sources of calcium include milk and most other dairy products, shellfish, egg yolk, canned sardines and salmon (with bones), soy beans, and many green vegetables. Adequate vitamin D is required for efficient absorption of calcium.

Copper. Copper-containing proteins in the body include ceruloplasmin, erythrocuprein, hepatocuprein, cerebrocuprein, cytochrome-C oxidase, tyrosinase, and monoamine oxidase. Copper depletion of a degree severe enough to cause hypocupremia has been observed in a few patients with iron deficiency anemia and edema, kwashiorkor, sprue, and the nephrotic syndrome. Anemia, neutropenia, and bone changes caused by copper depletion have been reported in Peruvian children.

A copper intake of 2 mg. per day appears to maintain balance in adults, and an intake of 0.08 mg. per kilogram per day is recommended.

Copper is widely distributed in foodstuffs, and a diet of even mediocre quality contains more than the recommended amount. The richest sources are liver, kidney, shellfish, nuts, raisins, and dried legumes. Milk is poor in both copper and iron.

Fluorine. Fluoride is incorporated into the structure of teeth and bone, and is necessary for maximal resistance to dental caries. In areas where natural water supplies do not contain this amount, the addition of fluoride to bring the concentration to 1 part per million has proved to be a safe, economical, and efficient way to reduce the incidence of dental decay. In communities where fluoridation has been introduced, the incidence of tooth decay in children has been decreased up to 50 per cent or more. The range of safety in fluoride intake is wide enough for safe accommodation to normal fluctuations in the fluoride content of foods among populations with fluoridated water supplies, without risk of inducing the first indication of an excess—slight mottling of the enamel. Some natural water supplies contain sufficient fluoride to induce mottling of the enamel, but no other associated adverse effects have been found.

Iodine. Iodine is an integral part of the thyroid hormones thyroxine and triiodothyronine, which have important metabolic roles. Dietary iodine deficiency leads to thyroid enlargement (goiter) as a result of increase in size and number of the epithelial cells in the gland (see Endemic Goiter in the section on Diseases of the Endocrine System).

Balance studies in adults indicate a daily requirement of 50 to 75 μg. of iodine, approximately 1 μg. per kilogram. Sources of iodine are food and water, but in large sections of the world, the amount of iodine in the water supply and locally produced foods is too low to meet human needs without hypertrophy and hyperplasia of the thyroid gland. Although today's wide diversification in the origin of foodstuffs has reduced the problem in many countries, iodization of salt is a desirable and effective measure of ensuring an adequate iodine intake for all segments of the population.

Iron. Iron is an essential constituent of hemoglobin and a variety of enzymes. An absolute deficiency owing to a low dietary intake, or a relative deficiency owing to high body losses of iron, results in the development of microcytic anemia and other clinical signs (see Hypochromic Anemias in the section on Hematologic and Hematopoietic Diseases).

Given sufficient available iron, the intestinal mucosa regulates absorption in a manner that keeps body iron constant. Available iron is dependent upon the amount of iron ingested, its chemical form, intake of other dietary substances such as phytates and oxalates that interact with iron to influence its availability, and gastrointestinal secretions that modify absorption. The recommended dietary intake is predicated on an average 10 per cent absorption of food iron, with a range of 2 to 20 per cent. Normal losses of iron from the body are small, but are significant in the menstruating woman and increase greatly in some pathologic states. The infant and the pregnant and lactating woman require proportionately larger quantities of iron.

Iron is widely distributed in both animal and vegetable foods, but intake estimates based on food iron values in food composition tables are of limited value. Foods lose iron during preparation, gain iron from cooking vessels or from other contamination, or have much of the iron in poorly utilized bound forms.

Magnesium. Magnesium appears to activate the enzymes that catalyze the transfer of phosphate from ATP to a phosphate receptor, or from a phosphorylated compound to ADP. It appears to be associated with thermoregulation, neuromuscular contraction, and protein synthesis. Magnesium deficiency disease in man is similar to hypocalcemic tetany, and is reversed by administration of magnesium sulfate. Low serum magnesium levels have been observed in a variety of clinical conditions including alcoholism, diabetes, malabsorption syndromes, kwashiorkor, neuromuscular conditions associated with parathyroid disease or without parathyroid disease, in surgical patients on restricted dietary regimens or parenteral feeding, and in patients receiving diuretic therapy.

The magnesium requirement of adult man has been estimated by balance techniques to lie between 200 and 300 mg. per day. Normal sweat losses of magnesium have been estimated to be about 15 mg. per day.

Magnesium is widely distributed in ordinary foods. For example, cocoa, nuts and soy flour, barley, lima beans, corn, whole wheat flour, and oatmeal all contain over 100 mg. per 100-gram edible portion.

Chromium, Cobalt, Manganese, Molybdenum, Selenium, and Zinc. Direct evidence for the essentiality of these trace or microelements in human nutrition is often difficult to obtain. Clear evidence that an element is required by mammals has provided a reliable index of a human requirement. Identification of elements in normal human enzyme systems has also afforded substantial evidence of a nutritional requirement.

There is evidence that *chromium* is a required nutrient. Continuing investigations of the relationship of this element to carbohydrate metabolism suggest its possible role in human nutrition.

Cobalt is an integral part of vitamin B_{12}. It is found in most common foods, and is readily absorbed from the gastrointestinal tract. Cobalt deficiency in man is unknown.

Manganese is an essential element, needed for normal bone structure, and is a part of enzyme systems that occur in man. A human deficiency has not been demonstrated, nor a recommended dietary allowance established.

Molybdenum and selenium have been shown to be essential in laboratory animals, and may also function nutritionally in man. There are insufficient data to establish a recommended dietary allowance. The close parallel of the functions of selenium and vitamin E in laboratory animals suggests a need for an evaluation of selenium in man.

Zinc has been recognized as an essential element in the nutrition of animals and humans, but the evidence for a primary zinc deficiency in man is limited. Patients exhibiting anemia, hepatosplenomegaly, short stature, hypogonadism, and geophagia have responded to zinc therapy when tissue levels of zinc and zinc intakes were low.

A mixed diet may be expected to supply adequate amounts of these microelements, and the risk of a deficiency in the United States is slight. Green leafy foods, fruit, whole grains, organ meats, and lean meats usually serve as generous sources of these elements.

At high levels of intake, all the elements are known to cause injury and to interfere with the utilization of other elements. Supplements should be used with caution and only with clear evidence of deficiency.

Beaton, G. H., and McHenry, E. W. (eds.): Nutrition: A Comprehensive Treatise, Vol. II: Vitamins, Nutrient Requirements, and Food Selection. New York, Academic Press, Inc., 1964.

Canadian Bulletin on Nutrition, Vol. 6, No. 1, Dietary Standard for Canada. Ottawa, Department of Public Printing and Stationery, March, 1964.

Department of Health and Social Security: Recommended Intakes of Nutrients for the United Kingdom (Report of the Panel on Recommended Allowances of Nutrients). Department of Health and Social Security Reports on Public Health and Medical Subjects No. 120. London, Her Majesty's Stationery Office, 1969.

Food and Agriculture Organization of the United Nations: Calorie Requirements: Report of the Second Committee on Calorie Requirements. FAO Nutritional Studies, No. 15. Rome, Italy, FAO, 1957. (Third printing, 1965.)

Food and Agriculture Organization of the United Nations/World Health Organization: Calcium Requirements; Report of an FAO/WHO Expert Group, Rome, Italy, 23 to 30 May, 1961.

Published jointly by FAO and WHO, FAO Nutrition Meetings Report Series No. 30 and World Health Organization Technical Report Series No. 230. Rome, FAO, 1962.

Food and Agriculture Organization of the United Nations/World Health Organization: Protein Requirements; Report of a Joint FAO/WHO Expert Group. Published jointly by FAO and WHO, FAO Nutrition Meetings Report Series No. 37 and World Health Organization Technical Report Series No. 301. Rome, FAO, 1965.

Food and Agriculture Organization of the United Nations/World Health Organization: Requirements of Vitamin A, Thiamin, Riboflavin and Niacin; Report of a Joint FAO/WHO Expert Group, Rome, Italy, 6-17 September, 1965. FAO Nutrition Meetings Report Series No. 41, World Health Organization Technical Report Series No. 362. Rome, FAO, 1967.

Food and Nutrition Board, National Research Council: Recommended Dietary Allowances, seventh revised edition, 1968. Publication 1694, National Academy of Sciences, 1968. Washington, D.C., Printing and Publishing Office, National Academy of Sciences.

ASSESSMENT OF NUTRITIONAL STATUS

Nevin S. Scrimshaw

The physician should always look for the clinical signs suggestive of nutritional disease in his patients. Inspection of those body areas in which signs of deficiency are most likely to be detected— the hair, eyes, lips, mouth, and skin of the face, neck, and arms—can be part of any examination, no matter how cursory, because neither formal examination facilities nor disrobing is essential. Suspicions aroused by clinical examination can then be verified by medical and dietary history and appropriate biochemical tests.

A manual of procedures developed primarily to guide surveys of the assessment of nutritional status in populations has been developed by the U.S. Interdepartmental Committee on Nutrition for National Development (ICNND, 1963); a more concise document was prepared by a committee of experts convened in 1962 by the World Health Organization (WHO, 1963).

Clinical Examination: Inspection and Measurement. The over-all nutritional appearance of each patient should be appraised before examination of specific areas. This will indicate whether a person is grossly overweight or underweight, or has excessive pallor, generalized skin lesions, or other indications of unsatisfactory health, possibly related to diet. Although simple inspection reveals obvious overweight and underweight in individuals, weight for height is a more reliable means of discrimination. Similarly, a gross subjective estimate of subcutaneous fat can be obtained by pinching a double fold of skin over the outer surface of the upper arm (mid-triceps region), but skin calipers provide a more precise estimate.

Hair. Protein malnutrition causes the hair to change color and become fine, dry, and brittle. Characteristically, the hair of persons with severe protein deficiency can be pulled out of the scalp without discomfort; whole tufts of hair come out readily by the roots. Since the hair is brittle, the tips also break off easily. In Caucasians, Indians, and Orientals who normally have brown or black hair, the change to a lighter color is readily detected, but without knowledge of prior hair color it might be thought to be genetic. The hair of Negroes tends to become reddish in cases of protein deficiency before becoming lighter. In persons with naturally light and fine hair, the change is more difficult to detect.

Eyes. Both vitamin A and riboflavin deficiencies are known to affect the eyes. The xerophthalmia due to avitaminosis A begins with a dryness of the bulbar conjunctiva, loss of the light reflex, lack of luster, and decreased lacrimation. It may proceed to keratomalacia, which is a softening of the cornea, and lead to ulceration, perforation, rupture, and destruction of the cornea. The final result is a scarred, opaque cornea and a sightless eye.

Bitot spots are often associated with vitamin A deficiency, although they cannot be regarded as specific to it. They appear as frothy, irregular, white or light yellow spots from one to several millimeters in diameter, most often on the conjunctiva lateral to the cornea. They look as if they could be wiped away, but are beneath the conjunctival epithelium. A small Bitot spot may consist of only a few tiny bubbles visible in the triangles, especially the outer ones. Both photophobia and the inability to see in dim light may be due to vitamin A deficiency.

The area of the eye between the sclera and the cornea is called the limbus. The circumcorneal injection seen in riboflavin deficiency consists of penetration of the corneal limbus and branching of the subconjunctival arterioles that normally terminate within 0.5 mm. of the limbus. However, proliferation and congestion of the blood vessels in the sclerae and their extension into the clear corneal tissue is by no means pathognomonic of riboflavin deficiency. Excessive exposure to sunlight, smoke, dust, and other irritants is a recognized conditioning factor even when riboflavin deficiency is present. Ariboflavinosis may also produce a moist, red lesion of the external angles of both eyes.

There are a number of other signs in the eye unrelated to nutrition which may be confusing to the examiner. For example, corneal scars, usually gray in color, are generally due to healed infectious conjunctivitis. Tiny hemorrhages at the end of the subconjunctival arterioles, as well as increased vascularization and pigmentation of the exposed part of the conjunctivae, are probably due to external irritants such as dust and smoke. Pinguecula, very small white or yellow subconjunctival cholesterol or lipid deposits, of no known nutritional significance, may be confused with Bitot spots. Another non-nutritional eye lesion is pterygium, a vascularized triangle of flesh which grows from either angle of the eye onto the cornea. Its cause is unknown.

Skin. The areas of the skin most affected by

nutritional deficiency usually are accessible to examination because they are also those most exposed to the environment. The skin of the face, neck, arms, and legs, and over pressure points such as the elbows, knees, and ankles is most likely to show positive findings in nutritional deficiencies.

Dyssebacea is the clinical term used to designate a series of disturbances of the sebaceous glands characterized by increased oiliness, dermatitis, fissuring, and exfoliation. For positive identification, the lesion must be red and moist. In riboflavin deficiency, it occurs at the external angles of the eye, the nasolabial fold, and behind the ears, and may appear in other skin folds of the body. The nasolabial lesions should not be confused with acne in adolescents or with the irritation from nasal discharge in small children.

Xerosis, or generalized dryness of the skin, is characteristic of vitamin A deficiency, but difficult to evaluate in the individual because the appearance of the skin is influenced so much by bathing habits and exposure to dust and sunlight. The follicular hyperkeratosis widely ascribed to vitamin A deficiency consists of a "goose flesh" appearance which is not altered by temperature or brisk rubbing, and is most prominent on the skin of the outer forearm and thigh. Fully developed lesions consist of symmetrically distributed, rough, horny papules formed by keratotic plugs projecting from hypertrophied hair follicles; they make the skin look and feel like coarse sandpaper. Several well conducted therapeutic trials have failed to demonstrate any relationship between this hyperkeratosis and vitamin A deficiency, even when dietary fat is sufficient, and its specific etiology is not yet understood.

It is important to differentiate follicular hyperkeratosis from the perifolliculitis of ascorbic acid deficiency. The latter consists of perifollicular congestion, swelling, and, eventually, hypertrophy of the follicles. Only in this late stage is the skin rough to the touch. Other skin changes observed in severe ascorbic acid deficiency include petechiae, purpura, and hematomas. Because of increased capillary fragility, they are readily caused by a blood pressure cuff, shoes, or accidental bruising. Obviously, other factors increasing capillary fragility or interfering with blood clotting, such as vitamin K deficiency, could cause these rare phenomena.

The cutaneous lesions of pellagra vary because of differences in the degree of deficiency, natural skin color, and conditioning factors, but they are sufficiently characteristic to be diagnostic in many instances. The most common chronic form is thickening, inelastic, fissured, and deeply pigmented areas of skin where exposed to sunlight or covering pressure points. Eventually, the skin in affected areas becomes dry, scaly, and atrophic.

Erythema upon exposure to sunlight is an acute manifestation, with subsequent vascularization, crusting, and desquamation out of proportion to the precipitating exposure. In intertriginous areas a common, acute, but highly nonspecific reaction is redness, maceration, abrasion, and superimposed infection. Heat friction and poor personal hygiene contribute importantly to these signs. The symmetrical distribution of pellagrous lesions over skin exposed to sunlight and over pressure points is the most characteristic feature. Casal's necklace is a virtually diagnostic distribution of pellagrous dermatitis which sharply follows the neckline when a low-necked dress or an open shirt collar is habitually worn outdoors by persons on a niacin-tryptophan–deficient diet.

In severe protein deficiency, the skin of the legs, arms, and thighs shows marked pitting edema (which is a *sine qua non* of the diagnosis), and a dermatosis characterized by hyperkeratosis, hyperpigmentation, and desquamation. Although often similar in appearance to the lesions of pellagra, they are not limited to the exposed areas, and often extend to the thighs and lower trunk.

Neck. Endemic goiter resulting from a deficiency of iodine available to the thyroid gland usually can be detected by inspection of the neck with the patient's head thrown back, and, in case of doubt, evaluated by simple palpation. If the goiter is visible when the head is in the normal position, its pathologic significance is beyond doubt, and it is Grade II according to the classification of the World Health Organization. Grade III goiter is one easily recognizable at a distance. The difficulty lies in the fact that in thin individuals not all thyroid glands that become visible with the head thrown back can be classified as being goiterous. As a rough guide, normal lateral lobe size corresponds to that of the thumbnail of the person being examined. When the volume of the lobe exceeds a lima bean–shaped object of this outline by four or five times, the goiter is classified as Grade I or higher. Parotid gland swelling is sometimes observed in patients with protein deficiency, and must be distinguished from mumps.

Mouth. The mouth is one of the areas most sensitive to nutritional deficiencies, but the changes are nonspecific, confusing, and difficult to evaluate. Pallor of the lips and mucous membranes, like pallor of the skin and fingernails, may be a consequence of anemia, but its clinical appraisal is so subjective as to be of little value unless the anemia is severe. The stomatitis which may be a consequence of riboflavin deficiency has already been mentioned. Angular scars may be the result of past episodes of acute ariboflavinosis, but may also be wholly non-nutritional in origin. Poorly fitting dentures are a common cause.

The gums may reflect any of a variety of nutritional deficiencies, but the changes are difficult to differentiate from those resulting from local irritants and poor hygiene. This is especially true because neglect of both diet and oral hygiene are likely in the same individual. Marginal gingivitis and periodontal disease are reported to be common in persons whose diets are deficient in ascorbic acid, but attempts to prove such a relationship by ascorbic acid therapy have been failures. On the other hand, engorged, dark red, and bleeding gums are almost pathognomonic of scurvy.

Marginal and generalized gingivitis may also be found associated wih deficiencies of vitamin A, niacin, and riboflavin. The problem is that many factors may play a causal role simultaneously so that the experimental correction of a single factor, even if contributory, does not necessarily effect a cure. General improvement of both diet and oral hygiene is usually required.

Marked hypertrophy of the filiform and fungiform papillae of the tongue is more frequently seen in populations in which vitamin B deficiencies, particularly of thiamin and riboflavin, are present. Papillary atrophy is sometimes related to niacin or iron deficiency, although any disease causing severe anemia will have this effect. For example, both nutritional megaloblastic anemia and the microcytic anemia of iron deficiency result in a smooth tongue. A markedly furrowed, so-called scrotal tongue is a possible manifestation of vitamin A deficiency.

Impression of the teeth on the borders of the tongue may be due to the edema resulting from protein deficiency as well as to defective dentures and a variety of other causes. When protein deficiency is the cause, evidence is likely to be present in the extremities as well.

Nutritional deficiencies may also cause changes in the color of the tongue, although they are usually difficult to evaluate. Reddening, either generalized or limited mainly to the distal third, may be associated with sprue. It affects first the tip and lateral margins, but may progress to include not only the entire tongue but all of the oral mucous membranes as well. A beefy red glossitis resembling raw beefsteak most frequently represents a deficiency of niacin, but other B vitamin deficiencies may be involved. Riboflavin deficiency is probably most often responsible for the purplish discoloration known as magenta tongue. Patchy areas of paler discoloration give rise to the name "geographic" tongue, which has no nutritional significance.

Teeth. The frequency and severity of dental caries is increased by a diet relatively high in soluble carbohydrates and decreased by adequate fluoride and phosphate intake. Any severe dietary deficiency in infancy and early childhood will delay tooth eruption and contribute to malposition of teeth. Malposition resulting from retarded mandibular development is a common sequela of early protein deficiency.

In children of many underdeveloped countries, a so-called hypoplastic line across the upper primary incisors has been described, in which a yellow or brown pigment becomes deposited. This is followed by the development of caries on the labial surface of the teeth. Subsequently, the teeth may break off along this line. A nutritional or febrile insult in the neonatal period is a probable cause.

Fluorosis, occurring in regions where the fluoride content of the water supplies is above about 2 to 6 parts per million of fluorine in drinking water, is characterized by mottled enamel and chalky white patches distributed over the surface of the teeth. In some cases, the entire tooth surface may be dull white and lusterless. Although cosmetically undesirable, the lesion is harmless, and such teeth are usually resistant to caries.

Edema. Edema of the lower extremities is characteristic of protein deficiency, and may also be seen in acute beriberi. In severe cases it becomes generalized.

Reflexes. Evaluation of knee and ankle jerk reflexes and a tuning fork test for vibratory sense add nothing to the physical examination for nutritional status unless there is a possibility of thiamin deficiency. They should be sought in people subsisting on rice diets and in alcoholics.

Evaluation of Signs. The signs suggesting nutritional deficiency are easier to evaluate and more specific in children than in adults. In adults, lesions from other causes, such as aging and repeated trauma, and confusing signs such as pinguecula, pterygium, and geographic tongue, are more likely to be present. The clinical signs which suggest more or less strongly the possibility of a nutritional deficiency are summarized in Table 2.

It must be emphasized again that the aforementioned signs are largely nonspecific. Moreover, they are more reliable in the assessment of nutritional status of population groups than of single individuals. Excellent color illustrations will be found in several of the references listed at the end of this article.

It should be clear from the foregoing that clinical examination alone will rarely be sufficient to establish a definite diagnosis. Many of the signs are so nonspecific that they cannot be relied upon in a given individual even when appropriate for population surveys. A medical history and confirmatory dietary and biochemical data are required when clinical examination raises the question of nutritional deficiency in the individual.

Physical Methods Complementary to Clinical Examination. Although routine roentgenographic studies are rarely possible, or indeed required, it is valuable to carry out roentgenographic examinations if physical signs and other circumstances suggest that rickets, osteomalacia, infantile scurvy, beriberi, fluorosis, or protein-calorie malnutrition is present. Such examinations also assist in the retrospective assessment of malnutrition, especially when there has been a history of rickets or protein-calorie malnutrition. In the latter, there may be transverse lines of growth disturbance at the epiphyses of the long bones and reduction in bone maturation best seen in wrist roentgenography.

The test of dark adaptation is sometimes used as a measure of vitamin A deficiency. It is, however, difficult to perform, and is influenced by factors other than vitamin A. The same appears to be true of electroretinography.

Biochemical Tests. A single biochemical determination, if accurate, may decisively confirm or deny the nutritional origin of an uncertain complex of clinical signs. Here again, biochemical

TABLE 2. SUGGESTED GUIDE FOR INTERPRETATION OF CLINICAL SIGNS*

Dietary Obesity
Excessive weight
Excessive skin folds
Excessive abdominal girth

Undernutrition
Lethargy, mental and physical
Low weight in relation to height
Diminished skin folds
Exaggerated skeletal prominences
Loss of elasticity of skin

Protein-Calorie Deficiency Disease
Edema
Muscle wasting
Low body weight
Pyschomotor change
Dyspigmentation of the hair
Thin, sparse hair
Moon face
Flaky paint dermatosis
Areas of hyperpigmentation

Vitamin A Deficiency
Xerosis of skin
Follicular hyperkeratosis
Xerosis conjunctivae
Keratomalacia
Bitot's spots

Riboflavin Deficiency
Angular stomatitis
Cheilosis
Magenta tongue
Central atrophy of lingual papillae
Nasolabial dyssebacea
Angular palpebritis
Scrotal and vulval dermatosis
Corneal vascularization

Thiamin Deficiency
Loss of ankle jerks

Sensory loss and motor weakness
Calf-muscle tenderness
Cardiovascular dysfunction
Edema

Niacin Deficiency
Pellagrous dermatosis
Scarlet and raw tongue
Tongue fissuring
Atrophic lingual papillae
Malar and supraorbital pigmentation

Vitamin C Deficiency
Spongy and bleeding gums
Folliculosis
Petechiae
Ecchymoses
Intramuscular or subperiosteal hematoma
Epiphyseal enlargement (painful)

Vitamin D Deficiency
1. *Active rickets* (in children)
   Epiphyseal enlargement (over 6 months of age), painless
   Beading of ribs
   Craniotabes (under 1 year of age)
   Muscular hypotonia
2. *Healed rickets* (in children or adults)
   Frontal and parietal bossing
   Knock-knees or bow legs
   Deformities of thorax
3. *Osteomalacia* (in adults)
   Local or generalized skeletal deformities

Iron Deficiency
Pallor of mucous membranes
Koilonychia
Atrophic lingual papillae

Iodine Deficiency
Enlargement of the thyroid

Excess of Fluorine (Fluorosis)
Mottled dental enamel

Adapted from World Health Organization Technical Report Series No. 258, Expert Committee on Medical Assessment of Nutritional Status. Geneva, WHO, 1963, pp. 59-61.

TABLE 3. TENTATIVE GUIDE TO THE INTERPRETATION OF SELECTED BIOCHEMICAL DATA USEFUL IN THE APPRAISAL OF NUTRITIONAL STATUS*

	Deficient	Low	Acceptable	High
Plasma protein: gram/100 ml.	< 6.0	6.0–6.4	6.5–6.9	≥ 7.0
Serum albumin (electrophoretic method): gram/100 ml.	< 2.80	2.80–3.51	3.52–4.24	≥ 4.25
Hemoglobin: gram/100 ml.				
Men	<12.0	12.0–13.9	14.0–14.9	≥ 15.0
Women (nonpregnant, nonlactating: ≥13 yr.)	<10.0	10.0–10.9	11.0–14.4	≥ 14.5
Children (3–12 yr.)	<10.0	10.0–10.9	11.0–12.4	≥ 12.5
Hematocrit (PCV): per cent				
Men	<36	36–41	42–44	≥ 45
Women (nonpregnant, nonlactating: ≥13 yr.)	<30	30–37	38–42	≥ 43
Children (3–12 yr.)	<30.0	30.0–33.9	34.0–36.9	≥ 37.0
Plasma ascorbic acid: mg./100 ml.	< 0.10	0.10–0.19	0.20–0.39	≥ 0.40
Plasma vitamin A: μg./100 ml.	<10	10–19	20–49	≥ 50
Urinary thiamine: μg./gram creatinine	<27	27–65	66–129	≥130
Urinary riboflavin: μg./gram creatinine	<27	27–79	80–269	≥270
Urinary N-methylnicotinamide: mg./gram creatinine	< 0.5	0.5–1.59	1.6–4.29	≥ 4.3

From Manual for Nutrition Surveys. 2nd ed. Bethesda, Md., Interdepartmental Committee on Nutrition for National Defense, National Institutes of Health, 1963.

measures vary in their reliability and specificity. Serum levels of vitamin A and ascorbic acid are quite useful, although very low levels may be present for some time before lesions appear.

For the B vitamins, blood serum levels are relatively insensitive, and measurement of thiamin, riboflavin, and niacin excretion in 24-hour urine samples is recommended.

Total serum protein and serum albumin are decreased markedly in protein deficiency, but only when the deficiency has progressed to the point at which it is beginning to be clinically evident. The ratio of urea to creatinine has been recommended recently as a measure of the loss of lean body mass in protein-calorie malnutrition. Anemia is also a laboratory-based diagnosis. A tentative guide to the interpretation of selected biochemical data is given in Table 3. It should be noted that most biochemical measures show only the current state of the patient, so that chronic nutritional lesions are possible even in those with normal serum levels of various nutrients.

Beaton, G. H., and McHenry, E. W. (eds.): Nutrition: A Comprehensive Treatise. Vol. III. New York Academic Press, Inc., 1966.
Davidson, S., and Passmore, R.: Human Nutrition and Dietetics. 4th ed. Baltimore, Williams & Williams Company, 1969.
Interdepartmental Committee on Nutrition for National Defense (National Institutes of Health): Manual for Nutrition Surveys. 2nd ed. Washington, D.C., Superintendent of Documents, U.S. Government Printing Office, 1963.
Jelliffe, D. B.: The Assessment of the Nutritional Status of the Community. World Health Organization Monograph Series No. 53. Geneva, World Health Organization, 1966.
Jolliffe, N.: Clinical Nutrition. 2nd ed. New York, A Hoeber Medical Book, Harper & Brothers, 1962.
World Health Organization Technical Report Series No. 258: Expert Committee on Medical Assessment of Nutritional Status. Geneva, World Health Organization, 1963.

NUTRITION AND INFECTION

Nevin S. Scrimshaw

Malnutrition in man is inseparable from the occurrence and effects of microbial disease. Infection precipitates nutritional disease in the malnourished, and malnutrition worsens the consequences of infection. The interaction between the two is synergistic. Both are major health problems wherever poverty and ignorance result in poor dietary habits, as well as inferior environmental sanitation and personal hygiene. The World Health Organization monograph, *Interactions of Nutrition and Infection*, provides extensive documentation for the statements and conclusions of this chapter.

EFFECT OF INFECTION ON NUTRITIONAL STATUS

General. One of the earliest and most constant consequences of infection is loss of appetite and a decrease in the amount of food tolerated. Another is the almost universal tendency to change the diet to one that is more liquid and higher in carbohydrates at the expense of foods that are good sources of protein and other essential nutrients. This is a particularly common practice in the feeding of young children in less developed areas. Often milk as well as solid food is removed from the diet in favor of starchy gruels and cooking water from cereal grains or plant leaves when a child has diarrheal disease or other acute infections. In addition, therapeutic agents such as purgatives may reduce intestinal absorption or, in the case of antimicrobial drugs, interfere with intestinal synthesis of some nutrients. The direct influence of fever in increasing both basal metabolism and the loss of nutrients in sweat must also be taken into account. Sweat losses may amount to as much as 4 grams of nitrogen per day, together with significant quantities of electrolytes and iron.

Protein. Acute infections cause a stress response qualitatively the same as that observed in states of pain, anxiety, fear, and other psychologic stress. The stress reaction, mediated by cortisone and insulin, mobilizes amino acids from skeletal muscle and other tissues from which they can be spared for gluconeogenesis in the liver. This is necessary because in man the contribution of liver glycogen to maintain blood glucose is relatively limited. The stress reaction undoubtedly arose to enable individuals to fight, flee from sudden danger, or recover from wounds and infections, regardless of the timing of meals. However, it necessarily depletes the body of protein because the amino acids thus mobilized are deaminated to provide the carbons of glucose, and the nitrogen is excreted in the urine, largely as urea.

Nitrogen losses during severe infectious diseases of bacterial origin such as typhoid fever, acute febrile tuberculosis, erysipelas, pneumonia, and pyelonephritis have long been recognized and can be equivalent to the nitrogen of 2 or 3 kg. of muscle during the acute phase of the illness. The effects of rickettsial diseases, such as Rocky Mountain spotted fever, and viral diseases, such as measles and chickenpox, are similar. It is now clear that even such mild infections as vaccination against smallpox and immunization with the 17-D strain of yellow fever vaccine, as well as tonsillitis, otitis media, bronchitis, and localized abscesses, will also provoke this stress reaction.

The duration of the metabolic effect of stress depends upon the nature and extent of the precipitating cause. If the stress is of short duration, it may be balanced by an increase in nitrogen retention during the same or succeeding 24 hours. The catabolic period associated with an infectious disease episode, however, is likely to last for several days, and the anabolic period of increased nitrogen retention is generally at least twice as long. After the acute stress is over, dietary amino acids are returned to the depleted tissues; hence protein intakes above maintenance levels are required at this time. In individuals already depleted by low levels of protein intake, the urinary loss of nitrogen measured during stress is less than that observed in those who are well nourished. Nevertheless, increases in urinary loss of nitrogen during minor infections have been found even in experimental subjects receiving a nitrogen-free diet.

In infections associated with diarrhea, reduced absorption of nitrogen and other nutrients adds to the nutritional consequences. However, even in severe diarrheal disease the drop in nitrogen absorption may be only 10 to 15 per cent, and seldom exceeds 50 per cent. *Thus, it is worthwhile to continue feeding persons with diarrhea even though stool volume may be increased.*

With so many factors adversely affecting protein nutritional status during infectious disease, it is not surprising that in underdeveloped countries the protein deficiency disease, kwashiorkor, is commonly precipitated by diarrheal disease, measles, or other infections in children who are already in a precarious nutritional state. Similarly, infections, especially of a chronic nature, are responsible for much of the protein deficiency seen in adults.

Vitamins. Blood levels of vitamin A are reduced in acute infections. Diarrheal and other infectious diseases, particularly measles, are frequently responsible for precipitating xerophthalmia and keratomalacia in children receiving diets deficient in vitamin A. It is probable that most clinical cases of avitaminosis A follow an acute infection. The absorption of vitamin A has been found to be reduced by severe *Giardia lamblia* infections. It is probable that other intestinal infections have this effect when sufficiently severe.

As was observed among prisoners of war of the Japanese during World War II, clinical beriberi is frequently precipitated in thiamin-deficient individuals by an infectious episode. Pneumonia and malaria have also been reported to be significant factors in the occurrence of beriberi in civilian populations. The synthesis of thiamin and other B vitamins by intestinal bacterial flora may also be affected by both intestinal infections and chemotherapy.

Spontaneous respiratory infections have been found to induce megaloblastic anemia in monkeys maintained on a diet low in folic acid. Also, the dietary intake of hemopoietic B vitamins is not low enough to account for the megaloblastic anemia seen in many patients with complicating infections.

Viral hepatitis has been specifically reported to increase dietary vitamin B_{12} requirement. Better confirmed is the appetite of the fish tapeworm, *Diphyllobothrium latum*, for vitamin B_{12}. These tapeworms are a significant cause of anemia in people infected from eating raw fresh-water fish, a common custom in Scandinavia and among persons of Scandinavian descent in the United States.

The role of infections in lowering serum ascorbic acid and increasing urinary excretion of this vitamin has been demonstrated by many experimental studies in guinea pigs. In poorly nourished children, otitis media, pneumonia, pyelonephritis, and other infections have long been recognized as precipitators of scurvy. Malaria, typhoid fever, influenza, measles, tuberculosis, and vaccination against smallpox are among other specific infections reported responsible for the appearance of scurvy in vulnerable children.

Minerals. It is well recognized that hookworm infection, if sufficiently severe, causes enough loss of blood to produce microcytic-hypochromic anemia even when dietary intakes of iron appear adequate. It should be noted, however, that mild to moderate hookworm infection is not likely to produce anemia and that iron deficiency anemia is common in populations not infected with hookworm.

There is evidence from experimental studies in rats, dogs, and cats that increasing protein and iron in the diets of infected and nutritionally deficient animals will decrease the hookworm burden as well as correct the anemia. Moreover, improving the iron intake of patients with hookworm disease cures the anemia without specific treatment to decrease or eliminate the worm burden. Chronic infections of almost any type are likely to produce the so-called anemia of infection by shortening the life span of erythrocytes and interfering with red cell production in the bone marrow. Increased losses of calcium and phosphorus have been reported for tuberculosis in both guinea pigs and man. Losses of sodium, chloride, potassium, and phosphorus, which are sometimes severe enough to cause death, occur in diarrhea of infectious origin.

Lipids. Marked increases in the concentrations of total serum lipids have been observed in patients with infection caused by gram-negative, but not gram-positive, bacilli. Patients with fever due to noninfectious disease and those with viral influenza have normal concentrations of total serum lipids and normal levels of the major lipid classes, but infectious or serum hepatitis causes heightened levels of serum triglycerides and cholesterol. Absorption of fat is decreased in infections which provoke diarrhea. Increases in liver fat and some degree of steatorrhea have also been reported in patients with influenza and pneumonia, and are probably associated with other infections.

EFFECT OF MALNUTRITION ON INFECTION

There are large numbers of laboratory, clinical, and field observations which demonstrate that the severity and outcome of infection are frequently worsened by malnutrition. The prevalence of diarrheal disease, both upper and lower respiratory infections, and some other types of microbial disease is also influenced by malnutrition. Moreover, much of the high infant and preschool mortality in developing countries attributed to microbial disease would not occur in well nourished children. The relative influence of the various potential mechanisms whereby nutritional deficiencies influence resistance to infectious disease under field conditions is not really known. The following must be considered.

Antibody Formation. Although other mechanisms may be equally important in defense against infections, formation of antibodies specific for infectious agents or their toxins has received the most attention. This is because there are excellent techniques for detecting the presence of antibodies, and protective immunizations have been developed against many infections. Severe deficiencies of protein, vitamin A, ascorbic acid, riboflavin, thiamin, pantothenic acid, biotin, and niacin-tryptophan in laboratory animals are known to interfere with antibody formation. A number of studies confirm that protein deficiency in man can interfere with formation of antibodies. There have been several reports of false-negative tuberculin reactions in malnourished patients with tuberculosis. In human volunteers, antibody formation has been suppressed by inducing metabolic deficiencies of pantothenic acid or pyridoxine by feeding the corresponding antimetabolites, desoxypyridoxine and omega-methylpyridoxine. The same effect has been observed in cases of severe pellagra and moderately severe deficiency of several of the B vitamins.

Phagocytic Activity. The macrophages and microphages of the reticuloendothelial system are important protectors of the body against microbial diseases, particularly those caused by bacteria. Nutritional deficiency can reduce both the number and the phagocytic capacity of these cells. Children with kwashiorkor have little or no leukocyte response to superimposed infections. Macrophage activity is decreased in the presence of vitamin A, ascorbic acid, thiamin, and riboflavin deficiency in laboratory animals. Both animal studies and clinical observations of folic acid deficiency have shown production of phagocytes in mammalian bone marrow to be depressed to the extent of nullifying the effect of protective antibodies.

Tissue Integrity. Both antibody formation and phagocytosis take place only after the microbial agent has entered the host. They do not prevent infection, but rather prevent or minimize possible pathologic consequences of infection. The integrity of the skin, mucous membranes, and other epithelial tissues helps to prevent entry of the infectious agent. Various pathologic changes occur in tissues, depending on the type and severity of the nutritional deficiency. Mucous secretions may be reduced or absent, mucosal surfaces may become easily permeable, changes may take place in intercellular substance, or there may be epithelial metaplasia, edema in underlying tissues, and accumulation of cellular debris to form a favorable culture medium for the infectious agent. Deficiencies in vitamin A, ascorbic acid, thiamin, riboflavin, niacin, and protein are especially likely to cause tissue changes that lower resistance.

Wound Healing and Collagen Formation. How long an infection will be disabling depends on how rapidly it can be localized and contained. Nutritional deficiencies affect not only tissue integrity, but also wound healing, fibroblastic response to trauma, walling off of abscesses, and collagen formation. In protein-deficient rats, the walls of induced sterile subcutaneous abscesses were much thinner than those of spontaneous or induced abscesses in well nourished animals. The fibroblastic response in the deficient rats was markedly reduced, and as a result fatal septicemia frequently developed. Protein deficiency, especially with an inadequate intake of methionine, interferes with conversion of procollagen to collagen and weakens the tensile strength of collagen fibers.

Ascorbic acid intake must be adequate for synthesis of the amino acids from which collagen is formed, particularly hydroxyproline and hydroxylysine, which are almost unique to collagen. The skin at the edges of wounds in scorbutic guinea pigs showed almost no hydroxyproline. Restoration of ascorbic acid to the diet induced rapid production of hydroxyproline and the onset of wound healing.

Nonspecific Resistance Factors. It is hard to assess the importance of various nonspecific mechanisms of resistance to infection, and the effect of nutritional deficiencies on most of them is not clearly understood. The so-called *lysozymes*, which help to destroy pathogenic micro-organisms, are found in tears, sweat, saliva, and other body fluids. Their activity is apparently reduced by generalized malnutrition, and particularly by vitamin A deficiency.

Properdin is a euglobulin found in the serum of all normal animals thus far tested, and is associated with natural resistance to many diseases of bacterial, viral, and even protozoal origin. The properdin system is vulnerable to nutritional deficiency in the formation of the compound itself, as well as in the presence of an appropriate complement of magnesium. The only published evidence of this to date, however, is the report of a marked reduction of properdin in the serum of pantothenic acid-deficient rats.

Interferon is a natural product of animal cells which supplements other mechanisms of resistance to viral and some other infections. It appears to act by uncoupling oxidation from phosphorylation, so that the production of adenosine triphosphate is inadequate for replication of the infectious agent. Since interferon is a protein molecule, it seems likely that its formation is depressed in deficiency states in which protein synthesis is impaired.

Destruction of Bacterial Toxins. Most of the destruction of bacterial toxins or resistance to them in the animal host occurs as the result of the toxins combining with specific antibodies. There is some evidence that other mechanisms may exist as well. For example, rats suffering from deficiencies of B vitamins or vitamin A are more susceptible than controls to diphtheria toxin, even though antitoxin titers and rate of disappearance of injected toxin are similar in the two groups. Probably because of the ethical difficulties of investigating the problem directly in man, there are no clinical observations of this phenomenon.

Intestinal Flora. There is evidence that changes

in the intestinal flora induced by diet can influence susceptibility to some intestinal pathogens. In kwashiorkor, there is a tendency for the bacteria of the lower intestinal tract to appear at a higher level. In milder degrees of protein malnutrition it seems likely that intestinal organisms which are not normally pathogenic to the well nourished host may cause diarrhea. Not only is no known pathogen identified in most diarrheal episodes in malnourished children, but also the frequency and severity of these episodes are decreased when dietary supplements are provided. Changes in gastrointestinal motility secondary to malnutrition may also play a role in the severity of protozoal and helminthic infections.

Endocrine Balance. Endocrine factors are intimately involved in a number of the mechanisms of resistance to infection already mentioned, although little is known of their precise role. Examples include the loss of resistance to infection in adrenalectomized animals and patients with Addison's disease and the serious problem of infections in poorly controlled diabetics. Prolonged adrenocorticotrophic hormone (ACTH) or cortisone therapy, however, increases the spread of many infections, presumably because these hormones inhibit local inflammatory reactions at the site of bacterial proliferation. These observations have a bearing on the question of how malnutrition influences resistance to infection, since protein deficiency, caloric deprivation, and a number of other nutritional deficiencies influence endocrine balance.

Chung, A., and Viščorová, B.: The effect of early oral feeding versus early oral starvation on the course of infantile diarrhea. J. Pediat., 33:14, 1948.

Gallin, J. I., Kaye, D., and O'Leary, W. M.: Serum lipids in infection. New Eng. J. Med., 281:1081, 1969.

Scrimshaw, N. S.: Protein deficiency and infective disease, *In* Munro, H. N., and Allison, J. B., (eds.): Mammalian Protein Metabolism, Vol. II. New York, Academic Press, Inc., 1964, chap. 23, p. 569.

Scrimshaw, N. S., Taylor, C. E., and Gordon, J. E.: Interactions of Nutrition and Infection, World Health Organization Monograph Series No. 57. Geneva, World Health Organization, 1968.

Taylor, P. E., Tejada, C., and Sánchez, M.: The effect of malnutrition on the inflammatory response as exhibited by the granuloma pouch of the rat. J. Exp. Med., 126:539, 1967.

KWASHIORKOR, MARASMUS, AND INTERMEDIATE FORMS OF PROTEIN-CALORIE MALNUTRITION

Nevin S. Scrimshaw

Definition. The clinical spectrum of protein-calorie deficiency ranges from forms characterized only by growth retardation to the extremes of kwashiorkor and marasmus. Kwashiorkor is due to a deficiency of protein relative to calories. It can be found in children whose caloric intake is adequate and even excessive, or it may be superimposed on a degree of protein-calorie deficiency which makes wasting of both adipose tissue and lean body mass a prominent feature. When protein and calories are equally limited, however, the clinical condition which develops is marasmus, characterized primarily by growth failure and severe tissue wasting. The principal features of kwashiorkor are edema, pellagroid skin lesions, hair changes, anorexia, apathy, diarrhea, fatty liver, and profound biochemical and physiologic alterations, none of which is seen in classic marasmus.

Pathogenesis. The various forms of protein-calorie malnutrition are of major public health significance in most underdeveloped countries. They result from two main factors: a diet that is quantitatively and qualitatively inadequate, and superimposed stress, usually of microbial origin. A deficient diet results in turn from varying combinations of low food production, inadequate preservation and distribution of foods, restricted purchasing power, poor food habits, and deficient knowledge of the relation between diet and health. The excessive incidence of infectious disease is a consequence of poor environmental conditions, inadequate knowledge of epidemiologic factors, poor personal hygiene, and insufficient health services. These factors are interrelated and act synergistically to the detriment of nutritional status.

The clinical result depends on many determinants — on the severity and duration of the nutritional deficiencies of protein and calories, on the relative importance of the deficiency of protein to that of calories, on the nature and severity of other associated nutritional deficiencies, on the age of the person affected, and on the presence of other complications. The mild and moderate forms in children, frequently unrecognized or misinterpreted, are primarily characterized by inadequate growth and development. In adults they reduce work performance and resistance to infection.

Mild to Moderate Protein-Calorie Malnutrition in Children. The period of retarded growth is from about the fourth month up to school age and this is when dietary inadequacy and frequency of infections are most pronounced. During the second six months of life, breast feeding continues, but with insufficient or improper supplementation. After weaning, the usual diet is cereal grains, starchy roots, overdiluted milk, or even cornstarch. In most cases this regimen not only fails to provide the needed calories but also is deficient in many essential nutrients, particularly proteins of high biologic value.

Although the diet may include some legumes, vegetables, and occasional meat, cheese, or other animal products, it is usually poor in proteins of high biologic value. Not until the third to fifth year of life is the usual child in underdeveloped countries permitted an adult type of diet. The period of greatest dietary inadequacy coincides in general with increased exposure to an unsanitary environment and a greater frequency of diarrheal and parasitic diseases, measles, whooping cough, and other diseases of childhood. By the time children enter school this critical period of high morbidity from infection is largely past because of an acquired immunity and better nutrition.

The assumption that reduced growth of children in underdeveloped countries is due more to environmental than to genetic factors is supported by observations of children of different races living under similar adverse conditions. Conversely, well nourished children of the same genetic origins usually follow the growth pattern of well fed North American or European children in a healthy environment.

Since growth retardation is most marked in the parts of the body with the highest rates of growth during the period of malnutrition, disproportions develop in anthropometric measures. The shorter limb-to-trunk ratio often observed in poorly nourished population groups is largely from this cause. Retarded growth is paralleled by retardation in bone maturation, as evidenced by the number and rates of appearance of ossification centers of wrist and hand in x-ray studies. There is also evidence that children with early retardation in growth experience a similar retardation of psychomotor development that persists at least through the school years.

Mild to Moderate Protein-Calorie Malnutrition in Adults. The consequences of the mild to moderate chronic protein-calorie malnutrition common among adult populations has been little studied. Adaptation to insufficient calories includes low weight for height and reduced caloric expenditure. Accordingly, it is probable that it seriously reduces work capacity and thereby contributes to the low social and economic development in these areas. The effects of such malnutrition on resistance to stress, particularly that resulting from infectious disease, also needs further attention. Pregnant women and lactating mothers are a particularly vulnerable segment of adult populations of underdeveloped countries. Many women do not gain a normal amount of weight during pregnancy, but average weights of children at birth are not much affected. The main effect is on the mothers. Breast-feeding often continues for as long as two years, and a further loss of weight with long lactation is usual. The consequences of repeated pregnancy and lactation on poorly nourished mothers have received too little attention. It is noteworthy that such women look older than their chronologic age.

MARASMUS

The extremely low calorie diets responsible for the syndrome of marasmus are obviously also deficient in proteins and many other essential nutrients. Since the number of calories is the main factor, the child utilizes amino acids from the skeletal muscles and other less essential tissues, as well as deriving energy from fat deposits. Growth stops, but the amino acids and other nutrients liberated from the child's own tissues make possible a continuing synthesis of serum albumin, enzymes, and other essential metabolites. For this reason, no serious metabolic disturbances are observed.

The child with marasmus looks and is emaciated owing to a loss of subcutaneous fat, extreme muscle wasting, and atrophy of most organs. Although the liver and other essential organs are much reduced in size, histologic changes are minimal. Despite the apt description of being reduced to "skin and bones," the child remains clinically alert, and maintains an appetite.

KWASHIORKOR

Clinical Characteristics. Clinically, the syndrome of kwashiorkor presents a pitting edema of varying degree, from a mild form localized in feet and ankles to severe, generalized edema, with eyelids swollen shut. Movement of the extremities may be limited, and fluid accumulates in the peritoneal cavity. Patients are usually extremely apathetic, with a weak, monotonous cry if disturbed. Anorexia is present in most of them, and is frequently severe; diarrhea is an almost constant finding. The characteristic alterations of the skin resemble the dermatosis of pellagra, with which they have been mistakenly identified. The lesions are pigmented, dry, hyperkeratotic, and sometimes desquamating and of a size varying from punctiform to large, confluent areas. They are most numerous where subject to irritation, especially in the perineal region. They frequently occur on the extremities and face, and may extend to the trunk.

Normally curly hair becomes dry, fine, brittle, and straight. It is easily pulled out or may even fall out. It may become reddish, yellowish, or even white. These pigmentation changes are often observed in stripes, indicating successive periods of normal and abnormal growth of the hair. The extremities are frequently cold and cyanotic. The abdomen may be distended owing to flaccid abdominal muscles and ascites. Hepatomegaly is sometimes found.

Biochemical Alterations. Protein. Low total serum protein is a diagnostic characteristic of kwashiorkor. It is due almost entirely to a low level of albumin, and is sometimes partially obscured by a relatively high level of gamma globulin resulting from a concurrent infectious process. There is a tendency for the beta globulin fraction to be both relatively and absolutely decreased; a relative increase in the alpha$_2$ globulin has also been found. Studies with I^{127}-labeled albumin indicate that the lowering of this fraction is due to a decrease in rate of synthesis and not to abnormal catabolism.

Total α-amino nitrogen in plasma is abnormally low because most amino acids are present in decreased amount. The greatest reductions are

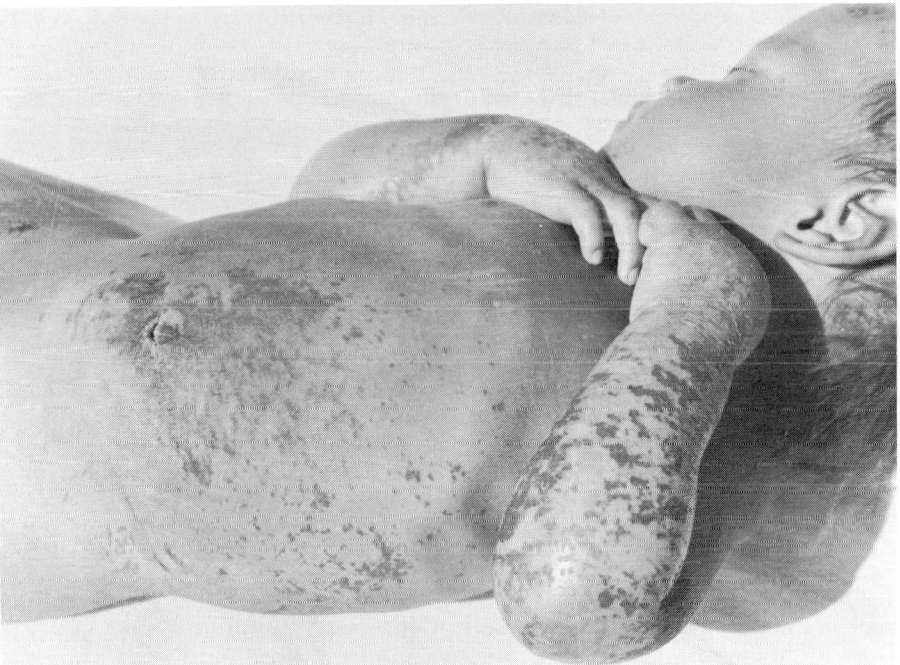

FIGURE 1. Edema and skin lesions in child with kwashiorkor. (Courtesy of Institute of Nutrition of Central America and Panama.)

found in tryptophan, cystine, valine, tryrosine, and methionine. Low levels of urea in both blood and urine indicate decreased protein metabolism. The synthesis of antibodies is also inhibited in kwashiorkor. A very marked increase in the proportion of urinary nitrogen excreted as purine derivatives has been taken as evidence of cellular breakdown in kwashiorkor. Other abnormal substances in the urine which indicate impairment of important metabolic pathways are β-aminoisobutyric acid and ethanolamine.

Although the liver protein in kwashiorkor is greatly diluted by fat, it is not decreased in absolute amount in relation to body size. However, a lowered ratio of nitrogen to deoxyribonucleic acid has been reported, suggesting a true loss of protoplasmic nitrogen. In any case, the level of nitrogen in the liver of children with kwashiorkor is markedly decreased over that for normal children of the same age. There is also a marked loss of muscle nitrogen in kwashiorkor, the degree depending largely upon the severity of pre-existing marasmus.

Lipids and Carbohydrates. All the lipid fractions which have been determined in the blood of children with kwashiorkor, including neutral fat, fatty acids, phospholipids, and cholesterol, have been found to be low, and levels of these substances rise rapidly in the course of treatment. An increase in fat content of the liver, found by gross and microscopic examination, is another diagnostic criterion. In true marasmus, on the other hand, the amount of liver fat is decreased. Blood glucose levels are generally low. Although glucose tolerance is sometimes reduced, so that the diabetic type of glucose tolerance curve is observed, this is not a constant feature of the disease.

Enzymes. In acute kwashiorkor, lipase, trypsin, and amylase activities in the duodenal secretion are lowered almost to zero, and marked reductions in serum pseudocholinesterase, amylase, carbonic anhydrase, and alkaline phosphatase are recognized characteristics. The activity of these enzymes returns rapidly to normal with the administration of an adequate diet. Alkaline phosphatase levels, however, show a slight further drop before rising with therapy.

The activity of a number of enzymes has also been measured in fresh liver tissue obtained by needle biopsy from children with kwashiorkor. The outstanding finding is a decrease in xanthine oxidase activity per unit of protein, although cholinesterase and D-amino acid oxidase activity are also definitely lowered. Alkaline phosphatase activity in the liver is generally increased. These findings suggest that, although the activity of many key enzymes is maintained even in the presence of extreme protein deficiency, some are sufficiently affected to initiate the train of events culminating in death.

Vitamins. Levels of vitamin A and carotene in the serum of children with kwashiorkor are extremely low. It was assumed that this was due to low intake of vitamin A, until studies demonstrated that children with acute kwashiorkor upon admission to the hospital did not have an increase in serum vitamin A after a 75-mg. oral dose of vitamin A palmitate. After three to five days of intensive protein therapy, however, a similar dose gave the same sharp increase in serum vitamin A that is found in normal children. It was also found that, in most cases, serum vitamin A levels rose with protein therapy, even when the diet contained no carotene or vitamin A.

Analysis of liver biopsy material demonstrated that this phenomenon occurred whenever there were adequate stores of vitamin A in the liver, and that in those few cases in which there was gross depletion of vitamin A in the liver, administration of protein alone produced no serum response. From this and similar studies, it appears probable that the *transport* of vitamin A and possibly of vitamin E, which also occurs in abnormally low amounts in blood plasma of children with kwashiorkor, is inadequate because of the lack of a protein carrier.

Blood levels of thiamin and riboflavin are within normal limits in children with kwashiorkor. Even though the pigmented skin lesions superficially resemble those of pellagra, there is no evidence of niacin involvement. The urinary excretion of N-methylnicotinamide, in cases in Central America at least, is within normal limits. Levels of serum ascorbic acid are relatively low, but are not in the range commonly associated with clinical deficiency. No significant alterations of levels of vitamin B_{12} in the blood have been found.

Electrolytes and Other Minerals. Potassium depletion is a major biochemical characteristic of kwashiorkor, and is a direct consequence of the protein deficiency. Other electrolyte changes are secondary consequences of diarrhea (a symptom almost always present in kwashiorkor) or vomiting, which may also accompany the deficiency. Interpretation and correction of electrolyte changes in kwashiorkor are complicated by the abnormal distribution of water and the severe degree of potassium depletion. Magnesium deficiency may occur and lead to tetany.

Endocrine Function. On the basis of observed normal function of the adrenal cortex in marasmus and decreased glucocorticoid production in kwashiorkor, the hypothesis has been proposed that the severe restriction of calories in children in whom marasmus develops results in increased production of ACTH by the anterior pituitary gland which in turn stimulates the adrenal cortex to produce more corticosteroids. These hormones assure catabolism of muscle and other labile proteins sufficient to furnish amino acids to the liver for gluconeogenesis and likewise provide the liver with amino acids for synthesis of metabolically essential proteins. This mechanism does not come into play when the child receives a diet with enough calories to meet minimal energy needs even though it is extremely deficient in proteins. Under these circumstances, children do not mobilize amino acids from their muscles, and instead present the serious metabolic disturbances of protein deficiency without further muscle wasting. The result is kwashiorkor. This hypothesis is now being tested experimentally.

Other Physiologic Changes. In the marasmic type of kwashiorkor seen in Central America, a relatively small heart, which rapidly increases in size with treatment, is found upon radiologic examination. Electrocardiographic findings have principally consisted of low voltage and minor abnormalities, including alterations in the T wave and changes in rhythm. To judge by the volume of feces excreted by children with kwashiorkor, these children suffer from a malabsorption syndrome which is not completely corrected even after some weeks of treatment. Good digestion and absorption of proteins still takes place during the acute state, but fat is poorly handled at first. Although fat absorption improves very rapidly as the child recovers, some degree of steatorrhea persists even into late recovery. Despite the marked histologic alterations in the liver, the common tests for liver function have been found to give results within normal limits, with the possible exception of Bromsulphalein retention, which is frequently high. A reduction in renal plasma flow has been reported; this is found particularly when there is dehydration, and therefore appears to be related to the diminished volume of circulation. The glomerular filtration rate, as indicated by clearance of inulin and endogenous creatinine, is also reduced. Although there is some evidence of reduced antidiuretic activity, the mechanism of water retention in kwashiorkor is not clear and may be primarily a physiologic response of the kidney to the electrolyte and water disturbances.

Electroencephalographic studies have shown diminished voltage and excessively slow rhythmic activity. Some authors have also reported abnormal focal activity and other alterations. These abnormalities tend to disappear as recovery progresses.

Pathology. The main pathologic alterations in kwashiorkor include fatty changes in the liver, of the large droplet type, beginning in periportal areas of the lobule and extending progressively to the central vein. The pancreas and other endocrine glands become atrophic, along with marked atrophy of the intestinal mucosa, to give changes like those in primary malabsorption. The skin shows atrophy of the epidermis, with varying degrees of hyperkeratosis and parakeratosis. Microbial diseases are common complications of severe protein-calorie malnutrition and are responsible for many deaths. Bronchopneumonia is the frequent final episode, often without the characteristic fever and leukocytosis. Respiratory insufficiency may suddenly occur, with death in a few hours, and only autopsy reveals the severe bronchopneumonia.

Coexisting Deficiencies. The clinical manifestations of protein-calorie malnutrition are further complicated by the presence of other nutritional deficiencies. Vitamin A deficiency with severe ocular lesions is frequent in both marasmus and kwashiorkor. Concurrent deficiencies of components of the vitamin B complex, particularly riboflavin, are also common. The mild normocytic, normochromic anemia attributable to protein deficiency is often complicated and becomes much more severe because of simultaneous deficiencies of iron, vitamin E, folic acid, and other hematopoietic factors of the B vitamins. A recent report suggests that vitamin E deficiency is sometimes responsible.

Dehydration and serious electrolyte imbalance are usual because of the coexisting diarrhea. Both present special features owing to the overhydration, sodium retention, potassium depletion, and renal disturbances present as a direct consequence of the deficiency in protein.

Treatment. The correction of dehydration and associated electrolyte imbalance and the treatment of infections are the immediate demands in management of protein-calorie malnutrition. The basic requirement, however, is a diet providing all essential nutrients. Three to 4 grams of protein of high biologic value and 100 to 140 calories per kilogram of body weight are useful in children with kwashiorkor, and up to 200 calories per kilogram in those with marasmus. All the forms of severe protein-calorie malnutrition just described are also observed in adults, although less commonly, and the principles of treatment are the same.

Prevention. The prevention of protein-calorie malnutrition depends upon teaching mothers how to feed their young children properly and the importance of doing so. Efforts should be made to increase the availability of low-cost protein foods suitable for feeding to infants and young children, ensuring that the mother can obtain them through either commercial channels or welfare programs. There must also be effective public health measures for reducing the burden of microbial disease in vulnerable populations.

Béhar, M., Viteri, F., and Scrimshaw, N. S.: Treatment of severe protein deficiency in children (kwashiorkor). Amer. J. Clin. Nutr., 5:506, 1957.

National Academy of Sciences–National Research Council: Pre-School Child Malnutrition: Primary Deterrent to Human Progress. An International Conference on Prevention of Malnutrition in the Pre-School Child, Washington, D.C., December 7-11, 1964. NAS–NRC Publication No. 1282, 1966.

Scrimshaw, N. S., and Béhar, M.: Protein malnutrition in young children. Science, 133:2039, 1961.

Scrimshaw, N. S., and Béhar, M.: Malnutrition in underdeveloped countries. New Eng. J. Med., 272:137, 193, 1965.

Viteri, F., Béhar, M., Arroyave, G., and Scrimshaw, N. S.: Clinical aspects of protein malnutrition. In Munro, H. N., and Allison, J. B. (eds.): Mammalian Protein Metabolism. Vol. II. New York, Academic Press, Inc., 1964, Chap. 22, p. 523.

Waterlow, J. C., and Alleyne, G. A. O.: Protein malnutrition in children: Advances in knowledge in the last ten years. Advances Protein Chem. (in press).

Waterlow, J. C., Cravioto, J., and Stephen, J. M. L.: Protein malnutrition in man. Advances Protein Chem., 15:131, 1960.

UNDERNUTRITION, STARVATION, AND HUNGER EDEMA

Nevin S. Scrimshaw

When a person's caloric intake is below his daily energy expenditure, he must either bring the two into balance by reduced activity or draw upon his own tissues for energy. Initially, tissue fat is a major energy source, but protein is also required as a source of amino acids for gluconeogenesis. Cahill has shown that after several weeks of fasting, dependence on endogenous amino acids decreases, because even the central nervous system can then utilize fatty acids.

A subject studied by Benedict who fasted completely for 31 days lost 13.2 kg. from a starting weight of 60.6 kg. He continued to excrete 7 to 10 grams of nitrogen daily in his urine, which corresponded to 15 to 18 per cent of his daily energy needs from endogenous protein, the remainder coming from adipose tissue. Thus, prolonged inadequate energy intake is accompanied by progressive loss of adipose tissue and lean body mass. Once adipose tissue has been exhausted, lassitude, loss of ambition, hypotension, collapse, and death follow if the caloric intake deficit continues. The late stages of this syndrome are also observed in anorexia nervosa, terminal carcinoma, and other wasting diseases.

Keys provides the most comprehensive review of the world literature on starvation, and adds important experimental observations of his own. Others have described severe malnutrition in the prisons and concentration camps of World War II and famines in many parts of the world.

Dependent edema often accompanies severe, prolonged undernutrition (starvation). The edema is soft and pitting, and usually disappears when the person is recumbent for some time, as during sleep. The causes of the edema are not entirely clear. Hypoproteinemia (specifically hypoalbuminemia, thus lowering the colloid osmotic pressure) is frequent but by no means invariable. Loss of fat and muscle, leaving a "loose sack" of skin with fluid filling the empty spaces, has been thought of as a contributing phenomenon. Diminished renal blood flow and glomerular filtration resulting from diminished cardiac output would presumably lead to sodium retention and edema.

Treatment of starvation demands caution. *In all forms of severe undernutrition, refeeding must be instituted slowly.* Overeating was a cause of shock and death of concentration camp victims at the end of World War II. Likewise in clinical medicine, e.g., esophageal carcinoma, sudden flooding of the intestine with rich food through a feeding jejunostomy or gastrostomy may produce shock and death. Graduated feeding similar to the feeding of newborn infants is essential. When sweetened water is shown to be tolerated, diluted milk is begun, and is followed by whole milk; only after this should simple foods be given.

Benedict, F. G.: A Study of Prolonged Fasting. Carnegie Institute of Washington, Publication No. 203, 1915.

Keys, A.: The Biology of Human Starvation. Minneapolis, University of Minnesota Press, 1950.

Mollison, P. L.: Observations on cases of starvation at Belsen. Brit. Med. J., 1:4, 1946.

Owen, O. E., Morgan, A. P., Kemp, H. G., Sullivan, J. M., Herrera, M. G., and Cahill, G. F., Jr.: Brain metabolism during fasting. J. Clin. Invest., 46:1589, 1967.

NUTRITIONAL ANEMIAS
Nevin S. Scrimshaw

Because dietary amino acids and nearly all of the vitamins are required for protein synthesis and cell multiplication, it is not surprising that a process of rapid cell production such as erythropoiesis would be affected by protein deficiency and most vitamin deficiencies when they become severe. In addition, because hemoglobin contains considerable iron, a deficiency of this nutrient will also affect red blood cell formation. It is increasingly recognized that nutritional anemias are probably the most widespread nutritional deficiency problem remaining in the world today.

Those anemias associated with deficiencies of vitamin B_{12}, folic acid, pyridoxine, and ascorbic acid are discussed under Megaloblastic Anemias in the section on Hematologic and Hematopoietic Diseases. Those associated with deficiency of iron are described in the section on Hypochromic Anemias in the same section. The anemia of protein deficiency is discussed above under Kwashiorkor, Marasmus, and Intermediate Forms of Protein-Calorie Malnutrition.

Recently, deficiency of alpha-tocopherol (vitamin E) has also been shown capable of producing anemia in man.

Harris, R. S., Wool, I. G., Loraine, J. A., and Thimann, K. V. (eds.): Vitamins and Hormones, Vol. 26. International Symposium on Vitamin-Related Anemias. New York, Academic Press, Inc., 1968.

ANOREXIA NERVOSA
Nevin S. Scrimshaw

Anorexia nervosa is a psychogenic disease in which distaste for food and refusal to eat lead to weight loss and, if protracted, to cachexia and death. For a more detailed discussion, see Anorexia Nervosa in Diseases of the Endocrine System. The differential diagnosis between anorexia nervosa and Simmonds' disease (panhypopituitarism) is described in Diseases of the Endocrine System.

DEFICIENCIES OF INDIVIDUAL NUTRIENTS: VITAMIN DISEASES
Nevin S. Scrimshaw

HYPOVITAMINOSIS A (INCLUDING XEROPHTHALMIA AND KERATOMALACIA)

Definition. Hypovitaminosis A is characterized by keratinizing metaplasia of both secretory and protective epithelial tissues and the development of night blindness. Lesions of the eye are the most serious, ranging from dryness of the conjunctiva (xerophthalmia) and Bitot spots, to softening and dissolution of the cornea (keratomalacia) in which the eye is permanently destroyed. The metaplasia may involve the linings of the respiratory, gastrointestinal, and genitourinary tracts, as well as the endocrine, salivary, sebaceous, and lacrimal glands.

Etiology and Distribution. The term vitamin A is used to include all compounds having vitamin A activity, but requirements are now expressed by the Food and Agriculture Organization and World Health Organization in terms of crystalline vitamin A_1 alcohol (retinol). The international unit, still used in many countries, is equivalent to 0.3 μg. of retinol (or 0.344 μg. of retinyl acetate) or to 0.6 μg. of the provitamin beta-carotene. The recommended intake for adults is 750 μg. of retinol per day, which will also meet requirements during pregnancy. During lactation 1200 μg. of retinol per day is recommended. For children the recommendations are estimated from expected body weight for age, ranging from 420 μg. per day at three to five months of age to the adult levels. Requirements are not influenced by physical activity or climate, but any pathologic condition which interferes with fat absorption is likely to impede vitamin A absorption, and infections can increase vitamin A needs.

Signs and symptoms of hypovitaminosis A are particularly common in Indonesia and most other countries of Southeast Asia and the Indian subcontinent, but are seen at least occasionally in nearly all economically underdeveloped countries. They are most often precipitated by infectious disease in infants and young children who already suffer from chronic malnutrition. Sporadic cases occur among particularly underprivileged infants in most of the industrialized areas of the world.

Clinical Manifestations; Pathology and Pathologic Physiology. The best known and generally the earliest physiologic effect of hypovitaminosis A is the loss of night vision (nyctalopia). The retinal rods responsible for vision in dim light contain a light-sensitive pigment, rhodopsin, an aldehyde of vitamin A which breaks down to retinine when light strikes a rod. In vitamin A deficiency rhodopsin regeneration fails.

Xerophthalmia is a dryness of the only transparent epithelial structures of the body which are exposed to air and light. The conjunctiva is affected earlier and more constantly than the cornea. Typical is a fatty dryness, most pronounced at the thickened wrinkles of the corners; the eye loses its porcelain aspect and looks muddy-greasy, like oil paint.

Bitot spots are often present, ranging in severity from a few tiny air bubbles visible on the exposed conjunctiva between the corneal rim and lumbus, to a frothy white coating which overflows onto the cornea. The meibomian glands sometimes enlarge to look like a string of beads along the margin of the eyelids. The cornea is more resistant, but becomes hazy, rough, and dry and insensitive to touch. Punctate superficial infiltrations or small erosions may be seen on the surface. As the disease progresses to *keratomalacia*, one of these erosions may enlarge rapidly, with protrusion and eventually prolapse of the iris and loss of the lens. Sometimes there is a rather sudden spongy swelling and melting down of the cornea, a colliquative necrosis, with subsequent shrinkage of the eyeball (Fig. 2).

The skin becomes dry as the sebaceous glands become covered with keratin, so that secretions are diminished. *Phrynoderma*, an elevated papular lesion caused by plugging of the mouth of the hair follicles with a dense keratotic mass together with hyperplasia of the epithelium lining the plugged follicles, has been mistakenly listed as a sign of vitamin A deficiency. This condition is not necessarily associated with low serum levels of vitamin A, and does not respond to prolonged vitamin A therapy. Moreover, it is different from the follicular lesion of vitamin A deficiency in laboratory animals, in which the upper third of the hair follicles contains loose keratin and becomes dilated.

An important clinical consequence of hypovitaminosis A is increased susceptibility to infection, resulting not only from reduced epithelial barriers to infectious agents, but also from direct impairment of such resistance mechanisms as antibody formation and leukocyte activity.

The small intestine is the main site of the conversion of active forms of carotene to vitamin A and its absorption. Therefore, when the intestine is affected by diseases such as sprue, fibrocystic disease of the pancreas, lymphomas, or lipodys-

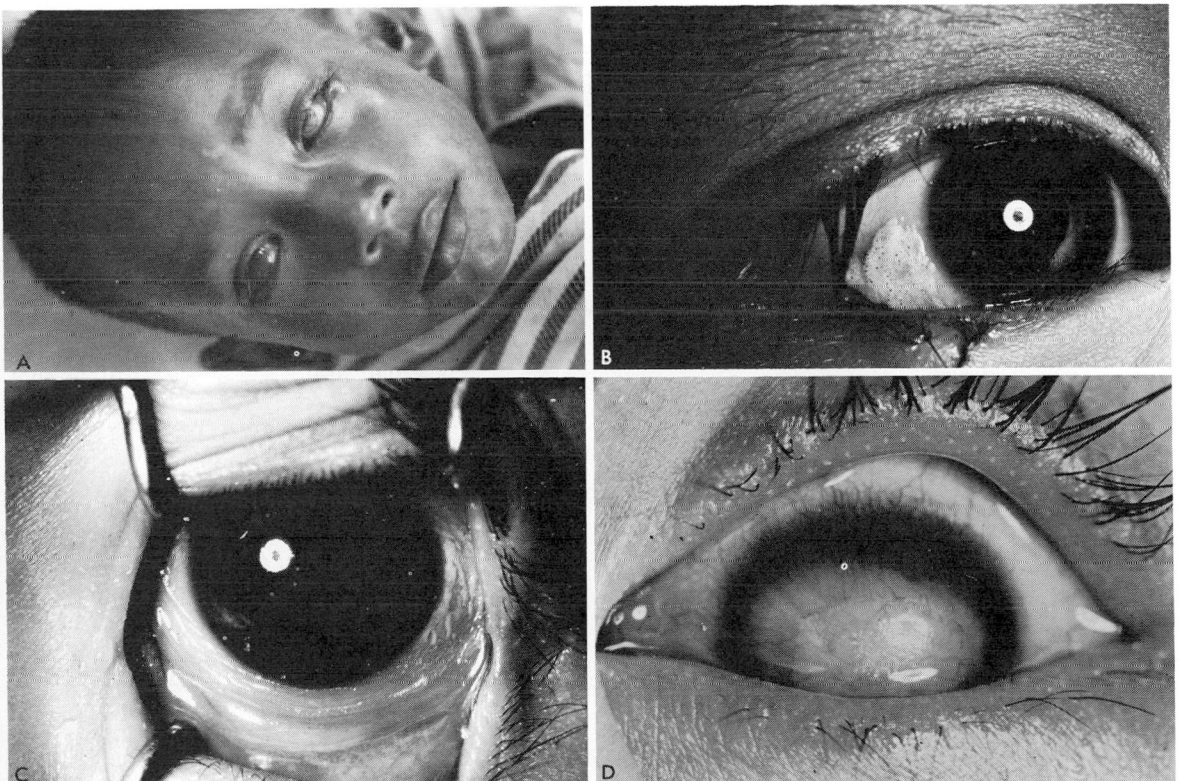

FIGURE 2. *A*, Keratomalacia in four year old boy. *Left eye:* Perforation of cornea, through which lens has escaped, with drop of vitreous substance visible on lower lid. *Right eye:* Necrosis of cornea with small ulcer. *B*, Bitot spot on transparent conjunctiva, nine year old child. *C*, Xerosis conjunctivae, showing Bitot spot and dryness of mucosal folds, four year old boy. *D*, Xerophthalmia with subtotal leukoma, after measles with perforating xerosis of cornea, in three year old child. (Courtesy of Dr. H. A. P. C. Oomen.)

trophy (Whipple's disease), hypovitaminosis A is likely to result. The liver contains 90 per cent of vitamin A stores, but these may be markedly reduced in some hepatic diseases.

Lowered dietary intake of preformed vitamin A or of an active carotene precursor is the most obvious and common factor in hypovitaminosis A, but any condition interfering with the intestinal absorption and conversion of carotene to vitamin A and its transport to the liver will contribute to deficiency of this vitamin. Surgical removal of sections of the small bowel or excessive consumption of mineral oil are in this category. So are massive intestinal infections with *Giardia lamblia* and probably also ascaris and hookworm. Severe protein deficiency (kwashiorkor) decreases the availability of transport protein.

Systemic infections precipitate clinical vitamin A deficiency in persons already in a borderline status, not only by further reducing appetite and dietary intake, but also by decreasing vitamin A levels in the blood and inducing vitamin A loss in the urine, which does not occur in healthy individuals. Dried skim milk fed to protein-deficient children in Indonesia increased the frequency of xerophthalmia, presumably by removing the limitation of protein and calories on growth and thereby increasing the need for vitamin A which the milk did not contain.

Treatment. Treatment consists of administration of therapeutic amounts of vitamin A, correction of the pattern of dietary intake, and, in cases of secondary deficiency, therapy of the underlying disease. In young children without serious eye involvement, the daily oral administration of 3000 μg. of retinol is recommended. When there is reason to suspect that dietary fat, including the fat-soluble vitamin A, is not properly absorbed, the new water-miscible vitamin A preparations are indicated rather than fish liver oil. If no response is observed, or signs of keratomalacia are present, doses of 15,000 to 25,000 μg. of retinol should be given intramuscularly for the first week in an attempt to prevent permanent impairment of vision. Improvement may be seen within a week, but maximal healing may take many weeks. If the lens is intact, residual corneal scarring can sometimes be treated by transplant.

When hypovitaminosis A is associated with protein deficiency, dietary protein alone will bring a prompt increase in serum vitamin A levels if the stores in the liver are adequate. Conversely, if protein deficiency is present, hypovitaminosis A will not respond to treatment with the vitamin alone owing to the lack of transport protein.

Prevention. Primary prevention depends upon assuring a diet with adequate vitamin A activity to meet all body needs and to maintain good stores of vitamin A in the liver. Foods of animal origin such as dairy products containing butter fat, egg yolk, liver, and fish liver oils are excellent sources. Sufficient quantities of the provitamin beta-carotene and other active carotenoids are also found in many vegetables and fruits. For populations in tropical and less developed countries, most of the vitamin A activity in the diet can come from fruits such as the mango and papaya. African palm oil, used in cooking in many parts of the world, is rich in vitamin A activity.

When processing has reduced the vitamin A activity of a food or when substitute foods of lower vitamin A content are introduced, fortification may be indicated. For example, margarine is routinely fortified with 10,000 I.U. of vitamin A per pound because it replaces butter, a good source of this vitamin. Similarly, skim milk for human consumption should be fortified with water-miscible vitamin A, because all vitamin A activity has been removed with the cream. Synthetic breakfast drinks replacing natural fruit juices can be made good sources of vitamin A.

Prevention of deficiency secondary to other disease requires measures to control the primary cause. Most important will be environmental sanitation and other public health measures to reduce the prevalence of infections.

Federation of American Societies for Experimental Biology: Nutritional Disease, Proceedings of a Conference on Beriberi, Endemic Goiter and Hypovitaminosis A, Held at Princeton, New Jersey, June 1-5, 1958. Fed. Proc. 17: Part II, Supplement No. 2, 1958, pp. 103-143.

McLaren, D. S.: Malnutrition and the Eye. New York, Academic Press, Inc., 1963.

Scrimshaw, N. S., Taylor, C. E., and Gordon, J. E.: Interactions of Nutrition and Infection. World Health Organization, Monograph Series No. 57. Geneva, World Health Organization, 1968.

RICKETS AND OSTEOMALACIA

Definition. Rickets is a disease of infancy and early childhood caused by deficiency of vitamin D. The characteristic rachitic deformities are caused by deficient calcification of growing cartilage and newly formed bone. As the body can obtain the vitamin either from absorption of ingested vitamin D or by synthesis in the skin under the influence of ultraviolet light, rickets occurs only when both diet and exposure to sunlight are insufficient. In the adult, vitamin D deficiency may result in osteomalacia, a generalized rarefaction and demineralization of bone sometimes seen in women in Eastern countries protected from sunlight by their customary clothing. (See article on The Osteomalacias in Diseases of Bone.)

ENDEMIC GOITER

Endemic goiter is a disease resulting from an absolute or relative lack of ingested iodine for the needs of the thyroid gland which therefore undergoes compensatory hypertrophy. Iodine administration returns the gland to normal size in a few weeks or months unless, as in cases of long-standing deficiency, the gland has undergone fibrosis. Severe iodine deficiency during pregnancy predisposes to cretinism, and probably also to deaf-mutism and feeblemindedness in the offspring. Iodization of salt is an inexpensive and effective way of eliminating endemic goiter as a public health problem. (See article on Thyroid in Diseases of the Endocrine System.)

ARIBOFLAVINOSIS

Definition. Ariboflavinosis is due to inadequate dietary intake of riboflavin or to some conditioning factor which impairs absorption or utilization of the vitamin, and is characterized by nonspecific lesions of the skin, lips, tongue, and eyes.

Etiology and Distribution. The intake of riboflavin must be low for many months before symptoms become evident. Among persons whose diets contain limited riboflavin, the disease often appears during periods of physiologic stress such as pregnancy and lactation, and during the rapid growth of childhood. Ariboflavinosis is so commonly associated with diets deficient in niacin and protein that for years it was considered part of the pellagra syndrome.

From published intake-excretion data obtained in subjects consuming abundant levels of riboflavin, infants have been calculated to require 0.1 and adults 0.75 mg. per kilogram to maintain tissue saturation. This amounts to 1.5 mg. per day for a 58-kg. female and 1.7 mg. per day for a 70-kg. male. For practical purposes, this does not differ from the FAO/WHO recommendation of 0.55 mg. of riboflavin per 1000 calories for persons of all ages. Characteristic deficiency signs appear in persons on deficient diets for three to eight months, depending upon the exact level of riboflavin and individual variation.

Low urinary riboflavin excretion levels and mild clinical signs of ariboflavinosis are common among the low-income populations of developing countries. Moderate to severe ariboflavinosis is usually seen only in association with other deficiency diseases such as pellagra and kwashiorkor. In the industrialized countries it is likely to be one of the deficiencies seen in alcoholics and persons with long-standing infections, malignancies, and other chronic debilitating diseases.

Clinical Signs. Signs seen in experimental riboflavin deficiency include cheilosis, redness of the lips, angular stomatitis, and denudation of the mucocutaneous junction, with maceration and fissures of the angles of the mouth. A seborrheic type of dermatitis involves the nasolabial folds, the alae nasi, the vestibule of the nose, and occasionally the ears and inner and outer canthi of the eyes.

Early symptoms of ariboflavinosis are soreness and burning of the lips, mouth, and tongue, and photophobia, lacrimation, burning, and itching of the eyes. The lesions of the lips described above may progress so that fissures extend from the angles of the mouth for a centimeter or more, and the lips themselves may appear dry and chapped. Shallow ulcerations and crusting sometimes de-

velop. Neither the cheilosis nor the angular stomatitis is pathognomonic of riboflavin deficiency, since similar lesions may result from deficiency of niacin, iron, or pyridoxine. Changes at the angles of the mouth may also be due to poorly fitting dentures, malocclusions, or unknown causes.

The seborrheic type of dermatitis has a scaly, greasy appearance and is associated with erythema. Hard sebaceous plugs or fine filiform comedones may be seen over the bridge of the nose and on the malar prominences and chin. Dermatitis of the scrotum and vulva may also appear. In some instances, the redness, scaling, and desquamation of the skin of the scrotum extend to adjacent areas of the thigh which become raw and weeping.

The tongue in ariboflavinosis is characteristically purplish red or magenta in color and often has deep fissures. The papillae may be swollen, flattened, or mushroom-shaped, giving a pebbled appearance. In chronic deficiency the papillae may become atrophic. The glossitis of riboflavin deficiency cannot be clearly differentiated from that caused by lack of niacin, folic acid, or vitamin B_{12}.

Eye signs responding to administration of riboflavin include diffuse inflammation of the conjunctivae, and red, swollen eyelids with a sticky exudate. Photophobia may be intense. Injection and proliferation of the capillaries of the limbic plexus may develop, but similar circumcorneal vascularization occurs with many types of trauma and infection and with other nutritional deficiencies.

Biochemical Function. Riboflavin functions as a coenzyme of the active prosthetic group of flavoproteins concerned with oxidative processes. Among these are cytochrome-c reductase, D- and L-amino oxidases, succinic dehydrogenase, diaphorase, and xanthine and aldehyde oxidases.

The concentrations of free riboflavin, flavin mononucleotide and flavin dinucleotide in plasma can be readily measured, but are not reliable indicators of deficiency, nor are white or red blood cell levels of riboflavin any more specific. Either 24-hour urinary excretion of riboflavin or the excretion four hours after subcutaneous administration of 1.0 mg. will be found reduced in those whose diets have been deficient in riboflavin for an extended period. Less than 50 mg. in 24 hours or 20 μg. in the four hours following the test dose indicate that prior intake has been inadequate.

Prevention and Treatment. Prevention requires a diet which includes foods that are rich sources of riboflavin such as milk, liver, other meats, eggs, and many green and yellow vegetables. For treatment, an adequate diet should be prescribed, and 5 mg. of riboflavin given orally twice a day. Symptoms disappear in a few days, and the lesions clear up in a few weeks. In general, it is better to give a multivitamin preparation in treating ariboflavinosis because of the frequency of simultaneous deficiency of other B vitamins. When signs sug-

gestive of such deficiencies are present, therapeutic doses of the appropriate vitamins should
also be given.

Goldsmith, G. A.: The B vitamins: Thiamine, riboflavin, niacin.
In Beaton, G. H., and McHenry, E. W. (eds.): Nutrition: A
Comprehensive Treatise. Vol. II. New York. Academic
Press, Inc., 1964, chap. 2, p. 145.

PELLAGRA

Definition. Pellagra is a deficiency disease
resulting from an insufficient dietary supply of
niacin and its precursor, tryptophan. It is characterized by a dermatitis on areas exposed to
sunlight and inflammation of mucosal surfaces.
Confusion, hallucination, and other mental abnormalities may be serious.

Etiology and Distribution. Although pellagra is
caused by a primary dietary deficiency of niacin,
the adequacy of dietary niacin is influenced by the
quantity and quality of dietary protein, and particularly by the availability of tryptophan, which
is a metabolic precursor of niacin. The term "niacin" is generic for both nicotinic acid and nicotinamide. One niacin equivalent is defined as
1 mg. of niacin or 60 mg. of tryptophan. The
minimum required to prevent pellagra is 4.4
niacin equivalents per 1000 kcal. per day, and a
recommended allowance of 6.6 niacin equivalents
per 1000 calories per day allows for individual
variation.

Pellagra is traditionally associated with maize
(corn) diets because this cereal grain has a low
tryptophan as well as niacin content. It does not
occur, however, where maize diets are supplemented with sufficient legume protein, as they are
in Central America. It is still seen in the Yucatan
peninsula of Mexico where the raising of hene-
quen, maguey, hemp, or sisal takes most of the
land, and in corn-eating populations of several
Middle Eastern and African countries, notably in
Egypt and Lesotho. In the 1930's it was still common in the southern United States among low-
income groups whose diets consisted mainly of
pork fat and hominy grits made from degerminated
corn, but the disease has now disappeared from the
United States except in alcoholics. Until recently
it was still seen among corn-eating populations
of rural Yugoslavia, Rumania, and Greece.

The pellagra common in Indian populations
subsisting on a diet of jowar (millet, *Sorghum
vulgare*) is reported to be influenced by the relative excess of leucine as well as the low tryptophan
and niacin of this cereal. Diets containing protein
of animal origin or vegetable proteins of good
quality contain enough tryptophan to prevent
pellagra even when niacin intakes are low.

Experimental niacin-tryptophan deficiency in
human subjects duplicates most but not all of the
features of pellagra as it occurs in populations,
because in the latter there are nearly always other
complicating diseases and deficiencies. Pellagra
in the industrialized countries at the present time
is generally a result of the vitamin- and protein-
deficient diets of chronic alcoholics.

Deficiency of folic acid probably accounts for the
frequency of megaloblastic anemia in pellagra.
The cheilosis, angular stomatitis, proctitis, scrotal
dermatitis, and vaginitis may be more related to
concomitant deficiency of riboflavin (vitamin B_2)
or vitamin B_6 than to that of niacin. The neurologic
and mental symptoms, especially the cord degeneration sometimes found, could possibly be
caused by poor vitamin B_{12} absorption. Reversible
achlorhydria often occurs. The peripheral neuropathy and occasional mental changes, suggesting
Korsakoff's psychosis, are possibly due to concomitant deficiency of thiamin or pyridoxine.
Since fatty liver may be present, deficiency of
protein and especially of choline and methionine
must also be considered.

Pellagra is encountered in patients with cirrhosis of the liver, chronic diarrheal disease,
diabetes mellitus, and neoplasia. Prolonged
infectious diseases such as tuberculosis, or thyrotoxicosis may lead to deficiency owing to an increase in niacin requirement. Pellagrous dermatitis has also been reported in patients with
malignant carcinoid, a rare tumor which may
convert as much as 60 per cent of the body's tryptophan to serotonin instead of the usual 1 per cent.
Decreased food intake and diarrhea presumably
contribute to the development of pellagra in this
condition.

Hartnup disease is a familial condition that
presents with a skin rash identical to that of pellagra in character and distribution. Mental
changes suggesting those seen in pellagra also
occur. The metabolic abnormality is not fully
known, but in addition to aminoaciduria there is
a pronounced excretion of indican and indolacetic
acid in the urine, both largely, if not entirely,
products of catabolism of tryptophan by intestinal
bacteria. A few studies of pellagra patients have
also revealed increased excretion of indole derivatives in the urine. The similarity of these two
diseases certainly suggests a common defect.

Clinical Manifestations. The early signs of pellagra are nonspecific and include lassitude,
anorexia, weakness, digestive disturbances, and
often anxiety, irritability, and depression. As the
deficiency progresses, soreness of the tongue gives
way to severe inflammation of mucous membranes
manifested by glossitis, stomatitis, esophagitis,
diarrhea, urethritis, proctitis, and vaginitis. The
mouth may be so painful that it is difficult to take
even liquids, and the mucous membranes become
bright red. The tongue is scarlet and swollen,
with atrophy of the papillae. Not surprisingly,
severe weight loss ensues.

The chronic dermatitis of pellagra may be difficult to distinguish from extensive exposure to
dust and sunlight. It varies with the acuteness and
severity of the deficiency state. At the earlier,
acute stages it resembles sunburn. In chronic
pellagra, which has developed more slowly, skin
changes include thickening, scaling, hyperkeratin-
ization, and pigmentation. Either type will usually

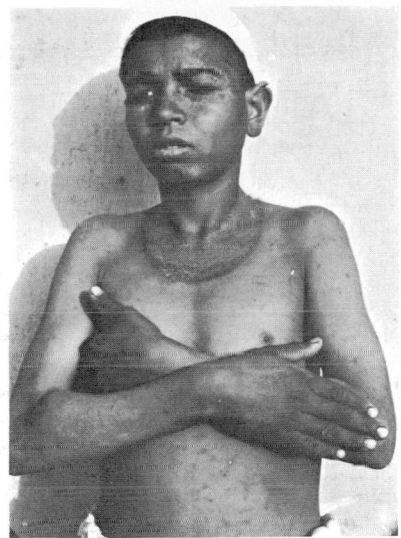 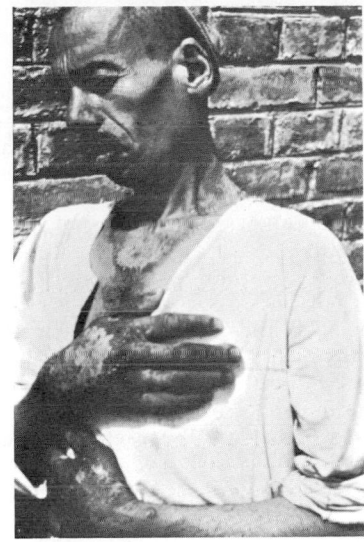

FIGURE 3. Modern pellagra. Egypt and the Balkans. (Courtesy of Dr. William J. Darby.)

be found on areas of skin exposed to sunlight—the backs of the hands and forearms, the anterior surfaces of the feet and lower legs, and the face and neck. Lesions following the sharp neckline of a dress or an open shirt are known as Casal's necklace. Other areas which may be involved are the axillae, groin, perineum, genitalia, elbows, knees, and skin under the breasts.

The early nonspecific psychic and emotional changes of early pellagra may, with increasing severity, progress to disorientation, delirium, and hallucination. The dementia may be hyperactive and manic or apathetic, lethargic, and stuporous. Other sensory and neurologic abnormalities and acute encephalopathy have been described in some cases. Anemia from associated deficiencies is common.

Biochemistry and Pathology. Nicotinamide functions in the body as the component of two important coenzymes, DPN (diphosphopyridine nucleotide) and TPN (triphosphopyridine nucleotide), which are functional groups in intracellular oxidation-reduction enzyme systems necessary for tissue respiration, glycolysis, and fat synthesis. In endemic pellagra the combined excretion of the niacin metabolites, N^1-methylnicotinamide and pyridone, seldom exceeds 2 grams daily.

The skin lesions are hyperkeratotic, often with vesicles containing erythrocytes, fibrin, and melanin pigment. Atrophy of the sebaceous glands and hair follicles and degeneration of the peripheral nerves of the skin are seen microscopically. Pathologic changes have also been reported in the brain, spinal cord, and peripheral nerves. Mucous membranes show inflammation and atrophy.

Treatment and Prevention. The treatment of pellagra is a diet adequate in niacin and tryptophan and the administration of therapeutic doses of the vitamin. The best food sources of niacin are yeast, liver, lean meat, poultry, peanuts, and legumes. Potatoes, other vegetables, and whole wheat cereal and bread are fair sources. Most of these are also good sources of tryptophan as well. Although milk and eggs contain little niacin, they are also protective against pellagra because of their high tryptophan content. Enrichment of cereal flours with niacin and other B vitamins is a simple and inexpensive way of ensuring an ample intake of these nutrients.

In severe deficiency, niacinamide may be given in divided doses of 50 to 100 mg. to a total of 300 to 500 mg. for the first few days and then decreased to 150 mg. daily. When circumstances make oral administration difficult, niacinamide can also be given intramuscularly in a dose of 100 mg. three times daily. In advanced pellagra, bed rest is essential, and calorie intakes up to 3500 per day may be required. Acute symptoms improve within a few days, but several weeks of therapy may be required for complete recovery. Because concurrent deficiencies of other B vitamins are generally present, a multivitamin tablet, which includes 5.0 mg. each of thiamin, riboflavin, and pyridoxine, should be given daily. Associated anemia may require either folic acid or iron therapy.

Goldsmith, G. A.: The B vitamins: Thiamine, riboflavin, niacin. *In* Beaton, G. H., and McIlenry, E. W. (eds.): Nutrition: A Comprehensive Treatise. Vol. II. New York, Academic Press, Inc., 1964, chap. 2, p. 161.

Goldsmith, G. A., Sarett, H. P., Register, U. D., and Gibbens, J.: Studies of niacin requirements in man. I. Experimental pellagra in subjects on corn diets low in niacin and tryptophan. J. Clin. Invest., 31:533, 1952.

Spies, T. D.: Niacinamide malnutrition and pellagra. *In* Jolliffe, N. (ed.): Clinical Nutrition. 2nd ed. New York, A Hoeber Medical Book, Harper & Brothers, 1962, chap. 18, p. 622.

Spies, T. D., Aring, C. D., Gelperin, J., and Bean, W. B.: The mental symptoms of pellagra. Their relief with nicotinic acid. Amer. J. Med. Sci., 196:461, 1938.

BERIBERI

Definition. Beriberi is the most common and important syndrome associated with thiamin deficiency. It occurs in both infants and adults as an acute disease with cardiac abnormalities, edema, altered tendon reflexes, and paresthesias. It may also be a more chronic disease in which peripheral neuropathy is the primary clinical feature. Wernicke's syndrome (see Nutritional Disorders of the Central Nervous System) is often associated with beriberi and responds dramatically to thiamin therapy; Korsakoff's psychosis found among alcoholics is closely related to it.

Etiology and Distribution. Beriberi occurs mainly in countries where polished rice provides a diet low in thiamin and high in carbohydrate. Among prisoners subsisting largely on polished rice in Japanese prison camps during World War II, beriberi developed when the thiamin supply was less than 0.3 mg. per 1000 nonfat calories, with the acute episode usually precipitated by dysentery or other infectious disease. Deficiency signs may be anticipated when dietary intakes are less than 0.2 mg. per 1000 calories, and intakes of 0.5 mg. or more per 1000 calories are recommended. Because it is possible that older persons utilize thiamin less efficiently, they should maintain an intake of 1.0 mg. per day, even when they are consuming less than 2000 kcal. daily. The allowance of 0.5 mg. per 1000 calories also applies to pregnant and lactating women and to children.

Beriberi is still seen occasionally in the rice-eating populations of Southeast Asia and the Indian subcontinent, and infantile beriberi has actually increased in some villages where newly introduced gasoline mills more completely separate the germ from the endosperm than traditional hand-pounding. Beriberi has been described in some populations of Brazil and Africa among persons consuming cassava as the primary source of calories. It may also occur in association with pathologic states which interfere with the ingestion or absorption of food, and it is the most important of the B vitamin deficiencies common to alcoholism.

Clinical Characteristics. The great majority of cases of beriberi are of the mild, subacute form, in which paresthesias and altered reflexes are the most characteristic findings. The muscle groups involved seem related to the length of the nerve controlling them, the amount of work they do, and possibly their blood supply. Laborers complain of disturbances of the lower legs, women more often of sensations in the fingers; other distributions can be related to the occupational use of muscle groups. Fullness or tightening of the muscles and fatigue pains resembling those of muscle ischemia are prominent, and, especially at night, muscle cramps occur.

In well developed cases, tachycardia is present, and the heart is enlarged. The edema may be generalized and massive or minimal without clear relation to the severity of the other symptoms. The most common characteristics of acute beriberi in prisoners of the Japanese in World War II were persistent tachycardia, symmetrical foot and wrist drop associated with muscle tenderness, mild disturbances of sensation over the outer aspects of the legs and thighs, and in patches over the abdomen, chest, and forearms. Most of these signs and symptoms have been reproduced experimentally in 30 to 120 days in adult subjects on thiamin intakes from 0.075 to 0.2 mg. per 1000 calories.

The acute fulminating form of beriberi has been called Shoshin; it is dominated by insufficiency of the heart and blood vessels. The milder forms may develop into this often fatal type, but more often it is of sudden onset. When nerve lesions develop early, the heart is saved from extreme insufficiency because the patient is forced to rest. In terminal cases, severe dyspnea and violent palpitations of the heart allow the patient no rest, and precordial pain may be intense. The patient tosses and turns about violently and complains of heaviness, constriction, oppression, and sometimes actual pain over the epigastrium. The moans and shrieks of the patient are distorted by the coincident hoarseness and sometimes aphonia. Pupils are dilated, and respirations are frequent and superficial. The liver and heart are enlarged and the heart action tumultuous. Cyanosis is obvious, and the pulse is weak but regular.

The chronic, dry, atrophic type—with wrist drop and foot drop—is generally found only in older adults. They no longer show the biochemical changes characteristic of acute beriberi, nor do they respond satisfactorily to therapy.

The beriberi seen in *infants*, particularly from one to four months of age, is associated with poor thiamin content of, and possibly abnormal metabolites in, the breast milk of mothers subsisting on a rice diet. It begins with vomiting, restlessness, pallor, anorexia, and insomnia, and evolves variously. In acute infantile beriberi, the infant develops cyanosis, dyspnea, and running pulse with cardiac crises which are often fatal. If the process is more chronic, the symptoms are vomiting, inanition, anorexia, aphonia, opisthotonos, edema, oliguria, constipation, and meteorism. A subacute form is also described which may evolve into either the acute or chronic type. The infant develops puffiness, vomiting, oliguria, abdominal pain, dysphagia, aphonia, and even convulsions. These forms are not really distinct, and the signs and symptoms may be present in almost any combination. Case fatality is very high unless treatment is given.

Biochemistry and Pathology. Thiamin functions in carbohydrate metabolism as a coenzyme in the decarboxylation of alpha-keto acids and in the utilization of pentose in the hexose-monophosphate shunt. Pyruvic acid tends to accumulate in the tissues in severe thiamin deficiency. Because thiamin pyrophosphate is a coenzyme in the reaction, reduced transketolase activity can be detected in the red blood cells of persons consuming diets low in thiamin. Urinary excretion of thiamin of 0 to 14 μg. in 24 hours has been reported in beriberi, and early signs have been observed with excretions of less than 40 μg. in 24 hours.

The pathology of thiamin-deficient states ranges from maximal disturbance of function with minimal histologic abnormalities in acute, severe deficiency to minimal biochemical changes and well defined peripheral nerve lesions in chronic deficiency. In fatal cases, hypertrophy of the heart is a constant finding.

Degeneration is found not only in peripheral, but also in cerebrospinal nerves, in terminal branches of the vagus and phrenic nerves, and sometimes in the spinal cord and fibers of the posterior root. In Wernicke's encephalopathy, histologic changes are found chiefly in the mamillary bodies, the related walls of the third ventricle, and the aqueduct and tegmentum of the medulla.

Treatment and Prevention. The treatment of beriberi consists of a balanced diet plus the administration of 5.0 to 10.0 mg. of thiamin three times daily. In severe beriberi the thiamin should be given parenterally for the first few days, but oral administration is satisfactory for the treatment of most cases. Delay in the treatment of Wernicke's syndrome may result in cardiac death or in permanent cerebral damage with signs of Korsakoff's syndrome. Because other B vitamin deficiencies are often present in beriberi, a multivitamin preparation is also advisable.

The biochemical lesions are rapidly reversed, but structural defects require long recovery periods. Signs of heart failure disappear within a few days; within a few weeks the heart returns to normal size, and electrocardiographic abnormalities disappear. In long-standing cases of advanced neuropathy, complete restoration to normal may be impossible, although improvement may continue for many months.

Prevention requires an increase in the intake of thiamin for persons consuming rice diets. Parboiling causes the thiamin to pass into the grain so that it is not removed in the milling process. In practice, efforts to encourage parboiling or the use of home-pounded and undermilled rice have not been successful. Enrichment of rice at the mill with thiamin, riboflavin, and niacin has not been adopted by those countries needing it most. A generally improved diet, containing foods which are good sources of thiamin, and extensive distribution of synthetic thiamin are the measures which have been most effective in Asia.

Federation of American Societies for Experimental Biology: Nutritional Disease, Proceedings of a Conference on Beriberi, Endemic Goiter and Hypovitaminosis A, Held at Princeton, New Jersey, June 1-5, 1958. Fed. Proc., 17: Part II, Supplement No. 2, September, 1958, pp. 3-56.

Goldsmith, G. A.: The B Vitamins: Thiamine, riboflavin, niacin, *In* Beaton, G. H., and McHenry, E. W. (eds.): A Comprehensive Treatise, Vol. II. New York, Academic Press, Inc., 1964, chap. 2, p. 109.

Spillane, J. D.: Nutritional Disorders of the Nervous System. Baltimore, Williams and Wilkins Company, 1947.

Weiss, S., and Wilkins, R. W.: The nature of the cardiovascular disturbances in nutritional deficiency states (beriberi). Ann. Intern. Med., 11:104, 1937.

SCURVY

Definition. Scurvy is a disease caused by prolonged deficiency of ascorbic acid (vitamin C). Infantile and adult scurvy have in common skin, hair, and gum changes, bleeding into the skin and deep tissues, impaired wound healing, mental depression, and, often, anemia. In infantile scurvy, rapidly growing bones are affected as well. Ascorbic acid is particularly needed for the formation of normal connective tissue (collagen and ground substance), and for resistance to infection.

Etiology and Distribution. Most mammals are able to synthesize ascorbic acid from glucose by way of glucuronic acid. Man and the guinea pig lack the enzyme required for conversion of gluconate to ascorbate. If dietary intake of the vitamin ceases for several months, clinical scurvy develops.

Scurvy has most commonly occurred in the spring in temperate climates or at the end of the dry season in tropical ones, because of the relative lack of fresh fruit and vegetables during the preceding months and because several months are required for the disease to become manifest. Although now rare, the disease is still seen in exceptional circumstances, and the treatment is specific and effective. The minimal daily requirement for ascorbic acid is controversial. A group of British volunteers remained in good health and had normal wound healing on a daily intake of 10 mg. for almost a year, although plasma and leukocyte ascorbic acid contents were very low. In a notable human experiment by Crandon, under controlled conditions with complete deficiency of the vitamin, the plasma level of ascorbic acid fell to zero by the forty-first day, but abnormal hair and hair follicles appeared only after four months. Perifollicular hemorrhages were not evident until after five months on the experimental diet. Subjective symptoms of a less specific nature — fatigability and anorexia — preceded the appearance of objective signs.

Biochemistry and Pathology. The effect of ascorbic acid on enzymes depends on its properties as either a strong reducing agent or the source of peroxide from its oxidation with air. It is a reactant with such well defined enzyme systems as hydroxylation to form norepinephrine, 5-hydroxylation of tryptophan, tyrosine oxidase, and a number of others. In the oxidation of p-hydroxyphenylpyruvic acid, it protects the enzyme involved from inhibition by its substrate, a necessary function when large amounts of tyrosine are being metabolized. It is also a specific reductant of the ferric ion in its transfer from plasma transferrin to liver ferritin.

It is needed also for the conversion of proline to hydroxyproline and the synthesis of chondroitin sulfate in the ground substance of collagen; hydroxyproline is an amino acid found only in collagen. Ascorbic acid is a necessary component of the mucopolysaccharides of ground substance. In the vitamin's absence, defective ground substance is formed, and can be seen by electron microscopy to have lost its characteristic periodicity. At any rate, scar tissue does not form. Ascorbic acid is involved in the preservation of folinic acid, the reduced form of folic acid. Perhaps this contributes to the occasional macrocytic anemia seen in scurvy by diminishing the amount of folinic acid available. There is no good evidence that ascorbic acid is itself required for erythropoiesis.

The pathologic changes in scurvy are predominantly in the mesenchymal tissues of the body, especially in collagen, growing bones, teeth, and blood vessels. In growing bones the histopathology of scurvy is distinctive: a suppression of the orderly growth process and of the normal calcification of the cartilage matrix. In addition, hemorrhages may be found in the interior of the bone at the cartilage-shaft junction, together with fractures of the minute columns of cartilage matrix and, at times, dislocation, separation, or impaction of the epiphyses.

Subperiosteal hemorrhages are relatively uncommon in the adult but frequent in infantile scurvy. Loosening of the periosteal attachment leads to capillary bleeding, which may dissect the periosteum free over a large area. Most frequently these subperiosteal hemorrhages are found at the lower end of the femur, the upper end of the humerus, both ends of the tibia, and the costochondral junctions of the middle ribs.

Capillaries in the skin become fragile, and petechiae, ecchymoses, and hematomas result. Hemorrhages into the gums lead to swelling, tissue friability, and even gangrene.

The teeth become loose because of resorption of alveolar bone. In children the teeth also show abnormalities of development, with poorly formed matrix and porous dentine.

The laboratory detection of this deficiency or confirmation of the clinical diagnosis of scurvy requires measurement of the plasma or leukocyte concentration of ascorbic acid, or the urinary excretion of the vitamin with or without a "loading" test. With low levels of dietary ascorbic acid intake, plasma ascorbic acid levels fall sharply, but even levels below 0.2 mg. may be associated with a wide range of tissue saturations, from 0 to approximately 50 per cent. At this level of nutriture, the white blood cell–platelet ascorbic acid level is most useful. It will average 20 to 30 mg. per 100 ml. in a well nourished subject, and on an ascorbic acid–free diet decrease to 0 to 2 mg. per 100 ml. in three to five months. Clinical scurvy usually appears shortly thereafter.

Clinical Manifestations. Malaise, weakness, and lassitude are early and constant symptoms. Shortness of breath and aching in the bones and joints follow. The most distinctive physical sign and one of the earliest is perifollicular hemorrhage, usually in hyperkeratotic hair follicles, appearing particularly on the posterior thighs, anterior

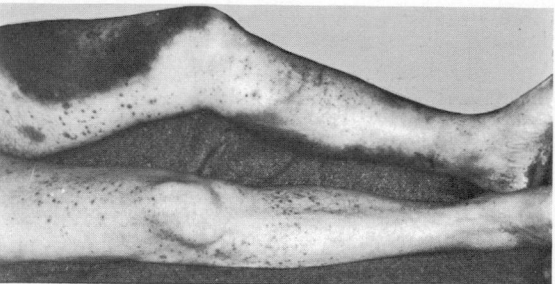

FIGURE 4. Ecchymoses, petechiae, and perifollicular hemorrhages on legs of patient with scurvy.

forearms, and abdomen. The hairs become fragmented, coiled, and buried in the follicles.

Petechiae are characteristic features of fully developed scurvy, and are usually most prominent in the same hair-bearing areas and in dependent parts of the body. Scorbutic petechiae are usually larger and more purplish than those in other forms of purpura, for example, in thrombocytopenia. Similarly, a tourniquet produces petechiae that are typically large and dark in color, appearing mostly on the hair-bearing areas of the forearm rather than on the flexor surface usually examined.

As scurvy becomes more advanced, ecchymoses appear, first at areas of irritation, pressure, or trauma. The "saddle area" and posterior thighs are the most frequent locations. Larger hemorrhages occur later in subcutaneous tissue, muscles, or joints, but are uncommon in the viscera, heart, or brain. Gums become swollen, inflamed, and "spongy," bleed easily, and are usually infected. Necrosis of gum tissue may follow. Gum changes are less pronounced in edentulous subjects.

In untreated disease of long duration, postural hypotension and syncope are common. They may be part of the preterminal state in which vomiting and frank hypotension occur, resembling an Addisonian crisis.

Anemia, normocytic or macrocytic, with resultant pallor, is frequent. Two major causes of anemia must be considered. First, and most important, is the blood loss into the skin and deeper tissues or, uncommonly, into the gastrointestinal tract. Second is the possibility that dietary intake of folic acid may also be deficient. Many foods are important sources of both folic acid and ascorbic acid, and the two deficiencies may potentiate one another.

Most cases of scurvy seen in infancy (*Barlow's disease*) develop six to twelve months after the institution of artificial feeding. A few examples have been reported in infants considerably younger, but in these instances the mothers habitually subsisted on a diet inadequate in ascorbic acid. The concentration of ascorbic acid in human milk, invariably higher than that in maternal plasma, closely reflects the mother's intake.

Loss of appetite, listlessness, and irritability are early and insidious signs of infantile scurvy. The bony lesions and subperiosteal hemorrhages lead to tenderness, swelling, and evidence of pain on movement. Bleeding into the costochondral junctions of the ribs is noted externally as swellings—the "scorbutic rosary." Purpura and gum changes are similar to those in the adult except that pre-existing gum infection is less common.

Significance of Ascorbic Acid in Clinical Medicine. Although scurvy is now a rare disease, in several important clinical situations the state of ascorbic acid nutrition is a significant consideration. Resistance to infection is reduced in ascorbic acid deficiency, and microbial diseases have long been recognized to precipitate scurvy in individuals on borderline intakes of this vitamin.

Healing of wounds is defective in scurvy because of poor collagen formation. Experimentally deficient subjects fail to form new collagen in experimental wounds until the vitamin is administered. Delayed healing of wounds, postoperative breakdown of incisions, and delayed union of fractures may sometimes be at least partly the result of unrecognized but severe ascorbic acid deficiency. It is also known that extensive trauma and infectious diseases lower the plasma concentration of the vitamin. Ascorbic acid appears to be transported to wounds soon after injury, its concentration rising there as the plasma concentration falls, perhaps because the vitamin is needed for new ground substance and collagen formation.

Patients with thermal burns may develop ascorbic acid deficiency, especially when the burns are extensive and deep. Large doses of the vitamin may be necessary to maintain even low-normal plasma concentrations. Such deficiency leads to delayed healing of burns and impaired skin graft "takes."

Attention to nutrient intake, including that of ascorbic acid, is an essential part of the medical care of many illnesses. For example, the diet prescribed for peptic ulcer may be almost free of ascorbic acid, a situation which favors bleeding rather than healing.

Treatment and Prevention. Small amounts of ascorbic acid will promptly reverse the florid clinical manifestations of scurvy. Even in severe scurvy, 100 mg. per day for several days, accompanied by a normal diet, usually produces rapid cure. Because retention is high in the deficient state, this is also sufficient to restore the normal 4- to 5-gram body content of the vitamin in a few weeks. Even if ascorbic acid is administered in very large amounts, i.e., several grams, the excess is harmlessly excreted in the urine.

Prevention requires a diet containing adequate ascorbic acid. The vitamin is present in most fresh fruits and vegetables, and in liver. Citrus fruits are particularly good sources. Synthetic ascorbic acid is chemically identical, and is very cheap.

Attention must be paid to the prevention of infantile scurvy, for the disease continues to occur sporadically in the United States in spite of our knowledge of prevention. At least 2 ounces of orange juice or its ascorbic acid equivalent should be given to all infants after the first month. All diets should either contain some fresh fruit and

vegetables as a source of ascorbic acid or be supplemented with synthetic vitamin C.

When extensive wounds, fractures, or chronic infections are treated, supplementary ascorbic acid should be given if any reasonable doubt exists regarding previous nutrition with this vitamin. Patients with deep and extensive burns may require large amounts of ascorbic acid (200 to 500 mg. daily) to maintain measurable blood concentrations.

Crandon, J. H., Lund, C. C., and Dill, D. B.: Experimental human scurvy. New Eng. J. Med., 223:253, 1940.
Levenson, S. M., Green, R. W., Taylor, F. H. L., Robinson, P., Page, R. C., Johnson, R. E., and Lund, C. C.: Ascorbic acid, riboflavin, thiamin, and nicotinic acid in relation to severe injury, hemorrhage and infection in the human. Ann. Surg., 124:840, 1946.
Sebrell, W. H., Jr., and Harris, R. S. (eds.): The Vitamins: Chemistry, Physiology, Pathology, Methods. New York, Academic Press, Inc., 1967. (See Chapter 2, Ascorbic Acid, p. 305.)
Woodruff, C. W.: Ascorbic Acid, In Beaton, G. H., and McHenry, E. W. (eds.): Nutrition, a Comprehensive Treatise. Vol. 2. New York, Academic Press, Inc., 1964, p. 265.

HYPERVITAMINOSIS A AND D

Nevin S. Scrimshaw

Vitamin A is not normally excreted except during disease states. Therefore, massive doses may lead to increased storage in the liver and hepatomegaly. Toxicity from hypervitaminosis A brought on by eating polar bear liver has been reported since 1596 by Arctic explorers. A 500-gram polar bear liver may contain over nine million I.U. of vitamin A, more than twenty times the total normal liver reserves in man. Toxic symptoms are drowsiness, irritability, severe headache, and vomiting within a few hours after ingestion. Acute hypervitaminosis A was reported in an infant given a single dose of 300,000 I.U. Drowsiness, hydrocephalus with protrusion of the fontanel, and vomiting ensued 12 hours after administration. Hepatosplenomegaly, hypoplastic anemia, leukopenia, precocious skeletal development, clubbing of the fingers, and coarse, sparse hair have been reported from long-continued high doses in children. Most symptoms, but not the hepatomegaly and abnormal bone growth, clear with discontinuation of the vitamin.

Overdosage of any form of vitamin D is dangerous. The syndrome of hypervitaminosis D is characterized by hypercalcemia and by generalized calcinosis (deposition of calcium phosphate in a matrix of mucoproteins) affecting joints, synovial membranes, kidneys, myocardium, pulmonary alveoli, parathyroid glands, pancreas, skin, lymph glands, arteries, conjunctivae and cornea of the eyes, and the acid-secreting portion of the stomach. In advanced stages, demineralization of the bones occurs.

The exact borderline between tolerable and

noxious doses is not known. Certainly the continuous ingestion of 150,000 I.U. per day may result in symptoms. It is possible that some infants may show hypercalcemia on relatively small doses of 2500 to 4000 I.U. per day. Retardation of linear growth in children has been reported with 1800 I.U. per day. Complete recovery usually occurs when vitamin D is withdrawn. Treatment should include lowering of the calcium intake and a generous fluid intake.

Dam, H., and Søndergaard, E.: Fat-soluble vitamins. *In* Beaton, G. H., and McHenry, E. W. (eds.): Nutrition, A Comprehensive Treatise. Vol. II. New York, Academic Press, Inc., 1964, pp. 34-35.
Sebrell, W. H., Jr., and Harris, R. S. (eds.): The Vitamins: Chemistry, Physiology, Pathology, Methods. Vol. I. 2nd ed. New York and London, Academic Press, Inc., 1967.
Stimson, W. H.: Vitamin A intoxication in adults. Report of a case with summary of the literature. New Eng. J. Med., 265:369, 1961.

OBESITY
Margaret J. Albrink

The differentiation of adipose tissue was a triumph of evolution. Phylogenetically the ability to store fat in true adipose tissue appeared first in the arthropods and became fully developed in birds and mammals; it was very likely an important factor in the liberation of life from the sea with its constant source of food. However, the ability to store fat in compact form, of great survival value when food was scarce, has become a handicap in affluent societies where overnutrition and underactivity have upset the ancient balance between caloric supply and demand. The consequence is obesity of epidemic proportions and the associated diseases of atherosclerosis, hypertension, and diabetes.

Definition. Obesity may be defined as excess adipose tissue. The dividing point between normal and excessive may be determined esthetically as fatness beyond the socially acceptable norms, or medically as adipose tissue in excess of that consistent with good health of mind and body. The latter definition includes the mild to moderate obesity characteristic of a large segment of our population, of paramount public health significance because of the associated toll of cardiovascular and other diseases.

Etiology. Obesity results from the relative excess of caloric intake over caloric expenditure. Most cases of obesity seen in common clinical practice are due to the interaction of cultural forces that encourage excess intake with genetic factors that, other things being equal, favor the synthesis of fat.

Cultural Factors. First the agricultural, then the industrial, and finally the computer revolution have all served to make food increasingly available and life livable with a minimum of physical exertion. An important cause of widespread moderate obesity in the United States is the plethora of purified foods of high caloric content but low nutrient value. International studies by Keys et al. have shown an inverse relationship between skinfold thickness and caloric intake, a clear indication of the importance of exercise.

Genetic Causes. Obesity, especially in its extreme form, tends to be familial. Obesity in children is much more common when both parents are obese than when neither parent is obese. Anabolic forces appear to be in operation from birth in very heavy people. (*Vide infra:* Central Nervous System Regulation.) Heavy children usually become heavy adults, and differ constitutionally from lean persons in being statistically of shorter stature and greater breadth of trunk and in having small hands and feet. The localization of extreme deposits of fat, such as the massive adipose tissue over the buttocks of certain Bushmen, the so-called "Hottentot bustle," is an instance of genetically determined localized adiposity. This extreme example suggests that a finite number of adipose cells may be allotted genetically to each individual and that the number and location of such cells or their precursors will determine in part the magnitude as well as the location of his obesity.

Endocrine Factors. Many endocrine and metabolic abnormalities have been reported in very obese persons. Whether they are cause or effect is not known. Insulin promotes the synthesis of fat. Large increases in postcibal insulin concentration are characteristic of obese persons, and are thought by some to be excessive in relation to the blood sugar level and to be the initiating event leading to obesity. Attractive as this theory is, the excess insulin is more likely the result than the cause of obesity.

A partial explanation for the hyperinsulinism of the obese may be found in the nature of the normal relationship between circulating insulin and glucose. A rise in plasma glucose in normal persons evokes a rise in circulating insulin, the insulin following the glucose in such a way that a linear relationship is maintained between the two when both are expressed on a logarithmic scale. A comparison of obese and thin persons with identical glucose tolerance reveals that the fasting insulin of the obese is slightly higher and the peak insulin considerably higher in arithmetic units than for the same points in the glucose tolerance curve for thin persons. The apparent excessive insulin rise above fasting is not excessive if the insulin is expressed on a logarithmic scale; rather, it is a normal log increase above the somewhat elevated fasting insulin levels. If the log of the fasting insulin is subtracted from the log of the postglucose insulins for both thin and obese, the resulting insulin values at each point of the glucose tolerance curve are identical for thin and obese. The increase in fasting insulin is thus the critical difference between thin and obese persons.

According to Felig and colleagues, the explanation for the elevated basal insulin may be the high fasting concentrations of those amino acids which stimulate the release of insulin and which are decreased in response to insulin. Insensitivity of the tissues to insulin, a basic characteristic of obese persons, accounts for the increase in insulin-sensitive substrates, such as certain amino acids as well as glucose and probably others. The fact of such insulin insensitivity is communicated to the pancreas by increased concentrations of such substrates, but the resulting increased insulin concentration is ineffective in restoring substrate levels to normal. The reason for the insulin insensitivity of the obese is not known. In the case of obese adipose tissue, insulin insensitivity is related to increased cell size. With weight reduction cell size returns to normal, and insulin sensitivity is restored.

The practical importance of even minor elevation in basal insulin for the obese is the burden on the pancreas of the resulting greatly increased postcibal demand for insulin. Over many years such increased insulin production may lead to pancreatic exhaustion and diabetes, accounting for the association between obesity and diabetes. When diabetes coincides with obesity, the rise of plasma insulin relative to plasma glucose following glucose ingestion is blunted, as in nonobese diabetics. The insulin increments, being superimposed on the increased basal levels, result in higher insulin values for each degree of glucose intolerance in the obese than in the nonobese. Weight loss greatly relieves the burden on the pancreas by decreasing both the basal and postcibal needs for insulin, with the result that glucose tolerance may become normal.

Adrenal Cortex. Although pathologic concentrations of various adrenal hormones are reported in obesity, overaction of the adrenal cortex is not implicated as the cause of simple obesity.

Pituitary. Several hormones of the anterior pituitary cause mobilization of fat from adipose tissue. The most important is growth hormone, which promotes mobilization and utilization of fat and conservation of protein and carbohydrate during caloric restriction. Hypoglycemia is the acute stimulus to growth hormone secretion. The increase of growth hormone in response to starvation is less marked in the obese than in the nonobese. The deficiency is secondary to the obesity and is corrected by weight loss. Although obese persons have elevated circulating free fatty acids after an overnight fast, they respond to prolonged fasting with a less than normal rise in free fatty acids, a phenomenon probably reflecting the deficiency of growth hormone response.

Sex Hormones. The sex hormones affect both the amount and distribution of fat. Women have a greater amount of subcutaneous fat than men. The relationship between parity and obesity and the frequent menopausal gain in weight, although difficult to document, suggest a possible role of female sex hormones in the regulation of fat metabolism. The obesity of eunuchs suggests further that absence of male sex hormones also promotes adiposity. The hypogonad obesity that occurs in children just prior to adolescence dis-appears with puberty, at which time the adult fat distribution of each sex takes place. The effect of sex hormones could be explained on the basis of emotional factors and physical activity rather than a direct effect on fat metabolism.

Thyroid. Thyroid function is normal in obese persons. Although thyroid hormone is commonly prescribed for obesity, weight loss is achieved only with toxic doses, and such treatment merely makes evaluation of thyroid function difficult because of resultant suppression of endogenous thyroid secretion. There is no evidence for a role of thyroid deficiency in the etiology of obesity.

Age. The tendency to gain weight with advancing age is associated with increased mortality from cardiovascular and other diseases, and can not be considered normal.

Central Nervous System Regulation of Food Intake. As the metabolic abnormalities of the obese turn out to be the result of the obesity rather than the cause, attention is increasingly turned to the central nervous system regulation of the intake of food. Knittle and Hirsch have shown that very early overfeeding in rats may "set" the regulatory centers in such a manner that obesity, manifest by an irreversibly increased number of adipose cells, persists in later life. The role of the central nervous system in controlling food intake resides chiefly in the hypothalamus. A satiety center in the ventral medial hypothalamus exerts an inhibitory influence on a neighboring feeding center. Destruction of the inhibitory center releases the feeding center, with resultant massive overeating and hypothalamic obesity. Brain injury in man on occasion causes obesity, but the extent to which variation in the balance between these centers contributes to ordinary obesity is unknown.

Behavioral and Emotional Aspects. Decreased activity rather than increased food intake is recognized in many obese persons, particularly obese women. Associated depression is a frequent concomitant of inactivity, and may be exaggerated by weight loss. The very obese person has a characteristic eating pattern in which the major caloric intake occurs at the evening meal or later. A distinctive personality type, if it exists, is more likely the result than the cause of obesity.

Like most of man's ills at one time or another, obesity has been blamed on the world's domineering mothers. The role of mothers in causing obesity in children can more likely be attributed to their enforcement in early life of patterns of overeating than to the psychologic effects of overprotection.

Pathology. Two general types of distribution of obesity are described. Obesity in the male is most pronounced in the upper trunk and spares the extremities. In the female, distribution is predominantly in the lower trunk and involves also the extremities, particularly the lower extremities. Obesity may be further divided into inherited obesity, which is generalized and involves the extremities as well as the trunk, and acquired obesity, which is localized mainly in the trunk.

Both the size of adipose cells and the number of cells are increased in obese persons. Obesity up to the time of maturity is due largely to increased numbers of adipose cells, and obesity acquired after maturity is due entirely to increased size of existing cells.

Excess adipose tissue is found subcutaneously, interspersed in muscle and about all organs. Extremely obese persons have generally enlarged organs; cardiac enlargement is mainly left ventricular, and may be due to the increased circulating blood volume and/or hypertension commonly present. The kidney, liver, and, indeed, the entire splanchnic area are of greater size than normal. Large fatty livers are frequently found in extreme obesity.

Pathologic findings may include those of the associated complications of hypertension and atherosclerosis.

Pathogenesis. The balance between fat synthesis and fat mobilization depends on several key reactions in the adipose cell and the influence of various hormones, as well as state of nutrition, on these reactions. A shift in the adipose cell toward increased synthesis of fat or decreased mobilization of fat would operate to cause obesity.

Synthesis of Triglyceride. Triglycerides are synthesized within the adipose cell from one alpha-glycerol-phosphate molecule and three fatty acid molecules. The latter may be synthesized within the adipose cell from glucose, a reaction favored by reduced nicotinamide adenine dinucleotide phosphate (NADPH) (reduced triphosphopyridine nucleotide), or may be derived from circulating triglycerides of dietary or endogenous origin. By contrast, the alpha-glycerol-phosphate must be derived from glucose metabolized within the adipose cell. The glycerol liberated from triglyceride breakdown cannot serve this purpose since adipose tissue lacks the enzyme, glycerol kinase, necessary for converting glycerol into alpha-glycerol-phosphate. The availability of carbohydrate thus determines the availability of alpha-glycerol-phosphate, which in turn is obligatory for triglyceride synthesis in adipose tissue.

Circulating triglycerides such as those present in chylomicrons are evidently available to the adipose cell only if they are first broken down into glycerol and free fatty acids, a reaction taking place at or near the adipose cell wall under the influence of the enzyme lipoprotein lipase. This enzyme is increased in the carbohydrate-fed state, decreased in starvation. Since the enzyme appears in the circulation after heparin injection, it is also called post-heparin lipoprotein lipase. The free fatty acids liberated by the action of lipoprotein lipase enter the adipose cell, where they are re-esterified into triglyceride, provided alpha-glycerol-phosphate is present. The latter must be derived from carbohydrate combustion. Carbohydrate combustion has the additional effect of generating NADPH via the pentose phosphate shunt, and NADPH favors the synthesis of fat from two-carbon precursors.

Insulin, through its stimulating action on carbohydrate metabolism, and possibly through a direct effect of inhibiting lipolysis, also favors the synthesis of fat in adipose tissue. Conversely, the lack of insulin or of carbohydrate causes impairment of lipogenesis and decreased lipoprotein lipase activity.

Fat Mobilization. Fat is mobilized entirely in the form of free fatty acids. The release of fat from the adipose cell is accomplished by activation of an intracellular lipolytic system different from lipoprotein lipase. The activation is dependent upon generation of cyclic adenosine monophosphate. This system splits triglycerides into free fatty acids and glycerol. The liberated free fatty acids are either re-esterified into triglyceride, provided conditions favor fat synthesis, or are transported into the circulation bound to albumin as free fatty acids, either to be utilized by tissue or transported to the liver for re-esterification into triglyceride and released as very low density lipoproteins. A rise in concentration of circulating free fatty acids is evidence of fat mobilization.

Fat mobilization is favored by various hormones that activate the lytic system, of which epinephrine, norepinephrine, and growth hormone are probably of the greatest physiologic significance. Factors that stimulate epinephrine secretion such as exercise and trauma thus activate mobilization of fat. The absence of carbohydrate combustion as in starvation or diabetic acidosis also results in fat mobilization either through activation of the lytic system or by prevention of re-esterification of fatty acids into triglycerides. Through these systems the deposition or mobilization of fat is regulated by the presence or absence of food, especially carbohydrate, and by the presence or absence of emergencies that require fat as fuel for sudden bursts of energy.

Obesity could result from primary defects in adipose tissue whereby lipolysis is diminished or lipogenesis increased. There is no convincing evidence for impaired lipolysis. Bray et al. have demonstrated a decreased mitochondrial oxidation of glycerol phosphate in the adipose tissue of obese humans. The resulting increased availability of glycerol phosphate for triglyceride synthesis could favor lipogenesis. Furthermore, oxidation of glycerol phosphate may regulate the efficiency with which oxidation and phosphorylation are coupled. Increase in the mitochondrial oxidation of glycerol phosphate, such as occurs with high caloric intake in normal persons, causes decreased caloric efficiency of food, more energy being lost as heat. Such a system might normally prevent excess weight gain with excess food intake by diverting calories to heat. A deficiency in the mitochondrial oxidation of glycerol phosphate in the obese might, by impairing ability to waste calories, cause weight gain. Although such a deficiency may be the exception, thus far the metabolic abnormalities appear to be the result rather than the cause of the obesity.

Manifestations and Complications. The sheer mechanical trauma of excessive body weight either aggravates or causes such troublesome ailments as osteoarthritis and flat feet, intertriginous dermatitis, varicose veins, ventral and diaphragmatic hernias. Cholelithiasis and cholecystitis are more common in the obese than in the lean.

Obesity — Hypoventilation Syndrome. Dickens' graphic description of Fat Joe, a character in *Pickwick Papers* who fell asleep at the most inopportune moments, led to the eponym "pickwickian syndrome." This condition, which appears in some very obese persons, is characterized by hypoventilation, somnolence, and carbon dioxide retention (Pco$_2$ values consistently elevated above 48 mm. of mercury). Decreased compliance of the thoracic wall and consequent increased work of respiration are thus evidently penalties of extreme obesity. Failure to make the necessary increased respiratory effort to move the ponderous thoracic wall initiates the syndrome. Possible underlying pulmonary disease may be a factor in some patients. Hypoxia, pulmonary hypertension, secondary polycythemia, and, eventually, cardiopulmonary failure ensue. All symptoms are improved by weight loss.

Hemodynamic Complications. Very obese persons have a greater than normal total circulating blood volume, probably because of the additional vascular bed of the excess adipose tissue. The blood volume per unit weight of adipose tissue, however, is less than that for lean tissue, with the result that the circulating blood volume per kilogram of body weight is less than for a lean person.

Hypertension. Studies around the world show a correlation between blood pressure and obesity. To a large extent the increased death rate of obese persons is due to hypertension. Increased stroke volume, a consequence of the increased cardiac output in the presence usually of a normal heart rate, may be in part responsible for the hypertension and left ventricular hypertrophy in obese persons.

Atherosclerosis. The urgency of the problem of obesity is the associated ischemic heart disease. Coronary artery disease occurs in America at an alarmingly high rate. The annual incidence estimated from the Framingham Study increases with age in males from less than 3.8 per 1000 at age 30, to 16 or more at age 55. The incidence is much lower in premenopausal females but ten years postmenopausally approaches that of men. The annual death rate from atherosclerosis and degenerative heart disease in the United States for men aged 50 to 59 is the highest in the world.

No single agent has been pinpointed as the causal agent of the *atherosclerotic plaque*. The lesions consist of subendothelial accumulation of cholesterol, triglyceride, and phospholipids that partially and at times completely occlude the lumen of the artery. Biochemical studies have demonstrated that cholesterol and triglyceride constituents are mainly derived from plasma lipids, whereas the phospholipids are at least partially synthesized in the vessel wall. The association between atherosclerosis and increased concentration of beta lipoproteins and very low density lipoproteins suggest that such triglyceride-rich giant molecules are particularly likely to become ensnared in the vessel wall.

A certain amount of lipid exchange between intima and plasma is normal, and such lipid is metabolized by the vessel wall. However, either because the entry of lipid becomes too great or because the metabolic processes by which it is normally removed are impaired, lipid accumulation becomes excessive, and plaque formation ensues. The lipid is at first present in foam cells. The early lesions consist chiefly of triglyceride and, according to some workers, cholesterol is not a prominent constituent of the early plaque. With time the triglycerides and phospholipids are metabolized, leaving behind cellular debris and the nonmetabolizable cholesterol as the chief constituents of the older plaque. Eventually fibrous tissue and calcium replace the lipids.

The localization of atherosclerotic plaques at sites of injury and at points of bifurcation of arteries and the greater incidence of atherosclerosis in hypertensive persons demonstrate that local injury and pressure relationships are important factors in plaque formation. Atherosclerosis is rare in pulmonary arteries unless pulmonary hypertension is present.

An alternative theory to the filtration theory attributes plaque formation to intravascular coagulation initiated by increased platelet stickiness and platelet agglomeration or by a shift in the balance between fibrin formation and fibrinolysis in the direction of fibrin deposition, with secondary enmeshment of circulating lipids. Increased coagulability, superimposed on underlying atherosclerotic disease, may be of importance in the 50 per cent of myocardial infarctions in which thrombosis is a prominent part of the pathologic change.

Although atherosclerosis is a generalized disease, coronary artery disease may occur without atherosclerotic involvement elsewhere. Such isolated coronary artery disease is a common cause of morbidity and mortality among younger men and is associated, more than is generalized atherosclerosis, with overnutrition. Cerebral atherosclerosis occurs in taller, thinner persons about 20 years later than coronary atherosclerosis.

Clinical and experimental evidence are sufficiently suggestive of the reversibility of the atherosclerotic lesion to justify efforts to correct the biochemical lesions associated with this disease.

Many studies indicate the importance of excess calories, either because of resultant obesity or because of specific dietary factors prevalent in fattening foods, in promoting susceptibility to coronary artery disease. Epidemiologic data show that members of ethnic groups with low incidence of ischemic heart disease, with a few unexplained exceptions, are leaner than Americans and do not gain significant weight after maturity. Among Americans, the prevalence of coronary artery disease is lowest in persons below normal weight, and increases proportionally with degree of overweight.

Obesity may hasten atherosclerosis by its influence on two critical causal agents, hypertension (see above) and concentration of serum lipids (see below). The effect of obesity when considered separately from the effects of hypercholesterolemia and hypertension is a markedly increased susceptibility to sudden death and to angina pectoris rather than to myocardial infarction, a finding suggesting that obesity predisposes to electrical abnormalities of the heart.

Diabetes. Diabetes is four times more common in obese than in lean adults (see above, section on Etiology), and with its toll of vascular disease accounts for some of the risk of obesity. Impaired glucose tolerance is one of the metabolic byproducts of obesity.

Diagnosis. The amount of body fat can be fairly accurately assessed from whole-body specific gravity or from the thickness of subcutaneous fat measured by skin-fold calipers or roentgenographically. The contribution of lean body mass to the total body mass can also be determined from whole-body radioactive potassium and the fat body mass indirectly calculated. The assessment of nutritional status earlier in this section contains further information on methods for evaluating nutritional state.

The most commonly used method, however, remains the height-weight tables. In Table 1 may be seen the ranges of the ideal weight, i.e., weight associated with lowest mortality according to insurance company data obtained from large numbers of policyholders. Ideal weight approximates that at age 25; this stresses the fact that weight gain during adult life is associated with increased mortality.

If a person weighs more than the upper limit of his ideal weight for his frame, he may be considered overweight, and if he is 20 pounds in excess of his ideal weight he is generally considered obese. Thirty per cent of men and 40 per cent of women over age 30 are 20 pounds or more above ideal weight.

Several height-weight indices are commonly used to express obesity, but, like other measures based on height and weight, actually measure body bulk rather than obesity. Of these indices the ponderal index, height/ $\sqrt[3]{\text{weight}}$, and the index weight/height² × 100 are best, the latter being most independent of height.

The chief drawback of height-weight indices is their failure to take into account the variable contributions of lean and fat body mass to total body weight. The measurement of subcutaneous fat with skin-fold calipers avoids this difficulty. Skin-fold thickness, preferably measured at several sites, correlates rather well with total body fat estimated from specific gravity, and has the advantage of ease and simplicity of measurement. Special calipers have been designed for the purpose. The results of the community-wide study of Tecumseh, Michigan, although not necessarily representative of the world, provide guide lines for comparison of individual readings (Table 2). Ideal standards for skin-fold thickness are not

TABLE 1. DESIRABLE WEIGHTS FOR MEN AND WOMEN ACCORDING TO HEIGHT AND FRAME, AGES 25 AND OVER*

Height (in shoes)†	Weight in pounds (in indoor clothing)		
	Small frame	Medium frame	Large frame
	Men		
5 ft. 2 in.	112–120	118–129	126–141
5 ft. 3 in.	115–123	121–133	129–144
5 ft. 4 in.	118–126	124–136	132–148
5 ft. 5 in.	121–129	127–139	135–152
5 ft. 6 in.	124–133	130–143	138–156
5 ft. 7 in.	128–137	134–147	142–161
5 ft. 8 in.	132–141	138–152	147–166
5 ft. 9 in.	136–145	142–156	151–170
5 ft. 10 in.	140–150	146–160	155–174
5 ft. 11 in.	144–154	150–165	159–179
6 ft. 0 in.	148–158	154–170	164–184
6 ft. 1 in.	152–162	158–175	168–189
6 ft. 2 in.	156–167	162–180	173–194
6 ft. 3 in.	160–171	167–185	177–199
6 ft. 4 in.	164–175	172–190	182–204
	Women		
4 ft. 10 in.	92–98	96–107	104–119
4 ft. 11 in.	94–101	98–110	106–122
5 ft. 0 in.	96–104	101–113	109–124
5 ft. 1 in.	99–107	104–116	112–128
5 ft. 2 in.	102–110	107–119	115–131
5 ft. 3 in.	105–113	110–122	118–134
5 ft. 4 in.	108–116	113–126	121–138
5 ft. 5 in.	111–119	116–130	125–142
5 ft. 6 in.	114–123	120–135	129–146
5 ft. 7 in.	118–127	124–139	133–150
5 ft. 8 in.	122–131	128–143	137–154
5 ft. 9 in.	126–135	132–147	141–158
5 ft. 10 in.	130–140	136–151	145–163
5 ft. 11 in.	134–144	140–155	149–168
6 ft. 0 in.	138–148	144–159	153–174

*Prepared by the Metropolitan Life Insurance Company. Derived primarily from data of the Build and Blood Pressure Study, 1959.

†1 in. heels for men and 2 in. heels for women.

yet available. Studies on the association between plasma triglycerides and skin-fold thickness suggest that scapular skin-fold thickness should not exceed 14 mm. in a naturally lean person or more than 23 mm. in a stocky person. As with weight, mean scapular skin-fold thickness at age 25 (12.4 mm.) might be considered desirable.

Differential Diagnosis. Hypothyroidism. The weight gain in hypothyroidism is usually only moderate, and is due in part to accumulation of myxedematous fluid as well as to adipose tissue. The reduction in caloric expenditure contributes to the obesity. The usual measurements of thyroid function such as PBI and I¹³¹ uptake are normal in ordinary obesity, and thus can be used to exclude hypothyroidism as a contributing cause of obesity. Hypothyroidism is rarely the cause of obesity.

Cushing's Disease. Hyperadrenocorticism causes moderate obesity that chiefly involves the face, causing the typical moon facies, the thorax, and abdomen, but spares the buttocks and extremities. The fat pad over the last cervical vertebra, the so-called buffalo hump, is characteristic, but may also occur in ordinary obesity, for example, the "dowager's hump" of the postmenopausal woman.

TABLE 2. SUBSCAPULAR AND TRICEPS SKINFOLD BY AGE AND SEX (VALUES IN MILLIMETERS)*

	Age (Yr.)	Male subjects, Percentiles			Female subjects, Percentiles		
		20	50	80	20	50	80
Subscapular	20–24	8.0	12.1	19.2	8.6	13.2	21.7
	25–29	8.0	12.4	20.9	9.1	13.2	20.4
	30–34	9.1	15.1	24.3	9.0	13.6	21.2
	35–39	8.9	14.7	21.4	9.7	16.9	24.8
	40–44	10.9	16.3	23.5	11.4	17.6	28.2
	45–49	11.0	17.3	25.9	13.0	20.8	29.1
	50–54	9.9	17.3	24.6	13.4	21.0	33.2
	55–59	11.8	18.8	30.7	13.5	22.3	32.0
	60–64	9.3	16.8	24.8	15.5	22.4	33.6
	65–69	8.0	12.5	17.4	13.0	20.9	30.0
	70–74	8.7	14.3	23.1	14.0	22.6	29.9
	75–79	9.9	14.8	20.8	10.0	21.6	31.2
Triceps	20–24	7.2	11.0	17.8	12.5	17.5	23.4
	25–29	7.1	10.4	16.7	12.1	17.5	23.8
	30–34	7.9	12.3	17.8	13.0	18.1	25.0
	35–39	7.4	11.8	17.3	14.1	20.0	26.0
	40–44	8.0	12.4	17.6	15.2	20.7	27.3
	45–49	8.6	12.5	17.3	16.3	22.1	27.7
	50–54	8.7	12.0	18.7	18.1	22.7	26.9
	55–59	9.9	14.0	18.7	17.3	22.9	28.8
	60–64	8.6	11.7	17.8	18.3	24.7	31.5
	65–69	7.1	10.9	15.4	17.2	21.8	26.6
	70–74	8.1	11.8	15.3	16.0	21.2	26.0
	75–79	7.4	13.5	17.2	12.2	20.0	26.0

*From Montoye, H. J., Epstein, F. H., and Kjelsberg, M. O.: The measurement of body fatness. A study in a total community. Amer. J. Clin. Nutrition, 16:417, 1965.

The presence of purple striae of the skin of the abdomen and elsewhere suggests Cushing's disease. However, striae are common in persons who gain weight rapidly. Obese adolescents frequently have striae of the upper arms, breasts, abdomen, hips, and thighs, although adrenal function is normal.

The differentiation of obesity with and without Cushing's disease may present difficulties because of the frequency with which the results of tests used to diagnose Cushing's disease are slightly abnormal in obesity. Elevated urinary 17-keto-steroids and 17-hydroxycorticosteroids as well as increased rate of cortisol secretion are common in obesity. The two most helpful tests for excluding Cushing's disease in obese patients are the diurnal variation in plasma cortisol concentration (usually lost in Cushing's disease but preserved in obesity) and the dexamethasone suppression test. Suppression is normal in the obese but impaired in Cushing's disease.

Stein-Leventhal Syndrome. In a women, obesity, hirsuitism, and infertility suggest this syndrome. The finding of large cystic ovaries on physical examination is confirmatory, although surgical exploration may be necessary for verification. Tests of adrenal cortical function are normal as a rule.

Insulinoma, Hyperinsulinism. The carbohydrate feeding necessary to counteract frequent hypoglycemic attacks may lead to obesity.

Treatment of Obesity. General Considerations. Reduction of excess weight in obese persons is associated with improvement in hypertension and diabetes as well as in amelioration of the mechanical effects of the adipose mass. Weight reduction is highly desirable for a large segment of our population, yet it is singularly difficult to achieve.

There is no satisfactory treatment for obesity. Once established, it is remarkably self-sustaining. Even if weight is temporarily lost, the former weight is regained with astonishing regularity within months as a rule, within five years almost certainly. A patient who has successfully lost weight must be prepared for a lifetime of vigilance if he is to maintain his success. Nonetheless, the benefits to be expected from weight loss justify the utmost effort on the part of both physician and patient to bring about and maintain optimal weight. If successful, such measures correct or improve the hypertension, the diabetes, and the abnormal serum lipids associated with excess calories, and relieve the mechanical injuries resulting from the increased adipose mass.

Of the three main approaches to obesity—drugs, diet, and exercise—diet is the mainstay of treatment. An understanding of the physiologic changes that accompany caloric restriction is essential if the patient's progress is to be understood. Under dietary treatment, the outlook for the extremely obese patient who has as much as a hundred pounds or more to lose is dismal. Perhaps the most hopeful outlook can be expected for the slightly obese patient who has only a few pounds to lose. Because such patients account for the great majority of cardiovascular disease victims in this country, every effort should be made to reach them and to achieve weight reduction.

Diet. *Effect of Caloric Restriction.* The seemingly simple and logical limitation of calories below caloric expenditure is often made difficult by the metabolic changes that occur in response to caloric restriction. After initial satisfactory weight loss of one to two or more pounds a week, a plateau is reached. The patient claims continued adherence to the diet, yet no further weight is lost. He finally yields to discouragement, abandons the diet altogether, and gains back all of the lost weight or even more.

One reason for this failure is that too much is expected of caloric restriction. Of the tissue lost, fat and protein tissue differ in their caloric density. Pure fat yields 9 calories per gram. Adipose tissue, consisting mainly of fat with little water, contains about 8 calories per gram of tissue. Protein, on the other hand, gives 4 calories per gram of protein, and carries with it about three or four times its weight in intracellular water. Protein tissue thus gives only about 0.8 caloric per gram, one tenth that of adipose tissue on a weight basis. If, for instance, a caloric deficit of 500 calories were derived only from protein tissue, it could be calculated that 620 grams or more than a pound a day would be lost. If only fat tissue were lost, a mere 62-gram tissue loss a day would account for the 500 calories.

Actually a mixture of protein and fat tissue is lost. Some nitrogen loss is acceptable since the excess tissue of obese persons contains 10 to 30 grams of nitrogen per kilogram of excess weight. The tendency for negative nitrogen balance in the early days of caloric restriction favors loss largely of protein tissue and thus large weight loss. However, particularly in the very obese, with continued caloric restriction the body reacts by defense of its nitrogen reserves, and the nitrogen balance becomes less negative. If nitrogen balance is established, weight loss then results only from loss of adipose tissue, and occurs very slowly. The nitrogen-conserving defense is so great that positive nitrogen balance can occur on the same diet that initially caused nitrogen loss. Conceivably, protein synthesis taking place concomitantly with loss of calories from adipose tissue could create new tissue that would more than equal in weight the adipose tissue lost, with resulting net weight gain despite continued caloric deficit. How long this state of affairs could last is not known, but the tendency toward positive nitrogen balance when undernourished persons are refed full diets may last for months.

The adaptation to caloric restriction includes a strong anabolic tendency that may be manifest not only as nitrogen retention but also as increased synthesis of fat from available carbohydrate. Adaptive hyperlipogenesis in laboratory animals is the greatly augmented synthesis of fat from carbohydrate on refeeding after a period of starvation. If this phenomenon occurs in humans, it would account further for the tendency to regain lost weight.

Not only do the logistics of weight loss from protein and fat tissue favor plateau and even weight gain in obese persons undergoing caloric restriction, but the tendency of such patients to retain sodium and extracellular water is further reason for weight gain. The resultant edema may be refractory to thiazide diuretics or salt restriction. The likelihood of depression, decreased activity, hunger, decreased metabolic rate, and weakness all operate against the successful continuation of a calorically restricted diet.

Specific Diets. A liberal diet with only a small caloric deficit is easier for the patient to accept than a rigidly restricted one. Conservative nutritionists recommend one gram of protein per kilogram of ideal body weight and fat roughly equal in weight to the protein, the remainder of the calories to be made up from carbohydrate. From 800 to 1800 calories are commonly recommended, depending on activity, size, and desired speed of weight loss. It must be recalled, however, that the few available long-term studies show discouraging results on all diets. There is no basis for recommending any one diet over any other.

Unbalanced Diets. A variety of unbalanced diets has been proposed. Such diets are so unpalatable in quantity that calories are automatically limited. Because they stimulate the patient's imagination, so-called "fad" diets, though the despair of dietitians, may elicit greater patient cooperation than conservative diets.

Low Protein Diet. On the assumption that a certain amount of excess tissue is nitrogen, and that the tendency of obese patients to retain nitrogen may defeat efforts at weight loss, some argument may be made for a low protein diet. The dangers of severe protein deficiency, especially liver disease, must be remembered.

Low Carbohydrate Diet. On theoretical grounds a low carbohydrate diet should be effective by discouraging lipogenesis and preventing reactive hypoglycemia with its attendant hunger. As noted in the section on pathogenesis, dietary carbohydrate favors lipogenesis at several steps. It is also required for the manifestation of salt and water retention so commonly encountered during weight reduction. Limitation of carbohydrate to 50 or 60 grams a day but with *ad libitum* intake of protein and fat causes initial rapid weight loss (largely water), mild ketosis, and absence of hunger, and is usually well tolerated. Total calories are voluntarily limited to 1300 or so because of reduced palatability of fat without carbohydrate.

Starvation. The treatment of obesity by total starvation is usually well tolerated for repeated periods of 10 to 15 days each, sometimes much longer, and causes an average weight loss of a pound a day. Complications include decreased uric acid excretion, and hyperuricemia, sometimes manifested as clinical gout. Postural hypotension, anemia, and cardiac irregularities may also occur. Upon refeeding, excess excretion of uric acid may cause uric acid nephropathy. Intense retention of sodium and water causes edema and weight gain. Both the uric acid excretion and sodium retention are dependent on dietary carbohydrate, as little as 40 grams a day being sufficient. Unless dietary supervision is continued, the lost weight is readily regained. Starvation is best reserved for hospitalized patients in whom rapid weight loss is mandatory, for some reason such as planned surgery.

Formula Diets. Prepared liquid diets of high satiety value have the advantage of simplicity but the drawback of monotony. Long-term studies indicate no greater success with these than with any other diets.

Drugs. Appetite-suppressant drugs of the amphetamine group are effective for only a few weeks. Dependence on their stimulatory effect occasionally makes withdrawal a problem. Such drugs have no demonstrated role in the long-term management of obesity.

Exercise. The notoriously poor state of physical fitness of Americans undoubtedly contributes to their problem of obesity. Exercise, in addition to its obvious effect of expending calories, engenders a state of physical fitness with an accompanying sense of well-being. A program of gradually increasing exercise is an important part of the treatment of obesity. The caloric expenditure resulting from various activities is presented in Table 3.

Dietary Treatment of Atherosclerosis. The problem of prevention or treatment of atherosclerosis is in part related to the treatment of obesity; in

TABLE 3. ENERGY COSTS IN SOME USUAL ACTIVITIES*

Normal Activity	Cal. Min. Sq. M.†	Sport	Cal. Min. Sq. M.†
Sitting, normal	0.70	Football	5.04
Sitting, reading	0.70	Basketball	4.31
Sitting, eating	0.80	Bowling	4.06
Sitting, playing cards	0.83	Swimming	6.06
Resting in bed	0.68	Golfing	2.76
Standing, normal	0.81	Tennis	3.50
Standing, light activity	1.41	Squash	5.00
Personal toilet	1.09	Table tennis	2.00
Shower	1.84	Badminton	1.91
Dressing	1.84	Rowing	4.00
Making bed	2.64	Sailing	1.30
Shining shoes	2.11	Snooker pool	1.50
Mopping floor	2.67	Dancing	2.00
Walking indoors	1.68	Riding	1.50
Walking outdoors	3.07	Boxing, sparring	5.00
Walking upstairs	10.00		
Walking downstairs	3.80		
Kneeling	0.68		
Squatting	1.12		
Washing clothes	1.46		

*From Pollack, H., Consolazio, C. F., and Isaac, G. J.: Metabolic demands as a factor in weight control. J.A.M.A., 167:216, 1958.
†Based on basal metabolic rate of 0.59 calorie per minute per square meter of surface area.

addition, special aspects require consideration because of the variable effect of diet on serum lipids. The identification of the lipid abnormalities associated with atherosclerosis has been simplified by Fredrickson's classification of the hyperlipoproteinemias into five electrophoretic patterns or types. Knowledge of the type permits prediction of response to diet. Type I, fat-induced lipemia, is a rare inherited type occurring most commonly in childhood; it is not associated with atherosclerosis, obesity, or diabetes (see article on Disorders of Lipid Metabolism). The remaining four types are all associated with increased susceptibility to atherosclerosis. They may be divided into two chief groups.

Hypercholesterolemia. The incidence of myocardial infarction increases as serum cholesterol concentration increases. Between the ages of 45 and 60, the annual incidence of coronary artery disease is about 0.4 per cent among men with cholesterol concentrations below 200 mg. per 100 ml.; this increases to about 1.8 per cent among men with cholesterol over 260 mg. per 100 ml. There is no low concentration below which absence of myocardial infarction can be guaranteed and no upper limit above which it is inevitable. The overlap is great between normal persons and those with coronary artery disease; however, a cholesterol below 200 mg. per 100 ml. may be considered desirable and one above 260 undesirable.

Pure hypercholesterolemia of the familial type (Fredrickson's familial type II) with or without xanthomatosis is characterized by a cholesterol concentration of 400 to 600 mg. per 100 ml. and by premature coronary artery disease. The serum triglyceride concentration is normal and the serum is clear. The plasma cholesterol is resistant to dietary or other treatment. However, this disease is uncommon and a rare cause of atherosclerosis. An acquired type II is much more common, and responds more readily to treatment.

Dietary Treatment of Hypercholesterolemia. Serum cholesterol is slightly influenced by total caloric intake, but is more influenced by the composition of the diet. In the United States the fat intake averages 140 grams or more a day (40 to 45 per cent of calories) and the serum cholesterol is usually over 200 mg. per 100 ml., whereas in Japan the fat intake is only 10 to 20 grams a day, and cholesterol is usually well below 200 mg. per 100 ml. However, variation in fat intake within the United States does not account for variations of the cholesterol in this country. Moreover, despite the low incidence of *coronary* artery disease in the fat-restricted Oriental countries, aortic and cerebral atherosclerosis, diabetes, and hypertensive vascular disease are as common as, or more common than, in the United States.

Reduction of dietary fat may cause a reduction in plasma cholesterol concentration proportional to the severity of fat restriction, but such a diet is unpalatable in the Western world and whether the beneficial effect is due to fat restriction or the associated loss of weight is difficult to determine. Furthermore, very low fat diets may be so high in carbohydrate that carbohydrate-induced lipemia may appear; this in turn is a possible cause of ischemic heart disease (*vide infra*), particularly if calories are not restricted at the same time. Diets containing less than 60 to 70 grams of fat are unpalatable to Americans and hence difficult to follow.

Type of Dietary Fat. The hypercholesterolemic effect of animal fat is attributed to the high degree of saturation of such fats. Vegetable oils that are rich in polyunsaturated fat have a cholesterol-lowering effect if substituted for animal fat in sufficient quantity. Reduction of animal fat by half with generous substitution of polyunsaturated oil such as corn oil or safflower oil in amounts of 60 to 90 ml. a day in place of more saturated fats has been recommended. According to the National Diet Heart Study such a diet produced only an 8 per cent reduction of serum cholesterol of free-living Americans if weight was stable. Those persons who lost weight on the diet showed a 14 per cent drop of cholesterol, although the control subjects who lost weight showed a 5 per cent decrease. The type of fat has no effect on serum triglyceride concentration.

Dietary Cholesterol. The amount of cholesterol in the diet has small influence on the serum cholesterol concentrations, particularly in the range of intake between 0 and 700 mg. of cholesterol daily. Further increase in dietary cholesterol above this critical level is less likely to be associated with further increase in serum cholesterol. The dietary cholesterol of most omnivorous peoples exceeds this amount, and may be well over 1000 mg. a day. A reduction to 200 mg. a day will effect a modest lowering of serum cholesterol concentration. Dietary cholesterol is derived entirely from animal sources. The important dietary sources of cholesterol may be seen in Table 4. Because one problem of cholesterol restriction is the maintenance of adequate protein intake, the protein values are also shown.

The elimination of eggs from the diet will do much to lower the cholesterol intake. Further reduction can readily be achieved by eliminating butter, shellfish, and organ meat, and by substituting skimmed milk for whole milk. Protein can then be supplied either by lean meat or by cheeses, as preferred, as well as by vegetable sources. Although even lean meat contains substantial amounts of cholesterol, meat is the mainstay of the American diet, the favorite food of many, and its elimination from the diet will jeopardize patient cooperation. If meat is the only significant source of cholesterol in the diet, as much as 8 ounces of meat a day can be permitted without exceeding the limit of 200 mg. of dietary cholesterol.

Hypertriglyceridemia. Carbohydrate-induced lipemia is frequently associated with coronary artery disease. Fasting serum triglycerides and the very low density lipoproteins in which they are transported are increased. The fasting serum may be slightly or moderately turbid, and the cholesterol concentration may be normal or may be increased. In the latter event the hypercholesterolemia may be at least in part due to the impaired fat transport and may respond to dietary measures aimed at correcting the triglycerides.

Serum triglyceride concentration expressed as triglyceride fatty acids (TGFA) exceeds the upper limit of normal, 5.4 mEq. per liter (about 150 mg. per 100 ml.), in as many as 40 per cent of apparently healthy middle-aged men, and in a considerably greater percentage of patients with coronary artery disease. An increase in triglycerides above this limit denotes the presence of large low-density lipoproteins, normally almost absent from the circulation. "Carbohydrate-induced lipemia" is better denoted as "endogenous lipemia" because the increased circulating triglycerides are thought to represent triglycerides endogenously synthesized from dietary carbohydrate by the liver. The triglycerides are released into the circulation as very low density lipoproteins for transport to the muscle for fuel if needed or to adipose tissue for storage if not needed. The endogenous lipemias consist of Fredrickson's Type III, IV, and V, Type IV being the most common. Type V represents abnormally increased concentration of both exogenous and endogenous triglyceride, but is probably best classed as an endogenous lipemia in which the lipid-removing mechanisms are so

TABLE 4. APPROXIMATE CHOLESTEROL CONTENT OF FOODS*

Item	Size Serving, Edible Portion as Purchased	Amount of Cholesterol (Milligrams)	Amount of Protein (Grams)
Milk, whole	One glass (200 ml.)	22	7
Milk, skim	One glass (200 ml.)	6	7
Whole milk cheeses, as American, Cheddar, and cream	100 gm.	85–100	21–36
Cheese, cottage	100 gm.	15	13
Butter	1 tablespoon (15 gm.)	38	0
Animal fat (lard)	1 tablespoon (15 gm.)	14	0
Egg yolk	1 egg	300	3
Egg white	1 egg	0	5
Lean cuts of any poultry, meat except organs, fish except shellfish	100 gm. of meat only	60–90	16–32
Shellfish and caviar	100 gm. of meat only	125–200	16–34
Organ meats	100 gm.	150–375	16–26
Brain	100 gm.	>2000	12

*Estimated from values listed in U.S. Department of Agriculture Handbook No. 8, Composition of Foods, 1963.

overloaded by the endogenous lipids that removal of exogenous lipids (chylomicrons) is also impaired.

Whether the endogenous lipemias result from increased synthesis of triglyceride, from abnormal circulating protein-triglyceride complexes which defy the usual means of removal, or from decreased ability of the tissues to remove the triglycerides from the circulation is not certain. Evidence for an abnormal lipoprotein is strongest in Type III.

Whatever the mechanism, the endogenous lipemias share certain metabolic characteristics, including obesity, frequently impaired glucose tolerance, insulin resistance, high basal insulin concentrations, and carbohydrate inducibility. In nondiabetics the postcibal rise in insulin being superimposed on an elevated fasting level may be high. In diabetics the insulin response is blunted. As in obesity the high insulin output may eventually lead to pancreatic exhaustion and low insulin-output diabetes, thus accounting for the frequency of impaired glucose tolerance. Also as in obesity, the insulin resistant state may be a fundamental aspect of endogenous lipemia.

The analogy to obesity is indeed close, yet the abnormalities of hypertriglyceridemia cannot be accounted for by associated obesity alone. The correlation between triglycerides and obesity is low grade at best. However, the correlation of both with circulating insulin is clear cut. Elevation of insulin may be the statistical link between obesity and hypertriglyceridemia. The causal sequences among obesity, hypertriglyceridemia, hyperinsulism, insulin resistance, and impaired glucose tolerance and ultimately atherosclerosis are not known. Empirically this cluster of abnormalities is exaggerated by factors which increase fat synthesis, specifically high carbohydrate diet and weight gain. All abnormalities are corrected or improved by low carbohydrate diet and weight loss.

Dietary Treatment of Hypertriglyceridemia. Endogenous lipemias (Fredrickson's Types III and IV) are exaggerated by a diet very low in fat (less than 20 grams a day) and high in carbohydrate, and are corrected or much improved by increasing fat to 70 per cent of calories. The amount of carbohydrate necessary to induce the lipemia is subject to marked individual variation. Obesity acts to accentuate the triglyceride-raising effect of a high carbohydrate diet. Conversely the triglyceride-lowering effect of a low calorie diet overrides the triglyceride-raising effect of a high carbohydrate diet. The low caloric intake of the Japanese compared to Americans, despite the very high proportion of the calories contributed by carbohydrate, probably accounts for the lack of hypertriglyceridemia in the Japanese. The first step in the treatment of hypertriglyceridemia is to obtain weight loss. A trial of weight reduction to or toward ideal weight (Table 1) or to weight at age 25 is desirable. If simple weight loss does not lower the serum triglycerides, moderate restriction of carbohydrate to 125 grams a day may be effective. In some instances restriction to 50 grams

a day is necessary. In Type V hyperlipidemia, the serum lipids may be lowered by the converse procedure of reducing dietary fat, an indication of the fact that such patients are intolerant to both dietary fat and carbohydrate. A minimum of 20 grams of fat a day should be given to allow adequate operation of the lipoprotein lipase system and thus efficient clearing of triglycerides from the circulation.

The response of serum cholesterol to such a diet is variable. With correction of lipemia or with weight loss, the cholesterol may be lowered, but occasionally it may become elevated. If it becomes elevated, avoidance of concentrated dietary sources of cholesterol is advisable (see Table 4).

Some evidence exists for the possibility that carbohydrate-induced lipemia is a response more to highly purified carbohydrates such as sucrose than to carbohydrate in general. For this reason it would be wise to eliminate sugar as such from the diet of obese or atherosclerotic patients, particularly if the triglycerides are elevated.

The treatment of the impaired glucose tolerance associated with hypertriglyceridemia is the same as of the hypertriglyceridemia itself; both probably share a common etiology.

Prevention. Prevention of weight gain after maturity is clearly more desirable than treatment of existing obesity. Once established, obesity seems to be self-perpetuating; the five-year cure rate is almost zero. Prevention means even further education of our already diet-conscious civilization. Such education might properly start with mothers who are responsible for establishing in their children life-long dietary patterns. Institutions, such as the army, that are responsible for feeding large segments of the population have an opportunity not only to establish restrained eating habits but to prevent weight gain in men during their tour of duty. Most important of all, and perhaps least achievable, would be the restraint by the food industry of its promotion of foodstuffs of high caloric but low nutritive value. The excess calories which contribute to mass obesity in the western world are derived mainly from products which the food industry has made too readily available. Purified fats and carbohydrates, either alone or combined in the form of rich pastries and other delicacies, are the worst offenders. Since an almost invariable result of food processing is the concentration of calories with loss of minerals and vitamins, a simple rule to apply would be to reduce the consumption of foodstuffs which require manufacturing at some stage of their preparation. The adoption in American homes of such simple diets with reservation of rich treats for special occasions would enhance appreciation of the special occasions and do much to eliminate obesity and its toll of vascular disease.

Amad, K. H., Brennan, J. C., and Alexander, J. K.: The cardiac pathology of chronic exogenous obesity. Circulation, 32: 740, 1965.

Bray, G. A.: Effect of diet and triiodothyronine on the activity of sn-glycerol-3-phosphate dehydrogenase and on the metabolism of obese patients. J. Clin. Invest., 48:1413, 1969.

Felig, P., Marliss, E., and Cahill, G. F.: Plasma amino acid levels and insulin secretion in obesity. New Eng. J. Med., 281: 811, 1969.

Heinle, R. A., Levy, R. I., Fredrickson, D. S., and Gorlin, R.: Lipid and carbohydrate abnormalities in patients with angiographically documented coronary artery disease. Amer. J. Cardiol., 24:178, 1969.

Kannel, W. B., LeBauer, J., Dawber, T. R., and McNamara, P. M.: Relation of body weight to development of coronary heart disease. The Framingham Study. Circulation, 35: 734, 1967.

Keys, A., et al.: Coronary heart disease in seven countries. Circulation (Supplement), Vol. 41, April, 1970.

Krittle, J. L., and Hirsch, J.: Effect of early nutrition on the development of rat epididymal fat pads: Cellularity and metabolism. J. Clin. Invest., 47:2091, 1968.

Symposium: Endocrine Aspects of Obesity. Amer. J. Clin. Nutr., 21:1397, 1968.

HEMATOLOGIC AND HEMATOPOIETIC DISEASES

Introduction

Carl V. Moore

Diseases of the blood and blood-forming organs may conveniently be divided into disorders affecting primarily the red blood corpuscles, leukocytes, cells of the reticuloendothelial system, platelets, and the coagulation mechanism. This classification permits an orderly presentation of clinical hematology even though it requires certain compromises because more than one type of cell is frequently involved. In aplastic anemia, for instance, failure of leukocyte or platelet production may be more pronounced than decreased erythropoiesis.

The principal hematopoietic organs are the bone marrow, liver, spleen, and lymph nodes. It is generally agreed that all blood cells are derived from reticuloendothelial cells, but there the agreement stops. Some histologists believe that a single multipotential stem cell or blast develops from reticulum cells and serves as the precursor of all blood cells, whereas others believe that several different blasts or stem cells are formed, each capable of producing two or more types of blood cells or each specific for a given cell line (myeloblast for granulocytes, lymphoblast for lymphocytes, monoblast for monocytes, etc.). Physiologic as well as advanced morphologic techniques have failed to identify the stem cell (or cells). New information of importance, however, has been added during the past few years. (1) Physiologic evidence indicates that erythropoietin stimulates the multiplication of stem cell precursors of the red blood cell series. That demonstration has intensified the search for leukopoietin(s) and thrombocytopoietin, but to date the efforts have been less fruitful. Their discovery would support the existence of at least several different stem (or blast) cells with limited potentiality for differentiation. (2) Lymphocytes serve important immunologic functions and can no longer be regarded as "resting cells," capable under appropriate stimulation of transforming into precursors of any of the cells of the bone marrow and blood. Although they superficially resemble each other, they are composed of at least two populations. The great majority of circulating lymphocytes and the bulk of those mobilizable from tissues are thymic dependent. These cells become immunologically competent either in the thymus or through the operation of a thymic humoral factor (thymopoietin). The majority are probably long-lived cells; they exercise immunologic functions related to cell-mediated immunity (delayed or bacterial allergies, certain homograft immunities, and the

graft-versus-host reactions). They are important in body defense against certain virus and fungal infections, in resistance to invasion by opportunistic invaders, and against malignant cell adaptation. By contrast, a few of the circulating lymphocytes and many located in lymphoid tissue and bone marrow are involved in the synthesis of immunoglobulins; they may be derived from the lymphoid tissue of the gut and probably give rise to plasma cells. Some but not all workers believe that a third population of lymphocytes in the peripheral blood is related to monocytes, macrophages, and fixed tissue phagocytes, i.e., Kupffer cells. However, when bone marrow and lymphoid tissue are made aplastic by high doses of total body irradiation, accelerated repopulation of marrow and nodes can be accomplished by transplanted marrow cells, but the injection of cells from the thoracic duct or lymph nodes of donor animals accelerates recovery of lymphoid organs only. Furthermore, if a single Peyer's patch is shielded during whole body irradiation, rapid repopulation occurs in lymphoid tissue but not in marrow. These observations suggest that lymphocytes are not capable of serving as precursors of granulocytes, erythroid elements, and megakaryocytes.

If one remembers that the liver, spleen, and lymph nodes are all sites of blood cell formation during fetal life, it is easier to understand why under appropriate stress these organs may regain this fetal function and become sites of extramedullary hematopoiesis. The bone marrow at birth is fairly uniformly red and active. As growth occurs, less of the marrow volume is required to meet physiologic demands; the shafts of the long bones become filled with fat and, even in the flat bones where blood cell formation remains most active, fat cells take up a portion of the marrow space. This fatty portion, however, remains as a reservoir into which active marrow can again expand when the need for hyperplasia occurs.

Cells of the blood, bone marrow, lymphoid tissues, and reticuloendothelial system are important in oxygen transport, resistance to infection, reaction to foreign substances of many kinds, hemostasis, production of antibodies, delayed hypersensitivity, and so forth. Cytopenia of a particular cell type can often be related to a corresponding derangement of function: severe anemia and inadequate oxygen supply to tissues; severe leukopenia and increased susceptibility to infection or defective immunologic response; thrombocytopenia and hemorrhage. Unfortunately, this kind of correlation cannot be carried very far because relationships are too complex, and our knowledge is too inadequate. Hemostasis, for instance, involves not only platelets, but capillary endothelium, fibrinogen, and a series of plasma and tissue enzymes of importance in both coagulation and fibrinolysis. We do not know with certainty all the jobs that are performed by lymphocytes, eosinophils, and basophils, although the importance of the lymphocytes in hypersensitivity or immune reactions is now more clearly established. Information has only recently been accumulated about the intracellular mechanisms that give neutrophils the ability to destroy phagocytized bacteria. Many more examples could be cited. Overproduction of blood cells may also lead to abnormalities: increased viscosity of the blood in polycythemia; infiltration or proliferation in many tissues with consequent organomegaly, pain, and disturbed function, as in leukemias and the lymphomas; or increased tendency to thrombosis from thrombocythemia of any cause. Dysfunction may be responsible for abnormal rates of blood cell destruction or for the production of abnormal proteins. These several considerations explain adequately why hematologic disorders affect every tissue or organ system in the body and why their clinical manifestations are protean.

The wide variety of pathogenic mechanisms responsible for hematologic dyscrasias includes simple blood loss, primary or conditioned deficiency states, toxicity by a wide variety of chemical substances, metabolic disturbances, the destructive effect of external irradiation, infections, immunologic abnormalities, acquired or genetically mediated biochemical lesions, malignant proliferation of cells, and accelerated destruction of cells by an enlarged spleen. In an embarrassing number of instances, however, the term "idiopathic" must still be applied, or admission of ignorance as to cause must be made.

In the laboratory, accurate blood counts and careful morphologic study of the cells in peripheral blood and bone marrow remain the foundation of hematologic diagnosis. Identification of young cells can tax the most experienced morphologists, but simple observations are often of great value. Too often the neophyte or technician, for instance, becomes preoccupied with the compulsion to count one hundred leukocytes on a blood film and ignores a telltale absence of platelets or a distinctive abnormality of erythrocytes. Bone marrow examination has at last become commonplace, and it should be done unless the diagnosis is otherwise obvious. If bone marrow aspiration results in a dry tap, trephine biopsy must be done. Biopsy of enlarged lymph nodes is an absolute requirement for the diagnosis of lymphomas. Basic morphologic data often are not sufficient for precise diagnosis, and must be supplemented by information that can now be obtained from a host of biochemical, physiologic, or immunologic procedures. Selection of additional diagnostic aids must be thoughtfully

and intelligently made to save time, inconvenience, and expense. In the study of anemias and polycythemia, for instance, valuable and necessary information may be obtained by determining the serum iron and saturation of the iron-binding protein, the hemosiderin present in aspirated bone marrow, the plasma folic acid and vitamin B_{12} level or the absorption of radioactively tagged vitamin B_{12}, the total circulating red blood cell mass, the arterial oxygen saturation, the rate of red blood cell destruction and whether erythrocytic destruction is selectively occurring in the spleen, the presence or absence of a positive Coombs test, the amount of free hemoglobin in plasma, the osmotic fragility, the electrophoretic pattern of the patient's hemoglobin, the presence or absence of sickling, or the erythrocyte enzymes that may be deficient in certain hereditary hemolytic anemias, i.e., glucose-6-phosphate dehydrogenase. For diseases of the white blood cells and platelets, many fewer such specialized techniques have so far been developed, but alkaline phosphatase staining of blood films, determination of chromosomal karyotypes, and methods for measuring platelet adhesiveness or survival have proved valuable. New procedures have added much greater precision to the differential diagnosis of coagulation disorders.

Treatment of the blood dyscrasias varies from specific to purely palliative. Administration of iron in iron deficiency anemias, vitamin B_{12} in pernicious anemia, and vitamin K in some forms of prothrombin deficiency corrects the hematologic abnormality, although the pathologic change that induced the deficiency may persist—either permanently, as in pernicious anemia, or to be dealt with separately. The very effectiveness of these antianemic agents has, however, led to the widespread but deplorable and to be discouraged practice of administering "shotgun" combinations of iron, vitamin B_{12}, and liver extracts indiscriminately to anemic patients. This practice is expensive, encourages shoddy diagnosis, leads to much disappointment—since most anemias are caused by factors other than deficiency of these nutrients—and may lead to harm by delaying other forms of therapy. Splenectomy for treatment of hereditary spherocytosis regularly eliminates the accelerated hemolysis characteristic of that disease so that red blood cell values are restored to normal, even though the spherocytosis persists. Splenectomy or corticosteroid therapy in acquired (Coombs positive) hemolytic anemia and in idiopathic thrombocytopenic purpura, and the administration of androgens in bone marrow failure and myelofibrosis may be cited as examples of therapeutic measures of inconstant or intermediate effectiveness. Although irradiation and chemotherapeutic agents in the treatment of the leukemias produce no cures, their intelligent use adds greatly to the comfort of patients, prolonging useful and probably total life. It now appears that properly administered irradiation therapy may produce cures in patients with localized Hodgkin's disease.

Transfusions of whole blood have become so commonplace that it is easy to forget what a boon the development of blood bank techniques has been during the last 30 years to the treatment of acute hemorrhage and to the support of patients with chronic anemias unresponsive to hematinic agents. It is difficult to mention the great value of intelligently employed transfusions, however, without bemoaning the unnecessary and careless use of blood, which too often leads to disastrous reactions. In the treatment of hemophilia, afibrinogenemia, and certain other coagulation disorders, the administration of properly prepared plasma or of appropriate fractions of plasma proteins can temporarily correct the clotting defect. Infections in patients with leukemia or severe neutropenia may often be brought under control with antimicrobial drugs. Many instances remain, however, in which attempts to control hemolysis, infection, or hemorrhage are still so ineffective that the few additional days or weeks of life that may be gained through the use of transfusions are miserable ones for the patient, the family, and the physician.

Good, R. A., et al.: The lymphocyte. Seminars Hemat. 6:1, 1969.
Leavell, B. S., and Thorup, O. A., Jr.: Fundamentals of Clinical Hematology. 3rd ed. Philadelphia, W. B. Saunders Company, 1971.
Mauer, A. M.: Pediatric Hematology. New York, Blakiston Division, McGraw-Hill Book Company, 1969.
McGregor, D. D.: Bone marrow origin of immunologically competent lymphocytes in the rat. J. Exp. Med., 127:953, 1968.
Smith, C. H.: Blood Diseases of Infancy and Childhood. 2nd ed. St. Louis, C. V. Mosby Company, 1966.
Tanaka, Y., Epstein, L. B., Brecher, G., and Stohlman, F., Jr.: Transformation of lymphocytes in cultures of human peripheral blood. Blood, 22:614, 1963.
Whitby, L. E. H., and Britton, C. J. C.: Disorders of the Blood. 10th ed. New York, Grune and Stratton, Inc., 1969.
Wintrobe, M. M.: Clinical Hematology. 6th ed. Philadelphia, Lea and Febiger, 1967.

The Anemias

INTRODUCTION

Carl V. Moore

Pathologic Physiology. The mammalian red corpuscle is an amazing cell since it serves its function, primarily that of oxygen transport, after its nucleus has been extruded. About 34 per cent of its mass is hemoglobin and about 65 per cent is water; the remaining small fraction is composed of stroma, electrolytes, glucose, vitamins, enzymes, and a number of other metabolically active substances. The time required for the maturation of reticulocytes from the earliest recognizable nucleated red blood cell precursor in the bone marrow is about three or four days; during this developmental period approximately three mitotic divisions occur; heme and the four polypeptide chains of globin (normally in adults, two alpha and two beta chains) are synthesized within the cell and united to form hemoglobin. From 10 to 15 per cent of cells probably die during some stage of development; in certain anemias, this ineffective erythropoiesis becomes much greater. The mechanism for delivery of cells to the peripheral circulation remains unknown. Although many of the corpuscles delivered to the peripheral blood are reticulocytes, others have apparently already lost the reticulum substance (ribonucleoprotein). Reticulocytes contain mitochondria and ribosomes, have synthetic activity, and demonstrate pronounced cellular movement; these properties are lost as the cell progresses within three or four days to a mature red corpuscle. When erythrocyte formation is greatly accelerated, reticulocytes are increased in number, nucleated red blood cells may be found in the peripheral blood, and some of the corpuscles may take a bluish hue with Wright's stain (basophilia) because of retained RNA. Control of the delivery mechanism is deranged in extramedullary hematopoiesis so that normoblasts in variable numbers are discharged into the blood stream. The normal corpuscle circulates for about 120 days; senescent red cells either are phagocytized and destroyed by the RE system (90 per cent) or are broken up intravascularly (10 per cent) as their membrane becomes less pliable and is less able to withstand the trauma of circulation. The normal steady state is maintained, therefore, by the daily formation and destruction of approximately 0.8 per cent of the red blood cell mass.

The physiologic mechanism responsible for maintaining the normal balance between erythrocyte formation and destruction is only partially understood. One of the controlling substances seems to be erythropoietin, apparently produced by the action of an enzyme elaborated by the kidney (renal erythropoietic factor) acting on a serum substrate. As erythropoiesis continues in anephric animals and man sustained by hemodialysis, however, there must either be an extrarenal source of erythropoietin or an additional erythropoietic stimulating mechanism. The site of action of erythropoietin appears to be primarily at the stem cell level, but some experimental work indicates that other stages in erythropoiesis may also be stimulated. Assayable levels of erythropoietin are increased by hypoxia and decreased by transfusion-induced polycythemia. Erythropoietin assays reported on human patients have revealed some surprises; they tend to be high in hypoplastic anemia and not increased in hemolytic states or polycythemia. To what extent these findings reflect poor utilization in hypoplastic anemia and active utilization when erythrocytosis is stimulated, rather than rates of production, is still uncertain.

The normal range of red blood cell values for adults is roughly:

	Men	Women
Erythrocytes	5.4 ± 0.8	4.8 ± 0.6 million/cu. mm.
Hemoglobin	16 ± 2	14 ± 2 grams/100 ml.
Packed cell volume	47 ± 7	42 ± 5 per cent

Values in children are approximately 10 to 20 per cent lower; differences between the sexes do not appear until after puberty. It would be more accurate to express corpuscular values as volume per kilogram of body weight (roughly 30.5 ml. for men and 23.5 ml. for adult women), but that is impractical. Variations in plasma volume do occur, however, that cause significant dilution or concentration of the red cell mass; as a result, instances have been recognized in which a normal circulating red cell mass may be associated with a hematocrit as low as 38 or as high as 60 per cent. The normal mean corpuscular volume (MCV) is 87 ± 5 cubic microns, and the mean corpuscular hemoglobin concentration (MCHbC) is 34 ± 2 per cent.

Anemia may be defined as a state in which the red blood cell values are less than normal. Because of variations in MCV and MCHbC, the values are not all equally abnormal. In a macrocytic anemia with an MCV of 120 cubic microns, for instance, the red blood cell count may be as low as 3.8 million per cubic millimeter with normal packed cell volume and hemoglobin levels; in hypochromic microcytic anemias the red blood cell count may remain normal while the hemoglobin and packed cell volume are depressed. Anemias may result from hemorrhage, decreased rates of erythropoiesis, accelerated destruction, or any combination of the three.

Ferrokinetic determination of hemoglobin synthesis and red blood cell survival measured with the radioactive chromium technique may be applied clinically to provide fairly accurate estimates of erythrocyte formation and destruction. These studies have demonstrated that (1) to a variable degree in different pathologic states, a portion of the red blood cells made in the bone marrow may be destroyed there without ever entering the circulation (ineffective erythropoiesis); (2) a mild to moderate shortening of erythrocyte life span is common to many anemias not previously suspected of having a hemolytic component; and (3) a normal marrow is capable of stepping up its rate of red blood cell formation six or seven times in response to a sustained demand. Consequently, erythrocyte survival in a chronic hemolytic anemia may be reduced from 120 to 20 days, and the bone marrow may be able to compensate sufficiently to maintain a normal total red blood cell count. More often, the marrow "decompensates," increasing its rate of production only three or four times when hemolysis is accelerated to a greater degree, and anemia results. These considerations help one think of anemias and of bone marrow function in physiologic terms.

Another illustration may be cited. A hypothetic patient has a normal red blood cell count of 5,000,000 per cubic millimeter and a circulating erythrocyte mass of 2400 ml.; with a corpuscular life span of 120 days, he would be destroying and making 20 ml. of erythrocytes per day. A disease now develops that causes his red cells to survive for only 40 days, so he begins to destroy 20 × 3 or 60 ml. of erythrocytes per day. Because the disease also affects his marrow, he is able to increase erythropoiesis to only 40 ml. per day. The corpuscular mass and count will gradually decrease until the circulating mass is down to 1600 ml. At this level, two thirds of the original, the volume of erythrocytes destroyed per day at a survival rate of 40 days will be 1600 ÷ 40 or 40 ml. A new equilibrium will now be set because the marrow is capable of producing this quantity of new cells per day. If the total blood volume has remained constant, the peripheral red blood cell count will now be 3,330,000 per cubic millimeter. The anemia in this hypothetic situation has resulted from increased hemolysis and failure of the marrow to compensate for a normally compensable rate of destruction—a state of relative bone marrow failure. True marrow failure, on the other hand, occurs when erythropoiesis falls below the normal rate for a given individual. In the past, it has often been difficult to understand why erythrocytic hyperplasia should be found in the bone marrow of anemic patients whose red blood cell formation was clearly inadequate; this finding can now be adequately explained in most instances as being due to relative marrow failure, to ineffective erythropoiesis, or to a combination of both.

Classification. Anemias are most frequently classified according to etiology or to morphology (MCV and MCHbC); neither classification is entirely satisfactory.

Anemias: Etiologic Classification

I. Loss of blood
  A. Acute
  B. Chronic
II. Excessive destruction of red corpuscles from
  A. Extracorpuscular causes
  B. Intracorpuscular defects
  C. Combination of both intra- and extracorpuscular influences (primaquine-sensitive hemolytic anemia, favism, lead poisoning, thermal injury)
III. Principally caused by impaired production
  A. Deficiency of substances essential for erythropoiesis (iron, vitamin B$_{12}$, folic acid, vitamin E, protein deficiency)
  B. Endocrine deficiency (pituitary, thyroid, adrenal, or testicular hormones)
  C. Physical or chemical injury (radiation, benzol, lead, and various other marrow toxins)
  D. Anemias associated with infection and various chronic diseases (renal, etc.)
  E. Myelophthisic anemias (leukemia, myelofibrosis, bone marrow involvement by Hodgkin's disease, metastatic carcinoma, granulomatous disorders, and so forth)
  F. Anemia associated with splenic disorders ("dyssplenism")
  G. Idiopathic bone marrow failure (aplastic, hypoplastic, sideroblastic, or refractory anemias)

Such an etiologic classification has many advantages, but fails by implying that mechanisms are purer than they really are; many of the hemolytic anemias are accompanied by defective erythropoiesis, at least in the sense that the rate of red blood cell production may be decidedly less than six or seven times the normal rate; greater than normal rates of red blood cell destruction are found in many anemias caused primarily by impaired production; and the anemia of chronic blood loss is essentially an iron deficiency anemia.

The morphologic classification is based on mean corpuscular size and hemoglobin concentration.

Anemias: Morphologic Classification

1. Macrocytic
    A. Megaloblastic (deficiency of vitamin B₁₂ or folic acid)
    B. Miscellaneous (chronic liver disease, hypothyroidism, normocytic anemias made temporarily macrocytic because of increased reticulocytes, etc.)
2. Normocytic
    A. Sudden loss of blood
    B. Hemolytic anemias
    C. Most of the anemias caused principally by impaired production (except deficiencies of vitamin B₁₂, folic acid, and iron)
3. Microcytic normochromic ("imperfect" formation of blood, as in subacute and chronic inflammatory conditions)
4. Microcytic hypochromic
    A. Iron deficiency anemia
    B. Miscellaneous (thalassemia major, pyridoxine-responsive anemia, sideroblastic refractory anemia)

The morphologic classification has the advantage that, if the MCV and MCHbC are determined with exacting care, the initial classification is automatic, a good start in differential diagnosis has been made, and a preliminary guide to therapy is provided. The megaloblastic macrocytic anemias respond to the administration of vitamin B₁₂ or folic acid, and the hypochromic anemias are usually caused by iron deficiency; for all the rest therapy is more difficult: treatment of the cause, transfusions, and in some cases splenectomy or corticosteroid or androgen administration. Disadvantages of the system are as follows: MCV and MCHbC must be calculated from values obtained with extreme care; crossovers between nonmegaloblastic macrocytic anemias and normocytic anemias are frequent; when a patient with megaloblastic anemia is also iron-deficient, the resulting mean corpuscular size may be normal.

Any system of classification, therefore, is a compromise. In the discussion that follows, a morphologic classification has been used, but only three main headings have been employed: megaloblastic, normocytic, and hypochromic. As a result, the nonmegaloblastic macrocytic and the microcytic normochromic anemias have been lumped with the normocytic anemias.

Physiologic adjustments to anemia include attempts to maintain a normal blood volume and to maintain the delivery of adequate amounts of oxygen to tissues. Plasma volume is increased to compensate for decreased red blood cell mass. Cardiac output is increased, circulation time becomes faster than normal, and respiration is stimulated. Exciting recent studies have also demonstrated an intraerythrocytic adaptation to anemia whereby the oxygen dissociation curve is shifted to the right so that hemoglobin has a decreased affinity for oxygen and more readily gives up its oxygen to tissues. This adjustment is mediated by a rise in erythrocyte organic phosphate, particularly 2,3-diphosphoglycerate; 2,3-DPG (and adenosine triphosphate) combines reversibly with deoxyhemoglobin, shifting the oxygen dissociation curve to the right. The increase in 2,3 DPG tends to be proportional to the degree of anemia, and frequently accounts for as much as half the compensation necessary to restore normal oxygen delivery to tissues.

Principles of Therapy. The therapeutic methods or agents available for treatment of anemia are comparatively few: vitamin B₁₂, folic acid, iron, transfusions, splenectomy, corticosteroids, androgens, recognition and removal of any bone marrow toxin, treatment of the cause (as in infection, rheumatoid arthritis, leukemia, etc.), replacement therapy in endocrine deficiency anemias, and in rare instances pyridoxine or crude liver extracts. Except under emergency conditions, therapy should be delayed until a diagnosis has been established. Diagnostic confusion and at times harm can result from indiscriminate use of vitamin B₁₂, folic acid, or iron; these substances are of great therapeutic value for the correction of specific deficiency states and should be so prescribed. "Shotgun" therapy of the anemias is indefensible. Transfusions must be wisely used; the incidence of serious reactions—even death—and of serum hepatitis is significant. When transfusions are given to older patients who are severely anemic, care must be taken to avoid circulatory overload. There is little reason to give transfusions when the hemoglobin is 10 grams per 100 ml. or more, or to raise the hemoglobin above that level. Reasonably fresh blood should be selected for administration to anemic patients, and the cross match should be checked with the indirect Coombs test. Splenectomy and administration of corticosteroids are valuable under very specific, select circumstances that will be stated in the discussion of specific diseases.

Crosby, W. H., and Akeroyd, J. H.: The limit of hemoglobin synthesis in hereditary anemia. Amer. J. Med., 13:273, 1952.

Gordon, A. S., Cooper, G. W., and Zanjani, E. D.: The kidney and erythropoiesis. Seminars Hemat., 4:437, 1967.

Harris, J. W.: The Red Cell—Production, Metabolism, Destruction: Normal and Abnormal. Cambridge, Mass., Harvard University Press, 1963.

Moore, C. V.: The concept of relative bone marrow failure. Amer. J. Med., 23:1, 1957.

Stohlman, F., Jr. (ed.): The Kinetics of Cellular Proliferation. New York, Grune and Stratton, Inc., 1959. Section V, Kinetics of the Regulation of Red Cell Production (by numerous authors).

Torrance, J., Jacobs, P., Restrepo, A., Eschbach, J., Lenfant, C., and Finch, C. A.: Intraerythrocytic adaptation to anemia. New Eng. J. Med., 283:165, 1970.

Wintrobe, M. M.: Clinical Hematology. 6th ed. Philadelphia, Lea and Febiger, 1967.

MEGALOBLASTIC ANEMIAS

INTRODUCTION

James H. Jandl

Definition. The megaloblastic anemias comprise a group of closely related disorders of hematopoiesis having in common the following cardinal features: (1) slowly progressive macrocytic anemia, leukopenia, and thrombocytopenia; (2) "megaloblastic" changes in the bone marrow; (3) frequent association of oral, gastrointestinal, or neurologic damage; and (4) in most instances, hematologic response to either vitamin B_{12} or folic acid.

Pathologic Physiology. The metabolic disturbance underlying various megaloblastic anemias is a disordered synthesis of deoxyribonucleic acid (DNA). An acquired general impairment in DNA synthesis is usually the result of a deficiency in one of two factors, vitamin B_{12} or folic acid, that are essential to the formation of DNA precursors. The similarity of the cellular lesions created by deficiencies in these vitamins is attributable to their similar sites of action, as will be discussed below. As the result of impaired formation of these precursors, proliferating cells that are preparing for division have difficulty in replicating their complement of DNA during the DNA synthetic (S) phase of the cell division cycle. The S phase is thereby prolonged, the cell cycle is disturbed, and cells accumulate in midcycle with an amount of DNA that exceeds that of a normal somatic cell (approximately 6×10^{-12} grams) but that is less than the doubled amount required for mitosis. Those cells that are eventually successful in reaching the phase of mitosis often manifest a variety of minor chromosomal errors, but actual mitotic arrest is not conspicuous. However, during each ensuing S phase the risk of a lethal delay in DNA replication is cumulative. In contrast to the slowed or interrupted synthesis of DNA, RNA synthesis seems to be disturbed little, if at all, in most megaloblastic anemias; accordingly, the RNA content of the cytoplasm may be very high, and in erythroblasts the main cytoplasmic function, hemoglobin synthesis, proceeds normally. The morphologic expression of these underlying disturbances is that red cell precursors in the marrow develop delicate sievelike chromatin patterns, enlarged deformed nuclei, and eventually the advanced changes of karyorrhexis and karyolysis. During the protracted cell cycle hemoglobin continues to accumulate, despite the arrested maturation of the nucleus; this asynchrony or "unbalanced growth" eventuates in large cells with young-appearing nuclei and old-appearing orthochromatic or eosinophilic cytoplasm. Most of the erythroblasts are permanently arrested during one or another of their several division cycles and are eventually destroyed within the marrow itself;

this process of intramedullary hemolysis, often termed "ineffective erythropoiesis," leads to increased erythrophagocytosis, heavy depositions of hemosiderin in the marrow, and heightened bile pigment excretion as the result of a marked increase in the second portion of the so-called "early-labeling peak" of bile pigments. Intramedullary hemolysis appears also to be responsible for the elevations, often high, in the serum levels of lactate dehydrogenase and α-hydroxybutyrate in patients with megaloblastic anemia. A few erythroblasts attain a level of maturity capable of producing red cells that can survive in the circulation. These cells nevertheless are bizarre: most are large and oval in shape, often containing nuclear remnants (Howell-Jolly bodies, Cabot rings), and some are small and deformed. It is probable that the characteristic oval macrocytosis of these "nutritional macrocytic anemias" results from the omission of one of the maturation divisions, whereby red cells having up to twice the normal cell volume are released from the marrow. The cell population is so replete with heterogeneous deformities, however, that the values for mean corpuscular volume may range from high normal to almost twice normal. Although less severely affected than those precursor cells that die in the marrow, the circulating red cells in patients with megaloblastic anemias do not survive normally, and many are sequestered prematurely in the spleen. Thus hemolysis, most of it in the marrow, may be regarded as the direct mechanism of anemia. However, the functional defect is the inadequate release of red cells from the marrow, reticulocyte levels therefore being low; accordingly, the megaloblastic anemias are best regarded as the result of underproduction, and should be classified among the disorders of erythropoiesis.

The disordered metabolism of DNA in the megaloblastic anemias also affects the maturation of granulocytes and of megakaryocytes, resulting in a moderate leukopenia, because of granulocytopenia, and in thrombocytopenia that is usually moderate but occasionally severe. Abnormal nuclear chromatin and cytomegaly are found in the granulocyte precursors, with giant metamyelocytes and giant band forms prevalent in marrow aspirates and hypersegmented polymorphonuclear leukocytes in the peripheral blood. Indeed, the finding of neutrophils with more than five lobes and an increase in the proportion of cells with four or five lobes, along with the presence of oval macrocytes, is often the first reliable indication that a megaloblastic anemia exists. The association of epithelial and, in some instances, neurologic damage with the megaloblastic anemias and the finding of giant epithelial cells in the mouth, stomach, and vagina of affected patients indicate that the metabolic disorders underlying the megaloblastic anemias are not confined to the blood cells.

The overwhelming majority of patients with megaloblastic anemia have a deficiency either of vitamin B_{12} or of folic acid; on recognizing that a megaloblastic process exists, one's chief diagnostic

ETIOLOGIC CLASSIFICATION OF THE MEGALOBLASTIC ANEMIAS

I. Vitamin B_{12} deficiency
  A. Defective diet (low in animal or bacterial products)
  B. Defective absorption
    1. Deficiency of intrinsic factor
      a. "Addisonian" pernicious anemia, adult onset and adolescent-onset ("juvenile")
      b. "Congenital" pernicious anemia
      c. Gastrectomy
    2. Competition for vitamin B_{12}
      a. "Blind-loop" syndrome
      b. Jejunal diverticula
      c. Fish tapeworm infestation
    3. Intestinal malabsorption (sprue; celiac disease; steatorrhea; resection, bypass, or disease of the ileum; "specific malabsorption")
  C. Deranged metabolism
    Increased requirement (pregnancy, ?thyrotoxicosis, ?neoplasia)

II. Folic acid deficiency
  A. Defective diet (low in vegetables and liver)
  B. Defective absorption
    Intestinal malabsorption (sprue; celiac disease; steatorrhea; resection of proximal small intestine; short circuits of the gastrointestinal tract; inhibition of intestinal deconjugating enzyme – ?Dilantin, ??oral contraceptives)
  C. Deranged metabolism
    1. Increased requirement (hemolytic anemia, pregnancy, neoplasia)
    2. Impaired utilization (administration of folic acid antagonists, ?liver disease, ?anticonvulsants, ?scurvy)

III. Miscellaneous and "refractory" megaloblastic anemias

problem is to discriminate between these two disorders. A deficiency of either vitamin B_{12} or folic acid may in turn arise in any of a number of ways, as indicated in the accompanying table. A small number of affected patients are not deficient in either of these vitamins and have a "refractory macrocytic anemia"; usually in these patients the morphologic changes described above are atypical or are less striking, and so-called "intermediate megaloblasts" may populate the marrow.

Deficiency of Vitamin B_{12}. Vitamin B_{12} is a reddish compound possessing a cobalt-containing ring (corrin) resembling the tetrapyrrolic ring of porphyrin. It is synthesized by certain micro-organisms and is principally available to man in diets containing the flesh of animals having access to bacterial products. The absorption of dietary vitamin B_{12} (extrinsic factor) requires its interaction with a mucoid secretion of the gastric fundus—the gastric *intrinsic factor* of Castle. This thermolabile substance, secreted in man by the gastric parietal cells, has an unusually strong binding affinity for vitamin B_{12} and facilitates its absorption by the ileum, apparently by attaching to specific Ca^{++}-dependent receptors on the intestinal wall at pH 6.5 or above. Intrinsic factor is essential to the absorption of normal dietary amounts of vitamin B_{12}; however, when unnaturally large amounts of vitamin B_{12} are ingested, a small portion will diffuse across the gut wall in the absence of intrinsic factor. After a delay of several hours in the gut wall the vitamin,

no longer associated with intrinsic factor, is carried through the blood stream by specific protein carriers (α_1 and β globulins), and most of it is deposited in the liver, which in normal adults contains about 1 μg. of vitamin B_{12} per gram of tissue. Thereafter the vitamin is apparently utilized by growing cells, in the form of cobamide derivatives that function as coenzymes or cofactors in various metabolic pathways. As noted earlier, the principal function of vitamin B_{12} with respect to blood formation is its role in the synthesis of DNA precursor compounds. Evidence in certain bacteria indicates that vitamin B_{12} is bound intracellularly to a special class of ribosomes that convert it to a coenzyme form. This coenzyme (5'-deoxyadenosyl cobamide coenzyme, or DBC coenzyme) is then released into the soluble cytoplasm to act as a cofactor for ribonucleotide reductase, promoting conversion of ribonucleotides to deoxyribonucleotides. Although an attractive explanation for defective DNA precursor synthesis occurring with vitamin B_{12} deficiency, this pathway has not been demonstrated in mammalian systems and is demonstrable in only certain micro-organisms. In man, two vitamin B_{12} coenzyme forms are known to exist. Methylcobalamin, probably produced in the liver from vitamin B_{12} and S-adenosylmethionine, may participate in DNA synthesis as an intrinsic component of the methyltetrahydrofolate-homocysteine transmethylase system, whereby it may be involved indirectly in the methylation of thymine to thymidine. The second, DBC coenzyme, is formed through adenosylation of the vitamin by ATP in the liver and kidney. This active cofactor is essential in the methylmalonyl CoA isomerase (or mutase) reaction of mitochondria, a function apparently unrelated to any role in cell proliferation. This key step in propionate metabolism, in which methylmalonyl CoA is converted reversibly to succinyl CoA, is vital to species such as ruminants, which rely heavily upon propionate as a primary nutrient. In man, impairment of this vitamin B_{12}-dependent isomerase (mutase) reaction, detectable by the accumulation and hyperexcretion of methylmalonate, appears to be considerably less damaging than in ruminants, but may be responsible for more subtle disturbances in lipid metabolism, possibly including metabolic abnormalities of the central nervous system. Recently an inborn error of metabolism appearing during infancy, characterized by methylmalonic aciduria and profound ketoacidosis without megaloblastic anemia, has been recognized. The defect appears to represent a mutation of methylmalonyl CoA isomerase, resulting in failure of conversion of methylmalonyl CoA to succinyl CoA. Parenteral administration of large doses of vitamin B_{12} results in reduction of methylmalonic acid secretion and clinical improvement in some patients. Requirements for the various vitamin B_{12} coenzymes are evidently greatest during the rapid growth period of infancy and childhood and during pregnancy and are probably increased in such disorders as thyrotoxicosis, infection, hemolytic anemia, and neoplasia. In the normal adult the average daily requirement of vitamin B_{12} is approximately 1 μg., although the liver normally contains a reserve of about 1 or 2 mg. that is sufficient for several years.

The causes of vitamin B_{12} deficiency are listed in the outline of etiologic classification of megaloblastic anemias (Table). Simple dietary deficiency of vitamin B_{12} is rarely responsible for megaloblastic anemia in temperate North America; it is found chiefly in strict vegetarians and occasionally in mild form in the chronically malnourished and the debilitated. In underdeveloped—particularly tropical—lands, in which diets low in animal protein prevail, deficiency of vitamin B_{12} is relatively common. Not uncommonly, mixed deficiencies of vitamin B_{12} and of folic acid are encountered, resulting in diagnostic confusion and in suboptimal therapeutic responses. Particularly troublesome is the combination of iron deficiency with deficiency either of vitamin B_{12} or of folic acid, for the morphologic changes in iron deficiency anemia are diametrically opposite to those of the megaloblastic anemias. Indeed it is quite probable that iron deficiency, by suppressing cytoplasmic function, acts to correct the "unbalanced growth" of the megaloblast. The result is that in such a mixed deficiency state morphologic study of the marrow and blood may show them to be remarkably normal, or there may appear to be two different populations of cells ("*dimorphic* anemia"). Usually the marrow is described as containing so-called "intermediate megaloblasts," and the deposits of marrow hemosiderin, characteristically heavy in megaloblastic anemias, may be scanty. Often the existence of one component of a mixed deficiency may become expressed morphologically during therapy with the other. A mixed deficiency of vitamin B_{12} and of iron is particularly encountered in pernicious anemia patients with bleeding gastric lesions (gastritis, polyps, and neoplasms).

PERNICIOUS ANEMIA

(Addisonian Pernicious Anemia, Biermer's Anemia, "Primary" Anemia)

James H. Jandl

Pernicious anemia is by far the most prevalent form of vitamin B_{12} deficiency in temperate North America. It is a "conditioned deficiency" of vitamin B_{12} arising from failure of the gastric fundus to secrete amounts of intrinsic factor adequate to ensure intestinal absorption of vitamin B_{12}. This failure of intrinsic factor secretion results from atrophy of the fundic glandular mucosa. The cardinal features of the disease are (1) chronic and progressive megaloblastic anemia of insidious onset; (2) achylia gastrica; (3) frequent occurrence of neurologic and, to a lesser extent, gastrointestinal damage; and (4) invariable benefit from parenteral administration of vitamin B_{12}.

True pernicious anemia is uncommon in persons less than 35 years old, but the incidence rises progressively thereafter with age. Both sexes are affected equally. Although found in all races, pernicious anemia may be particularly prevalent in people of northern European descent; it tends to affect blue-eyed persons of "bulky frame" with a propensity toward premature graying of the hair, and it is somewhat more frequent in people with blood group A. Although the essential lesion of pernicious anemia, failure of intrinsic factor secretion, may arise from many processes interfering with normal gastric secretory function (*vide infra*), in most patients the gastric lesion is idiopathic. About one in every five such patients gives a family history of pernicious anemia, but no clear mode of inheritance can be defined at present, presumably because a multiplicity of factors may lead to "spontaneous" gastric fundic atrophy. A small number of cases develop as the result of obvious damage to gastric secretory function, as by extensive neoplasia or gastrectomy. Vitamin B_{12} deficiency has been reported to occur in approximately 15 per cent of all patients after partial gastrectomy and gastrojejunostomy for peptic ulcer, a much higher incidence being recorded among patients who have been followed five years or more. Following total gastrectomy the syndrome of pernicious anemia is inevitable, its onset being delayed only by virtue of the pre-existing body stores of vitamin B_{12}. Whereas removal of the entire gastric fundus, as in total gastrectomy, deprives the patient of all intrinsic factor and predestines a deficiency of vitamin B_{12}, most patients with subtotal gastrectomy, even though extensive, usually retain sufficient fundic activity to avert vitamin B_{12} deficiency, provided the dietary intake, intestinal function, and body requirements are reasonably normal. It appears that the tendency for "pernicious anemia" to appear after partial gastrectomy is usually attributable not simply to inadequate secretion of intrinsic factor but also to dietary factors and to the impairment in intestinal function resulting from the duodenal bypass. There is some clinical and experimental evidence that protracted iron deficiency may predispose to pernicious anemia by causing gastric atrophy and curtailing the secretion of intrinsic factor. The secretion of intrinsic factor varies from person to person, and it is probable that an inborn tendency toward hyposecretion may be exacerbated by such factors, as well as by pregnancy and by aging. Indeed, a number of studies suggest that a state of "pre-pernicious anemia" may exist for years or decades before intrinsic factor secretion is so curtailed that tissue vitamin B_{12} levels fall and anemia develops. As little as 1 per cent of normal intrinsic factor secretion will likely prevent the development of pernicious anemia.

In recent years considerable evidence has accumulated implicating immunologic mechanisms in the pathogenesis of the gastric lesion of pernicious anemia. Most patients (about 90 per cent) with pernicious anemia possess defined serum antibodies that react specifically with the parietal cells of the gastric fundus. These complement-fixing, precipitating *parietal cell antibodies* are directed against microsomal antigens in the parietal cells and, like many organ-specific antibodies, are lacking in species specificity. Many patients with pernicious anemia, almost half, also have analogous antibodies against microsomal antigens of thyroid and, conversely, there is a high incidence of parietal cell antibodies in patients with thyroid disease, particularly in those with Hashimoto's thyroiditis. Relatives of patients with pernicious anemia, in addition to having an increased incidence of pernicious anemia and of achlorhydria, also have a comparatively high incidence of parietal cell antibodies, of thyroid antibodies, and even of antinuclear antibodies—a kind occasionally found in the patients themselves. Parietal cell antibodies are also found in most patients with chronic gastritis, and appear in from 5 to 10 per cent of normal people, the incidence increasing with age; most such "normal" people with parietal cell antibodies do in fact have chronic gastritis. In addition, roughly half of all pernicious anemia patients possess serum antibodies that appear to be directed specifically against human intrinsic factor, but that do not interfere with vitamin B_{12} absorption unless they leak into or are secreted into the gut. These IgG antibodies are detected by their ability to inhibit the formation of complexes to vitamin B_{12} with intrinsic factor ("blocking" antibodies) or to prevent the vitamin B_{12}–intrinsic factor complex from attaching to ileal receptor sites ("binding" antibodies). Unlike parietal cell antibodies, the antibodies to intrinsic factor are only rarely found in patients without pernicious anemia, their presence being virtually diagnostic of that disorder. The several findings that have been described, and the observation that prolonged administration of glucocorticoids to pernicious anemia patients may partially reverse the gastric lesion and enhance the absorption of vitamin B_{12}, have led to the view that autoimmune mechanisms may initiate, or at least perpetuate, the gastric lesion, either through the action of serum antibodies or more likely through associated cell-mediated hypersensitivity mechanisms. Indeed, the fact that parietal cell antibodies are more prevalent than gastric atrophy or achlorhydria in relatives of affected patients supports the hypothesis that an immunologic injury to the gastric mucosa is of primary pathogenic importance; the high incidence of these antibodies (about 20 per cent) among relatives and their distribution have led to the suggestion that pernicious anemia is the full and final expression of an immunologic process that is transmitted or controlled by a single-gene ("dominant") autosomal inheritance. An alternative view is that the antibodies described are associated, or secondary, manifestations having no essential part in the pathogenesis of the basic disease process.

Although pernicious anemia is characteristically a disease of older adults, occasionally a similar process is encountered in children. In some of these, in whom anemia is first manifest in late childhood or adolescence, the disease has the full clinical and pathologic picture of adult pernicious anemia: vitamin B_{12} deficiency, achlorhydria, and gastric mucosal atrophy ("adolescent-onset" or "juvenile" pernicious anemia). Most of these children also manifest multiple endocrine deficiencies. There is a high incidence of antibodies to intrinsic factor and to various endocrine gland acinar cells. In contrast to these, a number of patients have been reported who develop a megaloblastic anemia and vitamin B_{12} deficiency even earlier in childhood, commonly before two and a half ("infantile" or "congenital" pernicious anemia). These patients are lacking or severely deficient in the ability to secrete intrinsic factor, but they are not deficient in hydrochloric acid secretion, and their gastric mucosa remains histologically normal. It is of particular interest that these children, often the issue of consanguineous parents, lack antibodies either to parietal cells or to intrinsic factor, as do their relatives. Accordingly, it is generally believed that this rare and distinctive variant of pernicious anemia results from an inborn error in the formation of intrinsic factor, presumably the homozygous expression of an uncommon, "recessive" gene. These two entities affecting children or infants are sometimes referred to, without adequate distinction, as "juvenile pernicious anemia." A third group of young patients, who are selectively unable to absorb vitamin B_{12}, was first clearly defined by Imerslund and by Gräsbeck. These individuals manifest megaloblastic anemia, vitamin B_{12} deficiency, and proteinuria without other renal abnormalities, usually by two years of age. They appear to have "specific malabsorption" of vitamin B_{12} because of an intestinal defect, and thus are more correctly classified as having a form of intestinal malabsorption than as having pernicious anemia. Gastric mucosal histology, acid secretion, and intrinsic factor activity are normal. Evidence suggests autosomal recessive inheritance.

Clinical Manifestations. The clinical manifestations of pernicious anemia derive from the involvement of the blood, the nervous sytem, and the gastrointestinal system. When fully manifest, involvement of these three systems is sufficiently characteristic to permit an immediate diagnosis. In most, but not in all patients, symptoms arising from anemia appear at some time in the course of the disease. These include increased fatigability, weakness, faintness, pallor, and shortness of breath, usually progressing slowly and variably over the course of several months or even years. These symptoms are less dramatic than in persons with other anemias of comparable severity but of more rapid onset. Sooner or later neurologic complaints arise in most patients, and in some these may be the first symptoms. The earliest are symmetrical paresthesias of the toes or fingers, which may progress to feelings of numbness and weakness and to difficulty in walking or in performing such acts as buttoning clothing or holding utensils. Eventually incoordination, stiffness, weakness, and spasticity, particularly in the lower extremities, may cripple the patient severely. Loss of the senses of taste and smell may occur. Cerebral symptoms, not necessarily attributable to anoxia, are common and include dullness, apathy, irritability, loss of concentration, and sometimes—particularly in the elderly—frank psychoses. Some patients with pernicious anemia complain of a sore tongue; rarely there is soreness of the entire mouth. Epigastric discomfort and constipation or diarrhea are frequent but are seldom severe.

On physical examination the patient usually appears pale and may show an extreme waxy pallor, often tinged with jaundice or a "lemon yellow." Despite this appearance and the patient's history of pallor and weakness, he is not usually wasted and may be somewhat obese, or, in Addison's words, "flabby" and "bulky." The pulse is soft and bounding. There may be some fever, particularly with severe anemia. As in other severe anemias, retinal hemorrhages may be striking. Frequently the tongue is smooth and shiny, particularly at the tip and sides; in some patients it is beefy red as well, and rarely there may be ulcerations or vesicles. In at least half of the patients with pernicious anemia the tongue is of normal appearance; earlier descriptions of prevalent, marked glossal changes are attributable in part to later diagnosis and to complicating deficiencies of iron or of other B vitamins. The effects of anemia on the heart are manifest, with tachycardia and soft "hemic" murmurs audible. The liver may be somewhat enlarged. The spleen is probably enlarged in most patients, but it is seldom palpable. The various possible neurologic findings when fully manifest are sometimes given the pathologic terms "*combined system disease of the spinal cord*," "subacute combined sclerosis," or "posterolateral sclerosis." The most common and earliest of these neurologic changes is the loss of vibratory and, as time goes on, of position sense in the distal extremities. There may be loss of sensibility to touch, but often not to pain or temperature, over affected areas. Ataxia, positive Romberg's sign, diminished or heightened reflexes, flaccidity, extensor plantar responses and spasticity, and sphincter paralysis may be encountered in various patterns as the cord lesions progress. Visual defects and optic atrophy occasionally are observed. (For a full description of the clinical and pathologic features of combined system disease consult the appropriate article in the section on Disorders of the Nervous System and Behavior.)

Anemia eventually occurs in all patients although it may follow the neuropathy in onset in about one patient in ten. In neglected cases it may be extreme, red blood cell counts below 500,000 per cubic millimeter having been recorded. As in other megaloblastic anemias, the peripheral blood is characterized by oval macrocytosis, poikilo-cytosis, leukopenia with hypersegmented polymorphonuclear leukocytes, and usually a mild or moderate thrombocytopenia. Low-grade eosinophilia is not uncommon. On aspiration the bone marrow is voluminous and hypercellular; on removing the stylet from the inserted bone marrow needle, one often notes red marrow oozing over the needle hub. Microscopically, abnormal red and white blood cell precursors are seen. The serum bilirubin level is usually slightly elevated, and stool and urine urobilinogen levels are increased as is the serum concentration of lactate dehydrogenase (LDH), which may increase strikingly in the serum—particularly in serum obtained from bone marrow aspirates. Serum iron levels are elevated in relapse but fall abruptly between 12 and 24 hours after parenteral therapy.

In practically all adult patients with pernicious anemia the gastric juice lacks free hydrochloric acid even after subcutaneous injection of histamine (0.01 mg. per kilogram of body weight) or of its less toxic analogue, betazole. Characteristically, one can recover only small volumes of a mucoid secretion that lacks rennin and pepsin as well as hydrochloric acid and is described by the term "achylia." On gastroscopy, the mucosa appears gray and thinned out. Cells obtained by gastric lavage are large and reveal nuclear abnormalities. On histologic examination, whether before or after therapy, the mucosa of the gastric fundus usually shows marked thinning as the result of a diminished population of glandular epithelial cells. Parietal cells and chief cells are virtually absent, whereas mucus-secreting cells persist in relatively normal numbers. Usually the lamina propria is infiltrated to some extent with lymphocytes and plasma cells, and scattered islands of intestinal epithelial cells may appear as the result of intestinal metaplasia.

Diagnosis. Pernicious anemia should be thought of in any patient with megaloblastic anemia (or with the premegaloblastic blood changes described), particularly if the patient is over 40 years of age. The suspicion is increased if there is no history of antecedent malnutrition or of symptoms of general intestinal malabsorption, and it is practically certain if there are associated neurologic symptoms of the kinds described above. If, in addition, a histamine-fast achlorhydria exists, the diagnosis of pernicious anemia should be presumed. Clinical substantiation of this diagnosis requires evidence of a hematologic response to injected vitamin B_{12}. To be fully accepted, such a "therapeutic trial" should be preceded by a control period of a week or ten days during which reticulocyte levels remain fairly steady and low, and hemoglobin levels neither rise nor fall sharply. Usually, however, such a preliminary period is not feasible, and it may be necessary to proceed at once with a therapeutic trial. Large doses of vitamin B_{12} may occasionally induce partial responses in patients deficient only in folic acid (*vide infra*). Accordingly, if a therapeutic trial is to be conducted, the dose of vitamin B_{12} should not exceed

30 µg. daily and is best limited to daily parenteral doses of 1 to 5 µg. Ordinarily the reticulocyte concentration first rises appreciably on the third or fourth day of therapy, increases sharply to a "peak" value on the fifth to the eighth day, and then more gradually diminishes as the red cell count and hemoglobin rise to normal levels. The magnitude of the reticulocyte response is proportional to the severity of the anemia. The hematologic response to vitamin B$_{12}$ can also be judged by a conversion of the megaloblastic marrow to a normoblastic one, and, less reliably, by a rise in leukocyte and platelet levels. The limitations of the therapeutic trial are that a control period is necessary and that the therapeutic response may be stifled by complicating factors such as infection, concomitant iron deficiency, or uremia which may inhibit the marrow response. Vitamin B$_{12}$ deficiency can also be established by finding a low serum level of the vitamin by microbiologic assay, keeping in mind that the specific diagnosis of pernicious anemia requires also some evidence of deficiency of intrinsic factor. Although practicable only in specialized laboratories, determination of serum levels of vitamin B$_{12}$ has proved a highly reliable diagnostic technique; as assayed with *Euglena gracilis*, the sera of patients with pernicious anemia virtually always contain less than 100 micromicrograms of vitamin B$_{12}$ per milliliter. A biochemical indication of vitamin B$_{12}$ deficiency at the tissue level can be obtained by quantitating the urinary excretion of methylmalonic acid; an increased excretion of this metabolite reflects a block in the methylmalonyl CoA isomerase reaction described earlier, and is a highly specific indication of vitamin B$_{12}$ deficiency.

Deficiency of intrinsic factor may be suspected in patients with gastric achlorhydria, particularly in those with scanty volumes of gastric juice. In most instances the association of clinical or laboratory evidence of vitamin B$_{12}$ deficiency with gastric achlorhydria must suffice for the diagnosis of pernicious anemia. A more direct, albeit more sophisticated, test for the presence of intrinsic factor involves the oral administration of radioactive vitamin B$_{12}$, e.g., ^{60}Co- or ^{57}Co-labeled cyanocobalamin in a dose of 2.0 µg. In pernicious anemia very little of the labeled vitamin is absorbed, as determined by subsequently measuring the radioactivity of the stool, that over the liver, or, most commonly, that excreted in the urine after the patient is given a large parenteral "flushing" dose of unlabeled vitamin B$_{12}$ (the Schilling test). Since patients with vitamin B$_{12}$ deficiency caused by intestinal disease may have adequate intrinsic factor but may be unable to absorb the vitamin for other reasons, full confirmation of the diagnosis necessitates a second test in which labeled vitamin B$_{12}$ is given together with a preparation of intrinsic factor. In patients with pernicious anemia, even those in remission, the addition of intrinsic factor increases absorption of labeled vitamin B$_{12}$; in patients with primary intestinal malabsorption it does not. In performing the Schilling test in patients in hematologic relapse one should not overlook the fact that the "flushing" dose of vitamin B$_{12}$ eliminates any possibility of a subsequent therapeutic trial. Indeed, the Schilling test should be postponed until after a specific therapeutic effect has been established; it might be emphasized that this test does not detect vitamin B$_{12}$ deficiency, but is a measure of intrinsic factor function in vivo. In recent years several reliable methods have been devised for assaying gastric juice for intrinsic factor in vitro. Such methods, which make use of the strong binding of vitamin B$_{12}$ by intrinsic factor, have been used principally as investigative tools but may receive broader clinical application in the future.

Treatment. The treatment of pernicious anemia necessitates lifelong parenteral administration of vitamin B$_{12}$. Although animal liver extracts containing vitamin B$_{12}$ are still available for patients accustomed to such preparations, about 10 per cent develop local or general hypersensitivity reactions. It is preferable to use solutions of crystalline vitamin B$_{12}$, e.g., cyanocobalamin or hydroxocobalamin. A maximal hematologic response can be achieved with only 1 µg. of parenteral vitamin B$_{12}$ daily, and hematologic remission can be sustained by injection of as little as 20 to 30 µg. of vitamin B$_{12}$ monthly. However, with such doses the liver is unable to accumulate a reserve of the vitamin, and serum vitamin B$_{12}$ levels tend to be low. Accordingly, for the untreated patient whose diagnosis is considered established, or for whom a therapeutic trial with small "physiologic" doses is not practical, and for patients previously given a therapeutic trial, larger doses should be employed in an effort to build up some tissue reserve of vitamin B$_{12}$. A recommended practice is to give injections of 100 µg. of vitamin B$_{12}$ daily for approximately one week and at monthly intervals thereafter for the remainder of the patient's life. Oral therapy with massive doses of vitamin B$_{12}$ or with smaller doses in combination with animal intrinsic factor is less reliable.

For patients whose anemia is life-threatening, as when the hemoglobin concentration falls below 3 or 4 grams per 100 ml., it may be too risky to await hematologic remission, and transfusions may be judiciously employed in addition to vitamin B$_{12}$ therapy. If transfusions must be given, they should be administered slowly, preferably as packed cells. Ordinarily, one transfusion will suffice to avoid calamity; hurried or excessive transfusion to patients with pernicious anemia carries an exceptional risk of acute fatal pulmonary or cerebral edema.

The response of the patient with pernicious anemia to initial therapy with vitamin B$_{12}$ is usually dramatic. Within 24 to 48 hours there is often a change in mood and sense of well-being, followed shortly by increased appetite and strength. Associated with the characteristic hematologic response previously described (see accompanying figure), pallor and jaundice lessen,

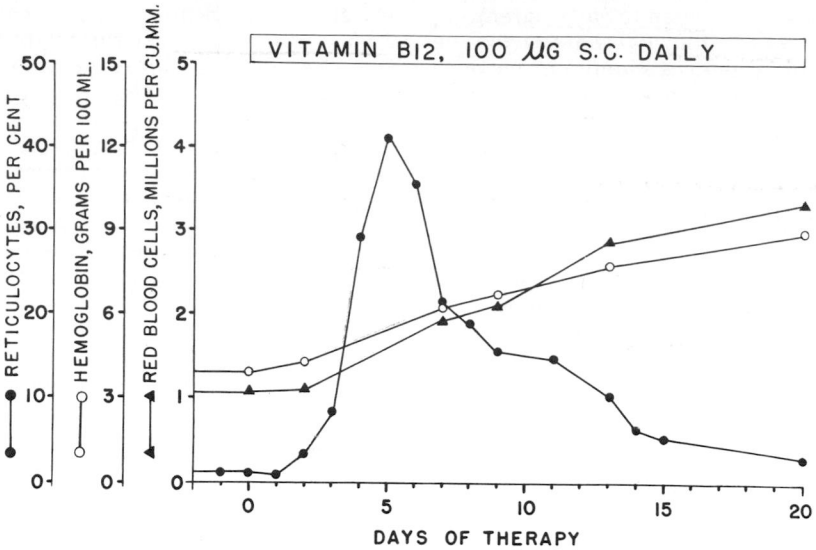

Response of the blood to therapy with vitamin B_{12} in a patient with pernicious anemia. In an uncomplicated, maximal response such as this, the reticulocyte concentration usually starts to rise on the third day of therapy and reaches a peak level on the fifth or sixth day, declining slowly thereafter. As the macrocytes are replaced by new red cells of normal size, there is a somewhat steeper increment in red count than in hemoglobin concentration or hematocrit.

the plasma volume increases, and transient water retention with dependent edema may be evident toward the end of the first week. A number of less striking metabolic changes may be detected, including acute hyperuricemia, hypoferremia, and decrease in urinary phosphorus levels. Mental changes, including psychotic manifestations, may or may not improve rapidly. The milder peripheral neurologic defects usually show significant improvement, whereas most manifestations of spinal cord injury are merely arrested, although functional improvement can occur with time. As the anemia gradually improves, there is a slow abatement of the cardiovascular symptoms.

Folic acid is closely related to vitamin B_{12} in its metabolic actions and, given in sufficient amounts, it will produce a partial, albeit impermanent, hematologic remission in most patients with pernicious anemia. Unlike vitamin B_{12}, folic acid does not arrest—and may possibly exacerbate—the neuropathy. Because folic acid is absorbed normally by patients with pernicious anemia, its oral administration in early, unsuspected cases, by ameliorating the hematologic changes, may cause the neuropathy to progress undiagnosed. It is probable that the danger of "masking" pernicious anemia is a function of folic acid dosage and that small daily doses of 0.1 to 0.2 mg., sufficient to correct a dietary deficiency of folic acid, may be employed safely for nutritional support to the undernourished. It may be emphasized that some patients with combined system disease of the spinal cord, whether or not folic acid had been administered, have little or no anemia. Virtually all such patients, however, do have some telltale morphologic abnormalities in their peripheral blood and bone marrow.

Prognosis. Prior to therapy with liver or vitamin B_{12}, pernicious anemia was an inexorable, fatal

disease; however, with appropriate and regular therapy the hematologic abnormalities are fully corrected, as are some of the epidermal changes. Much of the neurologic damage remains unchanged, although the more recent and peripheral damage may improve appreciably. On cessation of therapy, hematologic relapse or progression of the neuropathy may be expected to commence between two and three months or two and three years later. Presumably as an association with the chronic gastric atrophy, benign polyps and carcinoma of the stomach are relatively frequent in patients with pernicious anemia, occurring eventually in about one in ten. Accordingly, inquiries concerning gastric or constitutional symptoms are warranted at each examination, and stool examinations for occult blood should be made periodically.

INTESTINAL MALABSORPTION
James H. Jandl

Malabsorption of intestinal origin is a less common cause of vitamin B_{12} deficiency than achylia gastrica in temperate North America. However, in persons with long-standing intestinal disease that involves the ileum, or following ileal resection, vitamin B_{12} deficiency is common, as judged by serum levels of the vitamin, and megaloblastic anemia may be encountered. Thus, patients with idiopathic steatorrhea, sprue, celiac disease, regional enteritis, intestinal bypasses, and comparable disorders should receive parenteral vitamin B_{12} for the duration of their ileal dysfunction. Intestinal malabsorption of vitamin B_{12} may occur alone, unaccompanied by detectable malabsorption of other nutrients. *Competitive utilization of vitamin B_{12} by certain bacteria* appears to account for difficulty in absorbing the vitamin in the presence of intestinal blind loops, jejunal diverticula, and other causes of intestinal stasis; this particular type of absorption defect may be corrected by oral administration of a tetracycline. Intestinal infestation by the fish tapeworm *Diphyllobothrium latum* may cause vitamin B_{12} deficiency and megaloblastic anemia among peoples who eat uncooked fish. When a large worm is high in the intestine, it pre-empts dietary vitamin B_{12} and thereby deprives its host. Treatment consists of expelling the worm and temporarily administering parenteral vitamin B_{12}.

The propensity of a person to become deficient in vitamin B_{12} through any of the mechanisms described is undoubtedly influenced by the efficiency of the other mechanisms. Thus, in persons with incipient pernicious anemia the onset of the deficiency will be accelerated by dietary lack, partial gastrectomy, or infestation with *D. latum*. Similarly when assimilation of vitamin B_{12} is marginal, such increased demand as may be incurred during such diverse states as pregnancy, thyrotoxicosis, or neoplastic proliferation may precipitate frank deficiency.

DEFICIENCY OF FOLIC ACID*
Herman A. Godwin

Pathogenesis. Folic acid (pteroylglutamic acid) is synthesized by higher plants as well as by microorganisms and occurs richly in many vegetables, as well as in liver. A normal balanced diet contains 1.0 to 1.5 mg. of folic acid, although much of this may be destroyed by cooking. About 80 per cent of natural folic acid is conjugated with up to six additional glutamyl radicals, which must be split off by intestinal deconjugating enzymes (often termed "conjugases") for absorption to occur. Although relatively little is known about the efficiency with which such natural folic acid is absorbed and how much is required daily, synthetic pteroylglutamic acid is absorbed readily and rapidly, primarily in the jejunum, and therapy for the deficiency state can be provided with approximately 0.1 to 0.2 mg. of this material daily. After its absorption, folic acid is reduced through specific liver enzymes (folate reductases) to tetrahydrofolic acid, a compound that plays an essential part in the metabolism of "one-carbon fragments." Its most vital role is in the synthesis and transfer of methyl groups. Through a series of reactions, tetrahydrofolic acid catalyzes the transfer of the β carbon of serine (in the presence of pyridoxal) to homocysteine, forming methionine. A crucial

intermediate formed in this reaction sequence is N^5,N^{10}-methylenetetrahydrofolate, which, in the presence of thymidylate synthetase, is responsible for the methylation and conversion of deoxyuridylate to thymidylate, a precursor required for DNA synthesis. It is the deficiency of this metabolite that presumably underlies the defect of megaloblastic anemias. The further reduced, "end" metabolite, N^5-methyltetrahydrofolate, provides the methyl group for methionine synthesis and accounts for much of the folic acid activity of liver and of serum. In both transmethylation and thymine methyl synthesis, these tetrahydrofolate derivatives are closely linked to vitamin B_{12}-dependent reactions (*vide supra*). Accordingly, with respect to DNA synthesis and allied reactions, deficiencies of the two vitamins have very similar effects, and a deficiency of one may lead to biochemical aberrations devolving from faulty utilization of the other. Other important intermediate metabolites of reduced folic acid are the formylated derivatives, N^5-formyltetrahydrofolic acid (folinic acid, "citrovorum factor"), its unstable isomer, N^{10}-formyltetrahydrofolic acid, and the interconversion compound, N^5,N^{10}-methenyltetrahydrofolic acid. These derivatives participate as formyl donors in the de novo synthesis of purine nucleotides. Because of its relative stability, folinic acid is utilized as a pharmaceutical form of tetrahydrofolic acid that is principally of value in circumventing toxicologic blockade of dihydrofolate reductase. A metabolite of reduced folic acid having less importance is N^5-formiminotetrahydrofolic acid, an intermediate compound formed during the degradation of histidine; in the absence of tetrahydrofolic acid, formiminoglutamic acid accumulates and is excreted in the urine.

The body stores of folic acid and its derivatives in normally nourished persons are relatively less extensive or stable than are those of vitamin B_{12}. Total body stores of folic acid have been estimated to be approximately 5 or 10 mg., an amount roughly 50 to 100 times the normal daily requirement. By comparison, the normal stores of vitamin B_{12} amount to well over a thousand times the amount utilized daily. Perhaps for this reason folic acid deficiency is much more common among the malnourished. Symptoms of folic acid deficiency may commence within several months of dietary deprivation, as is true of scurvy, and, like scurvy, the deficiency state tends to appear in spring in cold climates, although it is found year-round among the consistently undernourished. Because of its more rapid turnover, folic acid deficiency is more frequently encountered in intestinal malabsorption states than is vitamin B_{12} deficiency and is a common complication of sprue, celiac disease, idiopathic steatorrhea, and intestinal short-circuits. Folic acid deficiency is occasionally seen in patients with partial gastrectomy, a patient group more often troubled by difficulty in assimilating vitamin B_{12}. A deficiency of folic acid is usually encountered in those gastrectomized patients whose course is complicated by

---

*The assistance of Dr. James H. Jandl in the preparation of this article and the one on Miscellaneous and Refractory Megaloblastic Anemias is gratefully acknowledged.

general malnutrition, faulty bowel function, or multiple surgical procedures. Conditions that increase general bodily requirements are prone to induce a folic acid deficiency state, particularly if the diet is marginal to begin with, and thus should in most instances be treated with supplemental folic acid to prevent the occurrence of deficiency. An example is the "*pernicious anemia of pregnancy*," a megaloblastic anemia appearing usually in the last trimester and frequently requiring bone marrow aspiration to establish the diagnosis; usually it is specifically responsive to folic acid, although in rare instances vitamin B_{12} deficiency is present. A more discrete increase in folic acid requirements is likely to occur in patients with chronic hemolytic anemia, wherein bone marrow failure and, in some, "aplastic crises" may develop, apparently as the result of a *relative deficiency of folic acid*. Impairment by a relative deficiency of folic acid of the erythropoietic response to anemia appears to be prevalent in chronic hemolytic anemias, and is not necessarily manifest by obvious megaloblastic changes in the marrow. Accordingly, patients with severe chronic hemolytic anemia should be given supplements of folic acid. Other proliferative disorders of long standing, including leukemia and polycythemia vera, also tend to be complicated by relative deficiency of folic acid; the desirability of therapy in these disorders is less certain. It is probable that the tendency of patients with alcoholic cirrhosis to develop folic acid deficiency and megaloblastic anemia is due to a direct metabolic antagonism by alcohol and possibly to inadequate hepatic conversion of folic acid to its active metabolites as well as to dietary inadequacies. A clear example of folic acid deficiency caused by impaired utilization is that occurring in some patients given "antifolic" compounds such as 4-aminopteroylglutamic acid (Aminopterin), 4-amino-N^{10}-methyl-pteroylglutamic acid (Amethopterin, Methotrexate), and the antimalarial agent pyrimethamine (Daraprim). These compounds inhibit the enzymatic reduction of folic acid, a block that can be circumvented by administering folinic acid. It is also probable that certain *anticonvulsant compounds*, such as diphenylhydantoin sodium (Dilantin), primidone (Mysoline), and the barbiturates, act as weak folic acid antagonists. Early evidence suggests that Dilantin may, in addition, inhibit the intestinal deconjugation of conjugated folate, resulting in malabsorption of this form of folic acid. Although only a small percentage of patients receiving Dilantin develop frank megaloblastic anemia, a great many show some cellular evidence of premegaloblastic arrest. Ascorbic acid may be involved in the stabilization of reduced folic acid, and occasionally patients with scurvy develop a folic acid deficiency that may be partly conditioned by the deficiency of ascorbic acid. The "*megaloblastic anemia of infancy*" arising from a dietary deficiency of folic acid may reflect such a mixed deficiency. This disorder is distinct from juvenile pernicious anemia and appears in infants fed on unsupplemented dried milk formulas or on goat's milk ("*goat's milk anemia*"), the latter milk being remarkably low in folic acid even when fresh.

Clinical Manifestations. The principal effects of folic acid deficiency are on the blood and the gastrointestinal tract. The anemia is indistinguishable from that caused by vitamin B_{12} deficiency and produces similar clinical effects. The gastrointestinal manifestations may be similar to those of pernicious anemia, but tend to be more widespread and severe, in part because of the greater likelihood of multiple B vitamin deficiencies. Cheilosis and glossitis are common in severely deficient patients and in patients receiving folic acid antagonists, and may proceed to a severe ulcerative stomatitis, pharyngitis, and esophagitis with dysphagia. Diarrhea is often present and may be accompanied by distention, meteorism, flatulence, and the roentgenologic picture of sprue. In some patients intestinal biopsy shows little or no change, whereas in others megalocytosis and spruelike changes are seen that are reversed by treatment with folic acid. Perirectal and perineal weeping and ulcerations may appear. There are, however, no specific neurologic abnormalities.

As in vitamin B_{12} deficiency, the peripheral blood in folic acid deficiency contains oval macrocytes and hypersegmented polymorphonuclear cells. Usually leukopenia and thrombocytopenia as well as anemia are found. The marrow is also richly cellular and megaloblastic, with severe abnormalities of granulocyte precursors, and has the attributes of ineffective erythropoiesis, including increased pigment excretion and hyperferremia.

Diagnosis. Folic acid deficiency is usually suspected either after exclusion of vitamin B_{12} deficiency or by the association of megaloblastic anemia with gross malnutrition, intestinal malabsorption, pregnancy, cirrhosis, chronic hemolysis, or anticonvulsant drug therapy, conditions in which a deficiency of folic acid is more common than one of vitamin B_{12}. As most patients with vitamin B_{12} deficiency have gastric achlorhydria, the finding of acid gastric secretion and megaloblastic anemia raises the suspicion of folic acid deficiency. On the other hand, patients with folic acid deficiency may also happen to have achlorhydria. Lack of the characteristic neuropathy of vitamin B_{12} deficiency and presence of severe oral or intestinal lesions also favor the diagnosis of folic acid deficiency. Confirmation of this diagnosis may be made with the therapeutic trial method: in folic acid deficiency physiologic doses of vitamin B_{12} of the order of 1 to 5 μg. parenterally daily are ineffective, whereas parenteral folic acid in doses of 0.1 to 0.2 mg. or more daily is usually effective in producing full hematologic and clinical response. Unlike the pernicious anemia patient, who is "isolated" from his dietary vitamin B_{12} by the deficiency of intrinsic factor, the folic acid–deficient patient is likely to have a "spontaneous" response to dietary folic acid unless the intake of vegetables and liver is strictly curtailed. Thus, a preliminary ten-day control period is necessary for definitive diagnosis by this method. In practice, such a control study is not usually possible, however, and potential therapy may have to be given at the outset and its results interpreted with less certainty. The diagnosis may be established more quickly by microbiologic assay of the serum for folic acid activity. Normally the serum level of folic acid (principally N⁵-methyl-tetrahydrofolate) as measured by the *L. casei* method is above 7 millimicrograms per milliliter; levels below 3 millimicrograms per milliliter indicate a deficiency. The urinary excretion of formiminoglutamic acid during oral "loading" with histidine has been measured as a metabolic indication of folic acid deficiency (urinary FIGLU test); unfortunately, the value of this test is diminished by the fact that increased excretion of formiminoglutamic acid is also found in many patients with vitamin B_{12} deficiency, with iron deficiency, or with liver disease, and it is no longer extensively used. These diagnostic techniques require specialized laboratories, and the diagnosis of folic acid deficiency usually must rest upon clinical suspicion and therapeutic response. It should be emphasized that folic acid in sufficient amounts will cause a hematologic response in vitamin B_{12} deficiency and that consequently therapeutic trials with folic acid should be conducted with daily doses not exceeding about 0.4 mg. daily.

Treatment. Hematologic, metabolic, and clinical effects analogous to those described with vitamin B_{12} therapy are induced by folic acid in patients who are deficient in this vitamin. Glossitis and stomatitis, when present, improve rapidly and, in contrast to that in most patients with primary intestinal disease, the diarrhea and malabsorption pattern by roentgenographic examination may disappear or improve rapidly. As intimated above, doses of about 0.1 to 0.2 mg. daily are probably adequate for most patients, and certainly tablets containing 5 mg. of folic acid will produce full therapeutic effects even in patients with intestinal malabsorption. Consequently, apart from its use in a therapeutic trial or in patients unable to swallow, folic acid need not usually be given parenterally. Folinic acid has no clear advantage over folic acid except for patients overdosed with folic acid antagonists such as Aminopterin, for which it is the specific antidote if given promptly. In dietary deficiency of folic acid a one- or two-week course of therapy and adherence to a normal diet should suffice. For patients with pernicious anemia of pregnancy, therapy should continue for several months after delivery. When deficiency is caused by underlying chronic or recurrent disorders such as sprue, surgical resection of the intestine, or chronic hemolytic anemia, folic acid administration should be continued accordingly. It should be emphasized that in providing general nutritional support to undernourished patients, multivitamin preparations containing doses of folic acid in excess of about 0.4 mg. daily are to be avoided because there is a danger that such doses might obscure the diagnosis in those patients with incipient or unsuspected pernicious anemia. However, this consideration should not deter the physician from judiciously employing smaller doses of folic acid (0.1 to 0.2 mg. daily) to protect undernourished patients from the common and debilitating complication of folic acid deficiency.

MISCELLANEOUS AND REFRACTORY MEGALOBLASTIC ANEMIAS

Herman A. Godwin

A relatively small proportion of patients with megaloblastic anemia are deficient in neither vitamin B_{12} nor folic acid and hence are sometimes referred to as "refractory." Megaloblastic or "megaloblastoid" changes with or without macrocytic anemia may be seen in the marrows of patients with a variety of disorders affecting the marrow, including invading neoplasms, leukemia, some infections, and in some patients with chronic azotemia. In about 15 per cent of patients with "*pyridoxine-responsive*" anemia, particularly the older ones, the bone marrow is megaloblastic, and often there are partial responses to therapy with folic acid as well as with pyridoxine. Although folic acid and pyridoxine overlap in at least one metabolic step ultimately affecting DNA synthesis (*vide supra*), there is presently no exact explanation for the occurrence of megaloblastic change in such patients. Because of the variable morphology and obscure pathogenesis of "pyridoxine-responsive" anemias, it is important that no patient with megaloblastic anemia be consigned to the "refractory" category without benefit of a therapeutic trial with pyridoxine (100 mg. daily intramuscularly or orally). Aplastic or hypoplastic anemias often show mild megaloblastic abnormalities. In the rare disorder *erythremic myelosis (DiGuglielmo's disease)* and in related syndromes, megaloblastic changes may be rather pronounced, and giant multinucleated red cells may be encountered in both the marrow and the peripheral blood. Splenomegaly and hepatomegaly, with erythroblastic infiltration, are seen, and in many patients a frank myeloblastic leukemia may supervene, creating a picture sometimes termed *erythroleukemia*. Although giant multinucleated erythroblasts are encountered in small numbers in pernicious anemia and related disorders, such cells are usually much more striking in erythremic myelosis. The observation that very similar morphologic abnormalities are encountered in patients who are exposed to ionizing radiation or who are undergoing combined treatment both with inhibitors of DNA synthesis and with stathmokinetic agents supports the presumption that erythremic myelosis involves a metabolic derangement of DNA. Many of these patients ultimately manifest myeloblastic leukemia, but some appear to have a primary neoplasm of the red cells. Several cases of megaloblastic anemia with *orotic aciduria* have been described in which there was an inborn defect in the conversion of orotic to orotidylic acid. Undoubtedly other examples of discrete defects, inborn or acquired, in nucleoprotein metabolism with megaloblastic anemia will be described in the future. Before accepting these miscellaneous disorders as being responsible for a megaloblastic anemia, every effort should be made to exclude deficiencies of vitamin B_{12} or of folic acid because these deficiencies are much more frequent and because they are correctible. Particular difficulty in doing so may arise in situations that compromise marrow proliferation, such as are found during infection and in mixed deficiencies.

Beck, W. S., and Goulian, M.: Drugs effective in pernicious anemia and other megaloblastic anemias. *In* DiPalma, J. R. (ed.): Drill's Pharmacology in Medicine. New York, McGraw-Hill, Inc., 1965, p. 817.

Castle, W. B.: A century of curiosity about pernicious anemia. Trans. Amer. Clin. Climat. Ass., 73:54, 1961.

Finch, C. A., Coleman, D. H., Motulsky, A. G., Donohue, D. M., and Reiff, R. H.: Erythrokinetics in pernicious anemia. Blood, 11:807, 1956.

Fisher, J. M., and Taylor, K. B.: A comparison of autoimmune phenomena in pernicious anemia and chronic atrophic gastritis. New Eng. J. Med., 272:499, 1965.

François, R., Revol, L., Germain, D., Bourlier, V., Karlin, Mme., Coeur, P., Pellet, H., and Manuel, Y.: Imerslund's syndrome. Ann. Pédiat. (Paris), 43:490, 1967.

Gräsbeck, R.: Intrinsic factor and the other vitamin B_{12} transport proteins. Prog. Hemat., 6:233, 1969.

Herbert, V. (ed.): Symposium on vitamin B_{12} and folate. Amer. J. Med., 48:539, 541, 549, 555, 562, 570, 580, 584, 594, 599, 609, 1970.

Herbert, V., and Castle, W. B.: Medical progress: Intrinsic factor. New Eng. J. Med., 270:1181, 1964.

Jandl, J. H., and Greenberg, M. S.: Bone marrow failure due to relative nutritional deficiency in Cooley's hemolytic anemia: Painful "erythropoietic crises" in response to folic acid. New Eng. J. Med., 260:461, 1959.

Johns, D. G., and Bertino, J. R.: Folates and megaloblastic anemia: A review. Clin. Pharmacol. Ther., 6:372, 1965.

McIntyre, O. R., Sullivan, L. W., Jeffries, G. H., and Silver, R. H.: Pernicious anemia in childhood. New Eng. J. Med., 272:981, 1965.

Rosenberg, I. H., Streiff, R. R., Godwin, H. A., and Castle, W. B.: Absorption of polyglutamic folate: Participation of deconjugating enzymes of the intestinal mucosa. New Eng. J. Med., 280:985, 1969.

NORMOCYTIC NORMOCHROMIC ANEMIAS

Carl V. Moore

ACUTE HEMORRHAGIC ANEMIA

Acute loss of a large volume of blood may result from trauma, ulcerative lesions, abnormal blood vessels, thrombocytopenia, or coagulation defects; it may occur from an obviously severed vessel, from the respiratory, gastrointestinal, or genitourinary tracts, or into certain body cavities or tissues (cysts, pleural or peritoneal spaces, retroperitoneally, or into a large muscle mass). The hemorrhage is grossly evident except when blood is lost into the alimentary canal, body cavities, or tissues. Clinical manifestations vary with the size, rate, and site of the hemorrhage, with the lesion responsible for the bleeding, and with the state of consciousness of the patient. The latter factor is of importance because of the natural apprehension anyone has when he knows he is losing blood.

A person may survive the gradual loss of half his blood volume over a period of 24 hours, but death may occur from the rapid loss of 33 per cent. The more severe degrees of hemorrhage cause prostration, restlessness, thirst, tachycardia, fall in blood pressure with a thready pulse, tachypnea, sweating, pallor, clamminess of the skin from the sweating and constriction of dermal blood vessels, often a pounding headache, and syncope. Mental confusion may result from cerebral anoxia. With lesser degrees of hemorrhage, the pulse may be full, bounding, and even slow. Manifestations are influenced by activity; for example, the blood pressure and pulse may be normal at rest, but hypotension, faintness, and tachycardia may develop when the patient gets out of bed and begins to move around. Hemorrhage into body cavities or tissues causes pain, fever, signs of serosal inflammation, displacement of organs, e.g., mediastinal shift from hemothorax, or limitation of motion, e.g., hemorrhage into a psoas muscle.

Because blood vessels of the skin and muscles constrict in an attempt to compensate for the decreased blood volume and to provide as much blood as possible for vital organs, and because restoration of plasma volume is slow, the blood count initially does not adequately reflect the size of the hemorrhage. The first change to occur is a rise in the platelets, often within the first hour, followed shortly thereafter by a polymorphonuclear leukocytosis with a white blood cell count as high as 20,000 per cubic millimeter or more; a few metamyelocytes and myelocytes may be found in the leukocyte differential. Gradually, fluid passes into the blood stream to restore the blood volume toward normal, and the erythrocyte values fall; this process continues for 24 to 48 hours so that, in the absence of further bleeding, the full extent of the resulting anemia is not evident until that time. The plasma iron falls during the first several days as erythropoiesis becomes stimulated; values do not usually return to normal levels until the patient has recovered from the anemia. Reticulocytes do not begin to increase for one to two days and reach peak levels of usually 5 to 15 per cent between the fourth and seventh days; a few normoblasts may also appear. Because reticulocytes tend to be larger than other cells, the MCV may be slightly greater than normal (up to 105 cu. μ) at the time of maximal reticulocytosis. The leukocyte count should be normal in three to four days and the reticulocytes in ten days. The time required for restoration of normal red cell values, from hemorrhages of varied size, is approximately five to six weeks, provided no further bleeding occurs. When blood is lost into the gastrointestinal tract, the blood urea nitrogen may rise moderately, particularly if renal function is impaired. Reabsorption of blood from body cavities or tissues may lead to moderate elevations of the indirect-reacting bilirubin with resultant icterus.

Treatment should be directed at stopping the hemorrhage, combating shock, and restoring blood volume. The patient should be kept warm and quiet, by sedation if necessary. If there are signs of shock or if the blood loss is estimated to be greater than 20 per cent of the blood volume, arrangements should be made immediately for transfusion with properly matched whole blood. In civilian practice, with the ready availability of blood banking services, it is rarely necessary or justifiable to resort to the use of unmatched universal donor blood. While blood is being cross-matched, 500 to 1000 ml. of one of the following solutions, arranged here in order of effectiveness and desirability, may be given intravenously if the patient's condition is sufficiently critical: human plasma or albumin, a plasma expander such as dextran, 0.9 per cent sodium chloride in water, or 5 per cent glucose in 0.9 per cent sodium chloride. The medical and surgical procedures necessary to control the hemorrhage will vary with its cause. If blood loss continues at a pace requiring replacement with 5000 ml. or more of blood per 24 hours, however, platelets tend to decrease rapidly so that thrombocytopenia may complicate the therapeutic problem. This fact must be one of the considerations that influence clinical judgment about when surgical intervention becomes necessary. After the emergency is over, the patient should be provided with a high-protein diet. Iron therapy may be given, but usually is not necessary because of the availability of iron from body stores; no other supplements are needed.

Coleman, D. H., Stevens, A. R., Jr., Dodge, H. T., and Finch, C. A.: Rate of Blood regeneration after blood loss. Arch. Intern. Med. (Chicago), 92:341, 1953.

Krevans, J. R., and Jackson, D. P.: Hemorrhagic disorder following massive whole blood transfusions. J.A.M.A., 159:171, 1955.

Pareira, M. D., Serres, K. D., and Lang, S.: Early response of plasma volume, red cell mass and plasma proteins to massive hemorrhage. Proc. Soc. Exp. Biol. Med., 103:9, 1960.

Schiødt, E.: Observations on blood regeneration in man. Amer. J. Med. Sci., 193:313, 327, 1937; ibid., 196:632, 1938.

ANEMIA ASSOCIATED WITH INFECTION AND CHRONIC SYSTEMIC DISEASES

(Simple Chronic Anemia)

Definition. Normocytic normochromic anemia develops during the course of most infections and chronic systemic diseases such as renal or hepatic disease, rheumatoid arthritis, the connective tis-sue disorders, malnutrition, malignancy, leukemia, the lymphomas, multiple myeloma, endocrine deficiencies, and gastrointestinal disorders. It is usually mild but may be severe, particularly in leukemia and severe renal failure. The red corpuscles may at times be larger or smaller than normal, but normocytosis is the rule; erythrocytes may occasionally be slightly hypochromic. The anemia is a manifestation of the underlying disease rather than a disease in itself, but it is one of the most common of all anemias as infections and the other systemic disorders are themselves so common. The causative factors vary with the disease. In general, however, the pathogenesis of the anemia can be explained by the combination of a frequently found mild, extracorpuscular hemolytic component together with decreased erythropoiesis or relative marrow failure—failure of the marrow to compensate for any mild increase in the rate of red blood cell destruction. The hemolysis is usually not severe enough to cause elevation of the serum bilirubin or clinically detectable icterus. Because the underlying disease may also produce chronic blood loss, anorexia with poor dietary intake, or malabsorption, the characteristics of the anemia may occasionally be altered by the concomitant development of deficiency of vitamin B_{12}, folic acid, or iron. The dominant manifestations are usually those of the disease causing the anemia. Treatment is that of the underlying disease plus administration of transfusions when necessary.

Mechanisms. At least three abnormalities are involved in the pathogenesis of the *anemia* of *infection, cancer,* and *rheumatoid arthritis:* (1) Moderate shortening of erythrocyte life span by an extracorpuscular mechanism; (2) failure of the bone marrow to compensate for the anemia; and (3) an unexplained impaired release of iron from RE cells that ingest and destroy erythrocytes. The latter change coupled with normal utilization of transferrin-bound plasma iron for hemoglobin synthesis leads to a decrease in plasma iron and of sideroblasts in the bone marrow, even though greater than normal amounts of hemosiderin iron may be found in marrow and other tissues rich in RE cells (sideropenic anemia with reticuloendothelial siderosis). Animals with experimentally induced anemia of infection will respond partially to hypoxia or to the administration of erythropoietin, but will not become polycythemic. Possible reasons for failure of the bone marrow to step up its production of erythrocytes and to compensate for the hemolytic component, therefore, include the defective release of iron from RE cells, impaired marrow response to erythropoietin, and lack of a compensatory increase in erythropoietin production. The nature of the extracorpuscular hemolytic factor has not been discovered. Bacterial and cold hemolysins, hemorrhage into and around tumor masses, hemolytic effects of metabolic products of tumor tissue, and stimulation of RE cell activity may provide partial explanation in some instances. Since the decrease in red cell survival is usually moderate, and since the impaired erythropoiesis usually represents failure of the marrow to *accelerate* its production, the anemia tends to develop rather slowly. After several months, a new equilibrium is established, and the anemia remains relatively steady; its severity often correlates with the debility and systemic involvement produced by the underlying disease, but the relationship is not constant. For instance, although anemia develops in more than 50 per cent of patients with malignant tumors, its occurrence cannot be correlated with the presence or absence of metastases.

Anemia is an inevitable complication of *renal failure*. Although there is no precise correlation with the degree of nitrogen retention, anemia tends to increase in severity as the level of blood urea nitrogen rises above 70 mg. pcr 100 ml. and may progress to hemoglobin levels as low as 5 grams per 100 ml. during the terminal stages. Erythrocyte survival may be shortened, sometimes by 50 per cent or more in patients with chronic renal disease and severe azotemia. The factor or factors responsible have not been identified, but probably are contained in plasma. Circulating erythrocytes in uremia frequently have spicules on their membrane. These "burr" cells become normal when suspended in normal serum, whereas normal cells become burred when suspended in uremic plasma. The "burr cell factor" is heat labile, is not removed by dialysis, persists after bilateral nephrectomy, but disappears from the plasma after a successful renal transplant. To what extent it is responsible for the hemolysis is unknown.

In patients with chronic renal failure hemolysis does not lessen when they are treated by chronic dialysis. The primary cause for the anemia of chronic renal disease, however, is either a true depression of erythropoiesis or failure of erythroid elements to increase production and compensate for the hemolysis. The number of nucleated red blood cells in the marrow is not clearly decreased until nitrogen retention is advanced; reticulocytes are normal or even slightly increased. Erythropoietin production is probably depressed, but evidence also suggests that uremic plasma has a "toxic" effect on erythrocyte production.

The anemia of *hepatic* disease is frequently complicated by chronic blood loss and, in patients with alcoholic cirrhosis, by folate deficiency. In these latter instances, the anemia may be megaloblastic. Alcohol, furthermore, has an inhibitory effect on folic acid. Consequently, alcoholic patients with cirrhosis of the liver may develop a reticulocyte response shortly after admission to a hospital caused both by cessation of alcoholic intake and the folate content of the hospital diet. After elimination of iron and folate deficiencies, a hard core of normocytic anemias remains, in some of which the red corpuscles, although normal in volume, are thin cells with an increased diameter. The plasma volume is often increased so that hemodilution exaggerates the depression of erythrocyte values; the degree of anemia cor-

relates roughly with the shortening of the corpuscular survival time; the spleen is usually a major site of erythrocyte destruction. Erythropoiesis tends to be increased, but is inadequate to compensate for the hemolysis. In general, the mechanism for the inadequate erythropoietic response found in hepatic failure, gastrointestinal disorders, and nutritional deficiencies (pellagra, kwashiorkor, scurvy) has never been determined. Protein malnutrition leading to decreased synthesis of globin may contribute, but can hardly be the sole explanation. Anemia is not a constant finding in scurvy. When it does occur, a hemolytic process, reversible by administration of ascorbic acid, can be demonstrated. Other deficiencies associated with clinical scurvy may be partly responsible.

A moderate normocytic anemia commonly appears during the course of various *endocrine deficiencies*: hypothyroidism, Addison's disease, hypopituitarism, and testicular failure. The red corpuscles in myxedema may be slightly macrocytic, but megaloblastic changes do not occur unless there is an associated deficiency of vitamin B_{12} or of folic acid. Deficiency of vitamin B_{12}, however, caused by decreased production of intrinsic factor, is more common than was formerly recognized. The anemia in endocrinopathies is often attributed to the incident general hypometabolism, but the regulatory influence of endocrine glands on erythropoiesis is really not understood.

Clinical Manifestations. The symptoms are primarily those of the underlying disease. The anemia may contribute to the patient's fatigue, anorexia, or dyspnea; it usually is too mild, however, to be troublesome except in chronic renal failure or in diseases like leukemia or the lymphomas. Pallor, tachycardia, and cardiac dilatation depend on the severity of the anemia. Lymph node enlargement, hepatomegaly, and splenomegaly are present only as manifestations of the pathologic process to which the anemia is secondary.

Diagnosis. Routine hematologic studies reveal little except the normocytic normochromic anemia. Anisocytosis may be moderate, but significant poikilocytosis is unusual (flat target cells in liver disease, "burr" cells in some patients with uremia and carcinoma). Reticulocytes may be normal or slightly increased; polychromasia or other evidence of red blood cell regeneration is rare. Any changes in leukocytes or platelets must be related to the causative disease or to concurrent deficiency, i.e., of folate. The serum bilirubin is usually normal unless there is associated hepatic dysfunction. The bone marrow most often appears qualitatively normal, although occasionally the number of nucleated red blood cells is decreased. Abnormalities related to the responsible disease may be found: increase in plasma cells or granulomatous lesions in infections, tumor cells in patients with carcinoma. The ineffective erythropoiesis and shortened corpuscular survival can be demonstrated only with special techniques (ferrokinetic studies, survival of chromium-tagged red corpuscles). In anemias caused by chronic infection, carcinoma, and rheumatoid arthritis, the following frequently found pattern is distinctive: plasma iron less than 40 μg. per 100 ml., total iron binding capacity less than 250 μg. per 100 ml., transferrin saturation of 10 to 15 per cent, reduction in the number of sideroblasts, and increase in reticuloendothelial iron. Demonstration of stainable iron in the bone marrow helps to rule out iron deficiency. Search to detect chronic blood loss should be made. At times, it may be necessary to do a Coombs test and to eliminate a concurrent vitamin B_{12} or folic acid deficiency. In the main, however, the diagnostic procedures of greatest value are those designed to detect and evaluate the primary disease.

Therapy. Treatment of the underlying cause— the infection, the endocrinopathy, the hepatic disease, or the tumor—is the most important therapy. When that is ineffective, transfusion of whole blood may be necessary, but is usually not required unless the hemoglobin falls below 8 or 9 grams per 100 ml. Patients with chronic renal disease fare best if their hematocrit levels are maintained between 25 and 30 per cent; at higher values, the renal plasma flow is decreased enough so that nitrogen retention may be further increased. Androgenic steroids may be of value in treatment of the anemia in patients with carcinoma, particularly of the breast, and corticosteroids may cause a therapeutic response in anemia associated with rheumatoid arthritis. Iron or folic acid should be given if deficiencies of these two nutrients coexist.

Cartwright, G. E.: The anemia of chronic disorders. Seminars Hemat., 3:351, 1966.
Eschbach, J. W., Jr., Funk, D., Adamson, J., Kuhn, I., Scribner, B. H., and Finch, C. A.: Erythropoiesis in patients with renal failure undergoing chronic dialysis. New Eng. J. Med., 276:653, 1967.
Harris, J. W.: The Red Cell Production, Metabolism, Destruction: Normal and Abnormal. Cambridge, Mass., Harvard University Press, 1963.
Loge, J. P., Lange, R. D., and Moore, C. V.: Characterization of the anemia associated with chronic renal insufficiency. Amer. J. Med., 24.4, 1958.
Merrill, J. P., and Hampers, C. L.: Uremia. New Eng. J. Med., 282:1014, 1970.
Wintrobe, M. M.: Clinical Hematology, 6th ed. Philadelphia, Lea and Febiger, 1967.

ANEMIA OF BONE MARROW FAILURE

Definition. Bone marrow failure has been variously called *aplastic anemia, hypoplastic anemia, primary refractory anemia,* and *aregenerative anemia.* These terms imply varying degrees of hypocellularity of the bone marrow or emphasize the relative refractoriness to therapy. At times, foci of hypercellularity may be found in an otherwise hypocellular marrow, or the over-all cellularity may be normal or hyperplastic. In these latter instances, ferrokinetic and erythrokinetic studies

have demonstrated that erythropoiesis is active but ineffective; the same probably applies to granulocytes and platelets, but methods for studying the kinetics of their formation are still too crude to tell. Remissions do occasionally occur either spontaneously after recognition and removal of a causative agent or in response to such therapy as splenectomy, adrenocorticosteroids, or androgens. For these reasons and because of its physiologic implication, "bone marrow failure" is a superior designation. All marrow elements may be involved, in which case pancytopenia is found in the peripheral blood, or there may be failure of only one or two of the cell types to give anemia without leukopenia and thrombocytopenia (*pure red blood cell aplasia*), anemia and leukopenia without thrombocytopenia, or anemia and thrombocytopenia without leukopenia. The disease may appear spontaneously without recognized cause, or it may follow exposure to ionizing irradiation or various chemical agents; rarely, it may be congenital (Fanconi syndrome) or may be found in association with thymic tumors (particularly true of pure red blood cell aplasia). The clinical course is prominently influenced by the degree of leukopenia or thrombocytopenia; if infections and hemorrhagic manifestations are not severe, patients can frequently be kept comfortable and active, with supportive care, for years.

Etiology. Under conditions of ordinary civilian medical practice, half or more of the cases of bone marrow failure develop without known cause. In addition, there are rare or unusual types, also of unknown causation: congenital or familial pancytopenia, which tends to appear in children (the Fanconi syndrome) and marrow failure associated with thymic tumors or with paroxysmal nocturnal hemoglobinuria. In the remaining patients, exposure to ionizing irradiation or to a possible offending chemical substance can be identified, although in the latter case it is often difficult or impossible to establish an etiologic relationship with certainty.

Agents responsible for the development of bone marrow failure may be divided into two categories: (1) Those that regularly produce bone marrow damage if a sufficient dose is given: irradiation from x-rays, radioactive elements, or nuclear explosions; benzene; agents used in the chemotherapy of malignancy, e.g., nitrogen mustard, cytoxan, busulfan, antimetabolites such as 6-mercaptopurine and methotrexate, antimitotic drugs. (2) Those that occasionally are associated with bone marrow failure. Some of these compounds have been reported to be responsible for 20 to 100 or more cases: chloramphenicol, sulfonamides, quinacrine (Atabrine), phenylbutazone (Butazolidin), diphenylhydantoin (Dilantin), methyl-phenyl-ethyl hydantoin (Mesantoin), trinitrotoluene, arsenobenzols, and gold preparations. Others have been suspected in only a few instances; the list is large and grows in size each year: antimicrobial agents (streptomycin, oxytetracycline, chlortetracycline), anticonvulsants (trimethadione, methyl-phenyl-hydantoin), anti-thyroid drugs (methimazol [Tapazole]), anti-histaminics (tripelennamine [Pyribenzamine]), insecticides (chlorophenothane or DDT, gamma-benzene hexachloride, lindane), dinitrophenol, chlorpromazine and promazine, meprobamate, tolbutamide and chloropropamide, acetazolamide and chlorothiazide, acetylsalicylic acid and phenacetin, cholchicine, Stoddard solvent, hair and aniline dyes, carbon tetrachloride, and certain heavy metals (arsenic, bismuth, mercury, colloidal silver).

Chloramphenicol is the agent most commonly associated with bone marrow aplasia in recent years. In the Registry on Adverse Reactions (Council on Drugs, American Medical Association), there are 771 cases of pancytopenia; 338 (44 per cent) of these followed the use of chloramphenicol, and in 154 chloramphenicol was the only drug administered during the previous six months. In many instances, pancytopenia appeared weeks after the last dose.

The suggestion has been made repeatedly that compounds containing the benzene ring are particularly likely to be bone marrow toxins. It is further suspected that idiopathic bone marrow failure may be due largely to exposure of the population to synthetic organic compounds used in industry, in food processing, in cosmetics, in farming or gardening, in the manufacture of cloth, and about the home. No satisfactory way of establishing or disproving these relationships has so far been discovered. A severe form of aplastic anemia has been observed in cattle or calves fed a soybean oil meal that had been extracted with trichlorethylene; the toxicity clearly developed during the extraction process.

Incidence. Idiopathic bone marrow failure is a comparatively rare disease; it tends to occur in young adults of either sex, but may appear at any age. The incidence of secondary cases depends largely on the current therapeutic popularity or industrial use of the responsible agents. It is estimated that one of every 20,000 to 30,000 patients who take chloramphenicol develops pancytopenia, a risk thought to be about 13 times greater than the risk of developing fatal idiopathic bone marrow failure. Irradiation damage was formerly limited to persons exposed industrially to radium or to patients being treated with some form of ionizing irradiation. As nuclear energy comes to be used more widely, reactor accidents will undoubtedly account for more instances of marrow damage. The two atomic explosions over Japan produced thousands of cases of hypoplastic anemia.

Pathology and Pathogenesis. The bone marrow may be hypocellular, normocellular, or hypercellular; when marrow aplasia is induced experimentally, as with benzene, hyperplasia is often the first change induced, followed by progressively severe hypoplasia. In any given case, not all the cellular elements of marrow are equally involved. Considerable immaturity, particularly in the granulocytic series, may be found so that differentiation from subleukemic myelocytic leukemia may at times be difficult; granulocytes tend to be deficient in granules. Erythroid elements may have nuclear chromatin patterns that resemble those of megaloblasts (megaloblastoid change); some of the normoblasts may contain two to four nuclei; megakaryocytes usually are sparse. The normo- or hypercellular marrows can probably be explained on the basis of ineffective hematopoiesis (formerly called "maturation arrest"). That certainly is true for the erythrocytic series of cells, but the balance between leukocyte and platelet production and destruction cannot yet be expressed in the same quantitative terms. The changes of hemosiderosis frequently are found in the liver and spleen, particularly in multitransfused patients. Under these circumstances, the spleen may gradually enlarge, and splenic stasis of red blood cells may become an increasingly important factor in causing accelerated destruction of erythrocytes. Areas of extramedullary hematopoiesis may be found in the liver and spleen, but are unusual. With severe degrees of anemia, cardiac dilatation and congestive heart failure may occur. The other pathologic changes are primarily those caused by infection or hemorrhage into tissues.

The mechanism by which irradiation or chemical agents damage cells is largely still obscure. Ionizing irradiation inhibits mitosis, probably by inhibiting the synthesis of deoxyribonucleic acid in nuclei. The antimetabolites used in the treatment of malignant disease interfere with the formation of purines or nucleic acids. Even more obscure is the effect of those agents that only occasionally cause marrow failure. The reaction may appear rather promptly or not until after months of therapy. Only rarely is there reason to suspect hypersensitivity in the sense of an antigen-antibody response. A more likely cause is individual susceptibility related to a biochemical defect involving some essential metabolic pathway. For instance, a significant inhibition of nucleic acid synthesis by pharmacologic concentrations of chloramphenicol has been observed in bone marrow from patients who have recovered from chloramphenicol-induced aplastic anemia. It is important to differentiate this serious but fortunately unusual susceptibility reaction to chloramphenicol from another hematopoietic effect of the agent that occurs in a very high percentage of all patients who receive the drug: vacuolization in the marrow erythroblasts and early granulocytes, a mild anemia occasionally associated with leukopenia and thrombocytopenia, reticulocytopenia, increased plasma iron, increased saturation of the plasma iron-binding protein, delayed plasma iron clearance, and other evidences of depressed erythropoiesis. These changes have been attributed to competition of chloramphenicol with messenger RNA for ribosomal binding sites and consequent inhibition of protein synthesis in marrow cells. Some workers regard these alterations as dose-dependent, promptly reversible when administration of chloramphenicol is discontinued, and unrelated to chloramphenicol-induced aplastic anemia; others believe them to be early and still reversible manifestations of the more severe toxic process. The author believes that the weight of evidence favors the former view.

"Pure" red cell anemia is frequently associated with a thymoma; recent work suggests that it may be initiated by an autoimmune mechanism with an antibody directed against developing erythroblasts.

Clinical Manifestations. Symptoms may appear explosively, particularly when marrow aplasia is secondary to large doses of ionizing irradiation or of drugs like nitrogen mustard, 6-mercaptopurine, or the folic acid antagonizing preparations. In idiopathic cases or bone marrow failure secondary to most chemical agents, the onset is usually insidious, symptoms often developing after exposure to the offending substance has ended. Manifestations depend to a large extent on the relative severity of the anemia, leukopenia, and thrombocytopenia. When the white blood cell and platelet counts remain above critical levels, weakness and fatigue are the chief complaints. As the hemoglobin level falls below 7 or 8 grams per 100 ml., dyspnea, pounding of the heart, headache, and fever become troublesome, but nutrition is usually well maintained. With the development of severe granulocytopenia, resistance is impaired, and infections become a serious problem: pyoderma, pneumonia, urinary tract infections, perirectal abscess, septicemia, and ulcerations in the oral cavity or around the nose, rectum, and vagina. These complications add greatly to the discomfort of the patient, particularly when the lesions make eating difficult and defecation painful. A low platelet count may occasionally be tolerated without serious hemorrhagic manifestations for weeks or months, but much more frequently it is attended by bleeding into skin and mucous membranes, oozing of blood from the gums, nose, vagina, or rectum, or hemorrhage into more vital areas like the subarachnoid space.

The pallor of patients with bone marrow failure tends to have a waxy appearance. After transfusion hemosiderosis develops, however, bronzing obscures the pallor except of mucous membranes, and can look deceptively like a fairly "healthy tan." Petechiae may be found on skin and mucous membranes, purpuric spots and ecchymoses on the trunk and extremities. Skin pustules may be surrounded by a cuff of darkly colored extravasated intradermal blood. Flame-shaped hemorrhages and occasionally Roth spots may be seen on funduscopic examination. Blood oozing from the nose or gums may make local hygiene difficult, and may cause the breath to be foul. Ulcerations on mucous membranes are usually covered by a dirty gray exudate, but true pus formation at sites of infection may not occur because of the neutropenia. If anemia is severe, the heart may be dilated and the rate rapid, systolic hemic murmurs may be heard, and dependent edema may be present. Lymph nodes and spleen are usually not enlarged, but splenomegaly may develop after many transfusions have produced the changes of transfusion hemosiderosis. The liver edge may often be felt several centimeters below the right costal margin. Neurologic examination is normal unless hemorrhage or infection has involved the brain, spinal cord, or peripheral nerves.

Diagnosis. A complete blood count, including reticulocyte and platelet counts, should be obtained. The anemia may be moderate or severe enough to give a red blood cell level of less than one million cells. The erythrocytes are usually fairly normal in appearance, but slight macrocytosis and anisocytosis may be found; significant poikilocytosis, polychromasia, or basophilic stippling is rare. Confusion about the level of reticulocytes sometimes results from the unfortunate habit of expressing these values in percentages rather than in number per cubic millimeter; the absolute number is almost always low, although 2 to 4 per cent of one million corpuscles may be reticulated. Nucleated red blood cells are only rarely found in the peripheral blood. Leukopenia and thrombocytopenia may also be moderate to severe. With white blood cell levels of 2000 to 3000 per cubic millimeter, the differential reflects primarily a decrease in the cells produced by the marrow so that the percentage of lymphocytes may be 90 per cent or more. If the count drops below 1000 cells per cubic millimeter, a lymphopenia is obviously also present. Neutrophils are often deficient in granules, but young forms are rare. Platelets may be larger than normal and bizarre in shape. When the platelet levels fall to 25,000 per cubic millimeter or less, the bleeding time becomes prolonged, tests for capillary fragility are abnormal, and prothrombin consumption and clot retraction are poor. The bone marrow must also be examined; aspiration can be done safely in spite of leukopenia and thrombocytopenia if careful aseptic technique is employed and gentle pressure is applied over the puncture site for at least 10 or 15 minutes. Changes in the marrow have already been described under Pathology and Pathogenesis.

The serum iron is elevated, and the iron-binding capacity is moderately reduced to about 200 to 250 μg. per 100 ml. Ferrokinetic studies are only rarely needed to establish a diagnosis, but when done they demonstrate a slow plasma iron turnover and very poor utilization of the tracer iron for hemoglobin synthesis. There are no signs of increased blood destruction even though chromium survival measurements may demonstrate moderate shortening of erythrocyte life span. Other laboratory tests are of no positive diagnostic value.

The diseases most likely to be confused with bone marrow failure or hypoplastic anemia are subleukemic leukemia and other forms of myelophthisic anemia. Differentiation is made largely on the basis of bone marrow examination, although the presence of young forms in the peripheral blood, of lymph node enlargement, of splenomegaly, or of abnormal elevations in plasma globulin should arouse suspicion. A preponderance of lymphocytes or of myeloma cells is usually easy to detect, but sometimes the differentiation between bone marrow failure and subleukemic myelocytic leukemia can be most difficult. Help can be obtained from alkaline phosphatase stains of peripheral blood films, particularly if most of the granulocytes are positive, and by determining the presence or absence of the Philadelphia chromosome. The task is made harder by the fact that a small number of patients with bone marrow failure develop, often after a period of years, the characteristic changes of acute myelocytic or monocytic leukemia. The relation between this preleukemic phase and the subsequent leukemia has not been established. It is difficult to believe that the process was leukemic from the onset, particularly as some patients have been carefully observed for five years or more before the leukemic change became evident. One is tempted to believe, rather, that the bone marrow damage in some way predisposes to the subsequent appearance of leukemia in much the same way as radiation damage from the atomic bomb explosions over Japan led to the development of leukemia some years later. If marrow aspiration results in a "dry tap," surgical biopsy should be done unless the condition of the patient is too critical to permit the procedure. Myelofibrosis, tumor metastases, granulomatous lesions, Hodgkin's disease, and other causes of myelophthisic anemia may be recognized in this manner.

When only erythropoietic elements are decreased (pure red cell anemia), caution must be used to make certain that one is not dealing merely with an anemia associated with infection or a chronic systemic disease.

Patients with bone marrow failure may, after a period of months to as long as six years, develop the manifestations of paroxysmal nocturnal hemoglobinuria. It is thought that the abnormal erythrocytes are formed from a mutant clone of stem cells. Even experienced hematologists may fail to detect the transformation until it has been present for a considerable period of time.

Therapy. Identification of exposure to a possible toxic agent, precautionary measures to prevent or minimize future exposure to this or other likely etiologic agents, general supportive care, and the intelligent use of transfusions constitute the basic treatment for bone marrow failure. In addition, the administration of corticosteroids and androgens may be tried; under carefully selected circumstances, splenectomy should be performed.

In a few patients, the temporal relationship between the anemia and exposure to ionizing irradiation or to a chemical marrow toxin permits identification of the etiologic agent. In most instances, however, the evidence on which a drug is incriminated is purely circumstantial; no tests exist whereby a causal relationship can be proved. The only safe thing to do is to prevent future contact if at all possible. Under these circumstances,

and in cases of the idiopathic form of bone marrow failure, the patient should be advised against the use of hair dyes, insecticides, plant sprays, volatile solvents, and all drugs except those specifically prescribed. The physician should keep medication simple and should avoid the use of potential marrow toxins unless a compelling reason exists for their administration.

Not enough attention is given to the details of supportive care although they may greatly influence the patient's comfort and ability to work and the duration of his disease. These details consist, for example, of caution against picking the nose, careful mouth hygiene with use of a soft tooth brush, warning that any dentist consulted should call the physician, avoidance of intramuscular or subcutaneous injections unless absolutely necessary, meticulous care of arm veins at the time of venipuncture, avoidance of constipation or of any trauma to the rectum in order to minimize the possibility of a perirectal abscess, caution about trauma to the head when the platelet count is low, and avoidance of any unnecessary exposure to infection. Mild antiseptic soaps and electric razors should be used. When the leukocyte count is less than 1000 per cu. mm., the danger of infection is particularly great; but unless there is reason to believe that the severe leukopenia will be transient, i.e., after chemotherapeutic drugs have been given, rigid "reverse" or protective isolation is not practical. Any well-balanced diet is adequate. Antimicrobial therapy should be reserved for the treatment of specific infections as they arise and should not be used prophylactically.

Blood selected for transfusions should be as type-specific as the available blood bank can make it, and should be stored for no longer than five to seven days before use. Unless transfusions are being given to combat shock or hemorrhage, they should be administered only when the hemoglobin level has dipped below 9 grams per 100 ml. A patient with 8.5 or 9 grams of hemoglobin can be given two or three 500-ml. units of blood on successive days and may be free of the need to receive blood for three or four weeks. In this way, his blood values are kept high enough to make him comfortable, yet the minimal number of transfusions is given. The inevitable development of transfusion hemosiderosis and of sensitization to minor blood groups, leukocytes, or platelets is thereby postponed as long as possible. Most patients tolerate remarkably well the iron overload inevitably produced by repeated transfusions, but a few develop manifestations indistinguishable from hemochromatosis. For this reason, attempts have been made to increase urinary iron loss by administration of desferrioxamine, but they have not been effective or practical.

Hemorrhagic manifestations are almost invariably due to thrombocytopenia. Corticosteroid therapy tends to increase capillary resistance and frequently diminishes bleeding abnormalities even though the platelet count remains unaltered. A satisfactory initial schedule is to administer prednisone, 20 mg. per day, increasing the dose if necessary, then gradually reducing it until the minimal effective level is attained. Bleeding not controlled by 50 mg. of prednisone per day is seldom benefited by larger doses. The precautions usually employed with corticosteroid therapy need to be observed. Platelet transfusions may also be tried; if the patient has previously received more than 10 to 20 transfusions, however, the platelets will probably be destroyed rapidly because of isosensitization.

Ideally, one would like not only to sustain the patient but to stimulate his bone marrow to produce more cells. Vitamin B_{12}, other B vitamins and crude liver extract are all without effect, but an occasional patient who survives for several years may become folate-deficient. Iron should not be administered; it is of no value, and would predispose to the more rapid development of iron overload. Even if erythropoietin were available for therapeutic use, it would almost certainly be ineffective because high levels of erythropoietin are usually found in the plasma. A therapeutic trial of corticotrophin (ACTH) or of a corticosteroid, i.e., prednisone, 20 to 40 mg. per day, is worth while because, *rarely*, a patient responds with a greatly increased number of nucleated erythrocytes in the marrow, a reticulocytosis, and either a rise in the red blood cell count or a decrease in transfusion requirement. When this result is obtained, the effect may not be sustained until after splenectomy. Occasionally, a patient also responds slowly over a period of two to three months to administration of pharmacologic doses of testosterone, i.e., testosterone enanthate, 600 mg. in sesame oil intramuscularly per week, often given in conjunction with a corticosteroid preparation. The anabolic steroid 2-hydroxymethylene-17 alpha-methyldihydrotestosterone (oxymethalone) has the advantages of less virilizing activity and less interference with bone maturation; it can be given orally (2 to 4 mg. per kilogram daily) either with or without corticosteroids, and has been reported to induce remissions even when equal doses of testosterone have failed. Oxymethalone has been at least partially effective in nearly half of some series of patients. Children seem to respond more frequently than do adults. The effect on red blood cells is apparently greater than on platelets or leukocytes. An oxymethalone-induced remission may or may not be sustained after discontinuance of therapy.

Splenectomy should be of value under two circumstances: (1) if the spleen is enlarged and is destroying cells at an accelerated rate, or (2) if a malfunctioning spleen is depressing marrow function. If a transfusion is required oftener than once every ten days, one can assume an increased rate of hemolysis. A more satisfactory evaluation can be made by tagging the patient's erythrocytes with radioactive chromium and then measuring both the half-life of the tagged cells and the increase in radioactivity over the spleen. If it increases to several times the activity over the liver, the assumption may be made that the spleen is at least partially responsible for the increased hemolysis. Splenectomy under these circumstances is often followed by a decreased transfusion requirement, and occasionally the red blood cells will even equilibrate at a level high enough to make further transfusions unnecessary. A depressive effect of an enlarged spleen on the marrow is more difficult to be sure of, but rarely splenectomy may be followed by a normoblastic hyperplasia in the marrow, reticulocytosis, and a rise in red cell values. It is difficult to explain such isolated experiences in any way other than by a depressive effect of the spleen on the marrow. Splenectomy in a patient with thrombocytopenia and hypoplasia of megakaryocytic elements is a hazardous procedure. Scott and his associates found shortened red cell survival and evidence of splenic destruction less helpful than we have indicated here, and concluded that splenectomy was most useful in those patients whose marrow function was sufficient to allow survival, but who needed repeated transfusions for the maintenance of life.

When thymoma and refractory anemia coexist, removal of the thymic tumor induces a remission in less than half the cases. Immunosuppressive agents given to several of these patients have induced partial or complete remissions, presumably by suppressing an autoimmune mechanism. Bone marrow transplants have so far not been successful unless an identical twin is available as the marrow donor.

Prognosis. Unlike most of the drug-induced hematologic syndromes, the pathologic changes of chronic bone marrow failure progress long after the drug has been discontinued; recovery, if it occurs, may require years. Spontaneous remissions are rare, but the patients most likely to improve are those with mild pancytopenia and a cellular marrow plus those in whom the causative agent can be identified. Death results primarily from infection and hemorrhage; prognosis is poor, therefore, when neutropenia or thrombocytopenia is severe. Those patients with leukocyte and platelet levels high enough to protect them from hemorrhage and infection may survive with reasonable comfort for a period of years. Scott found that roughly 50 per cent of such patients were alive at the end of one year and approximately 25 per cent at the end of three years. The survival time after splenectomy was distinctly better (about 80 per cent at one year and 50 per cent at three years); it must be remembered, however, that these figures are biased by the selection of patients for splenectomy. If transfusions continue to be necessary, reactions and hemosiderosis eventually become severe.

Allen, D. M., Fine, M. H., Nechles, T. F., and Dameshek, W.: Oxymethalone therapy in aplastic anemia. Blood, 32:83, 1968.

Bithell, T. C., and Wintrobe, M. M.: Drug-induced aplastic anemia. Seminars. Hemat., 4:194, 1967.

Huguley, C. M., Jr., Lea, J. W., Jr., and Butts, J. A.: Adverse hematologic reactions to drugs. *In* Brown, E. B., and Moore, C. V. (eds.): Progress in Hematology. Vol. 5. New York, Grune and Stratton, 1966.

Krantz, S. B., and Kao, V.: Studies on red cell aplasia. II. Report of a second patient with an antibody to erythroblast nuclei and a remission after immunosuppressive therapy. Blood, 34:1, 1969.

Loeb, V., Jr., Moore, C. V., and Dubach, R.: The physiologic evaluation and management of chronic bone marrow failure. Amer. J. Med., 15:499, 1953.

Mohler, D. N., and Leavell, B. S.: Aplastic anemia: An analysis of 50 cases. Ann. Intern. Med., 49:326, 1958.

Sanchez-Medal, L., Gomez-Leal, A., Duarte, L., and Rico, M. G.: Anabolic androgenic steroids in the treatment of acquired aplastic anemia. Blood, 34:283, 1969.

Scott, J. L., Cartwright, G. E., and Wintrobe, M. M.: Acquired aplastic anemia. Medicine, 38:119, 1958.

Wallerstein, R. O., Condit, P. K., Kasper, C. K., Brown, J. W., and Morrison, F. R.: Statewide study of chloramphenicol therapy of fatal aplastic anemia. J.A.M.A., 208:2045, 1969.

Yunis, A. A., and Bloomberg, G. R.: Chloramphenicol toxicity: Clinical features and pathogenesis. *In* Moore, C. V., and Brown, E. B. (eds.): Progress in Hematology. Vol. 4, p. 138. New York, Grune and Stratton, 1964.

SIDEROBLASTIC ANEMIAS

Sideroblastic anemias constitute a heterogeneous group of normocytic or slightly macrocytic anemias of multiple etiologies characterized by ineffective erythropoiesis, variable degrees of hypochromia as a manifestation of impaired hemoglobin synthesis, and the presence of *ringed sideroblasts* in the bone marrow. Ringed sideroblasts are nucleated red blood cells which contain a ring of siderotic granules surrounding the nucleus. Electron microscopic studies have demonstrated that the nonheme iron of these granules is (1) located between the cristae of perinuclear mitochondria, and (2) present both as ferritin and in an abnormal form as ferruginous micelles, dustlike or in plaques. These features suggest that the biochemical lesion responsible for the defective hemoglobin synthesis and resultant hypochromia may be located in mitochondria where protoporphyrin unites with iron to form heme. Sideroblastic anemias may be classified as follows:

I. Primary
   A. Acquired sideroblastic anemia in adults (chronic refractory anemia with sideroblastic bone marrow, refractory normoblastic anemia, sideroachrestic anemia, refractory sideroblastic anemia)
   B. Hereditary (sex-linked) sideroblastic anemia (anemia hypochromica sideroachrestica hereditaria)
II. Pyridoxine-responsive sideroblastic anemia
III. Secondary
   A. Sideroblastic anemia associated with rheumatoid arthritis, polyarteritis nodosa, carcinoma, myelofibrosis, leukemia, multiple myeloma, hereditary and acquired hemolytic anemias, malabsorption syndromes, thalassemia major, pernicious anemia, or chronic alcoholism
   B. Drug-induced sideroblastic anemia (isoniazid, cycloserine, and other antituberculous drugs)
   C. Lead poisoning

Primary sideroblastic anemia of adults is commonly regarded as a metabolic disorder of unknown cause, but some workers have favored the view that it is a form of erythroleukemia. Attempts to identify the biochemical defect in hemoglobin synthesis have yielded inconsistent results. It occurs most frequently in patients over the age of 60 years, has no distinguishing clinical features, is chronic in course, and rarely terminates as acute myelocytic or monocytic leukemia. Hereditary sideroblastic anemia is a rare disorder that occurs in males and is probably transmitted as a sex-linked recessive trait; affected males may survive for many years and tend to develop iron overload; terminal leukemia has not been described. Pyridoxine-responsive sideroblastic anemias occur among both the primary and secondary forms; they are apparently always sideroblastic, but only a portion of the patients with sideroblastic anemia are benefited by the administration of pyridoxine. Pyridoxal phosphate plays a role in heme synthesis (formation of aminolevulinic acid), but why very large doses are necessary for therapeutic effectiveness is unknown. The antituberculous drugs responsible for drug-induced sideroblastic anemia are pyridoxine antagonists; their effect on pyridoxine metabolism is synergistic, and usually two or more have been given simultaneously when the anemia is induced. Why secondary sideroblastic anemia occurs in some patients with the wide variety of disorders listed in the foregoing outline, and not in others, is a mystery. Lead produces sideroblastic anemia because of its toxic effect on heme synthesis.

The hemoglobin level may be as low as 5 grams per 100 ml., but more commonly is in the range of 7 to 10 grams. Some of the red blood cells have a normal amount of hemoglobin, whereas others are hypochromic. A few target cells, fragmented cells, siderocytes, and normoblasts may be seen; basophilic stippling is a feature of lead poisoning. Reticulocytes are normal or low. Osmotic fragility tends to be decreased. The plasma iron and transferrin saturation are normal to high. Leukocyte and platelet levels vary from normal to low. The bone marrow is characterized by intense erythroid hyperplasia, often associated with binucleated cells and a shift to younger megaloblastoid forms. Iron stains show many abnormal ringed sideroblasts and increased amounts of hemosiderin. Granulocytic precursors frequently are normal, but a shift to younger forms may occur. Erythrocyte survival is moderately shortened.

Therapy is the same as for bone marrow failure except that therapeutic trials with folic acid and with pyridoxine (50 to 200 mg. per day) should regularly be made. When therapeutic responses occur, they are usually only partial, but they may be great enough to obviate the need for continued transfusion or may significantly decrease transfusion requirement. In the case of drug- or lead-induced sideroblastic anemia, removal of the offending agent may be all that is required.

Griggs, R. C.: Lead poisoning: Hematologic aspects. *In* Moore, C. V., and Brown, E. B. (eds.): Progress in Hematology. New York, Grune and Stratton, 1964, Vol. 4, p. 117.

Horrigan, D. B., and Harris, J. W.: Pyridoxine-responsive anemia in man. *In* Vitamins and Hormones—Advances in Research and Applications. New York, Academic Press, Inc., 1968, Vol. 26, p. 549.

MacGibbon, B. H., and Mollin, D. L.: Sideroblastic anaemia in man: Observations on seventy cases. Brit. J. Haemat., 11:59, 1965.

Mollin, D. L.: Sideroblasts and sideroblastic anaemia. Brit. J. Haemat., 11:41, 1965.

MYELOPHTHISIC ANEMIAS

The term "myelophthisic anemia" is applied to those anemias associated with space-occupying lesions of the bone marrow. The anemia may be moderate to severe; the white blood cell count may be elevated or depressed; thrombocytopenia may or may not be present. Normoblasts are found in the peripheral blood, often in large numbers; young granulocytes may also be seen, but are less prominent. Red blood cell survival is shortened, and the anemia is caused because the bone marrow, although stimulated, does not increase erythrocyte production enough to compensate for the hemolysis. The old idea that normal marrow is crowded out by the invading tissue is no longer tenable.

Any cells or tissue that invade bone marrow may be responsible for the production of myelophthisic anemia: metastatic carcinoma, multiple myeloma, Hodgkin's disease and other malignant lymphomas, diffuse granulomatous involvement, the xanthomatoses, or myelofibrosis. Carcinomas of the breast, lung, prostate, stomach, kidney, and thyroid are malignancies that frequently metastasize to bone.

The clinical manifestations are primarily those of the disease causing the infiltration. Bone pain may be severe. At times the anemia may become great enough to contribute to the symptomatology, and bleeding may occur if the platelet count falls to critically low levels. Under some circumstances, particularly in myelofibrosis, extramedullary hematopoiesis may cause enlargement of liver and spleen.

The diagnosis should be suspected whenever nucleated red blood cells are found in the peripheral blood without obvious cause. The finding of normoblasts in a patient with known carcinoma is strong presumptive evidence of metastasis to marrow. With mild degrees of anemia the erythrocytes usually show little morphologic alteration, but as the anemia becomes more severe, considerable changes in size and shape occur together with polychromasia and basophilic stippling. Reticulocytes are frequently increased in number. The leukocytic forms found in the blood are usually mature cells even when the total white blood cell count is elevated to leukemoid levels; the occurrence of metamyelocytes and myelocytes, however, is not rare. The diagnosis is established by identifying the abnormal cells in the bone marrow; for this purpose, even with aspirated marrow, it is wise to save some of the aspirated material for the preparation of a paraffin block and sectioning. If no marrow can be aspirated, a trephine biopsy should be done. Except in some patients with myelofibrosis, fairly generous areas of active hematopoiesis can be found in addition to the abnormal invading tissue. Because involvement of the marrow may be spotty, more than one area may have to be examined before abnormal cells can be found.

Treatment and prognosis depend on the causative disorder. The same principles that govern general supportive care and the use of transfusions in bone marrow failure apply.

Wintrobe, M. M.: Clinical Hematology. 6th ed. Philadelphia, Lea and Febiger, 1967.

HEMOLYTIC DISORDERS

GENERAL CONSIDERATIONS
Lawrence E. Young

Definition. The essential feature of a hemolytic disorder is shortening of the life span of the red blood cells. The patient may have a compensated hemolytic state without anemia if the bone marrow responds adequately. As the marrow of adult man appears to be capable of increasing red blood cell production about eightfold, and as the normal life span of human red cells is about 120 days, anemia may not develop in some cases even if the average life span of the red cells is reduced to 15 to 20 days. The reserve capacity of the liver to excrete an increased quantity of bilirubin resulting from hemolysis may likewise result in maintenance of a normal concentration of bilirubin in the blood plasma. In a large proportion of the hemolytic states recognized clinically, however, patients are either anemic or mildly icteric, or both, so that the terms *hemolytic anemia* and *hemolytic icterus* are applicable.

Clinical Manifestations. In addition to pallor and mild icterus, the patient with a hemolytic disorder may present with fever, dyspnea, or shock if hemolysis is severe and anemia develops rapidly. The spleen is frequently enlarged but is by no means always palpable. In some instances, notably in hereditary spherocytosis, splenomegaly may be associated with accumulation of red cells in the splenic pulp; in others, enlargement may be due chiefly to proliferation of one or more cellular elements. The liver is also enlarged in many cases. Other clinical findings are related chiefly to the severity of the anemia and to the condition responsible for the hemolytic process. Chronic ulceration of the skin over or proximal to the malleoli may develop in sickle cell anemia, and rarely in hereditary spherocytosis and other chronic hemolytic disorders.

Gallstones containing chiefly bile pigment develop frequently in patients with chronic hemolytic disorders. Obstructive jaundice associated with choledocholithiasis or with cholestasis may develop rapidly and with extremely high concentrations of serum bilirubin because of the combination of excessive pigment production and biliary obstruction. Another major complication of chronic hemolytic disorders is rather sudden depression of erythropoiesis and fall in reticulocyte count, most often associated with acute infection. In such cases, the bone marrow may show hypoplasia or arrested maturation of erythroid cells. Folate deficiency may be demonstrable in some patients with chronic hemolytic anemia and may at times be associated with a megaloblastic marrow. Many of the "crises" in chronic hemolytic states are due chiefly to decrease in erythropoiesis for one reason or another. Anemia may suddenly become severe under these circumstances without significant increase in hemolysis above the patient's usual rate. Such episodes are often referred to as "hyporegenerative crises." Because folate requirement may be increased by persistent hemolysis, administration of 5 mg. of folic acid by mouth daily may be justified in chronic hemolytic states of any type to prevent deficiency of this vitamin.

Diagnosis. Persistent reticulocytosis, with or without nucleated red blood cells in the peripheral blood, in the absence of blood loss should arouse suspicion of hemolysis. Large, diffusely basophilic red cells, which appear as very immature reticulocytes on supravital staining, are especially indicative of heightened bone marrow response. Estimates of compensatory increase in rate of erythropoiesis by use of reticulocyte counts require calculation of the number per cubic millimeter (normal is about 60,000) and recognition of the fact that maturation time of reticulocytes in the circulation may increase two- to threefold as anemia becomes severe. The rate of red cell destruction can be estimated most conveniently by measuring the survival time of the patient's cells after tagging with radioactive chromium (Cr^{51}). Rapid disappearance of similarly labeled normal donor cells from the patient's circulation points to an extracorpuscular hemolytic mechanism. Measurement of fecal urobilinogen excretion, usually in four-day collections of stool, also provides an estimate of the rate of red cell destruction, but such estimates may be falsely low in some cases. Fecal urobilinogen determinations have been made much less frequently in most centers since isotopic tagging of red cells became available. Since the amount of urobilinogen excreted in the urine is affected by liver function, measurements of urinary urobilinogen are unreliable as indicators of the rate of red cell destruction. In the presence of modest hemolysis, urinary urobilinogen excretion may be normal if liver function is well preserved, or it may be greatly increased if liver function is impaired.

The concentration of bilirubin (predominantly unconjugated) seldom exceeds 8.0 mg. per 100 ml. of plasma. Hemolytic icterus has been recognized for many years as "acholuric"; little or no bilirubin is excreted in the urine unless liver function is impaired or the biliary tract becomes obstructed.

Since hemoglobinemia is largely the result of intravascular hemolysis, it is absent or minimal in many hemolytic states, especially those in which red cells are destroyed chiefly within the spleen, liver, and/or bone marrow. The renal threshold for hemoglobin depends on the capacity of plasma haptoglobins to bind hemoglobin (normally 100 to 150 mg. of hemoglobin per 100 ml. of plasma) and on the ability of renal tubular cells to remove hemoglobin from glomerular filtrate. The haptoglobins, which are alpha-2 globulins with remarkable capacity to bind hemoglobin, are markedly reduced in the plasma in most of the clinically recognized hemolytic states, acute and chronic, including those with little or no hemoglobinemia. The significance of methemalbuminemia, hemoglobinuria, and hemosiderinuria is discussed below.

Morphologic abnormalities of the red blood cells are best discussed in connection with the individual hemolytic disorders. In some examples of hemolytic disease, no abnormality of size or shape of the red cells is apparent. Fragmentation best observed with phase microscopy, but also evident in customary examination of stained blood smears, is recognized increasingly as a final common pathway in many hemolytic states. Platelets and granulocytes are usually present in normal or increased numbers, but either or both may be decreased in some instances. The bone marrow typically shows normoblastic hyperplasia in response to hemolysis except during hyporegenerative periods which are most commonly associated with infection.

Splenectomy. Since the estimated benefits and hazards of splenectomy must be weighed in the management of many patients with hemolytic disorders, certain general considerations can be presented to advantage at this point. Decision can often be reached easily on the basis of precise diagnosis and abundant documentation in the literature of favorable or unfavorable results with a given disorder. In some of the disorders to be described, decision regarding splenectomy may be influenced by measurements of radioactivity over the body surface above the spleen in comparison with counts above the liver after transfusion of autogenous or normal donated red cells tagged with Cr^{51}. Such measurements help to reveal the relative importance of the spleen in the hemolytic process. There are well-documented examples, however, of patients benefiting from splenectomy despite the fact that excessive splenic localization was not found in this type of preoperative study.

Immediate operative mortality from splenectomy performed primarily to relieve hemolytic disease is very low in the hands of experienced surgeons. Two possible sequelae of splenectomy deserve emphasis. Infants splenectomized during the first year or two of life probably have considerable reduction in resistance to infection. The risk thus imposed is sufficient to justify postponement of splenectomy in most cases until the age

CLASSIFICATION OF HEMOLYTIC DISORDERS

I. Intracorpuscular abnormalities (sometimes combined with extrinsic challenge)
  A. Membrane defects
    Spherocytosis
    Elliptocytosis
    Stomatocytosis
    Chronic hemolytic anemia with paroxysmal nocturnal hemoglobinuria
  B. Enzyme deficiencies
    Defect in Embden-Meyerhof pathway of glycolysis
      Pyruvate kinase
      Triosephosphate isomerase
      Glucosephosphate isomerase
      Hexokinase
      Phosphoglycerate kinase
      Phosphofructokinase
      2,3-Diphosphoglyceromutase
    Deficiency in enzyme activity or in cofactor related to the hexose monophosphate shunt pathway
      Glucose-6-phosphate dehydrogenase
      6-Phosphogluconate dehydrogenase
      Glutathione reductase
      Glutathione synthetase
      Glutathione peroxidase
  C. Hemoglobinopathies—qualitative defect in alpha or beta chains of globin
    Aggregating hemoglobins (S, C, D, I)
    Unstable hemoglobins (Zürich, Köln, etc.) with Heinz body formation
  D. Thalassemias—quantitative deficiency in synthesis of alpha or beta chains (may be combined with qualitative defect)
  E. Other types
II. Extracorpuscular abnormalities (hemolytic mechanisms and agents sometimes acting upon defective red cells)
  A. Deficiency of beta-lipoprotein in plasma
  B. Immune mechanism, idiopathic or associated with another disease
    Warm antibodies
      γG globulin, often with anti-Rh specificity
    Cold antibodies
      γM globulin with anti-I or -i specificity
      γG globulin with anti-P specificity
  C. Associated with other diseases (symptomatic, nonimmune)
    Splenomegaly from various causes
    Cancer
    Liver disease
    Renal disease
    Peripheral vascular disease
    Heart disease
  D. Introduction of agents or forces from outside the body
    Physical agents
    Infectious agents
    Chemical agents
    Antibodies passively acquired
      Hemolytic disease of the newborn
      Transfusion of incompatible plasma

of about four years. Another consequence of splenectomy is thromboembolism in patients with persistent thrombocytosis. Such patients are usually those who continue to have anemia and reticulocytosis as well as thrombocytosis for many years. The patient whose hemolytic anemia is not significantly relieved by splenectomy thus incurs the added risk of thrombophlebitis and embolic complications.

Classification. The classification in the accompanying table is based chiefly upon current concepts of pathogenic mechanisms. The disorders listed with intracorpuscular abnormalities of the red cell are hereditary except for that associated with nocturnal hemoglobinuria. Intrinsically defective red cells with shortened life span may be produced in patients with myeloid metaplasia, chronic myelocytic leukemia, deficiency of vitamin B_{12}, folate, or iron, and in patients with lead intoxication. These conditions will not be discussed here because other features of the respective illnesses are usually more important than the hemolytic component of the anemia.

INTRACORPUSCULAR ABNORMALITIES
Lawrence E. Young

Erythrocytes from patients with certain types of intracorpuscular abnormality have been found to disappear rapidly from the circulation after transfusion to normal recipients. Normal donor cells, on the other hand, survive normally in the circulation of such patients unless there are complicating hemolytic mechanisms such as hypersplenism or the development of immune isoantibodies as a result of previous transfusions. Although there are unmistakable abnormalities of the red blood cells in this group of patients, hemolysis may be dependent upon or heightened by the presence of environmental factors that provide a critical challenge to the defective cells. The sequence of events by which most recognized types of abnormal red cells are destroyed in vivo becomes clearer each year. This group of disorders provides excellent material for studies in cellular biology.

MEMBRANE DEFECTS

Hereditary Spherocytosis (HS)
(Congenital Hemolytic Anemia; Acholuric Jaundice)

Definition. This condition is inherited as an autosomal dominant disorder and is characterized by the presence of spherocytes or abnormally thick red blood cells in the circulation. It has been found in many populations, but appears to be most common in northern European stocks. In such populations, the incidence has been estimated from 200 to 300 per million.

Clinical Manifestations. Diagnosis may be made at birth if the condition is suspected, but in mild cases diagnosis may not be made until late in life. Moderate splenomegaly develops in nearly all cases. Leg ulcers are encountered infrequently. Roentgenographic examination reveals striation and thickening of the frontal and parietal bones in some cases. Anemia is rarely severe in the absence of hyporegenerative crises or other complications such as infection or hemorrhage.

Diagnosis. Spherocytosis is usually evident in blood smears or in wet preparations which show bizarre rouleaux formation. The increase in osmotic fragility provides a reliable measure of the degree of spherocytosis. Mechanical fragility of the red cells is also increased. Both types of fragility are increased by sterile incubation of the blood at body temperature for 24 hours, a procedure that may cause changes in red cells similar to those produced during sequestration within the spleen. Autohemolysis, or spontaneous lysis of red cells in defibrinated blood incubated at body temperature, is best measured at 48 hours and is markedly increased in most cases of HS. The percentage of lysis after incubation is computed by measuring the concentration of hemoglobin in the serum in relation to the hemoglobin content of the blood sample prior to incubation. Autohemolysis is strikingly inhibited by addition of glucose or by slight acidification of the blood from HS patients. Such inhibition of autohemolysis is less evident in other types of chronic spherocytosis, and is sometimes not demonstrable in HS until after splenectomy. In order to establish the diagnosis, similar abnormalities should be sought in relatives of patients with spherocytosis, even when there is no history of anemia, jaundice, or splenomegaly. In some cases only the measurements of fragility with incubated red cells are clearly abnormal. In instances of suspected low gene manifestation or gene mutation, both parents of patients with suspected HS may be hematologically normal by all available criteria.

Pathogenesis. Spherocytes are readily trapped, probably for variable periods of time, within the splenic pulp. When washed from that site after splenectomy, they show much greater osmotic fragility than do spherocytes in the peripheral blood, although normal donor cells in the splenic pulp show little increase in fragility. Transfused spherocytes are readily trapped and destroyed in the spleen of hematologically normal recipients but survive normally in splenectomized normal recipients.

The red cell membrane in this disease is less deformable and more permeable to sodium than the membrane of normal red cells. Trapping of HS red cells within the cords of Billroth of the spleen is probably related to cellular rigidity, which depends both on the decreased surface area to volume ratio and increased intrinsic rigidity of the cell membrane. Hereditary spherocytosis cells lose lipid and probably protein from the membrane surface as they make their way through the cords, with the result that they become more nearly spherical and still more rigid. Eventually the cells are unable to escape through the small openings into the venous sinusoids. Fragmentation of the rigid cells to the point of ultimate destruction has been observed by phase microscopy and electron microscopy in the spleens of mice afflicted with a comparable disorder. Hemoglobinemia is not encountered in HS patients, but plasma haptoglobin concentration is consistently low.

Treatment. Splenectomy is invariably effective

in lengthening the life span of the red cells to a nearly normal range. Anemia is fully corrected and there is a decrease to normal in reticulocytes and serum bilirubin concentration. Spherocytosis persists after splenectomy, but is less severe. All known abnormalities of the red cells, including the striking effects of in vitro incubation, persist but are of little or no consequence once the splenic trap is removed. Splenectomy can be recommended in most cases, even when well compensated, because of the threats of cholelithiasis and of severe anemia during periods of suppressed erythropoiesis. Splenectomy may prevent development of hemochromatosis, a recently reported complication in older patients. Operation is usually deferred during infancy for reasons explained previously. Transfusion of normal red blood cells is seldom indicated except during the periods of severe anemia associated with hyporegenerative bone marrow.

Hereditary Elliptocytosis

Hereditary elliptocytosis is similar to hereditary spherocytosis in many respects. It has been found in many populations, and may be encountered more frequently than spherocytosis in some localities. It is inherited as an autosomal dominant abnormality with wide variations in gene manifestation both within and between families. In some families there is evidence for location of the gene or genes determining elliptocytosis on the chromosome bearing genes for the Rh blood group system. The degree of elliptocytosis varies from person to person and also among the red cells of any affected person. A large number of the cells are usually abnormal in shape, some are greatly elongated, and others are slightly oval. There is no apparent relationship between the degree of elliptocytosis and the life span of the red cells. In the presence of active hemolysis, microspherocytes may be found in small numbers. Some affected persons have red cells with normal life span; others have a compensated hemolytic state; and a minority have overt hemolytic anemia. The very rare homozygous state is associated with severe hemolysis. Factors determining chronic hemolysis in the heterozygotes are unknown. Coexistence of elliptocytosis with hemoglobin S or hemoglobin C trait does not appear to cause an additive, deleterious effect on the red cells. Coexistence of elliptocytosis with heterozygous beta-thalassemia, on the other hand, may be associated with hemolysis.

Splenomegaly is common, and sequestration of red cells in the spleen is evident. Most patients splenectomized because of hemolysis associated with elliptocytosis have been benefited.

Stomatocytosis

Stomatocytosis, probably hereditary, is characterized by red cells with the appearance of a linear, mouthlike area of central pallor on stained films and with the appearance of bowls in wet preparations. The marked increase in osmotic fragility of these cells has been attributed to rigidity of the cell membrane. At least one variant of the cases first described has been reported. Response to splenectomy is variable.

Chronic Hemolytic Anemia with Paroxysmal Nocturnal Hemoglobinuria

Definition. This rare disorder has been encountered in many parts of the world. It occurs in both sexes, with onset most common during the third or fourth decade. There is no report of familial incidence.

Clinical Manifestations. The disease is characterized by chronic hemolysis, with hemoglobinemia and methemalbuminemia, usually increasing during sleep, regardless of the time when the patient sleeps. During the periods of hemolysis sufficient to cause hemoglobinuria, the urine passed on arising is usually brown or reddish brown. In severely affected patients hemoglobinuria may be continuous, with further darkening of the urine after sleep. Hemosiderinuria, a regular feature of the disease, results in considerable loss of iron from the body. Renal function is usually unimpaired, but there may be complications such as pyelonephritis. Hemosiderin is not found in any significant quantity in the body outside the cells of the convoluted tubules and ascending loops of Henle in the kidney, unless the patient has had frequent transfusions. The liver and spleen may be slightly enlarged. Neutropenia and moderate thrombocytopenia are commonly found. Alkaline phosphatase activity in the neutrophils is markedly decreased. Although erythroid hyperplasia of the bone marrow is usually present, marked hypoplasia of all elements is being recognized increasingly before, or rarely after, the hemolytic disorder becomes apparent. It has been suggested that in some cases the abnormal red cells may be derived from a mutant clone of precursors originating during a period of marrow aplasia even when the aplasia seems related to drug usage. The recently recognized development of stem cell or acute myelocytic leukemia in patients with antecedent nocturnal hemoglobinuria has led to the suggestion that this hemolytic disorder may represent a somatic mutation which at times involves the stem cells. Thrombotic complications are frequently associated with greatly accelerated hemolysis. Thrombosis may be accelerated, if not initiated, by liberation of phospholipids from hemolyzed cells, thus promoting a vicious cycle.

Pathogenesis. The red cells in the circulation of a patient at any time differ widely in susceptibility to lysis both in vitro and in vivo. No characteristic abnormality of the red cells is evident in blood smears or in tests of osmotic or mechanical fragility. There is nevertheless a consistent lesion, of unknown nature, in the red cell membrane which renders the cell highly sensitive to lysis by the final components of the complement sequence. Deficiency in red cell cholinesterase activity tends to be correlated with the severity of hemolysis in patients with this disorder, and the red cells most deficient in this enzyme can be shown to be most sensitive to lysis in acidified serum. Nevertheless, the significance of this enzyme deficiency is not known. It is noteworthy that familial deficiency of red cell cholinesterase has been demonstrated in some persons in the absence of hemolysis or other findings characteristic of nocturnal hemoglobinuria.

Ham's test, which reveals hemolysis of the patient's red blood cells in vitro in slightly acidified normal human serum, is nearly specific for this condition if the test is suitably controlled. Among the constituents of serum required for hemolysis in vitro are magnesium ions and all known components of the human complement complex. The sugar water test provides a simple screening procedure, consisting of mixing whole blood with nine volumes of 10 per cent sucrose in distilled water. After incubation of the mixture for 30 minutes, centrifugation reveals hemolysis in the supernatant portion if the test is positive. The mechanism by which the hemolytic system becomes more active in vivo during sleep remains to be determined. The degree of hemoglobinemia increases after administration of acid salts, and may be inhibited temporarily by alkalinization.

Treatment. Transfusion of washed, normal red blood cells is needed during periods of severe anemia. Transfusion of whole blood should be avoided in most cases, because constituents of normal plasma as well as leukocytes may accelerate hemolysis. Use of coumarin derivatives may be indicated in patients who have developed thrombosis, but it is difficult to justify for prevention of thrombosis. Their inhibitory effect on hemolysis is transient with tolerable doses. Use of heparin is controversial. Intravenous administration of 1000 ml. of 6 per cent dextran daily or at longer intervals may inhibit hemolysis during critical periods of the disease but is not recommended for sustained use. All operative procedures, including splenectomy, are to be avoided if possible. Administration of iron, preferably by mouth, may be beneficial for patients who are not transfused and who develop evidence of iron deficiency. Administration of androgens, such as fluoxymesterone, 20 to 30 mg. daily by mouth, may be beneficial by stimulating erythropoiesis and perhaps by reducing hemolysis. Folic acid, usually 5 mg. daily by mouth, is indicated to meet increased folate requirement.

Prognosis. This is a chronic disorder that terminates fatally in many cases. The patients may lead active lives between complicating episodes if suitably managed. Rarely, the abnormality of the red cells eventually disappears. A few women with this disease have borne normal children, but usually with complications during pregnancy or the puerperium.

ENZYME DEFICIENCIES

Defects in Embden-Meyerhof Pathway of Glycolysis

Hemolytic states associated with inherited deficiencies of seven enzymes involved in the Embden-Meyerhof pathway of anaerobic glycolysis in the red cells have been identified since 1962. The genetic pattern of pyruvate kinase (PK), triosephosphate isomerase (TPI), glucosephosphate isomerase, and hexokinase deficiency is that of autosomal recessive inheritance. Heterozygotes are phenotypically normal, but have measurable deficiency of enzyme activity in the red cells. Homozygotes have a lifelong hemolytic state of variable severity with splenomegaly and only partial relief from hemolysis after splenectomy. Spherocytosis is not prominent, but may be noted on close inspection of blood smears and wet preparations. Crenated red cells are frequently noted and are probably crenated spherocytes or irregularly contracted cells. Finding crenated spherocytes on the blood smear of a patient with splenomegaly and with a history suggesting hemolytic anemia since early childhood should stimulate the clinician to seek enzyme assays on the patient's red cells.

Available evidence suggests that phosphoglycerate kinase deficiency is X chromosome-linked. Studies on a single family with phosphofructokinase deficiency also suggest X-linkage. The hereditary pattern of 2,3-diphosphoglyceromutase deficiency is uncertain.

PK deficiency, the prototype of this group, is the most common within the populations thus far examined. Genetically determined heterogeneity of erythrocyte PK has been demonstrated, including evidence of kinetic abnormality of the enzyme and development of anemia in heterozygotes. Patients with such a variant may not be detectable by the usual assays of enzyme activity. Most patients with PK deficiency develop anemia and jaundice in the neonatal period. Anemia is usually more severe than in hereditary spherocytosis. Osmotic fragility of the red cells is normal with fresh blood but is abnormally increased after the blood has been incubated for 24 hours at 37° C. Autohemolysis is moderately increased except in patients with a presumed variant of PK and is usually not diminished when glucose is added to the blood. In some cases of PK deficiency, however, glucose may inhibit autohemolysis. Use of the autohemolysis test for differential diagnosis must take into account these exceptional cases of PK deficiency along with the exceptional cases of hereditary spherocytosis in which glucose fails to inhibit autohemolysis until after splenectomy.

Hemolysis in PK deficiency is generally attributed to impaired glycolysis and consequent reduction in adenosine triphosphate (ATP) generation. PK-deficient reticulocytes may be spared to some extent from destruction in the general circulation because their mitochondria provide ATP from aerobic metabolism. The PK-deficient reticulocytes, like normal reticulocytes, tend to be sequestered within the spleen. Within the hypoxic environment of the splenic pulp, aerobic metabolism, upon which the PK-deficient reticulocytes are dependent, is inhibited with consequent decrease in ATP content, increase in cellular rigidity, and irreversible sequestration of the reticulocytes. The partial relief of anemia and frequent reduction in transfusion requirement in this disorder after splenectomy may be attributable to removal of the hypoxic trap. Reticulocyte counts are frequently higher after splenectomy despite amelioration of anemia, thus reflecting the survival of reticulocytes which previously had been eliminated from the circulation by the spleen. Although splenectomy is much less effective than in hereditary spherocytosis, it can be recommended after infancy for patients requiring transfusions to maintain acceptable concentrations of hemoglobin.

In TPI deficiency, enzyme activity is also low in leukocytes, muscle, and cerebrospinal fluid. A severe, progressive neurologic disorder develops in addition to hemolytic anemia. The hematologic picture is similar to that of PK deficiency except that autohemolysis is more regularly inhibited by glucose.

Other examples of enzyme deficiency in the red cell related to anaerobic glycolysis are rare. In general, the clinical findings and course are similar to those of PK deficiency. Recent reports implicate deficiency of three additional enzymes of the glycolytic pathway in causing hemolytic anemia: phosphofructo-aldolase, glyceraldehyde phosphate dehydrogenase, and 2,3-diphosphoglycerophosphatase.

Deficiency in Enzyme Activity or in Cofactor Related to the Hexose Monophosphate (HMP) Shunt Pathway

GLUCOSE-6-PHOSPHATE DEHYDROGENASE (G-6-PD)

The enzyme G-6-PD is involved at the beginning of the oxidative HMP shunt pathway, which under usual conditions accounts for about 10 per cent of glucose metabolism of the red cell. In normal red cells the proportion of total glucose metabolized through the shunt pathway may be increased many-fold if the cells are subjected to oxidants such as those derived from certain drugs. The resulting increase in generation of the reduced form of nicotinamide adenine dinucleotide phosphate (NADPH) and consequently of reduced glutathione (GSH) helps to resist oxidant stresses. Otherwise, these stresses may inactivate essential thiol (SH) groups on membrane proteins, and within the cell may cause formation of methemoglobin and degradation of hemoglobin to form Heinz bodies. Drugs such as phenylhydrazine may overwhelm this protective mechanism, especially in older red cells because there is a decline in G-6-PD activity with aging of red cells in the circulation. Red cells with a genetically determined deficiency of G-6-PD are unable to withstand lesser oxidative stresses. The outcome in any given red cell is presumably determined by the amount of stress and the severity of enzyme deficiency, but predictions based on estimates of enzyme activity by the usual methods may nevertheless be inaccurate.

Studies on hemolytic disorders related to the HMP shunt pathway constitute one of the most fascinating and clinically significant chapters in the history of hematology. G-6-PD deficiency in red cells has been shown to be due to a wide range of genetic variants, each of which is X-linked. The defect is fully expressed in male hemizygotes and female homozygotes, but is variably manifest in female heterozygotes. It is not known whether the heterogeneity in G-6-PD formation is produced by different mutations at a single locus on the X chromosome or whether mutations at different loci affect the production and function of the enzyme. There are two common types of G-6-PD. Type A, moving rapidly on starch-gel electrophoresis, is found in about 35 per cent of American Negroes, including most of those who are enzyme deficient. Type B, moving more slowly on electrophoresis, is found in about 65 per cent of Negroes and in nearly all Caucasians.

Manifestations in Negroes. The most common type of G-6-PD deficiency is found in Negroes: about 10 per cent of American Negroes, 8 to 20 per cent of Negroes in West Africa, but in only 2 per cent of South African Bantus. Activity of this enzyme in the red cells is reduced to 7 to 15 per cent of normal in hemizygous males and homozygous females. Enzyme activity in heterozygous females ranges from normal to figures nearly as low as those obtained from homozygotes. Red cell life span is only slightly reduced in G-6-PD–deficient Negroes unless the cells are subjected to stress imposed by derivatives of certain drugs or by infection or diabetic ketoacidosis. More than 40 drugs have been found to produce hemolysis in G-6-PD–deficient persons. These include the antimalarial drugs primaquine and quinine (the latter also used in popular beverages), the antipyretics and analgesics acetylsalicylic acid and phenacetin, the nitrofurans, sulfones, many sulfonamides, chloramphenicol, para-aminosalicylic acid, probenecid, quinidine, phenylhydrazine, and water-soluble analogues of vitamin K. Naphthalene, of which moth balls are composed, is often ingested by children with effects similar to those of the drugs listed. Negroes whose G-6-PD–deficient red cells are challenged develop hemolytic anemia of varying severity, depending upon the dose and oxidative capacity of the derivatives of the chemical agent involved; in female heterozygotes the degree of enzyme deficiency appears also to influence the extent of hemolysis. Patients suffering from infection, acidosis, or impaired liver or kidney function, with consequent delay in drug excretion, may be more subject to hemolysis with a given dose of a potentially oxidant drug. Moreover, infection or acidosis may provoke hemolysis in the absence of an offending drug and they may in fact be the most common precipitants of hemolytic anemia in these individuals.

Hemoglobinemia and hemoglobinuria are usually of only moderate degree and short duration, and may not be observed. Plasma haptoglobin is usually reduced even in the cases of little or no hemoglobinemia. Many of the red cells may contain Heinz bodies during the first few days of hemolysis, but in typical cases most of the red cells containing Heinz bodies have been eliminated by the time the hematocrit reaches its lowest point. The red cells show fragmentation of widely varying degree from case to case prior to onset of the recovery phase. The cells may appear as though a portion had been torn away, but they do not as a rule show crenation or appear as irregularly contracted spherocytes. Careful inspection of the blood smear together with consideration of the patient's history and ethnic group help to differentiate this type of hemolytic anemia from that caused by a defect in the Embden-Meyerhof pathway within the red cell. Hemolysis is typically limited in duration because of the more nearly normal G-6-PD activity in younger red cells which become more abundant in the circulation in response to hemolysis. Consequently, the erythrocyte level may return to normal even though administration of the offending drug is continued. Diagnosis by estimates of enzyme activity in the red cells may be difficult at the time of acute hemolysis and reticulocytosis. Confirmation of the clinical diagnosis by enzyme assay often must await the return to normal of the red cell age distribution unless special methods are used.

Manifestations in Other Populations. G-6-PD deficiency in populations other than Negroes is usually more severe, with red cell enzyme activity in most cases in the range of 0 to 5 per cent of normal and with reduced G-6-PD activity in leukocytes and platelets as well as in red cells. At least 30 different forms of G-6-PD have been demonstrated among Caucasian and Oriental populations on the basis of kinetic properties of the enzyme. The incidence of G-6-PD deficiency is estimated at 5 to 20 per cent in non-Ashkenazic (Oriental) Jews, 2 to 9 per cent in Greeks, 0.5 to 1.0 per cent in Italians, 3 to 35 per cent in Sardinian groups, 2 to 4 per cent in Chinese, 1 to 5 per cent in Indians, and 12 per cent in Thais. Well documented examples of this enzyme deficiency have been found in other ethnic groups such as the English, Sicilian, and Ashkenazic Jewish, but the incidence is low. Studies of Caucasians with G-6-PD activity in the range of 0 to 18 per cent of normal have shown that about 20 per cent of the circulating red cells are destroyed after ingestion of a single standard prophylactic antimalarial dose of primaquine (45 mg.). The degree of hemolysis under these circumstances is not related to the estimated level of enzyme activity. G-6-PD–deficient Caucasians are generally more subject than are Negroes to hemolysis after use of potentially oxidant drugs or as a complication of infection or of diabetic ketoacidosis.

Chronic hemolytic anemia in the absence of drugs or other extrinsic challenge is encountered in Caucasian and occasionally in Oriental males with marked deficiency of G-6-PD activity. Hemolysis appears to be continuous from infancy, but may be accelerated by the same types of challenges causing acute hemolysis in the much more common, nonanemic G-6-PD–deficient Caucasian or Negro. Most of the G-6-PD variants associated with a chronic hemolytic state are abnormally labile at temperatures of 40 to 46° C. Osmotic fragility of the red cells in the chronic state is normal or nearly so. Autohemolysis is only slightly increased, and is usually inhibited by glucose. Ovalocytes are noted in some cases, but spherocytes are rarely seen. Data on spleen size and results of splenectomy are meager. Splenomegaly is not a regular feature as it is in hereditary spherocytosis and in PK deficiency. Studies with Cr^{51}-tagged red cells show no unusual concentration of radioactivity over the spleen.

Favism is an acute hemolytic anemia occurring after ingestion of fava beans or after inhalation of pollen from the plant, Vicia faba, by persons with G-6-PD–deficient red cells. Several other plants may have a similar effect. Favism has been observed only in Caucasians and is most common among certain groups of non-Ashkenazic Jews, Sardinians, Greeks, and Italians. Since many Caucasians with G-6-PD deficiency suffer no hemolysis after challenge by bean or plant, an additional mechanism is suspected. Studies on isolated populations with high incidence of favism suggest that the additional determinant may be inherited. Anemia may be very severe and accompanied by hemoglobinemia. During the early phase of an attack the hemoglobin appears to be concentrated on one side of some of the red cells, leaving the cell envelope visible on the opposite side. Heinz bodies and spherocytes may be seen, and osmotic fragility may be transiently increased. There is marked leukocytosis, often with transient eosinophilia.

Neonatal Jaundice. Neonatal jaundice with development of kernicterus is a hazard for infants, especially males, with G-6-PD deficiency. Hemolysis and hyperbilirubinemia can be induced in the newborn, particularly if premature, by use of drugs such as water-soluble, synthetic vitamin K preparations or by drugs given to the mother before delivery. Caucasian and Oriental infants, and perhaps Negro infants as well, may develop jaundice without exposure to drugs. In Hong Kong, for example, G-6-PD deficiency is claimed to be the most common cause of neonatal jaundice and kernicterus. Even in the presence of normal G-6-PD activity in the red cells, glutathione is unstable during the first few days of life. Since this instability can be corrected in vitro by addition of glucose, it is believed that hypoglycemia in the newborn may increase the risk of neonatal jaundice.

Use of Screening Tests. It is estimated from population surveys that at least 100 million persons in the world have red cells deficient in G-6-PD. Wide use of a simple screening test for this deficiency, such as that based on reduction of methemoglobin, is strongly indicated as a part of comprehensive health care for populations known to be at relatively high risk. Tests done when the patient is well serve to forewarn both patient and physician. Tests performed during or immediately after a period of hemolysis are unreliable because some genetic variants, especially Negroes, have a high activity of G-6-PD in reticulocytes; i.e., the tests may yield "false negative" results. As the transfusion of G-6-PD–deficient red cells creates a potential hazard for recipients, it should be avoided when possible under ideal circumstances by appropriate screening of donors. The potential hazard is maximal in a small child whose circulating red cells might be derived largely from a single donor with severe deficiency of G-6-PD.

Drug-Induced Hemolysis of Older Normal Red Cells. Since G-6-PD activity declines with aging of red cells in the circulation, even red cells with normal enzyme activity initially may become susceptible to hemolysis if challenged by large doses of a drug such as the commonly used phenacetin or by modest doses of a drug such as phenylhydrazine with high oxidizing potential. It seems likely that this type of drug-induced hemolysis of normal aging red cells would be accentuated in the presence of infection or of diabetic acidosis. This potential hazard should be kept in mind by the physician as he estimates the risk of contemplated therapy in many clinical situations.

OTHER DEFICIENCIES RELATED TO THE HMP PATHWAY

Deficiency of 6-phosphogluconate dehydrogenase has been the subject of recent studies revealing genetic polymorphism with respect to this enzyme; relationship to hemolysis is not yet clear.

Glutathione reductase deficiency, inherited as an autosomal dominant trait, is found in leukocytes and platelets as well as in red cells, and is associated with hemolytic anemia, thrombocytopenia, and, in some cases, with leukopenia. A neurologic disorder characterized by spasticity may develop in these patients. Use of oxidant drugs may cause severe pancytopenia.

Deficiency of red cell glutathione, which in turn is due to deficiency of glutathione synthetase, is probably inherited as an autosomal recessive trait. Affected persons have a compensated hemolytic state with acceleration of hemolysis after use of potentially oxidant drugs.

Deficiency of red cell glutathione peroxidase is associated with relatively mild hemolytic states. Since this enzyme normally helps to prevent peroxidative injury, increased susceptibility to hemolysis after use of oxidant drugs is anticipated but not yet demonstrated. Available data suggest that this deficiency is most likely an autosomal recessive trait.

OTHER INTRACORPUSCULAR ABNORMALITIES

The hemoglobinopathies and thalassemias, some of which are associated with a hemolytic state, are considered separately below. It is noteworthy that the Heinz body anemias associated with unstable hemoglobins are usually detectable by the simple procedure of heating hemolysate at 50° C., for one to two hours. The resulting turbidity owing to precipitation of unstable hemoglobin is not observed in the Heinz body anemias associated with deficiency in enzyme activity or in cofactor related to the HMP shunt pathway.

A large number of patients with erythropoietic porphyria have hemolytic anemia which is relieved to varying degree by splenectomy. Improvement both in the hemolytic state and in photosensitivity after splenectomy may be marked.

Other types of hereditary abnormalities of the red cell associated with hemolysis are not easily classified. An example is the familial occurrence of hemolytic anemia and increased red cell content of phosphatidyl choline that may be related to a defect in phosphatide metabolism in the cell membrane.

Patients have been described with hemolytic anemia associated with low ATP concentration in the red cells and very high glycolytic rate. Further studies on the metabolism and membrane characteristics of these cells are needed.

EXTRACORPUSCULAR HEMOLYTIC AGENTS AND MECHANISMS
Lawrence E. Young

In this large and heterogeneous group are included those states in which erythrocytes, presumably normal when synthesized in the patient, have shortened life span as a result of exposure to hemolytic substances or mechanisms. Normal red cells subjected to the same unfavorable environment after transfusion to the patient are usually destroyed with equal or even greater rapidity.

DEFICIENCY OF BETA-LIPOPROTEIN IN PLASMA

Acanthocytosis (thorny red cells) associated with marked deficiency of beta-lipoprotein in the plasma is described elsewhere in this textbook as a rare inborn error of metabolism. Abnormality in shape of red cells increases with aging of the cells as they circulate in the lipid-deficient plasma. This disease is classified with the extracorpuscular abnormalities, as the red cells are thought to be normal when released from the bone marrow to the circulation. The change in shape may be related to an increase in sphingomyelin and a decrease in the lecithin content of the cells. Decrease in life span of the red cells is variable; anemia in the few reported cases has been mild. Vitamin E normally present in the beta-lipoprotein fraction of plasma is lacking in these patients. In vitro autohemolysis of acanthocytes is markedly reduced by addition of α-tocopherol to the incubated blood, but therapeutic usefulness of tocopherol in this disorder is not determined.

HEMOLYTIC ANEMIAS WITH EVIDENCE OF IMMUNE MECHANISM

The distinguishing feature of this group of hemolytic anemias is the presence on the patient's red cells and/or in the serum of one or more globulins that appear to be involved in the hemolytic process. The complex serologic and immunochemical studies used to identify the various red cell reactive globulins in this group of disorders are described in detail in other sources. The reactivity of the globulins in serum is best studied with both the patient's own red cells and normal red cells having various combinations of antigenic determinants, at specified temperatures and pH, and in some instances after treatment of the normal red cells with enzymes such as trypsin. The proteins attached to the red cell are detected by antiglobulin (Coombs) reagents prepared by immunization of animals with whole human serum or with purified components. The antiglobulin serum is absorbed with normal human red cells before use. Additional absorptions with globulin fractions may be required to prepare reagents reacting specifically with immunoglobulins (γG, γA, or γM) or with complement components. Globulins attached to the patient's red cells may be eluted and subjected to both serologic and immunochemical study.

Autoimmune Hemolytic Disease Associated with γG Globulins Reacting with Red Cells at Body Temperature
(Warm Antibodies)

Definition. This group of hemolytic disorders is considered separately because the clinical features and management can be more clearly delineated than in cases in which only complement components are demonstrable on the red cells. The red cells of these patients react with antiglobulin reagents having anti-γG specificity; that is, the direct antiglobulin (Coombs) test is positive. In some cases, the red cells are also agglutinated by antiglobulin serum of anticomplement specificity, the significance of which will be discussed below. The antibody eluted from the patient's red cells or present in the serum can be shown to react in various ways in vitro with both the patient's red cells and normal red cells at body temperature.

Incidence. Five or six new cases of this type (with γG globulin on the red cells) are recognized annually in the University of Rochester Medical Center. About 40 to 60 per cent of the reported cases of this type appear to be idiopathic. The remainder are associated with other diseases, most commonly with chronic lymphocytic leukemia, lymphosarcoma, reticulum cell sarcoma, lupus erythematosus, and, rarely, with Hodgkin's disease, carcinoma, dermoid and ovarian cysts, sarcoidosis, ulcerative colitis, and periarteritis nodosa. The reported incidence of underlying disease is presumably dependent in part upon the interests of the investigator and upon the intensity and duration of clinical study. The idiopathic form is more frequent after the age of 40 years, but may be encountered at any age. The secondary cases tend to follow the age incidence of the associated disease. Additional cases of Coombs-positive hemolytic anemia related to drug administration will be considered separately.

Pathology. The bone marrow usually shows normoblastic hyperplasia. Erythrophagocytosis, chiefly in monocytes and tissue macrophages, may be evident in marrow, spleen, lymph nodes, and liver as well as in smears of peripheral blood. The spleen is often moderately enlarged, but is not always palpable even in patients with leukemia or lymphoma. Accumulation of red blood cells in the splenic pulp varies widely from patient to patient and is usually less marked than in hereditary spherocytosis. Findings characteristic of an underlying disease may also be present.

Pathogenesis. There is no clear genetic basis for this group of hemolytic disorders, but there are impressive reports of familial occurrence. Development of similar hematologic and serologic abnormalities in a very high proportion of an inbred strain of mice (NZB/BC) has been observed with great interest. Debate continues on possible changes in antigenic determinants of the red blood cells and in the capacity of the antibody-forming cells to respond to these determinants, thus causing apparent autoimmunization. In some cases, notably in disseminated lupus, demonstration of cryoglobulins, anticomplementary substances, hyperglobulinemia, false positive serologic tests for syphilis, and a variety of anti-tissue antibodies suggests a general disturbance in regulation of the immune system. In other patients, notably those with lymphocytic leukemia and lymphoma, the apparent autoimmunization is associated with reduced levels of the immunoglobulins and with impaired production of antibodies against most infectious agents.

The serologic characteristics of the autoantibodies in these patients vary widely. Recent studies with red cells lacking certain antigenic determinants in the Rh system, presumably as a result of gene deletion, reveal that the autoantibodies in most cases may have some degree of specificity for one or more components of the Rh complex. In a minority of cases the autoantibodies have more easily demonstrable specificity for a component of the Rh complex, most often e, c, C, or D. Most of the autoantibodies in this group are not hemolysins in the usual sense. The mechanisms by which hemolysis is initiated in vivo by these antibodies are not fully defined. Erythrophagocytosis may be readily observed in various parts of the reticuloendothelial system, but its relative importance is difficult to estimate. Partial phagocytosis of red cells coated with γG has been demonstrated in vitro, the remainder of the red cell having marked decrease in surface area–volume ratio. This phenomenon may account in part for the spherocytosis frequently noted in blood smears from patients with severe hemolysis. The spleen probably functions as both a site of antibody production and an organ contributing to the destruction of antibody-coated red cells.

It has been observed with great interest in recent years that patients treated for hypertension with α-methyldopa may develop hemolytic anemia with serologic findings identical with those of idiopathic autoimmune hemolytic disease. The direct antiglobulin test is positive, and the autoantibodies in most cases have Rh specificity; they do not react with α-methyldopa or its derivatives. Development of the abnormal antibodies is dose-dependent and usually requires at least three to six months of drug administration. About 20 per cent of patients taking the drug for this length of time develop a positive direct antiglobulin test, but of these as few as 1 per cent may have "overt" hemolytic anemia. The antiglobulin test does not become negative until 7 to 24 months after stopping use of the drug. Hemolytic anemia with similar autoantibodies has been observed after use of the antirheumatic drug, mefenamic acid. These experiences raise questions about the possible implication of still other drugs or chemical agents in the environment in initiating the production of autoantibodies reacting with red cells.

Clinical Manifestations. Symptoms and physical findings depend chiefly upon the severity of the hemolytic process and the status of any underlying disease. Onset may be gradual or abrupt, and may be accompanied by chills, fever, backache, and the usual manifestations of severe anemia. Hemoglobinuria occurs in a few of the most severe cases and may be followed by renal tubular necrosis, oliguria, and uremia, especially if serious hypotension develops during a period of rapid intravascular hemolysis. Mild jaundice and moderate splenomegaly are usually found, but either or both may be absent. Livido reticularis may be noted in some patients, especially in the lower extremities with dependency. In the experience of some observers, thrombophlebitis is a frequent complication.

The disorder in children tends to run an acute, self-limited course. The clinical course in adults covers a wide spectrum with regard to severity, duration, and frequency of recurrence in both idiopathic and symptomatic cases. Severe hemolysis of short duration may complicate chronic lymphocytic leukemia or lymphoma, and may antedate the diagnosis of lymphoma or disseminated lupus by months or years.

Diagnosis. The blood smear usually shows macrocytosis in proportion to the degree of reticulocytosis. Normoblasts may be seen in the peripheral blood and are usually numerous when hemolysis recurs after splenectomy. A relatively poor reticulocyte response in relation to the degree of anemia may be encountered in the more severely ill patients. Punctate basophilia is frequently noted. Spherocytosis is usually lacking when hemolysis is of only moderate degree, but may be marked and associated with increase in osmotic fragility of the red cells during periods of brisk hemolysis. Fragmentation of the red cells may be evident in some cases, perhaps most often in those with splenomegaly.

Thrombocytopenia sometimes develops prior to, during, or after bouts of hemolytic anemia, and may be associated with a bleeding tendency. Leukopenia may develop during periods of active hemolysis; however, leukocytosis with immaturity of the granulocytes is more common.

Clumping of erythrocytes is sometimes noted in blood drawn into bottles or tubes containing anticoagulant, and may be one of the first clues to a correct diagnosis. Aggregation of cells is best seen after the container has been tilted to cause a thin layer of blood to flow down the inside of the upper portion. Clumping of the red cells may persist even on washing with warm saline and may interfere with red cell counting, blood typing, and crossmatching. The antiglobulin test on the patient's red cells is positive, as explained above.

Treatment. Corticosteroids are effective in most cases, but the mechanism(s) of action is far from clear. Prednisone in an initial dose of 10 to 20 mg. every six hours or comparable doses of other corticosteroids will usually suffice. Doses several times larger may be indicated if hemolysis is severe and persistent. Patients with severe hemolysis should be treated initially with 100 mg. of hydrocortisone intravenously, usually given in 500 ml. of glucose and water over a period of several hours, and then repeated four times daily. Oral administration of prednisone should be started concurrently. As hemolysis subsides, the dose of corticosteroid is reduced, in most cases to about 30 mg. of prednisone per day by the time the hematocrit has risen to 30 per cent. If the course is favorable, the dose of prednisone should be reduced to 20 mg. per day by the end of the second month of treatment, and to 10 mg. per day by the end of the third month. Continuation of prednisone therapy in a dose of about 10 mg. per day for an additional period of one to three months may reduce the risk of relapse; more data are needed on this aspect of management. Larger doses of corticosteroid often produce undesirable side effects if given for more than a few months. Discontinuation of prednisone should be accomplished by tapering the dose from 10 mg. per day over a period of two to three weeks.

The first sign of response to corticosteroid therapy is usually a further increase in reticulocyte count, followed within several days by a rise in hematocrit. A reduction in titer of antibody free in the serum, often measured by agglutination of trypsin-treated normal red cells, tends to follow the clinical improvement, but the direct antiglobulin reaction of the patient's red cells may remain positive for months or years after a remission is obtained.

Splenectomy is advisable in patients—fortunately a minority—who respond unsatisfactorily to adequate corticosteroid therapy. Splenectomy may be indicated occasionally even during the first month or two of treatment, but seems especially advisable if the hematocrit falls significantly with each attempt to reduce the dose of corticosteroid after two to four months. Corticosteroid should be given if clinically significant hemolysis persists or recurs after operation. At the time of splenectomy the abdomen should be explored for accessory spleens, ovarian cysts, enlarged lymph nodes, and any other evidence of neoplasia. Histologic examination of the spleen or other tissue may provide unexpected evidence of an underlying disease. In the author's experience, patients without a palpable spleen have responded well to steroid therapy and have seldom been considered candidates for splenectomy.

Blood transfusion may be indicated if the hemoglobin falls to about 5 to 6 grams per 100 ml. or the hematocrit to about 15 to 18 per cent, and if the patient is poorly adjusted to the anemia or is being prepared for operation. Packed red blood cells are preferable to whole blood because the smaller volume of transfusion is less apt to overload the circulation. Cross-matching may be complicated by the coexistence of autoantibodies with specific isoantibodies in the patient's serum. Even "compatible" donor red cells may be destroyed more rapidly than the patient's own red cells, with resultant increase in hemoglobinemia after transfusion. The patient's own cells are relatively young during periods of marrow response to hemolysis, and may be more resistant to destruction than the older transfused cells, perhaps because of their immaturity or in some instances because of differences in antigenic determinants. In view of the hazards of transfusion and the likelihood of prompt response to administration of corticosteroid, transfusion can often be withheld if the patient is under close observation.

Immunosuppressive drugs may deserve trial in severe cases refractory to corticosteroid and splenectomy. Use of such drugs, with the risks of infection and of causing serious depression of bone marrow function at a time of great need for erythropoiesis, may be justified only occasionally in idiopathic cases as investigational therapy. Patients with chronic lymphocytic leukemia, lymphosarcoma, reticulum cell sarcoma, or disseminated lupus may be given a cytotoxic agent for the dual purpose of arresting the underlying disease and possibly reducing autoantibody formation.

There are reports of modest success in treatment of refractory autoimmune hemolytic anemia accompanying these diseases with 6-mercaptopurine and azathioprine in a manner like that used to suppress the immune response after renal allotransplantation. It is noteworthy that intensive therapy with 6-mercaptopurine in NZB mice immediately before onset of autoimmune hemolytic disease did not delay or modify the development of autoantibodies or hemolytic anemia. Evidence from animal studies suggests that cyclophosphamide may be a superior immunosuppressive drug, but the potential of this agent in clinical diseases has not been assessed.

Administration of heparin has been recommended because of its possible effect on red cell–antibody interaction as well as in preventing thrombotic complications. Use of this agent should be regarded as experimental at present.

Hemolytic Disease Associated with Complement Components on the Red Cells

In the recent experience of the Strong Memorial Hospital, more patients with hemolytic anemia have been found to have complement components on the red cells than either γG alone or both γG and complement. Most patients with only complement components on their red cells had evidence of an associated disease. This study did not include patients with high titer of cold hemagglutinins in the serum and with complement present on the red cells.

The complement component usually demonstrated on the red cells in these cases is C'3a. The means by which complement becomes attached to red cells having no γG on their surface detectable by the usual antiglobulin reactions is not clear. Hemolysis may or may not be associated with such attachment.

Although the clinical features are less well defined in this group than in the patients with readily demonstrable γG globulin on the red cells, they may follow similar patterns. The same principles of therapy can be applied as for the patients with demonstrable γG globulin; as a rule less vigorous treatment is indicated.

Autoimmune Hemolytic Disease Associated with Cold Antibodies

Cold autoantibodies of the γM type differ from the γG warm autoantibodies described above in the following respects: (1) Their specificity, like that of low-titer cold agglutinins present in many normal sera, most commonly is directed against the I antigen present on nearly all normal adult human red cells. Occasionally the specificity is anti-i, detected by tests with red cells from the umbilical cord of an infant or with red cells from the rare adults having only the reciprocal antigen on their red cell membranes. (2) The cold agglutinins directly agglutinate the patient's own red cells and normal group O red cells suspended in isotonic saline, the titer and degree of agglutination increasing markedly as the temperature of the reaction is lowered toward 0° C. By contrast, warm antibodies are maximally reactive at about 37° C., and, with occasional striking exceptions, they do not agglutinate normal red cells in saline unless the cells are pretreated with trypsin or another proteolytic enzyme. (3) The γM cold antibodies fix complement regularly and are therefore responsible for positive anti-complement Coombs tests on the patients' red cells. If present in high titer, the cold antibodies may hemolyze normal red cells in vitro. Most examples of γG warm antibody are incapable of hemolyzing normal red cells, although they may mediate binding of complement components, especially in patients with an associated disease, as explained previously.

High titer γM cold antibodies causing hemolytic anemia are seen most strikingly in chronic cold hemagglutinin disease, which has a lower incidence than autoimmune hemolytic disease of the γG warm antibody type. Chronic cold hemagglutinin disease occurs in both sexes, predominantly in the middle and older age groups. These patients may suffer from ischemia of exposed parts of the body at low temperature in addition to chronic or episodic hemolytic anemia. Except after prolonged exposure to low temperature, hemolysis is usually less severe than in patients with warm antibodies. Spherocytosis and splenomegaly are observed infrequently. An underlying lymphoma may become evident with continuing observation.

The anti-I cold agglutinins isolated from patients with the chronic hemagglutinin disease have a single light chain type, a finding consistent with the concept of monoclonal origin. Homogeneity of light chains is occasionally associated with a macroglobulin M component in the patient's serum. γM cold antibodies of modest titer and anti-I specificity develop frequently after pneumonia caused by *Myocoplasma pneumoniae*, but they are only rarely the cause of hemolytic anemia. The cold agglutinins developing after such pneumonia have both of the identifiable types of light chains, thus suggesting polyclonal origin. Cold antibodies of anti-i specificity develop occasionally in patients with infectious mononucleosis, but their association with hemolysis is probably rare except possibly in persons with thalassemia minor whose red cells are abnormally agglutinable by anti-i.

The γG type of cold antibody associated with paroxysmal cold hemoglobinuria of both acute and chronic forms has anti-P specificity and is best demonstrated by the Donath-Landsteiner test. In this test the patient's fresh serum is mixed with either the patient's or normal (usually group O) red cells, chilled to near 0° C. and then warmed to 37° C. and examined for hemolysis. The two-step reaction is required to permit antibody binding with complement fixation in the cold phase and complement-mediated lysis in the warm phase to proceed at optimal temperatures. The agglutinin titer is usually less than the hemolytic titer. The direct antiglobulin test is positive only during acute attacks of cold-induced hemolysis. As the P groups of these patients are found to be either P_1 or P_2, the antibodies are appropriately considered specific autoantibodies. Evidence of syphilis is now less frequently encountered than in the past among patients with serum giving a positive Donath-Landsteiner test.

Patients with either γM or γG type of cold antibody causing symptoms should avoid exposure to low temperatures. Splenectomy is not indicated, and the administration of corticosteroid is rarely helpful. Use of immunosuppressive agents must be considered experimental at this time, considerations listed above for γG warm antibodies being kept in mind.

HEMOLYTIC ANEMIA ASSOCIATED WITH OTHER DISEASES (SYMPTOMATIC, NONIMMUNE)

Splenomegaly

Hemolytic anemia may develop in patients with splenomegaly at any age without evidence of an immune mechanism and without introduction of hemolytic agents from outside the body. The clinical features of this group cover the same wide spectrum seen in patients with demonstrable autoantibodies. Most of the patients in this category have rather marked splenomegaly, which may be a feature of a neoplastic disorder such as chronic leukemia or lymphoma of any type or myeloid metaplasia, or of a non-neoplastic disorder such as sarcoidosis, portal hypertension, or Gaucher's disease.

Spherocytosis may be prominent during periods of brisk hemolysis or may be entirely lacking. The hemolytic state at times may be rather subtle and thus may pass without detection until an increasing requirement for transfusion is noted or until rapid disappearance of tagged donor or autogenous red cells is demonstrated. Leukopenia and thrombocytopenia commonly occur, and may be corrected, along with hemolytic anemia, by splenectomy in some cases. The pathogenic mechanisms in this heterogenous group of disorders are poorly understood.

Although corticosteroid may be less effective than in cases with demonstrable γG globulin on the red cells, a trial is frequently indicated, especially if treatment of the underlying disease does not arrest the hemolytic state. Because of the greater relative importance of the spleen in the hemolytic process, splenectomy is in general more frequently indicated in this group than in the patients with evidence of an immune mechanism. Accumulation of radioactivity in the splenic area after transfusion of chromium-tagged donor or autogenous red cells may help to determine the extent of participation of the spleen in hemolysis.

Carcinoma

The incidence of hemolysis associated with carcinoma is probably higher than that suggested by most available reports. When severe hemolysis occurs in patients with cancer, it is usually a terminal event. Reversal of hemolysis has been reported, however, after removal of pseudomucinous cystadenocarcinoma of the ovary. In patients with disseminated carcinoma, hemolysis, sometimes accompanied by thrombocytopenia, may be related to the effects of cancer cells on small blood vessels. (Note the discussion that follows on microangiopathic hemolytic anemia.)

Liver Disease

Evidence of hemolysis is occasionally encountered during or after acute hepatitis of presumed viral etiology. Reference has been made previously to the risk of hemolysis of G-6-PD–deficient red cells in patients whose elimination of oxidant drugs is delayed because of impaired liver function. Patients with G-6-PD deficiency may develop hemolysis as a complication of viral hepatitis, as with other infections and in the absence of oxidant drugs, possibly through interaction between virus particles and red cells with a faulty defense mechanism.

Transient hemolytic anemia with spherocytosis is sometimes associated with a fatty liver, hyperlipemia, and hypercholesterolemia after heavy consumption of alcohol (Zieve's syndrome). The hemolytic mechanism in these cases is not well understood. Splenic sequestration of red cells and significant shortening of the life span of both autogenous and normal donated red cells may be demonstrated frequently in patients with portal cirrhosis, especially in those with congestive splenomegaly. Relatively severe hemolytic anemia may be encountered in a small proportion of patients with advanced cirrhosis characterized by formation of "burr" and "spur" cells. Normal red cells incubated in the serum of some, although not all, of these patients develop similar abnormalities of shape, a phenomenon attributed to the presence of an abnormal serum protein, i.e., a low density lipoprotein or a factor transported on albumin.

Renal Disease

The anemia accompanying most forms of renal disease is predominantly due to impaired erythropoiesis. Hemolysis, when demonstrable, usually accompanies severe renal failure or severe vascular disease of the kidney, which may be the cause of the renal failure. Glucose utilization and ATP concentration are increased in the red cells of uremic patients and are highly correlated with the degree of increase in serum phosphorus concentration. Despite the increased ATP content, the red cells of uremic patients may have a shortened life span and may undergo autohemolysis in vitro at a significantly increased rate. Studies on dogs chronically intoxicated with methylguanidine or creatinine and the demonstration of in vitro auto-hemolysis in the presence of guanidine, creatine, and creatinine have suggested to some investigators that accumulation of these substances in uremic patients might be partly responsible for hemolysis. The rate of autohemolysis in these studies is much lower than that usually observed in red cells with hereditary membrane defects or in red cells with pyruvate kinase deficiency. The hemolytic mechanisms in uremia thus remain unclear except for those cases in which vascular disease may play a dominant role (see below).

Peripheral Vascular Disease

The term "microangiopathic hemolytic anemia" has been applied since 1962 to cases in which hemolysis, often with thrombocytopenia, is associated with thrombotic thrombocytopenic purpura, malignant hypertension, eclampsia, renal cortical necrosis, microscopic polyarteritis nodosa, or disseminated carcinoma. In these diseases fibrin thrombi develop within arterioles and capillaries with or without fibrinoid necrosis or inflammation of the arterioles. In the cases associated with carcinoma, tumor is found widely disseminated and invading the small blood vessels. The red cells appear fragmented, crenated, and irregularly contracted; "helmet" forms, "burr" cells, and microspherocytes are usually evident. Hemoglobinemia and hemoglobinuria of modest degree may be noted. Recent work with experimental models indicates that the red cells may be damaged as they make their way through small vessels partially occluded by fibrin clots. The similarity between the abnormalities in shape in these cases and those observed in patients with faulty cardiac prostheses or calcified heart valves suggests that mechanical forces may play a large role in the cellular damage. The mechanisms by which red cells may be injured from contact with necrotizing arterioles or with tumor cells deserve further study.

Since the patients presenting this type of red cell abnormality along with thrombocytopenia are quite likely to have "consumption coagulopathy," they may benefit, sometimes dramatically, from administration of heparin. Patients with thrombotic thrombocytopenic purpura may also benefit from splenectomy. The extent of the vascular lesions may be difficult to estimate in patients most dramatically improved after splenectomy and consequently not subjected to postmortem examination.

The term "hemolytic-uremic syndrome" has been applied to the hematologic picture of microangiopathic hemolytic anemia occurring in uremic patients, especially in young children and sometimes associated with pregnancy. The histologic findings are like those of thrombotic thrombocytopenic purpura with thrombosis, fibrinoid necrosis of renal arterioles and glomeruli, and both hypertrophy and hyperplasia of glomerular endothelial cells. Coxsackie virus has been isolated from one patient with this syndrome, and an unusual rickettsial organism classified as a microtatobiote has been isolated from two other as well as from a patient with thrombotic thrombocytopenic purpura.

The development of red cell deformation and hemolytic anemia may be one of the first clear indications of rejection of transplanted kidneys. This complication has been observed in patients who had no morphologic abnormality of the red cells during the uremic state prior to renal transplantation. It can, therefore, be argued that renal vascular disease alone, such as that demonstrated in the transplanted kidney during the early rejection phase, may be sufficient to cause a peripheral blood picture of microangiopathic hemolytic anemia.

Heart Disease

Hemolysis attributed to trauma inflicted upon red cells in the circulation has been recognized only in recent years in unoperated patients with aortic stenosis, and less commonly with severe aortic regurgitation and severe mitral stenosis. Calcification of the mitral and aortic valves has been a prominent finding in these cases. Hemolysis has been observed more commonly in patients with a defective aortic or mitral valve prosthesis or imperfect repair of a septal defect with a Teflon patch or other inert material. Hemolysis in the operated patients seems related to the effects of a regurgitant jet of blood or to shearing stress, and is accelerated with exercise, as is true of the unoperated patients having severe valvular heart disease.

Anemia and reticulocyte response in these patients vary from slight to marked. Serum haptoglobin is regularly reduced. Hemoglobinemia is commonly present, and hemosiderinuria is frequently found even in the absence of grossly evident hemoglobinemia. Iron loss as a result of persistent hemosiderinuria may be sufficient to cause iron deficiency. Deformities of the red cells are similar to those found in the microangiopathic hemolytic anemia. Thrombocytopenia may develop in the early postoperative period following open-heart surgery, but fibrin deposition within the heart and disseminated intravascular coagulation are not common features of hemolytic anemia owing to cardiac prostheses. The significance of positive direct antiglobulin tests obtained with the red cells of some patients with hemolysis after insertion of valvular prostheses is not clear.

HEMOLYTIC ANEMIA FOLLOWING INTRODUCTION OF AGENTS OR FORCES FROM OUTSIDE THE BODY

Physical Agents

Hemoglobinemia and hemoglobinuria, often referred to as "march hemoglobinuria," are the result of intravascular hemolysis following mechanical trauma sometimes inflicted upon red cells during their passage through the feet. Measurable hemolysis results only from running on a hard surface, and is prevented by use of resilient insoles in the shoes. The hemolytic mechanism is probably similar to that operating in patients with severe valvular heart disease or malfunctioning cardiac prostheses.

Extensive thermal burns may cause hemolytic anemia characterized by spherocytosis, fragmentation of the red cells, and hemoglobinuria. Hemolysis occurs chiefly during the first 24 hours, although spherocytosis may be evident for several days. Pertinent studies with dog red cells heated in vitro at 49° C. show that the cells become increasingly rigid and after return to the donor are subject to splenic sequestration; with longer periods of heating the red cells have increased osmotic fragility, and when returned to the donor are rapidly removed from the circulation with evidence of sequestration in both spleen and liver.

Infectious Agents

Infectious agents are capable of inducing hemolysis by various mechanisms, most of which are incompletely understood. Provocation of hemolysis by infection in patients with G-6-PD–deficient red cells, with or without concomitant drug usage, has been discussed previously. Development of autoantibodies in certain infections also has been discussed.

Bacterial endocarditis is sometimes accompanied by erythrophagocytosis in the circulation as well as in the spleen. Other infections such as *miliary tuberculosis, infectious hepatitis, infectious mononucleosis,* and *psittacosis* may be complicated by hemolysis associated with spherocytosis and splenic sequestration of red cells. This form of hypersplenism is encountered in infections capable of prolonged stimulation of the reticuloendothelial system. Hemolytic anemia in kala-azar may have a similar basis. The *beta-hemolytic Streptococcus* and other pyogenic cocci are rare causes of hemolysis. Meningococcemia may produce a blood picture like that of microangiopathic hemolytic anemia. Injection of meningococcal endotoxins into rabbits causes development of vascular lesions like those of thrombotic thrombocytopenic purpura.

Intravascular hemolysis is claimed by some observers to be a frequent complication, if looked for, during the bacteremic phase of *Salmonella typhi* infection. Severe hemolytic anemia with hemoglobinuria is reported in *cholera,* but the incidence is not known.

Clostridium welchii, usually in postabortal or puerperal infections, causes severe intravascular hemolysis with hemoglobinuria and spherocytosis by production of an α toxin acting as a lecithinase. Infection of red blood cells with *Bartonella bacilliformis* leads to sequestration of the red cells in the spleen and liver and to severe hemolytic anemia. The organisms are readily seen within the red cells.

Hemolytic anemia in *malaria* is probably due in part to the effects of red cell parasitism and in part to reticuloendothelial hyperplasia and hypersplenism. Acute hemolytic anemia with hemoglobinuria, known as blackwater fever, occurs chiefly in persons infected with *Pl. falciparum.* An immune mechanism has been suspected for many years but is unproved.

Chemical Agents

The inorganic chemicals arsine, sodium chlorate, and potassium chlorate cause severe hemolysis with hemoglobinuria. Hemolysis is a feature of acute lead poisoning, and may be demonstrable in chronic lead intoxication. With these inorganic substances, hemolysis is determined by dose rather than by idiosyncrasy.

Most of the organic chemicals and drugs causing hemolytic anemia do so by the oxidant effects of their derivatives or by an immune mechanism. The former mechanism has been discussed in the section concerned with the hexose monophosphate shunt pathway and related cofactors in the red cell.

Fuadin, quinine, quinidine, sulfonamides, phenacetin, and neoarsphenamine may produce hemolysis in susceptible persons by activation of an immune mechanism. Hemolysis occurs suddenly after administration of the drug to which the patient has been sensitized. Antibodies reacting in vitro with the patient's red cells in the presence of the drug have been demonstrated by various techniques. A popular hypothesis is that the antibodies are formed against a drug-protein complex and that the red cells are injured by passive adsorption of circulating complexes whenever the drug is administered. The damaged red cell is thus regarded as an "innocent bystander."

Brisk hemolysis may occur during and for several weeks after penicillin administration in large doses to patients developing circulating γG antipenicillin antibodies of unusual specificity. Red cells from such patients give a positive direct Coombs test, apparently because of the combination of antipenicillin antibody with a penicillin derivative adsorbed to the cells. The relatively common skin-sensitizing antibodies to penicillin, chiefly of the γA type, and the γM antibodies capable of agglutinating penicillinized red cells, do not appear to be involved in development of hemolytic disease.

Autoimmune hemolytic anemia developing in patients treated with α-methyldopa or mefenamic acid has already been discussed. Discontinuing the drug and/or administration of corticosteroid is followed by remission in most cases.

Antibodies Acquired Passively

Erythroblastosis fetalis or *hemolytic disease of the newborn* is due to the action of isoantibodies acquired by the fetus from the maternal circulation. The mother may be immunized by an antigenic determinant lacking in her own red cells but present in the fetal red cells as a result of inheritance from the father. About 0.5 per cent of newborn infants have significant anemia and hyperbilirubinemia associated with Rh incompatibility. Since fetal red cells enter the maternal circulation largely or entirely at the time of delivery as a result of transplacental hemorrhage, first-born babies rarely develop hemolytic disease caused by anti-Rh antibodies unless the Rh-negative mother has been transfused with Rh-positive blood. Administration of anti-Rh gamma globulin to the Rh-negative mother within three days after delivery of an Rh-positive child appears to prevent to a high degree the development of anti-Rh antibodies, thus protecting the mother's next Rh-positive child from developing hemolytic disease.

ABO incompatibility usually involves a group O mother with a group A, B, or AB infant; hemolysis in most but not all cases is less severe than that resulting from Rh incompatibility. Incomplete development of the A and B determinants in fetal red cells is presumed to be partly responsible for the usual mildness of hemolytic disease owing to anti-A and anti-B antibodies. Since a much higher proportion of first-born infants are affected by ABO incompatibility than by Rh incompatibility, it is believed that the entry of fetal red cells into the maternal circulation may be relatively unimportant in stimulating development of maternal anti-A and anti-B antibodies.

Hemolytic anemia of the newborn is accompanied by reticulocytosis and enlargement of the liver and spleen, caused chiefly by extramedullary erythropoiesis. Spherocytosis is a prominent feature in cases associated with ABO incompatibility but not in cases of Rh incompatibility. Tests with antiglobulin sera on the infant's red cells are usually positive when hemolytic disease is due to anti-Rh and other less common types of immune isoantibodies, but tests with most available antiglobulin sera are of less aid in diagnosis of ABO hemolytic disease. If the fetus is severely affected, hydrops develops and death may occur before or soon after delivery. The most serious complication that may develop during the neonatal period is kernicterus, a staining of the basal ganglia of the brain with bilirubin associated with degenerative changes in these centers.

Infants severely affected with hemolytic disease should be given exchange transfusions as soon as possible to remove bilirubin, isoantibodies, and incompatible red cells and to replace them with compatible plasma and red cells, i.e., Rh-negative cells. Intraperitoneal transfusion of the fetus in utero may be advantageous in carefully selected cases when the mother has had previous stillbirths caused by hemolytic disease. References should be consulted for many clinically important details regarding diagnosis and treatment, including the use of amniocentesis and measurement of optical density of amniotic fluid as a guide to early induction of labor in some cases.

Destruction of recipients' red cells after *transfusion of incompatible plasma* and the more common type of hemolytic transfusion reaction involving destruction of incompatible donor red cells are discussed above.

General

Beutler, E. (ed.): Hereditary Disorders of Erythrocyte Metabolism. New York and London, Grune and Stratton, Inc., 1968.
Dacie, J. V.: The Haemolytic Anaemias: Congenital and Acquired. 2nd ed. Part 1. The Congenital Anaemias. London and New York, J. & A. Churchill, Ltd. and Grune and Stratton, Inc., 1960; Part 2, The Auto-Immune Anaemias, 1962; Part 3, Secondary or Symptomatic Haemolytic Anaemias, 1967; Part 4, Drug-Induced Haemolytic Anemias, Paroxysmal Nocturnal Haemoglobinuria, Haemolytic Disease of the Newborn, 1967.
Dacie, J. V. (ed.): Haemolytic anaemias (British issue). Seminars Hemat., 6:109, 1969.
Jandl, J. H. (ed.): Symposium on disorders of the red cell. Amer. J. Med., 41:657, 1966.
Weed, R. I.: The importance of erythrocyte deformability. Amer. J. Med., 49:147, 1970.

Specific Hemolytic States

Burka, E. R., Weaver, Z., III, and Marks, P. A.: Clinical spectrum of hemolytic anemia associated with glucose-6-phosphate dehydrogenase deficiency. Ann. Intern. Med., 64:817, 1966.
Carlson, D. J., and Ham, T. H.: Physical properties of red cells as related to effects in vivo. III. Effect of thermal treatment on survival of red cells in the dog. Role of the spleen. Blood, 32:872, 1968.
Dacie, J. V., and Worlledge, S. M.: Auto-immune anemias. Progress in Hematology, 6:82, 1969.
George, J. N., Sears, D. A., McCurdy, P. R., and Conrad, M. E.: Primaquine sensitivity in Caucasians: Hemolytic reactions induced by primaquine in G-6-PD deficient subjects. J. Lab. Clin. Med., 70:80, 1967.
Mettler, N. E.: Isolation of a microtatobiote from patients with hemolytic-uremic syndrome and thrombotic thrombocytopenic purpura and from mites in the United States. New Eng. J. Med., 281:1023, 1969.

THE HEMOGLOBINOPATHIES AND THALASSEMIAS

C. Lockard Conley

INTRODUCTION

Inherited anomalies of hemoglobin synthesis are heterogeneously distributed among the populations of the world. Some are causes of important diseases, although many have little or no clinical effect. The primary abnormality can be identified in precise submolecular terms and by inference traced to a specific lesion in the genetic code itself. Abnormal molecular structure in many instances can be related directly to disordered function and in turn to the production of clinical manifestations. The hemoglobin of the normal adult (Hb A) contains four polypeptide chains, two alpha chains each with 141 amino acid residues, and two beta chains each with 146 residues; it is designated $\alpha_2\beta_2$. A heme group containing an iron atom is fixed to each chain. The predominant hemoglobin of the fetus and newborn (Hb F) contains pairs of alpha and gamma chains ($\alpha_2\gamma_2$). A minor component comprising 2 to 3 per cent of the hemoglobin is designated Hb A_2, consisting of alpha and delta chains ($\alpha_2\delta_2$). There are multiple differences in amino acid sequences of beta, gamma, and delta chains; but the physiologic properties of the hemoglobins are similar. The fashion in which the globin chains and their heme groups are bonded together provides the iron atoms with precisely the environment necessary for reversible combination with oxygen under physiologic conditions. If these stereochemical relationships are disturbed, oxygen binding may be abnormal, or there may be other deleterious effects on the hemoglobin molecule.

DEFINITIONS AND GENETIC CONSIDERATIONS

A *hemoglobinopathy* is an abnormality of hemoglobin synthesis manifested by the production of globin in which there is a structural abnormality. More than 100 genetically determined abnormalities of hemoglobin have been discovered. A separate gene determines the amino acid sequences of each of the globin chains. A single amino acid substitution in one type of polypeptide chain is accounted for by replacement of one nucleotide in an RNA codon. Thus the abnormality of sickle hemoglobin can be attributed to a change in a single purine base in the codon which specifies the sixth amino acid of the beta chain, with the result that glutamic acid is replaced by valine. Such a point mutation accounts for most of the inherited abnormalities of hemoglobin. Rarely two amino acid substitutions occur within a single polypeptide chain, as in Hb C$_{Harlem}$. In Hb Gun Hill and Hb Freiburg amino acid residues are missing from a globin chain, an abnormality that can be accounted for by loss of a segment of DNA ("deletion" of part of a gene) during nonhomologous crossing-over of genes. The hemoglobins Lepore consist of the amino-terminal portion of the delta chain and the carboxy-terminal portion of the beta chain, an abnormal structure that can be explained by loss of DNA from portions of closely linked genes, with formation of a "fusion" gene. *Thalassemia* is an inherited impairment of hemoglobin synthesis caused by retarded production of a specific type of globin chain, not associated with a primary structural abnormality. The mechanism is not clearly understood, but may be related to insufficiency of messenger RNA. *Hereditary persistence of fetal hemoglobin* is an anomaly in which beta and delta chains are not produced at all, perhaps because of deletion of closely linked genes or mutation of an operator gene. Complete compensation for the deficit is achieved by synthesis of gamma chains, and the homozygous carrier has exclusively Hb F but no anemia or other clinical manifestations.

The hemoglobinopathies are inherited as autosomal co-dominant traits; heterozygous carriers have both the normal and the abnormal hemoglobin in each red cell. The normal component almost always constitutes the larger fraction. The genes that determine the structure of one class of globin chains are alleles; thus a person heterozygous for Hb S and Hb C, both of which contain abnormalities of the beta chain, has no Hb A and transmits one or the other but never both of the abnormal hemoglobins to each child. Thalassemia is inherited as if closely linked to the structural gene for the same chain. The beta and delta chain genes are closely linked, but the alpha chain gene segregates independently; accordingly a person heterozygous for both Hb G$_{Philadelphia}$ (an alpha chain variant) and Hb S (a beta chain variant) may transmit either, both, or neither of the abnormal hemoglobins to a child.

Hemoglobinopathies and thalassemias occur as a result of genetic mutations. Very high gene frequencies for harmful mutants are maintained in some areas of the world, presumably by strong selection pressures. Hb S appears to protect infants against the lethal effects of falciparum malaria, accounting for the maintenance of a high frequency of this deleterious abnormality in Africa. What selective advantage is conferred by Hb C in Africa, by Hb E in Southeast Asia, and by thalassemia in several parts of the world is unknown.

Not all variations in hemoglobin are genetically determined. Increased levels of Hb F may occur in several acquired conditions, including aplastic anemia, leukemia, myeloproliferative disorders, and hemolytic anemias. Hemoglobin A$_2$ may be increased in pernicious anemia and decreased in iron deficiency and aplastic anemia. Hemoglobins with abnormal electrophoretic mobility have been encountered in lead poisoning and diabetes, presumably as a result of chemical alterations in Hb A induced by the metabolic disturbance.

CLINICAL SYNDROMES ASSOCIATED WITH HEMOGLOBINOPATHIES

Substitutions of amino acids in the globin chains do not necessarily cause untoward effects, and most of the known abnormal hemoglobins are not associated with disease. Two types of clinically important abnormalities have been identified: (1) Replacements on the surface of the molecule may cause abnormal *intermolecular* reactions, phenomena which explain the pathologic effects of Hb S and Hb C. Individual molecules function satisfactorily, and the peculiar interactions between molecules tend to occur only with the high intra-erythrocytic concentrations of the abnormal hemoglobin found in homozygotes. Therefore, the disease appears to be recessively inherited. When a red cell contains two major hemoglobin components (for example, Hb S and Hb C), interactions may occur that importantly influence the pathologic effects. (2) Replacements in critical areas of the molecule may lead to *intramolecular* abnormalities with resultant alteration in oxygen binding or in molecular stability. These effects, which are not dependent on hemoglobin concentration, are manifested in heterozygotes, and the clinical disorder appears to be dominantly inherited. Amino acid substitutions are likely to impair molecular function or stability when they occur in the area in which the heme group is attached, when they distort the conformation of the molecule, or when they occur at points of interaction between the polypeptide chains. The net result may be formation of methemoglobin, alteration of oxygen affinity, denaturation of the hemoglobin, or a combination of these effects.

Most of the known variant hemoglobins were discovered because of abnormal electrophoretic mobility under usual conditions of measurement. The electrophoretic method continues to be useful, but many amino acid substitutions do not alter net charge on the molecule and may be electrophoretically neutral. A number of abnormal hemoglobins have the same electrophoretic pattern. The method, therefore, has important limita-

CLINICAL DISORDERS ASSOCIATED WITH SOME ABNORMAL HEMOGLOBINS

Disorder	Abnormal Hb	Structural Change		Electrophoretic Mobility, Starch Alkaline pH*	Comments
	S	beta 6	glu→val	— —	Forms molecular aggregates when deoxygenated, producing sickle cell anemia in homozygotes
	C	beta 6	glu→lys	— — — —	Low solubility lessens plasticity of red cells, causing hemolytic anemia in homozygotes
	D_Punjab	beta 121	glu→gln	— —	Mechanism unknown
	E	beta 26	glu→lys	— — — —	
	Zürich	beta 63	his→arg	— —	Unstable hemoglobin precipitated by certain drugs, producing hemolytic anemia in heterozygotes
Hemolytic anemia	Köln	beta 98	val→met	— — —	Unstable hemoglobin causes congenital nonspherocytic hemolytic anemia in heterozygotes; precipitated hemoglobin tends to form inclusion bodies within red cells, under certain conditions
	Sydney	beta 67	val→ala	— —	
	Santa Ana	beta 88	leu→pro	— —	
	Philly	beta 35	tyr→phe	0	
	Gun Hill	beta deletion of 5 residues between 91 and 97		— — —	
	Wien	beta 130	tyr→asp		
	Torino	alpha 43	phe→val	0	
	Bibba	alpha 136	leu→pro	— —	
	Hammersmith	beta 42	phe→ser	0	
	Genova	beta 28	leu→pro	0	
	Sabine	beta 91	leu→pro	— — —	
	Borås	beta 88	leu→arg	—	
	Seattle	beta 76	ala→glu	0	
	Riverdale-Bronx	beta 24	arg→gly	— —	
	H	alpha₂beta₂→beta₄		+ + + +	Unstable hemoglobin occurring in some forms of alpha-thalassemia; precipitation of hemoglobin and hemolysis are accelerated by certain drugs
Cyanosis due to methemoglobinemia	M_Boston	alpha 58	his→tyr	0	Methemoglobin causes cyanosis in heterozygotes; some also have evidence of hemolytic anemia
	M_Iwate	alpha 87	his→tyr	0	
	M_Milwaukee	beta 67	val→glu	0	
	M_Saskatoon	beta 63	his→tyr	0	
	M_Hyde Park	beta 92	his→tyr	— — —	
	Freiburg	beta 23	val deleted	—	
Cyanosis due to increased deoxyhemoglobin	Kansas	beta 102	asn→thr	—	Decreased oxygen affinity of hemoglobin causes cyanosis in heterozygotes
Polycythemia (erythrocytosis)	J_Capetown	alpha 92	arg→gln	+ +	Increased oxygen affinity of hemoglobin hinders release of oxygen to tissues, causing compensatory polycythemia in heterozygotes
	Chesapeake	alpha 92	arg→leu	+ +	
	Yakima	beta 99	asp→his	—	
	Kempsey	beta 99	asp→asn	— —	
	Rainier	beta 145	tyr→his	0	
	Hiroshima	beta 143	his→asp	+ + +	
	Ypsilanti	beta 99	asp→tyr	—	
Hydrops fetalis	Bart's	alpha₂gamma₂→gamma₄		+ +	Unstable hemoglobin with high oxygen affinity occurring in high concentration in stillborn fetuses with homozygous alpha-thalassemia

*Symbols indicate relative mobility as compared with Hb A, less rapid (−), more rapid (+).

tions in the detection as well as in the recognition of mutant hemoglobins. Other types of investigation, including more detailed analysis of the hemoglobins, may be required for identification.

Sickling Disorders

The single amino acid substitution in the beta chain in Hb S, located on the surface of the molecule, has no significant effect on oxygen affinity or molecular stability. It causes a unique *intermolecular* reaction in which molecules of deoxygenated Hb S tend to form insoluble linear aggregates. These liquid crystals, or tactoids, distort the erythrocyte and increase its rigidity, causing the sickling deformation. The attractive forces between molecules operate only at short distances, so that the sickling phenomenon is markedly influenced by the concentration of deoxygenated Hb S in the red cell. Conditions influencing the intracellular concentration of deoxyhemoglobin, in particular oxygen tension and pH, are critical determinants of the degree of sickling. Sickling is not instantaneous when hemoglobin is deoxygenated, so that duration of exposure of red cells to low oxygen tension is also a conditioning factor. Whether intravascular sickling occurs depends on local conditions of blood flow, oxygen tension, and pH; on the concentration of Hb S in the red cell; and on the presence in the erythrocyte of another hemoglobin which may interact with Hb S to lessen or enhance sickling. Except for a few irreversibly sickled cells, erythrocytes quickly resume their normal shape when the hemoglobin is reoxygenated.

Manifestations of disease attributable to Hb S are caused by intravascular sickling of partially deoxygenated erythrocytes. The rigid sickle cells tend to be tangled, trapped, and fragmented in small vascular channels; in addition, the cell membrane may be damaged by the sickling distortion itself. Both factors shorten red cell survival with predominant destruction of erythrocytes within the RE system. The unyielding elongate and crescentic cells increase the viscosity of the blood, retarding flow, occluding small blood vessels, and producing infarcts and other lesions as a result of local anoxia.

Sickle Cell Anemia. Definition. Sickle cell anemia, the clinical expression of homozygosity for Hb S, is a serious disease characterized by unrelenting hemolytic anemia, recurrent episodes of pain and fever, and pathologic involvement of many organs. Affected persons are Negroes who have obtained the mutant gene from both parents. Since sickle cell trait occurs in about 8 per cent of American Negroes, about 16 per 10,000 are expected to be homozygous at the time of conception; the actual incidence of sickle cell anemia is lower because of its high mortality. First described by J. B. Herrick in 1910, the disease is of unique historic significance. Study of the sickling phenomenon led Hahn and Gillespie in 1927 to discover that the distortion of the red cells is related

to the state of oxygenation of the hemoglobin. Pauling and his associates in 1949 demonstrated the existence of an abnormal hemoglobin and developed the concept of "molecular" disease. Subsequently the investigations of Ingram and others showed that the abnormality in Hb S is limited to a single amino acid substitution within a polypeptide chain of globin. These discoveries initiated an unprecedented era of scientific advancement, with rapid evolution of knowledge pertaining to molecular biology, genetics, and pathophysiology.

Clinical Manifestations. Manifestations of the disease appear after the newborn period, when Hb F is replaced by Hb S. Persistent hemolytic anemia, although usually severe, is remarkably well tolerated and is not often the cause of the presenting symptoms. Many patients lead reasonably normal lives, at least for long intervals. Much of the havoc of the disease is related to the periodic occurrence of disabling "crises," acute self-limited episodes of pain and fever, usually incapacitating but often not associated with increase in the degree of anemia. Precipitating factors may not be apparent; but attacks tend to occur at night, on exposure to cold, or during infections, times at which erythrostasis may be enhanced. Pain frequently is experienced in the bones and large joints of the extremities and in the back. Agonizing pain of great severity may be localized to a single area, involve multiple sites, or have a migratory character. Episodes tend to subside within a few days, but some patients have more persistent grumbling discomfort. Dramatic episodes of severe abdominal pain and fever simulate acute appendicitis and other urgent intra-abdominal disorders.

Most patients have a characteristic asthenic habitus with disproportionately long extremities and "spider" fingers. Sexual maturation tends to be delayed, and fertility is reduced. Pregnancies often are concluded successfully, although maternal morbidity is increased. Susceptibility to infection is enhanced, and urinary tract infection and pneumonia are particularly common. A unique predisposition to salmonella osteomyelitis is a remarkable feature of the disease. Chronic ulcers of the legs, overlying the malleoli, tend to occur at puberty or later. Multisystem involvement is caused principally by anoxia resulting from erythrostasis and vascular occlusions. Segmentation of blood flow can be seen in conjunctival vessels, and the retinal vessels are tortuous, sometimes with peripheral vascular occlusions. Many symptoms are referable to bone involvement. In infancy the earliest manifestation may be the "hand-foot" syndrome, a painful swelling of the dorsa of hands or feet, associated with appearance in roentgenograms of rectangular deformities of metacarpals, metatarsals, and phalanges. Later avascular necrosis of the femoral or humeral head may cause permanent disability. Bone involvement is readily seen in dental films, which show radiolucency, abnormal trabeculation, and infarcts. Similar changes, including widening of marrow cavities and elevation of the periosteum, may be seen in other bones. Osteoporosis of the spine may be associated with a "fish vertebrae" deformity.

Repeated episodes of pneumonia tend to occur, sometimes in conjunction with painful crises. Infarction of the lung is responsible for many pneumonia-like illnesses. Pulmonary vessels are occluded by masses of sickled erythrocytes or by emboli arising in veins or in infarcted marrow. Rarely, repeated emboli lead to cor pulmonale. The heart is enlarged, and the dilated chambers and accelerated circulation give rise to impressive murmurs. These are most often systolic; they simulate the murmurs of valvular heart disease. Electrocardiographic abnormalities are not unusual. Congestive heart failure, uncommon in childhood, becomes more frequent as age advances. Vascular lesions in the nervous system may produce focal or multifocal neurologic manifestations, sometimes with convulsions. Hemolytic jaundice is persistent, and the chronic overproduction of bilirubin predisposes to formation of gallstones, cholecystitis, and obstruction of the biliary tract. The liver is usually enlarged. Erythrostasis in hepatic sinusoids causes necrosis of liver cells, leading sometimes to a peculiar cirrhosis. Marked jaundice with high levels of conjugated bilirubin and aberrations of liver function tests suggest both hepatocellular damage and intrahepatic biliary obstruction. Hepatitis may be acquired through blood transfusions. The spleen is enlarged in infancy, but infarctions lead to its shrinkage, often to a fibrous remnant, and splenomegaly is rare in adults. Hyposthenuria is the most common evidence of renal dysfunction. Infarcts of the kidney or papillary necrosis may cause hematuria, and recurrent infarction may lead to progressive renal insufficiency. Renal vein thrombosis may occur. Priapism is encountered predominantly in children.

Anemia is normocytic, with hemoglobin concentrations ranging between 5 and 10 grams per 100 ml. Reticulocytosis, polychromatophilia, stippling, and target cells are usual, and siderocytes and Howell-Jolly bodies may be seen. Sickled erythrocytes are not necessarily numerous in the blood smear, but in blood deoxygenated with sodium metabisulfite virtually all the red cells are sickled. In addition to hyperbilirubinemia, there is a slight increase in the plasma hemoglobin. Thrombocytosis and leukocytosis tend to persist but increase during crises, when leukocyte counts of more than 20,000 per cu. mm. are common. Profound anemia may be the result of "aplastic crises," transient episodes of retarded erythropoiesis occurring most often in children in association with infections. Folate deficiency, attributable in part to the high folate requirement of chronic hemolytic anemia, may lead to a superimposed megaloblastic anemia.

Diagnosis. In typical cases the diagnosis is readily established by the demonstration of hemolytic anemia, positive sickling preparation with sodium metabisulfite, and the abnormal mobility of the hemoglobin on electrophoresis. Anemia may

be overlooked in Negroes, and the dramatic non-hematologic manifestations can be misleading. Recurrent joint pain and striking cardiac abnormalities often suggest rheumatic fever. Differentiation between the painful abdominal crises and other intra-abdominal disorders may be extremely difficult. Differential diagnosis of marked jaundice in patients with sickle cell anemia may require meticulous evaluation, including liver biopsy in appropriate cases. Limitations of the electrophoretic method should be recognized. Sickle cell anemia is clearly distinguished from sickle cell trait by this procedure in untreated patients, but after transfusions the patterns may be similar. The electrophoretic pattern of hemoglobin in untreated sickle cell anemia may be indistinguishable from that of sickle cell–thalassemia, sickle cell–hemoglobin D disease, sickle cell–hereditary persistence of fetal hemoglobin, and homozygous sickle cell anemia with heterozygosity for hemoglobin Memphis, disorders which tend to be less severe. Accordingly, proof of diagnosis may require family studies and additional analysis of the hemoglobin. When the clinical disorder is atypical, for example, when splenomegaly persists into adult life, when anemia is mild or absent, or when the disease is unusually benign, special investigations are warranted.

Prognosis. The disease in the past has had a high mortality rate in early childhood, few patients reaching adult life. Recent decades have seen progressively increasing longevity, and some patients survive beyond the age of 50. This improvement in outlook is not attributable to advances in specific therapy, but is largely the result of better nutrition and more adequate prevention and treatment of infections. Infection remains the most common cause of death. Aplastic crises are a serious threat to life if not treated promptly. Death may result from renal or hepatic insufficiency, cardiac failure, or vascular occlusions in the nervous system. Widespread intravascular sickling is found in some patients dying suddenly or during a painful crisis.

Treatment. Specific therapy is not available. The painful episodes are self-limited; accordingly they appear to respond to a variety of therapeutic measures, but convincing evidence of efficacy is lacking. Severe pain justifies the use of narcotics, with care to avoid respiratory depression. Narcotic addiction is rare because the painful episodes are too short to induce dependence. Patients with sickle cell anemia should receive supplemental folic acid (0.5 mg. per day). Infections should be treated promptly. Transfusions may be life-saving in aplastic crises and in the shock of abdominal crises, but their use in other situations should be carefully considered. Administration of usual volumes of blood raises the hematocrit value without markedly diluting the sickle cells, increasing the viscosity of deoxygenated blood and potentially enhancing the production of vascular occlusions. Partial exchange transfusions are effective in preventing crises when about 50 per cent of the red cells are replaced by normal erythrocytes. This procedure is particularly useful in preparing patients for surgical operations, and may be used in other critical situations. Leg ulcers tend to heal with conservative measures, particularly during bed rest; however, they often recur even after grafting procedures. When anesthesia is administered, good ventilation and high oxygen tensions in the inspired gas mixture should be maintained. Surgical procedures can be safely performed in patients in good general condition; nevertheless, major elective procedures such as removal of asymptomatic gallstones appear to be unjustified.

Sickle Cell Trait. Persons heterozygous for hemoglobin S are said to have sickle cell trait, with rare exceptions innocuous and not associated with anemia. It occurs in Africa, the Mediterranean area, Arabia, and India. About 8 per cent of American Negroes are affected. As each erythrocyte contains both Hb S and Hb A, all the red cells sickle when deoxygenated; but the concentration of Hb S in the red cells is sufficiently low that intravascular sickling does not occur at physiologic oxygen tensions. Clinical manifestations may appear when unusual circumstances foster intravascular sickling. Hemolytic anemia simulating sickle cell anemia has been encountered in heterozygous carriers of Hb S with anoxemia owing to congenital heart disease. Infarction of the spleen has occurred during travel in unpressurized aircraft. Very rarely sudden death has been attributed to sicklemia, usually in patients with respiratory depression and acidosis. Hyposthenuria is more common. Unilateral renal hematuria appearing without demonstrable cause may persist for many weeks, and usually ceases without relation to therapeutic efforts, none of which are clearly effective. Recurrent bleeding from either kidney may occur, and nephrectomy is contraindicated. Infection of the urinary tract in pregnancy is reported to be increased in frequency in women with sickle cell trait.

Other Heterozygous Sickling Disorders. Persons heterozygous for hemoglobin S and for another abnormality of either the alpha or beta chain may have no evidence of disease. Thus, persons heterozygous for Hb S and J (an innocuous beta chain variant) have no Hb A in their red cell hemolysates, yet appear perfectly well. In certain other heterozygous states intravascular sickling of red cells is enhanced by the additional genetic abnormality.

Sickle cell–thalassemia resembles sickle cell anemia but is generally less severe, with atypical features including relatively mild anemia and persistent splenomegaly. It occurs in persons of Negro or Mediterranean ancestry. The beta thalassemia gene lessens production of Hb A, which occurs in low proportion. Electrophoresis of hemoglobin shows that the predominant hemoglobin is Hb S, with smaller fractions of Hb A and Hb F; sometimes Hb A cannot be detected, and family studies are required to differentiate the disorder from sickle cell anemia.

Sickle cell–hemoglobin C disease occurs in American Negroes with about one fourth the frequency of sickle cell anemia. Anemia tends to be mild, and some patients are asymptomatic. Splenomegaly is usual and may persist to old age; but atrophy of the spleen attributable to infarction occurs in some cases. The disease has special importance because of its predominantly nonhematologic manifestations. Symptoms may be referable to the eye, where peripheral vascular occlusions in the retina cause retinal avascularity and neovascular proliferations; these tend to bleed, producing vitreous hemorrhages with subsequent fibrosis and retinal detachment. Pain and dysfunction of the hip or shoulder are caused by avascular necrosis of capital epiphyses, especially the femoral head. Acute abdominal pain after anesthesia or during flight in unpressurized aircraft is the result of infarction of the spleen. Gross unilateral renal hematuria is not uncommon. Pregnancy may be complicated by severe anemia, infarcts of bone, and pulmonary emboli; but in most instances pregnancy is uncomplicated. Diagnosis is suggested by examination of the blood smear in which almost all of the red cells are target forms. Electrophoresis of hemoglobin shows two major components, Hb S and Hb C; Hb A is absent.

Sickle cell–hemoglobin D_{Punjab} disease has many of the features of sickle cell anemia and may be incapacitating because of vascular occlusive lesions, although anemia tends to be less severe. The rarity of the disease, its predominant occurrence in white persons, and the nonhematologic presenting manifestations obscure the diagnosis. Standard electrophoretic methods yield a pattern indistinguishable from that of sickle cell anemia, but Hb D separates from Hb S on agar gel at low pH.

Disorders Associated with Hemoglobins C, D, and E

Homozygous hemoglobin C disease is an uncommon disorder occurring in Negroes. Affected persons usually have few symptoms, but the spleen is enlarged. Chronic hemolytic anemia is rarely severe and is often discovered incidentally. Hb C is relatively insoluble and tends to crystallize in the red cell, causing increased rigidity with fragmentation and accelerated destruction. The blood film contains a double population of target cells and microspherocytes, the latter representing older fragmented cells. *Hemoglobin C–thalassemia* causes a similar disorder. Heterozygosity for Hb C, *hemoglobin C trait*, occurs with high frequency in some areas of East Africa and in about 2 per cent of American Negroes. Some target cells are seen in the blood smear without anemia or other evidence of disease.

Homozygous hemoglobin D_{Punjab} disease is a rare disorder causing mild or moderately severe anemia with numerous target cells in the blood smear. Hb D_{Punjab} occurs in India but also in many other parts of the world, and several instances of the disease have been encountered in Caucasian families. *Hemoglobin D–thalassemia* resembles the homozygous disorder but can be differentiated by family studies. Persons heterozygous for Hb D alone have no hematologic abnormalities.

Homozygous hemoglobin E disease is manifested by mild microcytic and normochromic anemia, usually without splenomegaly. Large numbers of target cells are seen in the blood smear. The disease has been encountered with considerable frequency in Orientals. Persons heterozygous for Hb E and beta thalassemia have a more severe anemia, and the spleen is usually enlarged. The high frequency of the genes for Hb E and various types of thalassemia in southeast Asia has led to the appearance of some complex genetic disorders, for example, hemoglobin E–alpha thalassemia disease, in which affected persons appear to have the characteristics of hemoglobin H disease in addition to hemoglobin E. Heterogeneity of the hemoglobin E diseases is related in part to the diversity of genetic factors.

Hemolytic Anemias Caused by Unstable Hemoglobins

Congenital hemolytic disorders attributable to unstable hemoglobin molecules have been discovered in a few widely scattered families. They present with anemia, which is usually mild and sometimes associated with splenomegaly. Affected persons are the heterozygous carriers of the abnormal hemoglobin, and homozygotes are unknown. Persons with *Hb Zürich* have no anemia except after administration of sulfonamides or during infections, when fulminant hemolytic anemia may occur. *Hb Köln* causes chronic hemolytic anemia, with recurring bouts of more severe anemia, jaundice, and dark urine; splenectomy has sometimes appeared to have a beneficial effect. Other unstable hemoglobins are not associated with distinguishing clinical features. Mild methemoglobinemia accompanies the hemolytic process, and the variant hemoglobin may have abnormal oxygen affinity. Increased oxygen affinity in Hb Zürich appears to have no clinical importance; reduced oxygen affinity in *Hb Seattle* is thought to increase anemia by lessening the stimulus for compensatory erythropoiesis. Diagnosis is suggested by demonstration of precipitates of denatured hemoglobin (Heinz bodies) in the red cells. In patients with Hb Zürich these may appear during hemolytic episodes as large globular inclusions. Heinz bodies are seen in many of the red cells of patients with Hb Köln after splenectomy. They can be demonstrated in other cases by incubating red cells with brilliant cresyl blue, a redox dye. The abnormal hemoglobin tends to precipitate when hemolysates are heated at 50° C. The dark urine contains a dipyrrole pigment thought to originate from heme groups dislodged from unstable hemoglobin molecules.

Disorders Caused by Hemoglobins with Abnormal Oxygen Affinity

Cyanosis is caused by methemoglobinemia in the heterozygous carriers of the hemoglobins M and *Hb Freiburg*. The concentration of methemo-globin is not sufficiently high to cause major symptoms. In some instances there is an associated hemolytic disorder (see Methemoglobinemia). Carriers of *Hb Kansas* also display cyanosis, in this instance caused by an increased concentration of deoxyhemoglobin in the blood in capillaries and venules. Hb Kansas has a low affinity for oxygen which facilitates the unloading of oxygen in the tissues, a phenomenon without apparent harmful effects.

Polycythemia (erythrocytosis) is the clinical expression of several abnormal hemoglobins with increased oxygen affinity. These variants have been discovered in scattered families, and it is noteworthy that they cause one form of familial polycythemia without leukocytosis, thrombocytosis, or splenomegaly. Hematocrit values of heterozygotes have not exceeded 65 per cent, and homozygotes are unknown. Impaired release of oxygen activates the erythropoietin mechanism, producing the compensatory erythrocytosis. These hemoglobins should be sought by direct measurement of oxygen affinity in cases of unexplained erythrocytosis; electrophoretic mobility of the variant hemoglobin is not always abnormal.

THE THALASSEMIA SYNDROMES

The thalassemia syndromes are a heterogeneous group of inherited disorders manifested in the homozygote by profound anemia or death in utero, and in the heterozygote by red cell abnormalities of relatively trivial significance. Two major categories are recognized: *alpha thalassemia*, caused by retarded production of alpha chains of globin, and *beta thalassemia*, caused by retarded production of beta chains. Delta thalassemia has been described but is of no clinical significance. Impaired hemoglobin synthesis causes anemia and microcytosis. In addition, unbalanced production of globin chains leads secondarily to accumulation of uncombined alpha chains in beta thalassemia and to formation of the abnormal molecules γ_4 (Hb Bart's) and β_4 (Hb H) in alpha thalassemia; these tend to precipitate within red cells, hastening their destruction. In rare instances a thalassemic disorder is associated with one of the Lepore hemoglobins.

Homozygous Beta Thalassemia

Definition. Homozygous beta thalassemia is the inherited disorder described by Cooley and Lee in 1925 and subsequently known as Cooley's anemia, Mediterranean anemia, target cell anemia, or thalassemia major. Occurring primarily in persons of Mediterranean ancestry, the disease is characterized by profound anemia, marked hepatosplenomegaly, and typically by death in childhood.

Clinical Manifestations. Anemia appears after the newborn period and thereafter is severe, with marked pallor and mild to moderate hemolytic jaundice. The spleen and liver become tremendously enlarged. Deformation of the bones, particularly those of the head, contributes to the characteristic "Mongoloid" facies, and distorts the mouth and disturbs the alignment of the teeth. Roentgenograms show a "hair-on-end" appearance of the skull, enlargement of other marrow cavities with thinning of cortical bone, and abnormalities of trabeculation related to the marked hyperplasia of marrow. Cardiac enlargement and failure are explained by the anemia and by the deposition of large amounts of iron in the myocardium. Hemosiderosis is largely the result of the many transfusions required to maintain life. The hypochromic microcytic red cells are flattened, usually with numerous target and stippled forms and variable numbers of nucleated erythrocytes, polychromatic cells, and reticulocytes. Inclusion bodies can be demonstrated in many normoblasts and reticulocytes when stained with methyl violet. Leukocytosis may be marked and persistent. Much of the hemolytic activity appears to be intramedullary with resulting ineffective erythropoiesis. Serum iron is elevated with increased saturation of iron-binding protein. The proportion of Hb F is usually between 20 and 60 per cent, but values as high as 90 per cent may occur. Hemoglobin A_2 is not increased.

Treatment and Prognosis. With frequent transfusions and appropriate prevention and treatment of infections, life may be improved and prolonged. Massive deposition of iron is often the cause of cardiac failure and death. In selected cases splenectomy is beneficial when the spleen is actively sequestering red cells, but susceptibility to infection may be enhanced. Supplemental folic acid (0.5 mg. per day) provides for the increased requirement.

Heterozygous Beta Thalassemia

Heterozygous beta thalassemia (thalassemia minor) is manifested by mild anemia, usually with microcytosis, hypochromia, stippling, and target cells. Most frequent in Mediterranean populations, it is widely distributed throughout the world, occurring not rarely in Negroes and less often in white persons from northern Europe. Symptoms are unusual, but some persons have anemia of moderate severity associated with jaundice and splenomegaly. Red cell abnormalities, which are variable and sometimes hardly detectable, are associated with resistance to osmotic lysis. Genetic heterogeneity is suggested not only by the clinical variability but also by differences in proportions of hemoglobins in hemolysates. Typically Hb A_2 is increased to about 5 per cent, sometimes with a slight increase in Hb F. But in some cases Hb F tends to be more elevated; in others Hb A_2 is reduced ($\delta\beta$ thalassemia). "Thalassemia intermedia," a term applied to instances of thalassemia which on clinical grounds appear to be intermediate between the typical heterozygous and homozygous disorders, has no specific meaning. Thalassemia minor is most often discovered during routine blood examinations and is usually mistaken for iron deficiency anemia.

Lead poisoning may be suggested by the numerous stippled cells, or other iron-refractory hypochromic anemias may be considered. Diagnosis is suggested by demonstration of the same blood abnormality in other members of the family. An elevated level of Hb A_2 is confirmatory.

Alpha Thalassemia

Homozygous alpha thalassemia is thought to be incompatible with life, and in a number of instances has appeared to be the cause of fetal death at about the thirtieth week. Most cases have been described in Orientals. The stillborn infant displays severe hydrops fetalis. Red cell hemolysates contain about 80 per cent Hb Bart's, a functionally inadequate hemoglobin with high oxygen affinity.

Heterozygous alpha thalassemia is manifested by very slight thalassemic abnormalities of the red cells with little or no anemia and by increased proportions of Hb Bart's (5 to 20 per cent) in cord blood. Identification is virtually impossible after the newborn period, although minor abnormalities of erythrocytes persist. It is widely distributed, occurring most frequently in Asiatic, African, and Mediterranean populations, and has been detected in almost 2 per cent of American Negroes at birth. Rarely, heterozygous alpha thalassemia has occurred in persons who also had an alpha chain structural abnormality. Hemoglobin Q–alpha thalassemia, described in Orientals, is manifested by severe anemia. Hemoglobin I–alpha thalassemia was encountered in a Negro with mild anemia.

Hemoglobin H disease is a chronic hemolytic anemia associated with splenomegaly and intermediate levels of Hb H in erythrocytes. It has been found in persons of various ethnic backgrounds, including persons of apparently north European origin. Hemolytic episodes may be precipitated by sulfonamides. Red cells are hypochromic and microcytic. Intracellular inclusions of Hb H appear in erythrocytes after splenectomy, and may be induced before splenectomy by incubating blood with brilliant cresyl blue. The disease is thought to occur in persons heterozygous for alpha thalassemia and for a different alpha thalassemia gene with milder effects. The resulting deficiency of alpha chains is not so severe as in homozygous alpha thalassemia, and the disease is compatible with long life.

Diggs, L. W.: Sickle cell crises. Amer. J. Clin. Path., 44:1, 1965.

Herrick, J. B.: Peculiar elongated and sickle-shaped red corpuscles in a case of severe anemia. Arch. Intern. Med. (Chicago), 6:517, 1910.

Huehns, E. R., and Bellingham, A. J.: Diseases of function and stability of haemoglobin. Brit. J. Haemat., 17:1, 1969.

Lehmann, H., and Huntsman, R. G.: Man's Haemoglobins. Philadelphia, J. B. Lippincott Company, 1966.

Pauling, L.: Abnormality of Hemoglobin Molecules in Hereditary Hemolytic Anemias. Harvey Lecture, 1953-1954. p. 216.

Perutz, M. F., and Lehmann, H.: Molecular pathology of human haemoglobin. Nature, 219:902, 1968.

Weatherall, D. J.: The Thalassaemia Syndromes. Philadelphia, F. A. Davis Company, 1965.

HEMOGLOBINURIA
Hugh Chaplin, Jr.

Definition and Mechanism. Hemoglobinuria (the presence of free hemoglobin in the urine) is a sign of variety of pathologic states and not a disease entity in itself. Hemoglobin generally finds its way into the urine by filtration from the plasma; uncommonly, it may be released from red cells which lyse within the kidney or urinary outflow tract. Normal human plasma contains an alpha$_2$ globulin, haptoglobin, present in amount sufficient to bind 75 to 175 mg. of hemoglobin per 100 ml. of plasma. The tightly bound hemoglobin-haptoglobin complex, which has a molecular weight above 280,000, is not filtered by the normal glomerulus but is metabolized independent of the kidney at a linear rate of approximately 10 mg. per 100 ml. of plasma per hour. The total plasma hemoglobin binding capacity of the average normal adult, e.g., 3 liter plasma volume, is 125 × 30 = 3750 mg. of hemoglobin, the amount contained in 11 ml. of red blood cells. When hemoglobin entering the total plasma pool exceeds this relatively modest amount, the pigment exists free in the plasma, and is either metabolized or filtered into the urine and excreted. During metabolism of free plasma hemoglobin, some of the heme moiety is split from the parent molecule and binds to albumin, forming methemalbumin, which is readily distinguishable chemically and spectroscopically from free hemoglobin and hemoglobin-haptoglobin complex, and which is relatively slowly metabolized over 24 to 48 hours.

It has been puzzling that free hemoglobin (m.w. 66,000) should pass so readily into the glomerular filtrate when albumin (m.w. 60,000) is filtered so poorly. Recent studies by Bunn et al. suggest that oxygenated hemoglobin in dilute solution physiologically and reversibly dissociates into two alpha beta dimers, and may thus be in the form of half-molecules at the moment of glomerular filtration. The kidney has a limited capacity for tubular reabsorption of filtered hemoglobin; free hemoglobin will be excreted in the urine when the plasma-free hemoglobin concentration exceeds 15 to 25 mg. per 100 ml.

Occurrence. Hemoglobinuria Following Intravascular Hemolysis. Lysis of red cells within the circulation may occur under a variety of circumstances. The plasma will appear pink or red (free and haptoglobin-bound hemoglobin) or brown (methemalbumin). *Isoimmune hemolysis* occurs in relation to transfusion when the patient's plasma contains antibodies to donor red cell antigens. Hemolytic transfusion reactions usually involve incompatibility within the ABO system, but may occur within the other blood group systems, especially when complement-binding antibodies are involved, e.g., anti-Jk^a. *Autoimmune hemolysis*, particularly when complement components are part of the erythrocyte-autoantibody complex, may result in massive hemoglobinemia

(as in "cold" autoimmune hemolytic anemia and in the rare condition of paroxysmal cold hemoglobinuria). It should be emphasized here that hemoglobinemia is not an inevitable accompaniment of severe iso- and autohemolysis; when red cell destruction occurs primarily extravascularly, i.e., by phagocytosis within the reticuloendothelial system (especially in the spleen), plasma hemoglobin levels will be low and haptoglobin levels normal or minimally depressed. Severe hemoglobinemia has also occurred in relation to certain *drug-antibody-erythrocyte complexes*, as in patients sensitized to fuadin and quinidine. A number of *intrinsic red cell defects* may result in massive intravascular hemolysis under appropriate conditions. The most striking example is the poorly understood cell membrane defect in patients with paroxysmal nocturnal hemoglobinuria (PNH); also important are the enzyme deficient cells, e.g., cells deficient in G-6-PD, which may lyse massively when exposed to sufficient concentrations of oxidant drugs or to components of the fava bean. Rarely, *mechanical damage* to red cells, as in severe microangiopathic hemolytic states or following extensive body surface burns, may cause gross hemoglobinemia; physical damage also accounts for the hemoglobinemia that accompanies many extracorporeal perfusion procedures. A number of *snake and spider venoms* contain enzymes that provoke rapid red cell lysis (lecithinase in the venom of the brown recluse spider, reported mainly in the south central United States). Massive destruction of red cells may result from direct *erythrocyte parisitism* in falciparum malaria. *Hypotonic red cell lysis* follows the intravenous infusion of distilled water, and may occur inadvertently when water is used to irrigate the bladder during exposure of the vascular prostatic bed in the course of transurethral resection procedures. A rare but interesting condition, *"march (or exertional) hemoglobinuria,"* has been described, wherein hemoglobinuria follows prolonged exercise (usually, running) in susceptible individuals. Because of the variety of conditions under which this poorly understood phenomenon has been reported, it is likely that multiple factors may be responsible for its occurrence. The condition is clearly distinguishable from myoglobinuria.

Hemoglobinuria Originating in the Urinary Tract. Hemoglobinuria may accompany *infarction of the kidney.* Presumably, red cells lyse in the infarcted tissue and the liberated hemoglobin "leaks" into the urinary outflow tract directly; cystostomy reveals the unilateral origin of the pigmenturia. Rarely, when *hematuria* occurs coincident with a very dilute urine (sp. gr. <1.006), hypotonic lysis of the cells occurs within the collecting system. In neither of the aforementioned conditions is hemoglobinemia found, and plasma haptoglobin levels are normal.

Clinical Manifestations and Implications. Hemoglobinemia and hemoglobinuria, when induced by the experimental infusion of hemoglobin, when occurring from nonimmune causes, and when unaccompanied by shock or dehydration, are asymptomatic and benign phenomena. Thus any symptoms occurring in association with hemoglobinuria are likely to be related to the cause of the hemolysis and not to the hemoglobinuria per se. Transient and reversible renal vasoconstriction and reduced glomerular filtration rate may be observed during intense hemoglobinemia, but there is no evidence that permanent renal damage occurs from the hemoglobinuria per se, even when it is severe and frequently recurrent, as in patients with PNH.

By contrast, hemoglobinuria can contribute importantly to severe renal damage when it occurs in association with a major antigen-antibody reaction, e.g., incompatible blood transfusion, and/or in association with markedly reduced renal blood flow, as in shock or severe dehydration. That hemoglobinuria per se is not necessarily the cause of renal shutdown following transfusion reaction has been demonstrated by Schmidt et al., who observed renal failure following the infusion of hemoglobin-free incompatible red cell stroma. Since hemoglobin and its breakdown products are relatively insoluble when in high concentration and at acid pH, the precipitation of hemoglobin products in the renal tubules will be favored by any condition that results in reduced urine volume and acid urine pH.

Diagnosis. Investigation of suspected hemoglobinuria should include studies of the plasma as well as of the urine. Plasma obtained at the time of active intravascular hemolysis will be pink or red; free hemoglobin and haptoglobin-bound hemoglobin (in acute hemolysis) will be demonstrable by electrophoretic and gel filtration methods. If a blood sample is not obtained until 18 to 48 hours after intravascular hemolysis has ceased, the plasma will have a brown discoloration, and the only heme-containing pigment present will be methemalbumin, demonstrable spectroscopically by Schumm's test (appearance of a sharply defined band at 558 mμ after treatment with one tenth volume of concentrated ammonium sulfide).

During acute hemoglobinuria, the freshly voided urine will be pink, red, or deep port wine in color, depending on the hemoglobin concentration. Over a period of hours (whether in the bladder or during storage after voiding) the color turns brownish red or almost black owing to the formation of reduced hemoglobin, methemoglobin, acid hematin, and other breakdown products. Differential diagnosis should include hematuria, myoglobinuria, porphyrinuria, bilirubinuria, melanuria, and alkaptonuria (darkens only after storage and at alkaline pH). Hematuria can be quickly ruled out by centrifugation of the specimen. Several techniques employing benzidine reagents (which react with the iron-containing heme portion of the molecule) will help to rule out porphyrinuria, bilirubinuria, melanuria, and alkaptonuria, each of which can be separately identified by appropriate laboratory tests. Benzidine reagents will not, however, make the important distinction between hemoglobinuria and myoglobinuria, as they react with the heme groups of both molecules. The excretion of myoglobin in the urine should be suspected on clinical grounds when pigmenturia follows extreme excessive exercise (especially in the untrained individual who complains of severe post-exercise muscle pain and weakness) and infarction of, or trauma to, a large muscle mass (crush syndrome). Although there are minor spectroscopic differences between hemoglobin and myoglobin, differentiation of these pigments is made easier by two physicochemical properties of myoglobin. Myoglobin does not bind to haptoglobin, and because of its small molecular size (m.w. 17,500), is rapidly excreted in the urine. Therefore, during acute myoglobinuria, the plasma will be only slightly discolored or normal in appearance, and plasma haptoglobin levels will be normal. Second, hemoglobin is essentially insoluble at 80 per cent saturation with ammonium sulfate, whereas myoglobin remains in solution under these conditions. Thus the addition of 2.8 grams of ammonium sulfate to 5 ml. of benzidine-positive red-brown urine will result in precipitation of the abnormal pigment if hemoglobinuria is present. Rarely, both pigments may occur together in the urine and may be identified by a variety of immunologic, electrophoretic, or gel filtration techniques.

Chronic hemoglobinuria, even at levels too low to discolor the urine, is always accompanied by *hemosiderin granules* in the urinary sediment. The hemosiderin is formed within tubular cells after reabsorption of hemoglobin, and is either released from the cells or appears within cells sloughed into the outflow tract. The brown granules are readily identified by the Prussian blue reaction with potassium ferrocyanide. Hemosiderinuria is a common accompaniment of many chronic hemolytic states, and is occasionally seen in patients with hemochromatosis.

Treatment. Therapy must be directed to the primary cause of the red cell lysis that is ultimately responsible for the hemoglobinuria. Assurance of adequate urine volume (by maintenance of adequate systolic blood pressure and good hydration) is essential. Special measures (including the use of mannitol and alkali) of importance in treating acute hemoglobinuria of isoimmune origin or under any circumstances, e.g., shock, in which acute renal shutdown is threatened are described in detail under Transfusion Reactions.

Allison, A. C., and Rees, W.: The binding of hemoglobin by plasma proteins (haptoglobins). Brit. Med. J., 2:1137, 1957.

Blondheim, S. H., Margoliash, E., and Shafrir, E.: A simple test for myohaemoglobinuria (myoglobinuria). J.A.M.A., 167:453, 1957.

Bunn, H. F., and Jandl, J. H.: The renal handling of hemoglobin. Trans. Ass. Amer. Physicians, 81:147, 1968

Ham, T. H.: Hemoglobinuria. Amer. J. Med., 18:990, 1955.

Lathem, W.: The renal excretion of hemoglobin: Regulatory mechanisms and the differential excretion of free and protein-bound hemoglobin. J. Clin. Invest., 38:652, 1959.

Schmidt, P. J., and Holland, P. V.: Pathogenesis of the acute renal failure associated with incompatible transfusions. Lancet, 2:1169, 1967.

HYPOCHROMIC ANEMIAS
Elmer B. Brown

IRON DEFICIENCY ANEMIA

Definition. Iron deficiency anemia occurs when the supply of iron is inadequate to support optimal erythropoiesis. In its fully developed form it is characterized by hypochromia and microcytosis of the circulating erythrocytes, low plasma iron, low transferrin saturation, and marked depletion of bone marrow and other body iron stores.

Prevalence. Throughout the world iron deficiency is almost certainly the most common cause of anemia. In parts of Africa and Asia, where marginal dietary intake and excessive iron loss owing to intestinal parasites occur together, more than 50 per cent of the population may suffer from iron deficiency anemia. Variable figures of the incidence of iron deficiency have been reported from surveys in temperate countries. Reasons for variation include the criteria used for detecting borderline iron deficiency as well as the nature of the population sampled in terms of age, sex, economic status, and local environmental factors. Fewer than 3 per cent of men are affected in most population surveys; 10 to 30 per cent of all women may show signs of iron deficiency; and 10 to 60 per cent of pregnant women and infants in the first year of life have iron deficiency anemia. Much more information is needed to define precisely the prevalence of iron deficiency in representative geographic and socioeconomic cross sections of the United States.

Iron Metabolism. Iron is essential to human life because of its central role in the heme molecule that permits oxygen and electron transport. The body's iron can be divided into two main categories: (1) an essential, functional component composed of hemoglobin, myoglobin, enzyme and cofactor iron, and plasma transport iron, and (2) a nonessential storage component made up predominantly of ferritin and hemosiderin, not required for health but providing a reserve of iron readily mobilizable into the essential functional component in time of need.

In the normal adult man there are about 50 mg. of iron per kilogram of body weight, approximately 70 per cent of which is in the functional category and 30 per cent in a storage form. Women with a smaller red blood cell mass and lower iron stores have a body iron concentration of about 35 mg. per kilogram. Total body iron ranges between 2 and 6 grams in small women and large men. Approximately 85 per cent of the functional iron in the body is present in the red blood cells as hemoglobin, which contains 0.34 per cent iron by weight. Divalent iron in each of the four heme groups binds oxygen reversibly for transport. Myoglobin, one fourth the size of hemoglobin and with one iron atom per molecule, accounts for about 5 per cent of the functional iron. Myoglobin is present in a concentration of 2 to 3 mg. per gram wet weight of human muscle and serves as a reservoir of oxygen for muscle metabolism. A small but extremely important component is the plasma iron, 4 mg. bound to transferrin, in transit from sites of hemoglobin destruction, absorption, or storage to bone marrow and other areas of utilization. Finally, intracellular iron of heme enzymes such as cytochromes, cytochrome oxidase, peroxidase, and catalase plus iron serving as a cofactor in other enzyme systems of all cells accounts for about 10 per cent of the essential body iron. Nonessential storage compounds that account for the remaining 30 per cent of body iron are (1) ferritin, composed of a large protein surrounding micelles of iron (up to about 20 per cent by weight), with a characteristic electron microscopic pattern and poor histochemical staining properties; and (2) hemosiderin, a water-insoluble protein containing higher concentrations of iron (up to 35 per cent by weight) and readily identified by Prussian blue staining of tissues.

Iron absorption assumes great importance in human iron metabolism, because iron balance is regulated by controlled absorption rather than by excretion. Despite intensive investigation many facets of the precise mechanism and control of iron absorption remain unexplained or controversial. Current information suggests that iron entering the stomach in organic compounds is digested to soluble ferric salts that may either be reduced to ferrous ions or chelated in either the ferric or ferrous valence state to promote absorption. Entry of iron at the brush border of mucosal cells appears to be by passive diffusion; exit from the cells to the plasma transferrin probably requires metabolic energy for active transport. Most of the iron destined to enter the blood stream traverses the mucosal cell rapidly in the form of small molecules, although a proportion of iron in excess of the rapid transport capacity is shunted into storage ferritin compounds that may be lost when the cell is desquamated at the end of its three- to five-day life span. Specific luminal factors of gastric or pancreatic origin that play a physiologic role in the control of iron absorption have been postulated, but remain elusive. The means by which the body's need for increased iron absorption is transmitted to the mucosal cell has not been completely defined. Multiple signals, including mucosal cell iron concentration, local hypoxia, plasma transferrin saturation, and perhaps humoral factors, have been suggested.

Studies of iron absorption can be divided conveniently into two groups: (1) those using simple iron salts such as ferrous sulfate or ferric chloride, which give information applicable to the behavior of iron given therapeutically; and (2) those measuring the absorption of iron from foods.

Ferrous salts are better absorbed than ferric compounds, and various agents such as ascorbic and succinic acids and sorbitol enhance iron absorption. Other substances suh as phytates, phosphates, and various antacid preparations bind iron and diminish its absorption. Maximal absorption occurs in the duodenum and upper jejunum, in which the luminal contents are acid; there is less absorption distally from a neutral or alkaline environment, although the potentiality for some iron absorption exists throughout the length of the gut from stomach to colon. Iron absorption is via intestinal capillaries with little lymphatic participation, and is virtually complete within an hour or two after ingestion. Uptake of iron is unidirectional without known back-flux except for iron lost into the gut lumen by cellular desquamation. Increasing doses of simple iron salts result in increasing absorption of iron until toxicity becomes the limiting factor. Conditions associated with increased iron absorption include iron deficiency, hemolytic and sideroblastic anemias, hypoxia, cobalt and erythropoietin administration, cirrhosis and portacaval shunts, some types of pancreatic insufficiency, and the later stages of pregnancy. Factors decreasing iron absorption include iron overload, erythroid hypoplasia, generalized malabsorption states, and possibly achlorhydria.

Less information is available about the absorption of food iron. Radioactive iron incorporated into foods or added as a simple iron salt to dietary food mixtures has allowed a comparison of dietary iron absorption with that of simple iron salts. Iron in hemoglobin, liver, meat, and fish is better absorbed than iron in cereals, vegetables, milk, and eggs. Iron added to "enriched" bread is absorbed best if added in soluble forms. Limited studies of the interactions of various foods and their effects on iron absorption have shown enhanced absorption with orange juice and reduced absorption when eggs were added to the test diet.

Iron is transported in plasma bound to a specific carrier protein, transferrin (siderophilin). This β-globulin is formed in the liver, and the 7 to 15 grams present in the body are almost equally distributed in the extravascular and intravascular spaces with plasma concentrations varying from 215 to 350 mg. per 100 ml. At least 19 genetic variants have been described, but all that have been studied appear to be identical in their iron-binding properties. One or two atoms of ferric iron can be bound to the transferrin molecule and are then released to specific receptor sites on erythroblast membranes. There is no exchange of iron from one molecule to another. Measurement of functional iron-binding capacity rather than direct determination of transferrin is employed clinically. Iron is present in equal amounts in plasma and serum, normal values ranging from 60 to 160 μg. per 100 ml., with a mean of 120 for men and 110 for women. Plasma transferrin is normally about one third saturated, and the total plasma iron binding capacity is 280 to 400 μg. per 100 ml. Plasma iron shows a diurnal variation, with morning values about 30 per cent higher than those in the evening. Menses, exercise, or normal meals have no appreciable effect on plasma iron concentrations; variations in a variety of disorders are shown in Figure 1.

Iron in excess of the needs for hemoglobin, myoglobin, and essential intracellular enzymes is stored as ferritin and hemosiderin. Major sites of storage iron are hepatic parenchymal cells and reticuloendothelial cells of the bone marrow, liver, and spleen. Precise measurement of iron stores is difficult, and estimates are usually based on histochemical appraisal of bone marrow or liver hemosiderin deposits. Iron in both storage forms is readily mobilized in response to need such as bleeding, although mobilization is somehow interfered with by infection, inflammation, and malignancy.

The body has a limited capacity to excrete iron except by means of hemorrhage. Normally, excretion balances absorption, because most of the iron released from hemoglobin of senescent red blood cells is conserved and reutilized. Total daily excretion amounts to slightly less than 1 mg. for men and postmenopausal women. Of this amount, approximately 0.1 mg. is excreted in the urine, and about 0.6 mg. in the feces from mucosal cell desquamation, bile, and small amounts of blood loss; the remainder is lost from skin as desquamated cells and in sweat. Approximately 0.5 mg. of iron is present per milliliter of blood. With normal menstrual blood losses of 25 to 60 ml. monthly, this normal bleeding accounts for an additional 12 to 30 mg. of iron monthly, or 0.4 to 1 mg. per day, in women during their reproductive years. Iron loss occurs in pregnancy and delivery in amounts totaling more than 500 mg. Obligatory daily iron losses are about 50 per cent less than normal in patients with iron deficiency anemia.

Since iron absorption must balance excretion for the body's iron stores to stay in balance, one may construct a table of iron requirements for different physiologic states (see accompanying table). In addition to the exceptional stresses on

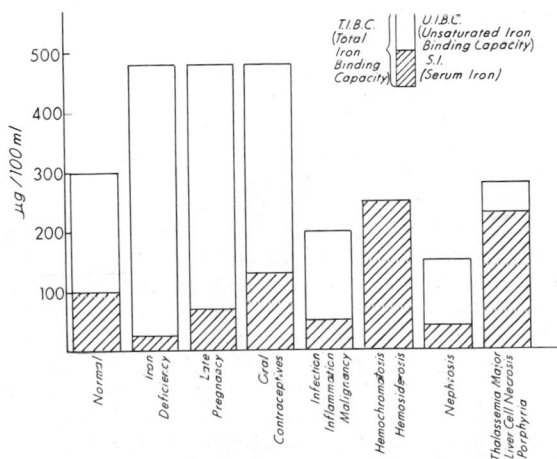

FIGURE 1. Representative serum iron and iron binding capacity values in a variety of conditions.

ESTIMATED DIETARY IRON REQUIREMENTS

	Absorbed Iron Requirement, mg./Day	Daily Food Iron Requirement,* mg./Day
Normal men and nonmenstruating women	0.5-1.0	5-10
Menstruating women	0.7-2.0	7-20
Pregnant women	2.0-4.8	20-48†
Adolescents	1.0-2.0	10-20
Children	0.4-1.0	4-10
Infants	0.5-1.5	1.5 mg./per kg.‡

*Assuming 10 per cent absorption.
†This amount of iron cannot be derived from diet and should be met by iron supplementation in the latter half of pregnancy.
‡To a maximum of 15 mg.

iron balance imposed by menstrual losses and pregnancy, one must also add the needs related to growth. These needs of iron to build hemoglobin, myoglobin, and other intracellular iron compounds are greatest at growth spurts of infancy and adolescence. An increment of 0.5 mg. per day is an acceptable estimate in the absence of precise measurements.

These requirements of iron to meet special circumstances can be translated into terms of nutritional iron intake to prevent a negative balance from occurring. Assuming that absorption of iron from food mixtures normally averages about 10 per cent, the figures for dietary iron intake can be derived (see table). Iron concentrations of foods in most western diets are related to calories, with about 6 mg. of iron per 1000 calories. Although iron absorption may increase to about 20 per cent with the onset of iron deficiency, it is obvious that pregnant women can hardly eat enough food to provide for their markedly increased iron needs and that they, with many menstruating women and adolescent girls, are likely to fall behind in meeting dietary iron needs.

Pathogenesis. Iron deficiency develops because of one or a combination of the following factors: inadequate dietary iron intake, malabsorption, blood loss, or repeated pregnancies. Since excretion of iron is limited, assigning the cause of iron deficiency in adults to inadequate intake or malabsorption implies chronicity measured in years. More important are iron losses which occur most often from the gastrointestinal tract of men and from abnormal menstrual bleeding in women. A convenient way to consider these causes of iron deficiency is to divide them into two categories—low intake and high output.

Low intake: Restrictions of dietary iron because of economic, religious, or cultural considerations lead to iron deficiency in many parts of the world. Economic and religious factors weigh heaviest in underdeveloped nations, whereas in the United States one might cite the inadequate meals of weight-conscious young women and mothers caught up in the harried pace of rearing children. In old age, absent or ill-fitting dentures combined with apathy, inactivity, and financial restrictions reduce the intake of foods with high iron nutritive

value. Continual refinement and cleanliness of our food supplies combined with the use of noniron cooking vessels may have the undesired effect of reducing our iron intake. Assimilation of iron is often reduced owing to interaction of phytates from cereals, phosphates, and other substances in the foods we eat. Malabsorption of iron rarely if ever occurs as an isolated absorptive defect, but is present in sprue syndromes and is associated with iron deficiency. (Surprisingly, the steatorrhea of pancreatic insufficiency allows normal or even increased iron absorption.) Abnormal gastrointestinal motility secondary to gastrectomy or to a variety of causes for diarrhea is usually associated with decreased iron absorption. Patients with achlorhydria have inefficient absorption of food iron, and cannot increase iron uptake effectively when they become iron deficient.

High output: Identification of the site of blood loss responsible for high output iron deficiency may be quite difficult. One reason for this difficulty is that increased menstrual blood loss, the single most common cause of iron deficiency in temperate countries, is often not recognized, and is difficult to quantitate. The best estimates of the frequency and extent of menorrhagia in randomly selected women indicate that the normal menstrual flow (25 to 60 ml.) is exceeded in about 20 per cent of women, with occasional blood losses as high as 500 ml. per month. Unfortunately, predictions of menstrual loss by the patient's account of the number and saturation of sanitary napkins and the number of days of flow are only partially successful. Iron loss associated with pregnancy is easier to estimate and totals about 500 mg. Unless iron supplementation is provided, repeated pregnancies are almost invariably accompanied by iron deficiency.

Blood loss from the alimentary tract is frequently occult and intermittent, and may elude careful search with a battery of sophisticated techniques. In a recent study no demonstrable source of blood loss could be found in 16 per cent of patients with gastrointestinal bleeding. In those whose bleeding could be explained, the cause was hemorrhoidal bleeding in 10 per cent, salicylate ingestion in 8 per cent, peptic ulceration and hiatus hernia in 7 per cent each, diverticulosis in 4 per cent, neoplasm in 2 per cent, and a sprinkling of additional cases of esophageal varices, hemorrhagic gastritis, regional enteritis, ulcerative colitis, hemorrhagic telangiectasia, and intestinal polyps. Hookworm and other intestinal parasites are important causes of blood loss and iron deficiency in many countries. Blood donation which must be specifically inquired about—doubles the amount of iron that must be absorbed when only three pints are removed per year. Blood removed for diagnostic studies from patients undergoing prolonged or repeated hospitalization is a cause for iron deficiency that can easily be overlooked. Rare causes of excess iron loss include the hemosiderinuria from chronic intravascular hemolysis of paroxysmal nocturnal hemoglobinuria and cardiac prostheses. One cannot overemphasize the dictum that iron deficiency anemia in the adult man and the postmenopausal woman is due to blood loss until proved otherwise.

The sequence of changes in slowly developing iron deficiency is fairly predictable. Initially iron stores in reticuloendothelial and parenchymal cells are mobilized to provide the metal for functional iron needs. When demands for functional iron cannot be met from the stores, a signal of some sort is transmitted to the intestine to increase iron absorption. Transferrin concentration increases while the plasma iron concentration falls as demands of the bone marrow exceed the supply of iron released from senescent erythrocytes and intestinal absorption. Anemia appears when the supply of iron restricts erythropoiesis. Distorted cells reflecting skipped divisions and hypochromic cells reflecting insufficient iron for heme synthesis gradually replace the normal cells of the circulating blood. Later, increased cell division or more severe maturation defects lead to microcytosis of the fully developed iron deficiency anemia. The extent of the depletion of cell enzyme iron is variable in different tissues sampled in man, and little is known of the rate of these changes.

Clinical Manifestations. Iron deficiency anemia is accompanied by a wide diversity of symptoms. Some patients have no awareness of ill health despite marked anemia which may be recognized by chance examinations. Symptoms usually appear insidiously and their onset is difficult to date. The gradual development of iron deficiency often allows remarkable adaptation, and may permit strenuous work with few symptoms. At the other extreme, marked tiredness, easy fatigability, dyspnea on exertion, palpitations, headache, irritability, paresthesias, lightheadedness, and other vague symptoms may trouble patients with borderline or mild anemia.

Examination usually discloses pallor, although on casual observation this finding may not be noticed. A peculiar greenish appearance of the skin of young girls, vividly described by careful observers before 1900 and termed chlorosis, has mysteriously disappeared. Vitiligo is a rare skin change in Negroes. Angular stomatitis—most marked in edentulous patients—frequent papillary

atrophy, and varying degrees of glossitis comprise the oral lesions associated with iron deficiency. Dysphagia resulting from postcricoid esophageal webs or strictures, associated with hypochromic anemia and achlorhydria, and most frequently seen in middle-aged women—the Patterson-Kelly or Plummer-Vinson syndrome—is rare in the United States, but is fairly common in the British Isles and Scandinavia. Whether this syndrome is due to iron deficiency or some associated disorder is not known. Multiple gastrointestinal complaints, such as anorexia, pyrosis, flatulence, nausea, eructation, and constipation, are common in association with iron deficiency. Occasionally bizarre cravings for cornstarch, ice, clay, and other substances may appear. These forms of pica are especially common in iron-deficient Negro women, but probably have a world-wide distribution. Gastritis, which is reversible after iron therapy, and permanent gastric atrophy have been described in numerous gastroscopic investigations of iron-deficient patients. Whether these gastric lesions are cause or effect of iron deficiency is debatable. Spoon nail (koilonychia) is the most advanced abnormality of the nails and is becoming very rare. Often, milder nail changes such as thinning, brittleness, lusterless appearance, longitudinal ridging, and flattening accompany prolonged iron deficiency, and are associated with depletion of cysteine in the nails. The frequent suggestion that these epithelial changes are related to the severity or chronicity of iron deficiency anemia may be questioned because of their virtual absence in patients with severe, lifelong iron deficiency owing to hookworm infestation. An attractive but unproved hypothesis is that the epithelial changes may reflect a chronically depressed intake of iron (and possibly other substances) rather than chronically increased loss of iron from bleeding.

Severe anemia often leads to cardiac dilatation, the occurrence of hemic murmurs, and, in older patients, the development of congestive heart failure. Enlargement of the spleen to slightly below the costal margin is observed in about 10 per cent of patients, and recedes after treatment. Claims of aggravation of menorrhagia by iron deficiency anemia and improvement after treatment are difficult to substantiate. Numbness and tingling without objective neurologic abnormalities are reported by about 25 per cent of patients. Extremely rare are the papilledema and increased pressure of cerebrospinal fluid that may be confused with intracranial tumors. Infants often show marked irritability and present difficulties in feeding.

Laboratory Findings. A number of laboratory procedures facilitate the identification of iron deficiency anemia. A well-stained blood film shows small erythrocytes (microcytosis) poorly filled with hemoglobin (hypochromia) with marked variation in size (anisocytosis) and shape (poikilocytosis). Mean corpuscular volume is less than 80 cu. μ and mean corpuscular hemoglobin concentration is less than 30 per cent. Plasma iron concentration is usually less than 80 μg. per 100 ml., associated with a total plasma iron-binding capacity of more than 400 μg. per 100 ml. Transferrin saturation (the product of plasma iron divided by total iron-binding capacity multiplied by 100) is 15 per cent or less. Examination of bone marrow particles shows normoblastic erythroid hyperplasia; sideroblasts and hemosiderin in macrophages are absent when the marrow particles are stained for iron. Defective heme synthesis is associated with elevated erythrocyte protoporphyrin concentration and decreased plasma bilirubin. Reticulocytes are present in normal numbers except for elevations secondary to recent hemorrhage. Erythrocyte osmotic fragility is decreased, reflecting the diminished hemoglobin concentration. The life span of erythrocytes is usually normal, although shortened survival has been reported. Thrombocytosis in the range of one million platelets per cu. mm., or less often thrombocytopenia, both of which return to normal after iron therapy, may be observed. Abnormalities of the leukocytes are rare and are usually confined to slight leukopenia and occasional hypersegmented neutrophils. Unfortunately there is no practical laboratory test to measure depletion of tissue enzyme iron.

Treatment. The two objects of treatment of iron deficiency anemia are (1) to replace the blood and tissue iron deficits, and (2) to recognize and, if possible, correct the underlying cause. Despite the vast array of therapeutic preparations containing iron, simple ferrous salts (ferrous sulfate, ferrous gluconate, and ferrous fumarate) given by mouth remain the mainstay of treatment for iron deficiency anemia. Large doses of ascorbic or succinic acid will increase iron absorption but only to a small extent that hardly warrants the extra expense. The addition of other substances found in "shotgun" mixtures such as copper, cobalt, molybdenum, intrinsic factor, and various B-vitamins is of no benefit. The use of these shotgun hematinics must be condemned, because they may obscure the correct diagnosis as indicated by a response to iron alone; further, they encourage sloppiness in diagnosis, and they are unnecessarily expensive. Enteric-coated and delayed release iron preparations are poorly designed to exploit the fact of maximal absorption in the upper gastrointestinal tract. All too often their delay in iron release serves to dump the metal in the lower intestine, in which absorption is greatly diminished. When iron medication is prescribed in tablet form, the physician should warn the patient to keep the tablets out of reach of small children to reduce the danger of severe iron intoxication. Suitable warnings on the label and the use of child-proof containers will further reduce this risk.

A total daily dose of iron in the range of 180 to 240 mg. provides for maximal rates of hemoglobin regeneration in adults. Three or four tablets of ferrous sulfate (60 mg. of elemental iron) or ferrous fumarate (66 mg. of iron) provide the requisite daily dose. Ferrous gluconate, with only 36 mg.

of elemental iron per tablet, requires a dosage of six tablets per day. These iron preparations are given in equal doses with or after meals and with a snack at bedtime. The advantage of increased absorption of iron salts taken on an empty stomach is overweighed by the undesirable side effects of gastrointestinal irritation.

Approximately one patient in ten will experience unpleasant side effects such as nausea, epigastric pain, abdominal cramps, diarrhea, or vomiting of sufficient severity to require discontinuation of treatment. No effective iron preparation is free from causing gastric or intestinal irritation. Gastric symptomatology is dose dependent, and may be minimized by a gradual buildup of the iron dose during the first three days of treatment. A few patients are completely unable or unwilling to take iron by mouth; patience and understanding on the part of the physician can keep this group small. Treatment with iron should be continued for four to six months and even longer in the face of recurrent bleeding. Restoration of iron stores to provide a buffer against recurrent iron deficiency is a slow process.

Infants and toddlers are best treated with liquid iron preparations. Infants should receive a total of 60 to 90 mg. of iron daily in water or fruit juices. Ferrous sulfate is available in concentrated drops containing 15 mg. of iron per 0.6 ml., as a syrup with 30 mg. of iron per 5 ml., or as an elixir with 44 mg. of iron per 5 ml. Transient staining of the teeth by liquid iron preparations can be prevented by using a dropper or a straw. Most children weighing 35 to 75 pounds can satisfactorily take iron tablets in half the adult dosage; larger children usually receive adult doses of iron.

Response to adequate doses of iron given to a patient with iron deficiency anemia is quite predictable (Fig. 2). An initial sense of well-being is often observed within 48 hours. This improvement appears to be more than a psychologic effect from taking medications, as infants often lose their irritability and begin to eat better. Because this response occurs before any change in blood values is measurable, it has been attributed, without any real evidence, to replenishment of some vital cellular iron compound. The height of the reticulocyte peak and the rate of hemoglobin regeneration are proportional to the severity of the anemia; maximal daily rates of hemoglobin regeneration are 0.3 gram per 100 ml.

Failure to respond to iron given by mouth should call forth the following considerations: (1) the patient failed to take the iron as prescribed; (2) the patient did not have iron deficiency anemia, and re-evaluation of the diagnosis is necessary; (3) blood loss exceeded new blood formation; (4) intercurrent infection, inflammation, or malignancy interfered with the response to iron; (5) the patient was unable to absorb the iron; and (6) an ineffective iron preparation was administered.

Parenteral administration of iron should be reserved for the following indications: (1) patients

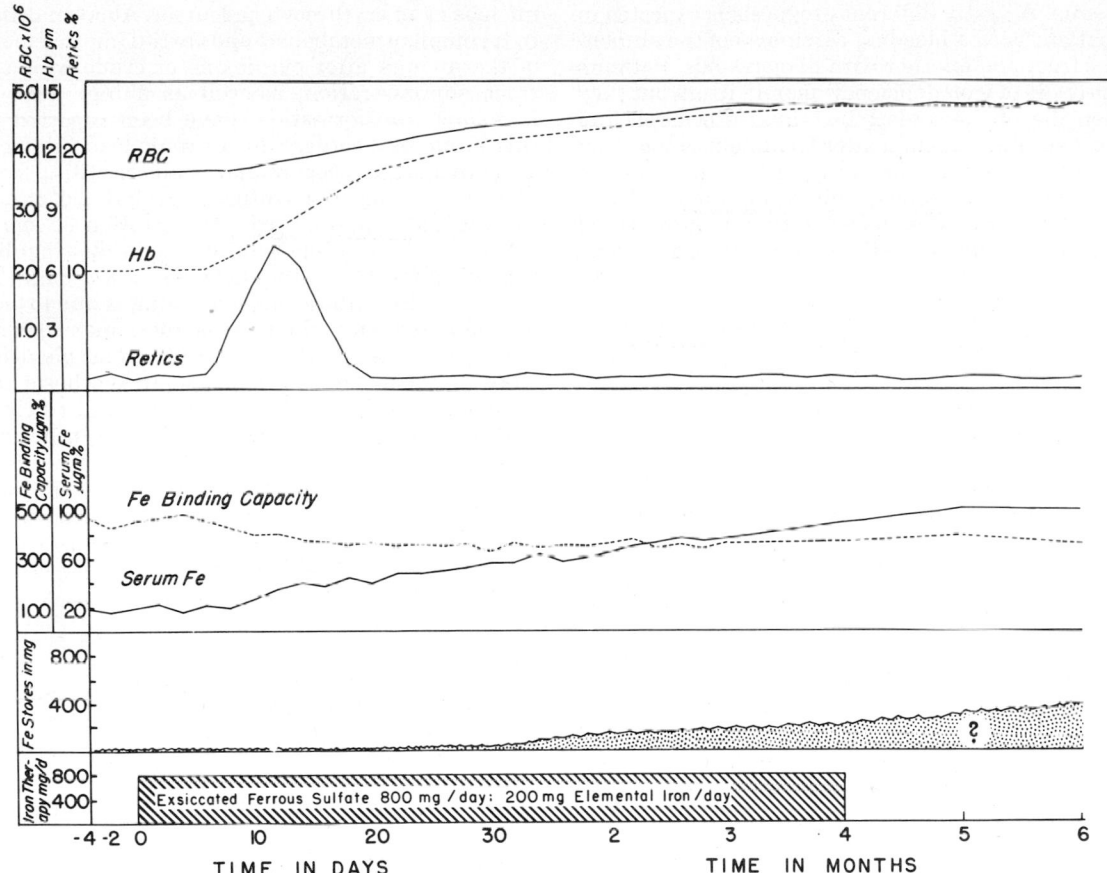

FIGURE 2. Schematized response to iron therapy. Reticulocytes begin to rise about the fifth to seventh day after iron therapy is started, reach a peak between the tenth and fourteenth days, and then fall to normal levels. Hemoglobin level begins to increase on about the seventh to tenth day. From four to eight weeks are required before normal values are attained. No accurate data are available to describe the reappearance of storage iron; its reaccumulation may be slower than shown; hence the question mark.

with malabsorption syndromes; (2) the relatively small group of patients who are unable or unwilling to take iron by mouth, including some people with ulcerative colitis, regional enteritis, and colostomies; (3) selected patients who prove unreliable in taking their prescribed iron; and (4) some patients with chronic uncorrectable bleeding with iron loss in excess of that which can be replaced by the oral route. Three satisfactory preparations are available for parenteral use. Iron dextran and iron sorbitex, each containing 50 mg. of iron per milliliter, are used for deep intramuscular injection into the buttocks, whereas iron dextrin (20 mg. of iron per milliliter) is injected intravenously. After an initial injection of 2 ml. of the intramuscularly administered preparations, 2- to 5-ml. doses are given daily into alternate extremities until a calculated total dose is administered. Dosage is calculated by the following formula: Normal Hgb (grams per 100 ml.) − patient's Hgb × 0.255 = iron dose in grams. This formula provides sufficient iron to replace the circulating hemoglobin deficit plus a 50 per cent excess for creation of tissue stores. Side effects such as local pain, lymphadenitis, headache, fever,

urticaria, arthralgias, and hypotension occur in about 5 per cent of patients; rare fatal anaphylactic reactions have been reported. Skin staining from reflux of iron along the injection path can be prevented by using a Z-shaped needle path. Black urine and urinary irritation may occur after injections of iron sorbitex, because one-third of the dose is excreted in the urine.

Preventive iron therapy for groups prone to develop iron deficiency (infants, pregnant women, and blood donors) requires special consideration. Fortification of foods seems a reasonable and effective way to provide the iron needs of infants. Pregnant women should be given iron during the last half of pregnancy after the early period of "morning sickness" that might erroneously be attributed to the iron tablets and influence the patient's subsequent willingness to take this medication. One tablet of ferrous sulfate (60 mg. of iron daily) is sufficient to provide for the iron needs of pregnancy. For repeated blood donors the dose of iron will depend on the rate of donation—one to three tablets daily may be required.

Prognosis. Prognosis in iron deficiency can only be applied to the underlying disorder causing the anemia. A vastly different prognosis is expected in a patient with a bleeding carcinoma of the alimentary tract and another with hemorrhoids. Patients rarely die of iron deficiency anemia itself, but they often die of the underlying cause. Recurrence of iron deficiency anemia after treatment is common; one third of women and one fourth of men have a recurrence in extended follow-up studies. These recurrence rates emphasize the importance of identifying and correcting the cause of iron deficiency.

Beutler, E., Fairbanks, V. F., and Fahey, J. L.: Clinical Disorders of Iron Metabolism. New York, Grune & Stratton, Inc., 1963.

Bothwell, T. H., and Finch, C. A.: Iron Metabolism. Boston, Little, Brown and Company, 1962.

Committee on Iron Deficiency: Iron deficiency in the United States. J.A.M.A., 203:407, 1968.

Gross, F. (ed.): Iron Metabolism — An International Symposium. Berlin, Springer-Verlag OHG, 1964.

Moore, C. V.: Iron nutrition and requirements. Scand. J. Haemat. (Series Haematologica), 6:1, 1965.

Wintrobe, M. M.: Clinical Hematology. 6th ed. Philadelphia, Lea & Febiger, 1967.

HYPOCHROMIC ANEMIAS NOT CAUSED BY IRON DEFICIENCY

Hypochromic anemia occurs predominantly when hemoglobin synthesis is interfered with out of proportion to defects in erythrocyte proliferation. Biosynthetic abnormalities have been identified at one or more stages of protoporphyrin synthesis, iron incorporation into the heme ring — the prime defect in iron deficiency anemia — or globin synthesis. Compared to iron deficiency anemia, these disorders of hemoglobin synthesis are rare. As a group they can be differentiated from iron deficiency anemia by increased body iron stores with increased hemosiderin in marrow particles, the presence of sideroblasts and siderocytes, and increased plasma iron and transferrin saturation. Special distinguishing features are included with the following list of these disorders. (1) By far the most common of the hypochromic anemias not caused by iron deficiency are thalassemia and its variants resulting from interaction with abnormal hemoglobins. The basic defect is in the synthesis of globin chains. Thalassemia and its variants can be distinguished from iron deficiency by hemoglobin electrophoresis and detection of elevated levels of hemoglobins A_2 and F. (2) Homozygous Hgb-C disease and Hgb-S-D are hypochromic anemias readily identified by appropriate hemoglobin electrophoresis. (3) Sideroblastic anemias can be subdivided into congenital, acquired, and pyridoxine-responsive categories. They share the common features of disordered heme synthesis with prominent ringed sideroblasts observable on iron staining of bone marrow particles. Electron microscopy discloses the siderotic granules to be diffuse iron aggregates in the intercristal spaces of mitochondria surrounding the nucleus of an erythrocyte precursor. Abnormalities in tryptophan metabolism and partial improvement of the anemia after pyridoxine or crude liver extract administration, as well as a high rate of leukemic transformation, have been reported in this group of disorders. (4) Chronic lead intoxication produces a hypochromic anemia resulting from defective hemoglobin synthesis. Stippling of erythrocytes and abnormal urinary excretion of coproporphyrin and aminolevulinic acid distinguish this disorder from iron deficiency, although in young children whose lead poisoning is due to pica of lead-based paint the two disorders may coexist. (5) Inadequate delivery of iron from plentiful stores to the marrow for hemoglobin synthesis has been observed in rare instances, such as in a child with congenital absence of transferrin, in pulmonary hemosiderosis, and in older people with an unexplained block in the release of iron from reticuloendothelial sites of hemoglobin catabolism.

Wintrobe, M. M.: Clinical Hematology. 6th ed. Philadelphia, Lea & Febiger, 1967.

HEMOCHROMATOSIS
(Iron Storage Disease)
Clement A. Finch

Definition. Hemochromatosis is a chronic disease characterized by the deposition of excess iron in parenchymal tissues of the body and eventual fibrosis and functional insufficiency of those organs severely involved.

Pathology. At autopsy the unique finding in hemochromatosis is bronze pigmentation of body tissues resulting from widespread deposition of hemosiderin. The iron deposits are heaviest in the liver and pancreas, in which the iron concentration is 50 to 100 times normal, but they are also prominent in other endocrine glands, cardiac muscle, and skin. The liver is sclerotic and usually large (average weight, 2400 grams). Iron deposits within the heart muscle cells are of particular significance because of the associated cardiac dysfunction.

Pathogenesis and Pathologic Physiology. Iron overload is the result of increased iron absorption and not of decreased excretion, as the amount excreted has been shown to be a negligible quantity in the adult male (about 1 mg. per day). Under ordinary circumstances the mucosa adjusts the amount of iron absorbed so as to maintain iron balance. There are five different circumstances in which mucosal regulation fails: (1) in idiopathic hemochromatosis, in which there is a genetic defect in regulation of absorption; (2) in certain anemic states, usually characterized by a block in heme synthesis (hypochromic anemia with hyperplastic erythroid marrow), in which an increase in erythropoiesis is associated with an increase in iron absorption; (3) with long-continued high iron intake, which occurs from alcoholic beverages in the Bantu or following may years of medicinal iron, in which normal mucosa appears unable to prevent excessive inflow of iron; (4) in certain patients with chronic liver disease, in whom both altered absorption and increased iron intake may play a role; and (5) in patients with cutaneous porphyria, in whom the amount of body iron is rarely enough to be of consequence. In all these conditions the rate of iron accumulation is no more than 2 to 4 mg. per day. Significant overload occurs then only after many years have passed. Thus 70 per cent of patients with idiopathic hemochromatosis present symptoms between the ages of 40 and 60 years. The greater frequency (over 80 per cent) in men as compared to women is explained at least in part by the increased iron losses through menstruation and pregnancy in the female. Iron overload may also be produced by parenteral iron injections, usually in the form of blood transfusions.

The location of iron in the hemochromatosis syndrome is in parenchymal tissue. A prerequisite for this pattern of distribution appears to be an elevated plasma iron and saturated plasma transferrin. In idiopathic hemochromatosis the elevation in plasma iron has been shown in some instances to precede significant iron loading. Iron deposits in the reticuloendothelium following transfusions appear innocuous so long as the iron is confined to these cells. Redistribution of iron into parenchymal cells occurs far more frequently when the erythroid marrow is hyperplastic than when it is aplastic.

Over a period of time large amounts of iron appear to produce tissue damage, because organ dysfunction correlates with parenchymal iron concentration and parenchymal iron overload of different causes produces the same clinical and pathologic picture. There is experimental evidence indicating that the effects of iron and other noxious agents are additive. The occurrence of alcoholism in one third of patients with idiopathic hemochromatosis is significant in this connection.

Clinical Manifestations. The presenting complaints in idiopathic hemochromatosis may relate to skin pigmentation, diabetes, hepatomegaly, symptoms of liver dysfunction, cardiac failure, or endocrine dysfunction. Pigmentation is either an addisonian-like bronzing resulting from increased melanin or a blue-gray color resulting from iron deposition. The pigment is distributed most prominently over the genitals, face, and arms, and in skin folds. Mucous membranes are involved in only about 15 per cent of the patients. The liver is usually palpable, and the spleen is palpable in about half of the cases. The enlarged liver may be associated with upper abdominal pain, occasionally excruciating and knifelike, simulating biliary colic or perforated peptic ulcer. Visible jaundice is unusual. Hemorrhage from a ruptured esophageal varix is less frequently encountered than it is in nonpigmentary cirrhosis, and evidence of increased collateral circulation is rare. Ascites may appear

as a terminal event. There is frequently no indication of the liver disease other than general body wasting. Many patients, as the result of some acute illness or stress situation, suffer acute liver decomposition, coma and death rapidly supervening. Sexual impotence is a common complaint in the later phase of the disease, but may occur when the patient is otherwise asymptomatic. Testicular atrophy, loss of axillary and chest hair, and occasional gynecomastia may be regarded as related to liver dysfunction. Hepatoma is an important complication in older patients. The diabetes of hemochromatosis is mild at the onset but progressively worsens. A few patients are sensitive to insulin, but a greater number are relatively resistant, occasionally requiring several hundred units a day. Cardiac deposits of hemosiderin are frequently associated with arrhythmias and congestive heart failure that respond poorly to conventional therapy. Chondrocalcinosis associated with iron deposits in the joints produces arthritic symptoms in some patients. Impairment of pituitary and other endocrine gland function has been described as another less frequent complication. A moderate macrocytic anemia is found only in the late stages of the disease. In the early phase the hemoglobin concentration is apt to be above normal.

Diagnosis. There is little difficulty in recognizing hemochromatosis in a patient with a classic tetrad of skin pigmentation, liver disease, diabetes, and heart failure. A high index of suspicion in the presence of any two of these four cardinal findings will frequently lead to the diagnosis. Laboratory studies center around the demonstration of increased iron stores and of functional impairment of the organs mentioned, i.e., liver, pancreas and heart.

The most important simple laboratory test in the diagnosis of hemochromatosis is the determination of *plasma iron and iron-binding capacity*, because a saturated transferrin appears to be prerequisite for parenchymal iron loading. A saturated transferrin, however, does not indicate how long the process has been present, how much iron deposition has occurred, or whether tissue damage is also present. The measurement is not entirely dependable, because high plasma iron levels may be transiently depressed if an inflammatory state is present. Excessive parenchymal iron deposits may be identified by *iron excretion after chelate injection*. A 24-hour urinary excretion in excess of 2 mg. of iron following an intramuscular injection of 0.5 gram of desferrioxamine indicates excessive parenchymal iron deposits; in untreated idiopathic hemochromatosis the amount will usually exceed 10 mg. *Liver biopsy* by needle aspiration is the definitive procedure in indicating the extent of iron deposition and the degree of tissue damage.

Once a diagnosis of hemochromatosis is made in an individual, attention should be directed to other family members. Approximately one half to one third of siblings of a person with idiopathic hemochromatosis have been shown to have iron overload, and an increased incidence is also found in certain hereditary anemias associated with disorders in hemoglobin synthesis (erythropoietic hemochromatosis).

Prognosis and Treatment. Hemochromatosis as a clinical disease should be preventable and, depending on its stage at the time of diagnosis, the tissue damage produced is partially reversible. Since iron deposits are chiefly responsible for tissue damage, specific therapy should be directed toward removal of iron by means of phlebotomy. In patients with idiopathic hemochromatosis weekly phlebotomies of 500 ml. are well tolerated. Each phlebotomy removes 200 to 250 mg. of iron from the blood, which is replaced by an equivalent amount of iron from tissue stores. In contrast to normal persons who rapidly become anemic on the regimen, patients with idiopathic hemochromatosis maintain their hematocrits at levels between 35 and 45 per cent. Over a period of two or three years the bulk of the iron deposits in the tissues will be mobilized for hemoglobin production and removed by bleedings. A fall in plasma iron level will signal the partial depletion of iron stores, and further phlebotomies are carried out as indicated by the plasma iron and hematocrit levels. The objective of therapy should be to maintain the plasma iron level within normal limits. When phlebotomy is not feasible, iron may be removed at about half the rate, i.e., 15 mg. per day, by continuous intramuscular administration of the chelate desferrioxamine. In addition to the removal of iron, the usual measures for management of hepatic dysfunction and diabetes are indicated. Testosterone and other endocrine supplements may also be useful as specific endocrine dysfunction can be demonstrated.

In the patient whose disease is recognized sufficiently early to permit iron depletion by phlebotomy, prognosis is excellent. In the series of 40 patients so treated, a five-year survival of 89 per cent was reported. Many of the deaths occur in patients in whom the diagnosis is not suspected. In patients younger than 40, most fatalities are ascribable to cardiac failure. In those between the ages of 40 and 60, hepatic failure and infection may cause death. In patients older than 60, hepatoma may develop. Under phlebotomy therapy pigmentation of the skin decreases and cardiac failure is reversed. Liver disease may improve, depending on the degree of existing damage, and diabetes appears to be ameliorated in about one third of the patients. Loss of libido is not affected, and hepatoma occurs as a late complication despite prior removal of excess iron.

Bothwell, T. H., and Finch, C. A.: Iron Metabolism. Boston, Little, Brown and Company, 1962.

Finch, S. C., and Finch, C. A.: Idiopathic hemochromatosis, an iron storage disease. Medicine, 34:381, 1955.

Harker, L. A., Funk, D. D., and Finch, C. C.: Evaluation of storage iron by chelates. Amer. J. Med., 45:105, 1968.

Williams, R., Smith, P. M., Spicer, E. J. F., Barry, M., and Sherlock, S.: Venesection therapy in idiopathic haemochromatosis. Quart. J. Med., 38:1, 1969.

TRANSFUSION REACTIONS

Hugh Chaplin, Jr.

General Considerations. The true frequency of untoward reactions to transfusions of whole human blood is unknown. Incidences varying from 10 per cent to less than 0.2 per cent have been reported; the wide variation reflects principally the care with which the observer followed the recipients and the strictness of the criteria employed for defining reactions. A conservative estimate would be that 2 per cent of all transfusions are accompanied by some sort of unfavorable response. Thus, with approximately 6 million units of whole blood administered annually in the United States, at least 120,000 recognizable reactions can be expected.

Caution must be exercised against erroneous diagnoses of transfusion reactions. Most of the symptoms of transfusion reactions are nonspecific (see accompanying table). Patients who receive transfusions are often seriously ill with disorders that themselves may be responsible for the acute onset of chills, fever, shock, or jaundice. The temporal association of the transfusion with the onset of symptoms certainly constitutes presumptive evidence of cause and effect, but important errors in patient care may result if wisdom and restraint are not exercised to assure a comprehensive consideration of possible causes other than transfusion.

Several complications of transfusions do not strictly qualify as transfusion "reactions," and thus are not included in the table. Among these are the *transmission of diseases* such as syphilis, malaria, and hepatitis, and the ultimate development of transfusion hemosiderosis in the chronically anemic patient who receives a great many transfusions (usually more than 50) over a period of months or years. The role of gamma globulin in prophylaxis against transmission of serum hepatitis via transfusion is controversial; its routine administration is not justified by existing evidence except possibly to "high risk" recipients, i.e., pregnant women, patients receiving more than 10 units of blood, elderly patients, and patients suffering from debilitating disease. Another recently recognized complication of transfusion is the *"post-pump syndrome,"* an infectious mononucleosis-like illness occurring in 5 to 10 per cent of patients approximately one month following open-heart surgery. Possible causes include transmission of infectious mononucleosis or cytomegalovirus organisms via the transfusions, or transient host vs. graft or graft vs. host reactions involving recipient and donor leukocytes (principally lymphocytes). There are several *complications of massive transfusion* (usually more than 3000 ml. to an adult recipient within 12 hours). Citrate

CATEGORIES OF TRANSFUSION REACTIONS

Cause of Reaction	Common Symptoms	Frequency	Shock	Prognosis
Contaminated blood	Chills, fever, headache, backache, delirium, bloody vomitus and diarrhea	Rare	Yes ("red shock")	Serious
Bacterial pyrogens	Chills, fever, headache, malaise	Rare	No*	Good
Circulatory overload	Dyspnea, cough, hemoptysis, tachycardia	Rare	Rare*	Good
Air embolism	Sudden onset of cough, cyanosis, syncope, convulsions	Rare	Yes	Serious
Allergy	Itching, urticaria, fever, angioneurotic edema, bronchospasm	Common	No*	Good
	Anaphylaxis	Rare	Yes	Serious
Red cell incompatibility	Chills, fever, headache, backache, hematuria, oliguria, jaundice	Moderate	Yes	Serious
Intravascular hemolysis				
Extravascular hemolysis				
Sensitivity to:	Chills, fever, headache, malaise, confusion			
Donor leukocytes		Common	Rare*	Good
Donor platelets		Rare	Rare*	Good
Donor plasma		Rare	Rare*	Good
Unexplained (febrile)	Chills, fever, headache, malaise	Common	No*	Good

*Although shock is absent or rare as a general feature of these types of reactions, in the seriously ill or injured patient shock may be precipitated by the added stress of the transfusion reaction.

toxicity may occur, particularly during rapid intra-arterial transfusion or in patients with hepatic insufficiency or shunt bypass of the portal venous circulation. At citrate concentrations higher than 100 mg. per 100 ml., skeletal muscle tremors may occur, along with prolongation of the QT segment of the electrocardiogram. Cardiac arrest may result if the citrate concentrations rise even higher. The manifestations of citrate intoxication can be prevented or eliminated by the simultaneous administration of calcium gluconate into another vein. Two other complications of massive transfusion are related to changes that take place in blood during storage in the blood bank. A hemorrhagic diathesis may develop, caused principally by the absence of viable donor platelets in blood stored more than 24 to 48 hours, even under ideal blood bank conditions. Depletion of the patient's own platelets by preceding massive blood loss is thus not compensated by the transfusion of viable donor platelets, and thrombocytopenia develops. Other causes for hemorrhagic tendency are deficiences of labile plasma coagulation factors in stored donor blood. The hemorrhagic complications can be largely prevented if every fourth unit of blood given within a 12- to 18-hour period is a "fresh" unit, i.e., drawn within three to four hours of administration. A less frequent complication of massive transfusion of stored blood is the occurrence of clinically significant hyperkalemia in the recipient. During storage in ACD preservative solution at 4° C., donor red blood cells continuously lose potassium ion; thus, the concentration of potassium in the suspending donor plasma will average 15 to 20 mEq. per liter after two weeks of storage and 25 to 30 mEq. per liter after three weeks. The danger of hyperkalemia is increased in the presence of impaired renal function. When renal insufficiency is known to exist, transfusion should employ blood stored less than five to seven days, and packed red cells should be used, whenever possible.

Contaminated Blood. The transfusion of banked blood contaminated by endotoxin-producing bacteria (usually gram-negative rods that grow well at refrigerator temperature) may give rise to extremely serious reactions in the recipient, with a fatal outcome likely in more than 50 per cent of the patients. Death usually results from profound and persistent vascular collapse. In addition to the symptoms listed in the table, a characteristic feature is the occurrence of "red shock": i.e., unlike the more common hypovolemic shock in which peripheral vasoconstriction results in cold, gray, clammy skin, endotoxin shock may be accompanied by marked peripheral vasodilatation so that the skin is dry, warm, and pink. Thus, it is essential that blood pressure be measured frequently in patients suspected of having reactions to contaminated blood, as dangerous hypotension may coexist with an outward appearance that belies the severity of the circulatory collapse.

Fortunately, with current blood banking procedures, contamination of stored blood rarely occurs. It is also fortunate that the diagnosis of significant bacterial contamination can be established within ten minutes. A small sample of residual donor blood from the container or tubing used for administration is centrifuged lightly (500 r.p.m. for two to three minutes); a drop of the supernatant plasma is smeared, fixed by heating, and Gram-stained. Unless most oil immersion fields contain several clearly definable organisms, contamination can be disregarded as the primary cause of the reaction. If the blood is cultured to confirm the diagnosis, incubation should be carried out at 30° C. as well as at 37° C., as some contaminants will not grow at temperatures as high as 37° C.

Because of the extreme gravity of reactions owing to contaminated blood, rapid institution of comprehensive supportive therapy is essential. Intravenous therapy should include sufficient vasopressor drug to maintain the systolic pressure above 100 mm. of mercury, corticosteroids (100 to 150 mg. of hydrocortisone), broad-spectrum antimicrobials in high dosage, and additional whole blood if the estimated blood loss has not been corrected. Special measures to mitigate renal complications are discussed later.

Pyrogenic Reactions. The term "pyrogenic reactions" should be reserved for reactions related to the presence of demonstrable bacterial pyrogens (endotoxins) in the infused blood or in the transfusion equipment. Now that commercially manufactured pyrogen-tested disposable transfusion equipment is widely employed, the frequency of pyrogenic transfusion reactions has diminished strikingly. When parenteral therapy equipment does contain pyrogens, febrile reactions are "epidemic" among patients receiving intravenous infusions, and the aid of a specialized laboratory qualified to demonstrate the presence of bacterial pyrogens should be sought. Treatment is symptomatic.

Circulatory Overload. The onset of acute left-sided heart failure during transfusion may reflect actual hypervolemia caused by administration of excessive amounts of blood to a patient whose volume deficit has been seriously overestimated. Even in the absence of hypervolemia, pulmonary edema may be precipitated by the too rapid administration of blood to a patient who is profoundly anemic (hemoglobin concentration less than 4 to 5 grams per 100 ml.) or in cardiac failure. A further cause for the symptoms of circulatory overload may be the presence of mechanical circulatory obstruction, e.g., mitral or aortic valve disease. Whatever the cause, treatment consists of slowing the rate of transfusion (cessation if necessary), changing to packed red blood cells, and digitalization. Rarely, a small phlebotomy is required. When the patient is elderly, severely anemic, or suffering from either cardiac or renal insufficiency, venous pressure should be monitored at frequent intervals during transfusion.

Air Embolism. Air embolism is rarely encountered as a life-threatening cause of transfusion reaction except when blood is being administered under air pressure following massive exsanguination. The accident occurs when all the blood in the container into which air has been pumped has been delivered and air is allowed to flow into the patient. The administration of pressure transfusions by means of air pumped into the blood container is extremely hazardous; transfusion from plastic bags to which external pressure can be safely applied without the possibility of air infusion should be substituted. When air embolism has occurred, the administration tubing should be immediately clamped and the patient turned on his left side in the head-down, feet-up position so that air in the right ventricle floats away from the pulmonary outflow tract.

Allergy. Allergic reactions are relatively common and are generally mild (hives, bronchial wheezing, and congestion of mucous membranes).

Treatment is symptomatic (antipyretics, antihistaminics). The drugs should be administered directly to the patient; under no circumstances should they be added to the container of blood. Marked angioneurotic edema or anaphylaxis may require prompt parenteral administration of epinephrine, vasopressor drugs, and corticosteroids.

Red Blood Cell Incompatibility. Incompatibility within the ABO system, with the resultant destruction of donor cells by isoantibodies in the recipient's circulation, is the most common cause of life-threatening reactions in contemporary transfusion practice. These preventable transfusion accidents almost always occur because of technical or logistic errors—the use of faulty techniques of blood typing and improper identification of blood samples, donor bottles, and patients. When the recipient's blood contains potent isohemolysins, acute intravascular hemolysis of the donor cells occurs. When the plasma hemoglobin concentration exceeds the hemoglobin binding capacity of the recipient's plasma (normally 75 to 175 mg. of hemoglobin per 100 ml. of plasma), *hemoglobinuria* occurs. Whereas many patients tolerate severe hemoglobinuria, e.g., paroxysmal nocturnal hemoglobinuria, without serious impairment of renal function, intravascular hemolytic reactions are potentially dangerous, especially when accompanied by shock, because of the possible development of oliguria, anuria, and uremia.

When donor red blood cell destruction occurs predominantly extravascularly, as for example in the presence of Rh antibodies demonstrable only by the indirect antiglobulin (Coombs) reaction, hemoglobinemia is generally much less severe, and jaundice is a more prominent feature, reflecting reticuloendothelial cell destruction of antibody-coated donor erythrocytes sequestered from the circulation predominantly in the spleen and/or liver.

Although the occurrence of an acute hemolytic transfusion reaction can generally be suspected on the basis of the symptoms and signs shown in the table, a special problem is presented by *anesthetized patients,* in whom the only sign of serious hemolytic reaction may be oozing of blood at the operative site. The bleeding tendency is generally associated with fibrinogen depletion thought to be the consequence of intravascular clotting in response to thromboplastic substances liberated from the hemolyzing cells, plus the added complication of increased fibrinolysis. A further contributing cause may be the severe transient thrombocytopenia that often accompanies erythrocyte incompatibility reactions.

To determine quickly whether acute intravascular hemolysis has occurred, a blood sample is drawn from the patient into a clean, dry syringe or a syringe rinsed with physiologic saline. The blood is mixed with an anticoagulant by repeated gentle inversion (with care to avoid foaming, which causes in vitro hemolysis) and immediately centrifuged. If the plasma is obtained within two to eight hours of massive intravascular lysis, it will appear frankly pink or red. Plasma examined 12 to 48 hours after intravascular lysis is more apt to be brown, reflecting the presence of methemalbumin, which can be confirmed by testing the plasma with ammonium sulfide (Schumm's test). When donor red blood cell destruction has been largely extravascular, the plasma will show increased indirect-reacting (unconjugated) bilirubin; peak levels generally occur four to six hours after the transfusion.

To ascertain the basis for incompatibility, blood freshly drawn from the recipient should be sent immediately to the blood bank along with the donor blood container so that a thorough serologic review can be carried out. Along with the conventional retesting of the recipient's serum for the presence of antibodies against donor erythrocytes, such a review should include search for antibodies in the *donor* plasma that might cause destruction of the patient's cells, or cells of the other donors in the case of multiple transfusions.

In addition to general supportive measures, therapy of acute hemolytic transfusion reactions should be especially directed to minimizing possible renal complications (*vide infra*).

Delayed hemolysis of donor cells may occur (usually three to ten days following the transfusion) as a result of post-transfusion sensitization of the recipient. Red blood cell destruction generally occurs by an extravascular mechanism, and is manifested principally by jaundice and progressive anemia. The latter, if severe, may be treated safely by further transfusion provided that serologic investigation has clarified the cause of the erythrocyte destruction so that repetition may be avoided.

Dangerous Universal Donor. A special instance of hemolytic transfusion reaction is the destruction of the Group A, B, or AB patient's cells by high-titer isoantibodies in the plasma of a Group O blood. In modern practice, every effort is made to screen Group O donor bloods so as to detect those with dangerously high titers of isoantibodies. Except under emergency conditions, Group O blood should be given to A, B, or AB recipients only if screening tests have defined the blood as "low titer." When a "dangerous universal donor" reaction does occur, its severity is usually tempered by the dilution effect of the recipient's plasma volume, the neutralizing effect of soluble group-specific A or B substance (or both) in the recipient plasma and the large recipient red cell mass. Nonetheless, hypotension, hemoglobinemia, hemoglobinuria, and renal shutdown may result. Clinical management is similar to that described above for hemolytic reactions resulting from destruction of donor cells.

When an A, B, or AB recipient must be transfused with multiple units (4 or more) of low-titer Group O whole blood, a cumulative effect of donor isoantibodies may result in relatively slow extravascular destruction of the patient's red blood cells. Jaundice and progressive anemia are the chief signs. If the patient requires further transfusions, it is advisable to continue with low-titer O blood and to resume type-specific blood only after two weeks have elapsed from the time of multiple Group O transfusions.

A special category of "dangerous donors" consists of those whose plasma contains isoantibodies (which may be of any blood group specificity) as a result of multiple transfusions received in the past. In many blood banks, donor isoantibodies against red cells will be detected by routine screening of all donor sera against commercially available cells containing all the clinically important erythrocyte antigens. Even when such screening has not been performed, the donor isoantibodies will be detected if a sensitive technique is employed for the minor cross-match. A particularly dangerous reaction may result when the plasma from multi-transfused donors contains antibodies to the recipient's platelets or leukocytes. Severe thrombocytopenia may be induced; and leukocyte antibodies may cause an anaphylaxis-like reaction, with hypotension, tachycardia, tachypnea, cyanosis, and the roentgenologic finding of "allergic pneumonia." Treatment is symptomatic.

Sensitivity to Donor Leukocytes, Platelets, or Plasma. Transfusion reactions in this category are observed in patients who have had multiple previous exposures to the homologous antigens either by repeated transfusions or by pregnancies. The aid of an experienced serologic laboratory should be sought to demonstrate the presence in the patient's plasma of antibodies to donor leukocytes and platelets. A provocative test for the extremely rare sensitivity to donor plasma may be performed by the slow intravenous administration (approximately 1 ml. per minute) of 15 to 20 ml. of donor plasma that has been centrifuged sufficiently to remove red cells, white cells, and platelets. A typical febrile reaction will occur within 90 minutes from the onset of injection if sensitization to plasma is present. Treatment of reactions caused by sensitization to donor leukocytes, platelets, or plasma is largely symptomatic. Similar reactions can be prevented subsequently by transfusing blood from which the offending antigen has been removed.

Unexplained Febrile Reactions. These continue to make up a large proportion of the febrile reactions observed on a busy hospital service. Incompatibility between recipient's plasma and donor's red cells, white cells, platelets, and plasma cannot be demonstrated, nor can pyrogens be detected. There have been several well documented reports of symptomatic reactions associated with rapid destruction of donor red cells in the absence of any evidence of incompatibility by an elaborate battery of in vitro serologic tests. Therefore, transfusion reactions that remain unexplained should be a source of continuing disquiet and a stimulus to persistent diagnostic investigation. Until the cause is found, the patient remains prey to recurring reactions with all subsequent transfusions.

Management of Renal Complications. A patient who has experienced severe hemorrhage with actual or impending hypovolemic shock, or who is suffering from bacteremia, may be precipitated into more severe circulatory collapse by any of the above described transfusion reactions. Under these circumstances the hazard of oliguric renal failure is ever present. The hazard is greatly increased when the reaction is of the acute hemolytic variety, in which the free hemoglobin that enters the urine may precipitate in the renal tubules.

The following recommendations for treatment of threatened or actual renal failure complicating transfusion reactions are based on a program developed by Barry and Crosby at the Walter Reed Medical Center. Urine flow, as a reliable indicator of renal function, is an important guide to management, and such measures as may be necessary should be taken to assure accurate measurement of urine volume at hourly intervals. The objective of treatment is to maintain a urine flow of at least 100 ml. per hour until the effects of the reaction have subsided. Systolic blood pressure should be maintained at a sufficient level (above 100 mm. of mercury) to assure adequate renal perfusion. As soon as the reaction has occurred, 20 grams of mannitol as a 20 per cent aqueous solution should be infused intravenously during a five-minute interval. This dose should initiate diuresis in the patient capable of responding to mannitol. In the event of an acute hemolytic reaction, the infusion of 45 mEq. of sodium bicarbonate subsequent to the test dose of mannitol may be indicated. Because some of the urine obtained at the end of the first hour may have been in the bladder before the reaction, an additional one-hour collection should be obtained to enable reliable evaluation of the patient's response to mannitol. If the urine flow is greater than 40 ml. per hour, intravenous fluid containing approximately 50 mEq. of sodium per liter as chloride or bicarbonate, e.g., 300 ml. normal saline plus 700 ml. 5 per cent dextrose in water, should be administered in sufficient volume to match the desired urine flow (100 to 150 ml. per hour) until the possibility of renal injury is past and the patient is able to take oral fluids in sufficient volume to maintain satisfactory urine flow. The original dose of mannitol may be repeated whenever urine flow drops below 100 ml. per hour for any two-hour period, but not more than 100 grams of mannitol should be administered in any 24-hour period.

If the patient does not respond to the above measures and renal shutdown has become established, Barry and Crosby recommend the following:

1. Restriction of fluid intake to 500 ml. plus visible output per 24 hours.

2. Provision of 100 grams of carbohydrate per day at a constant rate to avoid periods of hypoglycemia and to decrease catabolism.

3. Control of hyperkalemia by the administration of 15 to 30 grams of sodium polystyrene sulfonate resin every six hours by mouth or by rectum.

4. Transfer of the patient within the first few days of oliguria to a Renal Center. Prior to transport, any ECG abnormality associated with hyperkalemia should be corrected by the infusion of 25 per cent glucose in distilled water containing 25 units of regular insulin and 200 ml. of 10 per cent calcium gluconate per liter. An infusion rate of 3 ml. per minute or more may be required during the first 30 minutes to return the electrocardiogram to normal. Thereafter, during transportation, rates of 0.25 to 1 ml. per minute will usually protect the patient from cardiac arrest.

Subsequent Transfusion of the Reaction-Prone Patient. There is always an increased hazard in transfusing a recipient who has had a previous transfusion reaction. Therefore, the indications for subsequent transfusions in these patients should be subjected to especially critical scrutiny, and transfusion should be avoided whenever possible. On the other hand, the added hazard should not engender indecision and delay, to the detriment of the patient. Informed of the possible causes for transfusion reactions, supported by the results of thorough investigation of previous reactions in the patient, and possessing a variety of sensitive cross-matching procedures as well as methods for separating donor blood to provide only the components actually needed by the patient, the physician can proceed with confidence to meet such a patient's transfusion needs. The transfusion should be administered slowly, and the patient should be watched especially carefully to detect the earliest signs of recurrent reaction so that the procedure can be discontinued if serious symptoms develop.

Barry, K. G., and Crosby, W. H.: The prevention and treatment of renal failure following transfusion reactions. Transfusion, 3:34, 1963.

Cassell, M., Phillips, D. R., and Chaplin, J., Jr.: Transfusion of buffy coat-poor red cell suspensions prepared by dextran sedimentation. Transfusion, 2:216, 1962.

Chaplin, H., Jr., and Cassell, M.: The occasional fallibility of in vitro compatibility tests. Transfusion, 2:375, 1962.

Mirick, G. S., Ward, R., and McCollum, R. W.: Modification of post-transfusion hepatitis by gamma globulin. New Eng. J. Med., 273:59, 1965.

Strumia, M. M., Crosby, W. H., Gibson, J. G., Greenwalt, T. J., and Krevans, J. R.: General Principles of Blood Transfusion. Philadelphia, J. B. Lippincott Company, 1963.

Young, L. E.: Complications of blood transfusion. Ann. Intern. Med., 61:136, 1964.

Polycythemia

Edward H. Reinhard

Definition. Polycythemia is best defined as an abnormal increase in red blood cell mass rather than as an increase in the number of red blood cells; an abnormal increase in hemoglobin is invariably accompanied by an increase in erythrocytes, but the converse is not always so. Some writers apply the term *erythrocytosis* to polycythemias secondary to recognized causes, and the term *erythremia* to the idiopathic disorder otherwise known as *polycythemia (rubra) vera*. Polycythemic syndromes include those that are relative (owing to hemoconcentration), benign, secondary to a variety of causes, and primary.

RELATIVE POLYCYTHEMIA

Relative polycythemia occurs when there is a decrease of plasma without comparable decrease of red blood cells so that the erythrocytes become more concentrated. Restricted fluid intake alone may lead within a few days to lowered plasma volume. A more common mechanism in disease is increased loss of water and electrolytes because of diabetic acidosis, the postoperative state, diuretic therapy of congestive heart failure, vomiting, diarrhea, abnormal sweating, hyposthenuria, adrenal insufficiency, or excessive plasma loss owing to extensive burns or traumatic shock. The hemoconcentration accompanying dehydration rarely gives rise to more than a 25 per cent increase in hematocrit, but the leukocyte level may rise considerably more owing to mobilization from marrow and marginal leukocyte pools or stimulation of leukopoiesis by the disorder producing the dehydration. Restoration of fluid balance with appropriate amounts of water and electrolytes promptly abolishes the relative polycythemia. Release of erythrocytes from storage in the spleen in normal man is never sufficient to produce significant polycythemia.

GAISBÖCK'S SYNDROME, STRESS POLYCYTHEMIA, AND BENIGN POLYCYTHEMIA

Gaisböck in 1905 described 18 patients with hypertension associated with an elevated red blood cell count but without splenomegaly; subsequently this combination of findings became known as Gaisböck's syndrome. This term gradually fell into disuse, and some authors believed that these were patients in whom mild erythrocytosis and hypertension coexisted by coincidence.

In 1952 Lawrence and Berlin reported 18 patients with erythrocytosis in whom blood volume determinations revealed normal red blood cell mass and decreased plasma volume. It was thus apparent that these patients had relative polycythemia. Half of them had hypertension. The authors were so impressed by the anxiety-tension state of these patients that they attributed the relative polycythemia to "stress." Similar cases were described by other authors, and the diagnosis of "stress polycythemia" became popular. In 1964 Russell and Conley studied 25 patients with polycythemia who did not have the associated symptoms, the splenomegaly, the leukocytosis, and the thrombocytosis characteristic of polycythemia vera and in whom dehydration and arterial oxygen unsaturation were excluded. These patients formed a strikingly homogeneous group. They were predominantly white males with a mean age of 45 years, which was somewhat younger than that for patients with polycythemia vera. They tended to be moderately overweight and of stocky habitus. Slight plethora and suffusion of the eyes were common. Many of the patients were tense and nervous. Almost all of them smoked cigarettes. Twelve of the 25 patients had persistent hypertension. None of these patients had any demonstrable congenital heart disease, pulmonary disease, or vascular shunts. None had clubbing of the fingers or a palpable spleen. The highest documented hematocrit values for the group ranged between 54.5 and 65 per cent. Blood volume determinations were done on ten of the patients. Some had a mild absolute polycythemia, whereas others had only relative polycythemia. Seven of these 25 patients had had significant vascular disease (myocardial infarction, intermittent claudication, cerebrovascular accident, Leriche syndrome, or thrombophlebitis). Russell and Conley believed that the recurring pattern of manifestations justified the concept of a unique syndrome that they called benign polycythemia. They emphasized that this is the same syndrome described by earlier authors under the designations Gaisböck's syndrome or stress polycythemia. They doubted, however, that stress played any part in the etiology of the erythrocytosis, and were of the opinion that multiple features of the syndrome are of constitutional pathogenesis and, at times, of familial occurrence. Some patients with high hematocrit values are undoubtedly normal persons whose hematocrit and red blood cell counts fall rather far from the mean on the normal curves of distribution. The recognition of such persons and patients with the Gaisböck or benign polycythemia syndrome is important, because they should not be given radioactive phosphorus or alkylating agents. It is not established that venesection is of any value.

SECONDARY POLYCYTHEMIAS

A variety of conditions, most of which are associated with tissue hypoxia, may lead to the development of secondary polycythemia.

Pathologic Physiology. Sustained secondary polycythemia often occurs when there is prolonged lowering of the oxygen *tension* of the arterial blood despite a normal or elevated hemoglobin content. In polycythemia secondary to arterial anoxemia, the oxygen tension of the arterial blood is less than normal in spite of the increased oxygen-carrying capacity. This, together with increased viscosity of the blood and the underlying circulatory burden imposed by the primary cardiac or pulmonary disease, results in decreased delivery of oxygen to the tissues. The plasma of hypoxic animals and of man has been shown to produce accelerated erythropoiesis in recipient animals. The decreased delivery of oxygen to the tissues does not stimulate the bone marrow directly but rather acts on the kidneys, which mediate the release of the hormonal substance erythropoietin. Erythropoietin, in turn, stimulates increased erythropoiesis in the bone marrow. In almost all types of secondary polycythemia, increased levels of erythropoietin have been demonstrated in the plasma.

Situations and Disorders Causing Secondary Polycythemia. Polycythemia secondary to cardiac or pulmonary disease occurs when there is less than normal oxygen saturation of the blood entering the aorta because of short-circuiting of the pulmonary capillary bed by passage of part of the venous blood from the right directly into the left side of the heart or into the aorta, e.g., patent atrial or ventricular septum, dextroposition of the aorta, pulmonary arteriovenous fistula, or when the alveolar ventilation is restricted because of chronic pulmonary disease, e.g., emphysema or silicosis, or when there is thickening of the alveolar membranes, e.g., in mitral stenosis, or some other type of alveolar-capillary block preventing normal transfer of oxygen from the alveoli to the blood. Tremendous obesity (pickwickian syndrome), massive abdominal tumor, or ascites may decrease pulmonary ventilation and thus contribute to the development of secondary polycythemia. Healthy persons living at high altitudes have polycythemia proportional to the diminution in oxygen tensions of the inspired air (and hence in the arterial blood).

A high incidence of polycythemia in certain families has been recognized for many years. Recently it has been established that at least some *familial polycythemias* are the result of inherited hemoglobin abnormalities. The first such report involved an 81-year-old Caucasian man and 15 members of his family, in all of whom a new hemoglobin variant, hemoglobin Chesapeake, comprised about 30 per cent of the total hemoglobin. Hemoglobin Chesapeake has an abnormal alpha chain, the arginine residue at the ninety-second position being replaced by leucine (alpha$_2^{92}$ leu beta$_2$). This abnormal hemoglobin has an oxygen dissociation curve which is "shifted to the left"; it has an increased affinity for oxygen, and red blood cells containing such hemoglobin give up less oxygen to the tissues, with resultant stimulation of erythropoietin production. Since this initial report, familial polycythemia has been found to be caused by many other hemoglobin variants, including hemoglobins J Capetown, Yakima, Kempsey, Rainier, Hiroshima, and Ypsilanti. In all these familial polycythemias, the affected members of the families have had hematocrits in the range of 45 to 58 per cent with a proportionate elevation of the erythrocyte count and hemoglobin levels; none of them has had leukocytosis, thrombocytosis, or splenomegaly. There has been no associated disability.

A mild compensatory erythrocytosis may occur in patients with long-standing methemoglobinemia or sulfhemoglobinemia, particularly when the pigment abnormality is secondary to certain chemicals such as analine dyes or gum shellac. Methemoglobinemia associated with hemoglobin M is only rarely associated with erythrocytosis. Cobalt is thought to produce secondary polycythemia by direct stimulation of erythropoietin production.

Polycythemia occurs in association with primary aldosteronism, and may be induced by the administration of large doses of testosterone or vasopressin. Relative polycythemia is common in Cushing's syndrome, but a true polycythemia may occur if both corticosteroid and androgen production are increased.

Secondary polycythemia has also been reported in association with many types of cancer and a few benign tumors. The tumors which produce secondary polycythemia most frequently are malignant renal tumors and brain tumors; the brain tumors have usually been vascular tumors most commonly located in the posterior fossa. Papilledema was present in most of these cases. In one series of 37 cases of brain tumor (usually hemangioblastoma) with associated polycythemia, the hemoglobin returned to normal after removal of the tumor in 21 instances. Polycythemia has also been observed in association with carcinomas of the liver, prostate, lung, rectum, and breast, as well as with melanosarcomas, multiple myeloma, and pheochromocytoma. Secondary polycythemia also occurs in association with many types of renal disease other than tumors, including medullary cystic disease, renal tuberculosis, hydronephrosis, and renal artery stenosis, as well as after renal transplantation. There is evidence that many of the tumors and even some of the benign cysts of the kidneys elaborate a substance having erythropoietin-like activity that is responsible for the excessive erythropoiesis.

Clinical Manifestations. In contrast to the disabling acute symptoms that appear on ascent to an altitude of 10,000 feet or more, most permanent residents at such elevations make a satisfactory adjustment and are asymptomatic. By virtue of the increased oxygen-carrying power of the blood and an increase in erythrocyte 2,3-diphosphoglycerate, sufficient compensation for its lowered oxygen tension is achieved so that these people are able to carry on muscular work with comparative ease. However, Monge has described *chronic mountain sickness* in occasional persons living at such altitudes who presumably have chronic pulmonary disease as a superimposed additional cause of arterial anoxia. Recurrent bronchitis and laryngitis over a long period of time develop into an incapacitating illness characterized by headache, tinnitus, dyspnea, anorexia, vomiting, and lethargy. These symptoms are greatly aggravated by slight exertion. The chest is emphysematous, and the vital capacity is reduced. Cyanosis, clubbing of the digits, and congestion of the scleral capillaries are prominent. Examination of the blood reveals polycythemia that is severe relative to that of normal residents living at the same altitude. The blood volume is increased, and reticulocytosis, moderately increased bilirubinemia, and sometimes leukocytosis are found. Return to sea level promptly relieves the symptoms, and the polycythemia gradually subsides. *Brisket disease,* affecting 1 to 5 per cent of cattle grazing in certain areas at high altitudes in Utah and Colorado, is an interesting counterpart of chronic mountain sickness in man. Brisket disease affects young calves mainly and, unlike Monge's disease, is characterized by pulmonary hypertension followed by right heart failure. The animals do not have sustained arterial oxygen desaturation, and they do not develop significant polycythemia. All animals that have been studied show a thick muscular coat around the small pulmonary arteries; it has been postulated that excessive development of this muscular coat as well as excessive fluid and salt intake caused by grazing on marshy ground are factors that contribute to the pulmonary hypertension and cor pulmonale in the affected animals.

Polycythemias secondary to cardiac or pulmonary disease are accompanied by symptoms and signs characteristic of the primary disease. The patients are invariably cyanotic and often have clubbing of the digits. Cardiac failure is common. Slight splenomegaly may be due to congestive failure or chronic pulmonary infection. *Ayerza's syndrome* is a condition characterized by slowly developing symptoms of pulmonary insufficiency, cyanosis, and polycythemia owing to primary disease of the pulmonary artery and its branches (arterial and arteriolar sclerosis, syphilis, or congenital hypoplasia of the pulmonary artery), aggravated, in some cases, by emphysema and pulmonary fibrosis. In this condition right-sided heart failure eventually develops.

In these secondary forms of polycythemia the erythrocyte level often reaches 8 million and occasionally 10 million cells per cubic millimeter, usually with somewhat less than corresponding hemoglobin and hematocrit values. Reticulocytosis and slight hyperbilirubinemia are characteristic. Leukocytosis is absent except when resulting from associated infection, which also seems in some cases to restrict the polycythemic response to the arterial unsaturation. The essential diagnostic criterion of secondary polycythemia of this type is decreased oxygen saturation of the blood, which is almost always less than 90 per cent. The arterial oxygen saturation should always be determined at rest and following standard exercise; under the latter circumstances the arterial oxygen saturation remains approximately 95 per cent in normal persons and in most patients with polycythemia vera, whereas in patients with polycythemia secondary to anoxemia the arterial oxygen saturation following exercise always falls to less than 80 per cent and usually to much less than this (occasionally as low as 30 per cent).

Treatment. The treatment of secondary polycythemia is chiefly that of the underlying cardiac or pulmonary disorder or removal of the tumor. Elimination of the offending drug or toxic exposure relieves the polycythemia caused by methemoglobinemia, sulfhemoglobinemia, or carboxyhemoglobinemia. In acute episodes of cyanosis, oxygen administration may be helpful. The polycythemia with resultant increased oxygen-carrying capacity of the blood is a useful compensatory physiologic response. However, if the hematocrit value rises to levels above 65 or 70 per cent, phlebotomies may result in temporary relief of symptoms, perhaps because the bleeding lowers blood volume and viscosity.

PRIMARY POLYCYTHEMIA
(Polycythemia Vera, Erythremia)

Primary polycythemia is a chronic disease of unknown cause characterized by hyperplasia of all the cellular elements of the bone marrow, nucleated red blood cells being most prominently involved, with resultant sustained elevation of the red blood cell count and hemoglobin level and usually, to a lesser extent, leukocytosis and thrombocytosis. It has been regarded by many persons as a malignant neoplastic disease of the erythropoietic tissue analogous to leukemia. The relationship of these two diseases is emphasized by the fact that in primary polycythemia the leukocytosis is sometimes so pronounced as to suggest a diagnosis of chronic granulocytic leukemia, and many patients with well-established polycythemia eventually have developed blood and bone marrow findings, and even pathologic changes at autopsy, suggestive of leukemia even when no radiation therapy has been given. Conversely, several patients with typical granulocytic leukemia have been observed to develop polycythemia. Furthermore, in patients with primary polycythemia treated with radioactive phosphorus, the incidence of acute leukemia as a late manifestation has varied enormously in different series of cases (from 0 to greater than 20 per cent).

Aneuploidy and several other nonspecific chromosomal aberrations have been reported in untreated patients with polycythemia vera. In P[32]-treated patients, the frequency of these aberrations is moderately higher. According to a recent study, the one finding typical of P[32]-treated patients is the presence of dicentric chromosomes, and a dose response curve to the last P[32]-dose was demonstrated. A Philadelphia-like chromosome was observed in two patients with polycythemia vera and in one with benign erythrocytosis, all following P[32] therapy. These authors speculated whether the development of leukemia complicating P[32]-treated polycythemia might be dependent on the type and location of radiation-induced chromosomal damage, with the subsequent establishment of a clone of cells with a selective developmental advantage. There is no evidence that tissue anoxia or excessive production of any known endocrine or humoral factor, including erythropoietin, constitutes the stimulus to excessive blood cell production in primary polycythemia. When marrow from patients with polycythemia vera is incubated in vitro with erythropoietin, the rate of heme synthesis increases over the controls by only one tenth of the normal marrow response. Marrows from polycythemia vera patients in remission respond normally to erythropoietin. These data suggest that the disease is due to an abnormal cell line whose intrinsic stem cell defect does not allow normal control of erythrocytic production by the usual regulatory substance, erythropoietin.

It is now well established that many types of fowl and animal leukemia are due to viruses. Likewise, it has been observed that a "polycythemic virus" (a variant of Friend virus, or a passenger virus present in spleen filtrate prepared originally from mice infected with Friend virus) when injected into normal mice results in polycythemia and splenomegaly. Furthermore, this virus can initiate erythropoiesis in hypertransfused-polycythemic mice. The only other substance known to initiate erythropoiesis in a hypertransfused-polycythemic state is erythropoietin. The fact that this polycythemic virus causes an increase in proerythroblasts, erythroblasts, and reticulocytes and an increase in Fe[59] uptake in the bone marrow and spleen without detectable erythropoietin activity in the plasma and urine suggests that the virus acts directly on erythropoietic stem cells and not through the mediation of erythropoietin. It is not presently known whether these animal data have any applicability to human polycythemia vera.

It is now established that, in untreated polycythemia vera, the erythropoietic cells in the bone marrow do not respond normally to erythropoietin. The erythropoietin activity of plasma from patients with polycythemia is not increased, and no measurable level of erythropoietin can be found in the urine. However, when the hematocrits of patients with polycythemia vera are reduced to normal or anemic levels by bleeding, measurable amounts of erythropoietin appear in the urine. Patients with hypoxia-induced erythrocytosis have increased levels of urinary erythropoietin.

The incidence of this disease is high among Jews and low among Negroes. Men are more commonly affected than women. The usual age of onset is in middle or later life, although, rarely, young adults or children are affected. Familial polycythemia has been reported, and in these families onset of the disease in childhood is more common; as previously stated, at least some familial polycythemias are due to inherited hemoglobin variants.

Pathologic Physiology. In uncomplicated primary polycythemia the cardiac output and work are normal, but the velocity of blood flow is greatly slowed. Pulmonary functions are normal or nearly so. The arterial saturation of the blood is normal in most instances. Hypoxia has been demonstrated in some patients with polycythemia vera, but in such cases it has usually been attributed to unrelated coexisting cardiorespiratory disease. However, one study of 26 patients with polycythemia vera who had no evident heart or lung disease revealed that, although all of them had normal ventilatory function, 9 patients had an arterial oxygen saturation of less than 92 per cent and 11 patients had a mean arterial oxygen tension that was significantly lowered (that is, less than 80 mm. Hg). The diffusing capacity for carbon monoxide was significantly lower than normal in ten of these patients, and the defect in diffusing capacity appeared to correlate well with the level of hypoxia. It was suggested that these abnormalities might be due to widespread thrombosis in small pulmonary arteries. Whether this is the correct explanation or not, it is important to emphasize that many studies have confirmed the fact that *mild* hypoxemia is *not* uncommon in patients with well established polycythemia vera, and the arterial oxygen saturation is of little value in distinguishing between primary and secondary polycythemia unless the arterial saturation is less than 90 per cent.

Many of the clinical manifestations, as well as intravascular thrombosis, which is the most common complication of untreated primary polycythemia, can be attributed directly or indirectly to three factors: (1) increased total blood volume, (2) increased viscosity of the blood, and (3) thrombocytosis. The feeling of fullness and aching in the head and the fatigability characteristic of this disease can be relieved by phlebotomies so promptly and so consistently that it seems probable that the increased blood volume is a major factor in the pathogenesis of these symptoms. Some patients with this disease continue to have mild symptoms at times when the red blood cell level and the hematocrit value are in the upper portion of the normal range, and yet are completely asymptomatic when these values are reduced to the lower normal range. The extent to which the increased viscosity of the blood contributes to these symptoms and to the high incidence of intravascular thrombosis is not entirely clear, but the circulation time may be greatly prolonged with resultant visceral stasis; increased blood viscosity is at least a contributory factor. As the hematocrit level rises above normal there is a progressively more rapid increase in the blood viscosity; the higher the hematocrit rises above 60 per cent, the more imperative becomes the need to lower the hematocrit, and hence the viscosity, in order to relieve symptoms and minimize the danger of intravascular thrombosis. Paradoxically, when the hematocrit is greatly elevated, there is also a tendency to bleed excessively from minor injuries; this may be caused, in part, by the distention of the capillaries and veins required to accommodate the huge blood volume. However, there is a coagulation defect as well, because thromboplastin generation is abnormal and platelet factor 3 activity is reduced in the blood of patients with polycythemia vera who have thrombocytosis. The thrombocytosis may be pronounced, and is probably of more importance than the increased blood viscosity in the production of intravascular thromboses, as the incidence of thromboses is low in secondary polycythemia (high viscosity, normal platelet level).

In untreated polycythemia vera, the marrow iron stores are often depleted, and hypoferremia is not uncommon. Furthermore, as would be expected under these circumstances, the plasma iron disappearance time (T 1/2) is often markedly shortened. Following repletion of the iron stores by parenteral iron dextran administration, the plasma iron disappearance time increases toward normal. In uncomplicated *secondary* polycythemia, the marrow iron stores are normal or increased, and the plasma iron disappearance time is increased less than in polycythemia vera.

In polycythemia vera, there is very poor correlation between the hemoglobin value and the packed red blood cell volume on the one hand, and the total red blood cell mass on the other. This is due to the fact that the plasma volume in polycythemia vera may be normal, decreased, or increased.

The basal metabolic rate is frequently elevated. The increased production of blood cells results in an increased destruction of blood cells, and this in turn means increased nucleoprotein turnover. Since the end product of nucleoprotein degradation is uric acid, it is not surprising that hyperuricemia or increased urate excretion occurs in 75 per cent of cases of untreated polycythemia vera and that at least 5 per cent of patients develop clinical gout.

Clinical Manifestations. Symptoms may vary from none to so many that psychoneurosis is suspected. Common presenting complaints include headache or a feeling of fullness in the head, itching that is aggravated by a hot bath, paresthesias, dizziness, weakness, fatigability, dyspnea, and visual disturbances. A ruddy complexion usually of considerable duration, skin or mucous membrane hemorrhages, or awareness of a heavy sensation or fullness in the left side of the abdomen owing to enlargement of the spleen may be the initial manifestations. The plethora is especially noticeable in the face, mouth, neck, hands, and feet. The veins of the scleras and retinas are distended and dark. Elevation of the systolic pressure occurs in more than half the cases, but diastolic hypertension is no more common than in the general population. Hepatomegaly occurs in about half the cases and splenomegaly in over three fourths.

The red blood cells frequently number from 7 to 10 million or more per cubic millimeter when patients are first seen. The erythrocytes usually appear normal, but the hemoglobin value may be increased less, in proportion, than the erythrocyte level because of a low mean corpuscular volume and mean corpuscular hemoglobin. Sometimes there is hypochromia (low mean corpuscular hemoglobin concentration) in addition to microcytosis, especially after large hemorrhages or repeated phlebotomies. The reticulocyte percentage is usually normal, but the absolute number is increased. Reticulocytosis occurs, and normoblasts may appear in the blood, especially after hemorrhage. The leukocyte count is greater than 10,000 per cubic millimeter in more than half the patients; it is frequently over 25,000, and rarely as high as 50,000. Metamyelocytes and occasional myelocytes are seen in the blood. The platelets are usually increased in number, and counts as high as 3 million and even 6 million have been reported. The serum bilirubin levels, urine urobilinogen and stool urobilin values are commonly slightly increased.

Among the common complications of the disease are the vascular thromboses already referred to; the incidence of such thromboses can be greatly reduced by adequate therapy. Cirrhosis of the liver and occlusion of the hepatic veins (*Budd-Chiari syndrome*) have been observed. Hemorrhage from varices in the esophagus, stomach, bowel, or rectum may be massive, as may be bleeding from duodenal ulcers, which occurs in 8 to 16 per cent of cases. Many patients with polycythemia vera, after an extremely variable interval ranging from a few years to over 20 years, develop compensated myeloid metaplasia. During this phase they usually have severe splenomegaly and occasionally considerable leukocytosis with the appearance of increasing numbers of immature granulocytic leukocytes in the blood. The red blood cell count and hematocrit may remain perfectly normal without therapy. This phase may last from six months to several years, and is usually followed by the development of myelofibrosis, progressive myeloid metaplasia often with a leukemoid blood picture, and progressive anemia.

Treatment. The treatment of primary polycythemia is directed toward maintenance of a reasonably normal blood volume, viscosity, and thrombocyte level. When the hematocrit rises above 55 per cent, blood should be withdrawn. Myelosuppressive therapy should be employed (1) whenever, in order to keep the hematocrit below 55 per cent, it is necessary to withdraw blood so frequently that iron deficiency of sufficient degree to produce symptoms develops, or (2) when the platelet count rises significantly above normal. Radioactive phosphorus therapy is a very effective means of suppressing excessive hematopoiesis; 3.5 to 5 millicuries intravenously (or 4.5 to 6.5 millicuries by mouth) is a reasonable dose. If too much radioactive phosphorus is given, leukopenia, thrombocytopenia, anemia, or any combination of these may develop. Further treatment should not be given for at least two or three months, for this length of time is required before the red blood cell counts stabilize. An additional, somewhat smaller dose of P^{32} may then be necessary. Once the blood has been restored to normal by such treatment, it is desirable not to give further radiation therapy for at least one, and preferably, several years, occasional phlebotomies being resorted to in the meantime as necessary. It seems likely that such conservative therapy will minimize the danger of the patient's developing a radiation-induced acute leukemia. Control of the manifestations of polycythemia vera by radioactive phosphorus is so smooth that patients so treated have a greater number of symptom-free days than from any other form of treatment available. Nitrogen mustard, triethylene melamine, busulfan, chlorambucil, cyclophosphamide, and phenylalanine mustard have all been used successfully to reduce excessive hematopoiesis in this disease; the first two drugs are seldom employed for this purpose any longer, and there are insufficient data to indicate which of the latter four drugs is superior. If chemotherapy is being employed as the *only* form of therapy, busulfan should probably be avoided as it produces the most persistent and prolonged platelet depression. However, if the red blood cell level is being controlled by phlebotomies, and the only indication for drug treatment is control of marked thrombocytosis, busulfan may be the drug of choice. Any of these drugs may also be used as an adjunct to P^{32} therapy in the occa-

sional patient who develops severe thrombocytosis or progressive leukocytosis refractory to P^{32}. During therapy with any alkylating agent much closer supervision of the patient is necessary than when P^{32} is used. It is apparent that at present there are many different ways of treating this disease. The author believes that phlebotomy should be used as the primary method of control of the hematocrit; busulfan, chlorambucil, cyclophosphamide, or phenylalanine mustard should be used as an adjunct to phlebotomies when needed to control a markedly elevated platelet count; and P^{32} should be reserved for treatment of elderly patients, patients who cannot be seen by the physician at frequent intervals, and those rare patients who are refractory to other forms of treatment. Irradiation of the spleen, if it becomes uncomfortably large, may relieve the discomfort. Splenectomy is contraindicated, because an increase in the platelet level with resultant fatal thrombosis may result. Elective surgery of any sort should never be done until the platelet and hematocrit levels have been restored to normal. If emergency major surgery is unavoidable in a polycythemic patient with very high hematocrit and platelet levels, an immediate phlebotomy and P^{32} administration can be done within half an hour; rapid ambulation of the patient after surgery is imperative.

It is paradoxic that after blood has been withdrawn repeatedly over a period of many years, in the late stages of the disease transfusions are often necessary.

Erslev, A.: Erythropoietic activity of serum and bone marrow after time limited exposure to anemic and hypoxic anoxia. J. Lab. Clin. Med., 50:543, 1957.

Jepson, J. H.: Polycythemia: Diagnosis, pathophysiology and therapy. Canad. Med. Ass. J., 100:271, 1969.

Lertzman, M., Frome, B. M., and Israels, L. G.: Hypoxia in polycythemia vera. Ann. Intern. Med., 60:409, 1964.

Modan, B., and Lilienfeld, A. M.: Polycythemia vera and leukemia—The role of radiation treatment. Medicine, 44:305, 1965.

Reinhard, E. H., and Hahneman, B.: The treatment of polycythemia vera. J. Chron. Dis., 6:332, 1958.

Diseases of the White Blood Cells and Reticuloendothelial System

INTRODUCTION
Carl V. Moore

Information about the physiology, function, life span, and turnover rates for leukocytes is accumulating rapidly as the result of studies using biochemical, immunologic, and radioactive labeling techniques. Investigators are less preoccupied with unsolved questions about cell origins and have focused on physiologic problems that can be explored more profitably with current methods.

Leukocytes serve important functions in host resistance to infection and in reparative processes. Granulocytes contain at least three antimicrobial agents (phagocytin, lysozyme, and acid) that enable them to destroy ingested bacteria. Phagocytosis may be influenced by the presence of opsonins, but neutrophils may also engulf bacteria by trapping them against suitable surfaces (surface phagocytosis) even in the absence of antibody. As the bacterium is taken into the cell, it becomes encased in a coating of cellular membrane carried with it, and is outside the body of the cell just as intestinal luminal contents are "outside" the body. This particle ingestion is an energy-requiring process, utilizing ATP, and is dependent on active glycolysis within the cell; during phagocytosis, oxygen consumption of the neutrophil is accelerated, glucose is utilized, lactic acid and H_2O_2 are produced, and the number of granules decreases. The partial degranulation is of particular interest. Neutrophilic granules are lysosomes that contain phagocytin, several aldolases, and other proteolytic and hydrolytic enzymes. Within a short time after phagocytosis occurs, the lysosomes empty their content into and fuse with the phagocytic vacuole. As a result of the fusion, the enzymes reach the vacuole without gaining access to the cytoplasm of the cell proper.

The total life span of leukocytes is more difficult to measure than that of red blood corpuscles. Whereas the erythrocyte, once delivered to the peripheral blood, stays in the blood until it is destroyed, the white blood cell is merely transported by the blood from the bone marrow or other tissue of origin to tissues where it serves its function. Using isotopic techniques, investigators have demonstrated that the average granulocyte spends approximately 6 to 11 days in the bone marrow. During development, mitotic division occurs at the myeloblast, promyelocyte, and myelocyte stages before maturation is completed; the marrow contains a storage pool of granulocytes that is about 25 times greater than the number of circulating cells. In the peripheral blood, about half the granulocytes normally are freely circulating while the remainder are sequestered in capillaries as a marginated granulocyte pool, capable of being swept into circulation with exercise and other similar stimulation. The average blood transit time has been estimated to be about nine hours, with a few cells remaining in the peripheral blood long enough to develop pyknotic nuclei as a result of senescence (24 to 48 hours). Once granulocytes get out into tissues, they probably survive for only a few days, and apparently do not re-enter the circulating blood, at least not in large numbers. Some cells are lost in body secretions, but the majority probably disintegrate, particularly in liver, spleen, and lymph nodes.

Lymphocytes play a pivotal role in many immune functions. They recirculate through lymphoid tissues, lymphatics, and peripheral blood, and may be divided into two types. (1) The majority are dependent on the thymus for differentiation and development; they exercise functions related to cell-mediated immunities (delayed or bacterial allergy, certain homograft immunities, graft-versus-host reactions, and defense against malignant adaptation). (2) The remainder are a thymus-independent population capable of antibody and immunoglobulin synthesis. This type has been called the "gut-associated lymphoid line" because the cells come under the influence of the bursa of Fabricus in birds, and possibly of the appendix and Peyer's patches in mammals. The idea that the lymphocyte is a multipotential progenitor of other blood cells has become less popular. About one third of circulating lymphocytes apparently have a life span of less than two weeks; the remainder are long-lived cells with a mean life span of four to five years; some may survive as long as 20 years.

Mononuclear phagocytic cells exhibit physiologic properties of sticking to glass, membrane ruffling, and ingestion of fluid droplets (pinocytosis) or of particles (phagocytosis) from the environment. Recent studies favor the concept that these cells constitute a separate cell line that originates from a proliferating pool of promonocytes in the bone marrow, are transported as young adult forms (monocytes) in the blood, and then emigrate into tissues where they undergo further maturation to become macrophages. The ratio of tissue phagocytes to circulating monocytes has been estimated to be 400 to 1. Normally tissue macrophages undergo a slow turnover, i.e., 50 to 60 days for Kupffer cells and alveolar macrophages, and divide infrequently, but may multiply extensively under pathologic conditions. The factors that govern production, release, and turnover are unknown. The life history of mononuclear phagocytes differs from that of polymorphonuclear leukocytes in that (1) newly formed monocytes are released promptly from the marrow rather than being retained for several days in a maturation pool, (2) the average blood transit time is longer (about 32 hours), and (3) the sojourn in tissues is measurable in months rather than a few days. The so-called free macrophages of the serous cavities, lymph nodes, and spleen probably can be mobilized and transported by the blood to other organs. Many of the functions of mononuclear phagocytic cells are related to their endocytic activities (pinocytosis and phagocytosis) and the subsequent biochemical reactions that alter the ingested material; pinocytic vesicles contribute to lysosome formation by fusing with pre-existing lysosomes, and influence, by their content, the lysosomal enzymes that are induced. Known functions include phagocytosis of foreign particles, macromolecules, and collagen; phagocytosis of blood cells and degradation of hemoglobin; ingestion and destruction of susceptible bacteria; and important roles in cellular and viral immunity, delayed hypersensitivity, and antibody formation. A review of these latter relationships would require more space than is available here.

Unfortunately, the increased information about the biology and function of leukocytes cannot yet be translated into better methods for diagnosing or treating diseases of the white blood cells. Reliance for diagnosis must be based largely on the recognition of abnormal cells or pathologic changes in the peripheral blood, bone marrow, or other tissue. There are no practical ways to assay variations in the rates of leukocyte production or destruction. Diagnostic help can occasionally be obtained in the differentiation between chronic granulocytic leukemia and leukemoid reactions by determining leukocyte alkaline phosphatase, the blood vitamin B_{12} level, or the presence of the Philadelphia chromosome. Marked elevations in serum and urine lysozyme concentrations aid in the recognition of monocytic leukemia.

The etiologic factors or agents responsible for these diseases are known in only a few instances. Although therapy is still disappointing and only palliative in many instances, very significant progress has been made in the management of acute leukemia in children and of lymphomas. Hodgkin's disease can even be regarded as a potentially curable disorder.

Cline, M. J.: Metabolism of the circulating leukocyte. Physiol. Rev., 45:674, 1965.

Cronkite, E. P., and Fliedner, T. M.: Granulocytopoiesis. New Eng. J. Med., 270:1347; 1403, 1964.

Good, R. A.: The lymphocyte. Introduction. Seminars Hemat., 6:1, 1969.

Hirsch, J. G.: Cinemicrophotographic observation on granulocyte lysis in polymorphonuclear leukocytes during phagocytosis. J. Exp. Med., 116:827, 1962.

Perry, S.: Biochemistry of the white blood cell. J.A.M.A., 190:918, 1964.

van Furth, R.: Origin and kinetics of monocytes and macrophages. Seminars Hemat., 7:125, 1970.

Zucker-Franklin, D.: Electron microscopic studies of human granulocytes. Structural variations related to function. Seminars Hemat., 5:109, 1968.

THE LEUKOPENIC STATE AND AGRANULOCYTOSIS

William N. Valentine

THE LEUKOPENIC STATE

Leukopenia exists when a reduction below about 4000 per cubic millimeter occurs in the total blood leukocytes. In some instances the reduction in leukocyte numbers is balanced, and the differential count remains essentially normal. Much more frequently, the neutrophils are disproportionately low, in which case the term *neutropenia* or *granulocytopenia* is more accurately descriptive. *Lymphopenia* exists when the lymphocytes number below about 1400 per cubic millimeter in children, or 1000 per cubic millimeter in adults. Although severe leukopenia merges into agranulocytosis with its frequently fulminant clinical manifestations, the more moderate and usual degrees of leukopenia are often well tolerated. No hard and fast rule exists; many patients tolerate leukopenia as low as 1500 to 2000 per cubic millimeter without unusually severe or frequent infections, provided that the neutrophils constitute 15 to 20 per cent or more of the cells. With counts below this level and with more severe neutropenia, invasion of the mucous membranes, skin, and blood by micro-organisms becomes increasingly frequent and severe. However, there is considerable individual variability, and no precisely critical level can be accurately assumed.

Etiology of Leukopenia. *Infections* of various kinds are common causes: bacterial (typhoid and paratyphoid fever, brucellosis, at times tularemia, and overwhelming infections even with micro-organisms characteristically producing leukocytosis); viral (influenza, measles, dengue, infectious hepatitis, rubella, psittacosis); rickettsial (Rocky Mountain spotted fever, scrub typhus, typhus, rickettsialpox); protozoal (malaria, relapsing fever, kala-azar). *Diseases primarily involving the bone marrow* or interfering with its normal function are likewise frequently associated with leu-

disease, miliary tuberculosis, and bacterial endocarditis are also occasionally associated with extreme leukopenia. Such instances are not common, and the underlying disease is usually recognized on the basis of the other clinical findings. A carefully obtained history of drug or chemical exposure is often helpful.

Prognosis. Before the advent of antimicrobial drugs, mortality in well developed cases varied from 50 to 90 per cent, and approached 100 per cent in patients with counts below 1000 per cubic millimeter or in those over 60 years of age. At the present time, with early and proper antimicrobial management, most patients recover. Residual damage to leukopoietic tissue is usually not apparent.

Treatment. The fundamental basis of treatment is (1) immediate withdrawal of the offending agent, and (2) control of infection. Early cultures of the ulcerative mucous membrane lesions, the blood, the urine, and, if indicated, the cerebrospinal fluid are desirable and should be repeated as indicated by the clinical course. Antimicrobial therapy should be directed toward broad coverage and should not be withheld until the cultural results are known. However, therapy may require modification when the predominating organisms have been identified. It is, of course, important that all organisms cultured be tested for antimicrobial susceptibility. In many instances, the infecting organisms are those constituting "normal flora" rendered invasive by the presence of agranulocytosis in the patient. However, any micro-organisms may be offending, and the possibility of sepsis with gram-negative organisms such as Pseudomonas and Proteus or with penicillin-resistant staphylococci must be recognized by the treatment regimen. When agranulocytosis is detected, the writer prefers (1) immediate withdrawal of the offending medication, (2) hospitalization, (3) the administration of cephalothin (Keflin) intravenously in a dosage of 2 grams every four to six hours, combined with gentamicin intramuscularly, 1 mg. per kilogram of body weight every eight hours. The latter may be increased to 1.5 mg. per kilogram every eight hours when hypotension or other manifestations suggest severe sepsis. Because of its relative effectiveness against certain normal flora, some would favor the addition of penicillin G intravenously, 5 million units per day, to the aforementioned regimen if history of penicillin susceptibility is absent. If the offending agent is withdrawn, the clinician can take comfort that in most instances the agranulocytosis and, hence, need for antimicrobial therapy will be self-limited. The patient with agranulocytosis should be hospitalized in a single room, nurses or physicians with respiratory or other infections excluded, and visitors rigidly limited or excluded temporarily. The necessity for total "reverse isolation" with cap, gown, and mask precautions is advocated by some, but in the opinion of the writer it is of doubtful

report evidenc... or toxic factor... should be ma... This means w... sure consider... dance of subs... material, and... of improvemen... leukopenia.

AG...
(A...

Definition. ... in which the v... tously to low l... treme. Clinic... explosively; th... sion of tissue... ulcerations of... septicemia.

Etiology and ... instances agra... result of sens... fection then... cause, of the... cumstances, th... does not ordi... least 7 to 14... develop until... intermittent... rine, in which... able, a numbe... documented a... tosis in the... results in the... of patients re... tients who h... induced agra... of a small sin... experiments o... immune mech... tosis. He first... sensitive pati... amidopyrine. ... 300 ml. of blo... to a normal... 800 cells per... normal subje... about four ho... vitro of both l... cytes occurred... obtained from... after the cha... postulated th... destroyed and... Many of the... may do so by... that this is no... producing the... in certain pat... ing neutrope... develop gradu...

kopenia. These include aplastic and hypoplastic anemias, aleukemic leukemia, at times myelosclerosis and myelofibrosis, and widespread replacement of marrow such as occurs with lymphosarcoma. In this category must also be included hematopoietic depression associated with a wide and ever-increasing number of chemical and physical agents to which the population is exposed therapeutically, industrially, or environmentally. In certain instances, leukopenia is expected as a natural consequence of the therapeutic action of certain drugs such as the cytotoxic agent nitrogen mustard and its congeners, other alkylating drugs such as busulfan (Myleran), vinblastine and vincristine sulfate (Velban and Oncovin), and a wide variety of antimetabolites, including 6-mercaptopurine, the folic acid antagonists (Aminopterin, Amethopterin), 5-fluorouracil, and others. In other instances it develops as a side effect unrelated to therapeutic efficacy and with relatively high or low frequency. In some instances, the leukopenia appears to be associated with sensitivity or immunologic reactions engendered by drug administration. In other instances the mechanism is entirely unclear. The list of drugs producing leukopenia in certain patients is large and expanding. Those associated with a relatively or moderately high risk of leukopenia include the anticonvulsants methyl-phenyl-ethyl-hydantoin (Mesantoin) and trimethadione (Tridione); the antimicrobials chloramphenicol, arsenobenzol, and sulfonamides; the antithyroid agents thiouracil and, to a somewhat lesser extent, propylthiouracil and methimazole (Tapazole); the sedatives and analgesics allyl-isopropyl-acetylcarbamide (Sedormid) and amidopyrine; the phenothiazine antihistaminics; the antidiabetic drugs tolbutamide, chlorpropamide, and carbutamide; and such therapeutic agents as gold preparations and phenylbutazone (Butazolidin). Among other agents mentioned occasionally as apparent offenders are amphetamine, procaine amide, quinacrine (Atabrine), tripelennamine (Pyribenzamine), acetazolamide (Diamox), ethacrynic acid, hydroxychloroquine, and various antimicrobial drugs. The list is admittedly far from complete. Marrow depression and leukopenia also result from exposure to x-rays and other sources of external ionizing radiation and from the administration of radioactive material such as P^{32}. Exposure to benzol, to an unknown number of industrial chemicals and solvents, and to certain insecticides and sprays also carries the risk of leukopoietic depression. The hazards of benzol are particularly well recognized. *Splenic dysfunction* and almost any condition associated with splenomegaly may at times result in leukopenia alone or in combination with anemia or thrombocytopenia, or both. Thus leukopenia is frequently found in chronic congestive splenomegaly, in Gaucher's disease, in Felty's syndrome (rheumatoid arthritis, splenomegaly, and leukopenia), and in other splenomegalic states. Nutritional leukopenia may occur in deficiency of vitamin B_{12} or folic acid, in sprue, and

in a variety of chronic inanition states of multiple causes. It also occurs transiently as a component of anaphylactic foreign protein reactions. Leukopenia is also sometimes found for unknown reasons in disseminated lupus erythematosus and in paroxysmal nocturnal hemoglobinuria. In the latter disease, increased destruction of leukocytes by the unknown mechanism also responsible for hemolytic anemia may possibly occur.

Primary splenic neutropenia is a syndrome characterized by fever, pain over the spleen, variable splenomegaly, and neutropenia. In the few cases reported, manifestations varied from acute to chronic, and relief followed splenectomy. Doan regards this disorder as being due to splenic dysfunction ("hypersplenism"), resulting in selective, indiscriminate lysis of granulocytes by the spleen. In leukopenia associated with both idiopathic "hypersplenism" and that secondary to known disease, the bone marrow is normally cellular or hyperplastic, though with fewer mature granulocytes than usual.

Cyclic or periodic leukopenia is a poorly understood entity characterized by regular, recurrent diminution or disappearance of circulating neutrophils from the blood. The disease may persist for years, cycles of neutropenia occurring regularly, often with associated malaise and signs of infection. An average cycle is about 21 days, but variations from 14 to 45 days have been described. The cause is unknown. It may belong in the category of periodic disease.

Chronic hypoplastic neutropenia is a syndrome of unknown cause, having a chronic course usually associated with repeated infections, and sometimes with slight to moderate splenomegaly. It differs from primary splenic neutropenia in that *hypoplasia* of granulocytic precursor cells is found on marrow aspiration, and splenectomy is not beneficial. Rare cases have been described in which a strong predisposition to neutropenia appears familial (familial benign chronic leukopenia). A number of such cases have now been reported from Israel in Yemenite Jews, and similar cases have been seen in the United States and elsewhere. The disorder appears to be inherited as a non-sex-linked dominant characteristic, is relatively benign with little increased susceptibility to infection, and is associated with normal to modestly lowered total leukocyte counts and relative lymphocytosis and monocytosis. The marrow is cellular with abundant granulocytic precursors, though with greatly reduced band and segmented forms. Similar findings—but without a demonstrable familial instance—have been reported in certain chronic granulocytopenias in children and in adults under the name of chronic idiopathic neutropenia. In contrast, *infantile genetic agranulocytosis,* a rare disorder probably inherited as an autosomal recessive trait, is accompanied by severe infectious complications and early mortality. Of very considerable interest is the demonstration that *transitory neonatal neutropenia,* persisting for a few weeks, may occur as a result of maternal

isoimmu
a mann
erythro
challeng
with leu
chronic
a firm i
any cer
case of c
row con
high pr
ating. T
of gran
"myelok
   Althou
the tern
certain
with pr
lymphoc
aplasia
agamma
with aga
liable to
tibility t
death us
Less sev
documer
involvin
These i
ataxia t
"immun
depender
strated i
penia. I
related
immune
extremel
zoan, or
Hodgkin
and aner
   Pathog
is difficu
different
ations. T
more dif
those of
poiesis t
the circu
eral. The
ment con
postmitot
of matur
15 to 20
periphera
cular gra
twice tha
blood vol
walls, bu
circulatin
lating ha
to seven
the tissu
the intra
lar life sp

volved as causes of agranulocytosis include an
dopyrine, dinitrophenol, sulfonamides, thiouraç
and propylthiouracil, phenylbutazone, gold cor
pounds, organic arsenicals, trimethadione (Tr
dione), phenothiazine, tripelennamine (Pyribe
zamine), chloramphenicol, and chlorpromazin
Many additional agents, including procaine amid
barbiturates, quinine, acetanalid, pamaquir
(Plasmochin), hydralazine (Apresoline), mercuri
diuretics, ethacrynic acid, hydroxychloroquin
ampicillin, and DDT, have been reported to cau
the disorder.

Incidence. Agranulocytosis occurs in only
small number of patients exposed even to tho
drugs that cause the greatest number of case
The gravity of the complication, rather than i
frequency, accounts for its great importance. Fo
some reason agranulocytosis is more common i
females than in males in a ratio of two or three
one. Its distribution is worldwide, but its frequenc
parallels that of exposure of a population to offenc
ing agents.

Pathology. The ulcerative lesions in the mouth
rectum, skin, or elsewhere are necrotic and cor
tain large numbers of bacteria, but granulocyte
are conspicuously absent. If death occurs as th
granulocytic elements are returning to blood an
tissue, abscesses may make their appearance i
affected sites. The remaining pathologic change
aside from those of the bone marrow depend on th
localization of tissue reactions to invading micrc
organisms. The bone marrow changes vary wit
the stage of the disease. Megakaryocytes and ery
throid precursors are present in normal abur
dance. In severe cases, at the height of the disordε
granulocytic elements, including myelocytes an
metamyelocytes, are greatly reduced or absen
In later stages, or in milder cases, there may b
normal or hyperplastic granulopoiesis, with, how
ever, a preponderance of less mature precursc
cells and fewer than normal mature element:

Clinical Manifestations. The onset of the diseas
is sudden, usually with chills, high fever, and pros
tration. This pattern was initially regarded a
being due to bacterial invasion, but studies wit
amidopyrine indicate that these symptoms ma
follow a challenging dose of the medication withi
the hour, and may be associated with rapidl
developing neutropenia before sufficient time fo
significant bacterial invasion has elapsed. The
may, therefore, in this instance, initially be du
to an antigen-antibody reaction and to the perio
of rapid leukocyte lysis. Similar pyrogenic mani
festations occur in the absence of infection in cer
tain patients who have received repeated trans
fusions and who, as a result, develop antibodie
and reactions against homologous leukocytes i
transfused blood. The prodromal symptoms may b
either mild or severe, and are often followed by a
period of brief but variable duration in which
fatigue, prostration, and neutropenia persist, bu
no new symptoms develop. This second stage i
followed by return of fever, chills, and headache
frequently with ulceration of the oropharynx anc

that may involve any or all of the organs or tissues
of the body. Cells may proliferate at the site of
infiltration, causing tumors, pressure effects and
interference with organ function. Liver, spleen,
and lymph nodes are particularly common sites
of involvement. The pathologic aberrations are so
protean and so intimately related to the signs
and symptoms produced in leukemia that they will
be discussed along with the clinical manifestations
in order to avoid unnecessary repetition.

ACUTE LEUKEMIAS

Clinical Manifestations. Symptoms often appear abruptly in acute leukemia with fever, prostration, rapidly developing pallor, bone or joint
pain, bleeding from mucous membranes or into
skin, sudden enlargement of lymph nodes, or ulceration in the oral cavity. Frequently, however,
particularly in adults, the onset is more gradual,
the patient becoming aware during the course of
a month or two of progressive weakness, anorexia,
pallor and low-grade fever. With surprising frequency the patient traces his awareness of ill
health to an upper respiratory infection; instead
of rapid recovery, the sense of prostration increases
and the other symptoms appear.

The clinical manifestations of acute leukemia
are produced by proliferation and infiltration of
cells, anemia, hemorrhage, and infection; since
practically all organs and tissues may be affected,
the signs and symptoms are extremely varied.
Fever occurs almost invariably during the course
of the disease. The elevation of temperature may
be low-grade or high, continuous or spiking. In
most instances, a causative infection can be identified. Infections of the respiratory tract, pyelonephritis, septicemia, and ulcerative lesions or
abscesses, particularly in those areas heavily
populated by bacteria (oral cavity, rectum, skin),
are common. In addition to the usual pathogenic
bacteria, organisms that normally are relatively
avirulent may cause serious infections (proteus,
Ps. aeruginosa, etc.). Disseminated atypical mycobacterial and fungal infections, cytomegalic inclusion disease, *Pneumocystis carinii*, and generalized viral infections are recognized with increasing frequency, possibly because the use of
antimicrobial drugs, adrenal steroids, and antileukemic chemotherapeutic compounds may predispose to their development in patients with
diminished host resistance. In some patients in
whom no infecting organism can be isolated,
administration of antimicrobials may cause the
temperature to become normal. A few instances
remain in which infection cannot be proved, and
antimicrobial therapy is not beneficial; the fever
is then presumably caused by the general hypermetabolic state of the leukemic patients, by the
effect similar to tissue destruction produced by
the turnover of large numbers of leukemic cells,
by necrosis of normal cells destroyed by the infiltration, or by viral or other unrecognized infec-

tion. The anemia is caused by a combination of
factors: an absolute decrease in the rate of red
blood cell production or failure of erythropoiesis
to compensate for shortened erythrocyte survival,
a hemolytic component, and/or hemorrhage. Depending on its severity, the anemia is responsible
for pallor, much of the weakness, dyspnea, cardiac
dilatation, and even high output cardiac failure.
Bleeding can almost always be correlated with low
platelet counts (usually below 20,000 per cubic
millimeter), but coagulation abnormalities have
sometimes also been recognized: prolonged coagulation time, reduction in factor V, active fibrinolysis and hypofibrinogenemia (particularly in acute
myelocytic leukemia), and, rarely, the presence of
a circulating anticoagulant.

In approximately a third of patients, lymph
node enlargement is the first sign of acute leukemia. Generalized enlargement is particularly
common in the lymphocytic form, but may be conspicuous in acute myelocytic leukemia. The nodes
tend to be discrete, may be soft or firm, are often
tender, and usually do not become larger than 2
or 3 cm. in diameter unless they drain an area of
infection. When nodes are biopsied in patients
with acute myelocytic or monocytic leukemia,
touch preparations should be made and stained
with Wright stain; pathologists examining H
and E stained preparations may otherwise make
an erroneous diagnosis of lymphoma or anaplastic
carcinoma. Enlargement of tonsils, thymus, or
anterior mediastinal nodes may be so great in
lymphoblastic leukemia as to produce partial
obstruction; lymphatic tissue anywhere in the
body may become involved, causing local symptoms such as those simulating acute appendicitis.
The spleen usually increases enough in size to
extend several centimeters below the costal
margin, but may never become palpable during
the whole course of the disease; occasionally the
splenomegaly in acute lymphocytic leukemia may
be very great. Hepatic enlargement tends to be
moderate, the firm, often tender liver edge being
palpable several centimeters below the right
costal margin.

Petechiae, purpuric manifestations, and ecchymosis are common, sometimes associated with
blister formation or areas of necrosis. In acute
monocytic and myelocytic leukemia, particularly
the former, leukocytes deposited in the skin at
purpuric sites proliferate to form flat, elevated
plaques in which small abscesses may form.
Rarely, a generalized morbilliform rash or generalized exfoliative dermatitis may occur. Epistaxis, bleeding at the gingival margins of the
teeth, purpuric spots, and necrotic areas of ulceration in the nasal and oral cavities are frequent
manifestations. In acute monocytic leukemia,
leukemic infiltration causes the gums to become
spongy and so swollen or hyperplastic that the
teeth may become almost submerged; more rarely,
the same changes occur in acute myelocytic leukemia. With infection in the mouth, cervical and
submaxillary lymph nodes may become very large,

and cellulitis may involve the deep tissues of the face or neck. Retinal hemorrhages, either flame-shaped or rounded spots with a white central area, and white exudates are common; hemorrhage into the conjunctivae and eyelids may also be found. Unilateral or bilateral exophthalmos occurs in chloroma, when greenish masses or nodules of myeloblastic leukemic cells form in the retro-orbital space.

Miliary-like infiltrates of leukemic cells have been described in the lungs, but clinical interpretation of pulmonary infiltrates is difficult because bronchopneumonia is so frequent. Serous effusions, particularly in the pleural spaces, often develop. Leukemic infiltration of the stomach or other portions of the gastrointestinal tract is occasionally extensive enough to cause pain, ulceration, and signs of irritability. Severe gastrointestinal hemorrhage, usually from areas of hemorrhagic necrosis, mycotic infections involving any portion or all of the alimentary canal, and perforation of the appendix, cecum, or terminal ileum may occur. Perirectal abscess is a dreaded complication because the abscess seldom heals, tends to extend, and causes fever and much discomfort. Genitourinary manifestations include hematuria, bladder irritability from infiltration in the bladder wall, infection at any level, renal enlargement as the result of infiltration but usually without impairment of function, and, rarely, priapism. If pregnancy occurs during the course of acute leukemia, the fetus seldom survives.

Involvement of bones and joints may be very dramatic with constant or intermittent severe pain, tenderness, and signs of acute arthritis simulating acute rheumatic fever or Still's disease. These changes are usually due to subperiosteal infiltration or bone necrosis, or both. Leukopenia, bone pain, and bone necrosis constitute a clinicopathologic complex found in about 15 per cent of patients with acute lymphocytic leukemia; it is less frequent in other types. Secondary gout is an unusual cause of joint pain even though hyperuricemia is common and uric acid nephropathy is not rare (particularly during therapy). Nodules form in the subperiosteum along the shafts of bones, or marrow proliferation may lead to thinning of the cortex and resultant pathologic fractures. Sternal tenderness is often present.

Neurologic changes may be varied, depending on the nerves into which infiltration, hemorrhage, or direct extension of leukemic proliferation occurs. Cranial nerves may be affected, to produce abnormalities of ocular movement, disturbances of vision, deafness, vestibular symptoms, and facial paralysis. Involvement of the spinal meninges or spinal nerve roots and peripheral neuritis are not rare. Leukemic meningitis is most common in children, particularly among males with acute lymphocytic leukemia, and may occur even during the course of a therapeutically induced hematologic remission. The chemotherapeutic agents used to induce a remission fail to cross the blood-brain barrier, so leukemic cells may proliferate in the meninges although they are inhibited elsewhere. *Meningeal leukemia* is caused by arachnoidal infiltration, particularly along the brain stem, with resulting obstruction to the flow of cerebrospinal fluid, increased intracranial pressure, and even hydrocephalus. The principal clinical manifestations are nausea and vomiting, headache, lethargy, convulsions, papilledema, cranial nerve palsies, and other less specific neurologic signs. Kernig's sign is unusual. Skull suture lines are usually spread in children. Examination of the cerebrospinal fluid reveals increased pressure, pleocytosis of abnormal cells (25 to 11,000 per cubic millimeter), or both. Hyperphagia, pathologic weight gain, and behavioral disturbances (hypothalamic syndrome) have occasionally been observed in association with leukemic meningitis and leukemic infiltration of the hypothalamus.

Intracranial hemorrhage in patients with thrombocytopenia is a not uncommon terminal event; the hemorrhage is predominantly subarachnoid, although it frequently extends into the brain substance. Another kind of distinctive intracranial hemorrhage occurs in patients during blastic crises with leukocyte counts greater than 100,000 per cubic millimeter; the bleeding is into the cortex but, when massive, may extend into ventricles or the subarachnoid space. It is associated with nodules of leukemic cells within the areas of hemorrhage. Intracerebral leukostasis appears to result in localized proliferation, destruction of the vessel wall, formation of a leukemic nodule, and hemorrhage about the nodule. Coalescence of many such lesions results in the large hemorrhages seen grossly.

Diagnosis. The diagnosis of acute leukemia must be made by hematologic examination of the peripheral blood *and* bone marrow. Normocytic normochromic anemia and thrombocytopenia of moderate to severe degree are found in the majority of cases when patients first seek medical attention, or develop shortly thereafter. The total leukocyte count varies widely but is within normal limits in approximately 15 per cent, below normal to severely leukopenic in about 25 per cent, and elevated in 60 per cent of cases. Characteristically, very immature cells of the leukemic strain predominate and may constitute more than 90 per cent of all the leukocytes in the peripheral blood. With careless examination, they may erroneously be called normal lymphocytes. When the total white blood cell count is less than normal, however, the proportion of leukemic cells may decrease; at times only an occasional abnormal form can be identified. With few exceptions, the aspirated bone marrow samples consist of an almost solid mass of immature leukemic cells with very few normal granulocytes, nucleated erythrocytes, or megakaryocytes. The most common exception occurs early during the course of acute myelocytic and monocytic leukemia; the marrow may be hypocellular and a normal or nearly normal number of erythroid elements may be found, some of which may resemble megaloblasts (megaloblastoid). Differentiation among the types of acute leukemia is often difficult, requiring meticulous attention to cellular detail. For a detailed description of blasts and other immature forms of leukocytes, reference should be made to a text or atlas of hematology. Some hematologists believe that all forms can be classified, whereas others contend that the cells in an occasional patient are so immature that the designation "stem cell leukemia" should be used. Help in the identification of blast forms can be obtained from "the company they keep" — by the presence of intermediate and more mature forms of the leukocyte series. In acute myelocytic leukemia, for instance, one can usually identify promyelocytes or myelocytes with at least a few specific granules; the granules are more easily discernible in these immature cells with supravital or peroxidase stains than with Wright's stain. Similarly, in acute monocytic leukemia, the presence of early but definitely recognizable monocytes is helpful. Although Auer bodies have been described in a few questionable instances of fatal leukemoid reactions, they usually are found only in acute myelocytic or acute monocytic leukemia; these cytoplasmic inclusion bodies are rodlike, homogeneous crystalline structures that stain red with Wright's stain, sometimes have blunt and sometimes pointed ends so that they resemble acid-fast bacilli or needles, and are probably formed by coalescence of granules. It may be difficult at initial examination to differentiate between acute and chronic myelocytic leukemia because the manifestations of chronic myelocytic leukemia during severe relapse resemble those of the acute disease. Duration of symptoms for several months or more, the presence of a greatly enlarged spleen, the absence of hemorrhagic phenomena or of thrombocytopenia, and the presence of many myelocytes or more mature forms in the peripheral blood should make one suspect that the disease is chronic even though immaturity of cells in the bone marrow is advanced.

Very little practical diagnostic help can be obtained from other laboratory studies. The blood uric acid tends to be elevated. In monocytic or myelomonocytic leukemia, overproduction of lysozyme (muramidase) seems to be a consistent biochemical abnormality; detection of elevated serum and urine lysozyme is a valuable diagnostic test. A nonspecific rise in the plasma alpha-2 globulin is often found. The serum vitamin B_{12} binding capacity concentration and the serum vitamin B_{12} have been reported to be high in acute as well as in chronic myelocytic leukemia. Leukocytes may be found in increased numbers in cerebrospinal fluid even in the absence of recognizable involvement of the central nervous system.

When the white blood cell count is elevated significantly above the normal range, differentiation of acute leukemia from other diseases is usually not exceptionally difficult. In leukemoid reactions, the immaturity of cells in the peripheral blood and bone marrow tends to be modest. The hardest diagnostic problem occurs when lymphocytes are greatly increased as in infectious mononucleosis and in an occasional child with whooping cough, chickenpox, infectious lymphocytosis, or congenital syphilis; counts as high as 100,000 to 200,000 per cubic millimeter have been reported, nearly all lymphocytes. The bone marrow is usually affected to a lesser extent. Lymph nodes and the spleen may enlarge, but the course of the diseases causing lymphocytosis tends to be short. Detection of heterophil antibodies (Paul-Bunnell test) and recognition of the distinctive lymphocytic changes establish a diagnosis of infectious mononucleosis. In children, metastatic neuroblastoma may be especially difficult to differentiate from acute leukemia; bone changes similar to those of acute leukemia may be present, and the tumor cells, which bear a superficial resemblance to leukemic leukocytes, may be found in fairly large numbers in both the peripheral blood and the marrow.

Problems in differential diagnosis arise more frequently when the total white blood cell count in acute leukemia is within or below the normal range. With few exceptions, at least a few very immature leukemic cells can be found during the survey of a blood film; the bone marrow changes are usually as definite as when the count is high; anemia and thrombocytopenia develop early. Bone marrow failure or hypoplastic anemia with a cellular marrow is often the hardest to differentiate, as the leukocytic marrow elements may be relatively immature; furthermore, patients with these hematologic changes occasionally develop acute myelocytic or monocytic leukemia.

Myelophthisic anemias from any cause, the malignant lymphomas, multiple myeloma, and, rarely, agranulocytosis may cause confusion. In these diseases, clinical manifestations may include fever, enlargement of lymph nodes, spleen, or liver, bone pain, and ulceration of mucous membranes. Usually the uncertainty in diagnosis is of short duration, although lymph node biopsy may be required in addition to careful examination of the bone marrow. If the cells infiltrating or proliferating in the marrow are plasma cells, carcinoma cells, or fibrous tissue, they can be recognized by a trained cytologist. Anemia and thrombocytopenia are not features of agranulocytosis, and the course of the disease is short.

Treatment. During the last two decades, the treatment of acute leukemia has improved significantly, particularly for acute lymphocytic leukemia in children. Better supportive care, especially through the use of platelet transfusions and more effective antimicrobial therapy, has been partly responsible. Of even greater importance has been the development of a series of antileukemic chemotherapeutic agents that are more toxic to leukemic cells than to normal tissue; in many instances, however, the therapeutic index is narrow. Nine of the most effective are listed in the accompanying table, together with some of their properties and toxicities. The development, study, and clinical evaluation of these and other drugs

DRUGS OF PROVED EFFECTIVENESS IN THE TREATMENT OF ACUTE LEUKEMIA*

Drug	Drug Category	Mechanism of Action	Distribution	Major Method of Elimination	Major Toxicity
Prednisone, prednisolone	Adrenocorticosteroids	Lysis of lymphocytes and lymphoblasts; inhibition of cell cycle and DNA synthesis	Total body water; protein bound	Metabolism, renal excretion	Psychosis, hypertension, peptic ulcer, fluid retention, osteoporosis, immunodepression
Vincristine	Alkaloid of periwinkle	Metaphase arrest; inhibition of DNA and RNA synthesis	Unknown; does not enter CSF significantly	Metabolism, biliary excretion	Peripheral neuropathy, adynamic ileus, myopathy
Daunorubicin	Antimicrobial	Inhibition of DNA and RNA synthesis	Unknown; does not enter CSF	Unknown	Myelosuppression, cardiotoxicity
Asparaginase	Enzyme	Depletion of endogenous asparagine	Extracellular fluid; not in CSF	Metabolism	Defects in protein synthesis, hepatitis, pancreatitis, sensitivity reactions (anaphylaxis)
Methotrexate	Folic acid antagonist	Inhibition of dihydrofolate reductase and of DNA synthesis	Total body water, slow entry into CSF: protein bound	Renal excretion	Myelosuppression, gastrointestinal mucositis, hepatitis
6-Mercaptopurine (6-MP)	Purine antagonist	Inhibition of purine and of DNA synthesis	Total body water, slow entry into CSF	Metabolism, renal excretion	Myelosuppression, gastrointestinal mucositis, hepatitis
Cytosine arabinoside	Pyrimidine antagonist	Inhibition of synthesis of deoxycytidine, riboside, and DNA	Total body water, slow entry into CSF	Metabolism, renal excretion	Myelosuppression
Cyclophosphamide (Cytoxan)	Polyfunctional alkylating agent	Cross-linkage of DNA; metabolism required for activity	Total body water	Metabolism, renal excretion	Cystitis, alopecia
Methylglyoxal-bisguanylhydrazone (MeGAG)	Synthetic	Not known	Total body water, slow entry into CSF	Renal excretion	Myelosuppression, mucositis, polyneuropathy, arthritis, vasculitis, acroerythema, episcleritis

*After Henderson, E. S.: Seminars Hemat., 6:271, 1969.

are the product of an integrated program that involves the pharmaceutical industry and nearly every large hematologic service in this and other countries. Dosage schedules have been and continue to be manipulated in a systematic way in an attempt to determine the safest and most effective way to induce and maintain remissions. Because several drugs are often better than one when none is totally effective, because mechanisms of action differ, and because less toxic amounts of each might thereby be used, various combinations given either together or sequentially have also been tried. Several of the most widely used are prednisone and vincristine; prednisone and 6-MP; prednisone and methotrexate; prednisone, vincristine, and daunorubicin; vincristine, methotrexate, 6-MP, and prednisone (VAMP; the "a" comes from amethopterin as an alternate name for methotrexate); prednisolone, vincristine, methotrexate, and 6-MP (POMP, the "o" comes from Oncovin, a trade name for vincristine); cytosine arabinoside and cytoxan; cytoxan, vincristine, cytosine arabinoside, and prednisone (COAP); and so forth. Since cure has not been achieved, the search for new drugs and more effective combinations will continue. In general, life is prolonged by the duration of any remission induced; in the absence of a remission, little is gained by the therapy. The likelihood of inducing a remission increases if initial treatment can be given for a minimum of six weeks and if administration is pushed to the point of marrow depression. Consequently, severe degrees of thrombocytopenia and leukopenia with the attendant dangers of bleeding and infection are commonly encountered. If the chances for inducing a prolonged remission are high, as in acute lymphocytic leukemia of children, no one questions that the risk is worth taking.

When the likelihood of a remission is low and its duration is apt to be short, as in acute myelocytic or acute monocytic leukemia in older adults, the problem is more difficult, and some hematologists have argued that such patients should not routinely be treated. However, if untreated, their median survival, even with excellent supportive management, is probably only about two months, and nearly all are dead by six months. To withhold therapy, when the advances of chemotherapy are extolled almost daily in the news media, is psychologically devastating, and must seem like abandonment. It is much wiser for the physician to select and use one of the protocols whose effectiveness and relative safety have been established. Preferably, it should be a program that minimizes the need for hospitalization, provides maximal opportunity for personal happiness, and permits a patient to carry on his normal activities as long as possible. Investigative programs that explore new drugs, new combinations, and new dosage schedules designed to improve results or to attempt a total kill of all leukemic cells are of great importance. These efforts, however, should be clearly labeled as investigations, done under conditions in which ideal intensive care and isolation can be provided; the investigator has the responsibility for not letting his understandable enthusiasm imply that physicians are in error unless they treat every patient according to the last studied protocol.

Remissions can now be achieved in 85 per cent or more of children (2 to 19 years) with acute lymphocytic leukemia. In general, vincristine and prednisone can be used to induce a remission, and 6-MP or methotrexate may be employed to maintain it. One satisfactory treatment schedule provides for prednisone, 40 mg. per square meter of body surface per day orally, and vincristine sulfate, 2 mg. per square meter per week intravenously. The median time required is about four weeks. The temperature comes down to normal, the appetite and sense of well-being improve, hemorrhagic manifestations subside, enlarged lymph nodes and spleen recede, blood values return to normal, and leukemic changes in the marrow disappear. The remission is then maintained with injections of 30 mg. of methotrexate per square meter intramuscularly twice weekly.

Other acceptable treatment schedules are outlined in the review by Henderson. Some form of remission maintenance seems to be better than none. When a remission has been sustained for many months, it becomes difficult to decide when maintenance therapy should be discontinued; the advantage of continuing diminishes after about eight to ten months. Second and third remissions can often be induced. The median survival of children with acute lymphocytic leukemia who achieve complete remissions is about three years as opposed to four months for the few children failing to respond. Because most antileukemic drugs reach cerebrospinal fluid in very low concentrations (see Table), *leukemic meningitis* may occur while a remission is otherwise maintained; this complication can be treated by the intrathecal administration of 0.1 to 0.5 mg. of methotrexate per kilogram of body weight; the dose may need to be repeated once or twice at intervals of three or four days. Folinic acid may be given orally or parenterally at the same time to minimize bone marrow depression. Alternatively, the brain may be irradiated with 500 to 1000 r, but that method fails to destroy leukemic cells along the spinal cord. Adrenocorticosteroids have also been used successfully.

As previously stated, the response of adult patients with acute myelocytic and acute monocytic leukemia is much less satisfactory, particularly for those older than 60. Remissions occur less frequently and are of shorter duration. In the series by Boggs et al., 6-MP was administered orally in a daily dose of 2.5 mg. per kilogram; if toxic manifestations were encountered, the dose was reduced or omitted until the toxicity had subsided. In patients who were able to complete at least 6 weeks of therapy, remission (mean 8 months, range 2 to 18 months) developed in one third. Patients with initial leukocyte counts greater than 100,000 per cubic millimeter tended to do poorly. These results are somewhat better than have been achieved in other clinics with 6-MP alone, so that combinations such as VAMP have been tried. One variation has used 1.2 mg. of vincristine intravenously per week, 2.5 mg. of methotrexate by mouth daily, 100 mg. of 6-MP by mouth daily, and 60 mg. of prednisone by mouth daily. Of 23 patients treated, 14 were able to complete 6 weeks of therapy, and of these 10 developed remissions (median duration 13 weeks, range 4 weeks to 18 months). Currently, there is great interest in exploring the value of cytosine arabinoside in various combinations, e.g., COAP, for the treatment of acute myelocytic leukemia; it is too early to evaluate reports. In all regimens, injections of vincristine should be discontinued if paresthesias develop to avoid distressing neuropathy, and therapy is interrupted if bone marrow depression becomes severe.

During initial therapy of acute leukemia, allopurinol is frequently used to prevent nephropathy incident to hyperuricemia. This drug has a synergistic effect on 6-MP; consequently, the dose of 6-MP should be reduced to two thirds of the amount that otherwise would have been given.

Other measures contribute greatly to skillful clinical care of patients: (1) the judicious use of transfusions when anemia is troublesome or does not respond to the chemotherapeutic agents; (2) administration of platelet transfusions to help tide a patient over a bleeding episode; (3) meticulous care of veins at the time of venipuncture and avoidance of all unnecessary subcutaneous or intramuscular injections; (4) careful maintenance of oral hygiene, avoidance of all but the most urgent dental work, prevention of constipation, and gentle cleansing of the perianal region; and (5) early recognition and treatment of any infection.

Initial enthusiasm for attempts to cure leukemia by large doses of general body irradiation followed by bone marrow transplants has been dampened. When an identical twin has been the bone marrow donor and transplants have been successful, the leukemia has invariably recurred rather promptly even when the dose of general body irradiation has exceeded 1000 r. Remissions of relatively short duration may occur in a small number of patients after exchange transfusion of large volumes of blood. Spontaneous remissions are comparatively rare, usually last for only a month or two, but may persist for six months or longer. The hope of those workers who are trying to recover a human leukemogenic virus is that a way will be found to propagate the virus and prepare a vaccine. Its possible effectiveness could be proved within a few years by administering it to infants and determining whether the sharp peak in incidence among three- and four-year-old children could be eliminated.

Prognosis. With chemotherapy, transfusions, and appropriate use of antimicrobial drugs, the course of acute lymphocytic leukemia in children has been significantly and dramatically lengthened. The average duration of the disease for those children who develop a remission exceeds three years; a significant number have survived for more than five years, and a few for ten or more years. Therapeutic results achieved to date in adults with any form of acute leukemia are disappointing. Among adults with acute myelocytic leukemia treated by one of the Acute Leukemia Study Groups, the median survival was 11 months for those who had a complete remission, 5.5 months for those with a partial remission, and only 1 month for those who failed to respond. Even so, the total number of comfortable, useful days of life has been significantly increased.

The immediate causes of death in most patients are infection and hemorrhage. Antitumor agents impair host defense mechanisms and make the patients more susceptible to infection by agents that are normally of low virulence, e.g., Pseudomonas, cytomegalovirus, and fungi. The most common sites of fatal hemorrhage are in the central nervous system and the gastrointestinal tract.

Acute Leukemia Group B: New treatment schedule with improved survival in childhood leukemia. J.A.M.A., 194:187, 1965.

Boggs, D. R., Wintrobe, M. M., and Cartwright, G. E.: The acute leukemias. Medicine, 41:163, 1962.

Boggs, D. R., Wintrobe, M. M., and Cartwright, G. E.: To treat or not to treat acute myelocytic leukemia. II. Arch. Intern. Med. (Chicago), 123:568, 1969.

Bryan, W. R., Dalton, A. J., and Rauscher, F. J.: The viral approach to human leukemia and lymphoma: Its current status. In Brown, E. B., and Moore, C. V. (eds.): Progress in Hematology. New York, Grune & Stratton, Inc., Vol. 5, p. 137, 1966.

Dameshek, W., and Gunz, F.: Leukemia. 2nd ed. New York, Grune & Stratton, Inc., 1964.

Firkin, B., and Moore, C. V.: Clinical manifestations of leukemia. Amer. J. Med., 28:764, 1960.

Fraumeni, J. F., Jr., and Miller, R. W.: Leukemia mortality: Downturn rates in the United States. Science, 155:1126, 1967.

Freireich, E. J., and Frei, E., III: Recent advances in acute leukemia. In Moore, C. V., and Brown, E. B. (eds.): Progress in Hematology. New York, Grune & Stratton, Inc. Vol. 4, p. 187, 1964.

Hayhoe, F. G. J., Quaglino, D., and Doll, R.: The Cytology and Cytochemistry of Acute Leukaemias. Medical Research Council Special Report Series No. 304. London, Her Majesty's Stationery Office, 1964.

Henderson, E. S.: Treatment of acute leukemia. Seminars Hemat., 6:271, 1969.

Thompson, I., Hall, T. C., and Moloney, W. C.: Combination therapy of adult acute myelogenous leukemia. New Eng. J. Med., 273:1302, 1965.

Wintrobe, M. M.: Clinical Hematology. 6th ed. Philadelphia, Lea and Febiger, 1967.

CHRONIC LEUKEMIAS

Clinical Manifestations. The onset of chronic leukemia is frequently so insidious that it is accidentally discovered when a blood count is obtained for other reasons or when the patient reports to his physician that he has noted a few enlarged lymph nodes or felt, while bathing, a firm left upper quadrant abdominal mass. Constitutional signs early during the course of the disease are few, and the patient commonly appears healthy; gradually anorexia, weight loss, and weakness appear. Further manifestations are determined by the sites of proliferation and infiltration of the leukemic cells, the appearance of anemia and thrombocytopenia, and the general metabolic disturbance.

Lymph node enlargement occurs early in chronic lymphocytic leukemia. The nodes at all sites may be involved; they are firm, discrete, not tender, and rarely exceed 3 or 4 cm. in diameter. Enlarged mediastinal nodes may cause pressure symptoms. The tonsils may become huge. Proliferation of lymphocytes in lacrimal and salivary glands may cause bilateral painless enlargement (*Mikulicz syndrome*). In chronic myelocytic leukemia, lymphadenopathy is an unusual manifestation; when it occurs, it tends to be moderate but painful, and is associated with a relatively rapid course. Splenomegaly is almost constant, is usually more massive in chronic myelocytic leukemia, and usually causes no symptoms except for an uncomfortable heavy feeling in the upper abdomen. When infarction or perisplenitis occurs, however, pain in the region of the spleen may be intense, and is frequently accompanied by a friction rub. Hepatomegaly of moderate degree, caused by the leukemic infiltration, is also frequent; the liver is smooth, firm, and only rarely tender. Jaundice and ascites are unusual. Gastrointestinal symptoms, in addition to anorexia, include flatulence, occasionally diarrhea, and hemorrhage. Abdominal pain may be a late manifestation; its cause is unknown, but local areas of infarction or infiltration can sometimes be demonstrated. Infiltrative lesions may be extensive, involving any segment of the alimentary canal in chronic lymphocytic leukemia, but they are rare in chronic myelocytic leukemia. In the latter disease, peptic ulcer is not uncommon. Cardiovascular symptoms are usually secondary to anemia, but pericarditis with increased amounts of pericardial fluid and myocardial infiltration may occur. About one third of patients with chronic lymphocytic leukemia have symptoms from mediastinal lymph node enlargement, pulmonary infiltration, or pleural effusion; these changes are much less common in the chronic myelocytic form of the disease. Involvement of the genitourinary system may be manifested by hematuria (15 to 20 per cent of cases), priapism (especially in myelocytic leukemia), pain in the lumbar region apparently from renal infiltration, abnormal menstrual bleeding, or amenorrhea. Point tenderness over some spot on the sternum can be detected in about three fourths of all patients. Arthralgia and bone pain may occur, but they are unusual except during the blastic terminal phase of chronic myelocytic leukemia. Sclerosis and bony tumors are rare. Gout, as a reflection of the high uric acid, occurs but is uncommon.

Retinal hemorrhage, leukocytic infiltrates, and blurring of the optic disc cause visual disturbances. Leukemic nodules are occasionally found in the cornea and sclera. Hemorrhage or infiltration in the ear or along the course of the eighth nerve may produce deafness, otitis media, or

Meniere's syndrome. Any part of the nervous system may be affected because of infiltration, pressure from enlarged lymph nodes, or other tumor-like accumulations of leukemic cells, by interference with blood supply by pressure effects or thrombosis, or by hemorrhage. The resultant manifestations include cranial nerve palsies, absence of reflexes, pyramidal tract signs, paresthesias, signs of meningeal irritation, paralysis, tremors, and, in chronic lymphocytic leukemia, a syndrome that resembles amyotrophic lateral sclerosis.

Skin lesions occur frequently in chronic lymphocytic leukemia; they may take the form of nonspecific (leukemid) reactions or may be the result of specific nodular infiltrations. Nonspecific reactions include prurigo-like papules, vesicles, herpes zoster, exfoliative dermatitis, and a peculiar generalized lesion in which the skin is fiery red, leathery, and intensely pruritic (erythroderma). Skin involvement in chronic myelocytic leukemia is relatively rare but takes the form of sharply circumscribed cutaneous or subcutaneous plaques or nodules with a brownish, slate-gray, or bluish color.

Erythrocyte and platelet values may remain normal for a considerable period of time; early in the course of chronic myelocytic leukemia, even moderate polycythemia and thrombocytosis may be found. At some stage, however, normocytic normochromic anemia and thrombocytopenia appear and may become severe. Although a variable combination of impaired erythropoiesis, accelerated red blood cell destruction, and hemorrhage is responsible for the anemia, an interesting and decided difference exists between chronic myelocytic and lymphocytic leukemia. In the former, except during terminal stages, the anemia is corrected when antileukemic therapy induces a remission. By contrast, the anemia of chronic lymphocytic leukemia persists or improves but little with antileukemic therapy, the Coombs test is positive in about a third of the patients, and the anemia responds to the administration of corticosteroids; in other words, it resembles acquired hemolytic anemia (or "autoimmune" hemolytic anemia). The same generalization may be made about the thrombocytopenia in chronic lymphocytic leukemia; it responds to corticosteroid therapy rather than, as in chronic myelocytic leukemia, to treatment of the leukemia per se. Terminally, both the anemia and the thrombocytopenia become unresponsive in both forms of the disease.

Fever is a late manifestation; usually but not invariably an infectious cause can be demonstrated. About 30 to 60 per cent of patients with chronic lymphocytic leukemia have severe degrees of acquired hypogammaglobulinemia, and the lymphocytes have been suspected of being immuno-incompetent. As a result, immunity to bacteria, viruses, insect bites, and skin grafts may be greatly reduced. Patients are susceptible to infection with bacteria (particularly recurrent pneumonia), and may develop virulent reaction to viral infection: vaccinia gangrenosa after smallpox vaccination, widely disseminated lesions with herpes zoster, or rapid spread from herpes simplex lesions of the face. Smallpox vaccination is contraindicated in chronic lymphocytic leukemia. Mosquito bites may result in huge lesions. Somewhat paradoxically, patients with the disease may develop paraproteinemia, cryoglobulinemia with Raynaud's phenomenon, hypersensitivity to cold, and manifestations of autoimmune disease: hemolytic anemia, immuno-thrombocytopenic purpura, vasculitis, thyroiditis, rheumatoid arthritis, and Sjögren's syndrome. The incidence of associated malignant disease is higher in chronic lymphocytic leukemia than in the general population.

Clinically and hematologically, the terminal stage of chronic myelocytic leukemia closely resembles acute myelocytic leukemia. An acute terminal phase in chronic lymphocytic leukemia, by contrast, is very rare; anemia, infection, and hemorrhage dominate the last months of the disease.

Chronic monocytic leukemia is very rare. Normal to low white blood cell counts, cutaneous lesions, and bone pain have been prominent features in some of the few cases described.

Diagnosis. Although cases of chronic leukemia have been described in children, the disease predominantly affects adults. Diagnosis is established by examination of the peripheral blood and bone marrow. The total leukocyte count is usually high; levels above 100,000 per cubic millimeter are frequent, and the level may reach 500,000 or more. In chronic myelocytic leukemia, the granulocytes vary in maturity all the way from promyelocytes to the most mature neutrophils. Eosinophilic and basophilic elements are often increased; there are very few other conditions in which more than 5 per cent basophils are found, particularly with elevated total counts. Sometimes myelocytes contain mixed granules in the same cell: eosinophilic and basophilic, eosinophilic and neutrophilic, and so forth. Pelger-Huet-like granulocytes may be found. Nucleated red blood cells are seen occasionally. In chronic lymphocytic leukemia, on the other hand, the differential is much less varied; the lymphocytes frequently look like mirror images of each other, and constitute 75 to 99 per cent of all white blood cells.

Even though the diagnosis may appear to be definite from examination of the blood, confirmation should always be obtained by bone marrow study. In chronic myelocytic leukemia, one should look for hyperplasia of the granulocytic elements, high myeloid : erythroid ratio, some immaturity of the myelocytes, and increased percentage of eosinophilic and basophilic forms. The bone marrow in chronic lymphocytic leukemia contains a tremendous predominance of small lymphocytes, frequently more than 90 per cent of all cells. The marrow is so tightly packed that it aspirates with difficulty; even the most experienced hematologists may obtain a "dry tap" and find it necessary to resort to trephine biopsy. If any question about the diagnosis remains, biopsy of an enlarged lymph node is advisable; pathologists, however, are usually unable to distinguish the lymph node changes in chronic lymphocytic leukemia from those of small cell lymphosarcoma.

Of particular diagnostic value in untreated chronic myelocytic leukemia are an elevated serum vitamin B_{12} level (often greater than 1000 $\mu\mu g$. per milliliter) and the absence (or near absence) of granulocytes in the blood that give a positive staining reaction for alkaline phosphatase. In addition, a specific chromosomal abnormality has been found in the myeloid cells from 60 to 85 per cent of patients with chronic myelocytic leukemia: one of the acrocentric No. 21 chromosomes is abnormally small because of deletion of part of the long arms (Philadelphia or Ph^1 chromosome). Detection of this cytogenetic marker is hardly a routine procedure, but may be diagnostically useful when differentiation from myeloid metaplasia or leukemoid reaction is particularly difficult. It also has served to indicate that there are probably two types of chronic myelocytic leukemia: Ph^1-positive and Ph^1-negative. The latter tend to have lower leukocyte and platelet counts, respond less well to therapy, have an earlier onset of blastic crisis, and have a shorter mean survival time. The basal metabolic rate is commonly +20 to +40 per cent in both forms of chronic leukemia, and the blood uric acid tends to be high. Urinary excretion of uric acid is increased in chronic myelocytic leukemia and is usually normal in the lymphocytic disease.

The conditions most difficult to differentiate from chronic myelocytic leukemia are leukemoid reactions, myelofibrosis with myeloid metaplasia, and the late stages of polycythemia vera when the red blood cell count may be subnormal and the leukocytes increased. Recognition of abnormalities commonly responsible for leukemoid reactions (infections, metastatic carcinoma, and so forth) and identification of any abnormal infiltration of the marrow (tumor cells, granulomatous lesions, myelofibrosis) may be helpful. In these other conditions, the alkaline phosphatase staining reaction of blood granulocytes is usually greater (not less) than normal, the serum vitamin B_{12} level is not increased and the Ph^1 chromosome is not present (see above). Often the differentiation cannot be made with certainty, however, even at autopsy. When the white blood cell count in chronic myelocytic leukemia is within the normal range or is subnormal and anemia is present, it is also difficult to eliminate hypoplastic or refractory anemia with a cellular marrow as a possible diagnosis. Chronic lymphocytic leukemia must be differentiated from lymphocytic leukemoid reactions and from the malignant lymphomas. Greatest help comes from lymph node biopsy and from the fact that only in chronic lymphocytic leukemia is the marrow extensively replaced by lymphocytes. It is also difficult, and at times impossible, to distinguish between subleukemic lymphocytic leukemia and hypoplastic anemia in which 30 to 40 per cent of bone marrow cells may be lymphocytes. One should err on the side of conservatism. Much less harm is done by delaying a diagnosis of leukemia for several weeks than by making it erroneously.

Treatment. The same general comments made for the treatment of acute leukemia are applicable here. In chronic leukemia, it is particularly important to help the patient live a normal life, to keep him out of the hospital and at home as much as possible. Some hematologists prefer to treat patients with chronic leukemia only when symptoms develop; others attempt to maintain the peripheral blood and bone marrow as normal as possible at all times. The author prefers the latter approach because of the conviction that treated patients feel better, have a greater number of symptom-free days, and probably live somewhat longer.

Chronic myelocytic leukemia is most commonly treated with busulfan, radioactive phosphorus (P^{32}), or splenic irradiation; busulfan is currently considered the therapy of choice. When treatment is first begun with any of the three methods, urinary excretion of uric acid is greatly increased, and ureteral obstruction by uric acid crystals may result; for this reason fluid intake should be generous, urinary pH should be made alkaline, and allopurinol should be administered if hyperuricemia exists or the initial leukocyte count is above 100,000 per cubic millimeter.

Busulfan (1,4-dimethanesulfonyloxybutane, Myleran) is a polyfunctional alkylating agent that presumably exerts its effect by inactivating or destroying nucleic acids. A daily single dose of 60 μg. per kilogram of body weight (usual maximal dose is 4 mg., although some hematologists give as much as 6 mg.) is given before breakfast; treatment is continued until the leukocyte count, determined weekly, falls to between 15,000 and 20,000 per cubic millimeter, and is then stopped at least until the count stabilizes. The risk of irreversible bone marrow aplasia, if treatment is continued without interruption, is substantial; leukocytes will continue to fall for several weeks. The time required for production of a remission depends on the height of the original leukocyte level, the count being halved about every 21 days. The patient's sense of well-being returns, granulocytic elements in both blood and bone marrow return to normal or nearly normal, the enlarged liver and spleen decrease in size, and any anemia or thrombocytopenia tends to be corrected. Remissions may persist for as long as two years; during this time the leukocyte alkaline phosphatase may return to normal. In some clinics, maintenance doses of 2 mg. per day or 6 to 8 mg. on one day per week are given in the hope of prolonging the remission. Patients should be seen at intervals of one to two weeks; when it is established that the count has stabilized, the intervals can be extended to four to six weeks. Should the leukocyte or platelet counts fall, administration of the drug should be discontinued until levels have again returned to normal. Bone marrow aplasia is a constant threat with busulfan therapy. The aforementioned course should be repeated whenever the white blood cell count rises about 50,000 per cubic millimeter; subsequent remissions become progressively shorter. Patients who are Ph[1] chromosome-negative respond less well to chemotherapy than do those who have the marker (median survival of 8 to 18 months as compared with 40 to 45 months). Side effects of busulfan therapy, in addition to bone marrow aplasia, include interstitial pulmonary fibrosis, vomiting and diarrhea, anorexia, weight loss, amenorrhea, gynecomastia, testicular atrophy, and hyperpigmentation. When the hyperpigmentation occurs together with weakness, fatigue, anorexia, and weight loss, a syndrome is produced that resembles Addison's disease, but tests of adrenal cortical function remain normal. Cytologic dysplasia has been observed in cells obtained from bronchial washings and from the cervix; there is a superficial resemblance to carcinoma cells, but differentiation can be made by experienced pathologists. Busulfan therapy should be withheld during the first trimester of a pregnancy, but a number of normal infants have been born to mothers who took the drug without interruption throughout pregnancy.

P[32] has two important advantages over conventional radiotherapy: it can be given on an ambulatory basis at infrequent intervals, and produces practically no irradiation sickness. The dose must be highly individualized and must be controlled by following the changes in the peripheral blood. P[32] is administered as sodium acid phosphate either intravenously or orally. Oral doses are given while the patient is fasting to promote better absorption; approximately 75 per cent is absorbed. The following is one of several satisfactory schedules for parenteral administration; amounts should be increased by about one third for oral therapy. If the white blood cell count is above 50,000 per cubic millimeter, 1 to 2.5 millicuries is given initially depending on the degree of leukocytosis, and 1 to 1.5 millicuries two weeks later. If leukocyte levels are above 100,000 per cubic millimeter, the second dose may be administered at the end of one week. Blood counts should be obtained every two weeks, and additional injections of 1 to 1.5 millicuries should be given at the same time intervals until the white blood count falls below 20,000. It is important to "feel one's way" with dosage because the half-life of P[32] is about 14 days, and because severe degrees of bone marrow depression may be produced by overtreatment. An attempt should be made to obtain a normal blood count, but if that result is not achieved by 12 millicuries or less within several months, it is best to change to busulfan. The clinical and hematologic remissions induced by a course of P[32] therapy may persist for a year or more. Patients should be seen at intervals of one or two months, but should be advised to report promptly if symptoms recur. Whenever the white blood cell count rises above 25,000 per cubic millimeter, additional injections are given. Occasionally, readministration may be started cautiously with leukocyte levels below 25,000 if there

is increasing immaturity of leukocytes or clinical evidence of reactivation of the disease, i.e., enlargement of liver, spleen, or lymph nodes, or unexplained fever. P[32] provides general body irradiation and is less effective in reducing the size of a greatly enlarged spleen or of a group of lymph nodes than is local radiotherapy. Whenever there is local pain, particularly bone pain, or pressure from organ enlargement, roentgen irradiation is preferred.

If x-ray therapy to the spleen is employed, the clinician must work in close cooperation with the radiotherapist. Usually, a total of 400 to 500 r is administered in divided doses during the course of a week or ten days; the patient and his blood count are followed for several weeks, and additional irradiation is then given cautiously, if necessary, until a remission is induced.

The schedules described are designed for patients with elevated white blood cell counts; a special problem is posed when patients with subleukemic chronic myelocytic leukemia must be treated because of organ enlargement or other leukemic manifestations. The reluctance to treat such patients is irrational when one remembers that leukemia is a disease of the bone marrow, not of the blood; the marrow, however, must be examined to make certain that it shows the changes of leukemia untreated or in relapse. One must proceed with caution, using smaller doses. Frequently, symptoms, anemia, and thrombocytopenia can be relieved and the white blood cell count returned to normal values.

Eventually, with either busulfan or irradiation, therapy loses its effectiveness. If irradiation (P[32] or x-ray) has been used, substitution of busulfan may be tried, and vice versa. Prolonged remissions obtained by this change are unusual, but the response is occasionally gratifying. Other drugs that may be tried when resistance has occurred include 6-mercaptopurine, desacetylmethylcolchicine (Demecolcine), hydroxyurea, and dibromomannitol. For instructions about dose and methods of administration, reference should be made to a textbook of hematology. When the terminal blastic phase occurs, treatment is the same as for acute myelocytic leukemia; beneficial effects are usually of short duration.

Some patients with chronic lymphocytic leukemia run a very mild course with few symptoms, have leukocyte counts in the range of 20,000 to 30,000, and survive for many years with essentially no anemia or thrombocytopenia. They may do very well for long periods without any therapy at all. Moderately enlarged lymph nodes and spleen may cause no difficulty. Most affected patients, however, have a more aggressive form of the disease, and should be treated. P[32] used as described above is very effective. Chemotherapeutic agents of greatest value are chlorambucil, cyclophosphamide, and corticosteroids. Chlorambucil, an aromatic mustard (p-NN-di-2-chloroethylamino-phenylbutyric acid) is the mainstay at present for most hematologists. The initial dose range is 0.1 to 0.2 mg. per kilogram per day, or 6 to 12 mg. administered as one dose 30 minutes before breakfast. When the leukocyte count, determined weekly, decreases by half, the dose is reduced by half; when it reaches 15,000 to 25,000, administration is discontinued. Even though the total white blood cell level may become normal, the percentage of lymphocytes may remain high. Lymph nodes and spleen usually decrease in size, but frequently remain somewhat enlarged. If they are unsightly, produce symptoms, or interfere with function, it is safer to treat them further with local x-ray therapy (100 to 200 r) rather than to push chlorambucil and risk serious marrow depression.

Some hematologists prefer to withhold further therapy after a remission has been induced until the leukocytes rise to 25,000 or more, whereas others prefer to give a maintenance dose varying from 2 mg. every other day to 2 or 4 mg. per day. If a maintenance schedule is elected, the patient should be seen at weekly intervals until it is certain that the selected dose can be tolerated without inducing marrow depression. Thereafter, visits by the patient may be extended to once every two or three months unless symptoms recur during the interval. Toxic effects reported for chlorambucil in addition to marrow depression are dermatitis and several instances of jaundice with hepatomegaly. Precautions about administration during pregnancy are the same as for busulfan.

Remissions can also be induced with corticosteroids in many patients with chronic lymphocytic leukemia, even after they have become refractory to chlorambucil or P^{32}. Therapy is begun with daily doses of 60 to 100 mg. of prednisone for several weeks and then is continued by giving 100 mg. of prednisone, or its equivalent, on one or two days of each week. This type of intermittent dosage schedule minimizes the toxic effects.

The anemia in chronic myelocytic leukemia is almost always corrected when a remission is induced, and blood transfusions are rarely necessary until late in the course of the disease. By contrast, when anemia occurs in chronic lymphocytic leukemia it rarely responds satisfactorily to antileukemic therapy. Its mechanism is complex. The reticulocyte count may be elevated or very low. The Coombs test is positive in about one third of the cases, but even in the absence of a positive Coombs test, increased splenic sequestration and destruction of red blood cells can often be demonstrated. In the past, splenectomy and transfusions were the only effective therapy, but now very gratifying responses can usually be obtained with corticosteroids. A satisfactory initial amount is 40 to 60 mg. of prednisone, or its equivalent, daily in four equally divided doses, but in some instances several times this amount is required. After erythrocyte values have returned to normal, the dose can gradually be tapered to determine the minimal amount required for maintenance therapy; occasionally the drug can be discontinued altogether. If a maintenance amount is required, the secondary effects of continued corticosteroid therapy can often be minimized by giving a large dose, i.e., 60 to 100 mg. of prednisone, in divided doses one day per week. When corticosteroid therapy fails to correct the anemia, androgens are sometimes successful (for dosage schedule, see under bone marrow failure).

Although coagulation abnormalities may contribute to the hemorrhagic manifestations in chronic leukemia, abnormal bleeding is usually referable to thrombocytopenia. If a low platelet count occurs in chronic myelocytic leukemia while the disease is still responsive to therapy, the thrombocytopenia is usually corrected as a remission is induced. That is not commonly true in chronic lymphocytic leukemia, however, and therapy with corticosteroids, given as described for the anemia, is most effective. The thrombocytopenia eventually tends to become constant in both forms of the disease, unresponsive to any known therapy. Platelet transfusions provide transient relief.

Infections are treated when they occur rather than by the prophylactic administration of antimicrobials. Susceptibility to infection may be a particularly grave problem in patients with chronic lymphocytic leukemia who develop low levels of gamma globulin. When frequent, serious infections occur, it is justifiable to try antimicrobial drugs prophylactically or intramuscular injections of gamma globulin, 0.3 ml. per pound of body weight, followed by 0.15 ml. per pound every two weeks. Torula and other fungal infections occur with greater frequency than in the general population.

Associated surgical diseases should not be treated, unless an emergency exists, until a remission in the leukemic process can be induced. The patients should then be cared for so that the maximal degree of comfort and useful life can be obtained. There is no justification for failing to correct a troublesome hernia, for instance, just because the patient has chronic leukemia.

Prognosis. Leukemia is still a uniformly fatal disease; isolated reports of apparent cure are almost certainly the result of erroneous diagnosis or of death occurring during the course of a prolonged remission. No convincing statistical proof exists that therapy prolongs average survival, although it is difficult to believe otherwise, as there are so many specific instances in which correction of thrombocytopenia, successful treatment of serious infections, and so forth have relieved life-threatening situations. That life is made more comfortable and enjoyable by therapy cannot be doubted. The course of chronic leukemia and methods of clinical management vary so much that precise survival figures are not available. The longest median survival time (the time at which 50 per cent of patients are surviving) has been reported by Osgood and his associates: 54 months for patients with chronic myelocytic and lymphocytic leukemia grouped together, treated with regular titrated doses of radioactive phosphorus. In most other series, the median survival time for chronic myelocytic leukemia has varied from about 2½ to 3½ years; about 20 per cent survive for more than 5 years, and a few live for more than 10 years. The current median survival time of patients with chronic lymphocytic leukemia from diagnosis to death is approximately 4 to 6 years, and a few live for more than 20 years. Blast crises of the type seen in chronic myelocytic leukemia are very rare in chronic lymphocytic leukemia, although terminally large lymphocytes with less densely packed nuclear chromatin may appear.

The immediate causes of death are usually hemorrhage, infection, uncontrolled visceral involvement, and congestive heart failure.

Unusual Forms of Leukemia. In addition to the usual types of leukemia, a number of relatively rare forms have been described: eosinophilic leukemia, basophilic leukemia, mast cell leukemia, and Di Guglielmo's acute and chronic erythremic myelosis. The Di Guglielmo syndrome (erythroleukemia) is probably a variety of acute or subacute myelocytic and monocytic leukemia in which erythroid hyperplasia is particularly striking during the early stages of the disease. These rare syndromes are more properly a subject for discussion in a specialized textbook of hematology.

(See also references after article on acute leukemia.)

Ezdinli, E. Z., Sokal, J. E., Crosswhite, L., and Sandberg, A. A.: Philadelphia-chromosome-positive and -negative chronic myelocytic leukemia. Ann. Intern. Med., 72:175, 1970.

Haut, A., Abbott, W. S., Wintrobe, M. M., and Cartwright, G. E.: Busulfan in the long-term therapy of chronic myelocytic leukemia. Blood, 17:1, 1961.

Medical Research Council's Working Party for Therapeutic Trials in Leukaemia: Chronic granulocytic leukaemia: Comparison of radiotherapy and busulfan therapy. Brit. Med. J., 1:201, 1968.

Osgood, E. E., Seaman, A. J., and Koler, R. D.: Result of Fifteen-Year Program of Treatment of Chronic Leukemia with Titrated Regularly Spaced Total Body Irradiation with Phosphorus-32 or with X-ray. International Society of Hematology. Sixth International Congress, Boston, 1956. New York, Grune and Stratton, 1958.

Shaw, R. K., Szwed, C., Boggs, D. R., Fahey, J. L., Frie, E., III, Morrison, E., and Utz, J. F.: Infection and immunity in chronic lymphocytic leukemia. Arch. Intern. Med. (Chicago), 106:467, 1960.

Silver, R. T.: The treatment of chronic lymphocytic leukemia. Seminars Hemat., 6:344, 1969.

Tjio, J. H., Carbone, P. P., Whang, J., and Frei, E., III: The Philadelphia chromosome and chronic myelogenous leukemia. J. Nat. Cancer Inst., 36:567, 1966.

LEUKEMOID REACTIONS

Carl V. Moore

A leukemoid reaction may be defined simply as a syndrome in which morphologic changes resembling leukemia are found in the peripheral blood. The white blood cell count may be as high as 200,000 per cubic millimeter with moderate, minimal, or no immaturity of the cells; with normal or leukopenic leukocyte levels, resemblance to leukemia depends on the presence of immature leukocytes. Lymphocytic and myelocytic leukemoid reactions are common; monocytic leukemoid

reactions are rare. The conditions most frequently responsible for the various types are:

1. Myelocytic or granulocytic leukemoid reactions:
   a. Infections: pneumonia, tuberculosis, meningococcal meningitis, diphtheria
   b. Malignant disease: carcinoma or sarcoma, particularly but not necessarily with metastases to bone marrow; Hodgkin's disease; multiple myeloma
   c. Myelosclerosis with myeloid metaplasia
   d. Intoxications: severe burns, heavy metal poisoning, eclampsia, acute hepatic failure
   e. Stimulation of the marrow: severe hemorrhage; sudden hemolysis; thalassemia major; rarely, during the response to initial treatment of megaloblastic anemias with vitamin B_{12} or folic acid
   f. Polyarteritis
2. Lymphocytic leukemoid reactions:
   a. Infections: infectious mononucleosis, whooping cough, chickenpox, disseminated or miliary tuberculosis, infectious lymphocytosis (in children), toxoplasmosis
   b. Rarely, in patients with carcinoma or sarcoma
   c. Miscellaneous: Sézary syndrome; (?) erythrodermic mycosis fungoides
3. Monocytic leukemoid reactions:
   Rarely, in tuberculosis

The pathogenesis of leukemoid reactions is not understood. In many instances, the bone marrow and other blood-forming organs are directly affected: by direct involvement, as in infectious mononucleosis; by infiltration as with metastatic tumor cells or granulomatous lesions; by toxic effects on marrow cells; by extramedullary hematopoiesis; or by great stimulation of the marrow, as occurs after massive hemorrhage or a hemolytic crisis. Under these circumstances, derangement of the maturation and delivery of leukocytes may explain the appearance of young forms in the peripheral blood, but the leukokinetics of high white blood cell counts have not been worked out. Even more mysterious are the leukemoid reactions occurring in patients with cancer in whom careful search of postmortem specimens has failed to detect metastases to the bone marrow.

Reference has already been made to the fact that total white blood cell counts and degree of cellular immaturity may vary widely. Blast cells, usually in rather small numbers, may be found. Toxic granulation and vacuolization of granulocytes are common in the leukemoid reactions caused by infections or intoxications. Nucleated red blood cells are frequently present and may outnumber the leukocytes. Anemia and thrombocytopenia do not occur except as manifestations of the diseases responsible for the leukemoid reaction. Bone marrow changes are nonspecific. Myelocytic hyperplasia and a shift to younger forms are the rule in myelocytic leukemoid reactions with or without toxic changes in the individual cells; erythroid and megakaryocytic elements may be depressed, normal, or stimulated, depending on the cause. In lymphocytic leukemoid reactions, the number of lymphocytes in the bone marrow may be increased, but the almost total replacement of normal marrow cells by lymphocytes, so characteristic of lymphocytic leukemia, apparently does not occur.

Differentiation of leukemoid reactions from leukemia can be very difficult. In many instances the reaction is transient so that the clinical course alone may decide the issue. If the reaction persists until the patient dies, differentiation may be impossible even at postmortem examination. When granulocytic elements are hyperplastic and immature and erythroid cells are depressed, the morphologic appearance of the bone marrow closely simulates that of myelocytic leukemia. An alkaline phosphatase stain of the peripheral blood is often helpful because the mature granulocytes usually stain heavily in leukemoid reactions but give a negative reaction in granulocytic leukemia. The problem of differentiation is made even greater by reports that Auer bodies may rarely be found in granulocytic leukemoid reactions caused by tuberculosis. Infectious mononucleosis, a frequent cause of confusion, can be recognized by the characteristic lymphocyte morphology and the serologic changes found in that disease. In leukemoid reactions, leukemic infiltration of tissues does not occur. It is emphasized, however, that enough variations exist to make even the most experienced hematologic pathologist uncertain of the diagnosis in many instances.

Treatment should be directed toward the underlying cause of the leukemoid reaction. Severe bone marrow depression can result if vigorous antileukemic therapy is erroneously given to a patient with a leukemoid reaction. The isolated reports of patients said to have recovered from or to have been cured of leukemia are instances of incorrectly diagnosed leukemoid reactions.

Bichel, J.: Lymphocytic leukemia and lymphatic leukemoid states in cancer of the stomach. Blood, 4:759, 1959 (contains a review of lymphocytic leukemoid reactions occurring in patients with cancer).

Smith, C. H.: Blood Diseases of Infancy and Childhood. 2nd ed. St. Louis, C. V. Mosby Company, 1966.

Twomey, J. J., and Leavell, B. S.: Leukemoid Reactions to Tuberculosis. Arch. Intern. Med. (Chicago), 116:21, 1965.

Wintrobe, M. M.: Clinical Hematology. 6th ed. Philadelphia, Lea and Febiger, 1967.

THE CONCEPT OF MYELOPROLIFERATIVE DISORDERS
Carl V. Moore

Many students of hematology, stimulated largely by Dameshek, have become attracted to the idea that polycythemia vera, myelofibrosis with myeloid metaplasia, acute and chronic myelocytic leukemia, primary or essential thrombocythemia, and the Di Guglielmo syndrome should all be classified as myeloproliferative disorders. They involve, according to this concept, "proliferations of one, two, or several of the marrow cells, either within the marrow or in potential marrow (yellow marrow, embryonic rests such as spleen, liver), without discernible cause, and having a self-perpetuating character. Once the proliferation has begun, there is no tendency to revert to the original status." Because the proliferation may be confined to a single cell form, i.e., the megakaryocyte in essential thrombocythemia, or may involve several different strains of cells simultaneously or at different times, this "lumping" makes it possible to relate the overlapping and transitional forms that make precise "pigeonholing" difficult. For example, patients with chronic granulocytic leukemia may have areas of fibrosis in the marrow; polycythemic patients may, at different periods during their course, exhibit changes of essential thrombocythemia, myelofibrosis, or leukemia; and the Di Guglielmo syndrome fades almost imperceptibly into acute leukemia. The possible differences in etiology and pathogenesis are recognized. On the other hand, the evidence that such transitions occur is not universally regarded as convincing except for the frequent late development of myelofibrosis in polycythemia. Whether the concept of myeloproliferative disorders serves any purpose either in clarifying the physician's approach to the diagnosis and treatment of these disorders or in helping to guide further investigation of their nature and cause is debatable. A number of hematologists, however, find the classification useful and employ it in their writings. In the presentation of material in this text, the decision has been made to discuss these diseases under a more conventional outline, e.g., myelocytic leukemia under Leukemias; the designation "myeloproliferative disorders" has not been used.

Dameshek, W.: Some speculations on the myeloproliferative syndrome. Blood, 6:372, 1951.

Dameshek, W., and Gunz, F.: Leukemia. 2nd ed. New York, Grune & Stratton, Inc., 1964.

Glasser, R. M., and Walker, R. I.: Transitions among the myeloproliferative disorders. Ann. Intern. Med., 71:285, 1969.

MYELOFIBROSIS WITH MYELOID METAPLASIA

Definition. Myelofibrosis with myeloid metaplasia (agnogenic myeloid metaplasia, myeloid megakaryocytic hepatosplenomegaly, chronic nonleukemic myelosis) is an unusual but not rare disease characterized by varying degrees of fibrosis or osteosclerosis of the marrow cavity, extensive extramedullary hematopoiesis, particularly in the spleen, leukoerythroblastic changes in the peripheral blood, and usually a slow course. Although a few cases have been recognized in children, it is principally a disease of middle or advanced age, affecting both sexes approximately equally.

Etiology and Pathogenesis. Most instances of myelofibrosis are "primary" or of unknown cause. In a minority of patients, the disease appears secondary to: benzene or phosphorus poisoning; involvement of the marrow with tuberculosis, Hodgkin's disease, or metastatic carcinoma (prostate, stomach, breast, kidney, colon); or irradiation (radium dial workers, fourfold increased incidence in atomic bomb survivors). Myelofibrosis may develop during the course of acute or chronic myelocytic leukemia; conversely, patients with myelofibrosis may terminally have acute blastic crises similar to those of chronic myelocytic leukemia. Myelofibrosis with myeloid metaplasia occurs with considerable regularity late in the course of polycythemia vera, even when that disease is treated only by phlebotomy; occasional patients have some degree of myelofibrosis when the diagnosis of polycythemia is first established. Experimentally, myelofibrosis has been produced by exposure of animals to strontium or by the production of marrow infarcts. The pathogenesis of the disease is not known. The three most frequently advanced hypotheses, none of them really satisfactory, are (1) that myelofibrosis with myeloid metaplasia is a myeloproliferative disorder (see preceding article); (2) that it is a form of myelocytic leukemia; and (3) that fibrosis of the marrow occurs as a reaction to marrow injury and the extramedullary hematopoiesis represents a compensatory phenomenon. Objection to the third concept can be made because the extent of extramedullary hematopoiesis cannot be correlated with the degree of marrow replacement; extensive myeloid metaplasia and a very large spleen may be found with minimal fibrosis when the marrow is predominantly hypoplastic or hyperplastic as well as when it is predominantly fibrotic. The leukemia postulate does not explain the cases that seem to be secondary to granulomatous or tumor infiltration of the marrow or to other forms of injury; it ignores the facts that leukocyte alkaline phosphatase is usually normal or increased rather than low and that the cells are almost invariably negative for the Philadelphia chromosome. We know neither what sets off the proliferation of fibroblasts in the marrow nor what causes the extramedullary hematopoiesis; increased erythropoietin production does not explain the latter, because levels of erythropoietin do not correlate and are even higher in true bone marrow failure, in which extramedullary hematopoiesis is not a feature.

Pathology. The fibrosis or osteosclerosis of the marrow is by no means always uniform. It tends to be greatest in the flat bones, where the marrow normally is hematopoietically active; it may be associated with a variable amount of fat; it is often patchy, and may become more extensive with time, although it is not necessarily progressive. Early in the course, variable and sometimes large areas of hyperplastic marrow may be found. The spleen enlarges early and grows gradually to a huge size, filling most of the left side of the abdominal cavity and extending across the midline. Malpighian corpuscles tend to be preserved although reduced in size; the tremendous splenic enlargement is due to extramedullary hematopoiesis primarily in the red pulp; in large spleens, areas of fibrosis and infarction are common. Myeloid metaplasia causes moderate enlargement of the liver and may involve lymph nodes, kidneys, perirenal fat, the adrenals, and other tissues. Tumor-like masses of hematopoietic tissue may be found in the retroperitoneal area, epididymis, mediastinum, and elsewhere; they can be confusing if their nature is not realized. In all these areas (cellular portions of the marrow, extramedullarly hematopoiesis), the various cellular elements are represented without the dominance of granulocytic precursors that is characteristic of myelocytic leukemia; megakaryocytes may be very plentiful and grouped in small masses.

Clinical Manifestations. Weakness, fatigue, anorexia, weight loss, pallor, and awareness of a left upper quadrant mass are the most common initial complaints. Not infrequently these symptoms are so mild that they are tolerated for five to ten or more years before the patient seeks medical attention; in rare instances, the spleen is known to have been palpable for as long as 20 years prior to diagnosis. As the disease progresses, the enlarging spleen causes an uncomfortably heavy, dragging sensation in the left upper quadrant; infarction produces severe abdominal pain and a friction rub over the area of perisplenitis. Growth in the size of the liver is less dramatic, but the liver edge may extend as much as 8 to 10 cm. below the right costal margin. The combined hepatosplenomegaly produces an increase in abdominal girth which contrasts sharply with the gradual wasting of other tissues, particularly muscle mass. Increased portal pressure resulting from a variable combination of increased splenic blood flow, thrombosis in the portal vein, and intrahepatic obstruction from the extramedullary hematopoietic tissue may lead to ascites, esophageal varices, and gastrointestinal hemorrhage. Dependent edema, arthralgia, bone pain, and fever are other manifestations that may appear. Patients tend to be intolerant to heat because of their hypermetabolism, and may be found sleeping in a chilly room with practically all covers thrown off. When the platelet count is high, thromboses may be troublesome; when it is low, petechiae, ecchymoses, and bleeding from mucous membranes may be found. Anemia may be severe enough to produce symptoms of cardiac insufficiency; multiple transfusions result in transfusion hemosiderosis.

Diagnosis. Anemia, usually normocytic and normochromic, is frequently but not invariably found when patients are first seen; eventually it becomes a constant feature. Red blood cells vary considerably in size and shape; tear drop forms and polychromasia are common; normoblasts are usually found in the peripheral blood. The number of reticulocytes may be increased above normal. Erythrocyte survival is moderately shortened;

rarely the Coombs test becomes positive. The total white blood cell count is usually normal or slightly increased, but may be elevated (as high as 50,000 per cubic millimeter) or, in 20 per cent of cases, leukopenic. Most of the cells are mature granulocytes, but myelocytes are usually present, and promyelocytes or blasts may appear. Late in the course, the white blood cell count may rise above 50,000 per cubic millimeter, and the percentage of immature forms may increase. The mature neutrophils usually stain heavily with the alkaline phosphatase stain, but negative reactions may occur. Thrombocytosis commonly occurs early; moderate thrombocytopenia is more frequent later on. Platelets may be very large and bizarre in shape; megakaryocytes and megakaryocytic fragments are unusual in the peripheral blood. Bone marrow aspiration frequently results in a dry tap or a few drops of bloody material containing only a small number of marrow cells; a trephine biopsy is required to demonstrate the fibrosis. Needle biopsy of the liver is usually not necessary for diagnosis, but when done shows areas of extramedullary hematopoiesis. The basal metabolic rate is elevated, usually to values above +20 per cent. If electrolyte determinations are made, special care must be exercised in the collection of blood to avoid injury to the platelets; erroneously high values for potassium are otherwise obtained. The results of hepatic function tests depend on the degree of nutritional disturbance and the extent of the myeloid metaplasia. Blood uric acid is commonly elevated and may be associated with the manifestations of secondary gout. Roentgenographic changes of osteosclerosis can be demonstrated in about 33 to 50 per cent of patients.

Granulocytic leukemia is the most common disease confused with myelofibrosis and myeloid metaplasia; the alkaline phosphatase staining reaction and cytogenetic analysis for the Philadelphia chromosome help make the differentiation in difficult cases. Most of the confusion can be avoided if trephine biopsy of the marrow is done whenever an adequate specimen is not obtained by aspiration. A long prodromal period relatively free of symptoms is common in myelofibrosis, but very rare in granulocytic leukemia. Polycythemia as a forerunner of myelofibrosis is usually evident from the history. Unusual degrees of fever or the presence of tuberculosis elsewhere should alert one to culture the marrow as well as to stain it for acid-fast bacilli. Tumor cells in the marrow should be searched for.

Treatment. The disease runs a protracted, unrelenting course; patients often can be helped, however, to live a comfortable, productive life for years by directing therapy primarily at the anemia and the tremendous splenomegaly. Transfusions should not be given until the anemia becomes severe enough to cause discomfort (usually below 8 or 9 grams per 100 ml.). The anemia and thrombocytopenia in some patients with myelofibrosis respond to the administration of large doses of androgens (for dose, see Anemia of Bone Marrow Failure). Improvement, when it occurs, takes about six to ten weeks to become evident. Patients must be observed carefully because a few become worse rather than better. Folic acid deficiency may develop, primarily because of increased requirement for the vitamin; its recognition and correction may dramatically decrease the need for transfusion. Because the enlarged spleen sometimes is the site of excessive red blood cell destruction, patients with a large transfusion requirement should have a chromium[51]-tagged red cell survival performed with external counting over the liver and spleen to detect excessive splenic erythrocyte destruction. If the result is positive, attempts to reduce the size of the spleen by irradiation over the organ or by busulfan administration (2 mg. per day or three times a week) may be made; great caution must be used, however, to avoid severe depression of granulocyte and platelet production. Corticosteroid therapy is also occasionally beneficial and worthy of trial, particularly when the Coombs test is positive. In extreme situations, splenectomy may be done. During the immediate postoperative period, thromboses are common; they are difficult to control and cause high mortality. If the patient can be carried safely past the first very difficult few weeks, he may be able to compensate for the anemia and may not require transfusions for a long time. He relies on extramedullary blood formation in other organs to sustain his blood values. After splenectomy, however, the liver gradually becomes larger until it is huge; one merely buys a few extra years of fairly comfortable life. The decision to perform a splenectomy in patients with myelofibrosis should be made only in desperate situations, and then only by an expert after careful study.

Prognosis. A few patients with myelofibrosis and myeloid metaplasia succumb within the first year, the majority survive for three to five years after the diagnosis is made, and a few are able to live a decade or longer. Marked immaturity of granulocytes in the peripheral blood is usually associated with a shortened survival; blastic crises are essentially terminal events. Other causes of death include cardiac failure, hemorrhage, and infection.

Bouroncle, B. A., and Doan, C. A.: Myelofibrosis. Clinical, hematologic, and pathologic study of 110 cases. Amer. J. Med. Sci., 243:697, 1962.

Dameshek, W., and Gunz, F.: Leukemia. 2nd ed. New York, Grune & Stratton, 1964.

Gardner, F. H., and Nathan, D. G.: Androgens and erythropoiesis III. Further evaluation of testosterone treatment of myelofibrosis. New Eng. J. Med., 274:420, 1966.

Khumbananda, M., Horowitz, H. I., and Eyster, M. E.: Coombs positive hemolytic anemia in myelofibrosis with myeloid metaplasia. Amer. J. Med. Sci., 258:89, 1969

Pitcock, J. A., Reinhard, E. H., Justus, B., and Mendelsohn, R. S.: A clinical and pathologic study of seventy cases of myelofibrosis. Ann. Intern. Med., 57:73, 1962.

Shaldon, S., and Sherlock, S.: Portal hypertension in the myeloproliferative syndrome and the reticuloses. Amer. J. Med., 32:758, 1962.

Conditions Primarily Affecting
Lymph Nodes

Carl V. Moore

GENERAL CONSIDERATIONS

The conditions primarily affecting lymph nodes are often collectively called malignant lymphomas or lymphoproliferative disorders. The more general designation seems preferable at the present time because not all workers are agreed that they should uniformly be classified as malignant, and the designation "lymphoproliferative disorders" is variously used to include lymphocytic leukemia or to exclude Hodgkin's disease. The classification of these conditions has been confused because sharp histologic differentiation is often difficult; excellent pathologists often disagree about the interpretation of cytologic changes in abnormal lymph nodes, and about possible transitions from one type to another. Most agree (1) that each form of lymphoma exists in both a follicular and a diffuse form, and (2) that giant follicular lymphoma should no longer receive a separate pathologic designation. There is as yet no uniform acceptance of any of the new suggested classifications, but the following is illustrative:

1. Lymphocytic, well differentiated
2. Lymphocytic, poorly differentiated
3. Stem cell
4. Histiocytic
   ? Hodgkin's disease

Each form is divided into a diffuse and nodular type. Burkitt's lymphoma fits into the stem cell category, and most "reticulum cell sarcoma" into the histiocytic variety. Hodgkin's disease is placed in a questionable position because of its uncertain nature. In spite of the merits of this position, it is impractical to discuss the lymphomas clinically except under the designations lymphosarcoma, reticulum cell sarcoma, and Hodgkin's disease; descriptions of incidence, clinical manifestations, and response to therapy have, with few exceptions, been published under these titles. Follicular lymphoma is listed separately because of its usually more benign course and because the aforementioned position has not been universally adopted.

Diagnosis in all instances is a tissue diagnosis dependent on the recognition of histologic abnormalities. A disturbing problem confronts both the physician and the patient when a lymph node biopsy is obtained because of suspected lymphoma, and the biopsy report is returned as nondiagnostic—usually "reactive hyperplasia." In a recent follow-up study of a series of such patients, one of six eventually developed unequivocal changes of the suspected disease. Careful continued clinical observation and repeated biopsies are, therefore, necessary to avoid error.

LYMPHOSARCOMA AND RETICULUM CELL SARCOMA

The clinical manifestations, diagnosis, and treatment of lymphosarcoma and reticulum cell sarcoma are so similar that they will be considered together to avoid unnecessary repetition. The Burkitt or African lymphoma will be separately discussed at the end of this section.

Definition. Lymphosarcoma is a disease characterized by neoplastic proliferation of lymphocytes in lymph nodes, spleen, and the lymphoid tissue of other organs. It usually appears first in lymph nodes, but extranodal sites of origin are not uncommon (20 to 40 per cent). Controversy still exists about whether it is always unicentric in origin or can occasionally arise in several sites simultaneously (multicentric). Although lymphosarcoma often spreads first from the area of initial involvement to adjacent lymph node areas, distant (presumably blood-borne) metastases occur much more frequently than in Hodgkin's disease and in an unpredictable manner. The same comments apply to reticulum cell sarcoma except that the reticulum cell undergoes malignant transformation, and extranodal sites of initial lesions are even more frequent (30 to 60 per cent). Manifestations are determined largely by the tissues involved and by the structures subjected to pressure, obstruction, or infiltration by the sarcomatous growth. Terminally, cachexia, fever, anemia, hemorrhagic manifestations, and susceptibility to infections are common.

Incidence. Lymphosarcoma and reticulum cell sarcoma are not common, but neither are they rare diseases. Their distribution is worldwide, although their incidence seems to be somewhat less among nonwhite than among white races (except for African lymphoma; *vide infra*). Males are affected nearly twice as frequently as females; the ratio is highest in young people. Both diseases occur at all ages, but reticulum cell sarcoma in children and very young adults is unusual. A distinction must be made between the age distribution of these diseases and their incidence in the population at risk in any age group. The likelihood of developing lymphosarcoma or reticulum cell sarcoma increases as people grow older, reaching a peak incidence between the ages of 60 and 80 (roughly 30 per 100,000 for males and 20 per 100,000 for females). Because the population at risk decreases in later life, however, roughly 80 per cent of cases occur between the ages of 30 and 70. In most medical centers, lymphosarcoma is diagnosed two to four times more frequently than reticulum cell sarcoma.

Etiology. The etiology of these two diseases remains unknown, but the conviction that tumor viruses will ultimately be implicated continues to grow. Some of the forms of lymphosarcoma in animals have apparently been transmitted by cell-free extracts. The strong suggestion that the Burkitt or African lymphoma may be causally related to an infectious agent strengthens this belief. No predisposing factors have been recognized, although the familial incidence seems to be somewhat greater than would be expected on chance alone.

Pathology. The involved lymph nodes have a thickened capsule, are usually discrete, but may become matted, particularly in the retroperitoneal area where larger masses may form. The normal follicular pattern is partially or completely replaced by diffuse masses of sarcomatous cells. In lymphosarcoma, the predominant cell is a lymphocyte of varying degrees of immaturity, and the nodal changes are indistinguishable from those of lymphocytic leukemia. In reticulum cell sarcoma, the reticulum cell is predominant. Reticulin fibers may or may not be demonstrable with special staining techniques. In both types of lymphoma, mitotic figures are numerous, the marginal and medullary sinuses are invaded, and the cells may extend through the capsule to surrounding tissue. Similar changes may occur in any organs that normally contain lymphocytes or reticulum cells. In addition, the diseases may spread, apparently by metastasis, to any tissue. With serous membrane or meningeal involvement, the tumor may grow as thick sheets of cells rather than as nodular masses.

Confusion may occur in pathologic interpretation of the enlarged lymph nodes sometimes associated with anticonvulsant therapy, certain skin lesions like exfoliative dermatitis and erythroderma, toxoplasmosis, vaccinia, cat-scratch disease, and subleukemic acute granulocytic leukemia (often erroneously interpreted as reticulum cell sarcoma).

Clinical Manifestations. The most common and usually the earliest symptom is enlargement of lymph nodes in the cervical, axillary, or inguinal regions. The nodes are firm, discrete, and not painful unless growth has been rapid or an adjacent nerve is infiltrated. They often vary spontaneously in size. Involvement may at first be confined to one node or chain of nodes (unilateral), or it may occur in several areas at about the same time. Mediastinal or retroperitoneal nodes may be the first to enlarge so that the presenting symptoms may be those of mediastinal

obstruction, back pain, or abdominal discomfort. Experience with lymphangiography has taught that most patients who have several sites of involvement above the diaphragm will usually have areas of disease below the diaphragm as well. Extranodal lesions are frequently the primary sites of recognized involvement, particularly in the gastrointestinal tract, pharynx, skin, and bone. Many other areas or organs may be affected, such as the extradural space, lacrimal and salivary glands, thyroid, ovaries, testes, breast, lungs, pancreas, spleen, kidneys, and uterus. Primary lymphosarcoma or reticulum cell sarcoma of the stomach and rectum produces symptoms that may be clinically indistinguishable from those caused by carcinomas originating in these two organs. Systemic complaints (malaise, fever, weight loss, excessive sweating, pruritus) are the presenting manifestations in about one fifth of patients.

After an initial period, very brief or prolonged for many months, during which the disease seems to be fairly localized, involvement becomes more generalized, and the above-mentioned systemic complaints are more constant. More specific symptoms are extremely variable, being determined by the tissues infiltrated, compressed, or obstructed by the sarcomatous process. Enlarged mediastinal lymph nodes may produce cough, substernal pain, dysphagia, paralysis of the recurrent laryngeal nerve, and evidences of superior vena caval obstruction. Pulmonary involvement, nodular or of a diffuse miliary type, may cause atelectasis, cough, dyspnea, and cyanosis. Pleural effusion is relatively common, may be unilateral or bilateral, may be chylous or pseudochylous, particularly in lymphosarcoma, and is often incapacitating. Cardiac manifestations are rare, but there may occasionally be pericarditis with effusion or myocardial infiltration.

Lesions in the gastrointestinal tract may be secondary as well as primary. They may occur in the stomach, jejunum, ileum, cecum, appendix, and rectum. The nodular masses may be large enough to feel; pain, hematemesis or melena, weight loss, and evidences of chronic obstruction or intussusception are the principal manifestations. Rarely, malabsorption with steatorrhea may appear in patients with lymphomatous involvement of the small bowel; conversely, lymphoma of the jejunum has been described as developing in patients with typical adult celiac disease of many years' duration. Mesenteric nodes may become large enough to be palpated, and peritoneal infiltration may cause ascites. The liver may enlarge moderately. Tumor nodules are found in about half the patients at autopsy. When the nodules obstruct a segment of the liver or when nodes at the porta hepatis compress the common bile duct, obstructive jaundice may result. The spleen is often not palpable during the early stages of the disease, but later it usually enlarges enough to extend below the costal margin, and occasionally may become very large. Pain may occur in the left upper quadrant of the abdomen, and the spleen may temporarily become very tender as the result of splenic infarction or perisplenitis. Retroperitoneal nodes may become so large that they can be palpated as a nodular matted mass just beneath the anterior abdominal wall. They may then produce a sense of fullness in the abdomen, interfere with eating, cause severe pain by pressure on spinal nerves, cause partial obstruction of the inferior vena cava with resultant edema of the lower extremities, displace one or both kidneys, and occasionally obstruct the ureters. There may be infiltration of the kidneys, testes, bladder, or prostate, with enlargement, pain, hematuria, and retention of urine. Single or multiple nodules may be found in the breast or, more rarely, in the thyroid gland. The adrenal glands may become infiltrated so extensively that symptoms of adrenal cortical insufficiency are precipitated.

Osteolytic lesions have been described in 6 to 20 per cent of cases; the incidence at postmortem examination has been even higher. The lesions may result from metastases or from local extension in involved soft tissue. In order of diminishing frequency, the bones most commonly affected are vertebrae, femora, ribs, pelvis, and skull. Pain and tenderness, limited usually to the area involved, may be severe; localized enlargement and pathologic fractures may occur. Rarely, particularly in the younger patients, reticulum cell sarcoma may be primary in bone. In these instances, the disease seems to be localized initially, progresses very slowly, and bears a striking histologic similarity to Ewing's sarcoma. The femur, pelvis, tibia, humerus, and scapula are the most frequent initial sites of the disease. Primary reticulum cell sarcoma of bone is of special clinical importance because of its high degree of radiocurability if recognized and treated early.

Pruritus may be troublesome, but is less common than in Hodgkin's disease. Nodular infiltration in the skin or subcutaneous tissue is not unusual; there may be anywhere from one or two to hundreds of nodules scattered over a large portion of the body surface, particularly on the scalp. The nodules or plaques are usually dusky red or purplish; they may be small, discrete, and nontender, or they may enlarge to 5 cm. or more in diameter. In the latter case, they may extend several centimeters above the normal surface of the skin and may ulcerate and be painful.

All patients with lymphomas seem particularly susceptible to herpes zoster; those with lymphosarcoma and reticulum cell sarcoma are no exception. The pain may last for weeks or months, during which time it may overshadow all other clinical manifestations.

Progressive multifocal leukoencephalopathy, a rapidly progressive focal or asymmetric disorder of the brain unaccompanied by increased intracranial pressure or significant cerebrospinal fluid changes, has been described in a few cases. The central nervous system is affected in 10 to 14 per cent of patients; cranial nerve palsies are relatively common (external ocular palsies, facial nerve paralysis, sensory changes caused by invasion of the mandibular branch of the trigeminal nerve). Enlarged mediastinal nodes may involve the cervical sympathetics and produce Horner's syndrome, or the recurrent laryngeal nerve and induce vocal cord paralysis. Although peripheral neuropathy is usually caused by pressure or infiltration from adjacent lymph node masses, it may also be a manifestation of a demyelinating syndrome in the absence of local disease. Acute or subacute compression of the spinal cord, from collapse of an involved vertebra or from pressure by subdural or epidural tumor masses, is not at all uncommon. The paraplegia, sensory loss, and sphincter paralysis that follow may develop within a few days or may appear more slowly. Severe back pain often precedes the appearance of these symptoms. At times, the paraplegia comes on so quickly as to suggest interference with the blood supply to the cord; in these instances, return of neurologic function after appropriate therapy tends to be minimal or less complete than when the paraplegia has been gradual in onset. More rarely, there may be meningeal invasion, with or without cranial nerve paralysis, which causes headache, slight neck rigidity, evidences of increased intracranial pressure, mental changes, and even hemiparesis. A few instances have been reported of primary reticulum cell sarcoma of the brain; symptoms were those of a brain tumor and depended on localization. Retro-orbital or orbital involvement may cause proptosis. Infiltration of an eyelid or of the conjunctiva is an unusual manifestation.

Ultimately an anemia develops that contributes to the sense of weakness and exaggerates any shortness of breath that may otherwise be present. Petechiae and bleeding from mucous membranes may also occur as the result of thrombocytopenia.

Diagnosis. The diagnosis of lymphosarcoma and reticulum cell sarcoma can be established only by biopsy. Clinical manifestations are not sufficiently distinctive to permit differentiation from other diseases associated with lymph node enlargement. The lymph node to be removed for microscopic study should be selected with care and properly fixed and stained. If possible, the entire gland should be excised so that the peripheral sinuses in subcapsular areas will be available for study. Enlarged cervical, axillary, and femoral nodes are satisfactory, but those in the inguinal regions are so frequently the site of chronic inflammatory changes that they should be avoided if others are accessible. Nodes in the posterior cervical chain should also be avoided if possible because of the danger of cutting the spinal accessory nerve during their removal. When this happens, there may be enough pain and weakness of the shoulder girdle to be partially disabling. Early in the course of lymphosarcoma and reticulum cell sarcoma, the histologic changes may not be distinctive enough to permit a diagnosis. Under these circumstances, if there are nodes in other areas, a second biopsy should be done. When enlargement seems limited to mediastinal nodes, biopsy of scalene lymph nodes may be attempted, or a thoracic surgeon should be consulted about the possibility of obtaining tissue from the mediastinal lesion directly. If the only involved nodes are in the abdominal cavity, exploratory laparotomy should be done. Extranodal primary sites can be recognized only when enlargement of involved tissues or clinical manifestations occur that guide the alert clinician to have a biopsy performed. Unless the diagnosis is established before treatment is begun, other diseases that can be treated more satisfactorily will mistakenly be regarded as lymphomas, therapy will be less intense because of the uncertainty, and the patient or his family will be subjected to additional unnecessary anxiety.

It is no longer adequate, however, just to make a diagnosis. Treatment of lymphosarcoma and reticulum cell sarcoma, although not yet as successful as in Hodgkin's disease, has improved enough that the therapist should stage the disease to help him make the most intelligent decisions about treatment. The same guidelines designed for Hodgkin's disease can be used. It has been suggested that an adaptation be made, however, for lymphosarcoma and reticulum cell sarcoma to accommodate the more frequent incidence of patients who present with extranodal lesions. According to this modification involvement apparently limited to an extralymphatic primary site should be classified as Stage I when no lymph node enlargement can be detected, and as Stage II when lymphadenopathy is confined to the regional nodes draining the primary site. When local invasion has occurred beyond the extralymphatic site, the disease should be classified as Stage IV even in the absence of generalized lymph node enlargement.

Staging requires the use of diagnostic procedures to detect the extent of involvement. Roentgenographic studies of the chest, gastrointestinal tract, and skeletal system are particularly helpful. Lymphangiography permits detection of retroperitoneal disease. Pyelograms may help to define a retroperitoneal mass or to identify lesions in the genitourinary tract. Therapeutic results are not yet good enough to justify (as is often the case in Hodgkin's disease) exploratory laparotomy and splenectomy in patients who have no evidence of abdominal or retroperitoneal pathology, solely for the purpose of accurate staging. Cytologic examination of pleural or ascitic fluid may show great numbers of lymphocytes or reticulum cells.

Cerebrospinal fluid studies may reveal a block when there is compression of the cord, or pleocytosis when the meninges are infiltrated.

A clinical and pathologic syndrome closely mimicking malignant lymphomas can result from treatment of convulsive disorders with various hydantoin and hydantoin-like drugs. Clinically, the syndrome includes lymph node enlargement, fever, exanthema, eosinophilia, and, less frequently, hepatosplenomegaly. Pathologically, the nodes show obliteration of the normal architecture, hyperplasia of the reticulum cells, and other elements, with frequent mitoses, infiltration with eosinophilic leukocytes, focal necrosis, and phagocytosis. No Reed-Sternberg cells are present. Cessation of therapy with the offending drug results in remission of the clinical and pathologic manifestations.

Hematologic studies of the peripheral blood and bone marrow are usually of little diagnostic value except to rule out leukemia. In reticulum cell sarcoma reticulum cells may be found in increased numbers in the marrow, and a few young monocytes or reticulum cells may appear in the peripheral blood; the abnormalities, however, are usually not sufficiently definitive to be diagnostic. More frequently, in both lymphosarcoma and reticulum cell sarcoma the differential leukocyte count is normal except for an occasional myelocyte. The total white blood cell level is usually normal, but a slight leukocytosis or a slight leukopenia may be present. Platelet levels tend to be within the normal range. Normocytic, normochromic anemia of moderate degree is common. Its pathogenesis involves both a modest shortening of the red blood cell life span (hemolytic component) and depressed erythropoiesis.

There are two important exceptions to the above-mentioned statements that can best be classified as hematologic complications. Infrequently, late in the course of lymphosarcoma, peripheral blood and bone marrow changes similar to those of acute lymphocytic leukemia may appear. The bone marrow becomes heavily infiltrated by lymphosarcoma cells, the white blood cell count may rise to high levels, many of the leukocytes in the peripheral blood are abnormal lymphocytes, anemia becomes severe, and thrombocytopenia may be profound (leukosarcoma; changes are indistinguishable from acute lymphocytic leukemia). Of more practical therapeutic importance is the development of secondary dyssplenism. This complication may occur at any time in the course

TABLE 1. STAGING OF LYMPHOMAS

Stage I:	Disease limited to one anatomic region or to two contiguous anatomic regions on the same side of the diaphragm
Stage II:	Disease in more than two anatomic regions or in two noncontiguous regions on the same side of the diaphragm
Stage III:	Disease on both sides of the diaphragm, but limited to involvement of the lymph nodes, spleen, and Waldeyer's ring
Stage IV:	Involvement of the bone marrow, lung parenchyma, pleura, liver, bone, skin, kidneys, gastrointestinal tract, or any tissue or organ other than the lymph nodes, spleen, or Waldeyer's ring

All stages are subclassified as "A" or "B" to indicate the absence or presence, respectively, of systemic symptoms. Any of the following symptoms will be considered significant: documented and otherwise unexplained (1) fever, (2) night sweats, (3) pruritus, or (4) weight loss greater than 10 per cent of normal body weight.

of any lymphoma to cause hemolytic anemia, often severe, depression of the white cell count, thrombocytopenia, or any combination of the three. The spleen is enlarged and the bone marrow precursors of the involved cellular elements are normal or even increased in number. With hemolytic anemia, the Coombs test is frequently but not invariably positive.

Hyperuricemia, particularly after initiation of therapy and often associated with an elevation in the blood urea nitrogen, has been reported frequently. Hypercalcemia may occur when bone involvement is extensive or because the abnormal cells produce a parathormone-like substance. Myeloma-type paraproteins (IgG and IgA) have been recognized with increasing frequency in malignant lymphomas; Bence Jones proteinuria is rare.

Prognosis. Because of the propensity for lymphosarcoma and reticulum cell sarcoma to metastasize to distant sites, there is little immediate likelihood that cure rates comparable to those of Hodgkin's disease will be produced by radiotherapy alone, and available chemotherapeutic regimens have not succeeded in totally eradicating all abnormal cells. The survival rate when these diseases are still localized (Stages I and II) at the time treatment is begun with supravoltage irradiation, however, is about 50 per cent at five years, and 40 to 45 per cent at ten years; occasional cures are apparently obtained. After the diseases become generalized (Stages III and IV), therapy is much less satisfactory; comfortable life can often be extended in patients with lymphosarcoma for several years, but the majority of patients with reticulum cell sarcoma still die within 12 months.

Treatment. Stage I and Stage II lymphosarcoma and reticulum cell sarcoma should be treated by a tumoricidal dose of supravoltage irradiation. The clinician has the responsibility for staging the disease, for directing patients to a radiotherapy center where supravoltage equipment is used, for the management of any complications, and for the recognition of recurrent disease. Whether lymph node areas contiguous to the primary site of involvement should be treated is still not clear. Treatment of extranodal primary lesions may present special problems because of radiation damage to organs or tissues exposed, e.g., pulmonary fibrosis, radiation nephropathy, but can be of great importance because of the curability of the lesion, e.g., involvement of tonsil or the nasopharynx, primary reticulum cell sarcoma of bone. Recurrence of disease at a previously irradiated site does not necessarily imply resistance to irradiation or contraindicate another course. In general, if the total white blood cell count falls below 2000 or the platelet level below 50,000, therapy should be interrupted until the bone marrow can recover; exceptions to this rule are risky but occasionally justified.

Palliative irradiation is appropriate in patients with limited life expectancy in order to relieve local symptoms such as bone pain, nerve infil-tration, or spinal cord involvement. Roentgen therapy may cause edema of tissues for a day or two. For that reason, one must proceed very cautiously when treating mediastinal or spinal cord lesions for fear of inducing obstruction.

The clinical remissions produced by x-ray therapy vary greatly both in completeness and duration. At times, the patient may become asymptomatic for months or years; in other instances additional nodes enlarge before treatment at one site has been completed. When the remissions are good, the physician should observe the patient at intervals of one to two months in order that recurrences may be detected promptly.

Chemotherapeutic agents have their greatest usefulness (1) when the systemic manifestations are severe and the disease is widespread; and (2) when there is need to avoid the edema-producing effect of x-ray therapy or when roentgen irradiation is no longer effective. Nitrogen mustard (see article on Hodgkin's Disease) has largely been supplanted by other, more easily administered agents. Because of its prompt action, however, it is still useful in the treatment of mediastinal obstruction or spinal cord lesions. Cyclophosphamide (Cytoxan) produces remissions of three to six months in 50 to 60 per cent of patients when given orally in doses of 100 to 150 mg. Some chemotherapists begin with a loading dose of 20 to 40 mg. per kilogram intravenously in divided doses over two to five days; oral therapy (50 to 150 mg. per day) is then not started until the bone marrow recovers from the usually mild depression. Toxic manifestations include nausea and vomiting, hair loss, myelosuppression, and hemorrhagic cystitis. The latter effect is produced by a degradation product of Cytoxan that is excreted in the urine, and can be minimized by a high fluid intake plus frequent emptying of the bladder. Chlorambucil (0.1 mg. per kilogram given orally each day before breakfast) will induce a remission of five or more months in about half the patients with lymphosarcoma; the dose must be adjusted downward when marrow depression occurs; maintenance doses of 2 to 4 mg. daily may be tolerated for many months. The drug is less effective in reticulum cell sarcoma. Vincristine (1 mg. intravenously each 7 to 14 days) produces useful remissions in both lymphosarcoma and reticulum cell sarcoma, and is often effective when the aforementioned alkylating agents have lost their effectiveness. Toxic neuropathy is the most feared complication and may be incapacitating; it usually does not become severe until after 4 to 6 mg. has been given. Paresthesias, absent deep tendon reflexes, and marked weakness of the lower extremities are the principal manifestations. Pharmacologic doses of corticosteroids have a lympholytic effect in lymphosarcoma, and in doses of 50 to 150 mg. per day prednisone induces objective improvement in about 75 per cent of patients; prolonged remissions can occasionally be maintained on relatively modest doses (20 to 30 mg. of prednisone per day or 50 mg. every second or third day). Some therapists use prednisone and vincristine to induce remissions in both diseases, and attempt to maintain them with cyclophosphamide.

Experimental approaches being currently evaluated include whole body irradiation in an attempt to destroy occult as well as obvious lesions, and various combinations of chemotherapeutic agents (6-week course of cyclophosphamide, 15 mg. per kilogram per week intravenously; vincristine, 0.025 mg. per kilogram per week intravenously; and prednisone, 0.6 mg. per kilogram per day orally). Combinations of this type induce a higher remission rate than any single agent, but have not clearly prolonged survival beyond what can be accomplished by the judicious use of single drugs sequentially. In patients who have had prior chemotherapy or irradiation during the previous six months, severe marrow aplasia may result.

The serous effusions that may complicate lymphosarcoma or reticulum cell sarcoma are often distressing and difficult to treat. Quinacrine given intrapleurally (200 mg. per day for five successive days) or intraperitoneally (400 to 1000 mg. per day for two to four days) will produce control in about half the patients. Alternatively, one can drain the pleural fluid and instill either 100 millicuries of colloidal radioactive gold or 15 to 20 mg. of nitrogen mustard. When the latter is done, one hopes to eradicate the pleural cavity. It is desirable, therefore, to install a chest tube, drain the fluid, inject the mustard, clamp off the chest tube for 30 minutes, and then restart the drainage to keep the pleural surfaces approximated; the tube may be removed after 48 hours. Radiation therapy to the pleura is also sometimes effective, particularly when the fluid is chylous.

Anemia, thrombocytopenia, or leukopenia may occasionally develop as a manifestation of abnormal splenic function even when the sarcomatous process otherwise seems to have responded satisfactorily to treatment. Under these circumstances, steroid therapy (prednisone, 20 to 40 mg. or more per day as needed) or splenectomy may be followed by a return of the blood to normal, and may afford the patient additional months of comfortable, active life. The usual precautions for prolonged steroid therapy must be taken, including the administration of isoniazid. Anemia, not related to dyssplenism, may also appear late in the course of lymphosarcoma or reticulum cell sarcoma; if it does not respond to treatment of the lymphoma, transfusions should be given as necessary for general supportive care.

Kaplan, H. S., and Rosenberg, S. A.: Cure of Hodgkin's disease and other malignant lymphomas. Postgrad. Med., 43:146, 1968.

Johnston, R. E.: Modern approaches to the radiotherapy of lymphomas. Seminars Hemat., 6:357, 1969.

Lukes, R. J.: The pathologic picture of the malignant lymphomas. In Zarafonitis, C. (ed.): Proceedings of the International Conference on Lymphoma and Leukemia. Philadelphia, Lea and Febiger, 1968, p. 333.

Rappaport, H.: Tumors of the hematopoietic system. Atlas of Tumor Pathology, Section III, Fascicle 8. Washington, D.C., Armed Forces Institute of Pathology, 1966.

Richardson, E. P., Jr.: Progressive multifocal leukoencephalopathy. New Eng. J. Med., 265:815, 1961.

Rosenberg, S. A., Diamond, H. D., Jaslowitz, B., and Craver, L. F.: Lymphosarcoma: A review of 1269 cases. Medicine, 40:31, 1961.

Saltzstein, S. L.: The fate of patients with nondiagnostic lymph node biopsies. Surgery, 58:659, 1965.

Saltzstein, S. L., and Ackerman, L. V.: Lymphadenopathy induced by anticonvulsant drugs. Cancer, 12:164, 1959.

Ultmann, J. E., and Nixon, D. D.: The therapy of lymphoma. Seminars Hemat., 6:376, 1969.

BURKITT'S TUMOR OR AFRICAN LYMPHOMA

In 1958, Burkitt drew attention to an interesting form of lymphosarcoma in Negro children living in tropical Africa. The clinical distinguishing features are (1) high attack rate (accounting for 50 per cent or more of all childhood tumors found in some regions); (2) striking predilection for involvement of the maxilla or mandible, or both; (3) frequent occurrence of a retroperitoneal or abdominal mass, often affecting both ovaries or kidneys; (4) relative lack of involvement of peripheral lymph nodes and spleen; and (5) rarity of leukemic transformation. Other common sites of disease are the orbit, salivary glands, liver, and thyroid. Histologically the tumor has the characteristics of a poorly differentiated lymphosarcoma in which histiocytes are interspersed among the lymphocytes to give the sections a "starry-sky" appearance. The disease occurs with high frequency in a broad band extending across Africa adjacent to the equator, in areas where the minimum temperature is no less than 60° F. and the rainfall greater than 20 inches per year. In the same regions, the disease is rare at elevations greater than 5000 feet where the temperature falls below 60° F. This geographic distribution and apparent temperature and humidity dependence suggested that an infective agent, possibly transmitted by an insect vector, might be involved. Furthermore, the peculiar age distribution, climbing steeply after the age of two years and falling toward early adolescence, has suggested that the tumor might be an uncommon response to a common immunity-conferring virus infection. Two viruses have been isolated: a reovirus type 3 in approximately 25 per cent of tumors, and a herpes group virus (Epstein-Barr virus or EBV) in a large percentage of tissue cultures derived from Burkitt's lymphoma cells. The latter has attracted great interest because nearly all patients have a high titer of antibodies for the virus, and because EBV is apparently involved in the etiology of infectious mononucleosis. In addition, EBV is widespread, causing subclinical infections manifest solely by modest antibody response. Two questions arise: (1) Is EBV a passenger or a causative agent of the lymphoma? (2) If the latter, why should the same virus be related to both the etiology of infectious mononucleosis and a malignant lymphoma? Burkitt has suggested that geographic distribution of the lymphoma corresponds with the holoendemic distribution of malaria, that infection with plasmodia causes an intense and sustained lymphoreticular stimulation, and that the stimulated lymphatic tissues are more susceptible to neoplastic transformation in the presence of EBV. Whatever the correct answers to these questions turn out to be, many workers are currently impressed by the apparent relation of EBV to Burkitt's lymphoma.

Lymphosarcoma with the clinical and histologic changes of Burkitt's tumor has now been reported among children of several different races and in a number of countries: England, the United States, South America, Australia, other areas of Africa, and New Guinea. It has been argued with considerable effectiveness that the Burkitt lymphoma may not be a distinct disease entity, separate from conventional lymphosarcoma in children; instead, the unusually high incidence of the disease in equatorial Africa, the predilection for the bones of the jaw and face, and the unusually low incidence of leukemic transformation may reflect an altered host susceptibility in the African children.

Regression of the lesions of Burkitt's lymphoma has been observed in a few cases, occurring either spontaneously or after the administration of convalescent serum, as if host defenses or immunity were involved. Response to chemotherapeutic agents is unusually good, prolonged remissions often being produced by (1) cyclophosphamide in a total dose of 30 to 40 mg. per kilogram given in two divided doses intravenously, or orally in divided doses over three to four days; (2) two weekly injections of vincristine, 0.07 mg. per kilogram; or (3) methotrexate orally in a total dose of 4 to 5 mg. per kilogram distributed over three to four days. Maintenance therapy is apparently not required. Burkitt states that long-term remissions have been observed in more than 20 per cent of treated patients; some of the remissions are still in effect and may amount to cures.

Burkitt, D.: Long-term remissions following one- and two-dose chemotherapy for African lymphoma. Cancer, 20:756, 1967.

Burkitt, D. P.: Etiology of Burkitt's lymphoma—An alternate hypothesis to a vectored virus. J. Nat. Cancer Inst., 42:19, 1969.

Burkitt, D., and O'Connor, G. T.: Malignant lymphoma in African children—Clinical syndrome. Cancer, 14:258, 1966.

Dalldorf, G., Carvalho, R. P. S., Jamra, M., Frost, P., Erlich, D., and Marigo, C.: The lymphomas of Brazilian children. J.A.M.A., 208:1365, 1969.

Dorfman, R. F.: Childhood lymphosarcoma in St. Louis, Mo., clinically and histologically resembling Burkitt's tumor. Cancer, 18:418, 1965.

Henle, G., et al.: Antibodies to Epstein-Barr virus in Burkitt's lymphoma and control groups. J. Nat. Cancer Inst., 43:1147, 1969.

HODGKIN'S DISEASE

Definition. Hodgkin's is a disease of lymphatic tissue characterized by the presence of Reed-Sternberg cells and variable proliferation of lymphocytes and histiocytes. It is usually regarded as being neoplastic, but an inflammatory pathogenesis has not been excluded, and some investigators have suggested that the manifestations may represent a unique expression of an abnormal immune response. The disease is believed to have a unicentric origin. Involvement of lymph nodes in one or two adjacent areas, most often in the cervical region, is the most common type of initial involvement; dissemination usually occurs by spread to contiguous lymph node areas, but distant metastases are not infrequently found, particularly late in the course. The identity of the metastasizing "malignant" cell is not known. Long remissions and actual cures may be achieved when localized disease is properly treated with extended-field, high-dose megavoltage radiotherapy, and chemotherapists believe that eradication of disseminated disease may soon be possible. Systemic reactions, particularly fever, are more prominent than with lymphosarcoma and reticulum cell sarcoma. Other symptoms are determined largely by secondary effects from pressure, obstruction, or infiltration.

Incidence. Hodgkin's disease occurs among all races but seems to be more frequent among the white races. Males are affected almost twice as commonly as are females. Although the disease occurs in children, it is unusual before the age of 15. The greatest number of cases occurs in young adults (from 20 to 39 years of age); but if frequency is stated in terms of "population at risk," or the number of people living during any decade of life, then a bimodal curve is found with the first mode in those between 15 and 34 years, and the second, higher mode in those over 50 years of age; the peak annual incidence is about 50 to 60 per million during the seventh and eighth decades. In the United States, about 3400 deaths per year are due to Hodgkin's disease. More than one case has been observed in the same family; the chance of immediate relatives of a patient with Hodgkin's disease developing the disorder is about three times the expected rate.

Etiology. The cause of Hodgkin's disease is unknown. All attempts to transmit it have been unsuccessful. No animal counterpart of the disease has ever been recognized. The two principal opposing views are that it is an infectious granuloma or a true malignant neoplasm of lymphatic tissue.

Proponents of an infectious origin point to the similarity between the granulomatous changes found in Hodgkin's disease and those characteristic of tuberculosis, brucellosis, certain fungal infections like histoplasmosis, and other granulomas known to have an infectious origin. Various workers have cultured from affected lymph nodes tubercle bacilli, particularly of the avian strain, Brucella organisms, diphtheroids, *Histoplasma capsulatum*, and *Cryptococcus neoformans*. In each instance, however, subsequent work has indicated that the infectious agent was a contaminant, had secondarily invaded the involved tissue, or could not be established as the causative factor Evidence for a viral origin has been offered on the basis of experiments in which lymph node extracts were passed serially in embryonated chicken eggs and in suckling mice; the results, however, are not conclusive.

Greatest support for a neoplastic basis comes from the infiltrative character of the lesions late in the course of the disease, and from the morphologic similarity they have to reticulum cell sarcoma. It has been suggested that the variable histologic expression of the disease may result from an attempted host response to the factors responsible for the development of Reed-Sternberg cells.

Pathology. The lymph nodes in Hodgkin's disease are firm and are usually discrete until late in the disease, when invasion of the capsule causes them to become matted. Other tissues may become involved by direct extension or by development of lesions wherever accumulations of lymphocytes and reticulum cells are found; how distant metastases occur is not certain, although Reed-Sternberg cells are rarely found in the peripheral blood. The histologic pattern is complex. The definitive landmark is the Reed-Sternberg cell, a cell apparently of reticulum cell origin, 15 to 45 μ in diameter, with a folded or multilobulated nucleus, thick nuclear membrane, one or more prominent acidophilic nucleoli often surrounded by a clear zone of nucleoplasm, and abundant acidophilic or basophilic cytoplasm. Reed-Sternberg cells can be identified with greater confidence if they are bi- or multinucleated; the diagnosis should not be made unless they are present. In addition to these giant cells and lymphocytes, the nodes may also contain polymorphonuclear neutrophils, eosinophils, plasma cells, and a hyperplasia of reticulum cells. The normal architecture of the node is destroyed, and the capsule may be infiltrated. Necrosis and an increase in fibrous tissue are often present.

Various attempts to classify the types of histo-pathologic change have been made (Table 2). The most recent recommendation, by a committee of experts, is that four groups be recognized: (1) lymphocytic predominance; (2) nodular sclerosis; (3) mixed cellularity; and (4) lymphocytic depletion. Nodular sclerosis accounts for approximately 40 per cent of cases. In general, an inverse relationship exists between the frequency of lymphocytes and Reed-Sternberg cells. The lymphocytic depletion type includes cases of diffuse fibrosis and of the greatest number of Reed-Sternberg cells. The classification is of prognostic significance since median survival of patients with lymphocytic predominance and nodular sclerosis tends to be much longer than for patients with lymphocytic depletion and diffuse fibrosis. The natural evolution of the histologic process seems to be from lymphocytic predominance to mixed cellularity to lymphocytic depletion; nodular sclerosis is omitted from this chain because it seems frequently to represent a regional expression of Hodgkin's disease.

Clinical Manifestations. Painless enlargement of peripheral lymph nodes, with or without systemic symptoms, is usually the presenting complaint. The first nodes to be involved are most frequently those in the cervical region, axillary and inguinal nodes following in that order. They are initially discrete, may be enlarged only on one side, and may occasionally undergo spontaneous temporary regression in size; later they may become matted. The nodes feel firm or rubbery. If enlargement has been rapid, they may be tender. However, mediastinal or retroperitoneal lymph nodes may be enlarged before those in the peripheral areas; under these circumstances, the first symptoms may be those of mediastinal obstruction, substernal pain, abdominal pain, anorexia, or awareness of an abdominal mass. In Hodgkin's disease, lesions originate in extranodal sites less often than in lymphosarcoma or reticulum cell sarcoma.

Tonsillar involvement is unusual. Lesions within the chest occur at some time during the course of Hodgkin's disease in more than half the patients. In addition to mediastinal lymph node enlargement, there may be infiltration of the pulmonary parenchyma, pulmonary nodules in which cavitation may occur, pleural invasion with effusion, and, more rarely, myocardial invasion. Prom-

TABLE 2. CLASSIFICATIONS OF HODGKIN'S DISEASE

Jackson and Parker	Lukes, Butler, and Hicks	Nomenclature Committee
Paragranuloma	Lymphocytic and/or histiocytic (a) Nodular	
		Lymphocyte predominance
	(b) Diffuse	
	Nodular sclerosis	Nodular sclerosis
Granuloma	Mixed	Mixed cellularity
	Diffuse fibrosis	
Sarcoma	Reticular	Lymphocyte depletion

inent symptoms are cough, stridor, dyspnea, pain, cyanosis of the areas drained by the superior vena cava, and dysphagia. These symptoms may be incapacitating and so difficult to control that they overshadow all other manifestations of the disease.

The gastrointestinal tract is less frequently infiltrated in Hodgkin's disease than in lymphosarcoma and reticulum cell sarcoma, but lesions in the stomach and small intestine are not rare; they may produce the symptoms of partial obstruction, may cause diarrhea, or may ulcerate and bleed, sometimes profusely. A sense of fullness may result from pressure on the stomach by retroperitoneal nodes. The retroperitoneal mass may displace one or both kidneys, infiltrate spinal nerves or adjacent vertebrae, obstruct the ureters or the inferior vena cava, and grow so large that it is palpable in the epigastrium. Epigastric or back pain may be severe. A retroperitoneal mass, not otherwise palpable, can sometimes be felt by the examiner if the patient lies on his arms folded behind his back at the level of the upper lumbar vertebrae so that the vertebrae and retroperitoneal structures are forced anteriorly. The spleen becomes palpable in at least 50 per cent of cases. Hepatic enlargement is frequent. Jaundice may occur as the result of diffuse involvement and fibrosis of the portal triads, or more rarely because of obstruction by nodes near the hilum. Portal pressure may be increased enough to cause esophageal varices. Ascites may follow peritoneal invasion.

Lesions of Hodgkin's disease have been found in the uterus, breast, kidney, and prostate; symptoms are those of tumors occurring in these organs. Bone pain and tenderness may be very severe. Both osteoplastic and osteolytic changes can be demonstrated roentgenographically in about 15 per cent of patients; they most frequently occur in the pelvis, vertebrae, ribs, and femur.

Neurologic complications, observed in about 12 per cent of cases, have the following approximate frequencies: herpes zoster, 3 per cent; spinal cord compression, 3 per cent; peripheral nerve palsies, 3 per cent (including Horner's syndrome, involvement of brachial plexus, and phrenic nerve dysfunction); cerebral signs and symptoms, 1.5 per cent (convulsions, focal signs, progressive multifocal leukoencephalopathy, aseptic meningitis, pituitary involvement, and papilledema); cranial nerve palsies, 1 per cent; and central nervous system infections, 0.5 per cent (including *Cryptococcus neoformans* and other mycotic infections).

Cutaneous manifestations appear in about 25 per cent of patients with Hodgkin's disease. Pruritus is the most common and may be so severe as to be the major complaint. Its pathogenesis is unknown. Other lesions include hyperpigmentation (melanin deposition), intracutaneous nodules, acquired ichthyosis, exfoliative erythroderma, the eruption of herpes zoster, and alopecia.

Systemic manifestations are more prominent in Hodgkin's disease than in the other lymphomas. Anorexia, lassitude, weight loss, night sweats, fever, and chills may appear rather early. Fever unexplained by infection is regarded by some hematologists as a sign of relatively poor prognosis. It may be moderate or as high as 40° C. or more, irregular and continuous, but punctuated by afebrile periods of variable duration. In some instances the remittent or continuous pyrexia occurs in irregular waves of several days' duration separated by periods of remission (Pel-Ebstein type). Fever tends to be particularly troublesome when there is pulmonary or retroperitoneal involvement, and is sometimes a prominent symptom when no enlarged nodes can be located by physical examination or the usual roentgenologic techniques. At times, patients with Hodgkin's disease may have fever of 38 or 39° C. and be totally unaware of the temperature elevation. Tachycardia is often present. Anemia develops except during the early stages of the disease; its mechanism is that of variable shortening of erythrocyte life span coupled with relative failure of erythropoiesis. Petechiae and bleeding from mucous membranes appear if the platelet count falls to low levels. Patients in the advanced stages of Hodgkin's disease seem unusually susceptible to opportunistic infectious agents: fungi, atypical mycobacteria, *Pneumocystis carinii*, cytomegalovirus, herpes zoster, herpes simplex, and others. The adage that tuberculosis follows Hodgkin's disease like a shadow has merit. Patients, except possibly those with Stage I disease, demonstrate impaired delayed sensitivity: negative or poor reactions to delayed skin test antigens (cutaneous anergy), and delayed homograft rejection. The immunologic defect is not well understood but may be related to lymphopenia and a functional abnormality of circulating lymphocytes. Antibody production is relatively well preserved, and gamma globulin levels are often moderately elevated.

Alcohol-induced pain is a strange symptom of unknown mechanism that occurs with greater frequency in Hodgkin's disease than in other disorders, but is not peculiar to it. The pain appears at one of the sites of Hodgkin's involvement, such as the mediastinum or bone, shortly after the ingestion of even small amounts of alcohol, and persists for 30 to 60 minutes, i.e., until the greater part of the alcohol has been oxidized. The symptom tends to disappear when remissions are induced by x-ray therapy.

Secondary amyloidosis is a rare complication of Hodgkin's disease. Pregnancy is not unusual in young women during the early stages of the disease or during a therapeutically induced remission; there is no clear evidence indicating that it exerts a deleterious effect.

Diagnosis. Two things must be accomplished: the diagnosis must be established by biopsy, and the site or sites of involvement must be defined so that the disease can be staged. In selecting a node for biopsy, the same precautions as have been outlined for lymphosarcoma and reticulum cell sarcoma should be used. If several lymph nodes are enlarged in the area selected for biopsy, the surgeon should be urged to select not the most superficial, but one of the larger nodes, which may have been involved for a longer period of time. This recommendation is made because the microscopic diagnosis may be difficult early in the course of the disease, particularly in nodes that have only recently increased in size. An unequivocal diagnosis of Hodgkin's disease should not be made unless Reed-Sternberg cells can be identified. In some instances, two or three biopsies at intervals of several months may be required. The confusing lymphoma-like reaction to hydantoin drugs mimics Hodgkin's disease less commonly than lymphosarcoma or reticulum cell sarcoma. If the only detectable nodal involvement is in the mediastinum or retroperitoneal region, a decision must be reached about the advisability of an exploratory operation. Unless clear contraindications exist, it is usually wiser to proceed with the exploration and to establish the diagnosis with certainty because of the disadvantages of giving intensive irradiation therapy unless the diagnosis is certain.

The revised classification for the clinical staging of Hodgkin's disease is given in Table 3. Accurate staging is necessary as a guide to the radiotherapist and to the wise selection of those patients who will be treated by chemotherapy rather than irradiation. Careful clinical evaluation at the bedside will identify obvious areas of involvement, but must be supplemented by a blood count and urinalysis; roentgenograms of the chest, gastrointestinal tract, excretory urograms, and skeletal system; bone marrow examination (preferably trephine biopsy); and hepatic function tests. If the latter are abnormal or there is any other reason to suspect hepatic involvement (enlargement, right upper quadrant pain, or tenderness), needle biopsy of the liver should be done. A few years ago lower extremity lymphangiography was added to this battery of tests, because periaortic lymph node enlargement could often be detected when not otherwise evident. Reactions to the procedure are unusual (oil embolism to lungs, brain, and other organs; allergic reaction to the iodine-containing contrast media; fever). Inferior caval venography can be used as a less satisfactory alternate. Even these methods failed to provide the diagnostic

precision needed, and therapists are now evaluating the desirability of performing an exploratory laparotomy and splenectomy on patients before therapy is begun, unless (1) the liver biopsy is positive, (2) the bone marrow contains Reed-Sternberg cells, or (3) disease below the diaphragm has otherwise been unequivocally demonstrated. At first, this approach seems unduly radical, but surprising results have been obtained in pilot studies: no involvement has been demonstrated histologically in some patients whose lymphangiogram was read as positive for retroperitoneal nodes, and vice versa; retroperitoneal masses extended laterally farther than was indicated by lymphangiograms, and would not have been included in the irradiation field; the spleen has contained Hodgkin's tissue when there was no reason to suspect involvement and, conversely, has been normal when moderately enlarged; hepatic involvement has always been attended by disease in the spleen, but the reverse does not apply. As a result, some patients thought to be Stage III were reclassified Stage II; some thought to be Stage II were found to be Stage III. Splenectomy with the splenic pedicle identified by a surgically placed silver clip permits better shielding of the left lower lobe of the lung and of the upper half of the left kidney when irradiation is later given to nodes along the left pedicle. Further confirmation must be obtained before this radical approach to staging can be generally recommended, but it is likely to be much more widely applied. After a patient has been treated, the physician must be alert to detect recurrence or lesions at new sites.

Other laboratory procedures are of limited help. The differential leukocyte count most frequently shows an increase in granulocytes, lymphopenia, moderate monocytosis, and occasionally eosinophilia. The erythrocyte sedimentation rate is usually rapid. Plasma globulin may be elevated. Because the bone lesions are so frequently osteoblastic, they usually are associated with moderate increases in serum alkaline phosphatase and with normal blood calcium levels; hypercalcemia is rare. Pleural or ascitic fluid may have the characteristics of either a transudate or an exudate. With central nervous system involvement, spinal puncture may reveal a block, and/or the fluid may show both an elevation in protein and pleocytosis.

Prognosis. The few data available indicate that the duration of untreated Hodgkin's disease averaged approximately two years. With current therapeutic methods, particularly intensive irradiation, prognosis seems primarily related to the stage of the disease at which treatment is begun and to the histologic type. The best prognosis occurs among patients in Stage I and Stage II whose disease belongs to the lymphocyte predominance or nodular sclerosis categories: roughly 70 to 90 per cent survive for five years, 50 to 60 per cent for ten years, and roughly 40 per cent for twenty years. Some of these individuals are apparently cured. Ninety per cent of patients who relapse after therapy do so within three or four years; only infrequently does the initial recur-

TABLE 3.   REVISED CLASSIFICATION FOR CLINICAL STAGING OF HODGKIN'S DISEASE

Stage	Description
I	Disease limited to one anatomic region
II	(1) Disease limited to 2 contiguous anatomic regions on same side of the diaphragm
	(2) Disease in more than 2 anatomic regions or in 2 non-contiguous regions on same side of diaphragm
III	Disease on both sides of diaphragm but limited to involvement of lymph nodes, spleen, and Waldeyer's ring
IV	Involvement of bone marrow, lung parenchyma, pleura, liver, bone, skin, kidneys, gastrointestinal tract, or any tissue or organ other than lymph nodes, spleen, or Waldeyer's ring

All stages should be subclassified as "A" or "B" to indicate the absence or presence, respectively, of systemic symptoms.

rence appear after five years of continuously disease-free survival. A higher percentage of young people and of women fit into Stage I or Stage II and have, therefore, a better prognosis than the average. How serious a problem irradiation damage will become in future years is still unanswered; acute leukemia has now been diagnosed in a few. Five-year survival is about 20 to 40 per cent for patients with Stage III disease (those having systemic symptoms may do less well) and about 10 to 20 per cent for Stage IV disease. These figures will probably be affected favorably by the intensive combined chemotherapeutic programs currently being tried.

Treatment. If patients with Stage I and Stage II Hodgkin's disease are to be provided the maximal opportunity for cure, their treatment should be given and supervised by experts. They should be referred to a medical center where supervoltage therapy can be administered under the supervision of an experienced radiotherapist. Difference of opinion still exists about the optimal treatment factors (tumor dose, field size, duration of treatment), but in general a tumoricidal dose (3500 to 4000 rads) is given over a period of about four weeks to the lymph node area involved and to the adjacent proximal node-bearing areas. Thus, for unilateral cervical Hodgkin's disease, Stage I, both sides of the neck, both axillas, and the mediastinum would be included. Radiotherapists differ as to whether the retroperitoneal area should be treated if the mediastinum is involved, and some doubt the over-all necessity for treating lymph node areas contiguous to an area of known disease. Encouraged by the results in Stage I and II, several centers are currently applying the aforementioned principles to the treatment of Stage III disease. The area treated covers a large proportion of the active bone marrow and must be given cautiously to avoid severe bone marrow damage. Remissions lasting as long as several years, and continuing, have been produced in about 40 per cent of patients. Other workers, impressed with the possibility that distant metastases (noncontiguous spread) may occur more often than is indicated in the foregoing discussion, have been exploring the effectiveness of "total-nodal" therapy. The investigative activity in this field is intense, and modifications in current practices can be expected.

Chemotherapy has found its greatest usefulness in the treatment of widely disseminated disease or for recurrence after the maximal tolerable amount of irradiation. Single drugs have for the most part been used in the past, but combinations of drugs are now being tried not only to improve the remissions in Stage III and Stage IV Hodgkin's disease, but in the hope that they might equal or surpass the effectiveness of radiation in localized disease, or be combined with radiation to produce a higher percentage of cures. If patients have previously received intensive radiotherapy, their bone marrow reserves may have been sufficiently reduced to make them unusually vulnerable to the myelosuppressive effects of chemotherapeutic

agents. The extent of bone marrow irradiation and the interval from completion of radiotherapy to onset of chemotherapy are the principal factors that limit tolerance to drugs; tolerance improves when the interval is six months or longer.

With conventional therapy, the drugs used in the attempt to induce a remission are nitrogen mustard, cyclophosphamide, chlorambucil, vinblastine, and procarbazine. Cyclophosphamide and chlorambucil are administered as described under the treatment of lymphosarcoma; when given for the first time, cyclophosphamide produces objective improvement in about 70 per cent of patients, and chlorambucil in 50 per cent. Maintenance doses of these two drugs probably prolong remissions and provide patients with a greater number of days of comfortable life. Vinblastine is administered intravenously every 7 to 14 days; the starting dose of 0.1 mg. per kilogram is increased by 0.05 mg. per kilogram with each injection until leukopenia develops; maintenance dosage is determined by the response of the patient and the myelosuppression. Remissions are induced in about 65 to 80 per cent of patients and have a median duration of about seven months. Toxic reactions, in addition to leukopenia and thrombocytopenia, include phlebitis at injection sites, alopecia (15 per cent), and neurologic complications (8 per cent): peripheral neuropathy and constipation, occasionally with ileus, from involvement of the autonomic nervous system. Procarbazine (Natulan, a synthetic derivative of methylhydrazine) is given orally: 50 mg. on the first day, increasing by 50 mg. each day as tolerated (nausea and vomiting) or until a maximal daily dose of 300 mg. is attained. After remission occurs, a maintenance daily dose of 50 to 150 mg. is given. About 75 per cent of patients respond; the median duration of maintained remission is over five months. Side effects include significant myelosuppression (50 per cent), nausea and vomiting (50 per cent during induction), hyperirritability, ataxia, nystagmus, postural hypotension, accentuation of the effect of some drugs (chlorpromazine derivatives, alcohol, barbiturates), and a flush syndrome. The drug is particularly valuable in that patients resistant to irradiation and other chemotherapeutic agents may have a useful remission.

Nitrogen mustard, once the mainstay of chemotherapy for Hodgkin's disease, now finds its greatest usefulness—because of its prompt action—in the relief of urgent complications (obstruction of the airway or of the superior vena cava, compression of the spinal cord). Four-tenths of a milligram per kilogram of body weight given intravenously in two to four divided doses on successive days constitutes a course of therapy. The total amount given in a course should not exceed 40 mg. It is most easily administered in the following manner: An intravenous infusion of physiologic saline or of 5 per cent glucose in water is begun. The nitrogen mustard from one or two 10-mg. ampules is then dissolved in approximately 10 ml. of saline; the calculated dose is injected with-

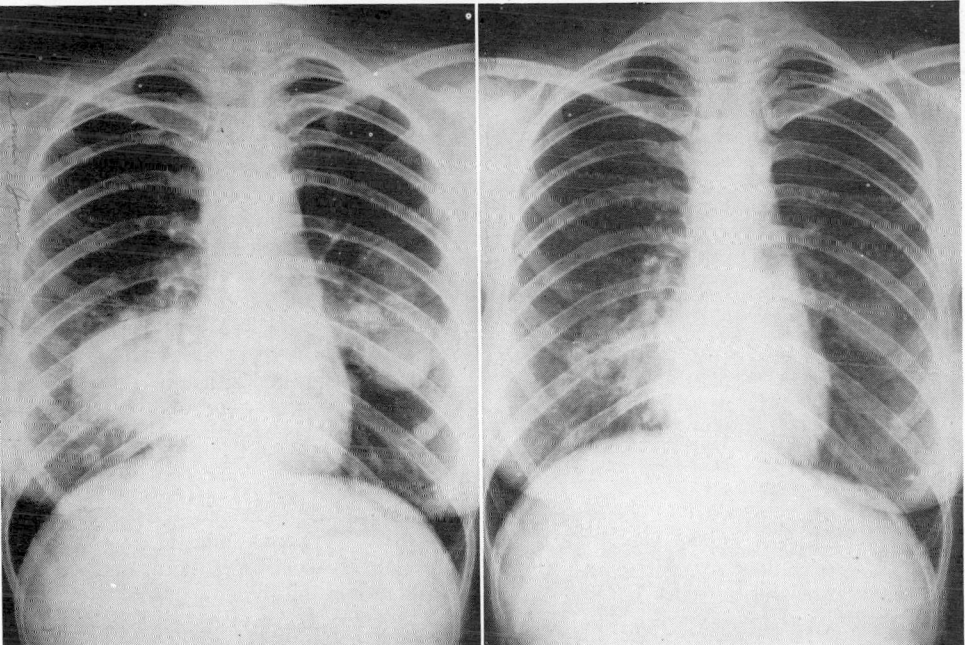

Pulmonary and mediastinal involvement by Hodgkin's disease in a girl 20 years of age. Pulmonary lesions had become refractory to x-ray therapy after having responded satisfactorily on several previous occasions. Roentgenogram at left was taken shortly after completion of last course of roentgen irradiation. There had been no decrease in the size of the infiltrations; cough, dyspnea, and fever continued. Nitrogen mustard therapy was followed by prompt symptomatic relief and diminution in the size of pulmonary infiltrate. Roentgenogram on right was made three weeks after nitrogen mustard had been given.

out delay into the tubing through which the saline or glucose solution is running. Because patients so frequently suffer from nausea and vomiting for 6 to 24 hours after the injection, one may minimize their discomfort by giving the nitrogen mustard at bedtime, approximately an hour after they have been given a sedative such as 0.1 to 0.2 gram of a rapidly acting barbiturate. In addition, several doses of chlorpromazine (25 mg.) may be administered. The therapeutic effects may be dramatic and prompt. Enlarged lymph nodes or infiltrating masses of tissue may seemingly melt away so that obstruction is temporarily relieved; fever that has been persistent for weeks may disappear within a few days. The remissions are not likely to be prolonged, however, so that as soon as the patient recovers from the leukopenia and thrombocytopenia that almost invariably follow administration of nitrogen mustard (usually three to four weeks), an additional form of therapy should be started. If desired or necessary, a second course of mustard can be given after an interval of five to six weeks. When enlarged lymph nodes are to be treated with irradiation but are so located that the edema that often follows x-ray therapy is likely to produce further damage—partial obstruction of respiratory passages or threatening obstruction of blood vessels—one may elect to give 0.2 mg. of nitrogen mustard per kilogram; that dose usually produces lesser degrees of myelosuppression, together with enough shrinkage to permit irradiation therapy after several days.

Corticosteroids frequently abolish fever, increase appetite, and produce a sense of well-being. In large doses (50 to 150 mg. of prednisone or its equivalent per day) they may cause objective improvement in the size of lymph nodes and in parenchymal lesions, but the favorable effect is usually of short duration. They are valuable when marrow suppression precludes the use of cytotoxic drugs, when rapid relief of symptoms is important in a severely toxic patient, when thrombocytopenia or hemolytic anemia occurs as a manifestation of hypersplenism, or when the Coombs test is positive. If the daily dose of prednisone required to control these hematologic complications is greater than 20 to 30 mg., and if the general clinical status permits, splenectomy may be effective.

By skillful manipulation of the aforementioned chemotherapeutic agents, life can often be appreciably prolonged and made much more comfortable. By combining three or four agents, therapists are attempting to prolong drug-induced remissions and to produce cures. Several of the combinations are vincristine, nitrogen mustard, and procarbazine; cyclophosphamide, vincristine, and prednisone; and nitrogen mustard, vincristine, procarbazine, and prednisone. Usually the drugs are given in cycles of several weeks each. Remissions of as long as four years have been reported. Details of dosage are not given here, because schedules are changing and because toxic complications can be severe; it is believed, therefore, that at present these kinds of programs should be confined to centers especially prepared to cope with the complications. Experiments in chemotherapy, however, are exciting and may well lead to further significant advance in treatment.

General supportive care should include transfusions and antimicrobial drugs when needed. Salicylates must be used with caution. Occasionally, aspirin even in low dosage will cause a sudden drop in temperature in patients with Hodgkin's disease from 40° C. to levels as low as 35° C. and precipitate a state of shock.

Curran, R. E., and Johnson, R. E.: Tolerance to chemotherapy after prior irradiation for Hodgkin's disease. Ann. Intern. Med., 72:505, 1970.

Diamond, H. D.: Hodgkin's disease: Neurologic sequelae. Missouri Med., 54:945, 1957.

Gladstein, E., Guernsey, J. M., Rosenberg, S. A., and Kaplan, H. S.: The value of laparotomy and splenectomy in the staging of Hodgkin's disease. Cancer, 24:709, 1969.

Johnson, R. E.: Modern approaches to the radiotherapy of lymphomas. Seminars Hemat., 6:357, 1969.

Kaplan, H. S.: Role of intensive radiotherapy in the management of Hodgkin's disease. Cancer, 19:356, 1966.

Kaplan, H. S.: Clinical evaluation and radiotherapeutic management of Hodgkin's disease and the malignant lymphomas. New Eng. J. Med., 278:892, 1968.

Keller, A. R., Kaplan, H. S., Lukes, R. J., and Rappaport, H.: Correlation of histopathology with other prognostic indicators in Hodgkin's disease. Cancer, 22:487, 1968.

Lowenbraun, S., Ramsey, H., Sutherland, J., and Serpick, A. A.: Diagnostic laparotomy and splenectomy for staging Hodgkin's disease. Ann. Intern. Med., 72:655, 1970.

Lukes, R. J., Craver, L. L., Hall, T. C., Rappaport, H., and Ruben, P.: Hodgkin's disease, report of Nomenclature Committee. Cancer Res., 26:1311, 1966.

Lukes, R. J., Butler, J. J., and Hicks, E. B.: Natural history of Hodgkin's disease as related to its pathologic picture. Cancer, 19:317, 1966.

Peters, M. V.: The place of irradiation in the control of Hodgkin's disease. In Fourth National Cancer Congress Proceedings, Philadelphia, J. B. Lippincott Company, 1961, page 571.

Peters, M. V., Alison, R. E., and Bush, R. S.: Natural history of Hodgkin's disease as related to staging. Cancer, 19:308, 1966.

Rubin, P.: Controversial issues in the treatment of Hodgkin's disease. In Brown, E. B., and Moore, C. V. (eds.): Progress in Hematology, New York, Grune & Stratton, Inc., Vol. 5, pp. 180–203, 1966.

Ultmann, J. E., and Nixon, D. D.: The therapy of lymphoma. Seminars Hemat., 6:376, 1969.

FOLLICULAR LYMPHOMA
(Giant Follicular Lymphoblastoma, Giant Follicle Lymphosarcoma, Brill-Symmers Disease)

Follicular lymphoma was originally described as a specific type of lymphoma characterized by the formation of multiple follicle-like nodules of various sizes in lymphatic tissue, a relatively benign course, and a propensity for eventual transformation into lymphosarcoma, reticulum cell sarcoma or, less frequently, Hodgkin's disease. The right of follicular lymphoma to be classified as a distinct entity has been questioned. The claim is made that any form of malignant lymphoma may have a nodular (follicular) as well as a diffuse pattern, that the follicular forms of lymphosarcoma and reticulum cell sarcoma are more closely related to their diffuse (nonfollicular) counter-

part than to each other, that nodular variants of Hodgkin's disease are responsible for the "misconception" that follicular lymphoma can undergo transition to Hodgkin's disease. Even though this concept may well be correct, clinicians are reluctant to abandon follicular lymphoma as a *syndrome* because of the relatively benign manifestations during most of its course.

Follicular lymphoma is distinctly less common than Hodgkin's disease, lymphosarcoma, or reticulum cell sarcoma. It is more frequent after the age of 40, although younger persons and even children are affected. Males predominate over females in an approximate ratio of 2 to 1.

The enlarged nodes may have a diameter of 5 cm. or more; they tend to be discrete and are not tender. Initially, the disease is usually (but not always) limited to one lymph node area; cervical, inguinal, and axillary nodes, in that order, are most frequently involved. Lymph follicles within a node are often large enough to be prominent when a microscopic section is examined without magnification. The follicles are more numerous than they normally are, vary in size and shape, are distributed throughout the substance of the node rather than being limited primarily to the cortex, and compress zones of mature lymphocytes and reticulum at their periphery. Fusion of follicles may occur. Trabeculae are obscured, lymph sinuses are narrowed or obliterated, and the capsule may be invaded. These changes are usually confined to lymph nodes and spleen, though rarely they may occur in other tissues and organs. Differentiation from reactive follicular hyperplasia is occasionally difficult.

Constitutional manifestations are infrequent. Skeletal and visceral involvement occurs less frequently than in the other lymphomas. Rarely, primary lesions may be found in the nasopharynx or the appendix. Hepatomegaly and splenomegaly are common; the latter may be of great degree. Retroperitoneal lymph nodes are frequently affected. Intracutaneous tumors and pruritus are not unusual.

Diagnosis can be established only by lymph node biopsy. Lymphocytes with distinctly notched or cleft nuclei may be found in the peripheral blood. The disease is best treated by x-ray therapy to areas of lymph node involvement, and remissions of long duration are often produced. All the information about response to modern supervoltage irradiation and to chemotherapeutic agents is contained, during most of the last decade, in the literature on Hodgkin's disease, lymphosarcoma, and reticulum cell sarcoma. In those reports, patients with the follicular lymphoma syndrome are found among the patients with nodular forms of the lymphomatous disorders, and usually among those who have responded most dramatically to treatment. In the presence of splenomegaly, hemolytic anemia, leukopenia, or thrombocytopenia may develop as a manifestation of dyssplenism. If these complications are severe, corticosteroid therapy or splenectomy may become necessary. In several instances, removal of massively enlarged spleens has been followed by long periods free of evident disease. The follicular or nodular pattern may be retained to death, but usually it gives way histologically to more malignant changes the diffuse pattern in lymphosarcoma or reticulum cell sarcoma, and the mixed cellularity or lymphocyte depletion form in Hodgkin's disease.

Hickling, R. A.: Giant follicle lymphoma of the spleen. Brit. Med. J., 2:787, 1964.

Rappaport, H., Winter, W. J., and Hicks, E. B.: Follicular lymphoma. A re-evaluation of its position in the scheme of malignant lymphoma, based on a survey of 253 cases. Cancer, 9:792, 1956.

Rosenberg, S. A., Diamond, H. D., Jaslowitz, B., and Craver, L. F.: Lymphosarcoma: A review of 1269 cases. Medicine, 40:31, 1961.

MYCOSIS FUNGOIDES

Mycosis fungoides is defined as an uncommon but not rare, chronic, poorly understood fatal disorder of the lymphoreticular system that is first manifested in the skin. Although lesions remain confined to the skin for many years, the disease eventually terminates in most but not all instances with the histopathologic changes of disseminated lymphoma. Prevailing opinion seems to be that mycosis fungoides is a peculiar form of lymphoma localized to the skin until dissemination occurs late in the course. Although that concept may be correct, it must be held suspect until more convincing evidence is provided that the lymphoreticular infiltration of the skin is neoplastic rather than inflammatory. If the latter, neoplastic transformation could eventually occur in a clone of the chronically stimulated cells to account for the lymphoma so frequently found terminally. Men are more frequently affected than women; the diagnosis is seldom made before the age of 40. Three stages can be recognized, although not all stages necessarily appear in a given patient:

1. Premycotic. Cutaneous eruptions resembling nonspecific dermatitis, psoriasis, eczema, neurodermatitis, and a fixed drug reaction may be present for many years before histologic changes appear that permit a diagnosis of mycosis fungoides.

2. Infiltration, lichenification, and plaque formation. At this stage, an eosinophil-rich pleomorphic intradermal cellular infiltrate is present, together with focal collections of reticular cells in the epidermis (Pautrier's abscesses), and a diagnosis can be made. When the infiltration is generalized, the patient's skin becomes thickened and has a dusky, red hue.

3. Tumor stage. With further progression, the cellular aggregates form skin tumors that may break through the epidermis and ulcerate or invade the subcutaneous tissue. The premycotic type of dermatitis may persist, but it often improves to a variable degree. In a small number of patients, cutaneous tumors develop without any prior eruption. The infiltrative tumors may bear a close histologic resemblance to reticulum cell sarcoma or Hodgkin's disease of the skin.

Erythrodermic mycosis fungoides is an interesting variant in which generalized erythroderma predominates. Patients look like boiled lobsters. Pruritus may be severe. Sezary described a syndrome of generalized erythroderma, lymph node enlargement, splenomegaly, elevated white blood cell count (10,000 to 50,000 per cubic millimeter), and a large percentage of abnormal lymphocytes. The bone marrow is not heavily infiltrated with lymphocytes so that the changes resemble a lymphocytic leukemoid reaction. The abnormal cell is characterized by a large convoluted nucleus with a narrow rim of cytoplasm frequently containing numerous vacuoles in a necklace-like arrangement around the nucleus. A periodic acid–Schiff-positive, diastase-resistant neutral polysaccharide can be stained within the vacuoles. Although opinion is not uniform, the Sezary syndrome is also probably a variant of mycosis fungoides.

Lymph node enlargement is the most common noncutaneous manifestation. The nodes are nontender, firm, and freely movable. The histologic changes in biopsy specimens may be those of simple hyperplasia, dermatopathic lymphadenitis, plasmacytosis only, a polymorphic cellular infiltrate similar to that seen in the skin, or lymphoma (lymphosarcoma, reticulum cell sarcoma). Occasionally, an initial biopsy may be nondiagnostic, whereas a subsequently removed node may be positive for lymphoma. Disseminated lymphomatous disease also occurs in the liver, spleen, lungs, heart, kidneys, gastrointestinal tract, endocrine glands, and central nervous system. Rarely, visceral manifestations may occur while the lymph nodes remain nondiagnostic.

Although the premycotic stage of the disease may be very prolonged, once the diagnosis is made and the lymph nodes enlarge, most patients succumb within three years. In a series of 165 patients, the mean duration of disease was 8.1 years for those who had died, (106), and 12.5 for those who were still living (59). The most frequent complication and the most common cause of death is infection (particularly skin infection, septicemia, and bronchopneumonia). Part of the confusion about mycosis fungoides being a form of lymphoma results from the fact that the lymph nodes and tissues of patients who die do not always show changes that permit a diagnosis of lymphoma; under these circumstances the designation depends on interpretation of the reticular histopathology in the skin. The most common types of visceral lymphoma diagnosed at autopsy of patients with mycosis fungoides are lymphosarcoma and reticulum cell sarcoma. In one series, 14 of 17 patients had visceral lymphomatous involvement at autopsy.

The results of treatment are usually not dramatic. Because good remissions are uncommonly obtained and therapy must be given for a long time, it is prudent to begin with the least toxic forms. Local therapy is effective in some instances: (1) painting the lesions with nitrogen mustard, i.e., weekly with freshly prepared 0.05 per cent solution; (2) topical corticosteroids; or (3) electron beam radiation. For systemic therapy, nitrogen mustard, cyclophosphamide, chlorambucil, methotrexate, and corticosteroids have all been used with variable effectiveness. In general, chemotherapeutic agents are employed only after local therapy is no longer able to provide relief or if there is evidence of lymph node or visceral involvement. The best responses (and a few complete remissions) have been reported after weekly intramuscular injections of methotrexate (37.5 to 75 mg.).

Block, J. B., Edgcomb, J., Eisen, A., and Van Scott, E. J.: Mycosis fungoides. Natural history and aspects of its relationship to other malignant lymphomas. Amer. J. Med., 34:228, 1963.

Bluefarb, S. M.: Is mycosis fungoides an entity? Arch. Derm. (Chicago), 71:293, 1955.

Cyr, D. P., Geokas, M. C., and Worsley, G. H.: Hematologic findings and terminal course. Arch. Derm. (Chicago), 94: 558, 1966.

Haynes, H. A., and Van Scott, E. J.: Therapy of mycosis fungoides. Progr. Derma., 3:1, 1968.

Pillsbury, D. M., Shelley, W. B., and Kligman, S. M.: Dermatology. Philadelphia, W. B. Saunders Company, 1956, pp. 1089–1093.

Taswell, H. F., and Winkleman, R. K.: Sézary syndrome—A malignant reticulemic erythroderma. J.A.M.A., 177:465, 1961.

Infectious Mononucleosis

William N. Valentine

Definition. Infectious mononucleosis is characterized typically by irregular fever, pharyngitis, lymph node enlargement, splenomegaly, absolute lymphocytosis with variably numerous morphologically atypical lymphocytes, the development in the patient's serum of abnormally high concentrations of heterophil antibodies against sheep erythrocytes, and the development of antibodies to the herpes-like Epstein-Barr virus (EBV) present in certain Burkitt-lymphoma cell lines. There is strong support for the etiologic role of the EB virus, but this is not unequivocally established.

History. Although the first account of the disease is generally credited to Emil Pfeiffer, who in 1889 described an epidemic in children that he termed "glandular fever," substantial clinical differences from the typical syndrome and absence of serologic or hematologic data render this assumption highly doubtful. Sprunt and Evans in 1920 first applied the name "infectious mononucleosis" to the disorder recognized as such today, and directed attention to the abnormal blood leukocytes. The latter were described in detail in 1923 by Downey and McKinlay. Paul and Bunnell in 1932 discovered the unusual concentrations of sheep cell agglutinins in the serum of subjects with the disease. In 1968, Gertrude and Werner Henle reported that patients with infectious mononucleosis acquired antibodies to EBV.

Etiology. Currently there is evidence supporting EBV, or a virus closely related to it, as the causative agent of infectious mononucleosis. In now relatively large numbers of typical, heterophil-antibody-positive cases of infectious mononucleosis, the presence of EBV antibody has been regularly demonstrated. In a number of patients, pre-illness serum lacked the antibody, and in all, antibody developed in high titer during typical infectious mononucleosis. In a smaller number of patients, rising EBV antibody titer has been observed during the illness, although in most, substantial titers are evident at the time of initial clinical manifestations. Moreover, in more than 300 college students tested on entry into college, infectious mononucleosis developed *only* in the EBV antibody-negative group. Over four years of college, the attack rate in this group was about 15 per cent. In contrast, a past history of typical clinical infectious mononucleosis was elicited only in students whose sera contained EBV antibodies. In none of these did clinically recognized infectious mononucleosis develop during their college years. EBV antibody persists for years, as would be expected of a true antibody in contrast to the transient life of the heterophil antibody. Antibodies to EBV have now been shown to develop in the course of infectious mononucleosis by both immunofluorescent and complement fixation techniques. Although the sero-epidemiologic evidence indeed very strongly supports the candidacy of EBV as the causative agent in infectious mononucleosis, the classic postulates of Koch are not thus far fulfilled. It should be noted that a number of lymphoblastic cell lines in culture (obtained not only from cases of Burkitt lymphoma, but from certain other malignant and benign lymphoproliferative disorders and from certain normal persons as well) contain EBV. Also, for example, antigenic stimulus for EBV antigens could occur if the abnormal cells associated with infectious mononucleosis, induced by some other agent, provided a substrate for EBV replication or altered a leukocyte-latent virus relationship. EBV appears probably to be more than a shared but unrelated antigen in infectious mononucleosis, but evidence of a more direct nature such as the isolation of the virus in a freely infectious state and the experimental production of the disease after its inoculation is essential to the establishment of the etiologic relationship which available evidence so strongly favors.

Incidence and Prevalence. Infectious mononucleosis is widely distributed, having been recognized in Europe, Asia, Australia, America, and elsewhere. Sporadic cases occur mainly, but not exclusively, between the ages of 15 and 30 years, with a slightly greater incidence in males. Epidemics have been reported chiefly in younger children, although in World War II a number of epidemics were observed in young adults. Unfortunately, in many reported epidemics clinical data fail to preclude other diagnoses, and hematologic and serologic data are inadequate or not convincingly confirmatory. Infectious mononucleosis has a low order of contagiousness, is rare in the endemic form among children, and most probably is largely, if not entirely, a sporadic disease. Large series of sporadic cases have been reported from college health dispensaries. Although earlier experience suggested the comparative rarity of the disease in Negroes, it is now clear that it is not uncommon in this race. A high incidence has been found among hospital personnel, nurses, and medical students, but it must be recognized that hematologic studies are more frequent with mild illnesses in this group. In Connecticut from 1948 to 1967 the reported incidence of the disease increased some 25-fold. Although the increase was in part undoubtedly related to better recognition and reporting, similar upward trends in various parts of the world suggest that a true increase in incidence may have occurred. At Yale University, about 75 per cent of entering students lacked EBV antibodies, and the annual student attack rate from 1962 to 1967 was 1.3 to 2.2 per cent.

Epidemiology. In the sporadic form of the disease, cases seldom appear in roommates, families, or other close contacts of patients with the disease. Evidence suggests that kissing may be one important mode of transmission. In epidemics reported before the development of the heterophil antibody test in 1932, serologic confirmation was unattainable, and those before about 1920 (and often later) were not substantiated by adequate hematologic studies. Variability in hematologic and serologic criteria for diagnosis in different reports, an unusual prevalence of atypical and subclinical cases in certain epidemics, and the handicap of the inability to demonstrate a specific etiologic agent combine to cast doubt upon whether reported epidemic and sporadic cases are necessarily the same disorder.

Pathology. The wide variety of clinical manifestations in infectious mononucleosis reflects the diffuse distribution of tissue lesions observed histologically. However, gross changes are confined almost exclusively to lymphoid tissues. Hyperplasia of nasopharyngeal lymphoid tissue is constant, and lymph node enlargement is present in varying degree. Histologically, lymph node reactions vary from a predominantly follicular hyperplasia to a blurred pattern, owing to proliferation of lymphocytic and reticuloendothelial elements in the medullary cords, and resemble malignant lymphoma in some instances. In properly prepared sections, the abnormal lymphocytes seen in the blood are also observed in nodal tissue. The spleen may be tense and swollen, the capsule and trabeculae being thinned and some-

times dissolved by lymphocytic infiltration. The normal splenic histologic pattern is usually partially effaced, with widely spaced follicles and with accumulations of normal and abnormal lymphocytes about the intratrabecular arteries, beneath the intima of veins, and in the blood sinuses. The changes in the spleen render it susceptible to rupture.

Other gross changes include hepatic enlargement and, occasionally, icterus and a skin rash. However, histologic lesions may be observed in virtually every body tissue, varying in distribution from case to case. These generalized lesions consist predominantly of perivascular aggregates of normal and abnormal lymphocytes, and resemble those of certain known viral diseases. Focal lesions are described in the myocardium, kidneys, lungs, skin, central nervous system, and elsewhere. The liver usually contains periportal lymphoid collars, and these occasionally attain the proportions seen in leukemia. Changes similar to those noted in the spleen are found in the capsule of the liver. Meningoencephalitis of mild to severe degree may be observed. In patients with severe nervous system involvement the meninges may be congested and edematous, and may contain increased numbers of mononuclear cells; perivascular cuffing with round cells may be found in brain tissue. Swelling and disruption of myelin sheaths and cellular infiltration of anterior nerve roots have been observed in patients with the Guillain-Barré syndrome associated with infectious mononucleosis. Custer and Smith are of the opinion that the widespread "infiltrates" of connective tissue and the cells composing the perivascular collars arise in situ from cells of the reticuloendothelial system rather than as cell migrations from distant locations. Particle sections of bone marrow fail to show lymphocytic infiltration, although smears of aspirates may contain increased mononuclear elements owing to dilution with peripheral blood. Granulomatous lesions have been described in particle sections on occasion.

Clinical Manifestations. The incubation period is uncertain, estimates varying from a few days to several weeks. Initial symptoms are nonspecific: malaise followed by fever, sore throat, and headache frequently appear with increasing intensity during the first five or more days of illness. Nearly all patients seeking medical advice experience fever, most commonly from 100 to 103° F., though sometimes higher. A variably severe pharyngitis is commonly present in the first week of illness, but onset may be delayed to the second week or very occasionally later. Fusospirochetal organisms and hemolytic streptococci are frequently secondary invaders (see Vincent's Angina). In some patients (with the so-called "typhoidal" type of the disease) sore throat is absent, though pharyngeal injection and lymphoid hyperplasia are almost invariably present. The throat may be diffusely injected, or membranous pharyngitis may be observed. A palatal enanthem consisting of sharply circumscribed red spots, probably petechial, appearing in crops of usually 6 to 20 lesions, is commonly seen between the fifth and twelfth days of illness.

Lymph node enlargement is present in virtually all cases, but it may be relatively transient in some. The cervical lymph nodes are almost always involved, and posterior cervical nodal enlargement is of value in differentiation from other forms of pharyngitis. Cervical adenopathy is generally moderate but may be massive, and there is little correlation with the severity of pharyngitis. Axillary and inguinal adenopathy are common but not invariable, and enlarged mediastinal nodes may be detected roentgenographically in rare instances. There is no correlation between degree of lymph node enlargement and severity of illness. The enlarged nodes are normally discrete, nontender, or slightly tender (unless they drain a secondarily infected area), firm, elastic, and nonsuppurating. Local heat and redness are not present. The spleen is variably enlarged in about 75 per cent of cases. Most commonly the enlarged spleen extends 2 to 3 cm. below the costal margin, but more severe enlargement has been recorded.

The liver is palpable less frequently, but jaundice with or without hepatomegaly may occur, most commonly between the fourth and fourteenth days of illness. It is usually mild to moderate and is associated with bilirubinemia, but only rarely with acholic stools. Anicteric hepatitis occurs in most cases.

Although this constellation of signs and symptoms usually predominates in varying degree, giving rise to classification into pharyngeal, typhoidal, and icteric types, involvement by the offending agent is diffuse, and may result in symptoms involving almost every body system. Skin rashes — most commonly transient maculopapular or faintly erythematous eruptions — have been described in different proportions of cases in different series. Their incidence and importance as a physical finding are in dispute, and evaluation is complicated by possible confusion of infectious mononucleosis with other diseases producing exanthems. The most frequently observed lesions are small (2 to 5 mm.), usually pinkish or pinkish-brown, and involve mainly the trunk and upper arms. In Hoagland's extensive experience skin rashes attributable to infectious mononucleosis itself occurred at the most in 3 to 4 per cent of cases. Neurologic manifestations indicative of involvement of the central and peripheral nervous systems may occur. Headache is common and frequently severe. Instances of isolated cranial and peripheral nerve palsies, nystagmus, papilledema, ataxia, skin hyperesthesia, paresis of an extremity, and toxic psychoses are recorded. Death from the Guillain-Barré syndrome, with ascending paralysis, involvement of multiple peripheral nerves, and high cerebrospinal fluid protein has occurred.

Electrocardiographic and pathologic evidence of focal cardiac or pericardial involvement may be noted, but clinically significant cardiac involvement or permanent cardiac damage appears to be very rare. Likewise, pulmonary symptoms in the form of cough, sputum, and parenchymal infiltrates demonstrable by roentgenographic examination are uncommon, but have been described. Clinically significant renal disease does not ordinarily occur, but red blood cells, leukocytes, and albumin are sometimes found in the urine. In this regard, however, it must be remembered that hemolytic streptococcal infections are common complications of the pharyngitis. In somewhat less than half of the cases, edema of the eyelids and a consequently narrowed ocular aperture are present. It should be emphasized, in addition, that, as with many illnesses, asymptomatic or subclinical cases occur and that the severity of the illness is extremely variable.

The characteristic "mononucleosis" most commonly appears by the fourth or fifth day of illness and persists two to eight weeks, occasionally for several months. Normal small lymphocytes and monocytes are found in abundance. The most common of these (Type I of Downey) has an oval, kidney-shaped, or lobulated nucleus with vacuolated, foamy, and usually nongranular cytoplasm. Others are larger with less condensation of nuclear chromatin and a nonvacuolated, more homogeneous cytoplasm (Type II of Downey), or may possess a finer chromatin pattern and one or two nucleoli, and may resemble lymphoblasts (Type III of Downey). Other forms of abnormal lymphocytes are also noted; the "Downey" cells individually are not specific for the disease. Their abundance in typical cases is characteristic, however. In the first two weeks of the disease, isotopic labeling evidence suggests that a high proportion of circulating lymphocytes are synthesizing DNA. The atypical lymphocyte in infectious mononucleosis is not only capable of in vivo proliferation, but has an increased potential for long term in vitro proliferation as well. Thus long-term cultures derived from peripheral blood may be established, whereas in normal persons such cultures usually fail to thrive. Although cytochemical studies indicate some differences from normal lymphocytes or monocytes, differences observed by electron microscopy are insufficient to classify three types of "Downey" cells by this modality. The total leukocyte count is usually 10,000 to 20,000 per cubic millimeter at some point in the disease, but may be normal or appreciably higher. In the fully developed disease, mononuclear cells usually comprise 60 per cent or more of the leukocytes, and values of more than 90 per cent have been reported. At the outset, counts in the normal or leukopenic range without lymphocytosis are often present. Anemia and clinically significant thrombocytopenia are normally absent, though both acute hemolytic anemia and thrombocytopenic purpura are observed in rare instances; in the former the Coombs test may or may not be positive.

Heterophil antibodies agglutinating sheep cells almost always appear in the first two weeks of illness, and persist from four to eight weeks up to several months. Highest titers are usually observed in the second and third weeks of illness. The characteristic heterophil agglutinins are absorbed by beef erythrocyte antigen, but not completely by guinea pig kidney. Differential absorption studies are imperative in atypical cases, and serve in most instances to differentiate infectious mononucleosis from other conditions in which occasionally increased heterophil antibodies are observed. In most of the latter the antibody present is of the Forssman type, and is absorbable by guinea pig kidney. In serum sickness, the heterophil agglutinins are absorbed by both guinea pig kidney and beef antigen. *In the presence of typical hematologic and clinical manifestations,* a heterophil titer of 1:224 or more (Wintrobe) or as low as 1:56 or more (Hoagland and Bender) has been regarded as presumptively diagnostic. However, a positive heterophil (Paul-Bunnell) test, even when confirmed by definitive absorption studies, may indicate acute infectious mononucleosis, persisting antibodies from an attack of the disease in the preceding few weeks or months or, rarely, a nonspecific anamnestic resurgence of heterophil antibodies during an unrelated illness.

In addition to agglutinins against sheep cells, hemolysins against ox cells develop and are the basis of an additional serologic test. A variety of nondiagnostic antibodies such as those responsible for biologically false positive tests for syphilis, cold agglutinins with anti-i specificity, and others may be observed in some cases. The immune globulins IgM and IgG increase in the course of the disease and return to normal, usually within three months. Although both the heterophil antibody and cold agglutinins are IgM antibodies, absorption of high titered sera indicates that less than 5 per cent of the increase in IgM is accounted for by these activities. As previously mentioned, the demonstration of the development of EBV antibodies is of great importance and current interest.

Hepatitis with or without icterus occurs in most patients. Cephalin flocculation, thymol turbidity, transaminase, alkaline phosphatase, and sulfobromophthalein retention tests for liver function are abnormal in a high proportion of cases. Elevations in SGOT and SGPT enzyme levels have been reported to be the most consistent abnormality. In one study the levels of both enzymes usually increased in the first week of illness, peaked in the second week, and returned to normal in about five weeks. Electrocardiographic changes such as abnormal T waves and prolonged P-R intervals are not uncommon. The cerebrospinal fluid may exhibit pleocytosis up to several hundred cells (chiefly lymphocytes). Moderate elevations in cerebrospinal fluid pressure have been observed.

Diagnosis. Diagnosis up to the present time has rested on the triad of (1) clinical features of fever, pharyngotonsillitis, lymph node enlargement, and splenomegaly; (2) absolute lymphocytosis persisting over a period of several days or longer and characterized by the presence of atypical lymphocytes, usually constituting 20 per cent or more of the leukocytes at some time during the acute stages; and (3) a positive heterophil agglutination test, with specific absorption studies when indicated. The recent findings of the association of EBV antibody with the disease may shortly provide new and still more precise diagnostic criteria. Typical cases are readily recognized. Atypical cases present substantial diagnostic problems. It must be remembered that transient lymphocytosis with a few atypical lymphocytes occurs in a number of febrile illnesses. A persisting negative heterophil antibody test has not been regarded by most observers to exclude the diagnosis completely, but a firm diagnosis in its absence throughout the entire course of the disease is regarded by Hoagland and Bender as dangerous and unconvincing. Recently, however, heterophil antibody negative cases, otherwise typical, have been shown in a few instances to develop EBV antibody during the course of illness. Conversely, for reasons previously discussed, a positive presumptive test, or even in some instances a positive test after specific absorption studies, is not ground for diagnosis in the absence of "mononucleosis" and appropriate clinical features. It is probably fair to state that the manifestations of infectious mononucleosis are protean; nonetheless reliance on incomplete criteria for diagnosis, or, indeed, at times on a single criterion, has resulted in diagnostic confusion and frequent inclusion of questionable illnesses as instances of the disease.

Infectious mononucleosis may be confused with a variety of febrile illnesses, particularly viral, accompanied by some degree of lymphocytosis and atypical cells. The prominent *pharyngotonsillitis* requires differentiation from streptococcal infections, Vincent's angina, diphtheria, aphthous stomatitis, and other causes of acute sore throat. Generalized infections such as typhoid fever, influenza, and brucellosis may be considered in the differential diagnosis in some cases. Constitutional symptoms associated with a skin rash may suggest a variety of exanthems. Adult *toxoplasmosis* may mimic the clinical syndrome of infectious mononucleosis, including the findings of pharyngitis, cervical lymphadenopathy, splenomegaly, fever, and lymphocytosis with atypical lymphocytes. No cross reaction has been found, however, between heterophil and Toxoplasma dye test antibodies. A syndrome resembling infectious mononucleosis may accompany infection with cytomegalovirus. CMV mononucleosis and infectious mononucleosis both may be characterized by indistinguishable hematologic abnormalities, protracted fever, hepatitis and abnormal liver function tests, splenomegaly, and a variety of nonspecific immunologic aberrations. CMV mononucleosis may occur occasionally in healthy individuals, or some 21 to 34 days after massive transfusion therapy for nonsurgical conditions, or after open-heart surgery with extracorporeal circulation. In CMV mononucleosis the heterophil test is negative, pharyngitis is ordinarily absent, and lymphadenopathy is often not present. With special studies the virus may sometimes be isolated and specific CMV antibodies demonstrated. Syndromes simulating infectious mononucleosis in many respects have also been reported in infection with adenovirus. The hepatitis of infectious mononucleosis may simulate *infectious hepatitis* or homologous serum jaundice, and indeed, lymphocytosis may also be observed in these disorders. Prominent neurologic features may simulate *encephalitis, poliomyelitis, Guillain-Barré syndrome,* or *lymphocytic choriomeningitis.* The abnormal blood picture may raise the question of *leukemia* or *infectious lymphocytosis.* The latter disorder is not accompanied by splenomegaly or lymph node enlargement, nor are the characteristic atypical lymphocytes or serologic features of infectious mononucleosis present. Hemolytic anemia and thrombocytopenia, when present, must be differentiated from similar findings in a variety of disorders.

Treatment. No specific therapy is available. Secondary bacterial invasion with streptococcal pharyngitis or Vincent's angina should be sought and treated with appropriate antimicrobial drugs and perborate mouth washes. Symptomatic treatment of the fever and pharyngitis with salicylates and sedation for pain is indicated when necessary. Splenic rupture occasionally occurs and may be heralded by abdominal pain and shock. This complication calls for prompt surgical intervention. Corticotrophin and 17-hydroxycorticosteroids have been reported to produce dramatic clinical improvements, but do not specifically influence the disease. They are not indicated except possibly for very ill patients, in extreme degrees of pharyngeal lymphoid hyperplasia or edema of the glottis threatening occlusion of the respiratory tract, and in rare instances of acute hemolytic anemia and thrombocytopenic purpura. They may be given to adults as a six-day course — prednisone, 80 mg. the first day, and 40 mg. a day for three additional days, followed by gradual reduction over the final two days of therapy. Although chloroquine has been advocated, there is little evidence of any significant effect on the basic disease. Very rarely, tracheostomy has been required for edema of the glottis or tracheal occlusion. The hepatitis is usually mild, and permanent sequelae are rare. However, it is probably wise to treat severely icteric patients with bed rest and close observation of liver function tests, as in other forms of hepatitis. Adequate rest and avoidance of activities in which splenic rupture may occur are important in the acute and convalescent period. The friability of the spleen is such that repeated or heavy-handed attempts at splenic palpation are to be avoided. The low order of contagiousness in sporadic cases precludes the necessity for strict isolation.

Prognosis. Infectious mononucleosis is essentially a benign disorder, although rare fatalities have occurred because of rupture of the spleen or severe neurologic involvement, particularly ascending paralysis with the Guillain-Barré syndrome. Very rarely myocarditis has been reported as a cause of death; also very rarely, edema of the glottis or secondary sepsis may be life-threatening.

In terms of morbidity, the prognosis is extremely variable. As with other disorders, some patients have clinically inapparent disease or mild, transient illnesses that may or may not be diagnosed. In the more severely ill patients, the febrile period is usually of one to three weeks' duration, and there is a variable but definite period of postconvalescent asthenia. Brief recrudescences are sometimes seen. Serologic and hematologic abnormalities can persist for some time after convalescence. Although long-standing "chronic" infectious mononucleosis has been reported, most observers are of the opinion that a true chronic form of the disease has not been definitely recognized. Clinically significant sequelae of hepatic or cardiac involvement are ordinarily not observed. Occasional focal neurologic residuals are reported, but complete recovery is the general rule.

Bender, C. E.: Interpretation of hematologic and serologic findings in the diagnosis of infectious mononucleosis. Ann. Intern. Med., 49:852, 1958.

Carter, R. L., and Penman, H. G. (eds.): Infectious Mononucleosis. Oxford and Edinburgh, Blackwell Scientific Publications, 1969.

Evans, A. S., Niederman, J. C., and McCollum, R. W.: Seroepidemiologic studies of infectious mononucleosis with EB virus. New Eng. J. Med., 279:1121, 1968.

Henle, G., Henle, W., and Diehl, V.: Relation of Burkitt's tumor-associated herpes-type virus to infectious mononucleosis. Proc. Nat. Acad. Sci., 59:94, 1968.

Klemola, E., von Essen, R., Wager, O., Haltia, K., Koivuniemi, A., and Salmi, I.: Cytomegalovirus mononucleosis in previously healthy individuals. Ann. Intern. Med., 71:11, 1969.

Remington, J. S., Barnett, C. G., Meikel, M., and Lunde, M. N.: Toxoplasmosis and infectious mononucleosis. Arch. Intern. Med. (Chicago), 110:744, 1962.

The Histiocytoses

HISTIOCYTOSIS X
(Reticuloendotheliosis, Eosinophilic Granuloma, Schüller Christian Syndrome, Letterer-Siwe Syndrome)

Carl V. Moore

Eosinophilic granuloma of bone and the Schüller-Christian and Letterer-Siwe syndromes are characterized by histiocytic proliferation of unknown etiology; the lesions in eosinophilic granuloma of bone are also infiltrated by eosinophils. Original descriptions regarded them as distinct entities, but subsequently many pathologists championed the view that they are interrelated manifestations of a single malady. Lichtenstein suggested that "histiocytosis X" be used as a generic name to cover all three. According to this concept, eosinophilic granuloma of bone is the mildest and most localized form of the condition, Schüller-Christian syndrome is its most chronic and protean expression, and Letterer-Siwe syndrome represents the gravest and most generalized form; transformation from unifocal to generalized disease could occur. Agreement has not been uniform, however, and the interrelationship has again recently been challenged. Lieberman and his associates re-examined the clinical and pathologic manifestations of 82 patients who bore one of these diagnoses; they concluded that 50 had unifocal eosinophilic granuloma, and 24 had multifocal eosinophilic granuloma. The remaining eight patients who died were infants or children; one had generalized viral and atypical mycobacterial infections; the remaining seven were thought to have malignant histiocytic neoplastic disorders. "Schüller-Christian syndrome" was regarded as a nonspecific designation for multifocal eosinophilic granuloma, "Letterer-Siwe syndrome" as a misnomer, and "histiocytosis X" as unnecessary. The debate is likely to continue until pathogenesis is defined.

Eosinophilic Granuloma. Eosinophilic granuloma is a moderately rare and comparatively benign disorder characterized usually by unifocal osteolytic skeletal lesions. It occurs chiefly in children or young adults, but may be found at all ages. It predominates in males in a ratio of 3:2 to 2:1. Only a few cases have been reported among Negroes. Histologically, the lesion consists primarily of proliferation of histiocytes with eosinophilic infiltration. It begins in the marrow but gradually erodes the cortex so that ultimately the bone expands at the area of involvement. Patchy areas of necrosis and hemorrhage are usually present. The granulomas may retain their original character for years, but eventually, at least in some of the foci, fibrosis occurs, the eosinophils diminish, and the histiocytes tend to be converted into lipophages. The lytic defects roentgenographically are usually within the medullary cavity, are commonly between 1 and 4 cm. in greatest diameter, and have a medullary border that tends to be less distinct than for bone cysts. In patients under the age of 20, lesions are found with equal frequency in the long (particularly femur and humerus) and the flat bones; in those over the age of 20, lesions are almost exclusively limited to flat bones; they have never been described in the hands or feet. Pain and swelling at the area of involvement are common complaints, but the foci may be silent. Pathologic fractures may occur. Patients are usually free of constitutional symptoms, although they may have mild degrees of fever. Eosinophilia in the peripheral blood is unusual. Solitary eosinophilic granuloma is best treated by curettement or excision; x-ray therapy should be reserved for surgically inaccessible lesions. Results are uniformly good, and prognosis is excellent.

Eosinophilic granulomatous lesions may occur in multiple osseous sites and in soft tissues: lung, pleura, gastrointestinal tract, lymph nodes, vulva, and skin. Pulmonary infiltration may appear before skeletal lesions can be identified; it is characterized by an interstitial infiltration by histiocytes and eosinophils with a fibrous tissue reaction. The granulomatous areas may become large enough to form nodules. The roentgenographic changes are usually those of a diffuse, bilateral, interstitial pulmonary infiltration, sometimes with honeycombing. Pulmonary symptoms are usually mild, but patients with severe respiratory insufficiency have been described; in these instances, administration of large doses of corticosteroids may afford dramatic subjective and objective improvement. Diabetes insipidus has been reported as a complication of eosinophilic granuloma. X-ray therapy of the multiple skeletal and soft tissue lesions is effective. Prognosis is good.

Schüller-Christian Syndrome. The classic triad of the Christian syndrome consists of single or multiple areas of "punched-out" bone destruction in the skull, unilateral or bilateral exophthalmos, and diabetes insipidus with or without other signs of pituitary failure; it is unusual, however, to find all three manifestations in the same patient. The syndrome is a relatively chronic disorder that affects children principally, but may be found in young adults and rarely in older people. The pathologic lesion is a histiocytic granuloma in which the histiocytes contain so much cholesterol that they become foam cells. Lichtenstein believes that the granulomas initially contain very little cholesterol, that eosinophils may at first be prominent, and that lipidization is a late, secondary change. The plasma cholesterol value is usually normal, although the tissue cholesterol content may be as high as eighteen times normal. Lesions are by no means limited to the skull;

they may appear in other bones, the skin, and the viscera. Otitis media is a common presenting complaint. Soft tissue nodules may be palpated in the scalp overlying cranial defects. Cutaneous involvement, often as a papular eczema-like eruption or as xanthomas, occurs in about one third of all cases. Ulcerative lesions may appear on the gums, and erosions of the tooth-bearing portions of the mandible cause loss of teeth. Visceral changes may be found in the lung, liver, spleen, kidneys, perirenal fat, walls of the larger blood vessels, lymph nodes, and in the brain (particularly in the hypothalamus and cerebellum). Any lymph node enlargement, hepatomegaly, or splenomegaly is usually modest, but may be striking. Pulmonary infiltration is bilateral, may be diffuse, but more commonly is perihilar or central. In children, growth may be retarded or puberty delayed. Anemia is rare and constitutes a grave prognostic sign. If new skeletal lesions are biopsied early, the histologic picture may at times be indistinguishable from eosinophilic granuloma. The disease can be treated by x-ray therapy to the areas involved. Although the response is often very satisfactory, new foci tend to appear elsewhere. Large doses of prednisone are capable of reversing all the skeletal and visceral manifestations. When large doses are administered for relatively short intervals, remissions are obtained and persist for periods of 12 to 30 months. From 15 to roughly 30 per cent of cases terminate fatally; apparently complete recovery does occur. Secondary changes caused by the disease often lead to difficult therapeutic problems, i.e., diabetes insipidus. Pulmonary fibrosis may cause alveolar-capillary block, pulmonary insufficiency, or right-sided heart failure.

Letterer-Siwe Syndrome. The Letterer-Siwe syndrome is more acute, is largely limited to young children below the age of three years, although occasional cases are observed in young adults, and is characterized by the development of multiple areas of proliferating histiocytes in the visceral organs. Secondary precipitation of cholesterol esters in the histiocytes to form foam cells usually does not occur. Clinical manifestations consist of an erythematous, papular, purpuric, or ecchymotic cutaneous eruption that sometimes ulcerates superficially, a persistent, spiking, low-grade fever, enlargement of liver, spleen, and lymph nodes, hyperplasia of the gums, and a progressive anemia. Normoblasts may be found in the peripheral blood. Skeletal lesions cause localized areas of bone destruction, have a predilection for the calvarium, and roentgenographically resemble those of Schüller-Christian syndrome. Histologic changes in lymph nodes and bone marrow resemble histiocytic lymphoma or monocytic leukemia. Therapy consists of supportive care, antimicrobial drugs to control secondary infection, the use of corticosteroids, roentgen irradiation to the skin and other areas of involvement, and possibly chemotherapy. The process is usually fatal, but an occasional patient diagnosed as having Letterer-Siwe syndrome has recovered or transformed into a more chronic phase resembling Schüller-Christian syndrome.

Avery, M. E., McAfee, J. G., and Guild, H. G.: The course and prognosis of reticuloendotheliosis (eosinophilic granuloma, Schüller-Christian disease and Letterer-Siwe disease). Amer. J. Med., 22:636, 1957.
Avioli, L. V., Lasersohn, J. T., and Lopresti, J. M.: Histiocytosis X (Schüller-Christian disease): A clinico-pathologic survey. Review of ten patients and the results of prednisone therapy. Medicine, 42:119, 1963.
Beard, W., Foster, D. B., Kepes, J. J., and Guillan, R. A.: Xanthomatosis of the central nervous system. Neurology, 20:305, 1970.
Lichtenstein, L.: Histiocytosis X. Integration of eosinophilic granuloma of bone, Letterer-Siwe disease and Hand-Schüller-Christian disease as related manifestations of a single nosologic entity. Arch. Path. (Chicago), 56:84, 1953.
Lieberman, P. H., Jones, C. R., Dargeon, H. W. K., and Begg, C. F.: A reappraisal of eosinophilic granuloma of bone, Hand-Schüller-Christian syndrome, and Letterer-Siwe syndrome. Medicine, 48:375, 1969.
Williams, A. W., Dunnington, W. G., and Berte, S. J.: Pulmonary eosinophilic granuloma: A clinical and pathologic discussion. Ann. Intern. Med., 54:30, 1961.

GAUCHER'S DISEASE AND NIEMANN-PICK DISEASE

Donald S. Fredrickson

GAUCHER'S DISEASE

Definition. Gaucher's disease is a relatively common familial disorder characterized by abnormal accumulation of glucocerebrosides in reticuloendothelial (RE) cells; the accumulation occurs because an enzyme necessary for the degradation of these glycolipids is deficient. The increasing mass of the storage cells accounts for most of the clinical manifestations of the disease, including hepatosplenomegaly, lymph node enlargement, and bone lesions owing to expansion of the involved marrow. At least three syndromes have been recognized: (1) a chronic non-neuronopathic or "adult" form, which is by far the most common, becoming evident at any age and associated with hypersplenism, bone lesions, skin pigmentation and pingueculae, and preponderance among Ashkenazic Jews; (2) an acute neuronopathic form, which is manifest in infancy, is associated with severe neurologic abnormalities, and is usually fatal by three years of age; and (3) a "juvenile" form, which may begin at any time in childhood, combining the features of the chronic form with slowly progressive neurologic dysfunction. At least three different mutations are represented by the different forms of Gaucher's disease. No specific treatment is available.

Pathologic Physiology and Pathogenesis. Cerebrosides are compounds that contain equimolar amounts of sphingosine, fatty acid, and hexose. In the brain the hexose component is galactose, and the galactocerebrosides form an essential part of the myelin in the white matter. In tissues outside the brain, except for the kidney, practically all the small amounts of cerebroside present contain only glucose. These glucocerebrosides arise mainly from the degradation of more complex sphingo-glycolipids, the most important source probably being the normal breakdown of both white and red blood cells. In Gaucher's disease there is a specific deficiency in the activity of glucosyl-ceramide-β-glucosidase (glucocerebrosidase), one of the acid hydrolases found in the lysosomes. Glucocerebroside, *a relatively* insoluble compound, then accumulates in RE cells.

The morphologic hallmark of Gaucher's disease is the *Gaucher cell*, a round or polyhedral pale reticulum cell 20 to 80 μ in diameter, with a small eccentrically placed nucleus and a wrinkled ("crumpled silk") cytoplasm that contains an irregular network of fibrils. With electron microscopy the fibrils are shown to represent tubules or strands of glucocerebroside contained within secondary lysosomes having a single limiting membrane. Evidence of active phagocytosis or pinocytosis is present at the cell border, and fragments of erythrocytes are often visible. A few cells may have two or more nuclei. The cytoplasm does not stain with fat stains, but numerous wavy fibrillae are stained deeply with the periodic acid–Schiff reaction or with Mallory's trichrome connective tissue stain. The cytoplasm also demonstrates strong acid phosphatase activity. Examination of unstained smears of aspirated bone marrow by phase microscopy affords the best visualization of the cells (see accompanying figure, part *A*).

Proliferation and expansion of the Gaucher cells are responsible for the enlargement of spleen, liver, and intrathoracic and intra-abdominal lymph nodes. The concentration of glucocerebrosides may be increased 50 to 100 times normal in these organs. The spleen may become tremendous in size. Hemosiderin may be increased in the skin and other organs. Gaucher cells are also scattered diffusely throughout the marrow, and in some areas form tumor-like accumulations that may expand, erode the cortex, and lead to pathologic fractures. Infiltration of the lungs, kidneys, thymus, tonsils, thyroid, adrenals, and lymphatic tissue of the intestinal tract also occurs. Functional impairment of these organs is unusual, except for the lungs. Serious pulmonary infections are common in children, and pulmonary hypertension may occur in adults. Pathologic changes in the brains of adults are restricted to the presence of perivascular adventitial cells swollen in the typical Gaucher configuration. In children with the acute neuronopathic type of disease, such "perivascular cuffing" is accompanied by acute nerve cell degeneration with active phagocytosis of the cellular remains by histiocytes and microglia, and cytoplasmic storage of periodic acid–Schiff positive lipid in either neurons or glial cells. These changes are distributed focally in the cerebrum, cerebellum, brainstem, and spinal cord. In the juvenile form the ballooning of neurons is

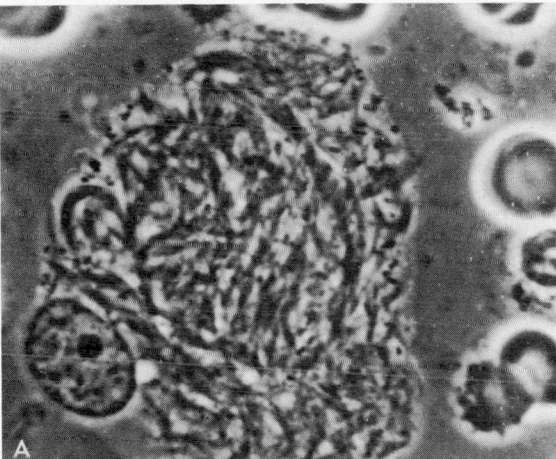

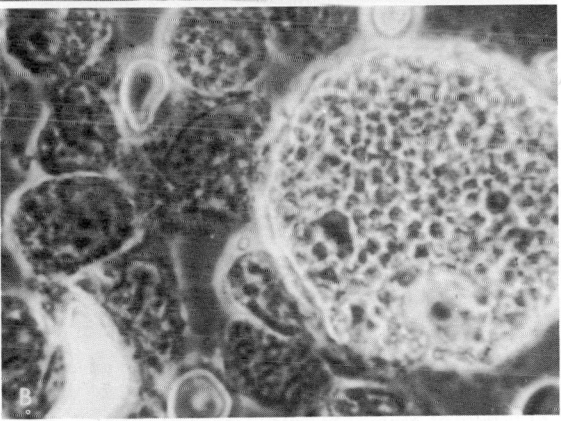

Appearance of the typical Gaucher cell (*A*) and a foam cell seen in Niemann-Pick disease (*B*). Both are viewed under phase microscopy in unstained smears of aspirated bone marrow. Magnification can be estimated from adjacent red cells.

accentuated. An accumulation of both glucocerebrosides and gangliosides has been reported in the brains of infants with the acute neuronopathic type. It is not known why the severity of the effect on the brain is so different in the several forms of the disease.

Acid phosphatase activity, not inhibited by L-tartrate (in contrast to the prostatic enzyme) is characteristically elevated in plasma and has diagnostic value. The enzyme is apparently spilled into plasma from the Gaucher cells. Plasma cerebroside concentrations are elevated after splenectomy.

Clinical Manifestations. *Chronic Non-neuronopathic Type.* The disease affects both sexes equally. It has been reported in Caucasians, Negroes, and Orientals; but a very high proportion of cases occurs among Ashkenazic Jews. Manifestations may appear at any age; the diagnosis has been made in the first month of life and past the age of 80 years. The course is extremely variable and tends to be more severe in affected children. Often, particularly in adults, the patient has no symptoms for a long time except awareness of a progressively enlarging mass in the left upper abdomen. The spleen may become very large; the liver is usually palpable. The second most common presenting abnormality is related to bone lesions. From 50 to 75 per cent of patients have roentgenographic changes, mostly asymptomatic. A common change is expansion of the cortex of the lower end of the femur, producing a characteristic radiolucent area with the configuration of an Erlenmeyer flask. The phalanges, long bones, vertebrae, ribs, and pelvis are more commonly involved than the skull. Bone pain or aching and pathologic fractures may appear at sites of skeletal lesions. With destruction of the head and neck of the femur, walking may become progressively more difficult. The hip abnormalities are sometimes confused with Legg-Perthes disease. In younger patients episodic attacks of bone pain simulating acute osteomyelitis are common. The long bones are usually affected; fever, joint tenderness, and redness occur, and draining sinus tracts may form. The cause is believed to be interference with the blood supply of the highly vascular metaphysis. Attacks usually last several weeks and no longer recur when growth is complete.

A diffuse yellowish-brown pigmentation is usually limited to exposed surfaces, but may be generalized or unilateral. Brownish, wedge-shaped thickenings of the subconjunctional fibrous tissue (pingueculae) often appear. The bases of these wedges are located near the cornea with the apices pointed toward the inner or outer canthi. Pingueculae tend to develop first on the nasal and later on the temporal side.

A high percentage of patients with Gaucher's disease develop hematologic changes of hypersplenism at some time during the course of their disease: hemolytic anemia, leukopenia, thrombocytopenia, or any combination of the three. The peripheral cytopenia is accompanied by a normal or increased number of the progenitors of the involved formed element in the bone marrow. Chronic Gaucher's disease usually involves only a single generation, but it has been observed in two generations. Otherwise normal parents, siblings, and other close relatives of patients sometimes have slight splenomegaly or small Gaucher cells in the marrow. An incompletely dominant transmission has not been excluded, and more than one mutation may be involved. Most patients probably are homozygous for an autosomal recessive allele or alleles.

Acute Neuronopathic Type. This "infantile" form of the disease is usually evident by three months of age but may become so any time between birth and 18 months. Among the earliest signs are splenomegaly, chronic cough, and psychomotor retardation. Other neurologic signs indicative of brain stem and cranial nerve involvement usually appear by the age of six months. The children have a stereotyped appearance: hepatosplenomegaly, strabismus, head retroflexed, lips retracted, and often spastic extremities held in flexion. The disease is fatal within three years; the average life span is about one year, respiratory infection and distress being the principal cause of death. Sex distribution is about equal. If one child in a family is afflicted, all other affected sibs will have the same form of disease. The disease appears to be transmitted as an autosomal recessive gene and is expressed only in the homozygote – double dose of a mutant allele. The mutation is present in low frequency in many ethnic groups. Four of about 70 reported cases have occurred in Jews.

Juvenile Type. About 25 examples of subacute neuronopathic Gaucher's disease have been described. Hepatosplenomegaly, hypersplenism, bone lesions, and other features of the chronic type appear from infancy onward. These are combined with mental retardation, behavioral problems, seizures, choreoathetoid movements, and sometimes strabismus, trismus, and other evidence of brainstem involvement. In several related Swedish families, glucocerebrosidase deficiency was demonstrated. Glycolipids other than glucocerebrosides may be stored in the spleen and liver, and a clear-cut phenotype has not been established.

Diagnosis. Gaucher's disease should be ruled out in any patient with unexplained splenomegaly, especially with elevated plasma acid phosphatase activity (not inhibited by L-tartrate). A presumptive diagnosis can be made from detection of Gaucher cells, usually in marrow aspirates. If there is doubt, liver biopsy with demonstration of glucocerebroside accumulation and deficient glucocerebrosidase activity provides a certain diagnosis. These analyses must be performed on tissues stored frozen in the absence of fixatives. Diagnosis is also possible through assay of cerebrosidase activity in white cells or fibroblasts in tissue culture.

Treatment and Prognosis. No specific therapy exists. X-ray therapy to bone lesions may alleviate pain, but usually does not arrest the destructive process. Bone pain may also respond well to corticosteroid therapy. Splenectomy corrects the manifestations of hypersplenism but does not otherwise influence the course of the disease. Because of the possibility that bone involvement may be accelerated by splenectomy, the indication for the procedure should be clear-cut. The course is protracted, often extending over many years. Most older patients die of intercurrent diseases rather than Gaucher's disease per se.

Fredrickson, D. S., and Sloan, H. R.: Glucosylceramide lipidoses: Gaucher's disease. *In* Stanbury, J. B., Wyngaarden, J. B., and Fredrickson, D. S. (eds.): The Metabolic Basis of Inherited Disease. 3rd ed. New York, McGraw-Hill Book Company, Inc., 1971 (in press).

Reich, C., Seife, M., and Kessler, B. J.: Gaucher's disease: A review and discussion of twenty cases. Medicine, 30:1, 1951.

Schettler, G., and Kahlke, W.: Gaucher's disease. *In* Schettler, G. (ed.): Lipids and Lipidoses. New York, Springer-Verlag, Inc., 1967, pp. 260–287.

NIEMANN-PICK DISEASE

Definition. The eponym Niemann-Pick disease refers to several rare disorders characterized by extensive tissue storage of sphingomyelin. All patients have hepatosplenomegaly and large macrophages filled with lipid droplets in the bone marrow (see accompanying figure, part *B*); some also have severe neurologic abnormalities. The "sphingomyelin lipidoses" fall into two major groups according to the tissue activity of sphingomyelinase. This enzyme catalyzes the hydrolysis of phosphorylcholine from sphingomyelin, an initial step in its catabolism. Sphingomyelinase deficiency is both severe and clearly inherited in the two most distinct forms of the disease: an acute neuronopathic form (type A) and a chronic non-neuronopathic form (type B). Both usually begin in infancy. Sphingomyelinase is normal or only slightly decreased in two other inheritable forms. These are types C and D, in which neurologic defects appear more slowly, and death occurs later than in type A. All affected members of the same family have the same type of disorder.

Pathophysiology. Sphingomyelin is normally found in most cells and in plasma and lymph. When sphingomyelinase activity is deficient, the phospholipid accumulates in RE cells, being sequestered there in residual bodies or secondary lysosomes. Unesterified cholesterol is also stored with the sphingomyelin. The swollen macrophages appear in every organ, and the sphingomyelin content of liver and spleen may increase 100 times or greater. When the central nervous system is affected, the neurons and glial cells are ballooned with lipid, the nuclei are pushed to one side, and Nissl substance disappears. Neuronal loss, gliosis, and demyelination are severe. It is not known why deficient activity of apparently the same enzyme causes brain damage in one form and not in another. Sphingomyelin accumulation is relatively less, and that of cholesterol greater, in those patients in whom sphingomyelinase activity is not clearly decreased. Although similar pathologic changes may be present, the lipidosis in these patients has no obious etiologic relationship to the enzyme-deficient disorders.

Clinical Manifestations. *Type A.* Type A is usually manifested by six months of age by abdominal enlargement and evidence of physical and mental retardation. Hepatosplenomegaly and roentgenographic evidence of diffuse pulmonary infiltration may be present as early as one month of age. Retinal degeneration in the macular area usually causes a cherry-red spot to appear. The disease progresses to a vegetative state, and death invariably occurs by the fourth year of life. Both sexes are affected. The disease occurs in all races; it is disproportionately frequent in Ashkenazic Jews.

Type B. Children with type B may develop evidence of visceral involvement as severe and as early as those with type A, but the central nervous system is spared, and mental development is normal. Chronic pulmonary infections and hypersplenism are sometimes life-threatening, but a reasonably normal life span may be possible. Sphingomyelinase activity in the liver and spleen is between 1 and 20 per cent of normal in both types A and B. The two types are distinguishable only by the presence or absence of neurologic involvement.

Forms Without Sphingomyelinase Deficiency. These children usually appear normal for one or more years before moderate hepatosplenomegaly is noted. Later neurologic abnormalities appear; these may include seizures, behavioral disorders, and mental retardation. Death usually occurs in childhood or adolescence. The increase in sphingomyelin in liver and spleen is less than in type A or B; cholesterol storage is proportionately greater. Sphingomyelinase activity is normal or only slightly decreased. The disorder is sometimes familial and is usually referred to as type C. A similar chronic neuropathic form occurring in related patients of Nova Scotian ancestry is designated type D because it appears to represent a distinctly different mutation.

Indeterminate Forms of Sphingomyelin Storage. There are occasional patients, usually adults, who have foam cells in the bone marrow in association with isolated clumps of macrophages containing excess sphingomyelin in the spleen, lung, or lymph nodes. Mild splenomegaly or roentgenographic evidence of localized pulmonary infiltration usually leads to their detection. These lesions have not been shown to be genetically determined. In a few instances sphingomyelinase has been measured and was normal. A relationship to other forms of Niemann-Pick disease is not established.

Diagnosis. The presence of foam cells in tissues that stain positively for phospholipids (Smith-Dietrich) and cholesterol (Schultz) and, often, for ceroid or lipofuscin pigments (a red periodic acid–Schiff reaction and autofluorescence under ultraviolet light) gives only a presumptive diagnosis of Niemann-Pick disease. The staining reactions and the appearance of the foam cells are not specific. Diagnosis must be confirmed by measurement of the sphingomyelin concentration in liver, lymph nodes, or spleen; sphingomyelinase activity should also be determined on the specimen. Tissue should be kept frozen in the absence of fixatives prior to chemical and enzymatic analyses. Sphingomyelinase deficiency may also be detected in tissue cultures of skin and bone marrow, and, probably, amniotic fluid. All the inheritable forms of Niemann-Pick disease seem to be inherited as autosomal recessive traits. No certain tests for the heterozygous phenotypes are available. There is no specific treatment.

Crocker, A. C., and Farber, S.: Neimann-Pick disease: A review of 18 patients. Medicine, 37:1, 1958.
Fredrickson, D. S., and Sloan, H. R.: Phosphorylcholine ceramidoses. Nicmann-Pick disease. *In* Stanbury, J. B., Wyngaarden, J. B., and Fredrickson, D. S. (eds.): The Metabolic Basis of Inherited Disease. 3rd ed. New York, McGraw-Hill Book Company, Inc., 1971 (in press).

Plasma Cell Dyscrasias

Elliott F. Osserman

GENERAL CONSIDERATIONS

Definition and Terminology. The term "plasma cell dyscrasia" is employed to encompass the wide range of pathologic conditions and biochemical abnormalities considered to represent unbalanced proliferative disorders of the cells that normally synthesize gamma (immuno-) globulins. The extent of the proliferative abnormality in the various plasma cell dyscrasias ranges from apparently autonomous, malignant proliferation (neoplasia) in typical multiple myeloma to apparently benign and stable dyscrasias manifested principally by their associated gamma globulin abnormalities. The plasma cell dyscrasias are characterized by (1) the proliferation of plasma cells in the absence of an identifiable antigenic stimulus; (2) elaboration of electrophoretically and structurally homogeneous, monoclonal, "M-type" (myeloma, macroglobulinemia) gamma globulins and/or excessive quantities of comparably homogeneous polypeptide subunits of these proteins, i.e., Bence Jones proteins, H-chains; and, (3) commonly, an associated deficiency in the synthesis of normal immunoglobulins.

The major clinical patterns associated with plasma cell dyscrasia are listed in the accompanying table. Certain of these categories, such as myeloma, macroglobulinemia, amyloidosis, and heavy chain diseases, have sufficiently well defined clinical patterns to permit precise diagnostic classification. With increasing use of electrophoresis, however, many cases of M-type gamma globulin abnormalities are being found that apparently do not represent typical plasma cell myeloma or primary Waldenström's macroglobulinemia at the time of initial study. The fact that some of these patients ultimately develop clinically typical myeloma or macroglobulinemia is well documented, but there are many cases (of the order of 20 to 30 per cent of patients with M-type gamma globulin abnormalities) that almost certainly do not belong in the diagnostic categories of myeloma or primary macroglobulinemia. Various designations have been given to these cases including premyeloma, essential hyperglobulinemia, essential benign hyperglobulinemia, essential macroglobulinemia, idiopathic or essential cryoglobulinemia, the dysgammaglobulinemic syndromes, idiopathic or essential monoclonal gammopathy, paraimmunoglobulinopathy, and others. The probable inaccuracies of all these terms are evident.

It is recommended that the inclusive term "plasma cell dyscrasia" be used, modified by the clinical pattern, e.g., myeloma, Waldenström's macroglobulinemia, or amyloidosis, when this is overt and evident. When no recognizable clinical pattern is associated with the finding of an M-type protein, the condition is classified as a plasma cell dyscrasia of unknown significance, since the ultimate course is not presently predictable. However, many, if not all, of the diagnostic categories listed in the table overlap. Thus, amyloidosis can either be the predominant feature of a plasma cell dyscrasia, in which case the diagnosis of "primary amyloidosis" is commonly, although inappropriately, applied, or the amyloid infiltrates can occur in association with otherwise typical myeloma. Also, a given case can progress from an asymptomatic status, i.e., plasma cell dyscrasia of unknown significance to symptomatic myeloma, macroglobulinemia, amyloidosis, and so forth. Accordingly, the categories listed in the table are tentative and somewhat indefinite diagnostic groupings in many instances.

In a significant percentage of cases the finding of an M-type protein abnormality is associated with another chronic disease such as recurrent cholecystitis and cholelithiasis, a chronic infection (particularly tuberculosis), or a nonreticular neoplasm (particularly rectosigmoid and biliary carcinoma). *These associations may not be coincidental,* but may represent plasma cell dyscrasias related to and possibly induced by these diverse chronic reticuloendothelial stimuli. For this reason, it is considered useful to document the associations by designations such as "plasma cell dyscrasia associated with chronic biliary tract disease" or "plasma cell dyscrasia associated with adenocarcinoma of the rectosigmoid."

Pathogenesis of Plasma Cell Dyscrasias. Although the etiologic factors responsible for production of plasma cell dyscrasias in man are still unknown, it is possible that some clues may have been provided by studies of experimental plasma cell tumors in mice. These studies have established the importance of genetic factors with the demonstration of the particular susceptibility of the inbred C_3H mouse strain and the F^1 hybrids of $CBA \times DBA/2$ mice to develop plasma cell tumors spontaneously. In an effort to document genetic factors, chromosome studies have been carried out in several of these murine tumors as well as in human myeloma and macroglobulinemia, but thus far no consistent karyotypic abnormalities have been documented.

The *interdependence of genetic and carcinogenic mechanisms* is apparent in the interesting group of experimental *plasma cell tumors* that have been induced in BALB/c strain mice. A variety of plasma cell neoplasms can be induced in this strain by the intraperitoneal implantation of plastics, mineral oil-adjuvant

PLASMA CELL DYSCHASIAS

Clinically overt
  Multiple myeloma
  Waldenström's macroglobulinemia
  "Primary" amyloidosis
  Lichen myxedematosus
  γG (Fc fragment) heavy chain disease
  γA (α chain) heavy chain disease
Clinically occult
  Plasma cell dyscrasia
    Of unknown significance
    Associated with chronic RES stimulation
    Associated with nonreticular neoplasms

mixtures, and mineral oil alone. The importance of genetic mechanisms is evident from the particular susceptibility in the BALB/c strain to develop plasma cell tumors in response to these forms of chronic peritoneal (reticuloendothelial) irritation. Significantly, strain C_3H mice, which develop spontaneous plasma cell tumors, are *not susceptible* to the induction of these tumors by intraperitoneal adjuvants and the like. With many other experimental tumors the intimate interaction of genetic factors, oncogenic viruses, and chemical and physical carcinogens has been established.

Cytology. The synthesis of specific proteins is the principal and probably the sole function of plasma cells. The abundant cytoplasmic RNA is responsible for the characteristic basophilia and pyroninophilia of plasma cells, and the highly developed Golgi apparatus is responsible for the typical paranuclear "halo" or clear zone. Electron microscopy of plasma cells has shown that the cytoplasmic RNA is organized in the form of granules (ribosomes) attached to a highly developed network of endoplasmic reticulum. All these structural features have now been related to the complex functions of protein synthesis and secretion. The nucleus of the plasma cell with its characteristically clumped chromatin (DNA) contains the genetic information that determines the structure of the protein to be synthesized. The synthesis of ribosomal RNA is carried out on DNA localized in the nucleolus. Messenger RNA's, which determine the structure of the specific proteins to be synthesized on these ribosomes, are derived from the non-nucleolar DNA's.

The different classes of immunoglobulins are probably synthesized by different cells. The possibility that a single cell may under certain conditions synthesize two types of immunoglobulins (e.g., γG and γM) either simultaneously or sequentially has not been excluded, but most studies have indicated the synthesis of only one type of immunoglobulin by a single cell. Immunohistochemical studies using fluorescein-labeled antisera specific for each of the immunoglobulin groups have generally shown γG globulin synthesis in typical, mature, Marshalko-type plasma cells. Gamma-A globulin has been localized in cells with relatively more abundant and vacuolated cytoplasm but still having the major features of plasma cells; gamma-M macroglobulin synthesis has been related to a population of somewhat smaller cells with proportionately less cytoplasm. These cells have been variously classified as lymphocytoid-plasma cells, plasmacytoid-lymphocytes, atypical plasma cells, and atypical lymphocytes.

Typical, ovoid plasma cells with eccentric nuclei, clumped chromatin, prominent nucleoli, paranuclear halo, and basophilic cytoplasm are widely distributed in lymph nodes, spleen, mar-

row, intestinal wall, and other tissues and organs. They constitute less than 5 per cent of the normal bone marrow population but increase significantly in association with infection, sensitivity reactions (particularly serum sickness), collagen diseases, cirrhosis, parasitism, and certain neoplasms. In these conditions, the increase in plasma cells includes both "typical" and "atypical" forms (including multinucleated cells and cells with prominent nucleoli), and there are *no reliable morphologic criteria to distinguish these reactive plasmacytic populations from the cells that are found in the plasma cell dyscrasias*.

Normal Immunoglobulins and the Paraproteins of the Plasma Cell Dyscrasias. The term "gamma" globulin strictly refers to the polydispersed group of proteins that occupies the most cathodal peak in the electrophoretic pattern of normal serum when separation is carried out under standard conditions (Veronal buffer, pH 8.6). Figure 1 is a schematic representation of this region of a normal serum electrophoretic pattern. As illustrated, it is now recognized that the broad gamma distribution actually extends anodally through the beta and into the alpha-2 mobility range. Within this area there are *at least five classes* of families of structurally distinct globulins, i.e., the γG, γA, γD, γE, and γM globulins, collectively termed the "immunoglubins." Each of these families is itself comprised of a large and as yet indeterminate number of individually specific proteins (specific antibodies) that share certain structural, physicochemical, and immunochemical properties, at the same time having *individual* structural and functional (antibody) specificities. The normal γG, γA, γD, γE, and γM globulins, and their counterparts in the plasma cell dyscrasias, are not distinguishable by electrophoresis alone because each family of immunoglobulins is distributed over a broad range of electrophoretic mobilities. These groups of immunoglobulins can be identified and distinguished only by specific immunochemical and physicochemical methods.

Figure 2 is a schematic summary of the present working hypothesis relating the synthesis of individual gamma globulin molecules (1, 2, 3, 4 . . . n) to specific plasmacytic clones. The normally broad, polydispersed serum gamma globulin peak represents the balanced synthesis of small quantities of a very large and presently indeterminate number (n) of individual and specific gamma globulin molecules by specific plasma cell populations. Normally, most of the proteins synthesized by these cells are complete immunoglobulin molecules, and there is only a small quantity of incomplete polypeptide subunits elaborated. These incomplete proteins, designated "gamma-u," are of low molecular weight constituents (M.W. 20,000 to 25,000) and closely resemble Bence Jones proteins. Because of their small molecular size, gamma-u polypeptides are rapidly excreted by

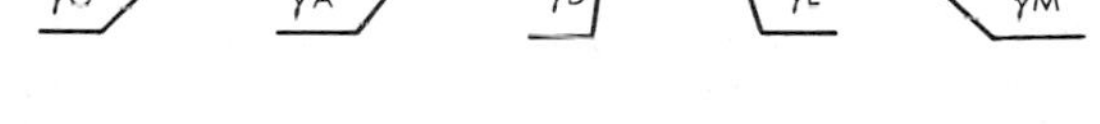

FIGURE 1. Schematic representation of the cathodal end of a normal serum electrophoretic pattern, showing the distribution of the five major classes of immunoglobulins (γG, γA, γD, γE, and γM) and certain of the physical and chemical properties of each class.

	γG	γA	γD	γE	γM
FUNCTION/ DISTRIBUTION	Circulatory Ab	Secretory	?	Reaginic Ab	? Early Ab
MOL. WT.	150,000	180,000 – 500,000	150,000	196,000	950,000
SEDIMENTATION	7S	7S (10 – 15 S polymers)	6S S	7.9S	19S
CARBOHYDRATE %	2.5 – 3.5	7 – 10	--	10.7	11.8
CONCENTRATION Normal Adult Serum (mg/100 ml)	800 – 1,600	50 – 200	< 1 – 40	.01 – .04	40 – 120

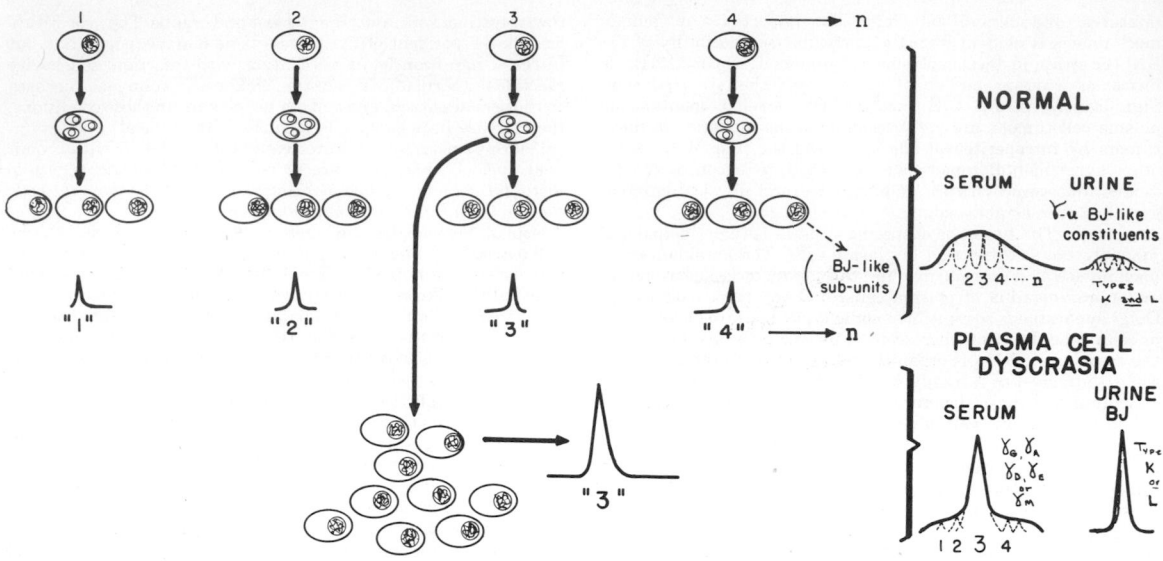

FIGURE 2. Schematic representation of the clonal hypothesis of immunoglobulin synthesis and the derangements in protein synthesis associated with plasma cell dyscrasias.

the kidney. Normally, 20 to 40 mg. of gamma-u are excreted per 24 hours.

A plasma cell dyscrasia is considered to represent the excessive proliferation of a single clone of plasma cells, resulting in the synthesis of large quantities of a single protein related to one of the major classes of immunoglobulins and/or the synthesis of excessive quantities of a constituent polypeptide subunit of one of these proteins, usually of the Bence Jones type.

The proteins elaborated in the plasma cell dyscrasias have been shown to be very closely related and structurally similar to the normal immunoglobulins. As large quantities of these single proteins are synthesized in the plasma cell dyscrasias, they are more suitable for structural studies than the heterogeneous and polydispersed normal immunoglobulins. Significantly, much of our present knowledge regarding the structure and properties of normal immunoglobulins has been obtained from studies of the M-type paraproteins. Since the normal gamma globulins and the paraproteins of the plasma cell dyscrasias are so closely related, their properties may be considered together.

As outlined in Figure 1, the γG globulins (syn., 7S γ, IgG) have molecular weights of the order of 160,000 and constitute about 80 per cent (800 to 1500 mg. per 100 ml.) of the electrophoretically defined gamma fraction of normal serum. Most acquired antibodies are in this immunoglobulin group, and approximately 70 per cent of myeloma serum globulins are γG globulins. The γG globulins contain approximately 2.5 to 3.5 per cent of conjugated carbohydrate. A small fraction of normal γG globulins (5 to 10 per cent) are euglobulins, i.e., relatively insoluble at low ionic concentrations. A comparable percentage of M-type γG globulins are euglobulins and can exhibit positive Sia reactions, i.e., precipitation when serum is added dropwise to distilled water. Certain γG globulins (5 to 8 per cent) exhibit a high intrinsic viscosity that is inversely temperature-dependent. Other γG globulins are relatively insoluble at temperatures below 37° C., i.e., cryoglobulins, precipitating when serum is cooled and redissolving on rewarming. Euglobulin, cryoglobulin and high viscosity properties are frequently but not invariably associated. These properties can be exhibited by either γG or γM globulins, but are extremely rare in γA globulins.

The γA globulins (syn., IgA) constitute a much smaller fraction of the total serum gamma globulin than the γG globulins and represent about 15 to 20 per cent (50 to 200 mg. per 100 ml.) of the normal immunoglobulins. Like γG globulins, γA globulins have molecular weights in the range of 160,000 with sedimentation constants of the order of 7S. Gamma-A globulins are distinguished by a high content of conjugated carbohydrate (10 to 12 per cent) and, possibly as a function of this carbohydrate, exhibit a tendency to form polymers with sedimentation constants of 9S, 11S, 13S, and 15S. Gamma-A globulins also tend to

form complexes (protein: protein interactions) with other serum proteins, including coagulation factors. A wide variety of antibacterial and antiviral antibody activities have been identified in γA fractions of normal and hyperimmunized subjects. Gamma-A globulins are the principal class of antibody present in external secretions, i.e., in saliva, intestinal and bronchial secretions, and colostrum. A specific transport mechanism for γA globulins, involving conjugation to another protein (so-called "secretory piece"), has been defined. Approximately 30 per cent of myeloma serum globulins are γA globulins.

The γD globulins (syn., IgD) constitute a very small fraction (1 to 3 per cent) of the serum immunoglobulins. The functional significance of γD globulins is entirely unknown at present. Approximately 40 cases of γD myeloma have been reported since the original description in 1965.

Gamma-E globulins are the most recently defined class of immunoglobulins. Reaginic antibody activities, responsible for immediate hypersensitivity reactions such as atopic dermatitis and allergic asthma, have been demonstrated to be associated with γE globulins. To date, there have been only two reported cases of γE plasma cell dyscrasia, and both exhibited the clinical pattern of myeloma and plasma cell leukemia.

The γM globulins (syn., 19S γ, IgM) comprise about 5 per cent of the normal serum immunoglobulins; their electrophoretic mobility, like that of the γA globulins, is somewhat faster, i.e., in the intermediate mobility range between beta and gamma globulin, than that of the γG globulins. Gamma-M macroglobulins have sedimentation constants of the order of 19S and molecular weights in the range of 1,000,000. Gamma-M macroglobulins can be dissociated by sulfhydryl reagents into subunits. Saline isohemagglutinins, saline Rh antibodies, cold hemagglutinins, and many of the heterophilic antibodies are γM globulins. The γM globulins, like the γA globulins, have a relatively high content of conjugated carbohydrate (10 to 12 per cent) and exhibit a similar tendency to form higher molecular weight polymers with sedimentation constants of the order of 23S and 35S.

A sixth group of proteins related to the gamma immunoglobulins is the low molecular weight constituents of the Bence Jones type. Small quantities are present in normal urine (gamma-u) and can also be demonstrated in normal serum by sensitive immunochemical methods. In approximately 50 to 60 per cent of cases of plasma cell dyscrasias, large quantities of these proteins are elaborated either alone or in association with a γG, A, D, E, or M paraprotein. Although normal gamma-u and Bence Jones proteins have been termed "micro-gamma-globulins," the available evidence indicates that they represent constituent polypeptide subunits of the immunoglobulins rather than complete molecules. The Bence Jones proteins have molecular weights in the range of 20,000 to 25,000 with sedimentation constants of approximately 2.5S, but are commonly excreted as dimers (M.W. = 40,000 to 50,000) with sedimentation constants of 3.5 to 4S. These dimers are linked by disulfide bonds and are dissociated by mercaptans.

Extensive studies of Bence Jones proteins and concomitant studies of the polypeptide subunits of the immunoglobulins obtained by either enzymatic (papain) or reductive cleavage of these molecules have led to the formulation of a schematic structure of an immunoglobulin molecule, which is shown in Figure 3. Present evidence indicates that immunoglobulin molecules are symmetrical and are comprised of two pairs of polypeptide chains designated, respectively, as the L (light) and H (heavy) chains interconnected by disulfide bonds. Cleavage of an immunoglobulin (γG) molecule by the enzyme papain yields subunits designated S and F fragments related but not identical to L and H chains obtained by reductive cleavage. The papain S fragment, also designated the Fab piece, is apparently comprised of an L chain plus a portion (the Fd piece) of the H chain. The papain F fragment is believed to represent the remaining portion of the H chain with its attached carbohydrate.

Considerable evidence indicates that immunoglobulins of all classes (γG, γA, γD, γE, and γM) contain L (light) chains of similar if not identical structure, i.e., that the L chains are common structural subunits of all immunoglobulins. The specific and distinct structural subunits that distinguish the major families of immunoglobulins are the H (heavy) chains. The Bence Jones proteins have been shown to be closely related and possibly identical to light chains. Two major structural (antigenic) types of Bence Jones proteins, designated K and L, respectively, have been identified, and corresponding structural types of light chains, designated by the corresponding Greek letters kappa (κ) and lambda (λ) have been identified in normal immunoglobulins and M-type serum paraproteins. The two light chains of any given immunoglobulin or paraprotein molecule are always of the same type, i.e., either κ or λ. In normal serum, approximately 60 per cent of γG globulins have κ light chains and 40 per cent have λ light chains. The low molecular weight gamma-u globulin in normal urine that resembles Bence Jones protein contains *both* Type K and Type L molecules, with a preponderance of Type K. It is believed that these constituents represent light chain subunits that have failed to become incorporated into complete immunoglobulin molecules. As previously noted, excessive quantities of these subunits, i.e., Bence Jones proteins, are elaborated in 50 to 60 per cent of cases of plasma cell dyscrasia. In any given case of plasma cell dyscrasia with Bence Jones proteinuria, the Bence Jones protein is *either* Type K *or* Type L, in contrast to excretion of small quantities of *both* Type K and Type L constituents in normal urine. In those cases of plasma cell

dyscrasia in which there is a synthesis of both an M-type serum paraprotein and a Bence Jones-type protein, the Bence Jones protein is apparently identical to the constituent light chains of the corresponding serum paraprotein. This evidence is interpreted as indicating that a portion of the abnormal cells have retained the capacity to elaborate complete molecules with light and heavy chains, whereas others are capable of synthesizing only one of the constituent polypeptide subunits, i.e., light chains.

The heavy (H) chains are the larger polypeptide subunits of the immunoglobulins to which the carbohydrate is attached and are the specific subunits that distinguish the major classes of immunoglobulins. The H chains are apparently responsible for some of the nonspecific functional properties of certain immunoglobulins, including skin fixation, placental transfer, and preferential secretion in certain fluids. This evidence has suggested that H chains and their diversity may reflect later developments in the phylogeny of immunity. L chains are possibly the more basic portions of the gamma globulin molecules, since these portions are almost invariably produced by normal as well as neoplastic plasma cells, either as constituent parts of complete gamma globulin molecules or as separate polypeptide subunits.

Recent studies of the amino acid sequences in both light and heavy chains have demonstrated that, in each instance, there is a variable sequence in one half of the molecule and a constant sequence, as compared with other molecules of the corresponding antigenic type, in the second half of the molecule. The structural diversity required for the functional specificity of individual antibodies is apparently derived from the variability in the amino acid sequence of the variable half of these polypeptide chains. Again, it should be emphasized that most of this information has been derived from the study of Bence Jones proteins and serum paraproteins from patients with myeloma and other plasma cell dyscrasias.

A fundamental question that remains unanswered is whether the proteins elaborated in the plasma cell dyscrasias are truly abnormal or whether they are, in fact, functional antibodies elaborated in great quantitative excess as a consequence of the proliferative abnormality. An increasing body of evidence obtained in recent years lends support to the latter hypothesis. Thus a number of human and mouse myeloma proteins and macroglobulins have been found to interact with a variety of synthetic haptens, polysaccharides, and bacterial antigens. The present consensus is that these reactions are probably cross-reactions between these proteins and antigens which are structurally related but not identical to the true antigens. Investigations are presently underway to identify the true antigens to which the myeloma proteins are directed, and this will unquestionably shed light on the pathogenic mechanisms responsible for plasma cell dyscrasias in man.

Electrophoretic Patterns of Serum and Urinary Proteins in the Plasma Cell Dyscrasias. As a result of the more general use of electrophoresis, increasing numbers of cases of plasma cell dyscrasia are being documented by the electrophoretic demonstration of M-type serum or urinary protein abnormalities, or both. These M-type abnormalities (Figs. 5 and 6) are best appreciated by comparison with the patterns of normal serum and urine and the serum in certain disease states affecting the reticuloendothelial system generally (Fig. 4). The electrophoretic analyses illustrated were performed by the Spinco cellulose acetate method, which has certain advantages over filter paper techniques. For diagnostic purposes, the *contours of electrophoretic patterns are more significant* than the precise quantitation of individual peaks. A careful appraisal of the contours of each peak, particularly distinguishing a diffuse gamma elevation from an M-type spike, in conjunction with a rough quantitative comparison of the patient's serum albumin, alpha-1, alpha-2, beta, and gamma globulins with a normal serum pattern will yield most of the clinically important information offered by this method.

In Figure 4, the normal serum pattern shows the characteristically broad contour of the major slow gamma peak, sometimes referred to as gamma-2, and a small secondary peak in the fast gamma region (between gamma and beta), which at times is designated gamma-1. The gamma-1 peak is detectable by cellulose acetate electrophoresis in most but not all normal sera. It is not resolved as a distinct peak by filter paper electrophoresis. The gamma-1 peak has been related to the faster migrating gamma-A and gamma-M globulins.

The electrophoretic pattern of the normal urinary proteins in

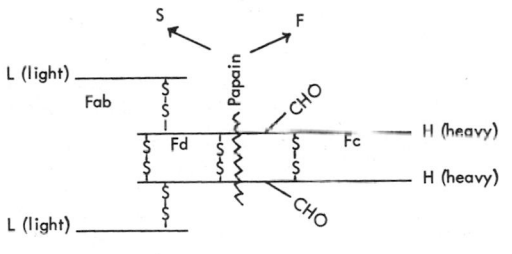

S   F

L (light) —————

Fab   Papain   CHO ——— H (heavy)

Fd   Fc ——— H (heavy)

CHO

L (light) —————

L (light)-Chains	H (heavy)-Chains
Common structural subunits of the γG, γA, and γM globulins.	Specific structural subunits of γG, γA, and γM globulins.
Related to the Bence Jones proteins.	Unrelated to the Bence Jones proteins.
Related to the papain S (slow) (Fab) fragment of γG globulin.	Related to the papain F (fast) (Fc) fragment of γG globulin.
M.W. ≅ 22,000	M.W. ≅ 55,000
Carbohydrate absent	Carbohydrate present

FIGURE 3. Schematic representation of the structure of an immunoglobulin molecule and certain properties of its constituent polypeptide subunits. The presumed site of papain cleavage of the molecule into the F (fast) and S (slow) fragment and their relation to the L (light) and H (heavy) chains obtained by reductive cleavage of interchain disulfide bonds is also indicated.

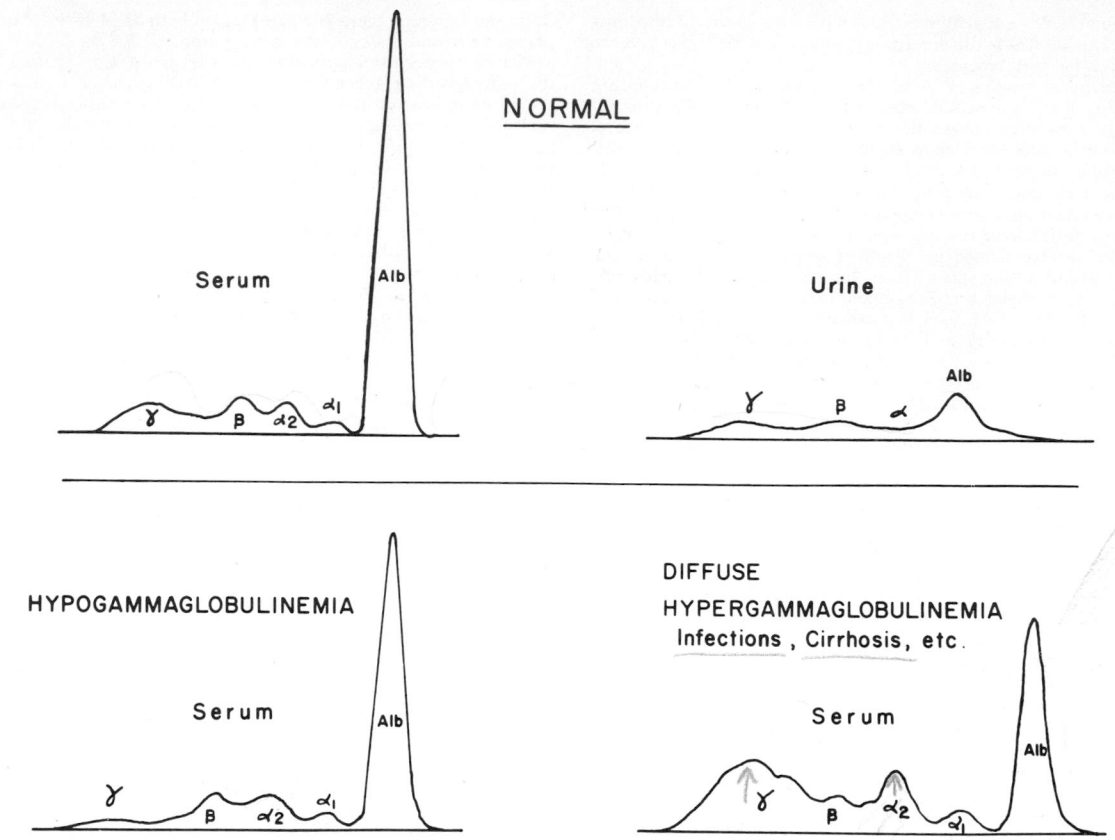

FIGURE 4. Representative electrophoretic patterns (Spinco, cellulose acetate system). *Top,* Normal serum and normal urinary proteins (concentrated 50×). *Bottom,* (Left) Hypogammaglobulinemia (adult, idiopathic); (Right) Diffuse hypergammaglobulinemia.

Figure 4 shows albumin to be the major constituent, with lesser quantities of alpha, beta, and gamma globulins. Because of the extremely low concentration of protein in normal urine, the sample must be concentrated 50- to 100-fold by dialysis against 25 per cent dextran or polyvinylpyrollidone (PVP) prior to electrophoresis. As in the case of serum proteins, the clinically important abnormal urinary proteins are detected as changes in the contours of the pattern and the relative concentrations of albumin and proteins of alpha, beta, and gamma mobility. Serial quantitation of 24-hour urinary protein excretion is useful for evaluating therapy but is not of particular importance diagnostically.

As illustrated in the lower patterns in Figure 4, the general suppression of plasmacytic function associated with the congenital and acquired forms of hypogammaglobulinemia is reflected in a *broad decrease* in gamma globulin, and, conversely, the generalized hyperactivity of the reticuloendothelial system associated with certain chronic infections, cirrhosis, collagen diseases, etc., is reflected in a *broad elevation* of gamma globulin. The pattern illustrating a diffuse hypergammaglobulinemia shows an elevation of the slow, major gamma (gamma-2) peak owing to an increase in gamma-G globulins, and also an increase in the fast gamma (gamma-1) peak, reflecting an increase in gamma-A and gamma M globulins.

The M-type serum and urinary protein abnormalities observed in myeloma, macroglobulinemia, and the other plasma cell dyscrasias are illustrated in Figures 5 and 6. In Figure 5, three sets of serum and urinary patterns from three cases of myeloma illustrate different combinations of abnormalities. Bence Jones proteinuria was present in all three cases of myeloma and was confirmed by the classic heat precipitation and re-solution at 90 to 100° C. Because of their small molecular size, the Bence Jones proteins are rapidly excreted, and their serum concentration is usually too low to be detected by conventional electrophoretic methods. Urine electrophoresis, however, demonstrates the Bence Jones proteins to have the same relative homogeneity as the myeloma serum globulins and electrophoretic mobilities, ranging from slow gamma through beta and into the alpha-2

mobility range. Urine electrophoresis is a more reliable method for the detection of Bence Jones proteins than the usual heat-precipitation procedure. *The finding in the urine of an electrophoretically homogeneous M-type component of gamma, beta, or alpha-2 mobility present in a concentration exceeding that of albumin indicates that the protein has a molecular size smaller than albumin (M.W. 70,000).* This is strong evidence in favor of Bence Jones proteinuria and can generally be confirmed by precipitation at 55 to 60° C. and re-solution at 90 to 100° C. *if the pH is carefully adjusted to 4.5 to 5.0.* False negative reactions will be obtained if inadequate attention is given to pH adjustment.

In the case of myeloma illustrated in Figure 5A, the serum pattern shows a large, electrophoretically homogeneous peak of slow gamma mobility, and the urine pattern shows a large, abnormal M-type peak with a somewhat faster (more anodally positioned) mobility than the serum M-type peak. The lack of correspondence in mobilities of the serum and urinary proteins establishes their *nonidentity.* Immunoelectrophoretically, the serum protein was identified as a γG globulin and the urinary protein as a Type K Bence Jones constituent.

In Figure 5B, the serum shows a small abnormal peak of slow gamma mobility and an obvious decrease in normal gamma globulin. The urine shows a very large abnormal peak of slow gamma mobility and a minimal amount of albumin. The serum and urinary protein were both identified immunoelectrophoretically as Type L Bence Jones protein. Bence Jones protein*emia* is usually not detectable by conventional electrophoresis, although it is almost always demonstrable by the more sensitive technique of immunoelectrophoresis when Bence Jones proteinuria is present.

In Figure 5C, the serum pattern shows two overlapping abnormal peaks of fast gamma (gamma-1) and beta mobility. The urine pattern has an abnormal beta peak along with significant quantities of albumin. In occasional cases of myeloma and other plasma cell dyscrasias, double peaks are found in serum patterns. Most frequently these have been shown to be due to an unusually high concentration of Bence Jones protein in the serum along

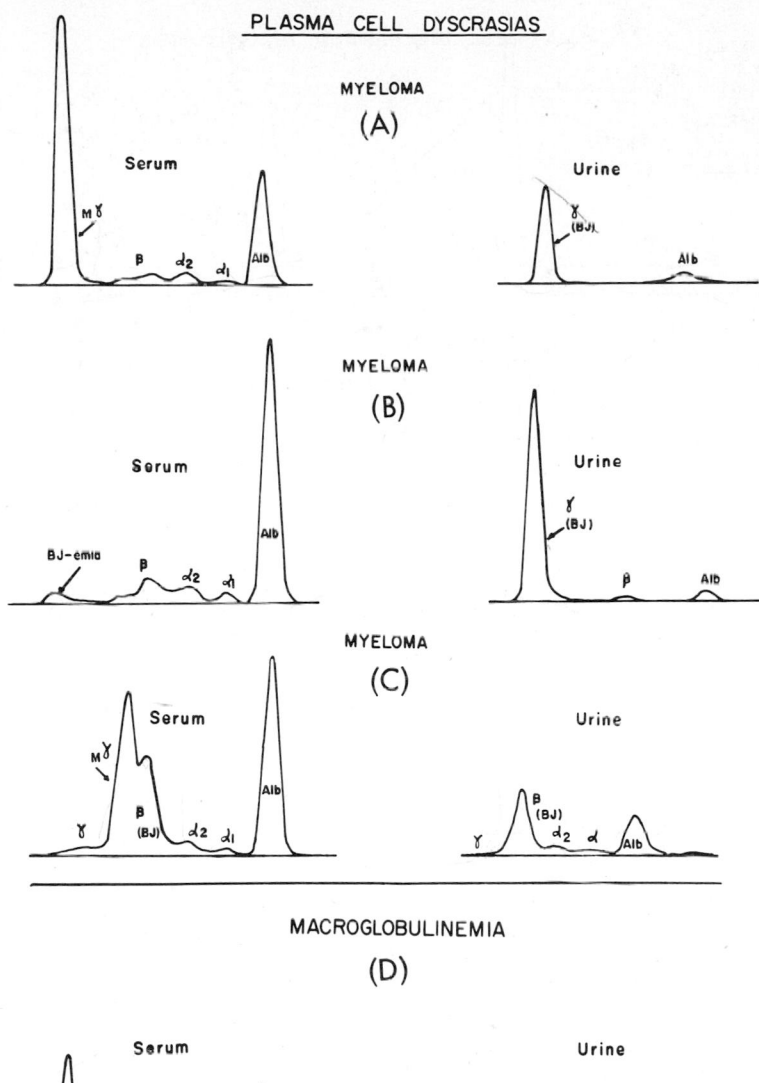

PLASMA CELL DYSCRASIAS

FIGURE 5. Serum and urinary protein patterns in three cases of multiple myeloma (*A, B, and C*) each with an M-type protein abnormality in the serum and Bence Jones proteinuria. *D,* Macroglobulinemia with nonspecific proteinuria.

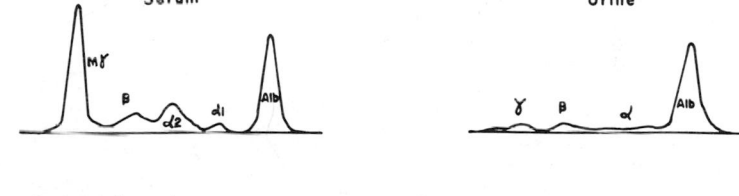

with an M-type γG or γA globulin. Rarely, two distinct γG or γA globulins or a γG *and* a γA, or γM globulin are found in the serum of a patient with a plasma cell dyscrasia. It is presumed that these doubled peaks indicate the simultaneous proliferation of more than one plasmacytic clone. In Figure 5C, the two serum peaks were immunoelectrophoretically identified, respectively, as a gamma-A globulin and a Type L Bence Jones protein. The abnormal urinary protein was identified as the same Type L Bence Jones constituent present in the serum. There was no detectable gamma-A globulin in the urine.

In Figure 5 *D* the serum and urinary patterns from a case of primary (Waldenström's) macroglobulinemia are illustrated. The serum has an M-type peak of slow gamma mobility indistinguishable from the gamma-C abnormality illustrated in Figure 5A. Definitive identification of the abnormal protein as a gamma-M macroglobulin in this as in all cases of macroglobulinemia was accomplished only by immunoelectrophoretic and ultracentrifugal analyses. The urinary protein pattern revealed nonspecific proteinuria with albumin as the predominant constituent. The virtual absence of the gamma-M macroglobulin from the urine is noteworthy. Bence Jones proteinuria occurs in a smaller percentage (10 to 20 per cent) of cases of macroglobulinemia than of myeloma (50 to 60 per cent).

Serum and urinary electrophoretic patterns from plasma cell dyscrasias other than typical myeloma and macroglobulinemia are illustrated in Figure 6. The patterns in Figure 6*A* are from a case of generalized amyloidosis with predominant involvement of the tongue, heart, and gastrointestinal tract, initially classified as primary atypical amyloidosis. There were no detectable skeletal lesions, but plasma cell dyscrasia was indicated by the finding of Bence Jones proteinuria, and was confirmed by the finding on marrow aspiration of abnormal numbers of plasma cells. The abnormal urinary protein was immunoelectrophoretically identified as a Type L Bence Jones constituent. The serum pattern shows an elevated alpha-2 globulin and a decreased gamma globulin, without an M-type peak.

In Figure 6*B*, the serum and urinary proteins from a case of γG heavy chain (Fc fragment) disease are shown. The protein elaborated in this condition has been characterized as representing the major portion (Fc fragment) of the γG H-chain with a molecular weight in the range of 50,000 to 55,000. Because these proteins are relatively larger than Bence Jones proteins, their renal clearance rate is relatively lower, and they are retained in the serum in sufficiently high concentrations to be detectable by conventional electrophoretic analysis. The abnormal serum and urinary protein peaks are of identical mobility and electrophor-

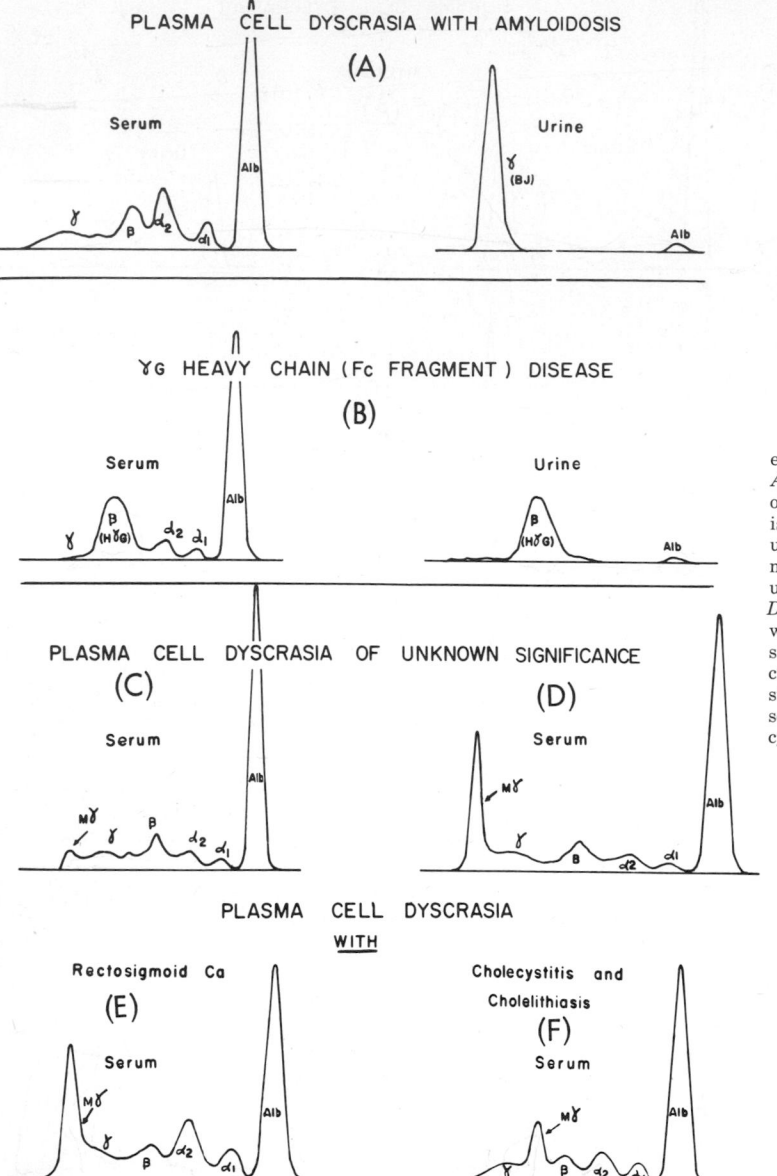

FIGURE 6. Representative electrophoretic patterns in plasma cell dyscrasias. *A*, Plasma cell dyscrasia and amyloidosis of "primary" distribution with a characteristic Bence Jones-type abnormality in the urine pattern. *B*, γG Heavy chain (Fc fragment) disease with corresponding serum and urinary M-type peaks of β mobility. *C* and *D*, Asymptomatic plasma cell dyscrasias with a small (*C*) and a large (*D*) M-type serum peak. *E*, Plasma cell dyscrasia associated with an adenocarcinoma of the rectosigmoid colon. *F*, Plasma cell dyscrasia associated with chronic and recurrent cholecystitis and cholelithiasis.

etically somewhat more polydispersed than the abnormal peaks in the other plasma cell dyscrasias. The urinary protein pattern, however, is indistinguishable from the patterns observed with Bence Jones proteinuria, and identification of the abnormal protein as related to the γG H-chain (Fc fragment) and unrelated to Bence Jones proteins and light chains must be accomplished by appropriate immunochemical and physicochemical studies.

The serum electrophoretic patterns illustrated in Figures 6*C* and 6*D* are from two cases in which M-type protein abnormalities were discovered in the absence of overt signs or symptoms of myeloma, macroglobulinemia, or any other recognizable disease. These cases are classified as "plasma cell dyscrasia of unknown significance." As will be noted subsequently, the clinical and pathologic significance of protein abnormalities of this type are presently still obscure. In some cases, progression to overt forms of plasma cell dyscrasia, such as myeloma, has been documented, but in many cases the protein abnormality has been found to persist for as long as 20 years without the development of clinically recognizable disease. Rarely, protein abnormalities of this type have been found on subsequent analyses to have disappeared—i.e., transient paraproteinemias—and these almost certainly represent examples of the synthesis of excessively large quantities of functional antibodies.

The M-type gamma globulin abnormalities illustrated in Figures 6*E* and 6*F* were found in association with clinical conditions that may have been related to the development of plasma cell dyscrasias, notably an adenocarcinoma of the rectosigmoid with an intense plasmacytic infiltration surrounding the tumor and in the resected nodes (Fig. 6*E*), and chronic and recurrent cholecystitis and cholelithiasis with extensive plasmacytosis in the gallbladder wall and along the biliary tract (Fig. 6*F*). Until a direct relationship is established between these conditions and the plasma cell dyscrasias, their association must be considered coincidental, but the relative frequency of these associations warrants the search for an occult neoplasm or biliary tract disease in patients found to have asymptomatic M-type gamma globulin abnormalities.

Bennich, H., and Johansson, S. G. D.: Studies on a new class of human immunoglobulins. II. Chemical and physical properties. *In* Killander, J. (ed.): Nobel Symposium on Gamma Globulins, 3. Stockholm, Almqvist and Wiksell, 1967, p. 199.

Edelman, G. M.: The antibody problem. Ann. Rev. Biochem., 38:415, 1969.

Heremans, J. F.: Les globulines sériques du système gamma:

Leur nature et leur pathologie. Brussels, Editions Arsia S. A., 1960.

Ishizaka, K., and Ishizaka, T.: Identification of γE-antibodies as a carrier of reaginic activity. J. Immun., 99:1187, 1967.

Metzger, H. M.: Editorial. Myeloma proteins and antibodies. Amer. J. Med., 17:837 1969.

Putnam, F. W.: Immunoglobulin structure: Variability and homology. Science, 163:633, 1909.

Young, V. H.: Transient paraproteins. Proc. Roy. Soc. Med., 62:778, 1969.

CLINICAL PATTERNS OF THE PLASMA CELL DYSCRASIAS

MULTIPLE MYELOMA
(Plasma Cell Myeloma, Myelomatosis)

Multiple myeloma is generally defined as a neoplasm of plasma cells manifested primarily by widespread skeletal destruction and frequently associated with anemia, hypercalcemia, renal functional impairment, and increased susceptibility to infections. Amyloidosis, coagulation defects and symptoms and signs related to cryoglobulins or increased serum viscosity are less commonly associated manifestations. Diagnosis depends upon the roentgenographic demonstration of diffuse osteolytic lesions and/or osteoporosis, documentation of increased numbers of plasma cells in the marrow, and the finding of M-type serum or urinary proteins.

The frequency of myeloma has apparently increased in recent years and now is comparable to that of Hodgkin's disease in many large clinics. Improved diagnostic techniques are unquestionably partly responsible for the apparent increase. Males and females are approximately equally affected. The age of onset of symptoms ranges from young adulthood to advanced years, the peak incidence being in the mid-fifties.

The symptomatic stage of myeloma is preceded by a significant asymptomatic or presymptomatic period in most and, perhaps, all cases. In this presymptomatic period, M-type serum and/or urinary proteins are demonstrable and are usually first suggested by the finding on routine examination of an increased erythrocyte sedimentation rate or unexplained and persistent proteinuria. Because intravenous pyelography may precipitate renal shutdown in the presence of Bence Jones proteinuria, the increased hazard of the procedure should be considered in planning the investigation of a case with unexplained proteinuria. The duration of the presymptomatic period in myeloma is impossible to define, but apparently can range up to 20 years. Repeated bacterial infections, particularly pneumonias, can occur during this period, presumably as a consequence of impaired immunologic mechanisms.

When myeloma becomes symptomatic, skeletal pains are the presenting and predominant manifestations in most cases. These may at first be mild and transient, or their onset may be sudden with severe back, rib, or extremity pain following an abrupt movement or effort. The abrupt onset of pain frequently indicates a pathologic fracture. With progression of the disease, more and more areas of bone destruction develop, frequently resulting in marked skeletal deformities, particularly of the sternum and rib cage, and shortening of the spine with as much as 5 or more inches decrease in stature. With earlier diagnosis and more effective chemotherapy and general management, these extreme degrees of skeletal deformity have become less common.

In most cases, multiple osteolytic ("punched-out") lesions are apparent on initial roentgenographic examination. The skull, spine, ribs, clavicles, sternum, pelvis, and proximal long bones exhibit the greatest destruction, but any part of the skeleton, including the phalanges, may be involved.

In many cases, the initial roentgenographic appearance of the skeleton is that of diffuse osteoporosis without discrete osteolytic lesions. Histologic studies demonstrate a diffuse infiltration of the marrow spaces by myeloma cells, with generalized thinning of trabeculae not detectable by standard roentgenographic techniques. Virtually all patients with this initial pattern of diffuse osteoporosis eventually develop osteolytic lesions as the disease progresses. Possibly the rarest finding in myeloma is an osteoblastic reaction in the absence of a pathologic fracture; there have been about 12 reported examples of this.

In occasional cases, myeloma presents as an *apparently single* skeletal lesion. Although these lesions are commonly designated as solitary plasmacytomas, most patients ultimately develop disseminated disease even if the original lesion is radically excised or irradiated. In cases of apparently solitary plasmacytomas, M-type protein abnormalities are almost invariably demonstrable.

Skeletal destruction results in the release of bone salts, negative calcium balance, and hypercalciuria in virtually all cases. This is generally well tolerated if adequate hydration is maintained. Hypercalcemia ensues, however, if the renal excretory capacity for calcium is exceeded, usually as a consequence of inadequate hydration and diminished urine output. All too frequently, there develops a menacing sequence of hypercalciuria → osmotic diuresis + impairment of renal tubular reabsorption → dehydration → diminished urine output → hypercalcemia + azotemia → anorexia, nausea, vomiting, and further dehydration. This set of circumstances constitutes a major threat requiring prompt therapeutic intervention with rehydration as the primary goal. Prednisone is a useful adjunct in the management of hypercalcemia, but other chemotherapy is contraindicated until hydration is accomplished and renal function restored.

In occasional cases, particularly those of diffuse osteoporosis rather than local skeletal destruction, the initial symptoms are the nonspecific gastrointestinal complaints related to hypercalcemia and the polyuria and polydipsia secondary to hypercalciuria.

Anemia of variable severity is present in virtually all cases, either at the time of diagnosis or developing subsequently as the disease progresses. It may remain moderate (hemoglobin in the range of 7 to 10 grams) and be well tolerated or become severe enough to require repeated transfusions. The anemia is usually normocytic and normochromic, but may be macrocytic. It is characteristically refractory to iron, vitamin B$_{12}$, folic acid, and liver therapy. In occasional cases a hypochromic anemia may be related to blood loss from the gastrointestinal tract, to a defect in coagulation, or to plasmacytic or amyloid infiltrates of the intestinal wall. Several factors participate in the production of anemia in myeloma, including marrow replacement, accelerated erythrocyte destruction, blood loss, renal insufficiency, the effects of radiotherapy and chemotherapy, associated infections, and nutritional factors.

Erythrocyte rouleau formation is observed in peripheral blood and marrow films, and in vivo erythrocyte aggregation ("sludged blood") is often demonstrable. This aggregation is probably due to erythrocyte coating by M-type proteins and may contribute to shortened red cell life span. Coombs' reactions, however, are usually negative.

Leukocyte and platelet counts are usually within normal limits prior to cytotoxic therapy. Occasionally, however, moderate to severe leukopenia or thrombocytopenia may be observed prior to treatment and, indeed, with therapy, the white cell and platelet counts may rise toward normal. Thrombocytopenia may contribute to a bleeding diathesis and leukopenia to an increased susceptibility to infection. The precise mechanisms responsible for leukopenia and thrombocytopenia in the plasma cell dyscrasias are unknown. The differential white cell count frequently reveals a relative lymphocytosis (40 to 55 per cent) with a variable proportion of immature lymphocytic and plasmacytic forms. Plasma cells in the peripheral blood have been reported in up to 70 per cent of cases. An outpouring of plasma cells into the peripheral blood is occasionally seen in the later stages of disease, and is considered to represent a displacement phenomenon.

A clinical pattern consistent with a diagnosis of plasma cell leukemia, with hepatosplenomegaly and white cell counts in excess of 15,000 and over 50 per cent plasma cells, is occasionally observed, with weakness, anemia, and bleeding manifestations. In the peripheral blood the cells range from typical plasmacytes to immature and atypical forms. Bence Jones proteinuria and abnormal serum globulins occur with the same frequency as in myeloma. The majority of these cases pursue an acute or subacute clinical course. It is of interest that the two known cases of γE myeloma exhibited the clinical pattern of plasma cell leukemia.

Eosinophilia, with eosinophil counts as high as 15 to 25 per cent, is observed in occasional cases of myeloma and somewhat more commonly in macroglobulinemia and γG heavy chain disease. The significance of eosinophilia in these diseases is unknown.

Marked elevation of the erythrocyte sedimentation rate (ESR) is found in most cases of myeloma. When the M-type serum proteins are cold-precipitable (cryoglobulins), the ESR may be markedly temperature-dependent, i.e., slower at room temperature or in the cold and accelerated when performed at 37° C.

Pathologic Effects of M-type Serum Globulins and Bence Jones Proteins. Each M-type protein must be recognized to be individually specific and to possess specific physicochemical properties, such as solubility, intrinsic viscosity, thermostability, and reactivity with other proteins. Certain of these properties can be correlated with specific clinical and pathologic manifestations. Thus, coagulation defects are related in certain cases to the interaction (protein:protein complexing) of specific M-type γG or γA globulins to specific coagulation factors, including fibrinogen, factors V, VII, prothrombin, and the antihemophilic globulin. Another group of protein-related symptoms are those produced by M-type γG globulins which are cold-precipitable, i.e., cryoglobulins. These include a Raynaud-type phenomenon, circulatory impairment, and, at times, occlusion and gangrene following relatively mild exposure to cold. Circulatory impairment, particularly in the central nervous system and retina, can also be related in certain cases to M-type γG globulins with a high intrinsic viscosity.

An association between Bence Jones proteinuria and renal functional impairment has long been implied, and is generally ascribed to the tubular precipitation of these proteins and blockage owing to cast formation. More recently, it has been found that Bence Jones proteinuria is occasionally associated with specific defects in renal tubular reabsorption mechanisms, including the adult Fanconi syndrome, indicating that certain Bence Jones proteins have the capacity to interfere with specific tubular transport mechanisms through direct (protein:protein) interaction with tubular cytoplasmic constituents. There is no evident correlation between the antigenic type of a Bence Jones protein and its nephrotoxic potential. The fact that a nephrotoxic potential is not common to all Bence Jones proteins is indicated by the persistence of apparently normal renal function in many cases with protracted and profound Bence Jones proteinuria. This is further evidence that several factors in addition to Bence Jones proteinuria, particularly hypercalciuria and dehydration, contribute to renal damage in myeloma.

Bence Jones proteins have also been implicated in the pathogenesis of amyloidosis. It is postulated that Bence Jones proteins traverse capillary beds because of their small molecular size and coprecipitate with as yet unidentified tissue proteins or polysaccharides, or both, to yield the complex proteinaceous tissue infiltrates, designated amyloid or paramyloid.

Additional Clinical Manifestations. Hyperuricemia and hyperuricosuria are observed in most cases as a result of increased turnover of nucleic acids in the proliferating cell population. Hyperuricosuria is not infrequently associated with renal functional impairment resulting from precipitation of urate crystals or stone formation, or both. The danger of increased urate excretion is particularly great in the initial stages of cytotoxic chemotherapy, and warrants special attention to the maintenance of adequate hydration and possibly therapy with allopurinol. Gouty arthropathy is a rare complication.

Neurologic manifestations may develop from direct pressure on the spinal cord, nerve roots, cranial or peripheral nerves, or as a result of a pathologic fracture of a vertebral body or long bone. Spinal cord compression leading to weakness and ultimately paraplegia is an especially serious complication because the osteoporosis and negative calcium balance produced by the myeloma is compounded by the osteoporosis of immobilization. Again, this complication of myeloma has become less common with improved therapeutic management.

Infiltration of peripheral nerves and nerve roots by amyloid can cause peripheral neuropathies or root symptoms that are usually symmetrical and are associated with other evidence of amyloidosis such as macroglossia, cardiac manifestations, and the carpal tunnel syndrome. Rarely, polyneuropathies develop in myeloma and the other plasma cell dyscrasias without demonstrable tumor or amyloid infiltration. The pattern of these polyneuropathies is nonspecific; apparently they are similar to the polyneuropathies of obscure origin occasionally associated with other neoplastic diseases.

Myopathies involving principally proximal muscle groups are also rarely associated with myeloma and other plasma cell dyscrasias and, again, the pathogenic mechanisms are completely unknown.

An apparent increase in the incidence of non-reticular neoplasms, particularly of bowel, breast, and biliary tract carcinomas, has been noted in association with myeloma in one comprehensive postmortem study (19 per cent) and in the author's series (22 per cent).

Immunologic Deficiency. Increased susceptibility to bacterial infections, particularly pneumococcal pneumonia, exists in many cases of myeloma and is at least partially the result of an impaired capacity for antibody formation. This is generally reflected in a decrease in the serum concentration of normal γG, γA, and γM immunoglobulins irrespective of the type of M-protein elaborated. The basis for these deficiencies is presently unknown, but available studies indicate that diminished production is a more significant factor than increased catabolism or loss. Herpes zoster and generalized varicella infections occur with increased frequency in myeloma and other plasma cell dyscrasias, but apparently no more so than in Hodgkin's disease and lymphosarcoma. Susceptibility to other viral infections apparently is not increased. Studies of the homograft rejection reaction have demonstrated a significant prolongation of rejection time, indicating that the immunologic deficiencies in myeloma may include cell-mediated immune mechanisms.

Treatment. Both the comfort and useful life of patients with myeloma can unquestionably be extended by proper management. The importance of *ambulation and adequate hydration* cannot be overemphasized. The constant threats of hypercalcemia, hypercalciuria, and hyperuricemia necessitate continual attention to these cardinal aspects of general care. Many patients are immobilized and bedridden with pain when first seen. In these circumstances, all effort should be made to achieve ambulation by a combination of analgesics, orthopedic supports (particularly Taylor spine bracing), and local radiotherapy, as indicated. Plasma cell tumors are characteristically radiosensitive, and x-ray therapy is of established value in the control of localized symptomatic lesions. The field of irradiation and the dosage should be limited in order to spare the marrow as much as possible. A total dose of 1200 to 1500 roentgens is usually adequate for symptomatic control and for the facilitation of ambulation. Pain relief is frequently noted after as little as 200 to 400 r. Salicylates and codeine are usually more effective analgesics for the pain of myeloma than meperidine (Demerol) or propoxyphene (Darvon). Prednisone, as previously indicated, is a useful agent in the management of hypercalcemia, but hydration sufficient to achieve a 24-hour urine output of over 1500 ml. is the principal need. Unless mobilization and hydration are accomplished by these measures, it is usually impossible to maintain a patient for the time required to accomplish a remission with chemotherapy.

Of the chemotherapeutic agents presently available, melphalan (l-phenylalanine mustard, Alkeran) and cytoxan (cyclophosphamide) are the two drugs most useful in the long-term management of myeloma. When properly administered, both agents can achieve significant objective and subjective remissions in approximately 60 per cent of cases. Although both melphalan and cytoxan are alkylating agents, their precise mechanisms of action must be different, because sensitivity or resistance to one agent does not necessarily imply the corresponding sensitivity or resistance to the other. Thus, the two agents can be used sequentially with an increased possibility of achieving a remission. As yet it is not known whether there is a preferential order, but melphalan is generally the first agent employed in the author's clinic. Therapy is usually initiated with an 8 to 10 day course of 8 to 10 mg. per day, i.e., an initial course of 64 to 100 mg., depending upon the patient's size, hematologic status, and general condition. Following this initial course, continuous maintenance therapy at a dose of 2 mg. a day is instituted. It is no longer considered necessary to interrupt therapy between the initial loading dose and institution of maintenance therapy. With this dosage regimen, it may be anticipated that the peripheral leukocyte count will fall to the range of 3000 to 4000 and be maintained in this range with continued therapy. This degree of marrow suppression is tolerated without complications and provides an index of the adequacy of dosage. In some cases, a decrease in white count below 3000 necessitates reducing the maintenance dose to 1 mg. per day. With cytoxan, therapy is initiated at a dosage level of 200 mg. a day for 7 to 10 days, following which the dose is reduced to 100 mg. a day for maintenance. Again, in some cases it is necessary to reduce the maintenance dose to 50 mg. a day because of leukopenia or thrombocytopenia, or both. With both melphalan and cytoxan, present evidence indicates that continuous drug administration is preferable to interrupted therapy.

With chemotherapy, the objective signs of improvement include a decrease in the concentration of abnormal M-type serum globulins, decreased Bence Jones proteinuria, hematologic improvement, cessation of further skeletal destruction, and occasionally recalcification of osteolytic lesions. In some cases, it has also been found that the concentrations of normal immunoglobulins increase, and this is associated with improved resistance to bacterial infections. It should be recognized, however, that several weeks may elapse between the institution of therapy and the first signs of improvement. Because of the rapid turnover of Bence Jones proteins, a decrease in Bence Jones proteinuria is the earliest objective sign of chemotherapeutic effect, and this has been noted within one week of initiating chemotherapy. A decrease in myeloma serum globulins is usually not observed until the fourth or fifth week. The duration of the remissions which can be achieved with chemotherapy has steadily increased in the past several years; there are now many patients who have been maintained in excellent clinical and functional remission for periods of six years or more. Thus, the prognosis in myeloma has greatly improved in the past several years with the introduction of these agents.

An attempt to increase skeletal density by inducing fluorosis with sodium fluoride has been made in some cases with generally equivocal results. At present, this therapy is not recommended. The maintenance of ambulation and the encouragement of exercise is equally as important in the long-term management of myeloma as it is in the initial phases of therapy. Patients should be encouraged to walk, swim, or engage in other forms of exercise to the extent of their ability, avoiding only those activities which involve excessive lifting and straining.

MACROGLOBULINEMIA
(Primary or Waldenström's Macroglobulinemia)

Macroglobulinemia is presently classified as a plasma cell dyscrasia involving those cell populations normally responsible for the synthesis of gamma-M macroglobulins. The excessive proliferation of these cells results in the elaboration of large quantities of electrophoretically homogeneous (M-type) γM globulins and a variable clinical pattern with anemia, bleeding manifestations, and symptoms related to the serum macroglobulins as the predominant features. Males and females are approximately equally affected. Symptoms generally begin in the fifth or sixth decade. As the disease slowly evolves, lymphadenopathy, splenomegaly, and hepatomegaly develop in a variable percentage of cases, producing a clinical pattern resembling a malignant lymphoma or lymphatic leukemia. Skeletal lesions of the type seen in myeloma do not occur.

Histologic studies of lymph nodes demonstrate a proliferation of lymphocytic-plasmacytic forms often arranged in a pattern of follicular hyperplasia. Immunofluorescent studies have confirmed the synthesis of γM globulin in these cells, as well as in the corresponding lymphocytic-plasmacytic forms demonstrable in peripheral blood and bone marrow preparations. It is generally impossible to ascertain whether the cellular proliferations observed in macroglobulinemia represent reactive responses or autonomous neoplasia. The possibility that initially benign and reactive proliferations may undergo transformation to neoplastic proliferations is suggested in many cases of macroglobulinemia as in other forms of plasma cell dyscrasia.

When macroglobulinemia becomes symptomatic, anemia is the most common presenting manifestation, and is frequently profound, with hemoglobin levels in the range of 4 to 6 grams per 100 ml. Usually the anemia is due to a combination of factors, including accelerated red cell destruction, blood loss, and decreased erythropoiesis. Coating of erythrocytes with γM macroglobulin is apparently responsible for the marked rouleaux formation, positive Coombs reactions, and cross-matching difficulties encountered in many cases.

As previously noted, a large percentage of γM macroglobulins have specific physicochemical properties that are responsible for specific symptom patterns in certain cases. These properties include cold-insolubility (cryoglobulins), high intrinsic viscosity, and the capacity to form complexes with coagulation factors and other plasma proteins. *Cryoglobulin-related symptoms* include Raynaud's phenomenon, cold sensitivity, cold urticaria, and vascular occlusion with gangrene following exposure to cold. *Viscosity-related manifestations* are most evident in the retinal vasculature, in which a pattern of patchy venous bulging and localized narrowing ("sausage-effect" or "fundus paraproteinemicus") develops, frequently associated with hemorrhages, exudates, and visual impairment. Circulatory impairment in the central nervous system owing to increased plasma viscosity produces changing patterns of neurologic signs and symptoms, e.g., transient paresis, reflex abnormalities, deafness, impairment of consciousness ("coma paraproteinemicum"), frequently terminating with cerebral vascular hemorrhage. Cardiac decompensation and pulmonary symptoms may also develop secondary to increased viscosity in the systemic and pulmonary vascular beds. *Protein:protein interaction* with formation of complexes between γM macroglobulins and coagulation factors (fibrinogen, prothrombin, factors V, VII, etc.) is an important contributing factor to the bleeding diathesis (particularly epistaxes, oral mucosal bleeding, and purpura) exhibited in many cases. Interference with platelet function (platelet agglutination) and capillary damage secondary to increased serum viscosity are additional factors contributing to bleeding manifestations. It must be recognized that all these symptom patterns are also observed in occasional cases of myeloma with M-type γG and γA globulins possessing similar physicochemical properties.

Bence Jones proteinuria is present in approximately 10 per cent of cases of macroglobulinemia, but renal functional impairment is much less common than in myeloma, presumably because of the absence of the contributing factors of hypercalcemia and hypercalciuria. Amyloidosis has been observed in only a few cases of macroglobulinemia, and in all of these, the liver, spleen, and parenchymal organs have been the major areas of involvement in contrast to the primary, atypical mesenchymal distribution of amyloid usually observed in myeloma.

Peripheral neuropathies (*Bing-Neel syndrome*) and myelopathy may be progressive and incapacitating. Circulatory impairment in vasa nervorum is a postulated but still unsubstantiated mechanism. Myopathies and rheumatoid-like arthropathies have also been observed.

In the author's series of 57 cases, 15 had clinical or postmortem evidence of an associated non-reticular neoplasm, and an additional 12 had a background of long-standing infection, particularly tuberculosis.

Many of the laboratory findings in macroglobulinemia have already been considered. The presymptomatic cases are usually detected initially as a result of finding an unexplained elevation of erythrocyte sedimentation rate on routine examination, followed by electrophoretic demonstration of an M-type serum protein (Fig. 5) and, finally, its characterization as a γM globulin by ultra-

centrifugation or immunoelectrophoresis, or both. The majority of γM globulins are euglobulins and give a positive Sia water-dilution reaction, but this is not specific for macroglobulins because certain γG globulins are also Sia-positive euglobulins. Approximately one third of macroglobulins are cryoglobulins, yielding a white precipitate or a thick clear gel on cooling. The temperature and duration of cooling needed for precipitation varies with individual cryoglobulins. With some cryoglobulins, precipitation or gel-formation occurs almost immediately following venipuncture, and a pre-warmed syringe is necessary for blood sampling. Others require several hours at 10° C. for precipitation. Similarly, the increased viscosity of serum containing a viscous M-type macroglobulin may be readily apparent when a tube of serum at room temperature is inverted, or viscosimetric determinations at different temperatures may be required.

Hematologic abnormalities, in addition to anemia, include an absolute lymphocytosis with "atypical, immature and plasmacytic" forms in many cases, occasionally reaching leukemic proportions. Polymorphonuclear leukopenia, thrombopenia, and eosinophilia are also observed. Bone marrow aspirations characteristically reveal an increase in lymphocytic-plasmacytic forms, accompanied by eosinophils and mast cells in many cases. The small lymphocyte, with a dense pyknotic nucleus, which has been considered most typical for macroglobulinemia, probably represents a degenerating cell undergoing cytoplasmic shedding (so-called "clasmatosis").

Additional laboratory abnormalities in certain cases of macroglobulinemia include positive flocculation reactions, false positive serologic reactions, and positive rheumatoid factors. The latter are occasionally associated with rheumatic symptoms and arthropathy.

Treatment. The principal indications for therapy in macroglobulinemia are anemia, bleeding manifestations, and symptoms related to increased plasma viscosity. When the latter symptoms are severe and threaten central nervous system function and vision, plasmapheresis is indicated as a temporary measure. Sufficient plasma should be removed to effect a lowering of viscosity, and the red cells should be returned. In certain cases, a prompt and dramatic improvement in clinical status follows the removal of as little as 500 ml. of plasma. Repeated plasmapheresis for a period of several weeks may be required until effective chemotherapy can be instituted.

Chlorambucil (Leukeran) is presently regarded as the chemotherapeutic agent of choice in macroglobulinemia. This should be administered continuously at a dosage level of 8 to 10 mg. daily. Although this dosage level is significantly higher than the average employed in most cases of lymphatic leukemia or lymphosarcoma, it is usually well tolerated in macroglobulinemia. A large number of patients have been maintained in objective and subjective remission for periods up to nine years with continuous chlorambucil therapy. More limited studies with melphalan indicate it to be less effective in macroglobulinemia than chlorambucil. Prednisone may be of some value in the control of capillary bleeding.

AMYLOIDOSIS

The term "amyloidosis" was introduced by Virchow over a century ago to describe the "starchlike" amorphous eosinophilic infiltrates that generally appeared in the liver, spleen, kidney, and adrenals as a secondary complication of a variety of chronic diseases, particularly chronic tuberculosis, osteomyelitis, leprosy, Hodgkin's disease, carcinomas, and so forth. Similar infiltrates were subsequently noted to develop in a somewhat different distribution pattern (mesenchymal tissue, tongue, heart, gastrointestinal tract) in certain cases in the absence of overt chronic suppuration or other apparent illness, and these cases were designated primary, idiopathic, or atypical amyloidosis. Amyloidosis was also recognized to develop in approximately 5 per cent of cases of myeloma but, somewhat paradoxically, the distribution and staining properties of the amyloid infiltrates in myeloma were generally more similar to those of the so-called primary, atypical form than to those of the typical secondary pattern.*

Extensive studies in recent years have begun to clarify some of the inter-relationships among these apparently diverse forms of amyloidosis. Chemical and histochemical studies have established that amyloid infiltrates are not simply "starchlike" but rather are protein:polysaccharide complexes of varying composition. Polarization microscopy and electron micrographic studies have shown that amyloid infiltrates are not amorphous, as originally concluded on the basis of conventional microscopy, but rather are deposited in a fibrillar pattern with a periodicity of approximately 100 Å. Experimental studies have established that amyloidosis of the secondary variety can be induced in several animal species by prolonged and excessive antigenic stimulation, apparently as a manifestation of exhaustion of the capacity of the reticuloendothelial system (RES) to elaborate complete antibody molecules. Immunohistochemical studies of experimental and human amyloid have shown the presence of antigenic determinants related to the immunoglobulins along with complement (C'3) and other plasma proteins, in addition to components unrelated to serum proteins. Which of these constituents are integral components of amyloid and which are simply trapped or adsorbed to a complex protein:polysaccharide matrix remains to be deter-

mined. Despite these limitations, however, most available evidence relates experimental amyloidosis to deranged RES function and abnormalities in immunoglobulin synthesis.

Clinical and biochemical studies of the various forms of amyloidosis in man have also provided considerable evidence of deranged plasmacytic function. Several studies have demonstrated a decrease in serum gamma globulin levels coincident with the development of amyloidosis in cases of chronic suppuration, etc., with initially elevated gamma globulin concentrations. Recent investigations in our laboratory have demonstrated that the decrease in serum gamma globulins is not simply due to excessive urinary loss caused by renal amyloidosis, but is more likely the result of decreased synthesis of complete immunoglobulin molecules. This is indicated by the immunoelectrophoretic demonstration of excessive quantities of low molecular weight, gamma-u fragments of the Bence Jones type in the urine of patients with secondary amyloidosis. It is, therefore, suggested that *secondary* amyloidosis, at least in certain cases, is associated with a plasmacytic dyscrasia according to the previously defined criteria.

In those cases in which amyloidosis is associated with overt myeloma, the criteria for plasmacytic dyscrasia are also met, and, significantly, a particular association with Bence Jones-type protein abnormalities has been well documented. Finally, in a series of 25 cases in which amyloidosis was considered to have been primary and idiopathic, Bence Jones-type protein abnormalities (Fig. 6A), decreased normal immunoglobulin levels, and abnormal numbers of plasma cells in bone marrow and tissue sections were demonstrated in 20 instances. The further observation of associated nonreticular neoplasms, chronic biliary tract disease, and occult infections (particularly pyelonephritis) in a large proportion of cases is also noteworthy and apparently similar to the increased frequency of these associated conditions in overt myeloma and the other plasma cell dyscrasias. Thus, evidence of a plasma cell dyscrasia can be found in the majority of cases of apparently "primary" amyloidosis, and the distinction between these cases and cases of amyloidosis with myelomatous skeletal destruction is considered to be quantitative (with respect to the extent of skeletal replacement) rather than qualitative. The possibility is also suggested that plasma cell dyscrasias may be induced by chronic and protracted RES stimulation in certain of these cases in a manner similar to that indicated in "secondary" amyloidosis.

The clinical manifestations of amyloidosis are determined by the distribution of the tissue infiltrates. In cases with involvement of parenchymatous organs and the so-called "typical" secondary distribution pattern, the principal manifestations are hepatosplenomegaly, the nephrotic syndrome, and, rarely, adrenal cortical insufficiency. In cases with the so-called primary "atypical" distribution pattern, the principal

---

*Several apparently hereditary forms of amyloidosis have been described, and amyloidosis has been observed in association with familial Mediterranean fever. These forms are considered elsewhere.

manifestations are referable to involvement of the heart (cardiac decompensation with narrowing of pulse pressure, low EKG voltage, arrhythmia), tongue and gastrointestinal tract (macroglossia, dysphagia, spruelike syndrome, gastrointestinal bleeding), nerves (peripheral neuropathy, dysesthesias, paresthesias), ligaments and periarticular tissues (carpal tunnel syndrome, arthropathy), and skin. The initial symptoms in a particular case may be referable to involvement of any one or a combination of these areas. To date there is no explanation for the differences in distribution patterns in different cases but it has been postulated that these may result from differences in the binding affinities of individual Bence Jones-type proteins.

Lichen myxedematosus (lichen amyloidosus, papular mucinosis) is a rare form of amyloidosis or tissue proteinosis characterized by the progressive deposition of amyloid deposits in the dermis of the face, trunk, and extremities. Recent studies have established that this form of amyloidosis is apparently consistently associated with the elaboration of unusually basic (cationic) M-type γG globulins. It has further been demonstrated in one case that the amyloid infiltrates of the skin were comprised, at least in part, by this specific protein, presumably deposited in combination with the acid mucopolysaccharides of the dermis. The possibility that lichen myxedematosus may be an autoimmune disease, in which a monoclonal antibody is directed against antigenic constituents of the dermis, has been suggested.

The diagnosis of amyloidosis depends upon the demonstration of the amyloid infiltrates. This is usually best accomplished by rectal mucosal biopsy, because amyloidosis involves the arterioles of the rectal submucosa in almost all clinical types. Following Congo red staining, amyloid deposits show a characteristic yellow-green birefringence when examined by polarization microscopy. This technique occasionally discloses amyloid deposits not revealed by the usual staining procedures. In all cases of amyloidosis, detailed examination of the serum and urinary proteins by electrophoresis and immunoelectrophoresis is indicated, along with bone marrow studies, to document a plasma cell dyscrasia. In a case of amyloidosis with proteinuria, the finding of a negative Bence Jones reaction on heat-testing does not exclude the presence of an abnormal constituent of the Bence Jones type, because albumin and other serum proteins in the urine may mask a Bence Jones reaction.

Treatment. There are no known methods to reverse the deposition of amyloid infiltrates except the identification and control of associated conditions, particularly osteomyelitis, pulmonary abscesses and tuberculosis. Several cases have been reported in which effective antimicrobial therapy or surgery, or both, for chronic suppurative processes has resulted in cessation of amyloid deposition and reabsorption of existing infiltrates. Unfortunately, this is rare; in most cases the amyloidosis continues despite apparently effective control of associated conditions.

Experience with melphalan therapy in cases of amyloidosis with overt myeloma or occult plasma cell dyscrasia is limited, but results have been generally discouraging. Most patients have continued to pursue a relentless downhill course, succumbing to cardiac decompensation or complications related to tongue and gastrointestinal involvement. Corticosteroids occasionally provide slight symptomatic benefit. In cases of macroglossia, careful attention to oral hygiene is important to avoid irritation and ulceration of the tongue.

γG HEAVY CHAIN DISEASE

Heavy chain (γG) disease is a relatively rare form of plasma cell dyscrasia characterized by the elaboration of excessive quantities of polypeptide related to the H(heavy)-chains (and, more specifically, to the Fc fragment) of γG globulin. The clinical pattern resembles a lymphoma with lymphadenopathy, splenomegaly, and hepatomegaly as the predominant manifestations associated with the nonspecific symptoms of weakness, fever, weight loss, and marked susceptibility to bacterial infections. Several patients have exhibited transient palatal erythema and edema resembling that of infectious mononucleosis, and in some there was transient spontaneous regression of the lymphadenopathy after an initially rapid onset. None have had clinical or roentgenographic evidence of skeletal destruction. Most have shown anemia, leukopenia, and thrombopenia, presumably owing to hypersplenism, and moderate to marked eosinophilia. Bone marrow aspirations and lymph node biopsies demonstrated proliferation of plasmacytic and lymphocytic forms along with eosinophils and large reticulum or reticuloendothelial cells.

Persistent proteinuria (4 to 15 grams per 24 hours) was generally the initial indication of an abnormality of protein metabolism. The characteristic serum and urinary protein electrophoretic patterns are illustrated in Figure 6B and have been described previously. Total serum protein concentrations were generally within normal limits. The serum concentration of the abnormal protein ranged from 2 to 4 grams per 100 ml. associated with marked decrease in the concentration of normal gamma globulin. Identification of the abnormal protein as related to the γG H-chain (Fc fragment) and unrelated to Bence Jones and L-chain polypeptides must be accomplished by immunochemical and physicochemical analyses.

In contrast to myeloma, erythrocyte sedimentation rates have been normal or only slightly elevated. Additional laboratory findings have included hyperuricemia with normal or only slightly elevated blood urea nitrogen levels and no other evidence of renal functional impairment.

Survival from the time of onset of symptoms has ranged from four months to over five years. Bacterial pneumonia and sepsis caused death in all cases.

Splenic radiation has produced temporary remissions with hematologic improvement. Limited trials of cyclophosphamide, melphalan, and steroids gave little or no benefit.

γA HEAVY CHAIN (α-CHAIN) DISEASE

γA heavy chain (α-chain) disease is the most recently identified plasma cell dyscrasia. As defined by Seligmann and his associates, the clinical pattern is that previously referred to as "Mediterranean-type abdominal lymphoma." The predominant features are a diffuse lymphoma-like proliferation in the small intestine and mesentery, chronic diarrhea, and malabsorption unresponsive to gluten withdrawal. Although all of Seligmann's cases were either non-Ashkenazi Jews or Israeli Arabs, we have recently documented the syndrome, with the specific α-chain abnormality, in a South American (Colombia) male of Spanish and Indian (Mestizo) descent. Thus, although genetic factors were considered to be of major importance, the disease is not exclusively restricted to the Mediterranean population.

Chronic diarrhea, malabsorption, and progressive wasting are the major clinical features. Small intestinal biopsies demonstrate a profound infiltration of the lamina propria with abnormal plasma cells. Intestinal absorption studies demonstrate impaired absorption of Vitamin B_{12}, glucose, lactose, and fat. Roentgenograms of the small intestines show thickened mucosal folds, segmentation, and dilated intestinal loops. Bone marrow aspiration reveals moderate increases in plasma cells, and skeletal roentgenograms show moderate diffuse osteoporosis but no destructive lesions.

On electrophoretic analysis of serum, the distinctive increase in γA heavy chains (α chains) has been evidenced by a markedly elevated, broad peak traversing the beta and alpha-2 mobility range. The electrophoretic polydispersity has been shown to be due to polymeric heterogeneity of the alpha chains. This tendency to polymerize also explains the relatively low concentration of alpha chains in the urine as compared with the excretion of gamma chains in γG heavy chain disease. Confirmation of the identity of the abnormal serum protein as free α-chains is accomplished by demonstrating the absence of associated light chains by appropriate immunologic and chemical analyses.

The association of this particular form of plasma cell dyscrasia with the small intestine is of particular interest in view of the known preponderance of γA-producing plasma cells in the intestinal tract. The possible role of antecedent chronic infection or irritation of the intestines in the pathogenesis of γA heavy chain disease cannot be presently defined.

PLASMA CELL DYSCRASIA OF UNKNOWN SIGNIFICANCE AND PLASMA CELL DYSCRASIA ASSOCIATED WITH CHRONIC INFECTIONS, BILIARY DISEASE, AND NONRETICULAR NEOPLASMS

Use of serum electrophoresis as a routine clinical laboratory procedure has resulted in the detection of M-type protein abnormalities, such as are illustrated in Figure 6C and D, in otherwise asymptomatic persons. As previously noted, certain of these later develop signs and symptoms of myeloma, macroglobulinemia, or amyloidosis after many months or years. A fundamental question is whether M-type protein abnormalities are invariably manifestations of plasma cell dyscrasia that will produce clinical symptoms if the patient survives "long enough" (possibly several decades), or whether certain M-type abnormalities are truly benign and "essential." Since this question is presently unanswerable, the term "plasma cell dyscrasia of unknown significance" is considered preferable to "premyeloma" or "essential or benign monoclonal gammopathy."

In general, asymptomatic M-type protein abnormalities are more commonly observed in older subjects. In many cases there is a background of tuberculosis, syphilis or other chronic infection, chronic biliary tract disease, or a nonreticular neoplasm, particularly large bowel, breast, oropharyngeal, and biliary tract carcinomas. Although a coincidental association cannot be excluded, particularly in older subjects, there is increasing evidence that certain plasma cell dyscrasias in man may be induced by diverse forms of protracted reticuloendothelial stimuli comparable to those described in mice. Because of the frequency of these associations, a careful search for an occult infection or neoplasm should be periodically carried out in all patients with asymptomatic M-type protein abnormalities, with particular attention to the bowel and biliary tracts.

To date, chemotherapy with melphalan or any other agent has not been deemed warranted in asymptomatic subjects, despite the knowledge that a certain percentage of them will later develop overt myeloma. Although there are obvious theoretical advantages to earlier chemotherapy, the unpredictability of the course in any one case and the significant toxicities of presently available agents are strong arguments against the institution of chemotherapy before a distinct clinical pattern is evident.

ASSOCIATION BETWEEN PLASMACYTIC AND MONOCYTIC DYSCRASIAS

A close functional relationship is known to exist between the monocyte-histiocyte-macrophage system and plasma cells in the processing of antigens and the synthesis of antibodies. As an apparently related phenomenon, there is a significant association between plasmacytic and monocytic dyscrasias in man. Thus, monocytic leukemia develops late in the course of a small but significant number of cases of long-standing plasma cell myeloma, generally after several years of effective chemotherapeutic control of the myeloma. In all cases, the monocytic leukemia is associated with markedly elevated serum and urine lysozyme levels. The onset of monocytic leukemia is usually abrupt, although in some cases transient episodes of peripheral monocytosis and fever precede the development of the terminal leukemic phase.

Additional evidence linking monocytic and plasmacytic dyscrasias has been the finding of M-type gamma globulin abnormalities or diffuse hypergammaglobulinemia, or both, in several cases of monocytic leukemia not associated with overt myeloma. Significantly, many of these latter patients have had protracted chronic illnesses, particularly chronic pulmonary infections, tuberculosis and osteomyelitis, similar to those associated with plasma cell dyscrasia. Thus, comparable pathogenic mechanisms may be operative, and may constitute a proliferative stimulus to both plasma cells and monocytes, either simultaneously or sequentially.

Cohen, A. S.: Amyloidosis. New Eng. J. Med., 277:522, 574, 628, 1967.

Hallén, J.: Discrete gamma globulin (M-) components in serum. Clinical study of 150 subjects without myelomatosis. Acta Med. Scand. (Suppl. 462, 127 pp.), 1966.

Korst, D. R., Clifford, G. O., Fowler, W. M., Louis, J., Will, J., and Wilson, H. E.: Multiple myeloma, II. Analysis of cyclophosphamide therapy in 165 patients. 189:758, 1964.

Osserman, E. F.: Clinical and biochemical studies of plasmacytic and monocytic dyscrasias and their interrelationships. Trans. and Studies, Coll. Phys. Phila., 36:134, 1969.

Osserman, E. F.: Plasma-cell myeloma: II. Clinical aspects. New Eng. J. Med., 261:952, 1006, 1959.

Osserman, E. F., and Lawlor, D. P.: Serum and urinary lysozyme (muramidase) in monocytic and mono-myelocytic leukemia. J. Exp. Med., 124:921, 1966.

Osserman, E. F., and Takatsuki, K.: Clinical and immunochemical studies of four cases of heavy (H₂) chain disease. Amer. J. Med., 37:351, 1964.

Osserman, E. F., and Takatsuki, K.: Considerations regarding the pathogenesis of the plasmacytic dyscrasias. Scand. J. Haemat., 4 (Suppl.): 28, 1964.

Osserman, E. F., Takatsuki, K., and Talal, N.: The pathogenesis of "amyloidosis." Studies on the role of abnormal gamma globulins and gamma globulin fragments of the Bence Jones (γ polypeptide) type in the pathogenesis of "primary" and "secondary amyloidosis," and the "amyloidosis" associated with plasma cell myeloma. Seminars Hemat., 1:3, 1964.

Seligman, M., Danon, F., Hurez, D., Mihesco, E., and Preud'homme, J. L.: Alpha-chain disease: A new immunoglobulin abnormality. Science, 162:1396, 1968.

Waldenström, J.: Studies on conditions associated with disturbed gamma globulin formation (gammopathies). Harvey Lect., Series 56:211, 1961.

Diseases of the Spleen
Carl V. Moore

INTRODUCTION

As information about the pathogenesis of the blood dyscrasias has increased, the number of disorders that can be classified as specific diseases of the spleen has gradually dwindled. The argument might be made that the list should include only such things as splenic abscesses, infarcts, or tumors because under other circumstances abnormal splenic function results from congestion, infiltration, or generalized involvement of the lymphocytic and reticuloendothelial cells. Even in hereditary spherocytosis, in which splenectomy is so effective, the enlarged spleen seems to be functioning normally when it traps and destroys the thick red blood cells found in that disease; spherocytes injected into a normal recipient are similarly removed by the spleen of the normal subject. There are circumstances, however, in which hematologic changes seem to be caused by or to be dependent on splenic malfunction. They may be classified as hypersplenism (dyssplenism) and congestive splenomegaly.

Circulation and Functions of the Spleen. The spleen holds a fascination for biologists because its circulation is unique, because its known functions are so varied, and because of a gnawing conviction that some of its functions are still unknown. It consists of a capsule and trabeculae enclosing the white and red pulp. The splenic artery branches into trabecular arteries. When the latter leave the trabeculi, they enter the white pulp (a periarterial sheath of lymphocytes with germinal centers and a variable number of monocytes, macrophages, and plasma cells enmeshed in a reticular framework), where some of their branches terminate. Those arteries that pass through the white into the red pulp (sinuses separated by cords composed of communicating compartments of reticulum containing phagocytic and other free cells) also terminate in arterial capillaries; only a few communicate directly with sinuses. For the most part, therefore, the circulation is open, so that cells from the blood are delivered to the pulp from which they must migrate through the white pulp and/or the cords of the red pulp, and then through the walls of the sinuses back into venous channels. This arrangement puts blood cells in intimate contact with phagocytic cells, causes sequestration within the pulp, and requires the cells to distort themselves as they squeeze through the cords and into sinuses on their way back to the circulation. It is estimated that blood may make about 500 passes through the spleen per day.

Known splenic functions include a role in *blood formation.* Lymphocytes, plasma cells, and probably monocytes are regularly produced. All blood cells are formed in the spleen, however, during a portion of fetal life, in diseases characterized by extramedullary hematopoiesis, and throughout the life of certain rodents. The spleen functions *immunologically* by making immunocompetent cells (lymphocytes, plasma cells, reticulum cells) of importance both in antibody production and delayed hypersensitivity reactions. It *sequesters* and serves as a *reservoir* for blood cells in some animals (sheep, dog, cat), but in man normally holds only 20 to 30 ml. The volume may be much greater in patients with large spleens; evidence indicates that a large percentage of peripheral blood platelets may be concentrated in a splenic platelet pool. *Cellular destruction* occurs as the result of phagocytosis, fragmentation, and metabolic changes incident to sequestration. When a red cell passes through the wall of a sinus, it must squeeze through an opening estimated to be 3 μ or less. Any abnormality that interferes with the distortability of the red cell can cause the membrane to fragment, and the loss of membrane leads to spherocytosis. Similarly, a cytoplasmic inclusion body, i.e., Heinz body, may be pinched off as the cell tries to pass through the basement membrane into a sinus (*culling* or *pitting* effect). Of special interest is the demonstration that macrophages have gamma globulin combining sites on their surface. A red cell coated with gamma globulin— as in autoimmune hemolytic anemia—will tend to stick to these combining sites. The macrophage partially engulfs the cell, bites off a portion of the membrane, and then releases the erythrocyte. Again the cell has lost more membrane than volume, tends to become more spherocytic, and is more easily trapped in the splenic cords, in which destruction may occur. Much less is known about the mechanisms for splenic destruction of leukocytes and platelets.

Fragments of experimental and clinical evidence exist suggesting that the spleen may also exert a *hormonal effect* on bone marrow function. Unexplained, for instance, is the clinical observation that modest doses of irradiation to the spleens of patients with chronic myelogenous leukemia may induce a clinical and hematologic remission that may persist for six months or more. If a similar amount of irradiation is given instead to the precordium or any other nonsplenic area, the results are much less dramatic and often minimal. Furthermore, an occasional patient with pure red cell anemia may improve dramatically after splenectomy, and erythropoiesis may be returned to normal. In these clinical situations as well as in the relevant experimental work, there are possible explanations other than hormonal control of marrow function, but neither has that possibility been eliminated. Unexplained also is the provision of nature which put the spleen in the portal circulation. That arrangement provides the liver with the opportunity to metabolize or detoxify products of splenic cellular destruction. Galen's designation of the spleen as an organ of mystery is still partially justified.

Several workers have attempted to define a state of *hyposplenism* after splenectomy or in children with congenital absence of the spleen, but no clear clinical pattern exists. Evidence has been presented to indicate that children (but not adults) have a greater susceptibility to infection after splenectomy. The injection of sheep erythrocytes into splenectomized persons causes the production of less antibody than in normal persons. After removal of the spleen, nucleated erythrocytes and red corpuscles containing Howell-Jolly bodies may be found in the blood for years; a mild leukocytosis and thrombocytosis may be present for months.

HYPERSPLENISM

At times the spleen performs abnormally or does its job too well. The resultant states of dyssplenism or hypersplenism are characterized by peripheral cytopenia which may involve red blood cells, leukocytes, and/or platelets in any combination. The abnormally functioning spleen produces these changes largely by destroying blood cells too rapidly—by changing from a graveyard to a slaughterhouse. Production of autoantibodies against cells and, possibly, depression of the marrow may occasionally contribute. Partial to complete recovery from the cytopenia frequently follows splenectomy. Acquired autoimmune hemolytic anemia and immune thrombocytopenic purpura might be included under this designation, because the spleen in these conditions is a principal site of cellular destruction and participates in the production of the "autoantibody" to red blood cells and platelets; these conditions, however, have been separately presented. The more usual examples are the following:

1. Hemolytic anemias caused primarily by accelerated red blood cell destruction in the enlarged spleens ("big-spleen syndrome") found in a variety of diseases: sarcoidosis, lupus erythematosus, malignant lymphoma, chronic lymphocytic leukemia, Gaucher's disease, myelofibrosis with myeloid metaplasia, and so forth. In some instances, erythrocyte sensitization (with a positive Coombs test) may also occur and may contribute

to the hemolysis. There are no distinctive clinical manifestations caused by the anemia per se, and jaundice is minimal unless related to the underlying disease process. The anemia may be moderate to severe, is usually normocytic, normochromic, or slightly macrocytic, and is often accompanied by a reticulocytosis of 5 to 10 per cent or more.

2. Neutropenia or thrombocytopenia associated with enlarged spleens and presumably with increased destruction of neutrophils or platelets; primary splenic neutropenia; Felty's syndrome (rheumatoid arthritis, splenomegaly, leukopenia); kala-azar. The neutropenia and thrombocytopenia may be moderate or severe (less than 2000 leukocytes per cubic millimeter with only 10 to 20 per cent granulocytes; less than 50,000 platelets per cubic millimeter). Patients may tolerate these low counts remarkably well for months or years, but mucous membrane ulcerations, frequent infections, and bleeding may be incapacitating.

3. Splenic pancytopenia (rare).

The marrow progenitors of the blood cells are usually increased in numbers, because production of cells is most often greater than normal even though the total response is less than would be expected of a normally functioning marrow. A valuable aid to diagnosis can be obtained for the hypersplenic hemolytic anemias by tagging a sample of the patient's erythrocytes with radioactive chromium, reinjecting the cells, and measuring the radioactivity over the surface of liver and spleen. A large stasis compartment will be manifest by two or three times more radioactivity over the spleen than over the liver one hour after the injection; increased splenic destruction is indicated when the radioactivity increases more over the spleen than over the liver during the subsequent four or five days. The hypersplenism may be corrected in some instances, when appropriate, by x-ray therapy to the enlarged spleen or by administration of corticosteroids (see discussion of chronic lymphocytic leukemia and the lymphomas). If these therapeutic approaches are inappropriate or ineffective, splenectomy will often at least reduce transfusion requirements or cause enough rise in leukocyte and platelet levels to relieve the manifestations of bleeding and infection; at times, the response is dramatic. Failure of splenic extirpation to relieve cytopenia, particularly neutropenia, however, is by no means unusual; there is no adequate way to predict which patients will respond.

One must be alert to the possibility that a left upper quadrant mass may not be spleen. For this purpose and to define splenic size, scanning over the spleen after injection of colloidal preparations of appropriate radioactive isotopes which are taken up by RE cells has proved most valuable.

CHRONIC CONGESTIVE SPLENOMEGALY

Chronic congestive splenomegaly (Banti's syndrome) is characterized by portal hypertension, splenomegaly, episodes of hemorrhage from the gastrointestinal tract, leukopenia, anemia, and moderate thrombocytopenia.

Pathogenesis. Direct measurement of portal pressure at the time of laparotomy has established the existence of portal hypertension (225 to 500 or more mm. of water). The cause is apparent in most but not all instances and may be intra- or extrahepatic. Cirrhosis of the liver and schistosomiasis are the common causes of intrahepatic obstruction; the liver is usually enlarged. Extrahepatic obstruction is often not associated with hepatomegaly and results from thrombosis or cavernous transformation of the portal vein, compression from pancreatic fibrosis or tumor, or compression from an aneurysm of the splenic artery. Thrombosis of the portal vein may occur subsequent to abdominal injury, umbilical venous catheterization, portal pyelophlebitis (particularly in infants and children), disorders associated with increased coagulability, pancreatic tumor, or during pregnancy; in about half of the cases, no etiologic factor is discovered. Cavernous transformation is probably a consequence of thrombosis. Gastrointestinal hemorrhage occurs principally from rupture of gastric or esophageal varices. The leukopenia, thrombocytopenia, and anemia may be related to splenic sequestration and destruction of cells, and to postulated but unproved splenic inhibition of bone marrow function. Any underlying disease responsible for the portal hypertension, i.e., cirrhosis of the liver or carcinoma, and chronic hemorrhage also contribute to the pathogenesis of the anemia.

Pathology. The spleen is enlarged, sometimes massively, has a thickened capsule often with adhesions to surrounding structures, distended veins in the splenic pedicle, and a rich supply of venous collaterals extending from its surface. Microscopic changes are principally distention of the sinuses, fibrosis, areas of hemorrhage, and siderotic nodules. The bone marrow is normally cellular to hyperplastic. Myeloid or erythroid hyperplasia may predominate, and moderate immaturity may occasionally be seen. Esophageal and gastric varices are prominent.

Clinical Manifestations. Any disease causing the portal hypertension may be responsible for most signs and symptoms exhibited by the patient. Manifestations related to the portal hypertension and chronic congestive splenomegaly include epistaxis, hematemesis and melena, episodes of abdominal pain thought to be caused by intermittent thrombosis of radicles of the portal vein, vague indigestion and flatulence, awareness of a left upper quadrant mass, and weakness from the anemia. The spleen may become so large that it extends below the pelvic brim and to the right of the umbilicus; it is usually very firm. Splenomegaly may be detected long before any other symptoms appear, but at times hemorrhage from the upper gastrointestinal tract occurs without previous warning. It may be so severe as to produce shock. Purpura and lymph node enlargement are not common.

When thrombosis of the portal or splenic vein occurs suddenly, as after injury to the upper abdomen, left upper quadrant pain may be very severe, the spleen rapidly becomes enlarged, and fever may be present.

Diagnosis. The recognition of chronic congestive splenomegaly requires the demonstration of an enlarged firm spleen and changes produced by portal hypertension. Gastric or esophageal varices can usually be seen by careful roentgenographic examination with barium, but endoscopic study may be required. Leukopenia of moderate degree affecting all types of white blood cells is frequent. The anemia is usually moderate (3 to 4 million cells per cubic millimeter) unless hemorrhage has occurred, in which case it is hypochromic in type. Because of the expanded plasma volume frequently found in patients with gross splenomegaly, the hematocrit may be reduced more than the total circulating red cell mass. Erythrocytes may be slightly macrocytic if liver disease is severe. The platelet count may be somewhat reduced, but severe thrombocytopenia is rare.

Medical evaluation should include a study of hepatic function and often biopsy of the liver. If these studies fail to provide a diagnosis and there is reason to suspect extrahepatic portal vein thrombosis, then splenoportal venography should be considered. That procedure should be done by specially trained personnel; in some centers it is performed only immediately prior to or at the time of laparotomy. Other diseases commonly associated wih splenomegaly, leukopenia, and anemia should be excluded. For this purpose, biopsy of any enlarged lymph nodes and examination of aspirated bone marrow are required.

Prognosis. The course depends largely on the underlying disease process. With uncomplicated portal vein thrombosis or cavernous transformation, manifestations may be largely relieved if a satisfactory shunt can be accomplished and the spleen removed.

Treatment. Some patients will tolerate chronic congestive splenomegaly without much difficulty. But if varices bleed or the hematologic manifestations of dyssplenism are severe enough to cause symptomatic anemia, increased susceptibility to infection, or thrombocytopenic bleeding, then splenectomy should be done. Removal of a large spleen with a blood supply that may be 10 to 20 per cent of cardiac output may cause a significant

decrease in portal pressure. Whether a portacaval or a splenorenal shunt should be performed at the same time is a difficult decision. The shunt often leads to metabolic changes similar to those of hepatic encephalopathy, but failure to reduce portal pressure sufficiently may result in continued hemorrhage. The best candidates for the procedure are patients with extrahepatic block of the portal vein or with cirrhosis who have reasonably good hepatic function and minimal or absent ascites and jaundice.

Iron deficiency that may have developed from chronic bleeding should be treated.

DeGruchy, C.: Diagnosis and treatment of Felty's syndrome. Geriatrics, 20:219, 1965.

Loeb, V., Jr., Moore, C. V., and Dubach, R.: The physiologic evaluation and management of chronic bone marrow failure. Amer. J. Med., 15:499, 1953.

McIntyre, P. A., and Wagner, H. N., Jr.: Newer tracer technics in hematology. *In* Brown, E. B., and Moore, C. V. (eds.): Progress in Hematology. Vol. 6, New York, Grune and Stratton, Inc., 1969, p. 305.

Motulsky, A. G., Casserd, F., Giblett, E. R., Broun, G. O., Jr., and Finch, C. A.: Anemia and the spleen. New Eng. J. Med., 259:1164, 1215, 1958.

Thompson, E. N., and Sherlock, S.: The aetiology of portal vein thrombosis with particular reference to the role of infection and exchange transfusion. Quart. J. Med., N. S., 132:465, 1964.

Turner, M. D., Sherlock, S., and Steiner, R. E.: Splenic venography and intrasplenic pressure measurement in the clinical investigation of the portal venous system. Amer. J. Med., 23:846, 1957.

Weed, R. I., and Weiss, L.: The relationship of red cell fragmentation occurring within the spleen to cell destruction. Trans. Ass. Amer. Physicians, 79:426, 1966.

MISCELLANEOUS ABNORMALITIES OF THE SPLEEN

Great need has existed for a method of visualizing the spleen so that large abscesses, infarcts, cysts, and tumors of the spleen can be detected. The development of isotopic techniques for radioscanning of the spleen, therefore, constitutes a significant diagnostic advance. Current methods include (1) damage and tag erythrocytes with mercurihydroxypropane (^{197}Hg-MHP), and (2) injection of colloids prepared with ^{99m}technetium or ^{113m}indium; the isotopes are taken up by the spleen so that its size and configuration can be outlined by surface scanning.

Infections. The spleen frequently enlarges during the course of many systemic bacterial and viral infections; there is hyperplasia of the lymphocytic and reticuloendothelial cellular elements, but the spleen does not necessarily harbor the infectious agent. On the other hand, direct infection is frequent with chronic infectious granulomatous lesions (tuberculosis, histoplasmosis, brucellosis) and with certain parasitic infections, particularly malaria and kala-azar. Under these circumstances, the spleen may become very large, and hematologic changes of dyssplenism may develop.

In many tropical areas, particularly where malaria is endemic, a *tropical splenomegaly syndrome* is recognized: chronic splenomegaly, elevated levels of macroglobulin, and normal transformation of lymphocytes under stimulation by phytohemagglutinin. A moderate lymphocytosis is frequent, and hepatic sinusoidal lymphocytosis may be found. The etiology is unknown; malaria and repeated antigenic stimulation by tropical infectious agents have been suspected. Patients apparently repond favorably to the administration of the antimalarial drug proguanil for six months or more.

Splenic abscesses are uncommon, are frequently multiple, and are usually secondary to pyemia with some other focus as the point of origin. They may result from some nearby bacterial infection in the upper abdomen, e.g., perforated peptic ulcer, or from septic thrombi of arterial or venous origin, or they may develop when a splenic hematoma becomes infected. Organisms responsible for the abscesses include staphylococci, pneumococci, salmonellae, and coliform bacilli. When small, they may run their course without being recognized, but if the infection fails to respond to antimicrobial therapy, one or more of the abscesses may enlarge, causing left upper quadrant pain, septic type of fever, chills, elevation of the left leaf of the diaphragm with splinting, a palpable mass, and leukocytosis. The omentum may attach itself to the surface of the spleen, thereby increasing the size of the left upper quadrant mass. An abscess may become so large that very little splenic tissue remains. It may rupture into the peritoneal cavity, causing generalized peritonitis, or beneath the diaphragm to form a left subphrenic abscess. In the latter case, empyema of the left chest may develop. Another complication of splenic abscesses is the discharge of infected venous thrombi into the portal circulation with resultant formation of liver abscesses. Treatment consists of broad-spectrum antimicrobial coverage, splenectomy, or surgical drainage of the abscessed cavity if adhesions make removal of the spleen impossible.

Splenic infarcts occur principally in hematologic disorders: in sickle cell anemia in children; in patients with sickle cell-hemoglobin C disease and sickle cell trait, particularly under conditions of relative anoxia as in airplane flights; in large spleens associated with polycythemia vera, leukemia, or malignant lymphomas; and in spleens with extensive extramedullary hematopoiesis, i.e., myelofibrosis. They cause sharp, intense pain over the area of infarction, often with radiation of pain to the left shoulder and splinting of the diaphragm and abdominal muscles. A friction rub may occasionally be detected. At autopsy one often finds in a greatly enlarged spleen more areas of splenic infarction than can be accounted for from carefully kept clinical records; some, therefore, must give few symptoms. The amount of pain is probably related to the extent of peritoneal irritation and perisplenitis produced by the infarction. The author has never seen a splenic infarct rupture, but that complication has been described. Conservative therapy with bed rest and sedation is usually all that is required; rarely, splenectomy may be necessary.

Splenic cysts may be classified as true, false, and parasitic; all forms are rare. Only about 200 cases of the two nonparasitic types have been reported. The true cysts, formed from embryonal defects or rests, are lined with flattened cuboidal or squamous epithelium; they include dermoids and mesenchymal inclusion cysts. False cysts are more common than the true, are usually single, are often associated with a history of trauma to the left upper abdomen, and tend to develop slowly but may attain a large size. It is thought that most of them originate in areas of intrasplenic hemorrhage. Their wall is composed of dense fibrous tissue, often with a lining of flattened squamous epithelium. The remainder of the splenic tissue may be normal or atrophic. Symptoms are minimal unless the cysts are large. There may then be a sense of heaviness or a dragging kind of pain. Pressure on the gastrointestinal tract may lead to epigastric discomfort when a large meal is eaten, and may sometimes cause either diarrhea or constipation. The left leaf of the diaphragm is elevated, and the lower left rib cage tends to flare outward. The left upper quadrant mass may have a doughy consistency, but often is difficult to identify as a cyst. Unless foci of calcification can be seen in the cyst wall, roentgenograms of the abdomen may contribute little to the differential diagnosis other than to show displacement of abdominal organs. Scans are much more valuable. Surgical removal constitutes the only treatment.

In those areas of the world where the disease is endemic, echinococcus cysts may be found in the spleen, but more rarely than in the liver. The wall is usually calcified and the blood shows varying degrees of eosinophilia.

Tumors of the Spleen. In order of decreasing frequency, tumors of the spleen may arise from (1) lymphoid elements (lymphosarcoma, reticulum cell sarcoma); (2) vascular or sinus endothelium (hemangioma, lymphangioma, endothelial sarcoma)—moderately rare; (3) capsular and trabecular framework (fibrosarcoma, leiomyosarcoma, myoma)—rare; or (4) embryonic inclusions—very rare. Primary lymphoma and reticulum cell sarcoma are being recognized with increasing frequency. Preoperative diagnosis of any splenic tumor is difficult but has been greatly facilitated by scanning procedures. Nodularity of the spleen can occasionally be detected by palpation. Frequent symptoms include left upper quadrant pain, anorexia, ulcer-like symptoms, and an impressive weight loss. Acute hemorrhagic shock occasionally results from rupture of a subcapsular cavernous hemangioma into the peritoneal cavity. Spread by local invasion of surrounding tissue has often occurred by the time splenectomy is attempted.

The spleen is an unusual site for metastatic carcinoma, but it may be involved either by direct extension, particularly from the stomach, or by hematogenous spread of any widely disseminated tumor. Metastatic lesions most commonly found are from carcinomas of the stomach, lung, pancreas, and breast and from malignant melanoma.

Rupture of the Spleen. Trauma to the upper abdomen, particularly crushing blows of the type suffered in automobile accidents, may cause the normal spleen to tear. Rupture may also occur spontaneously or during even gentle abdominal palpation of a spleen enlarged because of infectious mononucleosis, sepsis (acute splenic tumor), an abscess or, very rarely, leukemia (at the site of an infarct). There may be sharp pain in the upper abdomen at the onset, but signs of intra-abdominal hemorrhage with shock, tenderness, and muscle guard quickly predominate. The condition constitutes an acute surgical emergency. The clinician must be alert to the possibility of delayed rupture when subcapsular hemorrhage develops with the original trauma or tear, only to break through the capsule hours to several days later.

Splenic Artery Aneurysm. Aneurysms of the splenic artery are rare, are found predominantly in women, and occur most frequently after middle age. Congenital defects in the arterial wall, arteriosclerotic changes, trauma, infection, embolic phenomena, and portal hypertension have been considered the principal causative factors. Patients may be asymptomatic, may complain only of vague, crampy left upper abdominal pain, or may have symptoms referable to the stomach, duodenum, or gallbladder. Intermittent gastrointestinal bleeding has been reported in a few cases. The spleen is usually enlarged. Occasionally, the aneurysm is palpable, and a bruit may be heard. The diagnosis may sometimes be made roentgenographically when a calcific ring surrounded by scattered mottled densities is seen in the region of the splenic artery. Rupture may be suspected if there is initial sudden severe pain in the left upper quadrant with mild shock, followed by temporary improvement and then sudden collapse, with manifestations of massive intra-abdominal hemorrhage. In an impressive number of the reported cases, the splenic artery aneurysm has ruptured during pregnancy. If the patient is to be saved after rupture has occurred, massive transfusions must be given, and the spleen and the ruptured aneurysm must be removed promptly.

Splenosis is a term used to describe autotransplants of the spleen throughout the peritoneal cavity when rupture has seeded the cavity with small clumps of splenic cells. The growth of splenic tissue may increase to several centimeters in size; the nodules may number several hundred, and usually are asymptomatic. At times, however, they may cause irritation or pain. In several instances they have led to obstruction of the small intestine. Splenosis can be diagnosed only at the time of operation. The nodules of splenic tissue differ from accessory spleens in that the supporting framework is incomplete, and the blood vessels penetrate the capsule from around its circumference rather than enter through a hilus. It is said that splenosis rarely, if ever, follows rupture of a diseased spleen.

Ahmann, D. L., Kiely, J. M., Harrison, E. G., and Payne, W. S.: Malignant lymphoma of the spleen. Cancer, 19:461, 1966.

Bostick, W. L.: Primary splenic neoplasms. Amer. J. Path., 21:1143, 1945.

Das Gupta, T., Coombes, B., and Brashfield, R. D.: Primary malignant neoplasma of the spleen. Surg. Gynec. Obstet., 120:947, 1965.

Garamella, J. J., and Hay, L. J.: Autotransplantation of spleen: Splenosis. Ann. Surg., 140:107, 1954.

McIntyre, P. A., and Wagner, H. N., Jr.: Newer technics in hematology. *In* Brown, E. B., and Moore, C. V. (eds.): Progress in Hematology. Vol. 6. New York, Grune and Stratton, Inc. 1969, p. 305.

Moyer, C. A., Rhoads, J. E., Allen, J. G., and Harkins, H. N.: Surgery, Principles and Practice. 3rd ed. Philadelphia, J. B. Lippincott Company, 1965, pp. 890-910.

Sagoe, A. S.: Tropical splenomegaly syndrome: Long-term proguanil therapy correlated with spleen size, serum IgM, and lymphocyte transformation. Brit. Med. J., 3:378, 1970.

Sheps, S. G., Spittel, J. A., Jr., Fairbairn, J. F., II, and Edwards, J. E.: Aneurysms of the splenic artery with special reference to bland aneurysms. Mayo Clin. Proc., 33:381, 1958.

Hemorrhagic Disorders

INTRODUCTION

William J. Harrington

The term "hemorrhagic disorder" is applied to any generalized bleeding tendency; the site at which bleeding actually occurs, however, may be greatly influenced by local factors (e.g., menstruation, trauma, ulceration).

Man has many safeguards against abnormal bleeding. Of prime importance is the integrity of his vasculature. Injury normally sets in motion a remarkably integrated series of events leading to cessation of blood loss through all but large-caliber vessels. First, the local flow of blood quickly decreases because of reflex vasoconstriction of arterioles and metarterioles. Platelets promptly aggregate at the site of injury with hydrolysis of some of their rich supply of ATP to ADP. The latter promotes platelet clumping, whereupon the clumps undergo a transformation known as viscous metamorphosis, with local release in high concentration of the following constituents: vasoconstrictor catecholamines and serotonin, which supplement and sustain the initial vasoconstriction; glucocorticoids; procoagulants (discussed later) that accelerate clot formation; and a contractile protein, thrombosthenin, resembling actomyosin that retracts the fibrin mass into a firm hemostatic plug. Platelets thereby have a "homing instinct" and as "guided missiles" deposit their concentrate of hemostatic factors at points of need.

Inhibition of excessive coagulation by anticoagulants and ultimate dissolution of the clot by fibrinolytic enzymes as repair proceeds complete the cycle.

The adequacy of hemostasis is also influenced by the quality of perivascular support. Bleeding into solid structures is generally self-limited, as compression from extravasated blood impairs further loss. But because loose subcutaneous and submucosal tissues afford poor support, mucocutaneous signs of bleeding are common in all hemorrhagic disorders.

The rate of evolution and regression of ecchymoses and petechiae is modified by tissue macrophages that remove pigments from the breakdown of extravasated erythrocytes.

Any of the components in this elaborate design for hemostasis may singly or in combination be faulty. Because of the complementary character of many reactions, inadequacies may not be symptomatic; conversely, a demonstrated deficiency should not be faithfully accepted as sufficient cause for a given bleeding tendency.

As indicated in Table 1, hemorrhagic disorders may be primary or symptomatic of a variety of underlying diseases; they may be congenital, familial, or acquired; they may be acute or chronic. In all, intermittency of symptoms is common.

In the clinical work-up, particular attention should be given to the character of the bleeding. Lesions are generally most prominent on the lower extremities (increased hypostatic pressure). Petechiae indicate platelet or blood vessel defects; ecchymoses and hematomas may be caused by coagulation defects as well as platelet or blood vessel abnormalities; hemarthroses are most common in severe coagulation defects, especially the hemophilias. The cutaneous lesions are generally asymptomatic save for their cosmetic effects, but if they are characterized by premonitory or late-appearing paresthesias or discomfort, vasculitis and autoerythrocyte sensitization should be considered. Certain common challenges, e.g. menses, tooth extractions, tonsillectomy or other surgical procedures, merit special inquiry, because they are generally more provocative and provide a more reliable over-all assessment of the presence of a hemorrhagic disorder than do laboratory data. Family history and racial background may afford good diagnostic leads. Drug and chemical exposures may be relevant, both in causing some hemorrhagic disorders and in evoking bleeding crises in others. Finally, easy bruising may not be evidence of a definable hemorrhagic disorder, but rather a part of the spectrum of normality or a feature of no serious consequence related to character of skin, age, weight, and other variables.

Laboratory tests should include platelet count

TABLE 1. CAUSES OF PURPURA*

Extravascular Factors
  Congenital and Familial
    1. Ehlers-Danlos syndrome
    2. Pseudoxanthoma elasticum
    3. Hereditary hypoplasia of the mesenchyme
  Acquired
    1. Senile purpura
    2. Cachexia
    3. Cushing's syndrome
Vascular Factors
  Congenital and Familial
    1. Vascular pseudohemophilia
    2. Vascular hemophilia
    3. Hereditary hemorrhagic telangiectasia
  Acquired
    1. Trauma; purpura factitia
    2. Mechanical obstruction
    3. Scurvy
    4. Infectious diseases: embolic, toxic, purpura fulminans
    5. Neoplastic diseases
    6. Metabolic diseases: diabetes, uremia, (?) excess circulating histamine
    7. Associated with systemic vascular disease: hypertension, arteriosclerosis, polyarteritis, and hypersensitivity angiitis, other forms of vasculitis, amyloidosis
    8. Immunologic diseases: Schönlein-Henoch purpura, serum sickness, drug sensitivity, associated with autosensitization to erythrocyte stroma
    9. Toxins: venoms
   10. Unknown: devil's pinches, purpura simplex
Intravascular Factors: Platelets
  Thrombocytasthenia
    1. Congenital and Familial
       a. Qualitative: hereditary thrombocytasthenia and thrombocytopathia
    2. Acquired
       a. Thrombocytasthenia in uremia
       b. Cryoglobulinemia
       c. Macroglobulinemia
       d. Hyperglobulinemia
       e. Following infusion of synthetic macromolecules
  Thrombocytopenia
    1. Decreased production of platelets
    2. Increased destruction of platelets
  Thrombocytosis
Intravascular Factors: Blood Coagulation
  Defective synthesis of coagulation factors
  Accelerated utilization of coagulation factors (consumption coagulopathies)
  Circulating anticoagulants
  Accelerated proteolysis
Dermatologic Diseases That Simulate Hemorrhagic Disorders
  Purpura annularis telangiectodes, angioma serpinginosum, Schamberg's progressive pigmentary dermatitis, pigmented purpuric lichenoid dermatitis

*Those causes of special hematologic interest are concerned with platelet and primary vascular defects and abnormalities of blood coagulation.

and examination of a stained blood film for platelet morphology, determination of bleeding time, capillary fragility, coagulation time in glass and nonwettable tubes, clot retraction, and one-stage prothrombin time. Additional studies are required for precise definition of coagulation defects and mixed abnormalities. Methodology varies in different laboratories, depending upon personal preferences and available facilities, but generally includes a partial thromboplastin time, thromboplastin generation test, and assay for fibrinogen and fibrinolysis. It should be re-emphasized that misleading deviations from "normal values" may be found, especially in patients who are seriously ill with an underlying unrelated disease; this is often the case with the more quantitative and elaborate methods. When laboratory and bedside assessments are compared, the latter should receive at least equal weight.

DEFECTS IN HEMOSTATIC MECHANISMS

William J. Harrington

EXTRAVASCULAR HEMOSTATIC DEFECTS

The most common manifestations of extravascular hemostatic defects are easy bruising and spontaneous formation of ecchymoses; less frequently, hematomas and petechiae occur. Conventional assessments of hemostatic function are generally normal.

CONGENITAL AND FAMILIAL FORMS

Ehlers-Danlos syndrome is a rare dysplasia of mesenchyme with cardinal features consisting of hyperelasticity of skin, hyperextensibility of the joints, and formation of pseudotumors following trauma. It is transmitted as a dominant trait. Increased friability of the vessels coupled with excessive torsion accounts for the hemorrhagic manifestations.

Pseudoxanthoma elasticum is a rare familial disorder most often characterized by inheritance of abnormal recessive genes. In addition to cutaneous manifestations, bleeding may occur from any organ. In the skin, firm discrete waxy papules appear, especially in the folds. Surrounding the papules the skin is thickened, and may contain telangiectases. Angioid streaks are common in the retina. The basic lesion is thought to be a degeneration of elastic tissue or collagen.

Hereditary hypoplasia of the mesenchyme includes osteogenesis imperfecta and Marfan's syndrome. Blood vessels and their framework are involved. Bleeding from surgical intervention for hernia is a common complication, and is often the first event leading to diagnosis.

More detailed discussions of these defects are to be found elsewhere in this textbook.

ACQUIRED FORMS

Senile purpura reflects the loss of tissue succulence and elasticity of aging coupled with torpor of tissue macrophages. Violaceous subcutaneous extravasations of blood, slow to resolve, are seen most prominently on the dorsa of the hands and forearms of elderly persons; they are produced by minor trauma. *Cachexia* can result in a similar manifestation. *Cushing's syndrome* commonly is accompanied by easy bruising, most probably owing to the antianabolic effects of glucocorticoids on extravascular tissues. Administration of adrenocorticosteroids may cause purpura even in the absence of other evidences of iatrogenic Cushing's syndrome.

Diagnosis. The diagnosis of disorders of extravascular hemostatic mechanisms can be made only by clinical evaluation; the laboratory serves only to exclude other possibilities.

Treatment. Treatment, in general, is limited to minimizing chances of injury. Only in cachexia and Cushing's syndrome can more definitive measures be taken. Anabolic steroids have been of little value.

Prognosis. The prognosis is most often determined by factors other than the bleeding tendency in all save pseudoxanthoma elasticum, wherein fatal hemorrhage is common.

VASCULAR HEMOSTATIC MECHANISMS

Defects in vascular hemostatic mechanisms are characteristically manifested by either petechiae or ecchymoses and less commonly by hematomas. Prolongation of the bleeding time and a positive test for increased capillary fragility may occur but are not constant.

CONGENITAL AND FAMILIAL FORMS

Vascular pseudohemophilia is a disorder in which the blood vessels are thought to be inherently incapable of response to vasoconstrictor influences. Spontaneous bleeding may occur, but the greatest danger lies in trauma, e.g., tonsillectomy. Variation in the severity of symptoms is very characteristic. External blood loss, particularly uterine, may be a prominent complaint. A positive family history is often obtainable; the disorder appears to be transmitted as a dominant trait. Both sexes are affected. A prolonged bleeding time is the only abnormality found.

Vascular hemophilia (von Willebrand's disease) is a disorder with a dual defect: a deficiency in antihemophilic factor and a vascular abnormality. There is evidence, however, that the vascular lesion may be due also to lack of a specific plasma constituent distinct from antihemophilic factor and needed for response to injury. It is especially common in inhabitants of the Åland Islands. Both sexes are affected; transmission occurs as a dominant trait. The bleeding tendency may improve in middle and older age. The diagnosis should be made in patients with normal platelets but with (1) a prolonged bleeding time, decreased AHG, and an autosomal dominant inheritance; (2) a prolonged bleeding time with normal AHG but correction of the bleeding time with transfusion of normal plasma; or (3) normal bleeding time but decreased AHG, autosomal dominant inheritance, and correction of the decreased AHG by transfusion of hemophilic plasma. This paradoxic response to hemophilic plasma indicates that the regulation of plasma AHG activity is controlled by at least two genes, one of which is on the X chromosome—abnormal in classic hemophilia—and the other on an autosomal chromosome—abnormal in von Willebrand's disease.

Hereditary hemorrhagic telangiectasia (Sutton-Rendu-Osler-Weber syndrome) is transmitted as a simple dominant trait. Pathologically, the basic lesion is a defect in the vessel wall leading to visible dilatation of capillaries and arterioles and in some instances to the development of arteriovenous aneurysms. The typical lesions may assume the appearance of either small violaceous hemangiomas or spiders. Involvement of both skin and mucous membranes with lesions of various sizes is the rule, and, in certain families, there may be in addition visceral telangiectasia or even sizable aneurysms in the lungs, liver, spleen, and other sites. Although telangiectases may be found in childhood, they are found in increasing numbers as age advances. Bleeding is common only in adult life. Epistaxis and gastrointestinal bleeding are the most frequent symptoms. A stereotyped pattern of distribution and type of lesion is common among members of a family. Iron deficiency anemia is a nearly universal complication, although if cavernous hemangiomas appear in the lung secondary polycythemia may develop because of the shunt. All laboratory assessments of hemostasis are unrevealing, and direct visualization of the telangiectases is necessary.

ACQUIRED FORMS

Trauma is the most common cause of acquired purpura. The trauma may be self-inflicted and denied; a very perplexing syndrome can thereby be presented. *Mechanical obstruction* to venous return can cause purpura; tight garters, varicose veins, thrombophlebitis, vena caval obstruction, and paroxysms of coughing are a few examples. The only clearly established dietary deficiency associated with abnormal bleeding on a vascular basis is *scurvy.* Gingival and perifollicular bleeding are characteristic, but in childhood intramuscular and subperiosteal bleeding are also common. *Infectious diseases,* particularly when associated with a high fever, may induce purpura. Several factors are responsible. Fever alone can increase capillary fragility. In some infections minute thrombi with infarcts are seen, for example, as in rickettsial diseases. Furthermore, emboli may contribute to the picture: splinter hemorrhages of bacterial endocarditis. Thrombocytopenia occasionally plays a significant role. Some microorganisms elaborate enzymes that contribute to the friability of vessels. Some infectious agents, such as those of epidemic hemorrhagic fever and

Weil's disease, are extraordinarily damaging to endothelium. *Purpura fulminans* is a term applied to severe and usually fatal acute vasculitis, extensive infarction and tissue necrosis occurring during or immediately following acute infections, e.g., scarlet fever or the Waterhouse-Friderichsen syndrome. Depletion of blood coagulation factors may be superimposed. These most devastating examples of purpura in infection have pathologic features resembling the Shwartzman phenomenon. *Neoplastic disease* may cause vascular lesions with purpura through either tumor embolism or fibrin embolism secondary to aseptic fibrinous vegetations on heart valves, a phenomenon that may accompany any wasting disease. Here also abnormalities in blood coagulation, especially with dysproteinemia, or fibrinolysis may be noted. In some *metabolic disorders* the blood vessels are more fragile than normal. In diabetes, the reasons are unknown. Uremia is commonly accompanied by abnormal bleeding. A capillary defect is postulated, and recent studies have suggested that platelet phospholipids of importance in blood coagulation may be qualitatively or quantitatively abnormal or inefficiently released; guanidinosuccinate accumulated through disordered urea metabolism may handicap platelet function; there may be other coagulation abnormalities. Gastrointestinal bleeding is especially common. Purpura is occasionally noted during menses in girls and women in whom no hemostatic abnormalities can be detected. Purpura has been ascribed, rarely, to an excess of circulating *histamine.* Numerous *systemic vascular disorders* may induce an increase in vascular fragility. With hypertension alone, easy bruising may occasionally be seen. In polyarteritis, hypersensitivity angiitis, and other forms of vasculitis, purpura is sufficiently common to be of diagnostic value. In amyloidosis, particularly of the "primary" type, easy bruising is a feature. Infiltration of vessel walls is the chief etiologic factor, but impaired liver function may compound the tendency to bleed. *Anaphylactoid or Schönlein-Henoch purpura* is an acute or chronic generalized angiitis with predilection for cutaneous, joint, gastrointestinal, and renal involvement. Present evidence suggests that an immunologic reaction involves the host's endothelium. It is seen especially often in children or young adults, and usually occurs two to three weeks after a streptococcal infection. Other etiologic factors have also been implicated (see Table 2). The characteristic triad consists of purpura, abdominal and joint pains, and nephritis. Angioneurotic edema also may be noted. The skin lesions are generally macular or ecchymotic, varying in size and often confluent. A localized pinprick sensation often heralds the appearance of each lesion. Ultimate recovery is the rule, but deaths have been reported during the acute stage, and unremitting cases may occasionally evolve into a clinical picture indistinguishable from chronic glomerulonephritis or polyarteritis nodosa. A few instances have been described, in women only, of tender ecchymoses

TABLE 2. CAUSES OF ANAPHYLACTOID PURPURA*

Bacteria:	Especially streptococci; also tuberculosis and bacterial vaccines
Drugs:	Antimicrobial drugs (penicillin, streptomycin, sulfonamides, viomycin); antihistaminics; analgesics and antipyretics (aminopyrine, salicylates, phenacetin, acetophenetidin, phenylbutazone; sedatives (barbiturates, chloral hydrate, meprobamate, trifluoperazine, carbromal); antiepileptics (hydantoin, phenyl-ethyl-hydantoin); heavy metals (gold, bismuth, arsenic, mercury); agents employed in cardiovascular diseases (digitalis, quinidine, mercurials, thiosulfates, ephedrine, trichlormethiazide, merbaphen); agents employed in endocrine diseases (estrogens, iodides, insulin, thiouracil, carbutamide, tolbutamide); miscellaneous (quinine, thalidomide, menthol, cinchophen, dinitrophenol, ipecac, belladonna, atropine, copaiba)
Chemicals:	Coal tar derivatives?
Foods:	Wheat, eggs, chocolate, milk, beans, tomatoes, potatoes, onions, strawberries, blackberries, plums, nuts, pork, chicken, fish, crab
Physical agents:	Cold
Other causes:	Insect bites, serum sickness

*The table is merely a guide, since any agent to which history of exposure is elicited must be considered potentially responsible.

with surrounding erythema and edema; *autoerythrocyte sensitization* has been suspected, because either trauma or subcutaneous injections into the patient of a small volume of her own red blood cells or their stroma has reproduced the lesions. Once fully developed, the syndrome is chronic and debilitating. The suggestion has been made that this entity belongs in the realm of psychosomatic disease. Certain *toxins* regularly induce bleeding from vascular injury. Some snake and scorpion venoms contain endotheliotoxins; constituents more damaging to the patient, e.g., neurotoxins, are generally present also. *Purpura of unknown cause* includes "devil's pinches" and purpura simplex. Both are mild and of cosmetic significance only. They are especially common in obese, middle-aged women and consist of circumscribed ecchymotic patches most prominent on the trunk and lower extremities. The two syndromes are probably related, if not identical. A family history of similar manifestations may be elicited. These labels are too often applied in lieu of accurate diagnosis.

Diagnosis. In the hemorrhagic syndromes owing to vascular defects, laboratory diagnostic measures are, for the most part, inadequate. Concentrations of vitamin C should be assayed in scurvy. Vascular hemophilia can be well defined in the laboratory because of the deficiency of antihemophilic factor coupled with a prolonged bleeding time.

Treatment. Vascular hemophilia is managed much as is deficiency of antihemophilic factor. Data are too preliminary to evaluate the postulated value of the component in plasma said to correct the bleeding time specifically, but perhaps noteworthy is the claim that anti-Willebrand factor is increased in the plasmas of insulin-treated diabetic subjects. Vitamin C is useful only in scurvy. In every other syndrome no therapy directed primarily at the hemostatic defect is known. Hemorrhagic telangiectasia usually requires continual use of iron, often given parenterally, to compensate for blood loss. Epistaxes are best managed by instructing the patient in the use of a catheter with a small balloon tied on its end. This is coated with petrolatum, inserted into the nostril and inflated. Repeated cauterization or packing ultimately leads to atrophy, scarring, and more serious bleeding. Management of severe anaphylactoid purpura is similar to that of acute glomerulonephritis, but should be coupled with a search for allergens. Steroids have been of little value. In autoerythrocyte sensitization, trauma, including that of repeated testing, should be avoided.

DEFECTIVE INTRAVASCULAR HEMOSTATIC MECHANISMS INVOLVING PLATELETS

William J. Harrington

Platelet deficiencies may be either quantitative or qualitative. Their most typical clinical signs are petechiae and ecchymoses; menometrorrhagia and gastrointestinal bleeding are common, and occasionally are the only manifestations. Visceral bleeding is most ominous; intracranial hemorrhage is the usual cause of death. Characteristic laboratory abnormalities consist of prolonged bleeding time, positive test for increased capillary fragility, impaired clot retraction, and impaired prothrombin conversion. The clotting time is generally normal.

Single or multiple qualitative defects may occur; thrombocytasthenia is a term employed to designate these disorders. Thrombocytopathia (*q.v.*) is considered to be a special variety of congenital thrombocytasthenia. Anisocytosis and poikilocytosis of platelets occur following acute blood loss from any cause, in extramedullary hematopoiesis, and in diseases featured by accelerated platelet production, without apparent abnormalities in hemostasis; here the terms thrombocytopathia and thrombocytasthenia are not applicable.

THROMBOCYTASTHENIA

CONGENITAL AND FAMILIAL FORMS

Thrombocytasthenia is often difficult to distinguish from vascular pseudohemophilia. Defective clot retraction is a feature of one form known as Glanzmann's disease. Transmission appears to be as a dominant character. Adenosine triphosphate (ATP) is required for clot retraction, and defective glycolysis with impaired ATP generation has been demonstrated in these patients. Clumping of platelets in response to ADP may be impaired, and the concentration of platelet-bound fibrinogen may be low. *Thrombocytopathia* is a rare disorder wherein the platelets are almost the size of erythrocytes and have a more diffuse and fine granulation than normal. Megakaryocytes have similar atypical granulation. Although intermittent thrombocytopenia is characteristic, the bleeding manifestations occur without relationship to platelet levels because of the basic associated qualitative defects in these cells.

ACQUIRED FORMS

Acquired thrombocytasthenia has been found in uremia, in dysproteinemias, and following infusion of synthetic macromolecules, e.g., dextrans of the larger molecular species. In the last two instances adherence of the abnormal globulin or macromolecule to the platelet impairs its function. Of more common clinical importance is the handicap imposed on platelet function (release reaction) by aspirin. This handicap is especially significant in patients who have thrombocytopenia.

Diagnosis. Platelets are numerically adequate, but one or more of their functions are impaired; poor clot retraction, decreased prothrombin conversion, and a prolonged bleeding time with or without morphologic alterations are found.

Treatment. Therapy of thrombocytasthenias is unsatisfactory. Platelet transfusions in the hereditary syndromes soon lose their usefulness because of isoimmunization to these cells. In the acquired disorders, the abnormality in the patient's platelets would be expected to be conferred on the donor's platelets following transfusion. Glucocorticoids are also of little value. Aspirin should be avoided in patients with bleeding disorders, especially those related to platelet inadequacies.

THROMBOCYTOPENIA

Thrombocytopenia is the most common cause of hemorrhagic diatheses. The etiologic agents are listed in Table 3. The symptoms and laboratory findings are as given for thrombocytasthenia, but are generally of greater degree. Petechiae and ecchymoses, most prominent on the lower extremities, are generally present, but only menorrhagia or gastrointesinal bleeding may be observed. Subungual bleeding and blood loss into serosal cavities, including joints are very rare. In differential diagnosis the bone marrow should always be evaluated, even when the mechanism seems clear, e.g., in leukemia.

TABLE 3. CAUSES OF THROMBOCYTOPENIA*

Decreased Production of Platelets
1. Replacement of bone marrow: leukemia, carcinoma, sarcoma, lymphoma, granuloma, lipoidosis, sclerosis, fibrosis
2. Aplasia: due to known causes: chemicals, drugs, radiation, oncolytic agents; idiopathic
3. Deficiency diseases: megaloblastic anemias, scurvy
4. Some instances of idiopathic thrombocytopenia
5. Splenomegaly from any cause
6. Uremia?
7. Viremia, bacteremia?
8. Congenital defects: aplasia, lack of megakaryocyte-ripening factor, Hegglin's anomaly

Increased Destruction of Platelets
1. Splenomegaly
2. Stagnation of blood flow: extensive hemangioma, congestive heart failure, hypothermia
3. Massive blood loss with replacement by bank blood
4. Incompatible transfusion reactions
5. Accelerated intravascular coagulation: obstetric accidents, amniotic fluid embolism, premature separation of the placenta, eclampsia?, other consumption coagulopathies
6. Viremia, bacteremia
7. Onyalai?
8. Uremia?
9. Aldrich's syndrome
10. Thrombotic thrombocytopenia
11. Autoantibodies for platelets: most instances of idiopathic thrombocytopenia; neonatal thrombocytopenia, sensitization to certain drugs (Table 4), associated with certain diseases: lupus erythematosus, some instances of chronic leukemia, some carcinomas, infectious mononucleosis?, convalescent phase of acute exanthemas?, postpartum state

*Note that idiopathic thrombocytopenia is considered in some instances to be caused by deficient production and in other instances to accelerated destruction of circulating platelets.

DECREASED PRODUCTION OF PLATELETS

Most instances within this category require little comment. Included are all causes of *marrow replacement* and *aplasia*. In *megaloblastic anemias* and occasionally in *scurvy*, platelet production is impaired. *Splenomegaly* with thrombocytopenia may be due in part to inhibition of activity of megakaryocytes despite adequacy in their numbers. (Also involved, however, is an enlarged pool size, since one third of the circulating platelet mass may normally be temporarily sequestered in the spleen.) *Uremia* is at times featured by a low platelet count, with or without marrow hypoplasia. Thrombocytopenia during *acute infections* may be due in part to impaired thrombocytopoiesis. Rare instances of *congenital aplasia* and of *lack of a circulating megakaryocyte-ripening factor* have been described. Another constitutional disorder is *Hegglin's anomaly,* characterized by faulty maturation of platelets and granulocytes, with basophilic inclusions in the latter.

INCREASED DESTRUCTION OF PLATELETS

The normal life span of platelets (eight to ten days) is frequently shortened in patients with *splenomegaly,* presumably because of excessive sequestration of these cells. Closely related are other causes featured by stagnation of blood flow: extensive *hemangiomas* in infancy, severe *congestive heart failure*, and *hypothermia*. Platelets rapidly lose their viability on storage; *rapid replacement of massive blood loss* with large volumes of bank blood causes thrombocytopenia, owing in part to replacement of the recipient's viable platelets with nonviable ones. Exchange transfusion in infancy is an additional example. *Transfusion reactions* from incompatible blood induce thrombocytopenia, but the degree of thrombocytopenia is seldom sufficient to induce bleeding. *Accelerated intravascular coagulation* may be associated with profound thrombocytopenia ("consumption coagulopathies"). *Viremia and bacteremia* have been demonstrated to be capable of inducing acute depletion of circulating platelet numbers. Platelets adhere to one another and to the endothelium when micro-organisms or other particles are introduced into the blood stream. At times, the degree of thrombocytopenia must be held at least partially responsible for any hemorrhagic manifestations that may be present. *Onyalai* is a form of acute thrombocytopenia of unknown etiology observed in Africa and characterized by the presence of hemorrhagic bullae on the mucous membranes. Although its pathogenesis is unknown, the clinical picture suggests that increased destruction of platelets is taking place. The disorder is most common in young adult Bantu men and generally begins with a one- to three-day prodromal period of malaise, headache, and fever. Although an infectious etiology has been suspected, no causative organism has been demonstrated. *Uremia* is commonly associated with thrombocytopenia, in part probably because of accelerated thrombocytolysis. In eczema of baby boys, increased susceptibility to infection and thrombocytopenia may coexist (*Aldrich's syndrome*), a disorder transmitted as a sex-linked recessive characteristic. (This is also described in the article on agammaglobulinemia.)

Thrombotic thrombocytopenic purpura (TTP) is a microangiopathic disorder featured by hemolytic anemia, thrombocytopenia, bizarre neurologic abnormalities, renal dysfunction, and fever. Although described in all groups, its greatest frequency is in patients between 10 and 40 years of age, with nearly a 2:1 predominance in women. Although sometimes chronic, its most common course is acute, leading to death within a few weeks. The characteristic histologic abnormality is deposition of hyaline, acidophilic, PAS-positive material subendothelially and within the lumina of arterioles and capillaries. Endothelial proliferation is common, but inflammatory cell infiltrates are notably lacking. The hyaline deposits contain fibrin-like material, gamma globulin, platelet aggregates, and occasional erythrocytes. Although all tissues can be involved, the characteristic lesions occur with greatest frequency in heart, brain, kidneys, pancreas, and adrenals. The etiology of TTP is unknown. It is occasionally associated with lupus erythematosus. Recent

reports describe isolation of both viruses and Bartonella-like bacteria from the blood in TTP. Clinical features vary greatly. In its fully expressed form, there are usually purpura, slight jaundice, pallor, fever, fluctuations in consciousness with paresthesias, focal neurologic signs, and abdominal pain. Less common are renal failure and cardiac arrhythmias. The liver and spleen are seldom enlarged. Laboratory findings consist of anemia, reticulocytosis, thrombocytopenia (platelet counts most commonly range between 10,000 and 50,000 per cubic millimeter, and granulocytic leukocytosis. The bone marrow is hypercellular with respect to all elements. There is hyperbilirubinemia, a negative Coombs test and markedly shortened red cell and platelet life spans. The most notable hematologic feature, diagnostically, is the presence of "helmet" and other fragmented red blood cells—a finding required for the diagnosis, although mimicked in other hemolytic syndromes caused by red cell trauma. Proteinuria and microscopic or gross hematuria are seen in almost all instances. Slight to moderate elevations of blood urea nitrogen occur in more than half the patients. A probable variant is the "hemolytic uremic syndrome" of infancy, wherein renal failure is a cardinal feature. LE cells are demonstratable in approximately one fourth of the patients. A positive STS occurs in about 10 per cent of cases. Coagulation studies reveal little deviation from normal save for the thrombocytopenia, in contrast to findings in consumption coagulopathies. Diagnosis is based on demonstration of the characteristic microthrombi. Lymph node biopsy or paraffin section of marrow aspirations is diagnostic in 50 per cent or more of patients. Skin and muscle biopsies are positive in only 25 per cent of patients with TTP.

Certain drugs, chemicals, or foods may induce thrombocytopenia by depressing platelet production, by direct injury to platelets, or by immunologic mechanisms (Table 4). It has long been known that in a few persons acute "platelet crises" may occur on readministration of certain agents to which they have had previous uneventful exposure. The platelet count may fall from normal levels to nearly zero in one to three hours, indicating fulminant thrombocytolysis. Recent evidence has clearly established the immunologic nature of the clinical sequence. It has been demonstrated that the susceptible person has developed an antigen-antibody reaction that involves his own platelets and certain exogenous (and possibly endogenous) substances. If the responsible agent, usually a drug, is not present, the platelets are unaffected, but only a minute amount of agent, e.g., 0.5 mg. of drug given to a susceptible patient, can precipitate acute thrombocytopenia. In the bone marrow, megakaryocytes reflect the impact by a relative decrease in mature forms showing platelet formation. Because all three reactants are required (the platelet, the drug, and the antibody in the plasma) and because the body rapidly disposes of most drugs, recovery occurs within a few days unless contact with the responsible agent

TABLE 4. EXOGENOUS AGENTS CONSIDERED TO BE RESPONSIBLE FOR CERTAIN INSTANCES OF THROMBOCYTOPENIA

1. Decreased platelet production:
   Ethanol, estrogens, thiazides
2. Direct injury to circulating platelets:
   Ristocetin
3. Immunologic injury:

Agents	Definite*	Possible†
Sedatives	Carbamides, barbiturates, methylparafynol, 2-methyl-1-phenyl-3-butyne-1,2-diol	Paramethadione, thalidomide, hydantoins, trimethadione, meprobamate, desipramine, prochlorperazine
Analgesics		Phenylbutazone, procaine, acetaminophen
Antipyretics	Pyrazolon derivatives: amino-pyrine, phenyl-dimethyl-isopropyl-pyrazolon, phenyl-dimethyl-pyrazolon	Salicylates
Antimicrobials	Sulfonamides, arsenobenzols, para-amino-salicylic acid, stibophen, novobiocin, quinine, chloroquine	Streptomycin, isoniazid, penicillin, oxytetracycline, cephalothin
Antihistaminics	Chlorprophenpyridamine, 2-(N-phenyl-N-benzyl-aminomethyl)-imidazoline, diphenhydramine hydrochloride	
Agents employed in cardiovascular diseases	Digitoxin, quinidine, acetazolamide	Chlorothiazide, hydrochloro-thiazide, diazoxide, tetra-ethylammonium chloride, mercurials
Agents used in endocrinologic disorders	Chlorpropamide	Thioureas, insulin, estrogens, carbutamide tolbutamide
Heavy metals		Gold, silver, bismuth, copper
Food	Beans	Milk, potatoes, wheat, corn, eggs, citrus fruits, anchovies
Insecticides	Dichlorodiphenyltrichloroethane	2,2-Dichlorovinyl dimethyl phosphate
Miscellaneous	Chrysarobin, methyldopa	Tetraethylthiuram disulfide, toluene diisocyanate, viscum album, iodides, iopanoic acid, pertussis vaccine, tetanus toxoid, turpentine, organic hair dyes, leg stocking dye, mistletoe berries, insect bites, ergot, petroleum hydrocarbons

*Well established by clinical and/or serologic studies.
†Evidence incomplete, but sufficient to warrant suspicion of etiologic relationship.

continues. A rebound thrombocytosis characteristically follows the interval of platelet depletion. If there is no further exposure from the patient's plasma over a period of several months. It returns again within a few days if re-exposure takes place. This clinical sequence is to be distinguished from bone marrow aplasia resulting from marrow toxins.

IDIOPATHIC THROMBOCYTOPENIA

Idiopathic thrombocytopenia is most common in childhood and in premenopausal women, but may be seen in any age group. Except for symptoms and signs referable to blood loss or focal complications of bleeding, the patient seems to be well; the spleen is rarely palpable. Hematologic values of the peripheral blood are unremarkable except for thrombocytopenia and, if blood loss has occurred, anemia. Rarely an idiopathic autoimmune hemolytic anemia coexists, precedes, or follows the onset of the thrombocytopenia. Marrow aspiration reveals an abundance of megakaryocytes with a preponderance of immature forms.

In infancy and childhood an upper respiratory infection frequently antedates the onset of thrombocytopenia. It is probably not appropriate to classify these instances as "idiopathic" but rather to include them in the thrombocytopenias that follow recognizable infections, e.g., *rubella, varicella, mumps;* the child is convalescent or fully recovered from the acute viral infection when purpura abruptly appears. In some children, however, and in nearly all adults no inciting infection is apparent. Duration of disease also differs in the two age groups; in children the syndrome tends to be short-lived, whereas in adults it is nearly always chronic, relapsing, or recurrent.

In most cases, idiopathic thrombocytopenia appears to be an autoimmune disorder. The antibody appears to be directed against the platelet itself in that it does not seem to require added antigen as in the drug-induced syndromes. The spleen apparently plays a role by removing platelets modified by antibody. Since the antibody can traverse the placenta, if a pregnant woman has idiopathic thrombocytopenia with antiplatelet antibodies she will give birth to a thrombocytopenic infant, even if her purpura is in remission following splenectomy. On the other hand, if she does not have a circulating antiplatelet antibody, she will give birth to a normal infant, even though she herself may be purpuric. Finally, a mother may become isoimmunized to fetal platelets in a manner analogous to isoimmunization to erythrocytes in hemolytic disease of the newborn; the mother appears to be clinically normal but has an isoantibody for platelets, and thereby gives birth to a thrombocytopenic infant.

Idiopathic thrombocytopenia may be mimicked by many syndromes wherein platelet survival time is shortened, the marrow appears normal with adequate numbers of megakaryocytes, the spleen is not enlarged, and atypical clinical features are not readily appreciated. Warning has been given of the similarity of *drug-induced autoimmune thrombocytopenia*. Caution should be observed when a *viral infection* precedes the onset of purpura by one to two weeks. Some patients with idiopathic *cryoglobulinemia* present with "idiopathic thrombocytopenia." Occult *lymphomas* and *other malignant processes* may present with a syndrome indistinguishable from idiopathic thrombocytopenia; so also may *granulomatous diseases* without typical signs. Infrequently *systemic lupus erythematosus* may present with thrombocytopenia in advance of any other evidences of this disease. Occasionally thrombocytopenia develops one to two months post partum, and tends to last a few weeks or months only to recur after subsequent pregnancies.

Diagnosis. The most common sources of error are given in the preceding paragraph. A low platelet count, absence of other discernible cause, and a bone marrow with abundant megakaryocytes and no evidence of other dyscrasia are most critical. It is advisable to perform an LE test. Prolongation of the bleeding time, positive capillary fragility test, and impaired prothrombin conversion and clot retraction are of limited value when contrasted with accuracy in enumerating platelets.

Treatment. In addition to restriction of activity and protection from trauma, three measures are used in treatment of thrombocytopenia.

Glucocorticoid therapy may decrease the clinical severity of thrombocytopenic bleeding irrespective of etiology or effect on the platelet count. Prednisone, 0.5 mg. per kilogram per day, in divided doses, is probably adequate for this effect. In severe bleeding the dose should be increased two- to threefold if no contraindications exist. The larger amounts should also be given routinely as initial therapy in idiopathic thrombocytopenia.

Splenectomy is reserved for patients with readily demonstrable megakaryocytes in the bone marrow. It is undertaken most often in instances of splenomegaly not responsive to therapy for the underlying disease and when steroids are contraindicated or have proved ineffective in idiopathic thrombocytopenia and occasional instances of lupus erythematosus. In children the idiopathic disorder is usually self-limited, and surgery is deferred if possible for at least six months. Ultimately, most adults require splenectomy; most children do not. Therefore in adults surgical intervention is warranted earlier if the disease is poorly responsive to steroids or requires maintenance therapy of more than 15 mg. of prednisone

daily, and in severe fulminant thrombocytopenia it is justified without preliminary trial of glucocorticoids.

Platelet transfusions, although of no value in idiopathic thrombocytopenia, are useful in most other forms. Fresh whole blood is given, preferably collected into plastic equipment. Current studies suggest that an enriched ACD may be superior to other anticoagulants. Maintenance of the platelet count above 20,000 per cubic millimeter generally suffices except in instances of leukemia or infection; under ideal conditions a platelet transfusion given every three to four days should be adequate. However, platelets contain antigens, and isoimmunization usually develops over a period of weeks, making this measure subsequently useless. Therefore, platelet transfusions should be given only if the clinical status is alarming; in some patients, very low platelet counts may be tolerated with little or no purpura. Though many attempts have been made to develop a "platelet substitute," no clinically effective product is now known. The management of TTP, although still unsatisfactory, has improved with use of combined measures: large doses of glucocorticoids (up to 1000 mg. of prednisone daily), heparin, dextran, and splenectomy. Fibrinolytic agents, although promising, have had too limited use to be evaluated.

Prognosis. Approximately three fourths of patients with idiopathic thrombocytopenia have a prompt response to splenectomy, and in three fourths of these the remission lasts more than ten years. The initial remission rate is no better with glucocorticoids, is slower in onset, complications are more numerous, and in most patients relapse occurs after cessation of the treatment. In other forms of thrombocytopenia the prognosis generally depends on the cause. In drug-induced syndromes that mimic the idiopathic disorder, recovery is the rule within one week if exposure is stopped; platelet transfusions and steroids are both used. Most postviral thrombocytopenias last only a few days or weeks, although a few persist for months; steroids are employed. In lupus erythematosus, splenectomy can be undertaken if necessary, and lasting hematologic remission almost always follows. In thrombocytopenia with idiopathic cryoglobulinemia, splenectomy is more effective than steroid therapy. Splenectomy is contraindicated in Aldrich's syndrome because death from infection is a nearly uniform consequence; this is the only thrombocytopenia wherein splenectomy is known to be harmful. Remission rates in TTP may now exceed 50 per cent with combined therapy.

THROMBOCYTOSIS

Whenever the direct platelet count is above 1,000,000 per cubic millimeter, a bleeding tendency may occur; it is especially likely when levels twice this or greater are present. These very high platelet levels may occur in polycythemia vera, chronic myelocytic leukemia, myelofibrosis with myeloid metaplasia, after splenectomy for a variety of indications, and rarely in a syndrome (often the premonitor of leukemia or polycythemia) known as essential thrombocythemia. Thrombocytosis of similar degree is found, less commonly, in chronic granulomatous or malignant diseases. Mucocutaneous signs are most common Gastrointestinal bleeding may be massive. Thrombotic manifestations may coexist. Although various quantitative changes have been described in the platelets in thrombocytosis, these cells are effective in replacement therapy of thrombocytopenia. The excessive concentration of platelets probably interferes with the genesis of thromboplastin.

Accurate enumeration of platelets is necessary for diagnosis of this entity. The only problem presented is the determination of which primary disease the patient has. A note of caution is warranted. Since platelets disintegrate when blood clots, they release their soluble contents into the serum. Two spurious laboratory results may result: an increase in potassium and an increase in acid phosphatase. Both can be excluded by testing plasma instead of serum samples.

Radioactive phosphorus, as used in myelocytic leukemia and polycythemia vera, is often effective in treatment. Among the alkylating agents, busulfan is sometimes useful.

Harrington, W. J.: Purpura. Disease-a-Month, Chicago, Year Book Publishers, Inc., July, 1957.
Henry Ford Hospital International Symposium: Blood Platelets. Boston, Little, Brown and Company, 1960.
Hill, J. B., and Cooper, W. M.; Thrombotic thrombocytopenic purpura. Treatment with corticosteroids and splenectomy. Arch. Intern. Med. (Chicago), 122:353, 1968.
Hougie, C.: Fundamentals of Blood Coagulation in Clinical Medicine. New York, Blakiston-McGraw-Hill, Inc., 1963.
Marcus, A., and Zucker, M.: The Physiology of Blood Platelets. New York, Grune & Stratton, Inc., 1965.
Mettler, N. E.: Isolation of a microtatobiote from patients with hemolytic-uremia syndrome and thrombotic-thrombocytopenic purpura and from mites in the United States. New Eng. J. Med. 281:1023, 1969.
Ratnoff, O. D.: Bleeding Syndromes. Springfield, Illinois, Charles C Thomas, 1960.
Shulman, N. R., Marder, V. G., Hiller, M. C., and Collier, E.: Platelet and leukocyte isoantigens and their antibodies: Serologic, physiologic, and clinical studies. In Moore, C. V., and Brown, E. B. (eds.): Progress in Hematology. New York, Grune & Stratton, Inc., 1964, Vol. IV, p. 222.
Stefanini, M., and Dameshek, W.: The Hemorrhagic Disorders. 2nd ed. New York, Grune & Stratton, Inc., 1962.
Tocantins, L., and Kazal, L. A.: Blood Coagulation, Hemorrhage and Thrombosis. New York, Grune & Stratton, Inc., 1964.
Weiss, H. J.: Von Willebrand's disease – Diagnostic criteria. Blood, 32:668, 1968.

COAGULATION DEFECTS

INTRODUCTION
Oscar D. Ratnoff

A hemorrhagic disorder often appears when blood coagulation is impaired. Defective hemostasis may be caused by (1) inadequate production of one or more of the procoagulant substances of

blood, (2) depletion of components required for clotting as a result of increased utilization, (3) the presence in blood of inhibitors of coagulation, or (4) activation of proteolytic mechanisms of plasma. Blood normally contains a relative abundance of each clotting factor, and hemorrhage is rarely the result of deficiency of one of these substances unless its concentration has been reduced to less than 50 per cent of the normal value. Abnormal bleeding may result from lack of each of the known clotting factors, with two exceptions. Hageman factor (factor XII), a protein concerned with the initiation of blood clotting upon contact with foreign surfaces, is apparently not required for normal hemostasis. Depletion of calcium is not a cause of abnormal bleeding because the cardiovascular and neuromuscular effects of profound hypocalcemia are incompatible with life. Deficiency of a single clotting factor is usually the result of an inherited disorder. Acquired coagulation defects are more likely to involve multiple components of the clotting system. In some clinical situations several mechanisms operate to impair hemostasis, and the extent to which each contributes may be difficult to analyze.

A knowledge of the physiology of blood clotting is essential in interpreting the results of laboratory tests useful in the diagnosis of hemostatic defects. Blood clots when fibrinogen (factor I) is converted to insoluble strands of fibrin through the action of a proteolytic enzyme, thrombin (Fig. 1). The formation of fibrin is accelerated by calcium ions at physiologic concentrations, and probably by a heat-labile accelerator in normal plasma. Under physiologic conditions, the molecules of fibrin are chemically bonded to each other by a second enzyme, fibrin stabilizing factor (factor XIII), a transamidase which provides mechanical strength to the fibrin strands. Thrombin does not exist in detectable amounts in normal blood. When blood is shed, thrombin evolves through one or both of two sequences of chemical reactions, the extrinsic and intrinsic pathways. Presumably,

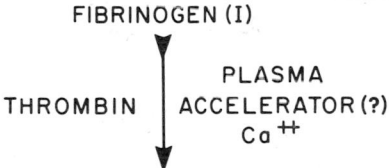

FIBRINOGEN (I)

THROMBIN | PLASMA ACCELERATOR (?) Ca⁺⁺

FIBRIN MONOMER + FIBRINOPEPTIDES (SOLUBLE)

THROMBIN + FIBRIN STABILIZING FACTOR (XIII) | Ca⁺⁺

FIBRIN POLYMER (INSOLUBLE)

FIGURE 1. Steps in the formation of fibrin. In this and the succeeding figures, Roman numerals are used to designate clotting factors as recommended by the International Committee for Haemostasis and Thrombosis.

similar mechanisms operate to induce clotting in vivo. Thrombin formation via the extrinsic pathway is initiated by components of tissue known as tissue thromboplastin which interact with several plasma agents, factor VII, Stuart factor (factor X), proaccelerin (factor V), and calcium ions, to bring about the formation of a prothrombin-converting principle (Fig. 2). Blood also clots without the participation of tissue thromboplastin upon contact with certain negatively charged surfaces such as glass; in vivo, collagen and sebum may serve this function. This intrinsic pathway requires the successive participation of Hageman

factor (factor XII), plasma thromboplastin antecedent (PTA, factor XI), Christmas factor (PTC, factor IX), antihemophilic factor (factor VIII), Stuart factor, and proaccelerin (Fig. 3). Some or all of these factors are "activated" during the clotting process. A prothrombin-converting principle, probably identical with that developed through the extrinsic pathway, evolves when calcium ions and phospholipids are available, the latter supplied by platelets and the plasma itself. Once the prothrombin-converting principle has formed, it liberates thrombin from its precursor, prothrombin (factor II), by an enzymatic process. Besides clotting fibrinogen, thrombin promotes clotting in several ways, liberating phospholipid from platelets, activating fibrin-stabilizing factor from an inert precursor, and altering antihemophilic factor and proaccelerin so as to heighten their activity. Plasma contains potent inhibitors of the clotting process, of which those inhibiting thrombin, tissue thromboplastin, and the activated forms of Hageman factor, PTA and Stuart factors are most clearly defined. It also contains the precursor of plasmin, a powerful proteolytic enzyme which can digest fibrinogen, fibrin and other clotting factors as well as certain other substrates. The sole or principal site of synthesis of several clotting factors—namely, fibrinogen, prothrombin, factor VII, proaccelerin, Stuart factor, and Christmas factor—is the hepatic parenchymal cell; the locus of synthesis of other factors is not certain.

The laboratory procedures used to differentiate disorders of blood clotting are based upon these physiologic considerations. Thus, defects in the

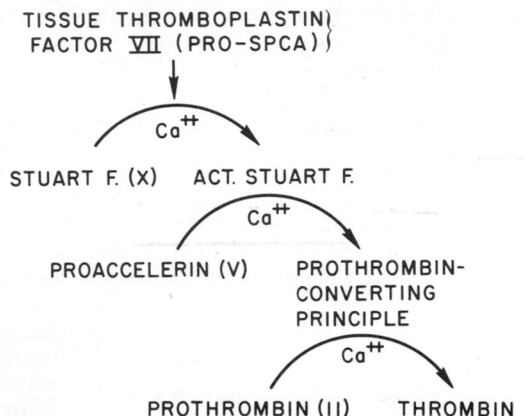

FIGURE 2. The extrinsic pathway for the formation of thrombin. Omitted from the diagram are inhibitors of the various steps and the alteration induced by thrombin in proaccelerin. The phospholipid portion of tissue thromboplastin may function in the formation and action of the prothrombin-converting principle.

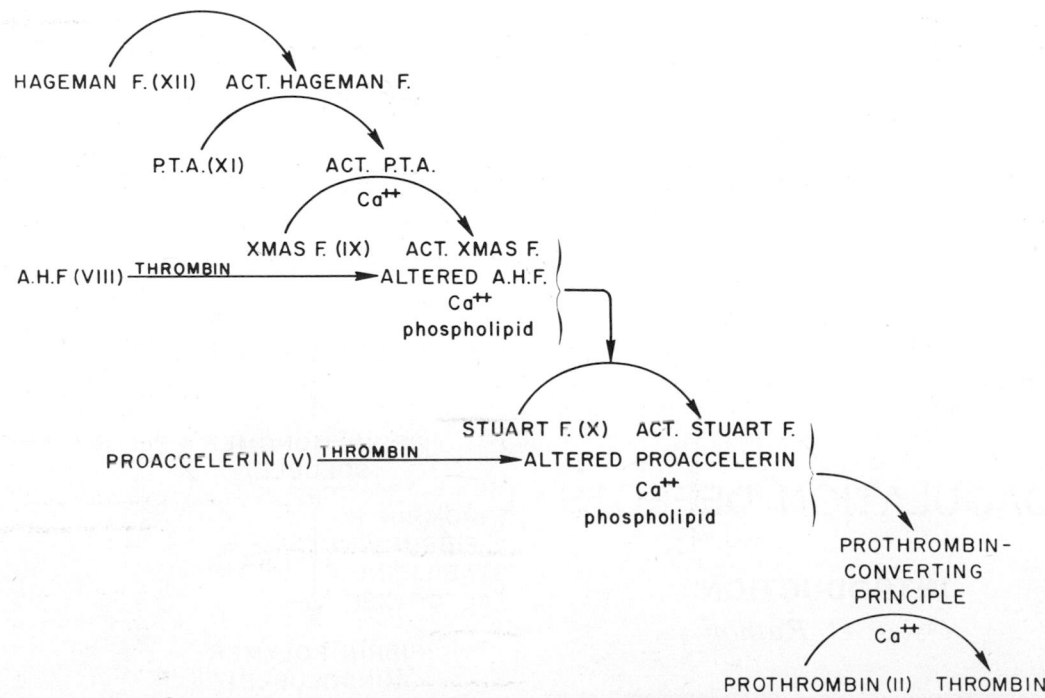

FIGURE 3. The intrinsic pathway of thrombin formation (PTA = plasma thromboplastin antecedent; AHF = antihemophilic factor). Omitted from the diagram are inhibitors of the various steps. The phospholipid is furnished by platelets and by the plasma itself.

extrinsic pathway of coagulation are readily detected by measuring the one-stage prothrombin time, in which tissue thromboplastin and calcium ions are added to decalcified plasma, and the interval of time elapsing until clotting takes place is measured. Defects in the intrinsic pathway are reflected in the test tube by delayed clotting of whole blood, retarded "thromboplastin generation" (a misnomer for the evolution of the prothrombin-converting principle), deficient conversion of prothrombin to thrombin, i.e., prothrombin consumption, and a prolonged partial thromboplastin time, i.e., the clotting time of recalcified plasma in the presence of phospholipid. The one-stage prothrombin time is normal in persons whose defect is restricted to the early part of the intrinsic pathway, before the participation of Stuart factor, but is prolonged if defects of the later parts of the pathway are present. Defects in the conversion of fibrinogen to fibrin are measured by testing the effect of preformed thrombin upon the clotting time of plasma, i.e., the thrombin time, whereas a deficiency of fibrin-stabilizing factor is detected by noting the solubility of fibrin in 5M urea or 1 per cent monochloroacetic acid, which cannot dissolve fibrin bonded by this factor.

The laboratory procedures available for investigation of defects of coagulation are often crude, nonspecific, and subject to influence by variations in technique. Accordingly, care is required in selection and performance of the tests and in interpretation of results. Assays for each of the known clotting factors are available. Final identification of a specific deficiency requires mixing of the patient's plasma with that of a patient with a known coagulation defect to determine whether correction occurs. Only fibrinogen can be measured in gravimetric terms, by its conversion to fibrin and by determination of the protein content of the clot.

HERITABLE DISORDERS OF BLOOD COAGULATION
Oscar D. Ratnoff

The familial occurrence of a deficiency of each of the organic clotting factors is well established. The cause is either deficient synthesis or the synthesis of functionally defective clotting factors. Transmission of the defect is genetically determined. In most instances, severe functional deficiency of a single clotting factor is encountered in homozygotes in autosomal recessive traits, and in male hemizygotes and female homozygotes in X-linked recessive disorders. In some cases, heterozygous carriers can be shown to have a reduced plasma level of the procoagulant, but, except in von Willebrand's disease, the deficiency is rarely sufficiently severe to impair hemostasis. In one anomaly, dysfibrinogenemia, an autosomal dominant gene appears to be responsible for the synthesis of a protein that may be normal in quantity but abnormal in structure and function. Familial deficiency of more than one clotting factor has been encountered. The genetic basis for multiple hemostatic defects is not understood.

CLASSIC HEMOPHILIA

Classic hemophilia, the best known of the familial disorders of blood coagulation, is the result of functional deficiency of antihemophilic factor (factor VIII). The plasma does not lack antihemophilic factor. Rather, it appears to contain a nonfunctional variant of this clotting factor. The abnormality is attributable to an X-linked recessive gene so that the disorder occurs almost exclusively in males. The sons of a male hemophiliac are unaffected and do not transmit the disease, although all his daughters are carriers. Heterozygous females do not bleed, but half their sons have hemophilia and half their daughters are carriers. Homozygous females, very rarely encountered, have the typical disease. The clinical manifestations of hemophilia vary from family to family, correlating with the intensity of the functional deficiency of antihemophilic factor, but within a family the degree of the bleeding tendency among affected members is about the same. A positive family history is obtained in only about two thirds of cases.

Clinical Manifestations. In severe hemophilia, in which virtually no antihemophilic factor is detectable in plasma, serious or lethal hemorrhage may occur in the neonatal period after circumcision, but bleeding from the umbilicus is unusual. In infancy, the bleeding tendency is frequently manifested by the appearance of cutaneous echymoses or hematomas in soft tissues, often after injuries so trivial as to be unnoted. Bleeding from the mouth, in particular from the frenulum of the upper lip, is sometimes encountered in young children. After the early years of life, hemorrhages into the joints are characteristic. Increasing deformity, limitation of motion, and destruction of joints result from repeated hemarthroses, commonly the most disabling manifestation of the disease. The ankles, knees, and elbows are particularly likely to be involved, whereas the hands are usually spared. Bleeding is limited by the tension of the joint capsule, and ceases when the synovial space becomes distended. Hemorrhages into soft tissues are not similarly restricted, and may extend widely, dissecting through subcutaneous tissue, along fascial planes, or into muscles. Even enormous hematomas are usually reabsorbed, but sometimes they persist, leaving firm masses that calcify. Pseudotumors can produce symptoms by pressure on other structures, or may erode bone and simulate neoplasms. Hemorrhages into the muscles sometimes cause contractures and deformities such as a claw hand. Bleeding into the lax tissues beneath the tongue, in the pharynx, or in the neck is particularly dangerous because it may interfere with swallowing or may occlude the respiratory passage. Retroperitoneal hemorrhage may produce symptoms simulating those of appendicitis, or may give rise to other manifestations such as obstructive jaundice owing to occlusion of the common bile duct or fulminant hypertension from compression of the kidneys. Hemorrhage into the mesentery can cause abdominal pain, digestive symptoms, or even avascular necrosis of the bowel. Episodes of hematuria, often accompanied by ureteral colic, are common and tend to persist for weeks if untreated. Hemorrhage into the gastrointestinal tract may occur. Excessive bleeding is the rule after dental extraction or minor surgery, and tonsillectomy or major operative procedures may lead to fatal hemorrhage. Subdural hematomas and other hemorrhages into the central nervous system, although uncommon, are an important cause of disability or death, and may result from relatively trivial injury. Hematomas encroaching on nerve trunks may cause sensory loss or paralysis.

Only about half of hemophiliacs present this grim picture. Such individuals have little or no functional antihemophilic factor in their plasma. In others, in whom the concentration of this factor may be as high as 30 per cent of normal, the symptoms are proportionately milder, and bleeding may occur only after such challenges as injury, operative procedures, or dental extractions.

Diagnosis. Specific diagnosis can be established only by laboratory tests of blood coagulation, although the character of the bleeding and the family history provide important clues. Tests that detect abnormalities in the intrinsic pathway of coagulation usually give abnormal results, but the clotting time of whole blood may be normal in mildly affected patients. The prothrombin time, thrombin time, and bleeding time are normal. Proof of diagnosis requires the use of appropriate tests to demonstrate the deficiency of antihemophilic factor, preferably including an assay using the plasma of a known hemophiliac. A normal bleeding time helps to differentiate mild cases from von Willebrand's disease; a careful analysis of the pattern of inheritance and tests of other relatives may be necessary. All patients deficient in antihemophilic factor must be tested for the presence of circulating anticoagulants directed against this substance.

Treatment. Patients with hereditary hemorrhagic disease often have difficulty adjusting to the problems inherent in a disorder that poses unexpected threats to normal behavior and to life itself. As soon as the diagnosis is made, the patient or his parents should be instructed concerning the care, prognostic implications, and hereditary nature of his disorder. The parents should be encouraged to rear their afflicted children in as normal a way as is consistent with safety, for emotional crippling is as devastating as that resulting from hemorrhage. While the patient is too young to guard himself, the parents should design his environment so that it is as danger-free as possible, in order to lessen the need to restrain his behavior. As he grows older, the patient should be advised to indulge in such sports as swimming, running, tennis, and golf, and to avoid those involving body contact or predisposing to injury. The hemophiliac should prepare for a vocation which is not inherently dangerous; he and his parents should be reminded that hemophilia does not preclude a useful life in business or the professions. The object of therapy is to allow the patient to become a self-supporting adult, capable of caring for himself and living as full a life as possible.

The mainstay of therapy for episodes of bleeding is the transfusion of normal plasma or fractions of plasma rich in antihemophilic factor to correct temporarily the patient's specific defect. The use of whole blood is restricted to the maintenance of blood volume after severe blood loss. Enough plasma or its fractions must be administered to raise the patient's blood level of antihemophilic factor sufficiently to permit normal hemostasis. Once transfused, antihemophilic factor disappears rapidly from the circulation, only about half remaining after 10 to 12 hours, so that repeated transfusions must be given until bleeding has been controlled. Therapy with plasma or its fractions carries with it risks of transmitting infectious hepatitis, and of inducing the formation of circulating anticoagulants that specifically inhibit antihemophilic factor.

In the event of major injury or in preparations for surgical procedures, the plasma level of antihemophilic factor must be raised to at least 30 or 40 per cent that of a normal individual; lesser amounts may be adequate to control bleeding into joints or minor soft tissue hemorrhage. When only fresh or fresh-frozen plasma was available as a source of antihemophilic factor, adequate plasma levels of this substance were difficult to achieve without danger of circulatory overload except by exchange transfusion. Fortunately, during the last few years concentrates of antihemophilic factor that can be administered in a small volume have become generally available. One preparation in wide use is cryoprecipitated antihemophilic factor, separated during the cold thawing of fresh-frozen plasma. Plasma levels sufficient for adequate hemostasis can be achieved with the administration of the cryoprecipitate of 1 unit of plasma for each 4 kg. of body weight, sustaining the plasma level of antihemophilic factor by administering half this amount every 12 hours. Another useful preparation is lyophilized antihemophilic factor, separated from plasma by the addition of glycine or other protein precipitants. Such material can be used under conditions in which cryoprecipitated antihemophilic factor is not available. No rule of thumb can be provided as to how long therapy should be continued. In general, after surgery, dental extraction, or severe bleeding, concentrated antihemophilic factor is administered in the manner described for at least two days after all signs of bleeding have ceased, and the dose is then gradually decreased over the succeeding three or four days. Shorter courses of therapy are used when the danger of renewed bleeding is less threatening, as in most instances of hemarthrosis.

The availability of concentrates of antihemophilic factor has made it possible to abort hemorrhage more readily than was formerly possible without circulatory embarrassment. It has reduced the risk of surgical procedures and dental extractions in hemophiliacs. Indeed, in many patients, elective surgical procedures may be carried out, although surgery should be performed only in hospitals equipped to deal with this special problem.

This optimistic picture must be tempered by the fact that in as many as 10 per cent of hemophiliacs a circulating anticoagulant appears in plasma that specifically inactivates antihemophilic factor. The presence of this agent, which is probably an antibody directed against antihemophilic factor, vitiates the beneficial results of transfusion. Patients in whom this complication is present should under no conditions be subjected to surgery.

If the bleeding site is accessible, hemostasis may be most effectively achieved by local measures. By appropriate use of local hemostatic agents such as bovine thrombin and the application of cold and gentle pressure, bleeding may often be controlled. These measures must be sustained, for recurrent bleeding is likely over a period of days. Dental extractions in particular require meticulous local measures. Extractions should be carried out only in the hospital and by dental surgeons with special training in the care of hemophiliacs. Except in patients with mild hemophilia, hemostasis should be enhanced by the transfusion of concentrates of antihemophilic factor.

The transfusion of concentrated antihemophilic factor is also useful in aborting bleeding into joints. Acutely swollen joints should be immobilized. Local chilling and application of elastic bandages may be beneficial, but the application of a constricting bandage is contraindicated. Aspiration of the joint is occasionally advantageous, and should be performed only after adequate transfusion therapy. Active motion without weight-bearing is essential after bleeding has stopped in order to prevent persistent limitation of motion. Careful use of physiotherapy, traction, and splints may be helpful in preventing and correcting deformities. Surgical correction of certain deformities has been successfully accomplished, but should be attempted only by experts and under the supervision of someone skilled in the transfusion therapy of hemophiliacs.

Other forms of bleeding require special types of care. Particularly hazardous is bleeding into the soft tissues of the neck, in which tracheostomy, performed under the cover of transfusion therapy, may be needed. Hemophiliacs should not be given intramuscular injections, but venipunctures are not hazardous if performed with care. Immunization against tetanus is important, because bleeders are particularly prone to infection with this organism, but this is wisely delayed in severe hemophiliacs until the first course of replacement therapy. Immunization may be carried out without such preparation in mildly affected patients. Regular prophylactic care of the teeth should be provided. Bleeders should avoid the use of salicylates, because these are thought to impair hemostasis.

Prognosis. The outlook for the hemophiliac has been greatly improved by modern methods of treatment. Those with moderately severe or mild hemophilia may seem so little affected that they live virtually normal lives, but even these patients may have exsanguinating hemorrhage after dental extraction, injury, or surgery. Those in whom the defect is more pronounced may require frequent admission to the hospital, and may be crippled by joint deformities. Some meet the challenge and are reasonably productive individuals, although others seem foredoomed to chronic invalidism. The life expectancy of hemophiliacs has lengthened with the availability of transfusion therapy, but death as the result of the complications of hemorrhage still occurs with disturbing frequency.

OTHER HERITABLE DISORDERS OF BLOOD COAGULATION

Von Willebrand's disease (vascular hemophilia) is a hemorrhagic disorder characterized by a long bleeding time and deficiency of antihemophilic factor (factor VIII). The disease is transmitted by a dominant autosomal mutant gene, but has been detected more often in women than in men. The severity of symptoms varies considerably among affected members of the same family, some of whom may be asymptomatic. Menorrhagia and postpartum bleeding are common. The patient may experience epistaxes and gingival bleeding in severe cases; cutaneous ecchymoses or hematomas may occur. Hemorrhage follows injury or surgical procedures. Hemarthroses are relatively uncommon, but visceral bleeding or severe and even lethal hemorrhage into the gastrointestinal tract have been observed. Occasionally, petechiae may be found.

A unique feature of von Willebrand's disease is the prolonged bleeding time, an abnormality not usually associated with other hemophilia-like diseases. The coagulation defect can be corrected in vitro by normal but not by hemophilic plasma. In contrast, transfusion of hemophilic as well as of normal plasma or serum is followed by a delayed but pronounced and protracted rise in the patient's plasma level of antihemophilic factor. A single unit of normal plasma may lead to the elevation of the antihemophilic activity of the patient's plasma to normal levels for many hours. These interesting observations are unexplained, although they suggest that the synthesis of antihemophilic factor takes place in at least two steps, the first of which is defective in von Willebrand's disease and the second in classic hemophilia. Whether the abnormality in the bleeding time is due to a second plasma defect is disputed; the administration of plasma, but not of purified antihemophilic factor, is reported to shorten the bleeding time. Diagnosis is readily made when a markedly long bleeding time is encountered in a patient with deficiency of antihemophilic factor. Additionally, adhesion of platelets to glass beads is often impaired, although the specificity of this test is doubtful. Sometimes, within a given family, affected individuals may be found in whom the bleeding time may be prolonged without significant deficiency of antihemophilic factor, or vice versa. A careful study of the patient's relatives may help to differentiate mild classic hemophilia from von Willebrand's disease. In cases in which the bleeding time is not significantly prolonged, recognition of the disease is facilitated by demonstration of the effectiveness of transfusion of relatively small amounts of normal plasma in raising the patient's antihemophilic factor titer; but this procedure carries the risk of transmitting homologous serum jaundice. Treatment of bleeding episodes consists of measures for local control of hemostasis and the administration of fresh blood, plasma, or cryoprecipitates of plasma, all of which contain the agent that induces synthesis of antihemophilic factor in von Willebrand's disease. Menorrhagia may be terminated by suppression of menstrual bleeding with hormonal preparations such as norethynodrel.

Christmas disease is attributable to functional deficiency of Christmas factor (factor IX, plasma thromboplastin component), an abnormality transmitted by an X chromosome-linked gene. In most cases, patients seem unable to synthesize Christmas factor, whereas in a minority nonfunctional Christmas factor is demonstrable in plasma. The disorder typically occurs in males, and is less common than hemophilia, from which it is clinically indistinguishable. All the clinical manifestations of hemophilia are encountered in patients with Christmas disease. The disorder varies in severity from family to family, symptomatology roughly paralleling the degree of the deficiency of Christmas factor measured in the laboratory. Heterozygous female carriers may have a partial deficiency of Christmas factor, and some have a mild bleeding tendency. A positive family history is obtained in only about two thirds of cases. Diagnosis is established by laboratory tests that demonstrate a defect in the early steps of the intrinsic pathway of thrombin formation, and by specific assay for Christmas factor, using a substrate plasma from a patient with known Christmas disease. Treatment is basically the same as for hemophilia, but cryoprecipitates of plasma lack Christmas factor. Christmas factor is relatively stable, so that the patient can be treated effectively with blood that has been stored under usual conditions in a blood bank. Large volumes of plasma are required to raise the level of Christmas factor sufficiently to provide normal hemostasis; thereafter smaller amounts will sustain the titer of this substance, because half the transfused Christmas factor is still present in the circulation after 20 or more hours. Concentrates of the vitamin K-dependent clotting factors, including Christmas factor, are now available, and can be used to provide large amounts of the missing factor without dangerous expansion of the circulating blood volume; these fractions may be contaminated with hepatitis virus. In a few cases, the beneficial effects of transfusion are vitiated by the presence in the patient's plasma of a circulating anticoagulant, presumably an antibody directed against Christmas factor.

Plasma thromboplastin antecedent deficiency, a rare familial hemorrhagic disorder encountered in both sexes, is attributable to deficiency of PTA (factor XI). The disorder is inherited in an autosomal recessive manner; in most reported cases, the patients have been Jewish. Bleeding episodes often follow trauma or surgical procedures, but spontaneous bleeding occasionally occurs. Hemorrhage is usually less severe than in hemophilia, and hemarthrosis is rare. Sometimes the disorder is asymptomatic. Laboratory tests demonstrate a defect in the early steps of the intrinsic pathway of clotting, but the specific diagnosis is often difficult to establish even with appropriate tests, and requires careful confirmation, including matching the plasma with that of a patient known to have PTA deficiency. Transfusion of blood or plasma is used in the treatment of bleeding episodes. Since half of the infused PTA is still present in the circulation 60 hours after transfusion, correction of the defect is relatively simple.

Hageman trait is the hereditary deficiency of Hageman factor (factor XII). It occurs in both sexes, and is inherited as an autosomal recessive defect. Hageman trait is usually asymptomatic, although minor bleeding has occasionally been encountered. The diagnosis may be suspected when the clotting time is prolonged and a defect in the early steps of the intrinsic pathway is detected, but it can be established only by comparison with plasma of patients known to have this disorder. No treatment has been needed in reported cases, but in the event of hemorrhage normal plasma should be efficacious.

Parahemophilia, a familial bleeding disorder affecting both sexes, is caused by a deficiency of proaccelerin (factor V). The disease is inherited in an autosomal recessive manner. Spontaneous bleeding may occur at numerous sites, but the joints are rarely involved. Menorrhagia and postoperative bleeding may occur, but in some patients the disease is mild or latent. The clue to diagnosis is provided by a prolonged prothrombin time which is not shortened by plasma deficient in proaccelerin. A presumptive diagnosis can be made by demonstrating that the prothrombin time is shortened by the addition of plasma from which the vitamin K-dependent clotting factors have been removed, but this test does not rule out a deficiency of fibrinogen. During surgical procedures or when abnormal bleeding is sufficiently severe to justify transfusion, fresh blood or plasma should be given in amounts adequate to maintain the plasma level of proaccelerin at about 25 per cent of normal; the amount of proaccelerin infused disappears from the circulation in 12 to 36 hours.

Congenital deficiency of factor VII is transmitted

in an autosomal recessive manner. Homozygous individuals of both sexes display a bleeding tendency of varying severity correlating with the severity of the deficiency. Numerous hemorrhagic manifestations have been encountered, including umbilical bleeding in the neonatal period, epistaxis, ecchymoses, hemarthroses, menorrhagia, and hemorrhages into the gastrointestinal tract and central nervous system. The one-stage prothrombin time is prolonged, an abnormality that is not affected by plasma or serum from patients known to have factor VII deficiency. Factor VII is stable so that stored plasma is of therapeutic value. Large volumes of plasma, infused repeatedly, are required for effective hemostasis because of the rapid disappearance of factor VII from the circulation, half of the amount infused being removed in only one or two hours; concentrates of the vitamin K-dependent clotting factors may also be used. Menorrhagia may be controlled by the administration of oral contraceptive agents.

Stuart factor deficiency, a rare congenital disorder of blood coagulation, is characterized by deficiency of Stuart factor (factor X), and is attributable to an autosomal mutant gene. Only homozygotes have a bleeding tendency, which is similar to that of congenital deficiency of factor VII. The prothrombin time is prolonged and is not shortened by plasma from patients with known Stuart factor deficiency. The clotting time of recalcified plasma is not shortened to a normal degree by the addition of Russell's viper venom, which requires Stuart factor for its procoagulant effect. Treatment is the same as that for factor VII deficiency, but transfusions have a much more prolonged action, half of the Stuart factor remaining in the blood after two or three days, so that transfusions need not be repeated as frequently.

Prothrombin deficiency, an extremely rare autosomal recessive trait, is clinically similar to factor VII and Stuart factor deficiencies. The prothrombin time is prolonged and is not shortened by the addition of normal serum or of plasma from which the vitamin K-dependent clotting factors have been removed. The treatment of bleeding is the same as that for factor VII deficiency; about half of infused prothrombin disappears from the circulation in nine hours.

A rare anomaly has been described in which individuals have unusual *resistance to coumarin-like drugs.* As much as 20 times the usual dose is required to achieve a therapeutic effect. The disorder is inherited in an autosomal dominant manner. The mechanism underlying the defect is unknown.

Congenital deficiency of fibrinogen, a rare disorder occurring in both sexes, is apparently transmitted as an autosomal recessive trait. Clinical manifestations may begin at birth with hemorrhage from the umbilicus. In general, bleeding is hemophilia-like except that permanent joint damage from hemarthroses is uncommon. Some patients have remarkably little bleeding, and even menstrual blood loss may not be excessive, but others have severe hemorrhages that are often fatal in early life. The blood does not clot even after the addition of thrombin, and little or no fibrinogen can be detected in plasma by chemical or immunologic methods. Bleeding episodes can be satisfactorily treated by intravenous administration of fibrinogen, either in the form of Cohn fraction I or of cryoprecipitates of plasma, in amounts sufficient to maintain a plasma fibrinogen level in excess of 100 mg. per 100 ml. Several instances in which therapy has been impeded by the development of antibodies against fibrinogen have been reported.

Congenital dysfibrinogenemia is a recently described group of familial disorders in which fibrinogen is usually present in normal amounts, but is abnormal in structure and coagulability. The abnormality has occurred in both sexes and in consecutive generations, suggesting autosomal dominant inheritance. The anomaly appears to be different in different families, but in almost all cases aggregation of fibrin monomers is impeded. The bleeding tendency is usually mild, although severe bleeding has been reported. In some patients, wounds have dehisced, whereas in others a paradoxic thrombotic tendency has occurred. Clots are small and friable and form slowly upon the addition of thrombin to plasma, but fibrinogen concentration as measured immunologically is usually normal.

Congenital deficiency of fibrin-stabilizing factor (factor XIII) is a rare disorder in which affected individuals have repeated episodes of serious bleeding after injury. Bleeding from the umbilicus is common. Hematomas, hemarthroses, hematuria, and habitual abortion have been described, and intracranial bleeding is a common cause of death. Sometimes, wounds appear to heal slowly, occasionally breaking down repeatedly. The plasma of affected persons contains nonfunctional material antigenically similar to fibrin-stabilizing factor. The mode of inheritance of fibrin-stabilizing factor deficiency is not certain. In some families, the disorder is attributable to autosomal recessive mutant genes, whereas in others the syndrome seems limited to males. Diagnosis is established by demonstrating that clots of the patient's plasma are soluble in 5 molar urea or 1 per cent monochloroacetic acid, in contrast to normal clots which are insoluble. More sophisticated tests of the transamidation function of fibrin-stabilizing factor are under study. Transfusion of normal blood or plasma transiently corrects the hemorrhagic tendency and facilitates the healing of wounds.

Simultaneous congenital deficiency of several clotting factors has been repeatedly described. Only the *coexistent deficiencies of antihemophilic factor and proaccelerin* appear well established. The defect is probably inherited as an autosomal recessive trait. The bleeding tendency is usually mild, but should treatment of hemorrhage be needed, fresh-frozen plasma should be effective.

ACQUIRED DISORDERS OF BLOOD COAGULATION
Oscar D. Ratnoff

VITAMIN K DEFICIENCY

Vitamin K is required for the synthesis of prothrombin, factor VII, Stuart factor, and Christmas factor. If the vitamin is not available in adequate amounts, the plasma levels of these procoagulant substances fall, and a hemorrhagic disorder ensues. The normal diet contains an abundance of vitamin K; deficiency rarely, if ever, can be attributed to inadequate diet alone. The bacteria of the intestinal tract synthesize relatively large amounts of the vitamin, which may contribute to the body's supply of this substance. Prolonged *oral administration of antibacterial agents* has been associated with depletion of vitamin K and a hemorrhagic disorder responsive to treatment with this vitamin. This syndrome is most likely to occur in patients undergoing parenteral feeding to whom no vitamin K is provided.

The infant at birth may be deficient in vitamin K and as a result may have *hemorrhagic disease of the newborn.* Melena is common, but bleeding may occur from numerous sites. In some cases transfusion is required, and hemorrhage may be fatal. The disorder is self-limited within a few days because the minute amounts of vitamin K needed by the infant are provided in milk; cow's milk contains more vitamin K than human milk. The establishment of intestinal flora may contribute to the supply, and the administration of antimicrobial drugs to infants requiring correction of congenital gastrointestinal lesions may precipitate hemorrhagic disease of the newborn. The frequency of this disease can be lessened by administration of small amounts of vitamin K to the mother before delivery or to the infant at birth.

Naturally occurring compounds with vitamin K activity are fat-soluble and are poorly absorbed from the intestine in the absence of bile salts. Bleeding that accompanies *obstructive jaundice* or *biliary fistula* is usually the result of impaired absorption of vitamin K and is promptly responsive to the parenteral injection of the vitamin. Vitamin K should always be given preoperatively in cases of biliary obstruction, for the first evidence of a hemorrhagic disorder often does not appear until the surgical procedure is performed. Deficiency of the vitamin of a degree sufficient to cause bleeding is encountered in *malabsorption syndromes* such as *sprue* or *celiac disease,* and is readily prevented by parenteral administration of vitamin K.

Derivatives of *coumarin* and *indandione* behave as antagonists of vitamin K. These substances, commonly employed in therapy of thromboembolic disease, impair synthesis of prothrombin and the other vitamin K-dependent clotting factors. *Salicylates,* related in chemical structure to coumarin, may produce the same effect when given in large amounts; possibly, *propylthiouracil* may have this action in rare instances. Hemorrhage associated with the administration of vitamin K antagonists is usually a complication of therapy. The possibility that hemorrhage complicating anticoagulant therapy is due to potentiation of vitamin K antagonists by other drugs, for example, phenylbutazone, chlofibrate, or anabolic steroids, must be kept in mind. Some patients with an obscure hemorrhagic disorder have been discovered to have taken coumarin compounds surreptitiously or because these agents were dispensed in error. A characteristic of the coagulation defects produced by vitamin K antagonists is failure to respond rapidly to injection of large amounts of menadione, a synthetic derivative of naphthoquinone, which ordinarily has potent vitamin K activity; in contrast, vitamin K_1 (phytonadione) is promptly effective. Psychiatric treatment of patients suspected of ingesting coumarin compounds surreptitiously is imperative, because this bizarre behavior may be a manifestation of depression, and the patient may seek more effective means of committing suicide.

Bleeding associated with deficiency of prothrombin and related clotting factors is similar to that occurring with other coagulation defects. Cutaneous ecchymoses, epistaxes, hematuria, gastrointestinal bleeding, and postoperative hemorrhage are common, and intracranial hemorrhage may occur. The hemorrhagic disorder may be fatal.

Diagnosis of vitamin K deficiency is established by the demonstration of a significantly prolonged prothrombin time that is shortened within a few hours after administration of vitamin K.

Treatment consists of oral or parenteral administration of a preparation of the vitamin. For most deficiency states, including those associated with biliary obstruction and malabsorption syndromes, water-soluble derivatives of menadione (menadiol sodium diphosphate or menadione sodium bisulfite) are rapidly and completely effective in correcting the abnormalities of coagulation. An injection of 10 mg. of the menadione preparation is adequate, but should be repeated at weekly intervals for patients with a persistent absorption defect. Menadione in moderate amounts can produce serious hemolytic anemia and kernicterus in the newborn, even if given to the mother before delivery. Vitamin K_1 (phytonadione) is preferable, and a single dose of 1 mg., given intramuscularly to the infant at the time of birth, is adequate to prevent hemorrhagic disease of the newborn. To overcome the effects of coumarin derivatives and related drugs, only vitamin K_1 is effective. It is given orally or intramuscularly in doses of 5 to 20 mg. Vitamin K_1 may be administered by slow intravenous injection, but this route should be avoided except in an urgent situation because of the possibility of untoward reactions. Immediate but transient correction of multiple deficiencies of the vitamin K-dependent clotting factors may be provided in life-threatening situations by the transfusion of plasma or of concentrates of these factors.

LIVER DISEASE

Diffuse hepatic disease often produces a hemorrhagic disorder. Ecchymoses and pretibial petechiae are common, and hemorrhage may occur from many sites; bleeding from surgical wounds is frequent. The bleeding tendency may have multiple causes, including vascular abnormalities, thrombocytopenia, and impairment of blood coagulation. Hypoprothrombinemia and deficiencies of the other vitamin K-dependent clotting factors are common; deficiencies of proaccelerin, antihemophilic factor, and PTA may contribute to the hemostatic defect. Rarely, when parenchymal disease is severe, fibrinogen may also be depleted. In cirrhosis of the liver, clots prepared from plasma or its euglobulin fraction dissolve abnormally rapidly, but evidence that this test tube phenomenon correlates with a bleeding tendency is insecure. Although the prothrombin time is usually prolonged in patients with hepatic disease who exhibit a bleeding tendency, the administration of vitamin K usually has little or no corrective effect. Transfusion of fresh blood or fresh-frozen plasma may provide transitory correction of the coagulative defect, but is usually not satisfactory in maintaining hemostasis. The use of currently available concentrates of the vitamin K-dependent clotting factors should be avoided, as fibrinolytic reactions have been described.

ACQUIRED HYPOFIBRINOGENEMIA AND SYNDROMES OF INTRAVASCULAR COAGULATION

Deficiency of fibrinogen of a degree sufficient to cause abnormal bleeding is encountered in a number of different clinical syndromes. It occurs only rarely because of retarded production of fibrinogen and more often as a result of rapid utilization. A bleeding tendency encountered in some patients with *cyanotic congenital heart disease* is attributable in part to the very high hematocrit; the fibrinogen concentration of whole blood is so low that an adequate clot cannot form. Although fibrinogen is synthesized in the liver, *hepatic disease* is seldom the cause of profound deficiency.

Hypofibrinogenemia or afibrinogenemia in many situations is thought to be due to intravascular conversion of fibrinogen to fibrin. In such cases, the depletion of fibrinogen is accompanied by other coagulation defects. Often the platelet count is reduced, and deficiencies of several clotting factors, particularly prothrombin, proaccelerin and antihemophilic factor, may be demonstrable. The factors that are reduced are those known to be depleted during clotting of blood, and intravascular coagulation is thought to be the mechanism by which the abnormalities are produced. Inconstantly, too, excessive plasma fibrinolytic activity may be observed and the plasma may acquire inhibitory properties directed against the clotting process. In rare instances, incoagulability

of the blood with marked thrombocytopenia follows *massive venous thrombosis*. Presumably the fibrinogen, platelets, and other clotting factors are depleted in the formation of thrombi. A similar coagulation defect may be encountered in cases of *purpura fulminans*, a disorder in which acute necrosis of superficial and peripheral parts of the body is associated with thrombosis in small blood vessels in the affected areas. Hypofibrinogenemia has been described in severe cases of *thrombotic thrombocytopenic purpura* in which fibrin is thought to be deposited at an accelerated rate. Afibrinogenemia may occur with *giant cavernous hemangioma*; the vascular tumor is filled with fibrin thrombi.

Hypofibrinogenemia or afibrinogenemia may be encountered in other disorders in which thrombosis may be difficult or impossible to demonstrate. In such cases, procoagulant substances are thought to be introduced into the blood stream sufficiently slowly that massive thrombosis does not occur. The fate of the fibrin that forms intravascularly is not clear. In laboratory animals, material antigenically resembling fibrin is found in reticuloendothelial cells. Perhaps fibrin is removed from the circulating blood by these cells. Alternatively, soluble fibrin monomers or polymers, perhaps complexed with fibrinogen, are cleared from the blood stream before insoluble fibrin strands can form, or fibrin is dissolved by plasmin, and the fibrin degradation products that result are removed by the reticuloendothelial cells. The clearest examples of defibrination by these mechanisms are *amniotic fluid embolism*, in which amniotic fluid and its contaminants enter the maternal blood stream during parturition, *envenomation* by the bite of snakes whose venom contains procoagulant agents, and the administration of several hundred milliliters of *incompatible blood*, an accident most likely to occur in an anesthetized or unresponsive patient. In this last circumstance, the products of lysis of the transfused cells may initiate intravascular coagulation and defibrinate the recipient's blood.

Similar mechanisms have been invoked to explain hypofibrinogenemia in other disorders. For example, hypofibrinogenemia may be encountered in patients with severe *sepsis,* particularly septic *abortion,* and *Waterhouse-Friderichsen syndrome,* in which the procoagulant may be derived from damaged vascular endothelium. Some cases of *premature separation of the placenta* may be complicated by hypofibrinogenemia; although introduction of highly thromboplastic placental tissue into the maternal blood stream has been invoked to explain the hypofibrinogenemia, other mechanisms, such as the formation of a retroplacental clot, may be operative. Hypofibrinogenemia, thrombocytopenia, and other coagulation defects have occurred during use of various types of *extracorporeal circulation*. The apparatus may defibrinate blood if insufficient heparin is employed. *Abnormal bleeding during cardiovascular surgical procedures* may have multiple causes, including the use of too much or too little heparin, as well as the operative procedure itself. Hypofibrinogenemia may accompany *aneurysm* of the aorta, presumably because the exposed subendothelial tissue is clot-promoting. The pathogenesis of hypofibrinogenemia in *prolonged retention of a dead fetus* or *neoplastic disease* is less clear, although in such cases intravascular coagulation by procoagulants introduced into the blood stream has been surmised. *Metastatic carcinoma of the prostate* is the most frequent of the neoplasms that produce hypofibrinogenemia, but it has also been encountered in patients with carcinoma of the stomach, gallbladder, pancreas, lung, and colon, and with leukemia, particularly of the acute promyelocytic type.

Bleeding associated with the defibrinating syndromes is often severe, but the character of the bleeding as well as the prognosis is influenced by the nature of the underlying disease. In women with *premature separation of the placenta* and *amniotic fluid embolism,* major hemorrhage is usually from the uterus, although a generalized bleeding tendency may be evident. The diagnosis of hypofibrinogenemia is suggested by the appearance of the coagulating blood in a test tube. A simple qualitative test is to add 1 ml. of blood to 0.1 ml. of bovine thrombin solution containing 1000 N.I.H. units per milliliter. Unless virtually no fibrinogen is present, the blood quickly clots. The size of the clot can then be estimated by tapping the tube and observing the degree to which the clot retracts. The retracted clot may be so small that it is difficult to find among the extruded red blood cells and serum, leading to the misinterpretation that fibrinolysis has occurred. The existence of hypofibrinogenemia is confirmed by additional tests, including a quantitative measure of fibrinogen concentration. A useful diagnostic adjunct is the demonstration of thrombocytopenia, often found in patients in whom other evidences of intravascular coagulation are present. Primary treatment is that of the basic disease; if the disease can be eradicated or improved, the coagulation defects are rapidly corrected. In patients with premature separation of the placenta or retention of a dead fetus, for example, recovery follows shortly after the uterus is emptied. Severe bleeding associated with carcinoma of the prostate may subside and the coagulation abnormalities may disappear within days of the institution of estrogen therapy. Transfusion of fresh blood is often required. Administration of fibrinogen may be of temporary value, but if the basic pathologic process continues, fibrinogen is rapidly removed from the circulation, and may participate in the formation of disseminated thrombi. In cases in which the primary disease cannot be treated, intravenous injection of heparin may impede intravascular defibrination and raise the levels of depleted clotting factors. This seemingly paradoxic approach to treatment is not likely to be effective unless the disease is self-limited, as in the case of extensive venous thrombosis or purpura fulminans.

Three advances have led to the view that still other pathologic states may induce widespread coagulation, perhaps insufficient in themselves to cause significant hypofibrinogenemia but adequate to bring about ischemic damage. First, material immunologically like fibrin has been demonstrated in the *serum* of individuals who have apparently undergone intravascular coagulation. Presumably, this material is either fibrin that has been degraded by plasmin or is insoluble, incompletely clotted fibrin. Second, the red blood cells of animals which have undergone experimental defibrination have the morphologic characteristics of erythrocytes observed in *microangiopathic hemolytic anemia,* a state seen pre-eminently in *thrombotic thrombocytopenic purpura,* suggesting that in these conditions intravascular coagulation has occurred. Finally, as has been noted, the administration of heparin has been effective in halting the progress of some cases of hypofibrinogenemia. These considerations have led to the view that disorders in which (1) material antigenically resembling fibrin is present in serum, (2) the characteristic cells of microangiopathic hemolytic anemia can be demonstrated, or (3) a therapeutic response follows the administration of heparin are complicated by intravascular coagulation. Such disorders include not only thrombotic thrombocytopenic purpura, but fulminant *eclampsia* with hemolytic anemia and thrombocytopenia, *malignant hypertension, renal cortical necrosis, cirrhosis of the liver, hyaline membrane disease, hemolytic uremic syndrome,* and *shock* as well. Intravascular coagulation may also be important in *rejection of organ grafts.* Evidence for the importance of intravascular coagulation in the pathogenesis of these different syndromes varies in the degree of conviction they carry.

ANTICOAGULANTS

The presence of an anticoagulant in the circulating blood causes a bleeding tendency that may be severe. This occurrence may follow parenteral administration of heparin, a substance that interferes with thromboplastin generation as well as with the conversion of fibrinogen to fibrin. Heparin rapidly disappears from the circulation so that the hemorrhagic disorder subsides within an hour or two after intravenous injection is terminated. Rarely, inadvertent administration of heparin may be responsible for sudden, unexpected bleeding. A number of hemorrhagic disorders have been attributed to the production of heparin in vivo, but there are few if any cases in which this claim is supported by convincing evidence. Antiheparin agents, including protamine sulfate and toluidine blue, effectively counteract the action of heparin when given intravenously in precisely calculated amounts. Bishydroxycoumarin (Dicumarol) and related compounds are often referred to as anticoagulants, but they interfere with the synthesis of clotting factors and do not retard coagulation directly.

Endogenously produced anticoagulants are encountered under several circumstances and may produce a hemophilia-like disease. These circulating anticoagulants appear to be complex proteins with the properties of gamma globulin, and they most often interfere with the early stage of coagulation. One frequently demonstrable in the plasma of patients with hemophilia specifically inactivates antihemophilic factor and is probably an antibody against factor VIII. An anticoagulant of similar nature and specificity sometimes occurs in the plasma of women following pregnancy, producing a hemophilia-like disorder. Hemorrhagic disease attributable to an apparently identical anticoagulant has appeared without obvious cause in persons who were previously healthy or who have a chronic disease. Comparable substances, specifically inactivating other clotting factors, have been encountered in patients with congenital deficiency of the clotting factor in question. A circulating anticoagulant occurring in the plasma of some patients with systemic lupus erythematosus is unusual because it interferes with the conversion of prothrombin to thrombin; less commonly, patients with this disease have circulating anticoagulants against antihemophilic factor.

The presence of an anticoagulant is detected by demonstrating the retarding action of small proportions of the patient's plasma on the coagulation of normal blood or recalcified plasma. Circulating anticoagulants may disappear spontaneously, sometimes after a period of many months or years, but therapy is difficult. Because of the anticoagulant effect of the patient's plasma, transfusions do not correct the clotting defect. When bleeding is life-threatening, exchange transfusion and the injection of massive amounts of the missing factor may be tried. The use of steroids or immunosuppressive agents has been disappointing. Patients with myeloma and with other diseases causing dysproteinemia may display impairment of blood coagulation attributable to the presence of the abnormal protein. However, the bleeding manifestations frequently associated with dysproteinemia are not clearly related to retarded clotting.

Barrow, E. M., and Graham, J. B.: Von Willebrand's disease. Progr. Hemat., 4:203, 1964.

Biggs, R., and Macfarlane, R. G.: Human Blood Coagulation and Its Disorders. 3rd ed. Philadelphia, F. A. Davis Company, 1962.

Biggs, R., and Macfarlane, R. G.: Treatment of Hemophilia and Other Coagulation Disorders. Oxford, Blackwell Scientific Publications, 1966.

Hardistry, R. M., and Ingram, G. I. C.: Bleeding Disorders. Investigation and Management. Philadelphia, F. A. Davis Company, 1965.

Jackson, D. P., Beck, E. A., and Charache, P.: Congenital disorders of fibrinogen. Fed. Proc., 24:816, 1965.

Margolius, A., Jr., Jackson, D. P., and Ratnoff, O. D.: Circulating anticoagulants: A study of 40 cases and a review of the literature. Medicine, 40:145, 1961.

McKay, D. G.: Disseminated Intravascular Coagulation: An Intermediary Mechanism of Disease. New York, Hoeber Medical Division, Harper and Row, Inc., 1965.

Poller, L. (ed.): Recent Advances in Blood Coagulation. London, J. and A. Churchill, Ltd., 1969.

Ratnoff, O. D.: Bleeding Syndromes. Springfield, Ill., Charles C Thomas, 1960.

Ratnoff, O. D. (ed.): Treatment of Hemorrhagic Disorders. New York, Harper and Row, Inc., 1968.

FIBRINOLYSIS AND FIBRINOLYTIC DISORDERS

Sol Sherry

Fibrinolysis in man is controlled and regulated by the activity of a proteolytic enzyme system termed the plasminogen-plasmin system. The naturally occurring precursor is a globulin, plasminogen, which can be converted by activators or kinases (streptokinase, urokinase, staphylokinase) to plasmin, a proteolytic enzyme, active at neutral pH and capable of digesting fibrin into a number of soluble fragments.

Plasminogen, normally present in all body fluids and secretions, has its highest concentration in plasma. Plasminogen activators, however, are concentrated in the body tissues and vascular endothelium; though not well characterized, they appear to be highly specific proteolytic enzymes capable of kinetically activating plasminogen into plasmin. Plasmin is an endopeptidase of relatively undifferentiated specificity. It has the capacity to hydrolyze peptide bonds adjacent to arginine and lysine residues, and extensively digests fibrinogen in a manner and rate similar to its action on fibrin; it rapidly attacks a great many other biologically important proteins, including antihemophilic (factor VIII) and accelerator globulin (factor V); and it hydrolyzes also many protein substrates commonly used in the laboratory, e.g., casein. In many respects plasmin has features similar but not identical to trypsin.

PHYSIOLOGIC FIBRINOLYSIS

For many years, the mechanism by which the organism utilized plasmin, an enzyme of such undifferentiated specificity, to lyse fibrin selectively without simultaneously destroying other susceptible plasma proteins of biologic significance posed problems of considerable importance, particularly because it was known that overactivity of this system in disease states was productive of severe coagulation defects and a sometimes catastrophic hemorrhagic diathesis. Rapid strides were made in understanding how this enzyme system worked in vivo when it was recognized that plasminogen was deposited in significant amounts whenever fibrin was laid down; this led to the development of a hypothesis that appears to account for the facts adequately, namely that, in vivo, plasminogen exists as a "two phase" system, as a soluble phase form in the body fluids, and as a gel phase form in thrombi and fibrinous deposits. The effect of activators on plasminogen in the two phases and the consequences of plasminogen activation in the two sites are dissimilar. In plasma, because of the presence of inhibitors, small to moderate amounts of plasminogen activator produce only minor or slow activation of plasminogen with little evidence of plasma proteolysis, because the plasmin formed is effectively inhibited.

However, in the presence of large amounts of activator, particularly when the concentration is sustained, rapid activation of plasma plasminogen ensues with the production of hyperplasminemia, excessive proteolytic activity, and extensive degradation of fibrinogen (the substrate most abundantly available). On the other hand, the diffusion of even small amounts of plasminogen activator into thrombi activates significant amounts of gel phase or clot plasminogen and produces fibrinolysis, for here the enzyme is protected by its close spatial relationship with fibrin, and the reaction appears, initially at least, to be independent of the inhibitors in body fluids.

Under physiologic circumstances, fibrinolytic phenomena are regulated by the release of a plasminogen activator, and the latter plays the key role in mediating fibrinolysis. The activator appears transiently in the circulation, following an appropriate stimulus, and directly raises the clot-dissolving activity of the plasma without invoking the consequences of increased plasma proteolysis. This fibrinolytic mechanism is particularly effective when significant quantities of activator are present at the time fibrin formation occurs; under these circumstances, the activator is incorporated throughout the clot while the latter is forming, and the subsequent widespread activation of clot plasminogen leads to very rapid fibrinolysis.

Recent observations have demonstrated that the fibrinolytic mechanism in vivo appears to be continuously active (particularly in the microcirculation) and dynamic in response to stimuli. The plasma of healthy adults normally contains significant but small amounts of plasminogen activator activity; this levels rises sharply whenever there is increased circulating fibrinolytic activity (accelerated euglobulin clot lysis time or whole blood clot lysis time). Increased fibrinolytic activity is observed frequently in certain diseases, e.g., hematologic malignancies, cirrhosis of the liver, and various infections. More striking changes are produced, however, by a great variety of physiologic and pharmacologic stimuli, e.g., electroshock, pneumoencephalography, hypoglycemia, ischemia, anoxia, intense exercise, and parenteral injections of epinephrine (Adrenalin), acetylcholine, nicotonic acid, and pyrogen. Current evidence indicates that the activator is released from the vascular endothelium into the circulation at sites of ischemia or other acute vascular changes either of a vasoconstrictive or vasodilatory nature. The lysosomal granules of tissue cells also appear to be rich in plasminogen activator, but the factors controlling the release from this site are less well understood.

FIBRINOLYTIC DISORDERS

Physiologically, fibrinolysis is accomplished without a significant increase in plasma proteolysis, but certain clinical situations arise in which there is excessive digestion of fibrin or fibrinogen; this state is associated with an acute or chronic coagulation disorder and, when the onset is sudden, a serious hemorrhagic diathesis may develop rapidly with severe bleeding, usually at the site of underlying disease or of previous surgery or trauma. Although the blood of patients suffering from this disorder frequently demonstrates multiple coagulation defects, the most striking finding is poor and slow blood clotting, even after the addition of thrombin, and the clot that forms is loose and friable. Subsequently, the clot may undergo spontaneous dissolution in a matter of minutes to hours; because of the latter phenomenon the syndrome is referred to as *pathologic fibrinolysis* or *fibrinolytic bleeding*. The severity of this disorder readily can be attributed to the particularly ineffective form of hemostasis present; clotting occurs slowly, with the formation of a very inadequate clot that may subsequently dissolve.

The understanding of this hemorrhagic diathesis has come from studies demonstrating that the products of the proteolytic digestion of fibrinogen and fibrin interfere with blood clotting and that the addition of such proteolysis products to normal blood reproduces, in vitro, the abnormal blood clotting seen in the fibrinolytic disorders. Further study of this problem has revealed that during the early phase of fibrinogen and fibrin digestion, fragments are released that readily complex with fibrinogen and are capable of interfering with both the action of thrombin and the ability of platelets to aggregate. Ultimately, however, several large fragments are formed that are incapable of being digested further by the action of plasmin. One of these fragments (sedimentation constant 5.27 S, molecular weight approximately 88,000), as well as its precursors, inhibits the interconversion of fibrinogen to fibrin; this inhibition does not appear to be on the thrombin reaction per se; rather, the effect is to inhibit the subsequent steps, i.e., the spontaneous polymerization of fibrin monomer (the subunit of the long, insoluble fibrin polymers of the normal clot). For this reason, these fragments are referred to as polymerization inhibitors, and, when present in large amounts, they delay normal polymerization and cause the formation of abnormal polymers that weaken and distort the final clot. The coagulation defects produced by the early and late fragments of fibrinogen or fibrin degradation, or both, have been shown to be primarily responsible for the impaired hemostasis seen in the clinically encountered fibrinolytic disorders. This abnormal clotting condition can be screened by measuring the thrombin clotting time; in the presence of excess thrombin, the thrombin clotting time is virtually a measure of the polymerization time, and the latter is significantly delayed in the pathologic fibrinolytic states. When desirable, quantification on the degradation products in serum can be accomplished through the use of a tanned red cell hemagglutination inhibition immunossay or by the ability of these fragments to clump staphylococci.

Pathogenically, two major types of fibrinolytic disorders exist, i.e., the primary and secondary forms. In the primary fibrinolytic disorders, the state is induced by a sustained increase in plasma proteolytic activity (hyperplasminemia) sufficient to digest large amounts of circulating fibrinogen (fibrinogenolysis), whereas, in the secondary form, the state appears either as a response to or in association (simultaneous release of tissue thromboplastin and tissue activator) with intravascular clotting or defibrination. In this latter type, the coexistence of clotting and fibrinolysis in large portions of the vascular bed results in the release of excessive amounts of fibrin breakdown products into the circulation.

Three mechanisms exist for the production of the primary disorders (excessive plasma proteolytic activity with fibrinogenolysis): First, inordinate amounts of plasminogen activator, e.g., urokinase, streptokinase, may be administered for therapeutic purposes or released endogenously from activator-rich neoplastic tissue, e.g., in metastic prostatic carcinoma, or in response to profound stimuli, such as severe anoxia or shock, or following extensive surgical procedures, particularly on the lung. This temporarily overwhelms normal plasma inhibitory mechanisms, sustaining free levels of plasmin in the circulation for significant periods of time. Second, deficiencies in inhibitory mechanisms may exist among patients with disease, e.g., in cirrhosis of the liver in which the ability to clear activator from the circulation is deficient. Under these circumstances, the body cannot cope adequately with the release of plasminogen activator in amounts ordinarily unlikely to produce significant hyperplasminemia. Finally, proteolytic enzymes, other than plasmin but also capable of degrading fibrinogen, may appear in the circulation and produce a similar state; such events have been described in the late stages of some leukemias.

Examination of the blood of patients with sustained increases in circulating plasmin frequently demonstrates the following: delayed clotting and abnormal appearance of the blood clot, prolonged thrombin clotting time, prolonged prothrombin time (two-stage prothrombin time usually normal), reduced fibrinogen level, immunologically identifiable fibrinogen breakdown products, moderate reductions of factors V and VIII, reduced plasminogen level, and increased fibrinolytic activity. Of these, the first five abnormalities can be traced to the effects of fibrinogen proteolysis; the other changes represent the proteolytic effects on other susceptible clotting components (factors V and VIII) and evidence for increased activity of the fibrinolytic enzyme system.

The secondary fibrinolytic disorders are seen in association with the disseminated intravascular coagulation syndromes: e.g., acute defibrination, as may occur in the obstetric catastrophies of placenta praevia, retained dead fetus and amniotic fluid embolism; or the more protracted or localized forms of widespread intravascular clotting as may be seen in purpura fulminans, the Waterhouse-Friderichsen syndrome, carcinomatosis, lymphoma, acute promyelocytic leukemia, thrombotic thrombocytopenic purpura, the Kasabach-Merritt syndrome, viper snake bites, and in gram-negative bacteremia with shock. These "coagulation consumption coagulopathies" also exhibit a hemorrhagic diathesis that is further complicated by evidences of secondary fibrinolysis, as demonstrated by the presence in the blood of immunologically identifiable breakdown products (presumably fibrin); however, the contribution of the latter to both the hemorrhagic diathesis and the laboratory findings varies greatly from case to case. In such instances, the problem of intravascular coagulation is the more serious one and can usually be recognized by the clinical or laboratory findings, but, on occasion, the presence of excessive evidences of fibrinolysis may mask the underlying thrombosing state. The latter instances may be difficult to unravel pathogenically, a consideration of particular importance because the therapeutic indications (anticoagulants vs. antifibrinolytic agents) depend on the nature of the primary insult. Noteworthy is the observation that the blood of patients with the secondary fibrinolytic disorders is usually accompanied by thrombocytopenia and is much less likely to demonstrate an increase in circulating fibrinolytic activity, because the extensive dissolution of fibrin is consequent to localized fibrinolytic phenomena rather than a heightened systemic activity of the fibrinolytic system.

Therapy of Fibrinolytic Disorders. Fortunately, the fragments formed during fibrinogen or fibrin proteolysis are spontaneously cleared from the circulation; their half-life is approximately nine hours. Thus, control of the underlying mechanism responsible for the fibrinolytic disorder is followed by spontaneous recovery; such recovery is usually rapid, because the severity of the disorder is critically dependent on the concentration of the breakdown products in the circulation.

Control of the primary fibrinolytic disorders can be accomplished rapidly by the administration of the synthetic amino acid epsilon aminocaproic acid, a potent inhibitor of plasminogen activators. Shortly after the oral or intravenous administration of this agent in appropriate dosage (loading dose of 5 grams followed by 20 to 30 grams per day), plasma plasminogen activation ceases, and the hemorrhagic diathesis usually subsides spontaneously, frequently very quickly. Such therapy need be carried out only as long as the underlying pathogenic mechanisms are operative. In most instances, two to three days of treatment are sufficient; however, in the fibrinolytic disorder occasionally encountered in metastatic carcinoma of the prostate, much longer periods of treatment are desirable. Epsilon aminocaproic acid also has proved very useful in the management of severe post-prostatectomy bleeding; here the agent, which is excreted rapidly into the urine following its oral or systemic administration, inhibits the action of urokinase, the naturally occurring urinary plasminogen activator that, by virtue of its ability to lyse clots, impairs hemostasis in the traumatized urinary tract. Amino-methylcyclohexane caproic acid, an analogue of epsilon aminocaproic acid, and trasylol, a plasmin and plasminogen activator inhibitor derived from ox lung, also have been claimed to be effective in the management of the primary fibrinolytic disorders.

At present, these antifibrinolytic agents are not recommended for use in the secondary fibrinolytic disorders, in which therapy is directed at controlling the intravascular coagulation; the use of antifibrinolytic agents in the absence of appropriate anticoagulation may prove hazardous by aggravating the underlying thrombosing tendency.

Fletcher, A. P., Alkjaersig, N., and Sherry, S.: Pathogenesis of the coagulation defect developing during pathological plasma proteolytic ("fibrinolytic") states. I. The significance of fibrinogen proteolysis and circulating fibrinogen breakdown products. J. Clin. Invest., 41:896, 1962.

Sherry, S.: Fibrinolysis. Ann. Rev. Med., 19:247, 1968.

Sweeney, W. M.: Aminocaproic acid, an inhibitor of fibrinolysis. Amer. J. Med. Sci., 249:576, 1965.

DISEASES OF METABOLISM

General Considerations

Nicholas P. Christy

The term "metabolism" used to be defined as the sum of the processes concerned in the building up and breaking down of living protoplasm, and as the chemical changes in living cells by which energy is provided for cellular work and for cellular repair (Webster, 1936). Such a definition depicts metabolism as a kind of cellular nutrition. Nowadays, the term is broadened to stand for "the sum of the processes by which a particular substance is handled . . . in the living body" (Webster, 1966), i.e., the processes that are essential for life, growth, maturation, and reproduction. Defined in this more general way, almost any disease is a "disease of metabolism" (from the Greek, μεταβολή, change; "metabolic" from μεταβολικόσ, changeable). After *trauma*, e.g., fracture of a hip, calcium may be lost from bone during prolonged immobilization, with accompanying hypercalcemia. An *infectious disease, chronic pyelonephritis,* may lead to renal insufficiency, uremia, and the familiar renal mismanagement of H^+, Ca^{++}, and other ions; cholera is associated with tremendous gastrointestinal losses of sodium and water. *Hereditary diseases* of several systems are characterized by disordered "handling" of particular substances: in congenital adrenal hyperplasia, deficiency of one or another adrenal cortical enzymes results in reduced synthesis of cortisol, excessive secretion of androgens, and precocious virilism; the disordered synthesis of hemoglobin in sickle cell anemia, the classic "molecular disease," results in the specific amino acid difference in the β chain that underlies the characteristically misshapen erythrocytes, the hemolysis and the micro-infarctions. A major clinical manifestation of a disease of *unknown etiology,* chronic pancreatitis, is steatorrhea with diarrhea, largely due to deficiency of pancreatic exocrine secretion and failure to hydrolyze triglycerides in the gut. Thus, diseases of all systems and of diverse etiologies are metabolic diseases, in the sense that they show some change in the way the body deals with (metabolizes) a particular chemical substance.

But metabolism itself must be changeable; the internal environment is only relatively constant. In his famous and much quoted generalization, Claude Bernard said: "All the vital mechanisms, varied as they are, have only one object: that of preserving constant the conditions of life in the *milieu intérieur.*" But, as the American physiologist L. J. Henderson wrote in 1926, "This should not be thought of as absolute constancy, and it should be understood that variations in the properties of the internal environment may be both cyclical and adaptive, that is, functional. . . ." Normal metabolism thus operates to keep the cellular environment in a state appropriate to constantly changing conditions: growth, reproduction, aging; changes in body temperature, hydration, nutrition. It is a mistake to think of the constancy of the *milieu intérieur* as simply a ceaseless struggle of the cells to return to some fixed and immutable baseline.

This section contains an account of hereditary and acquired diseases characterized by derangement of the internal environment, diseases which have in common *disordered production or fate of a well-defined, specific chemical substance.* Consequences of these disorders are an excess or deficiency of that substance or a substance closely related to it. The excess or deficiency gives rise to a well-defined, specific clinical syndrome which involves either predominantly one or in some cases several organs or systems. Assignment of disease entities to this category is somewhat arbitrary and therefore imperfect. For example, congenital adrenal hyperplasia and sickle cell anemia traditionally are more conveniently discussed in Diseases of the Endocrine System and in Hematologic and Hematopoietic Diseases, because the manifestations are chiefly endocrine and hematologic, respectively. The diabetes mellitus that is "genetic" rather than secondary, as in hemochromatosis or acromegaly, is generally agreed to be the result of an absolute or relative deficiency of pancreatic insulin; therefore, it might reasonably be placed in the section on Diseases of the Endocrine System. It seems wiser to include diabetes mellitus with the diseases of metabolism, because clinical features of *acute* diabetes have to be explained in terms of the characteristic derangements in carbohydrate, fat, and protein metabolism, derangements which are mutually interdependent and inseparable; and because the relation to simple insulin deficiency of some of the major manifestations of *chronic* diabetes mellitus, e.g., microangiopathy, is still not clear. The inclusion of diabetes in this section is certainly not made because we understand it so well—the reason regretfully ascribed by Albright in 1963: ". . . once some division of endocrinology is put on a firm footing, it is removed from the section of endocrinology to the section on metabolic diseases." Further, it might seem reasonable to place gout and alcaptonuria with diseases of the joints, but these disorders can only be thoroughly understood if one is familiar with the abnormalities in metabolism of uric acid and homogentisic acid. The reader may also wonder why certain diseases are placed in this section and others in the section on Miscellaneous Hereditary Diseases Affecting Multiple Organ Systems. The governing principle has been that the disorders in the latter group are chemically less well understood than those in this section; for example, the chemical lesion is not known in Laurence-Moon syndrome or dysautonomia and not completely characterized in porphyria or albinism. In future editions, as these disorders become better defined in biochemical terms, entities now grouped with Miscellaneous Hereditary Diseases will find their way into this section of the book.

The reader will observe the working of another governing principle, i.e., that in this section are placed most of the clinical conditions in which there is a demonstrated abnormality of a specific protein, either a "deficiency in a specific enzymatic activity . . . [or] a normal amount of a structurally abnormal protein" (See Inborn Errors of Metabolism and Molecular Disease in the section on Genetic Principles). Thus, the various forms of glycogen deposition disease, galactosemia, fructosuria and hereditary fructose intolerance, pentosuria, Type I hyperlipoproteinemia, Tangier disease, alcaptonuria, and xanthinuria are examples of the operation of the "one-gene, one-enzyme" hypothesis (Garrod, Tatum).

In diabetes mellitus and gout, two of the most common metabolic diseases, the exact mode of inheritance is not yet understood. In still other categories, most of the diseases are acquired, not hereditary (e.g., disorders of fluid, electrolyte and acid-base balance, and most of the many kinds of hypoglycemia). Here again the rationale

for classification in this section has been disordered metabolism of a *specific* substance: deficiency or excess of water or of Na^+, K^+, H^+, or HCO_3^- ion; depressed blood glucose concentration.

Finally, the reader will also observe that many of the diseases of metabolism are rare (not diabetes mellitus, with a prevalence in the United States of about 5 per cent, but, for example, primary hyperoxalemia, of which there are fewer than 100 reported cases) or of no clinical importance (fructosuria, pentosuria). If apologies are needed, one might offer these three: (1) study of rare diseases has very often made possible on understanding of normal metabolic processes; (2) discovery of some of these rare conditions early enough in life may lead to prevention of clinical disease simply by adjustment of the diet (galactosemia, phenylketonuria); (3) no disease is rare to the patient who has it or to the physician who has to manage it.

Albright, F.: Introduction: Diseases of the endocrine system. *In* Beeson, P. B., and McDermott, W. (eds.): Cecil-Loeb Textbook of Medicine. 11th ed. Philadelphia, W. B. Saunders Company, 1963, p. 1339.

Bernard, C.: An Introduction to the Study of Experimental Medicine (translated by H. L. Green). New York, Dover Publications, 1957, p. viii.

Bondy, P. K. (ed.): Duncan's Diseases of Metabolism. 6th ed. Philadelphia, W. B. Saunders Company, 1969.

Garrod, A. E.: Inborn errors of metabolism (Croonian Lectures). Lancet 2:1, 73, 142, 214, 1908.

Stanbury, J. B., Wyngaarden, J. B., and Fredrickson, D. S. (eds.): The Metabolic Basis of Inherited Disease. 2nd ed. New York, McGraw-Hill Publishing Company, Inc., 1966.

Tatum, E. L.: A case history in biological research. Science, 129:1711, 1959.

Disorders of Fluid, Electrolyte, and Acid-base Balance

William B. Schwartz

Fluid and electrolyte disturbances usually occur as complications of an underlying illness, and the disorders to be considered in this section must therefore be viewed not as isolated entities but in the context of the specific clinical settings in which they appear.

As general background to the following discussion, it should be recalled that the water content of the body (approximately 50 to 60 per cent of body weight) is distributed between the intracellular and the extracellular compartments. Approximately two thirds of the water is within cells, and the remaining third is divided between the interstitial space and plasma, which together comprise the extracellular compartment. Water

moves freely across cell boundaries, and for this reason changes in tonicity in one compartment induce a transfer of fluid that continues until a new steady state of osmotic equilibrium is established. By contrast, electrolytes are distributed in an asymmetric pattern, most of the ions in the extracellular fluid consisting of sodium, chloride, and bicarbonate and those in the intracellular fluid of potassium and organic anions. Except for the slight deviations attributable to the Donnan effect of the plasma proteins, the electrolyte compositions of plasma and interstitial fluid are virtually identical. Thus, for clinical purposes plasma composition can be taken as representative of the entire extracellular compartment.

The section on Renal Physiology and Tests of Renal Function summarizes the renal regulation of electrolyte and acid-base equilibrium, and in the present section relevant physiology will be presented entirely within the context of the clinical disorder under consideration.

DEPLETION OF VOLUME

The most common disturbance of fluid and electrolyte equilibrium is volume depletion. Loss of volume may occur from simple dehydration, but is seen more frequently in association with a combined loss of water and electrolytes.

Clinical Manifestations. The symptoms of volume depletion are few and nonspecific. The patient may complain of thirst, especially if the body fluids are hypertonic, but nausea, light-headedness, and weakness are perhaps the most frequent and troublesome manifestations. The major effects of volume depletion are on the circulation and on renal function. As plasma volume is diminished, blood pressure falls, heart rate rises, and a decrease in renal perfusion leads to oliguria and azotemia. When volume depletion is severe, profound shock becomes an immediate and serious threat to survival. The management of these clinical problems will be discussed after the individual causes of volume depletion have been considered.

Pathogenesis. The specific clinical circumstances in which volume depletion is encountered are listed in Table 1. These are discussed in the succeeding paragraphs.

Simple Dehydration (Loss of Water Without Electrolyte). The fluid requirement of the body is determined by the insensible losses through skin and lungs and by the amount of water that is required to excrete the daily solute load. Ordinarily the minimal intake that will serve to maintain water balance is 700 to 1000 ml. per day.

TABLE 1.   CAUSES OF VOLUME DEPLETION

SIMPLE DEHYDRATION
   (Loss of water without electrolyte)

COMBINED DEPLETION OF WATER AND SODIUM
   a. *Gastrointestinal losses*
       Vomiting
       Gastric or small bowel drainage
       Diarrhea
       Bowel fistulas (colostomy, ileostomy, etc.)

   b. *Renal losses*
       Chronic renal failure
       Diuretic phase of acute tubular necrosis
       Postobstructive nephropathy
       Adrenal insufficiency
       Osmotic diuresis
       Diuretics

   c. *Skin losses*
       Sweating
       Burns

   d. *Paracentesis*

Thirst ordinarily serves to maintain water intake well above this basal level; but, if weakness or disability sharply curtails fluid intake, dehydration will develop. The magnitude of the fluid deficit will be aggravated when insensible losses are increased by factors such as fever and hyperventilation or when urinary losses are abnormally large—for example, in uncontrolled diabetes insipidus.

Whenever water is lost without electrolyte, hypertonicity and elevation of the serum sodium concentration accompany the depletion of volume. The clinical features and consequences of hypernatremia are discussed later in this section.

Combined Depletion of Water and Sodium. Severe volume deficits occur most commonly in patients who have suffered a combined loss of water and sodium, usually from the gastrointestinal tract, the kidneys, or the skin.

Gastrointestinal Losses. Volume depletion may occur as the result of losses from any portion of the gastrointestinal tract. Gastrointestinal secretions normally amount to some 8 or 10 liters per day, and, if the body is deprived of a significant fraction of this total, severe dehydration will result. Depletion is most commonly the consequence of vomiting, gastric drainage, or diarrhea. It also is seen with small-bowel drainage, ileostomy, colostomy, and pancreatic or biliary fistulas. Most gastrointestinal secretions are either isotonic or slightly hypotonic and, for this reason, losses per se should not produce a striking change in serum sodium concentration. However, because serum sodium concentration is ultimately determined by over-all water balance (as influenced by fluid intake, skin losses, etc.), both hyponatremia and hypernatremia may be encountered.

Renal Losses. Patients with *chronic renal failure* commonly have a reduced ability to conserve sodium, but the sodium-wasting tendency is seldom severe enough to become apparent if dietary intake of salt is normal. If salt intake is restricted, however, continued excretion of sodium and the associated loss of water may produce severe depletion of extracellular volume. Contraction of volume, in turn, causes a further reduction in glomerular filtration rate, and may even precipitate frank uremia. Sodium intake in the azotemic patient should not be curtailed, therefore, without careful sequential observations of body weight and sodium excretion.

An occasional patient wastes sodium even while ingesting a normal quantity of salt; most of these appear to have *medullary cystic disease* as their underlying renal lesion. In such cases of severe salt-wasting, the diet must be supplemented with sodium chloride if volume depletion is to be avoided. It is important to remember that in the patient with renal disease volume depletion should always be considered as a possible explanation for a sudden, otherwise unexplained increase in azotemia.

During the *diuretic phase of acute tubular necrosis* a defect in the ability of the damaged tubules to reabsorb sodium may lead to a considerable loss of sodium and water. Sodium wasting does not usually persist for more than several days, and is not likely to become clinically significant if the patient is taking a diet of normal salt content. At times it may be difficult to distinguish between an abnormal diuresis and the physiologic diuresis that will occur if an excessive quantity of fluid and electrolyte has been administered during the oliguric phase of the disease. If one is uncertain about the cause, treatment can ordinarily be delayed for a day or two until the issue is resolved either by the cessation of the diuresis or by the appearance of early signs of volume depletion. In this way an unnecessary and prolonged cycle of saline loading and saline loss can be avoided.

Postobstructive nephropathy occasionally produces severe sodium and volume depletion in patients in whom complete or nearly complete obstruction has been present for a prolonged period. The defect in sodium reabsorption results from tubular damage, and becomes manifest promptly after the relief of obstruction permits the filtered load of sodium to increase. Loss of salt may lead to an obligatory diuresis of as much as 5 or 10 liters per day and, thus, to an acute contraction of extracellular and plasma volume. Just as with the diuretic phase of acute tubular necrosis, the disorder is self-limiting because the tubules generally recover their capacity to transport sodium within a few days.

Volume depletion consequent to excessive renal losses of fluid and electrolyte may also occur in the absence of structural renal disease. In patients with *adrenal insufficiency* (Addison's disease) a deficiency of salt-retaining steroids reduces the activity of renal transport mechanisms, and may allow large quantities of sodium and water to escape into the urine. Continued administration of *diuretics* to the patient who has been but is no longer edematous will also sometimes produce volume depletion.

Abnormal losses of sodium and water are also induced by the obligatory excretion of a large solute load. Such an osmotic diuresis is seen most frequently in association with the glycosuria of uncontrolled diabetes mellitus. A similar sequence of events sometimes occurs with administration of tube feedings containing large quantities of protein. Repeated infusions of *mannitol* may have the same effects.

Skin Losses. Large losses of water and electrolyte from the skin may result either from excessive sweating or from burns. *Sweat* is a hypotonic solution normally containing no more than 50 mEq. of sodium per liter, and for this reason sweating will produce a relatively larger deficit of water than of sodium. *Burns* can lead to two types of deficits: isotonic extracellular fluid may be lost by transudation; and water may be lost without electrolyte as the result of increased evaporation through damaged epithelium. An additional factor contributing to a severe depletion of circulating volume is the capillary damage that results in the interstitial accumulation of fluid, particularly during the first days after the burn

has occurred. Such fluid loss, because it takes place internally, can readily be overlooked.

Paracentesis. An occasional patient with cirrhosis and ascites has been noted to develop circulatory collapse after *paracentesis*. Reduction of pressure within the peritoneal cavity may allow transudation of a large quantity of fluid with consequent contraction of plasma volume. Clinically significant contraction is not likely to occur in patients who have a substantial amount of peripheral edema, apparently because plasma volume can be readily replenished by transfer of fluid from the expanded interstitial space.

Diagnosis. The *history* is frequently of great value in an appraisal of the origin and magnitude of a volume deficit. The patient should be questioned closely about fluid intake and about losses of fluid that may have resulted from vomiting, diarrhea, sweating, polyuria, or other disturbances. In many cases, particularly when a reliable history is not available, *physical examination* is the single most valuable diagnostic tool. Reduction in turgor of the skin, particularly over the arms, legs, and face, is the most characteristic finding, and is usually accompanied by postural hypotension. The facies are usually pinched, and the tongue is dry. Lowered tension of the eyeballs, a rapid resting pulse, and hypotension in the recumbent position may be observed when dehydration is severe.

Laboratory findings are likely to be of less value. The serum sodium concentration reflects only the ratio of sodium to water and, whether low, normal, or high, gives no insight into the total volume of extracellular fluid present. Elevated hematocrit and hemoglobin concentrations suggest that plasma volume is contracted, but, unless the values before the acute illness are known, the interpretation of these data is likely to be difficult. The plasma creatinine concentration is sometimes helpful because it may provide evidence of volume depletion and impairment of renal function even before the appearance of oliguria. The blood urea nitrogen level is a less useful index of renal dysfunction because the urea concentration can be elevated by external factors, such as fever or an excess of adrenal corticoids.

Once the diagnosis of a sodium and water deficit has been made, measurements of sodium excretion may help to identify the source of the losses. If the depletion is of *extrarenal* origin, the contraction in volume will normally lead to relatively prompt and efficient conservation of sodium by the kidney. Increased secretion of aldosterone, a fall in glomerular filtration rate, and other as yet undefined factors augment sodium reabsorption and reduce sodium excretion to less than 5 or 10 mEq. per day. If the excretion of sodium exceeds 30 to 40 mEq. per day, it can generally be concluded that the losses are of *renal* origin and are the result of primary renal disease, Addison's disease, or osmotic diuresis. It should be noted, however, that, if the contraction of volume is sufficiently severe to produce oliguria and marked reduction in filtration rate, sodium excretion will sometimes fall to a low level even in disorders in which the underlying abnormality is defective renal conservation of sodium.

Treatment. The most serious threat to the patient with severe volume depletion is circulatory collapse, and the most immediate concern in treatment is restoration of an adequate blood volume and blood pressure. This goal can be accomplished most effectively by the rapid infusion of plasma (if the hematocrit is elevated) or blood. If neither plasma nor blood is available, isotonic saline solution should be given instead; saline is not an entirely satisfactory substitute, however, because a large fraction of administered salt and water is promptly lost from the circulation as it diffuses into the interstitial space.

After shock has been corrected, the remaining fluid and electrolyte abnormalities can be repaired in a more leisurely fashion. Close observation of skin turgor, body weight, blood pressure, and serum creatinine concentration will, together with available information concerning the volume and composition of the losses, provide the most reliable guide to replacement therapy. In some cases as much as 4 or 5 liters of fluid will be required to correct the volume deficit. If serum sodium is within normal limits (indicating a virtually equivalent deficit of sodium and water), repair should be carried out largely with isotonic saline solution, water without electrolyte being given only as needed to replace insensible and renal losses occurring during the period of treatment. Even if serum sodium concentration is moderately abnormal (as low as 130 mEq. or as high as 150 mEq. per liter), the same approach to therapy can be employed as in the patient with isotonic contraction of extracellular volume. If physiologic saline solution and modest quantities of water are administered, the kidney can be relied upon for final adjustment of both volume and tonicity. With gross deviations in sodium concentration, more specific measures will be necessary. Severe hypernatremia will require the provision of considerably more water than salt and, conversely, severe hyponatremia (in the absence of edema) will call for correction, or partial correction, by administration of hypertonic sodium chloride solution. The management of hypernatremia and hyponatremia is discussed in detail later in this section.

The composition of the repair solutions must also allow for the presence of other electrolyte abnormalities. For example, if metabolic acidosis is present, the sodium deficit should be corrected in part with sodium bicarbonate rather than exclusively with sodium chloride.

HYPONATREMIA

Sodium is the ion present in highest concentration in the extracellular fluid, and sodium salts are thus the primary determinant of the osmolality (tonicity) of the extracellular compartment.

Changes in sodium concentration thus have a major influence on the distribution of water between the intracellular and extracellular spaces.

Normally, serum sodium concentration is stabilized at approximately 140 mEq. per liter by changes in water balance that occur in response to variations in plasma osmotic pressure. A slight increase in sodium concentration, and in osmotic pressure, leads to the release of antidiuretic hormone and to a retention of water that then restores normal tonicity. Conversely, a slight reduction in serum sodium concentration and osmotic pressure inhibits the release of hormone and permits any excess water to be excreted.

A variety of disturbances can lead to an abnormal and sustained reduction in serum sodium concentration. Retention of water without sodium, loss of sodium without a proportional loss of water, and redistribution of water between cells and extracellular fluid may each induce hyponatremia. As pointed out earlier, serum sodium concentration yields no direct information concerning the state of total sodium stores, but indicates only that there has been a disturbance in the ratio of sodium to water.

The specific causes of hyponatremia and the mechanisms that underlie their development are described in detail below. It is convenient, however, to consider first the clinical manifestations and the aspects of treatment that are common to all hypo-osmotic states.

Clinical Manifestations. The signs and symptoms of the hypo-osmotic state are those of *water intoxication,* and are apparently caused by movement of fluid from the extracellular space into the relatively more hypertonic cells. When serum sodium concentration falls to approximately 120 mEq. per liter, the patient frequently becomes irritable and confused. More serious disturbances are seen if the sodium concentration falls to 110 mEq. or below; the patient often becomes lethargic or comatose, and generalized convulsions develop. Death may result unless appropriate treatment is promptly instituted.

Treatment. Severe hyponatremia is best treated by the intravenous administration of hypertonic (5 per cent) sodium chloride. Elevation of serum sodium concentration to a level of 125 or 130 mEq. per liter will ordinarily suffice to eliminate all evidence of central nervous system dysfunction. Full correction of hyponatremia need not and should not be carried out over a short time because the sudden transfer of a large volume of fluid from the intracellular to the extracellular space is sometimes hazardous; an abrupt expansion of plasma volume may elevate central venous pressure and produce symptomatic pulmonary congestion, particularly in the patient with frank or latent heart disease.

Calculation of the amount of salt necessary to produce a given rise in sodium concentration must take into consideration the shift of water that will be induced by the increase in extracellular tonicity. As serum sodium concentration is elevated, water moves out of cells along the resulting osmotic gradient; the estimated sodium requirement must therefore be based on the need to restore tonicity throughout the total body water. The following is an illustrative example of this calculation, assuming an initial serum sodium concentration of 110 mEq. per liter, a final concentration of 125 mEq. per liter, and a body weight of 70 kg. Since approximately 50 per cent of the total body weight is water, the amount of sodium necessary to produce the desired change will be 35 liters × 15 mEq. per liter, or approximately 500 mEq. of sodium. The calculation can be summarized by the following equation:

$$[\text{Desired Na conc.} - \text{initial Na conc.}] \times 0.5 \text{ body weight} = \text{mEq. of Na}$$

Pathogenesis. Table 2 lists the specific clinical circumstances in which a low sodium concentration is encountered. These are discussed in the succeeding paragraphs.

Functional Disorders Leading to Defective Excretion of Water. Depletion of Sodium and Extracellular Volume. Significant impairment of water excretion often results from severe depletion of sodium and volume, thus predisposing to the development of hyponatremia. If water is ingested or infused without electrolyte, the retention of a portion of this water leads to a fall in serum sodium concentration. This sequence of events accounts for the frequent occurrence of hyponatremia in conditions such as vomiting or diarrhea. The exact mechanisms responsible for the failure of hypotonicity to induce a water diuresis in the patient with volume depletion are unknown, but a reduced delivery of sodium and water to the loop of Henle (where dilution occurs) appears to play an important part.

In most patients with volume depletion, the water intake is not large enough to produce hyponatremia of great severity, serum sodium concentration decreasing by no more than 10 or 15 mEq. per liter. In such cases the manifestations of volume depletion rather than hyponatremia usually dominate the clinical picture, and treatment should be aimed primarily at correction of extracellular volume rather than at elevating serum sodium concentration. As discussed earlier, if sodium concentration is only moderately reduced, correction of hyponatremia will occur as a by-product of expansion with isotonic saline solution; restoration of normal plasma volume will correct the renal defect in water excretion, and an augmented water output will then restore tonicity to normal.

Inappropriate Secretion of Antidiuretic Hormone. Water retention and hyponatremia may result from *inappropriate secretion of antidiuretic hormone.* This term is used to describe the condition in which hypotonicity fails to suppress the release of antidiuretic hormone, with the result that renal excretion of water is impaired. A notable feature of this syndrome is that the expansion of extracellular volume not only causes dilution but also induces a sodium diuresis and a negative sodium balance. The combination of water retention and salt wasting at times produces extreme hyponatremia, the sodium concentration occasionally decreasing to less than 100 mEq. per liter. The syndrome of inappropriate secretion of antidiuretic hormone has been noted most often in patients with bronchogenic carcinoma of the oat-cell type, but is also seen in a variety of other clinical settings, including pneumonia, meningitis, head injuries, porphyria, and myxedema.

The following features are virtually diagnostic of the syndrome: (1) hyponatremia with renal sodium wasting; (2) normal tissue turgor and normal blood pressure; (3) normal blood urea nitrogen and creatinine concentrations; (4) normal adrenal function; and (5) specific gravity of the urine inappropriately high for a hypotonic subject, that is, in excess of 1.002 or 1.003. Edema is not a usual feature because water retention does not ordinarily exceed 4 or 5 liters and because a large fraction of the retained fluid moves into cells.

Treatment consists of water restriction and the administration of sodium chloride. This disorder and its management are discussed in detail elsewhere.

Renal Disease with Defective Excretion of Water. During the oliguric phase of *acute renal failure* dilutional hyponatremia will regularly occur if fluid intake is not adequately restricted. The net loss of water from skin and lungs is normally about 400 to 500 ml. per day, and if severe oliguria or anuria is present, administration of significantly more than this quantity (for example, 1000 to 1200 ml.) will produce overhydration within a relatively short time.

Water intoxication is occasionally seen in *chronic renal failure,* and occurs primarily in patients who have been urged to ingest large quantities of fluid in an effort to increase urine volume and promote urea excretion. Such attempts to force a diuresis may not only be hazardous, but also appear to have little beneficial effect on the clinical course, even when they produce a slight reduction in blood urea concentration.

TABLE 2. CAUSES OF HYPONATREMIA

---

a. *Functional disorders leading to defective excretion of water*
    Depletion of sodium and extracellular fluid volume
    Inappropriate secretion of antidiuretic hormone
    Addison's disease

b. *Renal disease with defective excretion of water*
    Acute renal failure with oliguria
    Chronic renal failure

c. *Idiopathic hyponatremia*
    Congestive heart failure
    Cirrhosis of the liver

d. *Excessive water intake in the presence of normal renal function*
    Psychogenic polydipsia

e. *Hyponatremia without disturbance in water balance*
    Accumulation of solute in the extracellular fluid
    Pseudohyponatremia

Idiopathic Hyponatremia. Hyponatremia frequently appears without warning in the edematous patient entering the late stages of *congestive heart failure or cirrhosis of the liver*. In this setting it is an ominous prognostic sign that appears to be the reflection (rather than the cause) of an underlying clinical deterioration.

The factors responsible for this electrolyte disturbance have not been clearly defined. Salt depletion induced by diuretic therapy cannot be held accountable because the edematous patient has a larger than normal quantity of sodium in his extracellular space and, in theory, could readily restore plasma sodium concentration to normal simply by excreting surplus water. Furthermore, the disorder has been observed in patients who have not received diuretics or in whom diuretics have failed to promote salt excretion. In some cases it can be demonstrated that retention of water is responsible for the hyponatremic state, but in others measurements of body weight give no evidence that fluid was retained during the period that sodium concentration fell. In the latter circumstance it has been proposed that a primary reduction in intracellular osmolality allows water to shift into the extracellular space and that the lowered osmotic pressure of the plasma is simply a passive reflection of the change in cellular tonicity. According to this thesis, failure to increase the excretion of water is explained by the absence of an osmotic gradient between plasma and the osmoreceptors of the hypothalamus.

As noted above, the appearance of hyponatremia in the edematous patient is usually a grave prognostic sign. Even if the patient does not appear to be critically ill, prolonged survival is uncommon unless treatment directed toward improvement of the underlying cardiac or liver disease is successful. Elevation of the serum sodium concentration by either water restriction or the administration of hypertonic sodium chloride usually has no beneficial effect. Water restriction usually induces severe thirst before osmolality is restored to normal, and if the patient is then permitted to increase his fluid intake, he quickly re-establishes the hyponatremic state. The administration of hypertonic saline, although it may transiently elevate sodium concentration, appears to hasten rather than to retard the downward clinical course.

Hyponatremia of unknown cause is sometimes seen in seriously ill patients with a debilitating disease such as metastatic carcinoma or leukemia. Neither dehydration nor edema is present, and there is no evidence of extrarenal or urinary loss of sodium. The reason for this disturbance is obscure.

Excessive Water Intake in the Presence of Normal Renal Function (Psychogenic Polydipsia). A syndrome virtually identical to that already described for inappropriate secretion of antidiuretic hormone may be produced by the ingestion of more water than the normal kidney can excrete; that is, more than 1000 or 1200 ml. per hour. Intakes in excess of these amounts are unusual, but are occasionally seen in patients who have a severe psychiatric illness. In such cases the expansion of extracellular volume induced by the positive water balance leads to both hyponatremia and renal wasting of sodium. Characteristically, the urine is maximally dilute (specific gravity of 1.001), and it is this finding that unequivocally demonstrates that the syndrome is the result of excessive ingestion of water rather than of inappropriate secretion of antidiuretic hormone.

If signs of water intoxication are present, hypertonic saline solution should be given intravenously, but in most cases reduction of water intake and increased ingestion of salt will be the only treatment required.

Hyponatremia Without Disturbance in Water Balance. *Accumulation of Solute in the Extracellular Fluid.* Solutes such as glucose and mannitol, which do not distribute freely throughout body water, can accumulate in the extracellular space and create an osmotic gradient between cells and interstitial fluid. As a result, water shifts from the intracellular compartment, and the serum sodium concentration falls. Hyponatremia resulting from such a redistribution of fluid is a characteristic feature of the severe hyperglycemia seen in patients with uncontrolled diabetes mellitus; each 100 mg. per 100 ml. increment in blood sugar above normal represents the addition of slightly more than 5 milliosmoles of solute per kilogram to the extracellular compartment, and leads to a reduction in serum sodium concentration of approximately 3 mEq. per liter. A blood sugar of 600 mg. per 100 ml. (that is, an excess of 500 mg. per 100 ml.) can thus be expected to lower sodium concentration from 140 to 125 mEq. per liter. Failure to consider the role of hyperglycemia in the genesis of hyponatremia in the diabetic can lead to the administration of an excessive amount of sodium during the treatment of ketoacidosis.

The accumulation of mannitol in the extracellular fluid can also cause a shift of water sufficient to reduce serum sodium concentration. This problem is most likely to be encountered in the patient with acute renal failure in whom an unsuccessful attempt has been made to increase urine volume by repeated mannitol infusions.

Hyperosmolality will *not* produce hyponatremia if the solute distributes freely across cell membranes, and thus increases the osmolality of cells and interstitial fluid to a proportional degree. In uremia, for example, serum sodium concentration is unaffected by the hypertonicity induced by urea accumulation because urea penetrates cells readily, and its concentration is elevated throughout body water.

Pseudohyponatremia. Pseudohyponatremia refers to a spurious reduction in sodium concentration resulting from a displacement of some fraction of plasma water by an abnormal accumulation of lipid or protein. Although plasma sodium concentration is usually measured as milliequivalents per liter of plasma, the physiologically significant measurement is the sodium concentration expressed as milliequivalents per kilogram of plasma water. Thus, a sodium concentration of 140 mEq. per liter, as measured on whole plasma, reflects an actual concentration of 150 mEq. per kilogram of water in normal plasma containing 93 per cent water. Since the percentage of plasma that is water does not vary appreciably under most circumstances, reductions in plasma sodium concentration can generally be taken as reflecting a decrease in the sodium concentration per unit of plasma water and in the tonicity of extracellular fluid. On the other hand, if severe hyperlipemia (or hyperproteinemia) is present, the fraction of plasma that is water will be lower than normal, and a striking reduction in the sodium concentration per unit volume of plasma will be observed despite the absence of a significant change in the electrolyte concentration per kilogram of plasma water.

Hyperlipemia of sufficient magnitude to produce pseudohyponatremia occurs in a number of diseases, including diabetes mellitus, nephrotic syndrome, and biliary cirrhosis. In nearly all cases in which sodium concentration is reduced by lipidemia the plasma is frankly lactescent, and this will often be the first finding that points to the correct diagnosis. *Hyperproteinemia* severe enough to cause pseudohyponatremia is a rare occurrence, and has been seen only in multiple myeloma. In this disease the plasma sodium concentration may be lowered to a value of 125 or 130 mEq. per liter.

The contribution of an increased concentration of lipid or protein to a reduced plasma sodium concentration can be readily assessed by determination of plasma osmotic pressure (estimated from freezing-point depression). If osmotic pressure is normal despite the hyponatremia, it will be evident that the concentration of sodium in the aqueous phase of plasma is normal.

HYPERNATREMIA

Virtually all cases of hypernatremia result from a loss of water that produces a relative excess of sodium in the body fluids. Any hypotonic loss, such as that occurring with sweating or vomiting, will cause a modest degree of hypernatremia, which will persist if adequate fluid replacement is not provided. Extreme elevations of plasma sodium concentrations (160 mEq. per liter or above) are uncommon, however, and are usually encountered in only one of three clinical settings: decreased or absent fluid intake, diabetes insipidus, or osmotic diuresis. Such extreme increases in tonicity of the extracellular fluid, when they occur, lead to marked cellular dehydration.

The most common cause of hypernatremia is a fluid intake that is inadequate to replace urinary losses and the insensible loss of water from the skin and lungs. This problem is most frequently encountered in the patient who is stuporous or who has some other disability that prevents him from drinking normally. In the comatose patient in whom *diabetes insipidus* develops after a head injury or a neurosurgical procedure, a large negative water balance is likely to appear with unusual speed and severity. In most cases of diabetes insipidus, polyuria will quickly draw attention to the nature of the problem, but if solute intake is low, the diagnosis can readily be overlooked since urine volume may not exceed 2 or 3 liters per day.

Osmotic loading can also produce severe hypernatremia. During osmotic diuresis water is lost in excess of sodium, and with sustained or repeated diuresis the serum sodium concentration sometimes rises to values greater than 175 mEq. per liter. This sequence of events is most often observed in comatose patients who are confronted with a massive urea load as the result of being given tube feedings containing large amounts of protein. Such patients are entirely dependent on others to recognize and repair their water deficit, and maintenance of a normal urine volume by continued solute loading may sometimes obscure the fact that dehydration and hypertonicity are present. In such a circumstance, the progressive loss of weight, the physical signs of volume depletion, and the development of hypernatremia should draw attention to the correct diagnosis.

The specific signs and symptoms produced by a marked elevation of serum sodium concentration have not been clearly defined; most patients with hypernatremia are already seriously ill and the role of the hypertonicity, as distinguished from that of the underlying disease, is frequently difficult to evaluate. Clinical experience suggests, however, that when hypernatremia is encountered water should be administered (either orally or as 5 per cent glucose intravenously) in quantities sufficient to restore serum sodium concentration to normal. The quantity of water required must be calculated with an appreciation that hypertonicity is present not only in the extracellular fluid but throughout total body water. Thus, a 70-kg. man with a plasma sodium concentration of 170 mEq. per liter will require a 20 per cent expansion of body water, that is, 8 liters of fluid, to restore serum sodium concentration to a normal value of 140 mEq. per liter. Observations during the treatment of hypernatremia indicate that full correction should not be carried out over a short interval, e.g., a few hours, because a rapid reduction in tonicity may produce signs of water intoxication.

DISTURBANCES OF POTASSIUM EQUILIBRIUM

Potassium, the major intracellular cation, plays a significant part in control of osmotic pressure, and also serves as an essential activator in a number of enzymatic reactions. In addition, potassium concentration of body fluids has an important influence on the excitability of both skeletal and cardiac muscle and on the structure and function of the kidneys. Disturbances in potassium equilibrium may therefore produce a wide range of clinical disorders.

The potassium concentration in extracellular

fluid is normally 3.8 to 5 mEq. per liter and that in intracellular fluid approximately 150 mEq. per liter. Since about 20 per cent of body weight is extracellular fluid, it can readily be calculated that only a small fraction of the 2500 to 3000 mEq. of potassium within the body is contained in the extracellular space. On the other hand, changes in plasma potassium concentration often mirror changes in cellular potassium content, and plasma concentration thus provides a useful clinical guide to disturbances in potassium balance. Furthermore, relatively small absolute changes in extracellular concentration, by producing large differences in the ratio of intracellular to extracellular potassium, may have important effects on neuromuscular activity.

Despite the usual wide variations in dietary intake of potassium (40 to 120 mEq. per day), plasma potassium concentration is normally stabilized within the narrow range of 4 to 5 mEq. per liter by virtue of close renal regulation of potassium balance. As discussed earlier, renal potassium excretion is accomplished largely, if not exclusively, by a process of potassium secretion in the distal portion of the nephron; it has been demonstrated that essentially all filtered potassium is reabsorbed in the proximal tubule and that the potassium that appears in the urine is added to the filtrate by a distal process of sodium-cation exchange. Fecal excretion of potassium normally amounts to only a few milliequivalents per day and does not play a significant role in potassium homeostasis.

If a large potassium load is suddenly administered, renal mechanisms do not respond quickly enough to prevent a rise in serum potassium concentration to abnormal levels. Under such circumstances, sequestration of potassium within cells helps to prevent a dangerous degree of hyperkalemia. If renal function is normal, the elevation of serum potassium concentration usually persists only briefly.

The clinical aspects of disturbances in potassium metabolism will be considered under two headings, *potassium deficiency* and *potassium intoxication*.

Hypokalemia and Potassium Deficiency

Potassium deficiency may occur as the result of either *renal or extrarenal losses*. Typically, serum potassium concentration is reduced to a level of 2.5 to 3.5 mEq. per liter, but with severe potassium depletion it may fall below 2 mEq. per liter. In some circumstances, the reduction in potassium concentration is minimized or prevented by the concomitant presence of acidosis. Acidosis shifts the equilibrium between cells and extracellular fluid, tending to make serum potassium concentration high in relation to total body stores.

Pathogenesis and Diagnosis. Table 3 lists the common causes of potassium deficiency grouped according to whether the losses are of renal or extrarenal origin. As is evident from the table, a large variety of factors, including adrenal steroids, diuretics, and primary renal disease, may promote

TABLE 3. CAUSES OF POTASSIUM DEFICIENCY

A. *RENAL*
    a. *Adrenal steroids*
        Primary or secondary aldosteronism
        Cushing's syndrome
        Adrenal steroid therapy

    b. *Diuretics*
        Mercurials
        Ethacrynic acid
        Thiazides
        Furosemide
        Carbonic anhydrase inhibitors

    c. *Renal disease*
        Renal tubular acidosis
        Tetracycline (outdated)
        Diuretic phase of acute tubular necrosis

B. *EXTRARENAL*
    a. Vomiting
    b. Gastric drainage
    c. Diarrhea

abnormal renal excretion. Nearly all appear to increase sodium-potassium exchange in some fashion. *Adrenal steroids*, whether produced in excessive quantities by the body or given therapeutically, directly stimulate the sodium-cation exchange mechanism and thus induce a urinary potassium loss. *Diuretics* such as the mercurials, ethacrynic acid, and the thiazides act by increasing the delivery of sodium to distal exchange sites that are avid for sodium. The carbonic anhydrase inhibitors impair sodium-hydrogen exchange and thus favor the exchange of sodium for potassium.

The exact nature of the derangements that occur with *renal diseases* such as renal tubular acidosis and Fanconi's syndrome, or with renal damage induced by outdated tetracycline, is unknown. It is not clear whether potassium wasting is the consequence of defective proximal reabsorption, accelerated distal secretion, or some combination of the two.

The only significant *extrarenal* route of potassium depletion is through the loss of gastrointestinal secretions. Gastric juice contains potassium in a concentration somewhat higher than plasma and diarrheal fluid in concentrations as high as 50 to 60 mEq. per liter. As a result, an appreciable loss of potassium ensues during prolonged vomiting, drainage of the upper gastrointestinal tract, or diarrhea. If intake of potassium is poor, the severity of potassium deficiency is further aggravated by renal losses; inefficient renal conservation allows considerable quantities of potassium to escape into the urine for as long as ten days or two weeks after potassium intake is lowered sharply. As much as 150 or 200 mEq. can be lost before excretion is slowly reduced to a level of less than 10 or 15 mEq. per day.

In hypokalemia of unknown origin the quantity of potassium in the urine frequently provides the clue to the correct diagnosis. If a patient with persistent hypokalemia is excreting considerable quantities of potassium in the urine (30 mEq. or more per day), the deficit is clearly of renal origin, and attention can therefore immediately be focused on those disorders listed under Section A of Table 3. Ordinarily the history and other clinical findings will clarify the etiology because the distinction between renal losses resulting from adrenal steroid excess, diuretic therapy, and renal disease is, in most cases, not difficult. There are several exceptions to this statement, however. A common problem, for example, is the evaluation of hypokalemia in the hypertensive patient who has received an agent such as a thiazide as part of his antihypertensive regimen. In such patients it may be difficult to decide whether potassium deficiency is the result of diuretic therapy or is caused by primary aldosteronism. This question can usually be resolved by observation of the serum potassium level for at least several weeks after the drug has been discontinued.

The uncommon *syndrome of juxtaglomerular cell hyperplasia with secondary aldosteronism (Bartter's syndrome)* also may present a diagnostic problem. This disorder resembles both primary aldosteronism and Cushing's syndrome in that it is characterized by hypokalemia, renal potassium wasting, and metabolic alkalosis. It is distinguished, however, by a tendency to salt wasting, an excessive level of renin activity in the plasma, and the absence of hypertension. There is, in addition, a remarkable resistance of the hypokalemia and alkalosis to potassium therapy; often the diet must be supplemented by as much as 300 to 400 mEq. of potassium chloride per day in order to restore plasma values to normal or nearly normal levels. This finding alone should arouse suspicion of the diagnosis and lead to appropriate studies designed to elucidate the other characteristic features of the syndrome.

In the patient with hypokalemia in whom potassium excretion is low (less than 15 mEq. per day), the depletion is usually of extrarenal origin (Section B, Table 3). In nearly all such instances a history or other evidence pointing to gastrointestinal losses will easily be obtained, but sometimes the diagnosis is not easily discerned. Occasionally, a patient with *laxative-induced diarrhea* will deny both laxative ingestion and diarrhea, and it is often necessary to obtain the relevant history from members of the family. Similarly, some patients with *psychogenic* or *self-induced vomiting* do not readily admit to their difficulties. Patients with *villous adenomas of the rectum* may also pose a problem because they can have normally formed stools, and, unless asked specifically, may neglect to mention the nearly continuous rectal leakage of mucus-like material. Accordingly, whenever

unexplained chronic hypokalemia is associated with a low urinary potassium concentration, each of these uncommon disorders should be sought carefully.

Clinical Manifestations. The clinical effects of potassium deficiency may be manifested in one or more organ systems including skeletal muscle, heart, kidneys, and the gastrointestinal tract. Perhaps the most serious disturbances are those affecting the neuromuscular system. At serum potassium concentrations in the range of 2 to 2.5 mEq. per liter muscular weakness is likely to occur, and with more severe hypokalemia the patient may develop areflexic paralysis. In this latter state respiratory insufficiency is an immediate threat to survival. The severity of the neuromuscular disturbance tends to be proportional to the speed with which the potassium level has declined. In an occasional instance, *myoglobinuria* has been noted in association with marked hypokalemia.

It should also be noted that muscular weakness or frank paralysis may occur without loss of potassium from the body, as in *hypokalemic periodic paralysis*. In this unusual familial disorder a shift of potassium from extracellular fluid to cells is responsible for the fall in serum concentration.

Abnormalities in the electrocardiogram that commonly occur in hypokalemia are a sagging of the ST segment, depression of the T wave, and elevation of the U wave (Fig. 1). With marked reductions in serum concentration, the T wave becomes progressively smaller, whereas the U waves show increasing amplitude. In some cases the merging of a flat or positive T wave with a positive U wave may erroneously be interpreted as a prolonged QT interval. Ordinarily, there are no serious clinical consequences from the abnormalities in cardiac excitation, but in digitalized patients the sudden development of hypokalemia may precipitate serious arrhythmias.

Long-standing potassium depletion is apt to produce renal tubular damage—so-called *hypokalemic nephropathy*. This disorder is discussed in detail elsewhere. Potassium deficiency is believed to cause dysfunction of the smooth muscle of the gastrointestinal tract and in some patients has been held responsible for the development of *paralytic ileus*.

Potassium deficiency is also a regular concomitant of *metabolic alkalosis*. The role of potassium in the genesis and maintenance of alkalosis is considered later in this section.

Treatment. Under many circumstances potas-

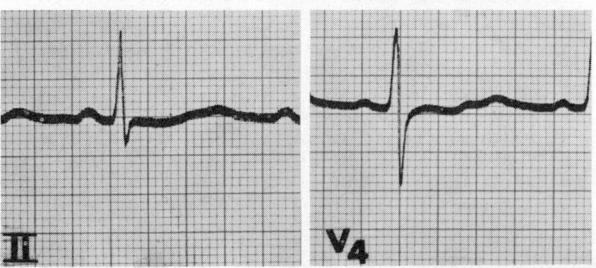

FIGURE 1. Typical electrocardiographic abnormalities induced by hypokalemia. (Serum potassium concentration 2.8 mEq. per liter.) Note in lead II how the merger of the T and U waves might lead to the erroneous interpretation that the Q-T interval is prolonged.

sium deficiency can be corrected by oral administration of potassium salts. The oral route should be used whenever feasible, since the relatively slow absorption from the gastrointestinal tract prevents a sudden large increase in serum potassium concentration and this avoids the risk of hyperkalemia which is attendant on administration of potassium intravenously. In this connection, it should be appreciated that restoration of a typical deficit of 200 to 500 mEq. requires the transfer through the extracellular compartment of a quantity of potassium that could raise serum concentration to well above lethal levels. For this reason, when potassium is administered intravenously, it should ordinarily be given at a rate not exceeding 15 to 20 mEq. per hour and at a concentration no higher than 40 to 60 mEq. per liter. It is also generally prudent to limit the supplement to 100 or 150 mEq. per day and to use the serum potassium concentration as a guide to the need for further replacement. If acidosis is present, the serum potassium may be higher than is appropriate to the degree of potassium deficiency, and this discrepancy must be taken into account when treatment is planned. As acidosis is corrected, a more accurate appraisal will be possible. Unfortunately, there is no way of directly calculating the quantity of potassium that will be required for full replacement.

The *electrocardiogram* does not provide a reliable guide to the need for replacement therapy, but is extremely useful as a convenient and rapid means for determining whether an excessive quantity of potassium has been given. The electrocardiogram in hyperkalemia and potassium intoxication is discussed later.

The chloride salt of potassium is used almost exclusively for intravenous therapy, but it has fallen into some disfavor for purposes of oral administration because it produces annoying and sometimes severe upper gastrointestinal symptoms. Such symptoms can be avoided if potassium chloride is used in the enteric-coated form, but this mode of administration occasionally creates other problems. Recent observations suggest that dissolution of the enteric coating in the small intestine and the resulting high local concentration of potassium on the mucosa may produce ulceration, obstruction, or bleeding. For this reason, organic potassium salts, which are more palatable than potassium chloride and which can be given without an enteric coating (and without untoward local effects on the intestine), have come into widespread use. Potassium gluconate and potassium "triplex" (citrate, acetate, and bicarbonate) are the most frequently employed, and are effective agents in patients who are not depleted of chloride. They are, however, relatively ineffective in repairing potassium deficiency when the patient is hypochloremic, alkalotic, and on a low-salt (low-chloride) intake. The explanation for this can be summarized as follows: In hypochloremic alkalosis a smaller than normal fraction of filtered sodium is reabsorbed with chloride and an increased fraction is reabsorbed by exchange with potassium and hydrogen. As long as hypochloremia persists, the accelerated rate of sodium-cation exchange forces a continued high rate of potassium excretion. For this reason, full repair of potassium deficiency cannot be achieved by administration of an organic potassium salt. Potassium must instead be provided as the chloride salt, or chloride must be made available in some other form, such as ammonium chloride or sodium chloride.

Hyperkalemia and Potassium Intoxication

Pathogenesis. Hyperkalemia is most often due to defective renal excretion of potassium. It may arise as the result of primary renal disease, deficiency of adrenal steroids, or the use of aldosterone antagonists (spironolactones) or other agents that inhibit sodium-potassium exchange by the tubule. Excessively rapid intravenous administration of potassium may also elevate plasma concentration to dangerous levels, as has been mentioned earlier in connection with the treatment of potassium deficiency. Potassium given by mouth rarely causes severe hyperkalemia unless renal function is severely impaired.

Hyperkalemia secondary to renal damage occurs frequently in *acute tubular necrosis* or any other form of acute renal failure that is characterized by severe oliguria or anuria. In *chronic renal failure* potassium intoxication is usually encountered only in the terminal stages of the disease, but is sometimes seen earlier as a sequel to the inadvertent administration of potassium supplements. Adrenal insufficiency, due either to *Addison's disease* or, in rare cases, to *primary hypoaldosteronism,* also impairs potassium secretion and may produce hyperkalemia.

The *spironolactones,* which are used in diuretic therapy for the purpose of antagonizing the sodium-retaining effects of aldosterone, do not usually cause significant elevation in serum potassium concentration. They do, however, impair the ability of the kidney to respond to a potassium load, and should not be given in conjunction with potassium supplements. The same caution concerning administration of potassium applies to patients receiving diuretic agents such as triamterene and amiloride, which also impair the exchange of sodium for potassium by the tubule.

Pseudohyperkalemia has been observed in a few patients with thrombocytosis secondary to a myeloproliferative disorder. The spurious elevation of serum concentration results from release of potassium from platelets during the coagulation process. Concentrations as high as 9 mEq. per liter can be found in the serum at a time when plasma (platelet-free) has a normal potassium level. Similar spurious elevations in serum potassium concentration resulting from the release of potassium from white blood cells have recently been reported in several patients with chronic myelogenous leukemia. The possibility that one is dealing with pseudohyperkalemia should be considered whenever an elevated serum potassium concentration cannot otherwise be explained.

Clinical Manifestations. The clinical manifestations of potassium intoxication are related primarily to the heart and the neuromuscular system. *Electrocardiographic abnormalities* are the earliest and most frequent sign of disturbed membrane excitability, and are characterized by the development of tall, "tent-shaped" T waves, by decreased amplitude of the P waves, and later by atrial asystole (Fig. 2). Intraventricular block, with widening of the QRS complex, may lead to the development of a sine wave pattern and ultimately to ventricular standstill. Changes in the electrocardiogram usually appear when the serum potassium concentration reaches 7 to 8 mEq. per liter, and cardiac standstill is likely to occur at a concentration of 9 to 10 mEq. per liter. *Weakness* and *flaccid paralysis* appear only in association with severe hyperkalemia, but are not always present even at plasma levels sufficiently high to produce serious deterioration in the electrocardiogram. Indeed, death from cardiac arrest may occur before muscular weakness is evident. For this reason the electrocardiogram is the single most important guide in appraising the threat posed by the hyperkalemia and in determining how aggressive a therapeutic approach is necessary.

Treatment. The treatment of severe potassium intoxication should be directed toward promoting rapid transfer of potassium into cells in order to lower serum potassium concentration and prevent cardiac arrest. Two approaches to this goal are likely to prove effective. Infusion of glucose and insulin induces the cellular deposition of glycogen and at the same time brings about a shift of potassium to the intracellular space; 1 liter of a 10 per cent glucose solution with 30 to 40 units of insulin is generally employed for this purpose. A further redistribution of potassium can be achieved in the acidotic patient by the administration of sodium bicarbonate (150 to 300 mEq.). In many cases these measures will induce a striking reduction in plasma potassium concentration and prompt improvement in the electrocardiogram. In some instances the administration of calcium (as 2 grams of calcium lactate) is also useful because calcium, though it has no effect on the plasma potassium concentration, opposes the cardiotoxic effects of potassium. It should be noted, incidentally, that calcium cannot be given in the same solution with sodium bicarbonate because precipitation of the calcium ion will result.

Because the techniques described above do not remove potassium from the body and may be only temporarily effective, longer-term effects should be directed toward promoting gastrointestinal losses of potassium. A cation-exchange resin in the sodium cycle, such as Kayexelate, will usually achieve this purpose if administered by mouth in a dose of 20 to 30 grams every six hours. Each gram of resin binds approximately 1 mEq. of potassium, and within 24 hours a significant effect on plasma potassium concentration should be achieved. To enhance potassium loss and assure the rapid movement of the resin through the gastrointestinal tract, sorbitol, a nonreabsorbable polyhydric alcohol, should be given in quantities sufficient to induce a soft or semiliquid bowel movement every few hours. The usual dose for this purpose is 20 ml. of a 70 per cent solution three or four times a day. If the patient is unable to take medication by mouth, the resin can be administered by rectum as a retention enema of 100 grams in several hundred milliliters of water.

Hemodialysis or peritoneal dialysis is efficient alternative means of removing the excess potassium, but usually will not be required if the program outlined above can be implemented.

DISTURBANCES OF ACID-BASE EQUILIBRIUM

The pH of extracellular fluid normally ranges between 7.35 and 7.45, and is stabilized within these limits despite wide variations in the dietary load of acid or alkali. A large number of body functions are importantly influenced by the pH of body fluids, disturbances in acid-base regulation often having serious effects on metabolic activity, on the circulation, and on the central nervous system.

As background to a discussion of the causes of acid-base disturbances, it is instructive to consider briefly the way in which the body deals with the *normal daily acid load* and thus maintains a steady-state of acid-base equilibrium. As food is oxidized, both carbon dioxide (carbonic acid) and nonvolatile acids such as sulfuric and phosphoric acids are added to the extracellular fluid. Immediate buffering within the interstitial fluid, plasma, and red blood cells minimizes the change in pH, and permits large quantities of acid to be

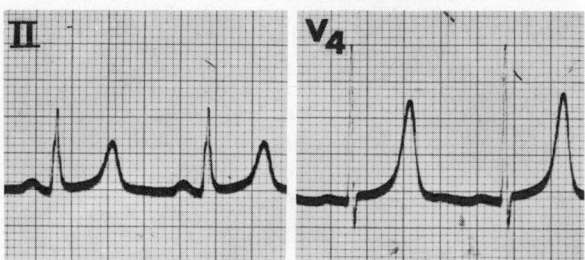

FIGURE 2. Typical electrocardiographic abnormalities induced by a moderate degree of hyperkalemia. (Serum potassium concentration 6.5 mEq. per liter.) Note the typical "tent-shaped" T waves.

transferred to lungs and kidneys for excretion. *Carbon dioxide* is excreted almost entirely by the lungs, and for this reason alveolar carbon dioxide tension is the prime determinant of P_{CO_2} in body fluids. With usual rates of carbon dioxide production, alveolar ventilation maintains the P_{CO_2} of blood at approximately 40 mm. of mercury, that is, 1.2 millimoles of dissolved carbon dioxide per liter of plasma.

Nonvolatile acids are excreted solely by the kidney. The process by which this is accomplished is complex because no significant fraction of the daily hydrogen ion load (some 50 to 100 mEq.) can be excreted in an unbuffered form at the minimal urinary pH of 4.0 that the kidney can establish. As discussed in detail in the article on renal physiology, virtually all hydrogen is removed as either *titratable acid* or *ammonium*. Acidification of the glomerular filtrate by a process of sodium-hydrogen exchange titrates buffers such as phosphate and also favors the diffusion of ammonia (NH_3) from the tubular cells to the lumen, where it reacts with hydrogen ions to form ammonium (NH_4^+). Bicarbonate generated in tubular cells as the result of acid excretion moves into peritubular blood and replenishes the bicarbonate stores that previously were depleted by the buffering of dietary acid. From all these considerations it is evident that derangements in either pulmonary or renal function, or the imposition of stresses that overwhelm normal regulatory mechanisms, can be expected to produce disturbances of acid-base equilibrium.

Because the carbonic acid-bicarbonate buffer pair is the major buffer system in the extracellular fluid, its parameters provide a meaningful and convenient expression of the acid-base status of the organism. The relation between pH and the bicarbonate and carbonic acid concentrations can be expressed in a general fashion according to the familiar Henderson-Hasselbalch equation,

$$pH = pK + \log \frac{HCO_3^-}{H_2CO_3} \quad (1)$$

where pK is the dissociation constant of carbonic acid. In the normal subject this expression will be

$$7.4 = 6.1 + \log \frac{24 \text{ mM/L}}{1.2 \text{ mM/L}} \quad (2)$$

Traditionally, disturbances in acid-balance equilibrium are considered in terms of a change in the ratio of bicarbonate to carbonic acid, but this approach, in the opinion of some, does not always provide the immediate and intuitive insight that can be derived from the following expression:

$$\begin{array}{c} 40 \text{ mm. Hg} \\ P_{CO_2} \\ \nwarrow \searrow \\ H_2CO_3 \rightleftarrows H^+ + HCO_3^- \\ 1.2 \text{ mM/L} \quad pH\ 7.4 \quad 24 \text{ mM/L}. \end{array} \quad (3)$$

This equation allows ready visualization of the directional changes that can be anticipated in

both metabolic and respiratory disturbances of acid-base equilibrium. It is apparent, for example, that a primary reduction in bicarbonate concentration (*metabolic acidosis*) will cause the reaction to shift to the right, thus increasing hydrogen ion concentration, whereas a primary elevation in bicarbonate concentration (*metabolic alkalosis*) will cause the reaction to shift to the left, thus decreasing hydrogen ion concentration. Respiratory disorders can be analyzed in the same fashion. A rise in P_{CO_2} increases the hydrogen ion concentration by shifting the reaction to the right (*respiratory acidosis*), and a fall has the reverse effect (*respiratory alkalosis*). In both metabolic and respiratory acid-base disturbances the widest range of pH values compatible with life is approximately 6.8 to 7.8.

Metabolic Acidosis

Metabolic acidosis results whenever acid is added to the body, alkali is lost from the body, or impaired renal function prevents the excretion of the normal endogenous acid load. In each case the reduction in bicarbonate concentration is accompanied by a rise in hydrogen ion concentration, that is, a decrease in pH.

Physiologic Considerations. The normal organism confronted with a large acid load has a remarkable ability to maintain hydrogen ion concentration within tolerable limits until augmented excretion of acid (and concomitant regeneration of buffer stores) allows restoration of a normal plasma bicarbonate concentration. This resiliency is explained by the magnitude of the total body buffer capacity and the prompt respiratory adjustment of P_{CO_2}.

Body buffers provide a large reservoir of hydrogen ion acceptors distributed through both the extracellular and intracellular compartments. In the extracellular space bicarbonate provides the bulk of the buffer capacity; hemoglobin and plasma proteins, though they make a significant contribution to the buffering ability of *blood*, are of little quantitative importance when viewed in terms of the entire extracellular compartment. Intracellular buffers, which consist largely of protein and organic anions, provide an additional buffer reserve that is responsible for sequestering half or more of an acid load and that serves the important function of protecting against lethal reductions in extracellular bicarbonate concentration and pH. As the price for maintaining electroneutrality during cellular accumulation of hydrogen, both potassium and sodium are forced out of cells. If renal function is normal, the displaced potassium is ultimately lost in the urine. On the other hand, if renal function is impaired or if dehydration has reduced urine volume to oliguric levels, potassium will be retained and potentially dangerous elevations of serum potassium concentration may occur.

Respiratory compensation takes place promptly after the development of metabolic acidosis, an increase in both depth and rate of respiration lowering alveolar and arterial Pco_2. The magnitude of the fall in Pco_2 becomes larger as the reduction in bicarbonate concentration becomes greater, but respiratory defense is never sufficient to restore pH to normal.

Even with the most severe metabolic acidosis, Pco_2 does not fall below 10 mm. of mercury because the physical effort required to produce a further increase in alveolar ventilation increases carbon dioxide production more rapidly than it does pulmonary gas exchange. For this reason, if bicarbonate concentration is very low and maximal reductions in Pco_2 have already been achieved, a slight further fall in bicarbonate concentration will produce a large decrement in pH.

The foregoing comments on respiratory defense have been based, of course, on the assumption that there will be a normal ventilatory response when metabolic acidosis occurs. Indeed, the clinical significance of a given reduction in plasma bicarbonate concentration is judged almost automatically (in the absence of pH measurements) on the basis of experience with the usual degree of respiratory compensation. In some circumstances, however, Pco_2 does not fall in the anticipated manner, and the increase in hydrogen ion concentration will therefore be far greater than is customary. This difficulty will be encountered if the respiratory center has been depressed by sedatives or other medications. It is also seen in the patient with pulmonary disease who, though able to maintain a normal Pco_2 under usual conditions, cannot increase alveolar ventilation to a significant degree under stress. In the patient with a plasma bicarbonate concentration of 10 mEq. per liter, for example, normal respiratory compensation will usually reduce the Pco_2 to approximately 25 mm. of mercury and keep the pH in the range of 7.20 to 7.25, whereas without a reduction in Pco_2 the pH would be 7.00. The measurement of pH, therefore, is often important even in circumstances in which the diagnosis of metabolic acidosis is not in question.

Renal compensation is the final step in the defense against metabolic acidosis, but takes place slowly and does not contribute to the immediate protection of pH. Several days are required before excretion of ammonium and titratable acid rises sufficiently to regenerate bicarbonate and restore plasma concentration to normal. If renal function is impaired, or if underlying renal tubular disease is present, an even longer period may be required for correction to take place.

Pathogenesis (Table 4). *Large Acid Loads as a Cause of Acidosis.* Probably the most frequent cause of metabolic acidosis is the addition of a large acid load to the body fluids. *Diabetic ketoacidosis* is a familiar example of such a disturbance. In diabetic acidosis there is an imbalance between the production and utilization of beta-hydroxybutyric and acetoacetic acids, with the result that both accumulate in the extracellular fluid. Because these acids are almost completely dissociated at the pH of body fluids, nearly 1 millimole of bicarbonate is dissipated by the addition of each millimole of ketoacid.

Accumulation of lactic acid also has recently been recognized as a relatively frequent cause of metabolic acidosis. *Lactic acidosis* is encountered most often under circumstances in which the circulation is compromised by dehydration or hemorrhage, or by inadequate perfusion during cardiopulmonary bypass. In these conditions the failure to supply sufficient oxygen to the tissues induces a shift from aerobic metabolism to anaerobic glycolysis, and produces a lactic acidosis analogous to that occurring with severe exercise. Lactic acidosis may also occur in the absence of any obvious predisposing cause such as hypotension or hypoxemia. The onset is usually abrupt and without warning, and the acidosis is often of great severity. This syndrome of *spontaneous lactic acidosis* is seen in association with a variety of major illnesses, including diabetes mellitus, hepatic failure, subacute bacterial endocarditis, and leukemia. The etiology remains obscure. Lactic acid may also accumulate in other conditions, but the only ones in which clinically significant acidosis occurs are *total fasting in the presence of obesity* and *glycogen-storage disease.*

Poisoning due to the ingestion of salicylates, methyl alcohol, ethylene glycol, or (occasionally) paraldehyde leads to the accumulation of relatively strong and highly dissociated organic acids in the body fluids and to marked reductions in plasma bicarbonate concentration. The specific organic acids responsible for the acidosis in these disorders have not been adequately identified.

Metabolic acidosis can also result from the ingestion of mineral acid such as *ammonium chloride.* The release of hydrogen, as ammonium is converted by the liver to urea, makes the administration of ammonium chloride analogous to the administration of an equivalent quantity of hydrochloric acid. *Lysine hydrochloride* and *arginine hydrochloride* have the same effect on acid-base equilibrium because they too deliver hydrochloric acid to the body fluids. Acidosis resulting from administration of acidifying salts is uncommon, however, because these agents are ordinarily used in conjunction with diuretic agents that tend to produce metabolic alkalosis.

Loss of Alkali as a Cause of Acidosis. Severe *diarrhea* frequently produces metabolic acidosis because liquid stools usually contain bicarbonate in concentrations considerably higher than those in extracellular fluid. Loss of *pancreatic juice,* another highly alkaline solution, also leads to a reduction in plasma bicarbonate concentration. Acidosis of this latter origin is encountered almost exclusively in patients who have undergone prolonged drainage of a pancreatic fistula or of the upper portion of the small bowel.

Transplantation of the ureters into the sigmoid colon for the purpose of urinary diversion (*ureterosigmoidostomy*) leads to pooling of urine in the bowel, and sets into motion two physiologic events that tend to produce metabolic acidosis: movement of bicarbonate from plasma to urine in exchange for chloride directly depletes bicarbonate stores; and reabsorption of ammonium, with the consequent addition of hydrogen ions to the body fluids, further reduces plasma bicarbonate concentration. The more prolonged the period during which urine is in contact with the colonic mucosa, the larger will be these exchanges. Acidosis can usually be avoided or minimized if the rectum is frequently emptied of urine, either voluntarily or by the use of a rectal tube.

Renal Dysfunction as a Cause of Acidosis. Inability of the diseased kidney to deal with the normal dietary load of nonvolatile acid will result in a positive acid balance and consequently in a reduction in plasma bicarbonate concentration. In *acute renal failure* the acid-base disturbance is usually transient and mild. In *chronic renal failure* metabolic acidosis is commonly present over an extended period and can be severe. In most patients with chronic renal failure the problem in acid excretion does not arise from any serious difficulty in acidifying the urine or in forming titratable acid, but is primarily the result of an inability to excrete normal quantities of ammonium. Defective renal reabsorption of bicarbonate is sometimes an additional contributory factor. Despite these abnormalities, plasma bicarbonate is usually stabilized at a level of 15 to 20 mEq. per liter. This new steady state is achieved in part by the enhanced excretion of acid that accompanies the fall in plasma pH and in part by buffering of some portion of the acid load, probably by alkaline bone salts. The equilibrium is precarious, however, and any factor that increases either the intake or the production of acid (or induces a loss of alkali) is likely to precipitate a dangerous degree of metabolic acidosis.

In the foregoing discussion of renal acidosis no mention has been made of the traditional view that retention of "acid anions" such as sulfate and phosphate is responsible for the reduction in plasma bicarbonate concentration. Such a view is obsolescent and is inconsistent with modern concepts of physical chemistry that define an acid as any substance that donates hydrogen ions and a base as any substance that accepts hydrogen ions. In these terms substances such as sulfate and dibasic phosphate are actually weak bases rather than acids, and accumulation of these ions could not be expected to have a significant influence on either bicarbonate concentration or pH. The tendency in many patients for bicarbonate to vary more or less reciprocally with the concentration of accumulated anions appears to be the fortuitous consequence of a parallel progression of glomerular and tubular damage, the reduction in filtration rate causing sulfate and phosphate retention and the damage to tubules impairing acid excretion. It should also be realized that such a parallel change is not inevitable. In some patients, particularly those with chronic pyelonephritis, tubular capacity for acid excretion may be impaired at a time when glomerular filtration rate is only slightly reduced; under these circumstances the fall in plasma bicarbonate concentration is accompanied by an increase in chloride reabsorption that produces a state of so-called hyperchloremic acidosis.

Hyperchloremic acidosis is also seen in an uncommon form of renal disease known as *renal tubular acidosis,* a disorder primarily affecting tubules rather than glomeruli. It is also observed in *Fanconi's syndrome,* a rare disease characterized by a multiplicity of tubular defects. Both these disorders are discussed in detail elsewhere in this volume.

Metabolic acidosis accompanied by hyperchloremia also follows the administration of *carbonic anhydrase inhibitors* such as acetazolamide. Carbonic anhydrase has an essential role in making hydrogen available for secretion by renal tubular cells, and inhibition of this enzyme impairs the cation-exchange process, and reduces both sodium reabsorption and acid excretion. Carbonic anhydrase inhibitors, because of their ability to increase sodium excretion, were at one time widely used as diuretics, but proved to be of relatively limited value because the modest diuresis which they produce is short-lived; the prompt development of metabolic acidosis quickly impairs the effectiveness of these agents, and a rest period of several days must then be allowed to permit regeneration of bicarbonate and restoration of a normal plasma bicarbonate concentration.

Diagnosis. Hyperventilation is the only clinical finding characteristic of metabolic acidosis, and even this sign is sometimes difficult to detect. Some patients with acidosis of long duration appear to be breathing nearly normally at a time when measurements of Pco_2 demonstrate a striking increase in alveolar ventilation. Other clinical disturbances such as lethargy and coma are frequently seen in the patient with severe acidosis, but it is frequently difficult to decide whether these abnormalities are a manifestation of the acidosis per se or of the underlying disease, for example, diabetic acidosis or uremia.

In most cases, the history, in conjunction with the low plasma bicarbonate concentration and other routine chemical studies, will provide the basis for a tentative diagnosis of metabolic acidosis. However, since plasma bicarbonate concentration can also be reduced by primary hyperventilation (*vide infra*), a measurement of pH will be necessary in order to distinguish with certainty between respiratory alkalosis and metabolic acidosis. Subsequent measurements of pH will also serve the important function of providing a guide to effective clinical management.

Once the presence of metabolic acidosis has been documented, it is important to determine the exact cause. In many cases the cause is obvious, but in other instances it is obscure, and some rapid and systematic approach to differential diagnosis is invaluable. Particularly helpful is the calculation of the so-called "anion gap," or concentration of unmeasured anions, in plasma. This value, which is estimated by subtraction of the sum of chloride and bicarbonate concentrations from that of sodium, is normally about 10 to 12 milliequivalents per liter (Fig. 3, column I), and represents negative charges contributed to plasma by ions other than chloride and bicarbonate (chiefly phosphate, sulfate, organic anions, and the anionic groups of plasma proteins).

In the patient with metabolic acidosis the reduction in bicarbonate concentration may or may not be accompanied by an increase in the "anion gap"; this distinction, which can be made on the basis of routine electrolyte measurements, immediately narrows the range of diagnostic possibilities (Table 4). If the concentration of unmeasured anions is increased (Fig. 3, column III), it can be concluded that hydrogen has been added to the body fluids with some anion other than chloride. This finding suggests a diagnosis of diabetic ketoacidosis, drug poisoning, renal failure, or lactic acidosis, and gives direction to further studies designed to identify the specific cause of the acid-base disturbance. Lactic acidosis is likely to pose the only special diagnostic problem because lactate determinations are not routinely available in most hospitals. In nearly all cases, however, a tentative diagnosis of lactic acidosis can be made by exclusion of the other disorders characterized by an increased concentration of undetermined anions.

If, on the other hand, the "anion gap" is not increased (Fig. 3, column II), the reduction in bicarbonate concentration can clearly be attributed either to the accumulation of hydrogen with chloride or to a loss of bicarbonate. With the spectrum thus narrowed, it should again be relatively

TABLE 4. CAUSES OF METABOLIC ACIDOSIS

With Increase in Unmeasured Anions	Without Increase in Unmeasured Anions
Diabetic ketoacidosis	Diarrhea
Salicylate poisoning	Drainage of pancreatic juice
Ethylene glycol poisoning	Ureterosigmoidostomy
Methyl alcohol poisoning	Carbonic anhydrase inhibitors
Paraldehyde (rarely)	Ammonium chloride
Lactic acidosis	Renal tubular acidosis
Renal failure	

easy to identify the underlying disorder. A history of diarrhea, or of the ingestion of an acidifying agent such as ammonium chloride or acetazolamide, will often clarify the problem. The finding of a relatively alkaline urine and of nephrocalcinosis on roentgenographic examination of the abdomen will strongly suggest the diagnosis of renal tubular acidosis.

In some patients, of course, several causes of metabolic acidosis may be present simultaneously, and this possibility should not be overlooked. If, for example, the disappearance of ketonemia during the treatment of diabetic acidosis is not accompanied by restoration of a normal plasma bicarbonate concentration, the presence of a coexistent disorder such as lactic acidosis should be suspected.

Treatment. General Principles. Treatment should ordinarily be directed toward any reversible abnormality, such as ketosis or shock, which may be responsible for the acidosis. However, if the underlying disturbance is not amenable to treatment, or if acidosis is life-threatening, alkali therapy will be necessary. Calculation of the amount of alkali to be administered must take into account not only the depletion of extracellular bicarbonate stores but also the magnitude of the intracellular acidosis. As mentioned earlier, a large fraction of an acid load is sequestered in cells, and restoration of normal acid-base equilibrium, therefore, involves repair of total body buffer stores. Estimates of alkali requirements should thus assume "distribution" of bicarbonate through a volume equivalent to 50 per cent of body weight. The calculation for full repair can be summarized by the following expression:

$$(25 \text{ mEq. per liter} - \text{observed plasma HCO}_3 \text{ conc.})$$
$$\times \ 0.5 \text{ body weight (kg.)} = \text{mEq. of alkali.}$$

The figure of 50 per cent for the distribution of bicarbonate is only approximate, but clinical experience has demonstrated that therapy based on this assumption usually induces a rise in plasma bicarbonate concentration close to the predicted level.

In most patients with severe acidosis immediate correction of the entire alkali deficit is unnecessary; if bicarbonate concentration is increased to 15 or 20 mEq. per liter, plasma pH will be returned to a safe level, and renal adjustments (or continued treatment of the underlying metabolic abnormality) can be relied upon to complete the corrective process. More rapid correction may, in

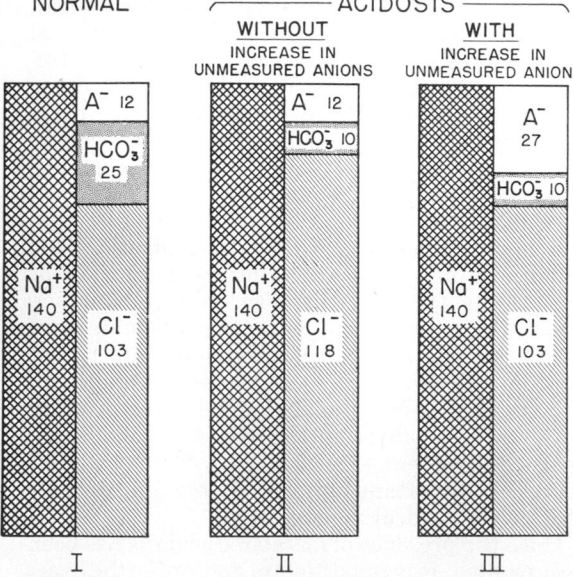

NORMAL   ——— ACIDOSIS ———
                WITHOUT   WITH
                INCREASE IN   INCREASE IN
                UNMEASURED ANIONS UNMEASURED ANIONS

Column I: A⁻ 12, HCO₃⁻ 25, Na⁺ 140, Cl⁻ 103
Column II: A⁻ 12, HCO₃⁻ 10, Na⁺ 140, Cl⁻ 118
Column III: A⁻ 27, HCO₃⁻ 10, Na⁺ 140, Cl⁻ 103

I   II   III

FIGURE 3. Composition of plasma in various forms of metabolic acidosis, with special reference to the concentration of unmeasured anions ("anion gap"). Column I shows that anions other than chloride and bicarbonate normally make up approximately 12 mEq. per liter of the total anion content of plasma. Columns II and III indicate that acidosis can develop with or without an associated increase in concentration of unmeasured anions. The various causes of acidosis that will produce these patterns are listed in Table 4, and the way in which the "anion gap" can be used in differential diagnosis is discussed in the text.

fact, be undesirable. If bicarbonate concentration is quickly restored to normal or nearly normal levels, blood pH may become frankly alkaline. This apparently paradoxical behavior is the consequence of persistent hyperventilation which often maintains a state of hypocapnia for as long as one or two days after bicarbonate stores have been replenished.

During the correction of metabolic acidosis, the movement of potassium into cells in exchange for hydrogen tends to lower serum potassium concentration. In the patient with hyperkalemia and potassium intoxication this serves a useful therapeutic purpose, as discussed earlier. If, however, serum potassium concentration is normal, the transfer of potassium from the extracellular fluid may produce hypokalemia and signs of potassium deficiency, including respiratory paralysis. This sequence of events has been noted with particular frequency during the correction of diabetic keto-acidosis, but it may also occur during the repair of other acidotic states. For this reason careful clinical observation and occasional measurements of serum potassium concentration should be carried out in the course of treatment to determine the need for replacement of potassium deficits.

Special Problems in Management. Some of the disorders that cause metabolic acidosis present particular problems in management. This discussion considers such problems as they occur in lactic acidosis, diabetic ketoacidosis, and renal acidosis; salicylate poisoning and methyl alcohol poisoning are dealt with in detail elsewhere in this volume.

In metabolic acidosis resulting from the accumulation of either ketoacids or lactic acid there is the potential for prompt and full correction of the bicarbonate deficit without administration of exogenous alkali. In both diabetic and lactic acidosis, the anion that has accumulated in the body fluids, if fully oxidized, will regenerate an equivalent quantity of bicarbonate, and will restore plasma bicarbonate concentration to normal. A familiar physiologic example of this behavior is seen with the lactic acidosis of exercise; after exertion is discontinued, acidosis is rapidly corrected according to the following reaction:

$$Na^+ + CH_3CH(OH)COO^- + HOH + 3O_2$$

$$\rightarrow \underbrace{Na^+ + OH^-}_{} + \underbrace{3CO_2}_{} + 3H_2O \qquad (4)$$

$$\underbrace{Na^+HCO_3^- + 2CO_2}_{}$$

In *diabetic ketoacidosis* full and rapid oxidation of the organic anion occurs promptly after the administration of adequate quantities of insulin and glucose, and it is for this reason that most patients with ketoacidosis do not require alkali therapy. On the other hand, it is reasonable to administer small quantities of alkali if, at the time of admission, the patient is found to have acidosis of life-threatening severity. Such treatment will have an important influence on pH at a time before insulin can exert a significant effect, and will lead to only an inconsequential degree of alkalosis after ketosis has been fully corrected.

The ease with which *lactic acidosis* can be corrected depends on the cause of the metabolic abnormality. If shock is responsible for the shift to anaerobic glycolysis, transfusions or other means of restoring blood volume and blood pressure will usually correct the acid-base disturbance. If the cause is inadequate perfusion during a cardiopulmonary bypass procedure, this difficulty can in most cases also be remedied. Lactic acidosis of unknown cause (*spontaneous lactic acidosis*) poses a completely different problem. Specific means for remedying the defect in lactate metabolism are not available, and one must therefore rely solely on alkali therapy. Treatment is often further complicated by the unpredictable response to administration of alkali; in some cases there is little or no rise in bicarbonate concentration despite administration of an amount of bicarbonate that, by usual estimates, would be more than sufficient to restore the plasma level to normal. The explanation for this "resistance" to therapy presumably lies in continued addition of lactic acid to the body fluids during the period of treatment. On the other hand, bicarbonate concentration will sometimes rise even without treatment as a spontaneous increase in the oxidation of lactate suddenly regenerates large quantities of bicarbonate. In the patient who has previously been given alkali, frank metabolic alkalosis may be the result. For these reasons the acid-base status must be monitored closely during the course of therapy. It should be emphasized that even when the acid-base disorder is well controlled, the majority of patients with spontaneous lactic acidosis do not survive. Any therapeutic approach directed toward the acid-base disturbance alone will obviously be far from satisfactory because it deals with effect rather than cause. In this connection it should be noted that problems analogous to those seen in spontaneous lactic acidosis were encountered in the management of diabetic acidosis during the preinsulin era; resistance to alkali therapy was common, and death frequently occurred even after plasma bicarbonate concentration was restored to normal.

Chronic *renal acidosis* poses still a different problem. There is no accumulation of organic anion from which bicarbonate can be regenerated, and irreversible renal damage ordinarily precludes correction of the underlying tubular abnormality responsible for the acid-base disturbance. For this reason, sole reliance must be placed on alkali therapy if plasma bicarbonate concentration is to be increased. Fortunately, in most patients with renal insufficiency the degree of metabolic acidosis is not sufficiently great to demand treatment; reductions in bicarbonate concentration to 16 or 18 mEq. per liter, which occur commonly, do not appear to cause symptoms or to aggravate the uremic syndrome. If, however, acidosis becomes sufficiently serious to warrant treatment, either sodium bicarbonate or sodium citrate can be given by mouth in doses of several grams per day; plasma bicarbonate concentration need not and, in fact, probably should not be raised to normal because of the risk of precipitating tetany if hypocalcemia is present. Sometimes the ingestion of alkali precipitates nausea or vomiting, and under these circumstances it may be necessary to discontinue treatment. Sodium bicarbonate is more likely than sodium citrate to produce gastrointestinal symptoms.

If the patient has a sodium-retaining state such as congestive heart failure, it is wise to defer administration of alkali as long as possible and, if treatment must be given, to restrict dietary sodium intake sharply.

The management of *renal tubular acidosis* and *Fanconi's syndrome* and the relation of renal acidosis to bone disease are discussed elsewhere.

Choice of an Alkalinizing Agent. Two agents, *sodium bicarbonate* and *sodium lactate* have been widely employed in patients requiring the intravenous administration of alkali. Until recent years only sodium lactate was readily available for intravenous therapy because packaging problems prevented the commercial preparation of suitable bicarbonate solutions. Sodium lactate is usually an effective and satisfactory means of treatment, but has the disadvantage that it depends on the intervention of oxidative processes to make bicarbonate available (Equation 4). Thus, if there is a defect in lactate metabolism, as in lactic acidosis, the prompt and quantitative conversion of lactate to bicarbonate cannot be relied upon. Bicarbonate, on the other hand, is ideally suited to the treatment of metabolic acidosis because it directly replenishes depleted buffer stores. Now that bicarbonate preparations for intravenous administration are readily available, it appears that tradition alone is responsible for perpetuating the use of lactate.

Bicarbonate can also be provided by the administration of *THAM* (tris-[hydroxymethyl]aminomethane), an organic buffer with a pK of 7.8, which reacts with carbonic acid according to the following equation:

$$THAM + H_2CO_3 \leftrightarrows THAMH^+ + HCO_3^- \quad (5)$$

It is not clear, however, that any advantage accrues from the administration of bicarbonate with, in effect, cationic THAM rather than sodium. THAM, or tris buffer, is toxic when given in large doses and furthermore may produce serious injury to tissue at the site of infusion because it is administered as an intensely alkaline solution (pH 10). Parenthetically, it should be noted that the slight and transient reduction in carbon dioxide tension that follows an infusion of THAM is of no clinical significance in the patient with metabolic acidosis. The possible role of THAM in the treatment of *respiratory acidosis* will be discussed later in this section.

Metabolic Alkalosis

Metabolic alkalosis results from either an abnormal loss of acid or an excessive retention of alkali. In each case the rise in bicarbonate concentration induces a fall in hydrogen ion concentration, that is, an increase in pH.

Physiologic Considerations. As in metabolic acidosis, pH is defended to a significant extent by *tissue buffering*. In response to alkalinization of the extracellular fluid, hydrogen ions migrate from cells to extracellular space (in exchange for sodium and potassium), and thus mitigate the severity of the acid-base disturbance.

Respiratory compensation may serve as an additional mitigating factor. Diminished ventilation and a resulting rise in Pco_2 tends to restore a more normal ratio between the concentrations of carbonic acid and bicarbonate. In contrast to metabolic acidosis, however, the magnitude of the respiratory compensation is usually small, and becomes significant only when plasma bicarbonate concentration rises to 35 or 40 mEq. per liter.

Renal excretion is the route for removal of excess alkali, and is thus ultimately responsible for the correction of metabolic alkalosis. Normally, the kidneys reabsorb approximately 25 mEq. of bicarbonate per liter of glomerular filtrate, and when plasma concentration is elevated above this level by ingestion or infusion of alkali, the excess bicarbonate is rapidly and quantitatively excreted. Thus, even a large alkali load can induce only a transient alkalosis so long as the bicarbonate threshold is not elevated. The following theoretical example will serve to illustrate this point. If plasma bicarbonate is raised from 25 mEq. per liter to 35 mEq. per liter, 10 mEq. of bicarbonate will be excreted each time a liter of glomerular filtrate is formed. With a glomerular filtration rate of 180 liters per day, daily excretion would thus be 1800 mEq. Maintenance of the metabolic alkalosis would therefore require either the daily administration of 150 grams of sodium bicarbonate or the loss per day of 18 liters of gastric juice containing 0.1N HCl. Although such circumstances are rarely, if ever, encountered clinically, sustained elevations of plasma bicarbonate concentration do occur with considerable frequency. Indeed, plasma concentrations of 40 to 50 mEq. per liter are seen even in patients who are neither receiving bicarbonate nor losing gastric juice. This finding clearly indicates that the renal threshold for bicarbonate must be abnormally high, a conclusion borne out by the fact that the urine of the alkalotic patient typically has a pH in the acid range and contains virtually no bicarbonate. The problem confronting the physician, therefore, is the identification and correction of the cause of the defect in bicarbonate excretion.

Before the causes of metabolic alkalosis are considered, it seems desirable to review briefly the mechanism of bicarbonate reabsorption, which has been considered in detail in the subsection on Renal Physiology. Reabsorption of bicarbonate takes place by an indirect process involving the transport of sodium from the glomerular filtrate and the secretion of hydrogen into the lumen in its place. The addition of hydrogen to the filtrate converts bicarbonate to carbonic acid, but at the same time generates an equivalent quantity of bicarbonate in the renal tubular cells; the subsequent diffusion of this bicarbonate into the peritubular blood serves as the mode of bicarbonate "reabsorption." It is evident that any stimulus that increases the rate of sodium-hydrogen exchange will also increase bicarbonate reabsorption, and will sustain a metabolic alkalosis.

Pathogenesis (Table 5). A variety of clinical disturbances can produce metabolic alkalosis, but most of these can be grouped under the general headings of *losses from the upper gastrointestinal tract,* *diuretic therapy,* or *hyperadrenocorticism.* To account for the alkalosis in each of these settings one must ascertain both the source of the bicarbonate that elevates plasma concentration and, as alluded to earlier, the mechanisms responsible for the persistently increased reabsorption of bicarbonate.

Ordinarily, the factor responsible for the generation of new bicarbonate is easily identified. With vomiting or gastric aspiration, for example, it is the loss of hydrogen as hydrochloric acid. Diuretics such as ethacrynic acid or the mercurials increase excretion of hydrogen by the kidney. Augmented renal excretion of hydrogen also accounts for the generation of bicarbonate by adrenal steroids; accelerated sodium-hydrogen exchange diverts abnormal quantities of acid into the urine and increases body alkali stores.

The second problem, that is, the explanation for the increased reabsorption of bicarbonate, is more complex and may involve many factors, including sodium depletion, dehydration, potassium depletion, and chloride deficiency. Loss of sodium and an associated contraction of extracellular volume restricts bicarbonate excretion by increasing the avidity of the renal tubule for sodium and thus accelerating sodium-hydrogen exchange. In the past it has generally been thought, however, that the single most frequent cause for maintenance of a high bicarbonate threshold is a deficiency of potassium. Potassium deficiency and hypokalemia are prominent features in nearly all cases of alkalosis, and the terms "metabolic alkalosis" and "hypokalemic alkalosis" have, in clinical parlance, come to be almost synonymous.

Potassium and hydrogen compete for exchange with sodium, and a deficiency of potassium is thought to enhance the rate of hydrogen ion secretion and of bicarbonate reabsorption.

Recent observations have suggested, however, that the importance of potassium deficiency may have been overemphasized, and it has been proposed that chloride depletion and hypochloremia, which are consistently present in metabolic alkalosis, are frequently the critical factors in maintenance of the high bicarbonate threshold. It has been shown, for example, that experimental alkalosis in man can be corrected by restoration of the chloride deficit even in the face of a considerable degree of potassium depletion. The influence of chloride on the regulation of acid-base equilibrium can be viewed as follows: Normally, that is, with a sodium concentration of 140 mEq. per liter and a chloride concentration of 105 mEq. per liter, about four fifths of the filtered sodium is reabsorbed with chloride, and the remainder by exchange with potassium and hydrogen. In the hypochloremic patient, less chloride is available for reabsorption with sodium, and an increased fraction of the sodium load is conserved by acceleration of sodium-cation exchange. As long as hypochloremia and a tubular avidity for sodium persist, the increased rate of cation exchange and bicarbonate reabsorption will continue. The interplay of potassium and chloride in the genesis and maintenance of various alkalotic states remains to be further clarified, but it is evident that the situation is more complex than has generally been thought.

Little is known about the mechanism responsible for the high bicarbonate threshold in *Cushing's syndrome* or *primary aldosteronism,* or during *administration of adrenal corticoids.* Patients with hyperadrenocorticism are depleted of potassium and are hypochloremic, but have persistent metabolic alkalosis despite a normal intake of potassium, chloride, and all other electrolytes. Alkalosis can be corrected, however, by administration of large amounts of supplementary potassium chloride. The alkalosis encountered in the *syndrome of juxtaglomerular hyperplasia with secondary aldosteronism (Bartter's syndrome)* has the special characteristic, as discussed earlier, of being quite resistant to correction by potassium chloride. Supplements of several hundred milliequivalents may be necessary to maintain a normal or nearly normal bicarbonate concentration. The nature of the abnormality in tubular function responsible for this behavior awaits further investigation.

Metabolic alkalosis has also been reported to occur with a small but significant frequency in patients with *hypercalcemia.* In some of the cases, however, vomiting or steroid therapy may have been responsible for the alkalosis, and in others the published data are not sufficient to permit critical evaluation of this possibility. At present, therefore, it is still not clear whether hypercalcemia per se does cause alkalosis in man. The syndrome of *posthypercapneic alkalosis* is discussed later under Respiratory Acidosis.

TABLE 5. CAUSES OF METABOLIC ALKALOSIS

Vomiting or gastric drainage
Diuretic therapy
    Mercurials
    Ethacrynic acid
    Thiazides
    Furosemide
Cushing's syndrome
Primary aldosteronism
Bartter's syndrome
Adrenal steroid therapy
Relief of chronic hypercapnia

Diagnosis. There are no signs or symptoms specific for metabolic alkalosis. The diagnosis is usually suspected because there is a history of vomiting, because therapy with diuretics or adrenal steroids has been given, or because the patient has undergone prolonged gastric drainage. Occasionally, an elevation of bicarbonate concentration is discovered accidentally when, for unrelated reasons, serum electrolyte concentrations have been measured. An unequivocal diagnosis of metabolic alkalosis can be made only after pH is shown to be increased, but, as a practical matter, an elevated bicarbonate concentration in a patient without significant pulmonary disease can be taken as virtually diagnostic.

The finding of unexplained metabolic alkalosis will sometimes lead to the diagnosis of *Cushing's syndrome* even when there are few, if any, clinical signs of the disease. This sequence of events is most likely to occur with adrenal hyperfunction associated with extra-adrenal neoplasms. The tumor most likely to produce this syndrome is bronchogenic carcinoma.

Treatment. The treatment of metabolic alkalosis (other than that due to an excess of adrenal steroids) consists of correction of dehydration and of the various ionic deficits. If sodium and volume depletion are present, they should be repaired by the administration of sodium chloride and water, either by mouth or by vein, depending on the state of the patient. The potassium deficit that regularly accompanies metabolic alkalosis should be repaired with potassium chloride. Organic potassium salts, for example, "triplex" and gluconate, are not effective in correcting either potassium deficiency or alkalosis unless adequate amounts of chloride are made available either in the electrolyte supplement or in the diet. As discussed earlier, in hypochloremic states there is a high rate of cation exchange, and neither the rate of potassium secretion nor that of hydrogen secretion can be reduced to normal until the chloride deficit has been remedied.

In most cases, correction of the volume and electrolyte deficits will increase alkali excretion and restore normal acid-base equilibrium within several days. On occasion, however, an extreme degree of metabolic alkalosis may necessitate a more direct and intensive approach to therapy. In the Zollinger-Ellison syndrome, for example, continuous and massive losses of hydrochloric acid may elevate the plasma bicarbonate concentration to 60 mEq. per liter or above, and direct titration of the excess bicarbonate by the intravenous administration of hydrochloric acid, as ammonium chloride or arginine hydrochloride, may be imperative.

If ammonium chloride is used, it must be given slowly and under close observation because, if the rate of infusion exceeds the capacity of the liver to convert ammonium to urea, lethal ammonium intoxication may occur. This risk will be greatly increased if there is any element of underlying hepatic disease. Arginine hydrochloride has recently come into favor as an alternative and

safer means of providing hydrochloric acid intravenously.

In treating patients who are receiving diuretics that tend to produce metabolic alkalosis, it may at times be desirable to administer an acidifying salt by mouth. Ammonium chloride is the agent most commonly used for this purpose, and can be given without hazard if liver disease is not present. It is usually administered as an enteric-coated form because otherwise it gives rise to unpleasant gastric symptoms. An amino acid salt such as lysine monohydrochloride is another useful vehicle for the oral provision of acid.

When metabolic alkalosis is due to primary adrenal disease, the definitive treatment consists of the surgical removal of the offending adrenal tissue. If steroid therapy is responsible for the acid-base disturbance, the dose of hormone should be reduced, or, if this is not feasible, potassium chloride should be given to supplement the normal dietary intake.

RESPIRATORY ACIDOSIS

Respiratory acidosis results from any disturbance in ventilation that increases arterial Pco_2. An elevation of Pco_2 shifts the normal equilibrium of the bicarbonate–carbonic acid buffer system and increases the plasma hydrogen ion concentration (that is, it decreases pH). This effect on pH is mitigated, however, by a secondary increase in plasma bicarbonate concentration that is dependent on two biologic mechanisms. During acute hypercapnia bicarbonate is generated by the titration of body buffers. With more prolonged elevation of Pco_2, additional bicarbonate is added to the extracellular fluid as the result of augmented renal acid excretion. A concomitant rise in the renal capacity for bicarbonate reabsorption permits conservation of the new bicarbonate and allows plasma concentration to be stabilized at an elevated level. Experimental studies indicate that the complete process of renal adaptation to hypercapnia requires several days or longer. It is apparent from these considerations that the extent of physiologic adjustment to a given degree of hypercapnia varies as a function of time and that intelligent appraisal of the acid-base changes in respiratory acidosis requires a knowledge of the duration of the ventilatory disturbance.

Pathogenesis. *Acute respiratory acidosis* occurs in a variety of clinical settings. Airway obstruction or hypoventilation resulting from anesthesia, neuromuscular disorders, or central nervous system disease are perhaps the most frequent causes. Abnormal ventilation-perfusion ratios and low compliance may also produce acute hypercapnia in disorders such as pneumonia, atelectasis, or pulmonary edema. Extreme respiratory acidosis is also often encountered in cardiopulmonary arrest.

Chronic respiratory acidosis is seen with progressive lung diseases such as emphysema or chronic asthmatic bronchitis. The disturbance in gas exchange results from alveolar hypoventilation secondary to unfavorable pulmonary mechanics and associated imbalance between distribution of ventilation and blood flow. Pulmonary diseases characterized primarily by diffusion abnormalities do not cause hypercapnia until late in the course of the illness.

Diagnosis. The tentative diagnosis of *acute respiratory acidosis* can often be made on clinical grounds alone if there is obvious impairment of ventilation. The definitive diagnosis depends, however, on demonstration that Pco$_2$ is elevated and that plasma pH is reduced. These measurements are of particular importance when clinical observation cannot be relied upon to reveal an impairment of gas exchange, as, for example, in the patient who is being artificially ventilated or who is suffering from intoxication with barbiturates or other central nervous system depressants.

Chronic respiratory acidosis should be suspected in any patient with the symptoms and physical findings of severe lung disease. Classically, the diagnosis rests on the finding of an elevated Pco$_2$ accompanied by a low pH. However, it is now recognized that in some patients with chronic pulmonary disease hypercapnia may occur in conjunction with a normal or even a high pH. This observation has sometimes been interpreted as indicating full compensation or even "overcompensation" for the respiratory acidosis, but it seems more likely that such a finding can best be attributed to a complicating metabolic alkalosis (*vide infra*). This difference in interpretation highlights the difficulty in deciding whether a patient with chronic pulmonary insufficiency is suffering from respiratory acidosis alone or from a mixed disorder in which metabolic components are also present. The answer to this dilemma is obviously of importance in both diagnosis and therapy.

Hypercapnia and Mixed Acid-Base Disorders. Just as a variety of illnesses, e.g., vomiting, diarrhea, may produce a metabolic acid-base disturbance in the normal subject, they can do the same in the patient with hypercapnia. To recognize and quantitate the magnitude of a complicating metabolic disturbance in pulmonary insufficiency, *one must have prior knowledge of the pH and bicarbonate concentration appropriate to the given degree of uncomplicated hypercapnia.* Recent observations on changes in plasma composition during exposure of normal subjects to various degrees of acute hypercapnia have provided a background for the appraisal of the acid-base status in *acute* respiratory acidosis. As shown in Figure 4, over a range of carbon dioxide tension up to 90 mm. of mercury there is only a slight rise in plasma bicarbonate concentration. From this response curve and other available information, it appears that in uncomplicated acute hypercapnia of mild or moderate severity the bicarbonate concentration should lie between 25 and 30 mEq. per liter. Concentrations above 30 mEq. per liter will indicate the presence of a complicating metabolic alkalosis, and those

below 25 mEq. per liter, the presence of a complicating metabolic acidosis.

Unfortunately, physiologic observations on the response to *chronic* hypercapnia are available only in the dog, but data on patients with chronic lung disease suggest that the pattern of response which has been defined experimentally is closely similar to that which occurs clinically. Figure 4 illustrates schematically how data on the adaptation to chronic hypercapnia can be utilized in the analysis of complex acid-base disorders. This figure contains four schematic diagrams depicting, by vectors, the ways in which the acid-base status in pre-existing chronic respiratory acidosis can be deranged. For purposes of discussion, the initial Pco$_2$ is assumed to be 65 mm. of mercury.

Figure 4a contains the vector for a superimposed metabolic alkalosis. The bicarbonate concentration lies above the level appropriate for chronic adaptation to a Pco$_2$ of 65 mm. of mercury, and indicates that there has been a pathologic loss of acid or retention of alkali. Such deviations of bicarbonate in the alkaline direction, occurring as a result of diuretics, steroid therapy, or vomiting, could have important clinical consequences since an inappropriately high pH may diminish respiratory drive and aggravate the pre-existing degree of hypoxemia.

Figure 4b shows the pathway of a superimposed metabolic acidosis. A mild degree of metabolic acidosis, as indicated by the solid portion of the vector, will produce bicarbonate concentrations in the zone lying between the acute and chronic response curves. With a more severe metabolic disturbance, as shown by the dotted extension of the vector, the bicarbonate concentration will be depressed to a level below even the acute response curve.

Figure 4c demonstrates the sequence that will ensue when an acute increase in Pco$_2$ is superimposed on chronic hypercapnia. This disturbance occurs in association with such common complications as pneumonia, heart failure, and excessive sedation, all of which may further compromise alveolar ventilation. As an element of *acute* hypercapnia develops, body buffers would be expected to generate only a small additional amount of bicarbonate, and, as indicated by the vector, plasma bicarbonate concentration should follow a course roughly parallel to the acute titration curve. For a period of several days—that is, until there is renal compensation appropriate to the new level of hypercapnia—the bicarbonate concentration will remain at a point below the chronic response curve. It should be noted in Figure 4 that when either mild metabolic acidosis (Fig. 4b) or acute hypercapnia (Fig. 4c) is superimposed on chronic respiratory acidosis, the bicarbonate values will lie between the acute and chronic response curves. Obviously, the acid-base parameters per se cannot be used to differentiate these two complications, and additional clinical information will be required.

Figure 4d contains the vector resulting from

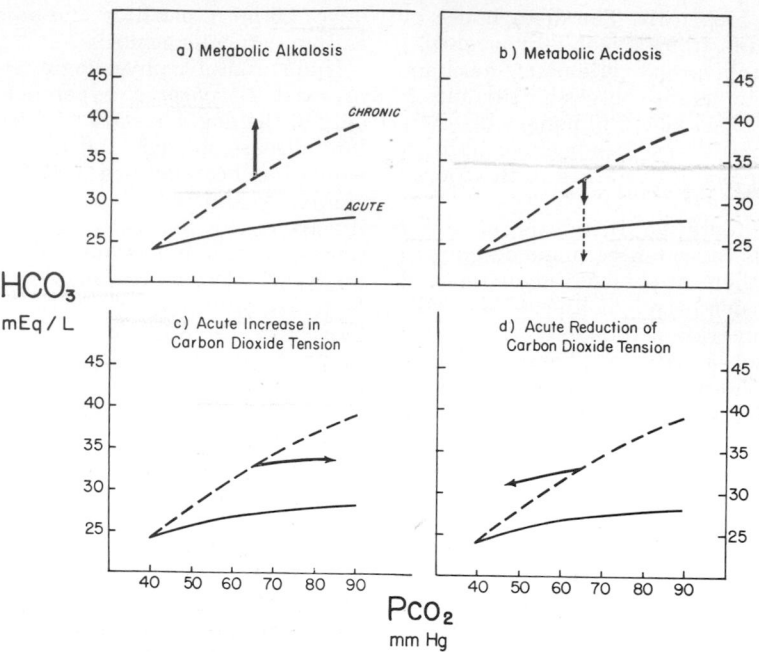

FIGURE 4. Schematic diagram of pathways followed by the acid-base disturbances that may complicate chronic respiratory acidosis. The *solid* lines represent the bicarbonate concentrations observed during acute hypercapnia in man and the *dashed* lines the bicarbonate concentrations seen during chronic hypercapnia in the dog. The origin of each vector has been placed arbitrarily at a point depicting physiologically complete adaption to a Pco_2 of 65 mm. of mercury. Each panel is discussed in detail in the text. (Reproduced by permission of the American Journal of Medicine.)

a recent improvement in alveolar ventilation. A sudden fall in Pco_2 will titrate body buffers toward normal and induce a fall in bicarbonate concentration. This titration would not be expected, however, immediately to erase the renal component of the initial increment in extracellular bicarbonate stores. Plasma bicarbonate concentration, therefore, will be high in relation to the Pco_2, a condition that has been termed "*posthypercapneic alkalosis.*" Under most circumstances the kidney will slowly excrete the excess bicarbonate and the condition will disappear within a day or two. In certain cases, however, the reabsorptive capacity for bicarbonate does not fall, and metabolic alkalosis persists for an extended period. A restricted intake of chloride (for example, in patients on a low-salt diet) probably has a key role in producing this syndrome; as discussed earlier, retention of chloride and correction of hypochloremia are prerequisites to reduction of an elevated bicarbonate concentration to normal levels.

Treatment. The treatment of *acute respiratory acidosis* should be directed toward the underlying cause of the impaired ventilation. The measures required obviously will depend on the nature of the clinical problem. If, for example, alveolar gas exchange is impeded by bronchospasm, bronchodilators should be used. If inadequate ventilation is the result of a neuromuscular disturbance, artificial ventilation may be necessary.

The treatment of *chronic respiratory acidosis* should also be directed primarily toward improving alveolar ventilation, not toward the restoration of a normal pH. Bronchodilators, adrenal steroids, antimicrobials, postural drainage, and artificial ventilation may all have a valuable place in therapy at one time or another in the course of the illness. The management of pulmonary insufficiency is dealt with in detail elsewhere, but a word of caution should be repeated here concerning the possible hazards of oxygen therapy in worsening chronic respiratory acidosis. In severe hypercapnia the sensitivity of the respiratory center to carbon dioxide may be diminished and, if this occurs, hypoxemia becomes the major stimulus to respiratory activity. If hypoxemia is then partially or totally corrected, ventilation often undergoes further serious impairment, hypercapnia becomes increasingly severe, and the patient can lapse into coma and die. Thus during oxygen therapy the patient must be watched closely to ensure that improvement in the degree of hypoxemia does not depress ventilation.

The use of an organic buffer such as THAM for the purpose of lowering Pco_2 (Equation 5) has little or nothing to recommend it; the rise in pH that follows the reaction of THAM with carbonic acid usually reduces minute ventilation and thus aggravates the pre-existing hypoxemia. This problem can be circumvented if the patient is given artificial ventilation, but even under such circumstances, THAM has little practical value; control of hypercapnia for more than one or two hours would require amounts of THAM far in excess of what can safely be administered.

Respiratory Alkalosis

Respiratory alkalosis results from any disturbance in ventilation that lowers arterial carbon dioxide tension. A reduction in P_{CO_2} shifts the normal equilibrium of the bicarbonate–carbonic acid buffer system and decreases the plasma hydrogen ion concentration (that is, it increases pH). This effect on pH is mitigated, however, by a secondary *decrease* in plasma bicarbonate concentration. During acute hypocapnia bicarbonate is removed from the extracellular fluid by a process of buffering in both blood and tissues, renal excretion of alkali playing only a minor role. During chronic hypocapnia there is a further reduction in bicarbonate concentration which is probably mediated largely if not entirely by the kidneys. If hyperventilation is sufficiently prolonged (as in persons living at high altitude), these adjustments are sufficient to restore plasma pH to normal or nearly normal levels.

Pathogenesis. Probably the most common cause of respiratory alkalosis is the hyperventilation resulting from extreme anxiety. Other causes are central nervous system injury involving the respiratory center, artificial ventilation, fever, hepatic coma, and salicylate intoxication. Hypocapnia is also encountered in the early phase of pulmonary disease if a disturbance in the relation between ventilation and perfusion has produced hypoxemia and hyperventilation.

Finally, as discussed earlier, the persistence of respiratory compensation after the correction of metabolic acidosis may produce a picture indistinguishable chemically from a primary respiratory alkalosis.

Diagnosis. The presence of hyperventilation in a patient suffering from any one of the disorders considered in the preceding section should suggest the diagnosis of respiratory alkalosis. In many cases characteristic signs and symptoms provide evidence that one is dealing with primary hyperventilation rather than respiratory compensation for metabolic acidosis. Respiratory alkalosis produces a typical clinical syndrome in which the cardinal features are lightheadedness, numbness, tingling of the extremities, and circumoral paresthesia. In some patients, frank carpopedal spasm occurs.

The finding of an abnormally low plasma bicarbonate concentration and P_{CO_2} does not in itself distinguish between metabolic acidosis and respiratory alkalosis; the measurement of plasma pH is often vital to the differentiation. The problem of diagnosis sometimes is further complicated by the presence of a mixed acid-base disorder— that is, one with both respiratory and metabolic components. This combination occurs very often in salicylate poisoning.

Treatment. The treatment of respiratory alkalosis should be directed toward correction of the underlying disturbance responsible for the hyperventilation. In the patient with salicylism the goal is to promote removal of the offending drug. One can accomplish this purpose either by augmenting the renal excretion of salicylate (by means of urinary alkalinization and the administration of osmotic diuretics) or by hemodialysis. With injury to the central nervous system or with liver failure, the ability to correct respiratory alkalosis will be determined by the effectiveness of therapy directed toward the underlying pathologic process. The hyperventilation syndrome resulting from anxiety can often be effectively controlled if the patient rebreathes into a paper bag. If this fails, sedation will usually put an end to the acute episode. Recurrences can sometimes be prevented by reassurance and by explanation of the nature of the disorder to the patient, but if these techniques fail, psychotherapy may be indicated.

Brackett, N. C., Jr., Wingo, C. F., Muren, O., and Solano, J. T.: Acid-base response to chronic hypercapnia in man. New Eng. J. Med., 280:124, 1969.

Leaf, A.: The clinical and physiologic significance of the serum sodium concentration. New Eng. J. Med., 267:24, 77, 1962.

Pitts, R. F.: Physiology of the Kidney and Body Fluids, Chicago, Year Book Medical Publishers, Inc., 1968.

Ross, E. J., and Christie, S. B. M.: Hypernatremia. Medicine, 48:441, 1969.

Schwartz, W. B., Van Ypersele de Strihou, C., and Kassirer, J. P.: Role of anions in metabolic alkalosis and potassium deficiency. New Eng. J. Med., 279:630, 1968.

Disorders of Carbohydrate Metabolism

DIABETES MELLITUS

Philip K. Bondy

Definition. Diabetes mellitus is a generalized chronic metabolic disorder usually developing in subjects with a hereditary predisposition and manifested in its fully developed form by weakness, lassitude, loss of weight, or failure to grow and by hyperglycemia, ketosis, acidosis, and protein breakdown. If the course of the disease is indolent, or if treatment prolongs the patient's existence, secondary abnormalities of small blood vessels appear and ultimately cause renal failure, blindness, hypertension, or congestive heart failure or some combination of these. Various neurologic disorders may also occur.

History. Although the disease undoubtedly has afflicted human beings for thousands of years, it was first clearly described in the first century A.D. by Aretaeus who described a "melting down of the flesh and limbs to urine," and named the disease "diabetes" from the Greek word for "siphon," because of the polyuria and polydipsia that characterize it. The sweetness of the urine was recognized by Susruta in the fifth century A.D., and the presence of sugar in the urine was recognized by Dobson in the 18th century. Von Mering and Minkowski, in 1889, produced the disease by pancreatectomy in dogs; and Banting and Best in 1921 produced a pancreatic extract capable, after appropriate purification, of maintaining life in pancreatectomized dogs and in human beings. The explanation of diabetes mellitus as a failure to produce enough of the pancreatic principle named "insulin" was gradually modified as investigations by Houssay, Long and Lukens, Renold, Randle, and others showed that many factors, endocrine, immunologic, and chemical, combine to regulate the blood glucose concentration, and that diabetic patients do not necessarily lack insulin. Even with these other factors in mind, however, diabetes is probably due to inadequate secretion of insulin.

Pathophysiology. The most obvious derangement in diabetes mellitus is that of carbohydrate metabolism; but the fates of protein and fats, of electrolytes and water are all so intimately intertwined with that of carbohydrate that it is impossible to discuss any single facet of the abnormal metabolism without implicating other areas.

Carbohydrates are ingested in the form of mono- or polysaccharides, but are digested in the intestinal tract to form glucose, fructose, galactose, or pentoses. The hexoses are absorbed, probably by an active process involving phosphorylation and, in the case of fructose, conversion to glucose. On entering the portal system they are carried to the liver, where fructose, galactose, and glucose may be transferred into the cells and converted into glucose-6-phosphate. Since the utilization of fructose and galactose by tissues outside the liver is negligible, peripheral carbohydrate metabolism can be considered entirely in terms of the metabolism of glucose.

Entry of Glucose into Cells. Under ordinary circumstances negligible amounts of free hexose exist within the cells. The movement of glucose across cell membranes is the slowest step in the metabolic process, and it may control the rate at which glucose is utilized. In many tissues, including skeletal and heart muscle and fat, the rate at which glucose enters the cell can be increased by insulin. Other tissues such as the nervous system and the gonads appear to be uninfluenced by insulin.

Once within the cell, glucose is immediately phosphorylated by combining with the terminal phosphate of adenosine triphosphate (ATP) under the influence of an appropriate enzyme. In muscle, fat, and liver the enzyme involved is known as *hexokinase*; but in the liver there is an additional enzyme, *glucokinase*. The activity of hexokinase is apparently uninfluenced by nutrition, insulin, or exercise; however, it is inhibited by glucose-6-phosphate. Since the hexokinase of liver works at close to full capacity at glucose concentrations lower than those usually found in plasma, increasing the blood glucose does not increase its activity. Glucokinase, on the other hand, is not saturated until concentrations far above normal are reached. As a result, increasing the blood glucose concentration causes an increased rate of glucose phosphorylation by glucokinase. This relationship probably provides a stabilizing mechanism for blood glucose by increasing hepatic glucose uptake. Glucokinase rapidly disappears from the liver when the animal is starved or when diabetes is produced. The absence of glucokinase activity in the starved animal may partly account for the fact that if an animal is given glucose after a period of starvation it is unable to utilize it efficiently, and a syndrome of "starvation diabetes" occurs temporarily. The increased secretion of growth hormone induced by starvation also contributes to this syndrome.

Regulation of Blood Glucose. The glucose concentration is normally held within rather narrow limits, seldom falling below 50 or rising above 150 mg. per 100 ml. When glucose determinations are made by methods that do not determine "true" glucose, the values may be 10 mg. per 100 ml. or so higher; and if the determination is made by automated methods that analyze plasma rather than whole blood, the values are 10 to 15 per cent higher. In the fasting subject, glucose is secreted into the blood by liver and kidney. In prolonged starvation, the latter organ may contribute as much as 50 per cent of the total glucose supply. In these organs, the presence of glucose-6-phosphatase permits glucose-6-phosphate derived from glycogen, from deamination of amino acids, or by assembly from smaller metabolic fragments to be dephosphorylated to release free glucose into the blood. Most of the glucose-6-phosphate in the fasting liver comes from glycogen by the action of the enzyme *phosphorylase*. This enzyme is activated by *glucagon*, a polypeptide hormone released by the alpha cells of the islets of Langerhans of the pancreas in response to hypoglycemia. A number of important adjustments help conserve the glucose thus liberated by reducing its utilization except in tissues that absolutely require it, such as the nervous system. Thus, entry of glucose into the peripheral muscles and fat cells is reduced by the secretion of anterior pituitary growth hormone and by a decrease in the secretion of insulin, which practically disappears from the blood. If the blood glucose drops below about 50 mg. per 100 ml., *epinephrine* is also released. These changes combine to promote mobilization of fat as a substitute substrate by mechanisms discussed below. On the other hand, since the ability of the brain to utilize glucose is not dependent on insulin, lack of this hormone does not prevent nervous tissue from receiving the amount of glucose it needs.

When glucose begins to enter the blood rapidly, the liver ceases secreting glucose and begins to take it up. Growth hormone is no longer secreted and is rapidly cleared from the plasma, and insulin appears within a few minutes. These factors cause glucose to enter the muscle, liver, and fat cells.

These events combine to reduce the release of fatty acids by the fat cells and thus to shift the metabolic mixture somewhat away from fat as a substrate and toward carbohydrate. Randle (1963) has shown that free fatty acids tend to reduce the entry of glucose into diaphragm and heart muscle, but, since voluntary muscle is not affected, this effect is of limited importance. In addition, the increased concentration of intracellular citrate resulting from augmented fatty acid oxidation may depress the activity of *phosphofructokinase*, a rate-limiting enzyme in glucose utilization. Even more important, the oxidation of fatty acids is required in order to maintain a high rate of gluconeogenesis, so reduced fat utilization causes a reduction in blood glucose, and fat mobilization tends to promote hyperglycemia.

As a result of these adjustments, the blood glucose rapidly falls to fasting levels. In normal persons, even after a large carbohydrate feeding, the blood glucose does not rise above 150 mg. per 100 ml., and within two hours it is normally below 100 mg. per 100 ml.

The Glucose Tolerance Test. The normal adjustments may be tested by standardized glucose loads and have been valuable in demonstrating abnormalities of carbohydrate metabolism. The blood glucose in the fasting person is normally between 60 and 95 mg. per 100 ml. After feeding glucose the blood glucose concentration rises to 120 to 150 mg. per 100 ml. The degree of elevation is independent of the dose, but a larger dose causes the elevation to persist longer. Most modern oral glucose tolerance tests utilize either 1 gram per kilogram or 100 grams of glucose. With this load the blood glucose should return to normal at two or occasionally three hours. Diabetics may have elevated fasting concentrations that rise to abnormally high levels, from which they descend abnormally slowly. In order to avoid distortion caused by "starvation diabetes" (see above), all patients should have received at least 150 grams of carbohydrate per day for at least three days before a glucose tolerance test.

The oral glucose tolerance test may be affected by abnormalities of glucose absorption. If the blood glucose fails to rise by at least 20 mg. per 100 ml., the results of the test must be questioned. In spite of this, the oral test is preferred for diagnostic purposes because it evaluates the entire range of physiologic stimuli to insulin secretion associated with entry of glucose into the gastrointestinal tract (see below). Measuring plasma insulin along with glucose has not yet proved of practical value. The sensitivity of the test may be increased by administering corticosteroids the night before and the morning of the test. Cortisone (100 mg.) often reveals mild diabetes in patients with a normal oral test. Some physicians measure the blood glucose two hours after a standard meal as a screening substitute for the glucose tolerance test. This is less accurate than the tolerance test but more valuable than the fasting blood level as a screening method.

Glucose may also be given intravenously to test glucose tolerance. Usually 25 grams is given, and the concentration is measured at two hours. This method is less sensitive than the oral method in detecting diabetes, but may be useful in patients with gastrointestinal disease (but beware of starvation diabetes).

Relationship of Carbohydrate and Fat Metabolism. Glucose is readily converted to fat by liver and adipose tissue cells. Biosynthesis of fatty acids from glucose is greatly inhibited in the absence of insulin. In the liver fatty acids thus formed are esterified with glycerophosphate to form triglycerides or phospholipids; or they may be esterified with cholesterol, vitamin A, or other acceptors. The cholesterol esters, triglycerides, and phospholipids are assembled with appropriate specific carrier proteins into lipoproteins that circulate in the plasma to provide a source of fat for energy or to be picked up by the adipose tissue cells for storage. Triglyceride fatty acids must be released as free fatty acids before they can enter cells. This occurs in plasma through the action of lipoprotein lipase, an enzyme which depends for its activity on the presence of insulin. Thus in insulin deficiency lipids are cleared from the blood more slowly than normal. The effect of fatty acid oxidation on glucose oxidation has already been mentioned.

In the *adipose tissue*, the fatty acids formed directly from glucose or obtained by the diet are assembled into triglycerides for storage. The only source of glycerophosphate for this reaction is glucose recently brought to the cell, since glycerol itself cannot be utilized by the fat cell. The triglycerides of the fat cell constantly break down to release three free fatty acid molecules and one glycerol molecule. Part of the free fatty acids normally is reincorporated into new triglycerides with glycerophosphate formed from glucose; the remainder leaves the cell to enter the plasma as a free fatty acid that is transported, associated with plasma albumin, to liver, muscle, myocardium, and other cells capable of using the fatty acid molecule as a major source of calories. The balance between synthesis and breakdown of triglycerides depends in part on whether the supply of glycerophosphate is sufficient to pick up the fatty acids released by spontaneous breakdown. Moreover, even in the absence of glucose, insulin inhibits release of free fatty acids directly. Epinephrine, adrenocorticotrophin, and growth hormone also stimulate fat mobilization directly.

In a very rare type of diabetes the metabolic lesion may be located primarily in the fat tissue. *Lipoatrophic diabetes* appears in infancy and is associated with widespread fat atrophy, severe insulin resistance, reduced lipid synthesis, cirrhosis, hyperlipemia, and often hypermetabolism. The diabetes may reflect failure to use carbohydrates for fat formation. There is little tendency to ketoacidosis. Although the cause is obscure, it is clearly a different disease from diabetes mellitus.

Progressive lipodystrophy may sometimes be confused with lipoatrophic diabetes. Lipodystrophy usually affects women, whose subcutaneous fat insidiously diminishes over part of the body until it has completely disappeared. The disorder usually involves the entire upper half of the body or, more rarely, the lower half. The loss of subcutaneous tissue causes the muscle masses to be clearly outlined, producing a bizarre appearance. Ordinarily there is no abnormality of carbohydrate metabolism, although in a few instances insulin-resistant diabetes has been described. It is distinguished from lipoatrophic diabetes because lipodystrophy begins in adult life and affects only part of the body, whereas lipoatrophic diabetes is present from birth and affects all the body fat. The cause is unknown and there is no treatment of the lipodystrophy.

Relationship of Carbohydrate and Protein Metabolism. Proteins are synthesized from dietary amino acids or from amino acids ("nonessential") formed by amination of fragments of carbohydrate and fat catabolism. This process requires large amounts of energy, made available as ATP. When energy supplies are limited, protein synthesis may be inhibited, and breakdown may predominate. In addition, insulin has a direct stimulating effect on protein synthesis, even in the absence of carbohydrate substrates, and it also inhibits gluconeogenesis. Thus in the presence of insulin, amino acids are conserved, and during insulin lack protein breaks down, and amino acids are deaminated and converted to glucose. This results in a negative nitrogen balance as protein is wasted.

Insulin. Insulin is a protein hormone with a molecular weight of 5734, consisting of two peptide chains linked by a pair of disulfide bridges. The sequence of the 50 amino acids in the protein is established for insulins from a number of species. Systematic experimental degradation of the molecule has shown that the core structure required for activity includes at least one disulfide bond and considerable fragments from both the A and B chains.

Insulin is synthesized in the beta cells of the islets of Langerhans as a single spiral polypeptide chain (proinsulin) in which the A and B chains of insulin are connected by a bridge of about 33 amino acids. Proinsulin is physiologically quite inactive. When the connecting chain is excised, the insulin thus formed is stored in granules in the cell. Release of the hormone is controlled by several factors. When the blood glucose concentration rises above 70 or 80 mg. per 100 ml., or when there is an increase in the concentration of certain amino acids (especially arginine), stored insulin is released. Glucose is a more potent stimulus when given orally than when given intravenously, probably because its presence in the duodenum stimulates secretion of a glucagon-like polypeptide which directly promotes insulin release. The intestinal hormone, secretin, also promotes insulin release. Beta adrenergic stimulation increases, and alpha stimulation decreases, secretion. Insulin secretion is controlled by two feedback loops. Increasing glucose concentration causes increased insulin secretion, which reduces

glucose concentration and thus reduces insulin secretion. A parallel loop exists for amino acids such as arginine.

Ordinarily little proinsulin is released, but after prolonged stimulation, the secretion of insulin is reduced and proinsulin increases. In the plasma, both insulin itself and a larger molecule, molecular weight of approximately 9000, are found. The latter may be proinsulin. Both molecules normally exist unbound in the plasma. The fasting concentration of insulin in normal plasma is between 10 and 20 μU. per ml.; during a glucose tolerance test it may rise to as high as 150 μU. per ml. Insulin enters the portal vein and is subject to metabolism by the liver, which contains enzyme systems capable of inactivating the hormone ("insulinase system"; glutathione insulin transhydrogenase). The portion that escapes destruction enters the peripheral circulation. In patients who have received exogenous insulin, the hormone binds to a beta globulin believed to be a non-neutralizing antibody. Diabetic patients with severe insulin resistance may have globulins capable of binding and neutralizing large amounts of insulin. In addition, a protein traveling near the albumin area ("synalbumin") is believed by Vallance-Owen (1962) to consist of the B chain of insulin attached to albumin and to act as a competitive inhibitor of insulin. However, the most recent data suggest that synalbumin is an artifact. Many observers doubt the importance of insulin antagonists in most diabetics.

The mechanism of action of insulin is not yet known. Undoubtedly it increases the permeability of certain cells to glucose and other monosaccharides of similar structure. This effect is rapid and is not dependent on biosynthesis of new enzymes or other proteins. In addition, it stimulates the formation of RNA and new proteins, especially in the muscle and myocardium. Zierler (1963) finds that the earliest effect of insulin detectable in human forearm muscle is the movement of potassium into the cells. No single one of these observations suffices to explain all the physiologic effects of the hormone, such as promotion of fat synthesis, growth, glycogen synthesis, and lowering of blood glucose; however, taken together these three mechanisms of action plus others not yet described may account for all the physiologic actions. Whether insulin actually has several kinds of primary effects or whether some still earlier primary action explains the three actions now known is still unclear. No effect of insulin has ever been demonstrated in the absence of intact cells.

Because insulin is a protein, it is ineffective if administered via the gastrointestinal tract. The rate of destruction of parenterally administered native insulin is very rapid, so that repeated injections are needed throughout the day. The hormone can be precipitated in crystals of controllable size, either by adding known amounts of protamine or globin, or by isoelectric precipitation. Such precipitates are absorbed slowly from the site of injection, and are therefore used most commonly for treating diabetes. The preparations usually available are mixtures of beef and pork insulin precipitated with protamine ("isophane" or "NPH" insulin) so as to have a maximal effect 10 to 12 hours after injection, or similar insulin precipitated isoelectrically ("lente") so as to have a similar rate of absorption, or soluble crystalline insulin (crystalline zinc or "semilente") with the maximal period of activity at about two hours. The application of these various time courses will be discussed later.

The Abnormality in Diabetes Mellitus. The patient with diabetes mellitus acts as though he had no insulin, or as though the insulin he has were insufficient for his needs. As a result, glucose enters the cells with difficulty, but the breakdown of proteins and conversion of amino acids to glucose by the liver are increased. The resulting increased secretion of glucose combined with reduced utilization raises the blood glucose concentration to abnormally high levels. As a result, so much glucose is filtered by the renal glomeruli that the tubules cannot absorb it all, and glycosuria occurs. At the same time, fatty acids are released in increased amounts by the adipose tissues. This promotes an increased use of fat as a metabolic substrate, but in the liver the rate of turnover becomes so large that two untoward effects occur. The fatty acids which enter the liver are converted, in part, to triglycerides, but reduced protein synthesis interferes with formation of lipoproteins, and the triglycerides accumulate to produce fatty liver. In addition, most of the fatty acids are oxidized to acetyl-coenzyme A, which is not able to follow its usual major pathway of conversion to fatty acids or cholesterol, and therefore tends to exceed the capacity of the tricarboxylic acid cycle. Accumulation of acetyl-coenzyme A is relieved by formation of four-carbon acids, the ketone bodies (Figs. 1 and 2). These enter the blood and go to the peripheral cells, where they are used for energy; but if the supply greatly exceeds the body's capacity to utilize them, the ketone bodies accumulate and ultimately provide an intolerable load of hydrogen ions, producing acidosis.

Osmotic Effects of Hyperglycemia. The high concentration of glucose in the extracellular fluids,

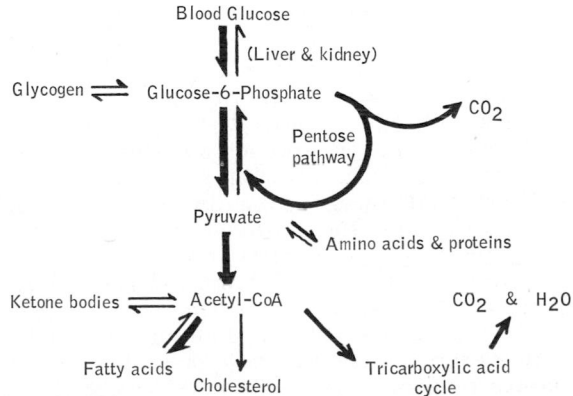

FIGURE 1. Diagram of normal carbohydrate metabolism. (Thickness of arrows indicates possible magnitude of reactions.)

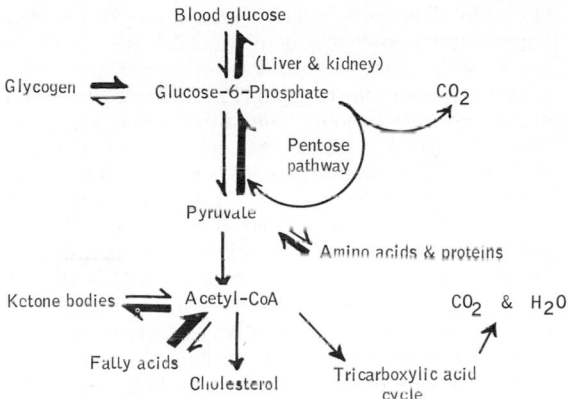

FIGURE 2. Diagram of carbohydrate metabolism in diabetes mellitus.

combined with virtual absence of glucose within the body cells, causes an osmotic imbalance across the cell membrane that is adjusted by movement of water out of the cell and into the extracellular fluid. This dilutes all of the solids in the extracellular fluids, an effect which is easily detected in the depression of the plasma sodium and chloride concentrations in the presence of very high glucose concentrations. The high concentration of glucose in the glomerular filtrate exceeds the capacity of the tubular cells to reabsorb it, and causes an osmotic diuresis, producing large volumes of urine of high total osmolarity or specific gravity but with a concentration of electrolytes lower than that of the extracellular fluid. Sustained osmotic diuresis therefore depletes the patient of water in excess of his loss of salt, an effect manifested clinically by intense thirst. The loss of glucose may be substantial, amounting to as much as 500 grams or 2000 calories per day. The combination of severe dehydration and hyperosmolarity may produce coma in some diabetic patients as a result of electrolyte changes, even though acidosis has not appeared. Sudden changes of blood glucose concentration cause temporary refractive errors in the eyes; the refractive indices of the lens and the aqueous and vitreous humors vary at different and asymmetrical rates because of the differences in the rate at which glucose concentrations come to equilibrium in these various tissues. By a similar mechanism, a rapid fall of blood glucose from a previous high equilibrium concentration may produce cerebral edema, as the movement of glucose and its metabolites (especially the hexitols) across the blood-brain barrier is slow.

Vascular Complications of Diabetes Mellitus. Although diabetic acidosis can kill rapidly and is therefore the most fearful complication of the disease, it is now less important as a cause of disability than the results of changes in the blood vessels. These can be divided into two groups of abnormalities: those affecting the large vessels and those affecting the small arterioles.

Diabetics are prone to develop atherosclerosis prematurely, an effect that doubtless reflects the elevation of plasma triglycerides and cholesterol when the disease is poorly controlled. The pathogenesis of atherosclerosis in this situation is therefore no different from that seen in patients with other forms of hypertriglyceridemia; it is discussed elsewhere in this book. The small vessel changes, however, are unique. They consist of thickening of the basement membrane as a result of excessive deposition of collagen and mucoproteins. Most parts of the body are affected, but especially important clinical effects are produced in the kidneys, retina, nervous system, and skin. Although the cause of these changes is completely unknown, several theories have been advanced to explain them. Since some of them can be demonstrated before the appearance of the carbohydrate abnormality in patients who will later develop diabetes, the vascular changes may be hereditary and a part of the diabetic picture independent of deranged carbohydrate metabolism. Indeed, some think that microvascular changes in the pancreatic islets may cause the derangement of insulin secretion. Another hypothesis blames deposition of an insulin-antibody complex in the vessel walls as the cause. Others believe that the vascular changes are a result of abnormal carbohydrate metabolism. Since the biosynthesis of the glucuronic acid derivatives of glucose, which may appear in the mucoproteins of the thickened basement membrane, depends on the concentration of glucose but not on the presence of insulin, whereas the utilization of glucose for energy and lipogenesis depends on the presence of insulin more than on the concentration of the hexose, the vascular changes may occur when hyperglycemia is combined with an insulin deficit. The argument has important clinical implications, as the physician who believes that the microvascular changes are not a result of hyperglycemia will not press for such rigid control of the blood glucose concentration as will one who fears that a high blood glucose concentration causes the vascular changes.

Pathology. The pathologic changes seen in diabetics can be divided into those possibly associated with the pathogenesis of the disease and those causing complications. Destruction of the islets of Langerhans surgically or by inflammation or tumor causes diabetes in a few patients. A syndrome superficially resembling diabetes may occur in patients with hyperadrenocorticism or acromegaly. In the former, the disease often persists after cure of Cushing's syndrome, suggesting that excess corticosteroids have merely unmasked an underlying diabetic tendency. In either case, the metabolic pattern produced by the hormones is different from that seen in insulin deficiency. Hemochromatosis is associated with diabetes, but the incidence of the disease is not correlated with the size of the iron stores, so the relationship is not clear. At least 90 per cent of diabetics have no recognizable associated causative lesion. Early in the course of diabetes the islets often are larger and have more beta cells than normal; after about five years the islets are reduced in size and there are fewer beta cells. About 40 per cent of diabetics

with long-standing disease have hyaline degeneration of the islets, and about 25 per cent have fibrosis. Lymphocytic infiltration and selective atrophy may also occur. In about a third of diabetics the islets appear essentially normal by light microscopy even late in the disease. The incidence of abnormal beta cells is higher with electron microscopy. Whether these changes cause diabetes or are a result of it is uncertain.

The insulin content of the pancreas is usually reduced, approximating zero in juvenile diabetics and about 50 per cent of normal in adult-onset diabetics. The insulin concentration parallels the estimated mass of beta cells.

Thickening of the basement membrane of muscle capillaries is found in all diabetics and in most persons with a genetic predisposition. In the preclinical phase and early in the disease this thickening may be demonstrable only in electron micrographs, but later the changes become visible under the light microscope. In the kidney the picture of intercapillary glomerulosclerosis results as the thickening progresses until large masses of hyaline material appear and ultimately cause sclerosis and destruction of the glomeruli. Similar changes are seen later in the skin, nerves, and other organs. In the retina these changes are accompanied by tiny aneurysmal dilations of the venules or venous ends of the capillaries, which may ultimately rupture and cause neovascularization of the vitreous with scarring and retinal detachment.

In addition to these specific changes, diabetics with poorly controlled disease often have enlargement of the liver with fat deposits in the cells. The liver glycogen is normal in well controlled diabetics, but may be depleted in acidotic patients; however, glycogen may appear in the nuclei of liver cells in diabetic acidosis. Glycogen is also deposited in large amounts in the renal tubular cells of diabetics with poorly controlled disease. All these changes reflect the metabolic alterations in carbohydrate and fat metabolism previously described. Premature atherosclerosis is frequent in all vessels, but especially in those of the legs and the coronary and cerebral vessels. It becomes more severe as the disease progresses, and its rate of development appears to be accelerated by poor control, especially when hypertriglyceridemia exists. Mönckeberg's sclerosis is also accelerated, producing premature calcification of the large and intermediate arteries.

Certain infections appear to be specifically aggravated in the presence of diabetes mellitus. Mucormycosis, especially of the nose and accessory sinuses, is almost entirely a disease of diabetics. Other infections, such as tuberculosis, pyogenic infections of skin and perineum, and pyelonephritis, are more aggressive than usual. Necrotizing papillitis may occur as a complication of pyelonephritis, and organisms that are ordinarily only weakly pathogenic may present with explosive violence.

Incidence and Heredity. Diabetes mellitus is a common disease. It rarely occurs in newborn infants, but appears with increasing frequency as the population ages. In over-all population surveys, Wilkerson (1952) estimates the prevalence at 1.4 to 1.7 per cent. In populations over the age of 60 years of age, however, the prevalence may be as high as 10 per cent. There is no apparent predilection for any nationality or racial stock. It is more common with increasing parity in women, and is more prevalent in women than in men in the United States until after the childbearing age. This sex distribution is reversed in certain parts of Japan, suggesting that the difference in rates of appearance between the sexes may reflect some other factor than sex hormones. Perhaps the tendency to obesity in multiparous Caucasian women affects the incidence in this group, since it is well known that obesity tends to aggravate or bring out latent diabetes.

These considerations make it difficult to find an acceptable pattern for the inheritance of the disease; indeed, not all observers agree that the disease is inherited. The most commonly held opinion is that it is transmitted as an autosomal recessive trait with varying degrees of expression that may be affected by environmental factors. The high concurrent incidence of the disease in identical twins supports this thesis. It has also been considered a multifactorial trait. If, as seems likely, the disease is inherited in a simple recessive fashion, it is difficult to account for the frequency of the disease unless heterozygotes enjoy a selective advantage.

Etiology. Diabetes can be divided into two categories: those few cases in which a clear cause can be found, discussed earlier, and those without known cause.

After the effects of pancreatectomy were demonstrated by von Mering and Minkowski (1893) and a corrective hormone was isolated by Banting and Best (1922), diabetes was considered a result of defective production of insulin. This point of view was undermined when it was shown that the pancreases of some adult diabetics contained insulin, although insulin was usually absent in the juvenile diabetic pancreas. In recent years, assays of plasma insulin, chiefly by immunoassay methods, have shown that virtually all diabetics, regardless of age, have a defect of insulin secretion. In juvenile diabetics this defect is often absolute, and no insulin is found in the fasting or postprandial plasma. Adult-onset diabetics usually have plasma insulin, and respond to a glucose load by secreting increased amounts of the hormone. In these patients, however, the rate of secretion is slower than normal and although the height of the curve may be greater than normal, the amount of insulin secreted is less than would be produced by a normal person with the same blood glucose concentration. In obese patients, whether diabetic or not, the fasting insulin level is increased, and the response to glucose feeding is exaggerated. A somewhat similar pattern is produced by pretreatment with adrenocorticosteroids.

These findings suggest that in spontaneous diabetes there is a defect in secretion of insulin by the beta cells. In obese patients who are not overtly diabetic and in patients treated with corticoids, the presence of high insulin levels when the glucose concentration is normal implies that the effectiveness of insulin is reduced. Thus diabetes may be considered a disease of relative or absolute deficiency of insulin. Very early in the disease, both in adult and in juvenile patients, the secretion of insulin may be normal or even somewhat increased. As a result, during the prediabetic period (defined later), glucose loading may result in late hypoglycemia. Later, as the lesion progresses, the secretion of insulin diminishes until ultimately, in severe cases, it ceases entirely.

It is not clear whether the primary difficulty in insulin secretion stems from abnormality of beta cell function, whether it is a result of secretion of an abnormal form of insulin, or whether there is increased demand for the hormone. Diabetes might occur if a mutation had resulted in synthesis of an insulin-like polypeptide which was immunologically indistinguishable from the hormone but was biologically ineffective. This might also occur if the enzyme necessary for removing the connecting bridge of proinsulin were defective, since proinsulin cross-reacts with insulin in immunoassay, but is physiologically very weak. Such an explanation would fit the genetic theory of the disease, but evidence to support it is inadequate. Finally, resistance of the peripheral cells to insulin action might underlie the disease. This type of resistance has been demonstrated in obesity. It is reversed when weight is lost. In other instances, there might be some extrapancreatic factor causing an increase in the requirement for insulin. This theory demands clarification of the cause for the increased need. Recent hypotheses have included the suggestion that insulin may be bound excessively by plasma proteins, but kinetic consideration of such binding shows that it could not cause insulin deficiency, because, once binding sites were filled, the demand for insulin would not be increased. It has also been suggested that insulin might be destroyed at an increased rate, but no evidence of this has been found. Plasma antagonists to insulin action have been sought with dubious success except in insulin-resistant diabetes and in acute ketoacidosis. Free fatty acids and some of the hormones appear to reduce the effectiveness of insulin, and corticoids and free fatty acids are elevated in the plasma of the uncontrolled diabetic. Recent interest in the autoimmune theory of the origin of certain diseases has led to the suggestion that diabetics may produce antibodies that inhibit the action of insulin. Although these have been clearly demonstrated in a few cases of severe insulin resistance, no such antibodies can be found in the ordinary patient with diabetes.

In summary, most cases of diabetes mellitus are of unknown cause, but an abnormality of insulin secretion or some imbalance between the production of insulin and the demand for the hormone may be responsible.

Precipitating Factors. Although the cause of the

disease is not known, many factors are recognized that tend to aggravate it or to produce clinically significant activity in patients whose metabolic defect had previously been undetectable. Any form of *physical stress,* including particularly infection and trauma, either accidental or surgical, may unmask or aggravate the disease. In addition, *emotional stress* is a frequent factor, especially in modifying the course of the disease. *Hyperthyroidism* may unmask or aggravate diabetes, as may *acromegaly.* The disease may first appear when a patient develops endogenous or exogenous *hyperadrenocorticism.* Possibly some of the effects of stress are mediated through increased adrenal activity, but other factors are also important. Adrenal activity is normal in well controlled diabetes, and therefore probably does not play a part in causing the disease. Women who have never previously demonstrated abnormal carbohydrate metabolism may have glycosuria during *pregnancy.* Care must be taken to be certain that normal lactosuria is not confused with glycosuria. Probably a decreased renal threshold plays some part in the glycosuria in pregnancy, but many pregnant women have abnormal oral glucose tolerance tests. In most cases the relatively insensitive intravenous glucose tolerance test is normal. Carbohydrate metabolism almost always returns to normal post partum. In spite of this, diabetes ultimately develops in a disproportionately large percentage of women who have previously had "benign" glycosuria of pregnancy. Moreover, the incidence of diabetes is progressively increased with each pregnancy after the third. Although pregnancy does not precipitate diabetes, therefore, it may unmask a diabetic tendency and, in some cases, may promote earlier appearance of the disease. The incidence of diabetes is increased in *obesity,* and the disease can often be controlled simply by weight reduction. (See above.) Obesity per se does not cause diabetes, however, since many severely obese persons never show signs of carbohydrate abnormality. Moreover, people with severe diabetes, especially those manifesting the disease in youth, are usually thin. In exceptional cases, a very *high intake of carbohydrate,* especially sucrose, has been associated with acute development of diabetes. On the other hand, countries in which starches represent a disproportionately high component of the diet do not have a higher incidence of diabetes. It has been suggested that sucrose is specifically toxic, but this is unproved. The most important diabetogenic *medications* in clinical use at present are the thiazide diuretics and their derivatives; lithium salts used in treating some psychiatric diseases also are diabetogenic. These substances apparently do not cause diabetes, but they may unmask it. Diazoxide, a nondiuretic derivative of the thiazide diuretics, can produce diabetes in laboratory animals, and may be useful in the treatment of spontaneous hypoglycemia. Diabetics receiving thiazide diuretics usually require more insulin.

Clinical Manifestations and Course. Assuming that diabetes is a genetic disease, its course can be divided into four stages, as recommended by the American Diabetes Association. *Prediabetes* consists of the period from birth until the first evidence of the disease. This diagnosis can be made clinically only when the person is assumed to be homozygous for the disease—in children of two diabetic parents and in identical twins of diabetics. *Suspected diabetes* means that the patient is usually normal in all respects, but responds to certain stressful influences, e.g., obesity, pregnancy, infections, trauma, pharmaceutical and hormonal agents, by developing an abnormal glucose tolerance test or even diabetic symptoms. When the precipitating agent is removed, the metabolism returns entirely to normal. During the first two phases, hypoglycemia may occur a few hours after eating as the first indication of a metabolic abnormality. The patient with *chemical or latent diabetes* has no signs or symptoms of the disease, but has an abnormal glucose tolerance test or an elevated fasting blood glucose when not under stress. The *overt diabetic* has symptomatic diabetes. These divisions depend on the changes in carbohydrate metabolism that occur as the disease manifests itself, and are therefore somewhat misleading. There is good evidence that changes in the basement membranes of the capillaries may be manifest in the glomerulus and muscle long before the best tests of carbohydrate metabolism now available produce abnormal results. Patients who will later develop overt diabetes may have elevated plasma lipids while the glucose metabolism remains normal, and women still in the prediabetic phase may bear abnormally heavy children.

Since diabetes may first become clinically manifest at any time in life, there is no theoretical justification for separating the disease into "juvenile" and "maturity-onset" forms, but these divisions have some practical value and will doubtless continue to be maintained. Juvenile onset implies that there is a long time available for the disease to develop and present its various vascular complications, whereas with later onset there may be less opportunity for the complications to appear. Moreover, the emotional instability common in childhood and adolescence, combined with the restrictive and unpleasant aspects of the treatment of the disease, tends to make children more difficult to manage. Finally, the progress of the disease may be more rapid in youth, so that insulin disappears from the body, and an absolute insulin requirement may occur more frequently among young people developing the disease than among adults over the age of 40. In spite of these differences, some people with adult-onset disease follow a course indistinguishable from that of children; and a few children may have very mild manifestations similar to those of the adult-onset type. Indeed, Fajans (1969) reports that some children may remain in the latent phase for years. The clinical separation of the disease into two categories is therefore a matter of probability and convenience rather than a dependable differentiation.

In some diabetics the disease is readily controlled; these patients are said to be "stable," whereas others have rapid and unpredictable swings from hypoglycemia to acidosis and are said to be "brittle." This classification also has no theoretical validity, although it is useful practically. However, under appropriate circumstances "brittle" patients may become stable, and vice versa.

It is natural to seek criteria that will permit prediction of the course of the disease. Patients requiring large amounts of insulin, those very prone to acidosis, or those developing the disease early in life are sometimes considered to have more severe diabetes than those who can be treated with sulfonylureas or who are not prone to develop acidosis and who manifest the disease late. The distinctions between "mild" and "severe" on these bases are also precarious, since "mild" diabetics may suffer from serious complications early in their course, whereas "severe" diabetics may have late development of vascular complications.

The onset may be so slow and subtle that the diagnosis is made only by the incidental demonstration of glycosuria or hyperglycemia on routine testing. In some patients the disease appears more aggressively, with symptoms of thirst, hunger, and polyuria but without other symptoms. The combination of increased appetite with weight loss should raise a suspicion of diabetes. Pruritus, especially of the vulva, is a common presenting symptom. As the disease becomes more severe, nocturia may be a major complaint, and the resumption of enuresis in a previously trained child is suggestive of the disease. With more severe decompensation, weight loss and profound weakness and malaise may develop. Later, acidosis produces dyspnea and anorexia, nausea and vomiting. Finally, mental depression progresses to coma; dehydration so depletes the blood volume as to produce shock, and the full-blown picture of diabetic ketoacidosis and coma appears. Any one patient may stop at any point in this progression; or the sequence may unfold over a period of months or years; but the picture may also develop with shocking speed, so that the transition from health to coma requires only a day or so.

Diagnosis. By definition the disease cannot be diagnosed in the prediabetic period, although it may be suspected from the family history. In this period, reversible episodes of glycosuria justify strong suspicion, but only the diagnosis of "suspected diabetes" is justified. Diabetes may be recognized with certainty when abnormal carbohydrate metabolism has been demonstrated in a nonstressed patient or when diabetic acidosis has occurred. The diagnosis may be made by demonstrating a "true" fasting blood glucose concentration over 120 mg. per 100 ml. (130 mg. per 100 ml. in serum) in a patient not under stress. In border-

line cases, or when the fasting blood glucose concentration is normal, a glucose tolerance test should be done as described previously. Some physicians consider the determination of a blood glucose level two hours after a high-carbohydrate breakfast to be as good as a glucose tolerance test. The two-hour postprandial blood glucose is better than a fasting blood sugar as a screening test, but is not nearly so specific or accurate as a true glucose tolerance test.

Rarely, glycosuria may occur when the glucose tolerance test is normal, because of a reduced renal threshold for glucose. Such "renal diabetes" is important because it may mislead the unwary physician into treating nonexistent diabetes mellitus, with disastrous results. It is often found in association with other renal functional defects such as aminoacidurias, which should be sought. Pure renal glycosuria is an inherited defect of tubular glucose transport. It does not affect the patient's health and does not indicate a diabetic tendency.

Treatment. Since cure of the disease is impossible at present, the objectives of life-long control must be recognized clearly. The minimal purpose of treatment is to prevent ketoacidosis and symptoms resulting from hyperglycemia. In most cases this is easy to attain, but some brittle diabetics may have trouble achieving even this limited objective. Prevention of complications, an obvious desideratum, can be achieved only partially. Finally, at least as important as the other two is the obligation to avoid damaging the patient by therapy. The modalities available for treating the patient include diet, insulin, exercise, and the oral hypoglycemic drugs. The progress of treatment is followed by measuring glycosuria, blood glucose, the progress of complications, and the state of the patient's nutrition.

Diet. The role of *diet* in treating diabetes has been greatly exaggerated. For obese diabetics, institution of a low-calorie reducing schedule is important, since weight reduction alone may control the metabolic defect. Diabetics have the same nutritional requirements as normal people, and these must be supplied. Adequate amounts of high quality protein (at least 1 gram per kilogram) are needed; and the balance of the calories should be supplied by carbohydrate and fat in a normal proportion. It is probably wise to hold ingestion of sucrose to a minimum, both because its rapid absorption causes exaggerated swings of blood glucose concentration and because it may elevate the plasma triglycerides in some patients. From this summary it is clear that there is no such thing as a "diabetic diet" and that a diabetic can be treated well on any nutritionally acceptable program of eating. In patients taking insulin, however, the pattern of distribution of calories and carbohydrate is critical. Since insulin secretion cannot respond to dietary stimuli in these patients, the diet must be adjusted to the availability of insulin. They should adhere to a standard pattern of food distribution from day to day, so that the interaction between insulin and the carbohydrate supply is predictable and reproducible. They usually require a mid-morning and mid-afternoon snack and almost always need a bed time feeding low in carbohydrate and high in protein.

Oral Hypoglycemic Agents. If diet alone does not control diabetes of the maturity-onset type, the physician may elect to use *oral antidiabetic* medications. These fall into two groups, the *sulfonylureas* and the *diguanides.* The sulfonylureas appear to work by promoting secretion of insulin by the pancreas or by releasing insulin previously bound in inactive form. Several preparations of sulfonylureas are available that differ chiefly in their duration of action and their toxicity. The least dangerous and shortest acting is *tolbutamide.* Treatment may be initiated with 2 to 4 grams per day in divided doses. The maintenance dose is usually 1 to 2 grams per day. Hypoglycemia may be produced with large doses or in patients with liver disease, in malnourished subjects, or in rare persons who lack the enzyme responsible for detoxifying the drug. Treatment is effective in 50 to 75 per cent of patients whose diabetes began after the age of 40, who are not prone to the development of ketoacidosis, and who have not required over 40 units of insulin for control of their diabetes. It is almost never effective in diabetes of juvenile onset or in patients who tend toward ketoacidosis.

Some patients not well controlled by tolbutamide may respond to *acetohexamide,* an intermediate-acting, or *chlorpropamide,* a long-acting sulfonylurea. The increased duration of action requires only a single dose each day, but hypoglycemia is more frequent and much more prolonged than with tolbutamide. Renal failure aggravates the hypoglycemic tendency by preventing excretion of the active drug. The range of doses for acetohexamide is 250 mg. to 1.5 grams per day and for chlorpropamide 100 to 500 mg. per day. Elderly patients are often unduly sensitive to sulfonylureas and should therefore be started on a low dose, which can be adjusted upward in small increments every three to four days. Sensitivity to sulfonylureas is also increased when salicylates, Coumadin anticoagulants, or phenylbutazone are given; moreover a disulfiram-like reaction of alarming proportions may occur if alcohol is taken by patients receiving sulfonylureas. All the sulfonylureas may produce sensitivity reactions, and jaundice has been reported with chlorpropamide and acetohexamide.

The diguanide most commonly used is *phenformin,* which is supplied in either ordinary or slow-release form. The mode of action is not clearly known, but it is not associated with release of insulin. Probably the effect is a result of some modification in the anaerobic dissimilation of carbohydrate, since it has been associated with lactic acidemia. Since phenformin may cause nausea, vomiting, a metallic taste in the mouth, lassitude, weakness, or drowsiness, it is best to try low doses first and gradually increase the dose to

tolerance or successful control. A starting dose of 25 mg. twice a day (or a single dose of 50 mg. of the slow-release form) is safe, and increments of 25 mg. per day may be added at two- or three-day intervals.

Some patients initially well controlled with sulfonylureas may develop late *"secondary failure."* In these patients, combinations of sulfonylureas and phenformin may be successful when either alone is inadequate. However, no combination of oral preparations should be used to treat diabetics in ketosis or those who are prone to develop this syndrome, or to maintain diabetics who are undergoing serious surgery or are suffering from infection or trauma.

Insulin. All whose diabetes cannot be controlled adequately with oral drugs or diet must use insulin. Many patients can be well controlled with a single injection of intermediate-acting insulin (isophane, globin, or lente) given about 30 minutes before breakfast. The insulin requirement cannot be predicted and must be determined empirically, usually by starting with a small dose (10 to 20 units) and gradually increasing every few days by 2 to 4 units until control is achieved or until hypoglycemic symptoms indicate overdosage. At doses over about 40 units per day it is often advantageous to add a small amount of rapidly acting insulin to obtain an effect on the breakfast load. Semilente may be mixed with lente insulin, or crystalline zinc with isophane. The decision to add rapidly acting insulin is made if hypoglycemia or normal blood glucose levels are achieved in midafternoon or evening by a dose of intermediate-acting insulin that does not prevent glycosuria or hyperglycemia before the midday meal. The relative proportions of the two types of insulin may be adjusted to provide the pattern of response desired. In some instances it may be best to give two doses of intermediate-acting insulin, one in the morning and one before the evening meal. This program is useful when study of the pattern of response of the blood glucose after a dose of intermediate-acting insulin shows that the major effect occurs 15 to 18 hours after injection rather than the usual 8 to 10 hours after.

The program outlined above is adequate and safe when the metabolic derangement does not immediately threaten the patient's life. In some instances it is necessary to bring the patient under control more rapidly. This may be achieved by giving short-acting insulin before each meal and at bed time, adjusting the dose according to the patient's response. When control has been established, the dose of intermediate-acting insulin needed can be estimated as approximately 75 per cent of the total units of short-acting insulin needed per day. It is not safe to estimate the insulin dosage by automatically prescribing a certain number of units for each "plus" of urine glucose, because patients differ greatly in their sensitivity to a given dose of insulin. Moreover, the urine glucose reflects the metabolic status during the entire period since the previous voiding (or even longer in patients who empty their bladder incompletely), rather than the situation at the time the insulin is given. In addition, overdosage with insulin may produce excessive compensatory activity with a "rebound" of glucose to high levels. Under these circumstances the proper adjustment for glycosuria would be a reduction in the insulin dose rather than an increase. When in doubt, the blood glucose should be the deciding factor.

In adjusting the dose of insulin it is important to follow the patient while he goes about his normal daily activities, since the protective atmosphere of the hospital may alter the insulin requirement. Although blood glucose determinations may be helpful in following a patient in the hospital, they are impractical with outpatients because a single determination is virtually useless, and repeated samples cannot be drawn without interfering with the patient's activities. The most convenient method of judging the adequacy of control, therefore, is to test the urine before each meal and at bed time. If the urine to be tested is collected half an hour after the previous urination, the test is more specifically applicable to the time of collection than if urine is tested that has been secreted over a period of several hours. Although glucose oxidase testing tapes are convenient, the range of their sensitivity is narrow; better quantitative data are given by Clinitest tablets. The pattern of insulin required can be judged from the distribution of glycosuria, and appropriate adjustments of insulin or diet may be recommended. There is considerable difference of opinion as to how closely the patient should be controlled. With most diabetics it is practical to prevent glycosuria without producing hypoglycemia, but with brittle diabetics it may be preferable to permit moderate hyperglycemia and glycosuria rather than run the risk of injury to brain and coronary circulation involved in severe hypoglycemic attacks. However, since the excellence of control may influence the rate of progression of complications, one should strive for the best control possible without inducing frequent hypoglycemia or interfering unreasonably with the patient's freedom to carry on a socially normal life. The combined use of insulin plus oral hypoglycemic agents has been suggested in an attempt to reduce the instability of brittle diabetics, but combined therapy does not usually improve control of the disease.

The insulin requirement may be greatly altered by other metabolic changes. Increased need for insulin suggests infection, hyperthyroidism, hyperadrenocorticism, and emotional stress. Chronic starvation, hypoadrenocorticism, hypopituitarism, hypothyroidism, and exercise reduce the insulin requirement. The reduced insulin requirement occasionally seen in uremic patients, e.g., those with terminal diabetic angiopathy, is probably a reflection of anorexia.

Instruction of the Patient. Because of the chronic nature of the disease, the physician merely acts as consultant, and the actual control of therapy lies in the hands of the patient. Education of the patient is therefore of paramount importance. He must learn the tools by which his disease is controlled and how to use them. Every diabetic who needs insulin should be able to give himself the hormone safely. He must learn how to rotate the site of injection to minimize local reactions. The important relationship between the timing of meals and the administration of hypoglycemic agents must be clearly understood. He must recognize that exercise reduces the requirement for hypoglycemic agents and must be prepared either to reduce his medication or to supplement his diet with carbohydrate if he exercises. He must know the importance of care of the skin, especially of the feet. He must learn the danger signs of impending acidosis, and must recognize hypoglycemia and understand how to cope with either of these emergencies. He should carry at all times some form of identification, preferably a bracelet or amulet, stating that he is a diabetic.

Most diabetics are psychiatrically disturbed by their disease, and may react by denying it, by defying it with reckless neglect of treatment, by becoming obsessed with the details of treatment until diabetes becomes a religion, by using the disease as a weapon with which to coerce friends and family, or by some combination of these. Often the difficulties experienced in controlling a patient's disease are not a result of poor biochemical control but reflect the patient's conscious or unconscious manipulation of the disease. The physician who recognizes these tendencies will attempt to control them by appropriate psychotherapeutic maneuvers, but such patients are hard to handle and may defy the best efforts of even a highly skilled therapist.

Complications. Although poor diabetic control produces mildly unpleasant symptoms or, if prolonged unduly, more serious complaints such as weakness, lethargy, and stunted growth, these abnormalities are so easily controlled by proper treatment that they rarely cause much trouble in practice. The major threats to the life and health of the diabetic patient arise from complications, especially those associated with severe metabolic abnormalities culminating in ketoacidosis, those resulting from lesions of the small blood vessels that lead to retinitis, renal failure, hypertension and neuropathy, and premature atherosclerosis (Table 1).

Ketoacidosis. The initial abnormality is usually a rise of blood glucose to high levels, with resulting severe osmotic diuresis and loss of water, sodium, potassium, chloride, calcium, and bicarbonate. Usually the electrolytes are lost in a solution that is hypotonic to plasma, so that relatively more water than electrolytes is lost. As abnormalities of lipid metabolism advance, there is a rise in concentration of acetoacetic and beta-hydroxybutyric acids in the plasma. These are first detected in the urine. Later, as the concentration rises higher, tests for acetone in the plasma become positive. The ketone bodies are themselves mildly toxic, tending to interfere with the excretion of uric acid and to produce mild depression of the central nervous system. More important,

TABLE 1. CAUSES OF DEATH IN DIABETIC PATIENTS*

Years	1914-1922	1923-1936	1937-1943	1944-1949	1950-1955	1956-1959	1960-1963
Clinical Factors	Pre-insulin	Regular Insulin	PZI Sulfonamides	NPH, Lente	Antimicrobials, Oral Diuretics		
Cause of Death (%)							
Coma	41	8	3	1.7	1.1	0.8	1.1
Cardiorenal	25	54	65	71.3	76.9	76.2	77.9
Infections	18	18	12	5.9	5.2	5.1	5.8
Cancer	4	9	9	9.7	10.1	11.0	9.5
Others	12	11	11	11.4	6.7	6.9	5.7
Total No.	836	3988	3234	4655	4148	4176	2634

*(Derived from data from the Metropolitan Life Insurance Co., and Root, M. F.: Med. Clin. N. Amer., 49:1147, 1965.)

however, is their ability to ionize to release hydrogen ions. It is possible for poorly controlled diabetics to excrete appreciable amounts of ketone bodies for months without becoming acidotic, but when the load of protons becomes more than the kidney tubules can handle, the plasma bicarbonate concentration and pH begin to drop. This is compensated to some degree by hyperventilation, which readjusts the pH by lowering the plasma Pco_2. Ultimately the loss of bicarbonate becomes so severe that even this adjustment is incomplete, and severe acidosis appears. After a certain point, the abnormality tends to become self-reinforcing because acidosis reduces the effectiveness of whatever insulin is present, and thus exaggerates the metabolic defect. Acidosis is also usually accompanied by vomiting, which aggravates electrolyte losses. Abdominal pain is often present. With severe acidosis the patient also develops impaired function of the central nervous system, culminating in coma. The combination of severe dehydration, deranged central nervous function, and cardiac dysfunction resulting from electrolyte abnormalities and acidosis causes shock, the usual terminal event in diabetic acidosis.

This syndrome may develop very gradually over a period of days or weeks, or it may strike rapidly, reaching life-threatening proportions in only a few hours. The *precipitating factors*, which should always be sought, include (1) failure to use insulin, either because the disease has not previously been recognized, or because some error on the part of the patient or his physician has reduced the insulin dose below necessary levels; (2) infection, which increases the need for insulin; (3) acute vascular accidents, especially myocardial or cerebral infarction; (4) trauma or surgery; (5) gastrointestinal upsets with vomiting or starvation (often complicated by the patient's ill-advised decision to stop insulin); (6) emotional disturbances; and (7) the appearance of severe insulin resistance.

The *severity* of an attack can be judged by the degree of disturbance of electrolytes, mental and vascular function. Thus a patient with plasma bicarbonate above 20 mEq. per liter who is alert and whose blood pressure is well maintained has mild ketoacidosis and has a good prognosis with proper treatment. In contrast, a patient with bicarbonate below 10 mEq. per liter who is obtunded but with reasonably well maintained blood pressure has a grave prognosis but should usually survive. A patient who has been in coma for many hours, who is in shock, or who has a very low bicarbonate may be difficult to save even with the best treatment. There are no good recent statistics pertaining to the prognosis of profound diabetic acidosis treated with the best modern methods. This may be partly because really severe acidosis has become a rare event in modern hospitals. Education of the public and of physicians has combined to bring most diabetics to treatment before they reach the most advanced stages.

The prognosis is also affected greatly by the nature of the precipitating factors. We have often found it difficult to determine whether a patient's shock was caused by his metabolic derangement or by the myocardial or cerebral infarct that produced it. Obviously, with such grave precipitating factors the patient's outlook may be poor.

The *diagnosis* is suggested by the appearance of the patient, who lies restlessly in bed with sunken, soft eyeballs, loose folds of skin and sunken cheeks, indicating the severity of dehydration. The tongue is dry, red and wrinkled; the "Kussmaul" breathing is rapid, deep, and labored and utilizes all the accessory muscles. The patient may be conscious although mentally dulled; or he may be unconscious. There is often evidence of vomitus, which may be black. The breath, however, is more likely to have the fruity-sweet smell of acetone than the usual odor of vomitus. Valuable help may be afforded by the presence of diabetic retinal or skin lesions. The elevated plasma lipids may produce lactescence of the serum, as well as the raspberry sherbet color of *lipemia retinalis* in the retinal blood vessels. The diagnosis must be confirmed by demonstrating elevated blood glucose and serum acetone levels. These determinations may be made by using bedside test strips and tablets or by more formal laboratory procedures. The *differential diagnosis* is that of acidosis and of causes of coma. Acidosis may be caused by renal failure or poisons (especially isopropyl alcohol, which also causes acetonuria, methanol intoxication, which causes severe overbreathing and acidosis, and salicylates, which cause hyperventilation and a false-positive test for acetonuria); coma may result from vascular lesions in the brain (often also associated with overbreathing), trauma, infection, drugs, or intracranial masses. Lesions causing central nervous system stimulation and hyperventilation, e.g., salicylate poisoning or brain disease, can be differentiated chemically from diabetic acidosis because they elevate the plasma pH and lower the Pco_2 as they cause respiratory alkalosis. A most important differential is that of hypoglycemia from insulin over-dosage. After severe hypoglycemia a compensatory overshoot of blood glucose may hide the previous low blood sugar level; or the urine in the bladder at the time the patient loses consciousness may have been formed in the previous hours when hyperglycemia was present. The most important differential points are that patients usually enter hypoglycemic coma rapidly; they are not dehydrated; they are not acidotic and therefore breathe normally or shallowly; they are often hypothermic; and they usually show some evidence of sympathetic discharge. In diabetic acidosis onset usually takes hours or days; the patient is severely dehydrated and acidotic and therefore breathes deeply and rapidly. It should be emphasized again that when diabetic patients become sick from other causes, their diabetes usually is aggravated. Thus, the common combination of infection or infarction with acidosis may tax the clinician's diagnostic ability, especially since the leukocyte count in uncomplicated ketoacidosis may be as high as 30,000 per cubic millimeter.

Treatment involves restoration of a normal metabolic state, replacement of electrolyte and fluid losses, and treatment of the precipitating or complicating factors. It is best considered in terms of the sequence that should be followed when the patient is first seen. If the diagnosis is first recognized outside the hospital, the patient should be transferred to the hospital. Before this he should be given a dose of insulin. If the acidosis is severe, at least 50 units of short-acting insulin should be given intravenously, and if he is in shock, at least 100 units should be given intravenously. Subcutaneously injected medications should not be used early in treating severe ketoacidosis because their effect is undesirably delayed. On arrival at the hospital blood should be drawn for determination of blood glucose, sodium, potassium, chloride, bicarbonate, and hematocrit. Some of the serum should be tested by serial dilutions for acetone by one of the spot test techniques. While these determinations are being performed, fluid restoration should be begun. It is almost always advisable to give fluids intravenously; only in exceptionally mild cases can the patient benefit from oral fluids, since most patients are nauseated and many have *acute gastric atony* which delays absorption of oral fluids. Since most patients have lost more water than electrolytes, and since hyperglycemia and resulting osmotic diuresis are deleterious, the ideal starting fluid contains no glucose and less electrolytes than isotonic. Several such fluids have been suggested.

One could simply dilute ordinary isotonic saline to half-isotonic with distilled water, but the use of such dilute solutions and the presence of distilled water itself on the ward are dangerous, since hemolysis can be produced by mistake. We preferred the use of a solution of 0.45 per cent NaCl and 2.5 per cent fructose. This is the equivalent of mixing isotonic saline and isotonic fructose in equal volumes. The main advantage of using fructose is that even in severe diabetes it is cleared from the blood in a normally rapid manner, chiefly by the liver. It does not, therefore, contribute to the osmotic diuresis, as would an equal amount of glucose, nor does it interfere seriously with the determination of the blood glucose concentration, since the contribution of fructose to the total reducing sugar content of the blood rarely rises above 30 mg. per 100 ml.

When the blood chemistry values are known, the fluid pattern may be modified. If the osmotic content of the plasma is essentially normal, isotonic electrolyte solutions may be used, whereas if the blood is hypertonic, the dilute fructose-saline mixture should be continued. An estimate of the osmotic level of the plasma is obtained by adding to the milliequivalents of sodium in the plasma the osmotic equivalent of half the glucose in excess of normal (the other half being applicable to the anionic osmotic balance). Since the molecular weight of glucose is 180, 360 mg. per liter is equivalent to 1 mEq. of sodium. Glucose concentrations are usually reported as milligrams per 100 ml., so 360 mg. per 100 ml. is equivalent to 10 mEq. of sodium. Two sample calculations are shown in Table 2. If the serum is severely lactescent, the lipids may displace enough water from the plasma to give spuriously low values for all water-soluble components, including electrolytes.

If the patient is severely acidotic, sodium bicarbonate should be added to the fructose-saline mix. As a general rule, a serum bicarbonate below 10 mEq. per liter is an indication for bicarbonate treatment. The total dose to be given can be calculated from the bicarbonate deficit in milliequivalents per liter, assuming a distribution of the bicarbonate in half of the body water, i.e., about 30 per cent of body weight. This calculation overestimates the required bicarbonate by the amount of bicarbonate that will be formed when the ketone bodies are oxidized. The calculated

TABLE 2

	Example 1	Example 2	Normal
Serum Na, mEq./L.	120	142	142
Blood glucose	890	890	100
Blood glucose in excess of normal	790	790	0
Osmotic equivalent of glucose, as mEq. of cation	22	22	0
"Corrected" Na, mEq./L.	142	164	142

In example 1 the sodium depression is balanced by the elevation of glucose, and the extracellular fluids are isotonic. In example 2, in spite of an apparently normal sodium level, the extracellular fluids are severely hypertonic.

bicarbonate should therefore be reduced by about 50 per cent. The amount to put in each liter of fructose saline depends on the severity of the acidosis, but usually 75 mEq. should be used. This results in a mixture that is now isotonic with respect to electrolytes, alkaline with respect to serum, and hypertonic as injected because of the extra fructose.

The need for potassium may sometimes also be estimated at this time. The serum potassium does not reflect the deficiency of this mineral; indeed, it is grossly misleading because in the presence of severe acidosis potassium leaves the cells and enters the extracellular compartment. Even in the presence of severe depletion, therefore, the serum potassium is usually normal or even a little elevated. If the serum potassium is low in the first sample analyzed, the potassium deficit may be assumed to be very large, and supplementation with potassium chloride can be started at once in doses of 40 to 60 mEq. per liter. Usually it is not necessary to start giving potassium until the third to sixth hour of treatment. At this time the serum potassium is usually depressed because restoration of normal pH and improved carbohydrate utilization continue to move potassium out of the extracellular fluid and into the cells. If shock has resulted in anuria, caution should be used in giving potassium, but the deficits involved are usually so large that some repletion is necessary even in this circumstance.

During the next several hours insulin administration should be continued, using 25 to 100 units per hour, depending on the severity of the derangement and the patient's response. If previous experience with the patient has shown him to be particularly sensitive to insulin, smaller doses may be used. If the circulation is well maintained, insulin may be given subcutaneously or intramuscularly, but it is best to give the insulin intravenously in a single rapid injection. Insulin should not be put in the bottle of intravenous fluids in treating acidosis, since the objective is to get a rapid effect.

The response to treatment is followed by half-hourly or hourly determination of the maximal dilution of plasma in which acetone can be detected. The first sign of improvement is usually a drop in this level; later blood glucose also begins to fall. Acetone clears from the urine rather late, after the undiluted plasma has become negative. Since changes in plasma acetone and glucose occur so much earlier than do changes in urinary excretion of these substances, urinalysis is a poor second choice for following the early progress of treatment. Later, when the plasma acetone is negative, urinalysis may be especially useful in following the final steps of treatment. In spite of these limitations, urinary output should be followed and tests for glucose and acetone performed as a check on the plasma tests and in order to keep track of the urinary output, so that renal shutdown may be recognized as early as possible. If the patient is unconscious or cannot void, an indwelling catheter may be used, with maximal precautions to prevent infection, but should be removed after a few hours. It is usually worth while to check the serum electrolyte pattern and glucose again after four or five hours of therapy. At this time the blood glucose should be appreciably lower and the bicarbonate considerably higher. If this response has failed to occur, the patient may have severe *insulin resistance* of the type that may require thousands of units to control. Under these circumstances the insulin dose may be doubled every hour until evidence of improvement begins to appear. It may also be worth while to give 100 to 200 mg. of a soluble cortisol preparation intravenously under these circumstances, since severe insulin resistance sometimes is lessened by the hormone.

When clear evidence of improvement appears, especially when the blood glucose begins to drop, the dose of insulin should be reduced or withheld for a while, and it may be advisable to begin using intravenous glucose infusions to avoid the rapid fall to hypoglycemia that sometimes occurs at about 12 to 18 hours after starting treatment. The most important mistake made early in treating diabetic acidosis is to give too little insulin, whereas the most serious error late in treatment is overuse of insulin, causing hypoglycemia.

It is useful early in treatment to estimate the total volume of fluid needed for replenishment. Severe dehydration represents loss of about 10 per cent of total body water (6 per cent of normal body weight). Thus one can estimate the deficit, to which should be added fluid losses from vomitus, urine, etc., during treatment. The average initial deficit is about 5 liters plus urinary losses (Table 3). Administration of much more fluid than this may overload the failing circulation in an aged diabetic.

The program outlined above may be modified for patients who are not very severely ill. When laboratory facilities are limited, especially at night, it may be justifiable to draw the appropriate chemical determinations but to set them aside in a refrigerator, after separating off the serum, for later study if the patient's progress is unsatisfactory. A great deal of information can be obtained by bedside tests for blood glucose and acetone, and these should be used freely. The insulin dose should be adjusted according to known variations in the sensitivity of a given patient. If renal shut-down or shock occurs, it may be advisable

TABLE 3. FLUID AND ELECTROLYTE DEFECT IN 8 PATIENTS WITH DIABETIC ACIDOSIS, AS JUDGED BY THE QUANTITIES RETAINED DURING THERAPY*

	Mean±S. D.	Range
Na+	601±497	201−1740 mEq.
K+	205±128	60− 461 mEq.
Cl−	625±615	25−1967 mEq.
H₂O	5.3±5	0.4− 13.6 liters
H₂O/Na†	3.42± 2.9	0.3− 9.1

*From Danowski et al., J. Clin. Invest., 28:1, 1949.

†Liters H_2O/140 mEq. Na retained. If the defect were equivalent to extracellular fluid (140 mEq. Na/L.), the ratio would = 1.0; a higher ratio represents disproportionate H_2O loss.

to use plasma expanders such as blood or albumin; the blood pressure should be maintained with isoproterenol. Digitalis therapy may be dangerous for patients in congestive failure as the potassium concentration of the serum drops under treatment, so caution should be exercised in rapid digitalization. The severe dehydration occurring early in the course of the disease may cause friction rubs and peritoneal or pleural signs without local disease; on the other hand, pulmonary consolidation may not be apparent early in treatment because the patient is so dehydrated that the usual physical signs cannot be detected. It is important to repeat the physical examination after a few hours of therapy to be sure that errors of this type have not been made.

Occasionally diabetic acidosis may occur in association with some other condition that urgently requires surgical treatment. The longer the surgeon can safely postpone operating, the better the chance of preparing the patient metabolically for surgery. If postponement is too dangerous, acidosis can be treated in the operating room as long as the physician has access to veins for intravenous medication and blood analyses. Under these circumstances treatment is usually pushed with the utmost vigor; but here as elsewhere the dangers of overtreatment and hypoglycemia should not be ignored.

Microvascular Complications. The pathologic appearance and pathogenesis of these abnormalities have already been discussed. In the *eye*, fluorescent retinography may show microaneurysms when diabetes is first diagnosed, but these are too small to see with an ophthalmoscope. The first manifestations of involvement on ordinary physical examination are tiny hemorrhages, which are usually punctate but may be flame-shaped. They may be seen to heal and disappear, only to reappear again over months of observation. After a time, white, shiny exudates, often with angular outlines, may appear. These are usually permanent, but may vanish slowly if the patient is treated with a very low fat diet. This diet has no advantage in preventing progress of hemorrhages, however. Later the hemorrhages become larger and begin to extend into the vitreous humor. It is usually at this point that the patient first notices impairment of vision. In the beginning, blood in the vitreous chamber is readily absorbed and even severe impairment of function may reverse completely. Later, tufts of blood vessels begin to invade the vitreous ("neovascularization"), and the hemorrhages heal by scarring, with permanent loss of vision. As the scar tissue retracts, it may detach the retina. About 70 per cent of all diabetics ultimately show evidence of retinopathy. In eyes observed from onset of minimal retinopathy, the rate of progression is about seven times more rapid in mature than in juvenile diabetics, in whom vision less than 20/200 occurs in only 3 per cent after the appearance of retinal changes. Once proliferation of blood vessels appears, about 75 per cent are blind within five years. Moreover, although the mean interval between discovery of diabetes and blindness is about 18 years, the mean survival after onset of blindness is only 5.8 years. The rate of progression may be slowed by *excellent* control of diabetes, but only questionable improvement in prognosis is provided by *good* vs. *poor* control. Of all "specific" methods for controlling progress of the lesions, only pituitary ablation and photocoagulation of early proliferative lesions offer hope; and even here the evidence is not entirely convincing. The subject has been discussed exhaustively in a symposium edited by Goldberg and Fine (1968).

The *kidneys* usually have microvascular changes on biopsy during the preclinical stage or very early after the disease is diagnosed. About 50 per cent of diabetics ultimately show clinical evidence of renal involvement. This usually appears in the first five to fifteen years after the metabolic defect is discovered. Proteinuria occurs initially, and the amount gradually increases. Later the blood urea nitrogen and the plasma creatinine gradually rise until clear-cut uremia develops. Associated with this, hypertension usually appears, and the proteinuria, together with the defective protein synthesis, may produce the nephrotic syndrome. The combination of proteinuria, hypertension, and edema is known as the *Kimmelstiel-Wilson syndrome,* and the microscopic lesions are known as *Kimmelstiel-Wilson lesions.* The lesions are often present when the syndrome has not developed. The susceptibility of diabetics to infection and the frequent catheterizations that have been performed on these patients in the past combine to produce a high incidence of *pyelonephritis,* which may complicate the diagnosis of diabetic nephropathy. A particularly progressive and dangerous complication of diabetic nephropathy is *papillary necrosis,* in which, to the accompaniment of high fever and flank pain, entire renal papillae slough out and may be recognized in the strained urine. This disease has previously been fatal, but with modern antimicrobial treatment it can sometimes be controlled. Its presence signifies very severe renal damage from infection as well as vascular disease, and indicates a poor long-term prognosis even if the acute infectious phase is controlled. The treatment of diabetic nephropathy is that of any chronic renal disease.

Involvement of the *neuromuscular system* produces several important syndromes. Early in the course of diabetes — or, indeed, as its presenting complaint — patients may develop ophthalmoplegias, especially of the lateral rectus muscle. These are transient and disappear without regard for the level of diabetic control. Other muscle weaknesses may also occur, involving the quadriceps or shoulder girdle muscles (amyotrophy). These are also self limited and, although alarming, produce little long-term disability. Less dramatic but more disabling is chronic neuritic involvement of the sensory nerves, especially to the extremities. Paresthesias, hypesthesias, hyperesthesias, and lightning-like pains may occur. Hyperesthesia may be so severe as to prevent walking or wearing shoes. The pain is often so severe that the patients demand narcotics for relief. Associated with these peripheral symptoms may be abdominal pain and autonomic paralyses leading to loss of bladder and bowel control, postural hypotension, and male impotence. The cerebrospinal fluid protein may be as high as 200 mg. per 100 ml. There is no very helpful treatment for these symptoms. Vitamins and other supportive measures have been useless. In some instances, improvement of diabetic control is associated with amelioration of symptoms, but in others stricter metabolic control is associated with exacerbation.

Atherosclerosis. Atherosclerosis occurs prematurely and causes the expected results in the heart. *Diabetic gangrene* of the toes and feet is common and distressing. Occasionally, measures that support or improve circulation to the legs, such as sympathectomy or plastic surgery on obstructed arteries, may help, but often the only recourse is amputation. This should be undertaken only when clearly needed and as conservatively as possible; but undue delay that causes prolonged pain and disability is also undesirable. The final decision requires expert judgment. Two types of "diabetic gangrene" that are not caused by major obstructions in the arterial supply must be differentiated from the type requiring amputation. One is the *penetrating ulcer of the foot,* usually painless as contrasted with the agonizing pain of atherosclerotic gangrene. Penetrating ulcer develops when neuropathic changes have so anesthetized the sole of the foot that the patient can injure himself and not be aware of it. The resulting trophic ulcer responds well to rest, elevation, and bland local treatment with cautious debridement, unless it has penetrated so deeply as to cause osteomyelitis. In this case, the surgical treatment should be very conservative, because the blood supply to the adjacent tissues is normal. Another type of gangrene occurs when microvascular changes in the skin cause *localized ischemic necrosis* of the skin, although the pulses in the foot continue to be palpable. In these cases conservative treatment may be justified if infection can be avoided, and, if amputation is necessary, usually the ankle can be spared.

Skin Lesions. Four types of skin lesions can be described: *infection, necrobiosis diabeticorum, cholesterol deposits,* and a peculiar *punctate depigmenting atrophy.* Although diabetics probably do not develop more infections than normal people, both bacterial and fungal invasions are likely to be more dramatic and dangerous. This may be related to the unusually high glycogen content of the skin of diabetics. *Necrobiosis diabeticorum* consists of plaquelike areas on the body or extremities, which begin as slightly elevated violaceous spots with an erythematous halo. As they spread with serpiginous borders, the centers become atrophic and white with dilated purplish blood vessels. They are not painful, but may become very unsightly (Fig. 3). In uncontrolled diabetes, the plasma lipid elevation may result in deposition of lipids in the skin. *Xanthelasma* is

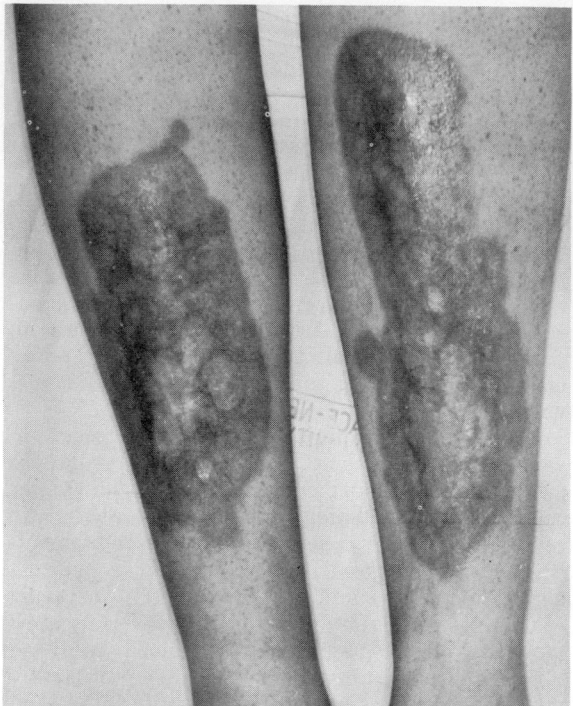

FIGURE 3. Necrobiosis diabeticorum in a 22-year-old woman.

common. *Eruptive xanthoma,* or *xanthoma diabeticorum,* which is more unusual, consists of the rapid appearance of firm, raised papules. At first these are erythematous, but as they grow larger, reaching a diameter of a few millimeters, the centers become pale yellow and very hard, and an erythematous halo persists. After the lipid disturbance has been corrected, the halo disappears rapidly, but reabsorption of the lipid deposits is slow, requiring weeks or months for completion. This eruption appears especially over pressure areas such as elbows, knees, and buttocks, and also on the dorsum of the arm. Its course and appearance suggest that similar, less innocent events may be occurring simultaneously in the arteries. Punctate or small round areas of depigmentation and atrophy, quite different in clinical appearance from necrobiosis, are also seen (*shin spots*). These changes are characteristic of diabetes, although similar changes are sometimes seen from trauma, heat, and other local influences.

As mentioned previously, *infections* are little more frequent in diabetics than in others, but they are likely to be more severe. Even ordinarily nonpathogenic organisms such as *C. albicans* or *E. coli* may become dangerous invaders in diabetes. *Escherichia coli,* for example, may cause a soft tissue infection clinically indistinguishable from gas gangrene. *Tuberculosis* has always been especially serious in diabetics. Modern methods of treatment have reduced this risk substantially. The prognosis of tuberculosis in diabetics is not affected by moderate degrees of hyperglycemia, so no special precautions need be taken in relation to treatment of the metabolic defect; however, young diabetics should have chest roentgenograms at least every two years. Genitourinary infections have already been mentioned. Candida infections of the vulva may be troublesome, especially when diabetes is poorly controlled. Both local and systemic fungus infections may be more persistent and dangerous in diabetics than in normal patients. This is most marked in the case of mucormycosis, an infection with a species of the fungus Mucorales, which is seen especially in patients with diabetes. It usually affects the nasal sinuses first and erodes and invades the soft tissues until involvement of the central nervous system causes death. Even with modern fungicidal medications, it is difficult to control, and the mortality of such infections is high.

Rapid fluctuations of the osmolarity of body fluids, produced by changing glucose concentrations in the extracellular fluid, alter the refractive index of the lens of the eye relative to the humors, and thus impair the visual acuity. Stability, whether at high or low glucose concentrations, restores the relative refractive index, as glucose diffuses equally into the lens and humors. Diabetics should therefore avoid refraction tests during periods of metabolic instability. The same rapid and repeated alterations of osmolarity may explain the tendency of diabetics to develop *premature cataracts* of the lens. Less clear is the reason for an increased tendency to *glaucoma* in diabetics.

Surgery in the Diabetic. Diabetes adds an extra dimension of risk to any surgical procedure. Ideally, an operation should be postponed until the diabetes is well controlled, and the patient is well nourished and properly hydrated. The normal diabetic regimen may be followed the day before surgery. The morning of the operation, oral intake will usually be prohibited, and the patient should receive fluids intravenously in such quantity as to provide at least 100 grams of glucose during the day of operation. In our experience it has been most convenient to add the necessary dose of insulin—usually 15 to 20 units per liter of 5 per cent dextrose—directly to the drip bottle, since this avoids the danger that subcutaneous insulin may not be balanced by adequate carbohydrate if the intravenous needle or tube becomes plugged or is inserted late. If the patient is particularly brittle, urine specimens may be obtained from an indwelling catheter and supplements of insulin given as needed; however, this is rarely required. Since patients previously adequately controlled with oral hypoglycemic agents usually need insulin during surgery, it is best to include them in this program. After minor surgical procedures, the patient may be placed on oral feedings that are covered with short-acting insulin during the first 24 hours; thereafter one can usually return to the preoperative schedule unless complications such as infection supervene. If feeding is impossible, a program similar to that used on the day of operation can be continued until feeding by mouth becomes possible. With prolonged parenteral feeding, the patient should receive vitamin supplements.

The nature of the electrolytes included with the glucose infusions will be determined by surgical and other medical factors.

Pregnancy and Diabetes. Patients who have had diabetes only a short time and who have no evidence of atherosclerosis or microvascular disease tolerate pregnancy well, although the insulin requirement is likely to increase during the second trimester. In spite of the bland course followed by most diabetic women, the fetal and neonatal mortality is high. Because the intrauterine mortality rises fairly steeply after the thirty-sixth to thirty-eighth week of gestation, delivery is commonly induced at this point, either medically or by cesarian section. The baby thus delivered may be heavy, but much of his weight is likely to be due to edema, and the baby should be treated as though he were premature in spite of his weight. The prognosis of the baby is worse if the mother has evidence of vascular disease, and it is also poor if ketoacidosis occurs during pregnancy. Since vascular lesions of the retina and kidneys frequently accelerate during pregnancy, it is unwise for diabetics with clearly established microvascular disease to become pregnant; and since repeated pregnancies aggravate these lesions, the diabetic woman should be content with a small family. Indeed, we believe that evidence of retinopathy or Kimmelstiel-Wilson disease is an adequate indication for interruption of pregnancy and sterilization of the mother.

Complications of Treatment. Characteristic areas of *fat atrophy* or *hypertrophy* may develop at sites of repeated insulin injection (Fig. 4). The cause of these rather unusual complications is not known, nor is any treatment available except systematic rotation of the sites of injection to avoid repeated trauma to any one area. Often atrophy or hypertrophy disappears spontaneously after several years. The atrophic change should be differentiated from *progressive lipodystrophy*, discussed earlier, because it is sharply demarcated, whereas lipodystrophy involves half the body. Fat hypertrophy must be differentiated from a benign lipoma. It may rarely be accompanied by local painful reaction to insulin injection, and thus superficially resemble the disease *adiposis dolorosa* of Dercum; but this disease usually manifests itself as scattered areas of painful nodules or fat accumulations in menopausal women. Insulin hypertrophy is usually present in only one or two locations where insulin is habitually injected. Some patients develop allergy to insulin, manifested by urticaria or local painful infiltrations at the sites of injection. Sometimes relief can be afforded by changing to insulin from another species, especially porcine, but usually antihistaminics are the best solution. One part of procaine can be added to four parts of the insulin suspension to provide relief.

Hypoglycemic attacks (insulin shock) may occur with overdoses of insulin or of the oral sulfonylureas. Although hypoglycemia may follow the usual clinical course seen when the disease occurs spontaneously (see below), it may develop very

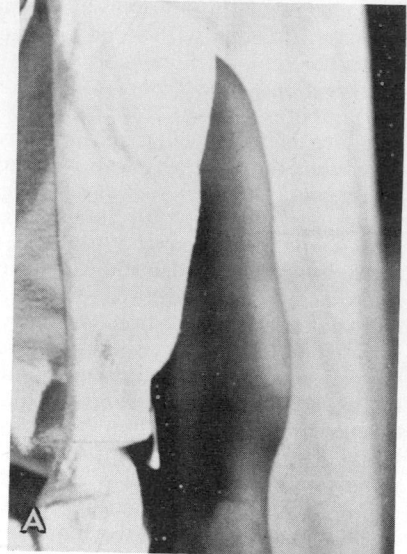
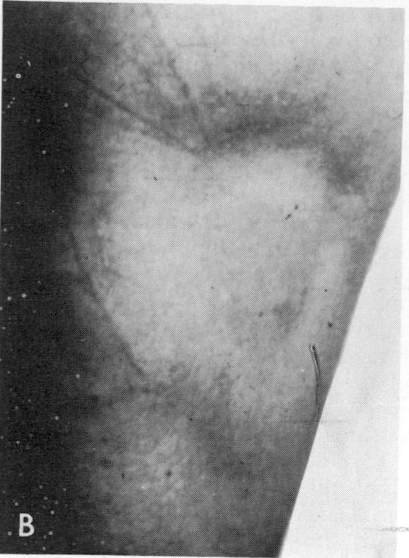

FIGURE 4.   *A,* Insulin hypertrophy in the upper arm. *B,* Fat atrophy induced by insulin in the upper thigh.

subtly, causing confusion and coma without the usual warning symptoms of fear, sweating, palpitation, and hunger. Some patients are nauseated by low blood sugar. Intermediate-acting insulins often cause hypoglycemia at night, when the only symptoms may be nightmares and sweating. If mild, the attacks can often be aborted by eating candy or drinking a sweet drink; however, sometimes the depression of blood glucose produces unconsciousness, so that intravenous glucose is required. In emergencies, 5 mg. of glucagon, subcutaneously or intramuscularly, may help. Repeated hypoglycemic attacks cause brain damage, resulting in personality changes, depressed intelligence, cerebral dysrhythmias, and sometimes epileptiform convulsions. In atherosclerotic patients, hypoglycemia may produce focal neurologic signs suggesting an area of locally defective circulation, or myocardial infarcts may occur. Retinal hemorrhages appear commonly after a hypoglycemic attack.

Prognosis. Although the metabolic defect can usually be controlled fairly successfully, most diabetics develop evidence of vascular complications after 15 years or more of the disease and ultimately succumb to renal failure, cerebral or myocardial infarction, or peripheral vascular disease with one of its complications. In spite of this, some patients (not necessarily those who have been best controlled) may live for 40 or more years with only minimal evidence of complications. From these considerations it is clear that the long-term outlook for patients who develop the disease in childhood and adolescence is poor, whereas the maturity-onset diabetic may live out the remainder of his life and die of some other disease. Although it seems sensible to control the disease as accurately as possible without harming the patient, the fact remains that such control does not predictably alter the prognosis.

Beaser, S. B.: A survey of current therapy of diabetes mellitus. Diabetes, 13:472, 1964.

Bondy, P. K.: Disorders of carbohydrate metabolism. *In* Duncan's Diseases of Metabolism. 6th ed. Philadelphia, W. B. Saunders Company, 1969, pp. 199–294.

Cameron, H. C., Lennard-Jones, J. E., and Robinson, M. P.: Amputations in the diabetic—Outcome and survival. Lancet, 2:605, 1964.

Chance, R. E., and Ellis, R. M.: Proinsulin. Single chain precursor of insulin. Ann. Intern. Med., 123:229, 1969.

Colby, A. O.: Neurologic disorders of diabetes mellitus. Diabetes, 14:424, 516, 1965.

Goldberg, M. F., and Fine, S. L.: Symposium on the Treatment of Diabetic Retinopathy. Public Health Service Publication No. 1890. Washington, D.C., U. S. Government Printing Office, 1969.

Gorden, P., and Roth, J.: Circulating insulins "big" and "little." Ann. Intern. Med., 123:237, 1969.

Kipnis, D. M.: Insulin secretion in diabetes mellitus. Ann. Intern. Med., 69:891, 1968.

Knowles, H. C., Jr., Guest, G. M., Lampe, J. R. N., Kessler, M., and Skillman, T. G.: The course of juvenile diabetes treated with unmeasured diet. J. Amer. Diabetes Ass., 14:239, 1965.

HYPOGLYCEMIC STATES
Philip K. Bondy

Definition. Hypoglycemia exists when the blood glucose concentration falls below 50 mg. per 100 ml. Since many factors may cause such a depression, hypoglycemia is a symptom, not a disease (see accompanying table). The major problem for the physician is to recognize the cause; the decision as to treatment is then usually self-evident.

Pathophysiology. Ordinarily the fasting blood glucose concentration is maintained within normal limits because the liver and kidneys convert amino acids to glucose, which is secreted at a rate equal to the rate of utilization. Hypoglycemia may occur either because glucose leaves the blood at an accelerated rate or because it is secreted too slowly, but in many instances both mechanisms obtain. Accelerated disappearance may reflect (1) increased utilization by muscles or fat tissue, usually a response to exogenous or endogenous insulin, muscular exercise, or failure of hypoglycemia to elicit secretion of pituitary growth hormone, epinephrine, or glucagon, (2) excessive uptake by massive tumors, or (3) inappropriate loss into the urine, which occurs only as a result of renal tubular poisons such as phlorhizin. Reduced entry of glucose into the blood may occur because of malabsorption or as a result of failure of gluconeogenesis. Reduced secretion of glucose by the liver may occur in *glycogenosis* because of enzyme defects preventing glycogen breakdown or hydrolysis of glucose-6-phosphate. Glycogen breakdown is also inhibited in patients with *hereditary fructose intolerance,* in whom defective function of the enzyme aldolase prevents conversion of fructose-1-phosphate to 3-carbon fragments. The resulting accumulation of fructose-1-phosphate appears to block the glycogenolytic effects of epinephrine and glucagon. As a result, feeding fructose causes the blood glucose concentration to fall to pathologic levels. *Insulin* reduces gluconeogenesis, as does the amino acid *tryptophan.* The oxidation of *ethanol* tends to tie up most of the hepatic NAD in reduced form. This promotes conversion of pyruvate to lactate, and also prevents oxidative reactions depending on NAD as a hydrogen receptor. As a result, the gluconeogenic pathway is deprived of its major sources of substrate. The resulting hypoglycemia is sometimes called *"smoke poisoning"* from the slang term for illicit alcohol in some localities. The *akee nut,* fruit of the tree *Blighia sapida,* contains, in its unripe form, a complex organic substance called *hypoglycin,* which is converted in the body to methylenecyclopropylacetic acid. This substance displaces fatty acids and acetyl-coenzyme A from carnitine, and thus prevents these substances from entering the citric acid and gluconeogenic pathways. As a result, fat utilization is inhibited, and glucose utilization is reduced, whereas gluconeogenesis is reduced. The resulting hypoglycemia is called *"Jamaican vomiting sickness."* Inadequate gluconeogenesis may also occur when *adrenocortical failure* reduces the rate of release of amino acids from body protein and thus reduces the substrate available for forming new glucose. Hepatic destruction may reduce the mass of live cells enough to cause hypoglycemia, but this rarely occurs except after exposures to poison such as *phosphorus* or *carbon tetrachloride,* or as a late complication of viral hepatitis progressing to *acute hepatic necrosis.* Ordinary viral hepatitis and cirrhosis do not usually cause hypoglycemia. Certain diguanidines depress the blood glucose by causing liver damage. Hypoglycemia is occasionally a complication of lesions of the hypothalamus, but the explanation is not known.

Clinical Classification. Although the various types of spontaneous hypoglycemia can be ex-

plained by underproduction or overutilization of glucose, or a combination of these, the clinician is best served by classifying patients according to whether the hypoglycemia is spontaneous, i.e., occurs while fasting, or induced by some external agent (Table 4). The agent may be a poison or drug; or, in susceptible persons, it may be a normal component of the diet such as *leucine, galactose, fructose,* or even *glucose.* The latter is especially likely to induce excessive insulin secretion when administered to persons after *gastrectomy* (since this permits a large concentration of glucose in the duodenum to stimulate excessive secretion of insulin-releasing gastrointestinal hormones) or in patients liable to develop diabetes, whose delayed but exaggerated insulin secretory response may result in hyperinsulinemia after the blood glucose has dropped to fasting levels. In some patients, feeding carbohydrate results in hypoglycemia after three or four hours, even without this mechanism (*"functional hypoglycemia"*). It is clear also that the age of the patient affects the type of hypoglycemia to be expected. Thus, in infants *glycogen storage disease,* leucine sensitivity *malnutrition,* and intolerance of galactose or fructose would be relatively common, whereas islet cell tumor is unusual and most of the other causes are very rare. When ketosis is associated with hypoglycemia in children, glycogen storage disease should be considered. Some patients with ketotic hypoglycemia also have fatty infiltration of the liver and a family history of siblings who have died with *Reye's syndrome.*

Clinical Manifestations. Hypoglycemia presents two separate but not exclusive patterns, one

TABLE 4. CLASSIFICATION OF HYPOGLYCEMIA

I. Spontaneous (Fasting) Hypoglycemia
  A. Excessive insulin
    1. Insulinoma or insulin-secreting carcinoma
    2. Erythroblastosis fetalis
  B. Nonendocrine tumor (usually large retroperitoneal sarcoma)
  C. Glycogen storage disease of the liver
  D. Malnutrition or malabsorption
  E. Adrenocortical or pituitary failure
  F. Liver necrosis
  G. Hereditary galactosemia
  H. Reye's syndrome and other forms of ketotic hypoglycemia in children
II. Induced Hypoglycemia
  A. Excessive insulin
    1. Overtreated diabetic
    2. Leucine (includes some islet cell tumors)
    3. Sulfonylureas
    4. Functional
      a. Prediabetic
      b. Postgastrectomy
      c. Hemodialysis with hypertonic glucose
      d. Idiopathic
  B. Reduced gluconeogenesis
    1. Ethanol
    2. Hypoglycin
    3. Hereditary fructose intolerance
    4. Failure of glucagon secretion
  C. Persistent increase of peripheral glucose uptake
    1. Failure of catecholamine secretion
    2. Propranolol blockade of catecholamine effect
  D. Cause uncertain
    Pentamidine

manifested by abnormalities of the nervous system and the other by adrenergic discharge. Reduction of the blood glucose to levels as low as 20 mg. per 100 ml. may be tolerated for brief periods by healthy persons without symptoms. If such low levels are sustained, inadequate amounts of glucose are available to the nervous system as its chief metabolic substrate, and symptoms of cerebral dysfunction develop. These may take the form of confusion, hallucinations, aimless hyperactivity, or even convulsions, but the ultimate result is deep coma. Hypothermia is common during unconsciousness. Persons with local restrictions of cerebral blood supply may have focal signs, either paralytic or convulsive, and these may recur in a characteristic pattern with each attack of hypoglycemia. The electroencephalogram in hypoglycemia shows slow regular waves, which promptly revert to normal when the blood glucose rises. The cerebral symptoms, however, may persist for hours or days before improving. If hypoglycemia is sufficiently prolonged, there is permanent cortical damage.

The normal response to hypoglycemia is a massive outpouring of epinephrine. A characteristic pattern in hypoglycemia, therefore, is tachycardia, anxiety, sweating, pallor, and rise of blood pressure. These effects may be minimized by drugs that block the sympathetic discharge, or in patients whose sympathetic nervous system has degenerated as a result of neuropathy, as in diabetes. When hypoglycemia develops slowly, there may be neurologic symptoms without detectable sympathomimetic response, and when the blood glucose falls rapidly, sympathetic discharge may occur before the blood glucose concentration has fallen low enough to interfere with normal cerebral function. Since eating carbohydrate can terminate hypoglycemia, hunger is often a symptom; however, some patients experience nausea rather than a desire for food. The patient subject to repeated attacks of hypoglycemia usually discovers that he can prevent or abort attacks by eating foods high in carbohydrate. Such patients therefore often gain weight.

Diagnosis. A suspicion of hypoglycemia should be entertained in the presence of unexplained coma or periodic episodes of confusion, convulsions, adrenergic symptoms, weakness, or inappropriate hunger. The history should explore possible exposure to hypoglycemia-inducing agents such as insulin, alcohol, etc. The relationship of symptoms to food intake is important since "functional" hypoglycemia occurs three to five hours after eating, whereas spontaneous attacks often occur on fasting or at night. It should be remembered that insulin is sometimes used for suicidal or homicidal purposes by persons who have access to it.

To establish a diagnosis of hypoglycemia, it is essential to demonstrate a depression of blood sugar, but, since the periods of hypoglycemia are often transient, special procedures must sometimes be used to detect them. Determination of blood glucose concentration during an attack is useful. However, if the episode is convulsive, the blood glucose may rise to normal levels toward the end of the attack.

The physician should first determine whether hypoglycemia occurs spontaneously or only after the action of a specific stimulus. In adults, spontaneous hypoglycemia is usually due either to an insulin-secreting tumor or a retroperitoneal sarcoma. The diagnosis is made by measuring the fasting blood glucose, but it may be necessary to prolong the fast up to 72 hours. In the Mayo Clinic series, 66 per cent of the patients had depressed fasting blood glucose concentrations, and 94 per cent of all insulinomas caused hypoglycemia after 48 hours of fasting. The diagnosis is made more secure if insulin is shown to be present in the plasma during hypoglycemia; but elevated levels are not required for the diagnosis, since even "normal" levels are abnormal in hypoglycemic patients. Prolonged hypoglycemia, remaining below 40 mg. per 100 ml. by three hours, is also induced by 1.0 gram of sodium tolbutamide given intravenously in about 75 per cent of these patients, and some show hypoglycemia after administration of 150 mg. of leucine per kilogram. The tumor can sometimes be localized by celiac angiography or, rarely, by scanning after administration of radioactive selenomethionine. Multiple benign tumors were found in 5 per cent and cancers in 10 per cent of the Mayo Clinic series. Insulinomas are often associated with tumors in other endocrine organs such as the parathyroid or pituitary glands. Hypoglycemia associated with tumors other than islet cell neoplasms occurs as a result of excessive utilization of glucose by the tumor or of release of excess amounts of a substance which suppresses gluconeogenesis (perhaps tryptophan). Such patients do not have abnormal plasma insulin levels. Since an elevated blood glucose concentration is the most potent known stimulus to insulin secretion, the glucose tolerance test is useful in precipitating attacks in patients with functional hypoglycemia, who usually develop symptoms three to five hours after the ingestion of 100 grams of glucose. Liver disease or prolonged starvation may give a false positive test both to a glucose load and to sodium tolbutamide. In some cases, in which demonstration of hypoglycemia has been difficult even after provocative tests, it may be useful to see whether the symptoms of the attacks can be reproduced by inducing hypoglycemia with insulin. Anxiety attacks, which may otherwise be difficult to differentiate from episodes of hypoglycemia, may be subjectively so different that the patient can distinguish them with ease. The diagnosis of most of the other types of hypoglycemia will be obvious from other manifestations such as severe liver disease, an odor of alcohol on the breath, and so on.

Treatment. When hypoglycemia is suspected as a cause of convulsions or coma, a blood specimen should be drawn immediately for determination of glucose, by chemical or spot-test, and glucose should then be given. The intravenous route is preferable, and at least 25 grams should be given rapidly; thereafter, a continuous drip of 5 per cent glucose can be maintained to provide about 12 grams of glucose per hour, a rate sufficient to sustain the blood glucose even in the absence of the liver. If glucose administration causes immediate improvement, subsequent treatment can be adjusted to the patient's needs; however, response to glucose may be slow, especially if hypoglycemia has been prolonged, and treatment should not be abandoned prematurely.

If facilities for intravenous glucose treatment are not available and the patient can swallow, any sort of drink sweetened with glucose or sucrose is useful. Fluids should not be forced on a comatose patient, however. In an emergency, epinephrine (1 mg. subcutaneously) or glucagon (5 mg. intramuscularly or intravenously) may be helpful.

When hypoglycemia is a result of endocrine or liver disease, the major therapeutic effort should be directed toward the primary disease. The treatment of functional hypoglycemia is based on the supposition that the attacks occur because of excessive and inappropriate secretion of insulin in response to hyperglycemia. A diet low in carbohydrate and high in fat and protein is therefore recommended to minimize fluctuations of blood glucose concentration and to supply (through the protein) adequate precursors of glycogen. Atropine or belladonna may also be useful in controlling the symptoms.

Hyperinsulinism demands removal of the secreting tumor, which is often small and difficult to find on exploration. If surgical exploration fails to reveal an adenoma, the body and tail of the pancreas should be resected arbitrarily, since over 70 per cent of benign insulinomas lie in this position. If this fails to control the disease, a second operation may be needed to remove the head of the pancreas. Immediately after the insulin-secreting tumor has been removed, the blood glucose often rises abruptly. This sign may be helpful to the surgeon in determining whether he has removed the offending portion of the pancreas. When carcinoma of the islet cells proves inoperable, one may be tempted to try to destroy the tumor with alloxan, but experience with this treatment has usually been unsuccessful. Diazoxide (up to 4 mg. per kilogram three times daily) may maintain the blood glucose in patients with inoperable insulinoma or idiopathic hypoglycemia. It has also been reported that streptozotocin can reduce the size of such tumors and control hypoglycemia.

Exploration may reveal a large fleshy tumor of the retroperitoneal or posterior mediastinal areas. Such tumors do not have the histologic characteristics of islet cell tumors, and attempts to extract insulin or insulin-like substances from them have usually been unsuccessful. The explanation of their hypoglycemia-producing effect is unclear, but removal of the bulk of the tumor usually terminates hypoglycemia. If the tumor returns, the blood glucose usually falls again.

Ernesti, M., Mitchell, M. L., and Raben, M. S.: Control of hypoglycemia with diazoxide and growth hormone. Lancet, 1:628, 1965.

Fajans, S. S., Schneider, J. M., Schteingart, D. E., and Conn, J. W.: The diagnostic value of sodium tolbutamide in hypoglycemia states. J. Clin. Endocr., 21:371, 1961.
Laroche, G. P., et al.: Hyperinsulinism. Surgical, results and management of occult functioning islet cell tumor. Review of 154 cases. Arch. Surg. (Chicago), 96:763, 1968.
Murray-Lyon, I. M., et al.: Treatment of multiple hormone-producing malignant islet-cell tumour with streptozotocin. Lancet, 2:895, 1968.
Pedersen, J., Lund, F., and Ringsted, J.: Hypoglycaemia in the presence of massive fibrosarcoma (mesenchymoma), Acta Endocr. (Kbh.), 34:148, 1960.
Symposium on Hypoglycemia. Diabetes, 14:333, 1965.
Unger, R. H.: The riddle of tumor hypoglycemia. Amer. J. Med., 40:325, 1966.

INBORN ERRORS OF CARBOHYDRATE METABOLISM

GALACTOSEMIA
Ernest Beutler

Definition. Patients with galactosemia have an inborn error of metabolism which results in a loss of their capacity to metabolize galactose. As a result, galactose accumulates in the blood when a substantial amount is absorbed from the gastrointestinal tract, and it may also appear in the urine.

Etiology. "Classic galactosemia" is due to a marked deficiency of the enzyme, galactose-1-phosphate uridyl transferase. A much rarer form of galactosemia, first described in 1965, is due to deficiency of the enzyme, galactokinase.

Incidence. Reliable estimates of the incidence of galactosemia have not been made. The best available data suggest that the incidence of classic galactosemia is approximately 1:100,000 births; only three families with homozygous galactokinase deficiency have been diagnosed, and it seems likely that the incidence of this disorder is less than 1:500,000 births.

Pathogenesis. The galactose molecule is identical to the glucose molecule except for the relative position of the hydroxyl and hydrogen groups attached to the 4-carbon. However, the body is unable to utilize this sugar until it has been converted to glucose. Only one pathway for the metabolism of galactose has been clearly established. First, galactose is phosphorylated in the 1-position by ATP through the mediation of the enzyme galactokinase:

$$\text{Galactose} + \text{ATP} \xrightarrow{\text{galactokinase}} \text{galactose-1-P}$$

Next, the galactose-1-P formed exchanges with the glucose-1-P moiety attached to a uridine diphosphate carrier. This reaction is catalyzed by galactose-1-phosphate uridyl transferase (transferase):

$$\text{Galactose-1-P} + \text{UDPG} \xrightleftharpoons{\text{transferase}} \text{glucose-1-P} + \text{UDPGal}$$

Finally, the uridine diphosphogalactose (UDPGal) formed may be converted to uridine diphosphoglucose (UDPG) through the action of epimerase:

$$\text{UDPGal} \underset{}{\overset{\text{epimerase}}{\rightleftharpoons}} \text{UDPG}$$

In galactokinase deficiency galactose accumulates in the body. This sugar may serve as substrate for aldose reductase, which oxidizes NADPH or NADH, converting some of the galactose to its polyol derivative, dulcatol, to which cell membranes are relatively impermeable. When this conversion occurs in the lens of the eye, it creates an unbalanced osmotic force in the lens, resulting in excessive hydration. At the same time it depletes the lens of its supply of NADPH which is required to maintain glutathione and the thiol groups of the lens crystallins in the reduced form. The result of these changes is irreversible precipitation of lens proteins with the formation of cataracts.

In "classic galactosemia," the absence of galactose-1-phosphate uridyl transferase results in accumulation of both galactose and galactose-1-P. The mechanism of cataract formation is probably the same in this disorder as in galactokinase deficiency. In addition, cirrhosis of the liver and mental retardation are characteristic of classic galactosemia. Since these changes do not occur in galactokinase deficiency it may be presumed that they are the result of galactose-1-P accumulation, but how galactose-1-phosphate damages the liver and the brain has not been elucidated.

Clinical Manifestations. Occasionally galactosemic infants may have cataracts at birth. More typically the symptoms of galactosemia begin within a few days or weeks of birth. The infant takes feedings poorly, vomits frequently, and may have diarrhea. The abdomen may enlarge owing to progressive hepatomegaly and ascites. Jaundice usually appears quite early, and the disorder has, at times, been mistaken for hemolytic disease of the newborn. Proteinuria and generalized aminoaciduria are constant findings. If they are not present at birth, cataracts may develop within a few weeks, or in some instances, not for many months. Mental retardation becomes evident as the infant matures. Administration of large galactose loads, given in connection with galactose tolerance tests, may produce dangerous hypoglycemia.

Cataracts and galactose intolerance are the only clinical manifestations of galactokinase deficiency.

Diagnosis. The diagnosis of galactokinase deficiency should be suspected in children with cataracts who manifest galactose intolerance and who excrete nonglucose-reducing substances in the urine. Definitive diagnosis is established by assaying galactokinase activity of the red blood cells.

Classic galactosemia is diagnosed by demonstrating that galactose-1-phosphate uridyl transferase activity is absent from the erythrocytes.

Treatment. The treatment of galactosemia consists of institution of a diet with a very low content of galactose as soon as the diagnosis is established. Because milk contains a high concentration of lactose, a disaccharide of glucose and galactose, a milk substitute such as Nutramigen must be fed during infancy. Although the effect of the galactose-free diet on infants is clearly established, no clear-cut data are available regarding the necessity for maintaining a galactose-free program after the first few years of life. It is likely that the ingestion of small amounts of galactose is relatively harmless after the fifth or sixth year of life. However, until further evidence is available regarding the possible harmful effects of galactose when fed to older galactosemic children and adults, it is probably wise to continue a moderate degree of dietary restriction throughout life.

Prognosis. Except for cataract formation, galactokinase deficiency is a relatively harmless disorder, compatible with long life. Untreated infants with classic galactosemia, however, rarely survive more than a few months. Only two cases have been described in which the diagnosis of classic galactosemia was first made in a severely mentally retarded adult. With the prompt institution of a galactose-free diet the development of galactosemic children appears to be normal or nearly so. If treatment is delayed, however, some degree of permanent mental retardation and irreversible cataracts is often present. Signs of liver failure and growth retardation appear to respond promptly to therapy in most instances, however, and treated galactosemics may live into adult life.

Prevention. Galactosemia itself can only be prevented through genetic counseling. Heterozygotes for galactokinase deficiency have half-normal galactokinase activity in their red blood cells. Heterozygotes for classic galactosemia have one half the normal galactose-1-phosphate uridyl transferase activity in their red cells. However, all persons with this level of enzyme activity are not carriers of galactosemia. Persons homozygous for another gene, that for the Duarte variant, also have one-half of normal transferase activity, but may be differentiated from those heterozygous for galactosemia on the basis of the electrophoretic properties of the red cell enzyme.

Prevention of the clinical sequelae of galactosemia by early diagnosis and prompt institution of treatment is the most practical means of control. Microbiologic and enzymatic methods for the detection of galactose in the blood or in the urine have been developed. These methods should detect most cases of galactokinase deficiency and of classic galactosemia. However, a considerable number of false positive results are encountered, and false negative results will be found in infants who are so ill as to refuse their feedings. A fluorescent screening test which depends directly upon galactose-1-phosphate uridyl transferase activity has been developed, and will detect classic galactosemia with few false positives and no false negatives. However, this procedure will not identify infants with galactokinase deficiency.

Mothers who have borne galactosemic children or who are at risk because of proved heterozygous status should not take milk during pregnancy. Their offspring should not be given milk until it has been established that they have normal galactose-1-phosphate uridyl transferase activity.

Beutler, E., and Mathai, C. K.: Genetic variation in red cell galactose-1-phosphate uridyl transferase. In Beutler, E. (ed.): Hereditary Disorders of Erythrocyte Metabolism. City of Hope Symposium Series Vol. I. New York, Gruno & Stratton, Inc., 1968, pp. 66-86.

Donnell, G. N., Bergren, W. R. and Ng, W. G.: Galactosemia. Biochem. Med., 1:29, 1967.

Hsia, D. Y. Y. (ed.): Galactosemia. Springfield, Ill., Charles C Thomas, 1969.

FRUCTOSURIA AND HEREDITARY FRUCTOSE INTOLERANCE

Howard H. Hiatt

Fructosuria (Essential Fructosuria). Fructosuria is a rare disturbance of carbohydrate metabolism, transmitted in autosomal recessive fashion and without known clinical consequence. Fructose, a hexose present in most fruits and in cane sugar, is assimilated via two pathways. The primary mechanism involves phosphorylation by a specific enzyme, fructokinase, to fructose-1-phosphate, which is then rapidly metabolized. Fructokinase is found in liver, kidney, and intestinal mucosa. The less efficient pathway of fructose metabolism involves phosphorylation by hexokinase (the same enzyme that phosphorylates glucose) to fructose-6-phosphate, which is an intermediate in the glycolytic pathway and is thus in the mainstream of carbohydrate metabolism. Under conditions of fasting, fructose is not detectable in urine, and is found in only very small quantity in blood. After intake of fructose or fructose-containing foods, however, as much as 15 to 25 mg. per 100 ml. can briefly be detected in the blood of normal individuals, and 1 to 2 per cent of a large administered load may be excreted in the urine. Identification of the sugar in body fluids can best be carried out chromatographically.

Subjects with fructosuria lack hepatic fructokinase, and because the hexokinase route of metabolism is much less efficient, their blood fructose rises to high levels after fructose ingestion (over 25 mg. per 100 ml. in a fructose tolerance test, in which 1 gram per kilogram of body weight is given orally or intravenously) and 10 to 20 per cent appears in the urine. The increased circulating fructose is, however, not harmful, and individuals with fructosuria are asymptomatic. Indeed, a principal hazard of fructosuria is that it may be confused with some other condition, particularly diabetes mellitus, and as a result inappropriate treatment may be initiated.

Hereditary Fructose Intolerance (Fructosemia). Hereditary fructose intolerance is the term applied to an infrequently occurring, serious genetically determined condition, which results from lack of fructose-1-phosphate aldolase activity, leading to a block at the second step in the principal pathway of fructose metabolism. Three phosphofructoaldolases (A, B, and C) have been described in animal tissues. Although all catalyze the conversion of both fructose-1-phosphate (F-1-P) and fructose-1, 6-diphosphate (FDP), an intermediate in the glycolytic pathway, to 3-carbon products, the relative affinity of each aldolase for the two fructose esters varies widely. Thus, phosphofructoaldolase B, the enzyme incriminated in hereditary fructose intolerance, is equally effective in metabolizing F-1-P and FDP, whereas aldolases A and C have perhaps 5 per cent as much affinity for F-1-P as for FDP. In order for F-1-P to accumulate, two conditions must be met—the enzyme specific for its production (fructokinase) must be present, and that required for its further metabolism (phosphofructoaldolase B) must be deficient. In patients with hereditary fructose intolerance these conditions prevail in liver, renal cortex, and intestinal mucosa, but not in other tissues tested. Ingestion of fructose by these persons leads to an accumulation of fructose in blood and urine and of F-1-P in liver, kidney, and intestinal mucosa, those tissues containing fructokinase. It is probably the high level of F-1-P to which the several harmful features of hereditary fructose intolerance can be ascribed. There is more than one genotype, but the most frequently reported variety of this rare disturbance is inherited in autosomal recessive fashion.

The F-1-P that is produced after fructose ingestion by normal persons is rapidly metabolized. However, the accumulation of F-1-P in subjects with hereditary fructose intolerance results in serious disturbances, including hypoglycemia (apparently caused by impaired glucose production and unresponsiveness to glucagon), nausea and vomiting, renal tubular acidosis with aminoaciduria, proteinuria, and impaired liver function. (In contrast, recall that the accumulation of fructose is harmless.) Continued intake of fructose, as may occur in infants before the problem is recognized, leads to inanition, hepatomegaly, liver failure, acidosis, and severe electrolyte disturbances, and may be fatal. The serious effects on blood sugar, liver, renal tubule, and gut have been shown to occur quickly after the administration of fructose and to be reversible, at least in early stages, upon fructose withdrawal. Thus, subjects with hereditary fructose intolerance who have avoided fructose through life seem to avoid the associated clinical problems. Administration of fructose to such individuals, however, rapidly brings on symptoms, and should be carried out only when deemed essential and with provision for managing at once the hypoglycemia that inevitably results.

Hereditary fructose intolerance can be diagnosed by demonstrating both abnormally high blood and urine fructose levels, as in fructosuria, and hypoglycemia and hypophosphatemia, which are not seen in fructosuria, following administration of fructose. Indeed, if this condition is suspected, the test dose of fructose administered intravenously should be very small, 0.25 gram per kilogram of body weight, an amount that may result in only a small rise in blood fructose, but that will generally produce a marked fall in blood glucose and phosphate. The abnormal fructosemia and fructosuria following fructose administration in hereditary fructose intolerance are believed to result from inhibition of fructokinase by F-1-P. The diagnosis has also been made by demonstrating in biopsy material a profound reduction or absence of hepatic or intestinal F-1-P aldolase (phosphofructoaldolase B) activity. The clinical picture resembles somewhat that seen in galactosemia, but differs in dietary history and in the absence of mental retardation and cataracts. Finally, hereditary fructose intolerance should be distinguished from the even rarer familial galactose and fructose intolerance, a condition in which both sugars produce hypoglycemia.

Froesch, E. R.: Essential fructosuria and hereditary fructose intolerance. *In* Stanbury, J. B., Wyngaarden, J. B., and Frederickson, D. S. (eds.): The Metabolic Basis of Inherited Disease. 2nd ed. New York, McGraw-Hill Book Company, 1966, p. 124.

Levin, B., Snodgrass, G. J. A. I., Oberholzer, V. G., Burgess, E. A., and Dobbs, R. H.: Fructosemia: Observations on seven cases. Amer. J. Med., 45:826, 1968.

Morris, R. C., Jr.: An experimental renal acidification defect in patients with hereditary fructose intolerance. I. Its resemblance to renal tubular acidosis. J. Clin. Invest., 47:1389, 1968.

PENTOSURIA
(Essential Pentosuria)
Howard H. Hiatt

Pentosuria is an innocuous, genetically determined error of carbohydrate metabolism characterized by urinary excretion of 1 to 4 grams of the pentose, L-xylulose, per day. It occurs infrequently, is seen almost exclusively in Jews, and is transmitted in autosomal recessive fashion. It is caused by a defect in the glucuronic acid oxidation pathway, at the step involving the conversion of L-xylulose to xylitol. Glucuronolactone administration leads to increased L-xylulose excretion in the pentosuric and permits recognition of the heterozygote, who under such conditions excretes very small amounts of the pentose. The glucuronic acid pathway apparently plays no important role in human metabolism. It may be slightly more active in patients with diabetes mellitus, although there is no relation between pentosuria and diabetes. The diagnosis is established by demonstrating chromatographically that the reducing substance in the urine is L-xylulose. The condition is thereby distinguished from diabetes mellitus, from alimentary pentosuria, the term applied to the excretion of very small (milligram) quantities of arabinose or xylose after intake of certain fruits, and from other states in which urinary sugar is demonstrable. The subject may then be reassured that he has a condition that

will result in lifelong urinary excretion of a sugar, but that will in no way affect his health.

Garrod, A. E.: Inborn Errors of Metabolism. London, Henry Frowde, 1909.

Hiatt, H. H.: Pentosuria. *In* Stanbury, J. B., Wyngaarden, J. B., and Frederickson, D. S. (eds.): The Metabolic Basis of Inherited Disease. 3rd ed. New York. McGraw-Hill Book Company, in press.

Wang, Y. M., and van Eys, J.: The enzymatic defect in essential pentosuria. New Eng. J. Med., 282:892, 1970.

GLYCOGEN STORAGE DISEASES
J. B. Sidbury, Jr.

Definition. The glycogenoses are a group of heritable disorders of glycogen metabolism which have in common a quantitative or qualitative aberration of tissue glycogen. Glycogen accumulation secondary to other factors such as excessive insulin administration, steroid therapy, or Mauriac's syndrome is thereby excluded. The glycogenoses are of historical interest in that the study of these conditions led to the first inborn errors of metabolism that were enzymatically defined. The original four glycogen storage diseases classified by Cori have been extended to eleven. The new types in the accompanying table have been added in the chronological order of their enzymatic definition. Subtypes are added to indicate different clinical manifestations involving the same altered enzyme, differences in tissue distribution of the altered enzymes, or altered function of the enzyme without demonstrated decreased activity in vitro.

Etiology. The best evidence available indicates that the several types of glycogen storage disease are transmitted as a recessive trait except for type IXa which is sex-linked. The symptoms of types O, I, III, VI, and IX derive basically from the inadequate availability of glycogen to modulate the blood glucose level. The symptoms of types V, VII, VIII, and X are related to the deficiency of glycolysis necessary for vigorous exercise. Type V has been called McArdle's syndrome. The findings in type II glycogenosis are related to muscle weakness, but the mechanism whereby glycogen accumulation in lysosomes gives rise to this state is not known. Type IV glycogen storage disease is characterized by cirrhosis of the liver which is suggested to result from the deposited insoluble glycogen which stimulates a foreign-body type response (fibrosis).

Clinical Manifestations. The deficiency of UDPG-glycogen transferase, type O, is characterized by hypoglycemia commencing shortly after birth, if feedings are withheld, or later when the frequency of feedings is reduced from every four hours. Types I, III, VI, and IX have very similar symptoms and may be indistinguishable clinically. Hypoglycemic seizures in the neonatal period may be the initial symptom, or an enlarged liver detected several months later may be the first sign noted. These children are often unusually susceptible to infec-

THE ENZYMATICALLY DEFINED GLYCOGENOSES

Type	Defect	Glycogen Structure	Tissue
0	UDPG-glycogen transferase	Normal	Liver, muscle
Ia	Glucose-6-phosphatase	Normal	Liver, kidney, GI tract
Ib	Functional G-6-p'tase deficiency	Normal	Liver
IIa	Lysosomal α-1,4-glucosidase	Normal	Generalized
IIb	Lysosomal α-1,4-glucosidase	Normal	Generalized, muscle
IIIa, b, c, d	Amylo-1,6-glucosidase and/or Oligo 1,4→1,4-glucantransferase	Limit dextrin or short chain	Liver and/or muscle
IV	Amylo-1,4→1,6-transglucosylase	Amylopectin-like	Generalized
V	Muscle phosphorylase	Normal	Muscle
VI	Liver phosphorylase	Normal	Liver, WBC
VII	Phosphofructokinase	Normal	Muscle, RBC
VIII	Phosphohexosisomerase (inhibitor?)	Normal	Muscle
IXa	Phosphorylase kinase	Normal	Liver, WBC
IXb	Phosphorylase kinase	Normal	Liver
X	Phosphorylase kinase	Normal	Muscle

tions. Infections are often associated with severe ketoacidosis which can lead to death if not treated promptly. When the infant is about 18 months or older the infections are often accompanied by troublesome epistaxes. Short stature becomes apparent at two or three years of age. Eruptive xanthomas may appear after three years. Gout, unique to type I, does not usually become symptomatic until after puberty despite the elevated serum uric acid. Types III, VI, and IX tend to improve with age. After puberty and in the absence of a previous history, the diagnosis is often not suspected. There is considerable variability in the severity of clinical expression both within a given type and between the several types of glycogen storage diseases involving the liver. Type IV glycogenosis, the other type primarily involving the liver from a clinical standpoint, is not distinguishable from cirrhosis in a child from any other cause except by special studies. These children have an enlarged nodular liver; furthermore this is the only type of glycogen storage disease in which the spleen is enlarged. Death ensues from the complications of elevated portal pressure.

Types V, VII, VIII, and X involve striated muscles. The symptoms may begin after several years of life (types V and VII) or in the third decade (types VIII and X). The symptoms from day to day are unimpressive and these patients are often labeled psychoneurotic. Vigorous exercise is associated with weakness, muscle cramps, and occasionally myoglobinuria. The symptoms tend to be slowly progressive in severity.

Type II glycogenosis is also primarily a muscle glycogen storage disease, but the symptoms are quite distinctive. Type IIa is the classic form originally described by Pompe. The infant has no symptoms at birth, but by three or four months of age shows signs of weakness and of exhaustion from feedings; a large heart can then be demonstrated. By five or six months the deep tendon reflexes are lost. The infant then exhibits a flaccid paralysis with pooling of saliva in the pharynx, and dies of pulmonary infection or heart failure usually before the first birthday. This condition must be considered in the differential diagnosis of the "floppy baby syndrome." Type IIb has the same enzymatic defect insofar as can be detected, but these children are distinguished by the fact that the heart is not clinically involved. The diagnosis is often missed because the presentation at three or four years of age so closely resembles that of muscular dystrophy. This form has been diagnosed as late as 35 years of age.

Diagnosis. The definitive diagnosis of glycogen storage disease is made by enzymatic assay of liver and/or muscle obtained by biopsy. The glycogen is characterized and the content determined. Enzymatic assays of leukocytes can be useful in types III, IV, VI, VIII, and IX. Skin fibroblasts grown in culture have been shown to be useful in diagnosis and in the determination of heterozygosity in types II and IV. The response of blood glucose and lactate to the glucagon tolerance test is useful in that the blood glucose usually does not respond in types I, III, and VI, and in type I the lactate is high in the fasting state with a further increase in response to the glucagon. The red cell glycogen may be elevated markedly in type III.

Types V, VII, VIII, and X are characterized by absence of rise in blood lactate consequent to anoxic exercise. This is performed by having the subject exercise the hand with the blood pressure cuff above the elbow inflated above systolic pressure and obtaining blood from the antecubital vein at intervals for several minutes. The normal individual will have a two- to fourfold rise, whereas the muscle glycogen patients will have none. Type II glycogenosis patients show no abnormality of carbohydrate metabolism that can be approached through blood sampling. Electromyography can be helpful. In type V and frequently in types VII, VIII, and X the signal becomes isoelectric after a period of vigorous exercise. The "dive bomber" effect is characteristically found in type IIb glycogen storage. Type IIa muscle does not demonstrate a characteristic finding.

Treatment. Type I glycogenosis is best treated by frequent feedings, for it is from this source that the patients must sustain their blood glucose. Allopurinol has been useful in lowering the uric acid in older patients. Type III responds best to a high protein diet, presumably through augmenting glucose from gluconeogenesis. Special care is usually needed only for the first four or five years. A high protein diet would also be advantageous to patients with types VI and IX if hypoglycemia was a problem. No treatment has been found of value for patients with types IIa, IIb, IV, V, VII, VIII, or IX. Fructose has been said to benefit the patient with type VIII glycogenosis. These individuals should have their condition explained to them and they should be trained for sedentary occupations.

Cori, G. T.: Glycogen structure and enzyme deficiencies in glycogen storage disease. Harvey Lect., 48:145, 1953.

Hers, H. G.: Glycogen Storage Disease. In Levine, R., and Luft, R. (eds.): Advances in Metabolic Disorders. New York, Academic Press, Inc., 1964, pp. 1-44.

Hug, G., Schubert, W. K., and Chuck, G.: Deficient activity of dephosphorylase kinase and accumulation of glycogen in the liver. J. Clin. Invest., 48:704, 1969.

Huijing, F., and Fernandes, J.: X-chromosomal inheritance of liver glycogenosis with phosphorylase kinase deficiency. Amer. J. Hum. Genet., 21:275, 1969.

Satoyoshi, E., and Kowa, H.: A myopathy due to glycolytic abnormality. Arch. Neurol. (Chicago), 17:248, 1967.

Strugalska-Cynowska, M.: Disturbances in the activity of phosphorylase kinase in a case of McArdle myopathy. Folia Histochem. Cytochem., 5:151, 1967.

Tarui, S., Okuno, G., Ikara, Y., Tanaka, T., Suda, M., and Nishikawa, M.: Phosphofructokinase deficiency in skeletal muscle: A new type of glycogenosis. Biochem. Biophys. Res. Commun., 19:517, 1965.

PRIMARY HYPEROXALURIA
Lloyd H. Smith, Jr.

Primary hyperoxaluria is a general term for two rare genetic disorders of glyoxylate metabolism productive of excessive synthesis and urinary excretion of oxalic acid. Both disorders are transmitted as autosomal recessive traits. The diseases are characterized by the onset in childhood of recurrent calcium oxalate nephrolithiasis or nephrocalcinosis, or both, usually leading to early death secondary to renal failure. At postmortem examination calcium oxalate may be found widely deposited in extrarenal sites, a condition known as oxalosis. More rarely, milder forms of the disease may be found in adults. Although oxalate is an important constituent in approximately two thirds of all kidney stones, most adult patients with calcium oxalate nephrolithiasis excrete normal amounts of urinary oxalate.

Primary hyperoxaluria Type I (glycolic aciduria) represents a genetic defect in the soluble enzyme α-ketoglutarate: glyoxylate carboligase. The resulting accumulation of glyoxylate leads to its excessive oxidation to oxalate and its reduction to glycolate, both of which are excreted in increased amounts in the urine (>60 mg. per 1.73 M.² per 24 hours each). In primary hyperoxaluria Type II (L-glyceric aciduria) there is a defect in the enzyme D-glyceric dehydrogenase. Hydroxypyruvate accumulates and is reduced by lactic dehydrogenase (LDH) to L-glyceric acid, a compound which is undetectable in normal urine. The reduction of hydroxypyruvate to L-glycerate is probably coupled to the oxidation of glyoxylate to oxalate, both catalyzed by LDH. Each disease can be diagnosed by the characteristic pattern of metabolites in urine: Type I, oxalate and glycolate; Type II, oxalate and L-glycerate. Pyridoxine deficiency in laboratory animals and man also leads to hyperoxaluria and even oxalosis with a urinary pattern similar to that of the genetic disease Type I. With the onset of renal failure the clearance of oxalate is reduced (normally about 1.2 times the creatinine clearance) so that its urinary excretion may return to normal. The diagnosis may then be difficult to establish because of the unreliability of current methods for measuring serum oxalate.

No specific methods of treatment are now available. Efforts are directed toward reducing the amount of oxalate excreted and increasing its solubility. Large amounts of pyridoxine (200 to 400 mg. per 24 hours) may decrease oxalate excretion in the Type I disease. Calcium carbimide has been introduced as an inhibitor of oxalate synthesis, but most investigators have not found it to be efficacious. Dilute urine should be maintained by forcing fluids, and a phosphate supplement seems to offer partial protection against stone formation. Attempts at renal homotransplantation have been disappointing because of rapid deposition of calcium oxalate in the transplanted kidney. A search for a more effective inhibitor of oxalate synthesis is being conducted.

Hockaday, T. D. R., Clayton, J. E., Frederick, E. W., and Smith, L. H., Jr.: Primary hyperoxaluria. Medicine, 43:315, 1964.

Williams, H. E., and Smith, L. H., Jr.: Primary hyperoxaluria. In Stanbury, J. B., Wyngaarden, J. B., and Frederickson, D. S. (eds.): The Metabolic Basis of Inherited Disease. 3rd ed. New York, McGraw-Hill Book Company (in press).

Williams, H. E., and Smith, L. H., Jr.: Disorders of oxalate metabolism. Amer. J. Med., 45:715, 1968.

Disorders of Lipid Metabolism

Richard J. Havel

TRANSPORT OF LIPIDS IN THE BLOOD

Because of their insolubility in aqueous environment, essentially all lipids in blood plasma are in complexes (lipoproteins) containing amphiphilic substances which permit their dispersal into small particles. The major lipids transported are fatty acids and cholesterol. Fatty acids exist as such in a complex with albumin and as esters of which the main transport form is triglyceride. The former are called free fatty acids (FFA) to indicate that their carboxyl groups are not in ester linkage. Cholesterol is also transported in the "free" state (alcohol group not in ester linkage) or esterified with fatty acids. The amphiphilic substances which coat the surface of microdroplets of the neutral lipids or form soluble complexes with them are mainly phospholipids and specific proteins.

Exogenous Fat (Triglyceride) Transport. Dietary fat, after hydrolysis to form partial glycerides and fatty acids, is absorbed from micelles containing conjugated bile acids. From these products, triglycerides are resynthesized in the mucosal cells of the small intestine, appear in particulate form in the Golgi region, and are secreted into the intestinal lacteals. In the lymph, they appear as chylomicrons and are delivered into the blood through the thoracic duct. Normally, chylomicrons are present only during active absorption of fat, since their life span in the blood is only a few minutes. Triglycerides in chylomicrons are removed primarily in tissues other than the liver which contain on the endothelial surface of their capillaries an enzyme, lipoprotein lipase, which hydrolyzes the triglycerides to FFA and glycerol. These products readily diffuse across the capillary and other cell membranes where they are stored or oxidized.

Endogenous Fat Transport. Triglycerides, derived from fat transported in the blood or synthesized from nonlipid precursors, are stored mainly in adipose tissue. Normally, these triglycerides are hydrolyzed at a variable rate controlled by the action of hormones and the adrenergic innervation of the tissue on a "hormone-sensitive" lipase. The FFA, as albumin complexes, are rapidly transported to various tissues to be oxidized or stored temporarily as lipid esters. They are also the major precursors of endogenous plasma triglycerides, secreted continuously by the liver in particles similar to, but smaller than, chylomicrons (very low density lipoproteins, VLDL; see Fig. 1). In the postprandial state, these triglycerides may be derived from fatty acids synthesized de novo in the liver, and this pathway appears to provide a mechanism for exporting excess fatty acids to sites of storage or oxidation. In the fasting state, triglycerides secreted by the liver in VLDL are derived mainly from FFA, but some VLDL may enter the blood through the lymphatic system as a result of continued absorption of lipids contained in bile. The metabolism of VLDL-triglycerides resembles that of chylomicrons, but their disposal is less efficient, and they remain in the blood for a considerably longer period.

Role of Other Lipoproteins. Incomplete evidence suggests that low density lipoproteins (LDL) are products of metabolism of chylomicrons and VLDL. The LDL contain a major peptide ("B") which appears to be essential for the formation of VLDL and chylomicrons. VLDL also contain other peptides ("C"). High density lipoproteins (HDL) also contain "C" peptides as minor protein constituents as well as "A" peptides as major constituents. Some of the "C" peptides may facilitate the formation of an enzyme-substrate complex of chylomicrons and VLDL with lipoprotein lipase. HDL are also the major site of action of the enzyme, lecithin–cholesterol acyl transferase, which is responsible for the formation of most cholesterol esters found in plasma lipoproteins.

CLASSIFICATION AND ANALYSIS OF PLASMA LIPOPROTEINS

Plasma lipoproteins can be separated by electrophoresis or in the ultracentrifuge into the four main classes shown in Figure 1. In most disorders involving plasma lipoproteins, these classes do not differ substantially from normal in gross chemical and physical properties so that they are classified as hyper- or hypolipoproteinemias. In some states, lipoproteins differing from those normally comprising the bulk of a given class may accumulate; these are classified as dyslipoproteinemias.

For most clinical purposes, relatively simple methods will characterize these states. Two general approaches are now generally used. In both, the concentration of cholesterol and triglycerides is measured in fasting serum or plasma. From the actual and relative values of these constituents, certain inferences can be made concerning the lipoprotein class or classes involved. For better subclassification of the hyperlipemias (increased concentration of triglycerides), it is necessary to establish whether their source is *exogenous* (chylomicrons), *endogenous* (VLDL), or *mixed* (chylomicrons plus VLDL). This can usually be achieved by evaluating lactescence of serum chilled overnight in a refrigerator, since chylomicrons tend to form a creamy layer spontaneously, while VLDL do not (see Fig. 2). Additional methods which can be used include electrophoresis on a supporting medium, such as

PROPERTIES OF PLASMA LIPOPROTEINS

CLASS	HDL	LDL	VLDL			CHYLOMICRONS		
· DIAMETER (Å)	100	200	300	500	800	800	2000	5000
· DENSITY	1.06-1.21	1.006-1.063	0.95 – 1.006			0.94		
· ELECTROPHORETIC MOBILITY	α_1	β	PRE-β			ORIGIN		
PER CENT · COMPOSITION								
· PROTEIN	50	20	15	7	4	4	2	1
· PHOSPHOLIPIDS	25	25	25	18	13	13	8	3
· CHOLESTEROL (FREE + ESTERS)	20	50	45	22	13	13	8	3
· TRIGLYCERIDES	5	5	15	53	70	70	82	93

FIGURE 1. Properties of plasma lipoproteins. (From Havel, R. J.: Adv. Intern. Med., 15:117, 1969.)

paper, agarose gel, or cellulose acetate, or measurement of light scattering before and after passing diluted serum through a microporous filter. The latter method has the advantage of simultaneously providing a quantitative estimate of triglyceride concentration. In some instances, particularly in certain dyslipoproteinemias, classification may be uncertain so that additional methods are needed. However, combined information gained from examination of the patient and from the simple laboratory tests will permit an accurate diagnosis in almost all cases.

NORMAL REGULATION OF PLASMA LIPOPROTEIN CONCENTRATION

Apart from chylomicrons, lipoproteins are present in blood plasma at all times. The concentration of VLDL, the carrier of endogenous triglyceride, is most variable and is a function of rate of hepatic triglyceride synthesis. This, in turn, depends upon rate of uptake of FFA from the blood or synthesis of fatty acids from glucose and upon the extent to which they are converted to triglycerides. Ingestion of glucose causes a rapid fall in level of VLDL initially, presumably related to the accompanying decrease in mobilization of fat from adipose tissue. After one to three days on a high carbohydrate, low fat diet, VLDL level tends to rise. The extent to which this reflects increased hepatic triglyceride synthesis or impaired removal of triglycerides in extrahepatic tissues is uncertain. Ingestion of foodstuffs in excess of need is accompanied by rapid increase in level of VLDL. In addition, in stable obesity, VLDL levels are increased. This has been equated with associated insulin resistance and hyperinsulinism, but the precise mechanism is not clear. Increased triglyceride and VLDL levels accompany several other states in which insulin resistance and hyperinsulinism are present. Plasma levels of LDL and HDL tend to fall as VLDL levels rise, presumably because some of these lipoprotein species also are constituent parts of VLDL. The concentration of HDL is regulated by sex hormones and, hence, is sex-dependent; increases are produced by estrogens and a fall by androgens. The level of LDL is also moderately sensitive to caloric intake, but is influenced more by specific dietary factors, particularly content of fats containing saturated fatty acids and of cholesterol. Substantial differences in lipoprotein

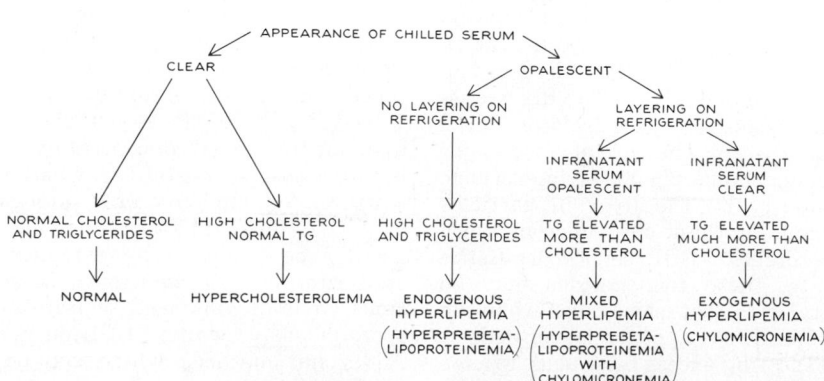

FIGURE 2. Evaluation of hyperliproproteinemias with simple techniques. (From Havel, R. J.: Adv. Intern. Med., 15:117, 1969.)

levels occur in various population groups throughout the world. The major cause of these differences, which occur predominantly in cholesterol-rich LDL, appears to be dietary and to relate to lesser consumption of all types of foods, but in particular saturated fats (mainly of mammalian origin) and cholesterol associated with animal fats.

HYPOLIPOPROTEINEMIAS

PRIMARY

The primary conditions are exceedingly rare, but have considerable importance for the light that they shed on normal functions of plasma lipoproteins.

Abetalipoproteinemia (Bassen-Kornzweig Syndrome). This disease, inherited as an autosomal recessive, is characterized by complete absence of LDL, VLDL, and chylomicrons. The absence of the "B" protein appears to be accompanied by virtually complete loss of ability to transport triglycerides in the blood. It is manifested by severe malabsorption, beginning in early childhood, followed by progressive ataxia, nystagmus, weakness, and visual impairment with scotomas. These are related, respectively, to inability to deliver triglycerides into the intestinal lymph, demyelination of spinocerebellar tracts, posterior columns and, occasionally, peripheral nerves, and pigmentary retinal degeneration ("atypical retinitis pigmentosa"). Other findings include peculiar thorny or spiny red cells (acanthocytes) and fatty liver (resulting from failure to export triglycerides in very low density lipoproteins).

Diagnosis is established by finding very low cholesterol concentration (about 50 mg. per 100 ml.) and almost no triglycerides in blood plasma in an individual with one or more of the characteristic symptoms. The disorder should be considered in any patient with hereditary ataxia. On paper electrophoresis, only alpha lipoproteins are present, and blood smears or wet preparations show the characteristic acanthocytes. Treatment is limited to restriction of ordinary fat and supplementation with fat-soluble vitamins. Medium-chain triglycerides are well tolerated. Such measures have not been shown to alter the progressive and disabling course of the disease.

Hypobetalipoproteinemia. A few families have been described with low concentrations of beta lipoproteins. Some patients have had acanthocytes and late onset of neuromuscular difficulties.

Tangier Disease (Alpha-lipoprotein Deficiency). This disorder, in the homozygous state, leads in childhood to diffuse deposition of cholesterol esters in reticuloendothelial tissues, with enlargement of liver, spleen, and lymph nodes, and especially to grossly enlarged tonsils with a characteristic orange color. Foam cells may be found in the bone marrow. In adults, flocculent corneal infiltrates may occur. Usually, the disorder does not affect growth, nutrition, or general health. Electrophoretic or ultracentrifugal examination shows almost no alpha lipoproteins or HDL. Immunochemical analysis demonstrates small quantities of protein similar to, but not identical with, normal "A" protein ("Tangier alpha"), and one of the polypeptides of HDL, with carboxy terminal threonine, is almost lacking. Heterozygotes have low concentrations of HDL but no other detectable abnormalities. In homozygotes, levels of LDL tend to be reduced, although those of triglycerides and VLDL are high. These various abnormalities suggest that HDL participate in transport of cholesterol and facilitate transport of triglycerides in the blood. No treatment is available. There is limited evidence that premature vascular disease may develop.

Lecithin-Cholesterol Acyltransferase Deficiency. This recently described disorder has been found only in a few individuals in Scandinavia. Affected subjects have proteinuria, anemia, and corneal deposits of lipid. HDL are almost absent, and moderate to large elevations of VLDL and chylomicrons are present. Cholesterol esters comprise less than 10 per cent of total cholesterol in plasma (normal value about 72 per cent) and are found almost entirely in the triglyceride-rich lipoproteins. Their fatty acids are much more saturated than those produced normally by the plasma-enzyme, lecithin-cholesterol acyltransferase, and this enzyme cannot be detected. Upon transfusion of normal plasma, the enzyme can be detected for several days, and progressive esterification of plasma cholesterol occurs, suggesting that deficiency of the transferase causes the disease. Other findings include foam cells in the bone marrow and renal glomeruli and increased concentration of cholesterol and lecithin in the red blood cells. The relationship between the enzyme deficiency and the various clinical and chemical abnormalities is uncertain, but may relate in part to the presumed function of the enzyme and HDL in transport of cholesterol. The hyperlipemia could be part of a nephrotic syndrome, but the proteinuria and albuminuria are mild, suggesting that other mechanisms, possibly related to the role of HDL in triglyceride transport, are involved.

SECONDARY

The secondary states are characterized chiefly by hypobetalipoproteinemia and are the result of malnutrition, malabsorption, or parenchymal liver disease. Presumably, they reflect decreased transport of exogenous and endogenous triglycerides, so that formation of LDL is decreased. Reduced concentrations of LDL also occur in healthy individuals when intake of calories and saturated fats is habitually low.

HYPERLIPO-
PROTEINEMIAS

PRIMARY

Familial Hyperbetalipoproteinemia (Hypercholes-terolemia, Type II Hyperlipoproteinemia). Familial hyperbetalipoproteinemia, inherited as a mendelian dominant trait, is characterized by increased concentration of LDL of normal composition. Xanthomas in the tendons, particularly the Achilles, plantar, patellar, and digital extensors of the hands, as well as tuberous xanthomas, xanthelasmas, and early onset of corneal arcus are frequently encountered. Because of the difficulty in establishing the normal values for serum cholesterol and the inconstant presence of xanthomas, its prevalence is not established, but it may occur in 1 per cent or more of the American population.

Etiology and Pathogenesis. The specific molecular or enzymatic defect responsible for the increased concentration of LDL is unknown, but recent studies suggest that the catabolism of the specific protein moiety may be impaired. It has not been established that the "B" protein is structurally normal.

Clinical Manifestations. The hyperlipoproteinemia is present from birth or shortly thereafter, and is generally detected as hypercholesterolemia with little or no increase in triglycerides; the xanthomas usually do not appear until after puberty. The patient may not be aware of the presence of large xanthomas in the Achilles or plantar tendons, and the latter may be missed by the physician unless they are put under tension by having the patient extend his toes. Small xanthomas of the extensor tendons of the hands are best detected by observing the tendon while the patient flexes and extends the finger, and small xanthomas in the Achilles tendon are detected by palpation of irregular contour, usually in the central region. Xanthelasmas (raised, yellow plaques about the eyelids near the inner canthus) and corneal arcus are not diagnostic, since they may also be seen in individuals with no discernible abnormality of plasma lipoproteins. The incidence of premature coronary heart disease is several times that of control populations in countries with a "Western" culture, and the incidence of peripheral atherosclerotic occlusive disease is also increased. In the homozygous states, the disease is much more severe with large xanthomas occurring in childhood, together with "malignant" atherosclerotic disease including calcific aortic stenosis. A possible variant of the disease is seen in the Near East in which early occurrence of large xanthomas is common.

Diagnosis. Hypercholesterolemia without hypertriglyceridemia in the absence of known cause, such as hypothyroidism, is not sufficient basis for making a diagnosis unless the cholesterol level exceeds 400 mg. per 100 ml. Presence of characteristic xanthomas is diagnostic, and demonstration of familial occurrence (at least one parent should have hyperbetalipoproteinemia) provides strong presumptive evidence. Some individuals or families may have moderate hypertriglyceridemia. This must be distinguished from familial dysbetalipoproteinemia, described below.

Treatment. No simple method has been devised to reduce lipoprotein levels to normal. Some reduction can be achieved by a diet restricted in saturated fats and cholesterol with sufficient polyunsaturated fats to provide a total fat intake of 30 to 35 per cent of calories. Nonabsorbable bile acid-binding substances, such as cholestyramine (15 to 30 grams daily in divided doses with meals), are more effective. Large doses of nicotinic acid (5 to 12 grams daily in divided doses) may also be effective. These drugs may in some cases reduce lipoprotein levels to normal. In postmenopausal women, estrogens may provide some improvement. Thyroxine and its analogues, especially d-thyroxine (4 to 8 mg. daily) and the ethyl ester of p-chlorophenoxyisobutyrate, occasionally give good results. Xanthomatous lesions regress slowly; tendinous lesions seldom disappear. It is reasonable to begin treatment in childhood, although it has not been established that reducing the lipoprotein level will prevent or delay onset of ischemic vascular disease.

Familial Dysbetalipoproteinemia (Broad-beta Disease, Type III Hyperlipoproteinemia). *Definition.* Familial dysbetalipoproteinemia, probably inherited as a recessive trait, is characterized by accumulation of abnormal beta lipoproteins, which resemble VLDL in size and flotation characteristics, but differ from them in composition. Planar xanthomas, particularly in the palmar and digital creases, are peculiar to this form of primary hyperlipoproteinemia, but tuberous, tubero-eruptive, and tendinous lesions also occur. It is much rarer than familial hyperbetalipoproteinemia; in the older literature, it was frequently called *xanthoma tuberosum.*

Etiology and Pathogenesis. The abnormal lipoprotein contains predominantly "B" peptide in particles with more cholesterol ester and less triglyceride than normal VLDL. Their electrophoretic mobility is also abnormal, encompassing the beta and extending toward the pre-beta region ("broad beta"). Whether the "B" peptide is itself abnormal is not known.

Clinical Manifestations. The disorder is seldom discovered before early adult life and is usually manifested by appearance of xanthomas when the patient gains weight. The patient may be unaware of the characteristic planar xanthomas which are yellow to orange and tend to fill the palmar and digital creases; they may also appear over the dorsal surfaces of the hands. The tuberous xanthomas tend to be smaller and more numerous than those in hyperbetalipoproteinemia and are often confluent and surrounded by an erythematous halo ("tuberoeruptive"). They occur most commonly over the knees and elbows and on the buttocks.

Tendinous lesions are usually in the extensors of the hands. Premature coronary and peripheral atherosclerotic vascular disease is fairly common. Overt diabetes mellitus is seldom seen, but slight degrees of glucose intolerance usually can be detected, as in the other forms of endogenous hypertriglyceridemia described below.

Diagnosis. Combined hypercholesterolemia and hypertriglyceridemia are always present, usually similar in extent, and they vary considerably with recent diet. Most patients have the characteristic planar xanthomas which, in the absence of obstructive biliary tract disease, are pathognomonic. The serum is usually lactescent. Lipoprotein electrophoresis shows a "broad-beta" pattern with normal or reduced content of alpha lipoproteins. Slight chylomicronemia is often present when hyperlipoproteinemia is severe. Spurious "broad-beta" bands may be seen in other states, particularly in some of the secondary hyperlipemias. Definitive laboratory diagnosis requires ultracentrifugation of serum at its own density to demonstrate "floating-beta" lipoproteins.

Treatment. The mainstay of treatment is diet. In obese subjects, caloric restriction is almost always very effective. The diet should be restricted in simple sugars and in cholesterol but not in fat, which should provide 40 to 50 per cent of calories. Concentration of cholesterol and triglycerides will usually fall almost to normal. For patients who will not adhere to a dietary program and for the few who respond inadequately, the ethyl ester of p-chlorophenoxyisobutyric acid, 250 mg. four times daily, will almost always produce a good response. Xanthomas invariably regress or disappear with effective reduction in lipid levels. Effect on atherosclerotic lesions is unknown, but treatment should be continued indefinitely (see article on Hyperlipoproteinemia and Atherosclerotic Vascular Disease).

Primary Hyperlipemias. *Exogenous Hyperlipemia (Bürger-Grütz Syndrome, Type I Hyperlipoproteinemia).* *Definition.* This rare disease, inherited as a recessive trait, is characterized by accumulation of chylomicrons proportional to intake of dietary fat and manifested by recurrent acute pancreatitis, usually beginning in childhood.

Etiology and Pathogenesis. Most if not all patients have deficient activity of lipoprotein lipase with resultant defective removal of triglycerides from the blood. It is not certain whether a structural abnormality causes the deficient activity or whether one of a family of enzymes is totally inactive, but limited hydrolytic activity against lipoprotein-bound triglycerides can usually be demonstrated in plasma taken a few minutes after intravenous injection of heparin. In one family, no lipoprotein lipase activity could be demonstrated in adipose tissue.

Clinical Manifestations. Chylomicronemia develops as soon as fat is ingested, and the disorder has been diagnosed during the first week of life. Pancreatitis is very common and many patients diagnosed in adult life have a history of bouts of abdominal pain in childhood. Abdominal pain, not definable as pancreatitis, has been reported frequently, but causes other than pancreatitis have not been established. Other complications described rarely include melena and pretibial ulcers. Like the pancreatitis, they may result from ischemia related to agglomeration of chylomicrons in capillaries. Hepatosplenomegaly, presumably the result of phagocytosis of chylomicrons by reticuloendothelial cells, is common, and hypersplenism has been described. Foam cells may be found in the bone marrow. The endogenous hyperlipemia occurring normally during pregnancy is greatly magnified, and may lead to repeated attacks of pancreatitis. In infants and children, eruptive xanthomas small yellow papules in the skin, surrounded by an erythematous halo—may occur when lipemia is severe. Lipemia retinalis—whitish reflection from retinal arterioles and venules—can usually be detected when triglyceride levels in plasma exceed 3000 mg. per 100 ml. and becomes florid with levels above 5000 mg. per 100 ml. Other xanthomas do not occur, and premature atherosclerotic vascular disease has not been described. Carbohydrate metabolism is normal.

Diagnosis. Markedly lactescent blood plasma in a young patient with severe midabdominal pain and no history of alcoholism is presumptive evidence for this disorder or one of the other primary hyperlipemias. In exogenous hyperlipemia, the chylomicrons rise to form a creamy layer when the serum is allowed to stand overnight in the refrigerator and the infranatant serum is limpid. Triglyceride concentration is increased far more than that of cholesterol and the chylomicron band predominates on electrophoresis. Triglyceride levels fall dramatically when intake of dietary fat is severely restricted for two to three days. Lipolytic activity, measured in blood plasma obtained ten minutes after intravenous injection of 0.1 mg. of heparin per kilogram of body weight, is reduced.

Treatment. The only established measure is restriction of dietary fat ("saturated" and "polyunsaturated" fats are equivalent) sufficient to reduce fasting triglyceride levels to 500 mg. per 100 ml. or less. This usually requires an intake of no more than 30 grams per day by adults. On this regimen, xanthomas disappear, and pancreatitis is uniformly prevented. Pretibial ulcers have also healed, and hypersplenism has subsided on this regimen. Once pancreatitis occurs, recurrence is very common when large amounts of fat are ingested—often within hours. During pregnancy complete elimination of fat from the diet may be necessary to control hyperlipemia and minimize the possibility of pancreatitis.

Endogenous Hyperlipemia (Type IV Hyperlipoproteinemia). *Definition.* Endogenous hyperlipemia is a common disorder of middle life, sometimes shown to be familial, characterized by accumulation of VLDL of normal composition and electrophoretic mobility and by insulin resistance, and occasionally accompanied by eruptive xanthomas and recurrent pancreatitis. The concentration of VLDL depends upon several environmental factors and the true prevalence is unknown.

Etiology and Pathogenesis. Secretion of hepatogenous triglycerides in VLDL varies with quantity and quality of food intake, including ethanol, and with neural and hormonal responses to stress. These responses are generally magnified in endogenous hyperlipemia, in which there is evidence for impaired catabolism of VLDL-triglycerides as well as increased hepatic secretion, but the nature of these abnormalities is not known. Evidence that severity of the hypertriglyceridemia is related to hyperinsulinism and insulin resistance, together with the fact that gain in weight, which increases insulin resistance, almost uniformly increases the hyperlipemia indicates a close relationship with disordered carbohydrate metabolism. It seems likely that, like diabetes mellitus, the disorder represents one or more genotypes which condition the response of VLDL to common environmental influences.

Clinical Manifestations. Most commonly, the disorder is detected when patients with ischemic vascular disease are screened for metabolic abnormalities. Although endogenous hyperlipemia is commonly found in those who develop such disease prematurely, the incidence of vascular complications has not been established. The great majority of patients are at least moderately obese when hyperlipemia is found, but only a few have fasting hyperglycemia. With severe hyperlipemia, eruptive xanthomas and pancreatitis may occur, as in exogenous hyperlipemia.

Diagnosis. The disorder should be suspected in obese subjects with premature vascular disease. It is diagnosed presumptively when fasting serum is lactescent with no layering on standing, and serum triglyceride level is increased more than that of cholesterol in the absence of known cause (see Secondary Hyperlipemias).

Treatment. Effective measures are available to reduce the level of VLDL, but it has not been shown that atherosclerotic lesions regress or that the progress of ischemic vascular disease is slowed. For obese patients, caloric restriction alone usually produces rapid reduction in serum triglycerides, often almost to normal. The diet should also be restricted in simple sugars as described for familial dyslipoproteinemia. Cholesterol levels often remain moderately elevated and may be reduced further by substitution of unsaturated for saturated fats. Ethyl ester of p-chlorophenoxyisobutyrate may be used for individuals with inadequate dietary response. When added after the patient has responded partially to a dietary program, it usually reduces triglycerides further, but cholesterol levels often remain unchanged, indicating an increase in level of LDL at the expense of VLDL. Since there is no evidence that such a change is beneficial, treatment with the drug should be discontinued in such patients.

Mixed Hyperlipemia (Type V Hyperlipoproteinemia). *Definition.* This is a rare disorder of adolescence and middle life, in which VLDL and chylomicrons of normal composition accumulate in the blood on ordinary diets. It is usually accompanied by overt, insulin-independent diabetes mellitus and often by eruptive xanthomas and recurrent acute pancreatitis.

Etiology and Pathogenesis. The metabolic abnormalities in this disorder partake of both endogenous and exogenous hyperlipemia. In familial cases, insulin resistance is usually accompanied by fasting hyperglycemia, and post-heparin lipolytic activity in plasma is often somewhat reduced. Possibly, multiple genetic defects are present which combine insulin resistance with defective activity of lipoprotein lipase. Some patients with endogenous hyperlipemia may accumulate chylomicrons when their lipemia is severe, particularly with ingestion of substantial quantities of ethanol; in these cases, the chylomicronemia may represent an "overload" phenomenon. In others, the distinction between endogenous and mixed hyperlipemia is blurred.

Clinical Manifestations. The disorder usually presents in adolescence or early adult life with recurrent attacks of obscure abdominal pain, sometimes definable as acute pancreatitis. At onset of pain, lipemia is usually severe. Eruptive xanthomas are often present and frequently are confluent. As in exogenous hyperlipemia, hepatosplenomegaly and lipemia retinalis are often found. Overt hyperglycemia is only occasionally severe enough to produce symptoms of diabetes, and evidences of microangiopathy are usually absent. Hyperuricemia is also common. Obesity is frequent, but by no means universal. In some patients, evidences of premature atherosclerotic vascular disease may be found, but incidence is not known to be increased.

Diagnosis. Markedly lactescent serum which separates into a creamy layer with persistent lactescence in the infranatant serum provides presumptive evidence for mixed hyperlipemia. This can be confirmed by nephelometry or electrophoresis. Alcoholic hyperlipemia must be considered, particularly in patients presenting with abdominal pain, and diabetic hyperlipemia must be ruled out when hyperglycemia is severe and accompanied by ketoacidosis. Differentiation from exogenous hyperlipemia usually presents no problem and depends on the accompanying severe endogenous hyperlipemia, hyperglycemia, and normal or slightly reduced lipolytic activity in post-heparin plasma.

Treatment. For obese patients, restriction of caloric intake and ethanol usually reduces levels of both chylomicrons and VLDL effectively. For patients of normal body weight, avoidance of intermittent excesses of sugars, fat, or ethanol generally provides some improvement. The hyperglycemia usually responds to the caloric restriction or to addition of sulfonylurea drugs. Neither the latter nor insulin, however, has a specific effect on the hyperlipemia. The ethyl ester of p-chlorophenoxyisobutyrate, given as described for familial dyslipoproteinemia, may be quite effective in patients not responding to diet. As in exogenous hyperlipemia, recurrent pancreatitis is prevented by effective reduction of lipoprotein levels and eruptive xanthomas disappear.

SECONDARY

These conditions are important as clues to diagnosis or because they may be associated with premature atherosclerotic vascular disease.

Hyperbetalipoproteinemia. *Hypothyroidism.* Hyperbetalipoproteinemia is a characteristic finding in myxedema, and hypothyroidism must be considered in all patients with this abnormality. All forms of hyperbetalipoproteinemia are accompanied by hypercarotenemia, but this is particularly striking in myxedema because of the additional defect in conversion of carotene to vitamin A. Occasionally, increased levels of VLDL are also present.

Dietary. Moderate degrees of hypercholesterolemia may occur in subjects ingesting large amounts of cholesterol, usually in eggs and dairy products.

Nephrotic Syndrome. Hyperbetalipoproteinemia is frequently observed in nephrotic states when serum albumin concentration falls below 3 grams per 100 ml. As the level of albumin falls below 1.5 grams per 100 ml., concentration of VLDL rises to produce the characteristic nephrotic hyperlipemia. Treatment is that of the underlying disorder.

Resolving Lipemias. As levels of chylomicrons or VLDL are reduced in various hyperlipemic states, the concentration of LDL usually rises, presumably reflecting the removal of triglyceride with liberation of constituent "B" protein and its associated lipids. Such hyperbetalipoproteinemia may persist for days to weeks, and can lead to confusion if the sequence is not appreciated.

Hyperadrenal Corticism. Hyperbetalipoproteinemia of moderate degree is commonly seen in Cushing's syndrome and subsides with appropriate treatment.

Endogenous and Mixed Hyperlipemias. *Diabetic Hyperlipemia.* Mixed hyperlipemia is characteristic of prolonged insulin deficiency with ketosis. It is generally accompanied by fatty liver and by weight loss and other evidences of a catabolic state. It is not ordinarily seen with acute diabetic ketoacidosis. Defective removal of triglycerides and reduced lipolytic activity in post-heparin plasma can be demonstrated. Eruptive xanthomas and lipemia retinalis are commonly seen. With administration of adequate insulin, triglyceride levels fall rapidly and cholesterol levels more slowly. Diabetic hyperlipemia must be differentiated from primary endogenous hyperlipemia and especially mixed hyperlipemia with its frequent associated hyperglycemia. These states are not accompanied by ketosis or wasting, and do not respond to insulin.

Alcoholic Hyperlipemia. The lipemia, usually mixed, is seen in chronic alcoholics with fatty liver and good hepatic function. Diversion of fatty acids entering the liver to triglyceride synthesis appears to be the most important abnormality, but decreased activity of lipoprotein lipase has also been implicated. Some of these patients have underlying primary hyperlipemias, and ingestion of ethanol is an important factor aggravating primary endogenous and mixed hyperlipemias. The association of jaundice and hemolytic anemia with hyperlipemia has been described in patients with alcoholism (Zieve's syndrome), but it has not been shown that the features of this triad are causally interrelated. Pancreatitis and hyperlipemia may also coexist. It is unlikely that pancreatitis causes the hyperlipemia since the association is confined almost entirely to alcoholics in whom these complications can occur separately. This situation must be clearly distinguished from occurrence of pancreatitis as a complication of one of the primary (usually exogenous or mixed) hyperlipemias.

In Glycogen Storage Disease Type I. Endogenous or mixed hyperlipemia is consistently found in children and adults. It is related to both increased hepatic secretion of triglycerides in VLDL and decreased activity of lipoprotein lipase. Measures decreasing delivery of absorbed carbohydrate to the liver may be helpful.

In Lipodystrophy. Hyperlipemia is consistently observed in generalized as well as in partial forms of lipodystrophy. The mechanism is not understood, especially in partial lipodystrophy but, as in primary endogenous hyperlipemia, insulin resistance and hyperinsulinism are associated phenomena.

Stress Hyperlipemia. In a variety of situations, increased secretion of catecholamines, together with growth hormone and corticotrophin, can lead to hyperlipemia by increasing mobilization of fatty acids from adipose tissue to liver with resultant increased secretion of triglycerides in VLDL. Such hyperlipemia, after myocardial infarction, can lead to confusion with primary endogenous hyperlipemia.

Administration of Contraceptive Steroids. Mild endogenous hyperlipemia is commonly produced by the estrogenic component of estrogen-progestagen mixtures, and is associated with insulin resistance, hyperinsulinism, and decreased lipolytic activity in post-heparin plasma.

Other Causes. Endogenous hyperlipemia has been described in uremia, after renal homotransplantation, and in hypopituitarism, Niemann-Pick disease, Gaucher's disease, Werner's syndrome, and hepatoma. The prevalence of hyperlipemia is increased in gout.

Dyslipoproteinemias. *Biliary Obstruction.* A low density lipoprotein which has not been detected in health appears in the plasma of patients with extrahepatic or intrahepatic biliary obstruction. The abnormal complex migrates with beta globulins on electrophoresis and contains large amounts of phospholipids and free cholesterol; its proteins consist of some of the normal "C" polypeptides of very low density lipoproteins together with albumin. The "obstructive lipoprotein" can be detected in most patients with biliary obstruction, but very high levels are most characteristic of the early stages of primary biliary cirrhosis and are frequently accompanied by eruptive and planar xanthomas and xanthelasmas. Bile acid-binding agents, such as cholestyramine, may reduce the concentration of the lipoprotein. Spontaneous subsidence of the hyperlipoproteinemia and disappearance of xanthomas usually signify failing hepatic parenchymal cell function.

Paraproteinemias. The abnormal globulins in patients with multiple myeloma and macroglobulinemia may rarely be associated with lipid. In some cases, lipoprotein-globulin complexes have been demonstrated with accompanying hyperlipemia and various xanthomas.

HYPERLIPOPROTEINEMIA IN ATHEROSCLEROTIC VASCULAR DISEASE

Levels of LDL, VLDL, or both tend to be elevated in patients with occlusive atherosclerotic disease, particularly before the sixth decade. The risk of developing coronary heart disease is directly proportional to the concentration of LDL in middle-aged men; this finding indicates that this abnormality precedes the symptomatic phase. Premenopausal women are relatively immune to complications of atherosclerosis, possibly because they have lower levels of LDL. Estrogens seem to account for this difference, which disappears after the menopause. The statistical association between hyperlipoproteinemia and atherosclerotic disease in a given population undoubtedly reflects the risk imposed by the heritable hyperlipoproteinemias, but may also be related to dietary and other influences on lipid transport. The relative importance of LDL and VLDL (or cholesterol and triglycerides) as risk factors is uncertain, but it is clear that both are important.

After myocardial infarction, the concentration of VLDL rises as a result of increased fat mobilization and secretion of "stress" hormones. Therefore, evaluation of the nature and magnitude of associated hyperlipoproteinemia should be postponed for two to three months after the acute episode.

The important question of whether reduction of lipoprotein levels will prevent progression or cause regression of atherosclerotic lesions has not been answered. Studies in animals demonstrate regression under some circumstances, and there is some indication that alterations of diet which decrease cholesterol levels may increase longevity of survivors of myocardial infarction. Thus, specific dietary or pharmacologic management of hyperlipidemia is probably indicated in coronary heart disease and peripheral atherosclerotic vascular disease as well as for prophylaxis.

Bagdade, J. D., Porte, D., and Bierman, E. L.: Diabetic lipemia. A form of acquired fat-induced lipemia. New Eng. J. Med., 276:427, 1967.

Fredrickson, D. S., et al.: Diseases characterized by abnormal lipid metabolism. *In* Stanbury, J. B., Wyngaarden, J. B., and Fredrickson, D. S. (eds.): The Metabolic Basis of Inherited Disease. 2nd ed. New York, McGraw-Hill Book Company, 1966, p. 429.

Fredrickson, D. S., Levy, R. I., and Lees, R. S.: Fat transport in lipoproteins—an integrated approach to mechanisms and disorders. New Eng. J. Med., 276:34, 1967.

Gjone, E., and Norum, K. R.: Familial serum cholesterol ester deficiency. Acta Med. Scand., 183:107, 1968.

Havel, R. J.: Pathogenesis, differentiation and management of hypertriglyceridemia. *In* Stollerman, G. H., (ed.): Advances in Internal Medicine, vol. 15. Chicago, Yearbook Medical Publishers, Inc., 1969, p. 117.

Havel, R. J., Balasse, E. O., Williams, H. E., Kane, J. P., and Segel, N.: Splanchnic metabolism in von Gierke's disease. Trans. Ass. Amer. Physicians, 82:305, 1969.

Seidel, D., Alaupovic, R., and Furman, R. H.: A lipoprotein characterizing obstructive jaundice: I. Method for quantitative separation and identification of lipoproteins in jaundiced subjects. J. Clin. Invest., 48:1211, 1969.

Slack, J., and Nevin, N. C.: Hyperlipidaemic xanthomatosis: I. Increased risk of death from ischaemic heart disease in first degree relatives of 53 patients with essential hyperlipidaemia and xanthomatosis. II. Mode of inheritance in 55 families with essential hyperlipidaemia and xanthomatosis. J. Med. Genet., 5:4, 8, 1968.

Inborn Errors of Amino Acid Metabolism

Charles R. Scriver

ALCAPTONURIA AND OCHRONOSIS

Definition. Alcaptonuria (homogentisicacid-uria) is a disorder of tyrosine metabolism which results from deficiency of the enzyme homo-gentisic acid oxidase. Alcaptonuria is the predecessor of ochronosis, the condition which results from chronic deposition of an oxidized brown-black pigment of homogentisic acid in connective tissue, causing spondylosis and arthropathy. Alcaptonuria is one of the inborn errors of metabolism originally described by Garrod, and the first disease for which autosomal recessive inheritance was proposed.

Pathogenesis. Homogentisic acid (2,5-dihydro-xyphenylacetic acid) is normally oxidized in liver and kidney to malylacetoacetic acid. In the absence of this reaction, homogentisic acid accumulates in tissues, and is secreted into urine by alcaptonuric subjects. There is no significant homogentisicacidemia because the compound is rapidly secreted by kidney, its renal clearance greatly exceeding the glomerular filtration rate. The damage to connective tissue characteristic of ochronosis results from prolonged exposure to homogentisic acid. Its oxidized pigment, benzoquinoneacetic acid, is believed to polymerize to form a melanin-like pigment, which binds irreversibly with collagen. It has been suggested that such binding cross-links collagen, thus altering its physicochemical properties, which in turn leads to the degenerative changes observed in ochronosis. Although alcaptonuria may be detected in the newborn period, changes in connective tissue do not appear until adulthood, perhaps because the enhanced remodeling of connective tissue during childhood and adolescence removes the chemically modified collagen.

Diagnosis. Homogentisicaciduria is present from birth onward, and its intensity is proportional to the dietary intake and catabolism of phenylalanine and tyrosine. With modern sanitation patients may not know for many years that their urine can darken on standing. Thus the diagnosis usually rests on clinical suspicion, a family history, and chemical tests.

Urine. Freshly voided urine is normal in appearance; darkening occurs slowly from the exposed surface downward on standing in air, and rapidly when made alkaline. Homogentisic acid reduces Benedict's reagent to a brown-black color, and produces a purple-black reaction with ferric chloride reagent. Large amounts of ascorbic acid may give false positive reactions with these chemical tests, and it will prevent spontaneous darkening. Coloration of urine caused by bile, porphyrins, myoglobin, and hemoglobin should be distinguished. Homogentisic acid can be confirmed by chromatography and a specific enzymatic method.

OCHRONOSIS

Deposition of brown-black pigment in connective tissue is the legacy of prolonged exposure to homogentisic acid. It can occur in dermis and sweat glands, conjunctiva and cornea, sclera, pinna, tympanic membrane, and ossicles of the middle ear, laryngeal and tracheal cartilages, heart valves, genitourinary tract, tendons, large diarthrodial joints, and spine. Pigment granules occur as both intracellular and extracellular deposits. Characteristically the pinna is stiff and opaque to transillumination; the corneas are black; conduction hearing loss may accompany involvement of tympanum and ossicles. Renal stones and prostatic calculi occur but usually do not cause renal disease, although prostatitis may be caused by alcaptonuria. Heart disease is not more frequent in alcaptonuria despite pigmentation of the endocardium and intima of the aorta.

Ochronotic Arthropathy. The most serious complication of ochronosis is arthropathy. Unlike rheumatoid disease, it spares the small joints of hands and feet. Onset of arthropathy is earlier and more severe in males, and the knee is the most frequently and severely affected peripheral joint. Spondylosis, which is very often present, appears slowly with pain and stiffness, usually in the low back. Ultimately involvement of the lumbar and thoracic spine results in loss of motion and disappearance of the normal lumbar lordosis. Herniation or calcification of the intervertebral discs is also characteristic. As a consequence of ochronotic arthropathy, the typical patient assumes a wide-based stance with forward stoop, rigid spine, and flexed hips and knees.

Roentgenographic examination reveals narrowing of the intervertebral spaces, disc calcification, and gradual fusion of vertebral bodies. However, the annular ossification ("bamboo spine") of ankylosing spondylitis is not seen. In the peripheral joints there may be evidence of synovial effusion and osteochondral bodies in the knee joint; the osteophytes and periarticular cystic changes of osteoarthritis are not prominent. With time, degenerative changes occur, with narrowing of the joint space, eburnation, sclerosis, and calcification of adjacent tendons.

Prognosis. Life expectancy is normal. Alcaptonuria and ochronotic pigmentation are symptomless manifestations of homogentisic acid accumulation. Patients with the disease usually marry noncarriers, and will transmit the trait, on the average, to 50 per cent of their offspring.

Treatment. There is no specific treatment for alcaptonuria. Limitation of phenylalanine and tyrosine intake would be of theoretical value to prevent homogentisic acid accumulation, but such life-long dietary treatment is not feasible. Large amounts of the reducing agent, vitamin C, impede oxidation and polymerization of homogentisic acid and might, therefore, delay ochronotic changes. Occupations which stress the spine and large joints should be avoided. Families expressing this autosomal recessive trait should be given appropriate genetic counseling.

Garrod, A. E.: The incidence of alkaptonuria. A study in chemical individuality. Lancet, 2:1616, 1902.

LaDu, B. N.: Alcaptonuria. *In* Stanbury, J. B., Wyngaarden, J. B., and Fredrickson, D. S. (eds.): The Metabolic Basis of Inherited Disease, New York, McGraw-Hill Book Company, 1966, pp. 303-323.

LaDu, B. N., Zannoni, V. G., Laster, L., and Seegmiller, J. E.: The nature of the defect in tyrosine metabolism in alcaptonuria. J. Biol. Chem., 230:251, 1958.

O'Brien, W. M., LaDu, B. N., and Bunim, J. J.: Biochemical, pathologic and clinical aspects of alcaptonuria, ochronosis and ochronotic arthropathy. Amer. J. Med., 34:813, 1963.

Stoner, R., and Blivaiss, B. B.: Reaction of quinone of homogentisic acid with biological amines. Arthritis and Rheum., 10:53, 1967.

THE HYPERPHENYL-ALANINEMIAS

Mass screening of newborn infants in recent years has shown that all that is hyperphenylalaninemia is not necessarily phenylketonuria. Hence this section has been broadened to include mention of several hyperphenylalaninemic phenotypes evident in the human race. As a position paper of its time, the Conference on Phenylketonuria and Allied Metabolic Disorders should be consulted to complement this brief discussion.

Metabolism of Phenylalanine. L-Phenylalanine is an essential amino acid for man. In infancy half or more of its dietary intake is used for protein synthesis, and the remainder is oxidized to tyrosine by hydroxylation in the liver. As body size increases, the phenylalanine intake increases from ½ gram per day at birth to as much as 4 grams daily in the older child and adult; at the same time that the rate of growth slows, a larger fraction of phenylalanine is catabolized to tyrosine, and the amount required for anabolism decreases proportionately. Any impairment of oxidation, without change in the other para-

meters, will cause the phenylalanine-free pool to enlarge, and its plasma concentration to rise above the normal maximum (1.2 mg. per 100 ml.). When this happens, other minor pathways of phenylalanine catabolism are called upon, and increased amounts of normal minor metabolites will appear in body fluids.

The key step in L-phenylalanine catabolism, namely, hydroxylation to tyrosine, has received much attention. The simple reaction of earlier texts has been replaced by the mechanism depicted in the accompanying figure. This complex reaction involves several alleles which control various components. Not surprisingly, several types of hyperphenylalaninemias are known: further variants will undoubtedly be discovered in the future.

CLASSIC PHENYLKETONURIA

Definition. The disease was first described by Følling in 1934. In its fully expressed form, there is persistent hyperphenylalaninemia in excess of 1 mMolar (16.5 mg. per 100 ml.), mental retardation (in most cases), and excessive urinary excretion of phenylpyruvic acid and other phenylalanine derivatives. The condition is autosomal recessive, being the result of complete absence of phenylalanine hydroxlase activity. If mass screening of newborn infants for this trait and genetic counseling are to be effective, the patient with classic untreated phenylketonuria should become an oddity, often mentioned but rarely seen in modern medical practice.

Prevalence. The homozygote occurs in about 1 in 10,000 to 20,000 live births in Caucasians; the exact frequency is still undetermined. The trait is also found in Orientals, but its prevalence is unknown. It is rare in the Negro and in the Ashkenazic Jew; in the latter cases, the mutation may not be allelic with the gene causing Caucasian phenylketonuria.

Clinical Manifestations. The most important and consistent feature is mental retardation. This becomes evident at six months of age, and in later childhood 98 per cent of untreated patients have an I.Q. below 70. Phenylketonuric patients are clinically normal at birth, distinguishable only by hyperphenylalaninemia, which is established in the first postnatal week. Other manifestations, such as seizures (often with the hypsarhythmic EEG pattern) psychotic behavior, eczema, dermatographia, "mousy" odor (owing to excretion of phenylacetic acid), and pigment dilution, are found in untreated patients. None of these are seen in patients who benefit from early diagnosis and proper treatment.

The Metabolic Error. Homozygotes are completely lacking in phenylalanine hydroxylase activity; heterozygotes have partial activity, sufficient to maintain normal phenylalanine metabolism under ordinary circumstances.

Phenylalanine accumulates when the catabolic

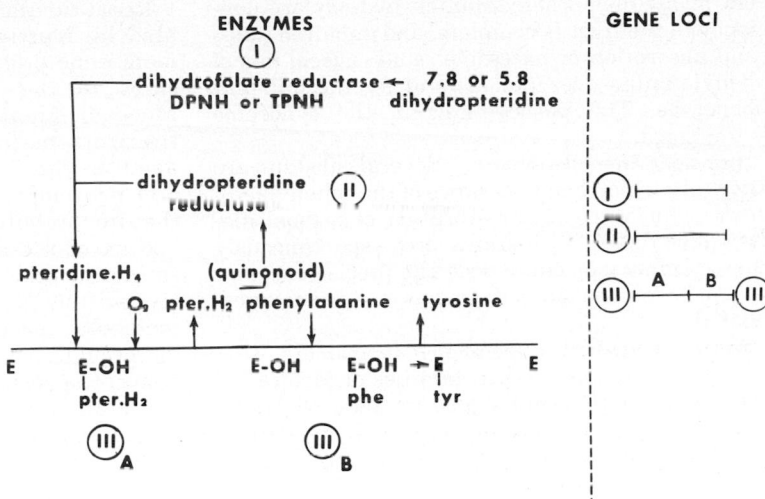

A model of phenylalanine hydroxylase, its cofactor system, and the presumed gene loci involved. (Based on the work of Zarrari and LaDu.)

pathway is blocked, and is found in excessive amounts in blood, urine, and cerebrospinal fluid. Minor pathways are then overutilized, and, characteristically, phenylpyruvic acid is formed and excreted in urine. Additional compounds such as the lactic and acetic derivatives and the glutamine conjugate are also formed and excreted. Orthohydroxylation can occur and the corresponding ortho series of metabolites may be present.

Excessive amounts of phenylalanine and its derivatives can inhibit other enzymes. As a result disturbances of tyrosine and tryptophan metabolism occur. Diminished formation of catecholamines, melanin, and serotonin is observed in untreated phenylketonuria.

The cause of mental retardation in phenylketonuria is still unknown. It is probably due to many chemical abnormalities which occur as a consequence of the disturbed chemical environment during the critical early postnatal stage of brain development.

Diagnosis. Recognition of the trait should result from early postnatal detection of hyperphenylalaninemia. Subsequent studies to assess the degree of hyperphenylalaninemia, the dietary phenylalanine tolerance, and the persistence of the trait will help to distinguish it from other genetic variants affecting phenylalanine metabolism. Testing of the urine with ferric chloride (a few drops of 5 per cent solution in 0.1N HCl added to 1 to 2 ml. urine) is not recommended for diagnosis in the newborn, since this test requires the excretion of phenylpyruvic acid, whose formation is dependent on transamination of phenylalanine; the latter function may not mature for at least three weeks after birth, even in full-term babies. All current newborn screening programs employ a specific microbiologic assay, fluorometric assay, or partition chromatography to detect excess phenylalanine in a few microliters of capillary blood collected from the heel of the infant.

Treatment. Replacement or induction of phenyl-alanine hydroxylase is not feasible. Partial liver transplantation from a normal homozygote or heterozygote would give the patient a stable source of enzyme, and perhaps this mode of treatment will be possible in the future. At present dietary restriction of phenylalanine is the only practical therapy. Special diets are available which provide 250 to 550 mg. of L-phenylalanine daily, plus the recommended amounts of other essential amino acids and of calories and other nutritional factors. Semi-synthetic foods low in phenylalanine are available in several countries. Supervision of this treatment is difficult, and is best performed at centers experienced with such regimens.

Restriction of phenylalanine intake and reduction of hyperphenylalaninemia to about 4 to 12 mg. per 100 ml. (relaxed regimen), when begun within 60 days of birth, will allow normal physical and mental development. Delayed or inadequate treatment impairs normal mental development. There is no agreement whether dietary treatment should be continued after the fifth year of life when human brain growth is complete. It is likely that female homozygous phenylketonurics should be treated during pregnancy to prevent harm to the fetus from intra-uterine hyperphenylalaninemia.

HYPERPHENYLALANINEMIC VARIANTS

The following phenotypes behave as independent autosomal recessive traits. Their recognition is important in order to avoid confusion with classic phenylketonuria and subsequent inadequate or even harmful treatment and counseling.

Atypical Phenylketonuria (Mild Variant). This variant is characterized by its high dietary tolerance for phenylalanine, which allows the patient to ingest between 700 and 2000 mg. of the amino acid in his diet. Phenylalanine hydroxylase deficiency in the liver is complete, and impaired intestinal absorption or excessive renal or fecal loss of phenylalanine does not account for the different phenotype. The pathogenesis of the syndrome is unknown.

Transient Phenylketonuria. Several sibships are known in which disappearance of the "phenylketonuric" phenotype and restoration of normal dietary phenylalanine tolerance occur spontaneously during infancy or childhood. The precise enzymatic basis for the phenotype has not been investigated.

Benign Persistent Hyperphenylalaninemia. This trait was first observed in families of Mediterranean origin but recently also in those of Anglo-Saxon lineage. The concentration of phenylalanine in plasma of homozygotes consuming normal diets is usually 4 to 12 mg. per 100 ml. Mental and physical development is normal without treatment in these subjects. Recognition of the trait is important, for it must not be confused with phenylketonuria.

Anderson, J. A., and Swaiman, K. F. (eds.): Proceedings of a Conference on Phenylketonuria and Allied Disorders. U. S. Department of Health, Education, and Welfare, Social and Rehabilitation Service, Children's Bureau. U. S. Government Printing Office, 1967-0-282-371.

Justice, P., O'Flynn, M. E., and Hsia, D. Y.: Phenylalanine-hydroxylase activity in hyperphenylalaninaemia. Lancet, 1:928, 1967.

Knox, W. E.: Phenylketonuria. In Stanbury, J. B., Wyngaarden, J. B., and Fredrickson, D. S. (eds.) The Metabolic Basis of Inherited Disease. 2nd ed. New York, McGraw-Hill Book Company, 1966, pp. 258-294.

Rosenberg, L. E., and Scriver, C. R.: Amino acid metabolism. In Bondy, P. E. (ed.): Duncan's Diseases of Metabolism. 6th ed. Philadelphia, W. B. Saunders Company 1969, pp. 366-515.

HYPERAMINOACIDURIA

General Comments. A certain amount of L-aminoaciduria, representing less than 2 to 3 per cent of the total urinary nitrogen, is a normal phenomenon. A small fraction, usually less than 5 per cent, of the filtered load of the amino acids in plasma is not absorbed completely by the proximal portion of the renal tubule and is excreted in the urine. In the healthy person, the efficiency of renal tubular transport for the individual amino acids is related to their chemical and steric structure, the load reaching the glomerular filtrate, the sex, age, and physiologic state of the subject. Data for normal range and mean values of endogenous renal clearance rates, plasma levels and urinary excretion rates of approximately 20 L-amino acids are now available for infants, children, and adults, both male and female, in fasting and nonfasting states. Advances in the knowledge of aminoaciduria have come primarily from the development of chromatographic methods, which allow rapid qualitative screening and reliable quantitative estimation of the complex amino acid composition of physiologic fluids.

Renal tubular absorption of amino acids is mediated by reactive sites which are believed to be membrane proteins, and whose catalytic relationships to the individual amino acids observe Michaelis-Menten kinetics. This means that the transport mechanism is both saturable (equivalent to the T_m) and susceptible to competitive and noncompetitive inhibition. The specificity of the site (protein) is genetically controlled.

Flux of the site–amino acid complex transfers the amino acid across the membrane (a directional process) by a mechanism which is coupled to metabolic reactions which produce energy (nondirectional reactions) or elicit coupled fluxes in the same or opposite direction of other solutes.

Abnormal aminoaciduria will result when there is an acquired or hereditary disturbance of cellular metabolism or transport of amino acids. The known hyperaminoacidurias (see accompanying table) can be classified according to four basic mechanisms:

1. *Saturation:* Substrate approaches and exceeds the capacity of the system ("overflow" aminoaciduria).

2. *Competition:* One substrate itself at elevated concentration competes with other members for access to the system ("combined" aminoaciduria).

3. *Modification of reactive site(s):* Substrate(s) not transported efficiently because access to the system is modified ("renal" aminoaciduria).

4. *Inhibition of substrate transfer:* Impaired energy-dependent processes, coupled to the transfer of substrates across membrane ("renal" aminoaciduria).

In some diseases, e.g., in Group III of the table, gene mutation affects amino acid transport in both the renal tubule and the intestine. Furthermore, it appears that the individual mechanisms required for transport of each amino acid can be grouped into at least five major gene-controlled and nonoverlapping systems, each having a particular preference for a group of amino acids normally found in plasma:

1. *The β-amino system:* β-alanine, β-aminoisobutyric acid, and taurine (viz., hyper-β-alaninemia).

2. *The α-amino systems:*
   a. "Basic" system: lysine, arginine, ornithine (and cystine, although not as a "basic" amino acid, viz., cystinuria).
   b. "Acidic" system: aspartic, glutamic (no disease yet demonstrated).
   c. Neutral-I system: proline, hydroxyproline, and glycine (viz., hyperprolinemia and renal iminoglycinuria).
   d. Neutral-II system: the remaining neutral α-amino acids (viz., Hartnup disease).

It is usually possible to classify the aminoaciduria by analyzing the amino acid content of plasma and urine collected conjointly. Chromatographic techniques will reveal the details of hyperaminoaciduria more accurately than any other method. The recognition of a specific aminoaciduria can provide an accurate clinical diagnosis for which there may be appropriate therapy.

HYPERAMINOACIDURIAS: CLASSIFIED ACCORDING TO MECHANISM

Group I-A: Saturation Mechanism (Low Clearance Group)

Disease	Amino Acids Elevated: In Plasma	In Urine	Abnormal Enzyme	Associated Symptoms and Additional Findings
1. Phenylketonuria	Phenylalanine	Same	Phenylalanine hydroxylase	Classic form: mental retardation, convulsions, pigment dilution, eczema. Responds to phenylalanine restriction in diet. Atypical form: same as classic, but dietary tolerance of phenylalanine two to three times greater. Transient form: begins like classic, but dietary tolerance increases to normal later in life.
2. Hyperphenylalanemia	Phenylalanine	Same	Unknown	Normal children(?). Ferric chloride negative.
3. Hypertyrosinemia i. Neonatal	Tyrosine	Same	Partially *inactive* para-hydroxy phenylpyruvic acid oxidase	Tyrosyluria; CNS depression if severe. Responds to ascorbic acid.
ii. Hereditary	Tyrosine (and methionine)	Same	p-HPPA oxidase activity greatly inactivated	Cirrhosis, developmental retardation; Baber's syndrome in older infants. Responds to tyrosine restriction in diet.
iii. "Oast-house" urine disease	Tyrosine, methionine, valine, leucine, isoleucine, and valine	Same	Unknown, may be like 3 ii	Mental retardation, white hair, edema, odor, convulsions.
iv. Tyrosinosis (Medes)	Tyrosine	Same	Tyrosine transaminase?	Single patient known; tyrosyluria and myasthenia gravis.
v. Supertyrosinemia (Oregon type)	Tyrosine	Same	Soluble (cytoplasmic) tyrosine transaminase	Single newborn patient with mental retardation and congenital anomalies.
4. Hyperhistidinemia	i. Histidine ii. Histidine plus alanine	Same Same	Histidase	Speech defect, mental retardation in some. Should respond to histidine restriction in diet.
5. Maple syrup urine disease (branched-chain ketoaciduria)	Valine, leucine, isoleucine, alloisoleucine	Same	Common branched-chain α-keto acid decarboxylase	i. Severe neonatal form; apnea and seizures, decerebrate rigidity, death or mental retardation. ii. Mild form: delayed mental and motor development. Both treatable by dietary restriction of leucine, isoleucine and valine.
6. Hypervalinemia	Valine	Same	Valine transaminase	Vomiting, irritability and mental retardation. Improvement with valine restricted diet.
7. a. Hypermethioninemia	Methionine (and tyrosine usually)	Same	Unknown for methionine defect	Methioninemia usually is secondary to acute liver disease. Treat primary cause.
b. Homocystinuria (see also I-B, 1)	Methionine and homocysteine	Methionine, homocystine	Cystathionine synthetase	Ectopia lentis, lax ligaments, mental retardation. Thromboembolic disease, malar flush. Treatable with methionine restriction, and cystine supplement.
8. Hyperglycinemia Type I	Glycine, serine, threonine, isoleucine, leucine, valine	Glycine predominantly	Propionyl CoA carboxylase	Vomiting, neutropenia, mental retardation, death. Responds to protein restriction.
Type II	Glycine	Same	Glycine "oxidase" or transaminase	Mild form of disease hypo-oxaluria, with mental retardation.
9. Sarcosinemia	Sarcosine, ethanolamine	Same	Sarcosine oxidase	No consistent findings
10. Hyperprolinemia (see also Group II) Type I	Proline	Proline, hydroxyproline, and glycine	L-proline oxidase	Sometimes associated with hereditary nephropathy.
Type II	Proline	Proline, hydroxyproline and glycine	Δ'-pyrroline-5-carboxylate dehydrogenase	Sometimes associated with mental retardation and seizures.
11. Hydroxyprolinemia	Hydroxyproline	Same (glycine and proline may ap pear.)	Hydroxyproline "oxidase"	Mental retardation.
12. Urea cycle diseases i. Hyperammonemia (2 types)	Glutamine (and ammonia)	Glutamine	a. Carbamyl phosphate synthetase b. Ornithine transcarbamylase	Vomiting, hepatomegaly, mental retardation. Diseases in this group (12, i-iv) respond to protein restriction.
ii. Hyperornithinemia	Ornithine, citrulline, ammonia	Citrulline	Unknown	Mental retardation, infantile spasms.
iii. Citrullinemia	Citrulline	Same	Argininosuccinic acid synthetase	Vomiting, hyperammonemia, hepatomegaly.
iv. Argininosuccinicaciduria	Argininosuccinic acid (see Group I-B, 3)	Same	Argininosuccinase	Mental retardation, trichorrhexis nodosum, convulsions, hyperammonemia.
13. Diseases of lysine metabolism i. Hyperlysinemia Type I	Lysine (and glutamine)	See Group II below	Unknown	Intermittent hyperammonemia; related to diet. Responds to protein restriction.
Type II	Lysine (and ornithine, arginine, glutamine)	Lysine, homocitrulline, homoarginine, ornithine and arginine	Lysine-ketoglutarate reductase (?)	Mental retardation and muscular hypotonia.
ii. Saccharopinuria	Citrulline, lysine, saccharopine	Same	Saccharopinase (?)	Mental retardation, short stature.
iii. Pipecolic acidemia	Pipecolic acid	Same	Pipecolate oxidase (?)	Demyelination of CNS, hepatomegaly.

HYPERAMINOACIDURIAS: CLASSIFIED ACCORDING TO MECHANISM (*Continued*)

Group I-B: (High Renal Clearance Group) (Detection in *Urine* Preferable)

Disease	Amino Acids Elevated: In Plasma	In Urine	Abnormal Enzyme	Associated Symptoms and Additional Findings
1. Homocystinuria	Methionine and homocysteine	Homocystine and methionine	Cystathionine synthetase	See Group I-A, 7b.
2. Cystathioninuria	Cystathionine	Same	Defective cofactor (pyridoxal phosphate) binding by cystathioninase	Mental retardation, plus various associated disorders. Biochemical response to pyridoxine therapy.
3. Argininosuccinic aciduria	– – – – (See Group I-A, 12 iii)– – – –			
4. Hypophosphatasia Type I	Phosphoethanolamine	Same	a. Alkaline phosphatase deficiency	
Type II (Pseudo–)	Phosphoethanolamine	Same	b. Normal alkaline phosphatase isozymes. Defect unknown.	"Rickets" (unresponsive to vitamin D), craniosynostosis, hypercalcemia.
5. β-aminoisobutyric acid excretor	β-aminoisobutyric acid	Same	Unknown	a. Example of genetic polymorphism (high excretors). b. Index of liver function and tissue catabolism.
6. Hyper-β-alaninemia	β-alanine	β-amino compounds (see II below) and γ-aminobutyric acid	(?) (β-alanine transaminase)	Somnolence, convulsions, γ-aminobutyric acid concentration in brain raised.
7. Ethanolaminuria	(?)	Ethanolamine	Unknown	Hepatic carcinoma (primary or secondary relation?).

Group II: Saturation and Competition

Disease	Amino Acids Elevated: In Plasma	In Urine	Abnormal Enzyme
1. Hyperprolinemia Types I and II	Proline	Proline, hydroxyproline and glycine	See I-A, 10
2. Hyper-β-alaninemia	β-alanine	β-alanine, taurine, β-aminoisobutyric acid	See I-B, 6
3. Hyperlysinemia	Lysine	Ornithine, arginine	See I-A, 13

Group III: Modification of Reactive Sites

Disease	Amino Acids Increased: In Urine	In Feces	Transport "System" Involved	Clinical Features
1. Cystinuria	Cystine, lysine, arginine, ornithine	Same in Type I and II only	Diamino monocarboxylic (+ cystine)	Genotypes Types I, II, and III. Renal calculi; severe rare cases also show growth retardation and malabsorption.
2. Iminoglycinuria	Proline, hydroxyproline and glycine	In one genotype	Neutral I (proline, hydroxyproline and glycine)	At least 2 genotypes. No abnormalities other than aminoaciduria.
3. Hartnup disease	Monoamino-monocarboxylic, α-aminoacids	Same in one genotype	Neutral II (excludes Neutral I)	Episodic pellagra-like state with psychosis and cerebellar signs. Two genotypes, only one has intestinal defect.
4. The glycinurias a. deVries type	Glycine	Unknown	Neutral I	a. Heterozygote of iminoglycinuria.
b. Dent type	Glycine and PO_4		Probably belong in Group IV of etiologic mechanisms	b. Rickets.
c. Scriver type	Glycine + PO_4 and glucose			c. Rickets.
d. Kaiser type	Glycine and glucose			d. Dominant inheritance without symptoms.
	Manifested in intestine primarily			
5. Blue diaper syndrome	Indole derivatives	Tryptophan	Subcomponent of neutral II?	Hypercalcemia. Autosomal recessive gene probably.
6. Methionine malabsorption	α-hydroxybutyric acid	Methionine and branch-chain amino acid	Subcomponent of neutral II?	(?) Like oast-house urine disease (Group I-A, 3 iv). Autosomal recessive trait.

HYPERAMINOACIDURIAS: CLASSIFIED ACCORDING TO MECHANISM *(Continued)*

Group IV: "Noncompetitive" Inhibition of Transport

Primary Abnormality	Aminoaciduria and Other Findings	Comment
1. Acquired e.g., Degraded tetracyclines, salicylates, heavy metals, vitamin D deficiency, scurvy, etc.	Generalized aminoaciduria, plus combinations of glucosuria, hyperphosphaturia, etc. (Fanconi syndrome)	Early removal of toxin or correction of deficiency usually followed by recovery of normal transport function
2. Hereditary Galactosemia	Generalized + galactosuria	Can be induced by galactose feeding and treated by removal of galactose.
Oculocerebro-renal syndrome	Generalized + phosphaturia and renal tubular acidosis	X-linked glaucoma, hypotonia and mental retardation; defect in ammonia synthesis?
Other Fanconi syndromes, related to:	Generalized + loss of glucose, phosphate, K, bicarbonate, water, etc.	Symptoms related to functional defect (Po₄ and K loss etc.) plus primary disease.
a Cystinosis		a. Cystine storage. Recessive gene.
b. Idiopathic (infants)		b. No cystine storage. Sporadic cases.
c. Idiopathic (adults)		c. Recessive inheritance. No cystinosis.
d. Luder-Sheldon variety		d. Onset in late childhood.
e. Secondary to Wilson's disease		e. Onset in late childhood.
f. Secondary to tyrosinemia (Baber's syndrome)		f. Onset usually in late infancy.
g Others		

OVERFLOW HYPERAMINOACIDURIAS

Branched-Chain Aminoaciduria

Maple Syrup Urine Disease. The colloquial term describes a characteristic odor of patients with *branched-chain ketoaciduria, and aminoacidopathy* (Group IA, 5 of the table). The disease is autosomal recessive and its apparent rarity may reflect, in part, missed diagnoses in patients dying in infancy. Severe hypotonia, apnea, feeding difficulty, and hypoglycemia appear in the first week of life, progressing to seizures, decorticate rigidity, severe mental retardation, and death. An episodic form of the disease with mild motor and mental retardation presenting in later infancy has been reported.

The primary enzymatic defect is a block in decarboxylation of branched chain α-keto acids; consequently leucine, isoleucine, alloisoleucine, and valine and their equivalent α-keto acids and α-hydroxyacids accumulate after birth; symptoms are primarily related to abnormal leucine metabolism. The aminoacidopathy can be detected in blood and urine within the first week of life; the enzyme defect can be assayed in leukocytes and in cultured skin fibroblasts.

The disease responds to dietary control of leucine, isoleucine, and valine intake, the best results following the earliest possible treatment.

Hypervalinemia (Group IA, 6 of the table). Symptoms of vomiting, blindness, and retardation of physical and mental development in a single Japanese infant were reported, which improved abruptly with a valine-restricted diet. Valine transaminase is the defective enzyme, hence only valine accumulates in body fluids.

HYPERHISTIDINEMIA

Many cases of this rare and apparently autosomal recessively inherited disease (Group I of the table) are now known. Inactivity of the enzyme histidase, which nonoxidatively deaminates histidine to uraconic acid, can be detected in skin biopsy material. Accumulation of histidine, (and sometimes of alanine) above normal levels and depressed serotonin levels are found in blood; increased excretion of imidazolepyruvic acid and a positive ferric chloride test are found in urine. Mild mental retardation and/or short auditory memory span, reflected as delayed speech development, usually occur.

THE HYPERPROLINEMIAS AND HYDROXYPROLINEMIA
(Iminoacidopathies)

Hyperprolinemias. *Type I* (L-proline oxidase deficiency) is a recessively inherited condition. Proline is the only amino acid elevated in plasma, but a "combined" aminoaciduria (Group II of the table) involving proline, hydroxyproline, and glycine is found. In *Type II* hyperprolinemia the block is at the second step in proline degradation (Δ'-pyrroline-5-carboxylate dehydrogenase); the pyrroline derivative is also excreted in urine. Type I hyperprolinemia is usually associated with familial hematuric nephropathy, but pedigree studies show that prolinemia and nephropathy are not the consequences of a single gene effect; seizures also occur in both disorders.

Hydroxyprolinemia. Mental retardation was the principal finding in the single patient described. The enzymes for free hydroxy-L-proline catabolism are distinct from those for L-proline, and the deficient enzyme is a hydroxyproline-specific "oxidase."

DISEASES OF THE UREA CYCLE

Argininosuccinicaciduria. This was the first reported hereditary impairment of the urea cycle; in subsequent years, four additional recessively inherited disorders of this cycle (*hyperammonemia* without aminoacidemia [two types], *hyperornithinemia*, and *citrullinemia*) have been recognized (Group IA, 12 of the table). Each causes hyperammonemia, which tends to be more severe the more proximal the defect is in the urea cycle, which in turn may determine the severity of signs and symptoms (convulsions, vomiting, failure to thrive, hepatomegaly) and degree of mental retardation. The concentration of blood urea and its renal excretion are both normal in each disease. The explanation for this paradox is found in the apparent phenotypic effect of the mutations on urea cycle enzymes. Studies of citrullinemic fibroblasts by Tedesco and Mellman showed partial activity of ASA synthetase with a new K_m about 25 times above normal. Substrate accumulation in this circumstance sustains formation of product, and thus urea.

Friable hair (trichorrhexis nodosum) is found in argininosuccinicaciduria during periods of poor nutrition, perhaps due to a conditioned deficiency of arginine. Symptomatic improvement in each disorder is reported with restriction of protein intake and specific management of hyperammonemia.

DISORDERS OF METHIONINE DEGRADATION

Homocystinuria. The clinical features of this increasingly recognized autosomal recessive disease (Group IB, 1 of the table) are diagnostic: ectopia lentis, mental retardation, lax ligaments, lengthened extremities, malar flush, and fine sparse hair; death from thromboembolic phenomena is frequent. Late-surviving patients have ocular, skeletal, and vascular changes likened to those of Marfan's syndrome. Cystathionine synthetase is deficient; its substrate, homocysteine, and the precursor, methionine, accumulate; the product, cystathionine, is deficient in brain. Homocysteine is oxidized and excreted in urine as homocystine, where it can be detected by the cyanide-nitroprusside test. Early dietary therapy with methionine restriction (and cystine supplementation) has apparent benefit. Some patients respond to large doses of pyridoxine (vitamin B_6).

Cystathioninuria. This condition (Group IB, 2 of the table) is transmitted in an autosomal recessive fashion. It appears to be a benign and not uncommon condition often found in patients with other diseases that attract attention first. Acquired cystathioninuria also occurs secondary to hepatic failure and neuroblastoma. In the hereditary form, the presumed heterozygote exhibits modest elevation, and the homozygote has marked elevation of cystathionine levels in body fluids related to a deficiency of cystathionine-cleaving enzyme activity. Frimpter, who observed biochemical improvement with pyridoxine therapy, demonstrated that the cleaving enzyme is present in the patient's tissues, but is inactive until an excess of pyridoxal-5-phosphate is available, indicating a specific defect in co-factor binding by the apoenzyme.

β-AMINOISOBUTYRICACIDURIA

β-Aminoisobutyric acid (βAIB) (Group IB, 5 of the table) is a derivative of thymine and valine metabolism. High urinary excretion (> 100 μM per gram total N) occurs in some humans who are probably homozygous for a gene controlling the activity of βAIB transaminase. In these subjects, plasma levels of βAIB are elevated; the renal clearance rate of the natural isomer, D-(-), βAIB, exceeds that for inulin, indicating net renal "secretion" of βAIB; probenecid can suppress excretion. Hyperexcretors are common in the Mongolian race and infrequent (approximately 5 per cent) in Caucasians; the adaptive significance for the mutation is unknown. Increased βAIB excretion can also be acquired under catabolic stress.

RENAL HYPERAMINOACIDURIAS

Certain hyperaminoacidurias reflect impairment of specific transport systems (Group III of the table); the transport lesion is frequently demonstrable in the gut as well as in the kidney. The renal clearance rates of affected amino acids are high, and their plasma levels are low or normal, rather than elevated.

Cystinuria (Group III, 1 of the table). Three cystinuric phenotypes are now recognized; in all, the homozygote has elevated urinary excretion of cystine, lysine, ornithine, and arginine. In type 1, gut transport of the four amino acids is also abnormal; the heterozygote has normal aminoaciduria (complete recessive). Type 2 has defective gut transport of the basic amino acids but not of cystine; the heterozygote has elevated urinary lysine and cystine (incomplete recessive). Type 3 has normal gut transport; the heterozygote phenotype is "incomplete." The exact mechanism of the hyperaminoaciduria is unclear; net tubular "secretion" of cystine found in most patients may reflect cellular cysteine efflux.

Urinary cystine calculi are the predominant clinical problem, related to the poor aqueous solubility of cystine. Prevention of calculi formation and attendant complications can be attained with copious free water excretion throughout day and night. Rapid solubilization of cystine by formation of a mixed disulfide with D(-) penicillamine (0.5 to 1.0 gram every six hours) may be useful in some patients. Cystinuric patients also have modest growth retardation, perhaps related to fecal and urinary loss of lysine. In a few children severe growth failure and generalized intestinal malabsorption occur with cystinuria as a particular syndrome.

Hartnup Disease (Group III, 3 of the table). Episodic clinical features include pellagra-like symptoms with photosensitive dermatitis, cerebellar ataxia, and psychosis; mental retardation is referred to, but is not a universal finding. Biochemical findings include reduced blood levels of tryptophan metabolites, e.g., nicotinic acid and serotonin, and a fluctuant increase in urinary excretion of indolic acids and derivatives. A constant transport defect for certain neutral α-amino acids is demonstrable in kidney and intestine. The abnormal "indoluria" is dependent on intestinal flora degrading unabsorbed L-tryptophan, with absorption and renal excretion of the products. Defective intracellular transport of tryptophan may account for the deficiency of its endogenous metabolites. Good protein nutrition, normal general intestinal health, and nicotinamide supplements (40 to 200 mg. per day) appear to improve the general health of the patient.

Proline-Hydroxyproline-Glycinuria (Iminoglycinuria) (Group III, 2 of the table). This finding is normal in early infancy. Failure of the specific transport system to develop has been observed as an autosomal recessive trait in otherwise healthy subjects of several pedigrees around the world. Presence or absence of an associated intestinal transport defect indicates at least two mutant genotypes.

THE HYPERGLYCINURIAS

Six forms of isolated hyperglycinuria are known:

1. Hyperglycinemia with "overflow" hyperglycinuria (Group IA, 8 of the table).

a. Type I: Vomiting, acetonuria, neutropenia, thrombocytopenia, and leucine intolerance occur in the neonatal period; retardation of growth and mental development follow if the infant survives. The missing enzyme is propionate CoA carboxylase. Restriction of dietary protein intake (1 gram per kilogram per day) is beneficial.

b. Type II: There are no severe symptoms, but mental retardation occurs. Conversion of glycine to serine is apparently impaired.

2. Renal glycinurias (Group III, 4 of the table).

a. Impaired renal conservation of glycine occurs as the heterozygous phenotype in one form of familial iminoglycinuria.

b. Resistant rickets and renal hyperglycinuria occur in association with: (i) hyperphosphaturia, (ii) hyperphosphaturia and glucosuria (both renal).

c. Dominantly inherited, asymptomatic renal glycinuria with renal glucosuria has been reported from Switzerland.

THE FANCONI SYNDROME

The term "Fanconi syndrome" (Group IV of the table) describes a disturbance of proximal renal tubular function of multiple causation and comprising generalized hyperaminoaciduria, renal glucosuria, and hyperphosphaturia, as well as renal loss of potassium, bicarbonate and water, and other substances conserved by the proximal tubule. The Fanconi syndrome should be considered as the final result of any one of many possible primary insults to proximal tubular function. The patient's symptoms reflect the disturbance of tubular function, in addition to the primary cause of the syndrome.

The Fanconi syndrome may be inherited or acquired. The various hereditary forms are predominantly recessive, different alleles being responsible for the different diseases causing the syndrome. For example, cystinosis is a recessive, inherited disease, with cystine accumulation occurring in tissues and accompanied by the syndrome that first appears about six months after birth. The idiopathic Fanconi syndrome in adults is a recessively inherited disorder of early middle age, with only the syndrome and its consequences. Acquired causes are numerous; deteriorated tetracycline (epianhydrotetracycline) is an interesting recent example.

The syndrome appears to be due to noncompetitive inhibition of cellular mechanisms sustaining transport function in the proximal tubule. As a result, the tubular capacity for transport is impaired. In severe cases, morphologic changes also occur, with reduction in cell organelles and cell mass of the proximal portion of the proximal convoluted tubule (swan-neck lesion).

The disturbance of proximal tubular function results in the alterations in urine and plasma composition referred to above. The final levels of expression of the syndrome are more peripheral, and are related to both the disturbances in renal physiology and the primary cause of the syndrome. Osteomalacia or rickets reflects the loss of inorganic phosphate; muscle weakness is symptomatic of potassium and phosphate loss; Pitressin-resistant diabetes insipidus is sometimes diagnosed in children before the syndrome is recognized. There may also be evidence for the primary cause of the syndrome, e.g., cystine crystals in the cornea, Kaiser-Fleischer rings of Wilson's disease, a history of exposure to antimicrobial drugs or toxins, or other affected family members.

Treatment. Attempt to eliminate the primary cause, e.g., removal of exogenous toxic agents or deficiency states. Other primary conditions may be ameliorated, e.g., removal of milk in galactosemia or chelation therapy in Wilson's disease.

Offset the disturbance in tubular physiology. Osteomalacia is readily treated, and prevented, with oral phosphate supplements (1.0 to 2.0 grams phosphorus per day, equivalent to 20 grams of "neutral" phosphate salt); vitamin D_2 may also be required in doses adjusted to the patient's need. Shohl's solution, 30 ml. three times daily for adults, usually controls the acidemia. Hypokalemia may be corrected with potassium salts (as phosphate or citrate). Adequate fluid intake is indicated to prevent dehydration.

Efron, M. L.: Aminoaciduria. New Eng. J. Med., 272:1058, 1107, 1965.

Frimpter, G.: Cystathioninuria: Nature of the defect. Science, 149:1095, 1965.

LaDu, B. N.: Genetic variation in metabolic disorders. In Nyhan, W. L. (ed.): Amino Acid Metabolism and Genetic Variation. New York, McGraw-Hill Book Company, 1966, pp. 121-130.

Nyhan, W. L. (ed.): Amino Acid Metabolism and Genetic Variation. New York, McGraw-Hill Book Company, 1967.

Rosenberg, L. E., and Scriver, C. R.: Amino acid metabolism. *In* Bondy, P. H. (ed.): Duncan's Diseases of Metabolism. 6th ed. Philadelphia, W. B. Saunders Company, 1969, pp. 366-515.

Scriver, C. R.: Inborn errors of amino-acid metabolism. Brit. Med. Bull., 25:35, 1969.

Tedesco, T. A., and Mellman, W. J.: Argininosuccinate synthetase activity and citrulline metabolism in cells cultured from a citrullinemic subject. Proc. Nat. Acad. Sci. U.S.A., 57:829, 1967.

Disorders of Purine Metabolism
Lloyd H. Smith, Jr.

GOUT

Definition. Gout represents a group of *genetic* diseases of purine metabolism or excretion ordinarily identifiable by *hyperuricemia*. When clinically manifest, gout presents as an acute inflammatory *arthritis,* the accumulation of sodium urate deposits as *tophi, uric acid nephrolithiasis,* or *renal failure*. These manifestations can occur in any combination. This definition, which must remain arbitrary until the pathogenesis of each gouty syndrome has been more firmly established, has several points of emphasis which will be discussed more fully later in this article. First, it emphasizes the genetic or familial origin of gout. This attribute has long been recognized. Galen attributed gout to "debauchery, intemperance, and an hereditary trait," and Sydenham emphasized its early occurrence in patients "when they have received the ill seeds of this disease from their parents by inheritance." Second, gout is defined here in terms of its chemical derangement, essential hyperuricemia. This is analogous to the diagnosis of diabetes mellitus, an essential hyperglucosemia. The clinical manifestations are complications of hyperuricemia (or hyperuricaciduria) which may or may not occur in the individual patient. It has been estimated that these complications in some combination occur in only 10 to 20 per cent of individuals with hyperuricemia, the incidence of increasing in rough proportion to the level of serum uric acid. Finally, the definition emphasizes the heterogeneity of gout. Several different diseases lead to the common feature of persistent hyperuricemia (see Pathogenesis and Table 1).

In a sense all of us have inappropriate hyperuricemia because of two errors in evolution. Uricase catalyzes the conversion of relatively insoluble urate to soluble allantoin, which would be a much more appropriate end product for the mammalian kidney. The evolutionary retention of this enzyme would have obviated both gout and uric acid nephrolithiasis. A second error compounds the first. The mechanism by which the human kidney excretes uric acid is complex, including glomerular filtration, tubular reabsorption, and tubular secretion. The net result is renal retention of more than 90 per cent of that filtered. At equilibrium, the same amount of uric acid is presumably excreted but at the cost of relative hyperuricemia. Renal tubular reabsorption of filtered uric acid is not present in other primates, which therefore have serum uric acid levels of less than 0.05 mg. per 100 ml. The suggestion has been made that renal retention might help to modulate bursts of uric acid excretion owing to purine ingestion, and also might shunt more urate into the gut for bacterial destruction. Whether this is true or not, it seems clear that gout represents an exaggeration of a genetic legacy of hyperuricemia common to all.

History. Gout has figured largely in history, perhaps rivaled only by pandemics of infectious diseases and mental illness. Its classic manifestations were noted in classical times, and the occurrence of osseous tophi and uric acid stones has allowed archeologic diagnoses to be made with confidence. Hippocrates, who recognized and described podagra, devoted three of his aphorisms to the disease, saying in effect: 28, Eunuchs do not take the gout, nor become bald; 29, Women do not take the gout until their menses be stopped; 30, Young men do not take the gout until they indulge in coition. Galen described tophaceous gout and commented upon the familial occurrence of the disease. The term gout, derived from the Latin word *gutta,* came into usage during the Middle Ages to reflect a theory of pathogenesis that this form of arthritis resulted from the "dropping" of a poisonous *"noxa"* into the joint. It is interesting to see the recent confirmation of this theory and the identification of sodium urate microcrystals as the *noxa*. In the seventeenth century, Thomas Sydenham (1683), sometimes called the Shakespeare of gout, wrote clinical descriptions of the disease which have yet to be improved on. He wrote with an authority based on intense personal experience with gouty arthritis and stones. Uric acid was first discovered as a component of stones by Scheele in 1776 (designated lithic acid), followed two decades later by its identification in tophi by Wallaston (1797). In the middle of the nineteenth century the elder (A. B.) Garrod developed a crude but ingenious method for estimating uric acid in serum (crystallization on a linen fiber), and found it to be elevated in patients with gout, demonstrating for the first time the chemical hallmark of the disease. His postulate that acute gouty arthritis was due to deposits of sodium urate was convincingly supported by the work of Freudweiler (1899), who demonstrated the inflammatory potential of sodium urate microcrystals and leukocytic phagocytosis of such crystals in such crystals in acute gout. This contribution was lost in the sediment of subsequent investigations, the phenomenon of *microcrystalline synovitis* being independently rediscovered within the past few years. In 1931, the younger (A. E.) Garrod proposed that gout should be classified as one of the inborn errors of metabolism. Over the past two decades studies in many laboratories, notably those of Buchanan (1960) and Greenberg, have elucidated the pathways of purine biosynthesis and degradation and the controlling mechanisms for modulating the appropriate rate control of purine metabolism. It is against this background that current studies of pathogenesis, to be reviewed below, are being conducted.

The history of gout has been intermingled with sociologic and cultural variables as well as the march of medical and biochemical progress. From earliest observations the disease has been associated with dissipation and venery. Even gouty Sydenham wrote, "the gout generally attacks those aged persons who have spent most of their lives in ease, voluptuousness, high living, and too free use of wine and other spirituous liquors." It gradually became a disease in caricature in the eighteenth and nineteenth centuries, used by novelist, satirist, and political cartoonist alike as symbolic of medical retribution for excessive indulgence of natural appetites. Ambrose Bierce defined gout as "a physician's name for the rheumatism of a rich patient." The disease gradually won grudging respect ("disease of kings and king of diseases") because of its remarkable association with men of genius and exceptional achievement. An incomplete list of those alleged to have suffered from the gout includes Alexander the Great, Louis XIV, Issac Newton, William Harvey, Martin Luther, John Calvin, Leonardo da Vinci,

Samuel Johnson, and Benjamin Franklin. It is an amusing sequel that several recent studies have confirmed positive statistical correlations of serum uric acid levels and intelligence or social status. In this context it is unkind to recall, with Hippocrates, that gout is rare in the premenopausal female.

Genetics of Gout. Family aggregation of clinical gout has been observed since the first clinical descriptions of the disease in antiquity. Gout has appeared in an irregular pattern both in successive generations and in sibships. A positive family history for clinical gout is found in about 10 to 20 per cent of patients with the primary disorder. Attempts have been made to use hyperuricemia as a more precise marker for the presence of the gouty trait. Within the restrictions imposed by the statistical uncertainties of the boundary between normal and abnormal serum urate levels (Fig. 1), hyperuricemia has been found in 15 to 25 per cent of close relatives of patients with clinical gout. It is sometimes stated that primary gout is transmitted as an autosomal dominant with incomplete penetrance. The pattern of inheritance of hyperuricemia has varied so widely that it may be polygenic in origin. Many variables affect the phenotypic expression of the gouty trait: age, sex, diet, and renal function. It is noteworthy that in the single form of gout in which a specific enzyme defect of purine metabolism has been established, the syndrome of hypoxanthine–guanine phosphoribosyltransferase deficiency, the genetic transmission has been established as that of a sex-linked recessive trait. Glycogen storage disease Type I, which is associated with a specific form of secondary renal gout, is transmitted as an autosomal recessive trait. It seems probable that the mode of inheritance of other forms of gout will not be clearly established until genetic markers more specific than hyperuricemia are available. This must await clarification of the pathogenesis

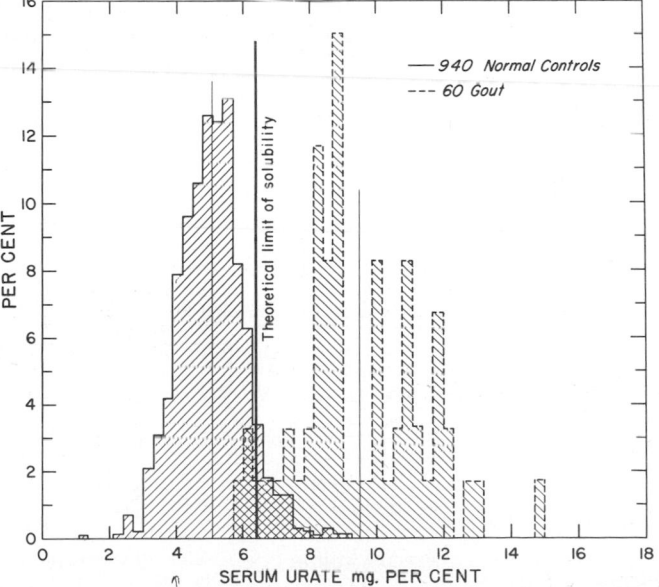

FIGURE 1. Distribution of serum urate concentrations in normal and gouty male subjects and calculated limit of solubility of sodium urate in serum. (From Seegmiller, J. E.: Diseases of purine and pyrimidine metabolism. *In* Bondy, P. K. [ed.]: Duncan's Diseases of Metabolism. 6th ed. Philadelphia, W. B. Saunders Company, 1969.)

of the various gouty syndromes in more specific phenotypic terms.

Pathogenesis. It has been established for over 100 years (A. B. Garrod) that the hallmark of gout is hyperuricemia. All the clinical manifestations of gout, with the single exception of uric acid nephrolithiasis, derive from the cystallization of sodium urate from extracellular fluids where it has accumulated in a supersaturated concentration. No one has shown that sodium urate in solution is toxic. There are several questions which relate to the pathogenesis of gout: What leads to the accumulation of urate in extracellular fluid? What are the variables in its precipitation? How do sodium urate crystals lead to inflammatory arthritis?

The Cause of Hyperuricemia. The accumulation of any metabolite in excess must result from one (or a combination) of three variables: increased absorption, decreased excretion, or increased biosynthesis. There is no evidence that gouty patients habitually ingest excessive purines or have an increased avidity for purine absorption. Elimination of purine ingestion usually results in a reduction of serum urate of about 0.6 mg. per 100 ml. in normal subjects and about 1.0 mg. per 100 ml. in gouty patients. Under experimental conditions, ingestion of a diet very high in nucleic acids may lead to hyperuricemia in normal subjects comparable to gouty levels. In summary, absorption of preformed purines from dietary sources may modify extracellular urate levels, but does not represent a primary cause of gout.

Uric acid is the end product of purine metabolism, most of it being excreted as free urinary urate. Recent studies have indicated at least two mechanisms by which it is partially destroyed in man. Leukocytes contain verdoperoxidases capable of degrading uric acid to allantoin and carbon dioxide. Of much greater importance quantitatively, uric acid is secreted into the gut where uricolysis is carried out by bacterial enzymes. Approximately one quarter of that synthesized daily is degraded through these mechanisms.

Studies in gout have not supported decreased uricolysis as a mechanism for hyperuricemia. In fact, with high urate concentrations, especially after the onset of renal insufficiency, excretion into the gut and uricolysis there may be enhanced as an important second line of defense. Particular attention has therefore been directed toward increased synthesis or decreased excretion as primary mechanisms for hyperuricemia in gout.

Uric acid is synthesized from xanthine and from hypoxanthine (via xanthine), these successive oxidations being catalyzed by xanthine oxidase (Fig. 2). The free purine bases bear complex metabolic relationships to various pools of purine nucleotides. In part the free bases are reutilized to form functioning nucleotides; in part they are converted to uric acid for excretion. Because of this reutilization, sometimes called "salvage synthesis," uric acid synthesis, as reflected in urinary excretion and intestinal destruction, represents only a part of the purine nucleotide turnover rate. At equilibrium, however, that part should approximate the *de novo* synthetic rate of purine nucleotides. Small amounts of hypoxanthine, xanthine, and other trace purines are normally excreted in the urine as well. Several methods have been widely applied in an attempt to determine whether there is excessive purine synthesis in gout: measurement of urate excreted on a low purine diet, use of isotopic urate to determine its pool size and turnover rate, and study of the time course of incorporation of a purine precursor, usually glycine, into urate (Fig. 3). Each of these methods is subject to limitations which cannot be detailed here. The following information has emerged from such studies. In normal man the daily rate of production of uric acid on a low purine diet averages about 750 mg. The miscible pool of uric acid is about 1.0 to 1.3 grams, so that two thirds to three fourths of the body pool turns over daily. Urinary excretion of urate varies widely even during dietary regulation, averaging in men 426 ± 81 mg. per 24 hours. The difference between the estimated production rate of urate and that excreted in the

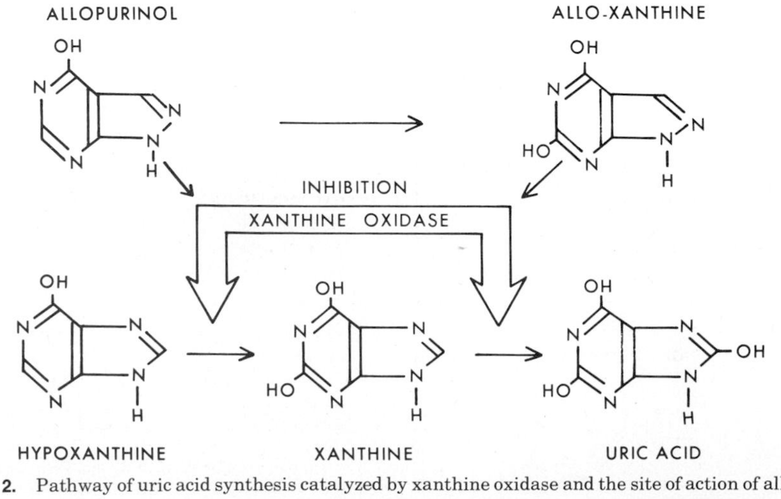

FIGURE 2.   Pathway of uric acid synthesis catalyzed by xanthine oxidase and the site of action of allopurinol.

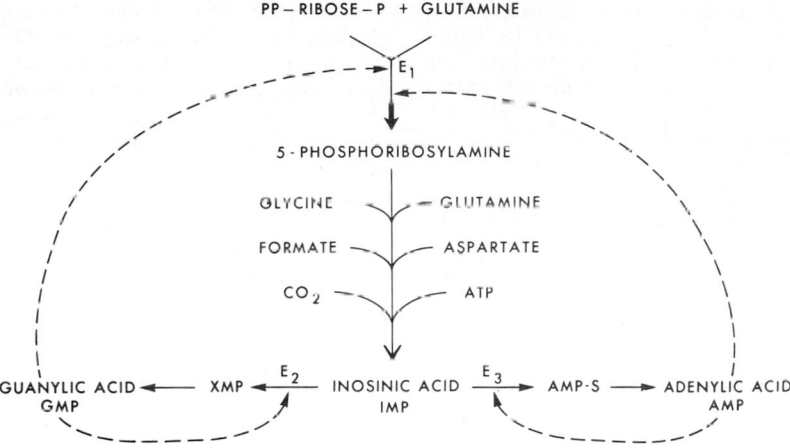

FIGURE 3. De novo pathway of purine nucleotide biosynthesis and the feedback control mechanisms $(- - - \rightarrow)$. E_1, Glutamine 5-phosphoribosylpyrophosphate amidotransferase; E_2, inosine 5'-phosphate dehydrogenase; E_3, adenylsuccinic acid (AMP-S) synthetase; XMP, xanthosine 5'-phosphate.

urine represents uricolysis, mostly by bacterial action in the gut.

By use of these methods, evidence for excessive synthesis of uric acid has been obtained in about two thirds of patients with primary gout. Overproduction is readily understood in patients with diseases resulting in increased tissue breakdown, e.g., myeloid metaplasia, polycythemia vera, and leukemia, With the exception of hypoxanthine-guanine phosphoribosyltransferase deficiency syndrome to be discussed later, the biochemical basis for excessive purine synthesis in other forms of gout has not been established. The first step unique to purine nucleotide biosynthesis and the major site of metabolic regulation is that of the synthesis of phosphoribosylamine, catalyzed by the enzyme glutamine 5-phosphoribosyl-pyrophosphate (PRPP) amidotransferase:

$$\text{Glutamine} + \text{PRPP} + H_2O \xrightarrow{Mg^{++}} \text{glutamic acid} + \\ \text{5-phosphoribosylamine} + \text{pyrophosphate}$$

There are several possibilities for loss of normal rate control at this regulatory site; these include excessive concentrations of the substrate glutamine or PRPP, or both, a genetic alteration in the enzyme rendering it less sensitive to normal feedback control by purine nucleotides, or a partial deficiency of one of the nucleotides (adenylic, guanylic, and inosinic acids) which, in concert, exert allosteric modulation of the enzyme (Fig. 3). Preliminary work has indicated defective feedback control in in vitro studies of fibroblasts from some patients with overproduction gout. Glutamate but not glutamine is raised in the plasma of a number of gouty patients. It can be anticipated that future studies will document further heterogeneity in the mechanisms by which purine synthesis is enhanced in various types of overproduction gout.

In about one third of patients with gout there is no evidence for overproduction of uric acid by any of the methods now available. Evidence suggests

that these patients have an inherited disorder (or group of disorders) of the renal tubule resulting in decreased urate clearance as the cause of hyperuricemia. Renal clearance of urate is a complex function of filtration, tubular reabsorption, and tubular secretion. The recent demonstration of partial binding of urate to plasma proteins has impaired the validity of some of the clearance studies reported. Using the assumption that urate is completely filterable at the glomerulus, there is net tubular reabsorption of 90 to 95 per cent. Urate which is excreted is in part and perhaps in toto that secreted by the tubule. Patients with "renal gout" exhibit reduced clearances of urate, the differences being most evident when compared to normal controls with dietary induction of comparable plasma levels of uric acid. The differences have not always been striking, and in some cases may be difficult to interpret because of early impairment of renal function by gout. Reduced net clearance could result from a genetic defect, leading to defective tubular secretion of urate or, less likely, to enhanced tubular reabsorption. An increase in the bound fraction of urate would also reduce clearance by reducing that filtered. An impaired tubular secretion of urate might be an intrinsic defect of the transport mechanism, which has not yet been clarified biochemically. It might also result from a genetic or acquired metabolic disorder in some other pathway which leads to the accumulation of a metabolite which secondarily interferes with tubular urate secretion. An example of this latter mechanism is the hyperuricemia associated with the lactic acidosis of Type I glycogen storage disease (q.v.). Idiopathic renal gout might similarly result from the accumulation of other uric acid transport inhibitors not yet identified. When overall reduction of renal function occurs, as it does not infrequently in gout, hyperuricemia is further exacerbated, and an increased percentage of urate is excreted into the gut for uricolysis.

In summary, the important causes of persistent hyperuricemia are those of excessive synthesis and decreased renal clearance. This allows for a rational classification of gout as shown in Table 1. Such a classification reflects only a progress report. Although hypoxanthine–guanine phosphoribosyltransferase deficiency represents the only type of metabolic gout for which a specific enzymatic defect has been established, new defects in the rate control mechanisms will almost certainly be established shortly, possibly as abnormalities of phosphoribosylpyrophosphate amidotransferase. Similarly, the genetic types of renal gout will probably prove to be more heterogeneous in future studies. A variety of drugs (notably the chlorothiazide diuretics) and metabolites (lactate, β-hydroxybutyrate) diminish urate clearance in the normal kidney, and may precipitate clinical gout.

Precipitation of Urate. Uric acid is not toxic to man in its soluble state. Although hyperuricemia has been associated epidemiologically with a number of conditions, e.g., coronary artery heart disease and hypertension, there is no evidence that it has any pathogenic relationship to those disorders. Uric acid seems to produce disease "physically" rather than "chemically" when precipitated as sodium urate at pH 7.40, or as uric acid in acidic urine. Its precipitation as amorphous sodium urate, which may occur in virtually any tissue in the body except for the central nervous system, results in tophi with tissue disruption and destruction but with minimal inflammatory response. Its precipitation as microcrystals of critical size in certain tissues, especially in synovial tissues and spaces, leads to an acute inflammatory reaction to be described below. Its precipitation in the renal distal collecting tubules as uric acid may rarely lead to acute renal failure. The precipitation of uric acid in a protein matrix in the renal pelvis, or more rarely in the ureter or bladder, leads to uric acid nephrolithiasis.

Sodium urate is soluble in human plasma to a concentration of only about 7 mg. per 100 ml. (of urate). Values above this denote supersaturated solutions, although sodium urate may remain in supersaturated solution with considerable stability. Why do some patients with serum uric acid levels of 9 mg. per 100 ml. have severe tophaceous gout or acute gouty arthritis or both, whereas others may maintain similar levels for years or even for life with no evidence of precipitation, i.e., of clinical gout? The reasons for these differences in threshold of precipitation are not known. One recently described variable is that of protein binding of urate in plasma to a specific α_1-α_2 globulin (Alvsaker) and to albumin. It has been reported that some patients with tophaceous gout have reduced protein-binding of urate. These interesting observations require further confirmation.

The solubility of urate in urine decreases with increasing acidity because of the shift to free uric acid. The titration curve is such that the undissociated uric acid increases to 85 per cent at pH 5.0. At this pH only 6 to 8 mg. of urate is soluble per 100 ml. of urine so that supersaturation is required to excrete an average uric acid load in a normal urine volume. The solubility increases 20-fold at pH 7.0 over that at pH 5.0. Three factors are therefore important in the urinary precipitation of uric acid: urine volume, the amount of urate excreted per 24 hours, and urine pH. It is possible that the availability of stone matrix and the level of stabilizing substances in urine may also play important roles.

Cause of Acute Gouty Arthritis. The four clinical manifestations of gout are those of tophaceous deposits, acute gouty arthritis, uric acid nephrolithiasis, and gouty kidney with various degrees of impairment of renal function. Of these clinical manifestations or complications associated with hyperuricemia, acute inflammatory arthritis is that which has been most obscure in its pathogenesis. Garrod the elder, in the second of his ten propositions on "the true nature or essence of gout" (1859) wrote: "Investigations recently made in the morbid anatomy of gout prove incontestably that true gouty inflammation is always accompanied with a deposition of urate of soda in the inflamed part." This proposition was strongly supported by the experimental work of Freudweiler (1899) who was able to produce inflammation with sodium urate crystals and observed their subsequent presence in leukocytes. For many years, however, this work was ignored because of evidence which seemed to indicate that retention of uric acid, the seemingly obvious basis of tophi, was unrelated to the sudden acute attacks of inflammatory arthritis. Several pieces of evidence supported that view. The onset of acute attacks bore no relation to changes in serum urate levels. Joints severely involved with tophaceous deposits were often free from acute attacks. Despite its almost specific therapeutic effectiveness, colchicine had no demonstrable effect on urate metabolism. During reductions of serum urate levels with uricosuric drugs, attacks of acute gouty arthritis were fairly often exacerbated. Because of these and other observations, major attention was directed toward alternative explanations, such as abnormalities in the metabolism of trace purines.

Within the past few years gouty arthritis has been clearly shown to be inflammatory reaction to microcrystals of sodium urate, mediated by a series of chemical changes accompanying phagocy-

TABLE 1. CLASSIFICATION OF HYPERURICEMIA AND GOUT

I. Metabolic gout — excessive synthesis
  A. Genetic
    1. Hypoxanthine–guanine phosphoribosyltransferase deficiency — Lesch-Nyhan syndrome or incomplete forms
    2. Other defects of rate control
  B. Acquired — excessive tissue turnover
II. Renal gout — reduced clearance
  A. Genetic — ↓ renal tubular secretion?
    1. Idiopathic
    2. Lactic acidosis — glycogen storage disease Type I
  B. Acquired
    1. Inhibition of urate transport — drugs, metabolites (lactic acid, β-hydroxybutyric acid)
    2. Renal failure

tosis of the crystals by leukocytes. The presence of sodium urate microcrystals in synovial fluid from gouty joints during acute inflammation, both free and in leukocytes, is so constant as to be of diagnostic value (Fig. 4). This was the key observation that led to the experiments supporting the early Garrod-Freudweiler concept. The injection of sodium urate microcrystals into joints of normal controls or gouty patients produces typical gout responsive to colchicine. Aspiration of these joints demonstrates phagocytosis of some of the injected crystals. In fact, no experimental gouty arthritis can be produced in laboratory animals in the absence of leukocytes. The inflammatory reaction of microcrystalline synovitis is a non-specific one, being produced by injection of other crystals of appropriate size and shape, such as sodium orotate or calcium pyrophosphate.

The exact mechanism by which sodium urate crystals initiate inflammation has not been established. The crystals can activate Hageman factor, and in this way initiate the chain of events resulting in bradykinin synthesis. Bradykinin levels are raised in synovial fluid from gouty joints, but injection of carboxypeptidase B, which destroys bradykinin, does not prevent experimental gout. The requirement for leukocyte-crystal interaction was noted above. Uric acid has been found to be leukotactic. Phagocytosis of the crystals leads to increased metabolic activity of the leukocyte, release of lysosomal enzymes, and increased

lactic acid production. Although the biochemical events of inflammation are poorly understood, the establishment of the general mechanism of microcrystalline synovitis has allowed a rational explanation of acute gouty arthritis. Still unexplained are the mechanisms by which the acute attack is initiated, i.e., what leads to the presumed burst of microcrystallization at a given time. How are the known precipitating events of acute gouty arthritis, which may be roughly grouped together as stresses, translated into microcrystallization?

The model of leukocyte-crystal interaction may offer an explanation for the action of colchicine. As stated, in the therapeutic range colchicine has no effect on net purine metabolism as reflected in levels of extracellular uric acid or in its excretion. On the other hand, colchicine diminishes leukocyte migration and modifies many of the metabolic concomitants of phagocytosis in the leukocyte. The use of such an in vitro model may allow the rational development of other therapeutic agents in the future.

Clinical Manifestations. As previously stated, the clinical manifestations of gout can be arbitrarily divided into four categories: acute gouty arthritis, tophaceous gout, uric acid nephrolithiasis, and gouty kidney. Although the basic metabolic abnormalities of genetic gout must be presumed to have been present since conception, clinical gout is extraordinarily rare before the rise in extracellular uric acid levels which accompany puberty in the male. Exceptions to this are seen in the juvenile gout of the Lesch-Nyhan syndrome and in glycogen storage disease Type I. Clinical gout usually makes its appearance in middle life in men, although the majority of patients with hyperuricemia never exhibit these complications. As observed by Hippocrates, clinical gout in women rarely occurs before the menopause, at which time there is a further rise in uric acid levels. In most series, gout in women accounts for only 5 to 10 per cent of cases.

The epidemiology of gout and hyperuricemia has received increasing attention beyond the genetic studies of families. The positive statistical correlation of uric acid levels with education, intelligence, and social status was pointed out above. Exceptionally high frequencies of hyperuricemia have been found in Filipinos (in the United States but not in the Philippines), in Maoris, and in the natives of the Marianas Islands. The over-all incidence of clinical gout in the United States has been estimated as 3 patients per 1000 population. As a generality it has been stated that gout makes up about 5 per cent of arthritis.

Acute Gouty Arthritis. Acute gouty arthritis is the most frequent first clinical manifestation of the disease. It has been eloquently described by many who have endured it, but by none more effectively than Sydenham, who wrote "it [the affected part] is not able to bear the weight of the cloths upon it, nor hard walking in the chamber." He further alluded to the pain as being "like the gnawing of a dog." Acute gouty arthritis often follows a precipitating event: surgery, injury,

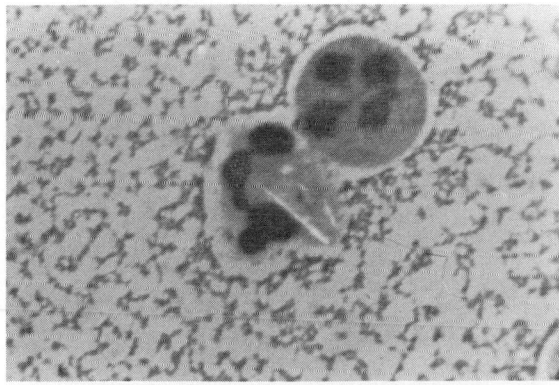
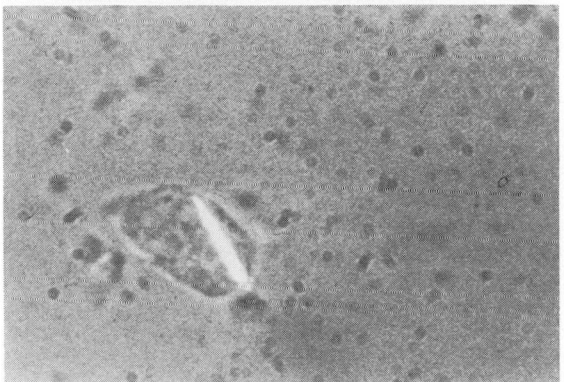

FIGURE 4. Sodium urate monohydrate crystals phagocytized by leukocytes in synovial fluid from acute gouty arthritis examined by polarized light. (Reproduced with permission of Dr. Daniel J. McCarty, Jr.)

alcohol ingestion, dietary excess, emotional stress, or even the minor stress of excessive walking. In view of the current concept of the pathogenesis as that of microcrystalline synovitis, such stress must somehow be translated into localized sodium urate crystallization, or must alter the tissue reaction to such crystals. Since sodium urate usually exists in a supersaturated solution in the gouty patient, the initiating event need introduce only a single crystal focus for seeding a cascade of precipitation. Similarly, a shift in protein binding might affect the concentration of free urate. Some of the precipitating events, such as starvation and alcohol ingestion, increase urate levels by inhibition of renal urate excretion through the accompanying ketosis and lactic acidosis, respectively. The particular association of gout with spirituous liquors, legendary in medieval history ("in the young wine goes to the head; in the aged it goes to the feet"), therefore finds some scientific basis at the level of the renal tubule. A particularly puzzling and important kind of exacerbation of acute gouty arthritis is that which frequently occurs during early stages of treatment designed to lower extracellular urate levels. This may complicate the use of uricosuric agents or of allopurinol, to the great distress of both patient and physician. It has been difficult to explain the exacerbation of gout in the face of a falling urate concentration. It is possible that mobilization of amorphous tophaceous deposits may allow for local precipitation of the microcrystals conducive to inflammation. The frequent occurrence of this complication may occasionally obviate or delay effective treatment.

Gout usually presents as a sudden, exquisitely painful arthritis. After a few premonitory twinges the onset of inflammation may occur within minutes with severe arthritis within a few hours. Typically a patient may retire for the night in good health, yet be awakened a few hours later with excruciating pain in the affected joint. He may develop podagra (gouty arthritis of the first metatarsophalangeal joint) with such rapidity that he is unable to remove his shoe in time. More rarely the warning signals of impending arthritis develop into a crescendo pattern ending in the acute attack.

Gouty arthritis exhibits a marked predilection for the larger joints, particularly in the feet and ankles. Hippocrates described podagra, which still represents the most frequent site of involvement (Fig. 5). This may reflect the trauma of weight-bearing which in the normal foot produces the greatest force per unit area (pressure) there. Other frequent sites of early attacks are the ankle, the instep, or occasionally the knee. Less frequently the elbow, wrist, or metacarpophalangeal joints are the sites of gouty arthritis. The hips, shoulders, and spine are very rarely the sites of microcrystalline synovitis, and almost never the sites of initial involvement. Gouty arthritis is usually monoarticular, especially in the earliest attacks. Some patients may have marked tophaceous gout with bone and articular destruction and few if any attacks of acute gout. Involvement of a joint by tophi does not seem to predispose that area to acute attacks, and some clinicians have even suggested that tophaceous areas enjoy relative immunity from acute inflammation.

Acute gouty arthritis is characterized by severe inflammation, not only in the joint itself but typically in the periarticular tissues and skin. The presence of heat, marked swelling, exquisite tenderness, and rubor extending well beyond the immediate vicinity of the joint capsule has often led to the erroneous diagnosis of septic arthritis or cellulitis. Occasionally lymphangitis may be evident. The skin over the area of inflammation is usually tense and shiny, and often subsidence of the attack undergoes superficial desquamation as is seen in erysipelas. Systemic signs of inflammation may include fever, leukocytosis, and elevation of the sedimentation rate which may further suggest an infectious etiology. The severity

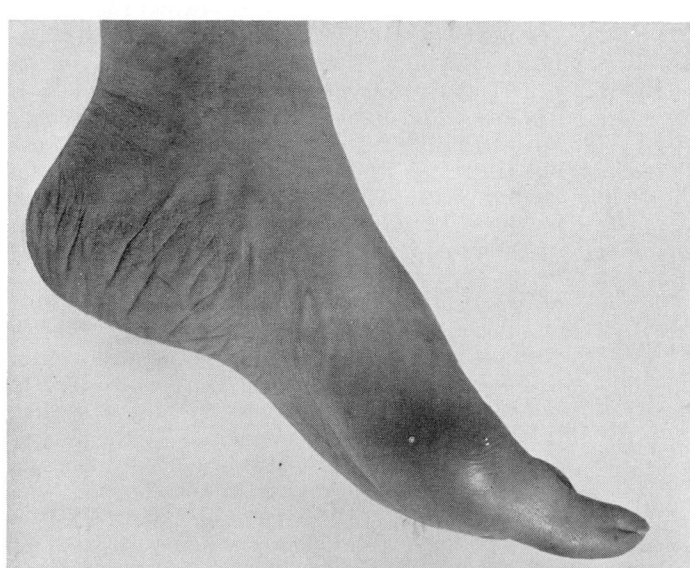

FIGURE 5. Acute gouty arthritis of great toe.

of the associated pain has been referred to above, and commands respect and attention rather than the traditional jocularity. When untreated, an attack of acute gouty arthritis usually subsides gradually over a period of one to two weeks. Generally there are no residual signs or symptoms; more rarely, stiffness persists, or a second flareup supervenes before there is complete recovery.

As stated, only about one of six patients with hyperuricemia will eventually have one or more of the complications of clinical gout. Moreover, the clinical course of gout following an initial attack of acute arthritis is highly variable. Some patients have only a single attack of monoarticular arthritis and then remain free of symptoms despite the persistence of hyperuricemia. More often, after a symptom-free interval, but usually within the first year, there is recurrence of an attack. In Gutman's series, 62 per cent have had recurrences within the first year, 16 per cent in one to two years, 11 per cent in two to five years, 4 per cent in ten years, and 7 per cent, no recurrence as yet during prolonged follow-up. In the usual pattern, subsequent attacks come with increasing frequency over the years unless prophylactic measures are taken, with gradual reduction in the duration of the symptom-free intervals (sometimes called intercritical gout). In about one third of patients, the number of attacks occurring each year has remained constant, and, rarely, there has been a spontaneous decline in frequency with increasing age of the patient. When attacks become more frequent they also tend to become more severe, both in the extent and duration of the inflammation and in the number of joints affected. The patient may reach a state at which he is rarely free of gouty inflammation, and at which even with subsidence of an acute attack there is enough residual swelling, stiffness, and pain in the involved joints to give permanent disability not responsive to the measures usually effective in acute attacks.

Tophaceous Gout. Sodium urate may accumulate in virtually any tissue in the body with the exception of the central nervous system, where the concentration is reduced by the blood-brain barrier. Tophi occur most often in and around joints in cartilage, bone, bursae, and subcutaneous tissue. As foreign bodies, these deposits elicit a low-grade chronic inflammatory process with disruption of tissues and fibrosis. Destruction of tissue is particularly evident in cartilage and bone, leading to radiolucent "punched-out" lesions of bone and gross deformities of joints (Figs. 6 and 7). Deposits of sodium urate may be massive, particularly in the hands and feet and around the olecranon bursa. Subcutaneous deposits may be easily visible as yellowish-white excrescences, which on occasion may erode through the skin and discharge a pale paste composed largely of crystalline needles of sodium urate. In advanced cases, deposits of several hundred grams may lead to grotesquely deformed extremities. Rarely, involvement of the heart has been observed with tophi causing conduction disturbances. A frequent site of tophaceous deposits is the external ear, especially in the helix and anthelix. The local factors that control the sites of crystallization are not known. Massive tophi may be found in the hands, feet, and elbows with none of the typical auricular deposits. Conversely, the external ear may be the only site of visible tophi over many years of the gouty diathesis. As stated above, some recent work suggests that patients most susceptible to tophi may have reduced protein binding of urate. This appealing concept is not yet firmly established.

About one half of all patients with clinical gout have visible tophi at some stage of their disease. Other patients may have more diffuse deposition

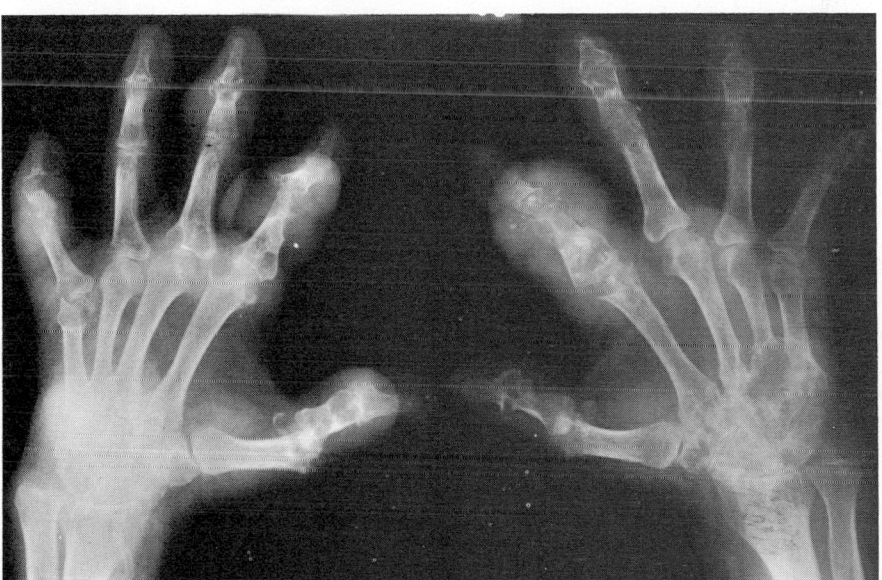

FIGURE 6.   Chronic gouty arthritis with tophaceous destruction of bone and joints.

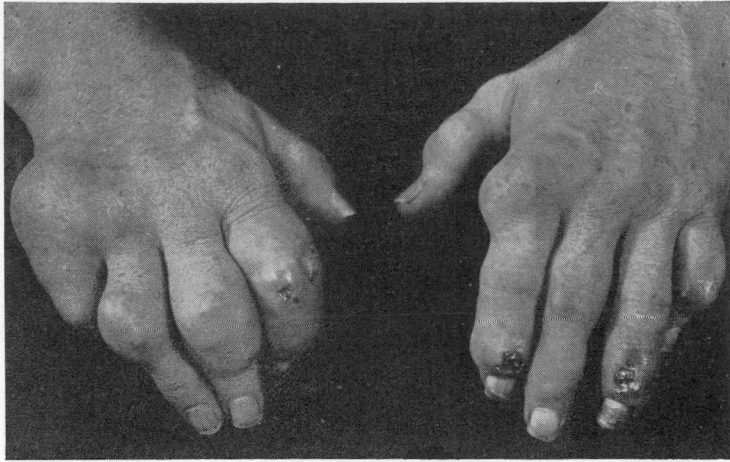

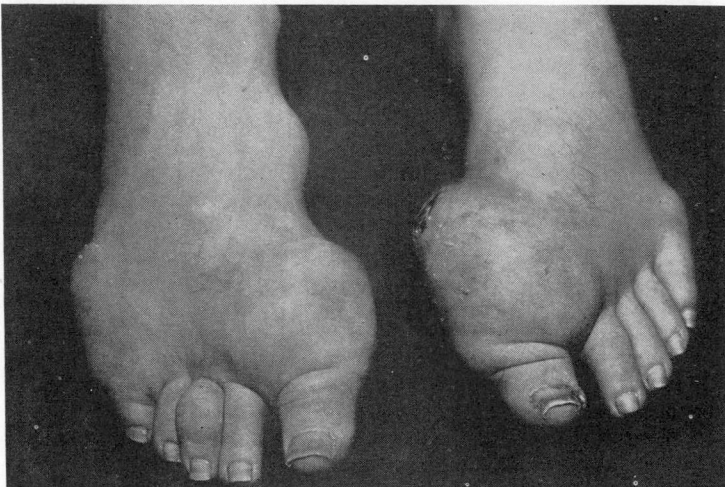

FIGURE 7. Advanced tophaceous gout, with ulcerations.

of sodium urate without local nodules or infiltrates demonstrable by physical or radiologic examination. The destruction and gross distortion of articular structures (cartilage, bone, capsule, synovial membranes) by tophi leads to a form of chronic gouty arthritis which compounds the stiffness, pain, and fibrosis that may follow repeated attacks of acute gouty arthritis. Although symptomatic and objective improvement may occur with proper therapy, this late stage of destructive gout cannot be completely reversed. One of the objectives of modern management is to prevent the excessive accumulation of urate that results in tophaceous destruction and connective tissue reaction.

Uric Acid Nephrolithiasis. Kidney stones are very common. It has been estimated that 1 in every 1000 inhabitants of the United States is hospitalized annually because of a kidney stone. This figure does not include those whose stones remain in situ or are passed without hospitalization. In large series it has been found that 5 to 10 per cent of all kidney stones in adults are composed mainly of uric acid deposits within a protein matrix. Uric acid may serve as the nidus for a stone of mixed composition, in particular in association with calcium oxalate. Pure uric acid stones are radiolucent, being demonstrable only by the use of contrast media. Other radiolucent stones, so-called matrix stones which are predominantly proteinaceous and xanthine stones, are extremely rare.

Most patients with uric acid stones do not have clinical gout. On the other hand, patients with gout are much more likely to have stones. The frequency of stones in primary or genetic gout has been estimated at 15 to 20 per cent, and in secondary overproduction gout (myeloid metaplasia, polycythemia vera, etc.) at 35 to 40 per cent. Stone formation may occur at any stage in the disease, as the first manifestation of gout or as a late complication in the course of crippling arthritis. Stones may be infrequent or, rarely, they may be the main problem, with almost constant uric acid gravel and superimposed episodes of acute renal colic from passage of larger stones.

As noted earlier, the absolute amount of uric acid excreted per 24 hours is only one of the factors conducive to stone formation. A concentrated acidic urine increases the likelihood of stones at any level of uricaciduria. Some investigators have reported that patients with gout, and certain other patients with uric acid stone diathesis, habitually excrete more acid urine. It is postulated that this reflects a shift toward increased titratable acidity rather than ammonia excretion because of a relative defect in renal ammonia production. These data have been both confirmed and denied, perhaps an indication of part of the difficulty in choosing proper controls.

Gouty Renal Disease. A selective defect in urate excretion may be the basic defect in possibly one third of all patients with gout. Extracellular urate rises nonspecifically in all patients with renal insufficiency, uric acid representing one component of nonprotein nitrogen. The onset of renal failure in gout tends to exacerbate the disease, especially the frequency and severity of tophaceous deposits. More generally, renal tubular reabsorption of urate in man, as opposed to other primates, leads to inappropriate urate retention without which there would be no gout. The kidney therefore plays a significant role in the pathogenesis and progression of gout.

Conversely, gout may impair renal function and lead to death in uremia. The so-called gouty kidney represents a variable mixture of factors. Sodium urate may crystallize in the renal interstitial tissue, especially in the pyramids, with tissue destruction and distortion, and a low-grade inflammatory reaction leading to fibrosis. In addition to this primary lesion, uric acid stones lead to obstruction with hydronephrosis and increased susceptibility to chronic pyelonephritis, a complication quite often found in late-stage gouty kidney. Finally, gout, or at least hyperuricemia, carries a statistical association with accelerated vascular disease and hypertension, so that nephrosclerosis may contribute in some measure to impairment of renal function. There are no characteristic clinical or laboratory findings to distinguish gouty kidney from chronic glomerulonephritis except for the association of the former with clinical gout. The question whether gout (i.e., hyperuricemia) ever leads to renal failure in the absence of the other three manifestations of the disease, i.e., arthritis, tophi, and stones, is pertinent to the prophylactic treatment of patients discovered to have essential hyperuricemia (considered here to be gout without complications). Gouty kidney in the absence of these manifestations of clinical gout is extraordinarily rare and even then the entity may be open to question because of variable interpretations of renal pathology. One unusual family has been described in which this syndrome occurred.

A particular form of uric acid nephropathy may be found in the absence of clinical gout. With sudden exceptionally high levels of uric acid excretion, seen almost exclusively after chemotherapeutic or radiation therapy of certain malignant myeloproliferative disorders, crystals may occlude the distal collecting tubules, leading to acute renal failure. These intraluminal crystals are uric acid rather than sodium urate, precipitate in the distal tubule in which maximal concentration and acidification occur, and lead to intranephronic hydronephrosis. This complication is easy to prevent with fluids, alkalinization of the urine, and allopurinol inhibition of urate synthesis. Oliguria, once established, usually follows a course similar to that seen with acute renal failure secondary to shock or to an incompatible blood transfusion.

Diseases Associated with Gout (Table 2). Several diseases have been described in association with gout. In some cases, the relationship seems to be clear pathogenically, as outlined in the classification of gout in Table 1. Some associations have not yet been so explained. Many diseases which lead to continued tissue synthesis and breakdown may produce hyperuricemia and clinical gout because of the resulting increased turnover of nucleic acids and functional nucleotides. This form of secondary or acquired metabolic gout is that seen with polycythemia vera, myeloid metaplasia, chronic leukemia, mast cell disease, extensive psoriasis, and sarcoidosis. The triad of sarcoidosis-psoriasis-gout has been described in a small number of patients, although this may represent the fortuitous coincidence of two quite common diseases, both of which may be productive of secondary gout. Severe gout may be a major complication in surviving patients with glycogen storage disease Type I because of the constant lactic acidosis which inhibits renal tubular urate secretion. Studies with isotopic glycine also suggest excessive synthesis of urate in this disease. It has been suggested that this may result from excessive synthesis of PRPP, one of the substrates for the rate-limiting initial step in purine synthesis catalyzed by glutamine 5-phosphoribosylpyrophosphate amidotransferase. The hyperuricemia of starvation has a similar mechanism in that β-hydroxybutyrate, as one of the ketone bodies, also inhibits renal urate excretion. The association of gout and diabetes mellitus is not a strong one. Three to 5 per cent of patients with gout have diabetes, but this figure is not far from that of the incidence of diabetes in the general population when adjusted for age. Some diabetic patients considered to have atypical gout in the past in fact have pseudogout, as described in this text. Over the last decade several clinics have documented a high incidence of hyperuricemia and clinical gout in patients with primary hyperparathyroidism even in the absence of renal failure. This relationship is obscure because the hyperuricemia has not always responded to successful surgical treatment of the hyperfunctioning parathyroid glands. Hyperuricemia may also be

TABLE 2. DISEASES ASSOCIATED WITH GOUT

1. Myeloproliferative disorders
2. Psoriasis
3. Sarcoidosis
4. Glycogen storage disease Type I (glucose 6-phosphatase deficiency)
5. Diabetes mellitus
6. Hyperparathyroidism
7. Chronic renal disease—glomerulonephritis, pyelonephritis, hereditary nephropathy
8. Lead poisoning

found in hypothyroidism. Renal insufficiency is a common cause of hyperuricemia. It is surprising how rarely this results in clinical gout in view of the high concentrations of uric acid which may be found. It may be that hyperuricemia in uremia does not have sufficient duration, i.e., time at risk, to result in a high incidence of sodium urate precipitation. Uremia may also interfere in some way with the crystallization potential of sodium urate, as it does for bone salts in osteoid, or diminish the inflammatory response to such crystals when they occur. Garrod commented upon the association of lead poisoning and gout in his treatise of 1876, and this has been repeatedly confirmed in subsequent reports. Saturnine gout, as it has been called, occurs late in the course of chronic plumbism. The mechanism has not been established but it has been supposed that enhanced breakdown of tissue, including the erythropoietic series, is the origin of excessive urate synthesis in lead poisoning. Hyperuricemia has also been described in Down's syndrome and in nephrogenic diabetes insipidus.

Pseudogout. The syndrome of pseudogout, also called *chondrocalcinosis articularis,* is considered as a separate entity elsewhere in this volume.

Hypoxanthine-Guanine Phosphoribosyltransferase (HG-PRT) Deficiency. The X-linked genetic disease HG-PRT deficiency is the only form of gout associated with overproduction of urate for which a specific enzymatic defect has been clearly established. It is important beyond its relative infrequency, because (1) the enzymatic defect can be demonstrated as a cause of excessive purine synthesis; (2) the mechanism of genetic transmission is known, in contrast to other forms of gout except for glycogen storage disease Type I; and (3) in its complete form it produces a distinct clinical picture with neurologic abnormalities: the Lesch-Nyhan syndrome.

In 1964, Lesch and Nyhan described a distinctive syndrome characterized by mental retardation, choreoathetosis, spasticity, weakness, and compulsive self-mutilation. Patients with this syndrome generally appear normal at birth but show evidence of neurologic deficits and retarded mental development within the first few months of life. Bizarre self-mutilation of extremities, lips, and other oral structures may require constant restraint of the patient, despite the evident pain which accompanies this uncontrollable self-destructive process (Fig. 8). These patients often develop uric acid stones and gouty nephropathy which may lead to death in uremia. In contrast, gouty arthritis rarely occurs despite very high levels of extracellular urate. The severity of the neurologic damage usually leads to institutionalization, and most patients with the Lesch-Nyhan syndrome die in childhood, although a few survive to early adult life. Some of the patients have had a megaloblastic anemia resistant to the usual hematinic agents. The enzyme HG-PRT is coded on the X chromosome and the disease is transmitted as an X-linked recessive with no clinical phenotypic expression in hemizygous females. As predicted in the Lyon hypothesis, mothers of children with the Lesch-Nyhan syndrome can be shown by tissue culture of their fibroblasts to exhibit mosaicism, with one cell population deficient in HG-PRT and one in which there is normal enzymatic activity.

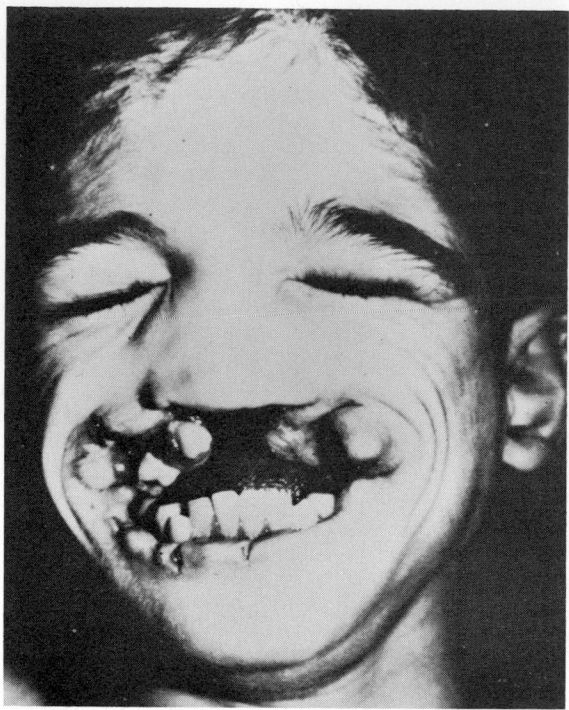

FIGURE 8.   Self-mutilation in a patient with the Lesch-Nyhan syndrome. (From Nyhan, W. L.: Fed. Proc., 27:1027, 1968.)

The Lesch-Nyhan syndrome as defined above represents one end of the clinical spectrum associated with HG-PRT deficiency. There are some patients who have some incomplete deficiency of HG-PRT with severe clinical gout, marked by excessive synthesis of urate, but without the characteristic mental and neurologic derangements. A minority of these patients have exhibited some neurologic abnormalities: mild spastic quadriplegia, cerebellar ataxia, dysarthria, and seizures. This group of patients, like those with the Lesch-Nyhan syndrome, have been particularly susceptible to uric acid stones as a consequence of the excessive uricaciduria. As might be anticipated, genetic transmission of partial HG-PRT deficiency resembles that of the Lesch-Nyhan syndrome, with relative constancy of phenotypic expression within a given family.

In the catabolism of purine nucleotides, free bases are released as adenine, guanine, and hypoxanthine. In part these undergo deamination and further oxidation to uric acid via hypoxanthine and xanthine, these oxidations being catalyzed by xanthine oxidase. In part, the free bases are reutilized, being coupled with PRPP to form purine nucleotides, a process sometimes described as "salvage synthesis" to distinguish it from de novo synthesis from simple precursors (Fig. 9). To the

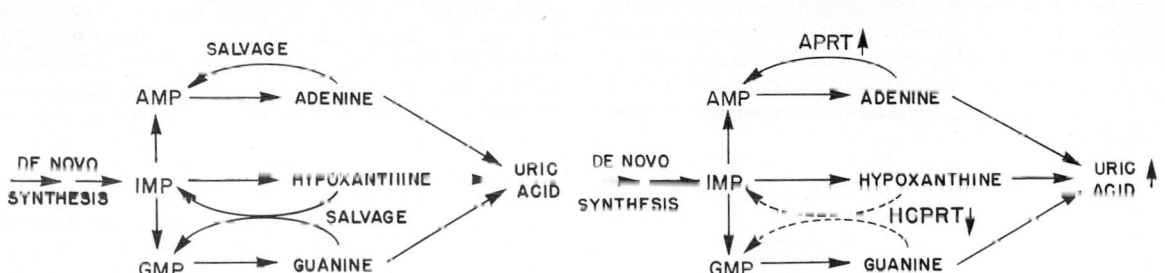

FIGURE 9. Pathways for salvage synthesis of purine nucleotides from free purine bases in normal subjects (left) and in the metabolic abnormality of hypoxanthine-guanine phosphoribosyltransferase (HG-PRT) deficiency (right). APRT, adenine phosphoribosyltransferase.

extent that salvage synthesis preserves the purine bases, the requirement for de novo synthesis is reduced, and at equilibrium urate synthesis and excretion are correspondingly reduced. One enzyme, HG-PRT, catalyzes the salvage synthesis of inosine-5'-phosphate and guanosine-5'-phosphate from hypoxanthine and guanine, respectively. A separate enzyme, A-PRT, catalyzes the synthesis of adenosine-5'-phosphate from adenine (and PRPP). The Lesch-Nyhan syndrome is secondary to a selective, almost complete deficiency of HG-PRT, the activity of adenine PRT being normal, or, more often, significantly increased. The defect, most conveniently shown in hemolysates of erythrocytes, has also been found in fibroblasts and brain. The enzyme activity is normally found in highest concentration in the basal ganglia, a major site of neurologic deficit in the Lesch-Nyhan syndrome. In HG-PRT deficiency, tissue levels of PRPP are increased. Uric acid synthesis is massively increased, with urinary excretion in the range of 50 mg. per kilogram per 24 hours (normal being about 6). Patients with partial deficiency of HG-PRT also have severe overproduction gout, with levels of uric acid excretion intermediate in amount between the normal range and those found in the Lesch-Nyhan syndrome (about 20 to 25 mg. per kilogram per 24 hours). This excessive purine synthesis probably results from inadequate allosteric inhibition of phosphoribosylamidotransferase, the rate-limiting first step in the biosynthetic sequence, because of reduced tissue levels of guanosine-5'-phosphate and inosine-5'-phosphate. The mechanism of neurologic injury has not been established. It may represent localized purine starvation owing to the inability of de novo synthesis to keep pace with the demands generated by failure of salvage synthesis. It is also possible that the resulting high levels of oxypurines (hypoxanthine and xanthine) in the central nervous system are injurious.

The diagnosis of the Lesch-Nyhan syndrome offers no difficulties when the typical neurologic and mental deficits are combined in a male with marked hyperuricemia, and in particular with grossly abnormal uricaciduria. Partial HG-PRT deficiency may be suspected in a male patient with severe gout, possibly with minor neurologic abnormalities, who excretes uric acid in an amount

greater than 0.75 times that of creatinine. The final diagnosis can best be made by enzymatic assay of a hemolysate preparation, preferably sent to one of the laboratories engaged in research on purine metabolism. Therapy is ineffective in preventing or reversing neurologic damage, but may reduce the complications directly related to urate accumulation and excretion, as described below.

Diagnosis. The diagnosis of acute gouty arthritis rarely offers difficulties when there is sudden onset of typical inflammatory involvement of a susceptible joint in a patient with hyperuricemia. Rarely, the serum uric acid concentration may be within the upper range of normal at the time of measurement (Fig. 1), or the arthritis may be atypical in its location or persistence. Rapid response of the pain and inflammation after administration of colchicine is so characteristic as to be of diagnostic usefulness. Some response of rheumatoid arthritis or sarcoid arthritis has been described with colchicine, but the effects are not so dramatic as those in gout. Demonstration of the typical needle-shaped birefringent crystals of sodium urate in leukocytes of synovial fluid is diagnostic of gout. With proper technique, intraleukocytic sodium urate crystals are found in over 95 per cent of aspirates from joints affected by acute gout (Fig. 4). Positive identification of the crystals may be achieved by incubation of the synovial fluid preparation with uricase. The particular characteristics of pseudogout or *chondrocalcinosis articularis* are described elsewhere in this text, as are the spectrum of disorders associated with hypoxanthine–guanine phosphoribosyltransferase deficiency. Occasionally, gout may simulate infectious arthritis or be confused with monarticular rheumatoid arthritis. Examination of the joint fluid measurement of serum uric acid, and response to colchicine should suffice to establish the diagnosis.

A classification of types of gout according to pathogenesis has been outlined in Table 1. It is clearly important to determine whether gout is secondary to a myeloproliferative disorder, renal failure, or drug or metabolite interference with renal tubular secretion of urate. In the study of the average patient with idiopathic gout, in the absence of the aforementioned disorders, it is not necessary to establish whether the disease is metabolic (overproduction) gout or renal (underexcretion) gout in order to institute proper treatment. In the absence of clear cut hyperuricaciduria on a low purine diet, this further classification is still a laborious procedure requiring isotopic studies.

Treatment. Genetic gout cannot be cured, but its phenotypic expression can usually be modified and progression of its clinical complications controlled or reversed. The therapeutic program differs according to the complications present. Generally, in the majority of patients, the treatment of gout is now quite adequate with the introduction of potent uricosuric drugs and allopurinol, and more skilled use of colchicine as a prophylactic agent. The purpose of every therapeutic program is to prevent the complications of gout or, failing complete prophylaxis, to treat each complication specifically when it occurs.

Acute Gouty Arthritis. Although acute gouty arthritis is self-limited in duration, the severity of the pain and the persistence of the untreated inflammatory process over one to two weeks call for early intervention. The earlier the onset of treatment, the more likely a rapid response. The affected joint should be placed at rest. Usually the degree of pain will demand this, and on occasion specific medication, i.e., a narcotic, for pain may be required. Four types of drugs have been utilized with repeated success in the treatment of acute gout: colchicine; phenylbutazone, indomethacin, and glucocorticoids (or ACTH).

Colchicine remains the most widely used and specific agent for the treatment of acute gout. A number of regimens can be used. It is recommended that an initial dose of 1.0 mg. be given orally, followed by 0.5 mg. every hour until the relief of pain or the onset of diarrhea. These responses often occur more or less spontaneously. No more than 6.0 mg. of colchicine should be given for an acute attack; no more than that should be given over a 72-hour period. Colchicine may also be given intravenously (2.0 mg. given in 20 ml. of saline over a ten-minute period) instead of orally, with less gastrointestinal reaction, and repeated if necessary after an interval of four to six hours. Not more than 5.0 mg. should be administered intravenously within a 24-hour period. Diarrhea is the most frequent complication of colchicine therapy and often requires treatment, e.g., paregoric, for rapid relief. Colchicine is excreted by the kidney and should be used cautiously in uremia. Large amounts of colchicine may cause transient leukopenia. The probable mechanism of action of colchicine has been discussed earlier.

Phenylbutazone (Butazolidin) or *oxyphenbutazone* (Tandearil) may be used as alternate antiinflammatory agents for the successful treatment of most patients with acute gout. Phenylbutazone is given in a dose of 200 mg. four times a day for two days, with rapid tapering to discontinuation over the following two days. With such brief therapeutic periods, toxicity is minimized. *Indomethacin* (Indocin) may be given in amounts of 50 mg. three times daily with early resolution of an acute attack, but it is less frequently effective than colchicine or phenylbutazone. Glucocorticoid (or ACTH) therapy is not recommended because of variability in response and the high incidence of rebound arthritis after its discontinuation.

When effective treatment has been given, improvement in symptoms usually begins within 6 to 12 hours, with virtually complete remission within 24 to 48 hours. In about 5 to 10 per cent of patients, no rapid relief is obtained, especially if treatment is begun late in the course, and the resolution of the inflammatory arthritis is more gradual. The use of uricosuric agents is not indicated in the management of acute gout.

One of the purposes of therapy is to prevent acute attacks of arthritis. By experience, patients may become aware of stressful experiences or dietary or alcoholic excesses which precipitate attacks, and in this way be able to avoid them. The proper use of uricosuric agents or allopurinol will lower urate levels below the saturation concentration over time, and in this way help to prevent the crystallization which precedes attacks. The short-term effect of such treatment, however, usually leads to exacerbation of gouty arthritis during periods of mobilization of urate deposits. Gutman (1955) has established the usefulness of daily colchicine (0.5 mg. once or twice a day) as a simple measure to prevent acute attacks in patients subject to recurrent arthritis. Colchicine prophylaxis is not recommended for patients with a single attack (which may never recur) but should be instituted for all patients with frequent attacks of arthritis. Finally, the importance of aborting acute attacks by the use of colchicine during the earliest premonitory symptoms should be stressed.

Tophaceous Gout. There are two ways to remove or reduce the size of tophi: surgical removal or redissolving sodium urate crystals. In extracellular fluid, sodium urate crystals can be dissolved only by lowering urate below the saturation level (approximately 7 mg. per 100 ml., assuming normal protein binding). The rate of redissolving sodium urate bears a direct relationship to the degree of unsaturation achieved, although it may be modified by blood supply, fibrosis, and the area of crystal surface exposed. Two methods are in general use to lower urate levels: the use of uricosuric drugs to increase renal clearance, and the use of allopurinol to inhibit urate synthesis. Dietary restriction may help to reduce urate synthesis from performed purines, but with the advent of the aforementioned methods of treatment it has become less important. In theory, an ideal approach to treatment would be to increase urate excretion into the gut (normally one fourth to one third of that synthesized) for bacterial uricolysis. No agent has yet been found which selectively increases gut excretion of urate.

Two uricosuric agents are most often employed, *probenecid* (Benemid) or *sulfinpyrazone* (Anturane). Either of these drugs should be started in small amounts with forced fluids and mild alkalinization of the urine (if no contraindications exist), in order to prevent uric acid stone formation. If the patient has been subject to acute arthritis, prophylactic colchicine should be administered simultaneously to anticipate the exacerbation of gouty arthritis during the early phases of uricosuric therapy. Probenecid should be started at a dose of 0.25 gram twice daily, gradually increasing over a two-week period to a maintenance dose of 0.5 gram two or three times daily. A few patients, particularly those with reduction in renal function, may require 2.5 to 3.0 grams daily in order to reduce serum urate to satisfactory levels, preferably lower than 6.0 mg. per 100 ml. Sulfinpyrazone may be used as an alternate in beginning doses of 50 mg. twice daily, gradually increasing to a maintenance dose of 100 mg. three to four times daily. Exceptionally, sulfinpyrazone may be required in doses of 200 mg. four times daily for effective uricosuria. In general, both drugs are well tolerated. The most frequently reported reactions are those of gastrointestinal intolerance and drug-induced dermatitis. Very rarely, marrow suppression and hepatic necrosis have been reported. Although uricosuric in large doses, salicylates should not be used in the treatment of gout. At usual therapeutic levels they may primarily inhibit renal tubular secretion of urate and therefore be uricoretentive.

The availability of *allopurinol* (Zyloprim) has introduced a new approach to the treatment of gout. This analogue of hypoxanthine and its oxidation product allo-xanthine competitively inhibit xanthine oxidase, and in this way reduce the oxidation of hypoxanthine to xanthine and of xanthine to uric acid (Fig. 2). The human kidney clears hypoxanthine and xanthine much more efficiently than uric acid, so that their extracellular fluid concentrations do not rise commensurately with the fall in urate. The total amount of purine bases excreted is generally somewhat reduced, owing probably to increased reutilization of the oxypurines for salvage synthesis of nucleotides. Furthermore, the more equitable distribution of purines excreted among the three metabolites reduces the tendency toward urinary saturation by either xanthine or uric acid (hypoxanthine being highly soluble). Allopurinol is usually given in divided doses of 300 to 800 mg. per day. As in the case of uricosuric drugs, its use may initially increase the number of acute attacks of gouty arthritis unless colchicine prophylaxis is used. The pharmacologic production of xanthinuria, an analogue of the genetic disorder, has not yet resulted in difficulties from xanthine stone formation except in two patients with the Lesch-Nyhan syndrome. The nucleotide of allopurinol is formed in vivo, and inhibits the enzyme orotidylic decarboxylase with secondary orotic aciduria and orotidinuria. This partial inhibition of pyrimidine synthesis has not been shown to be adverse, and no incorporation of allopurinol nucleotide into nucleic acid as a possible mutagenic agent has been found. Toxic effects of allopurinol are rare (3 to 5 per cent of patients), and consist of dermatitis, fever, headache, diarrhea, transitory leukopenia,

and elevation of serum transaminase enzymes of hepatic origin.

The availability of two general methods of treatment allows choice in the management of tophaceous gout or marked hyperuricemia productive of acute gout. It is recommended that uricosuric agents be given an initial trial in treatment, allopurinol being withheld for more specific indications. Probenecid has been widely used for over 20 years, whereas the use of allopurinol, although the known toxic effects are few and rarely severe, represents the introduction of a foreign purine base and nucleotide with which there has been extensive experience for only five or six years. Allopurinol is definitely indicated for certain patients: when uricosuric treatment proves ineffective in lowering the extracellular urate level sufficiently (to < 6 mg. per 100 ml.); when there are toxic reactions to uricosuric drugs; when tophaceous gout is particularly severe (which often accompanies some degree of renal functional impairment and poor response to uricosuric agents); or when there have been recurrent uric acid stones. In general, the allopurinol regimen is more effective in rapidly lowering urate levels without the added hazard of passing extra uric acid through the kidney and urinary tract. The resistance to use of allopurinol as the primary agent for lowering extracellular urate is diminishing as further experience has not yet documented late toxicity. Although a uricosuric drug may be used in conjunction with allopurinol, this is not usually wise because probenecid may increase urinary excretion of allopurinol and allo-xanthine, making it less effective, and may also decrease the excretion of the oxypurines. Combined treatment has been used successfully for patients with severe tophaceous gout with good renal function when neither drug alone has sufficed to lower urate levels adequately.

With prolonged treatment, remarkable reversal of tophaceous gout may be obtained. Treatment should then be continued for life to prevent recurrence of hyperuricemia and its complications.

Gouty Kidney. There is no specific way to treat gouty kidney when renal failure has occurred. There is rarely any evidence of improvement in renal function when urate values are reduced enough to mobilize tophaceous deposits. Treatment is limited to control of pyelonephritis if it exists, prevention of further stone formation, lowering extracellular urate levels by the methods previously described in order to prevent further injury, treatment of hypertension to modify the progress of nephrosclerosis, and the general metabolic measures used to treat any patient with diminished renal function. With early diagnosis and treatment, renal failure is becoming a much rarer complication of gout. With uremia, the dose of allopurinol used should be lower.

A particular form of gouty kidney, acute tubular blockade by uric acid with oliguria or anuria, can be prevented in patients being treated with cytotoxic agents by the use of fluids, alkalinization of the urine, and, in particular, full doses of allopurinol *before* the treatment of the myeloproliferative disorder. If anuria occurs, the usual measures for the treatment of acute renal failure should be instituted in anticipation of tubular regeneration over a 10 to 14 day period.

Uric Acid Stones. As previously described, the tendency to form uric acid stones is a function of the concentration of free uric acid, as opposed to sodium urate, in urine. Preventive measures attempt to reduce uric acid concentration by increasing urine volume (forcing of fluids, particularly at night), increasing urine pH (administration of sodium citrate or bicarbonate to maintain urine pH>6), or reducing urate excretion (allopurinol). In most patients, fluids and mild alkalinization suffice to prevent uric acid stones. When uricaciduria is marked, when excess sodium is contraindicated, or when these measures are not successful, the use of allopurinol offers a specific method for the prevention of uric acid stones. As stated, the theoretical possibility of substituting xanthine stones for uric acid stones exists, but this complication has so far occurred only in the Lesch-Nyhan syndrome.

Essential Hyperuricemia. In this article, essential hyperuricemia is considered to be gout without complications. The incidental discovery of elevated serum urate values in the absence of any of the clinical manifestations of gout has increased with the broader use of screening laboratory determinations. One of the most vexing problems facing the physician is whether asymptomatic hyperuricemia should be treated. There are few firm data on which to base a decision. Although hyperuricemia is associated epidemiologically with hyperlipidemia, hypertension, obesity, glucose intolerance, and accelerated vascular disease, there is no evidence that it is primary in any of these derangements, or that lowering uric acid levels affects their course. Similarly, gout may lead to renal failure, but documentation of gouty kidney in the absence of other clinical manifestations is exceedingly rare. Finally, only a minority of patients develop complications of gout despite a lifetime of hyperuricemia in the postpubertal period, although the incidence of complications is roughly proportional to the degree of sodium urate supersaturation in extracellular fluid. Because of these uncertainties, it does not seem justified to start therapy for life in essential hyperuricemia. On the other hand, when serum uric acid values are consistently above 9.0 mg. per 100 ml., the degree of supersaturation is such that the incidence of complications is perhaps 90 per cent. It would seem reasonable to treat such patients with uricosuric agents, or allopurinol, in order to maintain safer uric acid levels.

Garrod, A. B.: A Treatise on Gout and Rheumatic Gout. 3rd ed. London, Longmans, Green & Co., Ltd., 1876.

Gutman, A. B., and Yü Ts'ai-Fan.: Uric acid nephrolithiasis. Amer. J. Med., 45:756, 1968.

Kelley, W. N., Greene, M. L., Rosenbloom, F. M., Henderson, J. F., and Seegmiller, J. E.: Hypoxanthine–guanine phosphoribosyltransferase deficiency in gout. Ann. Intern. Med., 70: 155, 1969.

Seegmiller, J. E.: Diseases of purine and pyrimidine metabolism. *In* Bondy, P. K. (ed.): Duncan's Diseases of Metabolism. 6th ed. Philadelphia, W. B. Saunders Company, 1969, p. 516.

Wyngaarden, J. B.: Gout. *In* Stanbury, J. B., Wyngaarden, J. B., and Fredrickson, D. S. (eds.): The Metabolic Basis of Inherited Disease. 3rd ed. New York, McGraw-Hill Book Co. (in press).

XANTHINURIA

Xanthinuria is a rare genetic disorder secondary to deficiency of xanthine oxidase. Only nine cases have been described, and some of these have not been fully investigated. It is probably transmitted as an autosomal recessive trait, although this has not been firmly established and there is no method now available for detection of heterozygotes. Deficient activity of xanthine oxidase has been demonstrated in liver and gut mucosa in xanthinuria. The normal function of this enzyme is to catalyze the oxidation of hypoxanthine to xanthine and of xanthine to uric acid.

Most patients with xanthinuria have been asymptomatic, being discovered in the investigation of hypouricemia (serum urate <1 mg. per 100 ml.). Three of the nine patients had xanthine kidney stones, which resemble uric acid stones in their radiolucency. Two of the patients had muscle cramps, made worse by exercise, and were found on muscle biopsy to have intracellular crystals thought to be *xanthine* and *hypoxanthine*. Although one patient with xanthinuria had hemochromatosis, no other patients have shown abnormal avidity for iron absorption.

The diagnosis is established by hypouricemia and hypouricaciduria with increased excretion of hypoxanthine and xanthine. In xanthinuria these oxypurines are usually excreted in amounts somewhat less than the normal value for uric acid. Hypoxanthine is partially reutilized to form inosine-5'-phosphate, a reaction catalyzed by hypoxanthine guanine phosphoribosyltransferase, the enzyme which is deficient in the Lesch-Nyhan syndrome. Xanthinuria is simulated pharmacologically by the use of allopurinol which is a competitive inhibitor of, as well as a substrate for, xanthine oxidase. (See article on Gout.) The use of allopurinol has not yet resulted in xanthine kidney stones. Hypouricemia may also occur in proximal renal tubular disease (Fanconi syndrome, Wilson's disease) and during treatment with uricosuric agents. It has been described in one person who had an isolated defect in renal tubular reabsorption of urate (clearance of urate 1.3 times creatinine clearance), similar to that found in the Dalmatian coach hound and in primates other than man. Probably a few patients have had xanthine stones or mixed stones containing xanthine as one component in the absence of the genetic disease. The solubility of hypoxanthine prevents its precipitation in the urinary tract.

Treatment is usually not required. A program for the prevention of xanthine stones would be similar to that for uric acid stones, i.e., forcing fluids, alkalinization of the urine (to enhance solubility), and possibly a low purine diet if the above does not suffice. Despite the very low levels of xanthine oxidase, studies on a single patient suggest that allopurinol might increase the amount of oxypurine excreted as the more soluble hypoxanthine.

Engelman, K., Watts, R. W. E., Klinenberg, J. R., Sjoerdsma, A., and Seegmiller, J. E.: Clinical, physiological and biochemical studies of a patient with xanthinuria and pheochromocytoma. Amer. J. Med., 37:839, 1964.

Seegmiller, J. E.: Xanthine stone formation. Amer. J. Med., 45:780, 1968.

Seegmiller, J. E.: Hereditary xanthinuria. *In* Bondy, P. K. (ed.): Duncan's Diseases of Metabolism, 6th ed. Philadelphia, W. B. Saunders Company, 1969, p. 581.

MISCELLANEOUS HEREDITARY DISORDERS AFFECTING MULTIPLE ORGAN SYSTEMS

ALBINISM
(Oculocutaneous Albinism)
Alexander G. Bearn

Albinism is an autosomal recessively inherited disorder of melanin metabolism. It is characterized by a decrease of melanin in the skin, hair, and eyes, and is due to a failure of melanocytes to produce normal melanin. The biochemical block is not known precisely, but is probably related to defective synthesis of tyrosinase. Several independent genetic defects in tyrosine metabolism could theoretically lead to the same phenotypic effect. The existence of genetic heterogeneity is supported by the observation that, exceptionally, marriages between albinos have resulted in normally pigmented offspring. Albinism is not uncommon and occurs in all races with a frequency of about 1 in 10,000, with a carrier frequency for the abnormal gene of 1 in 50.

In Caucasians the skin is usually milk white, whereas the skin of the albino Negro is usually slightly darker than that of normal tanned Caucasians. Patients with albinism are sensitive to sunlight, and those who have been excessively exposed frequently develop precancerous keratoses. The hair of both Caucasians and Negroes is white; in the former the texture of the hair is usually fine, whereas that of the albino Negro is normal. Photophobia and defects in visual acuity are common. Horizontal nystagmus is almost invariable. The ocular fundus of albinos is bright orange-red, and the vessels are prominent.

The defect in *partial albinism* (*cutaneous albinism, piebald trait*) is limited to the skin and hair. The condition is inherited in a dominant fashion.

Ocular albinism is a very rare variety of albinism in which the defect in pigmentation is restricted to the eyes. Nystagmus, head-nodding, and defective vision also occur. It is probably inherited as an X-linked recessive trait.

Albinism must be distinguished from Chediak-Higashi syndrome, cutaneous albinism, Waardenburg's syndrome (albinism and cochlear deafness), and idiopathic vitiligo.

Fitzpatrick, T. B., and Quevedo, W. C.: Albinism. *In* Stanbury, J. B., Wyngaarden, J. B., and Frederickson, D. S. (eds.): The Metabolic Basis of Inherited Disease. 3rd ed. New York, McGraw-Hill Book Company (In press).

CHÉDIAK-HIGASHI SYNDROME
(Hereditary Leukomelanopathy)
Alexander G. Bearn

This rare, uniformly fatal, autosomal recessively inherited syndrome is characterized by decreased pigmentation of the skin, eyes, and hair, photophobia, shifting nystagmus on exposure to light, and cytoplasmic inclusions of the leukocytes. The cytoplasm of all the cells in the leukocytic series contains abnormally large peroxidase-positive lysosomal granules. Large eosinophilic inclusion bodies in myeloblasts and promyelocytes are found in the bone marrow, and enlarged melanin granules are frequently present in skin melanocytes. Histiocytic infiltration of the brain and other tissues has been reported in several cases.

Children with this syndrome show a markedly increased susceptibility to infections which is not due to a deficient production of antibodies. Indeed, most patients with this syndrome succumb to overwhelming bacterial infections; malignant lymphoma or leukemia may develop during the course of the disease. Survival beyond the first decade of life is extremely rare. Hepatosplenomegaly, anemia, leukopenia, and thrombocytopenia are common complications of the terminal stages of the disease. The presence of oculocutaneous albinism is a reminder that all patients with *albinism* should be examined for the presence of abnormal leukocytic granulations (see Albinism). A similar syndrome has been reported in Hereford cattle and mink.

Kritzler, R. A., Terner, J. Y., Lindenbaum, J., Magidson, J., Williams, R., Preisig, R., and Phillips, G. B.: Chédiak-Higashi syndrome. Cytologic and serum lipid observations in a case and family. Amer. J. Med., 36:583, 1964.
White, J. G.: The Chédiak-Higashi syndrome. A possible lysosomal disease. Blood, 28:143, 1966.

ACATALASIA
Alexander G. Bearn

Acatalasia is a rare, autosomal recessively inherited trait characterized by a deficiency of the enzyme catalase in many tissues of the body, including the erythrocytes, bone marrow, liver, and skin. The disease is common among Japanese and Korean populations, but has also been reported from Switzerland and Israel. Approximately 50 per cent of acatalasic subjects are asymptomatic. Symptoms are usually restricted to the oral cavity and are related to the increased susceptibility to tissue damage by normal oral flora. Oral sepsis may lead to severe gangrenous lesions, including alveolar destruction. When hydrogen peroxide is added, acatalasic blood turns a brownish black color owing to the formation of methemoglobin; by contrast normal blood bubbles vigorously and remains pink. An absence of catalase in individuals homozygous for the trait and intermediate values for catalase for the clinically normal heterozygous carriers of the trait are characteristic of the families reported from Japan, whereas those reported from Switzerland and Israel commonly show residual catalase activity. In some kindreds the heterozygote values for catalase may overlap with the normal. At least two forms of acatalasia exist in Japan where more than 50 patients with the disease have been reported. Genetic heterogeneity is also suggested from the variations in the clinical and biochemical expression of the disease in different populations. The estimated frequency of the disease in Japan is approximately 2 in 100,000, and the heterozygote frequency is 6 in 10,000. Variations in the gene frequency within Japan have been reported. Local surgical excision, extraction of teeth, and antimicrobial therapy have been employed. A similar disease occurs in mice, guinea pigs, dogs, and domestic fowl.

Aebi, H., Baggiolini, M., Dewald, B., Lauber, E., Sutter, H., Micheli, A., and Frei, J.: Observations in two Swiss families with acatalasia. Enzym. Biol. Clin. (Basel), 2:1, 1962.
Hamilton, H. B., and Neel, J. V.: Genetic heterogeneity in human acatalasia. Amer. J. Hum. Genet., 15:408, 1963.
Wyngaarden, J. B., and Howell, R. R.: Acatalasia. In Stanbury, J. B., Wyngaarden, J. B., and Frederickson, D. S. (eds.): The Metabolic Basis of Inherited Disease. 3rd ed. New York, McGraw-Hill Book Company (In press).

METHEMOGLOBINEMIA AND SULFHEMOGLOBINEMIA

Ernst R. Jaffe

METHEMOGLOBINEMIA

Definition. Methemoglobinemia occurs when the concentration of methemoglobin within circulating erythrocytes is increased above the normal level of about 1 per cent. Since the abnormal pigment is intracellular, methemoglobinemia is perhaps a misnomer, but methe-

moglobincythemia and methemoglobinia are too clumsy, and convention dictates the use of the former term. Methemoglobin (ferrihemoglobin, hemiglobin, ferric protoporphyrin IX-globin) is hemoglobin in which the ferrous (reduced) iron of the heme moiety is in the ferric (oxidized) state. Because of the additional positive charge, the sixth coordination position of iron is no longer available to bind molecular oxygen reversibly, but is occupied by water or forms complexes with anionic ligands such as cyanide.

Etiology and Pathogenesis. The intracellular environment of hemoglobin is such that some oxidation of heme iron might be expected. Although the intrinsic structure of hemoglobin shields the iron against oxidation, metabolic processes are also normally active to protect hemoglobin against oxidation or irreversible denaturation and to reduce any methemoglobin which is formed to hemoglobin. An increase in the concentration of methemoglobin above the normal level can result from (1) the presence of a hemoglobin with an abnormal structure that makes it more susceptible to oxidation and/or unsuitable for reduction, (2) deficiency in the ability to reduce methemoglobin, and (3) exposure to drugs or chemicals which increase the rate of oxidation beyond the protective and reductive capacities of the cell. Whereas the first two mechanisms are associated with inherited disorders, the latter occurs in toxic or acquired methemoglobinemia.

Hereditary Methemoglobinemia Due to an Abnormal Hemoglobin (Hemoglobin M; See Section on Hemoglobinopathies). Substitution of tyrosine for histidine occurs at or across from the heme-binding site in the α chains of hemoglobin M Iwate and M Boston and in the β chains of hemoglobin M Hyde Park and M Saskatoon. Glutamic acid replaces valine in the β chain of hemoglobin M Milwaukee-1 one helical turn away from, but still facing, the heme iron. These alterations in the primary structure of hemoglobin increase the tendency of the heme iron to be oxidized and/or stabilize the methemoglobin form so that the normal mechanism for the reduction of methemoglobin is ineffective. Thus, the methemoglobinemia does not respond significantly to conventional therapy (*vide infra*). As with other abnormal hemoglobins, hemoglobin M is transmitted as a codominant characteristic. Only heterozygotes for hemoglobin M have been identified, presumably because the homozygous state would be incompatible with life. Because only one pair of chains (either α or β) of a hemoglobin M is affected, and in the oxidized state, the concentration of methemoglobin does not exceed 25 to 30 per cent. Since α chains are already present in large amounts at birth, M hemoglobins with α chain substitutions are usually apparent immediately, whereas β chain abnormalities are often not manifest until later.

Hereditary Methemoglobinemia Due to a Deficiency in the Ability to Reduce Methemoglobin. The reduction of methemoglobin in human erythrocytes depends, primarily, on the activity of a reduced nicotinamide adenine dinucleotide (NADH or DPNH)-dependent methemoglobin reductase system. This system utilizes NADH generated by glyceraldehyde-3-phosphate dehydrogenase in the Embden-Meyerhof pathway of glycolysis to reduce methemoglobin to hemoglobin. Three other pathways capable of reducing methemoglobin are present in human erythrocytes, but are much less important: nonenzymatic reduction by ascorbic acid or reduced glutathione (GSH) and a reduced nicotinamide adenine dinucleotide phosphate (NADPH or TPNH)—methemoglobin reductase system, which requires an artificial electron carrier, such as methylene blue, to become effective in reducing methemoglobin. Significant methemoglobinemia is not observed in scurvy, glucose-6-phosphate dehydrogenase deficiency, marked GSH deficiency, or NADPH—methemoglobin reductase deficiency. Although other defects in the metabolic pathways of erythrocytes theoretically might lead to methemoglobinemia, they have not been identified.

The limited ability of erythrocytes from patients with hereditary methemoglobinemia not due to an abnormal hemoglobin to reduce methemoglobin in vitro has been demonstrated in numerous investigations. In most cases, this handicap has been traced to decreased activity of the NADH—methemoglobin reductase system. Methemoglobinemia as high as 40 to 50 per cent results from the accumulation of spontaneously formed methemoglobin in the absence of the normal mechanism for reduction. Data from family and biochemical studies are consistent with an autosomal recessive mode of inheritance. Marked deficiency in activity is seen in erythrocytes of affected homozygous patients, whereas approximately half normal activity is usually evident in cells from acyanotic, asymptomatic heterozygous subjects. Recent studies have demonstrated six different electrophoretic variants of NADH—methemoglobin reductase. One variant is associated with only a slight decrease in activity. Thus, as is true for hemoglobin and glucose-6-phosphate dehydrogenase, multiple aberrations in the NADH—methemoglobin reductase system apparently exist, some with and some without functional consequences.

Toxic (Acquired) Methemoglobinemia. Methemoglobinemia occurs when oxidative stress overwhelms the protective capacities of erythrocytes and exceeds the ability of the cells to reduce methemoglobin. Ferrous heme iron may be oxidized directly by ferricyanide, ferric tartrate, bivalent copper, chromate, chlorate, certain quinones, alloxans, and some dyes with a high oxidation-reduction potential. Nitrite, a powerful reducing agent and one of the most common methemoglobin-forming compounds, produces methemoglobinemia by a reaction that is not completely understood, although the generation of hydrogen peroxide has been suggested. Nitrates, upon conversion to nitrites, especially in the gastrointestinal tract of infants, can lead to toxic methemoglobinemia. Erythrocytes of newborns also are less able than adults' cells to protect hemoglobin against oxidation and to reduce methemoglobin, owing to decreased activities of NADH–methemoglobin reductase and other enzymes. More complex reactions are postulated to explain the methemoglobin-forming properties of aromatic amino and nitro compounds (acetanilid, phenacetin, nitrosobenzene, phenazopyridine, primaquine, sulfonamides, prilocaine, benzocaine) and of aniline dyes in laundry marks and wax crayons. These compounds may be converted to metabolites which either act as direct oxidants or participate in a coupled oxidation with oxyhemoglobin. In the latter reaction, generation of hydrogen peroxide, peroxyhemoglobin, or free radicals is thought to cause the formation of methemoglobin. In addition to producing methemoglobinemia, some of these agents also can induce alterations which lead to hemolysis, especially in erythrocytes deficient in glucose-6-phosphate dehydrogenase activity.

Incidence and Prevalence. Although hereditary methemoglobinemia is rare, over 350 probable cases have been recorded. It is impossible to determine accurately how many are the result of a deficiency in NADH–methemoglobin reductase activity and how many are due to hemoglobin M. Patients in whom complete biochemical studies have not been performed, but whose chronic methemoglobinemia responds to therapy, presumably have had an abnormality in erythrocyte metabolism. Most of these patients probably have a deficiency in NADH–methemoglobin reductase activity; about 200 examples can be cited. The abnormality has a worldwide distribution, and is particularly prevalent in inbred populations.

The M hemoglobins also have a worldwide distribution with about 150 examples. Although many patients are of Northern European origin, a number have been reported from Japan, and the patient with hemoglobin M Hyde Park is a 77-year-old Negro man.

There have probably been thousands of instances of acquired methemoglobinemia, but most have been transient and either clinically insignificant or coincidental complications of another disease. The chronic methemoglobinemia ("enterogenous cyanosis") which is believed to result from the absorption of nitrites produced in a gastrointestinal (or urinary) tract persistently infected with nitrite-producing bacteria is extremely rare. More than 700 cases of toxic methemoglobinemia have been reported in infants fed formulas prepared with well-water containing high concentrations of nitrate; the mortality has been as high as 10 per cent. The anticipated increase in susceptibility to toxic methemoglobinemia of individuals heterozygous for NADH–methemoglobin reductase deficiency is seen in such subjects while receiving prima-quine, chloroquine, or diaminodiphenylsulfone as malarial chemoprophylaxis.

Clinical Manifestations. The characteristic clinical picture of hereditary methemoglobinemia is presented by a patient with diffuse, persistent slate-gray cyanosis, often present from birth and not associated with clubbing of the fingers or evidence of cardiopulmonary disease. Concentrations of methemoglobin of 10 to 25 per cent are tolerated without apparent ill effect, but levels of 30 to 40 per cent may be associated with mild exertional dyspnea and headaches. These patients are really more blue than sick.

Toxic methemoglobinemia, especially if it develops rapidly, will produce symptoms of anoxia. Levels of 20 to 30 per cent methemoglobin are accompanied by dyspnea, tachycardia, headache, fatigue, fainting, nausea, anorexia, and vomiting. Some of these symptoms may reflect direct toxic effects of the causative agent. Lethargy and stupor may appear with methemoglobin concentrations above 55 or 60 per cent. The lethal concentration probably is greater than 70 per cent.

The decreased oxygen-carrying capacity resulting from untreated hereditary methemoglobinemia is sometimes associated with a mild compensatory erythrocytosis. This is often not as great as expected and is not observed with M hemoglobins. Segregation of methemoglobin in a population of older erythrocytes in NADH–methemoglobin reductase deficiency has been invoked to explain, in part, the absence of erythrocytosis. The heme groups of the normal hemoglobin chains in the M hemoglobins retain their capacity to bind oxygen, and normal oxygen affinities are observed with hemoglobin M Saskatoon and Hyde Park. The oxygen affinity, however, is decreased in hemoglobin M Boston, Iwate, and Milwaukee-1. This looser binding of oxygen may facilitate delivery to the tissues and may make an erythrocytosis unnecessary. In toxic methemoglobinemia, the methemoglobin not only decreases the available oxygen-carrying pigment, but also increases the affinity of the unaltered hemoglobin for oxygen, thereby further impairing the delivery of oxygen and enhancing symptoms.

Systemic effects usually do not occur in hereditary methemoglobinemia. A significant and unexplained association of severe mental retardation is seen in children from some families with NADH–methemoglobin reductase deficiency. Toxic methemoglobinemia may be associated with hemolysis, central nervous system depression, hepatic damage, or renal dysfunction, depending upon the causative agent or associated disease.

Diagnosis. Methemoglobinemia should be considered, even if only briefly, in the differential diagnosis of cyanosis. About 5 grams of deoxyhemoglobin per 100 ml. of blood are required to produce visible cyanosis, but a comparable discoloration is produced by 1.5 to 2 grams per 100 ml. of methemoglobin and by about 0.5 gram per 100 ml. of sulfhemoglobin (*vide infra*). The greater visible effect of these abnormal pigments is due to the alterations in the absorption spectra. Blood which contains more than about 10 per cent methemoglobin (or sulfhemoglobin) appears unusually dark red or even brown, and does not change color upon vigorous shaking with air. Addition and mixing of a few drops of 10 per cent NaCN or KCN results in the rapid formation of bright red cyanmethemoglobin, but has no effect on the color of sulfhemoglobin.

Determination of the absorption spectrum is required to define the nature of the abnormal pigment. Acid methemoglobin has a characteristic spectrum with peaks at 502 and 632 mμ that disappear upon the addition of cyanide. Sulfhemoglobin has a peak at 620 mμ that is not altered by cyanide. The absorption spectra of methemoglobin M variants differ from those of normal methemoglobin with displacement of the peaks at 502 and 632 mμ toward lower wavelengths. Sulfhemoglobin, however, may be difficult to differentiate from methemoglobin M. The rate of formation of a complex with cyanide, the resulting absorption spectrum and the electrophoretic migration of the methemoglobin form of hemoglobin M variants often differ from those of normal methemoglobin and help to establish the diagnosis.

NADH–methemoglobin reductase deficiency can be established by assay of this enzyme system in a hemolysate.

A careful history should provide clues to possible toxic methemoglobinemia. Parent to child transmission of congenital cyanosis should suggest the possibility of a hemoglobin M, whereas unexplained cyanosis in siblings but not in parents or offspring is more consistent with NADH–methemoglobin reductase deficiency.

Treatment. With toxic methemoglobinemia, concentrations of 20 to 30 per cent will disappear spontaneously in 24 to 72 hours after exposure to the offending agent terminates. More vigorous therapy is indicated if unconsciousness, stupor, or methemoglobinemia greater than 40 per cent supervenes. Oxygen administration and hemodialysis to remove the toxic agent may be helpful. Methylene blue, 1 to 2 mg. per kilogram given intravenously during five minutes, will often correct the methemoglobinemia within 30 to 60 minutes. Repeated doses may be needed. Toxicity from methylene blue is uncommon, but doses over 15 mg. per kilogram may cause hemolysis in infants. Individuals with glucose-6-phosphate dehydrogenase deficiency may respond suboptimally, and may develop hemolysis. Since neither methemoglobin M nor sulfhemoglobin will respond to methylene blue administration, failure to observe a significant change in color should alert the physician to the possibility of these abnormal pigments. Ascorbic acid has no place in the management of toxic methemoglobinemia because the rate at which it reduces methemoglobin is so much slower than that of the normal intrinsic mechanism.

Hereditary methemoglobinemia due to NADH–methemoglobin reductase deficiency usually does not require treatment except for cosmetic reasons. Intravenous methylene blue will reduce the methemoglobinemia rapidly, and daily oral administration of 100 to 300 mg. will maintain the concentration below 10 per cent. Somewhat less effective is oral administration of ascorbic acid, 500 mg. daily, to maintain the concentration of methemoglobin between 5 and 13 per cent. Despite good control of methemoglobinemia, therapy does not influence the mental retardation suffered by some patients.

Since the causal abnormality in the M hemoglobins resides in the structure of the hemoglobin, no effective form of therapy has been discovered.

Prognosis and Prevention. Methemoglobinemia, as an isolated alteration, does not have an adverse effect on the life expectancy of the patient or on the life span of the erythrocyte. The prognosis in toxic methemoglobinemia, once the acute episode is over, depends upon the precipitating circumstances. Toxic methemoglobinemia can be avoided by careful supervision of potential methemoglobin-producing drugs and chemicals, including thorough laundering of diapers to remove excess aniline dyes.

SULFHEMOGLOBINEMIA

Sulfhemoglobin, an incompletely characterized pigment not normally present, arises from the interaction of hemoglobin with soluble sulfides, especially hydrogen sulfide, in the presence of an oxidizing agent, usually hydrogen peroxide. Sulfhemoglobinemia is caused by the same aromatic amino drugs (acetanilid, phenacetin) that are associated with toxic methemoglobinemia. Why some patients develop methemoglobinemia and others have sulfhemoglobinemia is unknown. The concentration of GSH in the erythrocytes of some of the latter patients is elevated. Sulfhemoglobinemia may occur in patients with "enterogenous cyanosis," and has been attributed to the absorption of H_2S from the diseased gastrointestinal tract. The effect of sulfhemoglobin on the life span of human erythrocytes is uncertain, but many patients with sulfhemoglobinemia also have hemolysis. Since sulfhemoglobin cannot bind oxygen, the clinical effects are similar to those of methemoglobin. Sulfhemoglobin cannot be converted to hemoglobin, and there is no effective treatment. The pigment disappears when the erythrocytes containing sulfhemoglobin leave the circulation.

Cumming, R. L. C., and Pollock, A.: Drug-induced sulphaemoglobinaemia and Heinz body anaemia in pregnancy with involvement of the foetus. Scot. Med. J., 12:320, 1967.

Jaffé, E. R.: DPNH–methemoglobin reductase (diaphorase). In Yunis, J. J. (ed.): Biochemical Methods in Red Cell Genetics. New York, Academic Press, Inc., 1969, pp. 231-253.

Keitt, A.: Hereditary methemoglobinemia with deficiency of NADH–methemoglobin reductase. In Stanbury, J. B., Wyngaarden, J. B., and Frederickson, D. S. (eds.): The Metabolic Basis of Inherited Disease. 3rd ed. New York, McGraw-Hill Book Company (in press).

Kiese, M.: The biochemical production of ferrihemoglobin-forming derivatives from aromatic amines, and mechanisms of ferrihemoglobin formation. Pharmacol. Rev., 18:1091, 1966.

FAMILIAL MEDITERRANEAN FEVER
(Periodic Fever, Periodic Disease, Familial Recurrent Polyserositis, Benign Paroxysmal Peritonitis, Periodic Polyserositis, Recurrent Polyserositis)

Paul B. Beeson

Definition. Familial Mediterranean fever is a familial disease characterized by recurrent short attacks of febrile illness in which there are signs of peritonitis, pleuritis, and arthritis. It is especially common in people of Eastern Mediterranean or Middle East origin, i.e., Jews, Arabs, and Armenians, but because of their wanderings the disorder is now encountered in all parts of the world. In addition, cases which seem clinically indistinguishable from familial Mediterranean fever are sometimes encountered in persons of quite different ethnic background. The name familial Mediterranean fever will be employed in this edition of the textbook because of current usage, but it has undesirable features. Some of the synonyms, notably recurrent polyserositis, would seem preferable. The most definitive studies of the disorder have been carried out in Israel, and the review by Sohar and colleagues is the best single source of information.

Genetics. Extensive investigation of families in Israel has led to the conclusion that familial Mediterranean fever is inherited as a single recessive autosomal trait, although the somewhat higher incidence in males (3:2) has not been adequately explained.

Pathology. Exudates from the peritoneum, pleura, or joint cavities during acute attacks reveal a preponderance of polymorphonuclear leukocytes and no evidence of microbial invasion. Biopsies of inflamed serosal surfaces usually show mild acute inflammation without underlying vascular disease. The most serious pathologic lesion is amyloidosis, which affects arterioles throughout the body and can seriously injure the kidneys, liver, spleen, lung, and adrenals.

Clinical Manifestations. An affected person

shows no evidence of abnormality until the onset of the first attack, usually during the first or second decade of life. Between attacks, until amyloidosis becomes clinically manifest, the patient looks and feels well. Attacks are of short duration, usually one to four days, and consist of fever, which may be moderately high, together with manifestations of acute inflammation of the peritoneum, pleura, or synovial membranes. The peritoneal form is by far the most common, and consequently most sufferers have been subjected to laparotomy. Occasionally the joint manifestations assume more chronic form in which one or two large joints are the sites of painful swelling for weeks or months. Sometimes cutaneous lesions resembling erysipelas develop on the legs during an attack.

The serious hazard of this disease lies in the tendency to develop amyloidosis. This process is progressive, and most often causes death in renal failure. The rarity of familial Mediterranean fever in subjects over 40 years of age implies that amyloidosis develops in a high proportion of cases, causing death during adolescence or early adult life.

Differential Diagnosis. Inasmuch as a specific diagnostic test is lacking, the label of familial Mediterranean fever in an individual person must depend largely on ethnic background and the characteristic course of the disease. Obviously the disorder can mimic various infectious and "collagen" diseases, and a diagnosis of appendicitis is almost always considered at some time.

Treatment. No treatment other than symptomatic measures has been found effective in familial Mediterranean fever. Surprisingly, steroids, despite their antipyretic effects, seem to have little value in management of the acute bouts of illness. Nothing can be done to retard the progression of the amyloidosis which is the cause of death in a high proportion of cases.

SYNDROMES RESEMBLING FAMILIAL MEDITERRANEAN FEVER

Periodic Disease. Reimann has directed attention to a collection of syndromes which have the common features of periodic recurrence and intervals of well-being. He has laid emphasis on the tendency of these to recur at intervals of days which are multiples of the number seven; others have doubted the significance of the latter point simply because patients tend to estimate such time intervals in terms of x number of weeks. Among the syndromes Reimann has described are *periodic fever, periodic peritonitis* (familial Mediterranean fever?), *periodic neutropenia, periodic edema, periodic purpura, periodic arthralgia,* and *periodic psychosis.*

Etiocholanolone Fever. Bondy and Cohn have described a rare entity in which they postulate the pathogenic mechanism to be a recurrent aberration of steroid metabolism leading to the presence of excessive quantities of the pyrogenic steroid etiocholanolone. They described prompt subsidence of manifestations following a single administration of cortisone. The existence of such an entity has been challenged by George et al., who claim that by means of an improved assay method it is possible to show elevations of unconjugated etiocholanolone in the blood of patients with various febrile diseases; they find no clear correlation between temperature elevation and blood level of the steroid. Possible support for the concept of etiocholanolone fever has come from studies of a Lebanese family in which members had increased levels of plasma etiocholanolone and habitual fever (to 102°F.). Perhaps the best support for this concept would be identification of further cases in which symptoms and signs are "turned off" within hours by administration of hydrocortisone intravenously, since that is not the usual response in familial Mediterranean fever.

Bondy, P. K., Cohn, G. L., and Gregory, P. B.: Etiocholanolone fever. Medicine, 44:249, 1965.

George, J. M., Wolff, S. M., and Bartter, F. C.: Recurrent fever of unknown etiology: Failure to demonstrate association between fever and plasma unconjugated etiocholanolone. J. Clin. Invest., 48:558, 1969.

Herman, R. H., Overholt, E. L., and Hagler, L.: Familial lifelong persistent fever of unknown origin responding to dexamethasone and uronic acids. Amer. J. Med., 46:142, 1969.

Reimann, H. A.: Periodic Diseases. Philadelphia, F. A. Davis Company, 1963.

Reimann, H. A.: Perplexities of a periodic entity. J.A.M.A., 190:241, 1964.

Siegal, S.: Familial paroxysmal polyserositis: Analysis of fifty cases. Amer. J. Med., 36:893, 1964.

Sohar, E., Jafni, J., Pras, M., and Heller, H.: Familial Mediterranean fever. A survey of 470 cases and review of the literature. Amer. J. Med., 43:227, 1967.

LIPOID PROTEINOSIS
(Hyalinosis Cutis et Mucosae)
Alexander G. Bearn

This recently recognized rare autosomal recessively inherited disease, particularly common in South Africa, is characterized by the combination of a husky voice from birth and scarring maculopapular eruptions around the face, arms, and trunk. The mucous membranes of the mouth, tongue, and larynx are diffusely infiltrated with hyaline-like material. Recurrent painful parotitis may occur. Calcification of the hippocampal gyri is an inconstant but pathognomonic sign of the disease. No consistent biochemical abnormalities have been reported; the possibility that the disease is related to the mucopolysaccharidoses has been raised. The disease must not be confused with porphyria. Although there is no clear-cut evidence for their effectiveness, corticosteroids have been employed in the treatment of this disease.

Gordon, H., Gordon, W., and Botha, V.: Lipoid proteinosis in an inbred Namaqualand community. Lancet, 1:1032, 1969.

PORPHYRIA
Rudi Schmid

INTRODUCTION

Porphyrins are tetrapyrrole pigments in which four mono-pyrroles are linked by four carbon bridges. Each of the pyrroles in this planar ring structure has two substituent side chains, and the various porphyrins like uro-, copro-, and protoporphyrin differ only in the nature of these side chains. Their sequential arrangement in specific porphyrins determines the structural isomer type, numbered I to IV. In nature, only porphyrins of the isomer type I and III have been identified. With the exception of protoporphyrin III (9a), which in the form of ferroprotoporphyrin (heme) serves as the prosthetic group of hemoglobin and other essential heme proteins, porphyrins apparently neither possess physiologic functions nor act as metabolic intermediates. Rather, they are metabolic by-products that have escaped from the biosynthetic path to heme by irreversible oxidation of the corresponding reduced porphyrinogens (see accompanying figure). The latter are intermediates in heme biosynthesis and are formed from the monopyrrole porphobilinogen (PBG), which in turn is synthesized by condensation of 2 moles of δ-aminolevulinic acid (ALA). The over-all rate of heme and porphyrin biosynthesis is regulated primarily by the activity of ALA synthetase, which condenses glycine and succinyl-CoA to ALA. This mitochondrial enzyme system appears to be reversibly repressed and inhibited by the final product, heme, and it is likely that this and other regulatory mechanisms are responsible for preventing both overproduction of heme and accumulation of metabolic intermediates. In porphyria, the increased excretion of ALA, PBG, or porphyrins is a result of overproduction, because of an inherited defect or an acquired dysfunction of these biologic control systems.

Although all aerobic cells can synthesize heme-containing chromoproteins, heme formation is particularly active in the erythroid elements of bone marrow and in liver. The small quantities of porphyrins and porphyrin precursors excreted normally in urine and bile are derived primarily from these sources. Similarly, the metabolic defects in porphyria that result in the accumulation and consequent increased excretion of porphyrins or their precursors usually can be traced to the erythroid cells of the bone marrow or to the liver, or to both. This distinction serves as a convenient basis for the classification of the porphyrias as follows:

    A. Hepatic porphyria
        1. Acute intermittent porphyria
        2. Variegate porphyria
        3. Coproporphyria
        4. Cutaneous porphyria
            a. Hereditary
            b. Possibly genetically predisposed
            c. Acquired
    B. Congenital erythropoietic porphyria
    C. Protoporphyria

This classification indicates the site of the metabolic disturbance and separates the hereditary forms of porphyria from those with a possible but unproved genetic basis and from the few instances in which the disease appears to be acquired.

It should be noted that increased urinary excretion of porphyrins or precursors, including ALA and PBG, occurs in a variety of conditions other than porphyria. Chronic lead poisoning is commonly associated with increased ALA, and elevated PBG occasionally has been observed in carcinomatosis, Hodgkin's disease, cirrhosis, and affections of the nervous system. Normal urine contains only traces of uroporphyrin, but increased levels may be present in heavy metal poisoning and occasionally in parenchymal liver disease; gross uroporphyrinuria has been reported in a patient with a benign adenoma of the liver. Coproporphyrin frequently is increased in lead poisoning, hemolytic and refractory anemia, hepatitis, cirrhosis, infectious mononucleosis, and alcoholism. In liver disease, coproporphyrinuria may not indicate increased formation of the pigment, but rather its diversion from bile to urine. Protoporphyrin, which has only 2 carboxyl groups and consequently is poorly soluble in water, does not appear in urine, but is excreted exclusively in the bile. The feces regularly contain copro-, proto- and deuteroporphyrin, but these pigments may be derived in part from food, intestinal hemorrhage, and colonic microflora. Because of the wide range in fecal porphyrin concentration, values up to 200 mcg. per gram dry weight may not be indicative of porphyria without additional diagnostic evidence.

HEPATIC PORPHYRIA

Acute Intermittent Porphyria

Definition, Incidence, and Genetics.   Acute intermittent porphyria (synonyms: acute porphyria, porphyria hepatica, pyrroloporphyria, Swedish type) is an abnormality of pyrrole metabolism inherited as a dominant trait. It is associated with recurrent attacks of abdominal pain, gastrointestinal dysfunction, and neurologic manifestations. It is probably the most common form of porphyria, with an over-all incidence of approximately 1 per 100,000 population, but, because of its occurrence in large families, regional incidence may be much higher. The total number of reported cases suggests that people of Scandinavian, Anglo-Saxon, and German ancestry are affected more frequently, whereas the disease is very rare in Negroes.

Acute attacks are rarely seen before puberty; they most often begin in the third or fourth decade, and occur more frequently in women. Manifestations may appear only in later life, or recurrent symptoms may be so vague and protean as to escape recognition. Indeed, persons carrying the genetic abnormality may remain free of clinical manifestations throughout life; such latent porphyria tends to be more frequent in men. This probably accounts for the alleged preponderance of porphyria in women of childbearing age.

BIOSYNTHESIS OF HEME

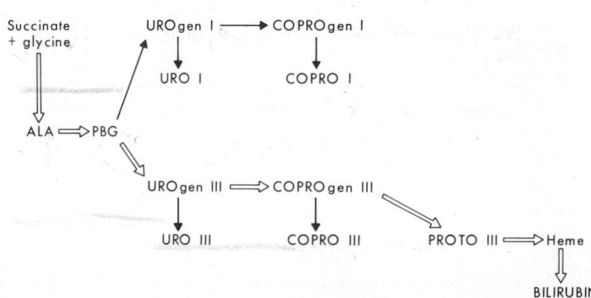

The metabolic pathway from glycine and succinate to heme.

Abbreviations: ALA, δ-aminolevulinic acid; PBG, porphobilinogen; UROgen, uroporphyrinogen; COPROgen, coproporphyrinogen; PROTOgen, protoporphyrinogen; URO, uroporphyrin; COPRO, coproporphyrin; PROTO, protoporphyrin; I, III, isomer types I and III.

Clinical Manifestations. Moderate to severe abdominal pain, often colicky, is frequently the initial or most prominent symptom. The pain may be localized, generalized or radiating to the back or loins, but the abdomen usually is soft. Abdominal tenderness and distention may exist, but are much less striking than would be expected from the intensity of the pain. Leukocytosis and mild fever may be present. Diarrhea occasionally occurs. Severe vomiting and persistent constipation are frequent and may be accompanied by lack of bowel sounds and dilatation of the stomach. Roentgenograms of the abdomen may reveal distended intestinal loops proximal to areas of spasm; volvulus and gangrene have been reported. Gastrointestinal complications commonly lead to weight loss and occasionally to severe emaciation. Prolonged vomiting may cause dehydration, oliguria, and azotemia.

Neurologic disturbances frequently, though not always, are associated with abdominal manifestations and may involve the peripheral, central, or autonomic nervous system. Peripheral neuropathy usually is predominantly motor, may be asymmetrical, and may vary from mild weakness in one extremity to complete flaccid quadriplegia. These motor disturbances may be preceded or accompanied by severe pain, particularly in the legs. Deep tendon reflexes are usually diminished or absent and, although subjective sensory symptoms are frequent, objective sensory loss is less common. Cranial nerve involvement leads to optic atrophy, ophthalmoplegia, facial palsy, dysphagia, and vocal cord paresis. Weakness of abdominal, intercostal, or diaphragmatic musculature may progress to respiratory paralysis, which has a poor prognosis and ranks as the chief cause of death. Wasting and contracture of affected muscles frequently occur but are reversible to a surprising degree during prolonged remissions.

Many patients have a long history of nervousness, emotional instability, and functional disturbances that may remain unexplained until an acute attack occurs. Striking psychiatric abnormalities include personality changes, hysteria, psychoses, and confusional states. With more severe central nervous system involvement, delirium, coma, and epileptic seizures may occur; on occasion they have followed ingestion of barbiturates or maladvised surgical exploration of the abdomen.

Sinus tachycardia frequently accompanies acute attacks, and the pulse rate has been found to be a good index of the activity of the disease. This is believed to be due to vagal neuropathy, and it may also account for nonspecific electrocardiographic abnormalities. Transient hypertension is often present, and on occasion spasm of retinal arteries has been observed. Frank photosensitivity does not occur in acute intermittent porphyria, but mild and apparently reversible pigmentation, particularly of exposed parts of the body, may accompany acute phases of the disease.

Acute episodes vary widely in duration and frequency. Some patients complain merely of occasional and intermittent abdominal pain, whereas in others the initial attack may begin almost explosively and may terminate fatally within days to several weeks. In the majority of cases, distinct attacks recur at irregular intervals over months or years, but tend to decrease in frequency and severity with age. There is strong evidence that attacks may be precipitated by a variety of drugs, including barbiturates, sulfonamides, griseofulvin, estrogens, and contraceptives, all of which are metabolized by the microsomal cytochrome system of the liver. Occasionally, periodic exacerbations are correlated with the menstrual cycle, or latent porphyria may become clinically manifest late in pregnancy or shortly after delivery.

Laboratory Findings and Pathogenesis. The most characteristic laboratory finding is excessive ALA and PBG in the urine. PBG is a colorless chromogen giving a red complex with Ehrlich aldehyde (p-dimethylaminobenzaldehyde in HCl) which after neutralization cannot be extracted with chloroform or butanol. During acute episodes the test is virtually always strongly positive; if the reaction is faintly pink or negative, the diagnosis remains doubtful. In latent porphyria and in patients recovered from an acute attack, urinary PBG excretion is less pronounced, though usually of sufficient magnitude to give a distinctly positive Ehrlich reaction. The red color produced by Ehrlich aldehyde with urobilinogen or indoles can be extracted with chloroform or butanol. Ingestion of antipyrine or admixture of methyl red (Zephiran) results in urine that turns red on acidification alone, whereas compounds of the phenolphthalein group show red only in alkaline urine. Occasionally, the qualitative Ehrlich test becomes negative, and urinary PBG can be demonstrated only by chromatographic methods, which usually but not invariably reveal increased PBG and ALA. Freshly passed urine may be normal in color and may contain relatively little preformed uro- and coproporphyrin. It darkens on standing because of conversion of PBG and other precursors to porphyrins and porphobilin, a dark brown pigment of unknown structure. Fecal porphyrins are within normal limits or moderately increased.

Hematologic abnormalities are absent, and conventional liver function tests frequently yield normal results. The urine may contain increased concentrations of amino acids and indoles; the latter sometimes give an atypical Ehrlich reaction. Elevated protein-bound iodine and cholesterol levels have been reported. During acute attacks hyponatremia may become an alarming complication; although this often can be ascribed to prolonged vomiting or excessive intravenous fluid replacement, inappropriate secretion of antidiuretic hormone has been demonstrated. The liver is microscopically normal or shows mild focal or centrolobular necrosis and fatty changes. It usually does not exhibit porphyrin fluorescence, but contains much PBG. Inconstant neuropathologic changes include patchy demyelination of the peripheral or central nervous system and chromatolysis of anterior horn cells.

The inherited biochemical defect almost certainly consists of increased formation of ALA in the liver, which results in elevated urinary excretion of this keto acid and its condensation product, PBG. Drugs and hormones known to aggravate the disease are believed to enhance further the activity of hepatic ALA synthetase. The pathogenesis of the abdominal and nervous manifestations is unknown; neither ALA nor PBG appears to have a direct toxic effect.

Diagnosis and Differential Diagnosis. The diagnosis rests on the demonstration of increased urinary excretion of ALA and PBG. As a screening procedure, the qualitative test with the Ehrlich aldehyde reagent usually is adequate, but for a definitive diagnosis, quantitative determination with chromatographic methods is essential. Lead intoxication may produce severe abdominal pain and neuropathy, but the urine rarely contains sufficient PBG to give a positive qualitative test, although ALA excretion frequently is increased.

The possibility of porphyria should always be considered in the presence of unexplained abdominal pain, since the disease has been mistaken for cholelithiasis, renal colic, peptic ulcer, appendicitis, bowel obstruction, pancreatitis, and pelvic disorders. Some patients have undergone several surgical procedures before the correct diagnosis was established. Acute attacks seldom last less than 48 hours, and very brief episodes of pain followed by complete remission are not suggestive of porphyria. Obscure neurologic disturbances, especially unexplained peripheral neuropathy, regional muscle weakness, flaccid paralysis, or bulbar palsy, should suggest the possibility of porphyria. Similarly, if hysterical behavior, psychoneurosis, psychosis, or unexplained epilepsy are aggravated by barbiturates, coincide with the menstrual cycle, or are noted in patients under treatment with contraceptives, porphyria should be suspected.

Persistent tachycardia, muscle weakness, and elevated protein-bound iodine may lead to confusion with hyperthyroidism. Occasionally weakness, abdominal pain, pigmentation, and hyponatremia may suggest Addison's disease. During the last trimester of pregnancy, hypertension, vomiting, and oliguria suggestive of eclampsia may in reality be due to porphyria. During clinical remission, when the qualitative test for urinary PBG may become negative, it is sometimes possible to support the diagnosis of porphyria by study of close family members. Provocative diagnostic tests by deliberate administration of barbiturates should be discouraged.

Treatment and Prognosis. There is no specific treatment for acute intermittent porphyria, and therapy remains symptomatic and prophylactic. Acute pain and psychic manifestations usually can be alleviated or controlled with phenothiazines, reserpine or meperidine. Oral phenothiazines, such as chlorpromazine (25 to 100 mg. four times daily) are the preferred treatment for abdominal and muscle pain. Neuropsychiatric manifestations frequently respond to relatively small doses of reserpine. Meperidine (Demerol) by intramuscular injection in doses of 50 to 100 mg. may give prompt though transient relief, but, in general, use of opiates should be limited because the severity and chronicity of the pain renders porphyric patients particularly susceptible to addiction. When recurrent manifestations are clearly related to the menstrual cycle, prolonged androgenic suppression has given promising results.

Acute attacks often can be aborted by prompt administration of carbohydrate ("glucose effect"). Intravenous infusion of glucose or fructose at a rate of 10 to 15 grams per hour for 24 hours, or comparable amounts of oral carbohydrates, may result in striking remissions, particularly in patients whose attacks were precipitated or aggravated by anorexia, nausea, and vomiting. In addition, supportive treatment is of great importance. Dehydration and hyponatremia should be prevented. If bulbar signs are present, respiratory paralysis should be anticipated and a mechanical respirator made available. When fever and leukocytosis in excess of 12,000 per cubic millimeter are suggestive of occult infection, most often of the respiratory or urinary tract, sulfonamides should not be used. Barbiturates, griseofulvin, estrogenic hormones, and contraceptives also should be avoided.

In the earlier literature, the prognosis of acute intermittent porphyria was considered grave, with a mortality of 80 per cent within five years of the first attack. This figure undoubtedly is high; indeed, more recent reports set it around 25 per cent. Death occurs most frequently during the second and third decades, although beyond this age manifestations tend to be less severe and the prognosis distinctly improves.

Variegate Porphyria

Definition, Incidence, and Genetics. Variegate porphyria (synonyms: porphyria cutanea tarda, protocoproporphyria hereditaria, mixed hepatic porphyria, South African genetic porphyria) is a hereditary abnormality of porphyrin metabolism associated with chronic cutaneous manifestations alone or in conjunction with acute, transient attacks of abdominal pain and neuropathy. The disease is inherited as a dominant trait and the sexes are equally affected. Because of its occurrence in large family groups, the incidence varies widely in different parts of the world. Among white settlers of South Africa it is estimated at 3 per 1000. It undoubtedly is very much less elsewhere, though reliable figures are not available.

Clinical Manifestations. Cutaneous symptoms consist of dermal abrasions, superficial erosions, and blister formation following trivial trauma, and commonly are first noted during the second or third decade. The excessive mechanical fragility is usually limited to exposed parts of the skin. The lesions tend to heal slowly, often leave pigmented or slightly depressed scars, and are subject to secondary infection. Direct sensitivity to sunlight is infrequent, but the distribution of the cutaneous lesions leaves little doubt that light exposure is an important pathogenic factor. Hyperpigmentation of face and hands is common, and women often exhibit hypertrichosis, particularly of the temporal margins. The extent of these manifestations varies considerably, but after increased fragility of the skin has developed, it rarely disappears completely. In some instances the abnormality is minimal and remains unnoticed, whereas in others chronicity and secondary infection lead to severe scarring and disfigurement. Cutaneous lesions are uncommon before puberty, are usually milder in women, but during pregnancy become more pronounced.

Although in many patients manifestations remain limited to the skin, acute episodes of abdominal pain, neuropathy, and encephalopathy, similar in all aspects to those in acute intermittent porphyria, are not uncommon. Barbiturates, sulfonamides, general anesthetics, and excessive amounts of ethanol and estrogens frequently appear to be precipitating or aggravating factors. During acute episodes mortality is approximately 25 per cent, but since many patients never develop acute manifestations, the over-all mortality of variegate porphyria is much lower. Genetic studies from South Africa suggest that before the widespread use of barbiturates and sulfonamides, kinships with porphyria survived and propagated as well as the unaffected population. Unless they terminate fatally, acute attacks commonly resolve completely, although neuropathy and muscle weakness may persist for several months. Evidence of hepatic dysfunction and histologic abnormality, including steatosis, fibrosis, or cirrhosis, is not uncommon, and biopsy material from the liver frequently shows extensive porphyrin fluorescence.

Laboratory Findings and Pathogenesis. The characteristic finding in variegate porphyria is the large amount of copro- and particularly protoporphyrin in the bile and feces. Fecal excretion of these pigments is continuous throughout the course of the disease, and takes place even in those patients with minimal cutaneous manifestations and in asymptomatic children with the genetic trait. PBG and porphyrin levels in the urine are usually slightly elevated, but the qualitative test for PBG is frequently negative. During acute attacks urinary excretion of ALA, PBG, and at times, uro- and coproporphyrin is greatly increased, and may reach values comparable to those in acute intermittent porphyria in relapse. Azotemia, hypochloremia, hyponatremia, and jaundice may be present but readily resolve as the acute attack subsides and the disease converts to its cutaneous form.

The exact nature of the inherited biochemical defect is unclear, but it undoubtedly involves increased formation of ALA, PBG, and porphyrins in the liver. Chronic exposure to sunlight is important in the pathogenesis of the cutaneous lesions, but the mechanism underlying the abnormal mechanical fragility of the skin is unclear.

Diagnosis and Differential Diagnosis. The diagnosis can best be established by demonstrating increased porphyrin in the feces. The following qualitative test frequently suffices: a small piece of stool is thoroughly mixed with four parts of ethyl ether and one part of glacial acetic acid, the mixture is filtered, and the filtrate is extracted with 5 per cent hydrochloric acid. Under ultraviolet light with a Wood's filter, extracts of porphyric feces exhibit intense red fluorescence, which is faint or absent with normal stool. In quantitative determinations, values in excess of 40 mcg. of coproporphyrin or 100 mcg. of protoporphyrin per gram of dry feces are suggestive of porphyria. During acute attacks the diagnosis can be ascertained by demonstrating increased ALA and PBG excretion in the urine.

Chronic cutaneous lesions limited to exposed parts, abnormal skin fragility, a positive family history, and increased fecal porphyrin excretion usually permit distinction of variegate porphyria from most other skin diseases. Erythropoietic protoporphyria is the only other light-sensitive dermatosis associated with increased fecal porphyrins, but in this condition erythrocyte or plasma protoporphyrin is usually increased, and the reaction to light is prompt and transient. During acute attacks it may be difficult to distinguish between variegate and acute intermittent porphyria except that the former diagnosis is suggested by concomitant skin involvement or a positive personal or family history of cutaneous manifestations.

Treatment. Treatment is symptomatic and prophylactic. Management of acute attacks is the same as for acute intermittent porphyria. Exposure to direct sunlight should be minimized and the hands protected from mechanical trauma by gloves. Of paramount importance is avoidance of drugs known to percipitate porphyria.

Coproporphyria

Hereditary coproporphyria was recognized only recently as a distinct entity. Clinically it resembles variegate porphyria except that a larger percentage of affected individuals remain asymptomatic, and photosensitivity is rare. As in acute intermittent and variegate porphyria, drugs may precipitate acute attacks which are associated with increased urinary excretion of ALA and PBG. The unique biochemical abnormality is the striking increase in fecal coproporphyrin excretion, whereas fecal protoporphyrin concentration usually is low. During acute attacks, urinary coproporphyrin excretion also may be very high. The disease is inherited as a dominant trait, and the sexes are equally affected. Treatment is the same as for acute intermittent porphyria.

Cutaneous Porphyria

Porphyria cutanea tarda hereditaria and protocoproporphyria hereditaria are names used to describe *familial and probably hereditary* forms of hepatic porphyria that symptomatically and biochemically resemble variegate porphyria except that abdominal and neurologic manifestations are uncommon or mild. It is unclear whether these represent different genetic defects or whether the rarity of acute episodes is due to other factors.

More frequent is a sporadic form of cutaneous porphyria, characterized by chronic skin lesions, hepatic dysfunction, and uroporphyrinuria (synonyms: porphyria cutanea tarda symptomatica; constitutional or idiosyncratic porphyria; symptomatic porphyria). The disease is more common in males and usually begins insidiously, most often in the fourth to sixth decade. It occurs in all parts of the world, but is most frequent in the Bantus of South Africa. Exposed skin shows abnormalities similar to those of variegate porphyria, ranging from slight dermal fragility to severe chronic scarring and disfiguration. The lesions often are more active in summer and tend to heal in winter. Hyperpigmentation and hirsutism are frequent and may be the presenting symptoms. Hepatomegaly with chemical and histologic evidence of liver disease, often due to chronic alcoholism, is present in the majority of patients. In addition to uroporphyrin, variable degrees of hemosiderosis are frequently found in the liver. Although hepatic hemosiderosis may not differ from that seen in nonporphyric patients with chronic liver disease, recent evidence suggests that cutaneous manifestations and porphyrin excretion may be improved by repeated venesection.

Urinary excretion of uroporphyrin and, to a lesser extent, coproporphyrin, is greatly increased, and urine may be pink or brownish. Fecal porphyrins are normal or slightly increased, and excretion of ALA or PBG is almost never elevated. The excreted porphyrins undoubtedly are derived from the liver, but the underlying biochemical defect is unknown. Because of the absence of a positive family history, the disturbance is generally assumed to be acquired, usually in association with some other form of liver disease, frequently one caused by alcoholism. However, since only a very small percentage of patients with chronic liver disease develop porphyria, the possibility of a genetically determined but normally undetected defect activated by hepatic injury cannot be ruled out. Treatment is symptomatic and directed toward the primary liver disease. Abstinence in alcoholic patients results in significant improvement or disappearance of the porphyria. Chloroquine and cholestyramine may be useful in reducing the photosensitivity, but both compounds need further clinical evaluation.

In rare instances, intoxications may lead to a form of hepatic porphyria that is *acquired*. A large number of persons in Turkey exposed to hexachlorobenzene developed porphyria with cutaneous manifestations, uroporphyrinuria and hepatic dysfunction.

CONGENITAL ERYTHROPOIETIC PORPHYRIA
(Congenital Photosensitive Porphyria, Günther's Disease)

This very rare disease is due to a hereditary defect of porphyrin metabolism in the erythroid cells that leads to chronic photosensitivity, hemolytic anemia and urinary excretion of uroporphyrin I. Only about 80 cases in both sexes have been reported. Inheritance is by autosomal recessive transmission; heterozygous individuals appear clinically normal.

Excretion of pinkish urine usually begins shortly after birth, although cutaneous lesions on exposed parts, increased hemolysis, and splenomegaly may not be detected until later. Hypertrichosis and erythrodontia are virtually always present. Urine contains high concentrations of uroporphyrin I and coproporphyrin I, but excretion of ALA and PBG is normal. Hemoglobin frequently is decreased, and reticulocytes and fecal urobilinogen are increased. Erythrocytes contain much uroporphyrin I, and normoblasts exhibit intense red fluorescence. The metabolic defect appears to involve faulty conversion of PBG to uroporphyrinogen in the maturing erythroid cells of the bone marrow. Death may occur in childhood, but if patients live to maturity, they usually exhibit severe scarring and mutilation of hands and face. Successful pregnancy with delivery of phenotypically normal children has been reported. Treatment is symptomatic and prophylactic, consisting essentially of rigorous protection from sunlight. In some instances hemolytic anemia, photosensitivity, and porphyrin excretion have been improved by splenectomy.

PROTOPORPHYRIA
(Erythropoietic Protoporphyria, Erythrohepatic Protoporphyria)

In this recently recognized form of porphyria, high concentrations of protoporphyrin in erythrocytes, plasma, and feces are associated with solar urticaria or solar eczema. Short exposure to sunlight results in intense pruritus, erythema, and edema of exposed skin. These lesions appear during or immediately after exposure, subside in 12 to 24 hours, and usually heal without significant scarring, atrophy, or pigmentation. Occasionally cutaneous manifestations develop only after prolonged exposure to sunlight, or the initial acute skin lesions may progress to a chronic eczematous stage persisting for weeks and healing with superficial scar formation. Skin manifestations commonly begin during childhood or adolescence, are more severe in summer, and recur throughout life. Affected skin shows neither abnormal mechanical fragility nor blister formation characteristic of the other forms of photosensitive porphyria. Erythrodontia, hirsutism, and hyperpigmentation are lacking. Photosensitivity is mediated by protoporphyrin in plasma or skin and is evoked by near-ultraviolet light in the 400 mμ range, in which porphyrins absorb maximally. The excessive protoporphyrin in plasma and feces is derived primarily from the liver, the erythroid cells serving as a minor source. Fasting increases the plasma protoporphyrin level, whereas carbohydrate administration reduces both protoporphyrin formation and photosensitivity. Urinary porphyrin excretion is normal.

The disturbance occurs in both sexes and appears to be inherited as a dominant trait. A significant percentage of persons carrying the genetic abnormality remain clinically asymptomatic, and detection may be possible only by repeated determination of erythrocyte and fecal protoporphyrin concentration. The disease has a good prognosis, and neither results in permanent disability nor influences normal life expectancy except for a high incidence of cholelithiasis. Treatment is prophylactic and consists largely in protection from direct sunlight.

Dean, G.: The Porphyrias. London, Pitman Medical Publishing Company, 1963.

Eales, L.: Porphyria as seen in Cape Town. A survey of 250 patients and some recent studies. S. Afr. J. Lab. Clin. Med., 9:151, 1963.

Goldberg, A., and Rimington, C.: Diseases of Porphyrin Metabolism. Springfield, Ill., Charles C Thomas, 1962.

Schmid, R.: The porphyrias. In Stanbury, J. B., Wyngaarden, J. B., and Frederickson, D. S. (eds.): The Metabolic Basis of Inherited Disease. 3rd ed. New York, McGraw-Hill Book Company (In press).

Taddeini, L., and Watson, C. J.: The clinical porphyrias. Seminars in Hematology, 5:335, 1968.

Tschudy, D. P.: Biochemical lesions in porphyria. J.A.M.A., 191:718, 1965.

Waldenström, J.: The porphyrias as inborn errors of metabolism. Amer. J. Med., 22:758, 1957.

Watson, C. J., Bossenmaier, I., and Cardinal, R.: Acute intermittent porphyria. Urinary porphobilinogen and other Ehrlich reactors in diagnosis. J.A.M.A., 175:1087, 1961.

THE MUCOPOLY-SACCHARIDOSES

Alexander G. Bearn

THE HURLER SYNDROME
(Mucopolysaccharidosis I, MPS I)

Definition. The Hurler syndrome is an autosomally inherited abnormality of mucopolysaccharide metabolism characterized by skeletal abnormalities, hepatosplenomegaly, corneal clouding, mental retardation, and an increased mucopolysaccharide excretion in the urine.

Etiology. The disease, which has a prevalence of approximately 1 in 40,000, is caused by an excessive intracellular accumulation of the mucopolysaccharides dermatan sulfate (chondroitin sulfate B) and heparan sulfate (heparatin sulfate). These substances are preferentially deposited in those tissues and organs in which they are normally found. An increased intracellular accumulation of glycolipid in several patients with the Hurler syndrome has been reported in addition to the increased mucopolysaccharides. Although the primary inherited defect in Hurler's syndrome is not yet known, the disease appears to be due to an imbalance in the synthesis and degradation of mucopolysaccharides. A recently described deficiency of β-galactosidase in the tissues of patients with Hurler's syndrome has raised the possibility that the primary defect may be due to faulty degradation of mucopolysaccharides, and, to a lesser extent, lipids. An increased intracellular deposition of mucopolysaccharides can be demonstrated in cultured fibroblasts derived from patients with Hurler's syndrome and their heterozygous relatives, using metachromatic dyes as well as chemical methods.

Pathology. The most characteristic pathologic feature of the disease is the excessive accumulation of intracellular mucopolysaccharides. Cells of the nervous system, liver, reticuloendothelial system, endocrine glands, cartilage, bone, and heart muscle are involved. Abnormal deposits are also present in the cornea, meninges, parenchymal and Kupffer cells of the liver, epicardium, pericardium, chordae tendineae, heart valves, tracheobronchial cartilages, upper air passages, and coronary and larger peripheral arteries. Distention of fibroblasts with this material causes the appearance of "clear" or "gargoyle" cells.

Clinical Manifestations. Although the patient

may appear normal at birth, the disease becomes evident during the first year or two of life and progresses during childhood and adolescence. In the full-blown disorder, the head is large, and there is hyperostosis of the sagittal suture that sometimes extends onto the forehead. The facial features are coarse and ugly because of a broad saddle nose and wide nostrils, thick lips, large tongue, open mouth, and noisy breathing. Skeletal abnormalities include short neck, dorsal and lumbar kyphosis with gibbus, short stature, and flaring of the costal margins. The hands are broad with stubby fingers, and there is a tendency for the fifth finger to bend radially. There may be deformity of joints such as genu valgus, coxa valga, pes planus, and talipes equinovarus. The skin, especially over upper extremities and thorax, is ridged and grooved, and may present nodular thickenings. Fine lanugo hairs are prominent over much of the cutaneous surface, and the extremities are likely to show profuse growth of large coarse hair. The heart is enlarged, and valvular involvement produces murmurs that may simulate those of rheumatic heart disease. Involvement of coronary arteries may give rise to angina or other evidence of occlusive disease. The abdomen is large and protuberant, and the liver and spleen are commonly enlarged. Umbilical and inguinal hernias are frequent. Clouding of the cornea is extremely common; slit-lamp examination of the eyes may be needed to detect the corneal opacification in the early stages of the disease. Mental deterioration is severe and progressive.

Abnormalities demonstrable by roentgenogram include large skull with frontal and occipital hyperostosis, hypertelorism, long shallow sella turcica with anterior pocketing, and deformities of the facial bones. Gibbus is associated with wedge-shaped deformities and anterior hooklike projections of the vertebral bodies. The ribs are broad, spatulate, and saber-shaped. The terminal phalanges of the hands are broad and short, and the long bones, especially of the arms, show swollen shafts from expansion of medullary cavities. The heart is often enlarged, and pulmonary congestion may be present.

Diagnosis. Diagnosis depends upon recognition of the characteristic clinical manifestations, biopsy, blood and bone marrow studies, and examination of the urine for increased mucopolysaccharide. A simple screening test for increased urinary mucopolysaccharides consists of adding acidified bovine serum albumin to the urine. A positive result is indicated by a dense white precipitate owing to the reaction of albumin and acid mucopolysaccharide at low pH. A more specific screening test can be performed by allowing urine to dry on filter paper and adding acetic acid and toluidine blue O. A purple color develops in the urine of patients with the Hurler syndrome. Metachromatic granules in the cytoplasm of circulating lymphocytes (Reilly bodies) are usually

demonstrable and are useful diagnostic adjuncts. An increased quantity of intracellular mucopolysaccharides can be demonstrated in cultured fibroblasts and white cells from affected individuals and those heterozygous for the abnormal gene using toluidine blue O. Detection of heterozygotes by this method requires skilled evaluation as other inherited traits may yield metachromatic fibroblasts.

The Hurler syndrome may suggest cretinism but differs in that bone age is normal, tests of thyroid function are normal, and the patient is active.

Treatment. No effective treatment is known.

THE HUNTER SYNDROME
(Mucopolysaccharidosis II, MPS II)

This is the only mucopolysaccharidosis which is known to be inherited in an X-linked recessive fashion. The disease is similar but clinically less severe than the classic Hurler syndrome, and is only one fifth as frequent. Clouding of the cornea is minimal or absent, and mental deterioration occurs more slowly. Nodular thickening of the skin and deafness are common. Cardiac enlargement and pulmonary hypertension may be features of the disease. An increased urinary excretion of dermatan sulfate and heparan sulfate is the rule. Abnormal accumulations of mucopolysaccharides can be observed in cultured fibroblasts from affected individuals and heterozygous carriers of the abnormal gene. Thus, unlike Hurler's syndrome and the other mucopolysaccharidoses, in which both parents are obligatory heterozygotes and yield metachromatic cultures, cultured fibroblasts derived from the mother of individuals with the X-linked Hunter syndrome are metachromatic, whereas cells derived from the father of the affected individual are normal.

SANFILIPPO SYNDROME
(Mucopolysaccharidosis III, MPS III)

Sanfilippo syndrome is rare and is characterized by severe progressive mental retardation with relatively minor somatic changes. Corneal clouding is rare, and dwarfism and hepatosplenomegaly only moderate. The disease is inherited as an autosomal recessive and occurs in approximately 1 in 10,000 to 1 in 200,000 individuals. Many patients languish in mental institutions undiagnosed. As in the other mucopolysaccharidoses, cultured fibroblasts from affected individuals and heterozygous carriers demonstrate increased mucopolysaccharides. An increased excretion of heparan sulfate, but not of dermatan sulfate, is diagnostic.

THE MORQUIO SYNDROME
(Morquio-Brailsford Syndrome,
Chondro-osteodystrophy, Mucopoly-
saccharidosis IV, MPS IV)

Patients with this recessively inherited syndrome are strikingly dwarfed. The characteristic radiologic features of the disease become evident after the age of two and consist of marked osteoporosis, platyspondyly, abnormalities of the femoral heads, and knock-knees. Severe skeletal changes may lead to symptoms of spinal cord or medullary compression. Intelligence is unimpaired or trivially decreased. The disease has an estimated frequency of 1 in 40,000 births. Although not invariably present, an increased excretion of keratosulfate in urine is diagnostic. The urinary excretion of dermatan sulfate and heparan sulfate is normal.

THE SCHEIE SYNDROME
(Mucopolysaccharidosis V, MPS V)

This rare autosomal variant of the Hurler syndrome is characterized by nearly normal intelligence, marked cloudy cornea, and the selective excretion of increased quantities of dermatan sulfate. Aortic regurgitation and the carpal tunnel syndrome are common features of this mucopolysaccharidosis.

MAROTEAUX-LAMY SYNDROME
(Mucopolysaccharidosis VI)

Early corneal clouding and a normal intelligence distinguish this rare autosomal variant of the Hurler syndrome. An increased excretion of dermatan sulfate can be demonstrated. Unlike the Scheie syndrome the skeletal abnormalities are severe, and aortic disease is absent.

I CELL DISEASE
(Inclusion Cell Disease, Mucopolysaccharidosis VII, Lipomucopoly-
saccharidosis)

This extremely rare variant of the classic Hurler syndrome is characterized by a notable increase in intracellular lipid, but the accumulation of mucopolysaccharides is less striking.

Danes, B. S., and Bearn, A. G.: Hurler's syndrome, a genetic study in cell culture. J. Exp. Med., 123:1, 1966.
Dorfman, A.: Heritable diseases of connective tissue: The Hurler syndrome. *In* Stanbury, J. B., Wyngaarden, J. B., and Frederickson, D. S. (eds.): The Metabolic Basis of Inherited Disease. 3rd ed. New York, McGraw-Hill Book Company (In press).
Hambrick, G. W., Jr., and Scheie, H. G.: Studies of the skin in Hurler's syndrome. Arch. Derm. (Chicago), 85:455, 1962.

Maroteaux, P., and Lamy, M.: Hurler's disease, Morquio's disease and related mucopolysaccharidoses. J. Pediat., 67:312, 1965.
McKusick, V. A.: Heritable Diseases of Connective Tissue. 3rd ed. St. Louis, C. V. Mosby Company, 1966, pp. 325-399.
Symposium on Mucopolysaccharidoses. Amer. J. Med., 47:661, 1969.

THE MARFAN SYNDROME
(Marfan's Syndrome, Arach-
nodactyly, Dolichostenomelia)
Alexander G. Bearn

Marfan's syndrome is a generalized disorder of connective tissue with skeletal, ocular, and cardiovascular manifestations. The molecular nature of the defect is not precisely known, and abnormalities of collagen as well as elastin have been implicated. The condition occurs equally in both sexes, and is inherited as a dominant trait with variable expression. The prevalence of the disease has been estimated to be 1.5 per 100,000 of the population, and approximately 15 per cent of all cases are due to new mutations.

Skeleton. The extremities are characteristically long and thin. The arm span is greater than the height, and the lower segment measurement (pubis to sole) is in excess of the upper segment (pubis to vertex). Excessive longitudinal growth gives rise to arachnodactyly, pectus excavatum or pigeon breast, dolichocephaly, a long narrow face, and a high arched palate. Weakness and reduplication of ligaments and joint capsules lead to "double-jointedness," backward curvature of the knees, flat feet, and recurrent dislocation of the hips, patella, and other joints. Cutaneous striae may be present, and probably reflect the abnormal elastic fibers. An unexplained sparsity of subcutaneous fat is said to be a feature in most cases. Femoral hernias are not uncommon.

Eyes. The eyes show subluxation of the lens (ectopia lentis). Although this is usually severe and bilateral, minor degrees of subluxation require careful slit-lamp examination. Diagnosis of the Marfan syndrome in the absence of subluxation or redundancy of the suspensory ligament and without affected family members should be made with extreme caution. Other ocular signs include tremor of the iris and glaucoma. Severe myopia, and spontaneous retinal detachment are common, and often lead to gross impairment of vision.

Cardiovascular Defects. A disruption and loss of the elastic fibers of the media, associated with an increase in collagen and smooth muscle, is the primary basic defect. The lack of elasticity results in progressive diffuse dilatation of the proximal segment of the ascending aorta and severe *aortic regurgitation*. The aorta is widest at the sinuses of Valsalva. Aortic regurgitation, owing to dilatation and stretching of the aortic cusps, may occur in the absence of roentgenographic evidence of aortic dilatation. An early systolic click is commonly heard at the apex as well as at the aortic area. Mitral regurgitation is being observed with increasing frequency, and appears to be due to stretching of the chordae tendineae. Myxomatous transformation of the mitral ring may occur. Heart failure and rupture of the aorta resulting from dissecting aneurysm are the most common causes of death. Prominence of the pulmonary artery is frequently seen, and is due to displacement of the dilated aortic ring as well as to dilatation of the pulmonary artery. Bacterial endocarditis may be superimposed on the cardiac lesion. Cystic disease of the lung may occur as an integral part of the Marfan syndrome.

Differential Diagnosis. The Marfan syndrome must be distinguished from *homocystinuria*, which clinically it may closely resemble. It has been estimated that 5 per cent of patients with nontraumatic ectopia lentis, one of the cardinal signs of classic Marfan syndrome, have homocystinuria. Ectopia lentis, pectus excavatum, and pigeon breast are common to both syndromes. Patients with homocystinuria, however, do not develop dissecting aneurysms; moreover, they can be distinguished from patients with the Marfan syndrome by the presence of a malar flush, generalized osteoporosis, and moderate to severe mental retardation. Homocystinuria is inherited as a recessive trait. The diagnosis can be made by a positive urinary nitroprusside test or, definitively, by paper electrophoresis of the urine. Rats given β-aminoproprionitrile (or seeds of *Lathyrus odoratus*) develop skeletal changes and dissecting aortic aneurysm reminiscent of some of the features of the Marfan syndrome.

McKusick, V. A.: Heritable Disorders of Connective Tissue. 3rd ed. St. Louis, C. V. Mosby Company, 1966.
Schimke, R. N., McKusick, V. A., Huang, T., and Pollack, A. D.: Homocystinuria. Studies of 20 families with 38 affected members. J.A.M.A., 193:711, 1965.

EHLERS-DANLOS SYNDROME

Clayton E. Wheeler, Jr.

Definition. The Ehlers-Danlos syndrome is an inherited systemic connective tissue disorder in which the major manifestations are fragility and hyperelasticity of skin, easy bruising, atrophic scars and soft pseudotumors, calcified cysts, hyperextensibility of joints with frequent luxations, bleeding tendency, and visceral anomalies.

Etiology. The chief abnormalities of connective tissue are increased fragility and friability and capacity to stretch to an unusual length and

return to the original position. Elastic tissue deficiency appears unlikely because the tissue returns to its original position after stretching. Since toughness and limited extensibility are characteristics of normal collagen, fragility and hyperelasticity seem to indicate a collagen defect. It is conjectural whether the defect is molecular or involves the arrangement of molecules into fibrils or fibrils into bundles. The condition is inherited as a dominant trait with somewhat variable expression. An uncommon x-linked form has been described.

Incidence. The Ehlers-Danlos syndrome is most prevalent among white persons of European ancestry, although dark-skinned people are occasionally affected. Males are involved slightly more often than females. Skin and joint changes usually appear at an early age, but may not be evident until adult life. The disorder, including mild and incomplete forms, is undoubtedly much more common than case reports in the literature indicate.

Pathology. No consistent abnormality of the corium has been demonstrated by microscopic examination. Normal, increased, or decreased amounts of elastic tissue or collagen, fragmentation of elastic tissue, and derangement of architecture of collagen have all been reported. Some of these findings may be late effects of overstretching and fragility rather than primary abnormalities. Limited study with the electron microscope has shown normal-appearing elastic tissue and collagen. No consistent microscopic abnormality has been found in blood vessels. Subcutaneous nodules are composed of encapsulated fat, which is often calcified. Pseudotumors show connective tissue proliferation, increased vascularity, islets of fatty degeneration, and cyst formation.

Pathogenesis. Defective, friable collagen that allows abnormal extensibility and normal elastic tissue that provides return to the original position explain many of the clinical features: hyperelastic skin, scars, pseudotumors, easy bruising, hyperextensibility of joints with luxations, hemarthroses and arthritis, rupture of the lung with emphysema, and fragility and bleeding from the bowel. Defective supporting tissue of vessel walls or surrounding structures account for much of the abnormal bleeding, but functional and structural abnormalities of platelets have been reported.

Clinical Manifestations. Clinical features are variable because of mild and incomplete forms of the syndrome. The facies may be normal, or there may be widely spaced eyes, epicanthal folds, broad nasal bridge, and "lop ears." Mentality is usually normal. The patient is likely to be small, short, and poorly developed.

The most striking feature of the soft, velvety skin is its capacity to be pulled abnormally far from underlying structures and to return promptly to its original position. The entire skin is usually hyperelastic, but some regions exhibit this property more than others. With age, elasticity of localized areas, especially about the elbows, may be lost so that the skin hangs in loose folds. Skin of the palms and soles is likely to become lax, furrowed, and redundant, and resembles loose-fitting gloves or moccasins. Despite increased elasticity, the skin is abnormally fragile or brittle, as shown by its tendency to bruise easily and by the development of scars and soft pseudotumors at sites of minor injury. Paper-thin atrophic scars develop over the elbows, knees, shins, and elsewhere. The scars are shiny, brown or red-violet, and often show telangiectasia. Subcutaneous spherules or nodules 2 to 8 mm. in size may appear on the legs and forearms. These are easily movable and often calcify. Minor blows result in purpura or hematomas that may organize to form tumors. Retraction of tissues prevents excessive bleeding from skin injury, but minor trauma or surgery produces a gaping, fish-mouth wound that is hard to close and heals slowly.

Hyperextensibility of joints is often striking; the head, extremities, and digits may be placed in abnormal positions ("India rubber men" and "human pretzels"). Because of hyperextensibility of the joints and poor muscular development or tone, infants may show delayed sitting or walking and unsteadiness that occasions frequent falling and subsequent fractures. Other consequences of loose joints and muscle atony or weakness are frequent joint effusions or hemarthroses, arthritis, and habitual dislocations of the hip, shoulder, patella, radius, and clavicle. In addition, flat feet, genu recurvatum, kyphoscoliosis, and loose-end clavicles are seen. Other musculoskeletal abnormalities that have been associated with the Ehlers-Danlos syndrome are spina bifida occulta, arachnodactyly, high arched palate, club foot, spondylolisthesis, pigeon breast, and osteolytic changes of distal phalanges. There may be too few, too many, or poorly formed teeth. Umbilical and inguinal hernias are common. Muscle cramps may involve the legs at night.

Recognition of internal manifestations will undoubtedly increase with further study. Dissecting aortic aneurysm, intracranial aneurysms, spontaneous rupture of large arteries, aneurysm of the sinus of Valsalva and aortic insufficiency, spontaneous rupture of the lung with mediastinal and subcutaneous emphysema, and fragility of the bowel with bleeding or perforation have been reported. Congenital anomalies of the heart, gastrointestinal, respiratory, or genitourinary tracts also occur. Bleeding may occur into the skin or from the lung, vagina, rectum, nose, gums, or tooth sockets, or after tonsillectomy, after operations on joints, or post partum.

Diagnosis. Two or more of the following clinical features usually suffice for diagnosis: (1) cutaneous hyperelasticity, (2) hyperextensibility of joints, (3) easy bruising, (4) atrophic scars and pseudotumors, (5) calcified subcutaneous cysts, and (6) typical cases in the family.

Cutis laxa is characterized by loose, inelastic skin that hangs in folds. In late stages of the Ehlers-Danlos syndrome, localized areas of skin may become lax, but otherwise there seems to be no relation between the two disorders. Hypermobility of joints occurs as a genetic trait distinct from the Ehlers-Danlos syndrome, and it is part of *Marfan's syndrome, osteogenesis imperfecta, mongolism, cretinism,* and *cachexia.* Blue sclerae are probably essential features of the Ehlers-Danlos syndrome and do not signify a relationship to osteogenesis imperfecta. Besides having hyperelastic joints and skin, patients with the *Bonnevie-Ullrich-Turner syndrome* show dwarfism, web neck, cubitus valgus, gonadal dysgenesis, and female phenotype with male genotype.

Treatment. There is no treatment for the basic disorder. Trauma to skin and joints should be avoided. Careful suturing, immobilization, and taping may promote wound healing. Hematomas occasionally require drainage. Orthopedic measures, including exercises, braces, reduction of dislocations, and drainage of hemarthroses, may be necessary. Dissecting aneurysm, hemorrhage, intestinal perforation, and various anomalies may require surgical intervention. Surgical procedures should be undertaken with great care because of the friability and hyperelasticity of skin and internal structures. Severed tissues separate abnormally, sutures are difficult to place and often do not hold, and wound dehiscence is a definite threat.

Prognosis. Prognosis for life is usually good, although deaths occur from various internal manifestations. Patients may be comfortable or may suffer considerable inconvenience and morbidity from cutaneous and musculoskeletal abnormalities. The joints tend to become more stable as the patient ages.

Beighton, P.: Obstetric aspects of the Ehlers-Danlos syndrome. J. Obstet. Gynaec. Brit. Comm., 76:97, 1969.
Beighton, P., and Horan, F. T.: Surgical aspects of the Ehlers-Danlos syndrome. Brit. J. Surg., 56:255, 1969.
Beighton, P., Price, A., Lord, J., and Dickson, E.: Variants of the Ehlers-Danlos syndrome. Ann. Rheum. Dis. 28:228, 1969.
Kashiwagi, H., Riddle, J. M., Abraham, J. P., and Frame, B.: Functional and ultrastructural abnormalities of platelets in Ehlers-Danlos syndrome. Ann. Intern. Med., 63:249, 1965.
McFarland, W., and Fuller, D. E.: Mortality in Ehlers-Danlos syndrome due to spontaneous rupture of large arteries. New Eng. J. Med., 271:1309, 1964.
McKusick, V. A.: Heritable Disorders of Connective Tissue. 3rd ed. St. Louis, C. V. Mosby Company, 1966.
Robitaille, G. A.: Ehlers-Danlos syndrome and recurrent hemoptysis. Ann. Intern. Med., 61:716, 1964.

PSEUDOXANTHOMA ELASTICUM
Clayton E. Wheeler, Jr.

Definition. Pseudoxanthoma elasticum is an uncommon, inherited disorder of connective tissue characterized by yellow skin lesions at flexural areas, retinal angioid streaks, chorioretinitis, arterial disease, and visceral bleeding tendencies.

The combination of cutaneous lesions and angioid streaks is called the *Grönblad-Strandberg syndrome.*

Etiology. The primary defect appears to be genetically determined premature degeneration and calcification of connective tissue of the skin, eyes, and cardiovascular system. Elastic tissue is probably the abnormal component, although abnormality of collagen has not been excluded. Autosomal recessive inheritance with partial limitation to the female is found most often, but dominant inheritance may occasionally occur.

Incidence. The disorder occurs in all races, in both sexes, and at any age. Skin lesions occur slightly more frequently in females, and angioid streaks more frequently in males. The disease may be present at birth or infancy, but the diagnosis is made most frequently in the third to fifth decades.

Pathology. The histologic picture of cutaneous lesions is diagnostic. The epidermis and upper corium are normal. Characteristic changes consist of granular or rodlike accumulations of basophilic material and calcium deposits in the middle and lower dermis. The basophilic material stains like elastic tissue but shows the periodicity of collagen when examined by the electron microscope. The eye shows basophilia and rents of Bruch's elastic lamina, sclerosis of choroidal vessels, and scleral changes that simulate those of the skin. Elastic tissue degeneration affects the media of vessels of medium and larger size. White plaques histologically resembling those in the skin have been found on the pericardium and endocardium of the ventricles and right atrium, and some investigators suspect specific involvement of the mitral valve.

Clinical Manifestations. The three major areas affected are skin, eyes, and cardiovascular system. Combined skin and eye changes are found in approximately 60 per cent of the cases, skin alone in 10 per cent, and eyes alone in 30 per cent. Cardiovascular abnormalities are present in nearly 80 per cent of the patients if careful search is made. The impression has been gained that the disorder is more severe when skin lesions are well developed, but instances of advanced cardiovascular or eye involvement occur in the absence of clinical cutaneous abnormalities.

Cutaneous lesions are small, soft, chamois-colored papules arranged parallel to skin lines and folds; the result is a crepelike or Moroccan leather appearance. A network of fine telangiectatic vessels sometimes outlines the papules. Coalescence produces circumscribed or diffuse plaques. In mild cases the lesions may be seen only after the skin is stretched. In advanced cases the skin is thickened, hangs in loose, inelastic folds, and resembles the skin of a plucked chicken. Sites of most frequent involvement are the sides of the neck, axillae, groin, cubital and popliteal fossae, and the periumbilical area, but the face, breasts, undersurface of the penis, and the perianal area may be affected as well as the mucosa of the mouth, palate, vagina, and rectum. Papular and

arcuate lesions of elastosis perforans serpiginosa may occur in pseudoxanthoma elasticum as well as in Ehlers-Danlos syndrome and other connective tissue diseases.

Angioid streaks of the retina are the most characteristic eye lesions. These lie behind the retinal vessels. They are most numerous around the optic disc, which they may encircle and from which they course like vessels over the fundus. They are flat, serrated streaks varying from narrow lines to three or four times the diameter of retinal veins. They are red, brown, gray, or black, and there may be hemorrhage or white areas of connective tissue proliferation along their course. The streaks are usually bilateral, although not symmetrical, and tend to progress slowly or to become stationary. When the streaks involve the macula, loss of vision occurs. Other eye changes are central chorioretinitis that may also involve the macula, pigmented stippling of the fundus, and hemorrhage from retinal vessels.

Patients often have premature and advanced arterial changes indistinguishable from arteriosclerosis or atherosclerosis with predilection for medium-sized arteries. These changes may result in weak or absent peripheral pulses of the arms or legs, easy fatigability of the legs, intermittent claudication, angina, arrhythmias, cerebrovascular accidents, and mental deterioration. Hypertension occurs in about half the cases. Renal hemangioma and abnormalities of renal arteries may be found. Left ventricular hypertrophy, congestive heart failure, and coronary thrombosis may occur, and mitral valvular disease has been reported. Pulse wave studies of involved extremities show decreased amplitude and velocity, and the dicrotic notch may be lost.

Internal hemorrhage is a special feature of the vascular disease. Bleeding from the gastrointestinal tract occurs in about 10 per cent of the cases, and it may be severe or fatal. Bleeding may arise in peptic ulcer, hiatal hernia, or ulcerative colitis, or its clinical origin may not be demonstrable. Other sites of hemorrhage are skin, subarachnoid space, kidney, uterus, bladder, nasal mucosa, and joints.

The association of thyrotoxicosis, diabetes mellitus, diabetes insipidus, low fertility, amenorrhea, and impotence with pseudoxanthoma elasticum has been suggested but seems doubtful.

Diagnosis. Cutaneous lesions are diagnostic, especially if confirmed by biopsy. Diagnostic histologic changes may be present when clinical findings are minimal or absent. Senile elastosis, a degenerative disease of dermal connective tissue, resembles pseudoxanthoma elasticum, but it affects only exposed sites. The histologic appearance rules out pseudoxanthoma. Angioid streaks are highly suggestive but not pathognomonic, since they are seen in sickle cell disease and in a small percentage of patients with Paget's disease of bone. Structures resembling angioid streaks occur in rupture of the choroid, choroidal arteriosclerosis, perivascular choroidal pigmentary atrophy, and pigmented streaks of retinal detachment. Cardiovascular changes must be accompanied by typical changes of the eye or skin before their association with pseudoxanthoma elasticum can be ascertained.

Treatment. There is no effective treatment of the basic disease. Symptomatic therapy is indicated for hypertension, congestive failure, subarachnoid or gastrointestinal hemorrhage, cerebrovascular accident, angina, and intermittent claudication. Plastic surgery is sometimes helpful for correction of cosmetic cutaneous defects.

Prognosis. Cutaneous lesions are usually of small consequence. The majority of patients develop angioid streaks, and approximately three quarters of these undergo visual impairment from damage to the macula. Complete blindness, which is unusual, results from glaucoma, vitreous hemorrhage, or retinal detachment. The life span is decreased by premature arterial disease; death may result from cerebrovascular accident, heart disease, or internal hemorrhage.

Farreras-Valenti, P., Rozman, C., Jurado-Grau, J., del Rio, G., and Elizalde, C.: Grönblad-Strandberg-Touraine syndrome with systemic hypertension due to unilateral renal angioma. Amer. J. Med., 39:355, 1965.

Flatley, F. J., Atwell, M. E., and McEvoy, R. K.: Pseudoxanthoma elasticum with gastric hemorrhage. Arch. Intern. Med. (Chicago), 112:352, 1963.

Huang, S., Kumar, G., Steele, H. D., and Parker, J. O.: Cardiac involvement in pseudoxanthoma elasticum. Amer. Heart J., 74:680, 1967.

McKusick, V. A.: Heritable Disorders of Connective Tissue. 3rd ed. St. Louis, C. V. Mosby Company, 1966.

Percival, S. P. B.: Angioid streaks and elastorrhexis. Brit. J. Ophthal., 52:297, 1968.

PIERRE ROBIN SYNDROME
(Primary Micrognathia)
Alexander G. Bearn

This syndrome is caused by a developmental anomaly characterized by micrognathia, cleft palate, and secondary glossoptosis. Inspiratory distress since birth, stridor, cyanosis, and failure to thrive are common presenting symptoms. The hypoplastic mandible is responsible for a characteristic "shrewlike" facies. Congenital heart disease occurs in about 10 per cent of cases. The occasional presence of accessory auricles and cerebral agenesis indicates the widespread nature of the developmental anomaly. Early recognition of the syndrome is imperative if patients are to survive the early months of life. Skilled nursing and tube feeding are the mainstays of treatment. Mandibular development occurs slowly and is accompanied by clinical improvement. Surgical correction may be needed to repair the cleft palate. The Pierre Robin syndrome superficially resembles trisomy 18 and the cri du chat syndrome, but can be distinguished by the normal karyotype.

Denison, W. M.: The Pierre Robin syndrome. Pediatrics, 36:336, 1965.

WILSON'S DISEASE
(Hepatolenticular Degeneration)
Alexander G. Bearn

Wilson's disease is a rare, autosomal recessively inherited disease characterized by degenerative changes in the brain, particularly in the basal ganglia, and cirrhosis of the liver. A brownish pigmented ring at the corneal margin, the Kayser-Fleischer ring, is pathognomonic of the disease.

Clinical Manifestations. The disease is frequently insidious in onset, manifesting itself as tremor and incoordination in the second or third decade of life. While the patients are at rest, the tremor is often minimal, and they are able to alleviate it by resting their hands on a table or placing them in their pockets; on purposive movement, however, a wild ataxia frequently develops. Rarely, symptoms may occur as early as four years of age or may be delayed until the fourth decade of life. In late childhood and early adolescence, the disease is more likely to be rapidly progressive, and rigidity, dysarthria, and dysphagia occur more frequently than tremor. Uncontrollable choreoathetotic movements and staggering may be particularly distressing. The sensory system is unaffected, and pyramidal signs are usually absent. In the terminal stages of the disease muscular rigidity and contractures dominate the clinical picture. The patient is frequently febrile and emaciated, shows marked mental deterioration, and finally becomes completely bedridden.

Although in adults the clinical signs of hepatic insufficiency are rare, cirrhosis can be recognized by liver biopsy, and there is usually a slight increase in Bromsulphalein retention. In childhood, however, the disease may present as severe juvenile cirrhosis with minimal or absent signs of central nervous system dysfunction. Signs of portal hypertension can frequently be demonstrated although ascites and hepatic coma are uncommon. Rarely, the presenting symptom is massive bleeding from esophageal varices. Jaundice may be an early symptom, and is frequently followed by several years of normal health.

Gross personality changes, acute schizophrenic episodes, transient hemiparesis, and unexplained hemolytic anemia may also occur early in the disease. Unusual pigmentation of the lower extremities, azure lunulae of the nails, and bone lesions may be found.

Genetics. The disease is ubiquitous but is particularly common in eastern European Jews, Italians from southern Italy and Sicily, and Japanese. These populations have a high inbreeding coefficient, which probably accounts for the apparent increase in the frequency of the condition. As anticipated in a rare autosomal recessive disease, an increased consanguinity in the parents of affected persons is common; in one series the frequency of marriages of first cousins was 36 per cent. The frequency of clinically normal heterozygous carriers of the abnormal gene has been estimated to be approximately 1 in 500.

Pathogenesis. An increase in the net absorption of copper is the primary disturbance in Wilson's disease and results in an accumulation of copper in the brain, liver, and other tissues, including Descemet's membrane of the cornea, where it gives rise to the Kayser-Fleischer ring. There is a decrease in the concentration of serum ceruloplasmin and total serum copper and an increase in the nonceruloplasmin copper. The excretion of copper in the urine is increased. Exceptionally, and particularly in girls with marked cirrhosis of the liver, the serum copper and ceruloplasmin levels are normal. Accumulation of copper in the kidneys may lead to damage to the proximal renal tubules, and aminoaciduria, glycosuria, phosphaturia, uricosuria, and calciuria may be present. The serum phosphate and serum uric acid may be decreased.

Pathology. Although it is assumed that the accumulation of copper in the tissues is responsible for the symptoms, the brain grossly may appear surprisingly normal at autopsy. Slight generalized atrophy is common, particularly of the basal ganglia. An accumulation of large astrocytes throughout the central nervous system, more marked in the basal ganglia and cerebral cortex, is usually observed. In the acute form of the disease, cavitation of the putamen, globus pallidus, candate nucleus, and cerebral cortex also may be evident. Cirrhosis of the liver is usually of the postnecrotic variety. Glycogen degeneration of hepatic cell nuclei, with the accumulation of cytoplasmic fat droplets, is frequently observed.

Diagnosis. The disease should be suspected in all cases of unexplained tremor and rigidity, particularly in early adult life. The differential diagnosis includes Parkinson's syndrome, cerebellar ataxia, chorea, and choreoathetosis. In children the disease may present with symptoms due to cirrhosis of the liver. The presence of Kayser-Fleischer rings is pathognomonic of the disease, but these may be absent in children under the age of 10. They are golden-brown or green-brown, and are located at the periphery of the cornea; examination with the slit-lamp helps to identify

them. Liver biopsy and determination of hepatic copper is a valuable adjunct to the other diagnostic tests in those cases in which there is no clinical evidence of hepatic dysfunction. In most patients with Wilson's disease the copper content of the liver is greater than 100 mcg. per gram dry weight. A decrease in serum ceruloplasmin (less than 20 mg. per 100 ml.) can nearly always be observed and, in the absence of malnutrition, sprue, or the nephrotic syndrome, is virtually diagnostic. The disease is difficult to diagnose in the first six months of life since a decreased ceruloplasmin and increased hepatic copper are commonly observed in normal children.

Treatment. Treatment is designed to decrease the total body copper. A high-protein, low-copper diet with the addition of potassium sulfide (20 mg. three times daily, with meals) is usually recommended. The administration of D-penicillamine, (β, β-dimethylcysteine) 1 to 2 grams a day, depending on body weight, is the treatment of choice and should be continued indefinitely. Occasional toxic reactions are seen. Some are due to sensitivity to penicillamine itself and include fever, maculopapular rash, nephrosis, and leukopenia. Pyridoxine deficiency, as a result of penicillamine treatment, may give rise to optic neuritis and can be prevented by administration of pyridoxine, 50 mg. daily. In the few patients who continue to be sensitive to penicillamine, BAL (2, 3-dimercaptopropanol), 2.5 mg. per kilogram of body weight, should be given twice daily for five days followed by two days' rest and continued as long as possible. A persistent decrease in serum ceruloplasmin accompanied by an elevated hepatic copper in an asymptomatic sib of an affected individual is certainly an indication to begin therapy. In newborn infants treatment should be delayed until it is apparent that the decreased serum ceruloplasmin and increased hepatic copper have persisted beyond the normal physiologic period of three to six months. When penicillamine treatment is started early and is continued indefinitely, improvement can be striking. In the absence of treatment the disease is progressive and invariably fatal.

Bearn, A. G.: Wilson's Disease. *In* Stanbury, J. B., Wyngaarden, J. B., and Frederickson, D. S. (eds.): The Metabolic Basis of Inherited Disease. 3rd ed. New York, McGraw-Hill Book Company (In press).

Scheinberg, I. H., and Sternlieb, I.: The dual role of the liver in Wilson's disease. Med. Clin. N. Amer., 47:815, 1963.

Scheinberg, I. H., and Sternlieb, I.: Wilson's disease. Ann. Rev. Med., 16:119, 1965.

Sternlieb, I.: Penicillamine therapy for hepatolenticular degeneration. J.A.M.A., 189:749, 1964.

LAURENCE-MOON SYNDROME

(Laurence-Moon-Biedl Syndrome, Laurence-Moon-Bardet-Biedl Syndrome)

Alexander G. Bearn

The salient features of this not uncommon recessively inherited syndrome are mental retardation, retinitis pigmentosa, hypogonadism, obesity, and polydactyly; the limits are poorly defined, and one or more of the diagnostic signs may be absent. The condition must be distinguished from familial polydactyly, Ellis–van Creveld syndrome, Froehlich's syndrome, and other causes of hypogonadism. A number of cases have been associated with sex chromosomal aneuploidy. The significance of this occasional association is not known.

Bell, J.: The Laurence-Moon syndrome. *In* Penrose, L. S. (ed.): The Treasury of Human Inheritance. Vol. 5, Part 3. London, Cambridge University Press, 1958.

Bowen, P., Ferguson-Smith, M. A., Mosier, D., Lee, C. S. N., and Butler, H. G.: The Laurence-Moon syndrome. Association with hypogonadotrophic hypogonadism and sex-chromosome aneuploidy. Arch. Intern. Med. (Chicago), 116:598, 1965.

DYSAUTONOMIA

(Riley-Day Syndrome)

Alexander G. Bearn

Dysautonomia is a rare familial disease of childhood occurring almost exclusively in Ashkenazi Jews. It is inherited in an autosomal recessive fashion. Clinically it is characterized by defective lacrimation, hyperhidrosis, vomiting, and episodic hypertension. Insensitivity to pain, dysphagia, and poor motor coordination are common. A markedly decreased taste discrimination resulting from an absence of the fungiform papillae is probably pathognomonic. An absence of pain following the intradermal administration of histamine, the occurrence of miosis following installation of methacholine into the eye, and the increased urinary excretion of homovanillic acid are useful diagnostic adjuncts.

Dancis, J., and Smith, A. A.: Familial dysautonomia. New Eng. J. Med., 274:207, 1966.

DISEASES OF THE ENDOCRINE SYSTEM

General Considerations

Nicholas P. Christy

FUNCTIONS OF THE ENDOCRINE SYSTEM

Like the nervous system, the endocrine system provides mechanisms by which the mammalian organism adapts itself to a constantly changing environment. Parts of the endocrine system may indeed be regarded as extensions of the nervous system: the adrenal medulla, which secretes epinephrine in response to environmental change, is of ectodermal origin, arising from the neural crest; many environmental stimuli cause cells in the hypothalamus to secrete neurohumoral peptides which are carried in the hypothalamic-hypophysial portal venous system to cells in the anterior pituitary, which then secrete growth hormone, adrenocorticotrophin, or gonadotrophins (*vide infra*, The Control of Anterior Pituitary Secretion). These two glands, the adrenal medulla and the anterior pituitary, are particularly clear examples of endocrine organs whose secretions mediate between the external and internal environments. Less dramatic but no less important examples are the neurohypophysial response to changes in hydration, and the fluctuations of adrenocortical secretion of aldosterone with changes in dietary Na^+.

These and the other endocrine glands, by steady or by waxing and waning secretion of hormones, wield an important regulatory influence on cellular metabolism (see the section on Diseases of Metabolism, especially Diabetes Mellitus). It is important to remember that hormones *do not initiate* cellular activity, but rather exert their effects by *influencing the rates of biochemical reactions.*

Again like the nervous system, the endocrine system has both *vegetative* and *adaptive* functions. The essential roles of pituitary growth hormone and thyroxine on normal growth, and the effects of the sex steroids, testosterone and estradiol, on the gradual and orderly maturation of the secondary sex characters are examples of *vegetative* activity. Rapid *adaptive* functions are numerous: insulin secretion in response to hyperglycemia; epinephrine secretion during profound hypoglycemia; antidiuretic hormone secretion in the presence of increased osmolarity of the plasma; and the instantaneous hypersecretion of pituitary adrenocorticotrophic hormone (ACTH) in response to many noxious stimuli, of growth hormone to severe muscular exercise, and of aldosterone to hemorrhage-induced hypovolemia. It is apparent that both the vegetative and adaptive, that is, the slowly acting and rapidly acting functions are in effect homeostatic (see General Considerations in the section on Diseases of Metabolism). However, it is probably a mistake to think of the endocrine system as a system in a rigid sense. It is true that the endocrine organs are all by definition ductless glands which secrete hormones that have many actions at sites remote from those glands. It is also true that several hormones may conspire to affect single, well-defined functions or substances. For instance, it can be shown that all these hormones have the capacity to influence the concentration of blood glucose: pituitary growth hormone, ACTH, thyroxine, cortisol, epinephrine, insulin, and glucagon. Pituitary growth hormone, ACTH, cortisol, aldosterone, and antidiuretic hormone all influence serum Na^+ concentration. But in any of these groupings, it is difficult to know in a given set of circumstances which hormone is quantitatively the most important and to calculate accurately how the several hormones, with their complementary, supplementary, synergistic, or opposing actions, operate together to regulate the serum concentration of glucose or Na^+. Further, it is hard to see how epinephrine secretion by the adrenal medulla relates to the secretion of parathyroid hormone, how growth hormone secretion bears on thyroxine secretion, and how aldosterone and gonadotrophins inter-relate. There are at least as many examples of independent as of interdependent functions among the endocrine glands. Therefore, it seems most reasonable not to regard the endocrine glands as quite such a tightly integrated system as the anatomically distinct nervous system, but rather as a loose group of secretory organs, arising from different embryologic sources, having arrived at different stages in evolution, and having a broad range of functions, some separate and distinct and some interdigitated. These regulatory functions are exerted by circulating chemical substances upon biochemical processes of all cells and tissues.

The *disorders of the endocrine glands* become clinically apparent through excessive, deficient, or untimely secretion of a hormone, owing either to primary disease of the endocrine gland or to an abnormal secretion by that gland in response to disease of some other organ (*vide infra*, Categories of Endocrine Disease). All endocrine diseases have this property in common: the secretion of the hormone is not regulated or is improperly regulated by the control mechanisms that operate under normal conditions; that is, the production of the hormone is *autonomous, anarchic,* or *inappropriate*, a state of affairs that leads to disordered homeostasis.

BIOCHEMISTRY AND MODE OF ACTION OF HORMONES

The *chemical nature* of human hormones is now well known. The substances are amines (epinephrine), amino acids (thyroxine), peptides (vasopressin or antidiuretic hormone), proteins (pituitary growth hormone, parathyroid hormone), and steroids (aldosterone). Many hormones have been chemically synthesized, e.g., epinephrine, thyroxine, most of the steroids, and even some of the peptides and proteins, as antidiuretic hormone, oxytocin, and ACTH. For some of the hormones of high molecular weight, e.g., growth hormone, amino acid sequences have been worked out; knowledge of the structures of thyrotrophin and the gonadotrophins is still not complete. Methods have now been developed for accurate measurement of nearly all the important human hormones. These chemical techniques, although difficult and time consuming, are enormously superior to the indirect or biologic assay methods investigators and clinicians used to rely on. The chemical methods, including the revolutionary radioimmunoassay techniques developed by Berson and Yalow, have now made it possible to quantify the plasma or urinary concentrations of virtually all the known hormones. These advances have put endocrine diagnosis on a firm footing, and have enabled workers in the field not only to measure blood levels but also to determine secretory rates or production rates of several classes of hormones. Thus, it is now possible to measure accurately the daily secretion rate of steroid hormones, e.g., aldosterone and cortisol, and even to estimate the daily turnover rate of such protein hormones as growth hormone and ACTH.

Despite intensive study by many workers, the mode of action of hormones is still not well understood. There is a good deal of information about the *structural determinants of hormonal activity*, e.g., the number, sequence, and identity of the amino acids that determine the immunologic reactivity and the biologic potency of the ACTH molecule (*vide infra*, Anterior Pituitary). Subtle changes in the molecular structure of hormones profoundly affect their biologic activity and metabolism, both qualitatively and quantitatively; for example, among the steroid hormones, cortisone, with a ketone group at the carbon-11 position of the steroid nucleus, is quite inactive in vitro, whereas cortisol, the principal adrenocortical glucocorticoid of man, which differs structurally from cortisone only by having a hydroxyl (–OH) instead of a ketone group (–O) at carbon-11, is highly active; among the thyroid hormones, L-

thyroxine has a half-time in plasma twice that of its stereoisomer, D-thyroxine, and ten times the calorigenic potency. What is not yet definitely known is the exact chemical form of any hormone that is active at the cellular level; it remains to be shown whether or not the known alterations of any hormone molecule brought about by peripheral metabolism are necessary steps in hormone action.

The significance of the *physical state* of a given hormone in the *plasma* is also not clear. The conventional view is that only the portion of a hormone that is *not* bound to a plasma protein is "active" in the sense that only the unbound, "free" form is available to cells. There is some evidence to support this view. Under various conditions, e.g., rare hereditary abnormalities in the serum concentration of certain α-globulins, pregnancy, estrogen therapy, nephrotic syndrome, severe hepatic disease, and several acute illnesses, there are definite changes in the plasma levels of thyroxine-binding globulin or of corticosteroid-binding globulin. Yet, although these changes give rise to easily measurable changes in *total* serum concentration of thyroxine or cortisol, there is no clinical evidence of an altered thyroid or adrenal state, presumably because the "free" thyroxine and "free" cortisol levels are normal.

The biochemical *mode of action of hormones* at the cellular level is not known. At the moment, there is *no unitary hypothesis* that can account for the biologic activity of all hormones, but many physical and biochemical actions of individual endocrine products have been reported. Some of these actions are the following: (1) *Effects on permeability of cell membranes.* Insulin increases the permeability of cell membranes to glucose, but may also act in other ways (Stanbury, Wyngaarden, and Fredrickson). (2) *Effects on amino acid transport.* Growth hormone stimulates the rate of transport of amino acids into cells. This effect is at least consonant with the hormone's known capacity to induce nitrogen retention and hypertrophy of organs in hypophysectomized man, but how the hormone produces the effect is not clear (*vide infra*, Anterior Pituitary). (3) *Effects on enzyme systems.* Many hormones have been shown to accelerate or inhibit enzymic reactions. For example, adrenocortical steroids of the cortisol type (glucocorticoids) affect the activities of more than 30 enzymes concerned in carbohydrate and amino acid metabolism (Janoski et al.). Aldosterone has been shown to accelerate enzyme synthesis in renal distal tubular cells, where the hormone appears to stimulate nuclear DNA-dependent formation of RNA with consequent synthesis of an enzyme essential for the energetics of sodium reabsorption. (4) *Effects on lysosomes.* Several workers have shown that corticosteroids may stabilize the surrounding membranes of intracellular organelles, lysosomes, which are "packets of enzymes." This stabilizing action may play a part in the anti-inflammatory effects of corticosteroids. (5) *Effects on cyclic AMP.* Several hormones have been shown to exert important biologic actions in which an early or even initial step is stimulation of the synthesis of intracellular cyclic 3′,5′-adenosine monophosphate (cyclic AMP). The glycogenolytic effect of epinephrine appears to depend on stimulation of cyclic AMP, which in turn activates the enzyme, liver phosphorylase. Protein hormones also stimulate cyclic AMP formation in specific organs: ACTH augments adrenal cyclic AMP, apparently a necessary precondition to certain of the enzymic reactions concerned with steroid biosynthesis, and parathyroid hormone stimulates cyclic AMP formation in the renal tubule, an effect that may be related to the phosphaturic effect of the hormone.

Many other effects of hormones on cells and tissues, e.g., imbibition of water by cells, H⁺ transfer, have been described. J. N. Loeb has comprehensively discussed current ideas about the mechanisms of hormone action.

UBIQUITY OF HORMONAL EFFECTS

Since all hormones circulate in the blood, their effects are to be found everywhere. Many acute and chronic diseases impinge on the endocrine glands, and the effects of disordered endocrine function impinge upon most systems and organs. In the first group are such changes as increased adrenocortical and adrenal medullary secretion of cortisol and epinephrine during *acute myocardial infarction*, increased aldosterone secretion in the accelerated phase of *hypertension*, decreased pituitary gonadotrophin secretion with hypogonadism accompanying the inanition and emotional disorder of *anorexia nervosa*, and the secondary hyperparathyroidism of renal insufficiency (see Diseases of Kidneys; also, Parathyroids). In the second group some examples are characteristic changes in the skin, central nervous system, muscles, gastrointestinal tract, heart, and blood vessels (increased susceptibility to atherosclerosis) in severe *hypothyroidism*; changes in the psyche, the eyes, the regulation of blood glucose, (hypoglycemia), the blood pressure, water metabolism, and the structure and function of the sexual apparatus in fully developed *pituitary insufficiency*; and the changes in the psyche, central nervous system (lethargy, coma), muscles, gastrointestinal tract (constipation, ileus), kidneys (stones), and skeleton that are characteristic of *hyperparathyroidism*.

Looking at endocrine disease from another point of view, many common symptoms and signs may be parts of endocrine syndromes. *Hypertension* is common in acromegaly and *Cushing's syndrome*; not all patients with these diseases can be diagnosed on inspection. Fixed hypertension is also present in *pheochromocytoma, aldosteronism, renal artery stenosis*, and in some patients with *congenital adrenal hyperplasia*. In the differential diagnosis of *coma*, one must at least consider the hypercalcemia of *hyperparathyroidism*, the hypoglycemia associated with *islet cell tumors* or *pan-*

hypopituitarism, and the sometimes severe water intoxication associated with the syndrome of *inappropriate secretion of antidiuretic hormone*. Serious *psychologic disturbances*, including psychosis, may be an important feature of *pituitary insufficiency, hypothyroidism, hyperthyroidism, hyperparathyroidism*, any of the *hypoglycemias, Addison's disease*, and *Cushing's syndrome*.

The aim here is to sensitize the reader to the systemic but less obvious signs of endocrine disease; he does not need to be reminded that the patient with precocious or greatly delayed puberty or with clear signs of hypercortisolism or thyrotoxicosis may have disease of an endocrine gland.

CATEGORIES OF ENDOCRINE DISEASE

In the light of the discoveries made during the last two decades, it is no longer enough to think of endocrine disease simply as too much or too little hormone. For clinical purposes, the following may be a helpful classification:

Primary Hyperfunction of Endocrine Glands. Most diseases in this group are due to benign tumors of endocrine glands, such as the eosinophilic *pituitary adenoma* of acromegaly, the "*toxic adenoma*" which produces hyperthyroidism, the *parathyroid adenoma* of hyperparathyroidism, the insulin-secreting *islet cell adenoma* of the pancreas, benign *pheochromocytoma*, and the *adrenal cortical adenoma* of Cushing's syndrome. There are hyperfunctional states not associated with endocrine tumors, e.g., that form of Cushing's syndrome which is associated with bilateral adrenocortical "hyperplasia"—something of a misnomer, as the glands are sometimes normal in weight and often appear normal histologically. This entity is probably the result of idiopathic oversecretion of endogenous pituitary ACTH (see Diseases of the Adrenals). Graves' disease, toxic diffuse goiter, formerly believed to be due to pituitary oversecretion of TSH, is not; plasma TSH levels are normal or low (see Diseases of the Thyroid). *Malignant* hormone-secreting tumors of the anterior pituitary and thyroid are extremely rare, but cancers of the parathyroids, islet cells, adrenal medulla, and adrenal cortex are occasional causes of severe and intractable endocrine disease. No more is known about the etiology of these endocrine cancers than about any other cancer, except in the case of virilizing neoplasms of the adrenal cortex which may rarely arise in hyperplastic adrenals overstimulated for long periods by endogenous ACTH.

Primary Hypofunction of Endocrine Glands. Primary glandular failure is the usual cause of endocrine deficiency syndromes. The etiology is often obscure. Fibrosis or even absence of the anterior pituitary has been discovered at autopsy *without anatomic evidence of any cause*. Destruction of a gland by formation of autoantibodies to that gland has been postulated as a cause of the hypothyroidism of chronic thyroiditis, and also as a cause of hypoparathyroidism and of "idiopathic" Addison's disease. Autoantibodies to thyroid, parathyroid, and adrenals have indeed been demonstrated in many patients with these disorders, but the significance of the observations is still in doubt. *Tumors* may destroy a gland. Breast cancer and lymphomas may metastasize or spread to invade the neurophypophysis or supraoptic nuclei, giving rise to diabetes insipidus; chromophobe adenoma is the most common cause of pituitary insufficiency. Several cancers, especially lung cancer, very often metastasize to the adrenals, but rarely cause enough destruction to produce adrenocortical insufficiency. *Infections* are not very common causes of glandular failure: tuberculosis and syphilitic gummas used to be occasional causes of pituitary destruction, but are now museum pieces; tuberculosis, histoplasmosis, and blastomycosis may destroy the adrenals with ensuing Addison's disease. *Chromosomal disorders*, such as Klinefelter's syndrome and gonadal dysgenesis, are not rare as causes of primary gonadal deficiency in phenotypic males and females (see The Gonads and Sexual Differentiation).

Secondary Failure of Endocrine Glands. This term means failure of the gonads, thyroid, or adrenals owing to *pituitary insufficiency*. Although it is true that the growth hormone-secreting and gonadotrophic functions of the pituitary are usually the first to drop out during the course of destructive pituitary disease, and, as a corollary, if only one function is affected it is likely to be either growth (hypopituitary dwarfism) or gonadal function, the other functions, i.e., thyrotrophic or adrenocorticotrophic, may fail singly or in any combination (see Anterior Pituitary). The key to diagnosis is to study the patient carefully for the presence of pituitary disease in every instance of growth failure, hypogonadism, hypothyroidism, or hypoadrenalism. There may be good clinical evidence to implicate or rule out pituitary involvement; but, if not, measurement of urinary gonadotrophins or response of the thyroid or adrenals to TSH or ACTH will clarify the diagnosis (see Anterior Pituitary).

Functional Disorders of the Endocrine Glands. The response of endocrine glands to certain disease states may be clinically important or clinically trivial. Important endocrine responses are the secondary hyperparathyroidism of renal failure, leading to renal osteodystrophy; the secondary aldosteronism of portal cirrhosis with ascites and edema, and of nephrotic syndrome—aldosterone is an important contributing factor in edema formation. Responses which are either trivial or not yet of proved clinical significance are altered metabolism of thyroxine in liver disease and in patients acutely ill from a variety of causes; the altered metabolism of cortisol in portal cirrhosis; the altered metabolic disposition of androgens in thyroid disease and acute intermittent porphyria; and many others.

Failure of an End-Organ to Respond to a Hormone. There are three good examples of this in human medicine: *failure to respond* by *linear growth or nitrogen retention* to administered *pituitary growth hormone*, which is endogenously secreted in normal amounts and which responds normally to the usual stimuli, as in the African pygmy; *pseudohypoparathyroidism*, a hereditary disease characterized by resistance to measurable effects of parathyroid hormone, which is secreted in normal amounts by normal or hyperplastic parathyroids; and the syndrome of *testicular feminization*, a developmental defect in which "target tissues" are unresponsive to endogenous or administered androgen. In none of these entities has the mechanism of failure to respond been worked out.

Production by an Endocrine Gland of an Abnormal or Unusual Hormone. Such lesions are characteristic of the inborn errors of metabolism. In *congenital adrenal hyperplasia*, deficiencies of C-21 and C-11 hydroxylases cause metabolic blocks in the synthesis of cortisol with the additional result that several cortisol precursors, e.g., pregnanetriol and 17α-hydroxyprogesterone, normally present in very small amounts, are secreted in amounts much greater than normal, as are C_{19} androgens. In *goitrous cretinism* enzymic blocks in the synthesis of thyroxine give rise to thyroidal secretion into the blood stream of large quantities of mono- and diiodotyrosines.

Further, it may be that, in the growth hormone–resistant forms of dwarfism, the pituitary is secreting a biologically ineffective growth hormone. Finally, an unusual form of hyperthyroidism is that associated with excessive secretion of L-triiodothyronine instead of the usual thyroxine.

Production of a Hormone by a Nonendocrine Organ. Cancers of many organs (lung, thymus, pancreas) may produce substances that cannot be chemically or immunologically distinguished from normal endocrine products, usually proteins, such as ACTH, MSH, gonadotrophins, erythropoietin, and others. The clinical features and hypotheses concerning the mechanisms by which these "hormones" are secreted are discussed in a succeeding article (Endocrine Syndromes Associated with Neoplasms of Nonendocrine Tissue).

Iatrogenic Endocrine Disease. By far the most common of these is iatrogenic Cushing's syndrome caused by administration of ACTH or cortisol and its derivatives in pharmacologic doses for many allergic, inflammatory, and neoplastic diseases. In the United States, there are hundreds of thousands of patients receiving long-term steroid therapy. An unknown number of these are getting very large doses (more than 50 mg. per day of cortisol, or equivalent), and an unknown fraction of them have overt hyperadrenocorticism. The features of this entity are the physical signs of spontaneously occurring Cushing's syndrome, but with a lesser incidence in the iatrogenic form of diabetes, hypertension, and psychosis, and a higher incidence of peptic ulcer and certain rarer untoward effects, e.g., pseudotumor cerebri, glaucoma, pancreatitis, and aseptic necrosis of the hip joint. In addition, an unpredictable and probably small number have enough suppression of pituitary-adrenal function to be important in times of intercurrent acute illness or surgical emergency. The writer has developed elsewhere the idea that these patients are addicted to corticosteroids (see References, also Anterior Pituitary and Adrenals below). The point is that one should be as ungenerous as possible in the dosage of corticosteroids.

Prescription of sex hormones and thyroid hormone to patients without gonadal or thyroidal deficiency rarely produces iatrogenic disease. Overenthusiastic use of estrogen may induce endometrial hyperplasia and breakthrough bleeding; some patients are apparently hypersensitive to methyl testosterone, which may cause cholestatic jaundice. The abnormalities in glucose tolerance, serum triglycerides, liver function tests, and plasma clotting factors associated with administration of oral contraceptives have become familiar. The writer once saw a patient, without hypothyroidism, who was genuinely addicted to thyroid hormone that had been prescribed for obesity.

The protein hormones are sometimes troublesome. There are more than 80 reported instances of anaphylaxis owing to ACTH. For further details of the toxicity of hormonal products, the reader is referred to textbooks of pharmacology. The keys to successful hormone therapy are accurate diagnosis and great restraint in dosage.

HORMONES AS MEDICINES

Hormones are legitimately given to patients in three sets of circumstances: (1) for replacement of lost functions, (2) as tests of endocrine function, and (3) to achieve a pharmacologic purpose.

Replacement Therapy. This is probably the most gratifying use of hormones both to patient and physician, and is the easiest to defend. So long as an endocrine deficiency is clearly and definitely demonstrated, in most instances a realistic goal owing to the availability of good chemical tests for most hormonal diseases, the physician can achieve brilliant clinical results with small doses of hormones. Cortisol for adrenal insufficiency, thyroid hormone USP or thyroxine for hypothyroidism, and human growth hormone for hypopituitary dwarfism are all given in amounts very close to the estimated daily production rates of the respective hormones. It is common practice to give too much cortisone to patients with primary or secondary adrenal insufficiency, i.e., enough to induce signs of mild Cushing's syndrome; daily doses of not more than 10 to 25 mg. per day are usually quite sufficient. With thyroid hormone replacement, restraint is also necessary, especially in older people with coronary artery disease, in whom the maintenance dose should be attained gradually. The writer believes that tri-

iodothyronine is almost never indicated for treatment of long-standing myxedema; too many older patients with atherosclerosis have had bouts of severe coronary insufficiency or even myocardial infarction when this rapidly acting hormone is given. Triiodothyronine may have a place in the treatment of myxedema coma (see Diseases of the Thyroid).

Replacement dosages of sex hormones have been arrived at by "clinical experience." In the writer's experience, treatment to develop deficient secondary sex characters is best given just before or at the expected time of puberty. If replacement therapy with estrogen or testosterone is delayed until late in the second or well into the third decade, the induced sexual development is suboptimal. This puts a premium on early diagnosis as the basis for early treatment.

Few protein hormones are used routinely in treatment. Although it would be theoretically most correct, say in hypopituitarism, to replace absent trophic hormones by giving gonadotrophins, TSH or ACTH, this is not practical, owing to antibody formation, short supply, and the need for parenteral administration. Gonadotrophins are given only in short courses to induce ovulation in women (see The Ovaries); to stimulate ovarian or testicular function is cumbersome, so sex hormones, which can be administered orally, are used instead. Treatment of secondary hypothyroidism and hypoadrenalism is much more easily done with thyroid hormone and cortisone; allergic reactions to ACTH have been alluded to above. Parathyroid hormone from human sources is not available; vitamin D and calcium salts are simpler to give. The only protein hormone other than insulin that is generally used as replacement therapy is human growth hormone, because there is still no satisfactory substitute for it.

Testing. TSH and ACTH are useful for assessing thyroidal and adrenal response in differentiating between primary and secondary deficiencies of these glands, and the triiodothyronine suppression test of thyroidal I^{131} uptake is a useful adjunct in diagnosis of some patients with hyperthyroidism. These testing procedures entail the direct chemical or physical measurement of a hormone or of a glandular function. Such methods have pretty completely superseded the older indirect methods of estimating endocrine activity, e.g., the BMR which is full of potential errors, and the eosinophil count. Some of the older techniques, being provocative tests, were potentially dangerous, e.g., the water-loading and salt withdrawal tests for Addison's disease. These should now be abandoned.

By testing, the writer does not mean the administration of a hormone as a *therapeutic trial*, that is, to determine by the patient's response whether he has or does not have an endocrine deficiency. This approach may be tolerable for a patient in acute shock when there seems to be some possibility of adrenocortical insufficiency and there is no time for careful chemical study. Under any other circumstances, failure to establish a diagnosis is an inexcusable basis for giving hormonal therapy.

Hormones Given to Achieve a Pharmacologic End. Hormones are given to patients in high doses to achieve some pharmacologic, not physiologic, goal in three sets of circumstances: treatment of diseases in which large doses of hormones are *often beneficial*; treatment of diseases for which larger doses of hormones are *possibly* or *sometimes* beneficial; and treatment of diseases for which large doses of hormones are *never beneficial* or of very doubtful value.

Beneficial Uses. The obvious examples are of course ACTH and cortisol and its congeners. Although ACTH is usually associated with fewer serious untoward effects and with less danger of a "withdrawal syndrome" when treatment is stopped, the corticosteroids are preferred because of the convenience of the oral route of administration, more flexibility in spacing of doses, shorter action, the larger doses attainable, and the absence of serious allergic reactions. The ideal use of high-dosage corticosteroids is in acute, self-limited diseases such as serum sickness owing to penicillin allergy or bouts of status asthmaticus. In serious inflammatory diseases such as pemphigus, ulcerative colitis, acute rheumatic fever, and lupus erythematosus, in hematologic disorders such as acute lymphoblastic leukemia of childhood, and in bronchial asthma of allergic origin, among other conditions, there is good evidence that corticosteroids often alter the course of the disease in a favorable direction. As in giving any other medicinal agent, the physician has to balance the probability of benefit from corticosteroid therapy against the disability or danger incurred by giving the patient corticosteroids with the attendant risk of iatrogenic Cushing's syndrome. To make this semiquantitative judgment, the doctor has to have the fullest possible knowledge of the *natural history* of what he proposes to treat, that is, the natural course of the disease untreated (Feinstein).

Possibly or Sometimes Beneficial Uses. The efficacy of corticosteroids in scleroderma and in endotoxin shock remains arguable. The same statement applies to the use of testosterone or estrogen, or both, in the treatment of postmenopausal osteoporosis (*q.v.*); the use of vasopressin or mineralocorticoids in the management of idiopathic postural hypotension; administration of small doses of corticosteroids to women with "acquired adrenal virilism," an entity which may or may not exist; and many others. In this group of diseases, further work is needed toward an understanding of pathogenesis; only this will provide a rational basis for giving or withholding treatment.

Uses That Are Never Beneficial. These uses are derived by the trial and error method, with emphasis on the latter. Examples are numerous: outstanding ones are the administration of thyroid hormone for obesity, for fatigability, and for infertility and menstrual disturbances when there is no firm proof of hypothyroidism; the use of estrogens to treat frigidity in the female when there is no evidence of deficient ovarian function; and the use of testosterone for male impotence, nearly always owing to psychologic disturbance, when hypogonadism is not proved. The major objection to such therapies is that they are ineffective. Further, they are often expensive and raise false hopes. The physician has to resist the temptation, which can be hard to resist, to keep trying one hormonal remedy after another in the hope that something will work. "The empiricist," said Claude Bernard, "is never at a loss." It is the patient who loses.

HORMONES AND MAGIC

By now, it is apparent to the reader that endocrinology is inseparable from the rest of internal medicine. Until the 1920's, endocrinology was entirely an empirical branch, not quite respectable, not quite accepted as professional, lurking on the outskirts of medicine. The endocrinologist dealt with patients who were too fat, too thin, too short, too tall, too tired, too hairy or not hairy enough, and patients with all sorts of sexual problems. With the discovery of insulin in 1922, the elucidation of the structures of thyroxine and the steroid hormones in the next decade, and with good studies of hormone metabolism in the period from 1950 to the present, there began to be a firm scientific basis for the practice of endocrinology. But two factors have contributed to the persistence of empiricism. One was the isolation and synthesis in the period from 1948 to 1956 of cortisone and cortisol and their derivatives; it is easier to list the diseases for which these compounds have *not* been given than those for which they have been at least tried. The other factor is that endocrine diagnostic procedures are time-consuming, technically difficult, and sometimes not available locally, and that the data produced are not always easy to interpret. The physician tends to become impatient. Enough has been said previously about the need for accurate diagnosis as an essential basis for endocrine replacement therapy. Accuracy is equally essential in establishing a diagnosis of glandular hyperfunction; since most of the treatments for such conditions are ablative, the physician has to be on solid ground before consigning the patient to such major surgical procedures as thyroidectomy, parathyroidectomy, partial pancreatectomy, or adrenalectomy. Fortified by accurate diagnosis, the endocrinologist no longer has any reason to treat blindly or to practice magic, as in the old days. He can do better by opposing the prevalent and growing views among patients that all diseases can be prevented or cured, and that people are immortal. In short, he can do as internists must: dispense the maximum of relief with a minimum of bedevilment.

Albright, F., and Reinfenstein, E. C.: The Parathyroid Glands and Metabolic Bone Disease. Baltimore, Williams & Wilkins Company, 1948.

Christy, N. P.: Iatrogenic Cushing's syndrome. In Christy, N. P. (ed.): The Human Adrenal Cortex. New York, Harper & Row, Publishers, Inc., 1970 (in press).

Feinstein, A. R.: Clinical Judgment. Baltimore, Williams & Wilkins Company, 1967.

Gray, C. H., and Bacharach, A. L. (eds.): Hormones in Blood, 2nd ed. Vols. 1 and 2. New York, Academic Press, Inc., 1967.

Haynes, R. C., Jr., Sutherland, E. W., and Rall, T. W.: The role of cyclic adenylic acid in hormone action. Recent Progr. Hormone Res. 16:121, 1960.

Janoski, A. H., Shaver, J. C., Christy, N. P., and Rosner, W.: On the pharmacologic actions of 21-carbon hormonal steroids ("glucocorticoids") of the adrenal cortex in mammals. In Deane, H. W., and Rubin, B. L. (eds.): Handbuch der experimentellen Pharmakologie: The Adrenocortical Hormones. Vol. XIV/3. Berlin, Springer Verlag, 1968, p. 256.

Jensen, E. V., and Jacobson, H. I.: Basic guides to the mechanism of estrogen action. Recent Progr. Hormone Res. 18:387, 1962.

Loeb, J. N.: Some models for hormone action. In Christy, N. P. (ed.): The Human Adrenal Cortex. New York, Harper & Row, Publishers, Inc., 1970 (in press).

Pincus, G., Thimann, K. V., and Astwood, E. B.: The Hormones. Vol. 5. New York, Academic Press, Inc., 1964.

Sawin, C. T.: The Hormones—Endocrine Physiology. Boston, Little, Brown and Company, 1969.

Stanbury, J. B., Wyngaarden, J. B., and Fredrickson, D. S.: The Metabolic Basis of Inherited Disease. 2nd ed. New York, McGraw-Hill, Inc., 1966.

Werner, S. C. (ed.): The Thyroid. 2nd ed. New York, Harper and Row, Publishers, Inc., 1962.

Wilkins, L.: The Diagnosis and Treatment of Endocrine Disorders in Childhood and Adolescence. 3rd ed. Springfield, Ill., Charles C Thomas, 1965.

Williams, R. H. (ed.): Textbook of Endocrinology, 4th ed. Philadelphia, W. B. Saunders, Company, 1968.

The Control of Anterior Pituitary Secretion

Seymour Reichlin

Although the anterior pituitary gland lacks a direct nerve supply, the secretion of each of its hormones is under the control of the central nervous system. Through specialized secretory neurons localized in the ventral hypothalamus, the function of the pituitary and, in turn, of its target glands becomes responsive to changes in the external and internal environment. In addition, the neurohumoral connections of the anterior pituitary are important in the feedback regulation of a number of hormones such as cortisol, the gonadal steroids, thyroxine, and prolactin, and serve as part of the integrated mechanism by which behavioral and metabolic adaptation to the external environment is accomplished.

During the last few years, as the importance of neural factors in the control of pituitary secretion has become increasingly apparent, a division of study of endocrinology has developed which is termed *neuroendocrinology*. This area deals mainly with the interaction of neural and hormonal factors in endocrine and metabolic control systems.

The pituitary gland and hypothalamus are closely related anatomically, as may be seen in the accompanying figure. This relationship has both embryologic and functional significance. The neural lobe develops as a downgrowth of axons from the diencephalon, whose cells of origin are located in the paraventricular and supraoptic nuclei of the hypothalamus. These nerve fibers pass as unmyelinated axons through the neural stalk and terminate in the neural lobe. Like neurons elsewhere, supraopticohypophysial and paraventriculo-hypophysial neurons are electrically excitable, conduct action potentials, and are responsive to neurotransmitters. Unlike most other neurons, these cells are *neurosecretory,* by which is meant that they synthesize hormonal substances which are released into blood vessels for action on a remote site rather than at synapses, as is characteristic of most neurons. Hormones of the neurohypophysis are synthesized mainly in cell bodies located in the hypothalamus and pass in granule form (associated with a protein carrier substance) to the nerve endings in the neural lobe where they are stored. Neurosecretory neurons thus manifest the properties of both nerve and gland. These cells, of which the neurohypophysial neurons are the classic example, have been termed by Wurtman "neuroendocrine transducers." Cells of this type are the major effector links between the nervous system and the endocrine glands.

Although the neural lobe lies close to the anterior lobe of the pituitary, the secretions of the neurohypophysis (oxytocin and vasopressin) have no local action in the pituitary but are released into the systemic circulation to affect remote tissues such as the kidney, breast, and uterus. The phylogenetically more primitive neuroendocrine "transducer" for anterior pituitary control is located within the median eminence of the hypothalamus. Nerve endings here are postulated to contain "hypophysiotropic" hormones; these substances, also called "releasing factors," reach the anterior pituitary through a specialized system of capillaries and veins (the hypophysial-portal circulation). The cells of origin of the median eminence neurons are clustered around the medial-basal hypothalamus in the so-called hypophysiotropic area. They resemble

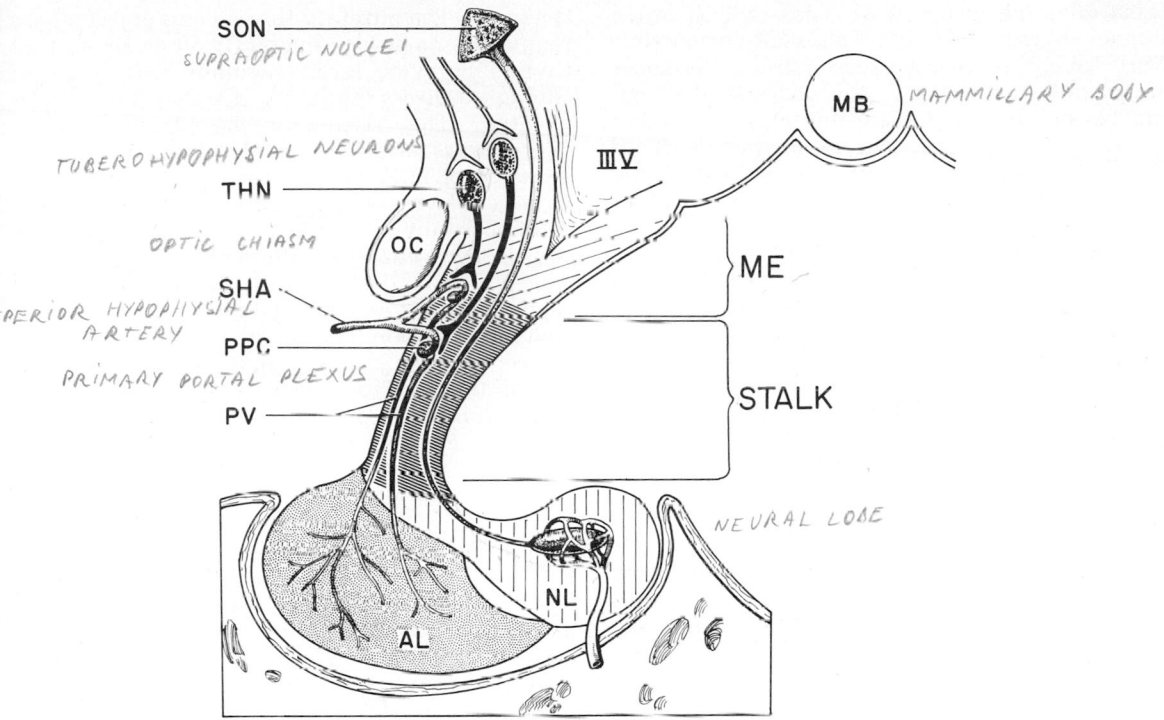

Hypothalamic-pituitary unit. This diagram of a sagittal section of the human brain demonstrates the anatomic relation between the base of the hypothalamus and the pituitary gland. The anterior border of the hypothalamus is limited by the optic chiasm (OC) anteriorly and by the mammillary body (MB) posteriorly. Two distinct and separate sets of neurosecretory neurons are illustrated. The first, the supraopticohypophysial cell bodies and axons, arise in the supraoptic nuclei (SON) and pass through the neurohypophysial stalk to terminate in dilated endings in the neural lobe (NL). Neurosecretory vesicles formed chiefly in the cell body carrying oxytocin and vasopressin pass down the axon, are stored in the nerve ending, and are released into the systemic circulation when activated by a propagated action potential. The second set of neurosecretory neurons illustrated are the tuberohypophysial neurons (THN). These lie clustered around the base of the hypothalamus and send short axons into the median eminence of the hypothalamus (ME) and the stalk, which terminate in the interstitial space of the stalk–median eminence region (ME) in relation to capillaries of the primary portal plexus (PPC). Blood destined to perfuse the anterior lobe of the pituitary comes from the superior hypophysial artery (SHA), which gives several branches to the stalk–median eminence. Capillaries formed here regroup into vessels (PV) and enter the sinusoids of the anterior pituitary. The base of the hypothalamus thus serves two roles. First, it is the site of transfer of hypophysiotropic hormones (releasing factors) from nerve endings to portal vessels. This complex of nerve endings and blood vessels is analogous to the posterior pituitary gland, and can be considered as a *median eminence gland.* The infundibulum also provides the structural support for the axons of the supraopticohypophysial tract which traverses this region without making functional contact with the primary portal vessels.

Not illustrated are the paraventriculohypophysial neurons and tracts which arise in cells situated adjacent to the third ventricle (III V), and pass, together with the supraoptic neurons, into the neural lobe. This diagram does not describe the detailed anatomy of the portal vessel system.

neurohypophysial neurons in being electrically active, pharmacologically excitable, and responsive to a wide variety of nerve impulses arising from other sites in the brain, and to feedback hormonal stimuli. Neuron endings of the stalk–median eminence region (tuberohypophysial neurons) and the associated blood vessels have been likened to the posterior lobe and can be looked upon as a "median eminence gland"; taken together these structures constitute the "final common pathway" for neural control of the anterior pituitary gland.

This outline of anterior pituitary regulation is the *portal-vessel chemotransmitter hypothesis.* According to this view, lesions of the hypothalamus (and of the portal vessel complex of the stalk) reduce most anterior pituitary functions by causing a deficiency of releasing factors. Direct electrical stimulation of the tuberohypophysial neurons, or reflex activation of these neurons, caused, for example, by emotional stress, acti-

vates the anterior pituitary by the release of hypophysiotropic hormones. Initially based on indirect physiologic experiments, this hypothesis has been reasonably well established by demonstration of hypothalamic substances which selectively affect each of the known pituitary hormones. These are CRF (corticotropin releasing factor), TRF (thyrotropin releasing factor), SRF (somatotropin releasing factor), LRF (luteinizing hormone RF), and FRF (FSH-RF). Because the existence of these substances seems so well established, it has been proposed that they be called releasing hormones. Physiologic studies have shown that two of the hormones of the pituitary, prolactin and MSH, are tonically *inhibited* by the hypothalamus. It is not surprising therefore to find that extracts of the stalk–median eminence region have prolactin secretion inhibitory (PIF) and MSH secretion inhibitory (MIF) effects. Beyond studies on laboratory animals, there is good evidence for an action in man. Human hypothalamic tissue contains releasing factors, TRF releases TSH in the human subject, and LRF releases LH and possibly FSH. That the other hypophysiotropic hormones act in man has not yet been demonstrated, but can be anticipated. Among the important consequences of these observations is the likelihood that the releasing factors can be used to test and control the secretion of each of the pituitary tropic hormones.

Based on the homology between median eminence and neurohypophysis, most workers had considered that the releasing hormones would prove to be polypeptides analogous to oxytocin and vasopressin, and the endocrine literature of the past decade is replete with conflicting claims about the nature and structure of the releasing factors, including the view that these materials are polyamines and not polypeptides. Prior reports to the contrary, there appears to be (at this this time of writing) only one reasonably well established hypophysiotropic hormone, TRF. Its structure was identified almost simultaneously in 1969 by workers in the laboratories of Guillemin and of Schally. It has now been synthesized and the synthetic material shown by both biologic and chemical tests to be identical with the native compound. TRF, which is a tripeptide amide (pyroglutamyl-histidyl-proline-amide) is now under clinical study as a test of pituitary TSH reserve.

The function of the hypophysiotropic neurons can be modified by neuropharmacologic agents such as reserpine, chlorpromazine, and alpha-methyl dopamine. This may explain why large doses of these drugs may cause irregular menstrual cycles or anovulation in the human female (owing to blockade of the cyclic discharge of LRF) or galactorrhea (owing to inhibition of PIF release). Recently, it has been shown that a certain proportion of axon endings of the median eminence contain dopamine and that dopamine itself acts to discharge releasing factors from median eminence neurons. The significance of this work has not been fully tested, but it seems likely that there are two mechanisms by which hypophysiotropic neurons are stimulated to secretion—one by direct nerve activation and another by dopamine release from adjacent cells.

The mechanism by which feedback control of anterior pituitary secretion is exerted probably differs from hormone to hormone, but for most hormones there appear to be both a pituitary and a hypothalamic component of action, with considerable variability in the relative importance of one or the other.

Cortisol feedback inhibition of the pituitary-adrenal axis appears to act primarily on the median eminence of the hypothalamus, but there is evidence for other neural sites of action, as well as for a direct pituitary effect. Similarly, pituitary-gonadal regulation is most sensitive to the effects of estrogens and progesterone on the hypo-

thalamus. The pituitary-thyroid axis appears to be regulated somewhat differently. It is likely that thyroid hormone levels regulate TSH secretion through a direct inhibitory effect on the anterior pituitary. The "setting" of the pituitary-thyroid axis appears to be determined by the hypothalamic secretion of TRF, which is in turn responsive to a variety of neural signals, including those involved in temperature regulation, and possibly also to a neurogenic sensor of thyroxine concentration. Analysis of TRF-thyroxine interactions is currently the best worked out model for neurohormonal integration. The pituitary thyrotrope cell is subject to two opposing influences. Neurogenic stimulation by TRF is opposed by thyroxine feedback inhibition. The inhibitory action of thyroxine on TRF effects is dependent upon thyroxine-induced changes in protein metabolism within the pituitary. This observation is important because it suggests (in the light of studies of thyroxine action on other tissues) that this hormone exerts its major actions in all systems on protein synthesis.

In the context of the foregoing comments on the portal-vessel chemotransmitter hypothesis, disorders of pituitary secretion can be viewed as occurring at many "levels" of function. Defects may arise resulting from destruction of the pituitary itself, as by a tumor, or from genetically determined deficiency of a particular type of pituitary cell, as in "ateliotic dwarfism." At a higher level, disorders may arise through disruption of the stalk-median eminence neurons or of their essential vascular channels to the anterior pituitary gland. Such destruction of the "final common path" of anterior pituitary regulation occurs after surgical stalk section, in tumors of the stalk region, e.g., craniopharyngioma, infundibuloma, or teratomas, and in such inflammations as sarcoidosis, tuberculosis, and abscess of the sphenoid sinus. Anterior pituitary hormone deficiency with associated prolactin hypersecretion is one consequence of this disruption of function.

At a higher level of control, the hypophysiotropic neurons themselves may be exposed to pathologic stimuli or may become pathologically responsive. For example, in neurogenic amenorrhea, the cycling stimulus to LH discharge is absent. In precocious puberty, the tonically active inhibitory system which determines the time at which the hypophysiotropic neurons will become active may be destroyed or inactivated too soon. In one form of hypogonadotropic hypogonadism (Kallman's syndrome) there appears to be a failure to develop normal hypophysiotropic-regulating neurons. At this level and also perhaps at higher levels are exerted the effects of neuropharmacologic agents like reserpine. A number of workers have speculated, but without adequate evidence, that at least two hypersecretory states of the pituitary, Cushing's disease and acromegaly, may be due to hypersecretion of releasing factors.

NEUROENDOCRINE DISEASES OF THE PITUITARY GLAND

It is apparent that any consideration of the neuroendocrine diseases of the pituitary overlaps the descriptions of diseases of the pituitary itself. This section emphasizes the primarily neuro-endocrine disorders of the anterior pituitary.

In the accompanying table the major endocrine diseases of hypothalamic origin are listed.

Hypophysiotropic deficiency can be induced by destruction of the hypophysiotropic area of the hypothalamus, or of the stalk, or of the vascular supply to the anterior pituitary. When fully man-

ENDOCRINE SYNDROMES OF HYPOTHALAMIC ORIGIN

Hypophysiotrophic Hormone Deficiency:
Surgical pituitary stalk section
Basilar meningitis and granuloma, sarcoidosis, tuberculosis, sphenoid osteomyelitis, eosinophilic granuloma
Craniopharyngioma
Hypothalamic tumor
  Infundibuloma
  Teratoma (ectopic pinealoma)
  Neuroglial tumors, particularly astrocytoma
Maternal deprivation syndrome

Disorders of Regulation of LRH and FRH:
Female
  Precocious puberty
  Delayed puberty
  Neurogenic amenorrhea
    Pseudocyesis
    Anorexia nervosa
    "Functional amenorrhea"
    "Functional oligomenorrhea"
    Drug-induced amenorrhea
Male
  Precocious puberty
  Frölich's syndrome
  Olfactory-genital dysplasia (Kallman's syndrome)

Disorders of Regulation of Prolactin-Inhibiting Hormone (Nonpuerperal galactorrhea):
Tumor
Sarcoid
Drug-induced
Reflex
  Herpes zoster of chest wall
  Post-thoracotomy
  Nipple manipulation
"Psychogenic"
Chiari-Frommel syndrome
Hypothyroidism
CO_2 narcosis

Disorder of Regulation of CRF:
Paroxysmal ACTH discharge (Wolff's syndrome)
Loss of circadian variation

Other than deficiency caused by destruction of the stalk or median eminence, no cases of TRF regulatory disease have yet been identified. Graves' disease, for many years attributed to TSH hypersecretion secondary to psychosomatic factors, has now been shown to be due to excessive quantities of a thyroid-stimulating material of nonpituitary origin (LATS). Two disorders have been postulated, without proof as yet, to be due to hypothalamic hyperactivity. These are Cushing's disease and some cases of acromegaly.

ifested (as in surgical stalk section) a moderate to severe degree of pituitary failure results, but the extent of the hormone deficiency is not so extreme as that seen after hypophysectomy. This residuum of function is thought to represent the "autonomous" activity of the pituitary gland. The main manifestations are moderate inhibition of TSH secretion and abolition of cyclic LH release with amenorrhea. Most patients lose the normal growth hormone secretory response to hypoglycemia. Circadian and tonic baseline corticotrophin secretion is abolished, as is feedback control by circulating cortisol levels, but the response to certain kinds of stress, pyrogen, for example, is retained. The deficiency of prolactin inhibitory hormone (PIH) leads to an increased prolactin secretion, with galactorrhea developing in as many as 25 per cent of women. Partial and selective hormone deficiencies may be observed. The most sensitive system to damage in most cases is that for reflex regulation of growth hormone; gonadotrophin regulation is also easily disturbed.

The concept of "levels" of neurogenic disruption of pituitary control is best illustrated in abnormalities of secretion of the gonadotrophins. Deficiency of both LH and FSH occurs after destruction of the hypophysiotropic neurons. But disturbances also occur if the hypophysiotropic neurons are themselves abnormally stimulated. The characteristic pattern of male gonadotrophin regulation is one of tonic low-level activity which leads to growth, development, and maturation of the spermatozoa, a process which takes place over a 70-day period. The characteristic pattern of human female regulation is that of the recurring menstrual cycle, in turn dependent upon a recurring surge of LH secretion. Animal experiments indicate that the fetal brain in both sexes possesses an intrinsic female type of cyclicity, but that the brain pattern is modified by exposure to testosterone from fetal or neonatal gonads at a critical time of brain development. The loss of the female type of LH cyclicity thus can be regarded as a secondary sexual characteristic. Similar mechanisms have not yet been definitely demonstrated in human beings. In certain forms of hypothalamic disease, the characteristic normally recurring cyclic pattern of LH secretion may be lost. Because this often occurs transiently in a setting of severe psychologic stress, as after incarceration in concentration camps, or in bombing attacks, or after minor stress, such as going away to school, and develops in the absence of evident structural disease of the pituitary or hypothalamus, it is probable that loss of LH cycling may be an acquired psychogenic disorder. A similar correlation appears likely in pseudocyesis, most often a manifestation of hysteria, and in anorexia nervosa. In about half the cases of anorexia nervosa, amenorrhea begins coincident with the disturbance in eating, and for this reason must be regarded as a concomitant rather than a consequence of inanition.

Besides these more obvious psychogenic changes in menstrual function, many women with "secondary" amenorrhea are encountered who have no apparent psychologic distress, but in whom the pattern of menstrual irregularity, amenorrhea, and oligomenorrhea is similar to that seen in the neurogenic syndromes. In one series, fully one fourth of the women in this category who were placed into a research study after one year or more of anovulation developed normal cycles within a month of their first visit to the gynecologist.

It is difficult to make a clear-cut differential diagnosis in some instances between functional amenorrhea and disease of the anterior pituitary or hypothalamus. Most helpful is the fact that, next to pregnancy, "functional" amenorrhea is the most common cause of secondary failure to menstruate. The patient with pituitary or hypothalamic disease most often has more than one tropic hormone deficiency, may have evidence of local pituitary damage, e.g., enlarged sella by x-ray, visual field defects, and behavioral or other neurologic abnormalities of the hypothalamus. Sixty to 80 per cent of patients with "functional" amenorrhea release luteinizing hormone following treatment with the drug clomiphene. In the future, it can be anticipated that pituitary failure as a cause of LH insufficiency may well be diagnosed by treatment with LH-releasing factor.

Drug-induced anovulation should be borne in mind as a cause of amenorrhea. Reserpine and phenothiazines are particularly common causes.

Gonadotrophin regulatory difficulties may arise from loss of hypophysiotropic function, from failure of the intrinsic cycling mechanism and, at a higher functional level, from precocious or delayed development of sexual maturation. The timing of the onset of puberty is a neural function, and involves a patterned development of brain function analogous to the patterns of development of other brain functions such as crawling, sitting, walking, and the development of abstract ability. Both delayed and accelerated puberty can be observed. When the sexual function is normal in other respects, the term precocious puberty is applied, in contradistinction to the condition arising from primary secretory abnormalities of the gonads, properly termed pseudoprecocious puberty. All true precocious puberty is neurogenic in origin. In males, more than half the cases are due to brain lesions which directly or indirectly impinge upon the hypothalamus. In girls, fewer than 10 per cent have demonstrable lesions, although a high proportion have EEG abnormalities and may be regarded as suffering from mild degrees of brain damage.

In the male, primary isolated gonadotrophin failure is a well recognized cause of delayed puberty. Whether the difficulty is due to failure to develop gonadotrope cells or failure to develop appropriate hypophysiotrophic neuron function is not known in most instances. In one group, there is an association with failure to develop rhinencephalic brain structures, manifested clinically by anosmia. Such cases have been termed olfactory-genital dysplasia (Kallman's syndrome), and appear to be due to failure to develop hypophysiotrophic function.

Many conditions cause lactation unrelated to pregnancy (nonpuerperal galactorrhea). Certain chromophobe pituitary tumors may secrete prolactin (Forbes-Albright syndrome) and induce lactation. However, hypothalamic disturbance or "psychogenic" factors are the most important cause of galactorrhea. Causes listed in the table have in common a presumed deficiency of prolactin-inhibitory hormone, whether due to irritation of the neural pathways involved in normal suckling reflexes, or to drugs, encephalopathy, hypothyroidism, or direct damage to the hypothalamus or stalk.

Bardin, C. W., Ross, G. T., Rifkind, A. B., Cargille, C. M., and Lipsett, M. B.: Studies of the pituitary–Leydig cell axis in young men with hypogonadotropic hypogonadism and hyposmia: Comparison with normal men, prepubertal boys, and hypopituitary patients. J. Clin. Invest., 48:2046, 1969.

Bowers, C. Y., Schally, A. V., Hawley, W. D., Gual, C., and Parlow, A.: Effect of thyrotropin-releasing factor in man. J. Clin. Endocr., 28:978, 1968.

Kastin, A. J., Schally, A. V., Gual, C., Midgley, A. R., Jr., Bowers, C. Y., and Diaz-Infante, A., Jr.: Stimulation of LH release in men and women by LH-releasing hormone purified from porcine hypothalami. J. Clin. Endocr., 29:1046, 1969.

Martini, L., and Ganong, W. F. (eds.): Neuroendocrinology. New York, Academic Press, Inc., vol. 1, 1966; vol. 2, 1967.

Martini, L., and Ganong, W. F. (eds.): Frontiers in Neuroendocrinology. New York, Oxford University Press, 1969.

McCann, S. Mc., and Porter, J. C.: Hypothalamic pituitary-stimulating- and inhibiting hormones. Physiol. Rev., 49:240, 1969.

Meites, J. (ed.): Hypophysiotropic Hormones of the Hypothalamus. Proceedings of the NIH Workshop. Baltimore, Williams and Wilkins Company, 1970.

Anterior Pituitary

(Adenohypophysis)

Nicholas P. Christy

Diseases of the anterior pituitary manifest themselves in two ways: mechanically, when space-occupying pituitary tumors impinge upon adjacent structures; and functionally, when there is deficient or excessive secretion of some or all of the several hormones secreted by the gland.

Functional Anatomy. For clinical purposes, the *gross anatomy* of the pituitary is the anatomy of the sella turcica; roentgenographic changes in that structure provide evidence of pituitary enlargement in the form of increase in the linear measurements of the sella, and erosion, demineralization, or displacement of its bony borders. The normal sella can be oval, round, or flat. In normal adults, the anteroposterior diameter (sagittal plane) should not exceed 17 mm., the vertical diameter should not be greater than 14 mm., and the normal width (frontal projection) is about 19 mm. Measured roentgenographically, the calculated lateral area of the normal adult pituitary does not exceed 130 sq. mm.; the volume is about 1100 cu. mm. Even when sellar measurements are normal, pituitary tumor is suspected if there is suprasellar calcification, elevation or destruction of the anterior or posterior clinoids, or "ballooning" of the fossa.

The pituitary fossa is enlarged in many but not all instances of intrasellar tumor; intrasellar calcification may be present. The fossa is also large in some suprasellar tumors with intrasellar extension, e.g., craniopharyngioma, metastases to the sella (as from carcinoma of the breast or prostate), long-standing increase of intracranial pressure from any cause, and hypothyroidism in early life. The fossa is often small in patients with postpartum pituitary necrosis (Sheehan's syndrome), hypopituitary dwarfism without pituitary tumor, and myotonic muscular dystrophy. Rarely observed in presumably normal people, the significance of the small sella is not clear. Roentgenographic changes in the base of the skull may involve the sella in several disorders, e.g., osteoporosis, Paget's disease, Hand-Schüller-Christian disease, and Hurler's syndrome.

When pituitary tumors extend upward through the diaphragma sellae they encroach upon the optic chiasm to produce the familiar bitemporal hemianopia and, more rarely, symptoms of hypothalamic involvement, e.g., diabetes insipidus. Such upward extensions can often be seen roentgenographically with the use of pneumoencephalography or carotid artery angiography.

The microscopic anatomy of the anterior pituitary is still debated. The classic concept of secretory, acidophilic (eosinophilic) and basophilic cells and functionless chromophobes has to be modified in the light of recent data. Without attempting to untangle the difficult problems of classification and nomenclature, it is possible to make these statements about pituitary cell types in man. There appear to be five or six distinct kinds of cells; it is probable that each pituitary hormone is secreted by one of the distinct cell types. Somatotrophic cells are acidophils which secrete growth hormone. The pituitary tumors associated with acromegaly (excessive secretion of growth hormone) are usually composed of acidophils; sometimes the tumors consist of acidophils mixed with chromophobes, or of cells which have features of both types of cell ("amphophils"). Another kind of acidophil, the lactotrophic cell, has been identified in the rodent pituitary; the picture is not yet clear in the human pituitary, which has not

been definitively shown to secrete prolactin as a separate hormone. A recognizable type of basophil secretes gonadotrophins; there is some evidence that two distinct subtypes of cells are associated with FSH and LH secretion. Gonadotrophin-secreting basophils are few or absent in childhood, but increase in number at puberty; there are subtle changes during the menstrual cycle; marked changes are observed after castration and menopause. The thyrotrophin-secreting cell is probably a basophil, but some workers consider it a specialized chromophobe. The number of these cells increases, and the morphology changes with thyroprivic states. The corticotrophin (ACTH)-secreting basophil probably also secretes MSH in man; the human pituitary lacks a definite intermediate lobe, the probable source of MSH secretion in lower animals. The pituitary tumors described by Cushing in hyperadrenocorticism are basophilic. In the absence of pituitary tumor, the most notable feature of pituitary cytology in patients with Cushing's syndrome is in the basophils; the cytoplasm becomes hyalinized ("Crooke's change"), a change also observed in patients whose hyperadrenocorticism is due to very large doses of administered adrenocortical steroids. In the pituitary tumors that develop after bilateral adrenalectomy in 10 to 15 per cent of patients with Cushing's syndrome associated with bilateral adrenal cortical hyperfunction (presumably owing to oversecretion of ACTH by the pituitary), the cell type is a distinctive kind of chromophobe which often has the capacity to secrete MSH as well as ACTH.

Daughaday, W. H.: The Adenohypophysis. In Williams, R. H. (ed.): Textbook of Endocrinology. 4th ed. Philadelphia, W. B. Saunders Company, 1968, p. 27.

Bergland, R. M., Ray, B. S., and Torack, R. M.: Anatomical variations in the pituitary gland and adjacent structures in 225 human autopsy cases. J. Neurosurg., 28:93, 1968.

Meador, C. K., and Worrell, J. L.: The sella turcica in postpartum pituitary necrosis (Sheehan's syndrome). Ann. Intern. Med., 65:259, 1966.

New, P. F. J.: The sella turcica as a mirror of disease. Radiol. Clin. N. Amer., 4:75, 1966.

Russfield, A. B.: Adenohypophysis. In Bloodworth, J. M. B. (ed.): Endocrine Pathology. Baltimore, Williams and Wilkins Company, 1968, p. 75.

Taveras, J. M., and Wood, E. H.: Diagnostic Neuroradiology. Baltimore, Williams and Wilkins Company, 1964.

THE HORMONES OF THE ANTERIOR PITUITARY

Ablation of the pituitary produces many defects in the organism; these can be corrected by administration of pituitary extracts. The defects and their repair are due to the influence of several distinct hormones secreted by the gland. Seven protein or peptide hormones have been isolated from anterior pituitary tissue: growth hormone, prolactin, follicle-stimulating hormone, luteinizing hormone, thyrotrophin, adrenocorticotrophin, and melanocyte-stimulating hormone.

GROWTH HORMONE

Pituitary growth hormone is the substance that, secreted or given in excessive amounts, induces gigantism and acromegaly in animals and man; its absence results in failure to grow. The hormone exerts a major influence on somatic growth in man from an early stage of infancy. It also has widespread metabolic effects in both young and adult subjects.

Chemically, human growth hormone is a single-chain peptide containing 188 amino acids whose sequence is now known; the molecular weight is 21,500 (C.-H.Li). Immunologically and electrophoretically, growth hormone is heterogeneous; different moieties may be responsible for different actions. Partial digestion by trypsin and several other enzymes does not diminish its activity. All human growth hormone preparations have prolactin activity. The chemical differences among growth hormones from different species partly account for the species specificity of these hormones. Whereas bovine and porcine growth hormones are active in lower orders, e.g., the rat, only primate growth hormone is active in man. The biologic specificity is to some extent reflected in immunologic specificity.

The physiologic effects of growth hormone are numerous. The salient action is anabolic. In the hypophysectomized, dwarfed animal, growth hormone administration induces symmetrical growth of the skeleton (chondrogenesis and osteogenesis), the musculature, and viscera. Optimal growth response requires the presence of thyroid hormone and insulin, which play incompletely defined roles. Growth hormone causes both cellular hypertrophy and hyperplasia; there is an increased rate of cellular mitosis, as well as an increase in tissue and organ weight. The mode of action of the hormone on protein anabolism is not understood. Growth hormone induces accelerated transport of specific amino acids into cells, stimulates synthesis of messenger and ribosomal RNA, and influences the activity of several enzymes. The primary site of action (or whether there is a single, primary action) is not known.

Growth hormone effects on protein anabolism are readily observed in hypophysectomized or hypopituitary human subjects. Intramuscular administration produces nitrogen retention within 24 to 48 hours; BUN concentration falls even earlier, within 12 to 24 hours. Nitrogen storage is very great (3 to 4 grams per day) for the first several days of treatment, then falls to an amount compatible with growth requirements, about 0.3 gram of nitrogen retained per day in children 9 to 13 years of age. The effective dose is 1 to 2 mg. per day. Linear growth can be induced in hypopituitary dwarfs (see Pituitary Insufficiency in Childhood).

Growth hormone brings about changes in electrolyte and water metabolism. Tissue protein and water are increased. Phosphorus and potassium are stored, the latter in amounts larger than can be accounted for by the estimated quantity of new tissue formed. Moderate sodium retention occurs; the role of aldosterone is probably minor. Hypercalciuria is the rule, but most studies of calcium metabolism suggest an over-all positive calcium balance.

The increase in tissue mass induced by administration of growth hormone is not accompanied by fat deposition. Growth hormone is in fact adipokinetic. Although many other pituitary hormones have fat-mobilizing properties, e.g., prolactin, thyrotrophin, corticotrophin, MSH, and several other peptides, growth hormone appears to be the major adipokinetic principle of the human anterior pituitary. Administration of this hormone to hypophysectomized man rapidly stimulates the release of fat from adipose tissue, with a rise in free fatty acids in the plasma. This growth hormone effect on fat metabolism may operate in the anabolic response by ensuring a supply of calories, yet sparing protein breakdown through gluconeogenesis. In acromegalic patients, fat deposition is notably absent; obesity is extremely rare.

Growth hormone also affects carbohydrate metabolism profoundly. The hormone is well known to be diabetogenic; many acromegalics have diabetes. The diabetic state is characterized by fasting hyperglycemia, impaired glucose tolerance, insulin resistance, lipemia, and ketosis. Growth hormone given to normal subjects produces only minor changes; in diabetics the diabetes is often substantially exacerbated. Nondiabetic and diabetic subjects are much more sensitive to this effect of growth hormone after hypophysectomy.

The closely interrelated effects of growth hormone on fat and carbohydrate metabolism may be of great importance in concert with insulin, not only in promoting growth, but in maintaining homeostasis during feast or famine.

Most important observations have followed the recent development of accurate methods for the measurement of human growth hormone in serum by radioimmunoassay (see Assessment of Pituitary Function). Normal values are less than 5 mμg. per milliliter of serum in the basal state. The mean daily production rate of the hormone is estimated at 0.5 mg. The findings have provided new insights into the role of the hormone in the growth of children. Basal serum concentrations are slightly higher in young children than in older children or adults. It is now clear that growth hormone is required for the normal growth rate of infants. Surprisingly, basal levels are not appreciably higher in adolescence; the contribution of growth hormone to the adolescent growth spurt is not known.

More surprising still is the extreme lability of the serum concentration of growth hormone in response to a great variety of stimuli in adults. Serum values vary during normal sleep. Rapid rises in the serum levels of growth hormone are induced by hypoglycemia, fasting, and exercise; in some obese subjects these responses are blunted. Growth hormone response to hypoglycemia is suppressed by corticosteroids. Hypoglycemia-induced rises in growth hormone level are quickly returned to normal when glucose is given. Ambulation raises the serum levels of growth hormone in women, not in men; estrogen administration reproduces this increase, so that the alleged beneficial effects of estrogen on acromegaly cannot be due to reduced secretion of growth hormone Increases in ambulatory (not basal) serum levels of growth hormone occur during the luteal phase of the menstrual cycle. Growth hormone also participates in the response to stress, e.g., surgery, but the pattern of response differs from that of ACTH; this suggests that the pathways influencing the two hormones are different.

Apart from the obvious value of measuring serum levels of growth hormone for the diagnosis of hypopituitarism and acromegaly (see Assessment of Pituitary Function), the above findings have clearly shown that growth hormone is not secreted at a uniform rate in adults. The lability of response to many metabolic events further suggests that the hormone is not functionless in adults, as formerly thought, but may actively participate in the day-to-day regulation of organic metabolism.

The use of human growth hormone as a growth-producing substance is discussed below (see Pituitary Insufficiency in Childhood).

PROLACTIN (LACTOGENIC HORMONE)

Prolactin stimulates the growth and development of the ducts and alveoli of mammary tissue in concert with several other hormones. In a few species, prolactin is also *luteotropic* (it induces the secretion of progesterone from the formed corpus luteum); in man there appear to be only two gonadotrophins (*vide infra*, FSH and LH). Prolactin has growth hormone-like effects in hypophysectomized animals and in human subjects with hypopituitarism. It evokes nitrogen retention, glucose intolerance, hypercalciuria, and skeletal growth, but not fat mobilization. The *physiologic* significance of prolactin in man is unknown. In animals, e.g., sheep, prolactin is a polypeptide with a molecular weight of about 23,000. It is not possible to separate completely growth hormone from prolactin activity in extracts of human pituitary. The questions of separateness, similarity or identity of human growth hormone and prolactin are not finally resolved at this time. Large amounts of prolactin have been isolated from the pituitary tumor of a patient with associated galactorrhea and amenorrhea (Forbes-Albright syndrome); the tumor contained no growth hormone. The observations raise the possibility that growth hormone and prolactin may be separate substances in man.

Purified animal prolactin evokes lactation in women in the prepared breast; it is not, however, an effective therapy for inadequate milk production. Very little is known about its function (if it is a separate hormone in man) in postpartum lactation of women. With the use of the standard biologic assay (increment in weight of the pigeon crop sac), it has recently been observed that there were *increased amounts of plasma prolactin* in five of six patients with *nonpuerperal galactorrhea*. Normal values are always less than 5, usually less than 1 milliunit per milliliter of plasma; the patients' levels were as high as 27 milliunits per milliliter. Confirmation of such results may be expected to elucidate many of the problems of nonpuerperal galactorrhea; heretofore, there has been no more than conjectural explanation for the galactorrhea associated with acromegaly, pituitary tumors with acromegaly, Cushing's syndrome, hyperthyroidism, adrenal carcinoma, testicular choriocarcinoma, myxedema, Chiari-Frommel syndrome, or phenothiazine administration. The interesting observation of galactorrhea after section of the pituitary stalk for metastatic carcinoma of the breast is now interpreted to mean that stalk section interrupts passage to the pituitary of a *hypothalamic prolactin-inhibiting factor* (see Section on Control of Anterior Pituitary Secretion).

FOLLICLE-STIMULATING HORMONE (FSH)

Follicle-stimulating hormone is a glycoprotein. It is the pituitary hormone essential for the normal cyclic growth of the ovarian follicle and for restoration of follicular growth in the hypophysectomized female; it stimulates spermatogenesis in the male without significant influence on the androgen-secreting interstitial cells of the testis. The molecular weight of human FSH is estimated at about 30,000. It contains 7 per cent carbohydrate. Sialic acid is an integral part of the molecule; biologic activity is lost on exposure to neuraminidase. It is difficult to separate FSH completely from luteinizing hormone (LH). The purest preparations contain virtually no LH activity, but are chemically heterogeneous. The point bears on the functional definition of FSH formerly regarded as incapable of eliciting follicular secretion of estrogen in the absence of LH. Highly purified human pituitary FSH not only stimulates the human ovary to polycystic enlargement but also evokes an increase in estrogen secretion in amenorrheic and postmenopausal women. The exact mechanism by which gonadotrophins stimulate steroidogenesis is unknown. Most workers agree that gonadotrophin exists as two separate chemical entities in man.

Gonadotrophins are absent or extremely low in the pituitaries and in the plasma and urine of infants and children. The hormones rise to reach detectable levels at the time of puberty, and remain fairly constant in adult males. In adult women, the values are about the same as those for men during the preovulatory (follicular) and postovulatory (luteal) phases of the menstrual cycle. Both FSH and LH rise sharply at mid-cycle, at the time of ovulation. (The role of the gonadotrophins in the regulation of the menstrual cycle is discussed in detail in the article on The Ovaries. The older view of this complex inter-relationship of pituitary and ovary is too simple.) Unopposed by ovarian secretion of steroid hormones, the values for gonadotrophins are very high in ovariectomized and postmenopausal women. For a similar reason, castrate males have raised levels of gonadotrophins. Administration of estrogen, testosterone, and estrogen-progesterone combinations, as antiovulatory contraceptive steroids, suppresses plasma and urinary values of both FSH and LH.

The *gonadotrophin of human urine* is a mixture of FSH and LH and should be designated simply "urinary gonadotrophin" rather than "FSH". Human urinary gonadotrophin is thought to consist of degradation products of human pituitary gonadotrophin. *Biologic assay* of human urinary gonadotrophin (also known as human pituitary gonadotrophin) is performed by measuring its potency in stimulating an increase in the ovarian weight of immature rats. The *unit* is usually defined as the quantity of extracted hormone required to elicit a 100 per cent increase in immature rat ovarian or mouse uterine weight in comparison with the corresponding organ weights of uninjected animals. The *unit of LH activity* of human urinary gonadotrophin is defined as the amount of hormone required to produce a 100 per cent increase in the weight of the ventral prostate of hypophysectomized male rats. LH can also be assayed by its capacity to deplete ovarian ascorbic acid in immature pseudopregnant rats. Potency of FSH and LH can also be expressed as "relative potency," or units per microgram as compared to accepted standards, such as those of the National Institutes of Health (FSH-NIH-Sl; LH-NIH-Sl). (See Assessment of Pituitary Function.)

In the *treatment of human infertility*, the FSH-like activity of urinary human menopausal gonadotrophin (HMG) not only induces estrogen secretion in amenorrheic women, but sequential use of HMG with human chorionic gonadotrophin (HCG) for periods of several days has induced *ovulation* in amenorrheic women, many of whom have then become pregnant. The method is apparently effective in many kinds of secondary ovarian failure, even when sterility and amenorrhea are of many years' duration; it is not effective in primary ovarian failure. The principal danger of treatment is overstimulation of the ovaries, with formation of large cysts. There seems to be no way to predict or control this complication. Very rarely, these cysts rupture and present surgical emergencies. In induced pregnancies, there is an extraordinarily high rate of multiple ovulations; viable quadruplets and quintuplets are reported.

Human gonadotrophin with HCG has also been used in the successful induction of spermatogenesis in hypophysectomized men. These therapeutic uses of FSH are limited by short supply.

LUTEINIZING HORMONE (LH) OR INTERSTITIAL-CELL-STIMULATING HORMONE (ICSH)

Luteinizing hormone is essential for ovulation and for the formation of the corpus luteum. It does not produce follicular growth; to be effective, LH requires the prior action of FSH on the follicle. Human LH is assumed to be the luteotrophic hormone; there is evidence that the corpus luteum has an intrinsic life span that is not much influenced by pituitary hormones. LH also stimulates the growth and secretory activity of the testicular interstitial cells. This interstitial-cell-stimulating activity is sufficient to correct the testicular endocrine defect of hypophysectomy, producing androgen secretion and maintenance of the secondary sex organs. Spermatogenesis in man requires the synergism of FSH.

Like FSH, LH is a glycoprotein. Human LH (ICSH) has a molecular weight estimated at about 30,000. The hormone has been little used therapeutically; the more readily available human chorionic gonadotrophin (HCG) has predominantly LH properties and is used instead. With the use of radioimmunoassay measurements, it has been calculated that about 30 μg. of LH is secreted daily in men; the value is the same in women except at mid-cycle, when the secretion rate increases 10 to 15 fold.

THYROTROPHIN (THYROTROPHIC OR THYROID-STIMULATING HORMONE, TSH)

Thyrotrophin repairs the atrophy of the thyroid gland that follows hypophysectomy. It is secreted by specific types of basophils of the anterior pituitary. Thyrotrophin also restores the ability of the thyroid to synthesize and secrete thyroxine and triiodothyronine. If given in large doses to normal or hypophysectomized animals or man, thyrotrophin evokes the morphologic and secretory changes of hyperthyroidism. Thyrotrophin elicits a rapid release of thyroxine and triiodothyronine from the gland; the content of colloid is reduced, and the quantity of organic iodine is decreased. Thyrotrophin stimulates many metabolic processes in the thyroid, e.g., the uptake and oxidation of glucose, the production of TPNH, and many others. As with other pituitary hormones, the primary mode of action is not known. The rapid discharge of thyroxine from the thyroid follicles is in part due to the action of TSH upon a proteolytic enzyme that accelerates the release of the hormone from the intrafollicular protein, thyroglobulin. Within 24 hours after the administration of thyrotrophin, hypertrophy and hyperplasia of the thyroid epithelium occur. The weight of the thyroid increases. Thyrotrophin augments the capacity of the thyroid to take up iodide, to convert iodide to organic iodine, and to synthesize thyroxine.

Thyrotrophin is a glycoprotein containing hexose and glucosamine. The molecular weight is not established; it is probably 26,000 to 30,000. A distinct pituitary principle, called exophthalmos-producing substance (EPS), acts on the orbital tissue to produce exophthalmos. The pathologic changes that can be induced by either administered thyrotrophin or EPS are similar to those observed in exophthalmic patients with Graves' disease. TSH and EPS are substances distinct from the so-called long-acting thyroid stimulator (LATS) found in plasma of some patients with Graves' disease, particularly exophthalmic patients. LATS has many of the properties of an antibody and is not detectable in the anterior pituitary. (See the Thyroid Gland.)

With the availability of highly purified human thyrotrophin, a useful radioimmunoassay for thyrotrophin in human serum has been developed. In normal men and women, serum contains less than 3.0 mμg. per milliliter. In primary myxedema, the values, as expected, are high, 10 to 150 mμg. per milliliter, and fall to normal when thyroid hormone is given. (These values can be expressed as less than 3 milliunits per 100 ml. and 10 to 150 milliunits per 100 ml.; [1 international unit of TSH is about equal to 1 U.S.P. unit].) Again, as expected, no thyrotrophin can be detected in the blood of hypophysectomized patients. Most interesting, the values of circulating TSH are normal or low in Graves' disease; these and other data about the role of the pituitary in the pathogenesis of Graves' disease are discussed in the article on the Thyroid Gland.

Bovine thyrotrophin is available for medical use; diagnostic TSH tests of thyroid function are discussed later (see Assessment of Pituitary Function).

ADRENOCORTICOTROPHIN (ACTH, CORTICOTROPHIN)

Adrenocorticotrophin repairs the adrenal cortical atrophy and failure to synthesize steroid hormones that follow hypophysectomy. In most species, ACTH administration causes hypertrophy and hyperplasia of the adrenal. The main effect appears to be upon the fascicular and reticular zones. The hormone stimulates the synthesis and release of cortisol, corticosterone, and androgens; it also elicits a moderate increase in the secretory rate of aldosterone, but this increase is not sustained. Large amounts of exogenous corticotrophin cause enlargement and hyperemia of the adrenal, and hemorrhagic infarction has been observed.

The chemical nature of adrenocorticotrophin is known. It is a single polypeptide made up of 39 amino acids. Smaller fragments of the ACTH peptide, e.g., that containing amino acids 1 to 20, have full biologic potency. The complete hormone has been synthesized; its molecular weight is 4567, its potency 100 to 140 units per milligram. One international unit, equal to 1 U.S.P. unit, is the biologic

activity of 1 mg. of international standard. Despite the availability of the pure hormone, the mode of action is not completely understood. The action of adrenocorticotrophin upon the adrenal cortex is complex. It stimulates an increased mitotic activity. The increase in steroidogenesis is the result of an increase in the rate of steroid biosynthesis, not simply of accelerated release of steroid into the blood stream. The precise point in the biosynthetic pathway at which corticotrophin acts is debatable; the increased steroid production may be mediated by ACTH stimulation of a particular messenger RNA. A possible primary mechanism by which ACTH may induce increased steroid synthesis resides in the capacity of the hormone to stimulate the synthesis of active adrenocortical phosphorylase by raising the concentration of cyclic AMP (adenosine-3',5'-monophosphate) in the gland. The increased phosphorylase activity makes available more glucose-6-phosphate from the hexose monophosphate shunt, thus providing larger quantities of NADH (TPNH), a compound essential for the synthesis and hydroxylation of steroids.

Corticotrophin, like TSH and many other pituitary peptides, also has extra-adrenal actions. For example, it stimulates the release of free fatty acids from adipose tissue; the importance of this effect is unknown. In large doses it causes darkening of the skin; this property may be related to a common sequence of seven amino acids in ACTH and β-MSH.

In man, the short-term administration of adrenocorticotrophin causes a rapid increase in the secretion of cortisol that is reflected in an abrupt rise in plasma cortisol concentration. This effect has proved useful in the diagnostic assessment of adrenocortical response, as has the biologic and immunologic assay of ACTH in human serum. Radioimmunoassay measurements of plasma ACTH concentration have confirmed earlier ideas about the extraordinary lability of this hormone in response to physiologic and pathologic stimuli. A diurnal rhythm of plasma ACTH is not so well marked as that of plasma cortisol, but, like plasma cortisol, ACTH levels tend to fall to a nadir in the late evening. Hospitalized patients not acutely ill often have ACTH concentrations higher than normal, and severely ill patients occasionally show extremely elevated levels. Plasma ACTH rises in response to metyrapone, and falls when suppressive doses of adrenocortical steroids, e.g., dexamethasone, are given (see Adrenal Cortex). Stressful stimuli, such as surgery under general anesthesia, electroshock, and hypoglycemia, and the administration of histamine and vasopressin are usually followed by raised plasma ACTH concentrations. The use of the radioimmunoassay method has yielded an estimate of ACTH turnover rate in normal human subjects of 7.2 μg. or 1 unit per day. (See Assessment of Pituitary Function.)

The long-term effects of adrenocorticotrophin in human subjects are the same as those produced by cortisone, cortisol, and their synthetic analogues. In contrast to the adrenal cortical steroids, corticotrophin evokes sensitivity reactions, but antihormone formation does not occur. Corticotrophin brings about a greater degree of sodium and water retention, more androgenicity, and a more constant elevation in serum cholesterol than do steroids. Large doses elicit the stigmata of Cushing's syndrome (osteoporosis, hyperglycemia, psychosis, etc.). The unpleasant symptoms associated with abrupt withdrawal of steroid therapy rarely occur after a course of corticotrophin. The use of corticotrophin in the management of steroid-induced hypopituitarism is discussed later (see Hormone-induced Hypopituitarism).

Adrenocorticotrophin regulates the growth, structural integrity, and steroid secretion of the adrenal cortex. This constantly changing regulatory influence is exerted by central nervous system control of the anterior pituitary and by a reciprocal relation between the amounts of circulating cortisol and ACTH (see Control of Anterior Pituitary Secretion). In man, noxious stimuli such as acute illness or emotional disturbance provoke an increased output of adrenocortical steroids, presumably mediated via an increased rate of endogenous corticotrophin release.

ACTH is available for *diagnostic* and *therapeutic* purposes in lyophilized and repository (with gelatin or zinc) forms (See Assessment of Anterior Pituitary Function). The diseases that respond to hyperadrenal therapy are more simply managed with corticosteroids than with ACTH.

MELANOCYTE-STIMULATING HORMONE (MSH)

Two MSH peptides have been identified in pituitary tissue. The smaller and more potent molecule, α-MSH, is made up of 13 amino acids and has a molecular weight of 1823; it is found in the pituitaries of pigs, cows, and monkeys, and may be present in the neurohypophysis of man. The characteristic human peptide, β-MSH, contains 22 amino acids and has a molecular weight of 2734. α-MSH has a 13-amino acid sequence with ACTH; β-MSH a 7-amino acid sequence. These common structural features may account for common physiologic properties among the three molecules: ACTH has a slight pigmentary effect on skin; MSH and ACTH are both adipokinetic. Studies of plasma β-MSH concentration in man have shown that the secretion of this hormone is regulated by the same factors that control ACTH. Normal subjects have values of 20 to 110 picograms per milliliter. Metyrapone raises and adrenocortical steroids depress plasma β-MSH levels. Plasma β-MSH undergoes a diurnal rhythm in normal subjects. The values are raised in untreated Addison's disease and congenital adrenal hyperplasia, and fall during corticosteroid administration. Plasma β-MSH is slightly elevated, as is plasma ACTH, in the "pituitary" form of Cushing's syndrome (see Adrenal Cortex), and very much elevated in patients who develop pituitary tumors and dermal hyperpigmentation after bilateral

adrenalectomy for this disease. Elevations of plasma β-MSH tend to parallel those of plasma ACTH, and similar amounts of each peptide have been found in extracts of hormone-secreting tumors (see Endocrine Syndromes Associated with Tumors of Nonendocrine Tissue). The functional significance of human β-MSH is unknown. Plasma values are the same in pigmented and nonpigmented races, and are normal in albinism and in several diseases characterized by increased skin pigment.

Abe, K., Nicholson, W. E., Liddle, G. W., Orth, D. N., and Island, D. P.: Normal and abnormal regulation of β-MSH in man. J. Clin. Invest., 48:1580, 1969.

Adams, J. H., Daniel, P. M., and Prichard, M. M. L.: Observations on the portal circulation of the pituitary gland. Neuroendocrinol, 1:193, 1965/66.

Berson, S. A., and Yalow, R. S.: Radioimmunoassay of peptide hormones in plasma. New Eng. J. Med., 277:640, 1967.

Berson, S. A., and Yalow, R. S.: Radioimmunoassay of ACTH in plasma. J. Clin. Invest., 47:2725, 1968.

Dixon, H. B. F.: Chemistry of pituitary hormones. *In* Pincus, G., Thimann, K. V., and Astwood, E. B. (eds.): The Hormones: Physiology, Chemistry and Applications, Vol. 5. New York, Academic Press, Inc., 1964, p. 1.

Engel, F. L., and Kostyo, J. L.: Metabolic actions of pituitary hormones. *In* Pincus, G., Thimann, K. V., and Astwood, E. B. (eds.): The Hormones: Physiology, Chemistry and Applications, Vol. 5. New York, Academic Press, Inc., 1964, p. 69.

Glick, S. M., Roth, J., Yalow, R. S., and Berson, S. A.: The regulation of growth hormone secretion. Recent Progr. Hormone Res., 21:241, 1965.

Harris, G. W., and Donovan, B. T. (eds.): The Pituitary Gland, 3 vols. Berkeley, University of California Press, 1966.

McCann, S. M., Dhariwal, A. P. S., and Porter, J. C.: Regulation of the adenohypophysis. Ann. Rev. Physiol., 30:589, 1968.

Ney, R. L.: The Anterior Pituitary Gland. *In* Duncan's Diseases of Metabolism, Vol. 2. 6th ed. Bondy, P. K. (ed.): Philadelphia, W. B. Saunders Company, 1969, p. 718.

Saxena, B. B., Demura, H., Gandy, H. M., and Peterson, R. E.: Radioimmunoassay of human follicle stimulating and luteinizing hormone in plasma. J. Clin. Endocr., 28:519, 1968.

Schalch, D. S., Parlow, A. F., Boon, R. C., and Reichlin, S.: Measurement of human luteinizing hormone in plasma by radioimmunoassay. J. Clin. Invest., 47:665, 1968.

Utiger, R. D.: Radioimmunoassay of human plasma thyrotropin. J. Clin. Invest., 44:1277, 1965.

Yalow, R. S., Varsano-Aharon, N., and Berson, S. A.: HGH and ACTH secretory responses to stress. Hormone & Metab. Res., 1:3, 1969.

ASSESSMENT OF ANTERIOR PITUITARY FUNCTION

Anatomic detection of pituitary disease has been touched upon above (*vide supra*, Functional Anatomy). Encroachment of a suprasellar or intrasellar mass on adjacent structures provides evidence of pituitary tumor. Since there is considerable anatomic variation in these adjacent structures, e.g., the optic chiasm, and in the thickness of the diaphragma sellae, clinical manifestations are correspondingly variable. It is uncommon for a pituitary tumor to produce *hypothalamic symptoms* by upward pressure on the diencephalon;

diabetes insipidus and disorders of sleep and of temperature regulation are rare and do not appear unless the diencephalon is grossly damaged. The classic sign of upward extension of a pituitary tumor is *bitemporal hemianopia*. Lesser degrees of damage to the optic chiasm evoke scotomata and *upper temporal defects* in the visual fields; serial tests disclose that loss of acuity for colored objects precedes that for white. Varying degrees of *optic atrophy*, unilateral or bilateral, may be observed on examination of the optic fundi. The *headaches* associated with tumors of this region are not characteristic enough to be of diagnostic value.

Roentgenographic detection (see Functional Anatomy) is ideally based on frontal as well as sagittal views of the skull and sella. In addition to changes in the length and depth of the pituitary fossa, the examiner looks for *erosion* or *destruction of the anterior and posterior clinoids* and of the *tuberculum sellae*, intrasellar or suprasellar *calcification* (chromophobe adenoma, craniopharyngioma), and *"double floor"* of the sella, seen when a tumor extends downward unevenly. *Laminagraphy* may show an *"empty sella"* or extension of a tumor into the sphenoid sinus. Carotid artery *angiography* and particularly *pneumoencephalography* may show quite accurately the degree of upward extension of an intrasellar tumor; these procedures, at least the latter, should always be done before craniotomy for pituitary tumor, and are also helpful guides in the design of a radiotherapeutic program. In *acromegaly*, plain films of the *skull* show not only enlargement of the sella turcica in more than 80 per cent of patients, but also thickening of the calvarium, enlargement of the paranasal sinuses, and widening of the mandibular angle with prognathism. Films of the *hands* disclose gross increase in the mass of soft tissue, a more characteristic finding than tufting of the distal phalanges. *Spine* films may reveal anterior lipping of vertebral bodies; lateral films of the *os calcis* often show thickening of the heel pad.

Functional detection of pituitary disease is based on measurement of hormones in plasma or urine. *Direct* measurement of pituitary hormones is made when possible, as for growth hormone and gonadotrophins; *indirect* measurement of the hormones of glands that are under pituitary trophic control is more generally available, e.g., thyroidal response to assess TSH function, adrenocortical response to assess ACTH (*vide infra*).

Radioimmunoassay of growth hormone is not yet a routine procedure, but can be done at many medical centers and commercial laboratories. This measurement is the most direct method for detecting *hypopituitary* states and *acromegaly*. In *hypopituitary dwarfism*, radioimmunoassay for growth hormone may be expected to supersede the crude indirect indices that clinicians have had to rely on, e.g., measurements of body proportions, chromosomal analysis, roentgenographic estimate of bone age, and laborious exclusion of all other causes of short stature. In several of the forms of pituitary dwarfism, *basal* serum growth hormone values of less than 1.0 mμg. per milliliter may be found; these low values are not diagnostic. It is necessary to demonstrate failure of growth hormone response to a stimulus, e.g., *hypoglycemia*. When suspicion is strong, the starting dose of insulin should be 0.05 units per kilogram, given intravenously; if the hypoglycemia is inadequate, the dose can be increased to 0.1 or even 0.15 units per kilogram, given under careful medical supervision to avoid prolonged hypoglycemia. Adequate stimulus requires a lowering of blood glucose to 40 mg per 100 ml. for at least 10 minutes; if this condition is satisfied, patients without growth hormone deficiency display a rise in growth hormone value of at least 10 mμg. per milliliter above the basal level. Failure of growth hormone response to hypoglycemia is the most common laboratory abnormality in adult hypopituitarism, and is characteristic only of the dwarfism associated with pituitary insufficiency. Certain amino acids also have the property of inducing growth hormone release; intravenous administration of neutralized *arginine* hydrochloride, 0.5 gram per kilogram, is preferred by some workers because one avoids possibly dangerous hypoglycemia. The rise in growth hormone value is again 10 mμg. per milliliter above the resting levels.

In *acromegaly*, growth hormone radioimmunoassay will soon supplant the highly unsatisfactory *indirect* methods clinicians have struggled with for years: histologic changes in the cartilage of the costochondral junction, measurement of serum phosphorus, PBI, urinary calcium, hydroxyproline excretion, etc. Basal serum growth hormone may be in the range of 50 to more than 100 mμg. per milliliter (normally not above 5). Many patients with untreated acromegaly fail to show a sharp drop in serum growth hormone concentration, as do normal people, after administration of glucose (given as for a standard glucose tolerance test, blood samples being taken for glucose and growth hormone determinations at 30-minute intervals for at least three hours). It will require protracted follow-up studies of acromegalic patients before and after treatment, and careful correlation with clinical findings, e.g., acral growth, to assess the usefulness of this *nonresponse to hyperglycemia* as an index of "acromegalic activity"; an ideal index has so far proved elusive.

Biologic assay of *prolactin* in the serum of patients with galactorrhea may prove to be helpful, but results are still controversial (*vide supra*, Prolactin).

Biologic assay of *urinary gonadotrophin* is useful in distinguishing primary from secondary gonadal failure *after* the expected age of puberty. In the first, urinary gonadotrophin titers are elevated; in the latter (resulting from pituitary deficiency) levels are not detectable. Results of urinary gonadotrophin (human pituitary gonadotrophin) assays, done by the mouse uterine weight or rat ovarian weight method (*vide supra*, FSH), are expressed in mouse uterine units (muu) or rat units (RU). In the *mouse assay*, a reported value of "positive at 20 muu" means that one twentieth of the extract of a 24-hour urine just produced a definite response in the injected mice. If one twentieth of a 24-hour urinary extract just produces a definite response in the *rat assay*, results are reported as "20 RU per 24 hours"; because of the more precise dose-response relationship in the rat assay, results may be reported as "25 RU per 24 hours," since the figure is read from a standard curve. The rat assay is the more sensitive; normal people occasionally have undetectable values in the mouse assay. There is no official reference standard for this bioassay. Representative mean values for the rat assay are: adult men, 10; women in the follicular and luteal phases, 7; women at mid-cycle, 15; postmenopausal women, 75 – all values being expressed in RU per 24 hours. Corresponding figures for the mouse assay are: 35, 20, 55, and 200 – all expressed in muu per 24 hours. In pituitary insufficiency, urinary gonadotrophins are usually undetectable; this abnormality is one of the earliest laboratory signs to appear in the course of the disease.

Urinary bioassays for FSH and LH are insensitive, and are not used for clinical purposes. The highly sensitive *radioimmunoassays* for *plasma FSH* and *LH* are not yet available for routine clinical use, but they may very well supplant the bioassay methods in time. As expected, values are low or undetectable in pituitary insufficiency. Representative mean *plasma* values for *FSH* are: in children, 4; adult men, 25; women in the follicular and luteal phases of the cycle, 25; midcycle, 40; postmenopausal women, 250 – all figures being expressed in micrograms per 100 ml. of plasma in terms of a standard human pituitary preparation. The corresponding mean values for *plasma LH* are 4, 12, 15, 50, and 60, expressed in micrograms per 100 ml. plasma as for FSH.

Radioimmunoassay for serum thyrotrophin is not yet available for general clinical use; normal and pathologic values are given above (*vide supra*, Thyrotrophin). The accepted method for distinguishing primary myxedema from secondary thyroid deficiency is the *thyrotrophin-stimulation test*. The most reliable technique seems to be measurement of 24-hour I[131] uptake by the thyroid before and after intramuscular administration of bovine TSH, 5 units per day for three days, or 10 units in a single dose in one day. In primary myxedema, there is no response; normal subjects respond briskly; patients with myxedema secondary to pituitary failure respond, but subnormally. Exceptions are some patients with Sheehan's disease of long duration, who may be unresponsive.

Measurement of the *ACTH secretion* of the pituitary is usually done *indirectly* by testing adrenocortical response. A safe and specific method is intravenous administration of 25 units of lyophilized ACTH in 500 ml. of 0.9 per cent saline over a four-hour period. Five per cent glucose in water should not be used as a diluent because it may aggravate pre-existing hyponatremia. In primary adrenocortical failure (Addison's disease) there is no response of plasma or urinary corticosteroids; in pituitary deficiency with secondary adrenal failure, response is present but subnormal. The nonspecific methods, insulin tolerance test and water loading, can be dangerous and are not recommended.

Four other methods have been used to assess pituitary ACTH release; like the ACTH-response test described above, the index is rise or failure to rise of plasma or urinary corticosteroid values. Three of the methods entail stimulation of ACTH release by giving a more or less noxious stimulus: *insulin-induced hypoglycemia, vasopressin,* and bacterial *pyrogen*. Although it is true that patients with hypopituitarism show absent or subnormal rises in plasma cortisol concentration after all three of these, there is no agreement about which is the most discriminating or the most sensitive. The insulin, vasopressin, and pyrogen tests have not found favor as clinical methods in this country. The fourth method, the *metyrapone test,* is a measure of pituitary ACTH reserve. Metyrapone, an adrenocortical 11β-hydroxylase inhibitor, partially inhibits adrenocortical biosynthesis of cortisol; its immediate biosynthetic precursor, 11-deoxycortisol (compound S) is secreted instead, and is a weak suppressor of endogenous pituitary ACTH secretion; ACTH secretion then increases, and in turn stimulates the adrenal cortex to secrete more steroid, measured in the urine as 17-hydroxycorticosteroids or 17-ketogenic steroids. In the normal subject, oral administration of 750 mg. of metyrapone every 4 hours for 24 hours is followed, on the day *after* the drug is given, by a rise in steroid excretion of 100 per cent or more over baseline values. In the patient with pituitary insufficiency with inadequate ACTH reserve, the rise in urinary corticosteroid excretion will be subnormal or absent. To exclude primary disease of the adrenal, i.e., to make certain that the adrenal has the capacity to respond to ACTH, a standard ACTH response test should be done *before* metyrapone is given. In a few patients with severe hypopituitarism, metyrapone blockade of adrenocortical biosynthesis coupled with poor or absent ACTH reserve has resulted in clinically significant adrenal insufficiency. In patients with possibly advanced hypopituitarism *caution* is therefore necessary.

Biologic assay and radioimmunoassay of plasma ACTH, although not yet applicable for clinical purposes, are *direct* techniques which have yielded valuable information about the fluctuations of this hormone (*vide supra*, ACTH). Normal values are a mean of about 0.3 mU. per 100 ml. by bioassay and a mean of about 22 $\mu\mu$g. per milliliter by radioimmunoassay. Values are occasionally 10 times higher than these in severely ill patients; as expected, levels are low or not detected in hypopituitarism. The changes in plasma ACTH concentration that occur in the various forms of

Cushing's syndrome are discussed in the article on the Adrenal Cortex.

For the design of an orderly clinical approach to the study of patients with hypopituitarism, the reader is referred to the general references below, particularly the paper by Lazarus.

General

Christy, N. P.: Pituitary insufficiency. In Astwood, E. B. (ed.): Clinical Endocrinology, I. New York, Grune & Stratton, Inc., 1960, p. 53.
Lazarus, L.: The investigation of hypopituitarism. Aust. Ann. Med. 16:107, 1967.
LeMay, M.: The radiologic diagnosis of pituitary disease. Radiol. Clin. N. Amer., 5:303, 1967.
Nieman, E. A., Landon, J., and Wynn, V.: Endocrine function in patients with untreated chromophobe adenomas. Quart. J. Med., 36N.S.:357, 1967.
Rabkin, M. T., and Frantz, A. G.: Hypopituitarism: a study of growth hormone and other endocrine functions. Ann. Intern. Med., 64:1197, 1966.

Growth Hormone

Beck, P., Schalch, D. S., Parker, M. L., Kipnis, D. M., and Daughaday, W. H.: Correlative studies of growth hormone and insulin plasma concentrations with metabolic abnormalities in acromegaly. J. Lab. Clin. Med., 66:366, 1965.
Frantz, A. G., and Rabkin, M. T.: Human growth hormone: Clinical measurement, response to hypoglycemia and suppression by corticosteroids. New Eng. J. Med., 271:1375, 1964.
Parker, M. L., Hammond, J. M., and Daughaday, W. H.: The arginine provocative test: An aid in the diagnosis of hyposomatotropism. J. Clin. Endocr., 27:1129, 1967.

Prolactin

Peake, G. T., McKeel, D. W., Jarett, L., and Daughaday, W. H.: Ultrastructural, histologic and hormonal characterization of a prolactin rich human pituitary tumor. J. Clin. Endocr., 29.1383, 1969.

Gonadotrophins

Northcutt, R. C., and Albert, A.: Laboratory tests for pituitary gonadotropins. J.A.M.A., 210:2386, 1969.

TSH

Bishopric, G. A., Garrett, N. H., and Nicholson, W. M.: Clinical value of the TSH test in the diagnosis of thyroid diseases. Amer. J. Med., 18:15, 1955.
Reichlin, S., and Utiger, R. D.: Regulation of the pituitary-thyroid axis in man: Relationship of TSH concentration to free and total thyroxine in plasma. J. Clin. Endocr., 27:251, 1967.

ACTH

Christy, N. P., Wallace, E. Z., and Jailer, J. W.: The effect of intravenously administered ACTH on plasma 17,21-dihydroxy-20-ketosteroids in normal individuals and in patients with disorders of the adrenal cortex. J. Clin. Invest., 34:899, 1955.
Liddle, G. W., Estep, H. L., Kendall, J. M., Jr., Williams, W. C., Jr., and Townes, A. W.: Clinical application of a new test of pituitary reserve. J. Clin. Endocr., 19:875, 1959.
Liddle, G. W., Island, D. P., and Meador, C. K.: Normal and abnormal regulation of corticotropin secretion in man. Recent Progr. Hormone Res., 18:125, 1962.

MSH

Abe, K., Nicholson, W. E., Liddle, G. W., Island, D. P., and Orth, D. N.: Radioimmunoassay of β-MSH in human plasma and tissues. J. Clin. Invest., 46:1609, 1967.

HYPOPITUITARISM

PITUITARY INSUFFICIENCY IN THE ADULT

Definitions. Hypopituitarism is the clinical condition resulting from destruction of the anterior pituitary; it is accompanied by secondary atrophy of the gonads, thyroid, and adrenal cortex. The term "panhypopituitarism" has been used to designate total absence of all the known pituitary secretions. "Simmonds' disease" is used synonymously. The term "Sheehan's disease" describes hypopituitarism due to postpartum necrosis of the gland. The designation "pituitary insufficiency" is inclusive.

Etiology, Pathology, and Pathogenesis. The most common cause of pituitary insufficiency in adult life is pituitary tumor, particularly chromophobe adenoma; the most common cause of very severe adult hypopituitarism is probably *postpartum necrosis* of the gland. The pathogenesis is debated. The common denominator is obstetric accident. According to Sheehan, peripheral vascular collapse is followed by *spasm* of local vessels, then thrombosis, then infarction. McKay holds that the primary event is not arteriolar spasm but thrombosis of pituitary vessels as part of *generalized intravascular coagulation*; he points out the frequent absence of severe hemorrhage, and indicates the association of pituitary necrosis with premature separation of the placenta and placenta previa. Neither view accounts for the peculiar susceptibility of the pituitary to damage in the postpartum period. The well-demarcated infarctions are small or nearly total. Sheehan and Summers have shown that pituitary insufficiency does not occur unless the lesion is very large. The late lesion is fibrosis with residual small nests of normal chromophils.

Other lesions are *fibrosis* of unknown cause and *granulomas*, which may be nonspecific, *syphilitic*, or *tuberculous*. Ischemic necrosis has occasionally followed *acute infection* (associated with diabetes mellitus), basal *skull fracture*, and *septic cavernous sinus thrombosis.*

Cysts and tumors within or outside the sella may compress and destroy the pituitary. The *chromophobe adenoma*, comprising 70 per cent of pituitary neoplasms, is the most common intrasellar tumor. Damage to the adenohypophysis is the result of mechanical compression. *These tumors are more likely to induce partial or mild degrees of pituitary insufficiency than panhypopituitarism.* A constitutional basis for chromophobe adenoma has been suggested because of the occasional occurrence of symptoms of hypogonadism long antedating the clinical onset of the tumor. Chromophobe adenomas are larger than the eosinophilic variety. Massive upward enlargement frequently involves the optic chiasm. Rapid expansion follows degeneration or hemorrhage, and increase in intracranial pressure may ensue. Remote extensions and metastases occur rarely. Extrasellar cysts and craniopharyngiomas cause pituitary insufficiency in childhood.

General pathologic findings in pituitary insufficiency include widespread *splanchnomicria* with particularly striking atrophy of the gonads, thyroid, and adrenal cortex.

Incidence. In several series, postpartum necrosis of the pituitary accounts for 30 to 50 per cent of the cases of pituitary insufficiency, extrasellar cysts, and tumors for 15 to 20 per cent, intrasellar tumors, cysts, and other types of necrosis and fibrosis for the rest.

Clinical Manifestations and Natural History. The speed of onset of pituitary insufficiency depends upon the nature and size of the lesion. When *postpartum necrosis* of the pituitary is extensive and severe, *acute* symptoms such as *diabetes insipidus* and *hypoglycemia* occur during the puerperium and may be only transitory; the patient may suddenly die within weeks, probably as a consequence of acute adrenocortical insufficiency. More commonly, the onset after obstetric accident is slow, occurring over months to years. The first symptom is usually failure to lactate; pubic and axillary hair fails to grow; menses do not return owing to gonadal failure, or the periods are scanty and transitory; amenorrhea follows. Libido is lost. Symptoms of *thyroid and adrenocortical failure* occur later as a rule than do those of ovarian deficiency, but *there is no set pattern*. General deterioration ensues. Patients become weak, easily fatigued, indifferent to their surroundings, slothful, and negligent of household duties. *Personality changes* range from mild idiosyncrasies through depression to frank psychosis. Intolerance of cold, as in primary hypothyroidism, may be extreme. *Hypopituitary coma* with hypotension and hypothermia, probably due in most instances to *hypoglycemia*, may have its onset gradually with no apparent cause, or rapidly in response to minor illness. At times collapse is preceded by clinical manifestations of *adrenal crisis* with nausea, vomiting, high fever, and hypotension. Although *anorexia* is a prominent feature in some patients, cachexia is uncommon and is a terminal event in the neglected patient. Pre-existing diabetes is on rare occasions ameliorated abruptly, with sudden lowering of the insulin requirement, after pituitary destruction ("Houssay phenomenon").

The *physical examination* discloses a fair state of nutrition as a rule (Fig. 1). The skin is thin, smooth, cool and pale, with fine wrinkling about the eyes (geroderma). The dry, scaly skin and puffy face of primary myxedema are unusual but occur on occasion. Pubic and axillary hair is absent or sparse. The pulse is slow and thin, the

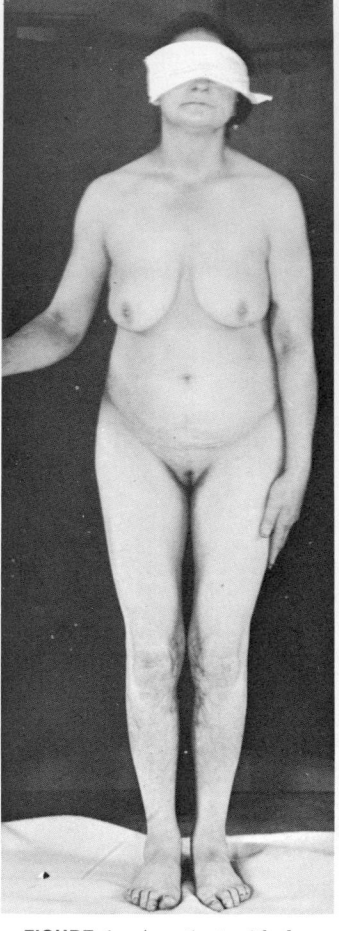
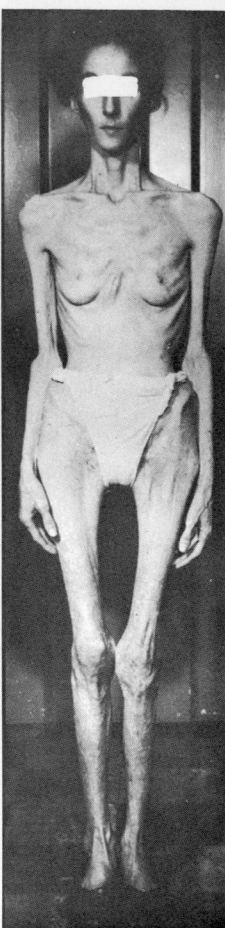

FIGURE 1. A patient with documented hypopituitarism 21 years after postpartum necrosis of the pituitary. Pubic and axillary hair are absent. Note the absence of cachexia. Compare with Figure 2. (Reproduced by permission from Sheehan, H. L., and Summers, V. K.: Quart J. Med., 42:319, 1949.)

FIGURE 2. The patient is a 30-year-old unmarried woman with anorexia nervosa who had lost 55 pounds (compare with the good nutritional state of the patient with hypopituitarism, Figure 1). Pubic hair was present and menses continued but were scanty and irregular. (Reproduced by permission from Bliss, E. L., and Branch, C. H. H.: Anorexia Nervosa. New York, Paul B. Hoeber, Inc., 1960.)

blood pressure low. Symptomatic hypotension on orthostasis is common. The breasts may appear well preserved, but genital atrophy is the rule.

General *laboratory examination* shows a moderate normochromic anemia that is less striking than the pallid appearance suggests. Roentgenogram of the skull is normal (there is no expanding intrasellar lesion). Blood glucose concentration is often low. The serum sodium concentration may be 120 mEq. per liter or lower without symptoms of adrenal insufficiency. Hyponatremia is probably related to hemodilution owing to inadequate excretion of water, which in turn is due to deficient cortisol secretion. Episodic hyponatremia in patients with pituitary insufficiency is correlated with measurable water retention (increased total body water), not with sodium depletion. The level of serum potassium is normal. As in the hypophysectomized animal or man, the aldosterone function of the adrenal cortex is fairly well preserved; the hypopituitary patient responds to salt withdrawal by a slow but adequate increase in aldosterone secretion and consequent retention of sodium. In very severe hypopituitarism with complete adrenal destruction, this capacity may be lost. The urinary 17-ketosteroids and corticosteroids are decreased. The basal metabolic rate is low, and serum protein-bound iodine is depressed; but thyroidal uptake of I^{131} is often inexplicably normal even when the patient is clinically hypothyroid.

The typical clinical picture becomes obvious as late as 15 to 20 years after the obstetric accident. Acute adrenocortical failure with or without superimposed infection is the chief cause of death in untreated patients.

Expanding intrasellar tumors— for example, chromophobe adenoma—may have a similar insidious onset. The symptoms of hypopituitarism are most often restricted to those of secondary gonadal failure. Symptoms and signs of the brain tumor (visual loss, increased intracranial pressure) may be absent or minimal, or may be so severe and so threatening that they completely dominate the clinical picture (*vide supra*, Assessment of Anterior Pituitary Function). In a recent large series, two thirds of the patients had visual symptoms, and about half had evidence of either gonadal or thyroid deficiency. In patients with intrasellar tumor, both the chief complaint and the ultimate cause of death are more commonly mechanical results of the adenoma than of pituitary failure.

Diagnosis. A history of postpartum hemorrhage, symptoms and signs of an intracranial tumor with chiasmal pressure, or evidence of multiple glandular deficiencies should raise the question of hypopituitarism. Diagnosis is difficult early in the course of the disease, before symptoms and signs of deficiency of more than one target gland are definite. Hypopituitarism should be suspected in patients with onset of gonadal failure in adult life. Amenorrhea occurring in a fertile woman before the expected age of menopause requires inquiry about obstetric hemorrhage in the past. Loss of axillary and pubic hair and atrophy of the external genitalia make hypopituitarism likely in a relatively young woman with amenorrhea. In men, loss of previously normal libido and potency and loss of body hair with or without genital atrophy are suggestive; roentgenogram of the skull shows sagittal stretching or ballooning of the sella if a chromophobe adenoma is present. Reduced visual acuity, optic atrophy, and bitemporal hemianopia provide evidence of suprasellar expansion of an intrasellar mass (*vide supra*, Assessment of Anterior Pituitary Function). Failure of sexual development late in the second decade raises the question of hypopituitarism in either sex.

In the *differential diagnosis*, pernicious anemia, primary gonadal failure, and primary hypothyroidism must be considered. The pallor and puffiness of the skin in *pernicious anemia* may be confused with pituitary failure, but the latter is not characterized by severe or megaloblastic anemia or by failure to absorb vitamin B_{12}. *Primary gonadal failure*, in the *male* especially, may resemble pituitary insufficiency. The degree of eunuchoidism (disproportionately long arms and legs) depends on the age of onset of hypoleydigism, being extreme if early, absent if late. Many males with gonadal failure have the fine, pale, wrinkled skin of hypopituitarism, but thyroid and adrenal function are normal.

Levels of urinary gonadotrophin are elevated in testicular deficiency, undetectable in pituitary failure. Klinefelter's syndrome (seminiferous tubule dysgenesis) is easily distinguished. In the *female* the same principles apply: The level of urinary gonadotrophin is undetectable in hypopituitarism, high in natural menopause. *Primary myxedema* is generally characterized by more noticeable dryness and puffiness of the skin, and the serum cholesterol tends to be higher. In hypothyroidism due to pituitary failure, other glandular deficiencies are often present and should be sought. Measurement of thyroidal response to thyrotrophin may be helpful (see discussion of Thyrotrophin). *Primary adrenal cortical failure* (Addison's disease) is not hard to differentiate. The skin is darkly tanned (MSH) rather than pale, gonadal function is often normal, and thyroidal function is unimpaired, unless Hashimoto's thyroiditis is associated. Diagnosis of this entity is discussed in the chapter on the thyroid. Primary adrenal failure is ruled out, and subtle adrenal insufficiency due to pituitary failure is diagnosed by measuring the response of plasma or urinary corticosteroids to intravenous corticotrophin. In Addison's disease there is no response. In hypopituitarism response is present but subnormal; this constitutes more specific evidence of adrenal deficiency than do low urinary steroid values, which are reduced in a great variety of chronic, debilitating diseases.

Treatment. If an intrasellar tumor is present, radiation is the usual treatment. The best results with respect to improvement in vision are obtained with a four- to five-week course in a dosage of 4000 to 5000 r tumor dose; more than 75 per cent of patients are benefited. Late complications of radiotherapy are few. Chromophobe adenomas are not extraordinarily radiosensitive, however, and large size, the presence of a cystic tumor, or serious or acute threat to vision requires surgical intervention. There is a fairly constant surgical mortality rate of about 9 per cent. Extirpation of the entire tumor is almost never possible. Even with relief of pressure symptoms, restoration of pituitary function is rare; operation is likely to be followed by more severe pituitary insufficiency. The best statistical results seem to follow partial surgical removal, then pituitary radiation. With surgery alone, the five-year control rate is about 60 per cent; with combined treatment, nearly 90 per cent. Small tumors, unless they are cystic, are well controlled by radiation alone.

Long-term medical management of the patient

with hypopituitarism consists of careful replacement of lost functions. Trophic hormones are not used because of expense and the bother of daily injections. By far the most important defect is that of the *adrenal cortex*; acute adrenal crisis may come on abruptly and without warning, and may lead to death. Under ordinary conditions, cortisone or hydrocortisone (10 to 25 mg. per day in two divided doses, by mouth) provides a sense of well-being and adequate protection against hypotension, hypoglycemia, and water and electrolyte imbalance. Small doses are preferred because patients with hypopituitarism have a peculiar susceptibility to the effects of larger doses of corticosteroids (peptic ulcer, facial rounding, psychosis). Added salt and a mineralocorticoid are only occasionally required. In the female, diethylstilbestrol, 0.5 to 1.0 mg. per day for 20 days of each month, provides good maintenance of developed secondary sex characters and, in time, leads to an artificial menstrual cycle. In the male, a fair degree of libido and potency can be conferred by androgens (methyl testosterone, 20 to 30 mg. per day orally; testosterone propionate, 25 to 100 mg. two to three times per week by intramuscular injection; or a long-acting ester once per month intramuscularly). Gonadal steroids are unnecessary in elderly patients. Thyroid replacement should be started with small doses (8 to 15 mg. per day of U.S.P. thyroid orally), which are gradually increased over a period of several weeks; for optimal effect a dose as large as 0.180 gram may be needed. Roughly equivalent doses of L-thyroxine are 0.1 to 0.2 mg. per day. It is probably wise to begin corticosteroid therapy first, since adrenal crisis has allegedly been precipitated by vigorous thyroid treatment.

Treatment of an acute illness or management during a surgical procedure, e.g., craniotomy for intrasellar tumor, is essentially that of adrenal crisis. Thyroid hormone is not necessary. *Corticotrophin should never be relied upon,* because the degree of endogenous adrenal response is unpredictable. Correct treatment is cortisone acetate (100 to 200 mg. intramuscularly per day) or hydrocortisone (100 to 300 mg. per day of a water-soluble ester in isotonic saline intravenously). It is better to err on the side of *moderately* excessive doses, since untoward reactions are not likely to occur during the few days of vigorous treatment generally required; the dose should be reduced as quickly as possible to the maintenance level. If in an emergency there is doubt concerning the presence of secondary hypoadrenalism, one should assume that it exists rather than attempt a time-consuming laboratory evaluation of adrenal status. If *diabetes insipidus* occurs postoperatively, treatment is as set out in the article on the Neurohypophysis (q.v.).

Brown, J., et al.: Purified human pituitary hormones: Treatment of pituitary insufficiency. Ann. Intern. Med., 66:594, 1967.

Chang, C. H., and Pool, J. L.: The radiotherapy of pituitary chromophobe adenomas. Radiology, 89:1005, 1967.

Fürst, E.: On chromophobe pituitary adenoma. Acta Med. Scand. (Suppl. 452), 1966.

Jenkins, J. S., and Else, W.: Pituitary-adrenal function tests in patients with untreated pituitary tumours. Lancet, 2:940, 1968.

Kernohan, J. W., and Sayre, G. P.: Tumors of the pituitary gland and infundibulum. *In* Atlas of Tumor Pathology, Section X, Fascicle 36. Washington, D.C., Armed Forces Institute of Pathology, 1956.

Levene, M. B.: Pituitary radiotherapy. Radiol. Clin. N. Amer. 5:333, 1967.

McKay, D. G.: Pituitary. Disseminated Intravascular Coagulation. New York, Hoeber Medical Division, Harper and Row, 1965, pp. 405, 460.

Nurnberger, J. I., and Korey, S. R.: Pituitary Chromophobe Adenomas. New York, Springer Publishing Company, 1953.

Purnell, D. C., Randall, R. V., and Rynearson, E. H.: Postpartum pituitary insufficiency (Sheehan's syndrome): Review of 18 cases. Mayo Clin. Proc., 39:321, 1964.

Ray, B. S., and Patterson, R. H.: Surgical treatment of pituitary adenomas. J. Neurosurg., 19:1, 1962.

Sheehan, H. L., and Davis, J. C.: Pituitary necrosis. Brit. Med. Bull., 24:59, 1968.

Sheehan, H. L., and Summers, V. K.: The syndrome of hypopituitarism. Quart. J. Med., 42:319, 1949.

Sheline, G. E., Boldrey, E. B., and Phillips, T. L.: Chromophobe adenomas of the pituitary gland. Amer. J. Roentgen., 92: 160, 1964.

DEFICIENCY OF SINGLE ANTERIOR PITUITARY HORMONES

It is hard to determine in an individual case whether there is isolated deficiency of a pituitary hormone or whether one is observing an early stage of what will ultimately be panhypopituitarism. The *hypogonadotrophic eunuchoidism* of Heller and Nelson seems a fairly well-established entity; the features are eunuchoidism with undetectable urinary gonadotrophin, but with normal thyroid and adrenal function. Stimulation of Leydig cells can be achieved with chorionic gonadotrophin and a degree of spermatogenesis by the addition of FSH. Isolated deficiencies of *thyrotrophin* and *adrenocorticotrophin* have been reported; in one instance of the latter, pituitary basophils were virtually absent. Isolated *growth hormone deficiency* is discussed under Pituitary Insufficiency during Childhood.

HORMONE-INDUCED HYPOPITUITARISM

Administration of gonadal, thyroidal, or adrenocortical hormones causes glandular hypofunction and atrophy because of reduction in the rate of synthesis and release of pituitary gonadotrophin, thyrotrophin, or adrenocorticotrophin; it has been shown experimentally that pituitary content and concentration of trophic hormones are sharply reduced after treatment with large doses of the respective target gland hormones. The reversible hypogonadotrophism brought about by treatment with small doses of estrogens is not of clinical importance. Prolonged suppression of ovulation by oral contraceptive agents (progestogens with estrogen added) is usually followed within one month by resumption of normal menstrual cycles, but in a minority of women there may be long delays until menses return.

The decrease in production of thyrotrophin that follows long-term administration of thyroid hormone to euthyroid subjects may cause symptoms. In such patients, withdrawal of thyroid hormone is sometimes associated with the appearance of transitory evidence of hypothyroidism (fatigue, lethargy, dry skin, intolerance of cold; low basal metabolic rate; thyroidal uptake of I^{131} and serum protein-bound iodine that are low or at the lower limits of normal). The syndrome is generally self-limited.

Pituitary-adrenal suppression after prolonged administration of adrenocortical steroids is occasionally of great clinical importance. Although there is controversy over which of three areas — the hypothalamus, the pituitary, or the adrenal — is principally deranged, there is no doubt that corticotrophin secretion is reduced and that adrenal atrophy results. Fraser and Salassa first reported postoperative shock and death associated with adrenal and pituitary atrophy in patients treated with large doses of cortisone (75 mg. or more per day) for 8 to 12 months. Many similar case reports have since appeared; several investigations have shown that adrenocortical response to exogenous corticotrophin may be reduced after as little as a week of steroid therapy. One may be faced with the paradoxical situation of a patient who looks clinically hyperadrenal ("cushingoid"), but whose adrenals are atrophic and whose ability to respond to an acute illness or to a surgical procedure is seriously impaired. Withdrawal of adrenocortical steroids, whether abrupt or gradual, may be followed by asthenia, fever, nausea, malaise, myalgias, slight hypotension, and, in some instances, brown dermal pigmentation and desquamation of the skin. In patients with these clinical manifestations, it is often difficult to distinguish between recurrent symptoms of the disease for which steroids were originally given and the so-called steroid withdrawal syndrome.

It is probable that intermittent injections of corticotrophin during prolonged periods of adrenal steroid therapy do not prevent the symptoms of corticoid withdrawal or the inadequate pituitary-adrenal response to stress. Corticotrophin therapy after a course of steroids is of little value. Postoperative shock, reversible by massive steroid therapy, has certainly occurred in patients treated with corticotrophin alone or in combination with steroids. Although there are data suggesting that recovery of normal pituitary synthesis and release of corticotrophin precedes structural and functional recovery of the adrenal, the total pituitary-adrenal response to stress may remain subnormal for more than a year after steroid withdrawal despite corticotrophin administration. Limited experimental data suggest that exogenous corticotrophin may actually interfere with pituitary release of endogenous corticotrophin.

The patient who is being treated with corticosteroids and who faces surgery or sustains an acute injury or infection should be treated with large doses of adrenocortical steroids like the patient with Addison's disease in crisis (see article on the adrenal cortex). The same approach is indicated for patients who have had clinical evidence of induced hyperadrenocorticism within one year preceding the acute emergency or who have been treated with doses the equivalent of more than 25 mg. per day of cortisone for ten days or more within one month. It is of utmost importance *not to rely on corticotrophin therapy for such patients*; their adrenal response to corticotrophin is unpredictable and is generally reduced. Proper replacement therapy is therefore the intravenous infusion of hydrocortisone (as the free steroid or the 21-phosphate or 21-hemisuccinate) in doses of 200 mg. or more per day during the acute episode, with gradual reduction of the dose to the baseline level over the next week or two.

Christy, N. P.: Iatrogenic Cushing's syndrome. *In* The Human Adrenal Cortex, New York, Hoeber Medical Division, Harper and Row (in press).

HYPOPHYSECTOMY-INDUCED HYPOPITUITARISM

Since 1952, *pituitary ablation* has been used in a large number of patients as a palliative treatment for *metastatic cancer* and for *diabetic retinopathy*.

The *metabolic consequences of hypophysectomy in man* are familiar. They are repaired by hormonal replacement therapy. If *diabetes insipidus* is present, it is treated with vasopressin as set forth in the article on the neurohypophysis. Loss of *gonadotrophic* function, observed as disappearance of detectable urinary gonadotrophin, occurs within a week after hypophysectomy. Gonadal steroids are not given, especially to patients with cancer, because hypogonadism may be an important part of the palliative therapy. Loss of *thyrotrophic* function is apparent from fall of serum PBI values to myxedematous levels one week, and of thyroidal uptake of I^{131} two weeks after pituitary ablation. If hypophysectomy is incomplete, these indices decline, only to return to normal within a month after surgery. Loss of *adrenocorticotrophic* function is notable only if hypophysectomy has been very nearly total. Some investigators believe that the metyrapone test is the most sensitive index of completeness of hypophysectomy; if response to metyrapone remains, pituitary ablation may be deemed inadequate.

Conventional treatment consists of thyroid U.S.P. in daily doses of 0.120 gram and cortisone acetate 25 mg. or less, both given by mouth.

Methods for pituitary ablation are numerous: intracranial and trans-sphenoidal hypophysectomy, cryosurgery, stereotaxic radiofrequency surgery, pituitary stalk section, implantation of radioactive gold or yttrium (Au[198], Y[90]), and external delivery of heavy particles (proton beam) from the cyclotron. It is not yet possible to decide which of these techniques is the safest or the most effective. It is also not clear why pituitary ablation is effective at all; there is evidence that adequate palliation is not closely or uniquely related to the degree of reduction in growth hormone secretion.

The present position can be summarized in this way. Carefully selected patients with advanced, widespread metastases from *cancer of the breast* have objective remissions in bony, cutaneous, and pulmonary metastases in about 50 per cent of cases treated with surgical hypophysectomy. Treatment at relatively early stages seems ineffective. Results are statistically better in patients who have had a prior remission from oophorectomy. In *metastatic prostatic cancer*, remissions occur in fewer than half the patients. Patients who respond well to pituitary ablation survive longer (as long as 20 months) than those who do not. The methods which bring about less complete ablation of the pituitary tend to be associated with lower remission rates.

In patients with *diabetic retinopathy* who have no operative contraindication (extreme old age, cardiac disease, severe renal disease, chronic infection), surgical hypophysectomy appears to halt visual deterioration in 20 to 40 per cent of cases; in some recent series, in which several different ablative methods were used, the rate of arrest of retinopathy was 60 to 80 per cent regardless of the technique. Further experience may be expected to clarify indications, contraindications, and the method of choice.

Goldberg, M. F., and Fine, S. L. (eds.): Symposium on the Treatment of Diabetic Retinopathy. Washington, D. C., U. S. Department of Health, Education, and Welfare, USPHS Publication No. 1890, 1969, pp. 147-436.

Juret, P.: Endocrine Surgery in Human Cancers. 2nd ed. Springfield, Ill., Charles C Thomas, 1966.

Leading Article: Pituitary ablation for diabetic retinopathy. Brit. Med. J. 1:254, 1968.

Ray, B. S.: Hypophysectomy as palliative treatment. J.A.M.A., 200:974, 1967.

ANOREXIA NERVOSA

The term "anorexia nervosa" defines the clinical state resulting from psychogenic aversion to food and consequent emaciation. Since the first medical description by Morton (1689) and the famous one by Sir William Gull (1874), a large and colorful literature has characterized the typical patient as an amenorrheic, hyperactive, vivacious, but emotionally disturbed adolescent girl whose frantic energy is in sharp contrast to her cadaverous aspect. Recent investigation has modified this stereotype. The *underlying emotional disorders* include nearly all psychiatric categories, ranging from neurotic overreaction to dieting for obesity to full-blown schizophrenic delusions. Developmental histories of patients show a wide variety of childhood traumas. Precipitating factors are similarly nonspecific. The unique psychodynamic features center about abnormal attitudes toward food and eating that predispose to anorexia as the cardinal symptom. These attitudes may derive from a parent's special preoccupation with eating or obesity, from feeding problems, or from notions in which food takes on bizarre symbolic significance. The three major areas of psychic disturbance appear to be abnormality of body image, which is reflected in a total lack of concern about emaciation, abnormality in perception, i.e., inability to recognize hunger or fatigue, and a sense of helplessness.

The incidence of severe psychic anorexia is low. The sex incidence is approximately 9 to 1 in favor of females. Onset may occur at any age, but the highest incidence is in the late teens and the twenties.

The *psychic origin* of anorexia nervosa is supported by the failure to find an organic basis for it either clinically or at autopsy. Despite earlier hypotheses that anorexia nervosa is primarily an endocrine disturbance, necropsy studies have not shown structural abnormalities in the anterior pituitary, thyroid, or adrenal cortex suggesting hypofunction. The only consistent glandular change appears to be atrophy of the ovaries, which contain few or immature follicles and often no corpora lutea.

The *clinical picture* is that of a patient who has lost a fourth, a half or even more of the total body weight (Fig. 2). Emaciation is variable, but may be extreme. The superabundance of energy (*vide supra*) is more correctly described as a degree of energy that seems out of proportion to the cachexia. Although the hyperactive, jaunty young woman is often encountered, many of the patients are fatigued or depressed, and in late stages there may be striking debility. Amenorrhea usually occurs, but may be independent of weight loss. In some series, more than half the patients have reported the onset of amenorrhea before substantial weight loss occurred; the change in sexual function is therefore not simply a result of malnutrition. Many gastrointestinal symptoms are observed, e.g., globus hystericus, dysphagia, epigastric fullness, constipation, nausea, and vomiting. Vomiting is especially likely to occur if food is forced. Some patients induce vomiting immediately after every meal so that food intake is effectively nil. If undue pressure to eat is exerted, the patient may resort to ingenious devices to avoid eating or may dispose of meals by subterfuge. The physical examination shows emaciation and hypotension, but not bradycardia. In contrast to hypopituitarism, sexual hair is usually not lost; some patients show a fine, generalized hypertrichosis. Anemia and hypoproteinemia may occasionally be found; the blood sugar tends to be at the lower limit of normal.

Laboratory data bear out the normal function of all the endocrine glands with the exception of the gonads. Vaginal smear usually shows absence of cornified cells, and urinary estrogens are low. The generally low or absent titer of urinary gonadotrophin suggests that the ovarian hypofunction is due to hypophysial rather than to primary ovarian failure. Urinary 17-ketosteroids and occasionally corticosteroids are low, as they are in most chronic, wasting diseases, but plasma cortisol levels and their response to administered corticotrophin are normal. Serum protein-bound iodine and thyroidal uptake of I^{131} are normal, although basal metabolic rate is usually low. In short, there is no evidence to support the notion of functional panhypopituitarism in anorexia nervosa.

The confusion about differentiating between anorexia nervosa and pituitary insufficiency has arisen mainly through historic overemphasis upon cachexia as a cardinal symptom of hypopituitarism. Cachexia is not common in pituitary deficiency. Sensible *diagnostic criteria* have been set out by Frazier. The history of severe emotional disturbance and the absence of clinical or laboratory evidence of *general* glandular failure make the diagnosis of anorexia nervosa fairly easy.

Treatment. Treatment, however, is difficult. The acutely ill, emaciated patient is never amenable to psychotherapy. Initial treatment has to be supportive. It is best not to nag the patient about eating; gentle persuasion is preferable. If this fails, tube feedings are necessary, but should be small at first. After the patient has gained weight to about 80 pounds, superficial psychiatric treatment is started. Since there is no fundamental endocrine disorder, endocrine therapy is not indicated; with recovery, the amenorrhea is usually corrected without specific hormonal treatment.

Prognosis. The prognosis is essentially that of the psychiatric disease. In a compilation of 500 cases from the literature, Bliss and Branch found that with various forms of somatic and psychiatric treatment, about 70 per cent of the patients recovered or were improved, 20 per cent showed no improvement, and 6 per cent died of the disease. In a more recent series, only a third of the patients were markedly better after treatment, a third were slightly improved, and a third were no better at all.

Bliss, E. L., and Branch, C. H. H.: Anorexia Nervosa. New York, P. B. Hoeber, Inc., 1960.
Bruch, H.: Perceptual and conceptual disturbances in anorexia nervosa. Psychosom. Med., 24:187, 1962.
Frazier, S.: Anorexia nervosa. Dis. Nerv. Syst., 26:155, 1965.

PITUITARY INSUFFICIENCY IN CHILDHOOD

Lesions involving the pituitary in childhood cause *dwarfism*; like that of gonadotrophin, secretion of growth hormone appears to be more sensitive to impairment than the thyrotrophic or adrenocorticotrophic functions of the pituitary. Pituitary insufficiency is an uncommon cause of dwarfism, accounting for fewer than 10 per cent of instances. About two thirds of pituitary dwarfs have no evidence of pituitary tumor; usually there is no evidence of an anatomic lesion. Idiopathic hypophysial *fibrosis* has been observed. Of the tumors, *craniopharyngioma* (adamantinoma) is the most common. This neoplasm arises from fragments of oral epithelium remaining from the embryologic invagination; the location is usually suprasellar, rarely intrasellar. The tumors become manifest, generally because of chiasmal involvement or symptoms and signs of intracranial pressure, before the onset of puberty. Most children with craniopharyngioma grow normally for the first few years, and the retardation becomes apparent only late in childhood. Suprasellar calcification is seen in roentgenograms of the skull in more than 80 per cent of patients; the sella may be normal in size or enlarged. Other causes are *suprasellar cysts* and *Hand-Schüller-Christian disease.*

Diagnosis of *pituitary dwarfism* is often difficult early in life. The infant's size may be normal at birth. Growth does not stop entirely, but is obviously retarded in early infancy. Evidence of thyroid and adrenocortical insufficiency, e.g., hypoglycemic attacks, is strongly suggestive, but may be subtle or absent. If, however, the patient reaches the early years of the second decade with continued retardation of growth and complete failure of sexual development, suspicion of pituitary dwarfism is raised. The physical examination discloses relatively normal proportions. The *facies* is childish, but the skin may become wrinkled early, imparting an incongruous aspect of aging. Laboratory study shows absence of urinary gonadotrophin, reduced concentration of serum protein-bound iodine and subnormal response of plasma corticosteroids to intravenous adrenocorticotrophin. Idiopathic hypopituitary dwarfism may occur either as an isolated, recessively inherited deficiency of growth hormone, or sporadically. When sporadic, the deficiency may involve growth hormone alone or several pituitary hormones.

The *differential diagnosis* of pituitary dwarfism includes constitutional retardation of growth and delay in the onset of puberty (see Pubertal Development in the Male); in the latter condition, the family history is often positive, evidence of thyroidal and adrenocortical insufficiency is lacking, and in time normal growth and maturation take place. *Systemic and other endocrine diseases* may cause dwarfism; among these are chondrodystrophy, rickets, Hurler's syndrome, intestinal malabsorption, chronic renal disease, hypoxia associated with congenital cardiac malformations, hypothyroidism, and sexual precocity with premature fusion of the epiphyses. These conditions are distinguished fairly easily by the inappropriately short extremities, osseous deformities, overt malnutrition and evidence of fat intolerance, gross proteinuria and nitrogen retention, cyanosis and heart murmur, mental deficiency and other stigmata of cretinism, or precocious development of the genitalia. D. W. Smith has presented a list of 52 conditions associated with short stature, some of which are recognized at a glance by seasoned pediatricians; Smith also lists the very numerous systemic diseases in which growth retardation is observed (*vide infra,* References).

One of the most difficult disorders to distinguish from pituitary dwarfism before puberty is *primordial dwarfism.* The patients, also known as sexual ateliotic (incomplete) dwarfs, become miniature adults, often capable of producing normal offspring. McKusick and his co-workers have shown that in some of these patients the failure to grow in association with normal gonadal and secondary sexual development and normal thyroid and adrenal function is due to a deficiency of end-organ response to growth. With radioimmunoassay measurements of serum growth hormone, it is possible to define four subgroups of ateliotic dwarfs. It is interesting that the African pygmy also has subresponsiveness to administered growth hormone, whereas endogenous growth hormone release is apparently normal. The differentiation of pituitary dwarfism in the female, and *gonadal dysgenesis (Turner's syndrome)* may be difficult before puberty; patients with this disorder are phenotypic females who often have associated congenital anomalies (webbed neck, coarctation of the aorta) and short stature; the distinguishing features are less immature facies, less delay in epiphysial closure, slight but definite growth of pubic hair at puberty, a frequently negative (male) chromatin pattern on buccal smear, and, after the age of 9 to 13, an elevated rather than absent titer of urinary gonadotrophin. Recognition of *progeria* is easy; this rare idiopathic condition is characterized by retardation of growth, baldness, loss of subcutaneous fat, premature fusion of epiphyses, and atherosclerosis or arterial calcification, all occurring within the first few years of life. The life span is short; there is no evidence of endocrine disease.

As indicated above (Assessment of Anterior Pituitary Function), the best way to detect growth hormone deficiency is to test the response of serum growth hormone values to insulin-induced hypoglycemia. If a metabolic ward is available, demonstration of a sharp increase in nitrogen retention in response to administered growth hormone is diagnostic. Analysis of the growth curve determines whether or not to subject the patient to elaborate testing procedures.

As to *treatment,* a moderate degree of linear growth can be achieved in pituitary dwarfs through the administration of thyroid hormone in combination with gonadal steroids. Impressive skeletal growth can be induced with the administration of purified human growth hormone. The optimal dose is about 20 to 45 mg. per month. This therapy is limited by the short supply of the hormone; if it is used, gonadal steroids should not be given until maximal linear growth is attained so that epiphysial closure will not occur; thyroid hormone augments the somatotrophic effects. Crawford and his colleagues have set out detailed criteria for diagnosis and treatment of pituitary dwarfism and have described the response to growth hormone. The hormone causes only minimal if any increase in linear growth rate in children whose short stature is not due to hypopituitarism. Since growth hormone should therefore be reserved for patients with growth hormone deficiency, a high premium is placed upon accurate diagnosis.

Goodman, H. C., Grumbach, M. M., and Kaplan, S. L.: Growth and growth hormone: II. A comparison of isolated growth hormone deficiency and multiple pituitary hormone deficiencies in 35 patients with idiopathic hypopituitary dwarfism. New Eng. J. Med., 278:57, 1968.

Henneman, P. H.: The effect of human growth hormone on growth of patients with hypopituitarism: A combined study. J.A.M.A., 205:828, 1968.

Martin, M. M., and Wilkins, L.: Pituitary dwarfism: Diagnosis and treatment. J. Clin. Endocr., 18:679, 1958.

Merimee, T. J., et al.: An unusual variety of endocrine dwarfism: Subresponsiveness to growth hormone in a sexually mature dwarf. Lancet, 2:191, 1968.

Merimee, T. J., Hall, J. D., Rimoin, D. L., and McKusick, V. A.: A metabolic and hormonal basis for classifying ateliotic dwarfs. Lancet, 1:963, 1969.

Prader, A.: Dwarfism, hypopituitarism, and growth hormone. Arch. Dis. Child., 42:225, 1967.

Rimoin, D. L., et al.: Peripheral subresponsiveness to human growth hormone in the African pygmies. New Eng. J. Med., 281:1383, 1969.

Root, A. W., Rosenfield, R. L., Bongiovanni, A. M., and Eberlein, W. R.: The plasma growth hormone response to insulin-induced hypoglycemia in children with retardation of growth. Pediatrics, 39:844, 1967.

Silver, H. K., and Finkelstein, M.: Deprivation dwarfism. J. Pediat., 70:317, 1967.

Smith, D. W.: Compendium on shortness of stature. J. Pediat., 70:463, 1967.

Soyka, L. F., Ziskind, A., and Crawford, J. D.: Treatment of short stature in children and adolescents with human pituitary growth hormone (Raben). New Eng. J. Med., 271:1754, 1964.

Wilkins, L.: The Diagnosis and Treatment of Endocrine Disorders in Childhood and Adolescence. 3rd ed. Springfield, Ill., Charles C Thomas, 1965.

HYPERPITUITARISM

ACROMEGALY

Definition. Acromegaly is a chronic disease of middle life characterized by overgrowth of bone, connective tissue, and viscera in response to prolonged and excessive secretion of adenohypophysial growth hormone. The term "acromegaly" denotes the typical enlargement of acral or distal parts of the body—the hands, feet, face, and head.

Etiology. The increased secretion of growth hormone results from overactivity of the acidophil cells of the pituitary. The evidence for excessive growth hormone is that (1) similar pathologic changes are produced in animals by administration of the hormone, and (2) increased concentrations of growth hormone have been detected in plasma of patients with acromegaly. Hyperactivity of the anterior pituitary is deduced from (1) the almost invariable necropsy finding of pituitary enlargement, (2) histologic observation of overgrowth of the acidophilic cells, and (3) the clinical improvement that frequently follows destruction of the gland.

Incidence and Prevalence. Acromegaly is a rare disorder (one in 5000 to 15,000 patients). The sexes are affected equally often. Acromegaly starts most commonly in the third and fourth decades; a few patients trace the start of acromegaly to adolescence. Some 30 acromegalic children have been reported.

Pathology and Pathogenesis. Acidophilic or mixed acidophilic and chromophobe adenoma is found in 75 per cent or more of autopsied patients with acromegaly. Rarely, acidophil cell hyperplasia is observed, malignancy almost never. The growth of the tumor may obliterate normal cells. The assumption is that if hypopituitarism occurs, it is a result of atrophy of normal pituitary tissue due to the pressure of the tumor. Over 80 per cent of adenomas cause sufficient enlargement of the sella turcica to be visible in roentgenograms of the skull. Sellar enlargement may be minimal or gross. Upward extension rarely produces clinical evidence of hypothalamic involvement, e.g., diabetes insipidus, but invasion of the optic tracts or chiasm is of clinical significance (visual field changes, optic atrophy) in about 60 per cent of patients.

The excessive secretion of growth hormone affects virtually all organs and tissues. The response of cartilage and bone is obvious and distinctive. The histologic appearance of chondrogenesis and osteogenesis is somewhat disorderly. The cartilaginous and bony response occurs at points of special sensitivity, e.g., mandible, zygoma, ribs, and clavicles. The uneven growth is thought to be due to the effect of pressure or of muscular traction. Increased *chondrogenesis* is most obvious in hypertrophy of the costal cartilages, which contributes to the increased circumference of the thorax. *Acromegalic arthritis,* affecting chiefly the large joints and the spine, resembles osteoarthritis and results from proliferation of deep layers of joint cartilage with thinning of articular cartilages. Hypertrophy of nasal and aural cartilage accounts for part of the enlargement of nose and ears. *Osteogenesis* from the thickened periosteum is accelerated; absorption of bone is also rapid; late in the disease *osteoporosis* may be striking. There is overgrowth of the supraorbital ridge. The anterior temporal ridge advances with forward growth of the lateral portions of the orbit, expansion of the frontal sinuses, and forward displacement of the zygoma. Overgrowth of the maxilla lengthens the face, and the teeth are separated by heaping up of alveolar bone. The ramus of the mandible grows longer; the angle between ramus and body opens out to produce mandibular prognathism. The ribs and clavicles widen and reach a length 2 to 3 inches greater than normal. The *long bones* thicken and become massive. The humerus and femur may be lengthened, and the latter may be deformed by bowing. The vertebral bodies are increased in the anteroposterior diameter; the greatest changes occur in the thoracic spine with deposit of new bone upon diaphyses, particularly anteriorly; this change makes forward flexion of the spine difficult.

The visible *enlargement of distal parts* is chiefly due to proliferation of soft tissue, not bone. Subcutaneous connective tissue is grossly increased, giving the characteristic thick and fleshy appearance of the *hands* and *feet*, enlargement of the *lips*, and *accentuation of skin folds*. The skin itself is greatly thickened; there are increased sweating and seborrhea; hirsutism occurs in a few female patients. The *tongue* may be so large as to protrude from the mouth.

Widespread splanchnomegaly is the rule. The heart, lungs, liver, spleen, and intestines are variously enlarged two- to fivefold. The kidneys are enlarged by the growth of individual nephrons; studies of renal function indicate increased glomerular filtration rate and proximal tubular activity. The endocrine glands participate in the splanchnomegaly. A possible role of accompanying oversecretion of trophic hormones is not proved. The gonads, although often functioning subnormally and showing histologic evidence of failure, may be large. The *adrenal cortex* is hypertrophied, and nodules are often found. The *thyroid* may be eight to nine times the normal size; goiters are diffuse or nodular. True hyperthyroidism is uncommon. The *parathyroids* are usually enlarged, and adenomas occur. Although there is generalized enlargement of tissues and organs and a considerable gain in weight, obesity is almost unknown, possibly because of the adipokinetic effect of growth hormone. The muscles enlarge somewhat but without conspicuous hypertrophy; edema and deposition of mucopolysaccharide in muscle have been reported; atrophy is a late finding.

Clinical Manifestations and Natural History. The onset of acromegaly is usually so insidious and so subtle that it escapes detection by the patient and his intimate associates. The gradualness and subtlety of onset are such that a third of the patients seek medical help for unrelated diseases, being unaware of their acromegaly. In Davidoff's series of 100 patients, the mean age of onset was estimated as 27 years, but the mean age at which the patients presented themselves was over 40; this average lapse of 13 or 14 years implies chronicity and a generally slow course. Careful analysis of the history reveals that early symptoms are related to peripheral effects of growth hormone or, much less commonly, to the mechanical pressure of the intrasellar tumor. Even before the obvious changes in appearance are noticed patients may complain of excessive sweating, paresthesias of the hands and feet, and pain and stiffness of the slowly expanding fingers and toes. Arthralgias are common. Accounts of hypersexuality and greatly increased muscular strength early in the course of the disease are rare. Complaints of hypogonadism (amenorrhea, loss of libido) are common. Headache may be extremely severe; the mechanism is not clear, since, in many instances, there is little clinically detectable enlargement of the pituitary tumor. Impairment of visual acuity or symptomatic encroachment upon visual fields occurs in over 60 per cent of patients at one time or another.

The *clinical picture* of advanced acromegaly is easily recognized on physical examination, but the changes are occasionally subtle. The typical acromegalic is large and burly; in late stages the forward carriage of the head, prognathism, kyphosis, bowing of the legs, and rolling gait are distinctive. The features are blunt and coarse, the nose and ears large, the brow is prominent and the jaw prognathous, the facial wrinkles are exaggerated, the lips are full. The skin is thick and hairy, the voice husky and cavernous. The hands and feet are enlarged; shaking hands with an acromegalic patient gives the startling impression of losing one's hand in a warm mass of rubbery dough. The superficial veins of the extremities are thick and prominent. The thoracic cage is widened and deepened and thoracic kyphosis is present. Galactorrhea is an occasional finding in men and women.

Most *laboratory data* are within normal limits. The basal metabolic rate is elevated in more than half the patients, but other evidence of hyperthyroidism (increased thyroidal uptake of I^{131} or level of serum precipitable iodine) is usually lacking even when the thyroid is palpably enlarged. Appraisal of adrenocortical function reveals normal plasma cortisol values, normal response to ACTH, occasionally increased excretion of urinary 17-ketosteroids or corticosteroids, and sometimes raised cortisol secretory rate and a degree of adrenal refractoriness to suppression by dexamethasone. Urinary gonadotrophin titer is normal or reduced; semen analysis generally shows oligospermia. Despite the reported increased insulin activity of acromegalic plasma, glycosuria or glucose intolerance is found in about a third of acromegalic subjects, frank diabetes in about one fifth. The diabetes is usually mild and somewhat resistant to insulin, but management of the diabetes presents no unusually difficult problems, and ketoacidosis is rare. Hypercalciuria is a common finding, and hypercalcemia occurs in a few patients; in some this abnormality is apparently due to hypersecretion of growth hormone, since it disappears with successful treatment of the acromegaly. However, in others the hypercalcemia persists and can be shown to be due to associated hyperparathyroidism as part of the syndrome of multiple endocrine adenomatosis.

As the disease progresses, muscular weakness supervenes; kyphosis increases, partly because of osteoporosis. Visual impairment may become aggravated to the point of blindness. Partial or total pituitary insufficiency may ensue. The course is extremely variable; it is hard to know with accuracy the natural history because the onset is usually so insidious and because most patients have received some sort of treatment. The course may be fulminant, resulting in death within three years (usually because of tumor growth in younger patients), or benign and intermittent, lasting 50 years or longer. Death comes from the tumor (expansion, hemorrhage into its substance, "pituitary apoplexy"), cardiac failure (owing to "acromegalic heart disease"), or the effects of hypertension (found in 20 to 50 per cent of patients) or degenerative vascular disease. The causes of death in years past were diabetes and hypopituitarism; these are now rarely lethal because of the availability of adequate treatment.

Diagnosis. The typical acromegalic is recognized at a glance. *The great need is a means of early diagnosis.* If acromegaly is suspected, a history of increasing size of gloves, shoes, and dentures provides useful clues. Tightness of old rings is suggestive; comparison of the patient's features with old photographs is helpful. Roentgenogram of the skull and tests of the visual fields usually give confirmatory evidence.

The differential diagnosis rarely presents difficulties. The large tongue, hoarse voice, and periorbital edema may suggest myxedema, but the other physical and laboratory abnormalities of hypothyroidism are absent. Patients with pachydermoperiostosis, some of whom look quite acromegalic, do not have involvement of the pituitary. The articular pains are usually distinguishable from those associated with other forms of arthritis by the typical acromegalic aspect.

There is no generally satisfactory method for the indirect assessment of the *secretory activity* of the adenoma. History of recent acral enlargement is the evidence of active secretion. Laboratory data are disappointing. Elevation of serum phosphorus follows administration of human growth hormone, but is an unreliable index of "activity" of the disease in acromegaly. The same may be said of the glucose tolerance test and basal metabolic rate. Some investigators consider the insulin tolerance test useful. Biopsy of costal cartilage may show active endochondral bone formation. Urinary excretion of hydroxyproline is increased. None of these laboratory indices has been conclusively proved to correlate closely with the clinical course of the disease. If plasma growth hormone measurements cannot be made, one must rely on a synthesis of historical, physical, and laboratory findings. Without documentary evidence of recent acral growth, judgment of secretory activity is highly subjective.

The use of *radioimmunoassay of plasma growth hormone* offers promise as a method of *direct* assessment of the secretory activity of the acidophilic tumor. It is known that most untreated acromegalics have high concentrations. After hypophysectomy these fall, often to normal, but sometimes they remain elevated, presumably when hypophysectomy is not complete. After pituitary radiation, levels often do not fall. Not enough data are yet available to allow a complete

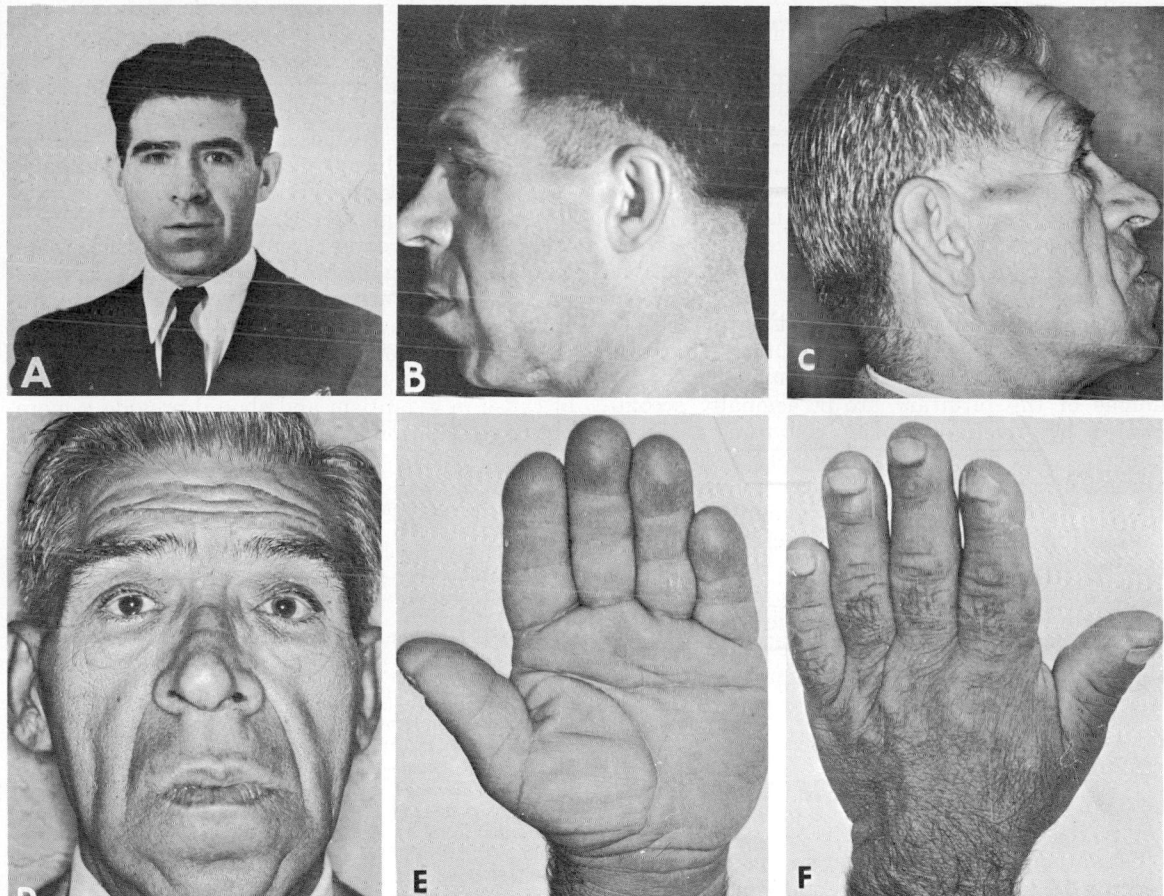

FIGURE 3. Evolution of acromegaly. *A,* Age 38, within a year after onset of the disease. *B,* Age 55, after two courses of radiation therapy to sella; disease has progressed with moderate coarsening of features: thickening of lips, enlargement of nose and ears, and prognathism. *C, D,* Age 64, 26 years after onset, after a third series of x-ray treatments to sella; nose and ears have enlarged further, supraorbital ridge and zygoma have become more prominent, and jaw is more prognathous, frontal view shows increasing wrinkling of the skin (temporary atrophy is a result of x-irradiation). *E, F,* Age 64, volar and dorsal aspects of hand, showing broadened fingers and characteristically "meaty" appearance owing to the gross increase in the soft tissue, not bone.

appraisal of growth hormone response to physiologic stimuli (hypoglycemia, glucose administration) as a measure of "activity" in acromegaly. What is needed is careful correlation (over a period of years) of plasma growth hormone levels with objective studies of acral growth. Such studies will reveal the value of plasma growth hormone measurements as indices of secretory activity. At the moment, it appears that sharp falls in basal plasma growth hormone value, or recovery of growth hormone responsiveness to administered glucose, should be related to clinically arrested disease. Further observations are required to confirm or refute this suspicion.

Treatment. Treatment is aimed at relief of the ocular and other local effects of the adenoma and at reduction of the secretory rate of growth hormone. Surgical extirpation is generally reserved for patients who have a visual acuity of 20/200 or less in one eye and a significant loss of acuity in the other. The acromegalic is a poor surgical risk; the slightest suspicion of adrenocortical insufficiency requires the use of cortisone. Improvement in vision is achieved in about half

the patients operated upon. Headache may or may not be relieved. Results are better if postoperative radiotherapy is used. X-radiation of the sella is the preferred treatment in the absence of serious visual loss. The standard dose is 3500 to 4500 r to the tumor. Side effects of radiotherapy are not trivial. Radiation sickness is rare, but lethargy is a common complaint; a few patients have transient worsening of ocular signs during therapy, and a small proportion of these may require operative intervention before the course of x-ray treatment is completed. Because of the extraordinary difficulty of evaluating the hormonal activity of the adenoma, results of radiotherapy are uncertain; estimates of its successful use (meaning arrest of growth and arrest of the progress of the tumor) range from 30 to 70 per cent, the percentage roughly paralleling the dose of x-ray used.

Hypophysectomy, when used in patients whose vision is threatened, affords good control of the secretory activity of the tumor only if pituitary tissue is totally removed. Other methods have been tried with some successful and even dramatic results: implantation of *radioactive substances* (yttrium-90, gold-198) directly into the tumor, cryosurgery, and *radiation with heavy particles* (alpha-particles, protons). With these more drastic methods recession in soft tissue and even in bony abnormalities has been observed. Although I believe that conventional pituitary radiation does not adequately control the oversecretion of growth hormone, tumor growth is probably arrested in about 70 per cent of patients. Since the disease is benign, slow-moving, and compatible with long life, one should be cautious in the use of radical treatments unless sight is threatened.

Acromegaly Associated with Other Endocrine Disorders. Eosinophilic or chromophobic adenomas of the pituitary are occasionally accompanied by functioning islet cell tumors of the pancreas and adenomas of the parathyroids and adrenals. Intractable peptic ulcer is often associated. The disorder is familial in many instances. Presenting symptoms may be those of hypoglycemia, hyperparathyroidism, e.g., renal colic, or gastrointestinal hemorrhage. It is probably more correct to regard *multiple endocrine adenomatosis* as a complex of separate genetic abnormalities than as a series of consequences of a single primary endocrine disease.

GIGANTISM

Gigantism is generally defined as height exceeding 78 to 80 inches or, in children, exceeding a height three standard deviations above the mean for age. This rare disorder has been conventionally regarded as the childhood counterpart of acromegaly, i.e., as oversecretion of growth hormone by a pituitary adenoma in a growing organism *before closure of the epiphyses.* However, acromegaly occurs in young children. It is reasonable to doubt a pituitary cause when (1) there is no evidence of acromegaly, (2) the sella is not enlarged, or (3) there is a strong familial history of unusually tall stature suggesting constitutional gigantism. A form of "cerebral gigantism" is described in children; associated features are macrocrania, large extremities, large hands and feet, evidence of cerebral dysfunction, and normal values and normal response of plasma growth hormone. An additional cause of tall stature is hypogonadism or late puberty, resulting in prolongation of the period of linear growth because of delayed epiphysial closure. In such patients, the bodily proportions are eunuchoidal, with a lower segment greater than the upper segment and arm span greater than height. In those giants who are acromegalic (about 50 per cent), management is that of acromegaly. Treatment of the pituitary adenoma should probably be more vigorous than it is. The radioimmunoassay for growth hormone should lead to more accurate assignment of cause in gigantism and should provide a more objective criterion as a guide to management.

Ballard, H. S., Frame, B., and Hartsock, R. J.: Familial multiple endocrine adenoma-peptic ulcer complex. Medicine, 43:481, 1964.

Boden, G., Soeldner, J. S., Steinke, J., and Thorn, G. W.: Serum growth hormone (HGH) response to IV glucose: Diagnosis of acromegaly in females and males, Metabolism, 17:1, 1968.

Davidoff, L. M.: Studies in acromegaly: III. The anamnesis and symptomatology in one hundred cases. Endocrinology, 10: 461, 1926.

Earll, J. M., Sparks, L. L., and Forsham, P. H.: Glucose suppression of serum growth hormone in the diagnosis of acromegaly. J.A.M.A., 201:628, 1967.

Forbes, A. P., Henneman, P. H., Griswold, G. C., and Albright, F.: Syndrome characterized by galactorrhea, amenorrhea, and low urinary FSH: Comparison with acromegaly and normal lactation. J. Clin. Endocr., 14:265, 1964.

Gordon, D. A., Hill, F. M., and Ezrin, C.: Acromegaly: A review of 100 cases. Canad. Med. Ass. J., 87:1106, 1962.

Hook, E. B., and Reynolds, J. W.: Cerebral gigantism: Endocrinological and clinical observations of six patients including a congenital giant, concordant monozygotic twins, and a child who achieved adult gigantic size. J. Pediat., 70: 900, 1967.

Kozak, G. P., Vagnucci, A. I., Lauler, D. P., and Thorn, G. W.: Acromegaly pre- and postpituitary irradiation. Metabolism, 15:290, 1966.

Roth, J., Gorden, P., and Brace, K.: Efficacy of conventional pituitary irradiation in acromegaly. New Eng. J. Med., 282: 1385, 1970.

Wermer, P.: Endocrine adenomatosis and peptic ulcer in a large kindred. Inherited multiple tumors and mosaic pleiotropism in man. Amer. J. Med., 35:205, 1963.

Wright, A. D., McLachlan, M. S. F., Doyle, F. H., and Fraser, T. R.: Serum growth hormone levels and size of pituitary tumour in untreated acromegaly. Brit. Med. J., 2:582, 1969.

Posterior Pituitary
Alexander Leaf

ANTIDIURETIC HORMONE

Normal Physiology. Antidiuretic hormone is produced in nuclei of the anterior hypothalamus. The major source of this hormone is the supraoptic nuclei, but contributions from the paraventricular and filiform nuclei are thought to be added. The hormone produced in these neural centers is transported by a process of neural secretion down the supraopticohypophysial tract to the neurohypophysis or posterior pituitary where the hormone is stored until released into the blood according to the state of hydration of the subject.

The antidiuretic hormone in man was identified by du Vigneaud as the octapeptide, arginine vasopressin. The hormone is released normally in response to osmotic stimuli; a rise in concentration of solute, largely the salts of sodium, in the plasma or extracellular fluid, serves as the stimulus for release of vasopressin from the neurohypophysis. The hormone circulates to the kidney where its major action is on the epithelium lining the collecting ducts. In the presence of vasopressin this epithelium becomes more permeable to water so that water is transported from the tubular lumen to the more concentrated peritubular fluids. This serves to reduce urine volume and increase its concentration, thereby conserving body water. Dilution of plasma or extracellular fluids, as occurs after water ingestion, inhibits release of antidiuretic hormone. The dilute luminal fluid entering the distal convoluted tubule is excreted with little modification in concentration, with the result that a copious flow of dilute urine characterizes the absence of antidiuretic hormone. This rids the body of any excess of water.

The thirst center is functionally and anatomically closely related to the antidiuretic mechanism. Andersson has shown that osmotic or electrical stimulation of the anterior portion of the supraoptic nuclei creates a sensation of thirst; dilution of plasma inhibits thirst. The integrated activity of thirst and antidiuretic mechanism serves to regulate the concentration of body fluids as follows:

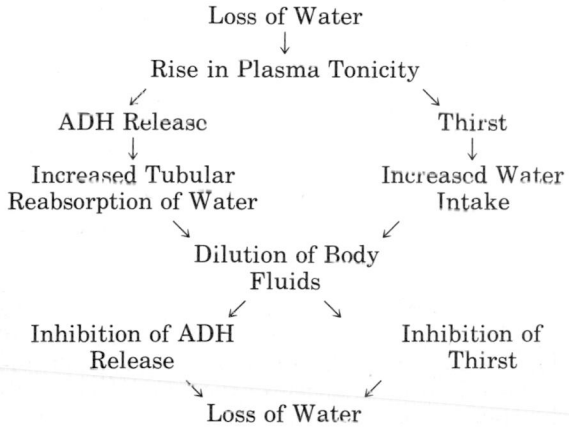

Loss of Water
↓
Rise in Plasma Tonicity
↙   ↘
ADH Release   Thirst
↓   ↓
Increased Tubular   Increased Water
Reabsorption of Water   Intake
↘   ↙
Dilution of Body
Fluids
↙   ↘
Inhibition of ADH   Inhibition of
Release   Thirst
↘   ↙
Loss of Water

This double negative feedback system works with remarkable effectiveness to preserve the concentration of sodium in the serum between some 136 and 143 mEq. per liter. Since intracellular fluids are in osmotic equilibrium with the extracellular fluids, this mechanism regulates the tonicity of the body fluid compartments.

In addition to the usual osmotic stimuli regulating release of vasopressin, other factors may affect this process. Pain and emotional states have been associated with antidiuresis as have a number of pharmacologic agents which act to release the hormone. These include cinchoninic acid, acetylcholine, nicotine, morphine, barbiturates, ferritin, and bradykinin. Alcohol may inhibit release of antidiuretic hormone, but the effect is weak and is often obscured. Physiologically, reduction in the effective plasma volume appears to be a stimulus for secretion of antidiuretic hormone;

at least this has been documented following acute large blood loss.

Andersson, B.: Polydipsia, antidiuresis and milk ejection caused by hypothalamic stimulation. *In* Heller, H. (ed.): The Neurohypophysis. London, Butterworth Scientific Publications, 1957.
du Vigneaud, V.: Hormones of the posterior pituitary gland: oxytocin and vasopressin. *In* The Harvey Lectures 1954–1955. New York, Academic Press, Inc., 1956.
Leaf, A.: The clinical and physiologic significance of the serum sodium concentration. New Eng. J. Med., 267:24, 77, 1962.
Verney, E. B.: The absorption and excretion of water: The antidiuretic hormone. Lancet, 2:739, 781, 1946.

DIABETES INSIPIDUS

Etiology. Diabetes insipidus is an uncommon disturbance resulting from any condition which damages the neurohypophysial system. Idiopathic cases constitute the major group, comprising approximately 45 per cent. The idiopathic condition may become manifest at any age and affect either sex. It is unusual in infancy, but may commence in early childhood. Familial diabetes insipidus is very uncommon, but may occur in infancy or childhood and affect either sex. The condition has been noted in seven generations of one family. Familial diabetes insipidus is to be distinguished from nephrogenic diabetes insipidus, which is a renal tubular defect, inherited largely by males, in whom the affected tubules are unresponsive to antidiuretic hormone.

Head trauma (accidental or neurosurgical) and neoplasms (primary or metastatic) are the major causes of acquired diabetes insipidus. Of the metastatic tumors, breast cancer seems to have a special predilection for the hypothalamic area. Other rarer etiologic factors include sarcoidosis, birth injuries, eosinophilic granuloma, and a variety of local infections. Even with lesions directly in the hypothalamus, diabetes insipidus is rare, because a small fraction of normal tissue suffices to protect against manifest dysfunction. Since the posterior and anterior pituitary have separate blood supplies, infarction of the latter need not be associated with failure of the former; a space-occupying lesion is suspect when insufficiency of both occurs.

Clinical Manifestations. The polyuria and polydipsia can be so dramatic that adult patients may remember an exact date or even hour when symptoms started. The fluid exchanges may reach the distressing proportions of 5 to 10 liters or more per 24 hours. The specific gravity of the urine is usually 1.001 to 1.005; corresponding concentrations will be about 100 to 200 mOsm. per liter. With restriction of fluid intake the specific gravity may reach 1.010, or even slightly higher with severe water lack, and urine concentration may increase to 300 mOsm. per liter. Urine slightly hypertonic to serum has been produced experimentally in the complete absence of antidiuretic hormone by greatly reducing the glomerular filtration rate. The elaboration of a hypertonic urine by a patient with diabetes insipidus during severe dehydration or with acute reduction of the glomerular filtration rate due to any cause need not, therefore, indicate the presence of residual neurohypophysial function.

Other than the annoyance of polyuria and polydypsia, there may be no evidence of ill health or of other physiologic disturbance associated with the condition, unless the patient suffers from the underlying local or systemic disease which has destroyed the neurohypophysial system. The assumption that patients with diabetes insipidus suffer from severe dehydration is not supported by measurements of serum sodium or total solute concentrations. A slight elevation of sodium and total solute concentrations of serum has been demonstrated statistically, but the overlap in individual cases is such as to make these determinations of little assistance diagnostically; 295 ± 15 mOsm. per liter (S.D.) for diabetes insipidus and 280 ± 60 mOsm. per liter (S.D.) for normal persons. As long as the patient's thirst center remains intact, the total solute concentration of the body fluids will be preserved close to normal values, but at the expense of polydipsia and the large fluid exchange characteristic of the condition. Following a period of water restriction, these differences may be accentuated and have greater diagnostic value.

With unconsciousness resulting from trauma or anesthesia, the inability of the patient to demand water may be fatal. This situation may occur at the onset of diabetes insipidus secondary to head injury or intracranial surgery, and is one of the causes of hypernatremia following trauma to the head. A careful record of urine volumes and urine and serum concentrations in patients with acute head trauma and coma will prevent the occurrence of severe dehydration.

Differential Diagnosis. A patient with persistent polyuria and urine of low concentration may have one or more of three basic disturbances: (1) inability of the kidney to elaborate a concentrated urine despite adequate vasopressin, (2) deficient vasopressin, or (3) persistent excessive water intake. Any condition which disturbs the renal concentrating mechanism, rendering it unresponsive to vasopressin, may produce polyuria. Hypercalcemia, potassium depletion, or renal failure (both chronic and acute) may impair maximal concentrating ability, but none of these conditions causes the urine to be persistently hypotonic, and in only a few patients does the resulting polyuria suggest diabetes insipidus. These conditions are readily excluded in establishing the diagnosis of diabetes insipidus. The rare nephrogenic diabetes insipidus results from a failure of the renal tubule to respond to vasopressin. Patients with uncontrolled diabetes mellitus may exhibit extreme polyuria and polydipsia, but the specific gravity of the urine is high, although its osmolality may not be over 300 mOsm. per liter; the large contribution which glucose makes to the specific gravity accounts for this seeming discrepancy.

Although it is evident that polyuria in diabetes insipidus is primary to polydipsia, compulsive water drinking may give rise to a condition which closely mimics diabetes insipidus. Chronic ingestion of large volumes of water impairs the renal concentrating mechanism, making it sometimes quite difficult to distinguish this psychogenic disturbance from true diabetes insipidus.

Several special procedures have been devised to assist in establishing the diagnosis of diabetes insipidus in patients with polyuria and polydipsia. They all test ability to respond to osmotic stimuli by elaboration of a concentrated urine, whether failure to do so is the consequence of a lack of endogenous vasopressin or of an inability of the renal tubules to respond to the hormone.

Water restriction with observation of urine volume and concentration constitutes the simplest test. Weight should be followed to avoid the hazards of incurring loss of more than 3 to 5 per cent of body weight. Small children and infants are especially liable to serious circulatory disturbances if dehydration is allowed beyond this limit. A normal subject may be expected to reduce urine flow to less than 0.5 ml. per minute and increase urine concentration to greater than 800 mOsm. per liter (corresponding to a specific gravity of 1.020 or above). In patients with diabetes insipidus, urine volumes well above this limit persist and urine concentration remains below 200 mOsm. per liter (specific gravities of 1.001 to 1.005) until advanced states of dehydration are present. Unfortunately, the differences are often not so clear, and patients with neurohypophysial insufficiency may concentrate their urine to 300 to 400 mOsm. per liter (specific gravities of 1.008 to 1.014) with marked dehydration.

Another means of increasing plasma osmolarity to test the release of antidiuretic hormone is by the infusion of hypertonic solutions. After an initial hydrated state is established, 2.5 per cent sodium chloride is infused intravenously at a rate of 0.25 ml. per minute per kilogram of body weight for 45 minutes. Urine flow is measured at 15-minute intervals. If neurohypophysial and renal functions are normal, urine flow will drop promptly to 25 per cent or less of control.

If either the water deprivation test or the infusion of hypertonic saline fails to reduce urine flow or to increase urine concentration, as expected, the ability of the patients' kidneys to respond to exogenous vasopressin must be demonstrated, in order to separate nephrogenic causes from hormone deficiency. For this purpose 5 mU. per minute of aqueous vasopressin (vasopressin injection, U.S.P.) may be administered intravenously for at least one hour by a slow drip, or 5 units of the long-acting vasopressin tannate in oil may be administered intramuscularly. An injection of the latter material in the evening, with urine samples collected on arising the following morning and hourly for three successive hours thereafter, should induce maximal concentration.

These simple measures will readily distinguish diabetes insipidus from nephrogenic causes of diminished response to vasopressin. To distinguish true diabetes insipidus from compulsive water drinking may be more difficult, because continued polydipsia lowers the maximal urinary concentrations achievable following dehydration, infusions of hypertonic saline, or exogenous vasopressin. In addition to the laboratory studies it should be remembered that compulsive water drinking to a degree which is confused with diabetes insipidus constitutes a severe psychogenic disorder. Clinical evaluation is usually rewarding in revealing other neurotic symptoms supporting the suspicion of a serious personality or behavioral disturbance.

Treatment. If symptoms are mild, no therapy may be warranted, although a thorough search for underlying causative factors should be conducted. When symptoms interfere with sleep or interrupt work, treatment is indicated. Replacement therapy intramuscularly with long-acting vasopressin in oil (1.0 ml. ampule contains 5 units per ml.; 0.5 to 1.0 ml. injected every 24 to 72 hours, as necessary to control polyuria) is generally reserved for the more severe cases, whereas a nasal spray, self-administered as necessary, every two to six hours may suffice to alleviate symptoms. Thiazide diuretics, 250 mg. chlorothiazide two or three times daily, presumably by sustaining a condition of persistent mild salt depletion, will blunt a water diuresis, and in patients with diabetes insipidus may reduce urine flow by some 50 per cent. In patients with nephrogenic diabetes insipidus this form of antidiuretic agent is also effective.

Barlow, E. D., and de Wardener, H. E.: Compulsive water drinking. Quart. J. of Med., 28:235, 1959.

Coggins, C. H., and Leaf, A.: Diabetes insipidus. Amer. J. Med., 42:807, 1967.

Leaf, A.: Diabetes insipidus. *In* Astwood, E. B. (ed.): Clinical Endocrinology, I. New York, Grune and Stratton, Inc., 1960.

Williams, R. H., and Henry, C.: Nephrogenic diabetes insipidus: transmitted by females and appearing during infancy in males. Ann. Intern. Med., 27:84, 1947.

THE SYNDROME OF INAPPROPRIATE SECRETION OF ANTIDIURETIC HORMONE

Inappropriate secretion of antidiuretic hormone, characterized by dilution of the body fluids, results from the presence of circulating antidiuretic activity in the absence of the usually recognized physiologic or pharmacologic stimuli for secretion of the antidiuretic hormone. The diagnosis of this condition, therefore, requires that osmotic stimuli for hormone secretion must not be present; nor can effective plasma volume or the circulatory system be insufficient. Furthermore, pharmacologic agents known to elicit antidiuresis, such as morphine or barbiturates, or psychic stimuli, such as pain, must be absent.

Pathophysiology. The syndrome can be easily reproduced in normal subjects by administration of a long-acting preparation of vasopressin. This will reduce urine flow and increase urine concentration, as expected. If fluid intake exceeds the sum of its losses, then a positive water balance ensues; there is a gain in body weight and dilution of body fluids with a fall in concentration of sodium. The water gained is shared by all body fluid compartments so that plasma volume and cardiac output are increased. The resulting increase in renal perfusion and glomerular filtration rate delivers more sodium into the renal tubules. Tubular reabsorption of sodium is diminished in the presence of an overexpanded plasma volume, and large amounts of sodium may be lost in the urine. This loss of sodium and chloride in the urine plus the dilution of body fluids leads to hyponatremia, with serum sodium concentrations in extreme cases falling below 100 mEq. per liter. The dilution is shared proportionately by serum chloride concentration, but does not detectably affect the concentration of the quantitatively minor extracellular ions, potassium, calcium, and so forth.

The clinical features of this syndrome are: (1) hyponatremia and hypochloremia; (2) normal cardiovascular function as indicated by normal blood pressure, normal skin turgor, and absence of edema or congestion; (3) normal renal function with low levels of blood urea nitrogen and of serum creatinine; (4) normal adrenal cortical function; and (5) urinary sodium excretion reflecting dietary sodium.

Etiology. This syndrome was first recognized by Schwartz and associates in 1957 in patients with bronchogenic carcinoma. Subsequently, it has been found in an increasing number of seemingly unrelated conditions. Patients with tuberculous meningitis, brain tumors, head trauma, pneumonia, pancreatic carcinoma, and intrathoracic tumors may all show this syndrome. Myxedema, acute intermittent porphyria, and cerebral dysrhythmia also have been associated with it.

What the nature of the antidiuretic substance is and whether it comes from neurohypophysial or other sources is not known in most instances. Assays of bronchogenic and pancreatic tumors have shown them to possess antidiuretic activity of considerable potency and indicate that they, rather than the neurohypophysis, were the sources of the antidiuretic activity.

Clinical Manifestations. Symptoms, when present, are related to dilution of the body fluids. Usually the hyponatremia is asymptomatic unless serum sodium concentrations fall below 120 mEq. per liter. Headache, mental sluggishness, nausea, and vomiting may occur, followed by blunting of consciousness, coma, generalized convulsions, and death. The severity of symptoms correlates only roughly with the degree of hyponatremia; the rate of dilution may be even more important. The author has seen one patient with a serum sodium concentration of 89 mEq. per liter who was alert and able to walk about the ward. With gradual development of dilution, symptoms may not appear. The osmotic derangements between brain and its extracellular fluid presumably are the causes of symptoms. Primary water retention in this syndrome, unassociated as it is with sodium retention, does not lead to clinically overt edema.

Differential Diagnosis. The hyponatremia without circulatory insufficiency, which characterizes this syndrome, must be differentiated from other causes of hyponatremia. Sodium depletion from any cause may be associated with hyponatremia. In the presence of suspected sodium loss, evidence of circulatory insufficiency should be sought: low blood pressure, loss of skin turgor, rapid pulse, postural tachycardia and hypotension, increased hematocrit, and elevated blood urea nitrogen. With such prerenal azotemia, the blood urea nitrogen is disproportionately high for the increase in serum creatinine concentration. Unless sodium depletion resulted from renal wasting of sodium, as in adrenal insufficiency, the urinary sodium is very low, generally less than 10 mEq. per 24 hours. In the syndrome of inappropriate secretion of antidiuretic hormone, sodium excretion may be very high during periods of positive water balance, but will in general reflect the level of sodium intake as the patient comes into water and sodium balance.

Patients with congestive heart failure, cirrhosis, or nephrotic syndrome may develop marked hyponatremia, especially if treated vigorously with restricted sodium intake and potent diuretics. Evidence for circulatory incompetence again should be sought, in spite of the overexpansion of the extracellular fluid volume. These patients also excrete urine which is essentially free of sodium. All patients with hyponatremia show inability to develop diuresis following water ingestion, and urine concentrations may be unremarkable even in the syndrome of inappropriate secretion of antidiuretic hormone, since maximal urine concentrations fall with dilution of the body fluids.

Treatment. Although the inclination may be to treat the hyponatremia by the administration of sodium chloride, this generally proves ineffective. As one might anticipate from the physiologic basis of this syndrome, the hyponatremia is very resistant to correction by administration of sodium chloride. The expanded state of extracellular fluid volume allows the patient to excrete promptly any administered sodium. If central nervous system symptoms of coma or seizures are present, hypertonic saline administered intravenously may give prompt but temporary relief. On the other hand, strict limitation of fluid intake will correct all the physiologic disturbances despite persistence of excessive antidiuretic activity.

Bartter, F. C., and Schwartz, W. B.: The syndrome of inappropriate secretion of antidiuretic hormone. Amer. J. Med., 42: 790, 1967.

Leaf, A., Bartter, F. C., Santos, R. F., and Wrong, O.: Evidence in man that urinary electrolyte loss induced by pitressin is a function of water retention. J. Clin. Invest., 32:868, 1953.

Schwartz, W. B., Bennett, W., Curelop, S., and Bartter, F. C.: A syndrome of renal sodium loss and hyponatremia, probably resulting from innappropriate secretion of antidiuretic hormone. Amer. J. Med., 23:529, 1957.

The Pineal

Seymour Reichlin

The pineal gland was discovered more than 20 centuries ago, and its function has long been a matter of scientific and philosophic speculation. Arising embryologically from ependyma lining the roof of the third ventricle, the pineal consists of parenchymal cells supported by a meshwork of neuroglia. In the adult, the gland weighs between 100 and 180 mg. and is a cone-shaped organ lying in the groove formed by the superior colliculi. Although connected to the epithalamus by a peduncle, the pineal does not receive a direct nerve supply from this source. Instead, it is innervated by postganglionic nerve fibers which arise in the cervical sympathetic ganglia and travel along the great vein of Galen. A number of humorally active substances have been isolated from the pineal. In addition to norepinephrine, which is located in the nerve endings of the sympathetic fibers and is the regulating neurotransmitter for the gland, serotonin, histamine, and melatonin are found. Melatonin is formed by an enzyme, 5-hydroxy indole-o-methyl transferase (HIOMT), which is found only in the pineal. Using the activity of this enzyme as an index of pineal activity in laboratory animals, the gland has been shown to be regulated by the sympathetic nervous system and to be responsive to alterations in the light-dark cycle. Although melatonin is a potent hormone in lower animals (it causes contraction of granules dispersed in melanocytes) and inhibits gonadotrophic and possibly thyrotrophic function, it has no known action in man. Lacking a method for measurement of melatonin in peripheral blood, there is no clear evidence for changes in pineal secretion of melatonin in the human subject under any of the conditions in which the activity of the pineal is altered in the laboratory animal.

The pineal gland has no known function in man but becomes of clinical significance because of the occurrence of calcification and of tumor formation. Calcific nodules termed *acervuli* form in a matrix of ground substance secreted by pinealocytes. This process begins in early childhood and becomes increasingly evident by roentgenography beginning in the second decade of life. Calcification has no known effect on pineal function, as inferred from the fact that the characteristic enzymes of the pineal (HIOMT, monoamine transferase, and histamine N-methyl transferase) maintain normal concentrations throughout life.

Pineal tumors are rare, and their classification and nature are still disputed by pathologists, some of whom believe that the pineal cell in situ or situated in ectopic regions of the brain (chiefly the infundibular area) can give rise to neoplasms. The most common pineal cell tumor is the parenchymal tumor, classified as a pineoblastoma or pineocytoma according to the degree of differentiation. Convincing evidence that at least certain of these tumors are truly of pineal origin comes from the finding by Wurtman and collaborators that tissue from a parenchymal and from an ectopic pinealoma contained the marker enzyme HIOMT. Pineal cell tumors may also resemble seminomas of the testis (seminomatous pinealomas); the relationship of these tumors to teratomas is not well understood. The pineal also gives rise to teratomas of dermoid type and to tumors of the supporting structures such as gliomas, astrocytomas, and endothelial tumors.

Pinealomas occur mainly in young males. The symptoms and signs of the tumor reflect both local effects on the brain and, in a minority of cases, more remote changes in sexual maturation. Enlargement of a mass in the pineal region compresses the aqueduct of Sylvius and distorts the quadrigeminal plate. Internal hydrocephalus gives rise to characteristic manifestations of increased intracranial pressure such as headache, vomiting, papilledema, and disturbance of sensorium. Pressure on the superior colliculi causes conjugate paralysis of upward gaze (Parinaud's syndrome). Disturbances of gait, resulting from either hydrocephalus or possibly cerebellar damage, are also observed.

Pineal tumors arising in male children may, in about one third of cases, cause precocious puberty, but over-all, pineal tumors are exceedingly rare and are therefore a relatively rare cause of sexual precocity. The mechanism of effect of the tumor on gonadotrophic function is controversial. It has been suggested that the pineal secretes a hormone which tonically inhibits onset of sexual maturation; destruction of the pineal permits the earlier development of puberty. In support of this hypothesis is the finding in laboratory animals that melatonin injections delay puberty, that tumors destroying the pineal are three times as likely to cause precocious puberty as are parenchymal tumors, and that some cases of precocious puberty occur in the absence of local brain damage.

On the other hand, there is impressive evidence that pineal tumors, like certain other types of hypothalamic tumors, cause precocious puberty by direct physical damage to the gonadotrophin-regulating areas of the brain. For example, Bing and co-workers found that whenever precocious puberty was caused by a pineal tumor, neuroanatomic evidence indicated extension beyond the pineal region with internal hydrocephalus or invasion of the third ventricle or hypothalamus. Clinical evidence of hypothalamic involvement, e.g., diabetes insipidus, polyphagia, somnolence, obesity, or behavioral disturbance, was observed in 71 per cent of cases. These clinicopathologic correlations strongly support the view that neoplasms of the pineal gland produce sexual precocity indirectly through involvement of the hypothalamus. In a few cases, precocity or infantilism (also reported to occur) may prove to be due to altered pineal hormone secretion, but convincing evidence of this occurrence has not yet been adduced.

A special type of pinealoma is sufficiently distinctive to be noted here. "Ectopic" pinealomas arising from pineal rests in midline areas most commonly occur in the region of the infundibulum, and produce diabetes insipidus, compression of the optic chiasm, and hypopituitarism. Precocious puberty may also occur in such patients.

Treatment of pineal tumors is generally unsatisfactory. Because of their critical location in the epithalamic region above the midbrain, or in the infundibulum, surgical removal is hazardous and usually impossible. Most of them are radiosensitive, and respond at least partially to deep x-ray therapy. A few apparent radiotherapeutic cures have been reported, but the long-range prognosis is poor.

Wurtman, R. J., Axelrod, J., and Kelly, D. E.: The Pineal. New York, Academic Press, Inc., 1968.

Diseases of the Thyroid
Leslie J. DeGroot

DEVELOPMENT AND ANATOMY

The embryonic thyroid gland develops from segments of the fourth pharyngeal pouches, joined by a midline anlage from the base of the tongue. By the end of the first trimester the gland has assumed its adult shape and position, concentrates iodide, and synthesizes thyroglobulin. During intrauterine life the gland can produce adequate hormone for the developing fetus or, if necessary, the fetus can derive hormone from the maternal circulation. During the first 18 or 20 years of life, the gland doubles in size three to four times to weigh 15 to 20 grams. In the absence of disease or alterations in iodine supply, the size and function of the gland remain relatively constant throughout life until advanced age, when hormone production gradually diminishes.

The normal thyroid gland is butterfly shaped, firm, smooth, and red-brown in color. It consists of two elongated lobes on either side of the trachea connected by a thin isthmus of tissue at or below the level of the cricoid cartilage. Often, a remnant of the lingual anlage, the pyramidal lobe, extends superiorly from one side of the isthmus. The fine structure consists of numerous follicles, each approximately 300 μ in diameter and made up of clusters of cells surrounding a colloid-filled luminal space. The colloid consists of a mixture of proteins, of which thyroglobulin comprises about 80 per cent.

The thyroid cells are 15 μ high; the borders facing the lumen have numerous microvilli, thought to be involved in secretory and resorptive activities. In hyperplastic glands the cells are taller, and colloid space is reduced. Certain cells do not contact the luminal surface and have slightly different staining properties; these secrete the hormone thyrocalcitonin and are involved in regulation of calcium metabolism. The parathyroid glands occur as two pairs, one posterior to the upper poles of the thyroid and the other below the lower poles, or imbedded in the substance of the lower pole of each lobe. The recurrent laryngeal nerves pass immediately beneath the lower poles of the thyroid, or are sometimes imbedded in the substance of the thyroid gland. Occasionally bits of normal-appearing thyroid tissue are present adjacent to the gland.

PHYSIOLOGY OF THE THYROID

It is best to view the thyroid gland as part of a system designed to provide hormone to somatic cells. In the peripheral tissues thyroid hormone produces its characteristic metabolic stimulation, and is in turn degraded. As the hormone is metabolized, more enters the cells from plasma. The thyroid gland replenishes this supply by se-

creting about 75 μg. of thyroxine (T_4), and 25 μg. of triiodothyronine (T_3) each day. If the hormone in blood is depleted, the alteration is sensed by the hypothalamus and pituitary, which increase the secretion of thyroid-stimulating hormone (TSH). TSH increases secretion of hormone by the thyroid gland, in a feedback control system, until the circulating supply of hormone returns to the original level.

Iodide Metabolism. Iodine bears a unique relation to thyroid physiology because the element is a major and characteristic constituent of the hormones. The average daily American diet contains 150 to 600 μg. of iodide, depending in part on the consumption of certain varieties of bread, which may contain much iodate, and milk, which may contain considerable iodide. Another major source is iodized salt. Most forms of ingested iodine are reduced to iodide in the gastrointestinal tract before absorption. Iodide is cleared from plasma by the salivary glands and gastric parietal cells, but normally this is returned to plasma (Fig. 1). Iodide is cleared unidirectionally by the kidney at a rate of about 30 ml. per minute. The normal thyroid clears plasma iodide at a rate of 12 ml. per minute. The TSH feedback control system regulates the clearance rate to provide the gland with enough iodide for hormone production. If iodide intake is low and thyroid uptake of iodide is diminished, thyroxine production is soon reduced, and the level of hormone in plasma falls. TSH secretion is then increased and augments iodide clearance by the thyroid gland. Under the influence of TSH, or in thyroid hyperactivity of thyrotoxicosis, clearance may be elevated 5 to 20 times the normal range. With augmented levels of iodide ion in the body, for example, during therapy with Lugol's solution, thyroid clearance falls to near zero.

Hormonogenesis. As rapidly as iodide is transported into the thyroid cell it is oxidized by a peroxidase and bound to tyrosine residues present in thyroglobulin (Fig. 2). This iodination process takes place near the apical cell border. The iodine

IODIDE METABOLISM

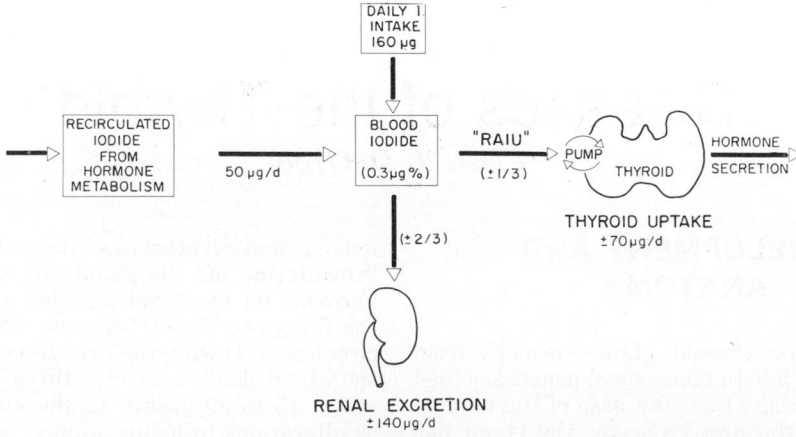

RENAL EXCRETION
±140 μg/d

FIGURE 1.

HORMONE FORMATION

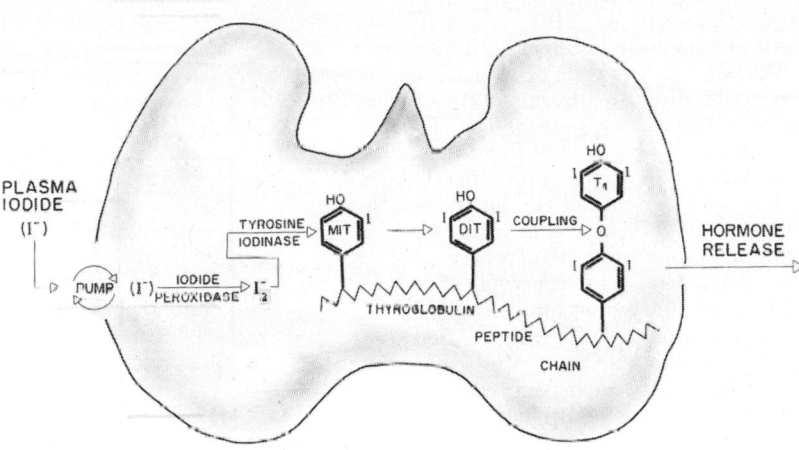

FIGURE 2.

acceptor protein, thyroglobulin, is a tetrameric structure of 650,000 molecular weight. Each thyroglobulin molecule contains approximately 120 tyrosine residues and 26 atoms of iodine. The iodination of the tyrosyl residues in thyroglobulin leads to the production of monoiodotyrosine (MIT) and diiodotyrosine (DIT) in the peptide chain. Then two iodotyrosyl groups couple to form an iodothyronine (T_3 or T_4), still within the peptide chain of thyroglobulin. In the iodine replete gland, each thyroglobulin molecule contains one iodothyronine. The ratio of T_4 to T_3 molecules is about 3 to 1.

Hormone Secretion. As thyroglobulin is iodinated and coupling occurs, some molecules are hydrolyzed, and others are secreted into the lumen and stored for days or weeks. Resorption occurs by pinocytosis; microvilli on the surface of the thyroid cell surround a small fragment of colloid, and a droplet is thus formed within the cell. The colloid droplet then fuses with a lysosome, producing a phagosome within which thyroid protease hydrolyzes thyroglobulin to its component amino acids (Fig. 3). MIT and DIT are deiodinated by a dehalogenase present in the microsomal fraction of the cell, and the liberated iodide is reincorporated into new MIT and DIT in thyroglobulin. The thyroxine and triiodothyronine released from thyroglobulin are secreted into plasma, along with some unhydrolyzed thyroglobulin, small amounts of iodotyrosines, and some iodide. The thyroid also iodinates plasma protein (primarily albumin) and returns the iodinated protein to the circulation. Other particulate iodoproteins are formed in the gland, but their metabolic role is unknown. Some thyroxine may be mono-deiodinated to form triiodothyronine within the thyroid cell.

Hormone Transport. The thyroxine and triiodothyronine secreted by the gland are transported

HORMONE RELEASE

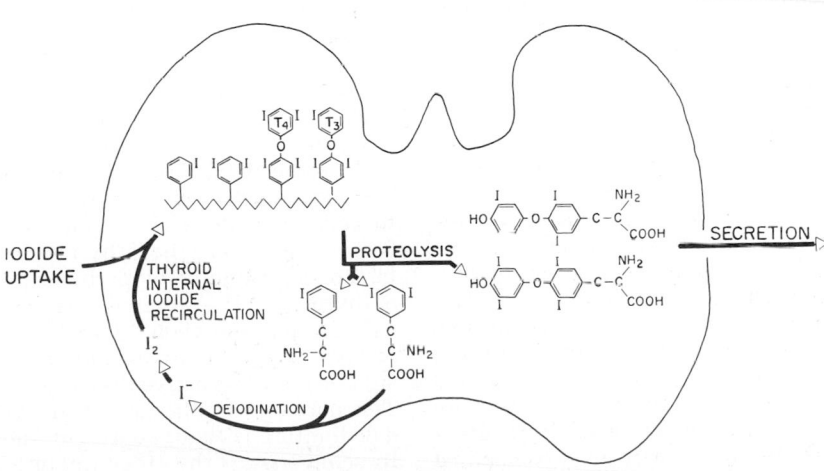

FIGURE 3.

in plasma largely bound by noncovalent bonds to plasma proteins. Of these, the main and most specific hormone-binding protein is thyroxine binding inter-alpha-globulin, or TBG. Approximately 70 per cent of thyroxine in blood is carried by this protein. Perhaps 15 per cent of thyroxine is bound to thyroxine-binding prealbumin (TBPA), and the remainder is bound to albumin. Triiodothyronine is less tightly bound to TBG and does not bind at all to TBPA. Thyroxine binds firmly to the proteins; only 0.05 per cent of the hormone exists free in solution at any one time (Fig. 4). The binding proteins probably control entry of the hormone into cells, serve as a reservoir constantly replenishing free hormone, and also prevent the iodinated thyronines from being excreted in urine. Free hormone gains access to cells and appears to be the metabolically important fraction. The level of thyroxine-binding globulin is elevated by estrogen treatment and depressed by testosterone. It is occasionally congenitally absent or present in excess, and its formation is depressed in serious malnutrition or liver disease. In these conditions there may be wide variations in the total thyroid hormone content of plasma, but since the absolute level of free hormone remains constant, the patients remain metabolically normal.

Free hormone penetrates cells and controls the feedback mechanism in the hypothalamus and pituitary. Approximately one third of the extrathyroidal hormone is loosely bound in the liver. The hormone slowly penetrates most other tissues, reaching an equilibrium within tissue such as muscle in two to three days.

Thyroxine leaves the blood with a disappearance half-time of about six days, and T_3 with a half-life of one to two days. The usual ratio of T_4 to T_3 in the thyroid is 3 to 1. Because of the difference in T_4 and T_3 binding and metabolism, the ratio of T_4 to T_3 in blood is about 20 to 1. Nevertheless, since T_3 is threefold as active (mol. per mol.) as T_4, its contribution to tissue metabolic stimulation is equal to that of T_4.

Metabolic Action. The exact metabolic action of the hormone is unclear. In animals made hypothyroid by ablation of the gland, administration of thyroid hormone is followed by stimulation of nucleic acid and protein synthesis and increased mitochondrial oxidative-phosphorylation, reaching a peak within two to seven days. Coincident with this increased synthetic and oxidative activity in the cell, the activity of many enzymes, including alpha-ketoglutarate dehydrogenase and isocitrate dehydrogenase, is stimulated.

Treatment of animals with large doses of thyroid hormone, or addition of thyroid hormone in vitro, can induce uncoupling of mitochondrial oxidative-phosphorylation. For years one theory of thyroid hormone action has centered around this phenomenon. However, the change from the sluggish metabolic activity of the hypothyroid state to the normal or mildly hyperactive state induced by administration of physiologic doses of thyroid hormone to animals is accompanied by an increased rate of oxidative-phosphorylation

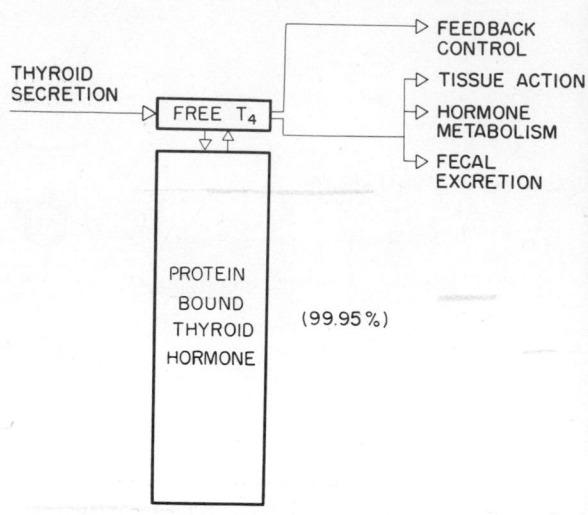

CENTRAL FUNCTION OF FREE-T₄

FIGURE 4.

with loss of efficiency. Another objection to this theory is raised by studies of mitochondria taken by biopsy from patients with severe hyperthyroidism. The preparations had increased metabolic activity, but normally coupled oxidative-phosphorylation.

Many other actions of thyroid hormone have been observed, including stimulation of protein synthesis in isolated mitochondria and microsomes, inhibition of pyridine nucleotide-linked dehydrogenases, and swelling of mitochondria. The hormone does not appear to act at the cell membrane as do certain of the peptide hormones, nor yet at the transcription level in the nucleus as do some steroid hormones. At this moment it can be said that the hormone modulates the level of activity of numerous intracellular processes, although its mode of action is unknown.

Usually several hours elapse before any action of the hormone is observed after administration to animals or man. After a single dose, peak action is seen within two to five days, and gradually decays over a period of two to three weeks. Triiodothyronine has a slightly more rapid onset of action than thyroxine, and its action is more rapidly dissipated. It is of interest that some tissues (brain, spleen, and testes) do not appear to respond to thyroxine.

Thyroxine Metabolism. It is possible that thyroid hormone must be altered in the tissues in order to carry out its action. One candidate for this "active" form is triiodothyronine; thyroxine can be monodeiodinated by peripheral tissues to triiodothyronine. The alanine side chain of the molecule is also metabolized to the acetic acid and pyruvic acid derivatives, but these analogues are significantly less active than the parent compound. The hormone is also metabolized extensively by deiodination without rupture of the ether linkage. In some tissues the ether linkage is broken with formation of hydroquinone and protein-bound DIT.

Some evidence suggests that thyroxine deiodination is a necessary part of hormone action, but this concept has not been proved. In any event, as a result of metabolism, the hormone is deiodinated and the iodide is returned to plasma to follow the same fate as newly absorbed dietary iodine.

Feedback Control. Each day the thyroid releases approximately 60 to 70 μg. of hormonal iodide, of which three fourths is thyroxine and one fourth triiodothyronine. If production falls because of inefficiency in the gland or diminished iodide supply, the level of free hormone in blood decreases, and this alteration is detected by the hypothalamus which secretes increased TRF (Fig. 5). It is presumed that T_3 and T_4 exert the same sort of metabolic activity on the tissues involved in feedback control as they do in other cells, and that this metabolic process constitutes the feedback signal. The hypothalamic control center, in response to a depression of free T_4, liberates a small molecule, pyro-glutamyl-histidyl-proline amide (thyrotrophin-releasing factor—TRF), which migrates from the median eminence through the hypophysial portal system to the anterior pituitary, and there stimulates synthesis and release of thyrotrophin. The anterior pituitary cell is also directly sensitive to the level of circulating thyroid hormone.

TSH Action on the Thyroid. Thyroid-stimulating hormone released by the pituitary binds to the thyroid cell membrane and initiates a sequence of reactions, including stimulation of adenylcyclase, formation of increased intracellular cyclic adenosine monophosphate, a colloid resorption, thyroglobulin proteolysis, and hormone release.

Other Controls of Thyroid Function. As described above, pituitary TSH is the main regulator of

thyroid function. The adrenal gland exerts some control; excess cortisol depresses pituitary production of TSH, and cortisol also directly depresses the level of binding proteins in plasma, and augments urinary excretion of iodide. Pregnancy, associated with its increased estrogen production, augments the level of circulating thyroxine-binding globulin, and increases the PBI level. However, the turnover rate of the hormone in blood is proportionately decelerated, so that net hormone utilization remains unchanged. Androgens have a converse effect. Severe illness and stress appear to accelerate thyroid hormone disappearance from plasma. Thyroid hormone utilization is also accelerated in animals by exposure to cold and in man by conditioning to strenuous exercise.

THYROID FUNCTION TESTS

In examining a patient with thyroid disease, one seeks to determine the level of metabolic activity and the nature of the thyroid abnormality. The most direct measure of metabolic activity is the basal metabolic rate (BMR). Unfortunately, the wide range of normal values and the alterations of the BMR resulting from nonthyroidal factors make the determination of limited diagnostic value. There is no other good approach to assaying the peripheral action of thyroid hormone, although numerous measurements can be made. Thus cholesterol is elevated in hypothyroidism and depressed in hyperthyroidism. The relaxation half-time of the deep tendon reflexes is sometimes shortened below 240 milliseconds in hyperthyroidism, and characteristically prolonged beyond 360 milliseconds in hypothyroidism. Plasma tyrosine levels are elevated in hyperthyroidism, urinary hydroxyproline excretion is depressed in hypothyroidism, and CPK, SGOT, and LDH are elevated in hypothyroidism. None of these tests is useful for definitive diagnosis.

Protein-bound Iodine. Lacking a good measure of hormone action in the tissues, most physicians turn to a measure of thyroid hormone in blood. The standard determination has for years been the protein-bound iodine (PBI), which measures all iodine in serum precipitable by protein-denaturing agents. Ordinarily this consists primarily of thyroid hormone, but if large quantities of iodide are present, or if any of the roentgenographic contrast medium used for gallbladder examinations, intravenous pyelograms, or arteriograms is present in plasma, the level is falsely elevated. Iodoproteins, formed by the thyroid in augmented amounts in some conditions, e.g. thyroiditis, are also precipitated. Nevertheless, the test is useful as a screening examination and is widely available. The normal range is 4 to 8 μg. per 100 ml. It is wise to determine total plasma iodine as well, and, if the level is no more than 2 or 3 μg. per 100 ml. above the PBI, it can be assumed that contamination with excess quantities of free iodide is not present. The butanol extract-

FEEDBACK CONTROL

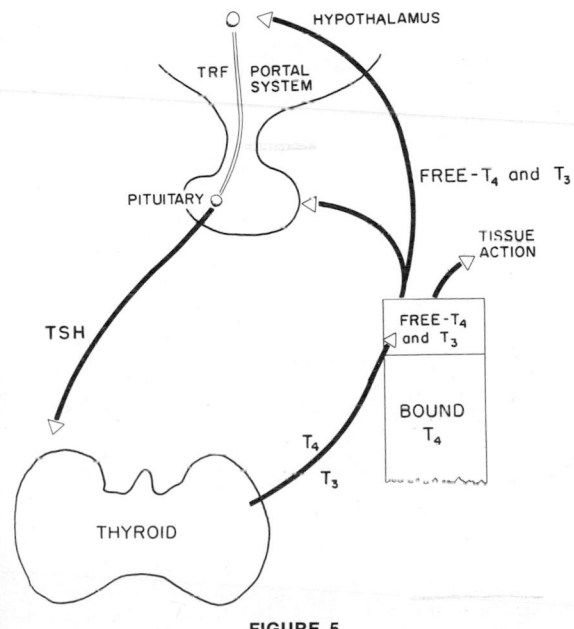

FIGURE 5.

able iodine (BEI) procedure is technically more sophisticated, and is more specific for thyroid hormone since it excludes iodoproteins. If the PBI exceeds the BEI by more than 20 per cent, iodoprotein may be present.

T$_3$ Resin Uptake. The T$_3$ resin uptake test measures the relative saturation of endogenous plasma-binding proteins by endogenous thyroid hormone. Alterations either in binding proteins or in hormone level can change the result, and in opposite ways. Elevation of binding proteins depresses the resin uptake. Increased free hormone in plasma, as in thyrotoxicosis, augments the resin uptake. The test is useful, although all answers must be carefully interpreted because of the two possible distinctly different causes of abnormal results.

Serum Thyroxine. Recently a competitive protein-binding assay for thyroxine, identical in principle to the radioimmunoassay of peptide hormones, has been developed. The technique is similar to the resin uptake test. Thyroxine extracted from a serum sample is added to a standard TBG-containing solution, and its capacity to displace some of the radioactive labeled hormone from the TBG is quantitated using a standard curve. The test is technically demanding, but is extremely useful because it is specific for tetraiodothyronine. If the patient's serum thyroxine level is multiplied by a "normalized" T$_3$ or T$_4$ resin uptake test (patient's resin uptake divided by a normal reference serum resin uptake), the free thyroxine index (FTI) is derived. This index is directly proportional to the level of free thyroid hormone in serum. It therefore will distinguish between patients who have a high thyroxine level owing to increased binding proteins and those in whom an elevation is caused by hyperthyroidism. Free thyroxine can also be measured by dialysis; the patient's serum, labeled with a tracer of radioiodinated thyroxine, is dialyzed against a salt buffer until equilibrium is approached. The dialyzable fraction, multiplied by the serum thyroxine, determines the free thyroid hormone. The range is 1.5 to 3.5 mμg. per 100 ml.

Radioactive Iodine Uptake. Another commonly used measure of thyroid activity is the thyroidal radioactive iodide uptake (RAIU). The patient is given a trace dose of radioactive iodide, and the fraction accumulated in the gland is determined at 2, 6, or 24 hours, the latter being the most widely used end point. The normal uptake is directly dependent upon available iodide supply. In areas where the iodide intake is 150 to 200 μg., it ranges from 20 to 50 per cent. In many parts of the United States, increased iodide in the diet has reduced the normal range to 14 to 35 per cent. This procedure measures the activity of the thyroid trapping and binding process, which can be augmented owing to excess TSH stimulation, or because of endogenous thyroid hyperactivity. The RAIU is characteristically elevated in areas of iodide deficiency.

Two problems must be remembered when performing function tests. Excess iodine in any form may elevate the PBI and BEI and depress the radioactive iodide uptake test. Roentgenographic contrast dyes may for a short time depress the radioactive uptake test, and for periods of weeks or months will falsely elevate the PBI and BEI. Alterations in binding proteins caused by heredity, hormones, illness, liver disease, or malnutrition can cause increases or decreases in the PBI, BEI, and serum thyroxine values without altering the level of free thyroid hormone.

Tests for Specific Conditions. The nature of the disease process affecting the thyroid can be evaluated by a number of other procedures. A high thyroid I^{131} uptake caused by TSH can be reduced to below the normal range by administration of 100 μg. of triiodothyronine daily for one week.

FACTORS AFFECTING THYROID FUNCTION TESTS

	PBI	T$_4$	T$_3$RU	FTI	RAIU	Scan	Antibodies
Normal	4–8 μg. per 100 ml.	3.5–10 μg. per 100 ml.	Usually 25–35%	Arbitrary, 4–10 units	Variable, 12–35%	Homogeneous	Absent
Hyperthyroidism	↑	↑	↑	↑	↑	N	+++
Primary hypothyroidism	↓	↓	↓	↓	↓	0	+++
Hashimoto's thyroiditis	V	V	V	V	V	Homogeneous	++++
Subacute thyroiditis	V	V	V	V	↓	Abnormal	0 or +
Multinodular goiter	N	N	N	N	N	Mottled	Absent
Thyroid cancer	N	N	N	N	N	Abnormal	0
Iodine deficiency	N, ↓	N, ↓	N, ↓	N, ↓	↑	N or mottled	0
Iodine excess	↑	N	N	N	↓	Absent	0
Estrogens, pregnancy, acute porphyria, hereditary excess TBG	↑	↑	↓	N	N	N	0
Androgens, steroids, (high doses), hereditary low TBG	↓	↓	↑	N	N	N	0
Cirrhosis, nephrosis	↓	↓	↑	N	N	N	0
Aspirin	↓ (2–4 μg. per 100 ml.)	↓	N, ↑	N, ↓	N	N	0
Diphenylhydantoin	↓ (3–4 μg. per 100 ml.)	↓	N	↓	N	N	0
L-Thyroxine therapy	↑	↑	↑	↑	↓	0	0
Triiodothyronine therapy	↓	↓	N	↓	↓	0	0
Desiccated thyroid or Liotrix therapy	N	N	N	N	↓	0	0

0 = absent; N = normal; V = variable (high, normal, or low).

This also will produce a depression in the thyroxine level. The presence of functioning thyroid tissue can be evaluated by administration of 5 units of TSH subcutaneously daily for three days, with a radioactive iodide uptake test before and after. TSH should raise the radioactive iodide uptake to a normal level or at least double it. Autoimmunity against thyroid antigens can be determined by the tanned red cell agglutination test, the immunofluorescent test measuring anticytoplasmic antibodies, or by bioassay of the long-acting thyroid stimulator, described below. Localization of radioisotope on scintiscan may provide evidence for areas of altered activity (inactive or hyperactive) in the thyroid tissue. The scan can locate adenomas and, if activity is found in areas outside the confines of the thyroid gland, may indicate the location of metastases from thyroid cancer. Needle biopsy of the thyroid is a useful procedure in properly selected cases, and can provide a histologic diagnosis when all other techniques fail.

Selection of Function Tests. In most thyroid diseases, careful history and physical examination lead to the diagnosis, and laboratory procedures serve to confirm the clinical impression. In the initial evaluation of most patients, it is useful to measure the PBI or serum thyroxine, the free thyroxine index, if available, and the radioactive iodide uptake test. A scan can be performed at the same time if there is a question of nonuniformity of gland function raised by history or examination of the neck. The tanned red cell agglutination test is also useful in the initial evaluation of many patients. To follow the progress of therapy, the most useful procedures are serial determinations of the PBI or serum thyroxine, or, if a good laboratory is available, the BMR. Frequent determinations of the patient's weight also constitute an excellent measure of whole body metabolism and are both quick and inexpensive.

GRAVES' DISEASE AND HYPERTHYROIDISM

Hyperthyroidism refers to a state of heightened thyroid gland activity associated with the production of excess quantities of thyroid hormone. The clinical state is also referred to as thyrotoxicosis. Most commonly hyperthyroidism is part of a syndrome which may include goiter, exophthalmos, and pretibial myxedema, known as Graves' disease (Basedow's disease). Thyrotoxicosis can also be caused by excess production of hormone by a single "toxic" nodule, by uncontrolled function of a toxic multinodular goiter, by functioning thyroid carcinomas (rarely), or by medication. Rarely, it is caused by a TSH-secreting pituitary adenoma, is associated with acromegaly, or occurs because of production of TSH-like material in chorioepithelial tumors or embryonal cell carcinomas.

Incidence. Hyperthyroidism is not a reportable condition, and thus exact data on incidence are unavailable. Prevalence is probably in excess of 3 per 10,000 adults per year. It is largely a disease of adult women, with a sex ratio of approximately 5 to 1. Peak incidence is between 30 and 50 years of age.

Etiology and Pathogenesis. The manifestations of endogenous hyperthyroidism fall in two categories: (1) the disease involving the thyroid (and eyes and skin in Graves' syndrome), which leads to production of excess hormone, and (2) all the other abnormalities, the circulatory, neurologic, and metabolic changes noted below, which are directly caused by excess thyroid hormone impinging on tissues. The mechanism of action of the hormone has been described previously. Here the underlying reasons for thyroid hyperfunction will be considered.

Two recurring themes relate to the etiology of Graves' disease: (1) It may be a manifestation of emotional trauma, or (2) it may be an "autoimmune" disease. The previous impression that the Graves thyroid was responding to excess TSH is erroneous, since TSH in plasma of patients with this disorder is characteristically reduced or absent, apparently suppressed by increased circulating thyroid hormone.

For decades it has been suggested that Graves' disease is induced by emotional stress, because of the frequency with which physicians obtain a history of emotional trauma occurring before the onset of hyperthyroidism. Characteristically the event is a marital problem or death of a loved one. Although such testimonials are frequent, the meager factual data available are inconclusive. Psychiatric evaluations indicate that there is nothing special about the individual who becomes a victim of Graves' disease, and that the incidence of emotional stress in these patients is comparable to that in a control population. Perhaps, in the individuals who report a stressful circumstance, Graves' disease was already present, and made the emotional reaction more dramatic. Also, the patient suffering from Graves' disease has anxiety and tremulousness as a result of the illness; these symptoms may be misinterpreted as the etiologic agent.

Antibodies directed against endogenous thyroid antigens were detected in patients with Hashimoto's thyroiditis in 1956, and several thyroid antibody-antigen systems have since been detected in patients with thyroiditis, idiopathic myxedema, and Graves' disease. This problem is reviewed in the section on thyroiditis. Sixty to 80 per cent of patients with Graves' disease have antibodies directed against thyroglobulin or against thyroid microsomes. Adams and Purves described in 1956 a factor (long-acting thyroid stimulator, LATS) present in the serum of about half the patients with Graves' disease which stimulated the release of hormone from the prelabeled thyroid of a test animal. LATS is now known to be a gamma globulin, an autoantibody probably directed against a component of the thyroid cell membrane. LATS can be neutralized by reacting with antibodies prepared against 7S human IgG. LATS adsorbs to thyroid microsomes, but the reaction is not entirely specific, and does not require complement. In addition to causing release of hormone, LATS stimulates increased synthesis of nucleic acids and proteins, increases incorporation of phosphate into phospholipids, stimulates glucose metabolism, and causes thyroid growth. A contemporary interpretation is that LATS is an autoantibody which stimulates the release of thyroid hormone. In patients whose thyroids are capable of responding to such a trophic stimulus, LATS may be the mediator of hyperthyroxinemia. LATS crosses the placenta and may be the cause of transient hyperthyroidism in neonates born to mothers who have high circulating levels of the antibody. Since no abnormal antigens have been detected in the thyroid cells in Graves' disease, and because of the association of thyroid autoimmunity with immunity against several other organs of the body, it seems possible that LATS is a manifestation of deranged immune homeostasis. Thus the body, for reasons quite unknown, produces organ specific autoantibodies. LATS does not seem to play a direct role in exophthalmos or pretibial myxedema, the other prominent characteristics of Graves' disease.

Much evidence indicates that a strong hereditary factor is involved in Graves' disease, Hashimoto's thyroiditis, and myxedema, and that the three diseases are intimately related. Patients with Graves' disease and thyroiditis usually have a family history positive for the same condition. Thyroid autoantibodies, including LATS, are found in relatives of patients with these diseases. The incidence of any one of the other two diseases is increased in relatives of patients who have one of the three. Some patients appear to have a combination of thyroiditis and Graves' disease that has been called "Hashitoxicosis."

Another intriguing bit of circumstantial evidence related to etiology is the frequently reported occurrence of Graves' disease after consumption of desiccated thyroid for weight reduction. It is as if the ingestion of thyroid hormone somehow conditioned the body to a high level of the substance and demanded continued thyroid hyperfunction after the exogenous hormone was withdrawn.

Iodine administration can occasionally induce hyperthyroidism. This Jod-Basedow phenomenon occurs in areas of endemic goiter when iodinization of salt is introduced. It apparently results because the thyroid was functioning at a hyperactive level before the introduction of iodine, but was unable to manifest hyperthyroidism owing to the limitation of hormone synthesis imposed by the low iodide intake.

Little is known about other causes of hyperthyroidism. Thus the etiology of the toxic nodular goiter, the toxic solitary nodule, or the hyperfunctioning thyroid carcinoma is related to the

problem of tumor formation. Hyperthyroidism is found in association with acromegaly, and may be due to increased TSH production, although this has not been established. Hyperthyroidism associated with choriocarcinoma may be due to the production of a trophic substance by the placenta. This material, placental thyrotrophin, is a normal placental product, but is formed in increased amounts in choriocarcinoma. It is immunologically related to bovine thyrotrophin, but does not cross-react with antibodies to human thyrotrophin.

Pathology. The main pathologic abnormality in Graves' disease is evident in the size of the thyroid cells. The cells are tall, and the size of the average follicle is reduced. Small amounts of colloid are present in the lumen. The picture is analogous to a gland under intense TSH stimulation. In addition there is characteristically an infiltration of mononuclear cells, primarily small lymphocytes and some plasma cells, and lymphoid germinal centers may be apparent. Sometimes the process shades into a picture characteristic of Hashimoto's thyroiditis. There is generalized lymph node hyperplasia, the thymus is enlarged, and the proportion of active thymic tissue is increased. Active germinal centers are also found in the thymus, and the histology is similar to that of myasthenia gravis or lupus erythematosus. The muscles are usually microscopically normal, but occasionally the cells are atrophic, multiple nuclei are present, striations are indistinct, and a lymphocyte infiltrate is apparent. The epidermis and dermis are thinned. Bones may show osteoporosis. Pathology of the eye and "localized myxedema" are described below.

Clinical Manifestations. The historical and physical findings are so obvious in many patients that the disease is easily recognized. The patient may note weakness, increased fatigue, insomnia, weight loss, or tremulousness. The skin becomes fine and moist, and there is excess perspiration. The hair thins, and the nails become thin and brittle. An increased tolerance to cold is noted. Friends note that the eyes are prominent, and the patient appears to be staring. Double vision, blurred vision, burning, tearing, and decreased visual acuity may occur. Often the patient notes a mass in the neck, although this produces few local symptoms. A hyperactive heart, palpitations, and dyspnea on exertion may be evident, usually in the absence of other symptoms of congestive failure. Weight loss occurs despite increase in appetite. There may occasionally be abdominal pain reminiscent of an ulcer and frequent loose bowel movements. Subdeltoid bursitis may occur. Menstrual periods become scant, the cycle is shortened, some periods may be missed, and fertility is reduced. Usually libido is not altered. Thirst and polyuria are occasionally noted. Weakness of the muscles is prominent. It may be the primary symptom in older persons who have had chronic low-grade thyroid hyperfunction for months or years. Such patients report that they cannot climb stairs or get easily from a chair. Pruritus is frequently noticed, and occasionally hives occur.

On examination the patient appears anxious and restless, and is typically quick to cooperate. The hair is fine and thin. The skin feels moist, thin, even silky, and pigmentation may be increased. Vitiligo, especially of the hands and feet, is present in about 7 per cent of cases. The nails are thin, and the hyponychium is often noted to have receded, forming an irregular concave erosion under the distal portion of the nail. This finding (onycholysis or Plummer's nails) is most typically found bilaterally on the fourth digit. The elbows are sometimes red, as are the palms. The eyes may appear prominent, and the sclera is visible above the iris on upward or downward gaze (lid lag). The lids may be grossly puffy. Proptosis (forward displacement of the globes in the orbits) may be evident, and if severe the lids may not close adequately. Edema of the scleral conjunctiva may form loose pockets filled with clear liquid (chemosis). Extraocular muscle function may be diminished, often first with a loss of upward gaze. In severe cases total loss of ocular motility and convergence are present. With proptosis the edge of the lacrimal gland may be felt bulging below the supraorbital ridge. The beefy red insertion of the lateral rectus can sometimes be seen. Depending on the severity of the process, there may be papilledema or hemorrhages and exudates in the retina. Visual acuity may be severely reduced.

The thyroid typically is enlarged, usually three to four times the normal size, although rarely the gland appears to be of normal dimensions. Usually the gland is symmetrically involved and may be lobulated. It characteristically feels rather firm and beefy, and often the pyramidal lobe is palpable. Lymph nodes are usually not present in the supraclavicular fossae. A systolic bruit may be heard over the thyroid or be palpated ("thrill") in very vascular glands.

The precordium is hyperactive, and the heart sounds are intensified. A systolic murmur is usually audible, and sometimes a scratching systolic sound (Lerman's sound) is heard in the second or third left intercostal space. Murmurs present before the onset of thyroid disease are intensified. Occasionally murmurs suggestive of mitral insufficiency or stenosis are audible, and disappear after hyperthyroidism is controlled. Tachycardia is usually present, and there is an increased propensity to auricular fibrillation. Axillary lymph nodes are frequently palpable, and on examination of the abdomen the spleen or liver or both may be minimally enlarged.

Rarely, typical attacks of hypokalemic periodic paralysis occur during severe hyperthyroidism, especially in young men.

Diagnosis. Occasionally patients develop severe hyperthyroidism, but present few classic manifestations. In this picture, termed *masked hyperthyroidism*, to which older people are most prone, the tremor, anxiety, and hyperkinesis may be lacking. Instead, the patient is apathetic, sometimes mentally confused, or obtunded. There may be extreme weakness and muscle atrophy. The skin may not be thinned, and the sweating and the eye signs may also be lacking. Usually, however, a tachycardia, goiter, and low-grade fever are present. A coincidental atrial fibrillation and weight loss should suggest this diagnosis.

The flagrant case with all the characteristic manifestations is usually recognized by laymen, who refer the patient to the physician for therapy. Other patients do not present with more than a few of the signs and symptoms of Graves' disease, and in these patients laboratory studies become critical. Diagnosis begins with the history and physical examination. Serial weights should be recorded, since progressive loss of weight is a strong clue to the diagnosis. To prove the diagnosis, a PBI or serum thyroxine (or better, the free thyroxine index), and RAIU are probably the most useful tests. The BMR, cholesterol, T_3 resin uptake, and reflex time may occasionally be helpful. The tanned red cell agglutination test may be useful, since a positive test indicates the patient has some thyroid autoimmune disease. Often patients develop a normochromic and normocytic anemia with 9 to 11 grams of hemoglobin. Alkaline phosphatase may be elevated, because of augmented bone turnover, and serum calcium, urinary calcium, and hydroxyproline excretion may be increased. Bilirubin is occasionally elevated. Roentgenograms of the skull and views of the orbits should be obtained if there is a question of an intracerebral or orbital space-occupying lesion, especially if unilateral exophthalmos occurs prior to the onset of hyperthyroidism. Determination of long-acting thyroid stimulator by bioassay is rarely necessary, but if present indicates that the patient has a characteristic feature of the Graves diathesis. All the tests must be carefully evaluated in the light of the patient's known iodide intake, exposure to radiographic contrast media, and medications. If there is doubt about the diagnosis, a T_3 suppression test may be useful. Nonsuppressibility of the thyroid is considered the most characteristic feature of Graves' disease. In some patients, who have clinical symptoms suggestive of hyperthyroidism, but in whom the radioactive iodide uptake and serum thyroxine are normal, measurement of elevated plasma triiodothyronine may confirm the condition known as "T_3—toxicosis."

It is especially important to consider this diagnosis in elderly patients who have fibrillation or congestive heart failure. Other diagnostic hints are unexplained diarrhea, severe muscle weakness, bursitis, and vitiligo of the hands and feet.

Severe pulmonary disease, anxiety, carcinoma,

malabsorption, cirrhosis, and myasthenia can have features similar to thyrotoxicosis, and must be considered in differential diagnosis.

Differentiation from other Mitochondrial Diseases. The symptoms and signs of thyrotoxicosis are due to hypermetabolism, and theoretically could be mimicked by any cause of uncontrolled mitochondrial function. In fact few conditions have been reported in which mitochondrial oxidative phosphorylation is disturbed, and only one case caused confusion in diagnosis. A unique syndrome suggestive of thyrotoxicosis was reported by Luft. Weakness, excessive perspiration, marked hypermetabolism, and weight loss led to thyroidectomy, but induction of overt myxedema failed to control the illness. Muscle mitochondria were unusually abundant and large, and had excessive crista formation. Respiration was not controlled as in normal tissues, and uncoupled oxidative phosphorylation was demonstrated. The cause of this illness is unknown.

Other cases that less clearly represent mitochondrial disease have been described. Abnormal, increased, diminished, and absent muscle mitochondria have been detected in various idiopathic myopathies, in steroid-induced myopathy, and in cardiac muscle in experimental left ventricular failure. Experimental iron deficiency can lower tissue cytochrome content, and copper deficiency may be associated with diminished cytochrome oxidase. The clinical correlates of these observations are unknown. Considering the importance of mitochondria in cell homeostasis, they so far appear to be remarkably immune from disease-related pathology.

Therapy. The choice of therapy for hyperthyroidism resulting from Graves' disease has been debated for three decades, and final resolution is not yet in sight.

Radioactive Iodide. For most adults older than 25, administration of radioactive iodide appears to be a satisfactory form of treatment. To date there is no evidence that this therapy is associated with an increased incidence of leukemia or significant somatic damage. Hypothyroidism, attributable to an "overeffective" treatment, is a problem, and will be discussed below. The radiation dose delivered to the gonads during treatment is similar to that given during an intravenous pyelogram or barium enema, and is probably inconsequential. Patients have now been treated with this agent for nearly three decades, and there is yet no evidence of I[131]-induced tumor formation. Evidence in regard to this problem must continually be accumulated, but for the moment it does not appear that radiation of the adult thyroid with I[131] leads to subsequent thyroid malignancy.

A major problem with radioactive iodine therapy has been the onset of hypothyroidism, either immediately or long after the treatment. The incidence of hypothyroidism may approach 40 to 60 per cent after ten years. Most patients are now treated with a dose of radioactive iodide

approximately half that used five or ten years ago, in an effort to diminish the incidence of hypothyroidism.

Therapy is planned to deliver a retained dose of 50 μc. per estimated gram of weight at 24 hours. With this dose, many patients do not achieve immediate euthyroidism, and require ancillary therapy such as administration of potassium iodide solution, or an antithyroid drug, if hyperthyroidism is not controlled within two or three months. These agents should be continued for 6 to 12 months, since the full effect of radiation is not obtained until then. At the end of 6 or 12 months the potassium iodide or the antithyroid drug is discontinued and, if hyperthyroidism recurs, a second treatment of radioactive iodide is administered. Thirty to 50 per cent of the patients need a second treatment, and occasionally a third dose is required. In selected individuals, in whom it is imperative that hyperthyroidism be rapidly controlled, a two to three times larger dose is administered, and re-treatment is given at three months if required. If prompt control is necessary, potassium iodide and antithyroid drugs can be instituted within 10 to 14 days of administration of the therapeutic dose without significant loss of the radiation effect.

All women in the reproductive age who are to receive radioactive iodide must be questioned for possible pregnancy. It is best to administer the radioactive iodide shortly after a menstrual period. Women should be advised to avoid pregnancy for a period of at least one year, because the possible need for re-treatment will not be eliminated before this time has elapsed.

Antithyroid Drugs. Children are best treated initially by a long-term course of antithyroid drug. Usually propylthiouracil, 100 mg. every eight hours, or methimazole, 10 mg. every eight hours, is given orally. If this is not effective within two to four weeks, the dose may be doubled. Rarely, a gram of propylthiouracil or 100 mg. of methimazole will be needed daily. It is imperative that the patient be instructed to take the medication at the time scheduled. Antithyroid drugs have a short duration of action, and one of the main causes of treatment failure is that patients do not adhere to a rigorous time schedule. As a response is obtained, the dose is progressively lowered to 50 or 100 mg. of propylthiouracil every 12 hours, or a comparable dose of methimazole. Some physicians prefer to maintain a higher dose of the antithyroid drug and to add replacement doses of thyroid hormone. Overtreatment with antithyroid drugs will of course block formation of thyroid hormone, lower the PBI, and cause a TSH response. This is usually evident by sudden enlargement of the thyroid.

Symptoms usually abate within two to six weeks, and the patient should be metabolically normal after this period of time. The thyroid gland, in the absence of induced hypothyroidism, either remains at the original size or gets smaller. The latter is a favorable prognostic sign. Another favorable prognostic sign is return of thyroid suppressibility, which has been documented in some patients as early as eight weeks after the onset of antithyroid drug treatment. The medication is continued for one to two years and then is gradually discontinued. Half the treated patients will enter a prolonged remission. Others will relapse within 1 to 12 months, and are either re-treated with the same drug or given an alternative form of therapy.

During antithyroid drug administration, patients must be carefully monitored for occurrence of side effects such as pruritus, rash, epigastric pain, and, with considerably less frequency, neutropenia or even agranulocytosis. A mild skin rash may disappear spontaneously. Pruritus can be treated by the addition of an antihistamine drug. A severe rash calls for discontinuation of the antithyroid drug. It is often useful to institute therapy with an alternate antithyroid medication since cross-reactions do not always occur. The leukocyte count should be checked at each visit during administration of antithyroid drugs. Occasionally, a count as low as 3500 cells per cubic millimeter may be observed spontaneously in patients with thyrotoxicosis. If, however, the blood count falls from a normal range down to a level of 3500 or lower during therapy, the antithyroid drug should be discontinued. Occasionally agranulocytosis develops, and this of course requires intensive care in hospital.

Surgery. Subtotal thyroidectomy performed by a skilled surgeon is also very useful. It is the preferred therapy in children who fail to respond to antithyroid drugs, in young adults who do not wish to pursue a prolonged course of treatment, in patients who are apprehensive of the possible adverse effects of radioactive iodide, in patients who have huge thyroids, and in patients whose glands are thought to possibly harbor a carcinoma. The procedure is accompanied by a mortality rate of less than 1 in 1000, an incidence of permanent hypothyroidism from 5 to 40 per cent, recurrence of thyrotoxicosis in 5 per cent or more (depending on the extent of the initial resection), and occasional instances of damage to the recurrent laryngeal nerves and parathyroids. Patients should be rendered euthyroid with an antithyroid drug in preparation for surgery, and should be given potassium iodide (saturated solution of potassium iodide, two drops twice daily) or Lugol's solution (ten drops twice daily) for a period of one to two weeks before the operation. Iodide decreases vascularity of the gland and makes the surgical procedure less difficult. Induction of euthyroidism before surgery is imperative, because cardiac arrhythmias are frequent during surgery of patients with thyrotoxicosis.

The choice of therapy in pregnancy is between antithyroid drug and surgery during the middle trimester. At present most patients are probably treated by administration of antithyroid drugs. It is advisable to use the smallest dose necessary to bring the PBI into the high normal range for pregnancy; that is, between 8 and 12 μg. per 100 ml., if this coincides with a remission of symptoms. This precaution is taken because induction of fetal hypothyroidism by the antithyroid drug could result in mental damage. An alternative, though not preferred, program is to continue the antithyroid drug and to institute coincident therapy with thyroid hormone.

Iodine. Iodine was introduced for control of hyperthyroidism 50 years ago but is rarely used today as the sole treatment. When given in doses greater than 6 mg. per day, iodide blocks further binding of iodide to form iodotyrosines (Wolff-Chaikoff effect), and diminishes release of thyroid hormone by inhibiting proteolysis of thyroglobulin. Most patients are benefited initially by iodide, although some respond only partially, and some have an exacerbation of their illness despite continuation of iodine. Iodine treatment may induce hypothyroidism, especially in patients who have previously been treated with surgery or radioactive iodine. Addition of iodine to the regimen of patients who are receiving antithyroid drugs has been known to induce a severe exacerbation of hyperthyroidism. At present the three more certain and well defined modes of treatment described above seem preferable to the use of potassium iodide, but it is probable that further study of this treatment will be forthcoming in future years, especially in treatment of mild hyperthyroidism.

Potassium perchlorate is rarely used at present for control of hyperthyroidism, because of its reported association with fatal aplastic anemia.

Prognosis. Untreated hyperthyroidism can result in death from inanition, congestive heart failure, and other causes. All three major forms of therapy described above should result in relatively prompt control of hyperthyroidism, and most patients subsequently lead a normal life. It is interesting to note that none of the treatments is directed toward the etiology of the illness. There is a tendency for a patient who responds to antithyroid drugs (less so to surgery) to have recurrence of the illness years later. This rarely if ever occurs in patients who have been adequately treated with radioactive iodide. Delayed onset of hypothyroidism must always be watched for, and therefore patients who have been treated with surgery or antithyroid drugs should be followed indefinitely at yearly intervals. The prognosis for the ophthalmologic and dermatologic complications of Graves' disease is not so sanguine. Often these complications persist for years or even decades, and may be incapacitating. As noted below, their course, strangely, seems to be uninfluenced by the course of hyperthyroidism.

COMPLICATIONS OF GRAVES' DISEASE

Exophthalmos. Lid retraction and stare are probably effects of hyperthyroxinemia and in themselves are inconsequential. The remaining abnormalities of Graves' ophthalmopathy described previously appear to be due to infiltration of the retro-orbital tissues, extraocular muscles, and lacrimal gland by lymphocytes, plasma cells, and polymorphonuclear leukocytes, as well as an increase in tissue water, mucopolysaccharides, and mucoproteins. The extraocular muscles are often swollen to five or ten times their normal diameter, and the muscle fibers may be largely destroyed, leading in time to contractures. The lacrimal gland may likewise be severely damaged, although keratitis sicca does not appear. Aside from the cosmetic defect and irritation, the patient's difficulties include diplopia and susceptibility to infection, and more severe complications such as loss of visual acuity, corneal ulceration, and panophthalmitis. Exophthalmos can occur at any time in relationship to hyperthyroidism of Graves' disease. Most typically it develops with the onset of hyperthyroidism, and subsides coincident with therapy. Changes of infiltrative ophthalmopathy are present in 10 to 20 per cent of patients with Graves' disease, and severe progressive ("malignant") exophthalmos occurs in 2 to 3 per cent.

The cause of this complication is unknown. Plasma of patients with progressive exophthalmos has been found to contain a factor which stimulates exophthalmos in certain test animals; the material is known as exophthalmos-producing substance (EPS). Some data suggest that EPS may be a fragment of TSH. Although LATS is present more frequently in patients with exophthalmos and typically in higher titers than in the average patient with Graves' disease, there is no evidence that LATS itself causes exophthalmos. No localization of gamma globulin in orbital tissue has been recognized, and retro-orbital tissue does not bind and neutralize LATS. Nevertheless, the suspicion remains that exophthalmos may be an autoimmune phenomenon and that the antigenic stimulus may reside in the thyroid gland. Although there is usually little confusion, some degree of exophthalmos may occur in Cushing's syndrome and cirrhosis. Orbital tumor, sphenoid ridge meningioma, and thrombosis of the cavernous sinus also must be considered in reaching a diagnosis.

Patients with any degree of exophthalmos should be reassured that the process almost invariably is self-limiting. The eyes usually return to an essentially normal condition, although some degree of proptosis may persist. Useful local measures include shielding the eyes from excessive light and dust, avoidance of smoke and other irritants, and instillation of 10 per cent methyl cellulose. Patients may find it useful to sleep with the head of the bed elevated, and to cover the eyes at night with cold saline compresses. If proptosis is severe, the lids may be taped together with cellophane tape which holds a piece of wet gauze and Saran Wrap over the eyelids. Diuresis (chlorothiazide, 500 mg. every day) may be useful. The difficulties of diplopia can be alleviated in part by covering one eye with a patch or obscuring one lens of the patient's glasses. Any sign of infection should be treated by appropriate antimicrobial ointments or, if necessary, by parenteral administration of antimicrobial drugs. If proptosis is severe, muscle function is progressively lost, or if vision deteriorates, administration of corticosteroid hormone may be helpful. Most patients who have active exophthalmos will respond, whereas those who have stable changes will not. A common starting dose is 20 to 40 mg. of prednisone daily in divided doses, although doses up to 120 mg. daily have been used. This medication will induce Cushing's syndrome. It should be given for a few weeks, after which an attempt should be made to gradually reduce the dosage. Sometimes improvement can be maintained in this way on 10 to 20 mg. of prednisone daily, or every other day. The response is variable, ranging from none at all to a complete remission of muscle paresis, papilledema, and recession of exophthalmos.

In patients resistant to steroid who require further therapy, a Kronlein lateral decompression may be useful. In some clinics other operative procedures such as the Naffzigger supraorbital decompression, or decompression into the antrum, may be performed. The results are unpredictable, but often some improvement is gained, and a few patients respond dramatically. In more chronic cases, operations on the muscles may restore binocular vision.

Lateral tarsorrhaphy is useful in patients whose eyes become damaged because the lids do not close during sleep. It provides some protection against corneal erosion and infection, but has little effect on the basic process.

When these procedures have been exhausted, therapy verges on the speculative. Some patients have been treated with azathioprine. Total ablation of the thyroid by surgery and by radioactive iodide has been proposed as being universally effective, but reports from several clinics indicate that it has no predictable effect on exophthalmos. Hypophysectomy, hypophysial stalk section, x-ray of the pituitary, and x-ray to the posterior aspects of the orbits have all been espoused, but none is of consistent usefulness.

The course and prognosis of this illness are difficult to predict. In general, patients whose thyroid disease is successfully controlled will in time do well, although they may go through a period of severe discomfort. Typically, in 6 to 18 months, the activity of the process appears to abate, and there is subsequent slow but progressive evolution toward normality. Rarely sight is severely impaired or even lost, despite the administration of steroids and use of local decompressive surgery. In general it is best to treat coincident hyperthyroidism by the most logical means irrespective of the ophthalmologic complication, and to maintain the patient in a euthyroid state after the initial control of the thyrotoxicosis.

Pretibial Myxedema. In the simplest form, pretibial myxedema presents as a firm bulging over the lateral aspect of the lower leg, just above the lateral malleolus. Often the skin is shiny and has an orange peel appearance. The deposits may extend from an area of a few centimeters to involve multiple areas or even the entire anterior leg and foot. Occasionally, similar deposits can be found on the abdomen, hands or face. Histologically there is an infiltration of mucopolysaccharide and mucoprotein material in the dermis, an increase in fluid, fraying of connective tissue fibers, and increase in collagen. The pattern is very similar to that observed in thyroid hormone deficiency, although there is no evidence that local thyroid hormone deficiency is present. There is a characteristic increase in hyaluronic acid in the lesions and also in uninvolved skin. The process almost invariably occurs in patients who have exophthalmos. It typically is first noted during the onset of hyperthyroidism, but may occur without associated hyperthyroidism and even in some patients whose thyroid appears to have been destroyed by thyroiditis and who are euthyroid or hypothyroid. Usually the process is not incapacitating and, except for its cosmetic detraction, requires no therapy. Topical application of triamcinolone ointment under Saran Wrap may be temporarily useful.

Thyroid Storm. Sudden severe exacerbation of hyperthyroidism may occur as a feature of the basic disease process or because of coincident infection, trauma, or surgery. In the absence of treatment, and even with therapy, the illness carries a high mortality. The patients develop severe hyperkinesis, tachycardia, hyperpyrexia, vomiting, and shock, and may drift into coma. Dehydration may be prominent.

Treatment of the hyperthyroidism should begin at once, using oral or parenteral blocking doses of an antithyroid drug, followed in one hour with potassium iodide. The latter agent should cause a rapid remission in the symptoms of hyperthyroidism, and it is active in the presence of a methimazole block. The prior introduction of an antithyroid drug block ensures that the gland will not be flooded with iodide, and guards against a subsequent flare of the illness. If the patient is not obtunded, sedatives such as phenobarbital (60 mg. intramuscularly every four to six hours) or reserpine (1 to 3 mg. every eight hours) should be given. Propranolol, 10 to 40 mg. every six hours orally, or 2 to 10 mg. every four hours intravenously, has recently been introduced for therapy of this condition and probably is useful, although experience is limited. This drug should be given with great caution in the presence of congestive heart failure. Dehydration should be treated by appropriate fluid supple-

mentation. Cultures should be taken to exclude infection, and antimicrobial therapy given as indicated. Adrenal steroids (50 to 100 mg. of hydrocortisone intramuscularly every six hours) are given if there is any suggestion of adrenal insufficiency. Occasionally plasma or blood or norepinephrine will be required to support the circulation. Hyperthermia can be treated by cooling. Digitalization may be required to control congestive heart failure.

THYROIDITIS

Chronic thyroiditis is not an infection, nor in the usual sense an inflammation, and therefore the name seems unsatisfactory. Two varieties are recognized by pathologists: In lymphocytic thyroiditis (Hashimoto's thyroiditis, struma lymphomatosa), the thyroid is replaced to a varying degree by lymphocytes and fibrous tissue, leading to goiter, parenchymal destruction, and thyroid hormone insufficiency. Reidel's thyroiditis (ligneous thyroiditis) is a possibly related, slowly progressive fibrosis of the thyroid, of great rarity. These two processes will be considered separately, with the main emphasis on Hashimoto's thyroiditis.

HASHIMOTO'S THYROIDITIS

Etiology and Pathogenesis. Hashimoto's thyroiditis is currently thought to be an autoimmune disease. In 1956, Doniach and Roitt, and Witebsky, coincidentally discovered antibodies to thyroid antigens in patients with this illness. The thyroid antibody-antigen systems that are now known include: (1) antibodies reacting with thyroglobulin, usually detected by the tanned red cell agglutination test; (2) antibodies reacting with a component of thyroid cytoplasm, detected by the immunofluorescent technique, or by a complement fixing reaction with thyroid microsomes; and (3) antibodies reacting with a colloidal antigen which is distinct from thyroglobulin. When both antibodies against thyroglobulin and thyroid cell cytoplasm are measured, more than 95 per cent of patients with Hashimoto's thyroiditis have a positive titer in one or both tests, and frequently the titers are extremely high. Further, thyroiditis with a similar histologic pattern can be induced by immunization of animals with thyroid tissue. It thus appears that the basic defect in this illness may lie in the production of autoantibodies directed against thyroid tissue components. The experimentally induced disease cannot be transferred from animal to animal by serum, but can be transferred in inbred guinea pigs by transfer of lymphocytes. This observation, and the poor correlation of circulating antibody titers with the course of the disease, suggests that a cell-mediated immunity may be important in the destruction of thyroid cells.

Why individuals should produce antibodies against thyroid antigens remains a mystery. It might be supposed that an abnormal antigen exists in the cells, but none has been found. It has been suggested that thyroglobulin is normally hidden from the organism during fetal life when immune tolerance is established, and that subsequent escape of the thyroglobulin from the thyroid follicle could induce immunity in the adult. This seems unlikely since thyroglobulin normally circulates in the blood of pregnant women and newborn infants. There is a strong hereditary pattern for the illness, and the propensity to produce antibodies is transmitted as a dominant trait. Further, thyroiditis is associated with a number of other possible autoimmune diseases, including pernicious anemia, idiopathic adrenal insufficiency, rheumatoid arthritis, Sjögren's syndrome, ulcerative colitis, lupoid hepatitis, disseminated lupus erythematosus, and hemolytic anemia. The relationship to pernicious anemia is especially prominent. Fifty per cent of patients with pernicious anemia have antibodies against thyroid tissue antigens, and the converse is likewise true. There is also an associated increased incidence of antibodies against parathyroid tissue, and possibly of antibodies against the pancreas and ovarian tissues.

Many have suggested that Graves' disease, Hashimoto's thyroiditis, and myxedema are variants of a common process. Among the relatives of patients with one of these three diseases, it is typical to find examples of the other two. The histology of Graves' disease shades into that of Hashimoto's thyroiditis, and the histology of idiopathic thyroid failure is interpreted by some as the end stage of lymphocytic and fibrotic replacement of the thyroid. Antibody titers against thyroid cell antigens are high in each condition. It is as if an abnormality in immune homeostasis were at the root of each illness, possibly triggered by some environmental factor. Perhaps with the development of antithyroglobulin and anticytoplasmic antibody, plus a cell-mediated response, Hashimoto's thyroiditis occurs. If the destructive cell-mediated response is severe, the process may go on to thyroid failure. If, in addition to, or in the absence of the other antibodies, the long-acting thyroid stimulator develops, and if the thyroid is capable of responding, thyroid hyperplasia and hypersecretion occur, with the picture of Graves' disease. Although this formulation is by no means universally accepted, it does embody the thinking of many students of these conditions.

Pathology. On gross inspection the thyroid appears pale yellow-tan and has a nubby surface. The normal thyroid structure is replaced with dense infiltration by lymphocytes, and lymphoid germinal centers are evident. The remaining thyroid tissue often shows hyperplasia, with small empty follicles. The cells frequently are enlarged and eosinophilic. In many specimens, fibrosis is prominent. The thymus is characteristically enlarged, and germinal centers are present. Lymph nodes showing reactive hyperplasia may be present in the area surrounding the thyroid.

Clinical Manifestations. Hashimoto's thyroiditis may present with thyroid enlargement or symptoms of hypothyroidism. The disease is 20 times as frequent in women as in men. The condition can occur even in young children, but is most common between ages 30 and 50. In children extensive destruction of the gland can lead to thyroid failure and growth retardation. Most characteristic is the thyroid enlargement, which varies from two to five times normal, averaging 30 to 50 grams. The gland may be soft, normal, or firm, and there is no thrill or bruit. The surface may feel lobulated, but distinct nodules are usually not found. Their presence suggests that a mass of lymph nodes is present or that a thyroid adenoma or malignancy is present. Typically the pyramidal lobe is palpable. Occasionally patients complain of difficulty swallowing or choking, or of a sensation of local pressure, but usually the goiter is asymptomatic. On rare occasions the illness seems to proceed more rapidly, and there is pain and tenderness in the thyroid gland. The trachea is characteristically midline. The remainder of the physical examination is unremarkable unless there are signs of hypothyroidism.

The presence of an asymptomatic diffuse thyroid enlargement (with a palpable pyramidal lobe) in a middle-aged woman who appears to be euthyroid is indicative of Hashimoto's thyroiditis. The serum thyroxine may be normal or depressed, depending on the stage of development of the process. The PBI may be elevated, normal, or depressed. Elevations of the PBI may be due to butanol-insoluble iodinated albumin in plasma. This can be detected by coincident determination of the PBI and BEI, or the PBI and serum thyroxine. The radioactive iodide uptake test may be elevated, normal, or depressed, but usually is normal unless the patient has developed hypothyroidism. Other tests of thyroid function reflect the ability of the thyroid to produce hormone. Characteristically, the scintiscan shows an enlarged thyroid with a smooth outline and diffuse distribution of the isotope. The diagnosis can be made if the tanned red cell agglutination titer is positive at greater than 1:2560 dilution, or if there is a very strongly positive complement fixation test for anticytoplasmic antibodies. However, only 60 per cent of the patients have a positive TRC, and only 95 per cent are positive if both tests are performed. If it seems imperative that the diagnosis be established and the antibody response is not in the diagnostic range, needle biopsy is both safe and effective. A diagnostic piece of tissue will be obtained in perhaps 80 per cent of the biopsies. Failure to augment radioactive iodide uptake after administration of TSH is also suggestive, indicating the syndrome of "low thyroid reserve." Further, some patients will manifest a positive perchlorate discharge test. Occasionally there are striking elevations of the gamma globulin.

Therapy. In patients with thyroid deficiency, therapy with thyroid hormone is indicated. It is also useful to give replacement therapy to euthyroid individuals who have developed a goiter causing a cosmetic defect or local symptoms, or to prevent further thyroid enlargement. In young patients therapy results in disappearance of the goiter, but in older persons whose thyroid enlargement has been present for a prolonged period, therapy may have little effect. When the thyroid is minimally enlarged, it is debatable whether therapy is indicated. Serial biopsies have shown that the histologic picture may not change over a decade. Further, there is no evidence that the process tends to spread to other organs.

Usually therapy is with thyroid hormone, although there are reports of other approaches. In children steroid therapy will cause diminution of goiter and suppress antibody titers, but the entire process recurs when therapy is withdrawn. This approach does not appear to have merit.

Prognosis. There is a tendency for the involved thyroid to enlarge slowly and for hypothyroidism to develop. Spontaneous thyroid atrophy may occur, and it is hypothesized that this sequence may be the cause of "idiopathic" myxedema.

RIEDEL'S THYROIDITIS

In Riedel's thyroiditis the gland is replaced by a mass of dense, infiltrative fibrotic tissue which extends into the capsule of the thyroid, the trachea, and the surrounding strap muscles. Patients seek attention because of local symptoms such as choking or difficult swallowing, because a small goiter is observed, or because of hypothyroidism. The disease is much more frequent in women than in men, and characteristically occurs after age 40. Some circumstantial evidence suggests that it is one of the variants of Hashimoto's thyroiditis. On examination, the thyroid is found to be of normal size, reduced in bulk, or moderately enlarged, and is unusually firm and densely adherent to the trachea. Thyroid function tests reveal normal function or hypothyroidism. There is no specific diagnostic test and antibody titers are not elevated in this condition as in Hashimoto's thyroiditis.

Diagnosis is usually made at operation, when the surgeon finds fibrotic thyroid tissue bound to the trachea. Often the process suggests a sclerosing carcinoma, and the diagnosis is made on frozen sections. The only known therapy is surgery, if pressure symptoms are sufficient to warrant this approach. The gland may be resected, or the isthmus may be exposed and divided, allowing the two halves of the gland to fall laterally, thus avoiding tracheal constriction. Since resection may cause loss of the parathyroids or recurrent laryngeal nerve, simple division of the isthmus and mobilization of the lateral lobes is the preferred approach. Thyroid hormone therapy may be required.

An association has been suggested between this process and sclerosing cholangitis, mediastinal fibrosis, and periureteral fibrosis. (See article on Fibrosing Syndromes.) Since some of these processes may respond to steroid administration, it is possible that this would be a useful therapy in Riedel's thyroiditis, although information on this therapeutic approach is not available.

ACUTE THYROIDITIS

Acute and subacute thyroiditis are etiologically unrelated. Both are transient inflammatory reactions involving the thyroid, and they are clinically distinct from chronic thyroiditis. Acute thyroiditis (acute infectious thyroiditis, suppurative thyroiditis) is used here to indicate the condition in which the thyroid gland is invaded by pathogenic bacteria. This rarity occurs as part of a cellulitis in the neck or because of infection of a cyst in a multinodular goiter. Usually the patient presents with fever, pain in the neck, and a mass involving the thyroid area. The area is erythematous and tender to palpation. Often only one portion of the thyroid is involved and contiguous infection is evident. The leukocyte count is elevated. The serum thyroxine is normal. There may be some depression of radioiodine uptake in a portion of the thyroid on scintiscan, but radioactive iodide uptake is usually normal.

Cultures should be taken and appropriate antimicrobials administered. With suitable therapy, there is rapid subsidence of the process.

SUBACUTE THYROIDITIS

Subacute thyroiditis (granulomatous thyroiditis, acute thyroiditis, DeQuervain's thyroiditis) is an inflammatory condition of the thyroid causing painful enlargement, lasting over a period of weeks or months, with prominent tendency to relapse.

Etiology. Subacute thyroiditis frequently occurs two to three weeks after viral upper respiratory infection. This association suggests that the thyroiditis represents an immunologic response to the viral infection. Other data imply that direct viral invasion of the thyroid may be the cause. Thyroiditis has occurred in outbreaks of mumps, and the mumps virus has been cultured from the thyroid. Numerous other attempts at viral culture have been negative. Volpé finds that most patients have antiviral antibody titers which are high at the time of diagnosis, and tend to fall progressively over subsequent weeks. Antibodies are frequently found against common pathogens such as echovirus, Coxsackie, and adenovirus, and often significant changes in titers are found against two or even three viral antigens. The reported occurrence with mumps virus or in mumps epidemics may represent one possible cause, but is not the most common. The causation remains obscure.

Pathology. The thyroid may be enlarged with dense infiltrate of polymorphonuclear cells, lymphocytes, and plasma cells. Fibrosis is prominent. Many pyknotic thyroid follicular cells are apparent. The follicular structure is often destroyed, and in its place are found small granulomas with giant cells. There is little correlation between the histologic aberration, which may be extreme, and the clinical picture.

Clinical Manifestations. Subacute thyroiditis can be painful and disabling, but fortunately it does not last forever. The patient usually notices gradual onset of severe pain and tenderness involving one or both sides of the lower neck, sometimes localized to the thyroid. There may be fullness and the sensation of pressure. Pain typically radiates up the lateral aspects of the neck and into the jaw and ear. Swallowing may be uncomfortable, causing the patient to choke over saliva. There is often mild fever, sore throat, malaise, and fatigue. Occasionally the process is entirely asymptomatic.

On examination the thyroid is enlarged and tender. The process may be restricted to one portion of a lobe or may involve the entire gland. Lymph nodes are usually not enlarged. Sometimes the patient develops symptoms and signs of mild hyperthyroidism, but usually the clinical status is that of euthyroidism or, rarely, hypothyroidism. The disease tends to remit spontaneously or because of therapy, only to recur after a period of two or three weeks, and this cycle may recur several times. Over the course of 4 to 12 months the process finally subsides.

Diagnosis. The typical history of pain and the tender enlargement of the thyroid are highly suggestive of subacute thyroiditis. The leukocyte count may be elevated to 15,000 to 20,000, or may be normal. The sedimentation rate is characteristically high, and may reach 100 mm. per hour by the Westergren method. Anemia is said to accompany the illness, although the cause is unknown. The PBI may be elevated because of iodoprotein or excess thyroid hormone released during the acute phase of the illness. In the latter case the patient may be thyrotoxic. There may be a transient depression of the PBI during recovery. Radioactive iodide uptake is suppressed in the involved portion of the gland, which may be one lobe or the entire thyroid, and the RAIU often is zero. During recovery the RAIU may be transiently elevated, and then over a period of two to three months fall to normal. Antibody titers against thyroid antigens may be transiently demonstrable, but rarely if ever reach the levels found in Hashimoto's thyroiditis, and the responses are not sustained.

This process can usually be differentiated from acute thyroiditis, because of the localization to the thyroid, absence of signs of infection, characteristically high sedimentation rate, and depressed radioactive iodide uptake. Occasionally, aspiration biopsy may be necessary to prove the diagnosis. Rarely, Hashimoto's thyroiditis presents with a rather acute and painful onset, and it may be difficult to make the distinction short of biopsy.

Therapy. In mild cases the inflammatory process subsides spontaneously, and all that is needed is mild analgesia. Aspirin, up to 6 grams daily, is useful in suppressing the pain. It is probably advantageous to give desiccated thyroid if the disease has gone on for more than a few days, because TSH stimulation may exacerbate the process. If the illness does not subside with these simple measures, corticosteroids are useful; 20 to 40 mg. of prednisone is given daily for a period of one to four weeks, with progressive diminution of the dose as symptoms are controlled. Often withdrawal of steroids is followed by exacerbation of the process, and such a cycle may recur several times before the illness eventually subsides. Rarely, a chronic, tender enlargement of the thyroid persists despite therapy, and requires surgical resection.

Prognosis. In the author's experience, all patients with subacute thyroiditis have eventually returned to normal thyroid function and become asymptomatic. It is reported, however, that up to 10 per cent of the patients develop permanent hypothyroidism.

HYPOTHYROIDISM AND MYXEDEMA

Hypothyroidism (Gull's disease) refers to the morbid state characterized by progressive slowing of all bodily activities, owing to deficiency in thyroid hormone. The severest form is known as myxedema, because of the characteristic infiltration of the skin by nonpitting, mucinous edema.

Etiology. Probably most cases of idiopathic hypothyroidism and myxedema develop as the end stage of Hashimoto's thyroiditis. The histologic pattern confirms this suggestion; antithyroglobulin and anticytoplasmic antibody are frequently present in high titers, and progress from Hashimoto's thyroiditis to hypothyroidism can be observed. More commonly, thyroid failure occurs because of administration of radioactive iodide to control Graves' disease, or following subtotal thyroidectomy for Graves' disease, multinodular goiter, or Hashimoto's thyroiditis. Hypothyroidism sometimes occurs as part of the presentation of Graves' syndrome, with coincident exophthalmos and pretibial myxedema. Less frequently, hypothyroidism occurs as a primary feature of panhypopituitarism, or because of isolated failure of the pituitary to produce TSH. Hypothyroidism is reported to occur in 10 per cent of patients who have had subacute thyroiditis. Some patients with multinodular goiter are hypothyroid. Hypothyroidism is also found in patients with congenital metabolic defects of thyroid hormone synthesis, is sometimes caused by severe iodine deficiency in areas of endemic goiter, and can be induced by medications such as the antithyroid drugs, resorcinol, PAS, and iodine. In some individuals, administration of iodine (more than 6 mg. per day) induces an inhibition of thyroid hormone synthesis and release, with the development of goiter and hypothyroidism.

Pathogenesis and Pathology. Whatever the cause of thyroid hormone deprivation, the effects are similar. Over a period of months and years, there is progressive infiltration of the skin by mucoprotein and mucopolysaccharides, giving a puffy appearance. Similar deposits of mucopolysaccharide are reported to occur under the sarcolemma of striated muscle. Muscle fibers become frayed, and the cells may become necrotic. There is a generalized decreased rate of nucleic acid and protein synthesis, and almost all enzyme systems are reported to be underactive.

In idiopathic myxedema the thyroid is replaced by scar tissue containing a few scattered thyroid cells and many lymphocytes. In secondary hypothyroidism, resulting from pituitary failure, the thyroid is small and inactive, with flattened, cuboidal epithelium and acini filled with colloid. In other conditions the pathology is that of the primary process. In goiter resulting from metabolic defects in hormone formation, or the action of thyroid blocking drugs or iodide, the characteristic picture is extreme hyperplasia, which may look much like papillary adenocarcinoma.

Clinical Manifestations. Quite typically the patient has no complaints. He, or more commonly she, may be brought to the doctor because someone else recognized unusual sluggishness, weight gain, or sleepiness. Sometimes the presenting symptom is edema, menorrhagia, or weight gain. The symptoms and signs are in proportion to the severity and length of duration of the illness. In advanced cases the diagnosis is obvious. The patient notes fatigue and sleepiness, often falling asleep at inopportune times. There is marked increase in sensitivity to cold. Hearing may be diminished. The eyes are puffy or watery. The hair is brittle, sparse, and coarse; curl tends to be lost. The eyebrows are sparse, and the outer third may be missing. The skin is thickened and dry, and sweating rarely occurs. There is generalized thickening and puffiness of the face and extremities; pitting is not characteristic, but may occur in the presence of fluid retention or congestive heart failure. The patients have a jocular air about them, their answers to questions often being delayed and seemingly humorously inappropriate. As a group they tend to be uncomplaining and hardly recognize the marked change that may have occurred in their appearance and behavior. The tongue is thick, and papillae may be atrophic, especially if there is coincident pernicious anemia, which occurs in 12 per cent of patients with idiopathic thyroid failure. The thyroid may be absent or palpable, depending on the etiology. The heart is quiet, the pulse is slow, and diastolic pressure may be elevated. Although pericardial effusion is frequently present, physical signs of tamponade rarely if ever occur. Pleural effusion may occur; and the abdomen may be distended by ascites. These fluids may have a high specific gravity. The patient complains of severe constipation, and ileus and megacolon are reported. Irregular menstrual pattern and severe menorrhagia frequently occur in younger women. Deep tendon reflex relaxation time is markedly prolonged. Other neurologic signs include diminished hearing, paresthesias, vertigo, and ataxia with lateral column signs. Often the skin shows perifollicular keratoses. The nails may be thickened. Joint stiffness, arthritis, and bursitis are occasionally seen.

Overt psychosis may develop as a manifestation of prolonged and severe myxedema. Hallucinations, disorientation, paranoia, and attempted suicide have been reported. With substitution therapy the psychosis usually clears, although some patients never regain sanity. The name *myxedema madness* has been applied.

The degree of abnormality is by no means always as great as that described. In mild hypothyroidism it may be impossible to make a clinical distinction from the normal state.

Diagnosis. In the classic case the diagnosis can be confirmed at the bedside by evaluation of the slow relaxation time of the Achilles tendon reflexes. Other tendon jerks are less reliable. The PBI and serum thyroxine are characteristically low, as is the radioactive iodine uptake test, except in individuals who have a block in thyroid hormone formation as a cause of their thyroprivia. Both the PBI and the radioactive iodine uptake tend to be less severely depressed in patients with pituitary failure as the cause of hypothyroidism, and in these subjects the values tend to overlap the normal range. The BMR is depressed, the serum cholesterol and carotene are elevated, and there may be marked elevation of the enzymes SGOT, LDH, and CPK. Uric acid is sometimes elevated. Most patients have anemia. This may be due to menorrhagia causing iron deficiency, coincident pernicious anemia, or may be normocytic or macrocytic and be related solely to hypothyroidism. Pernicious anemia, nephritis, uremia, and mongolism are occasional causes for confusion in differential diagnosis.

After the conclusion is reached that the patient is hypothyroid, it is imperative that the cause be evaluated. If there is atrophy of thyroid tissue, the presence of thyroiditis may be ascertained by the tanned red cell agglutination test and anticytoplasmic immunofluorescent test.

The $KClO_4$ discharge test may be positive. Pituitary dysfunction should be considered unless there is strong evidence incriminating some other cause of thyroid failure. In primary thyroid failure, the sella turcica is usually normal, but may be enlarged in cretins and in some adults with long-standing myxedema. Plasma cortisol is normal, although ketosteroid and hydroxycorticoid excretion is depressed, and the response to metapyrone may be delayed and low. Follicle-stimulating hormone is characteristically elevated in postmenopausal women with primary thyroid failure, but is occasionally low, returning to an elevated level after therapy with thyroid hormone has been initiated. Growth hormone should be present in primary thyroid failure, and the response to arginine is normal or depressed.

Therapy. Treatment with desiccated thyroid is a remarkably satisfactory therapeutic maneuver. Usually it is advantageous to initiate treatment with a low dose of hormone, such as 15 or 30 mg. of U.S.P. desiccated thyroid daily, with subsequent increments of 15 or 30 mg. at intervals of 7 to 14 days, until a full replacement dosage is reached in two to three months. Marked improvement should be seen with 30 mg. The usual replacement dosage is approximately 120 mg. of desiccated thyroid daily given in one dose, although a range of 60 to 300 mg. per day is found, with some dependence upon patient's size. Equivalent doses of thyroxine (100 μg. = 60 mg. U.S.P. desiccated thyroid), triiodothyronine (37.5 μg. = 60 mg. U.S.P. desiccated thyroid), or of one of the newer mixtures of thyroxine and triiodothyronine may be used for replacement therapy.

In patients who have congestive failure, previous myocardial infarction, or angina pectoris, it is best to initiate therapy very gradually. Often such problems are exacerbated by therapy, although some patients cease to have angina pectoris on replacement of the hormone. Although triiodothyronine is theoretically useful because of the more rapid disappearance of its effect should toxicity be encountered, in most patients replacement with desiccated thyroid, or one of the mixtures of synthetic hormones, is preferred since with the latter medications the PBI is within normal range during adequate therapy and is a useful guide. The best guide to treatment is the patient's and the physician's progressive re-evaluation of the clinical status. There should be a return to a normal and steady weight, a disappearance of all symptoms, and a feeling of well-being. Severe myalgias and arthralgias may occur during therapy, but disappear gradually if therapy is continued. It is sometimes useful to increase the dose until symptoms of thyroid hormone excess appear, and then return to a slightly lower dose, in order to be certain that sufficient medication is administered. Once the dosage is established, the patient may remain on this supply of exogenous hormone for years or decades without alteration. Patients must be cautioned to continue taking the medication indefinitely, for some will feel that once well-being has been restored, treatment is no longer needed. It is especially important that women be urged to continue the medication without interruption and at the same dosage level throughout pregnancy. Dosage need not be changed in preparation for or during surgery.

Prognosis. The prognosis for treatment of hypothyroidism in the ambulatory patient is excellent; usually there is a complete return to normal health.

SPECIAL PROBLEMS IN HYPOTHYROIDISM

Myxedema Coma. As myxedema worsens, the affected individual becomes more and more lethargic, and episodes of apparent sleep may become frequent, culminating in severe obtundation, or even in coma from which the patient cannot be aroused. In other instances coma develops abruptly during an intercurrent illness such as pyelonephritis, pneumonia, or cellulitis. Patients with severe myxedema may develop sepsis with minimal symptoms, no fever, and with little leukocytosis.

Typically, if a history is available, it is that the patient had previous surgery or radioactive iodide therapy for hyperthyroidism, did well for a number of years afterward, but then over five or ten years gradually lapsed into hypothyroidism, finally developing coma. Often such people have received replacement therapy with thyroid hormone, but have for some reason discontinued their medication.

The exact mechanism of this variety of coma is unknown. Blood flow to the brain is diminished, but oxygen consumption is allegedly not diminished. Altered cortical activity is apparent in the slowing of the alpha rhythm of the EEG and sluggish mentation. The pathologic correlates of these changes are not well known. Progressive hypothermia, hypoglycemia, and CO_2 retention may be specific causes of coma in some patients.

The clinical manifestations are fundamentally those of severe myxedema, as described before. Localizing neurologic signs are characteristically absent. The reflexes are symmetrical and depressed, and the relaxation time is delayed. Babinski reflex may be evident. Often the patients are severely obtunded, rather than comatose, and they are typically disoriented. It may be possible to arouse the patient from his stupor, only to have him immediately slip back into a depressed state. The temperature should be carefully recorded, and may be as low as 85 to 87° F.

The diagnosis is usually suggested by physical examination revealing signs of advanced hypothyroidism and cutaneous myxedema. The scar of a thyroidectomy, a history of previous thyroid surgery or radioactive iodide treatment, or a history of thyroid therapy are important diagnostic clues. The thyroid is impalpable or replaced by fibrous tissue. Careful search should be made for precipitating causes such as infection of the lungs or urinary tract, as well as other causes of coma such as cerebrovascular accidents, renal and hepatic failure, and drug ingestion. The latter is important because hypothyroid patients are excessively sensitive to ordinary doses of barbiturates and opiates. Diagnosis rests on finding abnormally low blood levels of thyroid hormone, but usually these tests are not immediately applicable. Clinical judgment is called for in the interim, and this can sometimes be supplemented by measurement of the deep tendon reflex relaxation time. Severe hyponatremia and hypoglycemia may occur as a manifestation of primary or secondary thyroid failure. Usual measures needed for differential diagnosis of primary and secondary thyroid failure, including the tanned red cell agglutination test, measurement of plasma cortisol, skull films, and measurement of FSH, should be carried out. Carbon dioxide retention should be excluded, if necessary by arterial gas determination, because hypoventilation may induce coma in some patients. If the diagnosis cannot be established at the time the patient is admitted, it is probably best to institute treatment without a diagnosis because of the urgency of the condition.

The appropriate treatment remains a matter of debate. Failure has consistently been reported in patients treated with very slow supplementation of thyroid hormone, and an impressive series of successes has been reported in patients given a massive intravenous dose of thyroxine in an attempt to return the circulating thyroid hormone to normal levels without delay. Approximately 300 μg. of thyroxine is administered intravenously and 100 to 200 μg. is given daily thereafter with monitoring of the plasma thyroid hormone blood levels. Hypothermia is best treated by covering the patient with warm blankets and allowing endogenous body heat to bring the temperature up gradually. Rapid warming by means of electrical blankets or hot baths has resulted in shock and death. Appropriate antimicrobial therapy should be given if there is evidence of infection. If there is CO_2 retention, the patient should be placed on a respirator to provide an adequate ventilatory exchange. If there is any suggestion of pituitary failure, shock, or hyponatremia suggestive of adrenal steroid insufficiency, the patient should be given cortisol. Occasionally blood pressure must be supported by transfusions or by use of norepinephrine. Fluid and electrolyte therapy should be given with caution. Since cutaneous and respiratory losses are extremely small, 600 to 1000 ml. of fluid per day, of which one third to one half is a balanced electrolyte solution, is sufficient. Overhydration is a common problem in therapy and often leads to congestive failure, cerebral edema, and death.

If the patient survives the critical first few days and is able to take medication orally, replacement therapy can be switched to any standard preparation of thyroid hormone. The blood thyroxine level should be checked to assay adequacy of replacement.

Despite some advances in understanding of the precipitating causes of this illness, therapy remains unsatisfactory, and mortality rates of 50 to 90 per cent are reported.

Myxedema Heart. Cardiomegaly and congestive failure frequently accompany myxedema. The EKG shows low voltage, flattened T waves, and occasionally first degree A-V block. Is there a specific variety of heart disease associated with thyroid hormone deficiency? Obviously patients who develop myxedema may be in the older age groups expected to have hypertension and coronary artery disease frequently. The coexistence of mild hypertension, which may be alleviated by therapy with thyroid hormone, has previously been noted. Another, and probably more common, cause of cardiomegaly is the frequent pericardial effusion found in this illness. The pericardial effusion is usually functionally insignificant, but instances of cardiac tamponade have been reported.

Atherosclerosis was for many years thought not to be accelerated by hypothyroidism, but present evidence indicates that there is an association between these two conditions.

In addition it appears that severe myxedema can be associated with a specific cardiac lesion, evident pathologically as an edema of the myocardium, deposition of mucopolysaccharides and mucoproteins between the cells, fraying of cardiac myofibrils, and death and necrosis of cells. Probably this represents a very advanced stage of myxedema, and these changes are not found in most patients dying of myxedema coma.

Although the effusion, decreased cardiac output, and EKG changes are manifestations of hypothyroidism per se, most instances of heart failure associated with myxedema are probably due to coexistent organic heart disease. Occasionally the problem may not be overt before institution of therapy because of the diminution in required cardiac output in the hypothyroid patient. With therapy, increased demands are put upon the heart, and congestive failure, angina, and even myocardial infarction may occur.

MULTINODULAR GOITER

Multinodular goiter refers to an enlargement of the thyroid associated with more than one identifiable nodule. In fact the condition more specifically refers to a replacement of the normal homogenous cyto-structure of the thyroid by a collection of nodules of variegated histologic pattern ranging from colloid-filled cysts and colloid adenomas to follicular and fetal adenomas.

There may be some residue of histologically normal thyroid between the lumps, but more typically the structure between the more discrete adenomatous nodules consists of follicles with distended colloid-filled lumina. Often there is considerable associated fibrosis, sometimes there is calcification in the fibrous tissue or in the nodules, and old hemorrhage into the nodules may be evident. Sometimes lymphocytic infiltration is present.

Etiology. The causation of this condition is not known with certainty, but there is strong evidence that iodide deficiency is at least one cause. In areas of iodide deficiency, children under age 10 typically have diffuse enlargement of the thyroid, which, on histologic examination, shows a pattern of follicles distended with colloid and low cuboidal epithelium. Between ages 10 and 20, there is a gradual transformation of the process into the multinodular structure. Alternate periods of iodide deficiency with thyroid hyperplasia, and iodide sufficiency with involution, may lead first to colloid goiter and subsequently to the typical multinodular goiter. Experimental proof of this theory in man is lacking. Presumably the hypertrophy of the thyroid in the iodide-deficient areas is due to TSH stimulation, but why this should lead to a colloid goiter rather than to hyperplasia is uncertain. Possibly the iodide-deficient gland forms poorly iodinated thyroglobulin which is resistant to hydrolysis by intrathyroidal proteases, and thus accumulates.

Another possible cause is an inherited partial defect in hormone synthesis. Some patients with typical multinodular goiter secrete a large proportion of the iodide from the thyroid in a butanol-insoluble form, apparently an iodinated protein. These patients are usually euthyroid. Multinodular goiter tends to occur with high incidence in some kindreds. It has been generalized from this evidence that mild forms of metabolic defects in hormone synthesis, or perhaps the heterozygous carrier state for such a defect, may lead to the development of sporadic multinodular goiter.

Incidence. The incidence of multinodular goiter is related to geography, age, and heredity, among other factors. In iodide-deficient areas, multinodular goiter may occur in most individuals. In the United States a conservative estimate of the incidence of palpable multinodular goiter among adults is 2 per cent, but this is probably low. Pathologic alterations in the thyroid that are identical, but which may not have produced gross enlargement of the gland, are present in a much higher proportion of individuals.

Clinical Presentation. Most commonly the condition exists throughout life and is not detected. In some patients enlargement and nodularity of the thyroid are found on routine physical examination. Since the incidence is 10 to 20 times as great in women as in men, and as it develops and progressively increases in size during life, it is often noted in females of 50 to 70. Usually the condition is asymptomatic, but with progressive growth there may be a visible enlargement

in the neck, tracheal compression producing a sensation of choking or coughing, and occasionally pressure on the recurrent laryngeal nerve or edema, producing hoarseness. Sometimes there is hemorrhage into a cyst, producing sudden enlargement and tenderness in one area of the goiter. The problems of thyrotoxicosis and malignancy are discussed below.

Diagnosis. The diagnosis of multinodular goiter is usually made on the basis of physical examination. In its most typical form, the goiter feels like a bunch of grapes. The nodules vary in size from one half to several centimeters in diameter and are of variable consistency. The patients are in most instances euthyroid on clinical examination, and this is confirmed by examination of the serum thyroxine or free thyroxine index and the RAIU. The most common source of confusion is between multinodular goiter, single nodule, and Hashimoto's thyroiditis. Extensive development of one portion of the gland may lead to the impression of a single nodule, and in fact half of all thyroid enlargements that are thought to be single nodules turn out at operation to be multinodular goiters. The gland of Hashimoto's thyroiditis may have a rather lobulated texture, making it impossible to distinguish from multinodular goiter. Thyroid scintiscan may be useful, if it shows a mottled distribution of radioisotope in the gland. Roentgenographic examination of the neck may give evidence of broad septate calcification or ringlike calcification in nodules. Often the trachea is deviated because of pressure by the goiter; this is rare in Hashimoto's thyroiditis. If diagnosis is imperative and cannot be made on the basis of the examinations already mentioned, needle biopsy is useful.

Therapy. Small nodular goiters in euthyroid subjects require no therapy. However, the natural history is progressive enlargement, and therefore it is usually appropriate to place the individuals on permanent therapy with desiccated thyroid in the hope that this will suppress TSH and prevent further enlargement of the gland. Some of the glands develop autonomy, and exogenous hormone occasionally causes thyrotoxicosis. If the gland is grossly enlarged and causing a cosmetic defect or tracheal compression, resection may be indicated. Subsequently such patients should be placed on replacement therapy, as there is a pronounced tendency for regrowth. Sudden swelling and pain in the gland owing to hemorrhage into a cyst usually subsides spontaneously over several weeks, and can be treated with analgesics. Nodular goiters that have progressively enlarged and have become displaced below the clavicles (substernal goiter) may cause tracheal compression and should be resected. Such lesions can usually be removed through a cervical incision. Long-term pressure on the trachea occasionally produces tracheomalacia. The cartilaginous rings of the trachea are destroyed, with a loss of normal rigidity. In such individuals it is imperative that the function of the trachea be examined during inspiration and expiration at operation. Occasionally it is necessary that a tracheostomy be performed. The tracheostomy tube is left in place for 10 to 14 days to induce a fibrous reaction in the trachea and give it some rigidity.

Prognosis. The prognosis in untreated multinodular goiter is for slow enlargement of the gland. Administration of thyroid hormone may prevent progressive growth. It is also typical for long-standing multinodular goiter to develop autonomy and produce clinical hyperthyroidism (*vide infra*).

COMPLICATIONS OF MULTINODULAR GOITER

Toxic Nodular Goiter. Many years ago Plummer observed that after nodular goiters had been present for an average of 17 years, thyrotoxicosis tended to develop. This may be due to the coincident occurrence of Graves' disease in the normal tissue between the nodules, but more frequently it is due to the uncontrolled hyperfunction of one or more nodules in the multinodular gland. In areas of endemic goiter this is the most common cause of hyperthyroidism. It is presumed that nodules developing because of TSH stimulation eventually become autonomous. Patients with toxic nodular goiter are typically elderly, and symptoms are often minimal. Although the pathophysiology does not differ from other forms of thyrotoxicosis, congestive failure, auricular fibrillation, and muscle weakness tend to be prominent. The diagnosis should be suspected in any individual with a multinodular goiter and symptoms suggestive of hyperthyroidism, especially if heart failure or auricular fibrillation is present. The RAIU and serum thyroxine may be in the high normal range or elevated. The diagnosis is further substantiated by a thyroid scan which localizes radioactivity to one or more of the nodules of the gland. In some of these individuals it has been shown that there is a preferential secretion of triiodothyronine leading to an increased ratio of T_3 to T_4 in blood. If the thyrotoxicosis is caused primarily by the excess triiodothyronine, the serum thyroxine level may be normal. This diagnosis can be partially corroborated by observing failure of suppressibility of the gland, but must be confirmed by a clinical trial of treatment or by direct measurement of triiodothyronine.

Toxic multinodular goiter may be treated either by thyroidectomy after appropriate preparation with antithyroid drugs and potassium iodide, or by administration of larger doses of radioiodine than are used in the treatment of Graves' disease, typically 10 to 15 mc. Hypothyroidism is rarely produced because the isotope is distributed unevenly throughout the gland, and some portions are spared from radiation. The gland usually shrinks, but does not disappear.

The Cancer Problem. The occurrence of sudden growth of one area of a multinodular gland, the palpation of an unusually firm area, or the development of hoarseness often raises the question of malignancy. Patients who come to surgery are obviously highly selected because they have developed symptoms that have brought them to a physician and that were considered of such significance that referral was made to a surgeon. The vast proportion of patients with multinodular goiter are never referred for evaluation or for surgery. Among those who are operated upon, the incidence of verified carcinoma, usually papillary adenocarcinoma, varies from 2 to 20 per cent. Because of this frequency, some physicians view the presence of multinodular goiter as sufficient indication for thyroidectomy.

The gross illogic of this reasoning can be seen by some simple calculations. If 2 per cent of the population have multinodular goiter, and 10 per cent of these have thyroid malignancy, at least 400,000 papillary cancers would be present in the United States. In fact it is known that the incidence of multinodular goiter is much greater than the figure used. In contrast only 5000 thyroid cancers are detected annually, and the majority of these are found in patients whose thyroids are normal except for the malignancy. Because of this, it seems more logical to accept multinodular goiter as a measure of assurance that malignancy is not present. In contrast, glands harboring a single nodule carry a certain increase in risk of thyroid carcinoma. Multinodular goiter should not be resected because of a general fear of malignancy, but thyroidectomy is logical in the presence of signs that in themselves are suggestive of malignant change.

ENDEMIC GOITER

In the United States, whether the average iodide intake is 150 μg. or more per day, detectable thyroid enlargement occurs in 2 to 4 per cent of adults. In contrast, in areas where iodide deficiency is present, as evidenced by urinary iodine excretion below 50 to 70 μg. per day, the incidence of palpable enlargement of the thyroid increases in inverse relation to the average urinary iodide excretion. Endemic goiter exists in numerous mountainous areas of the world, including the Andes, central New Guinea, and Switzerland, and as well in many lowland areas such as the Baltic Plains and the Belgian Congo. In almost all well-studied endemics, the cause is deficient iodide in the soil and water, leading to deficient iodide intake. Presumably iodide privation leads to diminished production of thyroid hormone, which is sensed by the hypothalamus and pituitary, resulting in augmented secretion of TSH, and thus to augmented thyroidal clearance of plasma iodide. With this there is also growth, both hyperplasia and hypertrophy, of the thyroid. The thyroid strives to gain the necessary 60 to

80 μg. of iodide needed daily for hormonogenesis, and does so by accumulating almost all the iodide ion entering the vascular compartment, either from the diet or from degradation of hormone within the body. The uptake of a radioactive tracer is 90 to 98 per cent in some endemic areas. Initially the gland is diffusely enlarged, and the histologic picture is a "colloid goiter" with large follicles and flat cuboidal epithelium. In time the picture changes into the multinodular goiter described previously; the histology is identical with that of sporadic multinodular goiter found in other regions. Usually diffuse goiter predominates in youth, and multinodular goiter in older persons. The incidence is higher in women than in men unless the endemic is unusually severe. In some areas, practically all adults have thyroid enlargement.

Pathogenesis. The biochemical abnormalities that lead to the formation of multinodular goiters in response to iodide deficiency are not known. Alternate periods of iodide deficiency and repletion may lead to hyperplasia and involution, and produce the picture of endemic goiter. Thyroid-stimulating hormone is elevated in some severe endemics, but in Argentina adults have been found to have endemic goiter in the presence of normal levels of plasma TSH. Possibly these people had elevated TSH levels earlier in their lives, or perhaps owing to iodide deficiency the gland is more sensitive to TSH. The thyroglobulin of endemic goiters is iodine poor and characteristically has an excess of MIT over DIT, and the content of thyroxine and triiodothyronine tends to be low. Possibly these alterations of iodide content or distribution in the amino acids of thyroglobulin lead to abnormalities in degradation of thyroglobulin and produce the picture of a colloid goiter.

Positive Goitrogens. In a few instances factors other than iodide deficiency operate to cause endemic goiter. Thus a factor present in water appears to be associated with an endemic in Colombia. Thiocyanates are found in some root plants eaten in Central Africa. Potent goitrogens related in action to the thioureas are found in some plant species and are transmitted through cow's milk to humans in Tasmania and Finland. As fascinating as the examples are, they account for a minute fraction of endemic goiter, a condition that involves many millions of people throughout the world.

Clinical Manifestations. Patients with goiter in endemic zones present with thyroid enlargements that may be diffuse or nodular, and vary in size from barely detectable to as large as the head. In some places monstrous enlargement of the thyroid is accepted as normal. Usually such individuals, when adult, are euthyroid, and thus appear to have adapted to iodide deficiency by growth of the goiter. All the problems related to thyroid enlargement, such as dysphagia, respiratory difficulty, tracheal deviation and compression, and cosmetic problems may of course be associated with the thyroid enlargement. Occasionally, in severe endemics, some individuals are hypothyroid clinically and by laboratory examination. In contrast to the condition known as endemic cretinism, described below, patients with endemic goiter do not manifest neurologic signs or mental retardation. Aside from what might be considered to foreigners a cosmetic problem, endemic goiter is relatively inconsequential to most adults with this condition.

Diagnosis. The diagnosis of endemic goiter is best made by study of a population group. The characteristic feature is reduced excretion of iodide in the urine. Iodide excretion is often 30 to 50 μg. per day, although values as low as 5 μg. per day have been recorded. Radioactive iodide uptake values are typically elevated to the 70 to 95 per cent range. Thyroid hormone in blood, as measured by the PBI, is normal, or rarely the PBI is depressed and the patients are hypothyroid. The PBI may be low in the presence of euthyroidism; possibly these patients secrete excess triiodothyronine. The findings of diminished urinary iodide, augmented thyroid uptake, and high incidence of goiter are sufficient to incriminate iodide as the cause of the endemic. If iodide intake is sufficient, i.e., above 100 μg. per day in the presence of endemic goiter, some other cause must be sought, such as a goitrogenic agent in foodstuffs.

Treatment. The best treatment for endemic goiter is prophylaxis with iodine applied to the population group. The most convenient approach is salt iodinization, adding about 50 μg. of iodide per gram of salt as iodate or as potassium iodide. Another approach is to inject population groups with iodinated poppyseed oil. This provides a depot of 1 to 2 grams of potassium iodide, and is sufficient to provide iodide for one to four years. Treatment with desiccated thyroid should prevent further enlargement of the goiters and suppress diffuse goiters in children. It usually has little effect on the multinodular goiters of adults. Local symptoms caused by massive enlargement of the thyroid may require thyroidectomy.

Thyrotoxicosis is rarely seen in areas of severe endemic goiter, apparently because the limitation of iodide supply prevents the development of hyperthyroidism. Occasionally it does occur, and may be difficult to recognize because radioactive iodide uptake values are elevated even in "normal" subjects. The PBI or serum thyroxine may be elevated, or may be normal if the patient secretes an excess of triiodothyronine. After administration of iodine in salt or by injection, some patients develop thyrotoxicosis. Sometimes this process (Jod-Basedow) is self-limiting, but therapy with antithyroid drugs, radioactive iodide, or surgery may be required.

There is no convincing evidence that carcinoma occurs with increased frequency in areas of endemic goiter.

ENDEMIC CRETINISM

This term refers to defective individuals having a typical constellation of signs and symptoms found with increased frequency in areas of severe endemic goiter. If recognized shortly after birth, the infants have a typical appearance with increased hair, low forehead, puffy features, umbilical hernia, enlarged tongue, and sluggish behavior. Later on, other abnormalities may be detected: retarded growth, deaf-mutism, mental retardation, and evidence of spastic paraplegia. If there is continued hypothyroidism, retarded bone age and epiphyseal stippling occur. The individual may be goitrous, or no thyroid tissue may be palpable. The syndrome of endemic cretinism is probably caused by severe iodide deficiency leading to hypothyroidism in both mother and fetus during the early stages of fetal development. Athyreotic individuals born to normal mothers in nonendemic zones rarely if ever develop the full-blown syndrome, apparently because significant quantities of thyroid hormone are transported to the fetus across the placenta from the mother. When investigated during childhood or adult life, endemic cretins may be hypothyroid or euthyroid. Treatment of adult cretins with thyroid hormone usually has had no beneficial effect. The only known therapy is prophylaxis, as described above for endemic goiter.

METABOLIC DEFECTS IN THYROID HORMONE FORMATION, TRANSPORT, AND ACTION

CONGENITAL METABOLIC DEFECTS IN THYROID HORMONE FORMATION
(Goitrous Hypothyroidism, Goitrous Cretinism)

The biosynthesis of thyroid hormone proceeds via transport of iodide into the thyroid, binding of iodide to tyrosine in thyroglobulin, coupling of iodotyrosines, subsequent proteolysis of thyroglobulin with release of iodotyrosines and thyronines, intrathyroidal deiodination of iodotyrosines and reutilization of their iodide, and release of thyroid hormone to the blood. Specific enzymatic defects causing diminished efficiency in the formation of thyroid hormone have been identified as several of these steps. The various genotypes usually produce a common phenotype,

characterized by the presence of a hyperplastic thyroid plus hypothyroidism or euthyroidism.

Etiology. It is simplest to categorize the defects in relation to their position along the biosynthetic sequence.

Defect in Iodide Trapping. A few patients have been recognized with hyperplastic thyroids and congenital hypothyroidism, associated with an inability to transport iodide into the thyroid. Thyroid tissue from such patients, studied in vitro, is unable to establish a concentration gradient. The patients also fail to transport iodide into saliva and gastric juice, and this observation forms the basis of a simple test for the defect. The concentration of iodide in saliva is compared with that in plasma two hours after administration of a radioactive iodide tracer. In affected individuals the ratio is 1, whereas in normal individuals and in presumed heterozygotes it is from 10 to 100. It should be remembered that the usual cause for failure of iodide uptake during a tracer test is that the gland is saturated by exogenous iodine, rather than a faulty iodide-concentrating mechanism.

Peroxidase Defect. The most common defect in hormone synthesis is at the iodide-binding step. The patients are able to transport iodide into the thyroid, but the iodide is not bound to tyrosine in thyroglobulin. A concentration gradient is achieved, but the iodide in the thyroid remains in equilibrium with that in plasma. Thus, as iodide in plasma is cleared in the urine, the free thyroidal iodide gradually returns to plasma. Such patients have an elevated uptake shortly after administration of a tracer and a low uptake at 24 hours. The iodide content of the gland is greatly reduced. No iodinated compounds are formed or released to plasma. PBI is low.

A defect in binding can be identified by administration of potassium perchlorate two hours after administration of a radioactive iodide tracer. The potassium perchlorate will effectively block the iodide transport mechanism. If there is a large pool of free intrathyroidal iodide, potassium perchlorate will cause a release of this material to plasma, with a dramatic drop in the thyroid iodide content. A release of 20 per cent or more of the iodide present at two hours is considered a positive test.

A variant of this condition is found in association with congenital nerve deafness (Pendred's syndrome). This condition is transmitted as a mendelian dominant, but is expressed to varying degrees. Deafness ranges from complete through nearly normal hearing, and hypothyroidism may be severe or thyroid function may be normal.

Coupling Defect. Some individuals with congenital goiter have large, hyperactive thyroids and low thyroid hormone in plasma. Large amounts of MIT and DIT are found in their thyroglobulin. An abnormality of the coupling process is implied by these observations, but it is by no means certain what this abnormality is. It could, for example, be an abnormality in energy supply, an abnormality in the structure of the thyroglobulin, or perhaps lack of an enzyme related to the coupling process. Although patients with congenital thyroid disease, hypothyroidism, low plasma PBI, and plentiful iodotyrosines in the thyroid must have a defect of the coupling process, a more exact definition will require new information about the normal synthetic process.

Iodotyrosine Dehalogenase Defect. Thyroglobulin is proteolyzed in the thyroid by a combination of protease and peptidases, and each amino acid of the thyroglobulin peptide chain is thus separated. Normally the iodotyrosines are deiodinated by a dehalogenase present in the microsomes. The liberated iodide is rebound to tyrosine to form more MIT and DIT. Each day about four times as much iodide goes through this cycle as enters the thyroid from the blood. Some patients have a specific defect of the dehalogenase. In the most carefully studied cases, the enzyme defect also exists in other tissues. Because of the defect in the thyroid, iodotyrosine is liberated from the gland into the blood. Because of lack of the enzyme in other tissues, iodotyrosines are not deiodinated, but are excreted in the urine. This iodide loss causes marked hypothyroidism and thyroid enlargement. The disease can be diagnosed by the identification of labeled iodotyrosines in plasma or urine after administration of a radioactive tracer. Also, infused iodotyrosine is not deiodinated, but is excreted unchanged in the urine. Parents of affected individuals, who are presumed to be heterozygous, often manifest a minor abnormality in their ability to deiodinate iodotyrosine.

Butanol-Insoluble Iodide Defect. Many patients with congenital or familial thyroid enlargement, often with hypothyroidism, have in their plasma iodine insoluble in acidified butanol, and thus not thyroxine or triiodothyronine. This material is formed in the thyroid, and is of heterogenous nature. Some glands secrete large amounts of iodinated albumin, prealbumin, or both. Others seem to secrete iodinated proteins that do not react with antihuman albumin serum; it is possible that these are subunits or fragments of thyroglobulin. The iodoproteins usually contain mainly MIT and DIT and no thyroxine or triiodothyronine.

This inefficient utilization of glandular iodide apparently restricts the formation of thyroxine and causes thyroid hyperplasia. The basic abnormality is poorly understood. There may be inadequate production of normal thyroglobulin. Other proteins may then gain access to the gland and be iodinated. Another possibility is an abnormality in the proteolytic enzymes of the thyroid so that iodinated subunits of thyroglobulin are released to plasma. Although this occurs in certain cattle and sheep, the anomaly has not been identified in humans, and attempts to identify defective protease activity have been inconclusive.

Epidemiology. The metabolic defects in hormone synthesis occur sporadically or in family groupings. Affected siblings may be identifiable, and occasionally parents are found to have a minor metabolic abnormality. Typically there is inbreeding in the family. The metabolic defects usually represent the expression of a homozygous recessive genetic abnormality. The exception to this is in Pendred's syndrome, which is inherited as a mendelian dominant.

Pathology. There is typically marked hyperplasia of the thyroid. The gland is beefy, the cells are columnar, there is little or no colloid, and there is marked hypervascularity. The extreme hyperplasia may take on the appearance of a papillary carcinoma. In other instances the long-standing thyrotrophin stimulation to the gland results in change into a carcinoma, metastases, and death. Disease other than in the thyroid depends upon the degree of hypothyroidism the patient manifests. In Pendred's syndrome, there is in addition nerve deafness, but information on the nature of the lesion is lacking.

Patients present a common phenotype. Usually the illness is not suspected at birth, but becomes apparent within the first few months or, more frequently, during childhood. If severe, the child will develop evidence of hypothyroidism. There is symmetrical enlargement of the thyroid from two to ten times normal size. The gland is usually very vascular, and typically a bruit and thrill are present. The signs and symptoms of hypothyroidism are those described previously. The presence of metastases, including pulmonary infiltrates, indicates malignant change in the goiter.

Diagnosis. The diagnosis is suggested by observation of a hyperplastic thyroid in an individual who is apparently euthyroid or hypothyroid. The iodide-trapping defect can be demonstrated by the inability of the gland to accumulate iodide during a tracer uptake study. A corroborative finding is lack of concentration of iodide in the saliva. The peroxidase defect can be shown by a positive perchlorate discharge test and hypothyroxinemia. A coupling defect is suggested by inability to form normal amounts of thyroxine in the presence of large quantities of glandular iodotyrosine, determined by chromatography on samples of the thyroid tissue. The iodotyrosine dehalogenase defect can be identified by chromatography revealing iodotyrosine in plasma and urine after administration of a tracer. The butanol-insoluble iodoprotein defect is detected by an abnormal difference between the PBI and BEI or between the PBI and serum thyroxine iodine. Ordinarily the difference is no more than 20 per cent. In patients with the syndrome, the BEI or thyroxine iodine may be only 30 or 40 per cent of the PBI. Identification of the labeled protein can be made by electrophoresis of plasma after administration of a tracer iodide.

Therapy. Since the patients have a goitrogenic response to TSH, caused by deficiency of thyroid hormone, the obvious therapy is to replace thyroid hormone. In children, this will usually result in complete regression of the goiter. In older individuals, in whom multinodular goiter has developed, there may be little change in size. In patients with the iodide trapping or dehalogenase defects, administration of a few drops of Lugol's solution daily will compensate for the defect.

Prognosis. It is imperative that individuals with these syndromes be treated with suppressive doses of thyroid hormone, or potassium iodide, as indicated, for the duration of their lives. Inadequate therapy will allow continued TSH stimulation of the gland, and malignancy and death may occur. In general the patients can be reassured that if the defect has been detected early so that there is no neurologic abnormality, treatment will result in normal health and longevity. Further, it is highly unlikely that progeny will be affected if there is no inbreeding.

DEFECTS IN HORMONE TRANSPORT

Occasionally patients have a great elevation or depression of blood thyroid hormone in the absence of corresponding clinical symptoms, owing to the presence of abnormal quantities of thyroxine-binding globulin. In well studied kinships, the abnormalities have been shown to be transmitted as X-linked traits. Thus the affected or "carrier" females are heterozygous and affected males are homozygous. In families with hypo-TBG-emia, the males typically have extremely low or undetectable levels of TBG, with protein-bound iodide or thyroxine values in the range of 1 to 2 μg. per 100 ml. Affected females usually have about half-normal PBI or serum thyroxine values. It is not certain whether the abnormality is in the production of an abnormal protein or the lack of a protein; the latter is favored. The decrease in total bound hormone in the plasma of such patients is counterbalanced by an increased fraction of free hormone. The absolute free hormone concentration is, however, normal, and the patients are eumetabolic. Aside from causing confusion in the interpretation of laboratory tests, there is no known physiologic abnormality associated with this defect.

A few individuals have been reported with elevations of TBG to approximately four times normal and gross elevation of serum thyroxine. Again this appears to be genetically X-linked; the patients are euthyroid, and no alteration in the availability of thyroid hormone to tissues can be demonstrated.

The possibility of genetically induced decreased, or infrequently increased, TBG should always be kept in mind when a thyroid hormone test reveals a level that appears to be discordant with the observed clinical state, and no hormonal or disease-related cause exists. Measurement of absolute free thyroxine content, or of the free thyroxine index, will indicate that the amount of functioning thyroid hormone in the plasma is normal. Another way to show the nature of the condition is by measurement of the T_4 carrying capacity of TBG; this can be done in commercial laboratories.

HEREDITARY RESISTANCE TO THE ACTION OF THYROID HORMONE

Three of eight children in one reported sibship have apparent resistance to the action of thyroid hormone. The children have a characteristic facial appearance, retarded growth, delayed bone age, stippled epiphyses, deaf-mutism, and elevated thyroid hormone level in blood. The hormone in blood is T_3 and T_4, and there is no abnormality of binding proteins. Their thyroids produce about five times the normal amount of hormone daily, and this quantity is likewise degraded in the peripheral tissues. They appear to be euthyroid. A large body of laboratory data supports the conclusion that these children are resistant to the action of thyroid hormone. In compensation, an increased quantity of hormone is made available to the peripheral tissues. Even with this, some organs (such as the ears and bones) receive an insufficient supply of hormone. It is hypothesized that the hypothalamus shares in the decreased sensitivity. Studies designed to identify the basic enzymatic defect have not been revealing, and no therapy has been devised. Conceivably, treatment of the mothers of such individuals with large doses of thyroid hormone during early pregnancy would be advantageous to the neurologic development of the fetus.

THYROID NEOPLASMS

Thyroid neoplasms are adenomas and malignant tumors. Pathologically, adenomas are classified into fetal, follicular, Hürthle cell, and papillary forms. Carcinomas are usually grouped into papillary, follicular, mixed, Hürthle cell, medullary, and anaplastic varieties. Lymphoma and lymphosarcoma are also found in the thyroid.

Etiology. As in all other neoplasms, the exact etiology is unknown. In the case of thyroid cells, it is certain that both radiation and TSH stimulation may be in some way involved. Following the original observation by Duffy, a relation between x-ray to the pharyngeal or thymic area in early childhood and subsequent development of thyroid carcinoma (usually papillary) was well documented. In children who develop thyroid carcinoma under the age of 20, this association is characteristically present. Although the tumors are presumed to occur because of x-ray damage to the thyroid, it is possible that the pathogenesis involves damage to the immunologic surveillance system of the thymus, or that the response is fundamentally due to x-ray damage to the thyroid with subsequent TSH hypersecretion. Another known relationship is between chronic TSH stimulation and the formation of invasive thyroid carcinoma, best identified in patients with congenital metabolic defects. A third relationship is to a variety of the multiple endocrine adenoma syndrome, involving pheochromocytoma and medullary thyroid carcinoma, which is transmitted as a genetic trait. The exact mode of inheritance is not yet clear. Multiple cutaneous neuromas are also seen in association with this syndrome, and occasionally parathyroid adenomas.

Many thyroid tumors are known to be TSH-dependent, in that administration of suppressive doses of thyroid hormone leads to decrease in or regression of the malignancy. The exact relation of x-ray or TSH to induction of autonomous growth is unclear, although it is presumed to involve a mutational change, with deletion of genes that restrict growth of the thyroid cells.

Little is known about the development of thyroid adenomas, although it may be presumed that the same sort of change that causes thyroid carcinoma is involved in the pathogenesis of adenomas. Thyroid adenomas, or at least nodularity, are present with increased frequency in patients who have received x-ray therapy to the thymus, and adenomas are produced in laboratory animals subjected to long-term TSH stimulation. Multiple follicular adenomas are occasionally found in family groups. Although adenomas may develop into thyroid carcinomas, direct proof of this is lacking.

A high incidence of thyroid carcinoma has been noted in patients coming to surgery with multinodular goiter. The reasons for this have been discussed in the article on multinodular goiter. It has been stated for years that the incidence of thyroid cancer in Graves' disease is diminished, but this is not certain. In a recently reported large series, 0.5 per cent of patients undergoing thyroidectomy for Graves' disease were found to have papillary thyroid carcinoma.

THYROID ADENOMAS

Pathology. Adenomas are new growths of thyroid tissue having a homogenous histologic pattern, surrounded by a capsule composed of fibrous tissue or compressed normal cells. They may present as single structures in otherwise normal glands, less frequently as two or three discrete adenomas, or may be a feature of the multinodular goiter. The most common variety is the follicular adenoma, composed of large colloid-filled follicles with flattened cuboidal epithelium. Occasionally there may be degeneration, and the adenoma is then cystic and filled with a gelatinous material. Evidence of old or recent hemorrhage into a degenerating adenoma is common. Some adenomas have the histologic appearance of normal thyroid tissue. Adenomas with smaller follicles and more cellularity are termed fetal or embryonal. In the Hürthle cell adenoma the cells are eosinophilic and have the appearance of liver cells. All are variants of the follicular adenoma. Papillary adenomas have characteristic fronds of cells projecting into a sparsely filled lumen.

Clinical Presentation. The clinical problem most often presented by the thyroid adenoma is management of a solitary thyroid nodule. This may be asymptomatic, or may be brought to attention because of hoarseness, pain, or difficulty in swallowing. Single nodules may be present in 2 per cent of the adult population. They are much less frequent in men than in women. It is certain that most remain without significant danger for long periods of time. The problem is in differentiation of such lesions from thyroid cancer. In the vast majority of persons, the clinical finding is limited to a nodule in an otherwise normal gland. On clinical and laboratory examination, most of them are euthyroid, although some are clinically toxic. Radioisotope uptake and scanning studies may show that the nodule is "cold" (most commonly), equal in uptake of radioactive iodide to that of the normal tissue, or that the nodule concentrates radioactive iodide selectively. Some of the latter "hot" nodules produce excessive hormone and suppress the normal gland, or produce clinical thyrotoxicosis. Nodules may be "cold" because they are biochemically unable to transport radioactive iodide into the thyroid or are unable to bind it, but most frequently are "cold" because they are cystic. If the nodule is "cold," is unusually firm, is fixed to the trachea or surrounding structures, is irregular in contour, or is known to have recently grown, or if cervical nodes are felt, the likelihood of malignancy is increased. However, it is certain that clinical examination and isotope scanning cannot segregate carcinomas from benign adenomas. Carcinoma may occur in nodules that are clinically "hot" on scanning; from 3 to 10 per cent of carcinomas actually are warm or hot by this technique. Solitary nodules in the thyroids of children and men are particularly dangerous. It cannot be taken for granted that a nodule known to have been present for a few years is benign. Further, it is probably not advantageous to treat such lesions for a long time with desiccated thyroid in an attempt to suppress their growth, since rarely does this cause disappearance of the nodule. Short-term therapy before surgery may be of value since it makes the lesion more discrete and facilitates a localized resection. Since clinical differentiation between benign and malignant lesions is very difficult, and since most physicians are reluctant to perform needle biopsy for diagnosis of possible neoplasm, a logical approach is to resect most single nodules unless there is a clear contraindication to surgery. The operative procedure is usually subtotal lobectomy if the lesion appears to be benign and if there are no observable lymph nodes. Frozen sections are made; if the diagnosis of adenoma is confirmed, no further procedure is done.

If the lesion is malignant, a more extensive procedure is carried out as discussed below. Patients who have a subtotal resection for a benign adenoma should be placed on permanent replacement thyroid hormone therapy. About half the "single nodules" subjected to surgery are found to be multinodular goiters, and from 10 to 20 per cent are diagnosed by the surgical pathologist as thyroid carcinoma.

THYROID CARCINOMA

Papillary Carcinoma. Nearly 80 per cent of thyroid carcinomas are papillary tumors, and there is debate over whether benign papillary adenoma exists. The tumors have fronds of cellular tissue projecting into slitlike lumina containing scant or no colloid. Other portions of the lesion may show differentiation into a relatively normal follicular structure. The lesions are frequently very small and often are found as incidentally observed microscopic tumors in glands removed for some other lesion. Papillary tumors tend to metastasize early to lymph nodes in the neck, often when the primary tumor cannot be detected by physical examination or by scanning. The tumor remains confined to cervical lymph nodes for a long period of time, but may invade locally into strap muscles and the larynx, and metastasize to lungs. The histologic pattern of the primary and metastatic disease may be quite different with follicular elements in either area. Growth tends to be partially dependent on TSH. The disease is less aggressive in individuals under age 40. Ten-year survival with various forms of therapy is 80 to 90 per cent.

Follicular Carcinoma. Follicular thyroid carcinoma varies in appearance from relatively normal-looking thyroid tissue to microfollicular structures or large follicles. Often some areas have Hürthle cell changes. These tumors metastasize early via the blood stream to lung and bones. The tumors are TSH responsive, tend to pick up and metabolize iodide, and to form thyroid hormone. Occasionally the unchecked biosynthetic activity of the tumor results in clinical thyrotoxicosis. The ten-year survival in patients with this illness is approximately 50 per cent.

Many of the thyroid tumors in the differentiated group cannot be categorized as purely papillary or follicular, but are mixed. It is impossible to tell which element has metastasized, and there may be major discrepancies in architecture and function between the primary and the metastatic deposits.

Hürthle cell carcinoma tends to invade and metastasize locally in the neck. It has a morbidity approximately like that of follicular carcinoma.

Medullary Carcinoma. Medullary cell carcinoma is derived from the "C" cells, or thyrocalcitonin-secreting parafollicular cells of the thyroid. These tumors form sheets of cells with large nuclei. There is usually extensive deposition of amyloid and considerable fibrosis, lymphocyte infiltration

may also be prominent. The tumors tend to metastasize locally to the neck and finally to the lungs and soft tissues. Their course is approximately like that of follicular carcinoma. The tumors are associated with pheochromocytoma and a variety of other endocrine syndromes. It is clear that they produce thyrocalcitonin and may cause hypocalcemia. In response to this they may induce parathyroid adenomas. The tumors also secrete polypeptides and through this mechanism may cause Cushing's syndrome.

Anaplastic Carcinomas. Anaplastic thyroid cancer ranges from small cell tumors through carcinosarcomas, giant cell tumors, and epidermoid tumors. These tend to invade locally and behave much as malignant neoplasms in any other portion of the body. Survival is usually less than 10 per cent after one year.

Lymphoma and lymphosarcoma may also involve the thyroid. It is dubious that this is related to the occurrence of Hashimoto's thyroiditis. The mortality rate depends upon the histologic nature of the lesion.

Treatment of Thyroid Cancer. The selection of patients for operation has been discussed above. Patients with a neck mass thought due to thyroid cancer, or those with a thyroid mass plus cervical nodes, should have thyroidectomy unless some contraindication to surgery is present. At surgery diagnosis is made on the basis of physical examination of the primary lesion, palpation of lymph nodes, and examination of frozen sections. If the lesion is differentiated (papillary or follicular cancer) and is confined to the thyroid, a total lobectomy is done on the involved side, resection of the lymph nodes in the tracheoesophageal groove is carried out, and a subtotal resection is performed on the opposite side. If there is evidence of multicentricity, a more radical resection is performed. If the lesion involves the thyroid and has metastasized to the neck, a total thyroidectomy is done, with preservation of the parathyroids by careful dissection, and a homolateral limited neck dissection is performed. Occasionally patients will present with metastatic disease. If there is proved thyroid cancer with a solitary metastasis, it may be profitable to extract both the thyroid and the metastasis, since some will survive for a comparatively long time.

If there is definite evidence of lymph node involvement or metastases, the patients are given courses of approximately 150 mc. of radioactive iodide[131] at intervals of three months in an attempt to ablate residual metastases. Except when receiving I[131] therapy, all should receive thyroid hormone in dosage sufficient to induce mild clinical hyperthyroidism.

Medullary thyroid cancer is treated by surgery followed by x-ray to the neck, since this tumor rarely concentrates radioactive iodide.

Anaplastic thyroid cancer is treated by local dissection to the extent possible. A radioactive iodide scan should be performed, but it is most unlikely that these tumors will concentrate radioactive iodide. Roentgen therapy is useful. Subsequent to surgery, patients are placed on suppressive doses of hormone. Patients with lymphoma or lymphosarcoma are usually treated by surgery combined with postsurgical radiotherapy. The long-term survival in the lymphomas is excellent, and is perhaps 50 per cent at ten years in lymphosarcoma.

DeGroot, L. J.: Current views on formation of thyroid hormones. New Eng. J. Med., 272:243, 1965.

Hoch, F. L.: Biochemistry of hyperthyroidism and hypothyroidism. Postgrad. Med. J., 44:347, 1968.

Irvine, W. J. (ed.): Thyrotoxicosis (Proc. Int. Symp., Edinburgh, May, 1967). Edinburgh, E. &. S. Livingstone, Ltd., 1967.

McKenzie, J. M.: Humoral factors in the pathogenesis of Graves' disease. Physiol. Rev., 48:252, 1968.

Means, J. H., DeGroot, L. J., and Stanbury, J. B.: The Thyroid and Its Diseases. 3rd ed. New York, McGraw-Hill Book Co., 1963.

Oppenheimer, J. H.: Role of plasma proteins in the binding, distribution and metabolism of the thyroid hormones. New Eng. J. Med., 278:1153, 1968.

Sisson, J. C.: Principles of, and pitfalls in, thyroid function tests. J. Nucl. Med., 6:853, 1965.

Stanbury, J. B. (ed.): Endemic Goiter (Report of PAHO Meeting, Puebla, Mexico, June, 1968). Washington, D.C., World Health Organization, 1969.

Stanbury, J. B., Wyngaarden, J. B., and Fredrickson, D. S.: The Metabolic Basis of Inherited Disease. 2nd ed. New York, McGraw-Hill Book Co., 1966.

Wolff, J.: Iodide goiter and the pharmacologic effects of excess iodide. Amer. J. Med., 47:101, 1969.

Adrenal Cortex

Grant W. Liddle

THE ADRENAL STEROIDS AND THEIR FUNCTIONS

The function of the adrenal cortex is to secrete hormonal steroids, and the major disorders of the adrenal cortex arise from deficiencies or excesses of one or another of the adrenal steroids. The accompanying table lists the major adrenal steroids, their most abundant metabolites, their functions, and the clinical consequences of steroid deficiencies or excesses.

It has been known since the publication of Thomas Addison's classic monograph in 1855 that the adrenal cortex is essential for life. The two essential hormones are cortisol and aldosterone. The former provides resistance to a variety of stresses and maintains the activity of a number of enzyme systems; the latter enables the organism to withstand salt deprivation. In the quantities normally secreted, all the other adrenal steroids may be regarded as relatively weak or inactive precursors, metabolites, or by-products of cortisol and aldosterone. Cortisol and aldosterone are, indirectly, self-regulating, since each one is capable of initiating a series of physiologic events that result in the suppression of their respective stimulators.

Although cortisol and aldosterone are essential for life, when secreted in excessive quantities they can be life-threatening. Beyond the scope of this article is the fact that supraphysiologic doses of cortisol and certain of its synthetic analogues can be used to modify the courses of a wide variety of nonendocrinologic disorders, particularly inflammatory and allergic processes.

Cortisol is the most important product of the human adrenal cortex in the sense that it is the one steroid that corrects most of the pathophysiologic effects of adrenalectomy when given in doses comparable to the amounts normally secreted. Cortisol is synonymous with hydrocortisone (the official pharmaceutical term) and, chemically, is 11β,17α,21-trihydroxy-pregn-4-ene-3,20-dione. It is closely related to cortisone, the steroid first produced synthetically on a large enough scale for widespread use as a therapeutic agent. Chemically, cortisone differs from cortisol in only one small detail: it has an 11-keto group instead of an 11β-hydroxyl group. This small chemical difference is extremely important biologically, however, for cortisone itself is lacking in biologic activity. It becomes effective in the body only because it can be converted to cortisol.

Cortisol is secreted by the zona fasciculata in response to adrenocorticotrophic hormone (ACTH). A specific biosynthetic step that is catalyzed by ACTH is the conversion of cholesterol to pregnenolone (3β-hydroxy-pregn-5-ene-20-one). Pregnenolone is then transformed by a series of adrenal enzymes to progesterone→17α-hydroxyprogesterone→11-deoxycortisol→cortisol. An inborn error in one of these enzymes or pharmacologic inhibition of one of them diminishes the efficiency of cortisol production and results in hypersecretion of the precursor occurring immediately before the inhibited step.

Upon entering the circulation, cortisol is reversibly bound to an α_2-globulin, transcortin. The major process of metabolic inactivation is carried out in the liver and involves reduction of ring A: Cortisol→dihydrocortisol→tetrahydrocortisol→tetrahydrocortisol glucuronide. The glucuronide is rapidly excreted by the kidneys. Some of the cortisol is oxidized to cortisone and then reduced and excreted as tetrahydrocortisone glucuronide. Tetrahydrocortisol and tetrahydrocortisone are the two most abundant end-products of cortisol metabolism; together, they account for almost 50 per cent of the total disposition of cortisol.

A widely used method for measuring cortisol in biologic fluids is the Porter-Silber reaction, utilizing the chromogenicity of the product resulting from the combination of phenylhydrazine

PROPERTIES OF THE MAJOR ADRENAL STEROIDS

Steroid	Regulated by	Major Metabolites*	Methods of Measurement	Major Actions	Clinical Consequences of Deficiency	Clinical Consequences of Excess
Cortisol	ACTH	Tetrahydro-cortisol Tetrahydro-cortisone	17-OHCS (Porter-Silber) Fluorogenic 17-KGS	Suppression of ACTH & MSH Protein catabolism Impairs glucose utilization Stabilizes lysosomes Suppresses inflammation Na retention K excretion	Hyperpigmentation (high ACTH, MSH) Fasting hypoglycemia Anorexia and vomiting Weight loss Apathy Impaired water excretion	Impaired glucose tolerance Thinning of skin Ecchymoses Poor wound healing Osteoporosis Weakness Hypertension Impaired growth
Aldosterone	Angiotensin K, Na ACTH Volume	Tetrahydro-aldosterone Aldosterone-18-glucuronide	Isotopic	Na retention K excretion	Hypotension Hyponatremia Hyperkalemia	Hypertension Hypokalemia
Deoxycorticosterone (DOC)	ACTH	Tetrahydro-DOC	Isotopic	Na retention K excretion		Hypertension Hypokalemia
Dehydrosio-androsterone	ACTH	Androsterone Etiocholanolone	17-KS	Weakly androgenic and anabolic	Lack of axillary hair in women	Virilization of women and children
Unidentified androgens	ACTH			Androgenic	Lack of axillary hair in women	Virilization of women and children
Unidentified estrogens	ACTH			Estrogenic		Feminization in men and children
Substance S	ACTH	Tetrahydro-S	17-OHCS 17-KGS			
17α-OH-pro-gesterone	ACTH	Pregnanetriol	17-KGS			

*Methods such as 17-OHCS, 17-KS, and 17-KGS are not specific; isotopic and chromatographic methods are used in specific identification of individual steroids.

with steroids having 17,21-dihydroxy-20-keto side chains (17-hydroxycorticosteroids, 17-OHCS). Normally, cortisol is the only major 17-OHCS in plasma, and tetrahydrocortisol and tetrahydrocortisone are the only major 17-OHCS in urine.

Another simple method for estimating plasma cortisol is based on the fact that it fluoresces; the fluorogenic steroid method is not applicable to the measurement of tetrahydrosteroids. Urinary tetrahydrocortisol and tetrahydrocortisone can be oxidized to 17-ketosteroids by bismuthate and are, therefore, 17-ketogenic steroids (17-KGS). This method is somewhat less specific than the Porter-Silber reaction; nevertheless, it is widely used for estimating cortisol metabolites.

Cortisol is ubiquitous as a physiologic regulator; hardly a tissue in the body is unaffected by this hormone. Cortisol influences the level of activity of certain enzymes. It restrains the secretion of ACTH and melanocyte-stimulating hormone (MSH) by the pituitary. It accelerates the catabolism of protein and the hepatic metabolism of amino acids. It increases the appetite and promotes the deposition of fat in the facial, cervical, and truncal portions of the body. It retards the uptake of glucose by muscle cells and promotes hepatic

gluconeogenesis from amino acids, pyruvate, lactate, and bicarbonate. It stabilizes lysosomes and suppresses a variety of inflammatory processes. It stimulates a number of electrolyte transport systems. As will become apparent in the discussions of Addison's disease and Cushing's syndrome, most of the manifestations of these clinical disorders can be understood in terms of inadequacies or exaggerations of the physiologic actions of cortisol.

Aldosterone is secreted by the zona glomerulosa in response to angiotensin, potassium, and ACTH. Like cortisol, it is metabolized by the liver to an inactive tetrahydro derivative; but, in addition, about 10 per cent is conjugated by the liver and kidneys to aldosterone-18-glucuronide. This is an acid hydrolyzable conjugate which recovers its identity as biologically active aldosterone when exposed to acid, a fact which has been exploited in the measurement of urinary aldosterone. Aldosterone is extremely potent, and the concentrations encountered in clinical situations are so low that they can be measured precisely only with highly sophisticated isotopic methods.

The physiologic effects of aldosterone stem from its property of stimulating transport of electrolytes by epithelial cells of the sweat glands, gastrointestinal tract, and, of greatest importance, the nephron. In response to aldosterone all these tissues tend to conserve sodium and lose potassium. Aldosterone deficiency leads to sodium depletion, loss of extracellular fluid, hypovolemia, and hypotension. An excess of aldosterone leads to sodium retention, expansion of extracellular volume, and hypertension.

11-Deoxycorticosterone (DOC) is normally secreted at about the same rate as aldosterone (of the order of 0.1 mg. per day), but since it has only about one thirtieth the mineralocorticoid potency of aldosterone it is usually of little physiologic importance. DOC normally occurs in the biosynthetic pathway as a precursor of corticosterone and aldosterone, but in certain varieties of congenital adrenal hyperplasia it may be secreted in quantities sufficient to cause hypertension. It is metabolized to tetrahydro-DOC, but the quantities of either DOC or its metabolite that appear in biologic fluids are so small that isotopic techniques are usually required to measure them.

Dehydroisoandrosterone, a weakly androgenic 17-ketosteroid, is the most abundant steroid secreted in response to ACTH. A small portion is excreted as such; some is excreted in the form of androsterone and etiocholanolone; a minute portion is converted to testosterone. Dehydroisoandrosterone is the major precursor of the urinary 17-ketosteroids. Except in states in which it is secreted in grossly excessive quantities, such as virilizing congenital adrenal hyperplasia, it is of little physiologic importance.

11-Deoxycortisol (Reichstein's substance S) is the immediate precursor of cortisol and is, therefore, produced in response to ACTH. Normally, it is retained by the adrenal long enough to undergo 11β-hydroxylation, resulting in formation of cortisol. Inefficiency of 11β-hydroxylase can occur as an inborn error of metabolism (hypertensive congenital adrenal hyperplasia), in carcinomatous adrenals, and as a consequence of treatment with an 11β-hydroxylase inhibitor (metyrapone). It has little biologic activity. Like cortisol it has a 17,21-dihydroxy-20-ketone side chain and is, therefore, measurable either as a 17-OHCS or as a 17-KGS.

17α-Hydroxyprogesterone is the cortisol precursor preceding the formation of 11-deoxycortisol and is under the regulatory control of ACTH. It has little biologic activity, and probably has no important role in the clinical manifestations of virilizing congenital adrenal hyperplasia. It is normally secreted in trivial quantities, but in the most common variety of congenital adrenal hyperplasia (21-hydroxylase deficiency) it is secreted in large amounts. This steroid is metabolized to a tetrahydro derivative, pregnanetriol, which is excreted in the urine and is of diagnostic value: a large excess of urinary pregnanetriol is practically pathognomonic of virilizing congenital adrenal hyperplasia owing to 21-hydroxylase deficiency. Although pregnanetriol is not a 17-OHCS by the Porter-Silber reaction, it is a 17-KGS and thus contributes to the nonspecificity of the latter as an index of cortisol production.

REGULATION OF ADRENAL STEROID SECRETION

The adrenal cortex may be regarded as two related but distinct organs. The inner portion of the cortex (zona fasciculata and zona reticularis) is under the control of ACTH and secretes all the adrenal steroids except aldosterone. The outer portion of the cortex (zona glomerulosa) secretes aldosterone in response to angiotensin, potassium, and ACTH.

ACTH activates adrenal adenyl cyclase, stimulating the formation of adenosine-3',5'-monophosphate (cyclic AMP). Cyclic AMP initiates the formation of a protein which directly or indirectly catalyzes the conversion of cholesterol to 20α-hydroxy-cholesterol, which in turn is converted to pregnenolone. The latter serves as a precursor for all hormonal steroids. The pattern of steroids secreted depends upon the enzymatic makeup of the adrenal cortex. Under normal circumstances the most abundant secretory products of the human adrenal cortex are cortisol and dehydroisoandrosterone, but a deficiency of one of the enzymes involved in the conversion of pregnenolone to its normal derivatives results in increased secretion of the biosynthetic intermediates occurring before the impaired step. Such distortions of adrenal secretory patterns are observed in congenital adrenal hyperplasia, in certain adrenal neoplasms, and during treatment with pharmacologic inhibitors of adrenal enzymes.

Since the secretory activity of the adrenal cortex is directly controlled by ACTH, many questions concerning the regulation of adrenal steroid secretion can be transformed into questions of what controls the secretion of ACTH. In brief, there are three major determinants of ACTH secretion in man. The *first* of these is the level of cortisol. Of all the products of the human adrenal cortex, only cortisol has significant ACTH-regulating potency. The higher the cortisol level, the greater is its restraining influence on ACTH secretion; the lower the cortisol level, the less the restraint on ACTH secretion. A *second* factor governing the secretion of ACTH is the sleep schedule. In people in the habit of sleeping at night, plasma ACTH (and cortisol secretion) begins to rise at about 2 A.M. It crests at about the time of awakening; then during the day it falls irregularly to low values during the evening. Thus, there is a "diurnal rhythm" in the secretion of ACTH. The *third* factor governing the secretion of ACTH has been referred to as stress. Such experiences as pyrogenic reactions, acute hypoglycemia, electroconvulsive treatments, and major surgical operations bring about increases in ACTH secretion. Whether various stresses influence ACTH secretion through a common mechanism or separate mechanisms is unknown.

For practical purposes, in people with normal adrenal responsiveness, the plasma cortisol concentration can be used as an indirect index of ACTH secretion. Within the physiologic range of ACTH concentrations the adrenal response is directly proportional to the amount of ACTH reaching it. The cortisol secretory response to ACTH begins within minutes and continues as long as the plasma ACTH concentration is maintained. Once ACTH secretion has ceased, the plasma ACTH concentration falls with a half time of about ten minutes; and once cortisol secretion has ceased, the plasma cortisol concentration falls with a half-time of one to two hours.

The secretion of aldosterone is only partially under the control of ACTH. Large amounts of ACTH induce increases in aldosterone transiently; but if ACTH is administered for more than two or three days, aldosterone secretion diminishes to pretreatment levels. Aldosterone is also influenced by potassium; depletion of bodily potassium diminishes aldosterone secretion. Impressive increases in aldosterone secretion can be brought about simply by depletion of bodily sodium, thus inducing hypovolemia. Hypovolemia of any cause induces renal production of renin, which catalyzes the generation of angiotensin; and angiotensin stimulates adrenocortical secretion of aldosterone. It is currently thought that the renin-angiotensin system is the principal regulator of aldosterone secretion, at least in most of the conditions grouped under the heading Secondary Aldosteronism.

DISORDERS OF THE ADRENAL CORTEX

ADDISON'S DISEASE
(Primary Adrenal Cortical Insufficiency)

Incidence and Etiology. Addison's disease has been estimated to occur with an incidence of 1 case per 100,000 population. It is usually caused by granulomatous destruction or idiopathic atrophy of the adrenal cortex. Clinical adrenal insufficiency usually does not occur unless at least 90 per cent of the adrenal cortex has been destroyed. The most common granulomatous disease destroying the adrenal cortex is tuberculosis, but, in certain regions, disseminated fungal infections are almost equally common. Idiopathic atrophy of the adrenal cortex is thought by some to be a consequence of an autoimmune process. All other causes of Addison's disease are decidedly rare. They include amyloidosis and destruction of the adrenal cortex by metastatic tumor.

Pathogenesis. From the foregoing comments, it should be apparent that Addison's disease commonly arises in association with other significant disease processes. Thus, the patient with Addison's disease resulting from granulomatous destruction of his adrenal glands should be considered to have had hematogenous spread of a tuberculous or fungal infection, and should be carefully surveyed for evidence of an active infection of other organs, particularly the genitourinary and respiratory systems. Patients with "autoimmune" atrophy of their adrenals have an increased probability of having other diseases such as diabetes mellitus, hypothyroidism, and hypoparathyroidism. Patients with Addison's disease preceded by the nephrotic syndrome should be suspected of having amyloidosis.

The pathology of the granulomatous adrenal was described in masterful detail in a monograph written in 1931 by Rowntree and Snell. Of interest to physiologists in later years was the fact that the few remaining adrenal cells were often "arranged in adenoma-like nodules . . . suggesting . . . compensatory hypertrophy." All the pathophysiologic consequences of Addison's disease can now be understood in terms of deficiencies of cortisol, aldosterone, and the adrenal androgen.

Cortisol deficiency results in increased pituitary secretion of ACTH and melanocyte-stimulating hormone (MSH), and these pituitary hormones are responsible for the mucocutaneous accumulation of melanin in classic Addison's disease. Cortisol deficiency also results in loss of appetite, loss of vigor, inability to maintain adequate blood glucose levels during prolonged fasting, inability to excrete a load of free water with normal rapidity, and inability to withstand severe or even rather minor stresses without going into shock.

Aldosterone deficiency renders the distal convoluted tubule of the nephron unable to carry out cation exchange at a normal rate. Consequently, there is failure to conserve sodium and excrete potassium normally. As a result of sodium wastage, there is depletion of extracellular fluid volume, blood volume decreases, blood pressure falls, cardiac output falls, and heart size diminishes. This process may culminate in peripheral vascular collapse, and is a prominent feature of addisonian crisis. Hyponatremia results from failure to conserve sodium and, as noted before, impaired ability to excrete a water load. Impaired ability to excrete potassium causes serum potassium concentrations to rise. If serum potassium concentrations exceed about 7 mEq. per liter, disturbances of cardiac electrophysiology occur, manifested by sharp peaking of the T-waves of the electrocardiogram and cardiac standstill in diastole.

Adrenal androgen deficiency is of no consequence in the male, because testicular androgen production suffices to induce adequate virilization. In women, however, the adrenal is responsible for a major portion of the total production of androgen, and loss of adrenal function results in a decreased growth of axillary and pubic hair.

The clinical manifestations of Addison's disease are usually insidious, and often exist in mild form for several weeks or months before correct diagnosis leads to proper treatment. Throughout this time, however, the patient with severely compromised adrenal function is in jeopardy of fatal addisonian crisis, through either progression of the chronic abnormalities or superimposition of some acute stress such as fasting (vomiting), injury (surgical operation), or infection.

The mechanisms of death are peripheral vascular collapse (shock) and hyperkalemic cardiac standstill; perhaps hypoglycemia plays a role in some cases.

Clinical Manifestations. One can hardly do better than to quote or paraphrase the clinical descriptions in the monographs by Addison and by Rowntree and Snell, written before synthetic steroids became available to alter the natural course of Addison's disease. Addison wrote:

> The patient, in most of the cases I have seen, has been observed gradually to fall off in general health; he becomes languid and weak, indisposed to either bodily or mental exertion; the appetite is impaired or entirely lost; . . . the pulse small and feeble . . . excessively soft and compressible; the body wastes . . . slight pain or uneasiness is from time to time referred to the region of the stomach, and there is occasionally actual vomiting . . . it is by no means uncommon for the patient to manifest indications of disturbed cerebral circulation. . . . We discover a most remarkable, and, so far as I know, characteristic discoloration taking place in the skin,—sufficiently marked indeed as generally to have attracted the attention of the patient himself, or of the patient's friends. . . . It may be said to present a dingy or smoky appearance, or various tints or shades of deep amber or chestnut-brown. . . . The body wastes . . . the pulse becomes smaller and weaker, and . . . the patient at length gradually sinks and expires.

In their experience with 108 cases of Addison's disease, Rowntree and Snell noted that asthenia, weight loss, gastrointestinal symptoms (anorexia, nausea, vomiting, and abdominal pain), and hypotension were almost always part of the syndrome. Hyperpigmentation was present in most cases and was described in such terms as "a suntan which does not wear off . . . tinged somewhat with blue or gray . . . dirty in appearance." The exposed portions of the body (hands, face, neck, and arms), points of pressure and friction, nipples, freckles, recently formed scars, genitalia, and creases of the palms often showed exaggerated pigmentation. Brown, blue, or gray spots on the lips and buccal mucous membranes were common.

Nowadays, earlier diagnosis and specific therapy make it possible to correct the compensatory hypersecretion of ACTH and MSH before development of prominent mucocutaneous hyperpigmentation, so that this manifestation may disappear in the patient who has been treated for a long time. Hyperpigmentation is not present in all untreated patients, so one should not take the position that the absence of characteristic hyperpigmentation rules out the diagnosis of Addison's disease.

The mental state of the untreated addisonian patient was frequently characterized as "asthenia, languor, exhaustion, or disinclination to physical or mental effort." Less frequently, irritability, confusion, and delusions were noted. Almost invariably the patients lacked the vigor to carry on productive lives.

Fever was not found in "uncomplicated" cases of Addison's disease. When it did occur it was attributable to coexisting infection.

It is of historical interest that the laboratory abnormalities of Addison's disease as listed by Rowntree and Snell were limited to such items as gastric achlorhydria, elevated serum urea, and delayed excretion of phenolsulfonphthalein and water. A later technical advance, in the form of flame photometry, made hyponatremia and hyperkalemia commonplace abnormalities in the chemical profile of Addison's disease.

It is important to remember that Addison's disease often occurs in association with other diseases. Since the clinical manifestations of Addison's disease are shared by many other debilitating disorders, it is easy to overlook the possible presence of Addison's disease while attributing all the manifestations to some coexisting condition. Fortunately, it is now possible to establish with certainty whether a patient has Addison's disease with a specific test for adrenocortical reserve, and this should be carefully performed without hesitation whenever the possibility of Addison's disease seems realistic.

Diagnosis and Differential Diagnosis. To establish the diagnosis of Addison's disease one should measure the steroid secretory response to a standard dose of ACTH. A standard test, which has a number of modifications, all valid in experienced hands, is to give 50 units of ACTH as a constant intravenous infusion for eight hours and measure the resulting rise in plasma cortisol. Individuals with normal adrenal glands should respond with increases in plasma cortisol to at least 30 μg. per 100 ml. Addisonian patients show little or no increase in plasma cortisol, which is usually less than 15 μg. per 100 ml. both before and during the infusion of ACTH. Intermediate (subnormal) responses are observed in patients with adrenocortical insufficiency secondary to hypopituitarism or prolonged corticosteroid therapy; these conditions can be distinguished from Addison's disease by demonstrating that repetitive treatment with ACTH, over several successive days, induces a stepwise increase in adrenal steroids until normal values are attained. Among the acceptable modifications of this standard test are procedures employing intramuscular injection of a good quality of depot ACTH and measurement of urinary 17-OHCS, 17-KGS, or 17-ketosteroids. The crucial point is that the patient with Addison's disease has little or no adrenocortical capacity to respond to ACTH.

Treatment. The most important principles to observe in the management of Addison's disease are (1) that only two adrenal hormones, cortisol and aldosterone, are vitally important; (2) that the physiologic requirements for these two hormones fluctuate; (3) that cortisol substitution therapy should never be totally withdrawn unless it can first be demonstrated that the diagnosis of Addison's disease was erroneous, and (4) that sodium chloride must be administered in liberal quantities in order to correct extracellular fluid depletion.

Treatment of Addisonian Crisis. The patient in addisonian crisis is in immediate danger of losing his life because of glucocorticoid deficiency, extracellular fluid depletion, and hyperkalemia. Without delay, he should be treated with an intravenous infusion of physiologic sodium chloride; the infusion should be given rapidly, on the assumption that the patient probably has a deficit of at least 20 per cent of his extracellular volume (at least 3 liters in the adult). A water-soluble glucocorticoid such as hydrocortisone phosphate, 100 mg., should be added to the infusion. Within a few hours, if the electrolyte imbalance is corrected, the endocrinologic crisis may be considered to be over, and therapy should be adapted to meet the patient's current needs; if there is no stressful complication, the dose of glucocorticoid may be reduced to the physiologic range of approximately 20 mg. of hydrocortisone daily; but, if the patient is stressed, larger doses will be required. An attempt should be made to determine whether the crisis might have been precipitated by some stress such as an infection, and if so, this should be treated specifically.

If the diagnosis of Addison's disease has not previously been established and the patient's illness is suggestive of addisonian crisis, one should without delay initiate therapy and, at the same time, carry out a definitive diagnostic test for Addison's disease. Physiologic sodium chloride solution should be administered as outlined above. Instead of adding hydrocortisone phosphate to the saline infusion, one should add the potent water-soluble glucocorticoid dexamethasone phosphate, 4 mg. This will be equivalent to 100 mg. of hydrocortisone in biologic potency, but will not obscure the adrenal response to an infusion of ACTH. To the intravenous infusion one may add ACTH in a dose sufficient to assure that the patient receives at least 5 units each hour for eight hours. Plasma cortisol should be measured prior to the addition of ACTH and again toward the end of the ACTH infusion. An adequate rise in plasma cortisol in response to ACTH excludes the diagnosis of Addison's disease; a negligible adrenal response confirms the diagnosis.

Chronic Treatment of Intercritical Addison's Disease. Therapeutic strategy in Addison's disease aims at simulating normal rates of secretion of cortisol and mineralocorticoid. Normal adults secrete about 20 mg. of cortisol per day, and adults with Addison's disease usually require approximately 20 mg. of cortisol (hydrocortisone) daily in the form of medication; it may be administered orally or parenterally in single or divided doses. Various synthetic glucocorticoids may be substituted for hydrocortisone, providing that proper adjustment is made for their differences in biologic potency.

Normal adults receiving unrestricted diets usually consume 100 to 300 mEq. of sodium daily, and while on such diets they secrete approximately 0.1 mg. of aldosterone daily. Aldosterone is not available for therapeutic use, but a synthetic mineralocorticoid, fludrocortisone (9α-fluoro-hydrocortisone), is available, and a tablet containing 0.1 mg. taken once daily usually suffices as an aldosterone substitute. Another useful preparation is *desoxycorticosterone trimethyl-acetate,* a slowly absorbed suspension given intramuscularly in doses of about 50 mg. (2 ml.) per month. A patient who has a history of hyperten-

sion prior to the onset of Addison's disease may not require mineralocorticoid replacement therapy as long as he receives glucocorticoids and ordinary amounts of dietary sodium. No addisonian patient will do well, however, without an ample intake of sodium chloride.

Children with Addison's disease require smaller doses of steroids than adults. The daily cortisol dose should be about 12 mg. per square meter of body surface. If the child's linear growth does not proceed normally, it should be assumed that the dose of cortisol might be excessive, and the dose should be adjusted downward. The dose of mineralocorticoid should be adjusted as necessary to maintain normal blood pressure.

Treatment During Stresses. The maximum response of the normal pituitary-adrenal system to extreme stress results in the secretion of 200 to 500 mg. of cortisol per day. This is the dosage range of hydrocortisone phosphate to be administered parenterally to patients undergoing bilateral adrenalectomy or to addisonian patients undergoing extensive surgical procedures. Hydrocortisone phosphate administered parenterally in doses of 100 mg. every four to six hours should suffice as glucocorticoid replacement therapy in any severely stressed addisonian patient. As the stress subsides, the dose of hydrocortisone should be diminished accordingly. For example, following a major surgical operation, the daily dose of hydrocortisone can usually be decreased by decrements of 50 per cent each day until the usual dosage employed in chronic substitution therapy is reached.

For one reason or another, severely stressed patients usually do not consume adequate diets. It is important that addisonian patients be given at least 1 liter of physiologic sodium chloride solution daily until they resume their normal diets; a particularly hazardous period in convalescence is that during which orders are ordinarily given for the patient to take a "soft diet" or "surgical liquids." During this period the patient often does not even take all that is offered, and may become depleted of extracellular fluid.

Mild stresses such as minor surgical operations and injuries require only minor increases in corticosteroid therapy. Usually a two- to fourfold increase in glucocorticoid treatment on the day of the stress will suffice. Oral medications may be used if they can be retained. Again, it is important that the addisonian patient who is fasting or vomiting be given parenteral sodium chloride solution.

Treatment in the Presence of Infection. In the presence of infection, it is particularly important that glucocorticoid dosage should simulate the cortisol secretion rate of the similarly infected but endocrinologically normal person. Overtreatment might impair the patient's mechanisms for defending against invading micro-organisms, whereas undertreatment might predispose the infection-stressed patient to addisonian crisis. As a rule, an endocrinologically normal person secretes no more than 20 to 100 mg. of cortisol per day in response to infection. This then is the hydrocortisone dosage range that is appropriate for the addisonian with an intercurrent infectious illness. A practical rule is to be guided by the patient's body temperature. If it is in excess of 102° F., the dose of hydrocortisone should be increased to whatever amount is needed to reduce the temperature to less than this level. If the temperature is normal, the hydrocortisone dosage should be lowered until maintenance doses are reached. If the temperature is between 99 and 102° F., it may be assumed that the dose of hydrocortisone is appropriate (presumably between 20 and 100 mg. per day). It is of utmost importance that infections be specifically diagnosed and specifically treated as quickly as possible.

Mineralocorticoid vs. Sodium Chloride Therapy. Mineralocorticoids are used in treating intercritical adrenal insufficiency in order to assist the well-fed patient in maintaining adequate sodium stores without taking supplemental sodium chloride. Ordinary doses of mineralocorticoids do not adequately protect the addisonian patient from sodium and extracellular fluid depletion during periods of fasting or vomiting. Once sodium depletion has occurred, it must be corrected by the administration of sodium chloride; if adequate attention is given to this matter, upward adjustment of mineralocorticoid dosage (simulating the normal aldosterone secretory response to sodium depletion) will be unnecessary. Patients who sustain losses of sodium chloride but who are still capable of retaining oral medication, e.g., patients who sweat excessively, may be given supplemental sodium chloride tablets in doses of 2 grams two to four times daily.

Identification Bracelet and Injectable Hydrocortisone. The patient with Addison's disease should wear an identification bracelet stating his name, nearest kin's name and telephone number, and physician's name and telephone number. It should also state: "I have adrenal insufficiency. In any emergency involving injury, vomiting, or loss of consciousness, the hydrocortisone in my possession should be injected under my skin, and my physician should be notified." The patient should carry a small, clearly labeled kit containing 100 mg. of hydrocortisone phosphate solution in a sterile syringe ready for injection. Even if never used, the bracelet and kit are of educational value to the addisonian patient who must understand that his survival depends upon the timely use of steroids.

Prognosis. With the advent of synthetic corticosteroids the prognosis of Addison's disease became radically altered from one of almost certain fatal termination within months (rarely years) to one of normal activity and life expectancy. The well-treated addisonian patient should have essentially normal steroid and electrolyte values under all circumstances; therefore, he should not be incapacitated or have his life expectancy shortened by the fact that he has Addison's disease. All of the author's addisonian patients are productively employed unless they suffer from some additional disorder which is in some way incapacitating. Addisonians must, however, face the perils of emergencies in which they are incapable of caring for themselves and in which they might depend upon the assistance of others to assure that the essential steroids and electrolytes are administered. Their prognosis might also be limited by other diseases sometimes associated with Addison's disease, such as tuberculosis, histoplasmosis, diabetes mellitus, or amyloidosis. Most of the addisonian patients who have been discovered since synthetic cortisone became generally available are still living, and there are no accurate data to indicate whether Addison's disease per se, when adequately treated, alters life expectancy.

ADRENAL INSUFFICIENCY SECONDARY TO BILATERAL ADRENALECTOMY

Adrenal insufficiency secondary to bilateral adrenalectomy is one variant of Addison's disease which should never present any diagnostic difficulty inasmuch as it is iatrogenic. Treatment is the same as that outlined under Addison's Disease.

ADRENAL APOPLEXY

Hemorrhagic infarction of the adrenal glands can occur in the course of meningococcal septicemia (Waterhouse-Friderichsen syndrome) or as a complication of anticoagulant therapy. The occurrence of hypotension in either of these clinical settings should alert the physician to the possibility of adrenal apoplexy, and treatment similar to that outlined under the heading Treatment During Stresses should be undertaken on an emergency basis. Specific treatment for the underlying disorder (meningococcemia or coagulation defects) should also be carried out without delay. If the patient survives, he may at some later date undergo a standard test for adrenocortical reserve in order to determine whether steroid replacement therapy can be withdrawn safely.

Although the adrenal glands are hemorrhagic in the Waterhouse-Friderichsen syndrome, hypotension, shock, and death in this condition are usually not attributable to adrenal insufficiency, since plasma cortisol levels are usually high. In most cases, the course of the disease is probably not altered by steroid therapy; nevertheless, cortisol should be given in large doses since it is impossible to rule out adrenal insufficiency within the time that is available to initiate decisive therapy; the occasional patient who might have true adrenal insufficiency in association with adrenal apoplexy should not be denied the benefits of adequate cortisol therapy.

ADRENAL INSUFFICIENCY SECONDARY TO HYPOPITUITARISM

Definition and Incidence. Since normal adrenal function is dependent upon the stimulatory action of ACTH secreted by the pituitary, it follows that any disorder in which the pituitary is damaged in such a way as to reduce ACTH secretion to subnormal values leads to secondary adrenocortical hypofunction. This situation is encountered in approximately 1 of 1000 patients admitted to hospitals. (See Anterior Pituitary.)

Pathogenesis. Whether associated with tumor or infarction, loss of pituitary function is attributable to loss of pituitary tissue or to interruption of the connections between the hypothalamus and the pituitary. The degree of hypopituitarism is variable from patient to patient, ranging from such profound deficiencies as to be incompatible with survival to such mild deficiencies that special tests of pituitary reserve are required to demonstrate an abnormality.

Absence of ACTH results in decreased secretion of cortisol and adrenal androgen, but aldosterone secretion remains relatively intact. Cortisol deficiency results in loss of appetite, loss of vigor, inability to maintain adequate blood glucose levels during prolonged fasting, inability to excrete free water with normal rapidity, and inability to withstand severe stresses without going into shock. Hyponatremia is commonly encountered in patients with hypopituitarism who have been given liberal amounts of fluid, but it is directly attributable to the difficulty these individuals have in excreting water rather than to impaired secretion of aldosterone. If they are given glucocorticoid so that they can excrete water adequately, they can be shown to have the capacity to withstand simple sodium chloride deprivation by increasing their aldosterone secretion sufficiently to enable them to excrete urine that is virtually sodium-free.

Absence of adrenal androgen is itself of little consequence; but when adrenal insufficiency is secondary to hypopituitarism, it is usually accompanied by a deficiency of gonadotrophins with secondary hypogonadism and a consequent decrease in testicular secretion of testosterone. Therefore, in contrast to Addison's disease, in which only the adult female shows evidence of androgen deficiency, in hypopituitarism, patients of either sex are likely to exhibit manifestations of androgen deficiency.

Clinical Manifestations. There are several similarities and a few important differences between hypopituitarism and Addison's disease with regard to their clinical manifestations. Like the addisonian, the patient with hypopituitarism "falls off in general health; he becomes languid and weak, indisposed to either bodily or mental exertion; the appetite is impaired . . . and there is occasionally actual vomiting." Fasting may lead to hypoglycemia, and hypoglycemic symptoms (including loss of consciousness) are probably more common in untreated hypopituitarism than in Addison's disease. A liberal intake of water may lead to severe hyponatremia and manifestations of water intoxication such as confusion, incoordination, stupor, and convulsions. Severe stress may precipitate peripheral vascular collapse.

In contrast to the addisonian, the patient with hypopituitarism does not show mucocutaneous hyperpigmentation (this abnormality, in Addison's disease, is a consequence of excessive secretion of the pituitary hormones ACTH and MSH). Unlike the addisonian, the patient with hypopituitarism can tolerate simple sodium deprivation without developing shock or hyponatremia. In addition to the manifestations of adrenal insufficiency, the patient with hypopituitarism usually exhibits manifestations of hypogonadism and hypothyroidism, and may show other evidence of pituitary or intracranial disease, e.g., erosion of the sella turcica and temporal visual field defects.

Diagnosis and Differential Diagnosis. The diagnosis of secondary adrenal insufficiency is established by the demonstration that cortisol levels in blood and cortisol metabolite levels in urine are subnormal and that they can be induced to rise to normal or above normal by repetitive treatment with ACTH over a period of one to three days. Urinary 17-ketosteroids are also subnormal, but rise in response to ACTH.

Primary adrenal insufficiency (Addison's disease) is easily differentiated from secondary adrenal insufficiency by the failure of steroids to rise substantially regardless of the dosage or duration of treatment with ACTH.

It is advisable to measure both plasma and urinary steroids in order to avoid pitfalls in differentiating secondary adrenal insufficiency from certain disorders of cortisol metabolism in which a normal relationship between plasma and urinary corticosteroids is lacking. Thus in primary hypothyroidism, hepatic insufficiency, and severe renal insufficiency, and during treatment with drugs that alter the extra-adrenal metabolism of cortisol (diphenylhydantoin, aminoglutethimide, amphotericin, o,p'-DDD, triparanol), the urinary 17-OHCS do not adequately reflect cortisol secretion rates and are falsely low in relation to plasma cortisol levels. In these situations, plasma cortisol concentrations accurately reflect cortisol secretion under basal conditions and in response to ACTH, whereas urinary 17-OHCS might falsely suggest the presence of secondary adrenal insufficiency. In contrast, there is a familial disorder in which plasma transcortin concentrations are subnormal, even though cortisol secretion rates, plasma free cortisol concentrations, and urinary 17-OHCS are all normal. In this situation, plasma cortisol concentrations alone might erroneously suggest the presence of secondary adrenal insufficiency.

Various clinical clues are also helpful in arriving at a correct diagnosis of secondary adrenal insufficiency, e.g., hypothyroidism with normal responsiveness to thyrotropin, hypogonadism with subnormal gonadotrophin levels in plasma or urine, or growth failure with consistently negligible levels of growth hormone in serum (even after provocative maneuvers such as arginine infusion or insulin-induced hypoglycemia). Other evidence of pituitary disease, such as erosion of the sella turcica or a history of postpartum hemorrhage, should also alert the physician to the possibility that the patient might have hypopituitarism, subnormal ACTH production, and secondary adrenocortical deficiency.

A mild degree of ACTH deficiency can exist with normal or slightly subnormal plasma and urinary corticosteroids and normal or slightly subnormal responses to ACTH. Such mild degrees of ACTH deficiency are referred to as limited pituitary reserve, and are characterized by failure of the pituitary to secrete normal quantities of ACTH (and, therefore, a failure of the adrenal glands to secrete normal quantities of corticosteroids) in response to stress or to standard test doses of metyrapone.

Treatment. Secondary adrenocortical insufficiency requires cortisol replacement therapy in the same doses and under the same conditions as outlined for Addison's disease. Mineralocorticoid therapy is unnecessary. An identification card and hydrocortisone phosphate for emergency use should be employed as in Addison's disease.

If the patient suffers from hypogonadism, hypothyroidism, or diabetes insipidus, these conditions should be treated with androgens or estrogens, thyroid, or pitressin, as outlined elsewhere (Anterior Pituitary, Posterior Pituitary).

Prognosis. As in the case of Addison's disease, the prognosis in secondary adrenal insufficiency is excellent if intelligent use is made of hormones for replacement therapy and if the primary basis for the hypopituitarism is not otherwise incapacitating or life-threatening. (See Anterior Pituitary.)

ADRENAL INSUFFICIENCY SECONDARY TO PITUITARY-ADRENAL SUPPRESSION BY CORTICOSTEROIDS

Prolonged administration of glucocorticoids or prolonged secretion of cortisol by an adrenal tumor in quantities sufficient to cause Cushing's syndrome consistently causes suppression of ACTH secretion and consequent adrenocortical atrophy. Withdrawal of steroid therapy or removal of the adrenal tumor results in adrenal insufficiency. Diagnosis should not be difficult in view of the physician's or surgeon's role in bringing about the condition. If the hypercortisolism has been severe and has existed continuously for at least one year, the course of pituitary-adrenal recovery may be slow, requiring several months for completion. Early in the course the basal corticosteroid levels, the adrenal response to ACTH, and the pituitary-adrenal response to metyrapone are all

subnormal, simulating adrenal insufficiency secondary to hypopituitarism. Treatment consists of giving a physiologic dose of hydrocortisone, 20 mg. once daily, to prevent symptoms of adrenal insufficiency. Over a period of months this dose can gradually be reduced to 5 mg. daily and finally withdrawn altogether as pituitary-adrenal function gradually returns to normal. Until pituitary-adrenal recovery is complete, one should treat the patient as if he had hypopituitarism during periods of stress or infection. (See Anterior Pituitary.)

CUSHING'S SYNDROME

Definition. Cushing's syndrome is the clinical and metabolic disorder resulting from a chronic excess of glucocorticoids. *Cushing's syndrome medicamentosus* is a common iatrogenic disorder caused by any of several synthetic glucocorticoids. Spontaneous Cushing's syndrome, on the other hand, is caused solely by cortisol, the only glucocorticoid produced in significant quantities by the human adrenal cortex.

Etiology. Normally, cortisol is not secreted except in response to ACTH, and ACTH is not secreted in the presence of supraphysiologic levels of cortisol. Therefore, the very occurrence of Cushing's syndrome implies a disorder in the regulation of cortisol or ACTH secretion: either the adrenal gland has acquired the capability of secreting cortisol in the absence of ACTH, or ACTH secretion is not normally suppressible by cortisol. There are three well-established causes of Cushing's syndrome. *First*, adrenocortical tumors can secrete cortisol autonomously, that is to say, in the virtual absence of ACTH. The tumors may be carcinomas, solitary adenomas, or (rarely) multiple adenomas. *Second*, certain nonpituitary neoplasms secrete ACTH, which stimulates the adrenal cortices to secrete supraphysiologic quantities of cortisol. This clinical entity is sometimes referred to as the ectopic ACTH syndrome. (See Endocrine Syndromes Associated with Neoplasms of Nonendocrine Tissues.) *Third*, pituitary function can become disordered so that ACTH is secreted in excessive quantities, thus stimulating excessive secretion of cortisol by the adrenals. This condition is referred to by the specific term Cushing's disease. The pituitary can be normal in appearance, contain a small basophil adenoma, or contain a large chromophobe adenoma; regardless of the morphologic appearance of the pituitary, virtually all patients with excessive pituitary ACTH show similar patterns of ACTH secretion. There is loss of normal diurnal rhythmicity, relative but not absolute resistance to suppression by glucocorticoids, and increased secretion of ACTH in response to a reduction of cortisol levels to normal.

Incidence. Cushing's syndrome resulting from adrenal tumor occurs in approximately 1 of every 10,000 hospital admissions. Cushing's disease occurs in approximately 1 of every 2000 admissions. The incidence of the ectopic ACTH syndrome is difficult to estimate since it is frequently overlooked. There is evidence that ectopic ACTH might be produced by as many as 8 per cent of visceral carcinomas. Careful screening of patients with nonpituitary tumors might reveal the production of ectopic ACTH to be the most common cause of hypercortisolism.

Pathogenesis. The major features of Cushing's syndrome are understandable in terms of the known actions of cortisol. When present in excessive quantities, this hormone accelerates the catabolism of protein and stimulates the hepatic uptake and deamination of amino acids. It also inhibits the transport of amino acids into extrahepatic tissues. As a consequence of these actions, prolonged high concentrations of cortisol cause clinical manifestations of protein wasting. Children show retardation of linear growth. Wasting of the integument and increasing capillary fragility result in ecchymoses. Cutaneous striae form in areas where the skin is stretched by an accumulation of adipose tissue. In extreme cases, wasting of muscle results in pronounced weakness. Wasting of bone matrix results in osteoporosis.

Abnormally high levels of cortisol alter the body's responses to injury and infection. Cortisol stabilizes lysosomal membranes, thus diminishing the tendency of injured tissues to perpetuate their own damage. It suppresses the sticking of leukocytes to endothelial surfaces, and diminishes the accumulation of leukocytes at sites of tissue injury. It inhibits the diapedesis of white blood cells and impairs their migration through tissues. In high concentrations over long periods of time, cortisol impairs antibody production and inhibits the proliferation of lymphocytes. Thus, almost every aspect of the normal cellular response to injury or infection is suppressed by high concentrations of cortisol, leaving the patient with impaired capacity to limit the spread of invading organisms.

Cortisol promotes potassium excretion and sodium retention by stimulating cation exchange by the distal convoluted tubules. A severe excess of cortisol can result in depletion of bodily potassium to such a degree that hypokalemia, electrocardiographic abnormalities, muscular weakness, and impairment of renal concentrating capacity develop. Retention of sodium and elevated blood pressure occur. Steroid hypertension, like other varieties of hypertension, leads to left ventricular hypertrophy and predisposes the patient to congestive heart failure and strokes. Even without frank congestive heart failure, some patients experience expansion of their extracellular fluid volumes to the point of edema.

In addition to stimulating the formation of new glucose from amino acids, lactate, pyruvate, and bicarbonate, cortisol impairs the action of insulin in transporting glucose across cell membranes. Consequently, abnormally high amounts of cortisol tend to raise the level of blood glucose; this is most readily apparent in the prolongation of hyperglycemia after a glucose load; a minority of patients with hypercortisolism have abnormally high fasting blood glucose levels.

Adrenal carcinomas that secrete cortisol usually secrete significant quantities of adrenal androgen as well. In men this is of no clinical consequence, but in women and children it gives rise to virilism. Benign adenomas that cause Cushing's syndrome are somewhat less likely to produce excessive quantities of androgen. Mild virilism, usually amounting to nothing more than acne, thinning of scalp hair, and some degree of facial hirsutism, is common in women with Cushing's disease or the ectopic ACTH syndrome. In these disorders the increased levels of ACTH result in increased production of adrenal androgens as well as cortisol.

Although Cushing's syndrome is due entirely to an excess of corticosteroids, one must realize that the clinical illness of the patient may be affected by other factors as well. This is readily apparent in the ectopic ACTH syndrome when the clinical picture is usually dominated by other effects of the ACTH-secreting tumor. These patients often have a degree of weakness out of proportion to the severity of their hypercortisolism, and they often lose weight, which is contrary to the course of patients with other varieties of Cushing's syndrome.

Clinical Manifestations. The clinical manifestations of Cushing's syndrome are familiar to every physician who has seen a patient treated with large doses of a cortisol-like steroid for several weeks or longer. The clinical picture of cortisol excess may be mixed with additional features of virilism and mineralocorticoid excess.

General Appearance and Physiognomy. The typical patient with Cushing's syndrome has central obesity, with rounding of the face, thickening of the fat pads in the supraclavicular fossae, and thickening of the thoracico-abdominal panniculus. In long-standing cases, the abdominal obesity can progress to grotesque proportions while the extremities remain remarkably slender. People with pre-existing obesity from other causes can, of course, develop Cushing's syndrome; under such circumstances it is difficult to decide on clinical grounds alone whether the patient has Cushing's syndrome and, if so, to what extent his obesity is attributable to the steroid excess. Patients with malignant tumors often show little or no obesity, even though their steroid levels are high and other features of Cushing's syndrome are fully expressed.

Cutaneous Manifestations. The face and neck often have a ruddy hyperemic appearance. Trivial trauma often results in ecchymosis. In advanced cases, the skin over the forearms and legs becomes thin, having the appearance of parchment. Slight injury to the skin can result in purpuric extravasation of blood; the sites of venipunctures sometimes show extensive subcutaneous hemorrhage. Removal of adhesive tape sometimes denudes the delicate skin of the patient with the advanced protein-wasting of Cushing's syndrome. Once formed, wounds heal slowly and often become the sites of indolent infections. In areas where the weakened skin is stretched by the underlying accumulation of fat (particularly the abdomen, shoulders, and hips), wide purplish striae may form.

The reaction to infection is attenuated in Cushing's syndrome. Superficial fungal infections, e.g., tinea versicolor, occur in about 20 per cent of cases. In more severe cases, bacterial infections are not well confined in the form of discrete abscesses of short duration, but are more likely to be chronic and to give rise to cellulitis and bacteremia. This is a dangerous situation which may escape notice because the patient with Cushing's syndrome often has less discomfort and experiences less of a febrile reaction than would ordinarily be expected with a given degree of infection.

Largely as a function of an associated excess of androgens, acne and hirsutism commonly occur in patients with Cushing's syndrome. The hirsutism is sometimes slight, downy, and distributed over the cheeks and shoulders, but sometimes coarse hairs appear in the beard area and on the chest and abdomen. In men, of course, this aspect of hyperadrenocorticism is unnoticed.

Reproductive Functions. Most women with Cushing's syndrome have oligomenorrhea. Although it is difficult to evaluate with certainty, many of them may have diminished fertility; however, this is by no means uniform. Men with Cushing's syndrome are sometimes said to be troubled with impotence; this is certainly not always so, and might not be related to the hyperadrenocorticism when it does occur. Infertility is probably not a feature of Cushing's syndrome in men.

Musculoskeletal Manifestations. Children with Cushing's syndrome experience arrest of linear growth. If obesity in a child is associated with growth arrest, the possibility of Cushing's syndrome should receive strong consideration; continued normal linear growth is strong evidence that the child's obesity is not due to Cushing's syndrome. Insidious atrophy of the skeleton results in mild hypercalciuria and, in time, in frank osteoporosis. Severe osteoporosis of the vertebral bodies may result in bulging of intervertebral discs, giving the appearance of codfish vertebrae in lateral roentgenographic views. Compression fractures with anterior wedging of the vertebral bodies result in kyphosis and loss of height. Pathologic fractures of ribs and hips occasionally occur.

In severe Cushing's syndrome, muscular atrophy may progress to such an extent that the patient is too weak to rise from a squatting position without assistance. Muscular weakness is usually not noticeable in milder cases.

Cardiovascular and Renal Manifestations. Most patients with Cushing's syndrome have hypertension, the course and complications of which are similar to those of essential hypertension.

Edema can occur as a manifestation of congestive heart failure, but in 10 to 20 per cent of cases, mild edema occurs in the absence of congestive failure.

Hypokalemia with hypochloremic alkalosis occurs spontaneously in about 10 to 20 per cent of the cases (usually those with the most severe excesses of steroid secretion), and may occur in others as a complication of diuretic therapy.

Renal lithiasis is a common occurrence in chronic cases of Cushing's syndrome.

Hematologic Features. Some patients with Cushing's syndrome have erythrocytosis, granulocytosis, lymphopenia, and eosinopenia.

Carbohydrate Tolerance. Impaired carbohydrate tolerance occurs in more than 90 per cent of cases of Cushing's syndrome. In the majority it is manifested merely by a failure of the blood glucose to return to normal fasting levels during the first three hours after a glucose load. In about 20 per cent it is manifested as clinical diabetes mellitus.

Psychologic Abnormalities. Alterations of mood are common in Cushing's syndrome. Many patients feel irritable and weep with little provocation. A few experience psychotic mentation with delusional content. A few patients are depressed, and some attempt suicide. Manic and hypomanic behavior may also occur.

Diagnosis and Differential Diagnosis. It is important for the physician to know when to suspect Cushing's syndrome and then how to prove or disprove the diagnosis, keeping in mind the need for economy and precision. Taken singly, the various clinical manifestations of Cushing's syndrome are not very specific. Thus, only a minute percentage of all hypertensive patients have Cushing's syndrome; only a minute percentage of diabetic patients have Cushing's syndrome; only a minute percentage of patients with renal lithiasis have Cushing's syndrome, and so forth. The coexistence of multiple clinical manifestations greatly increases the probability that a given patient might have hypercortisolism. If one encounters a patient with a single manifestation of Cushing's syndrome, he should always ask himself if hypercortisolism could be present; but if no other symptoms or signs of the syndrome can be found in the course of a complete medical evaluation, it will usually be unrewarding to pursue this line of investigation. Here we are discussing only probabilities, and should recognize that rare examples of hypercortisolism have been unequivocally diagnosed in the virtual absence of clinical manifestations.

Under certain conditions, one can make a clinical diagnosis quite confidently. For example, a patient with protein wasting (osteoporosis, easily denuded skin) and centripetal obesity probably has hypercortisolism. A child who simultaneously develops central obesity and experiences arrest of linear growth probably has Cushing's syndrome. Osteoporosis occurs commonly in patients beyond the age of 50 and is of limited value in diagnosis in this group; but osteoporosis in children and young adults should make one alert to the possibility of Cushing's syndrome. Although impaired glucose tolerance, taken by itself, is not especially suggestive of Cushing's syndrome, *normal* glucose tolerance is rare in Cushing's syndrome (about 10 per cent) and is therefore useful in discounting the probability of hypercortisolism. Patients with tumors of any organ and unprovoked hypokalemia should be suspected of having hypercortisolism, regardless of lack of obesity or signs of protein wasting.

Whenever the suspicion of Cushing's syndrome cannot be dismissed confidently, one should proceed with assays of plasma cortisol or urinary 17-hydroxycorticosteroids under basal conditions and during treatment with standard small doses of dexamethasone. At this point, a reliable laboratory with well-established ranges of normal values is indispensable. Equally important is close supervision of the patient so that specimens are collected properly, so that stresses or medications which might lead to high steroid values are avoided, and so that the physician knows that the dexamethasone is taken as prescribed.

Under basal conditions (in this context, "basal" means "in the absence of exogenous agents that stimulate or suppress ACTH or cortisol secretion"), nonstressed patients have plasma cortisol concentrations of 8 to 25 μg. per 100 ml. in the morning and less than 8 μg. per 100 ml. in the evening. Under the same conditions, patients with untreated Cushing's syndrome almost always have plasma cortisol concentrations in excess of 15 μg. per 100 ml. at all times. Under basal conditions, nonstressed patients have urinary 17-OHCS of 3 to 7 mg. per gram of urinary creatinine. Under the same conditions, patients with untreated Cushing's syndrome almost always have urinary 17-OHCS in excess of 10 mg. per gram of creatinine.

In response to small doses of dexamethasone (0.5 mg. every six hours for two days), nonstressed patients show decreases in plasma cortisol to less than 5 μg. per 100 ml. and excrete less than 2 mg. of 17-OHCS per gram of creatinine. Under similar conditions, patients with Cushing's syndrome almost always maintain plasma cortisol concentrations above 8 μg. per 100 ml. and excrete more than 3 mg. of 17-OHCS per gram of creatinine.

Having established the fact that a patient has hypercortisolism, the physician must then determine whether it is caused by autonomous adrenal function, ectopic secretion of ACTH, or inappropriate secretion of pituitary ACTH. There are many useful guides in making this differential diagnosis, but the most reliable approach is to perform a large-dose dexamethasone suppression test and then, if pituitary-adrenal suppressibility cannot be demonstrated, to perform an assay for plasma ACTH if this measurement is available. The purpose of the large dose of dexamethasone is to determine whether adrenal function is under pituitary control. In almost all cases of Cushing's syndrome caused by inappropriate secretion of ACTH by the pituitary, it is possible to suppress adrenal function distinctly and reproducibly

(though not necessarily profoundly) by administering dexamethasone in doses of 2 mg. every six hours for two days. If a distinct, reproducible decrease in adrenal function does not occur, one should assume that adrenal function is autonomous or that it is under the control of ectopic ACTH. The distinction between these two disorders can be made by assaying plasma ACTH. In patients with autonomous adrenal function, plasma ACTH concentrations should be subnormal; but in patients with the ectopic ACTH syndrome plasma ACTH is high normal or distinctly elevated. The reason for emphasizing the importance of reproducibility in the large-dose dexamethasone suppression test is to avoid diagnostic errors that might result if spontaneous decreases in tumor activity should occur, or if inadequate urine collections happen to be made at the same time as the administration of dexamethasone. Such coincidences should not be reproducible, but suppression of pituitary ACTH secretion should be. Frequently it is unnecessary to carry out the large-dose dexamethasone test since all the information one requires can be derived from an analysis of the results of the small-dose test. Many patients with an excess of pituitary ACTH show partial suppression of their steroid output in response to 0.5 mg. of dexamethasone every six hours. Definite, reproducible suppression of adrenal function with any dose of dexamethasone implies that adrenal function is under the control of the pituitary.

Blind reliance upon a single set of laboratory values is not to be recommended; for example, high levels of estrogen, such as those encountered in pregnancy or during treatment with oral contraceptives, lead to elevations of plasma cortisol by raising the concentration of cortisol-binding globulin, but there is no increase in cortisol secretion rate or in urinary 17-OHCS. Hyperthyroidism can lead to accelerated removal of cortisol from the circulation and a compensatory increase in cortisol secretion rate, accompanied by an increase in urinary 17-OHCS, but plasma 17-OHCS values are not elevated. Awareness of the total clinical condition and use of more than one dimension in evaluating adrenal function should protect one from making diagnostic errors.

Although the approach described above is the most economical and reliable method of establishing a definitive diagnosis of Cushing's syndrome, the following points may often offer additional help.

1. Patients with Cushing's disease almost invariably respond to metyrapone with increased secretion of ACTH and total 17-OHCS (the increase in 17-OHCS is attributable to a large increase in 11-deoxycortisol). Patients with Cushing's syndrome caused by adrenal tumor do not respond to metyrapone with increased 17-OHCS production. Patients with the ectopic ACTH syndrome vary in their responses; some show increases in 17-OHCS and others do not.

2. In patients with hypercortisolism, a grossly disproportionate elevation of urinary 17-keto-

steroids is highly suggestive of adrenal carcinoma. The same may be said if more than 30 per cent of the urinary 17-OHCS are made up of 11-deoxy-cortisol and its tetrahydrometabolite.

3. Virtually all patients with Cushing's disease respond to exogenous ACTH with large increases in cortisol secretion; this is also true of patients with the ectopic ACTH syndrome unless their basal levels of cortisol are very high. Patients with Cushing's syndrome resulting from adrenal carcinoma almost never respond to brief infusions of ACTH. Patients with cortisol-secreting adenomas vary in their responses; about half of them respond and half do not.

4. Adrenal carcinomas are usually so inefficient in producing steroids that they do not cause Cushing's syndrome until they have become large enough to be readily demonstrated by intravenous urography or arteriography; some are so large that they can be palpated through the anterior abdominal wall by the time the patient exhibits Cushing's syndrome.

Treatment.   The prime therapeutic objectives in Cushing's syndrome are to reduce cortisol levels to normal and to eradicate any associated tumors. Secondary objectives are to avoid producing hormonal deficiencies and to avoid making the patient chronically dependent upon medication. All these objectives can be achieved in some patients in each of the three categories of Cushing's syndrome. In many cases, however, compromises must be made. Good therapeutic strategy depends upon diagnostic precision.

In Cushing's disease, ideal therapeutic results can be achieved in only about 25 per cent of cases by irradiation of the pituitary with about 4500 r. Although this mode of therapy was abandoned in many medical centers when the availability of cortisone substitution therapy made it feasible to perform bilateral adrenalectomy, it remains the only form of therapy that offers the patient a chance of achieving all the therapeutic objectives listed above. The author has 19 patients who have been in remission from 1 to 14 years after pituitary irradiation. No serious side effects have been encountered, and none of the patients appears to have developed deficiencies of any pituitary hormones as a consequence of therapy. There are only three drawbacks to this therapeutic approach. First, one must be certain that his diagnosis is correct; pituitary irradiation is clearly inappropriate for patients with adrenal tumors or for patients with the ectopic ACTH syndrome. Second, 75 per cent of patients do not respond, and ultimately require other therapy. Third, the results of pituitary irradiation are not apparent for one to four months; and the patient with fulminant hypertension, rapidly progressive osteoporosis, or psychosis not well controlled by psychoactive drugs should be treated more aggressively.

Only three other modes of therapy have been consistently effective in Cushing's disease. With each of them, normalization of cortisol is usually achieved, but the patient incurs life-threatening

hormonal deficiencies which require lifelong substitution therapy. *Bilateral adrenalectomy* is most widely practiced. Subtotal adrenalectomy is not to be recommended because of the likelihood of recurrence of hyperadrenocorticism and the frequent impossibility of finding and removing all the regenerative remnant from a scarred mass of perinephric fat at a second operation. Substitution therapy with a glucocorticoid (and usually a mineralocorticoid) must begin at the time of adrenalectomy and continue for the duration of the patient's life. The principles of substitution therapy are outlined under Addison's Disease.

Hypophysectomy and subtotal ablation of the pituitary by means of cryosurgery or the implantation of radioactive gold or yttrium have been mastered in several medical centers, and destruction of the pituitary by sharply localized high-dosage irradiation has been achieved in at least two centers. Therapeutic success in Cushing's syndrome is likely to be accompanied by hypopituitarism, requiring substitution therapy with glucocorticoids, thyroid hormone, gonadal steroids, and occasionally antidiuretic hormone. This form of therapy is not to be recommended for the young patient to whom reproductive capacity and normal growth are, obviously, important matters.

Selective destruction of the zona fasciculata and zona reticularis without the induction of aldosterone deficiency can be achieved with prolonged administration of the adrenocorticolytic drug, o,p'-DDD. This mode of therapy is attended by at least minor gastrointestinal side effects and entails the risk of producing virtually complete loss of glucocorticoid secretory capacity, unless the physician is able to follow the patient closely enough to adjust the dose of o,p'-DDD so that plasma cortisol concentrations remain within the optimal range. The advantage of this form of treatment, apart from the avoidance of operative risks, is the preservation of the aldosterone secretory mechanism so that the patient is not so vulnerable to sodium depletion as is the totally adrenalectomized patient. Unfortunately, for the foreseeable future, the drug is to be available for only limited investigational use.

In the ectopic ACTH syndrome, ideal therapeutic results can be achieved only if the ACTH-secreting tumor can be completely removed. Thus far, this has been possible in only a score of cases. In the remainder, either the tumors have not been diagnosed before the death of the patient or they have not been completely resectable. In those cases in which the ACTH-secreting tumor cannot be removed, it is still possible to curtail the hypercortisolism by treatment with metyrapone. This drug inhibits the final step in cortisol synthesis and leads to secretion of the biologically weak precursor, 11-deoxycortisol. One can start with small doses of 250 mg. every eight hours and increase them if necessary to achieve the desired reduction of cortisol production (under these circumstances the simplest way to estimate cortisol levels is to measure plasma fluorogenic steroids). Doses in excess of 500 mg. every six hours are rarely required. Bilateral adrenalectomy or o,p'-DDD therapy might be employed in selected patients in whom the hypercortisolism offers a more immediate threat to life than does the ACTH-secreting tumor. It should be borne in mind that o,p'-DDD so alters the extra-adrenal metabolism of cortisol that the measurement of urinary 17-OHCS is unreliable in evaluating cortisol secretion; the patient's progress should be followed by measurements of plasma cortisol.

The only completely satisfactory treatment of Cushing's syndrome resulting from adrenal tumor is the surgical removal of the tumor. Most tumors are benign and unilateral, and removal of the tumor-bearing gland is curative. It is essential that the patient be supported with glucocorticoids during and for several days after the operation, because chronic suppression of ACTH production will have resulted in atrophy of the nontumorous adrenal. A regimen similar to that employed during bilateral adrenalectomy is appropriate. Postoperatively, glucocorticoid therapy should be progressively reduced so that within a week or so the patient receives only 20 to 30 mg. of cortisol per day. This supportive therapy should be withdrawn gradually over the ensuing year. It is possible during this period to give the entire daily steroid supplement as a single dose in the morning, thus permitting the pituitary-adrenal system to escape from the suppressive influence of cortisol for a portion of each day. On this schedule the daily dose of cortisol can gradually be reduced from 30 mg. to 5 mg. and then discontinued altogether. Throughout this first year the physician and patient should be alert to the possible need for increased cortisol dosage in the event of an acute stress. The principles of therapy in this situation are the same as those described for patients with adrenal insufficiency. After steroids have been withdrawn for a time, the patient's recovery of normal pituitary-adrenal function can be verified by a metyrapone test. A normal response should indicate that the patient no longer needs to be concerned about pituitary-adrenal insufficiency.

Approximately 5 to 10 per cent of patients with Cushing's syndrome resulting from benign adrenal adenomas have bilateral tumors. These patients require bilateral adrenalectomy followed by lifelong treatment, as for Addison's disease.

Although adrenal surgery is curative in some patients with adrenal carcinoma, a majority have either apparent or occult metastases by the time they seek medical attention. In about two thirds of these patients, the adrenocorticolytic drug o,p'-DDD will induce a temporary remission of hyperadrenocorticism, and about one-half of these experience regression of tumor mass for several months to a few years. The dose ranges from 3 to 10 grams per day, depending upon the severity of gastrointestinal side effects. If measures to control growth of the tumor are unsuccessful, it is still possible to control hypercortisolism with metyrapone given in divided doses totaling 1 to 2 grams daily. In patients with adrenal tumors, overtreatment with adrenal inhibitors can result in

adrenal insufficiency; this can be avoided by erring on the side of undertreatment or by giving 0.5 mg. of dexamethasone daily as a supportive measure.

Significance of Virilism in Association with Cushing's Syndrome. Clinical and chemical evidences of androgen hypersecretion are not uncommon in Cushing's syndrome. Although not a highly reliable rule, it is usually true that when a patient with Cushing's syndrome exhibits marked evidence of androgen excess, the cause is likely to be adrenocortical carcinoma. In other varieties of Cushing's syndrome, virilism is usually mild or inapparent.

The most important question to be settled early in the evaluation of any patient with virilism is whether or not this is associated with hypercortisolism, for virilism associated with hypercortisolism should be managed according to the principles outlined above for Cushing's syndrome, but virilism without hypercortisolism represents an entirely different group of disorders requiring drastically different treatment (cf. congenital adrenal hyperplasia, virilizing tumors, ovarian disorders, and precocious puberty).

PRIMARY ALDOSTERONISM

Definition, Etiology, and Incidence. Narrowly defined, "primary aldosteronism" is the constellation of chemical and clinical abnormalities resulting from the "autonomous" hypersecretion of aldosterone. The words "primary" and "autonomous" are employed to set this condition apart from "secondary aldosteronism," which refers to hypersecretion of aldosterone in response to a known stimulus such as angiotensin. Usually primary aldosteronism is due to an aldosterone-secreting adenoma (Conn's syndrome), but occasionally it is associated with adrenal hyperplasia or with morphologically normal adrenals (idiopathic hyperaldosteronism).

The incidence of primary aldosteronism is a subject of controversy. Conn has recently suggested that it might be present in 7 per cent of patients who otherwise appear to have essential hypertension. Others believe it to be less common, perhaps occurring in 1 per cent of the hypertensive population. It has been reported in about twice as many females as males.

Pathogenesis. Virtually all the features of primary aldosteronism are attributable to the fact that aldosterone promotes the conservation of sodium and the excretion of potassium.

Excessive conservation of sodium leads to expansion of extracellular volume, elevation of the blood pressure, and suppression of renin production. In the absence of circulatory insufficiency, modest expansion of extracellular volume leads to physiologic adjustments which enable the excretory system to come into equilibrium with the sodium intake; progressive expansion of extracellular volume is thus avoided, and overt edema is absent or only slight. (These adjustments are sometimes referred to in jargon as the escape phenomenon.)

Excessive excretion of potassium can result in potassium depletion, hypokalemic alkalosis, muscular weakness, areflexia, tetany, paresthesias, electrocardiographic abnormalities (S-T depression, flattening of T-waves, and appearance of U-waves), idioventricular arrhythmias, and kaliopenic nephropathy, with impaired renal concentrating capacity that cannot be corrected by vasopressin. Despite the hypokalemia, urinary potassium excretion usually exceeds 30 mEq. per day. Since potassium secretion in the distal convoluted tubule is, in part, a function of the quantity of sodium reaching that portion of the nephron, a high sodium intake tends to exaggerate the potassium-wasting process, and a low sodium intake tends to mask it.

The action of aldosterone in promoting the conservation of sodium and the rejection of potassium is observable not only in the kidney, but in all epithelialized organ systems which carry on cation exchange. Thus, in hyperaldosteronism one can often demonstrate depression of the sodium:potassium ratio in sweat, saliva, and gastrointestinal secretions.

Apart from the relatively rare patients who develop alarming ventricular arrhythmias or incapacitating muscular weakness as a result of potassium depletion, the great dangers of primary aldosteronism are the common complications of hypertensive cardiovascular disease: cardiac hypertrophy, congestive heart failure, strokes, and progressive impairment of renal function. Although uncommon, malignant hypertension can occur as a complication of primary aldosteronism and can be associated with either elevated or suppressed plasma renin activity.

Clinical Manifestations. All patients who have been proved to have primary aldosteronism have had hypertension. This is somewhat tautologic, since physicians do not usually consider the diagnosis in the absence of hypertension. Nevertheless, the clinical importance of primary aldosteronism is in the main related to hypertension and its sequelae. There are no characteristics of the hypertension of primary aldosteronism that are helpful in distinguishing it from "essential" hypertension.

The coexistence of hypertension and *unprovoked* hypokalemia is highly suggestive of primary aldosteronism. Indeed, in some studies as many as 50 per cent of patients with this combination of abnormalities have ultimately been shown to have primary aldosteronism. In a large percentage of patients the hypokalemia is asymptomatic. In an uncertain but probably small percentage it is not demonstrable at all. The clinical manifestations of potassium depletion have been summarized under Pathogenesis. Another possible consequence of potassium depletion in primary aldosteronism is impairment of carbohydrate tolerance.

Diagnosis and Differential Diagnosis. In practice, the diagnosis of primary aldosteronism usually begins with the recognition that the patient has hypertension. Serum potassium should be determined on several occasions while the patient is on a liberal sodium intake and is not receiving kaliuretic drugs (diuretics) or experiencing diarrhea or vomiting. The finding of unprovoked hypokalemia in association with hypertension calls for measurements of aldosterone and renin. If the aldosterone secretion rate is elevated, it may be assumed that the patient has either primary or secondary aldosteronism. If plasma renin activity is suppressed, one may assume that the patient has primary rather than secondary aldosteronism. Anecdotal evidence indicates that some patients have coexistent primary and secondary aldosteronism, but it is impossible to diagnose primary aldosteronism with certainty until the secondary aldosteronism has been corrected and it can be demonstrated that the hypersecretion of aldosterone persists in spite of subnormal plasma renin activity.

Hypokalemia is not an essential feature of primary aldosteronism, but the diagnosis is not easy to establish in its absence, when total reliance must be placed on the aldosterone and renin determinations. There is no substitute for a sophisticated and reliable laboratory if one is to practice competently in this area of medicine.

The differential diagnosis of primary aldosteronism is the differential diagnosis of hypertension itself. Thorough anamnesis, physical examination, and routine laboratory evaluation will sometimes reveal the underlying cause of hypertension, but often one is left with a diagnosis-by-exclusion of essential hypertension. This disorder (or group of disorders) can be distinguished from primary aldosteronism only by performing aldosterone and renin determinations. It should be borne in mind that about 20 per cent of patients with essential hypertension have profoundly suppressed plasma renin activity, so this determination alone will not designate which hypertensive patients have primary aldosteronism.

Conditions that can lead to concomitant hypertension and hypokalemia include malignant hypertension, Cushing's syndrome (especially the ectopic ACTH syndrome), congenital adrenal hyperplasia caused by 17-hydroxylase deficiency or 11-hydroxylase deficiency (see below), ingestion of large quantities of licorice, and a familial renal disorder simulating primary aldosteronism but with negligible aldosterone secretion (Liddle, Bledsoe, and Coppage). Except for the last condition, all these disorders should be recognizable in the course of a routine evaluation, which includes a determination of 17-OHCS.

A therapeutic trial with the aldosterone antagonist, spironolactone, in doses of 400 mg. daily for one month may indicate to what degree a patient's hypertension is aldosterone-dependent. Such a course of treatment has normalized the blood pressure and corrected the electrolyte abnormalities of several patients with primary aldosteronism. Precisely how reliable this approach will turn out to be in separating primary aldosteronism from other hypertensive disorders remains to be determined.

Treatment. Diagnostic precision is of utmost importance as a basis for definitive treatment of primary aldosteronism, since treatment ordinarily consists of a search for and resection of a small adrenal adenoma. Surgical exploration in primary aldosteronism should be performed not as an emergency but as an elective procedure, and preoperative preparation of the patient should include correction of any serious potassium deficiency and reasonable control of the hypertension. At the time of operation, both adrenal glands should be exposed through posterior incisions, giving the surgeon an opportunity to inspect and palpate both glands before removing any tissue. Any tumor should be resected. If no tumor can be found, one adrenal gland should be removed and serially sectioned. If no tumor is found, one half of the other adrenal gland should be removed and serially sectioned. At this point the operation should be terminated, leaving the patient a viable half-adrenal. If hypersecretion of aldosterone persists after the operation (or if a patient is unable or unwilling to undergo surgery), treatment with spironolactone may be instituted and continued indefinitely.

Prognosis. Without treatment, patients with primary aldosteronism will sooner or later have the disabling and fatal complications common to hypertensive cardiovascular disease in general; they have been known to die of strokes, congestive heart failure, and renal insufficiency. Within several days to several months after the successful removal of an aldosterone-secreting tumor, 70 per cent of the patients become normotensive, 25 per cent exhibit significant lowering of blood pressure but not to normal levels, and only 5 per cent are unimproved. Correction of the electrolyte disturbance is uniformly observed after correction of the aldosterone excess.

SECONDARY ALDOSTERONISM

The normal response of the adrenal cortex to increased stimulation by the renin-angiotensin system is to secrete increasing quantities of aldosterone. The aldosterone, in turn, promotes sodium conservation and potassium excretion. The retention of sodium results in expansion of extracellular volume and tends to restrain further production of renin. In many circumstances the renin–angiotensin–aldosterone–sodium-volume sequence can be viewed teleologically as a compensatory mechanism designed to support the blood flow to the kidney by expanding extracellular volume. Thus severe dehydration, sodium depletion, hemorrhage, hypoalbuminemic states, renal arterial constriction, and sequestration of blood on the venous side of the circulation are all conditions in which blood flow to the kidney is diminished, calling forth increased production of renin and

aldosterone. Secondary aldosteronism, then, is not a disease but, rather, is a response of the normal adrenal to physiologic demands arising in the course of a variety of disease processes, notably the nephrotic syndrome and hepatic cirrhosis.

CONGENITAL ADRENAL HYPERPLASIA

General Considerations, Definition, Etiology. Steroidal hormones are derived from cholesterol through a long series of enzymatically controlled steps. Each enzyme system carries the biosynthetic process one step along the pathway from ultimate precursor through an orderly series of intermediates to the final, biologically potent derivative. Many of these enzyme systems are common to both the zona fasciculata and zona glomerulosa and are important in the biosynthesis of gonadal androgens and estrogens as well as corticosteroids.

An inborn error in an adrenal enzyme system which impairs the efficiency of any step in the biosynthesis of cortisol or aldosterone can lead to congenital adrenal hyperplasia. Impairment of cortisol synthesis leads to a compensatory increase in ACTH secretion by the pituitary, and impairment of aldosterone synthesis leads to a compensatory increase in the production of renin and angiotensin. These trophic hormones stimulate the production of cortisol and aldosterone precursors and induce hyperplasia of the adrenal cortex. If the block in cortisol or aldosterone biosynthesis is not complete, and if the compensatory increase in ACTH or renin secretion is adequate, the resultant production of cortisol and aldosterone may be within the normal range. However, the chemical hallmark of an intra-adrenal enzyme deficiency would still be evident: a distortion of steroid secretory pattern with conspicuous overproduction of the intermediates that occur in the biosynthetic pathway immediately prior to the blocked step. The clinical manifestations of congenital adrenal hyperplasia are determined in part by the biologic properties of the biosynthetic intermediates which are excessively secreted and in part by the degree of deficiency of cortisol, aldosterone, or gonadal steroids.

Beyond the fact that the enzymatic defects that lead to congenital adrenal hyperplasia are genetically determined, little is known about their etiology. The pattern of familial occurrence is usually consistent with the view that congenital adrenal hyperplasia is inherited as a recessive trait. Within any one family, the same enzyme appears to be defective in all affected members.

Varieties of Congenital Adrenal Hyperplasia. Thus far, six varieties of congenital adrenal hyperplasia have been described, each due to impaired function of a different enzyme.

Deficiency of 21-Hydroxylase. The most common variety of congenital adrenal hyperplasia is attributable to a deficiency of 21-hydroxylase activity. This condition affects approximately one person in 10,000 of our general population. Cortisol synthesis is impaired at the step at which 17-hydroxyprogesterone should be converted to 11-deoxycortisol, and aldosterone synthesis is impaired at the step where progesterone is normally converted to 11-deoxycorticosterone. If the defect is severe, the patient during the first weeks of life may show signs of adrenocortical insufficiency such as salt-wasting, dehydration, hypotension, shock, prerenal azotemia, hyponatremia, hyperkalemia, vomiting, hypoglycemia, and poor tolerance to stress. Plasma ACTH and renin levels are high. Plasma concentrations of melanocyte-stimulating hormone (β-MSH) are also raised, and occasionally the patient may exhibit mucocutaneous hyperpigmentation. Hypersecretion of 17-hydroxyprogesterone is of no clinical consequence, but it results in the excretion of a diagnostically specific urinary metabolite, *pregnanetriol*.

Adrenal androgens do not require 21-hydroxylation for their synthesis, and as part of the adrenal response to high levels of ACTH they are produced in excessive quantities. Chemically, this is reflected in excessive levels of urinary 17-ketosteroids. The clinical consequence is virilization. The precise clinical manifestations of virilism depend upon the sex of the patient, the age at which the androgen excess occurs, and the severity of the androgen excess. In the male fetus, testicular production of androgen is sufficient to bring about completely masculine differentiation of the genitalia, and even a large excess of adrenal androgen has no obvious effect on genital differentiation or growth. The female fetus lacks gonadal androgen; in this circumstance, an excess of adrenal androgen results in partial masculinization of those portions of the genitourinary system that are the last to undergo differentiation. The abnormalities include the development of a urogenital sinus, fusion of labioscrotal folds, and hypertrophy of the clitoris. In extreme cases the external genitalia may be so ambiguous that on superficial examination the patient appears to be a male with hypospadias and bilateral cryptorchidism. In general, female infants with the most profound deficiencies of cortisol and aldosterone (the so-called salt-wasters) are likely to have conspicuous genital abnormalities, and the diagnosis should be suspected at birth, well in advance of any clinical difficulty from adrenal insufficiency. Salt-wasting males, on the other hand, lacking abnormalities of genital differentiation, are unlikely to attract special attention until they are in trouble with vomiting, dehydration, and other consequences of adrenal insufficiency. A positive family history, however, sometimes assists the pediatrician in considering the diagnosis before clinical complications arise.

Unless he or she succumbs or is treated, the patient with 21-hydroxylase deficiency grows rapidly and becomes quite muscular; at some time between two and ten years of age, pubic and axillary hair appear; this is followed by facial hirsutism and deepening of the voice. Investigation at this time reveals that the bone age is advanced beyond the height age, which, in turn, is advanced beyond the chronologic age. Early epiphyseal closure foredooms the patient to short stature during adult life.

Clinically, the male patient may appear normal except for precocious puberty. The untreated female patient, however, does not undergo true pubertal changes but simply shows slowly progressive virilization; she lacks the feminization, mammary development, uterine development, and menstrual cycles that are a part of true puberty in the female.

The definitive diagnosis of 21-hydroxylase deficiency is based upon the demonstration of excessive quantities of pregnanetriol in the urine together with *easy* suppressibility of pregnanetriol and 17-ketosteroids by administration of glucocorticoids. This maneuver aids in distinguishing patients with congenital adrenal hyperplasia from those with Cushing's syndrome and with adrenal tumors.

Deficiency of 11β-Hydroxylase. The second most common variety of congenital adrenal hyperplasia is attributable to a deficiency of 11β-hydroxylase. Fewer than 100 cases have been recognized thus far. The final step in cortisol synthesis is impaired so that cortisol secretion is subnormal, ACTH secretion is excessive, and *11-deoxycortisol* is secreted in large quantities. Normally, corticosterone is secreted by the zona fasciculata in quantities of the order of 2 mg. daily, but in patients with 11β-hydroxylase deficiency the final step in corticosterone synthesis is impaired so that large quantities of *11-deoxycorticosterone (DOC)* are secreted. DOC is a mineralocorticoid having about one thirtieth the potency of aldosterone. When secreted or injected in quantities of several milligrams daily, DOC induces hypertension. Renin and aldosterone levels are low.

Adrenal androgens do not require 11β-hydroxylation for synthesis, and they are produced in excessive quantities as part of the adrenal response to high levels of ACTH. The consequent virilization is similar in its pathogenesis to that observed in patients with 21-hydroxylase deficiency.

The clinical manifestations of 11β-hydroxylase deficiency are simply those of hypertension and virilism. Plasma and urinary 17-OHCS are elevated because 11-deoxycortisol and its tetrahydro derivative behave like cortisol and its tetrahydro derivatives in chemical tests based on the presence of the 17,21-dihydroxy-20-keto configuration. Despite the elevation of 17-OHCS, this condition should not be confused with Cushing's syndrome because plasma fluorogenic steroids should be normal or low in 11β-hydroxylase deficiency, the elevated steroids should be *readily* suppressible by the administration of glucocorticoids, and the clinical features of central obesity, protein wasting, and impaired carbohydrate tolerance are absent. The history of lifelong abnormalities together with *easy* suppressibility of the high steroid levels should distinguish 11β-hydroxylase deficiency from an adrenal tumor.

Deficiency of 17α-Hydroxylase. Congenital adrenal hyperplasia resulting from a deficiency of 17α-hydroxylase has only recently been described; it is undoubtedly a very rare disorder but is nevertheless important because it represents a curable cause of hypertension. Cortisol synthesis is impaired at the step where progesterone is converted to 17α-hydroxyprogesterone. Androgen and estrogen synthesis, whether by the adrenal, ovary, or testis, also depend upon hydroxylation at the 17α position prior to cleavage of the 17-20 carbon-carbon bond. Thus, impairment of 17α-hydroxylation leads to a deficiency of estrogen and androgen. The patient with 17-hydroxylase deficiency has subnormal cortisol production, a compensatory increase in ACTH, and a consequent increase in the secretion of 17-deoxycorticosteroids, the most prominent of which are DOC and corticosterone. The excessive mineralocorticoid results in hypertension and suppression of renin production; aldosterone production is subnormal. Estrogen and androgen deficiencies result in sexual infantilism and compensatory increases in gonadotrophin secretion.

Deficiency of 18-Hydroxysteroid Dehydrogenase. This rare disorder results in a selective impairment of the final step in aldosterone biosynthesis. As a consequence the patient suffers excessive sodium loss, dehydration, and hypotension; there is a compensatory increase in formation of the aldosterone precursor 18-hydroxycorticosterone.

Deficiency of 3β-Hydroxysteroid Dehydrogenase. This too is a rare disorder; it is characterized by genital ambiguity in infants of either sex. The explanation for this is that these patients have impaired capacity to transform Δ^5 steroids into Δ^4 steroids. Cortisol, aldosterone, and the potent androgens are all Δ^4 compounds; therefore, these hormones are subnormal in this disorder, and affected patients have clinical adrenal insufficiency. Males have inadequate genital differentiation owing to lack of testicular androgen during fetal life. In response to increased levels of ACTH, both males and females secrete superabundant amounts of the Δ^5 steroids, pregnenolone and dehydroisoandrosterone. Although the latter is not a very strong androgen, it is secreted in large enough quantities to cause partial masculinization of the external genitalia of the female fetus. Both males and females, therefore, have adrenal insufficiency, ambiguous genitalia, and elevated urinary 17-ketosteroids (derived from dehydroisoandrosterone).

Deficiency of 20α-Hydroxylase. The first step in the conversion of cholesterol into hormonal steroids is 20α hydroxylation. Impairment of this process results in clinical adrenal insufficiency and, in the male fetus, incomplete differentiation of the external genitalia. The adrenal glands are hyperplastic and contain high concentrations of cholesterol. This extremely uncommon disorder

has been fatal in infancy in all cases that have been reported thus far.

Treatment of Congenital Adrenal Hyperplasia. The major abnormalities in congenital adrenal hyperplasia stem from deficiencies of cortisol or aldosterone or both. Compensatory increases in secretion of ACTH or renin or both then stimulate overproduction of the precursors or by-products of these important steroids. The rationale of therapy is to provide physiologic quantities of glucocorticoid and mineralocorticoid, thus correcting the deficiency state, suppressing the trophic hormones, and curtailing the secretion of steroid precursors and by-products.

The technique of treatment is similar to that employed in adrenal insufficiency. For the first several days it is advisable to employ slightly greater than physiologic doses of glucocorticoid in order to hasten the involution of the hyperplastic, very responsive adrenal cortex. Thereafter, only physiologic doses are required, and overtreatment must be assiduously avoided so that growth will not be inhibited.

In those varieties of congenital adrenal hyperplasia that are characterized by the excessive excretion of 17-ketosteroids, glucocorticoid dosage should be adjusted from time to time so as to bring daily 17-ketosteroid excretion to approximately 1 mg. for each year of chronologic age, up to 12 years. More profound suppression of 17-ketosteroids is not necessary to prevent progression of virilism, but would be indicative of excessive glucocorticoid dosage. During intercurrent stressful illnesses, corticosteroid doses should be adjusted upward in the same manner and for the same reason as in treating adrenal insufficiency.

Several steroid preparations are available, and with proper consideration of relative potencies, effective routes of administration, and duration of effect, one can substitute one glucocorticoid for another and one mineralocorticoid for another at will. Many patients do well on approximately 12 mg. of hydrocortisone and 0.06 mg. of 9α-fluorohydrocortisone per square meter of body surface per day. In any case, the dosage must be adjusted to suit individual requirements; the objectives of therapy are to avoid adrenal insufficiency, to normalize 17-ketosteroid excretion, and to maintain normal blood pressure.

Certain therapeutic considerations are peculiar to the specific varieties of congenital adrenal hyperplasia. Mineralocorticoid therapy is required only for patients with salt-wasting varieties of congenital adrenal hyperplasia and not for those with the hypertensive varieties. Glucocorticoid therapy is not required in treating 18-hydroxysteroid dehydrogenase deficiency. Estrogen and androgen therapy may be needed to induce secondary sex characteristics in patients with 17α-hydroxylase deficiency and, if they survive to adult years, those with 20α-hydroxylase deficiency or those with 3β-hydroxysteroid dehydrogenase deficiency.

Plastic surgery to correct gross abnormalities

of the external genitalia should be carried out before the age of two years, by which time the child's psychosexual identity should be unambiguously established.

Prognosis. Without treatment, patients with various salt-wasting forms of congenital adrenal hyperplasia are unlikely to survive infancy. Probably the patients with the hypertensive varieties also have decreased life expectancy. The majority of the survivors (non-salt-losing 21-hydroxylase deficiency) usually have major psychosexual problems arising from pseudohermaphroditism in the females and precocious puberty in the males.

If recognized early and treated properly, patients with any variety of congenital adrenal hyperplasia should theoretically be able to live normal lives. This is true for the patients with 21-hydroxylase and 11β-hydroxylase deficiency, except that they have usually not attained normal height. It appears that reproductive functions will be normal if proper treatment is started before adulthood. It is of interest that a child whose bone age has advanced beyond about 13 years before suppressive treatment with glucocorticoids is instituted will exhibit adult pituitary-gonadal relationships (females will undergo breast development and establish their menstrual cycles) when glucocorticoid treatment is finally begun; this is true even if the chronologic age is only seven or eight years.

The other varieties of congenital adrenal hyperplasia have less favorable prognoses. In 17α-hydroxylase deficiency, reproduction will probably not be possible even though the hypertension can be controlled and all other clinical manifestations of steroid deficiency corrected. The survival of patients with deficiencies of 20α-hydroxylase or 3β-hydroxysteroid dehydrogenase has been unaccountably poor up to the present time.

VIRILIZING TUMORS

Adrenal tumors that produce a clinically significant excess of androgen along with cortisol have been discussed under the heading Cushing's Syndrome. Somewhat less common are adrenal tumors that secrete androgen without significant quantities of cortisol. Most of these tumors are malignant, and the majority are large and have metastasized by the time they are clinically apparent. The clinical hallmark of such tumors is virilization; this manifestation, of course, is limited to children and women; adult males usually recognize no increased virilization as a result of even large excesses of the relatively weak adrenal androgens. The common chemical hallmark of a purely virilizing tumor is the excessive excretion of 17-ketosteroids. This is a remarkably uniform characteristic of adrenal carcinomas. Several adrenal carcinomas have, probably erroneously, been reported as being non-

functioning simply because they did not give rise to clinical virilization. Evidence was inadequate to support this conclusion, however, whenever 17-ketosteroid excretion was not measured.

It is not sufficient just to measure urinary 17-ketosteroids; under basal conditions one should also carry out dexamethasone suppression tests and demonstrate that urinary 17-ketosteroids can reproducibly be reduced to less than 6 mg. per day within three days before concluding that an adrenocortical carcinoma is nonfunctioning.

Suprarenal "masses" that are discovered accidentally during roentgenographic examinations almost never prove to be adrenal cortical tumors if basal 17-OHCS and 17-ketosteroids are normal and normally suppressible, and they almost never prove to be adrenal medullary tumors if catecholamines are consistently normal.

Virilizing adrenal tumor must be differentiated from congenital adrenal hyperplasia, Cushing's syndrome with virilism, ovarian tumor, idiopathic hirsutism, and precocious puberty. This can be accomplished by a history of late onset of first clinical manifestations, absence of Cushing's syndrome, presence of a palpable abdominal mass, abnormal resistance to suppression of 17-ketosteroids with dexamethasone, absence of ovarian mass, and presence of an adrenal mass on urography or arteriography.

Treatment is with surgical resection and with o,p'-DDD. A sizable minority responds favorably to each mode of therapy, at least temporarily.

FEMINIZING ADRENAL TUMORS

Feminization as a clinical manifestation of adrenal tumor is exceedingly rare. The most common sign is gynecomastia, and this is one of the least common causes of gynecomastia. The diagnosis is made by the observation of other signs of adrenal overactivity, e.g., hypertension, demonstration of excessive estrogen in the urine, and demonstration of a suprarenal mass by intravenous urography or arteriography. If positively diagnosed, the tumor may be treated by surgical resection, and, if this fails, with o,p'-DDD. Experience is too limited to support a generalization as to prognosis.

Abe, K., Nicholson, W. E., Liddle, G. W., Island, D. P., and Orth, D. N.: Radio-immunoassays of β-MSH in human plasma and tissues. J. Clin. Invest., 46:1609, 1967.

Addison, T.: On the constitutional and local effects of diseases of the suprarenal capsules. London Med. Gaz., 43:517, 1849, 1855.

Bartter, F. C., Albright, F., Forbes, A. P., Leaf, A., Dempsey, E., and Carroll, E.: The effects of adrenocorticotropic hormone and cortisone in adrenogenital syndrome associated with congenital adrenal hyperplasia: An attempt to explain and correct its disordered hormonal pattern. J. Clin. Invest., 30:237, 1951.

Baulieu, E. E., and Robel, P. (eds.): Aldosterone: Prague Symposium. 1st ed. Oxford, Blackwell Scientific Publications, 1964.

Bongiovanni, A. M., Eberlein, W. R., Goldman, A. S., and New,

M.: Disorders of adrenal steroid biogenesis. Recent Progr. Hormone Res., 23:375, 1967.

Conn, J. W., Knopf, R. F., and Nesbit, R. M.: Clinical characteristics of primary aldosteronism from an analysis of 145 cases. Amer. J. Surg., 107:159, 1964.

Eisenstein, A. B. (ed.): The Adrenal Cortex, 1st ed. London, J & A Churchill, Ltd., 1967.

Graber, A. L., Ney, R. L., Nicholson, W. E., Island, D. P., and Liddle, G. W.: Natural history of pituitary-adrenal recovery following long term suppression with corticosteroids. J. Clin. Endocr., 25:11, 1965.

Liddle, G. W., Bledsoe, T., and Coppage, W. S., Jr.: A familial renal disorder simulating primary aldosteronism but with negligible aldosterone secretion. Trans. Ass. Amer. Physicians, 76:199, 1963.

Liddle, G. W., Island, D., and Meador, C. K.: Normal and abnormal regulation of corticotropin secretion in man. Recent Progr. Hormone Res. 18:125, 1962.

Liddle, G. W.: Tests of pituitary-adrenal suppressibility in the diagnosis of Cushing's syndrome. J. Clin. Endocr., 20:1539, 1960.

Rowntree, L. G., and Snell, A. M.: A Clinical Study of Addison's Disease. Mayo Clinic Monographs. Philadelphia, W. B. Saunders Company, 1931.

Gonads

DETERMINATION OF SEX AND SEXUAL DIFFERENTIATION

Melvin M. Grumbach

The diploid cells of man contain 46 chromosomes composed of 44 autosomes and one pair of sex chromosomes (XX in the female and XY in the male). It is now well accepted that the sex of the zygote at fertilization is established by a chromosomal mechanism that results in an unequal balance of sex-determining factors. In man, in contrast to Drosophila, evidence adduced from the detection of abnormal sex chromosome constitutions indicates that the Y chromosome has potent male determiners. With rare exceptions, in man an XY constitution is necessary for the development of testes and an XX constitution for the differentiation of functional ovaries. In all probability, the sex-determining genes control differentiation and development of the gonad through their action on specific chemical processes. Spontaneous and experimentally produced forms of ambisexual development provide evidence that this chromosomal mechanism of sex determination is not absolute, and may be modified by various genetic, hormonal, and environmental factors.

Sex differentiation takes place in three steps involving successively (1) the gonad, (2) the genital ducts, and (3) the urogenital sinus and external genitalia (Fig. 1). Normally, the pattern of all the sexual structures conforms to the genetic sex established in the zygote at the moment of fertilization.

Gonadogenesis. The primordial gonad arises in the urogenital ridge from intermediate mesoderm during the fifth week of gestation. Early in its development, the bipotential primitive gonad (Fig. 1) is composed of two unipotential mesodermal primordia, each with a distinct physiologic

as well as morphologic capacity: (1) a cortical component consisting of the germinal epithelium and (2) a medullary component made up of the primary sex cords (derived from the germinal epithelium) and mesonephric and blastemal elements. A third constituent, the primordial germ cell, which appears to be bipotential, arises from an extragonadal site. The cortical component can differentiate only as an ovary, and the medullary component only as a testis (Fig. 1); normally, the dominant element follows the genetic sex of the zygote, and the recessive element retrogresses.

When the gonad destined to become a testis begins to differentiate in a male direction during the seventh to eighth week of embryonic life, the cortical component involutes. Within the medulla, seminiferous tubules form from the primary sex cords and anastomose with the rete testis and testicular ducts, and Leydig cells develop. Leydig cells proliferate predominantly during the first half of gestation, but then gradually involute, persisting until shortly after birth.

Accessory Sex Structures. Fetal castration experiments in placental mammals have clarified the embryogenesis of the accessory sex structures. Jost and others demonstrated that castration of male fetuses at an early critical period prevented the differentiation of male structures and led to entirely female development of ducts, urogenital sinus, and external genitalia. These studies, in the light of recent observations of anomalies of sex in man, support the notion that fetal testicular morphogenetic substances are essential to prevent the inherent tendency of the fetus to feminize. It has been postulated that a secretion from the fetal testis leads to the regression of the müllerian (female) ducts and that testosterone secreted by the fetal Leydig cells, which does not have this property, brings about masculinization of the urogenital sinus and external genitalia.

Intrinsic or extrinsic factors that adversely affect any stage of the mechanisms of sex determination and sex differentiation (Fig. 1) can lead to sexual anomalies.

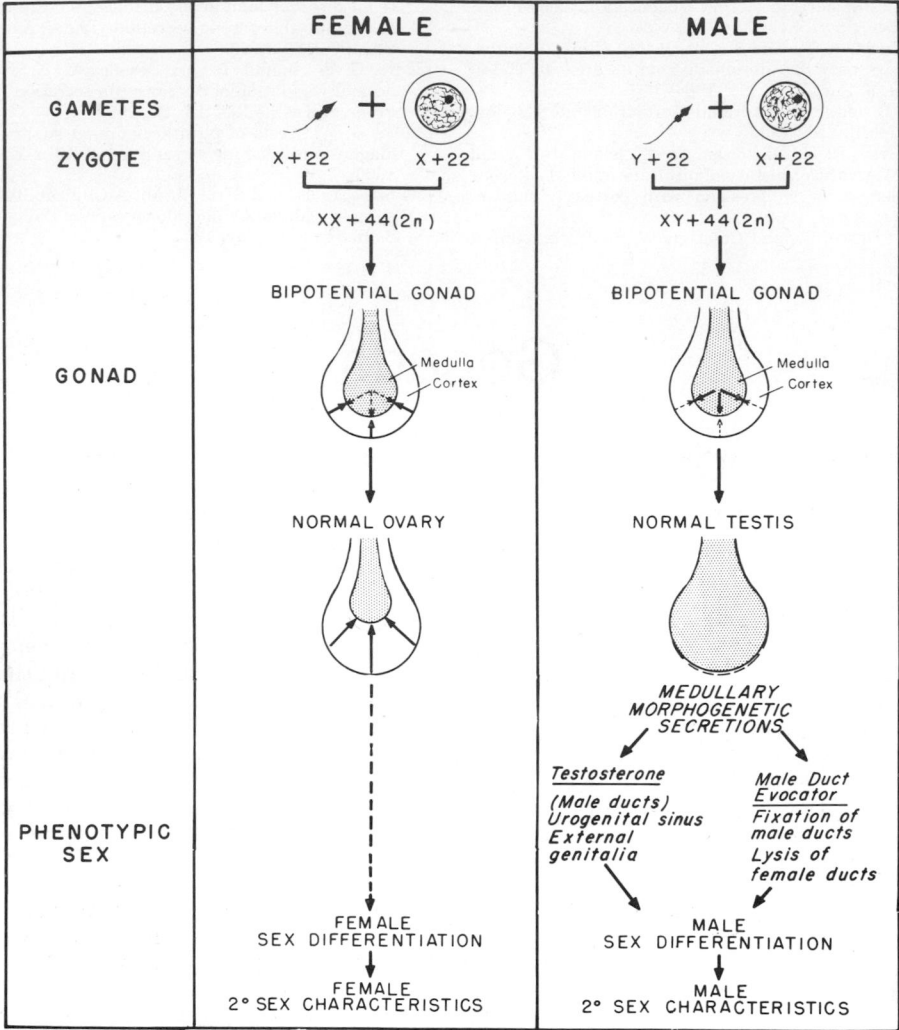

FIGURE 1. Diagrammatic scheme of human sex determination and differentiation. (Modified from Grumbach, M. M.: *In* Astwood, E. B. (ed.): Clinical Endocrinology I. New York, Grune and Stratton, Inc., 1960.)

HUMAN SEXUAL ANOMALIES

Melvin M. Grumbach

The terms *hermaphrodism* and *intersexuality* are commonly used to designate a group of congenital abnormalities characterized by a variable degree of ambisexual differentiation of the accessory sexual structures and gonads of one or both sexes. Intersexes may be further subdivided, depending upon the sex of the gonad, into male pseudohermaphrodites when the gonads are testes, female pseudohermaphrodites when the gonads are ovaries, and true hermaphrodites when both ovarian and testicular tissue are present. The application of the sex chromatin test of Barr and of cytogenetic techniques has brought to light two common anomalies of sex associated with an abnormal sex chromosome constitution, namely, the syndrome of gonadal dysgenesis or Turner's

syndrome in phenotypic females, and chromatin-positive seminiferous tubule dysgenesis or Klinefelter's syndrome in phenotypic males (Table 1). Postnatal virilization or feminization and psychiatric disorders, such as homosexuality, are not included among abnormalities of sex differentiation.

Anomalies of sex are not rare. They may result from genetic defects or from deleterious environmental factors.

THE SYNDROME OF GONADAL DYSGENESIS; TURNER'S SYNDROME

(Ovarian Dysgenesis, Bonnevie-Ullrich Syndrome)

The syndrome of gonadal dysgenesis, first defined clinically by Turner in 1938, is manifested in its typical form by female but infantile development of the accessory sex structures, including

TABLE 1. ANOMALIES OF SEX

Type	Sex Chromatin	Sex Chromosomes	Gonads	External Genitalia		Genital Ducts	2° Sexual Characteristics
				Phallus	Labioscrotal Fusion[1]		
Female Pseudohermaphrodism							
1. With adrenal hyperplasia	Positive	XX	Ovaries	Medium to large	0–3+	Female	Precocious male
2. Without adrenal hyperplasia	Positive	XX	Ovaries	Medium to large	0–3+	Female	Female
Male Pseudohermaphrodism							
1. Simulant female (syndrome of feminizing testes)	Negative	XY	Testes[2]	Female to slight clitoridal enlargement	0–1+	Usually male	Female Primary amenorrhea ±Absent or sparse sexual hair
2. External genitalia ambiguous or with large phallus	Negative	XY (XO/XY)	Testes[2]	Hypoplastic[3]	1 + –3+	Primarily male / Primarily female	Male ±Eunuchoid; female / Usually male ±Eunuchoid
True Hermaphrodism	Usually positive	XX>XY (XX/XY)	Ovotestis(es) or ovary and testis	Variable		Variable	Male or female
Syndrome of Gonadal Dysgenesis (Turner's Syndrome)	Negative (80%) / Positive	XO / XO/XX[4]	Vestigial streak[5]	Female (rarely slight clitoridal enlargement)		Female	Infantile
Seminiferous Tubule Dysgenesis (Klinefelter's Syndrome)	Positive / Negative	XXY[6] / XY	Small testes	Male		Male	Male ±Eunuchoidism ±Gynecomastia ±Mental deficiency

1. Degree of fusion: Absent = 0 to Extreme = 3+
2. Testes intra-abdominal, inguinal or labioscrotal
3. Usually hypospadiac penis; occasionally penile urethra, urogenital sinus, separate vaginal orifice.
4. Other sex chromosome abnormalities have been described in gonadal dysgenesis such as Xx, XX, XO/XXX, XO/XX/XXX in chromatin-positive individuals, and XO/XY, XO/XYY in chromatin-negative individuals.
5. Characteristically only mesonephric vestiges; occasionally varying degrees of cortical and medullary rudiments.
6. Other sex chromosome abnormalities which may be encountered in seminiferous tubule dysgenesis include XXYY, XXXY, XXXXY, XX/XXY, XY/XXY, XXXY/XXXXY.

the external genitalia, short stature, a characteristic habitus, and multiple congenital defects. The prevalence of this sporadic disorder is approximately 1 in 3000 phenotypic females; however, there is a considerable loss of XO embryos and fetuses (in one study 5 per cent of spontaneous abortuses had an XO karyotype). The most common associated anomalies include atypical facies, broad chest, low hairline over the back of the neck, webbed neck, coarctation of the aorta, lymphedema of the extremities, short fourth metacarpal ("metacarpal sign"), increased number of pigmented nevi and ocular, otitic, skeletal, and renal defects (especially horseshoe kidneys and duplication of the collecting system). Unexplained hypertension (not associated with coarctation of the aorta) and gastrointestinal bleeding secondary to intestinal telangiectasia are less common features. The incidence of mental deficiency is increased slightly, and, when present, is usually mild; impaired directional sense and space-form recognition are common. No true gonad is present as such; in each mesosalpinx there is a ridge of connective tissue devoid of ova, follicles, or seminiferous tubules. Except for the development of some pubic and axillary hair (in contrast to hypopituitary dwarfs), no secondary sexual development occurs, and these patients remain sexually infantile. The titer of urinary gonadotrophin is increased but rarely before nine years of age. A chromatin-negative (male) sex chromatin pattern has been found in about 80 per cent of patients with this syndrome, and is of diagnostic significance. In general, chromatin-positive patients exhibit fewer of the associated anomalies. Before the expected age of puberty, skeletal maturation is normal or slightly delayed, but epiphyseal fusion is often delayed. Rarefaction of the hands and feet, about the elbow joint, and about the upper femur is commonly observed in children; osteochondrosis-like changes in the spine are seen occasionally. In adults not treated with estrogen, the postmenopausal type of osteoporosis, which may be of sufficient severity to lead to collapse of vertebrae, has been described. A number of variant forms of this syndrome have been delineated which are associated with sex chromosome mosaicism or structural abnormalities of the X or Y chromosome. Rarely, the clitoris is enlarged.

The etiology of this disorder was clarified in 1959 when Ford and his associates reported an abnormal sex chromosome constitution. The typical finding in chromatin-negative gonadal dysgenesis is an XO sex chromosome constitution and a chromosome number of 45; the features of the syndrome are a consequence of the X chromosome monosomy. In rare instances sex chromosome mosaicism has been found in chromatin-negative gonadal dysgenesis, including patients with XO/XY or XO/XYY sex chromosome complements. The XO constitution may arise as a consequence of nondisjunction or chromosome loss in a parental gamete during meiosis, leading to the development of either a sperm or an ovum lacking a sex chromo-

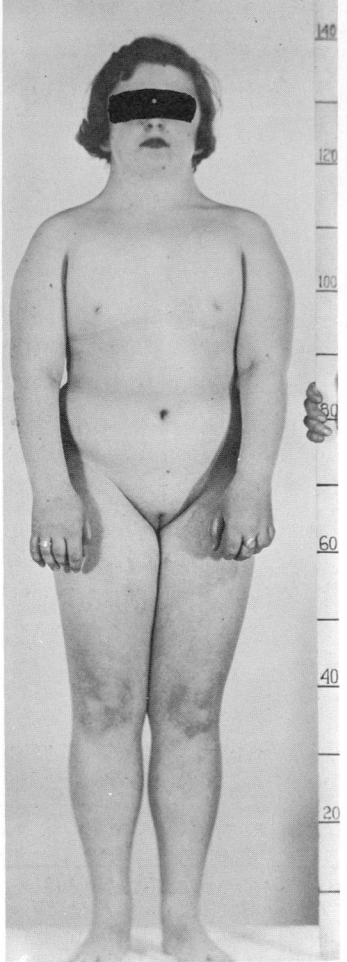

FIGURE 2.   Age 15⁷/₁₂ years; height age 9¹/₂ years.

some. It may also result from chromosome loss early in embryonic development between fertilization and the first cleavage division. The absence of a positive relationship between gonadal dysgenesis and advanced maternal age at conception and the prevalence of sex chromosome mosaicism in the chromatin-positive form (*vide infra*) suggest that a mitotic error, chromosome loss, in the zygote gives rise to at least a proportion of XO individuals. The chromosome abnormality leads to defective gonadal ontogenesis and provides an explanation for the multiplicity of associated somatic anomalies. The failure of gonadal differentiation results in female differentiation of the accessory sex structures (in keeping with the experiments of Jost). That failure of gonadal differentiation is not invariable is indicated by the report of a short, chromatin-negative XO woman who gave birth to a son and the occasional evidence of ovarian function in persons with the syndrome.

Two types of sex chromosome abnormalities have been described in chromatin-positive gonadal dysgenesis: sex chromosome mosaicism and structural anomalies of the X chromosome. (1) In the group of chromatin-positive subjects with mosaic-

ism, which can arise from a mitotic error in the zygote, e.g., nondisjunction at any stage following fertilization, a proportion of cells have an XO sex chromosome constitution and, in addition, one or even two or more cell lines with dissimilar sex chromosome complements. These include sex chromosome mosaics of the following types: XO/XX, XO/XXX, XO/XX/XXX. Here the relative number of chromatin-positive cells and the presence of cells with multiple sex chromatin bodies, or a discrepancy between the sex chromatin pattern in leukocytes and in epithelial cells of the buccal mucosa suggests the possibility of mosaicism. (2) Three structural alterations in an X chromosome have been described in chromatin-positive patients with gonadal dysgenesis having a chromosome number of 46. One of the anomalies is characterized by the presence of an exceptionally large X chromosome, thought to represent an isochromosome made up of the two long arms of the X chromosome and a normal-appearing X chromosome (XX), giving rise to an individual who is trisomic for the long arm and monosomic for the short arm. The second morphologic alteration is loss of a segment of either the long or short arm of one X chromosome (deletion) in an individual with a structurally normal X chromosome (Xx). A third abnormality is the X-ring-X constitution, which is associated with mosaicism (the XO/X-ring-X being the most common). Larger than normal sex chromatin bodies are found with an XX sex chromosome constitution and unusually small bodies in Xx and X-ring-X individuals. As mentioned previously, in general, fewer of the associated anomalies are found in the chromatin-positive form of the syndrome.

The typical phenotypic and gonadal findings in XO cases may be modified by mosaicism or by the presence of a structurally abnormal X or Y chromosome. For example, XO/XX or XO/XXX mosaicism may be associated with normal stature, minimal somatic features of Turner's syndrome, and functional ovaries. In other cases, the clinical picture is indistinguishable from classic gonadal dysgenesis. Similarly, the presence of a structurally abnormal X, e.g., deleted X, frequently modifies some features of the classic XO syndrome. When XO/XY mosaicism or a structurally abnormal Y chromosome is present, varying degrees of testicular differentiation are frequently found that may lead to a spectrum extending from a phenotypic male through pseudohermaphrodism to a phenotypic female, depending on the degree of fetal testicular insufficiency. Moreover, the beneficial effects of the normal XY cell line, or the presence of part of a Y chromosome may lead to normal stature and a modification of the somatic defects associated with XO monosomy. There is an increased prevalence of gonadal neoplasms in XO/XY mosaics; prophylactic ablation of intra-abdominal dysgenetic testes in this group warrants serious consideration.

The syndrome of gonadal dysgenesis is an X or Y chromosome-deficiency syndrome. Table 2 summarizes the correlation between partial sex

TABLE 2. RELATIONSHIP OF STRUCTURAL ABNORMALITIES OF THE X AND Y TO MANIFESTATIONS OF THE SYNDROME OF GONADAL DYSGENESIS

Type of Sex Chromosome Abnormality	Karyotypes	Phenotype	Sexual Infantilism	Shortness of Stature	Somatic Anomalies of Turner's Syndrome
Loss of an X or a Y	XO	Female	+	+	+
Deletion of short arm of an X	XX^I	Female	+ (occ. ±)	+	+
	XX^{SD}	Female	+ or (±, −)	+	+
Deletion of long arm of an X	XX^{SI}	Female	+	−	− or (±)
	XX^{LD}	Female	+	−	− or (±)
Partial deletion of both arms of an X	XO/XX^R	Female	− or (±)	I	+ or (±)
Complete deletion of short arm of a Y	XY^I	Female	+	−	−

X^I, Isochromosome for long arm of an X.
X^{SD}, Partial deletion of short arm of an X.
X^{SI}, Isochromosome for short arm of an X.

X^{LD}, Partial deletion of long arm of an X.
X^R, Ring chromosome derived from an X.
Y^I, Isochromosome for long arm of a Y.

chromosome deficiencies owing to structural abnormalities and the modifications in the cardinal features of the typical XO phenotype which may occur.

Several disorders are commonly associated with the syndrome of gonadal dysgenesis or its variants, including hypertension in the absence of coarctation of the aorta, Hashimoto's thyroiditis, thyrotoxicosis, diabetes mellitus, achlorhydria, and accelerated aging.

Therapy is directed toward the correction of sexual infantilism (see article on The Ovaries) and remediable congenital anomalies.

Chromatin-positive seminiferous tubule dysgenesis (Klinefelter's syndrome) and the XYY syndrome have been discussed under Hypogonadism in the Male.

It is noteworthy that a characteristic group of anomalies has not been found in females with either an XXX or XXXX sex chromosome constitution. Virtually all of the described patients have been mental defectives with functioning ovaries.

The management of patients with ambisexual development is greatly facilitated by early diagnosis; infants with anomalous development of the external genitalia deserve prompt investigation. The reader is referred to publications cited in the references for detailed discussions of diagnostic, therapeutic, and theoretical considerations and for additional references.

The articles on Cytogenetics and Numerical and Structural Aberrations of Chromosomes give a general discussion of methods of chromosome analysis and the mechanisms of nondisjunction and chromosomal rearrangements that lead to chromosomal disease.

SYNDROME OF FEMINIZING TESTES

(Testicular Feminization)

This relatively common form of familial male pseudohermaphrodism is characterized by female external genitalia, undescended or labial testes, a short blind vaginal pouch and absence of the uterus, male genital ducts, primary amenorrhea and frequently absence or sparseness of pubic and axillary hair, and a lack of end-organ response to testosterone. The sex chromosome constitution is XY. During puberty estrogenic steroids secreted by the testes lead to feminization of the habitus, breast development, and cornification of the vaginal mucosa. Castration is followed by a fall in urinary estrogens, a rise in gonadotrophins, and menopausal symptoms. The testes in this syndrome secrete testosterone and estrogens as in normal men. The disorder is transmitted either as an X-linked recessive or sex-limited autosomal dominant trait. The consequence of the mutant gene is failure of target organs to respond to testosterone, which in fetal life leads to female differentiation of the external genitalia and urogenital sinus and at puberty to the development of female secondary sex characteristics. The testes have the propensity to undergo malignant degeneration. Castration followed by estrogen substitution therapy is recommended in late adolescence or early adulthood. (See article on The Ovaries.)

REIFENSTEIN'S SYNDROME

This syndrome of familial male pseudohermaphrodism is associated with hypospadias, primary hypogonadism, postpubertal testicular atrophy and azoospermia, signs of testosterone deficiency, and often gynecomastia. The testicular lesion resembles that in myotonic dystrophy. The sex chromosome constitution is XY. It is transmitted as an X-linked recessive or a sex-limited autosomal dominant.

Court Brown, W. M., Harnden, D. G., Jacobs, P. A., Maclean, N., and Mantle, D. J.: Abnormalities of the Sex Chromosome Complement in Man. Medical Research Council, Special Report Series No. 305. London, H. M. Stationery Office, 1964.

Engel, E., and Forbes, A. P.: Cytogenetic and clinical findings in 48 patients with congenitally defective or absent ovaries. Medicine, 44:135, 1965.

Federman, D.: Abnormal Sexual Development—A Genetic and Endocrine Approach to Differential Diagnosis. Philadelphia, W. B. Saunders Company, 1967.

Ferguson-Smith, M. A.: Karyotype-phenotype correlations in gonadal dysgenesis and their bearing on the pathogenesis of malformations. J. Med. Genet., 2:142, 1965.

Grumbach, M. M.: Male reproductive system. *In* Cooke, R. E. (ed.): Biologic Basis of Pediatric Practice. New York, McGraw-Hill Book Company, 1968.

McKusick, V. A.: On the X Chromosome of Man. Washington, D.C., American Institute of Biological Sciences, 1964.

Moore, K. L. (ed.): The Sex Chromatin. Philadelphia, W. B. Saunders Company, 1966.

Morishima, A., and Grumbach, M. M.: The interrelationship of sex chromosome constitution and phenotype in the syndrome of gonadal dysgenesis and its variants. Ann. N.Y. Acad. Sci., 155:695, 1968.

Overzier, C. (ed.): Intersexuality. New York, Academic Press, Inc., 1963.

Van Wyk, J. J., and Grumbach, M. M.: Disorders of sex differentiation. *In* Williams, R. H. (ed.): Textbook of Endocrinology. 4th ed. Philadelphia, W. B. Saunders Company, 1968.

Wilkins, L.: Diagnosis and Treatment of Endocrine Disorders in Childhood and Adolescence. 3rd ed. Springfield, Ill., Charles C Thomas, 1965.

THE TESTES
Melvin M. Grumbach

CHEMISTRY AND PHYSIOLOGY OF THE TESTICULAR HORMONES

A wealth of knowledge has firmly established the primary role of testicular hormones (1) in the development and maintenance of the male accessory sex organs—including the penis and scrotum, Cowper's and preputial glands—and the secretion of semen, and (2) in the development of masculine secondary sexual characteristics. Substances with these properties are called androgens; the most potent produced by man is testosterone. Recent evidence suggests that the 5α reduced derivative of testosterone, 5α-dihydrotestosterone, is the active form of the hormone at the nuclear receptors within the male accessory sex structures, and has a principal role in androgen-induced growth of these organs.

All the properties of testicular androgen are shared by androgenic hormones derived from adrenocortical secretions. However, in the castrate male the latter are insufficient to prevent eunuchism.

It has been assumed since 1935 that testosterone is the principal testicular androgen, a contention borne out by the recent isolation of this steroid from human spermatic vein blood. It is estimated that in healthy young men the testes secrete about 7 mg. of testosterone per day and about one fourth this amount of androstenedione. From animal experiments in which the seminiferous tubules were destroyed without affecting the Leydig cells, it has been concluded that testicular androgen originates in the Leydig cells. Clinical signs of androgen deficiency are absent in certain testicular disorders in man associated with defective seminiferous tubules but with intact Leydig cells.

Recent studies have elucidated pathways for the biosynthesis of testosterone by the testis (see article on Steroid Metabolism). The Leydig cells are capable of synthesizing testosterone from available precursors such as cholesterol and acetate by the enzymatic conversion of these compounds to 17-hydroxypregnenolone and to 17-hydroxyprogesterone and then to testosterone and androstenedione. There is also good evidence that the testis can convert testosterone to the aromatic steroid, estradiol-17β. The estrogens, estradiol-17β and estrone, have been isolated from normal human testes and from testicular tumors. However, recent data indicate that in the adult male estradiol, the major estrogenic hormone, is derived partly from the conversion of secreted testosterone. On the other hand, the dominant source of circulating estrone is an adrenal precursor, not a testicular one, possibly estrone sulfate.

The liver is the main site of catabolism of testosterone and of the conjugation of its known metabolites with glucuronic or sulfuric acid; other tissues play a less important role in its metabolism. The major identifiable urinary metabolites are the 17-ketosteroids, androsterone and etiocholanolone, which are excreted principally as glucuronides and account for 20 to 40 per cent of the testosterone secreted. A small amount of testosterone (0.2 to 2 per cent) is excreted as testosterone glucuronide.

The testis is under the direct control of the anterior pituitary gland, which secretes follicle-stimulating hormone (FSH) and interstitial cell stimulating (ICSH) or luteinizing hormone (LH), both of which are glycoproteins. FSH stimulates growth of seminiferous tubules. Luteinizing hormone induces the Leydig cells to secrete testosterone and androstenedione, and together with FSH promotes the final stages of spermatogenesis. It has been shown that androgens can also stimulate and maintain spermatogenesis in hypophysectomized animals under certain experimental conditions, but in man FSH is necessary for maturation of spermatozoa. As is true of many other endocrine glands, there is a reciprocal relationship between the hypophysis and the hormonal secretion of the testis, mediated by the hypothalamus and its gonadotrophin-releasing neurohumors, FSH releasing factor (FRF) and LH releasing factor (LRF). The hypothalamus, through a neurohumoral control mechanism, regulates the secretion of FSH and LH. FRF and LRF pass from hypothalamic nerve endings at the level of the median eminence into the hypothalamic portal vessels, and are carried to the anterior pituitary gland. Certain organic lesions of the hypothalamus are associated with precocious puberty or sexual infantilism.

It has long been known that doses of testosterone sufficient to reverse signs of androgen deficiency in castrated animals and men lead to a fall in the high concentration of plasma LH and in the excretion of urinary LH over an interval of several days. There is a reciprocal relationship between the level of plasma testosterone and plasma LH. Although estrogen in physiologic doses suppresses secretion of both LH and FSH in castrates, the control of FSH secretion in the male is poorly understood. Destructive lesions or defects involving only the seminiferous tubules (without evidence of Leydig cell deficiency) are usually accompanied by elevated levels of FSH. However, the mechanism responsible for this rise in FSH secretion remains uncertain.

EVALUATION OF TESTICULAR FUNCTION

Clinical Assessment. A clinical estimate of the adequacy of androgenic function is obtained by ascertaining the degree of development of the penis and scrotum, the size of the prostate, the general maturity and status of male secondary sex characteristics, the habitus and skeletal proportions, muscular development, and potentia. Although of great value, this method of assessment has limitations, and can provide only a qualitative estimate of Leydig cell function. Once adult maturation has been attained, signs of androgen deficiency are difficult to detect by clinical means; even when there is complete loss of Leydig cell function in the mature male, e.g., after castration, regression of secondary sexual characteristics is a slow and selective process. Further, in addition to disease states that may alter the responsiveness of the target organs to hormone stimulation, it is well recognized that there are also racial, familial, and individual differences in the sensitivity of these structures. In this regard, the American Indian, African Negro, and some Orientals have sparse or absent facial and body hair despite normal testicular function.

Determination of Urinary 17-Ketosteroids and Androgen. It must be emphasized that steroids derived from the adrenal cortex comprise more than 80 per cent of the total 17-ketosteroids in urine (and a significant fraction of the androgenic activity). Less than 4 mg. daily are derived from Leydig cell secretions. Androsterone (an androgen) and etiocholanolone (a nonandrogenic steroid), the principal urinary metabolites of testosterone, are also metabolites of 11-deoxygenated adrenocortical steroids (see Steroid Metabolism). These facts limit the usefulness of measurement of 17-ketosteroid excretion for evaluation of Leydig cell function. Testosterone, which has an hydroxyl group at carbon atom 17, is not a 17-ketosteroid.

The normal range of 17-ketosteroid excretion in men is 8 to 25 mg. per day (mean, 15 mg.). Prior to puberty only small amounts of 17-ketosteroids and androgen are detectable in urine. In adult men (and women) there is a gradual fall with advancing age in the amount of 17-ketosteroids and androgen excreted, a fall which begins during the third decade. The excretion of 17-ketosteroids does not necessarily reflect biologic activity determined by animal assay, although the results tend to parallel one another. The excretion of 17-keto-steroids is generally reduced in eunuchoidism.

However, the values obtained in such patients may fall within the normal range or, occasionally, may even reach the upper limits of normal. In panhypopituitarism the function of both the testis and the adrenal cortex is impaired, and the level of urinary 17-ketosteroids is greatly decreased. Low values are also frequently obtained in chronic debilitating diseases and renal insufficiency.

Determination of Urinary Estrogen. It has been suggested by Maddock and Nelson that the increase in urinary estrogen following the administration of chorionic gonadotrophin (a placental gonadotrophin with luteinizing properties) is a useful index of Leydig cell function. This approach has not been used widely with the advent of methods for the determination of blood and urinary testosterone.

Determination of Plasma and Urinary Testosterone. The recent development of reliable methods for the measurement of plasma and urinary testosterone, the latter as the glucuronide conjugate, and for estimating the production rate of testosterone has facilitated more precise assessment of the androgenic function of the testis. Young adult males excrete 40 to 100 mcg. of testosterone as glucuronide; women excrete less than 10 mcg. per day, and boys before puberty less than 0.5 mcg. per day. The concentration of plasma testosterone in young adult males ranges from 0.44 to 0.96 mcg. per 100 ml. (mean 0.65 mcg. per 100 ml.), and the concentration in women varies from 0.034 to 0.101 mcg. per 100 ml. (mean 0.054 mcg. per 100 ml.). More than 95 per cent of testosterone in plasma is bound to a specific β-globulin. The administration of human chorionic gonadotrophin induces a rise in plasma and urinary testosterone values; this procedure has been utilized to assess Leydig cell reserve.

Determination of Plasma and Urinary Gonadotrophins. Gonadotrophic substances in the urine of normal men and nonpregnant women have been designated in the past as urinary FSH. However, since the urinary concentrate as prepared for routine bioassay contains a mixture of pituitary gonadotrophins, Albert has suggested the term HPG (human pituitary gonadotrophin). The excretion of gonadotrophin is not uniform, and spontaneous fluctuations in daily output must be considered in evaluating the results of random determinations. Further, only a small proportion of the FSH and LH secreted daily appears in the urine in a biologically active form. The normal range of HPG excretion by the mouse uterine weight method is 5 to 100 mouse units per day and by the rat ovarian weight method 5 to 30 rat units per day. HPG is detectable by bioassay in 15 per cent of samples obtained randomly from prepubertal children. HPG is absent or diminished in hypogonadism secondary to pituitary or hypothalamic disturbances and frequently in chronic debilitating diseases, malnutrition, and starvation. The excretion of HPG is increased in many, but not all, primary testicular disorders. In general, elevated levels appear to be related to the degree of damage to the seminiferous tubules.

The advent of radioimmunoassay procedures

has led to the development of sensitive, accurate, practical methods for the measurement of these glycoproteins in serum and urine. Determination of plasma or urinary FSH and LH is a useful diagnostic procedure which can be expected to replace the bioassay for general gonadotrophin (HPG) in urine. Since in most clinical situations parallel changes occur in the secretion of FSH and LH, assessment of either hormone usually suffices for most diagnostic purposes. The values obtained by immunoassay are expressed in terms of international units of the second international reference preparation (2nd IRP) of human menopausal gonadotrophin or in ng. of a human pituitary FSH and LH standard. According to Ross, the mean plasma FSH concentration in adult men is 9.6 mIU per milliliter (8.0 to 11.1 mIU per milliliter, 95 per cent confidence limits) and the mean plasma LH concentration 17.8 mIU per milliliter (15.7 to 19.9 mIU per milliliter, 95 per cent confidence limits) in terms of the 2nd IRP-HMG. (See Anterior Pituitary.)

Assessment of Hypothalamic-Pituitary Gonadotrophin Function. Clomiphene citrate, when administered by mouth, 100 to 200 mg. per day for five to seven days to normal men, evokes a mean increase in the concentration of plasma FSH of 130 per cent and of plasma LH of 160 per cent. It also induces a rise in urinary FSH and LH and of plasma testosterone. Clomiphene, an analogue of the nonsteroidal estrogen chlorotrianisene, is an estrogen antagonist, but its mechanism of action on the hypothalamus and the secretion of FRF and LRF is uncertain. No increase in FSH or LH secretion is elicited in men with gonadotrophin deficiency. This test is in a preliminary stage of evaluation. It is already apparent that the results in patients with delayed adolescence must be interpreted with caution as normal prepubertal boys and adolescents usually do not exhibit an increase in FSH and LH secretion.

Testicular Biopsy. This procedure is of great value in the diagnosis and prognosis of testicular disorders. It provides information concerning both the gametogenic and endocrine functions of the testis—the status of the seminiferous tubules and the Leydig cells. Biopsy examination of the testis is of use in differentiation of primary and secondary testicular failure, in determination of the specific nature of the testicular defect and its prognosis, and in distinguishing azoospermia due to obstruction in the passage of sperm from that due to other causes. Preferably, a specimen should be obtained from each testis.

Examination of Semen. Specimens of semen for analysis are usually obtained after an interval of three days following the last ejaculation. The volume of the specimen, the number of sperm per milliliter, and the motility and morphology of the sperm are determined.

Determination of the Sex Chromatin Pattern. The number of X chromosomes in the sex chromosome complex can be assessed indirectly by cytologic methods because of a sexual dimorphism in the nuclear structure of somatic cells, first described by Barr et al. Preparations suitable for examination can be obtained from smears of buccal mucosa, skin biopsy specimens, or blood. (See the article on Cytogenetics for a discussion of these methods.) This test is widely used in the investigation of abnormalities of sex differentiation, including males with defective testes and azoospermia or severe oligospermia. When a chromatin-positive (female-type) nuclear sex chromatin pattern is detected in a phenotypic male with bilateral testes, the test is indicative of a congenital primary testicular disorder (see Klinefelter's Syndrome, Seminiferous Tubule Dysgenesis).

Instances have been described in which a proportion of nuclei from phenotypic males or females contained two or more sex chromatin bodies. The maximal number of sex chromatin bodies in somatic nuclei is equivalent to one less than the number of X chromosomes in the sex chromosome complex. For example, XO and XY individuals have chromatin-negative (male-type) somatic nuclei, whereas a high proportion of diploid nuclei in individuals with XX or XXY sex chromosome constitution contain a maximum of one sex chromatin body. Similarly, in XXX females and XXXY males a maximum of two bodies are found in somatic nuclei. A small sex chromatin body in interphase nuclei has been associated with a deletion of the X and a large sex chromatin body with a large sex chromosome assumed to be an X isochromosome.

Accumulating evidence which indicates that only one X chromosome in somatic nuclei is fully genetically active, the other X or X's being in a heterochromatic state with the capacity to give rise to sex chromatin, has important genetic implications with respect to the expression and penetrance of X-linked genes in heterozygotes and to the severity of somatic anomalies in individuals with extra X chromosomes.

Recently, it has been found that quinacrine hydrochloride, an acridine derivative, when utilized as a stain produces intense fluorescence of the Y chromosome in interphase nuclei (Y chromatin body), in metaphase preparations, and in sperm. This discovery makes it possible to detect XYY, XXYY, and other double Y syndromes by the simple buccal smear technique.

Response to Chorionic Gonadotrophin. The effects of human chorionic gonadotrophin (HCG) on the immature testes are similar to those of LH. It induces differentiation and growth of Leydig cells, the secretion of testosterone, and an increase in plasma and urinary estrogen values. The clinical response to HCG has been used as an ancillary aid in differentiating between primary and secondary hypogonadism.

PUBERTAL DEVELOPMENT
IN THE MALE

There are wide variations in the age of onset, duration, and sequence of events that characterize the biologic pattern of male puberty. In normal boys signs of puberty may appear at any age between 10 and 17 years; the average age of onset is 12 to 13 years. Once initiated, the major changes are usually completed or well advanced in three to four years; in a small percentage of normal persons, adult maturity is not attained until the age of 21.

A substantial body of evidence suggests that the stimulus for release of pituitary gonadotrophin at puberty originates in the hypothalamus, and is mediated by a neurohumoral secretion. It seems likely that a certain level of physiologic maturation, presumably including the central nervous system, is necessary before this complex and incompletely understood mechanism is activated. This level of development is best reflected by the degree of osseous and epiphyseal development (bone age) rather than by the chronologic age. Of interest is the observation that small amounts of FSH and LH are secreted by prepubertal children. The hypothalamic–pituitary gonadotrophin–testicular negative feedback mechanism is operative but set at a low level.

The sequence of events that marks the pubertal period is initiated by an acceleration in the growth of the testes and scrotum. The initial increase in testicular size is largely attributable to changes in the seminiferous tubules, which occupy approximately two thirds of the mass of the testis. Following the initial acceleration of testicular growth, there is an increase in the size of the penis, the appearance of pubic hair, which has at first a transverse growth, gradual enlargement of the prostate and other accessory organs and glands, and areolar and subareolar enlargement of the breast.

Concomitantly, usually between the ages of 13 and 15, an acceleration of growth takes place, involving primarily the skeleton and muscles. More subtle changes occur elsewhere. The adolescent growth spurt is completed in about three years and, in boys, accounts for an average increment in height of about 8 inches (4 to 12 inches) and a gain in weight of about 40 pounds. Much has been written about the behavioral changes and the psychosexual dynamics of the adolescent period; the reader is referred elsewhere for a discussion of this subject.

It is necessary that the physician be cognizant of the wide range of normality in the pubertal process, in the time of onset, intensity and duration, and also of normal variations in the degree of development of the secondary sex characteristics. In normal men, the pitch of the voice, the size of the external genitalia, the amount of body hair, and the body habitus all vary from individual to individual, and are largely attributable to genetic factors and not to differences in the secretion of testosterone.

Delayed Adolescence. Commonly, failure to undergo sexual maturation by the average age is ascribable to an idiopathic normal variation in pubertal development; puberty occurs spontaneously, usually by the age of 16 years, but occasionally even later. Delayed adolescence, although inherently a benign condition, is often a severe psychologic handicap to the patient and a cause of much anxiety to his parents. Many of these boys are short, and a delay of several years in osseous development is not uncommon. Frequently there is a history of late onset of puberty in other members of the family.

In addition to "idiopathic" delay in sexual maturation, or pubertal failure or arrest in pubortal development secondary to gonadal or pituitary disease, retardation of puberty may be due to inadequate dietary intake and to chronic debilitating illness, since these may be associated with diminished secretion of pituitary gonadotrophin. Rare causes of delayed puberty are previously unsuspected hypothyroidism and regional ileitis.

Disorders involving the pituitary, hypothalamus, or testes must be excluded in instances of delayed puberty. Roentgenographic examination of the skull and careful examination of the fundi and visual fields are required, as well as search for other signs of neurologic involvement in all boys who are significantly delayed in their sexual development, particularly if this is accompanied by stunting of growth. It is advisable to assess other pituitary functions (see articles on pituitary disorders), especially if the delayed maturation is accompanied by short stature or a decreased rate of growth. In addition, a buccal smear for sex chromatin and determination of plasma testosterone and of plasma or urinary gonadotrophins may clarify the clinical situation. A therapeutic trial with chorionic gonadotrophin or testosterone may be of value. In boys with delayed adolescence, sexual maturation frequently continues after the cessation of hormone therapy; however, in pituitary hypogonadism the induced changes regress.

Treatment. If a cause of the delayed adolescence is found, treatment should be directed toward correction of the basic disturbance, e.g., measures to improve nutrition, surgical removal or irradiation of a pituitary neoplasm. If a lesion involving the hypophysis or testes is detected, it is advisable to institute substitution therapy with male sex hormone at about 13 or 14 years of age so that the onset of the patient's own puberty coincides with that of his coevals. Less well defined is the treatment of boys in whom no apparent etiologic factor is found. Many will mature spontaneously before 17 years of age and merely represent an extreme of the normal range. Indiscriminate use of hormonal treatment in this group is unwise, and a conservative approach is indicated. Nonetheless, at times, psychologic considerations may make it expedient to treat such boys. A therapeutic trial with human gonadotrophin, 500 to 1000 I.U. three times weekly injected intramuscularly, or with a testosterone preparation for three to four months, frequently initiates the physiologic reactions of puberty, and maturation will progress after treatment is discontinued.

SEXUAL PRECOCITY
IN THE MALE

Isosexual precocity in boys is defined as the occurrence of signs of masculinization before the age of ten years. Skeletal maturation is accelerated and the epiphyses fuse at a premature age, leading to short stature in adult life. On the other hand, mental and dental development are not precocious. Sexual precocity occurs about three times more frequently in girls than in boys. The main causes of isosexual precocity in boys can be divided into four groups: cerebral, adrenocortical, testicular, and extra-endocrine hormone-secreting tumors.

The cerebral causes of sexual precocity may be functional or organic. They are associated with premature activation of the hypothalamic-pituitary mechanism and the release of pituitary gonadotrophic hormones. This form, commonly designated *true precocious puberty* or *complete isosexual precocity,* is manifested by maturation of the testes and spermatogenesis.

Precocious puberty may be caused by organic lesions of the brain either directly or indirectly involving the posterior hypothalamus, such as hypothalamic and pineal tumors, hamartoma of the tuber cinereum, craniopharyngioma, hydrocephalus, postencephalitic lesions, congenital defects, tuberous sclerosis, and neurofibromatosis. The *McCune-Albright syndrome* of sexual precocity, polyostotic fibrous dysplasia, and pigmented areas of skin is rare in boys. When no organic cause is found, the condition is described as *idiopathic precocious puberty*; in some instances, it is transmitted as a sex-limited autosomal dominant trait. In the idiopathic cases, seizure disorders and abnormal electroencephalographic patterns are appreciably more frequent than in normal children. Cerebral lesions, particularly tumors, accompanied by precocious puberty may affect other hypothalamic functions, causing diabetes insipidus, bulimia, obesity, somnolence, emotional lability, or disturbances in temperature regulation. Diabetes insipidus in association with precocious puberty is a syndrome that tends to occur in the presence of an aberrant pinealoma. Involvement of the optic nerves or visual pathways causes visual disturbances. In some instances signs of puberty precede the onset of detectable neurologic involvement, and a prolonged period of observation with repeated careful neurologic examinations, roentgenograms of the skull, and determinations of the visual fields is necessary before it is possible to exclude cerebral neoplasm. In all varieties of true precocious puberty, the excretion of urinary 17-ketosteroids rises slowly to normal adolescent values; initially, levels between 2.5 and 4.0 mg. per day are usually found. Plasma and urinary testosterone values are increased. In contrast to precocious pseudopuberty, pituitary gonadotrophin (HPG) is excreted in the urine; frequently, however, this is not detectable early in the course, except by the more sensitive radioimmunoassay procedures for FSH and LH.

Recent evidence suggests that medroxyprogesterone acetate, administered intramuscularly, is of value in the management of patients with idiopathic precocious puberty by virtue of its capacity to inhibit pituitary LH secretion. Rarely, extrapituitary and gonadal neoplasms that secrete an LH-like gonadotrophin have been found, such as malignant hepatoma.

In other forms of isosexual precocity not related to intracranial causes, the testes remain more or less immature, in contrast to the enlarged phallus, and true puberty does not occur. Accordingly, this type has been called *incomplete sexual precocity* or *precocious pseudopuberty.*

The most common cause of *incomplete sexual precocity* in boys is adrenocortical hyperfunction due to congenital virilizing adrenal hyperplasia or a virilizing adrenocortical tumor. This is also the most common cause of isosexual precocity in males. With few exceptions the testes remain prepubertal in size despite enlargement of the penis and scrotum and development of other secondary sexual characteristics. An ectopic nodule of hyperplastic adrenal tissue is occasionally palpable in the testis, sometimes bilaterally, and may be confused with Leydig cell tumor, especially in rare instances in which striking enlargement of the testis is found. The excretion of 17-ketosteroids is profoundly increased in relation to chronologic age, and in adrenal hyperplasia an excessive amount of urinary pregnanetriol is detectable (see also under Adrenal Cortex, *supra*).

Interstitial cell tumor of the testis is an exceedingly rare cause of isosexual precocity. In 23 reported cases the tumor was unilateral, and the contralateral testis was immature. Gynecomastia was present in three patients. The excretion of 17-ketosteroids varied from 3 to 64 mg. per day. Exceedingly high values of plasma testosterone may be found.

Iatrogenic sexual precocity has been produced by the administration of male sex hormone and is seen frequently in boys who have been treated with large doses of chorionic gonadotrophin for cryptorchidism.

HYPOGONADISM IN THE MALE

Testicular insufficiency or hypogonadism is used here in its broader sense to denote a deficiency of either or both the endocrine and gametogenic functions of the testis. Depending upon the nature of the physiologic defect, hypogonadism can be divided into two categories. (1) Hypogonadism secondary to a deficiency of pituitary gonadotrophins, involving a lack of LH, or more commonly both LH and FSH, includes disorders characterized by small testes, androgen deficiency, and absent or low HPG excretion. (2) Hypogonadism of primary testicular origin includes disorders accompanied by normal or increased levels of urinary gonadotrophin and a variable degree of androgenic function from normal to deficient. Of common occurrence are primary lesions of the testes involving _only_ spermatogenic function that result in infertility. On the other hand, when androgenic function is deficient, usually but not invariably, spermatogenesis is impaired.

Androgen Deficiency. The clinical signs and effects of androgen deficiency depend upon the age of onset—prepubertal, pubertal, or postpubertal—and upon the severity and duration of the deficiency.

Total loss of testicular androgenic function, usually secondary to surgical castration, atrophy, or congenital defects of the testes, before the onset or at an early stage of puberty results in eunuchism in adulthood. Prepubertal castration is associated with disproportionate growth of the skeleton produced by the delay in epiphyseal closure. The span exceeds the measurement for height by several inches, and the distance between the symphysis pubis and the sole (lower segment) measures more than 55 per cent of the height. Tall stature is common, but not invariable. (The characteristic skeletal proportions of the eunuch are not pathognomonic and may be found in otherwise normal men.) The shoulders tend to be narrow and, although the habitus may be lean or obese, excessive fat deposition often occurs about the pectoral region, hips, thighs, and lower abdomen. Muscular development is poor, and strength is impaired. Except for the appearance of sparse pubic hair, secondary sex characteristics fail to appear, and the voice remains juvenile. True gynecomastia is commonly present. The skin exhibits a characteristic fine wrinkling about the face, especially in the perioral and periorbital regions, a generalized pale and sallow appearance, and increased distensibility. Acne and baldness do not occur. Sex drive and potentia are absent or greatly reduced. The basal metabolic rate is lower in many instances than in normal men. In some cases there is anemia, usually of a mild degree. The erythrocyte sedimentation rate characteristically rises after castration.

The effects on somatic and sexual development of partial loss of testicular androgenic function are less striking and vary greatly in degree. Characteristic of the milder forms of eunuchoidism are the scant growth of facial hair and a female distribution of pubic hair. In men who have attained sexual maturity, castration does not result in complete regression of secondary sexual characteristics, and the signs of androgen deficiency are less conspicuous. The most common signs are reduction in prostatic size, diminished growth of the beard and body hair, the appearance of fine wrinkles around the eyes, and a pasty, sallow complexion. Semen volume is reduced. Potentia and libido, though usually diminished, frequently persist. Vasomotor phenomena, including hot flushes, occur occasionally.

PRIMARY HYPOGONADISM
(Primary Failure of the Testis)

The problem of classification of primary hypogonadism has not been resolved entirely, mainly because the cause of many of the disorders in this group is uncertain. Primary hypogonadism may result from genetic and developmental defects, as in seminiferous tubule dysgenesis, Laurence-Moon Biedl syndrome, myotonia dystrophica, Werner's syndrome, thermal injury as in cryptorchidism, trauma, destruction and degeneration following orchitis or exposure to ionizing radiation, neoplasm, and surgical castration. Disorders in this group may or may not be accompanied by androgen deficiency, although in some, eunuchoidism is a constant or frequent feature. The excretion of gonadotrophin (HPG) is normal or increased, depending, apparently, upon the integrity of the seminiferous tubules. The application of the sex chromatin method and modern cytogenetic techniques to the study of testicular disorders has greatly advanced our knowledge.

Klinefelter's Syndrome; Seminiferous Tubule Dysgenesis

This syndrome, described in 1942 by Klinefelter, Reifenstein, and Albright and later modified by others, has been a subject of considerable interest and re-evaluation. The characteristic features, which become apparent during or after puberty, include a variable degree of eunuchoidism, azoospermia, gynecomastia, and small testes with atrophy and hyalinization of the seminiferous tubules in which Leydig cells are usually preserved but tend to occur in large clumps, and elevated urinary gonadotrophins. Some tubules are lined by Sertoli cells; rarely, germ cells are present in isolated tubules. In most instances, the cause is a developmental defect of the gonad owing to a sex chromosome abnormality; in others, the syndrome may be associated with a postnatal lesion. Although seminiferous tubule dysgenesis may occur in phenotypic males with either chromatin-positive or chromatin-negative nuclei, the chromatin-negative form is rare; in most instances the cause of Klinefelter's syndrome with a male chromatin pattern and XY sex chromosome constitution is uncertain.

Chromatin-Positive Klinefelter's Syndrome; Seminiferous Tubule Dysgenesis

The discovery in 1956 that most persons with Klinefelter's syndrome have a chromatin-positive sex chromatin pattern, followed by the detection of sex chromosome abnormalities, has served to identify an especially well-defined disorder due to a genetically determined gonadal defect at the chromosome level. In accordance with this observation and the histopathologic characteristics of the testicular lesion, the term "seminiferous tubule dysgenesis" has been suggested. This disorder, which occurs sporadically, is an important cause of male infertility and a common type of sexual anomaly. The results of several large surveys of newborns in nurseries indicate that the frequency of chromatin-positive seminiferous tubule dysgenesis is of the order of 1 in 500 newborn males. (All chromatin-positive male infants may not have Klinefelter's syndrome, since in one series in which karyotype analyses were performed, 5 of 18 chromatin-positive male infants had XY/XXY mosaicism, and some XY/XXY mosaics are fertile.) Familial cases are exceedingly rare.

The only constant clinical features of chromatin-positive seminiferous tubule dysgenesis are infertility and the small size of the testes (long diameter usually less than 3 cm.), which are often firmer than normal; in most instances testicular atrophy is severe. Gynecomastia (which occurs in less than 50 per cent of cases) and eunuchoidism are variable features and, when present, first appear during the pubertal period. Patients with this disorder are often tall. The skeletal proportions frequently are eunuchoid as a consequence of disproportionately long lower extremities, even though epiphyseal fusion is not delayed and skeletal maturation usually follows the normal male pattern (see Fig. 3). Cryptorchidism and hypospadias have been observed infrequently. Mental retardation and psychopathic behavior are not uncommon, and evidence of poor social adaptation is often obtained. This disorder has been reported in association with mongolism and with leukemia; it has been suggested that chronic pulmonary disease and varicose veins are more prevalent in affected adults. The frequency of im-

paired glucose tolerance and of mild diabetes is increased. A low radioactive iodine uptake over the thyroid and a diminished response to TSH have been described in a few patients.

The excretion of urinary gonadotrophin is almost invariably increased. In general, urinary 17-ketosteroids are within the normal range. However, the concentration of plasma testosterone may be low; if it is normal, it may not show a normal increase after the daily administration of chorionic gonadotrophin for four to five days. The histologic appearance of the testes is distinctive.

The presence of an abnormality of the sex chromosomes in chromatin-positive Klinefelter's syndrome, characterized by an XXY sex chromosome constitution and a chromosome number of 47, was first demonstrated in 1959 by Jacobs and Strong and by Ford and his associates. Subsequently, less common types of sex chromosome abnormalities have been reported in this disorder. These include phenotypic males with an XXYY, XXXY, or XXXXY sex chromosome constitution (Table 3), which have been found, so far, only in mentally retarded persons. Unusually tall stature has been found in the XXYY group and a tendency to more aggressive and delinquent behavior. The XXXY sex chromosome complex is associated with two sex chromatin bodies in a proportion of diploid somatic nuclei, and an XXXXY constitution with three sex chromatin bodies. In addition

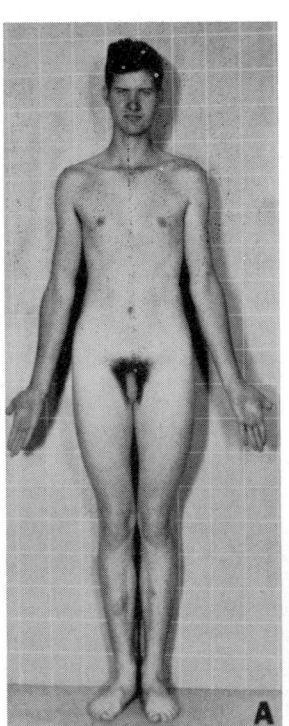
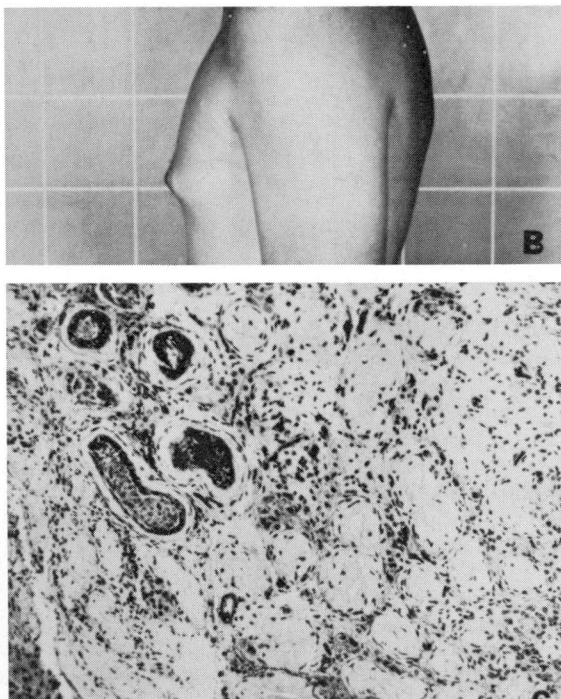
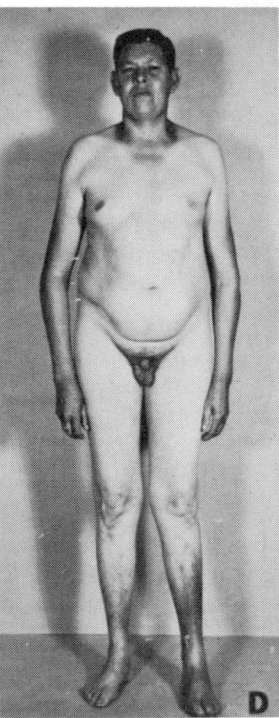

FIGURE 3. *A* and *B,* Typical 19-year-old phenotypic male with chromatin-positive seminiferous tubule dysgenesis (Klinefelter's syndrome). This patient had a positive sex chromatin pattern and an XXY karyotype. His 17-ketosteroid excretion was 11.2 mg. per 24 hours, and his urinary gonadotrophin excretion was more than 100 m.u. These patients vary widely in their habitus and degree of virilization. This patient is well virilized, but had long extremities with eunuchoidal proportions and exhibited gynecomastia. The testes measured 1.8 × 0.9 cm. and were small and firm. Testicular biopsy, *C,* revealed a severe degree of hyalinization of his seminiferous tubules and Leydig cell hyperplasia. *D,* Forty-eight-year-old man with chromatin-positive Klinefelter's syndrome who came to medical attention only because his severe leg varicosities were thought to reveal a "female trait." (From Van Wyk, J. J., and Grumbach, M. M.: Disorders of sex differentiation. *In* Williams, R. H. (ed.): *Textbook of Endocrinology.* Fourth edition, Philadelphia, W. B. Saunders Company, 1968, p. 537.)

TABLE 3. SEX CHROMATIN AND THE SEX CHROMOSOME COMPLEX IN PHENOTYPIC MALES WITH CHROMATIN-POSITIVE SEMINIFEROUS TUBULE DYSGENESIS

Maximum No. of Sex Chromatin Bodies in Diploid Somatic Nuclei	Sex Chromosomes	Chromosome No.
1	XX	46
1	XXY	47
1	XXYY	48
2	XXXY	48
2	XXXYY	49
3	XXXXY	49
Sex Chromosome Mosaics		
1	XY/XXY	46/47
1	XX/XXY	46/47
2	XY/XXXY	46/48
3	XXXY/XXXXY	48/49

to mental retardation, the XXXXY individuals have had severe manifestations of the syndrome, including very small, usually undescended testes, hypoplastic external genitalia, minor skeletal deformities including radioulnar synostosis, and other congenital anomalies.

Instances of sex chromosome mosaicism have also been described in which at least two populations of cells with different sex chromosome complexes were found in the same individual: e.g., XY/XXY (one cell line with an XY sex chromosome complex and another with an XXY sex chromosome complex), XY/XXXY, XX/XXY, XXXY/XXXXY. Sex chromosome mosaics arise from a mitotic error in an early division after fertilization in a zygote that originally had either a normal or an abnormal sex chromosome constitution. The detection of a chromatin-positive sex chromatin pattern on buccal smear should not by itself be used as incontrovertible evidence of sterility. Active spermatogenesis was found in the testes of an XY/XXXY mosaic, and additional examples of potential fertility may be found in chromatin-positive males with other forms of sex chromosome mosaicism, especially XY/XXY. In several carefully studied males with the syndrome, only an XX sex chromosome constitution was found. The maternal origin of the two X chromosomes demonstrated in one of these patients suggests that a Y chromosome was present early in ontogeny and was lost or more likely translocated to an X chromosome or autosome, or that these men were mosaics and the Y-bearing cell line has escaped detection.

The typical XXY sex chromosome constitution of seminiferous tubule dysgenesis may arise from an abnormality of meiosis during gametogenesis or from a mitotic error in the fertilized zygote (see the article on Cytogenetics and Figure 4). For example, nondisjunction of the sex chromosomes during gametogenesis in either parent may result in an XX ovum or an XY sperm. Fertilization of an aneuploid (XX) ovum by a Y sperm or of a normal X ovum by an aneuploid sperm (XY) would produce, in this instance, an XXY zygote.

The positive association of this disorder with advanced maternal age and the results of surveys of color-blindness (a sex-linked recessive trait) and of the Xg blood group suggest a maternal origin with nondisjunction during oogenesis, in some instances. Using X-linked markers, a paternal origin of one X has been established in several informative pedigrees, nondisjunction during spermatogenesis giving rise to an XY-bearing sperm (Fig. 4) and fertilization yielding an X^MX^PY zygote. The more complex sex chromosome anomalies listed in the table may arise from meiotic or mitotic errors, or a combination of both types.

The gonadal defect is a consequence of the abnormal sex chromosome constitution. The single Y chromosome is a sufficiently powerful male determiner to lead to suppression of the cortical component of the primordial gonad despite the presence of two (or even four) X chromosomes. The fetal testes that develop may have either an adequate number or a deficiency of germ cells, but bring about normal male differentiation of the genital tract. At puberty, if the function of the Leydig cells is adequate, male secondary sexual characteristics develop, but the seminiferous tubules lack or are severely deficient in germ cells. Tubular hyalinization does not begin until the late prepubertal period or the onset of puberty. It seems likely that the characteristic appearance of the testes in adolescent and adult cases depends on the action, either directly or indirectly, of pituitary gonadotrophins from the onset of puberty on an inherently defective testis, which, before this time, shows only subtle signs of an abnormal histologic structure.

In addition to the increased frequency of mental retardation and mental disorders—and quite likely epilepsy—it has been suggested that the abnormal sex chromosome constitution is associated with a susceptibility to certain diseases. This possibility clearly requires further study.

Treatment. The testicular lesion is irrever-

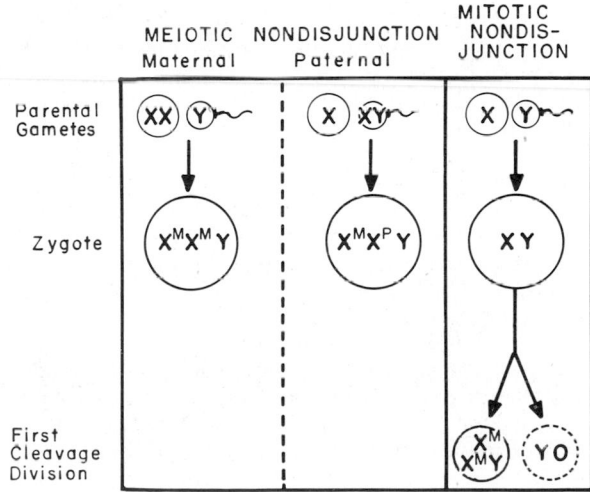

FIGURE 4. The origins of an XXY sex chromosome constitution. The superscripts M and P designate respective matriclinous and patriclinous X-chromosome. The interrupted circle indicates a nonviable cell line.

sible. If androgen deficiency is present, treatment with _male sex hormone_ is effective. The gynecomastia is not affected by hormonal treatment, and _mastectomy_ may be necessary in some patients for cosmetic reasons.

XYY Syndrome

The XYY syndrome is characterized by a chromosome complement of 47 with an extra Y chromosome and a sex chromatin–negative buccal smear that contains nuclei with two small fluorescent Y chromatin masses when stained with quinacrine hydrochloride. It is estimated to occur in 1 per 500 to 1 per 1000 male births. Newborn males and young boys with this syndrome have a normal phenotype. A number of associated characteristics have been reported in the adolescent and adult XYY male. These include tall stature (often over 6 fcct), severe acne, aggressive behavior, and, less often, hypogonadism, criminal tendencies, and skeletal abnormalities, e.g., radio-ulnar synostosis. On the other hand, some adult XYY males are physically and mentally normal.

This syndrome has raised important medicolegal issues. Do these individuals have a biologic predisposition for criminal behavior? If so, are they to be held accountable for their crimes? Several cases have reached the courtrooms and judges and juries are considering these issues. Until more data are available about this sex chromosome disorder and its behavioral manifestations, the controversy will remain disquieting. The only therapeutic approach is psychiatric counseling.

Germinal Aplasia
(Sertoli-Cell-Only Syndrome)

This condition is characterized by seminiferous tubules lined with Sertoli cells, little or no tubular fibrosis, and absent or rare germinal cells. Leydig cell function is usually normal. Azoospermia is an invariable finding. The testes are normal or moderately reduced in size. Urinary gonadotrophin is usually increased. However, only the concentration of plasma FSH and the excretion of FSH are increased; the level of LH is normal. The sex chromosome constitution is almost invariably XY. Although it has been suspected that in most instances germinal aplasia is a developmental defect, the lesion has also been described following exposure of the testes to ionizing radiation, in which case it may be reversible, and in some cryptorchid testes.

The histopathology and the clinical findings in patients with congenital defects of the testes (testicular dysgenesis) are highly variable. Male pseudohermaphrodism (_q.v._) may be a consequence of testicular dysgenesis.

Myotonic Muscular Dystrophy

Testicular atrophy is found in about 80 per cent of affected males who, in addition to myotonia and muscle wasting, often exhibit frontal baldness and lenticular opacities. In the series of Drucker et al., signs of androgen deficiency occurred in 18 per cent of the cases and gynecomastia in 12 per cent. The excretion of urinary gonadotrophin is usually normal. The testicular lesion is characterized by progressive tubular fibrosis and hyalinization and disordered spermatogenesis. Impaired glucose tolerance has been described despite an exaggerated insulin response to glucose and arginine.

Anorchia

Absence of both testes in phenotypic males is exceedingly rare; careful surgical exploration is required to establish the diagnosis. Unilateral anorchia is more common, and may result from testicular atrophy following herniorrhaphy or attempted orchiopexy, or from a developmental disturbance, in which case other anomalies of the genitourinary tract are not uncommon.

Infertility

In a variety of testicular lesions, the defect involves only _spermatic function_, and results in infertility. Endocrine manifestations are absent. Either the semen lacks sperm or the number or quality of sperm is impaired. _Testicular biopsy_ has assumed a major role in differentiating the various disturbances in spermatogenic activity and in determining prognosis. Azoospermia is usually associated with severe tubular fibrosis, germinal aplasia, or spermatogenic arrests, and oligospermia with germinal cell desquamation, hypospermatogenesis, incomplete spermatogenic arrest, and less severe forms of tubular fibrosis. In most cases the cause is unknown. Azoospermia may also result from obstruction in the excurrent ducts secondary to gonorrhea, tuberculosis, or a nonspecific infection. Absence or atresia of the vas deferens and a rudimentary epididymis are common bilateral lesions in boys with cystic fibrosis.

Sterility is a common sequel of bilateral cryptorchidism, being an almost invariable result of thermal injury to the germinal cells if the testes are not brought into the scrotum before puberty is well advanced. It may follow _orchitis_ caused by mumps, gonorrhea, brucellosis, leprosy, or occasionally some other severe systemic infection; it _may_ result from x-ray and other irradiation of the testes; or it _may_ be of developmental origin as in seminiferous tubule dysgenesis. Even relatively minor illnesses may be accompanied by a profound depression in sperm count. _Starvation_ and chronic debilitating diseases associated with _inanition_ adversely affect spermatic function. _Estrogen and large amounts of testosterone_ will also suppress spermatogenesis.

Treatment of Infertility in the Male. Although important advances have been made in the evaluation of spermatogenic function, treatment of the infertile male is, in general, both _difficult and unsatisfactory._ Only rarely is it possible to correct the underlying cause. The results of therapy of inherent testicular defects in spermatogenesis in noneunuchoidal men by the use of large doses of androgenic steroids, gonadotrophins, pregnenolone, thyroid, and vitamin preparations have been notably unsuccessful and, for all purposes, negligible. Although testosterone in massive dosage depresses spermatogenesis, intermittent treatment with relatively small doses may be of value in some patients with oligospermia. Some observers have attributed the beneficial effect to more efficient ejaculation and to improvement in the quality of the semen.

SECONDARY HYPOGONADISM

Secondary hypogonadism is due to pituitary gonadotrophic failure that may result from neoplastic, inflammatory, traumatic, vascular, and degenerative lesions involving the hypophysis or hypothalamus such as pituitary adenoma, craniopharyngioma, astrocytoma, infarction, carotid aneurysm, granulomas (especially tuberculosis and histiocytosis [Hand-Schüller-Christian disease and eosinophilic granuloma]), hemochromatosis, idiopathic atrophy, and developmental defects. In many instances, including the idiopathic and familial forms, the nature of the underlying lesion is not known. A functional and reversible depression of gonadotrophic activity occurs in malnutrition, in chronic disease states associated with inanition and nutritional deficiencies, and in some patients with myxedema. High concentrations of androgen and estrogen, as in the adrenogenital syndrome, may cause secondary hypogonadism. Excess estrogen, either from ingestion or endogenous, such as from a feminizing adrenal tumor, depresses the secretion of pituitary gonadotrophin. The testicular atrophy and gynecomastia that occur in some patients with severe liver disease have been ascribed by some to increased levels of estrogen. Irrespective of cause, *in almost all instances of secondary hypogonadism urinary gonadotrophin is absent or greatly diminished.*

The deficiency of pituitary gonadotrophic function occurs either as an isolated defect (hypogonadotrophic eunuchoidism, pituitary hypogonadism) or in association with a deficiency of other hormones of the anterior pituitary (hypopituitarism). On the other hand, hypoadrenalism or hypothyroidism secondary to pituitary failure is rarely found without concurrent involvement of gonadotrophin function and secondary hypogonadism. In some instances only the secretion of LH is impaired. Albert et al. have termed this "partial gonadotrophic failure." In any event, secondary hypogonadism is always accompanied by inadequate androgenic function of the testes and, with rare exceptions, absent or deficient spermatogenesis.

The clinical manifestations vary with age of onset, degree of the deficiency, and whether there is coexistent deficiency of other anterior pituitary hormones. Hypopituitarism occurring during childhood, commonly designated "pituitary dwarfism," results in proportionate dwarfism and complete sexual infantilism. The characteristic features of prepubertal or pubertal gonadotrophic failure (hypogonadotrophic eunuchoidism of Heller and Nelson), occurring as a selective and, in some instances, familial FSH and LH deficiency, include a eunuchoid habitus, small testes, lack of development of secondary sexual characteristics, an increased frequency of defective smell, absence of urinary gonadotrophin, low 17-ketosteroid excretion, a low plasma testosterone value, and failure of clomiphene to increase FSH, LH, and testosterone secretion. Kindreds have been described in which the pattern of inheritance was consistent with an X-linked or sex-limited dominant trait and with an autosomal recessive trait. The absence of gynecomastia, regarded by some as a salient feature, is of doubtful clinical value in differentiating primary from secondary hypogonadism. Deposition of fat in the pectoral region is common and, at times, may be difficult to distinguish from true gynecomastia. Isolated pituitary hypogonadism is relatively rare in adult men; a more frequent occurrence is a variable degree of panhypopituitarism (see articles on pituitary diseases).

It is essential in all instances to obtain roentgenograms of the sella turcica and to plot the visual fields. Testicular biopsy is useful, but considerable experience is necessary for adequate interpretation. When hypogonadism is accompanied by adrenal insufficiency, the excretion of 17-ketosteroids is usually less than 3.0 mg. per day, a level significantly below that found in castrate men. As previously emphasized, urinary gonadotrophin is absent (less than 6 mouse units).

A familial form of isolated hypogonadotrophic hypogonadism limited to males occurs in association with anosmia or hyposmia (*Kallmann's syndrome*) and is transmitted as either an X-linked or sex-limited dominant trait. Aplasia of the olfactory lobes has been found in autopsied cases. Both familial and sporadic forms of isolated FSH and LH deficiency are known, and these may be associated with a variety of somatic anomalies and neurologic defects. Of interest are patients who have a concomitant Leydig cell defect as evidenced by the impaired testosterone response to prolonged treatment with chorionic gonadotrophin.

Isolated LH Deficiency. Pasqualini and Bur described a group of eunuchoidal men with relatively intact spermatogenic function. Later, McCullagh applied the term "fertile eunuchs" to patients with this syndrome. The size of the testes is normal or only moderately reduced. Leydig cells are absent or hypoplastic, and androgen deficiency is always present. The excretion of urinary gonadotrophin (HPG) is usually normal. However, the concentration of plasma LH and the excretion of urinary LH is low or undetectable, whereas the secretion of FSH is normal. Chorionic gonadotrophin stimulates Leydig cell function and ameliorates the androgen deficiency. These patients have an isolated deficiency of LH, which may arise from an abnormality in the hypothalamus (and the synthesis or release of LRF) or in the pituitary gland. A kindred with two affected brothers has been reported. Similar findings have been reported in patients with arrest of puberty caused by a pituitary tumor and, rarely, in idiopathic delayed adolescence.

The pathogenesis of the testicular atrophy that follows traumatic injury to the spinal cord is uncertain. Both primary and secondary hypogonadism have been described in the Laurence-Moon-Biedl syndrome.

Treatment. A physiologic approach to the treatment of secondary hypogonadism necessitates the use of gonadotrophin therapy. Unfortunately, FSH preparations derived from animal sources are not consistently effective and when repeatedly injected stimulate immunologic mechanisms that reduce the effect of the hormones. Human pituitary FSH is not available commercially; however, gonadotrophin prepared from menopausal urine has been used successfully in combination with chorionic gonadotrophin to induce spermatogenesis in patients with secondary hypogonadism. Chorionic gonadotrophin, obtained for commercial use from human pregnancy urine, stimulates the Leydig cells to secrete androgen, but must be administered at frequent intervals (three to four times a week). It does not have a direct effect on the seminiferous tubules, although in a few instances of partial gonadotrophic failure, spermatogenic as well as Leydig cell function improved after its use. Because long-continued administration of chorionic gonadotrophin is expensive and, in general, impractical, substitution therapy with a testosterone preparation is usually advisable and effectively corrects the deficiency of androgen.

TREATMENT OF ANDROGEN DEFICIENCY

The most useful substances for the treatment of androgen deficiency are the preparations of testosterone that are available in forms suitable for intramuscular, oral, and buccal or sublingual administration, or as pellets for subcutaneous implantation. The mode of administration depends, for the most part, on the preference of the patient and the cost.

Esterification of testosterone with organic acids potentiates its activity when injected as an oily solution. Testosterone propionate in doses of 25 to 50 mg. by intramuscular injection twice or three times weekly is usually adequate for replacement therapy. However, longer-acting esters are available that can be administered less frequently. One dose of 200 to 400 mg. of testosterone cyclopentylpropionate or testosterone enanthate is highly effective when injected at two- to four-week intervals.

Methyltestosterone is an effective preparation for oral and buccal or sublingual use. It is usually administered in doses of 50 mg. (30 to 75 mg.) per day orally or about 25 mg. per day by sublingual absorption. It is not a natural compound and its metabolism differs from that of testosterone. Administration of the 17-methylated derivative does not cause an increase in 17-ketosteroid excretion; in addition, although a potent anabolic steroid, it frequently produces creatinuria rather than retention of creatine.

Pellets of testosterone implanted subcutaneously provide an efficient and economical method of administration. Implantation of 750 to 1000 mg. usually suffices for four to six months. However, patients usually prefer one of the slowly absorbed intramuscular preparations when a sustained androgenic effect is desirable.

No potent protein anabolic steroid lacking androgenic properties in man is available at present, although intensive efforts have been made to obtain one.

Undesirable effects include edema due to retention of extracellular electrolyte (an uncommon effect except with use of large doses or in elderly persons with diminished cardiac reserve), polycythemia, acne, gynecomastia, depression of spermatogenesis in some fertile men when administered in large doses, virilization in women, and premature closure of the epiphyses. Rarely, methyltestosterone causes intrahepatic cholestatic jaundice.

Androgen therapy is contraindicated in patients with carcinoma of the prostate.

CRYPTORCHIDISM

The terms "cryptorchidism" and "undescended testes" are used synonymously to designate testes that have never descended into the scrotum. Unilateral cryptorchidism is approximately four times as common as bilaterally undescended testes. A cryptorchid testis may be situated in the abdomen, within the inguinal canal, or in an ectopic position outside the scrotum and the normal pathway of descent. The majority of undescended testes are inguinal. To avoid needless treatment, it is essential to distinguish this condition from *migratory or retractile testes*, which lie in the lower or upper scrotum and with the slightest stimulus are withdrawn into the inguinal region and occasionally into the abdomen by contraction of the cremasteric muscles.

The testes usually descend into the scrotum at about the eighth fetal month; occasionally descent is delayed until or shortly after birth. Incomplete descent is common in premature male infants. Scorer found undescended testes at birth in 3.4 per cent of 1500 full-term male infants; during the first month of life 50 per cent of the undescended testes reached the scrotum. In a prospective study of the incidence of congenital anomalies by McIntosh and associates, only 0.5 per cent of 2793 live-born male infants had undescended testes at 12 months of age. The incidence of unilateral and bilateral cryptorchidism in large series of adult males has been variously estimated at 0.2 to 0.4 per cent. Spontaneous descent occurs frequently during the first year of life. It is probably less common after this age than was previously supposed.

The etiology is incompletely understood. Maldescent may be due to mechanical abnormalities that deter the passage of an otherwise normal testis or to imperfect development of the testis attributable to an inherent testicular defect, or to a deficiency of gonadotrophin. Not infrequently the ectopic testis resides in the superficial inguinal pouch, its descent arrested by Scarpa's fascia. Recent studies indicate that testicular dysgenesis is an important etiologic factor. In rare instances, unilateral or bilateral cryptorchidism is the only anatomic abnormality of the external genitalia in individuals with intersexuality.

Diagnosis. The most difficult aspect of diagnosis is distinguishing the true undescended testis from the more common retractile testis of childhood; repeated examinations may be necessary, especially in obese boys. It is important to ascertain by careful inquiry whether the testis at any time has been observed in the scrotum. In cryptorchidism the ipsilateral side of the scrotum is empty and poorly developed. The patient should be carefully examined in the erect and recumbent positions in a warm room and with warm hands. Bimanual examination and palpation while the patient performs the Valsalva maneuver or while the examiner applies pressure to the lower abdomen are useful procedures. In boys with retractile testes, elicitation of the cremasteric reflex often results in a localized puckering of the scrotal skin. If the testis is palpated in the normal pathway of descent, gentle manipulation should be used in an attempt to displace it into the scrotum. Such mobile testes do not require therapy and will remain in the scrotum with the advent of puberty. Failure to palpate a testis on multiple occasions suggests that the testis is intra-abdominal, atrophic, or absent. However, spontaneous descent may subsequently occur even in instances in which the testis is not felt.

Treatment. The treatment of undescended testes is a vexing and controversial subject; experienced observers differ in their approach to the problem. Though opinions are strong, there are too many gaps in our knowledge to justify dogmatism. Major considerations are (1) the potential fertility of the undescended testis, (2) the likelihood of spontaneous descent, and (3) the propensity of the undescended testis to undergo malignant change.

It is well established that during or after puberty the undescended testis shows degenerative changes that eventually proceed to atrophy. With good reason, these changes have been ascribed to the deleterious effect of the higher temperature of an extrascrotal environment on the testis, especially on the germinal epithelium. The tubules gradually undergo progressive fibrosis and loss of germinal elements, although androgenic function may persist for many years. Almost all *men*

with bilateral undescended testes are sterile. However, general agreement is lacking as to the age at which the fertility potential of the cryptorchid testis is impaired. Although Nelson and Robinson and Engle and others have observed a lag in development of the seminiferous tubules and in some instances a mild degree of fibrosis in testes retained after the age of six to ten years, the significance of these changes is uncertain; after puberty, irreversible degenerative changes frequently take place.

The incidence of cancer in undescended testes is considerably greater than in scrotal testes, and more so in abdominal than inguinal testes. Although precise statistics are not available, the over-all risk appears to be small with the exception of the dysgenetic, frequently undescended gonads of intersexes, which are especially prone to malignant degeneration.

The most important problem in the treatment of patients with cryptorchidism is the age at which it is advisable to attempt correction. Treatment consists of orchiopexy or of the administration of chorionic gonadotrophin followed by orchiopexy when necessary. It is generally agreed that therapy must be instituted before puberty is advanced if irreparable testicular damage is to be prevented, but opinions differ in regard to the optimal age for treatment. In the more common unilateral cryptorchid, the scrotal testis, if normal, is adequate for fertility. Treatment is recommended for cosmetic reasons, to facilitate examination for neoplasm, and as additional insurance against infertility in the event the scrotal testis is defective or impaired at a later age. In bilateral cryptorchidism preservation of fertility is the major consideration. Here the risk of damage to the testis by orchiopexy, which even in experienced hands is not negligible, must be weighed against the possibility of infertility if surgical treatment is delayed too long. When bilateral orchiopexy is followed by atrophy of the testes, the patient will be eunuchoid as well as sterile. Since most undescended testes descend before puberty, the writer believes it is justifiable to delay treatment until nine years of age unless the testis is ectopic or associated with a hernia.

Many workers recommend a course of treatment with chorionic gonadotrophin before orchiopexy. In some cases hormonal therapy is effective, and orchiopexy is unnecessary. It is the opinion of most that testes that descend with such therapy would have descended spontaneously at puberty under the stimulus of endogenous gonadotrophin. Testes that fail to descend are either inherently defective or mechanically retained. Some experienced workers believe that hormonal treatment should not be used for long periods because of the possibility of damage to the undescended testis from prolonged stimulation by chorionic gonadotrophin. To minimize this risk, a short intensive course is recommended of 4000 units of chorionic gonadotrophin administered intramuscularly daily for three days or 4000 units three times a week for three weeks. Hormonal treatment is contraindicated when the testis is ectopic (outside the normal pathway of descent, for example, in the superficial inguinal pouch) or associated with a hernia; in the latter instance, surgical correction is performed along with repair of the hernia.

If the undescended testis is atrophic and biopsy examination at the time of surgery shows irreversible changes, it is generally advisable to perform orchiectomy, provided the contralateral testis is in the scrotum. This also applies to a testis that, despite all attempts at mobilization, cannot be brought into the scrotum.

IMPOTENCE

Impotence is a complicated problem that may be either relative or complete and may involve any phase of the sexual act. Although it is a symptom of androgen deficiency and of genitourinary or neurologic disease, in many instances it is psychic in origin. Multiple sclerosis, tabes dorsalis, and diabetic neuropathy are commonly associated with impotence. Impotence without apparent impairment of libido has been described in patients with temporal lobe lesions. Ganglion-blocking agents, as used in the therapy of hypertension, are also a notable cause of impotence. When impotence is the principal complaint of a patient, it is usually the result of an emotional disturbance, in which case androgen therapy is valueless and at times may add to the psychic trauma.

"MALE CLIMACTERIC"

The spontaneous occurrence of a male climacteric is still controversial. Although in women during the fifth or sixth decade ovarian failure with a compensatory rise in gonadotrophin excretion is an anticipated and physiologic accompaniment of the aging process, spontaneous testicular deficiency of sufficient degree to produce symptoms is an exceedingly rare occurrence. Many of the symptoms ascribed to this syndrome are common in psychoneurotic syndromes in middle-aged and elderly men. The diagnosis should be documented by finding an increased excretion of gonadotrophin, by a low concentration of plasma testosterone, and by testicular biopsy, and should be confirmed by obtaining a therapeutic response to androgen therapy but not to placebos.

ORCHITIS

Acute orchitis, a common complication of mumps, is a rare occurrence in the course of other specific infectious diseases. (See article on Mumps in section on Microbial Diseases.)

Chronic orchitis is associated with painless, hard, sometimes nodular enlargement of the testis. Syphilis, the most common cause, may produce an interstitial orchitis in which the testis is characteristically smooth and wooden in consistency ("billiard ball" testis); involvement is frequently bilateral. Other causes include tuberculosis, leprosy, brucellosis, glanders, and certain parasitic infections such as filariasis and bilharziasis.

TUMORS OF TESTIS

Tumors of the testis are uncommon, comprising about 0.7 per cent of all forms of cancer in the male, occur in about 0.002 per cent, and frequently are malignant. The greatest incidence occurs in the third and fourth decades. The mortality rate for testicular carcinomas is lower among Negroes than among whites, and higher among Jews than among non-Jews. Testicular tumors may arise from any of the cellular components of the testis or their embryonal precursors.

Considerable uncertainty applies to classification, especially of those new growths whose origin has been ascribed to the potentially totipotent germ cell. Melicow has suggested the following classification:

A. Primary tumors
  I. Germinal
    1. Seminoma
    2. Embryonal tumors
      a. Embryoma
      b. Choriocarcinoma
      c. Embryonal carcinoma
      d. Teratocarcinoma
      e. Adult teratoma
    3. Combinations of 1 and 2 and of the various types of embryonal tumors
    4. Gonadal tumors in intersexes (gonadoblastomas)
  II. Nongerminal tumors
    1. Interstitial cell tumor
    2. Sertoli cell tumor
    3. Tumors of testicular stroma: fibroma, lipoma, etc.
B. Secondary tumors
  I. Lymphoma, plasmacytoma, leukemia, etc.
  II. Metastatic carcinoma

Germinal Tumors. Most common are germinal tumors, and, of these, seminoma exceeds in frequency all other testicular tumors. Seminoma, although usually fairly uniform in cellular architecture, may contain embryonal elements such as chorionic syncytium in the primary growth or in metastatic lesions. In contrast to the embryonal tumors, which tend to invade the spermatic cord and to metastasize early, especially to lung, seminomas in general are relatively slow growing and commonly invade the iliac and periaortic lymph nodes before generalized dissemination is demonstrable. In addition, seminomas are frequently highly radiosensitive, whereas embryonal tumors are usually resistant to radiotherapy. The significantly increased incidence of germinal tumors, particularly seminoma, in undescended testes and in the dysgenetic gonads of intersexes has been discussed above.

Many patients with germinal tumors excrete increased amounts of urinary gonadotrophin. The gonadotrophin may be pituitary in origin (HPG) and may show principally FSH activity on bioassay, or it may originate from tumor tissue, in which event chorionic gonadotrophin (HCG) and chorionic somatomammotrophin (HCS) are detectable in the urine and blood. Increased excretion of HPG is usually found in association with seminoma. The significance of this association is not clear, but it may reflect the increased incidence of this tumor in patients with certain inherent testicular defects or at times the augmenting effect of small amounts of HCG on the standard bioassay for urinary HPG. Excretion of chorionic gonadotrophin is most frequently associated with embryonal tumors, especially choriocarcinoma. However, neither increased levels of HPG nor detectable amounts of HCG are consistently found in patients with germinal tumors even when the involvement is widespread, nor is one type of gonadotrophin invariably associated with either seminoma or the embryonal tumors. This subject requires re-evaluation by modern methods of biologic and immunologic assay.

Interstitial Cell Tumors. Tumors of this type are rare, occur at any age, and are usually, but not invariably, benign. In boys interstitial cell tumors cause sexual precocity but not true puberty, since spermatogenesis is absent. Their only recognizable endocrine manifestation in the adult is gynecomastia, which has been observed in about 10 per cent of cases.

Clinical Manifestations. The most common and characteristic symptom is painless and frequently rapid enlargement of the testis. The swelling is firm, diffuse, and symmetrical in most instances, but may be nodular. Occasionally there is dull, dragging inguinal pain, and rarely flank pain, which has been attributed to involvement of the periaortic lymph nodes. Attachment of the testis to the scrotal skin is rare. The iliac, inguinal, and femoral lymph nodes may be enlarged; metastasis to a deep cervical node is sometimes found. Occasionally, tumors of the testis are associated with a coincident hydrocele. Gynecomastia may occur with germinal or interstitial cell tumors. Rarely, tumor cells may be identified in semen.

Tumor must be differentiated from tuberculosis, from syphilitic orchitis, from other forms of acute and chronic epididymo-orchitis, and from hydrocele, spermatocele, and adenomatoid tumor of the epididymis.

Management. The treatment is surgical removal of the involved testis and, depending upon the nature of the tumor, radical resection of regional lymph nodes and irradiation. The five-year survival rate for seminoma is greater than 75 per cent. The mortality rate is high for other germinal tumors with the exception of adult teratoma. In contrast to choriocarcinoma of the uterus, methotrexate therapy in metastatic choriocarcinoma in the male has been unsatisfactory. A significant remission rate has been reported with treatment of the radioresistant metastatic embryonal tumors by a combination of chlorambucil, methotrexate,

and actinomycin D. However, in a recent survey by Jacobs, few prolonged responses were observed.

Albert, A.: The mammalian testis. *In* Young, W. C. (ed.): Sex and Internal Secretions. 3rd ed. Vol. 1. Baltimore, Williams and Wilkins Company, 1961.

Bardin, C. W., Ross, G. T., and Lipsett, M. B.: Site of action of clomiphene citrate in men: A study of the pituitary–Leydig cell axis. J. Clin. Endocr., 27:1558, 1967.

Bardin, C. W., Ross, G. T., Rifkind, A. B., Cargille, C. M., and Lipsett, M. B.: Studies of the pituitary–Leydig cell axis in young men with hypogonadotropic hypogonadism and hyposmia: comparison with normal men, prepubertal boys, and hypopituitary patients. J. Clin. Invest., 48:2046, 1969.

Court Brown, W. M.: Males with an XYY sex chromosome complement. J. Med. Genet., 5;341, 1968.

Dorfman, R. I., and Shipley, R. A.: Androgens: Biochemistry, Physiology, and Clinical Significance. New York, John Wiley & Sons, Inc., 1956.

Drucker, W. D., Blanc, W. A., Rowland, L. P., Grumbach, M. M., and Christy, N. P.: The testis in myotonic muscular dystrophy: A clinical and pathologic study with a comparison with the Klinefelter syndrome. J. Clin. Endocr., 23:59, 1963.

Faiman, C., Hoffman, D. L., Ryan, R. J., and Albert, A.: The "fertile eunuch" syndrome: Demonstration of isolated luteinizing hormone deficiency by radioimmunoassay technique. Mayo Clin. Proc., 43:661, 1968.

Faiman, C., and Ryan, R. J.: Radioimmunoassay for human follicle stimulating hormone. J. Clin. Endocr., 27:444, 1967.

Gloyna, R. E., and Wilson, J. D.: A comparative study of the conversion of testosterone to 17β-hydroxy-5α-androstan-3-one (dihydrotestosterone) by prostate and epididymis. J. Clin. Endocr., 29:970, 1969.

Grumbach, M. M.: The male reproductive system. *In* Cooke, R. E. (ed.): Biologic Basis of Pediatric Practice. New York, McGraw-Hill Book Company, 1967.

Hand, J. R.: Treatment of undescended testis and its complications. J.A.M.A., 164:185, 1957.

Jacobs, E. M.: Combination chemotherapy of metastatic testicular germinal cell tumors and soft part sarcomas. Cancer, 25:324, 1970.

Landing, B. H., Wells, T. R., and Wang, C. I.: Abnormality of the epididymis and vas deferens in cystic fibrosis. Arch. Path. (Chicago), 88:569, 1969.

Lipsett, M. B.: The testis. *In* Bondy, P. K. (ed.): Duncan's Diseases of Metabolism. 6th ed. Philadelphia, W. B. Saunders Company, 1969.

Mancini, R. E., Seiguer, A. C., and Perez Lloret, A.: Effect of gonadotropins on the recovery of spermatogenesis in hypophysectomized patients. J. Clin. Endocr., 29:467, 1969.

Marshall, W. A., and Tanner, J. M.: Variations in the pattern of pubertal changes in boys. Arch. Dis. Childh., 45:13, 1970.

Martin, F. I. R.: The stimulation and prolonged maintenance of spermatogenesis by human pituitary gonadotrophins in a patient with hypogonadotrophic hypogonadism. J. Endocr., 38:431, 1967.

Moore, K. L. (ed.): The Sex Chromatin. Philadelphia, W. B. Saunders Company, 1966.

Nowakowski, H., and Lenz, W.: Genetic aspects in male hypogonadism. Recent Progr. Hormone Res., 17:53, 1961.

Odell, W. D., Ross, G. T., and Rayford, P. L.: Radioimmunoassay for luteinizing hormone in human plasma or serum: Physiological studies. J. Clin. Invest., 46:248, 1967.

Paulsen, C. A.: The testes. *In* Williams, R. H. (ed.): Textbook of Endocrinology. 4th ed. Philadelphia, W. B. Saunders Company, 1968.

Paulsen, C. A., Gordon, D. L., Carpenter, R. W., Gandy, H. M., and Drucker, W. D.: Klinefelter's syndrome and its variants: A hormonal and chromosomal study. Recent Progr. Hormone Res., 24:321, 1968.

Pearson, P. L., Borrow, M., and Vosa, A. G.: Technique for identifying Y chromosomes in human interphase nuclei. Nature, 226:78, 1970.

Peterson, N. T., Jr., Midgley, A. R., and Jaffe, R. B.: Regulation of human gonadotropins. III. Luteinizing hormone and follicle stimulating hormone in sera from adult males. J. Clin. Endocr., 28:1473, 1968.

Scorer, C. G.: The descent of the testis. Arch. Dis. Child., 39:204, 1964.

Swanson, D. W., and Stipes, A. H.: Psychiatric aspects of Klinefelter's syndrome. Amer. J. Psychiat., 126:814, 1969.

Van Wyk, J. J., and Grumbach, M. M.: Disorders of sex differentiation. *In* Williams, R. H. (ed.): Textbook of Endocrinology. 4th ed. Philadelphia, W. B. Saunders Company, 1968.

Whitmore, W. F.: Some experiences with retroperitoneal lymph node dissection and chemotherapy in the management of testis neoplasms. Brit. J. Urol., 34:436, 1962.

Wilkins, L.: The Diagnosis and Treatment of Endocrine Disorders in Childhood and Adolescence. 3rd ed. Springfield, Ill., Charles C Thomas, 1965.

THE OVARIES
Nathan Kase

OVARIAN STRUCTURE AND FUNCTION

The human ovary has a dual physiologic responsibility: (1) development and release of ova and (2) elaboration of estrogen and progesterone. From menarche to menopause both these activities are bound to the cycle of follicle development, ovulation, corpus luteum formation, and regression. In reality each ovary is a heterogeneous, cyclically changing tissue containing subunits with differing properties. During their brief interval of dominance each subunit defines the function of the total organ. The sequential appearance of each unit and their respective gametogenic and endocrine performances are directed by pituitary secretion of varying quantities of gonadotrophins: follicle stimulating hormone (FSH) and luteinizing hormone (LH). Release of these factors is controlled by specific neurosecretory substances originating in hypothalamic nuclei that are sensitive to "feedback" levels of circulating ovarian hormones.

The ovary contains specialized cells in the cortical and medullary areas that may contribute to abnormal ovarian function in certain pathologic conditions, but its major elements are the follicle and corpus luteum. The follicle consists of the ovum and two layers of tissue surrounding it: an inner band of granulosa cells without blood vessels, and an outer vascularized mantle of theca cells. At any given time in the preovulatory phase a number of follicles display varying degrees of developmental maturity, cystic changes, hormonal activity, and atresia. The factors responsible for the selection of one to attain full maturity and ovulation while others atrophy are unknown. Morphologic clues indicating development of a follicle are the degree of thecal proliferation and vascularity and the ratio of granulosa layer thickening and cystic dilation. The formation of a true corpus luteum is a direct consequence of final maturation and ovulation of the follicle. The ruptured follicle is transformed by proliferation, vascularization, and luteinization of the granulosa into the yellow body that characterizes the last two weeks of an ovulatory cycle. Contrary to evidence obtained in other mammals, the human corpus luteum appears to possess an inherent life span of two weeks, during which it is sustained by modest postovulatory pituitary secretion of LH. Following this period, the corpus luteum recedes unless renewed major trophic stimulation appears in the form of human chorionic gonadotrophin originating in an embedded trophoblast.

OVARIAN HORMONE FUNCTION— THE ENDOMETRIAL CYCLE

It is helpful to consider the function of ovarian hormones relative to their ability to provide an appropriate milieu for fertilization, implantation, and nutrition of the early embryo. Before menstruation has ceased, preparation for a more successful ovum is resumed. FSH and small quantities of LH renew follicle growth and augment estrogen secretion. Under the influence of estradiol and estrone, endothelial and mucosal repair takes place. In the ensuing fortnight continued estrogen stimulation produces growth of glands and spiral arterioles. These vessels remain unbranched to the periphery where a terminal capillary network is formed. Accompanying this proliferation, endometrial expansion is accomplished by accumulation of ground substance and modest edema of the stroma. This estrogen-induced phenomenon unfolds the collapsed stromal reticulum. In this way follicle estrogen produces an endometrium with sufficient height, vascularity, and concentrations of glycogen and protein to satisfy the early requirements of the anticipated embryo. Furthermore, estrogen-dependent changes in cervical mucus aid sperm migration.

The midcycle preovulatory peak of estrogen probably signals the release of pituitary LH. The brief surge of this gonadotrophin induces acute follicle distention. By unknown mechanisms necrosis of the thinned follicle wall occurs, leading to capsular rupture and permitting extrusion of the ovum. The corpus luteum is formed, and secretion of progesterone rapidly increases. This hormone and sustained levels of estrogen combine to inhibit further LH secretion.

In the absence of a conceptus, at day 12 post ovulation, the corpus luteum recedes and hormone levels wane. With stromal cell shrinkage and loss of ground substance, the endometrium thins. The vessels buckle, and diminished peripheral blood flow is reduced further by tonic vasoconstriction of spiral arterioles. Localized peripheral ischemia and fragmentation occur, with progressive hemorrhage and disruption of superficial zones of the endometrium. With the loss of the peripheral binding epithelium, menstruation begins.

OVARIAN STEROID BIOSYNTHESIS

It is clear that appropriate target organ processes are dependent on periodic variations in the

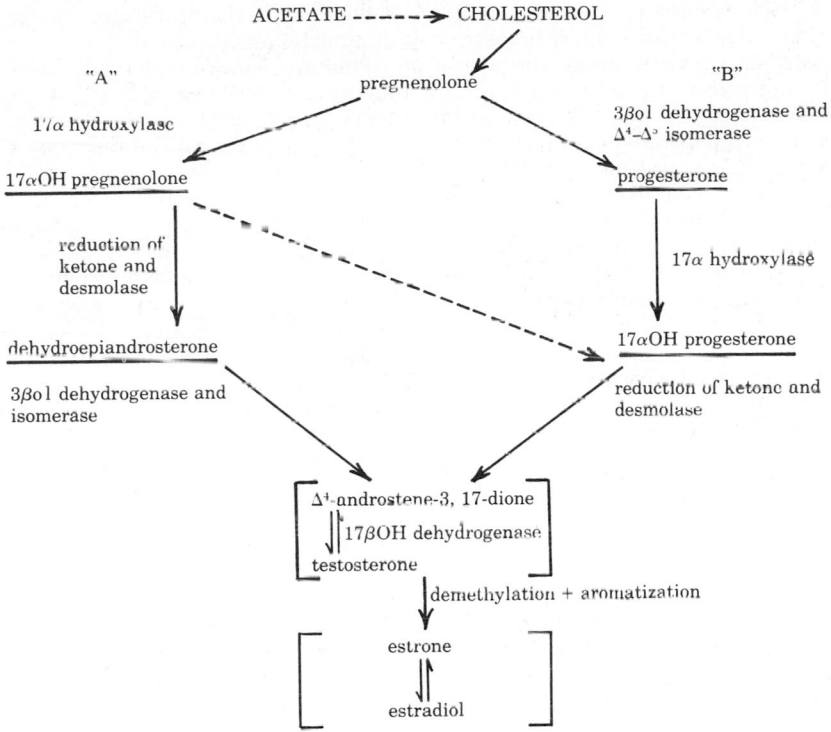

quantity and type of hormone emanating from the ovary. How does the ovary accomplish the initial production of microgram quantities of estrogen and then milligram secretion of progesterone? The in vitro analyses of Ryan, utilizing isolated follicles and corpora lutea and radioactive steroid precursors, have contributed significantly to the understanding of these processes. This work confirmed the accumulated evidence bearing on the dominance of two biosynthetic pathways leading to estrogen production in the ovary. These routes (A and B) are depicted in the accompanying scheme. Route A provides for conversion of pregnenolone to estrogen via a pathway in which the 3βol Δ⁵ characteristic is maintained to the C₁₉ stage. On the other hand, route B projects immediate conversion of pregnenolone to progesterone (change from Δ⁵-3βol to Δ⁴-3 ketone in ring A) prior to loss of sidechain and estrogen generation. Ryan's data suggest that, whereas the corpus luteum utilizes the pathway via progesterone ("B"), the follicle employs route "A," bypassing formation of this biologically active intermediate. Individual cell studies have shown that granulosa and theca cells have similar biosynthetic capabilities and that only quantitative differences exist between these tissues. Apparently both granulosa and theca cells are necessary for adequate steroid production in biologic studies.

There are broader endocrine implications in the biosynthetic mechanisms depicted in the figure. With certain notable exceptions, such as the 11 hydroxylation property of the adrenal cortex, it is apparent that all steroid-producing organs make steroids in roughly the same manner. The biosynthetic pathways require the presence

of biologically active steroids other than those typically secreted by a gland, but these are normally not apparent clinically. However, disordered activity of these pathways in certain ovarian disease leads to abnormal levels of secretion of these active intermediates with clinically demonstrable hormone effects.

Everett, J. W.: Central neural control of reproductive functions of the adenohypophysis. Physiol. Rev., 44:373, 1964.
Guillemin, R · The adenohypophysis and its hypothalamic control. Ann. Rev. Physiol. 29:313, 1967.
Hisaw, F. L.: Development of the graafian follicle and ovulation. Physiol. Rev., 27:95, 1947.
Rock, J., Garcia, C-R., and Menkin, M.: A theory of menstruation. Ann. N. Y. Acad. Sci., 75:831, 1959.
Ryan, K., and Smith, O. V.: Biogenesis of steroid hormones in the human ovary. Recent Prog. Hormone Res., 21:367, 1965.
Vande Wiele, R. L., et al.: Mechanisms regulating the menstrual cycle in women. Rec. Prog. Hormone Research. New York, Academic Press, Inc., 1970.

OVARIAN DISORDERS PERTINENT TO GENERAL MEDICINE

EVALUATION OF OVARIAN FUNCTION

The simple existence of ovarian function may be inferred from the development and maintenance of the breasts and the internal and external genitalia. However, a range of ovarian secretion essential to the full activity of these organs is more critically expressed by the periodic phenomenon of ovulatory menstruation. It is helpful to group disorders of ovarian function within the following descriptive categories:

Sexual precocity: the onset of menses prior to the age of ten years or development of breasts or pubic (not vulvar) hair growth before the age of eight years. Although these elements may appear as isolated manifestations, this general term usually applies to premature appearance of all three aspects of sexual maturation.

Primary amenorrhea: the delay of menarche beyond the age of 18. Statistically 5 per cent of girls initiate menses after 16 and 1 per cent after age 18. In the presence of breast development, pubic hair growth, and a normal adolescent growth spurt, diagnostic evaluation of delayed menarche may be postponed until 18.

Secondary amenorrhea: the cessation of uterine bleeding at any age in women who have previously menstruated. The elapsed interval of amenorrhea necessary for the diagnosis cannot be rigidly defined, and is often dictated by other clinical factors. However, if the patient has not bled within a length of time equivalent to three or four of her normal cycles, then investigation is warranted.

Oligomenorrhea: a recurrent prolongation of intermenstrual intervals leading to a decreased frequency of menses (three to six per year). This irregularity is commonly seen in postmenarchal and premenopausal women. In the absence of other signs and symptoms, intensive work-up is not required at these times. Evaluation is in order in other age groups because anovulatory infertility is frequently associated with this menstrual anomaly.

Hypomenorrhea: a diminution in the quantity of menstrual flow based on tampon or napkin requirement. It is of little diagnostic significance if found as a solitary problem. Investigation beyond a physical examination, which includes a pelvic examination and cytologic smear, is unnecessary.

Hypermenorrhea: a definite relative increase in duration and/or quantity of menstrual flow that occurs at normal cycle intervals. A subgrouping called *polymenorrhea* designates menstrual flow close to normal in quantity and duration but which recurs too frequently (less than 21 days apart). Each group requires immediate gynecologic assessment. Because each is frequently associated with anovulation, endocrine evaluation may also be in order.

AIDS TO DIAGNOSIS

The clinical categories just described represent a spectrum of abnormal ovarian function manifested in terms of sexual development, menstrual regularity, and ovulation. Such malfunction may be caused by primary ovarian disease, abnormal stimulation of the ovary by other glands, disease of target organs, or systemic disease. Steps to appropriate diagnosis begin with a complete history and physical examination, including careful examination of the pelvic organs and external genitalia. When properly selected, certain pro-

cedures and laboratory tests can be of considerable diagnostic assistance:

Pituitary Gonadotrophin Function. Depending on laboratory preference, the 24-hour urinary excretion of "total" gonadotrophin may be bioassayed in terms of the response of the immature mouse uterus or rat ovaries. Values are expressed in mouse uterine weight units (m.u.u.) or rat units (r.u.) with a normal adult range of 6.5 to 104 m.u.u. or 5 to 30 r.u. per 24 hours. Prepubertal girls excrete total gonadotrophin below detectable levels. Variations within normal range have no diagnostic significance. Values above normal support the diagnosis of ovarian failure. Repeated absence of gonadotrophins in urine implies hypogonadotrophism as a basis for hypogonadism. Although radioimmunoassay data on FSH and LH in serum in these categories are being accumulated, widespread clinical availability of these more specific tests is not yet realized.

Ovarian Function. Tests that are based on biologic effects of ovarian hormones are simply performed, providing immediate and valuable data at little cost to the patient. Therefore, more costly laboratory evaluation of hormone excretion is rarely required for clinical purposes.

Hormone Effects. *Cornification of vaginal epithelium.* The percentage of fully cornified cells is related to ovarian estrogen production. Because cytologic criteria and staining methods vary from center to center, no normal values can be given. However, because other factors affect this evaluation (progesterone, cortisone, and androgen diminish, although digitalis increases cornification), the stage of the cycle as well as current therapy must be considered in evaluation of test results.

Endometrial biopsy tests endometrial responsiveness as well as the existence of appropriate ovarian hormone secretion during the cycle. Evaluation must take into consideration the stage of the cycle when the biopsy specimen is taken.

In addition to the quantity and clarity of *cervical mucus,* the development of an arborization pattern in a dried specimen (*the "fern" test*) indicates the presence of estrogen. Correlation with cycle dates is essential, for secretion of progesterone inhibits this phenomenon.

The *basal body temperature* will demonstrate the occurrence of ovulation if serial readings are taken throughout a cycle. Based on the mild thermogenic properties of progesterone, a sustained postovulatory rise of temperature (0.4° F.) or more) of two weeks' duration indicates corpus luteum function. Retrospectively, the timing of ovulation in the cycle can be estimated from the date when the effect of progesterone first appeared.

Progesterone withdrawal bleeding. If menses can be induced following administration of progesterone or a nonestrogenic derivative, this event indicates prior ovarian estrogen secretion and its proliferative or "priming" effect on the endometrium.

Hormone Excretion. *Urinary pregnanediol.* In the absence of adrenal disease, excretion of this metabolite in excess of 2.5 mg. per 24 hours indicates the presence of a functioning corpus luteum or pregnancy.

Total urinary estrogens. The wide range of "normal" values (10 to 75 mcg. per 24 hours) reflects the variable functional capability of the ovary during the menstrual cycle. Because only serial determinations are informative, a single test has limited clinical value.

Other tests of importance include those that estimate *adrenal cortex and thyroid activity.* Specific details concerning interpretation of results and the diagnostic manipulations involved are given in other sections of this text. Dysfunction of either organ may have pronounced effects on ovarian and target organ physiology.

MENARCHE

The initiation of menstrual function in humans occurs with greatest frequency at age 12 or 13, but there is a considerable "normal" variation in the time of its onset. When menstruation begins before the age of 10 or after 16, a decision must be made whether the precocious or delayed menarche is a physiologic variant or whether it is due to some abnormality.

Certain aspects of the neuroendocrine mechanism involved in normal menarche have been uncovered. It has been shown that the anterior pituitary of infants contains adequate quantities of gonadotrophins and that an intact pituitary is essential for the prepubertal development and maintenance of the gonads. Removal of the ovaries in this age group is associated with increased gonadotrophin excretion, the formation of castration cells in the pituitary, and enlargement of the gland. These changes can be prevented by estrogen therapy in very low doses. Therefore, the small quantity of estrogen secreted prepubertally is sufficient to inhibit all but a small clinically undetectable quantity of gonadotrophin release. Further indirect evidence that this central inhibition is the critical mechanism in the *normal* delay of sexual maturation can be seen in the fully responsive competence of the premenarchal ovary to exogenous gonadotrophin therapy. Certain areas in the hypothalamus are believed to be responsible for this temporary extreme sensitivity to inhibiting levels of circulating steroids. Neoplastic and vascular disorders that alter hypothalamic function probably reverse this low threshold inhibition and lead to precocious puberty.

SEXUAL PRECOCITY

Precocity may be due to organic or constitutional (idiopathic) causes. Ninety per cent of patients with this symptom will fall in the latter category despite thorough evaluation. However, it is essential that these cases be distinguished from those with lesions of the brain or the rare diseases of ovary and adrenal that produce premature development.

Constitutional Sexual Precocity. This is due to the premature release of the adult sequence and levels of gonadotrophin, which are sufficient to initiate prematurely the normal physiologic and endocrine processes of breast development, appearance of pubic and axillary hair, and menstruation. Although it is assumed that hypothalamic inhibitory influences have been diminished, the precise inciting factor is unknown. Diminished secretion of inhibitory quantities of melatonin by the pineal gland is a suggested etiologic factor. Generally the normal, orderly, albeit more rapid appearance of breast development, pubic hair growth, and then menarche is found in the five- to eight-year age group. However, menarche may be the first symptom noted and may occur as early as three months of age. The usual sequential maturation pattern may be altered or only partially displayed. Although not all patients will ovulate, biologic manifestations of ovulation rule out precocity based on gonadotrophin-independent estrogen production by ovarian or adrenal disease. Estrogen production from any source is likely to induce accelerated linear growth and advancement of bone age, which is seen best in roentgenograms of carpal bones, knee, and elbow. Although these children are temporarily taller than their normal counterparts, premature closure of epiphyses produces a final height that is less than normal. Thus the diagnostic criteria for a constitutional etiology of precocity include: the sequence of secondary sex characteristics, advanced bone age, adult levels of estrogen and gonadotrophin, normal urinary adrenal metabolites, and normal neurologic examination and skull films. Optimal therapy (reversible suppression of gonadotrophins without peripheral target organ stimulation) may be achievable with long-acting nonestrogenic depomedroxyprogesterone acetate.

These children present a serious emotional and social problem not only because they are distinctly different from their contemporaries, but also because they are insufficiently mature emotionally to cope with the sexual interest they provoke in others. That they are capable of reproduction has been demonstrated many times, but most dramatically in the case of a Peruvian girl, Lena Medina, who was delivered of a normal child by cesarean section at five and a half years of age.

Precocity Due to Organic Causes. *Cerebral Lesions.* A variety of brain disorders produce sexual precocity secondary to premature gonadotrophin release, presumably by the abolition of the inhibitory effects of the hypothalamus. Although the anatomic location of these inhibitory centers is uncertain, three general groups of tumors may cause precocity: lesions in the tuber cinereum, lesions in the posterior hypothalamic mammillary body area, and lesions destroying the pineal. In addition, disorders indirectly affecting hypothalamic function (internal hydrocephalus, encephalitis, meningitis, and cranial trauma) may be associated with precocity. Differential diagnosis of this type of precocity from the constitutional variety cannot be achieved by endocrine survey. Only after intensive neurologic, roentgenographic, and pediatric evaluation and follow-up reappraisal will proper diagnosis be made.

Organic Precocious Pseudopuberty Due to Adrenal and Ovarian Hyperfunction. The term pseudopuberty defines the basic difference between precocity due to premature gonadotrophic activity (constitutional, central types) and those lesions in which adrenal and ovarian estrogen stimulates target organs. In the latter, gonadotrophin is absent, and therefore ovulation does not occur.

Although certain elements of premature maturation (pubic hair, bone age advancement) appear in adrenal disorders, the masculinization and rarity of vaginal bleeding (delayed menarche is usual) make the diagnosis relatively simple. Isosexual pseudopuberty is more commonly associated with estrogen-producing ovarian tumors. Although the diagnosis of tumor is always considered, it is rarely confirmed. Only 5 per cent of *granulosa tumors* occur before true puberty. The presence of a palpable adnexal mass and the absence of urinary gonadotrophin, ovulation, and regular cyclic bleeding support the diagnosis. In addition, the exceedingly rare *teratoma or dysgerminoma* of the ovary may be associated with pseudopuberty. However, these will sometimes pose a diagnostic complication. The production of chorionic gonadotrophin by these tumors will give falsely elevated adult levels of "FSH" in mouse uterine weight tests in addition to positive pregnancy tests. Absence of pubic hair and the finding of an ovarian mass call for laparotomy.

Albright's syndrome, consisting of cystic bone lesions, patchy skin pigmentation, and sexual precocity, is grouped with pseudopuberty in that gonadotrophin excretion and ovulation are absent. Normal puberty and ovulation follow and fertility is not decreased.

DISORDERS OF MENSTRUAL FUNCTION

Delayed Menarche and Primary Amenorrhea

Menarche may be delayed beyond the age of 16 years on a constitutional basis and often as a familial trait. In these instances there is no demonstrable organic lesion, and with time normal periods appear. However, some cases of delayed menarche are not benign, and these bring up the vexing problem of which patients in this age group require intensive work-up. In general, delayed menarche accompanied by any of the following signs requires full evaluation to prevent worsening of the underlying condition, which is only initially presenting as delayed menstruation: absence of other secondary sexual characteristics, symptoms and signs of outflow tract incompetence, systemic disorders (neurogenic, obesity, cachexia,

thyroid and adrenal disease), psychiatric disorders, signs of abnormal chromosomal constitution.

Lacking these associated conditions, delayed menarche may be managed by sympathetic reassurance of the likelihood of eventual establishment of normal menses.

Should menarche be delayed beyond the age of 18, *primary amenorrhea* is said to exist. The diagnostic investigation of this entity is best oriented to assessment of the various anatomic sites involved in the generation and transport of menstrual fluid. These include the vaginal tract, uterus, ovaries, the pituitary, and the hypothalamus.

Mechanical Obstruction. Mechanical obstruction at the hymen or in the vaginal or cervical canal will prevent drainage of uterine secretions. Such stenosis is usually congenital but may be secondary to infection. Outward signs of menses will be absent, but periodic vaginal or lower abdominal pain and the presence of a mass on rectal or vaginal examination will be noted. Depending on the site and duration of obstruction, hematocolpos, hematometra, and/or hematosalpinx will be present.

Absence or Unresponsiveness of the Endometrium. This will present as primary amenorrhea. Agenesis of the uterus is rare, as are the "acquired" lesions such as tuberculosis, radiation, and postsepsis obliteration of the endometrium and uterine cavity, which render this organ incapable of reacting to normal cyclic levels of estrogen.

Primary Hypogonadism. Amenorrhea is the basic symptom of primary hypogonadism. The most common cause of primary ovarian failure is *Turner's syndrome,* which can be recognized by associated anomalies, short stature, chromatin-negative buccal smear, XO karyotype, and castration levels of urinary gonadotrophin. However, in some instances the condition is not so obvious, there being reported exceptions and variations in each of the diagnostic criteria, including the temporary presence of menses. A disorder of ovarian function evidenced morphologically by polycystic changes, although more commonly associated with secondary amenorrhea (*vide infra*), may also produce primary amenorrhea.

Adrenal and Thyroid Disease and Diabetes Mellitus. These may be accompanied by primary amenorrhea or, more commonly, secondary amenorrhea, despite the presence of normal ovaries.

Inadequate Gonadotrophins. Although ovaries and external genitalia may be otherwise normal, menses will not appear if gonadotrophin stimulation of these organs is insufficient or absent. Causes of this hypogonadotrophic hypogonadism are best considered according to their anatomic distribution. Intrasellar lesions such as pituitary cysts, tumors, and infarction may interfere not only with gonadotrophin secretion but with the entire range of pituitary responsibilities. On the other hand, depending on a tumor's initial size and growth tendencies, amenorrhea may be the first sign of a disorder that by further encroachment gradually progresses to panhypopituitarism. Except for growth hormone, gonadotrophin secretion appears to be the most sensitive to adverse alterations in intrasellar pressures and blood flow.

Suprasellar disorders will also produce primary or secondary amenorrhea by diminishing gonadotrophin release. Aneurysm of the internal carotid artery, tumor, and internal hydrocephalus with expansion of the third ventricle are among the lesions reported. Hypogonadism, diminished adrenal and thyroid function, and short stature are seen in these conditions.

Amenorrhea due to isolated hypogonadotrophism without eventual impairment of other trophic hormones is common. The frequent association of this physiologic aberration (which reverses spontaneously in a high proportion of cases) with severe systemic illness, obesity, and emotional trauma should be noted.

"Testicular Feminization Syndrome." This syndrome consists of chromatin-negativity, primary amenorrhea, a mature feminine appearance, and abdominal, inguinal, or labial testes. The name is unfortunate, for Morris has shown that the basic defect is not in testicular steroid production, but is an interference in the mechanism of action of androgen at the target tissue level. Inability to form the biologically active dihydrotestosterone at the target is a suggested explanation for androgen insensitivity in these subjects. Thus, axillary and pubic hair are scant, the clitoris is small, and although only rudimentary oviducts are present and the uterus absent, nevertheless there is no wolffian duct stimulation. Exogenous androgen does not masculinize these patients. Differentiation of the complete syndrome from an incomplete type displaying clitoral enlargement, inactive gonads, and variably androgen-sensitive target tissue can be accomplished. Therapy in either form of the syndrome is castration and sufficient exogenous estrogen to maintain serviceable external genitalia in support of the female sex role with which these patients permanently identify.

Because the diagnostic evaluation and therapy of the lesions involved in primary and secondary amenorrhea are similar, these matters will be discussed in later paragraphs.

Secondary Amenorrhea

An alteration in the frequency of menstruation is a sensitive indication of ovarian dysfunction. Therefore, the most serious form of menstrual aberration is the appearance of secondary amenorrhea. Its onset may be marked by the abrupt cessation of previously normal cycles, or it may follow menses of diminishing frequency (oligomenorrhea). It is well to remember that certain physiologic states predispose to amenorrhea. Absence of periodic menstruation in any adult female should suggest the possibility of pregnancy. Furthermore, amenorrhea of varying length will frequently be associated with the puerperium and the immediate postmenarchal and premenopausal periods. Finally, the menopause is an irreversible state of ovarian inactivity and amenorrhea.

Not all instances of secondary amenorrhea have a hormonal basis. As noted in the discussion of primary amenorrheas, acquired anatomic disorders must be considered in the differential diagnosis of absent menstruation. Stenotic lesions obstructing the egress of uterine discharge may result from scarring induced by infection, chemical burns, and operative trauma. Similarly, endocervical carcinoma may diminish the caliber of the cervical canal. As always, pelvic examination is essential to proper evaluation of absent menses. Destruction of the endometrium will also produce amenorrhea despite the presence of normal cyclical ovarian hormone secretion. This condition may result from tuberculous endometritis or may be secondary to overzealous curettage performed to reverse unremitting hemorrhage occurring at abortion, post partum, or at withdrawal from prolonged anovulatory cycles. In the latter instances of iatrogenic endometrial failure, investigation of the uterine cavity by means of hysterography may reveal cavitary distortions and obliteration due to uterine synechia (*Asherman's syndrome*). Operative disruption of uterine defects and intensive estrogen therapy may reverse this situation. Finally, temporary endometrial inactivity may be inadvertently induced with the use of newer progestational agents, particularly of the long-acting intramuscular type (depo-medroxyprogesterone acetate). Protracted release of hormone leads to persistent amenorrhea and typical progestin-induced endometrial morphologic changes. Although most cases spontaneously reverse within a few months, periods may not recur for one or two years.

These local matters aside, the major diagnostic issues in secondary amenorrhea deal with evaluation of the integrity of the pituitary-ovarian servomechanism. Unfortunately, pituitary-ovarian relationships do not adhere to an "all or none" principle. If one assumes adequate gonadotrophin stimulation, it appears that not all cycles will be ovulatory or of equal length. Some cycles will be climaxed by ovulation only after a prolonged preovulatory phase. Other cycles may be anovulatory although cycle length displays no variation. The basic question in the pathogenesis of this relative hypogonadism is whether ovulation is due to inadequate or improper gonadotrophic stimulation or to an inherent unresponsiveness of certain follicles. As the follicle grows, additional intraovarian factors potentiate or diminish the response of the follicle to the stimulatory effect of FSH. Estradiol, by a local effect, stimulates the growth of the follicle even in the absence of FSH and also enhances its response to FSH. Inhibition of this reactivity is observed with androgens.

Although clinical experiments with exogenous

gonadotrophin therapy indicate some ovarian control over follicle maturation, most cases manifesting anovulatory amenorrhea and "normal" total gonadotrophins are probably ascribable to improper gonadotrophin stimulation. Abnormal quantity or sequence of gonadotrophin secretion may result from local disturbances of the hypothalamic-hypophyseal control mechanisms induced by emotional stress, precipitous weight changes, and systemic disease. On the other hand, these control centers may be misdirected by feedback levels of hormones of unusual type and quantity resulting from thyroid disease, adrenal disease, functioning ovarian tumors, and probably ovarian dysfunctions such as the Stein-Leventhal syndrome. Undoubtedly these conditions also affect ovarian reactivity to gonadotrophins, leading to disturbed or arrested follicle maturation seen in systemic disease as well as local pelvic disorders, including chronic pelvic infection, endometriosis, and uterine fibromyomas. Finally, absence of gonadotrophin secretion will result from a variety of insidiously destructive intrasellar and suprasellar disorders. As in primary amenorrheas, these lesions may produce isolated gonadotrophic insufficiency that may progress to diffuse panhypopituitarism.

Pituitary and Suprasellar Lesions. Altered menses may be the earliest sign of an otherwise asymptomatic pituitary tumor. At first, small lesions interfere with cyclic variations in gonadotrophin release, but urinary excretion of total gonadotrophin is unaffected. However, with increasing size and encroachment on production sites, diminished or absent gonadotrophin obtains. Eventually further enlargement leads to more obvious neurologic, ophthalmic, and roentgenologic signs. At this point other trophic hormone deficiencies occur, leading to the complex endocrine metabolic derangements of panhypopituitarism. Aneurysm of the internal carotid artery, tumor of the third ventricle, glioma of the optic chiasm, obstruction of the aqueduct of Sylvius, and meningioma of the floor of the anterior fossa may simulate pituitary tumor and produce amenorrhea. Similarly, functioning tumors of the pituitary will be associated with specific clinical patterns of acromegaly and Cushing's disease as well as amenorrhea. Extensive non-neoplastic pituitary damage may result from necrosis associated with postpartum hemorrhage or obstetric shock. In a series of studies concerning this entity spanning three decades, Sheehan has shown that almost total destruction of the anterior pituitary substance must exist before panhypopituitarism occurs. It is therefore understandable that a prolonged course of progressive deterioration is seen in a variety of lesions of the central nervous system. Gonadotrophic function is the first deficiency to appear clinically, although impaired growth hormone reaction to arginine or insulin-induced hypoglycemia is an earlier but usually occult event. Less often, only gonadotrophin inadequacy will exist. Although this may be associated with persistent lactation (*vide infra*), other patients display perfectly normal trophic responses save gonadotrophin inadequacy (psychogenic stress, obesity, and variants of anorexia nervosa).

Ovarian Lesions. Two major causes of ovarian amenorrhea are (a) inability of the ovary to react to appropriate gonadotrophic stimulation, (b) ovarian production of abnormal quantities of steroids, disrupting central nervous system control of cyclic gonadotrophin.

Irreversible ovarian failure is characterized by diminished ovarian steroid hormones and high total urinary gonadotrophins. *Premature menopause* exists when cessation of menses occurs prior to the age of 40 and is associated with the findings of hypergonadotrophic hypogonadism. The pathogenesis of this impairment of ovarian function is unknown. Somewhat better understood is the ovarian failure associated with the various forms of gonadal dysgenesis. In these instances reactive ovarian substrate is either absent or rapidly depleted, resulting in hypogonadism. In this regard, it is important to remember that not all of these patients have primary amenorrhea, and some (as many as 20 per cent) are chromatin-positive.

The *polycystic ovary syndrome (Stein-Leventhal syndrome)* is perhaps the best example of arrested ovarian follicle maturation associated with non-cyclic "dampening" of the pituitary-ovarian servomechanism. To be sure, infrequent anovulatory cycles may occur in normally menstruating, fertile women. As has been noted, some women will exhibit varying degrees of reversible hypogonadism characterized by limited fertility and irregular cycles. The Stein-Leventhal syndrome, therefore, is the severest form of a spectrum of ovarian follicle disorders associated with anovulation.

As originally described in 1935, this syndrome consists of menstrual abnormality, either oligomenorrhea or amenorrhea, anovulatory infertility, and the development of hirsutism, which occurs in about half the patients. Though insidiously progressive facial hirsutism and acne may exist, and a male pubic escutcheon may be noted, other signs of masculinization are absent. Obesity is no longer considered an important feature of the condition. The ovaries are bilaterally enlarged by the presence of multiple follicle cysts (never more than 1 cm. in diameter), which lie just beneath a thickened, smooth, and pale ovarian capsule. Each rotund, expanded ovary is equal in size to or is larger than the uterine fundus, which is often smaller than normal. Microscopically, the ovaries reveal hyperplastic fibrosis of the cortical stroma and unusual thickening and luteinization of the theca cells surrounding the ubiquitous follicle cysts. Evidence of ovulation (corpora lutea) is rarely found. This finding is reflected in the endometrium, which is proliferative or hyperplastic. Patients with concomitant endometrial carcinoma have been reported.

Although the structural changes of the ovary

were once thought to be pathognomonic of the syndrome, similar ovarian changes have been found in association with other disorders, such as adrenal hyperplasia, to which anovulatory amenorrhea is secondary. Because bilateral wedge resection of ovaries in properly selected patients leads to reversal of the syndrome in 90 per cent of cases, accurate differential diagnosis prior to surgery is the critical feature in the management of this syndrome. However, preliminary clinical classification is difficult to achieve, and diagnosis and therapy proceed by exclusion of other entities associated with amenorrhea.

The cause of the polycystic ovary syndrome is unknown. Originally it was believed that the thickened tunica presented a mechanical barrier to ovum extrusion, which was overcome by the wedge operation. However, it has been shown that removal of one ovary allows ovulation to occur in the remaining undisturbed ovary. Similarly, morphologically indistinguishable ovaries associated with adrenal hyperplasia readily ovulate when the primary disease is treated with cortisone.

A variety of evidence indicates that abnormal levels of a circulating biologically active androgen such as testosterone, regardless of organ source, are a factor in the production of the polycystic ovary syndrome. The association of polycystic ovaries with a virilizing syndrome of adrenal origin, the induction of polycystic ovaries in laboratory animals with exogenous testosterone, and the finding that the polycystic ovary itself is a potent source of this steroid support this thesis.

It may be concluded that wedge resection is effective if the procedure frees follicle maturation from the local suppressive effects of high concentrations of intraovarian androgen and decreases the secretion of androgen, permitting pituitary-ovarian relationships to return to normal cyclic secretion. Observations of LH excretion are in keeping with this view. Excretion patterns of this gonadotrophin are elevated and noncyclic in typical Stein-Leventhal cases as well as in cases of adrenal hyperplasia. Both conditions are characterized by excess androgen and anovulatory amenorrhea. A similar basis for contralateral ovarian dysfunction may be predicted for virilizing ovarian tumors such as arrhenoblastoma and hilus cell and adrenal rest tumors.

Consideration of the etiology of the Stein-Leventhal syndrome projects a differential diagnosis based on delineation of the source of excess androgen. Unfortunately, specific measurement of this steroid in blood or urine is not routinely available. Furthermore, the unusual biologic activity of testosterone allows considerable endocrine function to exist without alteration in androgen metabolite urinary excretion. For this reason the 17-ketosteroids are usually within normal limits. This characteristic assists in differentiating abnormalities of the adrenal cortex in which 17-ketosteroids, corticoids, pregnanetriol, 11-oxygenated 17-ketosteroids, and other metabolites specifically produced by the adrenal are elevated.

At the moment, the diagnosis (*vide infra*) of the Stein-Leventhal syndrome is made by exclusion of adrenal and pituitary abnormality.

Adrenal Disease. For more detailed description of these entities the reader is referred to other sections of this text.

Thyroid Disease. The practice of administering small doses of thyroid hormone preparations to basically euthyroid women with menstrual irregularities unfortunately is still prevalent. Delay of adequate work-up thus incurred compounds the basic physiologic irrationality of this approach. In fact, only patients with advanced thyroid disease display menstrual irregularities. In hyperthyroidism, as toxicity deepens the menses become less frequent, amenorrhea indicating a severe disorder. On the other hand, though oligomenorrhea is sometimes seen in hypothyroidism, menometrorrhagia is the rule, particularly in myxedema. In hypothyroidism secondary to hypopituitarism, of course, amenorrhea is a constant finding.

Systemic Disease. Throughout the discussion of the amenorrheas, it has been emphasized that details of the etiologic mechanisms involved are lacking. This issue is most acute in the consideration of the evolution of ovarian dysfunction secondary to chronic illnesses such as hepatic and renal disease, diabetes, anemia, etc. In addition to glands of internal secretion, the adequacy of organ systems involved in hormone conjugation, binding, and transport, extraction and excretion, inactivation by metabolism, interconversions of form, and interchange between anatomic pools of differing accessibility critically influence the total effective tissue concentrations of biologically active material.

Evaluation of Amenorrhea

Although understanding of the multiple interdependent factors that regulate menstrual function is admittedly incomplete, current concepts of neuroendocrine target organ relationships permit a relatively simple and precise localization of defective components. This program involves sequential testing of the major elements that produce a menstrual cycle: the endometrium, the ovary, and the hypothalamic pituitary unit. Estimates of modifying systems such as the thyroid and the adrenal cortex are also essential.

The determination of ovarian function can be achieved by a summation of information gathered from basal body temperature curves, appropriately timed cervical changes in mucus, vaginal cornification indexes, endometrial biopsy, and progesterone withdrawal bleeding. Fifty to 100 mg. of progesterone intramuscularly for two days or medroxyprogesterone acetate, 5 to 10 mg. orally for three days, will induce vaginal bleeding in a previously amenorrheic patient if the endometrium has been primed by ovarian estrogen. In this case the integrity of the entire system short of ovulation is confirmed. However, if progesterone withdrawal flow does not occur and the possibility of endometrial failure is eliminated by the appearance of vaginal bleeding following 20 days of diethylstilbestrol, 0.5 mg. twice a day orally, then the lack of estrogen production is due to either ovarian or pituitary failure. Should total urinary gonadotrophin be low or absent, pituitary failure is suggested, and neurologic, roentgenologic, ophthalmologic, and laboratory estimates of its competence are indicated. If gonadotrophins are high, reflecting diminished feedback inhibition, ovarian failure is diagnosed. If confirmation of the diagnosis is desired, challenge of the ovary with exogenous human gonadotrophin can be employed.

Utilizing this technique, amenorrheas can be classified according to the specific area of pituitary-ovarian derangement uncovered: (1) hypergonadotrophic hypogonadal amenorrhea (ovarian failure), (2) hypogonadotrophic hypogonadal amenorrhea (pituitary failure), (3) normogonadotrophic normoestrogenic amenorrhea (anovulation). With definition of these categories, appropriate therapy and management can be evolved.

Treatment of Amenorrhea

The therapy of inadequate ovarian hormone function depends not only on the degree of hormonal failure, but also on the therapeutic objectives. Certainly menstruation is not a necessity, for its absence does not represent a threat to the life expectancy of the patient. Therefore, except in the treatment of infertility, and possibly in rare psychologic situations, a patient need not be treated solely for the purpose of re-creating menstrual cycles. On the other hand, certain patients who show other evidence of estrogen deficiency, such as loss of secondary sex characteristics, deserve substitutive therapy. At no time should artificial cycles be instituted without preliminary investigation to uncover serious underlying lesions.

Hypergonadotrophic Hypogonadism. The patient with gonadal dysgenesis should be given cyclic exogenous estrogen therapy indefinitely for development and maintenance of adequate secondary sexual characteristics. The preliminary use of steroidal anabolic agents to induce growth prior to chronic administration of estrogen that will close epiphyses has been encouraging. The transformation induced by cyclic estrogen therapy in these otherwise anatomically, biologically, and cosmetically handicapped patients is particularly gratifying. Among the oral regimens available, stilbestrol, 0.5 mg. twice daily for 20 days, is satisfactory; during the last 5 days of stilbestrol treatment, the addition of 5 mg. daily of medroxy-progesterone acetate orally provides endometrial stability and controlled withdrawal flow.

The woman with premature ovarian failure (before the age of 40 years) presents a somewhat different therapeutic problem. In this situation replacement medication is required to sustain systems already developed and dependent upon ovarian hormone secretion. Patients of this type are concerned about not only secondary amenorrhea and the termination of their reproductive capabilities but also the usually severe vasomotor symptoms that attend this type of ovarian failure. It is of interest that these *hot flashes* are not seen in primary hypogonadism, although urinary gonadotrophins are elevated in both conditions. Probably as a consequence of these disabilities and the fear of further restrictions, there are various subjective symptoms such as depression, anxiety, and loss of libido. No satisfactory treatment of this condition exists at the present time except substitution therapy with estrogen. Control of vasomotor instability, preservation of a serviceable vagina, and maintenance of other feminine aspects including menses are possible with cyclic stilbestrol (0.5 mg. every day), Premarin (1.25 mg. every day), or Estinyl (0.05 mg. every day). Again, the terminal addition of progestin following 20 days of estrogen is advantageous. It should be noted that these doses of estrogen stimulate menstrual function and are higher than necessary for nonmenstrual metabolic requirements. This point comes into active consideration when determining what, if any, therapy should be given for ovarian failure occurring after the age of 40.

Menopause. The menopause is a physiologic and not a pathologic phenomenon. Menstruation ceases for a variety of reasons at other times of life, but after 40 the ovary becomes atrophic and ceases to respond to gonadotrophic stimulation. No amount of gonadotrophic stimulation can produce activity in the menopausal ovary. It becomes small, pale, and more wrinkled. The few remaining follicles undergo atresia so that none are found within a few years after cessation of menses. Diminution of all ovarian elements proceeds, producing a firm structure one third the size of the active organ.

Vasomotor instability is the only clinical symptom definitely associated with ovarian aging that occurs when otherwise the woman may be active, healthy, and vital physically, emotionally, and mentally. However, because of improved general health, women can expect to live for 20 to 25 years beyond the menopause, and interest has increased in the possible amelioration of certain disease states associated with the menopause by administration of exogenous estrogen therapy. Whether actual causal relationships exist between certain disorders and diminished estrogen secretion has not been established. Nevertheless, beneficial effects on extragenital organs and prevention of atherosclerosis and osteoporosis have been claimed.

A statistical rise in coronary atherosclerosis in postmenopausal women has been ascribed to estrogen deficiency. Castration performed before natural menopause also has been associated with increased coronary and peripheral vascular disease. The ability of estrogen to reverse abnormal serum lipids in laboratory animals as well as in human subjects is a possible mechanism by which treated castrates have a lower incidence of abnormal electrocardiograms and hypertension than untreated women.

Postmenopausal osteoporosis is also believed related to estrogen deficiency. Estrogen induces a positive calcium balance and continued osteoblastic activity, which may account for reports that osteoporosis does not develop in women receiving estrogen therapy. Appropriate diet and exercise are certainly also involved in bone matrix formation. Conclusive proof is lacking that diminished estrogen is a factor in this and other age-related disorders such as arthritis, muscular weakness, migraine headache, and stomatitis. On the other hand, atrophic changes in the distal urinary tract, particularly in the urethra, which results in urinary frequency, burning, and occasionally stress incontinence, are reversible by the administration of local or systemic estrogen. Finally, estrogen controls the often embarrassing and sometimes disabling irritations of atrophic vaginitis and vulvitis.

In the postmenopausal situation, in which menstrual function is not required, only small doses of cyclic estrogen are necessary for appropriate therapy. Stilbestrol, 0.1 to 0.2 mg. daily by mouth for three weeks of every four, is sufficient. Despite the ease of administration and its obvious physiologic and clinical value, estrogen therapy has often been limited in duration or actively avoided. The reason for this restraint is the concern that protracted estrogen treatment will induce neoplastic changes in estrogen-sensitive aging tissues. The contribution of endogenous estrogen to the pathogenesis of uterine and breast carcinoma is still speculative, but suspicion has been aroused, particularly as to the effects of unopposed estrogen in the stimulation of endometrial disease. Clearly, indiscriminate use of this hormone in high doses without periodic evaluation is condemned. On the other hand, if therapy is given within the restrictions stated, there is more evidence in favor of than against its use.

In this regard the importance of frequent medical evaluations in this age group should not be understated. In addition to the opportunities such interviews present for continual psychologic support of the apprehensive patient, the full physical examination performed on these occasions may uncover basic organic disease, the symptoms of which have been incorrectly minimized by the woman as further evidence of "a change of life."

Hypogonadotrophic Hypogonadism. Before embarking on a therapeutic program in this form of amenorrhea, the physician must have assured himself of the absence of various intracranial diseases that eliminate gonadotrophin secretion.

In the absence of neoplastic, vascular, or congenital anomaly to account for disruption in pituitary function, there is usually a history of some stressful circumstance as the precipitating event. Improved dietary habits or psychotherapy may result in return of ovulatory cycles. In fact, the frequency of spontaneous remission is so high that simple observation is often satisfactory. However, when amenorrhea is prolonged and is associated with incipient atrophy of dependent organs and infertility, or is accompanied by lactation, more active therapeutic measures must be undertaken.

Inappropriate Lactation Syndromes. *Galactorrhea* refers to the breast secretion of milky fluid that is persistent and unrelated to a recent pregnancy (although it may represent abnormal prolongation of lactation following a normal pregnancy). Among the common etiologic factors are all types of pituitary tumors (not necessarily eosinophil), as well as organic brain lesions of encephalitis, and trauma. The *Ahumada-del Castillo syndrome* is a particular type of segmental pituitary disorder unrelated to acromegaly or pregnancy in which an incidence of pituitary tumors approaching 50 per cent is found in association with lactation and amenorrhea. The *Chiari-Frommel syndrome*, on the other hand, which by definition always follows pregnancy, is only rarely associated with pituitary tumor, although profound but selective hypogonadotrophic hypogonadism is seen. The galactorrhea that is sometimes observed following castration is not understood. The lactation and amenorrhea seen in certain psychotic patients suggest hypothalamic involvement.

Not all instances of lactation are accompanied by evidence of gonadal failure. Patients receiving phenothiazine derivatives, Rauwolfia alkaloids, or meprobamates sometimes show galactorrhea. Similarly, cervical spine lesions, herpes zoster, chest operations, and prolonged suckling all can induce lactation, presumably by affecting the neural reflex involved.

Investigation of abnormal lactation and gonadal failure must rule out the presence of specific intracranial disease. In the absence of such lesions, management includes elimination of breast manipulation and direct therapy of gonadal failure by substitutive or stimulatory agents. Until recently no such choice was available. Only prolonged substitution with cyclic oral estrogen and progesterone could be offered. Although sporadic success occurred with a variety of agents (intravenous Premarin and thyroid hormone), the search continued for species-specific, nontoxic gonadotrophin with FSH activity for exogenous stimulation of otherwise competent ovaries. At the present time two materials have been shown to meet these requirements: human pituitary gonadotrophin (HPFSH or HPG) and human menopausal urinary gonadotrophin (HMG, Pergonal).

Gonadotrophin Therapy. *Human Pituitary Follicle Stimulating Hormone (HPFSH) and Human Chorionic Gonadotrophin (HCG) Therapy.* In 1958 Gemzell reported the use of a human pituitary preparation that stimulated follicular growth and estrogen production in amenorrheic women. The material was extracted from pituitary tissue collected at autopsy and partially purified by ammonium sulfate fractionation. When assayed against relatively specific standards, it revealed combined FSH and LH potencies, but with the former dominating the biologic activity. Ovulation occurs during HCG administration. Dose size and duration are adjusted according to the ovarian response noted. In limited trials it has been found that more than 90 per cent of patients ovulated once or several times, and more than 50 per cent became pregnant. The limited availability of material (requiring approximately 10 pituitaries to produce an ovulation with this system) has been its major disadvantage.

Human Menopausal Urinary Gonadotrophin (HMG-FSH, Pergonal). Although menopausal urine had been recognized as a potential source of gonadotrophins (FSH activity by animal studies) since 1930, toxic reactions precluded utilization in human investigations. Recently, however, workers have prepared acceptable material which, although variable in gonadotrophin content, has roughly the same biologic activity ratios as the pituitary substance. In one report of 70 infertile patients treated, two thirds conceived at least once. The program of drug administration is 8 to 12 days of HMG followed by 1 to 3 days of HCG.

Apparently species-specific FSH preparations obtained from menopausal urine are at least as efficient as the pituitary material. In view of the essentially unlimited source of supply, the clinical application of this product constitutes a major advance in the treatment of anovulation due to inappropriate hypothalamic-pituitary function.

Side Effects of Gonadotrophin Therapy. Certain side effects have been noted that may limit general application of these agents. The reactions encountered are attributable to the effects of ovarian enlargement and production of unusual quantities of ovarian hormones. These consist of abdominal pain, bloating, pressure, nausea, and general malaise. Acute distention can even cause ovarian rupture and hemorrhage. Because many of the reactions are self-limiting, nonsurgical supportive therapy is advised, laparotomy and conservative surgery short of castration being reserved for the deteriorating circumstance. In this regard hypovolemic shock due to a syndrome of severe ascites and hydrothorax has been recognized. More formidable expressions of ovarian hyperstimulation are the frequency of abortion and multiple pregnancy and the consequent diminution in fetal salvage noted in all series. Finally, it has become clear that gonadotrophin therapy is effective only during the treatment interval. Regardless of frequency of ovulation or the occurrence of pregnancy, patients revert to pretreatment hypogonadal status upon cessation of therapy or conclusion of pregnancy. For this reason gonadotrophin induction of ovulation is currently withheld until other modes of treatment have failed.

Normogonadotrophic Normoestrogenic Anovulation. In this type of amenorrhea, the chain of events leading to normal ovulation and menstruation is upset by the absence of the midcycle surge of LH. Lacking progesterone secretion, continued unopposed estrogen leads to hyperplasia of the endometrium. For this reason amenorrhea may be punctuated by prolonged, sometimes severe uterine hemorrhages (*metropathia hemorrhagica*) that require special attention. In addition, infertility further complicates this syndrome. Clearly the correction of both these circumstances is found in the return of recurrent ovulation.

Correction of Menstrual Pattern. There may be no specific requirement for reproductive function, but the inconvenience and uncertainty of the menstrual pattern prompts the patient to seek hormonal regulation of her cycle. In the absence of serious underlying disease, this may be accomplished by inducing progesterone withdrawal flow with an oral progestin such as 2.5 mg. of medroxyprogesterone acetate for five days after an interval of endogenous estrogen stimulation. Two to five days after progestin withdrawal, menses will appear. Re-treatment with progestin should be delayed for sufficient time (six weeks) to determine whether spontaneous ovulation will return. Only in cases of too frequent menstruation (polymenorrhea) is the disadvantage of complete cycle coverage by combined estrogen and progestin (such as Enovid, etc.) acceptable. Medication should be withdrawn periodically since spontaneous correction may have occurred during therapy.

When severe dysfunctional bleeding occurs, an effort must be made to obtain an endometrial biopsy, but curettage is not essential. Regardless of the duration or severity of flow, anovulatory bleeding of this type is treated by converting the proliferative endometrium to a secretory endometrium from which limited withdrawal flow will occur. Three to four times the contraceptive doses of oral 19-nor steroids will rapidly diminish dysfunctional bleeding with complete cessation within 12 hours. Therapy is then continued, and is gradually tapered to allow an interval for blood replacement as well as general, gynecologic, and hematologic evaluation. The possibility of underlying disorders of coagulation must always be considered. Following withdrawal flow, contraceptive doses of 19-nor steroids must be resumed for two to three cycles. The initial use of high doses of estrogen intravenously (Premarin, 20 mg.) prior to progestin conversion is limited to those cases in which bleeding has been prolonged or severe and immediate cessation is required. On the other hand, if agents such as 19-nor steroids do *not* control abnormal flow, then pathologic bleeding is diagnosed and curettage is mandatory.

Reversal of Anovulation. Obviously, correction of proved adrenal and thyroid disease will reverse associated anovulation. The drug Clomid (a synthetic nonsteroidal analogue of chlorotrianisene) has proved useful in therapy of diagnostically nonspecific anovulation. It has almost entirely replaced the low-dose corticosteroid regimens in this area. Using 50 to 100 mg. daily for five to seven days of each cycle, ovulation induction is achieved in patients with intermediate follicle maturation arrest but with sufficient function to secrete some estrogen. The drug's mode of action is not understood, though it appears to enhance both endogenous gonadotrophin secretion and ovarian synthesis of estrogen. The side effects are similar to those of the gonadotrophins and are related to increased ovarian size, hormone production, and multiple pregnancies. In the event that Clomid (after gradually increased doses over four to six months) is unsuccessful, then bilateral wedge resection of the ovaries or HMG plus HCG therapy is advised. Because all the therapies cited present some risk to the patient and none guarantee lasting results, other aspects of the fertility potential of the involved couple must be fully evaluated before ovulation induction is undertaken.

INVESTIGATION OF INFERTILITY

Approximately 15 per cent of married couples in the United States are unable to conceive. The cause of infertility varies with geographic and socio-economic factors, but some general statements can be made regarding the frequency of certain etiologic factors. Of 100 couples in whom a definite disorder is identified, approximately 40 will show a male factor deficiency, 20 a female hormonal defect, 30 a female tubal disorder, and in 10 a cervical defect. Because investigation of infertility in the female is time-consuming and expensive, prompt evaluation of the male factor is essential.

Male Factor. The most important procedure is the analysis of the semen. Although some estimate of sperm can be made from postcoital cervical examinations, before any final conclusion of deficiency is made, three separate masturbatory specimens should be examined for volume, sperm count, motility, morphology, and viability. A normal ejaculate is considered to have a volume not less than 2.5 ml. and not more than 6 ml., 60 per cent active forms after two hours, 60 per cent normal morphology, and at least 20 million sperm per milliliter. If counts are below 20 million, full urologic and medical investigation is warranted. Regardless of count, the male partner should be questioned and instructed when necessary in the development of appropriate sexual and social habits.

Female Factor. Once it is established that ovulation regularly occurs (by means of basal body temperature curves, appropriately timed examination of cervical mucus, endometrial biopsy, and pregnanediol excretion), investigation of the female attempts to certify functional and anatomic competence of the reproductive tract to permit union of sperm and ovum in the ampulla of the oviduct.

The postcoital test is performed at the expected date of ovulation, not less than two and not more than 16 hours following intercourse. A specimen of endocervical mucus is inspected for clarity, ferning, elasticity, and the number and activity of spermatozoa. In this way the adequacy of coital position, intromission, and ejaculate content, as well as the cervical environment, can be evaluated. Sperm survive in mucus that is abundant, clear, and elastic. The presence of this type of mucus is indicative of adequate local cervical and ovarian function. Repeatedly poor postcoital examinations, despite documented ovulation, make examination of the male factor and coital habits imperative. Furthermore, anatomic abnormalities of the cervix or hostile mucus resulting from erosions, infections, and other local disorders of the cervix should be investigated and specifically treated.

Tubal competence is evaluated by tubal insufflation with carbon dioxide (the Rubin test), roentgenographic demonstration of patency by hysterosalpingography, or by direct visualization by culdoscopy. Each serves distinct functions and should be included in the definitive infertility work-up.

The *Rubin test* is best performed prior to ovulation. It involves transcervical introduction of carbon dioxide under carefully monitored flow rate and pressures and insufflation of gas through the uterus and the ostia of the tubes into the peritoneal cavity. A positive test (indicating tubal patency) involves demonstration of gas under the diaphragm by the appearance of referred shoulder pain. The insufflation occurs at a gas pressure usually less than 120 mm. of mercury. If tubal blockade exists, escape of gas is prevented and the pressure readings rise continuously to above 200 mm. of mercury. At this point the test should be discontinued. It must be remembered that a single negative test is not diagnostic, as functional occlusion (tubospasm) is frequently encountered. Multiple studies are essential and may be undertaken with paracervical block local anesthesia. On the other hand, a positive Rubin test does not rule out the presence of distortions of the tube or tubal-ovarian junction secondary to pelvic adhesions. For this reason if infertility persists in the face of positive tubal insufflation, then ancillary tests of tubal competence are required.

Hysterosalpingography is ordinarily performed by instillation of 3 to 6 ml. of radiopaque oils into the uterine cavity and oviducts under fluoroscopic observation. In this way defects in the uterine cavity that may interfere with implantation and alteration in tubal architecture can be visualized and permanently recorded. The presence of peritubal adhesions may be diagnosed by the dye diffusion pattern about the tubal ostia at the time of examination and 24 hours later.

Culdoscopy accompanied by tubal insufflation with methylene blue is probably the most effective means of diagnosing peritubal and pelvic adhesions producing infertility. Combined with salpingography these procedures offer detailed information as to the feasibility and type of corrective adnexal surgery to be undertaken.

Uterine factors were once considered important elements in infertility. However, current views no longer give significance to the multiple anatomic variations in uterine displacement from the usual anterior position. However, abnormalities of the uterine cavity, such as congenital anomalies and submucous myomas, deserve surgical repair if associated with otherwise unexplained infertility.

FERTILITY CONTROL
(Population Control)

Discussion of the need for population control is beyond the scope of this text. Obviously, once the public health issues of the demographic gap and its consequences are put aside, the basic issue remains the acceptability of the form of fertility control offered to the individual couples. If 100 women of proved fertility are exposed to pregnancy for one year, approximately 80 pregnancies will result. Clearly, then, *any* method of contraception is more effective than none. It must be remembered that significant discrepancies always exist between the theoretical and practical effectiveness of any contraceptive method, as is illustrated by experience with the "rhythm" method. The fertile phase (requiring sexual continence) is estimated as extending from the eighteenth day before the onset of the earliest likely menstruation up to and including the eleventh day before the onset of the latest likely menstruation. The method assumes that ovulation occurs about 14 days before menstruation, that spermatozoa can fertilize for 48 hours after intercourse, and that the ovum can be fertilized for about 24 hours after it emerges from the ovary. The method depends on motivation to accumulate menstrual records for one year prior to use and to remain continent during the fertile period. Studies of the effectiveness of this method reveal pregnancy rates of about 15 conceptions per 100 years of exposure. Although this is about double the conception rates with mechanical devices (condom, diaphragm), it represents an important reduction compared with the projected rate of 80 which would have been expected. All physicians must be prepared to teach this method as long as a substantial proportion of the population is limited by religious belief to this method alone.

When considering the other available contraceptive modalities, it is apparent that with advancing scientific knowledge and public awareness the traditional, folklore-based methods (douche, withdrawal, household spermacides) have given way to proved methods of prevention. Vaginal jellies, foams, diaphragms, and condoms are all safe and fairly reliable. Their relative acceptability varies geographically and according to social class. Their application and use are described in Calderone's manual.

Two modern methods of contraception have altered world-wide concepts of conception control. These are the oral ovulation-inhibiting steroid "pill" and the intrauterine device (IUD).

Oral Hormonal Control of Ovulation. Whereas the inhibition of ovulation during pregnancy had been recognized, it was not until early 1950, when orally active progestins became available, that this known activity of progesterone could be tested in human beings. The most widely used oral progestins are norethindrone (17α-ethinyl-19-nortestosterone) and norethynodrel (17α-ethinyl-5, 10-estraenolone). Combined with estrogen, these remain the most reliable contraceptive steroids and therefore appear in a large variety of marketed items in varying ratios and in a variety of derivative forms. The reason for the continued proliferation of similar drugs, each with its own particular merits, relates to the severity of side effects and hence the restricted acceptability and usage that handicap all oral contraceptives currently available. Consequently, although they offer almost 100 per cent contraception, spontaneous withdrawal from their use is still commonplace. These side effects are related to the general metabolic and target organ effects of the progestin-estrogen combination.

Fifteen to 35 per cent of women experience unpleasant manifestations similar to early pregnancy during the first four months of drug use. Whereas the incidence of nausea, vomiting, breast fullness and tenderness, and headache decreases with use, in some patients they persist and recur cyclically. Furthermore depression and fatigue may worsen with prolonged use. Endometrial instability, reflected in intermenstrual spotting, is frequently seen. Switching drugs often relieves symptoms. Cessation of therapy produces remission. Chloasma, fluid retention, and weight gain are also noted during administration. Of greater concern are the reports of vascular changes and thrombophlebitis associated with oral contraceptives. A series of British studies reveals a 1 in 2000 incidence of thrombophlebitis and a 7 to 9 times greater risk of death as a result of pulmonary embolism in users versus nonusers. These steroids are wisely contraindicated in patients with known vascular disorders. An even rarer phenomenon, though more likely correlated to progestin administration, is the appearance of jaundice in some persons, particularly those who have noted similar findings during pregnancy. There appears to be no permanent liver damage, for the findings remit upon withdrawal of medication. The physician must remember that, as in pregnancy, the estrogen component of these drugs produces an elevated PBI.

The mechanism of contraception is probably selective inhibition of the midcycle LH surge with resulting anovulation as well as suppressed early cycle FSH. However, other sites of action are implicated. The cervical mucus does not develop the sperm-supporting qualities typical of the untreated ovulatory cycle. Furthermore, under the influence of these drugs the endometrium is rapidly transformed into predominantly pseudodecidual stromal tissue with sparse glands and vascularity. Implantation is unlikely under these conditions. Examination of the ovary during drug administration suggests local ovarian inactivity. Although follicle atresia proceeds at a normal pace (negating the possibilities of geriatric obstetrics), only the most minimal expressions of follicle maturation are found. Despite this inactivity, withdrawal of the drug even after prolonged treatment is associated with immediate and often dramatic return of ovulatory cycles and fecundity.

Progestins are administered from the fifth day of the menstrual cycle and are continued daily for 20- or 21-day courses. Cyclic reduplication achieves menstrual regularity, diminished menstrual flow, and decreased dysmenorrhea. In instances in which menses fail to appear, an interval of 7 days is allowed to elapse between the last medication and the resumption of the next 20-day cycle. Yearly examinations may be performed, but solely as an extension of good general medical care. A sequential program of oral hormonal contraception in which estrogen alone is administered for 15 days, followed by 5 days of combined estrogen and progestin, has also been used. In this regimen, the anti FSH aspect of the estrogen is responsible for contraception. It is claimed to be better tolerated by some patients.

Intrauterine Devices for Contraception. With increased use and experience, pregnancy rates in users of various intrauterine spiral or loop devices vary from 2 to 7.5 per 100 woman years, and therefore tend to be similar to rates observed for other mechanical contraceptives. Obviously the advantage of this mode of contraception is that it minimizes the factor of patient error and is therefore suited to large-scale application in the lower socioeconomic groups. A complicating factor is the often unnoticed expulsion of the device, with consequent loss of contraceptive protection. Pregnancy has occurred with the device in place. The disturbing incidence of intermenstrual spotting, menorrhagia, reproductive tract infection, and perforation of the uterus detracts from the acceptability of these devices. Furthermore, contraindications to their application include distorting fibromyomas and adnexal disease.

The mechanism of action is not understood. In rats they affect ovum transport, in rabbits implantation and postimplantation stages are affected, and in monkeys tubal ova are lost. Objective studies of associated alterations in human physiology have not appeared. Their usefulness to date has been in large-scale programs requiring minimal patient cooperation.

COUNSELING IN GYNECOLOGY

The emphasis in the preceding discussions has been directed to analysis of alterations of the primary ovarian function of ovulation. In these concluding paragraphs some mention of the physician's role in sexual counseling must be made.

Whereas deep-seated sexual problems are usually discussed in psychiatry teaching programs in the medical curriculum, ordinarily no instruction is given the medical student in the normal aspects of sexual life or in its commonly occurring abnormalities. The physician therefore enters practice without benefit of the usual guidelines of diagnosis and management that he has developed for all other disorders he will be called upon to see. However, because of his professional status he is often asked for advice in sexual matters and, owing to the uncertainty of applying his own intuitive perception to these matters, the physician usually avoids comment. Unfortunately, this attitude compounds the official silence with which these subjects are treated by schools, religious groups and families.

The physician may incorrectly assume that the "modern" girl is well versed in genital anatomy and physiology and the technique of the sexual act. Practical experience indicates that in many instances the young woman approaching marriage knows too little and has the disturbing notion, perhaps by conditioning from her mother's experience, that marital sex for the female is overrated, exploitative, and sinful. In such instances, without adequate counseling for both partners, repeated dissatisfaction may confirm these attitudes and set the pattern for a lifetime of maladjusted performance of a "wifely duty." Although it may appear too simple a solution for a problem of such magnitude, the physician can help the couple to avoid this situation by tactful and sympathetic review of basic facts during premarital examinations or any other occasion requiring medical consultation.

A detailed discussion of the myriad of potential sexual difficulties is beyond the scope of this text, but some of the common factors leading to female sexual anesthesia deserve comment.

The fear of genital injury or expectation of pain and hemorrhage due to rupture of the hymen during sexual intercourse poses a threat to achievement of vaginal-oriented orgasm. Such preconceived attitudes can be dispelled by the assurance of the physician that the pelvic examination just performed reveals anatomically adequate external and internal genitalia. Some pain is usually experienced on entry into the vagina, but lubrication, a considerate partner, and repeated experience favor prompt resolution of this difficulty.

Because mutual precoital sexual excitement is imperative, varying patterns of stimulation as well as coital techniques must be encouraged and instruction given. Every effort must be made to motivate both partners to seek this result by experimentation and frank discussion. In this situation affectation of false modesty or "man of the world" all-knowing attitudes should be discouraged.

It must be made clear that, no matter how satisfactory the circumstances, few women experience orgasm regularly. Often this misunderstanding, if uncorrected, provokes undue concern and tension that may produce further diminution in satisfaction, a change in coital frequency, substitution of clitoral orgasm, or pretending satisfaction when none occurs. Once these patterns are set, reconditioning for vaginal orgasm is possible but only after a long and difficult period of adjustment. Some of the factors leading to the initial lack of coital orgasm are fear of pregnancy, the possibility of discovery by parents or children, economic and social pressures, poor health, and fatigue. All these profoundly influence both partners' interest in and response to intercourse. Possibly the most common factor in the development of aversion to sexual intimacy in the somewhat older married woman is that over the years these intimacies have tended to follow a monotonous, routine sameness of time, place, and practice. Reluctance to discuss the matter with her husband or with her physician abets the situation. The alert physician can usually suspect this problem from the patient's response during history taking and the nature of her physical complaints. Again sympathetic but informative discussions will bring a more open and intelligent outlook on the part of the patient, and whereas no quick cure exists, reorientation of sexual practice and renewed motivation can occur, with an increasing degree of satisfaction derived. Coaching the couple in the recognition of the female indicators of sexual arousal and the sequence leading to achievement of orgasm is particularly helpful. Delay of coitus until extragenital and genital responses in the female (generalized skin flush, retraction of the clitoris, ballooning of the vagina, color changes in the labia) will increase the frequency of coital orgasm, release female sexual tension, and make the anxious, uncertain couple more confident and eager for sexual contact. The therapeutic use of testosterone and alcohol in the sexually frigid woman is not recommended. The effects are temporary and only serve to postpone the necessary personal examination that must be carried out. *Cantharis vesicatoria* (Spanish fly) is an undesirable irritant to the clitoris and has no place in therapeutics.

Sometimes problems appear to be so complicated and deep-seated that psychiatric help is worth while. Fortunately these are rare. However, if sexual frigidity appears to have the malicious motivation of deprivation, if sexual intercourse and practice are revolting prospects, or if the woman displays pronounced aggressive or homosexual tendencies, psychiatric evaluation is in order.

Bardin, C. W., and Lipsett, M. B.: Testosterone and androstenedione blood production rates in normal women and women with idiopathic hirsutism or polycystic ovaries. J. Clin. Invest., 46:891, 1967.
Calderone, M. S.: Manual of Contraceptive Practice. Baltimore, Williams & Wilkins Company, 1964.
Gemzell, C.: Induction of ovulation with human gonadotropins. Recent Prog. Hormone Res., 21:179, 1965.
Israel, S. L.: Diagnosis and Treatment of Menstrual Disorders and Sterility. New York, Paul B. Hoeber, Inc., 1967.
Masters, W., and Johnson, V.: Human Sexual Response. Boston, Little, Brown and Company, 1966.
Tait, J. F.: Review: Use of isotopic steroids for measurement of production rates in vivo. J. Clin. Endocr., 23:1285, 1963.
Vessey, M. P., and Doll, R.: Investigation of relation between use of oral contraceptives and thromboembolic disease. Brit. Med. J., 2:199, 1968.

Sympatho-Adrenal System

Albert Sjoerdsma

The cells of the adrenal medulla and other portions of the sympathetic nervous system are of ectodermal origin and arise from the primitive neural crest. The parent cells or sympathogonia may differentiate to form sympathoblasts or neuroblasts and finally mature ganglion cells, or, alternatively, they may give rise to chromaffin cells. The latter are so named because of intracellular granules that give a brown color on treatment with chromium salts.

Tumors may develop from any of these cell types and are usually classified according to the type that predominates. They occur not only in the adrenal medulla but also in adrenal cell rests in the renal areas, in the organs of Zuckerkandl at the origin of the inferior mesenteric artery, and in paravertebral and peripheral sympathetic ganglia. An understanding of the clinical syndromes produced by these tumors is obtained from consideration of the hormones they secrete.

THE SYMPATHO-ADRENAL HORMONES

The hormones of the adrenal medulla are epinephrine (Adrenalin) and norepinephrine (noradrenalin); the latter is also the neurohormone of the postganglionic sympathetic nerve fiber. Epinephrine was first identified as an active principle of the suprarenal medulla in 1901 by Takamine. Though both hormones were synthesized by Stoltz in 1904, it was not until 1949 with the work of von Euler, Goldenberg, and Tullar that norepinephrine was shown also to be an adrenal medullary hormone, as well as the peripheral transmitter of the sympathetic nervous system (von Euler, 1946–1948).

Biochemistry. The accepted pathway for synthesis of the hormones was first postulated by

Blaschko in 1939 and is shown in Figure 1. The rate-limiting step in the pathway is hydroxylation of the amino acid tyrosine to form DOPA; this reaction is under feedback control normally by end-product inhibition. DOPA is decarboxylated to dopamine, which is then hydroxylated on the β-position of the side chain to yield norepinephrine; the latter is N-methylated to form epinephrine. The last three compounds in this pathway are classified chemically as *catecholamines* (catechol = dihydroxybenzene), though in common usage this term refers only to norepinephrine and epinephrine. In sympathetic nerves and ganglia, synthesis terminates with norepinephrine, which is stored in amounts on the order of 5 to 10 μg. per gram of tissue. Human adrenal glands contain, on the average, 600 μg. of catecholamine per gram of tissue, 70 to 80 per cent of which is epinephrine and the remainder norepinephrine. The hormones are stored in intracellular granules in combination with adenosine phosphates and protein. At rest, concentrations of free catecholamines in plasma are extremely low, being less than 1 μg. per litor.

Physiologic inactivation of the catecholamines occurs through a combination of neurochemical binding and metabolism by enzymes. The metabolic fate of epinephrine and norepinephrine introduced into the circulation has been completely elucidated since the original demonstration by Armstrong, McMillan and Shaw (1957) that vanillylmandelic acid (VMA, 4-hydroxy-3-methoxymandelic acid) is a major urinary metabolite of these compounds. About 90 per cent of catecholamine metabolism is accounted for by the processes shown in Figure 2. For circulating catecholamines, the major route is by O-methylation followed by oxidative deamination. Approximately 5 per cent of a given intravenous dose is excreted in the urine as the catecholamine, 30 to 50 per cent as methoxy-analogue (normetanephrine or metanephrine), and 30 to 50 per cent as VMA. In the absence of pheochromocytoma, adult subjects (including hypertensives) excrete less than 100 μg. free catecholamines per 24 hours, of which 10 to 80 μg. per day is norepinephrine and 0 to 20 μg. per day is epinephrine. The preponderance of norepinephrine reflects liberation from sympathetic nerves; following adrenalectomy the excretion of epinephrine decreases, whereas that of norepinephrine is little changed. Normal excretion of normetanephrine plus metanephrine is less than 1.0 mg. per day and that of VMA is 2.0 to 6.5 mg. per day.

Pharmacology. The catecholamines are potent pharmacologic agents with cardiovascular and metabolic actions. Important qualitative differences between epinephrine and norepinephrine are observed when small doses (5 to 10 μg. per minute) are administered intravenously to humans. Though a potent direct vasoconstrictor, epinephrine infused in man produces over-all vasodilation and decrease in peripheral resistance, as well as striking increase in cardiac output and increase in heart rate. As a result, the systolic blood pressure is elevated, but the diastolic pressure remains unchanged or falls. In contrast, norepinephrine causes an increase of both systolic and diastolic blood pressure due to over-all vasoconstriction. Although norepinephrine is also a potent cardiotonic agent, the considerable rise in blood pressure leads to reflex slowing of the heart by the carotid sinus mechanism and, as a consequence, cardiac output is usually unchanged. Large doses of epinephrine also produce striking pressor effects, since vasodilation secondary to β-receptor stimulation and accumulation of lactic acid in vascular beds such as that of muscle is

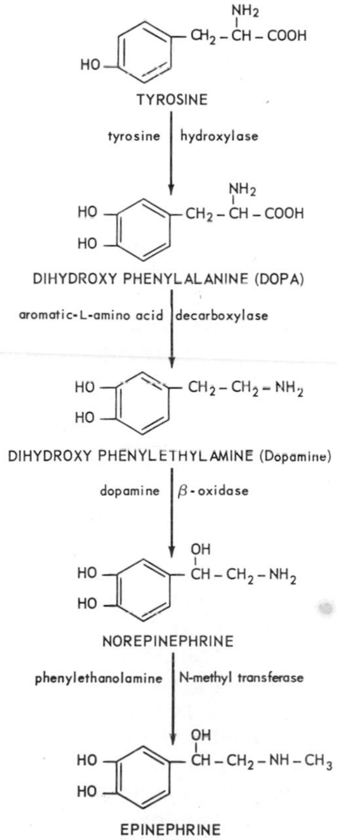

FIGURE 1. The catecholamine pathway of tyrosine metabolism.

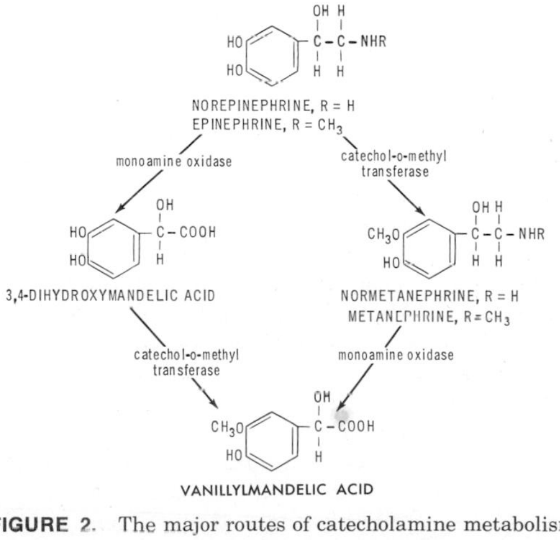

FIGURE 2. The major routes of catecholamine metabolism.

overcome by the potent vasoconstrictor and cardiac effects of the agent.

Both catecholamines have profound metabolic effects, epinephrine generally being more potent than norepinephrine. They cause increased oxygen consumption, elevation of body temperature, and hyperglycemia due to inhibition of insulin release as well as increased glycogenolysis and lipolysis. As shown by Sutherland and others, these latter effects are mediated by the adenyl cyclase system.

Secretion of epinephrine and norepinephrine by the adrenal under ordinary conditions is probably too small to have physiologic significance. However, increased synthesis and release of sympathoadrenal catecholamines during insulin hypoglycemia and situations of acute stress undoubtedly exert at least a metabolic effect and probably significant cardiovascular effects also. Release of norepinephrine at sympathetic nerve endings is essential to maintenance of blood pressure in the erect position.

PHEOCHROMOCYTOMA

The pheochromocytoma is a catecholamine-producing tumor arising from chromaffin cells of the sympatho-adrenal system. The first description of the syndrome of paroxysmal hypertension in association with pheochromocytoma is credited to Labbé and associates (1922). In 1927, C. H. Mayo successfully removed such a tumor, and Pincoffs in 1929 made the first correct preoperative diagnosis that was followed by successful excision.

Incidence. Pheochromocytoma is a relatively rare condition, accounting for less than 0.1 per cent of cases of hypertension. Its importance lies in its being a potentially lethal yet curable condition. Most cases appear sporadically, but a familial occurrence is being recognized more frequently, and a sufficient number of kindred have been observed to indicate a dominant mode of inheritance. In about 5 per cent of cases there is an associated neuroectodermal disorder, particularly neurofibromatosis. An unusual association also exists between pheochromocytoma (bilateral adrenal) and medullary carcinoma of the thyroid (a multifunctional tumor which secretes calcitonin and prostaglandins, and occasionally serotonin) occurring with a high familial incidence; such patients may also have hyperparathyroidism and mucocutaneous neuromas. There is no sex predilection or age exemption, though most cases occur during the second to sixth decades.

Pathology. About 80 per cent of pheochromocytomas originate in the adrenal glands, and more than 95 per cent of all the tumors are located in the abdominal and pelvic regions. The remainder occur in the paravertebral areas of the thorax and neck. Rarely, chemodectomas, e.g. carotid body tumors, produce pathologic quantities of catecholamines. Probably less than 5 per cent of pheochromocytomas are truly malignant, but in approximately 10 per cent of cases benign tumors may arise bilaterally in the adrenal areas or from multiple foci. Malignant disease cannot be determined on histologic grounds alone and must be judged on the basis of tumor invasion and true metastasis, usually to lymph nodes, liver, lung, and bone. The tumors vary in size but usually weigh less than 200 grams and may be very small. Some of the smallest may produce the most severe symptoms. Generally they are highly vascular and well encapsulated. The cut surface is yellowish brown and frequently shows evidence of hemorrhage or necrosis. Microscopically, the tumor cells are polygonal or spheroidal with granular cytoplasm, and are frequently arranged in alveolar cell masses separated by a delicate connective tissue stroma. The catecholamine content of tumor is generally higher than that of adrenal medulla, usually being 1 to 10 mg. per gram.

Clinical Manifestations. The manifestations of pheochromocytoma result from increased secretion of norepinephrine and epinephrine. Hypertension is the cardinal sign, being persistent though usually fluctuant in about half the cases and truly intermittent or paroxysmal in the others. Symptoms may be present for a few weeks or many years, and most patients complain of attacks. These vary considerably in frequency, severity, and duration in different patients. They may occur without warning or may be clearly precipitable by certain stimuli, such as emotional upsets, postural changes, and physical exertion. The most frequent symptoms during severe attacks are pounding headaches, sweating, palpitation, apprehension, tremulousness, pallor or flushing of the face, nausea and vomiting, pain in the chest and abdomen, and paresthesias in the extremities. During an attack the blood pressure may reach very high levels, hyperglycemia and glycosuria are present, and the patient appears acutely ill, has cold extremities and dilated pupils, and is drenched with perspiration. A feeling of prostration follows the attack. Since the effects of large doses of epinephrine and norepinephrine are similar, the clinical manifestations often do not yield an indication of which amine the tumor is producing predominantly. Death may occur in a shocklike state or from cerebral hemorrhage, cardiac failure, or hyperpyrexia.

Rarely, a pheochromocytoma may produce a picture closely simulating essential hypertension. However, as a rule patients with persistent hypertension have some manifestation that raises a suspicion of pheochromocytoma, such as excessive sweating (almost invariable), palpitations, wide fluctuations in blood pressure, an orthostatic fall in blood pressure (70 per cent of cases) owing to hypovolemia and defective arteriolar and venous reflexes, paradoxic response to autonomic blocking agents, impaired glucose tolerance, elevated basal metabolic rate, and weight loss. The disease may progress in a manner similar to essential hypertension, though severe impairment of renal function is unusual. Many patients with pheochromocytoma have cholelithiasis.

Diagnosis. Awareness is essential because pheochromocytoma may mimic a variety of conditions. The usual differentiation is from essential hypertension, hyperthyroidism, diabetes mellitus, and psychoneurosis. In many cases diagnosis may be established on the basis of history of typical attacks, palpable mass, blood pressure rise with position change or direct pressure over the tumor, displacement of renal tissue revealed by pyelography, and visualization of a tumor on laminagraphy of the adrenal areas. Although retroperitoneal CO_2 insufflation, arteriography, and adrenal venography may permit visualization of a tumor, such procedures are highly elective since a search for multiple tumors must always be made at operation. If such tests are done, the patient should be under pharmacologic control with phenoxybenzamine (cf. Treatment). The few tumors in the neck that have been reported have been palpable and those in the thorax have been visible roentgenographically (posteroanterior, lateral, and oblique views recommended). Certain pharmacologic and chemical tests are of considerable aid in diagnosis.

Pharmacologic Tests. Two types of tests have been used, provocative tests and blocking tests. Until ten years ago such tests were the major practical means of confirming the diagnosis. Provocative agents, which stimulate release of amines and thereby produce abnormal pressor responses in pheochromocytoma, include histamine, tetraethylammonium, methacholine (Mecholyl), and indirectly acting pressor amines such as tyramine. Contrariwise, adrenergic blocking agents such as piperoxan (a benzodioxan) and phentolamine HCl (Regitine) produce a selective decrease in blood pressure. Currently, these tests are of little importance, because reliable assays of catecholamines and their major metabolites in urine are generally available, and, regardless of the clinical impression or results of pharmacologic tests, no patient should be subjected to exploratory surgery in the absence of biochemical demonstration of catecholamine excess. However, even if physicians do not, patients unwittingly may continued to perform provocative tests by ingestion of foods or medicaments containing high amounts of tyramine (certain cheeses) and similar compounds. A striking personal case was that of a woman from Florida who reported postoperatively that she could now drink orange juice, whereas previously and embarrassingly it provoked attacks. Orange juice is rich in synephrine (sympatol).

Chemical Tests. Of the compounds shown in Figure 2, reliable assays are available for measurement in urine of the catecholamines (fluorometric or biologic assay), the metanephrines (fluorometric, colorimetric, and chromatographic assays), and VMA (colorimetric and chromatographic assays). Generally, all three urinary indices of catecholamine production are abnormal in patients with pheochromocytoma, catecholamines usually being

> 250 μg. per 24 hours, metanephrines > 2.0 mg. per 24 hours, and VMA > 10 mg. per 24 hours. In borderline cases, all three measurements should be made on a 24-hour collection of urine (15 ml. 6 N HCl in bottle as preservative).

Because catecholamines are cleared rapidly by the kidney, catecholamine assays may be employed to advantage on single voided specimens or preferably on a timed collection (two to four hours) in association with a spontaneous or provoked attack. Differential assay of norepinephrine and epinephrine in urine may be of value in predicting location of the tumor preoperatively. If the urine contains increased amounts of epinephrine as well as norepinephrine (40 per cent of cases), with rare exception (especially intrathoracic tumors) the tumor will be found in the adrenal areas or organs of Zuckerkandl. If the increased excretion of catecholamines is limited to norepinephrine (60 per cent of cases), the tumor may still be expected to be in or near the suprarenal area in two thirds of cases; in the remaining one third all possible sites must be considered. For the difficult case in which previous surgical exploration(s) has failed to reveal a tumor, catecholamine assays of blood collected by catheter at various sites in the venae cavae may localize the anatomic level of venous drainage from a tumor. Adrenal venography may produce high adrenal venous catecholamine levels in the absence of tumor. Although several drugs have been reported to produce spurious fluorescence in catecholamine assays, with proper use of the trihydroxyindole assay technique (employing oxidized sample blanks and internal and external standards) only the presence of exogenous compounds which are also catecholamines will produce false positive results. The most notorious offender has been the antihypertensive catechol–amino acid, methyldopa (Aldomet); recent application of DOPA in the treatment of parkinsonism may also be expected to cause diagnostic problems.

Measurements of the O-methylated urinary metabolites, i.e., total metanephrines and VMA, are more generally available (particularly VMA) than catecholamine assays, and are satisfactory for routine screening and diagnosis. Since the metanephrines are converted to VMA via monoamine oxidase (MAO), use of MAO inhibitors for treatment of hypertension or psychic depression in the patient will increase excretion of the metanephrines and decrease VMA excretion. Such therapy will increase normal metanephrine values into the range diagnostic of pheochromocytoma, but would be unlikely to reduce elevated VMA values to normal. VMA assay is preferred in most laboratories. Unfortunately, a number of the VMA tests used yield false positive results since they are merely screening tests for phenolic acids, many of which are ingested in food and drink, e.g., raw fruits, vanilla, coffee. If the results of such screening tests are quantified, the accepted upper limit of normal VMA for the particular laboratory will be in the range of 10 to 15 mg. per 24 hours, whereas comparable values using better tests are no more than 6 to 7 mg. per 24 hours. Since patients have been subjected erroneously to surgery on the basis of nonspecific VMA tests, such tests should be eliminated from clinical practice. Even with the better tests (specifically, those employing periodate oxidation), one may encounter interference from drug ingestion. The antibacterial agent nalidixic acid (NegGram) yields spuriously high values for VMA, whereas the cholesterol-lowering drug clofibrate (Atromid-S) spuriously lowers VMA values.

Treatment. Surgical excision results in a complete remission of symptoms except in metastatic disease, in cases of multiple tumors one or more of which were not removed, in cases of accidental ligation of renal artery (detected by radioactive renogram), and rarely in the presence of persistent renal damage. An anterior surgical approach should be used, consonant with body habitus, to permit exploration from the floor of the pelvis to the diaphragm. There are two serious hazards related to surgery: First, excessive discharge of pressor hormones may occur during induction of anesthesia or during manipulation of the tumor, leading to extreme rises in blood pressure and cardiac arrhythmias. Second, following resection the blood pressure may fall precipitously to shock levels. Preoperative control of hypertension with the experimental inhibitor of tyrosine hydroxylase, α-methyltyrosine, or the α-blocking agent, phenoxybenzamine hydrochloride (Dibenzyline) in single or divided daily dosage of 20 to 60 mg., may prevent many of the complications attendant on surgery. The β-blocking drug, propranolol hydrochloride (Inderal), 10 to 30 mg. orally every four to six hours, may be added to control arrhythmias, but otherwise probably should not be used preoperatively because of possible production of heart failure in patients with underlying catecholamine cardiomyopathy. Adequate preoperative sedation is important. Beginning before induction, continuous monitoring of intra-arterial pressure and the electrocardiogram (and central venous pressure after induction) is desirable. Thiopental (Pentothal)–ether, thiopental–nitrous oxide–oxygen–ether, thiopental–methoxyflurane, and thiopental–halothane anesthetic combinations have been used successfully. Halothane with muscular relaxants is recommended for deep anesthesia, but sensitizes to arrhythmias; Inderal, 1 to 5 mg. intravenously, should be available to combat these. Ligation of tumor blood supply before extensive manipulation may obviate hypertensive crises. These should be controlled with single intravenous doses of Regitine, 1 to 5 mg. Primary reliance should be placed on expansion of intravascular volume with 500 to 1500 ml. of blood (beyond replacement needs), and plasma, dextran, or 5 per cent albumin in iso-osmotic solution (Albumisol), to counteract the severe drop in blood pressure that follows interruption of the tumor's venous drainage. Generally, volume expansion obviates the need for pressor agents and is effective even in patients who do not have demonstrable hypovolemia preoperatively. Persistent hypotension should be handled promptly with norepinephrine (4 to 12 mg. per liter) via intravenous catheter. Postoperatively, the possibility of adrenal cortical insufficiency should be considered, especially in cases in which cortical tissue was resected. Most patients do well following the immediate postoperative period.

Prolonged therapy with Dibenzyline (up to 200 mg. daily) or α-methyltyrosine (0.5 gram every six hours), or both, is useful in controlling signs and symptoms in malignant pheochromocytoma and in preparing the seriously ill patient for operation. Inderal may be added to control arrhythmias and unopposed β-stimulation (by epinephrine) manifest as hypotension.

OTHER TUMORS ARISING FROM SYMPATHETIC AND MEDULLARY TISSUE

Two other main types of tumor may arise from cells of the sympathetic nervous system and adrenal medulla. These are the ganglioneuroma, which develops from mature cells, and neuroblastoma, which originates from primitive cells. Although these were formerly classed as nonfunctioning tumors because of apparent absence of chromaffin cells, it is now apparent that many of them, particularly the neuroblastomas, are functioning tumors. Occurrence of adrenergic symptoms depends on whether the tumors secrete predominantly catecholamines or less active (dopamine) or inactive precursors and metabolites. It would appear that the more primitive the tumor, the more primitive, in a sense, its chemistry. Chemical studies on the urine not only have diagnostic implications but may also lead to a new method of classifying the conditions. Recent exciting studies on serum levels of nerve growth factor (NGF) suggest a role in tumor sustenance and possibly pathogenesis, e.g., multicentric neuroblastoma. *Chronic diarrhea* occurs in some patients with catecholamine-producing ganglioneuromas and neuroblastomas, and all symptoms abate after removal of the tumor. The finding of prostaglandins in such tumors may account for the diarrhea noted here, as well as that in patients with medullary carcinoma of the thyroid (see previous article).

Ganglioneuroma. This small, well-encapsulated slow-growing tumor develops in youth and adulthood, and is often an incidental finding at autopsy. It has a wide distribution but is located most frequently in the posterior mediastinum. Microscopically, the ganglioneuroma is composed of differentiated ganglion cells in a neurofibromatous stroma containing nerve fibers. Some degree of anaplasia may be noted, and tumors of this type can assume all the characteristics of a malignant neuroblastoma. The treatment of ganglioneuroma is surgical extirpation.

Neuroblastoma (Sympathoblastoma, Sympathogonioma). This highly malignant tumor occurs for the most part in infancy and early childhood. Except for nephroblastoma (Wilms' tumor), it is the most common retroperitoneal malignant tumor of children. It arises most commonly from adrenal medulla, but also elsewhere retroperitoneally and retropleurally from sympathetic nerve elements. The tumor metastasizes early and widely, by permeation and embolic spread, to regional lymph nodes, liver, and other abdominal organs, bones, and orbit.

Pathologically, the tumors are large and highly cellular. The cut surface is firm and smooth with many areas of hemorrhage and necrosis. The cells are small and round and contain but little cytoplasm. They have large, central hyperchromatic nuclei. There may be distinctive rosettes. Otherwise, the structure varies in the extent to which nerve elements are developed. Neuroblastomas sometimes revert to benign ganglioneuromas, spontaneously or after therapy.

The early and widespread metastases developing from this deep-seated tumor produce protean and bizarre clinical expressions. The manifestations vary from those of a local tumor mass with abdominal enlargement, vomiting, and pain to those of a generalized malignancy with weakness, weight loss, fever, and anemia. Metastases may introduce the disease, and the child may present enlarged lymph nodes, swellings in the skull, or typical ocular signs with ecchymosis of the eyelids and proptosis. Careful observation will reveal signs and symptoms similar to those of pheochromocytoma in a significant percentage of patients. Urinary VMA is elevated in most cases.

Early and radical surgery, followed immediately by deep x-ray therapy, is the best treatment that can be offered. Additional benefit may be derived from chemotherapy. With skeletal metastases, the prognosis is poor. If tumor is confined to the abdomen, cure rates as high as 60 to 80 per cent may be achieved.

Conference on the Biology of Neuroblastoma. J. Pediat. Surg., 3:Part II, 1968.

Engelman, K., Horwitz, D., Jéquier, E., and Sjoerdsma, A.: Biochemical and pharmacologic effects of alpha-methyltyrosine in man. J. Clin. Invest., 47:577, 1968.

Gifford, R. W., Kvale, W. F., Maher, F. T., Roth, G. M., and Priestley, J. T.: Clinical features, diagnosis and treatment of pheochromocytoma: A review of 76 cases. Mayo Clin. Proc., 39:281, 1964.

Sandler, M., Karim, S. M. M, and Williams, E. D.: Prostaglandins in amine-peptide-secreting tumours. Lancet, 2:1053, 1968.

Second Catecholamine Symposium. Pharmacol. Rev., 18 Supp., March 1966.

Sjoerdsma, A., Engelman, K., Waldmann, T. A., Cooperman, L. H., and Hammond, W. G.: Pheochromocytoma: Current concepts of diagnosis and treatment. Ann. Intern. Med., 65:1302, 1966.

The Carcinoid Syndrome

Albert Sjoerdsma

Recognition of the endocrine properties of carcinoid tumors and the syndrome associated therewith occurred during the period 1953 to 1955. Waldenström and associates and, in part, Isler and Hedinger first described a constellation of signs and symptoms in patients with ileal carcinoid and hepatic metastases. The former workers, basing their studies on the findings by Lembeck of large amounts of serotonin (5-hydroxytryptamine) in carcinoid tumors, implicated overproduction of serotonin in pathogenesis of the syndrome. Sjoerdsma, Weissbach, and Udenfriend demonstrated the characteristic increased urinary excretion of 5-hydroxyindole acetic acid (5HIAA), and emphasized the metabolic and diagnostic significance of this finding.

With study of an increasing number of patients, it has been necessary to revise earlier concepts. Pharmacologically active substances other than serotonin are also produced by carcinoid tumors, and indeed the prime role of serotonin as the chemical mediator of the clinical syndrome has been questioned. Variant syndromes have been described, particularly in cases in which the primary tumors arise outside the small intestine. In some patients the tumors have been shown to be true carcinomas rather than carcinoids, thereby creating difficulties in nomenclature.

Pathology. Typically, functioning malignant carcinoid develops from a small primary in the distal third of the ileum. Other sites of origin include small bowel elsewhere, Meckel's diverticulum, stomach, colon, bronchus, bile ducts, pancreas, and ovary. Appendiceal carcinoids rarely metastasize, and rectal carcinoids are nonfunctional. Mesenteric and hepatic metastases are typical, but distant spread may occur. The tumors are yellow, firm on section, and consist of epithelial cells set in a fibrous stroma. Intracellular granules giving positive argentaffin reactions (hence, "argentaffinoma") reflect origin from specific cells of the intestinal mucosa.

Associated pathologic changes are found primarily in the skin and the heart. Greatly dilated capillaries and small veins are seen in the skin, representing telangiectasia during life. Cardiac involvement is predominantly, but not exclusively, right-sided, and consists of focal and diffuse collections of a peculiar type of fibrous tissue that is deposited on the endocardium of the cardiac chambers and valvular cusps. Major resulting valvular lesions are pulmonic stenosis, tricuspid regurgitation, and tricuspid stenosis, alone or in combination. The heart lesions associated with bronchial carcinoid may involve only the mitral and aortic valves. With ileal carcinoid, cardiac involvement is not observed in the absence of hepatic metastases.

Clinical Manifestations. A series of baffling illnesses extending over a period of years is typical, coinciding with slow growth of the tumor. Unfortunately, with the exception of some bronchial carcinoids and carcinoids developing in ovarian teratomas, metastatic spread usually precedes the development of symptoms. The clinical features are as follows:

Vasomotor. Frequent, brief episodes of cutaneous flushing, chiefly of the face and neck, are the most common and often the earliest manifestation. Remarkable change in color may be observed within a few minutes, ranging from bright red to violaceous to blanching white. Facial and periorbital edema, tachycardia, hypotension, and increased respiratory and intestinal distress may occur, with severe flushing. Precipitating stimuli include ingestion of food or alcohol, emotional upsets, defecation, physical activity, manipulation of the tumors, and intravenous administration of catecholamines. After several years, miliary and gross telangiectasia may develop and give an appearance of cyanosis in the absence of arterial O_2 unsaturation.

Gastrointestinal. There is usually a long history of abdominal discomfort in association with recurrent attacks of diarrhea. Nausea and vomiting develop, if there is frequent or prolonged flushing. Hyperperistalsis is often apparent at the bedside. Although the primary tumor is usually silent, hepatic metastases frequently undergo necrosis, leading to episodes of abdominal pain with fever and leukocytosis. There may be massive hepatomegaly with the usual clinical and laboratory evidence of neoplastic liver invasion. Increased incidences of peptic ulcer and intestinal malabsorption with steatorrhea have been noted.

Cardiopulmonary. The blood pressure is usually normal or low. Cardiac involvement is a late development and occurs in about half the cases. Right heart failure may supervene in association with pulmonary and tricuspid valve lesions. However, dependent edema is common even in the absence of cardiac disease. Clinical and laboratory findings relating to the heart are comparable to those seen in similar valvular lesions of rheumatic or congenital origin, and vary with the severity of involvement. Some patients have attacks of dyspnea and wheezing indistinguishable from bronchial asthma. Others experience constricting sensations in the chest and recurrent paroxysms of coughing.

Nutritional. Loss of weight occurs intermittently but is progressive. Cutaneous lesions and dementia resulting from pellagra have been encountered. Hypoalbuminemia is a frequent finding.

Pathologic Chemistry and Physiology. The major depot of serotonin in the body is the gastrointestinal mucosa. Smaller amounts are found also in the brain and blood platelets. This amine is derived from the essential amino acid tryptophan by hydroxylation and decarboxylation and is metabolized to 5-hydroxyindoleacetic acid (5HIAA), which is excreted in the urine (figure). In patients with malignant carcinoid, the tumor is the major body depot of serotonin and generally contains 1.0 to 3.0 mg. per gram. Hyperserotonemia is present, and the urinary excretion of 5HIAA is greatly elevated, usually being 50 to 600 mg. per day compared with 2.0 to 9 mg. per day in normal persons. As much as 60 per cent of dietary tryptophan may be diverted into the serotonin pathway by the tumor, whereas normally only about 1 per cent is metabolized in this manner. This diversion of tryptophan leaves less available for the formation of other substances such as niacin and protein and, along with diminished food intake and diarrhea, contributes to development of pellagra and protein deficiency.

The pharmacologic effects of serotonin on smooth muscle have long been considered to account for the vasomotor disturbances, hyperperistalsis, and bronchoconstriction. The acquired lesions of the heart have also been related to actions of serotonin. However, there are many reasons, e.g., flushing in some patients with only slightly elevated 5HIAA, to question the primacy of serotonin in producing these alterations. In many but not all patients studied, flushing is associated with

TRYPTOPHAN

Hydroxylase

5-HYDROXYTRYPTOPHAN

Decarboxylase

5-HYDROXYTRYPTAMINE
(Serotonin)

Monoamine Oxidase
Aldehyde Dehydrogenase

5-HYDROXYINDOLE ACETIC ACID
(5HIAA)

The 5-hydroxyindole pathway of tryptophan metabolism.

elevated blood levels of the vasodilator peptide bradykinin, produced by a proteolytic enzyme (kallikrein) released from tumor and acting on a circulating α_2-globulin (kininogen). Recently, prostaglandins have been identified in carcinoid tumors. The effects of prostaglandins and bradykinin on smooth muscle and that of the latter on endothelial permeability make plausible their involvement in many aspects of the syndrome. At this point the most defensible role for serotonin is in the production of diarrhea.

Variant Syndromes. Metastatic gastric carcinoids may secrete large amounts of histamine and 5-hydroxytryptophan (serotonin precursor), and produce vivid, patchy, red flushing, especially after eating, as the predominant symptom. Some bronchial and pancreatic tumors also may secrete more 5-hydroxytryptophan than serotonin. Other variations associated with bronchial tumors include: (1) excess serotonin production with elevated 5HIAA in patients with solitary tumors, (2) carcinomatous rather than carcinoid primary, (3) exclusively left-sided heart lesions, (4) concurrent endocrine disorders such as Cushing's syndrome and pluriglandular adenomatosis, (5) widespread metastases with osteogenic bone lesions, and (6) extremely severe flushing attacks with facial and conjunctival edema and excessive salivation and lacrimation. Additional variants include carcinomas and adenomas of the pancreas that produce flushing and diarrhea, with or without accompanying excess serotonin. Confusion about what should still be called the "carcinoid syndrome" is understandable, and must be viewed in the light of newer concepts of ectopic hormone production by tumors. The typical carcinoid tumor, in turn, may have multiple endocrine capacities.

Diagnosis. The diagnosis is suspected on appearance of one or more of the characteristic clinical features. Confirmation is achieved by examination of biopsy material or, preferably, by demonstration of increased urinary 5HIAA. Although slightly elevated levels occur in nontropical sprue, generally 5HIAA values above 15 mg. per 24 hours signify carcinoid. Since the qualitative screening test for 5-hydroxyindoles is positive only if daily excretion of 5HIAA exceeds 25 to 30 mg., specific quantitative tests should always be done in suspicious cases. Erroneously positive tests may occur in patients ingesting foods with a high serotonin content (bananas, pineapple, avocado, walnuts); spurious chromophores appear in tests on urine from patients receiving mephenesin or cough preparations containing glyceryl guaiacolate (a common medication in asthmatics!) and may be misinterpreted as positive tests. Phenothiazine drugs interfere with test reactants and may produce false negative tests. Indole chromatography is a useful adjunct, especially in the study of variant syndromes.

Prognosis. Patients with the full syndrome may survive beyond a decade but eventually succumb to nutritional, cardiac, or hepatic failure. In the interim there are periods of remission and exacerbation. A positive attitude by the physician, providing the patient with an understanding of his condition and involvement in its control, has proved beneficial.

Prevention and Treatment. The Tumor. Inspection of the terminal ileum during routine abdominal surgery, with excision of primary lesions, offers a means of prophylaxis. Surgical removal is curative of the syndrome only in the unusual case of a solitary bronchial or ovarian carcinoid. The results of partial hepatectomy have been disappointing. Probably the major indication for surgery is development of mechanical bowel obstruction secondary to primary or metastatic tumors. The surgeon should resect as little bowel (absorptive surface) as possible in his palliative procedure. Hypotension occurring during surgery is a serious problem since the usual vasopressor drugs often lower blood pressure further. However, methoxamine (Vasoxyl) and angiotensin (Hypertensin) may be used safely. Inhibition of serotonin synthesis by experimental drugs and pretreatment with corticosteroids may obviate hypotensive crises during operation.

Assessment of the results of tumor chemotherapy is difficult, although some moderate success and temporary improvement have been observed following oral administration of cyclophosphamide (Cytoxan) 100 to 150 mg. daily after a loading dose, or following hepatic artery perfusion with 5-fluorouracil. These and other chemotherapeutic agents often exacerbate the syndrome (with concomitant rises in 5HIAA) during the initial period of treatment. Generally, chemotherapy has taken a secondary role to pharmacologic control of symptoms. Radiation therapy has proved unsuccessful.

The Clinical Syndrome. An adequate diet tolerated by the patient, vitamin supplements, including niacin, and treatment of symptoms are important.

Flushing. Antiadrenergic and antikinin drugs, such as the phenothiazines prochlorperazine (Compazine), 5 to 10 mg., or chlorpromazine (Thorazine), 25 to 50 mg. orally every six hours, may be helpful; other antiadrenergic agents, including methyldopa (Aldomet), may be tried; anti-inflammatory steroids, e.g., prednisone, 5 mg. orally every six hours, may control uniquely the severe flushing in bronchial cases, but otherwise are reserved for tiding patients over periods of anorexia and inanition.

Diarrhea. Control of diarrhea and tenesmus may be achieved by use of either opium alkaloids or antiserotonin drugs given orally. Of the former, paregoric (5 to 10 ml. doses), opium tincture (6 to 15 drops), and the meperidine analogue diphenoxylate (Lomotil, 2.5 to 5.0 mg.) are useful. Of the serotonin antagonists, cyproheptadine (Periactin, 4 to 12 mg.) may be helpful, whereas methysergide (Sansert, 2 to 4 mg.), though highly effective in some patients, should be used only as a last resort because it produces vascular occlusive and fibrotic complications. Generally these drugs should be given on a regular daily schedule and individualized dosage. A new means of controlling gastrointestinal symptoms is provided by experimental drugs such as para-chlorophenylalanine (Fenclonine), which inhibit serotonin synthesis.

Adamson, A. R., Peart, W. S., Grahame-Smith, D. G., and Starr, M.: Pharmacological blockade of carcinoid flushing provoked by catecholamines and alcohol. Lancet, 2:293, 1969.

Engelman, K., Lovenberg, W., and Sjoerdsma, A.: Inhibition of serotonin synthesis by para-chlorophenylalanine in patients with the carcinoid syndrome. New Eng. J. Med., 277:1103, 1967.

Lotito, C. A., and Mengel, C. E.: Effect of melphalan in the malignant carcinoid syndrome. Arch. Intern. Med. (Chicago), 124:36, 1969.

Oates, J. A., Melmon, K., Sjoerdsma, A., Gillespie, L., and Mason, D. T.: Release of a kinin peptide in the carcinoid syndrome. Lancet, 1:514, 1964.

Sandler, M., Karim, S. M. M., and Williams, E. D.: Prostaglandins in amine-peptide-secreting tumours. Lancet, 2:1053, 1968.

Sjoerdsma, A., and Melmon, K.: The carcinoid spectrum. Gastroenterology, 47:104, 1964.

Sjoerdsma, A., Weissbach, H., and Udenfriend, S.: Simple test for diagnosis of metastatic carcinoid (argentaffinoma). J.A.M.A., 159:397, 1955.

Endocrine Syndromes Associated with Neoplasms of Nonendocrine Tissue

Nicholas P. Christy

Clinicians now recognize that neoplasms are often associated with systemic symptoms and signs not easily explained by local spread or distant metastases. Extreme cachexia in the presence of a small nonmetastatic tumor is familiar. Many other examples, involving various systems, can be cited (Table 1). These have been observed in all classes of neoplasms: carcinomas, sarcomas, lymphomas, and leukemias. It is not yet possible to ascribe all these effects to humoral agents elaborated by the tumors, although many substances have been postulated, including bradykinin, kallikrein, and others.

Owing to advances made in the 1960's, there are now plausible humoral explanations for certain quite well defined endocrine syndromes associated with cancer (Table 2). The weight of evidence is that the tumors themselves, although not arising from glandular tissue, secrete and release substances with the biologic properties of natural hormones. The syndromes are not always obvious. The hyperthyroidism that accompanies choriocarcinoma (Table 2) is more chemical than clinical, and many patients with oat cell carcinoma of the lung have laboratory evidence of hyperadrenocorticism, viz. elevated urinary and plasma 17-hydroxycorticosteroid values, exaggerated response of the latter to administrated ACTH, and abnormal diurnal variation of plasma corticoids, but do not have clinically detectable Cushing's syndrome. The point is that there probably are associated with cancer a great many biochemical abnormalities, still undetected, which probably will turn out to be useful as signals of clinically important problems.

The evidence that tumors secrete and release hormones is not perfect, but it is good. What is required for proof is roughly analogous to Koch's postulates as applied to the etiologic significance of a microbe. There must be (1) coexistence of tumor and an endocrine syndrome; (2) a demonstration in blood or urine of the causative hormone; (3) demonstration of large quantities of that hormone in the tumor and evidence that the hormone does not come from its "usual" glandular site; (4) ideally, demonstration in vitro of the tumor's capacity to make large amounts of the hormone; and (5) disappearance of, or definite improvement in, the endocrine syndrome upon removal of the tumor.

(1) Coexistence of neoplasms and endocrine syndromes is generally accepted; there are now several hundred reported cases, and the syndromes are of at least 11 distinct and recognizable types (Table 2). (2) Greatly elevated concentrations of hormone activity have been shown by biologic or radioimmunoassay in blood of patients with tumors, e.g., of ACTH in association with Cushing's syndrome, gonadotrophins with precocious puberty, TSH with hyperthyroidism, and erythropoietin with erythrocytosis (Table 2). One of the major imperfections in the data is that none of the hormones associated with tumors has been absolutely proved chemically to be identical with the natural product. However, the behavior of the best-studied hormones, e.g., ACTH, is so nearly that of the native substance in a large series of physical, chemical, immunologic, and biologic tests that there seems no good reason to doubt that most of the hormone-like materials presumably elaborated by the tumors are the same or nearly the same as those made by glands. (3) Very high concentrations of these hormones or hormone-like activities have been measured directly in tumors associated with endocrine syndromes, not in most other tumors: ACTH, MSH, gonadotrophins, chorionic gonadotrophin, TSH, ADH, parathyroid hormone, glucagon, gastrin, and erythropoietin. In one case of presumed gonadotrophin-secreting bronchogenic carcinoma, secretion was proved by showing a higher concentra-

TABLE 1. METABOLIC ABNORMALITIES ASSOCIATED WITH CARCINOMA*

Syndrome	Site of Tumor	Humoral Agent Shown To Be Secreted by Tumor
Dermatologic		
Acanthosis nigricans	Stomach, breast, lung	
Dermal hyperpigmentation	Lung, thyroid (see Table 2)	+
Herpes zoster	Lymphoma; breast, stomach, others	
Dermatomyositis	Stomach, breast, lung, ovary	
Neurologic		
Cortical cerebellar degeneration	Lung, breast, ovary, uterus	
Peripheral neuropathy	Lung, others	
Subacute spinocerebellar degeneration	Lung, breast	
Myopathies	Breast, lung, cervix, ovary, colon	
Myasthenia-like syndrome	Lung (oat cell type)	
Vascular		
Venous thrombosis	Lung, female reproductive organs, pancreas	
Marantic endocarditis	Stomach, lung, pancreas	
Fibrinogen deficiency	Prostate, bronchus	
Carcinoid syndrome	(See Table 2)	+
Hematologic		
Anemia (no blood loss, infection)	Many	
Eosinophilia	Colon, pancreas, stomach, breast	
Red cell aplasia	Thymus	
Erythrocytosis	(See Table 2)	+
Gastrointestinal		
Hepatomegaly without metastases	Kidney	
Zollinger-Ellison syndrome	Pancreas (see Table 2)	+
Metabolic		
Disturbances in protein metabolism		
Hypoalbuminemia, raised α-globulin	Many	
Amyloidosis	Several	
Cryofibrinogenemia (bleeding, thrombosis)	Prostate, others	
Macroglobulinemia, cryoglobulinemia, cold agglutinins	Several (mesothelioma)	
Hypoglycemia	Mesoderm, others (see Table 2)	
Hyperglycemia	Lung, pancreas, others	
Hypercalcemia	Lung, kidney, ovary, others (see Table 2)	+
Cushing's syndrome	Lung, thymus, others (see Table 2)	+
Gynecomastia	Lung, hepatoma	+
Inappropriate water retention	Lung, (see Table 2)	+
Skeletal		
Digital clubbing	Lung	
Pulmonary hypertrophic osteoarthropathy	Lung, mesothelioma of pleura (see Table 2)	±
Pachydermoperiostosis, acromegaloid features	Lung	

*Data from Greenberg et al., Amer. J. Med., 36:106, 1964. It is noteworthy that since these data were collected from the literature (1964), several of the syndromes have been shown to be due to the effects of hormone-like substances most probably secreted by the tumors.

tion of FSH in the venous effluent from the tumor than in its arterial supply. With respect to ACTH, high concentrations have been found in plasma and tumor, low concentrations in the pituitary; the inference is that the tumor secretes massive amounts of ACTH, adrenocortical hyperplasia follows, and the induced hypercortisolism suppresses synthesis of ACTH by the pituitary. Similarly, several patients have had tumors containing gonadotrophin, gonadotrophinuria, and reduced pituitary gonadotrophin. (4) In one malignant thymoma associated with Cushing's syndrome, cells propagated in tissue culture continued to produce ACTH for weeks. (5) There are now many instances of cure or definite remission of endocrine syndromes following successful removal of the

associated tumor. For example, Liddle et al. have reported nine surgical cures of Cushing's syndrome by removal of the "ACTH"-producing tumor. Dermal hyperpigmentation has disappeared after tumor removal in several cases of MSH-producing cancer. Radiation to a presumably ADH-secreting lung tumor has brought about temporary remission of inappropriate water retention in at least one case, and there are now 30 reported remissions of hypercalcemia after removal of a "parathyroid hormone"-secreting tumor. The primary role of the tumor in the secretion of the hormone is further strengthened by return of the hypercalcemia in ten of these patients when the tumor recurred.

Pathogenesis. The evidence for tumor secretion

TABLE 2. ENDOCRINE SYNDROMES ASSOCIATED WITH MALIGNANT DISEASE*

Syndrome	Hormone-like Activity	Sites of Primary Tumor
Cushing's syndrome	ACTH	Lung thyroid, thymus, pancreas, others
Dermal hyperpigmentation	MSH	Lung, thymus, pancreas
Precocious puberty, feminization	FSH, LH	Lung, liver
Precocious puberty, gynecomastia	HCG	Testis, pineal, liver, adrenal cortex
Hyperthyroidism	TSH	Trophoblast, testis
Pulmonary osteoarthropathy?†	GH, LH	Lung
Inappropriate antidiuresis	ADH	Lung, pancreas
Hypercalcemia	PTH	Lung, kidney, ovary, uterus, others
Hypoglycemia	Insulin-like	Mesenchyme, liver, adrenal, others
None recognized	Glucagon	Lung
Zollinger-Ellison syndrome	Gastrin	Pancreas
Erythrocythemia	Erythropoietin	Kidney, cerebellum, liver, uterus, adrenal medulla
Carcinoid syndrome	Serotonin	Pancreatic ducts, bronchus, lung
Spider angiomatosis	Estrogen?‡	Lung, liver

*Adapted from Lipsett, M. B., et al.: Ann. Intern. Med., 61:733, 1964, and Omenn, G. S.: Ann. Intern. Med., 72:136, 1970.
†A definite relationship between the observed elevated serum growth hormone or gonadotrophin concentrations and osteoarthropathy is not generally established.
‡There is not yet definite evidence that the tumors produce estrogen (see Ann. Intern. Med., 70:581, 1969).

and release of hormones, mostly polypeptides, is convincing. The mechanisms by which neoplastic tissue manages to synthesize complex molecules with hormonal activity are still conjectural. The prevailing view is that the neoplastic cells in a characteristic process of dedifferentiation lose certain genetic depressor mechanisms so that normally inhibited genetic information is expressed. This hypothesis now appears more tenable than the theory of the "sponge," i.e., the taking up of materials (hormones) from the circulation by the tumor; the matter is discussed in detail by Amatruda, by Bower and Gordan, and by Lipsett et al.

Terminology. These endocrine manifestations have been termed "ectopic," as in the "ectopic ACTH syndrome" (Liddle). The term is appropriate only when the site of the tumor presumably secreting the hormone is clearly not in the organ that ordinarily secretes that hormone, as in an oat cell carcinoma of the lung secreting ACTH, an ovarian tumor secreting parathyroid hormone-like peptide, or a pancreatic tumor secreting serotonin. The term is not appropriate in hyperthyroidism associated with TSH-secreting choriocarcinoma, since the normal placenta apparently synthesizes a TSH-like substance; in erythrocytosis associated with renal carcinoma or renal cyst, since the normal kidney synthesizes an erythropoietin; or in carcinoid tumors associated with argentaffin tumors of the small intestine, since this tissue is a normal site of serotonin production.

Clinical Manifestations and Treatment (Table 2). There are practical reasons for recognizing the associations of endocrine syndromes with neoplastic disease. (1) Frequently, the endocrinopathy antedates the appearance of the tumor, and thus may serve as a diagnostic clue to neoplastic disease. (2) The endocrine disorders may be life-threatening, as hypoglycemia or hypercalcemia, or severely disabling, as Cushing's syndrome, and yet amenable to palliative treatment. (3) Successful removal of tumor may cure the endocrine syndrome as well as the cancer. (4) Differences in clinical and biochemical behavior of these tumor-associated endocrinopathies from those associated with the classic glandular hyperfunctional states often make a differential diagnosis possible. The general characteristics of the tumor-associated endocrine syndromes are that the hormone is secreted in anarchic fashion, that is, secretion is not regulated by the normal control mechanisms; and, as indicated above, the locus of secretion is displaced to a site not ordinarily involved in hormonal synthesis.

In the discussion that follows, comparison with the classic syndromes of hormone overproduction is emphasized to facilitate differential diagnosis.

Cushing's Syndrome. Clinically evident hypercortisolism has been observed in association with oat cell carcinomas of the lung, thymomas, non-insulin-producing islet cell tumors of the pancreas, pheochromocytomas, and tumors of the thyroid, ovary, prostate, parotid, liver, and neural tissue. Perhaps 200 instances of this association have been reported, and subtle chemical evidence of hypercortisolism has been found in many more, especially with carcinoma of the lung (vide supra). Large quantities of ACTH have been thoroughly characterized in plasma and in some tumors. That the capacity to synthesize ACTH may be a more general property of tumors can be inferred from the finding of Liddle et al. that about 8 per cent of unselected visceral carcinomas not obviously associated with Cushing's syndrome contained considerable amounts of the hormone.

The most important point to be made about the clinical features of Cushing's syndrome associated with nonendocrine tumor is that they are often subtle. Patients may show the classic features, but most do not. The absence of obesity and striae is probably a function of the weight loss accompanying the cancer. Patients with all forms of Cushing's syndrome have an equal incidence of glucose intolerance and hypertension, about 90 per cent. But in the syndrome associated with tumor, the onset is faster and the sex incidence favors men, whereas the "pituitary" form of Cushing's disease and adrenal adenoma are far more common in women. Patients with the tumor-related form rarely have osteoporosis, probably because the clinical course of the tumor is short. Generalized dermal hyperpigmentation is common in the tumor form, probably because of the huge quantities of ACTH secreted by the cancer, or of MSH, which may also be produced in large amounts. Severe hypokalemia and weakness, as well as edema, are also more common in this form of the disease, and are best explained by the enormous quantities of cortisol secreted by the hyperplastic adrenals. Hypokalemia is not due to aldosteronism; the secretion of aldosterone is normal or low. In the other forms of Cushing's syndrome, the patients die of infection or the effects of hypertension; in the tumor form, the usual cause of death is the cancer. At necropsy, the adrenals are enormously hypertrophied, and the pituitary contains subnormal amounts of ACTH.

The laboratory evidence of hypercortisolism is definite and extreme. Plasma cortisol values (ca. 80 μg. per 100 ml.), and urinary 17-hydroxycorticosteroid and 17-ketogenic steroids may be ten times normal, all much higher than in the "pituitary" or adrenal adenoma forms of Cushing's syndrome. Provocative tests show autonomous cortisol secretion owing to autonomous ACTH secretion by the tumor; urinary steroids do not rise when metyrapone is given, and do not fall in response to dexamethasone. Differentiation from primary adrenocortical carcinoma, also characterized by very high steroid values, can be made by measuring plasma ACTH concentration; it is very low in adrenal cancer, very high in the presence of ACTH-secreting tumor (see article on the Adrenal Cortex).

To recapitulate: an ACTH-secreting tumor, most likely to be in lung, thymus, or pancreas, should be suspected in any patient with subtle or borderline clinical signs of Cushing's syndrome who has lost, not gained, weight, who has weakness and severe hypokalemia, and whose plasma or urinary corticosteroid values are extremely high.

Management, ideally, is total removal of the tumor, which has been followed by remission of the Cushing's syndrome in several cases. Therefore, a vigorous effort should be made to excise tumors completely; some are relatively benign, e.g., bronchial adenomas. If this is not possible, palliative x-radiation or chemotherapy of the cancer is carried out, and chemical palliation of the hyperadrenocorticism can be tried with o,p'-DDD, metyrapone, aminoglutethimide, or combinations of these drugs (see Cushing's syndrome in the article on the Adrenal Cortex). If the effects of hypercortisolism, e.g., hypokalemia, are incapacitating, bilateral total adrenalectomy may be done, and has in some cases provided good relief.

Dermal Hyperpigmentation. Generalized hyperpigmentation of the skin, resembling that of Addison's disease, may occur with oat cell carcinoma of the lung, thymoma, neurogenic tumors, or tumors of the ovary, pancreas, and prostate. Raised concentrations of α-MSH and β-MSH have

been measured in plasma by radioimmunoassay; most of the pigmentary effect is due to the β-MSH, which has also been found in the associated cancers. Some tumors in this group have been shown to secrete both excessive MSH and ACTH, with resulting Cushing's syndrome. Several patients have shown disappearance or diminution of dermal pigment when tumors were successfully removed.

Gynecomastia, Precocious Puberty. About 5 per cent of male patients with lung cancer have gynecomastia, but in only a few have elevated gonadotrophin values been detected in blood or urine. Tumor types are "large cell" carcinomas, epidermoid, anaplastic, and oat cell carcinomas, and adenocarcinoma. In some of the patients with gynecomastia, raised levels of urinary estrogens have also been found, possibly a result of adrenal or testicular stimulation by gonadotrophin secreted from the tumor; in some cases, striking hypertrophic pulmonary osteoarthropathy has also been present. Its relation to gonadotrophin or estrogen excess is not yet clear.

Evidence that the tumor is indeed the site of gonadotrophin secretion is convincing (*vide supra*). When analyzed by radioimmunoassay, the gonadotrophin has been usually LH, on one occasion FSH.

Spider angiomas and pulmonary osteoarthropathy may or may not accompany gynecomastia. In such cases, careful search for a pulmonary tumor by roentgenography should be done, and measurements made for urinary estrogens and for urinary gonadotrophins (by bioassay) or plasma LH (by radioimmunoassay). Failure to suppress high urinary or plasma gonadotrophin levels by administration of large amounts of estrogen for several days may turn out to be a useful diagnostic test.

Treatment is unsatisfactory. The tumors are very malignant and have not been surgically curable. Radiation and chemotherapy are ineffective. It remains to be seen whether methotrexate will reduce gonadotrophin production, as it does in trophoblastic tumors (*vide infra*).

Another group of tumors has been associated with secretion of HCG. In addition to benign or malignant tumors of the placenta, these are choriocarcinomas of the pineal or testis, hepatoblastoma of the liver, adrenal cortical carcinoma, carcinoma of the breast, and malignant melanoma. Again, the clinical manifestations are gynecomastia in the adult male and isosexual precocity in children. In boys, the testes have been enlarged in some, and all showed testicular interstitial cell hyperplasia histologically. The gonadotrophin has the characteristics of HCG, and has been found in high concentration in the urine, serum, and tumors. In a very few cases, gonadotrophin levels have been temporarily lowered by methotrexate which had variable effects on the tumor itself. So far, these tumors have all been fatal.

Hyperthyroidism. In addition to the rare association of hyperthyroidism with tumors of the gastrointestinal tract, hematopoietic system, lung, and other organs, eight recent patients have been identified in whom thyrotoxicosis coexisted with metastatic disease of trophoblastic origin (choriocarcinoma or hydatidiform mole) and, in one case, with metastatic embryonal cell carcinoma of the testis. Together with the expected finding of high titer of urinary HCG, some of these patients had elevated plasma TSH (bioassay), and TSH-like substance was detectable in tumor tissue. The *clinical manifestations* of hyperthyroidism were minimal; more than half the patients had no symptoms, and the rest had only mild symptoms of thyrotoxicosis. All had tachycardia, but other physical signs of the endocrinopathy, e.g., goiter, were generally absent, although laboratory evidence—raised serum PBI and high thyroidal uptake of I^{131}—was definite. These indices can be controlled with antithyroid drugs or iodides, but most striking is the favorable response of both clinical and laboratory signs of hyperthyroidism to treatment with methotrexate, which is capable of causing regression of these tumors. The presence of mild thyrotoxicosis, seen in fewer than 10 per cent of women with trophoblastic neoplasms, does not affect prognosis of the tumor.

Pulmonary Osteoarthropathy. Hypertrophic pulmonary osteoarthropathy has occurred accompanying gonadotrophin-producing cancers of the lung. The relation between the hormone and the skeletal abnormality is not clear, and the familiar remission of the latter on removal of such tumors does not establish the relation. A recent and intriguing finding is raised level of serum growth hormone in a patient with adenocarcinoma of the lung and painful hypertrophic osteoarthropathy. On removal of the tumor, joint pain and stiffness and swelling of the fingers disappeared, and the serum growth hormone value fell to normal. No data are available on growth hormone content of the tumor. In a few patients with lung cancer and digital clubbing, growth hormone values were essentially normal. Further studies must be aimed at growth hormone content of lung tumors associated with osteoarthropathy, especially when accompanied by pachydermoperiostosis or acromegaloid features.

Inappropriate Antidiuresis. Excessive sodium excretion in patients with lung cancer was first reported in 1938, but not until 1957 did Bartter and Schwartz and their co-workers attribute this abnormality to water retention resulting from abnormally regulated secretion of ADH. Studies done in the last decade have disclosed ADH-like activity in several tumors taken from patients with the syndrome of inappropriate ADH secretion; the tumors have been mostly oat cell carcinomas of the lung, with a few others, e.g. pancreatic and duodenal carcinoma. The ADH-like activity has not been completely characterized, but resembles in physical, chemical, and biologic properties human pituitary ADH, i.e., arginine vasopressin.

The clinical manifestations of hyponatremia may be minimal or absent, probably because the abnormality has developed slowly. Often, hyponatremia is a chance finding during routine study of a patient with lung cancer. To prove the entity, one has to show a urine hypertonic with respect to plasma, normal GFR, and normal adrenocortical function, i.e., absence of adrenocortical insufficiency. The extracellular space, if measured, is found to be expanded. The pathogenesis of this pattern of abnormalities is discussed in the article on Diseases of the Posterior Pituitary. Treatment with hypertonic salt is not useful; the only effective method is restriction of water intake to less than 1 liter a day. In a few patients, the water and electrolyte abnormality has undergone temporary remission with successful palliative treatment of the tumor by x-radiation or chemotherapy.

Hypercalcemia. The hypercalcemia of malignant disease may be due to three mechanisms: (1) osteolytic lesions of bone associated with widespread metastases, as from carcinoma of the thyroid, prostate, or lung, or lymphoma; (2) osteolysis in the absence of bony metastases, associated with some carcinomas of the breast which presumably elaborate sterols related to vitamin D; and (3) osteolysis in the absence of bony metastases, in association with tumors which appear to secrete a parathyroid hormone (PTH)-like substance. Tumors have been squamous cell carcinomas of the lung and other organs, and carcinoma of the kidney, ovary, uterus, pancreas, and colon. Evidence for primary secretion of parathyroid hormone by the neoplasm has come from demonstration of immunoreactive PTH in plasma of patients with nonparathyroid tumors and hypercalcemia, from the detection of PTH-like substance in the tumors, disappearance or diminution of hypercalcemia upon tumor removal, and reappearance of the electrolyte abnormality with recurrence of the cancer.

The clinical features of hypercalcemia are presented in detail in the article on the Parathyroids. The important clinical point is that the hypercalcemia associated with PTH-secreting tumor of nonendocrine tissue is more likely to manifest itself as lethargy, weakness, anorexia, nausea, and vomiting, and less likely to appear as renal stones or bone disease. Patients with the "ectopic PTH syndrome" are more apt to lose weight and to be anemic.

Separation of these patients from those with hyperparathyroidism by laboratory tests may be difficult. Both may have extreme hypercalcemia, low or normal serum phosphorus, elevated plasma values for PTH, and unresponsiveness of hypercalcemia to corticosteroids; but careful examination, laboratory study, and roentgenographic search, e.g., by chest films and intravenous pyelography, will disclose most of the nonparathyroid tumors.

The *treatment* of hypercalcemia is discussed in the article on the Parathyroids.

Hypoglycemia. The association of severe fasting hypoglycemia with certain neoplasms, especially very large retroperitoneal or intrathoracic tumors, is well established. Most of the tumors are fibromas or sarcomas, sometimes of huge size—up to 10 kg.; others are hepatoma, adrenocortical carcinoma, adenocarcinoma of stomach and colon, undifferentiated bronchial carcinoma, and bronchial carcinoid. As for the mechanism of hypoglycemia, there is evidence against excessive glucose utilization by the tumor and against stimulation by the tumor of insulin secretion by the pancreas, removal of which does not affect the hypoglycemia. The prevailing view is that the tumor secretes a hypoglycemia-producing substance, which, with only a few exceptions, is not demonstrable as high levels of immunoreactive insulin in plasma or tumor, but only as "insulin-like" activity. The secretory role of the tumor is affirmed by surgical "cure" of the hypoglycemia in about 20 patients whose tumors have been successfully removed.

The hypoglycemia is indistinguishable clinically and by most of the provocative tests from that associated with islet cell adenoma or carcinoma of the pancreas. However, almost all patients with nonpancreatic tumors lack high plasma insulin values, and the presence of a large tumor is usually apparent.

Treatment is best done by excising the tumor; even incomplete removal may relieve the hypoglycemia temporarily. Failing this, palliative measures must include continuous feeding of carbohydrate and administration of corticosteroids, diazoxide, and possibly glucagon (see the article on Hypoglycemia).

Zollinger-Ellison Syndrome. This entity, hypersecretion of gastric acid and intractable peptic ulceration, associated with noninsulin-secreting adenomas of the pancreatic islets, is discussed in the section on Diseases of the Digestive System. The responsible hormone is the gastric secretagogue gastrin, produced by the pancreatic tumor.

Erythrocythemia. Erythrocytosis, raised hemoglobin and hematocrit value, and increased red cell volume have occurred in nearly 300 reported patients with hypernephroma, benign renal lesions (polycystic disease, renal cysts, hydronephrosis), cerebellar hemangioblastoma, uterine fibroma, ovarian tumors, hepatoma, pheochromocytoma, and others. That the tumor produces an erythropoietic substance is indicated by presence of high concentrations of an erythropoiesis-stimulating factor in blood of patients, a similar substance in the tumors, and regression of erythremia upon removal of the tumor. The substance is indistinguishable from normal renal erythropoietin.

The clinical and laboratory features usually make possible the differentiation from secondary polycythemia and polycythemia vera. The erythremia is often asymptomatic and is found on routine study of blood. The splenomegaly and the thrombohemorrhagic complications of polycythemia vera are lacking, as are thrombocytosis and leukocytosis. Blood gases are normal, distinguishing tumor-related erythremia from secondary polycythemia. It is most important to search carefully for tumors when erythremia is present, since the neoplasms may be small or deep-seated and therefore occult. Because many of the tumors are relatively benign, surgical removal is often accompanied by long remissions.

Carcinoid Syndrome. This, the only definite example of an "endocrine" syndrome owing to production of a humoral agent that is not a polypeptide, is discussed in the article on the Sympatho-Adrenal System.

Multiple Hormones Produced by a Single Tumor. Several tumors have been reported which apparently secrete two or even three distinct hormones. The pulmonary and thymic tumors secreting both ACTH and MSH have already been mentioned. A few patients with hepatoma have had both hypoglycemia and polycythemia, and islet cell tumors of the pancreas have been described with hypoglycemia and carcinoid syndrome, and with Cushing's syndrome and carcinoid syndrome. Three hormones, ACTH, MSH, and gastrin, were found in a single pancreatic tumor. Glucagon has been detected in a few tumors (lung, pancreas), usually along with insulin or gastrin, but has not been identified with any clinical disorder. One may raise the question of whether the hyperglycemia of neoplastic disease is related to glucagon secretion by the cancer.

Amatruda, T. T., Jr.: Nonendocrine-secreting tumors. In Bondy, P. K. (ed.): Duncan's Diseases of Metabolism. 6th ed. Philadelphia, W. B. Saunders Company, 1969, p. 1227.

Amatruda, T. T., Jr., Mulrow, P. J., Gallagher, J. C., and Sawyer, W. H.: Carcinoma of the lung with inappropriate antidiuresis: Demonstration of antidiuretic hormone-like activity in tumor extract. New Eng. J. Med., 269:544, 1963.

Bower, B. F., and Gordan, G. S.: Hormonal effects of nonendocrine tumors. Ann. Rev. Med., 16:83, 1965.

Greenberg, E., Divertie, M. B., and Woolner, L. B.: A review of unusual systemic manifestations associated with carcinoma. Amer. J. Med., 36:106, 1964.

Liddle, G. W., Nicholson, W. E., Island, D. P., Orth, D. N., Abe, K., and Lowder, S. C.: Clinical and laboratory studies of ectopic humoral syndromes. Recent Progr. Hormone Res., 25:283, 1969.

Lipsett, M. B., Odell, W. D., Rosenberg, L. E., and Waldmann, T. A.: Humoral syndromes associated with nonendocrine tumors. Ann. Intern. Med., 61:733, 1964.

Meador, C. K., Liddle, G. W., Island, D. P., Nicholson, W. E., Lucas, C. P., Nuckton, J. G., and Luetscher, J. A.: Cause of Cushing's syndrome in patients with tumors arising from "nonendocrine" tissue. J. Clin. Endocr., 22:693, 1962.

Peart, W. S., Porter, K. A., Robertson, J. I. S., Sandler, M., and Bladock, E.: Carcinoid syndrome due to pancreatic-duct neoplasm secreting 5-hydroxytryptophan and 5-hydroxytryptamine. Lancet, 1:239, 1963.

Plimpton, C. H., and Gellhorn, A.: Hypercalcemia in malignant disease without evidence of bone destruction. Amer. J. Med., 21:750, 1956.

Unger, R. H.: The riddle of tumor hypoglycemia. Amer. J. Med., 40:325, 1966.

Parathyroid

G. D. Aurbach

PARATHYROID HORMONE AND CALCITONIN

Parathyroid hormone, a principal regulator of concentration of calcium in the extracellular fluid, has been isolated in pure form and characterized chemically as a polypeptide. Radioimmunoassays show that calcium is the primary factor controlling secretion of the hormone; phosphate is not a direct determinant of secretion. A fall in blood calcium effects secretion of the hormone which in turn causes an increased rate of removal of calcium from bone to the extracellular fluids. The hormone also enhances reabsorption of calcium from the glomerular filtrate and induces increased urinary excretion of phosphate by direct action (possibly inhibition of the reabsorption of phosphate) on the kidney. These physiologic effects on both calcium and phosphate are accounted for by a single hormonal molecule. The mechanism of action of parathyroid hormone is mediated by cyclic 3′,5′-adenosine monophosphate (3′,5′-AMP) produced through direct specific hormonal activation of the enzyme adenyl cyclase in bone and kidney. The consequent increase in concentration of 3′,5′-AMP in the renal cortex and bone activates other intracellular processes which account for the physiologic actions of the hormone. The increase in concentration of 3′,5′-AMP effected by parathyroid hormone in the renal parenchyma is also manifested by increased urinary excretion of 3′,5′-AMP.

A newly identified polypeptide, calcitonin, another hormone important in controlling blood calcium and bone metabolism, has been isolated, analyzed for structure, and synthesized. It is secreted from the parafollicular cells found in the mammalian thyroid but related embryologically to the ultimobranchial body of lower vertebrate species. The rate of secretion of calcitonin is a direct function of the concentration of calcium in plasma, whereas parathyroid hormone is secreted at a rate inversely proportional to calcium concentration. The hypocalcemic action of thyrocalcitonin is effected through an inhibition of resorption of mineral from bone. The precise biochemical mechanism involved is still unknown.

Diseases of the parathyroid gland include hyperparathyroidism and hypoparathyroidism. Pseudohypoparathyroidism encompasses the general clinical and laboratory features of hypoparathyroidism but is an abnormality not of parathyroid gland function but of the receptor tissues for parathyroid hormone. Excessive secretion of calcitonin is now recognized as a manifestation of some cases of medullary carcinoma of the thyroid. This syndrome comprises a complex pathophysiologic state in which hypocalcemia is rare even though there is excessive secretion of calcitonin, a high concentration of calcitonin in the plasma, and a compensatory increase in secretion of parathyroid hormone. Some cases are associated with primary hyperparathyroidism, pheochromocytoma, Cushing's syndrome, or multiple neuromas.

Aurbach, G. D.: Isolation of parathyroid hormone after extraction with phenol. J. Biol. Chem., 234:3179, 1959.

Aurbach, G. D., and Chase, L. R.: Cyclic 3′,5′-adenylic acid in bone and the mechanism of action of parathyroid hormone. Fed. Proc. 29:1179, 1970.

Aurbach, G. D., Potts, J. T., Jr., Chase, L. R., and Melson, G. L.: Polypeptide hormones and calcium metabolism. Ann. Intern. Med., 70:1243, 1969.

Chase, L. R., and Aurbach, G. D.: Renal adenyl cyclase: Anatomically separate sites for parathyroid hormone and vasopressin. Science, 159:545, 1968.

Copp, D. H., Cockcroft, D. W., and Kueh, Y.: Calcitonin from ultimobranchial glands of dogfish and chickens. Science, 158:924, 1967.

Deftos, L. J., Lee, M. R., and Potts, J. T., Jr.: A radioimmunoassay for thyrocalcitonin. Proc. Nat. Acad. Sci. USA, 60:293, 1968.

Hirsch, P. F., Gauthier, G. F., and Munson, P. L.: Thyroid hypocalcemic principle and recurrent laryngeal nerve injury as factors affecting the response to parathyroidectomy in rats. Endocrinology, 73:244, 1963.

Potts, J. T., Jr., Keutmann, H. T., Niall, H. D., Deftos, L., Brewer, H. B., Jr., and Aurbach, G. D.: Covalent structure of bovine parathyroid hormone in relation to biological and immunological activity. In Talmage, R. V., and Belanger, L. F. (eds.): Parathyroid Hormone and Thyrocalcitonin (Calcitonin). Amsterdam, Excerpta Medica Foundation, 1968, p. 44.

Hirsch, P. F., and Munson, P. L.: Thyrocalcitonin. Physiol. Rev., 49:548, 1969.

Potts, J. T., Jr., Niall, H. D., Keutmann, H. T., Brewer, H. B., Jr., and Deftos, L. J.: The amino acid sequence of porcine thyrocalcitonin. Proc. Nat. Acad. Sci. USA, 59:1321, 1968.

Sherwood, L. M., Mayer, G. P., Ramberg, C. F., Jr., Kronfeld, D. S., Aurbach, G. D., and Potts, J. T., Jr.: Regulation of parathyroid hormone secretion: Proportional control by calcium, lack of effect of phosphate. Endocrinology, 83:1043, 1968.

HYPERPARATHYROIDISM

Definition. Primary hyperparathyroidism is the clinical condition resulting from incompletely regulated excessive secretion of hormone from the parathyroid glands. The consequent pathophysiology, which may include hypercalcemia, tissue calcification, and osteitis fibrosa cystica, represents predominantly the result of excessive parathyroid hormone action on bone.

Etiology. Hypersecretion of parathyroid hormone as a manifestation of primary parathyroid disease may be caused by adenomas, single or multiple, primary chief cell or clear cell hyperplasia, or carcinoma of the glands. Secondary hyperparathyroidism develops as a compensatory mechanism in any abnormal physiological state tending to produce true hypocalcemia; this state may occur in hypovitaminosis D, vitamin D-resistant osteomalacia or rickets, malabsorption of calcium, chronic renal disease, or renal tubular acidosis. There are no known factors to which development of primary hyperparathyroidism can be attributed. There is a suggestion that prolonged, progressive secondary hyperparathyroidism may evolve into autonomous primary hyperparathyroidism in some cases of chronic renal disease, but there is no evidence that parathyrotropic substances exist in either normal or abnormal physiology. Several families with hyperparathyroidism have been reported, and a genetic factor may be involved in some cases of parathyroid adenoma or hyperplasia.

Incidence. Recent surveys validate earlier projections that better diagnostic methods and wider clinical awareness promote ready discovery of new cases. Automated laboratory facilities now make possible routine analysis of serum calcium for all patients in the clinic and hospital populations. In one center wherein routine analyses were performed, the incidence of hyperparathyroidism was as high as one case per thousand in the clinical population examined. Thus hyperparathyroidism is not so rare a disease as clinicians had believed. In over 80 per cent of the cases primary hyperparathyroidism is attributable to a single parathyroid adenoma, and in less than 2 per cent of the cases carcinoma of the parathyroid gland is the cause. Other cases are about equally divided in terms of primary pathology between clear cell hyperplasia, chief cell hyperplasia, and multiple adenomas.

Pathology. Usually parathyroid adenomas vary in size from 1 to 5 grams, but occasionally very large tumors, 50 grams or more, may develop. In general, large tumors are more likely to be associated with clinically evident bone disease, marked hypercalcemia, very high concentrations of parathyroid hormone in plasma, and a short interval between development of symptoms and establishment of diagnosis. Histologic examination usually shows chief cells and some water-clear cells; sometimes the latter are predominant. Rarely adenomas are composed of oxyphil cells. Hyperplasia may be of the chief cell or water-clear cell type. Occasionally adenomas of other endocrine glands are found in hyperparathyroidism (multiple endocrine adenomatosis; see Clinical Manifestations). The effect of the disease is manifested in the bones as osteitis fibrosa cystica generalista (see section on Diseases of Bone). When the kidneys are affected, nephrolithiasis or nephrocalcinosis is apparent; pyelonephritis often complicates the course of the kidney disease.

Pancreatitis, acute or chronic, is now recognized as a possible complication of hyperparathyroidism. About half of the patients with advanced hyperparathyroidism examined at autopsy show calcification in the pancreas. It is possible that chronic hypercalcemia contributes to the development of pancreatitis, but the actual cause of this association has not been established.

Pathologic Physiology and Chemistry. Hypersecretion of parathyroid hormone from adenomatous or hyperplastic glands is expressed in acceleration of the normal physiologic actions of the hormone on bone and kidney. The effect on bone is reflected in hypercalcemia, a consequence of increased resorption of calcium from bone, and in more severe cases in the pathologic development in bone of osteitis fibrosa cystica. The effect on the kidney is manifested by an increased rate of phosphate clearance from the plasma and hypophosphatemia. The urinary excretion of 3',5'-AMP is greater than normal, and increases further upon intravenous injection of parathyroid hormone.

The majority of cases of hyperparathyroidism now being recognized show little or no clinically detectable bone disease. This finding may be attributable to earlier recognition of the disease, detection of milder forms of the disease with more general appreciation of the problem, or possibly higher dietary intakes of calcium that are now widespread. Some early or mild forms of hyperparathyroidism may be recognized primarily by nephrolithiasis associated with hypophosphatemia, but little or no hypercalcemia or skeletal abnormality. It is conceivable that calcitonin elaborated as a compensatory mechanism partially protects against the hypercalcemic and skeletal effects of parathyroid hormone in some of these cases. There is suggestive evidence (although proof is lacking) that parathyroid hormone has a direct effect on the gastrointestinal tract to produce an increase in absorption of calcium. In any event, whether it is a primary or secondary manifestation, gastrointestinal absorption of calcium is increased in hyperparathyroidism.

Although hypercalcemia is primarily a manifestation of the effect of the hormone on bone, a renal mechanism may be involved also. Recent studies indicate that parathyroid hormone influences the renal absorption of calcium from the glomerular filtrate. Thus, at any given concentration of calcium in plasma the clearance of calcium is reduced when parathyroid hormone is being secreted.

The classic laboratory manifestations of primary hyperparathyroidism are low serum phosphate and high serum calcium. Frequently the 24-hour excretion of calcium is high because of significant hypercalcemia, even though the renal clearance of calcium is relatively reduced. Hypercalciuria, with calcium excretion in excess of intake, is particularly apparent when diets low in calcium are given. Generally the special diet is given for three days, and then total urinary calcium is determined for 24-hour periods. Normal subjects should not excrete in excess of 175 mg. per 24 hours when taking a diet containing 150 mg. of calcium. The alkaline phosphatase in plasma may be high in hyperparathyroidism when there is significant bone disease. The high alkaline phosphatase is probably a manifestation of increased bone formation compensatory for the high rate of bone resorption induced by excessive parathyroid hormone secretion. Other manifestations of increased bone resorption are increased urinary excretion of hydroxyproline and pyrophosphate. Kinetic studies utilizing radioactive calcium frequently show evidence of increased bone metabolism.

A number of tests have been described based on the known physiologic action of parathyroid hormone in causing increased phosphate clearance. In many of these tests results are expressed in terms of per cent tubular reabsorption of phosphate (TRP) by the kidney. Although these procedures are constantly modified in attempts to obtain greater diagnostic differentiation, none is sufficiently specific to distinguish uniformly between normal and hyperparathyroid subjects. One test based on determination of phosphate clearance with induced hypercalcemia shows better than average discrimination. Phosphate clearance is measured between 8 and 10 A.M., and calcium, 10 mg. per kilogram of body weight, is administered intravenously between 9 P.M. and midnight. The following morning phosphate clearance is measured again. In normal subjects phosphate clearance falls 40 per cent or more after infusion of calcium. This response reflects primarily diminished secretion of hormone by glands normally sensitive to the regulatory influence of calcium. Secretion of hormone ceases from the normal gland but not from the autonomous gland of primary hyperparathyroidism as serum calcium approaches 12 mg. per 100 ml.

A radioimmunoassay for bovine parathyroid hormone allows detection of the hormone in the circulation of ruminant species, but not always in man because the human hormone does not show complete immunologic cross-reactivity with antiserum to the bovine hormone. In many laboratories circulating parathyroid hormone cannot be detected uniformly in normal human subjects or even in some subjects with mild hyperparathyroidism, and the immunoassay is still to be regarded as an experimental procedure. Nevertheless, use of the assay has often shown abnormally high concentrations of hormone in the plasma of hyperparathyroid subjects. High concentrations of hormone have been found also in cases of hyperparathyroidism resulting from ectopic production of hormone by nonparathyroid tumors as well as in secondary hyperparathyroidism and pseudohypoparathyroidism. In the present state of development the hormone can be detected in venous effluent from the parathyroid gland, and the method could probably be adapted to measuring the hormone in concentrates of peripheral plasma. The problem of determining parathyroid hormone will undoubtedly be lessened by developing a more sensitive antibody, possibly one prepared against human parathyroid hormone. Ultimately it is likely that the radioimmunoassay will become the principle diagnostic test for hyperparathyroidism. In particular, measurement of the secretory response to induced hypo- and hypercalcemia should provide definitive differential tests for primary and secondary hyperparathyroidism. Clinical states showing high rates of parathyroid hormone secretion and the responses to induced hypercalcemia are listed in Table 1.

Clinical Manifestations. The symptoms and signs of primary hyperparathyroidism are in general relatable to the pathophysiologic effects of excessive secretion of parathyroid hormone. However, it should be emphasized that the disease may exist in apparently healthy subjects with no complaints. Recently, significant numbers of new cases have been recognized through routine measurement of serum calcium in the general clinic population. Hypercalcemia, a consequence of increased mobilization of calcium from the skeleton, may cause polydipsia, polyuria, anorexia, weakness, fatigability, nausea, vomiting, constipation, and hypotonicity of the muscles and ligaments. Sometimes the latter is manifested in unusual joint flexibility, or "double jointedness." Hypercalcemia may depress sensitivity to electrical stimuli of ganglia and peripheral nerves, and this effect can be examined by the use of Erb's test. Shortening of the Q-T interval in the electrocardiogram is found in some patients with hypercalcemia. Prolonged hypercalcemia may lead to calcification in the eye displayed as "band keratopathy," opaque material appearing in vertical lines parallel to and within the limbus, or as conjunctival crystals without the limbus or under the eyelids. These lesions may require examination by slit lamp for detection. Peptic ulcers are common in hyperparathyroidism, and may reflect a potentiating effect of hypercalcemia on acid secretion. An association between acute or chronic pancreatitis and hyperparathyroidism is recognized more and more frequently, and one should be aware that hyperparathyroidism may exist in any case of pancreatitis.

Bone disease in hyperparathyroidism, osteitis fibrosa cystica, may be recognized by roentgenographic examination; it sometimes causes symptoms of bone pain or pathologic fracture. Roentgenographically, bone disease may be evidenced by loss of the lamina dura about the teeth, erosion of the distal clavicle, bone cysts, "brown tumors" of bone, epulis of the jaw, or subcortical bone resorption, most readily observed in the phalanges

TABLE 1. CLINICAL STATES SHOWING HIGH RATES OF PARATHYROID HORMONE SECRETION

Syndrome	Secretion Suppressible by Hypercalcemia
Primary hyperparathyroidism	
Parathyroid adenoma	No
Parathyroid hyperplasia	No
Ectopic hyperparathyroidism (nonparathyroid tumors)	No
Secondary hyperparathyroidism	
Osteomalacia	Yes
Chronic renal disease	Yes
Pseudohypoparathyroidism	Yes

or distal clavicles. Intra-articular calcification of cartilage may also be found by roentgenography.

Hypercalciuria may lead to nephrolithiasis with or without episodes of renal colic and passage of calcium oxalate or calcium phosphate stones. In other instances nephrocalcinosis may develop, sometimes causing progressive renal failure. Infection may complicate the course with either type of renal disorder.

In some patients with hyperparathyroidism there are no symptoms. Still others show symptoms not readily attributable to hypercalcemia or the effects of parathyroid hormone on bone. There may be burning in the throat and abdomen, vague abdominal pain, nonspecific malaise, numbness, back pain, stiffness of the hands, coccygeal pain, mood variation with depression, dry skin or pruritus, and muscular weakness.

In addition to pancreatitis and peptic ulcer, several other diseases may be associated with primary hyperparathyroidism. There is an increased incidence of arthralgia of ill-defined nature as well as gout and pseudogout. The latter is associated with intra-articular deposition of calcium pyrophosphate crystals. The presence of pseudogout should suggest the coexistence of primary hyperparathyroidism. Primary hyperparathyroidism may exist as part of the multiple endocrine adenomatosis syndrome. In such cases pituitary and pancreatic tumors appear; the latter may secrete gastrin-like hormones (Zollinger-Ellison syndrome) or insulin, causing ulcers or hypoglycemia respectively. Hyperparathyroidism may also occur in another type of endocrine adenomatosis consisting of pheochromocytomas, parathyroid adenomas, and medullary carcinoma of the thyroid (see discussion of Medullary Carcinoma of the Thyroid). Each of the two types of multiple endocrine adenomatosis syndromes may be familial. In addition, hyperparathyroidism has been described in association with Cushing's syndrome, acromegaly, hyperthyroidism, sarcoidosis, Paget's disease, and malignancy.

Differential Diagnosis. Hypercalcemia, demineralizing disease of bone, and nephrolithiasis are clinical problems that commonly suggest the diagnosis of hyperparathyroidism. Hypercalcemia is discussed separately and a number of differential points are listed. Ectopic hyperparathyroidism caused by secretion of parathyroid hormone from nonparathyroid malignancies can be particularly difficult to diagnose. The laboratory findings do not differ from those of hyperparathyroidism caused by parathyroid adenoma or hyperplasia; blood calcium is high, blood phosphate is low, and the alkaline phosphatase may be elevated. This syndrome must be considered in any case of hyperparathyroidism in which there is a history of weight loss or other symptoms suggesting systemic malignancy. The suspicion of malignancy requires extensive studies to ascertain the true cause of the disease.

Paget's disease of bone, osteoporosis, osteomalacia, multiple myeloma, and malignancies metastatic to bone show varying degrees of skeletal demineralization. The roentgenographic appearance in each of these disorders, though, is more or less characteristic. In osteoporosis, the serum calcium, phosphate, and alkaline phosphatase are normal. Extensive Paget's disease is attended by an increase in serum alkaline phosphatase, but phosphate and calcium in blood are normal except during periods of immobilization, when hypercalcemia may develop. Examination of bone marrow is helpful in excluding the diagnosis of multiple myeloma, and is occasionally of value in diagnosing lymphoma or metastatic malignancy. Examination of plasma and urine for myeloma proteins should be routine in suspected cases. Osteomalacia may be caused by hypovitaminosis D, resistance to vitamin D, intestinal malabsorption syndromes, or renal tubular acidosis. In these conditions, serum calcium is normal or low, sometimes with tetany, blood phosphate is low, and the alkaline phosphatase is elevated.

Secondary hyperparathyroidism in chronic renal disease may produce the histologic picture of osteitis fibrosa cystica. In general, serum phosphate is high and there is a tendency to hypocalcemia. Occasionally, however, primary hyperparathyroidism may become superimposed upon chronic renal failure. This complication becomes evident by an increase in serum calcium to the high normal or hypercalcemic range. In this event the possibility of surgery should be considered for removal of hyperplastic or adenomatous parathyroid glands. Measurements by radioimmunoassay for parathyroid hormone combined with calcium infusion should ultimately be the best test in differentiating primary from secondary hyperparathyroidism (see Pathologic Physiology and Chemistry).

Nephrolithiasis with calcium phosphate or calcium oxalate stones, particularly when associated with hypercalciuria, should suggest the diagnosis of primary hyperparathyroidism. "Idiopathic hypercalciuria" with recurrent nephrolithiasis may be associated with hypophosphatemia, making the distinction more difficult. This latter category may still include some patients with bona fide hyperparathyroidism. Repeated tests for serum phosphate and calcium are essential in reaching the correct conclusion. In some cases in which the diagnosis has been dubious, hyperparathyroidism is obvious at the followup examination 6 to 12 months later.

Recent experience suggests that arteriography or venography is of value in localizing parathyroid adenomas. Selective injection of contrast dye into the thyrocervical trunk may show abnormal vessels or, more frequently, diffuse "staining," reflecting highly vascular adenomatous or hyperplastic tissue. Similarly, venography may outline abnormal vessels suggesting the existence of an adenoma. During venography, samples of plasma can be obtained selectively from particular vessels in the neck; radioimmunoassay for parathyroid hormone in these samples can give further important information on the location. Large adenomas have been identified prior to surgery by simply obtaining an esophagram during ingestion of barium.

Prognosis. Untreated, hyperparathyroidism with significant hypercalcemia may cause progressive renal impairment and ultimately death. Occasionally severe hypercalcemia develops rapidly ("hypercalcemic crisis") and causes an immediate threat to life (see discussion of Hypercalcemia). On the other hand, the disease may exist in mild form without symptoms, and it is probable that some patients in apparently excellent health harbor hyperfunctioning parathyroid adenomas for decades and die of unrelated causes.

Uncomplicated primary hyperparathyroidism responds favorably to surgery. Occasionally a second adenoma is discovered after initial resection was apparently successful. When primary hyperplasia of the parathyroid glands is the cause, and insufficient tissue has been resected, recurrence of the disease will be evidenced by return of preoperative symptoms and signs.

Treatment. Surgery is the only definitive treatment yet devised for primary hyperparathyroidism. It is essential that the highest possible rate of success be obtained at the initial surgical procedure. Best results are obtained in the hands of those with extensive experience in parathyroid surgery. Multiple explorations for parathyroid adenomas expectedly carry increased risk and expense, as well as causing greater difficulty for the surgeon, particularly when scarring from earlier surgery is significant. The surgeon must endeavor to identify all four parathyroid glands, and for this purpose should utilize biopsies with rapid histologic confirmation. Positive identification is important if subsequent surgical exploration becomes necessary, and also guards against the possible existence of diffuse hyperplasia, which is an indication for removal of seven eighths of all parathyroid tissue found. In rare instances there are more than four hyperplastic or adenomatous glands. Postoperatively tetany may be expected in patients who show significant bone disease. This requires treatment at intervals with 10 per cent calcium gluconate (*10* to *30* ml. in 500 to 1500 ml. of saline) intravenously, and the administration of vitamin D, 50,000 units or more daily by mouth, until severe hypocalcemia shows signs of control. Therapy should be withdrawn as rapidly as clinical progress allows. Almost invariably, remaining parathyroid tissue recovers normal function; definite signs of recovery are usual within seven to ten days. It is best to allow some degree of hypocalcemia during the recovery period as long as symptoms are controlled, in order to avoid hypercalcemia which would tend to inhibit recovery of remaining parathyroid tissue. Excessive therapy with calcium by vein or vitamin D by mouth is neither necessary nor desirable.

HYPERCALCEMIA

Hypercalcemia may be expressed in several metabolic, endocrine, or malignant diseases other than hyperparathyroidism. These include multiple myeloma, sarcoidosis, milk-alkali syndrome, vitamin D intoxication, hyperthyroidism, acute adrenal insufficiency, and a rare disease, hypophosphatasia. In Paget's disease or osteoporosis, hypercalcemia may develop upon prolonged bed rest. Malignancies with osteolytic metastases cause hypercalcemia through the resorptive influence of the lesions in bone. Another cause of hypercalcemia in malignancy is ectopic hyperparathyroidism; the problem of diagnosis and treatment of this syndrome is discussed under Hyperparathyroidism. The hypercalcemia of sarcoidosis and vitamin D intoxication is particularly amenable to correction with corticosteroid therapy; subjects with the milk-alkali syndrome respond frequently also. These observations form the basis of a test that is helpful in differentiating among several types of hypercalcemia. Usually either prednisone, 60 mg. daily, or hydrocortisone, 120 mg. daily, is given for ten days. The hypercalcemia of hyperparathyroidism, ectopic or primary, almost invariably is resistant to the effects of this treatment. However, this test, like the several empirical tests discussed under Hyperparathyroidism, is not uniformly dependable. The milk-alkali syndrome and hypervitaminosis D both respond to withdrawal of the offending agents, and the hypercalcemia of sarcoidosis may respond to therapy with chloroquine. Characteristic clinical, laboratory, and roentgenographic features cited under diagnosis of the particular disease should lead one to the proper diagnosis in the other disorders listed. Hypercalcemia in hyperthyroidism is best treated by correcting the hyperthyroid state. If hypercalcemia persists in the euthyroid state it suggests the coexistence, which is rare, of hyperparathyroidism and hyperthyroidism.

Treatment. Hypercalcemia that is neither severe nor progressive requires treatment directed only toward correction of the underlying disease state. On the other hand, progressive and severe hypercalcemia ("hypercalcemic crisis") leads to marked weakness, mental deterioration, coma, progressive uremia, and death within a short period. Several methods have been proposed for control of progressive hypercalcemia, which may be so severe as to require emergency attention. Intravenous infusions of EDTA, sodium sulfate, or phosphate salts have been recommended. Phosphate by mouth is effective in doses equal to those given intravenously, and there is probably less danger in this approach. Dehydration is often an important contributory factor in the development of progressive hypercalcemia and uremia. It is important, then, to restore extracellular fluids by giving intravenous saline or glucose or both, and at the same time to begin treatment with phosphate by mouth. For the first few days the equivalent of 2 grams of elemental phosphorus should be given in divided doses four times daily. Capsules can be prepared containing 190 mg. of potassium dihydrogen phosphate plus 800 mg. of disodium hydrogen phosphate. This provides approximately 0.22 gram of elemental phosphorus per capsule. After three to five days when control of hypercalcemia has begun to be effective, the dosage of phosphorus should be reduced to 1 to 1.5 grams daily. Calcium, phosphate, and blood urea nitrogen should be monitored daily to assure that the desired effect is being obtained. It is probably best not to allow the blood phosphorus to exceed 6 mg. per 100 ml. Some patients with primary hyperparathyroidism have been maintained with nearly normal blood calcium for periods up to six months pending clarification of other complications before parathyroidectomy. However, this form of treatment should be regarded as temporary; at the earliest possible moment, definitive therapy for the underlying disease should be instituted. Calcitonin may prove to be efficacious in controlling hypercalcemia, but its use is now considered experimental.

Albright, F., and Reifenstein, E. C., Jr.: The Parathyroid Glands and Metabolic Bone Disease. Baltimore, Williams & Wilkins Company, 1948.

Aurbach, G. D., and Potts, J. T., Jr.: The parathyroids. In Levine, R., and Luft, R. (eds.): Advances in Metabolic Disorders. New York, Academic Press, Inc., 1964, p. 45.

Berson, S. A., and Yalow, R. S.: Parathyroid hormone in plasma in adenomatous hyperparathyroidism, uremia, and bronchogenic carcinoma. Science, 154:907, 1966.

Berson, S. A., Yalow, R. S., Aurbach, G. D., and Potts, J. T., Jr.: Immunoassay of bovine and human parathyroid hormone. Proc. Nat. Acad. Sci, USA, 49:613, 1963.

Boonstra, C. E., and Jackson, C. E.: Hyperparathyroidism detected by routine serum calcium analysis. Ann. Intern. Med., 63:468, 1965.

Goldsmith, R. S.: Differential diagnosis of hypercalcemia. New Eng. J. Med., 274:674, 1966.

Goldsmith, R. S., and Ingbar, S. H.: Inorganic phosphate treatment of hypercalcemia of diverse etiologies. New Eng. J. Med., 274:1, 1966.

Kyle, L. H., Canary, J. J., Mintz, D. H., and De Leon, A.: Inhibitory effects of induced hypercalcemia on secretion of parathyroid hormone. J. Clin. Endocr., 22:52, 1962.

Moldawer, M. P., Nardi, G. L., and Raker, J. W.: Concomitance of multiple adenomas of the parathyroids and pancreatic islets with tumor of the pituitary: A syndrome with familial incidence. Amer. J. Med. Sci., 228:190, 1954.

Potts, J. T., Jr., Deftos, L. J., Buckle, R. M., Sherwood, L. M., and Aurbach, G. D.: Radioimmunoassay of parathyroid hormone: Studies of the control of secretion of the hormone and parathyroid function in clinical disorders. In Hays, R. L., Goswitz, F. A., and Murphy, B. E. P. (eds.): Radioisotopes in Medicine: In Vitro Studies. Oak Ridge, Tennessee, U.S. Atomic Energy Commission, 1968, p. 207.

Sherwood, L. M., O'Riordan, J. L. H., Aurbach, G. D., and Potts, J. T., Jr.: Production of parathyroid hormone by nonparathyroid tumors. J. Clin. Endocr., 27:140, 1967.

Wermer, P.: Endocrine adenomatosis and peptic ulcer in a large kindred. Inherited multiple tumors and mosaic pleiotropism in man. Amer. J. Med., 35:205, 1963.

HYPOPARATHYROIDISM

Definition. Hypoparathyroidism is the syndrome characterized by deficient secretion of parathyroid hormone, with consequent hypocalcemia.

Etiology. In most instances hypoparathyroidism is the consequence of mechanical injury to or removal of parathyroid glands during surgery for primary thyroid disorders or occasionally, parathyroid disorders. Idiopathic hypoparathyroidism is rare; approximately 100 cases are known. It is usually recognized in childhood or adolescence, and in distinction to pseudohypoparathyroidism may be associated with pernicious anemia, moniliasis, or Addison's disease; occurs with equal incidence in males and females; and rarely is familial.

Pathology. In postsurgical and most cases of idiopathic hypoparathyroidism there is complete absence of the parathyroid glands. There may be calcification in the basal ganglia and cataracts. The bones may be abnormally dense, and the calvarium may be thickened. It is possible that idiopathic hypoparathyroidism represents an autoimmune disease.

Pathologic Physiology and Chemistry. The physiologic consequences of insufficient secretion of parathyroid hormone are low blood calcium, high blood phosphate, and a low rate of phosphate clearance into the urine. Attendant upon hypocalcemia is a very low concentration of calcium in the urine. As a general rule, the clearance of calcium into the urine approaches zero as the concentration of calcium in blood falls below 7 mg. per 100 ml.

Hypocalcemia in hypoparathyroidism is a manifestation of the reduced rate of bone resorption in the absence of sufficient parathyroid hormone. The diminished concentration of calcium in the extracellular fluid leads to increased neuromuscular excitability and tetany. Hyperphosphatemia in this disorder is primarily attributable to lack of the hormone effect on phosphate clearance by the kidney. The rate of urinary excretion of 3',5'-AMP is also reduced, but in distinction to pseudohypoparathyroidism there is a normal response to exogenous parathyroid hormone.

Clinical Manifestations. The principal symptoms of hypoparathyroidism are due to a low concentration of calcium in the extracellular fluid. Hypocalcemic tetany is manifested by numbness and tingling in the fingers and toes and around the lips, and sometimes by laryngeal stridor with "crowing" inspiration, dyspnea, and cyanosis. In severe tetany, cramps of individual muscle groups occur in the hands and feet as carpopedal spasms. There may also be convulsions or abdominal pain, nausea, and vomiting. Epileptiform attacks are a striking and frequently described symptom of hypoparathyroidism. Usually the seizures are of a grand mal type, but are not always preceded by aura, loss of consciousness, involuntary trauma, or incontinence. Rarely the petit mal variant of epilepsy is expressed. The electroencephalogram shows abnormalities sometimes but not always typical of idiopathic epilepsy. The seizures and usually the abnormal electroencephalographic pattern associated with tetany respond to treatment with calcium, whereas the latter is without effect in idiopathic epilepsy. The differential diagnosis of tetany is discussed separately.

Mental abnormalities may occur in hypoparathyroidism. Irritability, emotional lability, moroseness, impairment of memory, mental confusion, lethargy, depression, and mental deficiency have been described.

Papilledema sometimes associated with increased intracranial pressure may also accompany the hypocalcemia of hypoparathyroidism. These manifestations as well as the electroencephalograms return to normal when hypocalcemia is corrected. Cataracts are a characteristic consequence of chronic hypoparathyroidism. Other forms of ectopic calcification may be exhibited in the basal ganglia or subcutaneous tissues. The calvarium may be thickened.

Patients with idiopathic hypoparathyroidism may display abnormalities of the ectodermal structures, including the teeth, skin, nails, and hair. A characteristic feature of hypoparathyroidism early in life is blunting of the roots of the teeth and dysplasia of the enamel. The nails may be malformed and brittle and show transverse grooves. In addition, there is a significant incidence of moniliasis in idiopathic hypoparathyroidism, and when this involves the nails they become pitted and flaky in appearance. The transverse grooves, but not moniliasis, disappear when the serum calcium is corrected toward normal. The hair is thin, there may be patchy alopecia, and the skin is sometimes coarse and dry.

Diagnosis. Complaints of numbness and tingling in the extremities and around the mouth should suggest tetany. "Latent" tetany may be detected by eliciting Chvostek's sign by tapping over the facial nerve. A positive response consists of twitching of the muscles about the mouth and sometimes the nose and eyelids. Trousseau's sign is sought by producing ischemia with a cuff inflated above systolic pressure for three minutes. Characteristically, carpal spasm becomes evident during the course of the test. In latent tetany one may find increased sensitivity to galvanic current in producing muscle contraction (Erb's sign). The electrocardiogram may show a prolonged $Q-_oT$ interval as a consequence of hypocalcemia.

Patients with atypical epilepsy, other manifestations of increased neuromuscular irritability, or bizarre mental symptoms should be investigated for possible hypoparathyroidism. Obviously a history of prior thyroid surgery should alert one to this possibility. Tetany associated with Addison's disease, pernicious anemia, or moniliasis should immediately suggest a diagnosis of idiopathic hypoparathyroidism.

Prognosis. Hypoparathyroidism following thyroid or parathyroid surgery may often be transient. Withdrawal of therapy should be tested in such cases before it is concluded that permanent hypoparathyroidism exists. The prognosis is excellent with full life expectancy in established cases adequately treated. Untreated, the subject with hypoparathyroidism may suffer the discomfort and morbidity of muscular spasms, convulsions, cataracts, and mental impairment. It is not certain that cataracts can be prevented in hypoparathyroidism by correction of hypocalcemia early in the course of the disease. Epileptiform seizures are generally alleviated as hypocalcemia is corrected.

Treatment. Acute hypocalcemic tetany requires treatment with intravenous calcium, for example, calcium gluconate, 10 per cent solution (10 to 30 ml. in 500 to 1500 ml. of saline) given as necessary to control the symptoms. At the same time vitamin D, 50,000 to 100,000 units daily by mouth, should be given. Adequate intake of at least 1 to 2 grams of calcium by mouth should be assured, and sometimes further supplementation with 15 grams of calcium lactate (equivalent to 2 grams of calcium) in divided doses is necessary. The amount of vitamin D and calcium should be gradually reduced as serum calcium approaches normal. Dihydrotachysterol has been used instead of vitamin D_2 or D_3 and would be advantageous in cases of toxicity because it is cleared more rapidly from the body. The commercial preparation "AT-10" shows variable potency and is not recommended for therapy. In the absence of parathyroid hormone, vitamin D may cause an inordinately high rate of excretion of urinary calcium with the danger of nephrolithiasis. If regulation is difficult by reduction of calcium and vitamin D intake, the hypercalciuria may be controlled by giving phosphate by mouth. The Sulkowitch test is not of value in the management of these patients; quantitative analyses for 24-hour excretion of calcium are required.

PSEUDOHYPOPARATHYROIDISM AND PSEUDOPSEUDO-HYPOPARATHYROIDISM

Definiton. *Pseudohypoparathyroidism* is a clinical state of hypoparathyroidism characterized by normal secretion of hormone from the parathyroid glands, but with a genetic defect in the receptor tissues so that there is little or no response to the action of the hormone. The defect is transmitted as a sex-linked dominant trait, and is associated with characteristic abnormalities of physiognomy and growth. The genetically related disorder *pseudopseudohypoparathyroidism* (see below) represents an incomplete form of the syndrome, shows the constitutional features without the chemical findings of hypoparathyroidism, and may occur in the same families with pseudohypoparathyroidism.

Etiology and Genetics. Recent clinical investigations in this disorder as well as current studies on the mechanism of action of parathyroid hormone have shed light on the pathophysiology in this syndrome. The original hypothesis of Albright and his associates that the receptor tissues, bone and kidney, are unresponsive to parathyroid hormone still best accounts for the endocrinopathy of this disorder. Other hypotheses such as secretion of a biologically inactive form of parathyroid hormone, circulating antibodies to the hormone, or secretion of excessive amounts of calcitonin have been tested without substantiation. The urinary excretion of cyclic 3',5'-AMP is an index of the direct action of parathyroid hormone on the kidney manifested by activation of the plasma membrane–bound enzyme adenyl cyclase in the tubular elements of the renal cortex. Pseudohypoparathyroidism is characterized by a defective response to exogenous parathyroid hormone in terms of urinary excretion of 3',5'-AMP. The most reasonable interpretation of this finding, and the probable explanation for the disorder, is the genetic transmission of defective or deficient receptor–adenyl cyclase complex in the kidney and bone of these subjects. It has been found that subjects with this disorder secrete parathyroid hormone at an increased rate and show higher than normal concentrations of the hormone in peripheral circulation. Secretion of the hormone in this disorder responds normally to blood calcium.

The genetics of the disorder is currently best explained by a sex-linked dominant mode of inheritance. The sex incidence ratio is female to male 2:1, and there are probably no cases of male to male transmission of the complete syndrome. Undoubtedly the short stature characteristic of the syndrome is also attributable to an abnormal X chromosome. Genetic studies of sex-linked disorders indicate that in order to achieve normal height two functional sex chromosomes are required; that is, both the X chromosomes in females or both X and Y in males must be normal in the segments controlling growth. Pseudopseudohypoparathyroidism, in females at least, may reflect genetic mosaicism with a relatively greater degree of inactivation of the abnormal X chromosome.

Incidence. Pseudohypoparathyroidism and its incomplete variant pseudopseudohypoparathyroidism are rare. The average case is recognized earlier in life than is idiopathic hypoparathyroidism. Approximately 100 cases of pseudohypoparathyroidism and still fewer cases of the variant have been reported.

Pathology. The parathyroid glands are normal or hyperplastic. Shortening of the carpal and metatarsal bones and metastatic calcification, including calcification of the basal ganglia, occur. Also, there may be thickening of the calvarium, defective enamel of the teeth, dental aplasia, coxa vara, coxa valga, and bowing of the long bones. Cataracts are common.

Pathologic Physiology and Chemistry. The clinical chemical findings, hypocalcemia, hyperphosphatemia, and a low urinary calcium, are qualitatively similar but sometimes milder than those found in idiopathic or postoperative hypoparathyroidism. However, in pseudohypoparathyroidism, biologically active hormone under normal secretory control is elaborated from the parathyroid glands, but the receptor tissues do not respond. Exogenously administered parathyroid hormone is without effect. Other endocrinopathies may coexist. Hypothyroidism (particularly that caused by selective pituitary TSH deficiency), diabetes mellitus, hypomenorrhea, or gonadal dysgenesis may be found associated with pseudohypoparathyroidism. Conversely, moniliasis, Addison's disease, and pernicious anemia, which may be associated with idiopathic hypoparathyroidism, have not been found in cases of pseudohypoparathyroidism.

Clinical Manifestations. The symptoms and signs of pseudohypoparathyroidism encompass those of hypoparathyroidism plus certain unique abnormalities of physiognomy and growth. Mental retardation, short, stocky, obese stature, and round facies are characteristic. The hands and feet are usually disproportionately short, resulting in about 75 per cent of cases from shortening of one or more metacarpal and metatarsal bones. This is readily recognized when the fist is clenched, thereby causing a dimple over the head of the affected bone. Less frequently, shortening of the phalanges or uniform brachydactyly may occur. The calvarium is thickened in over one third of the patients. There may be delayed dentition, defective enamel, or complete dental aplasia. Less common defects include abnormally dense or lucent bones, exostoses, coxa vara, coxa valga, bowing of the ulna, radius, tibula, and fibula, and loss of "tubulation" of the long bones. Calcification occurs in the basal ganglia and in the dentate nucleus, and there may be actual ossification as well as calcification in the skin, subcutaneous tissue, and deep connective tissues. Cataracts are also common. Rarely cases are found of true pseudohypoparathyroidism which show few or no abnormalities of growth, physiognomy, or ectopic calcification.

Diagnosis. The diagnosis is established by the characteristic constitutional changes, by the clinical and laboratory abnormalities of hypoparathyroidism, and by testing the response to purified parathyroid hormone or parathyroid extract given intravenously. The earlier test for pseudohypoparathyroidism based on measurement of urinary phosphate excretion did not allow clear-cut separation of pseudohypoparathyroidism from normal subjects who vary widely in response; determination of 3',5'-AMP in the urine affords virtually complete differentiation between the two groups. Normal subjects, but not those with pseudohypoparathyroidism, show a 20-fold rise in the rate of excretion of urinary 3',5'-AMP within 15 to 45 minutes after injection of hormone. There is no overlap of results between normal subjects and those with the disease. Baseline excretion of cyclic AMP is lower than normal in patients with idiopathic, postsurgical, and pseudohypoparathyroidism, but higher than normal in pseudopseudohypoparathyroidism. The latter group responds normally to injections of parathyroid hormone. Another distinguishing feature is the determination of parathyroid hormone in peripheral plasma which is found to be abnormally high (as long as hypocalcemia is not corrected) in pseudohypoparathyroidism, in contrast to other forms of hypoparathyroidism wherein it is undetectable. Some patients previously categorized as having pseudohypoparathyroidism associated with intestinal malabsorption syndromes and/or osteitis fibrosa cystica should be re-examined with the newer diagnostic procedures. It is the author's view that reservations must be held pending further tests before accepting a patient with atypical family history or clinical findings as a true example of pseudohypoparathyroidism.

Treatment. In general the treatment of pseudohypoparathyroidism is the same as that of hypoparathyroidism. Usually hypocalcemia is easier to control in pseudohypoparathyroidism, although there may be occasional patients requiring unusually large doses of vitamin D.

TETANY

Tetany may develop in hypocalcemia, alkalosis, potassium deficiency, and occasionally hypomagnesemia. The symptoms and signs of tetany are discussed under Hypoparathyroidism. In addition to the information obtained by clinical examination, the laboratory findings are particularly important in diagnosing the cause of tetany. Hypocalcemic tetany may occur in osteomalacia caused by hypovitaminosis D, resistance to vitamin D, intestinal malabsorption syndromes, renal tubular acidosis, and hypoparathyroidism. In hypoparathyroidism the serum phosphate is high, whereas in the hypocalcemic states of rickets, osteomalacia, or renal tubular acidosis serum phosphate is below normal. Except for renal tubular acidosis, the urinary calcium is low in all these states. The blood pH is normal except in renal tubular acidosis, and in this disorder the urinary pH remains high even after administration of ammonium chloride. Tetany caused by alkalosis is associated with normal serum phosphate and calcium and normal urinary excretion of calcium, but the blood pH is high. Alkalotic tetany may occur in hyperventilation, usually a manifestation of psychoneurosis, and can be corrected by inducing the patient to reduce the respiratory rate or breathe into a paper bag.

Metabolic alkalosis, caused by persistent vomiting, hypokalemic alkalosis, or excessive treatment with alkali, may also produce tetany. In the latter instance the serum calcium and phosphate are

TABLE 2. DIFFERENTIAL DIAGNOSIS OF TETANY

Cause	Serum			Urine	
	Ca	Pi	pH	Ca	pH
Hypocalcemia					
Hypovitaminosis D	↓	↓	N	↓	—
Resistance to vitamin D	N or ↓	↓	N	↓	—
Intestinal malabsorption syndromes	↓	↓	N	↓	—
Hypoparathyroidism	↓	↑	N	↓	—
Alkalosis					
Respiratory	N	N	↑	N	↑
Metabolic	N	N	↑	N	↑

Ca = Calcium. P_i = Phosphate. N = Normal.
(−) = Indeterminate. ↑ = High. ↓ = Low.

normal as long as there is no renal impairment, but the serum pH is high. Tetany is produced by overcorrection of acidosis in chronic renal disease. In the latter condition, there is a tendency to hypocalcemia as well as hyperphosphatemia. In respiratory alkalosis plasma bicarbonate is low or normal, whereas in metabolic alkalosis plasma bicarbonate is high. The history should suggest the appropriate diagnosis in cases of excessive intake of alkali or excessive loss of gastric acid. The diagnosis is supported by finding a high concentration of bicarbonate in the serum and an alkaline urine. Treatment is directed at checking the cause. Hypokalemic alkalosis may appear in primary aldosteronism or treatment with corticosteroid analogues, and calls for correction of hormone excess and repletion of body potassium. Hypocalcemia occurs in the neonatal period in the progeny of mothers with hyperparathyroidism. This is a transient phenomenon secondary to hypercalcemia attendant upon primary hyperparathyroidism in the mother. Hypomagnesemia is a rare cause of tetany refractory to treatment with calcium; magnesium deficiency in those instances should be corrected.

Albright, F., Burnett, C. H., Smith, P. H., and Parson, W.: Pseudohypoparathyroidism—an example of the "Seabright-Bantam syndrome." Endocrinology, 30:922, 1942.

Aurbach, G. D., and Potts, J. T., Jr.: The parathyroids. *In* Levine, R., and Luft, R. (eds.).: Advances in Metabolic Disorders. New York, Academic Press, Inc., 1964, p. 45.

Blizzard, R. M., Chee, D., and Davis, W.: The incidence of parathyroid and other antibodies in the sera of patients with idiopathic hypoparathyroidism. Clin. Exp. Immun., 1:119, 1966.

Bronsky, D., Kushner, D. S., Dubin, A., and Snapper, I.: Idiopathic hypoparathyroidism and pseudohypoparathyroidism: Case reports and review of the literature. Medicine, 37:317, 1958.

Chase, L. R., Melson, G. L., and Aurbach, G. D.: Pseudohypoparathyroidism: Defective excretion of 3′,5′-AMP in response to parathyroid hormone. J. Clin. Invest., 48:1832, 1969.

Harrison, H. E., Lifshitz, F., and Blizzard, R. M.: Comparison between crystalline dihydrotachysterol and calciferol in patients requiring pharmacologic vitamin D therapy. New Eng. J. Med., 276:894, 1967.

Tashjian, A. H., Jr., Frantz, A. G., and Lee, J. B.: Pseudohypoparathyroidism: Assays of parathyroid hormone and thyrocalcitonin. Proc. Nat. Acad. Sci. USA, 56:1138, 1966.

CALCITONIN AND MEDULLARY CARCINOMA OF THE THYROID

Description. Medullary carcinoma of the thyroid arises from the parafollicular cells of the thyroid which derive embryologically from the final or ultimobranchial cleft. In submammalian vertebrates the ultimobranchial cells remain as a separate body, the ultimobranchial gland, but in mammals the anlage merges with the thyroid. In either instance, the cells derived from the ultimobranchial cells constitute the gland that synthesizes and secretes calcitonin. Recently it has been discovered that some cases of medullary carcinoma of the thyroid in man cause a syndrome of excessive secretion of calcitonin. This syndrome is frequently familial and may encompass hyperplasia or adenoma of the parathyroid glands, sometimes expressed as primary hyperparathyroidism, pheochromocytoma, multiple neuromas, and Cushing's syndrome. Abnormally high concentrations of calcitonin have been detected in medullary thyroid tumors as well as in plasma taken from these patients.

Incidence. Medullary carcinoma of the thyroid accounts for 5 to 10 per cent of the cases of thyroid cancer. The syndrome can be familial with autosomal dominant form of inheritance. The frequency of associated hypersecretion of calcitonin is unknown.

Pathology. Histologically this tumor differs from other cancers of the thyroid in that the cells resemble those of parafollicular cells, there is often amyloid infiltration, and there are no papillary folds, follicles, or polymorphonuclear infiltrates in the tissue. (Sometimes artifacts of fixation appear like papillary folds in sections.) The tumor usually does not appear to be encapsulated, and may show areas of calcification. The tissue does not take up radioactive iodine. As noted above, pheochromocytoma or parathyroid hyperplasia or adenoma may be associated with medullary carcinoma of the thyroid.

Pathologic Physiology. Although many of these tumors elaborate calcitonin at a high rate, hypocalcemia is unusual, probably because parathyroid hormone is secreted as a compensatory mechanism (secondary hyperparathyroidism). Moreover, as stated above, there may be frequent occurrence of primary hyperparathyroidism in the syndrome. It is possible that the development of primary hyperparathyroidism represents induced autonomy in the glands as a consequence of prolonged chronic secondary hyperparathyroidism.

Measurements by radioimmunoassay or bioassay show that hypercalcemia induces secretion of calcitonin from normal parafollicular cells as well as from medullary carcinoma tissue. In addition, glucagon, in pharmacologic doses injected intravenously, causes secretion of calcitonin in some species as well as in the medullary carcinoma syndrome. Occasionally this effect of glucagon is manifested by transient systemic hypocalcemia. These responses to calcium and glucagon may be helpful eventually in conjunction with radioimmunoassay as diagnostic tests for the syndrome.

Clinical Manifestations, Prognosis, and Treatment. Medullary carcinoma may become evident simply by a mass in the thyroid or by the clinical expression of the associated endocrinopathies, pheochromocytoma, primary hyperparathyroidism, or Cushing's syndrome. The tumor, local or metastatic, may be hard and tender. Severe diarrhea may occur, possibly related to elaboration of prostaglandins or serotonin which can stimulate intestinal secretion. The tumor often spreads, and metastases may grow to huge size. There is not yet sufficient experience to project the natural clinical course in this disorder. The tumor is refractory to treatment with radioactive iodine, antithyroid drugs, or external radiation. At this time surgery represents the best approach, and should consist of wide excision, avoiding local seeding with tumor fragments. Isolated metastases may also be amenable to surgery.

Aurbach, G. D., Potts, J. T., Jr., Chase, L. R., and Melson, G. L.: Polypeptide hormones and calcium metabolism. Ann. Intern. Med., 70:1243, 1969.

Cunliffe, W. J., Black, M. M., Hall, R., Johnston, I. D. A., Hudgson, P., Shuster, S., Gudmundsson, T. V., Joplin, G. F., Williams, E. D., Woodhouse, N. J. Y., Galante, L., and MacIntyre, I.: A calcitonin-secreting thyroid carcinoma. Lancet, 2:63, 1968.

Foster, G. V.: Calcitonin (thyrocalcitonin). New Eng. J. Med., 279:349, 1968.

Hazard, J. B., Hawk, W. A., and Crile, G., Jr.: Medullary (solid) carcinoma of the thyroid—a clinicopathologic entity. J. Clin. Endocr., 19:152, 1959.

Hirsch, P. F., and Munson, P. L.: Thyrocalcitonin. Physiol. Rev., 49:548, 1969.

Melvin, K. E. W., and Tashjian, A. H., Jr.: The syndrome of excessive thyrocalcitonin produced by medullary carcinoma of the thyroid. Proc. Nat. Acad. Sci. USA, 59:1216, 1968.

Steiner, A. L., Goodman, A. D., and Powers, S. R.: Study of a kindred with pheochromocytoma, medullary thyroid carcinoma, hyperparathyroidism and Cushing's disease: Multiple endocrine neoplasia, type 2. Medicine, 47:371, 1968.

Tashjian, A. H., Jr., and Melvin, K. E. W.: Medullary carcinoma of the thyroid gland: Studies of thyrocalcitonin in plasma and tumor extracts. New Eng. J. Med., 279:279, 1968.

Tubiana, M., Milhaud, G., Coutris, G., Lacour, J., Parmentier, C., and Bok, B.: Medullary carcinoma and thyrocalcitonin. Brit. Med. J., 4:87, 1968.

DISEASES OF BONE
Robert P. Heaney

Bone Physiology and Calcium Homeostasis

Duality of Skeletal Function. Diseases that affect bone not only alter the supporting function of the skeleton but have far-reaching effects on the entire calcium-homeostatic system; conversely, derangements or alterations of calcium homeostasis are inevitably reflected in bone as a supporting tissue. Although terrestrial life as we know it could not be conceived without the mechanical, structural, and engineering aspects of the skeleton, bone as a tissue evolved in exclusively aquatic vertebrates, in which there probably was no selective advantage conferred by a rigid endoskeleton. Bone undoubtedly served a protective function (as dermal armor) in these very ancient forms, but its principal evolutionary significance lies in the fact that it has afforded higher vertebrates the ability to regulate the concentration of calcium and phosphate ions in body fluids. This primitive ability remains a fundamental property of the human skeleton, and reminds us of this by occasionally exerting its primacy over the much more obvious structural role of the tissue.

Whereas parathyroid hormone, discussed elsewhere in this text, exerts the primary endocrine control over calcium homeostasis, it is bone that provides the principal end-organ by which this homeostasis is effected. This action depends upon two fundamental properties of bone tissue: (1) the physical-chemical equilibrium between the solid phase bone mineral and calcium ions in the body fluids, and (2) the continuous structural remodeling of bone with its associated deposition and removal of large quantities of calcium and phosphorus.

Bone Structure and Composition. Bone consists of a highly organized system of cells surrounded by a matrix composed of a fibrous protein, collagen, encrusted with tiny calcium phosphate crystals. Cells occupy 2 to 3 per cent of the total volume, but are evenly distributed through the bone and interconnected by a series of canaliculi, so that no volume of interstitial bony material is more than a fraction of a micron from a cell or its processes, and no bone cell is more than 200 microns from a capillary. In fully mineralized bone the protein matrix accounts for half the volume and one third the weight of the intercellular material, and the crystals occupy most of the remainder. Mucopolysaccharides comprise about 5 per cent of the organic matrix, and although quantitatively a minor component of bone, they probably contribute significantly to matrix maturation and mineraliza-

tion. The collagen fibers in adult human bone are spatially highly organized, forming interlacing bundles and layers; this arrangement appears to be related to the direction and character of the mechanical forces which the organ must withstand. Furthermore, the intimate association of fibrous protein and ultramicroscopic crystals constitutes what, in materials engineering, has been termed a "two-phase" material. The breaking strength and elasticity of bones depend not only on their mass and shape, but as well on the intrinsic mechanical properties of this two-phase system and on changes that occur in those properties as the material ages. Although still poorly understood, it is probable that some of the symptoms and signs of the diseases to be described in the following pages represent qualitative abnormalities in the bone material itself.

The mineral component of bony material is a calcium-phosphate generally considered to possess the crystal structure of hydroxyapatite. There is an additional carbonate component which may comprise as much as 8 per cent of bone ash and which is currently believed to be present both as $CaCO_3$ and as limited carbonate substitution in or on the apatite crystal. The calcium carbonate phase is acid labile, even in vivo, and is depleted during systemic acidosis. When initially deposited, bone mineral appears crystallographically amorphous and gradually changes to the characteristic apatitic pattern with aging. It is not known how the physical properties of bone are influenced by the balance between these several mineral components. Understanding of mineralization of newly deposited matrix is particularly dependent upon elucidation of the nature of the mineral phase, and still unresolved questions concerning the pathogenesis of rickets and osteomalacia are largely attributable to this uncertainty.

Bone Formation. Bone is deposited on free surfaces by osteoblasts that synthesize collagen and secrete it onto the bone-forming surface. Soon after secretion the soluble collagen molecules aggregate into spatially oriented insoluble fibrils. The factors that control their orientation are not well understood, but bioelectrical fields of the magnitude known to be produced in bone by applied mechanical stress have been shown to influence the orientation of collagen fibrils in vitro. The layer of bone matrix thus deposited on a bone-forming surface is known as an osteoid seam, and in normal bone is about 10 microns thick. These seams are not immediately mineralizable. Under control of the parent osteoblast the matrix undergoes a complex series of biochemical changes, which ultimately render it capable of initiating crystal nucleation and growth. This process includes changes in the important mucopolysaccharide component of the matrix and appearance of lipid-staining material at the calcification front. These and other changes are reflected in distinct layers and sequences recognizable only by special stains. Alkaline phosphatase has long been associated with active bone formation and can be detected both within osteoblasts and extracellularly in the superficial layers of newly deposited matrix, but not more deeply at the calcification front itself. Despite many attractive hypotheses, no clearly definable role of this enzyme has been found, and its association with active bone formation remains largely circumstantial.

Matrix maturation requires periods of approximately ten days, is dependent upon active mediation of the osteoblast, and appears to proceed discontinuously, bursts of activity alternating with sometimes long periods of inactivity. Once maturation is complete, the collagen fibril becomes capable of initiating the deposition of mineral, in a specific crystalline pattern, from the ions present in the bathing fluid. These crystals are formed both within and upon the fibril and are oriented along its length. Crystal growth displaces the water that originally occupied 50 per cent of the volume of unmineralized matrix. There is almost no free water in mature bone, so that interaction between bone and body fluids is largely limited to free surfaces. (In the adult less than 1 per cent of total skeletal calcium exchanges with an intravenously injected tracer over periods measured in days.) Approximately three fourths of the ultimate mineral content may be deposited within a few hours. The remaining mineral enters more slowly, largely because the absence of free water severely limits diffusion, and thus completion of mineralization may sometimes require weeks or even months.

Once nucleation occurs, mineral is extracted from the surrounding fluid with great efficiency. This appears to be explained by the fact that the solubility product of hydroxyapatite is considerably lower than the Ca × P ion product in extracellular fluid, and thus crystal growth occurs as rapidly as blood flow can transport mineral to the site. On the other hand, spontaneous precipitation of calcium phosphates from the body fluids does not normally occur in other tissues because, though supersaturated with respect to the ultimate mineral phase of bone, these fluids are undersaturated with respect to the mineral crystalline forms that calcium phosphate is known to assume when precipitated at physiologic pH. The extraordinary beauty of this arrangement lies in the fact that mineralization thus occurs only at sites specifically rendered mineralizable by formation of an *improbable* nucleating configuration, and in the fact that one and the same body fluid carries a great surplus of mineral when in the presence of such a nucle-

ating center, but is indefinitely stable — indeed undersaturated — elsewhere.

An important consequence of this mineralization scheme is the demand for mineral created by nucleated, but as yet incompletely mineralized bone. This demand amounts to a kind of "mineralization debt," analogous to the lactic acid debt of anaerobic muscle work, and will inevitably lower the concentration of calcium in body fluids unless specifically offset by homeostatic adjustment. Indeed, this continuing demand, which cannot apparently be modulated after it is initiated, is quantitatively the largest single stress to which the calcium homeostatic system must respond. Normally new bone mineralization utilizes 300 to 500 mg. of calcium daily, an amount greater than the total calcium content of the entire blood volume. This demand may increase by as much as two orders of magnitude in diseases in which active bone formation occurs, such as severe osteitis fibrosa, and is responsible for the "bone hunger" and associated hypocalcemia that is sometimes seen following removal of a parathyroid adenoma.

Bone Resorption. Resorption occurs by virtually simultaneous dissolution of both mineral and matrix, and is usually associated with large multinucleated cells known as osteoclasts. These cells are not the only mediators of resorption, however; osteocytes are capable of enlarging their lacunae in response to parathyroid stimulation, and mononuclear cells on free surfaces may also participate in resorption. Osteoclasts are short-lived and do their work quickly. The space eventually to be filled by a new haversian system can be tunneled out of cortical bone in less than 10 per cent of the time required by osteoblasts to fill it in with new bone. This means that large quantities of mineral can be released from the skeleton in short periods of time. The mechanisms by which bone solids are solubilized are largely unknown. Collagenase and a variety of lysosomal proteases are involved in matrix hydrolysis, and large quantities of H^+ are consumed in solubilization of the mineral (approximately one proton for each calcium ion). The H^+ production derives from both organic acids and carbonic anhydrase, and is both dependent upon and stimulated by O_2 levels in the bathing fluids. Carbonic anhydrase has been specifically localized to osteoclasts, and its inhibitors can directly reduce bone resorption.

Control of Bone Remodeling. Teleologically, bone remodeling serves both homeostatic and structural needs. By processing large quantities of mineral each day it establishes an input-output system capable of being adapted to calcium deficiency or excess by comparatively minor adjustments of the balance between formation and resorption. Structurally it allows the bone to reshape itself to meet new forces and, even more fundamental, it continually renews its aging interstitial material and thus maintains optimal mechanical properties.

The control of bone formation and resorption, i.e., structural bone turnover, is exerted at two levels: in intrinsic bone cellular activity and responsiveness to applied stimuli, and in the superimposed systemic influences such as those produced by hormones, nutrition, and systemic disease. The former is the more important; unfortunately, it is still poorly understood.

Intrinsic Control. Apparently the two most important elements of local control are mechanical forces and local blood flow, the latter with its associated regulation of nutrient supply, pH, and O_2 tension. (Indeed, the two may be interrelated.) Increased blood flow is associated with osteoclastic resorption, and vascular stasis with increased osteoblastic activity. The effects of mechanical forces are profound. A bone or bony region subjected to heavy use will increase its mass and revise both its internal structure and external shape so as to resist applied forces; conversely, disuse leads rapidly to decrease in mass and loss of specific architectural features. Normally, muscle mass and skeletal mass maintain a ratio of approximately 10:1.

Both the nature of the signal that mechanical forces transmit to bone cells and the nature of the cellular response are largely unknown. However, bone exhibits many of the features of a semiconductor and has been shown to generate and maintain small electrical fields when deformed by externally applied forces. These fields are of the same magnitude as those shown to be capable of orienting collagen fibril aggregation and those controlling limb bud regeneration in amphibia. Thus it is possible that both cellular activity and extracellular organization of matrix fibrils may be determined by local electrical fields. It has long been assumed that the bone cell response to applied stress is a stimulation of osteoblastic activity. This is probably not true, or if it is true, it is only a minor feature of a much more complex response. The distribution of stresses within bone and associated induced electrical fields and altered blood flow are so complex and so heterogeneous that the process can be studied adequately only at the microscopic level. Bone turnover may be intense at one site and only a few millimeters distant may be virtually at a standstill. Available evidence obtained from macroscopic skeletal units suggests that *over-all* bone formation is little changed, at least quantitatively, by applied mechanical forces, whereas over-all bone resorption is decreased by mechanical stress and increased by disuse. It is not known whether this is true at the microscopic level as well, or whether it instead represents only the algebraic sum of locally different responses.

Systemic Control. Applied systemic control of the structural turnover of bone is better understood. Growth hormone and thyroid hormone stimulate osteoblast activity and osteoblastic recruitment from osteoprogenitor cells, whereas adrenal corticoids, malnutrition, fever, and a variety of systemic diseases decrease both new matrix production and the osteoblast-mediated ripening of the osteoid seam. Androgens and estrogens, previously thought to stimulate osteoblastic activity, have been shown to exert their effect, instead, by suppressing bone resorption, and if they have any effect on osteoblasts at all, probably suppress them to a minor extent. None of these effects can currently be considered homeostatic, either from the point of view of the skeleton as a structural unit or from the point of view of the extracellular fluid calcium ion level, simply because there exist no known feedback loops from the skeletal effects to the control of hormone secretion.

Homeostatic control of bone turnover is exerted by parathyroid hormone and calcitonin, which are concerned not with skeletal homeostasis, but with the maintenance of calcium ion concentration in the extracellular fluid. Parathyroid hormone secretion is inversely related to extracellular fluid calcium ion levels, and hormone action is exerted on at least three independent end-organs: bone, intestinal mucosa, and renal tubule. All three effects function to raise the concentration of calcium ion in extracellular fluid. In bone the most obvious effect of the hormone is a stimulation of bone resorption, with consequent release of calcium and phosphorus. In cases of severe parathyroid dysfunction there is commonly an increase or decrease of new bone formation that parallels the more immediate change in resorption, but it is not known whether this is due to a direct stimulation of osteoblastic activity by parathyroid hormone. In the intestinal mucosa parathyroid hormone stimulates calcium absorption. The efficiency of calcium absorption, which, in the adult, is about 30 per cent, may rise to over 90 per cent in hyperparathyroidism and fall to nearly zero in hypoparathyroidism. In the kidney parathyroid hormone effects are twofold: a decrease in tubular phosphate reabsorption (discussed elsewhere in this text) and an increase in tubular calcium reabsorption. The renal effects occur within minutes and the bone effects within hours, whereas the intestinal response requires days or even weeks to become apparent. Although all three responses have the same general effect, the renal response seems best suited for emergency adjustment, the bone response represents the largest reserve capacity of the three, and the intestinal response seems designed more to restore total body calcium balance than to adjust the level of calcium ion in extracellular fluid.

These homeostatic effects of parathyroid hormone are central to any consideration of metabolic bone disease for two reasons: (1) Calcium ion homeostasis takes precedence over the structural needs of the organism; by compensatory regulation of osteoclastic activity the system is capable of decreasing bone mass to the point of producing bone disease, if necessary, in order to maintain extracellular fluid calcium concentrations. (2) Primary, nonhomeostatic disruption of the balance between bone formation and bone resorption, such as that produced by inflammation, disuse, local bone disease, or systemic endocrinopathy, necessarily changes the calcium balance of the extracellular fluid and thus evokes secondary, compensatory adjustments in parathyroid hormonal control over calcium ion homeostasis.

A variety of factors modulate parathyroid hormone effects on bone resorption. Mechanical stresses, gonadal steroids, high concentrations of calcium or phosphate, calcitonin, fluoride, and the diphosphonate compounds all depress resorptive response to a given level of parathyroid hormone. Some act at the level of mesenchymal induction (such as the gonadal steroids), some at the existing resorptive cellular machinery (such as calcitonin), and some at the mineral level itself (such as the diphosphonates), but the ultimate effect of each is a shift in the dose response curve of parathyroid mediated bone resorption in the direction of resistance. On the other hand, disuse, heparin (both of exogenous and endogenous origin), increased oxygen tension, and local inflammation all enhance resorptive response to parathyroid hormone. The significance of these interactions lies not in calcium homeostasis (for plasma calcium regulation takes place despite these alterations of PTH responsiveness, simply by compensatory adjustment of parathyroid hormone secretion rate), but in the bone mass itself. Enhanced responsiveness leads to negative calcium balance, reduced responsiveness to positive balance.

Calcitonin suppresses bone resorption, both by inhibiting osteocytes and existing osteoclasts and by reducing mesenchymal production of new osteoclasts. Its immediate effect is reduction in release of calcium and phosphorus from bone; hence in the fasting state it produces a fall in both plasma calcium and phosphate. Although secreted in small quantities at normal plasma calcium levels, it is normally released in response to hypercalcemia and probably finds its chief role in normal physiology in moderating absorptive hypercalcemia. Its effect on skeletal mass in man is unknown, but it is to be expected that long-term overproduction or exogenous administration would lead to increased skeletal mass. (Calcitonin has, in fact, been indirectly implicated in the hyperostosis of bulls fed a milking ration.)

Vitamin D. Although one of the first of the vitamins to be characterized and identified, vitamin D has until recently eluded attempts to uncover its mode of action. It is now known that both the plant and animal D vitamins (ergo- and cholecalciferol, respectively) are first hydroxylated at the 25-position by a specific liver enzyme system, and that it is the 25-OH compound or a further, more polar derivative which is the active form of the vitamin. Calcium absorption from the intestine is associated with a transport protein with a high affinity for calcium (calcium-binding protein), and 25-OH vitamin D is necessary for production of this material in most species studied to date. Nevertheless, much uncertainty remains both as to the actual cellular mechanism of vitamin

D action and as to the tissues most affected by vitamin D deficiency. Plainly vitamin D is necessary for intestinal calcium absorption, and most particularly for the absorptive responses to low calcium intake or high parathyroid hormone levels. There is no general agreement, however, whether vitamin D is necessary for osteoclastic resorption, osteoid maturation, or epiphyseal cartilage growth and maturation, each of which is retarded in vitamin D deficiency states. Attempts to explain each of these effects as a result of calcium absorptive defects are unconvincing, and it seems safest to assume a direct dependence of each of these cell types on vitamin D until such is clearly shown to be unnecessary. In no case, however, does the vitamin actually control the process concerned. Thus no change in calcium absorption results from widely varying doses of vitamin D in normal people; only when administered in pharmacologic amounts does the vitamin exert a clear effect of its own on either intestinal absorption or bone resorption. Curiously, the renal tubular effects of parathyroid hormone seem to be independent of vitamin D.

Age Changes in Bone. After completion of epiphyseal closure and associated remodeling, bone enters a phase of relative quiescence. Structural turnover is low, and cortical bone is dense, thick, and fully mineralized. During the fourth decade, haversian remodeling increases and continues to rise slowly until death. This change is most apparent in the juxtamedullary regions of cortical bone. This bone becomes more porous, larger numbers of haversian systems are incompletely closed, and in some osteones mineralization is arrested short of the theoretical capacity. In addition, the number of plugged haversian canals increases and more and more osteocytes die, creating microscopic regions of dead bone. Associated with the increase in bone remodeling is a slight but continuous preponderance of bone resorption. After age 35 bone mass begins to decrease, and the decline continues steadily until death. Studies of many different bones in several racial groups suggest that the change is universal. Available estimates indicate that bone mass decreases by 5 to 10 per cent per decade. There is no satisfying explanation for any of these changes.

Bourne, G. H. (ed.): The Biochemistry and Physiology of Bone. New York, Academic Press, 1956.

Frost, H. M. (ed.): Bone Biodynamics. Boston, Little, Brown & Company, 1964.

Harris, W. H., and Heaney, R. P.: Skeletal Renewal and Metabolic Bone Disease. Boston, Little, Brown & Company, 1970.

McLean, F. C., and Urist, M. R.: Bone. 3rd ed. Chicago, University of Chicago Press, 1968.

Nordin, B. E. C., and Smith, D. A.: Diagnostic Procedures in Disorders of Calcium Metabolism. London, J. & A. Churchill, Ltd., 1965.

Vaughn, J.: The Physiology of Bone. New York, Oxford Univ. Press, 1970

The Osteoporoses

Definition. The term osteoporosis, literally "bone porosity," designates a deficiency of bone tissue per unit volume of bone as an organ. The deficiency relates only to the structural function of bone, not to its calcium homeostatic role. The bone that remains is considered to be normal by both chemical and ordinary histologic criteria. The fibrous and fatty marrow that fills the voids once occupied by bone is also normal, and there is no obvious morphologic evidence of osteoblastic or osteoclastic dysfunction. These requirements exclude many specific entities also associated with quantitative reduction in a qualitatively normal bone mass, such as hyperparathyroidism, multiple myeloma, and carcinoma metastatic to bone. Thus these features *describe* osteoporosis, rather than *define* it, because osteoporosis is not so much the presence of an abnormal bone condition as it is the absence of a normal quantity of bone.

Morphologic and Roentgenographic Characteristics. The decrease in bone mass expresses itself as loss of normal cortical thickness, increased porosity of normally compact cortical bone, and, in cancellous bone, thinning, fragmentation, and loss of trabeculae. The characteristic subperiosteal bone resorption of osteitis fibrosa is not seen and the external dimensions of the involved bone do not change (except as a consequence of fracture). The cortical thinning and porosity is usually readily visible on roentgenograms of long bones. Decreased roentgenographic density is an unreliable sign, and thus early changes in primarily cancellous bone, such as the pelvis and spine, are harder to evaluate. As the disease advances, one can discern increased contrast between the end plates and bodies of vertebrae, relative accentuation of vertical trabeculae, biconcave compression of the end plates (producing the characteristic "codfish" vertebrae), herniation of the nucleus pulposus into the bodies of the vertebrae (Schmorl's nodes), and, finally, vertebral compression fractures. The involved bodies are usually wedged anteriorly, especially in the thoracic region, but sometimes uniform collapse or even posterior body wedging is seen, depending on the region of the spine involved. The neural arch invariably remains intact.

Except for the purely local osteoporoses such as those associated with inflammation or disuse, most osteoporoses are generalized diseases involving the entire skeleton, and, if carefully sought, roentgenographic evidence of decreased bone mass can be found in all bones examined, including the skull, the long bones, and the hands and feet. Decreased cortical thickness of the femur and of the metacarpal, metatarsal, and phalangeal bones is a common accompaniment of vertebral osteoporosis and usually, though not always, parallels the latter in severity. The combined thickness of the two cortices usually amounts to more than 45 per cent of total shaft diameter in these bones; values less than this are indicative of decreased bone mass. When the degree of bone loss becomes extreme, macroscopic regions of cancellous bone may present a cystlike appearance roentgenographically.

Microscopically the bone shows no abnormalities by usual criteria. Increased marrow mast cell counts have been noted in all types of osteoporosis evaluated to date. This is of interest because of the known potentiation of endogenous parathyroid hormone by heparin and because the cortical thinning of osteoporosis occurs primarily by endosteal resorption (in contrast to the subperiosteal resorption characteristic of increased circulating levels of parathyroid hormone). However, it is not known whether the mast cells precede the onset of the osteoporotic process or are a response to it.

General Pathophysiologic Considerations. Many useful analogies can be drawn between osteoporosis and anemia. Like anemia, osteoporosis is not a specific disease entity but is instead a quantitative deficiency of a normal body constituent. It is the end result of many quite different pathophysiologic processes. The one element common to all these mechanisms is that, in the transition between normal bone and osteoporotic bone, the resorptive component of bone turnover must exceed new bone formation. But, again like anemia, this destructive imbalance can proceed at high, low, or normal rates of bone turnover. The osteoporosis of Cushing's syndrome develops at low rates of new bone formation; postmenopausal and senile osteoporoses usually develop at normal absolute rates of bone turnover; and disuse osteoporosis, peri-inflammatory osteoporosis, and the osteoporoses of acromegaly and hyperthyroidism develop at high rates of bone turnover. Indeed, the rate of bone turnover is largely an irrelevant consideration; the only important matter is why resorption is higher than formation. This problem is more difficult than it appears, because it implies a knowledge of the mechanisms by which formation and resorption are matched and bone mass is preserved in normal persons. This information is not yet available.

However, one thing seems certain: the elements of calcium ion homeostasis are involved in the pathogenesis of osteoporosis, at least as unwitting participants if not as originators of the process. Although not all bone resorption is controlled by parathyroid hormone, nevertheless parathyroid hormone is quantitatively the most important determinant of the amount of bone resorption, and thus parathyroid control of osteoclastic activity provides an important means of reducing *total* bone resorption whenever nonparathyroid mediated resorption rises. This occurs because the excess resorption elevates the extracellular fluid calcium ion concentration, which in turn reciprocally depresses parathyroid hormone secretion. This effect can be readily demonstrated in vivo by infusion of calcium, as well as in patients with severe osteolytic bone disease secondary to bone metastases, multiple myeloma, or immobilization, all of whom show evidence of depressed parathyroid hormone secretion. This is the normal and expected response to excess resorption. So long as parathyroid hormone secretion is not yet zero, there remains a mechanism for reflex reduction of bone resorption. This does not occur in most of the osteoporoses; parathyroid hormone secretion does not appear to be depressed, and in any event is certainly not zero. Thus parathyroid hormone secretion, responding to the needs of calcium ion homeostasis, is contributing to the excess bone resorption that produces the osteoporosis.

Rats, kittens, puppies, and lions in captivity all develop osteoporosis when placed on low calcium diets. The animals show clear evidence of increased parathyroid hormone secretion, and the osteoporosis can be prevented by prior parathyroidectomy. Nevertheless, histologic evidence of osteitis fibrosa is not seen, and the morphologic change is simply that of osteoporosis. The excess bone resorption and consequent osteoporosis are homeostatically mediated and represent not so much a homeostatic derangement as a quite appropriate consequence of normal calcium ion regulation. Bone is resorbed to meet mineral needs that the animal cannot obtain from its food. Comparable calcium-deficiency osteoporosis undoubtedly exists in man, but there is no evidence that it is common, and efforts to implicate calcium deficiency as a *primary* cause of most types of human osteoporosis have not been successful.

Nevertheless, the clear implication to be drawn from continued parathyroid secretion during development of most human osteoporosis is that this secretion is necessary to sustain normal calcium ion levels. Some fraction of the calcium resorbed from bone is lost from the body, not because it is present in excess, but for some other reason, and the extra resorption, mediated by parathyroid hormone, comes about precisely to compensate for this loss. It is in this fashion that the calcium homeostatic system becomes implicated in osteoporosis even when there is no evidence of absolute dietary calcium deficiency. The reasons for this calcium wastage are uncertain, but there is a growing body of evidence that changes in the intrinsic responsiveness of the three parathyroid hormone end-organs, and most specifically bone itself, to endogenous parathyroid hormone may account for inefficient calcium conservation. It is worth stressing that the sought-for effect need not be great; net calcium loss of as little as 50 mg. per day will reduce the skeletal mass by 15 to 20 per cent per decade.

POSTMENOPAUSAL AND SENILE OSTEOPOROSIS

Definition and Etiology. Postmenopausal and senile osteoporosis differs in no way from the foregoing general description. By definition it is found only in postmenopausal women and in elderly persons of both sexes. This is not an altogether arbitrary subdivision. These patients exhibit a remarkably homogeneous clinical picture and differ in several important respects from patients with specific osteoporoses in which known causal factors can be found. The cause of postmenopausal and senile osteoporosis is unknown. The temporal relationship to the menopause is probably fortuitous and can be found in any disease that has its peak onset after age 50. Gonadal hormone deficiency following the menopause was once implicated as the cause of the disorder; however, it probably plays no more than a secondary role. Because gonadal hormones depress bone resorption, their absence may aggravate an already existing tendency to excess resorption, but it has not been possible to find a relation between age at menopause and onset of osteoporosis, nor do surgical castrates clearly develop the disease sooner than their intact sisters. The common finding of osteoporosis in young women with gonadal agenesis (45,X syndromes) is now believed to represent an additional manifestation of the genetic defect rather than of endocrine deficiency.

Incidence. Postmenopausal and senile osteoporosis is the most common of all metabolic bone diseases. Satisfactory population studies have not yet been made, but available work suggests that approximately one fourth of all white females in the United States develop clinically significant osteoporosis. (By this is meant that they show the structural consequences of diminished bone mass: compression fractures, "codfish" vertebrae, Schmorl's nodes, dorsal kyphosis, and decreased stature). Furthermore, at least three fourths of all elderly people with fractures of the upper femur have pre-existing osteoporosis, presumably as the predisposing cause of fracture. The prevalence in elderly males, at about age 80, is similar, but in them the disease is usually less severe than in women. Thus in the two decades from age 50 to age 70 osteoporosis is predominantly a disease of women. Among women living in the United States, the disorder is most common in those of northern European extraction; it is less common in those of southern European ancestry and still less common in Negroes. Because of both racial and sexual protection, the disease is rare among Negro males of any age. Japanese living in the United States have a high incidence of osteoporosis. These racial differences appear to be related primarily to differences in normal adult bone mass, rather than to protection against age-related bone loss. Thus the adult Negro male has the largest initial bone mass and has therefore the largest structural reserve against the development of osteoporosis.

Pathogenesis. Many physiologic differences have been found between osteoporotics and comparable normal persons, but their relation to the pathogenesis of osteoporosis is uncertain. Studies of the population at risk have not been made, nor have individual women been studied long enough to determine whether these abnormalities precede the development of the disease. In comparison with normal persons, osteoporotics have been observed to consume 20 to 30 per cent less calcium in their diet, to absorb a smaller fraction of the ingested calcium, to have 40 per cent higher calcium requirements simply to achieve a balance between intake and output, to fail to reduce their urinary calcium normally when placed on low calcium diets, and to possess lower circulating vitamin D levels. In addition, alterations in the excretion pattern of steroid metabolites suggest a deficiency of secretion of androgen relative to corticosteroid. The significance of this hormonal change lies in the antiresorptive activity of androgens, their stimulation of the epidermal sebaceous secretion that provides the sterols activated to vitamin D, and their tonic effect on muscle mass and activity.

Although "normal" adults are able to adapt to calcium intakes below 500 mg. per day, some otherwise apparently healthy persons fail to achieve calcium balance on low intakes. There is no doubt that calcium deficiency can cause osteoporosis and that some of the patients in this group represent the end result of prolonged deficiency. Nevertheless, the disease occurs also in patients with higher than average intakes, and it seems safest to conclude that, in the group as a whole, inefficient calcium conservation serves as a contributory cause rather than as the primary factor in the development of osteoporosis.

All the changes cited above represent quantitative deviations from normal. Similar changes are found in normal men and women 20 to 30 years older than the osteoporotic patients, so that, in a sense, the typical osteoporotic patient can be considered to have a skeleton that appears to be a quarter of a century older than its chronologic age.

Clinical Manifestations. The principal manifestations of osteoporosis are vertebral compression with resultant kyphosis and loss of vertical height, back pain, and susceptibility to fractures (particularly fractures of the upper femur and distal radius). The vertebral compression is often asymptomatic, and probably no more than one third of all patients with the disease actively seek medical aid. The vertebral collapse and kyphosis exaggerate the downward angulation of the ribs and produce prominent horizontal skin folds over the lower chest and abdomen. These folds, particularly in thin people, are a clear indicator of vertebral collapse. The lower ribs may actually ride into the pelvic brim. Occasionally when this occurs the patient experiences severe flank pain, which is relieved by hyperextension of the spine or by surgical excision of the lower costal cartilages. Presumably the pain arises from the costal perichondrium.

Osteoporosis is an important predisposing factor in fractures, particularly those associated with minimal trauma. Hip fracture is a major cause of death and disability in the elderly, and it is probable that most such fractures are due to osteoporosis. Other bones are also more fragile, and fractures are often seen in the pubic and ischial rami, in the rib cage, and in the humerus. The fractures heal normally in all cases except those in which the original bone was so attenuated that the fracture completely destroyed the residual bony scaffolding. This sometimes happens in intertrochanteric and femoral neck fractures.

The back pain is of two types: an acute, sometimes severe pain, well localized to the midline over a restricted region of the spine, that disappears over a period of weeks, and a much more chronic, diffuse, aching pain. The former is related to new compression fractures or to extension of old collapse, and usually disappears as the associated soft tissue and periosteal damage heals. Occasionally the pain precedes roentgenographic evidence of fracture by several days or weeks. Patients commonly relate the attacks of pain to physical exertion, such as bending forward or lifting heavy objects, but weight bearing is not always found, and some patients incur fractures simply by turning over in bed. On physical examination, point tenderness can be found on percussion or pressure over the involved vertebrae. There are commonly associated paravertebral muscle spasm and tenderness. The more chronic pain is found only in a minority of patients, may not be related to the osteoporosis at all, or may be due to associated muscle spasm or to degenerative arthritis aggravated by malaligned weight-bearing forces. It is usually aggravated by prolonged standing or sitting and is relieved by lying down.

Diagnosis. The roentgenographic changes in postmenopausal and senile osteoporosis have been described. The plasma calcium, phosphorus, and alkaline phosphatase are normal, and the urine calcium is usually normal or low. Bone biopsy reveals only thinning of the cortex and attenuation and fragmentation of trabeculae, both of which are hard to evaluate in a single biopsy sample. The biopsy is of value, however, not because it is characteristic of osteoporosis, but because it excludes other disorders. The principal differential considerations include the specific osteoporoses such as that due to Cushing's syndrome, diffuse skeletal involvement with multiple myeloma, hyperparathyroidism, osteogenesis imperfecta (which in mild forms may first manifest itself in adult life), and metastatic malignancy. Despite a common misconception to the contrary, osteomalacia is not a cause of diffuse skeletal atrophy, and it does not present a clinical or roentgenographic picture similar to osteoporosis.

The clinical picture of Cushing's syndrome or of hyperthyroidism is usually sufficiently obvious so that little confusion with postmenopausal or senile osteoporosis should occur. Rarely, however, patients with these endocrinopathies may present with predominantly skeletal manifestations. Myeloma is excluded by examination of the bone marrow (which can be performed on the same specimen removed for bone biopsy), by electrophoretic separation of the plasma proteins, and by search for Bence Jones protein in the urine. Normal plasma calcium, phosphorus, and alkaline phosphatase serve to exclude hyperparathyroidism and those malignant conditions that mimic parathyroid hyperfunction. Metastatic malignancy presents a differential problem principally when it is a cause of vertebral compression fracture. In such patients, skeletal roentgenographic surveys may demonstrate more characteristic metastatic lesions in other bones. Further, the finding of apparently osteoporotic compression fractures in younger patients, particularly males, or of involvement of the neural arch should suggest a neoplastic cause for the lesion.

Treatment. Treatment in osteoporosis is directed at arresting and stabilizing the condition and at symptomatic relief, support, and rehabilitation of the patient. No form of treatment has been conclusively demonstrated to increase bone mass. Nevertheless, several forms of treatment have been shown to arrest the progress of the disorder, to decrease or eliminate further fractures, and to increase the functional capacity of the patient. Such treatment includes mineral supplements, gonadal hormones, and physical therapy. A number of other agents, including fluoride, phosphates, calcitonin, and the diphosphonate compounds, are still under investigation.

Because virtually all patients conserve calcium poorly, a high calcium intake must be the cornerstone of any therapeutic regimen. The risk of hypercalciuria with such treatment is negligible. Calcium intake should be at least 1500 mg. per day; if derived from the diet, this requires the ingestion of at least one quart of milk per day, which is more than most osteoporotic patients will accept. It is usually necessary to employ supplemental medicinal calcium, which is available in a variety of forms, including the gluconate, lactate, phosphate, carbonate, and glycerophosphate salts. All are absorbed equally well except for the carbonate, which is poorly absorbed in the presence of achlorhydria. There is suggestive, but still inconclusive, evidence that retention is better if supplemental phosphate is also provided; thus the phosphate salts may be preferable to the others.

Estrogens and androgens, alone or in combination, have been shown to improve calcium balance and to decrease the incidence of fracture. Dosage regimens vary greatly; adequate therapy is probably provided by ordinary replacement doses, i.e., 0.1 mg. of ethinyl estradiol or its equivalent. Androgen therapy in women is limited by its virilizing properties, and few patients will accept prolonged treatment at more than a few milligrams of methyltestosterone daily.

Intensive physical therapy is essential for successful treatment. The muscles of the back, hips, and thighs must be strengthened, and a lifelong program of exercise instituted. There is undoubtedly some component of disuse in most osteoporotics, and this must be abolished by a controlled sensible regimen of exercise. Patients must be taught to bend at the hips and knees and not to bend the back in order to pick up objects off the floor, and they must not carry or lift heavy objects. Bed rest is contraindicated except in the acute post-fracture period when it may be neces-

sary for pain relief. Patients should be up and about, and a physical therapy program should be started as soon as possible following an acute vertebral compression. Back braces are usually not indicated, but firm corsets or foundation garments are often very helpful.

Fluoride, given as the sodium salt in doses of 30 to 60 mg. daily, also improves calcium balance in many patients. This agent is still under intensive investigation but promises to be a useful adjunct to osteoporosis therapy. Fluoride is known to fit into the apatite crystal lattice in the place of hydroxyl radicals; the resulting fluorapatite is a more stable, less soluble mineral than hydroxyapatite. The bone is thus rendered more resistant to resorptive attack, and the calcium homeostatic system adapts by forcing more effective renal and intestinal calcium conservation.

Phosphate, given orally as a mixed neutral solution of sodium and potassium phosphates at a dose of 1 to 1.5 grams daily, has received limited trial. Such treatment reduces urine calcium during immobilization and is believed to retard bone resorption. Similarly calcitonin, with its known inhibitory effect on bone resorption, might be expected to increase bone mass, but adequate data are not available, and the necessity for parenteral administration makes this agent less attractive. Finally, the diphosphonate compounds (carbon analogues of pyrophosphate) have been shown to inhibit parathyroid mediated bone resorption, and because of their demonstrated ability to stabilize calcium phosphate crystals against resorptive attack and their apparent lack of toxicity, these compounds also offer considerable promise. Data concerning efficacy have not yet been provided for any of these agents, and it is not possible to say whether long-term treatment with any of them will lead to an increase in bone mass.

Prevention. The probable irreversibility of bone atrophy in the aged makes prevention all the more important. An adequate calcium intake ought to be urged on all postmenopausal and geriatric patients. Nevertheless, because the disease also develops in patients with higher than average intakes, additional investigation will be required before really satisfactory prevention is assured. There is suggestive evidence that prophylactic estrogen therapy retards postmenopausal bone loss. This effect is in keeping with what is known of estrogen action in bone resorption. Although adequately controlled prospective studies have not yet been performed, it seems likely that prophylactic estrogen therapy may be very useful. It would be particularly desirable to be able to select for such prophylaxis the 25 per cent of the white female population who constitute the high-risk group, but unfortunately this is not yet possible. The best one can suggest is to concentrate on small (less than 140 pounds), very fair-skinned women, with minimal body hair, and usually of Scotch, Irish, or Anglo-Saxon origin. All surveys to date suggest that such women have the highest risk of developing osteoporotic fractures.

Prognosis. There is little information about the natural history of the untreated disease. With adequate treatment, however, most patients can be stabilized and restored to useful functional activity. Hip fractures are probably the principal hazard of the disease; 10 to 15 per cent of patients are dead within three months of such fractures, and the associated enforced bed rest, trauma, and surgery markedly decrease the ultimate functional capacity of those who survive.

DISUSE OSTEOPOROSIS

Disuse osteoporosis is a local disorder confined to bones or regions subjected to immobilization or deprived of normal muscle pull. In severe lower motor neuron paralytic disease, such as quadriplegic poliomyelitis or the Guillain-Barré syndrome, virtually the entire skeleton may be involved, but, unlike other osteoporoses, the spine is less severely involved than are the long bones of the extremities. The effects of mechanical forces on the skeleton have been summarized elsewhere. The disease comes about because of a massive increase in bone resorption. This resorption does not appear to be systemically mediated or controllable, and is somehow a consequence of the local withdrawal of mechanical stress. Vascular engorgement within bone occurs during development of the disorder, but it is not known whether this change causes the resorption or is instead caused by it. The pathologic picture is otherwise no different from that of the other osteoporoses. Roentgenographic changes are also nondistinctive except for the localization of disease to the immobilized bones and for a zone of rarefaction in the region of the fused epiphyseal plate, which appears as the first detectable change in involved long bones.

Since immobilized bones are not subjected to mechanical stress, their fragility is of little structural consequence, and the principal significance of the disease lies in the hypercalcemia and hypercalciuria that may be produced by extensive resorption. In poliomyelitis this resorption begins almost immediately and reaches peak values four to five weeks after onset, with urine calcium values sometimes as high as 800 mg. per day. If care is not taken to keep these patients hydrated and to maintain a high urine flow, glomerular filtration falls, and hypercalcemia may result. Furthermore, stasis in the urinary tract predisposes to stone formation.

Comparable problems, though probably less severe, are believed to be a potential hazard of prolonged weightlessness, as in space flight. Such problems may be aggravated by the difficulty of maintaining a high fluid intake.

NUTRITIONAL OSTEOPOROSES

Osteoporosis is a frequent manifestation of many nutritional deficiency syndromes in patients of all ages. These include general protein and caloric malnutrition, kwashiorkor, scurvy, chronic alcoholism, and a variety of malabsorption syndromes as well as isolated calcium deficiency. These are specific osteoporoses, due to the malnutrition, and will heal both clinically and roentgenographically, at least in young people, if the underlying cause can be corrected. The osteoporosis is usually a minor part of the over-all syndrome.

Osteoporosis is a common finding in alcoholics of both sexes, and alcoholism should be suspected when osteoporotic fractures are found in men before age 65 and women before age 55. It is not known whether the disorder is due to the generally poor nutrition of alcoholics, to their usually very low calcium intakes, or to large endogenous losses of calcium. Its manifestations and consequences are the same as for ordinary postmenopausal or senile osteoporosis, but because of the coexisting alcoholism it is even harder to treat satisfactorily.

ENDOCRINE OSTEOPOROSES

Hyperthyroidism. Bone turnover is accelerated in hyperthyroidism. In some patients bone resorption may exceed formation sufficiently to produce significant osteoporosis. The same process, if still more severe, may mimic hyperparathyroidism. The difference seems to be only one of degree. The pathologic changes are usually the same as in the other osteoporoses. Plasma calcium, phosphorus, and alkaline phosphatase values may all be elevated, and the urine calcium may be normal or high. This too is a specific osteoporosis, treatable by recognizing and treating the hyperthyroidism. Roentgenographic improvement may occur, particularly in younger patients.

Cushing's Syndrome. Osteoporosis occurs in most patients with Cushing's syndrome and may be severe in approximately one third. It is associated with marked depression of osteoblast activity and with defective fracture healing. Similar changes can be produced by administration of glucocorticoids in high doses and are a complication of corticoid therapy, particularly in patients with rheumatoid arthritis. Except for depression of alkaline phosphatase activity, there are no distinctive plasma chemical changes. Urine calcium is usually only moderately elevated, and gastrointestinal calcium absorption is depressed. Improvement is poor, except in young patients, even with satisfactory control of the adrenal secretion.

MISCELLANEOUS OSTEOPOROSES

Idiopathic Osteoporosis. The term "idiopathic osteoporosis" was applied originally to young men or women in whom no demonstrable cause could be found, and who were not postmenopausal or senile (and hence were not considered to have gonadal deficiency as a causal factor). The disease has been described in adolescents and in pregnant women, is commonly more painful than usual postmenopausal osteoporosis, but differs in no other way from the latter. The cause remains unknown, but this is true as well for most of the postmenopausal cases, and it now appears probable that the disease does not differ significantly from the latter variety. The disease tends to stabilize with time, but does not heal, and except for physical therapy and rehabilitation no treatment has been of much value.

Sudeck's Atrophy. Following fracture in an extremity, structural turnover in adjacent bones increases markedly. Commonly, osteoporosis develops. Similar changes may also occur without fracture, sometimes following only minor injuries. The term "Sudeck's atrophy" refers to cases with or without fracture in which this osteoporosis comes on very acutely and is associated with severe pain and swelling, tenderness, and sweating in the overlying soft tissue. The disorder is most common in the wrists, hands, and feet, but may involve major portions of the skeleton. Abnormal autonomic vasomotor regulation has been implicated as the cause. Sympathetic block may produce profound relief. Although frequently disabling, the disease is usually self-limited and in most instances heals spontaneously over a period of several months to a few years. In particularly severe or protracted cases regional sympathectomy may be indicated.

Bassan, J., Frame, B., and Frost, H.: Osteoporosis: A review of pathogenesis and treatment. Ann. Intern. Med., 58:539, 1963.

Cooke, A. M.: Osteoporosis. Lancet, 1:877, 929, 1955.

deTakats, G.: Sympathetic reflex dystrophy. Med. Clin. N. Amer., 49:117, 1965.

Heaney, R. P.: A unified concept of osteoporosis. Amer. J. Med., 39:877, 1965.

Rich, C., Ensinck, J., and Ivannovich, P.: The effects of sodium fluoride on calcium metabolism of subjects with metabolic bone diseases. J. Clin. Invest., 43:545, 1964.

Rodahl, K., Nicholson, J. T., and Brown, E. M. (eds.): Bone as a Tissue. New York, Blakiston Division, McGraw-Hill Book Co., 1960, Part I: Osteoporosis, pp. 3–102.

Steinbach, H. L.: The roentgen appearance of osteoporosis. Radiol. Clin. N. Amer., 2:191, 1964.

Urist, M. R.: Osteoporosis. Ann. Rev. Med., 13:273, 1962.

The Osteomalacias

Definition. The term "osteomalacia," meaning softening of bone, was applied originally to a distinctive clinical syndrome consisting of severe bone pain, skeletal deformity, depressed plasma Ca × P ion product, and wide osteoid borders in bone, all associated with vitamin D deficiency. Although this complete picture still occurs occasionally, nutritional vitamin D deficiency is now rare in Europe and North America, and the term "osteomalacia" has been applied to a variety of conditions exhibiting some, but not all, of the features of the full-blown vitamin D deficiency syndrome. This has led to confusion and disagreement concerning the definition of the disorder. Some authorities confine the term to the *clinical syndrome* described above, irrespective of the cause; others choose to base their definition on *morphologic* criteria, i.e., the presence of wide osteoid borders on bone surfaces. For purposes of clarity in exposition, the latter course will be pursued in what follows.

The term "rickets" refers to a series of identical syndromes occurring in childhood, and adds to the picture of adult osteomalacia the features of retarded growth, abnormal proliferation and maturation of the epiphyseal growth plate, and associated periarticular pain.

Morphologic and Roentgenographic Characteristics. Grossly, the skeleton may show little abnormality. In severe cases, bowing of long bones is observed, the pelvic bones are deformed inward, and all bones convey the impression of plastic deformation in response to applied forces. Microscopically, osteoid seams are invariably increased in thickness and in number, both on trabecular surfaces and in newly forming haversian systems. This osteoid fails to show evidence of the normal maturation sequence that must precede mineralization. In some osteomalacias, particularly those with severe vitamin D deficiency, histologic changes of osteitis fibrosa may also be seen.

The principal roentgenographic changes are the deformities described above and, in rickets, widening, fraying, and cupping of all active growth plates. These rachitic changes are most apparent and most severe at sites of rapid growth, particularly the sternal ends of the ribs, the distal end of the radius and ulna, and the proximal ends of the tibia and humerus. In fact, the rachitic lesion is dependent upon growth for its expression. When growth slows or stops for any reason (such as intercurrent illness or increasing malnutrition), calcification of the disordered epiphyseal cartilage slowly occurs, and the roentgenographic lesion appears to heal, even though the basic abnormality remains unchanged. The bone of such persons then shows only osteomalacic lesions. In adults the only characteristic roentgenographic changes are the pseudofractures (Looser's zones, Milkman's lines). These lines are ribbon-like radiolucent zones, perpendicular to free bone surfaces, often bilateral and symmetrical, which give the appearance of incomplete fractures. They are found most commonly along the axillary border of the scapula, in the ischial and pubic rami, in the femoral neck, and in the ribs.

Generalized decrease in bone density is not a feature of osteomalacia per se. However, the disease commonly coexists with osteoporosis and hence may be found in skeletons that show decreased roentgenographic density. This decrease is not due to the osteomalacia. In fact, in many patients without pre-existing osteoporosis the spine may exhibit *increased* roentgenographic density.

General Pathophysiologic Considerations. The two features most characteristic of the osteomalacias are a low plasma Ca × P ion product and wide osteoid borders in bone. These have usually been considered to be related as cause and effect, and both have been attributed to poor intestinal calcium absorption. However, this simplified relationship is incorrect. As has been stressed before, defective calcium absorption leads to osteoporosis, not to osteomalacia; furthermore, in those osteomalacias due to vitamin D deficiency small doses of vitamin D sufficient to repair the absorptive defect do not heal the bone lesions; conversely, adequate vitamin D therapy will cure osteomalacia even on a calcium-poor diet.

There are two basic mechanisms that might lead to accumulation of unmineralized osteoid: (1) insufficient concentration of calcium and phosphorus in extracellular fluid to allow crystal nucleation and growth, and (2) abnormalities in the matrix that render it unmineralizable. These mechanisms are not necessarily distinct, for the osteoblasts may well be sensitive to the phosphate concentration of the extracellular fluid, and thus in some cases the matrix abnormality may be due to a metabolic consequence of osteoblast phosphorus deficiency. Probably both defects are involved to varying degrees in the different osteomalacias. Nevertheless, there are undoubted matrix abnormalities in most if not all of the osteomalacias. Both rachitic cartilage and osteomalacic osteoid fail to show staining reactions characteristic of normal premineralization ripening. Although the cartilage will mineralize when incubated in normal plasma, the osteoid will not, and the first detectable changes in vivo after vitamin D therapy are staining reactions indicative of matrix maturation. These occur prior to measurable changes in plasma calcium or phosphorus concentration. There can be little doubt that both new matrix

production and osteoblast-mediated ripening of osteoid seams are severely depressed. This decrease in individual osteoblast activity is usually compensated for by markedly increased numbers of osteoblasts, which, though working slowly, may succeed in blanketing every available bone surface with a thick layer of poorly mineralizable matrix. The ultimate rate of new bone formation may thus be normal or even high, even though individual osteoblast activity is severely retarded.

The depressed plasma Ca × P ion product is best explained by the combined effect of impaired bone resorptive response and normal renal tubular phosphate response to parathyroid hormone. As mentioned earlier, osteoclastic response to parathyroid hormone is vitamin D dependent, whereas renal tubular effects are not. There is invariably an increase in parathyroid gland weight and activity in rickets and osteomalacia, and the ultimate plasma calcium and phosphorus levels depend on both the final level of parathyroid hormone necessary to maintain calcium ion homeostasis and the residual responsiveness of vitamin D deficient osteoclasts to parathyroid hormone. Complete vitamin D deficiency is probably never seen in ordinary clinical situations; thus, these changes represent quantitative alterations in responsiveness rather than completely obstructed metabolic pathways.

RICKETS AND OSTEOMALACIA DUE TO VITAMIN D DEFICIENCY

Etiology and Incidence. At the turn of the century approximately 90 per cent of the children of northern European cities had clinical rickets secondary to vitamin D deficiency. For a time vitamin D deficiency became so rare that rickets and osteomalacia due solely to nutritional causes were almost unknown in Europe and North America. With the immigration of dark-skinned persons into the industrial cities of England and Scotland recently, there has been an increase in vitamin D deficiency disease. In general the disorder is still common in parts of the world where both diet and limited exposure to sunlight restrict vitamin D intake.

In the United States, vitamin D deficiency osteomalacia is virtually confined to patients with the various malabsorption syndromes, particularly idiopathic sprue. Curiously, it is unusual in patients with pancreatic disease, even though the efficiency of vitamin D absorption has been shown to be less in these patients than in those with sprue. This difference may be related to the generally much poorer nutrition in the sprue syndromes.

Pathogenesis. Vitamin D deficiency has two

main effects: it impairs the responsiveness of osteoclasts and intestinal mucosa to parathyroid hormone, and it leads to the defects in osteoblast activity mentioned earlier. The decreased sensitivity to parathyroid hormone is compensated for by increased parathyroid gland size and secretion, and this in turn produces markedly enhanced renal tubular responses, i.e., decreased calcium clearance and increased phosphate clearance. Augmented parathyroid hormone stimulation of intestinal mucosa and osteoclasts compensates with variable efficiency for the refractoriness of these end organs. Usually plasma calcium ion remains normal or nearly so, whereas plasma inorganic phosphate is reduced to low values, usually below 2 mg. per 100 ml. When skeletal demands for calcium are high, or osteoclast response is sharply reduced, plasma calcium may fall to tetanic levels.

Few patients with pure vitamin D deficiency are in significantly negative calcium balance. Although intestinal absorption is much reduced, it is not zero, and the limited absorption usually allows net recovery of most of the calcium of the digestive juices. Urine calcium is regularly reduced to extremely low values, often unmeasurably low. And thus, with no mechanism for losing calcium, it is not surprising that total bone mass remains essentially normal.

Clinical Manifestations. Early in their course, patients with osteomalacia superimposed on gastrointestinal disease may have few symptoms referable to the bone disease; the predominant clinical manifestations are those of the underlying disease. When the osteomalacia becomes more severe, typical symptoms related to the skeleton and the vitamin D deficiency become apparent. These include bone pain, waddling gait, muscle weakness, and anorexia. Aching bone pain is prolonged and is made worse on weight-bearing; the bones may be tender to pressure. Pseudofractures tend to occur in bursts and when present may be associated with severe muscle weakness and bone pain. Although hypophosphatemia is itself a cause of weakness, the weakness of clinical osteomalacia is better correlated with the appearance of pseudofractures than with any detectable change in phosphate levels. It seems probable therefore that the symptom is due largely to inhibition. If the serum calcium falls to low levels, typical hypocalcemic tetany may occur. Occasional patients may have osteomalacia secondary to gluten-sensitive enteropathy, without obvious nutritional or gastrointestinal complaints, and thus may present only with skeletal manifestations.

It should be stressed that the most common bone disease in malabsorption syndromes is osteoporosis, not osteomalacia, and that when osteomalacia occurs it does so not simply because of the malabsorption, but because the patient has become ill enough to lose even casual contact with direct sunlight, thus losing his last source of vitamin D. So long as vitamin D levels remain adequate, however, calcium ion homeostasis works efficiently, and the malabsorption of calcium simply leads to negative calcium balance, which in turn results in osteoporosis. It is for this reason that most of the osteomalacia seen in the United States occurs in patients with pre-existing osteoporosis and represents a combined deficiency state (calcium first, then vitamin D).

Diagnosis. The diagnosis rests securely on a tripod of biopsy, roentgenographic, and biochemical findings. Wide osteoid borders are found on biopsy in all cases. Pseudofractures, when seen in otherwise normal bone, are virtually diagnostic of osteomalacia. The characteristic chemical changes are a normal to low plasma calcium, low plasma phosphate, high alkaline phosphatase, and very low urine calcium. Furthermore, these changes are characteristically found in patients with steatorrhea and with more or less obvious evidence of malabsorption. Occasionally the osteomalacia will be more apparent than the underlying enteropathy, and the observation of the changes described above should lead to a search for an underlying cause. The only differential consideration of consequence relates to other causes of osteomalacia. These include vitamin D resistance, adult hypophosphatasia, and advanced renal disease, all of which will be discussed in succeeding sections.

Treatment. Treatment must be directed at both the vitamin D deficiency and any underlying gastrointestinal disease, which is the usual cause of the deficiency. Uncomplicated vitamin D deficiency responds well to the vitamin in daily doses of as low as 1000 units; the various malabsorption syndromes may require from 10,000 to 50,000 units daily. Requirements in excess of these levels suggest one of the vitamin D resistant forms of osteomalacia (vide infra). Therapeutic ultraviolet exposure may be particularly helpful in patients with malabsorption syndromes, since skin manufacture of vitamin D bypasses the intestinal absorption block. Healing may be expected to be complete. Any coexisting osteoporosis due to calcium malabsorption should be treated by means of a high calcium intake.

VITAMIN D RESISTANT RICKETS
(Familial Hypophosphatemia)

Definition and Inheritance. Vitamin D resistant rickets and osteomalacia are distinct syndromes, clinically similar to their vitamin D deficient counterparts, but different in that they fail to respond to usual therapeutic doses of vitamin D. The term "vitamin D resistance" is unfortunate, for there is little evidence of true biochemical refractoriness to the vitamin. The term "familial hypophosphatemia" is much more apt and describes the essential and invariable expression of the genetic defect that is responsible for the disorder.

This defect is most commonly inherited as a sex-linked dominant character with complete penetrance but widely varying expressivity. Other inheritance patterns probably reflect different genetic defects that express themselves as hypophosphatemia. In addition, sporadic cases of resistant rickets, otherwise indistinguishable from the inherited variety, also occur. It is not known whether such patients have offspring who inherit the disease. Furthermore, adults with no sign of childhood rickets or dwarfing can occasionally present with osteomalacia associated with renal tubular hypophosphatemia. These cases give no family history of renal disease. Several cases of severe hypophosphatemic osteomalacia associated with benign sclerosing hemangiomas have been described. Cure followed removal of the hemangioma.

Etiology and Pathogenesis. The nature of the genetic defect is unknown. The hypophosphatemia by which it is expressed is probably directly responsible for the osteomalacia. Although the matrix shows the same abnormal staining reactions as in vitamin D deficiency, simple elevation of the plasma phosphate by infusion or phosphate feeding will induce prompt healing and will lead to positive calcium balance. It cannot yet be decided whether the osteoid accumulates simply because there is inadequate mineral to allow crystal nucleation and growth or because the osteoblast suffers from an induced phosphate deficiency. The reason for the hypophosphatemia itself is also obscure. Defective tubular phosphate reabsorption has usually been implicated, and there is no doubt that renal phosphate clearance is greatly increased, but it has been established that tubular phosphate reabsorption in these patients responds normally to parathyroid hormone suppression; i.e., it can be returned to or toward normal by calcium infusion, by immobilization, or by any maneuver that reduces endogenous parathyroid hormone secretion. However, none of these increases the TM_p to normal. It has also been suggested that there is a primary defect in intestinal absorption of calcium leading to secondary parathyroid secretion, which in turn results in phosphaturia. However, it is common to find increased bone density in adults with the untreated disease (even to the extent that the axial skeleton can resemble osteopetrosis); this finding does not suggest lifelong inadequacy of calcium absorption.

Clinical Manifestations. Many affected persons have no demonstrable abnormality except for the hypophosphatemia. The expression of the defect ranges from simple hypophosphatemia without other abnormalities through histologically demonstrable osteomalacia without clinical symptoms, mild growth retardation, to typical, severe rickets and osteomalacia. The clinical features of the full-blown syndrome differ from ordinary vitamin D deficiency rickets in several respects. The disease is not common in early infancy and is seen most often after 18 months of age. The plasma calcium is almost always normal, whereas the plasma phosphorus is invariably low. The plasma alkaline phosphatase, although elevated, is rarely as high as in vitamin D deficiency. On biopsy the bone is essentially indistinguishable from that in vitamin D deficiency rickets, and, except for severity, roentgenographic changes do not distinguish between the two types of bone involvement. When the disease presents under the age of three, short stature and bowing of the legs is the characteristic deformity. With onset after three years, knock knee is usually seen. Muscle weakness is not observed in children with resistant rickets; but in adults, with either the acquired or the hereditary disease, severe weakness, especially of the lower limbs, is quite common and may even suggest a neurologic disorder. This is believed to be due to hypophosphatemia, but is rarely seen without pseudofractures and pain. Most of these children develop a coxa vara deformity and consequent waddling gait. The limb bones are short and often bowed and there is a tendency to hyperostosis at tendinous insertions which may suggest the diagnosis of achondroplasia. In adolescence the epiphyses close, alkaline phosphatase returns to normal, and the patients become asymptomatic. However, between 25 and 50 years pseudofractures may occur, especially in the femoral necks or over the convexity of the femoral shafts. These may not be associated with any rise in serum alkaline phosphatase activity.

In children, urinary calcium excretion is of the order of 10 to 20 mg. per 24 hours, whereas in adults urinary calcium excretion ranges between 50 to 120 mg. per 24 hours. These values are low, especially in children, but should be contrasted to the virtual absence of calcium in vitamin D deficiency rickets and osteomalacia.

Diagnosis. The diagnosis is based primarily on the observation of otherwise typical rickets and osteomalacia in patients without vitamin D deficiency or diseases predisposing thereto and without azotemia or other outspoken renal tubular defects, and on the failure of the bone disease to respond to usual vitamin D therapy. Commonly a positive family history or the familial occurrence of asymptomatic hypophosphatemia can be established. Quite similar bone disorders are seen in patients with multiple renal tubular reabsorptive defects. These defects include reabsorption of amino acids, bicarbonate, and glucose, as well as phosphate. In this group are included the Fanconi syndrome (vide infra) and renal tubular acidosis, as well as renal injury secondary to cystinosis and to lead or cadmium poisoning.

Treatment. Available treatment is not altogether satisfactory, and it is doubtful that asymptomatic patients need any treatment. The most widely used therapy has been vitamin D (ergocalciferol, 50,000 to 200,000 units daily). These doses will usually cause roentgenographic changes of the epiphyses to heal. The dose required to do this is always very close to a toxic one. Furthermore, serum levels of phosphorus can never be maintained at normal in these patients without toxicity from vitamin D. Finally, there is little evidence that such therapy improves the growth rate or prevents deformities, despite near toxic levels of vitamin D therapy over a prolonged period of time. The adult syndrome with pseudofractures is best treated by a balanced sodium phosphate mixture containing 1.5 to 2 grams of phosphorus daily. Intake is pushed to levels just short of a cathartic effect. There is a large but transient rise in plasma phosphate after each dose, and divided doses are necessary in order to sustain the effect for a sufficient fraction of each day. A combination of phosphate and vitamin D is commonly employed, but it is not known whether this is more effective than supplemental phosphate alone.

HYPOPHOSPHATASIA

Hypophosphatasia is a rare inherited disorder that expresses itself primarily as rickets and osteomalacia. It may be apparent soon after birth as severe infantile rickets, or it may present in adult life with fractures or pseudofractures. Adults are usually of short stature and give a history of rickets in childhood. The disease is transmitted as an autosomal recessive trait. The bone changes are similar to those of other patients with rickets or osteomalacia. Craniostenosis may occur in involved infants. A number of distinctive chemical abnormalities are found: most characteristic is a profound depression of plasma alkaline phosphatase. This deficiency is found also in osteoblasts, liver, kidney, and leukocytes, and undoubtedly reflects a general enzymatic defect. There is intermittent hypercalcemia in most patients, and both urine and blood contain excess quantities of phosphoethanolamine. Although the precise mechanism is unknown, it seems certain that the osteomalacic bone lesions in this disorder are due entirely to defective maturation of deposited osteoid. No treatment is effective, but the administration of corticosteroid drugs permits better mineralization of the growing epiphyses by slowing growth, and so seems to permit roentgenographic healing of the rickets. The prognosis in children who survive the neonatal period is good.

MISCELLANEOUS OSTEOMALACIAS

Bone changes typical of osteomalacia, but without clinical symptoms, may be observed in many bone diseases, and clinically significant rachitic and osteomalacic skeletal involvement may complicate a variety of disorders. Most important is the bone disease associated with chronic renal insufficiency (see below). Osteomalacic bone changes, with or without symptoms, may occasionally be seen in patients with other bone disorders, such as Paget's disease, hyperparathyroidism, and fluorosis, as well as in patients with neither biochemical changes in the circulating plasma nor predisposing disease. In all such instances osteoid accumulation must be presumed to be due to interference with normal matrix maturation. Only very rarely does such osteomalacia produce clinical symptoms, and it is mentioned here principally because it may present as an incidental finding on bone biopsy.

Fanconi Syndrome. The Fanconi syndrome consists of osteomalacic bone disease associated with renal tubular defect with respect to tubular reabsorption of glucose, amino acids, and phosphate. There may or may not be renal acidosis. The disease is commonly idiopathic, but may also result from renal tubular damage from cystine storage disease, in cadmium or lead poisoning, or from Wilson's disease (hepatolenticular degeneration). When renal acidosis occurs, hypocalcemia is common. Treatment is similar to that of resistant rickets except when acidosis complicates the picture and then it is important to correct acidosis with appropriate alkali therapy as well as to treat the patient with large doses of vitamin D.

Bartter, F. C.: Hypophosphatasia. *In* Stanbury, J. B., Wyngaarden, J. B., and Fredrickson, D. S. (eds.): Metabolic Basis of Inherited Disease, 2nd ed. New York, Blakiston Division, McGraw-Hill Book Co., 1966.

Frame, B., Smith, R. W., Jr., Fleming, J. L., and Manson, G.: Oral phosphates in vitamin-D-refractory rickets and osteomalacia. Amer. J. Dis. Child. 106:147, 1963.

Fraser, D.: Hypophosphatasia. Amer. J. Med., 22:739, 1957.

Hioco, D.: Osteomalacia. Paris, Editions Masson, 1966.

Stanbury, S. W., and Lumb, G.: Parathyroid function in chronic renal failure. Quart. J. Med., 35:1, 1966.

Williams, T. F., Winters, R. W., and Burnett, C. H.: Familial hypophosphatemia and vitamin D resistant rickets. *In* Stanbury, J. B., Wyngaarden, J. B., and Fredrickson, D. S. (eds.): Metabolic Basis of Inherited Disease. 2nd ed. New York, Blakiston Division, McGraw-Hill Book Co., 1966.

RENAL OSTEODYSTROPHY

Definition and Incidence. The bone disease of persons suffering from chronic uremia presents as a confusing variety of manifestations seemingly different from one part of the world to the next and depending as well on whether the patient is receiving hemodialysis. Typically the bone disease is a mixture of osteomalacia, osteitis fibrosa, osteosclerosis, and osteoporosis, the first two being the more important. Although it is not yet possible to predict which one of these will predominate in any individual, given time, some form of skeletal disease develops in all uremic patients.

Clinical Manifestations. Clinical manifestations include bone pain, deformity, fractures, and, in children, growth retardation. Since uremic patients are rarely in very negative calcium balance, total body calcium is usually normal or even high.

With the more severe cases of osteitis fibrosa and metastatic calcification there is usually an intra-body shift of mineral from bone to ectopic sites (such as bursae or vascular walls). Frequently the bone marrow is itself a site of metastatic calcification (as in vitamin D intoxication), and this phenomenon may produce or contribute to the roentgenographic appearance of osteosclerosis.

Pathogenesis and Diagnosis. There is resistance to the action of vitamin D in uremia, which begins to be manifest even at minor degrees of azotemia. At least some of this resistance appears to be due to an abnormality in the conversion of vitamin D to its 25-OH derivative. This resistance is associated with varying degrees of compensatory parathyroid hyperplasia and hypersecretion. The plasma calcium may be quite low but is more commonly in the low-normal range, and is presumably maintained at even this level only because of sometimes heroic levels of parathyroid hormone secretion.

The size of the parathyroid glands is invariably increased, and there appear to be at least a few cases of true autonomous hyperparathyroidism resulting from this long-continued hyperplasia. In general, gland hypertrophy is less severe in those patients with lesions that are predominantly osteomalacic and more severe in patients with predominant osteitis fibrosa and metastatic calcification. The level of phosphatemia depends on a combination of factors including the degree of renal failure, the level of parathyroid hormone secretion, the phosphate intake, and various therapeutic regimens (principally aluminum hydroxide gels) designed to lower effective phosphate intake. Nevertheless, the plasma phosphate is usually above normal, and the empirical $Ca \times P$ product correspondingly elevated. The alkaline phosphatase is usually elevated and roentgenograms demonstrate the features of the bone diseases listed above. It has been observed that, when the $Ca \times P$ product is below 70, the most prominent feature of the bone disease is likely to consist of rickets or osteomalacia, and when above 70, osteitis fibrosa together with varying degrees of metastatic calcification. There is broad overlap between these categories, and the distinction is further complicated by the fact that some degree of osteitis fibrosa, including typical roentgenographic features, is frequent in severe rickets and osteomalacia from any cause, including that seen in the uremic syndrome. The existence of rickets and osteomalacia in the presence of high mineral concentrations presents an interesting and as yet unsolved problem. There has been shown to be a circulating inhibitor of calcification in the plasma of uremic patients. Furthermore, the healing seen with high doses of vitamin D (which produces only trivial changes in $Ca \times P$ product in these patients) suggests either systemic removal of this inhibitor or direct vitamin D action on osteoblasts and growth cartilage.

Treatment. If the predominant bony lesion is rachitic (malacic) and if the $Ca \times P$ product is lower than 70, then the patient will very likely benefit from vitamin D, which must usually be given in large doses (50,000 to 500,000 units per day). Both the malacic lesions and any associated osteitis fibrosa may heal significantly with this regimen. On the other hand if there is little or no malacic component to the bone disease, vitamin D treatment will usually do no good and may, by raising the $Ca \times P$ product still further, aggravate an already dangerous propensity to metastatic calcification. It is thus important to evaluate both bone morphology and plasma calcium and phosphate levels before beginning vitamin D treatment. If roentgenographic findings of rickets or osteomalacia are not evident, a bone biopsy should be obtained and an undecalcified section examined for the presence of uncalcified osteoid.

Treatment directed at the uremia itself also has effects on the bone disease and on calcium homeostasis. In general, dialysis does little or nothing to alter the vitamin D resistance or the tendency to osteomalacia, and by prolonging life may allow osteodystrophy to develop to the point of producing significant disability. Successful renal transplantation, however, almost always leads to restoration of normal or nearly normal vitamin D sensitivity and corresponding healing of rickets and osteomalacia. Normal vitamin D metabolism returns well before the parathyroid glands can involute, and the sometimes huge residual mass of parathyroid tissue may thus oversecrete parathyroid hormone even when maximally suppressed, producing post-transplantation hypercalcemia. This phenomenon usually becomes apparent as the plasma phosphate falls, but may first make its appearance as much as six months following transplantation. This situation has been given the unhappy designation "tertiary hyperparathyroidism." It appears to be a true hyperparathyroidism, i.e., hypercalcemia caused by excessive secretion of parathyroid hormone, but in almost all cases is self-limited and subsides as the parathyroid glands complete their involution. In a small minority of cases autonomous parathyroid adenomas exist, and these must be removed surgically. In others the degree of hypercalcemia may be sufficiently severe or prolonged, or the risk of myocardial or pulmonary calcification considered so great, that subtotal parathyroidectomy may be warranted. Several authorities consider that extensive metastatic calcification is an indication for subtotal parathyroidectomy either prior to or soon after renal transplantation.

Kleeman, C. R. (ed.): Divalent ion metabolism and osteodystrophy in chronic renal failure. Arch. Intern. Med. (Chicago), 124:261, 389, 519, 649, 1969.

Osteitis Fibrosa

Definition. The term "osteitis fibrosa" is used to designate a pathologic rather than a clinical entity. It refers to the replacement of bone by a highly cellular fibrous tissue, associated with accumulations of osteoclasts, singly and in clumps, together with evidence of increased osteoblastic activity. The terms "dissecting osteitis" and "von Recklinghausen's bone disease" have also been used to describe this condition.

Etiology and Incidence. In most cases this morphologic picture comes about because of greatly exaggerated parathyroid hormonal stimulation It is found in 10 to 25 per cent of patients with primary hyperparathyroidism, is always found as a part of the picture of uremic osteodystrophy, and to variable degrees may be seen in patients with rickets and osteomalacia. In the latter disorders, the presence of osteitis fibrosa depends upon the degree of responsiveness to parathyroid hormone that the bone mesenchyme is able to manifest. However, the identical condition can be produced even without an excess of parathyroid hormone whenever bone turnover is exceedingly rapid, as in certain patients with hyperthyroidism, and locally in rapidly evolving Paget's disease (vide infra).

Pathogenesis and Pathology. In the typical case due to excess parathyroid hormone there is stimulation of all bone cells: osteocytes resorb their perilacunar bone; osteoclasts are found in large numbers and resorb bone on all available surfaces; osteoblastic new bone formation is also increased. However, osteoclasts predominate, and as a consequence there is usually a decrease in total skeletal mass. Resorption is particularly prominent in cortical bone immediately beneath the periosteum and is responsible for two typical and characteristic roentgenographic features of the disorder: (1) the presence of a fine lacy pattern of radiolucency at the outer edge of the cortex, particularly in the phalanges and metacarpals, and (2) the disappearance of the lamina dura (the equivalent of a bone cortex in the tooth socket). Undoubtedly the bony mesenchyme is itself stimulated by parathyroid hormone, and masses of growing fibrous tissue and osteoclasts may expand and destroy the bone cortex, giving rise to what appear, roentgenographically, to be large cystic tumors. Osteoclasts alone may form tumor-like masses that have been designated giant cell tumors. These produce discrete punched-out lesions roentgenographically, particularly in the jaw or facial bones, and in some cases such tumors may be the only roentgenographic manifestations of osteitis fibrosa. Such tumors are biologically benign and invariably regress if the underlying cause is removed.

Clinical Manifestations. The principal manifestations of osteitis fibrosa are bone pain and pathologic fractures. Early the pain is not distinctive and is easily mistaken for vague arthritic complaints. There may also be specific arthritides present: both gout and pseudogout have been described in association with osteitis fibrosa. Later the bones become tender to palpation, and in advanced cases the pain may become incapacitating. Pathologic fractures occur through areas weakened by general resorption or giant cell tumor formation, and may involve any bones of the body. Vertebral collapse is common, and compression fractures of the terminal phalanges may so shorten those bones as to simulate "clubbing" of the fingers.

Diagnosis. The generalized decrease in roentgenographic density must be distinguished from osteoporosis and multiple myeloma, and the cystlike lesions from fibrous dysplasia and true bone tumors. Bone biopsy establishes the true nature of the lesion, and plasma chemical determinations aid in determining its cause, e.g., primary hyperparathyroidism, uremia, and osteomalacia.

Treatment. In primary hyperparathyroidism, removal of the offending adenoma constitutes definitive therapy. Treatment in other conditions producing osteitis fibrosa is less certain or satisfactory. Chronic dialysis in patients with uremia may well provide the best treatment of uremic osteodystrophy, but current experience is inadequate for final evaluation. The bone lesions heal with great rapidity when the cause, such as a parathyroid adenoma, can be eradicated. For this reason, giant cell tumors, particularly in the facial bones, should not be treated by mutilating surgical operations until hyperparathyroidism has been excluded as a cause.

Johnson, L. C.: Morphologic analysis in pathology: The kinetics of disease and general biology of bone. *In* Frost, H. M. (ed.): Bone Biodynamics. Boston, Little, Brown & Company, 1964.

Weinmann, J. P., and Sicher, H.: Bone and Bones. St. Louis, C. V. Mosby Co., 1955, pp. 246–251.

Osteonecrosis

Definition. The term osteonecrosis is used here for the condition in the English literature called aseptic necrosis of bone or avascular necrosis of bone. The prefix aseptic no longer serves a useful function; similarly the prefix avascular should be dropped because it has no meaningful counterpart, and because it is by no means certain that the condition is "avascular."

Incidence. Osteonecrosis of bone occurs most commonly in the head of the femur, less commonly in the medial femoral condyle, and sometimes in the head of the humerus. This disease may be idiopathic or secondary to some precipitating cause. Primary osteonecrosis of the hip occurs in older adults, and 50 per cent of the cases are in chronic alcoholics.

Etiology. The cause of osteonecrosis is uncertain. Precipitating factors include systemic corticosteroid therapy, Gaucher's disease, sickle cell anemia, caisson disease, alcoholism, and systemic lupus erythematosus. Necrosis is believed to be due to obstruction of bony end-arteries by sludged red cells, gas bubbles, lipid droplets, and the like. In institutions dealing with patients who have renal homografts, osteonecrosis is becoming an increasing problem for those patients who survive this procedure.

Clinical Manifestations and Diagnosis. There is pain in the involved bony region. In the knee the onset is usually sudden and clear cut. Use of the affected part is painful, and patients frequently limp. Initially there are no positive physical findings, and roentgenograms reveal no abnormality. In the knee, where the natural history of the disorder has been most carefully studied, over a period of two or more months a small radiolucent zone may be seen on roentgenograms, followed by increased bone density, fragmentation, and collapse of the adjacent joint surface, ultimately progressing to changes indistinguishable from severe osteoarthritis. High resolution scanning with Sr^{85} invariably reveals a focus of intense isotope uptake at the involved site, well before roentgenographic changes appear. This technique should be employed to make the diagnosis without waiting for destructive changes to develop to the point of being roentgenographically demonstrable.

Treatment. If diagnosis is made before joint damage has occurred, weight-bearing should be stopped until the bone has had a chance to repair the defect. This may take many months. Once joint damage has occurred, the only treatment is surgical correction or prosthetic replacement. Early diagnosis is critically important if arthritis is to be prevented.

Ahlbäck, S., Bauer, G. C. H., and Böhne, W. H.: Spontaneous osteonecrosis of the knee. Arthritis Rheum., 11:705, 1968.

Bone Intoxications

FLUOROSIS

Fluoride is one of the more common constituents of the earth's crust, occurring particularly in association with phosphates, silicates, and calcium. It is abundant in sea water and in many fresh water supplies, and was undoubtedly a component of the environment in which life evolved. It probably functions as an important trace element in human nutrition, though a fluoride deficiency syndrome is not recognized. In optimal concentrations fluoride stabilizes the crystal structure of tooth enamel and probably also that of bone. In high concentrations fluoride acts as a general protoplasmic poison, resulting in death; but between toxic intake levels (> 100 mg.) and probably optimal intakes (about 1 mg. daily), chronic intake produces changes confined largely to the skeleton. Intoxication occurs because of accidental ingestion of fluoride-containing insecticides, chronic inhalation of industrial dusts (particularly in the aluminum mining and phosphate fertilizer industries), or prolonged drinking of certain fresh waters containing large amounts of fluorides. The skeletal lesions in man vary with the intake but consist of a combination of osteosclerosis and osteomalacia. The malacic lesions are more prominent at higher intake levels and represent interference with matrix maturation or crystal nucleation. Sclerosis consists of coarsening of trabeculae, periosteal new bone deposition, osteophyte formation, and ossification of tendons and ligaments. Severely fluorotic bone is chalky white in appearance and exhibits a crumbly consistency, cutting easily with a knife.

Early there are no specific complaints. As the skeletal disease advances there may be vague pains in the small joints of hands and feet. As osteophyte formation and periosteal bone growth progress, kyphosis, restriction of spine motion, flexion contractures of hips and knees, and ultimately nerve root and spinal cord compression develop. The neurologic involvement produces paresthesias, weakness, and ultimately paralysis. Early the neurologic involvement may simulate peripheral neuropathy, spinal cord tumors, or syringomyelia.

No municipal water supply in the United States contains more than 6 to 8 parts per million of fluoride, and this concentration, although sufficient to produce mottled tooth enamel, almost never produces bone disease. In certain regions of India and Arabia water-related fluoride intake reaches sufficient levels to produce fluoride intoxication. In the Punjab, for example, osteofluorosis is the most common form of bone disease. Deliberate osteofluorosis has sometimes been induced to halt the explosive skeletal demineralization of diseases such as multiple myeloma.

There is no effective treatment for the advanced syndrome except for orthopedic and supportive measures. Effort should be directed at prevention, particularly in the context of industrial exposure. Excess body burdens of fluoride are retained for years after exposure has terminated. Fluoride trapped in bone crystals is released only when bone resorption occurs, and some of the liberated ions are redeposited at sites of new bone formation. If the intake is low, however, urinary excretion will gradually lower the total body content.

VITAMIN A INTOXICATION

Although not confined to bone, the effects of chronic excessive vitamin A intake may be most apparent in the skeleton. Such intoxication is rare, and has occurred most frequently in young chil dren who received doses on the order of 100 times the normal daily vitamin requirement and in hunters who ingested large quantities of polar bear liver. The initial bony change is painful peri- osteal proliferation, particularly of the ulnae, clav- icles, and metatarsals. These are readily apparent on roentgenographic examination. Higher doses in small animals produce severe osteoporosis and multiple fractures. The diagnosis is suggested by a history of excessive vitamin intake, and by find- ing high vitamin A levels in the plasma. Bony healing is usually complete when vitamin expo- sure ceases.

VITAMIN D INTOXICATION

In the past intoxication with vitamin D occurred primarily because of inappropriate and massive vitamin therapy for diseases not caused by vitamin deficiency. The disease is still seen as a complica- tion of more appropriate vitamin D therapy for disorders such as osteomalacia or familial hypo- phosphatemia, and occasionally occurs in food fad- dists and in patients with an unusual sensitivity to doses usually considered to lie within the physio- logic range. Intoxication results in three principal and closely related effects: hypercalcemia, meta- static calcification, and osteitis fibrosa. The ulti- mate clinical picture varies, depending upon the relative importance of these effects.

In massive dosage the vitamin directly stimu- lates both gastrointestinal calcium absorption and osteoclastic bone resorption. Hypercalcemia ensues, and endogenous parathyroid suppression occurs. Plasma inorganic phosphate is therefore normal or high, and thus the $Ca \times P$ ion product may rise to extremely high values, probably reaching supersaturated levels in many normally unmineralized tissue regions. In any case large soft-tissue calcium deposits occur, particularly in already damaged regions such as the synovia of arthritic joints, as well as in arterial walls. Urine calcium is initially high, and the renal interstitium is particularly prone to calcification. Such renal calcinosis leads to deterioration of renal function, further phosphate retention, and inabil-

ity to excrete the excess plasma calcium load. This generates a vicious cycle which may lead to death from hypercalcemia or uremia. Metastatic calcifi- cation occurs also in the bone marrow of trabecular bone and may thus lead to the appearance of osteo- sclerosis. Osteitis fibrosa is usually seen as well, and the net roentgenographic appearance of bone depends on the balance between these two proc- esses.

Clinical manifestations are caused principally by the hypercalcemia and renal failure, and not by the bone disease itself. These are the same as those of hypercalcemia from any cause, and include anorexia, nausea, vomiting, lassitude, polyuria, dehydration, and ultimately fever, stupor, and death.

The diagnosis of vitamin D intoxication should be considered in the evaluation of patients with hypercalcemia or those found to have extensive soft tissue calcification. It is most readily con- firmed by obtaining a history of excessive vitamin D intake and by observing improvement when the vitamin is withdrawn. Treatment consists of man- agement of the hypercalcemia and stopping vita- min D ingestion; this is usually satisfactory unless irreversible kidney damage has occurred.

RADIONUCLIDE BONE TOXICITY

Many radioactive isotopes accumulate in the skeleton and, although ingested in doses too small to produce acute systemic effects, may lead years later to severe bone disease. Skeletal damage consists of (1) growth retardation if exposure oc- curred prior to epiphyseal closure; (2) aseptic necrosis, osteomyelitis, and bone abscess; (3) brittleness and tendency to fracture; and (4) osteogenic sarcoma. There are three categories of exposure: (1) strontium-90 and yttrium-91 from radioactive fallout of atom bomb fission products; (2) radium and thorium from industrial and medical exposure; and (3) uranium and the transuranic elements from processing of nuclear reactor fuel and wastes. Strontium and radium, like calcium, are alkaline earth elements and readily form phosphate salts. They are trapped in newly forming bone at the time of its mineraliza- tion. The localization of thorium, uranium, and the transuranic elements is less well understood, but appears to be predominantly on bone surfaces adjacent to the innumerable small vessels of bone. Radiation damage in each case is produced by the α and β particles, rather than by the γ radia- tion. Because of the extremely short range of these particles in bone, the damage is thus confined microscopically to the areas of isotope deposition. Cell death is the usual result, cell sensitivity varying with cell type, as follows: chondroblasts >

osteoblasts > osteocytes > osteoclasts. The surrounding bony material, deprived of continuing cellular influence, becomes hard and brittle. Ultimately it is subject to slow resorptive removal. The mechanism of sarcoma production is not known but is presumably the same as for radiation carcinogenesis elsewhere.

Clinical features are variable and not distinctive. Bone pain may be present, and spontaneous fractures may occur through bone that appears roentgenographically normal. Occasionally the long bones may present a punched-out appearance reminiscent of multiple myeloma. Radium dial painters frequently developed necrosis and osteomyelitis of the jaw, related to localization of radium in the periodontal tissues. Radiation damage, once it has occurred, is irrevocable, and no treatment is of any value. Bone localization following acute accidental ingestion of radium and strontium can be minimized by calcium infusion and deliberate production of sustained hypercalciuria.

Barnicot, N. A., and Datta, S. P.: Vitamin A and bone. *In* Bourne, G. H. (ed.): Biochemistry and Physiology of Bone. New York, Academic Press, 1956.

Harris, L. J.: Vitamin D and bone. *In* Bourne, G. H. (ed.): Biochemistry and Physiology of Bone. New York, Academic Press, 1956.

Hasterlik, R. J., and Finkel, A. J.: Diseases of bones and joints associated with intoxication by radioactive substances, principally radium. Med. Clin. N. Amer., 49:285, 1965.

Pugh, D. G.: Roentgenologic Diagnosis of Diseases of Bones. New York, Thomas Nelson and Sons, 1951.

Singh, A., Jolly, S. S., Bansal, B. C., and Mathur, C. C.: Endemic fluorosis; epidemiological, clinical and biochemical study of chronic fluorine intoxication in Punjab (India). Medicine, 42:229, 1963.

Vaughn, J. M.: The effects of radiation on bone. *In* Bourne, G. H. (ed.): Biochemistry and Physiology of Bone. New York, Academic Press, 1956.

Weinmann, J. P., and Sicher, H.: Bone and Bones. St. Louis, C. V. Mosby Company, 1955, pp. 246–251.

Osteomyelitis

Any of the bacterial or mycotic organisms that infect other tissues may produce localized infection in bone as well, as a consequence of penetrating wounds and ulcers, open surgery or compound fractures, or by means of blood-borne infection. Hematogenous osteomyelitis is predominantly a disease of children, in whom it involves primarily the metaphyseal regions of the long bones, and in the vast majority of cases is caused by the Staphylococcus (see section Staphylococcal Infections). In the adult, however, blood-borne osteomyelitis occurs most often in the pelvis and vertebral column, is an insidious and sometimes crippling disease, and may present few obvious evidences of pyogenic infection.

Etiology and Pathogenesis. Patients can usually be shown to have infection elsewhere, particularly in the skin or urinary tract, and the organism found in the involved bone is the same as that in the primary infection. As in osteomyelitis of childhood, *S. aureus* is probably the most common causative organism, but gram-negative infections are frequent, particularly following genitourinary tract infections or instrumentation. Negroes with sickle cell disease have a tendency to Salmonella osteomyelitis. Any region of the spine may be affected. There is a tendency for localization near the primary focus of infection, suggesting extension by way of venous plexuses or lymphatic communications. Both the vertebral bodies and the neural arches may be involved. When the infection is in the body, it usually arises in the region adjacent to an end plate. There is frequent extension to the body of the adjacent vertebra. Transcortical extension, as in juvenile osteomyelitis, is common and frequently leads to subperiosteal abscess formation, either in the anterior spinal ligaments or in the subdural space, with consequent neurologic and/or meningitic complications. Paravertebral abscess (Pott's abscess), once virtually synonymous with tuberculosis, is now more likely to be due to a pyogenic organism than to *M. tuberculosis*. The cancellous bone of the vertebral body is rapidly destroyed by the infection, and vertebral collapse may develop. However, reparative osteophytic response is usually exuberant and may completely bridge over defects before serious collapse occurs.

Clinical Manifestations. The onset is usually insidious and may be protracted over several months before the diagnosis is established. Fever, malaise, leukocytosis, and other constitutional manifestations of infection are usually absent or minimal. The predominant complaint is pain, which may ultimately become so severe as to be completely incapacitating. The pain is usually localized to the affected region of the back, but may sometimes be referred to trunk or extremities. It is constant, unrelenting, and not relieved by rest or usual analgesics, and is made worse by weight-bearing and motion. There are limitation of spine motion and severe muscle guarding. In many patients the disease resolves spontaneously after several months of activity, and undoubtedly the diagnosis is never made in a significant fraction of all cases.

Diagnosis. Initially no changes are visible roentgenographically, but within several weeks of onset localized destructive changes within the bone and narrowing of the intervertebral disc become apparent. The exuberant osteophytic reaction that follows is readily visible and serves to distinguish pyogenic osteomyelitis from tuberculous spondylitis, in which reparative reactions are minimal. Localized concentration of Sr[85] in a spine scan may be very helpful in confirming the existence of vertebral disease before roentgenographic changes are detectable, but this technique will not serve to distinguish most of the possible causes of such involvement. The principal diagnostic difficulties lie in the differentiation of osteomyelitis from other more common disorders involving the spine, particularly metastatic carcinoma, which may produce nearly identical clinical and roentgenographic findings. This is particularly important in cases of carcinoma of the prostate, in which vertebral osteomyelitis following prostate surgery may be mistaken for metastasis. Diagnosis is best confirmed by careful needle aspiration of the involved vertebra. Aspirated material should be submitted for both histologic and bacteriologic examination. Unfortunately the positive culture rate is low. Other laboratory studies are of little help. The erythrocyte sedimentation rate is high, and plasma globulins may be elevated.

Treatment. Appropriate antimicrobial therapy is frequently curative, but frank abscess formation may require surgical drainage.

Stone, D. B., and Bonfiglio, M.: Pyogenic vertebral osteomyelitis. Arch. Intern. Med. (Chicago), 112:491, 1963.

Congenital and/or Hereditary Disorders Involving Bone

OSTEOGENESIS IMPERFECTA

Definition. Osteogenesis imperfecta is an inherited disorder of collagen maturation and aggregation that results in defects in all collagen-containing connective tissues. The principal manifestations involve the skeleton and are responsible for the name given the disorder.

Incidence and Inheritance. The condition is generally transmitted as an autosomal dominant; the rate of spontaneous mutation is relatively high. There is also a recessive inheritance pattern. Children with this disorder are frequently stillborn or die soon after birth. The extremely wide variation in clinical expression has been responsible for considerable confusion in classification and terminology. The disease is relatively common, but no precise incidence figures are available.

Pathology and Pathogenesis. The basic chemical defect is unknown. Soluble collagen secreted by fibroblasts and osteoblasts fails to complete the normal sequence of extracellular changes necessary to convert it into a tough fibrous tissue. Total collagen is quantitatively deficient as well. As a result, tendons and ligaments are thin, translucent, unduly distensible, and subject to rupture; the skin is thin and translucent; the sclerae of the eyes are also thin and allow the choroidal pigment to show through, giving a blue color to the normally white sclerae; the bones are thin and fragile, bony architecture being more typical of a primitive or juvenile stage of development than of adult bone; osteons are more cellular than normal, and the ratio of mineral to matrix is lower than normal. Common associated abnormalities include an otosclerotic type of deafness and abnormal formation of dentin (dentinogenesis imperfecta).

Clinical Manifestations. Most important are the multiple fractures, often due to trivial trauma, blue sclerae, and lax ligaments. Because soft tissue damage is usually slight when trauma is minimal, the fractures are often much less painful than one might otherwise anticipate. Severely involved infants die in utero or at delivery because of lack of support for skull and rib cage. Somewhat less involved infants who survive delivery nonetheless experience frequent fractures during infancy and childhood; these are often produced by no more force than their own unbalanced muscular contractions. The sheer multiplicity of these fractures leads to deformities of long bones and, commonly, to growth retardation, the latter probably because of interference with blood supply to the epiphyseal growth plates. Generalized vertebral compression is common, and the torso is shortened by several inches as a consequence. Severity ranges from this extreme all the way to no signs other than blue sclerae and what might otherwise have passed for mild osteoporosis. Fractures heal well, sometimes with markedly exuberant callus formation. Plasma calcium, phosphorus, and alkaline phosphatase are normal.

Treatment. Except for proper orthopedic support, no treatment is of much value. Fracture incidence usually declines after puberty, but this may be because of cessation of growth rather than because of the gonadal hormones themselves. No good studies of hormone therapy have been reported.

OSTEOPETROSIS

The term osteopetrosis (Albers-Schönberg's disease, "marble bone" disease) has been applied to several probably unrelated hereditary syndromes characterized by increased mass and density of bones on roentgenographic examination. There are two main types of this disease. The first is a rare but clear-cut entity transmitted as an autosomal recessive trait. It is characterized by failure or delay of normal osteoclastic revision of bone, particularly resorption of the calcified cartilage columns and primary spongiosa beneath the growth plate. New bone apposition continues normally, and the metaphysis fills with a mass of calcified cartilage and superimposed bone. This primitive, unresorbed cartilage-bone admixture persists far down the shafts of long bones well into adult life. The marrow cavity is severely reduced, leading to anemia and extramedullary hematopoiesis with hepatosplenomegaly. Thus, these children present to pediatric hematologists in the first instance. Bony encroachment on cranial nerve foramina usually produces blindness, often deafness, and other cranial nerve palsies. Clublike deformities of the ends of the long bones are characteristic of this disorder and are due to failure of osteoclastic remodeling of the subepiphyseal cortical bone. Most patients die during infancy and childhood. Respiratory infections are common, and osteomyelitis of the skull results from nasal infections. Treatment is symptomatic with transfusions for anemia and antimicrobial drugs for infections.

The term osteopetrosis has also been applied to a disorder inherited as an autosomal dominant that expresses itself as an excess of bone that may appear qualitatively normal, much as if the disorder were the opposite of osteoporosis, but may also include abnormal persistence of the primary spongiosa, as in the recessive form of the disease. There may be no significant marrow cavity encroachment, and in these cases anemia and extramedullary hematopoiesis do not occur. Bone remodeling is probably normal. Onset occurs after infancy or childhood, and cranial nerve involvement may be the principal manifestation. The course may be protracted and mild. Albers-Schönberg's original case was of this type.

ELLIS-VAN CREVELD SYNDROME
(Chondroectodermal Dysplasia)

This syndrome is characterized by polydactyly of the hands and, rarely, of the feet, dwarfism, and dysplasia of the fingernails. It is inherited as an autosomal recessive trait. In contrast to classic *achondroplasia,* the shortening of the extremities is more marked proximally than distally. Fusion of the capitate and hamate bones of the wrist and a defect in the lateral aspect of the proximal part of the tibia, producing knock knees, are consistent features. Congenital heart disease is frequently present; atrial septal defect is the most common cardiac malformation. An abnormally short upper lip, bound down by multiple frenula, and premature eruption of the teeth are frequent features.

The disease is very rare, but it occurs as the main cause of dwarfism in the inbred socioreligious group known as the Old Order Amish, in Lancaster County, Pennsylvania, where it occurs with a frequency of 5 per 1000 births. One third of those afflicted die before two weeks of age. The condition must be distinguished from familial polydactyly and classic achondroplasia.

McKusick, V. A., Egeland, J. A., Eldridge, R., and Krusen, D. E.: Dwarfism in the Amish. I. The Ellis-van Creveld syndrome. Bull. Hopkins Hosp., 115:306, 1964.

OSTEOCHONDRO-DYSPLASIAS

ACHONDROPLASIA

Definition. Achondroplasia is a form of inherited dwarfism caused by retardation of endochondral bone formation. This relatively common disorder is inherited as an autosomal dominant trait. The disease is always apparent in utero, and many affected infants are stillborn.

Pathology and Pathogenesis. The abnormality is confined to cartilage and consists of failure or retardation of interstitial cellular proliferation and growth. As a result bones formed in cartilage models and dependent on cartilage proliferation for their growth are shortened. This is most apparent in the long bones of the extremities and in the bones of the base of the skull, and to a much lesser extent in the vertebrae. Membrane bone formation is normal; thus the bones of the cranial vault are able to grow normally and even accommodate themselves to the restricted growth of the base of the skull. Similarly, bone shafts enlarge normally. Microscopically there is a virtually complete lack of normal cartilage cell columns at the epiphyseal growth plates. Cell maturation is not apparent, and formation of the primary spongiosa proceeds very slowly and irregularly.

Clinical Manifestations. Clinically there is dwarfism, with disproportionate shortening of the extremities. Final height is usually less than 1.4 meters. The bridge of the nose is flattened and depressed, and the forehead may appear prominent and bulging. The hands and feet are short, and fingers tend to be nearly equal in length. The vertebrae are slightly and symmetrically flatter than normal. There is usually a dorsal kyphosis and compensatory posterior rotation of the sacrum and pelvis. The hip joints may thus be displaced backward and the pelvic inlet narrowed by the sacral promontory. Achondroplastic dwarfs exhibit entirely normal intelligence, endocrine function, and calcium metabolism, and, apart from their characteristic dwarfing and the problems it imposes, are able to live normal useful lives.

Diagnosis. Achondroplasia presents such a

typical picture that it is not usually confused with other causes of dwarfism. Occasionally patients with osteogenesis imperfecta may have very short extremities because of multiple fractures, but the true nature of the disease is immediately apparent roentgenographically. When diagnosis is difficult, measurement of the interpeduncular distance in the lumbar spine may be helpful. In normal people, interpeduncular distance increases (as one goes down) from T-12 to L-5, but in patients with achondroplasia T-11 or 12 are the widest vertebrae, while the lumbar interpeduncular distance either does not increase or actually decreases. Because of this restricted bony canal in the lumbar region, prolapsed intervertebral discs cause extremely severe symptoms, usually with neurologic sequelae. Paraplegia has been described in some cases. In addition, hydrocephalus is not uncommon and is usually of the communicating type, presumably because of bony restriction in the posterior fossa.

Treatment. There is no treatment.

OLLIER'S DYSCHONDROPLASIA; MULTIPLE ENCHONDROMATOSIS

Ollier's dyschondroplasia is a rare disorder in which projections or islands of epiphyseal cartilage proliferate down into the metaphysis. These cartilage remnants fail to undergo the changes required for mineralization but retain the growth potential of the epiphyseal plate, and under continued stimulation by growth hormone may expand slowly until much of the normal metaphyseal architecture is destroyed. There may be gross enlargement of the metaphysis. On the roentgenogram the lesions vary from elongated radiolucent patches to a fragmented, expanded picture that conveys the impression of a violent internal explosion within the metaphysis. Growth may cease and calcification may take place after puberty, but the inclusions may continue to enlarge throughout life, sometimes developing into chondrosarcomas. One side of the body is usually more severely involved than the other, but the lesions are fundamentally bilateral. The long bones and the ilia are most commonly involved, and when severe the disease may result in crippling and invalidism. The only treatment available consists of orthopedic procedures for correction of deformities and pathologic fractures.

HEREDITARY MULTIPLE EXOSTOSES

Probably the most common of the osteodyschondroplasias, the syndrome of hereditary multiple exostoses consists of irregular bony protuberances with a cartilage growth cap that project out from the subepiphyseal metaphyseal cortex and backward along the shaft. Lesions are bilateral, though not truly symmetrical, and represent more an abnormality of development of bony contour than a true exostosis. The metaphyseal cortex extends out around the periphery of the protuberances, and their trabecular structure and marrow spaces are continuous with that of the adjacent metaphysis. The disease occurs in families, but the mode of transmission is not known. Although the lesions begin to develop early in childhood, they rarely become apparent for several years. The basic abnormality is not known, but the disorder behaves as if portions of the zone of proliferating cartilage extended down the side of the metaphysis and in the process of growing split off from the growth plate and migrated back along the shaft, leaving a wake of normal endochondral bone behind them. The lesions are confined to the metaphyses of bones with active growth plates, and when severe may limit joint motion. Growth usually ceases when the epiphyses fuse. Very rarely the cartilaginous cap of an exostosis may develop into a chondrosarcoma.

MORQUIO'S DISEASE
(Morquio-Brailsford Syndrome, Morquio-Ullrich Syndrome)

Morquio's osteochondrodysplasia is a familial disorder of endochondral bone growth that may result in moderate dwarfing and sometimes severe deformity. Inheritance is as an autosomal recessive trait. In contrast to achondroplasia, the most severely involved bones are the vertebrae, which are flattened, irregular, and sometimes wedged anteriorly. Such wedged vertebral bodies may show an anterior tongue-like protrusion on lateral roentgenograms of the spine. The odontoid process is frequently hypoplastic. Long bone epiphyseal development is also abnormal; growth plates are widened and irregular, and growth may be asymmetrical. The femoral head is usually hypoplastic and irregular, and hip dislocation is common. Intelligence and general health are usually normal. There is frequently clouding of the cornea, aortic regurgitation, and excess urinary excretion of keratosulfate. The disease is now classified with the mucopolysaccharidoses, and is discussed in the article on those disorders.

McKusick, V. A.: Heritable Disorders of Connective Tissue. 2nd ed. St. Louis, C. V. Mosby Company, 1960.

Rubin, P.: Dynamic Classification of Bone Dysplasias. Chicago, Year Book Medical Publishers, Inc., 1964.

Paget's Disease of Bone: Osteitis Deformans

Definition. Paget's disease of bone is a chronic, progressive disorder of bone of unknown cause that is characterized grossly by deformity of both external bony contours and internal architecture and microscopically by replacement of normal structure by a morphologically and chemically abnormal bone.

Incidence. The disease is almost unknown before age 30; the incidence increases from 0.5 per cent at 40 to 10 per cent at 90 years of age. Men are affected twice as often as women. It is rare in Scandinavia and in Asia. Small described a 3 per cent prevalence in persons over 40. There appears to be a slight familial tendency, but the mode of genetic transmission (if such exists) is unknown.

Pathology and Pathogenesis. The disease is an essentially local, asymmetrical phenomenon, not a general metabolic or constitutional abnormality. It may, however, ultimately spread to involve a major fraction of the skeleton. It most commonly involves weight-bearing bones and is much more often seen on the right side than on the left. The sacrum and pelvis are most frequently involved, followed closely by the tibia and femur, and then in descending order by the lumbar, thoracic, and cervical vertebrae. Although the bones of the upper extremity are rarely involved, the skull is affected in a significant proportion of all cases.

The disease is characterized by extremely rapid bone formation and resorption in involved regions. It is commonly said that resorption and the consequent osteoporosis comprise the primary abnormality and that reparative processes simply follow along in their wake. This formulation is undoubtedly wrong. When the disease begins in the shaft of a long bone, the first detectable abnormality roentgenographically is indeed a zone of rarefaction, but microscopic examination of the roentgenographically normal bone into which the osteoporotic front is advancing reveals that this bone is already qualitatively abnormal. Furthermore, the repair is achieved by deposition of a primitive and, in some cases, highly abnormal bone that may amount to little more than a kind of metastatic calcification of an areolar, myxoid matrix. This is particularly true of rapid periosteal proliferation.

The replacement bone is thus architecturally and chemically abnormal and is subject to rapid, random remodeling and replacement. It is an unstable structure and may have little mechanical significance.

Microscopically the repeated waves of resorption and repair leave behind a bone with a striking mosaic appearance, created by the pattern of cement lines. There is little or no apparent structural orientation. Some of the repair bone may be osteomalacic, and thus wide osteoid seams are frequently found. Extremely rapid resorption may reproduce locally the picture of osteitis fibrosa.

Associated with the extensive remodeling there is usually a marked increase in local bony blood flow. This may render an involved bone, such as the tibia, distinctly warmer to the touch than its uninvolved mate.

Clinical Manifestations. Many patients with Paget's disease do not have symptoms. The principal clinical manifestation is bone deformity; much less common is pain. When Paget's disease occurs in the pelvis, osteoarthritis of the hip is a frequent association. The long bones are commonly enlarged, feel hot to the touch, and are bowed. Stress fractures are common along the convex borders of bowed long-bone cortices. Pathologic fractures may occur through these.

Enlargement of the skull, associated with headaches and sometimes cranial nerve palsies, especially nerve deafness, is common and typical. Vertebral enlargement and platyspondyly cause kyphosis and occasionally paraplegia. The course of the disease varies widely, but in most cases it is only very slowly progressive. Massive skeletal involvement is rare. When this occurs, however, serum alkaline phosphatase activity rises to very high levels, and because of the extreme vascularity of the bone, high output cardiac failure may develop. Indeed, when more than 30 per cent of the skeleton is involved, cardiac enlargement is the rule. The disease predisposes to two malignant bone tumors: malignant osteoclastoma and osteogenic sarcoma. Osteogenic sarcoma after age 40 is a rare disorder, and there is no doubt that most cases occurring in older patients do so in preexisting Paget's disease. The incidence is probably of the order of one per 4000 Paget patients per year.

Roentgenographic Manifestations. The first detectable change may be a sharply circumscribed zone of bone resorption. The lesion in the skull previously called osteoporosis circumscripta is now known to be an early manifestation of Paget's disease. Later the normal bony architecture of the skull is replaced by a greatly thickened, fluffy appearance. A roentgenographic characteristic of Paget's disease is replacement of normal bony architecture by coarse, abnormal-looking trabeculae, enlargement of the external contours of a bone, and flame-shaped lucent zones which start at the ends of the long bones and slowly progress up the shaft. Paget's disease of bone is occasionally the cause of so-called ivory vertebrae, the sclerotic end stage of Paget's disease.

Diagnosis. Except during periods of immobilization or markedly accelerated resorption, when hypercalcemia may occur, the plasma calcium and phosphorus and urine calcium are normal. However, the alkaline phosphatase is invariably high if any significant fraction of the skeleton is involved; indeed, it reaches higher values in this disease than in any other. Acid phosphatase values are also slightly elevated at times. Thus, without specific determination of prostatic acid phosphatase, this test may not be of much help in distinguishing Paget's disease from osteoblastic metastases of prostatic carcinoma. This differential problem arises chiefly when lesions are confined to the pelvis, for there carcinomatous infiltration beneath the periosteum may provoke a periosteal reaction that enlarges the contours of the pubic and ischial rami, thus simulating Paget's disease. In few other bony regions do osteoblastic metastases produce such change in external bony contour, and thus usually there is little diagnostic problem. The ordinary clinical and roentgenographic features are too distinctive to be confused with those of any other disease.

Treatment. In most cases no treatment is required. When progression is rapid, high doses of salicylates have been reported to arrest the progress of the disease. The same claim has been made for sodium fluoride. To date, however, there remains no generally accepted satisfactory treatment of the bone disease itself. Paraplegia or cauda equina compression can be successfully treated with laminectomy and decompression procedures. Pathologic fractures through pagetoid bone heal well but are technically difficult to deal with. Internal fixation is necessary, but is complicated by large marrow cavities, which often necessitate several rods being packed together, and by bowing which may prevent rods from being thrust down the femoral shaft, as well as by extreme vascularity of bone which causes severe hemorrhage. Sarcomas must be watched for carefully and treated surgically as soon as they become apparent.

Albright, F., and Reifenstein, E. C.: The Parathyroid Glands and Metabolic Bone Disease. Baltimore, Williams & Wilkins Company, 1958.

De Deuxchaisnes, C. N., and Krane, S. M.: Paget's disease of bone: Clinical and metabolic observations. Medicine, 43:233, 1964.

Johnson, L. C.: Morphologic analysis in pathology: The kinetics of disease and general biology of bone. In Frost, H. M. (ed.): Bone Biodynamics. Boston, Little, Brown & Company, 1964.

Pugh, D. G.: Roentgenologic Diagnosis of Diseases of Bones. New York, Thomas Nelson and Sons, 1951.

Snapper, I.: Bone Disease in Medical Practice. New York, Grune & Stratton, Inc., 1957.

Fibrous Dysplasia

Fibrous dysplasia, a developmental disorder of the bone mesenchyme, is characterized by replacement of bone by large masses of cellular fibrous tissue containing immature bone spicules and islands of cartilage. Except for the cartilage component, the histologic features are very similar to those of osteitis fibrosa, as is the roentgenographic appearance, but the two diseases differ in many respects. Fibrous dysplasia is a local disorder, and, although lesions may be widespread, there is always normal, uninvolved bone somewhere; furthermore, the disease is relatively slowly progressive and lacks the rapid bone resorption and formation of osteitis fibrosa. When the disease occurs in young girls, there are sometimes associated precocious puberty and patchy brownish skin pigmentation. This triad is known as "Albright's syndrome." Since large doses of estrogens produce a similar metaphyseal lesion in very young animals, it is not clear whether the precocious puberty of Albright's syndrome is simply a part of the picture or a contributing cause of the bone disease.

The cause is unknown. Snapper contends that the disorder is fundamentally a lipoid granuloma, others that it is a disturbance of mesenchymal differentiation.

The age of onset is usually unknown and the disease first becomes apparent between ages 5 and 15, commonly because of deformity or pathologic fractures. Typical roentgenographic changes are cystlike lesions of metaphyseal or shaft bone, with expansion of the cortex and sometimes severe destruction of bony architecture. Areas of increased density are frequently seen, and as the patient ages the lesions gradually acquire a uniform, ground-glass type of opacity. Plasma calcium and phosphorus are normal; the alkaline phosphatase is usually normal, but may be elevated when the disease is extensive.

Bone involvement is commonly unilateral. The femur and pelvis are frequently involved, as is the skull. In the skull, however, lesions are osteomatoid, rather than fibrous, and roentgenograms reveal dense, featureless opacification and distortion of the facial bones and the base of the skull. Encroachment on cranial nerves may produce neurologic symptoms.

Growth is slow throughout childhood and usually ceases entirely in adolescence. The principal significance of the disorder lies in the production of fractures and deformity. Except for indicated orthopedic procedures, no treatment is available.

See references for Paget's disease.

Hypertrophic Osteoarthropathy

Hypertrophic osteoarthropathy is a syndrome consisting of clubbing of the fingers, painful swelling and periosteal new bone deposition in the long bones of the extremities, and sometimes moderate joint swelling and tenderness. The disorder is almost always associated with disease elsewhere in the body. Over half the cases reported have been found in patients with pulmonary, mediastinal, or pleural disorders, either suppurative or neoplastic, and the remainder in patients with cyanotic heart disease, primary biliary cirrhosis, regional ileitis, and ulcerative colitis, as well as a large number of miscellaneous diseases. Very rarely it exists without apparent predisposing disease, and there is also a distinct hereditary form of the disorder (pachydermoperiostosis) associated with thickening of the skin of the scalp, face, and hands. In pachydermoperiostosis onset is usually at puberty. A family history of the disorder can be obtained in about one fourth of the cases.

In the finger tips the predominant changes are edema, hyperemia, and soft-tissue fibrous proliferation; bony changes are variable and usually not prominent. Grossly the finger tips appear bulbous, and there is increased curvature of the nails in all directions. The most typical bony lesions are found in the distal shafts of the bones of the forearm and leg, where there is distinct periosteal new bone deposition. Overlying tissues may be edematous, and the entire region is painful and tender to pressure. More advanced disease may involve the entire forearm and leg bones, and later the femur and humerus are affected.

The cause is unknown. The changes are probably mediated by alterations in periosteal blood flow. There is reason to suspect abnormal visceral reflex patterns, triggered by centrally located disease. Innominate artery aneurysms have been reported in association with osteoarthropathy confined to the involved extremity. In any case, surgical correction of lung lesions responsible for the disorder frequently produces dramatic relief of pain and swelling, and prompt healing on roentgenographic examination.

Early in the course of the disorder the arthritic complaints may be misdiagnosed as rheumatoid arthritis. The later periosteal manifestations must be differentiated from disorders such as scurvy, syphilitic periostitis, and progressive diaphyseal dysplasia. The skin changes of pachydermoperiostosis may suggest a diagnosis of acromegaly; however, neither the absence of facial bone changes nor the periosteal reaction is suggestive of this diagnosis, and thus the differentiation can usually be made by roentgenography.

The disorder is important for two reasons. It usually serves as an indicator of serious disease elsewhere in the body, and in many cases, particularly of pulmonary neoplasms, may be the first such sign. Second, it is usually painful and may contribute significantly to the over-all disability of the primary disease.

The treatment must obviously be directed at the underlying disease. Analgesics, and sometimes narcotics, are required for symptomatic relief. Vagotomy has also been reported to provide relief.

Fischer, D. S., Singer, D. H., and Feldman, S. M.: Clubbing, a review, with emphasis on hereditary acropachy. Medicine, 43:459, 1964.

Herman, M. A., Massaro, D., Katz, S., and Sachs, M.: Pachydermoperiostosis – Clinical spectrum. Arch. Intern. Med.: 116:918, 1965.

Pugh, D. G.: Roentgenologic Diagnosis of Diseases of Bones. New York, Thomas Nelson and Sons, 1951.

Tumors of Bone

PRIMARY BONE TUMORS

Primary bone tumors present some of the most difficult diagnostic and therapeutic problems in clinical medicine. Adequate treatment for the malignant lesions is almost always mutilating, and the decisions that must be made in order to determine appropriate surgery require the utmost skill and cooperation between surgeon, pathologist, and radiologist. These problems cannot be adequately summarized within the scope of a textbook of medicine. The reader is referred to texts dealing specifically with bone tumors, such as those listed at the end of this section.

METASTATIC BONE TUMORS

By far the most common malignant skeletal tumors are metastatic from primary sites elsewhere in the body. Virtually any malignant tumor may metastasize to bone, but there are a few that do so with such regularity that they constitute most skeletal metastatic lesions. In one autopsy series of 1000 cases, two thirds of all patients with breast cancer, one third with lung cancer, and one fourth with renal cancer had skeletal metastases. In addition, approximately one eighth of the patients with cancer of stomach, pancreas, colon, and rectum have bony metastases. More than half of the patients with carcinoma of the prostate have osseous metastases. Thyroid carcinoma frequently and characteristically metastasizes to bone. Thus, breast, lung, kidney, thyroid, and prostate account for the bulk of skeletal metastases. In addition leukemias and lymphomas commonly produce significant osseous involvement. Half the patients with Hodgkin's disease at autopsy are found to have osseous lesions.

Clinical Manifestations. Skeletal metastases present because of pain or pathologic fracture, or as an incidental finding on roentgenograms taken for another purpose. When lesions are widespread and related to a known primary site elsewhere, there is usually no diagnostic problem; but when an isolated lesion is discovered, the physician is faced with important differential considerations. He must decide whether the lesion represents a metastatic focus or a primary bone disorder. This may be just as important when the patient has a known primary malignancy as when he does not, for patients with cancer are as prone to unrelated bone disease as anyone else, and it is a serious mistake to assume the presence of metastatic spread if it does not really exist.

Similarly, it is a mistake to assume that the presence of skeletal metastases heralds a rapid, deteriorating course with prompt fatal termination. Many patients with bone metastases live for years, and whether those years are spent comfortably and productively will depend on the therapeutic approach taken by the physician. This is not usually true of lung cancer metastatic to bone, but it is true often enough of breast, prostate, kidney, and thyroid cancer to justify a positive therapeutic approach. It is worth stressing that such patients may have more years of useful productive life ahead of them than do many patients with diabetes, valvular heart disease, or emphysema, among others.

Most skeletal metastatic lesions are predominantly osteolytic. As tumors expand, the surrounding bone is destroyed, and the resulting focus appears roentgenographically as a radiolucent zone, sometimes sharply demarcated, sometimes with vague margins. These are referred to as osteolytic lesions. However, almost all tumors, except for multiple myeloma, provoke some degree of bone healing, and on microscopic examination new bone deposition and osteoblastic proliferation are frequently observed in and around metastatic foci. This osteoblastic activity is most pronounced in metastatic spread from cancers of prostate and breast, and to a lesser extent in spread from cancers of the urinary bladder. Breast lesions are fundamentally lytic, but superimposed bone reaction may predominate in many cases, producing patchy areas of increased roentgenographic density. These are referred to as osteoblastic metastases. Prostatic cancer, on the other hand, usually has no detectable lytic component. Metastatic cell clumps provoke such intense bone formation on trabecular surfaces that cancer foci literally have no room to expand peripherally, and instead they are pushed along bone tissue spaces by the evoked

closure of those spaces behind them. Leukemic infiltration produces bone pain, lytic lesions, and in some cases pathologic fractures. Involvement with Hodgkin's disease produces a combination of lytic and blastic responses, involves the pelvis, vertebrae, ribs and femora most commonly, and may sometimes evoke such an overwhelming osteoblastic response as to lead to near total opacification of involved regions.

Biochemical Manifestations. Plasma or urine biochemical changes reflect in general the extent and degree of activity of skeletal metastases. Quiescent or slowly progressive lesions usually produce no detectable change from normal values. Active or extensive osteolytic disease produces a large calcium load, which must be disposed of. This leads to hypercalciuria, hypercalcemia and secondary suppression of endogenous parathyroid activity; if not arrested, it may produce renal calcinosis, renal failure, and death. Prominent osteoblastic activity or healing of pathologic fractures is usually reflected in an elevated alkaline phosphatase (although this same change can be produced by liver metastases), and in prostatic carcinoma disease activity usually, but not always, produces a rise in acid phosphatase. Cancer not metastatic to bone may sometimes produce changes identical with primary hyperparathyroidism. This syndrome has been observed most often with breast, lung, and kidney tumors, and is in fact a true hyperparathyroidism, for the tumor produces a parathyroid hormone-like agent.

Diagnosis. Multiple lesions in patients with obvious primaries present no diagnostic problem, but isolated lesions, or lesions with uncertain relation to a possible primary, should be subjected to biopsy. This point cannot be stressed too strongly. Open surgical biopsy is preferable in most cases, but needle biopsy may be best for inaccessible lesions, such as involvement of vertebral bodies.

Persistent skeletal pain without obvious roentgenographic changes can frequently be investigated by isotopic techniques, employing bone-seeking isotopes such as fluorine-18, calcium-47, or strontium-85. The inevitable reparative reaction to tumor metastases is responsible for a striking increase in local uptake of these isotopes, and the finding of such tracer localization confirms the existence of real bone involvement, even though no changes are present roentgenographically.

Treatment. A significant fraction of patients with breast, prostate, kidney, and thyroid metastases can be helped by appropriate treatment. Hypernephromas exhibit a tendency toward apparently solitary metastases, and in some cases combined removal of the primary plus the metastatic focus may result in several years of symptom-free life before other metastatic lesions become apparent. Breast, prostate, and thyroid carcinomas commonly retain a dependency on their hormonal environment, and their growth can be controlled by manipulation of that environment. Breast cancer in women prior to the menopause, and even for a few years thereafter, responds to oophorectomy and hypophysectomy; prostatic cancer to orchiectomy and estrogen treatment; thyroid cancer to iodine-131 administration and TSH-suppression produced by exogenous thyroid hormone treatment. Estrogen-dependent metastases of breast cancer may also respond to androgens and to certain nonvirilizing experimental androgen analogues. The extreme virilization produced by ordinary androgens severely limits the acceptability and value of these agents. In older women with metastatic breast cancer high dosages of estrogens are frequently of value.

Other adjunctive treatment includes the use of radiation therapy to troublesome or isolated lesions, and sometimes regional perfusion with chemotherapeutic agents should be considered. Considerable relief of pain and healing of disabling pathologic fractures can be provided by such means.

Non-narcotic analgesics should be used as indicated for pain relief, particularly when more definitive treatment of the metastases fails. Narcotics should not be used until absolutely necessary, because the patient's course is commonly more protracted than the physician anticipates.

Dahlin, D. C.: Bone Tumors. Springfield, Ill., Charles C Thomas, 1957.

Lichtenstein, L.: Bone Tumors. 3rd ed. St. Louis, C. V. Mosby Company, 1965.

MacDonald, I.: Endocrine ablation in disseminated mammary carcinoma. Surg. Gynec. Obstet., 115:215, 1962.

Symposium on the Role of Hormones in the Origin and Control of Abnormal and Neoplastic Growth. Cancer Res., 17:421, 1957.

DISEASES OF JOINTS
William D. Robinson

Introduction

The term "rheumatism" embraces a variety of disorders that have in common pain and stiffness referable to the musculoskeletal system. When such symptoms are due to abnormality of the joint itself, the condition can be classified as arthritis. Nonarticular rheumatism includes those conditions in which the symptoms are produced not by pathologic changes in the joints proper, but in the structures contiguous to or related to the joints, such as bursae, tendons and tendon sheaths, nerves, muscles, and fibrous tissue.

Although arthritis occurs in a number of different forms, there are essentially two fundamental pathologic processes that affect the joints: (a) inflammation, which may be exudative or proliferative or a combination of each, and (b) degenerative changes, which are primarily dependent on the limited capacity of articular cartilage to repair itself. Varying degrees of these fundamental changes may be present in any example of joint disease. Arthritis may occur in either acute or chronic form. However, almost any type of acute arthritis may pass into a subacute or chronic stage, and many cases of chronic arthritis are subject to acute exacerbations. No classification of the rheumatic diseases can be considered entirely satisfactory while the causes of certain diseases in this group remain unknown. The following classification of diseases of the joints, somewhat abbreviated and modified, is based on that recommended by the American Rheumatism Association:

1. Polyarthritis of unknown etiology
   a. Rheumatoid arthritis (atrophic arthritis)
   b. Juvenile rheumatoid arthritis (Still's disease)
   c. Ankylosing spondylitis
   d. Psoriatic arthritis
   e. Reiter's syndrome
2. "Connective tissue" disorders
3. Rheumatic fever
4. Degenerative joint disease (osteoarthritis, osteoarthrosis, hypertrophic arthritis)
5. Arthritis associated with known infectious agents
6. Traumatic and/or neurogenic disorders
7. Gout and pseudogout
8. Tumor and tumor-like conditions

Arthritis Due to Specific Infectious Agents

Gonococcal Arthritis. This acute inflammation of one or more joints associated with genital gonorrhea has been described in the section of this textbook that deals with gonococcal infections.

Tuberculous Arthritis. Tuberculosis of the joints occurs most frequently in children, and is usually monoarticular. Almost any joint in the body may be involved, but the hip, spine, and knee are the most common sites. The manifestations are those of chronic inflammation with effusion, and the diagnosis may be suspected from the roentgenographic appearance of destruction of contiguous bone. The diagnosis is usually established by culture of aspirated joint fluid or by biopsy also supplemented with culture.

The treatment of tuberculous arthritis is largely surgical and orthopedic. Although the use of antituberculous chemotherapy has greatly simplified the management of these patients, orthopedic and surgical principles are still of greatest importance.

The reader is referred to a standard treatise on orthopedics for a full discussion of tuberculous arthritis.

Suppurative Arthritis. Purulent infections of the joints have been caused by almost every pathogenic micro-organism, but the most common are *Streptococcus hemolyticus*, *Staphylococcus aureus*, pneumococcus, and meningococcus. Infection may follow a penetrating wound of the joint or may develop as a secondary complication in bacteremia.

Suppurative arthritis begins in the synovial membrane, which rapidly becomes swollen and inflamed; an exudate rich in polymorphonuclear leukocytes forms in the joint cavity. Many patients give a history of trauma to the affected joint, followed in a day or two by sudden pain and swelling and excessive pain on motion. There is often an initial chill, followed by fever. The joint is hot, swollen, and tender, and in a short time shows fluctuation due to fluid accumulation. Aspiration yields purulent fluid, cultures of which usually show the causative organism.

Treatment consists of appropriate antimicrobial therapy and surgical drainage if necessary.

Syphilitic Arthritis. The joints may be affected in congenital syphilis and during either the secondary or tertiary stages of the disease. A mild, chronic effusion into the knee joints occurring at about the age of puberty in patients with congenital syphilis is known as "Clutton's joints." Secondary syphilis may be associated with arthralgia or with relatively transient swelling, tenderness, and limitation of motion of several of the larger joints. Gummatous involvement of the synovial membrane and joint capsule can occur in tertiary syphilis and closely resembles tuberculous arthritis. There is considerable swelling with effusion but no redness. An effusion of the knee joint associated with immediately adjacent periostitis is strongly suggestive of syphilis, particularly when there is no history of trauma to the joint.

The treatment is that of syphilis elsewhere in the body. Penicillin therapy usually yields excellent results unless the condition has been long neglected.

Charcot joint, a form of neurogenic arthropathy associated with tabes dorsalis, is discussed elsewhere.

Arthritis of Brucellosis. Generalized aches, backache, and joint pains are outstanding clinical manifestations of brucellosis. Definite tenderness and pain over bones and joints usually indicates localized involvement. The spine, the hip joints, and the sacroiliac joints are most frequently affected. The localized arthritis is usually purulent. Diagnosis and treatment are discussed in the article on brucellosis.

Arthritis of Typhoid Fever. This rare complication of typhoid fever most commonly affects the spine. It is described in the article on typhoid fever.

Arthritis of Bacillary Dysentery. Pain and swelling, most frequently involving the knees, sometimes develop after the acute stage of dysentery is over and are usually associated with recrudescence of the fever. The appearance of the joint fluid is that of a serous effusion. A similar clinical picture may develop in association with Salmonella infections.

Arthritis of Rubella. Polyarthritis occurs occasionally as a complication of German measles. The disease is self-limited, usually clearing in about one week.

Arthritis of Mycotic Disease. In the primary phase of coccidioidomycosis, transient joint symptoms including pain, tenderness, and slight swelling occur in about one third of the cases. This is "desert rheumatism," a self-limited disease that may persist for about one month and subsides without residual damage or deformity.

The much less common disseminated granulomatous form of coccidioidomycosis as well as histoplasmosis, blastomycosis, cryptococcosis, and actinomycosis can lead to joint involvement, usually by extension from granulomatous lesions in adjacent bony structures. The clinical and roentgenographic appearances resemble those of tuberculosis. Sporotrichosis may also simulate tuberculous involvement of the synovium, but without bony involvement.

Arthritis of Rheumatic Fever. The joint involvement of rheumatic fever is an excellent example of a purely exudative inflammation of the synovium. The inflammation is completely reversible. Clinically, the arthritis is characterized by its fleetingly migratory nature and the absence of permanent joint damage. Rheumatic fever is described in detail elsewhere.

Rheumatoid Arthritis
(Atrophic Arthritis)

Definition. Rheumatoid arthritis is a constitutional disease in which there are inflammatory changes throughout the connective tissues of the body. Most characteristic is the polyarthritis with a predilection for smaller joints, such as the proximal interphalangeal, the metacarpophalangeal, and the metatarsophalangeal, with a tendency for symmetric distribution after the disease has become established. The arthritis is produced by a chronic proliferative inflammation of the synovial membrane that has the potentiality of producing irreversible damage to the joint capsule and articular cartilage as these structures are replaced by granulation tissue. Both the constitutional manifestations and activity of the synovial inflammation are subject to variations in severity, with a strong tendency to unexplainable remissions and exacerbations.

Incidence. Rheumatoid arthritis is about three times as common in females as in males. Its onset can occur at any age, but it is largely a disease of young adults, the average age of onset being 35 years. Nevertheless, it is not uncommon to observe the onset of rheumatoid arthritis in the sixties or seventies.

Accurate surveys regarding incidence of rheumatoid arthritis in the general population are not available. Studies of selected populations in the United States and Canada indicate that about 2.5 to 3 per cent of the general adult population are afflicted. The disease is reputed to be rare in the tropics but has been found in any part of the world where search has been made.

Etiology and Pathogenesis. The cause of rheumatoid arthritis is unknown. Intensive efforts have failed to establish that it is caused by a specific infectious agent, by nutritional excess or deficiency, by metabolic aberrations, by faulty or unbalanced endocrine secretions, by a well defined mechanism involving dysfunction of the autonomic nervous system, or by the somatic reflections of emotional and personality disturbances. Although statistical considerations suggest an hereditary influence, critical genetic studies in selected population groups and in identical twins indicate clearly that heredity is not a dominant factor in rheumatoid arthritis. Impressive evidence is accumulating to suggest the importance of an immunologic mechanism in the pathogenesis of the disease, although the initiating events still remain obscure.

Hypotheses as to the cause of rheumatoid arthritis usually attempt to explain certain epidemiologic, clinical, pathologic, or laboratory findings characteristic of the disease, or are derived from evaluation of factors that appear to influence its course. Generally accepted facts regarding the disease include: its predilection for women and for temperate climates, its peak of onset between the ages of 20 and 50, the constitutional nature of the disease, the almost ubiquitous distribution of the inflammatory lesions in connective tissue, the self-perpetuating nature of the synovial inflammation, the tendency toward symmetrical distribution of the joint involvement, and the unpredictable course that the disease may follow in an individual patient, including exacerbation and remission without apparent rhyme or reason. Attention has been called to the frequency with which onset or recurrences are related to emotional shocks and acute illnesses; on the few occasions when the influence of these factors has been compared in an appropriate control group, it was concluded that any difference between sufferers and nonsufferers resides in some feature of the individual rather than in difference of stress and strains.

Ideas about the inciting events in rheumatoid arthritis are currently dominated by concepts of autoimmunity, or at least the role of the immune response in mediating tissue injury.

Characteristics of Rheumatoid Factor. For many years it has been recognized that the serum of some patients with rheumatoid arthritis could cause the agglutination of a number of different particles. These included certain strains of Group A streptococci, staphylococci, collodion particles and various erythrocytes, such as those of sheep coated with subagglutinating doses of rabbit antiserum. It was then demonstrated that the particle involved was nonspecific, and that the essential reaction was between the gamma globulin coating the particle and a factor in rheumatoid serum. It was shown that tanned sheep erythrocytes and inert particles such as latex and bentonite, when coated with normal gamma globulin, are agglutinated by rheumatoid sera. Under appropriate conditions, a precipitate forms when normal human gamma globulin is added to serum from certain patients with rheumatoid arthritis.

The substance in serum responsible for these reactions has been termed *rheumatoid factor*. It was characterized as a euglobulin with the electrophoretic mobility of gamma globulin and sedimentation constant in the ultracentrifuge of a macroglobulin (19S). It frequently is found in serum as a complex with 7S gamma globulin. The classic rheumatoid factor was defined as IgM with antibody binding sites directed toward determinants of IgG. Later, globulins of the IgG and possibly of the IgA classes were found to have anti-IgG activity, and polymorphism among rheumatoid factors is well established. Rheumatoid factors react most avidly with human IgG which has been denatured or aggregated.

As this information developed, there was difficulty in visualizing the role that rheumatoid factor would appear to play in the development of the symptoms and lesions of rheumatoid arthritis. Rheumatoid factor cannot be detected in the serum of some 30 per cent of patients diagnosed as having rheumatoid arthritis. It has been found in high titers in other disorders without arthritis, and in some normal subjects. In short-term studies, infusions of serum containing high titers of rheumatoid factor did not induce the disease in normal recipients. A rheumatoid arthritis-like disease occurs in patients with agammaglobulinemia, who lack rheumatoid factor.

Pathogenesis of Joint Inflammation. It has been postulated that the complex formed by rheumatoid factors and IgG is actively phagocytosed by the polymorphonuclear cells that characterize rheumatoid effusions. The lysosomal enzymes released in the process of phagocytosis enter into the inflammatory reaction either by producing direct tissue injury, or by activating substances such as kinins. Particulate cytoplasmic inclusions containing determinants of IgM and IgG have been demonstrated within the leukocytes of a high proportion of rheumatoid synovial effusions; this finding is not confined to rheumatoid arthritis, and is seen at times in other inflammatory states. Injection of autologous IgG into inactive or clinically uninvolved joints of patients with rheumatoid arthritis has produced acute inflammation in some, but not all, patients studied.

Other Factors. It is clear that several steps remain obscure in the elucidation of a completely satisfactory immunologic explanation of rheumatoid arthritis. If the rheumatoid factors are antibodies, presumably 7S gamma globulin should be the antigen. Several observations suggest that some alteration in the 7S gamma globulin molecule may be required to provide such antigenic properties. There are few clues to the nature of such alterations or the factors that could lead to them. Another possibility is that connective tissue components, such as proteinpolysaccharides, may be altered in such fashion that they may enter into the immunologic and inflammatory reaction.

The role of the immune response in the mediation of tissue injury does not preclude a possible genetic basis for a predisposition to rheumatoid arthritis. There is still a possibility that a microorganism is the actual inciting agent, constituting the antigenic challenge, and that the disease is perpetuated by the characteristics of the immune response. The overwhelmingly negative results of bacteriologic studies suggest strongly that rheumatoid arthritis is not attributable to an easily identified micro-organism. The search for an agent with more elusive properties that may play a role in the pathogenesis of the disease currently centers on viruses and Mycoplasma (formerly called pleuropneumonia-like organisms, or PPLO).

Pathology. Inflammation is the dominant pathologic change of rheumatoid arthritis. Although swelling of the joint, the most characteristic feature in the early stages, suggests predominantly an exudative inflammation, the proliferative type of inflammation is the outstanding characteristic of rheumatoid arthritis. The development of granulation tissue, which eventually is converted into dense fibrous scar tissue, dominates the later phases of the disease. Active inflammation is first seen in the synovial membrane and joint capsule. The synovial membrane is swollen, deep red in color, and the villous processes show hypertrophy. Microscopically the process is characterized by reduplication of lining cells, hypertrophy of the stroma (usually by increased vascularity), and infiltration with inflammatory cells (predominantly lymphocytes). Nodular collections of inflammatory cells in follicle-like arrangement are common. It should be recognized that nothing about the microscopic appearance of the synovitis is pathognomonic.

Pannus formation underlies the later changes in this disease. This is a layer of granulation tissue, derived from the synovial membrane, that extends over the surface of the cartilage as a reddish, roughened, tonguelike protrusion of tissue. The underlying cartilage is eroded and destroyed. Granulations from a pannus may adhere to similar structures on contiguous areas and may join with penetrating granulations derived from subchondral marrow. As the granulation tissue is converted to scar tissue, fibrous ankylosis with subluxation and distortion of the affected joints causes the deformities characteristic of the disease.

In addition to destructive changes in the joint itself, a certain amount of atrophy occurs in bones, muscles, and skin adjacent to the joint. In well-developed disease, the muscles adjacent to the joint are atrophic and the skin over the affected parts is thin, tight, and glossy.

Subcutaneous nodules, which occur in 20 to 30 per cent of patients at some time during their disease, are considered the most characteristic lesions of rheumatoid arthritis. Such nodules are usually located over bony prominences, but they can arise in connective tissue anywhere in the body. They may persist from weeks to months. Most characteristically they are attached to fibrous external portions of articular capsules, but they may be incorporated into periosteum, lie loose in subcutaneous tissue, or lie in the upper layers of the integument. Gross and microscopic characteristics are illustrated in Figures 1 and 2.

Focal collections of cells, predominantly lymphocytes, occur in the connective tissue between bundles of skeletal muscle and in connective tissue sheaths of the peripheral nerves. These are not specific for rheumatoid arthritis. Such nonspecific lesions also are encountered in the cardiac muscle. Fibrinous pericarditis and pleuritis are more common in patients with rheumatoid arthritis than in other people, and a chronic inflammatory and fibrotic involvement of the lungs is occasionally encountered.

Vascular lesions in rheumatoid arthritis have attracted considerable attention. Some workers believe that vasculitis is an important feature early in the formation of the subcutaneous nodule. In one series, evidence of arteritis was found in 15 per cent of muscle biopsies in patients with rheumatoid arthritis. A diffuse *arteritis*, at times difficult to distinguish from polyarteritis nodosa, may be encountered in severe cases; often such patients have been receiving long-term steroid therapy.

Inflammatory *ocular lesions*, affecting primarily the uveal tract or the scleral layers, present no characteristic pathologic findings. The one exception is *scleromalacia perforans*, which is a complication of rheumatoid nodules developing in the sclera.

Characteristic Serologic Reactions. The characteristics of rheumatoid factor or factors have been detailed under Etiology and Pathogenesis of Rheumatoid Arthritis. Tests for the detection of rheumatoid factor are most conveniently and commonly carried out by utilizing the sensitized or tanned sheep cell reaction, the latex flocculation test, or the bentonite agglutination test.

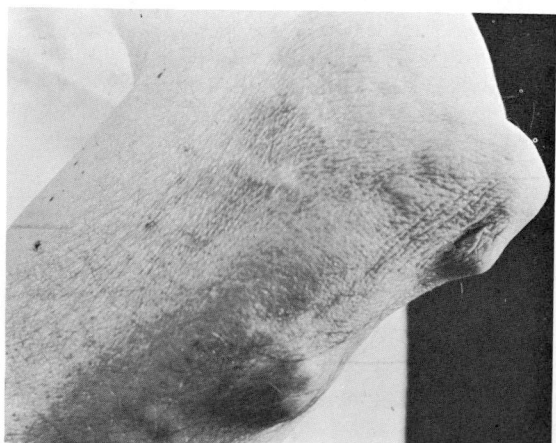

FIGURE 1.   Rheumatoid nodules in olecranon bursa and over upper portion of ulna in a patient with classic rheumatoid arthritis.

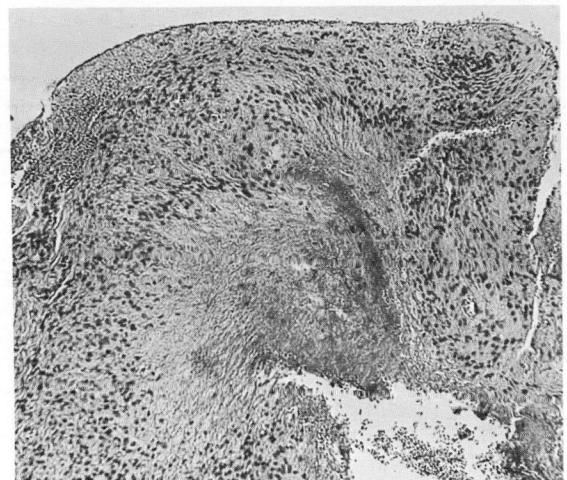

FIGURE 2. Microphotograph of a rheumatoid nodule. There is a characteristic histologic appearance with a central zone of fibrinoid necrosis surrounded by palisading cells, presumably young fibroblasts, arranged along the axes at right angles to the zone of central necrosis; this is in turn enveloped in a stroma of granulating fibrous tissue that may be densely cellular or sclerotic.

The percentage of patients with rheumatoid arthritis in which this factor can be detected ranges from 50 to 95, varying with the procedure used and the certainty with which the clinical diagnosis can be made. The techniques that give the highest percentage in patients with rheumatoid arthritis also appear to give the highest percentage of "false-positive" reactors in other diseases and in population groups. The percentage is highest among patients with classic rheumatoid arthritis or in those with nodules, who by most techniques will yield about 95 per cent positive reactions. The percentage of positive reactors is lower in cases classified as "probable" or "possible" rheumatoid arthritis.

Rheumatoid factor may be detected early in the course of the disease, and in general does not fluctuate with clinical activity of the process. A high titer is not necessarily associated with more chronic or fulminating forms of rheumatoid arthritis, but the highest titers are frequently found in patients with complications of rheumatoid arthritis, such as Felty's syndrome, peripheral neuritis, or arteritis. Positive tests are encountered in about 3 to 5 per cent of nonrheumatoid patients and in "normal" subjects in population studies. The incidence of positive reactions in population studies definitely increases with age and may reach as high as 15 per cent in the older age groups. Positive reactions are obtained in approximately 15 per cent of patients with other types of rheumatic diseases, particularly systemic lupus erythematosus. Positive tests are also encountered in nonrheumatic diseases, including liver disease, kala-azar, sarcoidosis, syphilis, bacterial endocarditis, tuberculosis, and acute viral infections.

Modes of Onset of Rheumatoid Arthritis. The clinical manifestations of this disease vary greatly from patient to patient, and in the same patient at different times. The degrees of severity of constitutional and articular manifestations do not necessarily parallel one another, and diverse modes of onset may present puzzling diagnostic problems early in the disease.

Prodromal symptoms may be found in about two thirds of patients. The most common are ease of fatigue, weakness, weight loss, and vasomotor disturbances with numbness and tingling of the hands and feet. Patients with rheumatoid arthritis often date the onset from disturbances that tend to deplete physical or emotional reserves, or both: acute infection, exposure, overwork, worry, and emotional strain.

A gradual, *insidious onset* is considered most characteristic, and this occurs in somewhat more than one half the patients. Pain on use and stiffness usually are noted in one or a few joints only, followed by swelling. Although almost any joint in the body may be initially involved, within a few weeks the smaller joints of the hands and feet are usually affected. The involvement is migratory but progressive. Once a joint develops objective evidence of inflammation, such evidence persists for at least a few weeks even though attention may be centered on the joints subsequently involved. Muscle aching without objective joint inflammation may occur in any part of the body and may last only a few hours or a few days. The temperature may be normal or only slightly elevated.

An *acute onset* is not uncommon, pain and swelling suddenly appearing in multiple joints, associated with chills, fever, and prostration. At times, particularly in children, the febrile reaction is the outstanding feature and may precede any articular involvement by several months.

An *episodic onset* may also occur, pain, swelling, and stiffness affecting one or several joints, persisting for a few days or weeks and then subsiding, only to recur after a few weeks or months. Careful examination will usually show some evidence of residual joint inflammation, even during asymptomatic periods. As time goes on the pain and swelling become more persistent, multiple joints are involved, and the signs and symptoms become characteristic of well-established rheumatoid arthritis.

A *monoarticular onset* can occur. Although involvement of a single joint may dominate the attention of both patient and physician, careful questioning and examination will often disclose abnormalities in other joints that are relatively asymptomatic. Nevertheless, rheumatoid arthritis may remain localized to only one joint for several months. Rarely, rheumatoid inflammation of tendon sheaths or bursae or development of rheumatoid nodules may precede articular involvement by months or even years.

Whatever the mode of onset, the disease sooner or later develops a characteristic chronic form that is still subject to exacerbations and remissions. The characteristic clinical features are the swelling of the joints, particularly of the hands, fingers, and knees; the symmetrical distribution of affected joints once the disease has become established; the tendency for successive and progressive involvement of multiple joints; and the tendency toward ankylosis and deformity of individual joints.

Clinical Manifestations. Symptoms. *Pain* in the affected joints varies considerably and is not always proportional to the degree of swelling. Pain at rest, unrelieved by heat and analgesics, is distinctly unusual except with severe acute inflammation. Pain on use is more persistent and is noted particularly with twisting motions of the hands and wrists, and in the feet and knees with weight bearing. *Stiffness* is perhaps the most constant symptom. Characteristically, the patient with rheumatoid arthritis is most uncomfortable on first arising in the morning, and requires a period of a half hour to several hours to "limber up." Such a patient is usually at his best late in the morning or in the early afternoon. There may be additional episodes of stiffening and aching after periods of rest later in the day, or with fatigue in the late afternoon or evening. Episodes of muscle aching and tenderness, particularly around the neck and shoulders, are frequent.

Constitutional symptoms vary greatly in severity. *Fatigability* and some degree of *weight loss* are most common; there are often associated malaise and actual weakness. *Fever* is usually low-grade, but instances of persistent daily temperature elevations to 102 to 104° F. with no alternative explanation have been well documented. On the other hand, there may be no elevation of temperature.

Vasomotor symptoms are not uncommon. Many patients complain of coldness of the hands and feet. Numbness and tingling of the hands and fingers should suggest the possibility of median nerve compression in the carpal tunnel. Flushing of the thenar and hypothenar eminences of the hands, resembling the "liver palm," is frequent. However, a true Raynaud's phenomenon is rarely seen.

Physical Signs. The cardinal objective joint findings are swelling, tenderness to pressure, and pain on motion. The skin over the affected joints is often warm, but rarely reddened. The swelling may be due to increased volume of synovial fluid (manifested by usual evidences of fluctuance), to thickening of the synovium and joint capsule (essentially the fact that there is an abnormal amount of soft tissue between the examiner's finger and the underlying bone), or to both. Tenderness to pressure is delineated by the attachments of the joint capsule. Pain on active or passive motion is usually noted first at the extremes of motion. Limitation of motion in early cases is usually due to pain, but later in the disease may be due to actual fibrosis of the joint capsule, to shortening of muscles, or to fibrous ankylosis as the articular cartilage is replaced by scar tissue. In the later stages the swelling may be less prominent, but some degree of thickening persists about the joint. Inside the joint the granulation

tissue may develop into adhesions that eventually lead to partial or complete fibrous ankylosis; bony ankylosis is less common, but it can occur. Atrophy of neighboring muscles may develop early and rapidly; it appears to be an integral part of the disease and cannot be attributed solely to disuse. The skin over the affected joints becomes smooth, shiny, and atrophic. Deformities, most commonly in flexion, develop with the ankylosis and associated cartilage destruction. Subluxations and joint instability frequently are prominent features.

In the majority of patients the hands are involved sooner or later and present a characteristic appearance. The swelling of the proximal interphalangeal joints gives the classic fusiform or sausage-shaped appearance to the fingers (Fig. 3). The terminal interphalangeal joints are rarely affected. The patient is unable to make a tight fist and the grip is weakened. The hands are often cold and clammy. As the disease progresses, many or all of the fingers may be affected, swelling appears in the metacarpophalangeal and wrist joints, and atrophy of the interosseous muscles becomes evident. Later, flexion deformities of the fingers and wrists develop, and lateral deflection and subluxation at the metacarpophalangeal joints produce the characteristic ulnar deviation of the fingers (Fig. 4).

Although any joint in the body may be affected, the knees, elbows, and ankles are often prominently involved. The entire ankle joint may appear swollen, but limitation of motion and deformity are especially evident in the subastragaloid articulation. Involvement of the metatarsophalangeal joints of the toes is more common than is generally appreciated; the chief evidences of this are pain on walking and tenderness to pressure early in the disease, and, later, a hammer-toe type of deformity.

On general physical examination, the typical arthritic patient usually appears chronically ill, undernourished, and possibly anemic. Some, however, are in an excellent state of nutrition. The *spleen* is palpable in 5 to 10 per cent of patients, and occasionally there is generalized lymphaden-

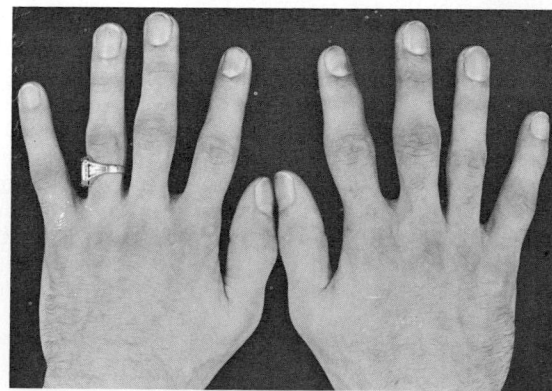

FIGURE 3. Hands of a patient with relatively early but definite rheumatoid arthritis. The swelling of the proximal interphalangeal joint is responsible for the characteristic fusiform appearance of the fingers.

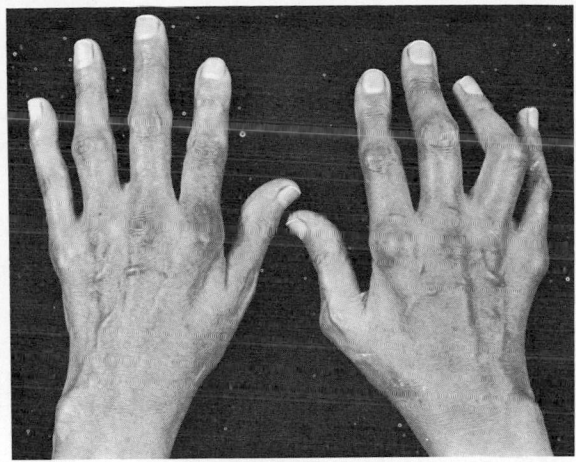

FIGURE 4. Hands of a patient in a more advanced stage of rheumatoid arthritis. Joint swelling is less prominent; atrophy of skin and interosseous muscles is evident; flexion deformities and subluxation have developed.

opathy. *Pedal edema*, distinct from joint swelling, is occasionally seen in the absence of cardiac, hepatic, renal, or nutritional explanations. It often appears to develop on a mechanical basis.

Three types of pulmonary lesions are found in patients with rheumatoid arthritis. Nodular lesions with the characteristic histologic appearance of rheumatoid nodules may be isolated, multiple or coalescent to produce a honeycombed *rheumatoid lung.* A type of progressive massive pulmonary fibrosis seen in miners with pneumoconiosis who also have rheumatoid arthritis or are positive reactors for rheumatoid factor is known as *Caplan's syndrome.* In addition, there appears to be a definitely increased incidence of idiopathic pulmonary fibrosis in patients with rheumatoid arthritis.

Clinical evidence of heart disease is uncommon, although *pericarditis* with effusion can be attributed to rheumatoid arthritis on occasion. *Iritis* or *uveitis* occurs in 3 to 5 per cent of patients at some time during their disease; *episcleritis* may also accompany rheumatoid arthritis. The pathogenesis of these ocular complications is not well understood. The most common renal complication is *amyloidosis.* Other complications are discussed under Variants of Rheumatoid Arthritis.

Clinical Course and Prognosis. Rheumatoid arthritis may run a comparatively short course of a few months, and there may be complete disappearance of symptoms for several months or even years. In the majority of patients, however, the disease returns and with each recurrence assumes a more chronic form. Even in those patients in whom the disease follows a chronic progressive course extending over years, there are often periods of comparative comfort alternating with periods of disease activity. With each exacerbation new joints may become involved, and further function may be lost in previously afflicted joints. Although the tendency toward loss of function and ankylosis is the rule, in some patients the

disease follows an undulating course characterized by joint swelling but little disability for years.

If the process is checked in its early stages, all the symptoms may disappear, and joint function may return entirely to normal. Even in well established disease, remission can occur either spontaneously or following treatment. In such cases the patient recovers partial or complete use of the affected joints, although swelling and deformity do not completely disappear. If the disease is not checked, the patient may eventually become a bedridden cripple, presenting a pitiful picture with his contracted deformed limbs and wasted muscles.

In any patient, the course of rheumatoid arthritis is unpredictable, but when a significant number of patients are followed for years, their status at the end of 5 to 10 years, as compared with that at the beginning of observation, is as follows: about 15 per cent are in remission; an additional 40 to 50 per cent are slightly to moderately improved; 10 per cent show no significant change; and 25 to 35 per cent are worse. After 15 years the total showing improvement drops to about 35 per cent, and 50 to 60 per cent are worse. Complete incapacitation leading to confinement in bed or in a wheel chair develops in a relatively small number. Patients who accept their limitations and live within them do better than those unable or unwilling to do so. It should be noted that the tendency toward remission is greatest early in the disease, and that in the first year of the disease two thirds or more of the patients can be expected to experience a significant remission.

Roentgenographic Findings. Roentgenographic abnormalities appear many months or even a few years after clinical evidences of soft tissue inflammation. Early in the disease roentgenograms of affected joints are usually negative, aside from evidence of soft tissue swelling. Later on there may be moderate osteoporosis of the bones adjacent to affected joints. Effusion may contribute to a haziness of the radiolucent structures around the joint. As granulation tissue erodes the cartilage, there is reduction in the apparent "joint space" (actually reduction in width of the radiolucent articular cartilages capping the bone ends), and when the cartilage is completely destroyed the bone ends appear to be in contact. At this stage there are atrophy and rarefaction of the cancellous bone, and often the appearance of small areas of bone erosion due to invasion of bone by the granulation tissue. Such "punched-out" areas of bone erosion are usually smaller than those that occur in gout. Late in the disease there is often gross distortion of the normal architecture due to subluxations, deformities, and bone resorption.

There is often great discrepancy between the functional state of the joint and its roentgenographic appearance. Progressive, though slow, deterioration of the joint may be demonstrated by serial roentgenograms even though the patient may appear clinically to be in remission.

Laboratory Findings. About 25 per cent of patients with rheumatoid arthritis have a normocytic normochromic anemia. This has characteristics of the anemia of chronic infection. The serum iron is reduced, but the iron transport and iron binding capacity of the serum are normal. The anemia is usually resistant to treatment with oral iron. A significant hemolytic factor has not been demonstrated, and studies of erythrocyte mass have yielded conflicting results. The anemia of rheumatoid arthritis can occasionally be severe, but it is well to search for additional causes if the hemoglobin is below 10 grams per 100 ml.

A moderate leukocytosis with increase in immature cells may be present in active cases. The urine shows no characteristic changes; proteinuria should suggest the possibility of amyloidosis as a complication.

Laboratory tests that may be helpful in diagnosis include tests for the rheumatoid factor and examination of the synovial fluid. As indicated previously, the sensitivity of tests for the rheumatoid factor varies with the technique used. The usual flocculation tests with latex, sheep erythrocytes, or bentonite particles are positive in approximately 70 per cent of adult patients with typical rheumatoid arthritis.

The synovial fluid in rheumatoid arthritis varies from clear to turbid and frequently clots on standing. The leukocyte count may be only slightly increased, but it usually is above 3000 per cubic millimeter, and may be as high as 100,000. The average is 14,000. Usually 70 to 95 per cent of the cells are polymorphonuclear. Protein content is elevated. The mucin clot, formed after addition of dilute acetic acid, ranges from good to poor in quality, and the viscosity of the joint fluid is characteristically decreased. Sugar content is reduced. The chief value of joint fluid examination is to place the rheumatoid fluid in the group of inflammatory effusions, separating it on the one hand from traumatic and degenerative effusions and on the other hand from frankly purulent joint fluids.

Certain other tests are nonspecific and are of value only in differentiating inflammatory arthritis from traumatic and degenerative joint disease. They may be useful, however, as *indicators of disease activity*, analogous to the "acute phase reactants" in rheumatic fever. The most commonly used is the erythrocyte sedimentation rate, which is accelerated in nearly all patients with rheumatoid arthritis. The test for C-reactive protein is usually positive. Serum protein electrophoresis frequently indicates a decrease in albumin and an increase in alpha-2 and gamma globulin. At times, the gamma globulin level may be as high as in systemic lupus erythematosus and other connective tissue diseases. The mucopolysaccharide and mucoprotein content of the serum are also elevated.

The erythrocyte sedimentation rate correlates in general with the clinical evidence of inflammatory activity, particularly during the first two or three years of the disease. The other "acute phase reactants" also appear to reflect rheumatoid activity. However, when rheumatoid arthritis has been present for several years, it is distinctly unusual for these indices to return to normal values.

Diagnosis. The diagnosis of rheumatoid arthritis can be made with ease in typical well-established disease, but recognition of an early, mild, or atypical case may present difficulties. The diagnosis is usually made on the basis of a combination of characteristic findings and the behavior of the disease over a period of time. Features important in diagnosis are the characteristic joint inflammation with swelling and tenderness, migratory progressive involvement of multiple joints, predilection for smaller joints, tendency to symmetrical distribution of affected joints once the disease is established, atrophy of neighboring muscle groups, and development of some degree of deformity and ankylosis in severe cases. Also important are the evidences of constitutional disease: clinically, the weight loss, ease of fatigue, etc.; in the laboratory, the accelerated erythrocyte sedimentation rate and other "acute phase reactants." The roentgenographic findings are not specific, but are helpful, particularly if the time relationships to the clinical manifestations are kept in mind. Serologic tests for rheumatoid factor are helpful if positive, but a negative test does not exclude the diagnosis.

Differential Diagnosis. Rheumatoid arthritis enters into the differential diagnosis of virtually every disease of the joints and of the connective tissue. The most common differentiation that must be made is between rheumatoid arthritis and osteoarthritis. In *osteoarthritis* the primary pathologic change is degenerative, and there is absence of inflammatory swelling. The disease affects a few larger joints, particularly weight-bearing joints, and does not spread. It is a local disease of the joints, and it does not present the clinical and laboratory evidences of a constitutional disease. Roentgenographically, osteoarthritis is characterized by hypertrophic lipping of bone around the joint margins. It rarely produces deformity and ankylosis. However, it must be kept in mind that rheumatoid arthritis and osteoarthritis may attack the same joint. In older persons, rheumatoid arthritis may be superimposed on a joint already showing degenerative changes. Conversely, the joint damaged by inflammatory arthritis is more susceptible to the subsequent development of degenerative arthritis.

Rheumatoid arthritis with an acute onset must often be differentiated from *acute rheumatic fever,* a distinction not always easy to make. In both conditions the patient may give a history of antecedent sore throat. However, in contrast to the progressive joint involvement of rheumatoid arthritis, the articular inflammation of rheumatic fever is fleetingly migratory, and a joint that had been acutely inflamed a few days before returns to normal both subjectively and objectively, even though at the same time other areas are acutely and painfully involved. Also in rheumatic fever the temperature usually rises higher, sweating is more profuse, and manifestations of cardiac involvement are more frequent. Serologic evidence of a recent streptococcal infection can usually be obtained by positive tests for antibodies to the Streptococcus. In rheumatic fever, adequate doses of aspirin or sodium salicylate (6 to 8 grams per day) usually result in prompt and complete relief of both fever and joint pain. These drugs produce a slower and less complete suppression of manifestations in rheumatoid arthritis.

Suppurative arthritis is usually recognized by association with disease produced elsewhere in the body by the gonococcus, the meningococcus, the Streptococcus, the Staphylococcus, the pneumococcus and, rarely, other organisms. A history of a true shaking chill, reflecting septicemia, may be useful. However, it is easy to mistake gonococcal arthritis for rheumatoid arthritis, particularly in women in whom the genital gonorrhea has not been recognized. Gonorrheal arthritis is frequently polyarticular, and the swollen painful joints may bear a close resemblance to those of rheumatoid arthritis or rheumatic fever. After two to three weeks of migratory involvement, the disease frequently settles down to a stubborn involvement of one or a few large joints. An adequate history, as well as examination of the genitourinary tract and appropriate cultures, is of prime importance in differentiation.

Rheumatoid arthritis involving only one joint may be confused with *tuberculous arthritis.* Roentgenographic examination and culture of the joint fluid can be of great assistance in making the distinction, but in some cases biopsy may be needed. *Traumatic joint disabilities* may also be mistaken for monoarticular rheumatoid arthritis. This is particularly true of internal derangements of the knee, such as torn semilunar cartilage, or of any joint in association with aseptic necrosis of bone. Accurate history, careful examination, and examination of the joint fluid usually permit a differentiation.

Gouty arthritis may easily be confused with rheumatoid arthritis, particularly if the latter has an acute or episodic onset. Classically, acute gout is characterized by sudden development of inflammation progressing in a few hours to an exquisitely painful inflammation of the joint and its surroundings, which subsides after a few days without leaving any residual pain or impairment. Gout is usually thought of as a possibility when the great toe is involved, but it should be borne in mind that about 25 per cent of initial attacks involve joints other than the great toe, and that in 10 per cent of patients classic podagra has not been experienced. Therefore, the characteristics of onset of the acute attack are often more helpful than the location of involvement. In nearly all cases of gout, the diagnosis can be made on the basis of the combination of the characteristics of the joint involvement, elevation of the serum uric acid, and response to colchicine properly administered. Demonstration of sodium monourate crystals in the joint fluid establishes the diagnosis of gout. Chronic gout can closely simulate the advanced deformities of rheumatoid arthritis. The presence of tophi in the helix of the ear or tophaceous deposits in the bone demonstrable by roentgenographic examination are helpful in differentiation, although punched-out areas in bone are found in both rheumatoid and gouty patients.

Rheumatoid arthritis also often has to be differentiated from other diseases of connective tissue. The most troublesome differentiation is encountered in some cases of *systemic lupus erythematosus.* The joint manifestations in this disease are more commonly arthralgia only, or articular or periarticular swellings that evolve and subside rapidly. In some patients, however, the arthritis follows a chronic destructive course indistinguishable from that of rheumatoid arthritis. In addition to the arthralgia and arthritis and the constitutional symptoms of fatigue, fever, and weight loss common to both diseases, clinical features of systemic lupus erythematosus include erythematous skin lesions; suppression of any or all of the formed elements of the blood with leukopenia, anemia, and/or thrombocytopenia; lymphadenopathy; polyserositis with pleural or pericardial effusion or, less commonly, peritonitis; nonbacterial endocarditis; and renal disease that may simulate nephritis or nephrosis. Rarely does a single patient present all the above manifestations at any one time, and the combination of findings in a given case may be extremely varied. Demonstration of the LE cell phenomenon is strong presumptive evidence for the diagnosis, but a negative test does not rule it out. Ten to 15 per cent of patients with manifestations only of rheumatoid arthritis exhibit a positive LE cell test.

Other conditions which on occasion need to be differentiated from rheumatoid arthritis include serum sickness, sarcoidosis, hypertrophic osteoarthropathy, polyarteritis nodosa, progressive systemic sclerosis, and polymyositis.

Prophylaxis. Until the cause of rheumatoid arthritis is established, prophylaxis for this disease will present a difficult problem. One of the most striking features of the disease is its tendency to relapse. Patients who recover completely from the first attack may remain free of symptoms for several years. The second or third attack is nearly always more stubborn in its course and often goes on to the chronic progressive form. Therefore, every effort should be made to prolong a remission and to prevent a relapse. The patient's life and personal hygiene must be carefully regulated to a point well within his capacity to function without fatigue. Every effort should be made to avoid exhausting his reserves, physical and emotional.

Treatment of Rheumatoid Arthritis. *Basic Principles.* Rheumatoid arthritis is a chronic systemic disease, and the physician should have this fact constantly in mind. Local treatment to painful joints often gives symptomatic relief, but much more is needed for successful results. The physician must also recognize that rheumatoid arthritis is subject to spontaneous remissions and exacerbations, a fact that may cause him to attribute therapeutic efficacy to useless agents.

It is important to use a well-rounded treatment program carefully adapted to the need of the individual patient, rather than to rely on any single measure. Methods of established value, all applicable to a greater or lesser extent to each patient with rheumatoid arthritis, can be summarized under the headings of (1) rest, (2) relief of pain, (3) maintenance of joint function by physical measures, (4) prevention and correction of deformities by application of orthopedic principles, and (5) correction of any factors that are deleterious to the health of the patient. The initiation of such a treatment program can often be best accomplished by a few weeks of hospital care. Hospitalization not only provides facilities for rest and nursing care and the opportunity to indoctrinate the patient in the use of relatively simple analgesics and physical therapy, but also permits careful appraisal of all factors bearing on his general health.

Rest. All students of rheumatoid arthritis are agreed that extensive and prolonged rest is the key to successful management. Particularly in the early treatment of the patient who is febrile or in whom there is acute inflammation in weight-bearing joints, complete bed rest is mandatory until these manifestations have subsided. Sometimes complete rest is difficult to enforce, chiefly because the patient is anxious to go on with his daily duties. Often for economic reasons the physician must compromise on the rest issue. Patients with rheumatoid arthritis should try to obtain 10, and if possible 12, hours of rest out of the 24. This can usually be accomplished by lengthening sleeping hours at night, using a mild hypnotic if necessary, and by establishing an afternoon rest period.

However, it should be pointed out that even if a patient is receiving hospital care, rest does not consist in lying in bed for 24 hours a day. Such "over-rest" encourages ankylosis and atrophy of the muscles in the back and legs. Attention must be given to the posture of the patient in bed, and a carefully balanced program of rest and exercise should be adapted to his individual needs.

Relief of Pain — Analgesics. For control of pain in rheumatoid arthritis, no drug stands up as well over a period time as salicylate. This may be administered either as *acetylsalicylic acid* or as *sodium salicylate*, in regular doses prescribed according to the needs of the patient. Doses may range from 0.6 gram three to four times a day for the average patient to as high as 0.9 to 1.2 grams every four hours while the patient is awake. There is less danger of gastric disturbance if the drug is combined with an antacid. Enteric-coated tablets may be useful, but in some patients gastrointestinal absorption from such enteric-coated preparations is incomplete. In our experience, combinations of salicylates with muscle-relaxing drugs and with para-aminobenzoic acid have not given better results than would be expected of the salicylates alone. When pain is not controlled by these drugs, addition of *codeine*, 30 mg., to the aspirin may be necessary as a temporary measure, but continued use of codeine is to be avoided. If its use appears necessary to control pain, this is usu-ally an indication for increasing the amount of rest and for more emphasis on physical therapy.

Phenylbutazone (Butazolidin) has value as an analgesic in rheumatoid arthritis, but in most cases of rheumatoid arthritis its effects are not clearly superior to those of the salicylates. The usual dose of phenylbutazone is 100 mg., two to three times daily. Its great disadvantage is a high incidence of toxic reactions, including gastrointestinal disturbances, exacerbation of gastric and duodenal ulcers, skin rashes, and occasionally bone marrow depression with leukopenia and agranulocytosis. Retention of sodium and water, which often occurs during the first ten days of administration of this drug, may prove deleterious for patients with cardiac or renal disease. In general, use of phenylbutazone should be reserved for patients in whom the desired analgesic effects cannot be obtained with safer drugs. Patients receiving this medication must be kept under medical supervision and should have frequent blood counts.

Indomethacin is chemically unrelated to other analgesics and exerts its analgesic, antipyretic, and anti-inflammatory effects independently of adrenal function. Although this compound may be useful in selected patients with ankylosing spondylitis and acute gout, the results in rheumatoid arthritis have been equivocal. An initial dosage of 50 to 100 mg. daily is recommended, with gradual increase not to exceed 150 to 200 mg. per day. Experience indicates that it cannot be considered a simple analgesic. Untoward reactions include headaches, nausea, epigastric pain, diarrhea, disturbances of equilibrium, and mild mental disturbances. Corneal deposits and retinal degeneration as well as bone marrow depression have been reported. The drug is contraindicated in patients under 14 years of age, during pregnancy, and in patients allergic to aspirin. Adverse reactions are more frequent in the elderly. Indomethacin also must be reserved for patients in whom the desired analgesic effect cannot be obtained with safer drugs and requires careful supervision by the physician. It cannot be recommended for long-term administration.

Physical Measures. Use of heat combined with a regular program of exercises constitutes the most important physical treatment of rheumatoid arthritis. The application of heat for a period of time should be followed immediately by range of motion or muscle-strengthening exercises. Massage is of no significant help in rheumatoid arthritis; it should be reserved for cases in which there is an unusual degree of muscle aching, and then it should be applied to the surrounding muscles instead of directly to the inflamed joint.

Heat can be applied either locally to the joint or to the entire body. Generalized heat is conveniently applied by means of a hot tub bath, a hot pack or steam cabinet, or an electric light bridge. Generalized heat is particularly advantageous for the patient with extensive joint involvement and has the advantage of stimulating the circulation, inducing copious perspiration, and elevating the body temperature slightly. Local application of heat is effectively carried out by the ordinary electric baker or by means of the infrared lamp. Some prefer moist heat in the form of hot towels, hot packs, or submersion of the joint in hot water. In general, diathermy and ultrasonic therapy has not proved superior to other effective methods of applying heat. The ordinary electric heating pad is not an effective means of applying heat in this disease. For both local and general application of heat, maximal benefit appears to be obtained in 20 to 30 minutes; more prolonged use of heat may have undesirable debilitating effects. Use of paraffin dips (see below) is an effective way of applying heat to the hands and wrists. Contrast baths, consisting of alternating immersion in hot and cold water, are useful for involvement of the hands and feet.

The primary objective of exercises is to maintain, insofar as possible, a normal or useful range of joint motion and to maintain the tone of the muscles that move the joints. Even acutely inflamed and painful joints should be put through as full a range of motion as pain permits a few times a day, if necessary by passive exercises. As soon as possible the patient should progress to active exercises so that muscle tone is maintained. The details of the exercises prescribed vary according to the part of the body affected. It is important that the patient clearly understand the need for purposeful use of his muscles. When lower extremity joints are involved, it is often necessary to make a sharp distinction between non-weight-bearing exercises and the amount of ambulatory activity permitted. Hydrotherapy in the form of supervised exercises in a warm pool, Hubbard tank, or bath tub plays an important part in the modern treatment of arthritis. The warmth relaxes the muscles, and the buoyant effect of the water makes movement easier. The best temperature for exercise under water is 98 to 100° F.

Of great importance are exercises that have to do with maintaining posture, including quadriceps drill. In this drill, the patient, lying supine in bed, contracts and relaxes the quadriceps muscles 20 times or more at least three times a day.

The use of physical medicine must be adapted carefully to the needs of each patient. For those with only hand and finger involvement, the use of paraffin dips or contrast baths followed by gripping exercises may suffice. In addition, hyperextension and separation of the fingers will tend to maintain function of the interosseous muscles and counteract the tendency to ulnar deviation. For patients with extensive involvement or those who have already developed deformities, a much more elaborate program with the advice of a physiatrist is often necessary. In the average case of rheumatoid arthritis, simple measures that the patient can use at home over long periods of time should be worked out. The value of written instructions with respect to exercises has been amply demonstrated. Many physicians and patients have found most helpful the instructions included in a pamphlet entitled *Home Care and Rheumatoid Arthritis* prepared by the Arthritis Foundation, and available at small cost from the regional and national headquarters of the Foundation.

Application of Orthopedic Principles. It is customary to think of orthopedic treatment only in advanced stages of the disease, after deformities have developed. However, certain simple orthopedic principles can be applied, to a greater or lesser extent, in nearly every case of rheumatoid arthritis. The arthritic should sleep on a flat bed with only one pillow. Placing a pillow under the swollen and painful knees should not be permitted because of the tendency to develop flexion deformity at this joint. A board at the foot of the bed may be needed to prevent foot drop. For patients with developing deformities, particularly of the wrists and knees, dynamic splints or half-shell molds constructed of plaster or plastics have definite advantages. The splint or mold should be removed at least twice a day for the application of physical therapy and exercises. The physician should know the positions for optimal function of joints threatened with ankylosis, particularly the knees, elbows, wrists, and fingers. When the feet are affected, a metatarsal pad or bar may be indicated to protect the inflamed metatarsophalangeal joints from the added trauma of weight bearing, and arch supports or even steel foot plates may be useful in preventing the common eversion deformity at the subastragaloid joint.

Surgical correction of ankylosed and deformed joints is beyond the scope of this discussion. Many excellent surgical procedures have been devised. Perhaps the most consistently successful are those designed to correct for ankylosis of the elbow, deformities at the metatarsophalangeal joints of the toes, and flexion contractures of the wrists.

Attention to General Health. Careful attention must be given to all factors, physical and psychologic, that can be deleterious to the general health of the patient. This presupposes a careful evaluation of such factors by the physician. Obviously, measures employed under this heading vary greatly from one patient to the next. However, certain problems are sufficiently frequent that they should be almost automatically checked off by the physician who is caring for such patients.

Diet. There is no special diet for the treatment of rheumatoid arthritis; rather the diet is indicated by the general nutritional state of the patient. Many affected persons are undernourished and underweight, with evidence of loss of body protein. For them a diet high in calories and protein and a liberal intake of vitamins and minerals are needed. An occasional overweight patient should be placed on a reduction diet. There is no evidence of specific value in the use of supplementary vitamins. That some patients feel better while taking vitamins is probably due to the suggestive effect of the medication. Many physicians prescribe vitamin concentrates or multivitamin capsules in order to ensure that their patients have an adequate vitamin intake. This apparently does no harm if the importance of an adequate caloric and protein intake is not neglected.

Correction of Anemia. The anemia of rheumatoid arthritis usually does not respond to hematinic agents. In some women, there may be coexistent iron deficiency anemia that will respond to oral administration of ferrous sulfate, 0.32 gram three times daily. Administration of folic acid and vitamin B_{12} is ineffective. Favorable reports have appeared on the use of intravenous or intramuscular iron therapy. The results have not been consistent, and as this form of treatment is not without danger it failed to achieve wide use. The most prompt and effective way of correcting a persistent anemia in rheumatoid arthritis is by transfusions. Even in patients who have persistent anemia, the transfusion gains are usually well maintained for several months. Occasionally, tranfusion may be followed by a general improvement considerably greater than can be explained by the correction of the anemia. Such results, however, are relatively infrequent, and in recent years tranfusions have become less popular because of the danger of transmitting serum hepatitis.

Psychotherapy. Once the disease has been established, the importance of emotional factors in rheumatoid arthritis and the need for psychological support cannot be overemphasized. Formal psychiatric management is rarely necessary or even successful. An understanding of the patient's personality and of his emotional reaction to his illness must enter into the all-important rapport between the patient and his physician. This relationship is best initiated when the physician takes the time to explain candidly, and in lay terms, the nature of the disease, its treatment, limitations of treatment, and outlook. Complete honesty, unshakable equanimity, unremitting patience in answering questions, and obvious willingness to keep the patient completely informed are needed to maintain and inspire confidence. Emotional rest is only one of many facets of therapy, but it must be supervised as conscientiously and judiciously as any physical support; motivation can sag easily if not propped with continual reassurance, and it is important to appreciate that without the patient's will to improve the program is doomed to failure.

If tenseness and emotional unrest are really interfering with management, and particularly if insomnia results, judicious use of phenobarbital or other barbiturates may be indicated. The so-called "tranquilizing agents" such as meprobamate, promazine derivatives, etc., are occasionally useful, but they are prescribed more frequently than is justified.

Certain measures of treatment that have had greater or less popularity in the past may occasionally be useful because they have a beneficial effect on the general health of the patient. Any infection, evident or "focal," should be treated by whatever means is necessary for its eradication.

It is rare indeed that a dramatic change in the course of the disease follows the treatment of such infection, and indiscriminate removal of teeth, tonsils and even internal organs because they might be sites of "focal infection" is to be condemned. The patient with definite hypothyroidism, or the woman with severe menopausal symptoms, may be benefited by the use of appropriate endocrine preparations; however, such treatment has no place in the management of the great majority of patients with rheumatoid arthritis.

Additional Measures. Many patients with rheumatoid arthritis respond to treatment based on the principles that have been outlined and do not require additional forms of treatment. All patients should be tried on such a regimen, carefully adapted to their needs and carefully supervised, for a period of three to six months before consideration is given to one of the special forms of treatment. For patients who do not respond satisfactorily, or in whom the disease progresses, many students of the disease believe that certain additional measures are helpful in inducing at least a temporary remission. At the present time, three groups of drugs appear to be helpful in this respect—soluble organic gold salts, adrenocortical steroids, and certain antimalarial agents. It must be appreciated that these represent additions to, not substitutions for, a sound basic program adapted to the needs of the individual patient.

Gold Salts. Soluble organic salts of gold have been used in the treatment of rheumatoid arthritis for forty years. Their use is strictly empirical, and the mode of action is not understood. There is evidence that these compounds can induce a remission of the disease more rapidly and in a higher percentage of patients than in a control group on conservative management. Such differences are most impressive in patients treated early, particularly in the first year after onset. On the other hand, evidence is lacking that these compounds are of value in preventing relapses after a remission has been obtained.

Studies on the rate of absorption and excretion of various gold salts indicate that about 75 per cent of the gold is retained in the body during the course of gold therapy and that excretion occurs largely through the kidneys. Gold salt continues to be excreted for months after the injections have ceased. This slow excretion of gold products is partly responsible for the toxic effects, which can occur any time during or after a course of gold therapy.

Forms of gold used in the United States are sodium aurothiomalate (Myochrysine) and aurothioglucose (Solganal). These are given by deep intramuscular injection at five- to seven-day intervals. The schedule most commonly used is as follows:

First injection	10 mg.
Second injection	25 mg.
Third and subsequent	
injections to sixteenth to twentieth	50 mg.

If there is no improvement after a total of 1000

mg., it is unlikely that further administration will be effective. If improvement has occurred, "maintenance therapy" is recommended in an effort to prevent relapse. Injections of 50 mg. are spaced at two-week intervals for four injections, then at three-week intervals for four injections, then at four-week intervals for an indefinite period.

Unfortunately, there are dangers in the use of gold therapy that have militated against its general acceptance. The most common toxic reactions are dermatitis and stomatitis. Renal damage, evidenced by either proteinuria or microscopic hematuria, may occur. Depression of bone marrow, with resulting thrombocytopenic purpura, aplastic anemia, or agranulocytosis is fortunately a much less common manifestation, but is by far the most serious, and it may be fatal. Patients receiving gold therapy should be watched carefully and questioned before each injection regarding itching or skin rash. The urine and blood count should be checked regularly, weekly at first and thereafter at least once a month. At the first suggestion of toxicity, treatment should be suspended. Dermatitis and urinary abnormalities usually subside in a few weeks, and severe exfoliative dermatitis can usually be avoided if attention is paid to the earliest cutaneous or mucosal lesions. However, the bone marrow depression can occur unpredictably and may be resistant to treatment.

BAL (British anti-lewisite, dimercaprol) is effective in the treatment of gold toxicity as well as other heavy metal poisonings. This compound successfully competes with the thiol groups in the tissues and accelerates excretion of gold from the body. Its efficacy is greater if it is used soon after the development of gold toxicity. The dose is 2.5 mg. per kilogram of body weight every four hours during the first and second days, and then two times daily for five to eight days. BAL itself may produce nausea, vomiting, and abdominal pain. Cortisone and related steroid compounds in doses equivalent to 10 to 25 mg. of prednisone are also effective in controlling the manifestations of gold toxicity, particularly the dermatitis. The chronic course of the complications is not necessarily shortened, however.

Improvement, when it occurs following gold therapy, is usually not apparent until the second or third month, or longer. Combinations of gold therapy with adrenocortical steroids, both measures of treatment being initiated at the same time, have been used in an attempt to obtain the more prompt effect of the adrenocortical steroids, which have been gradually withdrawn after two to three months in the hope that the somewhat longer-lasting effects of gold therapy would then keep the disease under control. The favorable results of such combined therapy have been no greater than those obtained with gold alone; an additional hazard was that occasionally gold toxicity was unmasked as the steroids were withdrawn.

The decision to use gold therapy obviously requires careful consideration whether the possible benefits justify the risks. Some students of the disease definitely question the value of gold therapy and believe that equally good results without toxic effects can be obtained by a conservative program of treatment. The majority of workers, however, endorse the use of gold therapy in carefully selected and properly supervised patients.

Systemic Use of Adrenal Corticosteroids. In 1949 Hench, Kendall, Slocumb, and Polley demonstrated the remarkable ability of cortisone to suppress the inflammatory manifestations of rheumatoid arthritis. Subsequent experience has shown that the effect of cortisone and related compounds is suppressive rather than curative, that the disease nearly always relapses when these agents are withdrawn, and that untoward effects directly related to their hormonal properties limit their use over long periods of time. The early enthusiastic and indiscreet use of these agents has given place to careful attempts to utilize them in a manner to provide optimal but not maximal relief, without the development of undesirable side effects, and at a dosage governed by the patient's tolerance to the steroids rather than by the severity of his symptoms.

Cortisol (hydrocortisone) is the major physiologic corticosteroid with anti-inflammatory properties. The synthetic compounds, prednisone and prednisolone, developed in 1954, do not produce significant effects on electrolyte metabolism. Therefore they do not cause the retention of salt and water and the occasional hypokalemia that was seen with cortisone and cortisol; however, the hormonal effect on organic metabolism is undiminished and can produce all of the other undesirable effects of corticosteroid administration, including suppression of the patient's own adrenal function. Synthetic steroids developed subsequently, including triamcinolone, methyl prednisolone, beta methasone, and dexamethasone, share essentially the same qualities as prednisone and prednisolone. Although the anti-inflammatory properties per milligram are increased in the latter compounds so that the effective dose is considerably smaller, there has been no significant diminution of the ability of these compounds to produce undesirable hormonal effects. These effects are essentially those of the hyperadrenocortical state as manifested in Cushing's disease, including weight gain, rounding of the face, hirsutism, unmasking of latent diabetes, increased incidence of peptic ulcer, masking of intercurrent infections, and development of osteoporosis.

It is now agreed that corticosteroids, systemically administered, should never be the initial agents used in the treatment of rheumatoid arthritis, but that they should be given only after a conscientious and adequate trial of the basic program described previously. Steroid treatment must not constitute the only measure but should be part of a comprehensive, carefully individualized program, and should be used only after a careful survey for the presence of contraindications. This form of therapy should be considered for those patients whose arthritis is moderate or severe and who have not responded satisfactorily to less toxic agents, and for patients who are threatened with disability or inability to carry on their occupational or household duties. It is often dangerous to give steroids to patients severely afflicted with the disease who are bedridden, ankylosed, and weakened by severe muscle atrophy. These people are prone to develop serious complications, such as fractures due to osteoporosis, and since the primary effect is suppression of inflammation without influence on previous damage, the risks outweigh the possible beneficial effects.

These hormonal agents can exert a beneficial effect on the clinical signs and symptoms of the disease and may result in inprovement of function. There is an initial decrease in subjective stiffness, diminution in tenderness over the joints, and a decrease in pain on motion, followed by a lessening of swelling. Sedimentation rate falls and the hemoglobin or hematocrit may rise. Accompanying these effects there is usually a feeling of wellbeing and an increase in appetite. This initial response is frequently not maintained even though the drugs are continued. After several months, signs and symptoms of active disease may return. Even though the clinical manifestations are suppressed over long periods of time, roentgenographic evidence of progressive destruction of articular cartilage, joint deformity, and other evidence of continued activity of the disease can often be demonstrated.

Before employing these agents, it is well to have a clear understanding with the patient that a trial is being undertaken to determine whether worthwhile suppression of symptoms and improvement of function can be obtained at a dosage that does not produce a significant degree of hyperadrenalism. The initial dosage is at or near the anticipated maintenance dose, 5.0 to 7.5 mg. of prednisolone, or its equivalent with the other preparations. The initial use of high doses and then gradual reduction to a maintenance level is not recommended, and may often be undesirable. Medication is usually given in three or four divided doses throughout the waking hours. Within two or three months it usually has become evident whether the use of these agents is a practical method of management for the specific patient. If it clearly is not, the corticosteroid can then be discontinued by gradual tapering of the dosage. It is much easier to discontinue steroids under these circumstances than after the patient has been on treatment for many months and complications may have developed. Patients receiving long-term steroid therapy should never have therapy terminated suddenly and should be warned not to discontinue treatment suddenly on their own initiative. Every effort should be made to keep the steroid dose at the lowest level effective in providing worthwhile relief of symptoms. This is accomplished by periodic decrease in dosage. Generally the decrements in dosage should be small, either when testing for effective level

of dosage or discontinuing treatment. The decrements should not exceed 5 to 10 per cent of the maintenance dose, and a period of five to seven days should be held at each step in the decrease.

The hyperadrenal state, manifested by "moon face" and hirsutism, may be tolerated without apparent untoward effects for a few weeks, but there are indications that further trouble can be anticipated if the medication is maintained for more than a few months. The physician responsible should be alert to the danger of peptic ulcer, osteoporosis, latent infection, and psychogenic disturbance. The incidence of *peptic ulceration* has varied greatly in cases studied, and it is not clearly greater than in patients with rheumatoid arthritis receiving other methods of treatment. However, some complication such as hemorrhage or perforation often is the initial manifestation.

Fractures of the long bones and particularly compression fractures of the spine due to osteoporosis are more likely to occur in postmenopausal women and in patients severely handicapped with respect to ambulation. Although this complication was thought to accompany high doses of steroids, with the longer use of these agents it has become apparent that osteoporosis also occurs in patients who have been taking low doses of steroids for years. Measures that should theoretically be effective in combating osteoporosis include calcium supplements and the use of anabolic sex hormones; however, their effectiveness in preventing this complication has not yet been proved.

The masking or aggravation of *infection* can be a serious side effect of corticosteroid therapy. Of particular concern is the activation and spread of tuberculosis. Therefore, every patient for whom steroid therapy is considered should have an initial chest roentgenogram. However, infection, including tuberculosis, is not a contraindication to the use of these agents, provided that the infection is recognized and treated by appropriate antimicrobial agents. The great danger is unrecognized infection.

Psychic disturbances, ranging from degrees of euphoria to severe psychosis with suicidal tendency, can develop. These have been less frequent in recent years with the use of smaller doses and possibly with greater use of the synthetic steroids.

It must also be appreciated that all the agents in use at the present time suppress the pituitary production of corticotrophin, with resulting atrophy of the patient's own adrenals. Such *adrenal atrophy* is reversible, and these glands respond to stimulation by exogenous corticotrophin. Gradual reduction of dosage permits the patient's self-regulatory mechanism to adjust, and symptoms of adrenal insufficiency are rarely seen when these agents are gradually withdrawn. However, both during therapy and for a period possibly of years after discontinuation of therapy, such glands may not be able to respond to the stress of a surgical procedure or intercurrent infection. Preparation of such patients for surgical procedures, usually with the parenteral use of cortisone or hydrocortisone, is necessary.

Conditions that increase the likelihood that one of the serious side effects of therapy will develop constitute the principal contraindications. These are peptic ulcer, osteoporosis, psychosis or psychoneurosis, and infections that cannot be readily controlled with antimicrobial therapy. Diabetes mellitus, renal insufficiency, and pregnancy are not absolute contraindications. Cardiovascular disease, congestive heart failure, and hypertension require caution and careful choice of appropriate steroid preparations.

Intra-articular Injections of Corticosteroids. A local anti-inflammatory effect is obtained when these steroids (with the exception of cortisone) are injected into an inflamed joint cavity. In rheumatoid arthritis the effect usually is temporary, lasting from a few days to 10 to 14 days. Occasionally longer remissions occur. These injections may be repeated many times without losing their effectiveness. The recommended dose for large joints, such as the knee, is 20 to 30 mg. of hydrocortisone T-butyl acetate or prednisolone T-butyl acetate. Before injecting these compounds into the synovial cavity, it is important to be sure that one is not dealing with an infectious arthritis. Aseptic precautions should be used.

From a practical point of view, intrasynovial treatment is most effective when combined with other measures. It is particularly helpful in controlling inflammation in the knee joint when mild flexion contractures are being corrected by physical or orthopedic procedures. It may be useful when persistent involvement of one or a few of the larger joints has not responded to other measures of treatment. Limitations of intrasynovial therapy stem from the fact that it is a local measure of treatment and that its effect is temporary and suppressive.

Antimalarial Therapy. Evidence has accumulated, particularly from double-blind studies, that certain antimalarial compounds have a moderate beneficial effect in rheumatoid arthritis and also in systemic lupus erythematosus. Their mode of action is not understood and their effectiveness varies greatly. An ameliorating effect is usually not seen until after one to three months of treatment. The drugs that have received the widest use are chloroquine (Aralen), in doses of 250 to 500 mg. daily, and hydroxychloroquine phosphate (Plaquenil), in doses of 200 mg. two to three times daily. Untoward reactions, particularly gastrointestinal disturbances, appear to be related to dosage. Other untoward reactions include skin eruption, headache, visual disturbance, loss of hair, blanching of hair color, and neurologic or mental disturbance. Bone marrow depression and macular retinopathy have been recorded. Since the retinal degeneration may be asymptomatic and can lead to irreversible loss of macular vision, ophthalmologic examination is advised

every three to four months during administration of these drugs.

VARIANTS OF RHEUMATOID ARTHRITIS

Felty's Syndrome. In 1924, Felty described the combination of rheumatoid arthritis with splenomegaly and lymphadenopathy, granulocytopenia, and usually anemia. The joint manifestations are indistinguishable from classic rheumatoid arthritis, and there is not necessarily a correlation between activity and severity of the joint disease and severity of the hematologic abnormality. The clinical significance of this combination rests on the evidence that the hematologic abnormalities are due to hypersplenism. Tests for the rheumatoid factor are nearly always positive. Frequently very high titers are obtained. The hematologic manifestations of the hypersplenism can usually be temporarily improved by the use of adrenocortical steroids, but invariably relapse occurs when treatment is discontinued. Splenectomy is the treatment of choice. Following removal of the spleen, the blood picture usually returns to normal, but there is no consistent effect on the course of the arthritis.

Sjögren's Syndrome. In 1933 Sjögren called attention to the combination of keratoconjunctivitis sicca, xerostomia, and rheumatoid arthritis. The term is applied when any two of these features are present. In some cases, lupus erythematosus, scleroderma, or polyarteritis nodosa may replace rheumatoid arthritis in the complex.

The joint involvement in this syndrome has no distinguishing characteristics. The lack of lacrimal and salivary secretions is due to inflammation and fibrosis in the salivary and lacrimal glands. Typically these consist of dense, intralobular infiltration of lymphocytes with atrophy of acinar tissue, and proliferation of the duct lining cells, resulting in narrowing or obliteration of the duct lumen. The pathologic changes have been compared with those seen in the thyroid gland in Hashimoto's struma.

Suspicion of this diagnosis should arise from the complaint of dryness of the eyes and mouth, and is confirmed by estimating the amount of tears produced, using the Schirmer test. Recent studies have revealed an abundance of diverse abnormal humoral antibodies to tissue components in the serums of patients with this syndrome. Nearly all patients show positive tests for the rheumatoid factor, but in addition there is a high percentage of positive tests for antinuclear antibody, thyroglobulin antibody, and complement-fixing antibodies to various human organs and tissues. Subsequent development of reticulum cell sarcoma has been noted.

Treatment of this condition is essentially treatment of the rheumatoid arthritis. No treatment is effective in restoring the lacrimal and salivary secretions. Use of artificial tears may be of symptomatic benefit and may prevent ocular complications due to the keratitis sicca.

Bernstein, C. A., and Freyberg, R. H.: Rheumatoid patients after five or more years of corticosteroid treatment: A comparative analysis of 183 cases. Ann. Intern. Med., 54:938, 1961.

Bunim, J. J.: A broader spectrum of Sjögren's syndrome and its pathogenetic implications. Ann Rheum. Dis., 20:1, 1961.

Christian, C. L., et al.: Eighteenth rheumatism review. Review of American and English literature for years 1965 and 1966. Arthritis Rheum., 11:525, 1968.

Empire Rheumatism Council, Research Subcommittee: Gold therapy in rheumatoid arthritis, final report of a multicentre controlled trial. Ann. Rheum. Dis., 20:35, 1961.

Hamerman, D.: New thoughts on the pathogenesis of rheumatoid arthritis (editorial). Amer. J. Med., 40:1, 1966.

Hollander, J. L., et al.: Arthritis and Allied Conditions. Textbook of Rheumatology. 7th ed. Philadelphia, Lea & Febiger, 1966.

Hollander, J. L., McCarty, D. J., Jr., Astorga, G., and Castro-Murrilo, E.: Studies on the pathogenesis of rheumatoid joint inflammation: I. The "R.A." cell and a working hypothesis. Ann. Intern. Med., 62:271, 1965.

Hollingsworth, J. W.: Local and Systemic Complications of Rheumatoid Arthritis. Philadelphia, W. B. Saunders Company, 1968.

Ruderman, M., Miller, L. M., and Pinals, R. S.: Clinical and serologic observations of 27 patients with Felty s syndrome. Arthritis Rheum., 11:377, 1968.

Short, C. L., Bauer, W., and Reynolds, W. D.: Rheumatoid Arthritis. Cambridge, Harvard University Press, 1957.

Vaughan, J. H., Morgan, E. S., and Jacon, R. R.: Role of gamma globulin complexes in rheumatoid arthritis. Trans. Ass. Amer. Physicians, 81:231, 1968.

Other Forms of Polyarthritis of Unknown Etiology

Juvenile Rheumatoid Arthritis. When rheumatoid arthritis occurs in children, certain features differ from the picture usually seen in adults. The constitutional symptoms, particularly fever, are likely to be more severe and may indeed precede the development of arthritis at times by several weeks or months. A variety of nonspecific skin rashes, usually of the erythema multiforme type, may be seen. Nodules are rare. Uveitis is frequent, and may lead to blindness. Evidence of cardiac involvement with pericarditis or valvular lesions is more common, as is also enlargement of the lymph nodes, liver, and spleen. The eponym *Still's disease* has been applied to juvenile rheumatoid arthritis in which such visceral involvement is prominent; there is general agreement that the range of manifestations in rheumatoid arthritis in children is just as varied as in the disease in adults and that separation of this combination as a disease entity is not justified. Monoarticular involvement at the onset of the disease is more frequent in children than in adults.

Certain skeletal abnormalities occur in children primarily because of interference with the normal rate of growth in secondary bone centers. The rheumatoid inflammation in proximity to these centers may temporarily accelerate their rate of growth and then may cause premature closure of the epiphysis. This may result in failure of certain bones, such as the mandible, to develop fully. Also particularly striking in juvenile rheumatoid arthritis is the predilection for involvement of the cervical spine, leading to ankylosis of the cervical vertebrae; other portions of the spine are spared. Tests for rheumatoid factor are positive in a lower percentage of children with rheumatoid arthritis than in adults.

Arthritis Associated with Agammaglobulinemia. Approximately one quarter of patients with congenital and acquired agammaglobulinemia develop a nonsuppurative form of arthritis with many features of rheumatoid arthritis. The joints exhibit effusion, slight increase in heat, pain and tenderness, and some limitation of motion. The joint involvement is usually asymmetrical and not associated with roentgenographic changes. The arthritis in most cases either has been transient, subsiding in a few weeks without evidence of residual damage, or has persisted for years with effusion and slight tenderness and little evidence of progressive change. Biopsy specimens of the synovial membrane have been indistinguishable from those obtained in rheumatoid arthritis. Usually the erythrocyte sedimentation rate is normal, other tests for "acute phase reactions" are negative, and tests for the rheumatoid factor are negative.

Although agammaglobulinemia is rare, the occurrence in this condition of arthritis closely simulating rheumatoid arthritis is of considerable interest because of its implications concerning the etiology of rheumatoid arthritis. The arthritis responds to salicylates and corticosteroids, but the latter should be avoided because of their tendency to aggravate infections. Treatment is directed at the underlying agammaglobulinemia and protection of the patient from intercurrent infection by antimicrobial drugs.

Palindromic Rheumatism. This term was applied by Hench and Rosenberg in 1944 to an unusual and often recurring form of arthritis. The outstanding features are multiple afebrile attacks of acute arthritis and periarthritis with pain, swelling, redness, and disability of one or more joints. The attacks appear suddenly and develop rapidly. Each attack is followed by a complete remission, and most attacks run their course within a few hours to a day or two. Any joint may be affected, but there is a distinct predilection for the finger joints. In spite of the frequent recurrences and the transitory but definite evidence of articular inflammation, there is little or no constitutional reaction, no persistent abnormality in laboratory tests, and no significant functional, pathologic, or roentgenographic residue even after years of the disease.

The cause of palindromic rheumatism has not been determined. Biopsies of acutely inflamed joints reveal exudation of polymorphonuclear leukocytes and thickening of the synovial villi. Some observers believe that it represents a prodrome or an atypical onset of rheumatic arthritis.

The differential diagnosis includes an episodic form of rheumatoid arthritis, gout, and systemic lupus erythematosus. Palindromic rheumatism affects males and females in equal numbers. Repeated attacks affect different joints. There is an absence of constitutional symptoms, and evidences of joint inflammation and discomfort subside completely between attacks. The serum uric acid is not elevated. Even if rigid criteria are adhered to, it appears that palindromic rheumatism cannot be distinguished from episodic rheumatoid arthritis or systemic lupus erythematosus early in the disease. The joint involvement characteristically does not respond to salicylates. Some of these patients have been benefited by gold therapy.

Intermittent Hydrarthrosis. This is an uncommon and chronic disorder characterized by periodic recurrences of joint effusion persisting for several days. The knees are most often affected; usually the condition appears in one knee, although it may be bilateral. Particularly characteristic is the regularity of recurrence; there is an average interval between attacks of seven to eleven days and a duration of the effusion for three to five days. During the attack the joint is distended with fluid, and the patient has pain on use of the extremity. There is no local inflammation, and there are no constitutional symptoms. In certain instances this syndrome may be the initial symptom of a definite rheumatoid arthritis. In others, the effusions may occur regularly for many years and then cease for no apparent reason.

The cause of the disease is unknown. Aspirated joint fluid is clear and may show considerable elevation of the leukocyte count, with as high as 50 per cent polymorphonuclear cells. A good mucin clot on the addition of dilute acetic acid and a high viscosity in relationship to hyaluronic acid concentration are in contrast to the findings in rheumatoid synovial fluid.

The results of treatment have not been impressive. Salicylates do not affect the appearance or duration of the effusion, and the response to intraarticular steroids has not been encouraging. Local discomfort may be relieved by hot applications and rest, and simple joint aspiration will relieve pressure if the joint becomes too uncomfortable. There is a spontaneous remission in a significant number of patients.

Ankylosing (Rheumatoid) Spondylitis (Marie-Strümpell Spondylitis; Von Bechterew-Strümpell Spondylitis). This disease is a chronic and usually progressive disease of the sacroiliac joints, the apophyseal joints (which are the synovial joints of the spine) and the adjacent soft tissues. The process begins nearly always in the sacroiliac joints and spreads upward to involve the synovial joints of the spine at increasingly higher levels. The costovertebral joints, the hips, and the shoulders are often involved. Pathologic changes are essentially those of chronic proliferative inflammation involving joint capsules and intervertebral ligaments; its outstanding characteristic is calcification in the outer layers of the anulus fibrosus of the intervertebral discs and in the overlying intervertebral ligaments. Ankylosis of the entire spine may occur, preventing motion in any direction. The chronic proliferative inflammatory changes of the synovium of the affected joints resemble closely those seen in rheumatoid arthritis; in addition, there is a greater degree of chondritis and osteitis. Arthritis of the peripheral joints, which coexists in 20 per cent or more of the cases, shows histopathologic changes indistinguishable from those of rheumatoid arthritis.

Although the pathologic features of ankylosing spondylitis closely resemble those of classic rheumatoid arthritis, there are sufficient differences so that many students of the disease regard it as a separate entity. Ankylosing spondylitis is essentially a disease of young men; about 90 per cent of cases occur in males, and the onset is frequently in the late teens or early twenties. Less than 10 per cent of patients with ankylosing spondylitis show positive tests for the rheumatoid factor. Subcutaneous nodules do not occur in ankylosing spondylitis. Episodes of uveitis or iritis occur in 10 to 15 per cent of patients, two to three times more frequently than in rheumatoid arthritis. The evidences of constitutional involvement are also less impressive in ankylosing spondylitis. Clinically, fatigue, weight loss, and anorexia are less common, and the sedimentation rate may be normal in 20 per cent of patients. The frequency and degree of abnormality in the electrophoretic pattern are less. When muscle biopsies are done, there is a lower incidence of inflammatory foci in the connective tissue between nerve and muscle bundles. An unusual type of heart disease with fairly specific characteristics has been described as a complication of ankylosing spondylitis. Clinically this is manifested as isolated *aortic insufficiency*. Pathologically, the typical lesion involves the aortic valve and the ascending aorta and can be distinguished from syphilitic aortitis and from rheumatic valvular disease.

The cause of the disease is unknown. Evidence for a genetic or hereditary factor in ankylosing spondylitis is somewhat more impressive than in rheumatoid arthritis of the peripheral joints. A positive family history of either ankylosing spondylitis or rheumatoid arthritis may often be obtained.

Clinical Manifestations. Initial symptoms are usually pain in the low back or in the hip and sciatic regions. The pain may awaken the patient in the early morning hours, and is nearly always associated with a considerable degree of morning stiffness referred to the back. As the disease progresses, symptoms referable to the lumbar and dorsal spine may develop, and pain on breathing and coughing may reflect involvement of the costovertebral joints. Involvement of the cervical spine usually occurs late in the disease. The symptoms are characteristically intermittent, attacks of aching and stiffness lasting a few days or weeks at a time and then subsiding almost completely. Less often the onset is acute, and progression is rapid. In one third to one half of the patients there may be involvement of the peripheral joints at some stage in the disease, and onset with peripheral joint involvement, particularly in the knees, is not uncommon. The peripheral arthritis may be relatively transient, clearing up spontaneously in a few months, or may be progressive and indistinguishable clinically and roentgenographically from rheumatoid arthritis without spinal involvement.

On physical examination in early cases the only finding may be tenderness to thumping over the sacroiliac joints and back pain when the lower extremities are flexed on the abdomen. Straightening of the lumbar spine, with loss of the normal lumbar lordosis, and limitation of flexion and extension are evidences of involvement of the lumbar spine. Impairment of rotary motion and of lateral bending, often associated with limitation of chest expansion, is evidence of thoracic spine involvement. Involvement of the cervical spine is manifested by pain and limitation of motion in all directions. In advanced cases, the entire spine may be fixed, with severe flexion and kyphosis, and the patient may be further handicapped by arthritis of the hips.

Roentgenographic Signs. The most important diagnostic procedure, even in early spondylitis, is adequate roentgenographic examination of the sacroiliac joints. The first changes consist of sclerosis of the subchondral bone and spotty demineralization of the juxta-articular portion of the ilium and of the sacrum. These changes are almost always bilateral, although not necessarily symmetrical in degree or extent. The margins of the sacroiliac joints appear blurred and indistinct (see Fig. 5). With further progression, fusion between the sacrum and ilium gradually develops over a period of two to five years, and, as ankylosis occurs, the subchondral bone sclerosis fades. Involvement of the apophyseal joints is difficult to demonstrate by roentgenographic means and is less constant than that in the sacroiliac articulations. Calcification of the outer layer of the intervertebral discs and the intervertebral ligaments is usually first seen in the lateral intervertebral ligaments near the dorsolumbar junction. Ligamentous calcification progresses until in

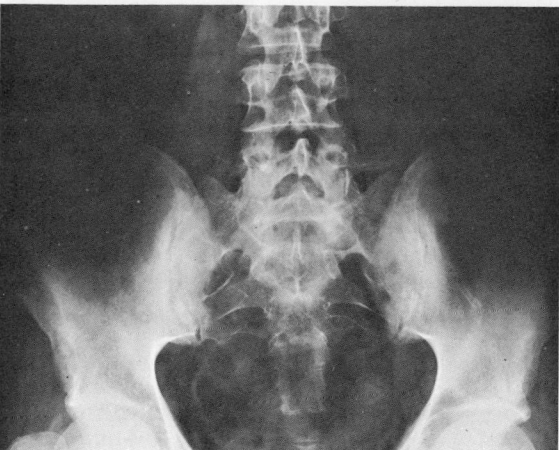

FIGURE 5. Roentgenographic appearance of sacroiliac joints in ankylosing spondylitis. The articular margins are irregular and indistinct. There is sclerosis of the subchondral bone.

advanced cases there appears the so-called "bamboo spine."

Diagnosis. The diagnosis is established by roentgenographic demonstration of the characteristic changes in the sacroiliac joints. Such changes precede intervertebral calcification by two to five years. Intervertebral disc diseases and traumatic and infectious disease of the spine may enter into the differential diagnosis.

Treatment. Therapy of this disease is subject to the same considerations that apply to rheumatoid arthritis. In both conditions it is highly important that the physician recognize the condition early and that proper treatment be instituted before irreversible deformities develop. In early stages treatment consists largely of adequate rest, use of boards under the mattress, elimination of a pillow to prevent flexion deformities of the cervical spine, and special postural and deep breathing exercises.

It is usually necessary to relieve the patient's pain and stiffness before he can cooperate effectively in exercises designed to maintain optimal posture and thoracic expansion. Again, salicylates are the safest analgesics and they are usually effective. However, phenylbutazone is particularly effective in controlling pain and stiffness of ankylosing spondylitis, and in some patients it is clearly superior to the salicylates. Because of potential toxicity, the patient must be observed carefully and the dose kept as low as possible. Initial dosage of phenylbutazone at 100 mg. three to four times a day is recommended, with subsequent decrease of the dose to 100 mg. once or twice daily. Indomethacin also appears to be superior to salicylates in relieving the discomfort in many patients, but has serious toxic hazards which require careful observation and use of minimal effective dosage.

Radiation therapy, although affording symptomatic relief, is rarely if ever justified. It does not affect the progression of the disease, and there is a well documented increase of malignant disease in patients who have received irradiation.

Corticosteroids will produce the same striking

benefit in ankylosing spondylitis that they do in rheumatoid arthritis. However, there is the same tendency to relapse when treatment with these agents is discontinued, and their use is subject to the same limitation as in rheumatoid arthritis. Gold therapy has no value in ankylosing spondylitis.

Every effort should be made to combat the tendency to flexion deformity of the spine by means of postural exercises and, if necessary, by orthopedic measures. Active and passive exercises are extremely important and should be supplemented by breathing exercises to maintain the capacity of the thorax. It is difficult to evaluate the long-term effects of therapy in this disease. The symptoms are characteristically intermittent, and the disease may become spontaneously arrested at any stage in its progression upward in the spine. The disease can progress insidiously, so that the spine gradually becomes stiff, without the patient's being aware of joint discomfort. Nevertheless, by conscientious attention to posture and exercise, the best possible position can be achieved even though the spine becomes fused.

Psoriatic Arthritis. Whether the joint disease that accompanies psoriasis should be regarded as a variant of rheumatoid arthritis or as a separate disease entity is a matter of controversy. Between 5 and 10 per cent of patients with rheumatoid arthritis also have psoriasis, and the coincidence of the two diseases is definitely higher than can be attributed to chance.

The skin disease usually antedates the joint manifestations by months or years, but at times the two systems are involved almost simultaneously, and occasionally joint involvement may precede skin disease. In the great majority of patients, the joint involvement cannot be distinguished by clinical examination, by roentgenographic findings, or by the histologic characteristics from rheumatoid arthritis occurring without psoriasis. The primary distinguishing clinical feature, which actually occurs in a minority of the patients with the two diseases, is inflammatory involvement of the terminal interphalangeal joint. For practical purposes such involvement occurs exclusively in patients with psoriasis, and some workers restrict the use of the term psoriatic arthritis or psoriatic arthropathy to cases of such involvement. There may or may not be psoriatic involvement of the corresponding nails. In some patients, remissions and exacerbations of the arthritis may be associated with remissions and exacerbations of the skin disease, but this is not always true. It is of interest that tests for the rheumatoid factor are rarely positive in psoriasis with arthritis; this is true regardless of involvement of the distal interphalangeal joint.

The treatment of this condition is essentially the same as for rheumatoid arthritis uncomplicated by psoriasis. In general, control of the psoriasis with corticosteroids requires larger doses than are needed to control the joint symptoms, and long-term treatment of the skin lesions with these agents is usually not practical. Antifolic acid agents have been used to treat severe and resistant psoriasis. When such patients also have arthritis, improvement occurs in both skin and joint manifestations.

Arthritis Accompanying Ulcerative Colitis. The incidence of inflammatory arthritis in patients with chronic ulcerative colitis ranges from as low as 5 per cent to as high as 30 per cent in various reported series; the same type of joint involvement occurs less frequently in regional ileitis. Careful study of the behavior of the joint disease accompanying ulcerative colitis shows that it takes the progressive course characteristic of classic rheumatoid arthritis in only 10 per cent of patients. The most striking difference is the tendency for the arthritis of the peripheral joints to be transient, lasting a few days to several months and clearing with little or no impairment of joint function. It is generally agreed that arthritis and colitis tend to flare together. The joints most commonly affected are the knees and ankles, and asymmetrical involvement is more common than in rheumatoid arthritis. Sacroiliac involvement can often be detected roentgenographically. In the majority of patients, the onset of the ulcerative colitis antedates the appearance of joint disease, but the two conditions can appear together. In a few cases arthritis may precede evident colitis by months or years. The joint manifestations may or may not be coincident with erythema nodosum. Tests for the rheumatoid factor are rarely positive and subcutaneous nodules are rarely seen.

Treatment is directed primarily to the chronic ulcerative colitis. The use of salicylate is usually sufficient to relieve the arthritis. Corticosteroids are seldom required for the joint disease, but, if they are indicated for the treatment of the colitis, the arthritis responds promptly also. When colectomy is indicated in severe progressive colitis, the arthritis clears rapidly in most instances.

Ankylosing spondylitis has also recently been reported in a significant number of patients with ulcerative colitis.

Reiter's Syndrome. The name of the German physician who described this combination in 1916 is attached to the triad of nongonococcal urethritis, conjunctivitis, and a subacute or chronic polyarthritis. Mucocutaneous lesions are very common and may be characteristic.

The disease occurs almost entirely in young male adults, although it has been observed rarely in women and in children. There may or may not be a history of antecedent sexual exposure. The British frequently regard Reiter's syndrome as a venereal disease in which gonococcal urethritis may occasionally coexist with the abacterial urethritis of Reiter's syndrome; many European authors regard this syndrome as a complication of bacillary dysentery. In this country the syndrome is usually observed in patients who deny sexual exposure, and antecedent diarrhea is infrequent.

Etiology. Features of the disease have led

many workers to believe that it is infectious in origin and that it should be regarded as a venereal disease. The infrequency of Reiter's syndrome among women and the absence of symptoms in female partners of men developing the disease would appear to challenge the venereal thesis. Usual bacteriologic studies have recovered no micro-organism consistently. Although pleuropneumonia-like organisms have been recovered from the genitourinary tract of several patients with Reiter's syndrome, they have also been found in persons who had no evident pathologic condition. It is well established that Reiter's syndrome may follow dysentery, but there is no evidence that the dysentery bacillus is the etiologic agent. Organisms of the psittacosis-lymphogranuloma venereum-trachoma group of microorganisms (Bedsoniae) have been isolated from tissues of some patients with Reiter's syndrome. Current information indicates that Bedsonia infection alone cannot explain all cases of this syndrome, and that there is as yet no proof of an etiologic role.

Clinical Manifestations. The syndrome is usually ushered in by urethritis, followed by conjunctivitis and then by arthritis. The urethral discharge may be scanty and serous or it may be profuse and bloody. The conjunctival inflammation is most often bilateral and also varies in severity; it may be mild and fleeting or profusely purulent. The arthritis dominates the clinical picture in both severity and duration. Although there is considerable variability, the complete triad is usually manifested within a period of three to four weeks. Constitutional symptoms often accompany the onset of the syndrome; these include malaise, anorexia, loss of weight, and recurrent moderate temperature elevations; chills do not occur.

The urethral and conjunctival signs tend to disappear within a few days or weeks, but the arthritis may persist for much longer periods of time. Recurrences occur in a high percentage of cases and may produce residual damage in any of the three systems.

Mucocutaneous lesions are seen most commonly on the glans penis, on the soles and the palms, and in the mouth. The most common lesion is a superficial moist ulceration on the glans penis, beginning as a small bleb. Its appearance is often independent of the presence or absence of urethritis. Oral lesions begin as tiny vesicles or papules and proceed to superficial ulcerations on the buccal mucosa, the palate, or pharynx. The lesions on the soles and palms appear as erythematous macules which later become hyperkeratotic waxy cones that may increase in number, coalesce, and form thick keratotic crusts or plaques. The lesions of the palms and soles are those of *keratosis blennorrhagica,* and cannot be differentiated from the lesions of pustular psoriasis.

Initially the joint involvement may be migratory, but in a few days it is confined to a few of the larger joints. Although the knees and ankles are most commonly affected, any joint in the body, including the small joints of the hands and feet, may be involved. These joints are usually hot, swollen, and tender, with demonstrable synovial thickening and accumulation of joint fluid. The acute inflammation commonly decreases after the first few weeks and is followed by slow regression in the joint symptoms and objective abnormalities. Remission usually occurs within a period of months but active arthritis has persisted as long as three and a half years.

The disease characteristically undergoes spontaneous remissions, but recurrences are common. Most patients apparently recover completely following one or several attacks, but residual joint damage and chronic arthritis do occur. Some authors have reported unusually high incidence of residual damage of the joints of the feet, and others have called attention to a high incidence of ankylosing spondylitis following typical attacks of Reiter's syndrome.

Laboratory Studies. Pathologic changes in joint tissue obtained from such patients show a consistent combination of acute and chronic inflammatory alterations, dependent somewhat on the duration and clinical course of the joint disease. These are concentrated chiefly in the superficial portions of the synovial membrane. The synovial histopathology has some of the characteristics of rheumatoid arthritis and some of the characteristics of infectious arthritis.

Laboratory findings are not diagnostic. A moderate leukocytosis of 10,000 to 20,000 per cubic millimeter, with an increase in polymorphonuclear cells, is common. The erythrocyte sedimentation rate is rapid and usually correlates with activity of the arthritis. Cultures of urethral, prostatic, and conjunctival exudates and of urine, synovial fluid, and blood show no consistent pathogens. Tests for rheumatoid factor are negative. The synovial fluid alterations are similar to those of mild infections or of early rheumatoid arthritis.

Treatment. Both favorable results and failures have been reported for almost all types of therapy. It is exceedingly difficult to evaluate the response to therapy of a disorder from which patients usually recover spontaneously. Consistently satisfactory results have not been obtained with any antimicrobial drug. The principles of the management of arthritis are the same as those recommended for the basic treatment of rheumatoid arthritis, and the simplest measures that relieve symptoms and minimize severity of sequelae comprise the treatment of choice. The joint manifestations can be suppressed by corticosteroids, but these agents apparently do not shorten the duration of the attack.

Kulka, J. P.: Lesions of Reiter's syndrome. Arthritis Rheum., 5:195, 1962.
Laaksonen, A-L.: A prognostic study of juvenile rheumatoid arthritis. Acta Paediat. Scand. (Suppl. 166), 1966.
Mattingly, S.: Palindromic rheumatism. Ann. Rheum. Dis., 25: 307, 1966.

McEwen, C., Lingg, C., and Kirsner, J.: Arthritis accompanying ulcerative colitis. Amer. J. Med., 33:923, 1962.

Schacter, J., Barnes, J. P., Engelman, E. P., and Meyer, K. F.: Isolation of Bedsoniae from the joints of patients with Reiter's syndrome. Proc. Soc. Exp. Biol. Med., 122:283, 1966.

Sharp, J.: Ankylosing spondylitis. Proc. Roy. Soc. Med., 59:453, 1966.

Ward, L. E.: Current methods of treatment: Rheumatoid spondylitis. Arthritis Rheum., 6:650, 1963.

Weinberger, H. W., Ropes, M. W., Kulka, J. P., and Bauer, W.: Reiter's syndrome, clinical and pathologic observations. Medicine, 41:35, 1962.

Wright, V.: Rheumatism and psoriasis; a re-evaluation. Amer. J. Med., 27:454, 1959.

Degenerative Joint Disease
(Osteoarthritis, Hypertrophic or Degenerative Arthritis)

Degenerative joint disease is characterized histologically by degeneration of articular cartilage, roentgenographically by hypertrophy of bone at the articular margins, and clinically by pain, which generally occurs on use and is relieved by rest. Changes in the synovial membrane are late and minor in degree. The disease affects chiefly older persons and usually involves weight-bearing joints, with the singular exception of frequent involvement of the terminal interphalangeal joints of the fingers. Characteristically it is not accompanied by systemic manifestations.

The cause is unknown. Its development is closely related to the normal processes of aging of articular structures. The term *primary osteoarthritis* has been used to designate those cases in which there is no apparent cause; the disease is regarded by some as the result of ordinary wear and tear. *Secondary osteoarthritis* can result from excessive or abnormal stresses and strains related to obesity or postural and orthopedic abnormalities; it may be a late result of trauma to the joint structures or of chronic irritation produced by internal joint derangements; it may appear in joints previously damaged by antecedent arthritis of other types and in joints in which the inherent integrity of the cartilage is weakened by metabolic abnormalities or hereditary factors.

Pathology. Understanding of the pathologic changes has been derived chiefly from study of the normal aging process in the joints. An excellent study of this type by Bennett, Waine, and Bauer reported the gross and microscopic appearance of knee joints obtained post mortem or following amputation in 63 cases. Abnormalities in the articular structures first appear in the second decade and increase with advancing age. First changes appear in the articular cartilage and consist of softening, roughening, and fibrillation. Later, clefts and pits appear, followed by erosion. Lipping at the margins of the joints is observed as early as the fourth decade and becomes increasingly evident in later years. As the cartilaginous surfaces become roughened and irregular, the cartilage is worn away, and the underlying bone is finally laid bare. The exposed bone becomes dense and hardened and takes on a highly polished, eburnated appearance. The synovial membrane is normal but may show thickening and hypertrophy of the villous processes. The joint cavity is never obliterated; the synovial membrane does not form adhesions, and ankylosis does not occur.

The gross and microscopic changes in the articular cartilage are preceded by submicroscopic alteration of alignment of the collagen fibrils and changes in the physical-chemical properties of the ground substance. As degenerative changes develop, the orderly pattern of the cartilage cells is disrupted, and large accumulations of cells appear in the vicinity of clefts and fissures, presumably due to increased cell division in an abortive attempt at regeneration. The bony marginal proliferation (spurs, osteophytes, lipping, exostoses) consist of spongy bone covered with cartilage. The stimulus for such spur formation is not clear.

These changes in normal and pathologic aging of the joints correlate well with most of the clinical characteristics of degenerative joint disease. It is important to appreciate that the extent of degeneration varies greatly among individuals and that some persons show more degenerative articular changes at 35 than others do at 60. It is clear that marginal proliferation is not an early sign of degenerative joint disease and that articular lipping is not a prerequisite for the diagnosis. It is also obvious that absence of roentgenographic abnormalities does not rule out degenerative joint disease, for the early changes in the articular cartilage are not visualized by roentgenographic examination.

Predisposing Factors. Age is obviously the most important predisposing factor. The disease occurs almost exclusively in middle-aged and elderly people. Occurrence of symptoms is particularly common in women at the time of the menopause.

Another important factor is trauma. This may be mild or long-continued irritation, or contusions, fractures, or dislocations of the joint. Among the most frequent causes of trauma is obesity. Postural or mechanical defects predispose to hypertrophic arthritis by putting an unnatural strain on the joint or by bringing about unequal pressure on the joint surfaces. Occupation may have an important bearing on the development of degenerative arthritis, for any joint which has been subjected to constant strenuous use is liable to develop such changes.

The most striking exception to trauma as a predisposing factor is seen in the predilection of osteoarthritis for the terminal interphalangeal joints, with the production of *Heberden's nodes.* In this condition, which is not necessarily associated with osteoarthritis elsewhere, there is impressive evidence of an important genetic factor.

Rare forms of degenerative joint disease with certain special features suggest that metabolic, endocrine, and dietary factors that influence the integrity of articular cartilage may predispose to the development of osteoarthritis. *Ochronosis* is often associated with unusually severe degenerative arthritis, presumably because the abnormal pigment deposited in the cartilage affects its physical properties. *Acromegaly*, in which there is excessive proliferation of cartilage, is associated with osteoarthritis with an unusual degree of bony overgrowth. *Kashin-Beck disease* is a chronic disabling degenerative disease of the peripheral joints and spine, occurring principally in childhood and endemic in eastern Siberia, northern China, and Korea. It is attributed to the ingestion of cereal grain infected with a specific fungus. In *hemophilia*, repeated hemorrhages into the joint eventually result in severe osteoarthritic change; an unusual feature is large cyst formation in the underlying bone.

Symptoms and Physical Signs. One of the baffling but fascinating aspects of osteoarthritis is lack of correlation between the symptoms and the degree of degenerative change, particularly as evidenced in the roentgenogram. A patient with advanced degenerative joint disease may have few or no complaints, whereas another patient showing only minor changes may be most uncomfortable. The most characteristic symptom in this disease is an aching pain, which occurs on use, is rarely intense, and is relieved by rest. Stiffness after sitting, and particularly with the first few motions involving use of the part, is a common complaint. However, such stiffness is relatively short in duration and rarely persists more than a few minutes, in contrast with stiffness in rheumatoid arthritis, which may persist for hours.

Objectively, the joints may appear normal, but crepitus, creaking, and grating are usually detected. There may be localized tenderness. When the joint is enlarged, the swelling usually feels hard. Increase in synovial fluid is uncommon, but may occur, particularly in the knees. In contrast to the effusion in rheumatoid arthritis, the increase in joint fluid in the synovial cavity disappears within a day or two if weight bearing is eliminated. The range of motion is usually not impaired, except in osteoarthritis of the hip. Ankylosis occurs rarely.

Diagnosis. The diagnosis of primary osteoarthritis can usually be made without difficulty. The age of the patient, the gradual onset of symptoms, and the characteristic stiffness in one or more joints, combined with absence of evidence of inflammatory disease, are the major points.

Clinical or laboratory evidence of a constitutional disease is lacking. Characteristic changes in the roentgenograms help to confirm the diagnosis.

Some judgment, however, is needed in correlating the roentgenographic findings with the patient's symptoms. It is important to remember that mild osteoarthritis can be present in a joint without causing symptoms. Some degree of senescent changes in the joints must be considered physiologic; the physician may prematurely attribute the patient's back symptoms, for example, to osteoarthritis of the lumbar spine when careful evaluation would indicate that the symptoms are related to poor posture, developmental abnormalities, or muscle strain.

Laboratory Findings. The erythrocyte sedimentation rate is normal, and tests for the other "acute phase reactants" are negative. The joint fluid in osteoarthritis characteristically has a low cell count, ranging from a few hundred to two or three thousand per cubic millimeter; the cells are predominantly mononuclear. The quantity and quality of the mucin is normal, and viscosity is not impaired.

Roentgenographic Findings. Many gradations of abnormality may be noted. Fairly characteristic findings early in the disease are sharpening of the articular margins. As cartilage degenerates and is eroded, the joint interspace appears narrow, and there may be erosion of the articular bone and alteration of the shape of the articulating surfaces. However, the bony surface remains well defined, and there is some condensation of subchondral bone. Later the periarticular lipping becomes more conspicuous. Bone cysts can occur.

Differential Diagnosis. Differential diagnosis of osteoarthritis from *rheumatoid arthritis* has been discussed in the section on rheumatoid arthritis. Osteoarthritis in some cases may be confused with *gout* if sufficient attention is not paid to the history of paroxysmal and intermittent attacks. Secondary osteoarthritis can occur in patients with chronic tophaceous gout. The differentiation of osteoarthritis from a *Charcot joint* is simple if the latter possibility is kept in mind. The physician should always be aware of the possibility that a *metastatic malignant disease* can cause pain in the cervical and lumbar spine or in the hips or pelvis. Routine roentgenographic studies will prevent attributing such pain to osteoarthritis.

Prognosis. There is no "cure" for osteoarthritis in the sense of reversal of the pathologic changes. The destruction of cartilage and the hypertrophic changes in the bone cannot be altered. However, the progress of osteoarthritis is slow, and the outlook for preservation of joint function is much better than in many other types of arthritis. In most cases the patient's discomfort can be completely relieved by proper treatment, even though the pathologic changes in the joints persist. This is particularly true when predisposing factors can be accurately evaluated and corrected by weight reduction, physical therapy, and orthopedic measures.

Treatment. It is always worthwhile to take the

time to explain the nature of the disease to the patient and to reassure him that the condition is relatively nonprogressive and will not result in deformity or incapacitation. Careful evaluation of predisposing factors and correction of postural defects and orthopedic abnormalities is often of great help. For obese patients with painful knees and hips, the most important aspect of treatment is weight reduction. Diet plays no part in the treatment of osteoarthritis except in relationship to obesity.

Physical therapy is particularly important in the management of symptomatic osteoarthritis. Heat relieves the aching and stiffness. Moist heat seems more effective than dry heat. Moderate exercises are helpful, particularly if distinction is made between non-weight-bearing and weight-bearing exercises. Patients whose symptoms are clearly related to overactivity must learn to live within tolerable limits. When lower extremity joints are involved, it may be particularly important to limit the amount of time the patient is on his feet. Several short periods of walking or standing are preferable to one long one.

Analgesics, particularly salicylates, are useful in controlling the symptoms of osteoarthritis. Phenylbutazone is sometimes helpful when salicylates have failed, but the potential toxic reactions rarely justify its use in such a mild disorder. Systemic corticosteroid therapy is not recommended for osteoarthritis. Intra-articular injections of hydrocortisone acetate or related steroids (with the exception of cortisone) may be helpful for joints which fail to respond to simpler measures. Painful knees are frequently benefited by this treatment, and sometimes relief persists for several weeks. However, such local use of steroids should be combined with physical therapy, and the patient must be instructed not to overuse the joints merely because his symptoms have been relieved.

SPECIAL FORMS OF DEGENERATIVE JOINT DISEASE

Heberden's Nodes. One of the most common manifestations of degenerative joint disease is a cartilaginous and bony enlargement of the terminal interphalangeal joints of the fingers. Women are affected about ten times as frequently as men. In large series of patients, Stecher has found this condition to occur twice as commonly in sisters of women affected as would be expected normally in the general population. The hereditary pattern is compatible with a genetic mechanism involving a single autosomal gene dominant in females and recessive in males. Similar nodes may develop soon after a specific injury; for example, in base-

ball players, and on the thumb, middle, and fourth fingers of bowlers.

Clinically, these enlargements often develop insidiously, without symptoms, and progress unnoticed for months or years. In other patients, they may develop rather rapidly, with swelling, local tenderness, and aching after use. The nodes may be particularly sensitive to pressure. Some patients complain of numbness and tingling of the finger tips and a sense of clumsiness on use. Such symptoms are usually of only a few months' duration and subside completely, although there may be no change whatever in the objective findings. Occasionally, the original swelling is preceded or complicated by the occurrence of small gelatinous *synovial cysts* on the dorsal aspect of the terminal interphalangeal joint or just proximal to it.

On examination, the terminal interphalangeal joints of one or several fingers present a hard swelling usually localized to the dorsal and lateral aspects of the joint, which may or may not be tender. When the changes are advanced, there may be flexion and lateral deviation at the terminal interphalangeal joint. Roentgenograms demonstrate enlargements of the ends of the bones, with distortion of the joint space, irregularities of the joint surface, and the development of lateral spurs as well as spurs at the attachments of the flexor and extensor tendons of the terminal phalanx. Since the palpable enlargement may consist of cartilage as well as bone, one is occasionally surprised to find that roentgenographic examination shows only minimal bony spurring.

Much less commonly, the proximal interphalangeal joints may be involved with the same type of changes; such involvement goes under the eponym of *Bouchard's nodes.*

Treatment. When Heberden's nodes are symptomatic, salicylates are helpful; use of the hands should be restricted as much as possible. Heat is particularly effective in relief of symptoms. The application of the paraffin bath is particularly useful in this condition. The method of applying paraffin is as follows:

Equipment: A candy or fat thermometer
    2 to 4 pounds of Parowax
    1 piece of silk cloth, 12 by 14 inches
    1 square of absorbent cotton or piece of wool
Parowax is melted gently and allowed to cool until the thermometer registers 110 to 120° F. The hands are soaked in hot water for about 3 minutes and, while still wet, are dipped into and out of the Parowax 12 to 15 times. The hands are then wrapped in oiled silk, over the accumulated Parowax, and then wrapped in the cotton or wool so that the heat may be retained. The pack can be left on for as long as an hour. The wax can then be removed and re-used at the next application. (Warning: the wax is flammable.)

Osteoarthritis of the Hip (Malum Coxae Senilis). This is the most disabling form of osteoarthritis. It results from degeneration of the articular cartilage both over the head of the femur and in the acetabulum, associated with or followed by changes in the underlying bone. Predisposing factors may include preexisting hip joint disease, such as trauma, slipped femoral epiphysis, developmental abnormalities of the femoral head and neck resulting in altered weight bearing, avascular necrosis of the head of the femur, or osteochondritis dissecans. Osteoarthritis of the hip occurs more frequently in men than in women. It is unilateral in about two thirds of cases.

In the early stages, pain is felt in the distribution of the sciatic, obturator, and anterior crural nerves, and is consistently related to weight bearing. Later, pain anteriorly and in the groin is prominent and may radiate to the knee joint. Occasionally, the symptoms in the knee joint are so prominent that the disease in the affected hip may be overlooked. The patient walks with a limp, and abduction and rotation of the hip become limited. In advanced cases, the leg is held in flexion, abduction, and external rotation, and the patient has an awkward, shuffling gait and experiences difficulty in sitting.

On examination of the joint, crepitation can usually be detected, and there is limitation of motion in the hip joint. On roentgenographic examination, the earliest evidence of the disease is increased density in the posterosuperior border of the acetabulum and the anterosuperior surface of the head of the femur. Decrease of width of cartilage is evident, especially in the weight-bearing portions of the femoral head and acetabulum. In well developed cases, roentgenographic examination shows loss of cartilage, sclerosis of the subchrondral bone, marginal extoses, and frequently bone cysts. The degree of pain varies widely and is not necessarily proportionate to the extent of bony change.

Treatment. Management of these patients is often difficult and unsatisfactory. Rest, particularly with limitation of weight bearing, and use of heat and non-weight-bearing exercises may be satisfactory as long as the pain is not too severe. Protection of the joint by the use of crutches or a cane is often helpful. Severe pain with muscle spasm may require use of traction. Intra-articular injection is usually disappointing in osteoarthritis of the hip. Surgery may be necessary in order to relieve severe pain and disability. Arthrodesis, when successful, gives complete relief of pain but leaves the patient with a stiff hip. Arthroplasty, usually with the insertion of a vitallium cup or prosthesis for the femoral head, preserves some motion but is less consistent in giving relief from pain. The type of surgery selected is usually adapted to the patient's occupation, temperament, and general condition.

Osteoarthritis of the Spine (Hypertrophic Spondylitis). The vertebral column can be affected by a variety of degenerative changes. Properly speaking, osteoarthritis as discussed previously in this section is a disease of synovial (diarthrodial) joints. Therefore, true osteoarthritis of the spine can occur only in the apophyseal and costovertebral joints. Such changes have been demonstrated in pathologic studies, but it is difficult to recognize them clinically or by roentgenographic examination.

The commonly recognized degenerative changes in the spine consist of lipping and spur formation (osteophytes) on the bodies of the spinal vertebrae. These changes clearly have their pathogenesis in a disorder of the intervertebral disc. Osteophytes do not form as long as the nucleus of the intervening disc is intact and the vertebral bodies are normally separated. However, when collapse of the disc follows degeneration or prolapse of the nucleus, the vertebra above tips forward slightly, and there is extrusion, usually forward, of the plastic disc substance. On either side of this extended disc osteophytes subsequently develop, presumably because the strain on the vertebral ligaments results in periosteal irritation and proliferation of bone. Disc collapse and osteophytosis of vertebral bodies lead to immobilization of the affected segments. To distinguish it from the usual type of osteoarthritis, some authors apply the name of *spondylosis* to this change in the vertebral column.

The vertebrae of most people past 50 years of age shows some evidence of this condition. It is important to realize that such findings may be asymptomatic and of no clinical significance. Many errors will be made if symptoms are attributed to osteoarthritis of the spine solely on the basis of reoentgenographic findings. Nerve root pain and paresthesias may be produced by the disc protrusion that precedes the formation of osteophytes; less commonly, it may be attributed to encroachment of the bony spurs on the intervertebral foramina. Conversely, back pain due to faulty posture, trauma, or muscular disorders may be incorrectly attributed to degenerative spinal changes that have been present for many years.

Osteoarthritis of the spine usually develops slowly, and in a great majority of patients it is manifested by gradual limitation of motion without significant pain. There may be aching and stiffness on motion, particularly when the patient is fatigued. Physical findings are usually meager. Tenderness over the spine is often not prominent. Limitation of motion, often with some degree of spasm of the paraspinal muscles, is a characteristic but not pathognomonic finding. Particularly in the cervical spine, an apparently good range of motion can coexist with a considerable degree of degenerative change. The diagnosis ultimately rests on careful appraisal of the patient's symptoms and the change demonstrated in roentgenograms.

Treatment. Treatment follows the principles of that of osteoarthritis in general. Rest is important. These patients should usually sleep on a firm mattress with a bed board beneath it. Faulty weight bearing, abdominal adiposity, and loss of tone of the back muscles should be corrected. Curtailment of activities that produce symptoms is usually indicated. Analgesics in the form of salicylates and application of heat and other forms of physical therapy are worthwhile symptomatic measures. If the patient fails to respond to these, orthopedic measures may become necessary. A strong back brace may afford relief of pain. When severe radicular pain is associated with degenerative changes of the cervical or lumbar spine, appropriate immobilization and traction are indicated.

Bennett, G. A., Waine, H., and Bauer, W.: Changes in the Knee Joint at Various Ages, with Particular Reference to the Development of Degenerative Joint Disease. Cambridge, Harvard University Press, 1942.

Collins, D. H.: The Pathology of Articular and Spinal Diseases. London, Edward Arnold and Company, 1949.
Heberden, W.: Commentaries on History and Cure of Diseases. London, T. Payne, 1802.
Hollander, J. L.: Arthritis and Allied Conditions. 7th ed. Philadelphia, Lea & Febiger, 1966.
Kellgren, J. H.: Current comment: Osteoarthrosis. Arthritis Rheum, 8:568, 1965.
Stecher, R. M.: Hereditary factors in arthritis. M. Clin. N. Amer., 39:499, 1955.

Neuropathic Joint Disease

(Charcot Joint)

Neuropathic joint disease is a chronic progressive degeneration of one or more joints that may develop as a complication of a variety of neurologic disorders leading to sensory disturbances. Classically, it occurs most frequently as a complication of tabes dorsalis. In recent years diabetic neuropathy is increasingly appreciated as a cause of Charcot joints. Involvement of the upper extremities is a complication of syringomyelia.

The pathogenesis of neuropathic joint disease is believed to depend on loss of proprioception and/or pain sensation, which leads to relaxation of supporting structures and chronic instability of the joint. Once the joint is deprived of the normal protective reactions, it is subject to severe and cumulative injury. The pathologic changes are a combination of degenerative and hypertrophic changes similar in many respects to those of non-neuropathic degenerative joint disease. The destructive changes include fragmentation, and bone production is excessive. There are fibrillation and erosion of articular cartilage, destruction of internal joint structures, formation of loose bodies, and exuberant marginal osteophytic growth. Subluxation and dislocation are common, as are intra-articular and juxta-articular fractures.

Charcot joints are encountered more often in men than in women and usually develop after the age of 40. The patient usually notes progressive enlargement of a single large joint, with effusion and instability. The degree of discomfort is unusually mild compared with the degree of distention and joint destruction that may be present. Sometimes a patient presents with dramatic symptoms due to intra-articular or juxta-articular fracture. The characteristic findings are relative absence of pain and remarkable hypermotility of the affected joint. Synovial effusions are persistent and, when there is extensive formation of loose bodies, the joint is described as feeling like a "bag of bones." The roentgenographic findings are characteristic in the well-developed case, showing various degrees of destructive and hypertrophic changes. The diagnosis is established by detecting the associated abnormal neurologic findings characteristic of the underlying disease. Monoarticular involvement in which there is considerable effusion and disproportionately little pain should be particularly suspected.

The Charcot joints associated with tabes dorsalis are most often the knee, hip, and ankle, and the lumbar and lower dorsal spine. Vertebral involvement may lead to kyphosis, but local symptoms may be lacking, and the diagnosis may be suspected only after roentgenograms are reviewed. In diabetic neuropathy, destructive changes occur chiefly in the tarsal and metatarsal joints, less commonly in the ankles, and rarely in the knees. In this variety, the destructive changes dominate, and there may be little or no new bone formation.

There is no satisfactory treatment. Syphilitic lesions are not influenced by penicillin therapy. Braces and splints are necessary to protect the joint against further damage. Surgical fusion may be successful, but it often fails because of infection or nonunion. When the ankle or foot is affected, amputation may be the only practical solution.

Pseudogout

(Articular Chondrocalcinosis, Calcium Pyrophosphate Crystal Deposition Disease)

Acute arthritis of the larger joints occurring at mid-life or beyond has been reported with associated characteristic roentgenographic findings of calcification in articular cartilage and fibrocartilage and with the presence of calcium pyrophosphate crystals in the synovial effusion. The knee is the joint predominantly affected, although attacks have been seen in the ankle, hip, shoulder, elbow, wrists, low back, cervical spine, the medial collateral ligaments of the knee, and the calcaneocuboid joints. Involvement of the great toe has been seen. Typical manifestations are stiffness, swelling, pain, local warmth, and joint tenderness requiring 12 to 36 hours to reach their maximal intensity. Erythema of the overlying skin may appear in severe attacks. The degree of pain varies greatly, but can be severe. The average duration of an attack is seven to ten days, and clustering of attacks is frequent. Low-grade fever and mild leukocytosis may occur. The roentgenographic features are specific, consisting of punctate calcium depositions, most frequently seen in the meniscus of the knee joint, the articular disc in the wrist joint, the articular cartilages in the knee and hip, the symphysis pubis, and the anulus fibrosus of the intervertebral discs. An arthritic may be satisfactorily "screened" for articular chondrocalcinosis with roentgenograms of the knees, pelvis, and both wrists. The diagnosis of pseudogout is established by aspiration of joint fluid and demonstration of characteristic crystals, which are frequently seen within synovial fluid leukocytes during an acute attack. In contrast to the crystals of sodium monourate which are linear or needle shaped and which exhibit strong negative birefringence under polarized light, the crystals of calcium pyrophosphate dihydrate are linear or rhombic in shape and either nonrefringent or weakly birefringent, usually weakly positive. Conclusive demonstration of the nature of the crystals can be established by the x-ray diffraction pattern.

As this entity has become more widely recognized, subacute and chronic arthritis, as well as acute forms, have been described in association with chondrocalcinosis. Association with a number of metabolic and degenerative diseases, such as diabetes and hypertension, is greater than might be expected. In some series hyperuricemia occurs in one third of patients, and the presence of both gout and pseudogout in the same patient is well documented. Aside from the occasional patient with hyperparathyroidism, serum values for calcium and phosphorus are normal.

The mechanism of calcium pyrophosphate crystal precipitation in the cartilage is unknown. The pathogenesis of the acute attack is explained on the basis of phagocytosis of the crystals, providing another example of "crystal-induced synovitis."

Thorough aspiration of the joint is recommended both for diagnostic purposes and for treatment. Injection of insoluble corticosteroids into the joint seems to hasten recovery. Salicylates in large doses and phenylbutazone are frequently helpful. The response to colchicine is usually not as dramatic as in true gout; indeed, this drug may have no effect.

McCarty, D. J., Jr., and Gatter, R. A.: Pseudogout syndrome (articular chondrocalcinosis). Bull. Rheum. Dis., 14:331, 1964.

Moskowitz, R. W., and Katz, D.: Chondrocalcinosis and chondrocalsynovitis (pseudogout syndrome). Analysis of 24 cases. Amer. J. Med., 43:322, 1967.

Mechanical Derangement of Joints

Traumatic Arthritis. Any one or several components of the joints and neighboring structures may be involved in trauma. The dominant injury may be a capsular or ligamentous tear or stretching, contusion of the synovia or juxta-articular bursa, meniscus tears or detachments, or splitting or detachment of the articular cartilage. Joint effusion results from contusion of the synovia, and is particularly common in the knee and ankle. When the degree and duration of the swelling and pain are disproportionate to the severity of the trauma, the possibility must be entertained that this may represent another form of arthritis that can be precipitated by trauma. Examination of the joint fluid may be helpful in such differentiation. Serous traumatic effusions show essentially normal joint fluid characteristics. The treatment of an injured joint consists of rest, physiotherapy, and orthopedic measures as necessary.

The late results of trauma to a joint may be manifested as a localized secondary osteoarthritis.

Internal Derangement of Joints. The knee is especially subject to injuries, with resulting instability of the ligaments and tears of the meniscus. Such injury may be characterized by pain and effusion simulating monoarticular arthritis. An accurate history and careful clinical and roentgenographic examination usually suffice to make the diagnosis. Treatment is orthopedic; surgical removal of damaged structures may be necessary to prevent development of secondary osteoarthritis.

Psychogenic Rheumatism and Fibrositis

Psychogenic rheumatism is the musculoskeletal expression of functional disorders, tension states, or psychoneuroses, equivalent to the functional symptoms that arise in many other systems. The degree of psychoneurosis may vary from a mild anxiety state to a major conversion hysteria. It is characterized by complaints of aching, stiffness, and pain that do not follow the pattern of organic rheumatic disease. The patients present a collection of subjective symptoms without objective manifestations. This was responsible for disability in a significant proportion of soldiers admitted to military general hospitals with musculoskeletal complaints during World War II.

Complaints are characteristically vague in regard to both quality and location of symptoms. The distribution of the pain may be bizarre and without respect for anatomic structures. Qualitatively, the pain does not correspond to that in rheumatic diseases. Such sensations as weakness, fatigue, paresthesias, numbness, deadness, fullness, and pressure may be described as constant, are uninfluenced by the application of heat and physical therapy, and are resistant to salicylates and other analgesics. When the discomfort shows a diurnal variation, it is usually more severe late in the day and exaggerated by fatigue. Physical examination may reveal nothing, or the patient may assume bizarre postures or positions of the extremities.

The diagnosis depends on (1) absence of organic disease, or of disease sufficient to account for the disability, (2) characteristics of the presenting complaints, and (3) evidence for a positive diagnosis of psychopathology. There are frequently associated psychoneurotic manifestations referable to other systems. At times, clear-cut evidence of coexisting psychoneurosis or previous neurotic traits can be elicited in the history. Careful search should be made for precipitating emotional factors by following the sequence of external events prior to onset of symptoms. The responsible precipitating factors most often are those which provoke a sense of grief, rage, or guilt, and there is usually restriction of outward expression of the conflict. A great majority of these patients can be classified as having psychoneurosis, most frequently of the conversion type. However, musculoskeletal complaints, particularly in the back and lower extremities, are occasionally an early manifestation of a serious depression.

The differentiation of psychogenic rheumatism from osteoarthritis and rheumatoid arthritis is usually easy. However, the manifestations of "fibrositis" are largely subjective, and the distinction is less clear. Primary fibrositis, however, follows a characteristic pattern of symptoms, which is lacking in psychogenic rheumatism. Victims of fibrositis are at the mercy of their external environment, whereas victims of psychogenic rheumatism are at the mercy of their internal environment.

Treatment must be directed at the relief of emotional conflict, rationalization of the problems, and correction of the psychoneurosis. The condition can be perpetuated by failure to recognize its fundamental psychogenic nature and by symptomatic treatment.

The term *fibrositis* was introduced to denote presumed chronic inflammatory changes in the white fibrous connective tissue occurring in all parts of the body and giving rise to pain, aching, and stiffness. The postulated pathologic changes have not been demonstrable. With better understanding of mechanical musculoskeletal derangements, many patients who in the past would have been said to be suffering from fibrositis are now recognized to have disc disease, muscle strains, bursitis, or tendinitis.

There remains a definite symptom complex designated as "primary fibrositis" or the "fibrositis syndrome." The chief symptoms are pain, stiffness, and soreness, and the usual signs are tenderness and perhaps some limitation of motion. The most frequent sites are in the neck, shoulder, lower back, and chest areas. There is little or no effect upon the general health of the patient, except at times complaints of easy fatigability. The distress is most often a dull ache, sometimes a burning sensation. Characteristically the symptoms are worse after rest, and particularly worse in the mornings. The muscles seem to jell with rest but the discomfort is definitely relieved by activity. Symptoms may be precipitated or made worse by cold, dampness, drafts, and emotional upsets. Apart from local tenderness, physical examination is entirely negative. The tenderness may be localized to a myalgic spot, the "trigger point" of fibrositis. Laboratory studies, including the sedimentation rate, are normal. Since similar symptoms may be secondary to other diseases, including early rheumatoid arthritis and other forms of joint disease, careful evaluation of the patient is necessary. Postural or muscular structural abnormalities resulting in unusual muscle strain must be evaluated.

Relief is often obtained, at least temporarily, by heat, salicylates, and mental and physical relaxation. Where "trigger points" are found, injection of a local anesthetic will occasionally give relief. The use of local heat followed by active exercises is recommended. These patients should be protected against an undue amount of chilling, dampening, and sudden changes in temperature. Fatigue and exhaustion should be avoided.

Weiss, E.: Psychogenic rheumatism. M. Clin. N. Amer., 39: 601, 1955.

Tumors and Tumorlike Conditions

Of the many swellings that are found in and around joints, very few are caused by new growth. However, when monoarticular swellings develop without definite traumatic history, or when they persist, neoplasia must be considered in the diagnosis. Benign soft tissue tumors include lipoma, hemangioma, exostoses and chondroma, and chondromyxoma. Osteochondroma acting as a cartilaginous rest, may cause symptoms similar to those of derangement, and should be removed. *Xanthomatous giant cell tumor* is a benign lesion, most commonly in the knee joint, with manifestations of effusion or of internal derangement.

Aspirated fluid may be dark or sanguineous and often contains a large amount of cholesterol crystals. This condition is very rarely diagnosed preoperatively.

Synovioma or *synovial sarcoma* is a highly malignant but fortunately rare tumor that may arise from joints or from bursas or tendon sheaths. Primary bone tumors occurring near the joints may cause stiffness, effusion, and limitation of motion. Metastatic tumors near the joints are rare. Probably the most common error is that of diagnosing metastatic carcinoma of the spine as osteoarthritis.

The Painful Shoulder

Pain in the shoulder may be caused by various conditions, including visceral disease. The shoulder can be affected by any of the types of arthritis described previously. Apart from acute traumatic lesions, 85 to 90 per cent of painful disability of the shoulder is due to nonarticular disorders of tendons, bursas, tendon sheaths, and the musculotendinous cuff that gives the shoulder joint its unusual anatomic characteristics.

Calcific Tendinitis (Subacromial Bursitis). Calcific depositis in and about the rotator tendons, and especially in the supraspinatus tendon, are the most frequent abnormality encountered in the subacute or acutely painful shoulder. However, similar calcifications are found in many asymptomatic patients. The commonly accepted pathogenesis of this disorder assumes that the increase in calcium content is an accompaniment of degenerative changes in the tendon. As the calcific granules accumulate, they cause no symptoms in the relatively avascular tendon. However, when they extend to vascular areas, and particularly to the underlying subdeltoid or subacromial bursa, they cause acute inflammation. When exposed at surgery, the calcific deposit has the appearance of a cyst or "sterile furuncle" in the floor of the subdeltoid bursa.

Symptoms. Cardinal symptoms are pain, tenderness, and limitation of motion. The onset may be sudden and the pain severe and agonizing. The pain is felt at the upper humerus and in the subacromial area, often radiates to the insertion of the deltoid, and, in severe cases, even up to the neck and downward to the fingertips. It is increased by motion, particularly abduction and external rotation. Tenderness is exquisite at the lateral area of the humeral head below the acromion and often at and above the insertion of the deltoid. Fever, leukocytosis, and elevated erythrocyte sedimentation rate are occasionally seen in a severe acute attack. Roentgenograms, particularly if taken in both slight internal and slight external rotation, usually reveal the calcific deposit in one of the rotator tendons; or a diffuse opacity in the bursal cavity, resulting from the rupture of the calcium into the bursa, may be visualized.

Acute symptoms may persist for several days and then diminish abruptly or gradually. Sometimes they assume a subacute form. Calcific bursitis in the acute form tends to be self-limited, a fact which makes evaluation of therapy difficult.

Treatment. Treatment consists of rest, with complete or partial immobilization if necessary, and the use of analgesics or other measures to relieve pain. As the pain subsides, physical therapy and exercises are introduced to restore function as rapidly as possible and to prevent residual subacute or chronic progression. Salicylates, in doses of 1 gram four to six times daily, may be useful. When symptoms are severe, the use of meperidine (Demerol) or codeine may be required. Phenylbutazone is considered by some to be a superior analgesic; initial doses are 200 mg. three times daily, later reduced according to response, and limited to a five- to seven-day period. Radiation therapy, local (subacromial) injection of hydrocortisone or other corticosteroid suspension, two-needle irrigation of a calcific deposit with local anesthetic solutions, systemic administration of corticosteroids or corticotrophin, and multiple needling of the calcareous deposits, all have their proponents. Surgical removal of the calcium deposit may be required. It is probably significant that the more acute the symptoms, the more satisfactory are the results reported for each of these forms of treatment. The essential features of management appear to be control of pain by whatever methods are necessary, and instituting range of motion exercises as soon as they can be tolerated.

Chronic Calcareous Bursitis. This is characterized by pain during certain motions, particularly those involving abduction and external rotation. The pain may be steady and nagging or only a sharp stabbing discomfort. Treatment centers primarily around the use of analgesics and physical therapy. The prognosis for recovery of normal shoulder motion is excellent.

Adhesive Capsulitis (Frozen Shoulder, Periarthritis of the Shoulder, Adhesive Bursitis, Adhesive Peritendinitis). Distinct from calcific tendinitis is the painful shoulder of gradual onset, with slowly increasing pain and stiffness, little or no localized tenderness, and progressive limitation of motion. The pathologic change is obliteration of the subdeltoid bursa and adhesive inflammation between the joint capsule and the peripheral articular cartilage. Some cases apparently follow calcareous tendinitis or inflammatory changes in the long head of the biceps tendon in the bicipital groove. In most patients no specific cause can be determined. Prolonged rest in bed or immobilization of the shoulder joint appears to be a predisposing cause. A considerable number of cases follow myocardial infarction or cerebrovascular accidents.

The most common history is of gradually increasing soreness of the shoulder, particularly during abduction and rotation, building up to a peak of constant pain, disability, and disturbed sleep. The pain may be at the upper humerus, may radiate along the arm to the forearm and sometimes posteriorly to the scapular area. There is limitation of motion, particularly in abduction and external rotation. Atrophy of the muscles of the shoulder girdle is almost always present. Roentgenographic examination may show demineralization of the head and upper portion of the humerus. A chronic course with prolonged disability is more common in adhesive capsulitis than in calcareous tendinitis and bursitis. In most cases the chronic disability persists for several months to two or three years.

Treatment. Treatment of this condition is the subject of considerable controversy. Physical therapy, with heat followed by assisted active exercises, is the mainstay. Analgesics are the same as for other forms of painful joints; it is often important to eliminate pain that keeps the patient awake at night. Radiation therapy is rarely as helpful as in acute calcific tendinitis. Systemic corticosteroid therapy is seldom beneficial. Local injection of hydrocortisone directly into the shoulder joint or over tender periarticular structures seems at times to be of value, but frequently is disappointing. In stubborn cases, manipulation of the shoulder under anesthesia may be necessary.

The Shoulder-Hand Syndrome (Reflex Dystrophy of the Upper Extremity, Postinfarctional Sclerodactylia). The shoulder-hand syndrome is a clinical entity characterized by painful disability of the shoulder closely associated with pain and puffy swelling in the homolateral hand, with associated vasomotor changes. Dystrophic changes in the hand and digital contractures may ensue.

Etiology. This syndrome is considered to be a reflex sympathetic dystrophy of the upper extremity, analogous to causalgia and Sudeck's atrophy in any extremity. It has been reported following myocardial infarction, and less commonly in association with other diseases of the thoracic viscera. Some cases are associated with cervical osteoarthritis. It has been described after hemiplegia, splinting of the arm after fracture, after manipulation of a shoulder, and in the convalescent period following an abdominal operation. It usually occurs in patients over the age of 50.

Clinical Manifestations. Symptoms and signs follow a rather typical pattern. Either the shoulder or the hand may be affected first, or the condition may develop in the two simultaneously. Bilateral involvement is seen in one quarter of cases. The shoulder exhibits generalized stiffness and moderate pain that becomes acute on attempted motion. The hand is subject to uniform generalized brawny thickening with edema, usually nonpitting. The pain has causalgic qualities; it is burning and nonsegmental in distribution. The fingers are held in partial flexion, with motion restricted in an effort to avoid pain. Although the patient may complain of pain radiating from the shoulder to the tips of the fingers, the elbow remains singularly unaffected objectively. As the edema spreads, the extremity shows cyanosis and becomes hard, brawny, and less tender. Thickening of the palmar fascia may be noted. The symptoms and findings may persist in this stage from six weeks to three months, and the painful dysfunction gradually subsides. The swelling of the hand also subsides, but stiffness and flexion deformities of the fingers are apt to become more pronounced, with atrophy of subcutaneous tissues and muscles of the hand. In this late stage, the skin of the hand is tight, smooth, and glossy. The muscles show atrophy, and the end stage may resemble Dupuytren's contracture. Roentgenograms reveal a diffuse osteoporosis.

Fortunately, all cases do not progress to deformity. Either spontaneously or as the result of treatment, the condition gradually subsides without evidence of ankylosis or deformity.

Diagnosis. Diagnosis is usually straightforward if the shoulder-hand syndrome is complete. At times the condition must be differentiated from adhesive capsulitis or subacromial bursitis, from a scalenus anticus syndrome and other syndromes of neurovascular compression of the thoracic outlet, and from scleroderma. Some cases of rheumatoid arthritis with acute onset are indistinguishable from typical shoulder-hand syndrome during the first four to six weeks of the disease. Then, as the diffuse edema subsides, persistent localized synovial swelling and development of arthritis in other joints indicate the true nature of the condition. In the typical shoulder-hand syndrome, systemic signs do not occur unless some complication is present. The sedimentation rate is increased in more than 20 per cent of patients. Usually this can be attributed to other disturbances.

Treatment. Most observers believe that early recognition and prompt treatment improve the outlook for resolution of symptoms and prevention of deformity. Exercises of the shoulder and hand, adjusted to the comfort and tolerance of the patient, are probably the most important measures.

For control of pain, large doses of salicylates in divided doses should be tried first. The administration of corticosteroids provides control of pain, but generally requires a somewhat larger dose than is used in rheumatoid arthritis, and it may have to be continued over a period of several months. The recommended initial dose is 20 mg. daily of prednisolone or its equivalent in other steroids, with adjustment of dose according to the response. Stellate ganglion blocks, repeated several times, have been reported effective in relieving pain and vasomotor symptoms in the acute phase.

Prevention. Prevention of the shoulder-hand syndrome may be possible. Avoidance of casts, splints, or manipulations in the management of painful symptoms associated with neurovascular features and effective control of pain in the conditions associated with the shoulder-hand syndrome are recommended. Particularly important may be avoidance of prolonged bed rest for middle-aged or elderly persons. The frequency of the shoulder-hand syndrome following myocardial infarctions appears to be decreasing as these patients are permitted earlier activity. Prophylactic range of motion exercises can be used for patients with myocardial infarctions or hemiplegia for whom prolonged bed rest is necessary.

Bateman, J. E.: The Shoulder and Environs. St. Louis, C. V. Mosby Company, 1955.

Bayles, T. B.: Current methods of treatment: The painful shoulder. Arthritis Rheum., 5:272, 1962.

Steinbrocker, O., and Argyros, T. G.: The shoulder-hand-syndrome: Present status as a diagnostic and therapeutic entity. Med. Clin. N. Amer., 42:1533, 1958.

Polychondritis

(Relapsing Polychondritis, Systemic Chondromalacia, Chronic Atrophic Polychondritis)

A distinctive though rare clinical syndrome is featured by an inflammatory and degenerative process in cartilaginous structures, including those of the nose, ears, laryngotracheobronchial tree, and joints. The disease occurs in both sexes over a wide age range. Its course is chronic with exacerbations and remissions. The acute inflammatory reaction causes pain, erythema, and swelling over the affected cartilage, which may suggest cellulitis of ear or nose, or arthritis. Fever and leukocytosis are usually present at this stage. Episcleritis is a common accompaniment. Diminished hearing, anemia, abnormalities of myocardium and liver, and aortic insufficiency have also been noted.

Following the acute stage, the destruction of cartilage leaves deformities, such as saddle nose

or floppy ear. Collapse of the tracheal or bronchial wall may favor acute respiratory complications; this has led to death in several reported cases. The changes in cartilage appear to be due to loss of chondroitin sulfate from the matrix, and these acid mucopolysaccharides can be recovered in the urine during acute exacerbations. Immunofluorescent studies suggest a possible immunologic mechanism in pathogenesis.

Corticosteroid therapy is the treatment of choice, with initial doses in the range of 20 mg. of prednisone (or its equivalent) daily. Maintenance therapy is nearly always necessary to suppress the inflammatory activity.

Dolan, D. L., Lemmon, G. B., Jr., and Teitelbaum, S. L.: Relapsing polychondritis. Analytic literature review and studies on pathogenesis. Amer. J. Med., 41:285, 1966.

Tietze's Syndrome
(Costal Chondritis, Chondropathia Tuberosa)

This syndrome of unknown cause, characterized by pain, tenderness, and fusiform or spindle-shaped swelling of one or more of the upper costal cartilages (most frequently that of the second rib) is seen in all age groups, most commonly in the fourth decade, with equal frequency in males and females. Roentgenograms are negative, and biopsies reveal no abnormality in the cartilage. Pain of sudden or gradual onset, accentuated by coughing and deep breathing, usually precedes the appearance of swelling. The presence of localized tenderness and swelling locates the disease process. Benign and malignant tumors and angina pectoris may simulate this lesion, which may persist for weeks or years. Treatment is symptomatic.

Levey, G. S., and Calabro, J. J.: Tietze's syndrome: Report of two cases and review of literature. Arthritis Rheum., 5:261, 1962.

Multicentric Reticulohistiocytosis
(Lipoid Dermato-Arthritis)

This is a rare systemic disease manifested by polyarthritis of the hands and large joints and the gradual development of nodules of scalp, ears, paranasal areas, sometimes upper extremities, and oral mucosa. The lesions of skin, mucosa, and synovia are characterized by the presence of lipid-laden histiocytes, including multinucleated giant cells. The lesions have been shown to contain a mixture of lipids. The cause is unknown.

The disease occurs worldwide, affects females three times more frequently than males, and usually begins in middle age. Polyarthritis, simulating rheumatoid arthritis, preceded the appearance of mucocutaneous nodules by months to a few years in two thirds of patients. Rapid progression of joint destruction, particularly in the finger joints, occurs in nearly half the patients. After an average of seven to eight years of waxing and waning, the disease usually becomes quiescent, leaving the patient with crippling arthritis and at times a leonine facies. Destruction of the terminal interphalangeal joints serves as a feature distinguishing it from rheumatoid arthritis. Histologic appearance of nodules is diagnostic and clearly distinct from that of the rheumatoid nodule. Treatment is essentially supportive.

Barrow, M. V., and Holubar, K.: Multicentric histiocytosis: A review of 33 patients. Medicine, 48:287, 1969.

NORMAL LABORATORY VALUES OF CLINICAL IMPORTANCE

Rex B. Conn

NORMAL HEMATOLOGIC VALUES

Acid hemolysis test (Ham)	No hemolysis
Alkaline phosphatase, leukocyte	Total score 14–100
Bleeding time	
Ivy	Less than 5 min.
Duke	1–5 min.
Carboxyhemoglobin	Up to 5% of total
Cell counts	
Erythrocytes: Males	4.6–6.2 million/cu. mm.
Females	4.2–5.4 million/cu. mm.
Children (varies with age)	4.5–5.1 million/cu. mm.
Leukocytes	
Total	5000–10,000/cu. mm.

Differential	Percentage	Absolute
Myelocytes	0	0/cu. mm.
Juvenile neutrophils	3– 5	150– 400/cu. mm.
Segmented neutrophils	54–62	3000–5800/cu. mm.
Lymphocytes	25–33	1500–3000/cu. mm.
Monocytes	3– 7	285– 500/cu. mm.
Eosinophils	1– 3	50– 250/cu. mm.
Basophils	0– 0.75	15– 50/cu. mm.

(Infants and children have greater relative numbers of lymphocytes and monocytes)

Platelets	150,000–350,000/cu. mm.
Reticulocytes	25,000– 75,000/cu. mm.
	0.5–1.5% of erythrocytes
Clot retraction, qualitative	Begins in 30–60 min.
	Complete in 24 hrs.
Coagulation time (Lee-White)	5–15 min. (glass tubes)
	19–60 min. (siliconized tubes)
Cold hemolysin test (Donath-Landsteiner)	No hemolysis
Corpuscular values of erythrocytes	
(Values are for adults; in children, values vary with age)	
M.C.H. (mean corpuscular hemoglobin)	27–31 picogm.
M.C.V. (mean corpuscular volume)	82–92 cu. micra
M.C.H.C. (mean corpuscular hemoglobin concentration)	32–36%
Fibrinogen	200–400 mg./100 ml.
Fibrinolysins	0
Hematocrit	
Males	40–54 ml./100 ml.
Females	37–47 ml./100 ml.
Newborn	49–54 ml./100 ml.
Children (varies with age)	35–49 ml./100 ml.
Hemoglobin	
Males	14.0–18.0 grams/100 ml.
Females	12.0–16.0 grams/100 ml.
Newborn	16.5–19.5 grams/100 ml.
Children (varies with age)	11.2–16.5 grams/100 ml.
Hemoglobin, fetal	Less than 1% of total
Hemoglobin A_2	1.5–3.0% of total
Hemoglobin, plasma	0–5.0 mg./100 ml.
Methemoglobin	0.03–0.13 grams/100 ml.

NORMAL HEMATOLOGIC VALUES (*Continued*)

Osmotic fragility of erythrocytes	Begins in 0.45–0.39% NaCl
	Complete in 0.33–0.30% NaCl
Partial thromboplastin time	60–70 sec.
Kaolin activated	35–45 sec.
Prothrombin consumption	Over 80% consumed in 1 hr.
Prothrombin content	100% (calculated from
	prothrombin time)
Prothrombin time (one stage)	12.0–14.0 sec.
Sedimentation rate	
Wintrobe: Males	0–5 mm. in 1 hr.
Females	0–15 mm. in 1 hr.
Westergren: Males	0–15 mm. in 1 hr.
Females	0–20 mm. in 1 hr.
(May be slightly higher in children and	
during pregnancy)	
Thromboplastin generation test	Compared to normal control
Tourniquet test	Ten or fewer petechiae in a
	2.5 cm. circle after 5 min.
	with cuff at 100 mm. Hg

Bone marrow, differential cell count	Range	Average
Myeloblasts	0.3– 5.0%	2.0%
Promyelocytes	1.0– 8.0%	5.0%
Myelocytes: Neutrophilic	5.0–19.0%	12.0%
Eosinophilic	0.5– 3.0%	1.5%
Basophilic	0.0– 0.5%	0.3%
Metamyelocytes ("juvenile" forms)	13.0–32.0%	22.0%
Polymorphonuclear neutrophils	7.0–30.0%	20.0%
Polymorphonuclear eosinophils	0.5– 4.0%	2.0%
Polymorphonuclear basophils	0.0– 0.7%	0.2%
Lymphocytes	3.0–17.0%	10.0%
Plasma cells	0.0– 2.0%	0.4%
Monocytes	0.5– 5.0%	2.0%
Reticulum cells	0.1– 2.0%	0.2%
Megakaryocytes	0.03– 3.0%	0.4%
Pronormoblasts	1.0– 8.0%	4.0%
Normoblasts	7.0–32.0%	18.0%

NORMAL BLOOD, PLASMA, AND SERUM VALUES

For procedures the normal values may vary depending
upon the methods used.

Acetone, serum	
Qualitative	Negative
Quantitative	0.3–2.0 mg./100 ml.
Aldolase, serum	
Male	Less than 33 units
Female	Less than 19 units
Amino acid nitrogen, serum	4–6 mg./100 ml.
Ammonia nitrogen, blood	75–196 mcg./100 ml.
plasma	56–122 mcg./100 ml.
Amylase, serum	80–160 Somogyi units/100 ml.
Ascorbic acid	See Vitamin C
Base, total, serum	145–160 mEq./liter
Bilirubin, serum	
Direct	0.1–0.4 mg./100 ml.

NORMAL BLOOD, PLASMA, AND SERUM VALUES (*Continued*)

Bilirubin (*Continued*)	
Indirect	0.2–0.7 mg./100 ml.
	(Total minus direct)
Total	0.3–1.1 mg./100 ml.
Calcium, serum	4.5–5.5 mEq./liter
	(9.0–11.0 mg./100 ml.)
	(Slightly higher in children)
	(Varies with protein concentration)
Calcium, serum, ionized	2.1–2.6 mEq./liter
	(4.25–5.25 mg./100 ml.)
Carbon dioxide content, serum	24–30 mEq./liter
	Infants: 20–28 mEq./liter
Carbon dioxide tension (Pco$_2$), blood	35–45 mm. Hg
Carotene, serum	50–300 mcg./100 ml.
Ceruloplasmin, serum	23–44 mg./100 ml.
Chloride, serum	96–106 mEq./liter
Cholesterol, serum	
Total	150–250 mg./100 ml.
Esters	68–76% of total cholesterol
Cholinesterase, serum	0.5–1.3 pH units
RBC	0.5–1.0 pH units
Copper, serum	
Male	70–140 mcg./100 ml.
Female	85–155 mcg./100 ml.
Creatine, serum	0.2–0.8 mg./100 ml.
Creatine phosphokinase, serum	Varies with method used
Creatinine, serum	0.7–1.5 mg./100 ml.
Cryoglobulins, serum	0
Fatty acids, total, serum	190–420 mg./100 ml.
Fibrinogen, plasma	200–400 mg./100 ml.
Folic acid, serum	7–16 nanogm./ml.
Glucose (fasting)	
blood, true	60–100 mg./100 ml.
Folin	80–120 mg./100 ml.
plasma or serum, true	70–115 mg./100 ml.
Haptoglobin, serum	40–170 mg./100 ml.
17-Hydroxycorticosteroids, plasma	8–18 mcg./100 ml.
Icterus index, serum	4–7
Immunoglobulins, serum	
IgG	800–1500 mg./100 ml.
IgA	50–200 mg./100 ml.
IgM	40–120 mg./100 ml.
Iodine, butanol extractable, serum	3.2–6.4 mcg./100 ml.
Iodine, protein bound, serum	3.5–8.0 mcg./100 ml.
	(May be slightly higher in infants)
Iron, serum	75–175 mcg./100 ml.
Iron binding capacity, total, serum	250–410 mcg./100 ml.
% saturation	20–55%
17-Ketosteroids, plasma	25–125 mcg./100 ml.
Lactic acid, blood	6–16 mg./100 ml.
Lactic dehydrogenase, serum	90–200 milliunits/ml. (I.U.)
Lipase, serum	Less than 1.5 units (ml. of N/20 NaOH)
Lipids, total, serum	450–850 mg./100 ml.
Magnesium, serum	1.5–2.5 mEq./liter
	(1.8–3.0 mg./100 ml.)
Nitrogen, nonprotein, serum	15–35 mg./100 ml.
Osmolality, serum	285–295 mOsm./liter
Oxygen, blood	
Capacity	16–24 vol. % (varies with Hb)
Content Arterial	15–23 vol. %
Venous	10–16 vol. %

NORMAL BLOOD, PLASMA, AND SERUM VALUES (*Continued*)

Oxygen, blood (*Continued*)	
Saturation Arterial	94–100% of capacity
Venous	60–85% of capacity
Tension, Po_2 Arterial	75–100 mm. Hg
pH, arterial, blood	7.95 7.45
Phenylalanine, serum	Less than 3 mg./100 ml.
Phosphatase, acid, serum	1.0–5.0 units (King-Armstrong)
	0.5–2.0 units (Bodansky)
	0.5–2.0 units (Gutman)
	0.0–1.1 units (Shinowara)
	0.1–0.63 unit (Bessey-Lowry)
Phosphatase, alkaline, serum	5.0–13.0 units (King-Armstrong)
	2.0–4.5 units (Bodansky)
	3.0–10.0 units (Gutman)
	2.2–8.6 units (Shinowara)
	0.8–2.3 units (Bassey-Lowry)
	30–85 milliunits/ml. (I.U.)
	(Values are higher in children)
Phosphate, inorganic, serum	3.0–4.5 mg./100 ml.
	(Children: 4.0–7.0 mg./100 ml.)
Phospholipids, serum	6–12 mg./100 ml. as lipid phosphorus
Potassium, serum	3.5–5.0 mEq./liter
Proteins, serum	
Total	6.0–8.0 grams/100 ml.
Albumin	3.5–5.5 grams/100 ml.
Globulin	2.5–3.5 grams/100 ml.
Electrophoresis	
Albumin	3.5–5.5 grams/100 ml.
	52–68% of total
Globulin	
$Alpha_1$	0.2–0.4 gram/100 ml.
	2–5% of total
$Alpha_2$	0.5–0.9 gram/100 ml.
	7–14% of total
Beta	0.6–1.1 grams/100 ml.
	9–15% of total
Gamma	0.7–1.7 grams/100 ml.
	11–21% of total
Pyruvic acid, plasma	1.0–2.0 mg./100 ml.
Serotonin, platelet suspension	0.1–0.3 mcg./ml. blood
serum	0.10–0.32 mcg./ml.
Sodium, serum	136–145 mEq./liter
Sulfates, inorganic, serum	0.8–1.2 mg./100 ml. (as S)
Thyroxine iodine (T_4), serum	2.9–6.4 mcg./100 ml.
Transaminase, serum: SGOT	5–40 units/ml.
	5–50 milliunits/ml. (I.U.)
SGPT	5–35 units/ml.
Triglycerides, serum	0–150 mg./100 ml.
Urea, blood	21–43 mg./100 ml.
plasma or serum	24–49 mg./100 ml.
Urea nitrogen, blood (BUN)	10–20 mg./100 ml.
plasma or serum	11–23 mg./100 ml.
Uric acid, serum	
Male	2.5–8.0 mg./100 ml.
Female	1.5–6.0 mg./100 ml.
Vitamin A, serum	20–80 mcg./100 ml.
Vitamin B_{12}, serum	200–800 picogm./ml.
Vitamin C, blood	0.4–1.5 mg./100 ml.

NORMAL URINE VALUES

Acetone and acetoacetate	0
Addis count	
Erythrocytes	0–130,000/24 hrs.
Leukocytes	0–650,000/24 hrs.
Casts (hyaline)	0–2000/24 hrs.
Alcapton bodies	Negative
Aldosterone	3–20 mcg./24 hrs.
Amino acid nitrogen	64–199 mg./24 hrs.
	(Not over 1.5% of total nitrogen)
Ammonia nitrogen	20–70 mEq./24 hrs.
Amylase	35–260 Somogyi units/hr.
Bence Jones protein	Negative
Bilirubin (bile)	Negative
Calcium	
Low Ca diet (Bauer-Aub)	Less than 150 mg./24 hrs.
Usual diet	Less than 250 mg./24 hrs.
Catecholamines	
Epinephrine	Less than 10 mcg./24 hrs.
Norepinephrine	Less than 100 mcg./24 hrs.
Chloride	110–250 mEq./24 hrs.
	(Varies with intake)
Chorionic gonadotrophin	0
Copper	0–30 mcg./24 hrs.
Creatine	
Male	0–40 mg./24 hrs.
Female	0–100 mg./24 hrs.
	(Higher in children and during pregnancy)
Creatinine	15–25 mg./kg. of body weight/24 hrs.
Cystine or cysteine, qualitative	Negative
Delta aminolevulinic acid	1.3–7.0 mg./24 hrs.
Estrogens	
Male	4–25 mcg./24 hrs.
Female	4–60 mcg./24 hrs.
	(Markedly increased during pregnancy)
Glucose (reducing substances)	Less than 250 mg./24 hrs.
Gonadotrophins, pituitary	5–10 rat units/24 hrs.
	10–50 mouse units/24 hrs.
	(Increased after menopause)
Hemoglobin and myoglobin	Negative
Homogentisic acid, qualitative	Negative
17-Hydroxycorticosteroids	
Male	5–15 mg./24 hrs.
Female	4–10 mg./24 hrs.
	(Varies with method used)
5-Hydroxyindole-acetic acid (5-HIAA)	
Qualitative	Negative
Quantitative	Less than 16 mg./24 hrs.
17-Ketosteroids	
Male	6–18 mg./24 hrs.
Female	4–13 mg./24 hrs.
Osmolality	38–1400 mOsm./kg. water
pH	4.6–8.0, average 6.0
	(Depends on diet)
Phenylpyruvic acid, qualitative	Negative
Phosphorus	0.9–1.3 gm./24 hrs.
	(Varies with intake)
Porphobilinogen	
Qualitative	Negative
Quantitative	0–0.2 mg./100 ml.
	Less than 2.0 mg./24 hrs.

NORMAL URINE VALUES (*Continued*)

Porphyrins	
Coproporphyrin	50–250 mcg./24 hrs.
Uroporphyrin	10–30 mcg./24 hrs.
Potassium	25–100 mEq./24 hrs.
	(Varies with intake)
Pregnanetriol	Less than 2.5 mg./24 hrs. in adults
Protein	
Qualitative	0
Quantitative	10–150 mg./24 hrs.
Sodium	130–260 mEq./24 hrs.
	(Varies with intake)
Solids, total	30–70 grams/liter, average
	50 grams/liter
	(To estimate total solids per liter, multiply last two figures of specific gravity by 2.66, Long's coefficient)
Specific gravity	1.003–1.030
Sugar	0
Titratable acidity	20–40 mEq./24 hrs.
Urobilinogen	Up to 1.0 Ehrlich unit/2 hrs. (1–3 P.M.)
	0–4.0 mg./24 hrs.
Vanillylmandelic acid (VMA)	1–8 mg./24 hrs.

NORMAL VALUES FOR GASTRIC ANALYSIS

Basal gastric secretion (one hour)

	Concentration Mean ± 1 S.D.	Output Mean ± 1 S.D.
Male	25.8 ± 1.8 mEq./liter	2.57 ± 0.16 mEq./hr.
Female	20.3 ± 3.0 mEq./liter	1.61 ± 0.18 mEq./hr.

After histamine stimulation		
Normal	Mean output = 11.8 mEq./hr.	
Duodenal ulcer	Mean output = 15.2 mEq./hr.	
After maximal histamine stimulation		
Normal	Mean output 22.6 mEq./hr.	
Duodenal ulcer	Mean output 44.6 mEq./hr.	
Diagnex blue (Squibb):	Anacidity	0–0.3 mg. in 2 hrs.
	Doubtful	0.3–0.6 mg. in 2 hrs.
	Normal	Greater than 0.6 mg. in 2 hrs.
Volume, fasting stomach content		50–100 ml.
Emptying time		3–6 hrs.
Color		Opalescent or colorless
Specific gravity		1.006–1.009
pH (adults)		0.9–1.5

NORMAL VALUES FOR CEREBROSPINAL FLUID

Cells	Fewer than 5 cu. mm., all mononuclear
Chloride	120–130 mEq./liter
	(20 mEq./liter higher than serum)
Colloidal gold test	Not more than 1 in any tube
Glucose	50–75 mg./100 ml.
	(20 mg./100 ml. less than blood)
Pressure	70–180 mm. water
Protein, total	15–45 mg./100 ml.
Albumin	52%
Alpha$_1$ globulin	5%
Alpha$_2$ globulin	14%
Beta globulin	10%
Gamma globulin	19%

NORMAL VALUES FOR SEMEN

Volume	2–5 ml., usually 3–4 ml.
Liquefaction	Complete in 15 min.
pH	7.2–8.0; average 7.8
Leukocytes	Occasional or absent
Count	60–150 million/ml.
	Below 60 million/ml. is abnormal
Motility	80% or more motile
Morphology	80–90% normal forms

NORMAL VALUES FOR FECES

Bulk	100–200 grams/24 hrs.
Dry matter	23–32 grams/24 hrs.
Fat, total	Less than 6.0 grams/24 hrs.
Nitrogen, total	Less than 2.0 grams/24 hrs.
Urobilinogen	40–280 mg./24 hrs.
Water	Approximately 65%

TOXICOLOGY

Arsenic, blood	3.5–7.2 mcg./100 ml.
Arsenic, urine	Less than 100 mcg./24 hrs
Barbiturates, serum	0
	Coma level: Phenobarbital approximately 11 mg./100 ml.; most other barbiturates 15 mg./100 ml.
Bromides, serum	0
	Toxic levels above 17 mEq./liter
Carbon monoxide, blood	Up to 5% saturation
	Symptoms occur with 20% saturation
Dilantin, blood or serum	Therapeutic levels 1–11 mcg./ml.
Ethanol, blood	Less than 0.005%
Marked intoxication	0.3–0.4%
Alcoholic stupor	0.4–0.5%
Coma	Above 0.5%
Lead, blood	0–40 mcg./100 ml.
Lead, urine	Less than 100 mcg./24 hrs.
Mercury, urine	Less than 10 mcg./24 hrs.
Salicylate, plasma	0
Therapeutic range	20–25 mg./100 ml.
Toxic range	Over 30 mg./100 ml.
Death	45–75 mg./100 ml.

LIVER FUNCTION TESTS

Bromsulphalein (B.S.P.)	Less than 5% remaining in serum 45 minutes after injection of 5 mg./kg. of body weight
Cephalin cholesterol flocculation	0–1 in 24 hours.
Cholinesterase (pseudo-cholinesterase), serum	0.5 pH units or more/hour.
Galactose tolerance	Excretion of not more than 3.0 grams galactose in the urine 5 hours after ingestion of 40 grams of galactose.
Glycogen storage	Increase of blood glucose 45 mg./100 ml. over fasting level 45 minutes after subcutaneous injection of 0.01 mg./kg. body weight of epinephrine.
Hippuric acid	Excretion of 3.0–3.5 grams hippuric acid in urine within 4 hours after ingestion of 6.0 grams sodium benzoate,

or

	Excretion of 0.7 gram hippuric acid in urine within 1 hour after intravenous injection of 1.77 grams sodium benzoate.
Thymol turbidity	0–5 units.
Zinc turbidity	2–12 units.

PANCREATIC (ISLET) FUNCTION TESTS

Glucose tolerance tests	Patient should be on a diet containing 300 grams of carbohydrate per day for 3 days prior to test.
Oral	After ingestion of 100 grams of glucose or 1.75 grams glucose/kg. body weight, blood glucose is not more than 160 mg./100 ml. after 60 minutes, 140 mg./100 ml. after 90 minutes, and 120 mg./100 ml. after 120 minutes. Values are for blood; serum measurements are approximately 15% higher.
Intravenous	Blood glucose does not exceed 200 mg./100 ml. after infusion of 0.5 gram of glucose/kg. body weight over 30 minutes. Glucose concentration falls below initial level at 2 hours and returns to preinfusion levels in 3 hours or 1 hour. Values are for blood; serum measurements are approximately 15% higher.
Cortisone-glucose tolerance test	The patient should be on a diet containing 300 grams of carbohydrate per day for 3 days prior to test. At $8\frac{1}{2}$ and again 2 hours prior to glucose load patient is given cortisone acetate by mouth (50 mg. if patient's ideal weight is less than 160 lb., 62.5 mg. if ideal weight is greater than 160 lb.). An oral dose of glucose 1.75 grams/kg. body weight, is given and blood samples are taken at 0, 30, 60, 90, and 120 minutes. Test is considered positive if true blood glucose exceeds 160 mg./100 ml. at 60 minutes, 140 mg./100 ml. at 90 minutes, and 120 mg./100 ml. at 120 minutes. Values are for blood; serum measurements are approximately 15% higher.

RENAL FUNCTION TESTS

Clearance tests (corrected to 1.73 sq. meters body surface area)

Glomerular filtration rate (G.F.R.) Inulin clearance, Mannitol clearance, or Endogenous creatinine clearance	Males	110–150 ml./min.
	Females	105–132 ml./min.
Renal plasma flow (R.P.F.) p-Aminohippurate (P.A.H.), or Diodrast	Males	560–830 ml./min.
	Females	490–700 ml./min.
Filtration fraction (F.F.) $$FF = \frac{G.F.R.}{R.P.F.}$$	Males	17–21%
	Females	17–23%
Urea clearance (C_u)	Standard	40–65 ml./min.
	Maximal	60–100 ml./min.

Concentration and dilution — Specific gravity > 1.025 on dry day

Specific gravity < 1.003 on water day

Maximal Diodrast excretory capacity T_{M_D}	Males	43–59 mg./min.
	Females	33–51 mg./min.
Maximal glucose reabsorptive capacity T_{M_G}	Males	300–450 mg./min.
	Females	250–350 mg./min.
Maximal PAH excretory capacity $T_{M_{PAH}}$		80–90 mg./min.

Phenolsulfonphthalein excretion (P.S.P.)

25% or more in 15 min.
40% or more in 30 min.
55% or more in 2 hrs.
After injection of 1 ml. P.S.P. intravenously

THYROID FUNCTION TESTS

Protein bound iodine, serum (P.B.I.)	3.5–8.0 mcg./100 ml.
Butanol extractable iodine, serum (B.E.I.)	3.2–6.4 mcg./100 ml.
Thyroxine iodine, serum (T_4)	2.9–6.4 mcg./100 ml.
Free thyroxine, serum	1.4–2.5 nanogram/100 ml.
T_3 (index of unsaturated T.B.G.)	10.0–14.6%
Thyroxine-binding globulin, serum (T.B.G.)	10–26 mcg. T_4/100 ml
Thyroid-stimulating hormone, serum (T.S.H.)	0 up to 0.2 milliunits/ml.
Radioactive iodine (I^{131}) uptake (R.A.I.)	20–50% of administered dose in 24 hrs.
Radioactive iodine (I^{131}) excretion	30–70% of administered dose in 24 hrs.
Radioactive iodine (I^{131}), protein bound	Less than 0.3% of administered dose per liter of plasma at 72 hrs.
Basal metabolic rate	Minus 10% to plus 10% of mean standard

GASTROINTESTINAL ABSORPTION TESTS

d-Xylose absorption test	After an 8 hour fast 10 ml./kg. body weight of a 5% solution of d-xylose is given by mouth. Nothing further by mouth is given until the test has been completed. All urine voided during the following 5 hours is pooled, and blood samples are taken at 0, 60, and 120 minutes. Normally 26% (range 16–33%) of ingested xylose is excreted within 5 hours, and the serum xylose reaches a level between 25 and 40 mg./100 ml. after 1 hour and is maintained at this level for another 60 minutes.
Vitamin A absorption test	A fasting blood specimen is obtained and 200,000 units of vitamin A in oil is given by mouth. Serum vitamin A level should rise to twice fasting level in 3 to 5 hours.

Castleman, B., and McNeely, B. U.: New Eng. J. Med., 276:167, 1967.

Davidsohn, I., and Henry, J. B.: Clinical Diagnosis by Laboratory Methods. 14th ed. Philadelphia, W. B. Saunders Company, 1969.

Henry, R. J.: Clinical Chemistry—Principles and Techniques. New York, Harper & Row, 1964.

Long, C.: Biochemists' Handbook. Princeton, D. Van Nostrand Company, 1961.

Miale, J. B.: Laboratory Medicine—Hematology. 3rd ed. St. Louis, C. V. Mosby Company, 1967.

Miller, S. E.: A Textbook of Clinical Pathology. 7th ed. Baltimore, Williams & Wilkins Company, 1966.

Stewart, C. P., and Stolman, A.: Toxicology, Mechanisms and Analytic Methods. New York, Academic Press, 1960.

Sunderman, F. W., and Boerner, F.: Normal Values in Clinical Medicine. Philadelphia, W. B. Saunders Company, 1949.

Wintrobe, M. M.: Clinical Hematology. 6th ed. Philadelphia, Lea & Febiger, 1967.

INDEX

INDEX

Note: In this index the expression "vs." has been used to denote "differential diagnosis." Thus, "Addison's disease, vs. acanthosis nigricans" is the equivalent of "Addison's disease, differential diagnosis from acanthosis nigricans." **Boldface entries and folios** in the index indicate main discussions in the text. *Italic folios* indicate illustrations and tables.